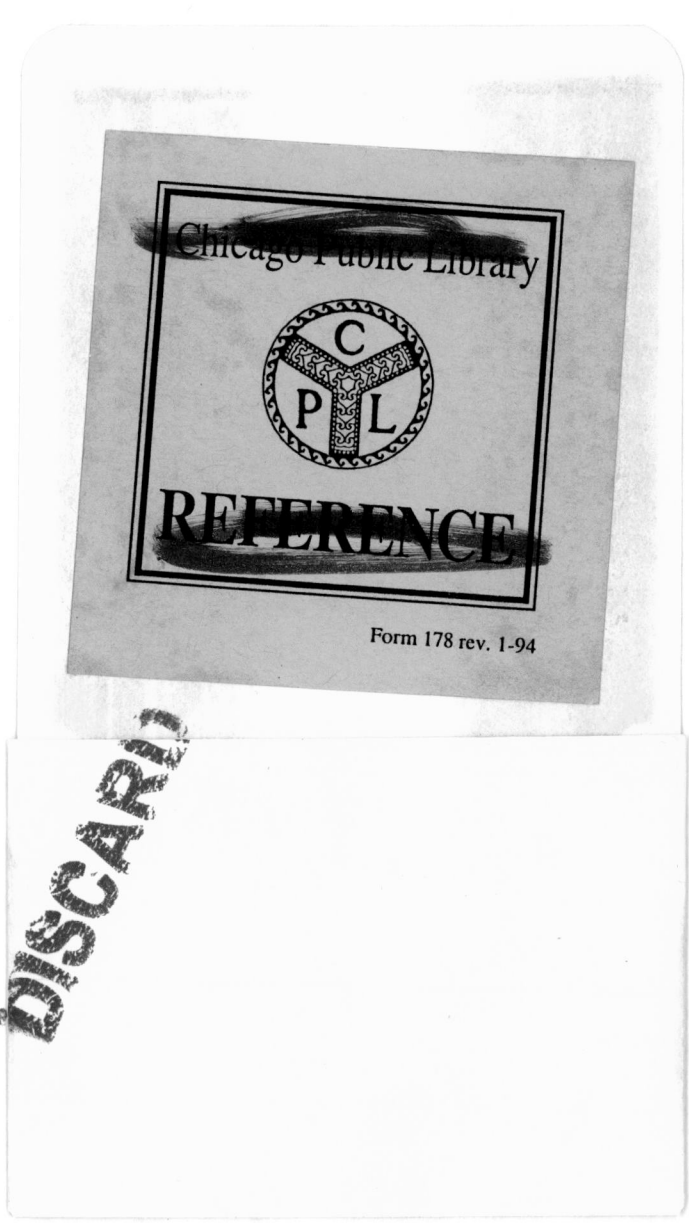

THE AMERICAN PSYCHIATRIC PRESS
TEXTBOOK OF PSYCHIATRY

THIRD EDITION

INTERNATIONAL ADVISORY BOARD

THE AMERICAN PSYCHIATRIC PRESS
TEXTBOOK OF PSYCHIATRY

THIRD EDITION

EDITED BY

ROBERT E. HALES, M.D., M.B.A.
Professor and Chair, Department of Psychiatry,
University of California, Davis School of Medicine;
Director, Behavioral Health Center, UC Davis Health System;
Medical Director, Sacramento County Mental Health Services,
Sacramento, California

STUART C. YUDOFSKY, M.D.
D. C. and Irene Ellwood Professor and Chairman,
Department of Psychiatry and Behavioral Sciences,
Baylor College of Medicine;
Chief, Psychiatry Service,
The Methodist Hospital,
Houston, Texas

JOHN A. TALBOTT, M.D.
Professor and Chairman,
Department of Psychiatry,
University of Maryland School of Medicine,
Baltimore, Maryland

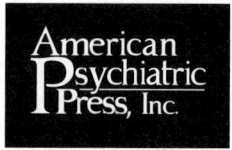

American Psychiatric Press, Inc.

Washington, DC
London, England

Third Edition   02   01   00   99   4   3   2   1

American Psychiatric Press, Inc.
1400 K Street, N.W., Washington, DC   20005
www.appi.org

Library of Congress Cataloging-in-Publication Data

The American Psychiatric Press textbook of psychiatry / edited by
   Robert E. Hales, Stuart C. Yudofsky, John A. Talbott. — 3rd ed.
      p.   cm.
   Includes bibliographical references and index.
   ISBN 0-88048-819-0 (alk. paper)
   1. Psychiatry.   I. Hales, Robert E.   II. Yudofsky, Stuart C.
III. Talbott, John A.   IV. Title: Textbook of psychiatry.
   [DNLM: 1. Mental Disorders.   2. Psychiatry.   WM 100 A5112 1999]
RC454.A197   1999
616.89—dc21
DNLM/DLC
for Library of Congress   98-43411
                                                                                                          CIP

British Library Cataloguing in Publication Data
  A CIP record is available from the British Library.

Dedicated to
Shervert H. Frazier, M.D.
and
Melvin Sabshin, M.D.

We thank you for being inspired teachers,
inspiring mentors, and devoted friends
over the entirety of our professional careers.

He shall be like a tree
Planted by the rivers of water
That brings forth its fruit in its season,
Whose leaf also shall not wither;
And whatever he does shall prosper.

—Psalm 1, verse 3

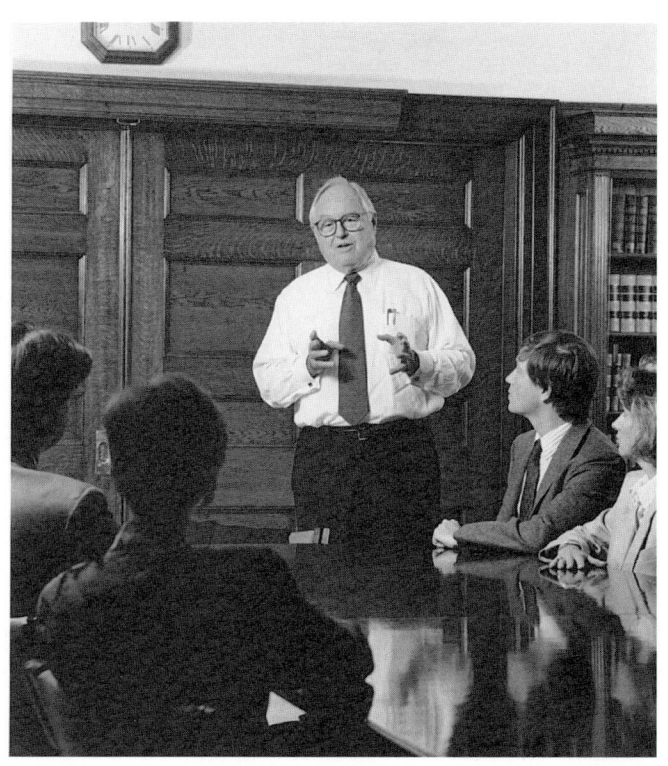

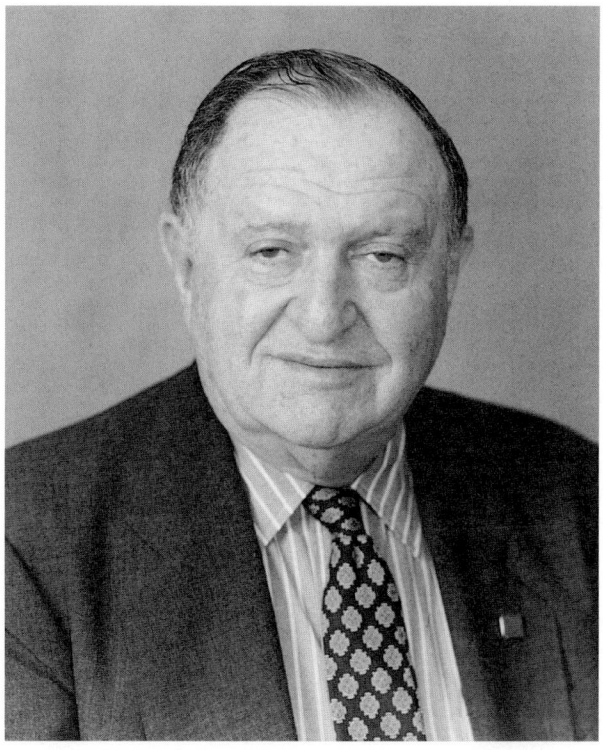

Shervert H. Frazier, M.D.
American Psychiatric Press
Founding Director
Editor-In-Chief, 1981–1986
Founder Consultant

Melvin Sabshin, M.D.
Founding Chairman of the Board,
American Psychiatric Press, 1981–1997
Medical Director, American Psychiatric Association
1974–1997

CONTENTS

SECTION I: THEORETICAL FOUNDATIONS

SECTION II: ASSESSMENT

SECTION IV: PSYCHIATRIC TREATMENTS

CONTRIBUTORS

W. STEWART AGRAS, M.D.
Professor of Psychiatry and Associate Chair, Department of Psychiatry and Behavioral Science, Stanford University School of Medicine, Stanford, California

NANCY C. ANDREASEN, M.D., PH.D.
Andrew H. Woods Chair of Psychiatry, Department of Psychiatry, University of Iowa College of Medicine; Mental Health Clinical Research Center, University of Iowa Hospitals and Clinics, Iowa City, Iowa

VICTORIA BALKOSKI, M.D.
Executive Associate Chairman and Chief, Division of Child and Adolescent Psychiatry, Department of Psychiatry, Albany Medical College, Albany, New York

AARON T. BECK, M.D.
University Professor, Department of Psychiatry, University of Pennsylvania, School of Medicine, Philadelphia, Pennsylvania

JUDITH V. BECKER, PH.D.
Professor of Psychiatry and Psychology, University of Arizona Health Sciences Center, Tucson, Arizona

ROBERT I. BERKOWITZ, M.D.
Associate Professor of Psychiatry, Division of Child and Adolescent Psychiatry, The University of Pennsylvania School of Medicine, The Children's Hospital of Philadelphia, Philadelphia, Pennsylvania

DONALD W. BLACK, M.D.
Professor, Department of Psychiatry, The University of Iowa College of Medicine, Iowa City, Iowa

DAN BLAZER, M.D., PH.D.
J. P. Gibbons Professor of Psychiatry, Dean of Medical Education, Duke University Medical Center, Durham, North Carolina

HOWARD C. BLUE, M.D.
Assistant Clinical Professor of Psychiatry, Department of Psychiatry, Yale University of Medicine, New Haven, Connecticut

JONATHAN F. BORUS, M.D.
Professor of Psychiatry, Harvard Medical School, and Psychiatrist in Chief, Brigham and Women's Hospital, Boston, Massachusetts

JACK D. BURKE, JR., M.D., M.P.H.
Professor and Head of the Department of Psychiatry and Behavioral Science, Texas A&M University Health Science Center; Chairman of the Department of Psychiatry at Scott and White Clinic and Hospital, Temple, Texas

VIVIEN K. BURT, M.D., PH.D.
Associate Professor of Psychiatry, UCLA School of Medicine; Director, Women's Life Center, UCLA Neuropsychiatric Institute and Hospital, Los Angeles, California

STEPHEN F. BUTLER, PH.D.
Research Associate, Innovative Training Systems, Newton Centre, Massachusetts

RANDALL BUZAN, M.D.
Assistant Professor of Psychiatry, Department of Psychiatry, University of Colorado School of Medicine, Denver, Colorado

JOHN F. CLARKIN, PH.D.
Professor of Clinical Psychology, Department of Psychiatry, Cornell University Medical College, New York Hospital–Cornell Medical Center, Westchester Division, White Plains, New York

PAUL D. COX, M.D.
Assistant Professor of Psychiatry, University of California, Davis School of Medicine, Sacramento, California

JOSEPH T. COYLE, M.D.
Eben S. Draper Professor of Psychiatry and Neuroscience, Chair of the Consolidated Department of Psychiatry, Harvard Medical School, Boston, Massachusetts

STEPHEN J. COZZA, M.D.
Chief, Division of Child Psychiatry, and Director, Clinical Psychiatry Residency Training, Department of Psychiatry, Walter Reed Army Medical Center, Washington, D.C.

C. DEBORAH CROSS, M.D.
Associate Professor of Psychiatry and Associate Chairman, Capital District Psychiatric Center, Department of Psychiatry, Albany Medical College; Assistant Psychiatrist, Albany Medical Center Hospital, Albany, New York

JEFFREY L. CUMMINGS, M.D.
The Augustus S. Rose Professor of Neurology and Professor of Psychiatry and Biobehavioral Sciences, UCLA School of Medicine, Los Angeles, California

STEVEN L. DUBOVSKY, M.D.
Professor of Psychiatry and Vice Chair, Department of Psychiatry, Professor of Medicine, Department of Medicine, University of Colorado School of Medicine, Denver, Colorado

MINA K. DULCAN, M.D.
Head, Department of Child Psychiatry, Osterman Professor of Child Psychiatry, Children's Memorial Hospital, Chicago, Illinois; Chief of Child and Adolescent Psychiatry, Northwestern University School of Medicine, Chicago, Illinois

ALLEN R. DYER, M.D., PH.D.
Professor of Psychiatry and Behavioral Sciences, James H. Quillen College of Medicine, East Tennessee State University, Johnson City, Tennessee

RICHARD J. FRANCES, M.D.
Medical Director and President of Silver Hill Hospital, Clinical Professor of Psychiatry, New York University Medical School, New York

JOHN E. FRANKLIN, JR., M.D.
Associate Professor of Psychiatry, Director Addiction Psychiatry, Northwestern University Medical School, Northwestern Memorial Hospital, Chicago, Illinois

GEORGE FULOP, M.D.
Assistant Professor, Division of Behavioral Medicine and Consultation Psychiatry, Department of Psychiatry, Mount Sinai School of Medicine, New York, New York

T. B. GHOSH, M.D.
Clinical Faculty, University of California San Francisco School of Medicine and California Pacific Medical Center, San Francisco, California

CARLOS A. GONZÁLEZ, M.D.
Assistant Clinical Professor of Psychiatry, Department of Psychiatry, Yale University School of Medicine, New Haven, Connecticut

JACK M. GORMAN, M.D.
Professor of Clinical Psychiatry; Director, Department of Clinical Psychobiology, Columbia University College of Physicians and Surgeons and New York State Psychiatric Institute, New York, New York

KEVIN F. GRAY, M.D.
Director, Memory Disorders Clinic, Veterans Affairs North Texas Health Care System; Assistant Professor, Departments of Psychiatry and Neurology, UT Southwestern Medical School, Dallas, Texas

EZRA E. H. GRIFFITH, M.D.
Professor of Psychiatry and of African and African American Studies, Department of Psychiatry, Yale University School of Medicine, New Haven, Connecticut

JOHN G. GUNDERSON, M.D.
Professor of Psychiatry, McLean Hospital, Belmont, MA; Harvard Medical School, Boston, Massachusetts

ROBERT E. HALES, M.D., M.B.A.
Professor and Chair, Department of Psychiatry, University of California, Davis School of Medicine; Director, Behavioral Health Center, UC Davis Health System; Medical Director, Sacramento County Mental Health Services, Sacramento, California

KATHERINE A. HALMI, M.D.
Professor of Psychiatry, Cornell University Medical College; Director, Eating Disorders Program, Cornell Medical Center—Westchester, White Plains, New York

VICTORIA HENDRICK, M.D.
Assistant Professor of Psychiatry, UCLA School of Medicine; Director, Pregnancy and Postpartum Mood Disorders Program, UCLA Neuropsychiatric Institute and Hospital, Los Angeles, California

MARGARET E. HERTZIG, M.D.
Professor of Psychiatry, Weill Medical College of Cornell University; Director, Child and Adolescent Outpatient Department, Payne Whitney Clinic, New York, New York

DONALD M. HILTY, M.D.
Assistant Professor of Clinical Psychiatry, University of California, Davis School of Medicine, Sacramento, California

ERIC HOLLANDER, M.D.
Professor of Psychiatry, Director, Clinical Psychopharmacology, Mount Sinai School of Medicine, New York, New York

STEPHEN W. HURT, PH.D.
Associate Professor of Clinical Psychology, Department of Psychiatry, Cornell University Medical College, New York Hospital–Cornell Medical Center, Westchester Division, White Plains, New York

STEVEN E. HYMAN, M.D.
Director, National Institute of Mental Health, Washington, D.C.

CHRISTINE A. INGRAHAM, PH.D.
Assistant Professor and Chief, Laboratory of Cellular and Molecular Neurobiology, Department of Psychiatry, Albany Medical College, Albany, New York

BRADLEY R. JOHNSON, M.D.
Professor, University of Arizona Health Sciences Center, Tucson, Arizona

LESLIE B. KADIS, M.D.
Private practice, Aptos, CA

CHARLES A. KAUFMANN, M.D.
Associate Professor of Clinical Psychiatry, Department of Psychiatry, Columbia University College of Physicians and Surgeons, New York, New York

RICHARD J. KAVOUSSI, M.D.
Assistant Professor of Psychiatry, Medical College of Pennsylvania, Philadelphia, Pennsylvania

STUART L. KEILL, M.D.
Clinical Professor of Psychiatry, New York University School of Medicine; Director of Forensic Services, Manhattan Psychiatric Center, Wards Island, New York, New York

STEVEN A. KING, M.D.
Director, Division of Pain Medicine, and Professor, Department of Psychiatry, Temple University School of Medicine, Philadelphia, Pennsylvania

JAMES A. KNOWLES, M.D., PH.D.
Assistant Professor of Psychiatry, Department of Psychiatry, and Columbia Genome Center, Columbia University College of Physicians and Surgeons; New York State Psychiatric Institute, New York, New York

DAVID J. KUPFER, M.D.
Professor and Chairman, Department of Psychiatry, University of Pittsburgh School of Medicine, Pittsburgh, Pennsylvania

H. RICHARD LAMB, M.D.
Professor of Psychiatry, Department of Psychiatry and the Behavioral Sciences, University of Southern California School of Medicine, Los Angeles, California

MARTIN H. LEAMON, M.D.
Assistant Professor of Clinical Psychiatry, Department of Psychiatry, University of California, Davis School of Medicine, Sacramento, California

HANNA LEVENSON, PH.D.
Clinical Professor, Department of Psychiatry, University of California School of Medicine, San Francisco; Director, Brief Psychotherapy Program, Department of Veterans Affairs Medical Center, San Francisco; Director, Brief Psychotherapy Program, California Pacific Medical Center, San Francisco; Director, Levenson Institute for Training in Brief Therapy, San Francisco and Oakland, California

JAMES L. LEVENSON, M.D.
Professor of Psychiatry, Medicine and Surgery, Medical College of Virginia, Richmond, Virginia

JOSE R. MALDONADO, M.D.
Assistant Professor and Chief, Medical Psychiatry Section, Department of Psychiatry and Behavioral Sciences, Stanford University; Medical Director, Consultation/Liaison Psychiatry Service, Stanford University Hospital; Director of the Medical Psychotherapy Clinic, Stanford University School of Medicine, Stanford, California

LAUREN B. MARANGELL, M.D.
Assistant Professor of Psychiatry, Director of Clinical Psychopharmacology, and Director of Mood Disorders Research, Baylor College of Medicine, Houston, Texas

STEPHEN S. MARMER, M.D., PH.D.
Assistant Clinical Professor, UCLA Neuropsychiatric Institute, Department of Psychiatry and Biobehavioral Medicine, University of California at Los Angeles; Senior Faculty, Southern California Psychoanalytic Institute, Los Angeles, California

RONALD L. MARTIN, M.D.[†]
Chairman, Department of Psychiatry, University of Kansas School of Medicine, Wichita, Kansas

STEVEN MATTIS, PH.D.
Psychological Services Director, Long Island Jewish–Hillside Hospital, Glen Oaks, New York

---

[†] Deceased.

RUTH MCCLENDON, M.S.W.
Private practice, Aptos, CA

J. STEPHEN MCDANIEL, M.D.
Assistant Professor of Psychiatry, Emory University School of Medicine, Atlanta, Georgia

JOHN S. MCINTYRE, M.D.
Chair, Department of Psychiatry and Behavioral Health, Unity Health System, Rochester, New York

MICHAEL G. MORAN, M.D.
Associate Professor of Psychiatry, University of Colorado School of Medicine, Denver, Colorado

JOHN M. MORIHISA, M.D.
Professor and Chairman, Department of Psychiatry, Albany Medical College; Psychiatrist-in-Chief, Albany Medical Center Hospital, Albany, New York

JEFFREY NEWCORN, M.D.
Division of Child and Adolescent Psychiatry, Department of Psychiatry, Mount Sinai School of Medicine, New York, New York

THOMAS C. NEYLAN, M.D.
Assistant Professor of Psychiatry, University of California San Francisco; Medical Director, Posttraumatic Stress Disorders Program, Veterans Affairs Medical Center, San Francisco, California

KATHARINE A. PHILLIPS, M.D.
Associate Professor of Psychiatry and Human Behavior, Brown University School of Medicine; Chief, Outpatient Services, Butler Hospital, Providence, Rhode Island

HAROLD ALAN PINCUS, M.D.
Deputy Medical Director, Office of Research, American Psychiatric Association, Washington, D.C.

JOHN PLEWES, M.D.
Lilly Research Labs, Indianapolis, Indiana

CHARLES POPPER, M.D.
Founding Editor, *Journal of Child and Adolescent Psychopharmacology*; Clinical Instructor in Psychiatry, Harvard Medical School, Boston, Massachusetts; Associate Child and Adolescent Psychiatrist, McLean Hospital, Belmont, Massachusetts

STEPHEN RACHLIN, M.D.
Clinical Director, Meadowview Psychiatric Hospital, Secaucus, New Jersey

DARREL A. REGIER, M.D., M.P.H.
Office of the Director, National Institute of Mental Health, Rockville, Maryland

CHARLES F. REYNOLDS III, M.D.
Professor of Psychiatry and Neurology; Director, MHCRC For Late-Life Mood Disorders, Department of Psychiatry, University of Pittsburgh School of Medicine, Pittsburgh, Pennsylvania

RONALD O. RIEDER, M.D.
Professor of Clinical Psychiatry, Vice Chair for Education, Department of Psychiatry, Columbia University College of Physicians and Surgeons, New York, New York

RICHARD B. ROSSE, M.D.
Associate Professor of Psychiatry, Georgetown University School of Medicine; Chief, Outpatient Mental Health Services, Washington Veterans Affairs Medical Center, Washington, D.C.

MELVIN SABSHIN, M.D.
Medical Director Emeritus, American Psychiatric Association, Washington, D.C.

STEPHEN C. SCHEIBER, M.D.
Executive Vice President, American Board of Psychiatry and Neurology, Inc., Deerfield, Illinois; Adjunct Professor, Department of Psychiatry, Northwestern University School of Medicine, Evanston, Illinois; Adjunct Professor, Department of Psychiatry, Medical College of Wisconsin, Milwaukee, Wisconsin

LESLIE SEIGLE, B.A.
Project Manager for Practice Guidelines, American Psychiatric Association, Washington, D.C.

BENJAMIN SELTZER, M.D.
Professor of Neurology and Psychiatry and Director of the Alzheimer's Disease and Memory Disorders Center, Tulane University School of Medicine, New Orleans, Louisiana

MARK E. SERVIS, M.D.
Associate Professor of Clinical Psychiatry, University of California, Davis School of Medicine, Sacramento, California

THEODORE SHAPIRO, M.D.
Professor of Psychiatry and Professor of Psychiatry in Pediatrics, Weill Medical College of Cornell University; Director, Child and Adolescent Psychiatry, Payne Whitney Clinic, New York, New York

EDWARD K. SILBERMAN, M.D.
Clinical Professor of Psychiatry and Human Behavior and Director of Residency Education, Jefferson Medical College of Thomas Jefferson University, Philadelphia, Pennsylvania

JONATHAN M. SILVER, M.D.
Associate Professor of Clinical Psychiatry, Columbia University College of Physicians and Surgeons; Director of Neuropsychiatry, Columbia-Presbyterian Medical Center, New York, New York

DAPHNE SIMEON, M.D.
Assistant Professor of Psychiatry, Director, Medical Student Education, Mount Sinai School of Medicine, New York, New York

ROBERT I. SIMON, M.D.
Clinical Professor of Psychiatry; Director, Program in Psychiatry and Law, Georgetown University School of Medicine, Washington, D.C.

WILLIAM H. SLEDGE, M.D.
Professor and Associate Chairman for Education, Department of Psychiatry, Yale University School of Medicine, New Haven, Connecticut

MIRIAM SOKOLYANSKAYA, B.A.
Research Assistant, Division of Behavioral Medicine and Consultation Psychiatry, Department of Psychiatry, Mount Sinai School of Medicine, New York, New York

DAVID SPIEGEL, M.D.
Professor of Psychiatry and Behavioral Sciences, Director of the Psychosocial Treatment Laboratory, Stanford University School of Medicine, Stanford, California

ALAN STOUDEMIRE, M.D.
Professor of Psychiatry, Emory University School of Medicine, Atlanta, Georgia

JAMES J. STRAIN, M.D.
Director, Division of Behavioral Medicine and Consultation Psychiatry, Department of Psychiatry, Mount Sinai School of Medicine, New York, New York

KENNETH TARDIFF, M.D., M.P.H.
Professor of Psychiatry; Payne Whitney Clinic, New York Hospital—Cornell Medical Center, New York, New York

JOHN G. TIERNEY, M.D.
Clinical Assistant Professor of Psychiatry, University of Texas Health Sciences Center; Medical Director, St. Luke's Psychiatric Behavioral Unit, San Antonio, Texas

MICHAEL R. TRIMBLE, M.D., F.R.C.P., F.R.C.PSYCH.
Professor of Behavioural Neurology, Institute of Neurology, London, England

ROBERT J. URSANO, M.D.
Professor and Chairman, Department of Psychiatry, F. Edward Hébert School of Medicine, Uniformed Services University of the Health Sciences, Bethesda, Maryland

BRUCE S. VICTOR, M.D.
Associate Clinical Professor of Psychiatry, University of California San Francisco School of Medicine; Director, Psychopharmacology Department, California Pacific Medical Center, San Francisco, California

SOPHIA VINOGRADOV, M.D.
Assistant Professor of Psychiatry, San Francisco VA Medical Center, San Francisco, California

SCOTT A. WEST, M.D.
President, Psychiatric Institute of Florida, Orlando, Florida

JANET B. W. WILLIAMS, D.S.W.
Professor of Clinical Psychiatric Social Work (in Psychiatry and Neurology), Department of Psychiatry, Columbia University College of Physicians and Surgeons; Biometrics Research, New York State Psychiatric Institute, New York, New York

MICHAEL G. WISE, M.D.
Clinical Professor of Psychiatry, Louisiana State University School of Medicine and Tulane University School of Medicine, New Orleans, Louisiana; Clinical Professor of Psychiatry, F. Edward Hébert School of Medicine, Uniformed Services University of the Health Sciences, Bethesda, Maryland

JESSE H. WRIGHT, M.D., PH.D.
Professor, Department of Psychiatry and Behavioral Sciences, University of Louisville School of Medicine; Medical Director, Norton Psychiatric Clinic, Louisville, Kentucky

IRVIN D. YALOM, M.D.
Professor of Psychiatry; Psyc, Group Therapy, and Existential Therapy Program, Stanford University School of Medicine, Stanford, California

STUART C. YUDOFSKY, M.D.
D. C. and Irene Ellwood Professor and Chairman,
Department of Psychiatry and Behavioral Sciences,
Baylor College of Medicine; Chief, Psychiatry Service,
The Methodist Hospital, Houston, Texas

SEAN H. YUTZY, M.D.
Assistant Professor of Psychiatry, Department of
Psychiatry, Washington University School of Medicine,
Washington University, St. Louis, Missouri

DEBORAH A. ZARIN, M.D.
Deputy Medical Director, Office of Quality
Improvement, American Psychiatric Association,
Washington, D.C.

DOUGLAS F. ZATZICK, M.D.
Assistant Professor of Psychiatry, Department of
Psychiatry, University of California, Davis School of
Medicine, Sacramento, California

The *American Psychiatric Press Textbook of Psychiatry* is a one-volume, clinically oriented, comprehensive textbook of psychiatry for use primarily by senior psychiatry residents and practicing psychiatrists. It is also a standard educational reference for physicians in other specialties, such as family practice, internal medicine, and neurology. Chapters are written to be scholarly and authoritative, yet of practical, clinical utility for treating patients.

We were extremely pleased with the enthusiastic reviews we received for the first two editions in *The New England Journal of Medicine*, *The Journal of the American Medical Association (JAMA)*, *The American Journal of Psychiatry*, *Academic Psychiatry*, and other publications.

We have maintained close contact with many of the professionals who purchased the 1988 and 1994 editions and have benefited from their periodic comments and suggestions.

Work on the third edition began in earnest in 1996. This edition represents a culmination of a 3-year effort to provide the latest and most up-to-date information in the field. New chapters have been added to address the following topics of current interest: psychiatry and primary care, managed care and psychiatry, practice guidelines in psychi-

atry and a psychiatric practice research network, neuropsychiatry, and the future of psychiatry. We also added 22 new contributors to this edition with an increase in the total number of contributors to 104. All chapters have been updated to include the latest references and research findings, and selected chapters have been completely rewritten by new authors.

In addition, two companion volumes are being published. *Essentials of Clinical Psychiatry*, which includes the 25 most clinically relevant chapters from the *Textbook*, is designed for third- and fourth-year medical students, junior psychiatry residents, and residents in other specialties, especially neurology, family practice, and internal medicine. To complement the *Essentials*, a *Study Guide to the Essentials of Clinical Psychiatry* is also being published. The *Study Guide* includes board-type questions that will test the reader's knowledge of the material contained within the chapters. This book is a valuable companion guide for medical students, psychiatry and neurology residents, and junior psychiatry and neurology attendings preparing for their board exams.

An online, interactive companion to the *Textbook* and *Study Guide* is planned for 1999. For this interactive work, now in the planning stages, we expect to provide the full text of the *Textbook* and *Study Guide*, with updates to chapters published online as they become available, instead of having to wait until the next print edition is published—a truly dynamic interactive publication. This online version will also include powerful search functions and hypertext links between chapters and to related Web sites, including Medline abstracts. The details of access, price, and so on will be announced later. Watch for news from American Psychiatric Press on this exciting development.

Many of the chapters in the third edition are contributions from leading scientists and investigators in their particular field, together with a younger faculty member who provides a fresh, clinical perspective. All chapters were reviewed by a member of our editorial board and by the editors. The *Textbook* has a distinguished editorial board from the United States that includes top psychiatrists who were actively involved in the chapters falling within their area of expertise. The book also includes a wonderfully written introduction by Herbert Pardes, M.D., Vice President for Health Sciences and Dean of the Faculty of Medicine at Columbia University College of Physicians and Surgeons, Past President of the American Psychiatric Association, and Past Director of the National Institute of Mental Health. For this edition we also added an international editorial advisory board because of the *Textbook's* popularity internationally and our desire to incorporate information and suggestions from distinguished colleagues from these countries.

This edition is approximately 10% larger than the second edition, even though we devoted a great amount of time to editing and paring down chapters to ensure that only essential material was included. The reality is that the knowledge base of psychiatry has continued to increase substantially since the second edition.

The outstanding American Psychiatric Press (APPI) leadership are congratulated for a unique development for this edition. In the first two editions, we included two appendixes: the complete diagnostic criteria from the fourth edition of the *Diagnostic and Statistical Manual of Mental Disorders* (DSM-IV) and excerpts from the *American Psychiatric Glossary*, Seventh Edition. However, as readers have reported to us, these appendixes added another 125 pages to an already big book, which we wanted to keep as a one-volume text. Consequently, readers who purchase the third edition will receive on CD-ROM the Electronic DSM-IV Plus, Version 3.0, which includes 1) the full text of DSM-IV, 2) all nine published APA Practice Guidelines, 3) the complete *American Psychiatric Glossary*, Seventh Edition, 4) the *Principles of Medical Ethics With Annotations Especially Applicable to Psychiatry*, 1998 Edition, and 5) *Opinions of the Ethics Committee on the Principles of Medical Ethics With Annotations Especially Applicable to Psychiatry*. The ad-

vantage of the CD-ROM is that the contents are fully searchable by disorder, code, or phrase and replete with cross-references and hypertext links. The CD-ROM will also give readers the ability to read through the text, print selected material, and add it to their own databases.

We thank many people for their invaluable assistance with the third edition of *The American Psychiatric Press Textbook of Psychiatry*. First, we are grateful to the outstanding authors who produced exceptional chapters and who labored to respond with good humor to our many editorial suggestions and critiques of their chapters. Our distinguished editorial board worked hard and closely with us in designing a clinically focused and educationally sound volume. In particular, Herbert Pardes, M.D., a true visionary and leader in the field, provided a conceptual framework for us to consider in organizing and updating the book and prepared a stimulating introduction that gives an overview of where psychiatry was, where it is today, and where it is going.

The outstanding staff at APPI has been highly encouraging and effective with all aspects of this project. Carol Nadelson, M.D., President, CEO, and Editor-in-Chief of APPI, and Chairperson of our International Editorial Advisory Board, and Ron McMillen, Director of Publishing Operations, have been perennially supportive, insightful, and invaluable to the concept, organization, and content of all editions of the *Textbook*. Claire Reinburg, Editorial Director, assisted us with key structural elements of the book and many related administrative matters. Pam Harley, Managing Editor, Books Department, coordinated the entire editorial process with Martin Lynds and Elizabeth Gould-Leger, Project Editors, who had the daunting challenge of overseeing the line-by-line editing of all the manuscripts. Special thanks also go to Anne Friedman, Prepress Manager, who designed and laid out the book, and Pam Maher, Production Manager, for getting the book to the printer on schedule. Thanks also go to Dick Bardes, the tough and highly competent former Business Manager, and the always pleasant and helpful Stacy Jobb, Acquisitions Assistant, who helped us with numerous administrative and technical requirements for the publication of this edition. Finally, Matthew Price, Director of Marketing, has organized an outstanding program for spreading the word about our textbook to the field through various promotional efforts.

The headquarters for this edition of *The American Psychiatric Press Textbook of Psychiatry* was located at the University of California, Davis in Sacramento. Tina Marshall handled all the correspondence and the majority of the calls to our authors and editorial board members. Her dedication and commitment to the publication of this edition are greatly appreciated and were invaluable. We don't know how we could have accomplished this project without her. We would also like to thank our wives, Dianne Hales, Beth Yudofsky, and Susan Talbott, for their support and understanding as we labored diligently on this project over the last 3 years, especially during evenings and on weekends.

Finally, we acknowledge the many people with psychiatric disorders, their families, and those who have dedicated their lives to caring for them through clinical service, research, and education. These people have provided the inspiration, motivation, and knowledge for publication of this textbook.

Robert E. Hales, M.D., M.B.A.
Sacramento, California

Stuart C. Yudofsky, M.D.
Houston, Texas

John A. Talbott, M.D.
Baltimore, Maryland

INTRODUCTION

The third edition of *The American Psychiatric Press Textbook of Psychiatry* has been conceptualized by its editors as a text to prepare students and to be used as a resource for practitioners for the care of patients in the twenty-first century. In addition, it is crafted to update both students and practitioners on the most promising, relevant, and current psychiatric research. It would be a useful and revealing exercise to review the standard psychiatric textbook at the turn of last century and compare its contents and emphases with this textbook. Perhaps, in this way, the changes and progress of psychiatry over the twentieth century can be highlighted.

The sixth edition of *Psychiatry, A Textbook for Students and Physicians*, by Emil Kraepelin, was published in 1899. The fact that the preeminent textbook of the era was published in German correctly indicates from whence the most prominent scholarship and academic leadership in our field emanated. Much of this tradition derived from the neuropsychiatrist disciples of Wilhelm Griesinger, who, in the middle of the nineteenth century, was professor of both neurology and psychiatry at the University of Berlin.

Kraepelin was born in northern Germany in 1856. He attended medical school at the University of Wurzburg and later studied and did research in psychopharmacology in the laboratories of Wilhelm Wundt. His first book was titled *On the Influence of Several Medications on Simple Psychic Processes.* In 1883, shortly before he was appointed the chief of staff of a mental hospital in Leubus, Germany, he wrote a small book titled *Compendium of Psychiatry for the Use of Students and Physicians.* Over the next 7 years, Kraepelin assumed several positions in more prominent institutions while he continued to expand his textbook in subsequent editions. By the sixth edition of *Psychiatry, A Textbook for Students and Physicians*, Kraepelin had achieved considerable influence as professor of psychiatry in Heidelberg, but the greatest source of his notoriety came from his textbook.

In the introduction to the sixth edition, Kraepelin defines psychiatry as "the science of mental illnesses and their treatment." He then decries the loss of the emphasis on the biologic sources of mental disorders, which had originally been appreciated by the ancient Greeks but by the Middle Ages had begun to be overlooked in favor of other theories and philosophies regarding the disorders:

Mental disorder was no longer considered an illness, but the work of the devil, punishment of heaven, sometimes even divine ecstasy. The doctor no longer dealt with the examination and treatment of the person suffering from psychic disorders, for it was the priest who tried to cast out the evil spirits; people worshiped the insane persons as a saint, and the judges of the witch trials made him do penance in the torture chamber and at the stake for his alleged, illusory sins . . . . Kant still held the opinion that it is rather the philosopher than the physicians who is qualified for judging pathologic mental states. Not until the establishment of special institutions for the mentally ill under medical supervision did a truly scientific view of insanity gradually develop.

Kraepelin thus clearly delineates the history of the origin of the stigmatization of the mentally ill in Western society, and he prescribes a powerful antidote to this disabling condition: the appreciation of the biologic bases of most severe mental illness and the application of the medical model to the treatment of psychiatric disorders. Kraepelin expressed optimism that the late nineteenth century focus of psychiatry on neurobiology would eradicate the stigmatization of the mentally ill; however, he was too optimistic. In the succeeding 100 years, neither the establishment of medical institutions to treat those afflicted with mental illness nor biologic treatment has succeeded in eradicating the stigmatization of the mentally ill and those who care for them.

A perusal of the first section of sixth edition, "The Causes of Insanity," reveals a remarkably modern approach to the understanding of mental illness. Kraepelin proposes a biopsychosocial approach to considering their etiologies. First among the so-called "physical causes" are "diseases of the brain." Included are strokes, tumors, infections, toxins, alcohol, and the like. Kraepelin also is aware of the effects of hormonal changes on brain functions such as mood regulation:

> In women the physiological process of menstruation is usually accompanied by a slight increase in nervous and psychic irritability, which in certain persons attains almost pathological states (severe irritability and great excitation). This influence is most evident at the onset of menses.

Next Kraepelin considers "psychic causes," which he conceptualizes as the influence of the emotions on the brain. Note how similar Kraepelin's approach to understanding mental illness is to that of psychiatrist and neuroscientist Eric R. Kandel as articulated in the April 1998 volume of *The American Journal of Psychiatry* in an essay entitled "A New Intellectual Framework for Psychiatry":

> We now need to ask, How do the biological processes of the brain give rise to mental events, and how in turn do so-

cial factors modulate the biological structure of the brain? In the attempt to understand a particular mental illness, it is more appropriate to ask, To what degree is this biological process determined by genetic and developmental factors? To what degree is it environmentally or socially determined? To what degree is it determined by a toxic or infectious agent? Even the mental disturbances that are considered to be the most heavily determined by social factors must have a biological component, since it is the activity of the brain that is being modified.

Kraepelin's consideration of social and cultural contexts of mental illness includes issues such as war, captivity, and suggestion. Of particular interest in Kraepelin's discussion of "The Causes of Insanity" is what he termed "predisposition," where he posited, among other predeterminants of mental disorders, the role of heredity:

> Taking into account that not only mental diseases strictly speaking but also a number of related states, alcoholism, neuroses, uncommon characteristics, criminal tendencies, and similar features are considered manifestations of pathological predisposition and are thus included in calculating the effect of heredity, the existence of such deviations among near relations can be ascertained on the average in at least 60 or 70% of all mental patients.

Kraepelin also wrote in eerily modern terms on what he called "disorders of development." He postulated,

> The influence on mental predisposition of injuries which, without being hereditary, concern the first period of development, is, until now, almost completely unknown, although such injuries are most probably of decisive importance in certain cases. Thus it is reported that drunkenness during the act of reproduction causes epilepsy in the offspring, that violent emotions in the mother during pregnancy induce a psychopathic predisposition in the child. No further explanation is required for the fact that all sorts of physical causes, insufficient nutrition, overage or underage parents, diseases of the parents or of the fetus may become of great importance for the cerebral development and thus for the psychic predisposition of the child.

The greatest emphasis of Kraepelin's textbook is on the manifestations of and classification of mental disorders. These general areas of interest are regarded as his most important contributions to our field. Approximately 75% of his two-volume textbook is devoted to these subjects. Remarkably, less than 5% (about 30 pages) of Kraepelin's work covers treatments, and this is the most telling revelation about the difference between psychiatry at the turn of the last century and today. On the other hand, many aspects of his textbook appear surprisingly modern and current. One example of the latter is Kraepelin's description and discussion of cocaine addiction: "Cocaine addiction is the most modern of the chronic intoxications." He explains that often the patient becomes addicted by physicians who use the drug to treat such maladies as morphine addiction and withdrawal:

> [C]ombating cocainism can only originate with the prevention of the same. Every not purely local application of the drug must be considered inadmissible, and its use in the withdrawal of morphine must be branded as downright irresponsible or, better still, be punished as malpractice. As doctors, we all have the duty to warn the public most insistently of the dangerous poison and denounce mercilessly the base exploitation of the sick by dealers and doctors.

Historian of psychiatry Jacques M. Quen, M.D., who edited and wrote a splendid introduction to the English translation of the sixth edition of *Psychiatry, A Textbook for Students and Physicians* (from which all the quotations in the preceding paragraphs have been taken), summarized the main contribution of the author and his textbook to the field of psychiatry:

> It is not unusual for Kraepelin to be referred to as the Father of Descriptive Psychiatry. However to do so is to misrepresent the state of earlier psychiatry, as well as to minimize and to misconstrue Kraepelin's actual contributions. "Descriptive" is a fair characterization of psychiatry as it was during the nineteenth century. It was in this period that psychiatric diagnoses were based upon the behavioral signs and symptoms at a given time. The description was the diagnosis. However it was Kraepelin who successfully and consistently used the late nineteenth-century medical model of study and classification in an entire nosologic system and thus incorporated the etiology, course, prognosis, and outcome in the definition of disease entities.

In their preface to the third edition of *The American Psychiatric Press Textbook of Psychiatry*, editors Hales, Yudofsky, and Talbott highlight the many changes and additions over the previous edition, which was published 5 years earlier. Content comparisons of corresponding chapters reveal the rapid pace at which our entire field is advancing. The new topics that have been added as chapters are a litmus of areas within our field of special currency: psychiatry and primary care, managed care and psychiatry, practice guidelines in psychiatry and a psychiatric practice research network, and the future of psychiatry.

One new chapter in the third edition of the textbook "completes the loop" with the nineteenth-century tradition from which Kraepelin emerged: neuropsychiatry. Neuropsychiatry has reemerged over the past decade; with the growth of the American Neuropsychiatric Association and scientific publications, including *The Journal of Neuropsychiatry and Clinical Neurosciences*, neuropsychiatry has now become sufficiently prominent to have earned its own chapter within the textbook. These additions and changes are as consequential as the disparities occurring in the 100 years between the sixth edition of Kraepelin's textbook and Hales et al.'s third edition. Nonetheless, I am struck by several fundamental similarities between the two books. Both books embrace a biopsychosocial model for understanding all people in health and disease. For much of this century, there has been an imbalance, wherein the psychological dimensions of a person's mental illness were prioritized at the expense of the biologic, social, and cultural aspects. Today, particularly in primary care settings operating under the severe fiscal and time constraints imposed by managed care, there are too many instances in which patients with severe psychiatric illnesses—such as major depression—are placed on medications without attention to intrapsychic, interpersonal, familial, occupational, dietary, or exercise components of causation and treatment. This biologic reductionism often results in treatment failures.

A second area of similarity between the two textbooks is the emphasis on careful clinical observation that buttresses precise classification of mental illnesses. I imagine that Kraepelin would have been most comfortable with Stephen C. Scheiber's chapter, "The Psychiatric Interview, Psychiatric History and Mental Status Examination." I believe, however, that he would have been most impressed by Janet B. W. Williams's chapter, "Psychiatric Classification," because this chapter exemplifies the remarkable progress our field has made in nontheoretically based classification as manifested by DSM-IV. Contemporary psychiatrist-historian Michael H. Stone summarizes Kraepelin's contributions and influences in this area:

> Kraepelin's systematization of psychiatric nosology was hardly limited to the psychoses. He studied thousands of patients during his lifetime, searching for commonalities, and the process brought clarity to the cluster of manic-depressive disorders as well as to what we now call (after Eugen Bleuler) "schizophrenia." Endowed with a subtler mind than he is sometimes given credit for, Kraepelin also described "borderline" variants of manic-depressive psychosis, created a whole catalogue of character types, and enumerated the traits peculiar to the temperaments associated with manic-depression: namely, the depressive, irritable, and manic temperaments, plus cyclothymic, a combination of the depressive and manic. Current editions of the American Psychiatric Association's

Diagnostic and Statistical Manual of Mental Disorders have often been called "neo-Kraepelinian," because of the profound influence Kraepelin exerted on contemporary biometricians.

Among the many advances in our field over the past century, as evidenced in the differences between the two texts, are the biologic bases of human behavior and mental disorders and psychopharmacology. Interestingly, these areas have also evidenced dramatic growth and change during the 5 years between the second and third editions of the *Textbook of Psychiatry*. As might be expected, Chapter 2, "Genetics," is an excellent example. Despite "pressure" from the editors to maintain the size of the third edition at the length of the previous edition, this chapter has grown by 5 pages, or about 14%. Even the most cursory review shows that more than half of the extensive list of scientific papers in the reference section are new. Encouraging are the recent discoveries made possible by linkage analysis, genetic association studies, and direct DNA sequencing. Drs. Marangell, Silver, and Yudofsky's chapter, "Psychopharmacology and Electroconvulsive Therapy," at over 100 pages, is one of the largest chapters in the textbook. It is comprehensively revised and demonstrates convincingly the advances that have been made over the past 5 years in the pharmacological treatment of manic depression and psychotic disorders and symptoms. It is curious to not that the terms *pharmacology*, *psychopharmacology*, or even *medicine treatments* are not referenced in the table of contents or the index of Kraepelin's sixth edition. Rather, only the occasional reference to medication treatment is made, such as *mercury treatment in paralysis*. In this realm of treatment we have certainly come a long way! And let us not forget the eight other chapters in the *Textbook of Psychiatry* that are devoted to treatments. Clearly, in 100 years, psychiatry has grown far beyond observation, categorization, and classification and has developed a robust therapeutic regimen.

Kraepelin did not, in his *Textbook*, consider service delivery or "the business" of psychiatry. This important area has also been underrepresented in previous editions of the *APP Textbook*. Dr. Melvin Sabshin, in his chapter, "The Future of Psychiatry," points out,

> Health care in the United States has changed from being offered through an almost free market to being heavily regulated. Today, for treatment to be reimbursed, approval of the treatment must be obtained in advance from the managed care company. Length of hospitalization is severely limited and alternative care systems are preferred. In the mental health field, an effort is often made by these intermediaries to have treatment conducted by psycholo-

> gists or social workers, who, it is assumed, will charge less than psychiatrists. (p. 1693)

Without question, these issues affect both the care of our patients and the professional satisfactions of psychiatrists. I expect even more extensive emphasis on economic considerations of mental health care and mental illness prevention in subsequent issues of the *APP Textbook*.

Finally, it is of interest that neither in Kraepelin's *Textbook* nor in any previous editions of the *APP Textbook* was there a special consideration of the evaluation of women who suffer from psychiatric disorders or of how psychiatric disorders differentially affect women. In the third edition of the *APPI Textbook*, Drs. Burt and Hendrick consider a broad range of women's issues in psychiatry. Topics such as premenstrual dysphoric disorder, the effects of hormones on the moods of women, treatments of mental illnesses in women who are pregnant, postpartum psychiatric disorders, and special issues involved in contraception, infertility, and menopause are included.

Although Adolf Meyer (1866–1950) was not born or trained in Germany, his medical education and early clinical experience in neuropsychiatry, which took place in Switzerland, France, and England, was strongly influenced by German scholarship and approaches to caring for patients with behavioral and emotional disorders. In 1893, Meyer immigrated to the United States, where, through prominent teaching and clinical positions in Illinois, New York City (the New York State Psychiatric Institute) and Baltimore (Johns Hopkins and the Henry Phipps Psychiatric Clinic) he strongly influenced American psychiatry at the turn of the century and over the next three decades. As an important bridge between European and American psychiatry, Professor Meyer can be credited with helping American psychiatry assume leadership in research, education and services related to the mentally ill. The first volume of Meyer's *Collected Papers* is entirely devoted to neurology, particularly the neuropathology of mental illness. In many subsequent writings, he critiqued Kraepelin's approach to understanding and conceptualizing mental illness. Meyer believed that Kraepelin depended too much on observation of the symptoms and course of psychiatric disorders to define the respective illnesses:

> Kraepelin subordinates the symptom complex to a broader clinical, or we might more properly say, to a more simply medical principle—that of evolution and outcome. To what extent has he created "diseases," or at least, to what extent are his diseases distinct entities from the point of view of pathology for pathology's sake, not pathology with undue reference to practical aims? (Vol. I, p. 352)

Kraepelin and Meyer, who both wished to link brain pathology with behavioral dysfunction—while keeping sight of the patient as a unique individual influenced by life experience and current social systems—would, most likely, be supportive of today's psychiatry. This progress is exemplified by the third edition of *The APP Textbook of Psychiatry* and its companion book, *The APP Textbook of Neuropsychiatry*. As evidenced in Drs. Black and Andreasen's chapter, "Schizophrenia, Schizophreniform Disorder, and Delusional (Paranoid) Disorder, modern technological advances such as functional magnetic resonance imaging (fMRI) are better able to link pathologic brain function with mental, emotional, and behavioral dysfunctions. Without question, subsequent editions of "The APP Textbook of Psychiatry will reflect our field's progress in elucidating the links between brain and behavior from genetic and subcellular levels to social, cultural, and spiritual representations. These advances will also bring more compassionate understanding of and more effective care to those suffering from psychiatric illnesses.

Herbert Pardes, M.D.
Vice President for Health Sciences
Dean, Faculty of Medicine
Columbia University College of Physicians and Surgeons
New York, New York

REFERENCES

American Psychiatric Association: Diagnostic and Statistical Manual of Mental Disorders, 4th Edition. Washington, DC, American Psychiatric Association, 1994

Kandel ER: A new intellectual framework for psychiatry. Am J Psychiatry 155:457–469, 1998

Quen JM (ed): Psychiatry: A Textbook for Students and Physicians, 6th Edition, by Emil Kraepelin. Canton, MA, Science History Publications, 1989

Stone MH: Healing the Mind: A History of Psychiatry From Antiquity to the Present. New York, WW Norton, 1997

Winters EE (ed): The Collected Papers of Adolf Meyer. Baltimore, MD, The Johns Hopkins Press, 1950

Yudofsky SC, Hales RE (eds): The American Psychiatric Press Textbook of Neuropsychiatry, 3rd Edition. Washington, DC, American Psychiatric Press, 1997

THEORETICAL FOUNDATIONS

CHAPTER 1

THE NEUROSCIENTIFIC FOUNDATIONS OF PSYCHIATRY

JOSEPH T. COYLE, M.D.
STEVEN E. HYMAN, M.D.

Advances in research on the brain have occurred with a rapidly increasing pace over the last 20 years and have reached the point that neuroscience can justifiably be considered the biomedical foundation of psychiatry. Logarithmic growth in our understanding of the organization and function of the brain has made it feasible to begin to analyze behavior at the systems, cellular, and molecular levels. Methodologies such as nuclear magnetic resonance imaging and spectroscopy and positron-emission tomography now permit us to characterize structural, metabolic, and physiological abnormalities in the brains of living psychiatric patients. Parallel advances at the cellular and molecular levels will permit us to define the genetic basis of vulnerability for disorders of behavior and, ultimately, to determine the molecular and cellular mechanisms responsible for psychiatric disorders. These developments are progressively narrowing the Cartesian separation between the mind and brain by improving our ability to correlate mental experience with brain processes.

Neuroscience research offers important opportunities to psychiatry in the interest of the care of patients and, in the long term, for the better understanding of human expe-rience and behavior. Thus, it is essential for psychiatry to harness this rapidly evolving area of knowledge. Accordingly, our purpose in this chapter is to review the molecular and cellular aspects of neuroscience research. It is not possible within this limited space to cover in depth the totality of the advances in brain research. Rather, in this chapter, we address major themes and critical research strategies in neuroscience that directly affect psychiatry. It is hoped that the review will serve as the foundation for understanding our current knowledge base and for critically evaluating future developments in neuroscience for psychiatrists.

FUNCTIONAL ANATOMY OF THE NEURON

The *neuron* is a cell type that is highly specialized, both anatomically and biochemically, to carry out the functions of information signaling and processing. Within the nervous system, there are hundreds of types of neurons, each subserving specialized functions. In contrast to many other cell types—such as those that make up the liver, the epidermis, or the hemopoietic system, which are capable of cell division throughout the life of the individual—neurons do not divide once they are fully mature. This inability of most mature neurons to undergo mitosis has obvious implications for the irreversible effects of damage to the nervous system.

The neuron can be divided into four distinct components: the *cell body* (or *perikaryon*), the *dendrites*, the *axon*, and the *presynaptic terminal* (Figure 1–1). The synthesis of proteins and other structural components of neurons generally occurs in the perikaryon, although there is growing evidence of specialized protein synthesis in dendrites. Situated within the perikaryon of the neuron is the nucleus, which contains the genetic material in the form of deoxyribonucleic acid (DNA). The information for protein synthesis is encoded by genes contained within the DNA; this genetic information is read out by a process called *transcription*, in which DNA serves as a template for the synthesis of ribonucleic acid (RNA). The resulting primary RNA transcripts are then processed to yield mature messenger RNA (mRNA) that is exported out of the nucleus into the cytoplasm of the perikaryon. There the mRNA is translated into proteins on organelles called *ribosomes*. The rich concentration of RNA-protein synthetic machinery surrounding the nucleus in the perikaryon accounts for the *Nissl substance* observed with certain classical stains of neurons in brain tissue. Protein translation occurs largely within the perikaryon, but active ribosomes have recently been detected in dendrites, raising the possibility that local control of protein translation by neural signaling processes may occur.

The size of the neuronal perikaryon is roughly proportional to the extent of the projections of dendrites and axons of the neuron. It should be emphasized that only a very small percentage of the neuronal volume is contained within the perikaryon; the bulk of cell volume is distributed throughout the axon and the dendritic arbor. For this reason, the metabolic and synthetic demands on the neuronal perikaryon are considerable, as the neuronal perikaryon sustains the rest of the neuron. Proteins synthesized within the perikaryon are transferred down the axons and dendrites by axoplasmic transport to replace inactivated components. Conversely, breakdown products of metabolic and structural proteins in the axons and dendrites are often transported back to the cell body for processing.

The *axon* is a fine tubular extension from the neuronal cell body down which electrical impulses are conducted to the nerve terminals. Neurons generally send out only a single axon, the length of which varies from less than a millimeter for interneurons to over a meter for motor neurons innervating the extremities. The axon, as it approaches its terminal field of innervation, branches to varying degrees, depending on the number of neurons with which it makes synaptic contact. Some neurons have very restrictive synaptic fields, whereas other neurons, such as the nigrostriatal dopaminergic neurons, have axons that may arborize tremendously to contact millions of neurons in their field of innervation.

Dendrites are multiple fine tubular extensions from the neuronal cell body that serve as the primary structure for the reception of synaptic contacts from other neurons. Neurons are generally involved in the integration of multiple synaptic inputs. Neurons such as the Purkinje cells in

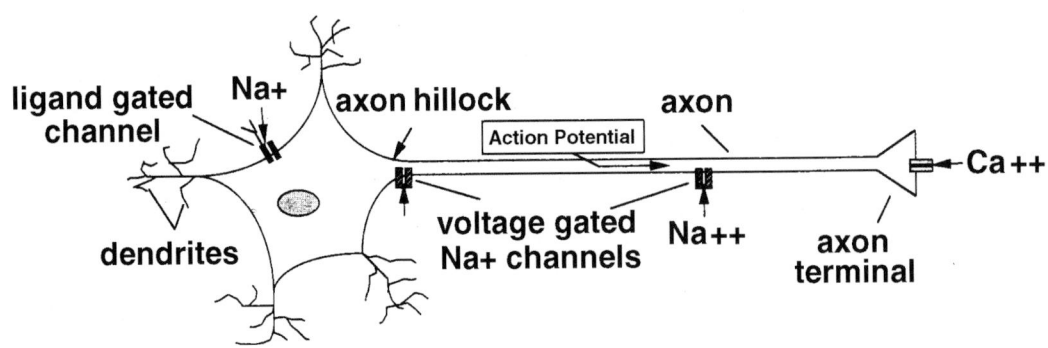

FIGURE 1–1. Schematic representation of a neuron. A ligand-gated channel, possibly a glutamate receptor, is shown permitting Na$^+$ entry into the cell body of a neuron. If the balance of positive to negative charges is adequate to depolarize the neuron to threshold in the region of the proximal axon or axon hillock, voltage-gated Na$^+$ channels will open, generating an action potential. The action potential propagates down the axon because of the sequential opening of Na$^+$ channels. When the action potential invades the presynaptic terminal, voltage-gated Ca^{++} channels open, and the entry of Ca^{++} causes neurotransmitter release (see discussion in text). Repolarization of the neuron results from the opening of voltage-gated K$^+$ channels in rapid succession after Na$^+$ entry.

the cerebellum and components of the reticular core of the brain stem, which have marked integrative functions, possess very extensive dendritic *trees* that receive synaptic input from thousands of neurons.

The *synapse* is a specialized structure involved in the transmission of information from one neuron to another; transmission is generally accomplished by chemical messengers called *neurotransmitters*, but in some cases it may be electrical. Structurally, the synapse consists of an outpouching of the terminal portion of the axon of the *presynaptic neuron* known as a *bouton*, which is firmly attached to the dendritic membrane of the adjacent *postsynaptic neuron* by specialized contacts. The dendritic membrane at the synapse is markedly enriched with receptors that respond to the neurotransmitter released by the terminal bouton of the presynaptic neuron. The presynaptic terminal contains a number of cellular structures that allow it to remain metabolically and functionally somewhat independent of the neuronal cell body. The terminal contains *mitochondria*—the power packs of the cell that generate adenosine triphosphate (ATP) from the aerobic metabolism of glucose—enzymes involved in the synthesis and degradation of neurotransmitters, and the storage vesicles that maintain substantial concentrations of the neurotransmitter in a protected state, awaiting release. When brain tissue is experimentally disrupted by gentle homogenization in properly buffered solutions, the synapse with the terminal bouton and the adjacent postsynaptic membrane specialization are sheared off to form *synaptosomes*, which have been exploited for studying biochemical aspects of synaptic functions such as the types and number of neurotransmitter receptors found within that region of the brain.

The fundamental property that permits neurons to function in information processing and signaling is the excitable nature of their membrane. This property derives from the membrane's specialized nature: it maintains a voltage gradient between the interior of the neuron and the extracellular fluid, and selectively gates the transmembranal flow of ions. Two types of proteins are primarily responsible for the regulation of ion distribution and hence voltage across the neuronal membrane. These are the transmembrane *ion pumps* and the *voltage-gated ion channels*. Based on the molecular cloning of DNA that encodes certain of these pumps and voltage-gated channels, it appears that each represents a gene family, each derived from its own common ancestral gene. More important, molecular cloning has initiated an era of detailed structure—activity analyses that will likely lead to the design of improved neuroactive medications.

Pumps critical in establishing the physiological gradient of ions found across the neuronal membrane are an energy (ATP)–dependent pump, the sodium-potassium ATPase, which moves two Na^+ ions out of the cell for every K^+ ion it allows in; and pumps that remove Ca^{++} from the cell. At rest, there are high relative concentrations of Na^+ and Cl^- outside the neuron and a high relative concentration of K^+ inside the cell. The major source of negative charge inside the cell is derived from negatively charged amino acids. Overall, the membrane is polarized, with a voltage difference across the membrane of about -70 mV with respect to the outside. This is called the *resting membrane potential*.

When the neuronal membrane is depolarized to about -35 mV, an *action potential* occurs, which represents cell *firing* and is the fundamental mechanism of neuronal signaling. Specifically, as the interior of the cell becomes more positive, specialized voltage-gated Na^+ channels open, permitting more positive ions to flow into the cell (Figure 1–1). The action potential represents the spread of depolarization by the vectorial opening of adjacent voltage-gated Na^+ channels. Because each Na^+ channel that opens in succession provides the positive charge to bring the next segment of the axon up to threshold for opening of its Na^+ channels, the action potential is self-regenerating, and once begun, it propagates down the axon without fail. When the action potential arrives in the presynaptic terminal, it causes opening of the unique voltage-gated Ca^{++} channels found there (denoted "N-type" Ca^{++} channels in contradistinction to the "L-type" channels blocked by the verapamil-like Ca^{++} channel blockers used clinically). Ca^{++} entry initiates a series of complex, but rapid biochemical processes that cause the neurotransmitter-containing vesicles to fuse with the presynaptic membrane and thereby release their contents into the synapse, thus permitting synaptic transmission. Because the entry of positive charge depolarizes the membrane, bringing the neuron closer to threshold for firing an action potential, neurotransmitter receptors that permit entry of cations such as Na^+ or Ca^{++} are excitatory, and those that cause entry of anions such as Cl^- or the exit of cations such as K^+ are inhibitory.

Neuronal dendrites and cell bodies are continuously summating excitatory and inhibitory inputs to determine whether a neuron will generate an action potential. The innervation of the neuron is not random but rather is highly organized. Excitatory inputs are generally concentrated at the distal end of dendrites, whereas inhibitory inputs are located primarily at the proximal end of dendrites and around the perikaryon. This spatial distribution means that inhibitory inputs play a predominant role in determining whether a neuron will generate an action potential. Because the action potential is self-regenerating, the decision to "fire" an action potential is an all-or-none process. Once the balance is struck toward adequate depolarization in the region of the proximal axon (i.e., axon hillock), where the density of voltage-gated Na$^+$ channels is high, an action potential is generated (Figure 1–1).

NEUROTRANSMITTERS

It is often not appreciated, but nevertheless appropriate, that psychiatry, the medical specialty most concerned with issues of communication, fostered much of the early research on the mechanisms of chemical communication among neurons in the brain. Notably, soon after the existence of brain neurotransmitters was first appreciated, Smythes hypothesized that schizophrenia resulted from an abnormality in the metabolism of the neurotransmitter epinephrine that would generate a psychotomimetic metabolite, which he called "adrenochrome." While this hypothesis did not ultimately prove to be true, it did prompt, during the 1960s, a number of studies to characterize the metabolic disposition of the catecholamines in the brain. More recently, attempts to understand neuronal communication in the brain have led to the identification of a rapidly expanding number of substances that serve as neurotransmitters. But in the mid-1960s, only a handful of substances were thought to satisfy the criteria for action as neurotransmitters in the brain with any certainty. Often the term *putative* neurotransmitter was used, to refer to the fact that it is exceedingly difficult to satisfy all the criteria that unequivocally establish a substance as a neurotransmitter in the brain (Table 1–1). Within the last decade, the number of putative neurotransmitters has increased nearly 10-fold (Tables 1–2 and 1–3). Furthermore, it has become increasingly clear that most neurons release more than one neurotransmitter, often a small molecule neurotransmitter and one or more peptides.

The following discussion focuses on representative

TABLE 1–1. Criteria for a neurotransmitter

1. The neuron contains the substance.[a]
2. The neuron synthesizes the substance.[a]
3. The neuron releases the substance upon depolarization.[a]
4. The substance is physiologically active on neurons.[a]
5. The postsynaptic physiological response to the substance is identical to that of the neurotransmitter released by the neuron.

[a]The criterion is satisfied by all substances listed in Tables 1–2 and 1–3.

TABLE 1–2. "Classical" neurotransmitters

Acetylcholine	Aspartic acid
Histamine	γ-Aminobutyric acid
Serotonin	Glutamic acid
Dopamine	Glycine
Norepinephrine	Homocysteine
Epinephrine	Taurine

TABLE 1–3. Selected neuropeptide neurotransmitter candidates

Adrenocorticotropic hormone (ACTH)
Angiotensin II
Atriopeptin
β-Endorphin[a]
Bombesin
Bradykinin
Calcitonin gene–related peptide (CGRP)
Carnosine
Cholecystokinin
Corticotropin-releasing factor
Dynorphin[a]
Galanin
Gastrin
Glucagon
Insulin
Leu-enkephalin[a]
Luteinizing hormone–releasing factor
Met-enkephalin[a]
N-acetylaspartylglutamate
Neurotensin
Neuropeptide Y
Somatostatin
Substance P
Thyrotropin-releasing hormone (TRH)
Vasoactive intestinal peptide (VIP)
Vasopressin

[a]Members of the endorphin family.

examples from the two major classes of neurotransmitters in the brain: the "classical" small-molecule neurotransmitters, such as norepinephrine, that are locally synthesized in nerve terminals, and the neuropeptide neurotransmitters, such as the endorphins, that are synthesized in the perikaryon. For detailed reviews, see Hyman and Nestler (1993) and Cooper et al. (1991).

CATECHOLAMINES

The best-characterized neurotransmitter system from the perspective of synthesis, storage, release, and metabolism is the catecholaminergic system. The principles established for catecholaminergic neurotransmission in the periphery and in the brain have general applicability to the other classical neurotransmitter systems. The catecholamine neurotransmitters include dopamine, norepinephrine, and epinephrine. Although each acts as a neurotransmitter in its own right, they are products of sequential steps in a single biosynthetic pathway (Figure 1–2). The enzymes responsible for catecholamine synthesis are synthesized in the cell perikaryon and are transported down axons to presynaptic terminals. Neurons that utilize dopamine as their neurotransmitter possess the first two enzymes in this pathway, tyrosine hydroxylase and dopa decarboxylase. Neurons that release norepinephrine express a third enzyme, dopamine β-hydroxylase, and neurons that produce epinephrine express a fourth enzyme, phenylethanolamine-*N*-methyltransferase (PNMT). Because tyrosine hydroxylase is a tightly controlled rate-limiting enzyme, important regulatory mechanisms that determine neurotransmitter availability are common to this entire group of neurotransmitters.

The synthetic pathways for classical neurotransmitters generally, although not invariably, involve the conversion of an informationally inert precursor to an informationally "charged" neurotransmitter. In the case of the catecholamines, the amino acid L-tyrosine serves as the precursor. Tyrosine hydroxylase, the rate-limiting enzyme in the synthesis pathway, is virtually saturated by the ambient levels of tyrosine in the brain. Therefore, increasing levels of this amino acid in the brain would not significantly affect catecholamine biosynthesis. Moreover, to prevent a

vicious cycle of catecholamine synthesis and degradation, tyrosine hydroxylase is subject to end-product inhibition. Accordingly, when the concentration of catecholamines in the nerve terminal exceeds its storage capacity, the excess catecholamines inhibit the activity of tyrosine hydroxylase, thereby preventing further synthesis of catecholamines. Thus, when the catecholaminergic neurons are not firing, further synthesis of catecholamines is arrested. On the other hand, when catecholamines are released and the stores are depleted, this inhibitory feedback is removed and the rate of synthesis increases.

With neuronal activity, however, other mechanisms come into play that are biologically even more significant. Repeated firing of the catecholamine neuron causes activation of second messenger systems and therefore of protein kinases (see below). Phosphorylation of tyrosine hydroxylase, by protein kinases, reduces its sensitivity to feedback inhibition and, in addition, increases its affinity for a critical cofactor, pterin (Nose et al. 1985). Periods of prolonged, increased catecholaminergic neuronal activity bring into play a second mechanism: the synthesis of additional enzyme molecules in the biosynthetic pathway for catecholamines. This second process is regulated at the level of the catecholaminergic cell body, where additional mRNA encoding for tyrosine hydroxylase is transcribed from the nuclear DNA. Thus, the synthesis of catecholamines is under dynamic regulation that is tightly coordinated by the activity of the catecholaminergic neuron.

After the enzymatic synthesis of catecholamines occurs within the cytosol of the nerve terminal, the catecholamines are concentrated in vesicles, small membranous sacs within the nerve terminal. Vesicular storage of catecholamines is an active process that consumes energy in the form of ATP, and is irreversibly inhibited by the antihypertensive drug reserpine. The storage vesicles serve two purposes. First, they protect the catecholamines from enzymatic degradation by the enzyme monoamine oxidase (MAO). This catabolic enzyme is localized on the outer membrane of the mitochondria. Interference with vesicular storage by treatment with reserpine releases catecholamines within the nerve terminal so that they are rapidly degraded by MAO. Second, the vesicles mediate the quantal release of catecholamines by exocytosis when an action potential reaches the nerve terminal.

In addition to the intracellular enzyme MAO, a second enzyme that inactivates catecholamines is located on the outer surface of the neuronal membrane as well as on the outer surface of many other cell types. This enzyme, catechol-*O*-methyltransferase (COMT), catalyzes the inactivation of catecholamines by methylating one of the ring hydroxyl groups.

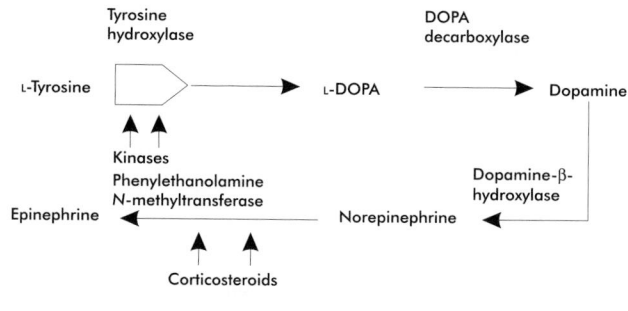

FIGURE 1–2. The biosynthetic pathway for catecholamines. Note that tyrosine hydroxylase is activated by phosphorylation by protein kinases, and the synthesis of phenylethanolamine-*N*-methyltransferase is regulated by corticosteroids.

However, enzymatic degradation is not the most significant mechanism by which the action of catecholamines in the synapse is terminated. The most critical mechanism is an active reuptake of the catecholamines into the nerve terminal that released them. Reuptake is mediated by a specific transporter protein that exchanges the catecholamine in an energy-dependent process that is driven by the gradient of sodium across the neuronal membrane (Pacholczyk et al. 1991). The dopamine and norepinephrine transporters are members of a large gene family of proteins that also includes the serotonin, glutamate and γ-aminobutyric acid (GABA) transporters (reviewed in Giros and Caron 1993).

The processes involved in the synthesis, storage, release, and inactivation of classical neurotransmitters are summarized in Figure 1–3. These interrelated processes ensure a ready availability of the neurotransmitter in the nerve terminals that can be regulated by neural activity and the inactivation of the released neurotransmitter in the synaptic cleft so that it does not produce undesired effects on neighboring neurons.

Similar mechanisms act, to a variable degree, for the other classical neurotransmitters, including serotonin, acetylcholine, and histamine. The amino acid neurotransmitters, however, represent an important exception from the principle that neurotransmitters are synthesized from neurophysiologically inactive precursors. The amino acid glutamate appears to be the predominant excitatory neurotransmitter in the brain; the amino acid glycine is a major inhibitory neurotransmitter. These molecules are present in plasma and are important precursors for protein synthesis, characteristics that would seem to be incompatible with the role of a neurotransmitter, which must have highly restricted spatial and temporal actions. However, the brain expends considerable energy on selective transport processes and catabolic enzymes to maintain extremely low

concentrations of these amino acid neurotransmitters in the extracellular space of the brain. The magnitude of this protection is exemplified by the fact that the intracellular concentration of glutamate in certain regions of the brain is as high as 10 mM, whereas its concentration in cerebrospinal fluid (CSF) is approximately 0.1 μM, which represents an extracellular-to-intracellular gradient of 100,000-fold.

NEUROPEPTIDES

The fact that small proteins (i.e., peptides) are used in the body as signals has long been known based on their role as hormones in the pituitary and other endocrine organs. The potential role of peptides as neurotransmitters came from the discovery that the releasing factors that control the secretion of several pituitary hormones were, in fact, peptides synthesized by neurons in the arcuate nucleus of the hypothalamus. However, the critical finding that provoked broad interest in peptides as neurotransmitters came from the discovery of the endorphins, endogenous opioid peptides that were found to have a widespread distribution in the central nervous system (CNS) (Hughes et al. 1975). Since the discovery of the endorphins nearly two decades ago, the number of peptides that are thought to serve as neurotransmitters in the brain has increased remarkably and exceeds threescore.

The research on neuropeptides (for review, see Hokfelt 1991) over the last decade has revealed a number of general principles. Unlike the small-molecule neurotransmitters that are synthesized by enzymatic processes located within the nerve terminal, the neuropeptides are synthesized within the neuronal cell body (Figure 1–4). This reflects the fact that synthesis of neuropeptides, which are small proteins, is directed by mRNA that has been transcribed from DNA within the nucleus. The levels of neuropeptides at the nerve terminal depend completely upon the synthesis, processing, and transport of the peptides from the neuronal perikaryon. Accordingly, it appears that peptidergic neurons may be less rapidly responsive to prolonged increases in the release because of the delay in the synthesis and transport of supplemental neuropeptides from the perikaryon.

One of the most striking findings concerning the synthesis of neuropeptides is that a single gene often gives rise to multiple active peptides and, further, that the array of peptides produced from a single gene may vary in different cell types. The generation of such diversity begins following transcription of the gene that encodes the peptide precursor. In eukaryotic cells most genes have their protein coding sequences (called *exons*) interrupted by noncoding

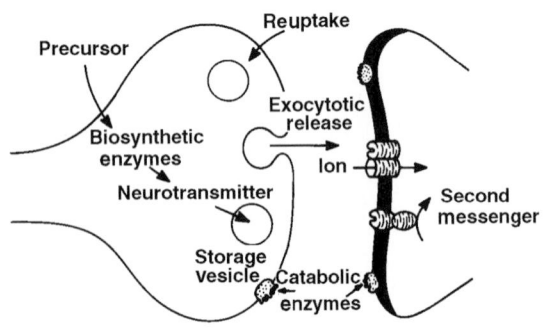

FIGURE 1–3. Schematic representation of the processes involved in the synthesis, synaptic action, and inactivation of classical neurotransmitters.

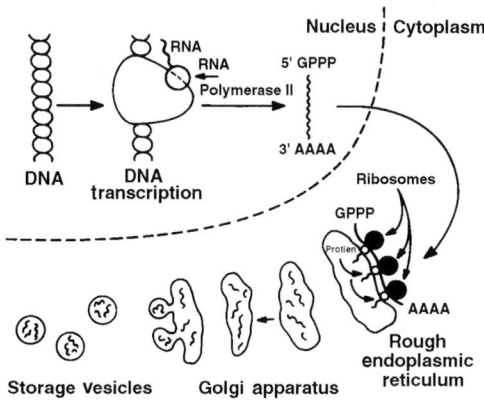

FIGURE 1–4. Sequence of neuropeptide synthesis. Within the nucleus, the gene for the precursor neuropeptide is transcribed into mRNA. The mRNA is transported from the nucleus into the cytoplasm, where it binds to ribosomes. The mRNA is then translated via protein synthesis on the ribosomes in the rough endoplasmic reticulum. Within the Golgi apparatus, the precursor peptide is enzymatically modified to yield the neuropeptide, which is packaged in storage vesicles for axoplasmic transport to the nerve terminal.

sequences (called *introns).* When a gene is transcribed, the primary transcript is colinear with the DNA and therefore contains both exons and introns. Before the RNA leaves the nucleus to be translated, the introns are removed and the exons are "spliced" to form a mature mRNA. It has been found that the primary transcript of certain neuropeptide genes is spliced in alternate ways in different cell types. By including or excluding particular exons in the mature cytoplasmic mRNA, mRNAs encoding distinctly different peptides can be produced. For example, calcitonin and calcitonin gene–related peptide are the products of the same gene derived by such alternate splicing.

The mature mRNAs encoding neuropeptides are translated on the rough endoplasmic reticulum (ER) to give rise to large precursors called *polyproteins.* These precursors (e.g., pre-pro-opiomelanocortin or pre-pro-enkephalin) contain a sequence, almost always at the amino terminus of the protein, that targets the protein to the neuron's secretory pathway. This *leader sequence,* or "pre" sequence, is rapidly cleaved by an endopeptidase, leaving the remainder of the precursor (e.g., pro- opiomelanocortin or pro-enkephalin). This precursor then undergoes further proteolytic cleavage and subsequent chemical modification (e.g., glycosylation, amidation, acetylation, or phosphorylation) within the ER and Golgi apparatus to yield numerous biologically active peptides for release.

Just as alternate splicing of mRNAs permits the generation of multiple signaling molecules from a single gene,

differential processing of peptide precursors permits the generation of multiple signaling molecules from a single peptide precursor. Within peptide precursors, pairs of basic amino acid residues (lysine or arginine) are recognized by processing enzymes as sites for cleavage. The family of enzymes responsible for processing within mammalian cells has only recently been discovered and remains incompletely characterized. However, it appears that certain enzymes have a greater affinity for some pairs of dibasic residues than for others. Thus, depending on which enzymes are expressed in a particular neuronal or endocrine cell type, the large precursor may be clipped into different active peptides that may have different physiological roles.

Among the peptide neurotransmitters, the endogenous opioid peptides are the most extensively studied and have clear relevance to psychiatry because of their role in the stress response, in motivated behaviors, and in analgesia. Hughes et al. (1975) identified the first endogenous opioids, Met- and Leu-enkephalin. Approximately 20 active opioid peptides have subsequently been isolated and characterized from mammalian brain and pituitary and adrenal glands. All of these endogenous opioids contain the same four amino acids at their amino terminus, Tyr-Gly-Gly-Phe, followed by either Met or Leu (Met-enkephalin, Leu-enkephalin). The opioid peptides all derive from one of three large polypeptide precursors, each encoded by a separate gene. The precursors are proenkephalin (which encodes six copies of the Met-enkephalin sequence and one of the Leu-enkephalin sequence), prodynorphin (which is the precursor of the endogenous opioid dynorphin and related peptides), and proopiomelanocortin. Proopiomelanocortin (POMC) is particularly interesting because it contains the sequences of active peptides with apparently different biological function, the opioid peptide β-endorphin and the nonopioid, adrenocorticotropic hormone (ACTH), and because it is processed to yield different active peptides in different tissues (Figure 1–5).

In the anterior lobe of the pituitary, only a subset of the dibasic cleavage sites within proopiomelanocortin are recognized by the processing enzyme that is present. In this tissue, the precursor yields an N-terminal peptide of unknown biological function along with ACTH and the hormone β-lipotropin. β-lipotropin is then further cleaved to yield the opioid peptide β-endorphin. Thus, whenever ACTH is released by the pituitary, β-endorphin is also released. Many mammals (but not humans) have a pituitary intermediate lobe that contains an additional processing enzyme. In the intermediate lobe, ACTH is therefore further cleaved to yield a peptide called *corticotropin-like intermediate-lobe peptide* and *melanocyte-stimulating hormone.*

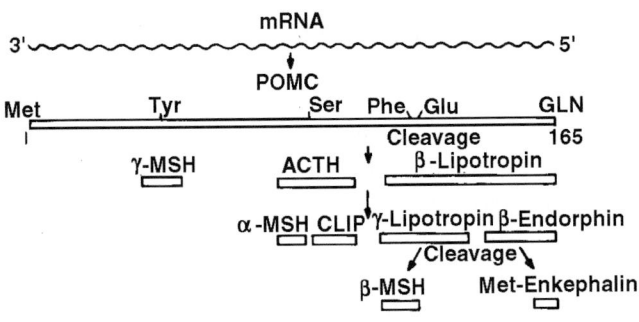

FIGURE 1–5. Processing of proopiomelanocortin (POMC). The precursor protein POMC, which contains 165 amino acids, is enzymatically cleaved to yield the physiologically active peptides indicated. Depending on the cellular localization (anterior pituitary, hypothalamus, midbrain nerve terminals), certain of these neuropeptides are expressed and others are not (see Watson et al. 1985).

This additional processing does not, however, occur within humans.

Although the N-terminal amino acids of β-endorphin are identical to the sequence of Met-enkephalin, the latter is not liberated from β-endorphin because there are no dibasic amino acid residues within β-endorphin that would permit peptidase cleavage to yield Met-enkephalin. Instead, Met-enkephalin is liberated from another precursor mentioned above, proenkephalin.

COLOCALIZATION

It was originally believed that a neuron uses one, and only one, neurotransmitter. However, during the last decade it has become apparent that in many, if not most, cases, neurons may release more than one neurotransmitter. Most cases that have been investigated have demonstrated colocalization of a classical neurotransmitter and one or more neuropeptides, but there are now even instances in which two classical neurotransmitters such as serotonin and GABA coexist in the same neuron. The same neurotransmitters are not always colocalized. For example, the opioid peptide enkephalin has been demonstrated to be colocalized in certain noradrenergic neurons in the sympathetic nervous system and in certain serotonergic neurons in the brain. In the brain, cholecystokinin has been demonstrated to be colocalized to the dopaminergic neurons innervating the corticolimbic system but not in the dopaminergic neurons innervating the striatum. With the large number of putative neurotransmitters in the brain, the number of possible combinations for colocalization is immense. Thus, colocalization suggests a much higher degree of complexity of synaptic neurotransmission than was appreciated heretofore.

The distinctly different mechanisms involved in the synthesis and release of neuropeptides versus small-molecule neurotransmitters suggest that the colocalized neurotransmitters may play somewhat different but complementary roles. Some studies indicate that neuropeptides are released only during periods of marked neuronal activity (i.e., only with repetitive firing), whereas the classical neurotransmitter is released in proportion to impulse flow. However, understanding of the mechanisms involved in shared communication remains rudimentary at present.

RECEPTORS

The identification, characterization, and, more recently, molecular cloning of neurotransmitter receptors constitute a major advance in neuroscience that has had considerable impact on the understanding of information processing in the brain and the sites of action of neuroactive substances, including psychotropic drugs. Although neurotransmitters are commonly described as excitatory or inhibitory, as if this action were inherent to their molecular structure, the nature of neuronal responses to a neurotransmitter ultimately depends on the presence of a receptor linked to a transducer. For this reason, depending on the receptors and transducers located on a given neuron, a neurotransmitter might exert inhibitory, excitatory, or more complicated "modulatory" effects.

Neurotransmitter receptors are proteins that span the neuronal membrane. These proteins have ligand binding regions that are accessible to extracellular messengers and other regions involved in transducing the binding interaction into an intercellular effect. The reversible binding of the neurotransmitter to the receptor causes a conformational change that triggers the transmembrane signaling event. The known neurotransmitter receptors can transduce neurotransmitter binding into one of two different general classes of effects: they can directly control or gate the opening of an ion channel that is an intrinsic part of the receptor molecule itself, or they can act by regulating the function of a signal-transducing G-protein (see below) that is associated with the inner surface of the membrane. Receptors that gate an intrinsic ion channel are called *ligand-gated channels;* receptors that act via G-proteins are called *G-protein–linked receptors.* As is the case for other important classes of molecules discussed earlier in this chapter, such as the voltage-sensitive ion channels and the neurotransmitter transporters, the ligand-gated channels, the G-protein–linked receptors, and the G-proteins themselves form independent large families of molecules with homologous structures. Each of these large *gene families* is thought to have begun with a single primitive ancestor (e.g., an ancestral ligand-gated channel) that, through gene duplication and mutation, gave rise to a large number of genes and hence proteins with specific but related functions, permitting increasing complexity of neural signaling during evolution.

LIGAND BINDING

Receptors bind their specific ligand in an avid, specific, reversible, and saturable (i.e., the number of receptor sites are limited) fashion. Neuroscientists have taken advantage of these characteristics to specifically label receptors with radioactive ligands. If the avidity of a specific interaction between radioligand and receptor is sufficiently high, the radioligand can be "caught in the act of binding" to the receptor long enough so that the radioactive complex can be isolated. This strategy has greatly facilitated studies to determine the characteristics of these neurotransmitter-receptor interactions and their localization within the nervous system. For example, the relative affinity of drugs or neurotransmitter analogs for a receptor can be determined by their potency at preventing the binding of the radioactive ligand to its receptor. With this strategy, Snyder and his colleagues demonstrated a compelling correlation between the affinities of antipsychiotic medications for dopamine D_2-like receptors and the clinical potency of these medications in treating psychotic disorders (Figure 1–6). Ligand binding methods combined with three-dimensional modeling of cloned receptors should facilitate understanding of the precise structure of molecules required for optimal recognition by the receptor site, and thus, eventually, rational drug design.

Because certain radioligands bind remarkably tightly to specific receptors, it has been possible to visualize receptor distribution in brain through autoradiographic techniques. With this method, thin slices of brain tissues are incubated in a physiological buffer with the radioactive ligand. Each slice is then washed free of the radioligand with buffer to remove nonspecifically and loosely bound radioligand. What remains in the tissue is the radioligand specifically associated with the receptor. This association can then be revealed by apposing the section to X-ray film, which results in the precipitation of silver grains in the photo emulsion at sites containing radioactive ligands. Figure 1–7 presents an autoradiogram of the distribution of muscarinic acetylcholine receptors as assessed by the binding of the very potent and specific muscarinic antagonist ^{3}H-labeled quinuclidinyl benzilate in a parasagittal section through the monkey brain.

With the development of computer-assisted imaging methods for localizing the source of radioactive emissions in three-dimensional space, it has become possible to exploit receptor-ligand binding techniques in vivo to determine neurotransmitter receptor distribution in the brain of the living human. For example, using ^{11}C-labeled positron-emitting spiperone, a neuroleptic with high affinity for D_2 family receptors, Wong et al. (1986) have visualized the distribution of these dopamine receptors in the human brain (Figure 1–8). As suitably avid positron-emitting ligands for other receptors are developed, they can be applied to visualizing other receptors in brain with positron emission tomography (PET) scanning techniques. Such technologies offer the possibility of studying changes in receptors in vivo in disease states and in response to drug administration.

NEUROPHYSIOLOGY

The transducers with which a neurotransmitter receptor interacts ultimately determine the physiological response resulting from neurotransmitter binding to the receptor. The relative ease of ligand binding studies for characterizing neurotransmitter-receptor interactions does not elim-

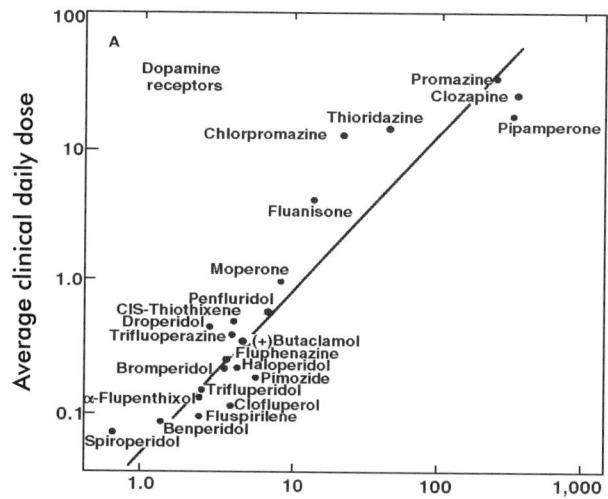

FIGURE 1–6. Correlation between the clinical potency of neuroleptics and their affinity for the dopamine D_2-like receptors. The ordinate presents the average daily dose of neuroleptic used to treat schizophrenia, and the abscissa indicates the affinity of the neuroleptics for the dopamine D_2-like receptors. It has recently been learned that there is a family of D_2-like receptors (see text). (Courtesy of S. Snyder.)

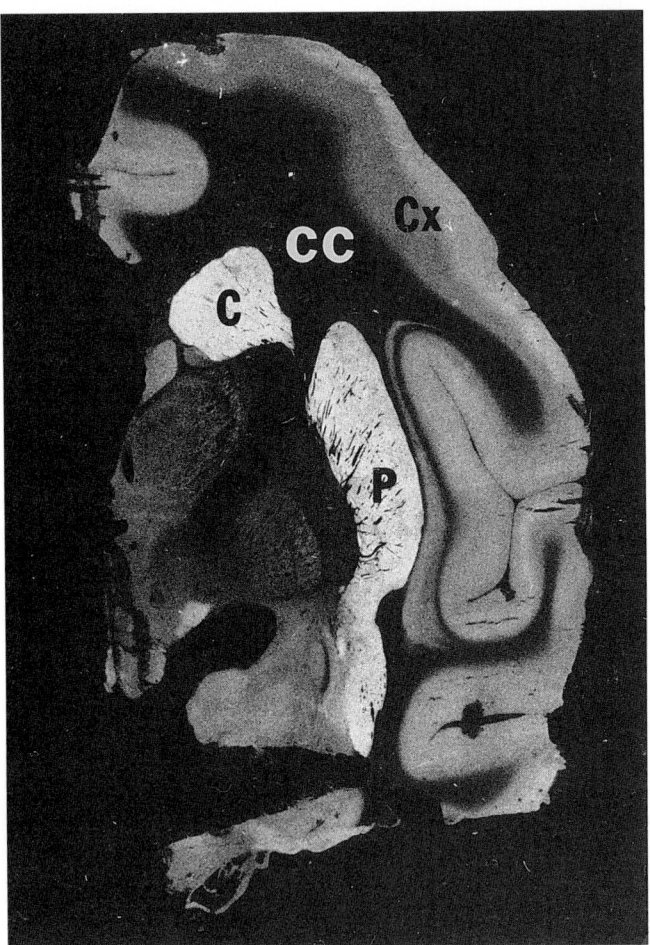

FIGURE 1-7. Coronal section through monkey brain showing the muscarinic receptors. The section was incubated with ³N-labeled quinuclidinyl benzilate, a potent muscarinic receptor antagonist. The section was then apposed to X-ray film to develop the autoradiogram. This negative image reveals muscarinic receptors as white dots; areas of high receptor density such as the caudate (C), putamen (P), and cortex (Cx) appear white, whereas areas of low receptor density such as the corpus callosum (cc) appear black.

cation of neurotransmitters on identified neurons. With multibarreled micropipettes, a recording electrode with an associated array of drug-filled pipettes can be apposed to a neuron in the brain. Neurotransmitter or drug is expelled from the micropipettes onto the neuron, and the consequences of the applied neurotransmitter or drug on the activity of the neuron can then be determined.

To obtain more rigorous information about the precise ion channels that might be involved in producing the electrophysiological response, investigators have increasingly relied upon intracellular recording techniques in which a fine micropipette is inserted into the neuronal cell body to assess voltage changes across the neuronal membrane in response to neurotransmitter application on the surface of the neuron. Intracellular recording studies in the intact animal are exceedingly difficult, analogous to attempting to skewer a grape on the tip of a 100-foot pole. Accordingly, investigators have developed preparations in

inate the more arduous task of defining the transducers coupled with specific receptors and the physiological effects of ligand binding on the target neuron. The difficulty derives from the fact that receptor-transducer interactions often cannot be assessed under conditions in which large populations of receptors are present, as is possible for ligand binding studies. This is because receptors may be associated with different transducers in different neurons and because these studies require technically more complicated measurements of the physiological response of activation of specific receptors on individual neurons.

A variety of approaches have been developed that measure the electrophysiological consequences of local appli-

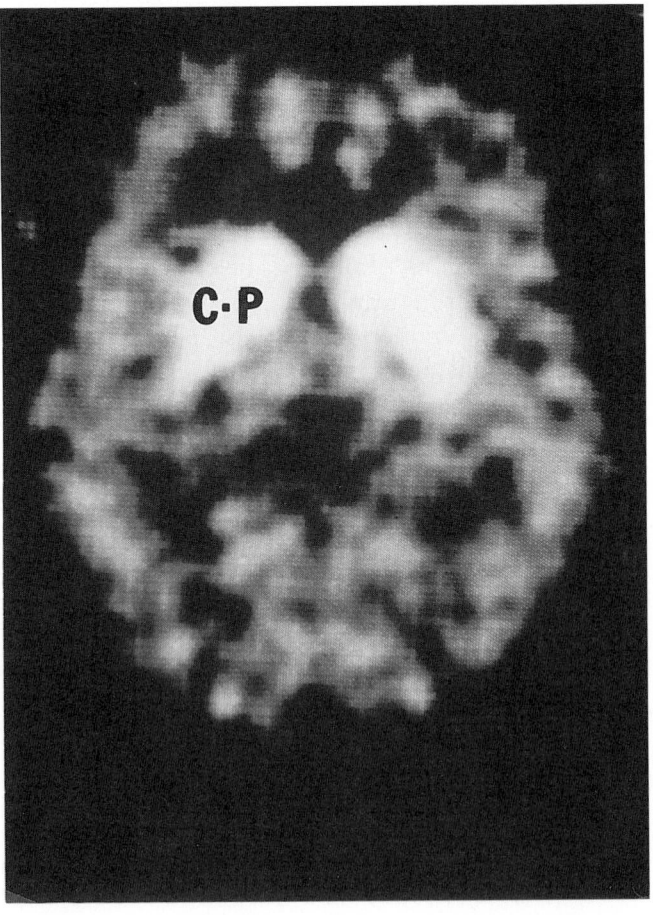

FIGURE 1-8. Positron-emission tomogram for the dopamine D₂ receptor in human brain labeled with [¹¹C]spiperone. Note the heavy labeling of the caudate-putamen (CP), a region markedly enriched with D₂ receptors. (Courtesy of L. Tune.)

which thin slices of brain tissue can be maintained viable for several hours in a bath by perfusion with oxygenated physiological medium. Neurons of interest can be directly visualized with phase-contrast microscopy, and the intracellular recording electrode can be inserted into identified neurons under direct visual control.

Finally, a newer procedure to provide the most precise information about the coupling of individual receptors with a single ion channel is *patch clamping*, wherein a microscopic piece of neuronal membrane is sucked onto the tip of a micropipette. With this method, the current flow through individual ion channels can be monitored following exposure of the "patch" of membrane to receptor agonists or other drugs. It is possible to determine which specific types of ion channels (sodium, potassium, calcium) are affected by the agonist and, indeed, to study in detail ionic conductances through single channels. Although ion channel properties may seem far removed from clinical psychiatry, they provide the physiological basis for neuronal signaling. Thus, channel function is an important consideration in thinking about the pathophysiology of psychiatric disorders and the overall effects of psychotropic drugs. Indeed, the anticonvulsant drugs carbamazepine and valproic acid, now used in the treatment of bipolar disorder, have as their primary action a direct effect on certain voltage- and ligand-gated Na^+ channels.

LIGAND-GATED CHANNELS

The ligand-gated channels are neurotransmitter receptor proteins that contain a neurotransmitter binding site and a channel pore. To form the pore, each subunit of the protein traverses the membrane four times. The receptors appear to be formed by five different subunits arranged in a barrellike conformation. Activation of this class of receptors, which contain rapidly responsive intrinsic ion channels, is responsible for fast "point-to-point" information transfer in the brain. The major excitatory neurotransmitter in brain is glutamate. A subset of its receptors directly gate Na^+ channels so that when glutamate binds to the receptor, the transmembrane channel within the receptor molecule opens to permit the influx of sodium, hence depolarizing the neuron. Other important excitatory ligand-gated channels in the nervous system include the nicotinic acetylcholine and serotonin (5-hydroxytryptamine [5-HT_3]) receptors. The major inhibitory neurotransmitter in brain is GABA and in the spinal cord the closely related amino acid glycine. The GABA and glycine receptor channels admit Cl^-, resulting in hyperpolarization of the neuronal membrane.

G-PROTEIN–LINKED RECEPTORS

Fast excitatory neurotransmission in the brain appears to be subserved by a small number of neurotransmitters, especially glutamate. In contrast, with only two known exceptions (the serotonin 5-HT_3 receptor and acetylcholine nicotinic receptors), the receptors for all of the monoamines and neuropeptides do not directly gate ion channels, but act via membrane-associated signal-transducing proteins called *G-proteins*. As will be seen, G-protein–linked receptors are involved in a constant process of modulation of the responsiveness of neural circuits. This adds a remarkable layer of complexity on top of the rapid transmission of excitatory and inhibitory impulses by glutamate, GABA, and related neurotransmitters throughout the neural network.

The G-protein–linked receptors that have been structurally analyzed to date in molecular cloning studies have a common overall structure, crossing the neuronal membrane seven times (Kobilka 1992). The ligand binding domain appears to be in a pocket produced by these transmembrane domains within the plane of the membrane. Coupling to intracellular signaling mechanisms occurs on the cytoplasmic side of the neuronal membrane. G-proteins, so named because they bind guanine nucleotides, are associated with the inside of the neuronal membrane. Binding of ligand to the receptor causes a change in receptor conformation that produces activation of the G-proteins. The G-proteins, in turn, transduce the receptor-mediated signal into intracellular effects.

G-proteins are heterotrimers (i.e., proteins made up of three different subunits), the subunits of which are denoted α, β, and γ. With few exceptions the α subunits, which are very diverse, are the specific effectors of G-protein activation (Simon et al. 1991; Figure 1–9). In the inactive state the α, β, and γ subunits are bound together, and a molecule of guanosine diphosphate (GDP) is bound to the α subunit. When activated by a receptor, the GDP is replaced by a guanosine triphosphate (GTP) on the α subunit, which then dissociates from its complex with β and γ. This active subunit remains associated with the membrane, where it can cause the opening or closing of specific voltage-gated ion channels or the activation or inhibition of enzymes that produce intracellular second messengers.

The particular action depends on which type of α subunit is activated by a given receptor. For example, β-adrenergic receptors and dopamine D_1 receptors activate a G-protein called G_s. The entire G-protein is named for its α subunit. Active α subunit can stimulate certain voltage-gated calcium channels (the L-type channels that are the type blocked by verapamil-like drugs) and activate

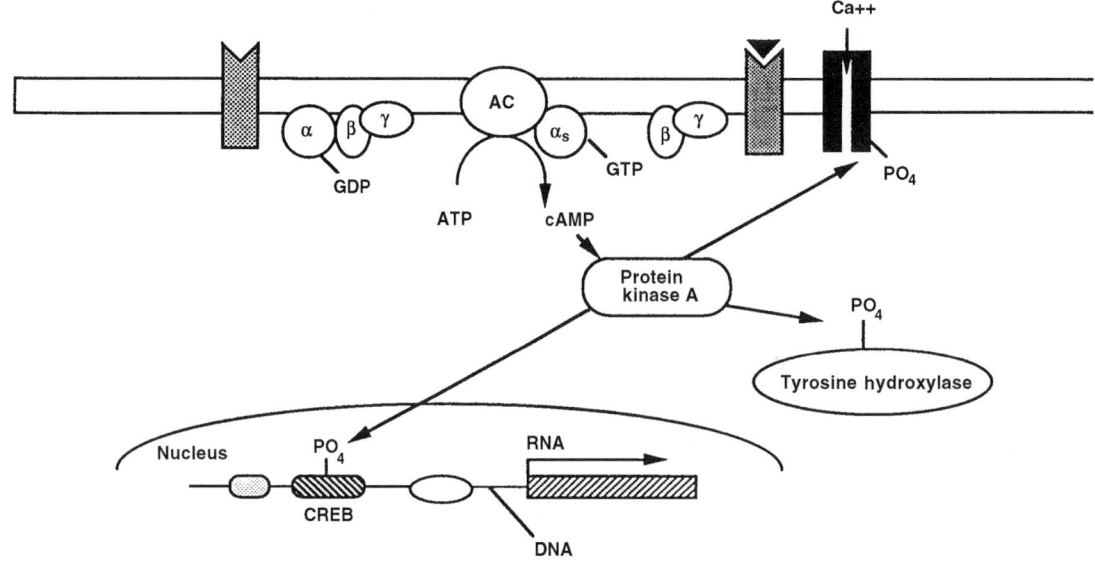

FIGURE 1-9.   The adenylate cyclase second messenger system. Shown at top is a schematic of a neuronal membrane. Neurotransmitter receptors (stippled), voltage-gated channels (a Ca^{++} channel is shown in black), and adenylate cyclase (AC) are integral membrane proteins. The subunits of heterotrimeric G-proteins (see text)—α, β, and γ—are associated with the inner surface of the membrane. An unoccupied receptor is shown at left; in this circumstance, the α subunit is bound to GDP and the G-protein subunits are fully associated. With binding of neurotransmitter (black triangle) shown at right, the receptor can activate the G-protein. GDP is exchanged for GTP, and the α subunit dissociates from β and γ. Here α$_s$ is shown at center activating adenylate cyclase that catalyzes the synthesis of the intracellular second messenger cyclic AMP (cAMP) from adenosine triphosphate (ATP). Cyclic AMP activates protein kinase A (which is shown phosphorylating the calcium channel), the neurotransmitter-synthesizing enzyme tyrosine hydroxylase, and the transcription factor CREB within the nucleus of the cell.

adenylate cyclase, an enzyme that catalyzes the production of the second messenger, cyclic AMP. The active α subunit has an intrinsic GTPase activity that leads to hydrolysis of GTP to GDP. When this occurs, the α subunit reassociates with β and γ and its action is terminated.

The effects of G-proteins on ion channels alter the responses of neurons to subsequent stimulation by excitatory or inhibitory neurotransmitters, such as glutamate and GABA. For example, endogenous opioid peptides can act via one type of receptor (designated μ) to activate a K$^+$ channel. Because the electrochemical driving force on K$^+$ is out of cells, these opioids decrease the net positive charge within target neurons. The neuron is therefore less responsive to glutamate (i.e., less likely to fire). This is one mechanism by which G-proteins can alter the responsiveness of neural circuits.

In addition to their effects on ion channels, G-proteins regulate enzymes that produce second messengers. As already described, G$_s$-linked receptors activate adenylate cyclase to increase cyclic AMP production. G$_i$-linked receptors inhibit adenylate cyclase. Another G-protein, designated G$_q$, activates the enzyme phospholipase C, which hydrolyzes certain membrane phospholipids to generate

two second messengers, diacylglycerol and inositol triphosphate (IP3) (Figure 1–10). Other important second messenger pathways appear to involve arachidonic acid metabolites and nitric oxide.

Although the number of second messengers found within cells is large, conceptually their mechanisms of action can be generalized. With few exceptions (e.g., cyclic AMP can independently gate certain ion channels within the olfactory system), second messengers exert their major biological effects via specific protein kinases. Protein kinases are enzymes that transfer phosphate groups from ATP to specific protein substrates. Based on their charge and size, phosphate groups alter the conformation of proteins and hence their function. Because phosphorylation is a covalent modification, it can act over a very long-time scale. Substrates for second messenger–activated phosphorylation include ion channels, receptors, neurotransmitter-synthesizing enzymes, cytoskeletal proteins, and proteins that control gene transcription. By activating protein phosphorylation, G-protein–linked receptors regulate diverse functions within the cell, and by regulating gene expression they even regulate the protein constituents of the cell. Phosphorylation, which may, for example,

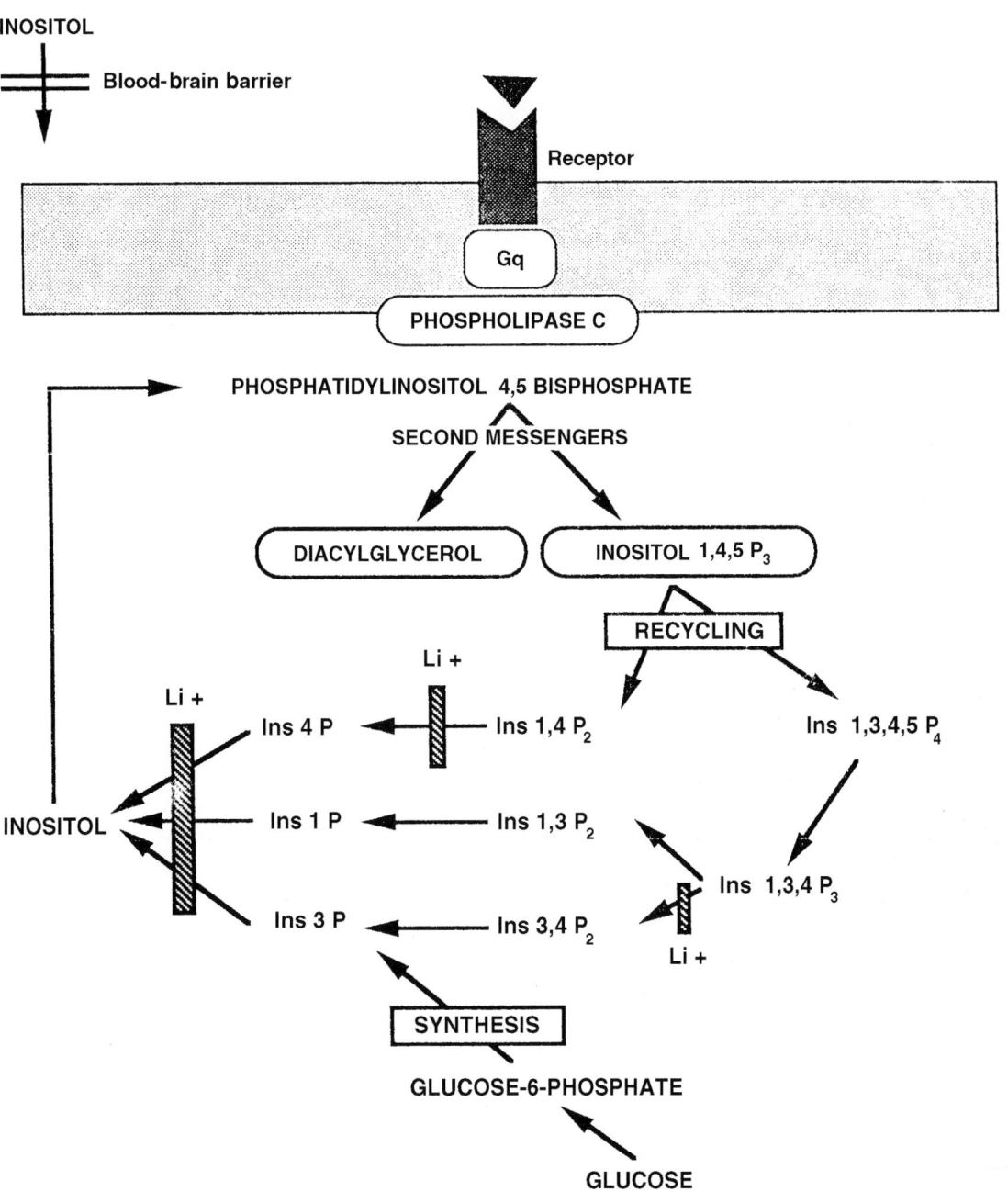

FIGURE 1–10. The phosphatidylinositol second messenger system. Many neurotransmitter receptors are linked via the G-proteins G_q and, occasionally, G_o to the enzyme phospholipase C, which hydrolyzes phosphatidylinositol 4,5-bisphosphate (PIP_2) to generate two second messengers, diacylglycerol and inositol 1,4,5-triphosphate (Ins 1,4,5 P_3, most often abbreviated as IP_3). IP_3 acts in cells by releasing calcium from intracellular stores. It is metabolized to forms that may be inactive, including inositol 1,3,4,5-tetraphosphate (Ins 1,3,4,5 P_4). These forms are eventually metabolized to produce three different inositol monophosphates that differ only by the carbon atom to which the phosphate group is linked. Synthesis of inositol from glucose-6-phosphate also must pass through an inositol monophosphate intermediate. All inositol monophosphates are metabolized by the enzyme inositol monophosphate phosphatase. This enzyme is inhibited by lithium at therapeutic concentrations. As a result, in the presence of lithium, inositol monophosphates cannot be dephosphorylated to yield free inositol, which is required to regenerate phosphatidylinositol 4,5-bisphosphate. Also shown in the figure is the ability of lithium to inhibit an additional enzyme in this cycle (inositol polyphosphate 1-phosphatase), which is required for two metabolic steps earlier in the recycling pathway.

Source. Adapted from Hyman and Nestler 1993.

inactivate receptors or increase or decrease the likelihood of voltage-gated ion channel opening, can alter the way that neurons process information and can therefore alter the behavior of brain circuits in significant ways. Clearly, then, the brain is not simply a hard-wired network relaying information via excitatory and inhibitory potentials. The brain is constantly modifying how the neurons within it can process information. Such plasticity of neural functioning is clearly required for processes such as learning and memory, but it is also likely involved in the onset of psychopathology (e.g., the state changes that occur with onset of depression) and, as will be described, the mechanism of action of many psychotropic drugs.

NEUROANATOMY

METHODS

Although a detailed description of the neuroanatomy of the brain is beyond the scope of this chapter, certain emerging themes and research strategies merit mention. Until 15 years ago, neuroanatomic procedures were restricted to staining techniques that revealed neurons primarily on the basis of peculiar chemical characteristics that were not unique to any particular class of neurons. The connections between neurons could be inferred only by indirect methods or by very laborious electron microscopic studies. Two major types of technical advances have permitted tremendous progress in understanding the functional organization of the brain. The first exploits specific methods to identify the unique chemical (protein and mRNA) constituents of neurons, and the second reveals neuronal connectivity.

The high degree of specificity of antibody-antigen interactions allows selective staining of elements of tissue such as neurotransmitters, enzymes, or surface markers against which antiserum has been raised. The efficiency and specificity of these techniques have been further enhanced by the ability to generate monoclonal antibodies, which recognize a single specific part of an antigen (i.e., an epitope).

With standard immunocytochemical procedures, antisera are prepared that recognize a larger number of epitopes. Although some specificity may be lost, the likelihood of detecting the antigen of interest may be increased. Whether monoclonal or polyclonal antibodies are used, they are incubated with tissue sections and bind to the antigen they recognize. This primary reaction is then visualized by incubating the section with a second antibody to which a visualizable marker has been attached, such as the enzyme peroxidase. The brain sections are then developed, and the presence of the antigen can be observed in particular neurons and their processes with light or electron microscopy.

The immunocytochemical approach has been exploited to a considerable degree to visualize the anatomy of neurons using specific neurotransmitters based on the development of antibodies against the neurotransmitter, against its specific synthesizing enzyme, or against a neuropeptide. As opposed to the traditional histological techniques that reveal neurons on the basis of common features such as the presence of nucleic acid in Nissl stains or the ability to be impregnated with silver ions as in the Golgi stain, the immunocytochemical staining for neurotransmitter-related antigens allows the visualization of a neuron and its axons on the basis of the neurotransmitter utilized (Figure 1–11).

The immunocytochemical approach is being expanded to identify other important components of the nervous system and to better understand its organization and function at the molecular level.

An additional method for identifying specific components of neurons is *in situ hybridization*. This technique exploits the principle of complementary base pairing that characterizes nucleic acids. Messenger RNAs encoding cellular proteins are single stranded. A radioactive single-stranded RNA or DNA "probe" hybridizes only to its complementary mRNA within a tissue section under the right experimental conditions. Much as in receptor autoradiography, described above, the section can then be apposed to film. Silver grains can be visualized over cells expressing the mRNA of interest. Combined with immunohistochemistry, in situ hybridization has revealed many of the molecular species that give particular neurons their specific identities.

A second type of method that has contributed considerably to the understanding of brain organization takes advantage of the process of axoplasmic transport, wherein substances are transported anterogradely from the neuronal cell body to the nerve terminal and retrogradely from the nerve terminal back to the neuronal cell body. Individual neuronal cell bodies may provide projections that innervate disparate areas of the brain. To understand the functional role of specific neuronal nuclei, it is essential to understand which neurons they innervate. This can be addressed through anterograde and retrograde tracing techniques.

With these methods, a highly discrete injection of a dye or other marker is made into a specific brain region. The dye is taken up by nerve terminals and then transported back to the neuronal cell bodies over 24–48 hours.

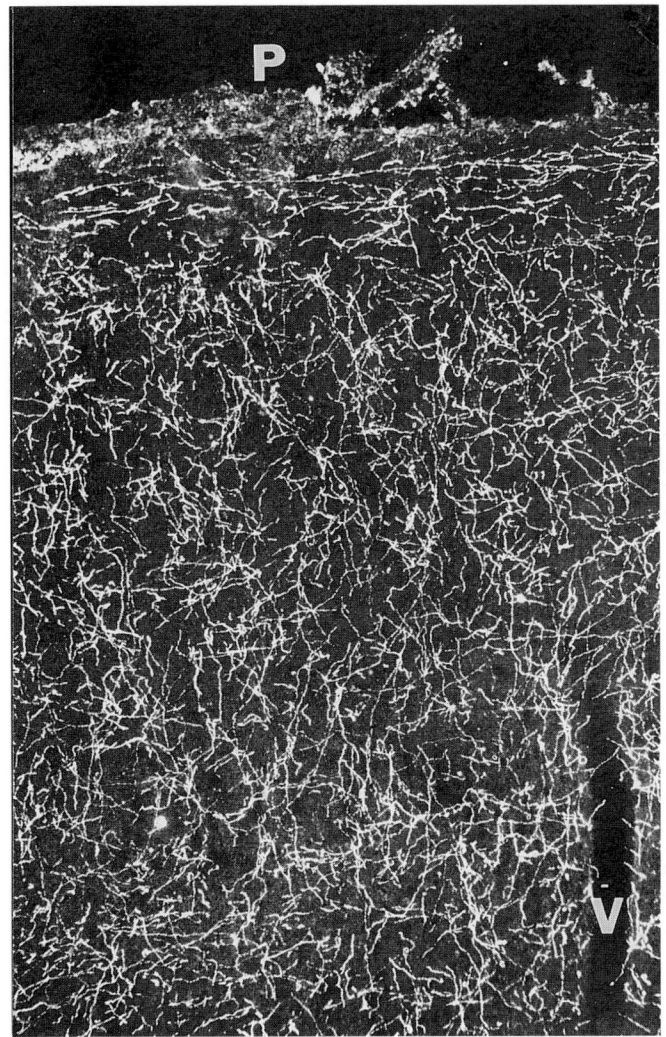

FIGURE 1–11. Immunocytochemical staining of serotonergic fibers in monkey somatosensory cortex. The fixed 10-μm section of monkey cortex was incubated with a guinea pig antiserotonin antibody. The antibody-serotonin complex within serotonergic axons is visualized by incubating with a fluorescein conjugated goat anti–guinea pig γ-globulin antibody. Note the dense meshwork of randomly arranged serotonergic axons in the field through layers I and II. P, pial surface; V, blood vessel. (Courtesy of M. A. Wilson and M. E. Molliver.)

Thus, after this delay, the neuronal cell bodies that send axons to innervate the injected area can be identified in the brain by the fact that they contain the dye. Conversely, a dye can be injected into the area of the neuronal cell body, and it will be transported in an anterograde fashion to illuminate the axons and terminals emanating from the neuron. Recently, these pathway-tracing techniques have been combined with immunocytochemical techniques to determine the precise neuronal circuitry of neurotransmitter-defined neuronal systems (Figure 1–12).

RETICULAR CORE

Among the neuronal systems likely to be directly relevant to psychiatric disorders are components of the reticular core of the brain stem and its rostral extension in the basal forebrain (Coyle 1986). The implication of these components in the pathophysiology of major mental disorders is based on the serendipitous discovery of several classes of effective psychopharmacological agents that have mechanisms of action that appear to alter synaptic neurotransmission of specific components of the reticular core.

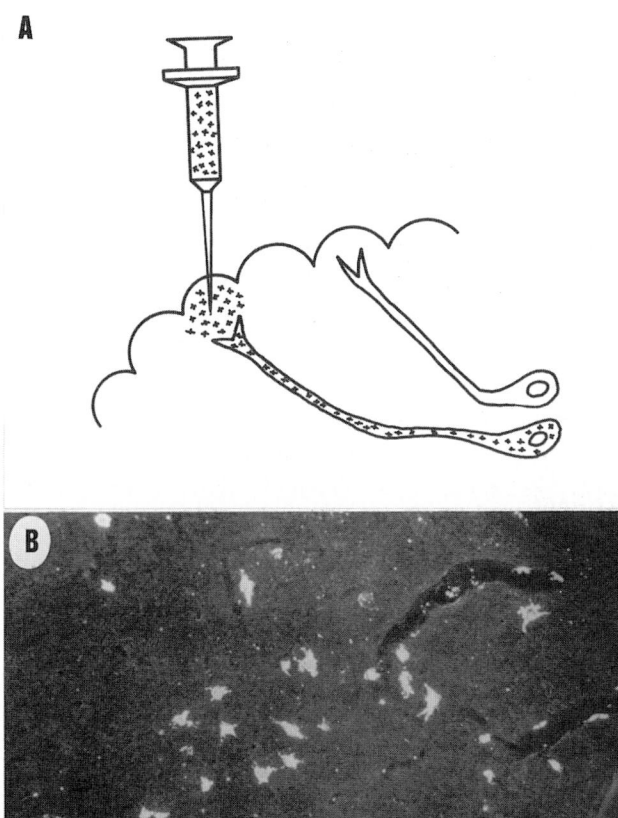

FIGURE 1–12. Retrograde neuron tracing technique. *A)* As schematically illustrated, a trace amount of marker substance (e.g., horseradish peroxidase) is injected in an area of neuronal innervation. After a suitable delay to allow for transport of the marker back to the neuronal cell body, histological sections through the neuronal cell bodies of interest are examined. If a neuron sends axons to innervate the injected area, it will contain the marker; otherwise, it will be devoid of marker. *B)* Medial septal cholinergic neurons as viewed by dark-field microscopy. These neurons were labeled with horseradish peroxidase by prior injection of the marker in the hippocampus, the region innervated by these septal neurons.

These findings have gained additional neurophysiological and neuroanatomic validation because of the unusual organization and function of reticular core neurons.

The reticular core neurons are not involved in conveying specific information but rather modulate neuronal function via G-protein–linked receptors throughout the nervous system, including cortical and limbic regions. Thus, disruption of their function is not generally associated with focal neurological signs typically associated with damage to "hard" information processing systems, such as ascending sensory systems or descending motor systems, but rather with abnormalities in drives, affects, arousal, and cognitive functions. Of course, these findings do not preclude the possibility that more localized abnormalities of neurons innervating or influenced by the reticular core projections might contribute substantially to the etiology or symptomatic manifestations of mental disorders.

Several components of the reticular core have been well characterized with regard to their neurotransmitters. Those of particular relevance to psychiatry are the noradrenergic, serotonergic, dopaminergic, and cholinergic pathways.

Noradrenergic Neurons

Norepinephrine is the principal neurotransmitter of an important class of neurons within the reticular core of the brain stem. The synthetic pathway for norepinephrine is shown in Figure 1–2. The principal noradrenergic nucleus is the locus coeruleus, so named because of its bluish color in fresh brain sections. The locus coeruleus is located bilaterally in the dorsal pons near the floor of the fourth ventricle (Figure 1–13). Additional noradrenergic (norepinephrine-releasing neuron) nuclei are scattered in the

medulla and pons and primarily innervate the brain stem. The estimated 40,000 neurons in the human locus coeruleus are the primary source of noradrenergic innervation for most of the CNS, including the forebrain, cerebellum, and spinal cord. Thus an extensive axonal arbor accounts for over 95% of the neuronal volume of individual coeruleus noradrenergic neurons. Like the other components of the reticular core, the noradrenergic axons are fine, unmyelinated processes that contain neurotransmitter throughout their extent. Beaded varicosities along the axons are sites of specialized synaptic contacts known as *synapses en passage*. As best exemplified in the cerebral cortex, individual noradrenergic axons make synaptic contacts with millions of neurons, and the axonal arbor appears as a dense meshwork ramifying throughout all cortical layers (Figure 1–13). Furthermore, individual noradrenergic neurons send axons that innervate functionally diverse regions of the brain (e.g., cerebral cortex and cerebellum).

The effects of norepinephrine are mediated in the brain by two classes of receptors: α- and β-adrenergic receptors (Table 1–4). These classes are further subdivided, based upon pharmacological characteristics and physiological effects, into α_1 (α_1) and α_2 (α_2), and β_1 (β_1) and β_2 (β_2) receptors. Stimulation of α_1 receptors results in activation of phosphoinositide turnover. α_2 receptors are linked via G_i/G_o to inhibition of adenylate cyclase and opening of a K^+ channel. These actions tend to decrease neuronal firing. The α_2 receptors on the noradrenergic cell body, which can be stimulated via recurrent noradrenergic collaterals, slow the firing rate of noradrenergic neurons. In addition, when activated, α_2 receptors on noradrenergic terminals decrease the amount of norepinephrine released, presumably by reducing the influx of calcium during the depolarization of the nerve terminal. Clonidine is an agonist at α_2 receptors and thus inhibits locus coeruleus firing. This accounts for its efficacy in attenuating physical symptoms of acute withdrawal from opiates.

β_1 and β_2 receptors are distinguished by the lower intrinsic activity of norepinephrine at the latter receptor and their differential sensitivity to certain antagonists. In brain, the β_1 receptors appear to have a high degree of localization on neurons, whereas the β_2 receptors are predominantly, although not exclusively, associated with nonneuronal elements such as the glial cells. Activation of β receptors results in stimulation of adenylate cyclase via G_s and the elevation of the intracellular levels of cyclic AMP. Thus, the cellular responses to β agonists reflect the activation of cyclic AMP–dependent protein kinases. Desensitization of cortical β-adrenergic receptors is a general effect of antidepressants.

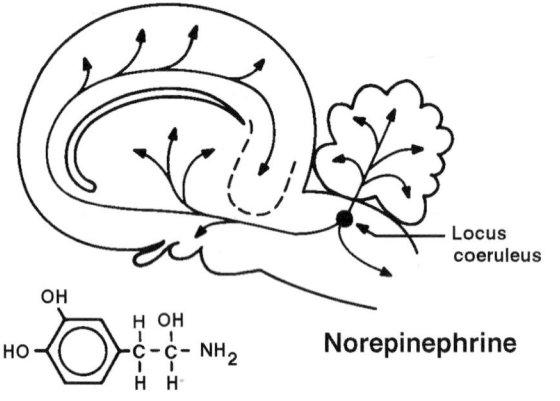

Norepinephrine

FIGURE 1–13.   The primary projections of the noradrenergic locus coeruleus.

TABLE 1-4. **Pharmacology of monoamine and acetylcholine receptors**

Receptor	Clinically relevant agonists	Clinically relevant antagonists	Coupling
Adrenergic receptors			
α_1-adrenergic (4 subtypes)	Phenylephrine	Prazosin	IP_3/DG
α_2-adrenergic (3 subtypes)	Clonidine	Yohimbine	cAMP⇓; K^+ channel ↑
β-adrenergic (3 subtypes: β_1 in heart; β_2 in lung)	Isoproterenol	Propranolol	cAMP ↑
Dopamine receptors			
D_1 (or D_{1A})	SKF38393	SCH39166	cAMP ↑
D_2 (or D_{2A})	Bromocriptine	Typical antipsychotics (raclopride selective)	cAMP⇓; K^+ channel ↑; Ca^{++} channel ⇓
D_3 (or D_{2B})	Quinpirole	Typical antipsychotics	Unknown
D_4 (or D_{2C})	Quinpirole	Clozapine	cAMP⇓
D_5 (or D_{1B})	SKF38393		cAMP ↑
Serotonin (5-HT) receptors			
5-HT_{1A}	Buspirone partial agonist; (8-OH-DPAT selective)		cAMP⇓ ; K^+ channel ↑
5-HT_{1B}			cAMP⇓
5-HT_{1D}	Sumatriptan		cAMP⇓
5-HT_{1E}			cAMP⇓
5-HT_{1F}			cAMP⇓
5-HT_{2A}	α-Methyl-5-HT	Ritanserin (selective) Clozapine (nonselective)	IP_3/DG
5-HT_{2B}	α-Methyl-5-HT		IP_3/DG
5-HT_{2C} (formerly 5-HT_{1C})	α-Methyl-5-HT	Clozapine (nonselective)	IP_3/DG
5-HT_3	2-Methyl-5-HT	Odansetron	Intrinsic cation channel
5-HT_4	5-Methoxytryptamine		cAMP ↑
Muscarinic receptors	Oxotremorine	Atropine	
M_1	Oxotremorine	Pirenzepine selective	IP_3/DG
M_2	Oxotremorine	Methoctramine selective	cAMP⇓; K^+ channel ↑
M_3	Oxotremorine	Hexahydrosiladifenidol selective	IP_3/DG
M_4	Oxotremorine	Tropicamide selective	cAMP⇓

Note. DG = diacylglycerol; 8-OH-DPAT = 8-hydroxy-2-(di-*n*-propylamino)tetralin.

Serotonergic Neurons

Serotonin-releasing neurons have their cell bodies located in the raphe nuclei found near the midline of the brain stem (Figure 1–14). Like the locus coeruleus noradrenergic neurons, the serotonergic neurons provide highly collateralized innervation to virtually all areas of the CNS. Nevertheless, components of the raphe nuclei provide more regionally discrete patterns of innervation.

The synaptic effects of serotonin are mediated by a large number of pre- and postsynaptic receptors (Table 1–4). Current pharmacological and cloning studies suggest at least four types of 5-HT receptors with multiple subtypes. The 5-HT$_1$ receptors relevant to human pharmacology are 5-HT$_{1A}$, a largely presynaptic receptor that is the site of action of the anxiolytic drug buspirone; the 5-HT$_{1C}$ receptor, which is both pre- and postsynaptic; and the 5-HT$_{1D}$ receptor, to which the new antimigraine drug sumatriptan is an agonist. The 5-HT$_2$ receptor is a postsynaptic receptor that appears to be the key site of ac-

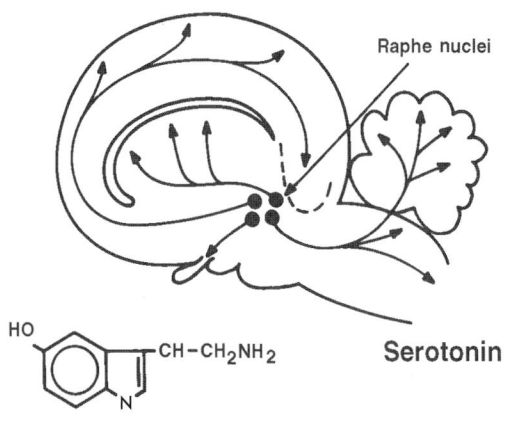

FIGURE 1-14. The pathways of the raphe serotonergic neurons.

tion of lysergic acid diethylamide (LSD), mescaline, and related hallucinogens. The 5-HT$_{1A}$ and 5-HT$_{1D}$ receptors inhibit adenylate cyclase and activate a voltage-sensitive K$^+$ channel via G$_i$. The 5-HT$_{1C}$ and 5-HT$_2$ receptors activate the inositol triphosphate/diacylglycerol second messenger pathways. The 5-HT$_3$ receptor is the only known monoamine receptor that is a ligand-gated channel. The novel antiemetic drug odansetron antagonizes the excitatory effects of serotonin at its 5-HT$_3$ reception in the chemotrigger zone of the medulla. (The other significant receptor type on these neurons is the dopamine D$_2$ receptor; thus older antiemetics are dopamine receptor antagonists.) The function of 5-HT$_4$ receptors is debated. Serotonergic neurons, through their innervation of the cerebral cortex, have been associated with regulation of alertness. Serotonergic effects in the limbic system may have a role in control of mood, anxiety, and aggression, and a role in the modulation of pain.

Dopaminergic Neurons

Three major dopaminergic systems have been of particular interest for psychiatric research (Figure 1–15). Large pigmented dopaminergic neurons located in the substantia nigra within the midbrain provide a remarkably dense innervation of the caudate and putamen that accounts for approximately 15% of the synapses in these structures. This highly collateralized pathway of unmyelinated axons arborizes into a fine filigree of varicosity-laden axons, providing thousands of *synapses en passage*. The nigrostriatal dopaminergic projection is intimately involved in the initiation and smooth execution of the motor activities and may play a comparable role in cognitive function, reflecting the major projection from the frontal cortex to the caudate. Degeneration of the nigrostriatal dopamine pro-

jections causes the symptoms of Parkinson's disease, and the blockade of dopamine receptors by neuroleptic drugs results in clinically similar extrapyramidal side effects, reflecting impaired striatal dopaminergic neurotransmission.

The more medially localized dopaminergic neuronal cell bodies in the ventral tegmental area (VTA) provide innervation to the nucleus accumbens, a pivotal arena of limbic circuitry, as well as to the neocortex, cingulate cortex, amygdala, and hippocampus. Whereas in the rat, dopamine innervation of the cortex is sparse and limited to prefrontal regions, in primates there appears to be significant innervation of the entire cerebral cortex by VTA dopaminergic neurons (Levitt et al. 1984). The dopaminergic projection of the VTA to the nucleus accumbens has been implicated as a "brain reward" circuit, mediating the positively reinforcing effects of drugs of abuse, including cocaine, amphetamine, and probably opiates. The cortical dopaminergic projections may be implicated in attention, "working memory," and, by inference, cognitive integration. Based on the dopamine antagonist properties of antipsychotic drugs (see below), dysfunction of mesocorticolimbic dopaminergic circuits has been hypothesized to occur in schizophrenia and other psychotic disorders.

Finally, a group of dopaminergic neurons located in the arcuate nucleus of the hypothalamus send axons that terminate in the venous sinuses of the pituitary. This tuberoinfundibular dopaminergic projection inhibits the release of the pituitary hormone prolactin. This physiological role has been widely exploited as a peripheral measure of altered central dopaminergic neurotransmission. Thus,

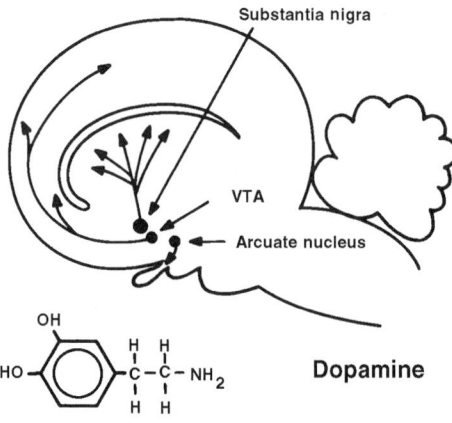

FIGURE 1-15. The three major dopaminergic pathways: the nigrostriatal pathway, the mesocorticolimbic pathway (originating in the ventral tegmental area [VTA]), and the arcuate nucleus pathway to the infundibulum.

the neuroleptics, as potent dopamine D_2 receptor blockers, augment prolactin release.

The synaptic effects of dopamine appear to be mediated by several pharmacologically and physiologically distinct receptors (Table 1–4). It is likely that not all dopamine receptor types have been discovered, and at present the nomenclature is unsettled. Based on their structure (deduced from molecular cloning) and their pharmacological properties, dopamine receptors can be grouped into two families, called D_1-like (the D_1 and D_5 receptors, also called D_{1A} and D_{1B} by some investigators) and D_2-like (the D_2, D_3, and D_4 receptors, also referred to as D_{2A}, D_{2B}, and D_{2C} by some investigators). In addition, a long form and a short form of the D_2 receptor have been found based on alternative splicing of the D_2 receptor mRNA, but no obvious functional differences between the forms have been elucidated. The different receptor types have overlapping but nonidentical distributions in brain regions innervated by dopaminergic fibers. The D_1 and D_5 receptors activate adenylate cyclase via G_s. The D_2 receptor inhibits adenylate cyclase and activates a voltage-sensitive K^+ channel via G_i. The precise second messenger effects of D_3 and D_4 receptors are not yet clear. The antipsychotic drugs are antagonists of D_2, D_3, and D_4 receptors. An intriguing observation, discussed further below, is that the atypical antipsychotic drug clozapine has a particularly high affinity for D_4 receptors (Van Tol et al. 1991). Its low affinity for the D_2 receptor probably explains its lack of extrapyramidal effects.

Cholinergic Neurons

The major source of cholinergic innervation to the cerebral cortex, hippocampus, and limbic structures is a complex of large neurons located in the basal forebrain (Figure 1–16). The nucleus basalis of Meynert, a somewhat dispersed group of cholinergic cell bodies located in the ventral and medial aspects of the globus pallidus, sends axons that innervate the cerebral cortex. The more anteriorly located diagonal band of Broca and medial septal nucleus innervate the hippocampal formation and cingulate cortex. The terminal arbor of the cholinergic afferents provides a meshwork of randomly oriented fibers distributed to all layers of the cerebral cortex, whereas in the hippocampal formation a much more laminar-specific distribution is apparent, especially in the dentate gyrus. The dense cholinergic innervation of the caudate and putamen is not provided by these ascending projections but by local circuit neurons the axonal arbors of which are restricted to the basal ganglia.

The postsynaptic effects of acetylcholine in the forebrain appear to be mediated by both muscarinic and nicotinic receptors. The nicotinic receptors in brain are ligand-gated channels, somewhat different from those mediating the effects of acetylcholine at the neuromuscular junction in that several brain-specific receptor subunits have been found. Aside from the central psychotropic effects of nicotine itself, the role of nicotinic receptors in the brain remains relatively poorly understood.

At least five types of muscarinic cholinergic receptors have been identified by pharmacological and cloning studies (M_1–M_4) (Table 1–4). The muscarinic receptors mediating the effects of acetylcholine for the cortical and hippocampal cholinergic projections play an integral role in higher cognitive functions, especially learning and memory. Drugs that block these receptors, such as scopolamine or atropine, and the destruction of the basal forebrain cholinergic projections in experimental animals produce selective deficits in memory functions. Notably, striking losses of cortical and hippocampal cholinergic axons seem to be a consistent defect in Alzheimer's disease and may contribute to the cognitive impairments in this disorder (Coyle et al. 1983). The cholinergic system has also been implicated in control of mood states, because muscarinic receptor antagonists have mood-enhancing effects in humans, whereas the centrally active acetylcholinesterase inhibitor physostigmine has been reported to provoke depressed mood. Finally, cholinergic projections have a role in sleep, especially rapid eye movement (REM) sleep. During REM sleep, locus coeruleus noradrenergic neurons are tonically inhibited, whereas cholinergic neurons are active. Cholinergic drugs promote REM, and anticholinergic drugs antagonize it. The observation that REM latency is decreased in major depression (consistent with hyperactivity of cholinergic neurons) is further evi-

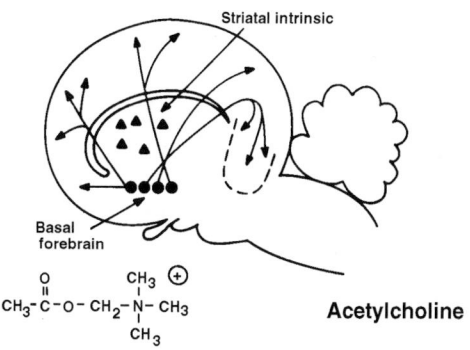

FIGURE 1–16. The forebrain cholinergic neurons. Cholinergic neurons in the basal forebrain, including the nucleus basalis of Meynert, the diagonal band of Broca, and the medial septal nucleus, innervate the cerebral cortex, hippocampus, and limbic structures. The striatum contains local circuit cholinergic interneurons.

dence that cholinergic systems may play a role in regulation of mood and mood disorders.

AMINO ACIDS

The primary excitatory and inhibitory neurotransmitters in brain are the amino acids L-glutamate and GABA. Their broad role in information processing indicates that they are localized to a large number of different neuronal systems throughout the brain, unlike the reticular core neurons, in which the cell bodies are restricted primarily to discrete nuclei within the brain stem.

GABA

GABAergic neurons are particularly relevant to psychiatry because the benzodiazepines, the barbiturates, and many anticonvulsants exert their primary effects through activation of the GABA receptors (see below). Within the cerebral cortex, hippocampus, and limbic structures, GABAergic neurons are predominantly local circuit neurons that have their cell bodies and axonal terminal arbors entirely contained within the structures (Figure 1–17). In fact, GABAergic inhibitory neurotransmission dominates in these structures, with pharmacological blockade of GABA receptors with bicuculline causing diffuse disinhibition and seizures. GABAergic neurons are also found as long projection neurons in other areas of the brain. For example, the main output of the caudate-putamen projecting to the globus pallidus and the substantia nigra consists of GABAergic neurons. The vulnerability of subsets of these striatal GABAergic neurons in Huntington's disease contributes to the abnormal movements

that characterize that disorder. The cerebellar efferent neurons, the Purkinje cells, are also long GABAergic projection neurons. The cerebellar signs such as ataxia that result from excessive doses of barbiturates or ethanol likely reflect potentiation of GABAergic neurotransmission via these cerebellar efferents.

Glutamate

Glutamate is the major excitatory neurotransmitter in the brain; well-studied examples of neurons that use glutamate include the pyramidal cells in the cerebral cortex and in the hippocampal formation (Figure 1–18), and primary sensory afferents. Most fast excitatory neurotransmission in the brain is subserved by glutamate receptors that are ligand-gated channels. These receptors have been named for their pharmacological agonists, kainate, α-amino-3-hydroxy-5-methyl-4-isoxazole propionic acid (AMPA), and N-methyl-D-aspartate (NMDA). The genes encoding the polypeptides that form the glutamate gated ion channels have been cloned (Seeburg 1993). There are also glutamate receptors that activate G-proteins, currently referred to as "metabotropic" glutamate receptors. Cloning studies have identified multiple subtypes of these receptors as well (Schoepp and Conn 1993).

Binding of glutamate causes kainate and AMPA receptors to open an intrinsic Na^+ channel, although certain subtypes may also admit Ca^{++}. NMDA receptors are unique in that their channel, which can permit both Na^+ and Ca^{++} entry, is blocked by Mg^+ at resting membrane potential (–70 mV). Activation of NMDA receptors can only occur when two events happen simultaneously: glutamate must bind to

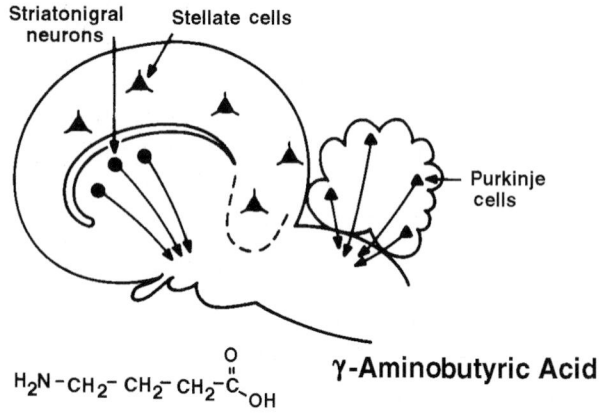

FIGURE 1-17. Major GABAergic pathways. The inhibitory neurotransmitter GABA is synthesized by local circuit stellate cells within the cerebral cortex, by the cerebellar Purkinje cells, and by striatonigral neurons.

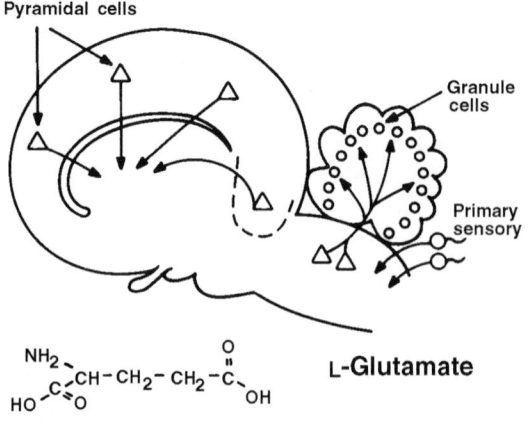

FIGURE 1-18. Major glutamatergic pathway. The excitatory neurotransmitter L-glutamic acid is released by a number of neurons including cortical and hippocampal pyramidal cells, cerebellar granule cells, cerebellar climbing fibers, and primary sensory afferents.

the receptor and the membrane must be depolarized (e.g., by activation of surrounding non-NMDA glutamate receptors), which permits Mg^+ to exit the channel. Because two simultaneous events are required for NMDA receptor activation (i.e., the receptor is a coincidence detector), NMDA receptors have been considered a possible substrate for associative learning through the process of long-term potentiation. Long-term potentiation refers to a persistent increase in synaptic efficacy that occurs as a consequence of a period of high excitatory presynaptic activity (Bliss and Collingridge 1993).

Glutamate has been implicated in an increasing number of neurological and psychiatric disorders. A striking finding relevant to psychiatry is that the psychotomimetic effects of phencylidine (PCP) and related compounds are due to the ability of these compounds to block the NMDA receptor channel (Martin and Lodge 1985). Because glutamate is the neurotransmitter of cortical and hippocampal pyramidal neurons, it has been hypothesized that the dissociative and psychotomimetic effects of PCP may reflect interference with glutamatergic neurotransmission in these brain regions.

Olney (1969) first demonstrated that peripheral injection of glutamate into neonatal animals produces a selective pattern of neuronal degeneration that affects neurons in the arcuate nucleus of the hypothalamus, the circumventricular organs of the brain, and the inner layers of the retina. He proposed that neurotoxicity of glutamate results from an overwhelming depolarization of the neurons mediated by excitatory glutamate receptors. Subsequent studies revealed that intracerebral injection of agonists at three major types of glutamate receptors—the kainate, AMPA, and NMDA receptors—killed neurons in proximity to the injection site but spared axons from distant neurons and nonneuronal elements such as glia. Depending on the site of brain injection, these "excitotoxins" can produce models of several neurodegenerative disorders including Huntington's disease, temporal lobe epilepsy, and spinocerebellar degeneration (Schwarz and Meldrum 1985).

These observations raised the question of whether glutamate and related endogenous excitatory neurotransmitters might cause neuronal degeneration in brain under certain circumstances as a result of excessive release or insufficient inactivation. With the development of potent and specific antagonists for NMDA receptors, recent findings have validated this hypothesis (Choi and Rothman 1990). Accordingly, treatment with NMDA antagonists prevents degeneration of neurons in the limbic system as a result of persistent seizures, degeneration of neurons in the striatum as a consequence of profound hypoglycemia, and prevention of degenerations of neurons in the hippocampus as a result of ischemia. These results hold promise for the development of new classes of "neuroprotective" medications that may prevent or markedly decrease brain damage consequent to hypoxemia and ischemia, the most frequent causes of morbidity and death following stroke and myocardial infarction (Robinson and Coyle 1988).

PURINES

Just as certain amino acid building blocks of proteins (e.g., glutamate, glycine) can act as signaling molecules in the nervous system, it has been found that certain purine building blocks of nucleic acids can also act as neurotransmitters. The purine *adenosine* acts via two types of G-protein–linked receptors. It has been established that the behavioral stimulant effects of caffeine result from its action as a competitive antagonist of adenosine receptors. In addition, it appears that ATP, the main source of energy for cells, may also act as a neurotransmitter. One type of ATP receptor has been shown to be a ligand-gated channel.

ENDORPHINS

As described earlier in this chapter, the neuropeptides best studied in relation to psychiatry are the endorphins. This family of neuropeptides was originally discovered in studies to determine whether there were endogenous substances in brain that served as agonists at opiate receptors. The pentapeptides Met- and Leu-enkephalin were the first endogenous opioid peptides discovered, although subsequent studies have revealed a family of these peptides with differential effects at subclasses of opioid receptors. Some of the opioid peptides that have been identified in brain are listed in Table 1–3.

The enkephalins are found primarily in local circuit neurons in several regions of the CNS, but they are also found in projection neurons. Enkephalin-containing interneurons within the periaqueductal gray matter, the raphe nuclei, and the dorsal horn of the spinal cord are critical components of endogenous analgesic systems. Enkephalin-containing interneurons that release VTA dopaminergic neurons from tonic inhibition by GABAergic neurons may present part of the substrate of opiate-induced brain reward and therefore of opiate abuse and addiction. Enkephalin neurons are also found in high concentrations in the caudate, putamen, and globus pallidus, where they appear to be involved in motor function.

The larger endogenous opioid peptide β-endorphin has a dual localization. β-Endorphin is contained within a group of neurons within the hypothalamus that send axons that project to limbic areas. In addition, as described earlier in this chapter, β-endorphin is also secreted by the corticotrophs in the anterior pituitary. The colocalization of ACTH and β-endorphin reflects the common source of these two peptides from the precursor, POMC. During periods of stress, the release of both ACTH and β-endorphin may contribute to stress-related analgesia. Furthermore, hypothalamic-pituitary-adrenal (HPA) dysregulation in major depressive disorder involves excess secretion of β-endorphin as well as ACTH and cortisol.

MOLECULAR NEUROBIOLOGY

Perhaps the most exciting recent development in neuroscience research has been the increasing exploitation of molecular biological techniques (Hyman and Nestler 1993). These strategies offer considerable hope of bridging the gap between clinical genetics in psychiatry and the molecular processes that regulate brain structure and function. These powerful methodologies include *linkage analysis* with *DNA polymorphisms* for localizing genes that may be responsible for psychiatric disorders; methods for identifying genes that code for proteins involved in brain structure and function; and methods for studying the regulation of gene expression by environmental stimuli, including drugs. With the rapidly increasing information about the location of genes relevant to brain function within the human genome, there will likely be a convergence of information that will clarify the molecular and cellular basis for a number of psychiatric disorders over the next decade and eventually for many nonpathological behaviors.

MOLECULAR CLONING

The most basic approach to the identification of neural genes involves purification of the protein of interest to homogeneity. The protein could be, for example, an enzyme involved in neurotransmitter synthesis, a receptor, a neuropeptide, or a transporter protein. A fragment of the protein is then sequenced to determine the series of amino acids. Because the genetic code is known, the protein sequence can be back-translated into a DNA sequence and used to generate synthetic radiolabeled DNA (i.e., oligonucleotide) probes that can be used to identify the gene of interest. This is accomplished by using the probe to hybridize with a *complementary DNA* (cDNA) fragment within what is called a *cDNA library.*

Briefly, the process of molecular cloning requires en-

zymes called *restriction endonucleases* that cut DNA at specific sequences, and enzymes called *ligases* that can join DNA fragments. A cDNA library contains a mixture of DNA fragments representing all of the genes expressed in a given tissue or cell type. To construct a cDNA library, a particular tissue (e.g., a brain region) is dissected and homogenized, and its mRNA is chemically extracted. A sample of the tissue's mRNA gives a representation of all of the genes within it that have been transcribed (i.e., expressed). Thus, for example, a sample of the striatum would contain mRNA encoding dopamine receptors but not mRNA encoding hemoglobin. Complementary DNA copies of each RNA are then produced in a process that includes the enzyme reverse transcriptase (so named because it "reverse transcribes" RNA into DNA).

Each of the resulting cDNAs must now be propagated (i.e., cloned) by inserting it into either a bacterial plasmid or into bacteriophage virus DNA. Either can serve as a vector that can replicate autonomously in bacteria such as *Escherichia coli.* Plasmids are small DNA circles that carry only a few genes; plasmids used in cloning were originally engineered from antibiotic-resistance plasmids found naturally in bacteria. Restriction endonucleases are used to cut open the cloning vector. Each vector is then made to reseal with ligase after a cDNA is introduced. The population of plasmids or bacteriophage, each containing a single cDNA copy of a gene expressed in the tissue of interest, is now reintroduced into *E. coli,* where it replicates. When these bacteria are grown on an agar plate, each bacterium will grow into a colony that contains multiple copies of a single cDNA, the so-called cDNA library. The library can now be screened for particular genes using probes that will detect particular sequences by complementary base pairing or with antibodies against the protein of interest.

An example of the power of this approach was the cloning of the gene encoding β-amyloid, the major constituent of senile neuritic plaques in Alzheimer's disease. The β-amyloid was purified from brains of patients with Alzheimer's disease, and the amino acid sequence was determined. From this sequence, a cDNA probe was synthesized and used to screen a human brain cDNA library. The power of these methods extends further, however. They can be used to clone cDNAs for proteins that never have been purified. As has been described above, many important proteins in the nervous system are members of evolutionarily related families. These include receptors, transporters, and ion channels. Recently the GABA and norepinephrine transporters were purified and cloned (Pacholczyk et al. 1991). It was then possible to compare their sequences and determine which regions were conserved between the two transporter proteins. Regions of sequence conservation shared by related protein generally represent critical functional domains that have been preserved from mutational drift by natural selection. Synthetic DNA probes that encode these conserved regions are then used to screen libraries under conditions that tolerate a small degree of mismatch between the probe and its complement; alternatively, the probe can be used in a process that amplifies cDNAs to which it binds in solution (a technique called the *polymerase chain reaction*, or PCR). Exploiting conserved transporter sequences derived from the GABA and norepinephrine transporters, the serotonin and dopamine transporters and several additional unknown transporters were cloned. Similar techniques were used to clone the entire family of dopamine receptors (e.g., Van Tol et al. 1991).

DNA POLYMORPHISMS

Recent advances have provided methods for localizing the genes that are responsible for inherited disorders without requiring any *a priori* knowledge of the defective protein responsible for the disorder (Wexler et al. 1991). Because so little is currently known about the defective gene products that may be responsible for psychiatric disorders such as bipolar disorder, schizophrenia, or Tourette's syndrome, for which there is evidence of genetic predisposition, this strategy represents a very powerful tool for clarifying the genetic mechanisms involved in these disorders. These techniques permit the identification of chromosomal loci closely associated with the phenotypic manifestation of a gene defect and therefore hold promise for the ultimate identification of defective genes conferring vulnerability for the disorders. Once a gene is identified, it becomes possible to characterize its function, which in many cases may involve a defective or altered gene product.

These methods represent a special type of genetic linkage analysis, except that the linkage is not to a phenotypic marker such as the HLA type, but to polymorphic DNA markers. These markers are detectable regions of chromosomes that contain variations in primary DNA sequence (i.e., polymorphisms) within the human population. Two of the major types of DNA polymorphisms in common use in linkage analyses are *restriction fragment length polymorphisms* (RFLPs) and polymorphisms in numbers of repeated sequences, most often *dinucleotide repeats*, but also longer sequences called *variable numbers of tandem repeats* (VNTRs). Polymorphic DNA markers can be used in linkage analysis by observing cosegregation of a trait of interest (e.g., bipolar disorder) within a pedigree with a particular marker.

In the RFLP method, demonstration of sequence variation among individuals depends on restriction endonucleases, the enzymes mentioned above that recognize particular sequences in DNA and cut the DNA within or near that sequence (Botstein et al. 1980). If sequence variation within the human genome occurs within the recognition sequence of a restriction enzyme, altering even a single base, the enzyme will no longer cut in that location. Alternatively, variation may create a recognition sequence where one did not exist previously. A loss or gain in a restriction site will lead to different-sized fragments when the DNA is digested by the enzyme. It is these different-sized fragments that are termed RFLPs.

In practice, a restriction enzyme is used to digest DNA from lymphocytes obtained from an individual subject. A given restriction enzyme may cut total human genomic DNA over a million times and produce an initially uninterpretable number of DNA fragments of widely varying sizes. However, the DNA fragments can be ordered according to size using gel electrophoresis. In electrophoresis, DNA, which is negatively charged, migrates toward a cathode in an applied electric field. Because the DNA is run through a gel that retards DNA movement, the smallest fragments of DNA migrate most quickly. Specific DNA fragments can then be identified by *Southern blotting*. In this procedure, DNA is transferred by capillary action from the gel to a membrane filter to which it adheres irreversibly. The filter is then incubated with a radioactively labeled DNA probe from a known chromosomal location that will hybridize only to those DNA strands on the filter that contain sequences complementary to the probe. The blot is then exposed to X-ray film, which reveals the location of the radioactively labeled DNA fragments. Gain or loss of a restriction site will change the migration pattern of the DNA visualized because it will change the length of the DNA fragments (i.e., the RFLPs) detected by the radioactive probe (Figure 1–19). By systematically hybridizing with a panel of probes that covers the human genome, it can be demonstrated that a particular RFLP (or, alternatively, dinucleotide repeat) pattern cosegregates with the disease in a given pedigree. If the linkage is tight, information can be obtained as to the general location of the disease vulnerability gene within the genome. The next step is isolating the gene and determining its function.

The power of this approach is that it does not require any prior knowledge about the pathophysiology of the disease, but rather depends on the inheritance of a polymorphism sufficiently close to the disease gene so that these alleles would cosegregate across generations. The systematic approach has been used successfully to find genes that cause Huntington's disease, cystic fibrosis, and now manic depressive disorder (Berrettini et al. 1994). This approach

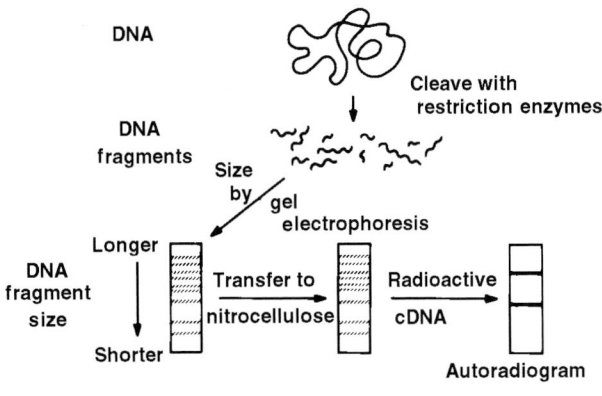

FIGURE 1–19.   Restriction fragment length polymorphism technique. The DNA isolated from lymphocytes is cleaved into fragments by incubating it with a specific restriction endonuclease. The fragments are then separated on the basis of size (i.e., length) by electrophoresis on an agarose gel. These DNA fragments are then transferred to nitrocellulose, to which they bind tightly, and are incubated with a radioactive cDNA probe. The cDNA probe will bind only to the fragment(s) to which it is complementary. The unbounded cDNA probe is washed off, and the band(s) to which the radioactive cDNA is bound is identified by autoradiography.

represents a prodigious amount of work, however.

An alternative strategy to identify disease genes can be employed if good pathophysiological information is available that provides clues as to the specific proteins that could potentially be abnormal in a particular disease. Genes encoding these proteins can be cloned and used as *candidate disease genes*. Polymorphisms are identified within or near the location of these genes that are then used in a linkage analysis. Not only is the initial linkage analysis more efficient, but if the candidate gene turns out to be the disease gene, no additional work is needed to move from the linked marker to the disease gene. In the case of Huntington's disease, the ongoing attempt to move from the tightly linked marker to the actual disease gene took a decade.

Once a disease gene is identified, its actions in the brain must be investigated. A number of approaches are possible, including the possibility of expressing the human gene in other species, most commonly mice, or of inactivating the implicated gene in a mouse model by a technique called *homologous recombination*. Such approaches are likely to permit a detailed study of the actions of the protein encoded by the gene, thus providing clues to the pathophysiology of the human disorder. Indeed, the mutant gene for amyloid precursor protein responsible for one type of hereditary Alzheimer's disease has been inserted in the mouse genome and causes the pathology of Alzheimer's disease in the transgenic mice.

REGULATION OF PROTEIN PHOSPHORYLATION AND NEURAL GENE EXPRESSION BY NEUROTRANSMITTERS AND DRUGS

One of the most important properties of the nervous system is its plasticity: it can adapt to changes in the environment, and it can form memories. A good example of adaptation was described above in the discussion of tyrosine hydroxylase, the rate-limiting enzyme in catecholamine biosynthesis. Under circumstances in which norepinephrine- or dopamine-expressing neurons must fire at high rates, they adapt by increasing the activity of tyrosine hydroxylase, and, in addition, they produce more molecules of tyrosine hydroxylase. The former adaptation is due to protein phosphorylation and the latter to regulation of gene expression. Together, these are the most significant mechanisms regulating long-term adaptation—and, in all likelihood, all forms of memory—in the nervous system. Regulation of neural gene expression by neurotransmitters, hormones, and drugs can potentially produce long-lasting alterations in virtually all aspects of a neuron's functioning by altering levels of neurotransmitter-synthesizing enzymes, peptide neurotransmitters, receptors, ion channels, signal transduction proteins, cytoskeletal components within the cells, and other critical neural proteins.

Protein phosphorylation and regulation of gene expression are often related. In most cases it is protein kinase–dependent phosphorylation that couples environmental stimuli to changes in neural gene expression. (Another important mechanism regulating neural gene expression is via steroid hormones, as described below.) Although gene expression is regulated at many levels, control of the initiation of transcription appears to be the major mechanism gating the flow of information from the genome into the production of cellular proteins. The regulation of transcription initiation involves two critical processes: 1) positioning of *polymerase*, the enzyme that transcribes DNA into RNA, at the correct start site of genes, and 2) controlling the efficiency of initiations to produce the appropriate transcriptional rate. These control functions are subserved by short stretches of DNA (*cis-regulatory elements*) within genes (Figure 1–20) that act as specific binding sites for proteins that regulate transcription, generally called *transcription factors*. Mutational analyses have shown that each gene has a particular combination of cis-regulatory elements. The nature, number, and spatial arrangement of cis-regulatory elements determine a gene's unique pattern of expression, including the cell types in which it is expressed, the times during development at which it is expressed, the basal levels at which it is expressed, and its responsiveness to environmental stimuli (Mitchell and Tjian 1989).

As described in an earlier section, stimulation of G-protein–linked receptors activates or inhibits second messenger systems and, in turn, protein kinases. When activated, certain protein kinases not only act in the cell cytoplasm but translocate into the nucleus of the cell where they can phosphorylate transcription factors. Those transcription factors that are activated (or inactivated) by phosphorylation can couple stimulation of neurotransmitter receptors with changes in gene expression.

Those cis-regulatory elements that bind transcription factors that are physiologically regulated (e.g., by phosphorylation) and that therefore confer neurotransmitter, hormone, or second messenger responsiveness on genes are often called *response elements*. Perhaps the best-characterized example of a second messenger response element is one that confers activation by cyclic AMP (and therefore cyclic AMP–dependent protein kinase) on those genes in which it is found (Comb et al. 1987). The discovery and analysis of *cyclic AMP response elements* (CREs) within many genes depend on the ability to mutate DNA sequences in vitro and then to reintroduce them into cells in culture (a process called *transfection*). The effects of the mutations in the DNA sequences on the ability of cyclic AMP to activate the gene could then be observed. By using such approaches, it was discovered that CREs contain the DNA sequence CGTCA or closely related sequences, and that this sequence of nucleotides could bind a protein called CREB (CRE-binding protein). When bound to a CRE, CREB activates transcription when it is phosphorylated by cyclic AMP–dependent protein kinase. Many additional response elements and transcription factors have been characterized.

STEROID HORMONE RECEPTORS

An important family of DNA response elements that do not necessarily involve phosphorylation are the glucocorticoid response elements (GREs) and other steroid hormone response elements. Unlike neurotransmitters or peptide hormones, which bind to cell surface receptors, glucocorticoids and other steroid hormones are fat soluble and directly enter cells. They act by binding to specific receptors within the cell cytoplasm. Cytoplasmic steroid receptors include glucocorticoid receptors, estrogen receptors, mineralocorticoid receptors, and the like. Because steroid hormones diffuse widely, the specificity of response depends on the presence or absence of specific receptors within particular cells. When activated by hormone binding, steroid receptors translocate into the nucleus, where they bind to GREs (or other steroid hormone response elements) contained within particular genes. The binding of the receptor to the DNA then increases or decreases the rate at which these target genes are transcribed. Thus steroid hormone receptors act as hormone-sensitive transcription factors. Most of the known effects of glucocorticoids, gonadal steroids, thyroid hormone, and vitamin D on cellular function are mediated via their actions on gene expression.

MOLECULAR PSYCHOPHARMACOLOGY

The discovery of drugs that selectively reduce the symptoms of psychiatric disorders has yielded a productive set of pharmacological probes to study the potential roles of specific neural systems in the pathophysiology of psychiatric disorders. Of course, it cannot be assumed that the molecular or cellular site of action of a psychotropic medica-

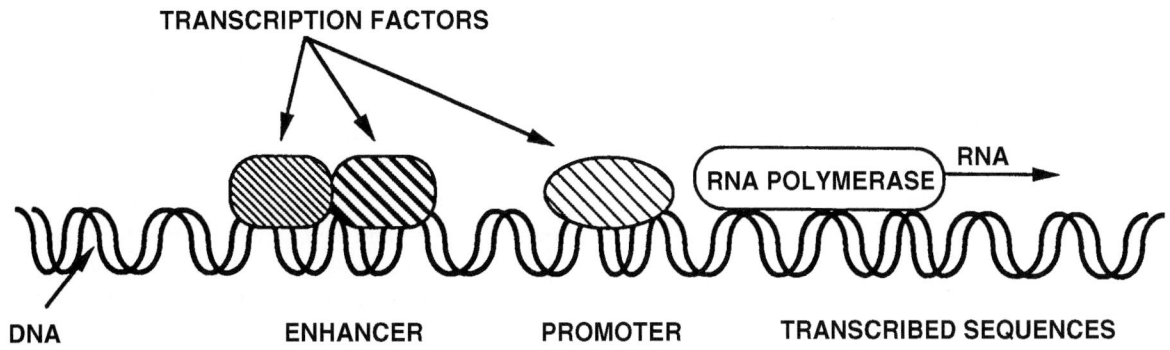

FIGURE 1–20. Regulation of gene expression. Certain regions of DNA, designated promoters and enhancers, are required for accurate transcription of genes and for determining the rates at which genes will be expressed. One specific function of the promoter of a gene is to set the precise site at which transcription by RNA polymerase begins. Promoters and enhancers are DNA sequences that function by serving as highly specific binding sites for proteins involved in the regulation of transcription (i.e., transcription factors).

tion localizes the pathophysiological defect responsible for the disorder. It is entirely possible that the neuronal system affected by the drug is only secondarily involved and that the pharmacologically induced alteration in its function compensates for a primary defect elsewhere in the nervous system. Nevertheless, our ability to identify the molecular targets and neural systems on which psychotropic drugs act has given rise to important pathophysiological theories and has provided the impetus for important discoveries in basic neuroscience. In this section, the current understanding of the mechanisms of action of major classes of psychotropic medications will be reviewed, with particular emphasis on the research strategies involved in clarifying their roles.

ANTIPSYCHOTIC DRUGS

The discovery that both reserpine and the phenothiazine chlorpromazine reduce the agitation, hallucinations, and delusions of psychotic patients ushered in the modern era of psychopharmacology 35 years ago. Over the subsequent decade, the pharmaceutical industry generated a substantial number of drugs that were thought to have antipsychotic effects. Whereas many of these drugs were variations on the structural theme of chlorpromazine, other novel structures were also developed such as the butyrophenone series as exemplified by haloperidol. Because the cause of schizophrenia and other psychotic disorders was unknown, and because the mechanism of action of the drugs was obscure, clinical use was largely based on empirical titration of symptoms against side effects.

In the early 1960s, the Veterans Administration and the National Institute of Mental Health (NIMH) undertook an ambitious study to demonstrate unequivocally the clinical efficacy of the antipsychotic medications. To guard against subjective biases, the strategy of the double-blind, placebo-controlled study was developed, a strategy that is now considered the gold standard to which most new medications are subjected (Kurland et al. 1961). Putative active drugs were compared with placebo to determine if the drug was more effective than an inert substance, a particularly important issue for a disorder in which symptoms wax and wane over time. To control for the possibility that the very fact of being treated might influence symptoms, the patients were "blind" to whether they were receiving active drug or placebo. To eliminate conscious and unconscious biases that may affect evaluation of treatment response, the clinicians and evaluators were also blind as to whether the patient was receiving placebo or active drug.

These studies generated a wealth of information that was essential for understanding the mechanism of action of antipsychotic medications. First, these studies established that sedation alone did not explain the therapeutic efficacy, because phenobarbital was ineffective. Second, these studies revealed that the phenothiazine structure was not sufficient, because promethazine was relatively ineffective compared with chlorpromazine. Third, these and subsequent studies, which compared other neuroleptics with chlorpromazine, revealed that all of the standard antipsychotic drugs were equally effective, although there was nearly a 50-fold range in clinical potency. Thus, these studies produced a critical tool, structure-activity relationships of antipsychotic medications, that could be exploited to investigate mechanisms of drug action and to design new active compounds.

Several disparate observations in the early 1960s implicated forebrain dopaminergic neurons in the mechanism of action of neuroleptics. Hornykiewicz (1966) had just demonstrated that Parkinson's disease was associated with a profound loss of dopamine in the substantia nigra and in the caudate-putamen. Reserpine, an antipsychotic that was structurally unrelated to the phenothiazines, was found to cause a marked depletion of biogenic amines, including dopamine, in the brains of experimental animals. Finally, the most common neurological side effects observed with all the effective antipsychotic medications were parkinsonian symptoms.

In studies done with chlorpromazine and haloperidol, Carlsson noted that although these antipsychotics did not deplete dopamine from the brain, as did reserpine, they did produce a marked increase in the turnover of dopamine. Tying these threads of evidence together, Carlsson first proposed that the antipsychotic medications may exert their therapeutic effects by blocking the brain receptors for dopamine (Carlsson and Lindqvist 1963). This hypothesis received support, albeit indirect, through behavioral psychopharmacological studies. Thus, behaviors such as stereotypies and emesis, which are induced in experimental animals by drugs that directly or indirectly enhance central dopaminergic neurotransmission, could be prevented by administration of neuroleptics.

Hypotheses about the interactions of antipsychotic drugs with dopamine receptors awaited validation until the methods for biochemically characterizing neurotransmitter receptors were developed in the 1970s. Following on the observation that the β-adrenergic receptor activates adenylate cyclase and thus stimulates cyclic AMP formation, Kebabian et al. (1972) demonstrated that dopamine stimulated the formation of cyclic AMP in homogenates prepared from the caudate-putamen, a brain area richly innervated by dopamine, but not by norepinephrine, fibers. In these homogenates the β-adrenergic receptor antagonist propranolol exhibited weak effects on blocking cyclic AMP formation, whereas phenothiazine neuroleptics were potent in blocking dopamine-stimulated adenylate cyclase activity. Moreover, because their potency in this assay was proportional to their clinical efficacy as antipsychotics, it was concluded that phenothiazines were acting on a dopamine receptor. The conclusion that this dopamine receptor mediated the antipsychotic effects of neuroleptics, however, was undercut by the observation that the potent butyrophenone neuroleptics such as haloperidol were weak as antagonists of cyclic AMP formation.

The use of radioactive haloperidol as a ligand to identify dopamine receptors by ligand binding techniques revealed that its lack of effect on adenylate cyclase reflected the fact that it was binding to a distinctly different dopamine receptor. ^{3}H-labeled haloperidol bound with high affinity to a population of recognition sites that were quite enriched in regions of the brain receiving dopaminergic innervation. Although dopamine itself had a 1,000-fold lower affinity for this site than did [^{3}H]haloperidol, dopamine nevertheless represented the most potent neurotransmitter active at the site. Furthermore, when the full range of clinically effective neuroleptics were examined, a remarkably high correlation was observed between their clinical potency as antipsychotics and their affinity for this novel receptor site, regardless of chemical structure (Creese et al. 1976). These two initially characterized dopamine receptors are now known to be structurally distinct: the former, which activates the adenylate cyclase via the G-protein G_s, was designated the D_1 receptor; and the latter, which binds neuroleptics with high affinity, is known as the D_2 receptor. The actions of phenothiazines on D_1 receptors reflected their lack of specificity rather than a critical therapeutic action. The D_2 receptor was subsequently shown to inhibit adenylate cyclase and activate a K^+ channel via G_i. As described in a previous section, however, recent molecular cloning studies have identified at least three additional dopamine receptors. These studies now call into question whether D_2 antagonism is necessary or even sufficient for antipsychotic drug action. This is because the atypical antipsychotic drug clozapine, which may have unique efficacy in schizophrenia but is relatively free of extrapyramidal effects, binds with low affinity to D_2 receptors but with high affinity to the newly discovered D_4 receptor. It turns out that almost all drugs that interact with D_2 receptors also interact with D_3 and D_4 receptors. Clozapine's uniquely low affinity for the D_2 receptor explains its lack of extrapyramidal side effects, and perhaps its unique efficacy in treating "negative" symptoms of schizophrenia, such as withdrawal, which may actually be caused by D_2 receptor antagonism. The relative importance of blocking D_2, D_3, D_4, or even as yet unknown dopamine receptors to antipsychotic drug action is currently a matter of intensive research.

There is one additional observation about antipsychotic drug action that is of critical importance in understanding the mechanism. All antipsychotic drugs require weeks of administration before achieving their maximum therapeutic effect. Patients on clozapine may even continue to improve for months. The implication is that blockade of dopamine receptors (of whatever type eventually turns out to be most important) represents the initial interaction of antipsychotic drugs with the nervous system. However, it is some as yet unknown slow-onset adaptive response of the nervous system to dopamine receptor blockade that represents the actual mechanism by which psychotic symptoms are relieved. Mechanisms thought most likely to be involved focus on the possibility that dopamine receptor blockade leads to significant changes in proteins (e.g., ion channels, receptors, enzymes) contained by target neurons (which may be the dopaminoceptive neuron itself or other neurons one or more synapses removed). Such changes are postulated to lead to altered functioning of critical limbic circuitry. Such delayed onset and long-lasting changes in neural functioning are likely to involve second messenger–mediated changes in gene expression.

ANTIDEPRESSANTS

The first clues to the mechanism of action of the antidepressant drugs resulted from the fundamental studies of Axelrod at the NIMH. In an experiment to monitor the catabolism of radioactive norepinephrine in vivo, Axelrod noted that a small portion of the systematically administered norepinephrine was retained, unmetabolized, in peripheral tissues (Axelrod et al. 1959). The amount of radioactive norepinephrine sequestered in these tissues was proportionate to the degree of sympathetic innervation. In subsequent studies, Axelrod demonstrated that noradrenergic neurons possess a high-affinity transport process to take up norepinephrine and that tricyclic antidepressant drugs are potent inhibitors of this transport process. Central noradrenergic, dopaminergic, and serotonergic neurons were subsequently found to possess specific transporter proteins for their neurotransmitters. These transporters, which have now been cloned, are the primary mechanism for the termination of action of these neurotransmitters after release into the synaptic cleft.

Detailed studies over the years have revealed that the tricyclic antidepressants are potent blockers of the norepinephrine and/or serotonin transporters and thereby potentiate the action of these two neurotransmitters in the synaptic cleft. More recently, selective serotonin uptake inhibitors such as fluoxetine and sertraline have been introduced. Studies of the tricyclic antidepressants and newer serotonin-selective reuptake inhibitors have verified the important distinction between identifying the initial site of action of a drug and understanding its mechanism of therapeutic action. Whereas the inhibition of reuptake and therefore potentiation of noradrenergic and serotonergic neurotransmission is a fairly immediate consequence of administration of antidepressants, there is substantial delay in the onset of symptomatic improvement in major depressive disorder. This delay is reminiscent of the action of antipsychotic drugs mentioned above.

The delay in onset of clinical effects prompted investigators to search for effects of antidepressants that only appeared with chronic drug administration. The first such delayed-onset effect to be observed was desensitization of β-adrenergic receptors in rat cerebral cortex. It is interesting that this desensitization occurs in response to virtually all effective antidepressant treatments, even antidepressants highly specific for the serotonin transporter and repeated electroconvulsive seizures. It was subsequently demonstrated that selective destruction of brain serotonergic neurons prevents antidepressant-induced β-receptor desensitization, demonstrating a functional linkage between the serotonergic and noradrenergic systems (Janowsky et al. 1982). Subsequently it has been shown that some, but not all, antidepressant treatments desensitize α_2-adrenergic receptors and 5-HT$_2$ receptors (see earlier subsection on serotonergic neurons for a review of serotonin receptors).

As evidence has accumulated, it appears likely that these alterations in receptor sensitivity are markers of chronic antidepressant effect but probably do not represent the mechanism of therapeutic action. The receptor findings, however, suggest feasible research strategies. For example, it is now known that β-adrenergic receptor desensitization is due to increases in activity of cyclic AMP–dependent protein kinase and other kinases with high specificity for the β receptor itself. Activation of these kinases probably results from increased noradrenergic stimulation of the β receptors themselves resulting from the initial actions of antidepressants (e.g., blockade of reuptake or inhibition of MAO). Thus β-receptor desensitization is a cellular marker showing that chronic antidepressant administration leads to increased activation of protein kinases within noradrenergically innervated neurons. We can now search for other important targets of these kinases, including transcription factors that may alter

neural gene expression. Complementary studies at the systems level are also needed—for example, analysis of the state of monoamine receptors in depressed patients that may be approachable with PET scanning techniques or eventually by magnetic resonance imaging. Together, these approaches promise exciting insights into the actions of antidepressants in the coming decade.

LITHIUM

The precise mechanism of action of lithium in treating manic-depressive illness is unknown, but there are scientifically compelling leads. In particular, it appears that uniquely among psychiatric drugs, lithium acts directly on G-proteins and second messenger systems. Many neurotransmitter receptors, including adrenergic and 5-HT$_2$ receptors, are linked via G-proteins (most likely G$_q$) to activation of phospholipase C, an enzyme that hydrolyzes a membrane phospholipid, phosphatidylinositol bisphosphate (PIP$_2$) to yield two second messengers, diacylglycerol and inositol triphosphate (IP$_3$). As shown in Figure 1–10, lithium inhibits certain steps in the phosphatidylinositol cycle, and some investigators have hypothesized that these actions are responsible for lithium's antimanic and antidepressant effects.

Phosphatidylinositol bisphosphate is synthesized from free inositol and lipid groups, and is subsequently phosphorylated. Most cells obtain inositol for this synthesis directly from the plasma, but neurons cannot because inositol does not cross the blood-brain barrier. As a result, neurons must either recycle inositol or synthesize it de novo from glucose-6-phosphate, a product of glycolysis. As shown in Figure 1–10, both recycling and synthesis require dephosphorylation of inositol phosphates; however, at therapeutically used concentrations, lithium inhibits several inositol phosphatases. Thus, lithium-exposed neurons have diminished ability to regenerate PIP$_2$ after it has been hydrolyzed in response to neurotransmitter receptor activation (Berridge et al. 1989). It has been hypothesized that when firing rates of neurons are abnormally high, lithium-treated neurons will become depleted of PIP$_2$ more rapidly, and neurotransmission dependent on this second messenger system will be dampened. This inositol-depletion hypothesis is attractive because the effects of lithium might become evident only in cells with abnormally high firing rates, and because lithium would dampen the effects of multiple neurotransmitter systems and therefore could treat both manic and depressive states. However, even if this hypothesis is correct, it remains incomplete. The critical cells in the brain that are targets of lithium's therapeutic action remain unknown, and it is unclear which of the many phosphatidylinositol-dependent neurotransmitter systems must be dampened for lithium to have its therapeutic effects.

In addition to its effects on the phosphatidylinositol cycle, lithium alters the coupling of a number of neurotransmitter receptors to G-proteins, thus altering the function of multiple neurotransmitter–signal transduction pathways in the brain (Avissar et al. 1988). Unlike the inositol-depletion hypothesis, however, there is presently no theory to explain how the effects of lithium on G-proteins would lead to specific effects on manic and depressed states.

Lithium also inhibits adenylate cyclase. However, the concentrations required to exert this effect in brain are higher than levels achieved clinically.

ANXIOLYTICS

Although the prototypical benzodiazepine chlordiazepoxide was discovered serendipitously, the remarkable properties of this benzodiazepine and subsequently synthesized benzodiazepines, and their superiority over barbiturates as sedatives and anxiolytics, soon became apparent. The benzodiazepines have a far more favorable ratio between anxiolytic action and sedative effects, a greater therapeutic index, and less risk for dependence and serious withdrawal symptoms than do the barbiturates.

The understanding of the molecular sites of action of benzodiazepines as well as barbiturates depended upon the elucidation of the physiological and receptor mechanisms mediating the effects of GABA, the major inhibitory neurotransmitter in brain. Local application of GABA to individual neurons results in inhibition of their firing, caused by opening of chloride channels in the neuronal membrane, thus hyperpolarizing the neuron. By using ligand binding techniques with radioactive GABA, a GABA receptor was detected within brain membranes. Moreover, by using radioactive diazepam, it was possible to directly label the recognition sites for the benzodiazepine. After additional investigation it was established that the benzodiazepine receptor represented a binding site on the GABA$_A$ receptor—a large multisubunit protein that serves as the main type of receptor for GABA in the CNS (Levitan et al. 1988). The GABA$_A$ receptor consists of multiple subunits, which have been denoted (based on cloning studies) α, β, γ, and δ. GABA$_A$ receptors are probably pentamers composed of two α, two β, and one γ or δ subunits. GABA$_A$-receptor subunits display an extraordinary degree of heterogeneity; to date, at least seven different α subunits, four different β subunits, and two different γ subunits have been cloned. The different subunits are differentially expressed in various regions within the CNS and display different functional properties.

The GABA$_A$ receptor contains at least three major binding sites relevant to psychopharmacology. The binding site for GABA is on the β subunit of the receptor; benzodiazepines bind to the α subunit. However, the α subunit is unable to bind benzodiazepines unless a γ subunit is present in the complex, presumably because of allosteric regulation of the α subunit by the γ subunit (Pritchett et al. 1989). Benzodiazepines do not directly open the receptor chloride channel. Rather, they act by increasing the affinity of the GABA binding site on the β subunit for GABA and thereby enhance the synaptic actions of GABA.

Barbiturates also bind to the GABA$_A$ receptor, but at a site that is physically distinct from that of benzodiazepines, and thus both drugs can be bound to the receptor at once. Barbiturates exert an influence on receptor function similar to that of benzodiazepines, increasing the affinity of the receptor for GABA and thereby increasing the ability of GABA to activate the receptor Cl⁻ channel. Unlike the benzodiazepines, however, barbiturates at higher doses can directly cause opening of the Cl⁻ channel in the absence of GABA. This may explain why barbiturates cause more serious CNS depression (with greater likelihood of lethality) than do benzodiazepines when taken in overdose. In addition to increasing the affinity of the GABA$_A$ receptor for GABA, benzodiazepines and barbiturates increase the affinity of the receptor for each other.

Ethyl alcohol produces its CNS effects at blood concentrations much higher than any other widely used psychotropic substance. At blood alcohol concentrations associated with intoxication, alterations in cell membrane properties are likely to affect the functioning of a wide range of membrane proteins such as receptors, channels, and transporters. There is increasing evidence, however, that a small number of neurotransmitter receptors and perhaps ion channels that are particularly susceptible to ethanol-induced changes in their membrane environment are responsible for ethanol's behavioral effects. In particular, at pharmacologically relevant concentrations, ethanol inhibits the actions of one type of receptor (i.e., the NMDA receptor) that mediates important effects of the brain's major excitatory neurotransmitter, glutamate (Tsai et al. 1996). At low concentrations, ethanol also alters GABA$_A$-receptor functioning much as do benzodiazepines and low-dose barbiturates: the receptor has a greater affinity for GABA. Like barbiturates, ethanol at high concentrations can cause opening of the chloride channel independently of GABA. Moreover, ethanol increases the apparent affinity of the receptor for both benzodiazepines and barbiturates. Thus, ethanol both attenuates excitatory neurotransmission and enhances inhibitory neurotransmission.

Our increasing understanding of the pharmacology of this receptor rationalizes a number of clinical observations. The similarity of actions among low-dose ethanol and anxiolytic and sedative drugs is consistent with the use of ethanol by many individuals to relieve anxiety, to overcome social inhibitions, and to put themselves to sleep. (This use is misguided, however, because as blood alcohol concentrations fall, rebound symptoms reflective of within-dose tolerance frequently occur. Thus anxiety may be worse than before alcohol was taken and sleep may be interrupted.) A common site of action for ethanol, benzodiazepines, and barbiturates also explains why these drugs produce cross-tolerance and cross-dependence, characteristics that are exploited in the use of benzodiazepines for detoxification from ethanol. It also explains why these drugs potentiate one another's effects, making combined overdoses so dangerous.

CONCLUSIONS

Psychiatry, as the medical specialty primarily involved in the diagnosis and management of behavioral disorders, must by necessity incorporate neuroscience into its scientific foundation. Based on the breathtaking growth in neuroscience research over the last decade, advances in the understanding of the structure, organization, and function of the brain promise to offer powerful new methods for diagnosing psychiatric disorders, clarifying their pathophysiology, and developing more specific and effective therapies.

Fears that these advances will undermine the humanistic tradition of psychiatry and negate the important relationship between physician and patient are unfounded. First, even when genetically based diagnostic techniques become feasible for identifying certain of the hereditary major mental disorders, the clinical method for developing provisional diagnosis that is used at present will still be necessary to determine which individuals warrant testing. Second, diagnoses should be neither offered nor accepted in a mechanical fashion; making a definitive diagnosis requires ongoing humane psychological management. Third, clinical research on psychopharmacological treatments for several psychiatric disorders is now demonstrating that pharmacotherapy alone is insufficient for the complete and effective management of many patients. To the contrary, evidence is growing that specific behavioral, psychological, and psychosocial strategies must often be coupled with pharmacotherapy to achieve optimal outcome in the man-

agement of psychiatric disorders. Fourth, the methods for rigorously establishing the efficacy of somatic therapies will have to be applied to behavioral and psychological therapies to determine the most effective interventions for particular disorders. Thus, clinicians will be able to tailor the treatments, be they somatic or psychological, with increasing confidence about their efficacy and specificity.

Although the advances in neuroscience and molecular biology can rightfully be seen as causing a paradigm shift in psychiatry, one must look beyond this to consider the next set of questions that this knowledge will foster. In dealing with the brain, an organ that is uniquely sensitive to life experience, it is likely that the intense interest in developmental life events will be rekindled, as these clearly play a critical role in the phenotypic expression of genes and ultimately affect brain neuronal systems that are involved in drives, affects, and cognitive functions. Furthermore, these sorts of questions will become accessible to rigorous study. Uncovering the molecular mechanisms involved in psychopathology will raise a host of questions about gene-environment interactions, including protective mechanisms that modify or prevent the expression of psychiatric disorders in those individuals who are genetically vulnerable. Thus, insights into the pathophysiology of mental illness and the disparity between phenotypic characteristics and genetic endowments will ultimately lead to a better understanding of factors that determine "mental wellness" as well as illness.

REFERENCES

Avissar S, Schreiber G, Danon A, et al: Lithium inhibits adrenergic and cholinergic increases in GTP binding in rat cortex. Nature 331:440–442, 1988

Axelrod J, Weil-Malherbe H, Tomchick R: The physiological disposition of 3H-epinephrine and its metabolite, metanephrine. J Pharmacol Exp Ther 127:251–256, 1959

Berridge MJ, Downes CP, Hanley MR: Neural and developmental actions of lithium: a unifying hypothesis. Cell 59:411–419, 1989

Berrittini WH, Ferraro TN, Goldin LR et al: Chromosome 18 DNA markers and manic-depressive illness: evidence of a susceptibility gene. Proc Natl Acad Sci U S A 91: 5918–5921, 1994

Bliss TVP, Collingridge GL: A synaptic model of memor: long term potentiation in the hippocampus. Nature 361:31–36, 1993

Botstein D, Whik R, Skolnick M, et al: Construction of a genetic linkage map in man using RFLPs. Am J Hum Genet 32:314–331, 1980

Carlsson A, Lindqvist M: Effect of chlorpromazine and haloperidol on formation of 3-methoxytyramine and normetanephrine in mouse brain. Acta Pharmacol Toxicol 20:140–144, 1963

Choi DW, Rothman SM: The role of glutamate neurotoxicity in hypoxic-ischemic neuronal death. Annu Rev Neurosci 13:171–182, 1990

Comb M, Hyman SE, Goodman HM: Mechanisms of trans-synaptic regulation of gene expression. Trends Neurosci 10:473–478, 1987

Cooper JR, Bloom FE, Roth RH: The Biochemical Basis of Neuropharmacology, 6th Edition. New York, Oxford University Press, 1991

Coyle JT: Aminergic projections from the reticular core, in Diseases of the Nervous System. Edited by Asbury A, McKhann G, McDonald W. Philadelphia, PA, WB Saunders, 1986, pp 880–889

Coyle JT, Price DL, DeLong MR: Alzheimer's disease: a disorder of cholinergic innervation of cortex. Science 219:1184–1190, 1983

Creese I, Burt DR, Snyder SH: Dopamine receptor binding predicts clinical and pharmacological potencies of antischizophrenic drugs. Science 192:481–483, 1976

Giros B, Caron MG: Molecular characterization of the dopamine transporter. Trends Pharmacol Sci 14:43–49, 1993

Hokfelt T: Neuropeptides in perspective: the last ten years. Neuron 7:867–879, 1991

Hornykiewicz O: Dopamine and brain function. Pharmacol Rev 18:925–964, 1966

Hughes JU, Smith TW, Kosterlitz HW: Identification of two related penta peptides from the brain with potent opiate agonist activity. Nature 258:577–579, 1975

Hyman SE, Nestler EJ: The Molecular Foundations of Psychiatry. Washington, DC, American Psychiatric Press, 1993

Janowsky AJ, Okada F, Applegate C, et al: Role of serotonergic input in the regulation of the beta-adrenoreceptor coupled adenylate cyclase system in brain. Science 218:900–901, 1982

Javitt DC, Zukin SR: Recent advances in the phencyclidine model of schizophrenia. Am J Psychiatry 148:1301–1308, 1991

Kebabian JW, Petzold GL, Greengard P: Dopamine-sensitive adenylate cyclase in the caudate nucleus of the rat brain and its similarity to the "dopamine receptor." Proc Natl Acad Sci U S A 79:2145–2149, 1972

Kobilka B: Adrenergic receptors as models for G protein–coupled receptors. Annu Rev Neurosci 15:87–114, 1992

Kurland AA, Hanlon TE, Tatom MH, et al: The comparative effectiveness of six phenothiazine compounds, phenobarbital and inert placebo in the treatment of acutely ill patients: global measures of severity of illness. J Nerv Ment Dis 133:1–18, 1961

Levitan ES, Schofield PR, Burt DR, et al: Structural and functional basis for GABA$_A$ receptor heterogeneity. Nature 335:76–79, 1988

Levitt P, Rakic P, Goldman-Rakic P: Region-specific distribution of catecholamine afferents in primate cerebral cortex: a fluorescence histochemical analysis. J Comp Neurol 227:23–36, 1984

Martin D, Lodge D: Ketamine acts as a non-competitive N-methyl-D-aspartate antagonist on frog spinal cord in vitro. Neuropharmacology 24:999–1006, 1985

Mitchell PJ, Tjian R: Transcriptional regulation in mammalian cells by sequence-specific DNA binding proteins. Science 245:371–378, 1989

Nose PS, Griffith LC, Schulman H: Ca^{2+}-dependent phosphorylation of tyrosine hydroxylase in PC 12 cells. J Cell Biol 101:1182–1190, 1985

Olney JW: Brain lesions, obesity and other disturbances in mice treated with monosodium glutamate. Science 164:719–721, 1969

Pacholczyk T, Blakely RD, Amara SG: Expression cloning of a cocaine- and antidepressant-sensitive human noradrenaline transporter. Nature 350:350–354, 1991

Pritchett DB, Sontheimer H, Shivers B, et al: Importance of a novel GABA$_A$ receptor subunit for benzodiazepine pharmacology. Nature 338:582–585, 1989

Robinson, Coyle JT: Glutamate and related acidic neurotransmitters: from basic science to clinical practice. FASEB J 1:446–455, 1988

Schoepp D, Conn DJ: Metabotropic glutamate receptors in brain function and pathology. Trends Pharmacol Sci 14:13–17, 1993

Schwarz R, Meldrum B: Excitatory amino acid antagonists provide a therapeutic approach to neurologic disorders. Lancet 2:140–143, 1985

Seeberg PH: The molecular biology of mammalian glutamate receptor channels. Trends Neurosci 16:359–366, 1993

Simon MI, Strathmann MP, Gautam N: Diversity of G proteins in signal transduction. Science 252:802–808, 1991

Tsai G, Gastfriend DR, Coyle JT: The glutamatergic bases of human alcoholism. Am J Psychiatry 152:332–340, 1995

Van Tol HMV, Bunzow JR, Guan HC, et al: Cloning of the gene for a human dopamine D$_4$ receptor with high affinity for the antipsychotic clozapine. Nature 350:610–614, 1991

Watson SJ, Kelsey JE, Lopez JF, et al: Neuropeptide biology: basic and clinical lessons from the opioids, in Psychiatry Update: American Psychiatric Association Annual Review, Vol 4. Edited by Hales RE, Frances AJ. Washington, DC, American Psychiatric Press, 1985, pp 83–96

Wexler NS, Rose EA, Housman DE: Molecular approaches to hereditary diseases of the nervous system: Huntington's disease as a paradigm. Annu Rev Neurosci 14:503–530, 1991

Wong DF, Wagner Jr HN, Tune LE, et al: Positron emission tomography reveals elevated D$_2$ dopamine receptors in drug-naive schizophrenics. Science 234:1558–1563, 1986

CHAPTER 2

GENETICS

JAMES A. KNOWLES, M.D., PH.D.
CHARLES A. KAUFMANN, M.D.
RONALD O. RIEDER, M.D.

The field of psychiatric genetics appears to be on the verge of several dramatic advances that should occur in the next few years. As will be described in this chapter, there are now several reports of genetic linkage that have been replicated when examined in some independent samples. These include, but are not limited to, linkages on chromosomes 5, 6, 8, and 22 in schizophrenia and chromosome 18 in manic-depressive (bipolar) illness. During the decade preceding these findings, most of the positive results in the field were not replicated in follow-up studies by either the original investigator or by other groups. As replication of a linkage finding is the best proof that it is real, the above findings represent a significant advance in the field and should lead to the isolation of gene products that, when mutated, increase an individual's risk of developing a psychiatric disorder. It is hoped that having such a gene product will facilitate a basic understanding of the pathogenesis of these disorders, enable investigators to conduct studies of the environmental factors that interact with each gene to modify an individual's risk to disease, and allow for rational drug design to develop better pharmaceutical treatments. In the more distant future, gene therapies for some of the disorders may be possible.

Underlying the recent successes in psychiatric genetics are advances in the field of human genetics. These advances are the following: the cloning by virtue of genomic position of many of the genes for the Mendelian disorders, the Human Genome Project, and the localization of loci for genes for the complex disorders. As of May 1997 there are 5,494 established gene loci and at least 1,489 genetic disorders that have been mapped to 1,205 genetic loci as described in the Online Mendelian Inheritance in Man (OMIM) (World Wide Web [WWW] URL: http://www3.ncbi.nlm.nih.gov/Omim/Stats/mimstats.html).

At the present time, most of the known genetic defects

This work was supported by National Institute of Mental Health (NIMH) Research Scientist Development Award K02 MH00682 (C.A.K.), NIMH Schizophrenia Research Training Grant MH18870 (R.O.R.), NIMH Research Training in Affective and Related Disorders, MH15144 (R.O.R.) and a NARSAD Distinguished Investigator Award (C.A.K.).

causing disease in humans are for disorders that are transmitted in patterns that can be predicted from knowledge of how genetic information is transmitted to offspring during meiosis (Mendel's laws). The identification of the genes that cause three relatively common diseases, cystic fibrosis (CF) (an autosomal recessive disease); neurofibromatosis, type I (NF1) (an autosomal dominant disease); and Duchenne muscular dystrophy (DMD) (an X-linked disease), illustrate the power of human genetics to determine the cause of human disease. In each of these Mendelian disorders, the techniques of molecular biology were used to 1) determine the chromosomal location of the disease gene, 2) isolate the gene itself, 3) identify the disease-causing mutation, and 4) produce the abnormal protein product of the disease gene in vitro for further study.

Unlike the Mendelian disorders mentioned above, the psychiatric disorders do not have clear-cut inheritance patterns and are therefore classified as some of the "complex" genetic disorders. In addition, the psychiatric disorders do not have etiological homogeneity, well-defined (or for that matter stable) phenotypes, or reproducibly associated chromosomal rearrangement syndromes, all of which make finding the disease genes considerably more difficult.

Help for this difficulty comes in the form of the Human Genome Project. Started in 1985 with the goal to determine the complete sequence of the human genome by 2005, the project has already provided many of the reagents and much of the information that will be required to find genes for the complex genetic disorders (Guyer et al. 1995). At the present time, approximately one-half of the genes in the human genome have been mapped (WWW URL: http://www.ncbi.nlm.nih.gov/SCIENCE96/), there are Yeast Artificial Chromosome (YAC) clones available that cover a majority of the genome (WWW URL: http://www-genome.wi.mit.edu/cgi-bin/contig/phys_map), and the complete DNA sequence of the genomes of several model organisms, including yeast and *E. coli*, have been determined (WWW URL: http://www.ncbi.nlm.nih.gov/Complete_Genomes/). In addition, there are now dense maps of highly polymorphic microsatellite markers available to facilitate the genetic linkage studies (explained below) (Dib et al. 1996; Sheffield et al. 1995).

By using these resources, genes responsible for several of the complex disorders have now been isolated or localized. The best success has been in the field of cancer genetics, in which multiple genes for the different forms of cancer have been isolated. For instance, analysis of families with multiple individuals who developed breast cancer revealed that the disorder had a complex mode of inheritance. However, when only those families with a young age

at onset were examined, an autosomal dominant mode of inheritance was observed (Newman et al. 1988). This lead to the linkage of the breast cancer 1 gene (BRCA1) to chromosome 17 (Hall et al. 1990), the subsequent cloning of the gene (Miki et al. 1994), and the detection of over 130 disease-causing mutations in the gene (Couch et al. 1996). Since then, a second breast cancer gene, BRCA2, has been localized to chromosome 13 and cloned (Wooster et al. 1994, 1995). There have also been several large-scale genome-wide scans for linkage to the complex disorders of diabetes (Davies et al. 1994), multiple sclerosis (Ebers et al. 1996; Haines et al. 1996b; Kuokkanen et al. 1996; Sawcer et al. 1996), and asthma (The Collaborative Study on the Genetics of Asthma [CSGA] 1997). In all these cases, there is a direct biological test for the presence or absence of the disorder (e.g., pathology, blood glucose). Genetic linkage studies in psychiatry are expected to be more difficult to because of the diagnostic uncertainties of our field. Nonetheless, there is great excitement over the prospects of the next few years.

PSYCHIATRIC GENETICS: AIMS AND METHODS

At the core of psychiatric genetics has been the investigation of the genetic contribution to psychiatric disorders. These core studies, however, have led researchers into many related areas, such as the search for environmental etiological factors, the refinement of psychiatric nosology, the investigation of normal and abnormal psychological/behavioral traits, and the development of effective methods for the prevention and treatment of psychiatric disorders.

AIMS

The goals of genetic investigation in psychiatry are as follows:

1. To establish and specify the genetic component of the etiology of psychiatric syndromes and thus determine a) to what extent a psychiatric disorder is genetically caused, b) the DNA rearrangement of the genetic contribution, c) the biopsychosocial abnormalities associated with the gene or genes involved, and d) the processes by which genetic abnormalities lead to symptoms.
2. To establish and specify the nongenetic component of the etiology of psychiatric syndromes and thus identify environmental factors that, acting inde-

pendently of or interacting with vulnerable genotypes, produce or increase the likelihood of a disorder.

3. To validate the boundaries of diagnostic entities and subtypes within entities by determining a) the genetic associations between disorders, or between subtypes of a disorder, to establish groupings of genetically related disorders (e.g., a schizophrenia spectrum), or to split disorders established on clinical phenomenology (e.g., different subtypes of schizoaffective disorder); and b) the characteristics (e.g., severity, subject's age at onset) of a disorder that increase its heritability, thereby helping to identify diagnostic boundaries that more closely correspond to biological boundaries.

4. To specify the genetic contribution to traits and psychological symptoms, independent of their role as components of defined psychiatric syndromes.

5. To develop methods of preventing or treating psychiatric disorders based on knowledge of genetic and environmental factors in their etiology. These methods include genetic counseling, alteration of the necessary/permissive environment for persons at risk, and gene therapy.

METHODS

Research methods have evolved for each of the aims of genetic investigation. Over the past two decades the methodologies have been especially productive in determining to what extent a psychiatric disorder is genetically caused (Table 2–1). New techniques hold the promise of determining the location, nature, and product of the genetic contribution to many disorders. Genetic investigation of a psychiatric disorder attempts to answer a sequence of questions:

■ Is the illness familial?
■ Is this familiality caused by genetic factors?
■ What are the various clinical expressions of the abnormal gene(s)?
■ What are the earliest manifestations of this predisposition to illness?
■ What environmental variables increase or decrease the chances of predisposed individuals developing the disorder?
■ What is the mode of transmission?
■ Where is (are) the abnormal gene(s)?
■ What is the biological, physiological, and psychological outcome of the genetic abnormality?

Different techniques, each with their own advantages and disadvantages, as described below, are used to attempt to answer these questions.

Is the Illness Familial?—Family Risk Studies and Epidemiological Studies

Family risk studies are designed to determine to what extent an illness runs in families, because all genetic illnesses have increased rates of illness among relatives (though not all familial traits are genetic [e.g., language]). Research by the pioneers of psychiatric genetics in the early part of the 20th century demonstrated that there were higher rates of schizophrenia and bipolar illness among family members of affected individuals than in the general population. As diagnostic criteria have been developed and validated, such studies have continued, both for the psychoses and for other diagnostic entities (schizophrenia [Kendler et al. 1985], affective disorders [Andreasen et al. 1987], panic disorder [Noyes et al. 1986], simple phobias [Fyer et al. 1990], anorexia nervosa [Gershon et al. 1984]).

The methodology of conducting such studies has developed to meet higher research standards. In those studies conducted in the early part of the century, nonrepresentative hospitalized cases were sampled, and the collection of data on family members was indirect. Diagnoses were made on the basis of global clinical impressions by investigators who were not blind to the diagnoses of other family members. The results were then compared with control subjects diagnosed by other investigators.

The current state-of-the-art family risk study involves the following:

1. Samples patients (termed *probands* or *index cases*) in a nonbiased way to obtain a sample representative of all patients with the disorder.

2. Either interviews family members directly or obtains detailed descriptions of a family member's illness through records and multiple informants.

3. Arrives at diagnoses while blind to the disease status of the index case.

4. Uses operationalized diagnostic criteria (such as those in the *Diagnostic and Statistical Manual of Mental Disorders*, 4th Edition [DSM-IV; American Psychiatric Association 1994]).

5. Demonstrates reliability in both the information gathering and the diagnostic processes.

6. Compares the data on familial psychopathology, using appropriate statistical analyses, with the rate of psychopathology in the family members of a matched control group investigated simultaneously using the same methodology.

TABLE 2–1. Evidence in support of genetic transmission of various psychiatric disorders

Illness	Genetic transmission supported by				Comments
	Family risk studies	Twin studies	Adoption studies	Linkage studies	
Schizophrenia	+	+	+	+	
Bipolar disorder	+	+	+	+	
Major depression	+	+	(+)		
Panic disorder and agoraphobia	+	+			Increased panic disorder among relatives of agoraphobic patients but not vice versa.
Generalized anxiety disorder	+	+			
Simple phobia	+	+			
Social phobia	+	+			
Obsessive-compulsive disorder	(+)				Familial increase of other disorders— anxiety and depressive disorders—and obsessive symptoms.
Posttraumatic stress disorder		+			
Anorexia nervosa	+	+			More relatives have affective disorders than eating disorders.
Briquet's syndrome/somatization disorder and sociopathy	+	(+)	+		Male family members tend to have sociopathy; female members, somatization disorder.
Alcoholism	+	(+)	+	+	Familial transmission more evident among males than females.
Personality disorders					
Antisocial	+				Schizotypal personality disorder is increased in relatives of schizophrenic probands, and perhaps in relatives of affective disorder probands as well.
Schizotypal	+	+			
Borderline	+	+			
Avoidant	+				
Dependent	+				
Huntington's disease	+	(+)		+	
Alzheimer's disease	+	(+)		+	Linkage studies show heterogeneity.

Note. Evidence discussed, with references, in text. + indicates most or all findings support genetic transmission; (+) indicates some findings support genetic transmission, but others do not.

Investigations employing these techniques not only have supported the original studies showing the familial nature of many psychiatric illnesses, but also have yielded much more precise estimates of the prevalence of various forms of psychopathology among relatives. From these studies the concepts of a spectrum of illnesses related to schizophrenia, an affective disorder spectrum, and associations between clinically distinct disorders such as anorexia nervosa and affective disorders have emerged.

Calculation of the extent of psychiatric disorders among the relatives of probands begins with the rates as determined through the process of family interviews. Because some family members will not have passed through the age of risk for the disorder, it would be an underestimate of the eventual rate of psychopathology among relatives to assume that these individuals will remain well. Therefore, the data are usually reported in terms of *lifetime morbid risk*, which is an estimate of the eventual rate of illness among relatives, were they to be followed through the age of risk. There are various methods of calculating lifetime morbid risk, all based on knowledge of the cumulative incidence of cases for a certain disorder through the life span. A simple method, the *Weinberg abridged method*, determines morbid risk by dividing the number of ill relatives by a new denominator (called a *bezugsziffern*). This denominator is determined by counting all relatives, then subtracting out the relatives below the age of risk, and subtracting out one-half of the number of relatives within the age of risk (Gottesman and Shields 1982). A more precise method used in modern studies is that of *survival analysis*, which is used to plot the time of onset of the disorder among relatives and, through this, to estimate the proportion of relatives who eventually will be affected (Kalbfeish and Prentice 1980). If the cumulative incidence of a disorder is not known, as is currently the case, for example, with most personality disorders, lifetime morbid risk calculations cannot legitimately be made.

When the lifetime morbid risks for first-degree relatives of ill and control probands are determined, a *relative risk* for first-degree relatives of ill probands can be calculated. As seen in Table 2–2, which is based on selected methodologically sound studies, this relative risk varies from approximately 3 to 25 for the psychiatric disorders studied, indicating significant familial aggregation for all of them. From these data it appears that bipolar disorder, schizophrenia, bulimia nervosa, panic disorder, and alcoholism are the most familial.

As noted above, however, such rates of illness may be influenced by environmental conditions shared by family members. Thus, the extent to which a disorder is familial cannot be immediately taken as an indication of the extent to which it is genetically determined. There also may be *assortative mating*, which is the tendency for those with a psychiatric disorder to mate preferentially, usually with those who have similar psychopathology, or in other nonrandom ways, thus increasing the likelihood of the children inheriting a genetic predisposition to the disorder beyond what would be the case were only one parent affected. Unless recognized, this could lead to a familial pattern that overestimates the genetic effect.

Large-scale epidemiological studies, such as the National Institute of Mental Health (NIMH) Epidemiologic Catchment Area (ECA) study (Robins et al. 1984), can contribute to the value and interpretation of the familial data. With the use of structured interview schedules and standardized diagnostic criteria, estimates of the population prevalence of disorders can be determined and compared with the data obtained from the family studies. Some studies blend the techniques of epidemiology and family risk, studying geographic, ethnic, or cultural isolates (Egeland et al. 1987; Gusella et al. 1983).

In isolated populations we expect greater genetic homogeneity for the psychiatric disorder present, because all or most cases of the disorder may stem from a common progenitor who is the single source of the pathogenic gene(s). There may also be a higher prevalence of certain disorders in such populations. These elevated rates may be caused by an increased frequency of the abnormal geno-

TABLE 2–2. **Relative risk for psychiatric disorders**

Disorder	Relative risk	Reference
Bipolar disorder	24.5	Weissman et al. 1984a
Schizophrenia	18.5	Kendler et al. 1985
Bulimia nervosa	9.6	Kassett et al. 1989
Panic disorder	9.6	Crowe et al. 1983
Alcoholism	7.4	Merikangas 1989
Generalized anxiety disorder	5.6	Noyes et al. 1987
Anorexia nervosa	4.6	Strober et al. 1985
Simple phobia	3.3	Fyer et al. 1990
Social phobia	3.2	Fyer et al. 1993
Somatization disorder	3.1	Cloninger et al. 1986
Major depression	3.0	Weissman et al. 1984a
Agoraphobia	2.8	Crowe et al. 1983

Note. Other studies may have relative risk ratios that differ considerably from those in these studies, especially if different diagnostic criteria were used. However, the methodological soundness of studies referenced here prompted our selection of them for discussion in the text and in this comparison.

type or a higher rate of expression of the gene (i.e., increased penetrance). Isolated kindreds showing a high incidence of the disorder provide the best samples for the segregation and linkage analytic techniques, described below, which can demonstrate and localize a potent genetic contributory factor.

Do Genetic Factors Contribute to the Illness?—Twin and Adoption Studies

After a psychiatric disorder has been found to be familial, twin and adoption studies are used to dissect the relative contributions of genetics and environment to the etiology of the disorder.

Twin studies.   Twin studies examine the concordance, or the co-incidence, of a disorder in monozygotic, genetically identical (MZ) and in dizygotic, fraternal (DZ) twins, the latter sharing, on average, one-half their genes, as do siblings.[1] One strategy involves comparing concordance in MZ pairs and same-sex DZ pairs. If only the rearing environment has predisposed an index case to illness, then the co-twin, whether MZ or DZ, should also be at risk, and the rates for both MZ and DZ twins should be elevated (compared with the population rate) and equal. If, on the other hand, pathogenic genes have predisposed the index twin to illness, then a MZ co-twin would be at a higher risk than would a DZ co-twin. The concordance rate for MZ twins would be higher than that for DZ twins, and the latter should be similar to the concordance rate for siblings.

One assumption of this strategy is that the MZ and DZ twins have the same degree of similarity of the familial environment—in other words, that MZ twins do not share more environmental similarity than do DZ twins in ways that would increase the MZ concordance for psychiatric disorders. It is obvious that in some ways MZ twins are treated more similarly (e.g., being dressed alike). It is also clear that in many families MZ twins receive very similar emotional and attitudinal input from their parents. However, to indicate the complexity of this issue, there is evidence that the temperamental characteristics of the MZ twins (which may be genetic in origin) generate this similarity in rearing.

Because it is difficult to determine the degree to which shared environment could account for the increased MZ concordance rates of twins raised in the same home, studies of twins raised apart in uncorrelated (i.e., randomly assigned) environments would be useful. Ideally, the concordance rates of MZ and DZ pairs raised apart could be compared, but even having only such a sample of MZ twins would allow for comparison of their concordance rates to those of MZ twins raised in the same home. Systematic samples of such twins are hard to obtain, however, and case reports of concordance are more likely to be noted and published than are those of discordant pairs.

A third way to use the concordance rates for twins to address the question of genetic versus environmental factors is to examine the extent to which MZ twins are discordant for a disorder. Given that MZ twins are genetically identical, any degree of discordance implies that there are nongenetic etiological factors that can either produce or unmask the disorder. For example, these findings could result from "phenocopies," cases that appear to have the disorder in question but have an environmentally determined, pathogenically distinct illness that mimics the genetically determined disease. Another possibility is that environmental conditions might be necessary to add to or to interact with genetic factors to produce the illness, leading to MZ twins being both predisposed genetically for the disorder but discordant on the basis of having experienced different environments. Huntington's disease has a nearly 100% MZ concordance rate, whereas common psychiatric disorders such as schizophrenia and bipolar disorder have rates that approximate 50% and 65%, respectively.

The twin strategies described above produce quantitative data that are tempting to translate into estimates of the extent to which a disorder is genetically or nongenetically caused. The *heritability* of a psychiatric disorder is defined as the portion of a trait's variation in the population that is accounted for by genetic factors's second law (Cox and Suarez 1985; Suarez and Cox 1985). This empirical observation, also known as the *law of independent assortment*, states that alleles (specific gene configurations) at different genetic loci are inherited in d_1b_1/a_2b_2), and the other who is homozygous at both loci (a_2b_2/a_2b_2). In the absence of crossing over, the gametes that are produced include only a_1b_1 and a_2b_2. If there is crossing over between loci A and B, two new gametes, known as *recombinants*, are produced by

---

[1] There are two methods of calculating concordance: pairwise and probandwise. In the pair method, every pair is counted only once; in the proband method, pairs are counted twice if each twin was an ill proband sampled for the study independently, and this usually results in somewhat higher concordances. Many geneticists regard the latter method as preferable, because the rates can be compared with population rates (Gottesman and Shields 1982). In this chapter, probandwise rates are given unless otherwise noted.

the mother (a_1b_2 and a_2b_1), and alleles at loci A and B may appear to be assorting independently in this family even though they are on the same chromosome.[2] Consequently, within a given pedigree, the parental gametes (in the example above, a_1b_1 and a_2b_2) will be disproportionately represented if loci A and B are located near each other, and alleles at these loci will appear to violate Mendel's second law. Loci A and B may then be said to be "linked" (see Figure 2–1). By extension, if linkage can be established between a hypothetical disease locus and a marker locus with known chromosomal location, then the approximate location of the disease locus can be inferred, and, ultimately, the disease gene can be isolated.

Several approaches are available for determining linkage between disease and marker loci. One approach, known as the *likelihood method* (Morton 1955), may be used to examine the co-segregation of the disease and marker phenotypes within a pedigree; determine the probability (likelihood [L]) of achieving the observed distribution of phenotypes, given estimates for the proportion of recombinant gametes among gametes (i.e., the recombination fraction), θ, ranging from 0.0 to 0.5 (the latter representing no linkage); and calculate the odds ratio (defined as the ratio $L[\theta]\backslash L[\theta = 0.5]$)—that is, the relative likelihood of the evidence for linkage versus the evidence for no linkage. By convention, the odds ratio is expressed as its base 10 logarithm (known as the *lod score*) so that linkage data from several families can be pooled and their respective contributions added to obtain a combined probability of linkage. For monogenic diseases that have Mendelian patterns of inheritance, when the lod score at the best estimate of θ (best being defined as that estimate that yields the highest lod score) is greater than +3, linkage is confirmed; when it is less than −2, linkage is rejected. The lod scores required to confirm or reject linkage for the psychiatric disorders need to be of greater magnitude because of the complex pattern of inheritance. Corrections for the testing of multiple disease models are also required.

If some, but not all, families have linkage to a marker, a statistical test can be performed to determine whether there is evidence for genetic heterogeneity within a disorder. This appears to be the case with Charcot-Marie-Tooth disease (peroneal muscular atrophy). Once linkage is established, knowledge of the genotype can then permit pre-

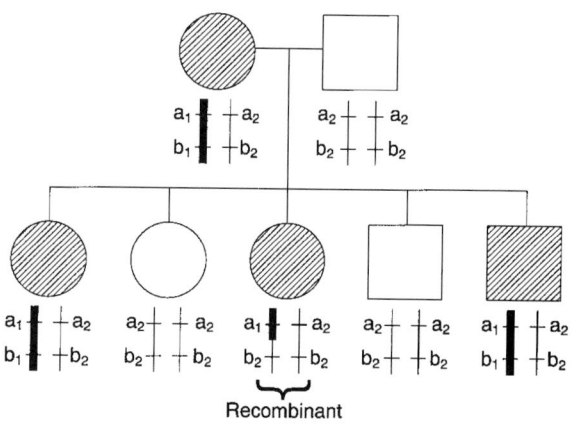

FIGURE 2–1. Genetic linkage and recombination. Depicted is a hypothetical family (circles: females; squares: males) transmitting an autosomal dominant disease. The disease locus A (containing either the defective allele a_1, or its normal counterpart a_2) lies close to a marker locus B (containing marker alleles b_1 and b_2). The mother is affected with the disease (solid symbol) and is heterozygous at both the disease and marker loci. The father is unaffected (open symbol) and is homozygous at both loci. Because the disease and marker loci are genetically linked (i.e., they lie near each other), crossing over rarely occurs between them. Most children who inherit the disease allele a_1 also receive the b_1 marker allele from their mother. Occasionally, a recombination event (i.e., "crossing over") occurs in the mother, and she transfers a chromosome bearing the b_2 marker allele along with the disease allele (as occurred in the daughter labeled "recombinant"). The frequency of such recombinants increases as the distance between the disease and marker locus

sumptive presymptomatic identification of affected persons in individual pedigrees at risk for the disease, given appropriate information about family members.

Although the likelihood method is a statistically powerful approach for detecting linkage, it relies on several assumptions that may not be warranted. These assumptions include random mating, no association between particular disease and marker alleles within the population, and genetic homogeneity of the illness across pedigrees. Also included is specification of genetic parameters (i.e., mode of inheritance, gene frequencies, and genotype penetrances) for both the disease and marker loci.

To circumvent these problems, several nonparametric methods for finding genetic loci have been developed. In

---

[2] However, crossing over rarely occurs between loci lying near one another. The frequency with which recombination results is roughly proportional to the distance between the affected loci. For example, a recombination frequency of 1% per meiosis corresponds to a functional distance of 1 centimorgan and a physical distance of approximately 1 million DNA base pairs.

general, these methods trade the need to specify a genetic model for the ability to detect linkage under a known model using the likelihood method.

The first of these, the *affected sib-pair method* (Suarez et al. 1978), posits that siblings who are both affected with a genetic disorder should be identical in the region of the genome that causes the disorder. In the other areas of the genome the siblings should, on average, share one-half of their genetic material. Multiple sib-pairs are tested, and the number of pairs who are identical for a given marker provides a statistical measure of support for linkage. This method makes no assumptions about mode of inheritance. By sampling only sib-pairs in which both members are clearly affected, it avoids considering either ambiguous cases or well individuals. (For disorders with reduced penetrance, the latter may be genetically vulnerable but are thought to represent instances of recombination.) The sib-pair method, despite its advantages, is also plagued with certain limitations. Although it can use information from sibships, it is forced to disregard other information present in extended pedigrees and does not provide an estimate of genetic distance to the disease. Although it is most powerful in detecting linkage in rare, recessive disorders, this technique may only be powerful enough to detect linkage in major psychiatric disorders if the illness is linked to a marker locus for the majority of families (Goldin and Gershon 1988).

In the likelihood and affected sib-pair methods, linkage refers to a correlation between two loci, not to their associated alleles within families. *Genetic association studies* look for correlations between certain alleles at a locus and the population of individuals with a disease. Although certain allele pairings of linked loci are likely to be disproportionately represented within any given kindred, as recombination occurs, this eventually will result in an even distribution of disease-marker allele combinations within the population at large. When the disease gene and marker loci are relatively far apart, such distribution will occur over the course of a few generations. On the other hand, if marker loci are close to a mutation that has spread through the population, this equilibrium may not have occurred.[3] Thus an association between a disease and a particular allele within the population (linkage disequilibrium) suggests that the location of the disease gene and the marker locus are within a small genetic region. The advantage of

this method over linkage analysis is that it may be sensitive to genes with small phenotypic effects. The drawbacks of this method are that the ability to detect a genetic association falls off rapidly as genetic distance increases and that this method, like linkage analysis, is affected by genetic heterogeneity. The choice of the genetic control group is also critical. If those with the illness are from different genetic backgrounds than the control subjects with whom they are compared, the observed differences in allele frequencies may be due to racial differences rather than to differences in disease status (population stratification). Newer statistical approaches have been developed to address this potential artifact.

Historically, a variety of marker loci have been used for genetic linkage mapping. The first markers were blood antigens from both erythrocytes (ABO, Rh, MNS) and leukocytes (HLA) that could be measured serologically; serum proteins and isoenzymes that could be measured electrophoretically; and common anomalies such as color blindness. The major shortcomings of these marker loci were their paucity (about 30 known) and their irregular distribution throughout the genome. In the early 1980s the first markers using DNA polymorphisms, the restriction fragment length polymorphisms (RFLPs), came into use. The RFLP markers detect variations in DNA sequence that cause the presence or absence of sites for enzymes that cut specific sequences of DNA (i.e., restriction endonucleases). Because a restriction endonuclease site is either present or absent in a given chromosome (i.e., there are only two possible alleles), the RFLP markers limit the frequency of heterozygotes to 50% (see below).

This limitation, and the cumbersome technique required to generate the RFLP data (i.e., Southern blots), have been the stimulus to develop the microsatellite markers. These markers utilize the naturally occurring variations in the length of dinucleotide (also tri-, tetra-, pentanucleotide) DNA repeat sequences. For example, an individual might have the DNA sequence GATT $(CA)_{12}$GCTA on one of his homologous chromosome pairs and the DNA sequence GATT(CA)16GCTA on the other. After these DNA fragments have been selectively amplified 105-fold by the polymerase chain reaction (PCR) using radioactive nucleotides, they can be separated by length (32 bp vs. 40 bp) and detected by autoradiography. The inheritance of these fragments can then be followed in fami-

---

[3] It has been estimated that approximately 69 generations, or 2,000 years, are necessary for the frequency of an allele combination to go to half of its equilibrium value for two loci that are separated by one centimorgan.

lies who have the disease of interest (Figure 2–2). The microsatellite markers have multiple alleles (e.g., $[CA]_{12}$ to $[CA]_{30}$) and therefore ensure that pedigree members are quite likely to be heterozygous for the marker loci. As illustrated in Figure 2–1, individuals who are heterozygous at a marker locus are essential for linkage studies. At the current microsatellite loci, 70%–95% of the individuals will be heterozygous. These markers are also widely and uniformly distributed in the human genome (approximately every 6 kilobases), and genotypes for the pedigree members can be determined rapidly with the PCR. Because incorrect linkage results may arise from misspecification of the parental origin of genotypes for critical members of pedigrees on whom marker data are uninformative, the availability of microsatellite markers should diminish the contribution of uninformativeness to unreplicable linkage findings (Baron et al. 1993; Kelsoe et al. 1989). In addition, the microsatellite markers are being used in the Human Genome Project to identify specific segments of each chromosome that have been cloned; the discovery of such linked markers will facilitate the physical isolation of the region of the chromosome containing the disease gene.

PROBLEMS OF DIAGNOSIS AND CLASSIFICATION IN GENETIC INVESTIGATIONS

Most genetic studies are greatly impeded by any ambiguity in knowing who has and who does not have the illness being studied. For example, accurate diagnosis of all family members is essential for all forms of segregation analysis and for almost all studies of linkage. (Changes in the diagnoses of pedigree members can have profound effects on the evidence for linkage, as described below for studies of bipolar disorder.)

The various versions of research diagnostic criteria developed for psychiatric disorders have not solved the diagnostic problems that exist for genetic investigation. These criteria often exclude ambiguous cases, rather than clarify their status. Also, although reliable criteria have been constructed for many psychiatric disorders, validation of the diagnostic categories as specific entities has not been established.

The high prevalence rates of psychiatric disorders and the existence of many known medical disorders that can produce the major psychiatric syndromes (e.g., the various "symptomatic schizophrenias") are reasons to believe that most psychiatric diagnostic categories are clinical syndromes, identifying patients with a variety of etiological abnormalities. A diagnosis of Huntington's disease or DMD is known to specify a group with a specific etiology and pathogenesis, whereas a diagnosis of schizophrenia or

major depressive disorder is not. If the diagnostic entities psychiatry has established are not etiologically homogeneous, then searching for the modes of transmission or genetic linkages of these disorders may be likened to the genetic study of pneumonia, renal failure, or dropsy. Thus, even the most reliable criteria available for psychiatric disorders, validated to the best of our current ability, may fail to identify certain individuals having the disease (especially those with milder or deviant forms) and may also fail by identifying as affected some individuals with a "similar disease" (if there are multiple diseases that lead to a common clinical picture).

Most psychiatric disorders are probably complex in origin, with multiple interacting genetic and environmental contributors (i.e., polygenetic or multifactorial inheritance). In these cases, for linkage studies to succeed, the diagnostic schema must identify a group in which most patients share some specific abnormal genetic component, and this may not be the case with the current nomenclature. Psychiatric nosology has of course aimed at identifying illnesses with the specificity needed by genetic analysis, and it has explored the validity of various diagnostic systems, using broad versus narrow definitions, exclusion criteria, definitions of "functional impairment" and "secondary cases," and correction factors for diagnostic instability. The relative failure of this attempt may be inevitable for a nosology based on clinical phenomenology, and greater knowledge of the biological pathogenesis of psychiatric disorders may be necessary. To make use of the new advances in genetic methodology, it may be necessary for psychiatry to discover subtypes of current diagnostic categories that have one or more specific measurable biochemical or physiological traits (e.g., precipitation of panic attacks with lactate infusion, association of schizophrenia with deviant eye tracking) in addition to the symptoms of the illness. This development may be fostered by the emerging advances in neuroradiography, neurophysiology, neurochemistry, and the specification of cognitive deficits.

However, certain aspects of psychiatric disorders will continue to make accurate diagnosis problematic, such as late age at onset, intermittent expression of symptoms, variation in symptomatology over time (e.g., major depressive disorder becoming bipolar disorder), and the influence of environmental factors on the emergence (i.e., penetrance) of these disorders or in producing phenocopies. Also, as discussed above under spectrum studies, there are mild or intermediate forms for all the major conditions (e.g., schizotypal personality disorder, schizoaffective disorder), and such cases may at times represent *formes frustes* that are genetically associated with the major disorder. There are benefits to counting these cases

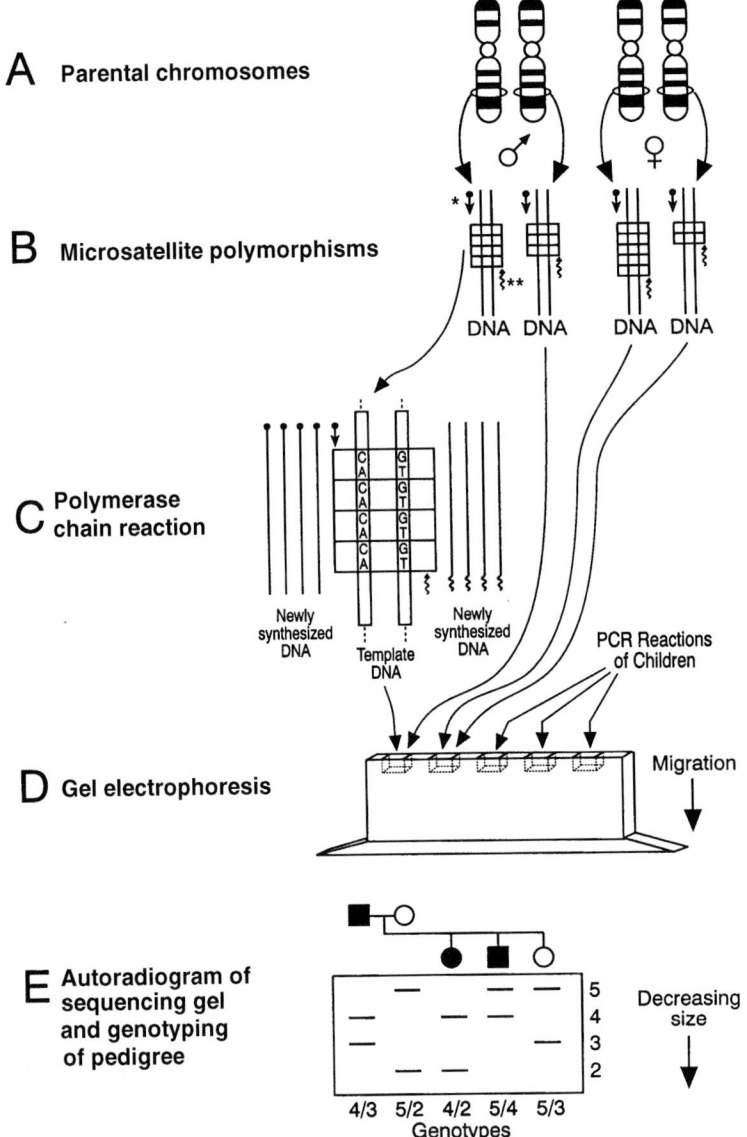

FIGURE 2–2. Schematic representation of a microsatellite marker. *A)* Autosomal homologous chromosome pairs from parents in a pedigree to be genotyped. *B)* The DNA sequence on the long arm of the chromosome is examined in greater detail, revealing the variable repeating DNA sequence termed a *microsatellite marker.* For a dinucleotide repeat each box represents two nucleotides (e.g., CA). Differing numbers of repeats of this dinucleotide are frequently found in different individuals. The example shows a father with four and three repeats, and a mother with five and two repeats. (This is a simplification; most commonly there are 15–20 repeats.) *C)* Using DNA primers (* and **), one of which is radioactivity labeled, and a heat-stable DNA polymerase, repetitive cycles of DNA denaturation and replication exponentially amplify (10^5-fold) the DNA sequence bound by the primers. This process is termed the *polymerase chain reaction,* or PCR, and is shown for only one of the two chromosomes of the father. Because the length of the fragment amplified is bounded by the primers, which are attached to nonrepeating sequences outside the microsatellite region, the length of the product of this reaction from each chromosome will be determined by the number of repeats. *D)* The amplified DNA fragments are separated on the basis of size by gel electrophoresis. *E)* The presence of the bands is determined by autoradiography. Individuals have two bands that correspond to the lengths of the amplified fragments. Each band is a marker for this region of the long arm of its own chromosome. The inheritance of these fragments can then be followed through all members of a pedigree whose DNA is available for the PCR reaction. Genotypes for each of the members of the hypothetical pedigree are shown under the autoradiogram. If an autosomal dominant disease is depicted by solid symbols, allele 4 would be linked to the disorder in this pedigree. This linkage, if statistically significant, indicates that the microsatellite marker is located close to the disease gene.

as affected in genetic studies, but there is likely to be even more etiological heterogeneity in these milder/intermediate syndromes than in the major ones, and considering such cases as affected can result in misleading results regarding specific genetic determinations (such as mode of transmission or linkage).

GENETICS OF PSYCHIATRIC DISORDERS

SCHIZOPHRENIA

Family Studies

Beginning with the pioneering work of Rudin (1916), Kallmann (1946), and others in the Berlin school, the past 80 years have witnessed over 20 studies examining the risk of schizophrenia in the relatives of over 5,000 affected individuals. These studies have consistently demonstrated elevated morbid risks for schizophrenia in the first-degree relatives of schizophrenic probands (parents, mean = 5.6%; sibs, 10.1%; children, 12.8%) compared with those in the general population (0.9%), which suggests that schizophrenia is familial (Gottesman and Shields 1982). Later studies that have satisfied modern criteria for the collection of family data have corroborated these earlier findings (Kendler 1986). The relatively lower risk to parents is at odds with Mendelian inheritance—all first-degree relatives, sharing 50% of their genes, should show equal risk—but may reflect the reproductive fitness effects.

It would appear that schizophrenia, both broadly and narrowly defined, is familial. Furthermore, schizoaffective disorder (as in DSM-III-R), paranoid disorder, atypical psychosis, and schizotypal personality disorder also aggregate in the relatives of schizophrenic probands, indicating the possible boundaries of the phenotypic spectrum (Kendler et al. 1985). Additional studies have extended this boundary to other clinical conditions (qualitative phenotypes) and clinical and subclinical signs (quantitative phenotypes). It appears that even bipolar disorder may be elevated in the relatives of schizophrenic probands, at least in some families (Pope and Yurgelun-Todd 1990)—possibly those with schizophrenia "spectrum conditions" (Baron and Gruen 1991)—or if the affective illness is associated with psychotic symptoms (Decina et al. 1991; Tsuang and Lyons 1989).

Quantitative, clinically apparent phenotypes that are elevated in the relatives of schizophrenic probands include 1) positive symptoms measured by the Thought Disorder Index (Shenton et al. 1989); 2) negative symptoms mea-

sured by the Scale for the Assessment of Negative Symptoms (Tsuang et al. 1991); 3) neuropsychological signs such as deficits in abstraction (as measured by the Wisconsin Card Sort Test [WCS]) and in short-term verbal memory (Franke et al. 1992; Tsuang et al. 1992); and 4) neurological soft signs (Kinney et al. 1991).

Subclinical phenotypes that are elevated in the relatives of schizophrenic probands include 1) disturbances in thinking, social relatedness, volition, and affective expressivity as measured by a psychometric index derived from the Minnesota Multiphasic Personality Inventory (MMPI) (Moldin et al. 1990a); 2) eye movement dysfunction on smooth pursuit (Clementz et al. 1990; Holzman and Levy 1977) and visual fixation tasks (Amador et al. 1995); 3) impairments in suppression of the 50 msec preattentional component (P50) of the auditory evoked potential in a conditioning testing paradigm (Waldo et al. 1991); and 4) attentional disturbances as measured by the Continuous Performance Task (CPT) (Keefe et al. 1997).

Family studies have also provided clues to the genetic boundaries of other psychotic and related disorders. Thus, both schizophrenia and bipolar disorder may be elevated in the relatives of probands with schizoaffective disorder (Coryell and Zimmerman 1988; Gershon et al. 1988); psychotic affective illness may be elevated in the relatives of patients with schizophreniform disorder (Pulver et al. 1991); and schizophrenia may be elevated in the relatives of patients with schizotypal personality disorder, especially if this disorder exists in the presence of comprehension impairments (Condray and Steinhauser 1992) and in the absence of other (non-Cluster A) personality disorders (Battaglia et al. 1991, 1995; Lyons et al. 1994).

Family studies may help in elucidating etiologically homogeneous subgroupings in schizophrenia. For example, specific environmental exposures, structural brain abnormalities and/or age at onset may predict more or less "familial" forms of the disorder: probands who suffered obstetrical complications may be at lower familial risk than those who did not (Bersani et al. 1995); likewise, male probands, especially those with ventricular enlargement, may have a lower family morbid risk than female probands, suggesting that there may be underrepresentation of "genetic" cases among the former (Goldstein et al. 1989; Vita et al. 1994; Wolyniec et al. 1992). One exception to this may be males with very early onset, who may be at elevated familial risk (Pulver et al. 1990). Similarly, females with especially early onset (< 22 years) may be at elevated familial risk (Sham et al. 1994). Age at onset has not been associated with familial risk of illness in all studies, however; for example, the epidemiologically based County Roscommon study found no such association (Kendler et al. 1996a).

Prognostic features may predict other types of familial risk: for example, probands with good social, occupational, and residential outcome may have elevated family risks for unipolar illness (Kendler and Tsuang 1988).

On the other hand, family studies may help to eliminate nongenetic subgroupings. For example, in one study paranoid versus nonparanoid subtypes of schizophrenia neither bred true nor could be distinguished by differential rates of schizophrenia or affective illness in the relatives of probands (Kendler et al. 1988). Likewise, there may be no individual symptoms in probands that result in differential risk for schizophrenia in relatives (Alda et al. 1989; Kendler et al. 1994).

Finally, family studies performed on special populations may shed light on (epigenetic) etiological factors contributing to disease expression. The recent observation of a 4- to 15-fold increase in the morbid risk for schizophrenia among siblings of (British-born) second-generation African Carribean schizophrenic probands compared with the siblings of their white counterparts (Hutchinson et al. 1996; Sugarman and Craufurd 1994) suggests the interaction of a particularly vulnerable genetic background with risk-conferring environmental factors, in a phenomenon known as phenotype amplification (Weiss 1993).

Thus, family studies have done much to define the (clinical and subclinical) schizophrenia spectrum, clarify the nosologic status of other psychotic disorders to schizophrenia, and address the issues of etiological heterogeneity and etiology. These studies have confirmed that schizophrenia is familial. It bears emphasizing, however, that even well-designed family studies cannot distinguish between genetic and environmental influences on familial aggregation of a disorder such as schizophrenia. Other strategies, including twin and adoption studies, are needed.

Twin Studies

If genetic factors are important in schizophrenia, we would expect that MZ and DZ co-twins of probands with schizophrenia would differ in their risk for the disorder. In fact, this has been consistently observed since the initial twin studies of Luxenberger conducted almost 60 years ago. In all, 817 MZ twin pairs and 1,016 same-sex DZ twin pairs have been studied, with weighted mean probandwise concordances of 59.2% and 15.2%, respectively, being reported (Kendler 1986). Nonetheless, estimates of probandwise concordance have varied, possibly reflecting differences in diagnostic criteria, case sampling, and zygosity assessment across studies (Walker et al. 1991). For example, broader diagnoses and more severe illness in probands—fewer positive symptoms, more negative symptoms, poorer premorbid social competence (Dworkin et al. 1988; Onstad et al. 1991)—both yield higher concordance rates.

In addition to establishing the importance of genetic factors, estimates of concordance may also shed light on the boundaries of schizophrenia: by identifying which operational definition of schizophrenia maximizes the difference between MZ and DZ concordance rates, investigators may determine a genetically validated definition of the disorder. A preliminary comparison has suggested that the RDC define the most heritable form of schizophrenia. Other definitions, which, unlike the RDC, rely exclusively on the presence or absence of psychotic symptoms, define a form of schizophrenia with limited heritability (McGuffin et al. 1984).

To summarize, the risk of schizophrenia in MZ co-twins of affected probands is at least three times that in DZ co-twins and some 40–60 times the risk in the general population. Just as noteworthy, however, is that only approximately half of MZ twin pairs are concordant for schizophrenia despite genetic identity. Monochorionic MZ twins are more likely to be concordant than dichorionic MZ twins, perhaps because the former share not only identical genetic, but a similar in utero environment (J. O. Davis et al. 1995). Although many nonschizophrenic MZ co-twins of affected probands show a variety of psychiatric disorders, including "neurotic" and character disorders and "schizoid" conditions, many (up to 43% in one series [Fischer 1971]) appear normal. Moreover, the offspring of nonschizophrenic MZ co-twins may be at as high a risk for schizophrenia as are the offspring of their affected sibs (Fischer 1971; Gottesman and Bertelsen 1989; Kringlen and Cramer 1989), implying that these co-twins carry the schizophrenic genotype despite their "normal" appearance. These findings argue against phenocopies as the sole explanation for MZ twin discordance in schizophrenia. (An additional argument against phenocopies is that discordant and concordant MZ twin pairs do not differ with respect to family risk, nor do they differ in birth order, birth weight, or condition at birth [Onstad et al. 1992].) These findings also suggest a range of phenotypes compatible with the schizophrenic genotype, and suggest an additive (or interactive) relationship between genes and epigenetic (environmental) factors in the pathogenesis of the disorder.

Discordant MZ twins also provide a clue to timing of these epigenetic factors and their effect on brain development. Differences between discordant MZ twins in dermatoglyphic patterns established in utero have suggested that a second-trimester environmental stressor combines with genetic risk in a "two-hit" model of disease pathogenesis (Bracha et al. 1992). Moreover, the affected members of discordant MZ twin pairs show left hemisphere hypodensity on computed tomography (CT) scan (Reveley et al. 1987), smaller anterior pes hippocampi on magnetic resonance imaging (MRI) (Suddath et al. 1990), and diminished activation of the dorsolateral prefrontal cortex while performing the WCS, as measured by regional cerebral flood flow (Weinberger et al. 1992).

Adoption Studies

All four varieties of adoption study have been applied to schizophrenia: adoptee study method, cross-fostering, adoptee's family method, and the study of MZ twins reared apart (see discussion of adoption studies earlier in this chapter). Despite varying methodology, these studies have consistently suggested a role for genetic influences in schizophrenia.

The adoptee study method was initially employed by Heston (1966), who found a significantly greater risk for schizophrenia among the offspring of schizophrenic mothers separated at birth than among the adopted-away offspring of control mothers. This finding was replicated in a Danish sample by Rosenthal et al. (1968), in a study that has withstood blind reanalysis using DSM-III criteria, and in a Finnish sample by Tienari et al. (1987), in a study that has incorporated such modern techniques as direct, blind interview of adoptees and detailed examination of adoptive families, the latter permitting an analysis of genotype-environmental interactions (Tienari 1991).

The sole cross-fostering study to date found equivalent rates of severe psychiatric illness among adoptees from biological parents without psychiatric illness, regardless of whether the adoptees were reared by adoptive parents with schizophrenia or without the illness: both adoptee groups had rates of illness significantly lower than those in a group of adoptees from biological parents with schizophrenia and related disorders (Wender et al. 1974). In addition to providing evidence for the etiological importance of genetic factors in schizophrenia, this cross-fostering study argues against a causative role for rearing factors associated with parent psychosis, except, perhaps, in the presence of a susceptible genotype.

The adoptee's family method has been employed in a series of studies conducted by Kety and colleagues in Denmark. They found that schizophrenia and related disorders were more common in the biological relatives of 34 schizophrenic adoptees (13/150 vs. 3/156, $P < 0.01$), whereas the rates for these disorders did not differentiate the adoptive relatives of either adoptee group, being low in both. The Danish adoption study has withstood reanalysis using

DSM-III criteria (Kendler and Gruenberg 1984) and has been replicated with a second cohort of 41 index and control adoptees (Kety 1988). The biological relatives of schizophrenic adoptees have shown higher rates not only of schizophrenia but also of DSM-III diagnosed schizotypal and paranoid personality disorders, again expanding the boundaries of the schizophrenic syndrome (Kendler and Gruenberg 1984). Overall, the biological relatives of schizophrenic adoptees have shown a 10-fold increase in risk for schizophrenia and "spectrum" disorders over the biological relatives of control subjects (Kety et al. 1994).

Finally, two studies of monozygotic twins reared apart have shown high pairwise concordance for schizophrenia, providing further evidence for a genetic component in the etiology of this disorder (Gottesman and Shields 1982).

High-Risk Studies

High-risk studies have examined both early characteristics that distinguish the offspring of schizophrenic parents from control subjects and premorbid features that predict which of those offspring will go on to develop schizophrenia. By 1 year of age, high-risk infants were more likely than control infants to show "anxious" attachment behavior and sensorimotor deficits. By 2 years of age, they were seen to be more passive and less attentive in play. Later, they had less social competence. These findings have been taken as evidence of an inherited neurointegrative defect in schizophrenia (Fish 1977, 1987; Fish et al. 1992; Marcus et al. 1987). Alternatively, the findings might reflect developmental delays caused by obstetrical complications (such as low birth weight), which frequently befall schizophrenic mothers. In fact, psychopathology at 6 years of age (especially among males) has been associated with low socioeconomic status, low Apgar score, and neonatal neurological abnormality (McNeil and Kaij 1987).

Older high-risk children have demonstrated defective emotional rapport and disturbed cognition in unblinded clinical interviews (Parnas et al. 1982), diminished attention on measures such as the Continuous Performance Test (Watt et al. 1984) and the digit cancellation task (Mirsky et al. 1995), and greater impairment on the aforementioned psychometric index derived from the MMPI (Moldin et al. 1990b). These abnormalities support the Bleulerian notion of a primary affective, associational, and attentional disturbance in schizophrenia. Moreover, because these abnormalities characterize high-risk individuals who go on to develop either schizophrenia or schizotypal personality disorder, they support the genetic relatedness of these disorders. Because the abnormalities described herein affect only about 10%–25% of high-risk offspring (Watt et al. 1984), they appear to be somewhat removed from a core monogenic defect (if present) in schizophrenia. On the other hand, smooth pursuit eye movement dysfunction has been reported to characterize approximately 50% of the teenage children of schizophrenic parents and thus may more closely reflect the schizophrenic diathesis (Mather 1985).

Premorbid psychosocial predictors of schizophrenia (versus schizotypal personality disorder) among adopted away high-risk children have included communication deviance within the adoptive family (Tienari et al. 1994). Such observations do not clarify, however, whether this intrafamilial deviance is causative of, or reactive to, greater psychopathology among juvenile adoptees destined to develop more severe psychopathology in adulthood. Premorbid physiological predictors of adult schizophrenia among high-risk children have included obstetrical complications; soft neurological signs such as impaired balance, left-right confusion, and motor overflow in childhood; and autonomic hypoarousal in adolescence (Cannon et al. 1990). Moreover, adult correlates of schizophrenia (versus schizotypal personality disorder) among high-risk offspring have included ventricular enlargement (especially of the third ventricle) on CT scan (Cannon et al. 1994; Dykes et al. 1992; Schulsinger et al. 1984). It is tempting to speculate that these clinical and radiological findings reflect a common perinatal neurological insult that contributes to disease expression. This speculation is supported not only by prospective studies of high-risk individuals but by retrospective studies of schizophrenic patients (Hultman et al. 1997) and by studies of discordant MZ twins. In these studies, poorer outcome has been associated with the triad of obstetrical complications, neurological dysfunction, and ventricular enlargement (the latter perhaps reflecting primarily enlargement ex vacuo of the temporal horn of the lateral ventricle in association with smaller anterior pes hippocampi). Nonetheless, many of these findings await replication and should be viewed with caution.

Mode of Inheritance

Several models for the genetic transmission of schizophrenia have been proposed, including monogenic/single major locus, oligogenic, and polygenic/multifactorial models. For example, Böök (1953) was able to account for observed frequencies of schizophrenia in a geographical isolate in northern Sweden by proposing a dominant gene (with gene frequency of 0.07) with homozygous penetrance of 100% and limited heterozygous penetrance

(20%). Similarly, Karlsson (1988) has suggested that a dominant gene with reduced penetrance (25%) could account for most cases of schizophrenia in Iceland. The reproductive disadvantage of schizophrenia (Larson and Nyman 1973), however, would seem to select strongly against a dominant gene.

A recessive monogenic model (with reduced penetrance) predicts that the incidence of schizophrenia among the offspring of two schizophrenic parents would be comparable to the probandwise concordance for MZ twins, and, in fact, this is what has been observed (Kringlen 1978). Similarly, a recessive model could allow for the maintenance of the abnormal gene in the population, despite reduced reproductive fitness of those individuals with the illness (Erlenmeyer-Kimling and Paradowski 1966). Normal rates of consanguinity in most families with schizophrenia, however, argue against recessive transmission of the disorder (Rosenthal 1970; but see Chaleby and Tuma 1987 regarding special populations).

Sex-linked models have been proposed by DeLisi and Crow (1989), who suggested that a schizophrenia susceptibility gene might reside on the X chromosome on the basis of gender differences in the clinical presentation of the illness, with a later onset and more benign course in women perhaps attributable to demonstration of random inactivation of X chromosomes carrying mutant alleles. Alternatively, these authors argued X chromosome inheritance on the basis of cytogenetic anomalies (including X chromosome aneuploidies—XXY, XXX—as well as a fragile site at Xq27) associated with schizophrenia-like psychoses. They attributed the observation that schizophrenia appears to be transmitted on the X chromosome in some families, and, given cases of male-to-male transmission, on an autosome in others, to be compatible with a susceptibility gene for the disorder residing in the "pseudoautosomal" region of the sex chromosomes (i.e., a region of sequence homology between X and Y chromosomes wherein recombination may occur during male meiosis [Burgoyne 1982]). "Pseudoautosomal" transmission would predict an increased frequency of same-sex sibling pairs affected with schizophrenia when illness is inherited through the paternal lineage, and, in fact, this has been observed (Crow et al. 1989).

Monogenic models, however, have difficulty accounting for the sharp drop in risk for schizophrenia as one moves from MZ twins to first- and second-degree relatives. Oligogenic models involving the epistatic interaction of two or three gene loci may better account for these data (Risch 1990). Likewise, monogenic models are hard pressed to account for the observed increased risk of schizophrenia in relatives, given either increased severity in the proband or a greater number of other affected relatives (Gottesman and Shields 1982). These observations, on the other hand, are compatible with a polygenic/multifactorial model. Furthermore, O'Rourke et al. (1982) have argued against a single-locus, two-allele model by citing its inability to account for the observed distribution in the rates of schizophrenia among four classes of relatives of schizophrenia probands (parents, siblings, MZ, and DZ co-twins) in 21 studies meeting criteria of adequacy. Finally, several segregation analyses have similarly rejected monogenic models or, at least, have been unable to reject polygenic models (Risch and Baron 1984; Tsuang et al. 1982; Vogler et al. 1990).

These results are compatible, however, with a so-called mixed model involving a major locus in the setting of a multifactorial background (Tsuang et al. 1991). Moreover, they do not preclude the possibility that major loci underlie certain aspects of the schizophrenia phenotype. Thus, admixture analysis, a strategy complementary to segregation analysis that examines the population distribution of a quantitative phenotype for multimodality (each mode presumably reflecting the mean phenotypic consequence of a particular genotype), has provided preliminary evidence for a major gene underlying the aforementioned psychometric index derived from the MMPI (Moldin et al. 1990c) and smooth pursuit eye movement dysfunction (Clementz et al. 1992).

Linkage Analysis and Association Studies

In the last few years, a number of genetic loci have been implicated in the pathogenesis of schizophrenia. There have been partially replicated findings of loci on chromosomes 5q, 6p, 8p, 13, and 22. In addition, there have been nonreplicated reports of linkage to loci on chromosomes 3p and 5p. Although none of these regions has yet to yield a gene for schizophrenia, the hopes are high that at least some of the regions contain genes for schizophrenia that will be isolated in the next several years. The replicated findings will be discussed in some detail below, followed by a brief mention of the nonreplicated findings. Numerous investigations have also been undertaken of various candidate genes for schizophrenia by linkage, genetic association, and direct DNA sequencing. Some of these studies will also be discussed. This area has also been the subject of several recent reviews (Karayiorgou and Gogos 1997; Murphy et al. 1996).

Chromosome 5q. Evidence for a locus that contribute vulnerability to schizophrenia in this region was first observed by a German research group during a genome scan for schizophrenia (Schwab et al. 1997). In their initial scan,

they observed a lod score of 1.8 for the marker IL9 on chromosome 5q in 14 German families. This was followed-up by examining 40 additional families with other markers in the region. Multipoint analyses of the affected sib-pairs in the sample gave a lod score peak of 1.8 at marker D5S399 (2 cM telomeric to IL9), which decreased to 1.3 when four families from the original 14 were removed (Schwab et al. 1997). By itself, this result is not suggestive of linkage, but additional support for a gene in the region came from a study of 265 Irish pedigrees by researchers at the Medical College of Virginia (MCV) (Straub et al. 1997). They obtained a pairwise lod score of 3.04 for marker D5S393 (same location as D5S399), using a recessive genetic model and assuming genetic heterogeneity. This locus (if it is real) appears to be segregating in 10%–25% of the Irish pedigrees. Analysis of the Irish data with multipoint methods gave a score of similar magnitude, but moved the most likely location of the gene 12 cM closer to the centromere (Straub et al. 1997). This entire region (5q21–q31) is distinct from the 5q11.2–13.3 linkage that was reported earlier (Sherrington et al. 1988) but was not replicated (Gurling 1992; McGuffin et al. 1990).

Chromosome 6p. In the summer of 1994, researchers at MCV informed other groups working on the genetics of schizophrenia that they had positive lod scores on chromosome 6p24–22, allowing many groups to publish their findings together in November 1995. The group at MCV found evidence for a locus that contributed to a vulnerability to schizophrenia in 15%–30% of their 265 pedigrees of Irish descent (Straub et al. 1995). They got their highest lod score (3.51) with D6S296, which is located telomeric to HLA, with an intermediate definition of affectedness (schizophrenia, poor outcome schizoaffective disorder, schizotypal personality disorder, and other nonaffective psychotic disorders).

As noted, several other groups reported their findings at the same time. Some of these studies found positive lod scores on chromosome 6p, although not with the same markers or phenotypic diagnoses as in the MCV study (Antonarakis et al. 1995; Moises et al. 1995a; Schwab et al. 1995a). Two other studies published at the same time did not find evidence of a gene for schizophrenia on 6p (Gurling et al. 1995a; Mowry et al. 1995), nor did two later studies (Garner et al. 1996; Riley et al. 1996). The genetic region that is positive in the original and replication studies spans about 40 cM of chromosome 6p that goes as far centromeric as the HLA locus. A critical appraisal of these findings has been published (Baron 1996).

In a large collaborative study designed to pool data from 14 research groups (713 pedigrees) with five microsatellite markers from the region, a suggestion of linkage to chromosome 6p was observed (Schizophrenia Linkage Collaborative Group for Chromosomes 3, 6, and 8 1996). A lod score of 2.19 was observed in the new sample using MAPMAKER/SIBS (a multipoint sib-pair analysis) and a narrow definition of affectedness (schizophrenia or schizoaffective disorder). When the MCV was added back in the score increased to 2.68. These scores are not conclusive for linkage to a schizophrenia gene in the region but are suggestive (Lander et al. 1995). Unfortunately, this large study only tested markers in the region that was positive in the original report (Straub et al. 1995) and hence did not cover the entire region flanking the HLA locus.

Chromosome 8p. During the course of a genome scan for genetic factors for schizophrenia using 520 markers, researchers at Johns Hopkins University (JHU) found evidence for loci on chromosomes 3 and 8 (Pulver et al. 1995). Markers D8S133 and D8S136 (9 cM apart) gave maximum lod scores of 2.35 with a dominant and 2.20 with a recessive "affected only" analysis model using a narrow diagnostic model (schizophrenia or schizoaffective disorder). Affected sib-pair analysis found four markers in the region that gave P values of < 0.001.

These findings have been replicated by other research groups (Kendler et al. 1996b; Kunugi et al. 1996) and in a large collaborative study (see chromosome 6 above) (Schizophrenia Linkage Collaborative Group for Chromosomes 3, 6, and 8 1996). In the collaborative study, a lod score of 2.22 was obtained in the replication sample using a recessive model and assuming genetic heterogeneity with marker D8S261. When the replication sample was combined with the JHU data, the score at this marker increased to 3.06 under the same analysis model. In both cases, the maximum lod score was obtained when the proportion of families linked to the marker was about 20%. A nonparametric sib-pair analysis gave a peak of 2.73 centered on marker D8S133 in the combined dataset.

Chromosome 13q. Positive lod scores have been observed on chromosome 13q14.1–q32 in a collection of 13 multiplex families (11 UK/2 Japanese) in the region of the 5-HT$_{2A}$ receptor gene locus (Lin et al. 1995). A lod score of 1.61 was obtained with marker D13S144 under a dominant genetic model and the assumption of genetic heterogeneity. About half of the families would appear to be linked to this locus. A multipoint analysis assuming 40% of the families are linked yielded a maximum lod score of 2.0 near marker D13S128 (about 30 cM telomeric from D13S144). A follow-up by the same group indicated that it is the Caucasian families that are linked to this re-

gion (Lin et al. 1997). Another group (JHU) has recently announced positive findings in the same region (Antonarakis et al. 1996). Using 54 families, they report a lod score of 2.54 with marker D13S128 with a dominant genetic model. Another marker in the region, D13S779 gave a score of 2.53 with a recessive genetic model.

Chromosome 22q. The first region of the genome that was found to contain replicable loci for potential genes for schizophrenia is chromosome 22q. Researchers at JHU obtained a lod score of 2.85 in 39 families using a dominant genetic model with marker IL2RB (Pulver et al. 1994b). At the same time, a group at the University of Utah had completed a genome scan for schizophrenia with 9 families and obtained a lod score of 2.07 with marker D22S276 and a recessive genetic model (Coon et al. 1994). An initial attempt to replicate the finding by the JHU and three other groups was unsuccessful (Pulver et al. 1994a).

Since that time, multiple groups have found some evidence for the presence of a locus for schizophrenia in the region (Moises et al. 1995b; Polymeropoulos et al. 1994; Schwab et al. 1995b; Vallada et al. 1995a, 1995b), whereas others have not (Kalsi et al. 1995). In the largest collaborative study, 11 research groups genotyped their samples for marker D22S278 (296 sib-pairs) and found evidence of allele sharing amongst affected siblings ($P = 0.001–0.006$) (Gill et al. 1996).

Other evidence supporting the presence of a gene for schizophrenia on chromosome 22q comes from the observation that affected individuals have a high rate of hemizygous microdeletions in the 22q11 region (Karayiorgou et al. 1995). In addition, these microdeletions overlap with the minimal genetic region containing the gene(s) for velocardiofacial syndrome (VCFS). This is of interest because individuals with VCFS have an extremely high rate of schizophrenia (Pulver et al. 1994c), and individuals with schizophrenia have a high rate of VCFS dysmorphic features (Beatty et al. 1996).

Nonreplicated regions reported. There have been several regions of the genome that have been implicated as harboring a gene for schizophrenia in individual studies. There was a report of positive lod scores on chromosome 3p (Pulver et al. 1995), but this finding appeared to be a false positive when the region was investigated in a large multicenter collaborative study (Schizophrenia Linkage Collaborative Group for Chromosomes 3, 6, and 8 1996). Examination of the short arm of chromosome 5 in a collection of 12 families revealed one large family, of Puerto Rican descent, that appeared to be linked to 5p14.1–p13.1. A two-point analysis using marker D5S111 gave a lod score of 3.72 for the family with an autosomal dominant genetic model. A multipoint genetic analysis with other markers in the region raised the score to 4.37. The other pedigrees in the collection did not support linkage to the region (Silverman et al. 1996).

Another linkage approach to the genetic dissection of the psychiatric diseases is to use physiological measures that correlate with the disorder. This has been done for two such measures related to schizophrenia, eye tracking dysfunction (ETD) and impaired inhibition of the P50 auditory-evoked response. Using 8 pedigrees, researchers from Germany found linkage of ETD to markers on chromosome 6p (lod score of 3.51 to D6S271) on the centromeric side of the HLA complex (most of the 6p findings described above find evidence of linkage telomeric to HLA), assuming autosomal dominant transmission (Arolt et al. 1996). Linkage analysis using various models of schizophrenia gave only moderately positive lod scores to 6p in this pedigree collection (Arolt et al. 1996). Similarly, strong evidence of linkage (lod score = 5.3) to the P50 response was found with a autosomal dominant to markers on chromosome 15q13–14 (which contains the α7-nicotinic cholinergic receptor gene) in 9 families (Freedman et al. 1997). Again, only moderately positive lod scores were observed if schizophrenia, rather than P50 status, was used as the phenotype for the analysis. If replicated, these studies may represent the future of psychiatric genetics as finding the genes for related phenotype that are inherited in a Mendelian manner should be straightforward.

Genetic Association Studies

A large number of candidate genes have been tested for linkage disequilibrium to schizophrenia in genetic association studies. There are currently well over one hundred published association studies. Most of these studies examine candidate genes in the dopaminergic and serotonergic pathways, and have not found convincing evidence of an association. As an example, one of the most studied loci, the dopamine D_3 receptor, has been observed to be associated with schizophrenia in some studies (Asherson et al. 1996; Crocq et al. 1992; Ebstein et al. 1997; Kennedy et al. 1995; Mant et al. 1994; Nimgaonkar et al. 1996; Tanaka et al. 1996), whereas no association is seen in others (Chen et al. 1997; Nothen et al. 1993; Rietschel et al. 1996; Sabate et al. 1994; Saha et al. 1994).

Molecular Approaches

Molecular studies of schizophrenia have included quantitation of known mRNAs for specific candidate proteins, screening of unknown mRNAs through in vitro translation and two-dimensional gel electrophoresis, and direct sequencing of genomic DNA. In an example of the first approach, Harrison et al. (1991) and Collinge and Curtis (1991) both found decreased non-NMDA glutamate receptor mRNA in the hippocampus of patients with schizophrenia, suggesting a role for aberrant glutaminergic function in the disorder. In an example of the second approach, Perrett et al. (1992) identified over 200 products coding for mRNA from postmortem tissue. One novel 26-kilodalton protein was specifically decreased in schizophrenia brain (18% of control level). In an example of the third approach, Sarkar and associates (1991) directly sequenced the dopamine D_2 receptor gene from 14 patients with schizophrenia and found no significant sequence differences in seven functionally significant regions (e.g., exons, splice junctions). Likewise, Jones and associates (1992) serendipitously identified a C-to-T nucleotide substitution producing an alanine-to-valine change in codon 713 of the amyloid precursor protein gene in one patient with schizophrenia. This substitution was not found in an additional 100 patients with schizophrenia, but given its critical location in a highly conserved portion of exon 17, which had previously been implicated in presenile dementia, it might prove to be a rare mutation of pathogenic significance in dementia praecox.

MOOD (AFFECTIVE) DISORDERS

Since the major mood disorders bipolar disorder and major depression (also called unipolar depressive disorder) were derived from the concept of bipolar illness 30 years ago, they have been found to be highly familial in a number of European and American studies. First-degree relatives of bipolar probands have an elevated morbid risk for both bipolar and major depressive illness, whereas relatives of major depression probands have an elevated risk for major depression but not bipolar disorder (Weissman et al. 1984a). In these studies there have been inconsistent findings of increased rates of alcoholism and sociopathy among relatives. Schizoaffective disorder, especially schizoaffective disorder with manic symptoms, also has frequently been found to be associated with a high rate of bipolar disorder among relatives.

In addition to finding these high familial rates of affective disorder, a number of studies have found that the risk for family members and the morbid risk in the population have increased for those born in later versus earlier decades of the 20th century (Gershon et al. 1987; Klerman et al. 1985). This has been termed an *age-period-cohort effect*, and it has been found to be present in many countries (Weissman et al. 1992). The cause of this ominous trend is undetermined.

The results of a very large NIMH collaborative study (2,226 interviewed relatives) using the RDC (Spitzer et al. 1978), as reported by Andreasen et al. (1987) for interviewed relatives, are summarized in Table 2–3. These data confirm the above findings. This study also found that schizoaffective probands with depressive features had a somewhat elevated rate (2.5%) of schizophrenia in first-degree relatives and a zero prevalence of bipolar-I disorder. These findings were quite different from those of schizoaffective disorder, bipolar type, providing evidence that certain types of schizoaffective disorder may not be related to bipolar disorder. In this study, the authors decided to report rates of illness rather than morbid risk figures, because the age and sex distributions across relative groups were similar and the presence of the age-period-cohort effect could prevent accurate morbid risk calculations.

Many other family studies have also attempted to use variations in the rate of affected relatives to validate subtypes of major depression. This is an effort, in part, to find a phenotype(s) that could be a discrete illness and correspond to Mendelian inheritance patterns or show linkage to genetic markers. This search has investigated various definitions of endogenous depression, pharmacological response, severity of illness, suicidality, the presence of psychotic features, rapid cycling, associated illnesses (e.g., alcoholism, anxiety disorder), decreased REM latency, and early age at onset. Most of these factors have not been consistently shown to increase familial risk. However, early age at onset (under age 20) has been shown, in more than six studies with depressed and/or bipolar probands, to be associated with an increased rate of illness among adult relatives 2- to 3-fold (versus relatives of other depressed probands). The increase is even greater for early onset cases among relatives (Kupfer et al. 1989; Rice et al. 1987b; Weissman et al. 1984b). The corresponding increase in a

study of prepubertal depression was 14-fold (Weissman et al. 1988). In two studies, reduced REM latency was also associated with higher familial rates (Giles et al. 1988; Mendlewicz et al. 1989).

Similar efforts to distinguish subtypes of major depression, but beginning with the differences in familial background rather than proband characteristics, were made by G. Winokur et al. (1975). In this work, patients with major depression who have a first-degree relative with bipolar disorder are considered bipolar disorder-related, whereas others with major depression are divided into *familial pure depressive disorder* (i.e., first-degree relative with affective illness), *depressive spectrum disease* (i.e., first-degree relative with alcoholism or antisocial personality), and *sporadic depressive disease* (i.e., no family history of depression, antisocial personality, or alcoholism). Additional studies using this typology have found a more favorable short-term (i.e., 6-month) outcome with pure depressive disorder, and those subjects with depressive spectrum disease were found to have less severe depression (but more alcoholism and social maladjustment) on long-term (i.e., 11-year) follow-up.

Twin studies have supported the importance of genetic factors in the transmission of the major affective disorders. Summed data from older twin studies give a 65% pairwise concordance rate for MZ twin pairs and a 14% rate for DZ pairs (Nurnberger and Gershon 1982). The MZ rate for bipolar disorder is higher than that for major depression. Older studies had an average MZ concordance of 72% for bipolar probands, with a Danish study, using strict criteria, finding an MZ rate of 79% versus 19% for DZ pairs (Bertelsen et al. 1977). This study found MZ and DZ rates of 54% and 24%, respectively, for major depression probands. Two newer twin studies of major depression by Kendler et al. (1992d) and McGuffin et al. (1991) both found substantial evidence for genetic factors, but differed

TABLE 2–3. **National Institute of Mental Health Collaborative Study of Affective Disorders: rates of illness in interviewed first-degree relatives**

| Diagnoses in relatives (%) | Diagnosis of proband | | | | | |
	Bipolar 1	Bipolar 2	Unipolar	Schizoaffective—depressive	Schizoaffective—bipolar	Schizophrenia
Bipolar 1	3.9	4.2	22.8	0.2	0.5	1.0
Bipolar 2	1.1	8.2	26.2	0	0.4	0.4
Unipolar	0.6	2.9	8.4	20.3	0.2	0.3
Schizoaffective—depressed	0	3.7	21.0	0	0	2.5
Schizoaffective—bipolar	3.6	5.8	25.4	0	0.7	0.7

Source. Data adapted from Andreasen et al. 1987.

on whether the environmental contribution to the disorder was from shared environmental (e.g., familial) factors or from experiences not shared by the twins.

The few adoption studies of major affective disorders have produced somewhat conflicting data that are confounded by differences in sampling. The one study of adopted-away offspring found that the children of mothers with bipolar disorder or major depression had a higher rate of major affective disorder than did the adopted-away children of mothers with other psychiatric conditions (Cadoret 1978).

Mendlewicz and Rainer (1977) found a significantly increased risk for affective illness in the biological parents of bipolar adoptee probands, compared with their adoptive parents or with the biological parents of control subjects. Wender et al. (1986) studied a group of adoptees with mixed affective disorder diagnoses (bipolar, unipolar, neurotic depression, "affect reaction") and found an increase in suicide and some affective disorders among their biological, but not their adoptive, relatives when each was compared with his or her corresponding control subject. Conversely, von Knorring et al. (1983), in a similar design, found no differences between the biological parent groups and noted an excess of psychiatric illness in the adoptive parents of the index cases, who were primarily adoptees with nonbipolar depression.

Many psychiatric disorders have been associated with bipolar disorder and/or major depression in family studies, so an "affective disorder spectrum" is thought to include dysthymia, cyclothymia, schizoaffective disorder (RDC criteria), alcoholism, and eating disorders. Newer studies convincingly add attention-deficit/hyperactivity disorder, and even migraine, to this list. In addition, certain personality traits, such as rigidity, appear to be increased among relatives (Maier et al. 1992). However, preferential mating between those persons with affective disorders, plus the frequency of secondary depressions complicating almost all severe illnesses, makes it difficult to determine whether these associations actually reflect joint etiological determinants.

High-risk studies of children of parents with major affective disorders have quite consistently found high rates of social and psychiatric impairment. Controlled studies of specific diagnoses have noted an increased prevalence of major depression, conduct disorder, attention-deficit/hyperactivity disorder, anxiety disorder, and substance abuse, as well as poorer social functioning and more school problems, among these children. The age at onset of depression in these high-risk offspring was earlier (mean ages 12–13) than among depressed control subjects whose parents were not depressed (mean age at onset of 16–17). Research on

the mode of transmission of the mood disorders is an area of great current activity and interest. One hypothesis that has been repeatedly tested is that major depression and bipolar disorder are, respectively, mild and severe forms of the same disorder, either by being on the same continuum of liability to illness (polygenic or multifactorial model) or by being phenotypic variants of the same (abnormal) genotype at a single major locus. The prevalence data from family studies have usually been consistent with multiple-threshold polygenic models, but some data sets have been equally consistent with multiple-threshold single major locus models.

Pedigree and segregation analysis, which are more powerful techniques, have tended to reject single autosomal locus transmission, but the best fitting genetic model in the largest segregation analysis was to a dominant, mendelian major locus (Spence et al. 1995). In contrast, a segregation analysis on the Amish pedigrees could rule-out autosomal dominant transmission under some circumstances (Pauls et al. 1995b). Data from the NIMH study cited above failed to correspond well to either multifactorial-polygenic or single major locus models, leading the authors to conclude that bipolar disorder, though highly familial, has a "complex" mode of transmission (Rice et al. 1987b). These analyses have been made more difficult by the observed increased rate of affective illness among relatives over the past three generations, and probably by the existence of genetic heterogeneity.

The first reported linkage findings in psychiatry used pedigrees collected from the Old Order Amish living in Lancaster County, Pennsylvania. They are a genetically bounded population descendant from 30 progenitors who emigrated from Europe in the early 18th century. Tight linkage was reported between a locus conferring a strong predisposition to bipolar disorder and two RFLP DNA polymorphisms located on chromosome 11p15, the cellular oncogene Ha-ras-1 and the insulin locus. The analyses showed lod scores of 3 or more for both of these markers within a wide range of penetrance and allele frequency values, further strengthening the findings (Egeland et al. 1987). Shortly after this study came a report of linkage of bipolar disorder to a region of the X chromosome (Xq28) (Baron et al. 1987), finding close linkage of bipolar disorder to the phenotypic markers color blindness and glucose-6-phosphate dehydrogenase in a series of Sephardic pedigrees from Israel. The maximum cumulative lod scores ranged from 7.52 (assuming homogeneity) to 9.17 (assuming heterogeneity). These findings confirmed some prior studies of bipolar disorder that had suggested linkage with the Xg locus and color blindness. Together, the Egeland and Baron studies indicated two separate genetic forms of the illness (i.e., heterogeneity).

Unfortunately, these promising early findings were reversed or have not been confirmed. A reanalysis of an updated and extended version of the Old Order Amish pedigree showed no evidence for linkage to the same *Ha-ras-1* and insulin loci on chromosome 11 (Kelsoe et al. 1989). Part of the change in lod score was the result of a key pedigree member developing bipolar illness. Numerous studies on other pedigrees for chromosome 11 linkage have similarly failed to find evidence for linkage, and a second Old Order Amish study concluded that it could exclude the possibility of linkage, at least for genes on the short arm of chromosome 11 (Pauls et al. 1991). Similarly, the existence of an X-chromosome-linked subtype of bipolar disorder has also not been upheld. One linkage report supported X linkage at Xq27 (Mendlewicz et al. 1987), however, an extension and reevaluation of the Israeli pedigrees using RFLP DNA markers found very little support for linkage to Xq28 and no support for linkage to Xq27 (Baron et al. 1993).

More recently, a Finnish research group has reported linkage of a large pedigree to markers on Xq24–q27.1 (Pekkarinen et al. 1995). They obtained lod scores between 1.3 to 3.54 depending on the phenotypic and genetic models used. In addition, they found a shared marker haplotype, 20 cM in length, in all members of the pedigree with bipolar or schizoaffective disorder. Lod scores between 1.23–1.34 have also been observed on the X-chromosome in a large collaborative study of bipolar illness (NIMH Genetics Initiative Bipolar Group 1997).

In the past several years, four other areas of the genome (chromosomes 18, 21q, 4p and 12q—in order of decreasing statistical support) have been implicated as containing genes for bipolar disorder by replicated linkage studies. During the course of a genome-wide search for loci for bipolar illness, Berrettini and colleagues noticed that markers in the pericentromeric region of chromosome 18 gave positive lod scores in some of their families (although the overall combined lod scores were negative) (Berrettini et al. 1994b). This occurred with both dominant and recessive genetic models. Analyses with nonparametric methods (affected sib-pairs and Affected Pedigree Member [APM]) gave positive results and suggested the presence of a locus in the region. Since then, multiple other groups have tested markers on chromosome 18. The data from some of these groups replicate the finding (De Bruyn et al. 1996; Maier et al. 1995; Stine et al. 1995), whereas others have not found evidence for genes on 18 when they specifically examined the region (Pauls et al. 1995c) or in the course of a genome scan (Blackwood et al. 1996; Ginns et al. 1996). Of note is the work of a group at JHU, who noticed an excess of ma-

ternally transmitting families (parent-of-origin effect) in their pedigree series (McMahon et al. 1995). When the group stratified their chromosome 18 linkage results on the basis on the sex of the transmitting parent they found evidence of linkage to the pericentromeric region in all pedigrees (thus replicating the initial finding) and evidence of a new locus on 18q in the paternal pedigrees (Stine et al. 1995). The pedigrees in the original report were then divided according to the sex of the transmitting parent and linkage was observed in the paternal but not the maternal (Gershon et al. 1996). Evidence for yet another locus on chromosome 18, this time much closer to the telomere (18q22–q23), was found in two pedigrees collected from Costa Rica (Freimer et al. 1996) and six pedigrees from Utah (Coon et al. 1996). In the Costa Rican study, seven markers in the 18q22–q23 region gave lod scores over 1.0 and a shared DNA marker haplotype was seen in 23 of 26 of the bipolar I individuals in the study. So, at this time, it appears likely that there is at least one, and possibly more, genetic loci for bipolar disorder located on chromosome 18. Close examination of one candidate gene in the pericentromeric region was negative (Ram et al. 1997).

At about the same time as the original chromosome 18 linkage report, researchers at Columbia University reported a lod score of 3.41 for one large family with bipolar disorder using marker PFKL, on chromosome 21q22.3 (Straub et al. 1994). Five of the other 46 families studied gave positive lod scores for markers in the region, but the total lod scores summed over all 47 families was negative. This was followed-up by Gurling and colleagues, who, using marker D21S171 (near PFKL), obtained a maximum lod score of 1.28 (with 35% of the families linked) in a collection of 23 pedigrees under the assumption of genetic heterogeneity (Gurling et al. 1995b). This group also saw moderately positive lod scores to the tyrosine hydroxylase locus (TH) on 11p15.5 (Smyth et al. 1996). Tyrosine hydroxylase is located near the *Ha-ras-1* locus implicated in the Amish study, and some (Meloni et al. 1995; Perez de Castro et al. 1995), but not all (Gill et al. 1991; Inayama et al. 1993; Korner et al. 1994; Souery et al. 1996), studies of the locus have found an allelic association to bipolar disorder. When an admixture analysis was performed that assumed that a family was linked to *either* TH or D21S171 locus, a lod score of 3.58 was obtained (Gurling et al. 1995b). Another group investigated the 21q region with 18 markers in 22 pedigrees and found significant sharing of alleles between affected sib-pairs for markers near PFKL (Detera-Wadleigh et al. 1996). In addition, the allele sharing was "more impressive" in the maternally transmitting pedigrees (Detera-Wadleigh et al. 1996). However, like all the other positive loci observed in psychiatric genetics, not every study of the region has been positive (Byerley et al. 1995).

Two other regions of the genome have been implicated as containing genes for bipolar disorder, 4p and 12q. In a study of 12 pedigrees, marker D4S394, gave a positive lod score (4.1) in one of the families under a dominant model (Blackwood et al. 1996). The score remained positive when the other families were added in, under the assumption of genetic heterogeneity, but did not increase further. Positive lod scores with affected sib-pair methods have also been observed in the 4p region in a separate set of 63 pedigrees (29). Similarly, positive lod scores have been observed by two groups for markers on chromosome 12q (Barden et al. 1996; Dawson et al. 1995b).

There have been numerous genetic association studies of bipolar illness. Besides the studies of the TH gene mentioned above, the dopaminergic (Adamson et al. 1995; Craddock et al. 1995b; De Bruyn et al. 1994; Di Bella et al. 1996; Lim et al. 1994; Parsian et al. 1995; Perez de Castro et al. 1995; Rietschel et al. 1993; Sasaki et al. 1996b; Shaikh et al. 1993) and serotonergic (Collier et al. 1996; Gutierrez et al. 1996; Ogilvie et al. 1996) systems, along with other potential candidate genes (Craddock et al. 1995a; Dawson et al. 1995a; Gutierrez et al. 1997; Kawada et al. 1995; Lim et al. 1995; Nothen et al. 1995; Rubinsztein et al. 1996b), have been tested without clear evidence of an association.

It has also been suggested that bipolar illness displays the phenomena of *genetic anticipation* (earlier onset or greater severity of illness with each succeeding generation in a pedigree) (McInnis et al. 1993; Petronis et al. 1995). However, it is always difficult to discern between genetic anticipation and an ascertainment bias. In disorders in which the molecular basis of the genetic anticipation is understood (i.e., Huntington's disease, fragile X syndrome, spinal and bulbar muscular atrophy), an expanding trinucleotide repeat sequence is responsible. This has prompted a search for evidence of expanding trinucleotide repeat sequences in bipolar illness (Jain et al. 1996; O'Donovan et al. 1995, 1996; Rubinsztein et al. 1996a; Sasaki et al. 1996a; Vincent et al. 1996). Although some of these studies are positive in populations, no study has demonstrated cosegregation of an expanding trinucleotide sequence in a pedigree.

ANXIETY DISORDERS

The NIMH epidemiological study of 1-year prevalence rates found anxiety disorders, at 12.6%, to be the most common category of illness (Regier et al. 1993). Diagnostic terms and concepts in the area of anxiety disorders have changed considerably over the past decade, diminishing the relevance of older studies in this area. However, whenever studied, "anxiety neurosis" was found to be highly familial, with up to two-thirds of families showing cases in first-degree relatives. Studies using DSM-III-R diagnostic categories have reported increased familial rates for panic disorder and agoraphobia, generalized anxiety disorder, simple and social phobias, and obsessive-compulsive disorder.

Panic Disorder

There have been several family studies that have found a higher rate of panic disorder in the relatives of probands who have the disorder than in the relatives of control subjects. This has been seen consistently in all studies, many of which are from different countries. The relative risk to first-degree relatives of panic disorder probands ranged between 2.6- to 20-fold (Crowe et al. 1980, 1983; Maier et al. 1993; Mendlewicz et al. 1993; Noyes Jr. et al. 1986; Weissman et al. 1993), with a median value of 7.8-fold (Knowles and Weissman 1995). Most of these studies were done on samples ascertained from treatment settings, and so this relative risk may reflect a more severe form of panic disorder. As an example of this type of study, Crowe et al. (1983) found a 17.3% risk for panic disorder in first-degree relatives and an additional risk of 7.4% for "probable panic disorder" (i.e., two or three rather than four criterion symptoms). Control rates were 1.8% and 0.4%, respectively. In a family study of agoraphobia, Noyes et al. (1986) found high risk for panic disorder (definite plus probable) both in the relatives of panic disorder probands (17.3%) and in the relatives of agoraphobic probands (8.3%), compared with 4.2% in the relatives of control subjects. They also found that the risk for agoraphobia was increased among the relatives of agoraphobic probands (11.6%), but not the relatives of panic disorder probands (1.9%), when compared with control subjects (4.2%). All agoraphobic probands and relatives had panic attacks as well. In both of these studies the risk of panic disorder and/or agoraphobia among female relatives was two to three times higher than that for male relatives. Neither study showed an increased rate of generalized anxiety disorder in the relatives of the index cases. Noyes and Crowe concluded that their findings are consistent with agoraphobia being a more severe variant of panic disorder, and that these two disorders are unrelated to generalized anxiety disorder.

The possibility of a genetic relationship between adult and childhood anxiety disorders has been prompted by the high rates of separation anxiety and school phobia reported by adults with panic disorder. No systematic, blind, case-control, high-risk study of the young children of parents with anxiety disorders has been published. Some available family studies have shown elevated rates of separation anxiety in the children of parents with panic disorder/agoraphobia, but others have concluded that childhood school phobias are related to adult neurotic illness in general rather than specifically to adult agoraphobia. There is likely to also be a genetic relationship between panic disorder and affective disorders, particularly bipolar disorder. Similarly, there is some evidence that there may be a higher rate of alcohol abuse in the relatives of panic disorder probands. The studies that have investigated the comorbidity between these disorders have not provided a clear answer to the degree of genetic overlap, and the final determination of this will probably await the cloning of disease genes for each of the disorders.

There have been several twin studies of panic disorder. A nationwide Norwegian study by Torgersen (1983) found that 4 of 13 MZ co-twins (31%) were concordant for panic disorder and/or agoraphobia, compared with 0 of 16 DZ co-twins. In a second study Torgersen concluded that mixed panic disorder-depression is genetically related to major depression but not to pure panic or other anxiety disorders (Torgersen 1990). A third study by the same group, using DSM-III-R criteria, found concordance rates of 42% in the MZ and 17% in DZ twin pairs for panic disorder (Skre et al. 1993). This study was not statistically significantly due to the small sample size. From these three studies by Torgersen, an estimate of broad sense heritability can be made. These estimates range from 30% to 62%. The higher estimates of heritability are likely to be overestimates because of the absence of observed DZ pairs concordant for panic disorder in the early studies.

The largest study of panic disorder in twins is a population-based study of 2,163 females (1,033 twin pairs) from the Virginia Twin Register with a mean age of 30 years (Kendler et al. 1993). Of the 2163 twins, 5.8%, 10.9% (166 twin pairs), 4.6%, and 7.6%, met lifetime criteria for clinician-narrow, clinician-broad, computer-narrow, and computer-broad diagnoses respectively. The estimate of narrow sense heritability was 46%, 32%, 0%, and 37%, for the clinician-narrow, clinician-broad, computer-narrow, and computer-broad diagnoses respectively. This estimate of narrow sense heritability for panic disorder (30%–40%) is markedly less than that observed for schizophrenia, autism, and major affective disorder (Plomin et al. 1994).

Several factors might account for the lower heritability observed in the Kendler study (Kendler et al. 1993) as compared with the Torgersen studies (Skre et al. 1993; Torgersen 1983, 1990). First, the Kendler sample was ascertained from the general population as compared with the Torgersen samples, which were treatment samples with a high proportion of inpatient probands. If more severe cases of panic disorder have a greater chance of entering treatment and have a higher familial loading for the disorder, the above results would be observed. Second, the Kendler sample was exclusively female, whereas the Torgersen sample was a mixture of same-sex twin pairs. If the male form of the disorder has a higher proportion of genetic loading it would account for some of the observed difference. Alternatively, the Torgersen studies may have found a falsely high estimate of heritability of panic disorder because the interviewers and/or diagnosticians were not blind to the diagnosis of the co-twin.

Of the anxiety disorders, only panic disorder has had findings from linkage studies reported in the literature. Crowe et al. (1990) used 29 serological polymorphisms to scan the genome for a gene for panic disorder in 26 pedigrees. One marker, α-haptoglobin (16q22), gave a lod score of 2.27. This locus was subsequently excluded by testing of additional families and the use of an RFLP DNA marker (Crowe et al. 1990). Several candidate genes have been examined (i.e., tyrosine hydroxylase, adrenergic receptors, proopiomelanocortin, DRD2 gene, and GABAB1R), and no evidence of genetic linkage has been found (Crawford et al. 1995; Crowe et al. 1987; Mutchler et al. 1990; Schmidt et al. 1993; Z. W. Wang et al. 1992). In one genomic scan for panic disorder a single autosomal dominant locus for the disorder could largely be excluded, and several loci gave lod scores over 1.0 (Knowles et al. 1998).

Obsessive-Compulsive Disorder

The results of family studies of obsessive-compulsive disorder (OCD) are inconsistent. No increase of OCD was found among relatives in studies by Hoover and Insel (1984), McKeon and Murray (1987), and Black et al. (1992). However, each of these studies found high family rates of other psychiatric disorders, described as depressive and neurotic disorders, anxiety disorders, or "a more broadly defined OCD." The one study that showed a significant familial increase in OCD began with child and adolescent probands and reported a 25% incidence among fathers plus 9% among mothers (Lenane et al. 1990). These findings raise the question of whether early-onset OCD, like early onset affective disorder, may be more highly familial. There are also studies linking OCD with Gilles de la Tourette syndrome (Leckman and Chittenden 1990). In contrast to the earlier studies, recent family studies of OCD do suggest a familial component to the disorder (Nicolini et al. 1993; Pauls et al. 1995a; Sciuto et al. 1995). In the largest and most methodologically sound of these, the relative risk of OCD to relatives of OCD probands was 5-fold higher than the risk to relatives of control subjects (Pauls et al. 1995a).

For OCD, Carey and Gottesman (1981) found significant MZ-DZ differences (87% vs. 47%, respectively), which is similar to results found earlier in a Japanese investigation. These twin studies of OCD indicate that genetic factors may be involved. Several studies of candidate genes for OCD have been performed, but all are negative (Altemus et al. 1996; Brett et al. 1995; Catalano et al. 1994; Di Bella et al. 1996). A genetic association between an allele at the catechol-*O*-methyltransferase (COMT) gene and males with OCD has been reported (Karayiorgou et al. 1997).

Other Anxiety Disorders (GAD, Phobias, and PTSD)

Family studies of generalized anxiety disorder, simple phobias, and social phobia, but not posttraumatic stress disorder (PTSD), have found familial aggregation. Noyes et al. (1987) noted that the increased rates of generalized anxiety disorder were specific and that they were not found among the relatives of panic disorder patients. Fyer et al. (1990) reported a rate of 31% for simple phobia in first-degree relatives, compared with 11% in control subjects (relative risk = 3.3). For social phobia, two studies (Fyer et al. 1993; Reich et al. 1988) found a threefold increase in this disorder in the relatives of probands, the latter reporting rates of 16% vs. 5% in the control group. Whether these disorders are separate at a genetic level is unknown at this time. There is extensive comorbidity of these disorders in probands (Goisman et al. 1995; Goldenberg et al. 1996), but the disorders "breed true" when the families of probands without comorbidity are studied (Fyer et al. 1995). Finally, no increase of PTSD was found in the families of PTSD probands studied (using family history methodology) by Davidson et al. (1989).

Kendler et al. (1992b) conducted a twin study of generalized anxiety disorder, finding MZ-DZ concordances of 28% and 17%, concluding that this disorder was moderately familial and heritable (heritability estimated at 30%). Kendler et al. (1992c) also found evidence for a significant genetic contribution to agoraphobia, social phobia, and animal phobia in a study of female twins (heritabilities of 30%–40%). The genetic contributions were greater for animal phobia and less so for agoraphobia. These authors also found evidence for the importance of environmental factors: some factors predisposed to all phobias, but other environmental experiences had a more specific effect, especially for simple phobias. In contrast to the family stud-

ies, True et al. (1993) reported that genetic factors provided a substantial contribution to all the symptoms of PTSD (but did not report MZ-DZ concordance rates). In addition, there is evidence that genetic factors may influence one's exposure to trauma (Lyons et al. 1993).

There are few molecular genetic studies of these disorders as yet. There is a unreplicated report of genetic association between PTSD and the A1 allele of the DRD2 gene (Comings et al. 1996).

EATING DISORDERS

Anorexia nervosa and bulimia nervosa have been studied with the techniques of psychiatric genetics, although not as extensively as have other major disorders. Family studies of anorexia nervosa have shown an increased rate of anorexia itself, as well as bulimia and subclinical anorexia nervosa. In one study, first-degree female relatives had lifetime risks for these disorders of 2.3%, 2.3%, and 5.4%, respectively, compared with control risks of 0.5%, 1.0%, and 0% (Strober et al. 1985). Most notably, however, many studies have found an increased risk for affective disorders among the first-degree relatives of anorexic patients, a risk exceeding that for eating disorders and equaling the risk among the relatives of patients with major depression (A. Winokur et al. 1980). Another study found a morbid risk of approximately 13% for major depression, plus a risk of approximately 8% for bipolar or schizoaffective disorder, in first-degree relatives of probands with anorexia nervosa, with control rates of 5.8% and 0.9%, respectively (Gershon et al. 1984). Family studies of bulimia have also found high rates of mood disorders and eating disorders (Kassett et al. 1989; Logue et al. 1989). A familial connection of both of these eating disorders with substance abuse has been reported, but not consistently (Kaye et al. 1996).

Twin studies have now been reported for anorexia and bulimia. Holland et al. (1988), in an expansion of their earlier study, found 56% of 25 MZ anorexic twin pairs and 5% of 20 DZ pairs to be concordant for the disorder. For bulimia, Kendler et al. (1991) found concordances of 23.9% for MZ and 8.7% for DZ twin pairs, as well as an increased risk for bulimia-like syndromes that appeared to be milder versions of the same illness caused by the same factors. Both research groups interpreted their data to show large genetic effects (heritability estimates for anorexia and bulimia of 55% and 80%, respectively). A twin study that explored the relationship of bulimia and major depression found some degree of genetic overlap and unique environmental risk factors for each disorder (Walters et al. 1992). Various studies have also reported increasing rates of both eating disorders, in the population and among family members, for those born later versus earlier in this century (i.e., an age-period-cohort effect similar to that reported for affective disorders). At present, there are no published molecular genetic studies of the eating disorders. However, a large multisite study has begun collecting pedigrees and will begin analysis with genetic markers in the near future.

ALCOHOLISM

The rates of alcoholism in the population vary greatly by definition and by sex. The 6-month prevalence rates found in the ECA study, in which broad criteria were used, were 8.2%–10.4% for males and 1.0%–1.9% for females (Robins et al. 1984). Alcoholism has been shown to be highly familial in many studies, which, as reviewed by Merikangas (1989), show the risk to first-degree relatives to be increased approximately 7-fold. For example, Pitts and Winokur (1966), using modern family study methods and strict diagnostic criteria for severe alcoholism, found a risk of 16% in the fathers and 7% in the sibs of alcoholic subjects, versus risks of 1.6% and 0.5% for the relatives of matched control subjects. As with mood disorders and eating disorders, the risk among family members, and in the general population, appears to be rising (Reich et al. 1988).

There have been several adoption studies that also provide evidence that genetic factors, as well as environmental ones, are involved in the etiology of alcoholism. Goodwin (1979) showed that alcoholism in the biological parents predicted alcoholism in their male offspring, even when the latter were raised by unrelated adoptive parents. Cadoret et al. (1980) reported similar results. The results for female offspring were less clear. Goodwin (1979) found elevated rates of alcoholism among both the adopted-away daughters of alcoholic persons and the control adoptees, whereas Cadoret et al. (1985) found higher rates in the daughters of the index cases compared with control subjects. Data from a large Swedish sample also support a genetic predisposition to alcoholism in both women and men (Bohman et al. 1981; Cloninger et al. 1981), as well as the possible importance of certain environmental factors (such as lower occupational status of the adoptive father). In all of these studies, alcoholism in the adoptive environment was not shown to increase the risk for alcoholism among the adoptees. However, one newer study (Cadoret et al. 1985) found that alcoholism in the adoptive family more broadly defined (to include all adoptive first- and second-degree relatives) increased the rates of alcohol abuse among adoptees. Because alcohol abuse frequently coexists with antisocial personality and depression, these studies examined the question of the specificity of inheritance. They suggest that one subtype of alcoholism may relate to criminality and antisocial personality, but that depression is not genetically related. Another adoption study suggested that there are two genetic paths to drug dependence: one transmitted from the biological parent's alcoholism to drug dependency, and a second that started as antisocial personality disorder in the parent and was transmitted as aggressivity and conduct disorder to the child which then became antisocial personality disorder leading to drug dependence (Cadoret et al. 1995).

Although there have been twin studies of alcoholism that do not suggest a genetic basis for the disorder, most studies are consistent with a significant genetic diathesis to the disorder. This inconsistency may be the result of the MZ-DZ concordance ratio being relatively low (1.0–2.0) and of variations in the severity of illness of probands in the various studies. Although some studies have found no differences in the concordance rate (e.g., 29% for MZ, 33% for DZ [Gurling et al. 1984]), Kaprio et al. (1984) found MZ concordances to be greater than DZ concordances for heavy alcohol use whether or not the twins were raised together. Pickens et al. (1991) found that for alcohol dependence these rates were 59% versus 36% for males and 25% versus 5% for females. A large twin-family study from the Virginia twin registry found estimated the heritability for the familial resemblance of alcoholism at 51%–59% (Kendler et al. 1994). A study of Swedish males found similar estimates of genetic liability to alcoholism (Kendler et al. 1997).

If alcoholism were heterogeneous, with a significant percentage of cases having a major genetic causative influence, then alcoholism in persons having alcoholic parents or other first-degree relatives ("familial cases of alcoholism") may differ from that in nonfamilial cases. Also, the offspring (sons) of alcoholic persons may differ from the offspring of nonalcoholic control subjects. Such studies have in fact shown that familial alcoholic persons have earlier and more severe alcoholic-related problems, early development of physical dependence, and poorer treatment outcome (Goodwin 1984). High-risk studies of sons of alcoholic persons, compared with control subjects, have shown a decreased intensity of subjective feelings of intoxication, reduced objective signs of intoxication, and differences in plasma cortisol and prolactin following ethanol challenge (Schuckit and Gold 1988). What has not been found are higher levels of personality disturbance, and this corroborates the findings of studies of the premorbid personality of alcoholic patients.

Most of the molecular studies in addiction genetics have focused on the candidate gene approach. An association of the illness (especially of alcoholism with severe medical complications) with the *Taq* A1 allele at the dopamine D_2 receptor locus (DRD_2) was reported (Blum et al. 1990) and confirmed in at least one study (Parsian et al. 1991). The association has also been observed in polysubstance abusers (Smith et al. 1992). These findings are controversial, as most other studies do not find a statistically significant association (Bolos et al. 1990; Chen et al. 1996; Cook et al. 1996; Gelernter et al. 1991; Heinz et al. 1996; Lu et al. 1996). Linkage analysis of the DRD_2 locus in two families excluded this region (Bolos et al. 1990), indicating that the gene is not necessary for alcoholism. It remains unclear whether the DRD2 locus acts as a modifier gene that increases the severity of alcoholism initiated through other means. Two meta-analyses of the data (Gelernter et al. 1993; Uhl et al. 1993) came to very different conclusions (i.e., the DRD2 locus accounts for one-half of the genetic variance vs. has no effect), because each group excluded a portion of the available data. DNA sequencing did not reveal any protein sequence polymorphism in the receptor itself that were in linkage disequilibrium with the *Taq* A_1 allele (Gejman et al. 1994). Several large collaborative genome scan projects looking for genetic factors for alcoholism are currently underway (Reich 1996).

An additional molecular genetic approach to that has worked particularly well in understanding the biology of substance abuse is the use of animal models. Berrettini and colleagues were able to map three loci in mice for oral morphine preference by breeding mice from progenitor strains that differed in their morphine preference (Berrettini et al. 1994a). The effect of one of these loci, on mouse chromosome 10, could be replicated in another sample and the linked region contains a good candidate gene, the μ opiate receptor (Alexander et al. 1996). Two sex-specific loci for alcohol preference in mice have also been mapped (Melo et al. 1996). Interestingly, the locus for alcohol preference in female mice demonstrates *genomic imprinting* (is only active when passed from one parental line-in this case from the mother). Neither locus for alcohol preference overlaps with the three loci for morphine preference, suggesting that the genetic basis for different addictive disorders is distinct.

SUICIDE AND IMPULSIVE BEHAVIOR

Many family studies have found familial clustering of suicide attempts and completions. This has been observed in studies of completers using either friends (Shafii et al. 1985), individuals from the community (Brent et al. 1996), or nonsuicidal diagnostically matched control subjects (Tsuang 1983). Although it is difficult to control for the psychiatric comorbidity that also runs in the families of the

victims, Brent and colleagues found a 4-fold increased risk of suicide attempts and completions in the relatives of suicide probands as compared to relatives of control subjects from the community (Brent et al. 1996). In the Amish, 73% of suicides occur in 16% of the pedigrees, even though some of the nonsuicide pedigrees are just as severely affected with bipolar disorder (Egeland et al. 1985). This pattern of increased risk to relatives of suicide probands as compared with relatives of control subjects, even beyond the risk conferred by an Axis I disorder, is also seen for relatives of suicide attempters.

Several lines of evidence suggest that a portion of this familial clustering is due to genetic factors. One study of 176 twin pairs found 11% (7/62) of MZ, and 2% (2/144) of DZ twin pairs to be concordant for suicide (Roy et al. 1991). Another study found concordance rates of attempted suicide among co-twins of suicide victims to be 38% (10/26) for MZ and 0% (0/9) for DZ twin pairs (Roy et al. 1995). Given the variability in these studies it is difficult to know what portion of the propensity to attempt or complete suicide is genetic, but it is unlikely to be zero. Adoption studies of suicide provide additional support for the hypothesis that there are genetic factors (Schulsinger et al. 1979; Wender et al. 1986).

Many studies have suggested that there is a disorder of serotonin metabolism in both, the trait of impulsivity, and suicidal behavior. With this theoretical basis, a two-allele polymorphism in an intron of the gene for tryptophan hydroxylase (TPH), the rate limiting enzyme in the synthesis of serotonin, was examined for genetic association to a group of violent alcoholic Finnish offenders and arsonists (Nielsen et al. 1994). The frequency of the "U" allele was 0.32 in the 36 individuals who had made a suicide attempt and 0.54 in the 34 who did not ($P = 0.016$), suggesting an association between the "L" allele a history of attempted suicide. This study also examined the relationship between CSF 5-HIAA concentration and TPH genotype and found a highly significant association ($P = 0.0036$) between the two in impulsive but not nonimpulsive or control subjects (Nielsen et al. 1994). Abbar et al. examined a different polymorphism in the TPH gene in 62 suicide attempters with affective disorder and 52 control subjects and no evidence of a genetic association (Abbar et al. 1995). This does not constitute a nonreplication of the earlier study given that a different polymorphism within the gene was examined. More recently, a strong association has been observed between TPH and suicide attempts but this time with U allele of the polymorphism (Mann et al. 1997). Clearly, more studies will have to be done to determine if there is another mutation in the gene in linkage disequilibrium with the intronic polymorphism.

Perhaps the clearest link between a genetic mutation and a human behavior causing a psychiatric illness comes from the study of Brunner's syndrome in a large Dutch family (Brunner et al. 1993b). This X-linked syndrome is characterized by borderline mental retardation along with aggressive and violent impulsive behavior in affected males. Some of these behaviors include arson, exhibitionism, and attempted rape and suicide. A linkage study of the X-chromosome found a lod score of 3.69 at the monoamine oxidase A (MAOA) gene locus, and 24-hour urinalysis of three affected males showed abnormal monoamine metabolism (Brunner et al. 1993b). Subsequent analysis of the MAOA gene revealed that affected males in the family have a C to T mutation at position 936, changing a glutamine codon to a termination codon, and cell culture assays demonstrated the lack of MAOA enzymatic activity in the affected males (Brunner et al. 1993a). Further proof of the effect of this gene on behavior comes from the finding of aggressive behavior in a transgenic mouse strain in which the MAOA gene is deleted (Cases et al. 1995).

SOMATOFORM DISORDERS AND SOCIOPATHY

Hysteria was not accepted as a diagnostic term in DSM-III, but most of the components of the concept were included in the DSM-III-R section on somatoform disorders, which includes somatization, conversion, and somatoform pain disorders, as well as hypochondriasis. Histrionic personality disorder, one of the most important "faces" of hysteria, was put into the personality disorders section, where it resides close to antisocial personality disorder but far from those disorders presenting medical symptomatology. Studies of hysteria as well as its component parts have continued, and the accumulated data on the genetic relationships of all these disorders and antisocial personality disorder will be considered here.

The DSM-IV criteria for somatization disorder are a shortened and simplified version of the criteria for *Briquet's syndrome*, a term coined by Samuel Guze and other researchers at Washington University (Guze 1970). These investigators attempted to delineate a syndrome of multiple somatic complaints that are without a demonstrable organic basis while avoiding the confusion and pejorative connotations of the term *hysteria*. Most of the studies to be reviewed here are of Briquet's syndrome rather than of somatization disorder, as this latter concept is relatively new. Studies have shown strong overlap of the two concepts but also the possibility of greater severity and/or greater homogeneity for patients meeting the full Briquet's criteria, as indicated by higher rates of familial aggrega-

tion. The prevalence of Briquet's syndrome in first-degree female relatives has been found to be 7.7%, compared with 2.5% in control subjects (Cloninger et al. 1986).

The connection between Briquet's syndrome and antisocial personality disorder was first recognized by finding the coincidence of these two disorders in many samples, especially among women. (Histrionic personality disorder has been associated with these two disorders as well.) Family studies have repeatedly shown a link, most consistently by finding Briquet's syndrome among female relatives of probands (male or female) who are sociopaths or criminals, but also by finding elevated rates of sociopathy in the first-degree relatives of Briquet's or somatization subjects (Lilienfeld et al. 1986).

Adoption studies have given support more to genetic than to environmental determinants of the intra-individual and familial associations between these disorders. Some studies, using the adoptee study method, have shown an increase of somatic symptoms without medical explanation, as well as antisocial symptoms, among female adoptees of biological parents having antisocial personality. The largest study, using the adoptee's family method, comprising 144 female adoptee "somatizers" (identified by having two or more sick leaves per year), identified two types of the disorder, each having a link to a form of criminality among the subjects' fathers. One type, termed *diversiform somatization*, was linked to a syndrome of alcoholism plus criminal behavior in biological fathers, with the finding of increased alcohol abuse among adoptive fathers as well. The other type, *high-frequency somatizers*, had biological fathers with a recurrent history of arrest for violent crimes but no history of alcoholism and no increase of psychopathology among adoptive fathers (Cloninger et al. 1984).

Older twin studies of hysteria found higher MZ than DZ rates of concordance, but the pairwise MZ rates were low enough (averaging 21%) to question the importance of genetic factors. A newer twin study examined a mixed group of somatoform disorders and found an MZ concordance of 29% and a DZ concordance of 10% for the group of disorders as a whole (Torgersen 1986). In this study, co-twins had an increased prevalence of generalized anxiety disorder as well, raising the question of a genetic connection between these disorders. Data on criminality or antisocial personality among the twins were not reported.

Multifactorial models of transmission allow for the possibility of linking clinically discrete illnesses on a continuum of shared liability. Such a model was proposed by Cloninger et al. (1975), in which Briquet's syndrome in women, sociopathy in men, and sociopathy in women were considered to be increasingly severe expressions of the same multifactorial determinants. This model adequately fits the available data on the risks to first-degree relatives of probands having the various disorders.

Most twin and adoption studies of criminality and antisocial personality have focused on the transmission of these conditions per se and their relationship with alcohol abuse, rather than on their relationship with somatization disorder. A genetic component has consistently been supported (Cloninger and Gottesman 1987), as well as environmental factors. The largest of these studies (Bohman et al. 1982) delineated two types of criminality, each showing genetic predisposition without significant overlap. One was associated with alcoholism and more violent, repeated offenses. The other, associated with petty crimes, appeared to be caused by a genetic predisposition independent of alcoholism as well as by environmental factors that differed for the two sexes. The specific nature of gene-environment interaction is now being investigated, revealing the importance of exposure to alcoholism, antisocial behavior, and other factors associated with low socioeconomic status for those who are genetically predisposed (Cadoret et al. 1990).

PERSONALITY DISORDERS AND QUANTITATIVE BEHAVIORAL TRAITS

There are many more genetic studies of Axis I disorders than of Axis II disorders and the two most extensively studied personality disorders, antisocial and schizotypal, have already been reviewed in this chapter. Because personality can be described by so many attributes, researchers have worked to condense these into a few "dimensions," usually by factor analytic techniques. Those that have emerged as most replicable and most used in genetic studies are extraversion and neuroticism, as originally derived by Eysenck (1981). The dimensions of *harm avoidance* (anxiety-proneness vs. risk-taking), *reward dependence* (social attachment versus disgust), and *novelty seeking* (impulsivity vs. slowness to anger), as defined by Cloninger (1986, 1987), plus the additional dimensions of persistence, self-directedness, cooperativeness, and self-transcendence added subsequently (Cloninger et al. 1993), as assessed by the Tridimensional Personality Questionnaire (TPQ) are also widely used. The seven dimension TPQ data can be associated with the respective DSM-III-R personality disorder diagnoses (Svrakic et al. 1993).

The extensive family, twin, and adoption studies of extraversion and neuroticism give strong evidence for a genetic effect, but the extent of the genetic contribution, measured as heritability estimates, is greater in twin studies (40%–60%) than in family studies, where values of approximately one-half those in twin studies have been reported.

A possible interpretation, as discussed by Plomin et al. (1990), is nonadditive genetic variance, an allelic interaction that makes identical twins quite alike but does not "breed true" for first-degree relatives, because only one of the alleles can be passed on from a parent.

Following the specification of diagnostic criteria for personality disorders in DSM-III and DSM-III-R, a few family studies have now been reported for the disorders. Reich (1989) found avoidant and dependent personality disorders to be significantly familial, and this held true for the disorders when grouped as Cluster C ("anxious cluster") as well. In a later report, Reich (1991) found that the increase in anxious cluster personality diagnoses among relatives was also found for probands with mixed anxiety and depression who did not have personality disorders. Relatives of Cluster B ("flamboyant cluster") personality disorders showed a high level of personality disorder psychopathology but of a diverse nature. Borderline personality disorder has also been found to be modestly familial. We have already discussed the familiality of Cluster A personality disorders in the section above on schizophrenia.

The large body of research on personality, personality disorders, and related psychophysiological and animal studies has been reviewed by McGuffin and Thapar (1992).

At present, there are no positive molecular genetic studies of the personality disorders, but there are now several reports of genes responsible for a portion of the genetic variance of some of the personality dimensions. Increased novelty seeking, one of the dimensions of the TPQ, has been associated with the 7 repeat allele in exon 3 of the dopamine D_4 receptor gene (DRD_4) in a study of 124 unrelated Israeli subjects (Ebstein et al. 1996). This has been replicated in a study of 315, mostly male, individuals from the United States, using data from the NEO personality index to reconstruct the TPQ scale (Benjamin et al. 1996). Variation at the DRD_4 gene was estimated to account for 3%–4% of the variance in the novelty seeking trait, which is estimated to about 40% genetic (Heath et al. 1994), therefore about 10% of the genetic variance has been accounted for. Loci for another dimension of the TPQ, harm avoidance, have been uncovered in a genome scan of 758 pairs of siblings in 177 nuclear families of alcoholics (Cloninger et al. 1998). A lod score of 3.2 was observed for a locus that accounted for 38% of the total variance to harm avoidance using markers on chromosome 8p21–23. Genetic interactions with loci on chromosomes 21q21–22.1, 11, and 20 were also observed and might account for most of the genetic variance of harm avoidance. One locus that was not observed in the genome scan was the gene for the serotonin transporter (SLC6A4) on chromosome 17q12.

An earlier study of 505 individuals had found a genetic association between a polymorphism in the regulatory region of the gene and the neuroticism scale of the NEO personality inventory ($P = 0.002$) and the anxiety scale of Cattell's personality inventory ($P = 0.023$) (Lesch et al. 1996). Both of these studies of "anxiety trait" await replication.

NEUROPSYCHIATRIC DISORDERS

The neuropsychiatric disorders—Gilles de la Tourette syndrome, Huntington's disease, Lesch-Nyhan syndrome, Parkinson's disease—are well covered in the companion *The American Psychiatric Press Textbook of Neuropsychiatry*, 3rd Edition (Yudofsky and Hales 1997). Alzheimer's disease is also well covered there but, because it is one of the "complex" genetic disorders and because there has been success in finding the disease genes for some forms of the disorder, it will be discussed here.

Approximately 10% of the population over age 65 and 45% of those over age 85 are affected with Alzheimer's disease. Epidemiological studies reveal an increased prevalence of dementia in the family members of Alzheimer's patients. Family studies are hindered by the late age at onset, because individuals can die from other conditions or develop a dementia from a different etiology. Family studies in Alzheimer's disease have been well reviewed by St. George-Hyslop et al. (1989): estimates of the increase in Alzheimer's disease risk to family members vary widely and may be small (10%–14.4% for parents; 3.8%–13.9% for siblings). Life table studies that adjust for deaths not due to Alzheimer's disease find that the risk of Alzheimer's disease may be as high as 50% in family members by age 90 and only 10% in control subjects (Breitner et al. 1986; Mohs et al. 1987). These analyses support the hypothesis that there could be an autosomal gene for Alzheimer's disease with an age-dependent penetrance. Farrer et al. (1989), however, who also factored in diagnostic uncertainties, found a risk of only 24% to first-degree relatives by age 93, and of 16% to control subjects by age 90. The increased family prevalence of Alzheimer's disease may occur predominantly in an early-onset group (Heston 1981), although it may be that such cases are just more easily ascertained.

Twin studies for Alzheimer's disease have been difficult to perform as the number of twin pairs that survive until the age of onset of the disorder is low. The concordance rates observed in a number of twin studies are quite similar in MZ and DZ pairs (about 40%) (Cook et al. 1981; Embry and Bruyland 1985; Jarvik et al. 1980; Nee et al. 1987). A more recent study of Veterans found concordance rates of 21% (4/19) for MZ and 11% (2/19) for DZ twin pairs, suggesting a small genetic component to the disorder (Breitner et al. 1995). These twin studies are much more supportive of a large environmental influence on the etiology of Alzheimer's disease.

The best support of a genetic diathesis on the predisposition to Alzheimer's disease comes from the finding of four genes, all of which affect the production or deposition of amyloid, that cause or influence the development of the disorder. Familial Alzheimer's disease (FAD) is classified as either early (mean family age at onset < 60 years, < 5% of all FAD) or late-onset disease. Early onset FAD tends to be transmitted in an autosomal dominant fashion and three genes that cause this form of the disorder have been found (APP, PS1, and PS2). The occurrence of neuropathological changes indicative of Alzheimer's disease by age 40 in individuals with Down's syndrome initially directed the search for an Alzheimer's disease locus to chromosome 21. The gene for amyloid precursor protein (APP), which has 19 exons, is located on this chromosome. Parts of exons 16 and 17 of the APP gene encode amyloid, a 39–43 amino acid peptide, which is the major constituent of the senile plaques of Alzheimer's disease. Several groups reported evidence for an Alzheimer's disease gene linked to the pericentromeric region of chromosome 21, especially in early onset families (David et al. 1988; Goate et al. 1989; St. George-Hyslop et al. 1987; Van Broeckhoven et al. 1988). However, linkage was not found in all pedigrees (Pericak-Vance et al. 1988; Roses et al. 1988; Schellenberg et al. 1988). Subsequently, Hardy and colleagues identified a mutation in the APP gene that cosegregated with Alzheimer's disease in two unrelated chromosome 21–linked early-onset families (Goate et al. 1991). A search of the early onset FAD pedigrees has lead to the identification of four disease mutations in APP. These mutations flank the amyloid peptide coding sequence suggesting that they cause improper cleavage of APP. Two mutations in the amyloid coding sequences cause cerebral hemorrhage either with or without dementia. The APP mutations are thought to account for about 5% of early onset FAD (St. George-Hyslop et al. 1990).

Presenilin 1 (PS1), located on chromosome 14, was the second gene for early onset Alzheimer's disease to be found. Schellenberg et al. (1992) initially described linkage to chromosome 14q in nine early-onset (mean age at onset < 52 years) pedigrees (maximum lod score = 9.15). This was quickly replicated by others (Mullan et al. 1992; St. George-Hyslop et al. 1992; Van Broeckhoven et al. 1992), and the gene was subsequently cloned (Sherrington et al. 1995). The PS1 gene is a 467 amino acid protein with 7–10 hydrophobic transmembrane domains. The coding sequence of the gene has been examined in over 30 families and greater than 25 different mutations have been described, most of which cause missense mutations (Levy-Lahad et al. 1996). Mutations in PS1 account for about 75% of early-onset FAD. The presenilin 2 (PS2) gene was cloned by homology to presenilin 1 and mapped to chromosome 1 (Levy-Lahad et al. 1995a), right into a region where a locus for Alzheimer's disease in the Volga Germans had been mapped (Levy-Lahad et al. 1995b). A missense mutation was then observed in the German pedigrees (Levy-Lahad et al. 1995a) and subsequently an Italian pedigree (Rogaev et al. 1995). Both of the presenilin gene products are thought to increase the production of the 42 amino acid form of the amyloid peptide. There is also evidence that PS1 is an essential gene in mice that is required for normal pattern formation during early development (Shen et al. 1997; Wong et al. 1997).

A susceptibility locus for late-onset Alzheimer's disease was localized to chromosome 19q13.2 by linkage analysis in a genome scan (Pericak-Vance et al. 1991). This region contained multiple candidate genes, and one of these, the APOE gene, was found to be associated with late-onset Alzheimer's disease. The frequency of the APOE ε4 allele was 0.50 in late-onset Alzheimer's disease cases as compared to 0.16 in age-matched control subjects (Saunders et al. 1993). This association has been replicated in over 100 laboratories (Roses 1996). Although a genetic association is a population correlation, and therefore not proof of causation, several aspects of the APOE ε4 allele support the hypothesis that it is the disease susceptibility locus. There is a dose effect of the ε4 alleles, there may be a protective effect of the ε2 allele, the association is seen in multiple ethnic groups, and APOE modifies the effect of some of the early-onset Alzheimer's disease genes (Levy-Lahad et al. 1996). Compared with the common ε3/ε3 genotype, individuals with one ε4 allele are at a 3- to 4-fold increased risk and individuals with two ε4 alleles are at 7- to 19-fold increased risk. This increased risk appears to act by causing an earlier age at onset of the illness, with each ε4 lowering the age of onset by 7–9 years in late-onset FAD (Strittmatter et al. 1993). However, individuals with one ε4 allele have only a 25%–40% chance of developing Alzheimer's disease. Likewise individuals with no copies of the ε4 allele are still at risk for developing the illness. This lack of sensitivity and specificity limit the use of APOE testing as a diagnostic or predictive test and it is not currently recommended (Jarvik et al. 1995).

A few other loci have been implicated in late-onset disease. A polymorphism in an intron of the PS1 gene has been associated with late-onset FAD (Wragg et al. 1996). This has been replicated in some (Higuchi et al. 1996a; Kehoe et al. 1996) but not all studies (Scott et al. 1996). Other groups have examined α 1-antichymotrypsin as a candidate gene for late-onset FAD, potentially as a modifier of the APOE locus. There has not been consistent replication (DeKosky et al. 1996; Gilfix et al. 1997; Haines et al. 1996a; Kowalska et al. 1996; Morgan et al. 1997; Muller et al. 1996; Murphy Jr. et al. 1996; Nacmias et al. 1996; Talbot et al. 1996) of the initial genetic association (Kamboh et al. 1995). Lastly, one group has observed mutations in the cytochrome c oxidase genes CO1 and CO2, which are encoded in the mitochondrial genome, in up to 70% of late-onset Alzheimer's disease cases examined (R. E. Davis et al. 1997). This study awaits replication.

PSYCHOPHARMACOGENETICS

Psychopharmacogenetics refers to the study of genetic differences in the behavioral response to pharmacological agents. Behavioral differences may result from both pharmacokinetic variability (i.e., genetic differences in the absorption and degradation of drugs) and pharmacodynamic variability (i.e., genetic differences in tissue sensitivity to drugs).

Pharmacokinetic studies have focused on antidepressants (both tricyclics and monoamine oxidase inhibitors [MAOIs]), neuroleptics, ethanol, and amphetamine. Plasma levels of one of the tricyclics, nortriptyline, appear to be under genetic control: MZ twins exhibit more comparable concentrations than DZ twins following identical oral doses (Alexanderson et al. 1969). The responsible genetic factor appears to be under polygenic control. Plasma levels of the MAOI phenelzine are also under genetic control: a polymorphism in the hepatic enzyme *N*-acetyltransferase that is responsible for degradation of the drug has been identified and appears to be inherited in a Mendelian fashion. Individuals with the less active isoenzyme ("slow acetylators") appear to be more prone to side effects from phenelzine (Price-Evans et al. 1965) and, in at least one study, have shown greater therapeutic response to moderate doses of the drug. There is also evidence to suggest that the tendency to respond to a specific class of antidepressants (tricyclic vs. MAOI) is familial (Pare et al. 1962). Although this might reflect the aforementioned pharmacokinetic differences in the rates of metabolism of these drugs, it is equally plausible that there are genetically distinct biological types of depression associated with different drug responses. Further family studies examining drug concentrations and therapeutic response are clearly needed.

Studies of neuroleptic response have suggested that among patients with schizophrenia, haloperidol nonresponders (Silverman et al. 1987) or delayed responders (Sautter et al. 1993) are more likely than other schizophrenic patients to have relatives with schizophrenia spectrum disorders. Genetic factors also appear to be important in the likelihood of developing an agranulocytotic reaction to the atypical neuroleptic clozapine. Lieberman et al. (1990) found increased frequencies of the HLA antigens B38, DR4, and DQw3 in Ashkenazi Jews who developed agranulocytosis.

Ethanol detoxification occurs via the oxidative enzyme alcohol dehydrogenase (ADH). This process may be under genetic control. Following a test dose of ethanol, relatives of alcoholic subjects show higher levels of the metabolic product of ADH, acetaldehyde, than do relatives of nonalcoholic subjects matched for drinking history (Schuckit and Rayses 1979). Moreover, there are significant ethnic differences in ADH activity between individuals of European or Asian ancestry, which may contribute to observed differences in their tolerance to ethanol. It has been reported that electroencephalographic changes following oral administration of ethanol are more similar in MZ than in DZ twins; blood ethanol levels, on the other hand, are not more similar in MZ than in DZ twins (Propping 1977).

Finally, Nurnberger et al. (1981) have indicated that psychiatrically normal MZ twin pairs show heritable differences in central nervous system noradrenergic function, as evidenced by differences in excitation, early morning motor activity, attention, and growth hormone and prolactin release following intravenous administration of amphetamine. These differences were not correlated with plasma amphetamine levels. Their study suggests that pharmacological probes, such as amphetamine, might be used to investigate genetically caused differences in neurophysiology that may be related to psychopathology.

GENETIC COUNSELING

With the increasing awareness among patients, families, psychiatrists, and the general public of the genetic aspects of psychiatric illness, interest in genetic counseling has developed. However, the aims of those seeking genetic counseling for psychiatric disorder are manifold, and these, as well as the data and techniques involved, must be understood by physicians before attempting such an endeavor or referring patients for it.

It is often not the patient who seeks genetic counseling; or, if such is the case, it may be at the insistence of others. Family members and prospective spouses frequently ask for genetic information 1) to learn about the risk for themselves or their offspring, 2) to obtain advice on decisions of marriage or pregnancy, 3) to gain an understanding of a devastating illness in a family member, or 4) to reduce their sense of guilt or to ascribe guilt to others. Patients themselves, when they do seek this type of help, usually do so in the context of an ongoing therapeutic relationship. They may be seeking to understand the cause of their illness, to discover the implications it has for their descendants (present and future), or to determine whether it is "curable."

The components, or stages, of counseling, as described by Tsuang (1978), are as follows:

- Diagnosis
- Family history
- Estimation of the risk of recurrence
- Evaluation of the aims, intelligence, and emotions of the counselee
- Helping the counselee understand the risk of recurrence in the context of the burden of the disorder
- Formation of a plan of action
- Follow-up

Accurate diagnosis is essential, and careful review of the patient's history as well as diagnostic interviews with relatives may reveal diagnostic issues that have genetic implications (e.g., depressive disorder with early onset, or "symptomatic schizophrenia" from temporal lobe epilepsy).

With the diagnosis established, there are various methods of estimating the risk of recurrence. Risk rates for siblings, offspring, and other classes of relatives, such as those presented in this chapter, are available. These, however, are averages that are known not to apply under certain circumstances. For example, the risk for schizophrenia is increased in families by severity of the proband's illness, the presence of schizophrenic relatives besides the proband, and psychiatric illness in the proband's mate (Gottesman and Shields 1982). More sophisticated analyses can take into account information such as the number of ill relatives, subclinical or "spectrum" illnesses, and the age of risk for onset of illness, but such computerized programs need to assume an underlying mode of transmission. The mode of transmission is not known for most psychiatric disorders, and such assumptions can affect risk estimates greatly (up to 10-fold). Thus, establishing accurate risk estimates in family members for most psychiatric disorders is not currently possible, and counseling must proceed in the face of considerable uncertainty.

Although we lack knowledge of the mode of transmission and the ability to identify family members at risk for most disorders, this is not true for all disorders. Before the gene for Huntington's disease was found, this disease was known to have autosomal dominant transmission and to be closely linked to a marker for a DNA polymorphism, G8 (or D4S10). It is illustrative to see how estimation of risk proceeded under these circumstances, which may apply to other late-onset disorders if efforts to establish linkage are successful. Although all individuals could be typed for the G8 marker, this by itself was not conclusive regarding risk status. It was necessary to know which G8 allele was linked to the Huntington's disease gene in the patient's parents. This determination was made by knowing the marker and illness status of parents, uncles/aunts, and members of a third generation (e.g., grandmother) who had lived through the age of risk. When this information was not available it could (at times) be reconstructed from the other family members. Even with full information on the pedigree, knowledge of the presence of the Huntington's gene was not assured, because of the possibilities of 1) recombination (crossover) occurring between the marker and the pathological gene, and 2) heterogeneity, in which case the marker is not informative regarding the presence of the gene. Thus, even in this disease with full penetrance, known dominant inheritance, and a closely linked marker, complicated calculations had to be done to determine the probability of being an affected individual. Fortunately, a computerized linkage program exists by which accurate assignments can be made, with the caveat that the program assumes no heterogeneity (Ott 1974).

The genetic counselor, especially one who is psychiatrically trained, has an opportunity to provide much important aid beyond estimating the risks of recurrence. This includes evaluating and helping the counselee, especially by reducing the amount of misinformation, confusion, guilt, and fear regarding the illness. The counselor may also be able to offer a plan with the potential for reducing or preventing the transmission of the illness but should recognize that counseling, though often successful in its educational goals, is unlikely to affect reproductive decisions (Kessler 1989). In doing this work, the counselor must combine the skills of geneticist, internist, psychiatrist, psychotherapist, marital counselor, and family therapist. Within psychiatry and in other fields, especially pediatrics, expertise, and training programs have developed in this area, and such specialized training is a prerequisite for success in this task.

TOWARD THE FUTURE

Over the past 5 years, we have witnessed the discovery of specific gene abnormalities underlying or associated with some neuropsychiatric disorders (such as presenilin and apolipoprotein 4 in Alzheimer's disease), as well as the detection of replicated linkage results in others (for example, the pericentric region of chromosome 18 in bipolar disorder and chromosomes 5q, 6p, 8q, and 22q in schizophrenia). Building on these promising results and on advances in clinical, molecular, and statistical genetics, we anticipate that over the next 5 years we will witness movement toward, or even realization of, a number of the goals of psychiatric genetics, including identification of specific susceptibility genes, clarification of the pathophysiological processes whereby these genes lead to symptoms, establishment of epigenetic factors that interact with these genes to produce disease, validation of nosological boundaries that more closely reflect the actions of these genes, and development of effective preventative and therapeutic interventions based on genetic counseling, gene therapy, and modification of permissive or protective environmental influences.

GENE DISCOVERY

Although genetically "simple" Mendelian disorders are usually associated with rare, disease-causing mutations in affected individuals, we have come to appreciate that genetically "complex" disorders, such as those in psychiatry, are likely associated with relatively common genetic variants, which enhance the likelihood of disease in affected individuals either by being more prevalent, by working in concert with common variants at other loci, or both.

We also have come to realize that the identification of common genetic variants that are neither necessary nor sufficient to produce disease may require different clinical resources than those that have been successfully employed in the identification of rare disease mutations. Linkage analyses may have to rely on very large samples (approaching several thousand affected subjects and/or affected sibling pairs); perforce this will lead to increasing reliance on collaboration among research groups. Significantly increased efficiency may be achieved by characterizing affected subjects by continuous, rather than categorical, phenotypes (Moldin et al. 1991) by selectively studying affected sibling pairs that are maximally discordant for the phenotype of interest (Risch et al. 1995), or by employing linkage disequilibrium strategies in genetically isolated and homogeneous populations (Risch and Merikangas 1996). Although relatively isolated populations, like that of Finland, have been a boon to the identification of genes underlying "simple" disorders (those with allele frequencies as large as 0.005) (Hastbacka et al. 1990), such populations still may have too many founders to assume that all individuals with a given "complex" disorder carry a specific, clonal disease predisposing allele, a necessary condition for linkage disequilibrium to be detectable (Weiss 1995). It may be necessary to study even more extremely isolated populations, in which the present day population can be thought of as one very large pedigree. In such a population, disease-predisposing alleles are likely to be clonal, and relatively few genetic and environmental factors may contribute to disease etiology.

Such studies will be facilitated by remarkable advances in molecular genetics. An important milestone in the Human Genome Project, the creation of a dense human transcript (gene) map, has been achieved (Schuler et al. 1996). The availability of this map has allowed a new approach to gene mapping, the "positional candidate" approach, to emerge. This strategy relies on using linkage (and/or linkage disequilibrium) information to localize a disease gene to a small chromosomal region, followed by a survey of all attractive candidate genes within that region (Collins 1995). The positional candidate approach already has led to the identification of fibrillin mutations in Marfan syndrome (Dietz et al. 1991) and KVLQT1 cardiac potassium channel mutations in the long QT syndrome (D. W. Wang et al. 1996), among many others. Recent advances in photolithography have made possible miniaturized arrays of densely packed oligonucleotide probes (DNA chips), which promise to greatly increase the speed of linkage and linkage disequilibrium scans, as well as DNA sequencing (Pease et al. 1994). Moreover, the rapid development of computational genomics should greatly facilitate the positional candidate approach: novel, uncharacterized sequences may be readily nominated as candidates based on their similarities to known genes or functional motifs and may be quickly voted up or down based on the ability to efficiently screen huge amounts of sequence data for transcriptional units and variations (Gaasterland et al. 1996).

Finally, developments in statistical genetics should help clarify the nonlinear relationship between genotype and phenotype in complex disorders. Established approaches like pedigree discriminant analysis (Goldin et al. 1980) can reveal the pleiotropic, multivariate effects of single genes, whereas evolving approaches like neural network analysis can reveal the epistatic, unique effects of multiple genes.

PATHOPHYSIOLOGY

Progress in molecular genetics and computational genomics also should help elucidate the complex pathophysiological links between genotype and phenotype. Approaches like differential display and 2-D gel electrophoresis may reveal coordinated changes in expression between a number of cDNAs or proteins following drug treatment or in the disease state. Once disease mutations are found, transgenic animal models not only serve to underscore a causal role for particular gene mutations, but should clarify the neuroanatomic, neurochemical, and neurophysiological concomitants of such mutations. Finally, computer-based approaches, such as the phylogeny metabolism alignment (PUMA) system under development at the Argonne National Laboratory, by interconnecting information about phylogenetic relationships and metabolic pathways, may very well reveal the complex pathophysiological connections among epistatic loci implicated in genome scans. These approaches should become increasingly tenable as we move from the gene mapping to the "complete genomics" era.

EPIGENESIS

Parallels between neuropsychiatric disorders and other medical conditions suggest potential mechanisms for gene-environment interactions and the methods by which such interactions might be elucidated. For example, schizophrenia bears many similarities to insulin-dependent diabetes (IDDM): viz. both disorders are associated with a modest increase in risk to first-degree relatives (λ_s of 15), an intermediate concordance among monozygotic twins (approximately 50%), and a combined effect of several major susceptibility loci. Perhaps the most important of these loci for IDDM is the class II MHC locus (Davies et al. 1994), governing, among other things, the host response to viral infection. Not surprisingly, infection by a common agent, *Coxsackievirus*, and molecular mimicry between viral and host antigens, has been implicated in the pathogenesis of IDDM (Solimena et al. 1995). Insofar as several studies have suggested a role for both the class II MHC locus (Nimgaonkar et al. 1995) and viral infection (Kaufmann and Ziegler 1987) in schizophrenia, a similar mechanism may be involved (Wright et al. 1995). The availability of suitable cohorts of subjects with schizophrenia, such as those originally identified through the landmark Child Health and Development Study (1959–1966), who have been followed since early in gestation, and on whom both subject DNA and maternal prenatal serum samples have been obtained, should permit questions of class II MHC variation and specific intrauterine viral exposure to be directly answered.

NOSOLOGY

As genetic variations underlying neuropsychiatric disorders are revealed, our notions of the boundaries between these disorders may need to be revised. With only linkage results in hand, we already have indications that disorders like bipolar disorder and schizophrenia, and bipolar disorder and panic disorder, once thought to be distinct, in fact overlap. Thus, some groups studying bipolar disorder have found linkage in the same region of chromosome 6 implicated in schizophrenia; conversely, other groups studying schizophrenia have found evidence for linkage in the same region of chromosome 18 implicated in bipolar disorder. Likewise, linkage analyses of both bipolar and panic disorders have demonstrated positive lod scores in similar chromosomal regions, corroborating path analyses that suggest an overlap between mood and anxiety disorders. The possibility of a continuum between bipolar disorder and schizophrenia has been debated since the time of Kraepelin. Perhaps these disorders do lie on a continuum, or share some, but not all, of a set of epistatic loci. Regardless of how, we can be certain that the lines between diagnostic categories will need to be redrawn as their molecular bases become clear.

PREVENTION AND TREATMENT

As the molecular mechanisms underlying neuropsychiatric disorders become clearer, points of potential clinical intervention will also become apparent. These may be divided into those involving primary, secondary, and tertiary prevention, referring to interventions that prevent disease, prevent its evolution, or prevent its complications, respectively. Among primary preventive interventions are genetic counseling and gene therapy. Preconceptional decision making will need to change, as genetic counseling takes stock of complex disorders for which risks are relative, susceptibilities are multiple, and outcomes are uncertain. Prospects for gene therapy of disorders that afflict the postmitotic brain, once thought impossible, now appear real. Highly selective, neurotropic, defective viral vectors (e.g., *adenoviruses* and *herpesviruses)* have emerged as likely agents for wild-type gene transfer into the nervous system (Kaplitt and Makimura 1997). The possibility that gene transfer into the central nervous system might be effective has gained support from the observation that certain "stemlike" neural cells retain their pleuripotentiality until late in development (Snyder et al. 1997). Among secondary preventive interventions are targeted environmental manipulations in at-risk subjects, that is, reductions in exposure to relevant epigenetic factors, be they viruses, nutritional deficiencies, or early losses, in individuals with particular genetic susceptibilities. Ironically, in this regard, the very complexities that vex the study of complex disorders bode well for their treatment. Finally, the long delay between in utero exposure and adult onset for many neuropsychiatric disorders provides a large window for tertiary preventive interventions. For example, pharmacological studies of animal models of schizophrenia, such as those involving perinatal damage to the anterior hippocampus, suggest that early intervention with anticonvulsants may forestall the development of limbic dopaminergic supersensitivity (and presumably "positive" symptoms), whereas epidemiological studies of patients with schizophrenia suggest that early intervention, after the development of "positive" symptoms, with neuroleptic or electroconvulsive therapy may forestall the development of "negative" symptoms.

Progress in human genetics in general, and psychiatric genetics in particular, is occurring at an ever increasing pace. No doubt, only some of the future developments that we have suggested will be borne out and other, unimagined developments will occur. We need only consider the disparity between the depiction of the late 20th century evident in early science fiction films and our current reality to know that prognistication is a clumsy art, at best. Nonetheless, we can be certain that the next few years will be enormously revealing and gratifying for psychiatric genetics.

REFERENCES

Abbar M, Courtet P, Amadeo S, et al: Suicidal behaviors and the tryptophan hydroxylase gene. Arch Gen Psychiatry 52:846–849, 1995

Adamson MD, Kennedy J, Petronis A, et al: DRD4 dopamine receptor genotype and CSF monoamine metabolites in Finnish alcoholics and controls. Am J Med Genet 60:199–205, 1995

Alda M, Dvorakova M, Zvolsky P, et al: Genetic aspects in chronic schizophrenia: morbidity risks and contributory factors. Schizophr Res 2:339–344, 1989

Alexander RC, Heydt D, Ferraro TN, et al: Further evidence for a quantitative trait locus on murine chromosome 10 controlling morphine preference in inbred mice (letter). Psychiat Genet 6:29–31, 1996

Alexanderson B, Price-Evans DA, Sjoqvist F: Steady-state plasma levels of nortriptyline in twins: influence of genetic factors and drug therapy. BMJ 4:764, 1969

Altemus M, Murphy DL, Greenberg B, et al: Intact coding region of the serotonin transporter gene in obsessive-compulsive disorder. Am J Med Genet 67:409–411, 1996

Amador XF, Malaspina D, Sackeim HA, et al: Visual fixation and smooth pursuit eye movement abnormalities in patients with schizophrenia and their relatives. J Neuropsychiatry Clin Neurosci 7:197–206, 1995

American Psychiatric Association: Diagnostic and Statistical Manual of Mental Disorders, 4th Edition. Washington, DC, American Psychiatric Association, 1994

Andreasen NC, Rice J, Endicott J, et al: Familial rates of affective disorder: a report from the National Institute of Mental Health Collaborative Study. Arch Gen Psychiatry 44:461–469, 1987

Antonarakis SE, Blouin JL, Pulver AE, et al: Schizophrenia susceptibility and chromosome 6p24-22. Nat Genet 11:235–236, 1995

Antonarakis SE, Blouin JL, Curran M, et al: Linkage and sib-pair analysis reveal a potential schizophrenia susceptibility gene on chromosome 13q32. Am J Hum Genet Suppl 59:A210, 1996

Arolt V, Lencer R, Nolte A, et al: Eye tracking dysfunction is a putative phenotypic susceptibility marker of schizophrenia and maps to a locus on chromosome 6p in families with multiple occurrence of the disease. Am J Med Genet 67:564–579, 1996

Asherson P, Mant R, Holmans P, et al: Linkage, association and mutational analysis of the dopamine D3 receptor gene in schizophrenia. Molecular Psychiatry 1:125–132, 1996

Barden N, Plante M, Rochette D, et al: Genome-wide microsatellite marker linkage study of bipolar affective disorders in a very large pedigree from a homogenous population in Quebec points to a susceptibility locus on chromosome 12. Psychiatr Genet 6:145, 1996

Baron M, Gruen RS: Schizophrenia and affective disorder: are they genetically linked? Br J Psychiatry 159:267–270, 1991

Baron M: Linkage results in schizophrenia. Am J Med Genet 67:121–123, 1996

Baron M, Risch N, Hamburger R, et al: Genetic linkage between X chromosome markers and bipolar affective illness. Nature 326:289–292, 1987

Baron M, Freimer NF, Risch N, et al: Diminished support for linkage between manic depressive illness and X-chromosome markers in three Israeli pedigrees. Nat Genet 3:49–55, 1993

Battaglia M, Gasperini M, Sciuto G, et al: Psychiatric disorders in the families of schizotypal subjects. Schizophr Bull 17:659–668, 1991

Battaglia M, Bernardeschi L, Franchini L, et al: A family study of schizotypal disorder. Schizophr Bull 21:33–45, 1995

Beatty B, Squires J, Weksberg R, et al: Velocardiofacial syndrome and schizophrenia. Am J Hum Genet Suppl 59:A87, 1996

Benjamin J, Li L, Patterson C, et al: Population and familial association between the D4 dopamine receptor gene and measures of Novelty Seeking. Nat Genet 12:81–84, 1996

Berrettini WH, Ferraro TN, Alexander RC, et al: Quantitative trait loci mapping of three loci controlling morphine preference using inbred mouse strains. Nat Genet 7:54–58, 1994a

Berrettini WH, Ferraro TN, Goldin LR, et al: Chromosome 18 DNA markers and manic-depressive illness: evidence for a susceptibility gene. Proceedings of the National Academy of Sciences of the United States of America 91:5918–5921, 1994b

Bersani G, Taddei I, Venturi P, et al: Familial occurrence and obstetric complications in siblings discordant for schizophrenia. Minerva Psichiatrica 36:127–132, 1995

Bertelsen A, Harvald B, Hauge M: A Danish twin study of manic-depressive disorders. Br J Psychiatry 130:330–351, 1977

Black DW, Noyes R Jr, Goldstein RB, et al: A family study of obsessive-compulsive disorder. Arch Gen Psychiatry 49:362–368, 1992

Blackwood DH, He L, Morris SW, et al: A locus for bipolar affective disorder on chromosome 4p. Nat Genet 12:427–430, 1996

Blum K, Noble EP, Sheridan PJ, et al: Allelic association of human dopamine D2 receptor gene in alcoholism. JAMA 263:2055–2060, 1990

Bohman M, Sigvardsson S, Cloninger CR: Maternal inheritance of alcohol abuse: cross-fostering analysis of adopted women. Arch Gen Psychiatry 38:965–969, 1981

Bohman M, Cloninger CR, Sigvardsson S, et al: Predisposition to petty criminality in Swedish adoptees, I: genetic and environmental heterogeneity. Arch Gen Psychiatry 39:1233–1241, 1982

Bolos AM, Dean M, Lucas-Derse S, et al: Population and pedigree studies reveal a lack of association between the dopamine D2 receptor gene and alcoholism. JAMA 264: 3156–3160, 1990

Böök JA: A genetic neuropsychiatric investigation of a North Swedish population. Acta Genetica Medica Statistica 4:1–100, 1953

Bracha HS, Torrey EF, Gottesman II, et al: Second-trimester markers of fetal size in schizophrenia: a study of monozygotic twins. Am J Psychiatry 149:1355–1361, 1992

Breitner JCS, Murphey EA, Folstein MF: Familial aggregation of Alzheimer dementia, II: clinical genetic implications of age dependent onset. J Psychiatr Res 20:45–55, 1986

Breitner JCS, Welsh KA, Gau BA, et al: Alzheimer's disease in the National Academy of Sciences—National Research Council Registry of Aging Twin Veterans, III: detection of cases, longitudinal results, and observations on twin concordance. Arch Neurol 52:763–771, 1995

Brent DA, Bridge J, Johnson BA, et al: Suicidal behavior runs in families. A controlled family study of adolescent suicide victims. Arch Gen Psychiatry 53:1145–1152, 1996

Brett PM, Curtis D, Robertson MM, et al: Exclusion of the 5-HT$_{1A}$ serotonin neuroreceptor and tryptophan oxygenase genes in a large British kindred multiply affected with Tourette's syndrome, chronic motor tics, and obsessive-compulsive behavior. Am J Psychiatry 152:437–440, 1995

Brunner HG, Nelen M, Breakefield XO, et al: Abnormal behavior associated with a point mutation in the structural gene for monoamine oxidase A. Science 262:578–580, 1993a

Brunner HG, Nelen MR, van Zandvoort P, et al: X-linked borderline mental retardation with prominent behavioral disturbance: phenotype, genetic localization, and evidence for disturbed monoamine metabolism. Am J Hum Genet 52:1032–1039, 1993b

Burgoyne PS: Genetic homology and crossing-over in the X and Y chromosomes of mammals. Hum Genet 61:85–90, 1982

Byerley W, Holik J, Hoff M, et al: Search for a gene predisposing to manic-depression on chromosome 21. Am J Med Genet 60:231–233, 1995

Cadoret RJ: Evidence for genetic inheritance of primary affective disorder in adoptees. Am J Psychiatry 135:463–466, 1978

Cadoret RJ, Cain CA, Grove WM: Development of alcoholism in adoptees raised apart from alcoholic biologic relatives. Arch Gen Psychiatry 37:561–563, 1980

Cadoret RJ, O'Gorman TW, Troughton E, et al: Alcoholism and antisocial personality: interrelationships, genetic and environmental factors. Arch Gen Psychiatry 42:161–167, 1985

Cadoret RJ, Throughton E, Bagford J, et al: Genetic and environmental factors in adoptee antisocial personality. Eur Arch Psychiatry Clin Neurosci 239:231–240, 1990

Cadoret RJ, Yates WR, Troughton E, et al: Adoption study demonstrating two genetic pathways to drug abuse. Arch Gen Psychiatry 52:42–52, 1995

Camachogamba J, Arenas J, Gomezvesga H: The Collaborative Perinatal Study: the first five years. Clin Pediatr (Phila) 66:553–554, 1964

Cannon TD, Mednick SA, Parnas J: Antecedents of predominantly negative- and predominantly positive-symptom schizophrenia in a high-risk population. Arch Gen Psychiatry 47:622–632, 1990

Cannon TD, Mednick SA, Parnas J, et al: Developmental brain abnormalities in the offspring of schizophrenic mothers, II: structural brain characteristics of schizophrenia and schizotypal personality disorder. Arch Gen Psychiatry 51:955–962, 1994

Carey G, Gottesman II: Twin and family studies of anxiety, phobic, and obsessive disorders, in Anxiety: New Research and Changing Concepts. Edited by Klein DF, Rabkin J. New York, Raven, 1981, pp 117–136

Cases O, Seif I, Grimsby J, et al: Aggressive behavior and altered amounts of brain serotonin and norepinephrine in mice lacking MAOA. Science 268:1763–1766, 1995

Catalano M, Sciuto G, Di Bella D, et al: Lack of association between obsessive-compulsive disorder and the dopamine D3 receptor gene: some preliminary considerations. Am J Med Genet 54:253–255, 1994

Chaleby K, Tuma TA: Cousin marriages and schizophrenia in Saudi Arabia. Br J Psychiatry 150:547–549, 1987

Chen CH, Chien SH, Hwu HG: Lack of association between TaqI A1 allele of dopamine D2 receptor gene and alcohol-use disorders in atayal natives of Taiwan. Am J Med Genet 67:488–490, 1996

Chen CH, Liu MY, Wei FC, et al: Further evidence of no association between Ser9Gly polymorphism of dopamine D3 receptor gene and schizophrenia. Am J Med Genet 74:40–43, 1997

Clementz BA, Sweeney JA, Hirt M, et al: Pursuit gain and saccadic intrusions in first-degree relatives of probands with schizophrenia. J Abnorm Psychol 99:327–335, 1990

Clementz BA, Grove WM, Iacono WG, et al: Smooth-pursuit eye movement dysfunction and liability for schizophrenia: implications for genetic modeling. J Abnorm Psychol 101:117–129, 1992

Cloninger CR: A unified biosocial theory of personality and its role in the development of anxiety states. Psychiatric Developments 4:167–226, 1986

Cloninger CR: A systematic method for clinical description and classification of personality variants: a proposal. Arch Gen Psychiatry 44:573–588, 1987

Cloninger CR, Gottesman II: Genetic and environmental factors in antisocial behavior disorders, in The Causes of Crime: New Biological Approaches. Edited by Mednick SA, Moffitt TE, Stack SA. New York, Cambridge University Press, 1987, pp 92–109

Cloninger CR, Reich T, Guze SB: The multifactorial model of disease transmission, III: familial relationship between sociopathy and hysteria (Briquet's syndrome). Br J Psychiatry 127:23–32, 1975

Cloninger CR, Bohman M, Sigvardsson S: Inheritance of alcohol abuse: cross-fostering analysis of adopted men. Arch Gen Psychiatry 38:861–868, 1981

Cloninger CR, Sigvardsson S, von Knorring A-L, et al: An adoption study of somatoform disorders, II: identification of two discrete somatoform disorders. Arch Gen Psychiatry 41:863–871, 1984

Cloninger CR, Martin RL, Guze SB, et al: A prospective follow-up and family study of somatization in men and women. Am J Psychiatry 143:873–878, 1986

Cloninger CR, Svrakic DM, Przybeck TR: A psychobiological model of temperament and character. Arch Gen Psychiatry 50:975–990, 1993

Cloninger CR, Van Eerdewegh P, Goate A, et al: Anxiety proneness linked to epistatic loci in genome scan of human personality traits. Am J Med Genet 81:313–317, 1998

The Collaborative Study on the Genetics of Asthma (CSGA): A genome-wide search for asthma susceptibility loci in ethnically diverse populations. Nat Genet 15:389–392, 1997

Collinge J, Curtis D: Decreased hippocampal expression of a glutamate receptor gene in schizophrenia. Br J Psychiatry 159:857–859, 1991

Collier DA, Arranz MJ, Sham P, et al: The serotonin transporter is a potential susceptibility factor for bipolar affective disorder. Neuroreport 7:1675–1679, 1996

Collins FS: Positional cloning moves from perditional to traditional. Nat Genet 9:347–350, 1995

Comings DE, Muhleman D, Gysin R: Dopamine D2 receptor (DRD2) gene and susceptibility to posttraumatic stress disorder: a study and replication. Biol Psychiatry 40:368–372, 1996

Condray R, Steinhauser SR: Schizotypal personality disorder in individuals with and without schizophrenic relatives: similarities and contrasts in neurocognitive and clinical functioning. Schizophr Res 7:33–41, 1992

Cook RH, Schneck SA, Clark DB: Twins with Alzheimer's disease. Arch Neurol 38:300–301, 1981

Cook CC, Palsson G, Turner A, et al: A genetic linkage study of the D2 dopamine receptor locus in heavy drinking and alcoholism. Br J Psychiatry 169:243–248, 1996

Coon H, Jensen S, Holik J, et al: Genomic scan for genes predisposing to schizophrenia. Am J Med Genet 54:59–71, 1994

Coon H, Hoff M, Holik J, et al: Analysis of chromosome 18 DNA markers in multiplex pedigrees with manic depression. Biol Psychiatry 39:689–696, 1996

Coryell W, Zimmerman M: The heritability of schizophrenia and schizoaffective disorder: a family study. Arch Gen Psychiatry 45:323–327, 1988

Couch FJ, Weber BL: Mutations and polymorphisms in the familial early onset breast cancer (BRCA1) gene; Breast Cancer Information Core. Human Mutation 8:8–18, 1996

Cox NJ, Suarez BK: Linkage analysis for psychiatric disorders, II: methodological considerations. Psychiatric Developments 3:369–382, 1985

Craddock N, Daniels J, Roberts E, et al: No evidence for allelic association between bipolar disorder and monoamine oxidase A gene polymorphisms. Am J Med Genet 60:322–324, 1995a

Craddock N, Roberts Q, Williams N, et al: Association study of bipolar disorder using a functional polymorphism (Ser311—>Cys) in the dopamine D2 receptor gene. Psychiatr Genet 5:63–65, 1995b

Crawford F, Hoyne J, Diaz P, et al: Occurrence of the Cys311 DRD2 variant in a pedigree multiply affected with panic disorder. Am J Med Genet 60:332–334, 1995

Crocq M-A, Mant R, Asherson P, et al: Association between schizophrenia and homozygosity at the dopamine D3 receptor gene. J Med Genet 29:858–860, 1992

Crow TJ, DeLisi LE, Johnstone EC: Concordance by sex in sibling pairs with schizophrenia is paternally inherited: evidence for a pseudoautosomal locus. Br J Psychiatry 155:92–97, 1989

Crowe RR, Pauls DL, Slymen DJ, et al: A family study of anxiety neurosis: morbidity risk in families of patients with and without mitral valve prolapse. Arch Gen Psychiatry 37:77–79, 1980

Crowe RR, Noyes R, Pauls DL, et al: A family study of panic disorder. Arch Gen Psychiatry 40:1065–1069, 1983

Crowe RR, Noyes R Jr, Persico AM: Pro-opiomelanocortin (POMC) gene excluded as a cause of panic disorder in a large family. J Affect Disord 12:23–27, 1987

Crowe RR, Noyes R Jr, Samuelson S, et al: Close linkage between panic disorder and alpha-haptoglobin excluded in 10 families. Arch Gen Psychiatry 47:377–380, 1990

David F, Clerget F, Lucote G: Familial Alzheimer's disease (FAD): cosegregation between alleles at the D21S11 DNA marker and the FAD gene in a particular pedigree. J Neurol 235:485–486, 1988

Davidson J, Smith R, Kudler H: Familial psychiatric illness in chronic posttraumatic stress disorder. Compr Psychiatry 30:339–345, 1989

Davies JL, Kawaguchi Y, Bennett ST, et al: A genome-wide search for human type 1 diabetes susceptibility genes. Nature 371:130–136, 1994

Davis JO, Phelps JA, Bracha HS: Prenatal development of monozygotic twins and concordance for schizophrenia. Schizophr Bull 21:357–366, 1995

Davis RE, Miller S, Herrnstadt C, et al: Mutations in mitochondrial cytochrome *c* oxidase genes segregate with late-onset Alzheimer disease. Proceedings of the National Academy of Sciences of the United States of America 94:4526–4531, 1997

Dawson E, Gill M, Curtis D, et al: Genetic association between alleles of pancreatic phospholipase A2 gene and bipolar affective disorder. Psychiatr Genet 5:177–180, 1995a

Dawson E, Parfitt E, Roberts Q, et al: Linkage studies of bipolar disorder in the region of the Darier's disease gene on chromosome 12q23-24.1. Am J Med Genet 60:94–102, 1995b

De Bruyn A, Mendelbaum K, Sandkuijl LA, et al: Nonlinkage of bipolar illness to tyrosine hydroxylase, tyrosinase, and D2 and D4 dopamine receptor genes on chromosome 11. Am J Psychiatry 151:102–106, 1994

De Bruyn A, Souery D, Mendelbaum K, et al: Linkage analysis of families with bipolar illness and chromosome 18 markers. Biol Psychiatry 39:679–688, 1996

Decina P, Mukherjee S, Lucas L, et al: Patterns of illness in parent-child pairs both hospitalized for either schizophrenia or a major mood disorder. Psychiatry Res 39:81–87, 1991

DeKosky ST, Aston CE, Kamboh MI: Polygenic determinants of Alzheimer's disease: modulation of the risk by alpha-1-antichymotrypsin. Ann N Y Acad Sci 802:27–34, 1996

DeLisi LE, Crow TJ: Evidence for a sex chromosome locus for schizophrenia. Schizophr Bull 15:431–440, 1989

Detera-Wadleigh SD, Badner JA, Goldin LR, et al: Affected-sib-pair analyses reveal support of prior evidence for a susceptibility locus for bipolar disorder, on 21q. Am J Hum Genet 58:1279–1285, 1996

Di Bella D, Catalano M, Cichon S, et al: Association study of a null mutation in the dopamine D4 receptor gene in Italian patients with obsessive-compulsive disorder, bipolar mood disorder and schizophrenia. Psychiatr Genet 6:119–121, 1996

Dib C, Faure S, Fizames C, et al: A comprehensive genetic map of the human genome based on 5,264 microsatellites. Nature 380:152–154, 1996

Dietz HC, Cutting GR, Pyeritz RE, et al: Marfan syndrome caused by a recurrent de novo missense mutation in the fibrillin gene. Nature 352:337–339, 1991

Dworkin RH, Lenzenweger MF, Moldin SO, et al: A multidimensional approach to the genetics of schizophrenia. Am J Psychiatry 145:1077–1083, 1988

Dykes KL, Mednick SA, Machon RA, et al: Adult third ventricle width and infant behavioral arousal in groups at high and low risk for schizophrenia. Schizophr Res 7:13–18, 1992

Ebers GC, Kukay K, Bulman DE, et al: A full genome search in multiple sclerosis. Nat Genet 13:472–476, 1996

Ebstein RP, Novick O, Umansky R, et al: Dopamine D4 receptor (D4DR) exon III polymorphism associated with the human personality trait of Novelty Seeking. Nat Genet 12:78–80, 1996

Ebstein RP, Macciardi F, Heresco-Levi U, et al: Evidence for an association between the dopamine D3 receptor gene DRD3 and schizophrenia. Hum Hered 47:6–16, 1997

Egeland JA, Sussex JN: Suicide and family loading for affective disorders. JAMA 254:915–918, 1985

Egeland JA, Gerhard DS, Pauls DL, et al: Bipolar affective disorders linked to DNA markers on chromosome 11. Nature 325:783–787, 1987

Embry C, Bruyland S: Presumed Alzheimer's disease beginning at different ages in two twins. J Am Geriatr Soc 33:61–62, 1985

Erlenmeyer-Kimling LE, Paradowski W: Selection and schizophrenia. American Naturalist 100:651–665, 1966

Eysenck HJ: A Model for Personality. New York, Springer, 1981

Farrer LA, O'Sullivan DM, Cupples A, et al: Assessment of genetic risk for Alzheimer's disease among first-degree relatives. Ann Neurol 25:485–493, 1989

Fischer M: Psychoses in the offspring of schizophrenic monozygotic twins and their normal co-twins. Br J Psychiatry 118:43–52, 1971

Fish B: Neurobiologic antecedents of schizophrenia in children: evidence for an inherited, congenital neurointegrative defect. Arch Gen Psychiatry 34:1297–1313, 1977

Fish B: Infant predictors of the longitudinal course of schizophrenic development. Schizophr Bull 13:395–409, 1987

Fish B, Marcus J, Hans SL, et al: Infants at risk for schizophrenia: sequelae of a genetic neurointegrative defect; a review and replication analysis of pandysmaturation in the Jerusalem Infant Development Study. Arch Gen Psychiatry 49:221–235, 1992

Franke P, Maier W, Hain C, et al: Wisconsin Card Sorting Test: an indicator of vulnerability to schizophrenia? Schizophr Res 6:243–249, 1992

Freedman R, Coon H, Myles-Worsley M, et al: Linkage of a neurophysiological deficit in schizophrenia to a chromosome 15 locus. Proceedings of the National Academy of Sciences of the United States of America 94:587–592, 1997

Freimer NB, Reus VI, Escamilla M, et al: An approach to investigating linkage for bipolar disorder using large Costa Rican pedigrees. Am J Med Genet 67:254–263, 1996

Fyer AJ, Mannuzza S, Gallops MS, et al: Familial transmission of simple phobias and fears: a prelimary report. Arch Gen Psychiatry 47:252–256, 1990

Fyer AJ, Mannuzza S, Chapman TF, et al: A direct interview family study of social phobia. Arch Gen Psychiatry 50:286–293, 1993

Fyer AJ, Mannuzza S, Chapman TF, et al: Specificity in familial aggregation of phobic disorders. Arch Gen Psychiatry 52:564–573, 1995

Gaasterland T, Sensen CW: MAGPIE: automated genome interpretation. Trends Genet 12:76–78, 1996

Garner C, Kelly M, Cardon L, et al: Linkage analyses of schizophrenia to chromosome 6p24-p22: an attempt to replicate. Am J Med Genet 67:595–610, 1996

Gejman PV, Ram A, Gelernter J, et al: No structural mutation in the dopamine D2 receptor gene in alcoholism or schizophrenia: analysis using denaturing gradient gel electrophoresis. JAMA 271:204–208, 1994

Gelernter J, O'Malley S, Risch N, et al: No association between an allele at the D2 dopamine receptor gene (DRD2) and alcoholism. JAMA 266:1801–1807, 1991

Gelernter J, Goldman D, Risch N: The A1 allele at the D2 dopamine receptor gene and alcoholism: a reappraisal. JAMA 269:1673–1677, 1993

Gershon ES, Schreiber JL, Hamovit JR, et al: Clinical findings in patients with anorexia nervosa and affective illness in their relatives. Am J Psychiatry 141:1419–1422, 1984

Gershon ES, Hamovit JH, Guroff JJ, et al: Birth-cohort changes in manic and depressive disorders in relatives of bipolar and schizoaffective patients. Arch Gen Psychiatry 44:314–319, 1987

Gershon ES, DeLisi LE, Hamovit J, et al: A controlled family study of chronic psychoses: schizophrenia and schizoaffective disorder. Arch Gen Psychiatry 45:328–336, 1988

Gershon ES, Badner JA, Detera-Wadleigh SD, et al: Maternal inheritance and chromosome 18 allele sharing in unilineal bipolar illness pedigrees. Am J Med Genet 67:202–207, 1996

Giles DE, Biggs MM, Rush AJ, et al: Risk factors in families of unipolar depression, I: psychiatric illness and reduced REM latency. J Affect Disord 14:51–59, 1988

Gilfix BM, Briones L: Absence of the A1252G mutation in alpha 1-antichymotrypsin in a North American population suffering from dementia. Journal of Cerebral Blood Flow and Metabolism 17:233–235, 1997

Gill M, Castle D, Hunt N, et al: Tyrosine hydroxylase polymorphisms and bipolar affective disorder. J Psychiatr Res 25:179–184, 1991

Gill M, Vallada H, Collier D, et al: A combined analysis of D22S278 marker alleles in affected sib-pairs: support for a susceptibility locus for schizophrenia at chromosome 22q12; Schizophrenia Collaborative Linkage Group (Chromosome 22). Am J Med Genet 67:40–45, 1996

Ginns EI, Ott J, Egeland JA, et al: A genome-wide search for chromosomal loci linked to bipolar affective disorder in the Old Order Amish. Nat Genet 12:431–435, 1996

Goate AM, Haynes AR, Owen MJ, et al: Predisposing locus for AD on chromosome 21. Lancet 1:352–355, 1989

Goate AM, Chartier-Harlin MC, Mullan M, et al: Segregation of a missense mutation in the amyloid precursor protein gene with familial Alzheimer's disease. Nature 349: 704–706, 1991

Goisman RM, Goldenberg I, Vasile RG, et al: Comorbidity of anxiety disorders in a multicenter anxiety study. Compr Psychiatry 36:303–311, 1995

Goldenberg IM, White K, Yonkers K, et al: The infrequency of "pure culture" diagnoses among the anxiety disorders. J Clin Psychiatry 57:528–533, 1996

Goldin LR, Gershon ES: Power of the affected-sib-pair method for heterogeneous disorders. Genet Epidemiol 5:35–42, 1988

Goldin LR, Elston RC, Graham JB, et al: Genetic analysis of von Willebrand's disease in two large pedigrees: a multivariate approach. Am J Med Genet 6:279–293, 1980

Goldstein JM, Tsuang MT, Faraone SV: Gender and schizophrenia: implications for understanding the heterogeneity of the illness. Psychiatry Res 28:243–253, 1989

Goodwin DW: Alcoholism and heredity: a review and hypothesis. Arch Gen Psychiatry 36:57–61, 1979

Goodwin DW: Studies of familial alcoholism: a review. J Clin Psychiatry 45:14–17, 1984

Gottesman II, Bertelsen A: Confirming unexpressed genotypes for schizophrenia: risks in the offspring of Fischer's Danish identical and fraternal discordant twins. Arch Gen Psychiatry 46:867–872, 1989

Gottesman II, Shields J: Schizophrenia: The Epigenetic Puzzle. Cambridge, UK, Cambridge University Press, 1982

Gurling HM: New microsatellite polymorphisms fail to confirm chromosome 5 linkage in Icelandic and British schizophrenia families. Paper presented at the American Psychopathological Association Meeting, New York, March 1992

Gurling HM, Oppenheim BE, Murray RM: Depression, criminality and psychopathology associated with alcoholism: evidence from a twin study. Acta Genet Med Gemellol (Roma) 33:333–339, 1984

Gurling H, Kalsi G, Hui-Sui Chen A, et al: Schizophrenia susceptibility and chromosome 6p24–22. Nat Genet 11:234–235, 1995a

Gurling H, Smyth C, Kalsi G, et al: Linkage findings in bipolar disorder. Nat Genet 10:8–9, 1995b

Gusella JF, Wexler NS, Conneally PM, et al: A polymorphic DNA marker genetically linked to Huntington's disease. Nature 306:234–238, 1983

Gutierrez B, Fananas L, Arranz MJ, et al: Allelic association analysis of the 5–HT2C receptor gene in bipolar affective disorder. Neurosci Lett 212:65–67, 1996

Gutierrez B, Bertranpetit J, Guillamat R, et al: Association analysis of the catechol O-methyltransferase gene and bipolar affective disorder. Am J Psychiatry 154:113–115, 1997

Guyer MS, Collins FS: How is the Human Genome Project doing, and what have we learned so far? Proceedings of the National Academy of Sciences of the United States of America 92:10841–10848, 1995

Guze SB: The role of follow-up studies: their contribution to diagnostic classification as applied to hysteria. Seminars in Psychiatry 2:392–402, 1970

Haines JL, Pritchard ML, Saunders AM, et al: No association between alpha 1–antichymotrypsin and familial Alzheimer's disease. Ann N Y Acad Sci 802:35–41, 1996a

Haines JL, Ter-Minassian M, Bazyk A, et al: A complete genomic screen for multiple sclerosis underscores a role for the major histocompatability complex; The Multiple Sclerosis Genetics Group. Nat Genet 13:469–471, 1996b

Hall JM, Lee MK, Newman B, et al: Linkage of early onset familial breast cancer to chromosome 17q21. Science 250:1684–1689, 1990

Harrison PJ, McLaughlin D, Kerwin RW: Decreased hippocampal expression of a glutamate receptor gene in schizophrenia. Lancet 337:450–452, 1991

Hastbacka J, Kaitila I, Sistonen P, et al: Diastrophic dysplasia gene maps to the distal long arm of chromosome 5. Proceedings of the National Academy of Sciences of the United States of America 87:8056–8059, 1990

Heath AC, Cloninger CR, Martin NG: Testing a model for the genetic structure of personality: a comparison of the personality systems of Cloninger and Eysenck. J Pers Soc Psychol 66:762–775, 1994

Heinz A, Sander T, Harms H, et al: Lack of allelic association of dopamine D1 and D2 (TaqIA) receptor gene polymorphisms with reduced dopaminergic sensitivity to alcoholism. Alcoholism, Clinical and Experimental Research 20:1109–1113, 1996

Heston LL: Psychiatric disorders in foster home reared children of schizophrenic mothers. Br J Psychiatry 112:819–825, 1966

Heston LL: Genetic studies of dementia: with emphasis on Parkinson's disease and Alzheimer's neuropathology, in The Epidemiology of Dementia. Edited by Mortimer JA, Schuman LM. New York, Oxford University Press, 1981, pp 101–117

Higuchi S, Muramatsu T, Matsushita S, et al: Presenilin-1 polymorphism and Alzheimer's disease. Lancet 347:1186, 1996a

Holland AJ, Sicott N, Treasure J: Anorexia nervosa: evidence for a genetic basis. J Psychosom Res 32:561–571, 1988

Holzman PS, Levy DL: Smooth-pursuit eye movements and functional psychoses: a review. Schizophr Bull 3:15–27, 1977

Hoover CF, Insel TR: Families of origin in obsessive-compulsive disorder. J Nerv Ment Dis 172:207–215, 1984

Hultman CM, Ohman A, Cnattingius S, et al: Prenatal and neonatal risk factors for schizophrenia. Br J Psychiatry 170:128–133, 1997

Hutchinson G, Takei N, Fahy TA, et al: Morbid risk of schizophrenia in first-degree relatives of white and African-Caribbean patients with psychosis. Br J Psychiatry 169:776–780, 1996

Inayama Y, Yoneda H, Sakai T, et al: Lack of association between bipolar affective disorder and tyrosine hydroxylase DNA marker. Am J Med Genet 48:87–89, 1993

Jacob HJ, Lindpauntner K, Lincoln SE, et al: Genetic mapping of a gene causing hypertension in the stroke-prone spontaneously hypertensive rat. Cell 67:213–224, 1991

Jacob HJ, Pettersson A, Wilson D, et al: Genetic dissection of autoimmune type I diabetes in the BB rat. Nat Genet 2:56–60, 1992

Jain S, Leggo J, Delisi LE, et al: Analysis of thirteen trinucleotide repeat loci as candidate genes for schizophrenia and bipolar affective disorder. Am J Med Genet 67:139–146, 1996

Jarvik LF, Ruth V, Matsuyama SS: Organic brain syndrome and aging: a six-year follow-up of surviving twins. Arch Gen Psychiatry 37:280–286, 1980

Jarvik GP, Wijsman EM, Kukull WA, et al: Interactions of apolipoprotein E genotype, total cholesterol level, age, and sex in prediction of Alzheimer's disease: a case-control study. Neurology 45:1092–1096, 1995

Jones CT, Morris S, Yates CM, et al: Mutation in codon 713 of the beta amyloid precursor protein gene presenting with schizophrenia. Nat Genet 1:306–309, 1992

Kalbfeish JD, Prentice RL: The Statistical Analysis of Failure Time Data. New York, Wiley, 1980

Kallmann FJ: The genetic theory of schizophrenia. Am J Psychiatry 103:309–322, 1946

Kalsi G, Brynjolfsson J, Butler R, et al: Linkage analysis of chromosome 22q12–13 in a United Kingdom/Icelandic sample of 23 multiplex schizophrenia families. Am J Med Genet 60:298–301, 1995

Kamboh MI, Sanghera DK, Ferrell RE, et al: APOE*4–associated Alzheimer's disease risk is modified by alpha 1–antichymotrypsin polymorphism. Nat Genet 10:486–488, 1995

Kaplitt MG, Makimura H: Defective viral vectors as agents for gene transfer in the nervous system. J Neurosci Methods 1:125–132, 1997

Kaprio J, Koskenvuo M, Langinvainio H: Finnish twins reared apart, IV: smoking and drinking habits. A preliminary analysis of the effect of heredity and environment. Acta Genet Med Gemellol (Roma) 33:425–433, 1984

Karayiorgou M, Gogos JA: Dissecting the genetic complexity of schizophrenia. Molecular Psychiatry 2:211–223, 1997

Karayiorgou M, Morris MA, Morrow B, et al: Schizophrenia susceptibility associated with interstitial deletions of chromosome 22q11. Proceedings of the National Academy of Sciences of the United States of America 92:7612–7616, 1995

Karayiorgou M, Altemus M, Galke BL, et al: Genotype determining low catechol-O-methyltransferase activity as a risk factor for obsessive-compulsive disorder. Proceedings of the National Academy of Sciences of the United States of America 94:4572–4575, 1997

Karlsson JL: Partially dominant transmission of schizophrenia in Iceland. Br J Psychiatry 152:324–329, 1988

Kassett JA, Gershon ES, Maxwell ME, et al: Psychiatric disorders in the first-degree relatives of probands with bulimia nervosa. Am J Psychiatry 146:1468–1471, 1989

Kaufmann CA, Ziegler RJ: The viral hypothesis of schizophrenia, in Receptors and Ligands in Psychiatry. Edited by Sen AK, Lee T. Cambridge, Cambridge University Press, 1987, pp 187–208

Kawada Y, Hattori M, Dai XY, et al: Possible association between monoamine oxidase A gene and bipolar affective disorder. Am J Hum Genet 56:335–336, 1995

Kaye WH, Lilenfeld LR, Plotnicov K, et al: Bulimia nervosa and substance dependence: association and family transmission. Alcoholism, Clinical and Experimental Research 20:878–881, 1996

Keefe RSE, Silverman JM, Mohs RC, et al: Eye tracking, attention, and schizotypal symptoms in nonpsychotic relatives of patients with schizophrenia. Arch Gen Psychiatry 54:169–176, 1997

Kehoe P, Williams J, Lovestone S, et al: Presenilin-1 polymorphism and Alzheimer's disease: the UK Alzheimer's Disease Collaborative Group (letter). Lancet 347:1185, 1996

Kelsoe JR, Ginns EI, Egeland JA, et al: Re-evaluation of the linkage relationship between chromosome 11p loci and the gene for bipolar affective disorder in the Old Order Amish. Nature 342:238–243, 1989

Kendler KS: Genetics of schizophrenia, in American Psychiatric Association Annual Review, Vol 5. Edited by Frances AJ, Hales RE. Washington, DC, American Psychiatric Press, 1986, pp 25–41

Kendler KS, Gruenberg AM: An independent analysis of the Danish adoption study of schizophrenia, VI: the relationship between psychiatric disorders as defined by DSM-III in the relatives and adoptees. Arch Gen Psychiatry 41:555–564, 1984

Kendler KS, Tsuang MT: Outcome and familial psychopathology in schizophrenia. Arch Gen Psychiatry 45:338–346, 1988

Kendler KS, Gruenberg AM, Tsuang MT: Psychiatric illness in first-degree relatives of schizophrenic and surgical control patients: a family study using DSM-III criteria. Arch Gen Psychiatry 42:770–779, 1985

Kendler KS, Heath AC, Martin NG, et al: Symptoms of anxiety and symptoms of depression: same genes, different environments? Arch Gen Psychiatry 44:451–457, 1987

Kendler KS, Gruenberg AM, Tsuang MT: A family study of the subtypes of schizophrenia. Am J Psychiatry 145:57–62, 1988

Kendler KS, MacLean C, Neale M, et al: The genetic epidemiology of bulimia nervosa. Am J Psychiatry 148:1627–1637, 1991

Kendler KS, Heath AC, Neale MC, et al: A population-based twin study of alcoholism in women. JAMA 268:1877–1882, 1992a

Kendler KS, Neale MC, Kessler RC, et al: Generalized anxiety disorder in women: a population-based twin study. Arch Gen Psychiatry 49:267–272, 1992b

Kendler KS, Neale MC, Kessler RC, et al: The genetic epidemiology of phobias in women: the interrelationship of agoraphobia, social phobia, situational phobia, and simple phobia. Arch Gen Psychiatry 49:273–281, 1992c

Kendler KS, Neale MC, Kessler RC, et al: A population-based twin study of major depression in women: the impact of varying definitions of illness. Arch Gen Psychiatry 49:257–266, 1992d

Kendler KS, Neale MC, Kessler RC, et al: Panic disorder in women: a population-based twin study. Psychol Med 23:397–406, 1993

Kendler KS, Neale MC, Heath AC, et al: A twin-family study of alcoholism in women. Am J Psychiatry 151:707–715, 1994

Kendler KS, Karkowski-Shuman L, Walsh D: Age at onset in schizophrenia and risk of illness in relatives. Results from the Roscommon Family Study. Br J Psychiatry 169:213–218, 1996a

Kendler KS, MacLean CJ, O'Neill FA, et al: Evidence for a schizophrenia vulnerability locus on chromosome 8p in the Irish Study of High-Density Schizophrenia Families. Am J Psychiatry 153:1534–1540, 1996b

Kendler KS, Prescott CA, Neale MC, et al: Temperance board registration for alcohol abuse in a national sample of Swedish male twins, born 1902 to 1949. Arch Gen Psychiatry 54:178–184, 1997

Kennedy JL, Billett EA, Macciardi FM, et al: Association study of dopamine D3 receptor gene and schizophrenia. Am J Med Genet 60:558–562, 1995

Kessler S: Psychological aspects of genetic counseling, VI: a critical review of the literature dealing with education and reproduction. Am J Med Genet 34:340–353, 1989

Kety SS: Schizophrenic illness in the families of schizophrenic adoptees: findings from the Danish national sample. Schizophr Bull 14:217–222, 1988

Kety SS, Wender PH, Jacobsen B, et al: Mental illness in the biological and adoptive relatives of schizophrenic adoptees. Replication of the Copenhagen Study in the rest of Denmark. Arch Gen Psychiatry 51:442–455, 1994

Kidd KK: Genetic models for psychiatric disorders, in Genetic Research Strategies for Psychobiology and Psychiatry. Edited by Gershon ES, Matthysse S, Breakefield XO, et al. Pacific Grove, CA, Boxwood Press, 1981, pp 369–382

Kinney DK, Yurgelun-Todd DA, Woods BT: Hard neurologic signs and psychopathology in relatives of schizophrenic patients. Psychiatry Res 39:45–53, 1991

Klerman GL, Lavori PW, Rice J, et al: Birth cohort trends in rates of major depressive disorder among relatives of patients with affective disorder. Arch Gen Psychiatry 42:689–693, 1985

Knowles JA, Weissman MM: Panic disorder and agoraphobia, in American Psychiatric Press Review of Psychiatry, Vol 14. Edited by Oldham JM, Riba MB. Washington, DC, American Psychiatric Press, 1995, pp 383–404

Knowles JA, Fyer AJ, Vieland VJ, et al: Results of a genome-wide genetic screen for panic disorder. Am J Med Genet 81:139–147, 1998

Korner J, Rietschel M, Hunt N, et al: Association and haplotype analysis at the tyrosine hydroxylase locus in a combined German-British sample of manic depressive patients and controls. Psychiatr Genet 4:167–175, 1994

Kowalska A, Danker-Hopfe H, Wender M, et al: Association between the PI*M3 allele of alpha 1–antitrypsin and Alzheimer's disease? A preliminary report. Hum Genet 98:744–746, 1996

Kringlen E: Adult offspring of two psychotic parents, with special reference to schizophrenia, in The Nature of Schizophrenia. Edited by Wynne LC, Cromwell RL, Matthysse S. New York, Wiley, 1978, pp 9–24

Kringlen E, Cramer G: Offspring of monozygotic twins discordant for schizophrenia. Arch Gen Psychiatry 46:873–877, 1989

Kunugi H, Curtis D, Vallada HP, et al: A linkage study of schizophrenia with DNA markers from chromosome 8p21–p22 in 25 muliplex familes. Schizophr Res 22:61–68, 1996

Kuokkanen S, Sundvall M, Terwilliger JD, et al: A putative vulnerability locus to multiple sclerosis maps to 5p14–p12 in a region syntenic to the murine locus Eae2. Nat Genet 13:477–480, 1996

Kupfer DJ, Frank E, Carpenter LL, et al: Family history in recurrent depression. J Affect Disord 17:113–119, 1989

Lander ES, Kruglyak L: Genetic dissection of complex traits: guidelines for interpreting and reporting linkage results. Nat Genet 11:241–247, 1995

Larson CA, Nyman GE: Differential fertility in schizophrenia. Acta Psychiatr Scand 49:272–280, 1973

Leckman JF, Chittenden EH: Gilles de la Tourette's syndrome and some forms of obsessive-compulsive disorder may share a common genetic diathesis. Encephale 16:321–323, 1990

Lenane MC, Swedo SE, Leonard H, et al: Psychiatric disorders in first degree relatives of children and adolescents with obsessive compulsive disorder. J Am Acad Child Adolesc Psychiatry 29:407–412, 1990

Lesch KP, Bengel D, Heils A, et al: Association of anxiety-related traits with a polymorphism in the serotonin transporter gene regulatory region. Science 274: 1527–1531, 1996

Levy-Lahad E, Wasco W, Poorkaj P, et al: Candidate gene for the chromosome 1 familial Alzheimer's disease locus. Science 269:973–977, 1995a

Levy-Lahad E, Wijsman EM, Nemens E, et al: A familial Alzheimer's disease locus on chromosome I. Science 269:970–973, 1995b

Levy-Lahad E, Bird TD: Genetic factors in Alzheimer's disease: a review of recent advances. Ann Neurol 40:829–840, 1996

Lieberman JA, Yunis J, Egea E, et al: HLA-B38, DR4, DQw3 and clozapine-induced agranulocytosis in Jewish patients with schizophrenia. Arch Gen Psychiatry 47:945–948, 1990

Lilienfeld SO, VanValkenburg C, Larntz K, et al: The relationship of histrionic personality disorder to antisocial personality and somatization disorders. Am J Psychiatry 143:718–722, 1986

Lim LC, Nothen MM, Korner J, et al: No evidence of association between dopamine D4 receptor variants and bipolar affective disorder. Am J Med Genet 54:259–263, 1994

Lim LCC, Powell J, Sham P, et al: Evidence for a genetic association between alleles of monoamine oxidase A gene and bipolar affective disorder. Am J Med Genet 60:325–331, 1995

Lin MW, Curtis D, Williams N, et al: Suggestive evidence for linkage of schizophrenia to markers on chromosome 13q14.1–q32. Psychiatr Genet 5:117–126, 1995

Lin MW, Sham P, Hwu HG, et al: Suggestive evidence for linkage of schizophrenia to markers on chromosome 13 in Caucasian but not Oriental populations. Hum Genet 99:417–420, 1997

Logue CM, Crowe RR, Bean JA: A family study of anorexia nervosa and bulimia. Compr Psychiatry 30:179–188, 1989

Lu RB, Ko HC, Chang FM, et al: No association between alcoholism and multiple polymorphisms at the dopamine D2 receptor gene (DRD2) in three distinct Taiwanese populations. Biol Psychiatry 39:419–429, 1996

Lyons MJ, Toomey R, Faraone SV, et al: Comparison of schizotypal relatives of schizophrenic versus affective probands. Am J Med Genet 54:279–285, 1994

Lyons MJ, Goldberg J, Eisen SA, et al: Do genes influence exposure to trauma? A twin study of combat. Am J Med Genet 48:22–27, 1993

Maier W, Lichtermann D, Minges J, et al: Personality traits in subjects at risk for unipolar major depression: a family study perspective. J Affect Disord 24:153–163, 1992

Maier W, Lichtermann D, Minges J, et al: A controlled family study in panic disorder. J Psychiatr Res 27 (suppl 1):79–87, 1993

Maier W, Hallmayer J, Zill P, et al: Linkage analysis between pericentrometric markers on chromosome 18 and bipolar disorder: a replication test. Psychiatr Res 59:7–15, 1995

Mann JJ, Malone KM, Nielsen DA, et al: Possible association of a polymorphism of the tryptophan hydroxylase gene with suicidal behavior in depressed patients. Am J Psychiatry 154:1451–1453, 1997

Mant R, Williams J, Asherson P, et al: Relationship between homozygosity at the dopamine D3 receptor gene and schizophrenia. Am J Med Genet 54:21–26, 1994

Marcus J, Hans SL, Nagler S, et al: Review of the NIMH Israeli Kibbutz-City Study and the Jerusalem Infant Development Study. Schizophr Bull 13:425–438, 1987

Mather JA: Eye movements of teenage children of schizophrenics: a possible inherited marker of susceptibility to the disease. J Psychiatr Res 19:523–532, 1985

Matthysse SW, Kidd KK: Estimating the genetic contribution to schizophrenia. Am J Psychiatry 133:185–191, 1976

McGuffin P, Thapar A: The genetics of personality disorder. Br J Psychiatry 160:12–23, 1992

McGuffin P, Farmer AE, Gottesman II, et al: Twin concordance for operationally defined schizophrenia: confirmation of familiality and heritability. Arch Gen Psychiatry 41: 541–545, 1984

McGuffin P, Sargeant M, Hetti G, et al: Exclusion of a schizophrenia susceptibility gene from the chromosome 5q11–q13 region: new data and a reanalysis of previous reports. Am J Hum Genet 47:524–535, 1990

McGuffin P, Katz R, Rutherford J: Nature, nurture and depression: a twin study. Psychol Med 21:329–335, 1991

McInnis MG, McMahon FJ, Chase GA, et al: Anticipation in bipolar affective disorder. Am J Hum Genet 53:385–390, 1993

McKeon P, Murray R: Familial aspects of obsessive-compulsive neurosis. Br J Psychiatry 151:528–534, 1987

McMahon FJ, Stine OC, Meyers DA, et al: Patterns of maternal transmission in bipolar affective disorder. Am J Hum Genet 56:1277–1286, 1995

McNeil TF, Kaij L: Swedish high-risk study: sample characteristics at age 6. Schizophr Bull 13:373–381, 1987

Melo JA, Shendure J, Pociask K, et al: Identification of sex-specific quantitative trait loci controlling alcohol preference in C57BL/ 6 mice. Nat Genet 13:147–153, 1996

Meloni R, Leboyer M, Bellivier F, et al: Association of manic-depressive illness with tyrosine hydroxylase microsatellite marker. Lancet 345:932, 1995

Mendlewicz J, Rainer JD: Adoption study supporting genetic transmission in manic depressive illness. Nature 268: 327–329, 1977

Mendlewicz J, Simon P, Sevy S, et al: Polymorphic DNA marker on X chromosome and manic depression. Lancet 1: 1230–1232, 1987

Mendlewicz J, Sevy S, deMaertelaer V: REM sleep latency and morbidity risk of affective disorders in depressive illness. Neuropsychobiology 22:14–17, 1989

Mendlewicz J, Papadimitriou G, Wilmotte J: Family study of panic disorder: comparison with generalized anxiety disorder, major depression, and normal subjects. Psychiatr Genet 3:73–78, 1993

Merikangas KR: Genetics of alcoholism: a review of human studies, in Genetics of Neuropsychiatric Diseases. Edited by Wetterberg I. London, Macmillan, 1989, pp 269–280

Miki Y, Swensen J, Shattuck-Eidens D, et al: A strong candidate for the breast and ovarian cancer susceptibility gene BRCA1. Science 266:66–71, 1994

Mirsky AF, Ingraham LJ, Kugelmass S: Neuropsychological assessment of attention and its pathology in the Israeli cohort. Schizophr Bull 21:193–204, 1995

Mohs RC, Breitner JCS, Silverman JM, et al: Alzheimer's disease: morbid risk among first-degree relatives approximates 50% by 90 years of age. Arch Gen Psychiatry 44:405–408, 1987

Moises HW, Yang L, Kristbjarnarson H, et al: An international two-stage genome-wide search for schizophrenia susceptibility genes. Nat Genet 11:321–324, 1995a

Moises HW, Yang L, Li T, et al: Potential linkage disequilibrium between schizophrenia and locus D22S278 on the long arm of chromosome 22. Am J Med Genet 60:465–467, 1995b

Moldin SO, Gottesman II, Erlenmeyer-Kimling L, et al: Psychometric deviance in offspring at risk for schizophrenia, I: initial delineation of a distinct subgroup. Psychiatr Res 32:297–310, 1990a

Moldin SO, Rice JP, Gottesman II, et al: Psychometric deviance in offspring at risk for schizophrenia, II: resolving heterogeneity through admixture analysis. Psychiatr Res 32:311–322, 1990b

Moldin SO, Rice JP, Gottesman II, et al: Transmission of a psychometric indicator for liability to schizophrenia in normal families. Genet Epidemiol 7:163–176, 1990c

Moldin SO, Gottesman II, Rice JP, et al: Replicated psychometric correlates of schizophrenia. Am J Psychiatry 148:762–767, 1991

Morgan K, Morgan L, Carpenter K, et al: Microsatellite polymorphism of the alpha 1-antichymotrypsin gene locus associated with sporadic Alzheimer's disease. Hum Genet 99:27–31, 1997

Morton NE: Sequential tests for the detection of linkage. Am J Hum Genet 7:277–318, 1955

Mowry BJ, Nancarrow DJ, Lennon DP, et al: Schizophrenia susceptibility and chromosome 6p24–22. Nat Genet 11:233–234, 1995

Mullan M, Houlden H, Windelspecht M, et al: A locus for familial early onset Alzheimer's disease on the long arm of chromosome 14, proximal to the alpha 1-antichymotrypsin gene. Nat Genet 2:340–342, 1992

Muller U, Bodeker RH, Gerundt I, et al: Lack of association between alpha 1-antichymotrypsin polymorphism, Alzheimer's disease, and allele epsilon 4 of apolipoprotein E. Neurology 47:1575–1577, 1996

Murphy GM Jr, Yang L, Yesavage J, et al: Rate of cognitive decline in Alzheimer's disease is not affected by the alpha-1-antichymotrypsin A allele or the CYP2D6 B mutant. Neurosci Lett 217:200–202, 1996

Murphy KC, Cardno AG, McGuffin P: The molecular genetics of schizophrenia. Journal of Molecular Neuroscience 7:147–157, 1996

Mutchler K, Crowe RR, Noyes R, Jr., et al: Exclusion of the tyrosine hydroxylase gene in 14 panic disorder pedigrees. Am J Psychiatry 147:1367–1369, 1990

Nacmias B, Tedde A, Latorraca S, et al: Apolipoprotein E and alpha 1-antichymotrypsin polymorphism in Alzheimer's disease. Ann Neurol 40:678–680, 1996

Nagler S: Overall design and methodology of the Israeli high-risk study. Schizophr Bull 11:31–37, 1985

Nee LE, Eldridge R, Sunderland T, et al: Dementia of the Alzheimer type: clinical and family study of 22 twin pairs. Neurology 37:359–363, 1987

Newman B, Austin MA, Lee M, et al: Inheritance of human breast cancer: evidence for autosomal dominant transmission in high-risk families. Proceedings of the National Academy of Sciences of the United States of America 85:3044–3048, 1988

Nicolini H, Weissbecker K, Mejia JM, et al: Family study of obsessive-compulsive disorder in a Mexican population. Arch Med Res 24:193–198, 1993

Nielsen DA, Goldman D, Virkkunen M, et al: Suicidality and 5-hydroxyindoleacetic acid concentration associated with a tryptophan hydroxylase polymorphism. Arch Gen Psychiatry 51:34–38, 1994

Nimgaonkar VL, Rudert WA, Zhang XR, et al: Further evidence for an association between schizophrenia and the HLA DQB1 gene locus. Schizophr Res 18:43–49, 1995

Nimgaonkar VL, Sanders AR, Ganguli R, et al: Association study of schizophrenia and the dopamine D3 receptor gene locus in two independent samples. Am J Med Genet 67:505–514, 1996

NIMH Genetics Initiative Bipolar Group: Genomic survey of bipolar illness in the NIMH genetics initiative pedigrees: a preliminary report. Am J Med Genet 74:227–237, 1997

Nothen MM, Cichon S, Propping P, et al: Excess of homozygosity at the dopamine D3 receptor gene in schizophrenia not confirmed. J Med Genet 30:708–709, 1993

Nothen MM, Eggermann K, Albus M, et al: Association analysis of the monoamine oxidase A gene in bipolar affective disorder by using family based internal controls. Am J Hum Genet 57:975–978, 1995

Noyes R Jr, Crowe RR, Harris EL, et al: Relationship between panic disorder and agoraphobia. A family study. Arch Gen Psychiatry 43:227–232, 1986

Noyes R Jr, Clarkson C, Crowe RR, et al: A family study of generalized anxiety disorder. Am J Psychiatry 144:1019–1024, 1987

Nurnberger JI Jr, Gershon ES: Genetics, in Handbook of Affective Disorders. Edited by Paykel ES. New York, Guilford, 1982, pp 126–145

Nurnberger JI Jr, Gershon ES, Jimerson DC, et al: Pharmacogenetics of D-amphetamine response in man, in Research Strategies for Psychobiology and Psychiatry. Edited by Gershon ES, Matthysse S, Breakefield XO, et al. Pacific Grove, CA, Boxwood Press, 1981, pp 257–268

O'Donovan MC, Guy C, Craddock N, et al: Expanded CAG repeats in schizophrenia and bipolar disorder. Nat Genet 10:380–381, 1995

O'Donovan MC, Guy C, Craddock N, et al: Confirmation of association between expanded CAG/CTG repeats and both schizophrenia and bipolar disorder. Psychol Med 26:1145–1153, 1996

Ogilvie AD, Battersby S, Bubb VJ, et al: Polymorphism in serotonin transporter gene associated with susceptibility to major depression. Lancet 347:731–733, 1996

Onstad S, Skre I, Torgersen S, et al: Subtypes of schizophrenia—evidence from a twin-family study. Acta Psychiatr Scand 84:203–206, 1991

Onstad S, Skre I, Torgersen S, et al: Birthweight and obstetric complications in schizophrenic twins. Acta Psychiatr Scand 85:70–73, 1992

O'Rourke DH, Gottesman II, Suarez BK, et al: Refutation of the general single locus model for the etiology of schizophrenia. Am J Hum Genet 34:630–649, 1982

Ott J: Estimation of the recombination fraction in human pedigrees: efficient computation of the likelihood for human linkage. Ann Hum Genet 26:588–597, 1974

Pare CMB, Ress L, Sainsbury MJ: Differentiation of two genetically specific types of depression by the response to antidepressants. Lancet 2:1240–1343, 1962

Parnas J, Schulsinger F, Schulsinger H, et al: Behavioral precursors of schizophrenia spectrum: a prospective study. Arch Gen Psychiatry 39:658–664, 1982

Parsian A, Todd RD, Devor EJ, et al: Alcoholism and alleles of the human D2 receptor locus: studies of association and linkage. Arch Gen Psychiatry 48:655–663, 1991

Parsian A, Chakraverty S, Todd RD: Possible association between the dopamine D_3 receptor gene and bipolar affective disorder. Am J Med Genet 60:234–237, 1995

Pauls DL: Behavioral disorders: lessons in linkage. Nat Genet 3:4–5, 1993

Pauls DL, Gerhard DS, Lacy LG, et al: Linkage of bipolar affective disorders to markers on chromosome 11p is excluded in a second lateral extension of Amish pedigree 110. Genomics 11:730–736, 1991

Pauls DL, Alsobrook JP, II, Goodman W, et al: A family study of obsessive-compulsive disorder. Am J Psychiatry 152:76–84, 1995a

Pauls DL, Bailey JN, Carter AS, et al: Complex segregation analyses of Old Order Amish families ascertained through bipolar I individuals. Am J Med Genet 60:290–297, 1995b

Pauls DL, Ott J, Paul SM, et al: Linkage analyses of chromosome 18 markers do not identify a major susceptibility locus for bipolar affective disorder in the Old Order Amish. Am J Hum Genet 57:636–643, 1995c

Pease AC, Solas D, Sullivan EJ, et al: Light-generated oligonucleotide arrays for rapid DNA sequence analysis. Proceedings of the National Academy of Sciences of the United States of America 91:5022–5026, 1994

Pekkarinen P, Terwilliger J, Bredbacka P, et al: Evidence of a predisposing locus to bipolar disorder on Xq24–q27.1 in an extended Finnish pedigree. Genome Res 5:105–115, 1995

Perez de Castro I, Santos J, Torres P, et al: A weak association between TH and DRD2 genes and bipolar affective disorder in a Spanish sample. J Med Genet 32:131–134, 1995

Pericak-Vance MA, Yamaoka LH, Haynes CS, et al: Genetic linkage studies in Alzheimer's disease families. Exp Neurol 102:271–279, 1988

Pericak-Vance MA, Bebout JL, Gaskell PC Jr, et al: Linkage studies in familial Alzheimer disease: evidence for chromosome 19 linkage. Am J Hum Genet 48:1034–1050, 1991

Perrett CW, Whatley SA, Ferrier I, et al: Changes in brain gene expression in schizophrenic and depressed patients. Schizophr Res 6:193–200, 1992

Petronis A, Kennedy JL: Unstable genes—Unstable mind. Am J Psychiatry 152:164–172, 1995

Pickens RW, Svikis DS, McGue M, et al: Heterogeneity in the inheritance of alcoholism: a study of male and female twins. Arch Gen Psychiatry 48:19–28, 1991

Pitts FN, Winokur G: Affective disorder, VII: alcoholism and affective disorder. J Psychiatr Res 4:37–50, 1966

Plomin R, DeFries JC, McClearn GE: Behavioral Genetics: A Primer, 2nd Edition. San Francisco, CA, WH Freeman, 1990

Plomin R, Owen MJ, McGuffin P: The genetic basis of complex human behaviors. Science 264:1733–1739, 1994

Polymeropoulos MH, Coon H, Byerley W, et al: Search for a schizophrenia susceptibility locus on human chromosome 22. Am J Med Genet 54:93–99, 1994

Pope HG Jr, Yurgelun-Todd D: Schizophrenic individuals with bipolar first-degree relatives: analysis of two pedigrees. J Clin Psychiatry 51:97–101, 1990

Price-Evans DA, Davison K, Pratt RTC: The influences of acetylator phenotype on the effects of treating depression with phenelzine. Clin Pharmacol Ther 6:430–433, 1965

Propping P: Genetic control of ethanol action on the central nervous system: an EEG study of twins. Hum Genet 35:309–334, 1977

Pulver AE, Brown CH, Wolyniec P, et al: Schizophrenia: age at onset, gender and familial risk. Acta Psychiatr Scand 82:344–351, 1990

Pulver AE, Brown CH, Wolyniec P, et al: Psychiatric morbidity in the relatives of patients with DSM-III schizophreniform disorder: comparisons with the relatives of schizophrenic and bipolar disorder patients. J Psychiatr Res 25:19–29, 1991

Pulver AE, Karayiorgou M, Lasseter VK, et al: Follow-up of a report of a potential linkage for schizophrenia on chromosome 22q12–q13.1: part 2. Am J Med Genet 54:44–50, 1994a

Pulver AE, Karayiorgou M, Wolyniec PS, et al: Sequential strategy to identify a susceptibility gene for schizophrenia: report of potential linkage on chromosome 22q12–q13.1: part 1. Am J Med Genet 54:36–43, 1994b

Pulver AE, Nestadt G, Goldberg R, et al: Psychotic illness in patients diagnosed with velo-cardio-facial syndrome and their relatives. J Nerv Ment Dis 182:476–478, 1994c

Pulver AE, Lasseter VK, Kasch L, et al: Schizophrenia: a genome scan targets chromosomes 3p and 8p as potential sites of susceptibility genes. Am J Med Genet 60:252–260, 1995

Ram A, Guedj F, Cravchik A, et al: No abnormality in the gene for the G protein stimulatory alpha subunit in patients with bipolar disorder. Arch Gen Psychiatry 54:44–48, 1997

Regier DA, Narrow WE, Rae DS, et al: The de facto US mental and addictive disorders service system: Epidemiologic Catchment Area prospective 1–year prevalence rates of disorders and services. Arch Gen Psychiatry 50:85–94, 1993

Reich JH: Familiality of DSM-III dramatic and anxious personality clusters. J Nerv Ment Dis 177:96–100, 1989

Reich J[H]: Using the family history method to distinguish relatives of patients with dependent personality disorder from relatives of controls. Psychiatr Res 39:227–237, 1991

Reich T: A genomic survey of alcohol dependence and related phenotypes: results from the Collaborative Study on the Genetics of Alcoholism (COGA). Alcoholism, Clinical and Experimental Research 20:Suppl:133A–137A, 1996

Reich T, Cloninger CR, Van Eerdewegh P, et al: Secular trends in the familial transmission of alcoholism. Alcoholism 12:458–464, 1988

Reveley MA, Reveley AM, Baldy R: Left cerebral hemisphere hypodensity in discordant schizophrenic twins: a controlled study. Arch Gen Psychiatry 44:625–632, 1987

Rice JP, Reich T, Andreasen NC, et al: The familial transmission of bipolar illness. Arch Gen Psychiatry 44:441–447, 1987b

Rietschel M, Nothen MM, Lannfelt L, et al: A serine to glycine substitution at position 9 in the extracellular N-terminal part of the dopamine D3 receptor protein: no role in the genetic predisposition to bipolar affective disorder. Psychiatr Res 46:253–259, 1993

Rietschel M, Nothen MM, Albus M, et al: Dopamine D3 receptor Gly9/Ser9 polymorphism and schizophrenia: no increased frequency of homozygosity in German familial cases. Schizophr Res 20:181–186, 1996

Riley BP, Rajagopalan S, Mogudi-Carter M, et al: No evidence for linkage of chromosome 6p markers to schizophrenia in southern African Bantu-speaking families. Psychiatr Genet 6:41–49, 1996

Risch N: Linkage strategies for genetically complex traits, I: multilocus models. Am J Hum Genet 46:222–228, 1990

Risch N, Baron M: Segregation analysis of schizophrenia and related disorders. Am J Hum Genet 36:1039–1059, 1984

Risch N, Merikangas K: The future of genetic studies of complex human diseases. Science 273:1516–1517, 1996

Risch N, Zhang H: Extreme discordant sib pairs for mapping quantitative trait loci in humans. Science 268:1584–1589, 1995

Robins LN, Helzer JE, Weissman MM, et al: Lifetime prevalence of specific psychiatric disorders in three sites. Arch Gen Psychiatry 41:949–958, 1984

Rogaev EI, Sherrington R, Rogaeva EA, et al: Familial Alzheimer's disease in kindreds with missense mutations in a gene on chromosome 1 related to the Alzheimer's disease type 3 gene. Nature 376:775–778, 1995

Rosenthal D: Genetic Theory and Abnormal Behavior. New York, McGraw-Hill, 1970

Rosenthal D, Wender PH, Kety SS, et al: Schizophrenics' offspring reared in adoptive homes. J Psychiatr Res 6:377–391, 1968

Roses AD: Apolipoprotein E alleles as risk factors in Alzheimer's disease. Annu Rev Med 47:387–400, 1996

Roses AD, Pericak-Vance MA, Dawson DV, et al: Standard likelihood and sib pair analyses in late onset Alzheimers disease, in The Molecular Biology of Alzheimer's Disease (Current Communications in Molecular Biology). Edited by Davis P, Finch C. New York, Cold Spring Harbor Laboratory, 1988, pp 180–186

Roy A, Segal NL, Centerwall BS, et al: Suicide in twins. Arch Gen Psychiatry 48:29–32, 1991

Roy A, Segal NL, Sarchiapone M: Attempted suicide among living co-twins of twin suicide victims. Am J Psychiatry 152:1075–1076, 1995

Rubinsztein DC, Leggo J, Crow TJ, et al: Analysis of polyglutamine-coding repeats in the TATA-binding protein in different human populations and in patients with schizophrenia and bipolar affective disorder. Am J Med Genet 67:495–498, 1996a

Rubinsztein DC, Leggo J, Goodburn S, et al: Genetic association between monoamine oxidase A microsatellite and RFLP alleles and bipolar affective disorder: analysis and meta-analysis. Hum Mol Genet 5:779–782, 1996b

Rudin E: Zur Vererbung und Neuenstehung der Dementia Praecox. Berlin, Springer-Verlag, 1916

Sabate O, Campion D, d'Amato T, et al: Failure to find evidence for linkage or association between the dopamine D3 receptor gene and schizophrenia. Am J Psychiatry 151:107–111, 1994

Saha N, Tsoi WF, Low PS, et al: Lack of association of the dopamine D3 receptor gene polymorphism (BalI) in Chinese schizophrenic males. Psychiatr Genet 4:201–204, 1994

Sarkar G, Kapelner S, Grandy DK, et al: Direct sequencing of the dopamine D2 receptor (DRD2) in schizophrenia reveals three polymorphisms but no structural change in the receptor. Genomics 11:8–14, 1991

Sasaki T, Billett E, Petronis A, et al: Psychosis and genes with trinucleotide repeat polymorphism. Hum Genet 97:244–246, 1996a

Sasaki T, Macciardi FM, Badri F, et al: No evidence for association of dopamine D2 receptor variant (Ser311/Cys311) with major psychosis. Am J Med Genet 67:415–417, 1996b

Saunders AM, Strittmatter WJ, Schmechel D, et al: Association of apolipoprotein E allele epsilon 4 with late-onset familial and sporadic Alzheimer's disease. Neurology 43:1467–1472, 1993

Sautter F, McDermott B, Garver D: Familial differences between rapid neuroleptic response psychosis and delayed neuroleptic response psychosis. Biol Psychiatry 33:15–21, 1993

Sawcer S, Jones HB, Feakes R, et al: A genome screen in multiple sclerosis reveals susceptibility loci on chromosome 6p21 and 17q22. Nat Genet 13:464–468, 1996

Schellenberg GD, Bird TD, Wijsman EM, et al: Absence of linkage of chromosome 21q21 markers to familial Alzheimer's disease. Science 241:1507–1510, 1988

Schellenberg GD, Bird TD, Wijsman EM, et al: Genetic linkage evidence for a familial Alzheimer's disease locus on chromosome 14. Science 258:668–671, 1992

Schizophrenia Linkage Collaborative Group for Chromosomes 3, 6, and 8: Additional support for schizophrenia linkage on chromosomes 6 and 8: a multicenter study. Am J Med Genet 67:580–594, 1996

Schmidt SM, Zoega T, Crowe RR: Excluding linkage between panic disorder and the gamma-aminobutyric acid beta 1 receptor locus in five Icelandic pedigrees. Acta Psychiatr Scand 88:225–228, 1993

Schuler GD, Boguski MS, Stewart EA, et al: A gene map of the human genome. Science 274:540–546, 1996

Schuckit MA, Gold EO: A simultaneous evaluation of multiple markers of ethanol/placebo challenges in sons of alcoholics and controls. Arch Gen Psychiatry 45:211–216, 1988

Schuckit MA, Rayses V: Ethanol ingestion differences in blood acetaldehyde concentrations in relatives of alcoholics and controls. Science 203:54–55, 1979

Schulsinger F, Kety SS, Rosenthal D, et al: A family study of suicide, in Origin, Prevention and Treatment of Affective Disorders. Edited by Schou M, Stromgren E. New York, Academic Press, 1979, pp 277–287

Schulsinger F, Parnas J, Petersen ET, et al: Cerebral ventricular size in the offspring of schizophrenic mothers: a preliminary study. Arch Gen Psychiatry 41:602–606, 1984

Schwab SG, Albus M, Hallmayer J, et al: Evaluation of a susceptibility gene for schizophrenia on chromosome 6p by multipoint affected sib-pair linkage analysis. Nat Genet 11:325–327, 1995a

Schwab SG, Lerer B, Albus M, et al: Potential linkage for schizophrenia on chromosome 22q12–q13: a replication study. Am J Med Genet 60:436–443, 1995b

Schwab SG, Eckstein GN, Hallmayer J, et al: Evidence suggestive of a locus on chromosome 5q31 contributing to susceptibility for schizophrenia in German and Israeli families by multipoint affected sib-pair linkage analysis. Molecular Psychiatry 2:156–160, 1997

Sciuto G, Pasquale L, Bellodi L: Obsessive compulsive disorder and mood disorders: a family study. Am J Med Genet 60:475–479, 1995

Scott WK, Roses AD, Haines JL, et al: Presenilin-1 polymorphism and Alzheimer's disease (letter). Lancet 347:1560, 1996

Shafii M, Carrigan S, Whittinghill JR, et al: Psychological autopsy of completed suicide in children and adolescents. Am J Psychiatry 142:1061–1064, 1985

Shaikh S, Ball D, Craddock N, et al: The dopamine D3 receptor gene: no association with bipolar affective disorder. J Med Genet 30:308–309, 1993

Sham PC, Jones P, Russell A, et al: Age at onset, sex, and familial psychiatric morbidity in schizophrenia: Camberwell Collaborative Psychosis Study. Br J Psychiatry 165:466–473, 1994

Sheffield VC, Weber JL, Buetow KH, et al: A collection of tri- and tetranucleotide repeat markers used to generate high quality, high resolution human genome-wide linkage maps. Hum Mol Genet 4:1837–1844, 1995

Shen J, Bronson RT, Chen DF, et al: Skeletal and CNS defects in presenilin-1--deficient mice. Cell 89:629–639, 1997

Shenton ME, Solovay MR, Holzman PS, et al: Thought disorder in the relatives of psychotic patients. Arch Gen Psychiatry 46:897–901, 1989

Sherrington R, Brynjolfsson J, Petursson H, et al: Localization of a susceptibility locus for schizophrenia on chromosome 5. Nature 336:164–167, 1988

Sherrington R, Rogaev EI, Liang Y, et al: Cloning of a gene bearing missense mutations in early onset familial Alzheimer's disease. Nature 375:754–760, 1995

Siever LJ, Silverman JM, Horvath TB, et al: Increased morbid risk for schizophrenia-related disorders in relatives of schizotypal personality disordered patients. Arch Gen Psychiatry 47:634–640, 1990

Silverman JM, Mohs RC, Davidson M, et al: Familial schizophrenia and treatment response. Am J Psychiatry 144:1271–1276, 1987

Silverman JM, Greenberg DA, Altstiel LD, et al: Evidence of a locus for schizophrenia and related disorders on the short arm of chromosome 5 in a large pedigree. Am J Med Genet 67:162–171, 1996

Skre I, Torgersen S, Lygren S, et al: A twin study of DSM-III-R anxiety disorders. Acta Psychiatr Scand 88:85–92, 1993

Smith SS, O'Hara BF, Persico AM, et al: Genetic vulnerability to drug abuse: the D2 dopamine receptor Taq I B1 restriction fragment length polymorphism appears more frequently in polysubstance abusers. Arch Gen Psychiatry 49:723–727, 1992

Smyth C, Kalsi G, Brynjolfsson J, et al: Further tests for linkage of bipolar affective disorder to the tyrosine hydroxylase gene locus on chromosome 11p15 in a new series of multiplex British affective disorder pedigrees. Am J Psychiatry 153:271–274, 1996

Snyder EY, Park KI, Flax JD, et al: Potential of neural "stem-like" cells for gene therapy and repair of the degenerating central nervous system. Adv Neurol 72:121–132, 1997

Solimena M, De Camilli P: Coxsackieviruses and diabetes [published erratum appears in Nature Med 1:272, 1995]. Nature Med 1:25–26, 1995

Souery D, Lipp O, Mahieu B, et al: Excess tyrosine hydroxylase restriction fragment length polymorphism homozygosity in unipolar but not bipolar patients: a preliminary report. Biol Psychiatry 40:305–308, 1996

Spence MA, Flodman PL, Sadovnick AD, et al: Bipolar disorder: evidence for a major locus. Am J Med Genet 60:370–376, 1995

Spitzer RL, Endicott J, Robins E: Research Diagnostic Criteria: rationale and reliability. Arch Gen Psychiatry 35:773–782, 1978

Squires-Wheeler E, Skodol AE, Bassett A, et al: DSM-III-R schizotypal personality traits in offspring of schizophrenic disorder, affective disorder, and normal control parents. J Psychiatr Res 23:229–239, 1989

St George-Hyslop PH, Tanzi RE, Polinsky RJ, et al: The genetic defect causing familial Alzheimer's disease maps on chromosome 21. Science 235:885–890, 1987

St George-Hyslop PH, Myers R, Haines JL, et al: Familial Alzheimer's disease: progress and problems. Neurobiol Aging 10:417–425, 1989

St George-Hyslop PH, Haines JL, Farrer LA, et al: Genetic linkage studies suggest that Alzheimer's disease is not a single homogeneous disorder. Nature 347:194–197, 1990

St George-Hyslop P, Haines J, Rogaev E, et al: Genetic evidence for a novel familial Alzheimer's disease locus on chromosome 14. Nat Genet 2:330–334, 1992

Stine OC, Xu J, Koskela R, et al: Evidence for linkage of bipolar disorder to chromosome 18 with a parent-of-origin effect. Am J Hum Genet 57:1384–1394, 1995

Straub RE, Lehner T, Luo Y, et al: A possible vulnerability locus for bipolar affective disorder on chromosome 21q22.3. Nat Genet 8:291–296, 1994

Straub RE, MacLean CJ, O'Neill FA, et al: A potential vulnerability locus for schizophrenia on chromosome 6p24–22: evidence for genetic heterogeneity. Nat Genet 11:287–293, 1995

Straub RE, MacLean CJ, O'Neill FA, et al: Support for a possible schizophrenia vulnerability locus in region 5q21–31 in Irish families. Molecular Psychiatry 2:148–155, 1997

Strittmatter WJ, Saunders AM, Schmechel D, et al: Apolipoprotein E: high-avidity binding to beta-amyloid and increased frequency of type 4 allele in late-onset familial Alzheimer disease. Proceedings of the National Academy of Sciences of the United States of America 90:1977–1981, 1993

Strober M, Morell W, Burroughs J, et al: A controlled family study of anorexia nervosa. J Psychiatr Res 19:239–246, 1985

Suarez BK, Cox NJ: Linkage analysis for psychiatric disorders, I: basic concepts. Psychiatric Developments 3:219–243, 1985

Suarez BK, Rice J, Reich T: The generalized sib pair IBD distribution: its use in the detection of linkage. Ann Hum Genet 42:87–94, 1978

Suddath RL, Christison GW, Torrey EF, et al: Anatomical abnormalities in the brains of monozygotic twins discordant for schizophrenia. N Engl J Med 322:789–794, 1990

Sugarman PA, Craufurd D: Schizophrenia in the Afro-Caribbean community. Br J Psychiatry 164:474–480, 1994

Svrakic DM, Whitehead C, Przybeck TR, et al: Differential diagnosis of personality disorders by the seven-factor model of temperament and character. Arch Gen Psychiatry 50:991–999, 1993

Talbot C, Houlden H, Craddock N, et al: Polymorphism in AACT gene may lower age of onset of Alzheimer's disease. Neuroreport 7:534–536, 1996

Tanaka T, Igarashi S, Onodera O, et al: Association study between schizophrenia and dopamine D3 receptor gene polymorphism. Am J Med Genet 67:366–368, 1996

Tienari P: Interaction between genetic vulnerability and family environment: the Finnish adoptive family study of schizophrenia. Acta Psychiatr Scand 84:460–465, 1991

Tienari P, Lahti I, Sorri A, et al: The Finnish adoptive family study of schizophrenia. J Psychiatr Res 21:437–445, 1987

Tienari P, Wynne LC, Moring J, et al: The Finnish adoptive family study of schizophrenia: implications for family research. Br J Psychiatry (supplement) 20–26, 1994

Torgersen S: Genetic factors in anxiety disorders. Arch Gen Psychiatry 40:1085–1089, 1983

Torgersen S: Genetics of somatoform disorders. Arch Gen Psychiatry 43:502–505, 1986

Torgersen S: Comorbidity of major depression and anxiety disorders in twin pairs. Am J Psychiatry 147:1199–1202, 1990

True WR, Rice J, Eisen SA, et al: A twin study of genetic and environmental contributions to liability for posttraumatic stress symptoms. Arch Gen Psychiatry 50:257–264, 1993

Tsuang MT: Genetic counseling for psychiatric patients and their families. Am J Psychiatry 135:1465–1475, 1978

Tsuang MT: Risk of suicide in the relatives of schizophrenics, manics, depressives, and controls. J Clin Psychiatry 44:396–400, 1983

Tsuang MT, Lyons MJ: Drawing the boundary of the schizophrenia spectrum: evidence from a family study, in Schizophrenia: Scientific Progress. Edited by Schultz SC, Tamminga CA. New York, Oxford University Press, 1989, pp 23–27

Tsuang MT, Bucher KD, Fleming JA: Testing the monogenic theory of schizophrenia: an application of segregation analysis to blind family study data. Br J Psychiatry 140:595–599, 1982

Tsuang MT, Gilbertson MW, Faraone SV: Genetic transmission of negative and positive symptoms in the biological relatives of schizophrenics, in Positive vs. Negative Schizophrenia. Edited by Marneros A, Tsuang MT, Andreasen N. New York, Springer-Verlag, 1991, pp 265–291

Tsuang MT, Faraone SV, Kremen W, et al: Familial connections with deficit syndrome. Paper presented at the annual meeting of the American Psychiatric Association, May 1992

Uhl G, Blum K, Noble E, et al: Substance abuse vulnerability and D2 receptor genes. Trends Neurosci 16:83–88, 1993

Vallada H, Curtis D, Sham PC, et al: Chromosome 22 markers demonstrate transmission disequilibrium with schizophrenia. Psychiatr Genet 5:127–130, 1995a

Vallada HP, Gill M, Sham P, et al: Linkage studies on chromosome 22 in familial schizophrenia. Am J Med Genet 60:139–146, 1995b

Van Broeckhoven C, van Hul W, Backhoven H, et al: The familial Alzheimer gene is located close to the centromere of chromosome 21 (abstract). Am J Hum Genet 43:A205, 1988

Van Broeckhoven C, Backhovens H, Cruts M, et al: Mapping of a gene predisposing to early onset Alzheimer's disease to chromosome 14q24.3. Nat Genet 2:335–339, 1992

Vincent JB, Klempan T, Parikh SS, et al: Frequency analysis of large CAG/CTG trinucleotide repeats in schizophrenia and bipolar affective disorder. Molecular Psychiatry 1:141–148, 1996

Vita A, Dieci M, Giobbio GM, et al: A reconsideration of the relationship between cerebral structural abnormalities and family history of schizophrenia. Psychiatry Res 53:41–55, 1994

Vogler GP, Gottesman II, McGue MK, et al: Mixed-model segregation analysis of schizophrenia in the Lindelius Swedish pedigrees. Behav Genet 20:461–472, 1990

von Knorring A-L, Cloninger CR, Bohman M, et al: An adoption study of depressive disorders and substance abuse. Arch Gen Psychiatry 40:943–950, 1983

Waldo MC, Carey G, Myles-Worsley M, et al: Codistribution of a sensory gating deficit and schizophrenia in multi-affected families. Psychiatr Res 39:257–268, 1991

Walker E, Downey G, Caspi A: Twin studies of psychopathology: why do the concordance rates vary? Schizophr Res 5:211–221, 1991

Walters EE, Neale MC, Eaves LJ, et al: Bulimia nervosa and major depression: a study of common genetic and environmental factors. Psychol Med 22:617–622, 1992

Wang DW, Yazawa K, George AL, Jr., et al: Characterization of human cardiac Na+ channel mutations in the congenital long QT syndrome. Proceedings of the National Academy of Sciences of the United States of America 93:13200–13205, 1996

Wang ZW, Crowe RR, Noyes RJ: Adrenergic receptor genes as candidate genes for panic disorder: a linkage study. Am J Psychiatry 149:470–474, 1992

Watt NF, Anthony EJ, Wynne LC, et al (eds): Children at Risk for Schizophrenia: A Longitudinal Perspective. Cambridge, UK, Cambridge University Press, 1984

Weinberger DR, Berman KF, Suddath R, et al: Evidence of dysfunction of a prefrontal-limbic network in schizophrenia: a magnetic resonance imaging and regional cerebral blood flow study of discordant monozygotic twins. Am J Psychiatry 149:890–897, 1992

Weiss KM: Genetic Variation and Human Disease. Cambridge, UK, Cambridge University Press, 1993, pp 229

Weiss KM: Genetic Variation and Human Disease: Principles and Evolutionary Approaches. Cambridge, UK, Cambridge University Press, 1995

Weissman MM, Gershon ES, Kidd KK, et al: Psychiatric disorders in the relatives of probands with affective disorders: the Yale University-National Institute of Mental Health Collaborative Study. Arch Gen Psychiatry 41:13–21, 1984a

Weissman MM, Wickramaratne P, Merikangas KR, et al: Onset of major depression in early childhood: increased familial loading and specificity. Arch Gen Psychiatry 41:1136–1143, 1984b

Weissman MM, Warner V, Wickramaratne P, et al: Early onset major depression in parents and their children. J Affect Disord 15:269–277, 1988

Weissman MM, Members of the Cross-National Collaborative Group: The changing rate of major depression: cross-national comparisons. JAMA 268:3098–3105, 1992

Weissman MM, Wickramaratne P, Adams PB, et al: The relationship between panic disorder and major depression: a new family study. Arch Gen Psychiatry 50:767–780, 1993

Wender PH, Rosenthal D, Kety SS, et al: Crossfostering: a research strategy for clarifying the role of genetic and experiential factors in the etiology of schizophrenia. Arch Gen Psychiatry 30:121–128, 1974

Wender PH, Kety SS, Rosenthal D, et al: Psychiatric disorders in the biological and adoptive families of adopted individuals with affective disorders. Arch Gen Psychiatry 43:923–929, 1986

Winokur A, March V, Mendels J: Primary affective disorder in relatives of patients with anorexia nervosa. Am J Psychiatry 137:695–698, 1980

Winokur G, Cadoret R, Baker M, et al: Depressive spectrum disease versus pure depressive disease: some further data. Br J Psychiatry 127:75–77, 1975

Wolyniec PS, Pulver AE, McGrath JA, et al: Schizophrenia: gender and familial risk. J Psychiatr Res 26:17–27, 1992

Wong PC, Zheng H, Chen H, et al: Presenilin 1 is required for Notch 1 and Dll1 expression in the paraxial mesoderm. Nature 387:288–292, 1997

Wooster R, Neuhausen SL, Mangion J, et al: Localization of a breast cancer susceptibility gene, BRCA2, to chromosome 13q12–13. Science 265:2088–2090, 1994

Wooster R, Bignell G, Lancaster J, et al: Identification of the breast cancer susceptibility gene BRCA2. Nature 378:789–792, 1995

Wragg M, Hutton M, Talbot C: Genetic association between intronic polymorphism in presenilin-1 gene and late-onset Alzheimer's disease: Alzheimer's Disease Collaborative Group. Lancet 347:509–512, 1996

Wright P, Takei N, Rifkin L, et al: Maternal influenza, obstetric complications, and schizophrenia. Am J Psychiatry 152:1714–1720, 1995

Yudofsky SC, Hales RE: The American Psychiatric Press Textbook of Neuropsychiatry, 3rd Edition. Washington, DC, American Psychiatric Press, 1997

SUGGESTED READINGS

Gottesman II, Shields J: Schizophrenia: The Epigenetic Puzzle. Cambridge, UK, Cambridge University Press, 1982

McKusick V: Mendelian Inheritance in Man, 11th Edition. Baltimore, MD, Johns Hopkins University Press, 1994

Ott J: Analysis of Human Genetic Linkage, Revised Edition. Baltimore, MD, Johns Hopkins University Press, 1991

CHAPTER 3

EPIDEMIOLOGY OF MENTAL DISORDERS

JACK D. BURKE, JR., M.D., M.P.H.
DARREL A. REGIER, M.D., M.P.H.

Psychiatric epidemiology is the quantitative study of the distribution of mental disorders in human populations. Embedded in this simple statement are several points that are especially important for clinical research on mental disorders.

The *population* has been the traditional concern of epidemiologists, especially in terms of large-population studies such as community surveys. More generally, though, epidemiology is unusual among clinical disciplines in focusing on populations rather than on individuals, and this characteristic has led it to be called the basic science of *public health*.

With this conceptual approach of studying defined populations, it has been possible to apply the population concept to clinical settings, an approach that has been called *clinical epidemiology*. By using the concept of a population as a starting point for investigations, clinical researchers can reduce, or at least identify, sources of selection bias. For example, studies of the co-occurrence of multiple disorders have been shown to suffer from potential "selection biases" under common conditions in clinical settings. By providing *quantitative* methods to study populations, epidemiology fosters precision in estimating the importance of risk factors, the performance of diagnostic tests, and the effectiveness of new treatments. These applications of epidemiological methods extend far beyond the traditional concern about the importance of measuring community rates of illness and assessing the extent of unmet need in the population.

Once the *distribution* of mental disorders in the population has been determined quantitatively, epidemiologists can identify high-risk groups in whom the study of risk factors may lead to important clues about the etiology of a disorder. An especially important aspect of the epidemiological method is that it does not impose any constraints on the type of risk factors that can be assessed, so it can accommodate both psychosocial and biological variables. Epidemiological techniques are powerful in dealing with multifactorial risks for clinical disorders; a new field of *genetic epidemiology* has grown in the past decade to combine molecular genetics and epidemiological studies of human populations. By taking *specific mental disorders* as the focus of study, psychiatric epidemiology deals with clinical entities that have immediate relevance to clinical research and practice whether the population is in the community or in clinical settings. Epidemiological studies are helpful in a clinical discipline that is concerned with improving its nosology, because it is a natural aim of epidemiological methods to examine the full spectrum of clinical illness, including subclinical variants, and to consider such problems as the threshold of severity to set for a disorder (i.e., number of symptoms for a diagnosis). Longitudinal epidemiological studies are useful in examining the course of illness, and epidemiology has developed experimental methods to test the effect of clinical or preventive interventions on the outcome of illness. For example, clinical trials were developed from experimental approaches in epidemiology to permit a quantitative assessment of the effectiveness of new medications.

For three decades after World War II, psychiatric epidemiologists were eager to apply these methods to studies of mental disorders, but it has not been until the rapid advances in clinical research over the past decade that the quantitative methods of epidemiology could be easily adapted to the study of mental disorders. In this chapter we provide an overview of the various uses of epidemiology followed by an explanation of the characteristic epidemiological methods. We then review the most important findings from contemporary studies in psychiatric epidemiology.

USES OF PSYCHIATRIC EPIDEMIOLOGY

Seven uses of epidemiology have been described by Morris (1964), and they are especially applicable to the current state of knowledge in psychiatry (Table 3–1). These types of studies can be broadly grouped according to the level of investigation of particular study designs. *Descriptive* studies provide estimates of the rate of disorder in a population; *analytic* studies explore variations in rates among different groups to identify risk factors; and *experimental* studies assess the effect of preventive or therapeutic interventions designed to alter the development or outcome of illnesses.

DESCRIPTIVE LEVEL

Community Diagnosis

For a broad range of purposes, from major policy decisions on providing community-based services for mentally ill individuals to more personal decisions such as locating a new private practice or hospital, some of the most impor-

TABLE 3–1. Uses of epidemiology

Descriptive studies
Community diagnosis
Completion of the clinical picture
Identification of syndromes

Analytic studies
Assessment of individual risks
Historical study

Experimental studies
Identification of causes
Assessment of the working of health services

tant questions about the nature of illness in the community population can be difficult to answer.

- How many people in the community have a clinically significant mental disorder?
- Which disorders are most common?
- To what extent are the treatment needs of these individuals being met?

When the President's Commission on Mental Health undertook a comprehensive study of the mental health needs of the nation in the late 1970s, questions of this sort were among its first concerns. At the time, the state of knowledge in psychiatric epidemiology did not permit confident answers to these questions. Rather, in 1978, educated guesses were made by consolidating information from a wide variety of sources. With data from studies conducted in the prior two decades, it was possible to construct a composite picture of the de facto United States mental health system. At that time, it was estimated that about 15% of the population, or 32 million Americans, had a mental disorder at some point during 1975 (Regier et al. 1978). Figure 3–1 depicts where these individuals were seen within the health or mental health system.

Completion of the Clinical Picture

Some aspects of mental disorders are difficult to study if the subjects can only be drawn from treatment settings. For example, careful study of the early development of mental disorders can usually best be accomplished before the individual has sought clinical care. For some disorders such as agoraphobia, which might reduce the likelihood that a person will be seen in treatment, epidemiological studies of the community appear to be especially important. Other questions of increasing importance, such as the co-occurrence of multiple disorders and the ascertainment of familial risks, can best be accomplished through an epidemiological framework. In some cases, especially for the co-occurrence of depressive and anxiety disorders, the relationship between panic disorder and agoraphobia, and the differentiation of serious psychotic illnesses, epidemiological studies have recently been undertaken and promise a new dimension of understanding for these conditions. In addition, some specific questions, such as the proper level of severity or symptomatology to set for the threshold between a subclinical case and a clinical disorder, can best be studied by including individuals who have not yet entered treatment settings (Boyle 1996).

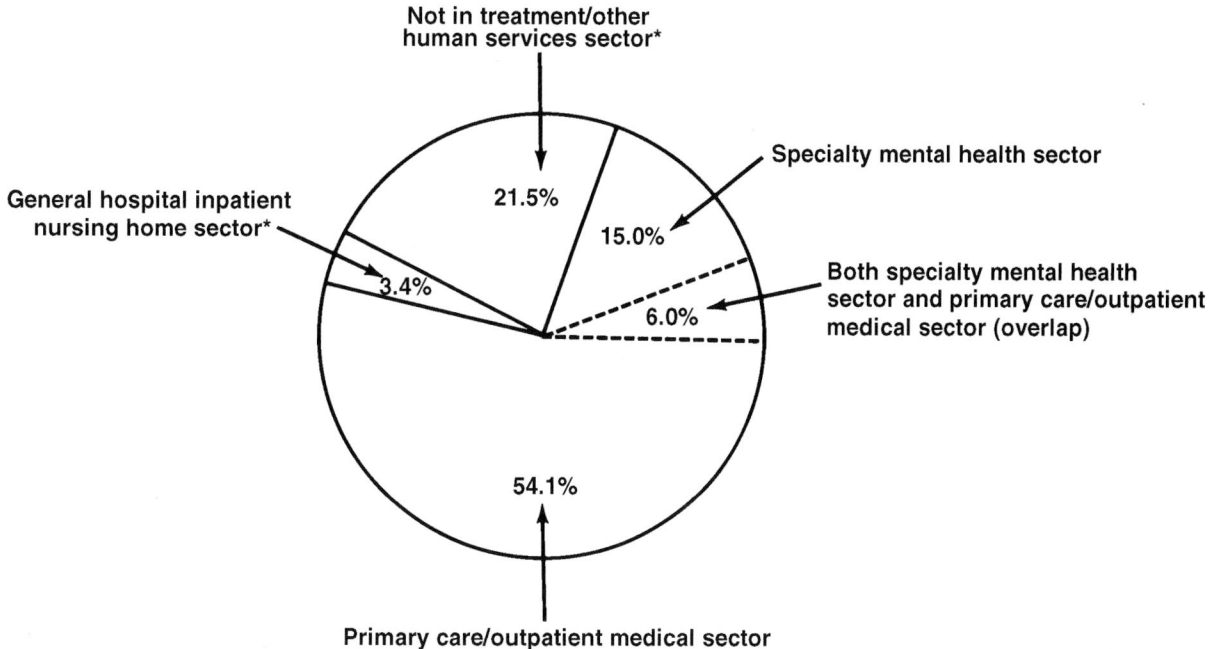

FIGURE 3–1. Estimated percent distribution of persons with mental disorders, by treatment setting, in the United States in 1975. Data relating to sectors other than the specialty mental health sector reflect the number of patients with mental disorder seen in those sectors without regard to the amount or adequacy of treatment provided. Asterisk denotes that sector excludes overlap of an unknown percentage of persons also seen in other sectors.

Identification of Syndromes

Ideally, epidemiological studies that use clinically based procedures for assessing potential cases can also contribute to clinical knowledge through identification of new, previously unrecognized conditions of clinical interest. With the increasing interchange between epidemiological studies and clinical methods, it may be that such payoffs will occur in psychiatry as well. More immediately, epidemiological studies are important for helping to determine the existence or relative importance of conditions that have been tentatively described in clinical settings. For example, epidemiological studies have provided evidence for disorders such as simple schizophrenia, introduced in ICD-10 (World Health Organization 1992), but omitted from DSM-III, DSM-III-R, and DSM-IV (Kendler 1994). Similarly, the decision not to include a category of "involutional melancholia" as a special form of affective illness in DSM-III (American Psychiatric Association 1980) was taken because of arguments based on epidemiological data.

ANALYTIC LEVEL

Assessment of Individual Risks

As individuals working in a public health field closely related to the overall goals of medical science, epidemi-

ologists are as interested in reducing the burden of illness in the population as clinicians are for individual patients. Knowing the rates of illness for the population at large provides the epidemiologist with a powerful springboard to identification of groups in that population who have especially high risks of developing the illness. Once these high-risk groups have been determined, it is possible to design more highly targeted studies to characterize the particular characteristics that place members of the group at higher risk. For this purpose, it is possible to investigate biological, genetic, environmental, infectious, or other factors that help explain the increased rate of illness in the more highly affected groups. An especially appealing feature of the epidemiological method is that a variety of different types of risk factors can be studied, so long as they can be measured in a reliable way in a population. In addition, statistical techniques developed by epidemiologists provide estimates of the magnitude of elevated risk and help establish the relative importance of individual risk factors when more than one factor has been identified.

Historical Study

In searching for possible risk factors and trying to establish their relative importance, investigators in psychiatric epidemiology have been especially interested in historical trends. For example, there has been some suggestive evidence that depressive illness may be occurring more commonly in younger generations, or perhaps having an onset at an earlier age, through the second half of this century (Klerman and Weissman 1989). Similarly, efforts to understand the apparent increase in adolescent drug abuse and adolescent suicide have used historical trends to try to elucidate specific risk factors. Another task will be to determine whether these apparent increases in rates of depressive illness, substance abuse, and suicide in adolescents and young adults are coincidental or linked in some way.

EXPERIMENTAL LEVEL

Identification of Causes

Once possible risk factors have been identified and a likely causal chain has been proposed, it is possible to design interventions and test how effective they are in reducing the clinical problem of interest. For example, in other fields of medicine, community-based interventions to reduce cigarette smoking may lead to a reduction in subsequent development of lung cancer; prophylactic use of aspirin may prevent recurrent myocardial infarction in those who have already had one infarct; and treatment of hypertension may reduce the development of cerebrovascular accidents. In psychiatry, two disorders that have been identified as particularly suitable for possible preventive interventions are depression and drug abuse. The methods for assessing a preventive intervention trial are analogous to those for determining therapeutic interventions. However, as a preventive effort becomes broader and more ambitious, it may be much more difficult to design systematic and rigorous studies of its effectiveness and a cost-benefit ratio.

Assessment of the Working of Health Services

Studies in all three categories—descriptive, analytic, and experimental—have been conducted to examine clinical care in psychiatry. At the broad descriptive level, epidemiological data on the rates of illness in a community can be combined with information about use of health services to determine the extent of untreated illness in the community population, to identify possible barriers to obtaining proper care, and to help in planning the most efficient allocation of public and private resources. At the analytic level, epidemiological methods have been used both to assess the performance of diagnostic tests and to identify patients who are at greatest risk of side effects (e.g., development of

tardive dyskinesia after neuroleptic medication). At the experimental level, controlled trials of therapeutic agents, including both medication and psychotherapy, are used to determine whether a particular treatment regimen has any significant beneficial effects. Epidemiologic concepts have been adapted to help clinicians estimate the impact of new interventions in their own practice, through a measure known as "number needed to treat" to achieve a specific outcome (Sackett 1991).

In addition to these aspects of clinical epidemiology, an analogous field of clinical services research has developed to determine whether there are population-based interventions that may improve the quality of care, such as the establishment of outpatient consultation-liaison services in general medical and primary care clinics, or the use of self-report questionnaires to screen for depression in primary care patients (Burke 1995).

EPIDEMIOLOGICAL METHODS

Although the proper application of quantitative techniques developed by epidemiologists and collaborating biostatisticians can become quite complex, the essential concepts underlying these techniques can be readily understood by clinicians. This overview of statistical and analytic methods will parallel the discussion of the three broad categories of epidemiological studies.

DESCRIPTIVE METHODS

Population Sampling

One distinguishing feature of epidemiological studies is the explicit use of a "population" from which the study subjects are drawn. Although the popular notion that epidemiologists deal with community populations is often correct, the epidemiological approach of using an explicit population can be demonstrated as easily in a clinical setting as in a community setting. For example, clinical research on schizophrenia may be conducted on patients who are most convenient for the research team to enroll in the study. Often these subjects may be those who are closest at hand, for example, long-term residents of a chronic state hospital. Or they may be those with particular relatives or other involved people who encourage the subject to participate in the study, or even those who feel most involved with the research or clinical team, for example, in gratitude for effective treatment. It is quite possible for such a study sample to be useful and to produce valid results. However, in such a sample of convenience there is always a danger of "selection bias," which arises when some particular characteristic associated with the variables of interest has led to higher or lower participation in the study. For example, discrepant results among early studies on computed tomography (CT) scans of schizophrenic patients were explained by a commentary in one research journal (Luchins 1982) as having been due to selection of different types of patients in different clinical studies. By contrast, a research study employing epidemiological principles would begin by asking not which cases are easiest to obtain but rather to what universe of patients should the study's results be applied. By asking this broader question first, the investigator can then determine what population is available for study that matches this desired universe so that a sample can then be drawn from this study population. Although selection bias may still exist, its discovery may be more straightforward within this explicit framework, and any limits on generalizability of the study will be addressed from the outset. Similarly, when different results are obtained from different studies, it may be easier to examine the relative impact of using different subject populations.

Technical aspects of drawing the sample are relatively easy to describe. The simplest case is the *simple random sample*, which consists of using random numbers to draw subjects from a list of the entire study population, for example, to select cases for a study from a series of consecutive admissions to a hospital.

A more complicated design includes drawing samples randomly from within different subgroups of the study population. For example, if men are much less commonly admitted to a particular hospital than women, it may be desirable to draw cases separately from male and female admissions. This technique, known as *stratified random sampling*, entails the use of an adjustment factor to correct for the fact that men and women will be sampled at different proportions. For example, 10% of female admissions but 50% of male admissions may be recruited into the study. The resulting sample needs to be adjusted by these different sampling fractions whenever the results are referred back to the study population of consecutive admissions to the hospital.

A third type of sampling design, called *cluster sampling*, is more convenient whenever individual cases cannot be easily rostered, for example, when patients are drawn from different clinics within a large medical center. Although this sampling technique is usually more economical, it provides for less precise estimates. Combinations of these methods, especially complex mixtures of stratified and cluster sampling, are often used for epidemiological surveys in the community. In such studies, elementary statistical techniques embodied in the routine computer software packages are not suitable for analyzing the data, and since 1980, sophisticated computer packages entailing the proper complex statistical approaches to analyze these data have been developed.

Whatever technique is used to draw the sample from the study population, the very fact of drawing a sample means that the study results are only estimates for the data that would have been obtained if the entire study population had been examined. For that reason, it is common to report whether results are statistically significant or only represent sampling variation. This report can be provided in terms of an interval showing how imprecise the sample estimate is or whether any differences observed are within the range expected for that study design. Well-known methods based on the standard error of a particular estimated value, such as a mean or a proportion, are used to derive either *confidence intervals* or *tests of statistical significance*. This application of a population-based approach to sampling in clinical settings illuminates the problems of selection bias and proper estimation of sampling errors for a particular study. An extension of this concept also demonstrates that for some purposes a clinical population may not be appropriate. For example, a topic of increased interest in psychiatry has been to examine the co-occurrence of multiple psychiatric disorders or of psychiatric disorders with medical or other conditions. However, estimates of the co-occurrence of disorders within clinical populations are difficult to make if the two conditions of interest are each likely to lead people to enter treatment settings. In that case, the apparent association between the two conditions will be exaggerated because the sample is drawn from clinical populations. It may be, for example, that the apparent close relationship between panic disorder and agoraphobia in clinical populations is made closer by sampling from clinical populations rather than from community populations. Similarly, if it is shown that women are more likely to enter psychiatric treatment than men, and if an illness such as depression leads people into psychiatric treatment, it may be that the apparent association between being female and being depressed could be overestimated if only clinical populations have been studied. This problem of examining the co-occurrence of disorders in clinical populations is known as *Berkson's fallacy*, after the biostatistician who first demonstrated it four decades ago (Berkson 1946).

Diagnostic Assessment

At the heart of any epidemiological study, whether within a community or a clinical population, is a determination of the disease status of the subjects in the study. Especially in a field like psychiatry, in which nosology has been one of the most vigorously pursued topics of research in the past decade, the question of what constitutes a case is a central one that ties together both epidemiological and clinical research studies (Wing et al. 1980). In the absence of any definitive standard for establishing the validity of a psychiatric diagnosis, it is difficult to judge the value of a diagnostic procedure. However, that uncertainty makes it even more important to describe any known sources of error in or flawed performance with a given diagnostic procedure. Four characteristics of diagnostic instruments are especially important.

1. The *safety* of any diagnostic procedure in human populations must be established, whether for psychiatric interviews or for more invasive procedures. At present, there is no evidence that psychiatric interviews themselves cause harm to any subjects, including children. However, this facet of a study design needs to be considered by researchers in the overall context of providing an opportunity for subjects to give informed consent to participate in a study. The essential uncertainty of the information needed for psychiatric diagnoses and ways of interpreting the information can sometimes lead to proposals for assessments that are comprehensive but much too complex for repeated administration even by highly trained and highly motivated clinician examiners.

2. The *feasibility* of a diagnostic procedure is especially important for investigators in terms of the proposed sample size and difficulty in gaining access to subjects. For example, in a large-scale community survey it may be quite difficult to obtain enough financial resources and skilled examiners to conduct a highly complex examination of subjects using board-certified psychiatrists. One impetus for increased clinical research in psychiatry in the past two decades was the earlier demonstration that psychiatric diagnoses were quite variable from one clinician to another, or sometimes in the same clinician's judgment over time for the same patient.

3. Demonstrating *reliability*, or consistency, in diagnostic assessment between examiners or between examinations has become a standard requirement that research assessments have been expected to meet.

4. Ideally, the diagnoses produced in any clinical or research setting would be accurate, that is, would demonstrate *validity*. However, the fact that there is no absolute standard for establishing a definitive diagnosis, and the fact that even skilled clinicians have low reliability for their routine diagnoses, make it difficult to know how to assess validity. At present, new assessment procedures are often tested by comparison to existing well-known procedures or to diagnostic judgments of "senior clinicians." However, it is generally recognized that neither of these comparisons provides an authoritative basis for assessing validity.

Measuring Reliability

Any diagnostic procedure should be able to produce consistent results when used to assess the same phenomena, either by different examiners or on different occasions. These measures of consistency, called *interrater reliability* and *test-retest reliability*, are essential characteristics of any diagnostic test, whether psychiatric interview, projective test, or chemical assay. Consistency is measured by assessing how well two examiners agree on their diagnostic judgments, or how well the test agrees on two different occasions (Figure 3–2).

The simplest measure of agreement is simply the percentage of times both tests agree that the subject is positive or that the subject is negative. This figure, known as *percentage agreement*, is commonly used but is no longer recommended. Because some agreements will occur by chance, the percentage agreement figure tends to overstate the reliability of a diagnostic procedure. The most widely used measure of agreement for reliability studies is *kappa* (κ),

	Examiner A		
	Positive	Negative	
Examiner B			
Positive	$a = 14$	$b = 16$	$B_1 = 30$
Negative	$c = 22$	$d = 148$	$B_2 = 170$
	$A_1 = 36$	$A_2 = 164$	$n = 200$

P_o = proportion of agreement observed

$$= \frac{a + d}{n} = 0.81$$

P_c = proportion of agreement by chance

$$= \left[\binom{A_1}{n} \right] \times \left(\binom{B_1}{n} \right] + \left[\binom{A_2}{n} \right) \times \binom{B_2}{n} \right]$$

$$= 0.724$$

$$\text{Kappa} = \frac{(P_o - P_c)}{(1 - P_c)}$$

$$= (0.81 - 0.724)/(1 - 0.724) = 0.31$$

FIGURE 3–2. Calculation of kappa.

a measure that corrects for the proportion of chance agreements to give an indication of agreement achieved beyond what would have occurred by chance alone. κ indicates what proportion of the potential agreement, beyond chance, was actually achieved. Calculations of κ have been described for a variety of situations, including those involving multiple examiners who produce multiple diagnoses for a given subject. Guidelines for interpreting κ suggest that values above 0.75 are excellent, values between 0.40 and 0.75 (inclusive) are good, and values below 0.40 are poor. One difficulty arises when the condition being assessed is rare; if this occurs, the κ value is attenuated. Several authorities suggest not calculating κ when the condition of interest occurs in fewer than 5% of the subjects. Suggestions have been made for alternative measures to substitute for κ in these situations but have been controversial, and some authorities use κ even for rare conditions (Fleiss 1981; Shrout et al. 1987; Spitznagel and Helzer 1985).

Validity

Several types of validity have been described (Table 3–2). *Face validity*, which refers to a judgment by "experts" that the items or procedure of a test "make sense," may be helpful in persuading clinicians to employ the test, but it may have no relationship to the accuracy of the test results. *Content validity* refers to a judgment by experts that the items of the test cover the appropriate domains of knowledge relevant for the test's purposes. On a psychiatric interview, for example, it would be important to determine that items are present for all of the specified DSM-IV criteria (American Psychiatric Association 1994) needed for a given disorder of interest. Although it is important to know if content validity does not exist, simply providing adequate coverage of relevant items does not guarantee that the test results will be accurate. In the absence of a definitive standard for establishing accuracy in an authoritative way, current practice in psychiatry is to use another, usually well-known, test with a similar purpose as a comparison instrument, for *criterion validity*. In assessing diagnostic interviews, for example, a comparison could be another psychiatric interview that has already been shown to have adequate reliability, or a panel of "expert clinicians" whose consensus judgment is considered the best composite picture of clinical knowledge for a given subject. Although it may be reassuring in such study designs to show that a new instrument is reasonably close to the judgment of another instrument or an expert panel, such procedures would not allow discovery of situations in which the new instrument, in fact, was superior to the criterion that had

been chosen for the study of interest.

In studies of criterion validity, several measures of interest have been developed. *Sensitivity* is a measure of the number of true cases who are detected by the instrument being evaluated; the false negative rate is generally considered the number of true cases who are missed by the instrument. *Specificity* is the number of true noncases who are accurately assessed by the new instrument; the false positive rate commonly is considered the number of true noncases who are mistakenly called cases by the diagnostic instrument (Figure 3–3).

Another measure, *positive predictive value*, is especially useful to clinicians who are assessing the potential value of a new test. This measure estimates the number of positive subjects on the new test who truly represent cases of the disorder.

Other forms of validity include *predictive validity*, which refers to an assessment of whether a test accurately identifies subjects who will at some future point be shown to have the disorder, perhaps by a more sophisticated diagnostic interview, or by accumulated evidence derived from course of the illness, response to treatment, family history, laboratory tests, and so forth.

Prevalence Rates

The *prevalence rate* is the proportion of a population who have the disorder at a given time. If the population sampling has been performed adequately, the sampling design allows estimation of the denominator for this proportion, and the case assessment procedure allows estimation of the numerator, or number of cases. Most commonly, prevalence rates are reported as of a given point, such as a day on the calendar or the day of interview in a study. In this case, the measure is known as the *point prevalence rate*. Another measure, *lifetime prevalence rate*, is the proportion of a pop-

TABLE 3–2. Types of validity

Face validity	Judgment by experts that the items make sense.
Content validity	Judgment by experts that the items cover the appropriate domains.
Criterion validity	Comparison with a similar, well-known test.
Predictive validity	Determination of whether a test accurately identifies subjects who will at some future point be shown to have the disorder.

"Truth"

	Disorder present	Disorder absent	
New instrument			
Positive	a = 70	b = 16	a + b = 86
Negative	c = 10	d = 104	c + d = 114
	a + c = 80	b + d = 120	n = 200

Sensitivity = a/(a + c) = (70/80) = 0.875

Specificity = d/(b + d) = (104/120) = 0.867

FIGURE 3–3. Calculation of sensitivity and specificity.

ulation who have ever had the illness at any point in their lives. This measure has been especially widely used in psychiatry, particularly for studies of genetics and family history, but it has drawbacks that limit its usefulness. As with any proportion from an adequate sampling design, it is possible to calculate the standard error, so prevalence rates should be accompanied by information about the confidence interval or the standard error to allow tests of significance for differences between prevalence rates.

ANALYTIC METHODS

To identify risk factors, a first step is to examine subgroups in the population to determine where the rates of illness are higher than usual. Although it would be relatively easy to use point prevalence rates for this purpose, the conclusions based from that kind of analysis would likely be flawed because these rates represent all subjects who are ill at a given time, regardless of how long they have had the disorder. As a result, chronic cases tend to be overrepresented in such a cross-sectional study, and some groups may have higher rates of illness because the disorder has been present for a longer time. For example, if those persons in lower socioeconomic classes have less access to effective treatment, the burden of illness may be greater simply because the condition has been untreated. To overcome the uncertainty introduced by chronic cases, risk factors for developing an illness are best examined by comparing rates of new cases, *incidence rates*, in the population. Study designs involving incidence rates need to be more complex than for prevalence surveys because the development of new cases usually requires passage of time. Although a variety of study designs have been developed to assess risk factors, two of them are particularly common.

Prospective Longitudinal Studies

An excellent way to assess incidence rates in a population would be to form a sample of persons from the population who are younger than the typical age at onset of the disorder of interest and to assess them for a variety of characteristics that are potential risk factors to be considered in the study. Diagnostic assessments, to exclude anyone from the sample who has already developed the illness, are undertaken also at the outset of the study. After a reasonable amount of time has passed, typically 1 year, subjects are reexamined to determine who has developed the illness. The incidence rate is calculated with the number of new cases in the numerator and the total number of persons at risk at the beginning of the time period in the denominator. For 1 year, this estimate would be the annual incidence rate. To assess elevated risks, the incidence rates in different groups could be compared. In this kind of study, if persons below the poverty line have twice the incidence rate of those above the poverty line, the ratio of incidence rates would be 2.0, and this ratio is taken as a measure of the *relative risk*. This figure indicates that those in the poverty group would have twice the rate of developing illness as those above the poverty line. Note that prevalence rates cannot be used to estimate relative risk for developing an illness, because prevalence includes both onset and duration; a chronic illness will have a higher prevalence than a short-lived one even if both have the same incidence rate.

Because it is unlikely that individuals would be followed for exactly 12 months, more complicated measures using the person-years of observation for each individual have been developed and are called *incidence density* measures. A ratio of these is also used to calculate relative risk estimates. Once an elevated relative risk has been established, further investigation can proceed to determine what factors place members of that group at a higher risk for developing the illness. In this hypothetical example, possible causal factors could include psychosocial problems associated with poverty, genetic or familial factors that cause families to "drift" downward in socioeconomic status, or infectious or toxic exposures that could be more likely for those living in impoverished areas.

Case Control Studies

Because prospective longitudinal studies are difficult and often expensive to conduct, and because they are even more difficult in the case of rare disorders, in which the incidence rate is low, an alternative study design is often used. This design is especially useful in the exploratory stage before putative risk factors have been identified well enough to justify undertaking a prospective longitudinal study. In this design, known cases are identified, for example, from hospital or medical records, and individuals who are similar in age, sex, socioeconomic status, or other relevant characteristics and are known not to have the illness are matched to these cases as a comparison group. Some assessment is then made of personal characteristics that existed before the time the cases would have developed the illness. For example, a common question in depression has been whether the death of a parent in the patient's early childhood is a risk factor for subsequent depressive illness. In this kind of study, depressed patients could be compared with other types of psychiatric or medical patients who are thought to provide a fair base of comparison, and their history of early parental death could be assessed retrospectively. A calculation similar to the one in Figure 3–4 could be made. In this case control design, however, the populations from whom the cases or the subjects in the comparison group have been drawn are not specified, and it is not possible to talk about these proportions as if they were incidence rates for risk and nonrisk groups. A satisfactory alternative measure to incidence rate ratios in most instances is the *odds ratio* (Figure 3–4). For most cross-sectional studies, such as this case control design, the odds ratio provides a reasonable estimate of relative risk.

Bias

Besides selection bias, these cross-sectional studies are subject to additional types of bias. First, the examiner who attempts to establish the risk factor status by inquiring about the subject's past history may have clues, perhaps even from the subject's clinical condition at the time, that the subject is in the case or comparison group; as a result, the examiner may probe more or less deeply to establish the presence of a particular risk factor and thus may inadvertently help to confirm the study's hypothesis. Such a possibility is called *observer bias* and is especially problem-atic for studies in which retrospective assessments are needed. Although observer bias should be the easiest source of bias to control, by requiring that examiners be blind to the subject's status and, ideally, blind to the study's hypothesis, it is often neglected. Another potential problem is *confounding bias*, which occurs when an unexamined characteristic is associated both with the suspected risk factor and with the disorder and is the true underlying cause of the disorder. For example, it could be that exposure to a particular toxin in some families resulted not only in the death of the parent but in the later vulnerability of the child to develop depression. Such unknown causes, as in this hypothetical example, could lead to misinterpretations of data from case control and other nonexperimental studies.

EXPERIMENTAL METHODS

Much epidemiological research is observational in nature, such as in the community surveys or prospective longitudinal studies previously described. At times, the opportunity to observe "natural experiments" in which some natural event intervenes in one group but not in a similar group arises. For example, it may be possible to observe the effects of a natural disaster (e.g., a tornado) on the children of one town and to use as a comparison group children of a nearby town who did not experience the disaster, if the exposure status of individual subjects can be verified. In such a design, it would be important to know the differences between the exposed and comparison groups.

However, the experimental method developed in the natural sciences has also been applied to study the onset and course of illness. The central feature of the experimental method is *random assignment* of subjects to either the experimental intervention group or the control group without the intervention. This process of assigning subjects at random is expected to prevent selection bias and also to reduce possible confounding bias, because any unknown underlying causes would be equally distributed between the control and experimental groups, at least when large enough numbers are considered. The practice of having examiners and subjects "blind" to their assignment in experimental or control groups is expected to minimize observer bias. This experimental methodology has been used in clinical trials of treatments, both pharmacological and psychotherapeutic, to determine their effectiveness for psychiatric patients. Similar methodology has also been developed for preventive interventions, to test the effectiveness of preventive programs in preventing the onset of illness in high-risk groups. One problem in designing these intervention trials is to determine how many subjects are needed

Disease status

	Cases	Noncases
Risk factor		
Present	a = 40	b = 75
Not present	c = 60	d = 225

$$\text{Odds ratio} = \frac{a}{b} \div \frac{c}{d} = \frac{ad}{bc} = \frac{(40)(225)}{(75)(60)} = 2.0$$

FIGURE 3–4.   Calculation of odds ratio.

to show that any differences in the two groups' outcomes are *true* differences, that is, statistically significant above the level expected from sampling variation. Because larger numbers of subjects provide more precise estimates from sampling, a key issue for clinical and epidemiological intervention trials is to estimate how many subjects are needed to be able to detect a true difference as large as the one expected by the investigator. Recent advances in biostatistics have made it possible to estimate the statistical power for different study designs, and epidemiological measures such as the *population attributable risk* (also called the "etiologic fraction") make it possible to estimate from descriptive studies what the likely proportion of cases is that can likely be attributed to a particular risk factor (Morgenstern and Bursic 1982).

Measures of attributable risk depend on rate differences, rather than rate ratios as in relative risk estimates. For example, if the rate of a disorder like generalized anxiety disorder is found to be 5% in a population of adolescents, and to be 15% in a similar population exposed to a tornado, it might be possible to estimate that the difference in rates (10%) is the risk attributable to tornado exposure, assuming bias in such a study design is not important. Similarly, in randomized clinical trials, the difference in mortality between a placebo-treated group (e.g., 30%) and the active treatment group (e.g., 10%) might be calculated as 20%. To make this figure more understandable in clinical situations, some clinical epidemiologists have found it helpful to take the reciprocal of this difference and calculate the "number needed to treat" to achieve a saving of one life. In this example, the clinician would need to treat 5 patients (1/0.2) with the experimental agent to save one life (Sackett et al. 1991).

Experimental epidemiology, particularly preventive trials designed to modify presumed risk factors in high-risk subjects, is one way to establish that an association observed in nonexperimental studies between a risk factor and an illness may be a true cause-and-effect relationship. This question of whether an observed association between a possible risk factor and an illness is truly one of cause and effect plagues many epidemiological studies. Short of conducting experimental interventions designed to reduce the impact of a potential risk factor, one may use other types of evidence to lend confidence that an observed association is meaningful.

First, the sequence of development of a risk factor and a disorder must indicate that the risk factor occurred before the disorder began; without this *temporal* sequence it would be hard to argue for causality. Unfortunately, in some instances the apparent temporal sequence is misleading. When there is a long delay between initiation of the disease process and the first manifestation of a disorder, for example, the relative order of exposure to the "risk" factor and development of illness may be misjudged.

Second, *replication* of the observed association across several studies using different designs or populations would strengthen belief that the association is likely to be a causal one. Replications of large-scale studies are increasingly expensive and difficult, although these factors make the development of commonly accepted methodologies, such as comparable methods of diagnostic assessment, especially important.

Third, the *magnitude* of the elevated risk would also tend to increase confidence that the association is a causal one. However, short of the experimental demonstration that changing the risk factor modifies the development of an illness, many skeptics will not accept arguments that epidemiological studies showing associations between putative risk factors and illnesses should be the basis for medical decisions or public policy; such arguments are used to bolster continuing commercial opposition to public health efforts to control cigarette smoking and dietary cholesterol, for example. The role of epidemiology in establishing causal relationships has been clarified recently by distinguishing *causative factors, etiologic agents,* and *pathogenic mechanisms* (Stallones 1987).

A classic example of the role of epidemiology comes from John Snow's quantitative analysis of the distribution of cholera cases in London from 1849 to 1854. Snow showed that contaminated water—not bad air, as had been thought—was the causative factor, and he helped stop the outbreak by removing the pump handles from affected wells and identifying the responsible water companies. Over the last century, *Vibrio cholerae* was identified as the waterborne etiologic agent. In the last decade, the pathogenic mechanism was shown to depend on an enterotoxin that stimulates adenylate cyclase in intestinal cells, creating persistent secretion of isotonic fluid throughout the small intestine and leading to severe hypovolemia. As this history illustrates, epidemiological studies are important both for preventive intervention and for stimulating clinical and biological research on basic mechanisms of disease.

ADVANCES IN PSYCHIATRIC EPIDEMIOLOGY: DIAGNOSTIC ASSESSMENTS

The field of survey sampling makes it possible to conduct highly sophisticated and complex sampling of household residents as well as residents of institutions of great interest to psychiatric epidemiologists, including prisons, state mental hospitals, and nursing homes. Advances in biostatistics have made it possible to estimate the sampling variation of these highly complex sampling designs so that accurate analyses can be conducted. Fortunately for psychiatric epidemiology, similar advances have been made in the technology of diagnostic assessments, so it has also been feasible to attempt to approximate clinical diagnoses in large-scale community studies and in large clinical studies.

Three major sources of potential error can make it difficult to achieve reliability in diagnostic assessments, both in clinical studies and in epidemiology. *Information variance* refers to the fact that different examiners, or even the same examiner on different occasions, may elicit different information from the subject and therefore use a different data base for assessing potential disorders and classifying them. *Observer variance* suggests that different examiners may interpret the same data differently, either reported symptoms such as depressed mood or clinical signs such as blunted affect. *Criterion variance* refers to the problem that different examiners, even when using the same data base, may have different criteria for assigning a subject to a particular diagnostic category.

One of the largest and best-known studies of variability of psychiatric diagnosis, conducted in the late 1960s in London and New York, was the U.S.-U.K. Diagnostic Project (Cooper et al. 1972). Its principal aim was to examine whether the apparently higher rates of schizophrenia in the United States represented a true difference from those in Europe or whether the apparent difference resulted only from variability in diagnostic practices. A major advance of that study was the application of standardized protocols guiding the psychiatric interview of subjects, such as the Present State Examination (PSE; Wing et al. 1974). These interview protocols specified exactly the information to be obtained by the examiner, and a glossary and full course of training were provided to ensure that examiners would be consistent in the way they interpreted the information from the psychiatric interview. In the diagnostic project, criterion variance was minimized by having panels of judges review all of the information available on cases to make consensus ratings of diagnosis.

In 1972, researchers from Washington University in St. Louis proposed a new way of controlling criterion variance in research by publishing a set of specified criteria to be used in assigning diagnoses to research subjects (Feighner et al. 1972).

These two approaches—an interview protocol and a set of explicit criteria—were linked in the mid-1970s by the development of a new set of criteria, the Research Diagnostic Criteria (RDC), and the simultaneous development of a standardized interview based on these criteria, the Sched-ule for Affective Disorders and Schizophrenia (SADS; Endicott and Spitzer 1978). This combined approach of using a standardized interview schedule with fully specified criteria guiding assignment to a particular diagnostic category made it possible for researchers to achieve a new standard of reliability in diagnostic assessments. This feature made its use widespread, a fact that also yielded the advantage of providing comparability in research studies across different centers and over time.

When DSM-III criteria were published in 1980, they represented an extension and elaboration of the approach of specifying criteria to be met for each psychiatric disorder. From the extensive experience with previous interview schedules, confidence developed that a fully specified set of questions for an interview schedule could be written so that even nonclinicians could administer them. With support from senior officials of the National Institute of Mental Health (NIMH), an interview schedule was commissioned that would be suitable for large-scale epidemiological studies in community populations. The resulting instrument, the NIMH Diagnostic Interview Schedule (DIS; Robins et al. 1981, 1982), contains the exact wording of questions intended to meet DSM-III criteria of the most important disorders thought to exist in community populations. A careful probe system was also developed for use with positive responses to be sure that the phenomenon being assessed was not attributable to drugs or alcohol or to medical illness or injury, and was significant enough that it could contribute toward accumulating evidence for a psychiatric disorder.

Computer scoring programs were developed to handle the large amount of data that would be gathered on each subject in the large-scale survey, and the resulting system was used as the basis for a new multisite epidemiological study called the NIMH Epidemiologic Catchment Area Program (ECA; Regier et al. 1984; Robins et al. 1981, 1982). Tests of the performance of the DIS were undertaken before the ECA began and during the course of the ECA itself. In addition, widespread use of the DIS in this country and abroad resulted in independent assessments of its performance (Burke 1986).

The difficulty in evaluating these "clinical comparison studies" is that the value of the independent clinical diagnosis is hard to determine. In many cases, even the reliability of the clinical diagnosis has not been established. However, the results are of great interest in determining how the diagnoses made by an instrument designed for epidemiological studies compare with diagnoses commonly given in clinical settings. Studies of three samples drawn from clinical treatment settings indicated acceptable κ values, with values for alcohol disorders ranging from 0.50 to 1.0, and those for major depression ranging from 0.72 to 1.0.

Studies undertaken with community populations demonstrated much greater variance, with two studies from the ECA showing κ values of 0.35 and 0.63 for alcohol disorders, and of 0.25 and 0.28 for major depression. (However, a community study in Germany using psychiatric diagnoses as a standard showed a κ value of 0.72 for major depression.) The lower results from community samples have provoked some discussion. For example, one interpretation of studies of community samples is that the κ values are artificially attenuated because of the rare occurrence of disorders in a population; an alternative explanation is that the κ values are legitimate, but that assessing subjects in the community is much more difficult, because either they are less seriously ill or they are less likely to report symptoms in an interview, for example. Perhaps the most skeptical interpretation is that the clinical diagnoses have little meaning in these comparison studies because the interrater reliability of the assessment instruments was often not demonstrated and because great variation can be expected in the application of DSM-III criteria (Burke 1986; Klerman 1985; Robins 1985).

Probably the most beneficial aspect of this controversy is to stimulate much more careful and systematic investigation of the nature of diagnostic assessments and the statistical techniques for analyzing them (Faraone and Tsuang 1994). That effort is also leading to several projects designed to produce a more advanced diagnostic interview schedule suitable for epidemiological surveys in different countries, as well as clinical interview protocols that are suitable for administration by psychiatrists. The Composite International Diagnostic Interview (CIDI) has been developed on the basis of the DIS and incorporates diagnostic criteria from DSM-IV as well as the new criteria for ICD-10. Its reliability has been tested in a preliminary study conducted among different cultures and language groups and has produced very high agreement in this first study (Robins et al. 1988; Wittchen et al. 1991). The Schedules for Clinical Assessment in Neuropsychiatry (SCAN) is a clinical interview that requires a trained clinical examiner to record information suitable for DSM-IV and ICD-10 diagnoses (Wing et al. 1990). The Structured Clinical Interview for DSM-IV (SCID), another clinical interview that allows one to assign DSM-IV diagnoses, has shown good reliability (Spitzer et al. 1992; Williams et al. 1992).

SURVEYS OF CLINICAL AND COMMUNITY POPULATIONS

The foundation for analysis of risk factors, etiological mechanisms, and the effectiveness of treatment and pre-ventive interventions is a confident level of knowledge about the basic rates of disorder in particular populations. Epidemiological surveys of patients seen in treatment settings as well as of the broader population of community residents have been conducted over the past four decades in the United States and abroad.

CLINICAL POPULATIONS

National Reporting Program

The National Reporting Program, conducted through 1992 by the NIMH and now by the Center for Mental Health Services (CMHS), is a series of periodic surveys of patients and facilities in the mental health delivery system. These surveys include an annual census of state and county mental hospitals, an inventory of specialty mental health facilities, and a sample survey of patients drawn from the universe of mental health facilities. Statistics of this sort provide a basis for following the marked decline in use of public inpatient services and the shift over the past five decades to private hospitals and to outpatient settings. The change among types of facilities also demonstrates the effects of changes in public policy, private resources (including coverage and health insurance), availability of facilities, and perhaps other uncertain characteristics, such as possible change in the relative proportions of different mental disorders (Witkin et al. 1990, pp. 36–37).

Social Class and Mental Illness

A classic study based on detailed information from mental health treatment settings in New Haven, Connecticut, was conducted by Hollingshead and Redlich (1958) in the 1950s. Within the New Haven area, every mental health facility and private office practice psychiatrist was surveyed to determine the number of patients seen in these different settings. The investigators estimated that patients in treatment within a 6-month period for any mental disorder represented 8 per 1,000 residents in the community. They demonstrated that the rate in the highest social classes ranged from 5 to 7 per 1,000, compared with 17 per 1,000 in the lowest social class, V. Although it was not possible to determine how reliably the diagnoses had been reported by the treating clinicians or whether social class was truly associated with prevalence of disorder or only with access to treatment, the study had a major impact on public policy makers and was one of the pieces of information lending support for the Community Mental Health Act of 1963.

Primary Care Settings

Studies conducted in the United Kingdom in the mid-1960s demonstrated that patients seen in general practice settings had high rates of diagnosable mental disorders, including as high as 15%. Studies conducted in the United States subsequently demonstrated that the rate of disorder among those visiting a general physician over a 3- to 6-month period of time were even higher (i.e., up to 28%) when standardized psychiatric interviews such as the lifetime version of the SADS (SADS-L) or DIS were used instead of relying on the chart diagnosis. The most common disorders in these primary care patients have been depressive illnesses, anxiety illnesses, and mixed conditions including substance abuse (Kamerow et al. 1986; Katon and Schulberg 1992). At the same time, more recent studies have demonstrated that the general physician commonly does not record a diagnosis of a mental disorder in the patient's chart, does not report it on special inquiries conducted during the research, and does not provide treatment or referral to a specialty mental health clinician.

As a result of the relatively high prevalence and the apparent underdetection and undertreatment, there has been a growing interest in ways to improve the recognition, diagnosis, and effective management through treatment or referral of patients with mental disorders seen in primary care settings. In 1986, the NIMH launched the Depression Awareness, Recognition, and Treatment Program (DART) to improve the detection, diagnosis, and effective treatment of depressive illnesses in the population, including general medical patients. This line of research demonstrates the immediate public health applications of epidemiological surveys in defined populations (Regier et al. 1988b).

COMMUNITY POPULATIONS

Classic surveys of community populations were conducted in the decade following World War II in the United States and Canada. Although these surveys were often characterized by extremely sophisticated efforts by the investigators to conduct appropriate sampling and to make reliable and clinically meaningful diagnoses, the relatively underdeveloped state of psychiatric nosology at that time, when the first edition of DSM-I (American Psychiatric Association 1952) had just been published, made it quite difficult to establish clinically relevant diagnoses in community studies. However, the studies established important baseline estimates that could not be improved upon until nearly 30 years of progress in other areas of psychiatric research enabled the next community studies to be launched.

Stirling County Study

Leighton and colleagues (1963) surveyed 1,010 adult residents in a rural Canadian county of 20,000 people. They estimated that 20% of the adult population were in need of psychiatric attention for a diagnosable mental disorder, although 57% had evidence of symptom patterns corresponding to the major categories of illness in DSM-I. One of the intriguing findings of that study was that high rates of illness were found in areas of social and economic deterioration, although the variables leading to this higher association were not identifiable. One of the important advances for the study was the careful effort to apply the implicit criteria of DSM-I in an explicit, systematic formulation of symptoms that could be documented through a structured psychiatric interview and with information from other informants such as the respondent's general physician. This interest in a careful delineation of explicit criteria for specific disorders foreshadowed the development of DSM-III and contemporary instruments like the DIS; it has also made possible an approximate comparison of findings from the Stirling County study to the more recent epidemiological studies using DSM-III criteria (Murphy 1980).

Midtown Manhattan Study

In an area of midtown Manhattan with 110,000 adults, Rennie, Srole, and their colleagues sampled 1,660 persons (Srole et al. 1962). Psychologists and social workers interviewed respondents according to a structured schedule, and the information was subsequently interpreted by two psychiatrists. There have been continuing controversies about the way this diagnostic information was presented, particularly because some observers have been concerned that it implied the existence of a single spectrum of illness, without allowance for specific psychiatric disorders. This impression was reinforced by the most widely publicized version of the findings, which noted that 81.5% of the population were shown to have at least mild impairment from psychological symptoms, although only 23.4% had significant impairment. There was widespread skepticism in both the scientific community and the public about a field that claimed that fewer than 20% of the population were "mentally healthy." Paradoxically, the negative reaction to this part of the study's findings also reinforced the need in both clinical psychiatry and epidemiological studies to develop explicit criteria that provided for consistency across raters and for clinically meaningful information.

Baltimore Morbidity Study

In Baltimore, household residents were interviewed by census interviewers, and a subsample of 809 individuals was determined for later examination by general physicians and pediatricians. The study was unusual in that it covered the entire age range of noninstitutionalized community residents, including children. For mental disorders, psychiatrists rated the interview protocols subsequent to the second examination according to the International Statistical Classification of Diseases (ISCD). A point prevalence rate of 10.9% was found for mental disorders, and 1.4% of the sample showed moderate to severe impairment (Commission on Chronic Illness 1957).

NIMH EPIDEMIOLOGIC CATCHMENT AREA PROGRAM

Evidence that a new effort to conduct a community survey of psychiatric disorders was timely came from a study conducted by Weissman and colleagues (1978). That study, which constituted a 7-year reexamination of a group of 1,000 community residents being followed over time in New Haven, Connecticut, demonstrated that the SADS-L could be administered reliably to 550 community respondents and that diagnostic assessments were feasible, because the respondents provided meaningful information in response to the lengthy psychiatric interview and history. This study, and another one using primary care patients in a large medical practice in Wisconsin conducted in 1978 (Hoeper et al. 1979), showed that the new generation of psychiatric interviews could be used outside specialty research settings. With encouraging results from these studies, development of the NIMH-DIS was undertaken, and plans were made to design, support, and conduct a large-scale multisite community survey of psychiatric disorders. The ECA was conducted at sites in five areas: New Haven, Connecticut; Baltimore, Maryland; St. Louis, Missouri; Durham, North Carolina; and Los Angeles, California. At each site, clearly specified geographic areas based on the catchment areas that had been developed through the Community Mental Health Act of 1963 were sampled so that a minimum of 3,000 adults aged 18 and older from each area would be interviewed at the initial examination. In addition, residents of institutions such as prisons, nursing homes, and chronic care hospitals were also sampled, and 500 respondents from these institutional settings were interviewed.

Besides the DIS, which was used to generate psychiatric diagnoses, extensive questions were asked about use of health and mental health services in the 6–12 months preceding the interview. Another interview 6 months after the initial examination, conducted by telephone in four of the five sites, inquired about subsequent use of health and mental health services after that first interview. A follow-up personal interview was conducted about 12 months after the initial visit, and the DIS and the Health Service questions were repeated at that time. These key features of the design were intended to 1) allow focus on specific mental disorders diagnosed by the then new DSM-III criteria using DIS information; 2) allow estimates of disorders for the total community population, including those persons in institutions; 3) provide data on incidence rates, as well as prevalence rates, obtained from the first interview; and 4) allow the integration of data on diagnostic status and use of treatment services (Robins and Regier 1991).

Prevalence Rates

The onset, recency, and clustering of symptoms were determined using the DIS, which made it possible to produce prevalence rates of disorders occurring in the past 1 month, 6 months, 1 year, and over the lifetime of all individuals in the sample. Because retrospective data on outpatient service use were obtained for the previous 6 months, 6-month period prevalence rate data have conventionally been presented when an analytic objective has been to compare prevalence and service use data. To generate estimates of mental illness in the community, data from the 18,572 subjects in the community samples at the five sites were pooled and standardized by age, sex, and race/ethnicity to the 1980 U.S. Census of the noninstitutionalized population. This effort produced estimates of DSM-III disorders in the general population and more detailed correlations with sociodemographic factors including age, sex, race/ethnicity, marital status, and socioeconomic status (Regier et al. 1988a; Robins and Regier 1991). For the major DSM-III disorders covered by the DIS, estimates for the 6-month prevalence rates from the pooled data, standardized to the U.S. population, are presented in Table 3–3 (Myers et al. 1984). Almost one in five persons, or 19.1%, in the population was found to have one or more DIS/DSM-III disorders, with a sampling standard error of 0.4%. As a group, the anxiety disorders were the most prevalent, with a rate of 8.9%—predominantly made up of the phobic disorders (7.7%) but also including panic disorder (0.8%) and obsessive-compulsive disorder (1.5%). Substance use disorders, which at 6.0% was the next most frequently found disorder group, consisted of alcohol abuse/dependence (4.7%) and drug abuse/dependence (2.0%), as well as the co-occurrence of both dis-

TABLE 3-3. **Estimate of 6-month prevalence of DIS/DSM-III disorders in the United States**

Disorder	Rate per 100 population	
Any DIS disorder covered	19.1%	(0.4)
Any DIS disorder except cognitive impairment and substance abuse	13.7	(0.4)
Substance use disorders	6.0	(0.3)
Alcohol abuse/dependence	4.7	(0.2)
Drug abuse/dependence	2.0	(0.1)
Schizophrenic/schizophreniform disorders	0.9	(0.1)
Schizophrenia	0.8	(0.1)
Schizophreniform disorder	0.1	(0.0)
Affective disorders	5.8	(0.3)
Manic episode	0.5	(0.1)
Major depressive episode	3.0	(0.2)
Dysthymia[a]	3.3	(0.2)
Anxiety disorders	8.9	(0.3)
Phobia	7.7	(0.3)
Panic disorder	0.8	(0.1)
Obsessive-compulsive disorder	1.5	(0.1)
Somatization disorder	0.1	(0.0)
Personality disorder (antisocial personality disorder)	0.8	(0.1)
Cognitive impairment[a] (severe)	1.3	(0.1)

Note. Data based on five Epidemiologic Catchment Area sites, standardized to 1980 U.S. census. DIS = Diagnostic Interview Schedule (Robins et al. 1981); DSM-III = *Diagnostic and Statistical Manual of Mental Disorders*, 3rd Edition (American Psychiatric Association 1980). Numbers in parentheses are standard errors.
[a]Because no recent information exists, the rates are the same for all prevalence time periods.

orders. The overall prevalence rate for affective disorders, at 5.8%, was not significantly different from those of the substance use disorders. A diagnosis of manic episode, necessary for meeting bipolar disorder criteria, was found in 0.5% of the population; major depressive episode in 3.0%; and dysthymia, requiring a 2-year duration of symptoms (without DIS onset information on the most recent occurrence), in 3.3%. Schizophrenia, requiring more than 6 months' duration of symptoms, was found in 0.8%, and schizophreniform disorder, requiring 2 weeks' to 6 months' duration, was found in 0.1%; an overall total for this group was 0.9%. Somatization disorder was the only somatoform disorder covered and was found almost exclusively in females and in just 0.1% of the total population. Antisocial personality disorder, the only personality disorder covered by the DIS, occurred at a rate of 0.8%, pre-

dominantly in young males under age 45. Finally, severe cognitive impairment on the Mini-Mental Status Examination component of the DIS was found in 1.3% of the total population, with rates rising from about 3% for those ages 65–74, and 7% for those ages 75–84, to almost 16% for those ages 85 and over (Regier et al. 1988a).

Use of Treatment Services

Use of health and mental health services for those persons with specific disorders and with any DIS disorder is represented in Table 3–4. For individuals with any DIS/DSM disorder in the past 6 months, 17.6% sought some type of mental health treatment from either a medical physician or a mental health specialist during the prior 6 months. For those without any mental disorder,

TABLE 3-4. **Estimate of any visit for mental health reasons to mental health specialist or medical physician over a 6-month period for persons with 6-month diagnosis of mental disorders**

Diagnosis	Any mental health visit	
No mental disorder	4.5%	(0.2)
Any DIS/DSM-III disorder	17.6	(0.9)
Any DIS/DSM-III disorder except cognitive impairment or substance abuse	22.0	(1.2)
Substance use disorder	12.4	(1.3)
Alcohol abuse/dependence	12.7	(1.5)
Drug abuse/dependence	11.0	(2.0)
Schizophrenia/schizophreniform disorders	48.1	(5.5)
Schizophrenia	48.6	(5.9)
Schizophreniform	43.8	(15.3)
Affective disorders	30.5	(2.1)
Manic episode	32.8	(6.9)
Major depressive episode	38.2	(2.8)
Dysthymia	24.2	(2.5)
Anxiety disorders	20.1	(1.3)
Phobia	18.6	(1.4)
Panic disorder	50.4	(5.4)
Obsessive-compulsive disorder	26.5	(4.2)
Somatization disorder	60.9	(9.0)
Personality disorder (antisocial personality disorder)	17.3	(4.0)
Severe cognitive impairment	6.6	(1.5)

Note. DIS = Diagnostic Interview Schedule (Robins et al. 1981); DSM-III = *Diagnostic and Statistical Manual of Mental Disorders*, 3rd Edition (American Psychiatric Association 1980). Numbers in parentheses are standard errors.

4.5% sought such mental health services.

There is marked variation in level of service use by type of mental disorder diagnosis. Individuals with alcohol abuse dependence or drug abuse dependence had a relatively low level of service use (i.e., 12.7% and 11%, respectively). Almost half (48.6%) of individuals with schizophrenia had received some type of mental health treatment in the prior 6 months. This level of service use was exceeded only by individuals with panic disorder (50.4%) and somatization disorder (60.9%). It should also be noted that 99% of individuals with somatization disorder had seen a general medical physician or mental health specialist during this 6-month period. Individuals with panic disorder had the second highest rate of overall medical/mental health utilization, with 85% having received some type of medical attention during the prior 6 months. This rate compares with an average overall rate of 55% for those with no mental disorder and 64% for those with any mental disorder. The affective disorders had intermediate levels of service use, with major depressive episode associated with a 38.2% level of service use, manic episode having a 32.8% level, and dysthymia having the lowest level of the affective disorders at 24.2%. As a group, the anxiety disorders have one of the highest levels of overall prevalence, as noted in Table 3–3, but are associated with one of the lowest service use rates. This low level of service use is primarily attributable to phobias, which have an 18.6% service use. Antisocial personality also results in a relatively low level of service use (17.3%), with severe cognitive impairment having the lowest level (6.6%), which is almost the same rate as that for those persons with no mental disorder (Shapiro et al. 1984).

To update the original 1978 estimate of mental health service use by the U.S. population (Figure 3–1), new estimates of the annual prevalence of mental disorders have been calculated based on the ECA data. Regier and colleagues (1993) estimate that 28.1% of the adult population have a mental disorder during any 1 year, compared with the earlier estimate of 15% of the population. Of this group with a 1-year disorder, only about one in four (28.5% of those with a 1-year DIS disorder) sought mental health or chemical dependency services. When the entire adult population is considered, 14.9% sought mental health or chemical dependency services.

Special Issues

In a reflection of the mutual interaction between epidemiology and nosology, Boyd and colleagues (1984) used the DIS information from the ECA to examine the co-occurrence of disorders. Their specific question was whether the pairs of disorders noted in DSM-III exclusion rules were more likely to occur than other pairs of disorders that had not been mentioned in DSM-III exclusion rules. The results indicated that although the hypothesized pairings from DSM-III were more likely to be demonstrated, pairings of all disorders were much more likely to occur than by chance, and a clear distinction between those disorders paired by DSM-III assumptions and those left unpaired in DSM-III could not be made.

One result of this demonstration was an effort to refine the exclusion rules in the revised version of DSM-III. Lifetime rates of mental disorders also demonstrated a decline in rates in older age groups, which occurred fairly constantly across specific disorder categories (Robins et al. 1984). Because those persons who are older have accumulated more experience and have passed through the age of risk for almost all disorders, it would be anticipated that their accumulated experience would be reflected in higher rates of lifetime illness than are found among younger subjects. Several possible explanations have been offered to account for this decline in lifetime prevalence rates with age. First, a tendency not to recall, or at least not to report, symptoms and other experience relevant to psychiatric disorders that occurred in younger life may be more common in older individuals than in younger ones. A second possible explanation is that those persons with severe psychiatric disorders have much higher mortality at younger ages, or other reasons to "leave the birth cohort," for example, by becoming homeless and much more difficult to track in a community survey. A third explanation, which is consistent with suggestive evidence from other studies, is that some disorders may be occurring more commonly in younger generations, such as possible increases of major depression as well as drug abuse and dependence. Analysis of reported onset of the major disorders covered by the DIS indicated that younger generations are experiencing earlier onset and higher rates of both major depression and drug abuse and dependence. This evidence is especially important in suggesting a possible causal link between adolescent depression and subsequent drug abuse. In fact, analysis of this link for young adults in the ECA suggested that early depression or anxiety doubled the subsequent risk of drug abuse/dependence (Christie et al. 1988).

The ECA data have also been used to identify population subgroups tending to have higher rates of disorders. Men and women were found to have approximately equal overall rates but to have significantly different rates of specific disorders. Rates of substance use disorders and antisocial personality disorder were significantly higher in males, whereas those for affective, anxiety, and somatization disorders were significantly higher in females. Because of the large contribution of the substance use, affective, and anxiety disorders, which are all found at higher rates under age 45, there is a significantly higher overall rate of disorders among the group under 45 years of age compared with the group 45 years and older. Evidence has also suggested that poverty is an independent risk factor for almost all of the specific mental disorders assessed in the ECA (Bruce et al. 1991).

Another striking finding has been the demonstration that for several disorders, peak onset occurs at earlier ages than had been thought. Although there are limitations to using retrospective recall of onset in a cross-sectional study, systematic examination of reported onset among ECA respondents with a history of a disorder suggests that adolescence and early adulthood are important time periods for development of many major mental disorders (Burke et al. 1990; Burke et al. 1994) (Table 3–5).

The early findings of increased co-occurrence of DSM-III disorders (Boyd et al. 1984) were amplified in an examination of the co-occurrence of mental disorders with alcohol and other drug use disorders. Among respondents with an alcohol disorder, 37% had a comorbid mental disorder; among those respondents with abuse or dependence of another drug besides alcohol, more than 50% had a comorbid mental disorder. In particular, respondents with schizophrenia, bipolar disorder, or antisocial personality disorder had elevated rates of both alcohol and drug use disorders. About 20% of individuals with a mental disorder who were seen in a specialty mental health clinic setting had a current diagnosis of substance abuse or dependence (Regier et al. 1990).

NATIONAL COMORBIDITY SURVEY

To examine the important finding from the ECA that co-occurrence of mental disorders was common, especially substance use disorders with other Axis I disorders, the U.S. Public Health Service funded a national survey to

investigate these associations further. This study, known as the National Comorbidity Survey (NCS) was conducted from 1990 to 1992 by investigators from the University of Michigan. The diagnostic instrument used was a modified version of the CIDI, the international interview schedule developed from the NIMH DIS, which allowed diagnoses to be generated using DSM-III-R criteria (American Psychiatric Association 1987). A sample representing the U.S. population from age 15 to 54 years was interviewed using this modified instrument, known as the CIDI-UM.

Prevalence Estimates

Findings from the NCS largely paralleled results from the ECA conducted a decade earlier using DSM-III criteria. But the most surprising difference was that NCS prevalence estimates using an interview designed for DSM-III-R are generally much higher than the ECA estimates. In the NCS, 48% of all respondents had a lifetime DSM-III-R disorder, and 29.5% had a disorder active in the 12 months prior to interview. The most common condition, major depressive episode, was found to occur on a lifetime basis in 17.1% of all NCS respondents, compared with 6.3% in the ECA. Prevalence rates for other common disorders in the NCS were alcohol dependence, found in 14.1% on a lifetime basis; social phobia, 13.3%; and simple phobia, 11.3% (Kessler et al. 1994).

To assess nonaffective psychoses, the NCS used a refined approach to diagnosis. Computer algorithms for diagnosis produced estimates of lifetime prevalence of 2.2% using broadly drawn categories and 1.3% for narrowly drawn categories. Clinicians then reviewed the data for NCS respondents who received a computer diagnosis of a narrowly defined category of nonaffective psychosis; of these, 10% were felt to have a "narrow" diagnosis of psychosis, and 37% were felt to have a broadly defined diagnosis. Final estimates of lifetime prevalence for nonaffective psychosis produced by these clinical reviewers ranged from 0.2% to 0.7% (Kendler et al. 1996).

For disorders whose prevalence estimates were generated by computer scoring, the high rates, compared with results from the earlier ECA study, have raised questions about variations in methods of assessment, and these methodologic questions are still unanswered.

Comorbidity

However, more striking than that disagreement on absolute prevalence rates is the confirmation of a high degree of comorbidity among various mental disorders. In the NCS, 56% of respondents with at least one lifetime disorder had

TABLE 3–5. **Median age at onset of selected mental disorders**

Disorder	Age (years)
Major depression (unipolar)	25
Bipolar illness	19
Panic disorder	24
Obsessive-compulsive disorder	23
Phobias	13
Drug abuse/dependence	18
Alcohol abuse/dependence	21

two or more disorders (Kessler et al. 1994). For major depressive disorder, only 26.0% of respondents with a lifetime history had this single diagnosis; for 61.8%, another DSM-III-R disorder had occurred before reported onset of the major depressive disorder. The most common type of disorder associated with major depressive disorder was an anxiety disorder, which was found in 58% of respondents with a history of major depressive disorder (Kessler et al. 1996a).

Comorbidity of mental and addictive disorders was also striking in the NCS, which found that 51% of those respondents with a substance use disorder on a lifetime basis also had a lifetime mental disorder. In most instances, for respondents with a lifetime history of co-occurring mental and substance disorders, the mental disorder occurred first (Kessler et al. 1996b).

Use of Services

As in the ECA, the NCS found that respondents with mental disorders, even those active in the past 12 months prior to interview, were unlikely to have received any professional attention. For respondents with a disorder reported active in the prior 12 months, only about 20% had received any professional help, only about 11% had received any help in the mental health sector, and only about 4% had received any help in a substance use treatment facility (Kessler et al. 1994).

In a comparison to population surveys conducted in Ontario, NCS investigators found that lifetime and 12-month prevalence estimates were higher for U.S. respondents than for Canadian respondents in the Ontario survey. They also found that use of outpatient services for any emotional problem was higher in the United States, particularly among those with no history of a mental disorder by the diagnostic interview used in the surveys. This difference suggests that in the United States, people with "low level of need for services" produce a higher probability of use of services compared with Canada (Kessler et al. 1997).

RISK FACTORS FOR SPECIFIC DISORDERS

Comparison of results is important in science generally, especially in epidemiological research. First, *replication* is a fundamental principle to confirm the validity of findings. Also, when there are *differences* in findings, and methodological variations are ruled out as the explanation, epidemiologists may be able to capitalize on these differences by identifying high-risk groups across studies, even

if group differences have not been found within a population studied. For both purposes, assessing replication and undertaking a search for differences, comparing epidemiological findings across sites and across studies is important in development of the field. In psychiatry, these comparisons have been hampered by the need to assume that diagnoses are comparable across studies, or at least that their differences are known, usually without clear evidence that this assumption is fully justified. Nevertheless, for several major groups of disorders, critical comparisons of epidemiological research in the past decade have helped identify high-risk groups, and sometimes the magnitude of associated risk factors has been quantified as well.

SCHIZOPHRENIA

In reviewing epidemiological studies of schizophrenia conducted in Europe, Jablensky (1986) concluded that point prevalence rates can be estimated to vary from 2.5 to 5.3 per 1,000, and annual incidence rates from 0.2 to 0.6 per 1,000. These figures represent a definitive summary of literature published in a variety of languages. Several studies outside Europe are consistent with these findings. An independent clinical examination of DSM-III schizophrenia in a sample derived from the NIMH ECA in Baltimore found a point prevalence of 6.4 per 1,000 adults, including both active and remitted cases at the time of interview (von Korff et al. 1985). In remote villages in Botswana, the annual period prevalence of DSM-III schizophrenia was estimated to be 4.3 per 1,000 adults (Ben-Tovim and Cushnie 1986). In a multinational study conducted in 10 countries, Sartorius and colleagues (1986) found an annual rate of first service contact for a "broad" definition of schizophrenia ranging from 0.15 to 0.42 per 1,000 population at risk, which is consistent with earlier estimates of annual disease incidence.

However, some pockets of increased prevalence appear to exist, based on studies reporting higher rates in Ireland, in arctic areas of Sweden, and in the Croatian areas of what was at that time Yugoslavia; some areas of lower prevalence, such as in the Hutterite community of the United States and in Papua, New Guinea, have also been reported. At present, it is not clear whether these reported geographic variations result from different study design, concentration through genetic transmission in isolated population groups, or some other influence; for example, reanalysis of data from some classic multinational studies conducted by the World Health Organization suggested that the risk of developing schizophrenia was positively related to mean environmental temperature (Gupta and Murray 1992). Other data have been difficult to interpret, and investigators disagree about the extent of any variation in Ireland, for example (Torrey 1994).

Considering these geographic variations as well as possible increases in the past two centuries, Torrey (1980) has suggested that the disorder may be related to some aspect of modern industrialized life (e.g., easier transmission of viruses). The evidence has been inconsistent, but an intriguing finding from some studies has been the suggestion that development of schizophrenia is related to maternal exposure to influenza in the second trimester (Mednick et al. 1988; O'Callaghan 1991b; Sham et al. 1992). Some studies have indicated that individuals with schizophrenia have a predominance of winter births (O'Callaghan et al. 1991a). Others have suggested that the apparent increase in recognition of the disorder over the past two centuries could be explained more easily as a result of the change in disease concepts, in both psychiatry and society (Jablensky 1986). In social terms, for example, Cooper and Sartorius (1977) have hypothesized that industrialization removes the relatively benign influence of preindustrialized life on the family and social structures that could support the individual with this disorder, so the disease becomes more apparent in industrialized societies.

In general, prevalence rates have been roughly equal for males and females, although there is evidence that males have an earlier age at onset (Flor-Henry 1985). In two reports of community populations other than those of the ECA, females have had a higher prevalence rate when remitted as well as active or treated cases are counted. Possibly the best-known risk factor is genetic, as first-degree relatives have been shown to have a higher risk of developing schizophrenia themselves. The genetic contribution was first distinguished from possible environmental influences by Kety and colleagues (1968), who used a case control design to study offspring of schizophrenic parents who had been adopted early and raised away from their biological parents. Even these genetic studies do not, however, provide an exhaustive explanation. Monozygotic twins share the illness in only about 40%–50% of cases, according to one of the most rigorous studies of this topic (Gottesman and Shields 1972).

DEPRESSIVE ILLNESS

Examining the world literature on prevalence of affective disorders just before the ECA began, Boyd and Weissman (1981) found generally consistent prevalence rates in studies within industrialized nations. They reported the point prevalence of unipolar depression as about 3 per 100 adult males and about 4–9 per 100 adult females. However, in a study of two Ugandan villages

based on results from the PSE (Orley and Wing 1979), much higher rates were found: 14.3 per 100 males and 22.6 per 100 females. To date, these higher rates in Africa have not been explained.

Although considerable research on risk factors and genetic transmission has been conducted in clinical populations for both unipolar depression and bipolar illness, epidemiological studies of community populations have suggested two intriguing leads for more research. In a variety of studies, prevalence rates of unipolar depression for females have been approximately twice as high as those for men. Because this female predominance is shown in community as well as in clinical settings, it cannot be attributed to a greater tendency for females to visit clinical facilities. At present, the range of possible explanations for this female predominance extends from hypotheses about the socioeconomic status of women in industrialized societies to hormonal, genetic, and other biological factors. Specific work by Brown and Harris (1978) has implicated the occurrence of adverse life events as a contributing factor to depression, and ECA data suggest an interaction between adverse events and early childhood experiences such as parental separation/divorce (Landerman et al. 1991). One analysis of ECA data has suggested that poor outcome in women, especially older women, may also contribute to the higher prevalence rates in women (Sargeant et al. 1990). In further analysis of the New Haven data, Weissman (1985) found the highest rates of depressive illness among unhappily married men and women, and Bruce et al. (1990) found higher rates of depressive episodes and dysphoria following conjugal bereavement.

A second hypothesis from epidemiological data is that depression may be increasing among younger generations. The suggestion was first made by Klerman (1976), and suggestive evidence has been offered by Hagnell and colleagues (1982) in Sweden, who examined trends over 25 years in a long-term community study of mental disorders. Skeptics have suggested that technical factors, such as poor reliability and growing sophistication of respondents in identifying and reporting their past symptoms, may at least partly explain the finding. Häffner (1985) has suggested that it is not illness that is increasing in the young but pessimism in their elders. However, analysis of several data sets has suggested that depressive illness has occurred more frequently, or has had onset at an earlier age, in generations born since World War II (Burke et al. 1991; Klerman and Weissman 1989).

Follow-up data on the original ECA samples in two sites have indicated that depressive illness may be a risk factor for heart disease (Pratt 1996) and for higher mortality in general (Bruce 1994).

ANXIETY DISORDERS

Recent epidemiological studies of anxiety disorders have provided evidence of their high frequency in the general population. In a comprehensive review of major community surveys conducted since 1969, Marks (1986) found that point prevalence rates for all anxiety disorders ranged from 2.9 to 8.4 per 100. In terms of specific disorders, the rates ranged from 1.2 to 3.8 per 100 for agoraphobia; 4.1 to 7.0 per 100 for simple phobia; 1.8 to 2.5 per 100 for obsessive-compulsive disorder; and 0.4 to 3.1 per 100 for panic disorder.

One striking point about these figures is that anxiety disorders appear to be more common in community populations than in clinical settings. This finding reflects evidence like that from the ECA indicating that only 15%–23% of those with an anxiety disorder in the prior 6 months received any clinical care for their condition. In the case of obsessive-compulsive disorder, for example, Karno et al. (1988) have noted that the epidemiological data suggest that this disorder is 25–60 times more common than had been thought on the basis of studies in clinical populations. In addition, the low rate of treatment changes the impression of the relative importance of particular anxiety disorders. For example, Marks notes that in one study agoraphobia accounted for 50% of cases of anxiety seen in treatment settings but only 8% of cases in the general population of that area. The existence of large groups of individuals with diagnosable anxiety disorders makes it difficult to generalize results from studies using only patient populations.

In particular, such questions as the extent of comorbidity (e.g., the extent to which panic disorder co-occurs with agoraphobia or with major depression) need to be studied in a community population. Initial findings suggested that panic disorder commonly occurs without agoraphobia, but later reappraisal of these findings led some investigators to suggest that the apparent lack of co-occurrence with agoraphobia resulted from misidentification of the disorders by the DIS (Horwath 1993). However, findings similar to those from the ECA were also obtained in the NCS, which reported that half the subjects with diagnosable panic disorder had no symptoms of agoraphobia (Eaton 1994). For obsessive-compulsive disorder, a prospective follow-up of a birth cohort to age 18 found that it was highly comorbid with major depressive disorder, which occurred in 62% of subjects with obsessive-compulsive disorder (Douglass 1995).

Another issue raised by the existence of large groups with disorders not yet well studied, such as phobia or generalized anxiety disorder, is whether these individuals need treatment. Diagnostic criteria such as those in DSM-III do not provide guidance for such questions of clinical judgment, and some doubt has been expressed about the meaning of high community rates of phobias in the ECA, for example. This point may become less controversial as therapeutic methods are employed more widely, such as behavior therapy for phobias. Analysis of ECA data on social phobia demonstrated that it causes distress and impairment and that 69% of respondents with this disorder also had another comorbid mental disorder on a lifetime basis. Recent population studies of social phobia have suggested that specific symptoms such as fear of public speaking may be highly related to school failure and dropout (Stein 1996). But this disorder is rarely treated by mental health professionals (Schneier et al. 1992).

An especially interesting aspect of anxiety disorders is the early age at onset reported in studies such as the ECA. Continuity of childhood disorders, such as separation anxiety and school phobia, with "adult" anxiety disorders that appear in adolescence or early adulthood seems a promising area for study.

SUBSTANCE ABUSE

Because drug abuse typically involves illicit use of drugs, some authorities believe that community surveys may have limitations in studying this problem. For some drugs, notably heroin, an alternative strategy has been to rely on treated incidence or prevalence rates. For some other drugs, such as marijuana, the interest of some investigators has centered on any reported use of the drug, both to assess exposure for possible chronic use and to determine the potential of moving from this "gateway" into a lifestyle of abusing other drugs as well. In terms of any reported use, studies would focus on single events, rather than a pattern of use that persists or otherwise crosses the threshold for diagnosis in the criteria for abuse and dependence in DSM-III.

Following such arguments, Kozel and Adams (1986) suggested that treated incidence of heroin abuse, as measured by first admissions to federally funded treatment programs, showed a large increase from 1965 to 1970, with a general decline since that time except for transient increases in the mid-1970s and around 1980. These authors used these data and other indirect measures to suggest that most heroin users in the mid-1980s were males in their mid-30s who began abusing the drug in the mid-1960s to mid-1970s. Using data from questionnaires administered to high school seniors, Kozel and Adams also estimated that daily marijuana use in the month prior to the survey steadily declined from a high of 10.7% in 1978 to 4.9% in 1985.

Several recent studies have attempted to identify risk factors for drug use and abuse. Adolescents with a cluster of interpersonal difficulties, such as social isolation, have been reported by Newcomb and colleagues (1986) to have higher rates of drug use than do their peers. Using data from the ECA, Christie and colleagues (1988) have shown that young adults with a history of major depression or anxiety disorders have about twice the risk of subsequent DSM-III drug abuse and dependence as do those without these prior disorders. By studying adoptees, Cadoret and colleagues (1986) provided evidence that adults with drug abuse were more likely to have had biological parents with alcohol problems or antisocial personality, or adoptive parents who divorced or had psychiatric problems. These early leads from studies conducted within a framework of analytic epidemiology suggest that further specification of risk factors for drug abuse and dependence may be possible despite the presumed difficulties of studying these conditions in traditional epidemiological designs.

In the NCS, Warner and colleagues (1995) found that the most recent birth cohort (aged 15–24 years) is less likely to use illicit drugs, but the users are more likely to become dependent. They also found that first use of drugs occurs most commonly in the age range of 15–19 years. These authors emphasize that different strategies may be useful in trying to reduce use, abuse, and dependence, because different mechanisms may lead to different stages in the progression from first use to dependence.

For alcohol abuse and dependence, Helzer and colleagues (1990) found wide variation among different cultures in the standardized lifetime prevalence of alcohol dependence (from 1.5% in Taiwanese metropolitan areas to 11.3% in Edmonton, Alberta, Canada). But they found similarity in age at onset, symptoms, and risk factors such as male gender, antisocial personality, and major depression.

PERSONALITY DISORDERS

Epidemiological study of personality disorders has been hampered by the difficulty in assessing these conditions, especially when using standardized instruments in nonclinical populations (Burke and Burke 1992; Widiger and Weissman 1991). The only personality disorder studied in the ECA was antisocial personality, as the original DSM-III criteria permitted assessment by a structured interview like the DIS. The 6-month prevalence rate was 0.8%, with predominance in males under age 45.

Risk factors for antisocial personality have been examined in a variety of longitudinal studies, especially in view of the probable but not inevitable continuity between childhood conduct disorder and adult antisocial personality (American Psychiatric Association 1987; Robins and Price 1991). Using data from the ECA, Robins and Price have suggested that a reported history of childhood conduct problems leads to higher rates of many psychiatric disorders in both men and women. Because the ECA also suggested that conduct problems in childhood have been more common in younger cohorts, these authors raised the possibility that increased rates of major depression may be related to the apparent rise in childhood conduct problems (Robins and Price 1991). Analysis of a Danish cohort of 18- to 21-year-old males born in the period from 1959 to 1961 suggested that having an alcoholic father did not raise the risk of adult antisocial personality, but that having been physically abused as a child was a risk factor for aggressive and antisocial behaviors (Pollock et al. 1990). Findings from these two studies suggest that interventions in childhood to reduce physical abuse and conduct problems may be helpful in reducing the development of antisocial personality disorder in adulthood.

Another disorder of major importance that has received much attention in clinical research is borderline personality disorder. Epidemiological data on this condition are sparse, especially because the disorder is difficult to assess on a cross-sectional basis in large community samples with nonclinician interviewers. (The ECA, for example, did not attempt to measure the occurrence of this disorder.) Widiger and Weissman (1991) have summarized existing studies that suggest a current prevalence rate between 0.2% and 1.8% in the general population. These authors reported that in clinical populations the rate may be about 15% for psychiatric inpatients and 50% for inpatients with a diagnosis of personality disorder. The diagnosis of borderline personality disorder is made more commonly in females, and about 73%–80% of patients are reported to be female (Widiger and Weissman 1991). In contrast, a recent Danish study of first-admission diagnoses from 1970 to 1985 showed no sex difference, but did suggest a cohort effect, with patients ages 15–34 showing the predominant increase. Whether these results reflect a true change in addition to changes in diagnostic practices is not certain (Mors 1988). Whether the diagnostic criteria permit clear delineation of a diagnostic condition has been questioned; for example, in one outpatient study in which a semistructured interview was used, the diagnosis of borderline personality was shown to have multiple overlaps with other personality disorders (Nurnberg et al. 1991). Without specific boundaries and useful criteria, diagnostic categories might be too diffuse to yield useful information about risk factors in epidemiological studies.

One Axis II disorder that may be specified well enough for epidemiological study is histrionic personality disorder.

Psychiatrists from the Baltimore ECA team conducted a separate interview with respondents chosen from the ECA sample, and reported a current prevalence of 2.1% for this disorder. They did not find any difference in rates between males and females, unlike in studies based on clinical samples. Women in this sample given diagnoses of histrionic personality disorder also had an elevated rate of major depression and of unexplained medical symptoms; men had elevated rates of substance use disorders (Nestadt et al. 1990). In the same study, obsessive-compulsive personality disorder was ascertained, and an overall rate of 1.7% was found. Males received the diagnosis five times more commonly than did females; the condition was found to be associated with anxiety disorders but was associated with a reduction in alcohol use disorders (Nestadt et al. 1991).

A 10-year follow-up study of children selected randomly from a community population showed that conduct problems were a strong predictor of later development of a personality disorder in any one of the three clusters used for classification by DSM-III-R. In boys, depressive symptoms predicted emergence of a Cluster A disorder, and in girls, immaturity predicted a Cluster B disorder (Bernstein 1996).

In Finland, a population based study of suicides by patients with personality disorders found that all of them had a coexisting Axis I disorder, and in 95% of them the disorder included major depressive disorder or a substance use disorder (Isometsä 1996).

CONCLUSIONS

As the improvements in nosology and diagnostic assessment have led to rapid progress in psychiatric research in the past 15 years, they have also provided the "missing ingredient" for which psychiatric epidemiologists have been searching for 30 years (Dohrenwend and Dohrenwend 1982). Now that large-scale community surveys have been able to lay a foundation of descriptive knowledge about basic distributions of specific mental disorders in the population, the field is poised for the next stage of research: to improve understanding of diseases by precise investigation of internal and external validating criteria of nosologic categories and elucidation of etiologic mechanisms (Freedman 1984). The unique contributions of epidemiological methods to these pursuits have been acknowledged in medicine as a whole by development of disciplines such as clinical epidemiology and genetic epidemiology (Feinstein 1985). In addition to its long-standing concern with improved public health through preventive efforts

and improved delivery of treatment services, psychiatric epidemiology has arrived at a point at which it can make substantial contributions to the most vital areas of psychiatric research and clinical practice in the next decade.

REFERENCES

American Psychiatric Association: Diagnostic and Statistical Manual: Mental Disorders. Washington, DC, American Psychiatric Association, 1952

American Psychiatric Association: Diagnostic and Statistical Manual of Mental Disorders, 3rd Edition. Washington, DC, American Psychiatric Association, 1980

American Psychiatric Association: Diagnostic and Statistical Manual of Mental Disorders, 3rd Edition, Revised. Washington, DC, American Psychiatric Association, 1987

American Psychiatric Association: Diagnostic and Statistical Manual of Mental Disorders, 4th Edition. Washington, DC, American Psychiatric Association, 1994

Ben-Tovim DI, Cushnie JM: The prevalence of schizophrenia in a remote area of Botswana. Br J Psychiatry 148:576–580, 1986

Berkson H: Limitations of the application of fourfold table analysis to hospital data. Biometrics Bulletin 2:47–53, 1946

Bernstein DP, Cohen P, Skodol A, et al: Childhood Antecedents of Adolescent Personality Disorders. Am J Psychiatry 153:907—913, 1996

Boyd JH, Weissman MM: Epidemiology of affective disorders: a reexamination and future directions. Arch Gen Psychiatry 38:1039–1046, 1981

Boyd JH, Burke JD Jr, Gruenberg E, et al: Exclusion criteria of DSM-III: a study of co-occurrence of hierarchy-free syndromes. Arch Gen Psychiatry 41:983–989, 1984

Boyle MH, Offord DR, Campbell D, et al: Mental health supplement to the Ontario Health Survey: Methodology. Can J Psychiatry 41:549–558, 1996

Brown GW, Harris T: Social Origins of Depression: A Study of Psychiatric Disorder in Women. Tavistock, London, 1978

Bruce ML, Kim K, Leaf PJ, et al: Depressive episodes and dysphoria resulting from conjugal bereavement in a prospective community sample. Am J Psychiatry 147:608–611, 1990

Bruce ML, Takeuchi DT, Leaf PJ: Poverty and psychiatric status: longitudinal evidence from the New Haven Epidemiologic Catchment Area Study. Arch Gen Psychiatry 48:470–474, 1991

Bruce ML, Leaf PJ, Rozal GPM, et al: Psychiatric Status and 9-Year Mortality Data in the New Haven Epidemiologic Catchment Area Study. Am J Psychiatry 151:716–721, 1994

Burke JD Jr: Diagnostic categorization by the Diagnostic Interview Schedule (DIS): a comparison with other methods of assessment, in Mental Disorders in the Community. Edited by Barrett JE, Rose RM. New York, Guilford, 1986, pp 255–279

Burke JD Jr, Burke KC: Diagnostic interviews in psychiatric epidemiology (Chapter 23), in Psychiatry. Edited by Michels R. Philadelphia, PA, JB Lippincott, 1992

Burke JD: Mental Health Services Research, in Textbook in Psychiatric Epidemiology. Edited by Tsuang MT, Tohen M, Zahner GEP: New York, Wiley-Liss, 1995, pp 199–209

Burke KC, Burke JD Jr, Regier DA, et al: Age at onset of selected mental disorders in five community populations. Arch Gen Psychiatry 47:511–518, 1990

Burke KC, Burke JD Jr, Rae DS, et al: Comparing age at onset of major depression and other psychiatric disorders by birth cohorts in five US community populations. Arch Gen Psychiatry 48:789–795, 1991

Burke JD, Burke KC, Rae DS: Increased Rates of Drug Abuse and Dependence After Onset of Mood or Anxiety Disorders in Adolescence. Hospital and Community Psychiatry 45:451–455, 1994

Cadoret RJ, Troughton E, O'Gorman TW, et al: An adoption study of genetic and environmental factors in drug abuse. Arch Gen Psychiatry 43:1131–1136, 1986

Christie KA, Burke JD, Regier DA, et al: Epidemiologic evidence for early onset of mental disorders and higher risk of drug abuse in young adults. Am J Psychiatry 145:971–975, 1988

Commission on Chronic Illness: Chronic Illness in the United States, Vol 4: Chronic Illness in a Large City. Cambridge, MA, Harvard University Press, 1957

Cooper JE, Sartorius N: Cultural and temporal variations in schizophrenia: a speculation on the importance of industrialization. Br J Psychiatry 130:50–55, 1977

Cooper JE, Kendell RE, Gurland BJ, et al: Psychiatric Diagnosis in New York and London: A Comparative Study of Mental Hospital Admissions. London, Oxford University Press, 1972

Dohrenwend BP, Dohrenwend BS: Perspectives on the past and future of psychiatric epidemiology (The 1981 Rema Lapouse Lecture). Am J Public Health 72:1271–1279, 1982

Douglass HM, Moffitt TE, Dar R, et al: Obsessive-Compulsive Disorder in a Birth Cohort of 18-Year-Olds: Prevalence and Predictors. J Am Acad Child Adolesc Psychiatry 34:1424–1431, 1995

Eaton WW, Kessler RC, Wittchen H-U, et al: Panic and Panic Disorder in the United States. Am J Psychiatry 151:413–420, 1994

Endicott J, Spitzer RL: A diagnostic interview: the Schedule for Affective Disorders and Schizophrenia. Arch Gen Psychiatry 35:837–844, 1978

Faraone SV, Tsuang MT: Measuring Diagnostic Accuracy in the Absence of a Gold Standard. Am J Psychiatry 151:650–657, 1994

Feighner JP, Robins E, Guze SB, et al: Diagnostic criteria for use in psychiatric research. Arch Gen Psychiatry 26:57–63, 1972

Feinstein A: Clinical Epidemiology. Philadelphia, WB Saunders, 1985

Fleiss JL: Statistical Methods for Rates and Proportions, 2nd Edition. New York, Wiley, 1981

Flor-Henry P: Schizophrenia: sex differences. Can J Psychiatry 30:319–322, 1985

Freedman DX: Psychiatric epidemiology counts (editorial). Arch Gen Psychiatry 41:931–933, 1984

Gottesman II, Shields J: Schizophrenia and Genetics: A Twin-Study Vantage Point. New York, Academic, 1972

Gupta S, Murray RM: The relationship of environmental temperature to the incidence and outcome of schizophrenia. Br J Psychiatry 160:788–792, 1992

Häffner H: Are mental disorders increasing over time? Psychopathology 18:66–81, 1985

Hagnell O, Lanke J, Rorsman B, et al: Are we entering an age of melancholy? Depressive illness in a prospective epidemiological study over 25 years: the Lundby Study, Sweden. Psychol Med 12:279–289, 1982

Helzer JE, Canino GJ, Yeh E-K, et al: Alcoholism—North America and Asia: a comparison of population surveys with the Diagnostic Interview Schedule. Arch Gen Psychiatry 47:313–319, 1990

Hoeper EW, Nycz GR, Cleary PD, et al: Estimated prevalence of RDC mental disorder in primary medical care. International Journal of Mental Health 8:6–15, 1979

Hollingshead AB, Redlich FC: Social Class and Mental Illness: A Community Study. New York, Wiley, 1958

Horwath E, Lish JD, Johnson J, et al: Agoraphobia Without Panic: Clinical Reappraisal of an Epidemiologic Finding. Am J Psychiatry 150:1496–1501, 1993

Isometsä ET, Henriksson MM, Keikkinen ME, et al: Suicide Among Subjects With Personality Disorders. Am J Psychiatry 1996; 153:667–673

Jablensky A: Epidemiology of schizophrenia: a European perspective. Schizophr Bull 12:52–73, 1986

Kamerow DB, Pincus HA, Macdonald DI: Alcohol abuse, other drug abuse, and mental disorders in medical practice: prevalence, costs, recognition, and treatment. JAMA 255:2054–2057, 1986

Karno M, Golding JM, Sorenson SB, et al: The epidemiology of obsessive-compulsive disorder in five US communities. Arch Gen Psychiatry 45:1094–1099, 1988

Katon W, Schulberg HC: Epidemiology of depression in primary care. Gen Hosp Psychiatry 14:237–247, 1992

Kendler KS, McGuire M, Gruenberg AM, et al: An Epidemiologic, Clinical, and Family Study of Simple Schizophrenia in County Roscommon, Ireland. Am J Psychiatry 151:27–34, 1994

Kendler KS, Gallagher J, Abelson JM, et al: Lifetime Prevalence, Demographic Risk Factors, and Diagnostic Validity of Nonaffective Psychosis as Assessed in a U.S. Community Sample. Arch Gen Psychiatry 53:1022–1031, 1996

Kessler RC, McGonagle KA, Ahao S, et al: Lifetime and 12-month prevalence of DSM-III-R psychiatric disorders in the United States: Results from the National Comorbidity Survey. Arch Gen Psychiatry 51:8—10, 1994

Kessler RC, Nelson CB, McGonagle KA, et al: Comorbidity of DSM-III-R Major Depressive Disorder in the General Population: Results frm the US National Comorbidity Survey. Br J Psychiatry 168 (suppl 30):17–30, 1996a

Kessler RC, Nelson CB, McGonagle KA, et al: The Epidemiology of Co-occurring Addictive and Mental Disorders: Implications for Prevention and Service Utilization. Am J Orthopsychiatry 66:17—31, 1996b

Kessler RC, Frank RG, Edlund M, et al: Differences in the Use of Psychiatric Outpatient Services Between the United States and Ontario. N Engl J Med 336:551—557, 1997

Kety SS, Rosenthal D, Wender PH, et al: The types and prevalence of mental illness in the biological and adoptive families of adopted schizophrenics, in The Transmission of Schizophrenia. Edited by Rosenthal D, Kety SS. Oxford, UK, Pergamon, 1968, pp 345–362

Klerman GL: Age and clinical depression: today's youth in the twenty-first century. J Gerontol 31:318–323, 1976

Klerman GL: Diagnosis of psychiatric disorders in epidemiologic field studies. Arch Gen Psychiatry 42:723–724, 1985

Klerman GL, Weissman MM: Increasing rates of depression. JAMA 261:2229–2235, 1989

Kozel NJ, Adams EH: Epidemiology of drug abuse: an overview. Science 234:970–974, 1986

Landerman R, George LK, Blazer DG: Adult vulnerability for psychiatric disorders: interactive effects of negative childhood experiences and recent stress. J Nerv Ment Dis 179:656–663, 1991

Leighton DC, Harding JS, Macklin DB, et al: The Character of Danger: Psychiatric Symptoms in Selected Communities. New York, Basic Books, 1963

Luchins DJ: Computed tomography in schizophrenia: disparities in the prevalence of abnormalities. Arch Gen Psychiatry 39:859–860, 1982

Marks IM: Epidemiology of anxiety. Social Psychiatry 21:167–171, 1986

Mednick SA, Machon RA, Huttunen MO, et al: Adult schizophrenia following prenatal exposure to an influenza epidemic. Arch Gen Psychiatry 45:189–192, 1988

Morgenstern H, Bursic ES: A method for using epidemiologic data to estimate the potential impact of an intervention on the health status of a target population. J Community Health 7:292–309, 1982

Morris JN: Uses of Epidemiology, 2nd Edition. Baltimore, MD, Williams & Wilkins, 1964

Mors O: Increasing incidence of borderline states in Denmark from 1970–1985. Acta Psychiatr Scand 77:575–583, 1988

Murphy JM: Continuities in community-based psychiatric epidemiology. Arch Gen Psychiatry 37:1215–1223, 1980

Myers JK, Weissman MM, Tischler GL, et al: Six-month prevalence of psychiatric disorders in three communities: 1980 to 1982. Arch Gen Psychiatry 41:959–967, 1984

Nestadt G, Romanoski AJ, Chahal R, et al: An epidemiological study of histrionic personality disorder. Psychol Med 20:413–422, 1990

Nestadt G, Romanoski AJ, Brown CH, et al: DSM-III compulsive personality disorder: an epidemiological survey. Psychol Med 21:461–471, 1991

Newcomb MD, Maddahian E, Bentler PM: Risk factors for drug use among adolescents: concurrent and longitudinal analyses. Am J Public Health 76:525–531, 1986

Nurnberg HG, Raskin M, Levine PE, et al: The comorbidity of borderline personality disorder and other DSM-III-R Axis II personality disorders. Am J Psychiatry 148:1371–1377, 1991

O'Callaghan E, Gibson T, Colohan HA, et al: Season of birth in schizophrenia: evidence for confinement of an excess of winter births to patients without a family history of mental disorder. Br J Psychiatry 158:764–769, 1991a

O'Callaghan E, Sham P, Takei N, et al: Schizophrenia after prenatal exposure to 1957 A2 influenza epidemic. Lancet 337:1248–1250, 1991b

Orley J, Wing JK: Psychiatric disorders in two African villages. Arch Gen Psychiatry 36:513–520, 1979

Pollock VE, Briere J, Schneider L, et al: Childhood antecedents of antisocial behavior: parental alcoholism and physical abusiveness. Am J Psychiatry 147:1290–1293, 1990

Pratt LA, Ford DE, Crum RM, et al: Depression, psychotropic medication, and risk of myocardial infarction: prospective data from the Baltimore ECA follow-up. Circulation 94:3123–3129, 1996

Regier DA, Goldberg ID, Taube CA: The de facto US mental health services system: a public health perspective. Arch Gen Psychiatry 35:685–693, 1978

Regier DA, Myers JK, Kramer M, et al: The NIMH Epidemiologic Catchment Area Program: historical context, major objectives, and study population characteristics. Arch Gen Psychiatry 41:934–941, 1984

Regier DA, Boyd JH, Burke JD Jr, et al: One-month prevalence of mental disorders in the United States—based on five Epidemiologic Catchment Area sites. Arch Gen Psychiatry 45:977–986, 1988a

Regier DA, Hirschfeld RMA, Goodwin FK, et al: The NIMH Depression Awareness, Recognition, and Treatment Program: structure, aims, and scientific basis. Am J Psychiatry 145:1351–1357, 1988b

Regier DA, Farmer ME, Rae DS, et al: Comorbidity of mental disorders with alcohol and other drug abuse: results from the Epidemiologic Catchment Area (ECA) Study. JAMA 264:2511–2518, 1990

Regier DA, Narrow WE, Rae DS, et al: The de facto US Mental and Addictive Disorders Service System: Epidemiologic Catchment Area prospective 1-year prevalence rates of disorders and services. Arch Gen Psychiatry 50:85–94, 1993

Robins LN: Epidemiology: reflections on testing the validity of psychiatric interviews. Arch Gen Psychiatry 42:918–924, 1985

Robins LN, Price RK: Adult disorders predicted by childhood conduct problems: results from the NIMH Epidemiologic Catchment Area Project. Psychiatry 54:116–132, 1991

Robins LN, Regier DA (eds): Psychiatric Disorders in America: The Epidemiologic Catchment Area Study. New York, Free Press, 1991

Robins LN, Helzer JE, Croughan J, et al: National Institute of Mental Health Diagnostic Interview Schedule: its history, characteristics, and validity. Arch Gen Psychiatry 38:381–389, 1981

Robins LN, Helzer JE, Ratcliff KS, et al: Validity of the Diagnostic Interview Schedule, Version II: DSM-III diagnoses. Psychol Med 12:855–870, 1982

Robins LN, Helzer JE, Weissman MM, et al: Lifetime prevalence of specific psychiatric disorders in three sites. Arch Gen Psychiatry 41:949–958, 1984

Robins LN, Wing J, Wittchen HU, et al: The Composite International Diagnostic Interview: an epidemiologic instrument suitable for use in conjunction with different diagnostic systems and in different cultures. Arch Gen Psychiatry 45:1069–1077, 1988

Sackett DL, Haynes RB, Tugwell P: Clinical Epidemiology: A Basic Science for Clinical Medicine. Philadelphia, PA, Lippincott-Raven, 1991

Sargeant JK, Bruce ML, Florio LP, et al: Factors associated with 1-year outcome of major depression in the community. Arch Gen Psychiatry 47:519–526, 1990

Sartorius N, Jablensky A, Korten A, et al: Early manifestations and first-contact incidence of schizophrenia in different cultures. Psychol Med 16:909–928, 1986

Schneier FR, Johnson J, Hornig CD, et al: Social phobia: comorbidity and morbidity in an epidemiologic sample. Arch Gen Psychiatry 49:282–288, 1992

Sham PC, O'Callaghan E, Takei N, et al: Schizophrenia following pre-natal exposure to influenza epidemics between 1939 and 1960. Br J Psychiatry 160:461–466, 1992

Shapiro S, Skinner EA, Kessler LG, et al: Utilization of health and mental health services: three Epidemiologic Catchment Area sites. Arch Gen Psychiatry 41:971–978, 1984

Shrout PE, Spitzer RL, Fleiss JL: Quantification of agreement in psychiatric diagnosis revisited. Arch Gen Psychiatry 44:172–177, 1987

Spitzer RL, Williams JBW, Gibbon M, et al: The Structured Clinical Interview for DSM-III-R (SCID), I: history, rationale, and description. Arch Gen Psychiatry 49:624–629, 1992

Spitznagel EL, Helzer JE: A proposed solution to the base rate problem in the kappa statistic. Arch Gen Psychiatry 42:725–728, 1985

Srole L, Langner TS, Michael ST, et al: Mental Health in the Metropolis: The Midtown Manhattan Study. New York, McGraw-Hill, 1962

Stallones RA: The concept of cause in disease. Journal of Chronic Diseases 40:279, 1987

Stein MB, Walker JR, Forde DR: Public-speaking fears in a community sample: prevalence, impact on functioning, and diagnostic classification. Arch Gen Psychiatry 53:169–174, 1996

Torrey EF: Schizophrenia and Civilization. New York, Jason Aronson, 1980

Torrey EF: The Prevalence of Schizophrenia in Ireland (letter, with reply by Kendler KS, Walsh D). Arch Gen Psychiatry 51:513–515, 1994

von Korff M, Nestadt G, Romanoski A, et al: Prevalence of treated and untreated DSM-III schizophrenia: results of a two-stage community survey. J Nerv Ment Dis 173:577–581, 1985

Warner LA, Kessler RC, Hughes M, et al: Prevalence and correlates of drug use and dependence in the United States: results from the National Comorbidity Survey. Arch Gen Psychiatry 52:219–229, 1995

Weissman MM: Presentation of the 1985 Rema Lapouse Mental Health Epidemiology Award at the special award session of the American Public Health Association Annual Meeting, Washington, DC, November 1985

Weissman MM, Myers JK, Harding PS: Psychiatric disorders in a U.S. urban community: 1975–1976. Am J Psychiatry 135:459–462, 1978

Widiger TA, Weissman MM: Epidemiology of borderline personality disorder. Hospital and Community Psychiatry 42:1015–1021, 1991

Williams JBW, Gibbon M, First MB, et al: The Structured Clinical Interview for DSM-III-R (SCID), II: multisite test-retest reliability. Arch Gen Psychiatry 49:630–636, 1992

Wing JK, Cooper JE, Sartorius N: Measurement and Classification of Psychiatric Symptoms. New York, Cambridge University Press, 1974

Wing JK, Bebbington PE, Robins LN: What Is a Case? London, Grant McIntyre, 1980

Wing JK, Babor T, Brugha T, et al: SCAN: Schedules for Clinical Assessment in Neuropsychiatry. Arch Gen Psychiatry 47:589–593, 1990

Witkin MJ, Atay JE, Fell AS, et al: Specialty mental health characteristics, in Mental Health, United States: 1990 (DHHS Publ No ADM-90-1708). Edited by Manderscheid RW, Sonnenschein MA. Washington, DC, U.S. Government Printing Office, 1990

Wittchen H-U, Robins LN, Cottler LB, et al: Cross-cultural feasibility, reliability and sources of variance of the Composite International Diagnostic Interview (CIDI). Br J Psychiatry 159:645–653, 1991

World Health Organization: International Classification of Diseases, 10th Revision. Geneva, World Health Organization, 1992

CHAPTER 4

NORMAL CHILD AND ADOLESCENT DEVELOPMENT

THEODORE SHAPIRO, M.D.
MARGARET E. HERTZIG, M.D.

The current focus in modern psychiatry on descriptive nomenclatures, diagnosis, and treatment does not necessarily include a developmental point of view. On the other hand, there are strong historical and clinical reasons why any student of personality and pathology within a medical framework should be interested in what is known about the normal developmental process—its stages, phases, inhibitions, impediments, and deviances. Moreover, the roots of the inquiry are within medicine and within psychiatry in particular.

HISTORICAL BACKGROUND

As far back as the Enlightenment, psychiatrists such as Pinel recorded longitudinal histories from patients in the French asylums in and about Paris. Pinel's understanding that psychopathology in adulthood may have something to do with life history or past social circumstance is deeply ingrained in the notion of "humane treatment" that followed. He struck the chains of the insane just as the ideas of the Quaker layman William Tuke, about treating patients without physical restraints, took hold in England. In the United States, Adolf Meyer, founder of the concept of

psychobiology, emphasized the life event chart as a mainstay of clinical knowledge.

While these trends in general psychiatry held sway, Freud (1905/1953), at the turn of the century, elaborated the idea that the first 5 years of life had a determining effect on later psychopathology and development. Whether one reads this as a strict rule of early influence or more loosely as a complementary series of intrinsic and extrinsic weightings, the view certainly echoed something that became a part of the medical mentality, adumbrated by the poet Wordsworth, who wrote "The child is father to the man."

From a more general medical vantage point, because there was so much to be learned about normal developmental processes for well baby care and so many skills to be gained in dealing with children of all ages, a more specialized training seemed to be required. As a result, pediatrics was split off from general medicine. Most pediatricians consider themselves practitioners of developmental medicine. Thus, the notions of developmental medicine and developmental psychiatry are the historical roots from which specific areas of knowledge and skill have grown. Such increased awareness has compelled us to look at normal growth and development as a key component of our work as well as an essential basis for etiological thought.

There are also important historical roots outside of medicine that have determined, in part, how we think about development. The language of developmental psychology derives from Darwin's linking of variation in forms of life to their survival value in evolution. Darwin's formulations then led to Ernst Haeckel's biogenetic law that "ontogeny recapitulates phylogeny." This series of events, barely skimmed here, served to turn biologists and physicians into students of embryology. Indeed, the language of embryology has been adopted in the literature of developmental psychology and medicine. Concepts such as maturation, development, differentiation, pleiomorphism, and organizers all have been borrowed from embryology and have enriched our understanding of how children start to be, beginning with gametization, embryogenesis, and then birth, and progressing to later developmental stages that can be observed and staged. In fact, the same terms used in embryology have been adapted for use in psychosocial development.

DEVELOPMENTAL PRINCIPLES

The starting point for our understanding of the general principles of development is the Darwinian notion of small brood in conjunction with prolonged caretaking because of the relative immaturity of those structures that permit independent survival. Freud (1905/1953), working from this viewpoint, was then able to conceive of the neuroses as an accrual of the prolonged dependency and caring necessary for the human infant before independence, and ultimately survival, could be ensured.

The terms *growth*, *maturation*, and *development*, although used imprecisely in common parlance, connote a direction from more global reactiveness to more specified reactiveness and from a less complex organization to a more complex state of organization (Table 4–1). *Growth* usually refers to the simple accretion of tissue (i.e., an increase in size or in the number of cells). Changes in height and weight are examples of growth. *Maturation* is a convenient fiction that has a somewhat teleological implication of a direction toward which the individual is headed in accord with his or her functions, abilities, structures, and competencies. In its most narrow meaning, the term suggests that there is a natural unfolding of genetic potential toward an end that is known as "maturity." This end can come about in average, expectable environments given the premise that the organism has average species-specific biological equipment. The concept does not invoke the variation that may occur in certain special ecologies. *Devel-*

TABLE 4–1.   Developmental principles (examples in each domain)

	Neurological	Biobehavioral	Intrapsychic	Social
Growth	Increasing length of neuronal axon; dendritic proliferation			
Maturation	Myelinization of axons	Palmar to pincer grasp; supine to prone; increasing axial control—sitting to walking	Fantasy level concerns—body themes to resolution of Oedipus complex; fearing loss of mother to fearing loss of love	Move from parent to peers and increasing intimacy
Development	Functional feedback of experience on selective dendritic proliferation	Acquisition of the speech of surround grafted on language universals	Using experience with others as feedback to relations, social referencing	Increasing arena of interactions, including peers
Differentiation	Neuronal specificity by regions: special senses: selective neurotransmitter areas	Pincer grasp; lexical discrimination and specificity	Appreciation of qualities of object that distinguish it from others; social smile to separation anxiety	Specificity of peer preferences, social group formation and selectivity
Integration	Increasing interhemispheric tracts; establishment of cerebral dominance	Grasp what is seen; syntactic organization; word-meaning	Good objects can be bad; affective regulation of impulse	Increasing capacity to adapt from one group to others

opment, on the other hand, includes whatever the maturational potential provides plus the variations in social and environmental influence. This concept refers to the changing structure of behavior and thought over time.

Many of the issues of developmental psychology and psychiatry concern the limiting factors that will prevent, alter, or render maturation sequences retarded or deviant. Normative studies suggest that there is a cephalocaudal developmental sequence, with the head end of the organism at the beginning of life being a more highly differentiated functional entity than the tail end. Biological forces such as myelinization of the central long tracts progressing from head to toe help us to understand that regardless of the cultural variation in the early months, most human children begin to walk between the ages of 10 and 18 months (Gesell and Amatruda 1947). This will occur whether the infant is bound to a pallet by its Native American mother or is permitted to kick free in an apartment in New York. Similarly, along with the achievement of that motor landmark, the landmarks of language development occur in a lockstep sequence. However, to add complexity, each line of development may mature independently, such as in a limited cerebral palsy affecting only the small section of the cortex that controls limb motor pathways.

Moreover, no matter what language is spoken by the parent, most 1-year-olds acquire the equivalent designations "Mama," "Dada," and one additional word. By 18 months the 20- to 50-word vocabulary is expressed in single-word utterances (Gesell and Amatruda 1947). By the time the child is 2 years old, he or she usually can string together two- and sometimes three-word utterances with some understanding of grammatical format. Such vocalizations appear as telegraphic utterances in which the small units of meaning that signify past, plural, etc., known as *grammatical morphemes*, are omitted. The addition of grammatical morphemes occurs next as toddlers take on the job of making sentences (Brown 1973). This maturational sequence does not mean that children do not make errors, but they do seem to be capable of forming the language units appropriately. The errors that are made derive from overgeneralization of grammatical rules and are not random.

From the developmental vantage, these maturational regularities are acted upon by social nurturing influences; the achievements are not entirely innate. For example, if a child is tied down or forced to remain recumbent, the maturational event of walking surely will be delayed because of muscular disuse. Nonetheless, walking is a somewhat irrepressible landmark given biologically normal equipment and the opportunity to exercise. Similarly, although the capacity for language and grammar may be built-in, children will not achieve speech and language in the usual manner if they are deaf or if they are not spoken to. Moreover, it is doubtful that children growing up in a German-speaking world, for example, will speak Italian or vice versa. Thus, environment has a significant influence on the developmental sequence of *what language* is spoken rather than *that a language is spoken*.

DIFFERENTIATION AND INTEGRATION

Maturation within individual systems also requires that we consider another central theme in development, *differentiation*. Just as the blastosphere differentiates into endoderm, ectoderm, and mesoderm, and these further mature into more highly differentiated tissues, so, analogously, do psychological and social systems differentiate. The newborn infant's grasp reflex traverses a known series of steps to its final form in the distinctively human function of pincer grasp. Although the newborn can distinguish between patterned visual stimuli, it is only later that colors, shapes, forms, and faces become meaningfully differentiated as familiar, hostile, friendly, or frightening. In a psychological sense, the general arousal of infants differentiates selectively into responses signifying that the child distinguishes between human and nonhuman, mother and nonmother, friend and foe.

Integration also emerges between and among the varying senses. In the beginning the eye sees what impinges on it; the hand grasps that which is put into it. At 3 or 4 months, if the child sees the hand and the thing to be grasped in the same visual field, he or she will grasp. It is not until some time later that the child reaches for that which he or she sees even if the hand is not in the visual field. The ultimate capacities to, for example, shoot a basket, hit a ball, draw in imitation of nature, and tap out a tune require higher levels of integration between and among the senses and the motor apparatus. At a psychological level, the capacity to put together good and bad experiences with a person and also to change set in relation to varying exposures requires integration. As the infant, showing more differentiated and integrated functioning, moves from the more global apprehension of the world, he or she may also lose some functions that were natively available. There is evidence, for example, that the infant can make distinctions between phonetic forms at 4 months, but he or she loses this ability when such forms become no longer useful in the language that is spoken (Eimas et al. 1971). By 6 months, infants pay special selective attention to phonemes that characterize the speech they hear (Kuhl 1992).

HIERARCHIC REORGANIZATION AND CRITICAL PERIODS

As each stage unfolds, the question arises as to whether it could unfold without the child having had to pass through the prior stage. *Epigenesis* is the concept of sequential steps influencing subsequent steps. Each stage in that model is highly dependent on resolution of the experiences of the prior stage. The epigenetic vantage point permits, but it does not necessarily include, another model that is known as *hierarchic reorganization*. Heinz Werner (1957) introduced this concept to indicate that development not only can be conceived of as linear, but perhaps also may involve changing structures over time that permit alterations in organization that are not the logical or necessary outcome of prior stages. Instead, each new integration of biological and neuronal function meshes with psychocognitive capacities that are more than the sum of their parts. Each stage is truly a new structure permitting functions and adaptations that are not easily predicted from their precursors. These reorganizations permit the next level of behavior and competence as the child pulls himself or herself along the chronological ladder. However, there is evidence to suggest both linear and discontinuous progression in the developmental course.

Invoking a hierarchically reorganized sequence permits consideration of a concept known as *critical periods*, which has been stressed by ethologists. Critical periods require that an environmental releaser stimulate the emergence of a developmental capacity that is inborn and ready for use only within a limited time period. If no release occurs, the function is said to *involute*. Such releasers may not adequately describe the way in which human biological development takes place (Schneirla and Rosenblatt 1961). The time lines are not as critically limited as in other mammals, and thus we should be cautious in applying data across species. Reorganization may occur in hierarchic fashion on the basis of independent neural and cognitive lines of maturation rather than by requiring that the organism must go through certain specific and critical experiences. Indeed, Schneirla and Rosenblatt indicate that some species require continuous biological influence to effect social behavior (which is known as *biosocial organization*). Other species obey rules of recency, and earliest experience may not be as prolonged in its influence (which is known as *psychosocial organization*). In one extreme case, a child who had not been spoken to from 18 months to 15 years was taught sufficient language to converse, to make her needs known, and to carry out basic communication (Curtiss 1981). However, in this cruel "experiment," the child had been bound and abused.

DEVELOPMENTAL PSYCHOLOGIES

It should be evident by now that there are various approaches to the study of development, each of which is based on different sets of data derived from looking at children using different observational techniques. All developmentalists explore questions of how children move from point A to point B over time. Indeed, what follows will necessarily indicate that the formulations available about developmental stages are all bound by a particular method. The empirical support for each stage is highly dependent on the experimental method used, and therefore there is not one developmental psychology, but rather a number of developmental psychologies, each of which is identified by the unique ideas of a particular investigator or technique of observation.

In terms of the psychiatric outlook, most psychiatrists are well versed in the retrospective reconstructive attitude of the Freudian developmental system. However, early psychoanalysts did not observe children, except as a derivative aspect of the genetic point of view. The *genetic point of view* was Freud's attempt to retrospectively divine the infantile roots of adult behavior and pathology. His assumptions of polymorphously perverse infantile sexuality and the maturational sequences described in libido theory were based on retrospective reconstructions of how men and women seem to organize their fantasy lives. Later psychoanalytic thinkers (e.g., Mahler et al. 1975; Spitz 1965) looked at children directly and created their own developmental systems that elaborated Freud's system.

The behavioral vantage point, which was well outlined in the initial work of Watson (1919) and then B. F. Skinner (1953), is based on learning theory and takes a Lockean philosophical position in which experience is said to be inscribed on a blank slate of mind, thereby transforming it. No competence becomes possible that is not learned. Furthermore, nothing can be learned that is not within the capacity of the species, which in turn determines the limits of responsiveness. The virtue of a learning model for development is that such a model can be empirically apprehended and there is little inferred substructure and very few intervening variables.

Jean Piaget, the most important progenitor of modern cognitive psychology, introduced a complex system during the first half of this century suggesting that experience alone cannot account for the child's understanding of the world (Piaget and Inhelder 1969). In fact, Piaget set out to determine how intelligent behavior evolves. Calling himself a "genetic epistomologist" concerned only with non–affect-laden behavior, he addressed the issue of how children strategically arrive at right or wrong answers utilizing their native capacities and regularized sequence of stages.

The normative developmental theory of Arnold Gesell (Gesell and Amatruda 1947) is more closely related to the learning theorists, but within the medical framework. Gesell attempted to unify the biological and neurodevelopmental principles that were available at that time from embryogenesis and the normative sequences of observed behaviors. His work was an important precursor to the concepts of normative stage–phase capacities and behaviors. Gesell's studies inspired others to examine large numbers of children "cross-sectionally" in order to find out what they do at each chronological age. These findings were then used to determine the limits of normal distribution and deviance within the range of the tasks presented. These cross-sectional, normative approaches established the essential empirical basis from which more highly theoretical proposals emerged.

Normative, cross-sectional studies, however, do not tell how one progresses (i.e., the process) throughout the longitudinal cycle from one stage to another. *Longitudinal* studies more easily address such issues. Although longitudinal studies are not generally reported in terms of how child A responds at point X and then at point Y, investigators in such studies do have the potential to do just that: to track developmental facts in individual subjects at varying stages, looking for outcomes from past behaviors and checking on retrospective suggestions.

Human development has always been studied by analogy. Investigators become impatient because of the longevity of humans and look for quicker ways of determining sequencing and invariance. Thus, animal models are employed, and in human development, analogy and homology to ethological studies of nonhuman species are sought. The effects of imprinting, inborn response systems, and species-specific releasers have been well studied in various animals. However, outside the ethological frame, other animal observers (Harlow 1960; Schneirla and Rosenblatt 1961) have questioned ideas such as critical periods and have produced more interesting models that do not depend as heavily on postulates of innateness. Rather, such models suggest that each emergent behavior can be tracked to precursor experiences and that the essence of a developmental analysis involves just such an exploration. However, a number of major human developmental theories, such as that of John Bowlby's (1969, 1973, 1980) attachment model, have grown out of work with nonhuman species.

Thus, in order to study normal development we have to inquire about developmental paths and investigative bi-ases, models, and tools. In this brief outline of the central developmental positions, our interest is in these issues in the context of the needs of physicians and psychiatrists. In addition, another matter will become apparent. Many mechanisms and processes are postulated as maturational, but a central concern remains for developmental psychology to determine *what* moves the individual from stage to stage—what pilot guides both biological and social adaptations. Such process variables tend to be less prominent than observed landmarks and behaviors.

The most influential points of view will now be described in their essentials to introduce the beginning developmentalist to some of the language and theory of each developmental system. We discuss as representative developmental positions the psychoanalytic perspective and the work of Piaget, Gesell, and Bowlby.

PSYCHOANALYTIC DEVELOPMENTAL VIEWPOINT

The psychoanalytic view of childhood (Table 4–2) derives from two sources. The first source (i.e., *genetic*) uses retrospective and reconstructive inferences about the patient's past to construct a coherent and plausible sequenced history. The other source (i.e., *developmental*), based on the prospective studies by psychoanalytically oriented observers, attempts to observationally flesh out the models of development derived from the genetic point of view. Thus, we can distinguish initially between genetic and developmental aspects of psychoanalytic theory.

The Freudian Perspective

Freud's initial view of childhood as a period of polymorphously perverse infantile sexuality grew out of his observation that adult disorder reveals certain constant, compelling features. Adult sexuality consists not only of coitus and gametization, but of erotic arousal that depends on stimulation of a variety of bodily zones. Perverse activity and normal foreplay both led to arousal and orgasmic behavior. Moreover, neurotic individuals did not dare think about the things that perverse individuals perpetrated. On these grounds, Freud suggested that repression was the prime mechanism that both hid and modified early sexual thoughts from the conscious minds of neurotic individuals. Libido theory was introduced to describe the maturational sequence that children were expected to traverse en route to adulthood. The theory included the active and passive aims of children seen retrospectively in relation to their primary objects, mother and father. These aims became what Erikson (1963) called the enactments and fantasies of the tragedies and comedies that occur around the orifices of the body.

TABLE 4–2.   **Psychoanalytic theories of development**

Period	Freud	Erikson	Spitz	Mahler	Stern
Infancy (approximately 0–12 months)	Oral	Trust vs. mistrust	Smiling response (1st organizer, 6 weeks); stranger anxiety (2nd organizer, 7 months)	Normal autism (0–2 months), normal symbiosis (2–6 months), separation-individuation; subphase 1, differentiation (6–10 months)	Sense of an emergent self (throughout life span); sense of a core self (2 months throughout life span); sense of a subjective self (7 months throughout life span)
Toddler (approximately 12–36 months)	Anal	Autonomy vs. shame and doubt	"No" (3rd organizer, 15 months)	Subphase 2, practicing period (10–15 months); subphase 3, rapprochement (16–24 months); subphase 4, consolidation and resolution (24–36 months)	Sense of a verbal self (15 months throughout life span)
Preschool (approximately 3–5 years)	Phallic Oedipal	Initiative vs. guilt Initiative vs. guilt			
School-age (approximately 5–12 years)	Latency	Industry vs. inferiority			
Adolescence (approximately 12 years and up)		Identity vs. role confusion			

Psychopathology was viewed by Freud as the result of either a fixation at (i.e., an arrest in the progress of psychosexual maturation) or a regression to (i.e., a symbolic or functional return to earlier ways of acting or thinking) one or another of these stages. As Erikson (1963), in his recasting of Freud, noted, the body zones and modes of function are analogous to other behaviors in life. For example, ingesting and spitting out as bodily acts were thought to become introjection and projection as mental defenses, and so forth. Although this sequence is looked at by many as the essence of Freudian psychology, it refers only to the content analysis of thought and fantasy and is, as Freud noted, his mythology and less significant to his later, more mature developmental theorizing.

Freud finally took up a strongly developmental position in response to the challenge thrown before him by Otto Rank, who wrote that birth anxiety was at the center of symptom formation. In 1926, Freud developed his last, and most sophisticated, major developmental theory (Freud 1926/1959). He suggested that anxiety only breaks through to consciousness when successful repression does not take place and that anxiety functions as a signal that a dangerous situation is at hand in response to the emergence of specific thoughts as they threaten to break into consciousness. Freud posited a hierarchy of threats that humans have to evaluate and cope with during early childhood. Helplessness is the first signal of danger. Separation occurring somewhere between 7 and 24 months follows, and then castration anxiety (or body integrity anxiety) takes over from the third to the sixth years. Finally danger of punishment by guilt ensues from an internalized value system embodied in the superego, which is an agency of the tripartite mind of the new structural model. Thus, at each stage of development the danger takes on a different configuration. The progression moves, as Freud (1926/1959) suggests, from fear of loss of the object to fear of loss of the love of the object, with, in this instance, the mental object being a representation of the mother. This progression from concrete to abstract is also consistent with cognitive models that do not derive from Freud's dynamic formulation.

It should be noted, however, that Freud recognized that the Oedipus complex consists of a recasting of the prior preoedipal determinants and considered it to be a nucleus of conflict around which neurosis forms. Thus, his model was both epigenetic, as Erikson noted, and discontinuous in its invocation of the principle of hierarchic reorganization. The Oedipus complex becomes a watershed of prior developmental lines because its formation takes into consideration the ambivalent love and hate, the active and passive aims, toward parents of a child growing up in a family. Boys in the oedipal phase unconsciously desire their mother's undivided love and attention and wish to dispense with their competitive father. This configuration in normal girls (the Electra complex) involves their wish for undivided love from their father and their disavowal of their mother. These configurations vary greatly, leading to other permutations and combinations that evolve into pathological personality formation.

The Perspective of Ego Psychology

Freud's work was followed by empirical observations by others who moved away from depth psychology toward what was called *ego psychology*. The observational model began to take hold around the work of Rene Spitz and then Margaret Mahler, each of whom was at the center of a larger array of contributors who observed children.

Spitz's genetic field theory. Rene Spitz's (1965) genetic field theory was derived from direct observation of infants. He invoked the concept of the "organizer" in the development of human behavior, of which three have significance for the differentiation process. The concept of an organizer was derived from the embryological model that prescribes a formative fixing element in maturation that interferes with the pluripotentiality of protoplasm. Although this theory has an essentially maturational thrust, there also are important considerations of how the environment interacts with the biological tendencies.

Spitz's first organizer, the *smiling response*, includes a consistent and repeatable social smile in response to a full face or a moving oval with darkened areas representing eyes. The format of the human face entailed here suggests that this is the first "not-me" object to be appreciated by an infant. This generalized other is smiled at sometime around 6 weeks. (Other psychoanalytically oriented observers [e.g., Emde and Harmon 1972], although not denying that smiles take place earlier or that responsiveness is possible earlier, contend that these earlier signs of responsiveness do not regularly elicit a repeated state of adaptiveness to this new human stimulus.) This maturational landmark links outside experience and autonomous function, supporting the notion of a regularly responsive internalization en route to what psychoanalysts call *object constancy*.

The next organizer, the *stranger response*, occurs at about 7 months. The child now turns away from the stranger with apprehension, terminating what Anna Freud (1965) has called the period of *need satisfying object*. This second organizer marks the attachment to a specific other.

The third organizer, the *development of the signal for no*, then signifies a fully internalized and individuated human toddler who now can undo with a verbal signal. According to Spitz, the toddler is now an agency and center of will separate from the mother.

Mahler's separation-individuation theory. Spitz's ideas have received further observational support in the later work of Margaret Mahler and colleagues (1975). Mahler's separation-individuation theory continues the process of development into the postuterine period, involving the "hatching" of human consciousness, with the toddler as a separate, discrete autonomous agency. In Mahlerian terms the child moves from an autistic to a symbiotic stage in which he or she is initially enmeshed psychologically with the mother as though he or she were not separate from the mother.

The separation-individuation process includes a number of substages that equip the child with various capacities that enable him or her to develop the ego strengths necessary for adaptation. During the *differentiation* subphase, psychological birth occurs under the rubric of hatching, which is characterized by a permanently alert sensorium in which visual and manual examination of the external world become central. Next emerges the *practicing* subphase, which is characterized by increased curiosity. In Greenacre's (1957) picturesque phrase, "the love affair with the world" begins. The child now appears as if he or she were omnipotent and as if an internal agency were not dissociated from an external agency. Only with the understanding that the mother is separate, during the next subphase, does the child arrive at what is called *object constancy*. Relative independent action can take place after the child is able to keep a stable mental image of the important caregiver.

Mahler's process of separation-individuation is an attempt to offer a psychoanalytic theory of development that is paralleled by fantasy formation matching the Freudian libido phases. When object constancy ensues at about 25 months to 3 years, the child is on his or her way toward independence, just as the three organizers proposed by Spitz provide the basis for later differentiation in that system.

Anna Freud's multilinear theory. Anna Freud (1974) described a series of developmental lines that are central to the modern psychoanalytic view. These developmental lines suggest multilinearity in development, as Heinz Werner posited, but also offer an easy clinical frame from which to look at development. Roughly summarized, the child moves 1) from being nursed to rational eating, 2) from wetting and soiling to bowel and bladder control, 3) from egocentricity toward companionship with peers, 4) from play to the capacity to work, 5) from physical to mental pathways of discharge of drives, 6) from animate to inanimate objects, and 7) from irresponsibility to guilt. One can infer from these observations and their variations that a central theme evolves concerning how the child organizes behavior in an affective climate and in relation to others. This has become the observational groundwork of what now is called *object-relations theory* in psychoanalysis, in which the object referred to is the child's mental representation of significant adults such as parents.

Other developmental frameworks do not consider these matters at such a molecular level of personal meaning. Cognitive and cross-sectional developmental schemes tend to exclude consideration of affect and conation (motive, will). (Later in this chapter the more recent nonpsychoanalytic theories of affect development will be considered.) Within Freudian theory, moral development was viewed as the resultant of Oedipus complex resolution. However, more recent work (Buchsbaum and Emde 1990) has clearly shown that even 36-month-old children make moral judgments and have various responses to narrative that was designed to stimulate conflict over negative parental injunctions.

NORMATIVE CROSS-SECTIONAL DEVELOPMENT

Cross-sectional developmental observers determine what children can do at varying ages and seek to construct sequential maps consisting of stages. Gesell's (see Gesell and Amatruda 1947) cross-sectional scheme (Table 4–3) is of interest because it was developed within a medical framework. Gesell divides behavior into four sectors: motor, adaptive, language, and personal-social. He tracked these behavioral observations over the long period of infancy and described a normative timetable. The essential question asked is does the child at age *x* achieve behavior in accord with what most children at age *x* can do? Gesell's organizing principle was neurodevelopmental integrity. He watched the child in the supine and prone positions give way to the sitting position and then to the standing and walking position. Nonetheless, Gesell matches Freud when he states that the developmental span that lies between birth and 5 years is formative and of major significance for the entire life of the human organism. He also avers strongly that prenatal fetal development has continuing relevance for the postnatal period and that the behaviors that one sees early can be organized into a developmental quotient for each sector. The developmental quotient (i.e., maturational age divided by chronological age and then multiplied by 100 [(MA/CA) × 100]) gives a rough index of what the child tested can do at each stage. These developmental quotients are only roughly related to later measures of IQ (intelligence quotient), but they are relevant for detecting retardation and also deviance during the first 3 years.

Other cross-sectional schemes of childhood pertain largely to the development of intelligence. At the turn of the century, the French sought to determine what sort of schooling children might best accommodate to if they were selected for some vital adaptive functions that could be called intelligence. Binet invented the IQ measure for that purpose. His test was revised in the United States as the Stanford-Binet Intelligence Test, which has been in continuous use as the IQ standard ever since. It has become, with revisions, a normative outline of what children are, on the average, capable of at each age.

Most studies of development rest on similar cross-sectional visions as the IQ and Gesell's developmental quotient, but the most recent studies of cross-sectional behavior have tried to include a large sector of behaviors other than verbal behavior. Thus, the Wechsler Intelligence Scale for Children (WISC; Wechsler 1949) was designed to include both verbal and performance scales. The most recent revisions (WISC-R [1974] and WISC-III [1991]) provide us with a broader understanding of the child's general adaptiveness that may be subsumed under intelligent behavior. The latest revisions provide updated norms for American youth whose primary language is English. The Wechsler Preschool and Primary Scale of Intelligence (WPPSI [1989]) is an adaptation of the WISC for children from 3 to 6 years of age.

PIAGETIAN COGNITIVE DEVELOPMENT

Intelligent behavior received a new definition from the pioneering work of Piaget (1952, 1969) during the 1920s

TABLE 4–3. Landmarks of normal behavioral development—the revised Gesell developmental schedules

Age	Motor (gross/fine)	Adaptive	Language	Personal/Social
4 weeks	Tonic neck reflex position; rotates head when prone; makes alternating crawling movements	Responds to sound; follows moving objects to midline	Small throaty noises	Regards face; reduces activity
8 weeks	Symmetric posture seen; head bobbingly erect	Follows moving objects past midline	Vocalizes in response to social stimulation; sustained "cooing"	Follows moving person; smiles responsively
16 weeks	Symmetric posture predominates; holds head balanced; hands engage in midline; rolls to prone	Looks at object in hand	Laughs and squeals; "talks" to people/toys spontaneously	Initiates social smile; smiles and vocalizes at mirror; discriminates strangers (20 weeks)
28 weeks	Sits unsupported with hands up (1 minute); gets to hands and knees	One hand reach and grasp of toy; transfers toy	Vocalizes "m-m-m-m" when crying; understands name (32 weeks)	Gets feet to mouth; tries to obtain toys out of reach
40 weeks	Sits indefinitely with hands free (36 weeks); pulls to stand (36 weeks); cruises; lets self down; inferior pincer grasp	Matches two objects in midline; uncovers toy (44 weeks)	"Mama" or "Dada" and 2 "words" with meaning; responds to "no-no"	Initiates "pat-a-cake" and "peek-a-boo"; holds own bottle (36 weeks); helps in dressing; gives toy on request (44 weeks)
52 weeks	Picks up object from floor from standing position; walks several steps; helps turn pages (56 weeks)	Releases toy; imitates scribble; puts round block in formboard spontaneously	6 "words"; uses jargon	Points for wants; hugs doll; offers toy to image in mirror
15 months	Walks alone, seldom falls; walks up stairs, 1 hand held; creeps down; hurls ball; builds tower of 3 blocks	Spontaneous scribble; gets toy with stick after demonstration	10–19 words; knows 1 body part	Feeds self with spoon (spills); says "Thank you"; seeks help; pulls adult's hand to show
18 months	Walks down stairs, 1 hand held; builds tower of 4 blocks	Imitates stroke of crayon; places 3 blocks in formboard after demonstration	20–29 words including names of siblings, friends, relatives; combines 2–3 words ("daddy go"); asks for more food and drink	Gets spoon to mouth right side up; hands empty dish; echoes 2 or more last words; imitates mother/father sweeping, hammering, etc.
24 months	Jumps, both feet off floor; kicks large ball on request; builds tower of 7 blocks	Imitates vertical stroke; imitates circular scribble; inserts circle, square, triangle in formboard spontaneously	50+ words; uses I and you; 3- to 4-word sentences; uses plurals	Occasionally indicates toilet needs; calls self or me; helps put things away
30 months	Alternates feet going up stairs; rides tricycle using pedals; turns pages singly; builds tower of 9 blocks	Names own drawing; imitates horizontal stroke; imitates circle, imitates circle, adapts to rotation of formboard; repeats 2 digits (1–3 trials)	8- to 9-word sentences; carries tune; uses be and she correctly; relates events of 2–3 days ago	Pours from glass to glass; keeps time to music; pulls up pants; puts shoes on; names self in mirror

(continued)

TABLE 4–3. Landmarks of normal behavioral development—the revised Gesell developmental schedules *(continued)*

Age	Motor (gross/fine)	Adaptive	Language	Personal/Social
36 months	Alternates feet going down stairs; throws ball overhand; builds tower of 10 blocks	Copies vertical and horizontal stroke; copies circle; imitates cross, repeats 3 digits (1–3 trials); imitates bridge	Uses *and* or *but*; recites all of a song; knows up and down; follows 3 commands (3 of the following: on, under, in back of, in front of, beside); knows 2 colors	Fully toilet trained; understands taking turns; plays with other children; washes and dries hands; knows front from back
48 months	Stands on 1 foot (4–8 seconds); skips on 1 foot only	Draws person with 2 parts; adds 3 parts to incomplete man	Follows 4 commands	Laces shoes; cooperates with children; goes on errands
60 months	Skips using feet alternately; walks on tiptoe	Adds 8 parts to incomplete man; copies square (54 months) and triangle; counts 10 objects pointing; prints first name	Names penny, nickel, dime; describes pictures; asks meanings of words; gives first and last name	Dresses and undresses with little assistance; dresses up in adult clothes; ties a bow

(Table 4–4). Piaget took a unique stance when he noted that getting the right answer is only one aspect of intelligence. He confessed that the affective component of development was of lesser interest to him; he wished instead to understand *how it is that children come to know what they seem to know.* In other words, what processes do children use to arrive at right or even wrong answers? Piaget found the regularities in sequence that permit abstract intelligent behavior. Piaget designated himself a "genetic epistemol-

TABLE 4–4. Piagetian stages of cognitive development

I. Sensory-motor intelligence
  A. Reflex looking and grasping (0–1 months)
  B. Primary circular reactions; the acquisition of new schemas centered on the infant's own body (1–4.5 months)
  C. Secondary circular reactions; new schema include events of objects in the external environment (4–9 months)
  D. Object permanence (9–12 months)
  E. Tertiary circular reactions; active searching for novel events (12–18 months)
  F. Beginning reasoning; mental trial and error replaces trial and error in action (18 months to 2 years)

II. Representative intelligence and the period of concrete operations
  A. Preoperational representations
    1. Appearance of symbolic function and the beginning of internalized actions (2–3.5 years)
    2. Representational organizations based on static configurations or on assimilation to one's own action (4–5.5 years)
    3. Meticulated representational regulation (5.5–7 or 8 years)
  B. Concrete operations
    1. Simple operations-classifications, seriations, term-by-term correspondence (8–9 to 10 years)
    2. Whole system—Euclidian coordinates, projective concepts, simultaneity (9–11 years)

III. Representative intelligence and formal operations
  A. Hypothetical deductive logic and combinatorial operations (11–12 to 13–14 years)
  B. Structure of lattice and the group of four transformations: identity, negation, reciprocity, and correlativity (13–14 years)

ogist," which clearly reflects his intention and his central triumph—that is, to make the emergence of intelligent behavior understandable.

Piaget proposes that the infant is born with two kinds of reflexes: those that remain fixed through life and those that are plastic in response to experience. The experiential world impinges on the child reflexively, and gradually a mental organization, called a *schema*, develops around repeated interactions. The *process* of development remains the same throughout life, but the *structures* change. The repeated process involves a reexperiencing in *assimilation*, but the assimilative schemas can change as they *accommodate*, leading to *adaptation*. For Piaget, assimilation is the incorporation of a structure of action that the subject judges to be equivalent into existing schemas. Accommodation, in turn, occurs when the schema must change to appreciate new objects and differentiate them from old assimilatory forms. Around this universal complementary functional format, the child then passes through four stages; sensory-motor, preoperational, concrete operational, and formal operational.

During the *sensory-motor stage*, no behavior and its schema is separated into sensory and motor components. A thing to be acted upon is appreciated as the thing acted upon. It does not exist as a sensorily discrete entity without action. It is as if the infant were constantly embedded in a trial-and-error world. Werner and Kaplan (1963) describe this as the period of "things of action."

As the infant strips away the motor component, he or she can, between the ages of 18 months and 2 years, maintain a stable mental representation and create a representational world. This inaugurates *the preoperational period*, during which things are worked upon in accord with how effective the child is.

The concrete operational *stage*, from 7 to 14 years, introduces a series of functional components suggesting that behavior becomes more rule-governed and that the rules permit decentering. When the child decenters he or she loses his or her literal egocentricity—that is, he or she can generalize. However, he or she cannot yet generalize from data. Conservation becomes possible, and change in surface appearance does not necessarily signify basic change as in the concepts of volume or weight. Reversal operations may become possible, and trial and error are superseded by mental work employed to solve problems in one's mind, as in equation reversibility.

The later stage, that of *formal operations*, involves reasoning from empirical observations that then can be abstracted as general rules which can be used to dictate future actions. The child is now sufficiently decentered to take on another's vantage point, and reversibility is well estab-

lished. The rules of logic of language are established. Piaget wrote also about imagination and dreams and about language itself. He looked at these functions as having various logical structures.

The intelligence of the mature human is a far cry from the intelligence described in the sensory-motor period. Most recently, neo-Piagetians have discovered that the stages outlined are not as rigid as stated and that empirical design may render some of the earlier judgments false, but that the regularities of sequence seem valid.

ETHOLOGICAL DEVELOPMENT

Bowlby (1969) was the first to build a human developmental psychology based on a melding of psychoanalytic and ethological literature. His exposure to children separated from parents during World War II provided the human impetus for his theoretical work (Bowlby 1952), as did his experiences with adolescents with conduct disorder. Bowlby recognized the nature of human ties as an organizing precursor to later mature development. His work paralleled the work of Spitz (1945) and Goldfarb (1955), who also studied separation, and extended his own earlier observations of affectively deprived delinquents who suffered early separation. Bowlby noted that there were strong reactive effects consequent to separation from the mother or her surrogate.

Bowlby (1969) reviewed the nature of the maternal tie, establishing what he called a component instinctual response system that bore some similarity to Freud's 1905 theory. The infant is described as having five components that make up attachment behavior. Experiences are integrated to create a unified mental representation. The activated reflexes of *sucking*, *clinging*, and *following* have representation in other species, but are also present in the human. *Crying* and *smiling* achieve their ends by reciprocal maternal behavior: they bring the mother to the child. Each of these component instincts is considered to be an inborn response that is activated by an external caregiver (e.g., the mother). The evolutionary basis for this attachment is accounted for in the survival value and the natural selection for these responses.

Borrowing from the work of Harlow, Lorenz, and Tinbergen, among others, Bowlby then suggested that the responses to separation could be systematized. *Protest, despair,* and *grief* were repeatedly observed upon separation, and then, if these responses were carried on too long, *denial* of need ensued. These behaviors serve as negative indicators that the normal process of the attached state has been interrupted. This work has been seminal in producing further empirical study of time of attachment, bonding and separation, and strange situation paradigms by which investigators explore attachment.

The research of Bowlby and others indicates that children who have been poorly attached later develop untoward consequences. Recent studies (e.g., Fonagy et al. 1991) have demonstrated that the mother's attachment profile extracted from a carefully structured interview (Main et al. 1985) is highly correlated with security of attachment of the child. This finding places great weight on the interactive nature of early behavior.

These major frames of reference for development have given rise to myriad further work. We will only touch on some new and derivative formats to alert the reader who may wish to pursue the topic further.

Longitudinal studies have been with us since the early diarists of language development. However, few of them have made as much impact as has the New York Longitudinal Study. This study group initially followed 133 middle-class children from 85 families, beginning in 1956. The observational data were organized in terms of nine variables: activity level, regularity, approach/withdrawal, adaptability, intensity, threshold, mood, distractibility, and persistence. Although somewhat removed from direct observation, the variables have good interrater reliability and give us a profile of reactivity for an individual child. The important work of relating these "temperamental variables," as they are called, to outcome in the "difficult child syndrome" or in relation to later personality development is ongoing (Thomas and Chess 1989). Such work holds promise as a developmental vantage point that should be integrated with later studies of character.

The work on affective development has provided yet another perspective (Lewis and Michelson 1983).

As noted earlier, although we have not exhausted the varying vantage developmental points that are currently used, those discussed provide a framework of empirically based or theoretically sound systems from which we can judge our new observations of developmental process.

We now will traverse the developmental span from birth to preadolescence, and then consider adolescence separately, in order to provide an overview of physical, neurological, sensory-motor, and cognitive development. Following this, we will then discuss the development of emotion in an interpersonal context. Finally, we will look at adolescence as a way station between middle childhood and adulthood that offers the integrations necessary for later life. Although we stress the early years, a truly developmental perspective includes the entire life span.

NORMAL GROWTH AND DEVELOPMENT: BIRTH TO PREPUBERTY

NEURODEVELOPMENTAL AND COGNITIVE ORGANIZATION

Biodevelopmental Reorganizations in the First Two Years of Life

According to recent findings, the human infant is born with a largely prewired nervous system, and many capacities designed for survival are already built into the organism (Stern 1985). The variations in the environment seem to influence the central nervous system (CNS) and neuronal networks largely through increases and decreases in the proliferation of synaptic connections and dendritic growth. We are accustomed to the idea that muscles grow stronger and senses are sharpened by use and that they atrophy by disuse. CNS growth during the early years seems to obey similar laws, with appropriate consideration for maturational differentiation and integration of pathways. While these processes are taking place, there also is evidence of discontinuities in neurodevelopment. There is a general proliferation of neural connections through the sixth and seventh year of life, followed by a decline, so that at puberty the network appears less dense (however, not as sparse as that found in the human brain at birth) (Huttenlocher 1979).

These recent discoveries at the cellular level also have their parallel at other levels on other measurements. Changes on the electroencephalogram (EEG), clinical neurological status, and cognitive levels also can be cited to document periods of radical change. These latter observations have led to formulations on the psychobehavioral level known as *discontinuities* in development, or as *biodevelopmental shifts* by other developmentalists intent on bringing the behavioral level into relation with the substrate (Emde and Harmon 1972; Emde et al. 1976; Shapiro and Perry 1976; Werner 1957). There is a correspondence between certain behavioral events at some stages and other parameters of biological study.

Neurological organization. The first suggestion of a biodevelopmental shift occurs at the time of the first social organizer, the social smile, described by Spitz as signaling the recognition of an external stimulus of the human face as a releaser. The EEG becomes reorganized at a physiological level. Moreover, the rapid heartbeat of early infancy during disposition of attention gives way to slowing of the heartbeat with attentive staring after 2 months. This biodevelopmental shift thus can be documented at a number of physiological levels as well as at the behavioral level.

Similar concepts have been promulgated regarding the variation in state in early development as measured in wake-sleep cycles and reflected in the organization of REM (rapid eye movement) patterns. The six or seven regularly recurring REM periods during adult sleep only gradually emerge, evolving from early infancy (less than 3 months), when light sleep (Stages 1 and 2) dominates the EEG (Roffwarg et al. 1966). Moreover, sleep EEGs of premature infants show that up to 70% of sleep time is spent in a Stage-1 REM pattern. Sleep spindles appear only at 3–4 months, and by 3 months the infantile form of going to sleep that is characterized by rapid shifts from Stage 1 to Stage 4 recedes. These changes parallel the behavioral characteristics known as *settling*, when 70% of babies become night sleepers, rescinding their former pattern of waking at 3- to 4-hour intervals. By the end of the first year of life, the adult pattern of sleep is established on a physiological level. This event has been matched on an observational level because of the concordance of rapid eye movements with restlessness and other motor and respiratory patterns that are associated with varying stages of sleep.

Motoric behavior. Gesell's observation of the functional significance of attaining upright posture derives from an evolutionary perspective. He emphasizes the capacity to turn over, sit upright, and, finally, use bipedal locomotion as developmental markers of maturation. These achievements are signs of the integration of CNS structures. Not only do they subsume the progression from cephalic dominance to the importance of manual dexterity and locomotion in human children, they also mark the growing capacity of the child to become separate from the caretaking parent on the grounds of motor competence and, later, linguistic abilities, which then provide the bases of psychological independence.

Behaviorally the infant at birth lies in a "fencer" position (tonic neck reflex) and during alert wakeful times can be stimulated to focus, grasp, and respond reflexively to rooting and sucking, all of which are adaptive for survival. These behaviors later give way to lying in a supine position and beginning to use both hands for grasping and mouthing objects as hand-mouth integrations become possible. The flailing hand sometimes scratches the infant's face as he or she tries to once again find his or her mouth. It almost seems as if there is an early dysmetria until the linkage becomes regular. Only by 10 months does the infant grasp objects in both hands and bring them to the midline. Symmetrical use of limbs and axial support become essential to the child's being able to turn over at 4 months and, ultimately, to achievement of the sitting position at 6 months. As these neuromuscular achievements take hold, other developing systems are also evident.

Linguistic behavior. The vocal apparatus is used to produce protolinguistic expressions attracting the environment to the child while the child is incorporating the vocalizations of the surround. Even at this stage, infants seem to be prepared to selectively attend to congruent visual and acoustic signals (MacKain et al. 1983). Infants' babbling begins to take on meaning and significance as it differentiates into the speech of their mothers. Sapir (1921) suggests that in the beginning the child is overheard. Overheard, expressive vocalizations in infancy, usually beginning with vowel sounds and gutturals, may seem simple to the external observer. They have been conveniently divided into comfort and discomfort series based on the assumption that they have social significance (M. M. Lewis 1936). The developmental psychologist Buhler (1934) suggests that the infant moves from expression to appeal to propositionalizing.

However, we now understand that the child is well prepared and that he or she can distinguish phonetic contrasts in a highly refined manner (Eimas et al. 1971). This refinement may undergo both specialization and involution as development proceeds so that appreciated distinctions that are important in one language involute if the infant hears another language (Kuhl 1992). For example, the r/l distinction in Japanese is lost, although it is available in infants, and can be retaught only with difficulty to adult native Japanese speakers. The t/d distinction is available in infancy but may be lost in some language groups. The outcome of the intrusion of experience on early language and speech competence guarantees that the phonetic shape of words becomes specialized in accord with the community heard by the child. Surprisingly, most languages are made up of only 20–30 discrete phonemes that serve as the building blocks of more complex forms (Shapiro 1979).

Cognitive behavior. On a cognitive level, infants of ages 3–6 months show evidence of interest in hidden objects that then reappear (Bower et al. 1970). However, the cognitive substructures that subsume representational reality and thus constancy are dependent upon the achievement of the passage through the Piagetian sensory-motor period to the preoperational and early concrete operational stages.

The earliest developmental models of differentiation and integration of cognition have been reconsidered in recent years, because there is reasonably firm evidence that many cognitive abilities are already available in infancy and that the developmental process is not just one of progression of function and structure. Progression may run hand in hand with involution of some capabilities, giving rise to accentuation of various capacities at each stage on the basis of the evolution of different substructures derived from substrate and experience.

During this first year of development, the child is undergoing major cognitive shifts in his or her capacity to apprehend the external environment in a manner consonant with commonsense cultural reality. As noted, the period from birth to 18 months, from the standpoint of the development of intelligent action, concerns the development of a representational reality that spans the six stages of sensory-motor intelligence, as described by Piaget and discussed below.

The first and second stages refer to *heterologous and practical groups* in which no behavior pattern relative to vanished objects is observed and each event in time and space does not seem to be connected to its contiguous event. The infant may focus on the red ball held in the air in a reflexive manner, but when the ball is dropped, he or she will focus at the first position rather than following the ball's trajectory. It is as if the experience is fragmented, or cut into frames. As noted, sensory impressions are intimately entwined with motor activity, hence the term *sensory-motor intelligence*. In fact, paradoxically, our adult concept of a distinctive perceptual sensory experience apart from motor activity should be viewed as an achievement of development. We would have to project ourselves into our distant past to realize the intimate entwinement of the two. An adult analogy to the infant's plight might be cited in the opposite sequence. We try to learn a new motor skill by first intellectually trying to grasp it. Only later do we do it as a motor automatism (e.g., our fingers "remember" the tune when we play a piano). Recent work indicates that earliest memories are stored as procedural sequences, only later to be translated into nominal and verbal propositions. The latter changes are related to hippocampal development (Cohen et al. 1985).

The third stage of cognitive development is presumed when the child *extends movements already started*, which indicates that there is some sense of "thing permanence" so that, for example, the child follows the trajectory of the dropped ball to a vanishing point.

The fourth stage is characterized by *reversible operations* of seeking and finding with an active search for the vanished object. However, the child is not yet able to take into account the *sequential displacements* that go on out of sight. Thus, the infant may search as an extension of the motor act already begun.

By the fifth stage, *objective groups* are established and

there is some sense of the permanence of the object that is extended into the sixth and final stage, that of *representative groups*. Only then can the child imagine invisible displacements. The "thing" finally exists as a mental property, naively but practically assumed to be in the world. Bishop Berkeley's demand that things exist only as they are perceived bears some resemblance to Piaget's notion of early developmental reality. Things thus become objectified as development proceeds, and during this last stage, from age 16 to 18 months, "things" are freed of their motor components. The child can begin to mentally retrace movements. The possibility of a mental world has become established on purely cognitive grounds.

Although Piaget's scheme does not refer to emotional systems, Heinz Werner, inferring a more holistic view of development, refers to the sensory-motor-affective world of the infant. More recent work on affect and attachment will be addressed in a later section of this chapter. It is sufficient at this juncture, however, to note that the establishment of a representational world has some bearing on other matters of representations that *do* indeed touch emotions. For example, how does the child represent the mother? How does the child keep an image alive as a mental property even in the absence of a stimulus? What are the precursors to fantasying, imagining, and, finally, projecting the future? These features are abstracted in Piaget's model into the minimum set of achievements that are required in the mental schemata that lead to the accession of well-established representations of the external world. The alternation between *assimilating* a new event into a preexisting mental schema and then having that schema *accommodate* as a new structure now ready to receive other experiences is a process that goes on throughout the life span, carrying the child to the *preoperational period* of 2–7 years.

Toddler and Preschool Years: Language and Cognition

A toddler's life is replete with rapid changes in phenomenal behavior. He or she is animated, lively, striking out for independence, beginning to speak, and certainly comprehending. Representational play begins to appear, as does rapidly advancing hand-eye manipulation. From 3 years of age on, the toddler can begin to copy geometric forms, name them, and progressively begin to represent the human figure. The 3-year-old, full of exuberance, is also a language user. He or she can participate at table and can behave in limited social situations. Attendance at nursery school, with its routinized group demands of sharing and taking turns, becomes possible. Fantasy pretend play emerges in the early socialization process as well.

During the preoperational period, the child is still not able to decenter or imagine the vantage point from different positions in a room. There is no conservation of weight or volume and no cardinality of number or reversibility.

Most recent studies of Piagetian concepts suggest good cross-cultural validity on Piaget's findings, although he was not much interested in normative support. Piaget instead concentrated on the regularities in sequence of developmental achievement. Moreover, he proposed that children are active in their learning and not passive. However, qualitative differences between stages may not be as clear-cut as formerly thought. An uncanny experiment suggests that some abilities are present early but must reemerge later during the age period of 2–6 years with new cognitive underpinnings. If one puts a cube in an infant's mouth and then presents different shaped objects visually, the child focuses on the cube. Other synesthesias have been described as well. For example, certain vowel sounds are regularly associated with certain colors (e.g., \a\ with red). The fact that these synesthesias do not last throughout the life cycle indicates some involution of inbuilt propensities. Certain children at 3 or 4 years of age can solve some conservation problems, but these problems must be presented in relatively simple terms. This indicates that perhaps some of the failures and difficulties of younger children are due to the kind of language that was used in the initial experiments. Egocentricity, too, in the taking of other vantages may be more confounded by the language of the experimenter than Piaget thought.

In summary, the general outline of cognitive development is in accord with the model proposed by the Geneva school. However, modifications in detail have been necessary to preserve the edifice. Other aspects of Piagetian staging have been modified to take into account the role of affects. Only a few aspects of staging—some of those having relevance for cognitive performance—will be discussed in this section.

For example, social referencing (Klinnert et al. 1986) is one area in which an early relationship influences cognitive performance. A young child who is capable of crawling (i.e., age 8 months and older) can recognize a "visual cliff" (i.e., an illusion that there is a drop-off, although a transparent Plexiglas plate covers the drop). The child stops crawling at the cliff margin. However, if the mother is at the other end encouraging him or her, the child will proceed in accord with the afforded confidence (perhaps a sign of Erikson's basic trust). This permission indicates that cognitive perceptual and neurodevelopmental capacity may be qualified on the grounds of early socialization. This hypothesis offers a fascinating possibility for a review of adaptation as an achievement not only of cognitive significance but of the emotional surround.

As the child moves into the toddler years, much of what takes place in the cognitive sphere well into the beginnings of school rests upon the acquisition of language and communicative ability. The emotional and social climate of learning also becomes very important, and we tend to take the neurodevelopmental aspects and cognitive aspects more for granted until the changes that occur at ages 6 and 7 years. Language competence and performance develop at a rapid pace. The 2-year-old rapidly achieves telegraphic speech of two words, which indicates his or her understanding that some words are more important than others when a message is to be conveyed. The child then adds grammatical morphemes (i.e., small endings on words that signify tense, person, etc.) (Brown 1973). These rapid shifts occur sequentially, in an orderly manner, in accord with the language that is spoken. By 3 years of age the child is a fairly competent speaker, with a three- to six-word mean length of utterance (MLU)—a circumstance that most competent adult speakers would be pleased to achieve if they were traveling in a foreign country and wished to have reasonable talking grasp of the commonplace aspects of living and expression of needs among that language group.

These linguistic feats have their precursors in the capacity to designate. Werner and Kaplan (1963) described the progression from reaching, to grasping, to pointing, and, finally, to designating verbally by single words. These early words may stand for full sentences. Indeed, it was formerly thought that the first 50-word corpus consisted of only nouns. However, some children have a higher concentration of prepositions and verbs that refer to rather complicated concepts (Nelson 1981). Moreover, what we thought of as concreteness during the 1- to 3-word stage may represent a more canny understanding of the world than our prior understanding would admit. It has been argued by some linguist-developmentalists that one-word utterances are indeed phrases (or at least refer to phrases), although the child has a constraint on his or her capacity to form longer phrases. Certainly there is general agreement that the child may imitate before he or she comprehends, and that production follows. Thus, there is a greater constraint developmentally on expression-production than on understanding. A most remarkable finding that undoes some of the mechanical presuppositions about language development concerns the early detection of narrative lines in children's learning, even with children at ages 2 or 3 years (Bretherton 1989; Nelson 1986). Events are organized into scripts that aid in mastery at each stage.

The remarkable achievement of deixis suggests a very early capacity to distinguish a "this" from a "that," or "I" from "you," from "me." These distinctions are regularly achieved by 2 years. Similarly, concreteness begs for explanation. The child of limited vocabulary who designates his or her dog "Rex" may then see a horse or a sheep and call either "Rex." The child is not acting concretely, nor is ignorance a factor. A more parsimonious explanation is that the child has an essential understanding of quadrupedia.

Nonetheless, the child may exhibit concreteness in other ways because of a limited understanding of the nuances of language. This is most apparent in the adult concept of the *joke*. Jokes told by 5- to 10-year-olds tend to be puns or restatements of naughty words and are not very funny to adults. The child practices with the laughter that goes with the presumed joke. He or she also seems to thrive on repetition, but it is certain that the adult sense of the word "joke" is not achieved.

Although the cognitive and neurodevelopmental capacities necessary for independence may be present before 7 years of age, the maturity of the mental apparatus and judgments about the world are not sufficient for the child to take his or her place in the larger social world. We have instituted nursery schools for day care and kindergartens since the late 19th century, but these are generally places where socialization occurs and manipulative skills are stressed. Even as such schooling has taken hold, we are forced to recognize variation in temperament as attributes to be considered in the interactive process. Kagan et al. (1989) have described quiet, vigilant, and restrained children at 2 years of age as constituting a distinctive group with physiological correlates. The children in this group negotiate the interpersonal world with more difficulty and require special attention lest they become anxious and, finally, ill. Although such variation is apparent early in life and may persist, most cultures have decided that formal schooling should take place somewhere between 6 and 7 years. This landmark, among others, marks the seventh year (plus or minus one) (Shapiro and Perry 1976).

The Second Biodevelopmental Shift

Every level of study, from the neurodevelopmental to the cognitive and social, suggests that there is a discontinuity at age 7 years that would correspond to a second biodevelopmental shift. The brain attains its adult format and reaches the asymptote of its maximum weight at 7 years. Neuronal dendrites are most dense at this age. Moreover, it is after age 7 that children begin to understand that their feelings, intuitions, and thoughts may be of interest to others and, more important, may be thought about by others. Recent work on the relevance of the concept of a theory of mind has been used to record phenomena related to our ability to conceptualize the other as different from ourselves. Children of age 7 have had the experience of viewing the actions of others in terms of separate motivation, and they can infer feelings. They also seem to begin to understand cause-and-effect relationships between objects, events, and situations, and they can begin to understand concepts such as ambivalence. Children at this age begin to show understanding of conservation and reversibility as noted earlier. They can grasp the concept of conservation of weight (despite how much a piece of clay is distorted in shape), of volume (despite container shape), or of number (despite, for example, the length of a line of coins).

Although children aged 7 years and older can do all these things, they may also develop rigidities. They become rule bound and even moralistic about rules, outreasoning their parents in accord with the rules they have been taught. They chastise parents for smoking or for minor infractions of the law. They make statements such as, "I didn't learn it this way!" Yet, although they expect devotion and rigor from their parents, children this age sometimes break rules too.

Children at this age are exceedingly fickle in friendships, but at the same time demand absolute allegiance. "Best friends" may turn out to be different individuals each day. Children during this period tend to set up clubs with complicated rule structures and debate (what would be the equivalent of Robert's Rules of Order). These clubs may consist of two or at most five individuals, thus making everyone a leader or officer.

Rituals are also rampant despite the achievement of formal cognitive landmarks. In their monumental work *Lore and Language of School Children*, Opie and Opie (1959) indicate how the development of children's games and jump-rope rhymes traversed the English-speaking world by oral transmission. The similarities in games across natural boundaries are remarkable. Latency is a period when games are paramount and when persistence at games and collecting are central concerns; 8- to 12-year-olds collect anything from baseball cards to paper clips, and commercial firms exploit that trait.

We know that in this stage inner life goes on, but it seems to become subsumed under tasks that are of highly practical and personal appeal. The period that Freud called *latency*, and is now more neutrally named *middle childhood*, becomes a time of mastering a great number of facts and skills. The period through fourth grade is considered by many educators to be a time of skill development in preparation for the application of reading, arithmetic, and writing to those creative activities that are to ensue. Self-righteousness and preoccupation with being admired and cared for, and acceptance of the ministrations of parents, are the hallmark of this stage in normal environments. On the other hand, persistence of difficulty in going to sleep, righteous indignation, and other irrationally dictated activities may be manifest in the same time period and setting in which these new maturities are developing.

Historically the period from age 7 years on has been recognized as a watershed. The Roman Catholic Church designated 7 years as the age of reason. It is a time when children in modern cultures begin first grade (or "real" school). During the 18th and 19th centuries this period was a time of apprenticeship away from the home. The language and motor capacities of these youngsters were so cultivated that during the Industrial Revolution heavy work and exploitation also were possible. Children were used for many tasks. Their size (cognitive capacities permitting) prompted their use as chimney sweeps and as laborers in mines, leading to the later development of child labor laws to legislate against the abuse that was permitted by such exploitation.

The beginning signs of puberty and the special socialization that Harry Stack Sullivan (1953, p. 245) called "chumship" (i.e., during the juvenile years between 10 and 14) mark the end of latency. The child then becomes ready to move on to adolescence. The physiological underpinnings of preadolescence and adolescence are marked by growth spurts, body configuration changes, and changes toward sexual readiness for procreation. The physiological and neurological bases are matched also by cognitive changes in the variable attainment of abstract reasoning. Thus, we have ample reason to believe that puberty is a biological event. Socialization changes also during this period. If one looks historically to the period prior to universal public education, many youngsters, barely pubescent, went off to the university or to seek their fortune or the like in the prepubertal era. For example, Benjamin Franklin at age 12 became an apprentice in a print shop in Philadelphia. Others went west to the Allegheny mountains and later to the Great Plains and the Rockies. The further characteristics of social maturation and development in this period will be dealt with later in the section on adolescence.

AFFECTIVE-INTERACTIVE ORGANIZATION

The Newborn Infant

The human infant is born into a social world. From the very first moments of life the infant's physical characteristics and behavioral patterns attract the caring attention of the people in its environment. Bowlby (1969), beginning with observations of children separated from their parents during World War II, has expanded our vision of the determinants of attachment between caregiver and child, in part through observations of humans but also of ethological systems across species. Drawing on work with primates, ungulates, and nonmammalian species, Bowlby proposed that attachment originates in inherited species-characteristic behavior called *inborn response systems.* The appeal of the very young—what Darwin (1872) called "babyness"—is universal. The infant's physical appearance—its tininess, largish head with prominent forehead, small face, big eyes, chubby cheeks and small mouth, coupled with its small body, uncoordinated movement patterns, occasional smiles, brightening of the eyes, and vocalizations and cries—stimulates the interest and concern of parents. By clinging, sucking, vocalizing, crying, smiling, and following, the infant brings or keeps the caregiver close. Human babies initially follow with their eyes and cling as part of a grasp reflex, and suck to obtain nutrition needed for survival. The behavioral patterns of the newborn ensure the proximity of the caretaker that is necessary for sheer physical survival. Indeed, it is the survival value of these systems that makes them relevant to the socialization process.

Among these inborn response systems, *affectivity* is essential. For the first 2 months of life, the care of the infant is primarily concerned with the regulation and stabilization of sleep-wake and hunger-satiation cycles. The parents of newborns are focused on the tasks of responding to signals of distress: of feeding, changing, and getting the infant to sleep. Parents accomplish these tasks through behaviors that are social as well as physical; they rock, stroke, talk, and sing to the baby in their efforts to comfort and soothe. These caregiving activities intensify parental attachment.

Recent research contributions have led to major revisions in our understanding of the capacities of the newborn to perceive, assimilate, organize, and respond to social stimuli. Rather than occupying a state of "normal autism," essentially unrelated to others (Mahler et al. 1975) and shielded by a "stimulus barrier" (Freud 1920/1959), it has become increasingly clear that the newborn infant seeks sensory stimulation in periods of quiet alertness. The world of the newborn is not the blooming, buzzing confusion postulated by William James. Between birth and 2 months of age, infants select out the movement and size attributes of visual stimuli. As noted earlier, these very young infants are capable of recognizing similarities and differences not only within sense systems but across sensory modalities as well. By 6 weeks of age babies tend to look more closely at faces that speak, and in experimental situations they focus longer on faces that move in ways consistent with, rather than discrepant from, a simultaneously presented auditory stimulus. Thus, infants appear to have an innate general capacity to take information received in one sensory modality and translate it into another sensory modality, a capacity referred to as *amodal perception* (Stern 1985; Karmiloff-Smith 1995).

Infants can perceive persons as unique forms from the very beginning. Newborns act differently when scanning live faces than when scanning inanimate patterns; they vocalize more and their movement patterns are smoother and more coordinated (Brazelton et al. 1974). Neonates have consistently been shown to be able to discriminate the mother's voice from that of another woman reading the same material (DeCasper and Fifer 1980), and infants as young as 2 days have been found to be able to reliably imitate an adult model who either smiled, frowned, or showed a surprise face (Field et al. 1982). Moreover, by 6 weeks of age infants display evidence of delayed imitation. Infants presented with a person who pulled his tongue in and out repeatedly, pushed out their tongues when viewing the same person, this time with lips closed, after an interval of 24 hours. Such behaviors were not generated in response to new faces seen for the first time (Meltzoff and Moore 1994).

Babies are particularly receptive to the ways in which people interact with them. When babies cry, fret, gaze, or vary their facial expressions, parents and other caregivers characteristically look with widened eyes and raised eyebrows (i.e., "baby faces") and speak in high-pitched voices with exaggerated rhythm (i.e., "baby talk" or "Motherese"). It is the rhythmic features of the acoustic signal itself, with its exaggerated prosodic contours, that initially holds the attention of infants (Kaplan et al. 1995). Mothers have little difficulty in deciding whether their babies are content or distressed, and only somewhat more difficulty in attaching specific affective labels to facial expressions (Emde and Harmon 1972; Pannabecker et al. 1980). Izard (1982), in analyzing film records of neonates, has reliably differentiated facial expressions of interest, joy, distress, disgust, surprise, and anger. The behavior repertoire of even the youngest of infants includes an emotional component (i.e., emotional expression).

Emergence of Emotional Experience

Modern theorists of emotional development distinguish between emotional state, emotional expression, and emotional experience. In the structural analysis of emotions proposed by Lewis and Michelson (1983), *emotional state* refers to internal changes in somatic and/or physiological activity, and *emotional expression* to observable changes in face, body, voice, and activity level that occur when the

CNS is activated by emotionally salient stimuli. *Emotional experience* refers to the consequences of the cognitive appraisal and interpretation of perceived emotional states and expression. Although some investigators have used emotional expression as an indicator of emotional state (Izard 1982), others have pointed out that the two are not necessarily congruent. However, neither state nor observable expression is connected in a one-to-one relationship with emotional experience. Emotional experiences require a sense of self—an "I" to evaluate changes in "me"—as well as the cognitive capacity to perceive, discriminate, recall, associate, and compare. From this perspective, the very young baby's emotional expressions tell us little of his or her emotional experience. Nevertheless, parents and others respond to the infant's emotional expressions as if they were reflections of subjective experience. By interpreting and evaluating emotional expression, the social environment provides the rules by which children come to learn to evaluate and interpret—in other words, to experience—their own behaviors and states.

Thus, the infant is a social being from the first moments of extrauterine life, with innate capacities that permit him or her to function as an active partner in the social interactions that occur within the context of the regulation of physiological functions. In Stern's (1985) view, an emergent sense of self—in relation to others—is present from birth: "[Infants] never experience a period of total self/other undifferentiation, [and] there is no confusion between self and other in the beginning or at any point during infancy" (p. 10). The affects, perceptions, sensorimotor events, memories, and other cognitions that accompany social interactions become increasingly integrated over time, providing a framework for the further elaboration of both a sense of self and an awareness of and attachment to others.

Even though newborn infants have the capacity to deal with the stimulation afforded by the external world, and can become deeply engaged in and related to social stimuli, their tolerance is limited. During the first 2 months of life, the baby is in a state of quiet alertness for only very short periods of time. Gesell and Amatruda (1947) noted that the 4-week-old child sleeps for as many as 20 hours each day. Often it is only in the late afternoon (typically between 4 and 6 o'clock) that there is a more sustained opportunity for social interaction.

By 2 months of age, biobehavioral transformations affecting the nature and quality of social interactions are well underway (Emde et al. 1976; Spitz 1965). Sleep and activity cycles have stabilized, motor patterns are more mature, and altered visual scanning patterns permit new strategies for attachment to the world. Symmetry, complexity, and novelty are becoming salient attributes of visual stimuli. Learning occurs more rapidly and more inclusively. The perceptual preferences for the human face and voice, present at birth, are fully operative. The social smile is well established, vocalizations directed at persons entering the infant's range of vision have begun, and mutual gaze is actively sought.

The period between 2 and 7 months is perhaps the most exclusively social period of life. The baby is described as liking people to pay attention, talk, or sing to him or her. The spontaneous behavior of adults—"baby talk" and "baby faces"—is well matched to the infant's perceptual biases, with the result that the infant can maximally attend to the adult social stimulus. Typically, caregivers repeat their exaggerated facial expressions, gestures, and vocalizations with minor variations, which serve to regulate the infant's level of arousal and excitation within a tolerable range. Infants, too, are able to regulate their level of social engagement, using gaze aversion to cut out stimulation that has risen above an optimal range, and vocalizations and alterations of facial expression to invite new levels of stimulation when excitation has fallen too low. As a consequence the baby gains experience with both self-regulation and the regulation of the behavior of others.

Infants draw upon these daily life experiences to consolidate a sense of a core self as a separate, cohesive, bounded physical unit. For Stern (1985) there is no symbiotic-like phase as Mahler has proposed. Between 2 and 6 or 7 months, babies come to recognize their own agency—that is, they are increasingly able to recognize relations between actions and reactions, to engage in voluntary activities, and to anticipate the consequences of such activities, both for themselves and for others. Moreover, the infant has a growing capacity to register motoric and perceptual events, together with their concomitant affects, in memory (Stern 1985).

Emergence of Seven-Month Wariness (Stranger Anxiety)

The development of a core sense of self is paralleled by an increasing ability to engage in social discriminations. Gesell notes that the 16-week-old baby displays a marked interest in the father and also in young children. Between 4 and 6 months the baby begins to respond to more than one person at a time, and appears to enjoy being handed from one familiar person to another.

At about this time a wariness of strangers first becomes apparent (Schaffer and Emerson 1964). The baby appears cautious and watchful in the presence of strangers. Often wariness is combined with expressions of interest and curiosity. Although facial expressions of fear begin to be noted at 6 months of age (Cicchetti and Sroufe 1978), outright fear in the presence of a stranger is not regularly observed until somewhat later (8–12 months), and even then it is dependent on the situation. Expressions of fear are least likely to occur if the infant is with a parent, if there is a familiarization period, and if the stranger's approach is mediated by a toy or game. Fear is most likely when strangers intrude rapidly and seek to pick up the infant (Bretherton and Ainsworth 1974; Horner 1980; Rheingold and Eckerman 1973).

Historically, expressions of wariness and fear in the presence of strangers have been referred to as "stranger anxiety." This has been designated as the second organizer by Spitz, as noted earlier. The baby is also beginning to be most demanding of attention from a particular person, most often, as Gesell points out, "the one who feeds him" (Gesell and Ilg 1949, p. 115), and is more readily comforted by this person when distressed.

Affective Attunement

When infants are between 7 and 9 months of age, Stern (1985) suggests, the sense of self undergoes further reorganization to include a capacity to share certain subjective experiences—in particular, attention, intention, and affective states. Infants of 9 months appear to be capable of joint attention. Not only will they visually follow the direction of the mother's pointing finger beyond her hand to the target, but after their gaze reaches the target they will look back at the mother and appear to use the feedback from her face to confirm that they have arrived at the intended goal. Similarly, babies at this time are increasingly capable of communicating intention and of sharing affective experiences.

Stern (1985) provides rich behavioral descriptions of the process of affective sharing that characterizes attunement. *Attunement* refers to that dimension of the caregiver's behavior that matches *not* behavior per se, but some aspect of the behavior that appears to underscore the baby's feeling state. In attunements, the matching is largely cross-modal—that is, the modality of expression used by the mother to match the infant's behavior is different from that used by the infant. For example, a 9-month-old boy bangs his hand on a soft toy, setting up a steady rhythm and smiling with pleasure and exuberance. Mother falls into his rhythm and says, "Kaaa-bam, kaaa-bam," with the "bam" falling on the stroke and the "kaaa" accompanying the upswing of his arm. These experiences play a role in the infant coming to recognize that internal feeling states are forms of human experience that are shareable with others. The baby's behavior is also beginning to be influenced by the emotional expressions of others—a phenomenon called *social referencing*. As noted above, investigators (Emde and Harmon 1972; Klinnert et al. 1986) have demonstrated that a baby of 8 months of age or older can be induced to cross a visual cliff if his or her mother smiles, but will turn away if she assumes a fearful facial expression. Taken together, Stern's sense of a core self and his sense of intersubjective self correspond to what self psychologists term the *subjective* or *existential self*—the "me" (Harter 1983).

Selective Attachment

By 10 months of age most infants not only exhibit wariness of strangers but also have developed selective attachments to a small number (usually three or four) of specific persons. Children become attached not only to their mothers, but to fathers, siblings, other relatives, baby-sitters, and family friends. However, there is usually a marked hierarchy among these various attachments, with the mother at top. Once attachment has developed, babies actively seek proximity and contact with the mother, particularly when faced with an unfamiliar or frightening situation. When they are with their mother they tend to comfortably play and explore the environment, but when mother is out of sight, the infants will very likely follow or protest, either immediately or after a short while. The term *separation anxiety* has been used to describe the distress exhibited by the baby when mother is unavailable. Also, according to Bowlby (1969), the visible distress of separation is a manifestation not only of anxiety but of depression occasioned by the loss of a love object. When this situation is considered in terms of the structural theory of emotions proposed by Lewis and Michelson (1983), it is not clear that the baby who exhibits wariness or fear of strangers, or protests the departure of an attachment figure, actually experiences anxiety and/or depression. The 10-month-old baby is just beginning to develop the capacity to engage in the cognitive self-appraisal of his or her emotional states and expressions.

The Strange Situation

Ainsworth and colleagues (1978) have developed a research method for assessing the quality of attachment in 12- to 18-month-old children. The *strange situation* procedure involves a set series of 3-minute separations and reunions with a caregiver and with a stranger in an unfamiliar room. Children who show mild protest following the departure, who seek the mother when she returns, and who are easily placated by her (about two-thirds of a sample of middle-class 1-year-old American children) are considered as the most *securely attached*. Infants who do not protest maternal departure and who do not approach the mother when she returns (about one-quarter of the sample) are characterized as *avoidant*. Children who become markedly upset by departure and who resist the mother's efforts to comfort them when she returns (about a tenth of the sample) are described as *resistant* or *anxiously attached*.

The classification derives from Bowlby's (1969) proposal that the biological "purpose" of attachment is to provide emotional security and social autonomy. Babies designated as showing "secure" attachments tend later to exhibit greater social competence and better peer relationships (Sroufe and Fleeson 1984). Reciprocally, it should be noted that the caregiver's own experience and attitude toward attachment are highly predictive of the toddler's security of attachment (Fonagy et al. 1991).

The behavior of children in the "strange situation" may also be considered from the perspective of individual differences in temperamental organization (Kagan 1984). In the New York Longitudinal Study, Thomas and Chess (Chess and Thomas 1984; Thomas and Chess 1977) have identified nine categories of temperament that describe how children behave in daily life situations:

1. Activity level
2. Rhythmicity (regularity of biological functions)
3. Approach or withdrawal to new situations
4. Adaptability in new or altered situations
5. Sensory threshhold of responsiveness to stimuli
6. Intensity of reaction
7. Quality of mood
8. Distractibility
9. Attention span/persistence

These categories cluster as follows:

1. The *easy child* pattern is characterized by regularity, positive approach responses to new stimuli, high adaptability to change, and expressions of mood that are only mild or moderate in intensity and predominantly positive.
2. The *difficult child* pattern, at the opposite end of the temperamental spectrum, is characterized by irregularity in biological functions, negative withdrawal responses to new situations, nonadaptability or slow adaptability to change, and intense, frequently negative expressions of mood.
3. The *slow-to-warm-up child* is characterized by a combination of negative responses of mild intensity to new situations with slow adaptability after repeated

contact. Kagan et al.'s (1989) inhibited child belongs in this group.

Although difficult children comprised only 10% of the New York Longitudinal Study sample, 70% of those who were classified as difficult during the first 3 years of life developed clinically evident behavior problems during early and middle childhood (Thomas and Chess 1977).

The 1-year-old child's behavior in the strange situation provides a prototype for many of the social developmental changes during the next 2 years. The child's capacity to physically explore the environment, to engage in social interactions, to comfort himself or herself, and to derive comfort from others in the absence of the mother increases dramatically. In Mahler's view (Mahler et al. 1975) these events occur as a consequence of a process of separation-individuation during which the mother comes to be perceived as a separate person while the child realizes his or her capabilities as an independent and autonomous entity who can function effectively in the mother's absence.

Separation-Individuation

In the period between approximately 10 and 16 months, the child devotes considerable energy to practicing locomotor skills and exploring the environment. Early in this period, the infant will search for the absent mother or repeat "Mama." Later the child shows a greater tolerance for separation and may seem unconcerned with the mother's whereabouts. Mahler calls this the *practicing subphase* (Mahler et al. 1975). Although having some mental representation of mother that is comforting in her absence, the infant also frequently seeks to reestablish bodily or visual contact with her. Mahler terms this behavior *refueling*, considering it a restorative process that provides the child with sufficient energy to further practice newly found skills and explore the environment.

Between 16 to 24 months, ambivalence is often intense. The child seems to want to be united with but at the same time be separate from the mother. Temper tantrums, whining, sad moods, and intense separation reactions are at their peak. Mahler suggests that during this *rapprochement subphase* the mental image of mother is considered to be insufficiently strong to provide comfort in periods of upset, leading the child to cling to the mother and to displace anger onto another caregiver.

Between 24 and 36 months, *negativism, willfulness,* and *contrariness* give way to a new realization of social demands. Disappointment, frustration, and absence of mother become better tolerated as the child's mental representation of the mother develops more stability. Not only is the mother clearly perceived as a separate person in the outside world, but the internal representations of her "good" and "bad" aspects are more solidly integrated. The availability of a secure and reliable internal representation of mother affords comfort when she is absent and facilitates the child's increasing ability to engage in independent activities and more flexible personal relations.

Between 18 months and 3 years, the development of language contributes to the further organization of the sense of self and the sense of others. Language provides the self and other with a new medium for exchange with which to create shared meanings. With the advent of what Stern (1985) refers to as the "verbal self," children begin to see themselves objectively. By 18 months of age they are able to recognize themselves in mirrors, still pictures, and videotapes (Lewis and Brooks-Gunn 1979). By 2 years they begin to use "I" to refer to themselves, and shortly thereafter to call other people "you" (see below). Genetic, prenatal-hormonal, pubertal-hormonal, and socialization factors all contribute to the determination of subsequent sexual status and orientation (Money 1987), but for most children, gender identity becomes established as well. Thus the achievements of locomotion, language, sense of self, and core gender all seem to coordinate a growing child's sense of separateness.

Lewis (Lewis and Michelson 1983; Lewis et al. 1989) suggests that the emergence of a categorical self and the corresponding ability to categorize others facilitate the acquisition of social knowledge of emotions and the development of the complex emotional experiences that accompany the social emotions of empathy, guilt, embarrassment, and shame. Children as young as 18 months display a beginning understanding of the goals and intentions of others (Meltzoff 1995), and by 2 years of age, some children are capable of empathic behavior and show some cognitive understanding of the emotions of others (Borke 1971).

Emotions in Toddlers and Middle Childhood

Children can discriminate among pictures depicting different emotions earlier than they can label them, although some 2-year-old children can produce verbal labels for emotional behaviors such as crying and laughter. The recognition and labeling of the basic emotions of joy, sadness, anger, and fear develop earlier than those of emotions such as contempt and shame. By 2 years of age, children can dissimulate emotions and pretend to assume emotional states. Between 2 and 4 years of age, children produce increasingly appropriate facial expressions when provided with a verbal label, whereas between 3 and 4 years they begin to be able to designate what emotions are appropriate to particular situations (Lewis and Michelson 1983). Emotional experiences become increasingly more clearly defined through the interaction of children with their social environment.

By 3 years of age, children have developed a well-articulated sense of both the subjective self and the objective self, or, to use the terminology of Lewis and Brooks-Gunn (1979), the *existential* self and the *categorical* self. Children at this age have well-established social relations with members of their immediate families, and are beginning to expand their social horizons beyond the confines of home. Nevertheless, if a stranger is present or the situation is otherwise stressful, children of 3 years may still become upset at separation from mother. The advent of language facilitates the capacity for symbolic play reflective of daily life experiences, as well as the identification and sharing of affective states. Affective displays come under increasing control. Affects are beginning to be socialized, and the complex experiences of guilt, embarrassment, and shame begin to be elaborated. Children come to know the names of their feelings and when to display what affects, and increasingly to experience empathy (Bretherton and Ainsworth 1974).

Between 3 and 5 years of age, the concept of a private self that is not observable by others begins to be elaborated. Expressed emotions, which encompass a full range of affects, fluctuate easily at age 4 but have become more stable by age 5. The ability to use language to distinguish among affects expands, as does the capacity to identify situation-appropriate emotions. Conversational reference to feelings and mental states expands during the preschool period (Brown et al. 1996). Children begin to elaborate a "theory of mind" as they become increasing adept at inferring what it is that others know and feel (Baron-Cohen 1989). As the capacity for "mindreading" develops, so does the ability to engage in deception, teasing, and cooperative play with a division of roles and a sharing of goals (Dunn 1996).

Relationship patterns become more complicated, and rivalries, jealousies, secrets, and envy begin to emerge. Fantasies become increasingly complex when compared with earlier scripts, and include aggressive and sexual elements as well as concerns about separation and loss of love. Behavioral differentiation of the sexes is minimal when children are observed or tested individually. Sex differences emerge primarily in social situations, and their nature varies with the gender composition of dyads and groups. Tendencies to prefer same-sexed playmates can be seen among 3-year-olds, and preferences increase in strength and are maintained at a high level between the ages of 6 and at least 11 (Maccoby 1990).

The period of middle childhood is marked by changes in the ability to regulate and modulate affects. Six-year-olds can be highly emotional, and angry outbursts are frequent. By age 7, children may appear to be moody and sulky, and complain that they are unliked and that people are mean and unfair. By age 8, children are described as impatient and demanding, frequently bursting into tears or laughing uproariously. Humor begins to play a role in the modulation of affects. A sense of right and wrong emerges, and children may feel guilty and inwardly unhappy and frankly sad if they have failed to live up to a standard. First-graders have come to appreciate that they cannot change—say, become an animal or a child of the opposite sex—and that the self is continuous from past to future (Guardo and Bohan 1971). As they progress through primary school, children become increasingly capable of emotional deceit—that is, the ability to display an emotion different from their underlying feelings (Saarni 1979).

During this period children are also interested in defining their place in the family and in relation to other family members. Children fluctuate between love for family and worries about not belonging. Fantasies of having been adopted and having rich and powerful natural parents are frequent. This is referred to as the *family romance* fantasy. The relationship between siblings is distinctive in its emotional power and intimacy. Studies of siblings throughout childhood and adolescence report a marked range of individual differences between sibling pairs in measures of friendliness, conflict, rivalry, and dominance. Moreover, such dimensions are relatively independent of one another. Maternal behavior (particularly *differences* in the mother's behavior toward her two children), the children's age, the difference in age between them, as well as their temperament, all contribute significantly to differences between sibling pairs (Stocker et al. 1989).

Not only do relationships between siblings differ in different families, but the personality characteristics of children growing up in the same family are also often strikingly dissimilar. Plomin and Daniels (1987) have suggested that within-family differences—the nonshared environment—may be more important than between-family differences in their effects on the developing child.

During middle childhood, interests in relationships with peers and teachers expand. Childhood games with rules emerge as does a capacity for intimacy with a "best friend." However, the two sexes engage in fairly different kinds of activities and games. Boys play in somewhat larger groups, on the average, and their play is rougher and more expansive. Boys more often play in streets and other public places, whereas girls more often congregate in private homes or yards. Girls tend to form close, intimate friendships with one or two other girls, and these friendships are marked by the sharing of confidences. Boys' friendships are more oriented around mutual interests in activities. The breakup of girls' friendships is usually accompanied by more intense emotional reactions than is the case for boys.

Different interactive styles develop in same-sex groups. Boys in their groups are more likely than girls in all-girl groups to interrupt one another, refuse to comply with another child's demand, heckle a speaker, or call another child names. Girls in all-girl groups are more likely than boys to express agreement with what another speaker has just said, pause to give another girl a chance to speak, and acknowledge a point made by another speaker. There is more conflict in boys' groups, and when conflict occurs, girls are more likely to use "conflict-mitigating strategies," whereas boys more often use threats of physical force. Although boys appear to be more concerned with issues of dominance, their confrontational style does not necessarily impede effective group functioning, as evidenced by their ability to cooperate with teammates in sports. Moreover, when interacting among themselves, girls are not unassertive. Rather, while pursuing their own ends, they simultaneously strive to tone down coercion and dominance to bring about agreement and restore or maintain group functioning (Maccoby 1990).

Between 9 and 10 years of age, children still define themselves in terms of concrete objective categories such as address, physical appearance, possessions, and play activities. Self-criticism is prominent, but children are also beginning to be able to accept jokes by others about themselves. The concept of family continues to be important to most children, although they often prefer to be either on their own, with friends, or with other adults who, like the parents, may serve as role models. There are well-developed capacities for empathy, love, compassion, and sharing, as well as outbursts of person-directed anger, self-evaluative depression, and self-centered righteousness. Children increasingly evaluate their own behavior; they may be disgusted or apprehensive about their own actions, and guilty and ashamed about past behaviors. New affects around sexual differences begin to emerge. Children begin to experience both excitement and shyness in relation to sexual themes, and shame becomes a prominent guide to action, heralding the onset of puberty and entry into adolescence.

ADOLESCENCE

WHAT IS ADOLESCENCE?

Adolescence has come to represent the developmental bridge between middle childhood or latency and adulthood. It also marks a discontinuity in development based upon biological, psychological, and social factors that set this period apart from both childhood and adulthood. Regrettably, in the minds of many, development ends here. However, modern theorists suggest that developmental processes continue throughout the life cycle and that each phase or period may be subjected to a developmental analysis. In that sense this chapter on development is incomplete. Among the developmental stages, adolescence has gathered a questionable, if not bad, reputation, second only in the terror that the "terrible twos" elicit in young parents. Adolescence stands out because of the disruptions in behavior, the moodiness, and the difficulties in living, as well as the conflicts and strife with families that have been considered normative.

These popular opinions are striking in view of the fact that adolescence is relatively new on the developmental scene, partly so because there remains some uncertainty as to how to define adolescence and whether adolescence existed in preindustrial society or exists in non-Western communities (Ariès 1962; Esman 1990; Stone and Church 1957). From a sociological vantage point, the rites of passage that mark the terminus of childhood are well known. They include initiation rights of religion and society in the form of confirmation, bar mitzvah, hunting tasks, scarification, and subincision that permit entry into the adult community of men and women in various cultures. These rituals mark entry into adulthood rather than into an intermediate phase. On the other hand, in some communities as distant as pre-Periclean Greece, there was a clear distinction between the young man (i.e., the *ephebus*) and the marriageable nubile girl, and those who became procreative members of the full community. Indeed, sociologists sometimes look at adolescence as consisting of an alienated group of a certain age who are defined by exclusion. Neither children nor adults, they are partially excluded from either of these more dominant communities. More recent work seeks to define adolescence as a distinct subculture with its own lore and rules.

Although some would like to see adolescence as equivalent to puberty (see below), it would be hard to justify that it simply is puberty. Nonetheless, growing into one's primary and secondary sexual characteristics is one of the essential tasks of adolescence. To this we might add the psychological and social adaptations that are secondary to external as well as internal biological demands. Thus, our definition of adolescence will have to be tailored to three factors: the biological, the social, and the psychological demands of the period.

PUBERTY

Biologically, *puberty* refers to attaining the capacity to procreate as a mature member of a species. The appropriate growth and development of the external genitalia and of the ovaries and testes and their products, the ovum and sperm becoming viable and ready for fertilization and the formation of a gamete, are essential for survival. The notion of puberty as a phase in the biological life cycle is more important from a psychosocial vantage point because the external characteristics (i.e., secondary sexual characteristics) of both sexes become prominent social signs. In females puberty occurs 2 years earlier than in males, and the first signs are breast buds, followed by the growth of pubic and axillary hair and the attainment of a feminine body habitus with broadening of the hips (Tanner 1968). In the United States, girls achieve menarche at a mean age of 12.7 years (Zacharias et al. 1970), with 5% beginning at 11–11.5 years, 25% at 12–12.5 years, and 60% by age 13. Nine percent of normal females experience menarche up to 5 years after the beginning of breast development. A height spurt also begins to take place at age 11 that peaks at 12 and then falls off at 14 or 15. Menarche is frequently followed by irregular anovulatory periods for 12–18 months, at which time a more regular menstrual cycle ensues. The task of adapting to the new bodily format soon encroaches on and influences psychological content and becomes an important feature of social adaptation (Tanner 1968).

In boys, the height spurt begins somewhat later, at age 12, peaking at around 14 years, and begins to fall by age 16 or 17. Correspondingly, the penis and the testes are already on their way to achieving adult size and form. Pubic and axillary hair likewise begin to be prominent, as does the masculine habitus, and there is deepening of the voice.

In both sexes these primary and secondary sexual changes correspond to activation of hypothalamic functions that in turn stimulate the gonadotropic hormones of the pituitary. These hormones stimulate both estrogen and luteinizing hormone at the periphery as well as testosterone, especially in boys. These changes are thought to be coordinated with maturation of the hypothalamic cells. They become less sensitive to the feedback dampening effect of circulating sex hormones. In males, nocturnal emissions are observed to occur about a year after the secondary sexual characteristics develop and mark the beginning of the capacity to procreate.

In the CNS, dendritic connections attain their adult levels, dropping back from the high density of proliferation seen at about age 7 (see subsection on second biodevelopmental shift earlier in this chapter). Encephalographic changes also occur by age 14 when mature alpha-rhythm patterns become well established.

The regular trend toward earlier puberty, especially in girls, in European and American populations has been attributed to better diet. There is also some suggestion that menarche and physical maturity may have long historical cycles so that the early onset of puberty in our time may be a temporary event. However, the data available do suggest that during the 1880s the average onset of menarche was 15–16 years; by 1925 it was 13–14.

COGNITIVE ORGANIZATION IN ADOLESCENCE

While these bodily changes are taking place, intellectual and cognitive developments keep pace. Piaget (1952) suggests that operational intelligence gained at age 7 is advanced *abstract* intelligence in adolescence. The adolescent is now ready to mature into formal operations, leaving concrete operations behind. For example, instead of the adolescent girl suggesting to her mother that she ought to be able to wear lipstick because all the other girls do, she could now argue that given her maturity, exemplified by new abilities, and her age, she ought to be able to make decisions about lipstick in the same way she is permitted to make other decisions. The march of sophisticated reasoning involving causal and combinatorial thought establishes the abstract attitude.

Achievement of the landmark of abstract intelligence, however, does not occur as uniformly at the age of 14 as previously thought. There are data to suggest that only 10% of 14-year-olds, and 35% of 16- to 17-year-olds, achieve formal operations. Sixty percent of those classified as gifted adolescents attain formal operations. This latter figure is in sharp contrast to the average adult population, in which 25%–33% attain formal operations (Dulit 1972). These developments in both cognitive and biological maturation provide the groundwork and raw material for varied psychosocial problems and have given rise to the many observations that make up the concept of adolescence.

SOCIAL DETERMINANTS OF ADOLESCENCE

The features to be discussed are more prominent now than in the early years of our nation. In the West, early in the history of the United States, formal education did not last into the young adult years for many. At the attainment of puberty, which coincided with the capacity to work or to become an independent earner, one could also start a new life. What we now consider the adolescent years coincided with young adulthood, and youths adopted the adventuresome spirit that has been romanticized in the popular history of this region. Moreover, the social significance of adolescence did not take hold until economic gain became attached to long periods of education and continuation of economic dependency.

Indeed, one of the by-products of adolescence is the conflict experienced by biologically mature organisms who are still dependent on family support both socially and psychologically. Such conflict does not seem to abate when education is financed by the state or by socialist governments. Thus, with the attainment of more leisure time, urbanization, and the increased need for a service work force over the need for manual labor, there has been an increasing necessity for specialized education and training. A full-blown "social adolescence" has been developed that implies psychological components as well.

Psychiatrists must attend to these issues not only because they may find themselves treating adolescents, but also because adolescent themes and conflicts persist into adulthood. Moreover, as we consider the social determinants of adolescence, we must also keep abreast of changing social patterns that may affect youngsters from ages 12 to 18. For example, what are the effects of a shift away from the nuclear family and a divorce rate that has exceeded 50%?

Directly related to the latter issue is the fact that there are more than 8 million one-parent families in the United States. In addition, divorce rates peak early in the first 2 years of marriage but then again just when families are rearing young teenagers. Other social forces involving the women's movement have changed family patterns, with both parents going out to work and women beginning or finishing their education just as their children can begin to be physically, but not psychologically, able to care for themselves. The latter condition shifts the time allotments of families so that time for intimacy, commiseration, and exchanges of all sorts may be curtailed. There is no doubt that poverty continues to have a major effect as well. Sociopathy, drug use, and legal entanglements associated with psychiatric disorder have much higher representation in the lower-socioeconomic-status classes.

Thus, biological and social factors converge to create adolescence. But how do these sectors affect the psychological unfolding of these older children?

PSYCHOLOGY OF ADOLESCENCE: NORMATIVE STUDIES

Among the earlier psychoanalytic writers, Freud himself described the treatment of a late adolescent (Freud 1905/1953). It was during treatment with this patient, as Freud later realized, that he developed the concept of *countertransference*. Perhaps it was apt that an adolescent

developmental process should have caused the early psychotherapist to have to ask about how his own feelings affected his actions.

Adolescence was largely ignored by analysts until Anna Freud (1936/1946) described a rapid oscillation between excess and asceticism during adolescence. She viewed the rapid swings of behavior and mood as secondary to the surgent effect on behavior of the drives stimulated by sexual maturity and the hormones of puberty. The instability of the newly stressed defenses against impulse was seen as the ego's contribution to the erratic behaviors being manifested.

This view of adolescence as tumult and turmoil colored the vantage point of subsequent investigators. In fact, Erikson's (1959) concept of *adolescent turmoil* and his concomitant notion of *identity diffusion* became the hallmarks of our view of normal adolescence. Although Erikson cautioned that diffusion was a maladaptive, temporary state, he implied that we all traverse the stage more or less. Later developmental normative studies employing the direct observation of adolescents have shown less turmoil and upheaval than formerly thought. Only now do we generally accept the formulations of Offer and Offer (1975), who showed that, by and large, adolescence is more quiescent than was formerly thought. Because their work is of landmark proportions, we will review it briefly.

Offer and Offer studied two Midwestern middle- and upper-middle-class community high schools. Their findings, although based on only adolescent males, were later extended and verified by others (see Emde 1985; Hauser et al. 1991; Oldham 1978). The young men in Offer and Offer's sample were 14 years old and entering high school in 1962. Those individuals who were within at least one standard deviation from the mean in 9 of 10 scales of personal and social adjustment were the subjects of the study. Sixty-one adolescents were then studied more intensively by a questionnaire technique and were followed well into later life to determine outcome. To convey the advantaged status of the sample, it is worth noting that 74% went to college during the first year after high school graduation. They came largely from intact families, and through the 8 years of study, from 1962 to 1970, there were no serious drug problems or any major delinquent activity, and no one was arrested for political sit-ins. The group showed no visible generational gap or difference in basic values from their parents. (An earlier study of young women at Bennington College in Vermont [Newcomb 1943] under the tutelage of their less-conventional teachers adopted radical political stances; however, 10 years later, having returned to their home communities, these women had reverted to conservative values similar to those of their parents.)

The findings from this study suggest that even after environmental influence from powerful social forces such as an educational milieu, early and long exposure to parental values has significant effects on long-term adaptation. Possibly relating to Offer's finding of stability, these effects on long-term adaptation are added testimony to the heightened impressionability of late teenagers under special cultural conditions that then give way, under the social temptations of middle-class ease, as new family responsibilities supersede more carefree adolescence.

VARIETIES OF ADOLESCENT PSYCHOLOGICAL DEVELOPMENT

The Offers found three developmental routes, which they designated as *continuous growth* (23% of the sample), *surgent growth* (35%), and *tumultous growth* (21%). The remaining 21% were not easily classified but were closer to the first two categories than the third. In the *continuous growth* group, major separation, death, and severe illness were less frequent. Parents were described as encouraging independence, and the adolescents showed a capacity for what was described as good human relationships. They were able to achieve Eriksonian intimacy and to display shame and guilt, and had few problems of major intrapsychic complexity as far as the methods of investigation could provide. The *surgent* group were "late-bloomers," as the term implies. They were not as action-oriented as the first group and were given to more frequent depressive and anxious moments. They were often successful but tended to be less introspective and reported more areas of disagreement between parents about child raising. Finally, the *tumultous group* reported recurrent self-doubt and conflict with their families and came from less stable backgrounds. Academically this group preferred the arts, humanities, and social sciences to professional and business careers.

The results of studies such as the Offers' (Offer 1969; Offer and Offer 1975; Offer and Sabshin 1974) and those of Block and Haan (1971), Levinson (1978), and Vaillant (1977) tend to negate the notion that turmoil is necessary for adolescent development.

Block (Block and Haan 1971) extended the observations of the earlier Berkeley longitudinal sample and showed a persistence of character style as individuals develop. A Q-sort technique was used as a study measure of repeat reliability. This approach showed repeated differences between men and women in those studies where both sexes were considered. However, certain important cohort effects and temporal cultural demands may have affected the outcomes. (For example, the Bennington study might be repeated during our current historical period to verify the effect seen in that group.) Block divided the data of the study sample into "changers" and "nonchangers" to refer to correlations across time, below and above the mean. Adolescent changers in their 30s appeared more unsure of themselves, were tenser and more guarded, and felt they were still working on problems. A factor-analytic approach was also used to render additional information. The 84 males and 86 females in the study were divided into five and six types, respectively. Among the males the following groups were isolated:

1. *Ego-resilient adolescents*
2. *Belated adjustors* (who seem very similar to Offer's surgent group)
3. *Vulnerable overcontrollers*
4. *Anomic extroverts* (who seem to have less inner life and relatively uncertain values)
5. *Unsettled undercontrollers* (who are given to impulsivity)

The categories represented by these individuals are not meant to refer to pathological entities but rather to styles of adaptation.

Block divided the cohort of females into the following:

1. *Female prototype* (obeying stereotyped descriptions of what the authors thought of as feminine in the 1980s)
2. *Cognitive type* (who tend to be intellectualized in the way in which they negotiate problems)
3. *Hyperfeminine repressors* (who are close in description to persons with hysterical personality disorders)
4. *Dominating narcissists*
5. *Vulnerable undercontrollers*
6. *Lonely independents*

As students of development, we can recognize the culture-bound stereotypes used.

There is some suggestion that identity formation in both boys and girls is the result of more than learning to be like mothers and fathers, and that sex-linked role characteristics result from how parents of one sex act toward the parents of the opposite sex as well. Most recently, Hauser and his colleagues (1991) at Harvard studied a sample of 133 14-year-olds longitudinally. Almost half the sample had been inpatients in a psychiatric hospital. However, these authors' mode of study did not show crucial differences in the outcome of this largely middle-class group through their teen years. An ego scale was used that describes stages in maturation with designations such as preconformist, conformist, and postconformist. The authors found three paths of progression from the steady conformist group: early, advanced, and dramatic. This central group of progressive development represents the "team players" of adolescence and constitutes one-third of the group. Only 6 teenagers attained the level designated as a stage of integrity and conscience, the highest level on the scale. Their parental environment was of a model sort, but as a group they did not differ significantly from the steady conformists in the measures taken.

The research of Hauser is based on Ericksonian and ego psychological constructs that have also been incorporated into further work concerning the role of the extended environment on identity formation in adolescence. A recent Dutch survey (Meeus and Dekoviic 1995) explores relational, school and occupational identity in 12- to 14-year-olds and 21- to 24-year-olds. Relational identity is the earliest to consolidate, while occupational roles follow. As one would expect in these age groups, peer influence is the most significant factor in role definition with only a minor influence from parents. The identity construct also has been studied in terms of competence in adolescents. Masten et al. (1995) have shown that romantic and job competence become important in the 17- to 23-year-old group in addition to school, social and conduct dimensions in the 8- to 12-year-old groups. Not surprisingly, antisocial behavior interferes with academic and job competence throughout adolescence. The longitudinal Duneden Study in New Zealand (1996) showed that the most resilient 16-year-olds studied had lower association with delinquent peers, higher IQ's and were less novelty seeking.

Studies such as those discussed above tend to emphasize the overriding effect of socioeconomic status, family intactness, and presumed genetic endowment as central to adequate adolescent progression.

DEVELOPMENTAL THEMES OF ADOLESCENCE

In addition to the data presented, clinical wisdom accumulated over three-quarters of a century suggests that adolescents must negotiate a series of issues before they emerge as adults. These issues can be grouped into eight themes in the developmental process, as shown in Table 4–5.

Dependence Versus Independence

The *dependence/independence* interaction refers to the intrapsychic struggle for a sense of emancipation from the nuclear family that permits goals to be formed as a personal claim. This struggle has both biological and social roots and has implications for the capacity for species survival

through procreation and the development of intimacy outside of the family. Adolescents feel that they must extricate themselves from the caretaking hold of parents. They see their elders as either exacting gratitude or inducing guilt and shame as internal controls over individual action. On the other hand, these actions may strike families as egocentric and selfish.

In contrast to nuclear families, children growing up in collectivist societies, where the group rather than the parents is the controlling social force, find it very difficult to move into the larger society where independent individualized action seems to be required (Ainsworth 1962). The notion of an individual achiever and self-starter seems to be related to social values, and these values then become the prominent dynamism in regard to what Blos (1985) called a *second separation-individuation phase*, in which biological, motor, and social equipment are developed to the point that a youth can take his or her place in society and begin to move away from the dependent relationships with parents. This is achieved only with ambivalence and conflict in many families, not only because of the actual social pull toward dependency, but because of the psychological pull that bespeaks the adolescent's wish for continued indulgence and caretaking without contingent sense of obligation.

License Versus Intellectualized Control

The conflict between *license* and *intellectualized control* is probably best exemplified by Anna Freud's descriptions during the 1930s of the oscillation in behaviors of adolescents. Adolescence may be a period of experimentation regarding sexuality, drug use, general disobedience, and other opportunities seen as temptations. Newly formed cognitive skills also permit intellectuality to be used as a controlling mechanism both on a defensive basis and as an interpersonal tool to resist indulgence of wishes and to help define one's goals during adolescence. It should be

TABLE 4–5. Developmental themes of adolescence

Dependence vs. independence

License vs. intellectualized control

Family vs. peer group

Normalization vs. privacy

Idealization vs. devaluation

Identity, role, and character

Sexuality: identity, role, and partner
  Masturbation/mutual pleasure

Reshuffling of defenses (style)

clear that these themes will of necessity overlap as they form an interpenetrating substrate for behavioral motives. Adolescents themselves have become fond of describing each other by employing distinctions that refer to various behavioral outcomes. The *nerd* and the *head* are most commonly employed. The *nerd* is typified as compliant, socially awkward, and overly intellectualized and is oblivious to temptations. In sharp contrast, the *head* is someone who has permitted himself or herself to drink or use drugs in excess or become oblivious to or defiant of external or internal controls supposedly defined for his or her well-being. In each of these extremes the adolescent is at the mercy of strong peer influence. Surveys such as Trent's et al. (1996) consistently show that external perceptions drive adolescents. However, they are more important for male scholastic and athletic performance, whereas young women maintain a stronger internal model, again reinforcing impressions about the psychological and personality differences between young men and women.

Family Versus Peer Group

The third theme, *group formation* in adolescence, is intimately related to the first two themes. Large or small peer group formation brings the adolescent's attempt at removal from family life into sharp focus. Whether this removal is used as a substitution for or regression from family life depends on how the group is used and how the adolescent determines his or her role in that group. During the juvenile period just prior to adolescence, or in early adolescence, Sullivan (1953) described the "chumship" as a time of same-sex social companionship and interest in which sharing and comparing of personal secrets take place. During this initial small group formation the adolescent is gradually made aware that companionship, companionableness, and the inner life can somehow now be translated into intimate relations with same-age, same-sex peers for developmental advantage. These small groups of two then gradually develop into larger groups during the early adolescent phase.

Phenomenologically, young women begin to wear the same clothes and share the same style, and young men belong to a team and exhibit the common expressions of individuality in pairs, bringing to light a kind of twinning effect (Burlingham 1945) that then proceeds into larger group formation. The larger groups may be clubs, teams, or social groups that are designed for the adolescent to share athletic or social interests. Such groups are usually self-governed as principles of self-determination and responsibility are learned. The resilient 16-year-olds in the Duneden Study mentioned previously (Fergusson 1996) had all the

prosocial traits that would exclude them from excessive novelty seeking and bad peers.

The generation of small groups into dispirited or isolated groups of individuals who seek mutual support as families begin to fail is an expression of both progressive socialization and sometimes antisocial forces. If these new social groups take on an antifamily stance or become indifferent to the values of the community, they may become degenerated groups or gangs. However, each adolescent in the group may then bolster his or her individual pride in the new group identity. New peer leadership is established as well that seems to the adolescent to be more caring and more responsive to his or her needs than parents have been in the past. This radical split occurs most commonly among those adolescents with disrupted families or in lower socioeconomic groups, or when social values have broken down. A recent study of 221 African American adolescents in 9th through 12th grade showed the important positive effect of peer support when stress was high. Racial identity seemed to be less significant in this study (McCreary et al. 1996). The issue of license for groups or gangs becomes a public concern when illicit drugs, drag racing, public sexual display, or harassment of "grownups" or elderly people are at the forefront. All of these activities bring youngsters together either in a common mockery of the adult community or in upholding the idea that there is adequate mutual support apart from one's family, sometimes mimicking a kind of Robin Hood mentality. The latter may be a distortion or a realistic protest taking the form of, for example, the following statement: "You have exploited us and have been indifferent to our needs for so long, we will now be indifferent to your values and exploit and confront you." The escape from conscience is thus justified. Among girls the adolescent breakaway from the family may center on romantic fantasies that another peer's parent(s) is more ideal than one's own parent(s). This *family romance* fantasy, which seems to be universal among both sexes at ages 6 and 7, is revived in adolescence. It may be expressed more prominently among girls in our culture, taking hold in the special chumship period during which younger adolescent woman engage in a twinning reaction with a same-sex peer. Together the young women plan together, discuss crushes, and plot strategies about romantic concerns. The sense of community that is generated sometimes expands into threesomes, foursomes, and small group formation, or is manifested in better-organized group activities such as dancing, gymnastics, or intellectual clubs. During the last quarter of the 20th century we have been witness to a greater tendency of opposite-sex friendships and chumships than earlier in this century and also to earlier incursion on groups by heterosexual pairing.

Normalization Versus Privacy

The *normalizing function of adolescent community* must be contrasted with the need for privacy. These two issues are sometimes, but not always, in opposition to each other. The normalizing function addresses issues of what the adolescent can tell a peer, what is private, and what the adolescent must feel is either sacred to the family or sacred to himself or herself. Recent studies of peer acceptance and friendships in 542 9th graders show that one friend is sufficient to ensure high self-esteem scores (Bishop 1995). However, such correlations do not attest to the priority of friendship or of self-esteem in this conjunction. The tempting possibility of sharing a special or "weird" fantasy with somebody involves risk taking for the adolescent and is an essential part of learning where he or she fits into the expanding world. The common language of adolescence (i.e., "sociolects") that becomes segregated from the adult's language (Shapiro 1985) is a startling representation of a search for group cohesion by excluding others. "Trading dozens" among ghetto blacks, and "Valley speak," imported from the West Coast, are examples of when adolescents try new forms that segregate themselves from an adult world that has not fully taken them in.

Even as the adolescent clings to groups, he or she also craves privacy. The closed door, secret telephone conversations, diaries, and music blasting through earphones are but a few examples of the need to counteract the adolescent's urge to tell with his or her need to hide. Being alone with one's thoughts, the sense of working one's problem through in one's head, writing poetry, and simply indulging one's feelings further exemplify how intellectualized or sentimental and brooding the adolescent may become.

We have ample recent examples from the Gay rights movement to suggest that some young men understand early—in their 11th to 15th year—that their homosexual impulses are dominant, and yet their ability to "come out" continues to be under social and familial constraints. Some of these children may become even more private for a time; yet others are able to find peers with whom they can express their interests and share their concerns. It is perhaps more the case than not that, whatever one's sexual preference, adolescence is a time for seeing how others feel about the same ideas or of becoming ashamed with the conviction that one's thoughts are unnatural.

Idealization Versus Devaluation

While attempting to normalize his or her experience, the adolescent often spends a great deal of time in *idealizing and devaluing adults or peers.* Crushes, pinups, and hero worship are the hallmark of the adolescent. Indeed, sometimes one's parent or parents may be temporarily idealized. The usual, expected adolescent sequence involves devaluing one's parents while idealizing a public figure or special teacher. Such idealization and devaluation, however, are fragile and frequently lose their power as rapidly as they are constructed. The slightest hurt or presumed injury is significant. A crush on a teacher or the longing wish to be a superstar quarterback or a prima ballerina may help the young adolescent to take the appropriate steps in the fulfillment of building ego ideals against which his or her own developmental progress may be measured. At the same time, the need to devalue parents permits a psychological means of discounting their authority, separating the adolescent from oedipal longing and also permitting him or her to move away from the family urgings and toward goals nourished and encouraged outside the family. As these processes are taking hold, the adolescent is also beginning to establish his or her own character or identity.

Identity, Role, and Character

Identity, role, and character have been associated in the developmental literature with the name of Erik Erikson (1963), who contended that "the sense of ego identity . . . is the accrued confidence that the inner sameness and continuity prepared in the past are matched by the sameness and continuity of one's meaning for others, as evidenced in the tangible promise of a 'career'" (pp. 261–262). The adolescent seeks to establish continuity with the past and to mentally work over the various and sometimes fragmentary idealizations and identifications to ultimately form a coherent unity in character. Thus, identity not only extends backward, but is projected forward in the form of establishment of goals, aims, and anticipated career and lifestyle. Sexual identity, sense of self, and role in the community are also part of the concept.

Identity usually is not viewed as being equivalent to character, but, on the other hand, it contains many of the elements that might be addressed under concepts such as character and personality. It is important to note that adolescence is a period involving the rapid establishment of these presumed structures. If a failure occurs, there may be a functional breakdown akin to what Erikson called *identity diffusion,* a condition that is marked by doubt, confusion, insecurity, and aimlessness. Once these particular structures become more consistently established, the adolescent may then move into the next stage of development to adulthood. Regrettably, concepts such as temperament have not been empirically well linked to later character and personality. Moreover, there is no strong evidence that Axis II personality disorder diagnoses are easily made in adolescence because of the rapid changes occurring.

Sexuality: Identity, Role, and Partner

Sexuality may be seen as a substructure of identity, but it is important during the adolescent period not only in terms of role establishment but in terms of matching one's core sexual identity with sexual role and sexual object choice. Blos (1985) posits, on clinical grounds, that the early phases of sexual functioning are characterized by a recrudescence of masturbation, especially in males. In fact, masturbation becomes a frequently used channel for discharge of tension as a generalized activity to relieve anxiety. It is only as the teenager moves into the second part of adolescence (ages 15–20) that this overuse of masturbation as a discharge channel gives way to more differentiated sexual activity that is guided by fantasies about others with a clearer determination of mental parties in pleasure. Whether this object is heterosexual or homosexual, the maturational thrust is in the direction of permitting one's sexuality to be expressed as a bid for an affiliation that ultimately will bind affection and bodily pleasure.

One of the important aspects of masturbatory activity in adolescence concerns the idiosyncratic establishment of the masturbation fantasy created to satisfy many features of past problems and current understanding. In short, the adolescent can in fantasy be active and passive, sadistic and compliant, tender and vigorous, male and female. In fact, he or she can be an observer or exhibitor as well. The imagery of the masturbation fantasy may make up a core personality feature, because the personal organization of the fantasy points to the central conflicts of that person's life. This view has been expressed specifically by Laufer (1976) in the notion of a *central masturbation fantasy.*

As adolescents move into the world and attempt to express their sexuality, they seek a person who more or less matches their mental object. Adolescents then attempt to work out the varying aspects of what is arousing and what creates a human interaction and brings the elements of satisfaction and security together. Sexual experimentation may take place. According to large epidemiologically based questionnaire studies, there seems to be an initial temporary homosexuality expressed transiently that then gives way to heterosexuality. Following this, a relative fixity of pattern of sexual choices is established. Adolescence is a time of dating, going together, and experimentation with others. Even if sexual intercourse or its arousing foreplay is not accomplished, it is on the mind of the adolescent. If the sexuality is enacted during adolescent turmoil and rebellion, developmental conflicts that correspond to issues concerning dependence and independence, license and intellectualization, and removal from family groups with sexual alliance are the themes of the enactment. For example, cohabitation in spite of family or religious restriction may be simultaneously a sexual act, a rebellion against authority, and a need for community. Choosing someone who is the opposite of one's mother or father in appearance or removed from one's ethnic group may be an example of reaction formation in the face of threatened oedipal impulses. Nonetheless, choices too close to home may have the same meaning of oedipal patterning and dependency. It is of maximum importance to understand that sexuality, like any other of the areas discussed, can be used in the service of either expression of wish or defense during the formative adolescent years.

As children move into adolescence, the patterns they developed in their childhood same-sex groups are carried over into cross-sex encounters. People of both sexes are faced with a relatively unfamiliar situation to which they must adapt. Young men, accustomed to counterdominance and competitive reactions to their own power assertions, may find themselves relating to women who agree with them and otherwise offer enabling responses. Young women, in interactions with men, are less likely to receive the reciprocal agreement and opportunities to talk that they have learned to expect from other women. Whereas the behavior of men in mixed-sex and same-sex groups tends to be similar, women's behavior in mixed groups is more complex. Some women become more like men—raising their voices, interrupting, and otherwise becoming more assertive than they would be when interacting with women only. Others appear to act as they do in same-sex groups, sometimes in exaggerated form, and may end up speaking less and smiling more than they would in a women's group.

Although patterns of mutual influence can become more symmetrical in intimate male-female dyads, the distinctive styles of the two sexes still persist (Maccoby 1990). On balance, the interactive styles of girls and women appear to put them at a disadvantage in cross-sex encounters, a factor of increasing importance as more and more women enter the workplace in traditionally male occupations. Moreover, the centrality of interdependence and caring relationships in the lives of girls and women tends to be viewed pejoratively by those persons, including many women themselves, who stress the importance of self-actualization through competitive success (Gilligan 1982).

Two recent surveys (De Gaston 1996; Harvey 1995) are relevant to our understanding: Among 1,800 junior high school students, females remain less likely than males to have had "sex" and show a greater commitment to abstinence and believe that early contact is more detrimental to future goal attainment. Moreover, a survey of 1,026 high school students suggests that sexually active males are also more likely to use alcohol, have higher levels of stress and were less likely to use seat belts and were more likely to engage in fist fights and worry about AIDS. Those girls who had engaged in sex also used alcohol and cigarettes and had higher levels of stress.

Reshuffling of Defenses (Style)

In the beginning of adolescence there is a tendency to project outward and to make adaptations that are alloplastic (i.e., externalized). The world, not the adolescent's inner wishes or aims, becomes the reason why the adolescent acts the way he or she does. Blame is placed outside of the individual; responsibility for actions are seen as exterior to the self. This tendency toward denial and projection has led some investigators to suggest that the adolescent acts in a way that may be dystonic to consensual reality. In other adolescents identifications take hold early in a firmer way, and reaction formations and repression begin to help the individual to cut loose from earlier oedipal ties. We begin to see in adolescents a clear establishment of defensive operations in line with productive work and adaptation using their idealized images as guides to planning future aims.

Style of functioning again may be related to temperament and how various traits help or hinder the adolescent's adaptive stance as he or she plans for the future. Thus, the characterizations of adolescence as a developmental step and a developmental epoch seem to be in line with the sum of developmental tasks that must be accomplished. Erikson suggested that adolescence is a time of life when work and sexuality must be linked and pregenital arousal and procreative aims converge. Others have described how reconciliations of the period concern not only the past and the future, but also the issues that are involved in identity formation and goal setting.

Erikson's contribution to our understanding that adolescence is not the end of the developmental line has been echoed by others as well (see, e.g., Vaillant 1977), producing more extensive visions of what development looks like *in later life*. These issues, which do not fall within the scope of this chapter, are discussed elsewhere in this textbook. Although this chapter ends with adolescence, developmental psychology is a state of mind of the observer—a point of view. Developmental analysis can be carried out to discover the stage-specific aspects of each age and how the individual enacts and experiences throughout the life cycle.

SUMMARY

There are strong historical and clinical reasons to recommend psychiatric interest in the process of normal development. General principles of development derive from the Darwinian proposal that small broods require prolonged caretaking. Growth, maturation, and development are the cornerstones of the process resulting in mature adaptive functioning and adult organization. The course of development is characterized by differentiation and by integrations among neurological, psychological, and social systems. Each new integration and hierarchic reorganization yields a new structure that offers new functions and adaptations. Development proceeds continuously, as well as discontinuously, as evidenced by biodevelopmental shifts. Rather than a single developmental psychology, the delineation of developmental process is method-bound. Psychoanalytic, Piagetian, Gesellian, and Bowlbyan stances are exemplars of representative positions. Any psychiatric problem can be approached from a developmental standpoint weighing risk and protective factors, as well as from a sequenced analysis of the evolution of disorder.

The psychoanalytic view of childhood initially derived from retrospective and reconstructive inferences. Freud suggested that repression was the prime mechanism that both hid and modified the postulated polymorphously perverse infantile sexual thoughts from the conscious minds of neurotic individuals. Freud introduced libido theory to describe the maturational mental sequence that children traversed. He also posited a hierarchy of danger signals that children have to evaluate and cope with: helplessness during the first months of life; separation between 7 and 12 months; castration or body integrity anxiety from ages 3–6 years; and, finally, danger of punishment by guilt ensued from an internalized value system (i.e., the superego). As development proceeds, the danger assumes a different configuration, progressing from *fear of loss of the object to fear of loss of the love of the object*. For Freud, the Oedipus complex represents a watershed of prior developmental lines and a focal configuration for conflict.

Later psychoanalysts directly observed children. Spitz postulated three organizers and their functions in the development of human behavior: 1) the smiling response linking external and internal events; 2) the stranger response marking attachment to a specific other; and 3) the development of the signal "No" reflecting a fully internalized and individualized human toddler who has become an agency of will separate from the mother. The separation-individuation process includes a number of substages that culminate in attachment and object constancy leading to independent action. Anna Freud posited developmental lines that describe how a child organizes behavior in an affective climate in relation to others.

Contributions from nonpsychoanalytic developmentalists include the following:

1. Gesell, in his normative developmental theory, attempted to unify principles derived from embryogenesis and normative sequences of observed behaviors. Four areas of behavior—motor, adaptive, language, and personal-social—were tracked during infancy and childhood, and a normative timetable was described that established an empirical basis for theory construction.

2. Piaget approached development from the perspective of understanding how it is that children come to know what they seem to know. He described the sensory-motor, preoperational, concrete operational, and formal operational stages through which the infant and child pass on the road to abstract intelligent behavior.

3. Bowlby constructed a human developmental psychology by melding psychoanalytic and ethological concepts, directing attention to both the biological and the social components of attachment, which have been expanded by a network of experimental paradigms.

These considerations provide a framework for the examination of the physical, neurological, sensory-motor, cognitive, and affective development from birth to preadolescence. Adolescence is considered as a way station to the further integrations necessary to adult life introduced by the Industrial Revolution.

The human infant is born with a largely prewired nervous system, and many capacities designed for survival are already built into the organism. Motor functions develop in a cephalocaudal direction. Reflexive behaviors gradually become reorganized so that by 10 months the infant grasps objects in both hands and brings them to the midline. Symmetrical use of limbs and axial support are essential precursors for the achievement of turning over at 4 months, sitting at 6 months, and standing and walking by the end of the first year of life. Motor and cognitive behaviors as well depend on maturation and feedback to the CNS. Although prewiring is the basis of some achievements, dendritic proliferation and pruning are also necessary, and these are dependent on experience.

During the first year of life the child undergoes major cognitive shifts in his or her capacity to apprehend the external environment on the way to the achievement of ob-

ject permanence. The vocal apparatus is used to produce protolinguistic expressions attracting the environment to the child. Infants selectively attend to congruent visual and acoustic signals. By the end of the first year of life the child can use several single words communicatively. Language competence and performance develop at a rapid pace. The 2-year-old rapidly moves from telegraphic speech of two-word phrases to the achievement of a three- to six-word mean length of utterance by 3 years of age.

Throughout the toddler and preschool years the child changes in behavior. A 3-year-old is a language user and can behave appropriately in limited social situations, attend nursery school, cooperate with routines and demands for sharing and taking turns, and participate in fantasy pretend play.

The human infant is born into a social world with capacities to perceive, assimilate, organize, and respond to social stimuli—capacities that permit him or her to function as an active partner in the social interaction. During the first year, caregivers regulate infants' level of arousal and excitation by varying facial expression, gestures, and vocalization. Infants regulate their level of social engagement through gaze aversion, vocalization, and facial expression. They gain experience with both self and other regulation and come to recognize their own agency.

By 7 months, wariness of strangers is apparent (so-called stranger anxiety). Between 7 and 9 months of age, joint attention emerges, as well as attunement and social referencing. By 10 months of age, selective attachments to specific individuals have developed. The Strange Situation Procedure has been used to assess the quality of attachment in 12- to 20-month-old children. Approximately two-thirds of children are securely attached, as evidenced by their seeking proximity with mother and using her as a source of comfort after separation. These children tend to exhibit greater social competence and better peer relationships during nursery school.

Between 10 and 16 months of age, the child devotes considerable energy and skill to locomotor activity and exploration. Infants will search for the absent mother or call for her (i.e., *refueling* in Mahlerian terms). Between 16 and 24 months, ambivalence is often intense. Later, as the child's mental representation of mother becomes more stable, separation is more easily tolerated. The availability of a secure and reliable internal representation of mother facilitates the child's increasing ability to engage in independent activities.

Data deriving from studies of neurodevelopmental cognitive and social organization suggest that there is a discontinuity at 7 years that corresponds to a second biodevelopmental shift. Neuronal dendrites are most dense at age 7. It is after age 7 that children begin to understand that their feelings, intuitions, and thoughts may be of interest to others. Children of this age begin to infer feelings and to understand cause-and-effect relationships between objects, events, and situations, and concepts such as ambivalence. Children of 7 years and older are initially rule-bound and even moralistic. Friendship patterns are frequently reorganized. The period of middle childhood is a time of skill development in preparation for application to the more creative aspects of learning in the future. Adolescence has come to represent the developmental bridge between middle childhood and adulthood. Biological, psychological, and social factors set it apart. Puberty refers to achievement of capacity to procreate as a mature member of a species. The external characteristics—secondary sexual characteristics—of both sexes become prominent social signs. Simultaneously, intellectual and cognitive capacities expand, too. Adolescents become capable of formal operations and the achievement of abstract intelligence.

Early psychoanalytically informed studies marked adolescence as a period of turmoil. Later developmental normative studies based on the direct observation of adolescents have identified developmental paths that are less dramatic. Nevertheless, adolescents must negotiate a series of issues before they can emerge as adults. The following themes characterize the developmental process during adolescence: dependence versus independence; license versus intellectualized control; family versus peer group; normalization versus privacy; idealization versus devaluation; the achievement of identity, role, and character; sexuality; and the reshuffling of defenses (style). Development does not stop with the attainment of adult status. Developmental analysis can be carried out at any age to discover the stage-specific aspects of each period and to define how the individual acts and experiences throughout the life cycle.

REFERENCES

Ainsworth MDS: The effects of maternal deprivation: a review of findings and controversy in the context of research strategy, in Deprivation of Maternal Care: A Reassessment of Its Effects. Public Health Papers No 14. Geneva, World Health Organization, 1962

Ainsworth MDS, Blehar MD, Waters E, et al: Patterns of Attachment: A Psychological Study of the Strange Situation. Hillsdale, NJ, Erlbaum, 1978

Ariès P: Centuries of Childhood: A Social History of Family Life. Translated by Robert Baldick. New York, Alfred A Knopf, 1962

Baron-Cohen S: The autistic child's theory of mind: A case of specific developmental delay. J Child Psychol Psychiatry 30:285–298, 1989

Bishop JA, Inderbitzen HM: Peer acceptance and friendship: an investigation of their relation to self-esteem. Journal of Early Adolescence 15:476–489, 1995

Block J, Haan N: Lives Through Time. Berkeley, CA, Bancroft Books, 1971

Blos P: Son and Father: Before and Beyond the Oedipus Complex. New York, Free Press, 1985

Borke H: Interpersonal perception of young children: egocentrism or empathy. Developmental Psychology 5:263–269, 1971

Bower T, Broghton J, Moore M: Infant responses to approaching objects. Perception and Psychophysics 9:193–196, 1970

Bowlby J: Maternal Care and Mental Health. Geneva, World Health Organization, 1952

Bowlby J: Attachment and Loss, Vol 1: Attachment. New York, Basic Books, 1969

Bowlby J: Attachment and Loss, Vol 2: Separation: Anxiety and Anger. New York, Basic Books, 1973

Bowlby J: Attachment and Loss, Vol 3: Loss: Sadness and Depression. New York, Basic Books, 1980

Brazelton TB, Koslowski B, Main N: The origins of reciprocity: the early mother-infant interaction, in The Effect of the Infant on Its Caregiver. Edited by Lewis M, Rosenblum L. New York, John Wiley, 1974, pp 49–76

Bretherton I, Ainsworth MDS: Responses of one-year-olds to a stranger in a strange situation, in The Origins of Fear. Edited by Lewis M, Rosenblum LA. New York, Wiley, 1974, pp 131–164

Bretherton I: Pretense: the form and function of make-believe play. Developmental Review 9:383–401, 1989

Brown R: A First Language: The Early Stages. Cambridge, MA, Harvard University Press, 1973

Brown JR, Donelan-McCall N, Dunn J: Why talk about mental states? The significance of children's conversations, with friends, siblings and mothers. Child Dev 67:836–849, 1996

Buchsbaum HK, Emde RN: Play narrations in thirty-six month old children: early moral development and family relationships. Psychoanal Stud Child 40:129–155, 1990

Buhler K: Sprachtheorie. Jena, Fischer Verlag, 1934

Burlingham DT: The fantasy of having a twin. Psychoanal Study Child 1:205–210, 1945

Cicchetti D, Sroufe LA: An organizational view of affect: illustration from the study of Down's syndrome infants, in The Development of Affect. Edited by Lewis M, Rosenblum LA. New York, Plenum, 1978, pp 309–335

Cohen NJ, Eichenbaum H, Deacedo BS, et al: Different memory systems underlying acquisition of procedural and declarative knowledge. Ann N Y Acad Sci 444:54–71, 1985

Curtiss S: Dissociations between language and cognition: cases and implications. J Autism Dev Disord 11:15–30, 1981

Darwin C: The Expression of the Emotions in Man and Animals. London, J Murray, 1872

DeCasper A, Fifer W: Of human bonding: newborns prefer their mothers' voices. Science 208:1174–1176, 1980

De Gaston JF, Week S, Jensen L: Understanding gender differences in adolescent sexuality. Adolescence 31:217–231, 1996

Dulit E: Adolescent thinking à la Piaget: the formal stage. Journal of Youth and Adolescence 4:281–301, 1972

Dunn J: The Emanuel Miller Memorial Lecture 1995: Children's relationships: bridging the divide between cognitive and social development. J Child Psychol Psychiatry 37:507–518, 1996

Eimas PD, Squeland ER, Josczyk P, et al: Speech perception in infants. Science 171:303–306, 1971

Emde RN: From adolescence to midlife: remodeling the structure of adult development. J Am Psychoanal Assoc 33 (suppl):59–112, 1985

Emde RN, Harmon RJ: Endogenous and exogenous smiling systems in early infancy. Journal of the American Academy of Child Psychiatry 11:177–200, 1972

Emde RN, Gaensbauer T, Harmon R: Emotional Expression in Infancy: A Bio-Behavioral Study. New York, International Universities Press, 1976

Erikson E: Growth and Crises of the Healthy Personality. New York, International Universities Press, 1959

Erikson E: Childhood and Society, 2nd Edition, Revised and Expanded. New York, WW Norton, 1963

Esman A: Adolescence and Culture. New York, Columbia University Press, 1990

Fergusson DM, Lynskey MT: Adolescent resiliency to family adversity. J Child Psychol Psychiatry 37:281–292, 1996

Field M, Woodson R, Greenberg R, et al: Discrimination and imitation of facial expressions by neonates. Science 218:179–181, 1982

Fonagy P, Steele H, Steele M: Maternal representations of attachment during pregnancy predict the organization of infant-mother attachment at one year of age. Child Dev 62:891–905, 1991

Freud A: The Ego and the Mechanisms of Defence (1936). Translated by Baines C. New York, International Universities Press, 1946

Freud A: The Assessment of Normality in Childhood. New York, International Universities Press, 1965

Freud A: A psychoanalytic view of developmental psychopathology. Journal of the Philadelphia Association for Psychoanalysis 1:7–17, 1974

Freud S: Three essays on the theory of sexuality (1905), in The Standard Edition of the Complete Psychological Works of Sigmund Freud, Vol 7. Translated and edited by Strachey J. London, Hogarth Press, 1953, pp 123–245

Freud S: Beyond the pleasure principle (1920), in The Standard Edition of the Complete Psychological Works of Sigmund Freud, Vol 18. Translated and edited by Strachey J. London, Hogarth Press, 1959, pp 1–64

Freud S: Inhibitions, symptoms and anxiety (1926), in The Standard Edition of the Complete Psychological Works of Sigmund Freud, Vol 20. Translated and edited by Strachey J. London, Hogarth Press, 1959, pp 75–175

Gesell AL, Amatruda CS: Developmental diagnosis, in Normal and Abnormal Child Development: Clinical Methods and Psychiatric Applications, 2nd Edition. New York, Hoeber, 1947, pp 3–14

Gesell AL, Ilg FL: Child Development: An Introduction to the Study of Human Growth. New York, Harper & Row, 1949

Gilligan C: In a Different Voice: Psychological Theory and Women's Development. Cambridge, MA, Harvard University Press, 1982

Goldfarb W: Emotional and intellectual consequences of psychologic deprivation in infancy: a reevaluation, in Psychopathology of Childhood. Edited by Hoch PH, Zubin J. New York, Grune & Stratton, 1955, pp 105–119

Greenacre P: The childhood of the artist. Psychoanal Stud Child 12:57–58, 1957

Guardo CJ, Bohan JB: Development of a sense of self-identity in children. Child Dev 42:1909–1921, 1971

Harlow HF: Primary affectional patterns in primates. Am J Orthopsychiatry 30:676–684, 1960

Harter S: Developmental perspectives on the self-system, in Handbook of Child Psychology, Vol 4: Socialization, Personality, and Social Development. Edited by Hetherington EM. New York, Wiley, 1983, pp 275–385

Harvey SM, Spigner C: Factors associated with sexual behavior among adolescents: a multivariate analysis. Adolescence 30:253–264, 1995

Hauser ST, Powers S, Noam GG: Adolescents and Their Families. New York, Free Press, 1991

Horner TM: Two methods of studying stranger reactivity in infancy: a review. J Child Psychol Psychiatry 21:203–219, 1980

Huttenlocher PR: Synaptic density in human frontal cortex: developmental changes and effects of aging. Brain Res 163:195–205, 1979

Izard CE: Measuring Emotions in Infants and Children. Cambridge, UK, Cambridge University Press, 1982

Kagan J: The Nature of the Child. New York, Basic Books, 1984

Kagan J, Reznick JS, Gibbons J: Inhibited and uninhibited types of children. Child Dev 60:838–845, 1989

Kaplan PS, Goldstein MH, Huckeby ER, et al: Habituation, sensitization, and infants' responses to Motherese speech. Dev Psychobiol 28:45–57, 1995

Karmiloff-Smith A: Annotation: the extraordinary cognitive journey from foetus through infancy. J Child Psychol Psychiatry 36:1293–1313, 1995

Klinnert MD, Emde RN, Butterfield P, et al: Social referencing: the infant's use of emotional signals from a friendly adult with mother present. Developmental Psychology 22:427–432, 1986

Kuhl P: Linguistic experience alters phonetic perception in infants by six months. Science 255:606–608, 1992

Laufer M: The central masturbation fantasy, the final sexual organization, and adolescence. Psychoanal Study Child 31:297–316, 1976

Levinson D: The Seasons of a Man's Life. New York, Ballantine Books, 1978

Lewis M, Brooks-Gunn J: Social Cognition and the Acquisition of Self. New York, Plenum, 1979

Lewis M, Michelson L: Children's Emotions and Moods: Developmental Theory and Measurement. New York, Plenum, 1983

Lewis M, Sullivan MW, Stanger C, et al: Self development and self consciousness emotions. Child Dev 60:146–156, 1989

Lewis MM: Infant Speech. New York, Harcourt Brace, 1936

Maccoby EE: Gender and relationships: a developmental account. Am Psychol 45:513–520, 1990

MacKain K, Studdert-Kennedy M, Spieker S, et al: Infant intermodal speech perception is a left-hemisphere function. Science 219:1347–1349, 1983

Mahler MS, Pine F, Bergman A: The Psychological Birth of the Human Infant: Symbiosis and Individuation. New York, Basic Books, 1975

Main M, Kaplan N, Cassidy J: Security in infancy, childhood and adulthood: a move to the level of representation, in Growing Points of Attachment Theory and Research (Monogr Soc Res Child Dev 50 [1–2, Ser No 209]). Edited by Bretherton I, Waters E, 1985, pp 66–106

Masten AS, Coatsworth JD, Neemann J, et al: The structure and coherence of competence from childhood through adolescence. Child Dev 66:1635–1659, 1995

McCreary ML, Slavin LA, Berry EJ: Predicting problem behavior and self-esteem among African American adolescents. Journal Adolescent Research 11:216–234

Meeus W, Dekoviic M: Identity development, parental and peer support in adolescence: results of a national Dutch survey. Adolescence 30:931–944, 1995

Meltzoff AN: Understanding the intentions of others: re-enactment of intended acts by 18-month-old children. Dev Psychol 31:838–850, 1995

Meltzoff AN, Moore MK: Imitation, memory and the representation of persons. Infant Behavior and Development 17:83–99, 1994

Money J: Sin, sickness, or status? Homosexual gender identity and psychoneuroendocrinology. Am Psychol 42:384–399, 1987

Nelson K: Individual differences in language development. Developmental Psychology 17:170–187, 1981

Nelson K: Event Knowledge: Structure and Function in Development. Hillsdale, NJ, Erlbaum, 1986

Newcomb TM: Personality and Social Change. New York, Dryden Press, 1943

Offer D: The Psychological World of the Teenager: A Study of Normal Adolescent Boys. New York, Basic Books, 1969

Offer B, Offer JB: From Teenage to Young Manhood: A Psychological Study. New York, Basic Books, 1975

Offer D, Sabshin M: Normality: Theoretical and Clinical Concepts of Mental Health, Revised Edition. New York, Basic Books, 1974

Oldham DG: Adolescent turmoil: a myth revisited, in Adolescent Psychiatry: Developmental and Clinical Studies, Vol 6. Edited by Feinstein SC, Giovacchini PL. Chicago, IL, University of Chicago Press, 1978, pp 267–279

Opie I, Opie P: The Lore and Language of School Children. London, Oxford University Press, 1959

Pannabecker BJ, Emde RN, Johnson W, et al: Maternal perceptions of infant emotions from birth to 18 months: a preliminary report. Paper presented at the International Conference of Infant Studies, New Haven, CT, April 1980

Piaget J: The Origins of Intelligence in Children. Translated by Cook M. New York, International Universities Press, 1952

Piaget J, Inhelder B: The Psychology of the Child. New York, Basic Books, 1969

Plomin R, Daniels D: Why are children in the same family so different from one another? Behavioral and Brain Sciences 10:1–16, 1987

Rheingold HL, Eckerman CO: Fear of the stranger: a critical examination, in Advances in Child Development and Behavior, Vol 8. Edited by Reese HW. New York, Academic, 1973, pp 186–223

Roffwarg H, Muzio J, Dement W: Ontogenetic development of the human sleep-dream cycle. Science 152:604–619, 1966

Saarni C: Children's understanding of display rules for expressive behavior. Developmental Psychology 15:424–429, 1979

Sapir E: Language: An Introduction to the Study of Speech. New York, Harcourt, Brace, and World, 1921

Schaffer HR, Emerson PE: The development of social attachments in infancy. Monogr Soc Res Child Dev 29 (3, Ser No 94), 1964

Schneirla TC, Rosenblatt JS: Behavioral organization and genesis of the social bond in insects and mammals. Am J Orthopsychiatry 31:223–253, 1961

Shapiro T: Clinical Psycholinguistics. New York, Plenum, 1979

Shapiro T: Adolescent language: a diagnostic clue to and group identity values and treatment, in Adolescent Psychiatry. Edited by Sugar M. Chicago, IL, University of Chicago Press, 1985, pp 297–311

Shapiro T, Perry R: Latency revisited: the age 7 plus or minus 1. Psychoanal Study Child 31:79–105, 1976

Skinner BF: Science and Human Behavior. New York, Macmillan, 1953

Spitz RA: Hospitalism: an inquiry into the genesis of psychiatric conditions in early childhood. Psychoanal Study Child 1:53–74, 1945

Spitz RA: The First Year of Life: A Psychoanalytic Study of Normal and Deviant Development of Object Relations. New York, International Universities Press, 1965

Sroufe LA, Fleeson J: Attachment and the construction of relationships, in Relationships and Development. Edited by Hartup W, Rubin Z. New York, Cambridge University Press, 1984, pp 51–71

Stern DN: The Interpersonal World of the Infant: A View From Psychoanalysis and Developmental Psychology. New York, Basic Books, 1985

Stocker C, Dunn J, Plomin R: Sibling relationships: links with child temperament, maternal behavior, and family structure. Child Dev 60:715–727, 1989

Stone L, Church J: Adolescence as a cultural phenomenon, in Childhood and Adolescence. New York, Random House, 1957, pp 438–443

Sullivan HS: Interpersonal Theory of Psychiatry. Edited by Perry HS, Gawel ML. New York, WW Norton, 1953

Tanner JM: Growth of bone, muscle and fat during childhood and adolescence, in Growth and Development of Mammals. Edited by Lodge ME. London, Butterworths, 1968

Thomas A, Chess S: Temperament and Development. New York, Brunner/Mazel, 1977

Thomas A, Chess S: Temperament and personality, in Treatment in Childhood. Edited by Kohnstamm GA, Bates JE, Rothbart MK. New York, John Wiley, 1989, pp 249–262

Vaillant GE: Adaptation to Life. Boston, Little, Brown, 1977

Vaughn BE, Stevenson-Hinde J, Waters E et al: Attachment security and temperament in infancy and early childhood: some conceptual clarifications. Dev Psychol 28:463–473, 1992

Wartner UG, Grossman K, Fremmer-Bombik E, et al: Attachment patterns at age six in South Germany: Predictability from infancy and implications for preschool behavior. Child Dev 65:1014–1027, 1994

Watson J: Psychology From the Standpoint of a Behaviorist. Philadelphia, PA, JB Lippincott, 1919

Wechsler D: Wechsler Intelligence Scale for Children. New York, The Psychological Corporation, 1949

Wechsler D: Wechsler Intelligence Scale for Children, Revised. New York, Harcourt Brace Jovanovich, 1974

Wechsler D: Wechsler Preschool and Primary Scale of Intelligence Manual. New York, Harcourt Brace Jovanovich, 1989

Wechsler D: Wechsler Intelligence Scale for Children, III. New York, Harcourt Brace Jovanovich, 1991

Werner H: Comparative Psychology of Mental Development. New York, International Universities Press, 1957

Werner H, Kaplan B: Symbol Formation. New York, Wiley, 1963

Zacharias L, Wurtman RJ, Shatzoff M: Sexual maturation in contemporary American girls. Am J Obstet Gynecol 108:833–846, 1970

APPENDIX: GLOSSARY

Accommodation A functional aspect of Piaget's model of cognitive development. Accommodation occurs when existing schemas (mental organization) differentiate into new structures ready for new psychic elements.

Assimilation A functional aspect of Piaget's model of cognitive development that refers to the incorporation of a sensorimotor schema that is repeated with new experiences judged to be equivalent into existing mental organizations.

Adolescence The developmental period between middle childhood (i.e., latency) and adulthood, characterized by puberty and psychological and social discontinuities in development.

Core self The self as a cohesive, bounded physical unit, a sense of which begins to emerge by 2 months of age (see Stern 1985).

Development The changing structure of behavior and thought over time. Development includes whatever is provided by maturational potential plus variations in social and environmental influences.

Differentiation The move from more global reactions to increasing individuated processes within systems that occurs in the course of maturation and development.

Epigenesis A description of how early sequential steps influence subsequent steps. In this linear model of development, each stage is dependent upon the resolution of the experiences of the prior stage.

Gender identity An individual's belief and self-awareness of being male or female. Gender identity is generally established by age 3 years and is usually determined by the sex in which an individual is reared independent of biological factors.

Growth Biologically simple accretion of tissue or increase in size or in the number of cells. Change over time in height and weight is an example of growth. Metaphorically used for describing development.

Hierarchic reorganization Changes in organization that are not the logical or necessary outcome of prior stages. In this nonlinear model of development, each new integration of biological and neuronal function meshes with psychocognitive capacities so that the result is more than the sum of the parts. Each new stage is a new structure that permits qualitatively different functions and adaptations (see Werner 1957).

Integration The increasing complexity of relations between and among the senses and the motor apparatus that occurs in the course of maturation and development. Can be applied to psychological functions as well.

Latency In psychoanalytic theory, the period between the resolution of the Oedipus complex and the onset of puberty during which the drives are quiescent. More neutrally described as middle childhood, this is a period of skill and social development and increasing ability to regulate and modulate affects.

Lines of development Anna Freud's proposal that in the course of development the child moves 1) from being nursed to rational eating; 2) from incontinence to bowel and bladder control; 3) from egocentricity toward companionship with peers; 4) from play to a capacity for work; 5) from physical to mental pathways of discharge of drives; 6) from animate to inanimate objects; and 7) from irresponsibility to guilt. Symptoms are viewed as regressors or arrests in these lines.

Maturation The natural unfolding of genetic potential toward an end characterized by full functioning.

Object constancy The capacity of the developing child (2–3 years) to maintain a stable mental image of the important caregiver in his or her absence.

Organizer A behavior identified by Spitz as being analogous to an embryonic organizer in general biology. These behaviors are the smiling response (2 months), the stranger response (7 months), and the signal for "No" (around 2 years).

Practicing Subphase of Mahler's theory of the process of separation-individuation (10–16 months) during which the child "practices" newly found locomotor skills and actively explores his or her environment with exuberance.

Puberty Attainment of the capacity to procreate as a mature member of a species (see Tanner 1968).

Rapprochement Subphase of Mahler's theory of the process of separation-individuation (16–24 months) during which temper tantrums, whining behavior, moodiness, and intense separation reactions are at their peak.

Separation-individuation Mahler's descriptive theory of the process by which the baby becomes a separate, discrete, and autonomous toddler.

Social referencing The ability of the baby, established during the final quarter of the first year of life, to respond behaviorally to the emotional expressions of others. Crawling babies can be induced to cross a "visual cliff" (i.e., an illusion that there is a drop-off, although a transparent plexiglass plate covers the drop) if their mother smiles in encouragement, and will turn away if the mother assumes a fearful facial expression. Eye gaze for permission is a later behavioral organizer.

Sensory-motor The first stage of Piaget's model of cognitive development in which the ability to maintain a stable mental representation and to create a representative world is established. During this stage, sensory and motor behaviors are fused.

CHAPTER 5

THEORIES OF THE MIND AND PSYCHOPATHOLOGY

STEPHEN S. MARMER, M.D., PH.D.

In this new era of scientific psychiatry, do we really need a theory of the mind? Is it not a hope that our field will soon have facts that will settle the claims of competing theories and resolve whether the concept of mind as apart from brain has a meaningful place in psychiatry?

Historians and philosophers of science such as Popper (1959, 1962), Kuhn (1970), and Fleck (1979) have written eloquently on the role of theory in all science. For them, the course of science is necessarily marked by communities of thinkers who invent hermeneutically useful theories or paradigms that reflect underlying world views. These paradigms determine ways to think about the topic in question.

Theories are not limited to subjects like psychiatry. Fleck points out that theories colored the perception of what we might otherwise think of as the hard science of bacteriology. For its ability to organize an approach to a field, theory is indispensable. In our era, theories are regarded as useful if they are confirmed by data, if they aid in our understanding of the subject being studied, or if they stimulate helpful questions, experiments, or observations. In this sense, theories are neither true nor false; instead they are more or less useful in interpreting available data, or in leading to new information.

In this chapter, I address psychological or mental theory. Current thinking in the biology of the mind or in the genetics of psychopathology is discussed elsewhere in this textbook (see Hyman and Coyle, Chapter 1; Knowles et al., Chapter 2). Since the last edition of this textbook, no new theories have risen to the top of our thinking. One older theory—on the role of trauma in shaping the mind and creating psychopathology—has received growing attention. Because of its importance, the discussion of repressed memory has been expanded for this edition. To put these theories into perspective, one can turn to the dawn of modern psychiatry, nearly 200 years ago.

At the beginning of the 19th century, psychiatric patients were just beginning to be considered legitimate "objects" of study. Personality was still viewed under one theory or another as an immutable matter of innate biology. Severe psychopathology was still treated mainly by sequestering patients, and milder psychopathology was still generally regarded as either moral weakness or malingering. Severe psychopathology was the focus of psychiatry, exemplified best by the work of Emil Kraepelin, who classified major mental disorders. Milder psychopathological states generally came to the attention not of psychiatrists but of general physicians and neurologists. This makes understandable the historical irony that the most influential theory of personality was created not by a psychiatrist but by a neurologist: Sigmund Freud.

The theories under discussion represent the ways ingenious investigators made sense out of human behavior. These theories emphasize various data, assume different notions of what constitutes proof or verification, reckon development of the personality according to different factors and timetables, place greater or lesser emphasis on either the biological sphere or the experiential sphere, offer different ideas about the mutability of personality and psychopathology, and therefore lead to different schools of treatment. A theory of the mind and its psychopathology in fact has several components, including concepts of development and of normality, ideas of how the mind works and even of what constitutes the mind, and determinations of treatment technique.

Theories of mind and psychopathology also position themselves variously along certain continua. For example, how much is psychopathology the result of deficiencies, or the absence of ingredients necessary for emotional health, and how much the result of conflict, whether between persons or within the individual? How much is psychopathology the result of actual historical events and how much the result of fantasy? How much influence shall be placed on constitutional factors, on the maturational stage of development, on ordinary learned experience, or on extraordinary traumatic events? How much is out of our awareness, and how much is within the realm of cognition? Answers to these questions lead in turn to treatment choices, and further questions: How much does treatment rely on interpretation, and how much on education, exhortation, or a nonspecific healing presence? How much is treatment dependent on the transference and how much on the real relationship?

In a brief chapter such as this, each point of view will be presented in an oversimplified, sometimes schematic manner that will not do justice to every subtlety. On the other hand, there may be some merit in surveying the entire forest. Although some theories are more ambitious than others, none can yet lay claim to explaining everything. Every generation accumulates experiences with patients that were not adequately addressed by the prior generation's theories. These various theories are best appreciated when the reader makes an effort to try to see the world through the eyes and theories of each theorist, on the assumption that no great thinker is either wholly right or wholly wrong.

It is the plan of this chapter to trace the development of the major modern theories of the mind, starting first with the mainstream of psychoanalysis, from Freud through those who questioned, revised, or modified his theories but stayed within the tradition of psychoanalysis.

Next the chapter turns to theories that offer notions of mental structure with a parallel psychodynamic tradition of their own, including the modern rediscovery of trauma.

The chapter will close with a look at some behavioral and cognitive theories that overlap but in many ways are different from the psychodynamic perspective.

THE PSYCHOANALYTIC TRADITION

FREUD'S THEORIES

So powerful is the influence of the theories of Sigmund Freud that it is nearly impossible to think about personality or about psychotherapy absent of Freudian considerations. Even the proponents of most alternative theories accept parts of the Freudian legacy that were hotly contested a century ago.

It is more proper to regard Freud as having offered a series of complementary theories, for while he revised his work often during his lifetime and corrected certain emphases, he never fully withdrew earlier versions of his work.

Prepsychoanalytic Theories

Many biographers have commented on the relevance of Freud's work in physiology and neurology to his psychoanalytic theorizing (Ellenberger 1970; Greenberg and Mitchell 1983; Grunbaum 1984; Jones 1953, 1955, 1957; Laplanche and Pontalis 1973; Ricoeur 1970; Wollheim 1971). Although Freud's teachers focused on physiology and not on personality, their metaphors became Freud's organizing principles for his studies of the mind. Strong influences were Helmholz, from whom Freud learned to pattern psychological theories after physical ones, and who particularly focused on matters of the distribution of energy; Brucke, who also emphasized the concept of conservation of energy; Meynert, who bridged Freud's interests in neuroanatomy and its behavioral consequences; and Charcot, whose work in hysteria opened for Freud the path that would eventually lead to psychoanalysis. Freud also borrowed heavily from the great neurologist Hughlings Jackson.

From Helmholz, Brucke, and Mynert Freud evolved his emphasis on discharge of drives, his principle of constancy, his notion of the theory of repression, and the concept of psychic energy, all anchored in the images of electrical and hydraulic science prevalent in that era. From Charcot he gained an interest in hysteria and hypnosis. From Jackson he gleaned an approach to the relationship between mental structure and function.

Charcot legitimized for Freud the study of patients suffering from hysteria. Older theories held that such patients were either malingering or had a "wandering uterus." Charcot rejected these in favor of an emphasis on the link between symptoms and traumatic events. He noted that hysterical symptoms followed popular rather than anatomically correct malfunction of sensation or movement. For example, a patient might develop numbness of the hand in the popular understanding of glove anesthesia, rather than the anatomically correct distribution of the median and ulnar nerves. This meant that symbolic factors were very important in hysteria. Further, Charcot demonstrated the role that hypnosis played in the treatment of hysteria. For him, hysteria was caused by trauma in susceptible individuals, yet because ideas rather than neuroanatomy determined the nature of the hysterical patients symptoms, the condition was also receptive to influence by treatment in the realm of ideas. Words, concepts, and symbols, which entered into the formation of symptoms, could therefore be curative.

The work of the great neurologist, Hughlings Jackson, constitutes a neglected inspiration for Freud's work in three critical areas. This can be seen in Freud's prepsychoanalytic monograph *On Aphasia* (1891/1953). From Jackson's thoughts on dynamic associationism grew the concept of psychoanalytic free association. From the maintenance of early memories in the brain grew the concept of regression. And from Jackson's evolutionary theories of brain development came Freud's own theory of psychological stages of development.

This protopsychoanalytic phase culminated with two major works. The first was *Studies on Hysteria* (1893–1895), which was coauthored with Josef Breuer (Breuer and Freud 1893–1895/1955). The second was *Project for a Scientific Psychology* (begun and largely left unfinished in 1895 but not published until 1950), Freud's ambitious attempt to link experience, behavior, memory, and motivation into a single neurophysiological system. Unfortunately, even the biology of our age is inadequate to explain such matters comprehensively, and Freud had to abandon his quest.

Freud's theory of hysteria at that time implied a theory of the mind. At first, Freud thought that hysteria was caused by actual events, generally traumatic, the memories of which do not fade away in the usual fashion. After a traumatic event, painful memory is repressed. However, because of a memory's powerful emotional charge, hysterical phenomena are the direct result of reproductions or enactments of the traumatic event. "Hysterics," Freud noted, "suffer mainly from reminiscences" (Breuer and Freud 1893–1895/1955, p. 71). Breuer and Freud employed hypnosis to help their patients rid themselves of pathological memories. They did so through a process called *abreaction*, the vivid reliving of the memories and emotions of a past, previously repressed event.

The results of abreaction however, forced Freud to expand his theory. First, cure rarely came from a single abreaction of a single memory. Every symptom had a multiplicity of "overdetermined" causes. This concept, which will be explained more fully below, means that most symptomatology stems from many layered causes rather than a single simple direct one. Second, Freud was an indifferent hypnotist, and some patients (Elisabeth von R. chief among them) found that talking freely was more effective. Some patients developed powerful emotional attachments to their doctors, which would eventually lead Freud to elaborate his theory of *transference*. Finally, Freud developed the theory that actual traumatic events, generally seductions, were not at the root of hysteria, although he never totally abandoned this view as a possibility in selected cases. This turned Freud from an exploration of actual traumatic experience toward an exploration of the world of inner fantasy. (For a vigorous dissenting minority view, see Masson 1984.) These latter two revisions, transference and fantasy, heralded central aspects of what was to become *psychoanalysis*.

Early theory of defense. In his early theories Freud made three important breakthroughs. First was his movement away from Charcot's trauma theory to one emphasizing fantasy. Second, Freud revised his thinking on the relationship between memory and symptoms. Charcot had emphasized that trauma itself caused hysteria in susceptible individuals. In "The Neuro-psychoses of Defence" (1894/1962), Freud stated that it was not the trauma itself, but rather the defense against the recollection of the memory of the trauma and its affects that caused neurotic symptoms. Predisposition or susceptibility was deemphasized. What was defended against was the linkage of the memory and the affect.

Third, Freud expanded the range of conditions that his method could study. For Charcot the field was limited to hysteria. Freud added obsessional neurosis to that list and soon expanded it to include phobia as well. He was then prepared to make certain distinctions between these conditions. In hysteria, Freud theorized that disturbing emotions or affects underwent a process he called *conversion* to a motor or sensory symptom. These symptoms were chosen symbolically so that the person could remove unpleasant or traumatic ideas from consciousness. In hysteria, the body did the talking and feeling so that the individual could forget. *Obsessional neurotics* used different defenses to solve the same problem of ridding their minds of unpleasant emotions or memories. Obsessional neurotics could not "convert" to body symptoms. Instead, in obsessional patients, both the affect and the memory data remained in consciousness. To rid them of their disturbing effect, they became separated from each other: the idea was rendered empty of affect, and the affect was displaced onto a different, "false" idea that became the clinical obsessional symptom. Freud moved from a simple trauma theory to a theory of defense that applied not just to hysteria but to a wide variety of symptomatic situations. Moving from a directly causal trauma theory to one that employed the concept of defense enriched Freud's notion of mental life as the arena in which psychopathology takes place (see also Freud 1896/1962).

Topographical Model

From his prepsychoanalytic era, Freud recognized that the bulk of psychic life lies outside of consciousness. It was his major contribution to psychiatric thinking to elaborate and illuminate unconscious mental life. Freud himself regarded this contribution as one of the two hypotheses fundamental to his psychoanalytic theory. The second, related hypothesis was that of *psychic determinism*, which held that all mental events were causally linked to others in an associative network. Both hypotheses trace their origins back to the *Project* and to the work on aphasia, which stressed associative links and considered the spatial topography of the brain. Freud's work with dreams bolstered and modified his topographic model. These were presented in a systematic way in the famous Chapter VII of *The Interpretation of Dreams* (1900/1953).

The *topographical model* introduces the three "areas" of the mind: conscious, preconscious, and unconscious (Table 5–1). The conscious mind was already conceptualized within existing psychiatric and neurological theories. The enduring significance of the topographical model was to define unconscious mental processes as the field of psychoanalytic investigation and treatment. Freud's first concept of unconscious processes has been called the *descriptive unconscious*. By this, Freud was referring to the fact that mental life could not be limited to conscious or cognitive processes alone. The fact that comatose patients could report registering events that took place while they had been unconscious was enough to suggest that mental life continued even during periods when consciousness was interrupted. Similar proofs included the phenomena of posthypnotic suggestion, the very act of dreaming, and patients with dual or multiple personality. The preconscious, which contained mental content that was not at that moment conscious, would be grouped with the unconscious, from this descriptive point of view. The concept of the *descriptive unconscious*, which filled in the gaps in mental life and accounted for well-observed phenomena such as sleep or coma, predates Freud and aroused relatively little controversy.

Elaborating on these concepts, Freud asserted that there are forces at work that keep mental processes and mental content unconscious, or that work to push the content of the unconscious into consciousness (Freud 1915b/1957, 1915c/1957). These forces constitute the *dynamic unconscious*. It is not merely that there is a neutral continuity of mental life at all times. Rather, the placement of mental content in consciousness or in the unconscious is a matter of the relative strength of powerful forces. Evi-

TABLE 5–1.   **The topographical model**

	Operating system	**Motivation principle**	**Descriptive position**	**Dynamic position**	**"System" position**
Conscious	Secondary process	Reality principle	Within awareness	Not repressed; easily accessible	Word oriented; denotative; linear; time bound; declarative
Preconscious	Secondary process	Reality principle	Outside of awareness	Not repressed; can have relatively easy access when attention is focused	Word oriented; denotative; linear; time bound; can be poetic
Unconscious	Primary process	Pleasure principle	Outside of awareness	Repressed; difficult access; available in dreams and symptoms	Image oriented; connotative; nonlinear; not time bound; symbolic

dence of the power of these forces could be taken from examples of what Freud called the "psychopathology of everyday life" in his work of the same name (Freud 1901/1960). Examples would be a slip of the tongue that betrays one's true feelings in a setting in which polite dissembling would be in order, or a behavior that reveals deeper disavowed feelings, such as a bridegroom stopping at a green light on the way to his wedding. In the clinical setting, Freud contended, resistance to remembering is evidence that forces are at work to keep mental content out of the patient's awareness. Yet the memories, ideas, and affects that are repressed exert their effect through symptoms that symbolically express what was to remain unconscious. The relationship of conscious, preconscious, and unconscious to each other is set forth in Table 5–1.

Here a number of questions arise. Does the barrier between consciousness and the dynamic unconscious lie in the unconscious or within consciousness? What is the content of the unconscious? Does energy flow toward keeping things unconscious, or does it flow in the direction of pushing toward emergence in consciousness? Herein lie some issues for psychoanalytic theory that caused Freud to expand and eventually revise his topographical model.

Freud was not completely consistent in his use of terms. At times it seems as though he asserts that only ideas, in the form of stored memory, exist in the unconscious, robbed of their energy by the fact of having been repressed. At other times Freud asserts that drives, wishes, and affects exist in the unconscious, with powerful energy that must be met by equally powerful repressive energy to keep them unconscious. At times it is only that which had once been conscious and was later repressed that fills the unconscious. At other times, Freud argued that most of mental content starts in the unconscious, with only a small portion emerging in consciousness. How Freud's later theory of drives and his eventual development of the structural model solve some of these questions will be seen in a subsequent section of this chapter.

Perhaps even more important than the dynamic unconscious is the theory of the *system unconscious*. The system unconscious, which Freud abbreviated as the system *UCs*, works by a different internal logic than does the conscious mind. In this theory, consciousness, or more properly the system conscious (system *Cs*), is linked to sensation and perception, as well as to speech and the association with words. The apparatus of perception records events, which are then stored as representations, or mnemic images. The storage system arranges these images in a chronological sequence and also into an associative system that connects related subjects. This unconscious storage system records *thing-presentations* that are related to, but are not exactly the same as, memory traces, but which may be linked to other thing-presentations according to the various affects and attributes that the thing-presentation possesses. In addition to mnemic images, mental representations of the drives, or instincts, may be stored. Associative links are made by means of a logic system specific to the system UCs, called *primary process*.

Primary process. Primary process is the set of rules that govern the workings of the system UCs. Primary process is motivated by what Freud first called the *unpleasure principle*, and later renamed the *pleasure principle* (Freud 1915c/1957). In the pleasure principle, unpleasure is avoided at all times, and drives seek to be discharged (i.e., satisfied or relieved). Thus, under the pleasure principle, the motivation of the system UCs is to fulfill wishes and to discharge instinctual drives. Attachment to a particular mental content moves freely from one association to another, in what is called a *mobile cathexis*, a terribly awkward neologism describing the concept of investment or binding of psychic energy. In primary process, time flows equally in both directions, permitting the blending of past, present, and future; an idea and its opposite may coexist, and mental contents are condensed and displaced freely.

Condensation is the representation of multiple ideas, memories, and affects in a single symbol. *Displacement* is the operation of taking attributes, affects, or aspects of one thing and attaching them to another. *Symbolization* is often listed as a third attribute of primary process. Because the system UCs operates on the basis of thing-presentations, symbols rather than words constitute its language.

Secondary process. The so-called system preconscious (or system *PCs*) and the system conscious (*Cs*) work by the rules of *secondary process*. The basic motivating force in secondary process is the *reality principle*, according to which gratification is delayed for other purposes. This delay of gratification required by the reality principle is made possible by, and in turn makes possible, delays in discharge of drives. Thus, psychic energy is more highly bound and less mobile. A consequence of this is that attention moves more slowly from one thing to another in the associative path of secondary process. What has come to be known as *Aristotelian logic* is followed: time moves in forward linear direction, contradictions may not exist simultaneously, and thinking is more concerned with the content and logic of ideas than with their emotional intensity. The vocabulary of the system PCs and the system Cs consists of both thing-presentations and *word-presentations*. Freud felt that an indispensable ingredient of consciousness was this linkage between the imagistic, visual thinking of thing-presentations and the linguistic, auditory thinking of word-presentations. This notion underlies the emphasis on psychoanalysis as a "talking cure," and on the power of verbal associations and verbal interpretations. It is precisely because thing-presentations, governed by the primary process in the system UCs, can be translated into verbal word-presentations, governed by secondary process in the system Cs, that conscious influences can gradually assert transforming control over the unconscious part of mental life.

The topographical model does not imply an anatomic correlation in the brain, although Freud always left that possibility open. It would be misleading, for example, to equate hemispheric specialization (i.e., right brain and left brain) with primary and secondary process, but it reminds us of the kind of metaphors Freud was using. One metaphor often used has to do with *topographical regression*. Because of their unique structure in which perception is stored what Freud called *mnemic images*, dreams reveal how topographical regression returns us to the imagistic unconscious mentation that resembles the original perception. Dreams give us special access to unconscious memories and feelings. This, in turn, leads us to a further consideration of dreams and dreaming.

Dreams and dreaming. Dreams have always had a special place in the development of psychoanalytic theory, and Freud said that whenever he began to doubt the direction of his work, he would return to the bedrock of dream theory for renewed certainty. He called dreams "the Royal Road to the Unconscious." Through the analysis and self-analysis of dreams, Freud discovered the main points of his theory.

Dreams, according to Freud (1900/1953, 1917[1915]/1957), were the outstanding example of unconscious mental activity. Dreamers reported what Freud called the *manifest dream:* the conscious rendition of what the dreamer had experienced during the act of dreaming. But even manifest dreams revealed imagistic content, with improbable actions, and frequent blending of past and present. Freud theorized that every dream contains several elements: *day residue*, which consists of the memories of events of the preceding day that retain unconscious emotional charge, and *nocturnal stimuli*, which may be noises within the area where the dreamer is sleeping, or may be enteroceptive awareness of bodily states (e.g., a full bladder). These relatively conscious elements are blended with *unconscious wishes* and the childhood memories associated with such wishes. Together, these constitute the *latent dream*.

In the process of sorting through the day residue and the nocturnal stimuli, the associative files to repressed un-

conscious childhood (or *infantile)* wishes are stimulated. With the ability of the system UCs to make rapid associative links via the mobile cathexis of primary process, elements from different periods can easily be mixed. Because the dreamer is asleep, motoric discharge for these infantile drives and wishes is blocked; topographical regression occurs, producing a dream experienced as a visual hallucination. The mere fact of exposure to these otherwise repressed wishes ordinarily would create anxiety, and in so doing might awaken the dreamer. The system UCs disguises the dream by using its intrinsic abilities of condensation and displacement, together with the symbolization inherent in dream images. The disguised dream affords the dreamer maximum expression of forbidden infantile wishes with minimum discovery. In this respect, dreams work the same way as Freud understood neurotic symptoms to work. They are both *compromise formations*, which simultaneously express and disguise, reveal and conceal, the underlying unconscious mental content, with its memories, associations, and drives.

The process of turning the latent dream into the manifest dream is called *dream work*. To the initial actions of condensation, displacement, and symbol formation is added the transformation of the dream after the dreamer awakens. This smoothing out of the logical contradictions in the dream to make it conform more to the rules of secondary process and conscious narration is called *secondary elaboration* or *secondary revision*.

Dream interpretation. The psychoanalytic approach to understanding a dream involves reversing the disguises of this dream work. Under the assumption of psychic determinism, every part of the dream comes into being for a reason related to the latent content of the dream and the dream censorship. Through the process of free association, the dreamer inexorably will be led back across the associative network to the original repressed memories and drives that stimulated the dream in the first place.

The reliance on free association to understand dreams places emphasis on the individual's personal use of symbols. Although dreamers from a common culture or era have similarities that would lead them to use common symbols, Freud emphasized that it was the individual's own personal free associations, not a standardized "dream dictionary," that would lead to the latent dream meaning.

Overdetermination. The emphasis on the overdetermined nature of the mind constitutes one of the most important differences between psychoanalysis and other popular theories of psychology. Psychoanalytic theory holds that no single explanation can account for what is seen in human behavior. Such matters as the stage of development, the symbolic meaning, the alignment of sibling order and parental unconscious issues, all go into determining whether a particular event will turn out the way it did. Kaufmann (1980) gives a particularly apt example when analyzing why an accident takes place:

> Why did it happen? The road was icy at that point. And the driver of the small car was in a great hurry because he was late for a crucial appointment, because the person who had promised to pick him up had not come. And his reflexes were slower than usual because he had had hardly any sleep that night because his mother had died the day before. And just before the accident his attention was distracted for one crucial second by a very pretty girl on the side of the road who reminded him of a girl he had once known. Yet he might have regained control of his car if only a truck had not come toward him just as he skidded into the left lane. The truck driver might have managed not to hit him, but . . . If we add that the truck driver had just gone through a red light and was, moreover, going much faster than the legal speed limit, [one] might discount as irrelevant everything said before the three dots and be quite content to explain the accident simply in terms of the truck drivers two violations. *He* caused the accident. But that does not rule out the possibility that the other driver had a strong death wish because his mother had died, or that he punished himself for looking at an attractive girl the way he did so soon after his mothers death, or that the person who had let him down was partly to blame. (pp. 279–280)

The overlapping of multiple causes, combining conscious and unconscious factors, mixing internal and external actions and motivations, is one of the hallmarks of the psychoanalytic view of the mind, originally forced on the theory by the failure of recovery of simple single memories to cure patients.

Instinctual Drives

Earlier in his work, Freud explained the cause of psychopathology in terms of his theory of trauma, particularly sexual trauma. When that theory was no longer tenable, Freud continued to preserve the central role of sexuality in the genesis of neurosis. He was able to reason that his patients had not universally been traumatized, but rather that they universally had sexual fantasies. This conclusion Freud deduced from his patients' dreams and associations and most importantly from the transference.

Transference, which is described more fully later on in this chapter, is the phenomenon whereby feelings and relationships from the past bend our perceptions and reactions in the present. For Freud, it was the capacity of individuals under the influence of transference to recreate their fantasies within the treatment situation that made him downplay actual trauma and emphasize fantasy in his theory of neurosis.

Some confusion has arisen over the terms *instinct* and *drive*. Outside of psychoanalysis the term *instinct* designates hereditary "prewiring" found in essentially the same form in all members of a given species; such "wiring" is highly specific and related to innate recognition patterns and trigger mechanisms. *Drive* indicates a general innate need that can induce a variety of pathways for satiation from a number of objects of satisfaction. The tendency to fly south for the winter would be an instinct, and hunger would be a drive in this usage. Freud himself preserves this distinction in the original German (see Freud 1915a/1957), but his translators elected to render *Trieb* as "instinct" rather than "drive," thus causing the aforementioned confusion. Many modern authors attempt to get around this by using the term *instinctual drives*.

Instinctual drives are the form that physiological forces take in mental life. When the organism is stimulated, instinctual drives must be discharged. Instinctual drives of all types become mentally significant as psychic energy. This energy has an innate tendency toward discharge, but may become attached (or *cathected*) to various mental representations on its way to achieving ultimate discharge, or may become bound or redirected.

Every instinctual drive has a pressure (or quantitative strength), a source, an object, and an aim. Because it was the maldischarge of sexual instinct that presented itself clinically in his earliest patients, Freud turned his attention to those instinctual drives first. Noting the frequency of childhood sexual fantasies, Freud postulated that sexuality begins not at puberty, as the then-prevailing view had it, but in childhood. For the adult, the source of sexual energy was excitation of the genital area, the aim was genital orgasm, and the object was a person who possessed the complementary genitals of the opposite sex. Matters were not so simple with childhood sexuality.

Sexuality can be broken down into component instincts (Freud 1905/1953). The first would be sucking. The pleasure that the infant gets from sucking is considered by Freud to be sexual in nature. The source is the sucking reflex and the aim is to suck. The object is at first the infant himself or herself, and the sucking is thus termed *autoerotic*. Soon the infant distinguishes the differences between sucking at the breast and autoerotic sucking. This is the phase of *orality*. In this phase the erotogenic zone is the mouth, and the aim is not only to nurse at the breast but to do all the things that a mouth is capable of doing, such as taking in, savoring, swallowing, digesting, and (later) biting, spitting, and remaining closed. As the child matures, the principal erotogenic zone moves to *anal* and *urethral* areas. Once again, what starts as direct pleasure in the sensation of urination and defecation generalizes to pleasure in what those zones can do, including such things as retaining, controlling, making orderly, expelling, and withholding. Sexuality next organizes in the *phallic stage.* This will be dealt with more fully in the section on development later in this chapter. Finally, childhood sexuality is bound during *latency,* when its energy is stripped for the next half-dozen or so years of its intense pleasurable affect and displaced onto other activities. It is this displacement that makes it possible for the child during latency to become absorbed with the cognitive tasks of school. Sexuality again reappears in its direct form in the true *genital phase,* which begins with puberty and goes on to adulthood.

Freud justified expanding his notion of sexuality beyond that of adult heterosexual intercourse for several reasons. There was the evidence of his early patients and their fantasies of childhood sexual experiences and yearnings. There also was evidence from such cases of child analysis as "Little Hans" (Freud 1909a/1955), whose overt interest in sexual matters and whose childhood sexual ideas seemed to confirm Freud's own views (see also Freud 1907/1959, 1908/1959). The transference, in which things that were not explicitly sexual in themselves took on intense sexual charge, also provided further evidence. Still further justification for Freud's expanded notion of sexuality could be found in the perversions, in which Freud asserted that the component instincts were displayed in variations of aim and object. In the perversions, oral and anal sexual component instincts and the variability of object choices could be seen clearly in the practices associated with adult perversions. Finally, Freud noted the component instincts in normal foreplay: *oral sexuality,* such as visual stimulation and kissing; *anal sexuality,* such as mastery, control, and domination, and the switching back and forth between activity and passivity; and *phallic sexuality,* with its focus on the penis itself, concomitant with exhibitionistic activity and an emphasis on exaggerated masculine and feminine roles. These component instincts seen in foreplay lead to and heighten genital sexuality if the participants are normally sexually healthy.

In expanding the concept of sexuality, Freud did not "make everything sexual." He was very explicit about the fact that his was not a theory of pansexuality. There was always an alternate category of instincts. In the earlier stages of Freud's work, the opposing categories of instincts were sexuality, also called *libido,* and life-preservation, also called *ego instincts.* At birth these two are joined in the *anaclitic* relationship between infant and mother. That is, the sexual pleasure in sucking is joined with the survival instinct in suckling. Freud hypothesized that, at first, the infant cannot distinguish between autoerotic sucking, the hallucination of the breast, and the real experience of sucking at the breast. As the infant makes this distinction, the survival ego-instinct and the pleasurable libidinal activity of the sexual instinct undergo a dysjunction, which, in turn, makes possible the beginnings of object relations (discussed later in this chapter).

Death instinct.   The subject of the *death instinct* has been difficult and controversial for the psychoanalytic tradition. Summaries of psychoanalysis (e.g., Brenner 1955; Fenichel 1945) generally give this concept a brief, dry dismissal. Because it was important to Freud (1920/1955), we will briefly attempt to see why he was drawn to proposing it and what he meant by it.

Freud acknowledges the hypothetical nature of his theory of instinctual drives: "The theory of the instincts is so to say our mythology. . . . In our work we cannot for a moment disregard them, yet we are never sure that we are seeing them clearly" (Freud 1933[1932]/1964, p. 95). But the view that instinctual life consisted of libido in opposition to ego-instincts was not satisfactory. It did not adequately explain such phenomena as sadism, masochism (Freud 1924a/1961), or negative therapeutic reaction (i.e., when the patient gets worse the closer the treatment gets to the heart of the patient's issues). Nor could such a view explain the extremes of melancholia, excessively aggressive behavior in patients, or the symptoms of traumatic neurosis.

To further understand the dilemma Freud faced, we should review his reliance on the pleasure principle as demonstrated in his theory of dreams. Recall that dreams were regarded by Freud as the disguised fulfillment of an infantile wish. According to the pleasure principle, unacceptable anxiety-producing wishes emerge from the unconscious during sleep and are transformed by the mechanism of dream work into a manifest dream that allows the dreamer to continue to sleep by taking anxiety below the threshold of awakening. The purpose of the dream is to bring pleasure through maximum tolerable expression of a wish. If dreams were under the influence of the pleasure principle alone, how then could we explain the persistent existence of painful traumatic dreams repeated over and over again? We cannot unless we go "beyond the pleasure principle" (1920/1955) to another principle. In this second principle, the *nirvana principle,* the individual uses drive discharge to reestablish quiescence, and erects barriers to stimuli to restore and maintain an undisturbed state. The pleasure principle explains the rules governing the operation of libido, and the nirvana principle explains and underlies the operation of the death instinct.

The new instinctual drive was unfortunately named the *death instinct*, but it actually consisted of three elements:

1. Aggression and the tendency to create destruction and disorder
2. The compulsion to repeat, which went beyond the notion of attempting mastery or restitution, but in which patterns and memories were repeated even without constructive purpose
3. The establishment of stimulus barriers to achieve a state of quiescence

All three elements were seen to arise independent of the pleasure principle, but, "luckily," as Freud (1933[1932]/1964) noted, "the aggressive instincts are never alone but always alloyed with the erotic ones" (p. 111).

The death instinct, then, is a broad concept that Freud used to explain the clinical phenomena of ambivalence, aggression, sadism, masochism, and severe melancholia. The death instinct is governed by the nirvana principle, which establishes stimulus barriers to create a state of quiescence. In the ultimate state of quiescence, of course, the individual would no longer be alive; hence Freud's ill chosen term, *death instinct.*

The role of instinct theory. Instinctual drives have had diminished importance within the psychoanalytic tradition, especially since the 1950s. The ego-instincts have resurfaced in some respects in the theories of ego psychologists and in Kohut's work on self psychology. Followers of those schools have tended to place the acquisition and maintenance of a coherent self in a position of primacy relative to the sexual or libidinal instinctual drives.

The notion of death instincts as a regulator of stimulus barriers of isolation and quiescence according to the nirvana principle has not been taken up as a major point by any of Freud's followers. The majority of them have also felt that the genesis of aggression did not require the existence of an independent instinctual drive. Some theorists view aggression as the natural forcefulness of any drive, and others view aggression as a secondary reaction to frustration. The death instinct expressed in terms of innate aggression has been most fully elaborated by Melanie Klein and her followers, who elevated it to a position of equality, or perhaps even primacy, and made it a centerpost of their theory.

The theory of instinctual drives led Freud back to the defenses, which had been known prior to 1900 but which were rediscovered as Freud studied the vicissitudes of instinctual drives (Freud 1915a/1957). His study of instinc-

tual drives also led to further investigation of the topics of narcissism and object relations.

Narcissism and Object Relations

The subjects of narcissism and object relations emerged naturally from Freud's instinct theory. Freud had indicated that every instinctual drive has a source, an aim, and an object. The object of an instinct is that through which the instinct is able to achieve its aim. It seems that Freud is implying that objects serve the purpose of providing satisfactory ways of achieving satisfaction for instinctual drives. Clearly the pleasure-seeking aspects predominate. However, as soon as we begin to look carefully at what is involved in satisfaction of instincts, the situation becomes more complicated, because our way of relating to objects, though initially instinctually driven, soon becomes separated from the initial instinctual need. For example, consider the fact that at the beginning the infant has a pleasure-seeking drive for oral sexual satisfaction by sucking at the breast and a survival need to suckle at the breast. Its way of relating to the breast is through the modality of swallowing or incorporation. Although things start this way, it soon becomes clear that the mode of oral incorporation is our way of relating to objects in the external world.

Instincts start out in their component forms. Sexuality, for example, is expressed orally, tactilely, and visually, and is only later consolidated into a multifaceted whole. By the same token, the objects of these component instincts also start out as *part objects*. In other words, mother, a whole object, is broken down by the infant into face, arms, breast, and so forth. These, in turn, are broken down further into good face, when mother is smiling, and bad face, when mother is scowling. Development progresses as drives become progressively more consolidated and objects also become progressively more whole. The biologically driven instinctual needs merge during the phase called *genital organization*. One of the most important signs of emerging maturity in childhood is the transformation of relations with part objects (breast, face, etc.) into relationships with complex whole objects (mother as total person) who can be understood and experienced to have both good and bad qualities.

Modern theories date these tasks earlier in development than did Freud, who conceived of component instincts as consolidating and of part objects as yielding to whole objects during the oedipal period. Most theorists now see these trends beginning by the second or third year of life, with some investigators arguing that the process starts within the first year.

The notion of object relations tends to emphasize the

interplay or interrelationship between the subject and the object. On the one hand, objects are entirely fungible. One is as good as another as long as it can fulfill an instinctual aim. Presumably for a newborn, any nipple would be equally as good and any bottle, any formula equally as good. On the other hand, during the course of development, the modes of relating to objects and our specific history with them leave a trail in our identity that is not at all fungible but highly particular. Freud, on the one hand, thought that objects were the easiest part of a drive complex to vary, and yet, on the other hand, he indicated that we never actually find objects but that we indeed only refind them. This is certainly true when we observe the ways that marital choices rework the object relations (part and whole) that we have with the internalized images of our parents, which affect our own identity and our ability to love others.

It is to be emphasized that the interest in object relations does not imply that everything is contained in the real relationship. The psychoanalytic tradition demands that object relationships be thought of in terms of internal fantasy life as well as the real relationship. This is a point of distinction between psychoanalytic and interpersonal schools.

In object relations the infant starts in a state of autoerotism, with all libido attached to the self and an obliviousness to external objects. As the ego develops, there is a stage of primary narcissism in which the individual is concerned with and in love with himself or herself. From this stage the child moves to a state of object relatedness that starts out as anaclitic or need related, but in the course of frustration of these needs returns for defensive purposes to a focus on the self, called *secondary narcissism*. In secondary narcissism, the individual makes object choices of persons like himself or herself. These later object choices are narcissistic object choices in that we are drawn to people who are like the way we would want to be, or who in some respect help define who we are. It is for this reason that in "Mourning and Melancholia" (1917[1915]/1957), Freud pointed out that when we lose a connection to a person in whom we had strong emotional investment, especially if that connection was ambivalent and our relationship narcissistic, "the shadow of the object falls upon the ego" (p. 249). We are then ever after influenced by our lost narcissistically held object.

Primary narcissism (Freud 1914a/1957) is a state in which the infant takes itself and its perceptions as a love object. This stage precedes the full acknowledgment of the external world as having a reality of its own beyond the infant. If development proceeds optimally, the child will become less self-absorbed and less omnipotent and will develop the capacity to love others for themselves. The child will also retain some reserve of primary narcissism to fuel self-confidence and self-esteem. In unfavorable development, which can come from neglect, conflict, or trauma, the child's ties to others will be narcissistic. In lieu of legitimate self-esteem, the child will develop narcissistic ties to others based on their ability to do things for the child or to maintain his or her self-esteem. Such a child grows into an adult who relies on others to define his or her self-image, indeed his or her very being.

Anxiety

As Freud originally conceived it, anxiety resulted from an accumulation of sexual tension or dammed-up libido. Freud then believed that neurosis originated in the holding back from libido. Observing that neurosis was accompanied by anxiety, he drew the conclusion that anxiety was transformed libido. And frequently when Freud found in his clinical experience that his patients had a more normal sexual life, indeed many of their symptoms did in fact disappear. Later in his thinking, Freud began to consider some of the differences between realistic anxiety and neurotic anxiety, anxiety as an affect, anxiety as a physiological reaction, and anxiety as connected with fear and fright. Anxiety can be bodily movements, an awareness of unpleasure, and an autonomic reaction.

Freud, in *Inhibitions, Symptoms and Anxiety* (1926/1959), concluded that psychological anxiety was in fact a signal phenomenon and that neurotic anxiety starts as the remembrance of realistic anxiety. A real danger is one that threatens a person with an external reality. A neurotic danger is one that threatens him or her from a fantasy or from an instinctual internal demand. If an individual feels overwhelmed, he or she is placed in a traumatic situation. Also if the person feels overwhelmed by an object on whom he or she depends for instinctual satisfaction or for survival, he or she is in a traumatic situation. Each stage of life has age-appropriate determinants of anxiety, beginning with the fear of birth and moving through the fear of separation from the mother and the fear of castration. The fear of the superego is experienced initially as fear of its anger or punishment, and then as fear of its loss of love, and ultimately as fear of death. Generally speaking, when faced with a realistic anxiety, we fight or we flee. Faced with an internal neurotic anxiety, we generally act against the internal source; thus, we displace the anxiety by doing something with the drive to make it no longer dangerous to us.

Various forms of neurotic anxiety express themselves as phase-appropriate or age-appropriate prototypes, but earlier ones continue to underlie later ones, and later fears can revive earlier ones. This accounts for great complexity in our neurotic lives and is in turn accounted for by the fact that time flows in both directions in primary process. Indeed, anxiety produces repression and other defenses, rather than repression producing anxiety. The various transference neuroses can be understood in terms of the type of neurotic anxiety from which they emerged. Freud, for instance, suggested that there was a connection between hysteria and the fear of loss of love, between phobia and the fear of castration, and between obsessional neurosis and the superego. Tracing the course of anxiety then became no less important than tracing the nature of the instinctual drives themselves. The shift of interest from the drive itself to the way in which the anxiety about the drive is handled laid the groundwork for the next main change in Freud's work, the structural model.

The Structural Model

In the structural model Freud proposed the division of the mind into id, ego, and superego. Why was it necessary to introduce this new theory? There had always been some sort of ego in prior theories, but its attributes and definition were different in various eras. The ego was a synonym for the mental self, the agency that exerted control over drives and defenses, including the ego-produced dream censorship and dream work. The ego was the organ of perception and the organizer of the filing system of mnemic images and memories, and, as we have seen, the ego was involved in primary and secondary narcissism. In addition, the ego was the source of the ego-instincts of self-preservation.

In the earliest days of psychoanalytic theory, the ego had at its command the ability to engage in a variety of defenses, but in the middle stages of his theorizing, Freud principally emphasized repression. In fleshing out his idea of repression, Freud saw that energy was needed to press against unconscious ideas in their striving to reach consciousness. Freud sometimes called this process *anti-cathexis* or *counter-cathexis*. In order to be most effective, this counter-cathexis had to operate out of awareness. But if it too was unconscious, what was doing the repressing? The question of the locus of the operation of repression, the awareness of the multiple forms of defense, early notions of the ego ideal and of identification, and the fact that psychopathology depended at least as much on management of instinctual drives as on the drives themselves—all converged to bring about a major rethinking of the operations of the mind. Structural theory is an attempt to find a better explanation for the various operations of the mind.

It should once again be emphasized that Freud never abandoned the topographical model. The structural and topographical points of view are neither incompatible nor exactly complementary. They are two different approaches to understanding the mechanisms of mental functioning.

What is the sense in which there could be mental structures? Freud certainly did not postulate that ego, id, and superego were physical or corporeal, having any particular locus. A good example of a noncorporeal structure from ordinary life would be the "free press." In the United States, there is a tradition of free expression and also specific provisions of the Bill of Rights that uphold a free press. The concept of a free press, however, goes beyond the physical structures of newspaper plants and radio and television studios, and goes beyond the words of the Constitution physically preserved in historical archives. Other countries may have the same hardware, and some even have the same words in their constitutions, but they do not have a "free" press. This noncorporeal structure is a combination of long-standing precedent, patterns of behavior, procedural mechanisms, symbolic meaning, and the interweaving of all of these into the definition of who we are as a country.

In like manner, the ego is heir to history—within a culture, within a specific family, and within an individual—which builds up over years. It is protected by defense mechanisms analogous to the procedural mechanisms of a country, which are institutionalized and become more than the materialist or corporeal reality upon which they rest. The ego is no more a collection of neurons than the free press is a collection of newspaper, ink, and metal; nor is the ego any more located in a specific area of the brain than could we identify the free press as existing in certain cities located on certain streets. Both are anchored in a corporeal, material reality, but both are noncorporeal structures or institutions.

According to the structural theory, the organism starts out as a poorly organized collection of drives. These drives are initially intensely physiologically driven. During this phase, the need to survive and the path to pleasure lean on each other. According to the original version of the structural theory, the ego does not exist at this phase, but the potential for the ego to exist begins immediately with perception. In fact, the ego owes its origin to and starts out from its activity of perception. In the course of perceiving, the ego discerns differences between internal and external; differences between pleasurable and unpleasurable; and differences between those perceptions that can be changed by body movement, those that can be made to disappear solely through mental acts, and those that the organism cannot influence. Thus the ego starts out as a function of the body that defines the mental image of the body, which is what Freud meant by saying that first and foremost the ego is a bodily ego.

One way the ego learns the difference between internal and external is through the sense of touch. This unique sensory modality is the earliest one in which the ego is simultaneously the organ that does the touching and the organ that is aware that it is being touched. Touching one's own skin thus becomes the beginning of learning who one is and what one's boundaries are. The distinction between the hallucinated dream or wish for the breast and the actual breast constitutes another way of distinguishing between internal and external, between real and hallucinated. The feeling of satiation that comes from the hallucinated breast does not last, in contrast to the feeling of satiation that comes from the real breast. Dreamed or wished mental content comes and goes for internal reasons. The mother and other objects in the world come and go of their own external volition. Thus the ego, in the course of its formation, begins to establish the *reality principle*. Rooted in perception, the ego is also anchored in reality, whereas the id, rooted in drives, is anchored in the pleasure principle.

The goal and mission of the id is to provide maximum pleasure through maximum fulfillment of the instinctual drives. The goal of the ego is to attain clarity of perception, accuracy of interpretation of the perceptions, and the greatest possible consonance with reality. Early on, the id learns, so to speak, that the hallucinations, dreams, and wishes of the pleasure principle are not ultimately as satisfying as the accuracy of the perceptions of the reality principle. The id forms an alliance with the ego, subordinating itself and its energy to the ego in return for the ego's help in focusing the organism's behaviors around the reality principle for maximum satisfaction of instinctual drives. Thus, during this period of cooperation, the ego gains enormous strength from the id.

The reality principle requires binding of cathexis, which is another way of saying that drive discharge must be postponed, deferred, or redirected in order to meet the constraints of reality. The pleasure principle works on the basis of primary process, with mobile cathexis and rapid movement from one strategy to another so as to get immediate gratification. Thus, although the ego and the id start out as allies, they frequently find themselves working at cross-purposes, with the impatient id wanting immediate results, and the cautionary ego insisting upon delay. The ego's "weapon" against the id could be the refusal to cooperate for the purpose of achieving the id's goals. To do so, however, would defeat the ego's goals as well. After all, the reality principle is also a more sophisticated and comprehensive version of the pleasure principle. The ego too wishes gratification. Through its capacity to understand time and to delay discharge, the ego understands that the shortest path is not always the most efficient one. The ego

then inflicts anxiety upon the id, creating pain (Freud preferred the term *unpleasure*) for the id. The avoidance of such unpleasure is a paramount consideration for the id. One can say, in somewhat anthropomorphic terms, that the id starts out wanting fulfillment; finds an ally in the ego, which has access to valuable perceptions; and engages in cooperation with the perceptual ego to accomplish its ends. However, the id, having soon enough given more power to the ego than it originally anticipated, now finds itself the recipient of unpleasure from its ally.

In the course of its evolution, the ego deals with an environment that more than any other single thing consists of the actions of the parents. The ego needs the parents and their cooperation and alliance every bit as much as the id needed the ego's perceptual cooperation. Thus, the successful pursuit of its mission to maximize pleasure according to the constraints of the reality principle requires that the ego understand and ultimately mold itself to the actions of the parents. In doing so, the ego becomes like the parents through identification. It needs the parents, but the parents, being separate individuals, are not always available. The ego takes the parents in and then has permanent mental representations of these important figures upon which it can rely in their absence.

The expectations of the parents for the organism and the ego's knowledge of what it needs to do to get the maximum cooperation from the parents form the basis of the *ego ideal*. The realistic awareness of those things that bring the ego unpleasure and diminish the cooperation between the ego and the parents becomes the basis of the *superego*.

The superego is initially an auditory superego, coming from the auditory perception of the word "no." The ego finds itself in relation to the ego ideal and superego in very much the position that the id found itself in relation to the ego earlier. The superego and ego ideal enforce a reality principle of an advanced form, a kind of moral reality principle rather than a purely perceptual reality principle, upon the ego. In similar fashion the ego offers some of its energy to the superego for maximum clarity of moral reality. The superego in turn uses its capacity to inflict anxiety to keep the ego in line. Thus, we have a finely tuned network: the ego relates to an id driven by the pleasure principle, to a super ego driven by identifications (mother, father, etc.), and to reality.

The superego starts out as harsh because the cognitive ability of the young child to understand the subtleties of the reason for prohibitions is absent. For example, the early, or "archaic," superego is extremely harsh because the small infant about to stick his finger into an electrical outlet is greeted with a loud "No!" from the parent, who might in addition slap the child's hand. The superego then is blunt, direct, harsh, and unequivocal. The archaic superego is incapable of a calm lecture on the dangers of electricity, but over the course of time a more mature superego might indeed function like that. It is postulated that in the resolution of the oedipal phase, the ego ideal and the harsh archaic superego blend to form a more mature superego, containing both punitive and loving elements, guiding the individual both for what not to do to avoid unpleasure and for what to do to gain maximum pleasure and self-regard.

The strength and harshness of the superego do not rest upon the actual harshness or gentleness of the parents during the oedipal period. Rather, the superego is an amalgam of real parental prohibitions, real parental approval, the ability of the child to overcome splitting defenses (see below), the nature and power of the child's drives and fantasies, and the style with which the child metabolizes those fantasies.

The foregoing account is highly simplified and somewhat anthropomorphic. It also conveys the impression that the ego, the superego, and the id become distinctly different from one another. This is extremely far from what Freud had in mind, as is evident in the following passage from *Inhibitions, Symptoms and Anxiety* (1926/1959):

> [Some misunderstanding] is due to our having taken abstractions too rigidly and attended exclusively now to the one side and now to the other of what is in fact a complicated state of affairs. We were justified, I think, in dividing the ego from the id, . . . *On the other hand the ego is identical with the id, and is merely a specially differentiated part of it.* . . . if a real split has occurred between the two, the weakness of the ego becomes apparent. But if the ego remains bound up with the id and indistinguishable from it, then it displays its strength. The same is true of the relation between the ego and the super-ego. In many situations the two are merged; and as a rule we can only distinguish one from the other when there is a tension or conflict between them. In repression the decisive fact is that the ego is an organization and the id is not. *The ego is, indeed, the organized portion of the id.* We should be quite wrong if we pictured the ego and the id as two opposing camps . . . (p. 97; emphasis added)

Freud was struggling to demonstrate that although there were in some respects no differences at all between ego and id, and that indeed they were parts of each other, a key difference had to do with the ways in which they were organized. The ego is the organized aspect of the id. The superego is a further organized aspect of the ego and thus the id too. At times it appears as though the ego is stronger than the id, in that it can cause repression and can inflict anxiety. Yet the ego is also powerless over the id. They react

against one another and yet they are the same as each other, one being organized more along the lines of secondary process and the reality principle, the other being organized more along the lines of primary process and the pleasure principle (Figure 5–1).

It is also important to remember that from the point of view of the descriptive unconscious, most of the functions of ego, superego, and id are unconscious. Occasionally, bits of the id emerge in consciousness and a bit more of the ego and the superego is also accessible to consciousness. From the point of view of the dynamic unconscious, ego, id, and superego also are largely unconscious. Their forces interact with one another out of ordinary awareness, although occasionally transparent dreams or the product of years of analysis results in some of that interaction reaching consciousness.

The concepts of the topographical model can be applied to the structural model. The ego operates mostly by secondary process (which is in the system Cs) even though most of the ego is out of daily awareness (which puts it in the descriptive preconscious). The id operates mostly by primary process (found in the system UCs) and is also unconscious from the descriptive point of view. The superego operates by both primary and secondary process. Figure 5–1 is an attempt to depict these relationships graphically.

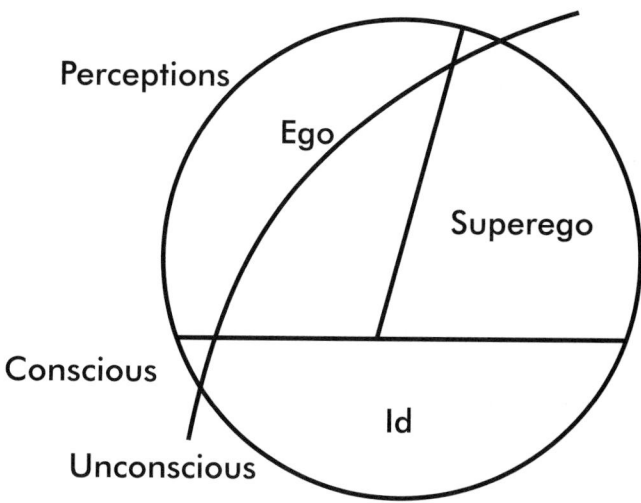

FIGURE 5–1. The structural model. The barriers between the three "structures" are semipermeable. Most of the id is unconscious, more of the superego is available to consciousness, and still more of the ego is conscious. However, for all three the bulk of activity goes on without consciousness. Because the ego has direct access to perception, it develops reality testing. However, it must serve "three harsh masters": the superego, the id, and reality.

Under the influence of the structural theory, the attention of psychoanalysis moved away from instinctual drives to the workings of each individual ego as it dealt with drives and anxiety to achieve maximum adaptation.

Mechanisms of Defense

It is a psychoanalytic cliché that the ego serves three harsh masters: the id, the superego, and reality. It is also emphasized that the ego is the executive of the organism in charge of the task of balancing the competitive needs of all of the other systems. In so doing, the ego acts as an organ of perception and of cognition, and as a regulator of internal mental life, all in the service of achieving the maximum amount of gratification consistent with its role as executor of the id. The ego itself grows largely as a result of layers of identifications and internal mental representations of the important figures to whom it has been exposed, particularly the parents and other members of the immediate family, who over the course of time and healthy development become *depersonified*, transforming their role from that of organized memory files of the original person to aspects of the ego itself.

To function smoothly, the ego has to have a set of automatic operations with which to deal with the competing memories, perceptions, external realistic needs, drives, and anxieties that it faces. These automatic operations by which the ego balances its competing interests are known as *defense mechanisms.*

In psychoanalytic theory, some confusion has arisen as to the differences among defense mechanisms, defenses, defensive operations, and defensive behaviors. Some authors have long lists, whereas others have short lists; some lists are simpler and more streamlined, whereas others are more highly elaborated and complex. For instance, the primary process rules of condensation, displacement, and symbolization could be viewed as defense mechanisms or alternatively as operations that permit defense mechanisms to function. The important concept is to remember that each defense mechanism employs capacities of the mind to alter mental content.

How many defense mechanisms are there? Some have contended that there is only one defense mechanism, namely repression, and that all other mechanisms are means by which repression is carried out. Authors add or subtract defenses according to the slant of their particular theoretical point of view.

Freud listed nine defense mechanisms, and Anna Freud (1936/1946) slightly modified the list, adding a 10th, "which pertains rather to the study of the normal than to that of neurosis: sublimation, or displacement of instinc-

tual aims. So far as we know at present the ego has these ten different methods at its disposal in its conflicts with instinctual representatives and affects" (p. 47).

Valenstein and his co-workers (Bibring et al. 1961) generated a "glossary of defenses" that contained 24 basic mechanisms and 15 more complex ones. Vaillant (1977) discussed pathological defense mechanisms and adaptive coping mechanisms, expanding the list manyfold.

However we organize the list, it is important to remember that defenses not only ward off unacceptable mental content but are themselves mental content with accompanying fantasies (Schafer 1968; Wallerstein 1983). Defenses also yield pleasure by allowing a degree of discharge while simultaneously warding off the drive through negation or fantasy. We must analyze in detail the fantasy contained within any particular defense, remembering as well that there can be defenses not only against unwelcome mental contents but against other defenses (Waelder 1936). Thus defenses exist in hierarchical layers.

Anna Freud attempted to correlate stages of psychic development with the coming into existence of different defenses but did not entirely succeed in her classification. Masterson and Rinsley, Kernberg, and others have attempted to continue this work. This approach is particularly important when each kind of psychopathology demonstrates its characteristic specific clusters of defenses. For example, in hysteria, repression and conversion are prominent defenses. In obsessive-compulsive disorder, isolation, reaction formation, regression, and undoing are the primary mechanisms. In paranoia and psychosis, introjection and projection are the primary mechanisms of defense. If one can know the diagnosis, one can infer the defense mechanisms most likely to be encountered in the treatment. Conversely, if one observes certain defensive operations in action, one can infer the diagnosis. One can also predict the form in which the transference will unfold by knowing the principal defense mechanisms used by a particular patient.

The classical defense mechanisms as enumerated by Freud are briefly discussed in the following subsections (Table 5–2).

Repression. Repression is the defense that keeps from consciousness unwanted affects, memories, or drives. Repression requires permanent energy against the emergence of unwelcome mental content into awareness. The counter-cathexis takes place on an unconscious basis. The equilibrium between the pressure of the repression to reach consciousness and the counter-cathexis to keep it unconscious is a fluid one, and the counter-cathexis of the ego is always in danger of being diminished, such as occurs

TABLE 5-2. **Classical defenses**

Repression	Keeping unwanted affects, memories, and drives from consciousness, allowing them to remain in our behavior outside of awareness. Mechanism by which we "forget" unpleasant information or feelings.
Regression	Returning to an earlier level of maturational functioning.
Isolation	Separating link between affect and memory. Often employed by obsessive-compulsive patients.
Reaction formation	Transforming affects into their opposites (e.g., "I don't love this; I hate it"). Often employed by obsessive-compulsive patients.
Undoing	Attempting to nullify or atone for forbidden fantasy, affect, or memory. Used by obsessive-compulsive patients.
Projection	Sending an unacceptable thought or feeling away and attributing it to an external source (e.g., "I don't hate him; he hates me"). Often used by paranoid patients. *Projective identification* is a more primitive version in which identity is ascribed to another, generally in a relationship in which the other accepts the projection.
Identification	Taking attributes of important others into our own selves. This can either be part of normal growth or be pathological, depending on maturational level. *Introjection* is the style of identification that takes in another person's identity as a foreign body. *Incorporation* is more advanced, taking on another's characteristics. Identification is most advanced; we become like others by acquiring their attributes, which we can then modify.
Turning against the self	Taking an impulse intended to be expressed toward someone else and directing it against oneself (e.g., biting your tongue by "accident" when you feel like saying something hostile toward another person).
Reversal	Taking an impulse and reversing its polarity (e.g., changing sadistic feelings into masochistic ones or transforming the active role into the passive role).
Denial	Invalidating an unpleasant or unwanted piece of information and living life as though it did not exist. Seen in many patients with addictions who do not acknowledge the consequences of their behavior. Differs from repression in that there is slight consciousness, but a piece of reality is being denied, not just mental content.
Splitting	Keeping "good objects," pleasurable affects, and good memories apart from "bad objects," unpleasurable affects, and bad memories. Early in life this defense keeps infants from having good experiences drowned out by bad ones. Later it prevents people from experiencing others as multifaceted, complex whole objects possessing both good and bad characteristics. Often seen in borderline personality disorder patients.
Sublimation	Turning our drives, affects, and memories into healthy and creative outcomes.

in sleep and which permits dreams to become part of mental content. When something is successfully repressed, it is barred from access to consciousness, but it is also no longer amenable to further modification by the ego and can take on a life of its own in the form of a symptom complex or a portion of character structure.

Regression.   When the defense of regression is employed, we return to an earlier level of maturational functioning. We see mild regression in medically ill patients and in college students when they return home on vacations. An example that Freud gives was that of a patient who transformed his phallic-level rivalry with his father into the fantasy of being orally devoured by a father figure in the children's story "The Gingerbread Man." In this

case the patient regressed to an earlier level of development and an earlier conceptualization of his interactions with the significant objects in his life in an effort to return to a state that was associated with less anxiety but in fact expressed his anxiety over his relationship in a more primitive way.

Isolation.   Isolation separates affect from memory. It is a defense mechanism that is frequently employed by obsessional persons and, in its more common form, consists of both ideational content and affect having access to consciousness, but not at the same time. What is blocked is the link between ideational content and affect. In its extreme forms, patients who utilize isolation may be unable to feel too much emotion of any kind.

Thoughts or affects are treated as though they were untouchable and therefore require distance. An example is a patient talking about a painful event with a bland emotional expression.

Reaction formation. In reaction formation, another defense mechanism frequently found in obsessional persons, affects are transformed into their opposites and ambivalence is resolved in the opposite manner from which it arises. For example, "I don't love this; I hate it," or, "I am not interested in gratifying a dangerous wish; I am interested in seeing to it that the fulfillment of these dangerous wishes never comes to pass." A historical example of reaction formation in action would be that of the 19th-century British statesman who, in reaction to his own lust, spent frequent evenings in the red-light district of London importuning prostitutes to give up their wayward lives. This outward set of behaviors permitted him to be in the company of prostitutes while denying forbidden desires by transforming them into what would look like their opposite.

Undoing. In undoing, a behavior is engaged in or a series of fantasies are indulged in that atone for a forbidden fantasy, affect, or memory (Freud 1909b/1955). A clinical example of undoing would be engaging in hand-washing rituals to atone for fantasies of soiling. The way in which undoing might enter character structure as a permanent defense is illustrated by the clinical vignette of a hyperconscientious physician who double and triple checked every detail of his patients' care with a devotion that made family life incompatible with professional life. During the course of analysis, it was discovered that this physician was spending a lifetime undoing the consequences of childhood murderous fantasies against his younger sibling during his mother's pregnancy. These fantasies had to be atoned for when the sibling was born with a severe birth defect. In this example, the defense became part of the character structure and had both an adaptive and a pathological meaning.

Projection. Projection is a complex defense mechanism that can operate at a more primitive or a more advanced level. Projection involves the fantasy of spitting, throwing, or in some other way hurling from ourselves some unacceptable mental content. The schematic prototype would be, "I don't hate him; he hates me," an example in which the affect is disowned and, through displacement, projected onto someone else (Freud 1911/1958, 1921/1955, 1922/1955). This defense mechanism is prevalent in paranoia. The advantage for the person who is using projection is that he or she rids himself or herself of unwelcome thoughts and affects; the disadvantage, however, is that the projecting person then lives in a merciless world in which others harbor the unacceptable affects and fantasies that he or she wishes to disown. They become purified of their bad fantasies, but then it appears that everyone else has those same bad intentions toward them. Once the affect is projected, one's ability to modify the content of the projection is severely diminished.

Projective identification. Projective identification is another form of projection, thought to be more primitive by Melanie Klein and her followers who elaborated it. It can best be understood by means of an example. A husband is plagued by feelings of incompetence. When he comes home he scans the house for any sign that it is his wife and not himself who has the identity of the incompetent one. He attacks her on flimsy pretext to attain the position of the self-righteously competent spouse stuck with an incompetent wife. He has projected an entire piece of his identity onto her. When projective identification occurs in an intimate or empathic relationship the recipient of the projection feels altered by it. In this example the wife may not only feel attacked but may actually take on the identity of incompetence projected upon her. When projective identification occurs in a treatment setting, the close and careful analysis of it within the transference, and the study of the countertransference reactions evoked in the analyst, form a significant portion of Kleinian theory and technique (Klein et al. 1973; Segal 1973).

Introjection and identification. Much confusion arises here because identification is both a defense and a normal mechanism of growth. Important objects are taken in to avoid the pain of losing or being separated from them. When the identification is primitive, it is called *introjection*, more closely resembling unconscious imitation. When a child develops a low frustration tolerance and becomes irritable as a result of an angry parent's interactions, the child is "swallowing whole" this image of the angry parent and growing into it himself or herself. When the characteristics of a parent become the child's own in a way that allows the child to modify them as he or she matures, this is *identification*. Incorporation entails partial blending of the external object and the self. Identification implies eventual depersonification in which the traits of the individual no longer remain bound to specific memories but are acquired as genuine traits of one's own. Thus, identification can be more or less healthy, more or less a part of normal growth and development, or more or less pathological, depending on its type.

Turning against the self.   As originally elaborated in the vicissitudes of the instincts, any drive can be directed toward its object or turned back against the self or both at once. This is the basis of secondary narcissism and explains how sadism and masochism can be two sides of the same coin. Turning against the self is illustrated in the following clinical vignette:

> A 5-year-old boy was bragging to his uncle about how superior his father was to his uncle. When the father showed disapproval, the boy became quiet. A few moments later, the boy, who was ordinarily quite well coordinated, tripped and hurt his head against the side of a table. Analysis of the event revealed that the boy's rivalry with his father had undergone a reaction formation and a projection as follows: "I'm not better than my father. My father is better than you. And it is not I who have a rivalry with my father; it is my uncle who has a rivalry with my father." When both of these mechanisms were not successful in binding the child's unacceptable thoughts because of the father's disapproval, the young boy turned his competitive aggression against himself and tripped.

This vignette also illustrates that defense mechanisms rarely appear in pure form and usually appear in clusters.

Reversal.   The difficult-to-understand defense of reversal is the process by which the aim of an instinct is transformed into its opposite, as in activity changing to passivity or passivity changing into activity. It is part of the elaboration of how sadism and masochism can alternate with each other. It is a defense very closely related to turning against the self.

Denial.   Denial is the invalidation of an unpleasant or unwanted piece of information and involves living one's life as though it did not exist. It is a more severe form of defense related to repression. It denies access to consciousness but is more thoroughgoing and costly in that a piece of reality has to be not only ignored as in repression but actually invalidated. Thus, reality testing is diminished. Milder forms of denial may exist in transient ways, as when one continues to refer to a recently deceased member of the family in the present tense. A patient who built a decorative fountain requiring strenuous work, the weekend after he was told that he had advanced coronary artery disease would be engaging in a stronger form of denial. Frequently denial is easiest to spot in its more nearly conscious forms, as in the case of the alcoholic person who denies the existence of the illness because he never drinks before 5:00 P.M. The persistent refusal to be swayed by the evidence of reality also is an indicator that the mechanism of denial is at work.

Splitting.   Another defense mentioned but not fully elaborated by Freud (1940a[1938]/1964, 1940b[1938]/1964), but regarded by modern psychoanalysis to be important, is splitting. In splitting, aspects of mental content are kept separate. Initially this consists of keeping pleasurable affects and memories, and the "good objects" with which they are associated separate from unpleasurable affects and memories, and the "bad objects" to which they are linked. At a phase when the infant would be overwhelmed by unpleasure, splitting helps the child form good objects and an idea of a good self. In adulthood, splitting severely interferes with all important ego functions. For example, splitting is used pathologically when a person loses access to any usable awareness of good history and loving feelings toward another when that other is felt to be disappointing or rejecting. Splitting creates "alternating univalences" rather than integrated ambivalence or a state of wholeness in which self and other can be seen as possessing good and bad aspects simultaneously. This defense is often seen in patients with borderline personality disorder as they alternate between overidealizing those who meet their needs and devaluing those who frustrate them. Splitting can also be observed in couples therapy. When happy, the couple ignore real flaws in each other. When frustrated, they forget why they ever fell in love, and regard each other as bitter enemies rather than as partners who have temporarily gotten off track.

Sublimation.   Anna Freud considered sublimation to be a normal part of defense mechanisms, revealing normal ego function. Sublimation occurs when the ego functions to achieve maximum satisfaction of drives with minimum anxiety and minimum disruption of the environment. The clinical vignette of the guiltily overconscientious physician presented above would have been an illustration of sublimation if the conscientiousness had existed in a moderate degree and had not disrupted the physician's ability to have a family life alongside his professional life.

Hierarchies of Defense

Kernberg (1976) has attempted to bring some clarity to the topic of defenses by clustering them in two hierarchies. There is the *splitting hierarchy of defenses*, which is more primitive, and the *repression hierarchy*, which is more advanced. Kernberg includes in his splitting hierarchy the mechanisms of projective identification, denial, and splitting. Into the repression hierarchy he places reaction formation, undoing, more mature forms of projection, and repression. More primitive forms of psychopathology employ the splitting hierarchy of defenses, whereas more neurotic or advanced forms of psychopathology employ the repression hierarchy of defenses. We will see this more fully elaborated in our discussion of psychopathology and character states.

In dealing with defenses and defense mechanisms in the psychoanalytic tradition, one understands that different defenses arise at different stages of development; that defenses are unconscious ways of getting rid of unpleasant mental content, whether it consists of memories, wishes, drives, or affects; that one can sometimes have defenses against defenses; that different pathologies are characteristically accompanied by certain clusters of defenses; and that one interprets defenses in the clinical setting. Defenses will unfold and find their replication in the transference. They are carried by the individual as internal automatic workings of the ego that reveal the style with which the individual copes with anxiety and with unwelcome mental content. Careful analysis of a defense must involve not only pointing out that the defense is being used and untangling what it is that is being defended against, but the careful analysis of the wishes and fantasies of the defense itself. In other words, psychoanalysis examines both what the defense mechanisms are defending against and the style with which they are working as important indicators of the coping style and adaptive capacity of the individual.

Technique

The discovery of the transference (defined below) stands alongside the discovery of the unconscious as Freud's most significant contributions to our understanding of the mind. If the cause of any psychopathology is the existence of unconscious forces at work, and if the mind, even under the structural model, works primarily in unconscious ways through unconscious defense mechanisms, then it stands to reason that to make proper diagnosis and treatment, one must look for ways in which unconscious forces reveal themselves to observation. It is in the transference that unconscious processes are revealed as indirect light reveals dust in a room or as a cloud chamber permits us to infer the existence of subatomic particles by the trail they leave behind (see Freud 1912/1958, 1913/1958, 1914b/1958; Gill 1979).

The psychoanalytic situation and the therapeutic alliance. Currently psychoanalysts emphasize that a precondition for treatment is the establishment of a psychoanalytic situation that includes the existence of a *working alliance* or *therapeutic alliance* (Greenson 1967). Such alliance was an aspect of the treatment that Freud recognized but tended to take for granted and sometimes considered to be a part of the positive transference. The capacity for a patient to develop a connection with the analyst was something Freud felt to be present in any of the transference neuroses. The analysis of transference is made possible by virtue of the unique psychoanalytic situation. In a psychoanalytic treatment, the patient is in a state of mild sensory deprivation caused by what some have referred to as *unilateral communicatory freedom*. The patient speaks freely and the analyst speaks rarely. The patient is encouraged to associate freely, and the analyst is encouraged to have free-floating attention but to reserve interventions to one kind only: interpretations. The function of the analyst is to listen, accept, and interpret. Analysis, then, is the interpretation of transference and resistance.

Transference. Transference is the set of feelings, beliefs, convictions, fantasies, and reactions that the patient brings into the analysis and reenacts in the therapeutic relationship. It can emerge in the analytic setting to fill the gaps of the mild sensory deprivation that occurs in the analyst's office. We know that in full-scale sensory deprivation people will hallucinate to fill the void. In the very mild, carefully titrated, unilateral communicative freedom that exists in the psychoanalytic situation, the patient supplies through fantasy the missing or withheld judgments of the analyst. By not discussing reality, personal opinions, private reflections, or details of personal biography, the analyst leaves the field open for the patient to supply the missing details, and the transference emerges like a projective test. The style with which the patient reports material to the analyst, therefore, becomes a clue about how the unconscious processes of that patient work. Some clinical vignettes will illustrate this process.

A colleague with an office that had a beautiful view of the mountains noted that on a day when snow covered the mountains and the air was especially clear, patients came to the office greeting her with their reactions to the view. The first patient said, "Good morning, Doctor. I could hardly wait to come to the office to see the beautiful view. I knew when it snowed last night that the view from your office would be especially beautiful." The second patient said, "Good morning, Doctor. You know, I was wondering what the view from your office would be like. It's not quite as good as what I remember when I was going to school in Switzerland." Another patient worried, "Good morning, Doctor. I think you'd better close the curtains. I'm afraid that you'll be distracted by the beauty of the scenery and won't listen to what I have to say." The stimuli were the same for all three cases. The patients supplied a fantasy in the transference that was then available for interpretation to reveal what they bring with them to important new situations in life.

Another example is illustrative. When reporting the details of a painful dental extraction, a patient took 20 minutes to explain and justify in meticulous detail the dose of analgesics that he had taken to relieve his pain. I was then able to make the interpretation that he was speaking as though awaiting a critical reaction to what he feared I might think was a self-indulgence in taking analgesics rather than enduring the pain. We were able to connect this interpretation to historical information about the patient's relationship with his father and the resultant harsh and demanding superego and ego ideal that made his life onerous and guilt-ridden.

The understanding of transference is a very powerful therapeutic tool. We can infer that patients bring their characteristic reactions to many important relationships and situations. Because of the analytic situation, the transference is allowed to flourish, is not diluted or diffused by ordinary conversation, and ultimately becomes the central focus of both the patient and the analyst in the form of the transference neurosis. This becomes the one event to which patient and analyst are witness in real time, giving it a status greater than either contemporaneous events of external life or the historical past. When present experiences and historical events of the patient's past are replicated in the analysis through the transference, one can have maximum confidence that one is dealing with the central and relevant features of that patient's mental structure.

Resistance. Resistance is the phenomenon by which the patient does not participate in the analysis. Originally this meant resistance to free association, when the patient would stop thinking and his or her mind would go blank. He or she would censor his or her thoughts or not talk because of embarrassment, fear of retribution, or some other fantasy, and then would not disclose that that was the reason why. Now resistance is less a noun and more a gerund. Resistance means that the patient is in the act of resisting (Schafer 1973). What is he or she resisting? The patient is resisting the ongoing nature of the analytic process of unfolding of the transference, free communication of mental content, and free flow of affect. Or he or she is trying to transform the relationship into something other than analysis by turning it into a friendship, into advice giving, or into problem solving.

Interpretation. Interpretation is the articulation on the part of the analyst, and eventually on the part of the patient, of the connections and meaning of what is going on during the process of analysis. Interpretations are strongest and most comprehensive when, as in the example given earlier, they link the historical past to the current life

situation and to phenomena within the analysis such as the transference.

To the extent that a treatment relies on the interpretation of transference and resistance, it comes closer to psychoanalysis. To the extent that it relies more on explanation, on theory, on construction of the historical past in lieu of the unfolding of the transference, on formulae for decoding rather than living through defense mechanisms, it moves into the realm of psychoanalytic psychotherapy or psychodynamic psychotherapy. To the extent that it focuses more on confrontation, on specific problem solving, or on teaching of techniques, it becomes more cognitive or behavior therapy. To the extent that the patient comes to treatment for direct solutions to problems, it most closely resembles counseling.

FOLLOWERS OF FREUD

There is by no means unanimity among current psychoanalysts. Intramural dispute has taken place among a profusion of schools of thought. While correcting and revising the work of Freud and adding new perspectives of their own, a large number of theorists have stayed within the psychoanalytic tradition, viewing themselves as resting upon the foundation of Freud's work and having the same ambitious goals to understand the entire structure of a person's mind. I therefore regard them as falling broadly within the psychoanalytic tradition.

We now turn to four areas of psychoanalytic theory left largely unfinished by Freud: *object relations and the self, development, character structure*, and the *rediscovery of trauma*. We will blend our historical approach with a survey of the modern state of affairs in each of these four main areas.

Object Relations and the Self

Freud had included a theory of object relations in his classical theory. Instincts had a source, an aim, and an object. The oedipal period depended on the actual relationship with the parents, and in "Mourning and Melancholia," Freud (1917[1915]/1957), attempting to distinguish between the depression of normal mourning and the pathological depression of melancholia, talked about the influence of object relations. The word *object* of course is in contrast to the word *subject*. Critics of psychoanalysis who point to use of the term *object relations* and contend that therefore psychoanalysis is not concerned with human beings simply misunderstand the usage of this term.

In "Mourning and Melancholia" Freud said that ordinarily when a significant object is lost to us, we enter a period of mourning, but that if the object relation was more of a narcissistic object choice than a true object relation, and if it was filled with intense ambivalence, then "the shadow of the object falls upon the ego." In other words, through identification we take in qualities of the object that then influence our ego state. To put it yet another way, the infant starts in an autoerotic state and moves through the anaclitic relationship to a state of object relation. The baby loves the mother. To the extent that the mother is excessively disappointing or to the extent that the baby is incapable of mastering its ambivalence, the baby will retreat into a state of secondary narcissism. In that case, its relationship with the mother confuses self and object. The mother is recognized only to the extent to which she fulfills the need of the baby. Thus a narcissistic object choice develops, in which others are not viewed in their own right but rather in terms of the extent to which they fulfill our needs. Thus, when they are lost, we have to incorporate them into ourselves in order not to feel that we are lost. Then the negative half of the ambivalence that we felt toward the object we now direct toward the self, hence melancholia.

Notwithstanding his acknowledgment of the importance of object relations, Freud primarily developed the instinctual drive portion of his theory to a greater extent, and he never completed the elaboration of his object-relational theory—a task that was left to his successors (Greenberg and Mitchell 1983; Sutherland 1980).

Melanie Klein.   Melanie Klein (see Klein et al. 1973) paid substantial attention to the process of pathological identification and to the fate of the incorporated object. In the strictest sense, she was not an object-relations theorist in that she still believed that the primary motive for human behavior was drive discharge. She placed her emphasis on the discharge of the aggressive drives and seemed to give them primacy over the libidinal drives, but, in any event, drives constituted the motivation for the individual. Klein was less concerned with the source and the aim and more concerned with the object of the drives. Noting the child's tendency to split experience into good and bad, Klein postulated that the child first has relations with part objects and that only later in development does the child have relations with whole objects. Her theory said that this tendency to engage in projective identification, to get rid of our unwelcome impulses and our unwelcome incorporation of part objects, causes our internal mental life to be populated by monstrous, distorted, and incomplete versions of objects. Thus, the more pathological splitting there was, the more split we would be in our internal mental life and the more vulnerable to ongoing distortion.

Fairbairn.   W. R. D. Fairbairn was the first true object-relations theorist insofar as he postulated that the primary drive was object seeking (Fairbairn 1972). Whereas Freud felt that the drive was primary and the objects were interchangeable, Fairbairn felt that the objects were primary and the drives were interchangeable. If for Freud anyone could satisfy the baby's hunger, for Fairbairn we were given hunger so that we could have a reason to make a human bond. For Fairbairn the ego is present at birth. Because it is immature and it cannot tolerate the intensity of stimuli, this pristine ego is then rendered asunder, splitting into a libidinal ego (which has an association with the exciting object) and an antilibidinal ego (which has an association with a rejecting object). The course of maturity, then, is to undo the split and reintegrate into a more robust central ego.

Winnicott.   D. W. Winnicott did not offer a full theory, but he is grouped with the object-relations theorists because of many important contributions. Winnicott points out that it is neither conceptually nor clinically proper to conceive of a baby without the mother as well. This viewpoint restores an interpersonal balance to psychoanalysis. A "good-enough" mother (Winnicott 1965) will respond to the baby's communications, meeting its needs within an optimal zone of frustration and gratification. Imposing her own needs, a pathological mother will force the baby to create a "false self" to protect its "true self." On the other hand, a mother who accepts increasing autonomy in gradual stages permits the child to have its own agenda while still remaining dependent on her. Under such circumstances the child can be himself in the presence of a mother who can be herself while they are still together. Winnicott called this "the capacity to be alone" in the presence of someone else.

Winnicott also postulated an intermediate stage of separation-individuation during which the infant relates to "transitional objects" (Winnicott 1953) that are neither self nor other but form an intermediate zone. This intermediate zone initially may take the form of a blanket or a toy but remains with us throughout life as a phenomenon to help us deal with our aloneness and separation in the universe. Thus, in mature adult life, music, scientific creativity, and religion constitute transitional phenomena or transitional experiences that are neither self nor object but act as a link between the two (see Winnicott 1966).

Kohut.   Although he would not have grouped himself in the object-relations school, Heinz Kohut also placed emphasis on the relationship between self and object. Kohut (1971) postulated two lines of development, one involving the libido and conflict, and the other involving the development of the self. Kohut stated that two kinds of transferences that are found in patients with narcissism are keys to the understanding of stages of development through which individuals pass on their way to developing a cohesive self. The development of a cohesive self requires optimal empathy that consists of mirroring and idealization. *Mirroring* is the experience wherein children define themselves by observing themselves in the gleam in their mother's eye. Kohut feels that the development of a cohesive self is more important than the vicissitudes of instincts. *Self psychology*, the school of thought that grew out of Kohut's theories, holds that the cohesive self can manage its drives.

Kohut's sensitivity to absences of phase-appropriate mirroring and idealization led him to emphasize deficiencies of emotional nutrients over conflicts as a cause of pathology. The narcissistic dilemma comes from object relations that were arrested in a phase during which others are seen in terms of how they help to define us. Kohut (1977) characterized this phase with the term *selfobjects*.

Kohut also stressed the paramount need for psychoanalysis to operate on the basis of empathy. Interpretations based on instinctual drives or ego structures are *experience-distant* and therefore not as useful as ones based on awareness of subjective feelings, especially of vulnerability, that are *experience-near*. Transference was not seen as a phenomenon whereby the patient distorts reality, but rather the way the patient experiences (perhaps with exaggerated intensity, but not without basis) the interaction between doctor and patient.

Kohut's earlier contributions described transferences that recapitulated deficient aspects of the child's development. With the introduction of selfobjects, a new school within psychoanalysis began. At first, Kohut tried to bridge earlier theories of libido with his newer theory of the self, by postulating two separate tracks for development. As time went on, this dual track theory was dropped, and the theory of the self took over.

As a theory, self psychology emphasized the absence of crucial "emotional vitamins" as the main pathogenic feature of childhood. On the assumption that "a well-regulated self can manage its drives," repair of an incoherent self was seen as the task of psychotherapy. Interpretation of childhood manifestations in adult action came to be seen as less important than empathic understanding of the transference-expressed needs of the patient at that moment. Affective attunement between patient and therapist superseded interpretations which looked for historical causes, and deficiency superseded conflict.

In an earlier era, psychoanalysis might not have been able to live harmoniously with self psychology. Just as Fairbairn had turned psychoanalytic theory upside down

when he made libido a derivative of object seeking, self psychology had the same effect when it made conflict and drives secondary to deficiency and the formation of a coherent self. However, by the 1970s, psychoanalysis had become a broader tradition and could embrace both object relations and self psychology.

As self psychology has matured, new emphasis has been focused on the intersubjective nature of psychotherapy (Kohut 1984; Stolorow and Brandschaft 1987; Stolorow and Lachmann 1980). This new focus has influenced technique. Therapists influenced by self psychology are more likely to take personal responsibility for their patient's negative affects in the transference and are more likely to address the patient's experience of hurt than the patient's active role in his or her life frustrations (Fine and Fine 1990). In an illustrative clinical vignette, a female patient was engaged to a man toward whom she felt extremely ambivalent. He reminded her of her father, with whom there was much conflict, and the death of her mother when the patient was quite young had made intimacy and commitment extremely difficult and frightening even as it was desperately sought. One day she returned in tears from a weekend with her fiancé: they had broken up after days of fighting, initiated largely by her. When the therapist interpreted her ambivalence, her conflicts over closeness, and her provocations that precipitated this breakup, the patient interrupted to say, "Everything you say may be true, but you could at least start by telling me you were sorry for the grief I'm suffering."

A theorist of self psychology might point to this vignette as an example of a patient's need for empathy to correct a childhood deficiency left by the death of her mother. A Kleinian might choose to emphasize the patient's hostility in provoking an argument with her fiancé or her wish to distance the fiancé to save both parties from the destruction inherent in intimacy. A more "classical" therapist might explore the patient's ambivalent relationship with her father and its influence on the relationship with the fiancé. These differences in emphasis and sequence have stimulated vigorous discussion among different subschools within the psychoanalytic tradition.

In another important distinction, a Kleinian would see aggression as a principle organizing force in character and psychopathology and would view aggressive drives as innate. Kohut and the self psychologists see aggression as the result of frustration and interpret the frustration rather than the aggression itself. This brings us to Kernberg, who sees affect and aggression as central to psychodynamics.

Kernberg.   One of Otto Kernberg's (1976) contributions to object-relations theory was to emphasize that affect, self-representation, and an object representation always appear together. One cannot analyze any one without knowing about the others.

The infant is born unable to distinguish between internal and external and is only able to distinguish between pleasurable and unpleasurable experience. This is the logical consequence of the fact that the infant spends the majority of the day sleeping and the majority of sleep dreaming. Therefore, at first the child has difficulty distinguishing between realistic experiences and dreamed or hallucinated experiences. However, the infant can distinguish between experiences that feel good and experiences that feel bad. This is the origin of what I term *passive splitting*, so called because it occurs as a result of the maturational phase of the infant rather than an affirmative mental effort. One of the positive consequences of passive splitting is that there is an opportunity for good images to be accumulated. For an infant, bad experiences feel more powerful than good experiences, and therefore passive splitting helps to preserve the integrity of good experiences. Eventually, as the infant begins to distinguish between inner and outer, he or she develops active splitting, based on the fear that if the good and the bad were to get too close together the bad would indeed destroy the good. Finally, the infant, growing into a child, begins to be aware of whole objects, to distinguish between internal and external (due to the ascendancy of the reality principle), and to fuse good and bad. This fusion into a whole self and a whole object coincides with the maturation of the superego and the fusion between the old, archaic superego and the ego ideal. Tremendous energy is liberated as a result of this fusion because the energy necessary to keep splits apart can now be employed for other purposes.

It is at this point coinciding with the end of rapprochement and beginning with the object-constancy phase, and also coinciding with the oedipal phase of classical theory, that the individual moves from the splitting hierarchy of defenses to the repression hierarchy of defenses. Kernberg's theory will be further elaborated on below in the subsection on character pathology.

Theories of Development

It is known that physically and cognitively the child grows in phases after birth until it reaches adulthood. Developmental theories assume that psychological growth also proceeds in phases, and the emotional capability of the child and his or her capacity for dealing with mental content, even the definition of what constitutes mental content, change according to the maturational stage. Developmental arrests, fixation points, and points of regression

have an impact on the development of the particular psychological system at greatest risk at any given age. The correlation of psychopathology in adults with the developmental stage of presumed trauma during childhood was an important extension of the concept that childhood events influence adult states.

A variety of developmental systems have been proposed by persons within the psychoanalytic tradition (Figure 5–2). Some of these systems have been full-fledged theories, and others have been simply limited observations or partial theories about substages of development. We introduce the main theories of development in this subsection and then discuss their application to adult psychopathology in the following subsection on character and psychopathology.

The classical theory of Freud and Abraham. The classical theory initiated by Freud (1905/1953, 1925/1961) and elaborated by Karl Abraham (1968) has already been alluded to and will be presented here briefly. At birth, the infant is in a state of autoerotism. The development of the libido at this point is such that the infant is attached only to itself, for a psychological sense of self per se does not yet exist. The ego instinct for survival and the libidinal instinct for pleasure are intertwined, and the child starts with an anaclitic relationship with the mother. In other words, libido leans on survival. Gradually, through the experience of frustration as well as the emergence of the ego and the beginnings of the reality principle associated with the maturation of perception, the child begins to recognize that there is a distinction between internal and external, and a rudimentary form of object relations emerges.

The child's first main modality for relating is oral, meaning literally the mouth, lips, and tongue importantly involved in nursing. But orality also includes taking in of perceptions and "swallowing" the world of sensory perceptions. If there is excessive frustration, the child will retreat from early object-relatedness and establish a state of secondary narcissism. If frustration is moderate and optimal, the child will begin to recognize bit by bit that the objects of the world are not under his or her full control, nor is he or she under their full control. As the organism matures, libidinal interest leaves the initial oral phase and enters an aggressive oral phase in which swallowing and taking in are replaced by biting and spitting. The child learns to say no, and this signals a crucial step in the differentiation of the child from others and the growing establishment of a sense of self (see Spitz 1965).

The libido then moves to the anal phase in which questions of control over bodily contents and the nature of

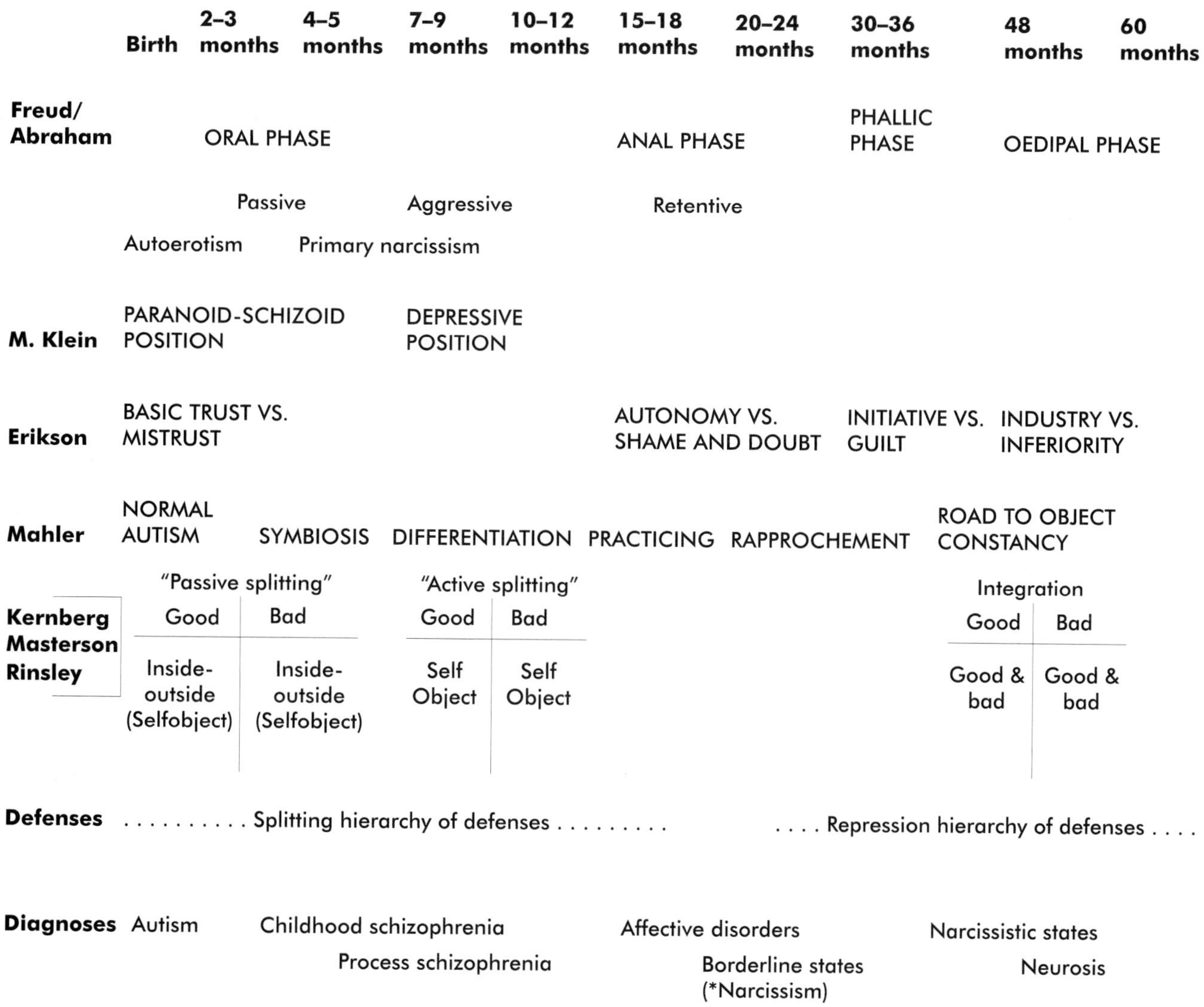

	Birth	2–3 months	4–5 months	7–9 months	10–12 months	15–18 months	20–24 months	30–36 months	48 months	60 months
Freud/ Abraham	ORAL PHASE					ANAL PHASE		PHALLIC PHASE	OEDIPAL PHASE	
		Passive		Aggressive		Retentive				
	Autoerotism		Primary narcissism							
M. Klein	PARANOID-SCHIZOID POSITION			DEPRESSIVE POSITION						
Erikson	BASIC TRUST VS. MISTRUST					AUTONOMY VS. SHAME AND DOUBT		INITIATIVE VS. GUILT	INDUSTRY VS. INFERIORITY	
Mahler	NORMAL AUTISM		SYMBIOSIS	DIFFERENTIATION		PRACTICING	RAPPROCHEMENT	ROAD TO OBJECT CONSTANCY		

Kernberg / Masterson / Rinsley

	2–3 months	4–5 months	7–9 months	10–12 months	30–36 months	48 months
	"Passive splitting"		"Active splitting"		Integration	
	Good	Bad	Good	Bad	Good	Bad
	Inside-outside (Selfobject)	Inside-outside (Selfobject)	Self Object	Self Object	Good & bad	Good & bad

Defenses . . . . Splitting hierarchy of defenses . . . . Repression hierarchy of defenses . . . .

Diagnoses	Autism	Childhood schizophrenia				Affective disorders			Narcissistic states	
			Process schizophrenia				Borderline states (*Narcissism)		Neurosis	

FIGURE 5–2. Theories of development. This figure is an approximate display of each listed author's developmental scheme for comparison with other authors schemes. The phases shown do not have exact correlation with age (i.e., this figure is not to be read in columns). The phases overlap, and neighboring phases may coexist. The theories of each author are not presented as exact equivalents of the similar-age stages of other authors. The diagnoses listed at the bottom are those that some developmental theorists believe match essential developmental fixations and arrests with future child and adult psychopathology.

bodily contents are paramount. These issues are both literal in terms of weaning and toilet training, and metaphorical in terms of the functions that an anus is supposed to fulfill, namely control of time, delay of discharge, containment, making sure that everything is in its proper place, yielding to authority, and making judgments about whether one's internal contents are good or bad. Difficulties in this area will result in fixation at the anal phase and yield an anal character type, with overemphasis on parsimony, orderliness, and obstinacy. Disorders characterized by obsessive-compulsive behaviors are thought to result from fixations at the anal phase.

The third phase of development is the phallic phase, expressed by means of interest in the penis itself, which, according to the classical theory, for boys results in exhibitionism and for girls a feeling of envy and inferiority. Most modern theorists working within the psychoanalytic tradition have importantly modified this aspect of the classical theory.

Exhibitionism and its grandiosity lead to a heightened rivalry with the same-sex parent and usher in the oedipal phase. This oedipal period shows its earliest beginnings in 3- to 4-year-olds and culminates in 5- to 6-year-olds.

The oedipal phase was seen as preeminent in neurosis

because it was 1) the culmination of childhood libidinal development, 2) a multiperson interaction on which future social relatedness would be based, and 3) the hypothesized period of solidification for the superego—the time when gender identity was fixed and sexual object choice was decided. Moving from a two-person to a three-person world was momentous because it prepared the child to relinquish the fantasy of centrality in the universe. Conventions of society, values of culture, the ability to share, the roots of sublimation—all converge at this time. Oedipal issues were felt to be universal and would eventually emerge in every psychoanalysis. Neurosis was believed to be crystallized at this time. A latency period follows, interrupted by puberty and followed by adolescence.

Klein and Fairbairn. Melanie Klein did not have a full-fledged theory of development; however, she took issue with the classical theory on some important points. Klein felt that the critical issue at birth was not autoerotism but what she originally called the paranoid position and what she later, under the influence of Fairbairn, renamed the *paranoid-schizoid position*. By that Klein meant that from birth the infant relies heavily on mechanisms of introjection, projective identification, and splitting, and sees the world in terms of what she called *part objects*. Aggression is preeminent and uncontrollable and cannot be neutralized. If successful, the child then moves to the depressive position by age 6 months when the realization occurs that objects are not entirely split but that they are indeed whole, and when the realization of the imperfection of the world and of the power of aggression takes hold. Thus the ego and superego are present, for Klein, at an extremely early age, as are precursors of the oedipal period. No stages of development are postulated beyond the depressive position of 6 months.

Fairbairn (1972) feels that the ego is present from birth and that the child is object seeking, not pleasure seeking. According to Fairbairn a child is born with a pristine ego, but owing to conflict the child is forced to split off the unacceptable object relations and ego states. Thus, an "id" is created as a result of splitting the pristine ego and repressing the libidinal ego and its associated exciting objects. A "superego" is created by splitting off the antilibidinal ego and its associated rejecting objects. To the extent that these splits are deep and profound, the remaining central ego is impoverished and depleted with little in the way of mature object relations. The task of treatment and of maturity becomes restoring as much as possible to the central ego and reducing the libidinal ego and its exciting objects and the antilibidinal ego and its rejecting objects.

Bowlby. John Bowlby is a British psychoanalyst whose interest in early development was heightened by his duties dealing with displaced children during World War II. Drawing on his knowledge and interest in ethology, Bowlby, agreeing with Fairbairn that the child at birth was object seeking, asserted that there was a primary independent bonding drive that was not anaclitic, leaning on physiological survival, but autonomous and independent and had phases of its own. Bowlby (1958) offers five responses that make up attachment behavior: sucking, clinging, following, crying, and smiling, which are behavior patterns specific to man. Working quasi-independently but synergistically, each one has a specific trajectory and reaches its height during different months of the first 3 years of life. The components of attachment behavior influence the development of the cognitive sphere as well as the formation of character structure.

In Bowlby's theory parent-child relationships are central and object relations have as much importance as instinctual drives.

Balint and Guntrip. Michael Balint described a stage of development in his more severely disturbed patients in which they developed a *basic fault* (Balint 1968). Balint adopted this term to indicate that some form of integration was missing in much the way an earthquake fault line would reveal the lack of integration of tectonic plates. The problem was one of integration, of something missing, rather than drives that were frustrated in their inability to find expression. Balint felt that this basic fault was caused by a failure of fit between the response of the mother and the needs of the child. Those persons who suffer from this basic fault will slip into one of two types of object relations: *ocnophilia*, in which the relations with others are filled with great intensity and deep dependence, or *philobatism*, in which objects are avoided and the inner world is intensely clung to. These two developmental alternatives then characterize the organizing principles for the reaction to the inadequate mother-child relationship.

Harry Guntrip (1974), the main disciple of Fairbairn, expanded the notion of philobatism in terms of his theory of schizoid phenomena. He also saw development as progressing according to degree and type of dependency, rather than drive discharge.

Erikson. Another ambitious theory of development was offered by Erik Erikson (1963). He postulated eight phases of development, spanning the entire life and serving as nodal points for adaptation to the age-appropriate requirements of any phase of development. He modified the concept of libidinal distribution by the concept of zones and modes. *Zone* refers to the organ system or cluster of physical and conceptual skills that the person has to deal with that particular phase of development. *Mode* refers to the manner in which the developmental task is undertaken. For example, applying Erikson's notion of zones and modes to Freud and Abraham's oral phase, one might say that the zone is the mouth and perhaps also the nerve endings of the perceptual system. The mode is that of taking in, of swallowing, and of digesting, spitting, or vomiting. When the oral mode is emphasized, we have issues of dependency and of neediness, hunger, and starvation that might operate quite independent of the oral zone.

Instead of using bodily zones to serve as signposts for his theory, Erikson chose the developmental task that exists at any particular age. *Basic trust versus mistrust* is the stage of acquisition of sense that the universe is reliable and that our most important object relations are consistent and available. *Autonomy versus shame and doubt* addresses the question of how much control of our body and our thinking can we attain and how much will we be a disappointment to those around us and to ourselves. The phase of *initiative versus guilt* coincides with the issues of the oedipal phase for Freud and Abraham. During the stage of *industry versus inferiority* the child deals with latency and school. During puberty and adolescence is the phase of *identity versus role confusion*, our opportunity to clarify issues of personal identity and owning our own internal representations. This is sometimes referred to as *depersonification*. Psychopathology around areas of identity confusion appears at this time. The young adulthood phase of *intimacy versus isolation* opens the task of rediscovering attachment and mature bonding. In midadulthood, the issue is *generativity versus stagnation*, and in maturity the questions concern *ego integrity versus despair*.

Another point that Erikson makes is the interactive nature between the child and the parent. Ordinarily it is assumed that it is the parent who raises the child, but Erikson emphasizes that the relationship goes in two directions:

> Babies control and bring up their families as much as they are controlled by them; in fact, we may say that the family brings up the baby by being brought up by him. Whatever reaction patterns are given biologically and whatever schedule is predetermined developmentally must be considered to be a series of *potentialities for changing patterns of mutual regulation.* (Erikson 1963, p. 69)

Erikson's phases of development were regarded as very important when initially promulgated but have not been given much attention by mainstream psychoanalysis in recent years.

Margaret Mahler. Probably the most influential and important developmental theory since Freud's and Abraham's is that proposed by Margaret Mahler (see Mahler et al. 1975). For Mahler, the issue was not the progress of libidinal development but rather phases of separation and individuation. The key question of development was, To what extent does the infant, who is originally born without identity, acquire a sense of separate identity? Mahler's early work with severely disturbed children led her to investigate this area. Her theory has become the modern classic theory of psychoanalysis, accepted in its essential form by most psychoanalysts, although current investigators are beginning to question certain aspects of it (see Stern 1985).

Normal autism. During the period from birth to 2 months, sleeplike states of the newborn and very young infant far outweigh states of arousal and are reminiscent of the primal states that prevailed during intrauterine life.

Symbiosis. The enhanced awakening and the increased perceptual experience of the infant permit a gradual distinction between what is inside and what is outside, and what is pleasurable and what is unpleasurable. Mahler feels that the mechanism of splitting arises in its first form during this phase. The essential feature of this phase is an omnipotent fusion with the representation of the mother and a delusion of a common boundary between two physically separate individuals. The symbiotic phase reaches its peak at about 4–5 months of age, when it starts to decline as the beginnings of differentiation emerge.

Differentiation. Differentiation coincides with a more permanently alert sensorium, as the infant awakens from its postnatal state and becomes more aware of the world. Mahler called this the *hatching process*. The infant's attention during the first few months had been primarily inward; now it becomes more outward. It is at this phase that transitional objects become important. At about 7–8 months, the baby is beginning to move away from the mother, but can do so only for brief periods of time and then has to check back with the mother visually or tactilely. At about 8 months the infant becomes acutely aware of the difference between familiar people like mother and those who are not familiar. This is called the *stranger reaction*, or in more severe cases, *stranger anxiety*. Its proper timing indicates progress of the differentiation phase.

Practicing. Practicing occurs from about 10 months to 16–18 months. As Mahler says, "During these precious six to eight months . . . the world is the junior toddler's oyster. . . . Narcissism is at its peak! The child's first upright independent steps mark the onset of the practicing period par excellence with substantial widening of his world and of reality testing" (Mahler et al. 1975, p. 71). The enormous expansion of the child's ability to be autonomous during this phase creates a state of imperviousness to disappointment that makes the child appear to be in love with the world.

Rapprochement. The child's ability to walk and to move away from the mother, together with the beginning of representational cognition (which is the precursor of speech), makes the child a much more separate and autonomous person. By 18 months, the infant has matured to a sufficient degree to recognize in a new way his or her helplessness and dependency. During the practicing phase, the child had been preoccupied with all of the new skills he or she was acquiring that permitted greater separation. Now there is a change in emotional life, with greater susceptibility to frustration, greater fears of object loss, and more awareness of separation and consequently greater anxiety. Mahler believes that the child alternates between periods of great need for closeness and periods of need for distance. During this subphase the child will need to be refueled by intimate bodily contact and also by language and other kinds of communication. He or she will shadow the mother and will dart away and then come back and dart away again.

Here the mother's attitude is extremely important, as well as that of the father, whose role expands considerably during this phase. The mother who rejects the child for having become more independent will make that child feel that further autonomy is dangerous. The child must not regard the mother as an extension of himself, nor must the mother regard the child as an extension of herself. It is in this phase that Mahler feels that there is a structuralization of the ego and the establishment of a coherent self. If mother and child have a fluent moving back and forth within an optimal range of closeness and distance, the child will gradually learn that it is safe and rewarding to move toward greater autonomy and that he can do so without fear of losing the relationship with the mother and father. Disturbances in this phase leave the child confused about autonomy; lacking a solid, cohesive self; and preoccupied with the dangers of separation—all of which might result in a clinging, dependent pattern or in a pattern of defiant, defensive disengagement.

Object constancy. The next subphase Mahler calls the consolidation of individuality and the beginnings of emotional object constancy. This stage begins at 24–30 months and lasts in a major way for 2–3 more years and in a subtler way for the rest of one's life. In this subphase the child takes the progressive steps toward object integration, affective stability, and a synthesis between the previously separated good and bad experiences.

Masterson (1981) and Rinsley (1980) have been important contributors in working out the correlation between Mahler's phases of separation-individuation and adult psychopathology.

Infant observation. Psychoanalytic theories of development come from two sources: reconstructions based on inferences made through interpretation of the transference in the psychoanalytic setting, and direct naturalistic and experimental observations of infants by a host of researchers. Compelling new work has emerged recently in this latter area and has been integrated by Daniel Stern (1985). He challenges some of Mahler's conceptions about symbiosis and autism, holding that even at birth the child is aware of surroundings and intensely interested in them. Stern postulates four senses of self that emerge during the first 12–18 months of life: a sense of an emergent self in the period from birth to about 2 months; a sense of a core self that arises from about 2–3 months to 7–9 months; a sense of a subjective self from about 9–15 months, with intersubjective relatedness; and a sense of a verbal self from about 15–18 months, with emphasis on verbal relatedness. Stern believes that there must be a greater correlation between the data of child observation and that of psychoanalysis.

Psychopathology and Character States

The weakest part of psychoanalytic theory is that of psychopathology. Psychoanalysts have generally striven to understand the entire workings of the mind. Symptoms are regarded as signs of malfunction of internal mental processes rather than as diagnostic entities themselves. Psychoanalysis attempts to understand and unravel the mysteries of the entire personality, not just seek symptomatic relief of the state for which the patient originally presented. Furthermore, the symptom may in itself be a defense against more severe underlying difficulties. Hence, a phenomenological approach has never played the important role for psychoanalysis that it has for psychiatry in general. Nevertheless, certain pathological states have been discussed at length and constitute clinical elaborations rather than a theory of psychopathology itself.

When Freud began treating patients, most of whom presented with hysteria (Freud 1905[1901]/1953), he found that the repression of unacceptable mental content was the central feature causing the symptoms. He postulated that the symptom was like a dream in that it was a compromise formation that allowed partial expression of a repressed idea or affect. The obvious therapeutic course, therefore, was to make the unconscious conscious. This Freud could do relatively quickly, and in the early days of psychoanalysis treatment was very brief, perhaps sometimes only a few weeks in length. Over time it became increasingly clear that symptoms could not be separated from character structure. The shift from analyzing id content to analyzing ego mechanisms solidified this change of emphasis from symptom neurosis to character.

Abraham (1968) attempted to organize character according to the presumed stage of development that was malformed. Wilhelm Reich (1972) tended to classify character according to the predominant form that the neurosis took. Thus, for Reich there were phallic characters, passive characters, dependent characters, obsessional characters, hysterical characters, etc. The goal, according to Reich, was to strive for a genital character. Reich's extremely important contribution to psychoanalysis was to emphasize the way in which character structure reveals itself directly and indirectly in the transference, which helped to shift psychoanalytic technique away from interpreting mental *content* in favor of interpreting mental *process*. The style with which the patient defends against mental content becomes equally important and in some cases more important than the content that is being defended against.

Anna Freud (1936/1946) attempted to link stages of development, clusters of defenses, and character types. Workers in the psychoanalytic tradition have isolated particular clusters of patients who were of interest to them and elaborated their character structure. For example, Balint and Guntrip were interested in patients with severe psychopathology and invented categories to describe them. Soon inconsistencies were found within seemingly similar psychopathology groups.

Hysterical neurosis was presumed to be based on repression of unwelcome sexual content. Obsessional neurosis was presumed to involve fixation at the anal phase and the development of symptoms that sought to get rid of unwelcome aggression and anal erotism. But individuals seeking treatment who come with apparently similar symptom pictures respond vastly differently to analysis. In the 1950s, patients diagnosed as suffering from hysteria were found to fall into at least two clusters, one of which had a more infantile or oral version and the other of which had the more classical oedipal disturbance. Similar confusion arose with patients who had an unusual degree of narcissism. Freud (1924[1923]/1961, 1924b/1961) had originally equated this condition with psychosis, indicating that the transference neuroses could be treated with analysis

but that the narcissistic neuroses were refractory to analysis because of an intractable inability to move from narcissistic object-choice to true object relations, a move that is a necessary precursor for development of the transference neurosis. However, some investigators began to have success with such patients, whereas others noted that narcissistic features emerged in treatment of patients who did not originally present with them. The same thing happened with severely regressed patients. In the 1950s and 1960s, psychoanalytic investigators believed that certain patients with psychotic symptoms were treatable with psychoanalysis; others felt that similar patients could be treated with modified psychoanalysis; still others maintained that such severe psychopathology was beyond the ken of psychoanalytic treatment. Clearly, there was some confusion in the psychoanalytic nomenclature to account for this disparity of findings.

The clarification of the borderline and narcissistic states, primarily by Kernberg and Kohut in the 1960s and 1970s, has been extremely helpful in reducing this confusion, although another decade or two may have to pass for accumulation of data not adequately explained by these theories. Nevertheless, it is one of Kernberg's greatest contributions to have rethought the question of character pathology and to have offered his scheme of hierarchies of character states.

Classification of character states. To understand an individual patient, one has to conduct a careful review of systems based on the patient's functional capacities and style of mental action. Within each of these categories one can make judgments about diagnosis and presumed underlying dynamics. There are six main areas that one must understand so as to classify properly a patient's character pathology (summarized in Table 5–3, as derived from Kernberg's [1976] work). As a commentary on this organization, Table 5–4 provides a "psychoanalytic review of systems" in the form of questions to be raised in evaluating a patient's character structure and psychopathology.

Diagnoses. Having done a review of systems, one will reduce the likelihood of mistakenly being drawn astray by overreliance on the presenting symptoms. There is a spectrum of character pathology, from the individual who is primarily psychotic through persons with low, medium, and high levels of character structure, up through persons in the normal range. Those persons with borderline and narcissistic disorders, those who have an infantile personality, those with multiple sexual perversions without stable object relations or ongoing partners, hypomanic persons, schizoid persons, those with a paranoid personal-

TABLE 5–3. A classification of character states

Category	Psychotic organization	Low level of organization	Medium level of organization	Higher level of organization	Healthy organization
Instinctual development		Preponderance of pathological condensation of genital and pregenital strivings, with excess primitive aggression.	Pregenital, especially oral; regression and fixation points predominate.	Genital primacy attained.	
Ego and its defenses	Lack of good, consistent reality testing.	Splitting and related defenses (e.g., primitive dissociation, denial, idealization, devaluation, omnipotence, projective identification). Excessive splitting impairs ego's synthetic function. Direct expression of instincts is linked with defenses. Self not cohesive or integrated; mix of grandiose, and contemptible and shameful.	Uses repression-type defenses, but reverts to splitting-type defenses under stress. Reaction formations coexist with partial expression of rejected impulses. Inconsistent self.	Repression and related defenses (e.g., intellectualization, rationalization, undoing, projection). Inhibitions and reactive traits predominate. Constricted ego.	Considerable conflict-free energy. Sublimation.
Superego		Archaic unintegrated superego precursors.	Lack of integration; sadistic, with overidealization in ego ideal.	Integrated, though severe, harsh, and perfectionistic.	Less severe superego, more realistic ego ideal, integration between them.
Internalized object relations	Difficulty distinguishing between self and object. Fusion, symbiosis, or autistic thinking.	Part objects predominate; object constancy not fully established. Inability to love an object who frustrates. Self not stable. Good and bad self images not integrated. Identity diffusion. Inner world inhabited by caricatures of good and bad aspects of important objects.	Stable self and object world, but with severe conflictual relationships. May fragment under severe stress.	Stable self, stable representational world. Whole objects predominate.	Mostly whole objects, and a consistent, cohesive self.
Affect		Impaired capacity for guilt or mourning. Basis for self-evaluation constantly fluctuating between harsh criticism and overidealized aspirations of grandiose notions.	Severe mood swings (according to relationship with superego and ego ideal).	Can experience guilt and mourning. Wider range of affects. Sexual and aggressive drives partially inhibited.	Wide range of possible affects. Excellent anxiety tolerance and frustration threshold.

	Good empathic powers. Able to love and to mourn.	Can have fairly deep and stable object relations, with genuine concern. Considerable empathy. Better anxiety tolerance.	"Structured impulsivity." Modest empathy. Slight anxiety tolerance.	Impulsive. Contradictory repetitive behaviors seen. Sadistic, polymorphously perverse infantile drives. Little empathy. Little conflict-free energy. Very poor tolerance of affects, especially anxiety.
Interpersonal		Moderate impairment of social adaptation. Problems may appear only in closest relationship (e.g., spouse, children).	Lasting, though turbulent relationships, sometimes promising intimacy that cannot be sustained.	Relationships tend to be need-gratifying or threatening. Chronic work failure and creative failure. Not nurturing to others when under stress.
Diagnostic groups		Hysterical characters, obsessive-compulsive, depressive-masochistic persons.	Passive-aggressive, sadomasochistic. Better-functioning infantile and hysteroid types. Many narcissistic, some borderline persons. Persons with stable sexual deviations with relatively stable object relations. Cyclothymic persons. Some persons who abuse substances (especially food and alcohol).	Infantile personality. Many of the narcissistic disorders. Most borderline patients. Antisocial, as-if, chaotic impulse-ridden, inadequate, and self-mutilating. Persons with multiple sexual perversions, especially those without stable object relations or ongoing partners. Paranoid personalities, hypomanic, schizoid. Some persons who abuse substances (including gambling, eating, alcohol and drugs).

TABLE 5–4. A psychoanalytic review of systems

Instinctual development

Where are the instinctual drives?

Is there a predominance of early oral or anal fixation?

Is the patient's experience oralized or analized?

Is there an enormity of aggression?

Is there a lack of fusion of aggression and libido, or has a degree of fusion of instincts been achieved?

Has the person made it to a primarily genital level?

To what extent has the individual attained primacy of secondary process?

Is the person capable of a bound cathexis, or is all psychic energy subject to mobile cathexis and the need for instantaneous discharge?

Has the capacity to delay been achieved?

Ego and defenses

Does the individual primarily use splitting and the related defenses of projective identification, primitive dissociation, denial, idealization, devaluation, and omnipotence?

Does excessive splitting impair the ego's synthetic function?

Do the defenses primarily express and only incidentally conceal the underlying drives? Or, does the individual use repression-type defenses, reverting to the splitting when only under stress? Or, does the person use primarily the repression defenses such as intellectualization, rationalization, undoing, projection, and reaction formation with primarily inhibitions and a constricted ego?

How much conflict-free energy is there?

To what extent is there a cohesive self?

How much does the individual vacillate between grandiose states and contemptible, shameful states?

Superego

Does the individual primarily demonstrate the features of an archaic, unintegrated superego precursor with extremely harsh prohibitions and an excessively lofty and grandiose ego ideal?

Is there a more integrated, still sadistic superego that is moderately harsh, and an overidealized ego ideal but not one that is too grandiose? Or, is there an integrated though harsh and perfectionistic superego? (In healthier states, the superego is less severe and more realistic, and there is considerable integration between the superego and the ego ideal. The person can feel praise for himself as well as punishment.)

Object relations

Does the individual have difficulty distinguishing between inside and outside, between self and object?

In the clinical setting or in the pathological situation of the symptoms, does one see fusion, symbiosis, or autistic defenses?

Do part objects predominate without object constancy being fully established?

Is there an inability to love an object who frustrates?

Is the self stable or not?

Do good and bad images become integrated?

How diffuse is identity?

To what extent is the inner world inhabited by caricatures or aspects of important objects rather than whole objects? (If there is primarily a whole object world and a consistent, cohesive self, then object relations have advanced to a more mature degree.)

Affects

Is there a wide range of affective expression or a very narrow one?

Is the individual impulsive?

Are contradictory repetitive behaviors seen?

Is the individual sadistic?

Does the affect fluctuate between overly harsh criticism and overly idealized grandiosity?

Is there cyclothymia?

Does the individual have empathy?

Can the individual experience guilt and mourning?

Can the individual have deep, stable object relations with genuine concern?

How much tolerance is there for anxiety, or to what extent must anxiety be instantaneously discharged?

Interpersonal relations

Is there an attainment of social adaptation?

Are there lasting relationships, or do the relationships promise intimacy but cannot be sustained?

Is the individual nurturing to others when under stress? Or do relationships constantly alternate between need gratification and threatening rejection?

---

ity, some persons who abuse substances, and those persons who are antisocial, chaotic, and impulse-ridden—all fall into the category of low character function and severe character pathology. Passive-aggressive persons, sado-masochistic persons, some of the better-functioning in-

fantile and hysteroid-type persons, many persons with narcissistic personalities, some persons with borderline disorders, some persons with some of the more stable sexual deviations with relatively stable object relations, some cyclothymic persons, and some persons who abuse substances, particularly those who abuse substances that are not illegal such as food and alcohol—all fall into the category of medium character function. The higher level of character function include the persons with hysterical characters, obsessive-compulsive persons, depressive-masochistic persons, and the assortment of neurotic persons whose complaints are lack of sufficient creativity, difficulties in achieving intimacy, and inability to sustain creativity.

Borderline and narcissistic states. Although there is general agreement that the borderline and narcissistic states are related to each other, investigators in the field nevertheless have considerable differences of opinion with regard to the details of these two states. Kohut writes almost as if to imply that in his conceptualization nearly all of these patients have narcissistic disorders, and the tiny few who are so badly damaged that they cannot be treated with psychoanalysis are consigned to the borderline category. Kernberg seems to conceptualize these persons primarily as suffering from the mechanisms of borderline personality organization and suggests that perhaps some of the most well-functioning group who have the lowest levels of aggression resemble those patients whom Kohut refers to as narcissistic. Masterson and Rinsley feel that there are many more borderline patients than there are narcissistic ones. Rinsley believes that the fixation point for narcissism is late in the rapprochement phase (18–30 months), because these are patients who generally have a higher level of function and more signs of maturity. Masterson feels that the predominance of grandiosity in these patients indicates that they are fixated in the practicing phase (10–15 months), as though stuck in the grandiose time warp characteristic of that phase.

The significance of one's point of view is that it will influence the sequence in which interpretations are given. For instance, Masterson advocates confrontation for borderline patients and interpretation for narcissistic patients, because the borderline patients lack a sense of identity and therefore will coalesce around the clarifying aspect of a confrontation, whereas the narcissistic patients will disintegrate if their fragile hold on well-being is punctured. Finally, the DSM system, starting with DSM-III (American Psychiatric Association 1980), which introduced the diagnosis of borderline personality disorder, merged the more descriptive approach of Gunderson (1976, 1984) with the more psychodynamic approach of Kernberg (1975) (Marmer and Fink 1994).

Two clinical illustrations. The following clinical vignettes illustrate the usefulness of Kernberg's review of systems approach for character pathology:

David was an extremely disturbed 23-year-old man when he first came into treatment. He appeared disheveled, his clothes did not match, and he had recently been fired from a menial job because he was unable to follow simple instructions. He had taken 5 years barely to graduate from the university with the lowest possible grade point average. At school he had spent most of his time cloistered in his room, even urinating in empty soda bottles that he would empty at 2:00 A.M. when he was confident no one would see him. He had a delusional numerology system for the date of his birth and fantasies that the clouds were giving him messages. He was in an extremely anxious state and appeared defiant and hostile when he first came to see me. Based on his symptoms, one might have wondered if he were either schizophrenic or severely borderline. However, a more careful evaluation revealed that he had a much wider range of affect, that he had a profound consistent relationship with mythical parents (humanistic authors whose works he had read and cherished throughout a very disturbed high school and college period), and that he had had several lifelong friends who had remained friendly with him through the course of his illness. In the sessions he displayed a warm, gentle sense of humor. All of these factors coexisted with the extremely severe psychopathology with which he presented. Consequently, I made the diagnosis of a medium level of character pathology and felt safe in initiating a psychoanalytic treatment.

In contrast, Peter was a successful musician and composer. He had had several hit songs and had written scores for television. His presenting symptom was panic attacks that began when his parents were given lifetime career achievement awards in a related profession. His own self-diagnosis was that of a severe anxiety reaction centered around oedipal issues. However, very early in the transference the predominance of severe splitting and projective identification and idealization was manifest. Both in the transference and in Peter's marriage, part objects predominated. Good and bad images of himself were not integrated, and his mood fluctuated in a cyclothymic manner according to whether he was in alignment with his grandiose ego ideal or his extremely harsh, punitive superego. Although he had occasional utilization of repression hierarchy defenses (such as intellectualization, reaction formation, and undoing), splitting predominated. He had an outwardly stable marriage, but his lack of ability to delay and the excess of primitive aggression were revealed both in the compulsive nature of his sexual behavior and in his inability to tolerate any frustration. Therefore, it was not surprising when in the second year of psychoanalytic psychotherapy a transference psychosis emerged with a full-fledged delusion regarding my influence over his mind and body, and in the office Peter experienced hallucinations of me in the appearance of the devil.

This latter case example demonstrates the converse of David's case: a patient whose underlying character structure was much more pathological than the apparent level of adaptation indicated by his initial presenting symptoms. These two cases also illustrate the kinds of patients that are addressed within the psychoanalytic tradition and the extent to which underlying character pathology is more important than phenomenological diagnosis.

The Rediscovery of Trauma

The most exciting development for theory of the mind and psychopathology in the 1980s and 1990s has been the rediscovery of the role trauma plays in shaping personality and creating symptoms. In some ways this represented a throw back to the 19th Century and the days of Charcot and Janet. Many authors (Davis 1990; Edelson 1990; Ellenberger 1970; Erdleyi 1990) have commented on the central role of trauma in the theories of the 19th century. The French, most especially Charcot and Janet, observed that acute and chronic trauma was responsible for a wide variety of psychopathology. This observation was the linchpin for Charcot's theory of hysteria and for Janet's notion of the role of dissociation in his theory of the mind. Even Briquet (1859, noted in Loewenstein 1990), whose name is not generally associated with psychodynamic thinking, noted that a substantial number of his patients with somatization disorder suffered histories of childhood physical and sexual abuse.

Certain characteristics of the 1980s seem to be responsible for this rediscovery. The posttraumatic stress disorders of the veterans of the war in Vietnam made a dramatic impact on American psychiatrists. The capacity of real trauma to have prolonged influence on symptoms and a debilitating effect on personality and adaptation forced us to rethink our assumptions about the relationship between trauma and the ability to function. Long-lasting dissociation and physiological instability in these patients could not be ascribed simply to preexisting conditions or to fantasy.

The recognition of the widespread prevalence of child abuse forced psychiatrists to review all of our former assumptions (Kluft 1990; McDougall 1982; Miller 1984, 1990). From the perspective of physical findings, pediatrics had become aware in the 1970s of the "battered child." In the 1980s, the awareness of the psychiatric findings exploded into public consciousness. Incest was found to be much more frequent than had been believed, and the results of childhood sexual and physical abuse were found to be longer lasting and more profound than previously thought. Several celebrated cases (e.g., the case of Sybil

[Schreiber 1973]) became widely known, and interest as well as the index of suspicion grew accordingly.

Terrorism and mind-controlling individuals and cults also drew the attention of psychiatrists worldwide. Whether the survivors of hijacking, hostage taking, kidnapping, or escape from religious or political cults, patients emerging from traumatic scenarios represented certain characteristic findings that challenged the field of psychiatry.

Both acute trauma (Herman 1992; Terr 1990; van der Kolk 1987) and chronic trauma (Fish-Murray et al. 1987; Goodwin 1985; Herman 1992; Horowitz 1991; Kluft 1985; Niedlerland 1974; Putnam 1985, 1989, 1990; Shengold 1989; Spiegel 1990a, 1990b; Wilbur 1985) can cause psychopathology, and both can warp the formation of personality. Acute trauma is more likely to be limited to the traditional symptoms of posttraumatic stress disorder: flashbacks, numbing, and hypervigilance. Chronic trauma leads to an increase in dissociative defenses that place the memory of the full impact of the trauma at a distance. Somatization may be one result, with physical symptoms expressing the psychic pain of the trauma, as in the phenomenon known as *alexithymia*. The alexithymic person is unable to feel affect as emotions and instead feels it in the form of body sensations. Memory problems ranging from reduced concentration to amnesia can be another response.

Repetition of the trauma in the form of seeking relationships that replicate abuse patterns constitutes an all too common pattern. For example, one patient who had been sexually abused by both mother and father married an alcoholic man who beat her when he was intoxicated. After her divorce, the patient became intimate with another psychiatric patient whom she had met during a hospitalization. He doused her with lighter fluid and threatened to ignite her when she tried to leave. Later, she married another man who did not abuse her, but who did molest the child they had together. Not until she was able to face the full impact of her own childhood was she successful in stopping this ongoing repetition.

Perhaps the most important finding in the rediscovery of trauma was the awareness of the profound impact and widespread nature of the defense of dissociation (see also Chapter 18 of this textbook). Dissociative responses can range from feelings of partial unreality in the form of depersonalization and derealization, all the way to such profound identity disturbances as dissociative identity disorder (also called multiple personality disorder) (Davis 1990; Edelson 1990; Erdleyi 1990; Kihlstrom and Hoyt 1990; Marmer 1980, 1991; Putnam 1985; Spiegel 1990a, 1990b; West 1967; Wilbur 1985). Although at times it appears that Freud (1920/1955) thought of dissociation as a basic defense unto itself, we now usually think of dissociation as a defense mechanism combining denial, repression, and isolation to detach the person from unbearable awareness—both ideational and emotional—of trauma and of the person's reaction to it. The effects of growing up in a dissociated state are severe and profound and can interfere with all aspects of cognitive and psychological development. Any part of the experience may be dissociated, or dissociation itself can become an organizing principle. In the latter case, thoughts, affects, body feelings, perceptions, memory, or concentration can be disconnected, singly or in combination. How the individual develops will depend on which combinations of the dissociative process predominate.

The thread that all these responses have in common is the organization of the mind that keeps the traumatic memory and its emotion out of awareness. All people develop the structure of their mind under the influence of nature, nurture, and fate (Masterson 1981; Winnicott 1988). Likewise, all people develop their personalities and their psychopathology in response to conflict, deficiency, and trauma. Traditional psychoanalytic theory emphasizes the concept of conflict, with different mental forces battling against each other, and fantasy struggling with reality. Self-psychology emphasizes deficiency, noting the effects on the formation of a coherent self when an insufficient supply of empathy is available during childhood. To these viewpoints is now being added an awareness of real trauma and the mind's reaction to it to form symptoms of somatization, alexithymia, flashbacks, numbing, hypervigilance, depersonalization, amnesia, dissociation, and repetition of trauma.

The pendulum of theory has a way of swinging too far in one direction, then too far in the other. Charcot and Janet focused on the innate vulnerability of some persons to real trauma. Freud called our attention to the complex way our fantasies can alter our perceptions and shape our personalities. Kohut and his followers make the question of lack of empathy their theory's fulcrum. Now a new wave of theorists in the tradition of Janet are again reminding us of the pivotal role of trauma. The student of psychiatric theory must remember that conflict and fantasy, deficiency and empathy, and trauma and dissociation are all present in everyone. The art is to see the correct proportion in each person.

The issue of repressed memory.   The renewed interest in trauma has brought about an increase in the reports of traumatic events. Some authors have wondered whether reports of previously repressed memories of trauma and abuse are iatrogenically engendered. For example, Loftus (1994) has argued that false memories can be implanted in normal college students, who later recall these memories as if they had happened. She contends that if false memories can be implanted, then patients' reports of childhood abuse that had previously been repressed might well be false also. This would occur in cases of excessive therapeutic zeal on the part of a therapist committed to the theory of trauma. On the other hand, Williams (1995) and her colleagues have demonstrated that repression of documented childhood abuse occurs approximately one-third of the time. She studied cases of childhood abuse seen in hospital emergency rooms. Nineteen years later the victims were interviewed. A third of them had nearly continuous memory of their abuse, a third had intermittently repressed the memories, and a third had no memory at all. At the present time, our theories of memory have not reconciled the Loftus and the Williams positions, nor has a complete theory of memory been integrated into our theories of the mind. Freud started out viewing repressed memories as causative for symptoms. Later he believed that defenses against memories caused symptoms. Still later, he believed that many memories were actually fantasies and that conflicts over fantasies and wishes or drives was the cause of psychopathology. Simple theories that ignore the layered overdetermination of both trauma and fantasy risk missing the richness of each particular patients presentation. Until we have a more complete theory of memory, the clinician is urged to avoid suggestive techniques when taking a trauma history but also to be open to traumas real role in psychopathology.

THEORIES OF DYNAMIC PSYCHIATRY

In the following section I discuss theorists of dynamic psychiatry whose interest included the total personality and character structure and the interplay of conscious and unconscious forces, but who either left the psychoanalytic tradition or never were part of it. The reader should be aware that the focus has been limited to a few representatives of each group. Many other important figures have not been mentioned. Within the psychoanalytic tradition, these figures include Alexander, Arlow, Bion, Brenner, Federn, Ferenczi, Hartmann, Kris, Loewenstein, Rapaport, Searles, Schafer, Spence, and Spitz. Kohut's and Melanie Klein's complex views have been highly condensed. In the psychodynamic tradition, the work of Allport, Bateson, Beck, Berne, Biswanger, Boss, Frankl, Fromm, Fromm-Reichman, Goldstein, Jackson, Jaspers, George Klein, Klerman, Lewin, Maslow, Masserman,

Meyer, Murray, Perls, Rodgers, and others has been omitted.

JUNG

Carl Jung is one of the most voluminous writers in dynamic psychiatry, with his collected works in the English edition nearly as extensive as those of Freud. Jung is perhaps the only theorist in this group to have a large international following that still refers to its school of thought by a term using his name. Jungians have had only an indirect influence on psychoanalysis, on general psychiatry, and on psychology, but have had a large influence in academic settings where psychoanalysis and depth psychology are taken seriously, as well as a substantial influence on psychotherapy in general and their own movement in particular.

Jung originally was a member of Freud's circle and was designated by Freud to be his successor as the leader of international psychoanalysis. However, several years after their collaboration began the two drifted apart permanently and irrevocably. Jung had had a wide background in philosophy, religion, and anthropology, as well as considerable psychiatric experience working with psychotic patients prior to and following his contact with Freud. The first significant difference between Freud (1925[1924]/1959) and Jung (1961) came on the question of libido and psychic energy. Freud had contended that libido was sexual, whereas Jung considered the libido to be the unitary force of psychic energy, not explicitly sexual, nor even limited to being sensual, but something closer to the *elan vital* of Henri Bergson. Both Freud and Jung believed in some kind of principle of constancy, which for Jung took the form of the principles of equivalence and entropy, indicating that psychic energy seeks an equilibrium and that if it is increased in one area it is depleted in another.

Freud and Jung also disagreed about the nature of the unconscious. For Freud, the content of the unconscious was the product of the individual's personal history. Although the unconscious contained innate drives, its specific content consisted of the introjects, identifications, fantasies, memories, affects, and associations accumulated over a life span. For Jung (1966b), the unconscious mind consisted of a collective unconscious, which was the storehouse of latent memories of our cultural past, our racial memory, the entire history of *homo sapiens*, and even prehuman memory. It was shared by all human beings as the psychic residue of evolution. Although Jung did not say that specific racial memories were inherited, the potential to revive them by means of symbols was always present. In contrast to Freud, Jung conceptualized the personal un-

conscious as constituting only a small portion of the total unconscious. In Jung's view, the ego was similar to the conscious mind.

The structure of the unconscious consisted of component archetypes. Jung (1964) conceptualized them as innate ideas (or preformatting) that ready us for real experiences. For instance, there is an innate idea of the mother that readies us for our real-life experience with our mother. There are innate ideas of father, of hero, of leader, and so forth. These archetypes originate in the mind as a permanent deposit accreted over the generations as the categories into which human symbolic thought is preordained to be experienced. Archetypes are also semiautonomous dynamic systems that can act with partial independence.

Five archetypes stand out and define personality organization. The *persona* is the outward mask by which the person balances the demands of society with other internal needs. An individual may have both a public and a private persona. *Anima* and *animus* are the feminine and masculine prototypes within each of us. On this issue Jung agreed with Freud about the innate bisexuality of humans, but elaborated it differently. Our understanding of men and women is the effect of the anima or animus in each of us that corresponds to the opposite gender. The *shadow* is the representation of animal instincts that human beings have as their legacy of evolution from lower animals. The shadow concept gives us passion, vitality, and zest as well as our concept of evil, devil, or enemy. The *self* holds everything together and attempts to produce unity, equilibrium, and stability by balancing various archetypes and complexes.

The mind has four functions or operations: thinking, feeling, sensing, and intuiting. These functions may be directed primarily to the inner world of subjective reality (i.e., introversion) or to the external world of objective reality (i.e., extroversion). *Thinking* is verbal and ideational, and consists of logic and reasoning. *Feeling* permits pleasure and pain, anger and joy, love and loss. It is also the faculty with which we make judgments about good and bad. Through *sensation* we acquire facts. *Intuition* is perception by means of unconscious processes, involving the essence of reality that lies beyond thoughts, perceptions, and feelings. In each individual, these four component functions may be ranked in order of superiority to inferiority according to the strength with which they are developed. Defense mechanisms are limited to repression and sublimation, which leads to the next concept.

Each faculty within the individual and each aspect are either in unity or in opposition, or each acts in compensation for weaknesses in another realm. Thus, the purpose of treatment is to restore balance and promote unity by means of understanding the component parts. In treatment, therefore, the focus is on understanding the various symbols, all of which are presumed to be present but out of balance in pathology.

In contrast to Freud's psychic determinism is Jung's own view of why events occur. *Causality* explains a present event in terms of the past, and *teleology* explains the present in terms of future potential. Synchronicity is a higher order of causation on the edge between the psychical and the physical worlds, and thus blends science with mysticism.

The theory of archetypes and the collective unconscious contrast with psychoanalytic theories in the interpretation of dreams. In keeping with the ontogenetic point of view emphasizing personal history, Freud holds that the dream is the unique idiosyncratic product of the dreamer and reflects an amalgam of current life situations, recent events, and infantile wishes from important periods of childhood. From the phylogenetic perspective, Jung contends that the dream reveals imbalances in the unity of the self and is understood by identifying the archetypal meaning of the symbols in question.

Critics point to the mystical and stereotyping aspects of Jung's theories, and to some of his controversial statements and actions (see Jung 1934/1966a; Carotenuto 1982). Adherents to Jung's theory see it as a comprehensive attempt to understand the individual's use of the universal characteristics of human beings. This theory has also been responsible for technical innovations and modifications practiced within Jungian therapy.

ADLER

Alfred Adler was another early member of Freud's circle who also differed with him on the subject of instinctual drives (Freud 1925[1924]/1959). He emphasized the importance of aggression and recognition, presaging some of Kohut's work on the self. Adler (1956) concluded that aggression was an innate drive, but one not used for the purpose of destruction, but rather with the emphasis on seeking power and recognition. Adler came to this position based on his studies of inferiority, which started out as a narrow concept of organ inferiority and was broadened to include the inevitable feeling of inferiority that every child has when faced with adults who have dominance or adults on whom the children depend. This situation stimulates a perpetual desire to overcome the feelings of inferiority and dependency.

Adler also emphasized that aggression and inferiority were not solely an intrapsychic issue. Every human is born into a family, and every child has a relationship with a mother; therefore, no human development can occur outside of a social context. Thus, for Adler, side by side with the striving for superiority and the innate assertiveness of aggression was also an innate drive for social cooperation and what he called social interest, which balances the personal and selfish interests.

Adler coined the term *style of life*, by which he meant pathways that each individual uses to balance social interest and personal striving. Style of life then is determined partly by the particular inferiorities that a child faced historically as well as the creative self, which also is an innate principle of human life helping the person transcend his or her physical and environmental beginnings.

Adler was particularly interested in the effects of birth order on personality and felt that the oldest, the middle, and the youngest children in a family were likely to be distinctive and predictable. Oldest children are given enormous attention and are suddenly dethroned when the second child is born. Second children are constantly striving to surpass older siblings. Youngest children tend to be spoiled. He also felt that earliest memories were capsulized versions of one's basic orientation in life.

In technique Adler differed considerably from therapists in the psychoanalytic tradition. For Adler the goal of treatment was the remaking of the patient's lifestyle, particularly balancing the sense of inferiority, the need to compensate for it, and the social feeling of cooperation. Great emphasis was placed on the therapeutic alliance, which in many respects was regarded as the most important aspect of the treatment. The therapist and the patient together then learned about the patient's history, mostly through reconstruction rather than through the transference. Adler relied a great deal on encouragement and on the nonspecific effects of the therapeutic alliance to reeducate the patient in a proper therapeutic environment, one in which he or she would feel totally accepted and that was felt would lead to a healthier style of life. Such a setting required an optimistic attitude, a belief in the possibility of change, encouragement to be responsible for one's actions, and a high degree of empathy and rapport between therapist and patient.

RANK

Otto Rank was yet another early follower of Freud who stayed within the psychoanalytic tradition for many years but eventually broke with Freud (Ferenczi and Rank 1956). Rank (1973) supplanted the centrality of the Oedipus complex in the formation of neurosis with the centrality of the birth trauma, which in his theory was the basic and original anxiety through which all subsequent anxieties were interpreted. Freud did not deny that there was birth anxiety, but he did not make it central to his theory. For Rank, the trauma of birth then became the paradigm for all separations, and separation anxiety became heir to primal birth anxiety. Infantile sexuality was subordinated to the birth trauma as well. Masochism was seen as the transmuting of the pain of birth into pleasure, and sadism as the expression of anger and retribution by one who has been traumatized by expulsion from the womb.

Individuation became a central principle for Rank. The individual has to define himself or herself and does so by saying no and asserting his or her will. However, the assertion of will results in guilt over the harm done to the person who formerly met the individual's dependency needs. Also, having remembered the trauma of birth, the individual has the fear that he or she will be expelled from the family if his or her individuality is too assertively revealed.

Development proceeds through three stages of individuation. During the first stage, the individual follows biological needs and the values of parents and society. In the second phase, there is a conflict of wills, and the individual seeks to construct his or her own standards. The third stage heralds an autonomous ego capable of creativity.

Rank felt that treatment could proceed more quickly than in traditional psychoanalysis, and in his treatment he emphasized the therapeutic relationship, especially the emotional dynamics revealed within the therapy and the development of new forms of behavior in the therapeutic setting. Rank also emphasized the value of setting time limits for treatment. Treatment goals are to help the patient overcome the birth trauma and all subsequent separations and be able to assert will without fear or guilt. It is recognized that every separation creates great anxiety and that acquisitions of autonomy create the fear of separation. Therefore, the therapist must accept negative reactions from the patient and gently encourage the acquisition of autonomy.

Because of the emphasis on the assertion of will in expressing autonomy, Rank felt that reality had to be introduced relatively early in treatment, and his theory emphasized realistic reexamination of the true life situation—past, present, and future. He also stressed realistic limitations on what the therapeutic situation could provide. Thus, the therapist and the patient learn through practice that it is safe to assert one's will and to be autonomous.

Rank's views addressed legitimate, unsolved problems that the psychoanalytic tradition has eventually addressed. The importance of separation and individuation and of separation anxiety was acknowledged by Mahler's theories. The role of the therapeutic alliance has been well documented by Greenson (1967) and others. The value of setting limitations for therapy is sometimes accepted in psychoanalytic psychotherapy, but not in psychoanalysis (but see also Freud 1937/1964). Rank's work

is an often unacknowledged source of relevant ideas for psychotherapy.

HORNEY

Karen Horney was trained in orthodox psychoanalysis and was a teacher at the traditional New York Psychoanalytic Institute. However, she broke with orthodox psychoanalysis, partly for reasons of organization and internal politics but largely for philosophical differences that she had with some of Freud's theories. In particular, she felt that classical psychoanalysis was too mechanistic, too biologically based, and insufficiently humanistic.

Horney (1937, 1950) also had specific differences with Freud regarding the psychology of women. She believed that the concept of penis envy, with its view that the psychology of women depended on their feelings of genital inferiority and jealousy of men, was ill-founded. Horney instead contended that feminine psychology overemphasized the love relationship and that it was not based on anatomy. She also felt that aggression was not innate, but was a self-protective mechanism that was stimulated by threats to one's security and added to by experiences of frustration.

Although she left the psychoanalytic tradition and modified psychoanalytic technique, Horney focused on unconscious forces and on the way in which unconscious factors create character structure. According to Horney (1950), neurosis originates in distorted parent-child relationships that are subsequently self-perpetuated throughout life. Neuroses are characterized by the repeated reaction in new situations to the same distortions or reactions that emanated from the original parent-child relationship. These neurotic strategies may involve pathological ways of moving toward people, of moving away from people, and of moving against people. Horney herself presented 10 neurotic needs that were manifestations of these three main ways of living. These were neurotic needs for 1) affection and approval, 2) a partner who will take over one's life, 3) restriction of one's own life, 4) power, 5) exploitation, 6) prestige, 7) admiration, 8) achievement, 9) self-sufficiency, and 10) perfection and unassailability. Three major character defenses result to reduce anxiety and resolve these neurotic needs: self-effacement, expansiveness, and resignation.

Horney's technique of treatment used modified psychoanalysis and psychoanalytic psychotherapy. She encouraged the patient to choose the couch or the face-to-face arrangement and analyzed the choice. Sessions could occur once a week or every day. Free association was important, but not central. Transference was still appreciated but stood on equal footing with the therapeutic alliance. Countertransference was regarded as an especially important clue and not simply a sign of an unanalyzed portion of the therapist's personality. Nonspecific factors in the therapeutic alliance, such as the analyst's mere presence, consistency, optimism, acceptance, lack of judgment, and sticking to the task, became therapeutic agents.

Horney's work brought psychoanalytic principles into psychotherapy settings and anticipated some of the modern work on narcissism, narcissistic defenses, and the transference/countertransference valences evoked when working with such defenses.

SULLIVAN

Harry Stack Sullivan is an important figure, in part, because he was the first altogether homegrown major theorist to start an American school of psychodynamic psychotherapy. For him, personality was a hypothetical construct; what was real and actual were relationships. Everything therefore had to be interpreted through the lens of interpersonal relations (Sullivan 1953). For Sullivan, anxiety is a product of interpersonal threats to security, and repeated experiences interpersonally between child and parent result in the formation of a good "me self" and a bad "me self."

Personifications, the internal representations of the self or other, include affects and grow out of need-satisfying relationships and anxiety in the pursuit of need-satisfying relationships.

In Sullivan's (1953) view the mind worked on the basis of three different cognitive processes. The earliest was called the *protaxic process*, which was that of raw perception. The *parataxic process* was the next to evolve, and it followed *post hoc ergo propter hoc* logic (i.e., things following each other in time are assumed to be causally related). This was the root of animistic superstitious thinking. The third form, *syntaxic thinking*, consensually validated reality with a symbolic content following something similar to the verbal logic of Freud's secondary process.

Motivations result from tension that arises both out of physiological need and out of anxiety related to maintenance of security. This sense of security was an important feature of Sullivan's work.

Sullivan had his own theory of development. During *infancy*, there is a period of apathy and detachment as well as connection. Good and bad personifications arise, the self

representation is formed, and thinking moves from a protaxic to a parataxic level. In the second phase, called *childhood*, language develops, playmates join parents as important interpersonal figures, gender takes shape, and the inner world is one of dramatizations and preoccupations, which are rehearsals for adulthood. The third phase, the *juvenile stage*, coincides with grammar school and is the period in which the child learns to expand the interpersonal world to group reactions and an orientation to living in society. The fourth phase is *preadolescence*. This very important phase introduces the special same-sex peer or "chum" form of interpersonal relating that becomes the first genuine human relationship not governed by excessive dependency. The fifth phase is that of *early adolescence*, in which heterosexuality and interpersonal gender questions are worked out. The sixth area of development is *late adolescence*, during which time adult responsibility is introduced. Finally, the organism emerges into *adulthood* and continues the cycle by reworking these themes in new interpersonal situations.

Sullivan's emphasis on interpersonal factors balanced the primary intrapsychic focus of Freud by underscoring that a baby cannot exist conceptually or in reality in the absence of the mother. One might say that Winnicott took some of the best points of Sullivan and elaborated them within the psychoanalytic tradition. On the other hand, the interpersonal focus may be criticized for neglecting the depth of fantasy that can take place on an intrapsychic level. Nevertheless, some followers of Sullivan, such as Searles, have become part of the psychoanalytic tradition.

BEHAVIORAL AND COGNITIVE THEORIES[1]

The next set of theories, those involving behavioral and cognitive principles, have evolved out of an entirely different tradition and are based on different notions of how the mind works and even what constitutes the mind. The learning theory that underlies these points of view arises from the laboratory setting of experimental psychology, generating applications for the clinical situation. This approach is in contrast to those of psychoanalysis and dynamic psychiatry, both of which arose in the treatment setting and rely on that same setting for confirmation. Although some philosophers of science (e.g., Grunbaum

---

[1] The behavioral and cognitive therapists are being reviewed as a group, with some of the important figures being examined but a considerable amount of detail being omitted, including the subtler differences among learning theorists such as Pavlov, Hull, Mowrer and Tolman, as well as the clinical innovations and contributions of Bandura, Dollard and Miller, and Wolpe, to name but a few.

1984) take psychoanalysis seriously enough to challenge it to seek independent settings for confirmation of its theories, learning theory has always based its idea of the mind on observation of performance and behavior.

Learning is itself an inference based on the observation of changes in the behavior of an organism. Learning may be inferred from permanent or quasi-permanent changes in behavior that occur under specific circumstances. An organism is influenced by the effect of its behaviors, and its responses reflect that learning. If the organism repeats a certain behavior to attain a particular state, or if the organism stops that behavior to avoid a particular state, then learning may be said to have taken place. This is known within learning theory as *Thorndike's law of effect.*

States associated with behaviors can become reinforcers. A *positive reinforcer* is the occurrence of an event that increases the probability that the antecedent behavior will be increased. A *negative reinforcer* is the occurrence of an event that decreases the probability that the antecedent behavior will be increased. *Punishment* is a special type of negative reinforcement that is intended to stop a specific behavior. Those behaviors that need periodic positive reinforcement to be maintained may slowly disappear by means of the phenomenon of *extinction*, if the positive reinforcer is removed (see Skinner 1938, 1953). Extinction essentially means that most conditioned responses will eventually fade away if they are not periodically reinforced.

Although some theorists believe that *classical conditioning* is a special case of *operant conditioning*, these two forms are traditionally regarded as separate. In classical conditioning, a stimulus not intrinsically or ordinarily associated with a response may be used to induce that response. The organism "learns" to take the once-neutral stimulus and respond according to the conditioning. Pavlov's famous experiment illustrates this type of conditioning. A dog will salivate when presented with food, because of an *unconditioned* physiological reflex response. If a bell, which has no intrinsic power to induce salivation, is rung before the food is presented, the dog will "learn" to salivate when it hears the bell.

Operant conditioning (or *instrumental conditioning*) occurs as the organism learns that behaviors are associated with positive or negative events. Behaviors in operant conditioning are initiated by the organism, and associated events are less directly linked to immediate physiological reflexes than in classical conditioning.

Behaviors may be "shaped" by means of introducing reinforcers for successive approximations of the desired behavior. Behaviors may be initiated by the presence of other incompatible states. For example, because anxiety and relaxation cannot occur simultaneously, behavior therapists link relaxation with stimuli that formerly produced anxiety. This method of reciprocal inhibition is used to desensitize phobic patients or persons suffering from post-traumatic states. Behaviors also may be linked in complex chains, by adding steps that the organism must perform to reach desired reinforcers. A clinical example might be the treatment of a person afraid of tall buildings. Under a psychoanalytic theory, the symbolic meaning of fear of heights might be explored; it might mean fear of success, fear of besting one's father, or some such thing. In a behavioral view of the mind, the underlying symbolic reasons are either thought not to exist or are not relevant to the treatment plan. In systematic desensitization the patient might first be taught how to relax and then to apply relaxation techniques to pictures of tall buildings. When this is mastered, they might be brought to the site of such a building to practice their relaxation. Then they might go to the second floor and do their relaxation exercises. Gradually they might make it up to the highest balcony.

When responding to stimuli during conditioning, the organism is capable of responding to other stimuli that resemble the original one. Stimulus generalization would explain how the dog who responded to a bell might respond similarly to a gong or a chime. Stimulus generalization may also be seen as the explanation learning theory gives to the psychoanalytic phenomenon of the transference. The transference would be an example of stimulus generalization gone amok, with an ordinarily innocuous stimulus from the analyst being erroneously generalized to a traumatic stimulus from the parent during childhood. The response then is the one that was originally "learned" in childhood and then inappropriately enacted in the present situation. For example, under psychoanalytic theory, a patient's overreaction to a doctor's 2-minute lateness might be a transferential recreation of panic at the chronic lateness of their mother during critical phases in childhood. Under learning theory, the same reaction might be seen as a case of stimuli from one circumstance (mother late during childhood) erroneously generalized to another circumstance (doctor 2 minutes late for appointment). From the perspective of learning theory, much psychopathology may be understood as based on errors in *stimulus discrimination* and *stimulus generalization.*

Drives are seen as propelling the organism to reduce its need by means of finding appropriate responses to stimuli. *Habits* are complex clusters of stimuli and responses. In behavior therapy, psychopathology is seen as persistent habits of learned unadaptive behavior acquired in anxiety-generating situations (Wolpe 1958). The need to respond to the anxiety and to avoid its negative effect maintains psychopathological behaviors.

Thus far, stimuli and responses, and behaviors and reinforcers, have been presented by a theory in which they are linked by contiguity or association. What an organism reacts to is association, not causality. Some learning theorists (e.g., Tolman, Bandura [1974], Dollard and Miller) believe that learning is more than reaction to association by contiguity. They believe that organisms form *cognitive maps* of the environmental situation by means of internal representations in the form of thoughts, signs, and symbols. Others (e.g., Skinner and Wolpe) feel that thoughts, perceptions, and even imagination are no different from the musculoskeletal responses and obey the same laws of stimulus, response, reinforcement, and conditioning.

For the first group, learning theory represents another level on which to explain the mind, much as physics may explain chemistry, or chemistry may explain biology. For the second group, the psychoanalytic and dynamic theories of this chapter represent unacceptable *mentalism*, or the inference about the existence of the mind in the absence of hard data. Members of the first group assume that there is a mind that organizes learned data. Members of the second group hold that it is not necessary to infer anything beyond complex chains of stimulus and response.

Behavioral and cognitive theorists focus their therapeutic strategies on the pathological behaviors themselves, using a variety of techniques to help the patient unlearn maladaptive behaviors and to inhibit unwanted states such as anxiety. They introduce new learning through such techniques as shaping and modeling, creating—through careful application of positive reinforcement, negative reinforcement, and extinction—new chains of habit and adaptive behavior.

CONCLUSIONS

In this chapter we have reviewed theories of the mind and psychopathology from the major psychotherapeutic schools. For most of these perspectives, Freud and psychoanalysis constitute a kind of "basic science" from which the schools make their modifications and their "applied science." Even when there are large differences in theory and practice, most psychotherapeutic schools grew out of or in reaction to that psychoanalytic beginning.

The behavioral and cognitive theories offer one pole that conceptualizes the mind as consisting of large chains of learned responses, and another pole that looks for internal cognitive maps. This latter pole is closer to psychoanalysis. It may even be possible to translate the data of the psychoanalytic and psychodynamic schools into learning theory language.

A large group of creative thinkers who were never a part of the psychoanalytic tradition, or else who left it, constitute a psychodynamic tradition of their own. These theories, which range from the more modest to the more ambitious, constitute the major theoretical foundation of eclectic psychotherapy.

The psychoanalytic tradition, although heavily indebted to Freud, is far from static. Major shifts have taken place over the decades, with emphasis on ego psychology, object relations, development, and the self. Reading about these theories can provide a theoretical basis for understanding patients. Studying these theories can provide a lifetime of deepening understanding of the mechanism of psychotherapy and the workings of the mind in normality and psychopathology.

REFERENCES

Abraham K: Selected Papers on Psychoanalysis. Translated by Bryan D, Strachey A. New York, Basic Books, 1968

Adler A: The Individual Psychology of Alfred Adler: A Systematic Presentation in Selections From His Writings. Edited by Ansbacher HL, Ansbacher RR. New York, Basic Books, 1956

American Psychiatric Association: Diagnostic and Statistical Manual of Mental Disorders, 3rd Edition. Washington, DC, American Psychiatric Association Press, 1980

Balint M: The Basic Fault. London, Tavistock, 1968

Bandura A: Behavior theory and the models of man. Am Psychol 29:859–869, 1974

Bibring GL, Dwyer TF, Huntington DS, et al: A study of the psychological processes in pregnancy and of the earliest mother-child relationship. Psychoanal Study Child 16:9–72, 1961

Bowlby J: The nature of the child's tie to his mother. Int J Psychoanal 39:350–373, 1958

Brenner C: An Elementary Textbook of Psychoanalysis. New York, International Universities Press, 1955

Breuer J, Freud S: Studies on hysteria (1893–1895), in Standard Edition of the Complete Psychological Works of Sigmund Freud, Vol 2. Translated and edited by Strachey J. London, Hogarth, 1955, pp 1–319

Briquet P: Traite de l'Hysterie. Paris, J Bailliere, 1859

Carotenuto A: A Secret Symmetry. New York, Pantheon, 1982

Davis PJ: Repression and the inaccessibility of emotional memories, in Repression and Dissociation: Implications for Personality Theory, Psychopathology, and Health. Edited by Singer JL. Chicago, IL, University of Chicago Press, 1990, pp 387–403

Edelson M: Defense in psychoanalytic theory: computation or fantasy? in Repression and Dissociation: Implications for Personality Theory, Psychopathology, and Health. Edited by Singer JL. Chicago, IL, University of Chicago Press, 1990, pp 33–60

Ellenberger H: The Discovery of the Unconscious: The History and Evolution of Dynamic Psychiatry. New York, Basic Books, 1970

Erdleyi MH: Repression, reconstruction, and defense: history and integration of the psychoanalytic and experimental frameworks, in Repression and Dissociation: Implications for Personality Theory, Psychopathology, and Health. Edited by Singer JL. Chicago, IL, University of Chicago Press, 1990, pp 1–31

Erikson E: Childhood and Society, 2nd Edition, Revised and Enlarged. New York, WW Norton, 1963

Fairbairn WRD: Psychoanalytic Studies of the Personality. London, Routledge and Kegan Paul, 1972

Fenichel O: The Psychoanlaytic Theory of Neurosis. New York, WW Norton, 1945

Ferenczi S, Rank O: The Development of Psycho-Analysis. New York, Dover, 1956

Fine S, Fine E: Four psychoanalytic perspectives: a study of differences in interpretive interventions. J Am Psychoanal Assoc 38:1017–1048, 1990

Fish-Murray CC, Koby EV, van der Kolk BA: Evolving ideas: the effect of abuse on children's thought, in Psychological Trauma. Edited by van der Kolk BA. Washington, DC, American Psychiatric Press, 1987, pp 89–110

Fleck L: Genesis and Development of a Scientific Fact. Chicago, IL, University of Chicago Press, 1979

Freud A: The Ego and the Mechanisms of Defence (1936). Translated by Baines C. New York, International Universities Press, 1946

Freud S: On Aphasia (1891). Translated by Stengel E. New York, International Universities Press, 1953

Freud S: The neuro-psychoses of defence (1894), in Standard Edition of the Complete Psychological Works of Sigmund Freud, Vol 3. Translated and edited by Strachey J. London, Hogarth, 1962, pp 41–68

Freud S: Further remarks on the neuro-psychoses of defence (1896), in Standard Edition of the Complete Psychological Works of Sigmund Freud, Vol 3. Translated and edited by Strachey J. London, Hogarth, 1962, pp 157–185

Freud S: The interpretation of dreams (1900), in Standard Edition of the Complete Psychological Works of Sigmund Freud, Vol 4. Translated and edited by Strachey J. London, Hogarth, 1953

Freud S: The psychopathology of everyday life (1901), in Standard Edition of the Complete Psychological Works of Sigmund Freud, Vol 6. Translated and edited by Strachey J. London, Hogarth, 1960

Freud S: Fragment of an analysis of a case of hysteria (1905[1901]), in Standard Edition of the Complete Psychological Works of Sigmund Freud, Vol 7. Translated and edited by Strachey J. London, Hogarth, 1953, pp 1–122

Freud S: Three essays on the theory of sexuality, I: the sexual aberrations (1905), in Standard Edition of the Complete Psychological Works of Sigmund Freud, Vol 7. Translated and edited by Strachey J. London, Hogarth, 1953, pp 135–172

Freud S: The sexual enlightenment of children (1907), in Standard Edition of the Complete Psychological Works of Sigmund Freud, Vol 9. Translated and edited by Strachey J. London, Hogarth, 1959, pp 129–139

Freud S: On the sexual theories of children (1908), in Standard Edition of the Complete Psychological Works of Sigmund Freud, Vol 9. Translated and edited by Strachey J. London, Hogarth, 1959, pp 5–226

Freud S: Analysis of a phobia in a five-year-old boy (1909a), in Standard Edition of the Complete Psychological Works of Sigmund Freud, Vol 10. Translated and edited by Strachey J. London, Hogarth, 1955, pp 1–149

Freud S: Notes upon a case of obsessional neurosis (1909b), in Standard Edition of the Complete Psychological Works of Sigmund Freud, Vol 10. Translated and edited by Strachey J. London, Hogarth, 1955, pp 151–318

Freud S: Psycho-analytic notes on an autobiographical account of a case of paranoia (dementia paranoides) (1911), in Standard Edition of the Complete Psychological Works of Sigmund Freud, Vol 12. Translated and edited by Strachey J. London, Hogarth, 1958, pp 1–82

Freud S: Recommendations to physicians practising psycho-analysis (1912), in Standard Edition of the Complete Psychological Works of Sigmund Freud, Vol 12. Translated and edited by Strachey J. London, Hogarth, 1958, pp 109–120

Freud S: On beginning the treatment (further recommendations on the technique of psycho-analysis I) (1913), in Standard Edition of the Complete Psychological Works of Sigmund Freud, Vol 12. Translated and edited by Strachey J. London, Hogarth, 1958, pp 121–144

Freud S: On narcissism: an introduction (1914a), in Standard Edition of the Complete Psychological Works of Sigmund Freud, Vol 14. Translated and edited by Strachey J. London, Hogarth, 1957, pp 67–102

Freud S: Remembering, repeating and working-through (further recommendations on the technique of psycho-analysis II) (1914b), in Standard Edition of the Complete Psychological Works of Sigmund Freud, Vol 12. Translated and edited by Strachey J. London, Hogarth, 1958, pp 145–156

Freud S: Instincts and their vicissitudes (1915a), in Standard Edition of the Complete Psychological Works of Sigmund Freud, Vol 14. Translated and edited by Strachey J. London, Hogarth, 1957, pp 109–140

Freud S: Repression (1915b), in Standard Edition of the Complete Psychological Works of Sigmund Freud, Vol 14. Translated and edited by Strachey J. London, Hogarth, 1957, pp 141–158

Freud S: The unconscious (1915c), in Standard Edition of the Complete Psychological Works of Sigmund Freud, Vol 14. Translated and edited by Strachey J. London, Hogarth, 1957, pp 159–215

Freud S: Mourning and melancholia (1917[1915]), in Standard Edition of the Complete Psychological Works of Sigmund Freud, Vol 14. Translated and edited by Strachey J. London, Hogarth, 1957, pp 237–260

Freud S: Beyond the pleasure principle (1920), in Standard Edition of the Complete Psychological Works of Sigmund Freud, Vol 18. Translated and edited by Strachey J. London, Hogarth, 1955, pp 1–64

Freud S: Group psychology and the analysis of the ego (1921), in Standard Edition of the Complete Psychological Works of Sigmund Freud, Vol 18. Translated and edited by Strachey J. London, Hogarth, 1955, pp 65–143

Freud S: Some neurotic mechanisms in jealousy, paranoia and homosexuality (1922), in Standard Edition of the Complete Psychological Works of Sigmund Freud, Vol 18. Translated and edited by Strachey J. London, Hogarth, 1955, pp 221–232

Freud S: Neurosis and psychosis (1924[1923]), in Standard Edition of the Complete Psychological Works of Sigmund Freud, Vol 19. Translated and edited by Strachey J. London, Hogarth, 1961, pp 147–153

Freud S: The economic problem of masochism (1924a), in Standard Edition of the Complete Psychological Works of Sigmund Freud, Vol 19. Translated and edited by Strachey J. London, Hogarth, 1961, pp 155–170

Freud S: The loss of reality in neurosis and psychosis (1924b), in Standard Edition of the Complete Psychological Works of Sigmund Freud, Vol 19. Translated and edited by Strachey J. London, Hogarth, 1961, pp 181–187

Freud S: Some psychical consequences of the anatomical distinction between the sexes (1925), in Standard Edition of the Complete Psychological Works of Sigmund Freud, Vol 19. Translated and edited by Strachey J. London, Hogarth, 1961, pp 241–258

Freud S: An autobiographical study (1925[1924]), in Standard Edition of the Complete Psychological Works of Sigmund Freud, Vol 20. Translated and edited by Strachey J. London, Hogarth, 1959, pp 1–74

Freud S: Inhibitions, symptoms and anxiety (1926), in Standard Edition of the Complete Psychological Works of Sigmund Freud, Vol 20. Translated and edited by Strachey J. London, Hogarth, 1959, pp 75–175

Freud S: New introductory lectures on psycho-analysis (1933[1932]) (Lectures XXIX–XXXV), in Standard Edition of the Complete Psychological Works of Sigmund Freud, Vol 22. Translated and edited by Strachey J. London, Hogarth, 1964, pp 1–182

Freud S: Analysis terminable and interminable (1937), in Standard Edition of the Complete Psychological Works of Sigmund Freud, Vol 23. Translated and edited by Strachey J. London, Hogarth, 1964, pp 209–253

Freud S: An outline of psycho-analysis (1940a[1938]), in Standard Edition of the Complete Psychological Works of Sigmund Freud, Vol 23. Translated and edited by Strachey J. London, Hogarth, 1964, pp 139–207

Freud S: Splitting of the ego in the process of defence (1940b[1938]), in Standard Edition of the Complete Psychological Works of Sigmund Freud, Vol 23. Translated and edited by Strachey J. London, Hogarth, 1964, pp 271–278

Freud S: Project for a scientific psychology (1950[1895]), in Standard Edition of the Complete Psychological Works of Sigmund Freud, Vol 1. Translated and edited by Strachey J. London, Hogarth, 1966, pp 281–397

Gill MM: The analysis of the transference. J Am Psychoanal Assoc 27 (suppl):263–288, 1979

Goodwin J: Post-traumatic symptoms in incest victims, in Post-traumatic Stress Disorder in Children. Edited by Eth S, Pynoos RS. Washington, DC, American Psychiatric Press, 1985, pp 155–168

Greenberg JR, Mitchell SA: Object Relations in Psychoanalytic Theory. Cambridge, MA, Harvard University Press, 1983

Greenson RR: The Technique and Practice of Psychoanalysis, Vol 1. New York, International Universities Press, 1967

Grunbaum A: The Foundations of Psychoanalysis. Berkeley, CA, University of California Press, 1984

Gunderson JG, Carpenter WT, Strauss JS: Borderline and Schizophrenic Patients: A Comparative Study. Am J Psyciatry 132:1257–1264, 1975

Gunderson JG, Kolb J: Discriminating Features of Borderline Patients. Am J Psychiatry 135:792–796, 1976

Gunderson JG: Borderline Personality Disorder. Washington, DC, American Psychiatric Press, 1984

Guntrip H: Personality Structure and Human Interaction. New York, International Universities Press, 1974

Herman JL: Trauma and Recovery. New York, Basic Books, 1992

Horney K: The Neurotic Personality of Our Time. New York, WW Norton, 1937

Horney K: Neurosis and Human Growth: The Struggle Toward Self-Realization. New York, WW Norton, 1950

Horowitz MJ (ed): Person Schemas and Maladaptive Interpersonal Patterns. Chicago, IL, University of Chicago Press, 1991

Jones E: The Life and Work of Sigmund Freud, Vol 1. New York, Basic Books, 1953

Jones E: The Life and Work of Sigmund Freud, Vol 2. New York, Basic Books, 1955

Jones E: The Life and Work of Sigmund Freud, Vol 3. New York, Basic Books, 1957

Jung CG: Memories, Dreams, Reflections. New York, Vintage, 1961

Jung CG: Man and His Symbols. New York, Dell, 1964

Jung CG: Zur gegenwartigen Lage der Psychotherapie (1934), qtd in Selesnick S: Psychoanalytic Pioneers. Edited by Alexander F, Eisenstein S, Grotjahn M. New York, Basic Books, 1966a, pp 63–77

Jung CG: Two Essays on Analytical Psychology. Princeton, NJ, Princeton University Press, 1966b

Kaufmann, W: Discovering The Mind, Vol 3. New York, McGraw-Hill, 1980, pp 279–280

Kernberg O: Borderline Conditions and Pathological Narcissism. New York, Jason Aronson, 1975

Kernberg O: Object-Relations Theory and Clinical Psychoanalysis. New York, Jason Aronson, 1976

Kihlstrom JF, Hoyt IP: Repression, dissociation and hypnosis, in Repression and Dissociation: Implications for Personality Theory, Psychopathology, and Health. Edited by Singer JL. Chicago, IL, University of Chicago Press, 1990, pp 181–208

Klein M, Heimann P, Isaacs S, et al: Developments in Psycho-Analysis. London, Hogarth/Institute of Psycho-Analysis, 1973

Kluft RP (ed): Childhood Antecedents of Multiple Personality. Washington, DC, American Psychiatric Press, 1985

Kluft RP: Introduction, in Incest-Related Syndromes of Adult Psychopathology. Edited by Kluft RP. Washington, DC, American Psychiatric Press, 1990, pp 1–10

Kohut H: The Analysis of the Self: A Systematic Approach to the Psychoanalytic Treatment of Narcissistic Personality Disorders. New York, International Universities Press, 1971

Kohut H: The Restoration of the Self. New York, International Universities Press, 1977

Kohut H: How Does Analysis Cure? Chicago, IL, University of Chicago Press, 1984

Kuhn TS: The Structure of Scientific Revolutions, 2nd Edition. Chicago, IL, University of Chicago Press, 1970

Laplanche J, Pontalis J-B: The Language of Psycho-Analysis. Translated by Nicholson-Smith D. New York, WW Norton, 1973

Loewenstein RJ: Somatoform disorders in victims of incest and child abuse, in Incest-Related Syndromes of Adult Psychopathology. Edited by Kluft RP. Washington, DC, American Psychiatric Press, 1990, pp 75–107

Loftus E, Ketcham K: The Myth of Repressed Memory: False Memories and Allegations of Sexual Abuse. New York, St. Martins Press, 1994

Mahler MS, Pine F, Bergman A: The Psychological Birth of the Human Infant: Symbiosis and Individuation. New York, Basic Books, 1975

Marmer SS: Psychoanalysis of multiple personality. Int J Psychoanal 61:439–459, 1980

Marmer SS, Fink D: Multiple personality disorder: a psychoanalytic perspective. Psychiatr Clin North Am 14:677–693, 1991

Marmer SS: Rethinking the Comparison of Borderline Personality Disorder and Multiple Personality Disorder. Psychitr Clin North Am 17:743–771, 1994

Masson J: The Assault on the Truth. New York, Farrar, Straus, & Giroux, 1984

Masterson JF: The Narcissistic and Borderline Disorders: An Integrated and Developmental Approach. New York, Brunner/Mazel, 1981

McDougall J: Theaters of the Mind: Illusion and Truth on the Psychoanalytic Stage. New York, Brunner/Mazel, 1982

Miller A: Thou Shalt Not Be Aware: Society's Betrayal of the Child. Translated by Hannum H, Hannum H. New York, Meridian, 1984

Miller A: For Your Own Good: Hidden Cruelty in Child-Rearing and the Roots of Violence. Translated by Hannum H, Hannum H. New York, Noonday Press, 1990

Niedlerland WG: The Schreber Case: Psychoanalytic Profile of a Paranoid Personality. New York, Quadrangle/New York Times Book Co, 1974

Popper KR: The Logic of Scientific Discovery. New York, Science Editions, 1959

Popper KR: Conjectures and Refutations: The Growth of Scientific Knowledge. New York, Basic Books, 1962

Putnam FW Jr: Dissociation as a response to extreme trauma, in Childhood Antecedents of Multiple Personality. Edited by Kluft RP. Washington, DC, American Psychiatric Press, 1985, pp 65–97

Putnam FW Jr: Diagnosis and Treatment of Multiple Personality Disorder. New York, Guilford, 1989

Putnam FW Jr: Disturbances of "self" in victims of childhood sexual abuse, in Incest-Related Syndromes of Adult Psychopathology. Edited by Kluft RP. Washington, DC, American Psychiatric Press, 1990, pp 113–131

Rank O: The Trauma of Birth. New York, Harper & Row, 1973

Reich W: Character Analysis, 3rd Edition. New York, Farrar, Straus and Giroux, 1972

Ricoeur P: Freud and Philosophy. New Haven, CT, Yale University Press, 1970

Rinsley DB: Treatment of the Severely Disturbed Adolescent. New York, Jason Aronson, 1980

Schafer R: The mechanisms of defence. Int J Psychoanal 49:49–62, 1968

Schafer R: The idea of resistance. Int J Psychoanal 54:259–285, 1973

Schreiber FR: Sybil. Chicago, IL, Henry Regnery Co, 1973

Segal H: Introduction to the Work of Melanie Klein. London, Hogarth/Institute of Psycho-Analysis, 1973

Shengold L: Soul Murder: The Effects of Childoood Abuse and Deprivation. New York, Fawcett Columbine, 1989

Skinner BF: The Behavior of Organisms. New York, Appleton-Century-Crofts, 1938

Skinner BF: Science and Human Behavior. New York, Macmillan, 1953

Spiegel D: Hypnosis, dissociation, and trauma: hidden and overt observers, in Repression and Dissociation: Implications for Personality Theory, Psychopathology, and Health. Edited by Singer JL. Chicago, IL, University of Chicago Press, 1990a, pp 121–142

Spiegel D: Trauma, dissociation, and hypnosis, in Incest-Related Syndromes of Adult Psychopathology. Edited by Kluft RP. Washington, DC, American Psychiatric Press, 1990b, pp 247–261

Spitz RA: The First Year of Life: A Psychoanalytic Study of Normal and Deviant Development of Object Relations. New York, International Universities Press, 1965

Stern D: The Interpersonal World of the Infant. New York, Basic Books, 1985

Stolorow R, Brandschaft B: Developmental failure and psychic conflict. Psychoanaltic Psychology 4:241–253, 1987

Stolorow R, Lachmann R: The Psychoanalysis of Developmental Arrests. New York, International Universities Press, 1980

Sullivan HS: The Interpersonal Theory of Psychiatry. Edited by Perry HS, Gawel ML. New York, WW Norton, 1953

Sutherland JD: The British object relations theorists: Balint, Winnicott, Fairbairn, Guntrip. J Am Psychoanal Assoc 28:829–860, 1980

Terr L: Too Scared to Cry: Psychic Trauma in Childhood. New York, Harper & Row, 1990

Vaillant GE: Adaptation to Life. Boston, MA, Little, Brown, 1977

van der Kolk BA: The psychological consequences of overwhelming life experiences, in Psychological Trauma. Edited by van der Kolk BA. Washington, DC, American Psychiatric Press, 1987, pp 1–30

Waelder R: The principle of multiple function: observations on over-determination. Psychoanal Q 5:45–62, 1936

Wallerstein R: Defense, defense mechanisms, and the structure of the mind. J Am Psychoanal Assoc 31 (suppl):201–225, 1983

West LJ: Dissociative reaction, in Comprehensive Textbook of Psychiatry. Edited by Freedman AM, Kaplan HI. Baltimore, MD, Williams & Wilkins, 1967, pp 885–899

Wilbur CB: The effect of child abuse on the psyche, in Childhood Antecedents of Multiple Personality. Edited by Kluft RP. Washington, DC, American Psychiatric Press, 1985, pp 21–35

Williams LM: Recovered Memories of Abuse in Women with Documented Child Sexual Victimization Histories. J Trauma Stress Vol 8:649–673, 1995

Winnicott DW: Transitional objects and transitional phenomena. Int J Psychoanal 34:89–97, 1953

Winnicott DW: The Maturational Processes and the Facilitating Environment. London, Hogarth/Institute of Psycho-Analysis, 1965

Winnicott DW: The location of cultural experience. Int J Psychoanal 48:368–372, 1966

Winnicott DW: Human Nature. New York, Schocken Books, 1988

Wollheim R: Sigmund Freud. New York, Viking, 1971

Wolpe J: Psychotherapy by Reciprocal Inhibition. Palo Alto, CA, Stanford University Press, 1958

SUGGESTED READINGS

Dollard J, Miller NE: Personality and Psychotherapy. New York, McGraw Hill, 1950 [Presents learning theory in a way that can be integrated with a psychodynamic approach.]

Freud S: Analysis of a phobia in a five-year-old boy (1909a), in Standard Edition of the Complete Psychological Works of Sigmund Freud, Vol 10. Translated and edited by Strachey J. London, Hogarth, 1955, pp 1–149

Freud S: Notes upon a case of obsessional neurosis (1909b), in Standard Edition of the Complete Psychological Works of Sigmund Freud, Vol 10. Translated and edited by Strachey J. London, Hogarth, 1955, pp 151–318

Freud S: The ego and the id (1923), in Standard Edition of the Complete Psychological Works of Sigmund Freud, Vol 19. Translated and edited by Strachey J. London, Hogarth, 1961, pp 1–66 [Demonstrates the applicability of learning theory to psychotherapy.]

Freud S: Inhibitions, symptoms and anxiety (1926), in Standard Edition of the Complete Psychological Works of Sigmund Freud, Vol 20. Translated and edited by Strachey J. London, Hogarth, 1959, pp 75–175 [These four papers by Freud demonstrate the breadth of his work. "Analysis of a Phobia in a Five-Year-Old Boy" (known as "Little Hans") and "Notes Upon a Case of Obessional Neurosis" (known as "The Rat Man") show Freud's clinical acumen. In The Ego and the Id, Freud clearly explains the structural model. Inhibitions, Symptoms and Anxiety, one of Freud's most important and interesting papers, exposes his thinking process at work.]

Greenberg JR, Mitchell SA: Object Relations in Psychoanalytic Theory. Cambridge, MA, Harvard University Press, 1983 [Presents the evolution of this line in psychoanalysis.]

Greenson RR: The Technique and Practice of Psychoanalysis, Vol 1. New York, International Universities Press, 1967 [A readable introduction to technique.]

Herman J: Trauma and Recovery. New York, Basic Books, 1992 [Despite its rather forceful rhetorical tone, the book offers an excellent presentation of the rediscovery of trauma in psychopathology.]

Jung CG: Man and His Symbols. New York, Dell, 1964 [Presents the Jungian viewpoint well.]

Kernberg O: Object-Relations Theory and Clinical Psychoanalysis. New York, Jason Aronson, 1976 [Dense and difficult reading, but presents the modern integration of drives, object relations, development, and psychopathology with great depth in all its complexity.]

Kohut H: The Restoration of the Self. New York, International Universities Press, 1977 [This important volume launched self psychology as a separate school within psychoanalysis.]

Mahler MS, Pine F, Bergman A: The Psychological Birth of the Human Infant: Symbiosis and Individuation. New York, Basic Books, 1975 [This work presents the modern view of development.]

Malcolm J: Psychoanalysis, the Impossible Profession. New York, Alfred A Knopf, 1981 [An outstanding exposition of the discovery of transference, and of the tension between more and less abstinent therapeutic technique.]

Strachey J: The nature of the therapeutic action of psychoanalysis (1934). Int J Psychoanal 50:275–292, 1969 [Discussion of how analysis works.]

Sullivan HS: The Interpersonal Theory of Psychiatry. Edited by Perry HS, Gawel ML. New York, WW Norton, 1953 [Sets forth the psychodynamic interpersonal view.]

ASSESSMENT

CHAPTER 6

THE PSYCHIATRIC INTERVIEW, PSYCHIATRIC HISTORY, AND MENTAL STATUS EXAMINATION

STEPHEN C. SCHEIBER, M.D.

The medical care health delivery system is changing in a revolutionary fashion. Rapid advances are being made in the understanding of the etiologies of mental disorders. The diagnosis of psychiatric disorders has been undergoing dramatic changes as a reflection of a better understanding of these disorders. Time allotted for diagnostic evaluations and for psychiatric treatments has been shortened. With all these changes, the psychiatric interview has remained the essential vehicle for the assessment of the psychiatric patient. The psychiatrist is the medical specialist in psychiatric diagnosis, psychiatric treatment, and understanding interpersonal relationships. The patient reveals what is troubling him or her in the context of a confidential doctor-patient relationship. The psychiatrist listens and responds, attempting to obtain as clear an understanding as possible of the patient's problems in the context of the patient's culture and environment. The psychiatrist encourages a free-flowing exchange with the patient, then, at the conclusion of the interview, arrives at a diagnostic formulation of the patient's problems. The more accu-rate the diagnostic assessment, the more appropriate the treatment planning (Halleck 1991).

The *psychiatric history* includes information about the patient as a person, the chief complaint, the present illness, premorbid adjustment, past history, history of medical illnesses, family history of psychiatric and medical disorders, and a developmental history of the patient. The psychiatrist obtains as much history as needed to arrive at a differential diagnosis. With subsequent interviews, the psychiatrist refines his or her working diagnosis and examines the influences of biological, psychological, cultural, familial, and social factors on the patient's life. During the course of a psychiatric history, the psychiatrist evaluates the patient's perceptions of himself or herself and his or her experiences, the patient's perspectives on his or her problems, the goals of treatment, and the desired treatment relationship.

The *mental status examination* is a cross-sectional summary of the patient's behavior, sensorium, and cognitive functioning. Information pertaining to the mental status of the patient is obtained informally during a psychiatric interview as well as through formal testing. Informal information is based on the psychiatrist's observations of the patient and his or her listening to what the patient says. Categories of such information include appearance and behavior, eye contact, mode of relating, mood, affect, quality and quantity of speech, thought content, thought processes, and use of vocabulary.

Formal testing considers orientation, attention and concentration, recent and remote memory, fund of information, vocabulary, abilities to abstract, judgment and insight, and perception and coordination. The need for and specificity of formal testing are based on information and clues derived from the psychiatric interview (Othmer and Othmer 1994).

THE PSYCHIATRIC INTERVIEW

PSYCHIATRIC DIAGNOSIS

The single most important method of arriving at an understanding of the patient who exhibits the signs and symptoms of a psychiatric disorder is by the psychiatric interview. Although having many features in common with a medical interview, the psychiatric interview has significant elaborations and departures from the medical interview. In addition to the descriptive features of psychiatric diagnoses, which are detailed in the fourth edition of DSM-IV (American Psychiatric Association 1994; see Chapter 7), the psychiatric interview serves as an entrée into a multidimensional understanding of the patient as a person.

The psychiatric interview is used to understand the following:

- The patient's psychological makeup
- How the patient relates to his or her environment
- The significant social, religious, and cultural influences on the patient's life
- The conscious and unconscious motivations for the patient's behavior
- The patient's ego strengths and weaknesses
- The coping strategies used by the patient
- The defense mechanisms that are predominant and under what conditions
- The available support systems and networks for the patient
- The patient's points of vulnerability
- The patient's areas of aptitude and achievement

The psychiatric interview is a creative act and is a study of movement and change (Fenichel 1984; Hartmann 1964; Havens 1984; Shea 1988). Common features of both the psychiatric interview and the medical interview include identifying data regarding the patient, the chief complaint, the history of the present illness, significant past history, social history, and family history.

Distinctive features of the psychiatric interview include examining feelings about significant events in the individual's life, identifying significant persons and their relationship to the patient in the course of his or her life, and identifying and tracing the major influences on the biological, social, and psychological development of the individual. The interviewer gathers cross-sectional data related to the signs and symptoms of primary psychiatric disorders, such as anxiety disorders, mood disorders, schizophrenic disorders, substance-related disorders and cognitive disorders—that is, those categorized under Axis I of the five axes of DSM-IV. The interviewer simultaneously examines for lifetime patterns of the individual's adaptation and relation to the environment in the form of character traits and, at times, character disorders that are described formally under Axis II of DSM-IV.

In the course of a thorough medical/psychiatric examination, the clinician elicits historical information, including genetic and family predispositions that may influence the type of problems the patient presents, and completes a physical examination with appropriate laboratory and roentgenographic examinations to ascertain the patient's medical problems, listed under Axis III of DSM-IV. This part of the examination aids the psychiatrist in assessing the influence of medical disorders on behavior, mood, and cognition. Axes IV and V are used to supplement the psychiatric diagnoses; they estimate, respectively, the severity of psychosocial stressors and the highest level of adaptive functioning currently and in the past year. These axes have potential value in planning treatment and assessing the prognosis of the patient's condition.

The psychiatrist in the course of the interview assesses whether the patient exhibits psychotic thinking and/or behavior and whether the patient is harboring suicidal or homicidal thoughts or plans. The patient's capacity to control impulses is also assessed. If in the course of an interview it is determined by the psychiatrist that a patient may be a danger to himself or herself or to others by virtue of a major mental disorder, the psychiatrist is obligated to consider psychiatric hospitalization to protect the patient and/or society. Some states mandate that a psychiatrist notify potential victims of threatened harm revealed during the course of an interview (Halleck 1991).

The psychiatric interview—in addition to eliciting information for the analysis of cross-sectional data to arrive at a formal diagnosis and to obtain information regarding the past growth and development of the individual—is also a potentially healing event in which a patient, a suffering individual with psychiatric signs and symptoms, gains relief from his or her symptoms by revealing himself or herself in the context of a trusting, nonjudgmental relationship with his or her psychiatrist. A variety of mechanisms may be used, including support, insight, and self-disclosure. Key elements in promoting therapeutic aspects of an interview are an openness to sharing information and the ability to listen empathetically within the context of a confidential doctor-patient relationship (Bird 1973; Shea 1988).

During the course of a diagnostic interview, the psychiatrist assesses which of several modalities of therapy could benefit the patient. This assessment is then periodically reviewed and updated. The psychiatrist brings to the interview an in-depth knowledge of normal and abnormal behavior and has a command of psychodynamic principles, using them as a theoretical framework to understand the complexities of the patient's unique personality patterns, major psychological conflicts, use of defense mechanisms, biological assets and deficits, and modes of adapting. The psychiatrist assesses the influences of genetic factors and organic processes on the patient's behavior, thinking, and feeling states. Psychopathology is evaluated as a product of the patient's entire being in the context of biological, social, economic, and cultural, as well as emotional, influences.

Psychiatric interviewing is an art that is learned over time, with practice under the tutelage of supervisors skilled and experienced in teaching the psychiatric interview. A careful, methodical review of interviewing style, technique, and process by a mentor or a peer augments the psychiatric resident/interviewer's learning. Audiovisual aids may also be used to facilitate the process of learning interviewing skills. In addition, educational guidelines, outlines, or manuals of principles and techniques help the resident. Among the topics discussed in training are general considerations about the interview, the physician/patient relationship, and specific interviewing techniques, all discussed below.

GENERAL CONSIDERATIONS

Initiation

The initial contact for psychiatric appointments is usually by telephone. Those receiving such calls must be attuned to recognizing psychiatric emergencies as well as be sensitive to issues of patient confidentiality. As much pertinent information as possible is obtained during the call. This includes the reason for the call, the location of the patient, how the caller can be reached by the psychiatrist, and the

urgency of the problem. When the recipient of the call assesses that a psychiatric emergency exists, the call should be transferred immediately to the psychiatrist, if he or she is available. If the psychiatrist is not available, the patient should be referred to an emergency psychiatric facility and the emergency room notified of the patient referral, with as much background information as was gleaned from the caller.

Most calls are not emergencies. The psychiatrist, when returning a call, allows sufficient time to determine the following:

- What are the circumstances that led to the patient's calling?
- What are the presenting complaints?
- Who referred the patient?
- Is (or was) the patient in treatment with another psychiatrist?
- What does the patient hope to gain by seeing a psychiatrist?
- Does the identified problem require the expertise of a psychiatrist?
- Does the caller need to be referred elsewhere?

The psychiatrist elicits enough information to determine whether the patient is in need of an immediate assessment and examination for a psychiatric hospitalization. If the psychiatrist judges that the patient may need hospitalization, the psychiatrist tells the patient to go to the emergency room. The psychiatrist then either goes to the emergency room or arranges for someone at the emergency room to evaluate (not admit) the caller.

If the patient is referred by his or her physician, the psychiatrist inquires about any current medical problems and about medications that the patient is taking. The psychiatrist requests permission to speak to the patient's physician to discuss reasons for the referral and to ascertain whether the physician is requesting consultation so as to better deal with a particular psychiatric problem (e.g., adjustment of dosage of antidepressant medication, compliance problems between the physician and his or her patient, level of depression of the patient) or whether the physician is requesting a thorough psychiatric evaluation and ultimate treatment by the psychiatrist.

Coordinating care with a referring physician is important, particularly when there are overlapping medical/psychiatric problems and when medications are prescribed. This coordination is critical in working with primary care physicians. When the patient is referred for a single visit or a limited number of visits, psychiatrists must determine whether it is reasonable to respond to the requests of the referring physician within the time limits that have been predetermined, often by third-party payers. Complicated problems typically require extended evaluations. Many medications will alter the mental status of the patient (e.g., antianxiety agents, antihypertensive agents, anticholinergic drugs). Psychotropic medications can influence medical conditions (e.g., lithium and renal disease). The patient's physician is also an excellent resource for obtaining objective information. The psychiatrist should welcome as much data as the primary physician can offer regarding the patient's history and mental status. The psychiatrist assures the primary care physician that the patient will be referred back to the physician on conclusion of the evaluation. If the patient agrees to psychiatric treatment, the primary care physician is informed. On conclusion of the evaluation, the psychiatrist sends the referring physician a summary of his or her clinical findings, conclusions, and recommendations.

In initial contacts with a patient, the psychiatrist should ascertain whether the patient's presenting problems are appropriate for the psychiatrist's field of expertise. A patient may call inquiring whether the psychiatrist uses a specific therapeutic method to treat a specific complaint, such as nicotine patches for smoking addictions, hypnosis for memory lapses, or health food store natural herbs or vitamins as substitutes for prescribed medications for depression. If responding "No" to the specific inquiry, the psychiatrist inquires whether he or she may be of help in some other way. If the patient requests a particular treatment and the psychiatrist does not have experience with or believe in the efficacy of that treatment, he or she offers to refer the patient to a colleague with specific expertise. Consumer-minded patients may request an interview with several psychiatrists to assess which one they believe will be most helpful to them.

Initial telephone contacts set the stage for subsequent psychiatric interviews. The psychiatrist exhibits the capacity to be an expert listener who will work to understand the patient and his or her problem. Rapport with a patient begins with the initial contact. In addition to listening to the patient's problems, the psychiatrist advises the patient about what to expect when coming for an interview. The patient is told the minimum amount of time that the psychiatrist expects will be needed to do a complete assessment, how much time will be allowed per visit, over what period of time the assessment will be conducted, what the hourly cost will be, the charge for missed appointments, and whether the psychiatrist anticipates being available to treat the patient when the assessment is completed. The psychiatrist inquires about when the patient would be available to come for an evaluation and sets up a time that

is mutually agreeable (Table 6–1).

Requests for appointments with a psychiatrist are also initiated by third parties, who can include relatives, treating physicians, judges, lawyers, staff of employee health services or student health services, staff of disability evaluation organizations, and others. In every instance, it is essential for the psychiatrist to learn what the patient has been told about requests for a psychiatric consultation or evaluation and to find out what the patient expects from seeing a psychiatrist. The purpose of the examination should be explicit. If the purpose is to advise an employer about the patient's psychiatric fitness to continue employment, the psychiatrist advises the employer to inform the patient that this is the purpose and to make sure the patient knows that the psychiatrist's conclusions will be shared with the employer.

If a relative is calling, it is important not only to ascertain what the patient knows of the call but to find out the reasons why the patient is not calling directly. The psychiatrist does everything possible to dissuade a family member from using deception in getting the patient to agree to an appointment. An example of deception would be a parent advising a youngster that he is going for a doctor's appointment to have a thorough examination without mentioning that it is a psychiatric examination (Leventhal and Conroy 1991) or a grown child bringing an elderly parent to a psychiatrist after telling the parent that she is going to have her back pain checked out by a doctor.

Third-party callers should also be advised of what information they can expect following a psychiatric examination. In most instances, no information will be shared with-

TABLE 6–1. Initial steps of the psychiatric interview

Background information

Reason for call

Location of patient

How caller can be reached

Presenting complaints

Referral source's name and telephone number

Treatment history

Concurrent medical conditions

What patient hopes to gain

Determination of urgency

Primary physician's name and phone number

Expectations

Time for assessment

Cost of evaluation

Purpose of assessment

Psychiatrist's availability for treatment

out the patient's consent. In the case of a minor, the information may be shared with the parent. If the purpose of an examination is to collect information as an expert witness in a court of law, the patient is advised at the onset of the interview that everything he or she says may be used as part of the psychiatrist's expert testimony in court. In this instance, the usual doctor-patient confidentiality is not in force.

Time

The amount of time set aside for an initial psychiatric outpatient evaluation varies, ranging from 45 minutes for some evaluations to 90 minutes for others. If the evaluation is conducted at the bedside on a medical service, the length of the interview is often shorter because of the patient's medical condition, and more frequent, brief visits may be necessary. In emergency room settings, the evaluation may be prolonged, particularly if hospitalization is in question and supporting data are needed from resources not immediately available, such as from relatives and treating physicians who have to be reached by telephone. If a patient is exhibiting psychotic behaviors during an outpatient appointment, the interview may be abbreviated if, in the judgment of the psychiatrist, prolonging the interview will aggravate the patient's condition. When possible, the psychiatrist should have some flexibility in his or her schedule at the time of an initial interview. In most instances, evaluations for treatment require scheduling additional meetings beyond the initial hour.

Among the psychiatrist's first observations of the patient will be the patient's handling of time. A patient who arrives an hour early for an appointment is usually very anxious. Those arriving very late are often conflicted about coming. Psychiatrists can learn much about patients' handling of time by exploring with patients the reasons for their tardiness. For the patient who is very late, it is important for the psychiatrist not only to explore reasons for tardiness but also to discourage the patient from introducing emotionally charged issues at or near the conclusion of an initial visit, unless the psychiatrist is prepared to stay with the patient beyond the scheduled hour.

Psychiatrists need to be aware and conscious of their own handling of time as well. The psychiatrist, if he or she anticipates being late, should contact the patient, and, as a minimum, the patient should be informed of when he or she may expect the psychiatrist to arrive. If not able to contact the patient beforehand, the psychiatrist after arriving should acknowledge the tardiness and apologize for the delay. Repeated violations of appointment hours by psychiatrists suggest an unresolved problem for them in the doctor-patient relationship and one that they need to explore and correct.

Setting

The most important space consideration for a psychiatric interview is establishing privacy so that the interview proceeds in a setting where confidentiality can be ensured. In academic settings, where audiovisual equipment and one-way viewing mirrors are used for teaching, the patient is owed an explanation by the resident about the purposes for which recording devices are being used. The patient has the right of refusal regarding the use of such devices. Most patients attending a clinic in a teaching institution expect that part of going to such an institution for help will involve using them as teaching aids for residents. The resident's dealing directly and honestly with a patient's questions and concerns is essential and also will enhance the doctor-patient relationship. The resident learns the importance of being sensitive to the patient's reactions to the use of such equipment. For instance, adolescent patients may be reluctant to discuss negative feelings toward their parents or other authority figures in the face of a camera or recording device until they are ensured that such data will not be shared with the parents.

The psychiatrist does everything possible to put the patient at ease during the interview. The setting should be one that promotes comfort for both patient and psychiatrist. The height of chairs should be approximately equal in size so that neither party is looking down on the other. There should be no barriers between the patient and doctor such as a desk, and there should be sufficient light to maximize the psychiatrist's visual observation without glaring light that would disturb the patient. Background sounds should be minimized. Noisy distractions such as bubbling fish tanks, which psychiatrists may like for aesthetic reasons, should not mar the quiet of an interview room, as it may interfere with the patient's concentration.

Special populations and settings require variations from an office setting with comfortable chairs. Hospital bedside consultations are difficult to conduct while ensuring privacy. The psychiatrist should check with the nursing staff to see whether the patient's medical condition will permit his or her being moved to a quiet room to avoid multiple interruptions at the bedside by hospital personnel, visitors, shared bedside telephones, and roommates in semiprivate rooms and ward settings.

For young children, a playroom setup, with toys that children can express themselves with, is preferable for diagnostic interviewing. Much formal training, skill, and experience are needed to appropriately evaluate a child in a playroom setting (Greenspan and Greenspan 1991; Kestenbaum 1991; Robson 1986; Rutter et al. 1988).

In hospital emergency room settings, a quiet room should be available with a mattress and no removable (and potentially dangerous) objects. Such a room will prove to be the safest setting in which to interview a psychotic patient who has exhibited out-of-control behaviors. In addition to privacy and comfort, safety is an important consideration. With a potentially agitated paranoid patient, it is important for the psychiatrist to have unimpeded access to an exit door.

Note Taking

The purpose of taking written notes during a psychiatric interview is so that the psychiatrist has accurate information for preparing the report of the interview. Neophyte interviewers tend to take extensive notes, because they are lacking in knowledge and experience about what is relevant and what is not. For the neophyte who often uses audiovisual aids such as audio- or videotape recorders for supervisory review, these same devices can be used for reviewing databases and can substitute for note taking. Any recording devices need to be in clear view of the patient, and an explanation must be given to the patient such as "I use this audiotape in lieu of written notes, and after reviewing the tapes, I erase them."

The greatest limitation in excessive note taking is that it can inhibit the free flow of exchange between patient and doctor. If preoccupied with taking notes, the psychiatrist will often miss the patient's important nonverbal messages and will not pursue important leads in the interview. The psychiatrist might not observe, for example, the patient's tears when the patient is discussing the loss of an important object in his or her life. The psychiatrist would then miss the opportunity to reflect, "You seem sad when talking about your sister." Another problem with extensive note taking is the failure to notice important aspects of the mental status examination, such as appearance and behavior. The psychiatrist may not notice the patient's becoming fidgety in his chair, tapping his right index fingers on his knees, and exhibiting a malar flush when describing the first date with his girlfriend at age 16 (Edelson 1980).

If the patient's resentment about note taking interferes with the interview, the psychiatrist should refrain from doing so. Patients may react to the relative absence of note taking as well. They may comment, "How can you remember everything I have to say?" Such patients are concerned about whether the psychiatrist values them and cares about what they are saying. The psychiatrist then reflects these concerns, for example, by commenting, "You wonder whether I value what you are saying."

Notes help psychiatrists remember information accurately. The psychiatrist should summarize his or her notes, observations, and conclusions as soon after the interview as possible. Prompt recording of data and information while still fresh in the psychiatrist's mind maximizes the accuracy of the information and minimizes distortions and gaps in the database that will result when the psychiatrist delays his or her recording. The psychiatrist should set aside time at the conclusion of the interview to accomplish this task. For the experienced psychiatrist, 5 to 10 minutes at the conclusion of a 45- to 50-minute interview usually suffices. The neophyte will require additional time.

The notes that are incorporated in the patient's record are necessarily more comprehensive following initial interviews than subsequent ones, because all the data constitute new information. With subsequent interviews, only new, pertinent information needs to be recorded. Psychiatrists need to be particularly sensitive to what information is incorporated into a general hospital chart that is available to multiple caretakers and to third-party reviewers. Only essential information for the overall care of the patient should be included in a general medical chart.

Interruptions

The time set aside and agreed upon for a patient interview is viewed as sacred and protected time for the patient. Calculated measures are taken to discourage interruptions. If the door to the interview room is in an area where others may knock, a sign should be hung on the door with an instruction such as "Do not disturb" or "Interview in progress" or "In session." If someone does knock and the psychiatrist chooses to respond, he or she should go to the door and open it only wide enough for the other party to hear. The psychiatrist positions himself or herself to protect the patient from being seen. The interaction with the person knocking should be as brief as possible.

Incoming telephone calls are screened by a secretary and the callers informed that the psychiatrist is with a patient. Sessions are interrupted only for emergencies. If the psychiatrist must leave, the patient should be informed of when the psychiatrist anticipates returning, if the absence is expected to be brief. Otherwise, the psychiatrist advises the patient when to return. If, at the beginning of an interview, the psychiatrist anticipates that an urgent call may be received during the hour, he or she informs the patient at the beginning of the interview that an interruption may occur and that the psychiatrist will ask the patient to leave during the telephone call. Most patients understand interruptions for emergencies and appreciate feeling that if they were in an emergency situation, the psychiatrist would respond immediately (Bernstein and Bernstein 1980).

Relatives or Friends Accompanying the Patient

When relatives arrive with the patient, the psychiatrist always interviews the patient first and tells relatives that he or she may want to talk with them later. (An exception would be a couple coming for couples' evaluation and possible couples' therapy.) In the course of the patient's interviews, the psychiatrist can indicate his or her desire to speak with the relatives and can explore the patient's feelings about the psychiatrist's doing so. The patient must grant permission before relatives are interviewed. If the patient refuses, the psychiatrist must respect the patient's wishes. By doing so, the psychiatrist demonstrates that the most valued part of his or her relationship with the patient is confidentiality. Patients must also grant permission before the psychiatrist discusses their case with any other party.

An exception to this rule occurs when the psychiatrist judges the patient to be in imminent danger of hurting self or others and when the patient refuses voluntary hospitalization. In such an instance, the patient must be told why the psychiatrist is obliged to talk to a third party without the patient's permission.

If the psychiatrist wants to meet with the patient's relatives, he or she must advise the patient whether the meeting will take place with or without the patient present. If in doubt, the psychiatrist chooses to have the patient present. This signals to the patient that the psychiatrist does not want to jeopardize the patient-doctor relationship. This relationship is more important than obtaining additional information that relatives may not want to reveal in the patient's presence. Another advantage of having the patient present is that the psychiatrist can observe the interactions of the patient with the relative(s). The patient's presence also discourages a relative from trying to reveal any information that he or she would prefer that the patient not know and thus avoids the situation in which the relative wants the psychiatrist to keep secrets from the patient. It is possible to enhance the accuracy of diagnoses by a best-estimate procedure. This involves diagnosis made by one clinician on the basis of diagnostic information from a direct interview conducted by another clinician, plus information from medical records and reports from family members. Such an approach may be especially applicable for enhancing the diagnosis of antisocial personality disorder and of alcoholism (Kosten and Rounsaville 1992).

If the psychiatrist chooses to see relatives without the patient present, the ground rule needs to be established with relatives that the psychiatrist is not at liberty to share, without the patient's permission, any information obtained from the patient in confidence but is at liberty to share with the patient any information that relatives reveal. This principle extends beyond the initial visit to subsequent telephone calls that relatives may initiate. If relatives call after an initial visit, it is best for the psychiatrist to inquire first whether the patient has given permission for relatives to call. If not, the psychiatrist suggests that the patient's permission be granted before proceeding. At the beginning of the next contact with the patient, the psychiatrist informs him or her that relatives called.

Sequence

The psychiatrist's first impressions of the patient begin with the initial telephone contact. The formal assessment of the patient begins with the psychiatrist's initial observations of the patient. The psychiatrist observes the patient's appearance and behavior in the waiting area, who is with the patient, how the patient responds when the psychiatrist greets him or her by name, and how the patient responds to a handshake. It is preferable with adult patients to refer to them by their last names during the initial encounter, and then, when they are in the interview room, to inquire what the patient's preference is regarding first- or last-name usage. Referring to geriatric patients by first names without the patients' permission is particularly demeaning and infantilizing.

The psychiatrist then walks with the patient to the interview room and indicates interest in the patient by being friendly but does not make any clinical inquiries or comments until the interviewing room door is closed. The psychiatrist indicates which seat he or she will sit in while offering the patient a choice if there is more than one seat present.

At the beginning of the interview, the psychiatrist encourages the patient to speak as spontaneously and openly as possible about the reasons for his or her coming at this time. The psychiatrist can facilitate this process by briefly summarizing what he or she has learned about the patient and the patient's problems and then saying that he or she would like to hear in the patient's own words what is troubling the patient. An opening inquiry such as "Tell me what brings you here today" encourages the patient to express what currently is troubling him or her. The psychiatrist establishes a primary posture of listening, allowing the patient to tell his or her story with minimal interruptions or direction. In the early part of the interview, if the patient stops talking, the psychiatrist encourages him or her to continue, using comments such as "Tell me more about [a particular incident]." If the patient describes a significant event in his or her life and expresses no emotion, the psychiatrist inquires, "How do you feel about this?" If the patient describes a disturbing event and starts clenching his or her fists and exhibiting flushing, the psychiatrist inquires about the patient's feelings at the moment. If the patient denies any feelings, the psychiatrist advises him or her that most people would react to similar circumstances with anger. Thus, in the initial part of the interview, the psychiatrist establishes that he or she is interested in not only the chronology of events that led to the patient's coming, but also the feelings that accompany such events, and encourages the patient's expression of these feelings. At times, when the expression of feelings is too overwhelming for the patient, the psychiatrist must not push the patient beyond his or her tolerance for expressing them. If the patient has had one or more psychiatric hospitalizations, the psychiatrist should learn details about each hospitalization and most particularly the events leading up to the initial hospitalization. It is also key to inquire what was most helpful during a patient's hospitalization as well as what follow-up care was most beneficial.

Throughout the interview the psychiatrist tries to learn how the patient experiences life events and to understand the patient's perceptions of how such events evolve. Once the psychiatrist has a grasp of the essentials of the present illness and accompanying feelings, he or she then shifts the focus to other subjects.

In the middle portion of the interview, the psychiatrist tries to learn about the patient as a person. There are numerous areas of the patient's life to explore: significant relationships, multigenerational family history, current living situation, occupation, avocations, education, value systems, religious and cultural background, military history, social history, medical history, developmental history, sexual history, and legal history, to name a few. The breadth of material requires several interview sessions for the psychiatrist to gather the pertinent data.

The patient will frequently be asked to describe a typical day in his or her life. The psychiatrist tries to establish the patient's highest level of functioning and assesses when current symptoms began to interfere with the patient's functioning. The decision regarding the order in which the psychiatrist inquires about these data is a matter of clinical judgment. The patient usually signifies his or her comfort with particular subjects by raising them in the interview, and the psychiatrist then follows up with questions to get more in-depth information.

As a rule, the psychiatrist moves from areas assumed to be of positive value to those of neutral interest and, finally, to those that the psychiatrist anticipates will be more emotionally charged for the patient. For example, in interviewing an adolescent, the psychiatrist may begin with inquiries regarding activities that the patient enjoys by asking, "What do you do for fun?" The psychiatrist may choose to begin his or her inquiries about school with, "Tell me about your favorite subject in school." Inquiries about relationships may be made by starting with a request such as "Tell me about your best friend." The psychiatrist then may proceed to inquiries about family members by saying, "Tell me about your family."

Throughout these initial inquiries, the psychiatrist is ascertaining the patient's strengths and weaknesses and is monitoring the responses to ascertain potential areas of conflict for the patient. The psychiatrist's follow-up inquiries will be guided by the responses to the initial questions. Inquiry may then be made about specific relationships, for example, "How do you get along with your mother? your father? your brother? your sister?" With the latter, the psychiatrist is advised to ask for names and to refer to the siblings in subsequent inquiries by name.

Again, the psychiatrist is guided by the patient's responses in terms of inquiring about areas in which the patient may be reluctant to respond. When inquiring about a sexual history with a boy or man, the psychiatrist begins with, "Do you have a girlfriend?" If yes, the psychiatrist follows with "Tell me about her" and can then inquire about the nature of the relationship. The psychiatrist follows up by asking about specific areas of sexual conduct. Beginning with questions regarding kissing and then petting and then sexual intercourse, the psychiatrist then asks about the patient's feelings in regard to various sexual activities, inquiring about both heterosexual and homosexual interests and relationships. Histories of sexual abuse should be elicited (Morrison 1993).

In the concluding portion of the interview, the psychiatrist notes for the patient the remaining time left. The patient is asked whether there are any important areas that he or she has not talked about. The psychiatrist asks whether the patient has any questions, then answers each of the patient's questions. If the psychiatrist has insufficient information to answer a question, he or she tells the patient just that.

At this time the psychiatrist shares with the patient his or her clinical impressions in words that the patient understands, avoiding psychiatric jargon. The psychiatrist then presents a treatment plan to the patient. It is important to ascertain the patient's fiscal status as well as to understand the third-party insurance that will cover the patient's care. It may be that, under the limitations of a managed-care situation, the psychiatrist will have to advise the patient that the tried and true treatment modalities may not be available to certain patients because of the limitations of the patients' reimbursement system. Psychiatrists have the ethical responsibility to try to assist patients to receive optimal care. On the other hand, patients must decide within the limitations of their fiscal abilities what is feasible for themselves and their families.

If records and information are available from other sources, the psychiatrist requests written permission to obtain medical records from hospitals or other physicians. If the psychiatrist wants to contact others by telephone, he or she obtains permission from the patient before doing so. If the patient is receiving medical care from other physicians, the psychiatrist obtains consent to contact them. If the patient is reluctant to grant permission, the psychiatrist explains his or her reasons for wanting to initiate these contacts. For example, the psychiatrist may want to prescribe medications but before doing so wants to be sure that there are no medical contraindications. If the patient was referred by another physician, it is important for the psychiatrist to call the referring physician. The patient may want the psychiatrist to advise him or her about what information the psychiatrist will share with the referring physician. Most patients understand the importance of their care being coordinated by the two physicians when assured that information that is best kept in confidence will not be shared.

For example, a 58-year-old depressed male patient with hypertension and cardiac arrhythmia reveals that he had homosexual relations when he was a teenager. The psychiatrist advises the patient that she would like to prescribe antidepressant medications but, before doing so, wants to confer with the patient's primary physician about the type of cardiac arrhythmia he has had and the current treatment of his cardiovascular problems. The psychiatrist wants to ascertain which antidepressants may be contraindicated because of the patient's cardiac problems and wants to avoid any adverse drug reactions as well as to choose the most appropriate medication, given the patient's combined medical/psychiatric problems. At the same time, the psychiatrist assures the patient that his past sexual life will not be revealed to the primary care physician.

It is important to solicit patients' reactions to as well as agreement with a given treatment plan. Patients are entitled to know the various treatments available for their disorder. The psychiatrist shares with the patient his or her specific recommendations for treatment and responds to the patient's questions about why the psychiatrist believes these suggestions are best for the patient. If the patient wants an alternative plan, it is best for the psychiatrist to postpone implementation of specific treatment until there is mutual agreement. There is a better likelihood for patient compliance when the patient understands a treatment plan and agrees to it (Table 6–2) (Garrett 1942; Gill et al. 1954; Group for the Advancement of Psychiatry 1961; Leon 1982; Nurcombe and Fitzhenry-Coor 1982; Rutter and Cox 1981; Strupp and Binder 1984; Sullivan 1954; Whitehorn 1944).

THE PHYSICIAN-PATIENT RELATIONSHIP

Transference

Transference is a process whereby the patient unconsciously projects his or her emotions, thoughts, and wishes related to significant persons in his or her past life onto people in his or her current life and, in the context of the psychiatrist-patient relationship, onto the psychiatrist. The patient is reacting to the psychiatrist as if the psychiatrist were part of the patient's past. Whereas the reaction patterns may have been appropriate in an earlier life situa-

TABLE 6–2. **Phases of the psychiatric interview**

Initial
Chief complaint
Present illness
Feelings about significant events
Middle
Patient as a person
Multigenerational family history
Current living situation
Occupation
Avocations
Education
Value systems
Religions and cultural background
Military history
Social history
Medical history
Developmental history
Sexual history
Typical day
Strengths and weaknesses
Concluding
Time remaining
Important areas not covered
Patient's questions
Sharing clinical impressions
Permission to obtain records
Permission to speak with others

tion, they are inappropriate when applied to figures in the present, including the psychiatrist. This theoretical construct is borrowed from the psychoanalytic literature.

For example, a 24-year-old male patient notices the long braided hair and blue eyes of the psychiatrist. He starts making several demands of the psychiatrist using a whining voice, without being consciously aware that he is doing so. Such demanding behavior replicates how he behaved in the presence of a significant aunt in his youth with similar physical features, with whom he had a highly dependent relationship and in whose presence he had exhibited similar whining voice intonations.

It is important for the psychiatrist to recognize these patterns and to treat them as distortions, not to respond in kind. An ultimate understanding of such unconscious behaviors is one of the goals of insight-oriented psychotherapy. In the early training of a psychiatrist, the psychiatric supervisor devotes considerable time to the resident's understanding of the process of transference so that the resident will not treat these reaction patterns as personal assaults.

Countertransference

Countertransference is a process whereby the psychiatrist unconsciously projects emotions, thoughts, and wishes from his or her past onto the patient's personality or onto the material that the patient is presenting, thus expressing unresolved conflicts and/or gratifying the psychiatrist's own personal needs. These reactions are inappropriate in the patient-doctor relationship. In this instance, the patient assumes the role of an important person from the psychiatrist's earlier life. This construct is also gleaned from the psychoanalytic literature. In such instances, the psychiatrist mistakenly attributes to the patient feelings and thoughts that are based on the psychiatrist's own life experiences, which can interfere with his or her understanding of the patient.

For example, a male psychiatrist responds inappropriately to an internist's consultation request on a 76-year-old dying hospitalized female patient. The psychiatrist has been making twice-daily hourly bedside visits followed by frequent calls to the patient's internist. The psychiatrist questions the internist's medical care of the patient and recommends anti-anxiety agents to treat the patient's presumed anxiety. As a child, the psychiatrist had experienced strong attachment to his grandmother, who had died in his childhood home. He unconsciously retained guilt feelings for not doing something to prevent her death. The psychiatrist's handling of the consultation is in essence an attempt to cope with his own anxieties and guilt about his grand-

mother's death without consciously realizing that he was doing this or being cognizant of the inappropriateness of his behavior.

The psychiatrist in this case would benefit from consultation with a colleague, who could help clarify the psychiatrist's reaction patterns and guide him toward more appropriate professional behavior.

One of the values of personal psychoanalysis for psychiatrists is to enhance their awareness of their unconsciously motivated behaviors so that they can better use their countertransference reactions to understand their patients. In their training, residents will be helped by a supervisor to examine their countertransference reactions so that these reactions will not interfere with patients' treatment but will aid the residents in understanding their patients.

Therapeutic Alliance

The therapeutic alliance, a third theoretical construct from the psychoanalytic literature, is a process whereby the patient's mature, rational observing ego is used in combination with the psychiatrist's analytic abilities to advance the psychiatrist's understanding of the patient. The basis for such an alliance is the trusting relationship established in early life between the child and the mother, as well as other significant trusting relationships from the patient's past. The psychiatrist encourages the development of this alliance, and both persons must invest in cultivating the alliance so that the patient can benefit. The psychiatrist enhances this alliance by his or her professional conduct and attitudes of caring, concern, and respect.

Psychiatrists accept and respect patients' value systems and their integrity as persons. Without a therapeutic alliance, patients cannot reveal their innermost thoughts and feelings. It is unethical for psychiatrists to exploit patients sexually or to exploit them for personal financial gain by inquiring about investment opportunities from patients knowledgeable about such matters. These are violations of the doctor-patient relationship. Psychiatrists must never victimize patients by exploiting their roles as physician healers (American Psychiatric Association 1995).

Resistance

Resistance is a theoretical construct that reflects any attitude or behaviors that run counter to the therapeutic objectives of the treatment. Understanding resistances is critical to the conduct of dynamic psychotherapy. Freud described several types of resistance, including conscious resistance, ego resistance, id resistance, and superego resistance.

Conscious resistance by patients occurs for a variety of reasons, such as lack of trust of psychiatrists, shame on the part of patients in revealing certain events and aspects of themselves or feelings that they are experiencing, or fear of displeasing or risking rejection by psychiatrists. One form of resistance by patients is silence. The psychiatrist must acknowledge the difficulties the patient is experiencing and encourage the patient to verbalize material that is difficult to express. This should be done in a tactful, sensitive manner.

One form of *ego resistance* is *repression resistance*, whereby, for mostly unconscious reasons, the same forces that led to the patient's symptoms keep him or her from developing an awareness of the underlying conflicts. A second type of ego resistance, *transference resistance*, can take many forms. Such resistance may occur when the patient projects undesirable feelings onto the psychiatrist and ascribes these feelings to the psychiatrist. This, in turn, can lead to the patient's attacking the psychiatrist, and a negative transference can result. It is critical that the psychiatrist understand the underpinnings of such a transaction and, rather than retaliate, treat the patient's expressions as a resistance. A third type of ego resistance is *secondary-gain resistance*. A patient's symptoms will elicit nurturing responses from significant figures and will gratify his or her dependency needs. Manifestations of this phenomenon are common on inpatient services. For example, the patient who has been hospitalized 7 days for a cerebral hemorrhage secondary to a cerebral aneurysm shows gradual improvement in healing and has decreased complaints of headaches for 6 days. However, he resumes his complaints to the nurse in the 24 hours before his proposed discharge from the hospital. In addition to gratifying dependency needs, symptoms also serve as attention-seeking devices. Patients unconsciously resist giving up their symptoms. Such resistances must be understood by the patients' caregivers.

Id resistance occurs in psychoanalytic practice when the patient repeatedly brings up the same material in the face of repeated interpretations of the behavior.

Superego resistance occurs most frequently with obsessional, depressed patients who, by virtue of their guilt feelings and self-defeating behaviors, exhibit a need for punishment. Thus, patients continue to exhibit symptoms that serve as punishment, and they are resistant to relinquishing them (Luborsky 1984).

Resistance takes many forms. They include patients' censoring of what they are thinking, intellectualization, generalization, preoccupation with one phase of life, concentration on trivial details while avoiding important topics, affective displays, frequent requests to change appointment times, using minor physical symptoms as an excuse to avoid sessions, arriving late or forgetting appointments, forgetting to pay bills, competitive behaviors with the psychiatrist, seductive behaviors, asking for favors, and acting out (MacKinnon and Michels 1971).

Confidentiality

Psychiatrists are bound by medical ethical principles to not divulge any information revealed to them unless they have patients' consent. They must protect patients and assume responsibility for seeing that no harm will come to patients by virtue of the patients' revealing information about themselves. If patients refuse to give permission to psychiatrists to reveal information, whether it be to a referring physician or for filling out an insurance form, psychiatrists must respect the patients' wishes.

For example, a 32-year-old female patient with borderline personality disorder is referred to a psychiatrist by her internist for evaluation of depressive symptoms. The psychiatrist learns that the patient episodically abuses diazepam, prescribed by her internist, along with alcohol when she is feeling upset. The psychiatrist's assessment is that the combination of these two chemical depressants is contributing to her depressive symptoms. The psychiatrist requests permission to share this assessment with the referring internist, but the patient refuses. The psychiatrist abides by the patient's wishes while advising the patient that this combination is likely to be responsible for contributing to her depressive symptoms. He also suggests that the patient reconsider the refusal to let him share his findings with her internist.

In hospital or clinic settings, the patient is told about the types of information that will be recorded and who may have access to the information. When psychiatrists record information in the general hospital record, they record only data pertinent to the overall care of the patient, such as medications prescribed, and minimize recording personal information that has no relevance to the general medical care of the patient. In general hospital settings, it is preferable to have separate psychiatric records that can be housed and locked in an area separate from the general hospital records, to which only trained psychiatric personnel will have access.

Only when patients are in danger of hurting themselves or others by virtue of their mental illness is the psychiatrist obliged to reveal such information in order to institute involuntary hospitalization.

When third-party carriers are seeking psychiatric information, psychiatrists review with patients the information that has been prepared for the carrier and obtain patients' permission to submit reports.

INTERVIEW TECHNIQUE

Facilitative Messages

The most important component in the psychiatrist-patient relationship is the interest psychiatrists show in their patients. The most important element in the psychiatric interview of patients is for psychiatrists to allow patients to tell their stories in an uninterrupted fashion. Psychiatrists assume an attentive listening posture; they do not ask excessive questions that would interrupt the flow of the interview. Throughout the interview, patients will experience resistances to revealing themselves that are based on the realities of the interview situation as well as on transference issues.

Neophyte residents often mistakenly believe that sitting in an unresponsive, silent posture emulates a psychoanalyst's approach to a patient and that this is the optimal way to interview a psychiatric patient. On the contrary, residents need to learn a repertoire of interviewing techniques that will facilitate communications as much as possible (Table 6–3). Some of these techniques are described below.

Open-ended questions.   An open-ended question reflects a topic that the psychiatrist is interested in exploring but leaves it to the patient to choose the areas he or she believes are relevant and important to share.

Examples of open-ended questions by the psychiatrist are as follows:

> **Psychiatrist:** Can you tell me about your depression?
> **Patient:** I've been having crying spells.
> **Psychiatrist:** Can you describe them?
> **Patient:** They come on during certain times of the month.
> **Psychiatrist:** Can you say more about them?
> **Patient:** They've been troubling me since I was a teenager.
> **Psychiatrist:** They seem to have been bothering you for a long time; tell me more.

The psychiatrist attempts to get the patient to relate in his or her own words, as much as possible, the most significant aspects of his or her depression. The psychiatrist may return later in the interview to fill in specific details if the patient fails to do so spontaneously. In the example above, the psychiatrist would want to know more about the patient's symptoms, the times of the month that the symptoms appear, and what precipitated their onset when the patient was a teenager, among other issues.

Reflections.   The psychiatrist often wants to draw patients' attention to the affective concomitants of their verbal productions. One way of doing this is by rephrasing what the patient has stated and stressing the feelings that accompany a reported event. By restating the patient's verbalizations, the psychiatrist provides the patient with an opportunity to correct any misconceptions that the psychiatrist may have about the patient's condition. This technique is referred to as *reflections*. Examples of reflective responses are as follows:

> **Patient:** I've been concerned about my job. I used to be able to keep up with my fellow workers. But in the last 3 months they seem to be handling the adjustments to the new computer and I have been unable to do so.
> **Psychiatrist:** You're concerned about keeping up with new demands and about retaining your job.
> **Patient:** That's right. You know that at 58 you can't concentrate on those new manuals the way the younger people can, and I've been experiencing butterflies in my stomach and sweaty palms these last 3 months.
> **Psychiatrist:** You've been anxious since these changes occurred at work?
> **Patient:** You better believe it! I have not been myself. I've

TABLE 6–3.   Facilitative messages

Type	Example
Open-ended questions	"Tell me about . . ."
Reflections	"You're anxious about succeeding."
Facilitation	"Uh-huh."
Positive reinforcement	"Good. That helps me understand you."
Silence	Long pause allowing patient to take distance from verbal material.
Interpretation	"When you can't perform the way you think you should, you try to do something to please."
Checklist questions	"When you feel nervous, do you develop sweaty palms? heart palpitations? rapid breathing? butterflies in your stomach?"
"I want" messages	"We should explore other topics besides your depression. Tell me about your family."
Transitions	"Now that you've told me about your job, tell me what a typical day is like."
Self-disclosure	"When I've been in similar situations, I feel terrified."

had heart palpitations, shakiness all over my body, and occasionally I've been stuttering.

Psychiatrist: So you'd like help in dealing with your anxieties?

Patient: I sure would.

By reflecting the patient's recent life events and by drawing attention to the principal affective component, in this case anxiety, the psychiatrist demonstrates his or her capacity to understand what the patient has been experiencing and is able to help the patient define the areas they will work on together in treatment.

Facilitation.   The psychiatrist uses body language and minimal verbal cues to encourage and reinforce the patient's continuing along a particular line of thought with minimal interruptions in the patient's flow of verbalizations. Examples of these cues include attributes that are frequently ascribed to psychiatrists, such as the nodding of their heads or comments such as "Uh-huh." Other examples of facilitations include raising of eyebrows, cocking of head, leaning toward patients, and verbalizations from the psychiatrist such as "I see," "Go on," "What else?" "Anything more?" and "Proceed." Facilitations indicate to the patient that the psychiatrist is interested in the particular train of thought and that he or she is attentive to what the patient is saying. Excessive reliance on a single facilitation will, however, approach the parody of a psychiatrist and become counterproductive.

Positive reinforcement.   The subjects that the psychiatrist explores with the patient are frequently ones that the patient is unaccustomed to talking about and finds difficult to explain. When the patient has struggled with a particular topic and is then able to communicate clearly, the psychiatrist signals his or her approval by using positive reinforcement. An example of such reinforcement would be the following:

Psychiatrist: How do you feel when you can't have an erection?

Patient (*blushes*): You know—it just doesn't get hard.

Psychiatrist: Do you experience anything else?

Patient (*long pause*): How do I feel?

Psychiatrist: Yes.

Patient: Oh! I get terribly frustrated and then I get angry.

Psychiatrist: Good. Those are the kinds of feelings I was asking about. That helps a lot for me to better understand what you experience.

In this manner, the psychiatrist encourages the patient to describe sensitive topics and feelings without demeaning the patient for his or her initial response. Positive reinforcement will then encourage the patient to verbalize other emotional states as he or she, along with the psychiatrist, explores other areas of his or her life.

Silence.   The judicious use of silence when interviewing a patient is an important component of the psychiatrist's repertoire of interviewing techniques. Silences allow patients to create some distance from what they have been saying and can help them put their thoughts in order or enable them to understand better the psychological meaning and context of what has happened in the interview.

Neophyte psychiatrists are frequently anxious when interviewing patients. One way they deal with their own anxiety is to try to fill any voids in the flow of conversation by asking questions or making comments before patients have had time to digest and process what has been said and to determine what they think or feel. In this situation, patients are denied an opportunity to reflect and to gain an understanding of what they have experienced.

In a similar fashion, patients often try to please the psychiatrist by continuously verbalizing, in the belief that the psychiatrist wants to have them speak continuously. It is often necessary for the psychiatrist to educate patients that silences are desirable. The psychiatrist must also keep in mind that silences can be a form of resistance, and, in such instances, he or she needs to encourage patients to proceed by responding to those silences with "Tell me what you are thinking."

Interpretation.   The psychiatrist works with patients to try to help them understand their motivations and the meanings of their thoughts, feelings, and actions. The psychiatrist examines repeated patterns of behaviors and draws inferences regarding these patterns. Such inferences are called *interpretations*. Several interpretation techniques may be used to help patients. The psychiatrist may lead the patient in the direction of self-interpretation by taking certain pieces of data that the patient assumes are unrelated and helping him or her identify certain patterns. The patient can then piece together these seemingly unrelated events and feelings and draw inferences. In another way of interpreting, the psychiatrist both presents the patterns of behavior and draws the inferences for the patient as a tentative hypothesis, which the patient can then either accept or reject. The following are examples of interpretations:

Patient: Based on what I've been telling you, it seems that every time I face new situations, I develop symptoms that reflect my anxieties.

Psychiatrist: Yes, that's what I've observed.

Psychiatrist: You've just shared with me how upset you are when you can't please your mother. What do you make of that?

Patient: Yeah, every time I try to do something to please someone I want to get strokes from and they don't respond the way I want them to, I get frustrated and angry.

Psychiatrist: It appears that when you can't get your own way with women, you resort to seductive behaviors and then you engage in activities that you later regret. How do you see these patterns?

Patient *(long pause)*: I've never realized that before, but it sure seems to fit.

Interpretations allow patients to advance their understanding of their own behaviors and, by helping them to be more conscious of their patterns of behavior, give them the opportunity to choose to behave or react differently when similar events occur in the future. Neophyte psychiatrists, in their anxiety to please patients and show they understand them, will often overinterpret patients' behavior and reassure them inappropriately and unnecessarily. The timing and appropriate use of interpretation are best learned under supervision.

Checklist questions. The psychiatrist spells out a list of potential responses for a patient when the patient is unable to describe or quantify to the degree of specificity that the psychiatrist believes is important to know in particular situations, as in the following examples:

Patient: This makes me feel dizzy.

Psychiatrist: Can you tell me what you experience? [*open-ended*]

Patient: You know—I don't like the dizzy sensation.

Psychiatrist: Do you feel light-headed, or do you experience your head spinning, or do you feel that the room is spinning?

Patient: It's more light-headed—like I'm going to faint.

Patient: I get this pain in my stomach.

Psychiatrist: What seems to bring it on? [*open-ended*]

Patient: It just seems to come any time.

Psychiatrist: Do you experience pain when you have an empty stomach, or is it after meals, or when you feel anxious?

Patient *(pause)*: It seems to be when I'm experiencing tension.

The psychiatrist uses a checklist of questions when open-ended questions do not yield the necessary information and when more specific information than what has been obtained with the open-ended questions is needed.

The checklist format is often helpful for elucidating medical problems.

"I want" messages. When the psychiatrist senses that an interview has failed to progress because of the patient's need to focus on a single theme, the psychiatrist asserts that they need to move on to other areas of inquiry. The psychiatrist is firm with the patient that sufficient information has been obtained about the single theme and that he or she understands the patient's concerns and feelings about that particular topic.

Patient *(for the fourth time)*: These voices—do you know what they're doing to me?

Psychiatrist: Yes, I understand how terrifying they are to you, but we must move on to talk about other areas now, and we can return at another time to discuss the voices. How would that be for you?

By asserting his need to move on, the psychiatrist avoids building up his own resentments and averts acting on his own frustrations with the patient.

Transitions. Once sufficient information regarding a particular part of a patient's history is obtained, the psychiatrist then signals to the patient his or her satisfaction with the understanding of that portion of the interview and invites the patient to move on to another area. This technique is referred to as *transitions*, an example of which is as follows:

Psychiatrist: I understand what it is that brings you here. Now, I'd like for you to tell me something about yourself.

Once the psychiatrist believes he knows about the patient as a person, the next transition would be

Psychiatrist: I have a sense of what you're like as a person; tell me how you get along with people.

This could then lead to the next transition:

Psychiatrist: Now that you've told me about your friendships, please tell me about your family.

These transitions allow the psychiatrist to guide the patient from one significant topic to another while signaling to the patient the areas that are important for the psychiatrist to learn about. Once the patient has given clues that he or she is prepared to talk about a particular area, the choice of ordering of topics is best dictated by the patient.

The psychiatrist, by keeping attuned to the patient's readiness to discuss a topic, will orchestrate a smooth transition from one topic to another.

Self-disclosure.   The psychiatrist, at times, will judge that it is in the patient's best interest for the psychiatrist to disclose certain thoughts, feelings, or actions about himself or herself. This self-disclosure may be in response to the patient's questions, or it may occur when the psychiatrist believes that sharing his or her own experiences will benefit the patient:

> **Patient:** I am uncertain about whether a counselor or a psychiatrist is best suited for treating my problems. What kind of training did you have?
>
> **Psychiatrist:** I am a graduate of Northwestern Medical School, where I also completed 4 years of residency training, and I'm certified by the American Board of Psychiatry and Neurology.

or

> I've experienced similar problems in dealing with what my doctor should reveal to my health insurance carrier about my history. This is how I handled the situation . . . .

Requests on the part of patients for the psychiatrist to reveal himself or herself are best treated in the context of understanding the individual patient. In the first example, the patient may have been exhibiting a resistance to treatment, in which case the psychiatrist's response would have been very different. If judging the patient's question in that way, the psychiatrist would have responded, "You're wondering whether I'm able to help you with your problems." Such resistances will often be presented by the patient in the form of questions such as "How old are you?" Residents need to understand that the patient's meta-message is, "Are you experienced enough to treat me?" Residents need to learn to reflect the patient's underlying concerns back to the patient; in the case above, a resident's self-disclosure that he is 28 years old is not going to be helpful and will be counterproductive.

Obstructive Messages

Obstructive messages tend to interfere with the uninterrupted flow of the patient's verbalizations and stand in the way of the establishment of a trusting relationship between psychiatrist and patient (Table 6–4). These communications are interview techniques that should be avoided. Some were learned in medical school, and psychiatric residents need to be coached in how to avoid using them.

Excessive direct questions.   Excessive direct questions represent the antithesis of open-ended questions. They occur when the psychiatrist directs the patient to a single response. This technique does not allow the patient to choose those areas that are of greatest concern to him or her. An example of an excessive number of direct questions is as follows:

TABLE 6–4.   **Obstructive messages**

Type	Example
Excessively direct questions	**Psychiatrist:** What's making you sad? **Patient:** I've lost a girlfriend. **Psychiatrist:** Do you cry a lot? **Patient:** Probably not. **Psychiatrist:** Did you grieve inadequately? **Patient:** I'm not sure.
Preemptive topic shifts	**Patient:** I feel suicidal. **Psychiatrist:** Are you feeling despondent? **Patient:** I'm terribly depressed. **Psychiatrist:** Are you having trouble with your marriage? **Patient:** I can't say.
Premature advice	**Patient:** I have an upset stomach. **Psychiatrist:** You may want to try antacids and warm milk at bedtime and six meals a day.
False reassurance	**Psychiatrist:** You need not worry about your phantom pains—lots of persons with amputations experience the same problem.
Doing without explanation	**Psychiatrist:** I know what your problem is. You're suffering anxiety from too much stress. Cut back your hours of study. Take these pills three times a day. Start eating three meals a day.
Put-down questions	**Psychiatrist:** How can you continue to complain about your academic inadequacies when you have all A's and just made Phi Beta Kappa?
"You are bad" statements	**Psychiatrist:** You keep crying when you mention your mother—hysterics are known to do that.
Trapping patients with their own words	**Psychiatrist:** You just said you were pleased with your progress; now you're complaining that you're still depressed.
Nonverbal messages of resentment	Psychiatrist turns away from patient, shuffles papers on desk, and closes eyes when patient repeats same verbalization.

Psychiatrist: Are you a sad person?
Patient: I think so.
Psychiatrist: Have you been sad since you were a little boy?
Patient: Perhaps.
Psychiatrist: Do you lose your appetite when you're sad?
Patient: Yes.
Psychiatrist: How much weight do you lose?
Patient: Around five pounds.
Psychiatrist: Does being thin make you sad?

The excessive use of direct questions lends itself to the patient's answering only what is on the psychiatrist's list of questions. It presupposes that the psychiatrist alone knows the issues, priorities, and relevant information. The patient thus becomes a passive recipient of the psychiatrist's inquiries and fails to become an equal partner with the psychiatrist.

Run-on questioning.   Rather than giving the patient a chance to respond to a single question, the psychiatrist asks several questions at one time. The patient may not know which question to answer or attempt to condense all the questions into one and respond with a yes or no response. For example:

Psychiatrist: Now that we have discussed your depression, have you ever felt the opposite of depressed—where you had racing thoughts, where others have trouble keeping up with your thinking? Have you had spending sprees where you run up huge bills on a credit card? Have you had feelings of euphoria, where you feel happier than everyone around you? Have you gone 36 or more waking hours without requiring sleep?
Patient: No.

The psychiatrist is lumping together for the patient a series of hypomanic signs and symptoms without giving the patient an opportunity to respond to each one. Such run-on questions suggest that there is no interest in the answers to each of the questions being posed.

Preemptive topic shifts.   Rather than responding to the patient's cues about meaningful events, the psychiatrist moves from one topic to another, seemingly insensitive to what is important to the patient, as in the following example:

Patient *(tremulously)*: I'm feeling very shaky inside.
Psychiatrist: Tell me how you get along with your mother.
Patient: I've been having troubles trusting her lately.
Psychiatrist: And your father?
Patient: I don't see that much of him.

Rather than focusing on the patient's shaky feelings and exploring this area in depth, the psychiatrist shifts to other areas that he or she wants to cover and fails to investigate issues that are of immediate concern to the patient. The patient is left feeling that the psychiatrist is unconcerned about the patient's troubles. Preemptive topic shifts may be a conscious or unconscious defense by the psychiatrist when he or she is threatened or unhappy with the topic.

Premature advice.   The psychiatrist may assert his or her authority by telling the patient what to do without sufficient information and without engaging the patient in seeking solutions to his or her own problems. The following exchange demonstrates premature advice:

Patient: I've been having trouble getting to sleep.
Psychiatrist: You ought to try running 2 miles each evening and drink a warm glass of milk before retiring, and then read a book that doesn't excite you when you go to bed.

Rather than pursuing what may be the etiology of the patient's complaint and getting details of what may be going on in the patient's life, the psychiatrist advances a series of solutions that may be totally inappropriate for the patient. Such premature advice leads the patient to react with resentment and hinders his or her relationship with the psychiatrist (Balint 1972).

False reassurance.   When the psychiatrist tells the patient that something will or will not occur, and either he or she has insufficient information to draw that conclusion or the clinical situation suggests that just the opposite may happen, the psychiatrist is giving the patient false reassurance. Examples of such an obstructive message are as follows:

Patient: I've been having trouble with my memory.
Psychiatrist: That occasionally happens with someone your age, and I know it will improve.

Patient: I've been hospitalized four times in the last 2 years for my schizophrenia. Will it ever go away?
Psychiatrist: Lots of people get over their schizophrenia, and you need not worry.

In the first instance, the psychiatrist has no basis for knowing that the patient's memories will improve, but tells the patient something that the psychiatrist thinks the patient would want to hear in order to feel better. In the second example, the psychiatrist is advising the patient of something the patient knows is unlikely to happen, and the admonishment not to worry accentuates rather than alleviates the patient's concerns. Such responses serve to undermine the patient's trust in the psychiatrist.

Doing without explanations.   When psychiatrists do something to or for patients without reviewing their rationale and without getting the patients' consent, they falsely assume that patients accept their authority without question and are passive recipients of their ministrations. An example of doing without explanations is as follows:

> **Patient:** So you believe my problem is depression.
>
> **Psychiatrist:** Yes, and I'm writing you a prescription for some pills that you should take twice daily for a week and then increase to three a day for the second week. I will have my secretary set you up for a follow-up appointment in 2 weeks. Call me if you have any problems.

The psychiatrist in this example assumes that the patient implicitly trusts the psychiatrist's clinical judgment about diagnosis and about the precise treatment that will aid the patient without any questioning of authority. Other than in life-threatening emergency situations, psychiatrists as physicians are obligated to describe what they plan to do for or to patients and not only to obtain consent in advance but to elicit patients' cooperation as well.

Put-down questions.   Although the psychiatrist may pose a question, the underlying message is one of criticism, derision, or annoyance with the patient. Examples of put-down questions include the following:

> **Patient** (*appears disheveled*): I can't seem to find work.
>
> **Psychiatrist:** How can you expect any employer to hire you when you're dressed that way?

> **Patient:** I forgot to take my pills.
>
> **Psychiatrist:** Don't you ever want to get better?

In the first example, the psychiatrist is expressing his own displeasure with the patient's dress. Although there is no justification for ever attacking a person's appearance, couching disapproval in the form of a question is an indirect way for the psychiatrist to express his own feelings. In the second example, the psychiatrist misuses the questioning mode as a way of dealing with his frustration at the patient's noncompliance with treatment. By virtue of patients' showing up for their appointments, psychiatrists should assume patients want to get better.

"You are bad" statements.   In another form of derision of a patient, the psychiatrist, falsely believing that he or she is making an interpretation, makes a statement critical of the patient:

> **Patient:** You don't seem to know what's wrong with me.
>
> **Psychiatrist:** You keep trying to put the burden of your problem on me; you're a passive-dependent personality, and that's how you deal with all your relationships.

The psychiatrist, in this case, uses a diagnostic term to label the patient, which in turn signifies to the patient that being passive-dependent is bad. The psychiatrist places the patient in a defensive posture while falsely believing that he or she is interpreting the patient's behavior. The psychiatrist in this example is also encouraging the patient to play "word games," which often leads to adversarial jousting.

Trapping patients with their own words.   The psychiatrist may focus on contradictions in the patient's verbalizations to the point of trapping the patient. An example would be a patient who protests that he is very fond of a teacher whom he describes as not treating him fairly in the classroom. The psychiatrist then traps him in the following manner:

> **Psychiatrist:** And how do you feel about this teacher who treated you unfairly?
>
> **Patient:** I am furious with him.
>
> **Psychiatrist:** Now you're contradicting yourself. Before you said how fond you were of him, and now you claim you're furious.
>
> **Patient:** You're wrong—I never said that.

At this point, the flow of the interview stops. The patient gets angry and upset that the psychiatrist has trapped him in a contradiction. The patient was initially denying his angry feelings. Confronting the patient with a contradiction in his verbalizations is counterproductive.

Nonverbal messages of resentment.   A psychiatrist may be annoyed at or disapprove of a patient's behaviors. Rather than dealing directly with the patient, he or she uses body language to signal disapproval. For example, a patient walks into the psychiatrist's office and ignores "No Smoking" signs. The patient lights up a cigarette. Instead of confronting the patient's behavior, the psychiatrist begins coughing frequently and frowning at the patient. The patient picks up from these nonverbal cues that the psychiatrist is signaling disapproval. The patient believes that the psychiatrist disapproves of her as a patient. Because of the psychiatrist's behavior, the patient experiences diminished self-esteem and feels demeaned (Platt and McMath 1979; Strayhorn 1977).

SPECIFIC INTERVIEWING SITUATIONS

Psychiatrists learn to adapt their interviewing methods and styles on the basis of multiple variables that any individual patient presents, including particular psychiatric problems.

Interviewing the Delusional Patient

A delusion is a fixed, false belief that the patient holds to even though it has no basis in reality. There are several types of delusions: delusions of persecution, delusions of grandiosity, erotomania, delusions of jealousy, delusions of reference, and somatic delusions. The psychiatrist inquires whether the patient has ever acted on a delusional belief or has plans to do so.

The psychiatrist's examination of the patient's delusional beliefs will yield significant information regarding the patient's underlying psychodynamic conflicts. The psychiatrist can also observe how the patient defends against painful realities in his or her life and uses his or her delusional system as a form of protection. The psychiatrist looks for the precipitating stresses in the patient's life that led to the formation of these delusions.

The delusional patient is most often brought to treatment by third parties against his or her will. It is important for the psychiatrist to empathically acknowledge the patient's wishes not to be a patient, but also to point out how the psychiatrist may be helpful to the patient and to encourage the patient to communicate with him or her.

The most common error for the neophyte resident is to try to convince the patient with delusions that his or her false beliefs make no logical sense. Such an approach is counterproductive. Instead, the psychiatrist takes a neutral stance with the patient and neither agrees with a delusional belief nor openly challenges its verity. Only at such a point that the patient expresses doubt about a delusion should the psychiatrist support this doubt. Patients usually do not consider their delusions to be a clinical problem. It is preferable for the psychiatrist to focus on other signs and symptoms for which the patient may want help.

Very often, as the patient's overall clinical condition improves, he or she stops talking about his or her delusional beliefs. It is not necessary for the psychiatrist to raise questions about the delusions, even though he or she may be curious about how steadfast the patient is in retaining the delusions.

Interviewing the Depressed and Potentially Suicidal Patient

Depression, one of the most common problems that psychiatrists evaluate and treat in their practice, can be either a primary psychiatric disorder or secondary to medical disorders or other psychiatric disorders. It is frequently part of a dual diagnosis. For every depressed patient, it is imperative that psychiatrists explore the risks of suicide.

The assessment of depression begins with the patient's appearance and behavior. The psychiatrist observes the patient's general demeanor and posture to be slowed. The patient walks slowly, holding his or her head down, and lacks in spontaneity. Some patients present with an anxious or an agitated depression, with the wringing of hands and pacing. Others exhibit a retarded depression, with a paucity of spontaneous movements. The pace of the interview itself is usually slow, with the patient responding to questions with long pauses and short answers. Very often there is a blunted range of facial expressions, and, at other times, the patient may cry or fight back tears. Not all patients will verbalize feeling depressed. They will often give clues through their verbalizations that indicate a sense of giving up and of not wanting to go on. A depressed patient's thinking and verbalizations are also slowed. Voice intonation patterns are often monotonal. Thinking often reveals excessive guilt, feelings of loss of self-esteem and self-confidence, and a general lack of interest in activities that the patient had previously participated in. These patients exhibit low energy, and their social contacts are diminished as well.

Because the patient often has a number of physical manifestations that are part of the depression, the psychiatrist explores problems with sleep, appetite, bowel habits, sexual functioning, and pain syndromes, among others. The psychiatrist explores the nature of these disturbances and how they have interfered with the patient's functioning. The patient is helped to understand that these physical changes are part of the depression. Because the patient often does not associate the physical complaints with depression, this new knowledge can be a relief.

In exploring the origins of a depression, the psychiatrist looks for significant losses and separations in the patient's life. Death or separation from a loved one often leads to depression. The onset of the syndrome of depression is often times delayed following a significant loss. The psychiatrist should also explore anniversary phenomena—depression that occurs on the anniversary of a significant loss.

The psychiatrist takes an active role when interviewing the depressed patient. The patient is encouraged to verbalize what he or she is experiencing. The psychiatrist empathizes with the patient's pain and mental anguish. Prolonged silences on the part of the psychiatrist are rarely helpful with these patients and should be discouraged.

The neophyte psychiatrist is often reluctant to inquire about suicide with a depressed patient, fearing that he or she may be planting an idea that the patient may not have had, or fearing that the patient will take offense. Psychiatrists' inquiries about suicide are, on the contrary, a relief to patients. It is essential that the psychiatrist find out what kinds of thoughts the patient has had regarding suicide and whether the patient has ever acted on these thoughts, what plans he or she currently has, and what has kept him or her from acting on these plans.

The subject of suicide is introduced with such questions as "Have things ever gotten so bad that you've had thoughts of ending your life?" If the patient answers in the affirmative, the psychiatrist follows with "Tell me about them." In inquiring about past suicidal behavior, the psychiatrist asks, "Have you ever done anything to hurt yourself?" Again, the psychiatrist pursues details. If all the responses are about the past, the psychiatrist inquires about the present with "Have you had any thoughts of ending your life lately?" The interest here is not only in thoughts or actions but also in the patient's ability to control these impulses. To assess this, the psychiatrist inquires, "What is it that has kept you from carrying out your plans?"

By pursuing the topic of suicide, the psychiatrist arrives at a clinical judgment about the imminent danger of suicide in the patient's life. He or she also learns about what suicide means to an individual patient.

Interviewing the Psychosomatic Patient

Patients with psychosomatic illnesses are usually referred by their primary care physician and rarely seek psychiatric consultation on their own. Their greatest fear is that psychiatric consultation is being sought because they are "crazy" or because the primary physician does not believe that they have a legitimate reason for their complaints. Psychosomatic patients may interpret psychiatric consultation as a signal that their primary physician has given up on them. It is important for the psychiatrist to discuss with the referring physician what the patient has been told about the consultation and to ascertain what clinical questions the referring physician wants the psychiatrist to address in the consultation. Before seeing the patient, the psychiatrist reviews the patient's medical history, including medications and medical procedures and the results of any tests given.

After introducing and identifying himself or herself as a psychiatrist, the consultant psychiatrist reviews with the patient the complaints that led to the patient's seeking care. The psychiatrist then explores with the patient his or her understanding of the reasons for the primary physician's wanting a psychiatric consultation. The psychiatrist establishes his or her interest in the patient's physical complaints

as well as any emotional concomitants and also follows up with the patient in clarifying any misunderstandings about the psychiatrist's role as a consultant.

While reviewing the patient's medical history with the patient, the psychiatrist looks for clues to any psychological stresses that may be accompanying the patient's physical symptoms. The psychiatrist checks for autonomic signs of distress during the interview and inquires about the patient's feelings at these points. As the interview progresses, the psychiatrist reviews the specific circumstances that were occurring in the patient's life when he or she first became symptomatic, any significant antecedent events, and the range of feelings that the patient experienced with the onset of the illness.

The psychiatrist inquires about how the patient's symptoms may be interfering with the patient's level of functioning and looks for both the primary and the secondary gains of the symptoms. The psychiatrist explores what the patient feels is wrong with himself or herself, what he or she fears will happen as a result of the illness, and in what ways the symptoms will interfere with the patient's future life.

Because the patient's presenting complaints are physical, the psychiatrist establishes that he or she is interested in these complaints and that in no way is his or her intention to minimize the significance of the complaints. The psychiatrist acknowledges that subjective complaints are real and that his or her inquiries about emotional concomitants are necessary to gain a better understanding of the patient.

The psychiatrist leaves time at the end of the psychiatric consultation visit to answer specific questions that the patient may have or to clarify any misunderstandings. The psychiatrist also summarizes his or her findings and shares any specific recommendations, including return visits to further explore areas not covered in the initial visit. Usually several visits are needed before patients are ready to accept the importance of the impact of emotional reactions on their physical complaints.

Interviewing the Elderly Patient

Elderly patients often need special attention during a psychiatric interview. Psychiatrists usually need to slow the pace of the interview and may need several short interviews instead of one prolonged interview. They need to pay special attention to any physical limitations, whether sensory, motor, coordination, extrapyramidal, or other. For example, hearing-impaired individuals might need to be seated closer to the psychiatrist. The psychiatrist must speak in clear, loud tones for a hearing-impaired elderly patient to be able to understand him or her. Visual impairments such as cataracts and macular degeneration may lead to elderly patients' not being able to clearly see those interviewing them. Unlike younger patients, with whom an initial handshake may and should be the only physical contact, elderly patients may need to have psychiatrists assist with the patients' safely walking in and out of the room, and a gentle pat on the shoulder or a grasping of elderly patients' hands as a signal of reassurance is often indicated.

The physical status of elderly patients needs special attention so that those with cardiac or respiratory limitations are not overly stressed in an individual interview session. The psychiatrist needs to review medications prescribed and those taken over the counter so that he or she is especially attuned to any drug interactions and aware of the influences of these medications on the elderly patient's mental status and behavior.

Interviewing the Violent Patient

Patients exhibiting violent behavior are most frequently seen in a hospital emergency room setting. The police often bring violent patients to the hospital. One of the first judgments that a psychiatrist must make is the safety of removing physical restraints from patients. Before the police remove handcuffs, the psychiatrist makes contact with the patient to assess his or her reality testing and ability to verbalize. If the patient is judged to be unable to communicate verbally or to be out of touch with reality, the psychiatrist, before proceeding with the interview, requests that the patient be placed in a quiet room where he or she may be restrained. Restraints can be physical or chemical. The psychiatrist first talks with a patient who can communicate verbally about whether to remove restraints. If the patient exhibits any hostile or belligerent behavior when the restraints are being removed, the psychiatrist requests that the restraints remain in place until the patient is calmer. The interview is often conducted with a security officer present, as the officer's uniform is often a deterrent to patients' acting out their impulses. The psychiatrist emphasizes to the patient that the restraints are needed for both the patient's safety and for the safety of persons in the immediate area.

The psychiatrist never confronts or challenges a violent patient. The psychiatrist lets the patient know when the psychiatrist is frightened by the patient's behavior, and he or she seeks assistance in placing a potentially violent patient in a safe setting. On inpatient units, a seclusion room is used as a temporary placement for violent patients until their behavior is judged not to be dangerous to themselves or others.

The key factor in the approach to violent patients is

safety. The psychiatrist works with available staff to maintain the safety of the patient, the staff, and other patients. At no time should the psychiatrist resort to individual heroics in trying to subdue a violent patient. Each hospital is advised to have an emergency plan of action for the management of violent patients, with nursing personnel trained to respond to help control violent patients' behavior. This plan should be rehearsed at staff meetings from month to month, because personnel may change or may forget procedures (Slaby et al. 1981).

Interviewing Relatives

The importance of obtaining consent from the patient before interviewing relatives was addressed earlier in this chapter. Interviewing relatives can serve several useful functions. The relatives' observations of the patient's presenting problems, their impressions of his or her current living situation, their understanding of the family, their knowledge of the patient's past history, and their recital of developmental milestones can aid in the diagnosis and add to the psychiatrist's understanding of the patient. Relatives can also serve as valuable allies in the treatment process. They can learn to recognize early signs of decompensation and to seek help to prevent further decompensation. They can participate in treatment and aid with compliance, such as with medications, and they can work with the patient and psychiatrist in noting significant changes in the patient's condition. Such changes can include the onset of manic symptoms, suicidal thoughts or behaviors, and psychotic behaviors. The psychiatrist can assess whether couples or family therapy may benefit the patient. The more serious the psychiatric condition, the more likely that the patient will benefit from a relative's participation in assessment and/or treatment. The relative's participation is contingent on the knowledge and agreement that the psychiatrist cannot, without obtaining consent, divulge to a relative any material that the patient presented in confidence to the psychiatrist. On the other hand, the psychiatrist can share any material with the patient that a relative presents. It is of vital importance to consider involving family members and other significant persons in the treatment of most (although not all) patients.

PAST HISTORY

The previous section on interviewing emphasized the importance of the psychiatrist's pursuing a patient's history according to the leads that the patient presents. However, when recording the material, a specific format is used.

This section provides an outline of such a format for the patient's record.

IDENTIFICATION OF THE PATIENT

The psychiatrist begins with a brief report of who the patient is, including the following:

- Full name
- Age
- Race
- National/ethnic origin
- Religious affiliation
- Marital status and number of children
- Current employment (past employment, if the patient is unemployed)
- Living situation
- Total number of hospitalizations (and in each case the name of the hospital), including nonpsychiatric hospitalizations
- Total number of hospitalizations *for the presenting problem* (if the patient has been hospitalized)
- Names and phone numbers of the patient's primary physicians
- Name and phone number of the nearest living relative

CIRCUMSTANCES OF REFERRAL

The psychiatrist describes how the patient came to see him or her, who referred the patient, and how the patient was transported. If a patient is referred by a professional, the name and phone number of the referring agent are recorded. If a third party brought the patient, the psychiatrist notes the third party's name and relationship to the patient. The psychiatrist records his or her judgment of the reliability of the third-party informant.

CHIEF COMPLAINT

The psychiatrist records verbatim the patient's reasons for seeking help at the time of the initial interview. If the patient is too disturbed to verbalize his or her reasons for being seen, a statement from a third party is recorded and the informant is identified. The chief complaint is not always evident in the first interview, particularly in patients with long, complex histories.

HISTORY OF PRESENT ILLNESS

The psychiatrist records the chronology of events from the onset of symptoms up to the present. With patients who can give a coherent account of their problems, the psychiatrist inquires when the symptoms began. The patient's highest level of functioning is established, and a description is made of how the patient's problems are interfering with his or her optimal functioning. The psychiatrist examines the patient's functioning in the biological, psychological, and social spheres. The psychiatrist documents all the relevant symptoms with which the patient presents. For psychotic patients, psychiatrists need to structure the interview in a way that will obtain the necessary data and to record them in an organized fashion.

The psychiatrist also notes the precipitating stressors at the time the patient became symptomatic. For psychosomatic patients, a "parallel history" is a useful technique and is considered when patients are unable to make connections between emotional factors and physical complaints. The psychiatrist draws inferences about the influence of emotional factors on the physical symptoms but does not confront the patient with these inferences. Only when the patient gives clues that he or she is ready to look at the influence of emotional factors does the psychiatrist encourage the patient in this direction.

The psychiatrist also assesses the secondary gains of the patient's symptoms but, again, does not confront the patient with his or her findings.

PSYCHIATRIC HISTORY

The psychiatrist inquires about the first time the patient was aware of any psychiatric problems. The psychiatrist asks whether any help was sought at that time, and, if help was sought, he or she notes the following:

- Who saw the patient and for how long
- The nature of the treatment
- Medications, if any, that were prescribed
- Modality that was helpful (i.e., individual therapy, group therapy, psychopharmacological interventions)
- Length of treatment
- Reason for discontinuing treatment

Significant events such as hospitalizations, as well as information on where they took place, which treatment modalities were used in these settings, and the length of stay, should also be noted. Contact with previous treating psychiatrists is most helpful in assisting with understanding past evaluations and treatments.

ALCOHOL AND DRUG HISTORY

The psychiatrist obtains a history from the patient on the consumption of alcohol and drugs. Inquiries are made about the precise amounts that are consumed and the method of administration, whether it be oral (alcohol), by sniffing (cocaine), or by injections (heroin). The frequency of use is noted. The social setting in which the substances are used is recorded. The psychiatrist learns about the patient's reasons for using drugs—that is, for recreational purposes, to treat or mask one's symptoms (e.g., hallucinations or depression), to succumb to peer pressure, or as part of an addiction pattern. Tolerance for drugs such as sedatives or narcotics is ascertained. The psychiatrist asks whether the patient has ever considered drug taking or alcohol consumption a problem. If so, the psychiatrist learns whether the patient has 1) overdosed on drugs, 2) lost consciousness in the past, and 3) ever suffered from withdrawal effects from drugs. Medical, orthopedic, and surgical complications (including head trauma) as a result of drug consumption are recorded. Any previous efforts toward withdrawal from addicting substances are noted, including problems such as delirium tremens with alcohol withdrawal. The psychiatrist also notes whether the patient has been in psychiatric treatment or has been treated in separate chemical dependency programs, including self-help groups.

The effects of alcohol consumption and drug taking on the patient's life are also evaluated. These effects include the patient's ability to maintain employment, his or her ability to maintain social relationships, and whether the patient has had any trouble with the law, such as charges of driving while intoxicated.

The effectiveness of previous therapeutic interventions is assessed. The consideration of dual diagnoses with other DSM-IV Axis I diagnoses is reviewed, along with Axis II considerations.

Collateral histories are often vital, since drug- and alcohol-consuming populations are notorious for historical distortions.

FAMILY HISTORY

The psychiatrist reviews and records a family tree and lists names and ages of living relatives and names, ages, and time of death of deceased relatives. Any emotional problems as well as organic diseases in family members are indicated. Specifically, the psychiatrist notes the following:

- Who had sought psychiatric help and their diagnosis, if known

- Psychiatric hospitalizations, if any
- What treatment modalities were administered
- The names of specific drugs taken, if known
- The outcome of treatment
- Suicidal behaviors or death by suicide

Family histories are particularly useful in families who seem to have a genetic vulnerability for psychiatric or organic diseases, including schizophrenia, major affective disorders, Huntington's chorea, and epilepsy.

The family history also describes who the significant relatives in the patient's life have been, what they were like as persons, how the patient related to them, and what roles they played in the patient's upbringing, as well as a description of current significant relationships. When obtaining information about the family from relatives, the psychiatrist notes the sources and reliability of each of the historians. The psychiatrist is also interested in assessing who the supportive figures currently are in the patient's life.

PERSONAL HISTORY

The psychiatrist obtains information on the patient's personal history in order to help determine a psychodynamic formulation of the patient's problems. The psychiatrist seeks to understand the critical past events that have led the patient to be the way he or she is today as a person. The clues regarding relevant areas to explore are gleaned from the patient's presentations of the present illness.

A patient's history is never complete. The organization of the data follows a chronology of life events.

Prenatal Period

The psychiatrist records information on the patient from conception to birth. The principal family members are described, and the environment and the household before the patient was born are noted. Significant data include whether a pregnancy was "planned," whether the baby was "wanted," what the toxicological and nutritional status of the mother was during pregnancy, whether the mother had any medical problems such as infections or obstetrical complications, and what type of prenatal care she received. Particular prenatal wishes are noted, such as whether the parents wanted a boy or a girl, what the parental expectations were for the child when he or she was growing up (e.g., to be an astronaut), whether the child was replacing one lost through a miscarriage or childhood death, and any other special characteristics that were expected of the child. Learning how names were selected and whom the child was named after (if anyone) can give important clues as to parental expectations. The recording of the father's role during the pregnancy and delivery can also yield helpful information. Data about any problems with the delivery, such as a cesarean section and the reasons for it, and any defects at birth are also important to record. Drugs taken by the mother, whether prescribed, over the counter, or illicit, are important to know.

Infancy and Early Childhood Development

The psychiatrist describes the early infant-mother relationship, noting any problems in feeding and sleep patterns, as well as development milestones such as smiling, sitting, standing, and walking. Infantile illnesses or illnesses of the infant's caregivers are noted, as well as how such illnesses may have affected the development of the baby. The psychiatrist also ascertains who the significant people were in the caregiving of the baby and what particular influences each individual had on the child's development.

Symptoms of unusual rocking behaviors, head banging, screaming, thumb sucking, temper tantrums, bed wetting, and nail biting are explored and recorded in detail. Delays of motor activities, speech development, and socialization are noted.

A description is given of each of the siblings at home and of how the early sibling relationships developed. The psychiatrist looks for the caregiving roles of siblings as well as roles in which rivalries developed.

To assess social development, the psychiatrist examines the child's play activities. Independent behaviors and the capacity to concentrate and to look for social interactions are assessed. The patient's earliest memories and the events and feelings associated are important to record. The psychiatrist also explores favorite childhood stories and the patient's associations with them, as well as favorite activities and favorite people.

Middle Childhood (Ages 3–11)

The psychiatrist, who is interested in the intellectual development of the child, inquires about nursery school experiences and how the child adapted to social situations. The child's reactions to first going off to school and leaving home are noted. The psychiatrist inquires about important figures in the patient's life: schoolteachers, ministers, camp counselors, and childhood friends. The child's recreational, athletic, and cultural activities are explored, as well as how the child would spend a typical day. Explorations regarding academic development include the child's favorite subjects, subjects that he or she excelled in, and those that he or she found difficult. If the child repeated any grades, the reasons for having done so are noted.

The psychiatrist also records any prolonged illnesses, surgeries, and accidents with injuries and the influence of these medical/surgical events on the patient's life. In children who were "accident prone" or had multiple soft-tissue injuries and multiple fractures, the psychiatrist is alerted to the possibility of child abuse.

Areas that relate to discipline and the types of punishment that were used are also explored. The psychiatrist learns who the figures were who meted out punishment and assesses the effects that these behaviors had on the child's development. The psychiatrist also explores any significant personal losses or separations during this period, such as the death of significant figures and whether there were any parental separations or divorces and remarriages. The emotional impact of these events is also recorded.

Symptoms reflecting emotional distress are noted. These would include enuresis, nail biting, night terrors, and excessive masturbation.

Late Childhood and Adolescence

The teenage years are important transitional years in the development of the individual from those of a dependent child to an independent adult. The psychiatrist traces biological development in terms of major body changes and their influence on the individual, as well as the child's psychological development and social development. The psychiatrist inquires about the child's interests and activities, participation in organized sports, hobbies, church activities, introduction to civic responsibilities, work history (often beginning with baby-sitting and newspaper delivery routes), social network, and the influence of religious instruction and the commonalities and differences of the child's belief systems with those of his or her family. In addition to noting the grades and achievements in academic work, the psychiatrist further studies the child's academic potential and his or her areas of special interest and the child's relationship with his or her peer group and with people whom the child likes and wants to emulate, such as teachers, coaches, or public figures.

The psychiatrist examines areas that have led to psychological stress, such as problems in relationships with authority figures, with peers, and with siblings. The psychiatrist also inquires about eating disorders, sleep disturbances, periods of depression, self-mutilation, suicidal ideation, alcohol and drug intake, and problems that relate to the personal identity of the teenager.

Adulthood

The psychiatrist explores the patient's capacities for intimacy, development of friendships, social networks, adult educational history, employment record, intellectual pursuits, recreational activities, and avocational interests. The patient's military history, civic responsibilities, religious affiliations, value systems, political involvements, fiscal security, vacation habits, and relationship with his or her family are also reviewed. The psychiatrist documents what the patient's plans are for the future, whether such plans are achievable, and how the patient intends to implement them. The psychiatrist then records the impact of illnesses, both the patient's own and those affecting close relationships and affecting the patient's life.

SEXUAL HISTORY

The psychiatrist inquires about the patient's early life experiences related to sexual development. The patient's childhood sexual playing experiences, such as playing "doctor" and "nurse," observing the genitalia of other children, and fantasies about sexuality as a child, are explored. The psychiatrist notes not only the child's reactions to these fantasies and play activities but also how family members reacted when the child revealed them or was found engaged in them.

The psychiatrist inquires about what and how the patient learned about sexual activities, conception, and pregnancy and who was responsible for the learning. The reactions of the patient's parents to the patient's inquiries about how babies are born are elicited. The psychiatrist also inquires about a history of sexual abuse.

The psychiatrist asks both male and female patients about their experiences in puberty. With female patients, the inquiries begin with menarche. The female patient is asked about who prepared her for menses, what she was told about what to expect, what the meaning of menses was to the patient, and what the parents' reactions to the menarche were. For both male and female patients, a masturbatory history is obtained with explorations about fantasies that accompanied masturbation. Descriptions of sexual experiences, both heterosexual and homosexual, are elicited, including activities such as kissing, necking, petting, and sexual intercourse.

Attitudes of the patient toward heterosexual and homosexual fantasies and experiences are noted. The psychiatrist also records parental and sibling responses to the adolescent's activities.

The psychiatrist then explores adulthood attitudes and behaviors: the patient's choice of partner, how the couple met, their courting history, their engagement history, premarital sexual activities, their marriage, and (with traditional marriages) their honeymoon. Also recorded are the couple's expectations regarding children, as well as the cou-

ple's reactions to childbearing and child rearing and to different stages of development of their children. Marital crises and threats, or actual separations and/or divorces, are also subjects of inquiry. Similar inquiries are made for patients with nontraditional relationships.

Areas of sexual conflict or sexual dysfunctions are examined, such as loss of sexual desire, inability to perform, difficulties with erections and ejaculations, and problems of pain with intercourse or failure to achieve orgasm. The biological, psychological, and social factors influencing these dysfunctions are sought.

Patients will often be reluctant to discuss some, if not all, of these topics regarding sexuality because of accompanying shame, embarrassment, or discomfort. Psychiatrists learn to be nonjudgmental and supportive in exploring the sexual history of their patients.

MEDICAL HISTORY

The psychiatrist reviews the patient's medical history, including common as well as chronic childhood illnesses, conditions leading to frequent medical consultation and treatment, and those requiring emergency room visits as well as those leading to hospitalizations. The psychiatrist also reviews the patient's surgical experiences and those requiring the administration of anesthesia. The history of accidents and orthopedic interventions is recorded. In addition to the nature and course of each illness, the psychiatrist reviews the impact of these illnesses on the child's growth and development. Inquiries are made about the patient's attitudes toward the professionals who cared for him or her as a child as well as family attitudes toward his or her medical problems.

The psychological meaning of illnesses and interventions is explored in terms of the patient's feelings about injury to body parts, effects on body image, and fears and concerns about invalidism and death. The psychiatrist reviews adult-onset illnesses, medical interventions, and surgical and obstetrical events. The effects of these on the patient's functioning at work and at play, on the families, and on interpersonal relationships are noted. The psychiatrist also assesses the patient's motivations for and capacities to assist in recovery, his or her levels of denial of the effect of serious illnesses on functioning and longevity, and the coping mechanisms that the patient employs. Inquiries are made about support systems that the patient has used to aid in the recovery from past illnesses, including the availability of these systems and the willingness of the patient to use them to help with the current situation (Table 6–5).

TABLE 6–5.   Order of recording psychiatric history

1. Patient identification
2. Circumstances of referral
3. Chief complaint
4. History of present illness
5. Past psychiatric history
6. Alcohol and drug history
7. Family history
8. Past personal history
   a. Prenatal history
   b. Infancy and early childhood development
   c. Middle childhood
   d. Late childhood and adolescence
   e. Adult history
9. Sexual history
10. Medical history

PROBLEMS WITH PSYCHIATRIC HISTORY TAKING

One of the most difficult challenges for the neophyte resident in psychiatry is learning how to conduct a smoothly flowing interview that allows patients to unfold their stories in such a fashion that they feel they are understood. Simultaneously, the psychiatrist is examining for patterns of behaviors so that he or she can construct a multidimensional formulation of the patient's problems while accumulating the necessary facts and chronology of events to arrive at a cross-sectional diagnosis. In addition to a formal diagnosis, the psychiatrist attempts to obtain a keen understanding of what renders the patient unique and individual in terms of personality patterns and how the patient relates to his or her social setting and environment. Therefore, it is essential for psychiatrists not only to learn pertinent facts in patients' histories but also to learn about patterns of behavior.

The art of psychiatric interviewing develops with practice and supervision by skilled mentors. Psychiatric supervisors are well advised not only to listen to residents' verbal reports of their clinical findings but to experience firsthand how residents conduct themselves in interviews with patients. The interviewers may do this by sitting in the room with residents and patients, or they may elect to observe behind a one-way viewing mirror or review video- or audiotapes of an interview. Telemedicine should add another dimension to this type of learning in the future. The supervisors not only coach the residents about transference and countertransference issues but critique the residents' interviewing style and methods and share with residents

their observations of the residents' interviewing strengths and areas that need improvement. It is also important for supervisors to review the recording of observations and to critique the residents' record-keeping abilities (MacKinnon and Yudofsky 1986).

MENTAL STATUS EXAMINATION

The mental status examination is a description of all the areas of mental functioning of the patient. It serves the same function for psychiatrists as the physical examination does for the primary care physician. Psychiatrists follow a structured format in recording their findings. These descriptive data are then used to support the psychiatrists' diagnostic conclusions. An outline of the component parts of the mental status examination follows (Engel 1979; Keller and Manschreck 1981; Lewis 1943; Masserman and Schwab 1974; Menninger 1952; Reiser and Schroder 1980; Small 1981; Stevenson 1969; Tilley and Hoffman 1981; Trzepacz and Baker 1993; Weitzel et al. 1973).

GENERAL DESCRIPTION

Appearance

The psychiatrist records in detail the prominent physical features of an individual such that a portrait of the person could be painted that highlights his or her unique aspects. Included are facial features; hair color, texture, styling, and grooming; height; weight; body shape; cleanliness; neatness; posture; bearing; clothing; jewelry; skin texture, scar formation, and tattoos; level of eye contact; eye movements; facial expressions and mobility; tearfulness; degrees of friendliness; and an estimate of how old the patient looks compared with chronological age. In the report of these findings, poetic license can be used in painting a picture of the person.

Motor Behavior

The psychiatrist describes the patient's gait and freedom of movement, noting the firmness and strength of handshake. The psychiatrist observes any involuntary or abnormal movements such as tremors, tics, mannerisms, lip smacking, akathisias, or repeated stereotyped movements. The pace of movements, whether accelerated or retarded, is also noted. The psychiatrist comments on the purposefulness of movements and takes note of degrees of agitation of the patient as reflected in pacing and hand wringing.

Speech

The psychiatrist listens for the patient's rate of speech, the spontaneity of verbalizations, the range of voice intonation patterns, the volume in terms of loudness, defects with verbalizations such as stammering or stuttering, and any aphasias.

Attitudes

The psychiatrist routinely summarizes how the patient related to him or her in the course of the interview. The psychiatrist not only notes general impressions such as "friendly and cooperative" but focuses on any shifts or changes in attitude during particular points in the interview. An example would be the psychiatrist's noting that when inquiring about a patient's relations with authority figures, the patient related in a "belligerent, hostile, and threatening manner."

It is also helpful for the psychiatrist to keep track of his or her own attitudes toward the patient, whether they be "warm, caring, concerned, and empathic" or "frustrated and angry." Such a summary of the psychiatrist's attitudes can often help in diagnostic formulations as well as in planning treatment strategies.

EMOTIONS

Mood

Mood is the sustained feeling tone that prevails over time for a patient. At times the patient will verbalize this mood. At other times, the psychiatrist will have to inquire about it and even infer the patient's mood from observations of the patient's nonverbal body language. When describing a mood, the psychiatrist records how deeply it is felt, the length of time that it prevails, and how much it fluctuates. Anxious, panicky, terrified, sad, depressed, angry, enraged, euphoric, and guilty are moods frequently described.

Affective Expression

The psychiatrist records his or her observations regarding the range of expression of feeling tones. The predominant expression is described. This may include flat affect, in which there is virtually no visible expression of feelings during the relating of emotionally charged material. This mode of expression has been classically associated with schizophrenia. The incongruity of the expressions with the verbalizations is most striking in schizophrenia and other psychotic disorders. Constricted affects are often seen with depression, lability of mood may be associated with cognitive disorders, and blunting of affect is often seen with dementia. The psychiatrist observes and records the patient's nonverbal behaviors, such as facial mobility, voice intonation patterns, and body movements, to assess affective expression.

Appropriateness

The psychiatrist judges whether the affective tone and expression are appropriate to the subject matter being discussed in the context of the patient's thinking. Disharmonies between affective expression and thought content are worthy of exploration with the patient.

PERCEPTUAL DISTURBANCES

Hallucinations and Illusions

A *hallucination* is a perceptual distortion that a patient experiences for which there is no external stimulus. These hallucinations may be auditory (hearing noises or voices that nobody else hears), visual (seeing objects that are not present), tactile (feeling sensations when there is no stimulus for them), gustatory (tasting sensations when there is no stimulus for them), or olfactory (smelling odors that are not present). Hallucinations during the hypnagogic state (the drowsy state preceding sleep) and the hypnopompic state (the semiconscious state preceding awakening) are experiences associated with normal sleep and with narcolepsy.

An *illusion* is a false impression that results from a real stimulus. An example of an illusion is driving down a dry road and observing "water patches" several hundred feet ahead of you, then driving closer and having them disappear.

Depersonalization and Derealization

Depersonalization describes patients' feelings that they are not themselves, that they are strange, or that there is something different about themselves that they cannot account for. The symptom is associated with a variety of psychiatric disorders.

Derealization expresses patients' feeling that the environment is somehow different or strange but they cannot account for these changes. This perceptual distortion is frequently seen in schizophrenic patients.

THOUGHT PROCESS

The psychiatrist assesses how well a patient formulates, organizes, and expresses his thoughts. Coherent thought is clear, easy to follow, and logical. A formal thought disorder includes all disorders of thinking that affect language, communication of thought, or thought content. Such disorder is often ascribed to the disordered thinking of schizophrenic patients.

Stream of Thought

The psychiatrist records the quantity and rate of the patient's thoughts. The psychiatrist looks for the two extremes, whether a paucity or a flooding of thoughts. He or she also notes whether there is retardation or slowing or whether there is acceleration or racing. When thoughts are so sped up that the psychiatrist has difficulty keeping up with the patient, it is termed a flight of ideas.

The psychiatrist also examines the patient for the goal directedness and continuity of the patient's thoughts. Disturbances include circumstantiality, tangential thinking, blocking, loose associations, and perseveration. *Circumstantiality* is a disorder of associations in which the patient exhibits lack of goal directedness, incorporates tedious and unnecessary details, and has difficulty in arriving at an end point. *Tangentiality* describes a thought process in which the patient digresses from the subject under discussion and introduces thoughts that seem unrelated, oblique, and irrelevant. An example of *blocking* is a sudden cessation in the middle of a sentence, at which point a patient cannot recover what he or she has said or complete his or her thoughts. *Loose associations* refers to a jumping from one topic to another with no apparent connection between the topics. *Perseveration* refers to the patient's repeating the same response to a variety of questions and topics, with an inability to change his or her responses or to change the topic.

Marked abnormalities of thought processes include neologisms, word salad, clang associations, and echolalia. A *neologism* is a word that a patient makes up—often a condensation of several words that is unintelligible to another person. *Word salad* is an incomprehensible mixing of meaningless words and phrases. In *clang associations*, the connections between thoughts may be tenuous, and the patient uses rhyming and punning. *Echolalia* describes a patient's irrelevant parroting of what another person has said.

Thought Content (Delusions, Obsessions, Compulsions, Preoccupations, Phobias)

Thought content refers to what the patient talks about. There are specific areas that the psychiatrist inquires about if they are not brought up by the patient. One important area is whether the patient has suicidal thoughts. This is particularly important in patients who signal feelings of helplessness, hopelessness, worthlessness, or giving up.

Delusions are false fixed beliefs that have no rational basis in reality and are deemed unacceptable by the patient's culture. Delusions that cannot be understood by other psychological processes are referred to as *primary delusions*. Examples include thought insertion, thought broadcasting, and beliefs about world destruction. *Secondary delusions* are based on other psychological experiences. These include delusions derived from hallucinations, other delusions, and morbid affective states.

Types of delusions include those of persecution, of jealousy, of guilt, of love, of poverty, and of nihilism.

In addition to the description of delusions, the psychiatrist assesses the degrees of organization of the delusion. The psychiatrist notes ideas of reference and ideas of influence.

The psychiatrist notes any *obsessions* the patient may have. These are marked by repetitive, unwelcome, irrational thoughts that impose themselves on the patient's consciousness and over which he or she has no apparent control. These thoughts are accompanied by feelings of anxious dread and are ego-alien, unacceptable, and undesirable. They are strongly resisted by the patient.

Compulsions, a closely parallel phenomenon, are repetitive, stereotyped behaviors that the patient feels impelled to perform ritualistically, even though he or she recognizes the irrationality and absurdity of the behaviors. Although no pleasure is derived from performing such an act, there is a temporary sense of relief of tension when it is completed.

In addition to describing obsessions and compulsions, the psychiatrist discusses the degree of interference with the patient's functioning. *Preoccupations* are also noted. These reflect the patient's absorption with his or her own thoughts to such a degree that the patient loses contact with external reality. The degree of preoccupation is also observed. Mild forms are reflected in absentmindedness; severe forms can involve suicidal or homicidal ideation and the autistic thinking of the schizophrenic patient.

Phobias are morbid fears that are reflected by morbid anxiety. They are often not spontaneously conveyed in the interview, and the psychiatrist should make specific inquiries about their presence (Campbell 1981; Stone 1988; Thompson 1979).

Abstract Thinking

Abstract, or categorical, thinking is formed late in the development of thought and reflects the capacity to formulate concepts and to generalize. Several methods are used to test this capacity. These include testing similarities, differences, and the meaning of proverbs. The inability to abstract is referred to as concreteness, which in turn reflects an earlier childhood development of thought. Concreteness of responses on formal testing reflects intellectual impoverishment, cultural deprivation, and cognitive disorders such as dementia. Bizarre and inappropriate responses to proverbs reflect schizophrenic thinking.

An example of testing for similarities is the psychiatrist's asking a patient how a peach and a plum are alike. The patient who responds "They are both fruit" reflects her ability to abstract. The patient who responds "You bite into each of them" exhibits a form of concreteness. A bizarre response would be "Juice, plum, like peach, you know."

In testing with proverbs, psychiatrists begin with "Do you know what proverbs are? They are sayings that have different meanings for different people. I will tell you a proverb and ask what it means to you. For instance, 'A bird in the hand is worth two in the bush.' What does that mean to you?" A patient's explanation, "It's preferable to gamble on something small that you know you can win than to take the chance of losing it all by going for a long shot" is an example of an abstract response. A response such as "Having one bird in your hand—you know—is better than having two birds in a bush" is an example of a concrete response. An inappropriate response would be "Birds fly—one bird flies, two birds fly—fly away birdy—chirp, chirp."

Education and Intelligence

Intelligence is best measured in the clinical interview by the patient's use of vocabulary. The expectations of levels of intelligence are influenced by the level of education of the patient. If the patient had dropped out of grade school and exhibits an advanced vocabulary, the psychiatrist concludes that the patient's intelligence exceeds his or her scholastic achievement. Specific testing for intelligence is used only when deficits are anticipated on the basis of the interview.

Concentration

Concentration reflects the patient's ability to focus and to maintain his or her attention on a task. In the interview, troubles with concentration are reflected in the patient's inability to pay attention to the questions that he or she is being asked. He or she may be distracted by external or internal stimuli. When the patient's concentration is impaired, the psychiatrist often has to repeat the questions.

Formal testing for concentration includes serial 7s, in which the patient is asked to subtract 7 from 100 and keep subtracting 7 from each answer. Serial 3s or counting backward from 20 can be substituted if the patient has cognitive

difficulties performing serial 7s. If the patient has been asked to do serial 7s repeatedly, he or she should start subtracting from 101 rather than 100 to avoid giving learned responses.

Immediate recall and concentration abilities often overlap. One way to test for immediate recall is to ask the patient to repeat digits forward and backward.

The patient is instructed that the psychiatrist is going to recite numbers and then ask the patient to repeat them. The psychiatrist tells the patient, "I am going to recite the numbers 3, 8, 7, and I want you to repeat 3, 8, 7." The psychiatrist recites the numbers 1 second apart and then asks the patient to repeat them. Once the patient understands the instruction, the psychiatrist recites three other numbers, increasing by 1 the number he or she recites until the patient fails to repeat them accurately. If the patient fails to repeat six numbers forward, the psychiatrist then gives a different series of six numbers. If again the patient fails to repeat them, the psychiatrist stops the exercise and records that the patient was able to repeat five digits forward.

The psychiatrist then conducts an exercise with repeating digits backward. The patient is instructed that when the psychiatrist says, "4, 9, 2," he or she wants the patient to respond, "2, 9, 4." Again, the difficulty is increased by adding one digit at a time until the patient fails to repeat the numbers backward on two trials. The psychiatrist then records how many numbers the patient can recite backward.

ORIENTATION (TIME, PLACE, PERSON, SITUATION)

Orientation reflects patients' capacities to know who they are, where they are, what date and time it is, and what their present circumstances are. Patients who have deficits in three spheres are commonly suffering from cognitive disorders. Testing for time includes asking the patient the month, the day of the month, the year, the day of the week, and the time of day and the season of the year. Orientation to place includes the patient's knowing the name of the place where he or she is currently located and the name of the city and state. Orientation to person includes the patient's knowing his or her own name and the names and roles of persons in his or her immediate surroundings. Orientation to situation indicates the patient's present circumstances and why he or she finds himself or herself in such circumstances. This is often an important clue toward the competency of individuals to give informed consent. In reversible cognitive disorders such as delirium, the reorientation to person precedes that of place, and the last function recovered is time.

Psychiatrists introduce orientation testing with a question such as "Do you have any difficulties keeping track of time?—For instance, do you know what today's date is? the month? the year? What day of the week is this? Do you know the name of this place? What is your full name? Do you know my name?"

MEMORY

Remote Memory

Remote memory is the recollection of events from earlier in life. The psychiatrist tests for this function by asking where the patient grew up, where he or she went to school, and what his or her first job was and inquires about significant people from the past (e.g., naming of presidents) and also significant events (e.g., World War II, the Korean War, the Vietnam War).

Recent Past Memory

Recent past memory refers to recalling verifiable events from the past few days. To test for this, the psychiatrist inquires about what the patient ate for breakfast or what he or she read in the newspaper or asks for details about what the patient watched on television the night before.

Recent Memory

Recent or short-term memory is gauged by the patient's capacity to recount what he or she was told 5 minutes after hearing it and being coached to remember it. The psychiatrist tests this capacity by asking the patient to repeat the names of three unrelated objects, then informing him or her that they will go on to discuss other subjects and that in 5 minutes the patient will be asked to name the three objects (Albert 1984; Folstein et al. 1975; Gurland et al. 1976; Taylor et al. 1980; Yudofsky and Hales 1992).

IMPULSE CONTROL

Impulse control is "the ability to control the expression of aggressive, hostile, fearful, guilty, affectionate, or sexual impulses in situations where their expression should be maladaptive" (MacKinnon and Yudofsky 1986, p. 74). Manifestations of this phenomenon are verbal and/or behavioral. A loss of control can reflect a low frustration tolerance (MacKinnon and Yudofsky 1986; Yudofsky et al. 1986).

JUDGMENT

Judgment refers to the patient's capacity to make appropriate decisions and appropriately act on them in social situations. An assessment of this function is best made in the course of obtaining the patient's history. There is no necessary correlation between intelligence and judgment. Formal testing is rarely helpful. An example of testing would be to ask the patient "What would you do if you saw a train approaching a broken track?"

INSIGHT

The capacity of the patient to be aware and to understand that he or she has a problem or illness and to be able to review its probable causes and arrive at tenable solutions is referred to as insight. Emotional insight refers to the patient's awareness of his or her motivations, and, in turn, his or her feelings, so that the patient can change longstanding, ingrained patterns of behavior. Self-observation alone is insufficient for insight. Emotional insight must be applied for change to occur (Donnelly et al. 1970; Ross and Leichner 1984).

RELIABILITY

Upon completion of an interview, the psychiatrist assesses the reliability of the information that has been obtained. Factors affecting reliability include the patient's intellectual endowment, his or her honesty and motivations, the presence of psychosis or organic defects, and the patient's tendency to magnify or understate his or her problems (Table 6–6).

PSYCHODYNAMIC FORMULATION

At the conclusion of the interview, history taking, and mental status examination, the psychiatrist documents a psychodynamic formulation of the patient. The psychiatrist describes the key elements of the patient's personality structures, principal psychological conflicts, and healthier, adaptive abilities.

The psychiatrist assesses the ego functions of the patient, including defense mechanisms used, regulation and control of drives, relationships to others, self-representation, stimulus regulation, adaptive relaxation, reality testing, and synthetic integration. By reviewing the patient's developmental history, the psychiatrist assesses the patient's typical drives, impulses, wishes, and anxieties at each stage of development. The psychiatrist can then establish the origins of each of the patient's conflicts and how they carry over to successive periods of development. The psychiatrist focuses on the major adaptive problems of the patient and on how earlier developmental deficits help ex-

TABLE 6–6.   The mental status examination

1. General description
   a. Appearance
   b. Motor behavior
   c. Speech
   d. Attitudes
2. Emotions
   a. Mood
   b. Affective expression
   c. Appropriateness
3. Perceptual disturbances
   a. Hallucinations
   b. Illusions
   c. Depersonalization
   d. Derealization
4. Thought process
   a. Stream of thought
   b. Thought content
   c. Abstract thinking
   d. Education and intelligence
   e. Concentration
5. Orientation
6. Memory
7. Impulse control
8. Judgment
9. Insight

plain the patient's current difficulties (Freud 1936/1946; Pruyser 1979; Wallerstein 1983; Yudofsky et al. 1986).

Psychiatrists thus trace from early development to the present patients' major conflicts, evolving symptoms, character traits, and defenses. They then organize these data in a psychodynamic formulation (MacKinnon and Yudofsky 1986).

REFERENCES

Albert M: Assessment of cognitive function in the elderly. Psychosomatics 25:310–313, 316–317, 1984

American Psychiatric Association: Diagnostic and Statistical Manual of Mental Disorders, 4th Edition. Washington, DC, American Psychiatric Association, 1994

American Psychiatric Association: The Principles of Medical Ethics With Annotations Especially Applicable to Psychiatry, Washington, DC, American Psychiatric Association, 1995

Balint M: The Doctor, His Patient and the Illness, 2nd Edition. New York, International Universities Press, 1972

Bernstein L, Bernstein RS: Interviewing: A Guide for Health Professionals. New York, Appleton-Century-Crofts, 1980

Bird B: Talking With Patients. Philadelphia, PA, JB Lippincott, 1973

Campbell RJ: Psychiatric Dictionary, 5th Edition. New York, Oxford University Press, 1981

Donnelly J, Rosenberg M, Fleeson WP: The evolution of the mental status—past and future. Am J Psychiatry 126: 997–1002, 1970

Edelson M: Language and medicine, in Applied Psycholinguistics and Mental Health. Edited by Rieber RW. New York, Plenum, 1980, pp 177–204

Engel IM: The mental status examination in psychiatry: origin, use and content. Journal of Psychiatric Education 3: 99–108, 1979

Fenichel O: Ego strength and ego weakness, in Collected Papers (Series 2). New York, WW Norton, 1984

Folstein MF, Folstein SW, McHugh PR: "Mini-Mental State": a practical method of grading the cognitive state of patients for the clinician. J Psychiatr Res 12:189–198, 1975

Freud A: The Ego and the Mechanisms of Defense (1936). New York, International Universities Press, 1946

Garrett A: Interviewing: Its Principles and Methods. New York, Family Service Association of America, 1942

Gill M, Newman R, Redich FC: The Initial Interview in Psychiatric Practice. New York, International Universities Press, 1954

Greenspan SI, Greenspan NT: The Clinical Interview of the Child, 2nd Edition. Washington, DC, American Psychiatric Press, 1991

Group for the Advancement of Psychiatry: Initial Interviews. New York, Group for the Advancement of Psychiatry, 1961

Gurland BJ, Copeland L, Sharpe J, et al: The Geriatric Mental Status Interview (GMS). Int J Aging Hum Dev 7:303–311, 1976

Halleck SL: Evaluation of the Psychiatric Patient: A Primer. New York, Plenum, 1991

Hartmann H: Essays on Ego Psychology: Selected Problems in Psychoanalytic Theory. New York, International Universities Press, 1964

Havens LL: The need for tests of normal functioning in the psychiatric interview. Am J Psychiatry 141:1208–1211, 1984

Keller MB, Manschreck TC: The bedside mental status examination—reliability and validity. Compr Psychiatry 22:500–511, 1981

Kestenbaum CJ: The clinical interview of the child, in Textbook of Child and Adolescent Psychiatry. Edited by Wiener JM. Washington, DC, American Psychiatric Press, 1991, pp 65–73

Kosten TA, Rounsaville BJ: Sensitivity of psychiatric diagnosis based on the best estimate procedure. Am J Psychiatry 149:1225–1227, 1992

Leon RL: Psychiatric Interviewing: A Primer. New York, Elsevier/North Holland, 1982

Leventhal BL, Conroy LM: The parent interview, in Textbook of Child and Adolescent Psychiatry. Edited by Wiener JM. Washington, DC, American Psychiatric Press, 1991, pp 78–83

Lewis NDC: Outlines for Psychiatric Examinations, 3rd Edition. Albany, NY, New York State Department of Mental Hygiene, 1943

Luborsky L: Principles of Psychoanalytic Psychotherapy: A Manual for Supportive-Expressive Treatment. New York, Basic Books, 1984

MacKinnon RA, Michels R: The Psychiatric Interview in Clinical Practice. Philadelphia, PA, WB Saunders, 1971

MacKinnon RA, Yudofsky SC: The Psychiatric Evaluation in Clinical Practice. Philadelphia, PA, JB Lippincott, 1986

Masserman JH, Schwab JJ: The Psychiatric Examination. New York, Intercontinental Medical Books, 1974

Menninger KA: A Manual for Psychiatric Case Study. New York, Grune and Stratton, 1952

Morrison J: The First Interview: A Guide for Clinicians, New York, NY, Guilford Press, 1993

Nurcombe B, Fitzhenry-Coor I: How do psychiatrists think? clinical reasoning in the psychiatric interview: a research and education project. Aust N Z J Psychiatry 16:13–24, 1982

Othmer E, Othmer SC: The Clinical Interview Using DSM-IV, Vol. 1: Fundamentals. Washington, DC, American Psychiatric Press, 1994

Platt FW, McMath JC: Clinical hypocompetence: the interview. Ann Intern Med 91:898–902, 1979

Pruyser PW: The Psychological Examination: A Guide for Clinicians. New York, International Universities Press, 1979

Reiser DE, Schroder AK: Patient Interviewing: The Human Dimension. Baltimore, MD, Williams & Wilkins, 1980

Robson KS (ed): Manual of Clinical Child Psychiatry. Washington, DC, American Psychiatric Press, 1986

Ross CA, Leichner P: Residents training in the mental status examination. Can J Psychiatry 29:315–318, 1984

Rutter M, Cox A: Psychiatric interviewing techniques, I: methods and measures. Br J Psychiatry 138:273–282, 1981

Rutter M, Tuma AH, Lann IS: Assessment and Diagnosis in Child Psychopathology. New York, Guilford, 1988

Shea SC: Psychiatric Interviewing: The Art of Understanding. Philadelphia, PA, WB Saunders, 1988

Slaby AE, Lieb J, Tancredi LR: Handbook of Psychiatric Emergencies: A Guide for Emergencies in Psychiatry, 2nd Edition. Garden City, NY, Medical Examination Publishing, 1981

Small SM: Outline for Psychiatric Examination. East Hanover, NJ, Sandoz Pharmaceuticals, 1981

Stevenson I: The Psychiatric Examination. Boston, MA, Little, Brown, 1969

Stone EM: American Psychiatric Glossary, 6th Edition. Washington, DC, American Psychiatric Press, 1988

Strayhorn JM Jr: Talking It Out: A Guide to Effective Communication and Problem Solving. Champaign, IL, Illinois Research Press, 1977

Strupp HH, Binder JL: Psychotherapy in a New Key: A Guide to Time-Limited Dynamic Psychotherapy. New York, Basic Books, 1984

Sullivan HS: The Psychiatric Interview. Edited by Perry HS, Gawel ML. New York, WW Norton, 1954

Taylor MA, Abrams R, Faber R, et al: Cognitive tasks in the mental status examination. J Nerv Ment Dis 168:167–170, 1980

Thompson MGG (ed): A Resident's Guide to Psychiatric Education. New York, Plenum, 1979

Tilley DH, Hoffman JA: Mental status examination: myth or method? Compr Psychiatry 22:562–564, 1981

Trzepacz PT, Baker RW: The Psychiatric Mental Status Examination. New York, Oxford University Press, 1993

Wallerstein RS: Defenses, defense mechanisms, and the structure of the mind. J Am Psychoanal Assoc 31 (suppl):207–225, 1983

Weitzel WD, Morgan DW, Guyden TE, et al: Toward a more efficient mental status examination. Arch Gen Psychiatry 28:215–218, 1973

Whitehorn JC: Guide to interviewing and clinical personality study. Archives of Neurology and Psychiatry 52:197–216, 1944

Yudofsky SC, Hales RE (eds): American Psychiatric Press Textbook of Neuropsychiatry, 2nd Edition. Washington, DC, American Psychiatric Press, 1992

Yudofsky SC, Silver JM, Jackson W, et al: The Overt Aggression Scale for the objective rating of verbal and physical aggression. Am J Psychiatry 143:35–39, 1986

SUGGESTED READINGS

Cameron N: Personality Development and Psychopathology: A Dynamic Approach. Boston, MA, Houghton-Mifflin, 1963

Endicott J, Spitzer RL: A diagnostic interview: the Schedule for Affective Disorders and Schizophrenia. Arch Gen Psychiatry 35:837–844, 1978

Enelow AJ, Swisher SN: Interviewing and Patient Care, 2nd Edition. New York, Oxford University Press, 1979

Spitzer RL, Williams JBW: Instruction Manual for the Structured Clinical Interview for DSM-III (SCID). New York, Biometrics Research Department, New York State Psychiatric Institute, 1984

APPENDIX: GLOSSARY

Abstract thinking   The capacity to formulate concepts and to generalize.

Affect   Range of expression of feelings.

Categorical thinking (*see* Abstract thinking)

Compulsions   Repetitive stereotyped behaviors that patients feel they must perform in a ritualistic fashion even though they are consciously aware of the irrationality and absurdity of the behaviors.

Concentration   Ability to focus and maintain attention on a task.

Concrete thought   Inability to abstract.

Countertransference   A process whereby psychiatrists unconsciously project their emotions, thoughts, and wishes from their past life onto patients' personalities or onto other material that patients are presenting, thus expressing unresolved conflicts and gratifying their own personal needs.

Delusions   Fixed false beliefs that patients hold to even though the beliefs have no basis in reality.

Depersonalization   Patients' feelings that they are not themselves, that they are strange, or that there is something different about themselves for which they cannot account.

Derealization   Patients' feelings that the environment is somehow different or strange in a way for which they cannot account.

Echolalia   Irrelevant parroting of another person's words.

Hallucinations   A perceptual distortion for which there is no external stimulus.

Illusion   False impression resulting from real stimuli.

Impulse control   Ability to keep in check the expressions of aggressive, hostile, fearful, guilty, affectionate, or sexual impulses in situations when their expression would be maladaptive.

Insight   Capacity to be aware of and understand a problem or illness and be able to review probable causes and arrive at tenable solutions.

Interpretations   Inferences that psychiatrists draw from examination of repeated patterns of behavior.

Judgment   Capacity to make appropriate decisions and act upon them appropriately in social situations.

Mood   Sustained feeling tone that prevails over time for patients.

Neologism   Words made up or a condensation of several words that are unintelligible.

Phobia   Marked fear reflected by intense anxiety.

Preoccupations   Absorption with one's own thoughts to the extent of losing contact with external reality.

Resistance   A reflection of any attitudes or behaviors that run counter to the therapeutic objective of treatment.

Therapeutic alliance   A process whereby a patient's mature rational observing ego is used in combination with the psychiatrist's analytic abilities to advance the latter's understanding of the patient.

Word salad   Incomprehensible mixing of meaningless words and phrases.

CHAPTER 7

PSYCHIATRIC CLASSIFICATION

JANET B. W. WILLIAMS, D.S.W.

A 25-year-old married insurance salesman is admitted to the medical service of a hospital by his internist when he [the patient] arrives at the emergency room, for the fourth time in a month, insisting that he is having a heart attack. The cardiologist's workup is completely negative.

The patient states that his "heart problem" started 6 months ago when he had a sudden episode of terror, chest pain, palpitations, sweating, and shortness of breath while driving across a bridge on his way to visit a prospective client. His father and uncle had both had heart problems, and the patient was sure he was developing a similar illness. Not wanting to alarm his wife and family, he initially said nothing; but when the attacks began to recur several times a month, he consulted his internist. The internist found nothing wrong and told him he should try to relax, take more time off from work, and develop some leisure interests. In spite of his attempts to follow this advice, the attacks recurred with increasing intensity and frequency.

The patient claims that he believes the doctors who say there is nothing wrong with his heart, but during an attack he still becomes concerned that he is having a heart attack and will die.

How would one diagnose this patient? Does he have myocardial infarction? depression? anxiety neurosis? If you saw this patient in an emergency room, you would probably order an electrocardiogram (ECG) and perhaps other tests to rule out myocardial infarction. Once this was ruled out, if the year were 1975, you would probably diagnose the condition as anxiety neurosis and prescribe either psychotherapy alone (some would even treat this patient with psychoanalytically oriented psychotherapy or psychoanalysis) or psychotherapy and an anxiolytic such as diazepam. Over time, the anxiety symptoms would resolve or not, but in any case the patient would probably not get immediate relief.

Since 1980, however, the diagnosis and treatment of this case would be a different story. According to DSM-IV (American Psychiatric Association 1994) and its immediate predecessors, the diagnosis of panic disorder would clearly account for this patient's symptoms of sudden discrete periods of extreme fear, accompanied by physical symptoms such as chest pain, heart palpitations, sweating, shortness of breath, and a fear that he will die during the attack. Further, these symptoms seem to occur at times other than during life-threatening circumstances, and they are not precipitated just by exposure to a circumscribed phobic stimulus. The diagnosis of panic disorder indicates specific and often dramatically effective treatment: an antidepressant medication combined with behavior therapy if there is anticipatory anxiety and avoidance. This treatment works in a very high percentage of cases.

This case illustrates, as well as any case can, the importance of accurate diagnosis and also the great strides that have been made in psychiatric classification in the last 20 years. In this chapter, I discuss the general principles guiding DSM-III (American Psychiatric Association 1980), DSM-III-R (American Psychiatric Association 1987), and DSM-IV; discuss strategies useful to the clinician in making diagnoses; and review features of the major categories themselves.

GENERAL PURPOSES OF CLASSIFICATION SYSTEMS

There are three general purposes to having a diagnostic classification system, as well as many specific clinical, administrative, legal, and research purposes. First, such a system provides a language with which all mental health professionals can communicate. Generally-agreed-upon names for the various mental syndromes serve as a shorthand way of describing the entities that mental health professionals deal with, enabling professionals to make efficient communication. For example, instead of one telling a colleague that "I am seeing a patient who has depressed mood and has lost interest in things; she also has trouble sleeping, has lost her appetite, has trouble concentrating, and thinks about suicide," one is able to say that "I am seeing a patient who has major depressive disorder." Certainly the former description conveys more specific information and may in some settings be a more useful description, but in most instances the abbreviated diagnostic term is all that is required to make a particular point.

Second, in order to study the natural history of a particular disorder and develop an effective treatment, it is necessary to define the characteristics of that disorder and have an understanding of how it differs from other, similar disorders. To the extent that a relationship between diagnosis and treatment has been established for a particular category, the proper diagnosis of a person's condition can indicate the most effective treatment. The discussion above on panic disorder is an excellent example of this, illustrating that the former broad diagnostic grouping of anxiety neurosis (DSM-II; American Psychiatric Association 1968) included a heterogeneous group of conditions, each of which might have called for a different treatment. As our diagnostic classification system has become refined over time, correlations between diagnoses and treatments have increased. Unfortunately, even with DSM-IV, relatively few diagnoses are directly associated with specific effective treatments, although the most progress in this regard has been made for major and common categories such as mood disorders and anxiety disorders.

Finally, the ultimate purpose of classification is to develop an understanding of the causes of the various mental disorders. Knowing the cause of a disorder usually leads to the development of an effective treatment. The etiology or pathophysiological process for most of the mental disorders in DSM-IV is unknown, except for disorders that are due to a general medical condition and the few disorders (e.g., posttraumatic stress disorder, adjustment disorder) for which the etiology is included in the definition. For most of the DSM-IV disorders, however, etiological theories abound, formulated by clinicians and researchers of differing theoretical orientations. For example, phobic disorders are believed by many investigators to represent a displacement of anxiety resulting from the breakdown of defense mechanisms that keep internal conflicts out of consciousness. Others explain phobias on the basis of learned avoidance responses to conditioned anxiety. Still others believe that certain phobias result from a dysregulation of basic biological systems mediating separation anxiety. However, despite differing etiological theories about how these disorders come about, it has become clear that clinicians and researchers can agree on what the disorders look like. Therefore, in DSM-III, DSM-III-R, and DSM-IV, a descriptive approach to classification has been taken that includes definitions of the various disorders without reference to their etiology, except for disorders for which the etiology or pathophysiological process is known. This largely atheoretical approach has enabled clinicians of varying theoretical orientations to use this descriptive classification; in other words, clinicians can identify these conditions and still preserve their own approaches to understanding and treating them.

MENTAL DISORDER: DEFINITION

To develop and refine a diagnostic classification system of mental disorders, it is necessary to have some definition of the concept *mental disorder*. For many years, sociologists, psychologists, philosophers of science, and members of the legal profession have struggled with defining the concept (Spitzer and Williams 1982). It was not until the early 1970s, when the issue of whether or not to classify homosexuality as a mental disorder was confronted, that psychiatry began to struggle with the issue. This effort eventually resulted in a definition of mental disorder in DSM-III that has been retained, in refined form, in DSM-III-R and DSM-IV:

In DSM-IV, each of the mental disorders is conceptualized as a clinically significant behavioral or psychological syndrome or pattern that occurs in an individual and that is associated with present distress (a painful symptom) or disability (impairment in one or more important areas of functioning) or with a significantly increased risk of suffering death, pain, disability, or an important loss of freedom. In addition, this syndrome or pattern must not be merely an expectable and culturally sanctioned response to a particular event, e.g., the death of a loved one. Whatever its original cause, it must currently be considered a manifestation of a behavioral, psychological, or biological dysfunction in the individual. Neither deviant behavior, e.g., political, religious, or sexual, nor conflicts that are primarily between the individual and society are mental disorders unless the deviance or conflict is a symptom of a dysfunction in the individual, as described above. (American Psychiatric Association 1994, pp. xxi–xxii)

It is recognized that more precise boundaries for the concept *mental disorder* cannot be specified, just as they cannot for *physical disorder*. However, the above definition was helpful in guiding the development of the later DSM editions, as a basis for deciding which syndromes should be included as mental disorders and determining how they should be defined. More recently, Wakefield (1992) has criticized the DSM definition as lacking precision. He has offered his own revised definition, which specifies that the dysfunction in all mental disorders is of a psychological or behavioral system that has developed through evolution because of its survival value. He argues that the DSM definition, as well as many of the DSM diagnostic criteria, insufficiently distinguish normal distress from true disorder (Wakefield 1992).

A common misunderstanding about the disorders in DSM-IV is that each category represents a discrete entity with distinct boundaries between it and other mental disorders, and between it and normality. Although the disorders by necessity have been defined as distinctly as possible, there are continuing controversies about the relationships among many of the categories. For example, although DSM-IV defines two specific depressive disorders, major depressive disorder and dysthymic disorder, many believe that these two disorders represent merely different points on a continuum of depressive symptoms rather than two distinct entities. Also, many posit that the personality disorders defined in DSM-IV are only points on a continuum of personality traits. Future research will have to answer the question of whether it would be more useful to adopt an approach in which scaled ratings of disturbance, rather than discrete diagnoses, are made in certain areas of psychopathology.

It must be made clear that the objects of the classification are conditions that persons have, rather than the persons themselves (Spitzer and Williams 1979). Thus, for example, there should be no reference to "a schizophrenic" or "a depressive," but rather to "a person with schizophrenia," or someone "who has depression." This avoids the mistaken connotation that someone with a mental disorder has only that, and not also other attributes and roles in life. It also does not imply that all persons with a particular mental disorder are alike; on the contrary, they may differ in many important ways that can affect treatment and outcome.

DEVELOPMENT OF THE DIAGNOSTIC AND STATISTICAL MANUAL SYSTEM: PROCESS AND CONTROVERSIES

BACKGROUND

Official classifications of mental disorders first came into use in the United States in 1840, with the adoption of a one-item classification scheme. "Idiocy (insanity)" was the single category used to categorize mental illness in the census of 1840. By the 1880 census, however, eight categories were listed, suggesting a significant increase in the attention paid to and understanding of mental disorders. This trend continued in the United States and abroad, eventually resulting in the World Health Organization's revisions of the mental disorders chapter of the *International Classification of Diseases* (ICD) and the American Psychiatric Association's *Diagnostic and Statistical Manual of Mental Disorders* (DSM).

DSM-I

The first version of the diagnostic manual was published by the American Psychiatric Association (APA) in 1952 and was called at that time *Diagnostic and Statistical Manual: Mental Disorders* (American Psychiatric Association 1952). It was not until later, when it became clear that revision was needed, that this volume came to be known as DSM-I. The major significance of this book was that, for the first time, it provided descriptions for the mental disorder categories it listed.

DSM-II

In 1965 the APA decided that a new edition of DSM should be published to coincide with the eighth revision of the World Health Organization (WHO) international system, ICD-8 (World Health Organization 1969). Therefore, although it did not differ substantially from the first DSM, DSM-II was published in 1968. Although many believed it would be ideal to have one international diagnostic system, the publication of DSM-II, with its accompanying definitions of the disorders, was necessary, because ICD-8, when initially published, did not contain such a glossary.

DSM-III

Because ICD-9 was scheduled to go into effect in 1979, the APA appointed the Task Force on Nomenclature and Statistics in 1974 to begin work on the development of DSM-III. Although representatives of the APA had worked closely with the WHO on the development of ICD-9 (World Health Organization 1977), there was concern that the ICD-9 classification and glossary would not be suitable for use in the United States. Most important, many specific areas of the classification did not seem sufficiently detailed for clinical and research use. For example, the ICD-9 classification contains only one category for "frigidity and impotence"—despite substantial work in the area of sexual dysfunctions that has identified several specific types with different clinical pictures and treatment implications. In addition, the glossary of ICD-9 was believed by many to be less than optimal in that it had not made use of such recent major methodological developments as specified diagnostic criteria and a multiaxial approach to evaluation. For these reasons, the task force was directed to prepare a new classification and glossary that would, as much as possible, reflect the most current state of knowledge regarding mental disorders, yet maintain compatibility with ICD-9.

In the years since DSM-II was published, a major revolution had taken place in psychiatry with the development of diagnostic criteria. Although it is hard for some to imagine what diagnosis was like without specified criteria, this concept was introduced in psychiatry only in the 1970s, and then only for a few categories in research classifications. Beginning in 1972 with the publication of what have come to be known as the Feighner criteria (Feighner et al. 1972), research was greatly enhanced by the availability of specific and detailed definitions of diagnostic categories. Further, it was demonstrated that such criteria increased the reliability with which these diagnoses could be identified (Spitzer et al. 1978a). The Feighner criteria covered 16 diagnostic categories. These were revised and expanded in 1978 into the Research Diagnostic Criteria (RDC; Spitzer et al. 1978b), covering 21 categories. The greatest challenge to the developers of DSM-III was the creation of specified criteria for over 150 diagnostic categories! This constituted the major work of the Task Force on Nomenclature and Statistics and its advisory committees and was undoubtedly the

single most significant achievement of DSM-III.

Successive drafts of DSM-III were prepared by 14 advisory committees comprised of professionals with special expertise in each substantive area. In addition, a group of consultants provided advice and information on a variety of special subjects. The final product included an increased list of mental disorder categories and greatly expanded descriptions of each of them. In addition to the specified diagnostic criteria that were provided for each of the categories, for the first time a multiaxial system for evaluation was included (see below). Table 7–1 demonstrates, as an example, the great improvements made from DSM-I through DSM-IV in the definition of a major category, obsessive-compulsive disorder, in the first (DSM-I), second (DSM-II), and most recent (DSM-IV) of these manuals. (The description of this category in DSM-III and DSM-III-R is similar to that in DSM-IV.)

For the first time in the development of a standard diagnostic manual, an extensive field trial was conducted to try out the proposed DSM-III prior to its final adoption (Spitzer and Forman 1979; Spitzer et al. 1979). In the course of this project, more than 12,000 patients were evaluated. Clinicians prepared diagnostic reports for each patient that listed their complete multiaxial evaluation and provided feedback about any difficulties the clinicians encountered in using the draft of DSM-III. In addition, 670 adults and 126 children were evaluated by two clinicians in a test of the reliability of the drafted diagnostic criteria. Although the method of this reliability study was less than ideal because of the uncontrollable field conditions, the study did demonstrate that improvements had been made in our ability to reliably diagnose most of the major mental disorders.

The impact of DSM-III was remarkable. Soon after its publication, it became widely accepted in the United States as the common language of mental health clinicians and researchers for communicating about the disorders for which they have professional responsibility. All major textbooks of psychiatry and other textbooks that discuss psychopathology either made extensive reference to DSM-III or largely adopted its terminology and concepts, and it was used as a major teaching tool in medical student education and residency training programs (Williams et al. 1985). In the 10 years following the publication of DSM-III, several thousand articles that directly addressed some aspect of it had already appeared in the scientific literature. Although DSM-III was intended primarily for use in the United States, it also had considerable influence internationally (Spitzer et al. 1983). In addition to fairly widespread use of DSM-III abroad, many of its basic features, such as the inclusion of specified diagnostic criteria, were adopted for in-

TABLE 7–1.   Comparison of DSM definitions of obsessive-compulsive disorder

DSM-I: Obsessive Compulsive Reaction

In this reaction the anxiety is associated with the persistence of unwanted ideas and of repetitive impulses to perform acts which may be considered morbid by the patient. The patient himself may regard his ideas and behavior as unreasonable, but nevertheless is compelled to carry out his rituals.

The diagnosis will specify the symptomatic expression of such reactions as touching, counting, ceremonials, hand-washing, or recurring thoughts (accompanied often by a compulsion to repetitive actions). This category includes many cases formerly classified as *psychasthenia.*

DSM-II: Obsessive Compulsive Neurosis

This disorder is characterized by the persistent intrusion of unwanted thoughts, urges, or actions that the patient is unable to stop. The thoughts may consist of single words or ideas, ruminations, or trains of thought often perceived by the patient as nonsensical. The actions vary from simple movements to complex rituals such as repeated handwashing. Anxiety and distress are often present either if the patient is prevented from completing his compulsive ritual or if he is concerned about being unable to control it himself.

DSM-IV: Diagnostic Criteria for Obsessive-Compulsive Disorder[a]

A.   Either obsessions or compulsions:

Obsessions as defined by (1), (2), (3), and (4):

(1)   recurrent and persistent thoughts, impulses, or images that are experienced, at some time during the disturbance, as intrusive and inappropriate and that cause marked anxiety or distress

(2)   the thoughts, impulses, or images are not simply excessive worries about real-life problems

(3)   the person attempts to ignore or suppress such thoughts, impulses, or images, or to neutralize them with some other thought or action

(4)   the person recognizes that the obsessional thoughts, impulses, or images are a product of his or her own

mind (not imposed from without as in thought insertion)

Compulsions as defined by (1) and (2):

(1)   repetitive behaviors (e.g., hand washing, ordering, checking) or mental acts (e.g., praying, counting, repeating words silently) that the person feels driven to perform in response to an obsession, or according to rules that must be applied rigidly

(2)   the behaviors or mental acts are aimed at preventing or reducing distress or preventing some dreaded event or situation; however, these behaviors or mental acts either are not connected in a realistic way with what they are designed to neutralize or prevent or are clearly excessive

B.   At some point during the course of the disorder, the person has recognized that the obsessions or compulsions are excessive or unreasonable. **Note:** This does not apply to children.

C.   The obsessions or compulsions cause marked distress, are time consuming (take more than 1 hour a day), or significantly interfere with the person's normal routine, occupational (or academic) functioning, or usual social activities or relationships.

D.   If another Axis I disorder is present, the content of the obsessions or compulsions is not restricted to it (e.g., preoccupation with food in the presence of an eating disorder; hair pulling in the presence of trichotillomania; concern with appearance in the presence of body dysmorphic disorder; preoccupation with drugs in the presence of a substance use disorder; preoccupation with having a serious illness in the presence of hypochondriasis; preoccupation with sexual urges or fantasies in the presence of a paraphilia; or guilty ruminations in the presence of major depressive disorder).

E.   The disturbance is not due to the direct physiological effects of a substance (e.g., a drug of abuse, a medication) or a general medical condition.

Note.   The description of obsessive-compulsive disorder in DSM-III and DSM-III-R is similar to that in DSM-IV and for the purposes of this table has been omitted.
[a]In addition to these diagnostic criteria, a full description of the clinical features of the category is included in DSM-IV.

clusion in the mental disorders chapter of ICD-10 (World Health Organization 1992).

DSM-III-R

Work on DSM-III-R was begun in 1983, just 3 short years after the publication of DSM-III. Although at the time some questioned the seeming haste shown in working on a revision, the scientific literature, as mentioned above, was already replete with articles reporting the results of studies

using the DSM-III diagnostic criteria to select samples of patients and articles reporting studies of the reliability and validity of the categories themselves. New data had accumulated that indicated the need for changes in some of the DSM-III definitions, and experience with the criteria had revealed many instances in which they were not entirely clear, were inconsistent across diagnostic categories, or were even contradictory. Although originally intended to be merely a refinement of DSM-III, some sections of DSM-III-R underwent more significant changes (Spitzer and Williams 1988; Widiger et al. 1988; Williams 1985a, 1985b).

DSM-IV

When work began on ICD-10, the President of the APA appointed Dr. Allen Frances to chair the development of DSM-IV. Thus, in 1988, Dr. Frances selected the new task force, made up of 25 individuals, many of whom also served as the chair of a work group focused on a particular aspect of the classification or the manual. There were 13 work groups, each of which had five to eight members. In addition, each work group consulted an extensive list of advisors and consultants both in the United States and abroad.

Work on DSM-IV proceeded in three major phases. First, each work group developed comprehensive literature reviews bearing on controversial issues in its area of focus and considered recent scientific findings that might suggest changes in the classification, text, or criteria for DSM-IV (Widiger et al. 1990, 1994, 1996, 1997). Second, a series of analyses of data from studies that had already been completed or were in progress was funded by the John D. and Catherine T. MacArthur Foundation to answer specific nosological questions. Finally, 12 field trials were funded by the National Institute of Mental Health (NIMH), the National Institute on Drug Abuse (NIDA), and the National Institute on Alcohol Abuse and Alcoholism (NIAAA), to study the impact of changes that were being considered for inclusion in DSM-IV (Frances et al. 1991). (Descriptions of the DSM-IV categories are provided later in this chapter.)

DIAGNOSTIC RELIABILITY

The reliability of a diagnostic category puts an upper limit on its usefulness (i.e., validity). The extent to which a diagnostic category is reliable is the extent to which clinicians can agree with each other on the identification of the disorder; this includes agreement on when the disorder is or is not present. A series of cases with different diagnoses is necessary in order to assess reliability, and the degree to which clinicians can correctly discriminate the diagnostic differences is measured.

ASSESSMENT METHODS AND SOURCES OF UNRELIABILITY

There are several methods for testing reliability, each having its own advantages and disadvantages. The easiest but least powerful way is to ask two clinicians to diagnose independently a series of cases based on written case records or on audio- or videotapes of diagnostic interviews with the subjects.

There are two methods of assessing "live" reliability. This is the hardest test of diagnostic reliability, but the one that can be argued to approximate real life most closely, because it is applied to live patients. The first is the *joint method*, so named because it involves two or more clinicians jointly observing the same interview. One of the clinicians conducts the interview, and often the other may ask additional questions. In the *test-retest method*, each clinician independently conducts his or her own interview, one after the other. An advantage of this procedure is that it more closely approximates the model of interchangeable interviewers, because a reliable diagnosis is one that can be made in the same patients by different people. As expected, reliability assessed by this method is generally lower than that obtained by joint assessments because of the increase in information variance (i.e., variability in the information available to each clinician) (Spitzer and Williams 1985). Despite the fact that the test-retest method requires subjects to undergo more interviews and may be more difficult to coordinate logistically, this expense is usually worth the increase in generalizability of the results.

When reliability is assessed on the basis of written case material, it is generally lower than that assessed on the basis of "live" interviews (Hyler et al. 1982). The reasons for this are not clear, since the complete standardization of material guarantees the elimination of information variance. A reliability study based on audio- or videotapes may more closely approximate the "live" situation, although in such a study, as in a case record reliability study, information variance is eliminated.

Even when both clinicians observe the same patient interview, they may pay attention to different things, resulting in *observation variance*. For example, one clinician may notice that the subject has psychomotor agitation, whereas the other clinician may not. *Interpretation variance* means that clinicians differ in the way they interpret the signs and symptoms exhibited by the patient. An example of this would be differing interpretations of the content of a patient's delusions: one clinician decides the delusions are bizarre, and the other does not. Observation variance can be minimized with training; interpretation variance is minimized when both clinicians use the same definitions of psychopathological symptoms.

A final source of variance that affects diagnostic reliability is *criterion variance*, resulting when clinicians use differing rules for combining their observations into diagnoses. As discussed above, standard sets of specified diagnostic criteria have been available since the early

1970s. Criterion variance is minimized when clinicians use the same diagnostic criteria.

STATISTICAL INDICES OF RELIABILITY

Generally, one is interested in knowing the reliability of a single diagnostic category (e.g., how good is agreement on the diagnosis of schizophrenia?), a diagnostic class (e.g., how good is the agreement on a diagnosis of any mood disorder?), or an entire classification of disorders (e.g., what is the average reliability of all DSM-IV Axis I disorders?). One way of calculating agreement is simply to calculate the percentage of cases in the sample on which there is agreement. For example, a pair of clinicians might jointly assess 100 patients on an inpatient unit that specializes in the treatment of psychotic disorders. As shown in Table 7–2, the overall agreement on the diagnosis of schizophrenia might be 70% (40% agreement on who has the diagnosed disorder and 30% agreement on who does not have the diagnosed disorder)—seemingly quite satisfactory. However, much of the apparent agreement was actually due to chance alone. Agreement by chance alone would be calculated by summing the products of the clinicians' base rates of diagnosis and nondiagnosis ($[0.55 \times 0.55] + [0.45 \times 0.45] = 0.51$).

In 1960, Cohen proposed the use of the *kappa statistic* for indexing agreement among clinicians, correcting for chance agreement (Cohen 1960). The values of kappa vary from –1.0 (total disagreement) to +1.0 (perfect agreement), with a kappa of 0 indicating no more than chance agreement. It is generally agreed that a kappa value of 0.70 and above is quite good, between 0.50 and 0.70 fair, and below 0.50 poor (Perry 1992; Spitzer and Fleiss 1974). Kappa is calculated as follows:

$$\text{kappa} = \frac{P_{observed} - P_{chance}}{1 - P_{chance}}$$

TABLE 7–2. **Mock results of reliability study**

| Clinician 1 | Clinician 2 | | |
	Schizophrenia present	Schizophrenia absent	Total
Schizophrenia present	40	15	55
Schizophrenia absent	15	30	45
Total	55	45	100

In our case of joint assessment by 2 clinicians of 100 inpatients, $P_{observed}$ was .70 and P_{chance} was .51. Therefore, kappa is only 0.39—considerably lower than the original 70% overall agreement. By correcting for chance agreement, kappa provides a truer estimate of diagnostic reliability and has become the standard method for indexing diagnostic agreement in psychiatry (Shrout et al. 1987).

TYPES OF VALIDITY

DIAGNOSTIC VALIDITY

The *validity* of a diagnosis is the extent to which it serves the multiple purposes for which it is intended. Four major types of validity are applied to psychiatric diagnoses: face, descriptive, predictive, and construct.

Face validity is the extent to which, on the face of it, the definition of a disorder seems reasonable as a description of a particular clinical entity and allows professionals to communicate about the disorder. For example, the list of symptoms that define the DSM-IV category *major depressive disorder* has significant face validity because clinicians generally agree that these are the signs and symptoms they see in their patients who are very depressed.

Descriptive validity is the extent to which the defining features of a diagnostic category are unique to that category. For example, the DSM-IV category of manic episode has a great deal of descriptive validity because its clinical features clearly distinguish it from other categories (i.e., euphoric mood and decreased need for sleep are rarely seen in other disorders). On the other hand, the category of generalized anxiety disorder has less descriptive validity because its essential features, excessive anxiety and worry, are often present in persons with other mental disorders.

If a diagnosis has high *predictive validity*, it is useful for predicting the natural history and treatment response of a person with the disorder. For example, the category of panic disorder has high predictive validity because there is a high likelihood that a person with this disorder will develop agoraphobia as a complication, and, as described previously, there is a high probability that there will be a good response to certain treatments.

Finally, *construct validity* is the highest form of validity and the form for which most of the mental disorders have the least evidence. Construct validity is the extent to which we understand the etiology or pathophysiological process of a disorder. Evidence for the construct validity of a disorder includes evidence of a genetic factor, a biological mechanism, and social and environmental factors that cause the disorder.

In a classic article describing a method for establishing the validity of a diagnostic category, Robins and Guze (1970) discussed demonstrating a distinct clinical picture of subjects with the disorder, the presence of any distinguishing laboratory findings (granted, these are rare in psychiatry), the occurrence of the disorder in the subjects' relatives, and the consistency of the disorder over time. Klein et al. (1980) addressed "pharmacological dissection" in adding differential response to psychopharmacological agents. These factors all contribute to the validity of a diagnostic category.

PROCEDURAL VALIDITY

When evaluating the usefulness or accuracy (i.e., validity) of a particular diagnostic test or procedure, it is necessary to evaluate it against some standard procedure assumed to be valid. This is referred to as *procedural validity* and should not be confused with diagnostic validity (discussed previously) (Spitzer and Williams 1985).

There are basically three important indices with which a new test or procedure can be evaluated, using some standard test or procedure as the criterion: sensitivity, specificity, and predictive power. (These concepts are fully described and illustrated in a classic paper by Baldessarini et al. [1983].) The *sensitivity* of a diagnostic procedure is calculated as the percentage of "true" cases it correctly identifies as having the diagnosed disorder (i.e., its *true-positive* rate). The *specificity* is the percentage of noncases that it correctly identifies as *not* having the diagnosis (i.e., its *true-negative* rate). Finally, the *predictive power* of a test is the percentage of total cases in which the test agrees with the standard—that is, the total number of cases that both tests agree have the diagnosed disorder plus the total number of cases that both tests agree do not have the diagnosis, all divided by the total number of cases. The predictive power of a test can be broken down into positive predictive power and negative predictive power. A test's total predictive power is equivalent to overall agreement.

An example may be helpful in illustrating these concepts. An investigator is developing a self-report rating scale that makes a DSM-IV diagnosis of generalized anxiety disorder. Unfortunately, because of the lack of confirmatory diagnostic laboratory tests in psychiatry, it is not always clear what the standard of comparison should be. However, for better or worse, the investigator has chosen to compare the new rating scale with an expert clinician's diagnosis. She plans a study in which both the rating scale and an expert clinician's acumen are applied to a series of 100 cases that are being evaluated for admission to an anxiety disorders clinic. The results that might have been obtained are presented in Table 7–3. The sensitivity, specificity, and predictive power of the rating scale prove to be only modest. A next step might be for the investigator to examine, case by case, the reasons for the disagreements so that her rating scale can be revised and retested.

CROSS-NATIONAL STUDIES

In the 1960s two major cross-national studies were conducted that bear on the validity of psychiatric diagnoses. The purpose of the first of these, the United States–United Kingdom Diagnostic Project (which is referred to as the US-UK study), was to explore the reasons for the facts that affective disorders were much more commonly diagnosed in England than in the United States and that the reverse was true for schizophrenia. A group of psychiatrists evaluated patients in both countries, using a structured diagnostic interview. The results indicated that the international diagnostic differences were mainly due to differing clinical concepts in the two countries rather than to differences in the characteristics of patients in the United States and the United Kingdom (Cooper et al. 1972).

In the second study, the International Pilot Study of Schizophrenia (IPSS), diagnoses made by clinicians working in less-developed countries were compared with those made by clinicians in developed countries, with both sets of clinicians using standardized diagnostic assessment instruments. The results indicated that schizophrenia, narrowly defined, could be identified in nine countries that differed significantly in culture and level of development (World Health Organization 1973).

STRUCTURED INTERVIEWS

In recent years, psychiatric research has been greatly facilitated by the evolution of specified diagnostic criteria

TABLE 7–3. **Mock results of validity study**

Rating scale	Expert's diagnosis		
	Positive	**Negative**	**Total**
Positive	40	15	55
Negative	15	30	45
Total	55	45	100

Note. Sensitivity of rating scale: 40/55 = 0.73. Specificity of rating scale: 30/45 = 0.67. Overall predictive value of rating scale: 70/100 = 0.70.

(American Psychiatric Association 1980, 1987, 1994; Feighner et al. 1972; Spitzer et al. 1978b) and by structured diagnostic interviews keyed to these criteria (e.g., Endicott and Spitzer 1978; First et al. 1997a; Pfohl et al. 1997; Robins et al. 1995; Spitzer et al. 1992b). Such interviews have many advantages: 1) they enhance the reliability with which diagnoses are made, 2) they facilitate the recording of which specific symptoms are present and which are absent, and 3) they enable even relatively junior clinicians to make relatively reliable psychiatric diagnoses.

The use of standardized psychiatric assessment instruments began in this country in 1961 with Spitzer et al.'s Mental Status Schedule (Spitzer et al. 1964), and in England a few years earlier with Wing's Present State Examination (PSE; Wing and Giddens 1959). Since that time, a large number of standardized interview schedules for psychiatric assessment have been developed (Guy 1976; Hedlund and Vieweg 1981; Thompson 1989; van Riezen and Segal 1988). However, most of these standardized interview schedules yield scores on one or more symptom dimensions and do not yield psychiatric diagnoses.

Standardized interview schedules specifically designed to yield a range of the major psychiatric diagnoses represent a more recent advance. Those in most widespread use are described below; all have been adapted to accommodate DSM-IV criteria. A growing number focus on one or more personality disorders (see Chapter 22; see also Baron et al. 1981; Clark 1993; First et al. 1997b; Pfohl et al. 1997; Zanarini et al. 1987). It should also be noted that similar interview guides have now been developed to cover diagnoses often made in children and adolescents (Gutterman et al. 1987; Hodges 1993).

PRESENT STATE EXAMINATION

The PSE, the "grandparent" of structured diagnostic interviews, was initially developed 20 years ago by a group in England headed by Dr. John Wing (Wing et al. 1967). It consists of a structured interview schedule that generally focuses on symptoms that have occurred during the past month. Diagnoses are made by a computer program called CATEGO. The latest version of this interview schedule, PSE-10, has been incorporated into a new system known as Schedules for Clinical Assessment in Neuropsychiatry (SCAN; Wing et al. 1990). SCAN is a comprehensive procedure that enables a clinician to assess many of the ICD-10 and DSM-IV categories, with optional sections for further characterizing certain aspects of psychopathology and other clinical variables. Its development was sponsored by the WHO, and it was specifically designed for worldwide use.

SCHEDULE FOR AFFECTIVE DISORDERS AND SCHIZOPHRENIA

The Schedule for Affective Disorders and Schizophrenia (SADS; Endicott and Spitzer 1978) has been widely used in this country and abroad for making diagnoses according to the RDC described in an earlier section of this chapter. Diagnoses are made by the clinician following the interview, in consultation with the RDC criteria. Mini 6-point rating scales are provided for most of the symptoms, which generate extensive descriptive information and a mechanism for charting change over time but make the administration of the instrument lengthy.

Several versions of the SADS have been developed, including the SADS-L (Lifetime Version), which is used for community subjects and patients' relatives (Endicott and Spitzer 1978), and the SADS-LA[R] (Revised Lifetime Version for anxiety disorders specifically), which focuses on a detailed history of anxiety symptoms (Mannuzza et al. 1989; Schleyer et al. 1990).

NIMH DIAGNOSTIC INTERVIEW SCHEDULE AND WHO-ADAMHA COMPOSITE INTERNATIONAL DIAGNOSTIC INTERVIEW

The Diagnostic Interview Schedule (DIS; Robins et al. 1981, 1995) was explicitly developed for use by nonclinicians to facilitate the screening of a large number of community subjects in the Epidemiologic Catchment Area survey described in Chapter 3 (Regier et al. 1984). The Composite International Diagnostic Interview (CIDI), by WHO and the U.S. Alcohol, Drug, and Mental Health Administration (ADAMHA) (Robins et al. 1988), a revision and expansion of the DIS, was developed for international cross-cultural epidemiologic studies and comparative studies of psychopathology. Diagnoses are made by a computer algorithm according to the DSM-III, DSM-III-R, and ICD-10 criteria. Although these instruments have been used in some studies by clinical interviewers, they are fully structured to minimize the amount of judgment required to administer them; thus they do not make use of the skills of an experienced clinical interviewer, which many believe is essential to ensuring the validity of diagnostic assessments (Spitzer 1983).

STRUCTURED CLINICAL INTERVIEW FOR DSM-IV (SCID)

The Structured Clinical Interview for DSM-IV (SCID) is designed to enable clinicians to gather the appropriate information for making Axis I and II diagnoses according to

DSM-IV (First et al. 1997a; Spitzer et al. 1992b; Williams et al. 1992). Modeled on a clinical diagnostic interview, SCID begins with an overview of the present illness and past episodes of psychopathology. It then proceeds to inquire systematically about specific symptoms, beginning with screening questions to rule in or rule out specific disorders. SCID is designed for use in a modular fashion so that a clinician or investigator can select for a particular study only the diagnostic modules that are of interest or relevant to the sample of subjects in a particular study.

Two main versions of SCID for DSM-IV Axis I disorders have been developed: a Clinician Version (SCID-CV) and a Research Version (SCID). SCID-CV covers only the DSM-IV diagnoses most commonly seen in clinical practice and excludes most of the subtypes and specifiers included in the Research Version. SCID-CV can be used in at least three ways. In the first, a clinician conducts his or her usual interview, then uses a portion of SCID-CV to confirm and document a suspected DSM-IV diagnosis. For example, the clinician, hearing the patient describe what appear to be panic attacks, may use the Anxiety Disorder module of SCID-CV to inquire about the specific DSM-IV criteria for panic disorder. In this instance, SCID-CV provides the clinician not only with the actual DSM-IV criteria for panic disorder, but also with the SCID questions, which are efficient ways of obtaining the information necessary for judging the diagnostic criteria. In the second, the complete SCID-CV and SCID-II (for Personality Disorders) are administered as an intake procedure, ensuring that all the major Axis I and Axis II diagnoses are systematically evaluated. SCID has been used in this way in hospitals and clinics by mental health professionals of varying backgrounds, including psychiatry, psychology, psychiatric social work, and psychiatric nursing. Finally, SCID-CV can be helpful in improving the interview skills of students in the mental health professions. SCID-CV can provide them with a repertoire of useful questions for eliciting information from a patient that will be the basis for making judgments about the diagnostic criteria. Through repeated administrations of SCID-CV, students become familiar with DSM-IV criteria and at the same time incorporate useful questions into their interviewing repertoire.

The Research Version includes details about the symptoms present that are generally more useful to researchers than to clinicians. The Research Version is much longer than SCID-CV because it includes ratings for a number of subtypes, severity and course specifiers, and disorders that are diagnostically useful for researchers but that may not be of general interest to clinicians. Two versions of the Research Version are available: SCID-P for use with psychiatric patients, and SCID-NP for community subjects, patients' relatives, primary care patients, and other persons not identified as psychiatric patients.

SCID-II, for making personality disorder diagnoses, is designed to be used with a self-report questionnaire that the subject completes just before the interview (First et al. 1997b). The clinician then focuses on the positive responses to the questionnaire in reviewing the personality disorder symptoms. SCID-II covers 12 personality disorders: 10 of them appear in the Personality Disorders section of DSM-IV; 2 of them (negativistic personality disorder and depressive personality disorder) appear in Appendix B of DSM-IV ("Criteria Sets and Axes Provided for Further Study"). SCID-II is published as a separate instrument with a separate instruction manual available from American Psychiatric Press (First et al. 1997b).

PRIMARY CARE EVALUATION OF MENTAL DISORDERS

The Primary Care Evaluation of Mental Disorders (PRIME-MD) system is a new standardized but brief and easy diagnostic assessment procedure designed for primary care clinicians and researchers, but also potentially useful for mental health practitioners and researchers (Spitzer et al. 1994). PRIME-MD evaluates mood, anxiety, alcohol, and somatoform disorders—the four groups of mental disorders most commonly encountered in the general population and primary care settings—and eating disorders, which have more recently been shown to be common in the general population.

PRIME-MD has two components: a 1-page Patient Questionnaire (PQ) that is completed by the patient prior to the interview with the clinician, and a 12-page Clinician Evaluation Guide (CEG), which is a structured interview form that the clinician uses to follow up positive responses on the PQ. The PQ, then, serves as an initial symptom screen for the mental disorders covered by the CEG evaluation. The PQ consists of 26 yes/no questions about symptoms present during the past month, divided into the five diagnostic areas just listed, plus 1 question about the patient's overall health. Patient responses to the PQ indicate to the clinician which, if any, of the five diagnostic modules in the CEG should be used. Using the CEG, the clinician determines the presence or absence of 18 possible current mental disorders in the five broad categories by asking specific questions based on the diagnostic criteria contained in DSM-IV (often simplified for primary care use). The final diagnostic findings are recorded on a summary sheet that can be included in the patient's chart.

In a field test of 1,000 primary care patients, PRIME-MD administered by primary care physicians was found to have good to excellent agreement with independent mental health clinicians evaluating the same patients (via a telephone interview). Patients with PRIME-MD mental disorders also had significantly impaired functioning and greater health care use compared with patients without PRIME-MD diagnoses. In addition, the PRIME-MD facilitated first-time recognition of mental disorders in patients who were already known to their doctors. The physicians found the information to be "very" or "somewhat" valuable for 61% of patients given the CEG and for 83% of those with a PRIME-MD diagnosis (Spitzer et al. 1994).

The data from this study of 1,000 primary care patients provide considerable support for the utility and validity of the PRIME-MD system, which allows the clinician, in a relatively short period of time (an average of 8.5 minutes), to actually screen and complete a differential diagnosis of the major classes of mental disorders commonly seen in primary care settings. However, although this study suggests that PRIME-MD may be both accurate and efficient, it is still perceived by many to take too long to fit into a busy primary care office practice. Therefore, a self-report version of PRIME-MD is currently being field tested. If such a procedure is successful, patients will be able to provide sufficient information in a self-report format for clinicians to review and more quickly make a diagnosis.

DSM-IV: GENERAL FEATURES

Many of the general features of DSM-IV are similar to those of DSM-III and DSM-III-R and are further described in the introduction to DSM-IV.

DIAGNOSTIC CRITERIA

As mentioned in a previous section, specified diagnostic criteria are included in DSM-IV for every specific category. These criteria have been revised from those in DSM-III-R on the basis of continued clinical experience and new empirical findings.

DESCRIPTIVE APPROACH

One of the most important and successful features of DSM-III was its generally atheoretical, or descriptive, approach to defining the mental disorders. For a few of the DSM-III mental disorders, notably the organic mental disorders, the etiology or pathophysiologic process is known, presumed, or included in the definition (as in adjustment disorder). For most of the disorders, however,

the etiology is unknown, although there may be many theories about their causes. The developers of DSM-III recognized that, by and large, clinicians could agree on the defining features of most of the mental disorders despite disagreement about their causes. For this reason, except for the disorders for which the etiology is known, the mental disorders in DSM-III, DSM-III-R, and DSM-IV are defined without reference to etiological theories. This approach does not inhibit the belief in specific etiological theories or the creation and study of new ones, and it does at least encourage the study of homogeneous groups of patients in the pursuit of data supporting such theories.

DIAGNOSTIC HIERARCHIES

In the DSM-III classification, the diagnostic categories were arranged hierarchically, on the principle that disorders higher in the hierarchy often had symptoms found in disorders lower in the hierarchy, but not the reverse. This hierarchic structure was operationalized in the diagnostic criteria: a diagnosis lower in the hierarchy was not given (even if its diagnostic criteria were met) if the criteria for a diagnosis higher in the hierarchy were also met for the same symptomatology. For example, in DSM-III the diagnosis of panic disorder was not given if the panic attacks occurred only in the course of major depression, a disorder that was higher in the hierarchy. In such a case, the panic attacks were judged to be "due to," or merely associated symptoms of, the major depression, and it was only the major depression that was then diagnosed. In this case, the patient was not considered to have two separate disorders.

After the publication of DSM-III, however, data from several studies called into question the fundamental assumptions on which the DSM-III hierarchies had been based. Leckman et al. (1983) conducted a large study of the relatives of persons with major depression; some of the persons with major depression had had panic attacks at the same time as the major depression, and others had had panic attacks at other times. These investigators demonstrated that the relatives of both groups had an increased risk of both anxiety disorders and depression, suggesting that the panic attacks should be diagnosed separately, whether or not they are associated with major depression. Another study found that the presence of *any* DSM-III disorder increased the likelihood of another DSM-III disorder (Boyd et al. 1984). These studies indicated that research and clinical practice would be improved by eliminating many of the DSM-III diagnostic hierarchies that prevented giving multiple diagnoses when different syndromes occurred together in one episode of illness. Therefore, in DSM-III-R most of the diagnostic hierarchies were removed. Those that remain in DSM-IV largely follow two principles:

1. Disorders due to a general medical condition and substance-induced disorders preempt the diagnosis of any other disorder that could produce the same symptoms, if an etiological general medical condition or substance can be identified. For example, a patient with a major depressive syndrome could be diagnosed as having either major depressive disorder, mood disorder due to hypothyroidism, or hallucinogen-induced mood disorder. If the patient's history or laboratory tests reveal that the depression began during the course of hypothyroidism, or during hallucinogen intoxication, the clinician should consider one of the two latter diagnoses rather than major depressive disorder. However, if no etiological general medical condition or specific substance intoxication or withdrawal is identified, and the criteria for major depressive disorder are met, it is the mood disorder that should be diagnosed.

2. When a more pervasive disorder commonly has essential or associated symptoms that are the defining symptoms of a less pervasive disorder, only the more pervasive disorder is diagnosed, if its diagnostic criteria are met. For example, when chronic mild depression is present only when the essential features of schizophrenia are also present, only schizophrenia is diagnosed rather than schizophrenia and dysthymic disorder (to account for the chronic mild depression), because depressive symptoms are commonly associated with schizophrenia.

The decisions of which diagnostic hierarchies to impose and which to abandon were not easy ones. It was necessary to balance competing goals of clinical validity (i.e., not preempting the diagnosis of disorders with differential predictive validity) and parsimony (i.e., not encouraging a diagnosis for every symptom present). If all the hierarchies had been suspended, many individuals would have received many diagnoses. For example, in many cases of schizophrenia there are also depression, anxiety, and often somatoform symptoms. Without any diagnostic hierarchies, an approach advocated by some, such cases could receive diagnoses of major depressive disorder, dysthymic disorder, generalized anxiety disorder, social phobia, and undifferentiated somatoform disorder, as well as schizophrenia. Such a list might distract the treating clinician from concentrating on treatment of the schizophrenia, when many of the other symptoms might resolve on their own once the acute phase of schizophrenia resolved.

MULTIAXIAL SYSTEM FOR EVALUATION

DSM-III took a major step forward by incorporating, for the first time in an official diagnostic manual in this country, a multiaxial system for evaluation. The basic concept of such a system is that several different domains of information assumed to be of high clinical value are evaluated for each person. Ideally, each of these domains is assessed independently of the others, although in practice they are often related. Together, they represent a view of the person's condition that is more comprehensive than an evaluation limited to mental disorder diagnoses. Use of a multiaxial system ensures that attention is given to certain types of disorders, aspects of the environment, and areas of functioning that might be overlooked if the focus were on assessing a single presenting problem. Although not empirically demonstrated, it is assumed that a multiaxial evaluation is more useful for treatment planning and evaluating prognosis, because it better reflects the interrelated complexities of the various biological, psychological, and social aspects of a person's condition (Williams 1985a, 1985b).

After 10 years of experience and one revision, however, there was disappointment about the relatively infrequent use of the multiaxial system in clinical and research settings. The DSM-IV Multiaxial Issues Work Group considered possible reasons for this lack of use, including that 1) the system was too complex and clinicians had not received adequate training in how to make ratings on Axes IV and V, 2) no prototypical recording form had been provided for agencies to adopt that would facilitate the systematic inclusion of all five axes in regular clinical evaluations, and 3) the multiaxial system was not useful for facilitating a comprehensive evaluation. Revisions made in DSM-IV reflect consideration of all these possibilities.

The DSM-IV multiaxial system consists of five axes, as was also the case in DSM-III and DSM-III-R. All the mental disorders are included on the first two axes: Axis I is entitled "Clinical Disorders [and] Other Conditions That May Be a Focus of Clinical Attention" (see below), and Axis II is entitled "Personality Disorders [and] Mental Retardation." The provision of a separate axis for personality disorders and mental retardation ensures that consideration is given to the possible presence of such disorders, which might otherwise be overlooked when attention is directed to the usually more florid Axis I disorders. For example, in a patient with both major depressive disorder with psychotic features and paranoid personality disorder, the clinician might inadvertently overlook the personality disorder because its features are so overshadowed by the psychotic symptoms associated with the depression. In many instances, disorders will be present on both Axes I and II, and, in such cases, all appropriate diagnoses should be recorded. This Axis I/Axis II convention has undoubtedly been at least partially responsible for the tremendous increase in research and clinical attention that has been directed to the personality disorders in the last 10 to 15 years.

Axis III is for listing current general medical conditions that the clinician believes are potentially relevant to the understanding or management of the case. In ICD-9-CM (ICD-9, Clinical Modification), these conditions are classified outside the mental disorders section. General medical conditions can be related to mental disorders in a variety of ways. In some cases it is clear that the general medical condition is directly etiological to the development or worsening of a mental disorder (e.g., anxiety disorder due to hyperthyroidism), and that the mechanism for this effect is physiological. In other instances, the general medical disorder may not seem to be etiological but is important in the overall management of the case (e.g., a person with diabetes mellitus, admitted to the hospital for an exacerbation of schizophrenia, for whom insulin management must be monitored). Sometimes a general medical disorder has important prognostic or treatment implications for the mental disorder, as, for example, a case involving both major depressive disorder and arrhythmia, in which the choice of pharmacotherapy is influenced by the general medical condition.

Axis IV provides a checklist for recording psychosocial and environmental problems that may affect the diagnosis, treatment planning, and prognosis of the individual's mental disorders (on Axes I and II). A psychosocial or environmental problem may be a negative life event, an environmental difficulty, an interpersonal stress, inadequacy of social supports or personal resources, or another problem that describes the context in which a person's difficulties have developed. The list of problem categories to be considered on Axis IV includes problems with one's primary support group, problems related to the social environment, inadequate access to health care services, problems related to interaction with the legal system, and educational, occupational, housing, economic, and other psychosocial problems. In general, only problems that have been present during the year preceding the evaluation should be noted; in many cases it is appropriate to record more than one problem. When a psychosocial or environmental problem is the primary focus of clinical attention, it is also recorded on Axis I with its corresponding conditions from the section "Other Conditions That May Be a Focus of Clinical Attention."

This formulation of Axis IV represents a change from DSM-III and DSM-III-R, in which quantitative rating scales were provided for rating the overall severity of psychosocial stressors. Although the DSM-IV axis may not be as useful for researchers, since it lacks a way to quantify the severity of psychosocial and environmental problems, it will undoubtedly be simpler for clinicians to use.

The Global Assessment of Functioning (GAF) Scale on Axis V, from DSM-IV, as shown in Table 7–4, summarizes psychological, social, and occupational functioning on a continuum of mental health–illness. Studies have shown that clinical ratings of overall severity of disturbance are reliable and are related to treatment use (Curran et al. 1980; Fenichel and Murphy 1985; Gordon et al. 1985a, 1985b; Husby 1985; Mezzich et al. 1984). The GAF ratings are made for current functioning (at the time of evaluation) and generally reflect the present need for treatment or care. Ratings may be made for other periods (e.g., past year) for special purposes.

Although there are surely many other areas of functioning that are important for clinicians to consider in planning for treatment, a multiaxial system, in order to have maximal clinical usefulness, must have a limited number of axes. These five axes were selected to represent the minimal number of areas of clinical information that would be of maximal clinical utility regardless of treatment approach and treatment context (i.e., what basic information every clinician would want to consider about every case). It is hoped that changes made in the various axes will make the system more useful for comprehensive evaluations. A prototypical recording form (Figure 7–1) has been included in DSM-IV to facilitate the use of all five axes. The reliability and validity of the DSM-III multiaxial system have been studied by a number of groups and reviewed by Williams (1985b) and Skodol (1997). It is hoped that research studies using the DSM-IV system will reveal improved reliability and validity.

SYSTEMATIC DESCRIPTIONS

The DSM-IV, like its immediate predecessors, includes standard categories of information in order to offer a complete description of the features of the various disorders (Table 7–5). The description of each category begins with its *diagnostic features*, the clinical signs and symptoms that are required for making the diagnosis. This is followed by a discussion of the disorder's *associated features and disorders*, which can include 1) descriptive features and mental disorders that are often associated with the disorder but are not essential for making the diagnosis; 2) associated laboratory findings that may be diagnostic (as in some sleep disorders), confirmatory of the construct of the disorder, or merely associated with the complications of the disorder;

TABLE 7-4.   Global Assessment of Functioning Scale (GAF Scale—Axis V)

Consider psychological, social, and occupational functioning on a hypothetical continuum of mental health–illness. Do not include impairment in functioning due to physical (or environmental) limitations. (Note: Use intermediate codes when appropriate, e.g., 45, 68, 72.)

Code

100   Superior functioning in a wide range of activities, life's problems never seem to get out of hand, is sought out by others because of his or her many positive qualities. No symptoms.

91

90   Absent or minimal symptoms (e.g., mild anxiety before an exam), good functioning in all areas, interested and involved in a wide range of activities, socially effective, generally satisfied with life, no more than everyday problems or concerns (e.g., an occasional argument with family members).

81

80   If symptoms are present, they are transient and expectable reactions to psychosocial stressors (e.g., difficulty concentrating after family argument); no more than slight impairment in social, occupational, or school functioning (e.g., temporarily falling behind in schoolwork).

71

70   Some mild symptoms (e.g., depressed mood and mild insomnia) **OR** some difficulty in social, occupational, or school functioning (e.g., occasional truancy, or theft within the household), but generally functioning pretty well, has some meaningful interpersonal relationships.

61

60   Moderate symptoms (e.g., flat affect and circumstantial speech, occasional panic attacks) **OR** moderate difficulty in social, occupational, or school functioning (e.g., few friends, conflicts with peers or co-workers).

51

50   Serious symptoms (e.g., suicidal ideation, severe obsessional rituals, frequent shoplifting) **OR** any serious impairment in social, occupational, or school functioning (e.g., no friends, unable to keep a job).

41

40   Some impairment in reality testing or communication (e.g., speech is at times illogical, obscure, or irrelevant) **OR** major impairment in several areas, such as work or school, family relations, judgment, thinking, or mood (e.g., depressed man avoids friends, neglects family, and is unable to work; child frequently beats up younger children, is defiant at home, and is failing at school).

31

30   Behavior is considerably influenced by delusions or hallucinations **OR** serious impairment in communication or judgment (e.g., sometimes incoherent, acts grossly inappropriately, suicidal preoccupation) **OR** inability to function in almost all areas (e.g., stays in bed all day; no job, home, or friends).

21

20   Some danger of hurting self or others (e.g., suicide attempts without clear expectation of death, frequently violent, manic excitement) **OR** occasionally fails to maintain minimal personal hygiene (e.g., smears feces) **OR** gross impairment in communication (e.g., largely incoherent or mute).

11

10   Persistent danger of severely hurting self or others (e.g., recurrent violence) **OR** persistent inability to maintain minimal personal hygiene **OR** serious suicidal act with clear expectation of death.

1

0   Inadequate information.

Note.   The rating of overall psychological functioning on a scale of 0–100 was operationalized by Luborsky in the Health-Sickness Rating Scale (Luborsky L: "Clinicians' Judgments of Mental Health." *Archives of General Psychiatry* 7:407–417, 1962). Spitzer and colleagues developed a revision of the Health-Sickness Rating Scale called the Global Assessment Scale (GAS) (Endicott J, Spitzer RL, Fleiss JL, et al: "The Global Assessment Scale: A Procedure for Measuring Overall Severity of Psychiatric Disturbance." *Archives of General Psychiatry* 33:766–771, 1976). A modified version of the GAS was included in DSM-III-R as the Global Assessment of Functioning (GAF) Scale.

MULTIAXIAL EVALUATION REPORT FORM

AXIS I: CLINICAL DISORDERS

            OTHER CONDITIONS THAT MAY BE A
            FOCUS OF CLINICAL ATTENTION

DSM-IV code   DSM-IV name

— — • — — —   _____

— — • • — — —   _____

— — • — — —   _____

— — • — — —   _____

AXIS II: PERSONALITY DISORDERS
            MENTAL RETARDATION

DSM-IV code   DSM-IV name

— — • — — —   _____

— — • — — —   _____

— — • — — —   _____

AXIS III: GENERAL MEDICAL CONDITIONS

ICD-9-CM code   ICD-9-CM name

— — • — — —   _____

— — • — — —   _____

— — — • — — —   _____

AXIS IV: PSYCHOSOCIAL AND ENVIRONMENTAL
            PROBLEMS

Check:

____ Problems with primary support group.
      Specify:_____

____ Problems related to the social environment.
      Specify:_____

____ Educational problems. Specify:_____

____ Occupational problems. Specify:_____

____ Housing problems. Specify:_____

____ Economic problems. Specify:_____

____ Problems with access to health care services.
      Specify:_____

____ Problems related to interaction with the legal
      system/crime. Specify:_____

____ Other psychosocial and environmental problems.
      Specify:_____

AXIS V: GLOBAL ASSESSMENT OF
            FUNCTIONING SCALE

                              Score:__ __

                              Time frame:__

FIGURE 7–1.   Multiaxial Evaluation Report Form.

TABLE 7–5. **Categories of information included in the DSM-IV text**

Diagnostic features

Associated features and disorders

Specific age, culture, or gender features

Prevalence and incidence

Predisposing factors

Course

Complications

Familial pattern

Differential diagnosis

and 3) associated symptoms, physical examination signs, and general medical conditions that may be of diagnostic significance but are not essential to the diagnosis (e.g., dental erosion resulting from vomiting associated with bulimia nervosa), or that are merely associated conditions.

A section addressing *specific age, cultural, or gender features* provides guidance for the clinician concerning variations in the presentation of the disorder that may be attributable to the individual's developmental stage (e.g., infancy, childhood, adolescence, late life), cultural setting, or gender. This section also includes information on differential prevalence rates (e.g., sex ratio).

Under *prevalence and incidence* are provided data on point and lifetime prevalence and incidence of the disorder. These data are provided for different clinical settings (e.g., inpatient, outpatient) when known.

The section on *predisposing factors* describes the characteristics of a person that can be identified before the development of the disorder and that increase the risk of that person's developing the disorder.

The section on *course* describes the typical lifetime patterns of presentation and evolution of the disorder. This may include information on the usual age at onset, mode of onset (e.g., abrupt or insidious), chronicity, typical duration of episodes, and progression over time (e.g., stationary, worsening, improving).

Under *complications* is a description of the types of serious morbidity that may occur as a result of having the disorder (e.g., suicide, violence, school suspension).

The *familial pattern* section provides data on the frequency of the disorder among first-degree biological relatives of persons with the disorder as compared with the general population.

Finally, each category also includes a discussion of *differential diagnosis*, describing how to distinguish the disorder in question from other disorders that have some similar presenting characteristics.

An interim revision of the DSM-IV text has now begun. Comprehensive literature reviews are being conducted in each area to identify new findings that have been reported since DSM-IV was first published. These literature reviews will guide changes that will be made in the text; the diagnostic criteria will be left unchanged. This interim volume is expected to become available in the year 2000. Also at this time, a clinical modification of ICD-10 (ICD-10-CM) that will replace the ICD-9-CM currently in use is expected to be implemented in the United States. The names, terminology, and definitions of the mental disorders in ICD-10-CM will closely resemble those in DSM-IV.

CROSS-CULTURAL CONSIDERATIONS

DSM-III has been translated into many languages and has been widely used in other parts of the world. Somewhat surprisingly, its use in cultures vastly different from those of most of the people who were mainly responsible for developing it was generally successful (Spitzer et al. 1983). During the development of DSM-III-R, however, an advisory committee was formed specifically to consider cross-cultural issues, and some improvements were made in the classification and criteria in order to increase the value of DSM-III-R in other cultures. Further, the introduction to DSM-III-R contained a discussion about the use of DSM-III-R in different cultures.

In DSM-IV this issue received even more attention, supported by a Conference on Culture and DSM-IV, held specifically to address needed changes in the text and criteria to make them more useful and accurate across cultures (Mezzich et al. 1996). Further, three additional innovative features were added to DSM-IV. First, because of evidence suggesting that the symptoms and course of a number of DSM-IV disorders are influenced by local cultural factors, a new section that describes specific cultural features was added to the text for many disorders. Second, descriptions of some "culture-bound syndromes" were added as examples to "not otherwise specified" categories (e.g., possession trance added as an example to the section on dissociative disorder not otherwise specified). Finally, an appendix to DSM-IV provides a guideline for cultural formulation and a glossary of culture-bound syndromes.

RELATIONAL DISTURBANCES

An often-made criticism of DSM-III focused on the fact that it included only mental disorders that were conceptualized as occurring in the individual. This feature restricted the usefulness of the system in the diagnosis and treatment of problems that occurred in the family and other relational units (Wynne 1987). Early in the development of DSM-IV, a Coalition on Family Diagnoses was formed by professional groups dealing with these issues to consider possible changes that might be made in DSM-IV. This collaboration resulted in several new features, including the addition of a group of "relational problems" to the section entitled "Other Conditions That May Be a Focus of Clinical Attention." This new grouping includes relational problems related to a mental disorder or a general medical condition, parent-child relational problems, partner relational problems, sibling relational problems, and relational problems not otherwise specified. In addition, an optional axis, called the Global Assessment of Relational Functioning (GARF) Scale, appears in an appendix to DSM-IV.

APPENDIXES

DSM-IV contains a number of appendixes, many of which are designed to make the manual more user-friendly (i.e., to facilitate its use by clinicians and researchers). As in DSM-III and DSM-III-R, a small forest of decision trees is provided to make the differential diagnostic process easier. Using one of these trees, a clinician can follow a series of questions to rule in or out various disorders. The decision tree for mood disturbance is presented in Figure 7–2. A glossary of technical terms included in the criteria of DSM-IV has been retained as an appendix. To highlight the changes made in DSM-III-R, an annotated listing of changes made for DSM-IV specifies the corresponding categories in each manual, with a brief discussion of the reasons for major changes. A numerical listing of the codes and an alphabetical listing of the diagnostic categories are included as separate appendixes, as are listings of selected ICD-9-CM codes for general medical conditions and corresponding ICD-10 codes for DSM-IV disorders.

DSM-IV: OVERVIEW OF THE MAJOR CLASSES

In the following subsections, the major classes of DSM-IV are described. Categories that were added to DSM-IV and deleted since DSM-III-R are discussed further in Appendix D of DSM-IV, "Annotated Listing of Changes in DSM-IV."

DISORDERS USUALLY FIRST DIAGNOSED IN INFANCY, CHILDHOOD, OR ADOLESCENCE

The disorders usually first diagnosed in infancy, childhood, or adolescence are divided into a number of classes:

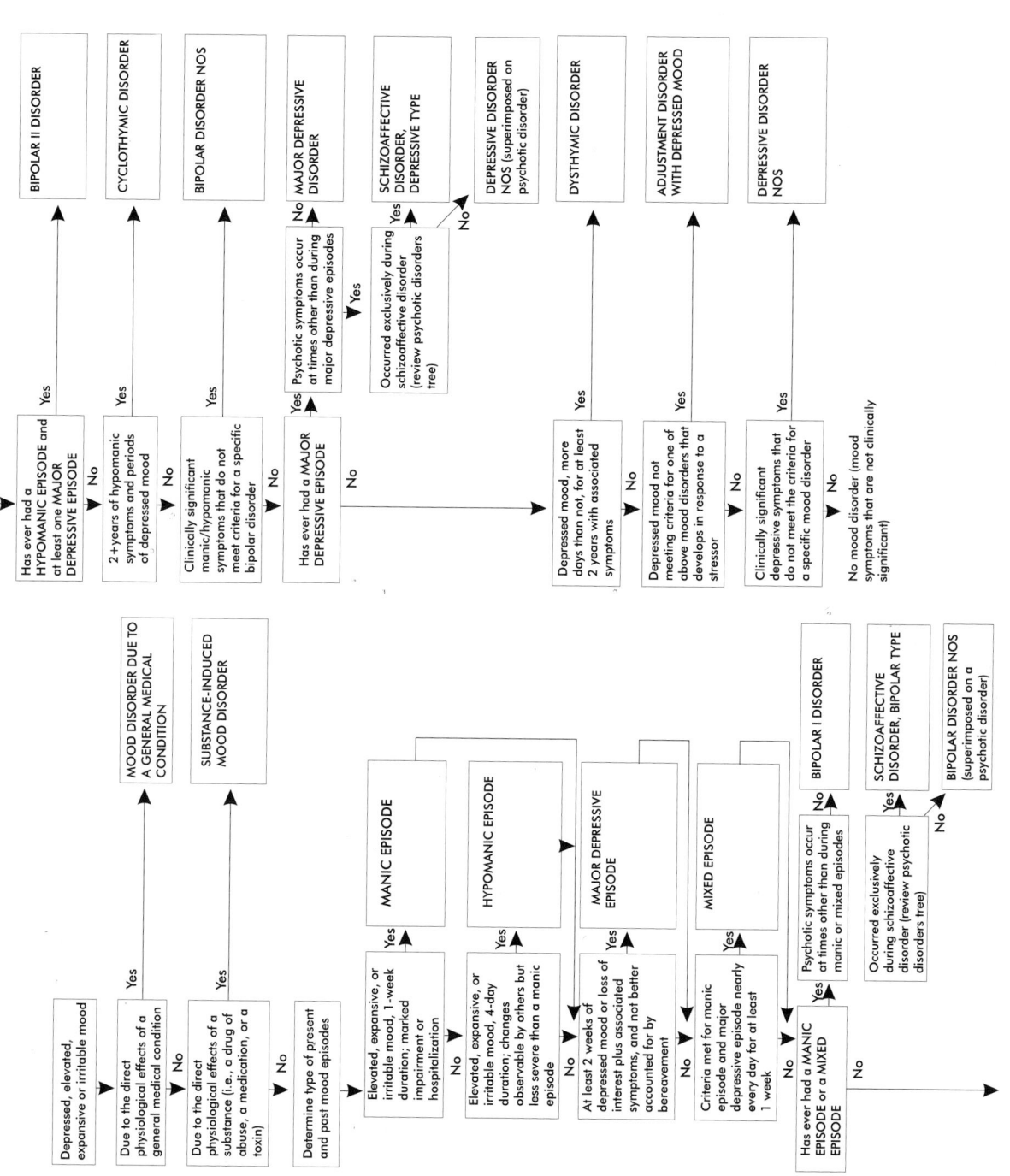

FIGURE 7–2. DSM-IV decision tree for differential diagnosis of mood disturbance. NOS = not otherwise specified.

mental retardation, learning disorders, motor skills disorder, pervasive developmental disorders, attention-deficit and disruptive behavior disorders, feeding and eating disorders of infancy or early childhood, tic disorders, communication disorders, elimination disorders, and other disorders of infancy, childhood, or adolescence. All the childhood disorders are recorded on Axis I, except mental retardation, which is recorded on Axis II.

DELIRIUM, DEMENTIA, AMNESTIC DISORDERS, AND OTHER COGNITIVE DISORDERS

The next three sections in DSM-III-R were grouped together as "organic mental disorders." However, this term is not used in DSM-IV, because it implies that the "nonorganic" mental disorders in DSM do not also have a biological basis. Instead, the so-called cognitive disorders are grouped together (see description below). The mental disorders due to general medical conditions and the substance-related disorders are referenced and described within the diagnostic classes with which they share phenomenology. So, for example, anxiety disorder due to a general medical condition and substance-induced anxiety disorder in DSM-IV are both listed within the class of anxiety disorders. This makes the classification more user-friendly because it references in one place all the disorders that a clinician must consider when making a differential diagnosis, for instance, of anxiety symptoms (Spitzer et al. 1989, 1992a).

The cognitive disorders include deliria, dementias, and amnestic disorders due to general medical conditions and substances. A category of cognitive disorder not otherwise specified (NOS) has been added for disorders that are characterized by cognitive dysfunction presumed to be due to either substance use or a general medical condition, but that do not meet criteria for any of the specific categories for delirium, dementia, or amnestic disorder.

It has often been noted that Alzheimer's disease is not included as a mental disorder in DSM-IV, even though many persons with the disease are psychiatric patients. Technically, Alzheimer's disease is a general medical condition listed in the neurological disorders section of ICD, as are Pick's and Creutzfeldt-Jakob diseases. It is the behavioral syndrome, the dementia, that results from having Alzheimer's disease that is classified as a mental disorder within DSM-IV. Thus, when making a diagnosis in a person with Alzheimer's disease, the clinician should list "dementia of the Alzheimer's type" on Axis I as the mental disorder and "Alzheimer's disease" on Axis III as the general medical disorder.

MENTAL DISORDERS DUE TO A GENERAL MEDICAL CONDITION

This section of DSM-IV includes categories for catatonic disorder, personality change, and mental disorder NOS, each due to a general medical condition.

SUBSTANCE-RELATED DISORDERS

This major class of disorders includes categories for (when applicable) dependence, abuse, intoxication, and withdrawal for the specific substance groups, as well as the criteria for hallucinogen persisting perception disorder. The text descriptions and criteria for substance-induced delirium and dementia, as well as those for substance-induced amnestic, psychotic, mood, anxiety, sexual dysfunction, and sleep disorders, appear in the sections for disorders with which they share phenomenology (e.g., substance-induced mood disorder is contained in the "Mood Disorders" section).

Single sets of criteria for dependence and abuse apply across all the substance groups. *Substance dependence* is a maladaptive pattern of substance use leading to clinically significant impairment or distress. This maladaptive use may include tolerance or withdrawal and other symptoms that indicate loss of control of substance use and continued use of the substance despite adverse consequences. *Substance abuse*, which describes the consequences of maladaptive substance use, is defined with a lower threshold than substance dependence and is appropriate only when the criteria for substance dependence have never been met. The substances themselves are divided into 11 specific groups: alcohol, amphetamine, caffeine, cannabis, cocaine, hallucinogens, inhalants, nicotine, opioids, and phencyclidine; and sedatives, hypnotics, or anxiolytics. A category for polysubstance dependence is also included.

SCHIZOPHRENIA AND OTHER PSYCHOTIC DISORDERS

This major class includes schizophrenia and its subtypes, schizophreniform disorder, schizoaffective disorder, delusional disorder, brief psychotic disorder, shared psychotic disorder, psychotic disorder due to a general medical condition, substance-induced psychotic disorder, and psychotic disorder not otherwise specified (NOS).

The diagnosis of *schizophrenia* requires both a period of active symptoms (delusions, hallucinations, disorganized speech, grossly disorganized or catatonic behavior, and negative symptoms) and a total duration of the disturbance of at least 6 months. This duration usually includes a period of prodromal symptoms in which there is deterioration in functioning, an active phase of psychotic symptoms, and a residual phase during which there is impairment in functioning but not the florid psychotic symptoms characteristic of the active phase. The symptoms of the active phase must be present for a significant portion of time during a 1-month period, unless they are successfully treated. If the active phase lasts longer than 6 months, identification of a distinct prodromal or residual phase is not necessary, even though such phases are usually present. The most common course of schizophrenia is one of recurrent exacerbations and remissions; full recovery, although it does occur, is not as common. Often, the challenge to the clinician is to distinguish schizophrenia from a psychotic disorder due to a general medical condition, a psychotic mood disorder, or schizoaffective disorder.

This concept of schizophrenia represents a narrowing of the boundaries of the disorder since DSM-II in an effort to identify a more homogeneous population with regard to a tendency toward onset in early adult life, recurrent episodes, an increased prevalence among family members, severe functional impairment, and differential response to somatic therapies (Endicott et al. 1986; Helzer et al. 1981, 1983; Stephens et al. 1982). In DSM-IV the following phenomenological subtypes of schizophrenia are recognized and defined by their cross-sectional picture: paranoid, disorganized, catatonic, undifferentiated, and residual. In addition, the course of the illness may be described as in partial or full remission after a single episode, continuous, episodic with or without interepisode residual symptoms, other pattern, or period of observation less than 1 year.

Schizophreniform disorder is phenomenologically the same as schizophrenia, except that the disturbance has had a duration of less than 6 months (but of at least 1 month). There is a provision for clinicians to indicate whether the condition is associated with good prognostic features (e.g., good premorbid functioning, acute onset). Such cases are particularly unlikely to go on to meet the criteria for schizophrenia.

In *schizoaffective disorder* there is an uninterrupted period of illness during which, at some time, there is a major depressive, manic, or mixed episode concurrent with psychotic symptoms characteristic of schizophrenia, and during the same period of illness there have been delusions or hallucinations for at least 2 weeks in the absence of prominent mood symptoms. Further, symptoms meeting criteria for a mood episode are present for a substantial part of the total duration of the active and residual periods of the illness. Schizoaffective disorder must be distinguished from schizophrenia on the one hand and psychotic mood disorders on the other.

The essential feature of *delusional disorder* is the presence of nonbizarre delusions of at least 1 month's duration that are not due to any other mental disorder, such as schizophrenia or a mood disorder, or to a general medical condition or use of a substance. The following delusional types are recognized: erotomanic, grandiose, jealous, persecutory, somatic, mixed, and unspecified.

Brief psychotic disorder may occur following a marked stressor (in which case it is equivalent to the DSM-III-R category of brief reactive psychosis) or without a marked stressor. This disorder is characterized by psychotic symptoms lasting from 1 day up to 1 month, with the person's eventual full return to his or her premorbid level of functioning.

In *shared psychotic disorder* there is a delusion that develops in one person in the context of a close relationship with another person who has an already established delusion. The same delusion is at least partly shared by both persons.

Psychotic disorder due to a general medical condition has been added to this group of disorders. Although the general medical condition is listed on both Axis I and Axis III, it should be coded only on Axis III. *Substance-induced psychotic disorder* has also been added to this part of the classification.

Finally, the category of *psychotic disorder NOS* is used when psychotic symptoms are present but there is inadequate information to make a more specific diagnosis, when there is contradictory information, or when none of the full criteria for any of the specific psychotic disorders above are met.

The diagnoses for several common patterns of psychotic symptoms and mood syndromes have been depicted in Figure 7–3 to help the reader understand the relationships among schizophrenia, psychotic mood disorder, and schizoaffective disorder, because these disorders are often included in the same differential diagnosis.

MOOD DISORDERS

The mood disorders are divided into depressive disorders (i.e., major depressive and dysthymic disorders) and bipolar disorders (i.e., bipolar I, bipolar II, and cyclothymic disorders). The depressive disorders are characterized by one or more periods of depression and the absence of a history of manic or hypomanic episodes. Major depressive episodes can be further specified as having melancholic features (a subtype that may be more severe, associated with classic vegetative signs, and particularly responsive to somatic therapy [Skodol et al. 1987]), atypical features (characterized by mood reactivity, overeating, oversleeping, leaden paralysis, and interpersonal rejection sensitivity), and catatonic features. The longitudinal course of *major depressive disorder* can be described on the basis of its episodicity, its chronicity, and

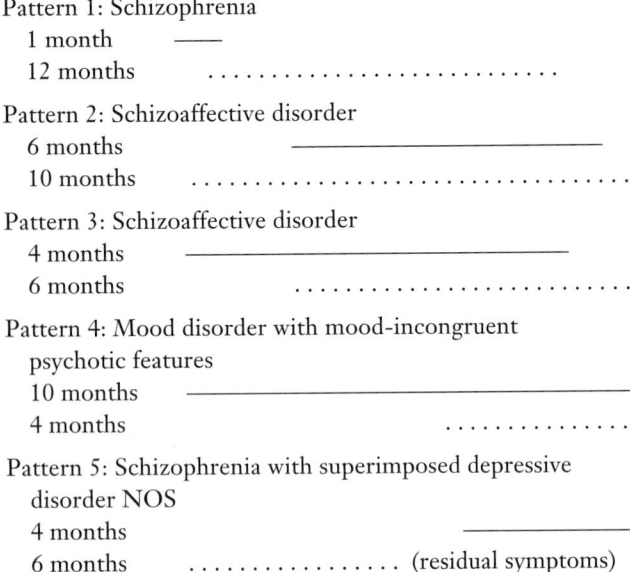

Pattern 1: Schizophrenia
  1 month
  12 months

Pattern 2: Schizoaffective disorder
  6 months
  10 months

Pattern 3: Schizoaffective disorder
  4 months
  6 months

Pattern 4: Mood disorder with mood-incongruent
  psychotic features
  10 months
  4 months

Pattern 5: Schizophrenia with superimposed depressive
  disorder NOS
  4 months
  6 months .... (residual symptoms)

FIGURE 7–3. Differential diagnosis of several common patterns of psychotic symptoms and mood syndromes. Solid lines indicate a full mood syndrome (depressed or manic); dotted lines indicate schizophrenic-like psychotic symptoms. The number of months is the duration of symptoms; the position of the mood syndrome (solid) line indicates the relative time of onset and end of the mood syndrome in relation to the psychotic symptoms (dotted line).

whether it is superimposed on dysthymic disorder.

Dysthymic disorder is a form of chronic depression of at least 2 years' duration that is distinguished from a chronic major depressive disorder by its lesser severity. The age at onset is specified as either early (before age 21) or late, because of evidence suggesting that early onset characterizes a more homogeneous group (Akiskal et al. 1981).

In *bipolar I disorder* there are one or more manic episodes or mixed episodes, and although the diagnosis does not require a history of a major depressive episode, in virtually all cases such an episode eventually develops (Nurnberger et al. 1979). *Bipolar II disorder*, newly added to the classification, does require one or more major depressive episodes, at least one hypomanic episode, and the absence of a history of manic or mixed episodes (Endicott et al. 1985). Manic episodes are distinguished from hypomanic episodes by their duration and marked impairment in social or occupational functioning or the need for hospitalization. The course of bipolar I and II disorders may be indicated as "with rapid cycling" if there have been at least 4 episodes of the mood disturbance in the previous 12 months. Further, the longitudinal course of bipolar I disorder may be specified as single-episode or recurrent.

Cyclothymic disorder is a chronic mood disturbance of at least 2 years' duration that involves numerous periods with hypomanic symptoms and numerous periods with depressed mood or loss of interest or pleasure.

A "seasonal pattern" can be indicated for major depressive episodes when there is a regular temporal relationship between the onset of the mood episodes and a particular time of the year; full remissions also must occur at a characteristic time of the year. This specification makes use of the accumulated evidence regarding the validity of a seasonal subtype of mood disorder (Rosenthal et al. 1984; Terman et al. 1989). Clinicians can also indicate whether a major depressive or manic episode developed within 4 weeks after giving birth ("with postpartum onset").

ANXIETY DISORDERS

In DSM-IV the disorders in which anxiety is experienced directly, or in which there is avoidance behavior due to anxiety, are grouped together in the class of anxiety disorders.

In *panic disorder* there are recurrent unexpected panic attacks, at least one of the attacks followed by a month or more of persistent concern about having additional attacks, worry about the implications of the attack or its consequences, or a significant change in behavior related to the attacks. Many cases of panic disorder are complicated by the presence of agoraphobia, which is anxiety about being in places or situations from which escape might be difficult or in which help might not be available if one has another panic attack; in such cases the diagnosis of *panic disorder with agoraphobia* is made.

Agoraphobia without history of panic disorder is exceedingly rare in clinical settings, because agoraphobia typically develops out of fear of having another panic attack and the resulting avoidance behavior.

Specific and social phobias both involve marked and persistent fear of a situation or stimulus with consequent avoidance behavior (or intense anxiety or distress when enduring the situation or stimulus). They are included as separate categories because of their different clinical pictures and treatment responses (Marks 1969).

In *obsessive-compulsive disorder* there are either true obsessions or compulsions that cause marked distress, are time consuming, or significantly interfere with daily functioning.

Posttraumatic stress disorder follows a traumatic event in which the person has experienced an event that involved actual or threatened death or serious injury or a threat to the physical integrity of himself or herself or others. This event is reexperienced by the person, along with other characteristic symptoms, for more than a month. Examples of symptoms specific to children are included. *Acute stress disorder* is a new category added to DSM-IV for a posttraumatic syndrome that lasts for at least 2 days but no longer than 4 weeks.

Finally, *generalized anxiety disorder* involves excessive anxiety and worry, lasting at least 6 months, about a number of events or activities. The person finds it difficult to control the worry, and it is associated with physical symptoms of anxiety, such as restlessness, difficulty concentrating, and sleep disturbance. The prevalence and validity of this diagnosis are unclear (Brown et al. 1994).

Categories for *anxiety disorder due to a general medical condition, substance-induced anxiety disorder,* and *anxiety disorder NOS* also appear in this section.

SOMATOFORM DISORDERS

Somatoform disorders all involve physical symptoms that, although suggesting a general medical disorder, cannot be accounted for by any known general medical condition. Thus, this diagnostic class includes *somatization disorder,* a chronic illness with recurrent and multiple physical complaints; *conversion disorder,* in which there are one or more symptoms or deficits affecting voluntary motor or sensory function; *hypochondriasis,* a preoccupation with fears of having, or the idea that one has, a serious disease, which is based on the person's misinterpretation of bodily symptoms; *body dysmorphic disorder,* in which there is preoccupation with an imagined defect in appearance; *pain disorder,* in which pain is the predominant focus of the clinical presentation and psychological factors are judged to have an important role in the onset, severity, exacerbation, or maintenance of the pain; and *undifferentiated somatoform disorder,* which is characterized by one or more chronic physical complaints that cause clinically significant distress or impairment in social, occupational, or other important areas of functioning.

FACTITIOUS DISORDERS

Individuals who simulate physical or psychological symptoms in such a way that their simulation is not discovered, and who therefore appear to voluntarily produce illness, have disorders that are classified as *factitious disorders.* These individuals' actions are compulsive and voluntary in the sense that they are intentionally produced or feigned, but not in the sense that they can be controlled. The prototypical *factitious disorder with predominantly physical signs and symptoms* is also referred to in the literature as Munchausen syndrome. Factitious disorders are dis-

tinguished from *malingering* (classified in the DSM-IV chapter "Other Conditions That May Be a Focus of Clinical Attention"), which, in addition to the symptoms' being under voluntary control, involves an external incentive, such as avoiding military duty or obtaining financial compensation.

DISSOCIATIVE DISORDERS

Dissociative disorders all involve a disturbance or alteration in the normally integrative functions of identity, memory, or consciousness. The disturbance or alteration may be sudden or gradual, and transient or chronic. If it occurs primarily in identity, the person's customary identity is temporarily forgotten and a new identity is assumed or imposed (as in *dissociative identity disorder,* formerly called "multiple personality disorder"), or the customary feeling of one's own reality is lost and is replaced by a feeling of unreality (as in *depersonalization disorder*). If the disturbance occurs primarily in memory, important personal events cannot be recalled (as in *dissociative amnesia* and *dissociative fugue*).

SEXUAL AND GENDER IDENTITY DISORDERS

Sexual dysfunctions, paraphilias, and gender identity disorders are included in this diagnostic class. In the *sexual dysfunctions* there is inhibition in sexual desire or in the psychophysiological changes of the sexual response cycle. *Paraphilias* all involve sexual arousal in response to objects or situations that are not part of normative arousal-activity patterns. Further, the behavior, sexual urges, or fantasies cause clinically significant distress or impairment in social, occupational, or other important areas of functioning. Finally, in *gender identity disorder* there is a strong and persistent cross-gender identification, with persistent discomfort with one's sex or a sense of inappropriateness in that gender role.

EATING DISORDERS

Anorexia nervosa and bulimia nervosa are the two specific categories in this class of disorders. In *anorexia nervosa* there is a refusal to maintain one's body weight at or above a minimally normal weight for age and height, along with an intense fear of gaining weight or becoming fat. This fear is accompanied by a disturbance in the way in which the individual experiences his or her body weight or shape. *Bulimia nervosa* is characterized by recurrent episodes of binge eating accompanied by recurrent inappropriate compensatory behaviors in order to prevent weight gain, such as self-induced vomiting, fasting, or excessive exercise.

SLEEP DISORDERS

This diagnostic class includes disorders of sleep that are chronic, rather than the transient disturbances of sleep that are commonly experienced. Sleep disorders are divided into the *dyssomnias*, in which there is a disturbance in the amount, quality, or timing of sleep; the *parasomnias*, in which the hallmark is an abnormal event that occurs either during sleep or at the threshold between wakefulness and sleep; *sleep disorders related to another mental disorder*, in which insomnia or hypersomnia is judged to be related to another Axis I or II disorder, but is sufficiently severe to warrant independent clinical attention; and *other sleep disorders*, which include sleep disorder due to a general medical condition and substance-induced sleep disorder.

The dyssomnias include *primary insomnia*, in which there is difficulty initiating or maintaining sleep, or there is nonrestorative sleep, for at least 1 month, with consequent clinically significant distress or impairment in functioning; *primary hypersomnia*, characterized by complaint of excessive sleepiness for at least 1 month, also resulting in clinically significant distress or impairment in functioning; *narcolepsy* (added in DSM-IV), with irresistible attacks of refreshing sleep occurring daily over at least 3 months, cataplexy, and intrusions of REM sleep into the transition between sleep and wakefulness (e.g., sleep paralysis); *breathing-related sleep disorder*, in which there is sleep disruption leading to excessive sleepiness or insomnia that is due to a sleep-related breathing disorder such as sleep apnea; and *circadian rhythm sleep disorder*, a persistent or recurrent pattern of sleep disruption leading to excessive sleepiness or insomnia that is due to a mismatch between the sleep-wake schedule required by a person's environment and his or her circadian sleep-wake pattern (subtypes are delayed sleep phase type, jet lag type, shift work type, and unspecified).

The parasomnias include the following: *Nightmare disorder* is characterized by repeated awakenings from sleep with detailed recall of extended and extremely frightening dreams. *Sleep terror disorder* also includes recurrent awakenings from sleep, but they are accompanied by intense anxiety and signs of autonomic arousal such as tachycardia and sweating; yet no detailed dream is recalled. *Sleepwalking disorder* is one in which the individual repeatedly walks about during sleep and is relatively unresponsive during the episodes. In both sleep terror and sleepwalking disorders, there is later amnesia for the episode. Finally, *insomnia or hypersomnia related to [Axis I or Axis II disorder]* may be diagnosed when the sleep disturbance is sufficiently severe to cause clinically significant distress or impairment in social, occupational, or other important areas of functioning.

IMPULSE CONTROL DISORDERS NOT ELSEWHERE CLASSIFIED

The impulse control disorders not elsewhere classified involve disturbances in impulse control that do not satisfy the criteria for other diagnostic categories (e.g., substance-related disorders or paraphilias). These disorders are characterized by 1) recurrent failure to resist an impulse, drive, or temptation to perform some act that is harmful to oneself or others; 2) an increasing sense of tension before committing the act; and 3) a sense of either pleasure, gratification, or relief at the time of committing the act. Included in this class of disorders are *intermittent explosive disorder*, *kleptomania*, *pyromania*, *pathological gambling*, and *trichotillomania* (a disorder characterized by impulsive pulling out of one's own hair).

ADJUSTMENT DISORDER

Adjustment disorder is a clinically significant reaction to an identifiable stressor that occurs within 3 months of the onset of the stressor and persists for no longer than 6 months after the termination of the stressor or its consequences. This category is not diagnosed if the disturbance meets the criteria for another specific Axis I disorder or is merely an exacerbation of a preexisting Axis I or Axis II disorder. Five specific types of adjustment disorder are included: adjustment disorder with anxiety, with depressed mood, with disturbance of conduct, with mixed disturbance of emotions and conduct, and with mixed anxiety and depressed mood. Adjustment disorder may also be qualified as acute or chronic, depending on whether the symptoms have persisted for 6 months or longer.

PERSONALITY DISORDERS

Each of the diagnostic criteria for the 10 specific personality disorders is in the form of a brief summary description of the disorder followed by an index of specific behaviors, no single one of which is required for making the diagnosis. The personality disorders, all recorded on Axis II of the multiaxial system, are grouped into three clusters based on common behavioral features (Kass et al. 1985). Cluster A includes paranoid, schizoid, and schizotypal personality disorders; people with these often appear odd or eccentric. In Cluster B, comprising antisocial, borderline, histrionic, and narcissistic personality disorders, there is usually dramatic, emotional, or erratic behavior. Finally, Cluster C includes avoidant, dependent, and obsessive-compulsive personality disorders, all of which usually involve anxiety or fearfulness. A residual category, personality disorder NOS, is provided for 1) disorders of personality functioning that do not meet the criteria for any specific personality disorder and 2) other specific personality disorders not included in this classification (such as passive aggressive personality disorder, included in DSM-III-R but not in DSM-IV).

It is not uncommon for several personality disorder diagnoses to be made for a single person. Many of the categories have overlapping behaviors, and many people have disturbances in more than one area of personality functioning. When several personality disorders are diagnosed concurrently, there is probably severe personality disturbance, and this should be taken into account when treatment is planned.

It is sometimes difficult to determine whether a disturbance is best diagnosed as an Axis I disorder or as a personality disorder on Axis II. In differentiating a personality disorder, the clinician must consider several factors. First, a personality disorder is characteristic of the person's current and long-term functioning and is not limited to episodes of illness; that is, it represents a pervasive pattern of disturbance that is present in a variety of contexts in the person's life. Therefore, an individual who is excessively perfectionistic in her work life may have an obsessive-compulsive personality trait, but not the corresponding personality disorder unless her excessive perfectionism is associated with other types of inflexibility and is apparent in several other areas of her life (e.g., with her friends, at home, and in leisure activities). Second, in distinguishing a personality disorder from a personality trait, the clinician must determine that the behaviors are above a certain threshold in terms of causing either subjective distress or significant impairment in social or occupational functioning, and in terms of having enough criteria met. Using the same example, if the person's perfectionism at work does not impair her work functioning to a significant degree and is not associated with a lot of other features, the diagnosis should not be given. Finally, the disturbance must begin by early adulthood and usually is apparent by adolescence.

OTHER CONDITIONS THAT MAY BE A FOCUS OF CLINICAL ATTENTION

Other conditions may be a focus of clinical attention but are not considered mental disorder diagnoses. A list of such conditions (e.g., medication-induced movement disorders, relational problems, problems related to abuse or neglect, bereavement, occupational problems, malingering, and phase-of-life problem) is included for use when no mental disorder diagnosis is appropriate but help is needed, or when there is a mental disorder related to one of these conditions but the condition is sufficiently severe to warrant independent clinical attention. In addition, there are codes for indicating that the diagnosis is deferred on Axis I or Axis II or that there is no diagnosis or condition on these axes.

CRITERIA SETS AND AXES PROVIDED FOR FURTHER STUDY

During the development of DSM-IV, there were proposals for many new categories. The advisory committees that worked on the definitions of these disorders and the task force believed that there was sufficient research and clinical evidence regarding the validity of each of these categories to justify their inclusion in the revised manual, although not as full-fledged disorders and axes. Table 7–6 lists the categories for which criteria sets are included in

TABLE 7–6. List of DSM-IV criteria sets and axes provided for further study (DSM-IV Appendix B)

Postconcussional disorder

Mild neurocognitive disorder

Caffeine withdrawal

Alternative dimensional descriptors for schizophrenia

Postpsychotic depressive disorder of schizophrenia

Simple deteriorative disorder (simple schizophrenia)

Premenstrual dysphoric disorder

Alternative Criterion B for dysthymic disorder

Minor depressive disorder

Recurrent brief depressive disorder

Mixed anxiety-depressive disorder

Factitious disorder by proxy

Dissociative trance disorder

Binge-eating disorder

Depressive personality disorder

Passive-aggressive personality disorder (negativistic personality disorder)

Medication-induced movement disorders

    Neuroleptic-induced parkinsonism

    Neuroleptic malignant syndrome

    Neuroleptic-induced acute dystonia

    Neuroleptic-induced acute akathisia

    Neuroleptic-induced tardive dyskinesia

    Medication-induced postural tremor

    Medication-induced movement disorder not otherwise specified

Defensive Functioning Scale

Global Assessment of Relational Functioning (GARF) Scale

Social and Occupational Functioning Assessment Scale (SOFAS)

Appendix B of DSM-IV. Also listed are three optional axes that may be useful to clinicians and researchers.

THE FUTURE

It is clear that both DSM-III and DSM-III-R have had a major impact on psychiatry in this country and abroad. The tenth revision of ICD (ICD-10) has incorporated many of the most important and unique features that were first included in DSM-III, such as the provision of diagnostic criteria and the grouping together of disorders on the basis of shared clinical features rather than presumed etiology, indicating international acceptance of these advances. DSM-IV maintains compatibility with ICD-10 while incorporating innovative features that are leading psychiatry in new directions.

REFERENCES

Akiskal HS, King D, Rosenthal TL, et al: Chronic depressions, I: clinical and familial characteristics in 137 probands. J Affect Disord 3:297–315, 1981

American Psychiatric Association: Diagnostic and Statistical Manual: Mental Disorders. Washington, DC, American Psychiatric Association, 1952

American Psychiatric Association: Diagnostic and Statistical Manual of Mental Disorders, 2nd Edition. Washington, DC, American Psychiatric Association, 1968

American Psychiatric Association: Diagnostic and Statistical Manual of Mental Disorders, 3rd Edition. Washington, DC, American Psychiatric Association, 1980

American Psychiatric Association: Diagnostic and Statistical Manual of Mental Disorders, 3rd Edition, Revised. Washington, DC, American Psychiatric Association, 1987

American Psychiatric Association: Diagnostic and Statistical Manual of Mental Disorders, 4th Edition. Washington, DC, American Psychiatric Association, 1994

Baldessarini RJ, Finklestein S, Arana GW: The predictive power of diagnostic tests and the effect of prevalence of illness. Arch Gen Psychiatry 40:569–573, 1983

Baron M, Asnis L, Gruen R: The Schedule for Schizotypal Personalities (SSP): a diagnostic interview for schizotypal features. Psychiatry Res 4:213–228, 1981

Boyd JH, Burke JD Jr, Gruenberg E, et al: Exclusion criteria of DSM-III: a study of co-occurrence of hierarchy-free syndromes. Arch Gen Psychiatry 41:983–989, 1984

Brown TA, Barlow DH, Liebowitz MR: The empirical basis of generalized anxiety disorder. Am J Psychiatry 151:1271-1280, 1994

Clark LA: Schedule for Nonadaptive and Adaptive Personality. Minneapolis, MN, University of Minnesota Press, 1993

Cohen J: A coefficient of agreement for nominal scales. Educational and Psychological Measurement 20:37–46, 1960

Cooper JE, Kendell RE, Gurland BJ, et al: Psychiatric Diagnosis in New York and London. London, Oxford University Press, 1972

Curran JP, Miller IW, Zwick WR, et al: The socially inadequate patient: incidence rate, demographic and clinical features, and hospital and posthospital functioning. J Consult Clin Psychol 48:375–382, 1980

Endicott J, Spitzer RL: A diagnostic interview: the Schedule for Affective Disorders and Schizophrenia. Arch Gen Psychiatry 35:837–844, 1978

Endicott J, Nee J, Andreasen N, et al: Bipolar II: combine or keep separate? J Affect Disord 8:17–28, 1985

Endicott J, Nee J, Cohen J, et al: Diagnosis of schizophrenia: prediction of short-term outcome. Arch Gen Psychiatry 43:13–19, 1986

Feighner JP, Robins E, Guze SB, et al: Diagnostic criteria for use in psychiatric research. Arch Gen Psychiatry 26:57–63, 1972

Fenichel GS, Murphy JG: Factors that predict psychiatric consultation in the emergency department. Med Care 23:258–265, 1985

First MB, Gibbon M, Spitzer RL, et al: Structured Clinical Interview for DSM-IV—Clinical Version (SCID-CV). Washington, DC, American Psychiatric Press, 1997a

First MB, Gibbon M, Spitzer RL, et al: Structured Clinical Interview for DSM-IV Axis II—Personality Disorders (SCID-II). Washington, DC, American Psychiatric Press, 1997b

Frances A, Davis WW, Kline M, et al: The DSM-IV field trials: moving towards an empirically derived classification. European Psychiatry 6:307–314, 1991

Gordon RE, Jardiolin P, Gordon KK: Predicting length of hospital stay of psychiatric patients. Am J Psychiatry 142:235–237, 1985a

Gordon RE, Vijay J, Sloate SG, et al: Aggravating stress and functional level as predictors of length of psychiatric hospitalization. Hosp Community Psychiatry 36:773–774, 1985b

Gutterman EM, O'Brien JD, Young JG: Structured diagnostic interviews for children and adolescents: current status and future directions. J Am Acad Child Adolesc Psychiatry 26:621–630, 1987

Guy W (ed): ECDEU Assessment Manual for Psychopharmacology (DHEW Publ No ADM 76-336). Rockville, MD, U.S. Dept of Health, Education, and Welfare, 1976

Hedlund JL, Vieweg BW: Structured psychiatric interviews: a comparative review. Journal of Operational Psychiatry 12:39–67, 1981

Helzer JE, Brockington IF, Kendell RE: Predictive validity of DSM-III and Feighner definitions of schizophrenia: a comparison with Research Diagnostic Criteria and CATEGO. Arch Gen Psychiatry 38:791–797, 1981

Helzer JE, Kendell RE, Brockington IF: Contribution of the six-month criterion to the predictive validityof the DSM-III definition of schizophrenia. Arch Gen Psychiatry 40:1277–1280, 1983

Hodges K: Structured interviews for assessing children. J Child Psychol Psychiatry 34:49–68, 1993

Husby R: Short-term dynamic psychotherapy, V: Global Assessment Scale as an instrument for description and measurement of changes for 33 neurotic patients. Psychother Psychosom 43:28–31, 1985

Hyler SE, Williams JBW, Spitzer RL: Reliability in the DSM-III field trials: interview v case summary. Arch Gen Psychiatry 39:1275–1278, 1982

Kass F, Skodol AE, Charles E, et al: Scaled ratings of DSM-III personality disorders. Am J Psychiatry 142:627–630, 1985

Klein DF, Gittelman R, Quitkin F, et al: Diagnosis and Drug Treatment of Psychiatric Disorders: Adults and Children. Baltimore, MD, Williams & Willkins, 1980

Leckman JF, Merikangas KR, Pauls DL, et al: Anxiety disorders and depression: contradictions between family study data and DSM-III conventions. Am J Psychiatry 140:880–882, 1983

Mannuzza S, Fyer AJ, Martin LY, et al: Reliability of anxiety assessment, I: diagnostic agreement. Arch Gen Psychiatry 46:1093–1101, 1989

Marks I: Fears and Phobias. New York, Academic Press, 1969

Mezzich JE, Evanczuk KJ, Mathias RJ, et al: Admission decisions and multiaxial diagnosis. Arch Gen Psychiatry 41:1001–1004, 1984

Mezzich JE, Kleinman A, Fabrega H, Parron DL: Culture and Psychiatric Diagnosis: A DSM-IV Perspective. Washington, DC, American Psychiatric Press, 1996

Nurnberger J Jr, Roose SP, Dunner DL, et al: Unipolar mania: a distinct clinical entity? Am J Psychiatry 136:1420–1423, 1979

Perry JC: Problems and considerations in the valid assessment of personality disorders. Am J Psychiatry 149:1645–1653, 1992

Pfohl B, Blum N, Zimmerman M: The Structured Interview for DSM-IV Personality (SIDP-IV). Washington, DC, American Psychiatric Press, 1997

Regier DA, Myers JK, Kramer M, et al: The NIMH Epidemiologic Catchment Area program: historical context, major objectives, and study population characteristics. Arch Gen Psychiatry 41:934–941, 1984

Robins E, Guze SB: Establishment of diagnostic validity in psychiatric illness: its application to schizophrenia. Am J Psychiatry 126:983–987, 1970

Robins LN, Helzer JE, Croughan J, et al: National Institute of Mental Health Diagnostic Interview Schedule: its history, characteristics, and validity. Arch Gen Psychiatry 38:381–389, 1981

Robins LN, Wing J, Wittchen HU, et al: The Composite International Diagnostic Interview: an epidemiologic instrument suitable for use in conjunction with different diagnostic systems and in different cultures. Arch Gen Psychiatry 45:1069–1077, 1988

Robins LN, Cottler L, Bucholz K, et al: Diagnostic Interview Schedule for DSM-IV (DIS-IV). St. Louis, MO, Washington University, 1995

Rosenthal NE, Sack DA, Gillin JC, et al: Seasonal affective disorder: description of syndrome and preliminary findings with light therapy. Arch Gen Psychiatry 41:72–80, 1984

Schleyer B, Aaronson C, Mannuzza S, et al: SADS-LA[R]. New York, Anxiety Disorders Clinic, New York State Psychiatric Institute, 1990

Shrout PE, Spitzer RL, Fleiss JL: Quantification of agreement in psychiatry diagnosis revisited. Arch Gen Psychiatry 44:172–177, 1987

Skodol AE: Axis IV, in DSM-IV Source Book, Vol. 3. Edited by Widiger T, Frances AJ, Pincus HA, et al. Washington, DC, American Psychiatric Press, 1997

Skodol AE, Zimmerman M, Hirschfeld RMA: Affective and adjustment disorders, in An Annotated Bibliography of DSM-III. Edited by Skodol AE, Spitzer RL. Washington, DC, American Psychiatric Press, 1987, pp 95–109

Spitzer RL: Psychiatric diagnosis: are clinicians still necessary? Compr Psychiatry 24:399–411, 1983

Spitzer RL, Fleiss JL: A re-analysis of the reliability of psychiatric diagnosis. Br J Psychiatry 125:341–347, 1974

Spitzer RL, Forman JBW: DSM-III field trials, II: initial experience with the multiaxial system. Am J Psychiatry 136:818–820, 1979

Spitzer RL, Williams JBW: Dehumanizing descriptors? (letter) Am J Psychiatry 136:1481, 1979

Spitzer RL, Williams JBW: The definition and diagnosis of mental disorder, in Deviance and Mental Illness (Sage Annual Reviews of Studies in Deviance, Vol 6). Edited by Gove WR. Beverly Hills, CA, Sage, 1982, pp 15–31

Spitzer RL, Williams JBW: Classification of mental disorders, in Comprehensive Textbook of Psychiatry/IV, 4th Edition, Vol 1. Edited by Kaplan HI, Sadock BJ. Baltimore, MD, Williams & Wilkins, 1985, pp 591–613

Spitzer RL, Williams JBW: Revision of DSM-III: process and changes, in International Classification in Psychiatry: Unity and Diversity. Edited by Mezzich JE, von Cranach M. London, Cambridge University Press, 1988, pp 263–283

Spitzer RL, Fleiss JL, Burdock EI, et al: The Mental Status Schedule: rationale, reliability and validity. Compr Psychiatry 5:384–395, 1964

Spitzer RL, Endicott J, Robins E: Reliability of clinical criteria for psychiatric diagnosis, in Psychiatric Diagnosis: Exploration of Biological Predictors. Edited by Akiskal H, Webb W. New York, Spectrum, 1978a, pp 61–73

Spitzer RL, Endicott J, Robins E: Research Diagnostic Criteria: rationale and reliability. Arch Gen Psychiatry 35:773–782, 1978b

Spitzer RL, Forman JBW, Nee J: DSM-III field trials, I: initial interrater diagnostic reliability. Am J Psychiatry 136:815–817, 1979

Spitzer RL, Williams JBW, Skodol AE (eds): International Perspectives on DSM-III. Washington, DC, American Psychiatric Press, 1983

Spitzer RL, Williams JBW, First MB, et al: A proposal for DSM-IV: solving the "organic/nonorganic" problem (editorial). J Neuropsychiatry Clin Neurosci 1:126–127, 1989

Spitzer RL, First M[B], Williams JBW, et al: Now is the time to retire the term "organic mental disorders." Am J Psychiatry 149:240–244, 1992a

Spitzer RL, Williams JBW, Gibbon M, et al: The Structured Clinical Interview for DSM-III-R (SCID), I: history, rationale, and description. Arch Gen Psychiatry 49:624–629, 1992b

Spitzer RL, Williams JBW, Kroenke K, et al: The PRIME-MD 1000 Study: Description, validation, and clinical utility of a new procedure for diagnosing mental disorders in primary care. JAMA 272:1749–1756, 1994

Stephens JH, Astrup C, Carpenter WT Jr, et al: A comparison of nine systems to diagnose schizophrenia. Psychiatry Res 6:127–143, 1982

Terman M, Terman JS, Quitkin FM, et al: Light therapy for seasonal affective disorder: a review of efficacy. Neuropsychopharmacology 2:1–22, 1989

Thompson C (ed): The Instruments of Psychiatric Research. Chichester, UK, Wiley, 1989

van Riezen H, Segal M: Comparative Evaluation of Rating Scales for Clinical Psychopharmacology. Amsterdam, Elsevier, 1988

Wakefield JC: The concept of mental disorder: on the boundary between biological facts and social values. Am Psychologist 47:373–388, 1992

Widiger TA, Frances A, Spitzer RL, et al: The DSM-III-R personality disorders: an overview. Am J Psychiatry 145:786–795, 1988

Widiger TA, Frances AJ, Pincus HA, et al: DSM-IV literature reviews: rationale, process, and limitations. J Psychopathology and Behavioral Assessment 12:189–202, 1990

Widiger TA, Frances AJ, Pincus HA, et al: DSM-IV Sourcebook, Vol I. Washington, DC, American Psychiatric Press, 1994

Widiger TA, Frances AJ, Pincus HA, et al: DSM-IV Sourcebook, Vol II. Washington, DC, American Psychiatric Press, 1996

Widiger TA, Frances AJ, Pincus HA, et al: DSM-IV Sourcebook, Vol 3. Washington, DC, American Psychiatric Press, 1997

Williams JBW: The multiaxial system of DSM-III: where did it come from and where should it go? I: its origins and critiques. Arch Gen Psychiatry 42:175–180, 1985a

Williams JBW: The multiaxial system of DSM-III: where did it come from and where should it go? II: empirical studies, innovations, and recommendations. Arch Gen Psychiatry 42:181–186, 1985b

Williams JBW, Spitzer RL, Skodol AE: DSM-III in residency training: results of a national survey. Am J Psychiatry 142:755–758, 1985

Williams JBW, Gibbon M, First MB, et al: The Structured Clinical Interview for DSM-III-R (SCID), II: multisite test-retest reliability. Arch Gen Psychiatry 49:630–636, 1992

Wing JK, Giddens RGJ: Industrial rehabilitation of male chronic schizophrenics. Lancet 2:505–507, 1959

Wing JK, Birley JLT, Cooper JE, et al: Reliability of a procedure for measuring and classifying "present psychiatric state." Br J Psychiatry 113:499–515, 1967

Wing JK, Babor T, Brugha T, et al: SCAN: Schedules for Clinical Assessment in Neuropsychiatry. Arch Gen Psychiatry 47:589–593, 1990

World Health Organization: International Statistical Classification of Diseases, Injuries, and Causes of Death, 8th Revision. Geneva, World Health Organization, 1969

World Health Organization: Report of the International Pilot Study of Schizophrenia, Vol 1. Geneva, World Health Organization, 1973

World Health Organization: International Classification of Diseases, 9th Revision. Geneva, World Health Organization, 1977

World Health Organization: International Classification of Diseases, 10th Revision. Geneva, World Health Organization, 1992

Wynne LC: A preliminary proposal for strengthening the multiaxial approach of DSM-III: possible family-oriented revisions, in Diagnosis and Classification in Psychiatry: A Critical Appraisal of DSM-III. Edited by Tischler GL. Cambridge, UK, Cambridge University Press, 1987, pp 477–488

Zanarini MC, Frankenburg FR, Chauncey DL, et al: The Diagnostic Interview for Personality Disorders: interrater and test-retest reliability. Compr Psychiatry 28:467–480, 1987

CHAPTER 8

PSYCHOLOGICAL AND NEUROPSYCHOLOGICAL ASSESSMENT

JOHN F. CLARKIN, PH.D.
STEPHEN W. HURT, PH.D.
STEVEN MATTIS, PH.D.

The current methodology and content of psychiatric diagnosis, the level of sophistication of treatment planning in regard to both medication and psychosocial interventions, and the nature of the health care delivery system all influence the context that determines the use of psychological tests and rating scales to inform treatment planning. Two major forces have influenced treatment planning in the recent past: 1) the use of a diagnostic system, since 1980, which has been strong on reliability and relatively uneven and weak on validity, and 2) the impact of managed care, with its emphasis on cost saving and delivery of services deemed "medically necessary." These forces have shaped the use of psychological and neuropsychological assessments. Developments that are relatively new are 1) the use of instruments to provide data on patients in a managed care system and 2) the assessment of systems of care as a whole.

DEFINITION AND DEVELOPMENT OF PSYCHOLOGICAL ASSESSMENT

INSTRUMENTS

Three types of instruments are currently used in the assessment of patient functioning: psychological tests, rating scales, and semistructured interviews (Table 8–1). Psychological tests are standardized methods of sampling behaviors in a reliable and valid way. The test stimuli, the method of presenting these stimuli, and the method of scoring the responses are carefully standardized to ensure reliability. The actual test stimuli can be constructed in numerous ways. For example, test items on the Wechsler Adult Intelligence Scale—Revised (WAIS-R; Wechsler 1981), a widely used intelligence test, include factual questions (e.g., "What does *ponder* mean?"), and each answer is scored 2 (e.g., to contemplate), 1 (e.g., to wonder), or

Table 8–1. Three types of psychological assessment instruments

Type of test	Example
Psychological tests	Wechsler Adult Intelligence Scale—Revised (WAIS-R)
	Minnesota Multiphasic Personality Inventory–2 (MMPI-2)
Rating scales	Brief Psychiatric Rating Scale (BPRS)
Semistructured interviews	Structured Clinical Interview for DSM-IV (SCID)
	Personality Disorders Examination (PDE)

0 (e.g., to fret). The restandardized Minnesota Multiphasic Personality Inventory—2 (MMPI-2; Butcher et al. 1989), a highly developed and widely used symptom and personality test, consists of questions about the presence or absence of feelings, thoughts, and experiences (e.g., "I usually feel that life is worthwhile," an item on Scale 2 in a true/false format. Test stimuli on the Rorschach Inkblot Test (Rorschach 1949), a widely used projective test of personality styles and characteristics, are amorphous inkblots (Figure 8–1). The patient is asked to tell the examiner what it looks like or what it reminds the patient of. The response is recorded verbatim and scored with a standardized system.

Behavior rating scales are standardized devices that allow various informants or observers (e.g., therapist, nurse on a clinical inpatient unit, relatives, trained observers) to rate the behavior of the patient in specified areas. To aid the observer in a reliable rating of the behavior, anchor points are provided in one of several ways. For example, on the Brief Psychiatric Rating Scale (BPRS; Overall and Gorham 1962), somatic concern, defined as the "degree of concern over present bodily health," is rated by the interviewer on a 7-point scale from "not present" to "extremely severe." Commonly used rating scales, to be discussed later in this chapter, include the BPRS, the Hamilton Rating Scale for Depression (Ham-D; Hamilton 1960, 1967), and the Katz Adjustment Scales (KAS) (Katz and Lyerly 1963).

Semistructured interviews are standardized by controlling the questions, including specifying what kind of probes can be used, and standardizing the scoring of the patient's response, often by using rating scales as described above. Although developed for research, these interviews have clinical usefulness in the reliable assessment of diagnostic criteria. As an example of a semistructured interview item, the following is a question from the Structured Clinical Interview for DSM-IV Axis I Disorders (SCID): "In the last month, has there been a period of time when you were feeling depressed or down most of the day nearly every day?" The subject's response is rated on a scale from 1 (absent or false), to 2 (subthreshold) to 3 (threshold or true). Useful semistructured interviews include the Schedule for Affective Disorders and Schizophrenia (SADS), the Structured Clinical Interview for DSM-IV Axis I Disorders (SCID; First et al. 1996), and the International Personality Disorders Examination (IPDE; Loranger 1995).

The science of assessment depends on the development of instruments that meet certain standards. Chief among these standards are those for reliability and various types of validity.

Standardization of administration and scoring to minimize the influence of factors unrelated to the area of assessment is essential for establishing reliability. The degree to which a test meets acceptable standards for reliability is evaluated by 1) readministering the test at later times to determine if individual scores remain stable, 2) developing alternate forms of the test that, when compared, provide roughly equivalent scores for an individual, and 3) demonstrating that any subgroup of items from the test yields a score comparable to an equivalent number of items in any other subgroup of items. These procedures for establishing reliability are generally referred to as test-retest reliability, alternate form reliability, and split-half reliability, respectively (Table 8–2).

Demonstration of adequate test reliability is only the first step in test development. It establishes that the test items are sufficiently closely related to one another to provide relatively stable measurements. However, a test's reliability does not guarantee its validity. Establishing validity

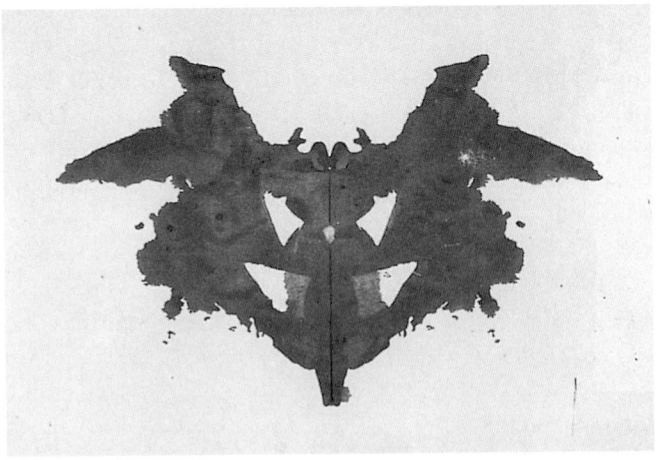

Figure 8–1. Rorschach, Card I.
Source. Reprinted with permission from Rorschach H: Rorschach-Test. Copyright 1921, 1948, 1994, Verlag Hans Huber, Bern, Switzerland.

TABLE 8–2. Types of reliability and validity

Type	Description
Reliability	
Test-retest	Test yields comparable scores at two proximate points in time.
Alternate form	Two forms of the same test yield comparable scores.
Split-half	Subgroups of items yield scores comparable to those of other subgroups of items.
Validity	
Content	Items adequately sample the content area.
Criterion-related	Test score correlates with other measurements of the same area of activity.
Construct	Test measures a theoretical construct and is unrelated to similar but different constructs.

requires a demonstration that a test measures what it is intended to measure. Three major types of validity can be assessed: 1) content validity, 2) criterion-related validity, and 3) construct validity.

Content validity can be achieved only if the content of the test can be said to adequately sample the area of interest. For example, an intelligence test must contain items that tap several areas of intellectual functioning, such as knowledge of words, arithmetic ability, abstracting ability, knowledge of social conventions, and so forth, in order to meet acceptable standards for content validity. Criterion-related validity refers to the test's relationship to independent criteria of an individual's ability in a particular area (called concurrent validity) or to the ability of the test to make predictions about future behavior (called predictive validity). For example, a test of the severity of depressive symptoms would achieve concurrent validity if scores on the test were closely related to a trained observer's rating of the severity of the depression; it would achieve predictive validity if scores on the test were found to be related to the likelihood that a given individual would respond to a specific treatment for reducing depressive symptoms. Construct validity can be achieved only by demonstrating that the test specifically measures a theoretical construct of interest and that scores on the test are unrelated to similar areas.

For further information on the general principles of assessment, tests, and test construction, one can consult Anastasi (1982). Also, the Mental Measurements Yearbooks, edited by Buros (1971, 1978), provide excellent reviews of existing instruments. One can also consult Newman and Ciarlo (1994) for criteria that can be used to select instruments for various tasks.

GOALS OF ASSESSMENT

The role of assessment has always been closely linked to the need to conceptualize and implement successful intervention strategies for the remediation of psychological disorders. As a consequence, the goals of assessment should constantly be revised as new treatment methods are developed. Common assessment goals are listed in Table 8–3.

Diagnostic assessment remains the primary reason for clinical psychiatric referral. DSM-IV (American Psychiatric Association 1994) provides a focus for diagnostic issues and simultaneously capitalizes on and fuels a growing interest in the issues of accurate diagnosis. Much of the research stimulated by the development and implementation of DSM-III and its successors focused on the sensitivity and specificity of the diagnostic criteria, with the aim of identifying groups of symptoms that are optimally responsive to a growing armamentarium of psychiatric and psychological interventions. This kind of research represented a shift from the idiographic approach, typical of earlier psychiatric research, to a more nomothetic approach. In the latter approach, the goals of assessment are to relate the individual features of test performance to patterns of performance typical of certain diagnostic groups rather than to highlight the unique aspects of any one individual's performance (see Hurt et al. 1991).

For the clinical psychologist, this shift in emphasis suggests that assessment is much more likely to be tailored to specific aspects of the referral and to the salient dimensions of information that constitute the differential. For example, depressed mood is featured as a criterion for a number of DSM-IV disorders, including major depression, atypical depression, bipolar disorder, dysthymia, adjust-

TABLE 8–3. Specific objectives of assessment

1. To clarify diagnostic uncertainty following the clinical interview
2. To specify the severity of symptoms and other difficulties
3. To assess patient strengths (e.g., intelligence, personality traits)
4. To inform differential treatment assignment
5. To develop a role consistent with a therapeutic alliance
6. To monitor the impact of treatment

ment disorder with depressed mood, schizoaffective disorder, and borderline personality disorder, among others. Because these different disorders are optimally responsive to different treatments, or because attempts to ameliorate the depressed mood itself may require different intervention strategies for some of these disorders, the goal of differential diagnosis takes on added value. The clinical psychologist, therefore, must carefully choose the instruments for the assessment in light of the need for distinguishing among these disorders.

Differential treatment planning, then, is at the heart of the assessment process and provides the rationale for the diagnostic effort. In the absence of treatment specificity, there is little justification for an intensive focus on diagnosis. Although the science of differential therapeutics is in its infancy, the proliferation of medication and treatment approaches and modalities has spawned a growing literature on the assessment of various characteristics and dimensions thought to be essential to the understanding of and rational treatment planning for the various disorders.

A ready example of this kind of development can be found in the literature on depression. Drawing on the infrahuman learning literature, Beck and Young (1985) have argued that cognitions such as hopelessness, helplessness, and worthlessness are essential for understanding depression. This cognitive theory of depression has been sufficiently well elaborated to lead to the development of rating scales that are sensitive to these cognitions and to lead to the design of an appropriate treatment approach.

MAJOR AREAS OF ASSESSMENT

To further the overall goal of clinical assessment—differential treatment planning—one must consider the most important content areas of assessment. The assessment procedures chosen should depend on the nature of the patient's difficulties revealed or suspected during routine psychiatric examination. They should be carried out in the context of the major dimensions of human functioning relevant to diagnosis and treatment planning. The areas or dimensions of human functioning that seem most central

to diagnosis and treatment planning include 1) symptoms and related Axis I disorders, 2) cognitive functioning, 3) personality traits and disorders, 4) psychodynamics, and 5) environmental demands and social adjustment. In the sections that follow we review the best available instruments in each of these five areas.

ASSESSMENT OF AXIS I CONSTELLATIONS AND RELATED SYMPTOMS

As psychiatric nomenclature has undergone revision, assessment tools have been developed that rely on interviews and self-reports (Table 8–4), providing data that are immediately relevant to diagnosis.

SADS represents this tradition. Developed in the 1970s at the New York State Psychiatric Institute, SADS was designed as a semistructured interview instrument to gather information pertinent to the classification of psychiatric disorders. Its primary purpose was to provide information sufficient for classifying patients into relatively homogeneous subgroups for the purposes of research (Endicott and Spitzer 1979). These classifications were explicated by using the Research Diagnostic Criteria (RDC; Feighner et al. 1972), which specified explicit symptomatic criteria for 23 psychiatric disorders. These criteria served as the forerunner to DSM-III and have, in the main, been incorporated into that version of psychiatric nomenclature. Using the same semistructured interview format and item rating procedures, Spitzer and his associates developed the Structured Clinical Interview for DSM-IV (SCID; First et al 1997), which directly orients the diagnostic process to the Axis I and Axis II categories of the DSM system.

With their explicit focus on psychiatric classification, SADS and SCID have acquired all of the problems inherent in adopting the present psychiatric nomenclature as the reference point for assessment. Chief among these problems is the insufficient validation of the diagnostic categories themselves. However, as tools for investigating the range, severity, frequency, and duration of symptomatic disturbance and for training in the formal interview assessment of psychopathology, these instruments are an important part of the assessment armamentarium.

TABLE 8–4. Assessment of DSM-IV Axis I disorders

Instrument	General classification	Description	Scoring features
Structured Clinical Interview for DSM-IV Axis I Disorders, Clinician Version (SCID-IV)	Semistructured interview	3-point rating scales of symptoms	Oriented to diagnosis using DSM-IV

Omnibus Measures of Symptoms

A number of instruments have been developed for the assessment of a wide variety of symptoms (Table 8–5). These measures depend on either self-report or interview methods for data collection.

Minnesota Multiphasic Personality Inventory. The Minnesota Multiphasic Personality Inventory (MMPI; Hathaway and McKinley 1967), and its successor, the MMPI-2, are probably the most widely used assessment instruments in existence. There are a number of reasons for its extensive use, including its efficiency (the patient spends 1 to 2 hours taking the test, which can then be computer scored), the extensive data accumulated with the test, its normative base, and the use of validity scales that indicate the patient's test-taking attitude. Although labeled as a personality test, the MMPI was constructed to assess what are now categorized as Axis I conditions and, to a lesser extent, a few dimensions of personality that are not represented on Axis II.

The MMPI was developed in the 1940s by J. Charnley McKinley, a psychiatrist, and Starke R. Hathaway, a psychologist. Items were generated from lists of psychiatric symptoms and complaints found in the current textbooks of psychiatry and previously constructed personality inventories. Beginning with a large pool of such items, McKinley and Hathaway used the method of contrasting criterion groups to construct several psychopathological scales. For example, a hypochondriasis scale measuring the degree of concern with bodily health was developed on the basis of items frequently endorsed by patients with hypochondriasis uncomplicated by psychosis or other psychiatric disorders. The patients' responses to the MMPI items were contrasted to those of friends or relatives who visited the University Hospitals in Minneapolis. Using this method of criterion-keyed scoring, McKinley and Hathaway constructed nine clinical scales: hypochondriasis (Hs, or Scale 1), depression (D, or Scale 2), hysteria (Hy, or Scale 3), psychopathic deviance (Pd, or Scale 4), masculinity-femininity (Mf, or Scale 5), paranoia (Pa, or Scale 6), psychasthenia (Pt, or Scale 7), schizophrenia (Sc, or Scale 8), and mania (Ma, or Scale 9). Items were worded so that persons with an elementary school education could take the test, and norms were established for determining the degree of disturbance typical of psychopathological groups. For example, an item on Scale 2 (i.e., depression) reads as follows: I find it hard to keep my mind on a task or job (True).

In addition to the clinical scales, validity scales were developed to assess the test-taking attitudes of the patient. McKinley et al. (1948) focused on the assessment of defensiveness or of minimizing symptoms and problems (faking good) and maximizing or exaggerating problems (faking bad). Validity scales were constructed to evaluate these dimensions, which are helpful in interpreting the severity of symptomatic complaints on the clinical scales.

The MMPI has been revised and restandardized as the MMPI-2 (Butcher et al. 1989). Revisions include the deletion of objectionable items and the rewording of other items to reflect more modern language usage, as well as the addition of several new items focusing on suicide, drug and alcohol abuse, Type A behavior, interpersonal relations, and treatment compliance. Restandardization of the norms was based on a randomly solicited national sample of 1,138 males and 1,462 females.

Clinical interpretation of the MMPI-2 is not, however,

TABLE 8–5. **Instruments for the assessment of symptom patterns**

Instrument	General Classification	Description	Scoring Features
Minnesota Multiphasic Personality Inventory-II	Self-report	566-item checklist, true/false format	T-scores for 13 criterion scales
Hopkins Symptom Checklist—90(SCL-90)	Self-report	90-item checklist, 5-point intensity scales	T-scores for 9 symptom clusters
Brief Psychiatric Rating Scale(BPRS)	Clinical interview	16 items, 7-point severity scales	5 factor scores and total scores
Personality Assessment Inventory (PAI)	Self-report	344 items, true/false format	4 validity scales, 10 clinical scales covering symptoms and severe personality disorders
Millon Clinical Multiaxial Inventory—II (MCMI-II)	Self-report	175 items, true/ false format	3 validity scales, 22 clinical scales covering Axis I and II areas

simply a matter of noting a scale that is high relative to these norms and assigning that diagnosis to the patient (e.g., in a patient with a high Sc, or Scale 8, score, schizophrenia would not necessarily be diagnosed). Instead, relying on an extensive clinical database, typical symptomatic and personality dysfunctions are described on the basis of 2- and 3-point codes (Dahlstrom et al. 1972; Greene 1991; Marks et al. 1974). For example, individuals with a three-point code of 2-4-8 (scores above 70 on Scales 2, 4, and 8) are described as typically distrustful of people, keeping others at a distance, afraid of emotional involvement, using projection and rationalization as defenses, argumentative and sensitive to anything that can be construed as a demand, and unpredictable and changeable in behavior and attitudes (Marks and Seeman 1963). Research has indicated that many patients with this code exhibit symptoms that fulfill the DSM-III criteria for borderline personality disorder (Hurt et al. 1985).

The MMPI-2 is an excellent example of a psychological test, because it was developed with careful attention to issues of reliability and validity. Both the severity and the pattern of symptomatic disturbance are considered, and a large body of literature relevant to the test's predictive validity has developed. Moreover, the MMPI-2 provides information on the response style of the individual taking the test, a personality attribute that is essential in interpreting the clinical scales.

Personality Assessment Inventory. A relatively new instrument, the Personality Assessment Inventory (PAI; Morey 1991), focuses on clinical syndromes that have been staples of psychopathological nosology and have retained their importance in contemporary diagnostic practice. Items were written with careful attention to their content validity, which was designed to reflect the phenomenology of the clinical construct across a broad range of severity. An initial pool of 2,200 items was generated from the research literature, classic texts, the DSM, and other diagnostic manuals and from the clinical experience of practitioners who participated in the project. This pool of items was finally reduced to 344 items covering 4 validity scales, 11 clinical syndromes, 5 treatment planning areas, and the 2 major dimensions of the interpersonal complex. All items are rated with a 4-point Likert-type response format. (For example, on the borderline scale is the following item: "I'm too impulsive for my own good.") Final clinical validation was carried out on the data from 235 subjects from 10 clinical sites and 2 community and 2 college student samples.

Hopkins Symptom Checklist—90. The Hopkins Symptom Checklist—90 (SCL-90; Derogatis 1977) is an-

other example of a self-report instrument designed to provide information about a broad range of complaints typical of individuals with psychological symptomatic distress. Briefer than the MMPI-2 and the PAI, the SCL-90 contains only 90 items and can be administered in 30 minutes and scored by computer. These items are combined into nine symptom scales: 1) somatization, 2) obsessive-compulsive behavior, 3) interpersonal sensitivity, 4) depression, 5) anxiety, 6) hostility, 7) phobic anxiety, 8) paranoid ideation, and 9) psychoticism. In addition, three global indices are compiled: 1) general severity, 2) positive symptom distress index, and 3) total positive symptoms. The criterion group method was not used in the development of this test. Rather, the content validity and internal consistency of the items guided the construction of the scales.

A companion instrument, the Hopkins Psychiatric Rating Scale (HPRS; Derogatis et al. 1974), can be used to rate material obtained through direct interview of the patient on each of the nine symptom dimensions of the SCL-90. No structured interview procedure is associated with the HPRS, so formal training in the interview assessment of psychopathology is essential to the accuracy of the assessment. Eight additional dimensions are covered in the interview.

Brief Psychiatric Rating Scale. Another widely used rating scale for a range of psychiatric symptoms is the Brief Psychiatric Rating Scale (BPRS; Overall and Gorham 1962), which was developed mainly for the assessment of symptoms with an inpatient population. Areas rated include somatic concern, anxiety, emotional withdrawal, conceptual disorganization, guilt, tension, mannerisms and posturing, grandiosity, depressive mood, hostility, suspiciousness, hallucinatory behavior, motor retardation, uncooperativeness, unusual thought content, blunted affect, excitement, and disorientation.

The MMPI-2, PAI, SCL-90, HPRS, and BPRS represent efforts to develop procedures for the general assessment of psychopathology that meet standards of test construction. These procedures provide coverage of symptomatically distressing areas that are independent of psychiatric classifications. However, through the extensive use of these procedures in psychiatric settings, a large body of literature has developed that relates the findings of these tests to diagnostic categories favored in such settings.

Specific Areas of Symptomatology

In addition to the omnibus measures of symptomatology, there are a number of instruments that assess one area of symptomatology in depth (Table 8–6). The major constellations of symptoms that may require assessment are 1) substance abuse, including abuse of food, alcohol, and drugs, 2) affects such as anxiety, elation, and depression, 3) thought disorder, and 4) suicidal intentions and behaviors.

Substance abuse. Psychological distress and dysfunction arising from the abuse of a wide variety of substances is perhaps the chief reason for seeking psychological or psychiatric treatment. The treatment of alcoholism, drug abuse, and eating disorders, combined with the income lost, probably consumes more health dollars than does any other group of disorders. Thus, the identification of these disorders deserves careful attention. The threat to the va-

lidity of self-report screening instruments for detecting substance abuse is such that these instruments should be buttressed by urine screens and interview (Greene and Banken 1995). However, it is helpful to review the instruments that have been used for this purpose. The prominent instruments in this area are the MacAndrew Alcoholism Scale (MacAndrew 1965), the Addiction Potential Scale from the MMPI-2 (Weed et al. 1992) and scales B and T from the Millon Clinical Multiaxial Inventory—II (MCMI-II).

The assessment of substance abuse potential is reflected in omnibus symptom rating scales such as the MMPI-2, which contains an item key, the MacAndrew Alcoholism Scale (MacAndrew 1965), for identifying patients who have histories of alcohol abuse or who have the

TABLE 8–6. Instruments for the assessment of specific symptom areas

Instrument	General classification	Description	Scoring features
Substance abuse			
Alcohol Use Inventory (AUI)	Self-report	228 items rated on 2- to 6-point scales	17 primary scales in four areas and 7 second-order factor scales
Eating Disorders Inventory–2 (EDI-2)	Self-report	91 forced-choice items rated on 6-point frequency scale	8 subscales and 3 provisional scales for issues and features pertinent to eating disorders
Affects			
State-Trait Anxiety Inventory (STAI)	Self-report	Two 20-item scales, 4-point frequency ratings	Total scores for state and trait anxiety
S-R Inventory of Anxiousness	Self-report	14-item responses on 5-point severity scales to 11 situations	Focus on intensity and quality of situations arousing anxiety
Fear Questionnaire	Self-report	17 items reflecting specific phobias rated on 9-point avoidance scales	Total scores for agoraphobia, social phobia, and blood and injury phobias
Beck Depression Inventory	Self-report	20 items, 4-point intensity scales	Total score
Hamilton Rating Scale for Depression (Ham-D)	Clinical interview	17–24 items, 3- to 5-point severity scales	Total score
Manic-State Rating Scale (MSRS)	Observer rating	26 items, each scored for frequency and intensity	Total score
State-Trait Anger Inventory (STAXI)	Self-report	44 items	Total scores for state and trait anger
Suicidal behavior			
Suicide Intent Scale (SIS)	Self-report	15 items, 3-point categorical scales	Total score
Index of Potential Suicide	Self-report or semi-structured interview	50 items, 5-point severity scales	Total score and 6 subscores
Reasons for Living Inventory (RFL)	Self-report	6 factors	Total score
Thought disorder			
Thought Disorder Index	Content rating	22 categories at 4 levels of severity	Total score

potential to develop problems with alcohol (Hoffmann et al. 1974). A more thorough instrument, the Alcohol Use Inventory (AUI; Horn et al. 1986), is a self-administered test standardized on over 1,200 admissions to an alcoholism treatment program. It contains 24 scales that measure alcohol-related problems and considers the subjects' responses in four separate domains: benefits from drinking, style of drinking, consequences of drinking, and concerns associated with drinking.

Garner has developed an inventory to assess attitudes and behaviors associated with anorexia nervosa. This inventory, the Eating Disorders Inventory—2 (EDI-2) (Garner 1992) consists of 91 items rated on 6-point frequency scales. The items were chosen to reflect important clinical aspects of anorexia and were retained if they successfully discriminated between anorexic, normal-weight, and obese males and females. Internal reliability, construct validity, and treatment response data have been reported, and the EDI-2 can be a useful screening instrument for identifying inpatients with potentially serious eating disorders.

Affects. The content, range, and management of emotional expression constitute a symptomatic area of focus for the evaluation of psychopathology and are important in the differential diagnosis of a wide variety of psychiatric disorders. The main affects of interest are anxiety, depression, and elation.

As one factor in the larger context of the total personality, anxiety can be assessed with the 16-Personality Factor Inventory (16-PF; Cattell et al. 1970), the Eysenck Personality Inventory (EPI; Eysenck and Eysenck 1969), and the Taylor Manifest Anxiety Scale (TMAS; Taylor-Spence and Spence 1966), a scale derived from the MMPI.

Other instruments assess only anxiety or other forms of fearfulness and thus may be more clinically useful as dimensional measures of the severity of anxiety or in identifying specific situational anxiety that will become the focus of intervention. The Anxiety Status Inventory (ASI) is a rating scale for anxiety developed for clinical use following an interview guide, and the Self-Rating Anxiety Scale (SRAS) is a companion self-report instrument, both developed by Zung (1971). Both scales assess a wide range of anxiety-related behaviors: fear, panic, physical symptoms of fear, nightmares, and cognitive effects. These scales are recommended for the serial measurement of the effects of therapy on anxiety states. Hamilton (1959) has devised an anxiety rating scale parallel to the Ham-D but less frequently used.

The State-Trait Anxiety Inventory (STAI; Spielberger et al. 1976) is a self-report instrument in which the patient is asked to report on anxiety in general (i.e., trait) and at particular points in time (i.e., state). The Endler S-R In-

ventory of Anxiousness (Endler et al. 1962) is a self-report measure of the interaction between the patient's anxiety and environmental situations such as interpersonal, physically dangerous, and ambiguous situations. This instrument has been widely used as a therapy outcome measure and is recommended as an instrument that may be helpful in tailoring treatment to the specific circumstances of the patient's anxiety.

The Beck Depression Inventory (BDI) is probably the most widely used self-report inventory of depression. The original scale was administered in an interviewer-assisted manner, but a later version is completely self-administered. The 21 items of the inventory were selected to represent symptoms commonly associated with a depressive disorder. The rating of each item relies on the endorsement of one or more of four statements listed in order of symptom severity. Item categories include mood, pessimism, crying spells, guilt, self-hate and accusations, irritability, social withdrawal, work inhibition, sleep and appetite disturbance, and loss of libido. The content of the BDI emphasizes pessimism, a sense of failure, and self-punitive wishes. This emphasis is consistent with Beck's cognitive view of depression and its causes. This self-report instrument is frequently used in conjunction with Ham-D, which allows a clinician to rate the severity of depressive symptoms during an interview with the patient. In contrast to BDI, Ham-D is more systematic in assessing neurovegetative signs. There are only rough interview guidelines for using Ham-D, but interrater reliability is generally good.

The Manic-State Rating Scale (MSRS; Beigel et al. 1971) is a 26-item observer-rated scale that is useful with patients who have bipolar depression. Eleven items reflecting elation-grandiosity and paranoid-destructive features of manic patients have been applied successfully in the prediction of inpatient length of stay (Young et al. 1978). The scale has demonstrated adequate reliability and concurrent validity, and reflects clinical change (Janowsky et al. 1978). Secunda et al. (1985) used similar item content from several instruments employed in the National Institute of Mental Health Clinical Research Branch Collaborative Program on the psychobiology of depression to develop indices for responsiveness to lithium treatment in manic patients. A newer rating scale, the Internal State Scale (ISS; Bauer et al. 1991), is a self-report instrument that allows individuals to rate the present state of 17 items reflecting bipolar symptomatology on a 100-millimeter line.

Aggressive behavior, including aggressive imagery and hostile affect, is an important area in treatment planning, both for the individual patient and for the general concepts that the inventory assesses. The Buss-Durkee Hostility Inventory (Buss and Durkee 1957) is a 75-item self-report questionnaire that measures aspects of hostility and aggression. There are eight subscales: Assault, Indirect Hostility, Irritability, Negativism, Resentment, Suspicion, Verbal Hostility, and Guilt. Some norms exist for clinical populations. Megargee et al. (1967) developed an overcontrolled hostility scale using MMPI items. A review of the number of studies involving this scale (Greene 1991) suggests that it can be used to screen for patients who display excessive control of their hostile impulses and are socially alienated. Spielberger has developed a State-Trait Anger Expression Inventory (STAEI; Spielberger 1991; Spielberger et al. 1976) that takes about 15 minutes to complete. This 44-item scale divides behavior into state anger (i.e., current feelings) and trait anger (i.e., disposition toward angry reactions), and the latter area has subscales called Angry Temperament and Angry Reaction. (Sample items: "How I feel right now: I feel irritated"; "How I generally feel: I fly off the handle").

Suicidal behavior.   The suicide potential of patients has obvious treatment and management implications for the clinician. Suicidal threats, suicidal planning and/or preparation, suicidal ideation, and recent parasuicidal behavior are all direct indicators of current risk and should be assessed thoroughly and specifically in the clinical interview. In addition, self-report instruments that focus specific and detailed attention on known predictors of suicidal behavior are sometimes clinically useful. Thus, it is recommended that the assessment of suicidal behavior be embedded in an assessment package that involves interview and use of instruments (Bongar 1991).

With that caveat in mind, suicidal assessment instruments that are frequently used include the Beck Hopelessness Scale (Beck et al. 1974b) and the Beck Suicide Intent Scale (SIS; Beck et al. 1974a). In addition, it should be noted that the Koss-Butcher critical item set revised on the MMPI is a list of 22 items related specifically to the depressed, suicidal ideation. These critical items should not been seen as scales, but rather as markers of particular item content that might be significant in assessing the individual patient (Butcher 1989).

SIS, the Index of Potential Suicide (Zung 1974), and the Suicide Probability Scale (SPS; Cull and Gill 1986) are three widely used instruments. A complementary approach has been taken, culminating in the development of the Reasons for Living Inventory (RFL; Linehan et al. 1983). Of practical interest is that the fear-of-suicide subscale in the RFL differentiates between those who have only considered suicide and those who have made previous suicide attempts. Individuals scoring high on reasons for living and on subscales measuring survival and coping skills, respon-

sibility to family, and child-related concerns were less likely to attempt suicide.

Thought disorder.   One approach to the reliable assessment of cognition is the use of semistructured interviews such as SADS and SCID. The presence or absence of disorders of thinking, such as thought derailment or frank hallucinations or delusions, is determined during the course of an extensive interview. There are obvious problems with this approach. Many individuals may not want to reveal frank delusional experiences, or they may be unaware of the presence of more subtle varieties of disordered thinking. To avoid these pitfalls, an alternative approach is to obtain a sample of the thought process. The test most widely used in examinations for thought disorders has been the Rorschach Inkblot Test, developed by the Swiss psychiatrist Hermann Rorschach (Rorschach 1949). In this test, a relatively ambiguous stimulus (a colored or achromatic inkblot) is used, and, without additional instruction, individuals are asked to state what the blot looks like to them. Responses are scored for location (the area of the card that elicits a response), determinants (form, movement, color, and shading), form quality (the degree to which percepts are congruent with the area chosen), and content (e.g., human, animal, object). Exner (1974, 1978) has developed a scoring system that attempts to integrate the best aspects of prior systems.

Holzman and his colleagues have published extensively on the relationship of various forms of thought disorder and its severity to psychiatric diagnosis and treatment (Hurt et al. 1983; Johnston and Holzman 1979; Solovay et al. 1986). Although the scoring scheme can be applied to any record of verbal production, its most frequent application has been in the context of verbal records from the administration of such tests as WAIS and the Rorschach. In its present version, the Thought Disorder Index considers 22 forms of thought disturbance ranging across four levels of severity as the basis for a total score. The total score has been found to distinguish psychotic from nonpsychotic patients, and more severe forms of thought disorder have been most frequently associated with schizophrenic disorders. A recent report indicates a strong relationship between the degree of hypertrophy of the left posterior superior temporal gyrus, noticeable with magnetic resonance imaging (MRI), and the severity of thought disorder in patients with schizophrenia (Shenton et al. 1992).

In addition to the work of Holzman and his colleagues, Harrow and associates have developed another battery, consisting of three tests, to quantify thought disorder. This work has considered patients with clinical diagnoses of schizophrenia, affective disorder, and schizoaffective disorder. In a series of studies, these investigators addressed the persistence of thought disorders in treated groups who had been followed for a period of 2–4 years (Harrow and Quinlan 1985; Marengo and Harrow 1985).

ASSESSMENT OF COGNITIVE FUNCTIONING

The development of clinical assessment procedures for the investigation of brain-behavior relationships has been an active area of psychological investigation. Because impairment of various areas of the brain results in disorders in higher cortical functions in humans, clinical neuropsychology has been able to develop assessment procedures that consider both the localization and the degree of functional impairment as the focus for test development. Present-day neuropsychological assessment procedures in the United States can be traced to the pioneering work begun in the 1930s by such investigators as Ward Halstead and Joseph Wepman at the University of Chicago. These early investigators were concerned with the localization and degree of functional impairment in neurologically impaired populations. In recent years, these neuropsychological assessment procedures have been extended to the assessment of less clearly anatomically based functional disorders characteristic of clinical psychiatric populations (Clarkin and Mattis 1991).

Application of these procedures beyond the arena in which they were first developed has introduced difficulties in the interpretation of the results of such procedures. These procedures are sensitive to abnormalities of brain function due to the direct alteration of brain tissue. For example, among chronically schizophrenic patients, the degree of neuropsychological dysfunction has been found to be correlated with structural abnormalities on computed tomography (CT) scan (Seidman 1983). In other psychiatric groups in which the evidence for structural abnormalities is less clear, the degree to which these disorders interfere with performance on these tests by mechanisms other than structural abnormalities of brain tissue is as yet unclear. There is increasing evidence that some schizophrenic and affective disorders that were traditionally considered functional psychoses may result from as yet poorly understood abnormalities of brain biochemistry (Barchas et al. 1977), and modern imaging techniques such as positron-emission tomography (PET) and MRI have begun to produce evidence of alterations in brain functioning that may be relatively specific to traditional functional psychiatric diagnoses. The relationships between these biochemical and neurophysiological findings and the quality and severity of functional impairment identified through neuropsychological assessments remain to be clarified.

In general, one assesses specific cognitive abilities in psychiatric patients for one of two reasons: 1) to document disorders in cognitive skills referable to primary or concomitant neurogenic disorder (e.g., to discriminate between a thought disorder and a language disorder or the mnemonic deficits of depression versus those of dementia), or 2) to document a specific disorder in cognition referable to a specific class of psychiatric disorders (e.g., the intrusion into thought of task-irrelevant items in patients complaining of delusional or obsessive ideation, or disturbances in recall in patients with major affective disorders).

Common clinical questions in a psychiatric setting with a neuropsychological focus include 1) differentiating between early dementia, mild delirium, and depression, 2) toxicity in substance-abusing individuals, 3) cognitive and affective status of an individual after head injury (Mattis and Wilson, in press), and 4) specific learning disabilities in children and adolescents. In clinical psychiatric populations, the possibly confounding influences of behavioral impairment because of the nature and severity of the emotional disturbance and the effect of concurrent pharmacological treatments must be carefully assessed to reduce the rate of false-positive diagnoses of organic mental disorder. These factors should be carefully weighed in scheduling the timing of the assessment and in interpreting the results. Heaton and Crowley (1981) provided a thorough review of the literature on neuropsychological testing and organic mental disorder in psychiatric patients, in which the above issues are considered. Their review is particularly useful because of its attention to the issue of the effects of somatic treatments on neuropsychological functioning in psychiatric populations.

Although the fields of cognitive and experimental psychology may offer an almost limitless number of cognitive functions capable of being defined and measured in the adult, only a finite number appear, at present, to be clinically useful. In one form or another, most neuropsychological assessments of cognitive processes evaluate the presence of disorders in the following abilities:

- General intelligence
- Attention and concentration
- Memory and learning
- Perception
- Language
- Conceptualization
- Constructional skills
- Executive motor processes
- Affect

In many clinical settings, the areas of higher cortical functions of interest are assessed by a formal battery of tests. Two such standardized batteries are the Halstead-Reitan (Boll 1981) and the Luria-Nebraska (Golden et al. 1978) neuropsychological batteries (Table 8–7).

The Halstead-Reitan is a composite battery of tests originally developed by Ward Halstead and his former student, Ralph Reitan. In its present form, the Halstead Neuropsychological Test Battery consists of five tests that yield seven summary scores and a total impairment index. The five tests are a category test, a tactile perception test, a speech sounds perception test, the Seashore rhythm test, and a finger oscillation test. A group of tests referred to as the allied procedures are frequently included as a part of the total examination. The entire examination typically takes from 4 to 6 hours, depending on the number of ancillary procedures (i.e., intelligence and academic performance) included. The reliability and validity of the tests are well established, and normative data for most comparisons of interest in clinical psychiatric populations are available.

A second widely used battery of procedures has been developed from the work of Luria (1966, 1973). Christensen (1975) was instrumental in bringing Luria's stimuli and procedures to the attention of neuropsychologists outside the former Soviet Union. Golden and his colleagues (1978) have been the primary proponents and developers of a standardized neuropsychological instrument using Christensen's published material. In its present form, the Luria-Nebraska covers the areas of 1) motor function, 2) rhythm (and pitch) skills, 3) tactile and visual functions, 4) receptive and expressive speech, 4) writing, reading, and arithmetic skills, 5) memory, and 6) intelligence. The complete examination consists of 269 items that yield raw scores in each area. Three additional scores for right- and left-hemisphere impairment and a pathognomonic score are also computed. These 14 raw scores are plotted as T scores for interscale and interindividual comparison. The current literature on the Luria-Nebraska includes studies of groups of subjects with brain damage and chronic schizophrenia and medical control subjects. The results of these studies have established the preliminary validity of the battery; no reliability data have been published.

Both the Halstead-Reitan and the Luria-Nebraska batteries are oriented toward an extensive evaluation of neuropsychological functioning, and in clinical practice they are typically supplemented with instruments that allow a more flexible test approach and a more intensive focus on areas of possible dysfunction. The neuropsychological areas of interest and appropriate assessment procedures for detailed examination of these processes are given below.

Premorbid Intelligence

A number of inferences as to the presence of neuropsychological deficits are based on observed discrepancies between present functioning and estimated premorbid abilities. Premorbid intelligence may be estimated by assessing those cognitive abilities that do not rapidly deteriorate with dementing processes. These include the general fund of information and vocabulary as measured by the respective subtests of the WAIS, or reading recognition as measured by the Wide Range Achievement Test reading subtest (Jastak and Wilkinson 1981) or the Nelson Adult Reading Test (Nelson 1982), which has new North American norms and for which reasonable validity has been demonstrated. It is also common to estimate premorbid intelligence on the basis of educational and vocational background. The validity of a number of different estimates of premorbid intelligence based on demographic data has been demonstrated (Karzmark et al. 1985).

General Intellectual Abilities

The most frequently used instrument, the WAIS-R, has been described in an earlier section. Because of the length of administration, abbreviated versions of this measure are often employed, either by using only some of the subtests or by using fewer of the specific items and weighting each response. Alternatively, different, briefer measures may be employed—for example, the Ammons Quick Test (Ammons and Ammons 1962) or the Shipley-Hartford Test (Shipley 1946).

Most tests of general intellectual abilities obtain normative data from an unimpaired population and therefore are sensitive instruments in detecting individuals whose performance lies at the extremes of the normal range. Such instruments lose sensitivity to discriminate among patient populations whose performance falls outside this range. There are a number of instruments in broad use for the assessment of general cognitive abilities in patient populations. All such instruments have skewed distributions in normal populations (i.e., a decided floor effect) but distribute well in the atypical population. Perhaps the most commonly used instrument in a psychiatric setting is the Mini Mental Status Exam (MMSE) (Folstein et al. 1975), a 10-minute test generating 30 points, in which a score below 24 is considered to be good evidence of clinically significant cognitive impairment. A commonly used instrument is the Dementia Rating Scale (Mattis 1988), a 20- to 30-minute instrument generating 144 points, with sensitivity at the upper levels that provides detection of progressive changes of dementia over several years (Haxby

TABLE 8-7. Instruments for the assessment of cognitive functioning

Instrument	Focus of assessment	Description	Scoring features
Wechsler Adult Intelligence Scale—III	General intellectual abilities	166 items sampling intellectual skills	Full scale, verbal, and performance IQs
Wechsler Intelligence Scale for Children—Revised	General intellectual abilities	187 items sampling intellectual skills	Full scale, verbal, and performance IQs
Wechsler Preschool and Primary Scale of Intelligence	General intellectual abilities	Taps 6 verbal and 5 performance areas	Full scale, verbal, and performance IQs
Halstead-Reitan Neuropsychological Battery	Items sampling intellectual, tactual, auditory, and kinesthetic functions	7 summary sources for clinical interpretation	
Luria-Nebraska	Neuropsychological battery	269 items sampling intellectual, motor, sensory, and expressive skills	14 T-scores for clinical interpretation
Mini Mental State Exam	Brief assessment of general cognitive impairment	30 items sampling orientation, memory, and drawing skills	Total number correct
Dementia Rating	Brief assessment of general cognitive impairment	144 items sampling attention, memory, abstraction, drawing, and executive motor skills	5 subscale scores, total scores, percentile score relative to dementia patients
Wide Range Achievement Test	Academic achievement	Reading, spelling, arithmetic achievement	Standard score
Continuous Performance Test	Attention	Test of vigilance	Hits, false alarms, reaction time
Wechsler Memory Scale—Revised	Memory	Attention, verbal, nonverbal memory	Subscale scores on attention, verbal memory, and nonverbal memory
Benton Test of Visual Retention	Memory	Reproduction of geometric figures	Total number correct, total number errors
Benton Line Orientation Test	Perception	Target lines at given orientations detected from among a radial display of lines	Total number correct
Benton Face Recognition Test	Perception	Target face detected from among similar faces	Total number of correct detections
Goldman-Fristoe-Woodcock Auditory Battery	Perception	Auditory perception measured under three different conditions of ambient noise	Total number correct
Category Test (Booklet)	Conceptualization	Concept formation task	Total number of errors
Wisconsin Card Sorting Test	Conceptualization	Concept formation task	Total number of categories obtained, total number of perseverative errors
Conceptual Level Analogies Test	Conceptualization	Verbal analogies	Number correct
Raven Progressive Matrices Test	Conceptualization	Spatial analogies test using patterned visual stimuli	Number correct
Trail Making Test	Set sequencing	Connect dots in ascending numeric order, then in alternating alphanumeric order	Time to completion
Purdue Pegboard	Fine motor	Fine motor task	Number of pegs placed in 30 sec

et al. 1992; Vitaliano et al. 1984).

Within the neuropsychological literature there exists a vast armamentarium of tests of specific neurocognitive processes validated within neurological and neurosurgical populations. There is a smaller number of instruments that are useful in a psychiatric setting, but even this number is too large to itemize within the scope of this chapter. Research concerning the neuropsychology of psychiatric disorders is relatively new. It should therefore be noted that the tests presented below are examples of widely used measures of cognitive processes and do not constitute an exhaustive list and that these tests are expected to be replaced as new data accrue.

Attentional Disorders

Attentional disorders are among the most common findings in psychiatric patients, because attention and concentration will be affected both by psychologically determined processes, such as anxiety, depressive mood, and/or rumination, and by neurogenic compromise of brain stem and limbic structures due to toxic-metabolic disorders or direct structural impairment. Attentional processes are most commonly measured by the WAIS-R subtests constituting the "distractibility" triad (i.e., Digit Span, Mental Arithmetic, and Digit Symbol). In Digit Span, the patient is asked to repeat a string of digits of increasing length and then, in a separate administration, repeat a string of digits in reverse of the order in which they were presented. The digit string cannot be repeated by the examiner, so lapses in attention by the patient result in repetition of only the shorter strings. In the Mental Arithmetic subtest, the patient is asked to solve arithmetic problems of increasing difficulty without the aid of pencil and paper. Selection and monitoring of the appropriate arithmetic operation while storing partial solutions are easily disrupted by alterations in arousal and attention. The Digit Symbol subtest presents the patient with the digits 1 through 9 and matches each digit with a separate, very simple geometric design. The digits are then randomly sequenced in rows across the page, and the patient, who may refer to the designs, must draw the appropriate design beneath each digit. The number of designs correctly drawn in 90 seconds is noted. This task not only is affected by impairment of the attentional system but is very sensitive to fine motor tremor and extrapyramidal impairment secondary to neurotoxins.

In addition to the above, a number of variants of these procedures and specialized procedures are in common practice. Cancellation tasks are available, in which the patient is required to cross out a given letter or design presented within rows of randomly distributed other letters or designs (Mesulam 1985). An advantage of such tasks is that they can be strung together to form a lengthy, continuous performance task of 10 to 15 minutes and that variation in accuracy across discrete 20-second periods can be determined.

With increasing use of computer-assisted examinations, a popular continuous-performance test developed by Rosvold can be employed (Mirsky and Kornetsky 1964; Rosvold et al. 1956). In this task, the patient is presented with a randomly selected letter in midscreen at fixed intervals and directed to push a button (or press the space bar) when a given letter is presented. The number of hits (i.e., correct responses), misses, false alarms (i.e., the number of times the bar is pressed in response to a nontarget item), and correct rejections is then noted. The advantage to this computer-assisted approach to the measure of attention lies in its flexibility and the accuracy with which stimuli can be presented and responses can be recorded. The reaction time of each response can be measured and fluctuations in reaction time noted over the duration of the task. Stimulus characteristics such as stimulus duration, speed of presentation, or even size of target and duration of task can be systematically altered. A good deal of clinical research has been conducted using such a procedure to explore the attentional characteristics of children with attention-deficit/hyperactivity disorder.

Research in attentional processes has demonstrated the efficacy of a procedure called "dichotic stimulation" (Kimura 1967), which presents dissimilar auditory stimuli simultaneously to each ear and requires the patient to report both stimuli. Thus the patient might simultaneously hear the number "1" in the right ear and "4" in the left ear. Strings of three such pairs might be presented to the adult patient and he or she asked to report all six digits. The competing stimuli can be matched for such stimulus characteristics as time of onset, offset, peak amplitude, and so forth, making it a very difficult task of discriminating speech sounds as well as an attentional measure.

Memory Disorders

The memory disorder of particular interest to the clinician is the one that affects recent memory and that is generally referable to impairment of limbic system functioning. Operationally, one seeks to present the patient with a specific set of information or events, then divert attention so that it cannot be rehearsed, and then require the patient to demonstrate that the target information has been encoded and stored by either reproducing the material or recognizing it among distractor items. Thus recall of brief paragraphs or reproduction of geometric designs from memory is often used to assess mnemonic processes. Among the most commonly used standard tests of memory are the Wechsler Memory Scale—Revised (Wechsler 1987), which presents both verbal and nonverbal material as the items to be remembered, and the Benton Test of Visual Retention (Benton 1955), which presents only geometric designs.

Free recall of recent events has been found to be among the most sensitive functions of the memory process. Unfortunately, in many instances free recall has been found to be quite fragile and vulnerable to disruption because of affective arousal, depression, and motivational factors and therefore may present many "false positives" when being used to discriminate between neurogenic and psychogenic diagnostic considerations. It has been suggested that mechanisms other than free recall might be employed to assess the integrity of encoding and storage processes. Recognition memory techniques, in which the patient is asked to detect a recently presented word or design from among distractor items, have been successfully used to discriminate patients with major affective disorders from those with organic amnesias such as progressive dementia. In patients presenting with major depression, for example, free recall might be quite consonant with recall in patients with Alzheimer's disease, but recognition memory in patients with major depression remains relatively intact.

Well-designed instruments assessing both recall and recognition memory generally present the patient with a list-learning task requiring free recall and, subsequent to that, a recognition memory probe in which the patient must detect the target among distractor items. Most of the instruments introduce either an interpolated list or a significant time delay before presentation of the final recall and recognition trials. Among the most widely used instruments are the Rey Auditory Verbal Learning Test (Geffen et al. 1990; Rey 1964) and the California Verbal Learning Test (Delis et al. 1987). Several instruments have multiple forms that are useful in the serial examination of patients, for example, the Hopkins Verbal Learning Test (Brandt 1991) and the Mattis-Kovner Verbal Learning Test (Mattis et al. 1978).

It should be noted that neurology patients with focal lesions might present a recent memory defect that is only verbal or only nonverbal, depending on the locus of the lesion. It is therefore only in patients with bilateral or diffuse neurogenic impairment that one finds amnesic disorders in both realms. Thus, both verbal and nonverbal memory must be assessed independently; the finding of asymmetric dysfunction strongly suggests focal neurological impairment.

Perceptual Disorders

Very little evidence exists for a significant prevalence of perceptual deficits in a psychiatric population when care is taken to exclude significant problem-solving components from the task and the presence of concurrent toxic metabolic disorders in the patients. Nonetheless, it is probably a good idea to rule out the presence of perceptual deficits. Visual-perceptual processes can be assessed with tasks such as the Benton Line Orientation Test (Benton et al. 1975), which requires the patient to match a target line at a given orientation to true vertical with alternative lines presented at various orientations. Another such test is the Benton Face Recognition Test (Benton and Van Allen 1968), in which a photograph of a face is presented as the target and the patient is requested to detect this face among alternatives. In this task the correct face is presented as an identical photograph as well as photographs of the same individual in various profiles. Both of these tests have good validation as measures of the integrity of posterior cerebral, primarily nondominant hemisphere, functioning.

Auditory perception tends to be difficult to assess without hardware. However, the fidelity available in some small portable tape recorders with earphones affords the clinician a wide range of excellent auditory stimuli. Tests such as the Goldman-Fristoe Test of Speech Sound Discrimination (Goldman et al. 1976) allow for the assessment of the efficiency of speech sound detection with and without background noise. The use of dichotic stimulation tests as measures of speech sound discrimination has already been mentioned in the discussion of attentional disorders. Subtests of the Seashore battery of tests of musical abilities (Seashore et al. 1960), especially the timbre discrimination and tonal memory subtests, have been used as measures of auditory perception of nonverbal material.

The study of disorders of somatosensory perception has a long history in the field of psychophysics, and the techniques evolved from this early literature constitute a large part of the standard neurological examination for peripheral and central nervous system (CNS) disorder. Measures of pressure threshold (Von Frey hairs and Semmes-Ghent-Weinstein pressure esthesiometer), two-point discrimination, joint position sense, finger agnosia, finger order and differentiation, graphesthesia, and stereognosis are common assessment procedures for the presence of disorders of parietal lobe functioning.

Language Disorders

Perhaps the most specific index of neurogenic impairment is the presence of a language disorder. For almost all right-handed persons and half of left-handed persons, focal or diffuse impairment of the left hemisphere is likely to result in aphasia (i.e., a disorder of language comprehension and/or usage). The relationship between the nature of the aphasia (e.g., fluent vs. nonfluent) and the locus of cerebral impairment is among the most well documented of brain-behavior relations (Mesulam 1985). Thus, the examination for the aphasias can provide the hardest evidence in the mental status exam of the presence and locus of brain impairment. There are, needless to say, many well-constructed tests for aphasia. In general, the aphasia examination consists of specific measures of disorders of linguistic processes well correlated with focal brain lesion. Most such batteries will contain measures of verbal labeling or word-finding skills, language comprehension, imitative speech, and motor-expressive speech. Many such tests also include specific measures of reading and writing. Among the most commonly used multifactorial instruments are the Multilingual Aphasia Examination (Benton and Hamsher 1976), the Neurosensory Center Comprehensive Examination for Aphasia (Spreen and Benton 1977), and the Boston Diagnostic Aphasia Examination (Goodglass and Kaplan 1972). Among the most widely used screening instruments for the assessment of aphasia is the Halstead-Wepman Aphasia Screening Test (Halstead and Wepman 1959).

Conceptualization Disorders

The question of whether the patient can assume an abstract attitude is often critical to diagnosis and to treatment planning. The question arises most often when the considerations of differential diagnosis include diffuse brain damage and, to some degree, schizophrenia. Perhaps the most direct measure of the concept of abstract or categorical thinking is the similarities subtest of the WAIS-R, which presents the patient with perceptually dissimilar items and asks him or her to determine the category to which they both belong (e.g., "How are North and West alike?"). Proverb explanation has a long history in the psychiatric mental status examination as a task designed to measure abstract reasoning and is included among the items of the comprehension subtest of the WAIS-R (e.g., "Shallow brooks are noisy"). However, some consider explanation of proverbs too dependent on general intellectual abilities and sociocultural factors to be a specific measure of concretization of thought. Analogical reasoning can also be gauged with such tasks as the Conceptual Level Analogies Test (Willner 1971) for verbal reasoning and the Raven Progressive Matrices Test (Raven 1960) for nonverbal or spatial analogical reasoning.

Two measures of concept formation arising from the neuropsychological literature have recently been applied to psychiatric patients. The data thus far indicate that schizophrenic patients, like patients with frontal lobe lesions, have particular difficulty with the booklet form of the Category Test (DeFillipis et al. 1979) and the Wisconsin Card Sorting Test (Berg 1948; Heaton and Crowley 1981). Both tests require the patient to induce a concept or rule of organization from patterned visual stimuli. In the Wisconsin Card Sorting Test, which has received the most recent programmatic research attention, the patient is shown a pack of cards depicting colored geometric figures. The patient is required to match the top card with one of four cards that vary as to color, number, or form. As the patient matches the card to one of the alternatives, the examiner informs him or her about the correctness of the sort, and the patient then attempts to match the next card correctly. The rule of sorting—in color, form, or number that the examiner reinforces is changed after the patient correctly sorts 10 cards in a row (indicating he or she has grasped the rule). The examiner notes the number of concepts correctly induced and the number of perseverative errors in matching.

Constructional Disorders

Perhaps the quickest estimate of the integrity of the CNS can be obtained by asking the patient to draw a complex figure. Posterior sensory, central spatial, and anterior planning, monitoring, and simple motor skills must all be intact, integrated, and appropriately sequenced for this task to be successfully completed. One can alter the degree to which psychological and dynamic factors and initiative or executive planning play a role by modulating both task structure and design complexity. For example, asking the patient to draw a person in his or her family requires a maximum level of planning, initiative, and decision making; does not put any limit on the degree of complexity of the figures; and involves a subject matter fraught with complex feelings and attitudes. Patients without structural impairment but with conflictual feelings about family or disordered thinking that affects planning and execution will have difficulty with such tasks. However, asking a patient to draw a clock, setting the hands to a specific time (e.g., 10 minutes to 11), also requires complex planning and initiative but without the conflictual overlay. Similarly, asking the patient to copy a complex design (e.g., the Rey-Osterreith figure [Rey 1941]) minimizes initiative and limits (although it does not eliminate) planning, but maintains assessment of high levels of spatial constructional skills. Contrasting the patient's figure drawing to his or her clock and copy of geometric figures often allows valid inferences about the presence and locus of CNS impairment and the degree to which affective and psychiatric factors impair otherwise intact cognitive skills. Quite often, construction tasks other than drawing, such as the WAIS-R subtests of block design and object assembly, are used for the same assessment goals.

Disorders of Executive Motor Skills

In general, in assessing disorders in executive skills, one is alert to the presence of perseveration in motor activity, thought, and affect. Perseveration of motor activity is often elicited by starting the patient on a simple repeated task and then altering one of the motor components. Thus, having the patient perform a simple diadochokinetic task such as alternating palm up/palm down and then presenting as the next task palm up/palm down/fist, may result in repeated performance of only two components of the task. Similarly, asking the patient to write, in script, alternating m's and n's will also elicit simple motor perseveration. Perseveration of thought or set is often quickly elicited by shifting task instruction. For example, in a task developed by Luria (1966) for the assessment of frontal lobe dysfunction, the examiner tells the patient, "When I raise one finger, then you raise one finger, and when I raise two fingers, you raise two fingers." After a number of successful completions, the patient is told, "Now when I raise one finger, you raise two fingers, and when I raise two fingers, you raise one." Patients with dorsal lateral frontal lobe lesions have a great deal of trouble with such tasks. The Trail Making Test (Lezak 1969) is a "connect the dots" type of task in which the patient must first connect the dots in ascending numerical order (Trails A), and then connect the dots in an alternating sequence of numbers and letters (e.g., 1 to A to 2 to B to 3 to C, etc.; Trails B). Note is made of both the time to completion and the number of errors.

Disorders in evolving or shifting more complex ideas can also be measured quite accurately. Concept formation tasks such as the booklet form of the Category Test and the Wisconsin Card Sorting Test differ in specific directions and stimuli but present a series of specific examples of a class of events and require the patient to induce the concept or rule of which they are an exemplar. The rule changes over time. Thus, one might observe the failure of the patient to induce the first concept or the perseveration in the same rule well past its utility. The number of perseveration errors is among the scores obtained on both tests.

Disorders in Motor Skills

Disorders in simple motor skills are among the common concomitants of most toxic-metabolic disorders and of structural lesions of both the extrapyramidal and the pyramidal systems. Examination is usually exceptionally brief, and the results are quite reproducible and valid. One can measure line quality parameters of copied geometric drawings (Mattis et al. 1975). One can, in addition, present simple fine-motor coordination tasks such as those performed with the Purdue Pegboard (Costa et al. 1963) or the Grooved Pegboard. The Purdue Pegboard test measures the number of slim cylinders (pegs) the examinee can insert in a row of holes in 30 seconds. One notes the number of 1) pegs placed with the right hand alone, 2) pegs placed with left hand alone, and 3) pairs of pegs placed with both hands simultaneously. The number of pegs placed simultaneously has proved a sensitive measure of frontal dysfunction. The Grooved Pegboard has pegs containing a flange on one side so that the pegs fit into a keyhole-shaped opening. The keyholes are placed in differing orientations on the board. One notes the total time needed to place all the pegs with each hand alone. Given the greater fine-motor component of the Grooved Pegboard test, it tends to be a more sensitive measure of tremor than is the Purdue.

ASSESSMENT OF PERSONALITY TRAITS AND DISORDERS

In developing a treatment plan for a specific patient, the psychiatrist must assess personality traits for various reasons: personality traits or disorders may 1) be the focus of intervention, 2) exacerbate or be related to the incidence of certain symptoms (e.g., depression), or 3) either help or hinder the development of a therapeutic relationship with the patient.

Dimensional Assessment of Personality

The dimensional assessment of personality using psychological tests has been characterized by a nomothetic approach in which specific personality dimensions (e.g., introversion) are assessed. The dimensions chosen for assessment are typically derived from a personality theory, and individuals are expected to show quantitative differences on these various dimensions. The number of items relevant to a particular dimension that are endorsed is thought to reflect important aspects of that individual's personality style. Within the field of personality measurement, much attention has been paid to the generalizability of such measures. Efforts to investigate the relationship between self-report measures of interpersonal behavior and actual behavior in interpersonal situations continue to contribute to the refinement of this important area of psychological assessment. Just as the levels of distress and of awareness of specific problems are insufficient for determining the capacity to profit from any specific treatment, so too is general knowledge about the reported style of interpersonal behavior insufficient for determining the reaction to various interpersonal situations or the ability to modify the style under certain circumstances.

Several widely used and psychometrically sound instruments are available for the assessment of personality (Table 8–8). Such tests include the 16-PF, the EPI, and the California Psychological Inventory (CPI; Gough 1956). These instruments were designed for the validation of personality constructs rather than for the assessment of psychopathology, although they have been employed in clinical settings with limited success. These instruments and their designers, however, have not been oriented toward psychopathology, and there is no explicit theory of personality disorder that underlies the interpretation of results from these tests.

The NEO–Personality Inventory–Revised (NEO-PI-R; Costa and McCrae 1992), a carefully constructed instrument measuring five central facets of personality, has gained in recognition (Wiggins and Pincus 1992), and its clinical use will probably increase. The revised version, the NEO-PI-R (Costa and McCrae 1992), provides a measure of five facets of personality: Neuroticism, Extraversion, Openness, Agreeableness, and Conscientiousness. Each of the facets also includes six subscales. For example, the six facets of Neuroticism include Anxiety, Anger/Hostility, Depression, Self-Consciousness, Impulsiveness, and Vulnerability. The revised version completes the earlier instrument by providing the facet scales Agreeableness and Conscientiousness.

In this era of searching for efficient care, some consideration should be given to the use of screening instruments that can be administered rapidly to assess for the potential for personality disorders, disorders that retard and compli-

TABLE 8–8. **Instruments for the assessment of personality traits and disorders**

Instrument	General classification	Description	Scoring features
NEO—Personality Inventory—Revised (NEO-PI-R)	Self-report	240 items, 5-point scale	Five domain scales and 30 facet scales
6-Personality Factor Inventory	Self-report	3 equivalent forms of 106–187 items each	Scaled scores for 16 personality traits
Eysenck Personality Inventory(EPI)	Self-report	57 yes/no items, parallel forms	Scores on extraversion and neuroticism
Schedule for Nonadaptive and Adaptive Personality (SNAP)	Self-report	12 primary traits and 3 temperament dimensions	Scores on 15 scales
Dimensional Assessment of Personality Pathology—Basic Questionnaire (DAPP-BQ)	Self-report	18 scales	Scores on 18 scales
California Personality Inventory (CPI)	Self-report	468 items	Scores on 18 scales and 4 special scales
Millon Clinical Multiaxial Inventory—II (MCMI-II)	Self-report	175 items, true/false format	Base rate scores on 22 clinical scales
Structural Interview for the DSM-IV Personality Disorders	Semistructured interview	3-point rating scales	Yields DSM-IV Axis II diagnoses
Personality Disorder Examination	Semistructured interview	Semistructured interview for patient and self-report by family member on patient	Dimensional and categorical scales on DSM-IV Axis II personality disorders
Structured Clinical Interview	Semistructured interview	3-point rating scales of personality traits	Yields Axis II diagnoses
Structural Analyses of Social Behavior	Self-report	36–72 statements of interpersonal behavior rated true/false	Internalized attitudes regarding self and significant others

cate the treatment of Axis I disorders. Four screening instruments deserve consideration: the International Personality Disorder Examination DSM-III-R Screen (IPDE-S) (Lenzenweger et al. 1997), the Iowa Personality Disorder Screen (Pfohl and Langbehn 1994), the Self-Directedness subscale from the Temperament and Character Inventory (Cloninger et al. 1993; Svrakic et al. 1993), and a screen for personality disorders developed from the Inventory of Interpersonal Problems (IIP) (Pilkonis et al. 1996).

Interpersonal Aspects of Personality

One particular school of personality research that has concerned itself with pathological expressions of personality factors has focused explicitly on interpersonal behavior. Adherents to this view of psychopathology emphasize the centrality of the problems that people experience with others, for, in this school of thought, it is in the interpersonal area that all symptoms are activated, reinforced, and (for some persons) caused. The assessment of interpersonal behavior can be central to understanding the patient's social world with its pleasures and disappointments, as well as barriers to success in love and work, and it can be used as a forecast of the kind of relationship the patient will form with the clinician.

This interpersonal tradition dates back to psychologist Timothy Leary's circumplex model (Leary 1957). Underlying the expression of all interpersonal styles are the two major, orthogonal axes of power and affiliation. Each interpersonal style is seen as involving varying degrees of the expression of power and affiliation, leading to 16 modes of interaction. These 16 modes are organized along the circumference of a circle defining eight broad categories that are used in interpersonal diagnosis: Ambitious-Dominant, Gregarious-Extraverted, Warm-Agreeable, Unassuming-Ingenuous, Lazy-Submissive, Aloof-Introverted, Cold-Quarrelsome, and Arrogant-Calculating. This system is more than merely descriptive. Theoretically, one is able to predict not only the kind of interpersonal style that the patient expresses but also the kind of behavior that this style tends to elicit from others. Behavior on one side of the circle tends to elicit from others behaviors on the opposite side of the circle. For example, a patient who is Ambitious-Dominant tends to elicit Lazy-Submissive behavior from others. In terms of differential therapeutic treatment planning, this model suggests not only that the patient will behave in a certain fashion, but also that this behavior will elicit therapist behavior found on the opposite side of the circle. It has been suggested that interpersonal diagnosis can thus highlight transference and possibly counter-

transference reactions in therapies that are interpersonal in orientation. Furthermore, the theory indicates what kinds of counterbehavior the therapist should engage in to dislodge the patient from his or her predominant mode of interaction.

Several instruments have been developed from this basic interpersonal theory. In a series of investigations, Lorr and McNair (1965) generated the latest version of the Interpersonal Behavior Inventory (IBI). The IBI has been judged to be psychometrically sound and a useful clinical device for the assessment of patient characteristics and therapy outcome (Wiggins 1982). The instrument is a clinical rating by professionals but in principle could be employed in a self-report format. The Interpersonal Style Inventory (ISI; Lorr and Youniss 1973) is a self-report instrument for persons 14 years old and older. A large number (300) of true-false statements is employed to assess interpersonal involvement, socialization, self-control, stability, and autonomy. Techniques of rational scale construction were employed, including validity factor analyses. Norms are based on 1,500 college and high school students.

Also in the same tradition, Benjamin (1974) developed an instrument for the assessment of interpersonal behavior, the Structural Analysis of Social Behavior (SASB), and a computer-based scoring system marketed under the trade name INTREX, which is self-administered. The SASB can also be used by clinicians to record their impressions about the patient. A related coding scheme has been developed for use by trained observers to record the patient's actual interactions with others, such as family members, during the course of treatment.

Assessment of Personality Disorders

A relatively new approach to the assessment of personality disorders is to construct instruments, either self-report or semistructured interviews, that evaluate the presence or absence of specific personality traits described in Axis II of DSM-IV. DSM-IV neither defines nor develops from any particular theory of personality. Instead, it identifies clusters (in most cases, clusters with little empirical validation) of personality traits considered sufficiently maladaptive to warrant the designation *personality disorder*. Personality traits are described as enduring patterns of perceiving, relating to, and thinking about the environment and oneself that are exhibited or manifested in a wide range of important social and interpersonal contexts. When these traits are inflexible and maladaptive and cause either significant impairment in social or occupational functioning or subjective distress, they are defined as a personality disorder in

DSM-IV. The most useful instruments of this type include the Personality Diagnostic Questionnaire–4 (PDQ-4; Hurt et al. 1984; Hyler 1994), the Millon Clinical Multiaxial Inventory (MCMI; Millon 1983), the SCID, the Personality Disorders Examination, and the Structural Interview for the DSM-IV Personality (SIDP-IV; Pfohl et al. 1997).

The PDQ-4 is a self-report inventory of Axis II traits, and the test yields scores on each of the personality disorder categories of DSM-IV. Preliminary investigation of the instrument suggests that patients typically report a number of traits and will often meet criteria for several diagnostic categories; the PDQ may, however, be useful for screening (Hurt et al. 1984).

The MCMI is a 175-item true-false self-report instrument that yields scores on 11 personality disorder dimensions closely related to the personality disorder diagnoses of DSM-III Axis II, and 9 clinical syndromes. Probably the major difficulty with this instrument is psychometric, because there is much item overlap in the scales (Wiggins 1982). In the MCMI-II (Millon 1987), a revision of the original scale, two new personality disorder scales were introduced and two prior personality scales were modified. An item-weighting system has been introduced into the MCMI-II to reflect item differences related to the strength of each item's supporting validation data.

There are several self-report questionnaires assessing personality and personality pathology that have been carefully constructed with attention to psychometric properties. These questionnaires include the Schedule for Nonadaptive and Adaptive Personality (SNAP; Clark 1993) and the Dimensional Assessment of Personality Pathology—Basic Questionnaire (DAPP-BQ) (Schroeder et al. 1994).

There are three semistructured interviews that have been designed to assess, via the patient's report and the clinical judgment of the interviewer, the presence of Axis II disorders: the IPDE, the Structural Interview for the DSM-IV Personality (SIDP-IV), and the Structured Clinical Interview for DSM-IV.

The IPDE (Loranger 1995) is a semistructured interview that yields both dimensional and categorical scores for DSM-IV Axis II criteria. An important feature of this semistructured interview, which takes approximately 1–2 hours to administer, is that the criteria are assessed in related clusters such as self-concept, affect expression, reality testing, impulse control, interpersonal relations, and work. The interview goes beyond a simple listing of the criteria and in many cases provides multiple questions designed to help the interviewer gain a broad appreciation of the criterion under assessment. A parallel version of the interview has been constructed for use with informants, recognizing

that information from patients themselves, especially around personality issues, may be distorted. Initial reliability data are impressive and validity studies are under way. The instrument is likely to be widely used. In fact, it has been translated into several languages and was used in an international study approved by the World Health Organization and the then Alcohol, Drug Abuse, and Mental Health Administration (Loranger et al. 1991).

SIDP consists of a semistructured interview form that provides 160 questions pertinent to the diagnostic criteria of Axis II of DSM-III. The questions are organized into 16 assessment areas, such as low self-esteem/dependency, egocentricity, ideas of reference and magical thinking, and hostility/anger. The questions are keyed to DSM-III criteria for Axis II disorders. A rating form provides a 3-point rating scale for each criterion. Ratings are based on the clinical assessment of the interview data. The authors of the interview recommend that it be used in conjunction with a general psychiatric interview in which major (i.e., Axis I) psychiatric disorders have been diagnosed so that lifelong personality traits can be distinguished from episodic psychiatric disorders. The authors also recommend gathering information from an informant who knows the patient well.

SCID-II is concerned with the assessment of Axis II personality disorders. The interview format is determined by DSM-IV disorders and provides no guide for elaborating the assessment of the criteria.

There are several problems with this relatively new approach of assessing personality disorders guided solely by DSM-IV. First, Axis II is neither an empirically nor a theoretically derived compilation of personality traits that lead to, cause, or constitute psychopathology. Rather, it is a somewhat arbitrary collection of traits that are thought to be important markers of pathology. Thus, any instrument guided solely by DSM-IV will leave serious questions of internal consistency, content validity, and construct validity largely unanswered. Most probably, attempts to assess these important test characteristics within the context of DSM-IV are likely to be carried out with these instruments.

ASSESSMENT OF PSYCHODYNAMICS

The assessment of factors relevant to psychodynamic and psychoanalytic theory and treatment approaches has a long history in the clinical psychological literature. The development of the "standard battery," including the WAIS, Rorschach, and Thematic Apperception Test (Table 8–9), has its origins in the efforts of clinical psychologists to provide an assessment of such psychodynamic factors as drives, unconscious wishes, conflicts, and defenses.

Table 8–9. Instruments for the assessment of personality traits and disorders

Instrument	General classification	Description	Scoring features
Rorschach Inkblot Test	Unstructured or projective text	10 ambiguous inkblots, responses scored on multiple criteria	Accuracy of form, location, use of color, shading, etc., provide summary scores
Thematic Apperception Text	Unstructured or projective test	30 ambiguous scenes	Affects, outcomes, and other qualities
Minnesota Multiphasic PersonalityInventory—II	Self-report	566-item checklist, true/false format	T-scores for 13 criterion scales
Symptom Checklist—90	Self-report	90-item checklist, 5-point intensity scale	T-scores for 9 symptom clusters
Millon Clinical Multiaxial Inventory—II	Self-report	175 items, true/false format	Base rate scores for 22 clinical scales

For clinicians committed to the psychodynamic model, assessments that focus exclusively on overt behaviors will be less than totally satisfactory.

The importance of providing information about personality dynamics and structure that are outside the conscious awareness of the examinee has been the single most important rationale for the continued use of projective tests. In part, therefore, the value of such assessments varies directly with the degree to which maladaptive and symptomatic behaviors are presumed to be beyond the conscious control of the examinee. There is a second rationale for the continued use of these tests: their unstructured nature provides a singular opportunity to assess the degree to which organization of behavior depends on a high degree of structure in the examination procedure itself. The assessment of both these factors is of clear relevance to a treatment method that attempts to explore and alter unconscious determinants of behavior and that depends for its success on introducing as little structure into the treatment as is realistically possible.

The most widely used assessment procedure for the examination of patients over a range of ego functions and dynamic factors is the Rorschach Inkblot Test, described earlier. Scoring systems have been developed by many authors; Exner (1974, 1978) developed a scoring system that attempts to integrate the best aspects of the prior systems. From these scores, inferences are drawn concerning the patient's self-image, identity, defensive structure, reality testing, affective control, amount and degree of fantasy life, degree of thought organization, and potential for impulsive acting out.

The Thematic Apperception Test (TAT) is another widely used projective process for assessing the patient's self-concept in relation to others. Originally developed by Murray (1943), the test consists of a set of 30 pictures de-

picting one or more individuals (Figure 8–2). The patient is asked to make up a story based on each picture. The stories generated are then scored for the individual's needs as reflected in the feelings and impulses attributed to the major character in each story and the interactions with the envi-

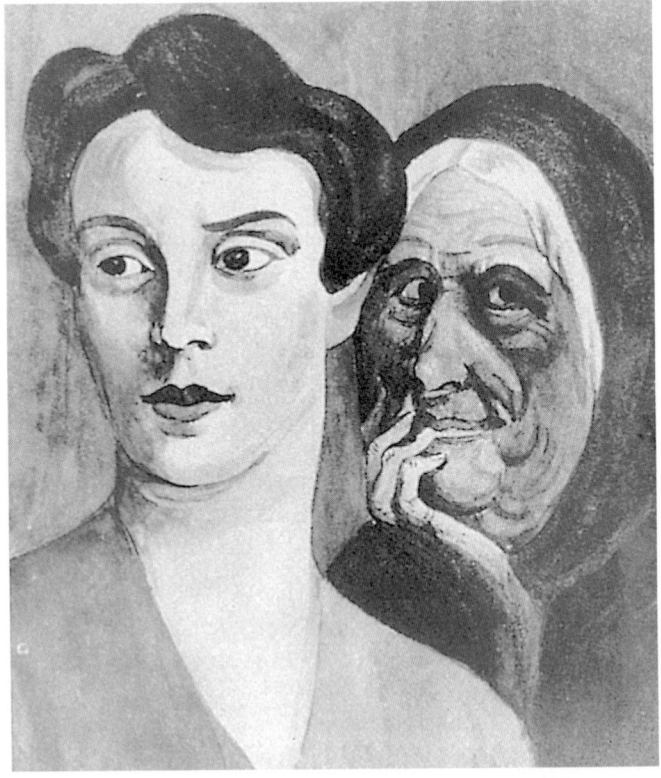

Figure 8–2. Thematic Apperception Test, Card 12F.
Source.   Reprinted by permission of the publisher from Murray HA: *Thematic Apperception Test.* Cambridge, MA, Harvard University Press. Copyright 1943 by the President and Fellows of Harvard College; copyright 1971 by Henry A. Murray.

ronment leading to a resolution. As currently used, the stories are most often examined for the patient's self-other concepts as revealed in the interaction and outcome of the story line.

ASSESSMENT OF ENVIRONMENTAL DEMANDS AND SOCIAL ADJUSTMENT

The interaction between the patient and the pressures of the environment is now acknowledged in the standard diagnostic system (DSM-IV) by a rating on Axis IV. Probably the most substantiated area with empirical data indicating the effect of the patient-environment interaction is the investigation of expressed emotion (EE) and its influence on the course of schizophrenia. This work suggests that certain elements in the home environment of a schizophrenic patient can adversely affect the course of the illness. EE can be assessed by the Camberwell Family Interview (Brown and Rutter 1966), a 1-hour semistructured interview of a relative of the patient. The scoring scheme for this instrument is not readily accessible and is therefore not usable in standard clinical situations.

In measuring both stress and the patient's ability to cope with stress, one can assess the stimuli, the individual's response to the stimuli, or the interaction of the person with stressful stimuli (see (Table 8–10). The Jenkins Activity Survey (JAS; Jenkins et al. 1967) is the prototype of an interaction-based measure of stress, focusing on the cognitive and perceptual characteristics of the individual that mediate responses to stress. This instrument has been shown to have predictive validity in studies of reaction to coronary heart disease. The Derogatis Stress Profile (DSP; Derogatis 1982) is useful in evaluating stimuli from work and home and can be used to assess health, as well as characteristic attitudes and coping mechanisms.

We use the term *social adjustment* to indicate the skill of the individual in handling interpersonal situations, whether at home, in school, or in the work setting. The term *social adjustment* has been used more narrowly to indicate the community and social adjustment of diagnosed psychiatric patients, who

often have severe illnesses such as schizophrenia and major affective disorder (Weissman and Sholomskas 1982). Notable assessment instruments in this area include the Katz Adjustment Scale—Relative's Form (KAS-R; Katz and Lyerly 1963), the Social Adjustment Scale—Self-Report (SAS-SR; Weissman and Bothwell 1976), and the Dyadic Adjustment Scale (DAS) (Spanier 1976).

The KAS-R is a relative's self-report inventory of the patient's symptomatic behavior and social adjustment in the community. The scale has sections on symptoms and social behavior, performance of socially expected tasks, the relative's expectation for the performance of these tasks, the patient's free-time activities, and the relative's satisfaction with the performance of these free-time activities.

The SAS-SR contains 42 questions covering instrumental and affective qualities in role performance, social and leisure activities, relationships with extended family, marital role, parental role, family unit, and economic independence. Norms are available for nonpatient community samples, acute and recovered depressed outpatients, schizophrenic patients, and drug-addicted patients. The Social Support Questionnaire (SSQ) (Sarason et al. 1983) is an efficient method for assessing social satisfaction. This instrument provides information about available resources for support and the patient's level of satisfaction with this support system.

The area of the quality of marital adjustment is relevant to treatment planning for married individuals with psychiatric disorders such as phobias and mood disorders (Clarkin et al. 1992), as well as couples who present with marital difficulties. Several useful self-report instruments in this area are the DAS and the Marital Satisfaction Inventory (Snyder et al. 1981).

ASSESSMENT OF THERAPEUTIC ENABLING FACTORS

Accurate diagnosis is not sufficient for determining optimal specific treatments. Although the patient's diagnosis

TABLE 8–10. **Instruments for the assessment of environmental stressors**

Instrument	General classification	Description	Scoring features
Social Adjustment Scale—Self-Report	Self-report	42 questions, rated on 5-point scale of severity	Mean score for 7 areas and an overall score
Dyadic Adjustment Scale	Self-report	31 items, 4 dimensions	Total score
Marital Satisfaction Inventory	Self-report	280 items	T-scores on 11 scales

helps to narrow the focus, optimal treatment planning depends on nondiagnostic factors such as characteristics of the patient that will affect the acceptance, use of, and absorption of the treatment recommended. Psychological tests can be useful in assessing these dimensions. From a review of the comparative psychotherapy outcome research data (Beutler 1983; Beutler and Clarkin 1990; Gaw and Beutler 1995) one can isolate five areas of assessment: 1) problem severity, 2) motivational distress, 3) problem complexity, 4) resistance potential or reactance level, and 5) coping style. These areas are discussed in the following paragraphs.

Problem severity is defined as a continuum of functioning ranging from little impairment to incapacitation. Instruments reviewed in this chapter assessing symptoms and general functioning are appropriate measures of problem severity. Motivational distress is the degree of subjective disturbance experienced by the patient in reference to his/her problems. Motivational distress is important because it motivates help-seeking activity such as psychotherapy in order to reduce discomfort. The Brief Symptom Inventory (BSI; Derogatis 1992) is an efficient method of assessing aspects of a patient's self-defined problem severity. The Global Severity Index (GSI) from the BSI can be used as an estimate of subjective or motivational distress. It is suggested that when the GSI value exceeds a T score of 63, a treatment that is designed to reduce subjective distress is indicated (Derogatis 1992). If distress levels are low, the clinician must consider confronting the patient with the contradiction of low distress in the face of impairment. The MMPI-2 can also be used to assess motivational distress. For example, scale 7 is an index of psychological turmoil and discomfort (Graham 1990). Scores above 70 on the F subscale may suggest good motivation for treatment. Those whose high scores on the F scale are matched with elevations on L and K tend to resist and react to authority and, inferentially, to therapists. Problem complexity relates to the pervasiveness and the endurance of the problem. A complex problem is pervasive and enduring; that is, it is chronic and trans-situational rather than specific to the situation. The BSI offers information on the degree to which the problem spreads across symptom domains, as this is one aspect of complexity. The MMPI-2 two-point code types (Graham 1990) and the Axis II indicators from the MCMI-II may also shed light on the spread and chronicity of problems.

Reactance, a construct that comes from social psychology, indicates the degree to which an individual is resistant or oppositional to interpersonal demands such as the recommendations or advice of a mental health professional. One of the most promising instruments for assessing reactance is the Therapeutic Reactance Scale (TRS) (Dowd et al. 1991). It is a 28-item self-report instrument, and there have been two normative studies.

Coping style refers to the manner in which an individual manages or deals with anxiety arising from interpersonal or intrapersonal conflict. The MMPI-2 is useful in defining the patient's coping styles along an internalizing-externalizing dimension. Externalizing patterns are indicated by the Hy, Pd, Pa, and Ma scales. Internalizing coping styles are indicated by the Hs, B, Pt, and Si scales.

CLINICAL DECISION TREE

The indications for assessment vary with the setting in which the assessment is conducted and the typical patient encountered in such a setting. In clinical psychiatric settings, assessment is most often requested to aid in reducing uncertainty about diagnosis and in evaluating the severity of specific symptoms or symptom complexes (e.g., depression, suicide intent, or thought disorder). Such an assessment plays an important role in providing information on patients that can be usefully generalized by facilitating comparisons between patients or by tracking the severity of symptoms under the impact of treatment. This assessment may form the basis for recommended treatments, help in establishing goals for the general treatment plan, or help in determining treatment progress and the need for further intervention.

Inpatient settings have focused historically on the questions of differential diagnosis, and a recent survey indicates that this trend continues: referrals for assessment of DSM-III Axis I disorders are the most frequent (69%) and those for Axis II disorders the next most frequent (15%) (Clarkin and Sweeney 1992). In hospital settings, referrals often emphasize the need for the assessment of specific cognitive, vocational, and social assets that can be adaptively employed in helping the patient return to full participation in community life. Behavior therapists working in a phobia clinic may be particularly interested in the interaction between fear and situation so as to successfully plan a program of desensitization. A psychoanalyst may refer a patient early in treatment to determine the patient's capacity for long-term, insight-oriented psychotherapy and to assess the status of various transference paradigms that would help the analyst to tailor the patient's treatment. In neurology clinics, referral for assessment is frequently made to more specifically identify the nature, degree, and localization of impairment, particularly in children and in elderly persons.

With medical care costs soaring, in part because of an indiscriminate use of laboratory tests, psychiatrists should be clear about the precise areas needed for assessment before referring a patient for testing. Likewise, the clinical psychologist should pursue the testing with efficiency and use instruments that will answer the referral questions with precision, reliability, and validity. Both psychiatrist and psychologist should use a clinical decision tree that informs their differential therapeutic procedures.

In the present state of knowledge, we suggest that in referring a patient for assessment the psychiatrist have already completed a semistructured interview (or methodical clinical interview) that provides knowledge of which DSM-IV criteria (on both Axis I and Axis II) the patient meets. With this diagnostic information, the clinical psychologist can pursue questions about the patient along any one or mix of the axes that we have described in this chapter—symptoms, personality traits, cognitive functioning, psychodynamics, and environment and social adjustment—by the selection and administration of tests, interviews, and rating scales with the overall goal of informed differential therapeutics. Which of the five axes the psychologist pursues will depend on which DSM-IV criteria the patient meets and the nature of the pathology that needs further explication.

ASSESSMENT OF PATIENT IN SYSTEM OF CARE; ASSESSMENT OF SYSTEM OF CARE

What is relatively new is the standard, routine assessment of each patient in a system of care and the assessment of the system of care itself. The Integra outpatient mental-health tracking system called Compass is one of the most developed tracking systems and one based upon a model of patient treatment response (Howard et al. 1993). By gathering systematic and sequential data from both patient and therapist, the system provides information for utilization review regarding the need for additional treatment. It can also be a tool for evaluating the therapists' performance in relation to cost and identifying therapists who are effective or ineffective in treating the various patient types. The instrument focuses on patient outcomes of interest to employers: alleviation of symptom distress, reduction of medical expenses, and reduction of absenteeism. Thus, the instrument focuses on three main areas: symptoms, functioning, and the patient's sense of well-being. The patient fills out an instrument with 111 items at the initiation of treatment and 83 items at regular intervals during the treatment. In parallel fashion, the clinician fills out an

11-item assessment of patient functioning. Items filled out by the patient cover demographics, treatment motivation, presenting problems, sense of well-being, current life functioning, current symptoms, and perception of the therapist.

REFERENCES

American Psychiatric Association: Diagnostic and Statistical Manual of Mental Disorders, 4th Edition. Washington, DC, American Psychiatric Association, 1994

Ammons RB, Ammons CH: The Quick Test (QT): provisional manual. Psychol Rep 11:111–161, 1962

Anastasi A: Psychological Testing, 5th Edition. New York, Macmillan, 1982

Barchas JD, Berger PA, Ciaranello RD, et al: Psychopharmacology: From Theory to Practice. New York, Oxford University Press, 1977

Bauer MS, Crits-Christoph P, Ball WA, et al: Independent assessment of manic and depressive symptoms by self-rating: scale characteristics and implications for the study of mania. Arch Gen Psychiatry 48:807–812, 1991

Beck AT, Young JE: Depression, in Clinical Handbook of Psychological Disorders. Edited by Barlow DH. New York, Guilford, 1985, pp 202–244

Beck AT, Schuyler D, Herman I: Development of suicidal intent scales, in The Prediction of Suicide. Edited by Beck AT, Resnick HLP, Lettieri DJ. Bowie, MD, Charles Press, 1974a, pp 45–56

Beck AT, Weissman A, Lester D, et al: The measurement of pessimism: The Hopelessness Scale. J Consult Clin Psychol 42:861–865, 1994b

Beigel A, Murphy DL, Bunney WE Jr: The Manic-State Rating Scale: scale construction, reliability, and validity. Arch Gen Psychiatry 25:256–262, 1971

Benjamin LS: Structural analysis of social behavior. Psychol Rev 81:392–425, 1974

Benton AL: Visual Retention Test. New York, Psychological Corporation, 1955

Benton AL, Hamsher K: Multilingual Aphasia Examination. Iowa City, IA, University of Iowa, 1976

Benton AL, Van Allen MW: Impairment in facial recognition in patients with cerebral disease. Cortex 4:344–358, 1968

Benton AL, Hannay HJ, Varney NR: Visual perception of line direction in patients with unilateral brain disease. Neurology 25:907–910, 1975

Berg EA: A simple objective test for measuring flexibility in thinking. J Gen Psychol 39:15–32, 1948

Beutler LE: Eclectic Psychotherapy: A Systematic Approach. New York, Pergamon, 1983

Beutler LE, Clarkin JF: Systematic Treatment Selection: Toward Targeted Therapeutic Interventions. New York, Brunner/Mazel, 1990

Boll TJ: The Halstead-Reitan Neuropsychology Battery, in Handbook of Clinical Neuropsychology. Edited by Filskov SB, Boll TJ. New York, Wiley, 1981, pp 577–607

Bongar B: The Suicidal Patient: Clinical and Legal Standards of Care. Washington, DC, American Psychological Association, 1991

Brandt J: The Hopkins Verbal Learning Test: development of a new memory test with six equivalent forms. The Clinical Neuropsychologist 5:125–142, 1991

Brown GW, Rutter M: The measurement of family activities and relationships: a methodological study. Human Relations 19:241–263, 1966

Buros OK (ed): The Seventh Mental Measurements Yearbook. Highland Park, NJ, Gryphon Press, 1971

Buros OK (ed): The Eighth Mental Measurements Yearbook. Highland Park, NJ, Gryphon Press, 1978

Buss AH, Durkee A: An inventory for assessing different kinds of hostility. Journal of Consulting Psychology 21:343–349, 1957

Butcher JN: The Minnesota Report: Adult Clinical System MMPI-2. Minneapolis MN, University of Minnesota Press, 1989

Butcher JN, Dahlstrom WG, Graham JR, et al: Manual for the Restandardized Minnesota Multiphasic Personality Inventory (MMPI-2): An Administrative and Interpretive Guide. Minneapolis, MN, University of Minnesota Press, 1989

Cattell RB, Eber HW, Tatsuoka MM: Handbook for the Sixteen Personality Factor Inventory. Champaign, IL, Institute for Personality and Ability Testing, 1970

Christensen AL: Luria's Neuropsychological Investigation: Manual. New York, Spectrum, 1975

Clark LA: Manual for the Schedule for Nonadaptive and Adaptive Personality (SNAP). Minneapolis, MN, University of Minnesota Press, 1993

Clarkin JF, Mattis S: Psychological assessment, in Inpatient Psychiatry: Diagnosis and Treatment, 3rd Edition. Edited by Sederer LI. Baltimore MD, Williams and Wilkins, 1991, pp 360–378

Clarkin JF, Sweeney JA: Psychological testing (Chapter 7), in Psychiatry, Vol 1. Edited by Michels R, Cavenar JO Jr, et al. Philadelphia, PA, JB Lippincott, 1992

Clarkin JF, Haas GL, Glick ID: Family and marital therapy, in Handbook of Affective Disorders, 2nd Edition. Edited by Paykel ES. London, Churchill Livingstone, 1992, pp 487–500

Cloninger CR, Svrakic DM, Przybeck TR: A psychobiological model of temperament and character. Arch Gen Psychiatry 50:975–990, 1993

Costa LD, Vaughan HG, Levita E, et al: Purdue Pegboard as a predictor of the presence and laterality of cerebral lesions. Journal of Consulting Psychology 27:133–137, 1963

Costa PT, McCrae RR: NEO PI-R: Professional Manual. Odessa, FL, Psychological Assessment Resources, 1992

Cull JG, Gill WS: Suicide Probability Scale (SPS) Manual. Los Angeles, CA, Western Psychological Services, 1986

Dahlstrom WG, Welsh GS, Dahlstrom LE: An MMPI Handbook, Revised Edition, Vols 1 and 2. Minneapolis, MN, University of Minnesota Press, 1972

DeFillipis NA, McCambell E, Rogers P: Development of a booklet form of the Category Test: normative and validity data. Journal of Clinical Neuropsychology 1:339–342, 1979

Delis DC, Kramer J, Kaplan E, et al: California Verbal Learning Test (CVLT), Research Edition Manual. New York, Psychological Corporation, 1987

Derogatis LR: The SCL-90R. Baltimore, MD, Clinical Psychometric Research, 1977

Derogatis LR: Self-report measures of stress, in Handbook of Stress. Edited by Goldberger L, Breznitz S. New York, Free Press, 1982, pp 270–294

Derogatis LR: BSI: Administration, Scoring and Procedures Manual-II (2nd ed.). Baltimore, Clinical Psychometric Research, 1992

Derogatis LR, Lipman RS, Rickels K, et al: The Hopkins Symptom Checklist (HSCL): a measure of primary symptom dimensions, in Psychological Measurements in Psychopharmacology, Vol 7: Modern Problems of Pharmacopsychiatry. Edited by Pichot P. Basel, S Karger, 1974, pp79–110

Dowd ET, Milne CR, Wise SL: The Therapeutic Reactance Scale: A measure of psychological reactance. J Consult Clin Psychol 69:541–545, 1991

Endicott J, Spitzer RL: Use of the Research Diagnostic Criteria and the Schedule for Affective Disorders and Schizophrenia to study affective disorders. Am J Psychiatry 136:52–56, 1979

Endler NS, Hunt J McV, Rosenstein AJ: An S-R inventory of anxiousness. Psychological Monographs: General and Applied 76 (17):1–31, 1962

Exner JE Jr: The Rorschach: A Comprehensive System, Vol 1. New York, Wiley, 1974

Exner JE Jr: The Rorschach: A Comprehensive System, Vol 2. New York, Wiley, 1978

Eysenck HJ, Eysenck SB: The Structure and Measurement of Personality. San Diego, CA, RR Knapp, 1969

Feighner JP, Robins E, Guze SB, et al: Diagnostic criteria for use in psychiatric research. Arch Gen Psychiatry 26:57–63, 1972

First MB, Spitzer RL, Gibbon M, et al: User's Guide for the Structured Clinical Interview for DSM-IV Axis II—Research Version (SCID-II, Version 2.0, February 1996, Final Version). New York, New York State Psychiatric Institute, 1996

First MB, Spitzer RL, Gibbon M, et al: Structured Clinical Interview for DSM-IV Axis I Disorders (SCID-I), Clincal Version, New York, New York State Psychiatric Institute, 1997

Folstein MF, Folstein SE, McHugh PR: Mini-mental state: a practical method for grading the cognitive state of patients for the clinician. J Psychiatr Res 11:189–198, 1975

Garner DM: Eating Disorder Inventory 2: Professional Manual. Odessa, FL, Psychological Assessment Resources, 1992

Gaw KF, Beutler LE: Integrating treatment recommendations, in Integrative Assessment of Adult Personality. Edited by Beutler LE, Berren MR. New York, Guilford, 1995, pp 280–319

Geffen G, Moar KJ, O'Hanlon AP, et al: Performance measures of 16- to 86-year-old males and females on the Auditory Verbal Learning Test. The Clinical Neuropsychologist 4:45–63, 1990

Golden CJ, Hammeke TA, Purisch AD: Diagnostic validity of a standardized neuropsychological battery derived from Luria's neuropsychological tests. J Consult Clin Psychol 46:1258–1265, 1978

Goldman R, Fristoe M, Woodcock RW: Auditory Skills Test Battery. Circle Pines, MN, American Guidance Service, 1976

Goodglass H, Kaplan E: Assessment of Aphasia and Related Disorders. Philadelphia, PA, Lea and Febiger, 1972

Gough HG: California Psychological Inventory. Palo Alto, CA, Consulting Psychologists Press, 1956

Graham JR: MMPI-2: Assessing Personality and Psychopathology. New York, Oxford University Press, 1990

Greene RL: The MMPI-2/MMPI: An Interpretive Manual. Needham Heights, MA, Allyn & Bacon, 1991

Greene RL, Banken JA: Assessing alcohol/drug abuse problems, in Clinical Personality Assessment: Practical Approaches. Edited by Butcher JN. New York, Oxford University Press, 1995, pp 460–474

Halstead WC, Wepman JM: The Halstead-Wepman Aphasia Screening Test. Journal of Speech and Hearing Disorders 14:9–15, 1959

Hamilton M: The assessment of anxiety states by rating. Br J Med Psychol 32:50–55, 1959

Hamilton M: A rating scale for depression. J Neurol Neurosurg Psychiatry 23:51–56, 1960

Hamilton M: Development of a rating scale for primary depressive illness. Br J Soc Clin Psychol 6:278–296, 1967

Harrow M, Quinlan D (eds): Disordered Thinking and Schizophrenic Psychopathology. New York, Gardner Press, 1985

Hathaway SR, McKinley JC: Minnesota Multiphasic Personality Inventory Manual, Revised Edition. New York, Psychological Corporation, 1967

Haxby JV, Raffaele K, Gillete J, et al: Individual trajectories of cognitive decline in patients with dementia of the Alzheimer type. J Clin Exp Neuropsychol 14:575–592, 1992

Heaton RK, Crowley TJ: Effects of psychiatric disorders and their somatic treatments on neuropsychological test results, in Handbook of Clinical Neuropsychology. Edited by Filskov SB, Boll TJ. New York, Wiley, 1981, pp 481–525

Hoffmann H, Loper RG, Kammeier ML: Identifying future alcoholics with MMPI alcoholism scales. Quarterly Journal of Studies on Alcohol 35:490–498, 1974

Horn JL, Wanberg KW, Foster FM: Alcohol Use Inventory. Minneapolis, MN, National Computer Systems, 1986

Howard K, Lueger R, Maling M, et al: A phase model of psychotherapy outcome: Causal mediation of change. J Consult Clin Psychol 61:678–685, 1993

Hurt SW, Holzman PS, Davis JM: Thought disorder: the measurement of its changes. Arch Gen Psychiatry 40:1281–1285, 1983

Hurt SW, Hyler SE, Frances A, et al: Assessing borderline personality disorder with self-report, clinical interview, or semistructured interview. Am J Psychiatry 141:1228–1231, 1984

Hurt SW, Clarkin JF, Frances A, et al: Discriminate validity of the MMPI for borderline personality disorder. J Pers Assess 49:56–61, 1985

Hurt SW, Reznikoff M, Clarkin JF: Psychological Assessment, Psychiatric Diagnosis, and Treatment Planning. New York, Brunner/Mazel, 1991

Hyler SE: Personality Diagnostic Questionnaire–4. New York, New York State Psychiatric Institute, 1994

Hyler SE, Rieder R, Spitzer RL, et al: Personality Diagnostic Questionnaire (PDQ). New York, New York State Psychiatric Institute, Biometrics Research Division, 1978

Janowsky D, Judd L, Huey L, et al: Naloxone effects on manic symptoms and growth hormone levels. Lancet 2:320, 1978

Jastak S, Wilkinson GS: The Wide Range Achievement Test—Revised. Wilmington, DE, Jastak Associates, 1981

Jenkins CD, Rosenman RH, Friedman J: Development of an objective psychological test for the determination of the coronary-prone behavior pattern in employed men. J Chronic Dis 20:371–379, 1967

Johnston MH, Holzman PS: Assessing Schizophrenic Thinking. San Francisco, CA, Jossey-Bass, 1979

Karzmark P, Heaton RK, Grant I, et al: Use of demographic variables to predict full scale IQ: a replication and extension. J Clin Exp Neuropsychol 7:412–420, 1985

Katz MM, Lyerly SB: Methods for measuring adjustment and social behavior in the community, I: rationale, description, discriminative validity and scale development. Psychol Rep Monograph 13:503–535, 1963

Kimura D: Functional asymmetry of the brain in dichotic listening. Cortex 3:163–178, 1967

Leary T: Interpersonal Diagnosis of Personality. New York, Ronald Press, 1957

Lenzenweger MF, Loranger AW, Korfine L, Neff C: Detecting personality disorders in a nonclinical population: application of a two-stage procedure for case detection. Arch Gen Psychiatry 54:345–351, 1997

Lezak M: Neuropsychological Assessment. New York, Oxford University Press, 1969

Linehan MM, Goodstein JL, Nielson SL, et al: Reasons for staying alive when you are thinking of killing yourself: the Reasons for Living Inventory. J Consult Clin Psychol 51:276–286, 1983

Loranger AW: International Personality Disorder Examination (IPDE) Manual. Geneva, Switzerland, World Health Organization, 1995

Loranger AW, Hirschfeld RMA, Sartorius N, et al: The WHO/ADAMHA international pilot study of personality disorders: background and purpose. Journal of Personality Disorders 5:296–306, 1991

Lorr M, McNair DM: Expansion of the interpersonal behavior circle. J Pers Soc Psychol 2:823–830, 1965

Lorr M, Youniss RP: An inventory of interpersonal style. J Pers Assess 37:165–173, 1973

Luria AR: Higher Cortical Functions in Man. New York, Basic Books, 1966

Luria AR: The Working Brain: An Introduction to Neuropsychology. Translated by Haigh B. New York, Basic Books, 1973

MacAndrew C: The differentiation of male alcohol outpatients from nonalcoholic psychiatric patients by means of the MMPI. Quarterly Journal of Studies on Alcohol 26:238–246, 1965

Marengo J, Harrow M: Thought disorder: a function of schizophrenia, mania, or psychosis? J Nerv Ment Dis 173:35–41, 1985

Marks IM, Seeman W: The Actuarial Description of Abnormal Personality. Baltimore, MD, Williams & Wilkins, 1963

Marks IM, Seeman W, Haller DL: The Actuarial Use of the MMPI With Adolescents and Adults. Baltimore, MD, Williams & Wilkins, 1974

Mattis S: Dementia Rating Scale: Professional Manual. Odessa, FL, Psychological Assessment Resources, 1988

Mattis S, French JH, Rapin I: Dyslexia in children and young adults: three independent neuropsychological syndromes. Dev Med Child Neurol 17:150–163, 1975

Mattis S, Kovner R, Goldmeier E: Different patterns of mnemonic deficits in two organic amnestic syndromes. Brain Lang 6:179–191, 1978

McKinley JC, Hathaway SR, Meehl PE: The MMPI, VI: K scale. Journal of Consulting Psychology 12:20–31, 1948

Megargee EI, Cook PE, Mendelsohn GA: Development and validation of an MMPI scale of assaultiveness in overcontrolled individuals. J Abnorm Psychol 72:519–528, 1967

Mesulam M-M: Principles of Behavioral Neurology. Philadelphia, PA, FA Davis, 1985

Millon T: Millon Clinical Multiaxial Inventory, 3rd Edition. Minneapolis, MN, Interpretive Scoring Systems, 1983

Millon T: Millon Clinical Multiaxial Inventory—II: Manual for the MCMI-II. Minneapolis, MN, National Computer Systems, 1987

Mirsky AF, Kornetsky C: On the dissimilar effects of drugs on the Digit Symbol Substitution and Continuous Performance Tests: a review and preliminary integration of behavioral and physiological evidence. Psychopharmacologia 5:161–177, 1964

Morey LC: Personality Assessment Inventory. Odessa, FL, Psychological Assessment Resources, 1991

Murray HA: Thematic Apperception Test Manual. Cambridge, MA, Harvard University Press, 1943

Nelson HE: National Adult Reading Test (NART) Test Manual. Berkshire, MA, NFER-Nelson, 1982

Newman FL, Ciarlo JA: Criteria for selecting psychological tests/instruments, in Use of Psychological Testing for Treatment Planning and Outcome Assessment. Edited by Maruish M. Malvern, PA, LEA Publishers, 1994, pp 98–110

Overall JE, Gorham DR: The Brief Psychiatric Rating Scale. Psychol Rep 10:799–812, 1962

Pfohl B, Langbehn D: Iowa Personality Disorder Screen (Version 1.2). Iowa City, University of Iowa, Department of Psychiatry, 1994

Pfohl B, Blum N, Zimmerman M: Structured Interview for DSM-IV—Personality. Washington, DC, American Psychiatric Press, 1997

Pilkonis PA, Kim Y, Proietti JM, et al: A screen scale for personality disorders developed from the Inventory of Interpersonal Problems. Journal of Personality Disorders 10:355–369, 1996

Psychological Corporation: Wechsler Adult Intelligence Scale—3rd Edition (WAIS-III): Technical Manual. San Antonio, TX, Harcourt Brace, 1997

Raven JC: Guide to the Standard Progressive Matrices. London, HK Lewis, 1960

Rey A: L'examen psychologique dans les cas d'encephalopathie traumatique. Archives de Psychologie 28:286–340, 1941

Rey A: L'Examen Clinique en Psychologique. Paris, Presses Universitaires de France, 1964

Rorschach H: Psychodiagnostics. New York, Grune & Stratton, 1949

Rosvold HE, Mirsky AF, Sarason I, et al: A continuous performance test of brain damage. J Consult Clin Psychol 20:343–350, 1956

Sarason IG, Levine HM, Basham RB, et al: Assessing social support: the Social Support Questionnaire. J Pers Soc Psychol 44:127–139, 1983

Schroeder ML, Wormworth JA, Livesley WJ: Dimensions of personality disorder and the five-factor model of personality, in Personality Disorders and the Five-Factor Model of Personality. Edited by Costa PT, Widiger TA. Washington DC, American Psychological Association, 1994, pp 117–127

Seashore CE, Lewis D, Saetveit DL: Seashore Measures of Musical Talents, Revised Edition. New York, Psychological Corporation, 1960

Seidman IJ: Schizophrenia and brain dysfunction: an integration of recent neurodiagnostic findings. Psychol Bull 94:195–238, 1983

Shenton ME, Kikinis R, Frenc AJ, et al: Abnormalities of the left temporal lobe and thought disorder in schizophrenia: a quantitative magnetic resonance imaging study. N Engl J Med 327:604–612, 1992

Shipley WC: The Institute of Living Scale. Los Angeles, Western Psychological Services, 1946

Snyder DK, Wills RM, Keiser TW: Empirical validation of the Marital Satisfaction Inventory: an actuarial approach. J Consult Clin Psychol 49:262–268, 1981

Solovay MR, Shenton ME, Gasperetti C, et al: Scoring manual for the Thought Disorder Index. Schizophr Bull 12:483–496, 1986

Spanier GB: Measuring dyadic adjustment: new scales for assessing the quality of marriage and similar dyads. Journal of Marriage and the Family 38:15–28, 1976

Spielberger CD: State-Trait Anger Expression Inventory, Revised Research Edition. Odessa, FL, Psychological Assessment Resources, 1991

Spielberger CD, Gorsuch RL, Luchene RE: Manual for the State-Trait Anxiety Inventory. Palo Alto, CA, Consulting Psychologists Press, 1976

Spitzer RL, Williams J, Gibbon M, et al: Structured Clinical Interview for DSM-III-R (SCID): User's Guide. Washington DC, American Psychiatric Press, 1992

Spreen O, Benton AL: Neurosensory Center Comprehensive Examination for Aphasia. Victoria, BC, University of Victoria, 1977

Stangl D, Pfohl B, Zimmerman M, et al: A structured interview for the DSM-III personality disorders: a preliminary report. Arch Gen Psychiatry 42:591–596, 1985

Svrakic DM, Whitehead C, Przybeck TR, et al: Differential diagnosis of personality disorders by the seven-factor model of temperament and character. Arch Gen Psychiatry 50:991–999, 1993

Taylor-Spence JA, Spence KW: The motivational components of manifest anxiety: drive and drive stimuli, in Anxiety and Behavior. Edited by Spielberger CD. New York, Academic Press, 1966, pp 291–326

Vitaliano PP, Breen AR, Russo J, et al: The clinical utility of the Dementia Rating Scale for assessing Alzheimer patients. Journal of Chronic Disease 37:743–753, 1984

Wechsler D: Wechsler Adult Intelligence Scale-Revised. New York, Psychological Corporation, 1981

Wechsler D: The Wechsler Memory Scale-Revised. New York, Psychological Corporation, 1987

Weed NC, Butcher JN, McKenna T, et al: New measures for assessing alcohol and drug abuse with the MMPI-2: the APS and AAS. J Pers Assess 58:389–404, 1992

Weissman MM, Bothwell S: Assessment of social adjustment by patient self-report. Arch Gen Psychiatry 33:1111–1115, 1976

Weissman MM, Sholomskas D: The assessment of social adjustment by the clinician, the patient, and the family, in The Behavior of Psychiatric Patients: Quantitative Techniques for Evaluation. Edited by Burdock EI, Sudilovsky A, Gershon S. New York, Marcel Dekker, 1982, pp 177–209

Wiggins JS: Circumplex models of interpersonal behavior in clinical psychology, in Handbook of Research Methods in Clinical Psychology. Edited by Kendall PC, Butcher JN. New York, Wiley, 1982, pp 183–221

Wiggins JS, Pincus AL: Personality: structure and assessment. Annu Rev Psychol 43:473–504, 1992

Willner AE: Towards development of more sensitive clinical tests of abstraction: the analogy test. Proceedings of the 78th Annual Convention of the American Psychological Association 5:553–554, 1971

Young RC, Biggs JT, Ziegler VE, et al: A rating scale for mania: reliability, validity and sensitivity. Br J Psychiatry 133:429–435, 1978

Zung WWK: A rating instrument for anxiety disorders. Psychosomatics 12:371–379, 1971

Zung WWK: Index of Potential Suicide (IPS): a rating scale for suicide prevention, in The Prediction of Suicide. Edited by Beck AT, Resnick HLP, Lettieri DJ. Bowie, MD, Charles Press, 1974, pp 221–249

CHAPTER 9

LABORATORY AND OTHER DIAGNOSTIC TESTS IN PSYCHIATRY

JOHN M. MORIHISA, M.D.
RICHARD B. ROSSE, M.D.
C. DEBORAH CROSS, M.D.
VICTORIA BALKOSKI, M.D.
CHRISTINE A. INGRAHAM, PH.D.

The increased use of biological therapies in psychiatry a has resulted in a parallel enhanced interest in the application of laboratory and diagnostic test evaluations for psychiatric patients. The reasons for this growing interest include an expanding awareness of physical conditions that can produce psychiatric symptoms and the need to use the laboratory to monitor certain psychopharmacological interventions. Additionally, psychiatrists have been accumulating evidence of subtle neurophysiological dysfunction in many psychiatric disorders, and an effort is being made to try to characterize some of these abnormalities. Such research findings have significantly expanded the scope of thinking concerning many disease processes and have raised the hope that if these pathophysiological abnormalities can be clearly elucidated, new and more useful laboratory tests for psychiatry might be developed.

The laboratory and diagnostic test procedures used by psychiatrists today range from those commonly used by physicians (e.g., complete blood count [CBC], chemistry panels, electrocardiography) to those employed mainly in psychiatric research (e.g., positron emission tomography [PET]). However, the reader should be aware that the field of laboratory and diagnostic testing in psychiatry will not only be determined by research findings in clinical psychiatry and the neurosciences but will probably also be influenced by changing economic realities and by quality assurance and liability issues. Furthermore, medical science is constantly evolving, and no consensus has been achieved concerning many diagnostic approaches. The reader must ultimately use good clinical judgment in determining an appropriate, comprehensive evaluation for each patient. No chapter or table can provide complete or exhaustive protocols for every patient; rather, this information is meant to be a starting point from which the reader can begin the complicated, complex, and demanding task of customizing the appropriate evaluation for each patient.

The use of laboratory and other diagnostic tests in the evaluation and treatment of psychiatric patients must ultimately be determined by each physician, who can consider the entire unique constellation of clinical elements that characterizes each individual patient. No text or protocol can replace the clinical judgment required of each physician in determining the appropriate selection and interpretation of such tests in the development of an effective diagnostic and therapeutic strategy.

USE OF DIAGNOSTIC TESTS IN DETECTING PHYSICAL ILLNESS IN PSYCHIATRIC PATIENTS

The most recent edition of the *Diagnostic and Statistical Manual of Mental Disorders*, DSM-IV (American Psychiatric Association 1994) has for many psychiatric diagnoses a common criterion: the necessary exclusion of any underlying physical condition that might account for the patient's symptomatology. Indeed, several studies have found that physical illnesses are quite common among psychiatric patients. In addition, many of these physical disorders have been thought to be causative or exacerbating factors in patients' psychiatric presentation (Hoffman and Koran 1984). Furthermore, it has been suggested that many psychiatric patients with concomitant medical disorders are particularly vulnerable to excessive morbidity because of their medical conditions (Dvoredsky and Cooley 1986).

Initial suspicion of a possible organic component in a patient's psychiatric presentation can come from clues provided by a careful history taking and physical examination. Although there is no complete consensus about which signs and symptoms are most suggestive of organic conditions, a number of investigators have proposed criteria that they feel might implicate an organic mental disorder. For example, Hoffman and Koran (1984) outlined a table of clues "suggestive" of organic mental disorders (Table 9–1). In addition, Hall et al. (1978) reported that when a review-of-symptoms checklist was used in psychiatric outpatients, patients with four or more positive responses on the checklist had a much higher incidence of abnormal laboratory results than did those who were symptom negative. Many of these abnormal laboratory results were felt to reflect physical conditions that influenced the patients' psychiatric presentation.

For patients known to have (or who are suspected of having) a medical illness, one orders the laboratory tests necessary to work up or follow up the physical condition (Hales 1986). Physical conditions not thought to be con-

tributing to the psychiatric presentation also need to be appropriately evaluated, because psychiatric patients with concomitant medical problems have been reported to demonstrate increased mortality secondary to their medical conditions (Dvoredsky and Cooley 1986; Karasu et al. 1980; Koranyi 1979). In addition, there is the possibility that some of the physical conditions initially considered only coincidental to the psychiatric illness might later prove to be etiological or to exacerbate the psychiatric condition. Consultation from other medical specialists might be necessary, but the consultants' impressions and recommendations all require careful scrutiny by the attending

TABLE 9–1. Some clues suggestive of organic mental disorders

1. Psychiatric symptoms after age 40
2. Psychiatric symptoms
    a. During a major medical illness
    b. While taking drugs that can cause mental symptoms
3. History of
    a. Alcohol or drug abuse
    b. Physical illness impairing organ function (neurological, endocrine, renal, hepatic, cardiac, pulmonary)
    c. Taking multiple prescribed or over-the-counter drugs
4. Family history of
    a. Degenerative or inheritable brain disease
    b. Inherited metabolic disease (e.g., diabetes, pernicious anemia, porphyria)
5. Mental signs including
    a. Altered level of consciousness
    b. Fluctuating mental status
    c. Cognitive impairment
    d. Episodic, recurrent, or cyclic course
    e. Visual, tactile, or olfactory hallucinations
6. Physical signs including
    a. Signs of organ malfunction that can affect the brain
    b. Focal neurological deficits
    c. Diffuse subcortical dysfunction, such as slowed speech/mentation/movement, ataxia, incoordination, tremor, chorea, asterixis, dysarthria
    d. Cortical dysfunction (e.g., dysphasia, apraxias, agnosias, visuospatial deficits, or defective cortical sensation)

Source.   Reprinted with permission from Hoffman RS, Koran RM: "Detecting Physical Illness in Patients With Mental Disorders." *Psychosomatics* 25:654–660, 1984. Copyright 1984.

psychiatrist, who holds the ultimate responsibility for fitting together the pattern of specialized opinions. Decisions to continue or extend laboratory evaluation are often complex and generally include some type of risk-benefit analysis, as well as consideration of prevailing economic and liability issues. This is not to suggest that a laboratory test that a physician believes might be useful should or should not be employed because of primarily economic or legal considerations. Good clinical judgment needs to be the final arbiter for all clinical decisions regarding choice of laboratory and diagnostic testing. Test risks that should be considered (and weighed against the potential benefits of obtaining the test) include possible physical complications, pain, or discomfort (e.g., from repeated venipuncture).

Most clinicians must limit studies according to some assessment of their likely utility in each individual case. Some studies of the use of rather extensive laboratory testing strategies in psychiatric patients have reported that such approaches yield a relatively small amount of useful new information for the clinician (see, e.g., Dolan and Mushlin 1985). However, it can be argued that subclinical physical disorders can cause or possibly exacerbate psychiatric symptoms. Cognitive or behavioral symptoms usually do not signal a specific type of underlying organic problem, but rather suggest an often extensive differential diagnosis.

Studies of medically ill patients and anecdotal reports in the literature have described a wide range of different psychiatric symptoms or syndromes caused by different neuromedical conditions (e.g., Giannini et al. 1978). Additionally, psychiatric symptoms alone are usually inadequate for differentiating the type of underlying medical problem present. For instance, Asaad and Shapiro (1986) outlined a number of organic conditions that can be associated with hallucinations. These organic conditions can include substance abuse disorders, medication psychotoxicity (e.g., secondary to such agents as propranolol and atropine), neurological disorders (e.g., partial complex seizures, central nervous system [CNS] infections), and endocrine and metabolic abnormalities, as well as hallucinations associated with eye and ear diseases (e.g., bilateral hearing loss). Furthermore, many specific organic factors can cause a myriad of different psychiatric symptom pictures in different patients.

Specific laboratory protocols for a number of common psychiatric complaints, such as schizophrenia, bipolar disorder, depression, and anxiety, have been proposed (e.g., Expert Consensus Panel for Bipolar Disorder 1996; Expert Consensus Panel for Schizophrenia 1996). The protocols would provide the psychiatric clinician with thorough laboratory and diagnostic tests based on the possible differential diagnosis for the patient's psychiatric complaints. Note

that the patients would generally not have any obvious physical signs or symptoms of the possible organic disorder to be evaluated in the laboratory screen. Many of the diagnostic tests ordered would be part of a search for various areas of possible organic dysfunction. The use of these laboratory screening test protocols would require the clinician to become familiar with the often complex organic differential diagnoses for various psychiatric symptoms so that he or she could more meaningfully interpret any discovered laboratory test abnormalities and proceed appropriately. A possible general algorithm for laboratory and diagnostic testing in psychiatric patients is outlined in Figure 9–1.

SCREENING TESTS IN PSYCHIATRY

There is incomplete agreement as to what should constitute a "routine" screening laboratory and diagnostic test battery (see Tables 9–2 and 9–3). Some investigators recommend a very brief and selective laboratory and diagnostic test evaluation in patients with no obvious signs or symptoms of physical disease; the choice of tests in this situation is generally based on clinical relevance to the patient's particular condition. Hoffman and Koran (1984) proposed a somewhat more extensive screening battery based on a selection of the available studies of physical disorders in psychiatric patients (see, e.g., Hall et al. 1980). The recommendations include a CBC; automated chemistry panels (including electrolytes, glucose, renal and hepatic functions, and calcium and phosphate levels); thyroid function tests; a screening test for syphilis and for B_{12} and folate levels; and a urinalysis. Specific thyroid function tests that have been recommended in the past include T_3 resin uptake (T_3RU), T_4, and thyroid-stimulating hormone (TSH); however, other thyroid function tests are also available (e.g., T_3 radioimmunoassay [RIA]). Hoffman and Koran (1984) further recommended an electrocardiogram (ECG) and chest X ray as part of the workup, because possible cardiopulmonary dysfunction detected by these screening tests could be particularly relevant to an evaluation of a possible organic mental disorder. Additional suggestions for tests to be included in routine screens are a slide test of stool for occult blood, tuberculin skin tests, and an electroencephalogram (EEG) (Hoffman and Koran 1984). Other tests sometimes added to this routine laboratory workup include an erythrocyte sedimentation rate, serum proteins, serum protein electrophoresis, and tests for lupus erythematosus (LE) cells or antinuclear antibodies, as well as urine examinations for substances of abuse, porphyrins, and heavy metals (see Table 9–3). Finally, periodic Pap smear tests and mammogra-

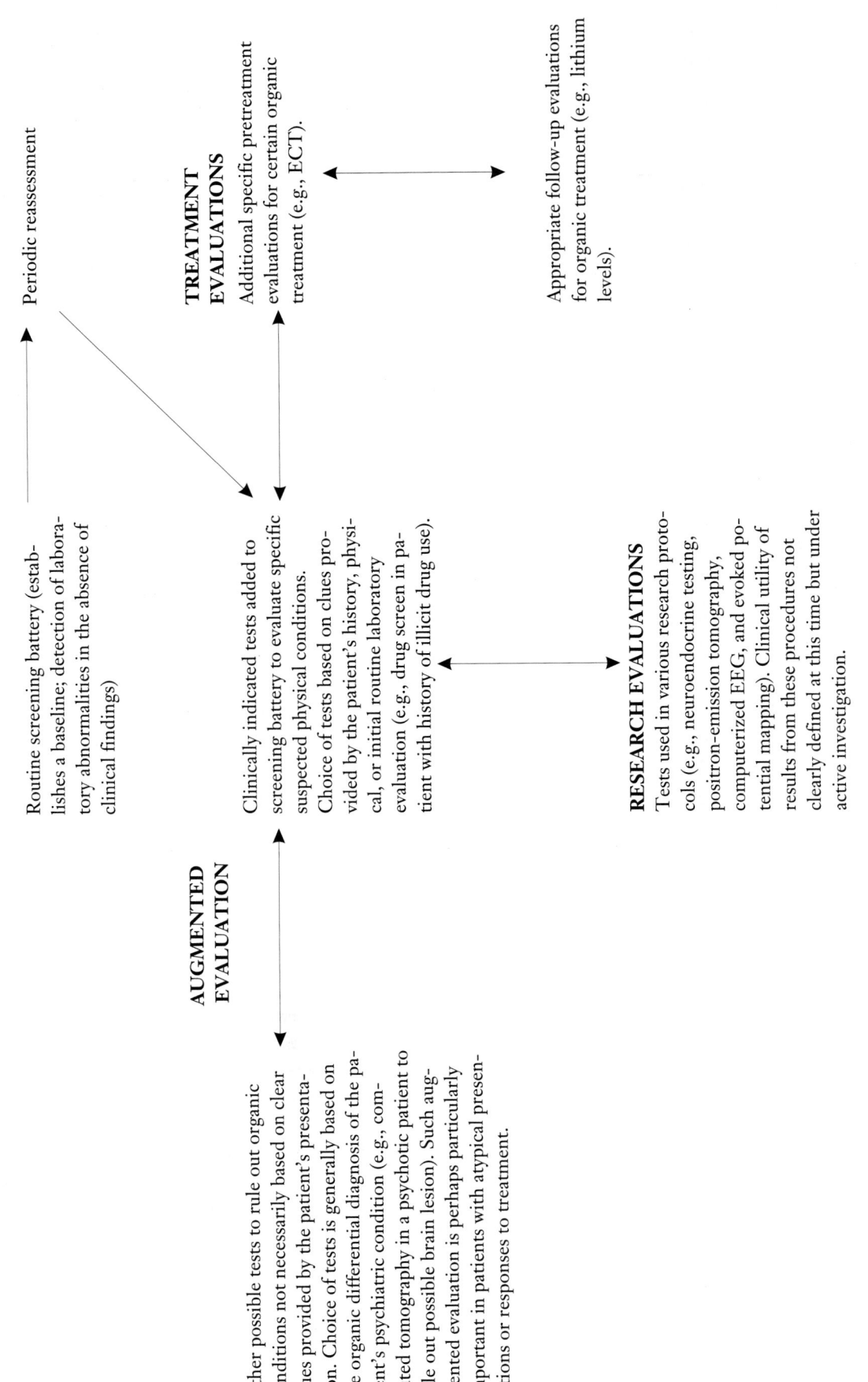

FIGURE 9–1.   General guidelines for the use of diagnostic testing in psychiatry.

Periodic reassessment

TREATMENT EVALUATIONS

Additional specific pretreatment evaluations for certain organic treatment (e.g., ECT).

Appropriate follow-up evaluations for organic treatment (e.g., lithium levels).

Routine screening battery (establishes a baseline; detection of laboratory abnormalities in the absence of clinical findings)

Clinically indicated tests added to screening battery to evaluate specific suspected physical conditions. Choice of tests based on clues provided by the patient's history, physical, or initial routine laboratory evaluation (e.g., drug screen in patient with history of illicit drug use).

RESEARCH EVALUATIONS

Tests used in various research protocols (e.g., neuroendocrine testing, positron-emission tomography, computerized EEG, and evoked potential mapping). Clinical utility of results from these procedures not clearly defined at this time but under active investigation.

AUGMENTED EVALUATION

Other possible tests to rule out organic conditions not necessarily based on clear clues provided by the patient's presentation. Choice of tests is generally based on the organic differential diagnosis of the patient's psychiatric condition (e.g., computed tomography in a psychotic patient to rule out possible brain lesion). Such augmented evaluation is perhaps particularly important in patients with atypical presentations or responses to treatment.

TABLE 9–2. Laboratory and diagnostic tests useful for detecting physical disease in psychiatric patients

Complete blood count (CBC)[a]

Chemistry panel, including serum electrolytes,[a] glucose,[a] albumin, total protein, blood urea nitrogen,[a] creatinine,[a] calcium, phosphate, aspartate aminotransferase (SGOT),[a] alanine aminotransferase (SGPT),[a] alkaline phosphatase,[a] γ-glutamyltransferase,[a] bilirubin,[a] iron, magnesium, serum cholesterol, and triglycerides

Thyroid function tests[a]

Screening test for syphilis (VDRL or RPR)[a]

Human immunodeficiency virus (HIV) serology in potentially high-risk patients

Serum vitamin B$_{12}$ and folate levels[a]

Urinalysis (with dipstick for protein and glucose)[a]

Urine toxicology (e.g., for abuse substances, heavy metals, anabolic steroids)

Urine for uroporphyrins and porphobilinogen

Erythrocyte uroporphyrinogen-1-synthetase

Serum ceruloplasmin

Chest X ray

Electrocardiography

Electroencephalography[a]

Computed tomography or magnetic resonance imaging[a]

Note. The important principles of informed consent should always be applied. Tables 9–2 and 9–3 are not meant to be mutually exclusive.
[a]These tests are included in the recommended screening battery for patients with new onset of dementia. Tests considered "supplemental" to the core battery are computed tomography, magnetic resonance imaging, electroencephalography, and lumbar puncture studies. National Institutes of Health Consensus Development Panel: "Differential Diagnosis of Dementing Disease." National Institutes of Health Consensus Development Conference Statement 6:1–9, 1987.
Source. Based on Rosse et al. (1989), Koran et al. (1989), and Sox et al. (1989).

TABLE 9–3. Supplemental laboratory and diagnostic tests for evaluating physical conditions in psychiatric patients

Computerized tomographic scan

Magnetic resonance imaging scan

Skull films

Electroencephalography

Blood or breath alcohol level

Drug screen (e.g., thin layer chromatography) and possible confirmatory test(s) for positive results (e.g., chromatography-mass-spectroscopy)

Heavy-metal screen

Blood levels of medications

Sedimentation rate

Antinuclear antibodies

Lumbar puncture with cerebrospinal fluid studies

Serum and urine copper levels

Serum ceruloplasmin

Human immunodeficiency virus testing

Monospot test

Blood cultures

Skin test for tuberculosis or brucellosis

Pregnancy tests

Urine for uroporphyrins

Urine and serum osmolality

Polysomnography

Nocturnal penile tumescence

Evoked potentials

Stool tests for occult blood

Arterial blood gases

Note. The important principles of informed consent should always be applied. Tables 9–2 and 9–3 are not meant to be mutually exclusive.

phy for women in appropriate age groups represent important screening procedures for all physicians to remember.

As alluded to earlier, some investigators have argued for less extensive, more selective routine screening batteries for psychiatric patients who have no signs or symptoms of physical illness. These investigators would probably recommend that many of these previously described laboratory and diagnostic tests be ordered only if indicated by the history, clinical, or initial laboratory evaluation. For instance, Dolan and Mushlin (1985) studied 250 psychiatric inpatients who had a mean number of routine admission laboratory tests of close to 30. They found that the mean percentage of true positive results from all the laboratory

tests performed was only 1.8%, and that for only 11 patients (4%) were important medical problems discovered through the routine laboratory testing described by the investigators. Dolan and Mushlin reported that a routine battery—consisting of only a CBC (hemoglobin, hematocrit, white blood cell [WBC] count, and mean cell volume); serum levels of thyroxine, calcium, aspartate aminotransferase (AST), alkaline phosphatase, and syphilis serology; and a urinalysis—would have identified all 11 psychiatric patients whose diagnoses had been made on the basis of the screening laboratory examination and who required further evaluation.

The reader should note, however, that Dolan and Mushlin addressed only some of the clinical laboratory and diagnostic testing procedures that we have described so far.

For instance, their study did not address the value of routine screening with such tests as sedimentation rate, vitamin B_{12} and folate levels, stool tests for occult blood, ECG, EEG, skin testing (e.g., purified protein derivative), or chest X ray. It is hoped that future epidemiological research on large numbers of psychiatric patients will help settle the debate about a selective versus a nonselective screening battery, which should help clinicians better decide which tests would be most appropriate in a "routine" screen for psychiatric patients.

Economic factors and cost-benefit analyses for populations of patients are often taken into consideration in this debate (especially with the increasing emphasis on cost containment in health care). Until some consensus is reached, the psychiatrist must use his or her judgment in selecting screening protocols for patients who present without symptoms that mandate a specific laboratory strategy.

DIAGNOSTIC SCREENING BATTERIES FOR GERIATRIC PSYCHIATRIC PATIENTS

Regarding the most useful diagnostic test screening battery for geriatric patients, no complete consensus yet seems to exist. For instance, Kolman (1985) reported on a study that attempted to determine whether the number of routine laboratory tests ordered for a geriatric patient population could be decreased without compromising quality of care. The admitting psychiatrist's judgment in deciding which laboratory and diagnostic tests should be performed for a particular patient was evaluated. In this study, Kolman found that the admitting physicians tended to underestimate the number of tests that would yield an abnormal result.

For a geriatric population, Kolman suggested the use of a fairly extensive routine admission screening protocol: serum hemoglobin; a WBC count; sedimentation rate; serum vitamin B_{12} and folate levels; a biochemical profile, including serum sodium, potassium, bicarbonate, blood urea nitrogen (BUN), calcium, phosphate, alkaline phosphatase, bilirubin, thyroxine, and glucose; a urinalysis (with bacteriological culture, if appropriate); a chest X ray; a skull X ray; and an ECG.

The National Institute on Aging Task Force recommended a similar test battery for the evaluation of dementia. Their recommendation included a CBC, erythrocyte sedimentation rate, serum electrolytes (sodium, potassium, bicarbonate, chloride, calcium, phosphorus), BUN and glucose, serum bilirubin, serum vitamin B_{12} and folate, thyroid screen, serological test for syphilis, urinalysis (including albumin, glucose, and ketone levels and microscopic examination), stool examination (including a test for occult blood), chest X ray, ECG, and computed tomography (CT) scan of the brain.

On the other hand, Larson et al. (1986) suggested that a fairly selective test-ordering strategy in the evaluation of dementia in elderly patients might not significantly compromise care and would be more cost effective. These authors' strategy used a careful history and physical examination, with blood tests that initially included only a CBC, a blood chemistry battery (including sodium and other electrolytes, calcium, and creatinine), and TSH level. They suggested that other tests be selectively ordered: for example, in a patient with anemia and/or macrocytosis, vitamin B_{12} and folate levels; in patients with an elevated TSH, T_4, and T_3RU. So what constitutes a routine diagnostic test for some clinicians in certain clinical situations might be a supplementary, follow-up test for others (and vice versa). Again, it seems at this time that the clinician must use his or her own careful judgment in choosing a screening battery for a particular patient. Some useful guidelines are presented here.

SUPPLEMENTARY TESTS TO EVALUATE PHYSICAL CONDITIONS IN PSYCHIATRIC PATIENTS

Some commonly considered supplementary laboratory and other diagnostic tests that can at times be useful to screen and evaluate physical conditions in psychiatric patients are outlined in Table 9–3. Supplementation of the routine screening battery is indicated when there are specific clues in the patient's history, physical, or laboratory examination of an underlying physical condition. For instance, in a young psychotic patient with a movement disorder, a serum and urine copper and serum ceruloplasmin might be ordered to help rule out Wilson's disease.

Sexually active women of childbearing age should probably have a pregnancy test, especially if there is the possibility of pregnancy as well as a possibility of psychotropic medications being employed in their treatment. Patients at high risk for acquired immunodeficiency syndrome (AIDS) with some unexplained intellectual and behavioral symptoms might benefit from testing for blood human immunodeficiency virus (HIV), because the AIDS virus affects the CNS even in the absence of other signs and symptoms of the disease (Perry and Jacobsen 1986). Organic mental disorders related to AIDS include syndromes manifested by cognitive decline as well as chronic mild depression, acute psychosis, and mania (Gabel et al. 1986; Perry and Jacobsen 1986). Some other viral syndromes (e.g., influenza, Epstein-Barr virus, cytomegalovirus, viral-induced hepatitis) have been associated with asthenia and/or depression.

Many other possible clinical situations exist in which the psychiatrist might need to order additional laboratory tests. For instance, in the case of a patient taking prescribed or over-the-counter medications, the physician might order a blood level for the medications that have meaningful therapeutic or toxic ranges. Researchers have outlined attempts at providing recommendations for thorough laboratory test evaluations for many possible physical problems that can masquerade as psychiatric illness (see, e.g., Giannini et al. 1978). The psychiatrist needs to be sensitive and knowledgeable about physical disorders that can mimic psychiatric conditions.

A note about using supplemental tests to evaluate physical conditions in psychiatric patients: any laboratory abnormality noted on a routine or supplemental laboratory screen needs to be thoughtfully evaluated and the need for possible follow-up carefully considered. Consultation with other specialists might at times be required. Some additional tests commonly employed in the workup of some physical conditions include lumbar puncture, urine or blood toxicology determinations, CT and magnetic resonance imaging (MRI), and EEG. In the following subsections these procedures are described in greater detail.

Examination of the Cerebrospinal Fluid

Any physician attempting to perform a lumbar puncture needs to 1) be aware of the possible complications of the procedure and 2) possess the requisite technical competence. The lumbar puncture, with subsequent examination of the obtained cerebrospinal fluid (CSF), can aid in the diagnosis of a number of important neurological diseases that can have psychiatric symptoms, including CNS syphilis, meningitis, encephalitis, and subarachnoid hemorrhage. Feinsilver (1984) discussed possible indications for a lumbar puncture, including sudden changes in mental status associated with fever or signs of meningeal irritation (e.g., Kernig's sign or Brudzinski's sign). Jenike (1985) outlined similar indications for the role of the lumbar puncture in the workup for dementia, which in some settings is becoming increasingly the responsibility of the psychiatrist. Physicians should carefully consider the indications for performing a lumbar puncture in a particular patient, because the procedure is associated with potential risks and discomfort. Some possible contraindications to a lumbar puncture include situations involving raised intracranial pressure, the presence of an intracranial mass lesion (e.g., brain tumor, brain abscess, subdural hematoma, intracerebral hemorrhage), skin infection around the lumbar puncture site, and the patient's use of anticoagulants (Pryse-Phillips and Murray 1986). Com-

mon examinations of the CSF include a WBC count; sugar, protein, and chloride determinations; serology; and bacteriological studies. A full, careful discussion of the lumbar puncture procedure and subsequent CSF examination and interpretation of the findings is beyond the scope of this chapter. Normal values for some commonly evaluated CSF parameters are given in Table 9–4. For this and all other laboratory tests, clinicians should be familiar with the normal values delineated by their specific laboratory and patient population. Reference to some of the possible CSF markers of psychiatric disease currently being investigated can be found later in this chapter in the section on biochemical markers.

Laboratory Evaluation of Suspected Drug Abuse

In certain patient populations (e.g., adolescents), illicit drug use is reported to be quite high, and it is probably best for the clinician to have a relatively low threshold for ordering a drug screen in high-risk patients with unexplained behavioral symptoms (M. S. Gold and Dackis 1986). Some clinicians argue that an illicit-drug screen should almost always be a part of the routine screening battery for psychiatric patients, because substance-induced psychiatric disorders are quite common and can mimic or exacerbate idiopathic psychiatric illness. Patients with a history of illicit-drug abuse or dependence need some type of laboratory evaluation for drug use (e.g., blood alcohol levels, urine drug screens). Historical information obtained from patients regarding recent drug use is often unreliable, and the clinician might not be able to base his or her decision to order a drug screen solely on a patient's history. In addition, routine follow-up monitoring for illicit drug use is often a necessary part of the treatment of the drug-abusing patient. Periodic repeat drug screens can provide a gauge of the effectiveness of the treatment intervention.

The clinician should be aware that different laboratory test methodologies exist for the detection of illicit drugs and that the various methodologies might have differing

TABLE 9–4. **Characteristics of normal cerebrospinal fluid (CSF) (obtained via lumbar puncture)**

Opening pressure (patient reclining)	70–200 mm of water (average 125 mm)
Appearance	Clear, colorless
Glucose	40–85 mg/dL (60%–80% of the blood glucose)
Protein	15–45 mg/dL
Cells	0–5 mononuclear cells/mm^3

sensitivities and capacities for drug detection. Some of the various laboratory methodologies used in the evaluation of illicit drug abuse are outlined in Table 9–5. Different laboratories might use different techniques for drug screening and confirmation of positive results. Furthermore, the clinician should note that some of the laboratories using these procedures might be more reliable than others. Gas chromatography–mass spectroscopy (GC-MS) is perhaps the most sensitive and reliable test, but it also is usually the most expensive.

Detection tests for illicit drugs are available either 1) in the form of broad drug screens, which evaluate the presence of any number of multiple drugs (e.g., ethanol, barbiturates, amphetamines, cocaine, opiates, methadone, marijuana, phencyclidine, benzodiazepines, mescaline, and the indole hallucinogens such as lysergic acid diethylamide [LSD]), or 2) in the form of individual tests for specific drugs, which might be designed to detect lower levels of substance use than do the tests employed in the broad drug screen (M. S. Gold and Dackis 1986). The number of drugs included in a broad screening test varies from laboratory to laboratory, and the specimens (e.g., urine versus blood) best used by any particular test can also be different. The number of positives detected in routine drug screens can often be increased by using more specific and sensitive measurement techniques, such as gas chromatography, high-performance liquid chromatography (HPLC), or GC-MS. A preliminary drug screen might use a less expensive laboratory test, such as an immunoassay method, and the test results can be confirmed by a different and more sensitive test (also generally more complex and expensive), such as GC-MS.

Specimens for the analysis of possible recent alcohol or substance use can include a patient's urine, blood, breath, and saliva, and, in certain instances, a piece of the patient's hair (Sramek et al. 1985). The most common specimens used are urine and blood. Breath analysis is frequently used to screen for recent alcohol intake (e.g., by police officers for individuals suspected of driving under the influence of alcohol, or for psychiatric inpatients returning from a pass outside the hospital when it is suspected that they recently ingested alcohol). Different types of breath alcohol instruments exist (e.g., chemical reagent tube tests, tests using an electrochemical cell that generates a voltage in response to alcohol vapor, and tests that use infrared detectors). Finally, it is often helpful to consult with staff from the laboratory used by the physician about which drug screening and follow-up confirmation tests might be ordered and which specimens should be sent in a specific clinical situation.

Laboratory Evaluation for Environmental Toxins

Exposure to a number of different environmental toxins has been associated with various behavioral abnormalities. Possible environmental toxins with behavioral consequences include the heavy metals, such as mercury, lead, manganese, thallium, and arsenic. In the case of suspected heavy-metal exposure (e.g., through industrial or toxic waste contamination), a determination of blood or urinary concentrations of these metals might be helpful (DeLisi 1984). The clinician should remain alert to the possibility of poisoning by these metals as well as other environmental toxins (e.g., organophosphate insecticides) associated with behavioral aberrations. The appropriate laboratory tests should be ordered when the possibility of such environmental toxin exposure is high. Care must be taken to avoid possible artifactual contamination of the sample. For instance, if capillary blood is drawn from the fingertips of small children in the evaluation of possible lead poisoning, the risk of contamination from the skin is reduced if proper washing procedures are used.

Computed Tomography and Magnetic Resonance Imaging in Clinical Psychiatry

Computed tomographic scanning of the head offers the clinician cross-sectional X ray images of the brain from multiple brain levels (both cortical and subcortical). The procedure has been available for general clinical use by psychiatrists since the mid-1970s and is most often employed in the evaluation of patients with suspected structural brain abnormalities (e.g., tumor, subdural hematoma, stroke, abscess). An example of a single cross-sectional CT scan image is presented in Figure 9–2. Guidelines to help clinicians in deciding when to order structural brain-imaging studies such as a CT scan for psychiatric patients have ranged from very specific, limited indications to a broad spectrum of symptoms and presentations (see Table 9–6). Larson et al. (1986) recommended

TABLE 9–5.   Laboratory methods used in the evaluation of suspected illicit drug abuse

Thin-layer chromatography

High-performance thin-layer chromatography

Enzyme multiplied immunoassay technique

Radioimmunoassay

Gas-liquid chromatography

High-performance liquid chromatography

Liquid chromatography–mass spectrometry

Gas chromatography–mass spectroscopy

ordering a CT scan in psychiatric patients with focal neurological findings, whereas others have felt that the presence of an abnormal EEG in psychiatric patients would also be a good indication for ordering a CT scan. Weinberger (1984) has expanded on these two possible indications and recommends obtaining a CT scan in psychiatric patients whose clinical presentation includes any of the following: confusion, dementia of unknown cause, a first episode of a psychosis of unknown etiology, a movement disorder of unknown etiology, a diagnosis of anorexia nervosa, prolonged catatonia, or a first episode of major affective disorder or personality change after age 50. Emsley et al. (1986) extended these recommendations to include ordering CT scans for any patient with a history of alcohol abuse, craniocerebral trauma, or seizures.

Magnetic resonance imaging of the brain (Figure 9–3) can usefully supplement and/or replace CT in certain clinical situations, because some lesions are better appreciated on MRI than on CT scan (Table 9–7). The MRI is usually superior to CT scan when there is suspicion of lesions in the posterior fossa, brain stem, or temporal and apical areas of the brain, because the surrounding bone can distort the CT image (Jaskiw et al. 1987) or obstruct visualization (Figure 9–4). Indeed, the CT scan, with its excellent visualization of bone and calcifications, has an important utility in the evaluation of trauma and pathological processes involving calcification. The ability to differentiate between gray and white matter, as well as CSF, gives MRI a distinct advantage over CT. Furthermore, MRI provides superior delineation of the pathology of and changes associated with demyelinating disease and is, as well, of special value in the investigation of pathology in the cervical spinal cord and the cervicomedullary junction (Jacobson 1988). MRI has an advantage for patients who require multiple scans over time, because there is no ionizing radiation and there are no known adverse effects of MRI studies at present. However, MRI is contraindicated in patients with ferromagnetic structures or devices that may be adversely affected by powerful magnetic fields, such as aneurysm clips (Morihisa 1991). In addition, because of the length of time needed to complete the scan and the confining nature of the machine, some patients may be psychologically or medically unable to tolerate the procedure.

Electroencephalogram

The EEG measures brain electrical activity from electrodes placed on the scalp in standardized positions (usu-

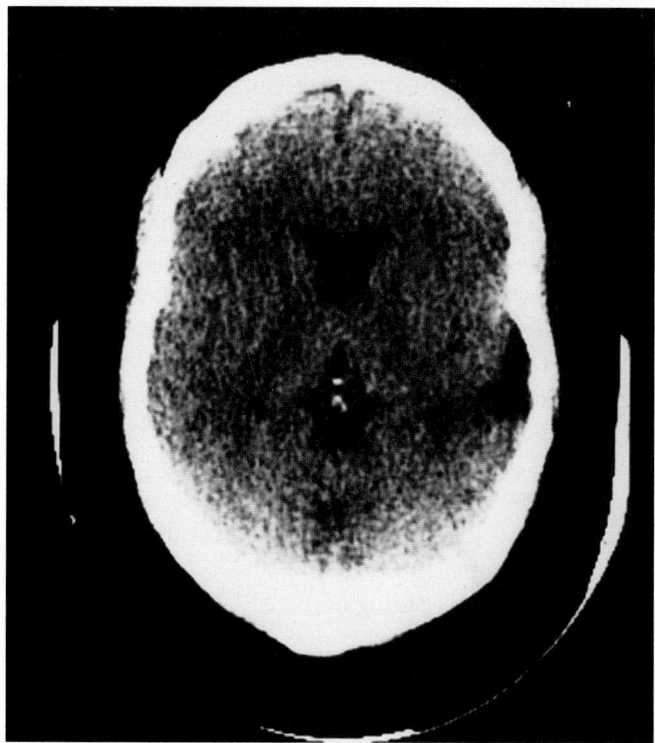

FIGURE 9–2. Computed tomographic scan of the head without contrast material. Image for a single brain level shown. Note hypodense area in the left temporal region adjacent to the skull. Intravenous injection of a standard roentgenographic contrast medium may be used to enhance a computed tomographic study for improved visualization of certain brain lesions (e.g., recent stroke, tumors, infections, abscesses).

Table 9–6. Possible indications for structural brain imaging procedure (computed tomography [CT] or magnetic resonance imaging [MRI]) in psychiatric practice

Focal neurological findings

Abnormal electroencephalogram (EEG)

Unknown etiology in cases of

    Confusion

    First episode of psychosis

    Movement disorder

    Anorexia nervosa

    Prolonged catatonia

    First affective episode after age 50

    Personality change after age 50

Alcohol dependence

History of head trauma

History of seizures

Impaired cognition on mental status examination

Source. Based on table in Rosse et al. 1989, p. 85.

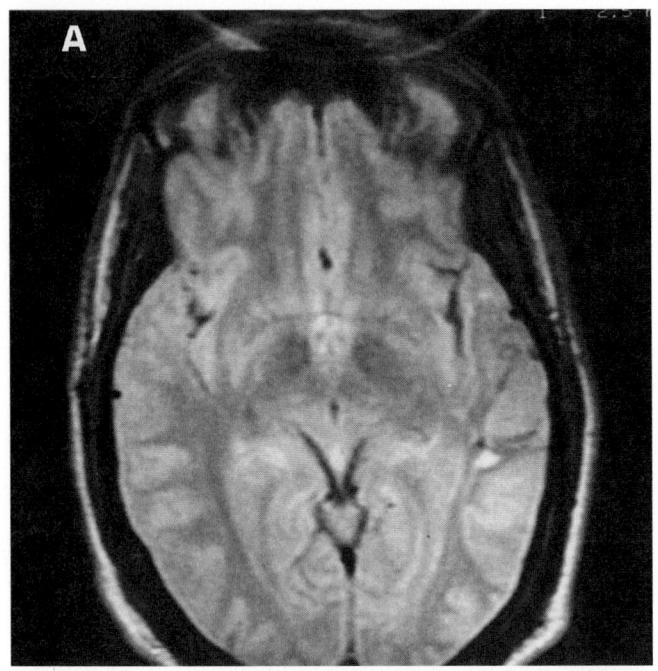

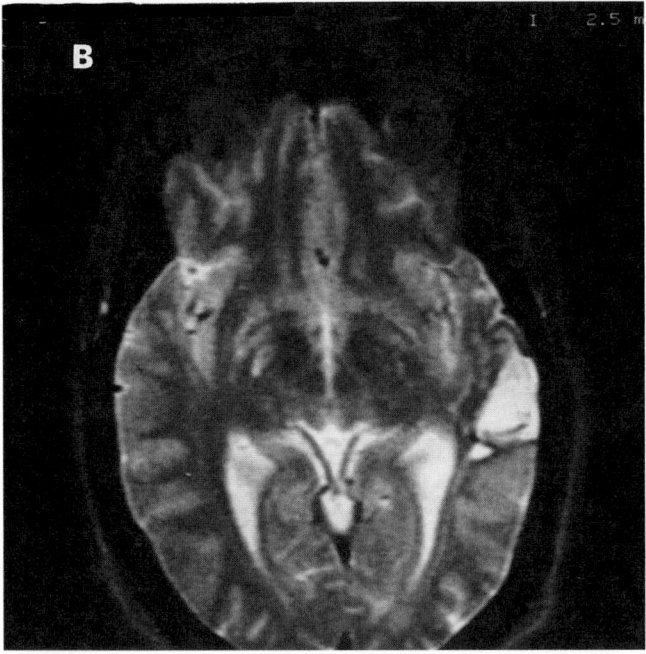

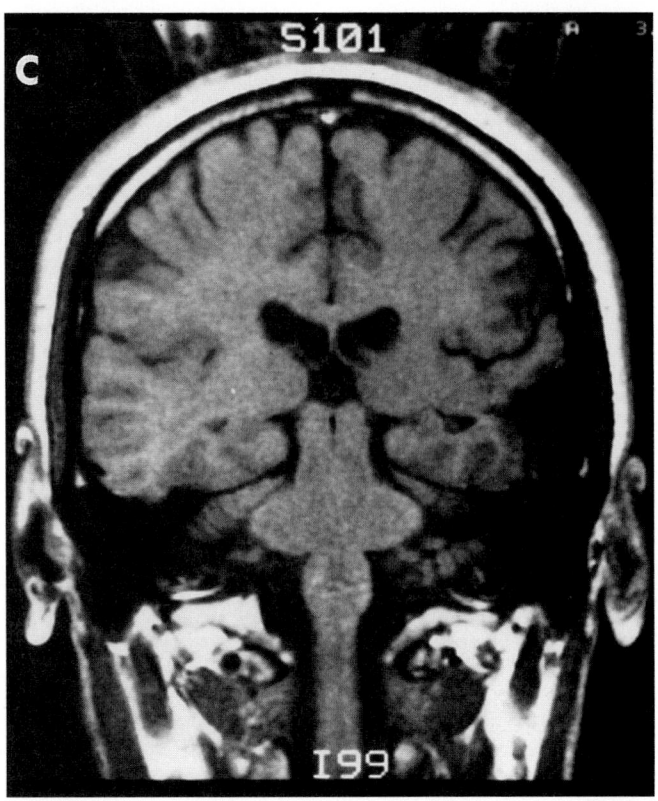

FIGURE 9-3. Three magnetic resonance imaging (MRI) scans from the patient depicted in Figure 9–2. Each MRI here was obtained by a different scanning mode. (A) An axial "spin-echo intermediate" image. (B) A T_2-weighted image. (C) A coronal T_1-weighted image. MRI images can appear to be different, depending on the scanning mode used. The signal properties of the left temporal region lesion shown in these scans suggest encephalomalacia. An MRI scan can be useful in helping to further characterize a lesion detected by computed tomography.

ally conforming to the International 10-20 system of scalp electrode placement). The electrical activity that can be detected by the EEG scalp electrodes is presumed to originate primarily in neurons in the uppermost cortical cell layers. The amplitude and frequency of the electrical activity are graphically recorded on paper by ink markers for multiple areas of the brain surface as oscillating lines with different peaks and troughs, giving rise to the EEG tracing. The EEG frequencies have been divided into the following bands: beta activity (equal to or greater than 13 Hz), alpha rhythm (between 8 and 13 Hz), theta activity (between 4 and 8 Hz), and delta activity (less than 4 Hz) (see Figure 9–5). The EEG is used primarily in the evaluation of epilepsy and other neurological disorders (e.g., neoplasm, trauma, stroke, metabolic or degenerative disease). The clinical reading of the EEG involves the visual inspection of, usually, large amounts of EEG tracings for certain EEG abnormalities, which can be divided as follows (Figure 9–5):

1. Dysrhythmias, such as isolated bursts of slow activity or spikes, as can be seen in the epilepsies
2. Asymmetries of the EEG recording from comparable parts of the head
3. Suppression of EEG amplitude (as in subdural hematoma or brain death)
4. EEG slowing (e.g., delta activity in an awake tracing, as can be seen in delirium; see Nunez 1981)

Table 9–7. Some issues to consider in the decision whether to order a computed tomography (CT) or a magnetic resonance imaging (MRI) brain scan

CT advantages

Is less expensive than MRI.

Provides better detection of calcified brain lesions.

Can be, under some circumstances, more useful when differential diagnosis includes the possibility of some meningeal tumors, pituitary disease.

Can be used when the imaging subject has a pacemaker.

Does not raise concern about the potentially dangerous "projectile effect" associated with MRI, in which metal objects (e.g., pens, paper clips, or even oxygen tanks) can be rapidly pulled onto the MRI magnets.

Can be used in patients with metal in their heads (e.g., surgical clips, metal skull plates, shrapnel). Not only can such metal be pulled toward the magnet, but it can heat up.

Imaging procedure and device typically induce less anxiety than an MRI.

Procedure and device typically require a shorter period of patient cooperation than the MRI.

Can have a uniquely useful role in the evaluation of central nervous system trauma.

MRI advantages[a]

Provides better visualization of lesions in the posterior fossa, brain stem, temporal and apical brain areas (i.e., areas closely surrounded by skull bone) (Jaskiw et al. 1987)

Provides better visualization of demyelinating disease (considered the best method of detecting brain lesions associated with multiple sclerosis).

May be superior to CT in detecting brain abnormalities related to seizure foci.

Is considered better at detecting neoplasms (other than certain meningeal tumors) or vascular malformations (even when angiographically occult).

Does not require use of X rays. (However, the long-term biological effects of magnetic fields on patients are unknown).

Note. When weighing the decision to order a CT scan versus an MRI scan in a psychiatric patient, it is often useful to consult with the neuroradiologist who will be involved in the study.
[a]Note that an MRI brain study might be ordered after an equivocal or unrevealing CT scan study (and when brain pathology is still suspected).
Source. Based on Garber et al. 1988.

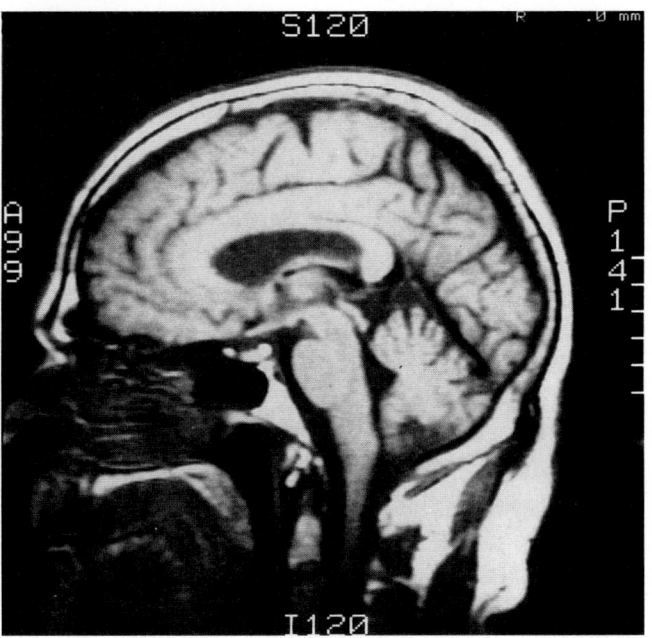

Figure 9–4. Sagittal T_1-weighted magnetic resonance imaging (MRI) scan. Note the clarity of the anatomic structures visualized (e.g., brain stem, cerebellum). Scanning modes that are best for depicting structure might not always be best for visualizing certain types of normal or abnormal tissue.
Source. Veterans Administration Medical Center, Washington, D.C.

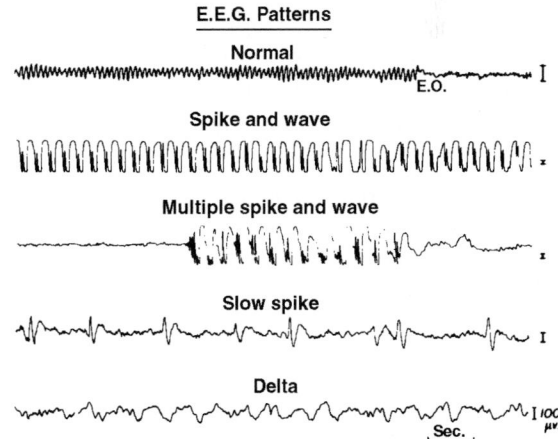

FIGURE 9–5. Some examples of electroencephalogram (EEG) abnormalities. Top tracing demonstrates alpha rhythm, which attenuates with eye opening (E.O.) and is then replaced by lower amplitude beta rhythm.
Source. Reprinted with permission from Nunez PL: *Electric Fields of the Brain.* New York, Oxford University Press, 1981, p. 234. Copyright 1981, Oxford University Press.

Most important, it should be noted that the effective use of an EEG recording depends on the skill and training of the electroencephalographer who reads and interprets the EEG data.

Some investigators have recommended that the EEG be a part of the routine screening battery for psychiatric patients (e.g., Hoffman and Koran 1984), especially patients with suspected organic mental disorder. In cases where the patients have episodic behavioral disturbances that are possibly epileptic in nature, Goodin and Aminoff (1984) noted that a normal initial EEG alone cannot be used to completely exclude a diagnosis of epilepsy. Repeat EEGs or 24-hour ambulatory recordings can be obtained. Hall et al. (1980) suggested the utility of the sleep-deprived EEG, which they believe is more sensitive than a routine EEG. The role of augmenting the EEG with nasopharyngeal (NP) leads is unclear. Some researchers and clinicians, such as Sternberg (1986), have suggested that NP leads can increase the diagnostic yield of the EEG, but a study by Ramani et al. (1985) called into question the value of the EEG supplemented with NP leads in psychiatric patients. In patients with a possible diagnosis of schizophrenia, a protocol described by Grebb et al. (1986) suggests obtaining a sleep-deprived EEG, preferably with NP leads, especially if it is the patient's first episode of psychosis, if the psychotic patient is young (e.g., under 25), or if there is a history of possible brain injury (e.g., accidents, infections, birth complications).

An increased number of various EEG abnormalities have been noted in a variety of psychiatric disorders, especially schizophrenia, although none can be considered diagnostic at this time. It is hoped that computerized analysis of EEG data will enhance the utility of the EEG for both the psychiatric clinician and the research neuroscientist. Computerized EEG mapping is discussed later in this chapter in the section on brain imaging.

Further Tests

Polysomnography.   Polysomnography involves the recording of EEG activity during sleep (or attempts at sleep) and is usually performed at night. In addition, other physiological functions that might be relevant to the evaluation of a patient's symptoms are monitored, such as electromyographic, electrooculographic, and electrocardiographic activity, as well as measurements of respiratory effort, airflow, and blood oxygen saturation. Polysomnography is used in the evaluation of certain sleep disorders (e.g., narcolepsy, sleep apnea, treatment-resistant insomnias). Patients being evaluated for excessive daytime sleepiness might require special daytime sleep evaluations. For example, polysomnography used in the assessment of narcolepsy (i.e., the multiple sleep latency test [MSLT]) is performed during the day. Important determinations about sleep disorders (e.g., the differentiation between central and peripheral sleep apnea) can be obtained by polysomnography.

Nocturnal penile tumescence studies.   Nocturnal penile tumescence (NPT) studies can be used in the evaluation of impotence. NPT is often useful, although not absolutely reliable, in helping to differentiate between organic and functional causes of impotence (Williams 1985). The NPT procedure usually involves quantification of such variables as penile circumferential changes (expansion) and frequency of penile tumescence during sleep at night. In addition, the adjunctive assessment of penile rigidity is thought to be important, because normal nocturnal penile expansion is reportedly not always associated with normal penile rigidity. Computerized tumescence monitoring devices are available that quantitate both penile base and tip expansion as well as rigidity (Bradley et al. 1985). NPT studies can be a part of a polysomnographic evaluation. The absence of adequate erectile function during nocturnal sleep lends some diagnostic support to an organic etiology of a patient's impotence. However, abnormal NPT studies suggestive of an organic etiology have been reported in association with major depression (Thase et al. 1987).

Evoked potentials.   Evoked potential (EP) testing involves the measurement of specific brain electrical responses to discrete sensory stimuli. The evoking stimulus can be visual (VEP), auditory (AEP), or somatosensory (SEP). In the process of EP testing, the subject is repeatedly exposed to certain stimuli (e.g., flashing lights), and the evoked brain electrical responses are added together and averaged by a computer to remove background, non-stimulus-related activity. The result is a characteristic waveform (the EP), which generally consists of negative and positive peaks spread along a time axis, measured in milliseconds (msec). The "early" peaks (or components) are often defined as peaks occurring within the first 50 msec poststimulus. Middle peaks occur 50 to 250 msec poststimulus, and late peaks encompass those occurring after 250 msec. At this time, EP testing can theoretically help the psychiatrist in differentiating between some organic and functional complaints (e.g., in the evaluation of hysterical blindness using VEP). A brain stem auditory evoked potential (BSAEP) might be ordered in cases of suspected psychogenic deafness or used in the evaluation of an unresponsive, mute, catatonic patient. Such a study would assess the integrity of the brain stem structures involved in the processing of auditory stimuli. Demyelinating conditions such as multiple sclerosis can also be usefully evaluated using certain EP testing procedures.

Various abnormalities of different EPs in certain psychiatric disorders have been described, including abnormalities of the early, middle, and late EP components (Shagass 1977; Buchsbaum 1977; Roth 1977, respectively). However, none of these findings have been clearly demonstrated to be characteristic of any specific psychiatric disorders, and their diagnostic potential is the subject of investigation. Evoked potential studies are unique in their ability to provide information on certain aspects of cortical processing that occur on the order of milliseconds.

LABORATORY EVALUATION OF SOME PSYCHIATRIC ORGANIC THERAPIES

As Hall and Beresford (1984) pointed out, one of the goals of the initial laboratory workup is to help provide useful baseline information for the patient who is likely to receive psychotropic medications. Many of the organic treatments are associated with adverse reactions that might be detected by changes in certain laboratory or other diagnostic test values (e.g., increasing liver function test values suggesting hepatotoxicity from a medication, or electrocardiographic changes reflecting potential cardiac toxicity from a psychotropic agent). It is therefore important to have baseline test values on a patient who is about to be exposed to an organic therapy so that future changes from these baseline values, possibly reflecting drug toxicity, can be properly assessed.

When using a specific psychotropic agent, more information regarding potentially useful laboratory tests, drug-drug interactions, and possible side effects and contraindications should be reviewed in other more comprehensive publications, such as the *Physicians' Desk Reference* and textbooks of psychopharmacology.

TRICYCLIC ANTIDEPRESSANTS, ANTIPSYCHOTICS, AND BENZODIAZEPINES

In general, there is no absolute consensus concerning standardized protocols for the pretreatment evaluation of most biological treatments in psychiatry. However, some important examples will be presented. For instance, because of the risk of agranulocytosis with clozapine, patients on this medication must have baseline and weekly WBC counts. Another example would be that for patients about to be started on tricyclic antidepressants (TCAs),

antipsychotics, or benzodiazepine medications, Gelenberg (1983) recommended laboratory tests only as clinically indicated, based on consideration of each patient's past medical history, physical examination, previous history of adverse drug reactions, and knowledge of the potential adverse effects from the biological therapy to be used. For example, an ECG should be ordered in a patient with a significant history of cardiac pathology who is about to be started on an antidepressant or some of the antipsychotics, because some of these medications have been associated with potentially significant ECG abnormalities (especially the TCAs and the antipsychotic thioridazine). In the absence of a history of cardiac pathology, one might consider obtaining an ECG in a man older than 30 or a woman older than 40 who has not had one in the past year and is about to start taking a psychotropic medication that has been associated with potential cardiotoxicity (Gelenberg 1983). In addition, it seems advisable to order liver function tests in patients with a history of liver disease who are about to start taking certain psychotropics metabolized by the liver. The clinician might need to have a lower threshold for ordering diagnostic tests in patients belonging to populations at greater risk for adverse reactions from some of the organic therapies (e.g., pediatric, geriatric, or chronically ill patients). Likewise, the follow-up laboratory evaluation for some of these organic therapies might also need to be more extensive in such vulnerable patient populations. Again, the clinician needs to be aware of the major potential adverse reactions of the organic therapies he or she employs and should use this knowledge to help guide the pretreatment and follow-up laboratory test evaluations. For instance, because of the risk of seizure for patients on clozapine, some clinicians obtain EEGs on these patients before treatment. Furthermore, an EEG study might be of particular value during the course of treatment if high dosages of clozapine are contemplated.

In the following subsections are presented more specific guidelines for the pretreatment and follow-up evaluations of the patient about to begin treatment with lithium carbonate, an anticonvulsant, or electroconvulsive therapy (ECT). Of course, many of the broad principles previously described for choosing appropriate diagnostic tests for a particular patient also apply to the patient about to begin each of these treatments.

TRICYCLIC ANTIDEPRESSANT BLOOD LEVELS

There seems to be incomplete agreement concerning the usefulness of plasma TCA levels (Kocsis et al. 1986; Simpson et al. 1983). The American Psychiatric Association (APA) Task Force on the Use of Laboratory Tests in Psychiatry (1985) concluded that plasma-level measurements of imipramine, desmethylimipramine (desipramine), and nortriptyline are unequivocally useful in certain situations. Situations in which a TCA blood level might be ordered include those involving 1) patients with questionable compliance, 2) patients with a poor response to a "typical" antidepressant dose, 3) patients who experience side effects at a very low dose, 4) patients who are potentially very sensitive to side effects (e.g., medically ill or geriatric patients), and 5) patients for whom treatment is urgent and who require potentially therapeutic blood levels in as short a time possible (e.g., the severely suicidal patient). Therapeutic blood levels described by the APA Task Force (Table 9–8) are as follows:

1. For imipramine, when a combined plasma level of imipramine plus its metabolite, desmethylimipramine, exceeds 200 ng/mL.
2. For nortriptyline, a "therapeutic window" of plasma levels between 50 ng/mL and 150 ng/mL. (Levels below 50 ng/mL or above 150 ng/mL have been reported to be less effective.)
3. For desipramine, when plasma levels are above 125 ng/mL.

It should be noted that TCA blood levels are generally obtained about 9 to 12 hours after the last dose (usually in the morning after a nighttime dose). In addition, steady-state blood levels of the TCA are reportedly not achieved until about 5 days after either initiating the medication or changing the medication dose. The utility of plasma level determinations for antidepressants other than those just outlined is still under investigation.

TABLE 9–8. Tricyclic antidepressant (TCA) therapeutic blood levels suggested by the American Psychiatric Association Task Force on the Use of Laboratory Tests in Psychiatry

TCA	Blood levels
Imipramine	Total of imipramine and desmethylimipramine (desipramine) should exceed 200 ng/ml
Nortriptyline	50–150 ng/ml (therapeutic window)
Desipramine	> 125 ng/ml

Source. Based on data in American Psychiatric Association Task Force on the Use of Laboratory Tests in Psychiatry 1985.

PRETREATMENT LITHIUM EVALUATION

Lithium can have several potentially significant adverse affects, including those on the thyroid gland, kidney, heart, and developing fetus, as well as a usually benign elevation of the WBC count. Recommended pretreatment diagnostic evaluations often include a CBC, serum electrolytes, BUN, serum creatinine, thyroid function tests, urinalysis, an ECG, and, sometimes, a 24-hour urine test for creatinine clearance. Thyroid function tests commonly employed include a TSH as well as possibly a T_3RU and T_4. Other tests that have been suggested include a fasting blood sugar, urine for glucose and ketones, a 24-hour urine volume test, and a 12-hour dehydration test for urine osmolality. For potentially pregnant patients, a pregnancy test should be ordered to clarify the patient's childbearing status. Some of the important laboratory studies often ordered before a patient is started on lithium therapy are outlined in Table 9–9.

LITHIUM BLOOD LEVELS

Therapeutic and toxic blood levels for lithium in the treatment of bipolar affective illness have been approximated. For acute mania, Jefferson et al. (1987) reported therapeutic lithium levels from a lower range of 0.8 to 1.0 mEq/L to an upper range of 1.4 to 1.5 mEq/L. Amdisen (1980) characterizes a range from about 1.2 to 1.5 mEq/L as a "warning range." Clinicians with patients who have serum lithium levels in this upper range should be alert for possible early signs of lithium toxicity. Of course, this does not preclude the individual patients who have idiosyncratic therapeutic responses outside the generally accepted response range or patients who become toxic at relatively low serum lithium levels.

Stable, steady-state lithium levels are generally obtained about 4–5 days after either initiating lithium or adjusting the dose. Nevertheless, it is sometimes recom-

TABLE 9–9. Some important laboratory determinations to be made before treatment with lithium

Complete blood count (CBC)

Serum electrolytes

Blood urea nitrogen (BUN)

Serum creatinine

Thyroid function tests

Urinalysis

Electrocardiogram

Pregnancy test in potentially childbearing patients

mended that blood samples for lithium be drawn a couple of times a week when first initiating lithium therapy to help prevent lithium toxicity in patients requiring only small amounts of lithium to achieve therapeutic levels. Of course, blood levels should also be drawn if the patient demonstrates any signs of possible toxicity. Blood samples for lithium determinations are generally drawn about 12 hours after the last dose of lithium.

After resolution of an acute manic episode, maintenance therapy is generally prescribed at a lower lithium level than that required for the treatment of acute mania. Levels of 0.6–0.9 mEq/L have been advocated (Jefferson et al. 1987), although effective maintenance has been reported at lower levels. During maintenance therapy, lithium levels should be drawn periodically (e.g., every 1 to 3 months, but more often if clinically indicated). Other proposed methods for monitoring lithium therapy have included measuring salivary lithium levels or red blood cell/plasma lithium ratios. The utility of these methods is still under investigation.

The clinician needs to be sensitive to situations in which the serum lithium level can dramatically change—for example, in patients who are pregnant or immediately postpartum, patients who are on thiazide diuretics or are dehydrated, or patients with deteriorating renal function. If any of these or other similar situations are encountered, lithium levels might have to be drawn more frequently.

OTHER LABORATORY TESTS DURING LITHIUM THERAPY

Other follow-up tests during maintenance therapy with lithium might include periodic CBCs, thyroid function tests, BUN, serum creatinine, and possibly an ECG. Thyroid function tests that might be employed include a TSH assay, followed up by a T_4 or a T_3RU should the TSH assay results be abnormal. Generally, these follow-up tests for patients on lithium therapy might be performed as frequently as every few months or as infrequently as about once a year (generally depending on the clinical situation). Pregnancy tests for potentially childbearing women might also have to be done on occasion. Hypoparathyroidism has been reported to be rarely associated with lithium therapy, so the clinician should remain aware of the fact that a periodic serum calcium determination might also be needed if clinically indicated.

PRETREATMENT ANTICONVULSANT EVALUATION

Certain anticonvulsants, such as carbamazepine, valproic acid, and clonazepam, are being increasingly employed in the treatment of patients with certain psychiatric disorders, such as lithium-resistant or lithium-intolerant manic patients. Before the clinician uses any of these medications to treat a psychiatric illness, he or she should be fully aware of each of their potentially adverse effects and how they might be reflected in laboratory and other diagnostic test evaluations.

For instance, when carbamazepine is used, because of the reported risk of certain hematologic abnormalities such as aplastic anemia, leukopenia, thrombocytopenia, and anemia, it is recommended that the clinician obtain some baseline hematologic indices, which might include a CBC and platelet count. A serum iron assay and a reticulocyte count might also be included (Hart and Easton 1982). It should be noted, however, that clinically important hematologic toxicity with carbamazepine is felt by some to be a relatively uncommon occurrence (Hart and Easton 1982). Gelenberg (1985) recommended that a baseline laboratory screen for a patient about to start carbamazepine therapy should include a CBC, platelet count, and creatinine and liver function tests. Because carbamazepine has been reported to slow atrioventricular conduction, a pretreatment ECG might be useful in patients with a history of cardiac pathology, especially in patients with a history of heart block (Table 9–10).

In patients taking valproic acid preparations, baseline liver function tests are recommended because of this anticonvulsant's potential for hepatotoxicity. In patients with a clear history of liver disorder who are going to begin taking either carbamazepine or valproic acid, baseline liver function tests should always be on record. The necessary follow-up evaluation for patients on carbamazepine or valproic acid is discussed in the next section.

Pregnancy tests should probably be obtained in potentially childbearing women about to receive any of these anticonvulsant drugs, because there have been reports that suggest an association between the use of anticonvulsant drugs by pregnant women and an elevated incidence of birth defects in the children born to these women. For patients about to be started on an anticonvulsant for a

TABLE 9–10. **Possible laboratory evaluation prior to treatment with carbamazepine**

Complete blood count (CBC)

Platelet count

Reticulocyte count

Liver function tests

Electrocardiogram

Serum electrolytes

psychiatric indication, a pretreatment EEG is not necessarily mandatory, since it has not been established whether the presence of minor EEG abnormalities is a biological marker for anticonvulsant efficacy in these psychiatric patients.

ANTICONVULSANT BLOOD LEVELS

It has been reported that when carbamazepine or valproic acid is used in the treatment of mood disorders, the effective plasma levels are similar to those employed in the control of seizures. For valproic acid, serum levels shown to be of therapeutic efficacy for the treatment of mania are 45–100 µg/mL (Expert Consensus Panel for Bipolar Disorder 1996). Monitoring serum carbamazepine and valproic acid levels is important for predicting adverse effects secondary to toxicity from the medications, because side effects tend to be more prominent when the blood levels reach the upper limits of the established therapeutic ranges.

OTHER LABORATORY TESTS DURING ANTICONVULSANT THERAPY

Because of the relatively rare, but medically significant, incidence of hematologic disturbance associated with carbamazepine use (as described earlier in this chapter), periodic follow-up of hematologic function is felt to be necessary.

When carbamazepine was first introduced for treatment of psychiatric patients, weekly hematologic evaluations (CBC) for the first 3 months with monthly follow-up thereafter for the first 2–3 years had been recommended (Physicians' Desk Reference [PDR] 1986). Hart and Easton (1982) suggested that CBCs be performed only biweekly for the first 2 months of carbamazepine therapy. They suggested that if no abnormalities appeared during this time, counts could be obtained quarterly. However, there is no consensus concerning a protocol for hematologic evaluation; each clinician must carefully assess cost-risk-benefit considerations. Of course, blood counts should be immediately obtained should signs or symptoms of bone marrow suppression be present (e.g., petechiae, pallor, undue weakness, fever, infection). If hematologic abnormalities appear on the laboratory examination, the hematologic studies should be repeated more often until the results approach baseline.

Minor decreases in the WBC count are often seen in patients taking carbamazepine. Post (1984) suggested guidelines for carbamazepine discontinuation that include a WBC count of less than 3,000, erythrocyte count of less than $4.0 \times 10_6$ mm$_3$, hemoglobin less than 11 mg/dL, platelets less than 100,000, reticulocyte count of less than 0.3%,

and serum iron greater than 150 mg/dL. It should be noted that the hematologic thresholds for drug discontinuation outlined in the PDR are more conservative. Hyponatremia has been associated with carbamazepine therapy, so the clinician might need to order serum electrolytes if the clinical situation so warrants. Furthermore, periodic monitoring of hepatic function might be required, especially in patients with known hepatic dysfunction. Patients on valproic acid need evaluation of their hepatic function (e.g., liver function tests) before initiating treatment and frequently thereafter, particularly in the first 6 months of therapy (Physicians' Desk Reference 1998, p. 425). Finally, carbamazepine blood levels should be carefully monitored, because this drug can increase its metabolism through induction of liver enzymes (Schatzberg et al. 1997, p. 210).

ANTIPSYCHOTIC BLOOD LEVELS

Methodologies for the laboratory measurement of blood antipsychotic levels include gas-liquid chromatography (GLC), HPLC, GC-MS, fluorimetry, RIA, and radio-receptor assay (Creese and Synder 1977). Therapeutic levels and ranges for some of the antipsychotics have been reported (Van Putten et al. 1992), but a clear consensus concerning therapeutic levels or ranges has not yet been achieved using any measurement methodology. Interesting findings relevant to the clinical use of antipsychotic blood levels include the reports of low correlations between prescribed neuroleptic dose and subsequent serum neuroleptic levels, and reports that low neuroleptic levels for any given neuroleptic often help identify those patients who are most likely to relapse. However, patients with persistent psychotic symptoms have been reported to generally demonstrate neuroleptic levels indistinguishable from those of patients who are in remission (Brown and Laughren 1983).

Clear guidelines for the use of antipsychotic blood levels have not been established. Examples of possible current uses of this laboratory test might include the assessment of patient compliance or the evaluation of patients taking medication but possibly achieving only low serum levels. There may be some other specific situations in which antipsychotic blood levels might be of some value, such as the assessment of certain drug interactions. An example of this was described by Arana et al. (1985), who noted a decrease in plasma haloperidol levels in patients taking both haloperidol and carbamazepine. These authors therefore suggest that blood haloperidol level monitoring might be useful for patients taking both haloperidol and carbamazepine, especially in the context of clinical deterioration after the initiation of carbamazepine.

ELECTROCARDIOGRAPHIC MONITORING OF PATIENTS ON PSYCHOTROPICS

Psychotropic medications, including the TCAs, antipsychotics, and carbamazepine, have been associated with various electrocardiographic changes. The most frequently alluded to changes are those representing a slowing of atrioventricular conduction in the heart—for example, as reflected by a widening of the QT or QRS interval on the ECG. Significantly, malignant arrhythmias have been reported in some patients taking TCAs and thioridazine. It has been suggested that a lengthening of the QT interval may prolong the period of cardiac vulnerability to potentially life-threatening arrhythmias. Patients who seem at particularly high risk of developing these potentially lethal arrhythmias are those with preexisting "excessively" prolonged QT intervals or those who develop "excessive" QT prolongation during drug treatment (Flugelman et al. 1985), as well as patients with already compromised cardiac function. It is perhaps in these cases that ECGs obtained both before and during administration of certain psychotropic drugs associated with electrocardiographic changes would be most important. Schwartz and Wolf (1978) reported that when the QT interval corrected for rate (QTc) exceeds 0.440 seconds, there is an increased risk of sudden cardiac death due to ventricular tachycardia or ventricular fibrillation. Beresford et al. (1986) have argued that it is difficult to predict which psychiatric patients taking psychotropic medications will develop widened QT intervals. They suggest that the clinician must evaluate each patient case by case and maintain a low threshold for seeking cardiology consultation.

Some other applications of the ECG for psychiatric patients are worth mentioning. In the situation of TCA overdose, it has been reported that a widened QRS interval (e.g., greater than 0.10 seconds) is more reliable for determining the degree for potential TCA-induced cardiac morbidity and toxicity than is an antidepressant blood level (Boehnert and Lovejoy 1985). Additionally, with the increasing use of β-blockers for certain psychiatric conditions, the clinician should realize that β-blockers are contraindicated in patients with sinus bradycardia or evidence of certain cardiac conduction abnormalities.

LABORATORY EVALUATION PRIOR TO ELECTROCONVULSIVE THERAPY

Certain laboratory and diagnostic tests are commonly completed before a patient begins ECT. The pretreatment workup often includes a CBC, blood chemistries (for example, chem-20 profile), urinalysis, chest X ray, spinal X rays, and ECG (Sakauye 1986). In addition, a CT scan and EEG might also be ordered if indicated by medical history or by the physical, neurological, or mental status examination. Spinal X rays are currently ordered less often than in the past because of the reportedly lower incidence of orthopedic complications associated with the contemporary administration of ECT (e.g., with the routine use of succinylcholine as part of the ECT procedure). Routine pre-ECT screening for abnormal pseudocholinesterase activity is probably not mandatory, because inherited or acquired deficiency of pseudocholinesterase is reportedly quite rare. Indications for possibly obtaining measures of plasma pseudocholinesterase activity include a past history of prolonged succinylcholine-induced apnea in the patient or in a blood relative (Nelson and Burritt 1986). A possible pre-ECT laboratory evaluation is outlined in Table 9–11.

BIOLOGICAL MARKER RESEARCH

Neuroscience investigators continue to search for meaningful laboratory and diagnostic tests for *functional* psychiatric disorders. These functional, or idiopathic, disorders are psychiatric conditions for which a clear causative or contributing neuropathophysiological lesion has yet to be identified. The proposed tests are also referred to as "biological markers," and these markers might have a number of potential future uses to psychiatrists and neuroscientists, including assistance in improving our understanding of the underlying neurobiology of functional disorders, in making an accurate psychiatric diagnosis, in arriving at the most appropriate treatment plan, in assessing prognosis, and in identifying patients who are at potential risk of developing a psychiatric disorder who might benefit from preventive measures. These biological marker tests have been receiving increasing attention in

---

TABLE 9–11. Suggested laboratory evaluation before administering electroconvulsive therapy

Complete blood count

Blood chemistries (Chem-20 profile)

Chest X ray

Spinal X ray

Urinalysis

Electrocardiogram

the psychiatric literature. The tests encompass a wide range of procedures, including neuroendocrine challenge tests, brain-imaging techniques, and the quantitative and qualitative laboratory evaluation of CNS active substances or other relevant samplings obtained from the urine, blood, cerebrospinal fluid, and peripheral tissues. Some difficulties associated with the markers studied to date have been problems with sensitivity, specificity, reliability, and possible contamination from artifactual influences (e.g., concurrent illnesses, medication effects, and normal individual variation among patients). Currently, because of these and other problems, none of the markers yet seem to have the sensitivity and specificity that would make them clearly useful in routine clinical practice.

NEUROENDOCRINE TESTING

Neuroendocrine testing research in psychiatry currently includes measurements of basal hormone levels as well as neuroendocrine challenge tests. Basal endocrine evaluation includes blood measurements of certain hormone levels (e.g., thyroid function testing or serum cortisol levels) or measurement of certain hormone metabolites in the urine (e.g., urine ketosteroid measurements). Although frank endocrine dysfunction (as manifested by blood hormonal levels outside norms accepted by most endocrinologists) is known to be associated with various organic mental disorders, demonstration of a clear relationship between subtle differences in basal measurements (still within established normal ranges) in psychiatric patients remains an elusive goal of ongoing research. Of course, thorough endocrine laboratory testing should be performed if the clinician suspects underlying endocrine disease. A possible example of the utility of basal hormonal measurements to the psychiatric clinician is the patient with a rapid-cycling bipolar disorder. Both clinical and subclinical hypothyroidism (e.g., as manifested by an elevated serum TSH level) have been reported to be associated with a significant proportion of these patients (Cho et al. 1979; Cowdry et al. 1983). In addition, severe depression has been associated with a hypersecretion of cortisol (i.e., hypercortisolism) as well as a possible loss of the normal diurnal variation of cortisol secretion (Allen et al. 1987). A lower prevalence of hypercortisolism has been reported in patients with schizophrenia (Roy et al. 1986).

Dexamethasone Suppression Test

The dexamethasone suppression test (DST) has been one of the most actively investigated of the neuroendocrine challenge tests used in psychiatric research. In fact, this test enjoyed a brief period during which it was employed by some psychiatrists in their routine clinical practice, outside an established research setting. This was the result of the considerable excitement surrounding the possibility that the DST might be a useful marker for endogenous melancholic depression (Carroll 1984). It was proposed by some investigators that the DST could detect some of the subtle abnormalities of the hypothalamic-pituitary-adrenal axis that had been hypothesized to be present in patients with depression.

In a commonly described version of the DST (Allen et al. 1987; Carroll 1984), the patient received 1 mg of dexamethasone orally at 11:00 P.M. Blood was drawn over the next 24 hours, generally at 8:00 A.M., 4:00 P.M., and 11:00 P.M. The test was considered abnormal, or positive, if the postdexamethasone serum cortisol level equaled or exceeded approximately 5 mg/dL, although this cutoff point varied somewhat among different laboratories and investigators. In addition, different laboratories used different cortisol measurement methodologies with different accuracies and reliability for measuring serum cortisol.

Although extensive research has been devoted to the evaluation of the clinical application of this test, its role in clinical psychiatry is unclear. When it has been used to try to assist in the diagnostic assessment of melancholic depression, major limitations in the use of the DST have included problems with test sensitivity (reflecting accurate identification of those with depression) and specificity (reflecting correct identification of those who do not have major depression). Significant limitations in specificity have been noted when the DST is used in patients with other psychiatric disorders. Moreover, artifactual contamination has been reported from such variables as weight loss, certain medical illnesses (e.g., uncontrolled diabetes mellitus), acute psychiatric hospitalization, certain medications (e.g., steroids, estrogens, phenytoin, carbamazepine, indomethacin, barbiturates), and individual differences in the metabolism of dexamethasone (Allen et al. 1987; Arana et al. 1985; Carroll 1986). Such confounding variables will greatly limit any potential clinical application that might be delineated for this test. The DST does not appear to be appropriate for routine screening of psychiatric patients (Carroll 1986). Indeed, it remains to be demonstrated whether this test can increase incrementally our ability to diagnose or treat patients with depression. Moreover, a normal DST result is probably without specific clinical utility.

In conclusion, the DST remains a research tool, and attempts to delineate a specific clinical application will require further investigation. One possible use of the DST may lie in its potential for providing biological subtypes and prognostically meaningful subgroups. For example, preliminary evidence has suggested that the DST may prove useful in predicting relapse in some patients treated for depression (Nemeroff and Evans 1984).

Thyrotropin-Releasing Hormone Stimulation Test

The thyrotropin-releasing hormone stimulation test (TRHST) has been proposed as a potential biological marker of mood disorders (Loosen and Prange 1982). In a commonly described version of this test, an endocrine challenge of 500 μg of TRH was administered intravenously to a patient. Serum values of TSH were obtained just prior to the TRH administration, as well as 15, 30, 60, and 90 minutes after the TRH was given. (TRH normally stimulates the pituitary to release TSH.) A change in the TSH serum value from before TRH administration (i.e., baseline TSH) to after TRH administration was determined (called TSH). A "blunted" response was regarded as a change in TSH values (or ΔTSH)/5–7 μIU/mL.

In major depression, a blunted TSH response to TRH has been reported to occur about 25% of the time (Loosen and Prange 1982). Similar responses have also been noted in patients with alcoholism, bulimia, borderline personality, and panic disorder, all of which are illnesses that have been hypothesized as possibly being related to affective disorders (Roy-Byrne et al. 1986). The reader should note that hyperthyroidism is also associated with a blunted TSH response to TRH, although there are generally also abnormalities of some of the baseline thyroid function tests (e.g., TSH, T_4, T_3RU). In another possible use of the TRHST, Targum et al. (1984) suggested that treatment-resistant depressed patients with an "augmented" TSH response (e.g., greater than 30 μIU/mL) might benefit from thyroid hormone medication added to their antidepressant regimen. Targum and associates (1992) also reported variability of responses to the TRH test in depressed and nondepressed elderly subjects.

In addition, there has been the suggestion that the TRHST combined with the DST might be able to identify more patients with affective disorder than would either test used alone (Extein at al. 1981). More research will be required to clarify whether this is so. Like the DST, the TRHST is a useful research approach, but its clinical utility requires further investigative clarification.

Other Neuroendocrine Challenge Tests

Other neuroendocrine research diagnostic tests include serum growth hormone responses to such pharmacological challenges as dopamine, apomorphine, dextro-amphetamine, clonidine, and insulin-induced hypoglycemia, as well as serum prolactin changes secondary to challenges by such substances as apomorphine, TRH, and methadone. A sample of findings in this area includes the reports of blunted growth hormone responses to insulin-induced hypoglycemia in patients with major depression and reports that apomorphine-induced prolactin suppression is greater in depressed patients than in patients with schizophrenia or in psychiatrically normal control subjects (Allen et al. 1987; Meltzer et al. 1984). Another neuroendocrine challenge test perhaps related to the DST is the corticotropin-releasing hormone (CRH) stimulation test. CRH is normally released by the hypothalamus and acts on the pituitary to cause a release of adrenocorticotropin (ACTH). P. W. Gold et al. (1986) reported that depressed patients had basal hypercortisolism that was associated with a decreased responsiveness of ACTH to an intravenous challenge with CRH. Roy et al. (1986) reported that patients with schizophrenia generally had basal cortisol blood levels as well as ACTH responses to CRH challenge that were similar to those of psychiatrically normal control subjects.

All of these tests remain research tools at this time. Their most significant potential contribution to our understanding of psychiatric disorders may lie in their possible utility in the development of biologically based diagnostic and prognostic subtyping strategies.

BRAIN IMAGING

Whereas the proposed neuroendocrine tests largely provide an indirect measure of brain activity (e.g., through central effects on endocrine function), brain-imaging techniques have the potential for providing a more direct window on the functioning of the living human brain. Functional brain-imaging techniques include computerized electroencephalography and evoked potential mapping, positron-emission tomography (PET), single-photon emission computed tomography (SPECT), and regional cerebral blood flow (rCBF). Magnetic resonance imaging and computed tomography are structural brain-imaging techniques that can provide an anatomic view of the living human brain. Of special note, software and technical advances in MRI have allowed this technique to "evolve" into new functional brain-imaging approaches: magnetic resonance spectroscopy (MRS), blood-oxygenation-level-dependent functional magnetic resonance imaging (BOLD fMRI), and dynamic fMRI. Another promising application of brain-imaging technology will be the combined use of complementary brain-imaging techniques (e.g., using a functional brain-imaging technique such as computerized EEG mapping with a structural brain-imaging technique such as CT) (Morihisa and McAnulty 1985). Recent advances have made possible the coregistration of functional and structural brain images.

Positron-Emission Tomography

Whereas computerized EEG mapping provides information about brain electrical activity presumably arising from only the uppermost cortical cell layers, PET allows for the direct visualization of both cortical and subcortical (e.g., limbic system) brain functioning. Different aspects of brain functioning can be evaluated, including cerebral blood flow (CBF), brain oxygen use, and certain aspects of brain glucose metabolism, as well as some specific CNS neurotransmitter systems function.

In preparation for a PET scan, a positron-emitting element (e.g., fluorine-18 [^{18}F], carbon-14 [^{14}C], carbon-11 [^{11}C]) is incorporated into a biologically significant compound, which is introduced into the body (usually intravenously). The compound used determines which brain function will be visualized. For example, when ^{18}F-labeled deoxy-D-glucose is employed, it allows for the visualization of certain aspects of brain glucose metabolism. Other examples of radionuclides used include etorphine or carfentanil citrate labeled with ^{11}C, which allows for the visualization of brain opiate receptor activity, as well as ^{18}F-labeled N-methylspiroperidol, ^{11}C-labeled ^{3}N-methylspiperone, and ^{11}C-labeled raclopride, which permit the visualization of dopamine receptor function. The evaluation of the utility and accuracy of using different radiopharmaceuticals to assess certain neurotransmitter system functions is an area of very active investigation and some controversy. In addition, inhalation of the radionuclide oxygen-15 allows for the direct visualization of oxygen use in the brain.

The distribution of these compounds after they enter the brain is determined by an array of detectors that surround the head. The detectors are sensitive to gamma rays that are formed after the positrons emitted by the radionuclides collide with electrons in the brain, resulting in the generation of coincident gamma rays in opposite (180°) directions. Data collected by the detectors are relayed to a computer, which uses the detection of these two coincident gamma rays to calculate the amount of radionuclide at different locations in the brain and produce the PET brain image.

Some PET findings in patients with schizophrenia and bipolar disorder have included reports of abnormalities of the anteroposterior gradient of glucose use (Buchsbaum 1986; Buchsbaum et al. 1984), as well as decreased absolute glucose use in the frontal lobes in schizophrenia (Wolkin et al. 1985). R. E. Gur et al. (1987) did not find "hypofrontality" in the schizophrenic patients studied, but reported higher subcortical/cortical glucose metabolism ratios for patients with schizophrenia as compared with psychiatrically normal control subjects. In another study, using radioisotopes capable of binding to brain dopamine D$_2$ receptors, D$_2$ receptors in the caudate nucleus were found to be elevated in patients with schizophrenia compared with psychiatrically normal control subjects (Wong et al. 1986), although there is a lack of consensus in the literature concerning this finding. In another PET study, Tamminga and associates (1992) reported abnormalities of the limbic system, in particular the hippocampus, in schizophrenia. More recently, R. E. Gur and associates (1995) found that left midtemporal metabolism was relatively higher in schizophrenic patients and that this finding varied with clinical subtypes. These PET findings in schizophrenia are generally consistent with a theory of dysfunction of neural networks involving temporal limbic structures and associated prefrontal cortex. However, attempts to correlate metabolic findings with clinical variables have thus far failed to achieve any consensus. The disparity in research design and focus has contributed to the difficulty in comparing and integrating the wide spectrum of findings. The multiplicity of findings in brain-imaging research in schizophrenia may also reflect the heterogeneity of this disorder. Furthermore, in affective disorders, there have been functional imaging reports of abnormalities of temporal lobes and in particular the prefrontal cortex (Ketter et al. 1994). PET studies have not yet demonstrated sufficient sensitivity or specificity to elaborate a definitive role in psychiatric practice. As is the case for most brain-imaging applications, PET is most accurately considered a research tool in the investigation of classical psychiatric disorders.

Single Photon Emission Computed Tomography

SPECT can generate cross-sectional images from multiple levels of the brain and can therefore visualize the CNS in three dimensions (as can PET). SPECT uses radionuclides that emit gamma radiation (i.e., photons). These photons are measured by gamma detectors containing sodium iodide scintillation crystals. Information may then be calculated about the location in the brain and the relative amount of radionuclide at that locus. Different radiopharmaceuticals can be used to investigate different parameters of brain function. For example, qualitative measures of rCBF have been obtained with ^{123}I-labeled iodoamphetamine, and quantitative measures of rCBF with xenon-133. ^{99}mTc-hexamethylpropylene amine oxime (HMPAO) has been used in SPECT rCBF studies as well. One radiopharmaceutical presently being evaluated as a putative window on muscarinic receptor activity is ^{123}I-labeled 3-quinuclidinyl-4-iodobenzilate (QNB). Weinberger and associates (1992b) studied patients with Alzheimer's disease with both [^{123}I]-QNB SPECT, a measure of muscarinic receptor availability (Figure 9–6), and [^{18}F]-2- fluoro-2-deoxyglucose PET in order to investigate the potential utility of using both types of functional brain-imaging approaches in the study of this disorder (Figure 9–7). Knable et al. (1995) evaluated iodine-123-IBZM ([^{123}I] IBZM) as a putative in vivo window on dopamine receptor availability.

For classical psychiatric disorders there is insufficient evidence that SPECT can yet provide the sensitivity or specificity that will be required for the development of new diagnostic or prognostic approaches (Morihisa 1991). One of the confounding variables in any attempt to consolidate SPECT findings into clinically meaningful protocols is that there is a significant discrepancy between the investigational capabilities of many SPECT systems presently in use. Nevertheless, recently developed research-grade SPECT systems feature improved resolution that can rival that of PET scans, and preliminary investigations have suggested that this modality may provide valuable research information in some disease entities.

Regional Cerebral Blood Flow

In rCBF, blood flow to various regions of the brain is evaluated. To accomplish this, a metabolically inert radioactive substance (usually xenon-133) is introduced into the body

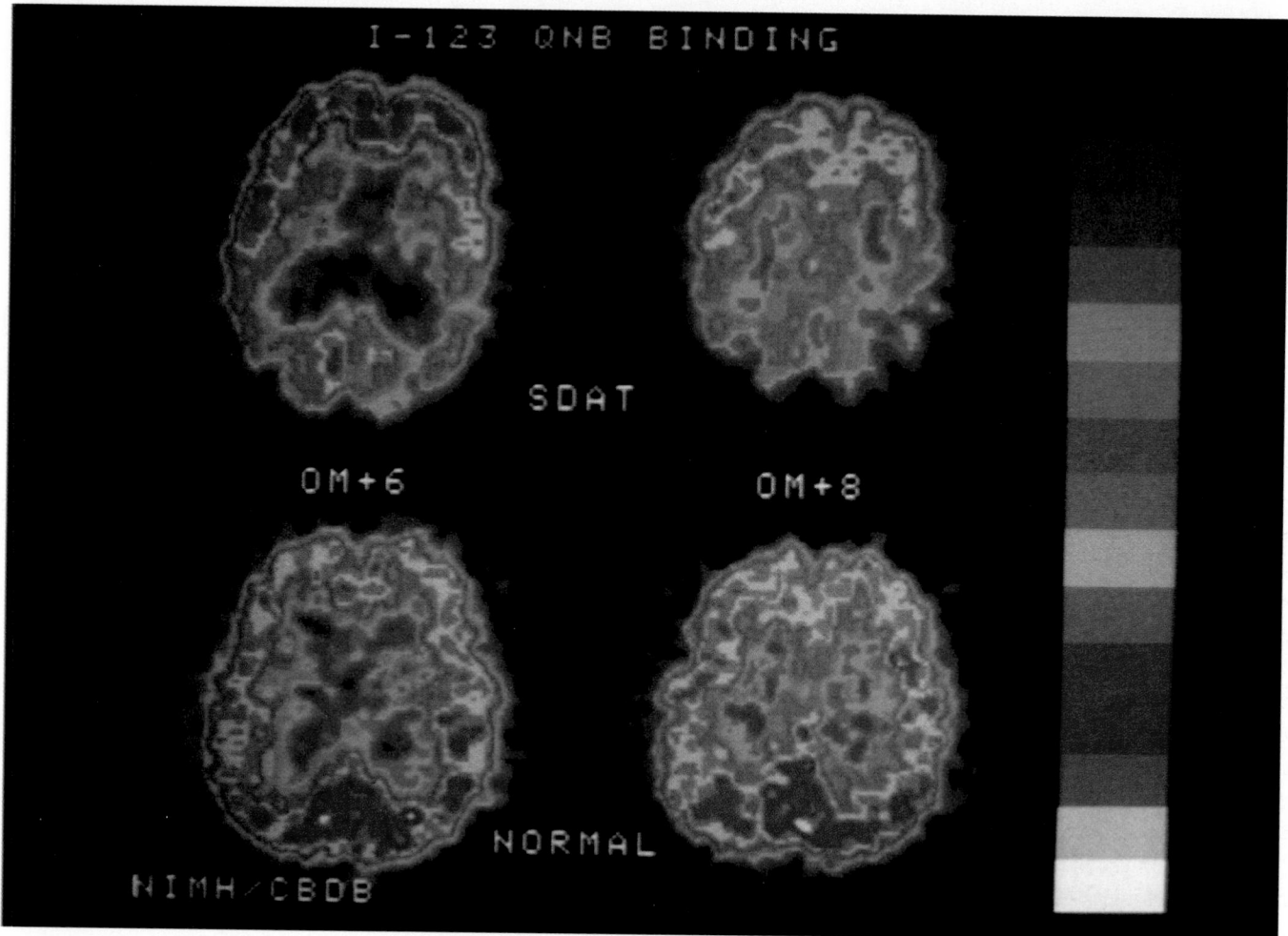

FIGURE 9–6. A single photon emission computed tomographic (SPECT) image of two subjects using the radiopharmaceutical ^{123}I-labeled 3-quinuclidinyl-4-iodobenzilate (QNB). The bottom two images represent a normal control subject, and the top two images represent a subject with primary degenerative dementia of the Alzheimer type.
Source. Courtesy of Daniel R. Weinberger, M.D., Clinical Brain Disorders Branch, National Institute of Mental Health, Bethesda, Maryland.

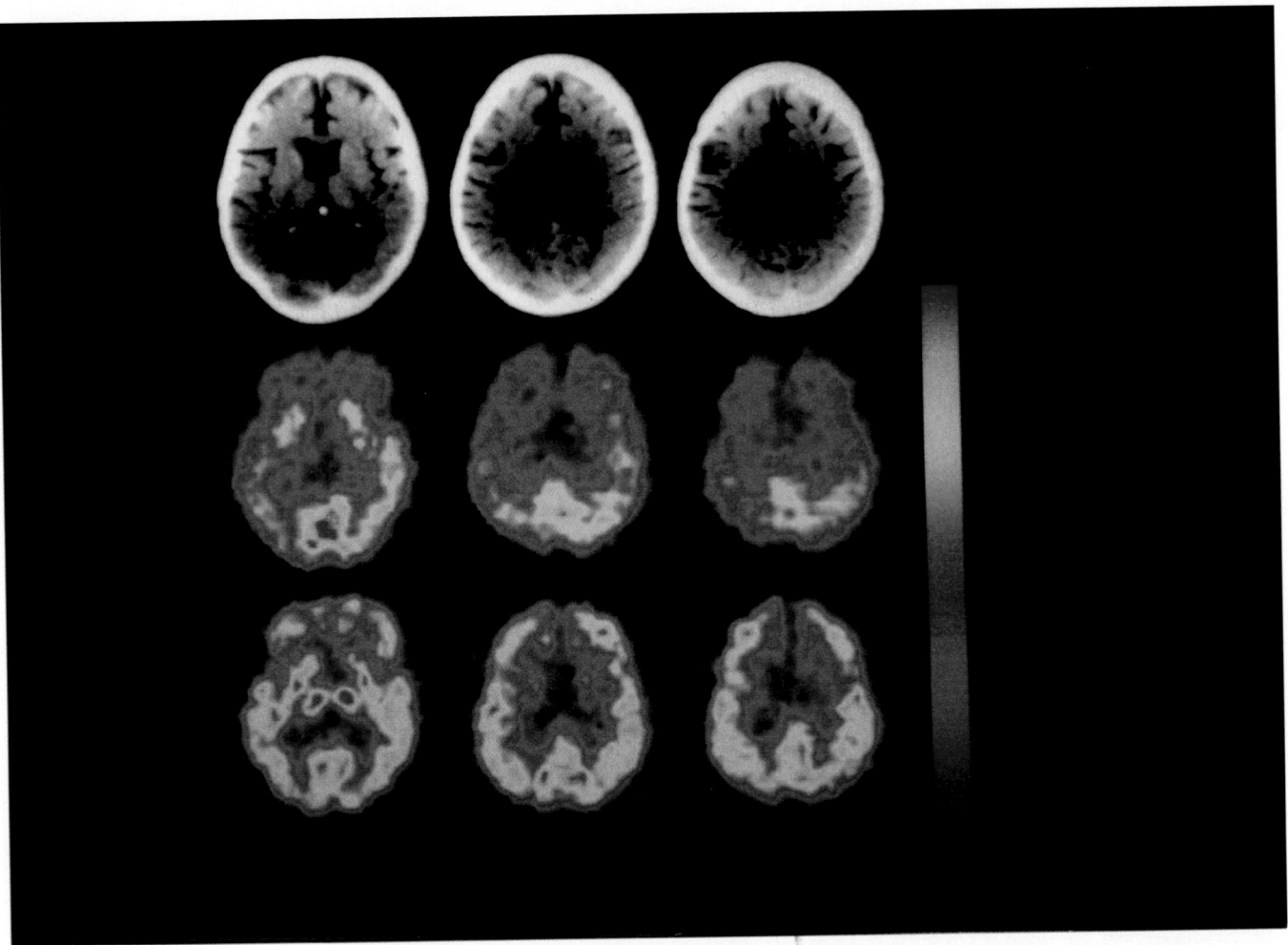

FIGURE 9–7. Magnetic resonance imaging, ^{123}I-labeled 3-quinuclidinyl-4-iodobenzilate (QNB) single photon emission computed tomography (SPECT), and ^{18}F-labeled fluorodeoxyglucose positron emission tomography (PET) are demonstrated for a subject with a clinical diagnosis of Pick's disease–type dementia. Note the relative hypoactivity of the prefrontal and temporal regions.
Source.   Courtesy of Daniel R. Weinberger, M.D., Clinical Brain Disorders Branch, National Institute of Mental Health, Bethesda, Maryland.

(usually through inhalation). The radioactive substance is carried by the blood to various parts of the brain, and radiation emanating from the brain is picked up by detectors surrounding the skull. This method of investigation of brain function depends on the close linkage between cerebral blood flow and cerebral metabolism (i.e., increased activity of a certain part of the brain is normally associated with an increase in blood flow to the area). The procedure can be performed with the subject at rest or engaging in mental activity (Figure 9–8). Unfortunately, unlike PET or SPECT, rCBF using the xenon-133 inhalation technique cannot delineate blood flow in subcortical structures.

Ingvar and Franzen (1974) reported on rCBF studies in patients with schizophrenia. They found decreased blood flow in frontal brain regions in these patients, which

they did not find in their alcoholic control subjects. More recently, Weinberger et al. (1986) reported that schizophrenic subjects failed to show increased blood flow to the dorsolateral prefrontal cortex (DLPFC) during challenge by the Wisconsin Card Sorting Test, a task that is felt to require the functional integrity of the DLPFC and has been shown to be associated with increased blood flow to the DLPFC in normal subjects (see Figure 9–8). This work has provided the basis for an exciting neurodevelopmental theory for the pathogenesis of schizophrenia (Weinberger 1987) and focused investigational interest on the DLPFC (Morihisa and Weinberger 1986). Furthermore, work by Weinberger and associates (1992a) has extended this theory to implicate dysfunction of a prefrontal-limbic neural network in schizophrenia.

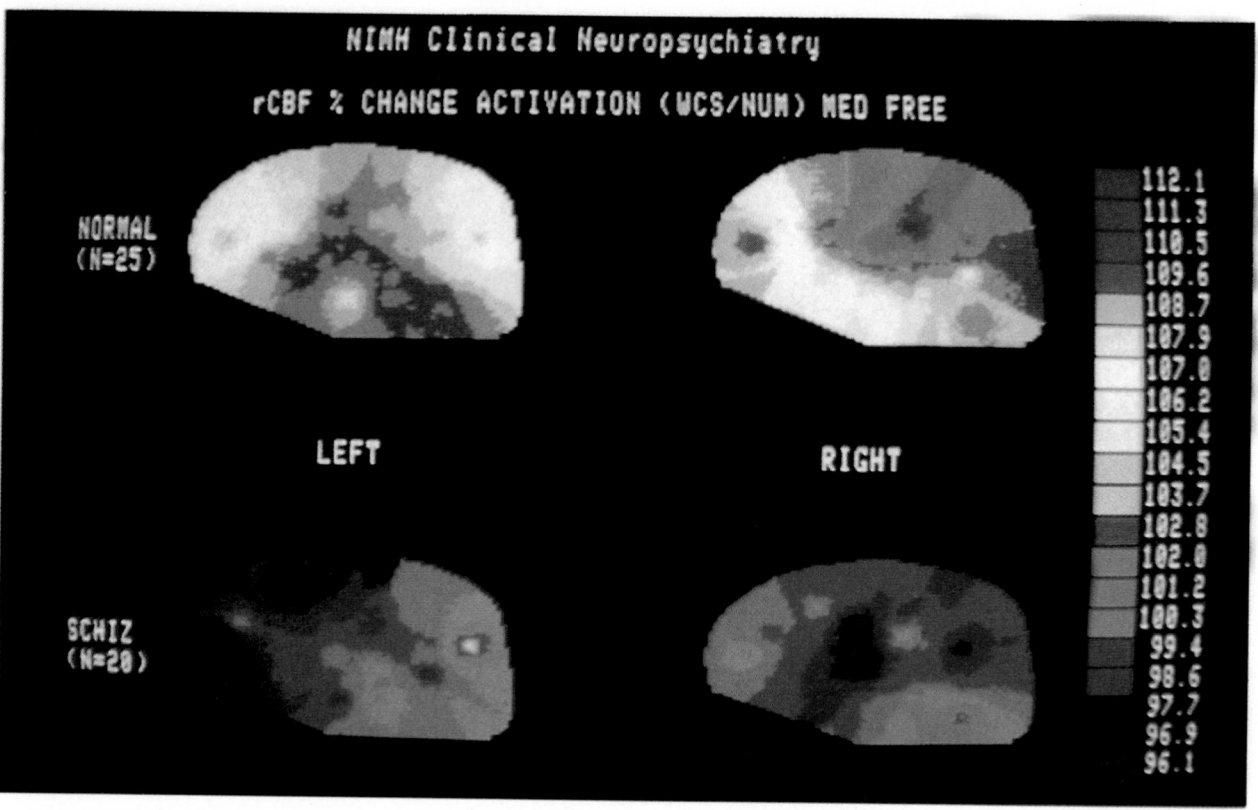

FIGURE 9–8. Topographic map of the regional distribution of cerebral blood flow (CBF) percent change in a group of patients with schizophrenia *(bottom)* versus control subjects *(top)*, comparing two cognitive challenge tasks: a number-matching task and the Wisconsin Card Sorting (WCS) Test. Note that, in the control group, blood flow to the frontal cortex is increased during the WCS, whereas in the schizophrenic patients it is not. Red denotes the greatest amounts of CBF change from the baseline number task that controls for CBF during a cognitive activation task.
Source. Courtesy of Daniel R. Weinberger, M.D., Clinical Brain Disorders Branch, National Institute of Mental Health, Bethesda, Maryland.

Computed Tomography

In CT, multiple X rays are taken through the CNS that provide the basis for the elaboration of cross-sectional images of the brain. Possible indications for the use of CT in the organic workup of psychiatric patients have already been described in this chapter. Again, when CT is employed in this manner, it is generally in an effort to rule out neurological lesions, such as CNS neoplasms, that might be causing or contributing to the psychiatric symptomatology. Indeed, it would appear that it is in the evaluation of classically neurological disease processes that structural imaging techniques such as CT and MRI demonstrate their most significant utility in clinical psychiatry (Morihisa 1991).

Scientific investigators have employed CT to identify a number of subtle structural abnormalities in the CNS of patients with primary psychiatric disorders. Findings have included increased ventricular-to-brain (VBR) ratios in pa-

tients with schizophrenia (Weinberger et al. 1979), cortical atrophy, and third ventricle enlargement in schizophrenia (Nasrallah et al. 1985). There is a growing body of research that suggests that the structural findings in schizophrenia are the result of abnormal neurodevelopment (Weinberger 1987, 1995).

An extensive scientific effort has been under way to attempt to correlate these structural findings with clinically relevant variables, but it has thus far failed to delineate clearly any parameters that can significantly enhance our present diagnostic or treatment approach to classical psychiatric disorders. It has been suggested that there may be an association between enlarged ventricles in schizophrenia and a number of variables including medication response, negative symptoms (Pearlson et al. 1984), and cognitive impairment (Johnston et al. 1976). The attempt to elaborate the clinical meaning of these findings is further confounded by the fact that enlarged ventricles have been reported in other psychiatric illnesses, including eating disorders, alcoholism, bipolar disorder, dementia (Coffman 1989; Fogel and Faust 1987), and depression (Nasrallah et al. 1989). Thus, it is clear that this finding is neither pathognomonic nor even characteristic of a single psychiatric disorder (Morihisa 1991). Further research will be required to move us from our present stage of reporting statistically significant findings, based upon intergroup comparisons, to the next stage of clearly established clinical correlates before we can achieve a consensus concerning the use of these data in the clinical practice of psychiatry.

Magnetic Resonance Imaging

The technique of MRI provides three-dimensional visualization of the brain's structure in axial, sagittal, and coronal planes by measuring the differential distribution of hydrogen nuclei, mainly in the water and fat of the brain. In the MRI technique, a magnetic field (usually 0.5–1.5 tesla in strength) is applied to the brain, and the spinning nuclei of hydrogen become aligned in accordance with this field. These nuclei are then exposed to brief pulses of a second field created by a radio frequency (RF) coil that causes nuclei to precess as well as spin. These pulses must "broadcast" on the characteristic resonant frequency (Larmor frequency) of hydrogen. Following the pulse, the nuclei return to their previously aligned positions and in doing so emit a characteristic electromagnetic pattern. MRI detects this characteristic signal with a radio frequency receiver. The imposition of a magnetic gradient allows spatial information to be acquired. The return over time of these hydrogen nuclei to their previously aligned positions is termed relaxation. T_1 and T_2 (relaxation times) are measures of the rate of this return of nuclei to their original state. Adjustments in transmission parameters can emphasize (i.e., weight) certain informational characteristics in the image. For example, a T_1-weighted scan generally provides the best gray/white matter differentiation, whereas a T_2-weighted scan generally provides superior discrimination of brain tissue abnormalities (Morihisa 1991).

MRI studies of schizophrenia have successfully replicated the work of previous CT investigations, extending findings of frontal lobe abnormalities (Andreasen et al. 1994) and significantly highlighting a compelling focus on regional abnormalities of the temporal lobes (Suddath et al. 1989).

It has been thought that only a subpopulation of all patients with schizophrenia demonstrate significantly enlarged ventricles compared with a psychiatrically normal control population. However, MRI research on monozygotic twins discordant for schizophrenia (Suddath et al.

1990) has raised the possibility that enlarged ventricular size may be found to be more pervasive than originally thought. In this research, the twin with schizophrenia usually demonstrates ventricular enlargement when compared to his or her unaffected twin, a uniquely powerful control who shares the same genome (Weinberger 1995; Figure 9–9). Thus, it is possible that with appropriate controls or sufficiently elegant research paradigms, ventricular enlargement may be found to be present in a greater percentage of patients with schizophrenia than previously reported. A related finding in monozygotic twins discordant for schizophrenia was found by employing $H_2^{15}O$ PET rCBF, in which the twin with schizophrenia demonstrated decreased metabolic activity in the DLPFC compared to the unaffected twin (Figure 9–10) (D. R. Weinberger, personal communication, July 1997).

In patients with mood disorders there have been structural research reports of increased ventricular size and reductions in the temporal lobe and the prefrontal region (Ketter et al. 1994). In addition, there have been reports of subcortical leukoencephalopathy or periventricular hyperintensities seen in some patients with affective disorder. The significance of these findings have yet to be elucidated (Nasrallah et al. 1989). Nevertheless, exciting efforts are being made (Steffen and Krishman 1998) to delineate the potentially meaningful clinical correlates of MRI findings in affective disorders with intention of further expanding the frontiers of psychiatric classification by proposing new biologically based diagnostic subtypes.

Advances in technology use MRS to image brain function, as reflected by differences in brain chemistry, for compounds that contain phosphorus-31, carbon-13, sodium-23, fluoride-19, and hydrogen, as well as the element lithium-7. In this manner, in vivo investigations of certain neurotransmitters, lipid metabolism, electrolyte balance, amino acid metabolism, high-energy phosphate metabolism, and carbohydrate metabolism may be pursued (Keshavan et al. 1991). In addition, drug studies of compounds incorporating carbon-13, lithium-7, or fluoride-19 may be possible (Guze 1991). An MRS study using phosphorus-31 (Pettegrew et al. 1991) has investigated CNS membrane phospholipid metabolism as well as high-energy phosphate metabolism in the dorsal prefrontal cortex in schizophrenia. The authors interpreted their results as suggestive of hypoactivity in this region and also speculated that abnormalities of cell membranes may play a role in the pathogenesis of schizophrenia (Pettegrew et al. 1991). More recently, a multislice proton magnetic resonance spectroscopy imaging (H-MRSI) study (Bertolino et al. 1996) investigated the regional

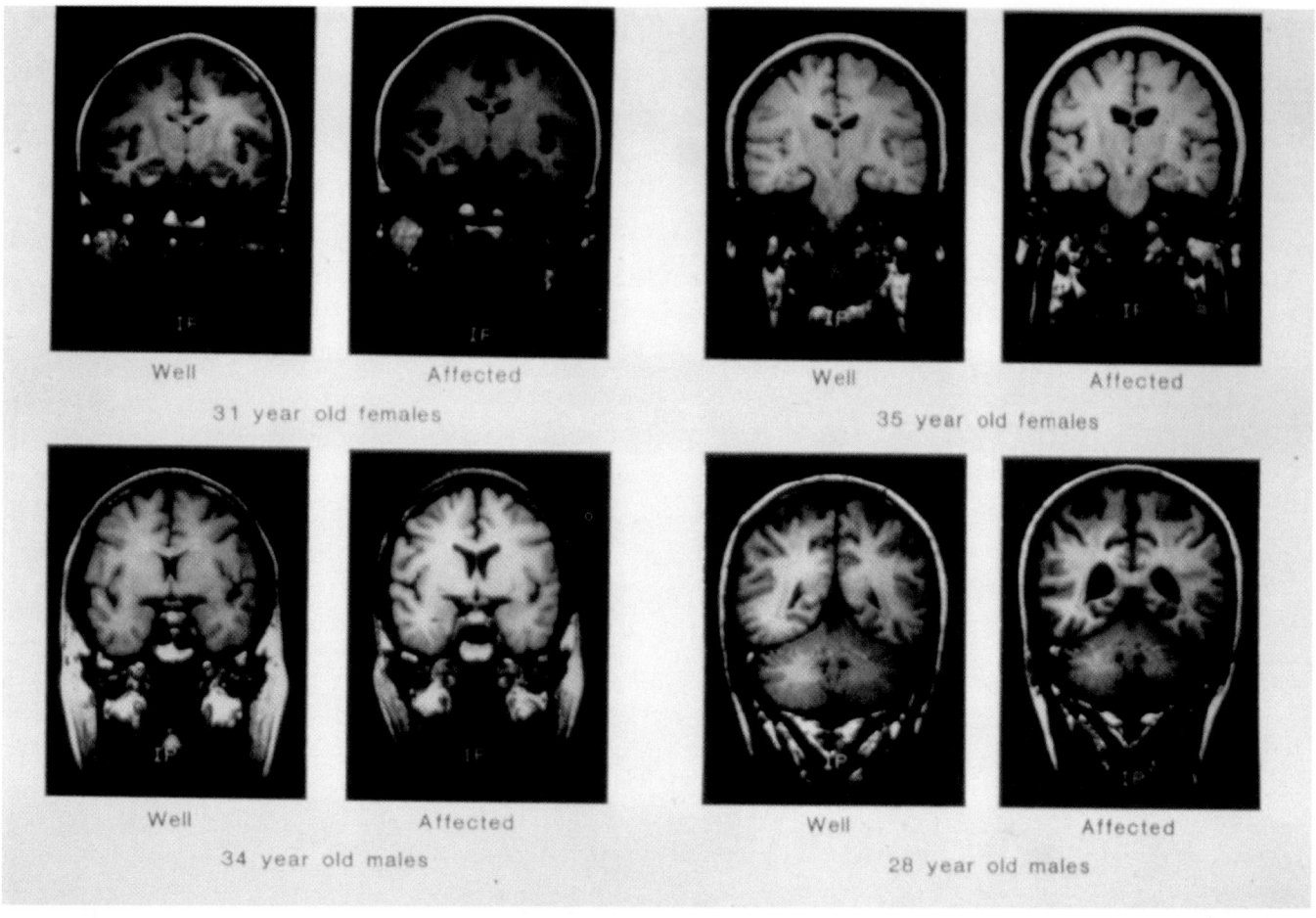

FIGURE 9–9. Paired magnetic resonance imaging (MRI) scans from four sets of monozygotic twins discordant for schizophrenia. Note that in each case the affected twin demonstrates greater ventricular size than does the affected twin.
Source. Reprinted with permission from Weinberger DR: "From Neuropathology to Neurodevelopment." *Lancet* 346:552–557, 1995.

neurochemical concentrations of N-acetyl aspartate (NAA), choline-containing compounds (CHO), and creatinine/phosphocreatinine in schizophrenia. These investigators (Bertolino et al. 1996, 1998) reported reductions of relative signal intensities of NAA in the dorsolateral prefrontal cortex (DLPFC) and hippocampal regions and interpreted (Bertolino et al. 1996) these findings as suggestive of neuronal pathology, consistent with a neurodevelopmental theory of dysfunction in temporal limbic and associated prefrontal cortical neural networks in schizophrenia. Figure 9–11 demonstrates MRS data of a psychiatrically normal control subject with the associated MRI structural image.

A new functional imaging approach using magnetic resonance (fMRI) has been developed that avoids exposure to ionizing radiation and offers superior spatial/temporal resolution compared to SPECT and PET. One such fMRI approach, blood-oxygenation-level-dependent (BOLD) MR imaging, exploits the paramagnetic properties of deoxygenated hemoglobin (David et al. 1994). Another approach, dynamic MR imaging, employs signal enhancement by use of contrast materials such as gadopentetate dimeglumine. A recent study (Ramsey et al. 1996) compared a PET technique ($H_2{}^{15}O$ PET rCBF) to a three-dimensional (3D) BOLD fMRI technique in order to investigate the potential utility of this new functional MR imaging approach. Such studies have opened a new era of functional brain-imaging investigations in psychiatry.

GENETIC MARKERS

A rapidly developing area of biological research is the field of genetic markers of psychiatric illness. Markers have recently been described for Huntington's disease (Gusella et al. 1984), and numerous reports raise the possibility of

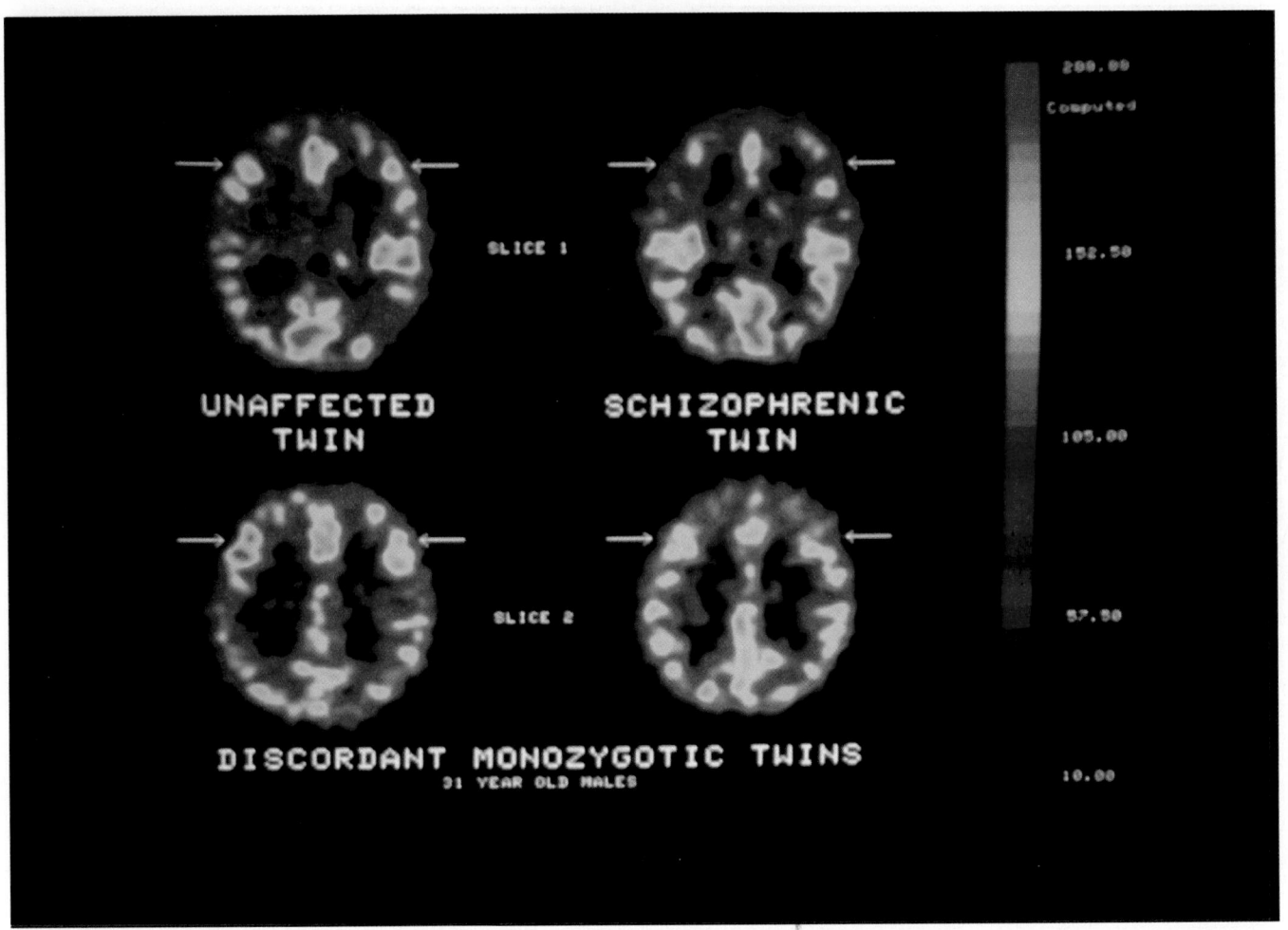

FIGURE 9–10. $H_2{}^{15}O$ positron emission tomography (PET) regional cerebral blood flow (rCBF) scan of a pair of twins discordant for schizophrenia. Note that the area of the dorsolateral prefrontal cortex (DLPFC) (see arrows) is relatively decreased in the twin with schizophrenia compared to the unaffected twin.
Source.   Courtesy of Daniel R. Weinberger, M.D., Clinical Brain Disorders Branch, National Institute of Mental Health, Bethesda, Maryland.

identifying clinically relevant genetic markers for neuropsychiatric disorders at some time in the future. For instance, the presence of an apolipoprotein E4 (apo E4) allele is reported to be associated with an increased risk of dementia of the Alzheimer's type (DAT). Individuals with two copies of the apo E4 allele (i.e., persons homozygous for apo E4) appear to have an especially increased risk (Reiman et al. 1996). For instance, by late middle age, persons homozygous for apo E4 but still cognitively normal have been reported to show evidence of reduced glucose metabolism on PET in the same regions of the brain as do patients with DAT. These findings have been interpreted as being supportive of the notion that apo E4 is an important risk factor for DAT (National Institute on Aging/Alzheimer's Association Working Group 1996; Reiman et al. 1996).

BIOCHEMICAL MARKERS

The laboratory has been increasingly used by physicians from all specialties to help detect, confirm, or rule out diagnoses of various physical conditions. There has also been the hope that the quantitative laboratory could similarly be used by psychiatrists and neuroscientists to help in the evaluation of patients with functional disorders. Research scientists have employed various strategies in their search for quantitative laboratory applications to psychiatry, including the examination of various potentially relevant compounds found in the blood, urine, and spinal fluid, as well as the examination of CNS enzyme and receptor systems also found in tissues outside of the brain (e.g., blood platelets, lymphocytes, skin fibroblasts). An example of a spinal fluid marker for dementia of the Alzheimer's

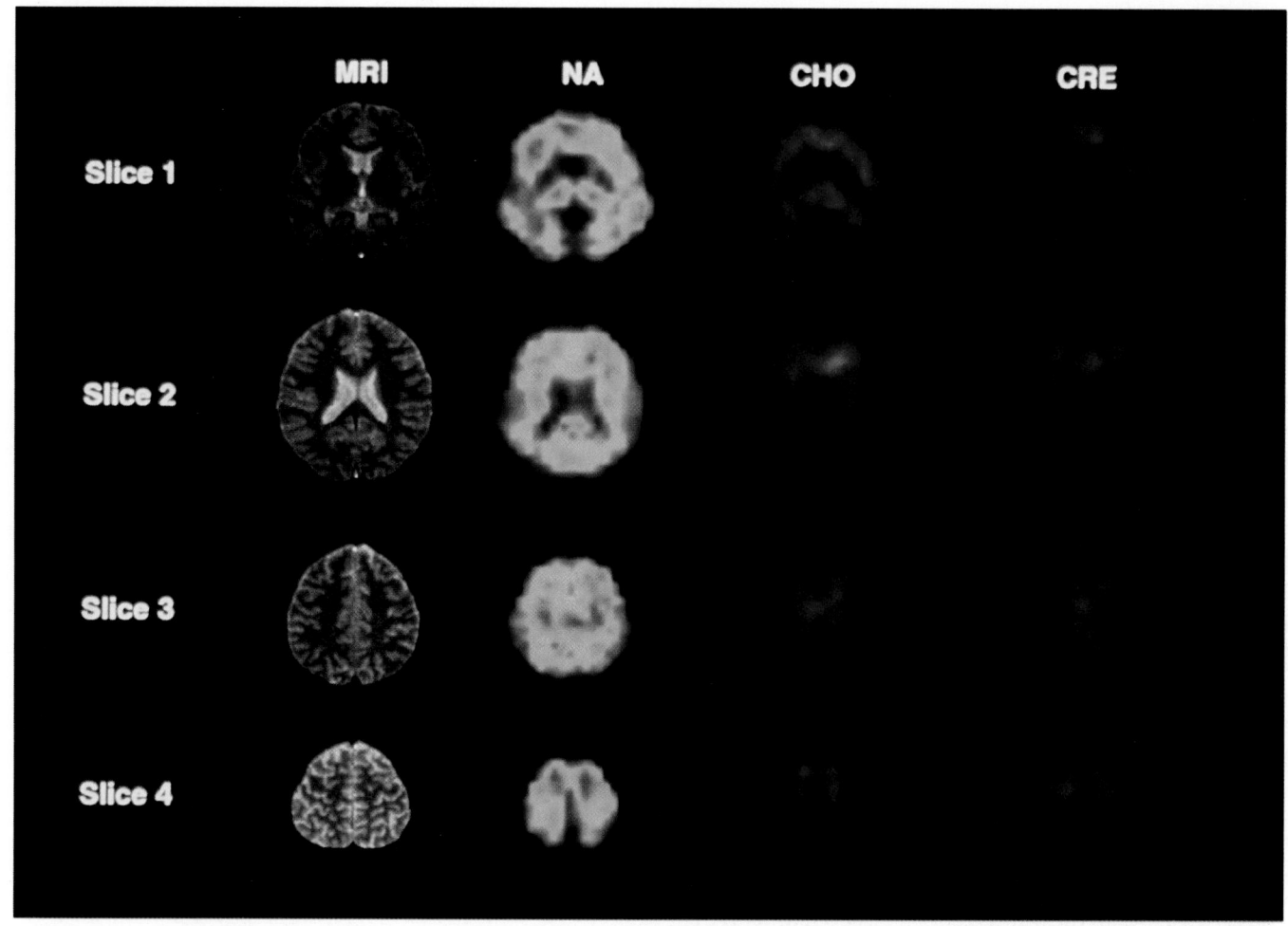

FIGURE 9-11. Magnetic resonance spectroscopy (MRS) data of a psychiatrically normal control subject at four slice levels with the associated magnetic resonance imaging (MRI) structural image. Signal intensities for *N*-acetyl aspartate (NA), choline-containing compounds (CHO), and creatinine/phosphocreatinine (CRE) are shown.
Source. Courtesy of Daniel R. Weinberger, M.D., Clinical Brain Disorders Branch, National Institute of Mental Health, Bethesda, Maryland.

type (DAT) is the CSF test for neural thread protein (NTP). The test measures an approximately 20 kD protein which is reported to be increased in DAT compared to normal controls (de la Monte et al. 1992). Other potential CSF tests for DAT include measurement of tau protein (e.g., Jensen et al. 1995) and amyloid beta-protein (Pirttila et al. 1994).

Body Fluid Markers

Body fluid markers include molecular compounds found in the plasma, serum, urine, and CSF that are of particular interest to psychiatrists. Some of the biochemical markers that have been studied include neurotransmitter substances felt to be relevant to the pathogenesis of some psy-

chiatric disorders (e.g., dopamine, serotonin, and norepinephrine), their metabolites (e.g., homovanillic acid [HVA], 5-hydroxyindoleacetic acid [5-HIAA], and 3-methoxy-4-hydroxyphenylglycol [MHPG]), various neuropeptides (e.g., endorphins, enkephalins), and biological compounds such as immunoglobulins (e.g., IgM) and plasma melatonin. Overall, most of the studies are either preliminary or have yielded mixed results.

Among some of the interesting research findings are the reported association between reduced CSF 5-HIAA and suicidal behavior (Asberg et al. 1976) and the possibility that unipolar depressed patients may be partly differentiated from bipolar depressed patients by a lower 24-hour urinary MHPG reportedly found in some of the bipolar patients (Muscettola et al. 1984; Schildkraut et al. 1978). On this latter point, however, Davis and Bresnahan (1987) did not believe that the differences are great enough to be of significant utility. An interesting finding concerning learned helplessness and urinary MHPG levels in unipolar depression was reported by Samson et al. (1992).

PROVOCATIVE TESTS FOR PANIC DISORDER

Intravenous lactate infusions have been reported to induce panic attacks in many patients with histories consistent with panic disorder. A commonly described procedure for this test involves the intravenous infusion of 10 mL of 0.5 M/kg of body weight sodium lactate over a 20-minute period (Liebowitz et al. 1985). It has been reported that approximately 70%–90% of patients with panic disorder, compared with only 0%–30% of control subjects, will experience a panic attack with such an infusion (Rainey and Nesse 1985). It should be noted that Cowley et al. (1986) have described similar rates of lactate-induced panic in both patients with "primary" panic disorder (i.e., only panic disorder, or panic attacks and agoraphobia) and those with secondary panic disorder (i.e., primary depression associated with panic attacks). Thus, the lactate infusion test might not be specific for patients with only a primary panic disorder. Other provocative tests of panic disorder include patient challenge with such substances as carbon dioxide, isoproterenol, β-carboline, yohimbine, and caffeine. All of these tests remain research tools at this time.

ADDITIONAL RESEARCH DIAGNOSTIC STUDIES IN PSYCHIATRY

Polysomnography

Polysomnography, besides having demonstrated utility in the evaluation of sleep disorders (e.g., narcolepsy, sleep apneas), has also been used in the search for potential biological markers of psychiatric disorder. An interesting example of a research finding in this area includes the report by Kupfer et al. (1978) of an increase in the overall amount of rapid eye movement (REM) sleep and a shortened REM latency period in patients with major depression. Polysomnographic findings in schizophrenia include reports of decreased amounts of stages 2, 3, and 4 sleep (Grebb et al. 1986).

Neuro-Ophthalmological Markers

The study of unusual eye movement patterns found more commonly among psychiatric patients than among psychiatrically normal control subjects has also been an area of research for potential biological markers. One measure of an abnormal voluntary eye movement has been the evaluation of smooth pursuit eye movement (SPEM). The SPEM abnormality consists of a larger number of jerky eye movements (saccades) during the tracking of a smoothly moving object. Various eye-tracking tasks and recording techniques have been used. SPEM dysfunction has been reported in up to 85% of schizophrenic patients, 40% of bipolar patients, and about 8% of the psychiatrically normal population (Holzman 1985; Holzman et al. 1984).

Computerized Electroencephalography and Evoked Potential

In computerized EEG and evoked potential mapping, computers are used to amass and process large quantities of electrophysiological data. The computers analyze the data in various ways and graphically present the data in two-dimensional, color-coded maps of brain electrical activity. The brain electrical activity is measured in a manner similar to that used in the conventional EEG, although extra scalp electrode positions might be employed to augment the conventional International 10-20 system of electrode placement depending on the type of computerized topographic system employed. Computerized topographic systems can generally display data within a graphic outline of the head as if viewed from above or in profile. (Separate maps for the left and right hemispheres are produced.) Computerized EEG and EP have yet to demonstrate clear clinical utility in the diagnosis of classical psychiatric illnesses such as schizophrenia and major depression, and they are most appropriately considered research tools at this time. Research investigations using computerized EEG and EP approaches have added to the body of evidence suggesting brain abnormalities in schizophrenia (Morihisa 1990).

Although this brain-imaging technique has high chronological resolution (a window measured in milliseconds for evoked potentials), it is limited by a relatively poor spatial resolution for data collected from electrodes placed on the scalp and by vulnerability to a variety of artifacts (e.g., medication, muscle, and eye movement artifacts). However, ongoing advances in computer applications and the use of specialized test paradigms may enhance the utility of this research approach.

Magnetoencephalography

Magnetoencephalography (MEG) is a technique for measuring brain electrical activity (Lopes da Silva and Van Rotterdam 1982). The MEG exploits the fact that the electrical activity of the neurons of the brain generates very weak magnetic fields. When a very sensitive instrument is used to measure these generated magnetic fields, the magnetic energy is converted back into an electrical signal. The detection of these very weak fields currently requires the use of a super quantum interference device (SQUID) that must be cooled to 260°C.

The MEG can measure electrical activity in all areas of the brain (e.g., both cortical and subcortical brain tissues), in contrast to the conventional EEG and computerized EEG and EP, which are thought to reflect largely cortical surface electrical activity. The MEG is totally noninvasive, and the patient is exposed to no gamma or X irradiation. Despite innovative investigations, major advances in the widespread application of this approach in psychiatric research may need to await significant refinements in MEG technology.

CONCLUSIONS

The use of laboratory and diagnostic tests in psychiatry is a rapidly evolving area. This process is most clear in the evaluation of possible organic disorders of the CNS in psychiatric patients as well as in patients who are beginning or continuing treatment with a psychotropic medication. However, controversies exist concerning the extent to which screening batteries should be employed in psychiatric patients who do not have signs or symptoms of an organic condition, as well as the exact clinical utility of some psychotropic drug levels. Nevertheless, regardless of the type or number of tests used, the clinician should be sensitive to the fact that many of these tests are associated with varying degrees of discomfort, expense, and risk of adverse effects. In addition, abnormal laboratory results can at times lead to other procedures that might be associated with unnecessary danger and expense. Good clinical judgment needs to be the final arbiter when choosing any laboratory or other diagnostic tests for a particular patient.

No biological markers for any classical psychiatric disorders (such as major depression, schizophrenia, or bipolar disorder) have yet been demonstrated as having a clearly defined utility in routine clinical practice. Nevertheless, psychiatrists and clinical neuroscientists continue their search for biological markers that will be useful to clinicians in making diagnostic, treatment, and prognostic determinations for psychiatric patients. The promise of research involving potential biological markers is that they may help elucidate the underlying pathophysiology of psychiatric illness, suggest useful new diagnostic approaches and subtyping strategies, and lead to more efficacious

treatment approaches. However, while rapidly evolving technical advances have provided a wealth of new data, many new challenges in the areas of managing and interpreting this information have been created. Innovative software developments (e.g., Andreasen et al. 1992) have extended the utility of many of these techniques. However, major advances in new technologies, such as MRS and fMRI, represent a new leading edge in the normal maturational process of applying brain imaging techniques to psychiatry.

CAVEATS

When assessing research reports in brain imaging and laboratory testing it is useful to view the findings as only statistically significant. Often these abnormalities are subtle and can only be appreciated when a group of patients are compared to a group of matched controls. The findings should therefore be seen primarily as possible evidence that the measured phenomenon is relevant to the specific disease process. These exciting investigational achievements through laboratory and brain-imaging research, however, have not as yet been able to provide an innovative new basis for the diagnostic categorization of classical psychiatric disorders such as schizophrenia and unipolar depression. Indeed, we have not yet even achieved incremental validity. In other words, there is as yet no definitive evidence that any psychiatric laboratory test or brain-imaging measure can provide a clearly incremental improvement to the existent approach to the clinical diagnosis of classical psychiatric illnesses (Morihisa 1991). (This caveat, of course, excludes the important use of these tests to rule out or identify organic processes such as are associated with classical neurological disorders—e.g., dementia, CNS neoplasms, and demyelinating disorders—endocrine disorders, or general medical disorders, as well as the workup and monitoring of biological therapies). Further, one of the most significant obstacles in psychiatric research in this area is our inadequate investigation and understanding of the range of normal brain function. For example, the finding in normal adults of gender differences in resting regional cerebral glucose metabolism (R. C. Gur et al. 1995) has significant ramifications for the interpretation of functional studies of psychiatric disorders.

Finally, the danger exists that if immature technology is too quickly embraced, frustration and possibly premature abandonment of such technology will occur (Morihisa 1990). Indeed, the recent developmental evolution of the field of immunology may provide an instructive warning against any expectation of quick, clear, and concise clinical applications. The explosion of research investigations in the immunological sciences has led to a rapidly expanding knowledge base concerning disease processes, which has made the clinical practice of medicine far more complex and demanding rather than providing simplification or rapid definitive therapeutic interventions (Morihisa 1991). In a similar fashion, we should expect that findings in the clinical neurosciences will raise far more questions in the short run than they will provide immediate, clear resolution of vexing diagnostic and therapeutic challenges.

REFERENCES

Allen CB, Davis BM, Davis KL: Psychoendocrinology in clinical psychiatry, in American Psychiatric Association Annual Review, Vol 6. Edited by Hales RE, Frances AJ. Washington, DC, American Psychiatric Press, 1987, pp 188–209

Amdisen A: Monitoring lithium dose levels: clinical aspects of serum lithium estimation, in Handbook of Lithium Therapy. Edited by Johnson FN. Lancaster, UK, MTP Press, 1980, p 179

American Psychiatric Association Task Force on the Use of Laboratory Tests in Psychiatry: Tricyclic antidepressants-blood level measurements and clinical outcome: an APA Task Force report. Am J Psychiatry 142:155–162, 1985

American Psychiatric Association: Diagnostic and Statistical Manual of Mental Disorders, 4th Edition. Washington, DC, American Psychiatric Association, 1994

Andreasen NC, Cohen G, Harris G, et al: Image processing for the study of brain structure and function: problems and programs. Journal of Neuropsychiatry and Clinical Neurosciences 4:125–133, 1992

Andreasen, NC, Flashman L, Flaum M: Regional brain abnormalities in schizophrenia measured with magnetic resonance imaging. JAMA 272:1768–1769, 1994

Arana GW, Baldessarini RJ, Ornsteen M: The dexamethasone suppression test for diagnosis and prognosis in psychiatry: commentary and review. Arch Gen Psychiatry 42:1193–1204, 1985

Asaad G, Shapiro B: Hallucinations: theoretical and clinical overview. Am J Psychiatry 143:1088–1097, 1986

Asberg M, Träskman C, Thorén P: 5-HIAA in the cerebrospinal fluid: a biochemical suicide predictor? Arch Gen Psychiatry 33:1193–1197, 1976

Beresford TP, Wilson F, Hall RCW, et al: Q-T prolongation in psychiatric outpatients. Psychosomatics 27:497–500, 1986

Bertolino A, Nawroz S, Mattay V, et al: Regionally specific pattern of neurochemical pathology in schizophrenia as assessed by multislice proton magnetic resonance spectroscopic imaging. Am J Psychiatry 153:1554–1563, 1996

Bertolino A, Callicott JH, Elman I, et al: Regionally specific neuronal pathology in untreated patients with schizophrenia: a proton magnetic resonance spectroscopic imaging study. Biol Psychiatry 43:641–648, 1998

Boehnert MT, Lovejoy FH: Value of the QRS duration versus the serum drug level in predicting seizures and ventricular arrhythmias after an acute overdose of tricyclic antidepressants. N Engl J Med 313:474–479, 1985

Bradley WE, Timm GW, Gallagher JM, et al: New method for continuous measurement of nocturnal penile tumescence and rigidity. Urology 26:4–9, 1985

Brown WA, Laughren T: Serum neuroleptic levels in the maintenance treatment of schizophrenia. Psychopharmacol Bull 19:76–78, 1983

Buchsbaum MS: The middle evoked response components and schizophrenia. Schizophr Bull 3:93–104, 1977

Buchsbaum MS: Brain imaging in the search for biological markers in affective disorder. J Clin Psychiatry 47 (no 10, suppl):7–10, 1986

Buchsbaum MS, DeLisi LE, Holcomb HH, et al: Anteroposterior gradients in cerebral glucose use in schizophrenia and affective disorders. Arch Gen Psychiatry 41:1159–1166, 1984

Carroll BJ: Dexamethasone suppression test, in Handbook of Psychiatric Diagnostic Procedures, Vol 1. Edited by Hall RCW, Beresford TP. New York, SP Medical and Scientific Books, 1984, pp 3–28

Carroll BJ: Informed use of the dexamethasone suppression test. J Clin Psychiatry 47 (no 1, suppl):10–12, 1986

Cho JT, Bone S, Dunner DL, et al: The effect of lithium treatment on thyroid function in patients with primary affective disorder. Am J Psychiatry 136:115–116, 1979

Coffman JA: Computed tomography in psychiatry, in Brain Imaging: Applications in Psychiatry. Edited by Andreasen NC. Washington, DC, American Psychiatric Press, 1989, pp 1–65

Cowdry RW, Wehr TA, Zis AP, et al: Thyroid abnormalities associated with rapid-cycling bipolar illness. Arch Gen Psychiatry 40:414–420, 1983

Cowley DS, Dager SR, Dunner DL: Lactate-induced panic in primary affective disorder. Am J Psychiatry 143:646–648, 1986

Creese I, Synder SH: A simple and sensitive radioreceptor assay for antischizophrenic drugs in blood. Nature 270:180–182, 1977

David A, Blamire A, Breiter H: Functional magnetic resonance imaging (editorial). Br J Psychiatry 164:2–7, 1994

Davis JM, Bresnahan DB: Psychopharmacology in clinical psychiatry, in American Psychiatric Association Annual Review, Vol 6. Edited by Hales RE, Frances AJ. Washington, DC, American Psychiatric Press, 1987, pp 159–187

de la Monte SM, Volcier L, Hauser SL, et al: Increased levels of neuronal thread protein in cerebrospinal fluid of patients with Alzheimer's disease. Ann Neurol 32:733–742, 1992

DeLisi LE: Use of the clinical laboratory, in Biomedical Psychiatric Therapeutics. Edited by Sullivan JL, Sullivan PD. Boston, MA, Butterworth Publishers, pp 89–119, 1984

Dolan JG, Mushlin AI: Routine laboratory testing for medical disorders in psychiatric inpatients. Arch Intern Med 145:2085–2088, 1985

Dvoredsky AE, Cooley HW: Comparative severity of illness in patients with combined medical and psychiatric diagnoses. Psychosomatics 27:625–630, 1986

Emsley RA, Gledhill RF, Bell PSH, et al: Indications for CAT scans of psychiatric patients (letter). Am J Psychiatry 143:1199, 1986

Expert Consensus Panel for Bipolar Disorder: Treatment of Bipolar Disorder. J Clin Psychiatry 57 (suppl 12A), 1996a

Expert Consensus Panel for Schizophrenia: Treatment of Schizophrenia. J Clin Psychiatry 57 (suppl 12B), 1996b

Extein I, Pottash ALC, Gold MS: Thyrotropin-releasing hormone test in the diagnosis of unipolar depressives. Psychiatry Res 5:311–316, 1981

Feinsilver DL: Psychiatric diagnostic procedures in the emergency department, in Handbook of Psychiatric Diagnostic Procedures, Vol 1. Edited by Hall RCW, Beresford TP. New York, SP Medical and Scientific Books, 1984, pp 315–330

Flugelman MY, Tal A, Pollack S, et al: Psychotropic drugs and long QT syndromes: case reports. J Clin Psychiatry 46:290–291, 1985

Fogel BS, Faust D: Neurologic assessment, neurodiagnostic tests, and neuropsychiatry in medical psychiatry, in Principles of Medical Psychiatry. Edited by Stoudemire A, Fogel BS. Orlando, FL, Grune and Stratton, 1987, pp 37–77

Gabel RH, Barnard N, Norko M, et al: AIDS presenting as mania. Compr Psychiatry 27:251–254, 1986

Garber HJ, Weinberg JB, Buonammo FS, et al: Use of magnetic resonance imaging in psychiatry. Am J Psychiatry 145:154–171, 1988

Gelenberg AJ: Laboratory tests for patients taking psychotropic drugs. Massachusetts General Hospital Newsletter 6:5–7, 1983

Gelenberg AJ: Carbamazepine (Tegretol) for manic depressive illness: an update. Massachusetts General Hospital Newsletter 8:21–24, 1985

Giannini AJ, Black HR, Goettsche RL: Psychiatric Psychogenic and Somatopsychotic Disorders Handbook. Garden City, NY, Medical Examination Publishing, 1978

Gold MS, Dackis CA: Role of the laboratory in the evaluation of suspected drug abuse. J Clin Psychiatry 47 (no 1, suppl):17–23, 1986

Gold PW, Loriaux DL, Roy A, et al: Response to corticotropin-releasing hormone in the hypercortisolism of depression and Cushing's disease: physiologic and diagnostic implications. N Engl J Med 314:1329–1335, 1986

Goodin DS, Aminoff MJ: Does the interictal EEG have a role in the diagnosis of epilepsy? Lancet 1:837–839, 1984

Grebb JA, Weinberger DR, Morihisa JM: Electroencephalogram and evoked potential studies of schizophrenia, in Handbook of Schizophrenia, Vol 1: The Neurology of Schizophrenia. Edited by Nasrallah HA, Weinberger DR. Amsterdam, Elsevier, 1986, pp 121–140

Gur RE, Resnick JM, Alavi A, et al: Regional brain function in schizophrenia, I: a positron emission tomography study. Arch Gen Psychiatry 44:119–125, 1987

Gur RC, Mozley LH, Mozley PD, et al: Sex differences in regional cerebral glucose metabolism during a resting state. Science 267:528–531, 1995

Gur RE, Mozley PD, Resnick SM, et al: Resting cerebral glucose metabolism in first-episode and previously treated patients with schizophrenia relates to clinical features. Arch Gen Psychiatry 52:657–667, 1995

Gusella JF, Tanzi RE, Anderson MA, et al: DNA markers for nervous system diseases. Science 225:1320–1326, 1984

Guze BH: Magnetic resonance spectroscopy: a technique for functional brain imaging. Arch Gen Psychiatry 48:572–574, 1991

Hales RE: The diagnosis and treatment of psychiatric disorders in medically ill patients. Mil Med 151:587–595, 1986

Hall RCW, Beresford TP: Laboratory evaluation of newly admitted psychiatric patients, in Handbook of Psychiatry Diagnostic Procedures, Vol 1. Edited by Hall RCW, Beresford TP. New York, SP Medical and Scientific Books, 1984, pp 255–314

Hall RCW, Popkin MK, Devaul RA, et al: Physical illness presenting as psychiatric disease. Arch Gen Psychiatry 35:1315–1320, 1978

Hall RCW, Gardner ER, Stickney SK, et al: Physical illness manifesting as psychiatric disease, II: analysis of a state hospital inpatient population. Arch Gen Psychiatry 37:989–995, 1980

Hart RG, Easton JD: Carbamazepine and hematological monitoring. Ann Neurol 11:309–312, 1982

Hoffman RS, Koran LM: Detecting physical illness in patients with mental disorders. Psychosomatics 25:654–660, 1984

Holzman PS: Eye movement dysfunctions and psychosis. Int Rev Neurobiol 27:179–205, 1985

Holzman PS, Solomon CM, Levin S, et al: Pursuit eye movement dysfunctions in schizophrenia: family evidence for specificity. Arch Gen Psychiatry 41:136–139, 1984

Ingvar DH, Franzen G: Abnormalities of cerebral blood flow distribution in patients with chronic schizophrenia. Acta Psychiatr Scand 50:425–462, 1974

Jacobson HG: Magnetic resonance imaging of the central nervous system: Council on Scientific Affairs Report of the Panel on Magnetic Resonance Imaging. JAMA 259:1211–1222, 1988

Jaskiw GE, Andreasen NC, Weinberger DR: X-ray computed tomography and magnetic resonance imaging in psychiatry, in American Psychiatric Association Annual Review, Vol 6. Edited by Hales RE, Frances AJ. Washington, DC, American Psychiatric Press, 1987, pp 260–299

Jefferson JW, Greist JH, Ackerman DC: Lithium Encyclopedia for Clinical Practice, 2nd Edition. Washington, DC, American Psychiatric Press, 1987

Jenike MA: Should lumbar puncture be part of the workup for dementia? Massachusetts General Hospital Newsletter: Topics in Geriatrics 4:21–23, 1985

Jensen M, Basun H, Lannfelt L: Increased cerebrospinal fluid tau in patients with Alzheimer's disease. Neurosci Lett 186:189–191, 1995

Johnston EC, Crow TJ, Frith CD, et al: Cerebral ventricular size and cognitive impairment in schizophrenia. Lancet 2:924–926, 1976

Karasu TB, Waltzman SA, Lindenmayer J-P, et al: The medical care of patients with psychiatric illness. Hosp Community Psychiatry 31:463–472, 1980

Keshavan MS, Kapur S, Pettegrew JW: Magnetic resonance spectroscopy in psychiatry: potential, pitfalls, and promise. Am J Psychiatry 148:976–985, 1991

Ketter TA, George MS, Ring AA: Primary mood disorders: structural and resting functional studies. Psychiatric Annals 24(12):637–642, 1994

Knable MB, Jones DW, Coppola R, et al: Lateralized differences in iodine-123-IBZM uptake in the basal ganglia in asymmetric Parkinson's disease. J Nucl Med 36:1216–1225, 1995

Kocsis JH, Hanin I, Bowden C, et al: Imipramine and amitriptyline plasma concentrations and clinical response in major depression. Br J Psychiatry 148:52–57, 1986

Kolman PBR: Predicting the results of routine laboratory tests in elderly psychiatric patients admitted to hospital. J Clin Psychiatry 46:532–534, 1985

Koranyi EK: Morbidity and rate of undiagnosed physical illnesses in a psychiatric clinic population. Arch Gen Psychiatry 36:414–419, 1979

Kupfer DJ, Foster FG, Coble P, et al: The application of EEG sleep for the differential diagnosis of affective disorders. Am J Psychiatry 135:69–74, 1978

Larson EB, Reifler BV, Sumi SM, et al: Diagnostic tests in the evaluation of dementia: a prospective study of 200 elderly outpatients. Arch Intern Med 146:1917–1922, 1986

Liebowitz MR, Gorman JM, Fyer AJ, et al: Lactate provocation of panic attacks, II: biochemical and physiological findings. Arch Gen Psychiatry 42:709–719, 1985

Loosen PT, Prange AJ Jr: Serum thyrotropin response to thyrotropin-releasing hormone in psychotic patients: a review. Am J Psychiatry 139:405–416, 1982

Lopes da Silva F, Van Rotterdam A: Biophysical aspects of EEG and MEG generation, in Electroencephalography: Basic Principles: Clinical Applications and Related Fields. Edited by Niedermeyer E, Lopes da Silva F. Baltimore, MD, Urban and Schwarzenberg, 1982, pp 15–26

Meltzer HY, Kolakowska T, Fang VS, et al: Growth hormone and prolactin response to apomorphine in schizophrenia and the major affective disorders: relation to duration of illness and depressive symptoms. Arch Gen Psychiatry 41:512–519, 1984

Morihisa JM: Brain-imaging approaches in psychiatry: early developmental considerations. J Clin Psychiatry 51 (no 1, suppl):44–46, 1990

Morihisa JM: Advances in neuroimaging technologies, in Medical Psychiatric Practice. Edited by Stoudemire A, Fogel BS. Washington, DC, American Psychiatric Press, 1991, pp 3–28

Morihisa JM, McAnulty GB: Structure and function: brain electrical activity mapping and computed tomography in schizophrenia. Biol Psychiatry 20:3–19, 1985

Morihisa JM, Weinberger DR: Is schizophrenia a frontal lobe disease? an organizing theory of relevant anatomy and physiology, in Can Schizophrenia Be Localized in the Brain? Edited by Andreasen NC. Washington, DC, American Psychiatric Press, 1986, pp 17–36

Muscettola G, Potter WZ, Pickar D, et al: Urinary 3-methoxy-4-hydroxyphenylglycol and major affective disorders: a replication and new findings. Arch Gen Psychiatry 41:337–342, 1984

Nasrallah HA, Jacoby CG, Chapman S, et al: Third ventricular enlargement on CT scans in schizophrenia: association with cerebellar atrophy. Biol Psychiatry 20:443–450, 1985

Nasrallah HA, Coffman, JA, Olson SC: Structural brain imaging findings in affective disorders: an overview. J Neuropsychiatry Clin Neurosci 1(1):21–26, 1989

National Institute on Aging/Alzheimer's Association Working Group: Apolipoprotein E genotyping in Alzheimer's disease. Lancet 347:1091–1095, 1996

National Institute on Aging Task Force: Senility reconsidered: treatment possibilities for mental impairment in the elderly. JAMA 244:259–263, 1980

Nelson TC, Burritt MF: Pesticide poisoning, succinylcholine-induced apnea, and pseudocholinesterase. Mayo Clin Proc 61:750–755, 1986

Nemeroff CB, Evans DL: Correlation between the dexamethasone suppression test in depressed patients and clinical response. Am J Psychiatry 141:247–249, 1984

Nunez PL: Electric Fields of the Brain: The Neuroleptics of EEG. New York, Oxford University Press, 1981

Pearlson GD, Garbacz DJ, Breakey WR, et al: Lateral ventricular enlargement associated with persistent unemployment and negative symptoms in both schizophrenia and bipolar disorder. Psychiatry Res 12:1–9, 1984

Perry S, Jacobsen P: Neuropsychiatric manifestations of AIDS-spectrum disorders. Hosp Community Psychiatry 37:135–142, 1986

Pettegrew JW, Keshavan MS, Panchalingam K, et al: Alterations in brain high-energy phosphate and membrane phospholipid metabolism in first-episode, drug-naive schizophrenics: a pilot study of the dorsal prefrontal cortex by in vivo phosphorus 31 nuclear magnetic resonance spectroscopy. Arch Gen Psychiatry 48:563–568, 1991

Physicians' Desk Reference, 52nd Edition. Montvale, NJ, Medical Economics Company, 1998

Pirttila T, Kim KS, Mehta PD, et al: Soluble amyloid beta-protein in the cerebrospinal fluid from patients with Alzheimer's disease, vascular dementia and controls. J Neurol Sci 127: 90–95, 1994

Post RM: Clinical approaches to the treatment resistant manic and depressive patient, in Psychopharmacology in Practice: Clinical and Research Update 1984. Bethesda, MD, Foundation for Advanced Education in the Sciences, 1984, pp 23–54

Pryse-Phillips W, Murray TJ: Essential Neurology, 3rd Edition. New York, Medical Examination Publishing Company, 1986

Rainey JM Jr, Nesse RM: Psychobiology of anxiety and anxiety disorders. Psychiatr Clin North Am 8:133–144, 1985

Ramani V, Loewenson RB, Torres F: The limited usefulness of nasopharyngeal EEG recording in psychiatric patients. Am J Psychiatry 142:1099–1100, 1985

Ramsey NF, Kirby BS, Gelderen PV, et al: Functional mapping of human sensorimotor cortex with 3D BOLD fMRI correlates highly with H_2 ^{15}O PET and CBF. J Cereb Blood Flow Metab 16:755–764, 1996

Reiman EM, Caselli RJ, Yun LS, et al: Preclinical evidence of Alzheimer's disease in persons homozygous for the episolon 4 allele for apolipoprotein E. N Engl J Med 334: 752–758, 1996

Rosse RB, Giese AA, Deutsch SI, et al: Concise guide to laboratory and diagnostic testing in psychiatry. Washington, DC, American Psychiatric Press, 1989

Roth WT: Late event-related potentials and psychopathology. Schizophr Bull 3:105–120, 1977

Roy A, Pickar D, Doran A, et al: The corticotropin-releasing hormone stimulation test in chronic schizophrenia. Am J Psychiatry 143:1393–1397, 1986

Roy-Byrne PP, Uhde TW, Rubinow DR, et al: Reduced TSH and prolactin response to TRH in patients with panic disorder. Am J Psychiatry 143:503–507, 1986

Sakauye KM: A model for administration of electroconvulsive therapy. Hosp Community Psychiatry 37:785–788, 1986

Samson JA, Mirin SM, Hauser ST, et al: Learned helplessness and urinary MHPG levels in unipolar depression. Am J Psychiatry 149:806–809, 1992

Schatzberg AF, Cole JO, DeBattista C: Manual of Clinical Psychopharmacology, 3rd Edition. Washington, DC, American Psychiatric Press, Washington, DC, 1997

Schildkraut JJ, Orsulak PJ, Schatzberg AF, et al: Toward a biochemical classification of depressive disorders, I: differences in urinary excretion of MHPG and other catecholamine metabolites in clinically defined subtypes of depressions. Arch Gen Psychiatry 35:1427–1433, 1978

Schwartz P, Wolf S: QT interval prolongation as prediction of sudden death in patients with myocardial infarction. Circulation 57:1074–1077, 1978

Shagass C: Early evoked potentials. Schizophr Bull 3:80–92, 1977

Simpson GM, Pi EH, White K: Plasma drug levels and clinical response to antidepressants. J Clin Psychiatry 44 (no 5, sec 2):27–34, 1983

Sox HC Jr, Koran LM, Sox CH, et al: A medical algorithm for detecting physical disease in psychiatric patients. Hospital and Community Psychiatry 40:1270–1276, 1989

Sramek JJ, Baumgartner WA, Tallos JA, et al: Hair analysis for detection of phencyclidine in newly admitted psychiatric patients. Am J Psychiatry 142:950–953, 1985

Steffens DC, Krishnan KRR: Structural neuroimaging and mood disorders: recent findings, implications for classification, and future directions. Biol Psychiatry 43:705–712, 1998

Sternberg DE: Testing for physical illness in psychiatric patients. J Clin Psychiatry 47 (no 1, suppl):3–9, 1986

Suddath RL, Casanova MF, Goldberg TE, et al: Temporal lobe pathology in schizophrenia: a quantitative magnetic resonance imaging study. Am J Psychiatry 46:464–472, 1989

Suddath RL, Christison GW, Torrey EF: Cerebral anatomical abnormalities in monozygotic twins discordant for schizophrenia. N Engl J Med 322:789–94, 1990

Tamminga CA, Thaker GK, Buchanan R, et al: Limbic system abnormalities identified in schizophrenia using positron emission tomography with fluorodeoxyglucose and neocortical alterations with deficit syndrome. Arch Gen Psychiatry 49:522–530, 1992

Targum SD, Greenberg RD, Harmon RL, et al: Thyroid hormone and the TRH stimulation test in refractory depression. J Clin Psychiatry 45:345–346, 1984

Targum SD, Marshall LE, Fischman P: Variability of TRH test responses in depressed and normal elderly subjects. Biol Psychiatry 31:787–793, 1992

Thase ME, Reynolds CF, Glanz LM, et al: Nocturnal penile tumescence in depressed men. Am J Psychiatry 144:89–92, 1987

Van Putten T, Marder SR, Mintz J, et al: Haloperidol plasma levels and clinical response: a therapeutic window relationship. Am J Psychiatry 149:500–505, 1992

Weinberger DR: Brain disease and psychiatric illness: when should a psychiatrist order a CAT scan? Am J Psychiatry 141:1521–1527, 1984

Weinberger DR: Implications of normal brain development for the pathogenesis of schizophrenia. Arch Gen Psychiatry 44:660–669, 1987

Weinberger DR: From neuropathology to neurodevelopment. Lancet 346:552–557, 1995

Weinberger DR, Torrey EF, Neophytides AN, et al: Lateral cerebral ventricular enlargement in chronic schizophrenia. Arch Gen Psychiatry 36:735–739, 1979

Weinberger DR, Berman KF, Zec RF: Physiologic dysfunction of dorsolateral prefrontal cortex in schizophrenia, I: regional cerebral blood flow evidence. Arch Gen Psychiatry 43:114–124, 1986

Weinberger DR, Berman KF, Suddath R, et al: Evidence of dysfunction of a prefrontal-limbic network in schizophrenia: a magnetic resonance imaging and regional cerebral blood flow study of discordant monozygotic twins. Am J Psychiatry 149:890–897, 1992a

Weinberger DR, Jones D, Reba RC, et al: A comparison of FDG PET and IQNB SPECT in normal subjects and in patients with dementia. J Neuropsychiatry Clin Neurosci 4:239–248, 1992b

Williams W: Psychogenic erectile impotence a useful or a misleading concept? Aust N Z J Psychiatry 19:77–82, 1985

Wolkin A, Jaeger J, Brodie JD, et al: Persistence of cerebral metabolic abnormalities in chronic schizophrenia as determined by positron emission tomography. Am J Psychiatry 142:564–571, 1985

Wong DF, Wagner HN, Tune LE, et al: Positron emission tomography reveals elevated D2 dopamine receptors in drug-naive schizophrenics. Science 234:1558–1563, 1986

SECTION III

PSYCHIATRIC DISORDERS

CHAPTER 10

DELIRIUM, DEMENTIA, AND AMNESTIC DISORDERS

MICHAEL G. WISE, M.D.
KEVIN F. GRAY, M.D.
BENJAMIN SELTZER, M.D.

DELIRIUM

Delirium was one of the first mental disorders described in medicine and is the most common psychiatric syndrome found in a general medical hospital (Lipowski 1990). It is especially common among elderly persons who are hospitalized (Francis 1992). The presence of delirium signifies impending death in 25% of identified cases (Rabins and Folstein 1982). In addition, patients with dementia or brain damage have a lower threshold for developing delirium and do so with greater frequency (Lipowski 1990; Miller et al. 1991; O'Keeffe and Lavan 1997). Although it is commonly seen by physicians and is associated with high mortality and morbidity, delirium remains an under-recognized, underresearched phenomenon (Inouye 1994).

A conceptual overview of delirium is presented in Figure 10–1. A large number of diverse physiological insults can produce the delirium syndrome. Delirium can manifest clinically as a hypoactive state (i.e., decreased arousal and psychomotor activity), a hyperactive state (i.e., increased arousal and psychomotor activity), or a mixed form with fluctuations between hypoactive and hyperactive states. Accurate identification of the cause or causes for the delirium must precede treatment. Without proper diagnosis and treatment, the prognosis for patients with delirium is poor.

DEFINITION

More than 30 diagnostic terms have been used to describe this clinical syndrome (Francis 1992). In addition, the diagnostic criteria for delirium have changed several times since DSM-I was first published in 1952 (American Psychiatric Association 1952). In DSM-I and DSM-II (American Psychiatric Association 1968), the categorization was "acute [reversible] organic brain syndrome" of either a psychotic or a nonpsychotic type. In DSM-III (American Psychiatric Association 1980), delirium was grouped with other "global" disorders of cognitive function, such as dementia, and its core or essential features were listed as "clouding of consciousness" and "disorientation and memory impairment." In DSM-III-R (American Psychiatric Association 1987), the core aspect of the diagnosis was changed to "reduced ability to maintain attention to external stimuli" and "disorganized thinking" (p.103). In the most recent diagnostic manual, DSM-IV (American Psychiatric Association 1994), the diagnostic criteria

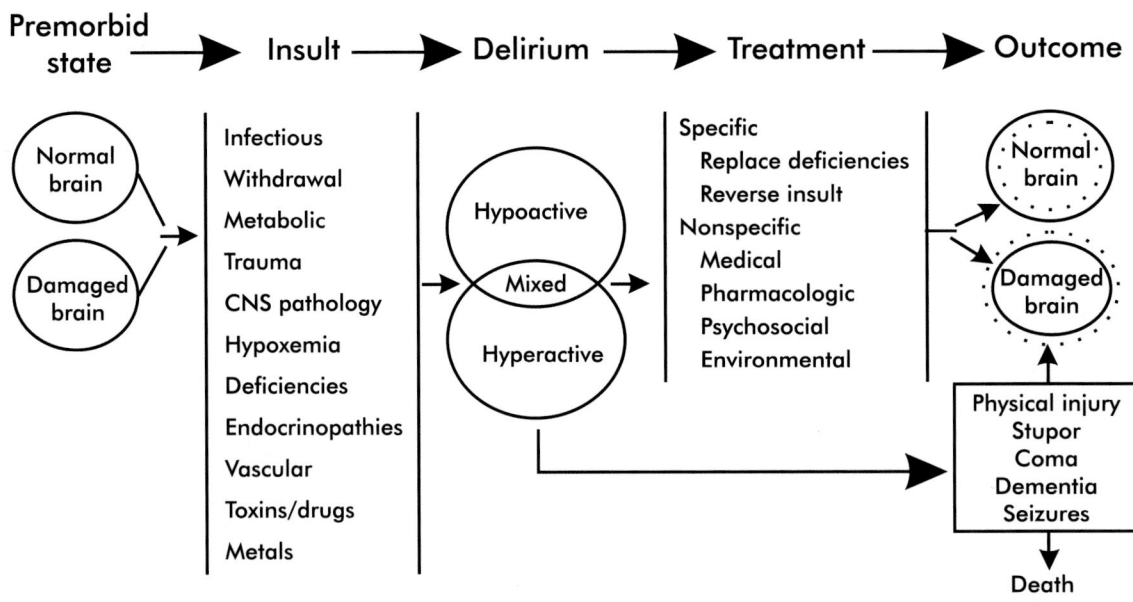

FIGURE 10–1.   Conceptual overview of delirium.

(Table 10–1) again were altered, and reduced level of consciousness (difficulty keeping awake), sleep disturbance, psychomotor changing, and disorganized thinking were eliminated from the list of criteria.

In DSM-IV, like its predecessors, different clinical presentations (i.e., hypoactive, hyperactive, and mixed states) are considered aspects of one entity called delirium. This conceptualization is not accepted by some physicians, who believe that the diagnosis of delirium should be reserved for confused patients with agitation, autonomic instability, and hallucinations (Adams and Victor 1989). Delirium tremens (DTs) is used as the model for delirium.

TABLE 10–1.   DSM-IV diagnostic criteria for delirium caused by a general medical condition

A. Disturbance of consciousness (i.e., reduced clarity of awareness of the environment) with reduced ability to focus, sustain, or shift attention.

B. Change in cognition (such as memory deficit, disorientation, language disturbance, perceptual disturbance) that is not better accounted for by a preexisting, established, or evolving dementia.

C. The disturbance develops over a short period of time (usually hours to days) and tends to fluctuate during the course of the day.

D. There is evidence from the history, physical examination, or laboratory findings of a general medical condition judged to be etiologically related to the disturbance.

Patients who acutely become quietly confused, incoherent, and disoriented, but without autonomic instability and hallucinations, would be diagnosed with an "acute confusional state," not delirium. These classification disparities are rooted in the history and evolution of the concept of delirium (Berrios 1981; Lipowski 1980b, 1990).

Pending further research, it seems appropriate to consider both hyperactive and hypoactive presentations as forms of a single syndrome, delirium. This unified concept received early support from the pioneering research of Engel and Romano (1959), who hypothesized that the delirium syndrome was caused by a metabolic derangement of central nervous system function. Several other aspects of the syndrome deserve mention. Delirium typically has a sudden onset and a brief duration, and it is usually reversible, although individual symptoms of delirium may linger (Levkoff et al. 1992; Rockwood 1993). Therefore, delirium is herein defined as *a transient, usually reversible dysfunction in the cerebral nervous system that has an acute or subacute onset and is manifest clinically by a wide array of neuropsychiatric abnormalities.*

EPIDEMIOLOGY

Past research was confounded by the following: 1) lack of diagnostic criteria before the publication of DSM-III in 1980; 2) changing diagnostic criteria since 1980; 3) lack of reliable tools to ascertain the diagnosis; 4) studies of heterogeneous populations in which individual risk factors for delirium, such as dementia or age, were not considered;

5) studies that relied on retrospective chart review; and 6) missed diagnoses owing to the patient's lucidity when examined (rapid fluctuations in cognitive status are typical of delirium). Although more recent prospective studies using instruments specifically designed to evaluate delirium have improved the understanding of this syndrome, much research remains to be done (Inouye 1994).

Incidence and Prevalence

The frequency of delirium found within a particular population depends on the predisposition of the individuals within that population. It has been estimated that 10%–15% of patients on acute medical and surgical wards have delirium (Engel 1967). The increasing age of the population may make this estimate low (Lipowski 1990). The diagnostic criteria for delirium in DSM-III, although difficult to operationalize, and those in DSM-III-R provide more reliable guidelines for research. As a result, the literature now contains numerous prospective studies that provide data on the prevalence and incidence of delirium in hospitalized medically ill and surgical patients (Table 10–2).

Predisposing Factors

Certain groups of patients are at increased risk to develop delirium. These include: 1) the elderly, 2) individuals recovering from surgery, 3) burn patients, 4) patients with preexisting brain dysfunction (e.g., dementia, stroke), 5) patients with drug dependency who are experiencing withdrawal, 6) patients with acquired immune deficiency syndrome (AIDS), and 7) those with high illness burden (Table 10–3). Individual patients may have multiple risk factors for developing delirium (e.g., an elderly, cognitively impaired patient recovering from surgery). Advancing age increases the risk of delirium, with an age of 60 or older usually cited as associated with the highest risk (Francis 1992; Lipowski 1980a, 1990). In a study of the natural history of mental disorders in older people, Sir Martin Roth (1955) reported acute confusional states in 7.5% of psychiatric patients ages 60–69, 9% of those ages 70–79, and 12% of those older than 80. A recent review of delirium in elderly patients attributes the increased frequency of delirium in the elderly to severe medical illness, impaired physical function, chronic brain disease, and increased numbers of medications (Francis 1992).

Delirium is a frequent finding in the postoperative state. Although the syndrome can follow any type of surgical procedure, postcardiotomy delirium has been investigated the most. Dubin et al. (1979), in a thorough review of postcardiotomy delirium, reported that the frequency across studies varied from 13% to 67%. A more recent study revealed a lower frequency of delirium: delirium developed in 8.6% of patients who received narcotic anesthesia and 5.6% who received barbiturate coma (Nussmeier et al. 1986). Although there is a generally held belief that the frequency of postcardiotomy delirium has declined with experience and improved technology, a meta-analysis of 44 studies revealed that the prevalence has remained constant at 32% (Smith and Dimsdale 1989).

TABLE 10–2. Epidemiology of delirium using DSM-III or DSM-III-R criteria

Reference	No. of patients	Type of patient	Frequency	Prevalence	Incidence
Erkinjuntti et al. (1986)	2,000	Medical, age 55 or older		15%	—
Cameron et al. (1987)	133	Medical, age 32 to 97		11.3%	4.2%
Gustafson et al. (1988)	111	Femoral neck fracture, age 65 or older			
		Before surgery	33%		
		After surgery	42%		
Rockwood (1989)	80	Medical, age 65 or older		16%	10.4%
Johnson et al. (1990)	235	Medical, age 70 or older		16%	5%
Francis et al. (1990)	229	Medical, age 70 or older		15.7%	7.3%
Schor et al. (1992)	325	Medical/surgical, age 65 or older		11%	31%
Rockwood (1993)	168	Geriatric		18%	7%
Marcantonio et al. (1994)	134	Post-surgical (elective non-cardiac)			9%
Pompei et al. (1994)[a]	432	Medical/surgical, age 65 or older		5%	10%
	323	Medical/surgical, age 70 or older		15%	12%
O'Keeffe (1997)	225	Acute-case geriatric		18%	29%

[a]Lower rates in this study may be explained by exclusion of patients with severe cognitive impairment.

TABLE 10–3. Patients with high risk for developing delirium

Elderly patients

Postcardiotomy patients

Burn patients

Patients with cognitive dysfunction

Patients in drug withdrawal

Patients with acquired immune deficiency syndrome (AIDS)

Patients with a high illness burden

In addition to increased age and preexisting brain dysfunction, the following factors may increase the risk of postcardiotomy delirium: time on bypass (Heller et al. 1970; Kornfeld et al. 1974), severity of postoperative illness (Kornfeld et al. 1974), serum levels of anticholinergic drugs (Tune et al. 1981), increased levels of central nervous system (CNS) adenylate kinase and subclinical brain injury (Aberg et al. 1984), decreased cardiac output (Blachly and Kloster 1966), complexity of the surgical procedure (Dubin et al. 1979), complement activation (Chenoweth et al. 1981), embolism (Nussmeier et al. 1986), and nutritional status as measured by albumin levels (Wise 1987). Despite these numerous potential organic etiologies, preoperative psychiatric interviews may reduce postoperative psychosis by 50% (Kornfeld et al. 1974; Layne and Yudofsky 1971). Smith and Dimsdale (1989) found that preoperative psychiatric intervention correlated with a decreasing occurrence of postcardiotomy delirium, which suggests that a preoperative psychiatric interview may offer some protection against delirium.

About 30% of adult burn patients have symptoms of delirium, and the "frequency increases with both the age of the patient and the severity of the burn" (Andreasen et al. 1972, p. 68). Other researchers have described an incidence of delirium in burn patients of 18% (Blank and Perry 1984) and an incidence of burn encephalopathy in children of 14% (Antoon et al. 1972). However, in the latter study, *burn encephalopathy* was defined as "neurologic disturbances ranging from hallucination, personality changes, and delirium to seizures and coma" (Antoon et al. 1972, p. 609), so that the frequency of delirium was probably lower.

The presence of preexisting brain damage, whether focal CNS neurological abnormalities (Folstein et al. 1991; Layne and Yudofsky 1971) or dementia, lowers the patient's threshold for developing delirium (Lipowski 1990). Koponen et al. (1989c) found that 81% of patients with delirium in their study had dementia. A 90% frequency of organic mental disorders was reported in patients with AIDS-associated delirium (Perry 1990), which is the most frequent neuropsychiatric complication of AIDS (Fernandez et al. 1989). In another study, 30%–40% of medically hospitalized patients with AIDS developed delirium (Brietbart et al. 1996). An additional risk factor for the development of delirium is the rapid withdrawal of a drug in a patient who is physiologically dependent; this is a particular risk in individuals who have chronically abused alcohol or benzodiazepines. Severe chronic illness, with its associated functional impairment, also predisposes patients to delirium. Numerous other risk factors for delirium have been postulated (Inouye 1994; Pompei et al. 1994).

A final consideration concerns the role of psychosocial factors, sensory deprivation, and sleep deprivation as predisposing factors to delirium (Inouye 1994; Rabins 1991). Sleep-wake abnormalities undoubtedly are common features of delirium, but how critical sleep deprivation is to the development of delirium remains an unanswered question. One study found that sleep disturbance developed after the score on the Mini-Mental Status Examination (MMSE) decreased (i.e., after the delirium developed) but not before (Harrell and Othmer 1987). The crucial issue in sensory deprivation and sensory overload may not be the quantity of stimuli but rather the quality. It is known, for example, that the electroencephalogram (EEG) of a subject exposed to monotonous stimuli shows more slowing than does the EEG of a sensory-deprived subject (Zubek and Welch 1963). Patients in an intensive care unit (ICU) do not lack stimulation; rather, they lack the kinds of stimuli that orient people to time and environment. Lipowski (1990) pointed out that "there is no evidence that sensory deprivation alone can cause delirium" (p. 128). Personality and psychological variables have been investigated as well, but no specific personality profile has been found to correlate with delirium (Dubin et al. 1979). Lipowski (1980a) agreed, reporting that "it may be stated that so far not a single psychological variable has been conclusively shown to predispose one to delirium" (p. 115).

CLINICAL FEATURES

Prodrome and Rapid Onset

Patients often manifest symptoms such as restlessness, anxiety, irritability, and sleep disruption before the onset of delirium. Review of the hospital medical chart of a patient with delirium, particularly the nursing notes, often reveals these prodromal features. The time between the appearance of the first symptom and the diagnosis of delirium is relatively short. In a prospective study by Levkoff et al. (1992), 50% of patients met criteria for delirium on the same day they developed their first symptom, and 86% met the criteria within 2 days.

Fluctuating Course

The clinical features of delirium are protean (Table 10–4) and, to complicate the picture further, vary rapidly over time. The variability and fluctuation in clinical findings are characteristic of delirium but can lead to diagnostic confusion among clinicians. For example, the surgery team sees Mr. Jones on early-morning rounds and finds him friendly, sleepy, and noncomplaining. The psychiatric consultant later that day finds Mr. Jones grossly confused, paranoid, agitated, uncooperative, and visually hallucinating. The surgeons, when approached by the psychiatrist about Mr. Jones's worrisome mental status (delirium), may believe that the psychiatrist is more confused than the patient. The appearance of lucid intervals in the clinical course of a patient is an important observation. However, there is a subgroup of patients who manifest what has been called "reversible dementia" (Task Force Sponsored by the National Institute on Aging 1980) who lack the dramatic fluctuations so typical of delirium.

Attentional Deficits

Some authors maintain that inattention is the core neuropsychological feature of delirium (Levkoff et al.

TABLE 10–4.   Clinical features of delirium

Prodrome (restlessness, anxiety, sleep disturbance, irritability) and rapid onset

Rapidly fluctuating course

Attention decreased (easily distractible)

Altered arousal and psychomotor abnormality

Disturbance of sleep-wake cycle

Impaired memory (cannot register new information)

Disorganized thinking and speech

Disorientation (very rarely, if ever, to person)

Perceptions altered (misperceptions, illusions, delusions [poorly formed], hallucinations)

Neurological abnormalities

    Dysgraphia

    Constructional apraxia

    Dysnomic aphasia

    Motor abnormalities (tremor, asterixis, myoclonus, reflex, and tone changes)

    Electroencephalogram (EEG) abnormalities (almost always background slowing)

Other features (sadness, irritability, anger, or euphoria)

1991; Seltzer and Mesulam 1988); this concept was adopted in DSM-III-R. Patients often perform poorly on bedside tests of sustained attention, such as giving the months of the year backward. In addition, patients with delirium are easily distracted by incidental activities in the environment. For example, if one were interviewing such a patient in a hospital room and someone walked by in the corridor, the patient might lose interest in the interview and attend to the distraction. When the patient looks back at the examiner, he or she may say, "Did you ask me a question?" This inability to sustain attention undoubtedly plays a key role in memory and orientation difficulties.

Arousal Disturbance and Psychomotor Abnormalities

Some patients with delirium appear apathetic, somnolent, and quietly confused, whereas others are agitated and hypervigilant and exhibit psychomotor hyperactivity. Some patients swing back and forth between hypoactive and hyperactive states (so-called mixed delirium); however, as Lipowski (1990) noted, "the frequency of the respective variants in clinical practice is unknown" (p. 65). The patient with a hypoactive type of delirium is less apt to be diagnosed as delirious and is often mislabeled as depressed or uncooperative, or as having a character disorder. The diagnosis of depression in an apathetic, quietly confused patient can lead to inappropriate treatment with an antidepressant, which, in turn, adds unnecessary side effects that may worsen brain function (e.g., resulting from the anticholinergic potency of many tricyclic antidepressants). In addition, the failure to diagnose and treat the potentially lethal causes of delirium increases morbidity and mortality.

It is not clear whether the type of delirium the patient exhibits (i.e., the hyperactive or hypoactive form) gives the clinician any clues concerning etiology. It is said, however, that patients with delirium caused by hepatic failure are virtually always hypoactive and without visual hallucinations (Ross et al. 1991). In contrast, patients with delirium secondary to sedative hypnotic withdrawal, especially alcohol withdrawal, are typically agitated, hyperactive, and hallucinating.

Sleep-Wake Disturbance

Sleep-wake disturbance is an important symptom of delirium. The sleep-wake cycle of delirious patients is often reversed. The patient may be somnolent during the day and active during the night, when the nursing staff is reduced. Restoration of the normal diurnal sleep cycle is an important part of treatment, because sleep deprivation may worsen the confusion.

Impaired Memory

The ability of patients with delirium to register events into memory is severely impaired. Whether because of attentional deficits, perceptual disturbances, or other neuropsychological dysfunction, patients fail tests of recent memory. Following recovery from delirium, some patients are amnestic for the entire episode; others have islands of memory for events during the episode. Whether these islands of memory correspond to the previously described "lucid intervals" is unknown.

Disorganized Thinking and Impaired Speech

The thought patterns of patients with delirium are disorganized, and reasoning is defective. A patient presumptively diagnosed with delirium might be asked to explain the following story: "I have a friend by the name of Frank Jones whose feet are so large he has to put on his pants by pulling them over his head. Can Mr. Jones do that?" Typical responses from patients with delirium, usually given with a smile and a laugh, are "Sure, as long as he unzips his fly" or "I guess so, if he does one leg at a time." The patient does not understand the problem at hand and is unable to reason normally. In addition, as the severity of delirium increases, spontaneous speech becomes "incoherent, rambling, and shifts from topic to topic" (Cummings 1985a, p. 68).

Disorientation

Except for lucid intervals, patients with delirium are usually disoriented to time, often disoriented to place, but rarely, if ever, disoriented to person. It is not unusual for a delirious patient to feel he or she is in a familiar place (e.g., "a room in the attic of my house") while also nodding agreement that he or she is being monitored in a surgical intensive care unit. The extent of the patient's disorientation fluctuates with the severity of the delirium.

Altered Perceptions

Virtually all patients with delirium have misperceptions, often involving illusions, delusions, and hallucinations. Patients often weave these misperceptions into a loosely knit delusional, usually paranoid, system. The patient may, for example, overhear a nurse say, "We're going to move him out" (i.e., move the patient to another room). The patient may then hear a postoperative patient moaning, hear a chart fall on the floor, and conclude that he has heard a shot fired. The patient may then put these events together and suspect that he is about to be transferred to a torture chamber and be killed.

Visual hallucinations are common, ranging from simple visual distortions to complex scenes. Visual hallucinations occur more frequently than auditory hallucinations. Tactile hallucinations occur least frequently. In our experience, most auditory and tactile phenomena that are labeled hallucinations are, in fact, illusions. For example, intravenous tubing that brushes against the skin may be perceived as a crawling snake.

Neurological Abnormalities

A number of neurological abnormalities are found in delirium. Testing for these signs at the bedside not only strengthens the clinician's suspicion of the diagnosis but, when added to the chart, helps other physicians recognize the presence of a confusional state. One of the most pathognomonic neuropsychological signs is attentional deficit (O'Keeffe and Gosney 1997). This can be assessed by asking the patient to repeat a series of digits or count from 20 back to zero. Another simple test is to present verbally a series of random letters of the alphabet, including a stimulus letter (e.g., A), and ask the patient to indicate each time he or she recognizes the A. Patients with delirium frequently fail to indicate the target letter. Individuals with normal brain function virtually never make errors on this task. Inability to draw the face of a clock (Figure 10–2) and to perform other constructional tasks are sensitive indicators of the presence of a confusional state delirium. One may ask the patient to name objects (testing for dysnomia) and to write a sentence (testing for dysgraphia). Dysgraphia is one of the most sensitive indicators of delirium. In Chedru and Geschwind's study (1972), 33 of 34 acutely confused patients had impaired writing. Writing shows motor impairment (from minor awkwardness owing to tremor to illegible scribble), spatial impairment (letter malalignment and line disorientation), misspellings, and linguistic errors. It must be stressed, however, that constructional difficulty, dysnomia, and dysgraphia are not specific to delirium and can occur with dementia and other organic mental disorders (Patten and Lamarre 1989).

Patients with delirium may not have motor system abnormalities, although many patients manifest tremor, myoclonus, asterixis, or changes in reflex and muscle tone. Myoclonus and asterixis (so-called liver flap) occur in many toxic and metabolic conditions. Symmetrical reflex and muscle tone changes can also occur.

Other Features

Emotional disturbances are common in patients with delirium. The intensity of the patient's emotional response to

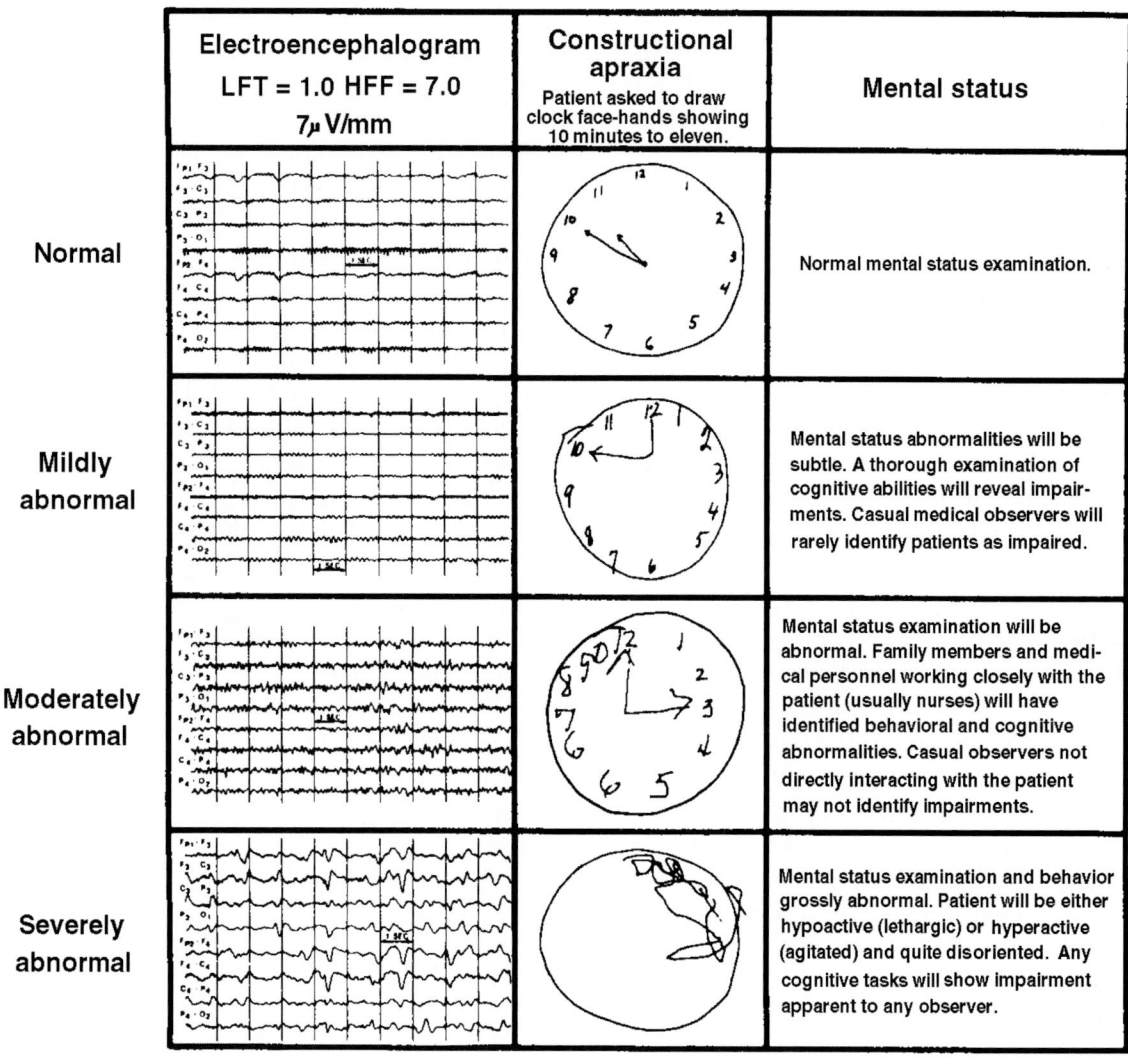

Electroencephalogram LFT = 1.0 HFF = 7.0 7μ V/mm	Constructional apraxia Patient asked to draw clock face-hands showing 10 minutes to eleven.	Mental status
Normal		Normal mental status examination.
Mildly abnormal		Mental status abnormalities will be subtle. A thorough examination of cognitive abilities will reveal impairments. Casual medical observers will rarely identify patients as impaired.
Moderately abnormal		Mental status examination will be abnormal. Family members and medical personnel working closely with the patient (usually nurses) will have identified behavioral and cognitive abnormalities. Casual observers not directly interacting with the patient may not identify impairments.
Severely abnormal		Mental status examination and behavior grossly abnormal. Patient will be either hypoactive (lethargic) or hyperactive (agitated) and quite disoriented. Any cognitive tasks will show impairment apparent to any observer.

FIGURE 10-2.   Comparison of electroencephalogram, constructional apraxia, and mental status in delirium.

mental confusion may fluctuate relatively rapidly and may also change in character with the passage of time (e.g., from fear with associated hyperarousal to apathy with hypoarousal). Therefore, patients with delirium are sometimes described as emotionally labile.

The emotional responses seen in patients with delirium include anxiety, panic, fear, anger, rage, sadness, apathy, and rarely—except in steroid-induced delirium—euphoria. Medical caregivers may identify the emotional or behavioral disturbance of the critically ill patient without recognizing the underlying confusional state. The determinants of the individual's response to delirium are personality structure, the nature of the underlying illness, the content of thoughts and hallucinations, and the characteristics of the environment (Lipowski 1967, 1980a).

PATHOPHYSIOLOGY AND ELECTROENCEPHALOGRAPHIC ABNORMALITIES

Significant information about the pathophysiology of delirium was provided by early EEG investigators (Engel et al. 1947; Romano and Engel 1944). Indeed, in their classic paper "Delirium, a Syndrome of Cerebral Insufficiency," Engel and Romano (1959) proposed that the basic etiology of all delirium was a derangement in functional metabolism, manifested at the clinical level by characteristic disturbances in cognitive functions and at the physiological level by characteristic slowing of the EEG. Their clinical research established the following:

1. "The degree of slowing of the EEG corresponds best with the disturbance of consciousness" (p. 267).

2. Changes on the EEG were reversible to the extent that the clinical delirium was reversible.

3. The character of the EEG changes appeared to be independent of the specific underlying disease process.

4. The character of the EEG changes was determined by the strength, duration, and reversibility of the noxious factors, as well as the integrity of the CNS.

5. Clinical interventions (e.g., administration of oxygen in congestive heart failure and pulmonary insufficiency) improved (i.e., normalized) the EEG and also the mental status.

Spectral EEG analyses, which measure the quality of alpha, beta, theta, and delta background activity, have further supported Engel and Romano's proposed correlation between EEG slowing and cognitive deterioration (Koponen et al. 1989d). Quantitative measurement of brain electrical activity offers advantages over visual interpretation of EEG tracings. Specifically, the former is "much more sensitive to changes in power than [is] visual analysis" (Leuchter and Jacobson 1991, p. 244), and as little as 30 seconds of quantitative data can produce results representative of background frequency. This is certainly a benefit over standard EEG techniques, which require the agitated or confused patient to lie still for 30 minutes.

Delirium is virtually always accompanied by EEG changes (Pro and Wells 1977), but the changes are not always slowing of brain rhythms. The pattern can be low-voltage fast activity, as in delirium tremens (Kennard et al. 1945). Low-voltage fast activity is usually found in hyperactive, agitated patients with heightened arousal (Pro and Wells 1977). EEG slowing may be found in lethargic, anergic, abulic patients. Koponen et al. (1989d), who looked at EEG slowing in delirium using quantitative methods, did not, however, find differences in mean EEG frequencies between "hyperactive" and "hypoactive" patients. The EEG slowing illustrated in Figure 10–2 is typical for delirium when there is a toxic-metabolic etiology.

A patient's EEG can have significant slowing but can still be read as normal if the baseline background activity is 12 cycles/second and during a metabolic encephalopathy the background slows to 8 cycles/second. Significant slowing has occurred, even though the reported rate, 8 cycles/second, still falls within the "normal" range and the EEG could be read as normal. Documentation of the encephalopathy might occur only if the patient has a previous EEG on record or if a second EEG is obtained once the patient is again cognitively normal. EEG abnormalities also can occur before and linger after the occurrence of the clinical manifestations of delirium (Andreasen et al. 1977).

Since the hypothesis that delirium represents a metabolic derangement was proposed, little additional research on pathophysiology has been forthcoming (Engel and Romano 1959). There are reports of a correlation between decreased MMSE scores in delirium and decreased somatostatin and β-endorphin-like immunoreactivity in the cerebrospinal fluid (CSF; Koponen et al. 1989a, 1989b). Recent research has also led to speculation about the role of γ-aminobutyric acid (GABA) in delirium caused by hepatic failure as well as by other conditions (Basile et al. 1991; Ross et al. 1991). GABAergic transmission in hepatic failure may be increased because of endogenous benzodiazepine-like compounds that cause the hypoactive type of delirium; on the other hand, GABAergic transmission may be decreased in sedative-hypnotic withdrawal, resulting in hyperactive delirium. Other investigators have speculated about the importance of the cholinergic system in delirium, pointing particularly to this system's vulnerability to metabolic insults, aging, and anticholinergic drugs (Gibson et al. 1991).

Although most cases of delirium occur in the setting of some systemic illness or metabolic derangement, in a small proportion of patients the syndrome results from focal CNS disease. The most consistent localization is the cortex and subcortical white matter supplied by the right middle cerebral artery (Mori and Yamadori 1987). Strokes in that region disrupt neural systems that are important to the maintenance of directed attention (Seltzer and Mesulam 1988).

DIFFERENTIAL DIAGNOSIS

The differential diagnosis of delirium is so extensive that there may be a tendency to avoid the search for etiologies. In addition, confusional states, particularly in elderly persons, may represent the response of the CNS to multiple abnormalities. For example, an elderly patient with delirium is found to have a low hematocrit, to have multiorgan system disease (e.g., pulmonary insufficiency, cardiac failure, or dementia), and to take multiple medications. Each potential contributor to the delirium needs to be pursued and addressed independently.

Nonspecific terms such as *ICU psychosis* are sometimes used as an explanation for delirium, when, in fact, these terms simply mask ignorance. Koponen et al. (1989c) found clear organic etiologies in 87% of delirious patients and also found that patients who became confused because of environmental events had severe cases of dementia. The task for the clinician is to organize the wide array of potential causes of delirium into a usable diagnostic system. The following is an attempt to present a systematic approach to the differential diagnosis of delirium.

Emergent Items

A two-tiered differential diagnostic system is helpful for evaluating a patient with delirium. The first level of this diagnostic system is represented in Table 10–5 by the mnemonic WHHHHIMP and discussed in the following sections. These diagnoses must be discovered early in the course of a delirium because failure to do so may result in irreversible damage to the patient. The mnemonic can help clinicians to recall these critical items. Table 10–5 also contains many of the questions that clinicians must ask to investigate the etiology.

Wernicke's encephalopathy or withdrawal. A patient with Wernicke's encephalopathy has the triad of confusion, ataxia, and ophthalmoplegia (usually lateral gaze paralysis). If Wernicke's encephalopathy is not promptly treated with parenteral thiamine, the patient will develop Korsakoff's psychosis, which is a permanent amnestic disorder. A precise history of alcohol intake is critical for the diagnosis of alcohol withdrawal and/or DTs. Other findings that increase the suspicion of alcohol withdrawal/DTs are a history of alcohol-related arrests, alcoholic blackouts, medical complications associated with alcohol abuse, liver function abnormalities, and elevated red cell mean corpuscular volume (MCV). Hyperreflexia and increased sympathetic tone (e.g., tachycardia, tremor, sweating, hyperarousal) at the time of examination should lead the clinician to suspect a hyperadrenergic withdrawal state.

Hypertensive encephalopathy, hypoglycemia, hypoperfusion, or hypoxemia. A check of the arterial blood gases and current and past vital signs should quickly establish whether hypoxemia or hypertensive encephalopathy is present. The patient with hypoglycemia-induced delirium almost always has a history of insulin-dependent diabetes mellitus. Hypoglycemic delirium also presents as a hyperadrenergic state. There are a number of clinical phenomena that can singularly or collectively decrease brain perfusion. These cause "relative" hypoperfusion (relative to usual perfusion pressures), such as decreased cardiac output from a myocardial infarction, cardiac failure, arrhythmias, or anemia.

Intracranial bleeding or infection. It is important to determine whether the patient has had a subarachnoid bleed or any other type of CNS hemorrhage. If the patient had a brief period of unconsciousness, with or without headache, and is now delirious, or if the patient had or now has focal neurological signs, an intracranial bleed is suspected. Immediate neurological/neurosurgical evaluation

TABLE 10–5. Differential diagnosis for delirium: emergent items (WHHHHIMP)

Diagnosis	Clinical questions
Wernicke's encephalopathy or **W**ithdrawal	Ataxia? Ophthalmoplegia? Alcohol or drug history? Increased mean corpuscular volume? Increased sympathetic activity (e.g., increased blood pressure or sweating)? Hyperreflexia?
Hypertensive encephalopathy	Increased blood pressure? Papilledema?
Hypoglycemia	History of insulin-dependent diabetes mellitus? Decreased glucose?
Hypoperfusion of central nervous system	Decreased blood pressure? Decreased cardiac output (e.g., myocardial infarct, arrhythmia, cardiac failure)? Decreased hematocrit?
Hypoxemia	Arterial blood gases (decreased Po$_2$)? History of pulmonary disease?
Intracranial bleeding or infection	History of unconsciousness? Focal neurological signs?
Meningitis or encephalitis	Meningeal signs? Increased white blood count? Increased temperature? Viral prodrome?
Poisons or medications	Should toxic screen be ordered? Signs of toxicity (e.g., pupillary abnormality, nystagmus, or ataxia)? Is the patient on a drug that can cause delirium?

is necessary. Signs of an infectious process, such as elevated white blood cell count or fever, must be sought. One must look especially for urinary tract infections in a confused, elderly patient.

Meningitis or encephalitis. Meningitis and encephalitis are typically acute febrile illnesses (vital signs must be checked for fever) and usually have either nonspecific localizing neurological signs (e.g., meningismus with stiff neck) or more focal neurological signs.

Poisons or medications. When a patient with delirium is encountered in the emergency room, the clinician must consider a toxic organic reaction and order a drug screen. Pesticide or solvent poisoning is less likely but should be considered. In hospital and emergency room patients, a common cause of delirium is prescribed medications (Table 10–6). Medications were reported to contribute to delirium in 22%–39% of studies reviewed by Inouye (1994). The importance of taking a thorough medication history cannot be overemphasized. For hospitalized patients who become delirious, the examiner must thoroughly review the patient's medication records. The doctor's order sheets can be misleading because drugs may have been ordered but not given. Correlation of behavior with medication administration or discontinuation is often extremely helpful in sorting through a difficult case.

Critical Items

The I WATCH DEATH mnemonic (Table 10–7) represents a comprehensive list of insults that can cause delirium. Because the list is lengthy, it may be helpful for the clinician to carry a card containing the entire differential diagnosis of delirium. The mnemonic I WATCH DEATH may sound melodramatic, but this is not the case. The appearance of delirium, which is equivalent to acute brain failure, should marshal the same medical forces as failure

TABLE 10–6. Drugs that can cause delirium

Antibiotic
Acyclovir (antiviral)
Amphotericin B (antifungal)
Cephalexin (Keflex)
Chloroquine (antimalarial)

Anticholinergic
Antihistamines
Chlorpheniramine (Ornade and Teldrin)
Antiparkinson drugs
  Benztropine (Cogentin)
  Biperiden (Akineton)
Antispasmodics
Atropine/homatropine
Belladonna alkaloids
Diphenhydramine (Benadryl)
Phenothiazines
  (especially thioridazine)
Promethazine (Phenergan)
Scopolamine
Tricyclic antidepressants
  (especially amitriptyline)
Trihexyphenidyl (Artane)

Anticonvulsant
Phenobarbital
Phenytoin (Dilantin)
Sodium valproate (Depakene)

Anti-inflammatory
Adrenocorticotropic hormone
Corticosteroids

Ibuprofen (Motrin and Advil)
Indomethacin (Indocin)
Naproxen (Naprosyn)
Phenylbutazone (Butazolidin)

Antineoplastic
5-Fluorouracil

Antiparkinsonian
Amantadine (Symmetrel)
Carbidopa (Sinemet)
Levodopa (Larodopa)

Antituberculous
Isoniazid
Rifampin

Analgesic
Opiates
Salicylates
Synthetic narcotics

Cardiac
β-blockers
Propranolol (Inderal)
Clonidine (Catapres)
Digitalis (Digoxin and Lanoxin)
Disopyramide (Norpace)
Lidocaine (Xylocaine)
Mexiletine
Methyldopa (Aldomet)
Quinidine (Quinaglute and Duraquine)

Drug withdrawal
Alcohol

Barbiturates
Benzodiazepines

Sedative-hypnotic
Barbiturates (Miltown and Equanil)
Glutethimide (Doriden)
Benzodiazepines

Sympathomimetic
Amphetamines
Phenylephrine
Phenylpropanolamine

Over-the-counter
Compoz
Excedrin P.M.
Sleep-Eze
Sominex

Miscellaneous
Aminophylline
Bromides
Chlorpropamide (Diabinese)
Cimetidine (Tagamet)
Disulfiram (Antabuse)
Lithium
Metrizamide (Amipaque)
Metronidazole (Flagyl)
Podophyllin by absorption
Propylthiouracil
Quinacrine
Theophylline
Timolol ophthalmic

TABLE 10–7. Differential diagnosis for delirium: critical items (I WATCH DEATH)

Infectious	Encephalitis, meningitis, and syphilis
Withdrawal	Alcohol, barbiturates, sedative-hypnotics
Acute metabolic	Acidosis, alkalosis, electrolyte disturbance, hepatic failure, and renal failure
Trauma	Heat stroke, postoperative, and severe burns
CNS pathology	Abscesses, hemorrhage, normal-pressure hydrocephalus, seizures, stroke, tumors, and vasculitis
Hypoxia	Anemia, carbon monoxide poisoning, hypotension, and pulmonary or cardiac failure
Deficiencies	Vitamin B$_{12}$, niacin, and thiamine and hypovitaminosis
Endocrinopathies	Hyper- or hypoadrenocortisolism and hyper- or hypoglycemia
Acute vascular	Hypertensive encephalopathy and shock
Toxins or drugs	Medications (see Table 10–6), pesticides, and solvents
Heavy metals	Lead, manganese, and mercury

of any other vital organ. The morbidity and mortality that result from untreated or undertreated delirium are substantial and should not be ignored.

COURSE AND PROGNOSIS

The clinical course of a patient with delirium is variable. The possibilities include 1) full recovery, 2) progression to stupor and/or coma, 3) development of seizures, 4) progression to chronic brain syndromes, 5) death, and 6) associated morbidity, such as fractures or subdural hematomas from falls. The majority of patients who experience delirium probably have a full recovery, although the statistical probability of this outcome is questioned (Levkoff et al. 1992). Levkoff et al. (1992), in a prospective study of 325 elderly patients, found a minority of patients had full resolution of symptoms by 6 months. Patients who progress to stupor and/or coma either recover (with or without chronic brain injury), become chronically vegetative, or die. Seizures can accompany delirium and are more likely to occur with drug withdrawal, particularly alcohol, and

burn encephalopathy (Antoon et al. 1972). Finally, a number of patients do not completely recover and have residual deficits. The resultant chronic brain syndrome may be global or focal (e.g., amnestic syndrome, secondary personality disorder).

Morbidity

Research indicates that hospitalization is prolonged (Cameron et al. 1987; Francis et al. 1990; Kay et al. 1956; Levkoff et al. 1992; O'Keeffe and Lavan 1997; Pompei et al. 1994). In one study, 38.9% of patients with acute brain syndromes developed chronic brain syndromes (Titchener et al. 1956). In another study, 15% of postcardiotomy patients with delirium had persistent neurological signs at discharge (Tufo et al. 1970). Fernandez et al. (1989) found that only 37% of patients with AIDS who became delirious had a complete recovery of cognitive function.

Patients who undergo orthopedic procedures provide fertile ground for research in delirium. Rogers et al. (1989) reported that patients who were cognitively normal when tested preoperatively and then developed delirium showed no improvement in level of physical function 6 months postoperatively. In other words, patients who became delirious postoperatively gained no functional benefit from the surgery. Delirium seems to be the best predictor of outcome in patients who present with femoral neck fractures (Gustafson et al. 1988); Gustafson et al. reported that 37 of 111 patients were delirious preoperatively and another 31 became delirious postoperatively. Patients without dementia who became delirious had longer hospital stays (21.7 days for patient with versus 13.5 days for patients without delirium) and were more likely to require walking aids, be bedridden, require rehabilitation, or die. The patients with delirium spent four times as long in recuperation before discharge. In a study comparing 50 elderly patients with and 50 patients without delirium, the patients with delirium were more likely to die (39% versus 23% over 2 years), lose independence, and experience future cognitive decline (Francis and Kapoor 1992). In a prospective study by Murray et al. (1993), a strong association was found between delirium and functional decline.

Any clinician who performs hospital consultations has seen patients, as Moore (1977) described, who "became agitated, struck a nurse, and pulled out his nasogastric tube" (p. 1431). Patients with delirium pull out intravenous lines, nasogastric tubes, arterial lines, nasopharyngeal tubes, and intra-aortic balloon pumps. Inouye et al. (1989) reported that the risk of complications such as decubiti and aspiration pneumonia was more than six times greater in elderly hospital patients with delirium than in similar patients without delirium. Levkoff et al. (1986) projected a $1–2 billion savings in the United States if the hospital stay of each patient with delirium could be reduced by 1 day.

Mortality

Many physicians underestimate the mortality associated with delirium. Of 77 patients who received a DSM-III diagnosis of delirium from a consulting psychiatrist, 19 (25%) died within 6 months (Trzepacz et al. 1985). Three months following diagnosis, the mortality rate for delirium was found to be 14 times greater than the mortality rate for affective disorders (Weddington 1982). A patient diagnosed with delirium during a hospital admission has a hospital mortality rate that is 5.5 times greater than a patient diagnosed with dementia (Rabins and Folstein 1982). Furthermore, elderly patients who develop delirium in the hospital have a 22% (Rabins and Folstein 1982) to 76% (Flint and Richards 1956) chance of dying during that hospitalization. Cameron et al. (1987) reported that 13 of 20 (65%) patients with delirium died during hospitalization. Patients who survive hospitalization have a very high death rate during the months immediately following discharge. Patients with a diagnosis of delirium followed for several months showed a mortality rate equal to that of patients with dementia followed for several years (Roth 1955; Varsamis et al. 1972). Pompei et al. (1994) confirmed the increased risk of death in patients with delirium; however, O'Keeffe and Lavan (1997) did not find this association when confounding factors, such as severity of acute illness and extent of comorbid disease, were considered.

MAKING THE DIAGNOSIS OF DELIRIUM

Regardless of the suspected diagnosis, the evaluation of a patient follows a particular generic process. A specific diagnosis such as delirium follows from an appreciation of the clinical features of the syndrome (Table 10–4) and a thorough examination of the patient's mental and physical status (Table 10–8). In addition to the usual mental status examination, the examiner should, at a minimum, test for constructional ability (see Figure 10–2), writing ability, and the ability to name objects. If delirium is present, the examiner should make every effort to identify the specific etiology or etiologies. In one study, 56% of patients with delirium had a single definite or probable etiology, and the remaining 44% had an average of 2.8 etiologies per patient (Francis et al. 1990). When no apparent etiology is identified initially, the etiology often "declares itself" within a few days.

The gold standard for diagnosis is the clinical evaluation, and the most useful diagnostic laboratory test is the EEG. Several paper-and-pencil tests exist to aid the clinician in diagnosis. The MMSE (Figure 10–3) provides a screening tool for organicity and is also used to follow the patient's clinical course serially (Folstein et al. 1975). The major problem with the MMSE is its lack of sensitivity (i.e., high rate of false negatives). For example, in a recent study, a number of patients who had slowed background activity on the EEG at the time of evaluation scored in the mid to

---

TABLE 10–8.   Neuropsychiatric evaluation of the patient

Mental status

Interview (assessment of level of consciousness, psychomotor activity, appearance, affect, mood, intellect, and thought processes)

Performance tests (memory, concentration, reasoning, motor and constructional apraxia, dysgraphia, and dysnomia)

Physical status

Brief neurological exam (reflexes, limb strength, Babinski reflex, cranial nerves, meningeal signs, and gait)

Review of past and present vital signs (pulse, temperature, blood pressure, and respiration rate)

Review of chart (check laboratory results [e.g., VDRL and FTA-ABS], abnormal behavior after medication is started or stopped)

Laboratory examination—basic

Blood chemistries (electrolytes, glucose, calcium, albumin, blood urea nitrogen, ammonia [NH_4^+], and liver functions)

Blood count (hematocrit, white count and differential, mean corpuscular volume, sedimentation rate)

Drug levels (need toxic screen? medication blood levels?)

Arterial blood gases

Urinalysis

Electrocardiogram

Chest X-ray

Laboratory—based on clinical judgment

Electroencephalogram (seizures? focal lesion? or confirm delirium)

Computed tomography (normal-pressure hydrocephalus, stroke, and space-occupying lesion)

Additional blood chemistries (heavy metals, thiamine and folate levels, thyroid battery, lupus erythematosus prep, antinuclear antibodies, and urinary porphobilinogen)

Lumbar puncture (if indication of infection or intracranial bleed)

Note.   VDRL = Venereal Disease Research Laboratory; FTA-ABS = fluorescent treponemal antibody absorption.

MINI-MENTAL STATE EXAM AND INSTRUCTIONS

Patient _____

Examiner _____

Date _____

Maximum score	Score	Orientation
5	( )	What is the (year) (season) (date) (day) (month)?
5	( )	Where are we: (state) (county) (town) (hospital) (floor)?

Registration

3	( )	Name 3 objects: 1 second to say each. Then ask the patient all 3 after you have said them. Give 1 point for each correct answer. Then say them until he/she learns all 3. Count trials and record.
		Trials _____

Attention and Calculation

5	( )	Serial 7s. 1 point for each correct. Stop after 5 answers. Alternatively spell "world" backwards.

Recall

3	( )	Ask for the 3 objects repeated above. Give 1 point for each correct.

Language

9	( )	Name a pencil, and watch (2 points)
		Repeat the following "No ifs, ands, or buts." (1 point)
		Follow a 3-stage command:
		"Take a paper in your right hand, fold it in half, and put it on the floor." (3 points)

Read and obey the following:

Close your eyes (1 point)

Write a sentence (1 point)

Copy design (1 point)

Total score

Assess level of consciousness along a continuum

Alert   Drowsy   Stupor   Coma

(continued)

FIGURE 10–3.   Mini-Mental State Exam and instructions.

Source.   Reprinted with permission from Folstein MF, Folstein SE, McHugh PR: "Mini-Mental State: A Practical Method for Grading the Cognitive State of Patients for the Clinician." *Journal of Psychiatric Research* 12:198, 1975. Copyright 1975 by Pergamon Press, Ltd., Headington Hill Hall, Oxford 0X3 0BW, UK.

INSTRUCTIONS FOR ADMINISTRATION OF MINI-MENTAL STATE EXAM

Orientation

1. Ask for the date. Then ask specifically for parts omitted, e.g., "Can you also tell me what season it is?" One point for each correct.

2. Ask in turn "Can you tell me the name of this hospital?" (town, county, etc.). One point for each correct.

Registration

Ask the patient if you may test his memory. Then say the names of 3 unrelated objects, clearly and slowly, about one second for each. After you have said all 3, ask him to repeat them. This first repetition determines his score (0–3) but keep saying them until he can repeat all 3, up to 6 trials. If he does not eventually learn all 3, recall cannot be meaningfully tested.

Attention and Calculation

Ask the patient to begin with 100 and count backwards by 7. Stop after 5 subtractions (93, 86, 79, 72, 65). Score the total number of correct answers.

If the patient cannot or will not perform this task, ask him to spell the word "world" backwards. The score is the number of letters in correct order, e.g., dlrow = 5, dlorw = 3.

Recall

Ask the patient if he can recall the 3 words you previously asked him to remember. Score 0–3.

Language

Naming: Show the patient a wrist watch and ask him what it is. Repeat for pencil. Score 0–2.

Repetition: Ask the patient to repeat the sentence after you. Allow only one trial. Score 0 or 1.

3-Stage command: Give the patient a piece of plain blank paper and repeat the command. Score 1 point for each part correctly executed.

Reading: On a blank piece of paper print the sentence "Close your eyes," in letters large enough for the patient to see clearly. Ask him to read it and do what it says. Score 1 point only if he actually closes his eyes.

Writing: Give the patient a blank piece of paper and ask him to write a sentence for you. Do not dictate a sentence; it is to be written spontaneously. It must contain a subject and verb and be sensible. Correct grammar and punctuation are not necessary.

Coding: On a clean piece of paper, draw intersecting pentagons, each side about 1 in., and ask him to copy it exactly as it is. All 10 angles must be present and 2 must intersect to score 1 point. Tremor and rotation are ignored.

Estimate the patient's level of sensorium along a continuum, from alert on the left to coma on the right.

FIGURE 10-3.   Mini-Mental State Exam and instructions. *(continued)*
Source.   Reprinted with permission from Folstein MF, Folstein SE, McHugh PR: "Mini-Mental State: A Practical Method for Grading the Cognitive State of Patients for the Clinician." *Journal of Psychiatric Research* 12:198, 1975. Copyright 1975 by Pergamon Press, Ltd., Headington Hill Hall, Oxford 0X3 0BW, UK.

---

upper 20s (out of a possible 30) on the MMSE (M. G. Wise, unpublished data, 1989).

More than 18 scales are now available to help the clinician or researcher detect delirium (Inouye 1994): examples include the Delirium Rating Scale (DRS; Trzepacz et al. 1988), Confusion Assessment Method (Inouye et al. 1990), Confusion Rating Scale (Williams et al. 1986), NEECHAM Confusion Scale (Champagne et al. 1987), Global Accessibility Scale (Anthony et al. 1982), Delirium Symptom Interview (Levkoff et al. 1991), and High Sensitivity Cognitive Screen (Faust and Fogel 1989). With these assessment instruments, an attempt has been made to operationalize the DSM diagnostic criteria for delirium.

There are two levels of laboratory evaluation of a delirious patient. The basic laboratory battery listed in Table 10-8 is ordered for virtually every patient with a diagnosis of delirium. When information concerning the patient's history and mental and physical status is combined with the laboratory results, the specific etiology or etiologies are often apparent. If it is not, the clinician should review the case and consider ordering additional diagnostic studies.

TREATMENT

There are two distinct issues in the management of delirium. The first is treatment of the underlying medical condition causing the delirium, and the second is treatment of inappropriate behaviors that endanger medical care.

The clinician must systematically attempt to establish a diagnosis, because many causes of delirium have specific treatments. The goal of diagnosis is to discover reversible causes for delirium. For example, the delirious patient who has a blood pressure of 260/150 and papilledema must immediately receive antihypertensive medication. The alcoholic patient having withdrawal symptoms must receive appropriate intervention with thiamine and a drug such as a benzodiazepine. Without an organized approach to diagnosis, one might incorrectly treat the agitation and hallucinations of the patient having DTs with chlorpromazine, which would increase the likelihood of seizures. In some instances, the exact reason for a delirious episode cannot be ascertained. Nevertheless, the general measures described in the following sections are applicable to these patients as well. Furthermore, whether or not an etiology is determined, some patients require pharmacological treatment for agitated behavior.

Medical and Nursing Care

In addition to ordering the laboratory tests essential for identifying the cause of a delirium, one of the important roles of the psychiatrist is to raise the level of awareness of the medical and nursing staff about the morbidity and mortality associated with delirium. The patient should be placed in a room near the nursing station, and vital signs should be closely monitored. Increased observation of the patient ensures awareness of medical deterioration and dangerous behaviors such as trying to crawl over bed rails or pulling out intravenous lines. Fluid input and output must be monitored and good oxygenation ensured. All nonessential medications should be discontinued.

It must be remembered that the brain is a sensitive forecaster of upcoming medical perils. When an etiology for the confusional state is not immediately identified, vigilance, frequent laboratory examinations, and daily physical examinations are essential.

Pharmacological Treatment

There is no consensus concerning whether delirium should be treated pharmacologically. Neuroleptic prescribing practices in delirium remain controversial; issues concerning the rapid administration of neuroleptics and appropriate dosage levels continue to be debated. The critical clinical issue, however, is the individual patient's situation and response to medications. Because delirium is defined by its variability, a one-time assessment will evoke management and medical recommendations that are

time-limited in efficacy. Therefore, only constant follow-up of the patient will suffice, with modification in the treatment plan when appropriate.

The clinician must rely on experience, known properties of drugs (particularly side effects), and anecdotal reports of various treatments. The scenario for pharmacological intervention often involves consultation concerning an agitated, combative, hallucinating, and paranoid medically ill patient whose behavior is a threat to continuing medical treatment.

A drug used to control agitated psychotic behavior in an ICU should calm the patient without obtunding consciousness and stop hallucinations and paranoid ideation. The drug should not suppress respiratory drive, cause hypotension, or worsen delirium (e.g., it should not be anticholinergic). The drug should be available in a parenteral form. Review of the literature and clinical experience indicate that haloperidol comes closest to meeting these criteria and is the drug of first choice for treating patients with agitated delirium of unknown etiology (Lipowski 1980b, 1990). Haloperidol is a potent antipsychotic with virtually no anticholinergic or hypotensive properties, and it can be given parenterally. Although haloperidol is not approved by the U.S. Food and Drug Administration (FDA) for intravenous use, intravenous haloperidol has been used in very high doses for many years in seriously ill patients without harmful side effects (Fernandez et al. 1988; Sos and Cassem 1980; Tesar et al. 1985). Severe refractory agitation has also been controlled with a continuous intravenous infusion of haloperidol (Fernandez et al. 1988). Although extrapyramidal side effects are more likely with the higher potency antipsychotic drugs, their occurrence rate in medically ill patients, particularly when the drug is administered intravenously, is strikingly low. When extrapyramidal symptoms of oral versus intravenous haloperidol were measured in a blind fashion, intravenous administration of haloperidol was associated with fewer and less severe extrapyramidal symptoms (Menza et al. 1987). Rare cases of QT prolongation or torsades de pointes were reported with overdoses of haloperidol taken orally and with administration of intravenous haloperidol (Metzger and Friedman 1993).

Other antipsychotic medications found useful in treating the positive symptom of delirium are thiothixene (Navane) and droperidol. Droperidol is used by anesthesiologists as a preanesthetic agent and by other physicians for the control of nausea and vomiting. Like haloperidol, it is a butyrophenone and has comparable antipsychotic potency. Droperidol is approved for intravenous use but is more sedating than haloperidol and has a slight risk of provoking hypotension. In a double-blind study in which haloperidol (im) was compared with droperidol in actively agitated patients, droperidol appeared to give more rapid relief (Resnick and Burton 1984). Antipsychotic medications that are less potent, such as chlorpromazine and thioridazine, are not recommended because they are more likely to cause hypotension and anticholinergic side effects.

Regardless of the route of administration, the usual initial dose of haloperidol in younger agitated patients is 2 mg for mild agitation, 5 mg for moderate agitation, and 10 mg for severe agitation. The initial dose for elderly patients is 0.5 mg for mild agitation, 1 mg for moderate agitation, and 2 mg for severe agitation. Following administration of haloperidol intravenously, the Q-T interval on the electrocardiogram (ECG) should be checked for prolongation. The intravenous or intramuscular dose is repeated every 30 minutes, and the oral dose is repeated every hour, until the patient is sedated and/or calm. After the confusion has cleared, the medications are continued for 3–5 days. Abrupt discontinuation of medication after improvement may be followed by recurrence of the delirium within 24 hours. A more rational approach is to taper the medication over a 3- to 5-day period, administering the largest dose of the medication before bedtime to help normalize the sleep-wake cycle.

The use of benzodiazepines in delirium has its proponents. Although benzodiazepines are the drugs of choice in DTs, the sedation that accompanies benzodiazepines may further impair the sensorium in patients with delirium. In addition, some patients may be further disinhibited when given benzodiazepines. In a double-blind trial of haloperidol, chlorpromazine, and lorazepam in the treatment of delirium in patients with AIDS, Breitbart et al. (1996) discontinued the lorazepam arm of the protocol because patients developed treatment-limiting adverse effects. Therefore, with the exception of drug withdrawal states, benzodiazepines are not recommended as the sole agent in the treatment of patients with delirium. Benzodiazepines have been used with success as adjuncts to high-potency neuroleptics such as haloperidol (Adams 1984; Garza-Trevino et al. 1989). Intravenous lorazepam in doses of 0.5–2.0 mg, particularly in patients who have not responded to haloperidol alone, is quite useful.

Psychosocial Support

The psychological support of a patient both during and after an episode of delirium is important. For the paranoid, agitated patient, having a calm family member remain with the patient is reassuring and can prevent mishaps (e.g., pulling out arterial lines, falling out of bed). In lieu of a family member, close supervision by reassuring nursing staff is crucial.

After the delirium has resolved, helping the patient understand the bizarre experience can be therapeutic (Mackenzie and Popkin 1980). An explanation of delirium to the family can reduce anxiety and calm fears. Although many patients who remember the delirious period are reluctant to discuss their experiences, they should be encouraged to do so. A simple explanation of delirium is usually all that is required to reduce posttraumatic morbidity.

Environmental Intervention

Environmental interventions are sometimes helpful but should not be considered the primary treatment. Both nurses and family members can reorient the patient to date and surroundings. Placing a clock, calendar, and familiar objects in the room may be helpful. Adequate light in the room during the night usually decreases frightening illusions. Despite recommendations to the contrary, a private room for patients with delirium is appropriate only if adequate supervision can be assured. A common error occurring on medical and surgical wards is to place patients with delirium in the same room. This makes reorientation impossible and often leads to confirmation, on the basis of conversations with a paranoid roommate, that strange things are indeed happening in the hospital. A room with a window may be helpful to orient the patient to normal diurnal cues (Wilson 1972). If the patient normally wears eyeglasses or a hearing aid, return of these devices to the patient may help him or her better understand the environment.

DEMENTIA

Dementia is an emerging major health challenge, not only for clinicians but for society as a whole. The dementia syndrome affects 5%–8% of individuals older than age 65, 15%–20% of individuals older than age 75, and 25%–50% of individuals older than age 85 (American Psychiatric Association 1997).

The term *dementia* is often used to describe chronic, irreversible, and progressive conditions. It must be emphasized that this diagnosis is nonspecific and should not automatically imply irreversibility. Indeed, an early review suggested that one-third of the demented patients presenting for initial evaluation have reversible syndromes (Rabins 1983); however, more recent reviews find that reversible dementia occurs in as few as 1% of outpatients (Arnold and Kumar 1993; Clarfield 1995; Weytingh et al. 1995). For the purposes of this chapter, *dementia* is defined as a syndrome of acquired, persistent intellectual impairment with compromised function in multiple spheres of mental activity, such as memory, language, visuospatial skills, emotion or personality, and cognition (Cummings et al. 1980). The principal causes of dementia are listed in Table 10–9.

A diagnostically useful way to categorize dementing disorders is into *cortical* and *subcortical* types. The clinical findings in the cortical dementias reflect dysfunction of the cerebral cortex and are characterized by amnesia, aphasia, apraxia, and agnosia. Alzheimer's disease is the classic example of a cortical dementia. The signs and symptoms found in patients with subcortical dementias are caused by dysfunction of the deep gray and deep white matter structures, including the basal ganglia, thalamus, brain stem nuclei, and frontal lobe projections of these structures. Injury to subcortical structures often disrupts arousal, attention, motivation, and the rate of information processing; this manifests clinically as psychomotor retardation, defective recall, poor abstraction and strategy formation, and mood and personality alterations such as depression and apathy. Dementias caused by human immunodeficiency virus (HIV) disease, Huntington's disease, and Parkinson's disease are examples of subcortical dementias (Mandell and Albert 1990).

NORMAL AGING

The changes seen in patients with dementia reflect the impact of significant brain pathology, *not* normal aging.

TABLE 10–9. **Etiological classification of the principal dementia syndromes**

Degenerative disorders	*Dysmyelinating*	Whipple's disease
Cortical	Metachromatic leukodystrophy	Acquired immunodeficiency syndrome (AIDS)
Alzheimer's disease	Adrenoleukodystrophy	Jakob-Creutzfeldt disease
Lewy body disease	Cerebrotendinous xanthomatosis	Subacute sclerosing panencephalitis
Pick's disease	**Traumatic conditions**	Progressive multifocal leukoencephalopathy
Frontal lobe degeneration of non-Alzheimer type	Posttraumatic encephalopathy	**Toxic conditions**
Subcortical	Subdural hematoma	Alcohol-related syndromes
Parkinson's disease	Dementia pugilistica	Polydrug abuse
Huntington's disease	**Neoplastic dementias**	Iatrogenic dementias
Progressive supranuclear palsy	Meningioma (particularly subfrontal)	Anticholinergic agents
Spinocerebellar degenerations	Glioma	Antihypertensive agents
Idiopathic basal ganglia calcification	Metastatic deposits	Psychotropic agents
Striatonigral degeneration	Meningeal carcinomatosis	Anticonvulsant agents
Wilson's disease	**Hydrocephalic dementias**	Miscellaneous agents
Thalamic dementia	*Communicating*	Metals
Vascular dementias	Normal-pressure hydrocephalus	Industrial solvents
Multiple large vessel occlusions	*Noncommunicating*	**Metabolic disorders**
Lacunar state (multiple subcortical infarctions)	Aqueductal stenosis	Cardiopulmonary failure
Binswanger's disease (white matter ischemic injury)	Intraventricular neoplasm	Uremia
	Intraventricular cyst	Hepatic encephalopathy
Strategic infarctions	Basilar meningitis	Endocrine disorders
Mixed cortical and subcortical infarctions	**Inflammatory conditions**	Thyroid
	Systemic lupus erythematosus	Adrenal
Cerebral autosomal dominant arteriopathy with subcortical infarcts and leukoencephalopathy (CADASIL)	Antiphospholipid syndrome	Parathyroid
	Temporal arteritis	Anemia and hematological conditions
	Sarcoidosis	Deficiency states (vitamin B$_{12}$, folate)
Myelinoclastic disorders	Granulomatous arteritis	Porphyria
Demyelinating	**Infection-related dementias**	**Psychiatric disorders**
Multiple sclerosis	Syphilis	Depression
Marchiafava-Bignami disease	Chronic meningitis	Mania
	Lyme disease	Schizophrenia
	Postencephalitic dementia syndrome	

Studies have confirmed that memory decline in normal aging is distinct from that seen in dementia (Bamford and Caine 1988; Crook et al. 1986); research criteria for age-associated memory impairment (AAMI) are shown in Table 10–10. To date, studies have shown a high prevalence for AAMI in individuals age 80 or older, ranging from nearly 40% to 85% (Larrabee and Crook 1994). AAMI appears to be a stable heterogeneous condition associated with normal aging and does not represent the earliest stages of a dementing illness, such as Alzheimer's disease (Hanninen and Soininen 1997). Newly proposed, more comprehensive diagnostic criteria will further characterize and refine aging-associated cognitive decline (Levy 1994).

Two diagnoses in DSM-IV (1994) can be used to describe mild or normal cognitive decline often observed with aging. Age-related cognitive decline (DSM-IV code 780.9) denotes mild cognitive changes that are within normal limits for age and are not due to a medical disorder. Mild neurocognitive disorder (DSM-IV code 294.9) is used when a medical illness causes an individual to have mild impairment in two or more cognitive areas. Exclusion criteria for this diagnosis include delirium, dementia, and amnestic disorder, and the cognitive dysfunction must not be better accounted for by another mental disorder.

Neurobiological data suggest that frontal-subcortical systems are the most vulnerable to aging, with prominent neuronal cell loss in the frontal cortex and basal ganglia. In addition, many nondemented elderly patients have ischemic changes in the deep white matter and basal ganglia that result in loss of brain tissue and ventricular enlargement; small decreases in total brain weight typically occur with advancing age. Neuropsychology research has

TABLE 10–10. Diagnostic criteria for age-associated memory impairment

Patients at least 50 years of age

Subjective complaints of *gradual* onset of memory dysfunction in daily life activities (e.g., difficulty remembering names, misplacing objects, forgetting phone numbers)

Psychometric evidence of memory failure, as measured by a performance at least one standard deviation below the mean established for young adults on a well-standardized test

Intact global intellectual function

Absence of dementia

Absence of any current or past medical, neurological, or psychiatric illness known to produce cognitive impairment, including the effects of psychotropic or other medications, drug or alcohol use, and any history of head trauma resulting in a period of unconsciousness for 1 hour or more

Source. Adapted from Crook et al. 1986.

suggested that psychomotor slowing, lowered arousal, diminished performance on nonverbal tasks, forgetfulness for nonverbal information, and poor performance on tasks of cognitive flexibility are associated with normal aging (Van Gorp and Mahler 1990). These findings must be interpreted with caution because the assessment of neuropsychological functions in the "normal elderly" is complicated by the effects of illness and medications. Recent studies of optimally healthy elderly persons have shown only slowed information processing and some signs of inefficiency in finding correct problem-solving strategies (Boone et al. 1990). Naming, attention, and verbal neuropsychological tasks appear to be relatively insensitive to aging.

DEMENTIA OF THE ALZHEIMER'S TYPE

In 1907, Alois Alzheimer reported "a peculiar disease of the cerebral cortex" in a 51-year-old woman. The patient displayed the clinical and pathological features of the dementing illness that came to bear Alzheimer's name (Wilkins and Brody 1969). The patient exhibited a progressive, deteriorating course, memory loss, delusions of persecution and jealousy, hiding of objects, disorientation, naming difficulties, paraphasias, and a tendency to perseverate. Her neurological examination was unremarkable. At the time of death, the patient was stuporous and lay in bed with her legs drawn into a fetal position. Autopsy revealed brain atrophy without macroscopic lesions. Microscopic inspection demonstrated the neurofibrillary tangles and "miliary foci" (plaques) associated with Alzheimer's disease (Wilkins and Brody 1969). These characteristic lesions of the brain parenchyma are shown in Figure 10–4.

Epidemiology

Dementia of the Alzheimer's type (DAT) is the most commonly occurring dementia, accounting for approximately 50% of patients evaluated for progressive cognitive decline. Perhaps an additional 15%–20% of these patients have a combination of Alzheimer's and vascular pathology at autopsy (Cummings and Benson 1992; Tomlinson et al. 1970).

The risk of developing DAT increases with age. A recent community survey showed annual incidence (i.e., new cases of DAT each year) of 0.6% for ages 65–69, 1% for ages 70–74, 2.0% for ages 75–79, 3.3% for ages 80–84, and 8.4% for individuals of 85 and older (Hebert et al. 1995). As a general rule, the risk for DAT is 1% at age 60, and this prevalence doubles with every 5-year increase in age (Jorm et al. 1987). It remains unknown whether this risk ulti-

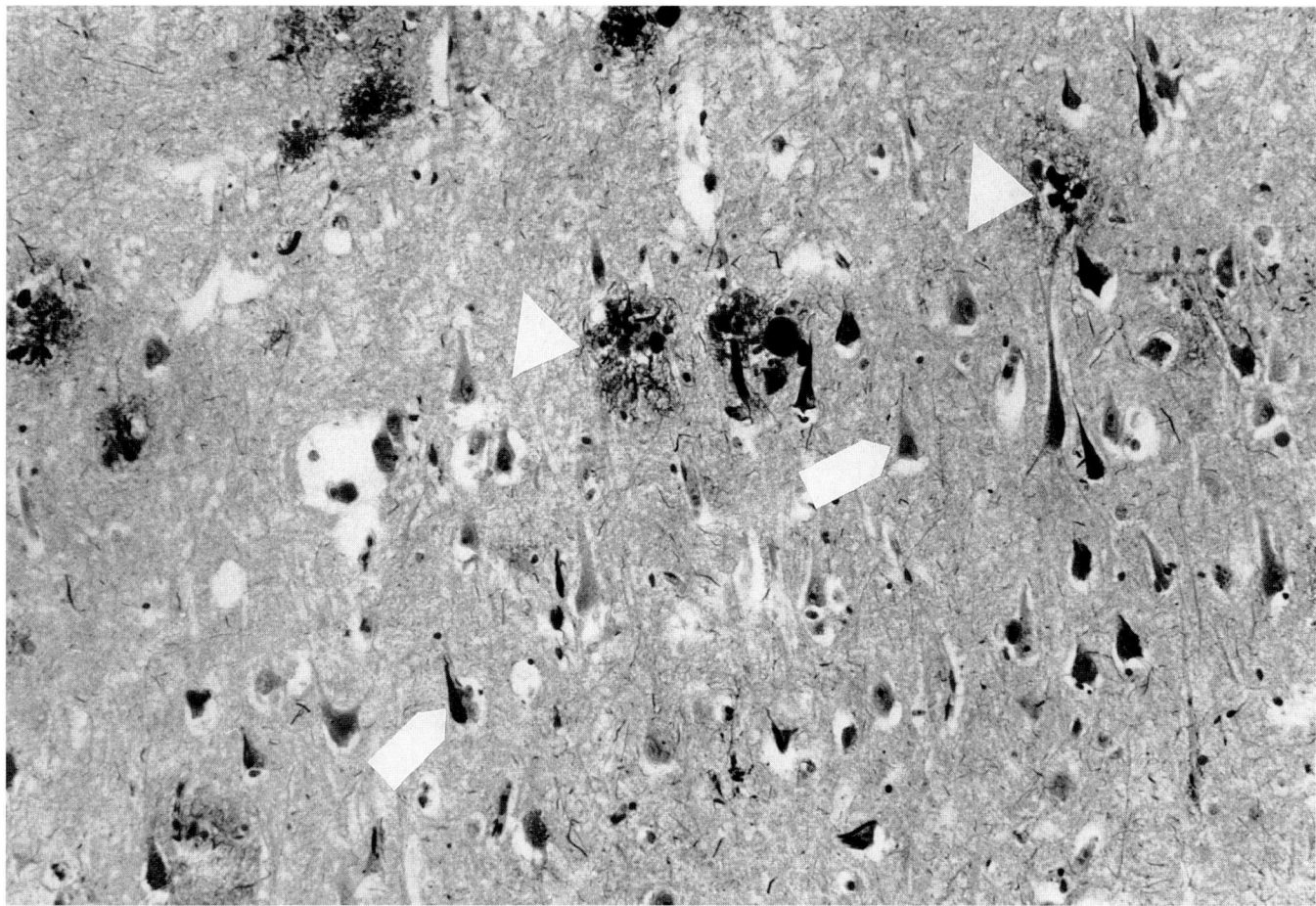

FIGURE 10–4. Alzheimer's disease. Microscopic brain section showing pyramidal cell layer of hippocampus with numerous triangular intraneuronal neurofibrillary tangles [⇨] and several senile plaques [▷] (Bielschowsky stain; original magnification ×190).
Source. Figure provided by Dr. H. V. Vinters, Section of Neuropathology, UCLA Medical Center, Los Angeles, CA. Reprinted with permission from Vinters HV, Miller BL, Pardridge WM: "Brain amyloid and Alzheimer disease." *Ann Intern Med* 109:41–54, 1988.

mately plateaus, continues to increase, or finally declines in the oldest old population (Fratiglioni et al. 1997; Ritchie and Kildea 1995). Currently, DAT is the fourth leading cause of death among elderly persons.

Whereas advanced age remains the one undisputed risk factor for DAT, several others have been proposed. For example, women are overrepresented in the DAT population. This may occur because more women live to the age of increased risk, although genetic and other factors appear to put women at higher risk for DAT (Fratiglioni et al. 1997; Mendez et al. 1992; Payami et al. 1996a, 1996b). Low educational level may increase risk for developing DAT and other dementias; certainly greater education appears to increase reserve and confer protection against detection until more advanced stages of neuropathology (Alexander et al. 1997; Stern et al. 1994). Proposed exogenous risk factors

for the development of DAT include head trauma with loss of consciousness (Schofield et al. 1997; Van Duijn et al. 1992), a history of depression, late maternal age, occupational and environmental exposures (e.g., to aluminum), electroconvulsive therapy, alcohol abuse, analgesic abuse, long-standing physical inactivity, and other medical conditions (Henderson 1991; Mendez et al. 1992; Speck et al. 1995; Van Duijn et al. 1994).

Compelling data now exist to implicate endogenous, specifically genetic, factors in the etiology of at least some cases of DAT. Down's syndrome patients inevitably develop neuropathological features indistinguishable from those of DAT as they grow older. Chromosome 21, the chromosome known to be abnormal in Down's syndrome, is the location of the gene for the amyloid precursor protein (Whatley and Anderton 1990).

Approximately 5% of DAT cases are clearly familial in nature. Familial DAT is more likely to have an early age at onset than sporadic DAT (Lendon et al. 1997). In several affected pedigrees, mutations occur within the amyloid precursor protein gene on chromosome 21 (Chartier-Harlin et al. 1991; Goate et al. 1991; Hendriks et al. 1992; Mullan et al. 1992; Murrell et al. 1991). In other families, the responsible mutations are found at loci on chromosomes 14 and 1 that code for the proteins presenilin-1 and -2, respectively (Levy-Lahad et al. 1995; Schellenberg et al. 1992; Van Broeckhoeven 1995). Mutations in each of these three genes presumably lead to elevated levels of a fragment of the amyloid precursor protein that is deposited in the brains of DAT patients (Lendon et al. 1997). Efforts to unravel genetic contributions to late-onset familial DAT are ongoing; a new locus found on chromosome 12 and mutations found in mitochondrial cytochrome c oxidase genes may prove promising (Davis et al. 1997; Pericak-Vance et al. 1997).

Most cases of DAT are sporadic. Patients have either no affected relatives or only a few, without the dramatic clustering of cases seen in familial DAT. Nevertheless, genetic factors may play a role in predisposing to sporadic DAT. The epsilon 4 allele of the apolipoprotein E (APOE) gene on chromosome 19 increases the risk of developing the disease (Chartier-Harlin et al. 1994; Roses 1994; Strittmatter et al. 1993). The effect is dose dependent (Corder et al. 1993). Individuals homozygous for the epsilon 4 isoform have a greater chance of developing DAT, and at an earlier age, than those who are heterozygous and have only one copy. The latter, in turn, are more likely to develop DAT, and at an earlier age, than individuals without the epsilon 4 allele. Nevertheless, not all individuals who possess the epsilon 4 allele are affected by DAT, and at least 35%–50% of persons with DAT do not carry an epsilon 4 allele. Therefore, the APOE genotype is a risk factor for DAT but not a direct cause, and use of APOE genotyping is not recommended either for routine clinical diagnosis or for predictive testing (American College of Medical Genetics/American Society of Human Genetics Working Group 1995; National Institute on Aging/Alzheimer's Association Working Group 1996; Post et al. 1997).

The APOE epsilon 4 isoform and other, as yet undetermined, genetic factors likely interact with environmental risk factors such as head trauma (Katzman et al. 1996; Mayeux et al. 1995) in producing the disease. The biological basis for the association between the epsilon 4 allele and DAT is unclear, but it has been suggested that APOE isoforms may differentially affect the deposition of β-amyloid (Lendon et al. 1997). In fact, Selkoe (1997) postulates that all known genetic alterations underlying DAT increase the production or deposition (or both) of amyloid β protein.

Pathophysiology

On gross inspection, the brain of a patient with DAT is characterized by cortical atrophy, widened sulci, and ventricular enlargement. Microscopic examination reveals neuronal loss, neurofibrillary tangles, neuropil threads, neuritic plaques, dystrophic neuronal processes, granulovacuolar degeneration, and amyloid angiopathy. The most severe pathological changes occur in the medial temporal lobe, including the hippocampus, amygdala, entorhinal cortex, and parahippocampal gyrus; areas of the parietotemporal and frontal lobes are involved to an intermediate degree (Pearson and Powell 1989). The first changes are seen in the entorhinal cortex, then spread in a predictable, nonrandom manner across other portions of the brain. These sequential changes in the distribution pattern of the lesions provide the basis for a staging procedure that provides accurate neuropathologic diagnoses in the initial stages and even reveals brain changes developing prior to the appearance of clinical symptoms (Braak and Braak 1997). Tangles are located within neurons and are composed primarily of paired helical filaments that contain abnormally phosphorylated microtubule-associated tau proteins. Plaques are located extracellularly and consist of a core of amyloid peptide and aluminosilicates, surrounded by dystrophic nerve processes, terminals, and organelles (Matsuyama and Jarvik 1989). Granulovacuolar degeneration consists of intracytoplasmic vacuoles, particularly in neurons of the hippocampus. Amyloid angiopathy is present in nearly all cases of DAT. The amyloid found in the cerebral vasculature is identical to that in neuritic plaques; it is also present in extracerebral vessels in skin, subcutaneous tissue, and intestine (Cummings and Benson 1992; Vinters et al. 1988). Recent findings have indicated that the amyloid β-peptide of DAT is produced by normal cell metabolism. The abnormal accumulation of amyloid implies chronically enhanced production and/or decreased clearance mechanisms (Haass et al. 1992).

It is important to remember that all the neuropathological changes in DAT are found in the brains of clinically normal, nondemented individuals; the location and number of these lesions determine the postmortem histological diagnosis (Khachaturian 1985; Vinters 1991).

Clinical Features

Dementia of the Alzheimer's type typically begins after age 50 and is associated with an insidious and gradually progressive decline in mental abilities. Often the patient and family members are unaware of the evolving cognitive impairment, and the onset of the illness is identified only in retrospect. Memory difficulties are manifest by the patient's forgetting tasks, repeating questions, or losing the thread of a conversation or a television program. The patient may complain about memory problems early in the course of the disease, but insight is rapidly lost. In fact, the patient's lack of insight in the face of gross cognitive impairments is characteristic of DAT. Family members may notice that the patient is more rigid and inflexible, less adventurous, more irritable, and less spontaneous.

Job performance declines, and the person is less productive, misses appointments, fails to return phone calls, and may be forcibly "retired." More and more of the patient's responsibilities are assumed by colleagues, secretaries, and family members, who do not realize this person has a progressive disease and may feel only that the patient is "slipping" with age. Individuals also may neglect to pay bills, pay the same bill several times, fail to balance the checkbook, incorrectly follow recipes, or get lost while driving. Alcohol may produce an exaggerated emotional response, and any disruption in the person's routine is poorly tolerated. A family vacation or trip to visit relatives often reveals problems with orientation and memory. Intercurrent illness that requires hospitalization or anesthesia may provoke episodes of "sundowning" or delirium.

Deterioration progresses over months and years. Studies of patients with DAT have consistently shown a decline of 3–4 points per year on the MMSE (Folstein 1997a, 1997b). This decline in cognitive function occurs regardless of the patient's age, sex, or educational level, or whether or not the patient resides in a nursing home (Katzman et al. 1988). Individual patients may vary in their rate of deterioration, but a dramatic decline in MMSE warrants investigation for underlying medical illness.

Tasks performed independently in the past, such as grocery shopping, preparing meals, and selecting appropriate clothing to wear, become impossible for the patient with DAT. Driving may become especially problematic, even though the patient insists he or she is competent in an automobile. Personal hygiene and grooming are neglected; the patient is no longer able to shave, bathe, or use the toilet properly. The ability to dress also fails; the patient may wear the same clothes for days at a time or may wear several layers of clothes improperly buttoned or fastened.

Delusional beliefs often develop (Burns et al. 1990a, 1990b). Patients with DAT commonly are convinced that others are trying to steal from them or harm them, that their spouse is unfaithful, that family members have been replaced by impostors (Capgras's syndrome), that their house is not really their home, or that family members are plotting to abandon them. Hallucinatory experiences may occur, with the patient hearing or talking to people who are not there. The patient may cling to family members, often not letting the caregiver out of his or her sight. The patient will pace around the house without apparent purpose, engaging in repetitive, stereotyped activities such as opening and closing drawers, putting on and taking off clothing, handling buttons, turning doorknobs, picking at clothing, or wrapping and unwrapping balls of string. The patient may wander from the house and get lost in familiar surroundings or become more and more reclusive.

As family members and caregivers become concerned and attempt to reassure the patient or assist with activities of daily living, the patient's responses become increasingly erratic and exaggerated. Well-intended attempts to assist or "force" the patient to perform tasks such as bathing or getting into a car may precipitate catastrophic reactions. These are abrupt, possibly even violent outbursts of verbal and/or physical aggression. The overreaction in these episodes may be misinterpreted by caregivers as stubbornness, criticism, or ingratitude. The episodes may cease almost as abruptly as they arose, a situation that can confuse and frustrate caregivers (Mace and Rabins 1991).

Eventually, patients become unable to recognize close family members and may even misidentify their own reflection in a mirror. Late-onset seizures may appear (Romanelli et al. 1990). Primitive reflexes emerge, such as the grasp, snout, and suck reflexes. In the final stage of the illness, the patient becomes incontinent of urine and feces, loses all intelligible vocabulary, and is unable to walk or to sit up (Reisberg 1988). Death from pneumonia or another infectious process frequently occurs during a period of total confinement in bed.

Diagnosis

The clinical diagnosis of DAT requires the gradual, progressive development of multiple cognitive deficits, including both memory impairment and cognitive disturbances (American Psychiatric Association 1994). The DSM-IV diagnostic criteria are shown in Table 10–11.

It is recommended in DSM-IV that clinicians record the type of onset as "early" (i.e., age 65 or younger) or "late" (i.e., older than age 65). Although the pathology is indistinguishable, nevertheless there are clear clinical differences between patients with early- versus late-onset DAT (Amaducci et al. 1986; Seltzer and Sherwin 1983). Early-onset patients perform more poorly on measures of language, praxis, and concentration, whereas late-onset patients perform more poorly on measures of memory and orientation. Early-onset patients demonstrate a signifi-

TABLE 10–11. DSM-IV diagnostic criteria for dementia of the Alzheimer's type

A. The development of multiple cognitive deficits manifested by both

    (1) Memory impairment (impaired ability to learn new information or to recall previously learned information)

    (2) One (or more) of the following cognitive disturbances:

        (a) Aphasia (language disturbance)

        (b) Apraxia (impaired ability to carry out motor activities despite intact motor function)

        (c) Agnosia (failure to recognize or identify objects despite intact sensory function)

        (d) Disturbance in executive functioning (i.e., planning, organizing, sequencing, abstracting)

B. The cognitive deficits in Criteria A1 and A2 each cause significant impairment in social or occupational functioning and represent a significant decline from a previous level of functioning.

C. The course is characterized by gradual onset and continuing cognitive decline.

D. The cognitive deficits in Criteria A1 and A2 are not due to any of the following:

    (1) Other central nervous system conditions that cause progressive deficits in memory and cognition (e.g., cerebrovascular disease, Parkinson's disease, Huntington's disease, subdural hematoma, normal-pressure hydrocephalus, brain tumor)

    (2) Systemic conditions that are known to cause dementia (e.g., hypothyroidism, vitamin B_{12} or folic acid deficiency, niacin deficiency, hypercalcemia, neurosyphilis, HIV infection)

    (3) Substance-induced conditions

E. The deficits do not occur exclusively during the course of a delirium.

F. The disturbance is not better accounted for by another Axis I disorder (e.g., major depressive disorder, schizophrenia).

---

cantly faster rate of progression for all neuropsychological measures (Koss et al. 1996).

In the past, the diagnosis of DAT was one of exclusion. Fortunately, the refinement of diagnostic criteria enables clinicians to use specific clinical features to identify the disease (McKhann et al. 1984). The application of modern criteria, such as the NINCDS-ADRDA criteria (Table 10–12), yields an accuracy rate approaching 85% when compared with a postmortem diagnosis of DAT (Joachim et al. 1988).

The memory impairment found in patients with DAT

TABLE 10–12. NINCDS-ADRDA criteria for definite, probable, possible, and unlikely dementia of the Alzheimer type (DAT)

Definite DAT

Clinical criteria for probable DAT

Histopathological evidence of DAT (autopsy or biopsy)

Probable DAT

Dementia established by clinical examination and documented by mental status questionnaire

Dementia confirmed by neuropsychological testing

Deficits in two or more areas of cognition

Progressive worsening of memory or other cognitive functions

No disturbance of consciousness

Onset between ages 40 and 49

Absence of systemic or other brain diseases capable of producing a dementia syndrome

Possible DAT

Atypical onset, presentation, or progression of a dementia syndrome without a known etiology

Presence of a systemic or other brain disease capable of producing dementia but not thought to be the cause of the dementia

Gradually progressive decline in a single intellectual function in the absence of any other identifiable cause

Unlikely DAT

Sudden onset

Focal neurological signs

Seizures or gait disturbance early in the course of the illness

---

Note. NINCDS-ADRDA = National Institute of Neurological and Communicative Disorders and Stroke—Alzheimer's Disease and Related Disorders Association.
Source. Reprinted with permission from McKhann G, Drachman D, Folstein M, et al: "Clinical Diagnosis of Alzheimer's Disease: Report of the NINCDS-ADRDA Work Group Under the Auspices of the Department of Health and Human Services Task Force on Alzheimer's Disease." *Neurology* 34:939–944, 1984. Copyright 1984, Springer-Verlag.

is manifested by disorientation for time and place, and failure to remember three unrelated words for 3 minutes, even with cues. The language disturbance is a fluent aphasia with anomia; speech has an empty quality and lacks specific content words. Naming and comprehension are progressively impaired, whereas the ability to repeat is relatively preserved; paraphasic errors are common (Cummings and Benson 1986). The gradual development of an isolated, progressive aphasia is often the precursor of a more generalized dementia syndrome (Green et al. 1990). Agnosia and apraxia in DAT are difficult to distinguish from disabilities related to aphasia, amnesia, and visuospatial impairment.

Patients can often recognize objects and use them appropriately even though they can no longer name them accurately (Cummings and Benson 1992; Rapcsak et al. 1989).

Executive cognitive functions help individuals to orchestrate and maintain goal-directed behavior. Problems in executive function commonly occur in patients with DAT, such as difficulties with planning, organizing, sequencing, and abstracting. These may manifest clinically as apathy, distractibility, purposeless stereotypies, overreliance on environmental cues, disinhibition, and a tendency to perseverate (Royall et al. 1992). The stages, or progression, of DAT are summarized in Table 10–13.

With no laboratory tests yet available for DAT, diagnosis is often aided by the use of neuroimaging techniques. Atrophy is usually present on computed tomography (CT) and magnetic resonance imaging (MRI) in patients with DAT; however, brain atrophy of similar magnitude is sometimes found in nondemented individuals. In addition, patients in the early stages of DAT can have normal CT scans (DeCarli et al. 1990). In general, DAT patients have significantly larger ventricles than age-matched control subjects; correlations between ventricular enlargement (especially the temporal horns) and cognitive function are stronger than those between cortical atrophy and cognition (Burns 1990; Frison et al. 1996). Functional imaging using single photon emission computed tomography (SPECT) characteristically shows bilaterally decreased cerebral blood flow in the parietal and posterior temporal lobes in patients who have DAT; frontal lobe blood flow declines in the later stages of the illness. Primary motor, sensory, and visual cortices and basal ganglia maintain normal blood flow (Geaney and Abou-Saleh 1990). SPECT images of a normal patient and a patient with DAT are shown in Figure 10–5.

Positron emission tomography (PET) also consistently shows an early and progressive hypofunction of the posterior temporoparietal cortex and later involvement of the frontal cortex; the primary motor and sensory areas appear normal (Bench et al. 1990; Benson et al. 1983). It must be emphasized that currently both SPECT and PET remain research, rather than clinical diagnostic tools for DAT (Bergman et al. 1997; Santens and Petit 1997).

Treatment

Therapy for DAT is divided into three main categories: 1) control of abnormal behavior associated with the illness, 2) attempts to restore cognitive function, and 3) attempts to delay cognitive decline. Behavioral disturbances such as agitation, insomnia, wandering, suspiciousness, hallucinations, and hostility often arise during the course of dementia. Psychotic symptoms are generally treated with low-dose neuroleptic medication (Schneider et al. 1990); initial treatment with low doses of a high-potency agent such as haloperidol 0.5–2 mg/day is typically recommended. If more sedation is required, a trial with a low-potency agent such as thioridazine is recommended;

TABLE 10–13. Principal clinical findings in each stage of dementia of the Alzheimer type (DAT)

Stage I *(duration of disease 1–3 years)*

Memory: new learning defective, remote recall mildly impaired

Visuospatial skills: topographical disorientation, poor complex constructions

Language: poor word list generation, anomia

Personality: indifference, occasional irritability

Psychiatric features: sadness or, in some cases, delusions

Motor system: normal

EEG: normal

CT/MRI: normal

PET/SPECT: bilateral posterior parietal hypometabolism/ hypoperfusion

Stage II *(duration of disease 2–10 years)*

Memory: recent and remote recall more severely impaired

Visuospatial skills: poor constructions, spatial disorientation

Language: fluent aphasia

Calculation: acalculia

Praxis: ideomotor apraxia

Personality: indifference or irritability

Psychiatric features: delusions in some cases

Motor system: restlessness, pacing

EEG: slowing of background rhythm

CT/MRI: normal and ventricular dilatation and sulcal enlargement

PET/SPECT: bilateral parietal and frontal hypometabolism/ hypoperfusion

Stage III *(duration of disease 8–12 years)*

Intellectual functions: severely deteriorated

Motor: limb rigidity and flexion posture

Sphincter control: urinary and fecal incontinence

EEG: diffusely slow

CT/MRI: ventricular dilatation and sulcal enlargement

PET/SPECT: bilateral parietal and frontal hypometabolism/hypoperfusion

Note. EEG = electroencephalogram; CT = computed tomography; MRI = magnetic resonance imaging; PET = positron emission tomography; SPECT = single photon emission computed tomography.

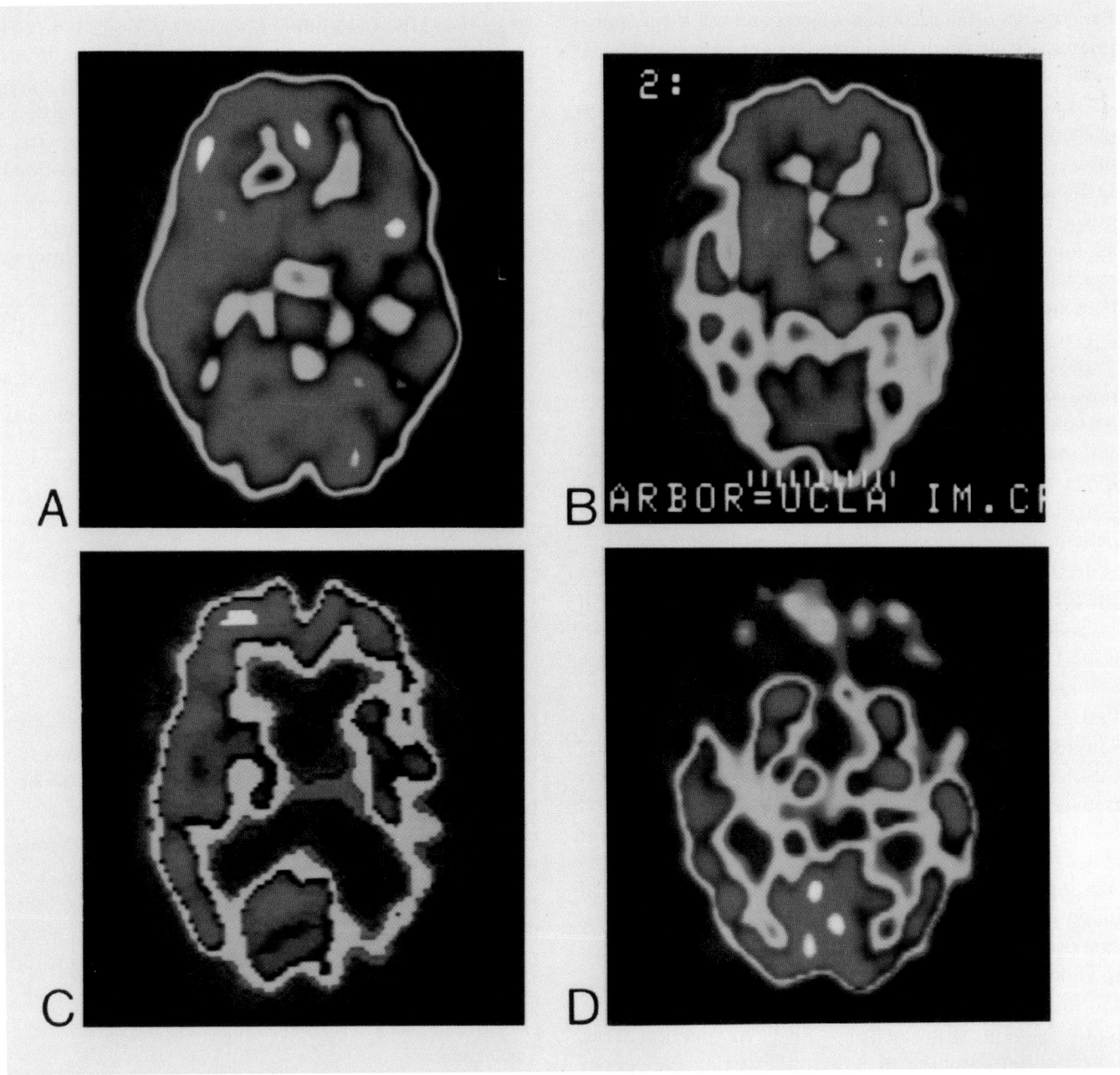

FIGURE 10-5. ^{99}m-Tc-HMPAO transaxial SPECT images. *A)* Individual with normal brain. *B)* Patient with Alzheimer's disease shows characteristic bilateral temporal-parietal hypoperfusion. *C)* Patient with vascular dementia shows asymmetrical unilateral hypoperfusion in anterior and posterior regions. *D)* Patient with frontal lobe degeneration shows marked frontal hypoperfusion with preservation of posterior perfusion.
Source.   Figure provided by Drs. Ismael Mena and Bruce L. Miller, UCLA Harbor Medical Center, Los Angeles, CA. Used with permission.

in dosages below 75 mg/day, this medication usually produces no detectable anticholinergic effects (Steele et al. 1986). A medication must be scheduled properly to produce the desired effects (e.g., 1 hour before bedtime to improve sleep, 1 hour before bathing to diminish agitation). Use of prn, or "as needed," medication should be avoided, because this method of administration medicates the patient's agitation after the fact. Instead, caregivers should be helped to recognize times during the day when problems regularly arise, so that patients can be medicated in anticipation of agitation. This helps to minimize the total amount of medication required.

The cautious, adjunctive use of low doses of short-acting benzodiazepines, such as lorazepam or oxazepam, may also prove beneficial. Other medications recently reported to help modify agitated behavior include trazodone, buspirone, valproate, carbamazepine, risperidone, and gabapentin (Kopala and Honor 1997; Lund and Manchester 1994; Regan and Gordon 1997; Schneider and Sobin 1991; Sultzer et al. 1997; Tiller et al. 1988). Sexual aggression responds well to medroxyprogesterone (Weiner et al. 1992). Creative use of medications often leads to control of an individual patient's target symptoms. The physician must always be on the lookout for medical illnesses, such as urinary tract infections or electrolyte disturbances, that might cause sudden changes in behavior or mental status (Small 1988).

Control of unwanted behavioral symptoms is the key to helping patients with dementia remain with their families (Zubenko et al. 1992). The clinician must pay close attention to the patient's environment; too much or too little stimulation may result in withdrawal or agitation. Patients with dementia do best with regular daily routines conducted in a familiar and constant environment. Clocks, calendars, night-lights, checklists, and diaries all aid in orientation and memory during the early phase of the illness. Caregivers must display a pleasant tone and a pleasant countenance during their interactions with the DAT patient, and must learn their patients' (and their own) limitations. Caregivers should be urged to simplify tasks and to avoid rushing or forcing patients to attempt things beyond their ability (Mace and Rabins 1991; Small 1989).

The discovery of profound cholinergic deficits in the brains of DAT patients led to the formulation of a "cholinergic hypothesis" analogous to the dopamine deficiency hypothesis in Parkinson's disease (Davis and Mohs 1982). As a result, various cholinomimetic treatment strategies have been tried, including the use of acetylcholine precursors, cholinergic agonists, and cholinesterase inhibitors. Several centrally active cholinesterase inhibitors, including donepezil, metrifonate, and tacrine, have produced modest cognitive improvement in controlled trials (Becker et al. 1998; Davis et al. 1992; Rogers et al. 1996) and are currently available for use in DAT.

Deficits in multiple other neurotransmitters are present in DAT, including norepinephrine and serotonin; thus, the usefulness of single neurotransmitter replacement therapy appears limited. Future strategies for cognitive restoration likely will target multiple neurotransmitter systems, using drug combinations (Schneider et al. 1993). To date, clinical trials of psychostimulants, cerebral vasodilators, and nootropics such as piracetam and ergoloid mesylates (Hydergine) have not shown consistent beneficial effects. A placebo-controlled, randomized trial of Ginkgo biloba has shown modest cognitive enhancement (Le et al. 1997). Early and more accurate identification of patients with DAT will allow therapeutic intervention before the degenerative processes are advanced beyond the brain's reserve capacity (Stern and Davis 1991). Protective therapy aimed at retarding neuronal degeneration and preventive therapy to eliminate neuronal degeneration entirely will likely be the ultimate treatment strategies (Growdon 1992).

Several treatments may delay or slow the progress of DAT. α-Tocopherol (vitamin E) and selegiline may significantly delay the decline in patients with DAT (Sano et al. 1997). A lowered risk of acquiring DAT may be associated with use of anti-inflammatory medications (Aisen and Davis 1994), such as nonsteroidal anti-inflammatory drugs (MacKenzie and Munoz 1998; Stewart et al. 1997), and with use of estrogen by postmenopausal women (Tang et al. 1996; Yaffe et al. 1998).

VASCULAR DEMENTIA

Vascular dementia (VaD) is the diagnostic term used when cerebral injury from vascular disease leads to multiple cognitive impairments. There is considerable heterogeneity in both the pathological and the clinical expression of VaD. Cerebral infarctions can accumulate and produce the progressive cognitive impairment called *multi-infarct dementia*. Alternatively, chronic ischemia without infarction can impair cognition, or ischemic injury can coexist with other neuropathology, such as DAT (Chui et al. 1992). Although ischemia, hemorrhage, and anoxia all can cause dementia, VaD is most often associated with ischemic vascular disease.

Epidemiology

Vascular dementia is the second most common cause of dementia. It occurs in 15%–30% of patients with dementia and is mixed with DAT in an additional 15%–20%. The frequency of VaD syndromes reported in the literature ranges from 1.5% to 65%, figures that either underestimate (O'Brien 1988) or overestimate (Brust 1988) the true prevalence of VaD (Roman et al. 1993). The prevalence of cerebrovascular disease increases with age, and VaD is most commonly encountered after age 60. Men are affected more often than women. Whereas hereditary factors play a major role in DAT, environmental factors appear to dominate in VaD (Bergem et al. 1997). Almost invariably, VaD is associated with stroke risk factors: hypertension, heart disease, cigarette smoking, diabetes mellitus, excessive alcohol consumption (more than three drinks per day), and hyperlipidemia. Several of these risk factors are often present in the patient with VaD (Meyer et al. 1988; Skoog 1998).

Pathophysiology

Strokes cause dementia through several mechanisms that are related to the location of cerebral injury, the volume of cerebral tissue involved, the number of cerebral insults, and the co-occurrence of VaD and DAT (Tatemichi 1990). Subcortical lacunar infarctions are found in approximately 70% of patients with VaD. Therefore, a "lacunar state" is the most frequent cause of VaD; it is produced by multiple small infarctions involving the basal ganglia, thalamus, and internal capsule. VaD may also result from the cumulative effects of watershed or border zone infarctions caused by critical reductions of cerebral perfusion in patients who have severe extracranial atherosclerosis; this pathology is seen in up to 40% of patients with VaD, making it the second most frequent etiology for VaD (Meyer et al. 1988). A diagnosis of Binswanger's disease is made on the basis of extensive ischemic white matter damage in the subcortical periventricular regions of the centrum semiovale. These periventricular regions are susceptible to hypoperfusion from the blood vessels supplying the deep white matter (Tatemichi 1990). VaD may also result from the cumulative effects of multiple cerebral emboli; these embolic infarcts are found in approximately 20% of patients with VaD and represent the third most frequent cause of this dementia. Embolic infarcts are usually larger than lacunae and have a bilateral hemispheric distribution. An identifiable cardiac source for the emboli is found in one-fourth of these patients. A mixture of two or more different types of strokes is common, occurring in nearly one-third of VaD patients (Meyer et al. 1988). Additional, less common causes of VaD include the hypercoagulopathy associated with antiphospholipid antibody syndrome, and the recently identified familial syndrome of cerebral autosomal dominant arteriopathy with subcortical infarcts and leukoencephalopathy (CADASIL) (Gorman and Cummings 1993; Ruchoux and Maurage 1997). These syndromes should be considered when the patient who has suffered a stroke either is young or has few other known risk factors.

Both the volume of cerebral injury and the number of infarctions have considerable face validity as mechanisms of VaD. Although recent findings indicate that the total infarction area correlates with dementia following stroke, the location of cerebral infarction (especially cortical loca-

tion and left hemispheric laterality) appears to be more critically correlated with the development of VaD than does the total volume of infarcted brain (Liu et al. 1992; Meyer et al. 1988).

Clinical Features

Vascular dementia is characterized by abrupt onset, stepwise progression, fluctuating course, depression, pseudobulbar palsy, a history of hypertension, a history of strokes, evidence of associated atherosclerosis, focal neurological symptoms, and focal neurological signs (Hachinski et al. 1975). These features constitute an ischemia score (Table 10–14) that helps differentiate VaD from DAT (Molsa et al. 1985; Rosen et al. 1980). Unfortunately, the ischemia score does not differentiate VaD from VaD plus DAT (Erkinjuntti et al. 1988).

The clinical presentation of VaD depends on the location of cerebral injury. Deep hemispheric infarction or ischemia can cause a lacunar state or Binswanger's disease and produce a subcortical dementia with pseudobulbar palsy, spasticity, and weakness. Superficial cortical infarctions can produce cortical dementia with hemimotor and hemisensory dysfunction. Left hemispheric insults produce aphasia, acalculia, apraxia, and verbal amnesia, whereas right hemispheric damage causes aprosodia; disturbances in recognition of face, voice, and place; nonverbal amnesia; visuospatial deficits; and neglect of left visual field (i.e., left hemineglect). Mixed cortical and subcortical syndromes are not uncommon (Cummings 1987). The mechanical aspects of speech are more abnormal in VaD,

TABLE 10–14.   Hachinski ischemia score

Abrupt onset	2
Stepwise progression	1
Fluctuating course	2
Nocturnal confusion	1
Relative preservation of personality	1
Depression	1
Somatic complaints	1
Emotional incontinence	1
History of hypertension	1
History of strokes	2
Evidence of associated atherosclerosis	1
Focal neurological symptoms	2
Focal neurological signs	2
Alzheimer's disease if scores total	4 or less
Vascular dementia if scores total	7 or more

whereas linguistic changes are more profound in DAT. The presence of an articulatory deficit and abnormal speech melody supports the diagnosis of VaD; VaD patients have more information content in spontaneous speech and are less anomic than DAT patients (Powell et al. 1988). Neither the nature and prevalence of delusions nor the occurrence of hallucinations distinguishes VaD from DAT (Cummings et al. 1987). Depression is extremely common following stroke and occurs most often with left cortical and subcortical lesions. The severity of depression is positively correlated with proximity of the lesion to the left frontal pole. Preexisting cortical atrophy and previous strokes may be important risk factors for the subsequent development of poststroke depression (Robinson and Starkstein 1990).

Diagnosis

The DSM-IV diagnostic criteria for VaD are listed in Table 10–15. Neuroimaging plays an especially important role in the diagnosis of VaD, with MRI being the most sensitive structural imaging technique (Kertesz et al. 1987). T_2-weighted MRI images are best for the detection of white matter hyperintensities that represent ischemic changes and dysmyelination (Figure 10–6; Gupta et al. 1988; Kertesz et al. 1988). These white matter changes are not specific to VaD and may occur to some extent in DAT patients, as well as in healthy elderly control subjects. Clinical correlation is therefore essential for diagnosis (Erkinjuntti et al. 1987; Hunt et al. 1989).

Computed tomography detects infarctions in less than half of patients with clinical evidence of VaD (Radue et al. 1978). Nonetheless, areas of decreased lucency in the white matter, called leucoaraiosis, are seen on CT in the majority of patients with VaD. Enlargement of the lateral and third ventricles correlates significantly with severity of cognitive impairment in VaD (Aharon-Peretz et al. 1988).

SPECT images in patients with VaD typically show a pattern of diffusely diminished cerebral blood flow with focal areas of severe hypoperfusion (see Figure 10–5). This pattern theoretically could mimic patterns seen in other diseases; however, the presence of scattered perfusion defects (either unilateral or bilateral) located in primarily cortical areas is suggestive of VaD, especially if perfusion deficits correlate with cerebral infarcts seen on CT or MRI scans (Geaney and Abou-Saleh 1990). PET studies in patients with VaD show global reductions in cerebral metabolism, with additional focal and asymmetrical areas of hypometabolism that are not limited to specific cortical or subcortical brain regions (Benson et al. 1983; De et al. 1998). This suggests that a single lesion may have extensive

and distant metabolic sequelae (Metter et al. 1985). Severity of dementia correlates with the global hypometabolism and frontal cortex deficits seen on PET (Bench et al. 1990).

Treatment

The goals of treatment in VaD are to halt the progression of cognitive deterioration and to optimize remaining cognitive capacity. Therefore, therapy is focused on the management of risk factors, disease-specific interventions for medical conditions, and treatment of psychiatric illness such as depression or psychosis. Individual patients may benefit from speech therapy or physical therapy (Cummings and Benson 1992). Use of daily aspirin therapy (325 mg/day) to inhibit platelet aggregation is recommended (Meyer et al. 1989). In a paper titled "Preventable Senility: A Call for Action Against the Vascular Dementias," Hachinski (1992) outlined the following therapeutic measures: smoking cessation, exercise, diet (control of diabetes, obesity, hyperlipidemia), estrogen re-

TABLE 10–15. DSM-IV diagnostic criteria for vascular dementia

A. The development of multiple cognitive deficits manifested by both:

   (1) Memory impairment (impaired ability to learn new information or to recall previously learned information)

   (2) One (or more) of the following cognitive disturbances:

      (a) aphasia (language disturbance)

      (b) apraxia (impaired ability to carry out motor activities despite intact motor function)

      (c) agnosia (failure to recognize or identify objects despite intact sensory function)

      (d) disturbance in executive functioning (i.e., planning, organizing, sequencing, abstracting)

B. The cognitive deficits in A1 and A2 each cause significant impairment in social or occupational functioning and represent a significant decline from a previous level of functioning.

C. Focal neurological signs and symptoms (e.g., exaggeration of deep tendon reflexes, extensor plantar response, pseudobulbar palsy, gait abnormalities, weakness of an extremity) or laboratory evidence indicative of cerebrovascular disease (e.g., multiple infarctions involving cortex and underlying white matter) that are judged to be etiologically related to the disturbance.

D. The deficits do not occur exclusively during the course of a delirium.

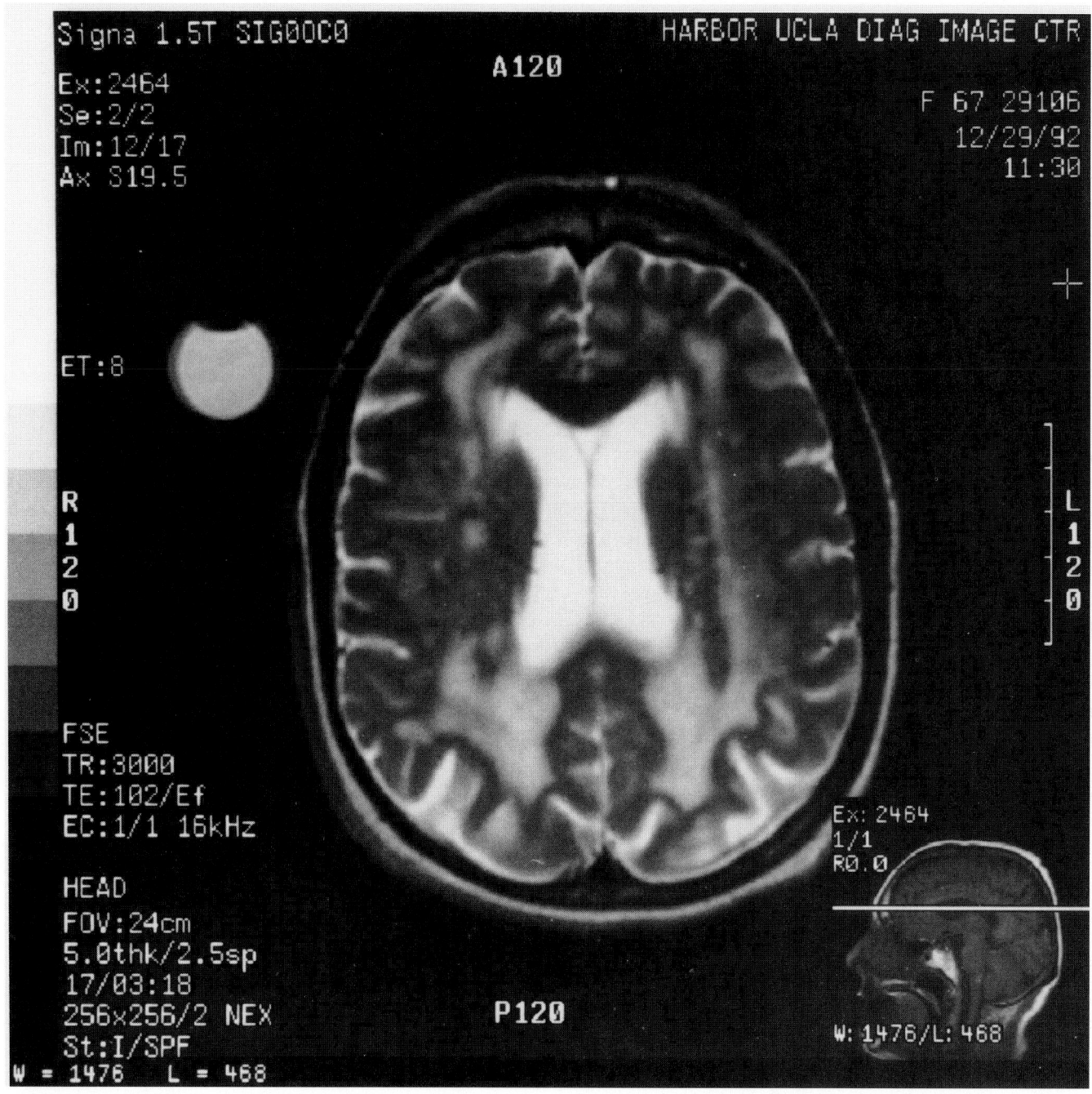

Figure 10–6. T_2-weighted magnetic resonance imaging of a patient with vascular dementia shows extensive white matter hyperintensities.
Source. Figure provided by Dr. Bruce L. Miller, UCLA Harbor Medical Center, Los Angeles, CA. Used with permission.

placement, antihypertensive and lipid-lowering agents, anticoagulants (in atrial fibrillation), and aspirin.

DEMENTIA DUE TO PICK'S DISEASE

Pick's disease is a progressive, degenerative disorder of the frontal lobes or frontal and temporal lobes, and is perhaps the best known type of frontotemporal dementia (FTD). FTD is more common than previously recognized, accounting for 13%–16% of dementias in some studies. Perhaps 20% of FTD cases are diagnosed as Pick's disease; the remaining 80% are designated as frontal lobe degeneration (FLD) of the non-Alzheimer's type. Pick's disease is diagnosed by the presence of distinctive intraneuronal Pick bodies and ballooned Pick cells on microscopic examination; FLD lacks these distinctive histological features (Brun 1987).

Patients with Pick's disease are clinically indistinguishable from other patients with FTD. Patients with FTD present with marked personality changes that may precede obvious cognitive decline by at least 2 years. Disinhibition and irritability are common, as are wandering, impulsivity, and poor judgment. In some patients the first symptoms are social withdrawal, loss of drive, or major depression. Features of Klüver-Bucy syndrome, including hyperorality, hypersexuality, compulsory exploration of the environment, and visual agnosia, are not uncommon. Impairments in frontal executive skills are demonstrable on neuropsychological testing. The clinical presentation, with progressive reduction of speech, loss of insight and stereotyped, perseverative behaviors, together with the relatively late onset of memory and visuospatial disturbances in FTD helps distinguish FTD from DAT (Kertesz et al. 1997; Miller et al. 1997). Recently a temporal lobe variant of FTD has been distinguished, with prominent aphasia in addition to the behavioral disturbances typical for FTD (Edwards-Lee et al. 1997). Frontal atrophy on CT or MRI is sometimes not apparent until late in the course of FTD, making SPECT (see Figure 10–5) or PET imaging extremely useful in separating these patients from patients with DAT (Miller et al. 1991).

DEMENTIA DUE TO CREUTZFELDT-JAKOB DISEASE

Creutzfeldt-Jakob disease (CJD) is an uncommon neurodegenerative disease caused by a transmissible infectious agent, the prion. Prions are proteinaceous particles devoid of nucleic acid. Most cases of this disease arise sporadically; familial forms, following an autosomal dominant pattern of inheritance, constitute 5%–15% of cases. Direct transmission has been thought to occur only iatrogenically, for example from corneal transplants or contaminated neurosurgical instruments. However, there is now considerable concern that prion diseases may be more infectious than previously recognized, and there remains the possibility that bovine prions may have been passed to humans, resulting in a new variant form of CJD (Prusiner 1997; Will et al. 1996). Microscopic neuropathology includes neuronal loss, astrocytic proliferation, and spongiform change in the cells of the cortex, striatum, and thalamus (Masters and Richardson 1978).

Clinical deterioration is extremely rapid, with progressive decline and death within 1 year. Patients show intellectual devastation, myoclonic jerks, muscle rigidity, and ataxia. The EEG frequently shows an intermittent periodic burst pattern that is suggestive of the disease (Brown et al. 1986; Cummings and Benson 1992). Neuroimaging is nondiagnostic; functional imaging techniques may help identify sites for brain biopsy (Miller et al. 1998).

DEMENTIA DUE TO HUNTINGTON'S DISEASE

Huntington's disease (HD) is an idiopathic neurodegenerative disorder inherited as an autosomal dominant trait with complete penetrance. Average age at onset is 40 years, with gradual progression and death about 17 years later. The prevalence of HD has been estimated at from 5 to 7 per 100,000 population (Folstein et al. 1990). Pathologically, there is atrophy of the caudate nucleus and loss of the GABAergic interneurons from the striatum. The clinical triad of dementia, chorea, and a positive family history should suggest the diagnosis of HD. Definitive, presymptomatic diagnosis of HD is now possible using polymerase chain reaction analysis of a CAG repeat sequence in the HD gene (International Huntington Association and World Federation of Neurology Research Group on Huntington's Chorea 1994). Personality changes, such as irritability or apathy, commonly occur before the onset of chorea, and recent work indicates that cognitive deficits may be the very first symptoms of HD (Hahn-Barma et al. 1998). Depression is quite common in HD, and mania and schizophrenia-like persecutory delusions are also seen (McHugh and Folstein 1975). HD is a subcortical dementia, with diminished cognitive speed, a memory retrieval deficit, frontal executive dysfunctions, and motor symptoms. The absence of aphasia and other cortical features helps to distinguish HD from DAT (Cummings and Benson 1992). CT or MRI can demonstrate gross atrophy of the caudate nucleus in HD; functional imaging with PET shows marked caudate hypometabolism before there is any detectable loss of tissue volume (Young et al. 1986).

DEMENTIA DUE TO PARKINSON'S DISEASE

Parkinson's disease (PD) is characterized by progressive loss of dopaminergic neurons in the substantia nigra and other pigmented brain stem nuclei. PD is an example of a long-latency neurological disease, because the tremor, rigidity, bradykinesia, and postural instability emerge when the nigrostriatal system is already 70% damaged. The prevalence of PD is approximately 1 per 1,000, with usual onset between the ages of 50 and 65 years; no definitive role for heredity in PD is known (Cummings and Benson 1992; Koller et al. 1991). The pathological hallmark of PD is the presence of Lewy bodies in the cytoplasm of the remaining nigral neurons; they likely represent an early marker for neuronal cell degeneration (Gibb 1989).

Assessment of intellectual function in patients with PD is difficult, because the clinician must consider the effects of age, depression (in perhaps half of all PD patients), and chronic disability, as well as profound motor deficits. Current estimates suggest that significant neuropsychological deficits are present in at least 60% of PD patients (Mahler and Cummings 1990); however, studies that apply rigorous diagnostic criteria estimate the prevalence of dementia at 25% (Aarsland et al. 1996).

The presentation and course of dementia in PD are complex and reflect degeneration of subcortical ascending systems with neuronal losses in dopaminergic, noradrenergic, serotonergic, cholinergic, or multiple systems. Various combinations of limbic and/or cortical Alzheimer and/or Lewy body pathologies with loss of synapses and neurons are found in more severely demented cases (Jellinger 1997). Later age at onset of PD (> 60 years) and prominent executive and visuospatial deficits predict subsequent development of dementia. Neither depressive symptoms nor severity of motor impairment are predictive of dementia (Mahieux et al. 1998). MRI studies have not demonstrated any specific pattern in patients with dementia caused by PD (Huber et al. 1989); functional imaging techniques may aid in identifying concomitant DAT (Brooks 1997).

DEMENTIA DUE TO HUMAN IMMUNODEFICIENCY VIRUS DISEASE

Infection with the human immunodeficiency virus–type 1 (HIV-1) produces a dementing illness initially called the AIDS dementia complex (Navia 1990; Navia et al. 1986). A more recent designation is HIV-1-associated cognitive/motor complex (American Academy of Neurology AIDS Task Force 1991). HIV disease is pandemic, with an estimated 1.5–2 million Americans already infected. Two high-risk groups for HIV infection are bisexual/homosexual men (70% of HIV cases) and persons who abuse drugs intravenously (15%–20% of cases; Faulstich 1987). With changes in lifestyle, teenagers and females are emerging as new high-risk groups, and HIV infection is the most common cause of dementia in children, young adults, and middle-aged people (Nath and Geiger 1998).

HIV-1-associated cognitive/motor complex is separated into two disorders: a more severe form known as *HIV-1-associated dementia complex* and a less severe form termed *HIV-1-associated minor cognitive/motor disorder*. In the latter group, only the most demanding activities of daily living reveal mild impairments in cognition, motor abilities, or behavior.

The dementia is caused by HIV itself, and HIV proteins may themselves be either directly toxic to brain cells or may, through their actions on glial cells or macrophages, release neurotoxic products coded by the host cell genome. The severity of clinical dementia generally correlates with the severity of brain pathology; the strongest predictors for developing dementia are low CD4+ T-lymphocyte count, anemia, and exhibiting AIDS-defining infections or cancer (Qureshi et al. 1998). Some degree of cerebral atrophy is present in almost all HIV patients with dementia. Histological examination demonstrates diffuse pallor of the centrum semiovale with a mononuclear inflammatory response in the white matter and the deep gray nuclei (Navia 1990). HIV-1-associated dementia complex is the most frequent neurological complication of HIV infection; in some patients it is the earliest or only clinical manifestation of HIV-1 infection. Neuropsychological deficits include impaired attention and concentration, psychomotor slowing, poor reaction time, memory disturbance, and personality/mood alterations such as apathy and irritability. This combination of cognitive impairment, motor dysfunction, and behavioral change is typical for a subcortical type of dementia. There is evidence for three distinct subtypes of individuals seropositive for HIV-1: 1) a "subcortical, depressed" group, with depressed mood, psychomotor slowing, and forgetfulness; 2) a "cortical" group, with verbal and visuospatial deficits, some psychomotor slowing, and euthymic mood; and 3) an "unimpaired" group, with normal findings on neuropsychological assessment. Thus, patients with HIV-1 may not always demonstrate a subcortical presentation (Van Gorp et al. 1993). HIV-1-associated dementia complex is not invariably progressive; it can remain static or fluctuate (American Academy of Neurology AIDS Task Force 1991). Structural imaging studies using CT or MRI show atrophy and demyelination of subcortical white matter. In the early and middle stages of HIV infection, PET studies demonstrate relative hypermetabolism of the thalamus and basal ganglia. As the dementia worsens, the temporal lobes become metabolically hypoactive (Bencherif and Rottenberg 1998; Van Gorp et al. 1992). Treating the dementia involves treating the HIV infection with zidovudine and other antiviral agents (Melton et al. 1997). Nonsedating antidepressants and psychostimulants are useful for treating the dysphoric mood symptoms in HIV patients (Holmes et al. 1989).

SUBSTANCE-INDUCED DEMENTIA

The DSM-IV diagnostic criteria for substance-induced dementia are listed in Table 10–16. The majority of patients with this diagnosis are alcoholic, although younger patients may acquire this form of dementia from chronic exposure to solvent vapors, such as spray paint that contains toluene (Filley et al. 1990).

Alcoholic dementia is present in about 3% of alcoholic inpatients and is diagnosed in 7% of patients evaluated for cognitive impairment. Risk factors include female gender; age greater than 50; and continuous, rather than periodic, drinking (Cutting 1982). The clinical and pathological delineation of a persistent dementia attributable to the direct toxic effects of alcohol on the brain remains ambiguous. Four distinct brain diseases—Wernicke-Korsakoff, Marchiafava-Bignami, pellagrous encephalopathy, and acquired hepatocerebral degeneration—are associated with chronic alcoholism. Each is characterized by a distinctive

---

TABLE 10–16. DSM-IV diagnostic criteria for substance-induced persisting dementia

A. The development of multiple cognitive deficits manifested by both:

   (1) Memory impairment (impaired ability to learn new information or to recall previously learned information)

   (2) One (or more) of the following cognitive disturbances:

      (a) Aphasia (language disturbance)

      (b) Apraxia (inability to carry out motor activities despite intact motor function)

      (c) Agnosia (failure to recognize or identify objects despite intact sensory function)

      (d) Disturbance in executive functioning (i.e., planning, organizing, sequencing, abstracting)

B. The cognitive deficits in criteria A1 and A2 each cause significant impairment in social or occupational functioning and represent a significant decline from a previous level of functioning.

C. The deficits do not occur exclusively during the course of a delirium and persist beyond the usual duration of substance intoxication or withdrawal.

D. There is evidence from the history, physical examination, or laboratory findings that the deficits are etiologically related to the persisting effects of substance use (e.g., a drug of abuse, a medication).

Code [Specific substance]-induced persisting dementia: Alcohol; inhalant; sedative, hypnotic, or anxiolytic; other (or unknown) substance.

---

pathology, however, in each the role of alcohol is secondary (Victor 1994). At autopsy, chronically alcoholic persons have cortical atrophy and nerve fiber disintegration with dissolution of myelin sheaths (Lishman 1981). Neuropsychological deficits include difficulty with many aspects of memory and new learning, visuospatial functions, and tests of frontal lobe function. These deficits improve with abstinence, most dramatically in the first 10 days, with some additional limited improvement measured at 6 months (Hambidge 1990). CT imaging in abstinent chronically alcoholic persons demonstrates lateral ventricular enlargement with widening of the cortical sulci; this atrophy does not correlate with intellectual impairment and may improve in some patients with abstinence (Carlen et al. 1978).

DEMENTIA SYNDROME OF DEPRESSION

Depression is often encountered among patients evaluated for impaired cognition. For example, in one large series, 27% of patients referred to a dementia clinic met criteria for a depressive disorder (Reding et al. 1985). Several potential relationships exist between depression and dementia: 1) depression can occur in response to the onset of cognitive impairment; 2) depression and dementia can be produced by the same underlying condition, such as stroke or Parkinson's disease; 3) symptoms of dementing illnesses may mimic those of depression and lead to the misdiagnosis of a mood disorder; and 4) depression can cause a dementia syndrome (Cummings 1989). The term *pseudodementia* is sometimes used to refer to dementia caused by depression (Caine 1981; Wells 1979). Authors who use this term describe a reversible syndrome of cognitive impairment indistinguishable from "organic" brain disease. However, there is nothing "pseudo" about the cognitive impairment demonstrable in some depressed patients. In these patients, the term *dementia syndrome of depression* (DSD) is more accurate (Folstein and McHugh 1978). Currently, DSD can be established only retrospectively, when the patient recovers intellectual function following successful antidepressant therapy. Outcome of DSD remains uncertain: in one study of 44 patients treated for DSD, all reverted to premorbid levels of cognitive function; subsequently, at an average follow-up period of 8 years, 89% developed a DAT-like dementia (Kral and Emery 1989). A more recent study found 43% of successfully treated DSD patients had developed DAT within 3 years (Alexopoulos et al. 1993).

Clinical features of DSD reviewed by Emery and Oxman (1992) include the following:

1. In contrast to primary dementia, the elapsed time between onset and seeking medical help is shorter in DSD.
2. A history of previous affective disorder is reported more frequently in DSD than in primary dementia.
3. Patients with DSD manifest depressed mood and delusions more than do patients with primary dementia.
4. Behavioral deterioration in patients with primary dementia is more consistent with the severity of cognitive dysfunction than in patients with DSD.
5. Sleep disturbance in DSD is more severe and involves early morning awakening.

Neuropsychological features that distinguish DSD from DAT include memory and language impairments. Unlike patients with DAT, those with DSD retain self-awareness, have intact recognition, and improve their memory performance with prompting and organization of material. DAT patients manifest a characteristic "empty" speech, often with paraphasic errors not typically seen in DSD (Cummings 1989). Structural imaging studies have shown that patients with DSD have diminished brain density and increased ventricular brain ratio values similar to those in patients with organic dementias (Pearlson et al. 1989). The prognostic significance of these findings remains unclear. Although functional imaging studies in DSD have not been reported, PET in depressed patients shows asymmetrical frontal hypometabolism, which is greater on the left. Results normalize with successful therapy (Martinot et al. 1990). This hypofrontality with depression is distinct from the biparietal hypometabolism of DAT and may prove helpful in distinguishing these disorders in elderly patients. Application of newer techniques such as polysomnographic sleep studies may eventually also prove useful (Buysse et al. 1992).

Antidepressant or electroconvulsive therapy for DSD should be initiated on the basis of findings of intrapsychic depressive symptoms and characteristic sleep disturbance, rather than for the mere complaint or presence of cognitive impairment (Emery and Oxman 1992). Evidence of confusion in DSD patients taking low doses of tricyclic antidepressants may identify those who are at high risk to develop primary dementia (Reding et al. 1985). However, the availability of newer antidepressant agents (with more favorable side-effect profiles) should prompt a medication trial in cognitively impaired patients whenever the relative contribution of depression to the overall clinical picture remains uncertain.

DEMENTIA CAUSED BY OTHER CONDITIONS

Serious head trauma can cause dementia and other neuropsychiatric signs or symptoms. Amnesia is the most common neurobehavioral sequela after traumatic brain injury (TBI); recovery of memory function is not always complete, and a degree of permanent disturbance may persist (Levin 1989). Aphasia can occur in up to 30% of patients after TBI (Jennett and Teasdale 1981). In addition, personality changes, attentional disturbances, and other cognitive impairments suggestive of frontal lobe damage are common (Mattson and Levin 1990). TBI also increases the risk for developing psychiatric disorders such as depression, mania, and psychosis (McAllister 1992). Posttraumatic seizures occur in 2%–5% of patients with TBI and often begin within 7 days of the trauma (Slagle 1990). Even after mild head trauma, subjective symptoms such as headache, dizziness, easy fatigability, and disordered sleep persist in some patients for several months; this "postconcussional syndrome," referred to in DSM-IV as *postconcussional disorder* (DSM-IV code 294.9), is a complex blend of physiological and psychological factors that result in chronic disability for a small proportion of patients (Lishman 1988). Repetitive head trauma, such as that experienced by boxers, can lead to *dementia pugilistica*, a syndrome characterized by ataxia and dysarthria that can progress to dementia with Parkinson-type extrapyramidal features (Jordan 1987).

A potentially reversible cause of dementia that may occur after head trauma is *subdural hematoma*. This condition may present as delirium or psychosis (Black 1984), and the history of head trauma may be minimal or entirely absent, especially in elderly patients. MRI is the best procedure available for diagnosis (Cummings and Benson 1992). Another uncommon but potentially treatable dementia associated with head trauma is *normal-pressure hydrocephalus* (NPH). NPH may also develop as a late complication of subarachnoid hemorrhage or intracranial infection. NPH produces a triad of clinical symptoms: 1) a gait disturbance, often described as "magnetic," that appears early; 2) a subcortical dementia; and 3) urinary incontinence that may appear late (Benson 1985). This triad is not specific to NPH; VaD occurs more frequently and is likely to present with these features. MRI is becoming the primary diagnostic test for NPH and can demonstrate CSF flow disturbance within the internal ventricular system (Kunz et al. 1989). Surgical shunting of CSF produces improvement in 40%–50% of cases; dementia is the least likely of the triad to improve with shunting, whereas the gait disturbance has the best outcome. No guidelines exist that accurately identify patients for shunting; however, patients with a good outcome usually present with the full clinical triad and with a short duration of symptoms, and they do not have idiopathic NPH (Clarfield 1989; Friedland 1989).

Of the remaining dementia syndromes listed in Table 10–9, several are potentially reversible. These etiologies include vitamin B_{12} deficiency (O'Neill and Barber 1993), hypothyroidism (Whybrow et al. 1969), and brain tumor (Barry and Moskowitz 1988). When rare or complicated dementia syndromes are encountered, a systematic approach to diagnosis is essential; neuroimaging studies, specific enzymatic or immunological assays, or biopsy of extraneural tissues is sometimes required for diagnosis (Reichman and Cummings 1990).

AMNESTIC DISORDERS

Amnestic disorders are characterized by an inability to learn new information despite normal attention and an ability to recall extremely remote information, with no other cognitive deficits (Benson 1978). Although anything that damages the hippocampus–fornix–mammillary body–thalamus circuits can produce an amnestic disorder, the principal causes of amnesia include head trauma, Wernicke-Korsakoff syndrome, stroke, neoplasm, herpes encephalitis, anoxia, hypoglycemia, and surgical procedures that disrupt medial temporal structures. Causes of transient amnesia include epileptic convulsions, ischemic episodes, and the syndrome known as *transient global amnesia* (Benson and McDaniel 1991). Exaggerated or simulated amnesia is uncommon outside of forensic settings and is generally detected using neuropsychological methods (Leng and Parkin 1995). Psychogenic causes of amnesia are not discussed in this chapter.

AMNESTIC DISORDERS CAUSED BY A GENERAL MEDICAL CONDITION

The DSM-IV diagnostic criteria for amnestic disorders caused by a general medical condition are listed in Table 10–17. Clinical features and pathophysiology vary according to the specific cause of the amnestic disorder.

Posttraumatic Amnesia

Head trauma is easily the most common cause of amnesia, with 400,000–500,000 patients hospitalized in this country each year for head injuries. Four to five times that number of head injuries occur without hospitalization (U.S. Department of Health and Human Services 1989). Rapid acceleration or deceleration of the brain stretches and twists neuronal

TABLE 10-17. DSM-IV diagnostic criteria for amnestic disorder due to a general medical condition

A. The development of memory impairment as manifested by impairment in the ability to learn new information or the inability to recall previously learned information.

B. The memory disturbance causes significant impairment in social or occupational functioning and represents a significant decline from a previous level of functioning.

C. The memory disturbance does not occur exclusively during the course of a delirium or a dementia.

D. There is evidence from the history, physical examination, or laboratory findings that the disturbance is the direct physiological consequence of a general medical condition (including physical trauma).

Specify if:

Transient: if memory impairment lasts for 1 month or less.

Chronic: if memory impairment lasts for more than 1 month.

axons. The resulting damage ranges from a brief disruption of physiological function with no obvious anatomic disruption to frank axonal tearing (Graham et al. 1987).

Posttraumatic amnesia (PTA) is the summation of several factors including unconsciousness caused by the injury, retrograde amnesia (RGA) for a period that ranges from a few minutes to a few years before the injury, and anterograde amnesia (AGA) that lingers from hours to months following recovery from unconsciousness (Levin et al. 1982). Patients with ongoing amnesia have a long period of RGA as well. As patients recover the ability to learn new information (i.e., AGA, or ongoing amnesia, resolves), RGA remains only for the short period from seconds or minutes before the injury. Thus, the presence of a prolonged period of RGA indicates ongoing amnesia, whereas a short period of RGA indicates recovery (Benson and McDaniel 1991). Lishman (1968) studied the relationship between the duration of PTA and subsequent psychiatric disability. He found that severe psychiatric disability was rare when PTA lasted less than 1 hour, but common when PTA lasted longer than 24 hours. Patients with PTA that lasted from 1 to 24 hours had a variable outcome.

Poststroke Amnesia

Amnesia can occur when a stroke damages the fornix or hippocampus. Bilateral posterior cerebral artery involvement with damage to the medial temporal regions commonly causes amnesia; unilateral infarction of the language-dominant hemisphere can also produce amnesia (Benson et al. 1974). Posterior cerebral artery occlusion frequently produces some degree of visual field disturbance and may produce Anton's syndrome, in which the patient dramatically denies blindness (Benson and McDaniel 1991). There are reports of amnesia following rupture of an anterior communicating artery aneurysm (Alexander and Freedman 1984) and following bilateral medial thalamic infarction (Graff-Radford et al. 1990).

Other Causes

There are several other important clinical causes of amnesia. Both intracerebral and extracerebral *neoplasms* affecting structures critical for memory function can produce amnestic disorders. Gliomas are common and typically involve the thalamus, hippocampus, splenium, and third ventricle (Meador et al. 1985; Rudge and Warrington 1991; Williams and Pennybacker 1954; Ziegler et al. 1977). *Anoxia* causes a breakdown of energy-dependent membrane functions, with loss of ionic homeostasis and eventual neuronal death (Espinoza and Parer 1991). Hippocampal neurons are extremely vulnerable to anoxic injury (Zola-Morgan et al. 1986). Cerebral anoxia, whether occurring as the result of an accident or attempted suicide or during the course of cardiopulmonary resuscitation, can produce a profound amnesia; gradual recovery is often seen over a period of months, but some residual amnesia is almost always present (Benson and McDaniel 1991).

Herpes simplex encephalitis, the most common nonepidemic encephalitis, has a unique tendency to involve the medial temporal areas of the brain. Onset is abrupt, with fever and coma evolving gradually into neurological deficits such as aphasia, hemiparesis, and a dense amnesia that persists after other deficits have cleared (Cermak and O'Connor 1983). Other evidence of temporal lobe dysfunction such as the Klüver-Bucy syndrome may be present in these patients (Lilly et al. 1983). Poorly controlled insulin-dependent diabetic individuals are at risk for amnesia because repeated or severe episodes of *hypoglycemia* can produce permanent brain injury (Sachon et al. 1992). Hypoglycemia has its greatest impact on hippocampal neurons and therefore affects cognitive processes much more than motor or sensory function (Blackman et al. 1990; Chalmers et al. 1991). *Surgical procedures*, including temporal lobectomy, cingulectomy, sectioning of the fornices, and injury to the mammillary bodies during removal of pituitary tumors, can result in amnestic syndromes (Cummings 1985b).

Transient Amnestic Syndromes

Epileptic convulsions are a significant source of acute amnesia encountered in clinical practice. Amnesia is a consis-

tent finding in the postictal state and is almost always transient. Temporal lobe status epilepticus can produce prolonged amnestic periods, and the phenomenon known as *poriomania*, an ictal or interictal state of wandering, may last for hours or even days (Benson and McDaniel 1991; Mayeux et al. 1979). Electroconvulsive therapy (ECT) produces a period of confusion immediately following the seizure, with AGA and RGA during the course of treatment. These side effects gradually resolve over a period of weeks following cessation of treatment (Sackeim et al. 1986; Weiner et al. 1986). There may be permanent loss of specific memories for events in the months immediately preceding, during, and following a course of ECT; however, objective testing does not demonstrate that the ability to acquire new information or to remember information from the past is persistently impaired by ECT (Squire 1986). Bilateral electrode placement, excessive electrical current, closely spaced treatments, and high doses of barbiturate anesthesia all may increase the severity of cognitive side effects with ECT (American Psychiatric Association 1990b).

Transient global amnesia (TGA) is characterized by the abrupt onset of severe AGA that lasts for a period of hours. The patient returns to normal except for a dense amnestic gap during the episode (Fisher and Adams 1958). TGA occurs in middle-aged or elderly patients; focal neurological and epileptic features are absent. The etiology of TGA remains unknown, although a variety of clinical conditions have been implicated, including thromboembolic cerebrovascular disease, epilepsy, migraine, brain tumors, cerebral hemorrhage, and drug overdosage (Hodges and Warlow 1990a). Widespread use of formal diagnostic criteria should help to clarify the TGA syndrome (Table 10–18).

Transient global amnesia is more common in men and most often occurs between the ages of 50 and 80. Duration of the amnestic period is brief, with a mean of 4.2 hours; periods greater than 12 hours are exceptional. Most patients also have a permanent RGA gap for events occurring before the onset of TGA. Prognosis is good for TGA, with perhaps 8% having another episode (Hodges and Warlow 1990b). CT scans are normal, although cerebral blood flow studies have revealed diminished blood flow in the posterior hemispheric or inferior temporal regions (Crowell et al. 1984). A history of migraine headaches is significantly more common in patients with TGA; further evidence for the role of arterial spasm comes from case reports of TGA following cerebral angiography (Jackson et al. 1995). In one series, 7% of strictly diagnosed TGA patients developed epilepsy, most within 1 year of presentation. Two important clinical features that predicted the development of

TABLE 10–18.   Proposed diagnostic criteria for transient global amnesia

Attacks must be witnessed by a capable observer who is present for most of the attack.

Clear-cut anterograde amnesia must be demonstrated during the attack.

Clouding of consciousness and loss of personal identity must be absent; cognitive impairment is limited to amnesia. No accompanying focal neurological symptoms occur during the attack, and no significant neurological signs are found afterward.

Epileptic features must be absent.

Attacks must resolve within 24 hours.

Patients with active epilepsy (either taking medication or have had one seizure in the past 2 years) or with recent head injury are excluded from this diagnosis.

Source.   Adapted from Hodges and Warlow 1990b.

epilepsy were multiple previous episodes and episodes lasting less than 1 hour. A thromboembolic etiology for TGA now appears unlikely, although cases with additional focal neurological deficits probably represent transient ischemic amnesia. Alcohol does not appear to play an etiological role in TGA, and the role of physical and emotional stress in precipitating TGA remains unsettled (Hodges and Warlow 1990a).

SUBSTANCE-INDUCED AMNESTIC DISORDER

The DSM-IV diagnostic criteria for substance-induced amnestic disorder are listed in Table 10–19. The two most commonly encountered substances responsible for this amnestic disorder are ethyl alcohol and benzodiazepines.

Alcohol Persisting Amnestic Disorder

Alcohol persisting amnestic disorder, also known as Korsakoff's syndrome, is among the most common causes of amnesia and is due to thiamine deficiency associated with prolonged, heavy ingestion of alcohol (Victor et al. 1989). Korsakoff's syndrome is the chronic amnestic phase of the Wernicke-Korsakoff syndrome (WKS) and is characterized by a complete inability to learn new material and by relative sparing of remote memories. Confabulation is common in the early phases of the illness, and a variable degree of loss of insight and initiative frequently accompanies the amnesia. Other mental functions are relatively preserved. The acute phase of WKS, Wernicke's encephalopathy, is characterized by ophthalmoplegia, ataxia, and confusion; perhaps only 25% of patients who

eventually develop the chronic amnesia of WKS have a previous clinical diagnosis of Wernicke's encephalopathy (Blansjaar et al. 1992a). The characteristic pathology of WKS involves punctate lesions of the gray nuclei in the periventricular regions surrounding the third and fourth ventricles and the Sylvian aqueduct (Victor et al. 1989). Using this distinctive pathology as a diagnostic marker for WKS, Bowden (1990) comprehensively reviewed the WKS literature and concluded the following:

1. Postmortem studies reveal a high incidence of WKS undiagnosed while the subjects were living, implying that the classic neurological diagnosis cannot be relied on as a guide to the presence of WKS pathology.
2. The clinical and cognitive manifestations of acute WKS are highly variable, and the most commonly recorded clinical sign in WKS is a vaguely defined disorder of mentation.
3. The disorder appears to be relatively common, with WKS pathology detected in 12.5% of all alcoholic persons.
4. The majority of WKS cases appear to follow an insidious, progressive course in which each clinical or subclinical episode gives rise to cumulative damage.
5. The clinical distinction between the acute and chronic phases of WKS is unjustified, because WKS most commonly is chronic in nature and is frequently labeled as "dementia."
6. The established neuropsychological profile of Korsakoff's syndrome as a discrete amnestic disorder is misleading, because it may be characteristic of only a proportion of the clinically diagnosed group and

TABLE 10–19.   DSM-IV diagnostic criteria for substance-induced persisting amnestic disorder

A.   The development of memory impairment as manifested by impairment in the ability to learn new information or the inability to recall previously learned information.

B.   The memory disturbance causes significant impairment in social or occupational functioning and represents a significant decline from a previous level of functioning.

C.   The memory disturbance does not occur exclusively during the course of a delirium or a dementia and persists beyond the usual duration of substance intoxication or withdrawal.

D.   There is evidence from the history, physical examination, or laboratory findings that the memory disturbance is etiologically related to the persisting effects of substance use (e.g., a drug of abuse, a medication).

only a fraction of the pathological group with WKS.

7. With abstinence from alcohol, a significant proportion of WKS patients show improvement in cognitive deficits, usually within the first year, refuting the widespread view that WKS is permanent and irreversible (Bowden 1990).

Clearly, further clinical refinement of the WKS diagnosis is needed. To date, MRI studies have been unable consistently to distinguish patients with WKS from chronic alcoholic persons without cognitive impairment (Blansjaar et al. 1992b; Jernigan et al. 1991). There seems to be no objective basis for the widespread assumption of site-specific effects, namely, that thiamine deficiency acts primarily on periventricular gray matter, whereas ethanol neurotoxicity acts primarily on cerebral cortex (Bowden 1990). Given the insidious course of WKS and the high prevalence of missed WKS diagnoses, all alcohol-dependent patients should be treated with thiamine (Blansjaar and van Dijk 1992).

Benzodiazepine Persisting Amnestic Disorder

Benzodiazepines are among the most widely prescribed medications in the world. These drugs have valuable sedative, hypnotic, and anxiolytic properties; however, they impair memory in two distinct ways: 1) AGA may occur following benzodiazepine administration, and 2) benzodiazepines may cause impairment of memory consolidation and subsequent memory retrieval (American Psychiatric Association 1990a). AGA is seen following high-dose acute intravenous benzodiazepine administration, as used in presurgical anesthesia. Amnesia is also reported following oral doses of high-potency, short-half-life benzodiazepines such as triazolam, especially when taken with alcohol (Linnoila 1990; Roth et al. 1984). Benzodiazepines impair memory consolidation and delay recall without affecting memory acquisition or short-term memory (Angus and Romney 1984). This memory impairment is not associated with the degree of sedation and psychomotor impairment (Roache and Griffiths 1985).

Benzodiazepines have no effect on the retrieval of information learned before the drug is taken (Petersen and Ghoneim 1980). High-potency, short-half-life benzodiazepines are more likely to impair memory, even after a single dose (Scharf et al. 1987). Memory impairment depends on the dose and the route of benzodiazepine administration, with higher doses and intravenous administration causing the greatest impairment. Duration of benzodiazepine treatment is also a significant factor; this is especially true in elderly patients, who may experience an insidious, gradual decrement in memory function, even at a constant benzodiazepine dose (American Psychiatric Association 1990a).

MENTAL DISORDERS DUE TO A GENERAL MEDICAL CONDITION

In DSM-III-R, a single category, Organic Mental Syndromes and Disorders, was used to encompass all "organic" disorders. Because use of the term *organic* implies that mental disorders not found in this section have no biological basis, in DSM-IV the "organic" label was eliminated and the "organic" diagnoses were divided into three sections: Delirium, Dementia, Amnestic, and Other Cognitive Disorders; Substance Related Disorders; and Mental Disorders Due to a General Medical Condition. The latter category contains diagnostic criteria for three disorders: 1) catatonic disorder due to a general medical condition, 2) mental disorder not otherwise specified due to a general medical condition, and 3) personality change due to a general medical condition. The types of personality change specified in DSM-IV include labile, disinhibited, aggressive, apathetic, paranoid, other (e.g., associated with a seizure disorder), combined (in which more than one of the preceding features predominate), and unspecified.

Catatonic disorder due to a general medical condition must be considered in every patient with catatonic features: immobility, staring, mutism, withdrawal, refusal to eat, posturing, grimacing, and rigidity. Medical conditions associated with catatonic disorder include dystonia, HIV encephalopathy, progressive multifocal leukoencephalopathy, encephalitis, and renal failure. The majority of patients have multifactorial etiologies, yet most respond dramatically to 1–2 mg lorazepam treatment. A beneficial response to lorazepam is not limited to patients with pure psychogenic catatonia (Carroll et al. 1994; Rosebush et al. 1990). Specific details about other mental disorders caused by medical conditions, such as psychotic disorders, mood disorders, anxiety disorders, sexual dysfunction, and sleep disorders, are found in other chapters in this textbook.

CONCLUSIONS

As the number of older individuals in the population rapidly increases, psychiatrists will see more patients who suffer from delirium, dementia, amnesia, and other cognitive disorders. These cognitive disorders occur commonly and are particularly prevalent in geriatric patients. Delirium is the most common psychiatric syndrome seen in a general medical hospital. Dementia is a rapidly growing major health problem, with upward of 9 million people in the United States currently affected. Amnestic disorders, although seen somewhat less frequently, commonly occur after severe head trauma, strokes, alcohol abuse, and other disorders.

In summary, patients with delirium, dementia, amnestic, and other mental disorders caused by medical conditions, are often encountered in medical and psychiatric settings, and their numbers are growing as the population ages. Clinical comfort in the diagnosis, management, and treatment of these disorders is essential for a psychiatrist.

REFERENCES

Aarsland D, Tandberg E, Larsen JP, et al: Frequency of dementia in Parkinson disease. Arch Neurol 53:538–542, 1996

Aberg T, Ronquist G, Tyden H, et al: Adverse effects on the brain in cardiac operations as assessed by biochemical, psychometric, and radiologic methods. J Thorac Cardiovasc Surg 87:99–105, 1984

Adams F: Neuropsychiatric evaluation and treatment of delirium in the critically ill cancer patient. Cancer Bulletin 36:156–160, 1984

Adams RD, Victor M: Principles of Neurology, 4th Edition. New York, McGraw-Hill, 1989

Aharon-Peretz J, Cummings JL, Hill MA: Vascular dementia and dementia of the Alzheimer type. Arch Neurol 45:719–721, 1988

Aisen PS, Davis KL: Inflammatory mechanisms in Alzheimer's disease: implications for therapy. Am J Psychiatry 151:1105–1113, 1994

Alexander GE, Furey ML, Grady CL, et al: Association of premorbid intellectual function with cerebral metabolism in Alzheimer's disease: implications for the cognitive reserve hypothesis. Am J Psychiatry 154:165–172, 1997

Alexander MP, Freedman M: Amnesia after anterior communicating artery aneurysm rupture. Neurology 34:752–757, 1984

Alexopoulos GS, Meyers BS, Young RC, et al: The course of geriatric depression with "reversible dementia": a controlled study. Am J Psychiatry 150:1693–1699, 1993

Amaducci LA, Rocca WA, Schoenberg BS: Origin of the distinction between Alzheimer's disease and senile dementia: how history can clarify nosology. Neurology 36:1497–1499, 1986

American Academy of Neurology AIDS Task Force: Nomenclature and research case definitions for neurologic manifestations of human immunodeficiency virus–type 1 (HIV-1) infection. Neurology 41:778–785, 1991

American College of Medical Genetics/American Society of Human Genetics Working Group: Consensus statement on use of apolipoprotein E testing for Alzheimer disease. JAMA 274:1627–1629, 1995

American Psychiatric Association: Diagnostic and Statistical Manual: Mental Disorders. Washington, DC, American Psychiatric Association, 1952

American Psychiatric Association: Diagnostic and Statistical Manual of Mental Disorders, 2nd Edition. Washington, DC, American Psychiatric Association, 1968

American Psychiatric Association: Diagnostic and Statistical Manual of Mental Disorders, 3rd Edition. Washington, DC, American Psychiatric Association, 1980

American Psychiatric Association: Diagnostic and Statistical Manual of Mental Disorders, 3rd Edition, Revised. Washington, DC, American Psychiatric Association, 1987

American Psychiatric Association: Benzodiazepine Dependence, Toxicity, and Abuse: A Task Force Report of the American Psychiatric Association. Washington, DC, American Psychiatric Association, 1990a

American Psychiatric Association: The Practice of Electroconvulsive Therapy: Recommendations for Treatment, Training, and Privileging: A Task Force Report of the American Psychiatric Association. Washington, DC, American Psychiatric Association, 1990b

American Psychiatric Association: Diagnostic and Statistical Manual of Mental Disorders, 4th Edition. Washington, DC, American Psychiatric Association, 1994

American Psychiatric Association: Practice guideline for the treatment of patients with Alzheimer's disease and other dementias of late life. Am J Psychiatry 154:5 (suppl):1–39, 1997

Andreasen N[J]C, Noyes R, Hartford C, et al: Management of emotional reactions in seriously burned adults. N Engl J Med 286:65–69, 1972

Andreasen NJC, Hartford CE, Knott JR, et al: EEG changes associated with burn delirium. Diseases of the Nervous System 38:27–31, 1977

Angus WR, Romney DM: The effect of diazepam on patients' memory. J Clin Psychopharmacol 4:203–206, 1984

Anthony JC, LeResche L, Niaz U, et al: Limits of the "Mini-Mental State" as a screening test for dementia and delirium among hospital patients. Psychol Med 12:397–408, 1982

Antoon AY, Volpe JJ, Crawford JD: Burn encephalopathy in children. Pediatrics 50:609–616, 1972

Arnold SE, Kumar A: Reversible dementias (review). Med Clin North Am 77:215–230, 1993

Bamford KA, Caine ED: Does "benign senescent forgetfulness" exist? Clin Geriatr Med 4:897–916, 1988

Barry PP, Moskowitz MA: The diagnosis of reversible dementia in the elderly: a critical review. Arch Intern Med 148:1914–1918, 1988

Basile AS, Hughes RD, Harrison PM, et al: Elevated brain concentrations of 1,4-benzodiazepines in fulminant hepatic failure. N Engl J Med 325:473–478, 1991

Becker RE, Colliver JA, Markwell SJ, et al: Effects of metrifonate on cognitive decline in Alzheimer disease: a double-blind, placebo-controlled, 6-month study. Alzheimer Dis Assoc Disord 12:54–57, 1998

Bench CJ, Dolan RJ, Friston KJ, et al: Positron emission tomography in the study of brain metabolism in psychiatric and neuropsychiatric disorders. Br J Psychiatry 157 (suppl 9):82–95, 1990

Bencherif B, Rottenberg DA: Neuroimaging of the AIDS dementia complex. AIDS 12:233–244, 1998

Benson DF: Amnesia. South Med J 71:1221–1228, 1978

Benson DF: Hydrocephalic dementia, in Handbook of Clinical Neurology, Vol 2: Neurobehavioral Disorders. Edited by Vinken PJ, Bruyn GW, Klawans HL. New York, Elsevier, 1985, pp 323–333

Benson DF, McDaniel KD: Memory disorders, in Neurology in Clinical Practice, Vol 2. Edited by Bradley WG, Daroff RB, Fenichel GM, et al. Boston, MA, Butterworth-Heinemann, 1991, pp 1389–1406

Benson DF, Marsden CD, Meadows JC: The amnestic syndrome of posterior cerebral artery occlusion. Acta Neurol Scand 50:133–145, 1974

Benson DF, Kuhl DE, Hawkins RA, et al: The fluorodeoxyglucose ^{18}F scan in Alzheimer's disease and multiinfarct dementia. Arch Neurol 40:711–714, 1983

Bergem ALM, Engedal K, Kringlen E: The role of heredity in late-onset Alzheimer disease and vascular dementia. Arch Gen Psychiatry 54:264–270, 1997

Bergman H, Chertkow H, Wolfson C, et al: HM-PAO (CERETEC) SPECT brain scanning in the diagnosis of Alzheimer's disease. J Am Geriatr Soc 45:15–20, 1997

Berrios GE: Delirium and confusion in the 19th century: a conceptual history. Br J Psychiatry 139:439–449, 1981

Blachly PH, Kloster FE: Relation of cardiac output to postcardiotomy delirium. J Thorac Cardiovasc Surg 52:423–427, 1966

Black DW: Mental changes resulting from subdural hematoma. Br J Psychiatry 145:200–203, 1984

Blackman JD, Towle VL, Lewis GF, et al: Hypoglycemic thresholds for cognitive dysfunction in humans. Diabetes 39:828–835, 1990

Blank K, Perry S: Relationship of psychological processes during delirium to outcome. Am J Psychiatry 141:843–847, 1984

Blansjaar BA, van Dijk JG: Korsakoff minus Wernicke syndrome. Alcohol Alcohol 27:435–437, 1992

Blansjaar BA, Takens H, Zwinderman AH: The course of alcohol amnestic disorder: a three-year follow-up study of clinical signs and social disabilities. Acta Psychiatr Scand 86:240–246, 1992a

Blansjaar BA, Vielvoye GJ, van Dijk JG, et al: Similar brain lesions in alcoholics and Korsakoff patients: MRI, psychometric and clinical findings. Clin Neurol Neurosurg 94:197–203, 1992b

Boone KB, Miller BL, Lesser IM, et al: Performance on frontal lobe tests in healthy, older individuals. Developmental Neuropsychology 6:215–223, 1990

Bowden SC: Separating cognitive impairment in neurologically asymptomatic alcoholism from Wernicke-Korsakoff syndrome: is the neuropsychological distinction justified? Psychol Bull 107:355–366, 1990

Breitbart W, Marotta R, Platt MM, et al: A double-blind trial of haloperidol, chlorpromazine, and lorazepam in the treatment of delirium in hospitalized AIDS patients. Am J Psychiatry 153:231–237, 1996

Brooks DJ: PET and SPECT studies in Parkinson's disease. Baillieres Clin Neurol 6:69–87, 1997

Brown P, Cathala F, Castaigne P, et al: Creutzfeldt-Jakob disease: clinical analysis of a consecutive series of 230 neuropathologically verified cases. Ann Neurol 20: 597–602, 1986

Brun A: Frontal lobe degeneration of non-Alzheimer type, I: neuropathology. Archives of Gerontology and Geriatrics 6: 193–208, 1987

Brust JCM: Vascular dementia is overdiagnosed. Arch Neurol 45:799–801, 1988

Burns A: Cranial computerised tomography in dementia of the Alzheimer type. Br J Psychiatry 157 (suppl 9):1015, 1990

Burns A, Jacoby R, Levy R: Psychiatric phenomena in Alzheimer's disease, I: disorders of thought content. Br J Psychiatry 157:72–76, 1990a

Burns A, Jacoby R, Levy R: Psychiatric phenomena in Alzheimer's disease, II: disorders of perception. Br J Psychiatry 157:76–81, 1990b

Buysse DJ, Reynolds CF, Hoch CC, et al: Rapid eye movement sleep deprivation in elderly patients with concurrent symptoms of depression and dementia. J Neuropsychiatry Clin Neurosci 4:249–256, 1992

Caine ED: Pseudodementia: current concepts and future directions. Arch Gen Psychiatry 38:1359–1364, 1981

Cameron D, Thomas R, Mulvihill M, et al: Delirium: a test of the Diagnostic and Statistical Manual III criteria on medical inpatients. J Am Geriatr Soc 35:1007–1010, 1987

Carlen PL, Wortzman G, Holgate RC, et al: Reversible cerebral atrophy in recently abstinent chronic alcoholics measured by computed tomography scans. Science 200:1076–1078, 1978

Carroll BT, Anfinson TJ, Kennedy JC, et al: Catatonic disorder due to general medical conditions. J Neuropsychiatry ClinNeurosci 6:122–133, 1994

Cermak LS, O'Connor M: The anterograde and retrograde retrieval ability of a patient with amnesia due to encephalitis. Neuropsychologia 21:213–234, 1983

Chalmers J, Risk MT, Kean DM, et al: Severe amnesia after hypoglycemia: clinical, psychometric, and magnetic resonance imaging correlations. Diabetes Care 14:922–925, 1991

Champagne MT, Neelon VJ, McConnell ES, et al: The NEECHAM Confusion Scale: assessing acute confusion in the hospitalized and nursing home elderly. The Gerontologist 27:4A, 1987 (special issue)

Chartier-Harlin MC, Crawford F, Houlden H, et al: Early-onset Alzheimer's disease caused by mutations at codon 717 of the beta-amyloid precursor protein gene. Nature 358:844–846, 1991

Chartier-Harlin MC, Parfitt M, Legrain S, et al: Apolipoprotein E epsilon 4 allele as a major risk factor for sporadic early- and late-onset forms of Alzheimer's disease: analysis of the 19q13.2 chromosomal region. Hum Mol Genet 3:569–574, 1994

Chedru F, Geschwind N: Writing disturbances in acute confusional states. Neuropsychologia 10:343–353, 1972

Chenoweth DE, Cooper SW, Hugli TE, et al: Complement activation during cardiopulmonary bypass. N Engl J Med 304:497–502, 1981

Chui HC, Victoroff JI, Margolin D, et al: Criteria for the diagnosis of ischemic vascular dementia proposed by the State of California Alzheimer's Disease Diagnostic and Treatment Centers. Neurology 42:473–480, 1992

Clarfield AM: Normal-pressure hydrocephalus: saga or swamp? JAMA 262:2592–2593, 1989

Clarfield AM: Reversible dementia (letter). Neurology 45:601, 1995

Corder E, Saunders A, Strittmatter W, et al: Gene dose of apolipoprotein E type 4 allele and the risk of Alzheimer's disease in late onset families. Science 261:921–923, 1993

Crook T, Bartus RT, Ferris SH, et al: Age-associated memory impairment: proposed diagnostic criteria and measures of clinical change— report of a National Institute of Mental Health work group. Developmental Neuropsychology 2:261–276, 1986

Crowell GF, Stump DA, Biller J, et al: The transient global amnesia-migraine connection. Arch Neurol 41:75–79, 1984

Cummings JL: Acute confusional states, in Clinical Neuropsychiatry. Edited by Cummings JL. Orlando, FL, Grune & Stratton, 1985a, pp 68–74

Cummings JL: Amnesia, paramnesia, and confabulation, in Clinical Neuropsychiatry. Edited by Cummings JL. Orlando, FL, Grune & Stratton, 1985b, pp 36–47

Cummings JL: Dementia syndromes: neurobehavioral and neuropsychiatric features. J Clin Psychiatry 48 (No 5, suppl):3–8, 1987

Cummings JL: Dementia and depression: an evolving enigma (editorial). J Neuropsychiatry Clin Neurosci 1:236–242, 1989

Cummings JL, Benson DF: Dementia of the Alzheimer's type: an inventory of diagnostic clinical features. J Am Geriatr Soc 34:12–19, 1986

Cummings JL, Benson DF: Dementia: A Clinical Approach, 2nd Edition. Boston, MA, Butterworth-Heinemann, 1992

Cummings JL, Benson DF, LoVerme S Jr: Reversible dementia. JAMA 243:2434–2439, 1980

Cummings JL, Miller B, Hill MA, et al: Neuropsychiatric aspects of multi-infarct dementia and dementia of the Alzheimer's type. Arch Neurol 44:389–393, 1987

Cutting J: Alcoholic dementia, in Psychiatric Aspects of Neurologic Disease, Vol 2. Edited by Benson DF, Blumer D. New York, Grune & Stratton, 1982, pp 149–165

Davis KL, Mohs RC: Enhancement of memory processes in Alzheimer's disease with multiple-dose intravenous physostigmine. Am J Psychiatry 139:1421–1424, 1982

Davis KL, Thal LJ, Gamzu ER, et al: A double-blind, placebo-controlled multicenter study of tacrine for Alzheimer's disease. N Engl J Med 327:1253–1259, 1992

Davis RE, Miller S, Herrnstadt C, et al: Mutations in mitochondrial cytochrome c oxidase genes segregate with late-onset Alzheimer disease. Proceedings of the National Academy of Sciences of the United States of America 94:4526–4531, 1997

De RJ, Decoo D, Marchau M, et al: Positron emission tomography in vascular dementia. J Neurol Sci 154:55–61, 1998

DeCarli C, Kaye JA, Horowitz B, et al: Critical analysis of the use of computer-assisted transverse axial tomography to study human brain in aging and dementia of the Alzheimer's type. Neurology 40:872–883, 1990

Dubin WR, Field NL, Gastfriend DR: Postcardiotomy delirium: a critical review. J Thorac Cardiovasc Surg 77: 586–594, 1979

Edwards-Lee T, Miller BL, Benson DF, et al: The temporal variant of frontotemporal dementia. Brain 120:1027–1040, 1997

Emery VO, Oxman TE: Update on the dementia spectrum of depression. Am J Psychiatry 149:305–317, 1992

Engel GL: Delirium, in Comprehensive Textbook of Psychiatry. Edited by Freedman AM, Kaplan HI. Baltimore, MD, Williams & Wilkins, 1967, pp 711–716

Engel GL, Romano J: Delirium, a syndrome of cerebral insufficiency. Journal of Chronic Diseases 9:260–277, 1959

Engel GL, Romano J, Ferris EB: Effect of quinacrine (Atabrine) on the central nervous system: clinical and electroencephalographic studies. Archives of Neurology and Psychiatry 58:337–350, 1947

Erkinjuntti T, Ketonen L, Sulkava R, et al: Do white matter changes on MRI and CT differentiate vascular dementia from Alzheimer's disease? J Neurol Neurosurg Psychiatry 50:37–42, 1987

Erkinjuntti T, Haltia M, Palo J, et al: Accuracy of the clinical diagnosis of vascular dementia: a prospective clinical and postmortem neuropathological study. J Neurol Neurosurg Psychiatry 51:1037–1044, 1988

Espinoza MT, Parer JT: Mechanisms of asphyxial brain damage and possible pharmacologic interventions in the fetus. Am J Obstet Gynecol 164:1582–1591, 1991

Faulstich ME: Psychiatric aspects of AIDS. Am J Psychiatry 144:551–556, 1987

Faust D, Fogel BS: The development and initial validation of a sensitive bedside cognitive screening test. J Nerv Ment Dis 177:25–31, 1989

Fernandez F, Holmes VF, Adams F, et al: Treatment of severe, refractory agitation with a haloperidol drip. J Clin Psychiatry 49:239–241, 1988

Fernandez F, Levy JK, Mansell PWA: Management of delirium in terminally ill AIDS patients. Int J Psychiatry Med 19:165–172, 1989

Filley CM, Heaton RK, Rosenberg NL: White matter dementia in chronic toluene abuse. Neurology 40:532–534, 1990

Fisher CM, Adams RD: Transient global amnesia. Transactions of the American Neurological Association 83:143–146, 1958

Flint FJ, Richards SM: Organic basis of confusional states in the elderly. BMJ 2:1537–1539, 1956

Folstein MF: Differential diagnosis of dementia, in Geriatric Psychiatry: What's New About the Old. Psychiatric Clinics of North America. Philadelphia, PA, Saunders, March 1997

Folstein MF: Differential diagnosis of dementia: the clinical process. Psychiatr Clin North Am 20:45–57, 1997

Folstein MF, McHugh PR: Dementia syndrome of depression, in Alzheimer's Disease, Senile Dementia and Related Disorders. Edited by Katzman R, Terry RD, Bick KL. New York, Raven, 1978, pp 87–93

Folstein MF, Folstein SE, McHugh PR: "Mini-mental state": a practical method for grading the cognitive state of patients for the clinician. J Psychiatr Res 12:189–198, 1975

Folstein SE, Brandt J, Folstein MF: Huntington's disease, in Subcortical Dementia. Edited by Cummings JL. New York, Oxford University Press, 1990, pp 87–107

Folstein MF, Bassett SS, Romanoski AJ, et al: The Eastern Baltimore Mental Health Survey. Int Psychogeriatr 3:169–176, 1991

Francis J: Delirium in older patients. J Am Geriatr Soc 40:829–838, 1992

Francis J, Kapoor WN: Prognosis after hospital discharge of older medical patients with delirium. J Am Geriatr Soc 40:601–606, 1992

Francis J, Martin D, Kapoor W: A prospective study of delirium in hospitalized elderly. JAMA 263:1097–1101, 1990

Fratiglioni L, Vitanen M, von Strauss E, et al: Very old women at highest risk of dementia and Alzheimer's disease: incidence data from the Kungsholmen Project, Stockholm. Neurology 48:132–138, 1997

Friedland RP: "Normal" pressure hydrocephalus and the saga of the treatable dementias. JAMA 262:2577–2581, 1989

Frisoni GB, Beltramello A, Weiss C, et al: Linear measures of atrophy in mild Alzheimer disease. AJNR: AJNR Am J Neuroradiol 17:913–923, 1996

Garza-Trevino E, Hollister LE, Overall JE, et al: Efficacy of combinations of intramuscular antipsychotics and sedative-hypnotics for control of psychotic agitation. Am J Psychiatry 146:1598–1601, 1989

Geaney DP, Abou-Saleh MT: The use and applications of single-photon emission computerised tomography in dementia. Br J Psychiatry 157 (suppl 9):66–75, 1990

Gibson GE, Blass JP, Huang HM, et al: The cellular basis of delirium and its relevance to age-related disorders including Alzheimer's disease. Int Psychogeriatr 3:373–395, 1991

Goate A, Chartier-Harlin MC, Mullan M, et al: Segregation of a missense mutation in the amyloid precursor protein gene with familial Alzheimer's disease. Nature 349:704–706, 1991.

Gorman DG, Cummings JL: Neurobehavioral presentations of the antiphospholipid antibody syndrome. J Neuropsychiatry Clin Neurosci 5:37–42, 1993

Graff-Radford NR, Tranel D, Van Hoesen GW, et al: Diencephalic amnesia. Brain 113:1–25, 1990

Graham DI, Adams JH, Gennarelli TA: Pathology of brain damage in head injury, in Head Injury, 2nd Edition. Edited by Cooper PR. Baltimore, MD, Williams & Wilkins, 1987, pp 72–88

Green J, Morris JC, Sandson J, et al: Progressive aphasia: a precursor of global dementia? Neurology 40:423–429, 1990

Growdon JH: Treatment for Alzheimer's disease? N Engl J Med 327:1306–1308, 1992

Gupta SR, Naheedy MH, Young JC, et al: Periventricular white matter changes and dementia: clinical, neuropsychological, radiological and pathological correlation. Arch Neurol 45:637–641, 1988

Gustafson Y, Berggren D, Brannstrom B, et al: Acute confusional states in elderly patients treated for femoral neck fracture. J Am Geriatr Soc 36:525–530, 1988

Haass CH, Schlossmacher MG, Hung AY, et al: Amyloid beta-peptide is produced by cultured cells during normal metabolism. Nature 359:322–325, 1992

Hachinski V: Preventable senility: a call for action against the vascular dementias. Lancet 340:645–648, 1992

Hachinski VC, Iliff LD, Zilhka E, et al: Cerebral blood flow in dementia. Arch Neurol 32:632–637, 1975

Hahn-Barma V, Deweer B, Durr A, et al: Are cognitive changes the first symptoms of Huntington's disease? A study of gene carriers. J Neurol Neurosurg Psychiatry 64:172–177, 1998

Hambidge DM: Intellectual impairment in male alcoholics. Alcohol Alcohol 25:555–559, 1990

Hanninen T, Soininen H: Age-associated memory impairment: normal aging or warning of dementia? Drugs Aging 11:480–489, 1997

Harrell RG, Othmer E: Postcardiotomy confusion and sleep loss. J Clin Psychiatry 48:445–446, 1987

Hebert LE, Scherr PA, Beckett LA, et al: Age-specific incidence of Alzheimer's disease in a community population. JAMA 273:1354–1359, 1995

Heller SS, Frank KA, Malm JR, et al: Psychiatric complications of open-heart surgery. N Engl J Med 283:1015–1020, 1970

Henderson AS: Epidemiology of dementia: the current state. Eur Arch Psychiatry Clin Neurosci 240:205–206, 1991

Hendriks L, van Duijn C, Cras P, et al: Presenile dementia and cerebral hemorrhage linked to a mutation at codon 692 of the beta-amyloid precursor protein gene. Nat Genet 1:218–221, 1992

Hodges JR, Warlow CP: The aetiology of transient global amnesia. Brain 113:639–657, 1990a

Hodges JR, Warlow CP: Syndromes of transient amnesia: towards a classification. A study of 153 cases. J Neurol Neurosurg Psychiatry 53:834–843, 1990b

Holmes VF, Fernandez F, Levy JK: Psychostimulant response in AIDS-related complex patients. J Clin Psychiatry 50:5–8, 1989

Hsich G, Kenney K, Gibbs CJ, et al: The 14-3-3 brain protein in cerebrospinal fluid as a marker for transmissible spongiform encephalopathies. N Engl J Med 335:924–930, 1996

Huber SJ, Shuttleworth EC, Christy JA, et al: Magnetic resonance imaging in dementia of Parkinson's disease. J Neurol Neurosurg Psychiatry 52:1221–1227, 1989

Hunt AL, Orrison WW, Yeo RA, et al: Clinical significance of MRI white matter lesions in the elderly. Neurology 39:1470–1474, 1989

Inouye SK: The dilemma of delirium: clinical research controversies regarding diagnosis and evaluation of delirium in hospitalized elderly medical patients. Am J Med 97:278–288, 1994

Inouye S, Horwitz R, Tinetti M, et al: Acute confusional states in the hospitalized elderly: incidence, factors, and complications. Clin Res 37(2):524A, 1989

Inouye S, van Dyck C, Alessi C, et al: Clarifying confusion: the confusion assessment method. Ann Intern Med 113:941–948, 1990

International Huntington Association, World Federation of Neurology Research Group on Huntington's Chorea: Guidelines for the molecular genetics predictive test in Huntington's disease. Neurology 44:1533–1536, 1994

Jackson A, Stewart G, Wood A, et al: Transient global amnesia and cortical blindness after vertebral angiography: further evidence for the role of arterial spasm. AJNR: AJNR Am J Neuroradiol 16 (suppl):955–959, 1995

Jellinger KA: Morphological substrates of dementia in parkinsonism. A critical update. J Neural Transm Suppl 51:57–82, 1997

Jennett B, Teasdale G: Management of Head Injuries. Philadelphia, PA, FA Davis, 1981

Jernigan TL, Schafer K, Butters N, et al: Magnetic resonance imaging of Korsakoff patients. Neuropsychopharmacology 4:175–186, 1991

Joachim CL, Morris JH, Selkoe DJ: Clinically diagnosed Alzheimer's disease: autopsy results in 150 cases. Ann Neurol 24:50–56, 1988

Jobst KA, Barnetson LP, Shepstone BJ: Accurate prediction of histologically confirmed Alzheimer's disease and the differential diagnosis of dementia: the use of NINCDS-ADRDA AND DSM-III-R criteria, SPECT, X-ray CT, and APO E4 medial temporal lobe dementias: the Oxford Project to Investigate Memory and Aging. Int Psychogeriatr 9 (suppl 1):191–222, 1997

Jordan BD: Neurologic aspects of boxing. Arch Neurol 44:453–459, 1987

Jorm AF, Korten AE, Henderson AS: The prevalence of dementia: a quantitative integration of the literature (review). Acta Psychiatr Scand 76:465–479, 1987

Katzman R, Brown T, Thal LJ, et al: Comparison of rate of annual change of mental status score in four independent studies of patients with Alzheimer's disease. Ann Neurol 24:384–389, 1988

Katzman R, Galasko D, Saitoh T, et al: Apolipoprotein epsilon 4 and head trauma: synergistic or additive risks? Neurology 46:889–891, 1996

Kay DWK, Norris V, Post F: Prognosis in psychiatric disorders of the elderly. Journal of Mental Science 102:129–140, 1956

Kennard MA, Bueding E, Wortis SB: Some biochemical and electroencephalographic changes in delirium tremens. Quarterly Journal of Studies on Alcohol 6:4–14, 1945

Kertesz A, Black SE, Nicholson L, et al: The sensitivity and specificity of MRI in stroke. Neurology 37:1580–1585, 1987

Kertesz A, Black SE, Tokar G, et al: Periventricular and subcortical hyperintensities on magnetic resonance imaging. Arch Neurol 45:404–408, 1988

Kertesz A, Davidson W, Fox H: Frontal behavioral inventory: diagnostic criteria for frontal lobe dementia. Can J Neurol Sci 24:29–36, 1997

Khachaturian ZS: Diagnosis of Alzheimer's disease. Arch Neurol 42:1097–1105, 1985

Koller WC, Langston JW, Hubble JP, et al: Does a long preclinical period occur in Parkinson's disease? Neurology 41 (suppl 2):8–13, 1991

Kopala LC, Honer WG: The use of risperidone in severely demented patients with persistent vocalizations. Int J Geriatr Psychiatry 12:73–77, 1997

Koponen H, Stenbäck U, Mattila E, et al: Cerebrospinal fluid somatostatin in delirium. Psychol Med 19:605–609, 1989a

Koponen H, Stenbäck U, Mattila E, et al: CSF beta-endorphin-like immunoreactivity in delirium. Biol Psychiatry 25:938–944, 1989b

Koponen H, Stenbäck U, Mattila E, et al: Delirium among elderly persons admitted to a psychiatric hospital: clinical course during the acute stage and one-year follow-up. Acta Psychiatr Scand 79:579–585, 1989c

Koponen H, Partanen J, Paakkonen A, et al: EEG spectral analysis in delirium. J Neurol Neurosurg Psychiatry 52:980–985, 1989d

Kornfeld DS, Heller SS, Frank KA, et al: Personality and psychological factors in postcardiotomy delirium. Arch Gen Psychiatry 31:249–253, 1974

Koss E, Edland S, Fillenbaum G, et al: Clinical and neuropsychological differences between patients with earlier and later onset of Alzheimer's disease: a CERAD analysis, Part XII. Neurology 46:136–141, 1996

Kral VA, Emery OB: Long-term follow-up of depressive pseudodementia of the aged. Can J Psychiatry 34:445–446, 1989

Kunz U, Heintz P, Ehrenheim C, et al: MRI as the primary diagnostic instrument in normal pressure hydrocephalus? Psychiatry Res 29:287–288, 1989

Larrabee GJ, Crook TH: Estimated prevalence of age-associated memory impairment derived from standardized tests of memory function. International Psychogeriatrics 6:95–104, 1994

Layne OL, Yudofsky SC: Postoperative psychosis in cardiotomy patients: the role of organic and psychiatric factors. N Engl J Med 284:518–520, 1971

Le BL, Katz MM, Berman N, et al: A placebo-controlled, double-blind, randomized trial of an extract of Ginkgo biloba for dementia: North American EGb Study Group. JAMA 278:1327–1332, 1997

Leng NR, Parkin AJ: The detection of exaggerated or simulated memory disorder by neuropsychological methods. J Psychosom Res 39:767–776, 1995

Leuchter AF, Jacobson SA: Quantitative measurement of brain electrical activity in delirium. Int Psychogeriatr 3:231–247, 1991

Levin HS: Memory deficit after closed-head injury. J Clin Exp Neuropsychol 12:129–153, 1989

Levin HS, Benton AL, Gassman RG: Neurobehavioral Consequences of Closed Head Injury. New York, Oxford University Press, 1982

Levkoff SE, Besdine RW, Wetle T: Acute confusional states (delirium) in the hospitalized elderly. Annual Review of Gerontology and Geriatrics 6:1–26, 1986

Levkoff SE, Liptzin B, Cleary P, et al: Review of research instruments and techniques used to detect delirium. Int Psychogeriatr 3:253–271, 1991

Levkoff SE, Evans DA, Liptzin B, et al: Delirium: The occurrence and persistence of symptoms among elderly hospitalized patients. Arch Intern Med 152:334–340, 1992

Levy R: Aging-associated cognitive decline. Int Psychogeriatr 6:63–68, 1994

Levy-Lahad E, Wijsman EM, Nemens E, et al: A familial Alzheimer's disease locus on chromosome 1. Science 269:970–973, 1995

Lilly R, Cummings JL, Benson DF, et al: The human Klüver-Bucy syndrome. Neurology 33:1141–1145, 1983

Linnoila MI: Benzodiazepines and alcohol. J Psychiatr Res 24 (suppl 2):121–127, 1990

Lipowski ZJ: Delirium, clouding of consciousness and confusion. J Nerv Ment Dis 145:227–255, 1967

Lipowski ZJ: Delirium: Acute Brain Failure in Man. Springfield, IL, Charles C Thomas, 1980a

Lipowski ZJ: Delirium updated. Compr Psychiatry 21:190–196, 1980b

Lipowski ZJ: Delirium: Acute Confusional States. New York, Oxford University Press, 1990

Lishman WA: Brain damage in relation to psychiatric disability after head injury. Br J Psychiatry 114:373–410, 1968

Lishman WA: Cerebral disorder in alcoholism: syndromes of impairment. Brain 104:1–20, 1981

Lishman WA: Physiogenesis and psychogenesis in the "postconcussional syndrome." Br J Psychiatry 153:460–469, 1988

Liu CK, Miller BL, Cummings JL, et al: A quantitative MRI study of vascular dementia. Neurology 42:138–143, 1992

Lott AD, McElroy SL, Keys MA: Valproate in the treatment of behavioral agitation in elderly patients with dementia. J Neuropsychiatry Clin Neurosci 7:314–319, 1995

Lund and Manchester Groups: Clinical and neuropathological criteria for frontotemporal dementia. J Neurol Neurosurg Psychiatry 57:416–418, 1994

Mace NL, Rabins PV: The 36-Hour Day: A Family Guide to Caring for Persons With Alzheimer's Disease, Related Dementing Illnesses, and Memory Loss in Later Life. Baltimore, MD, Johns Hopkins University Press, 1991

MacKenzie IR, Munoz DG: Nonsteroidal anti-inflammatory drug use and Alzheimer-type pathology in aging. Neurology 50:986–990, 1998

Mackenzie TB, Popkin MK: Stress response syndrome occurring after delirium. Am J Psychiatry 137:1433–1435, 1980

Mahieux F, Fenelon G, Flahault A, et al: Neuropsychological prediction of dementia in Parkinson's disease. J Neurol Neurosurg Psychiatry 64:178–183, 1998

Mahler ME, Cummings JL: Alzheimer disease and the dementia of Parkinson disease: comparative investigations. Alzheimer Dis Assoc Disord 4(3):133–149, 1990

Mandell AM, Albert ML: History of subcortical dementia, in Subcortical Dementia. Edited by Cummings JL. New York, Oxford University Press, 1990, pp 17–30

Martinot JL, Hardy P, Feline A, et al: Left prefrontal glucose hypometabolism in the depressed state: a confirmation. Am J Psychiatry 147:1313–1317, 1990

Masters CL, Richardson EP Jr: Subacute spongiform encephalopathy (Creutzfeldt-Jakob disease)—the nature and progression of spongiform change. Brain 101:333–344, 1978

Matsuyama SS, Jarvik LJ: Hypothesis: microtubules, a key to Alzheimer disease. Proc Natl Acad Sci USA 86:8152–8156, 1989

Mattson AJ, Levin HS: Frontal lobe dysfunction following closed head injury: a review of the literature. J Nerv Ment Dis 178:282–291, 1990

Mayeux R, Alexander MP, Benson DF, et al: Poriomania. Neurology 29:1616–1619, 1979

Mayeux R, Ottman R, Maestre G, et al: Synergistic effects of traumatic head injury and apolipoprotein-epsilon 4 in patients with Alzheimer's disease. Neurology 45:555–557, 1995

McAllister TW: Neuropsychiatric sequelae of head injuries. Psychiatr Clin North Am 15:395–413, 1992

McHugh PR, Folstein MF: Psychiatric syndromes of Huntington's chorea: a clinical and phenomenologic study, in Psychiatric Aspects of Neurologic Disease, Vol 1. Edited by Benson DF, Blumer D. New York, Grune & Stratton, 1975, pp 267–286

McKhann G, Drachman D, Folstein M, et al: Clinical diagnosis of Alzheimer's disease: report of the NINCDS-ADRDA Work Group under the auspices of the Department of Health and Human Services Task Force on Alzheimer's Disease. Neurology 34:939–944, 1984

Meador KJ, Adams RJ, Flanigin HF: Transient global amnesia and meningioma. Neurology 35:769–771, 1985

Melton ST, Kirkwood CK, Ghaemi SN: Pharmacotherapy of HIV dementia. Ann Pharmacother 31:457–473, 1997

Mendez MF, Underwood KL, Zander BA, et al: Risk factors in Alzheimer's disease. Neurology 42:770–775, 1992

Menza MA, Murray GB, Holmes VF, et al: Decreased extrapyramidal symptoms with intravenous haloperidol. J Clin Psychiatry 48:278–280, 1987

Metter EJ, Mazziotta JC, Itabashi HH, et al: Comparison of glucose metabolism, x-ray CT, and postmortem data in a patient with multiple cerebral infarcts. Neurology 35:1695–1701, 1985

Metzger E, Friedman R: Prolongation of the corrected QT and torsades de pointes cardiac arrhythmia associated with intravenous haloperidol in the medically ill. J Clin Psychopharmacol 13:128–132, 1993

Meyer JS, McClintic KL, Rogers RL, et al: Aetiological considerations and risk factors for multi-infarct dementia. J Neurol Neurosurg Psychiatry 51:1489–1497, 1988

Meyer JS, Rogers RL, McClintic K, et al: Randomized clinical trial of daily aspirin therapy in multi-infarct dementia: a pilot study. J Am Geriatr Soc 37:549–555, 1989

Miller BL, Cummings JL, Villanueva-Meyer J, et al: Frontal lobe degeneration: clinical, neuropsychological, and SPECT characteristics. Neurology 41:1374–1382, 1991

Miller BL, Ikonte C, Ponton M, et al: A study of the Lund-Manchester research criteria for frontotemporal dementia: clinical and single-photon emission CT correlations. Neurology 48:937–942, 1997

Miller DA, Vitti RA, Maslack MM: The role of 99m-Tc HMPAO SPECT in the diagnosis of Creutzfeldt-Jacob disease. AJNR: AJNR Am J Neuroradiol 19:454–455, 1998

Molsa PK, Paljarvi L, Rinne JO, et al: Validity of clinical diagnosis in dementia: a prospective clinicopathological study. J Neurol Neurosurg Psychiatry 48:1085–1090, 1985

Moore DP: Rapid treatment of delirium in critically ill patients. Am J Psychiatry 134:1431–1432, 1977

Mori E, Yamadori A: Acute confusional state and acute agitated delirium. Arch Neurol 44:1139–1143, 1987

Mullan M, Crawford F, Axelman K, et al: A pathogenic mutation for probable Alzheimer's disease in the APP gene at the N-terminus of beta-amyloid. Nat Genet 1:345–347, 1992.

Murray AM, Levkoff SE, Wetle TT, et al: Acute delirium and functional decline in the hospitalized elderly patient. Journal of Gerontology 48:M181–M186, 1993

Murrell J, Farlow M, Ghetti B, et al: A mutation in the amyloid precursor protein associated with hereditary Alzheimer's disease. Science 254:97–99, 1991

Nath A, Geiger J: Neurobiological aspects of human immunodeficiency virus infection: neurotoxic mechanisms. Prog Neurobiol 54:19–33, 1998

National Institute on Aging/Alzheimer's Association Working Group: Apolipoprotein E genotyping in Alzheimer's disease. Lancet 347:1091–1095, 1996

Navia BA: The AIDS dementia complex, in Subcortical Dementia. Edited by Cummings JL. New York, Oxford University Press, 1990, pp 181–198

Navia BA, Jordan BD, Price RW: The AIDS dementia complex, I: clinical features. Ann Neurol 19:517–524, 1986

Nussmeier N, Arlund C, Slogoff S: Neuropsychiatric complications after cardiopulmonary bypass: cerebral protection by a barbiturate. Anesthesiology 64:165–170, 1986

O'Brien MD: Vascular dementia is underdiagnosed. Arch Neurol 45:797–798, 1988

O'Keeffe S, Gosney MA: Assessing attentiveness in older hospital patients: global assessment versus tests of attention. J Am Geriatr Soc 45:470–473, 1997

O'Keeffe S, Lavan J: The prognostic significance of delirium in older hospital patients. J Am Geriatr Soc 45:174–178, 1997

O'Neill D, Barber RD: Reversible dementia caused by vitamin B_{12} deficiency (letter). J Am Geriatr Soc 41:192–193, 1993

Patten SB, Lamarre CJ: Dysgraphia (letter). Can J Psychiatry 34:746, 1989

Payami H, Montee K, Grimslid H, et al: Increased risk of familial late-onset Alzheimer's disease in women. Neurology 46:126–129, 1996a

Payami H, Zareparsi S, Montee KR, et al: Gender difference in apolipoprotein E-associated risk for familial Alzheimer disease: a possible clue to the higher incidence of Alzheimer disease in women. American Journal of Human Genetics 58:803–811, 1996b

Pearson RCA, Powell TPS: The neuroanatomy of Alzheimer's disease. Reviews in the Neurosciences 2:101–122, 1989

Pericak-Vance MA, Bass MP, Yamaoka LH, et al: Complete genomic screen in late-onset familial Alzheimer disease: evidence for a new locus on chromosome 12. JAMA 278:1237–1241, 1997

Perry SW: Organic mental disorders caused by HIV: update on early diagnosis and treatment. Am J Psychiatry 147:696–710, 1990

Petersen RC, Ghoneim MM: Diazepam and human memory: influence on acquisition, retrieval, and state-dependent learning. Prog Neuropsychopharmacol Biol Psychiatry 4:81–89, 1980

Pompei P, Foreman M, Rudberg M, et al: Delirium in hospitalized older persons: outcomes and predictors. J Am Geriatr Soc 42:809–815, 1994

Post SG, Whitehouse PH, Binstock RH, et al: The clinical introduction of genetic testing for Alzheimer disease. An ethical perspective. JAMA 227:832–836, 1997

Powell AL, Cummings JL, Hill MA, et al: Speech and language alterations in multi-infarct dementia. Neurology 38:717–719, 1988

Pro JD, Wells CE: The use of the electroencephalogram in the diagnosis of delirium. Diseases of the Nervous System 38:804–808, 1977

Prusiner SB: Prion diseases and the BSE crisis. Science 278: 245–251, 1997

Qureshi AI, Hanson DL, Jones JL, et al: Estimation of the temporal probability of human immunodeficiency virus (HIV) dementia after risk stratification for HIV-infected persons. Neurology 50:392–397, 1998

Rabins PV: Reversible dementia and the misdiagnosis of dementia: a review. Hosp Community Psychiatry 34:830–835, 1983

Rabins PV: Psychosocial and management aspects of delirium. Int Psychogeriatr 3:319–324, 1991

Rabins PV, Folstein MF: Delirium and dementia: diagnostic criteria and fatality rates. Br J Psychiatry 140:149–153, 1982

Radue EW, duBoulay GH, Harrison MJG, et al: Comparison of angiographic and CT findings between patients with multi-infarct dementia and those with dementia due to primary neuronal degeneration. Neuroradiology 16:113–115, 1978

Rapcsak SZ, Croswell SC, Rubens AB: Apraxia in Alzheimer's disease. Neurology 39:664–668, 1989

Reding M, Haycox J, Blass J: Depression in patients referred to a dementia clinic: a three-year prospective study. Arch Neurol 42:894–896, 1985

Regan WM, Gordon SM: Gabapentin for behavioral agitation in Alzheimer's disease. J Clin Psychopharmacol 17:59–60, 1997

Reichman WE, Cummings JL: Diagnosis of rare dementia syndromes: an algorithmic approach. J Geriatr Psychiatry Neurol 3:73–84, 1990

Reisberg B: Functional assessment staging (FAST). Psychopharmacol Bull 24:653–659, 1988

Resnick M, Burton BT: Droperidol vs haloperidol in the initial management of acutely agitated patients. J Clin Psychiatry 45:298–299, 1984

Ritchie K, Kildea D: Is senile dementia "age-related" or "ageing-related"?—evidence from meta-analysis of dementia prevalence in the oldest old. Lancet 346:931–934, 1995

Roache JD, Griffiths RR: Comparison of triazolam and pentobarbital: performance impairment, subjective effects, and abuse liability. J Pharmacol Exp Ther 234:120–133, 1985

Robinson RG, Starkstein SE: Current research in affective disorders following stroke. J Neuropsychiatry Clin Neurosci 2:1–14, 1990

Rockwood J: Acute confusion in elderly medical patients. J Am Geriatr Soc 37:150–154, 1989

Rockwood K: The occurrence and duration of symptoms in elderly patients with delirium. J Gerontol 48:M162–M166, 1993

Rogers MP, Liang MH, Daltroy LH: Delirium after elective orthopedic surgery: risk factors and natural history. Int J Psychiatry Med 19:109–121, 1989

Rogers SL, Doody R, Mohs R, et al: E2020 produces both clinical global and cognitive test improvements in patients with mild to moderately severe Alzheimer's disease: results of a 30-week Phase III trial. Neurology 46:A217, 1996

Roman GC, Tatemichi TK, Erkinjuntti T, et al: Vascular dementia: diagnostic criteria for research studies: report of the NINDS-AIREN International Workshop. Neurology 43:250–260, 1993

Romanelli MF, Morris JC, Ashkin K, et al: Advanced Alzheimer's disease is a risk factor for late-onset seizures. Arch Neurol 47:847–850, 1990

Romano J, Engel GL: Delirium, I: electroencephalographic data. Archives of Neurology and Psychiatry 51:356–377, 1944

Rosebush PI, Hildebrand AM, Furlong BG, et al: Catatonic syndrome in a general psychiatric inpatient population: frequency, clinical presentation, and response to lorazepam. J Clin Psychiatry 51:357–362, 1990

Rosen WG, Terry RD, Fuld PA, et al: Pathological verification of ischemic score in differentiation of dementias. Ann Neurol 7:486–488, 1980

Roses A: Apolipoprotein E affects the rate of Alzheimer disease expression: beta-amyloid burden is a secondary consequence dependent on APOE genotype and duration of disease. J Neuropath Exp Neurol 53:429–437, 1994

Ross CA, Peyser CE, Shapiro I, et al: Delirium: phenomenologic and etiologic subtypes. Int Psychogeriatr 3:135–147, 1991

Roth M: The natural history of mental disorder in old age. Journal of Mental Science 101:281–301, 1955

Roth T, Roehrs R, Wittig R, et al: Benzodiazepines and memory. Br J Clin Pharmacol 18S:45–49, 1984

Royall DR, Mahurin RK, Gray KF: Bedside assessment of executive cognitive impairment: the Executive Interview. J Am Geriatr Soc 40:1221–1226, 1992

Ruchoux MM, Maurage CA: CADASIL: Cerebral autosomal dominant arteriopathy with subcortical infarcts and leukoencephalopathy. Journal of Neuropathology and Experimental Neurology 56:947–964, 1997

Rudge P, Warrington EK: Selective impairment of memory and visual perception in splenial tumors. Brain 114:349–360, 1991

Sachon C, Grimaldi A, Digy JP, et al: Cognitive function, insulin-dependent diabetes and hypoglycaemia. J Intern Med 231:471–475, 1992

Sackeim HA, Portnoy S, Neeley P, et al: Cognitive consequences of low-dosage electroconvulsive therapy. Ann NY Acad Sci 462:326–340, 1986

Sano M, Ernesto C, Thomas RG, et al: A controlled trial of selegiline, α-tocopherol, or both as treatment for Alzheimer's disease. N Engl J Med 336:1216–1222, 1997

Santens P, Petit H: Positron emission tomography in dementia. Acta Neurol Belg 97:192–195, 1997

Scharf MB, Saskin P, Fletcher K: Benzodiazepine-induced amnesia: clinical laboratory findings. J Clin Psychiatry Monogr 5:14–17, 1987

Schellenberg GD, Bird TD, Wijsman EM, et al: Genetic linkage evidence for a familial Alzheimer's disease locus on chromosome 14. Science 258:668–671, 1992

Schneider LS, Sobin PB: Nonneuroleptic medications in the management of agitation in Alzheimer's disease and other dementia: a selective review. International Journal of Geriatric Psychiatry 6:691–708, 1991

Schneider LS, Pollock VE, Lyness SA: A metaanalysis of controlled trials of neuroleptic treatment in dementia. J Am Geriatr Soc 38:553–563, 1990

Schneider LS, Olin JT, Pawluczyk S: A double-blind crossover pilot study of Ldeprenyl (Selegiline) combined with cholinesterase inhibitor in Alzheimer's disease. Am J Psychiatry 150:321–323, 1993

Schofield PW, Tang M, Marder K, et al: Alzheimer's disease after remote head injury: an incidence study. J Neurol Neurosurg Psychiatry 62:119–124, 1997

Schor JD, Levkoff SE, Lipsitz LA, et al: Risk factors for delirium in hospitalized elderly. JAMA 267:827–831, 1992

Selkoe DJ: Alzheimer's disease: genotypes, phenotype, and treatments. Science 275:630–631, 1997

Seltzer B, Mesulam MM: Confusional states and delirium as disorders of attention, in Handbook of Neuropsychology, Vol. 1. Edited by Boller F, Grafman J. Amsterdam, Elsevier, 1988, pp 165–174

Seltzer B, Sherwin I: A comparison of clinical features in early and late onset primary degenerative dementia: one entity or two? Arch Neurol 40:143–146, 1983

Skoog I: Status of risk factors for vascular dementia. Neuroepidemiology 17:2–9, 1998

Slagle DA: Psychiatric disorders following closed head injury: an overview of biopsychosocial factors in their etiology and management. Int J Psychiatry Med 20:1–35, 1990

Small GW: Psychopharmacological treatment of elderly demented patients. J Clin Psychiatry 49:5 (suppl):8–13, 1988

Small GW: Dementia and amnestic syndromes, in Treatments of Psychiatric Disorders: A Task Force Report of the American Psychiatric Association, Vol 2. Edited by Karasu TB. Washington, DC, American Psychiatric Association, 1989, pp 815–831

Smith LW, Dimsdale JE: Postcardiotomy delirium: conclusions after 25 years? Am J Psychiatry 146:452–458, 1989

Sos J, Cassem NH: Managing postoperative agitation. Drug Therapy 10:103–106, 1980

Speck CE, Kukull WA, Brenner DE, et al: History of depression as a risk factor for Alzheimer's disease. Epidemiology 6:366–369, 1995

Squire LR: Memory functions as affected by electroconvulsive therapy. Ann NY Acad Sci 462:307–314, 1986

Steele C, Lucas MJ, Tune L: Haloperidol versus thioridazine in the treatment of behavioral symptoms in senile dementia of the Alzheimer's type: preliminary findings. J Clin Psychiatry 47:310–312, 1986

Stern RG, Davis KL: Treatment approaches in Alzheimer's disease: past, present, and future, in The Dementias: Diagnosis and Management. Edited by Weiner MF. Washington, DC, American Psychiatric Press, 1991, pp 227–248

Stern Y, Gurland B, Tatemichi TK, et al: Influence of education and occupation on the incidence of Alzheimer's disease. JAMA 271:1004–1010, 1994

Stewart WF, Kawas C, Corrada M, et al: Risk of Alzheimer's disease and duration of NSAID use. Neurology 48:626–632, 1997

Strittmatter WJ, Saunders AM, Schmechel D, et al: Apolipoprotein E: high-avidity binding to beta-amyloid and increased frequency of type 4 allele in late-onset familial Alzheimer's disease. Proc Natl Acad Sci USA 90: 1977–1981, 1993

Sultzer DL, Gray KF, Gunay I, et al: A double-blind comparison for trazodone and haloperidol for treatment of agitation in patients with dementia. Am J Geriatr Psychiatry 5:60–69, 1997

Tang MX, Jacobs D, Stern Y, et al: Effect of oestrogen during menopause on risk and age at onset of Alzheimer's disease. Lancet 348:429–432, 1996

Tariot PN, Erb R, Podgorski CA, et al: Efficacy and tolerability of carbamazepine for agitation and aggression in dementia. Am J Psychiatry 155:54–61, 1998

Task force sponsored by the National Institute on Aging: senility reconsidered. JAMA 244:259–263, 1980

Tatemichi TK: How acute brain failure becomes chronic: a view of the mechanisms of dementia related to stroke. Neurology 40:1652–1659, 1990

Tesar GE, Murray GB, Cassem NH: Use of high-dose intravenous haloperidol in the treatment of agitated cardiac patients. J Clin Psychopharmacol 5:344–347, 1985

Tiller JWG, Dakis JA, Shaw JM: Short-term buspirone treatment in disinhibition with dementia. Lancet 2:510, 1988

Titchener JL, Swerling I, Gottschalk L, et al: Psychosis in surgical patients. Surg Gynecol Obstet 102:59–65, 1956

Tomlinson BE, Blessed G, Roth M: Observations on the brains of demented old people. J Neurol Sci 11:205–242, 1970

Trzepacz PT, Teague GB, Lipowski ZJ: Delirium and other organic mental disorders in a general hospital. Gen Hosp Psychiatry 7:101–106, 1985

Trzepacz PT, Baker RW, Greenhouse J: A symptom rating scale for delirium. Psychiatry Res 23:89–97, 1988

Tufo HM, Ostfeld AM, Shekelle R: Central nervous system dysfunction following open-heart surgery. JAMA 212:1333–1340, 1970

Tune LE, Damlouh NF, Holland A, et al: Association of postoperative delirium with raised serum levels of anticholinergic drugs. Lancet 2:651–653, 1981

U.S. Department of Health and Human Services: Interagency Head Injury Task Force Report. Washington, DC, U.S. Department of Health and Human Services, February 1989

Van Broeckhoeven C: Presenilins in Alzheimer's disease. Nat Genet 11:230–232, 1995

Van Duijn CM, Tanja TA, Haaxma R, et al: Head trauma and the risk of Alzheimer's disease. Am J Epidemiol 135:775–782, 1992

Van Duijn CM, Clayton DG, Chyandra V, et al: Interaction between genetic and environmental risk factors for Alzheimer's disease: a reanalysis of case-control studies. EURODEM Risk Factors Research Group, Genet Epidemiol 11:539–551, 1994

Van Gorp WG, Mahler M: Subcortical features of normal aging, in Subcortical Dementia. Edited by Cummings JL. New York, Oxford University Press, 1990, pp 231–250

Van Gorp WG, Mandelkern MA, Gee M, et al: Cerebral metabolic dysfunction in AIDS: findings in a sample with and without dementia. J Neuropsychiatry Clin Neurosci 4:280–287, 1992

Van Gorp WG, Hinken C, Satz P, et al: Subtypes of HIV-related neuropsychological functioning: a cluster analysis approach. Neuropsychology 7:62–72, 1993

Varsamis J, Zuchowski T, Maini KK: Survival rates and causes of death in geriatric psychiatric patients: a six-year follow-up study. Canadian Psychiatric Association Journal 17:17–22, 1972

Victor M: Alcoholic dementia. Can J Neurol Sci 21:88–99, 1994

Victor M, Adams RD, Collins GH: The Wernicke-Korsakoff Syndrome and Related Neurologic Disorders Due to Alcoholism and Malnutrition, 2nd Edition. Philadelphia, PA, FA Davis, 1989

Vinters HV: Pathologic issues in the diagnosis of Alzheimer disease. Bulletin of Clinical Neurosciences 56:39–47, 1991

Vinters HV, Miller BL, Pardridge WM: Brain amyloid and Alzheimer disease. Ann Intern Med 109:41–54, 1988

Weddington WW Jr: The mortality of delirium: an underappreciated problem? Psychosomatics 23:1232–1235, 1982

Weiner RD, Rogers HJ, Davidson JR, et al: Effects of electroconvulsive therapy upon brain electrical activity. Ann NY Acad Sci 462:270–281, 1986

Weiner MF, Denke M, Williams K, et al: Intramuscular medroxyprogesterone acetate for sexual aggression in elderly men. Lancet 339:1121–1122, 1992

Wells CE: Pseudodementia. Am J Psychiatry 136:895–900, 1979

Weytingh MD, Bossuyt PM, van Crevel H: Reversible dementia: more than 10% or less than 1%? A quantitative review. Journal of Neurology 242:466–471, 1995

Whatley SA, Anderton BH: The genetics of Alzheimer's disease. International Journal of Geriatric Psychiatry 5:145–159, 1990

Whybrow PC, Prange AJ Jr, Treadway CR: Mental changes accompanying thyroid gland dysfunction: a reappraisal using objective psychological measurement. Arch Gen Psychiatry 20:48–63, 1969

Wilkins RH, Brody IA: Alzheimer's disease. Arch Neurol 21:109–110, 1969

Will RG, Ironside JW, Zeidler M, et al: A new variant of Creutzfeldt-Jakob disease in the UK. Lancet 347:921–925, 1996

Williams M, Pennybacker J: Memory disturbances in third ventricular tumors. J Neurol Neurosurg Psychiatry 17:115–123, 1954

Williams MA, Ward SE, Campbell EB: Confusion: testing versus observation. Journal of Gerontological Nursing 14:25–30, 1986

Wilson LM: Intensive care delirium: the effect of outside deprivation in a windowless unit. Arch Intern Med 130:225–226, 1972

Wise MG: Delirium, in American Psychiatric Press Textbook of Neuropsychiatry. Edited by Hales RE, Yudofsky SC. Washington DC, American Psychiatric Press, 1987, pp 89–105

Yaffe K, Sawaya G, Lieberburg I, et al: Estrogen therapy in postmenopausal women: effects on cognitive function and dementia. JAMA 279:688–695, 1998

Young AB, Penney JB, Starosta-Rubinstein S, et al: PET scan investigations of Huntington's disease: cerebral metabolic correlates of neurological features and functional decline. Ann Neurol 20:296–303, 1986

Ziegler DK, Kaufman A, Marshall HE: Abrupt memory loss associated with thalamic tumor. Arch Neurol 34:545–548, 1977

Zola-Morgan S, Squire LR, Amaral DG: Human amnesia and the medial temporal region: enduring memory impairment following a bilateral lesion limited to the CA1 field of the hippocampus. J Neurosci 6:2950–2967, 1986

Zubek JP, Welch G: Electroencephalographic changes after prolonged sensory and perceptual deprivation. Science 139:1209–1210, 1963

Zubenko GS, Rosen J, Sweet RA, et al: Impact of psychiatric hospitalization on behavioral complications of Alzheimer's disease. Am J Psychiatry 149:1484–1491, 1992

CHAPTER 11

ALCOHOL AND OTHER PSYCHOACTIVE SUBSTANCE USE DISORDERS

JOHN E. FRANKLIN, JR., M.D.
RICHARD J. FRANCES, M.D.

Accounts of use and abuse of psychoactive substances, including alcohol, coca leaves, opium, and cannabis, are as old as civilization. Dependence on drugs and alcohol was described by Greek, Roman, and biblical authors. Physicians, philosophers, theologians, poets, and politicians have long debated the merits and harmful effects of psychoactive substance use (Edwards et al. 1982). Production of beer in Africa, medicinal use of opium in ancient Mesopotamia and Egypt, and use of cannabis in an early Hindu religious context date back more than 3,000 years. Use of plant stimulants and hallucinogens by Native Indian tribes in the Americas has had cultural, religious, and medical connections.

Two international "opium wars" were fought between Great Britain and China in the 1800s because opium was forced upon the Chinese by the British in exchange for commercial trade (Suwanwela 1979). Morphine was used widely during the American Civil War, and the turn of the century found hundreds of thousands of middle-class white individuals addicted to ubiquitous opium products. Widespread opioid use decreased after the 1914 Harrison Act, which made nonmedical use of narcotic drugs illegal. After interdiction, abuse of opioids remained endemic in certain populations. The 1960s found heroin abuse spreading from urban ghettos to middle-class suburbs.

In recent decades, advances in communication, technology, and medicine have led to the production of new drugs, wider distribution and marketing of drugs produced in many parts of the world, and new routes of administration of drugs that have long been available. Fueled by widespread demand in the United States, there has been increased cocaine production and distribution from Latin America. Insufflation of heroin has increased in the mid-1990s as a result of the availability of more potent heroin. Debates on the value of legalization of narcotics has intensified in recent years (Grinspon and Bakalar 1994; Kinsbourne 1994). Analogs of plant-derived psychoactive drugs have been designed in the laboratory and have had epidemic use. Industrial volatiles such as gasoline, cleaning fluid, paint, and aerosols also have been used to produce psychoactive effects.

Tobacco companies have only recently begun to acknowledge the medical complications and addictive aspects of tobacco use. Major legal efforts are underway to address possible tobacco company compensation to states and individuals.

Alcohol has long played an important economic, social, cultural, and religious role in Europe. Efforts at worldwide marketing of alcohol and tobacco have contributed to an increase in health-related problems, especially in developing countries. Alcohol control policies in the United States continue to be complex (Gordis 1997). Alcohol continues to be the psychoactive substance most frequently used and abused and, along with tobacco, poses the greatest health hazard.

WHAT IS A SUBSTANCE USE DISORDER?

The study of disorders resulting from psychoactive substances has made remarkable strides and produced promising leads for understanding the biological and psychosocial aspects of psychoactive chemical dependency. The dimensions of worldwide public health problems associated with alcoholism and other addictive drugs have recently become more amenable to study, with the development of instruments for measuring agreed-upon criteria for diagnosis of levels of severity of psychoactive substance use disorders (Helzer et al. 1986). It is difficult, however, to develop a nomenclature that is consistent across cultures and across substances and that can validly describe the clinical phenomena.

In DSM-III (American Psychiatric Association 1980), an effort was made to operationalize criteria for diagnosis that could be used to form research instruments for measuring substance abuse and dependence across populations. Substance use disorders can be diagnosed along with other disorders on Axes I, II, and III to allow for greater examination of the interaction between diagnoses. The term *substance abuse* was introduced in DSM-III to designate a pattern of pathological use of at least 1 month's duration that leads to impairment in social or occupational functioning. It was distinguished from substance dependence, which required the presence of tolerance or withdrawal symptoms.

The classification of substance use disorders in DSM-III underwent revision in DSM-III-R (American Psychiatric Association 1987) (Williams 1986). In DSM-III-R, the term *psychoactive* was added to substance abuse and substance dependence disorders in order to differentiate psychoactive substance abuse and dependence from nutritional or other adverse drug-related problems (Rounsaville et al. 1986). The DSM-III-R advisory committee proposed that the definition of psychoactive substance dependence be broadened to include at least three significant behaviors out of a nine-item list that includes psychosocial problems indicating a serious degree of involvement with a psychoactive substance. DSM-III-R criteria were designed with help from Robins and Helzer to overcome problems in operationalizing each item for use in diagnostic interviews based on these criteria. The substance-specific patterns of tolerance and withdrawal, which were both listed as criteria, were no longer the sole criteria for dependence. Severity criteria were included to indicate whether the dependence is mild, moderate, severe, in partial remission, or in full remission.

The disorder of psychoactive substance abuse became a residual category for those who continued substance use despite existence of problems caused by the use. Field tests showed that most of what was diagnosed as substance abuse by DSM-III was diagnosed as psychoactive substance dependency by DSM-III-R (Williams 1986). These changes were suggested because of the difficulty in distinguishing clear set points at which risk factors (hazardous use), abuse (harmful use), and dependence develop in an individual's history of use. The question of what level of problem or potential problem should constitute a disorder has been hotly debated. Both tolerance and withdrawal symptoms are graded phenomena, and psychosocial aspects of dependence for some drugs may contribute to major morbidity and mortality.

A World Health Organization (WHO) work group has made preliminary proposals for classification of alcohol- and drug-related problems in the *International Classification of Diseases*, 10th Revision (ICD-10; World Health Organization 1992) (Edwards et al. 1982). In ICD-10, a wider spectrum of problems is included that might be viewed as being relevant to prevention and early detection of potential problems compared with DSM-III-R, in which risk factors are clearly separated from diagnoses of a disorder. The notion of a general drug dependency syndrome was endorsed by the WHO work group, and the criteria largely overlap with DSM-III-R (Edwards et al. 1982) and DSM-IV (American Psychiatric Association 1994) criteria.

In DSM-III-R, organic mental disorders that are associated with psychoactive substance were moved and grouped with other disorders involving psychoactive substances (Williams 1986). An organic flashback syndrome was included that is caused by phencyclidine and hallucinogens. This syndrome is defined as the reexperiencing of one or more of the perceptual symptoms that the patient had experienced while intoxicated (e.g., hallucinations or derealization), resulting in marked distress. In DSM-III-R, organic disorders such as cannabis delirium and cocaine withdrawal, delirium, and delusional disorder were also included. Several new categories were added to cover dependence on cocaine, phencyclidine, hallucinogens, and inhalants. The DSM-III category "Barbiturate and Similarly Acting Sedative or Hypnotic" was changed to "Sedative, Hypnotic, or Anxiolytic."

In DSM-IV the term *substance-related disorders* replaces psychoactive substance use disorders. This change broadens the concept to include not only substances taken by individuals to alter mood or behavior but also substance-induced conditions that occur as a result of the unintentional use of a substance or as a side effect of a medication. Such cases are classified using an "Other (or Unknown) Substance Use Disorders" category. In DSM-IV the substance-related disorders place dependence, abuse, intoxication, and withdrawal syndromes in a "Substance Use Disorders" section. Disorders that were formerly in a "Psychoactive Substance-Induced Organic Mental Disorders" section, such as substance-induced delusional disorders and substance-induced mood disorders, have been moved to sections with which they phenomenologically overlap. For example, substance-induced mood disorder is placed in the "Mood Disorders" section.

Because, increasingly, patients are using combinations of psychoactive substances, drug interactions and polysubstance use are discussed throughout this chapter. For a list of classes of substances, see Table 11–1.

Specific substance-induced disorders have a three-part name (e.g., "Cocaine, Intoxication, Mood Disorder, With Manic Features") that includes the name of the substance, occurring with intoxication or withdrawal or beyond, and the phenomenological presentation, and are located both in the substance-related section and in the mood disorders section.

In DSM-IV, substance dependence has not been markedly altered even though criteria related to physiological dependence have been grouped differently, and there is a subtyping method of noting whether physiological dependence is part of the substance dependence (see Tables 11–2 and 11–3).

TABLE 11–1. DSM-IV substance-related disorders

- Alcohol use disorders
- Amphetamine (or related substance) use disorders
- Caffeine use disorders
- Cannabis use disorders
- Cocaine use disorders
- Hallucinogen use disorders
- Inhalant use disorders
- Nicotine use disorders
- Opioid use disorders
- Phencyclidine (or related substance) use disorders
- Sedative, hypnotic, or anxiolytic substance use disorders
- Polysubstance use disorders
- Other (or unknown) substance use disorders

In DSM-IV an effort is made to make a clearer distinction in the boundaries between nonpathological substance use, abuse and dependence, specific terms defining substance abuse, and the influence of cultural and situation-specific factors that impact on the definition (see Table 11–4). In DSM-IV, abuse depends on social difficulties and use in hazardous situations. DSM-IV abuse criteria may increase case finding when compared with DSM-III-R criteria (Hasin and Grant 1994). This increase may have profound effects on insurance and other public health concerns.

TABLE 11–2. DSM-IV criteria for substance dependence

A maladaptive pattern of substance use, leading to clinically significant impairment or distress, as manifested by three (or more) of the following, occurring at any time in the same 12-month period:

(1) Tolerance, as defined by either of the following:

   (a) A need for markedly increased amounts of the substance to achieve intoxication or desired effect.

   (b) Markedly diminished effect with continued use of the same amount of the substance.

(2) Withdrawal, as manifested by either of the following:

   (a) The characteristic withdrawal syndrome for the substance (refer to criteria A and B of the criteria sets for withdrawal from the specific substances).

   (b) The same (or a closely related) substance is taken to relieve or avoid withdrawal symptoms.

(3) The substance is often taken in larger amounts or over a longer period than was intended.

(4) There is a persistent desire or unsuccessful efforts to cut down or control substance use.

(5) A great deal of time is spent in activities necessary to obtain the substance (e.g., visiting multiple doctors or driving long distances), use the substance (e.g., chain-smoking), or recover from its effects.

(6) Important social, occupational, or recreational activities are given up or reduced because of substance use.

(7) The substance use is continued despite knowledge of having had a persistent or recurrent physical or psychological problem that is likely to have been caused or exacerbated by the substance (e.g., current cocaine use despite recognition of cocaine-induced depression, or continued drinking despite recognition that an ulcer was made worse by alcohol consumption).

Specify if:

With physiological dependence: evidence of tolerance or withdrawal (i.e., either item (1) or (2) is present).

Without physiological dependence: no evidence of tolerance or withdrawal (i.e., neither item (1) nor (2) is present).

TABLE 11–3. DSM-IV course specifiers for substance dependence

Six course specifiers are available for substance dependence. The four remission specifiers can be applied only after none of the criteria for substance dependence or substance abuse have been present for at least 1 month. The definition of these four types of remission is based on the interval of time that has elapsed since the cessation of dependence (early versus sustained remission) and whether there is continued presence of one or more of the items included in the criteria sets for dependence or abuse (partial versus full remission). Because the first 12 months following dependence is a time of particularly high risk for relapse, this period is designated early remission. After 12 months of early remission have passed without relapse to dependence, the person enters into sustained remission. For both early remission and sustained remission, a further designation of full is given if no criteria for dependence or abuse have been met during the period of remission; a designation of partial is given if at least one of the criteria for dependence or abuse has been met, intermittently or continuously, during the period of remission. The differentiation of sustained full remission from recovered (no current substance use disorder) requires consideration of the length of time since the last period of disturbance, the total duration of the disturbance, and the need for continued evaluation. If, after a period of remission or recovery, the individual again becomes dependent, the application of the early remission specifier requires that there again be at least 1 month in which no criteria for dependence or abuse are met. Two additional specifiers have been provided: on agonist therapy and in a controlled environment. For an individual to qualify for early remission after cessation of agonist therapy or release from a controlled environment, there must be a 1-month period in which none of the criteria for dependence or abuse are met.

The following remission specifiers can be applied only after no criteria for dependence or abuse have been met for at least 1 month. Note that these specifiers do not apply if the individual is on agonist therapy or in a controlled environment (see below).

Early full remission.   This specifier is used if, for at least 1 month, but for less than 12 months, no criteria for dependence or abuse have been met.

Early partial remission.   This specifier is used if, for at least 1 month, but less than 12 months, one or more criteria for dependence or abuse have been met (but the full criteria for dependence have not been met).

Sustained full remission.   This specifier is used if none of the criteria for dependence or abuse have been met at any time during a period of 12 months or longer.

Sustained partial remission.   This specifier is used if full criteria for dependence have not been met for a period of 12 months or longer; however, one or more criteria for dependence or abuse have been met.

The following specifiers apply if the individual is on agonist therapy or in a controlled environment:

On agonist therapy.   This specifier is used if the individual is on a prescribed agonist medication, and no criteria for dependence or abuse have been met for that class of medication for at least the past month (except tolerance to, or withdrawal from, the agonist). This category also applies to those being treated for dependence using a partial agonist or an agonist/antagonist.

In a controlled environment.   This specifier is used if the individual is in an environment where access to alcohol and controlled substances is restricted, and no criteria for dependence or abuse have been met for at least the past month. Examples of these environments are closely supervised and substance-free jails, therapeutic communities, or locked hospital units.

In DSM-IV the diagnosis of idiosyncratic alcohol intoxication was eliminated because it was found to be poorly researched, rare, ill defined, and overused in forensic cases.

Although a good argument could have been made for combining amphetamines and cocaine into a single, large category labeled "Stimulants," it was decided to keep independent categories to maintain compatibility with ICD-10 and consistency with DSM-III-R.

ALCOHOL ABUSE AND DEPENDENCE

DEFINITION

In DSM-IV the definitions of alcohol abuse and dependence closely follow and parallel those for other substance disorders, as described in Tables 11–2, 11–3, and 11–4. People vary a great deal in their tolerance to alcohol, and tolerance is difficult to measure. For example, if a 180-lb. man can consume five drinks in an hour and does not develop signs of intoxication, that would be evidence of considerable tolerance to alcohol. Similarly, use of one quart of spirits, one gallon of wine, or one case of beer per day or a finding of blood alcohol concentration (BAC) over 0.15 mg% demonstrates tolerance and may be almost pathognomonic for alcoholism. Withdrawal starts within several hours of stopping prolonged heavy drinking and is defined by at least *two* of the following: autonomic hyperactivity (e.g., sweating or pulse rate greater than 100); increased hand tremor; insomnia; nausea or vomiting; transient visual, tactile, or auditory hallucinations or illusions; psychomotor agitation; anxiety; or grand mal seizures.

TABLE 11–4.   **DSM-IV criteria for substance abuse**

A.   A maladaptive pattern of substance use leading to clinically significant impairment or distress, as manifested by one (or more) of the following, occurring within a 12-month period:

   (1)   Recurrent substance use resulting in a failure to fulfill major role obligations at work, school, or home (e.g., repeated absences or poor work performance related to substance use; substance-related absences, suspensions, or expulsions from school; neglect of children or household).

   (2)   Recurrent substance use in situations in which it is physically hazardous (e.g., driving an automobile or operating a machine when impaired by substance use).

   (3)   Recurrent substance-related legal problems (e.g., arrests for substance-related disorderly conduct).

   (4)   Continued substance use despite having persistent or recurrent social or interpersonal problems caused or exacerbated by the effects of the substance (e.g., arguments with spouse about consequences of intoxication, physical fights).

B.   The symptoms have never met the criteria for substance dependence for this class of substance.

EPIDEMIOLOGY

The vast impact that alcohol and alcoholism have as a public health problem can be measured by per capita consumption, lifetime prevalence, the number of current cases, morbidity and mortality, the rate of fetal alcohol syndrome, health care costs, and total cost of lost work time. Although recently there may have been a slight decline of total alcohol consumption in the United States, alcohol remains the most used and abused psychoactive chemical, with a per-person average annual consumption of 2.43 gallons of absolute alcohol by individuals age 15 and older. This is decreased from a high of 2.76 gallons in 1980–1981 (U.S. Department of Health and Human Services 1993).

PREVALENCE

Studies of the incidence and prevalence of alcoholism are often hard to evaluate because of the lack of clear criteria for diagnosis of alcoholism, variations in subpopulations studied, and tolerance of a particular culture or subculture for alcohol-related behaviors. In the National Institute of Mental Health Epidemiologic Catchment Area (ECA) study, which involved the use of standardized interviews in three U.S. cities (Robins et al. 1984), investigators found that psychoactive substance use disorders ranked first among 15 DSM-III diagnoses, with an average of 13.6% of the general population sampled having a lifetime prevalence of alcohol abuse or dependence (Myers et al. 1984). Using data from the same study, Blazer et al. (1985) reported that alcohol abuse or dependence was significantly more prevalent in more rural regions and in less educated persons. Kessler et al. (1994), using the National Comorbidity Survey data, estimated the lifetime and 12-month prevalence of alcohol abuse as 9.4% and 2.5%, respectively. The lifetime prevalence of alcohol dependence is 13.6% (Robins et al. 1984). In most cultures, men are more likely to be problem drinkers and heavy drinkers than are women, with studies showing a ratio of 4 to 1 in the United States and up to 28 to 1 in Korea (Helzer et al. 1986). Most alcohol-related problems begin between the ages of 16 and 30, with the lowest percentage of problems in persons older than 50. Onset of alcohol problems have been found to be later in African Americans and women (Caetano and Schafer 1996). Alcoholism is associated with high levels of divorce and separation, and the greatest number of problems occur in persons who are not presently married. Alcoholism rates have been found to be high in some cultures, such as the countries of the former Soviet Union, France, Scandinavia, Ireland, and Korea, and lower in other cultures, such as Asian, Islamic, and Mediterranean countries. Helzer et al. (1986) used the Diagnostic Interview Schedule (DIS) in five countries and found that whereas schizophrenia has a consistent cross-cultural prevalence, alcoholism prevalence varies with cultural context; the symptoms, however, are similar across culture.

MORBIDITY AND MORTALITY

In the U.S. Department of Health and Human Services' *Eighth Special Report to the U.S. Congress on Alcohol and Health* (1993), it was estimated that 100,000 deaths per year are alcohol related. Death rates of patients with primary alcoholism have been threefold greater than those of a control group. Liver disease ranks as the fourth leading cause of death, and alcoholism presents as a major cause of liver disease. Although less than 10% of alcoholic individuals develop cirrhosis, this disease accounts for 31,500 deaths annually in the United States, with alcohol being the leading associated factor. Alcohol cirrhosis accounts for 23.4% of the approximate 4,000 liver transplants performed in the United States each year (Belle et al. 1997).

There is an association between alcohol use and violent crime, including assault, rape, child molestation, and attempted murder (Collins 1991). Among male alcoholic violent offenders, low cerebrospinal fluid (CSF) 5-hydroxyindoleacetic acid (5-HIAA) and homovanillic acid concentrations have been found to be strongly associated with family history of paternal violence and alcoholism (Virkkunen et al. 1996).

Each year 25,000 people die and 150,000 are permanently disabled because of alcohol-related traffic accidents. One study of 2,095 trauma victims found that 41% had been drinking prior to their injury (Meyers et al. 1990). Soderstrom et al. (1997) report that 54.2% of 1,220 level 1 trauma victims have a lifetime diagnosis of psychoactive substance use disorders using the Structured Clinical Interview (SCID). The usual legal standard for drunken driving, a BAC of 0.10 mg%, can be reached after five to six drinks in the 2 hours before driving (see Figure 11–1). However, even lower BAC levels (0.05 mg%) increase risk up to three times. A 120-lb. person who has two drinks within 2 hours may not be aware of an impairment that could lead to driving problems.

Alcohol morbidity and a disproportionate number of hospital inpatient days are associated with the effects of intoxication, overdose, withdrawal, and chronic use. Withdrawal syndromes can be life threatening and are most dangerous when accompanied by medical problems such as

pneumonia, liver failure, and subdural hematomas. Common alcohol-related medical complications include gastritis, ulcers, pancreatitis, liver disease, cardiomyopathy, anemia, peripheral neuropathy, organicity, sexual dysfunction, cancer, and fetal alcohol syndrome. Korsakoff's psychosis and alcoholic dementia occur in approximately 2% of patients with alcohol dependence.

Recent reports suggest a cardiovascular benefit to light to moderate alcohol intake, however, new risks linked to breast cancer and stroke are also being reported (Chou et al. 1996). The risk of developing acute respiratory distress syndrome has also been reported to be increased with alcohol abuse (Moss et al. 1996).

ECONOMIC COSTS

Total economic losses in the United States in 1990 due to alcohol have been estimated to be 98 billion (Rice 1993). Costs due to alcohol-related cases include lost work production, lost future earnings secondary to excess mortality, health care costs, motor vehicle accident costs, highway safety program costs, crime and fire losses, police activity, prison costs, and judicial costs. Alcohol contributes to impairment in work function in industry, sports, medicine, and the military. For example, with 12% of military personnel impaired by alcoholism, human errors caused by intoxication or organicity can lead to catastrophic results. Reports of ships grounded off course and airplane crashes highlight the dangers of serious lapses in job function.

CLINICAL FEATURES

General

The early detection and treatment of alcohol abuse and dependency are complicated by denial, which tends to manifest itself in the individual, in the family, and in society as a whole. Diagnosis of alcoholism (or psychoactive substance abuse) for the patient and the physician is easier late in the course of the illness, although treatment at that point may be more complicated. Because of the widespread prevalence of alcoholism and the protean forms in which it presents, the diagnostician should always have a high index of suspicion and awareness of its signs and symptoms. Often underdiagnosed and undertreated, patients with alcoholism may resist and avoid doctors because of embarrassment, problems with authority figures, and poor self-care. The components of a basic alcohol and substance use history are listed in Table 11–5.

Clinicians should be alert to the subtle signs and symptoms of early alcohol problems, including loss of commu-

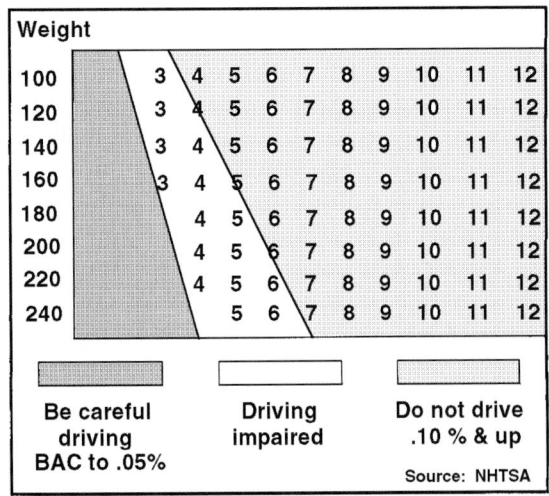

FIGURE 11–1. Intoxication from number of drinks (1.2 oz. 80-proof liquor or 12 oz. beer) in a 2-hour period. The chart shows average responses. Younger people generally become impaired sooner, whereas older people have more vision problems at night. Tests show a wide range of responses even for persons of the same age and weight. For some persons, one drink may be too many.

TABLE 11–5. Components of a basic alcohol and substance use history

- Chief complaint
- History of present illness
- Current medical signs and symptoms
- Substance abuse review of symptoms (ROS) for all psychoactive substances
- Dates of first use, regular use, heaviest use, longest period of sobriety, pattern, amount, frequency, time of last use, route of administration, circumstances of use, reactions to use
- Medical history, medications, human immunodeficiency virus (HIV) status
- History of past substance abuse treatment, response to treatment
- Family history, including substance abuse history
- Psychiatric history
- Legal history
- Object-relations history
- Personal history

Source. Reprinted with permission from Frances RJ, Franklin JE: *A Concise Guide to Treatment of Alcoholism and Addictions.* Washington, DC, American Psychiatric Press, 1989, p. 62. Copyright 1989, American Psychiatric Press.

nication in a marriage, frequent temper flare-ups, belligerent demands, and a loss of overall interest in the marital relationship. Alcohol may be used either to decrease sexual inhibition or to avoid sexual life.

The three self-administered brief screening tests most widely used for alcoholism are the Michigan Alcoholism Screening Test (MAST; Selzer 1971), a 25-question form that is 90% sensitive (Table 11–6); the CAGE questionnaire (Ewing 1984) (Table 11–7), a four-item test; and the Alcohol Use Disorders Identification Test (AUDIT) (Allen et al. 1997; Saunders et al. 1993).

Personality change detected at work in the form of irritability, inability to complete projects on time, lateness, and absence may be noted. Before there are severe accidents or loss of a driver's license because of driving while intoxicated, the person may have had complaints by passengers about his or her driving. Drinking may be used to cope with depressed mood or anxiety, or as an aid to sleep. Early medical problems include morning vomiting, abdominal pain, diarrhea, gastritis, and enlarged liver. There may be an increased tendency toward accidents, bruises, blackouts, and seizures; an increase in infection; and, in those persons who smoke, the occurrence of cigarette-burned fingers. An evidence of family history should be looked for, and the possible vulnerability on a genetic basis can be explained to patients.

The longer-term effects of chronic alcoholism are

much more obvious and severely affect every aspect of a person's life. Long-term alcohol dependence has effects on personality, mood, and cognition and leads to social stigma. It also becomes more difficult to separate alcohol effects that may be superimposed on preexisting psychiatric disorders. Awareness that alcoholism is a chronic, relapsing disease and that suicide potential increases over time is important in designing treatment programs.

Adverse Physical Effects

Ethyl alcohol content in alcoholic beverages can range from 12% in wine products to 75% in distilled spirits. Alcohol is primarily absorbed in the small intestine and is metabolized in the liver. Alcohol dehydrogenase (ADH), a liver enzyme, metabolizes alcohol to toxic acetaldehyde. Aldehyde dehydrogenase (AldDH) completes the transformation of acetaldehyde to acetic acid. Lactic acid, uric acid, and fat accumulation in the liver are hazardous by-products. Alcohol dehydrogenase metabolizes 1 ounce of 86-proof spirits (or 43% alcohol) in approximately 1 hour.

Progression of alcoholism leads to associated medical problems regarding the brain, the digestive tract, the heart, other muscles, blood, hormones, and pregnancy. Alcohol, heavy tobacco use, and deficiency of vitamins A and B all contribute to high cancer rates in the mouth, tongue, larynx, esophagus, stomach, liver, and pancreas (Lieber et al. 1995). Alcohol dissolves mucus and irritates gastric lining, contributing to bleeding. Seventy-five percent of patients with chronic pancreatitis have alcoholism. Liver problems range from fatty liver to alcoholic hepatitis to cirrhosis, which is life threatening. Lieber (1977) found that given a nutritious diet, some baboons who were chronically force-fed with alcohol developed cirrhosis, indicating that alcohol has direct toxic effects on the liver. Blass and Gibson (1977) reported a familial transketolase deficiency in humans that causes a vitamin B deficiency in a subgroup at risk for Korsakoff's syndrome. The question of whether alcohol has direct toxic effects on the liver, the cortex, and the fetus, or whether these effects are primarily due to malnutrition or other variables, has not been fully answered. Most likely, the combined effects of alcohol, diet, and heredity are important.

In one prospective study, 50% of individuals with alcohol liver cirrhosis died within 4 years of diagnosis (Chedid et al. 1991). The development of diabetes can also be enhanced with alcohol use, and alcohol is a major risk factor for hypertension.

Alcoholic cardiomyopathy can develop after 10 or more years of drinking. Abstinence contributes to recovery in those cases in which damage is not too extensive. Alcohol

TABLE 11-6. Michigan Alcoholism Screening Test (MAST)

Points			Yes	No
	0.	Do you enjoy a drink now and then?		
(2)	1.	Do you feel you are a normal drinker? (By normal we mean you drink less than or as much as most other people.)		
(2)	2.	Have you ever awakened the morning after some drinking the night before and found that you could not remember a part of the evening?		
(1)	3.	Does your wife, husband, a parent, or other near relative ever worry or complain about your drinking?		
(2)	4.	Can you stop drinking without a struggle after one or two drinks?		
(1)	5.	Do you ever feel guilty about your drinking?		
(2)	6.	Do friends or relatives think you are a normal drinker?		
(0)	7.	Do you ever try to limit your drinking to certain times of the day or to certain places?		
(2)	8.	Have you ever attended a meeting of Alcoholics Anonymous?		
(1)	9.	Have you gotten into physical fights when drinking?		
(2)	10.	Has your drinking ever created problems between you and your wife, husband, a parent, or other relative?		
(2)	11.	Has your wife, husband (or other family members) ever gone to anyone for help about your drinking?		
(2)	12.	Have you ever lost friends because of your drinking?		
(2)	13.	Have you ever gotten into trouble at work or school because you were drinking?		
(2)	14.	Have you ever lost a job because of drinking?		
(2)	15.	Have you ever neglected your obligations, your family, or your work for two or more days in a row because you were drinking?		
(1)	16.	Do you drink before noon fairly often?		
(2)	17.	Have you ever been told you have liver trouble? Cirrhosis?		
(2)*	18.	After heavy drinking have you ever had Delirium Tremens (DTs) or severe shaking, or heard voices or seen things that really weren't there?		
(5)	19.	Have you ever gone to anyone for help about your drinking?		
(5)	20.	Have you ever been in a hospital because of drinking?		
(2)	21.	Have you ever been a patient in a psychiatric hospital or on a psychiatric ward of a general hospital where drinking was part of the problem that resulted in hospitalization?		
(2)	22.	Have you ever been seen at a psychiatric or mental health clinic or gone to any doctor, social worker, or clergyman for help with any emotional problem, where drinking was part of the problem?		
(2)**	23.	Have you ever been arrested for drunk driving, driving while intoxicated, or driving under the influence of alcoholic beverages? (If YES, how many times? _____)		
(2)**	24.	Have you ever been arrested, or taken into custody, even for a few hours, because of other drunk behavior? (If YES, how many times? _____)		

*5 points for Delirium Tremens   **2 points for *each* arrest

SCORING SYSTEM: In general, Five points or more would place that subject in an "alcoholic" category. Four points would suggest alcoholism, three points or less would indicate the subject was not alcoholic.

Programs using the above scoring system find it very sensitive at the 5-point level, and it tends to find more people alcoholics than anticipated. However, it is a screening test and should be sensitive at its lower levels.

Source. Adapted with permission from Selzer ML: "The Michigan Alcoholism Screening Test: The Quest for a New Diagnostic Instrument." *American Journal of Psychiatry* 127:1653–1658, 1971. Copyright 1971, American Psychiatric Association.

TABLE 11–7. "CAGE" screen for diagnosis of alcoholism

Have you ever:

C   thought you should CUT back on your drinking?

A   felt ANNOYED by people criticizing your drinking?

G   felt GUILTY or bad about your drinking?

E   had a morning EYE-OPENER to relieve hangover or nerves?

Note. A score of 2 or 3 indicates a high index of suspicion of alcohol dependence, and a score of 4 is pathognomonic for dependence.
Source. Adapted with permission from Ewing JA: "Detecting Alcoholism: The CAGE Questionnaire." JAMA 252:1905–1907, 1984. Copyright 1984, American Medical Association.

has chronic effects on other muscle and nerve tissue and reduces white blood cell count, which may affect the body's immune response. Infectious diseases have been common in this group.

Alcohol interferes with male sexual functioning and fertility through direct effects on testosterone levels and testicular atrophy. Increased levels of female hormones lead to the development of a feminine pubic hair pattern and breast enlargement in 50% of male alcoholic individuals. Sexual functioning is affected indirectly through alcohol's impact on the hypothalamus and pituitary. Alcohol can affect sexual desire by toxic effects on the limbic system and hypothalamic-pituitary axis. Sexual distress (impotency) can result from neuropathy of the peripheral parasympathetic autonomic nerves involved in penile erection. In alcoholic females, severe gonadal failure, with inability to produce adequate amounts of female hormones, may also occur, affecting secondary sexual characteristics, reducing menstruation, and producing infertility.

Alcohol abuse is a significant risk factor for trauma. Alcohol abuse is associated with an increased risk for readmission for trauma and hospital complications (Jurkovich et al. 1993; Rivera et al. 1993). Arrests for drunken drinking increase risk for mortality from automobile accidents (Brewer et al. 1994).

Comorbidity

Depression, anxiety, personality disorders, and drug abuse have all been associated with alcohol abuse. Regier (1990), also using ECA data, found that in a community sample of those with an alcohol disorder and drug abuse, 53% also had a comorbid mental disorder. The most common comorbid disorders for women were anxiety and affective disorders, whereas with men other substance abuse disorders, conduct disorder, and antisocial personality disorder

was more prevalent (Kessler et al. 1997). Alcoholic subjects have a greater than twofold comorbidity of other psychiatric disorders compared with nonalcoholic subjects. Significant secondary depressions may occur in between one-quarter to two-thirds of alcoholic persons over a lifetime (Schuckit 1985). Secondary alcoholism is particularly associated with bipolar illness (Winokur et al. 1995). The comorbidity of major depression and alcoholism in women appears substantial and may be related to genetic and environmental factors (Kendler 1993). Depressive symptoms secondary to alcoholism will generally remit in 3 weeks (Brown et al. 1995). Alcoholism has been found in prospective studies to have deleterious effects on recovery from major depression (Mueller et al. 1994).

Alcoholism is as high a risk factor for suicide as depression, with rates between 60 and 120 times that of persons without psychiatric illness (Murphy and Wetzel 1990); the lifetime risk of suicide is 2%–3.4%, and 25% of all suicides are related to alcoholism. Alcoholic persons who attempt suicide may have more severe alcohol problems and greater comorbidity than those who do not attempt suicide (Roy et al. 1990). There appears to be a disproportionate rate of suicidality with persons with major depression and alcoholism (Cornelius et al. 1995). Continued drinking, major depression, suicidal communication, poor social support, serious medical illness, unemployment, and living alone are identified risk factors (Murphy et al. 1992). Those alcoholic persons who also have comorbid anxiety disorder are at high risk for suicide (Johnson et al. 1990).

Alcohol use is common in schizophrenia and may be related to poorer outcome (Drake et al. 1989). High rates of alcohol and other drug abuse occur in schizophrenic persons, and alcohol use may be related to subjective decreases in social anxiety, dysphoria, insomnia, and other nonpsychotic but unpleasant experiences (Noordsy et al. 1991). In a study of acute general hospital patients with a diagnosis of borderline personality disorder, 67% also had a substance abuse diagnosis (Dulit et al. 1990). Antisocial personality has been related to higher rates of alcohol abuse (Nestadt et al. 1992). Antisocial personality disorder has been the only personality feature in prospective studies that has been predictive of future alcoholism (Schuckit et al. 1994). Several investigators are attempting to subtype substance-abusing individuals with antisocial personalities into symptomatic psychopathic persons with little psychopathy and true psychopathic persons (Gerstley et al. 1990). True, early-onset antisocial personality that fulfills childhood antisocial criteria may be more associated with criminal and violent behavior (Cacciola et al. 1994).

Kushner et al. (1990) reviewed the clinical relationship between alcohol problems and anxiety disorders. Their review suggests that agoraphobia and social phobia appear to predate chronic alcohol use, and panic attacks and generalized anxiety disorder tend to follow pathological alcohol consumption. Evidence still suggests that heavy alcohol use causes and exacerbates general psychiatric distress, and baseline levels of high stress are predictive of poorer outcome (Dryman and Anthony 1989).

EFFECTS OF ALCOHOL ON PREGNANCY

Maternal alcohol misuse can lead to *fetal alcohol syndrome*, which consists of growth retardation before or after birth; abnormal features of the face and head, such as unusually small head circumference and/or flattening of facial features; and evidence of central nervous system (CNS) abnormalities (e.g., mental retardation and abnormal behavior). Characteristic craniofacial malformation may diminish in time, however, microcephaly persists (Spohr et al. 1993). Fortunately, the prevalence of drinking during pregnancy has decreased in recent years (Serdula et al. 1991). The question of whether low doses of alcohol consumption may increase risk of decreased birth weight and of increased spontaneous abortions has been debated; regardless, the National Institute on Alcohol Abuse and Alcoholism (NIAAA) recommends no use of alcohol during pregnancy.

Abel and Sokol (1991) estimate the rate of fetal alcohol syndrome in the general population to be 0.33 cases per 1,000 births and the risk of an alcoholic women having a child with fetal alcohol syndrome to be 6%. Rates of fetal alcohol syndrome vary from 1 in 1,000 live births in the general population to as high as 1 in 100 in some Native American Indian and Eskimo societies.

INTERACTION OF ALCOHOL WITH DRUGS

The interaction of ethanol with other drugs may lead to lethal overdoses or undermedication through effects on drug or alcohol metabolism, absorption, or action ("Interaction of Alcohol With Drugs" *Medical Letter* 1977; see Table 11–8). Alcohol is partly metabolized through the hepatic microsomal enzyme system that metabolizes many other drugs. Acute effects may slow metabolism and increase blood levels of drugs such as oral anticoagulants and phenytoin, and chronic effects may lead to increased metabolism and decreased blood levels. Severe cirrhosis and liver failure may also slow drug metabolism and slow detoxification of diazepam. Conversely, drugs can affect alcohol's metabolism, and mild disulfiram-like reactions can occur with oral hypoglycemics (e.g., tolbutamide, chlorpropamide), griseofulvin, metronidazole, and quinacrine hydrochloride.

TABLE 11–8.   Effects of some drug interactions with alcohol

Drug	Effect with alcohol
Disulfiram (Antabuse)	Flushing, diaphoresis, vomiting, confusion
Anticoagulants (oral)	↑ Effect with acute; ↓ intoxication effect after chronic use
Antimicrobials	Minor Antabuse reactions
Tranquilizers, narcotics, antihistamines	Increased central nervous system depression
Diazepam	↑ Absorption
Phenytoin	↑ Anticonvulsant effect with acute intoxication; alcohol intoxication or withdrawal may lower seizure threshold after chronic alcohol abuse
Salicylates	Gastrointestinal bleeding
Chlorpromazine	↑ Levels of alcohol
Monoamine oxidase inhibitor	Adverse reactions to tyramine in some alcoholic beverages

Chlorpromazine increases blood alcohol levels through inhibiting alcohol dehydrogenase. Alcohol enhances absorption of diazepam, which decreases its safety margin and increases chance of overdose. In addition to the above effects, alcohol has additive effects with other CNS depressants, narcotics, and antihistamines, and unpredictable effects with CNS stimulants. Additive effects with salicylates can occur, leading to gastrointestinal bleeding. Because many alcoholic beverages contain tyramine, use of monoamine oxidase inhibitors (MAOIs) is relatively counterindicated in active or recovering alcoholic persons and should be avoided except when indicated in closely managed, very reliable patients for whom the benefits may outweigh the risks.

LABORATORY TESTING IN ALCOHOLISM

Standard Tests

Standard laboratory tests include

- Complete blood count with differential
- Serum electrolytes
- Liver function tests
- Bilirubin
- Blood urea nitrogen
- Creatinine

- Fasting blood sugar
- Prothrombin time
- Cholesterol
- Triglycerides
- Calcium
- Magnesium
- Albumin with total protein
- Hepatitis B surface antigen, hepatitis C
- B_{12} and folic acid levels
- Stool guaiac
- Urinalysis
- Drug and alcohol urine screen
- Chest X ray
- Electrocardiogram

Ancillary tests such as an electroencephalogram (EEG) and a computed tomography (CT) scan series may be ordered as indicated.

Serum γ-glutamyltransferase (SGGT) is a sensitive test for chronic, heavy alcohol intake and is increased in more than 50% of patients with an alcohol problem and 80% of those with liver problems (Trell et al. 1984). Liver function test such as aspartate aminotransferase (AST) and alanine aminotransferase (ALT) are frequently elevated with heavy drinking and markedly elevated with alcohol hepatitis. Increased mean corpuscular volume, decreased white cell count and platelets, and increased levels of uric acid, triglyceride, and urea are also common in alcoholism (see Table 11–9). A fingerprint of commonly available blood chemistry tests using quadratic discriminant analysis may be specific for recent heavy drinking; however, its usefulness in detecting alcoholism is limited by false negatives

TABLE 11-9. Laboratory findings associated with alcohol abuse

- Blood alcohol level
- Positive breathalyzer
- Elevated MCV
- Elevated SGOT (AST), SGPT (ALT), LDH
- Elevated SGGT (particularly sensitive)
- Decreased albumin, B_{12}, folic acid
- Increased uric acid, elevated amylase, evidence of bone suppression

Note. MCV = mean corpuscular volume; SGOT = serum glutamic-oxaloacetic transaminase; AST = aspartate aminotransferase; SGPT = serum glutamic pyruvic transaminase; ALT = alanine aminotransferase; LDH = lactate dehydrogenase; SGGT = Serum γ-glutamyltransferase.
Source. Reprinted with permission from Frances RJ, Franklin JE: *A Concise Guide to Treatment of Alcoholism and Addictions.* Washington, DC, American Psychiatric Press, 1989, p. 74. Copyright 1989, American Psychiatric Press.

and false positives (Goodwin 1985a). Receiver operating characteristics (ROC) can also show the percentage of true positives versus true negatives.

Two new promising markers for recent alcohol use are 5-hytroxytryptophol (5-HTOL) and fatty acid ethyl esters (FAEEs). Urinary 5-HTOL rises in a dose-dependent fashion after acute ingestion. The 5-HTOL/5-HIAA ratio can detect relatively small amounts of drinking for a 7–10 hour period after last alcohol ingestion (Voltaire et al. 1992). Elevated FAEEs can detect recent use intake up to 24 hours after ethanol intake (Doyle et al. 1996).

Carbohydrate-Deficient Transferrin

The search for markers of recent heavy alcohol use has led to the finding that carbohydrate-deficient transferrin is a valuable aid in identifying alcohol use and may be a tool in monitoring relapse. Kapur et al. (1989) earlier confirmed the marker as 86% sensitive for daily intake of at least 80 grams for a minimum of 3 weeks, and 98% specific. Clinical limitations of this marker appear to be its low sensitivity with short lived or low alcohol consumption (Salmela et al. 1994). There is some evidence that carbohydrate-deficient transferrin (CDT) may have some benefit in moderate consumption (Huseby et al. 1997). Further, differences in sensitivity and specificity have been reported with sex, age, ethnicity, and medical status (Allen et al. 1994). However, CDT remains useful in the context of liver damage unless the liver disease is severe. Two recent studies suggest that CDT is more sensitive than serum SGGT as an indicator of treatment outcome (Anton et al. 1997b; Schmidt et al. 1997). Combining CDT and SGGT may increase diagnostic performance.

Biological Markers

As in other areas of psychiatry, the search for biological markers that may help in the primary prevention of alcoholism continues. Early studies found platelet monoamine oxidase levels are low in alcoholic individuals, first-degree relatives of alcoholic individuals, bipolar affective disorder patients, schizophrenia patients, and mountain climbers, and therefore too broad to be of much use (Alexopoulos et al. 1983). Porjesz and Begleiter (1981) found that the male offspring of alcoholic males have an increase in the P3 wave of evoked potentials, indicating a possible marker, and that neuropsychological problems may occur prior to the onset of alcoholism. Schuckit has found differences in the way corticosteroids and prolactin levels, body sway, P3 amplitude and subjective intoxication differ in 20-year-old biologic sons of alcoholic individuals compared with control subjects in response to an alcohol challenge (Schuckit et al. 1988). Schuckit has followed the 227 biologic sons of alcoholic individuals and 227 matched control subjects for over 10 years. Low level of response to alcohol at baseline, more prevalent in sons of alcoholic individuals, predicted a fourfold increase rate of alcohol dependence 10 years later (Schuckit 1994). Other studies, however, have reported family history positive individuals to be more sensitive to alcohol (McCaul et al. 1991; O'Malley and Maisto 1985). Nonalcoholic men at high risk for alcoholism may have a relatively lower plasma γ-aminobutyric acid (GABA) level than do control subjects (Moss et al. 1990). EEG response, 5-HIAA levels, and β endorphin differences have been associated with high risk (Fils-Aime et al. 1996; Gianoulakis et al. 1996; Volavka et al. 1996). Currently, however, the these biological markers for alcoholism have had limited clinical usefulness.

CAUSES OF ALCOHOLISM

Alcoholism is the final result of a complex interaction between biological vulnerability and environmental factors such as childhood experience, parental attitudes, social policies, and culture. A series of twin and adoption studies have found that genetic variables significantly influence causation, although the mechanism of genetic transmission is not known (Goodwin 1985b). Monozygotic twins have a two-times higher rate for the concordance of alcoholism compared with dizygotic twins, and the incidence of alcoholism is four times higher among male biological offspring of alcoholic fathers compared with offspring of nonalcoholic fathers, regardless of whether they are raised by foster parents or their own biological parents. Kendler (1997) recently examined the Swedish Temperance Board twin registrations between 1929 and 1974. The genetic versus familial-environmental risk for alcoholism was estimated at 54% and 14%, respectively. Hereditary factors among women are less clear. However, some twin studies have found genetic vulnerability in females (Kendler et al. 1992) (Table 11–10).

Several studies have subtyped alcoholic persons building on the early work of Jellinek (1960). The most prominent is the Type 1 versus Type 2 described by Cloninger (Bohman et al. 1987). The Type 1 milieu-limited prototype is characterized by onset of alcoholism after the age of 25; the presence of only isolated alcohol-related difficulties with health, marital relationships, or self-care; behavior inhibition; anticipatory worry; rigidity; reflectiveness; and sparse histories of arrests, violence, or abuse of other drugs. The Type 2 prototype is characterized by being a relative of an alcoholic man; onset of alcohol problems before the age of 25; antisocial traits, including histories of violence,

TABLE 11–10.   Characteristics of familial alcoholic individuals

- Earlier onset of problem drinking
- More severe social consequences
- Less consistently stable family involvement
- Poor academic and social performance in school
- More antisocial behavior
- Poorer prognosis in treatment

Source.   Reprinted with permission from Frances RJ, Franklin JE: *A Concise Guide to Treatment of Alcoholism and Addictions.* Washington, DC, American Psychiatric Press, 1989, p. 74. Copyright 1989, American Psychiatric Press.

arrests, and illegal drug abuse; and risk taking, impulsiveness, and quick temper. Type 2 alcoholism is associated with a stronger genetic propensity for the disorder. Cloninger associated Type 1 alcoholic individuals with personality traits of low novelty seeking, high harm avoidance, and high reward dependence. Type 2 alcoholic individuals were high novelty seeking, low harm avoidance, and low reward dependence. Differences in novelty seeking, harm avoidance, and reward dependence reflect variation in dopaminergic, serotonergic, and noradrenergic brain function. However, several negative studies have shown no differences in these personality traits between sons of alcoholic individuals and sons of control subjects (Howard et al. 1996), and many questions remain as to what is the best criteria to subtype. Age at onset of alcoholism may overlap with primary/secondary typology (Anthenelli et al. 1994). Irwin et al. (1990) hypothesized that Type 2 might be more closely aligned with antisocial personality and not the severity of alcohol abuse. Buydens-Branchey et al. (1989) suggest that onset of alcohol problems in persons before the age of 20 is associated with higher paternal alcoholism, antisocial behavior, and serotonin deficit. George et al. (1997) have reported reduced 5-HT$_{2A}$ receptor sensitivity in alcoholics and a differential clinical response to a mixed serotonin agonist/antagonist between Type 1 and Type 2 alcoholic individuals.

A similar Type A/Type B typology exists that differs by eliminating "loss of control" and neurotic attributes from the Type 1 subgroup and "inability to abstain" from the Type 2 subgroup (Babor et al. 1992). Type A is characterized by later onset, fewer indicators of vulnerability, less psychiatric disturbance, a more benign alcohol-related problem profile, and better prognosis. Type B is characterized by early onset of problem drinking, rapid progression, indicators of childhood and familial vulnerability, more psychiatric disturbance, greater symptom severity, and poor prognosis. The two types may differ in respect to outcome, and attempts have been made to differentially apply treatments to subtypes. Litt et al. (1992) found that coping skills training had a better outcome with Type B persons and interactional therapy had a better outcome with Type A persons.

In a prospective study, Vaillant (1984) found that there may not be any personality style predictive of alcoholism. McCord and McCord (1960) found aggressive and impulsive problems in adolescents with future drinking problems. Although Cloninger et al. (1979) reported that alcoholism, sociopathy, and depression are genetically distinct, other authors, such as Winokur et al. (1974), found that a broad-based genetic vulnerability may end up being expressed in either alcoholism or depression. Loranger and Tulis (1985) found a greater family history of alcoholism in borderline patients compared with bipolar or schizophrenic patients.

Alcoholism has been associated with other disorders such as somatization disorder and childhood minimal brain disorder. Childhood attention-deficit/hyperactivity disorder (ADHD) has been associated with antisocial personality and drug abuse disorders; it seems, however, to be mediated by the development of conduct disorders in childhood (Mannuzza et al. 1993). In one study, monozygotic twins raised apart were found to have high heritability for drug abuse and antisocial personality, but, surprisingly, the results did not confirm earlier risk factor studies that found at least mild heritability for alcohol abuse (Grove et al. 1990). Tarter (1982) found that primary alcoholic persons reported a history of the prevalence of minimal brain disorder and had poorer performance on psychological tests. The mechanisms for risk factors such as positive family history of alcoholism, gender, or hyperactivity in childhood are currently not known.

The search for a gene for alcoholism led to a report by Blum et al. (1990) of an A1 allele linkage of the dopamine D_2-receptor gene and alcoholism. This specificity of this finding has not been confirmed (Bolos et al. 1990; Uhl et al. 1992). The effort to map the genes for addictive disorders using candidate probes is a high research priority. The Cooperative Study of the Genetics of Alcoholism, sponsored by NIAAA, is using statistical genetics and molecular biology to further understanding of what is inherited in alcoholism.

PATHOPHYSIOLOGY

With increasing evidence that alcoholism is inherited, there has been growing attention to the question of exactly what is inherited. A number of hypotheses have been brought forward that are currently being studied (Table 11–11):

TABLE 11–11. Hypotheses concerning role of inheritance in alcoholism

- A deficiency of some factor such as serotonin or prostaglandins may occur, with levels at first increased and then decreased by alcohol.
- Alcohol could lead to increased activity of endorphins or morphine-like substances such as tetrahydroisoquinalone.
- Alcohol may at first increase relaxation in susceptible individuals, such as sons of alcoholic persons, as evidenced by slow-wave alpha activity on the EEG.
- Sons of alcoholic persons may be particularly prone to high tolerance in early stages of the problem.
- Unpleasant physiological reactions to alcohol such as the "oriental flush" might be protective against alcoholism.

1. Alcoholic individuals may have reduced serotonergic function.
2. Alcoholic individuals have depressed activity of endogenous opiates.
3. Alcohol may increase relaxation in susceptible individuals, as evidenced in increased slow-wave alpha activity on the EEG during alcohol use.
4. Sons of alcoholic fathers may be particularly prone to high tolerance in early stages of the problem (see Table 11–12).

Unpleasant physiological reactions to alcohol such as the "oriental flush" might be protective against alcoholism (Goodwin 1985a). (It is interesting that a high percentage of Chinese react to alcohol with a cutaneous flush, queasiness, tachycardia, and decreased blood pressure. However, Koreans also have a flush response and yet have a high incidence of alcoholism, indicating that low rates of alcoholism in Chinese may have to do with cultural factors in addition to the flush response [Helzer et al. 1986]. The interaction of biological protective factors with physiological and sociocultural variables needs to be further researched.)

Strains of rats (HS/lbg) and mice have been produced that either will or will not drink alcohol, and it has been controversial whether this constitutes an animal model for studying the effects of alcoholism (Dole 1986). Lower levels of neurotransmitters such as serotonin and endorphins in the brains of these mice may give information about genetic transmission. Long-sleep and short-sleep mouse lines have been developed with differential CNS sensitivity to the sedative-hypnotic effects of alcohol (McClearn and Erwin 1982). The rate of tolerance development and the severity of physical dependence caused by chronic alcohol ingestion have been found to be determined genetically in mice and possibly in humans.

TABLE 11–12.   **Possible markers of alcoholism in biological sons of alcoholic individuals**

- Decreased subjective feelings of intoxication
- Less impairment of motor performance
- Less body sway
- Less static ataxia
- Less change in cortisol and prolactin levels
- Low P3 amplitude (electroencephalogram)
- Increased alpha wave activity

Source.   Reprinted with permission from Frances RJ, Franklin JE: *A Concise Guide to Treatment of Alcoholism and Addictions.* Washington, DC, American Psychiatric Press, 1989, p. 74. Copyright 1989, American Psychiatric Press.

DIFFERENTIAL DIAGNOSIS

It can be difficult to differentiate the effects of alcohol intoxication, overdose, and withdrawal; the effects of chronic use; and the complex interaction of alcoholism with other psychiatric disorders. Alcohol and alcoholism may mask or mimic a variety of other clinical syndromes. In any patient who presents intoxicated or in a coma it is important to consider the possibility of overdose. In any individual who is unconscious, signs of alcohol and drug abuse should be looked for: a red nose, red palms, skin tracks, scars, spider nevi, erythema, cigarette burns between the index and middle fingers, poor dental care, jaundice, enlarged liver, abdominal pain, reduced sensation, and muscle weakness. When patients present severely intoxicated, comatose, or semicomatose, other complications should be ruled out, including head and spinal cord injuries, hypoglycemia, diabetic coma, hepatic coma, cardiac arrhythmias, myasthenia, and other drug overdose.

Differential diagnosis of withdrawal symptoms from other medical causes, psychiatric disorders, other alcohol-related psychosis, alcohol idiosyncratic intoxication, alcoholic hallucinosis, and alcoholic paranoidal state depends on careful history taking and evaluation of signs and symptoms. In delirium other than that which is alcohol induced, there is frequently less autonomic hyperactivity, less disorientation, a more fixed delusional system, and less memory loss following the psychosis than in alcohol withdrawal syndrome. Syndromes associated with sedative-hypnotic withdrawal resemble alcohol withdrawal but occur more rapidly and with greater severity, except for withdrawal from minor tranquilizers, which may be protracted. Depression, anxiety, and attentional problems may either lead to or be caused by drinking. An alcohol paranoidal state can develop in males over age 45 and may begin 1–2 weeks after the last drink. It may be persistent and is marked by suspicion, distrust, jealousy, highly developed fixed paranoid delusions, a history of homosexual feelings, inappropriate violent behavior, and amnesia.

ALCOHOL-INDUCED ORGANIC MENTAL DISORDERS

Alcohol Intoxication

Alcohol intoxication, the most frequently induced organic mental disorder, is time limited and, depending on individual variation and tolerance, may occur with varying amounts of alcohol use (see Table 11–13). Stages range from mild inebriation to anesthesia, coma, respiratory depression, and, rarely, death. A CNS depressant, alcohol may in low doses produce clinical excitement. In those who have not built up tolerance, BACs of 0.03 mg% can lead to euphoria, and those of 0.05 mg% can cause mild coordination problems. First pass metabolism by gastric tissue has been found to be lower in alcoholic women patients compared with men, and this may explain the increased bioavailability of alcohol in women and the increased rates of hepatic injury (Frezza et al. 1990).

Intoxication leads to disinhibiting behavioral changes including inappropriate sexual or aggressive behavior, mood lability, impaired judgment, and impaired social or occupational functioning. Ataxia is present at 0.1 mg%. Confusion and decreased consciousness can occur at 0.2 mg%. Anesthesia, coma, and death can occur with BACs of greater than 0.4 mg% (Adams and Victor 1981). Because of tolerance, chronic heavy drinkers may reach high blood levels (> 500 BAL) with fewer of these effects (Minion et al. 1989).

In addition to producing euphoria, alcohol leads to impaired motor performance, poor muscular control, slurred speech, flushed face, ataxia, slower thinking, and poor concentration, reasoning, attention, and ability to form word associations (Lishman 1978). Changes in heart rate, nystagmus, electromyographic activity, and EEG, and slowed reaction times occur (Cohen et al. 1983). Acute alcohol intoxication produces deficits in functions associated with the prefrontal and temporal lobes (Peterson et al. 1990). Tiihonen and colleagues (1994), using single-photon emission computed tomography (SPECT), found alcohol intoxication euphoria is associated with activation of the prefrontal cortex and medicated through the endogenous opioid system.

Alcohol activates GABA inhibitory systems, inhibits excitatory *N*-methyl-D-aspartate (NMDA) systems, potentiates serotonin function, stimulates opiate receptors, and indirectly increases dopamine turnover. Alcohol effects on second messenger systems and other intracellular

TABLE 11–13. **Alcohol-induced organic mental disorders**

Disorder	Onset	Treatment
Alcohol intoxication	Depends on tolerance of individual, amount ingested, amount absorbed over time period; pathological intoxication may be evident with small amounts	Time; protective environment; hemodialysis can be attempted in potentially fatal overdoses
Alcohol withdrawal	Several hours; peak symptoms 24–48 hours after last drink	See Table 11–17
Alcohol seizures	6–48 hours after cessation of alcohol	Diazepam, phenytoin; maintenance phenytoin activity; prevent seizures by chlordiazepoxide detoxification
Alcohol withdrawal delirium (DTs)	Gradual onset 2–3 days after cessation of alcohol; peak intensity at 4–5 days; may fluctuate over several weeks	Chlordiazepoxide detoxification; haloperidol 2–5 mg orally twice daily for psychotic symptomatology
Alcohol hallucinosis	Usually within 48 hours or less of last drink; may last several weeks	Haloperidol 2–5 mg twice daily for psychotic symptoms
Wernicke's encephalopathy	Abrupt onset; ataxia may precede mental confusion	Thiamine 100 mg intravenously with $MgSO_4$ 1–2 mL in 50% solution; should be given prior to glucose loading

functions have been implicated as mediating factors (Franklin and Frances 1992; Nestler et al. 1995). Chronic alcohol use produces neuronal adaptation in these systems and cessation after chronic use results in rebound activation. The glutamatergic hypothesis of alcoholism proposes that there is a range of neuropsychiatric disorders that are the result of the alcohol related dysfunction in NMDA receptors (Tsai et al. 1995).

Substance-Induced Amnestic Disorder (Wernicke-Korsakoff Syndrome)

The Wernicke-Korsakoff syndrome classically begins with abrupt-onset encephalopathy, with truncal ataxia, ophthalmoplegia, and mental confusion. Several authors (e.g., Brew 1986) have suggested that the diagnosis should not rely on the presence of all three criteria and that the presence of two of the three criteria is suggestive of limited forms of the disorder. The etiology of the syndrome involves thiamine deficiency due to dietary, genetic, or medical factors. Wernicke's encephalopathy may result in death or, more commonly, Korsakoff's psychosis, a chronic amnestic disorder. Approximately 80% of patients with Wernicke's encephalopathy who survive will develop Korsakoff's psychosis (Reuler et al. 1985). Korsakoff's psychosis is classically a severe anterograde amnesia in which memory is not transferred from short- to long-term memory storage. Structural deficits on postmortem examinations have been reported in the brain stem and the diencephalon regions of the brain (Victor et al. 1989).

Alcohol Withdrawal

Alcohol withdrawal symptoms relate to a relative drop in alcohol blood levels and therefore may occur during continuous alcohol consumption. Increased duration of drinking and binge patterns of alcohol ingestion are tied to an increase in withdrawal phenomena. A coarse, fast-frequency generalized tremor that is made worse by motor activity or stress is observed when the hand or the tongue is extended, with peak symptoms occurring 24–48 hours after the last drink and subsiding in 5–7 days, even without treatment, although irritability and insomnia may last 10 days or longer. Patients show signs of autonomic hyperactivity, including increased blood pressure, pulse rate greater than 100, sweating, malaise, nausea, vomiting, anxiety, tactile illusions or hallucinations, and disturbed sleep. These symptoms frequently lead to rapid return to drinking in order to reduce the withdrawal symptoms. Biological studies suggest altered hypothalamic-pituitary-adrenal axis activation and dysfunction during withdrawal (Adinoff et al. 1990, 1991), decreased regional brain metabolism as measured by positron emission tomography (PET) (Volkow et al. 1992), and persistent low metabolic levels in the basal ganglia of detoxified alcoholic individuals (Volkow et al. 1994).

Alcohol Withdrawal Seizures

Withdrawal seizures may occur 7–38 hours after last alcohol use in chronic drinkers, peaking at approximately

24 hours (Adams and Victor 1981). In some series, 10% of patients with chronic alcoholism have recurrent seizures, and a considerably higher number have had solitary seizures (Espir and Rose 1987). Alcohol intoxication may also precipitate seizures by lowering seizure threshold. Ng et al. (1988) concluded that alcohol, in a dose-related fashion, can independently induce seizures outside the normal withdrawal period. Hypomagnesemia, respiratory alkalosis, hypoglycemia, and increased intracellular sodium have been associated with alcohol seizures (Victor and Wolfe 1973).

Alcohol Withdrawal Delirium (Delirium Tremens)

One-third of patients with seizures go on to develop alcohol withdrawal delirium, or *delirium tremens* (DTs) characterized by confusion, disorientation, fluctuating or clouded consciousness, and perceptual disturbances, in addition to the usual withdrawal symptoms (Adams and Victor 1981). DTs is the prototypical hyperactive delirium. Typical signs and symptoms are delusions, vivid hallucinations, agitation, insomnia, mild fever, and marked autonomic arousal, which may appear suddenly but can develop 2–3 days after cessation of heavy drinking, with peak intensity on the fourth or fifth day. Patients frequently report visual hallucinations of insects, small animals, or other perceptual distortions, along with terror and agitation. Patients may show similar patterns of behavior each time they withdraw from alcohol (Turner et al. 1989). Although DTs may last as long as 4–5 weeks and can wax and wane, the majority of cases subside after 3 days of full-blown DTs and have a mortality rate that in recent years has decreased to less than 1% when treated (Gessner 1979). Cause of death in DTs is usually infections, fat emboli, and cardiac arrhythmias, which are usually associated with hyperkalemia, hyperpyrexia, and poor hydration. DTs occur more frequently and are most dangerous in those who have associated infection, subdural hematomas, trauma, poor nutrition, liver disease, or metabolic disorder.

Alcohol-Induced Psychotic Disorders (Alcohol Hallucinosis, Alcohol Paranoia)

Alcohol hallucinosis is associated with vivid auditory hallucinations lasting at least 1 week and occurring shortly after the cessation or reduction of heavy ingestion of alcohol. The hallucinosis can develop in a clear sensorium with a lower amount of autonomic symptoms than is typical in DTs. The hallucinations may include familiar noises or clear voices, which may be responded to with fear, anxiety, and agitation (Lishman 1978). The diagnosis is usually based on heavy alcohol use, lack of formal thought disorder, and lack of schizophrenia or mania in past or family history (see DSM-III-R [American Psychiatric Association 1987], pp. 131–132).

Alcohol paranoia is prominent paranoid delusions secondary to substance abuse. Alcohol hallucinosis and paranoia is subsumed under alcohol-induced psychotic disorder in DSM-IV.

TREATMENT OF ALCOHOL-INDUCED ORGANIC DISORDERS

Intoxication

Intoxication is managed supportively by decreasing external stimuli, interrupting alcohol ingestion, and protecting individuals from damaging themselves and others. In potentially fatal cases, hemodialysis has been attempted; otherwise, careful observation is all that is indicated. There is no proven amethystic agent despite several experimental approaches (Litten et al. 1996). Laboratory research is still focusing on pharmacologic agents effecting the GABAergic and glutamatergic systems. Flumazenil, a benzodiazepine antagonist, has been used in clinically settings to reverse coma in alcohol and benzodiazepine intoxication. General overdose elimination methods and management of overdose are presented in Tables 11–14 and 11–15, respectively. Biological markers for prediction for relapse have been reported (Gillin et al. 1994).

Withdrawal Syndrome

The choice of inpatient versus outpatient treatment depends on the severity of symptoms, the stage of withdrawal, medical and psychiatric complications, polydrug abuse, patient cooperation, the patient's ability to follow instructions, social support systems, and past history. In the era of managed care, criteria for inpatient admission has been largely limited severely to persons in considerable risk of medical complications. Level of care criteria, such as the American Society of Addiction Medicine (ASAM) criteria are being widely applied by clinical, managed care, and governmental agencies. In addition to risk for seizures or DTs other considerations for inpatient placement might include organic brain syndrome, low intelligence, Wernicke's encephalopathy, dehydration, history of head trauma, neurological symptoms, medical complications, DTs, alcoholic seizures, alcohol-induced psychosis, or psychopathology that requires rapid administration of psychotropic medications. Inpatient detoxifi-

TABLE 11–14. Overdose elimination methods

	Ipecac syrup	Forced diuresis	Gastric lavage	Activated charcoal	Hemodialysis	Hemoperfusion
Acetaminophen	Yes	Yes (alkaline)	Yes	No	No	No
Alcohol	No	No	Yes	Yes	Yes	No
Amphetamine	Yes	Yes (acid)	Yes	Yes	Yes	
Barbiturates		Only long		Yes		Yes
Benzodiazepines	Yes	No	Yes	Repeated		
Carbon monoxide	No	No	No	No	No	No
Cocaine	No	No	No	No	No	No
Hypnotics	Yes	No	Yes	Yes		
Hydrocarbons	Yes		Yes			
Opioids	(Treat with naloxone, 0.4–2 mg)					
Phencyclidine	Only severe	Not with rhabdomyolysis (may precipitate renal failure)	Only severe	Yes		
Phenothiazines	Yes		Yes	Yes		
Salicylates	Yes	Yes (alkaline)	Yes	Yes	Yes	
Tricyclics				Repeated	No	No

Source. Adapted with permission from Frances RJ, Franklin JE: *A Concise Guide to Treatment of Alcoholism and Addictions.* Washington, DC, American Psychiatric Press, 1989, p. 107. Copyright 1989, American Psychiatric Press.

cation is best done in a structured, supportive atmosphere that avoids overstimulation and provides frequent orientation and a nonjudgmental approach. Patient's vital signs and behavior should be carefully watched every 4 hours for symptoms of withdrawal or overdose. A good medical workup for alcohol withdrawal is essential (Table 11–16).

Nonpharmacological detoxification for mild to moderate withdrawal is usually uneventful (Naranjo et al. 1983). However, animal and clinical studies suggest that repeated, untreated alcohol withdrawal may promote "kindling" and hypercortisol states and may lead to severe withdrawal and cognitive damage (Booth and Blow 1993).

Nutritional deficiencies in B_{12}, thiamine, and folic acid can be corrected with multivitamins, oral thiamine (100 mg), folic acid (1 mg), plus adequate nutrition. Thiamine, 100–200 mg administered intramuscularly or intravenously, may be necessary in cases of very poor nutrition and should be given prior to any situation in which glucose loading is required, because glucose infusion can affect stores of thiamine. Patients with a past history of alcohol withdrawal seizures should be given magnesium sulfate, 1 g/2 mL (50%) four times a day intramuscularly, for 2 days. Usually, intravenous fluid replacement is not needed, and overhydration may occur. However, in cases in which sweating, fever, or vomiting has caused severe dehydration, careful rehydration and attention to electrolyte replacement should be effected with medical supervision.

Detoxification strives for adequate sedation of the patient and the substitution and gradual withdrawal of medications to prevent complications of withdrawal. A variety of agents have been used including alcohol, carbamazepine, clonidine, propranolol, paraldehyde, chloral hydrate, calcium antagonists, chlormethiazole, piracetam, lofexidine, benzodiazepines, calcium channel agents, and long-acting barbiturates. The β_2 agonists clonidine and carbamazepine may be useful adjuncts for symptomatic relief of alcohol withdrawal, however, they are limited in preventing severe complications such as DTs (Baumgartner and Rowen 1991; Hillbom et al. 1989; Malcolm et al. 1989; Stuppaeck et al. 1992; Worner 1994).

Benzodiazepines are preferred for withdrawal symptoms because of a relatively high therapeutic safety index, oral and intravenous routes of administration, anticonvulsant properties, and good prevention of DTs. Although patients with severe liver disease and elderly patients may be best detoxified with intermediate-acting benzodiazepines such as lorazepam (Ativan) or oxazepam (Serax), with their added advantage of renal versus liver

TABLE 11–15.   Management of overdose

	Major medical complication	Antidote	Potentially lethal dose
Acetaminophen	Liver toxicity (peak, 72–96 hours)	Acetylcysteine 140 mg/kg po followed by 70 mg/kg every 4 hours × 17 doses	140 mg/kg
Alcohol	Respiratory depression	None	350–700 mg/blood level
Amphetamine	Seizures	None	20–25 mg/kg
Barbiturates	Respiratory depression	None	
Short			Short > 3 g
Long			Long > 6 g
Benzodiazepines	Sedation		
Carbon monoxide	Oxygen in tissue, neuro-psychiatric sequelae	Hyperbaric oxygen	
Cocaine	Seizures, acidosis	None	
Hypnotics	Delirium, extrapyramidal side effects	None	May vary with tolerance
Hydrocarbons	Gastrointestinal, pulmonary, central nervous system side effects	None	
Opioids	Miosis, respiratory depression, decreased mental status	Naloxone 0.4–2 mg initially, up to 10 mg (half-life 60 minutes)	May vary with tolerance
Phencyclidine	Hypertension, nystagmus, rhabdomyolysis	None	
Phenothiazines	Anticholinergic, extrapyramidal cardiac side effects	None	150 mg/kg
Salicylates	Central nervous system side effects, acidosis	None	500 mg/kg
Tricyclics	Cardiac side effects, hypotension, anticholinergic side effects	None	35 mg/kg

Source.   Reprinted with permission from Frances RJ, Franklin JE: *A Concise Guide to Treatment of Alcoholism and Addictions.* Washington, DC, American Psychiatric Press, 1989, pp. 110–111. Copyright 1989, American Psychiatric Press.

excretion, there are no clear advantages to any one benzodiazepine. Diazepam (Valium) and chlordiazepoxide (Librium) are most commonly used. Because of its greater anticonvulsant effects, diazepam is used in cases in which there is a history of seizures or cross-addiction with other depressant drugs.

Saitz et al. (1994), in a double blind, randomized controlled trial, compared a fixed dose of chlordiazepoxide versus a symptom triggered prn regimen. The severity of withdrawal was measured by the Clinical Institute and Withdrawal Assessment for Alcohol, Revised (CIWA-AR; Sullivan 1991). Both groups were effective in preventing seizures and DTs. The mean duration of treatment (9 versus 68 hours) and dose (100 versus 425 mg) of the medication were lower in the symptom triggered group.

Loading of long-acting benzodiazepines and medication self taper has also been successfully employed for alco-hol withdrawal (Sellers 1983). Salloum et al. (1995) effectively used diazepam 20 mg doses every 2 hours with CIWA-AR scores above 15 points. Forty percent of patients required only a single 20-mg diazepam dose.

Outpatient detoxification with close follow-up, daily visits, and observation for complications is preferable for the majority of patients with mild withdrawal symptoms. In uncomplicated outpatient withdrawal, 25–50 mg of chlordiazepoxide to be taken orally four times a day should be prescribed on the first day, with a 20% decrease in dose over a 5-day period (see Table 11–17). Standard fixed dose inpatient detoxification is accomplished with chlordiazepoxide, 25–100 mg orally four times on first day, with 25–50 mg every 2 hours as needed, with nurses carefully watching for agitation, tremulousness, or change of vital signs. Doses should be held if the patient appears to be sleepy or intoxicated. The total 24-hour dose should be

TABLE 11-16. Medical workup for alcohol withdrawal

Medical history and complete physical examination

Routine laboratory tests

Complete blood count with differential
Serum electrolytes
Liver function tests (including bilirubin)
Blood urea nitrogen
Creatinine
Fasting blood sugar
Prothrombin time
Cholesterol
Triglycerides
Calcium
Magnesium
Albumin with total protein
Hepatitis B surface antigen
B_{12} and folic acid levels
Stool guiac
Urinalysis
Urine drug and alcohol screen
Chest X ray
Electrocardiogram

Ancillary tests

Electroencephalogram
Head computed tomography
Gastrointestinal series

tapered over 3–5 days in equally divided dosages per day. Patients who have had a history of epilepsy may require additional anticonvulsant medication such as phenytoin; however, in uncomplicated withdrawal seizures, adding anticonvulsants to benzodiazepines may not be needed. Diazepam, 10 mg intravenously, usually aborts status epilepticus; however, loading with phenytoin may be necessary.

Alcohol-Induced Psychotic Disorder (Alcohol Hallucinosis)

Appropriate withdrawal treatment should be given to any patient with alcohol hallucinosis. A potent antipsychotic such as haloperidol (Haldol), 2–5 mg orally or intravenously twice a day, may be needed for patients with extreme agitation and hallucinations. Medications should be reassessed shortly after cessation of symptoms and need not be continued.

Alcohol-Induced Amnestic Disorder (Wernicke's Encephalopathy and Korsakoff's Psychosis)

Treatment of Wernicke's encephalopathy with parenteral thiamine, 100 mg with titration upward until ophthal-moplegia has been resolved, may prevent dangerous progression of the illness. Magnesium sulfate should also be administered. Thiamine should be given prior to any glucose loading. Ophthalmoplegia usually responds fairly quickly, but truncal ataxia may persist. Abstinence is the primary treatment for Korsakoff's psychosis. Pharmacological approaches—including the use of clonidine to improve recent memory recall, and propranolol to control rage attacks—have been tried but are not especially effective. More recently, fluvoxamine has shown some promise in reducing memory deficits, a reduction that is hypothesized to occur through the serotonergic effects of this agent (Martin et al. 1989).

Alcohol-Induced Delirium

Sedation with benzodiazepines and treatment with neuroleptics are the standard pharmacological treatment of DTs. Diazepam, lorazepam, and midazolam all have certain advantages and disadvantages for use in DTs. Lorazepam tends to result in less oversedation; midazolam, a short-acting benzodiazepine, can be useful as a continuous drip; and diazepam has rapid onset and smooth self-taper. Massive doses of diazepam, as high as 2,640 mg, have been reported to have been administered to patients with DTs; this high dosage may represent cellular resistance. Droperidol and propofol (an ultra short-acting alkylphenol) and in extreme cases paralysis and mechanical ventilation are other approaches.

Summary

In general, organicity needs to be taken into account in treatment planning and may make educational programs

TABLE 11-17. Standard treatment regimen for alcohol withdrawal

Outpatient

Chlordiazepoxide 25–50 mg orally, four times on first day; 20% decrease in dose over a 5-day period

Daily visits to assess symptoms

Inpatient

Chlordiazepoxide 25–100 mg orally four times on first day; 20% decrease in dose over 5–7 days

Chlordiazepoxide 25–100 mg orally every 6 hours in addition to standing dose as needed for agitation, tremors, or change in vital signs

Thiamine 100 mg orally four times daily

Folic acid 1 mg orally four times daily

Multivitamin one per day

Magnesium sulfate 1 g intramuscularly every 6 hours for 2 days (if status postwithdrawal seizures)

in inpatient rehabilitation treatment more difficult. Interaction between alcohol-related organic brain syndromes and psychiatric, neurological, and medical conditions increases the complexity of differential diagnosis and affects treatment planning.

REHABILITATION AND TREATMENT OF ALCOHOLISM

Once the diagnosis and treatment of intoxication and withdrawal syndromes have been accomplished, the greater challenge is tailoring the right longer term treatment or the right combination of treatments to meet each patient's needs.

Brief physician interventions such as motivational therapy, advice, and physician warnings are proving to be effective especially in early cases of alcoholism (Babor and Grant 1992; Walsh et al. 1992). Case management and network therapy may be more useful for indigent patients (Galanter 1993). Careful psychiatric diagnosis and sorting of primary and secondary conditions are of crucial importance. Differential therapeutics for the two-thirds of patients with alcoholism who have additional psychiatric diagnoses such as depression, anxiety disorders, and ADHD used a wide range of advances in the field of alcoholism. Patients with both primary and secondary affective illness have an increased suicide rate, and recognition and appropriate treatment of the depression are important, even if no medication is indicated with secondary depression.

Indications for inpatient treatment are described above in the subsection on treatment of the withdrawal syndrome. Most alcohol inpatient treatment services in the United States have emphasized a combination of psychoeducation, 12-step programs, disulfiram, naltrexone, and individual, group, and family counseling for 1–2 weeks to 1 month, modeled after Hazelton and the Naval Alcohol Treatment Centers (see Table 11–18). Some centers also emphasize psychiatric treatment with evaluation and with appropriate use of other modalities such as psychotherapy and pharmacotherapy, especially for the dual-diagnosis patient. Disulfiram is thought by many therapists to be an important adjunct to treating patients with alcoholism, and early studies report favorable results. The patient has only to make the decision about not drinking once per day when taking medication and to provide time to deal with situations that increase the impulse to drink; he or she also is cautioned to avoid any substance that may have alcohol in it in order to prevent a disulfiram-alcohol reaction. Family members, including the spouse, can be enlisted to help monitor the taking of medication. A well-designed study (Fuller et al. 1986) found that the disulfiram group

reported fewer drinking days than did a control group, but the two groups had no significant difference in total abstinence. Although disulfiram is not recommended to be used routinely, it can be useful in selected highly motivated individuals.

The search for pharmacological treatments for alcoholism continues, and some promising drugs include naltrexone, acamprosate, selective serotonin reuptake inhibitors (SSRIs), 5-HT antagonists, and buspirone. Opiate dysregulation in animal and human studies has been implicated in the preference for alcohol intake and craving. In a seminal human study in VA patients, Volpicelli et al. (1992) found naltrexone, a opiate antagonist, reduced relapse in alcoholic patients. The study was a 12-week trial of 50 mg of naltrexone in intensive outpatient treatment. The naltrexone decreased drinking days 0.57 days per week with 54% abstinence to 0.11 days per week and 31% abstinence. Mediating factors may involve decrease in subjective intoxication, decrease relapse with slips, and decreased craving (O'Malley et al. 1996a). O'Malley et al. (1996a) also found that rates of continuous abstinence were higher when naltrexone was combined with supportive therapy versus coping skills therapy. In subjects who "slipped," coping skills appeared superior. After 6 month follow-up of not taking naltrexone, initial benefits waned, suggesting that continued treatment with naltrexone may be warranted (O'Malley et al. 1996b). In addition, compliance with naltrexone and completing psychosocial treatment appear to be crucial variables to the clinical effectiveness of the opiate antagonists (Volpicelli et al. 1997). Studies to attempt to increase compliance are warranted. Naltrexone appears relatively safe, with no significant effects on liver function tests. Nausea and headache appear to be the most

TABLE 11–18. Inpatient treatment rehabilitation modalities for psychoactive substance use disorders

- Diagnostic evaluation
- Drug-free periods
- Medication trials
- Team approach
- Group therapy
- Psychoeducation
- Family evaluation and treatment
- 12-step programs (e.g., Alcoholics Anonymous, Narcotics Anonymous)
- Individual counseling
- Activity therapy
- Urine testing—abstinence orientation
- Discharge planning
- Follow-up treatment

common side effects (Croop et al. 1997).

Several early studies have suggested that selective serotonin reuptake inhibitors may be effective in alcoholism (Naranjo et al. 1990, 1992). Kranzler et al. (1995) and Kabel and Petty (1996) reported they found no benefit of fluoxetine in alcoholics who did not suffer from depression. Kranzler et al. (1995) have also suggested negative effects of fluoxetine in type B alcoholics. Alcoholics with comorbid alcohol dependence and major depression may prove to show both improvement with alcohol consumption and depression with SSRI therapy (Cornelius et al. 1997).

Acamprosate (calcium acetylhomotaurinate), an analogue of GABA, is actively being investigated as a treatment of alcohol dependence and has shown promising results (Paille et al. 1995; Sass et al. 1996). Carbamazepine and dopaminergic agents such as tiapride are also showing promise in preliminary human trials (Mueller et al. 1997; Shaw et al. 1994). Several other novel approaches are being explored in animals (Litten et al. 1996).

Buspirone treatment of anxious alcoholics has shown to decrease alcohol consumption and treating depression secondary to alcoholism with antidepressants may be beneficial for the depression and alcohol use (Kranzler et al. 1994; Malec et al. 1996a; Mason et al. 1996; McGrath et al. 1996).

The team approach and biopsychosocial model lead to a sophisticated understanding of the physiological, hereditary, congenital, developmental, psychological, familial, social, and cultural contributions to the etiology and manifestations of alcoholism. Assessment of ego functions includes object relations, impulse control, reality testing, and defenses. A central feature of dynamically oriented treatment is an awareness of the therapist-patient relationship. When patients are identically treated regardless of diagnosis or special problems, many treatment "failures" may end up being attributed simply to "lack of motivation." A consensus has developed among experienced therapists that abstinence be required during treatment, for both diagnostic and therapeutic reasons (Frances and Alexopoulos 1982a).

Chemical aversive conditioning with emetine has been used in several hospital chains and is used widely in the Soviet Union. Administration of an aversive chemical to induce vomiting and discomfort is paired with the smell and taste of alcohol, leading to extinction of alcohol-seeking behavior. Although treatment effectiveness for chemical aversive conditioning has been found in several studies to be equal to that of other modalities of treatment, its relatively greater risks, including cardiac toxicity and possible Mallory-Weiss syndrome, compared with other treatments, limit its usefulness and warrant trials with other forms of treatment first. At present, emetine is not approved by the U.S. Food and Drug Administration (FDA) for chemical aversive conditioning.

Evaluation and treatment of the families of patients with alcoholism are essential. A family system that has been altered to accommodate the patient's drinking may also reinforce it. Frequently it is a family crisis that brings the patient to treatment, and including the family in treatment planning increases the chances that the patient will engage in treatment. An emphasis on group and self-help aspects of treatment aids in a patient's resocialization and practicing of object relatedness, impulse control, and acceptance of an identity as a recovering person. Setting limits and providing structure serve as auxiliary superego supports until the patient is able to be his or her own social director and policeman.

As the patient comes closer to meeting ego ideals associated with sober living, he or she gains pleasure from being able to function again, with a concomitant return of self-esteem. Primitive defenses such as denial, splitting, projection, and projective identification are likely to be more prominent in the initial stages of treatment and may be similar to those frequently seen in depressed and borderline patients. Object-relations regression is seen in selfish use of others as part objects or need-satisfying objects. Frequently, patients with alcoholism have suffered major recent losses and have unresolved problems in individuation and separation from parents. Reality testing and sense of reality may be affected, and temporary psychotic phenomena that are substance related may occur.

Individual supportive or dynamically oriented therapy may be especially needed in patients who through embarrassment or need for privacy refuse to accept Alcoholics Anonymous (AA), group, or family treatment. Adolescents and young adults sorting out identity issues, problems in individuation, and needs for independence may also especially benefit from individual therapy. Candidates especially suitable for dynamic therapy include those with a capacity for honesty, insight, intimacy, and identification with the therapist; average or superior intelligence; and the time, money, and motivation needed to change not just the drinking but other aspects of conflict that lead to distress in the person's life. Relative counterindications to outpatient therapy are when a patient will not accept abstinence as a precondition for treatment and when a period of hospitalization or crisis work is needed to prepare the patient for treatment.

The initial focus of treatment is on conflicts about acceptance of the diagnosis of dependency, the need for help, and the loss of loved ones and friends, jobs, health, and even alcohol. Gradually confronting other problems in self-care, self-esteem, assertiveness, the handling of aggression, and alcohol's role in allowing or distancing oneself from sexual life and issues around control may become important. Support is usually needed at first, with gradual increase in clarification, confrontation, and interpretation of denial, lying, splitting, and projective defenses. Helping patients express their feelings openly and appropriately in a sober state is a major goal of treatment.

Patients may enter treatment as a result of coercion by family, employer, physician, or probation officer. A thorough understanding of alcoholism and an empathic approach to the patient's resistances help the therapist form a working alliance with the patient who is initially hostile. Other positive therapist characteristics are listed in Table 11–19. Confrontation of lying and denial is important and may be aided by family meetings and the use of laboratory aids. Because alcoholism is a chronic, relapsing illness, a nonjudgmental approach aids in patients' willingness to talk openly about "slips."

Countertransference problems on the part of therapists most frequently occur either in response to patients' transferences of rebelliousness, dishonesty, or aggression; therapists' lack of knowledge about alcoholism or its treatment; or problems that the therapists have had with alcohol either themselves or in their close relationships. Many therapists are attracted to the psychoactive substance abuse field because they are either recovering from the problem themselves or have had experience with a relative who has had a problem. For this group there is a special danger of an unconscious collusion between patient and therapist to avoid certain unconscious issues that may be painful to both of them. Silber (1974) has emphasized beginning therapists' problems in dealing with their own fear of alcohol.

TABLE 11–19. Attributes of therapists that facilitate substance use disorder treatment

- Caring relationship
- Informed optimism
- Capacity to tolerate anxiety, depression
- Flexibility
- Knowledge of addictions
- Intellectual curiosity
- Wisdom
- Persistence and patience
- Capacity to listen
- Honesty and integrity

Source. Reprinted with permission from Frances RJ, Franklin JE: *A Concise Guide to Treatment of Alcoholism and Addictions.* Washington, DC, American Psychiatric Press, 1989, p. 2. Copyright 1989, American Psychiatric Press.

holic patients' aggression, which when understood leads to an improved therapeutic alliance.

Alcoholics Anonymous is a worldwide self-help group of recovering alcoholic individuals started in 1936 by Bill Wilson. Meetings provide members with acceptance, understanding, forgiveness, confrontation, and a means for positive identification. In a program of 12 steps, new members are asked to admit to a problem, give up a sense of personal control over the disease, do a personal assessment, make amends, and help others. Telephone numbers are exchanged, and new members pick "sponsors" (i.e., more experienced members who guide them through the process). Though not tied to any religion, AA also allows for spiritual reevaluation. Members continue their involvement with AA, frequently for many years, to maintain sobriety. Regular AA attendance is associated with favorable outcome (Vaillant 1984).

Professional treatment programs can work very well in concert with self-help groups. A study of employed alcoholic individuals found that treatment plus AA was more effective than AA alone in helping employed alcohol-abusing persons to attain and continue abstinence (Walsh et al. 1991). Other 12-step programs, such as Overeaters Anonymous, Gamblers Anonymous, and Narcotics Anonymous, are modeled on the AA program.

Although attention has been devoted to children of alcoholics (COA) and adult children of alcoholics (ACOA), there has been relatively little scientific study of the experience of having an alcoholic parent who is frequently inconsistent and emotionally depriving. The nonalcoholic parent is also affected by alcoholism and may have had difficulty protecting the child from neglect or sexual and aggressive abuse by the alcoholic parent. These children often feel forced into parental roles with respect to the alcohol-dependent parent and have special problems with sexual identity, loss, abandonment, and neglect. Parental inconsistency leads to a distrust of authority figures and a greater tendency to depend on peers or on psychoactive substances. Siblings have to care for each other and tend to pick friends who come from similarly troubled families. The COA peer group grows up protesting their parents' behavior but developing the same problems. The lack of trust is brought into the treatment situation and is experienced with teachers, nurses, and other professionals who represent authority figures. Interpretation of this resistance may help in forming a therapeutic alliance. Self-help groups, group therapy, and family approaches are especially useful alone or in conjunction with individual therapy in part because the ACOA participant can turn to peer support, this time with friends and family working at obtaining sobriety together. Discussing these issues at a peer level first may lead to being able to deal with authority issues better later in individual therapy.

The treatment of the patient with alcoholism and psychiatric disorders has been made difficult by the lack of integrated psychiatric and substance abuse approaches in many facilities. Many psychiatric inpatient units, psychiatric halfway houses, outpatient clinics, and other support systems in the community are often unable or unwilling to treat psychiatric patients with an alcohol problem. Patients with alcoholism and additional psychiatric problems are unlikely to get these attended to in free-standing alcohol and drug rehabilitation facilities that are generally not equipped to deal with psychopathology. In these facilities, there is often minimal contact with a psychiatric consultant and relatively greater input by alcoholism counselors who rarely have had psychiatric training.

In patients with dual problems, if the need for medication is not well explained and accepted, the abstinence emphasis of alcohol programs can work antithetically to prescribed psychotropic medication compliance. Many alcohol halfway houses will not accept patients on any medication. Confrontational methods found in some self-help groups may be detrimental to some psychologically ill patients. Facilities that treat dual-diagnosis patients with combined psychiatric treatment and substance disorder rehabilitation are expensive and have yet to demonstrate that tailoring treatment to the patient is cost-effective; however, at present, they provide state-of-the-art treatment in the field.

TREATMENT OUTCOME

Any discussion of treatment outcome must address the methodology of how and what is being measured. There is a large body of research evidence that treatment for alcohol and substance abuse can be effective (Crits-Christoph and Siqueland 1996). Vaillant has recently reported data from his four-decade natural history of alcoholism study, that after 5 years of sobriety relapse is rare (Vaillant 1996). Treatment outcome studies in alcoholism indicate that a variety of treatment programs yield benefit and may be cost-effective; however, few studies exist that differentiate which treatments are best for which kinds of patients. In one large multicenter study initiated by NIAAA, Project Match Research Group (1997), 12-step facilitation, cognitive-behavioral, and motivational therapy were matched to certain types of patient characteristics. Only 1 match out of 10 (12 step better than cognitive-behavioral with minimal psychiatric comorbidity), improved outcome. Others, such as McLellan et al. (1997), have found improved outcome by tailoring treatment to individuals'

needs. In one well-designed outcome study, Woody et al. (1984) treated patients who had an additional psychiatric diagnosis along with a psychoactive substance use disorder(s) and found improved outcome of these poor-prognosis patients. The outcome literature continues to reflect that patient factors such as a stable family, stable job, less sociopathy, less psychopathology, and a negative family history for alcoholism are more powerful predictors of positive prognosis than is the type of treatment used. Studies that test various treatment alternatives that are well controlled, well designed, implemented by good clinicians, or manual driven with good follow-up, are expensive and difficult to do (Kranzler et al. 1996a).

SEDATIVE, HYPNOTIC, OR ANXIOLYTIC ABUSE AND DEPENDENCE

Benzodiazepines and barbiturates are useful medications with potential for abuse and dependence. In the early 1980s, 15% of the United States population used a benzodiazepine during a 1-year period. The ratios of female-to-male use and white-to-black use are approximately 3:1 (Gottschalk et al. 1979). Only a minority (16%) of users abuse sedatives (Rickels et al. 1983). Alprazolam abuse is more prevalent among women with family histories of alcoholism (Ciraulo et al. 1996). Abuse may be iatrogenically caused or intentional. Emergency visits secondary to barbiturate overdoses have decreased because of the waning popularity of barbiturate use. Benzodiazepines have a higher index of therapeutic safety and produce less respiratory depression than barbiturates. However, they potentiate the CNS depression and euphoria of other sedatives and opioids. Physicians prescribing these medications should be skilled in their prudent use and be aware of individuals susceptible to abuse.

DEFINITION

Diagnosis of sedative abuse may be difficult. Such abuse may start in the context of treatment for anxiety, medical disorders, or insomnia. Individuals prone to polysubstance abuse may use sedatives for their calming effects or for their ability to potentiate euphoric effects of other drug classes such as opioids, or to self-medicate overwhelming affects including anxiety. DSM-IV definitions of sedative, hypnotic, or anxiolytic abuse and dependence are presented in Tables 11–1, 11–2, and 11–3. Physical dependence can develop to low-dose use (10–40 mg per day) over several years or high-dose use over weeks to months (Dietch 1983). Individuals may develop tolerance to extremely high doses (up to 1,000 to 1,500 mg per day) of diazepam. Tolerance to sedative-hypnotic effects can develop in 2–3 weeks; however, antianxiety effects may persist. Intoxication, withdrawal, withdrawal delirium, and amnestic disorder symptoms are similar to those found with alcohol. Benzodiazepines, however, have a much longer half-life. Diazepam withdrawal may not be evident until 7–10 days after cessation of use. In high-dose withdrawal, seizures may be the first heralding sign and are a prominent component of unexpected or poorly managed benzodiazepine withdrawal. Severe withdrawal may produce anxiety, psychosis, and possibly death from cardiovascular collapse.

CLINICAL FEATURES

Benzodiazepines are useful short-term adjuncts in therapy for insomnia, medical disorders such as postmyocardial infarction, and anxiety in selected cases (O'Brien and Woody 1986). Indiscriminate use of benzodiazepines prescribed by physicians may contribute to abuse. A patient may become tolerant to considerable benzodiazepine dosages without showing behavioral pathology. In individuals with generalized anxiety, panic attacks, agitated depression, or personality disorders, in whom affect regulation is impaired, benzodiazepines may serve as self-medication, and alarmingly high doses of benzodiazepines may be used. These individuals may be prone to behavioral disinhibition, especially when alcohol, opioid, or cocaine abuse is also present. Social and legal consequences of abuse may present similarly to those of alcohol, opioid, and cocaine abuse. In a study of long-term benzodiazepine use with a mean daily use of 14.1 mg of diazepam equivalents, subjects had significant residual symptoms of anxiety and depression (Rickels et al. 1990). Patients are often exposed to the risks of long-term use without significant benefits. Long half-life benzodiazepines have been associated with motor vehicle accidents and hip fractures in the elderly (Cummings et al. 1995; Hemmelgarn et al. 1997).

ADVERSE EFFECTS

Chronic sedative abuse may lead to neuropsychological impairment (Bergman et al. 1980). Deficits in memory (verbal and nonverbal), concentration, motor coordination, and speed have been described (O'Brien and Woody 1986). Overdose secondary to brain-stem depression is possible with little warning when benzodiazepines are used at extremely high dosages because of a patient's high tolerance to sedation. Enlargement of CSF spaces in long-term abuse of benzodiazepines has been described (Schmauss and Krieg 1987).

It may be difficult to distinguish withdrawal symptoms and side effects from presumed underlying anxiety symptoms, and prognosis for benzodiazepine abuse is guarded. The primary sedative-hypnotic–abusing patient should be viewed with a high suspicion of underlying psychiatric symptoms. Baseline personality traits such as dependency, neuroticism, depression, and anxiety have been associated with higher daily use (Rickels et al. 1990). Eighty-four percent of primary sedative-hypnotic–abusing patients 4–6 years after hospital discharge had resumed use of sedative-hypnotics; physical signs of alcoholism had developed in 22%, and 8% committed suicide (Allgulander et al. 1984). In a longer term follow-up of subjects with primary sedative-hypnotic dependence, 46% continued to abuse drugs (Allgulander et al. 1987). Alcohol and opioid CNS depression may interact with sedative-hypnotics with potentiation of depressive actions. Thus, additional small amounts of alcohol or opioids may precipitate overdose. Complex perceptual and motor tasks, such as driving, may be negatively affected because of acute neuropsychological impairment. Prescription-induced sedativism may become a lead-in to alcoholism, especially in women.

TREATMENT

The treatment of sedative, hypnotic, and anxiolytic withdrawal is similar to that of withdrawal from alcohol. A cross-tolerant sedative is given to prevent withdrawal symptoms and is gradually decreased. Long-acting barbiturates or benzodiazepines are preferred. Clonazepam (Klonopin) has an extremely long half-life and has shown some promise in alprazolam (Xanax) withdrawal, which has proven to be a benzodiazepine that is particularly difficult to taper after long-term use or high-dose abuse. For inpatient detoxification of high-dose benzodiazepine–abusing patients, a benzodiazepine or pentobarbital challenge test may help determine starting dose of medication, usually diazepam, 15–25 mg four times daily (see Tables 11–20 and 11–21). The most important factor in keeping complications to a minimum is to decrease dose by approximately 10% per day, with the terminal 10% dosage tapered slowly to zero over a 3- to 4-day period. Orders for as-needed dosages should be available for vital sign or marked subjective changes.

Generally, detoxification can be accomplished in a 10- to 14-day period, but longer detoxification may be required in certain individuals. For outpatient detoxification, a taper (25% a week) is generally well tolerated; however, more discomfort may be evident at the end of the taper. Factors such as neuroticism, female sex, and history of alcohol abuse may contribute to a patient's difficulty with

TABLE 11–20. Benzodiazepine detoxification

1. Estimate usual maintenance dose by history or pentobarbital challenge test (see Table 11–21).
2. Divide maintenance dose into equivalent as-needed dose of diazepam and administer first 2 days.
3. Decrease diazepam 10% per day.
4. Administer diazepam 5 mg orally every 6 hours in addition to as needed for signs of increased withdrawal (increased pulse, increase in blood pressure, diaphoresis).
5. When the diazepam dose approaches 10%, reduce dose slowly over 3–4 days and discontinue.

TABLE 11–21. Pentobarbital challenge test: clinical responses to 200-mg test dose of pentobarbital

Patient's condition after test dose	Degree of tolerance	Estimated 24-hour pentobarbital requirement
Asleep, but arousal	None or minimal	None
Drowsy; slurred speech; ataxia; marked intoxication	Definite but mild	400–600 mg
Comfortable; fine lateral nystagmus is only sign of intoxication	Marked	600–1,000 mg
No signs of drug effect; abstinence signs may persist	Extreme	1,000–1,200 mg or more

withdrawal (Schweizer et al. 1990). Because of potential medical complications of detoxification, especially with high-dose abuse, initial inpatient treatment is preferred. Detoxification with shorter-acting benzodiazepines such as oxazepam or lorazepam is indicated in patients with liver or pulmonary disease. Carbamazepine has also recently been reported to be useful in discontinuing long-term benzodiazepine therapy (Schweizer et al. 1991).

A major aspect of primary prevention is prevention of habituation to prescription drugs. Although a minority of patients under medical care abuse benzodiazepines, certain precautions may further minimize such abuse. Paternal alcoholism in a recent study was a risk factor for benzodiazepine abuse, thus indicating a possible higher potential for abuse for sons of alcoholic fathers (Ciraulo et al. 1989).

Generally, benzodiazepines should be targeted to specific symptoms or avoided in addicted or alcoholic individuals and used only for short periods of time. When indicated for dual-diagnosis patients with anxiety disorders and after other behavioral and pharmacological treatments have failed, use of benzodiazepines can be tried with patients who are abstinent and are not escalating doses and with close monitoring of the patient and family (Dupont and Saylor 1991). Excuses of lost prescriptions, requests for dosage increase, or suspicion of doctor shopping are tip-offs of possible abuse. Rehabilitation treatment strategies generally proceed in a fashion similar to those for other substance abuse. Because of the potential medical complications of detoxification, especially when abuse has been at high doses, initial inpatient treatment is preferred.

ILLICIT DRUG USE

Major federal commitment to research and treatment in opioid abuse in the early 1970s gave way to a period of relative public inattention even though the number of addicted individuals remained fairly stable. In 1987, a renewal of significant federal funding for drug abuse resulted from public concern about an epidemic of cocaine addiction and the spread of AIDS in addicted persons, and significant White House interest. Public awareness of the harmful effects of drugs led to a drop of drug use between 1985 and 1988, however the report of an increase in past month illicit drug use among African Americans between 1988 and 1991 was alarming. The National Household Survey on Drug Abuse (SAMSA 1995) showed past month use of any illicit drug is highest for whites between the ages of 12 and 25 and highest for African Americans above the age of 26. There were an estimated 476,000 hard-core drug users. Apparent differences in racial groups may be more a factor of economic deprivation, racism, and availability of drugs than issues intrinsic to race (Lillie-Banton 1993).

Polysubstance abuse has increased, with combined use of heroin, cocaine, and methadone, and the frequent addition of alcohol and tobacco. "Speedballing" with heroin and cocaine is one of the most frequent ways to take the edge off of a cocaine high. Although cocaine deaths have captured more headlines, deaths related to heroin and ethanol, taken separately or in combination, are far more frequent. Purer forms of heroin have been surfacing on the streets of many Northeastern cities. These purer forms can be snorted. This alternative route of administration, which is attractive to some addicts who fear HIV contraction, has contributed to heroin's surge in popularity. A subset of heroin-abusing individuals has been described among working middle- and upper-class individuals. In addition, synthetic opiates such as fentanyl have been abused among high-access individuals such as nurses and physicians.

OPIOID DEPENDENCE

Consistent with that of other psychoactive substance dependence, the definition of diagnosis of opioid dependency in DSM-IV includes psychosocial factors, and the concept of abuse has been made more specific (see Tables 11–1, 11–2, 11–3, and 11–4 presented earlier in this chapter). Frequently tolerance and withdrawal are present with dependence.

EPIDEMIOLOGY

There were approximately 492,000 opioid-addicted individuals in the United States in 1980 (National Institute on Drug Abuse 1981). Recidivism rates as high as 90% contribute to this number's stability in the 1990s. Estimates of opioid use come from overdose reports, surveys, prevalence of medical complications, arrests, and admissions into treatment programs. The majority of opioid-dependent individuals are not in treatment, and recent attempts have been made to characterize this group. Smart and Murray's (1985) survey of 152 countries does not support the contention that technologically developed societies are more prone to narcotic drug abuse. Availability of opioids is an important factor in the incidence.

Heroin abuse occurs more frequently in males than in females (3:1) in urban areas, and it is more common among the 18- to 25-year-old age group. In the United States overall, nonmedical use of opioids other than heroin is more frequent among whites (12% versus 7% for African Americans and other minority groups). Some databases suggest that minority groups have twice the prevalence of individuals abusing heroin as is found in the general population. These figures may be skewed, however, because they are based on admissions to public treatment facilities and may exclude substantial numbers of white middle-class addicted individuals who are less likely to be admitted to those facilities. Hanson (1985) suggested that further studies should focus on improvement of minority employment and vocational status, which are significant predictors of treatment outcome. Racial consciousness, church involvement, and drug intolerance have been reported to be factors preventive of opioid abuse. Puerto Rican opioid-addicted men more frequently are unemployed and have higher prevalence of depression and anxiety (Kosten et al. 1985b). Although opioid use is overrepresented in minority groups, recently heroin use has increased in affluent populations. When heroin abuse is less endemic to a cultural group, greater psychopathology may be found in those who use the drug (Kosten et al. 1985b).

CLINICAL FEATURES

Intravenous heroin intoxication produces a subjective euphoric "rush" that can be highly reinforcing. Tolerance to this high develops with repeated use over time. Physical signs of intoxication include pupillary constriction, decreased gastrointestinal motility, marked sedation, slurred speech, and impairment in attention or memory. There is a clear association between heroin use and crime. Daily use of opioids over days to weeks, depending on dose and potency of the drug, will produce opioid withdrawal symptoms upon cessation of use. Rather intense but generally non–life-threatening withdrawal syndromes start approximately 10 hours after the last dose of short-acting opioids such as morphine and heroin. The onset of opioid withdrawal depends on the half-life of the opioid and the chronicity of use.

Mild opioid withdrawal presents a flulike syndrome with symptoms of anxiety, dysphoria, yawning, sweating, rhinorrhea, lacrimation, pupillary dilation, piloerection, mild hypertension, tachycardia, and disrupted sleep. Severe symptoms include hot and cold flashes, deep muscle and joint pain, nausea, vomiting, diarrhea, abdominal pain, weight loss, fever, and waves of gooseflesh. Kosten et al. (1985a) have found that self-reports of severity of withdrawal symptoms in treatment settings are as important as observer ratings and that inadequate coverage of withdrawal symptoms can be associated with treatment failure. Subacute, protracted withdrawal symptoms may extend for several weeks.

ADVERSE PHYSICAL EFFECTS

Contaminated needles and impure drugs can lead to endocarditis, septicemia, pulmonary emboli, and pulmonary hypertension. Contaminants can cause skin infections, hepatitis, and HIV spread. Intravenous drug abuse, needle sharing, and sexual contact are significant vectors for the spread of HIV. Twenty-five percent of AIDS cases involve persons who abuse intravenous drugs. Some Northeast cities report HIV positivity of 60%–65% among persons who abuse intravenous drugs. Death rates in young addicted individuals are increased 20-fold by infection, homicide, suicide, overdose, and AIDS. Opioid overdose should be suspected in any undiagnosed coma patient, especially when accompanied by respiratory depression, pupillary constriction, or the presence of needle marks. In any suspected opioid overdose, naloxone (Narcan), 0.4 mg, should be given immediately and may need to be repeated, and it may be lifesaving.

A syndrome of narcotic abstinence is reported in 68%–94% of neonates of mothers addicted to narcotics. Methadone doses above 20 mg per day in the mother are associated with moderate to severe withdrawal (Ostrea et al. 1991). Total detoxification of pregnant women on methadone is not recommended (Harris-Allen 1991). Stimmel et al. (1982–1983) found outcome of withdrawal in infants to be improved in women supervised in methadone maintenance programs. Although the baby may appear normal at or shortly after birth, symptoms may appear 12–24 hours later, depending on the half-life of the opioid, and may persist for several months. The full-blown syndrome can include hyperactivity, tremors, seizures, hyperactive reflexes, gastrointestinal dysfunction, respiratory dysfunction, and vague autonomic symptoms such as yawning, sneezing, sweating, nasal congestion, increased lacrimation, and fever. Total perinatal mortality has been reported to be as high as 10.7%, with 4% stillbirths and 6.7% neonatal deaths. Long-term residual features include infants appearing anxious, hard to please, hyperactive, and emotionally labile. Camphorated tincture of opium (paregoric) is the oldest treatment, but no specific dosage is cited in the literature. There have also been reports of babies of intravenous opioid-addicted individuals born HIV-positive and having congenital features similar to those of fetal alcohol syndrome.

ETIOLOGY

Pathophysiology

Basic research advances in the identification of distinct subtypes of opioid receptors have provided increased understanding of the mechanism of endogenous opioid neuroregulation and physiology. Cellular mechanisms of opioid neuroadaptation are being explored in relation to characteristics of opioid receptors and intracellular modulators of opioid action. Multiple subtypes of opioid receptors, designated μ, δ, κ, σ, and ϵ, have been described (Redmond and Krystal 1984). Neuroadaptive changes at receptor sites have been hypothesized to produce tolerance and dependence. The μ receptor is the classic morphine receptor and has selective affinity for heroin, meperidine, hydromorphone (Dilaudid), and methadone. It is highly sensitive to naloxone (an opioid antagonist) and mediates analgesia, euphoria, sedation, meiosis, hypothermia, bradycardia, respiratory depression, and increases in release of prolactin and growth hormone. δ receptors are

more sensitive to endogenous enkephalins. κ-sensitive opioids such as pentazocine (Talwin) and butorphanol (Stadol) produce analgesia but reduced respiratory depression and no euphoria at this receptor; however, Talwin is clinically euphoric and may act at other receptor sites. Mild classic withdrawal symptoms may result after cessation of chronic use. However, dependence on nasal spray butorphanol is being reported.

Certain individuals may be more prone to opioid addiction because of a hypothesized lack of endogenous opioid peptide homeostasis. Other models have linked opioid tolerance and dependence to a disruption of balance between endogenous opioids and contraopioid ligands such as adrenocorticotropic hormone (ACTH). ACTH may interact with endogenous endorphins in a mutually antagonistic manner (Hendrie 1985).

Neuroadaptation leads to tolerance of opioid effects, especially respiratory depression. Removal of opioid drug from receptors produces rebound withdrawal symptoms. Neuroadaptation appears to be a result of intracellular modulations that may affect the numbers or conformation of opioid receptors. Redmond and Krystal (1984) have reviewed the effects of opioids on intracellular systems of cyclic adenosine 3′,5′-monophosphate (cyclic AMP), acetylcholine, GABA, serotonin, dopamine, and norepinephrine. Kosten (1990) reviewed the synaptic mechanisms of opiate action and opiate effects on second messenger systems, G proteins, and regulatory phosphoroproteins. Alterations in the coupling of G-protein subunits may be involved in opioid dependency, tolerance, and withdrawal. "Resetting" of second messenger systems may aid in opioid detoxification. Escriba et al. (1994) describe alterations in the G proteins as being clinically relevant to opiate tolerance, dependence, and abstinence based on postmortem brain findings.

Nestler et al. (1995) reviewed the role of altered gene expression as the ultimate expression of neuroadaptation in opiate, cocaine addiction and the importance of the dopamine reinforcement system substate for most drugs of abuse.

Important clinical tools have resulted from basic research into opioid-norepinephrine interaction. The locus coeruleus is the primary source of noradrenergic interaction of the limbic system, cerebellar, and cerebral cortices. Endogenous opioid receptors have been found in the locus coeruleus, and the chronic administration of opioids inhibits the firing rates of the locus coeruleus noradrenergic system, probably through inhibitory action on common second messenger systems. Opioid withdrawal symptoms are mediated by noradrenergic activity in the locus coeruleus. 3-methoxy-4-hydroxyphenylglycol (MHPG) levels in the

CNS increase after naltrexone-precipitated withdrawal and correlate positively to the signs and symptoms of withdrawal (Charney et al. 1984). These findings have led to the use of clonidine, a noradrenergic α_2-receptor agonist, to suppress and inhibit narcotic withdrawal symptoms.

Psychosocial Factors

Etiological hypotheses of opioid use must take into account social and psychodynamic factors in addition to the pharmacological addictive properties of the drug. With the burgeoning of research into opioid receptors, future biological markers may be developed to identify individuals predisposed to opioid abuse. Some studies suggest that the dopamine marker D_2 may be more frequent in substance-abusing persons in general and may confer genetic vulnerability (Smith et al. 1992). However, complex gene-environmental interactions are more likely to be useful models for drug abuse vulnerability (Cadoret et al. 1995). Different subpopulations may be differentially affected by specific contributing factors. Although drug use/experimentation has declined in middle- and upper-class communities, it has remained endemic and has had increasing social consequences in recent years.

In blacks, less psychopathology has been found among persons who use opioids compared with white persons who use opioids; therefore, psychoactive self-medication may be less frequent and social factors may play a larger role in opiate use by African Americans (Kosten et al. 1985b). However, affective and organic disorders tend to be underdiagnosed in African Americans. Inner-city children are exposed to increased availability of drugs in economically disadvantaged communities with high unemployment, low family stability, increased tolerance of criminality, and increased hopelessness. These social stressors may result in further hopelessness, low self-esteem, poor self-concept, and identification with drug-involved role models, and may be intervening variables in the increased opioid dependency rates in minorities. Entire communities may be corrupted by the economic power and criminal activity that keep demand for drugs high. Where poverty and high unemployment are prevalent, many individuals feel they have little to lose with drug experimentation, and conventional "scare tactics" have little impact. Alienation from social institutions such as school, increased social deviancy, and impulsivity are high-risk characteristics. The overwhelming majority of inner-city community members, however, are not opioid users. Research into the factors that are protective for individuals at high risk is important.

Severe stress and conditioned response may also play a role. U.S. soldiers in Vietnam faced the major stressors of loneliness, fear, and social disruption along with availability, and had high rates of opioid and other psychoactive substance dependency. In most instances, when factors favorable for extinction of the behavior were present, the prognosis for abstinence was good.

Yamaguchi and Kandel (1984) have extensively studied patterns of psychoactive substance use in adolescence through young adulthood and found a progression from tobacco, alcohol, and marijuana to sedatives, cocaine, and finally opioids. Regular marijuana use, depressive symptoms, lack of closeness to parents, and dropping out of school may predispose the adolescent to later narcotic use. Low sensation-seeking scores have been found in opioid-dependent subjects, whereas highly sensation-seeking individuals have been found to use cocaine (Galizio and Stein 1983). Avoidance of excessive internal or external arousal may be a factor in opioid preference.

Khantzian (1985) has found a strong interaction between dominant dysphoric feelings and drug preference. The self-medication hypothesis postulates that individuals self-select drugs on the basis of personality and ego impairments. Khantzian emphasizes an "anti-rage" property to opioids that provides a pharmacological solution to an overwhelming affect that is due to either deficient ego defenses or low frustration tolerance. Patients may seek mastery over pain through self-administered drug titration of withdrawal and dysphoria. Khantzian and colleagues have discussed the "self-care deficits" that many of these individuals suffer from and has described group psychotherapeutic treatment approaches (Brehm et al. 1993).

Spotts and Shontz (1985), in their study of individuals associated with heavy drug abuse, found that opioid-addicted persons had difficulty in maintaining intimate relationships, partly related to their social withdrawal and avoidance of sexual and aggressive conflict. Blatt et al. (1984) noted that the primary disturbance in opioid-addicted individuals appeared to be social perceptual difficulties. Compared with normal subjects, addicted individuals experienced people to be less stable in affect; involved in less meaningful, purposeful, and constructive activity; and less well differentiated as persons.

DUAL DIAGNOSIS

Impressions that addicted individuals are likely to have a comorbid psychiatric disorder(s) have been supported empirically. In a diverse sample of 133 narcotic-addicted persons, there was a 93% rate of other diagnosable DSM-III psychiatric disorders, including depression in 60%, antisocial personality disorder in 35%, and other personality disorders in 30% (Khantzian and Treece 1985). It is often hard to separate out the influence of symptoms of chronic intoxication and withdrawal from other Axis I and Axis II pathology. Several studies have questioned the utility of DSM-III-R criteria for antisocial personality disorder in substance-abusing individuals, particularly in those who abuse intravenous drugs (Alterman and Cacciola 1991; Brooner et al. 1992; Gerstley et al. 1990). Diagnosis of true early-onset antisocial personality disorder may require antisocial behaviors independent of substance abuse, as well as childhood antecedents, and may be associated with greater psychopathy and poorer prognosis. Rounsaville et al. (1982) found that 80% of a sample of outpatients on methadone had lifetime histories of psychiatric disorders, with 74% meeting a lifetime diagnosis of affective disorder. Although depressive symptoms generally develop in those who chronically use depressants and psychotic symptoms develop in those who use stimulants at high doses, those persons who regularly use opioids have shown no change in psychopathology over time (Perkins et al. 1986). Rounsaville and Kleber (1985) have found that those addicted individuals who sought treatment in community programs were comparable to untreated addicted individuals in duration and severity of opioid activity but that those seeking treatment had more depression, poorer social functioning, nonspecific anxiety symptoms, and more drug-related legal problems. Brooner et al. (1997) reports a 47% comorbidity rate among 716 opioid abusers seeking methadone maintenance. Antisocial personality and major depression were most frequent. These factors may facilitate crises that lead patients to treatment sooner. Although frank schizophrenia is uncommon, there have been case reports of psychotic episodes following methadone discontinuance.

TREATMENT

General

Approaches to treatment of opioid addiction can be grouped into opioid substitution or maintenance versus abstinence approaches. Methadone maintenance and therapeutic community programs were developed in the 1960s. Currently, work is being done to improve therapists' diagnostic and prognostic skills with patients in these programs. New pharmacological tools such as clonidine (Catapres) and naltrexone (Trexan) allow a select minority of patients to be detoxified as outpatients. Novel approaches to detoxification such as buprenorphine and clonidine-naltrexone combinations are being developed and will be described further in this section. The value of

psychotherapy in appropriate patients is being increasingly recognized as an important adjunct. Optimal setting and length of rehabilitative treatment have important prognostic value. Family therapy, vocational training, and respect for indigenous community sensitivities and needs are factors that have received attention (Dembo et al. 1983; Kosten and Kleber 1984). Choice of the proper treatment or combination of treatments depends on patient characteristics, and few good outcome studies exist in the differential therapeutics of opioid addiction (Woody et al. 1983). Further research may clarify the genetic, psychological, social, economic, and political variables that may affect primary, secondary, and tertiary prevention.

Maintenance Versus Detoxification

The course of heroin addiction typically involves a 2- to 6-year interval between regular heroin use and the seeking of treatment. Early experimentation with opioids may not lead to opioid addiction, but once addiction develops, a lifelong pattern of use and relapse frequently ensues. A preexisting personality disorder may be a factor in drug use progression. The need to secure the drug predisposes the addicted individual to participate in illegal activities or complicates an already existing tendency toward criminality. Attitudes toward one's self, society's attitudes toward addicted individuals, personality problems, unemployment, and empathic impairments are not responsive to psychopharmacological treatment alone; thus treatment almost always involves psychosocial rehabilitation.

Methadone Maintenance

Dole and Nyswander (1965) first postulated that problematic drug-seeking behavior would diminish, personal productivity would increase, and illicit activities would be hampered if wide fluctuations in opioid blood levels could be inhibited. They reported that 80% of unreachable heroin-addicted individuals improved with methadone maintenance therapy. Although methadone maintenance is now widely available, its merits and drawbacks are still hotly debated, and new pharmacological approaches are still sought.

Methadone is a relatively long-acting (half-life of 24–36 hours), cross-tolerant opioid that mutes extreme fluctuation in opioid blood level and blunts euphoric response to illicit heroin. Unlike heroin, which has a shorter half-life of 8–12 hours, methadone can be administered once daily without causing withdrawal and provides a treatment structure for rehabilitation without the need for illegal activities to support a costly habit.

A patient who gives a history of heroin use two or more

times per day for several weeks and is unemployed has a moderate to severe degree of opioid dependence and warrants methadone maintenance. Methadone is administered orally and is most often reliably absorbed; it binds nonspecifically to body tissues and therefore maintains a fairly steady blood concentration. The slow onset of subjective effects decreases reinforcing euphoric peaks and diminishes acute withdrawal symptoms. Acute decreases in follicle-stimulating hormone and luteinizing hormone, and EEG abnormalities have been reported. Subjectively, common side effects are sedation, mild euphoria, constipation, and reduced sweating if the dosage is too high. These symptoms usually remit after the first few weeks. Occasionally, transient ankle edema, skin problems, and reduced libido have been reported. Long-term euphoric effects persist in some patients, but many find methadone relatively dysphoric. Although a mainstay treatment, this therapy reaches only 20%–25% of addicted individuals, with retention rates of 59%–85% (Stimmel et al. 1977).

Methadone maintenance programs are required to be registered and follow a variety of federal, state, and local regulations. Patients substitute for their current addiction an addiction to methadone, which leads to a close attachment to treatment programs. Controversy exists as to the efficacy of high versus low methadone schedules, with higher doses leading to better program retention. Dole and Nyswander (1965) advocate starting at 20–40 mg the first day, with gradual increase up to a total of 120 mg a day in certain individuals, on a chronic basis to adequately suppress opioid hunger and block any response to illicit heroin. Other programs approach methadone maintenance not as a lifelong substitution but as a transitional phase toward total abstinence, and use doses of 20 mg to 60 mg per day. Large doses of heroin with this regimen may result in euphoria. Poor retention rate in low-dose programs is a critical factor in leading experts to favor higher doses (Brown et al. 1982). Some programs offer take-home medications for methadone patients who have had long-term success, and this is very appropriate for a subset of methadone maintenance clients; however, this can result in diversion to illegal methadone markets. Carefully selected patients may be able to have less frequent monitoring (Novick et al. 1988). Behavioral contingency contacting based on urine monitoring in methadone clients may play a role in reducing illicit drug use while the patient is on methadone and may improve compliance (Calsyn et al. 1991; Stine et al. 1991). Illicit use of drugs such as cocaine and alcohol continues to be a problem among individuals who use methadone. Methadone use may have drug interactions with medications used in substance abuse treatment, such as in a recent study which shows that

desipramine plasma concentrations are affected by methadone usage (Kosten et al. 1990).

The optimal length of methadone maintenance treatment is difficult to predetermine. Advocates for long-term maintenance cite the benefits as a decrease in opioid drug use (if not total abstinence), less criminal behavior, less unemployment, and reduced sharing of needles with consequent lower risk of contracting HIV infection (Metzger et al. 1991). Methadone detoxification is a viable option for patients who have better pretreatment functioning, long successful maintenance at low-dose methadone, less psychosocial connection to a "street culture," and/or addiction to opioids other than heroin. Ethical, cultural, and political objections have been raised concerning the addictive aspect of methadone maintenance. Some have questioned the effectiveness originally reported by Dole and Nyswander (1965). Ausubel (1983) describes a chronic subliminal type of euphoria in which methadone is seen as an iatrogenic pharmacological defense system. He gives examples of patients who report that methadone can be overridden with high doses of heroin or enhanced by methadone abuse. Despite these objections, long-term methadone maintenance remains the leading modality of treatment for hard-core addiction. Patients who are abstinent 3 years after stopping methadone maintenance range from 12% to 83% in different studies (Stimmel et al. 1977). In general, patients with better pretreatment functioning and shorter drug histories do better.

Methadone maintenance patients often have the added problem of polysubstance use. Cocaine and alcohol are frequently combined with or used instead of opioids. Cocaine itself has been linked to criminal activity and an addictive lifestyle. Strug et al. (1985) reported that approximately 20% of methadone clients have abused cocaine and that 63% of methadone-addicted persons not in treatment use cocaine and heroin (i.e., "speedball"). For patients on methadone maintenance, cocaine may provide the substitute high that is no longer available with heroin. Alcoholism is a factor in 26% of terminations from methadone treatment and may be abused by 14%–40% of all opioid patients (Joseph and Appel 1985). The majority of polysubstance-using individuals have had problems with alcohol prior to methadone treatment, and they frequently increase their alcohol use after methadone detoxification. The dual addiction of methadone and alcohol decreases survival rates and increases the chances of overdose and medical complications. Treatment should target both problems and may involve a variety of approaches. Urine samples aid in the detection of abuse of other substances.

Detoxification from multiple drug dependence is best achieved by beginning with sedative-hypnotic withdrawal while maintaining methadone. Combined use of methadone and benzodiazepines must be very carefully monitored because of the interaction of the two drugs and the greater danger of overdose. Methadone tends to potentiate the sedative effects of benzodiazepines. The naloxone challenge test using 0.8 mg of naloxone may help to determine the degree of dependence and predict treatment outcome (Jacobsen and Kosten 1989).

A recently clinically approved long-acting opioid agonist has some advantages over methadone. L-Alphacetylmethadol (LAAM), an agonist similar to methadone, has a longer half-life, providing suppression of withdrawal symptoms for from 72 to 96 hours (Jaffe and Martin 1985). Therefore, LAAM can be given just 3 days per week, making take-home privileges unnecessary. Because of LAAM's slow induction, the potential for abuse is less. Generally LAAM compares favorably to methadone, but decreased retention rates and mood side effects may be drawbacks. LAAM has a delayed onset of action and clinicians should be especially wary of potential for relapse in the first 3 weeks. Lofexidine hydrochloride is also undergoing FDA review for treatment of opiate dependence.

Buprenorphine (Temgesic) is a mixed μ-receptor agonist/antagonist. In experimental settings, patients who use heroin have sharply decreased their intake when started and maintained on subcutaneous buprenorphine. This agent may have the advantage of lower abuse and overdose potential. With increasing dose, it exhibits less intense agonist properties. Buprenorphine at high doses (8–12 mg daily) compares favorably with standard doses of methadone in promoting opioid abstinence (Johnson et al. 1992; Schottenfeld et al. 1997). Buprenorphine may have the added advantage of attenuating the high of the "speedball" effect of opiates and cocaine (Kosten et al. 1991).

However, there is a recent negative study that does not support the superiority of buprenorphine compared with methadone for reducing cocaine use (Schottenfeld et al. 1997).

McLellan et al. (1993) randomly assigned methadone maintenance clients to methadone alone, methadone plus standard methadone counseling, and methadone plus enhanced treatment. The enhanced group showed the most improvement, however, recent analysis suggest that enhanced treatment may be less cost effective than standard counseling for individuals without major psychopathology (Kraft et al. 1997).

Opioid Detoxification

Methadone detoxification.   Recent studies have suggested a 76% success rate of completion for methadone detoxification (Milby 1988). When attempted, detoxification should be very slow, because abstinence symptoms may be protracted. Some patients in methadone maintenance programs (15%–34%) may not have a true opioid dependence when tested with antagonist challenge.

Conservative detoxification of methadone is achieved through decreasing doses by 10% per week until the 10-to-20 mg range is reached, and then decreasing by 3% per week (Table 11–22). This slow detoxification regimen is used to reduce relapse rates. This method is also appropriate for detoxification from equivalent dosages of heroin. Detoxification of weak opioids such as codeine conservatively can be achieved by starting methadone at 20 mg and then decreasing this dosage by 1 mg per day over a 14- to 21-day period.

Although it is frequently easy to decrease methadone level dose to 20 mg per day, it is hard to go lower because subsequent mild withdrawal symptoms may be conditioned to fear of being off drugs in opioid-addicted individuals. Hall (1984) has proposed a concept of an opioid abstinence phobia. Double-blind studies show that patients' expectations of difficulties with decreased dosages produce profound withdrawal symptoms. Opioid use is reinforcing by its pharmacological avoidance of painful and conflictual situations. Anxiety may be paired with conditioned abstinence stimuli and cues. Deficient social and interpersonal skills may be a component to this abstinence-connected anxiety.

Unless there are complications, deaths are not reported from methadone withdrawal, although patients may suffer extreme discomfort upon sudden withdrawal. Controversy still exists on whether pregnant opioid-addicted women should be completely detoxified from methadone. Many authors recommend decreasing methadone to at least less than 20 mg.

Clonidine.   Two recent advances in opioid detoxification and abstinence-oriented treatment have been the introduction of clonidine and naltrexone. Clonidine has

TABLE 11-22.   Opiate detoxification

Methadone
Outpatient: Decrease methadone 10% per week until 10–20 mg range, then decrease 3% per week
Inpatient: 1 mg/day over 20 days

Clonidine
After patient stabilized at 20 mg of methadone, can abruptly switch to clonidine 0.1–0.3 mg three times daily for 2 days, then third day 0.2–0.7 mg three times daily for 8 to 14 days, then discontinue.

been found to be a nonopioid suppressor of opioid withdrawal symptoms.

Gold et al. (1978) decided to test clonidine clinically as a method for opiate withdrawal based on the hypothesis that many signs and symptoms of withdrawal are mediated by the locus coeruleus and that clonidine, as an α-adrenergic antagonist, acts to suppress locus coeruleus activity and reduce symptoms. Several studies have confirmed the usefulness of clonidine detoxification for inpatient detoxification of methadone and heroin (Charney et al. 1981), but less success has been reported in outpatient populations (Kleber et al. 1985; Washton and Resnick 1981). Clonidine generally provides good suppression of autonomic signs of withdrawal but may be less effective at relieving subjective discomfort (Jasinski et al. 1985). Withdrawal symptoms may be more prominent with clonidine in the early phase of withdrawal compared with methadone. Patients do better with an abrupt switch to clonidine if the methadone dose is first stabilized at 20 mg or less. Rounsaville et al. (1986) found outpatient detoxification failure in both clonidine- and methadone-assisted withdrawal. In both groups, high psychiatric severity ratings were evident before withdrawal.

Clonidine for heroin withdrawal can be given in doses starting at 0.1–0.3 mg tid, which may be increased to 1.2 mg total per day. Typical opiate detoxification with clonidine is 3–5 days. Sedation and hypotension are common side effects. Clonidine should be held if the blood pressure is less than 85/55. Clonidine patches may also be used but may require oral prn. Clonidine's main benefit may prove to be the period of 5–7 days in which the patient is opioid free, making it easier for the patient to be started on an opioid antagonist. Although approved for other uses, clonidine is not currently FDA approved for opioid detoxification. Lofexidine and guanabenz are other α-antagonists receiving trials.

Naltrexone. Naltrexone is an opioid antagonist that blocks opioid receptors, preventing the reinforcing euphoric effects of opioids. Its long-term use results in gradual extinction of drug-seeking behavior, and consequently it is a tool in abstinence-oriented treatment (Greenstein et al. 1984). Naltrexone does not produce dependence, has few side effects, reduces the chance of overdose when narcotics are used, and is FDA approved for this use. Because of its antagonist properties, naltrexone can precipitate withdrawal symptoms if receptors are not clear of opioids. Dysphoria may result from naltrexone use in formerly opioid-addicted individuals long after use of opioids is stopped and also occurs in normal subjects (Crowley et al. 1985). Naltrexone is usually given as a 25- to 50-mg daily dose over a 5- to 10-day period after last opioid use, and then is gradually increased to 100–150 mg three times a week. Two cc of naloxone (0.8 mg), which is short-acting, can be given intravenously to test whether an individual is opioid free.

The clinical effectiveness of naltrexone has varied greatly according to the population studied and the degree of patient motivation for treatment (Kosten and Kleber 1984). High refusal rates of 70% and dropout rates of 90% in 9 months with naltrexone were found in urban outpatient clinic populations, indicating limited usefulness for most cases of hard-core addiction (Resnick et al. 1980). Washton and Resnick (1981) reported a 70% 1-year abstinence rate in an outpatient naltrexone program for highly motivated patients with families and jobs whose incomes averaged $40,000 per year and who had strong reasons to continue the treatment. Clonidine-naltrexone combinations, contingency contracting, family therapy, and lifestyle changes have aimed at enhancing retention and success rates. It is unlikely that any abstinence-oriented treatment will ever approach the outpatient retention rates that are found in programs that use addicting substances such as methadone.

Clonidine and naltrexone. Abrupt switch to clonidine may be started along with gradual low-dose naltrexone (antagonist) administration. The combination appears to shorten the withdrawal period to 3–4 days without increasing symptomatology and can be used successfully on an outpatient basis (Kleber et al. 1987). Stine and Kosten (1992) and Kleber (Kleber and Gawin 1996) provide an excellent review of combination strategies. The naltrexone may serve to "reset" the opioid homeostasis. Higher doses of naltrexone may speed withdrawal duration but require higher dose levels of clonidine to suppress symptoms.

Buprenorphine and others. Buprenorphine treatment uses a strategy of using a mixed opioid agonistic/antagonist that precipitates a mild withdrawal by its antagonist activity. Doses of 2–4 mg are generally agonistic, whereas doses of more than 8 mg are more purely antagonistic. Patients can be abruptly switched from heroin to buprenorphine and then detoxified (Margolin et al. 1991). Kosten et al. (1991) have described a protocol of abruptly switching from heroin or methadone to buprenorphine 2–6 mg per day for 1 month and then maintaining on naltrexone. Retention in the study was 72%, and withdrawal symptoms were mild. The 1-month stabilization may have the benefit of providing time for psychosocial engagement in treatment. Rapid detoxification strategies using short-acting sedatives (e.g., midazolam) in combination with opiate antagonists and enkephalinase inhibitors (e.g., acetorphine) have recently been described (Loimer et al. 1991). Useful adjunctive therapies for opiate withdrawal are nonsteroidal anti-inflammatory drugs (NSAIDS) for muscle ache, benzodiazepines for sleep and anxiety, and bentyl for gastrointestinal distress. Mild dependence may be treated by nonopioid alternatives such as acupuncture, clonidine, and major and minor tranquilizers. The rapid detoxification program (CITA-UROD), a 6-hour detoxification program done under anesthesia, is controversial and has not to date been subject to good research.

PSYCHOSOCIAL TREATMENT OUTCOME

Treatment outcome factors have included a variety of measures involving choice of drug of abuse, employment, psychosocial adjustment, degree of sociopathy, and severity of psychopathology. Psychosocial therapy strategies have included therapeutic communities, Narcotics Anonymous, and psychotherapy. The prognosis of opioid-addicted patients is inversely related to severity of psychopathology; however, if psychotherapy is added, psychiatrically ill patients do better than they would otherwise have done (Woody et al. 1985). Antisocial personality alone is a negative predictor of psychotherapy outcome, but additional presence of depression improves therapy outcome considerably as measured by drug use and functioning (Woody et al. 1985). Rounsaville et al. (1986) found that a high psychiatric severity index scale rating in methadone patients best predicts poor functioning at 2.5-year follow-up. The ability to form a meaningful relationship in therapy is a positive prognostic factor. Woody et al. (1985) found that professional psychotherapy was associated with greater benefits than was drug counseling alone, especially in those patients with severe psychiatric symptoms. Treatment goals other than illicit drug use need to be assessed. Good patient-therapist alliance and purity of technique may predict better therapy outcome (Luborsky et al. 1985).

Kosten et al. (1986) found depression and life crises to be predictors of poor outcome in drug programs at 2.5-year follow-up. Major depressive symptoms need special attention in that adjunct medication trials with antidepressants and lithium may be indicated. Rounsaville and Kleber (1985) suggest that better results are achieved when therapists 1) are physically near the treatment facility, 2) treat depression early in its course, and 3) pay close attention to attendance.

Therapeutic communities remove the addicted individual from the drug environment, confront his or her attitudes with peer support, and emphasize assumption of personal responsibility. Only the highly motivated patients stay in treatment, with estimated dropout rates of 50% at 6 months and 90% at 12 months (Deleon et al. 1982). Select patients who do stay in treatment 3–6 months have a relatively good prognosis (Simpson 1981). These programs are generally drug free and highly structured, although alcohol may be tolerated. Overall success rates in therapeutic communities have not been impressive.

Total abstinence is often used as the only measure of success, but decreased opioid use and fewer episodes may have very positive effects on life quality. In an 11-year follow-up of 83 addicted subjects in England, 29 were still using drugs, 37 were not using drugs, and 17 had died (Cottrell et al. 1985). HIV seroprevalence has begun to stabilize in New York City (Des Jarlais 1994). However the trend toward intranasal use could eventually lead to wider transmission of HIV. Needle exchange programs, although controversial, may show promise in further decreasing HIV transmissions among intravenous drug users (Watters et al. 1994).

Recently, a new drug-resistant strain of tuberculosis has once again raised concerns among high-risk individuals such as AIDS patients, substance-abusing individuals, homeless persons, prisoners, and health care workers.

COCAINE

HISTORY

Cocaine is derived from the coca plant *Erythroxylon coca*, indigenous to Peru, Bolivia, Ecuador, and Colombia, and has been used for more than 2,000 years by Native American Indian tribes and civilizations.

Sixteenth-century observers reported use of the coca plant by Peruvian Inca high society in religious and social rituals. Coca leaves were placed in burial tombs for passage to the next world and were an element in the decorative arts (Mortimer 1974). Cocaine's analgesic properties apparently were exploited during the process of extirpation, when holes were drilled into skulls to let evil spirits out. The plant was also used as a folk remedy for physical disorders and as a source of vitamins (B_1, C, and riboflavin).

The Spanish Inquisition had a devastating effect on Incan society, and Catholic religious leaders initially associated coca use with sin. However, coca use appeared to aid in the hard work needed in the gold mines by increasing endurance, reducing fatigue, and decreasing hunger. Coca leaves were chewed, and only recently has the smoking of coca paste in South America become a problem. The coca leaves brought back to Europe lost potency on the long journey and did not grow well.

Modern interest in cocaine started with its chemical isolation from the coca plant by the German chemist Albert Newman in 1882 (Nicholi 1984). At the end of the 19th century, Montegazza extolled its pleasurable effects. Sigmund Freud personally experimented with cocaine and was impressed with its effects on mood and work. After one of his patients had a cocaine-related death and a friend developed problems with cocaine, Freud closed this chapter in his work with regrets. However, Freud's writings about the analgesic properties of cocaine were applied successfully to eye surgery by Dr. Carl Koller, who operated on Freud's father using this technique.

In the United States, interest in cocaine remained intense. Cocaine extract was used in a variety of elixirs such as Vin Mariani and in the original Coca-Cola® formula. Eminent physicians such as Hammond, Mortimer, and Halstead all published extensively on the benefits of cocaine; and some, like Halstead, the father of modern surgery, became dependent on cocaine themselves. In scientific and newspaper reports, cocaine was increasingly implicated in deaths, mental problems, and addiction. Anecdotal reports of heavy use among black persons may have been exaggerated by prejudice.

Congress responded to an alarmed public sensitized to the general dangers of cocaine use by proclaiming cocaine an illegal narcotic in the Harrison Act of 1914. Cocaine decreased in availability but continued to be used by avant-garde groups. In the 1960s drug use increased generally in the United States. Because of the high cost of the crystal form, cocaine was available mainly to the affluent and increasingly was considered fashionable. Historically, societies have had an alternating fascination with and abhorrence to cocaine.

DEFINITION

Whereas DSM-III includes a diagnosis only of cocaine abuse, DSM-III-R includes cocaine dependency, which has a broad definition, including a pattern of social or occupational problems (see Tables 11–1, 11–2, 11–3, and 11–4 presented earlier in this chapter). In DSM-IV, cocaine-related problems are discussed in relation to intoxication, cocaine intoxication paranoia, uncomplicated withdrawal, dependence, and abuse, and are similar to behavior found with amphetamine and other similarly acting stimulants.

Diagnosis of intoxication requires recent use (within minutes to hours) and a "high" with euphoria, hyper-

alertness, grandiosity, and, often, impaired judgment. Chronic use may result in affective blunting, fatigue, and sadness. Individuals may be more gregarious or socially avoidant and may have increased anxiety, restlessness and hypervigilance, and stereotypical behavior. Physical symptoms include two or more of tachycardia, bradycardia, dilated pupils, elevated or lowered blood pressure, perspiration or chills, nausea or vomiting, weight loss, chest pain or cardiac arrhythmias, confusion, seizures, dyskinesia, or dystonias.

Cocaine intoxication paranoia occurs with high-dose, chronic, or binge use and is usually of short duration. It is associated with aggression and violence, and distortion of perceived threat.

Uncomplicated withdrawal occurs with decrease or cessation of regular high-dose use accompanied by dysphoric mood, including sadness or anxiety, and two or more rebound physiological symptoms such as fatigue, drug craving, disturbed dreams, sleep problems, increased appetite, psychomotor retardation, or agitation.

In DSM-IV, *dependence* is defined as compulsive self-administration of high doses of cocaine and the involvement with the drug to the exclusion of other important activities and responsibilities such as work, eating, and family, with adverse consequences to work, health, legal, and social relationships. Dependence may be episodic or continuous (daily).

In DSM-IV, *abuse* is defined as repetitive self-administration of high doses of cocaine with consequent social or medical problems, without the compulsive quality that is present with dependence.

Because of the high cost of cocaine, financial difficulties, legal problems, and prostitution may be early signs of trouble before other stigmata of dependence develop. Loss of control, exaggerated involvement, and continued use despite adverse social, occupational, and health effects are diagnostic criteria for cocaine dependency.

EPIDEMIOLOGY

During the 1970s, experimentation with cocaine was considered relatively safe, and even some addictions experts thought it not to be very dangerous. Major complications such as cocaine psychosis were said to be extremely rare occurrences. In the 1980s, market demand led to an increased availability of cocaine in new, purer, more potent forms at low prices. In addition, more rapid routes of administration were developed, contributing to more frequent severe complications, telescoping of the course, and wider problems across social class and race.

The extent of the cocaine problem can be estimated

through national surveys, hotlines, emergency room visits, and reports from treatment facilities, although the full impact is hard to measure because use is illegal. The National Institute on Drug Abuse estimated that 5.4 million Americans had tried cocaine at least once by 1974, 21.6 million by 1982, and perhaps 25–40 million by 1986 (National Institute on Drug Abuse 1986). Bachman et al. (1990) traced lowering of cocaine and drug abuse in 3,000 high school seniors to perceived risk of physical and other harm and to disapproval. Cocaine use dropped dramatically after the deaths of a college basketball star, Len Bias, and, a week later, professional football player Don Rogers, and after the subsequent heavy media coverage dramatizing the dangers of drug use. Demand reduction programs have impacted cocaine and marijuana epidemics in youth but have not been as effective with poor, disadvantaged groups, who have maintained high levels of "crack" addiction.

Pope et al. (1990) found that seniors in college had reduced drug use in 1989 compared with seniors in 1969 and 1978. Cocaine use peaked in 1978 at 25% and was reduced to 20% in 1989. Weekly marijuana use fell to 5.7% in 1989 from 26% in 1978. These trends indicate attitudinal changes in young Americans about drugs in the last decade. Recent surveys (Johnston et al. 1996) of junior high school students report, however, a reversal in the 3-year trend in decrease of psychoactive substance use. Crack cocaine is used by a small subset of the general population; however, it is more popular among younger, more serious cocaine users (Smart 1991). There has been a recent decline in cocaine use, especially among middle-class and affluent populations and among students (Bachman et al. 1990; Perlstadt et al. 1991; Pope et al. 1990). Reasons given for the decline include students being better informed about the risk and consequences of cocaine use; health promotion; and the need to remain competitive in today's society. Cocaine use tends to decrease in social users as they assume adult responsibility. Kandel and Raveis's (1989) longitudinal study of nonclinical populations of teenagers found, however, a subset of users characterized by greater involvement with drug-using friends, more antisocial behavior, and increased dependence on marijuana. These teenagers were more likely to be involved with drugs at age 28 or 29. High school students who use crack have low levels of psychosocial functioning compared to other drugs of abuse (Kandel and Davies 1996). Cocaine remains a significant problem, especially in underprivileged environments where availability of drugs persists and less opportunities to enter into the mainstream society are available. According to the latest Drug Abuse Treatment Outcome data (National Institute on Drug Abuse 1997), 54.8% of clients in drug treatment programs (i.e., methadone, long-term residential, outpatient drug-free, and short-term inpatient programs) are dependent on cocaine, thus cocaine continues to be the prominent drug of abuse. DAWN (1990) data also signal that cocaine emergencies are still prevalent and overrepresented by African Americans. Cocaine has been highly associated with homicide, HIV transmission (especially in women who smoke crack), early sexual intercourse, and low birth weight (Edlin et al. 1994; Racine et al. 1993; Tardiff et al. 1994). Current controversy surrounds the federal sentencing laws that allow possessing 100 times the amount of power cocaine compared with crack cocaine to trigger mandatory sentencing. This law is thought to discriminate against the poor and minorities (Hatsukami and Fischman 1996). Cocaine abuse in adolescents leads to more rapid and severe consequences than it does in adults. The time lapse from first use to addiction is reduced from 4 years in adults to 1.5 years in adolescents (Washton et al. 1984).

Ultimately, reduced availability in the United States will continue to depend on intergovernmental cooperation and diminished demand on the part of individuals in the United States. So far, law enforcement efforts alone have not reduced the production and distribution of drugs.

Cocaine's functional affordability has dramatically risen, with the potent, almost instantaneous high of cocaine freebase distributed in vials of "crack" selling for as little as $10. The majority of those persons who use cocaine casually (especially intranasally) do not become dependent, but the widespread thinking in the late 1970s that cocaine is not addictive is mistaken.

CLINICAL FEATURES

General

Effects of intoxication depend on the dose and administration of the drug and include euphoria, hyperalertness, perceptual changes, disinhibition, enhanced sense of mastery, sexual arousal, and improved self-esteem (Kleber and Gawin 1986). This "rush" experience may be greatly intensified with intravenous or freebase use. Maladaptive behavioral changes include fighting, grandiosity, hypervigilance, psychomotor agitation, impaired judgment, and impaired social or occupational functioning. Tachycardia, pupillary dilation, elevated blood pressure, perspiration or chills, nausea or vomiting, and visual or tactile hallucinations are signs that may present within 1 hour of use.

Frequently, the symptoms of cocaine toxicity resemble a hypomanic state. Tolerance to the euphoric effects develops during a binge; however, there is decreased tolerance for adverse experiences such as increasing anxiety, panic, or frank delirium. With prolonged cocaine administration, a transient delusional psychosis, simulating paranoid schizophrenia, can be seen. In one study, experienced cocaine-using individuals given cocaine intravenously were uniformly paranoid (Sherer et al. 1988). Usually these symptoms remit, although heavy prolonged use or predisposing psychopathology may result in persistence of psychosis. Generally, higher doses distinguish overdose from simple intoxication. Cocaine abuse tends to occur in binge patterns. In humans, cocaine binges can last a few hours to several days, are highly reinforcing, and may lead to psychosis or death. Dopamine can increase psychomotor activity, induce stereotypical behavior, and decrease food consumption. When given free access to cocaine, monkeys have been found to self-administer continuously until death results from cardiorespiratory collapse or infection. Lack of control over excessive cocaine use may result from this highly positively rewarding property of cocaine.

Pharmacology

Cocaine hydrochloride is a white crystal powder derived from coca leaves and coca paste. It is usually diluted, or "stepped on," to 20% pure by mixing it with other local anesthetics such as lidocaine, procaine, and various sugars. Cocaine freebase is a by-product in which the hydrochloride salt is removed by various substances. Freebasing is smoking the fumes of the 80% pure alkaloid form of cocaine. This preparation of cocaine has a lower volatile temperature, which prevents the destruction of its psychoactive properties when smoked. "Crack" or "rock" is a prepackaged freebased derivative ready for smoking. Intranasal cocaine's half-life is less than 90 minutes, with euphoric effects lasting 15–30 minutes. Most cocaine is hydrolyzed in the body to benzoylecgonine, which can be detected in the urine for up to 36 hours. Repeated doses are self-administered in lines of 25–50 mg as rapid tolerance builds up to the euphoric effects. Smoked freebase cocaine has a rapid onset of intense euphoria within seconds because it passes directly from the lungs through the heart to the brain and does not have to pass the liver first. Euphoric effects depend on concentration and on the rate of increase of the peak concentration.

Cocaine blocks neuronal dopamine, serotonin, and norepinephrine reuptake. It is clear cocaine has a specific activating effect on mesolimbic or mesocortical dopaminergic pathways as do other drugs of abuse. Dopaminergic pathways involving the ventral tegmental area, frontal lobe, septum, amygdala, and particularly the nucleus accumbens are important in reinforcing behavior.

Second, third, and fourth messenger intracellular systems and target gene transcriptional effects can produce short- and long-term gene expression (Nestler et al. 1995). The importance of neurotransmitter transporters and their genes are appearing to be crucial substrates for addiction to cocaine (Giros et al. 1996).

With repeated cocaine use, tolerance to cocaine's effect develops that may be due to hypothesized decreases in reuptake inhibition, decreased release of catecholamines, or catecholamine receptor sensitivity changes, either postsynaptic desensitization or presynaptic supersensitization. PET studies suggest that postsynaptic dopamine receptor availability decreases with chronic cocaine abuse (Volkow et al. 1990). There is also reduced glucose utilization (London et al. 1990) and higher dopamine concentration at receptor sites (Schlaepfer et al. 1997) after cocaine administration.

Reduced blue cone electroretinograms and noradrenergic dysregulation has been reported in cocaine-dependent subjects (McDougle et al. 1994; Roy et al. 1997). Perventricular brain damage produces a relative insensitivity to cocaine euphoria (Morgan et al. 1993). Sensitization and "kindling" phenomena have been linked to cocaine craving (Halikas et al. 1991).

Abstinence Symptomatology

Efforts have been made to systematically study and correlate abstinence phenomena with neurobiological findings. Using structural diagnostic interviews in a longitudinal fashion, Gawin and Kleber (1986a) studied 30 chronic cocaine-abusing subjects. The authors identified three phases of abstinence symptomatology, with possible implications for intervention and future biological research.

Phase 1 consisted of the immediate postuse cocaine dysphoria known as "the crash." During prolonged intoxication, subjects reported receiving diminished euphoric effects from larger doses. Subsequent use served only to avoid the crash, which consisted of depression, anhedonia, insomnia, anxiety, irritability, and intense cocaine craving. Major depressive features and suicidal ideation can be prominent. Gradually, cocaine craving subsided and the desire for sleep superseded cocaine craving. Sedative agents such as benzodiazepines and alcohol were used as self-medication in attempts to sleep. This partially explains the associated sedativism that was frequently found with cocaine dependency. Phase 1 lasted up to 3 days.

In Phase 2, low-level cocaine craving continued, with irritability, anxiety, and decreased capacity to experience pleasure. Over several days, the memory of the unpleasant cocaine effect waned, some normalization returned, and craving for cocaine increased, especially in the context of environmental cues. Frequently, this led to another binge cycle, which sometimes repeated itself every 3–10 days.

If the first two phases were successfully completed, Phase 3, a period of milder episodic craving lasting several weeks, developed in a context of conditioned environmental stimuli. Many patients appeared to have a major depressive disorder shortly after cocaine cessation, but most of these symptoms eventually cleared.

A more recent study of 12 subjects who used cocaine intravenously longitudinally found the greatest craving for cocaine during the 24 hours just before admission and the greatest severity of mood distress on the first day of admission. Mood states, craving, and sleep symptoms improved gradually yet persistently during the 28-day stay (Weddington et al. 1990).

Adverse Medical Sequelae

Cocaine has been associated with acute and chronic ailments. Chronic intranasal use can lead to septal necrosis due to vasoconstriction and subsequent dilation, producing nasal stuffiness and "the runs." The anesthetic properties of cocaine may lead to oral numbness and dental neglect. Malnutrition, severe weight loss, and dehydration often result from cocaine binges. Intravenous cocaine use complicated by impurities may produce endocarditis, septicemia, HIV spread, local vasculitis, hepatitis B, emphysema, pulmonary emboli, and granulomas. Freebase cocaine has been associated with decreased pulmonary exchange, and pulmonary dysfunction may persist (Itkomen et al. 1984). Intravenous cocaine injection sites are characterized by prominent ecchymosis, whereas those persons using opioids intravenously more frequently show needle scars.

Positive cocaine urine test results have been found increasingly in homicide victims, those arrested for murder, and those who die by overdose. Autopsies of 33 deaths secondary to acute cocaine intoxication showed that most of these individuals used cocaine intravenously as well as using other toxic substances (McKelway et al. 1990). In New York City, one out of every five persons who had completed suicide during a 1-year period had used cocaine immediately prior to committing suicide (Marzuk et al. 1992), and high rates of death by homicide among African Americans and Latinos have been associated with cocaine and firearms (Tardiff et al. 1994). Cocaine-induced fatalities have an average blood concentration of 6.2 mg per liter (Spiehler and Reed 1985). Congenital deficiency of pseudocholinesterase may slow down metabolism and result in toxic levels, sudden delirium, and hypothermia. Deaths among persons

who use cocaine recreationally in low doses have been reported. Acute agitation, diaphoresis, tachycardia, metabolic and respiratory acidosis, cardiac dysrhythmia, and grand mal seizures can lead ultimately to respiratory arrest. Treatment of seizures and acidosis is essential, and intravenous propranolol and diazepam have been helpful adjuncts (Jonsson et al. 1983). Recurrent myocardial infarction in cocaine use associated with tachycardia and coronary vasoconstriction has been reported. Myocarditis, myocardial ischemia, and acute rhabdomyolysis have all been reported to be associated with cocaine use (Nadamanee et al. 1989; Roth et al. 1988; Virmani et al. 1988). Subarachnoid hemorrhage may be precipitated in patients with underlying arterial venous malformations (Lichtenfeld et al. 1986).

Early studies reported that pregnant women who used cocaine were found to have increased abruptio placentae, and their babies had decreased interactive behavior on the Brazelton scale (Chasnoff et al. 1985). However, the methodology of the studies has been in question. Maternal cocaine use may be a predictor of preterm birth and lower birth weight even after controlling for prematurity (Singer et al. 1994). Further research may uncover teratogenicity in infants born to cocaine-using mothers.

INTERACTION WITH OTHER DISORDERS

Because of the lack of prospective studies, it is very difficult to differentiate cocaine-induced psychiatric disorders from interaction with preexisting disorders. There may be a significant subset of patients with underlying affective mood disorder (cyclothymic or dysthymic); narcissistic, borderline, or antisocial personality disorder; other Axis I substance abuse; or ADHD (Weiss and Mirin 1986). Weiss et al. (1988) have reported lower levels of affective disorders. In cocaine-using subjects who sought treatment, 55% had a current psychiatric diagnosis other than substance abuse, and 73% had a lifetime diagnosis (Rounsaville et al. 1991). These subjects may differ from untreated cocaine-addicted individuals. Carroll and Rounsaville (1992) found that untreated cocaine-abusing subjects had higher levels of polysubstance abuse, fewer negative consequences of cocaine use, lower levels of participation in adult social roles, greater involvement with the legal system and with illegal activities, and a diminished sense of negative consequences of their use despite comparable severity of abuse and psychiatric symptomatology. Affective disorders and alcoholism usually followed the onset of drug abuse, whereas anxiety disorders, antisocial personality disorder, and ADHD preceded drug abuse.

Women, when compared with men, have been found

to have greater rates of major depression, residual depressive symptoms, and job dissatisfaction (Griffin et al. 1989). Depressed cocaine-addicted subjects in one study had started to use tobacco, marijuana, and cocaine at a significantly earlier age (Kleinman et al. 1990). Dysthymic patients may use cocaine to avoid depressive affect. Cyclothymic patients may use cocaine to heighten or maintain elevated mood. Patients with ADHD may, when not diagnosed or treated with methylphenidate, self-medicate with cocaine, which paradoxically sedates, decreases stimulation, and improves concentration. The majority of persons using cocaine do not have Axis I diagnoses other than those related to substance abuse. Several studies have highlighted the use of cocaine in schizophrenia (Salloum et al. 1991; Schneier and Siris 1987; Sevy et al. 1990). Compared with other psychiatric patients, schizophrenic patients seem to have higher rates of stimulant use and lower rates of alcohol abuse. Cocaine continues to be underrecognized among schizophrenic patients (Shaner et al. 1993). This suggests that many schizophrenic individuals may be treating negative symptoms of their disease, despite the fact that stimulant abuse may worsen their prognosis (Brady et al. 1990). Persons using cocaine heavily who experience transient paranoia while intoxicated may be at higher risk for development of psychosis than those cocaine-using individuals who do not experience paranoia (Satel and Edell 1991).

The role of the relationship of personality factors to choice of drug continues to be debated. Spotts and Shontz (1984) have reported that users of low doses take cocaine to support defenses, bolster courage, and provide stimulation and excitement. High sensation-seeking individuals may be attracted to cocaine. Khantzian (1985) proposes that certain individuals use cocaine to augment 1) hyperactive restless lifestyles, 2) an already exaggerated need for self-sufficiency, and 3) flight from depression. Narcissistically impaired individuals may have a strong attraction to cocaine, which further heightens grandiosity.

TREATMENT

The principles of cocaine rehabilitation are similar to treatment of alcoholism or sedativism, although new approaches have taken into account unique features of cocaine dependency. Patterns of use, administration, and psychopathological features are the main determinants of treatment choice.

Psychological Treatment

Kleber and Gawin (1986) recommend an initial trial of outpatient nonpharmacological treatment, especially for those who have passed the initial cocaine crash and craving. In uncomplicated cases, outpatient treatment has the advantage of keeping patients in their natural environment, allowing them to better master everyday temptations and conflicts. Inpatient hospitalization may be needed for severe crash symptoms, suicidal ideation, or psychotic symptoms. Washton (1990) recommends inpatient treatment for 1) chronic freebase or intravenous use, 2) concurrent dependency on other addictive drugs or alcohol, 3) serious medical or psychiatric problems, 4) severe impairment of psychosocial functioning, 5) insufficient motivation for outpatient treatment, 6) lack of family and supports, or 7) failure in outpatient treatment. Under managed care, prior recommendations, however, are generally not being necessarily tailored to individuals as aggregate studies have not supported the costs of the most intense interventions. There is presently underway a national cocaine treatment collaboration study that will answer, it is hoped, some of these treatment matching questions (Crits-Christoph et al. 1997). Cocaine rehabilitation is usually structured along the same general principles of rehabilitation as those that are described in the alcohol treatment section earlier in this chapter, with emphasis on Cocaine Anonymous and Narcotics Anonymous.

Because of adverse consequences of his or her cocaine use, a patient may be coerced into treatment by family, employer, physician, or the law, or he or she may willingly seek refuge from the physical, emotional, or financial consequences of abuse. Treatment outcome is affected more by such factors as employment status, family support, and degree of antisocial features than by initial motivation for treatment. Initial strategy focuses on confronting denial, teaching the disease concept of addictions, fostering in the patient an identification as a recovering person, rediscovering shades of affect, helping the patient to recognize the ambivalent relationship with cocaine, helping the patient to avoid situational and intrapsychic cues that stimulate craving, and formulating support plans. The euphoria and satisfaction that cocaine provides need to be replaced with more realistic and ultimately fulfilling achievements. Association with an identified cocaine-using peer group needs to be replaced by a search for another identity as a recovering person.

Carroll et al. (1991a) compared two purely psychotherapeutic treatments of cocaine abuse: relapse prevention and interpersonal psychotherapy. Those subjects with severe abuse who received relapse prevention treatment achieved abstinence significantly better than did those who received interpersonal therapy (59% versus 9%). Individuals with lower severity abuse had no difference in outcome. One-year follow-up suggests a delayed improvement response for patients who received cognitive-behavioral relapse prevention (Carroll et al. 1994). Relapse prevention addresses ambivalence and strives to reduce cocaine availability, minimize high risk situations and develop coping strategies, recognize conditioned cues to craving, recognize decision patterns that can lead into actual use, obtain a lifestyle modification with behavioral alternatives to cocaine use, and avoid an abstinence violation effect that says to the addicted individual who relapses, "All is lost and I might as well go all the way" (Carroll et al. 1991b).

Behavior therapy contingency contracting is a treatment tool described by Anker and Crowly (1982). There is both positive and negative contingency contracting. One form of aversion conditioning is "Ulysses contracting," in which the patient thinks of the worst scenario of continued cocaine use. This adverse effect is then structured by written agreement with the therapist to occur after the next use of cocaine. This often takes a form of letters to employers or family members. Drug urine tests are given to ensure compliance. The constant reminder of the adverse consequences of cocaine is the most salient feature of this approach. Aversive contingency contracts may be criticized as unnecessary in good prognosis patients and as impractical or overly punitive in severe habitual users.

Higgins et al. (1991) describe a modified positive contingency model involving cooperation with nonabusing spouses and psychosocial changes. Clean urine results are tied to points toward vouchers to purchase retail items. In a later study, 75% of the voucher group completed 24 weeks of treatment compared with the 40% of the control group (Higgins et al. 1994). There was also a higher average of continuous abstinence in the voucher group. This approach compared favorably to 12-step counseling.

On follow-up, the therapist must be watchful for return of cocaine-related activities, attitudes, friendships, and paraphernalia. Alcohol and other mood-altering drugs should be avoided, because they may disinhibit behavior and lead to relapse. Concurrent Axis I or II psychiatric disorders should be treated, with attention to the interaction with cocaine disorder. Treatment of clearly defined ADHD or bipolar or unipolar depression should proceed along with attention to the addiction. Treatment of additional psychoactive disorders will be impossible if the addiction is not addressed.

Rounsaville et al. (1985) have studied the use of interpersonal psychotherapy (IPT) adapted for ambulatory cocaine-abusing individuals. Devised by Klerman et al. (1984), IPT is based on the premise that psychiatric syndromes (and cocaine abuse) are related to disturbances in interpersonal functioning. The therapy, which is brief and focused on current interpersonal functioning, is similar to supportive and exploratory psychotherapies. Goals include acceptance of the need to stop, management of impulsiveness, and recognition of the context of cocaine use and of supply. Close attention is paid to affective and cognitive factors in relapse and the interaction between drug use and relationships with others. Interpersonal role disputes, role transitions, grief work, and interpersonal deficits are the four focus interventions. Relapse is destigmatized and becomes important information to be explored by patient and therapist for cues to the attitudes, circumstances, and emotions that preceded drug use (Rounsaville and Carroll 1993).

Kang et al. (1991) compared the efficacy of once-weekly psychotherapy, family therapy, and group therapy led by paraprofessionals in a largely blue-collar population. In this outpatient population, group therapy was associated with significant improvement in psychological functioning and family/social functioning in the 19% who were not using cocaine at 6- to 12-month follow-up. The once-weekly outpatient psychotherapy was not especially effective.

Pharmacological Treatment

Cocaine intoxication, agitation, and anxiety can be treated with diazepam or, in persistent cases, propranolol. If cocaine psychosis persists, haloperidol or the more sedating chlorpromazine is effective. A schizophreniform picture may develop in some cocaine-using individuals, requiring continuing neuroleptic use.

Mirin and Weiss (1991) have proposed four classes of pharmacological treatment for cocaine abuse: 1) antagonists, 2) aversive agents, 3) drugs that treat premorbid coexisting psychiatric disorders, and 4) drugs that treat cocaine-induced states such as intoxication, withdrawal, and craving. Kosten and Kosten (1991) have reviewed blocking agents for cocaine and other stimulants. Work in this area is still in its early stages, and no blocking has been found to be definitely effective. Mazindol, a competitor for the catecholamine reuptake carrier, and haloperidol, a D_2-receptor blocker, in theory could act as cocaine antagonists but have not been found to be clinically useful. Aversive agents have received scant attention.

Experimental treatments of cocaine withdrawal, anhedonia, and craving have been based on neurobiological findings in cocaine use. More recently, dopamine autoreceptor supersensitivity has been related to the cocaine withdrawal syndrome. Dopamine agonists such as bromocriptine and amantadine have been tested in cocaine withdrawal to improve dopaminergic functioning during the withdrawal period. Clinically the findings have been mixed (Giannini et al. 1989; Kosten 1990; Weddington et al. 1990, 1991), and these drugs cannot be recommended for routine clinical use at this time. Flupentixol decanoate, a dopamine-blocking agent that is an antidepressant at low doses, in a preliminary study was found to have promise in decreasing craving in crack cocaine use (Gawin et al. 1989a).

The monoamine precursors tryptophan and tyrosine had been used to attempt to treat the "crash" symptoms by replenishing neurotransmitter stores (Gawin and Kleber 1986b; Kleber and Gawin 1984). One recent study did not find this approach to be clinically effective (Chadwick et al. 1990).

Imipramine and amitriptyline are potent serotonin reuptake blockers. Serotonin has been implicated in sensitization to cocaine and its related negative symptoms such as anxiety. More specific serotonergic agents may have some role in the pharmacological treatment of cocaine withdrawal states in the future.

Desipramine and nortriptyline are more potent norepinephrine reuptake blockers. Antidepressants have been proposed to effect change by down-regulating norepinephrine (p-adrenoceptor) or serotonin receptor density by an as yet unclear mechanism of presynaptic inhibition. The interaction between these neurotransmitter systems is complex, and further research is needed to determine how antidepressants work. Tricyclics have been used to treat the severe anhedonia resembling depressive illness and cocaine craving that may be related to β-adrenergic and dopaminergic receptor supersensitivity. Compared with cocaine, tricyclics appear to have an opposite effect on urinary MHPG levels. Gawin et al. (1989b) conducted a double-blind, random-assignment 6-week comparison of desipramine, lithium, and placebo in 72 cocaine-abusing outpatients. Cocaine craving and use were significantly reduced in the desipramine group. More recently, Fischman et al. (1990) found that cocaine administration was not attenuated by desipramine and was associated with irritability and cardiovascular toxicity. The pharmacological agents carbamazepine, bupropion, and buprenorphine have also had trials in the treatment of cocaine abuse.

Until positive findings are well replicated and safety is well established, clinicians should be cautious about the use of antidepressants as an adjunct analogous to naltrexone in patients who are actively abusing cocaine and other substances. Low-dose desipramine has been found to be useful in the treatment of cocaine-related panic attacks (Bystritsky et al. 1991). Lithium has been reported to block cocaine's euphoric effects, although recent evidence suggests that lithium carbonate is effective only in bipolar or cyclothymic patients. Neuroleptic dopamine antagonists are being tested as euphoric blocking agents. Methylphenidate has not been found to be useful in those individuals abusing cocaine who do not have preexisting ADHD.

AMPHETAMINES

Amphetamines, or "speed," are compounds with stimulant and reinforcing effects similar to those of cocaine. Central stimulant drugs such as dextroamphetamine (Dexedrine) and methylphenidate (Ritalin) are manufactured for the treatment of medical conditions such as narcolepsy and ADHD. Illegal "black market" diversion and abuse peaked in the late 1960s. Because of more careful prescription of this drug class, legal use has declined.

The signs and symptoms of amphetamine use include tachycardia, elevated blood pressure, pupillary dilation, agitation, elation, loquacity, and hypervigilance. Adverse side effects may include insomnia, irritability, confusion, and hostility. Amphetamine psychosis can resemble acute paranoid schizophrenia, but visual hallucinations are common. As in cocaine use, binge episodes or runs may alternate with severe crash symptoms (Table 11–23).

Amphetamines block reuptake of dopamine, serotonin, and norepinephrine similarly to cocaine but produce more profound effects on dopamine storage release. Amphetamines share many similar signs, symptoms, and long-term sequelae with cocaine, but further work is needed to clarify the differences.

Amphetamine abuse may start in conjunction with weight-loss treatment, energy enhancement, or more serious intravenous use. Amphetamines abused intravenously can present with complications that are similar to those seen with intravenous cocaine and heroin abuse. Patients who use amphetamines daily or intravenously may require a period of inpatient hospitalization for depression, suicidal ideation during withdrawal, psychosis, or violence during intoxication. In suspected overdose, acidification of the urine may help with elimination. Antipsychotic medication such as haloperidol may be needed to treat paranoid or delusional symptoms. Rehabilitation should include a comprehensive treatment approach, as described in the alcohol and cocaine sections earlier in this chapter.

PHENCYCLIDINE ("ANGEL DUST")

Phencyclidine (PCP) is an anesthetic that was initially manufactured for use in animal surgery. Street use of PCP

TABLE 11–23. DSM-IV criteria for amphetamine (or a related substance) intoxication

A. Recent use of amphetamine or a related substance (e.g., methylphenidate).

B. Clinically significant maladaptive behavioral or psychological changes (e.g., euphoria or affective blunting; changes in sociability; hypervigilance; interpersonal sensitivity; anxiety, tension, or anger; stereotyped behaviors; impaired judgment; or impaired social or occupational functioning) that developed during, or shortly after, use of amphetamine or a related substance.

C. Two (or more) of the following, developing during, or shortly after, use of amphetamine or a related substance:

(1) Tachycardia or bradycardia
(2) Pupillary dilation
(3) Elevated or lowered blood pressure
(4) Perspiration or chills
(5) Nausea or vomiting
(6) Evidence of weight loss
(7) Psychomotor agitation or retardation
(8) Muscular weakness, respiratory depression, chest pain, or cardiac arrhythmias
(9) Confusion, seizures, dyskinesias, dystonias, or coma

D. The symptoms are not due to a general medical condition and are not better accounted for by another mental disorder.

Specify if:
With perceptual disturbances

first appeared in the 1960s and extended to widespread use in the 1970s. Phencyclidine abuse is still epidemic in certain urban areas of the eastern United States (Caracci et al. 1983). Street samples sold as PCP may vary greatly in dose and purity. Smoking marijuana cigarettes laced with PCP is the most common form of administration.

DEFINITION

Phencyclidine has been reported to be reinforcing in animals (Grinspoon and Bakalar 1986). Although the mechanism of action is unclear, PCP has been known to affect several neurotransmitters and to affect the σ opiate receptor. The DSM-IV definition of PCP abuse and dependence is defined as for other drugs (see Tables 11–1, 11–2, and 11–4 presented earlier in this chapter). Phencyclidine induces several organic mental disorders including intoxication, delirium, and delusional, mood, and flashback disorders.

ETIOLOGY

Phencyclidine abuse may occur in conjunction with multiple substance abuse and be associated with similar risk factors. Cases of pure PCP abuse have been reported. In our experience, these individuals appear to have significant psychopathology; however, it is difficult to distinguish drug effects from premorbid personality.

CLINICAL FEATURES

Psychoactive effects generally begin within 5 minutes and plateau at 30 minutes. Volatile emotional affects are the predominant behavioral presentation. Affects range from intense euphoria to anxiety, stereotypical repetitive behavior, and bizarre aggressive behavior. Violent murders have been attributed to complications of PCP abuse. Distorted perceptions, numbness, and confusion also are common. Physical signs include high blood pressure, muscle rigidity, ataxia, and, at higher dosages, hypothermia, involuntary movements, and coma. Rhabdomyolysis in overdoses may lead to acute renal failure. Dilated pupils and nystagmus, particularly vertical nystagmus, may heighten suspicion of use. With the unpredictability of the experience, it is difficult to explain the appeal of this substance in certain individuals. Chronic psychotic episodes are reported following use. In contrast to use of hallucinogens (see next section), use of PCP may lead to long-term neuropsychological deficits (Davis 1982).

TREATMENT

Acute adverse reactions generally require pharmacological adjuncts to control symptoms. Intravenous diazepam is the drug of first choice, but antipsychotics may occasionally be necessary as long as they are used with caution, because of the possibility of anticholinergic psychosis in unknown cases. When the diagnosis is unclear, other causes of delirium need to be considered. Because other supportive treatment may be necessary, treatment in a medical setting is preferred. Urine testing for PCP can remain positive for 7 days, and false negatives can occur. Phencyclidine elimination should be enhanced by ammonium chloride in the acute stage and by ascorbic acid or cranberry juice later on (Aronow et al. 1980).

HALLUCINOGENS

Hallucinogens were popular in the 1960s and 1970s for their psychoactive effects and because of the cultural setting at the time. The mind-expanding properties of psychedelics were romanticized and became a symbol for a cultural movement. The psychedelic psilocybin had long been used in religious ceremonies by Southwest Native American Indians. The synthetic drug lysergic acid diethylamide (LSD) is the psychedelic most available. New synthetic derivatives such as 3,4-methylenedioxyamphetamine (MDA) and 3,4-methylenedioxymethamphetamine (MDMA) have been promoted as "mood drugs" without the distracting perceptual changes (Grinspoon and Bakalar 1986; Kosten and Price 1992; Liester et al. 1992). Dangerous side effects such as parkinsonian syndromes have been reported. Psychedelics generally have been decreasing in popularity since 1979. In 1979, 7.1% of the 12- to 17-year-old age group and 25.1% of the 18- to 25-year-old age group had tried a psychedelic at least once. In 1982, the rates for these same age groups dropped to 5% and 21%, respectively (Miller 1983).

DEFINITION

Hallucinogens have not been reported to be reinforcing in animal studies. In humans, actual psychedelic use is infrequent, and psychedelic use greater than 20 times is considered chronic abuse. The DSM-IV definition of abuse and dependence is presented in Tables 11–1, 11–2, and 11–4. Hallucinogen intoxication (DSM-IV) is defined in Table 11–24. Other disorders included in DSM-IV are hallucinogen persisting perception disorder (flashbacks); hallucinogen delirium; hallucinogen psychotic disorder, with delusions; hallucinogen psychotic disorder, with hallucinations; hallucinogen mood disorder; hallucinogen anxiety disorder; and hallucinogen use disorder not otherwise specified.

CLINICAL FEATURES

LSD and related drugs produce changes in perception that vary greatly with setting and user's personality. Rather intense perceptual changes in time, space, and body image can occur. Illusions and pseudohallucinations, primarily visual, can predominate in conjunction with intense emotional or mystical experiences. Generally, overall reality testing and orientation are preserved.

Proposed mechanisms of action have centered on disrupted serotonin action on the raphe nucleus, producing a disinhibition of cerebral occipital and limbic structures. Physical signs of intoxication include increased heart rate, dilation of pupils, and sweating. Adverse experiences, or "bad trips," can present with marked anxiety or paranoia. The chance of a bad trip may be increased by emotional dis-

TABLE 11–24. DSM-IV criteria for hallucinogen intoxication

A. Recent use of a hallucinogen.

B. Clinically significant maladaptive behavioral or psychological changes (e.g., marked anxiety or depression, ideas of reference, fear of losing one's mind, paranoid ideation, impaired judgment, or impaired social or occupational functioning) that developed during, or shortly after, hallucinogen use.

C. Perceptual changes occurring in a state of full wakefulness and alertness (e.g., subjective intensification of perceptions, depersonalization, derealization, illusions, hallucinations, synesthesias) that developed during, or shortly after, hallucinogen use.

D. Two (or more) of the following signs, developing during, or shortly after, hallucinogen use:

(1) Pupillary dilation

(2) Tachycardia

(3) Sweating

(4) Palpitations

(5) Blurring of vision

(6) Tremors

(7) Incoordination

E. The symptoms are not due to a general medical condition and are not better accounted for by another mental disorder.

tress before use, reluctant use, or an aversive setting.

"Flashbacks" are psychedelic drug experiences that occur spontaneously in the absence of concurrent use. These may occur in as many as 25% of users (Naditch and Fenwick 1977). Large numbers of prior psychedelic experiences, marijuana smoking, and emotional stress are common precipitating factors.

CHRONIC ADVERSE PSYCHIATRIC EFFECTS

Chronic delusional and psychotic reactions, and rarely schizophreniform states, have been reported in a minority of persons who use psychedelics (Vardy and Kay 1983). In the vast majority of users, no characteristic personality is evident. Most use can be classified as experimental. Individuals who develop prolonged psychiatric syndromes tend to have schizophrenic susceptibility based on genetic or personality vulnerabilities. Clearly, psychedelics can precipitate psychotic episodes in vulnerable individuals.

TREATMENT

Generally, intoxicated patients can be "talked down" from frightening experiences in a quiet setting with minimal stimuli, stressing the time-limited extent of the drugs. Occasionally, diazepam is used as an adjunct, and rarely antipsychotics are needed in the case of marked disturbance.

CANNABIS

Cannabis sativa is an India hemp plant known to have been used for medicinal purposes since the third century B.C. in China. Marijuana is a varying mixture of the cannabis plant's leaves, seeds, stems, and flowering tops. It has been used recreationally throughout the world, and recently it is being bred to be more potent. Delta-9-tetrahydrocannabinol (THC), one of 60 cannabinoids, has been identified as the main psychoactive constituent of marijuana, which may contain 0.1%–10% THC (Turner 1980). Hashish preparations consist of the resin from the cannabis plant and contain a higher percentage of THC. Abuse of marijuana in the United States peaked in the 1960s and 1970s; controversy surrounds its medical and psychological risks.

DEFINITION

Three cannabis-related organic disorders are listed in DSM-IV: 1) cannabis intoxication, 2) cannabis delirium, and 3) cannabis delusional disorder. Definitions of cannabis abuse and dependence follow definitions of other psychoactive substances (see Tables 11–1, 11–2, 11–3, and 11–4). There is no cannabis withdrawal diagnosis in DSM-IV.

Based on case reports, withdrawal symptoms in persons who chronically use high doses of cannabis have included anxiety, dysphoria, insomnia, anorexia, tremulousness, and sweating. However, no stereotypical syndrome develops, and there is no specific DSM-III-R category for withdrawal from cannabis (Mendelson et al. 1984). Specific factors associated with marijuana abuse have been daily use, greater amounts of use, and problematic behavior.

EPIDEMIOLOGY

In 1979, more than 50 million people had used marijuana at least once. The number of regular marijuana users (i.e., once weekly or more) was estimated by the 1993 National Institute on Drug Abuse Household Survey to be 5.1 million (National Institute on Drug Abuse 1993). Alcohol, tobacco, and marijuana are the most frequent substances of abuse among adolescents. Adolescence and early adulthood are the peak ages of prevalence for marijuana abuse, and risk factors for this period have been most studied.

A 1982 NIDA survey revealed that 21% of young teenagers, 40% of young adults ages 18–25, and only 10% of older adults had tried marijuana (Miller 1983). It is generally acknowledged that marijuana use among adolescents peaked in the late 1970s, and, possibly because of less peer approval, regular marijuana use dropped from 51% to 42% between 1979 and 1983. Alarmingly, perceived danger about drug use dropped among high school students in the mid-1990s (Johnson et al. 1995). Prevention efforts have been aimed at the high school level, although risk factors in latency and at the junior high school level need to be addressed. Unfortunately, marijuana use for many teenagers may still be a rite of passage to adulthood.

CLINICAL FEATURES

Peak intoxication with smoking generally occurs after 10–30 minutes, when THC levels are maximal. Highly lipid soluble, THC and metabolites tend to accumulate in fat cells and have a half-life of approximately 50 hours. Most marijuana cigarettes (i.e., "joints") contain 5–20 mg of THC (Jaffe 1980). Intoxication usually lasts from 2 to 4 hours depending on the dose used; however, behavioral and psychomotor impairment may continue several hours longer.

The interaction of drug and setting of use appears to have a considerable influence on the psychoactive effects of the drug. Inexperienced and first-time users may not experience a marked change in subjective state (i.e., the "high"), even if they smoke correctly (Weil et al. 1968). Marijuana users may have to learn to appreciate the subtle psychoactive effects most associated with intoxication. Chronic users conversely may learn to suppress undesirable behavioral responses with long-term exposure. Intoxication generally involves characteristic physiological, behavioral, subjective, and neuropsychological findings.

Intoxication can produce many subjective psychoactive effects that become the "high" experience repeatedly sought (Halikas et al. 1971). Persons who use marijuana experience slowed time; increased appetite; increased thirst; a keener sense of color, sound, pattern, textures, and tastes; euphoria; heightened introspection; ability to be absorbed in sensual experiences; feelings of relaxation and floating; and increased self-confidence. Other subjective symptoms include heightened sexual desire, transitory illusions, hallucinations, and increased interpersonal sensitivity. Conjunctivitis (i.e., red eyes), strong odor, dilated pupils, tachycardia, dry mouth, and coughing are physical signs of immediate use.

Adverse effects such as mild anxiety, depression, and paranoia are infrequently treated in a medical setting and usually are not a deterrent to further use. Behavior may be marked by passivity and sedation or by hyperactivity and marked hilarity.

Numerous studies have outlined the neuropsychological changes and deficits related to marijuana intoxication, although effects can be highly variable. Decreases have been found in complex reaction time and digit code memory tasks, concept formation, memory, tactile form discrimination, motor function, time estimation, and the ability to track information over time (Clark and Nakashima 1968; Klonoff et al. 1973; Melges 1976). In one study, 33% of reckless drivers intoxicated with alcohol also were positive for marijuana (Brookoff et al. 1994). Psychosis, derealization, and aggression have been described to occur rarely. Weller and Halikas (1985) followed 97 persons who regularly used marijuana over a 5- to 6-year period. Continued use was associated with a decrease in pleasurable effects. Undesirable effects persisted, but decreases were found in tachycardia, dry mouth, and lightheadedness. Numerous studies have demonstrated that marijuana intoxication impairs automobile driving, airplane flying, and other complex skilled activities through impaired attention span, motor coordination, and depth perception for up to 10 hours or more after use.

In school, jobs, or any situation in which clarity of mind is required, marijuana may have detrimental effects. Even after acute intoxication effects recede, a morning "hangover" may interfere with functioning. Ability to speak coherently, form concepts, concentrate, and transfer material from immediate to long-term memory is impaired. EEG studies have had inconsistent findings of both a decrease and an increase in alpha rhythm patterns (Low et al. 1973). Milder symptoms of anxiety, confusion, fear, and increased dependency can progress to panic and paranoid symptomatology and depressive reactions. Personality, past experience with the drug, and setting can alter the experience dramatically, although higher doses of THC will increase the chance of toxic reactions.

THC-induced acute toxic psychosis has been described in first-time users and chronic users and may include organic features or persist in a clear consciousness (Spencer 1970; Talbott and Teague 1969; Weil 1970). Psychosis can present suddenly with first-rank Schneiderian symptoms, agitation, and amnesia for toxic events. Thacore and Shukla (1976) found that, compared with paranoid schizophrenia, cannabis psychosis is characterized by agitation, violence, flight of ideas, and less thought disorder. Prolonged psychotic episodes may herald residual psychopathology. Cannabis can precipitate "flashbacks" or psychotic experiences from past psychedelic or marijuana experiences.

Several authors have warned about marijuana use in preexisting psychiatric disorders. Treffert (1978) identified marijuana as the independent variable for psychosis in previously well-controlled schizophrenic individuals over time. Melges (1976) proposed that paranoid ideation induced by marijuana use may be a product of loss of information tracking about the environment, which prompts paranoid ideas to fill in the gaps in order to decrease the threat of loss of control. This process may be magnified with schizophrenia.

Differential diagnosis of cannabis psychosis and schizophrenia can be difficult; however, assessment of past history, urine testing, and the short-lived nature of toxic symptoms usually help in making the diagnosis. Millman and Sbriglio (1986) suggest that by attributing their symptoms to marijuana abuse, some schizophrenic individuals may distance themselves from their underlying illness. In summary, marijuana use should be especially cautioned in individuals prone to psychotic illness.

ETIOLOGY

Studies on the etiology of marijuana abuse have tended to focus on adolescent developmental issues and have not found simple generalizable factors. Kandel and Faust's (1975) longitudinal studies of drug use progression found that teenage use of liquor and cigarettes is associated with the highest rates of future marijuana abuse. The temporal order between alcohol and marijuana may be stronger than that between tobacco and marijuana. Marijuana use was found to be a key stepping-stone to other illicit drugs, and progression to harder drugs was directly related to the intensity of marijuana use. Recently, adolescents have increasingly proceeded to using cocaine without extensive marijuana use. Experimentation with marijuana may not have produced warned adverse effects, and adolescents may be less fearful of experimentation with other drugs. Marijuana introduces youth to drug subcultures and lowers inhibition to use of other drugs. Peer drug use, parents' substance use, and low parental monitoring are risk factors for marijuana abuse. Delinquency is a risk factor for abuse of marijuana and other substances; however, peer group choice is usually with other drug-using individuals more so than with delinquent persons. Marijuana abuse frequently starts in junior high school. Difficulty or boredom in school may contribute to its use with friends as a social alternative.

The myth that adolescence is a "time-limited psychosis" has recently given way to the recognition that for the majority of adolescents this is not a period of marked turbulence or marked parental rejection. Rebelliousness, depression, poor school performance, and self-destructive acts may be a sign of underlying disturbance. Depression in marijuana-using adolescents may be a further risk factor for progression to other drugs. Some adolescents may use marijuana to avoid normal conflict resolution. Teenagers who abuse marijuana frequently have loss of communication with family, with erratic mood changes, deterioration in moral values, apathy, change in friends, truancy, academic underachievement, denial of use even when found with drug paraphernalia, and obvious signs of intoxication (Niven 1986). Kandel (1984) suggests that marijuana use in young adulthood is associated with a social context favorable to its use and with disaffection from social institutions. High-risk factors may operate independent of personality.

PSYCHOPATHOLOGY

Psychopathology in individuals prior to marijuana abuse has been difficult to assess. Curiosity and conformity are principal reasons for starting, although a desire for a marked change in consciousness may be associated with continued marijuana use. Some writers have argued for a specific antirage or antianxiety effect of marijuana, whereas others report high incidences of aggression in chronic abusers. Marijuana has a sedating effect and may be used as a "self-medication" by anxious individuals. It can potentiate other CNS depressants such as alcohol and increase cognitive deficit. Linn (1972) suggests that an introspective psychological orientation may make marijuana appealing to certain individuals. Weller and Halikas (1985) found that, compared with control subjects, persons using marijuana exhibited more antisocial personality but no other significant differences in psychopathology. Cannabis can be a trigger for relapse in schizophrenia (Linszen et al. 1994).

Physiological explanations of marijuana effects have ranged from a hypothesis concerning a shift in hemispheric dominance from left to right brain, to disinhibition of paleocortex limbic-lobe primitive brain functions (Cohen 1986). THC may act to alter the normal functional relationship between the limbic system and the neocortex. Specific EEG changes have been found in the septal regions during marijuana intoxication. PET scans and other dynamic brain studies may help determine marijuana brain effects.

PATHOPHYSIOLOGY AND ADVERSE PHYSICAL EFFECTS

The exact physiological action of marijuana is not known; however, several biochemical findings have been reported.

THC has been noted to affect synthesis of proteins and nucleic acids, disrupting cell metabolism and DNA/RNA formation (Nahas 1977). In vitro studies have reported abnormal cell division and abnormal spermatogenesis, resulting in decreased sperm counts. High THC exposure has been associated with birth and reproductive abnormalities in animals, and decreases in female sexual and reproductive hormones have been found in humans. However, marijuana's effect on human male or female fertility remains controversial.

The report of the National Academy of Sciences, Institute of Medicine, Committee to Study the Health-Related Effects of Cannabis and Its Derivatives (1982) on the long-term effects of marijuana was inconclusive. There was no convincing evidence that marijuana produces permanent changes in the CNS or in behavior. Patients with underlying cardiovascular disease may not tolerate the increased heart rate and blood pressure that marijuana causes. Marijuana may have a mild immunosuppressant effect. Cannabis smoke contains carcinogens similar to those in tobacco smoke, and chronic heavy marijuana use may predispose to chronic obstructive lung disease or pulmonary neoplasm.

Controversy has surrounded the concept of a chronic cannabis behavioral syndrome. Much of this work was done in Jamaica, India, and Egypt, where heavy, chronic use of powerful cannabis derivatives was studied. Classically, this "amotivational syndrome" is characterized by passivity, decreased drive, diminished goal-directed activity, decreased memory, fatigue, problem-solving deficits, and apathy, and is described as a "fog" that lasts several weeks after abstinence. A recent study conducted in Costa Rica found long-term cannabis use was associated with disruption of short-term memory, working memory, and attentional skills in older long-term users (Fletcher et al. 1996). Heavy marijuana use is associated with residual cognitive deficits in college students 24 hours later (Pope et al. 1996).

Amotivational syndrome research has been plagued by methodological problems including selection bias and lack of controls. It is very difficult to determine predating personality factors and the effects of oppressive environmental factors. Similar findings in chronic marijuana users in the United States have been described, although a full-blown amotivational syndrome has not been clearly established. Kupfer et al. (1973) compared chronic heavy and light marijuana smokers and found no overall increase in psychopathology, although depressive features and organicity were found to be increased in both groups. One hypothesis is that the subset of amotivational patients in both groups may have had underlying depressive tendencies. A spectrum of cognitive and behavioral difficulty may result secondarily to long-term cannabis abuse. Apathy and lack of motivation in these patients may represent one pole of the spectrum and may be the result of multiple factors (Millman and Sbriglio 1986).

THERAPEUTIC POTENTIAL

THC has been used in medical settings to combat nausea and vomiting, mainly in association with cancer chemotherapy agents and in glaucoma. Bronchodilation, anticonvulsant, and antispasmatic effects have also been reported but not proved (Cohen 1986). THC has been reported to decrease intraocular pressure by 30% in normal subjects, which makes it a useful agent in patients with glaucoma. However, lifelong use is often necessary, which exposes patients to long-term THC health hazards. Despite recent press and resolution that passed in California that marijuana can be used for medicinal purposes, the NIH says more study is needed to assess marijuana's medicinal uses (Medical News and Perspectives 1997).

TREATMENT

Acute Treatment

Usually adverse effects of marijuana intoxication do not lead to professional attention. Support, reassurance, and reality testing by friends or family usually suffice. Physical symptoms such as tachycardia may contribute to a "fight-or-flight syndrome." Pointing out that marijuana can cause these symptoms and reassurance that they will pass usually helps these individuals. Anxiolytic agents occasionally are needed, and neuroleptics can be used in cases of protracted psychosis.

Treatment of Chronic Use

The treatment of marijuana abuse follows the general principles for that of other substance abuse, with special attention to developmental issues affecting adolescence. Marijuana may be one of many drugs abused, and total abstinence from all psychoactive substances is the goal.

Interventions need to be made early in adolescent drug careers, as severe disruption in developmental milestones occur. Complete psychiatric evaluation includes a school and family assessment. Denial of health and psychological risks often needs to be confronted, especially in patients forced into treatment. Many times it is not until the patient stops using the drug and notices the cognitive improvement that self-motivation ensues. Lifestyle changes such as avoiding those persons, places, and things related to use should be encouraged. Poor self-esteem, depression, severe family problems, and learning disorders may emerge and need to be addressed. Parental counseling may be very effective in resolving disturbed family interaction and boundary issues. In very young teenagers, involvement, concern, and control by parents have a strong influence on behavior. Several years later, parental influence may wane and peer-group identification may increase.

Inpatient Treatment

Pure marijuana abuse rarely requires inpatient treatment, and detoxification is not necessary. Occasionally with severe abuse or behavioral problems, especially in teenage populations, inpatient intervention is needed.

Outpatient Treatment

Outpatient treatment consists of self-help 12-step groups, group and individual therapy, family therapy, and periodic urine testing to monitor abstinence. Adolescent drug programs may concentrate on promoting age-related behavior and increasing communication through various verbal and nonverbal modalities. Families need to become aware of how they can help or hurt the treatment process. Generally, a nonjudgmental, honest, steady, and firm approach is needed with adolescents.

Cannabinoids can be detected in the urine up to 21 days after abstinence in chronic abusers due to fat redistribution; however, 1–5 days is the normal urine positive period (Schwartz and Hawks 1986). Thus, beginning drug monitoring needs to be interpreted accordingly. The primary method for urinalysis detection is enzyme immunoassay or radioimmunoassay. This method is quick, relatively inexpensive, and fairly accurate (95% level). Chromatography studies are more expensive but increase sensitivity and specificity. Only blood samples can be used as indicators of acute levels of intoxication. Unless assays are standardized across laboratories, results can be variable.

NICOTINE

Tobacco addiction is the number one preventable health problem in the United States. Awareness of the health risk factors associated with tobacco use has existed since the 1950s. Tobacco companies have been pressured into admitting medical consequences and addiction potential of tobacco products. A deal is presently in discussion to have the tobacco companies settle with states for medical costs of care. Despite the attempts of educational campaigns, self-help groups, self-help literature, treatment facilities, and governmental legislation to decrease the numbers of smokers, tobacco addiction remains a significant but scientifically neglected area of research and treatment.

DEFINITION

Starting with DSM-III and continuing with DSM-IV, tobacco has been listed under psychoactive substance use disorders. Tobacco's main psychoactive substance is nicotine. Nicotine is a psychoactive substance as evidenced by euphoric effects and by placebo and positive reinforcement properties similar to those of cocaine and opiates (Henningfield 1984). Tolerance develops to the effects of nicotine, and mild withdrawal syndromes have been described. Hughes and Hatsukami (1986) tested the signs and symptoms of DSM-III tobacco withdrawal criteria for validity, magnitude, and clinical significance. Craving for tobacco, irritability, anxiety, difficulty concentrating, and restlessness were validated. Decreased heart rate, increased eating, increased sleep disturbance, and decreased alcohol intake were also found. Subjects with higher nicotine tolerance had more withdrawal discomfort, and nicotine withdrawal symptoms simulated a "rebound" nicotine effect.

EPIDEMIOLOGY

Approximately 60 million Americans smoke tobacco, and $23 billion yearly is spent on its use. Cigarette sales, curiously, have been a direct revenue generator for government. For example in 1980, tobacco sales yielded $8 billion a year in tax revenues. In the United States, cigarette use among men has decreased to approximately 35% and increased in women to 30%. The biggest drop in cigarette smoking has been in the higher socioeconomic groups. Negative publicity and legal threats have moved the tobacco industry to curb marketing to teenagers and away from dependency on tobacco profits in this country. Cigarette smoking is the chief preventable cause of cancer in the United States and is responsible for 30% of cancers (Centers for Disease Control and Prevention 1993).

ETIOLOGY

Cigarette smoking generally begins in the teenage years and may be associated with peer tobacco use, parental tobacco use, and other substance abuse. Individuals may smoke for a period of time, attempt to quit, and then relapse. Tobacco addiction has many properties that are similar to those of opioid addiction. There is great similarity between cigarettes, alcoholism, and opioids in the temporal pattern of relapse, and circumstantial evidence suggests that tobacco use is usually an addictive form of behavior. High stress, poor social support, maladjustment, anxiety, and low self-confidence have been associated with poor treatment outcome, and these factors may play a part in promoting continued use. Psychological characteristics such as extraversion, anxiety, and anger have been proposed to be associated with tobacco use. However, individuals in more intensive treatment facilities may be more recalcitrant smokers and present with less overall adjustment. There is a strong association between alcohol and smoking, especially in women and alcoholic persons.

CLINICAL FEATURES

Tobacco use can produce a calming, euphoric effect on chronic users, more characteristic after a period of tobacco deprivation. Acute nicotine poisoning consists of nausea, salivation, abdominal pain, vomiting, diarrhea, headaches, dizziness, and a cold sweat. Inability to concentrate, confusion, and tachycardia may also result.

ADVERSE MEDICAL SEQUELAE

There are well-known associations between tobacco use and chronic obstructive lung disease, lung cancer, stroke, cardiovascular disease, oral cancers, and hypertension. Tobacco use may complicate prescribed psychiatric medication by increasing liver drug metabolism and lowering neuroleptic and antidepressant levels. The combination of cocaine and cigarette smoking may promote coronary-artery vasoconstriction and have a marked deleterious effect on myocardial oxygen supply (Moliterno et al. 1994). Low birth weight has been associated with smoking in pregnant mothers. This information has led to a decrease in smoking in pregnant women.

TREATMENT

Various treatment approaches, including behavioral, cognitive, educational, self-help, and pharmacological, have been applied to tobacco addiction. Yet the vast majority (95%) of abstainers receive no formal intervention, and research is needed to clarify how and why these individuals ceased use. Tunstall et al. (1985) reviewed factors that influenced treatment outcome. Environmental stress; poor social support, including having family members who continue to smoke; lack of exposure to educational information; being female; poor overall adjustment; low self-confidence; poor motivation; and high pretreatment cotinine (a metabolite of nicotine) levels were associated with poor long-term outcome. Numerous studies have highlighted the genetic and clinical treatment implications of the association between depressive disorders and nicotine dependence (Breslau et al. 1992; Covey et al. 1997; Fergusson et al. 1996; Glassman 1993; Kendler et al. 1993). Major depression and smoking tends to be genetically linked in women. Major depression can be a relapse risk for smoking and may be more prevalent in vulnerable ex-smokers.

It is evident that public information campaigns have had some impact on cigarette use. Decreased tolerance in society and legislation may be intervening variables. Self-help books are best received in the context of therapist intervention. Self-help groups, primary physician involvement, and contingency contracting may also be useful. In individuals with higher tobacco use, poor social adjustment, and other substance abuse, more intensive treatment programs should be available. Overall, intensive treatment generally produces better results. Intensive programs may borrow successful treatment techniques from other substance abuse programs.

The Agency for Health Care Policy and Research has issued a recent clinical practice guideline for physicians to perform smoking cessation interventions in their offices (Agency for Health Care Policy and Research Consensus Statement 1996). The guideline—in which all English-language, peer-reviewed literature on the treatment of nicotine addiction was reviewed—provides recommendations for primary care doctors to feel comfortable and knowledgeable with office-based smoking cessation. It reviews the optimal number and length of smoking cessation sessions for specialists and recommends strategies for health care administrators to better identify users. Disseminating educational information regarding smoking cessation to medical students and trainees is also crucial.

Nicotine gum is a pharmacological substitution approach in which smoking behavior is interrupted while blood levels of nicotine are maintained to minimize withdrawal (Raw 1985). Three-month success rates of 76% and 1-year success rates of 50% have been reported. Effectiveness is maximized with therapeutic contact. However, considerable relapse after gum use is terminated has been found (Hall et al. 1985). Hypnosis, rapid smoking, or aversive treatment and nicotine blockade with mecamylamine are other alternative treatments. The 1-year postintervention effectiveness of most intensive smoking cessation programs is between 25% to 40%, which roughly parallels the postintervention effectiveness of programs for other substance abuse.

Nicotine patches are now available over the counter.

Fiore et al. (1994) conducted a meta-analysis of the double-blind randomized controlled trials of 4-week duration or longer. The abstinence rates were 27% for the active patch versus 13% for placebo patch during treatment; and 22% and 9% at 6 months. These findings suggest that at least in experimental settings a nicotine patch roughly doubles the chance of quitting. This general trend seems to hold true even without behavioral counseling, although behavioral counseling improves quit rates.

The FDA in 1997 approved the use of Wellbutrin sustained release capsules (Zyban) for smoking cessation. Data presented to the FDA suggested that Wellbutrin was at least equal to the patch as an aid for smoking cessation and is well tolerated. Wellbutrin may be particularly useful for patients with depression and smoking in cardiac settings. The most serious potential side effect is seizures, which is minimal if the dose is kept below 300 mg. Nicotine inhalers have demonstrated similar success and may play a role for individuals who need to do something with their hands.

INHALANTS

Inhalants include substances with diverse chemical structures such as gasoline, airplane glue, aerosol (spray paints), lighter fluid, fingernail polish remover, typewriter fluid, a variety of cleaners, amyl and butyl nitrates, and nitrous oxide. Hydrocarbons are the most active ingredients. In 1980, 10% of 12- to 17-year-olds had reported using inhalants at least once, but the vast majority did not report abuse patterns (National Institute on Drug Abuse 1981). The definition of inhalant intoxication is presented in Table 11–25.

The majority of people who use inhalants are socioeconomically deprived young males ages 13–15 years (Watson 1980). A high prevalence of abuse is found among Native American and Mexican Indians (Reed and May 1984). Amyl nitrate use was popular in the 1970s in a subset of the homosexual community, and nitrous oxide abuse may be predominant among health personnel with easy access, such as dentists. Typical signs and symptoms of intoxication may include grandiosity, a sense of invulnerability, immense strength, euphoria, slurred speech, and ataxia. Visual distortions and faulty space perception are also common.

There is a fairly strong association between aggressive, disruptive, and antisocial behavior and inhalant intoxication. Inhalants are usually easily and cheaply obtained and can be inhaled from a variety of containers. Intoxication

TABLE 11–25. DSM-IV criteria for inhalant intoxication

A. Recent intentional use or short-term, high-dose exposure to volatile inhalants (excluding anesthetic cases and short-acting vasodilators).

B. Clinically significant maladaptive behavioral or psychological changes (e.g., belligerence, assaultiveness, apathy, impaired judgment, impaired social or occupational functioning) that developed during, or shortly after, use of or exposure to volatile inhalants.

C. Two (or more) of the following signs, developing during, or shortly after, inhalant use or exposure:

    (1) Dizziness

    (2) Nystagmus

    (3) Incoordination

    (4) Slurred speech

    (5) Unsteady gait

    (6) Lethargy

    (7) Depressed reflexes

    (8) Psychomotor retardation

    (9) Tremor

    (10) Generalized muscle weakness

    (11) Blurred vision or diplopia

    (12) Stupor or coma

    (13) Euphoria

D. The symptoms are not due to a general medical condition and are not better accounted for by another mental disorder.

can last from a few minutes up to 2 hours. Impaired judgment, poor insight, violence, and psychosis may be psychological sequelae (Cohen 1984). Inhalant abuse among adolescents has been associated with arrests, poor performance in school, increased family disruption, and other drug abuse (Santos de Barona and Simpson 1984). Deaths have been reported from central respiratory depression, cardiac arrhythmia, and accidents (King et al. 1985). Long-term damage to bone marrow, kidneys, liver, neuromusculature, and brain has also been reported. The course of inhalant abuse is unclear. Incidence reports suggest that inhalants are primarily abused in youths who may move on to other substances in later life.

CONCLUSIONS

Psychoactive substance use disorders are major public health problems that are frequently underdiagnosed and undertreated. Increased public awareness is leading to promising efforts at locating high-risk populations, providing early treatment, designing effective social policies aimed at prevention, and improving differential therapeutics. Solutions to the myriad physiological, cultural, and psychological intervening variables that contribute to substance use and dependence are unlikely to be fast in coming, and there are likely to be changing patterns of use of old and new substances.

REFERENCES

Abel E, Sokol R: A revised conservative estimate of the incidence of FAS and its economic impact. Alcohol Clin Exp Res 15:514–524, 1991

Adams RD, Victor M: Principles of Neurology. New York, McGraw-Hill, 1981

Adinoff B, Martin PR, Bone GHA, et al: Hypothalamic-pituitary-adrenal axis functioning and cerebrospinal fluid corticotropin releasing hormone and corticotropin levels in alcoholics after recent and long-term abstinence. Arch Gen Psychiatry 47:325–330, 1990

Adinoff B, Risher-Flowers D, De Jong J, et al: Disturbances of hypothalamic-pituitary-adrenal axis functioning during ethanol withdrawal in six men. Am J Psychiatry 148:1023–1025, 1991

Alexopoulos GS, Lieberman KW, Frances RJ: Platelet MAO activity in alcoholic patients and their first-degree relatives. Am J Psychiatry 140:1501–1504, 1983

Allen JP, Litten RZ, Anton RF, et al: Carbohydrate-deficient transferrin as a measure of immoderate drinking: remaining issue. Alcohol Clin Exp Res 18:799–812, 1994

Allen JP, Litten RZ, Fertig JB, et al: A review of research on the Alcohol Use Disorders Identification Test (AUDIT). Alcohol Clin Exp Res 21:613–619, 1997

Allgulander CS, Borg S, Vikander B: A 4–6-year follow-up of 30 patients with primary dependence on sedative and hypnotic drugs. Am J Psychiatry 141:1580–1582, 1984

Allgulander CS, Ljungberg L, Fisher LD: Long-term prognosis in addiction on sedative and hypnotic drugs analyzed with the Cox regression model. Acta Psychiatr Scand 75:521–531, 1987

Alterman AI, Cacciola JS: The antisocial personality disorder diagnosis in substance abusers: problems and issues. J Nerv Ment Dis 179:401–409, 1991

American Psychiatric Association: Diagnostic and Statistical Manual of Mental Disorders, 3rd Edition. Washington, DC, American Psychiatric Association, 1980

American Psychiatric Association: Diagnostic and Statistical Manual of Mental Disorders, 3rd Edition, Revised. Washington, DC, American Psychiatric Association, 1987

American Psychiatric Association: Diagnostic and Statistical Manual of Mental Disorders, 4th Edition. Washington, DC, American Psychiatric Association, 1994

Anker AL, Crowly TJ: Use of contingency contracting in specialty clinics for cocaine abuse, in Problems of Drug Dependence 1981 (NIDA Drug Res Monogr No 41). Edited by Harris LS. Rockville, MD, National Institute on Drug Abuse, 1982, pp 452–459

Anthenelli RM, Smith TL, Irwin MR, et al: A comparative study of criteria for subgrouping alcoholics: the primary/secondary diagnostic scheme versus variations of the type 1/type 2 criteria. Am J Psychiatry 151:1468–1474, 1994

Anton RF, Moak DH, Latham P: Carbohydrate-deficient transferrin as an indicator of drinking status during a treatment outcome study. Alcohol Clin Exp Res 20:841–846, 1996

Aronow R, Miceli JN, Done AK: A therapeutic approach to the acutely overdosed PCP patient. J Psychoactive Drugs 12:259–267, 1980

Ausubel DP: Methadone maintenance treatment: the other side of the coin. International Journal of Addictions 18: 851–862, 1983

Babor TF, Grant M: Programme on Substance Abuse: Project on Identification and Management of Alcohol-Related Problems. Report on Phase II: A Randomized Clinical Trial of Brief Interventions in Primary Health Care. Geneva, World Health Organization, 1992

Babor TF, Hofmann M, DelBoca FK, et al: Types of alcoholics, I: evidence for an empirically derived typology based on indicators of vulnerability and severity. Arch Gen Psychiatry 49:599–608, 1992

Bachman JG, Johnston LD, O'Malley PM: Explaining the recent decline in cocaine use among young adults: further evidence that perceived risks and disapproval lead to reduced drug use. J Health Soc Behav 31:173–184, 1990

Baumgartner GR, Rowen RC: Transdermal clonidine versus chlordiazepoxide in alcohol withdrawal: a randomized, controlled clinical trial. South Med J 84:312–321, 1991

Belle SH, Beringer KC, Detre KM: Liver transplantation for alcoholic liver disease in the United States: 1988 to 1995. Liver Transpl Surg 3:212–219, 1997

Bergman H, Borg S, Holin L: Neuropsychological impairment and exclusive abuse of sedatives or hypnotics. Am J Psychiatry 137:215–217, 1980

Blass JP, Gibson GE: Abnormality of a thiamine-requiring enzyme in patients with Wernicke-Korsakoff syndrome. N Engl J Med 297:1367–1370, 1977

Blatt SJ, Berman W, Bloom-Feshbach S, et al: Psychological assessment of psychopathology in opiate addicts. J Nerv Ment Dis 172:156–165, 1984

Blazer D, George LK, Landerman R, et al: Psychiatric disorders: a rural/urban comparison. Arch Gen Psychiatry 42:651–656, 1985

Blum K, Noble EP, Sheridan PJ, et al: Allelic association of human dopamine D$_2$ receptor gene in alcoholism. JAMA 263:2055–2060, 1990

Bohman M, Cloninger CR, Sigvardsson S, et al: The genetics of alcoholism and related disorders. J Psychiatr Res 21:447–452, 1987

Bolos AM, Dean M, Lucas-Derse S, et al: Population and pedigree studies reveal a lack of association between the dopamine D$_2$ receptor gene and alcoholism. JAMA 264:3156–3160, 1990

Booth BM, Blow FC: The kindling hypothesis: further evidence from a U.S. national study of alcoholic men. Alcohol Alcohol 28:593–598, 1993

Brady K, Anton R, Ballenger JC, et al: Cocaine abuse among schizophrenic patients. Am J Psychiatry 147:1164–1167, 1990

Brehm N, Khantzian EJ, Dodes LM: Recent developments in alcoholism: psychodynamic approaches. Recent Dev Alcohol 11:453–471, 1993

Breslau N, Kilbey M, Andereski P: Nicotine withdrawal symptoms and psychiatric disorders: findings from an epidemiologic study of young adults. Am J Psychiatry 149:464–469, 1992

Brew BJ: Diagnosis of Wernicke's encephalopathy. Aust N Z J Med 16:676–678, 1986

Brewer RD, Morris PD, Cole TB, et al: The risk of dying in alcohol-related automobile crashes among habitual drunk drivers. N Engl J Med 331:513–517, 1994

Brookoff D, Cook CL, Williams CL, et al: Testing reckless drivers for cocaine and marijuana. N Engl J Med 331:518–22, 1994

Brooner RK, Schmidt CW, Felch LJ, et al: Antisocial behavior of intravenous drug abusers: implications for diagnosis of antisocial personality disorder. Am J Psychiatry 149: 482–487, 1992

Brooner RK, King VL, Kidorf M, et al: Psychiatric and substance use comorbidity among treatment-seeking opioid abusers. Arch Gen Psychiatry 54:71–80, 1997

Brown BS, Watters JK, Iglehart AS: Methadone maintenance dosage levels and program retention. Am J Drug Alcohol Abuse 9:129–139, 1982

Brown SA, Inaba RK, Gillin JC, et al: Alcoholism and affective disorder: clinical course of depressive symptoms. Am J Psychiatry 152:45–52, 1995

Buydens-Branchey L, Branchey MH, Noumair D, et al: Age of alcoholism onset, II: relationship to susceptibility to serotonin precursor availability. Arch Gen Psychiatry 46:231–236, 1989

Bystritsky A, Ackerman DL, Pasnau RO: Low dose desipramine treatment of cocaine-related panic attacks. J Nerv Ment Dis 179:755–758, 1991

Cacciola J, Rutherford MJ, Alterman A, et al: An examination of the diagnostic criteria for antisocial personality disorder in substance abusers. J Nerv Ment Dis 182:517–523, 1994

Cadoret RJ, Yates WR, Troughton E, et al: Adoption study demonstrating two genetic pathways to drug abuse. Arch Gen Psychiatry 52:42–52, 1995

Caetano R, Schafer J: DSM-IV alcohol dependence in a treatment sample of white, black, and Mexican-American men. Alcohol Clin Exp Res 20:384–390, 1996

Calsyn DA, Saxon AJ, Barndt DC: Urine screening practices in methadone maintenance clinics: a survey of how the results are used. J Nerv Ment Dis 179:222–227, 1991

Caracci L, Migone P, Dornbush R: Phencyclidine in an East Harlem psychiatric population. J Natl Med Assoc 75:869–874, 1983

Carroll KM, Rounsaville BJ: Contrast of treatment-seeking and untreated cocaine abusers. Arch Gen Psychiatry 49:464–471, 1992

Carroll KM, Rounsaville BJ, Gawin FH: A comparative trial of psychotherapies for ambulatory cocaine abusers: relapse prevention and interpersonal psychotherapy. Am J Drug Alcohol Abuse 17:229–247, 1991a

Carroll KM, Rounsaville FJ, Keller DS: Relapse prevention strategies for the treatment of cocaine abuse. Am J Drug Alcohol Abuse 17:249–265, 1991b

Carroll KM, Rounsaville BJ, Nich C, et al: One-year follow-up of psychotherapy and pharmacotherapy for cocaine dependence. Arch Gen Psychiatry 51:989–990, 1994

Centers for Disease Control and Prevention: Cigarette smoking: attributable mortality and years of potential life lost—United States, 1990. MMWR Morb Mortal Wkly Rep 42:645–649, 1993

Chadwick MJ, Gregory DL, Wendling G: A double-blind amino acids, L-tryptophan and L-tyrosine, and placebo study with cocaine-dependent subjects in an inpatient chemical dependency treatment center. Am J Drug Alcohol Abuse 16:275–286, 1990

Charney DS, Sternberg DE, Kleber HD, et al: The clinical use of clonidine in abrupt withdrawal from methadone: effects on blood pressure and specific signs and symptoms. Arch Gen Psychiatry 38:1273–1277, 1981

Charney DS, Redmond E, Galloway MP: Naltrexone precipitated opiate withdrawal in methadone addicted human subjects: evidence for noradrenergic hyperactivity. Life Sci 35:1263–1272, 1984

Chasnoff IJ, Burns WJ, Schnoll SH: Cocaine use in pregnancy. N Engl J Med 313:666–669, 1985

Chedid A, Mendenhall CL, Gartside P, et al: Prognostic factors in alcoholic liver disease: VA Cooperative Study Group. Am J Gastroenterol 86:210–216, 1991

Chou SP, Grant BF, Dawson DA: Medical consequences of alcohol consumption—United States, 1992. Alcohol Clin Exp Res 20:1423–1429, 1996

Ciraulo DA, Barnhill JG, Ciraulo AM: Parental alcoholism as a risk factor in benzodiazepine abuse: a pilot study. Am J Psychiatry 146:1333–1335, 1989

Ciraulo DA, Sarid-Segal O, Knapp C, et al: Liability to alprazolam abuse in daughters of alcoholics. Am J Psychiatry 153:956–958, 1996

Clark LD, Nakashima EN: Experimental studies of marijuana. Am J Psychiatry 125:379–384, 1968

Cloninger RC, Reich T, Wetzel R: Alcoholism and affective disorders: familial associations and genetic models, in Alcoholism and Affective Disorders. Edited by Goodwin DW, Erickson CK. Jamaica, NY, Spectrum, 1979, pp 57–86

Cohen MJ, Schandler SL, Naliboff BD: Psychophysiological measures from intoxicated and detoxified alcoholics. J Stud Alcohol 44:271–282, 1983

Cohen S: The hallucinogens and the inhalants. Psychiatr Clin North Am 7:681–688, 1984

Cohen S: Marijuana, in Psychiatry Update: American Psychiatric Association Annual Review, Vol 5. Edited by Frances AJ, Hales RE. Washington, DC, American Psychiatric Press, 1986, pp 200–211

Collins JJ (ed): Drinking and Crime. New York, Guilford, 1991

Cornelius JR, Salloum IM, Mezzich J, et al: Disproportionate suicidality in patients with comorbid major depression and alcoholism. Am J Psychiatry 152:358–364, 1995

Cornelius JR, Salloum IM, Ehler JG, et al: Fluoxetine in depressed alcoholics. Arch Gen Psychiatry 54:700–705, 1997

Cottrell D, Childs-Clarke A, Ghodse AH: British opiate addicts: an 11-year follow-up. Br J Psychiatry 146:448–450, 1985

Covey LS, Glassman AH, Stetner F: Major depression following smoking cessation. Am J Psychiatry 154:263–265, 1997

Crits-Christoph P, Siqueland L: Psychosocial treatment for drug abuse. Arch Gen Psychiatry 53:749–756, 1996

Crits-Christoph P, Siqueland L, Blaine J, et al: The National Institute on Drug Abuse Collaborative Cocaine Treatment Study. Arch Gen Psychiatry 54:721–726, 1997

Croop RS, Faulkner EB, Labriola DF: The safety profile of naltrexone in the treatment of alcoholism. Arch Gen Psychiatry 54:1130–1135, 1997

Crowley TJ, Wagner JE, Zerbe G, et al: Naltrexone-induced dysphoria in former opioid addicts. Am J Psychiatry 142:1081–1084, 1985

Cummings SR, Nevitt MC, Browner WS, et al: Risk factors for hip fracture in white women. N Engl J Med 332:767–773, 1995

Davis BL: The PCP epidemic: a critical review. Int J Addict 17:1137–1155, 1982

Deleon D, Weiller HK, Jainchill N: The therapeutic community: success and improvement rates five years after treatment. International Journal of Addictions 17:703–747, 1982

Dembo R, Ciarlo JA, Taylor RW: A model of assessing and improving drug abuse treatment resource use in inner city areas. International Journal of Addictions 18:921–936, 1983

Des Jarlais DC, Friedman SR, Sotheran JL, et al: Continuity and change within an HIV epidemic. JAMA 271:121–127, 1994

Dietch J: The nature and extent of benzodiazepine abuse: an overview of recent literature. Hospital and Community Psychiatry 34:1139–1145, 1983

Dole VP: On the relevance of animal models to alcoholism in humans. Alcoholism 10:361–364, 1986

Dole VP, Nyswander ME: A medical treatment of heroin addiction. JAMA 193:646–650, 1965

Doyle K, Cluette-Brown JE, Dube DM, et al: Fatty acid ethyl esters in the blood as markers of ethanol intake. JAMA 276:1152–1156, 1996

Drake RE, Osher FC, Wallach MA: Alcohol use and abuse in schizophrenia: a prospective community study. J Nerv Ment Dis 177:408–414, 1989

Dryman A, Anthony JC: An epidemiologic study of alcohol use as a predictor of psychiatric distress over time. Acta Psychiatr Scand 80:315–321, 1989

Dulit RA, Fyer MR, Haas GL, et al: Substance use in borderline personality disorder. Am J Psychiatry 147:1002–1007, 1990

Dupont RL, Saylor KE: Sedatives/hypnotics and benzodiazepines, in Clinical Textbook of Addictive Disorders. Edited by Frances RJ, Miller SI. New York, Guilford, 1991, pp 69–102

Edlin BR, Irwin KL, Farque S, et al: Intersecting epidemics: crack cocaine use and HIV infection among inner-city young adults. N Engl J Med 331:1422–1427, 1994

Edwards G, Arif A, Hodgson R: Nomenclature and classification of drug and alcohol-related problems: a shortened version of a WHO memorandum. Br J Addict 77:3–20, 1982

Escriba PV, Sastre M, Garcia-Sevilla JA: Increased density of guanine nucleotide-binding proteins in the postmortem brains of heroin addicts. Arch Gen Psychiatry 51:494–501, 1994

Espir ML, Rose FC: Alcohol, seizures and epilepsy. J R Soc Med 9:542–543, 1987

Ewing JA: Detecting alcoholism: the CAGE questionnaire. JAMA 252:1905–1907, 1984

Fergusson DM, Lynskey MT, Horwood LJ: Comorbidity between depressive disorders and nicotine dependence in a cohort of 16-year-olds. Arch Gen Psychiatry 53: 1043–1047, 1996

Fils-Aime ML, Eckardt MJ, George DT, et al: Early onset alcoholics have lower cerebrospinal fluid 5-hydroxyindoleacetic acid levels than late-onset alcoholics. Arch Gen Psychiatry 53:211–216, 1996

Fiore MC, Smith SS, Jorenby DE, et al: The effectiveness of the nicotine patch for smoking cessation. JAMA 271: 1040–1047, 1994

Fischman MW, Foltin RW, Nestadt G, et al: Effects of desipramine maintenance on cocaine self-administration by humans. J Pharmacol Exp Ther 253:760–770, 1990

Fletcher JM, Page JB, Francis DJ, et al: Cognitive correlates of long-term cannabis use in Costa Rican men. Arch Gen Psychiatry 53:1051–1057, 1996

Franklin JE Jr, Frances RJ: Alcohol-induced organic mental disorders, in The American Psychiatric Press Textbook of Neuropsychiatry, 2nd Edition. Edited by Yudofsky SC, Hales RE. Washington, DC, American Psychiatric Press, 1992, pp 563–583

Frezza M, di Padova C, Pozzato G, et al: High blood alcohol levels in women: the role of decreased gastric alcohol dehydrogenase activity and first-pass metabolism. N Engl J Med 322:95–99, 1990

Fuller R, Branchey L, Brightwell DR, et al: Disulfiram treatment of alcoholism: a Veterans Administration cooperative study. JAMA 256:1449–1455, 1986

Galanter M: Network therapy for addiction: a model for office practice. Am J Psychiatry 150:28–36, 1993

Galizio M, Stein FS: Sensation seeking and drug choice. International Journal of Addictions 18:1039–1048, 1983

Gawin FH, Kleber HD: Abstinence symptomatology and psychiatric diagnosis in cocaine abusers. Arch Gen Psychiatry 43:107–113, 1986a

Gawin FH, Kleber HD: Pharmacologic treatments of cocaine abuse. Psychiatr Clin North Am 9:573–583, 1986b

Gawin FH, Allen D, Humblestone B: Outpatient treatment of "crack" cocaine smoking with flupenthixol decanoate: a preliminary report. Arch Gen Psychiatry 46:322–325, 1989a

Gawin FH, Kleber HD, Byck R, et al: Desipramine facilitation of initial cocaine abstinence. Arch Gen Psychiatry 46:117–121, 1989b

George DT, Benkelfat C, Rawlings RR, et al: Behavioral and neuroendocrine responses to M-chlorophenylpiperazine in subtypes of alcoholics and in healthy comparison subjects. Am J Psychiatry 154:81–87, 1997

Gerstley LJ, Alterman AI, McLellan AT, et al: Antisocial personality disorder in patients with substance abuse disorders: a problematic diagnosis? Am J Psychiatry 147:173–178, 1990

Gessner PK: Drug therapy of the alcohol withdrawal syndrome, in Biochemistry and Pharmacology of Ethanol, Vol 2. Edited by Majchrowicz E, Noble E. New York, Plenum, 1979, pp 375–434

Giannini AJ, Folts DJ, Feather JN, et al: Bromocriptine and amantadine in cocaine detoxification. Psychiatry Res 29:11–16, 1989

Gianoulakis C, Krishman B, Thavundayil J: Enhanced sensitivity of pituitary B-endorphin to ethanol in subjects at high risk of alcoholism. Arch Gen Psychiatry 53:250–257, 1996

Gillin JC, Smith TL, Irwin M, et al: Increased pressure for rapid eye movement sleep at time of hospital admission predicts relapse in nondepressed patients with primary alcoholism at 3-month follow-up. Arch Gen Psychiatry 51:189–197, 1994

Giros B, Jaber M, Jones SR, et al: Hyperlocomotion and indifference to cocaine and amphetamine in mice lacking the dopamine transporter. Nature 379:606–612, 1996

Glassman AH: Cigarette smoking: implications for psychiatric illness. Am J Psychiatry 150:546–553, 1993

Gold MS, Redmond DE, Kleber HD: Clonidine in opiate withdrawal. Lancet 1:929–930, 1978

Goodwin DW: Alcoholism and alcoholic psychoses, in Comprehensive Textbook of Psychiatry/IV, 4th Edition, Vol 1. Edited by Kaplan HI, Sadock BJ. Baltimore, MD, Williams & Wilkins, 1985a, pp 1016–1026

Goodwin DW: Alcoholism and genetics: the sins of the fathers. Arch Gen Psychiatry 42:171–174, 1985b

Gordis E: Alcohol problems and public health policy. JAMA 278:1781–1782, 1997

Gottschalk L, McGuire F, Haser F, et al: Drug abuse deaths in nine cities: a survey report (NIDA Res Monogr No 29). Rockville, MD, National Institute of Drug Abuse, 1979

Greenstein RA, Arndt IC, McLellan AT, et al: Naltrexone: a clinical perspective. J Clin Psychiatry 45 (No 9, Sec 2):25–28, 1984

Griffin ML, Weiss RD, Mirin SM, et al: A comparison of male and female cocaine abusers. Arch Gen Psychiatry 46:122–126, 1989

Grinspoon L, Bakalar JB: Psychedelics and arylcyclohexylamines, in Psychiatry Update: American Psychiatric Association Annual Review, Vol 5. Edited by Frances AJ, Hales RE. Washington, DC, American Psychiatric Press, 1986, pp 212–225

Grinspoon L, Bakalar JB: The war on drugs—a peace proposal. N Engl J Med 330:357–360, 1994

Grove WM, Eckert ED, Heston L, et al: Heritability of substance abuse and antisocial behavior: a study of monozygotic twins reared apart. Biol Psychiatry 27:1293–1304, 1990

Halikas JA, Goodwin DW, Guze SB: Marijuana effects. JAMA 217:692–694, 1971

Halikas JA, Crosby RD, Carlson GA, et al: Cocaine reduction in unmotivated crack users using carbamazepine versus placebo in a short-term, double-blind crossover design. Clin Pharmacol Ther 50:81–95, 1991

Hall SM: The abstinence phobias: links between substance abuse and anxiety. International Journal of Addictions 19:613–631, 1984

Hall SM, Tunstall C, Rugg D, et al: Nicotine gum and behavioral treatment in smoking cessation. J Consult Clin Psychol 53:256–258, 1985

Hanson B: Drug treatment effectiveness: the case of racial and ethnic minorities in America: some research questions and proposals. International Journal of Addictions 20:99–137, 1985

Harris-Allen M: Detoxification considerations in the medical management of substance abuse in pregnancy. Bull N Y Acad Med 67:270–276, 1991

Hasin D, Grant B: Draft DSM-IV criteria for alcohol use disorders: comparison to DSM-III-R and implications. Alcohol Clin Exp Res 18:1348–1353, 1994

Hatsukami DK, Fischman MW: Crack cocaine and cocaine hydorchloride: are the differences myth or reality? JAMA 276:1580–1588, 1996

Helzer JE, Camino GJ, Hwu H, et al: Alcoholism: a cross-national comparison of population surveys with the DIS, in Alcoholism: A Medical Disorder. Edited by Rose RM, Barrett J. New York, Raven, 1986

Hemmelgarn B, Suissa S, Huang A, et al: Benzodiazepine use and the risk of motor vehicle crash in the elderly. JAMA 1:27–31, 1997

Hendrie CA: Opiate dependence and withdrawal: a new synthesis. Pharmacol Biochem Behav 23:863–870, 1985

Henningfield JE: Pharmacologic basis and treatment of cigarette smoking. J Clin Psychiatry 45 (No 12, Sec 2):24–34, 1984

Higgins ST, Delaney DD, Budney AJ: A behavioral approach to achieving initial cocaine abstinence. Am J Psychiatry 148:1218–1224, 1991

Higgins ST, Budney AJ, Bickel WK, et al: Incentives improve outcome in outpatient behavioral treatment of cocaine dependence. Arch Gen Psychiatry 51:568–576, 1994

Hillbom M, Tokola R, Kuusela V, et al: Prevention of alcohol withdrawal seizures with carbamazepine and valproic acid. Alcohol 6:223–226, 1989

Howard MO, Cowley DS, Roy-Byrne PP, et al: Tridimensional personality traits in sons of alcoholic and nonalcoholic fathers. Alcohol Clin Exp Res 20:445–448, 1996

Hughes JR, Hatsukami D: Signs and symptoms of tobacco withdrawal. Arch Gen Psychiatry 43:289–294, 1986

Huseby NE, Bjordal E, Nilssen O, et al: Utility of biological markers during outpatient treatment of alcohol-dependent subjects: carbohydrate-deficient transferrin responds to moderate changes in alcohol consumption. Alcohol Clin Exp Res 21:1343–1346, 1997

Interaction of alcohol with drugs. The Medical Letter on Drugs and Therapeutics 19:47–48, 1977

Irwin M, Schuckit M, Smith TL: Clinical importance of age at onset in Type 1 and Type 2 primary alcoholics. Arch Gen Psychiatry 47:320–324, 1990

Itkomen J, Schnoll S, Glassroth J: Pulmonary dysfunction in freebase cocaine users. Arch Intern Med 144:2195–2197, 1984

Jacobsen LK, Kosten TR: Naloxone challenge as a biological predictor of treatment outcome in opiate addicts. Am J Drug Alcohol Abuse 15:355–366, 1989

Jaffe JH: Drug addiction and drug abuse, in Goodman and Gilman's Pharmacological Basis of Therapeutics, 6th Edition. Edited by Gilman AG, et al. New York, Macmillan, 1980, pp 535–584

Jaffe JH, Martin WR: Opioid analysis and analgesics and antagonists, in Goodman and Gilman's The Pharmacological Basis of Therapeutics, 7th Edition. Edited by Gilman AG, Goodman LS, Rall TW, et al. New York, Macmillan, 1985, pp 491–531

Jasinski DR, Johnson RE, Kocher TR: Clonidine in morphine withdrawal: differential effects on signs and symptoms. Arch Gen Psychiatry 42:1063–1066, 1985

Jellinek EM: The Disease Concept of Alcoholism. New Haven, CT, Hillhouse, 1960

Johnson J, Weissman MM, Klerman GL: Panic disorder, comorbidity, and suicide attempts. Arch Gen Psychiatry 47:805–808, 1990

Johnson RE, Jaffe JH, Fudala PJ: A controlled trial of buprenorphine treatment for opioid dependence. JAMA 267:2750–2755, 1992

Johnson L, O'Malley P, Bachman J: National Survey Results on Drug User From the Monitoring the Future Study, Vol 1 (Secondary Students) 1989–1995 (DHHS Publ No 96-4139). Washington, DC, National Institute on Drug Abuse, U.S. Department of Health and Human Services, 1996

Jonsson S, O'Meara M, Young JB: Acute cocaine poisoning. Am J Med 75:1061–1064, 1983

Joseph H, Appel P: Alcoholism and methadone treatment: consequences for the patient and program. Am J Drug Alcohol Abuse 11:37–53, 1985

Jurkovich GJ, Rivera FP, Gurney JG, et al: The effect of acute alcohol intoxication and chronic alcohol abuse on outcome from trauma. JAMA 270:51–56, 1993

Kabel DI, Petty F: A placebo-controlled, double-blind study of fluoxetine in severe alcohol dependence: adjunctive pharmacotherapy during and after inpatient treatment. Alcohol Clin Exp Res 20:780–784, 1996

Kandel DB: Marijuana users in young adulthood. Arch Gen Psychiatry 41:200–209, 1984

Kandel DB, Faust R: Sequence and stages in patterns of adolescent drug use. Arch Gen Psychiatry 32:923–932, 1975

Kandel DB, Davies M: High school students who use crack and other drugs. Arch Gen Psychiatry 53:71–80, 1996

Kandel DB, Raveis VH: Cessation of illicit drug use in young adulthood. Arch Gen Psychiatry 46:109–116, 1989

Kang S-Y, Kleinman PH, Woody GE, et al: Outcomes for cocaine abusers after once-a-week psychosocial therapy. Am J Psychiatry 148:630–635, 1991

Kapur A, Wild G, Milford-Ward A, et al: Carbohydrate deficient transferrin: a marker for alcohol abuse. BMJ 299:427–431, 1989

Kendler KS, Heath AC, Neale MC, et al: A population-based twin study of alcoholism in women. JAMA 268:1877–1882, 1992

Kendler KS, Heath AC, Neale MC, et al: Alcoholism and major depression in women. Arch Gen Psychiatry 50:690–698, 1993

Kendler KS, Prescott CA, Neal MC, et al: Temperance board registration for alcohol abuse in a national sample of Swedish male twins, born 1902 to 1949. Arch Gen Psychiatry 54:178–184, 1997

Kessler RC, McGonagle KA, Zhao S, et al: Lifetime and 12-month prevalence of DSM-III-R psychiatric disorders in the United States. Arch Gen Psychiatry 51:8–19, 1994

Kessler RC, Crumb, Warner LA, et al: Lifetime co-occurrence of DSM-III-R alcohol abuse and dependence with other psychiatric disorders in the National Comorbidity Survey. Arch Gen Psychiatry 54:313–321, 1997

Khantzian EJ: The self-medication hypotheses of addictive disorders: focus on heroin and cocaine dependence. Am J Psychiatry 142:1259–1264, 1985

Khantzian EJ, Treece C: DSM-III psychiatric diagnosis of narcotic addicts: recent findings. Arch Gen Psychiatry 42:1067–1071, 1985

King GS, Smialek JE, Troutman WG: Sudden death in adolescents resulting from the inhalation of typewriter correction fluid. JAMA 253:1604–1609, 1985

Kinsbourne M: Sounding board: U.S. drug laws—an introduction. N Engl J Med 330:355–356, 1994

Kleber HD, Gawin FH: The spectrum of cocaine abuse and its treatment. J Clin Psychiatry 45 (No 12, Sec 2):18–23, 1984

Kleber HD, Riordan CE, Rounsaville B, et al: Clonidine in outpatient detoxification from methadone maintenance. Arch Gen Psychiatry 42:391–394, 1985

Kleber HD, Topazian M, Gaspari J, et al: Clonidine and naltrexone in outpatient treatment of opioid withdrawal. Am J Drug Alcohol Abuse 13:1–18, 1987

Kleinman PH, Miller AB, Millman RB, et al: Psychopathology among cocaine abusers entering treatment. J Nerv Ment Dis 178:442–447, 1990

Klerman GL, Weissman MM, Rounsaville BJ, et al: Theory and Practice of Interpersonal Psychotherapy for Depression. New York, Basic Books, 1984

Klonoff H, Low M, Marcus A: Neuropsychological effects of marijuana. CMAJ 108:150–157, 1973

Kosten TA, Kosten TR: Pharmacological blocking agents for treating substance abuse. J Nerv Ment Dis 179:583–592, 1991

Kosten TR: Neurobiology of abused drugs: opioids and stimulants. J Nerv Ment Dis 178:217–227, 1990

Kosten TR, Kleber HD: Strategies to improve compliance with narcotic antagonists. Am J Drug Alcohol Abuse 10:249–266, 1984

Kosten TR, Price LH: Phenomenology and sequelae of 3,4-methylenedioxymethamphetamine use. J Nerv Ment Dis 180:353–354, 1992

Kosten TR, Rounsaville BJ, Kleber HD: Comparison of clinician ratings to self-reports of withdrawal during clonidine detoxification of opiate addicts. Am J Drug Alcohol Abuse 11:1–10, 1985a

Kosten TR, Rounsaville BJ, Kleber HD: Ethnic and gender differences among opiate addicts. International Journal of Addictions 20:1143–1162, 1985b

Kosten TR, Rounsaville BJ, Kleber HD: A 2.5-year follow-up of depression, life crises, and treatment effects on abstinence among opioid addicts. Arch Gen Psychiatry 43:733–738, 1986

Kosten TR, Gawin FH, Morgan C: Evidence for altered desipramine disposition in methadone-maintained patients treated for cocaine abuse. Am J Drug Alcohol Abuse 16:329–336, 1990

Kosten TR, Morgan C, Kleber HD: Treatment of heroin addicts using buprenorphine. Am J Drug Alcohol Abuse 2:119–128, 1991

Kraft MK, Rothbard AB, Hadley TR, et al: Are supplementary services provided during methadone maintenance really cost-effective? Am J Psychiatry 154:1195–1197, 1997

Kranzler HR, Burleson JA, Del Boca FK, et al: Buspirone treatment of anxious alcoholics: a placebo-controlled trial. Arch Gen Psychiatry 51:720–731, 1994

Kranzler HR, Burleson JA, Korner P, et al: Placebo-controlled trial of fluoxetine as an adjunct to relapse prevention in alcoholics. Am J Psychiatry 152:391–397, 1995

Kranzler HR, Escobar R, Lee DK, et al: Elevated rates of early discontinuation from pharmacotherapy trials in alcoholics and drug abusers. Alcohol Clin Exp Res 20:16–20, 1996a

Kranzler HR, Burleson JA, Brown J, et al: Fluoxetine treatment seems to reduce the beneficial effects of cognitive-behavioral therapy in type B alcoholics. Alcohol Clin Exp Res 20:1534–1541, 1996b

Kupfer DJ, Detre T, Koral J, et al: A comment on the "amotivational syndrome" in marijuana smokers. Am J Psychiatry 130:1319–1322, 1973

Kushner MG, Sher KJ, Beitman BD: The relation between alcohol problems and the anxiety disorders. Am J Psychiatry 147:685–695, 1990

Lichtenfeld J, Rubin DB, Feldman RS: Subarachnoid hemorrhage precipitated by cocaine snorting. Arch Neurol 41:223–224, 1986

Lieber CS: Medical disorders of alcoholism. N Engl J Med 333:1058–1065, 1995

Liester MB, Grob CS, Bravo GL, et al: Phenomenology and sequelae of 3,4-methylenedioxymethamphetamine use. J Nerv Ment Dis 180:345–352, 1992

Lillie-Blanton M, Anthony J, Schuster CR: Probing the meaning of racial/ethnic group comparisons in crack cocaine smoking. JAMA 296:993–997, 1993

Linn LS: Psychopathology and experience with marijuana. Br J Addict 67:55–64, 1972

Linszen DH, Dingemans PM, Lenior ME: Cannabis abuse and the course of recent-onset schizophrenic disorders. Arch Gen Psychiatry 51:273–279, 1994

Lishman WA: Organic Psychiatry. Philadelphia, PA, JB Lippincott, 1978

Litt MD, Babor TF, DelBoca FK, et al: Types of alcoholics, II: application of an empirically derived typology to treatment matching. Arch Gen Psychiatry 49:609–614, 1992

Litten RZ, Allen J, Fertig J: Pharmacotherapies for alcohol problems: a review of research with focus on developments since 1991. Alcohol Clin Exp Res 20:859–876, 1996

Loimer N, Lenz K, Schmid R, et al: Technique for greatly shortening the transition from methadone to naltrexone maintenance of patients addicted to opiates. Am J Psychiatry 148:933–935, 1991

London ED, Cascella NG, Wong DF, et al: Cocaine-induced reduction of glucose utilization in human brain: a study using positron emission tomography and [fluorine 18]-fluorodeoxyglucose. Arch Gen Psychiatry 47:567–574, 1990

Loranger AW, Tulis EH: Family history of alcoholism in borderline personality disorder. Arch Gen Psychiatry 42:153–157, 1985

Low M, Klonoff H, Marcus A: The neurophysiological basis of the marijuana experience. CMAJ 108:157–165, 1973

Luborsky L, McLellan AT, Woody GE, et al: Therapist success and its determinants. Arch Gen Psychiatry 42:602–611, 1985

Malcolm R, Ballenger JC, Strugis ET, et al: Double-blind controlled trial comparing carbamazepine to oxazepam treatment of alcohol withdrawal. Am J Psychiatry 146:617–621, 1989

Malec E, Malec T, Gagne MA, et al: Buspirone in the treatment of alcohol dependence: a placebo-controlled trial. Alcohol Clin Exp Res 20:207–312, 1996

Mannuzza S, Klein RG, Bessler A, et al: Adult outcome of hyperactive boys. Arch Gen Psychiatry 50:565–576, 1993

Margolin A, Kosten T, Petrakis I, et al: An open pilot study of bupropion and psychotherapy for the treatment of cocaine abuse in methadone-maintained patients, in Problems of Drug Dependence 1990 (DHHS Publ No ADM-91-1753). Rockville, MD, National Institute on Drug Abuse, 1991, pp 367–368

Martin PR, Adinoff B, Eckardt MJ, et al: Effective pharmacotherapy of alcoholic amnestic disorder with fluvoxamine: preliminary findings. Arch Gen Psychiatry 46:617–621, 1989

Marzuk PM, Tardiff K, Leon AC, et al: Prevalence of cocaine use among residents of New York City who committed suicide during a one-year period. Am J Psychiatry 149:371–375, 1992

Mason BJ, Kocsis JH, Ritvo EC, et al: A double-blind, placebo-controlled trial of desipramine for primary alcohol dependence stratified on the presence or absence of major depression. JAMA 275:761–767, 1996

McCaul ME, Turkan JS, Svikis DS, et al: Alcohol and secobarbital effects as a function of familial alcoholism: extended intoxication and increased withdrawal effects. Alcohol Clin Exp Res 15:94–101, 1991

McClearn GE, Erwin V: Mechanisms of genetic influence on alcohol-related behaviors, in Alcohol Consumption and Related Problems (DHHS Publ No ADM-82-1190). Rockville, MD, National Institute on Alcohol Abuse and Alcoholism, 1982

McCord W, McCord J: Origins of Alcoholism. Stanford, CA, Stanford University Press, 1960

McDougle CJ, Black JE, Malison RT, et al: Noradrenergic dysregulation during discontinuation of cocaine use in addicts. Arch Gen Psychiatry 51:713–719, 1994

McGrath PJ, Nunes EV, Stewart JW, et al: Imipramine treatment of alcoholics with primary depression. Arch Gen Psychiatry 53:232–240, 1996

McKelway R, Vieweg V, Westerman P: Sudden death from acute cocaine intoxication in Virginia in 1988. Am J Psychiatry 147:1667–1669, 1990

McLellan AT, Arndt IO, Metzger DS, et al: The effects of psychosocial services in substance abuse treatment. JAMA 296:1953–1959, 1993

McLellan AT, Grissom GR, Zanis D, et al: Problem-service 'matching' in addiction treatment. Arch Gen Psychiatry 54:730–735, 1997

Medical News and Perspectives: NIH panel says more study is needed to assess marijuana's medicinal use. JAMA 277:867–868, 1997

Melges FT: Tracking difficulties and paranoid ideation during hashish and alcohol intoxication. Am J Psychiatry 133:1024–1028, 1976

Mendelson JH, Mello NK, Lex BW, et al: Marijuana withdrawal syndrome in a woman. Am J Psychiatry 141:1289–1290, 1984

Metzger D, Woody G, De Philippis D, et al: Risk factors for needle sharing among methadone-treated patients. Am J Psychiatry 148:636–640, 1991

Meyers HB, Zepeda SG, Murdock MA: Alcohol and trauma: an endemic syndrome. West J Med 153:149–153, 1990

Milby JB: Methadone maintenance to abstinence: how many make it? J Nerv Ment Dis 176:409–422, 1988

Miller JD: National Survey on Drug Abuse, Main Findings, 1982. Rockville, MD, National Institute on Drug Abuse, 1983

Millman RB, Sbriglio R: Patterns of use and psychopathology in chronic marijuana users. Psychiatr Clin North Am 9:533–545, 1986

Minion GE, Slovid CM, Boutiette L: Severe alcohol intoxication: a study of 204 consecutive patients. Clinical Toxicology 27:375–384, 1989

Mirin SM, Weiss RD: Substance abuse and mental illness, in Clinical Textbook of Addictive Disorders. Edited by Frances RJ, Miller SI. New York, Guilford, 1991, pp 271–298

Moliterno DJ, Willard JE, Lange RA, et al: Coronary-artery vasoconstriction induced by cocaine, cigarette smoking, or both. N Engl J Med 330:454–459, 1994

Morgan MJ, Cascella NG, Stapleton JM, et al: Sensitivity to subjective effects of cocaine in drug abusers: relationship to cerebral ventricle size. Am J Psychiatry 150:1712–1717, 1993

Mortimer WG: History of Coca, The Divine Plant of the Mind (Fitz Hugh Ludlow Memorial Library Edition). San Francisco, CA, And/Or Press, 1974

Moss HB, Yao JK, Burns M, et al: Plasma GABA-like activity in response to ethanol challenge in men at high risk for alcoholism. Biol Psychiatry 27:617–625, 1990

Moss M, Bucher B, Moore F, et al: The role of chronic alcohol abuse in the development of acute respiratory distress syndrome in adults. JAMA 275:50–54, 1996

Mueller TI, Lavori PW, Keller MB, et al: Prognostic effect of the variable course of alcoholism on the 10-year course of depression. Am J Psychiatry 151:701–706, 1994

Mueller TT, Stout RL, Rudden S, et al: A double-blind, placebo-controlled pilot study of carbamazepine for the treatment of alcohol dependence. Alcohol Clin Exp Res 21:86–92, 1997

Murphy GE, Wetzel RD: The lifetime risk of suicide in alcoholism. Arch Gen Psychiatry 47:383–392, 1990

Murphy GE, Wetzel RD, Robins E, et al: Multiple risk factors predict suicide in alcoholism. Arch Gen Psychiatry 49:459–463, 1992

Myers JK, Weissman MM, Tischler GL, et al: Six-month prevalence of psychiatric disorders in three communities: 1980–1982. Arch Gen Psychiatry 41:959–967, 1984

Nadamanee K, Gorelick DA, Josephson MA: Myocardial ischemia during cocaine withdrawal. Ann Intern Med 111:876–880, 1989

Naditch MP, Fenwick S: LSD flashbacks and ego functioning. J Abnorm Psychol 86:352–359, 1977

Nahas G: Biomedical aspects of cannabis usage. Bull Narc 29:13–27, 1977

Naranjo CA, Sellers EM, Chater K, et al: Nonpharmacologic intervention in acute alcohol withdrawal. Clin Pharmacol Ther 34:214–219, 1983

Naranjo CA, Kadlec KE, Sanhueza P, et al: Fluoxetine differentially alters alcohol intake and other consummatory behaviors in problem drinkers. Clin Pharmacol Ther 47:490–498, 1990

Naranjo CA, Poulos CX, Bremner KE, et al: Ctalopram decreased desirability, liking, and consumption of alcohol in alcohol-dependent drinkers. Clin Pharmacol Ther 51:729–739, 1992

National Academy of Sciences, Institute of Medicine, Committee to Study the Health-Related Effects of Cannabis and Its Derivatives: Marijuana and Health. Washington, DC, National Academy Press, 1982

National Institute on Alcohol Abuse and Alcoholism: Eighth Special Report to the U.S. Congress on Alcohol and Health (NIH Publ No 94-3699). Bethesda, MD, National Institutes of Health, 1993

National Institute on Drug Abuse: Client Oriented Data Acquisition Process (CODAP), Annual Data and Quarterly Reports, Statistical Series D and E. Rockville, MD, NIADA/MHA, 1981

National Institute on Drug Abuse: Drug use among American high school students and other young adults: national trends through 1985 (DHHS Publ No ADM 86-1450). Rockville, MD, National Institute on Drug Abuse, 1986

National Institute on Drug Abuse: Semiannual report trend data through December 1989: data from the Drug Abuse Warning Network (DAWN) (statistical series GG, No 24, DHHS Publ No ADM-90-1664). Washington, DC, U.S. Government Printing Office, 1990

National Institute on Drug Abuse: NIDA Notes, Vol 12 (NIH Publ No 97-3478). Washington, DC, U.S. Department of Health and Human Services, 1997

Nestadt G, Romanoski AJ, Samuels JF, et al: The relationship between personality and DSM-III Axis I disorders in the population: results from an epidemiological survey. Am J Psychiatry 149:1228–1233, 1992

Nestler EJ, Fitzgerald LW, Self DW: Neurobiology, in American Psychiatric Press Review of Psychiatry, Vol 14. Edited by Oldham JM, Riba MB. Washington, DC, American Psychiatric Press, 1995, pp 51–81

Ng SKC, Hauser WA, Brust JCM, et al: Alcohol consumption and withdrawal in new-onset seizures. N Engl J Med 319:666–673, 1988

NIAAA Project MATCH Research Group: Matching alcoholism treatments to client heterogeneity: project MATCH posttreatment drinking outcomes. J Stud Alcohol 90:1179–1188, 1997

Nicholi AM: Historical perspective: the long and colorful history of erythoxylon coca. J Am Coll Health 32:252–257, 1984

Niven RG: Adolescent drug abuse. Hospital and Community Psychiatry 37:596–607, 1986

Noordsy DL, Drake RE, Teague GB, et al: Subjective experiences related to alcohol use among schizophrenics. J Nerv Ment Dis 179:410–414, 1991

Novick DM, Pascarelli EF, Joseph H: Methadone maintenance patients in general medical practice: a preliminary report. JAMA 259:3299–3302, 1988

O'Brien CP, Woody GE: Sedative-hypnotics and antianxiety agents, in Psychiatry Update: American Psychiatric Association Annual Review, Vol 5. Edited by Frances AJ, Hales RE. Washington, DC, American Psychiatric Press, 1986, pp 186–199

O'Malley SS, Maisto SA: Effects of family drinking history and expectancies on responses to alcohol in men. J Stud Alcohol 46:289–297, 1985

O'Malley SS, Jaffe AJ, Rode S, et al: Experience of a "slip" among alcoholics treated with naltrexone or placebo. Am J Psychiatry 153:281–283, 1996a

O'Malley SS, Jaffe AJ, Chang G, et al: Six-month follow-up of naltrexone and psychotherapy for alcohol dependence. Arch Gen Psychiatry 53:217–224, 1996b

Ostrea EM Jr, Yee H, Thrasher S: GC/MS analysis of meconium for cocaine: clinical implications (abstract). Pediatr Res 29:63A, 1991

Paille F, Guelfi JD, Perkins AC, et al: Double-blind randomized multicentre trial of acamprostate in maintaining abstinence from alcohol. Alcohol Alcohol 30:239–247, 1995

Perkins KA, Simpson JC, Tsuang MT: Ten-year follow-up of drug abusers with acute or chronic psychoses. Hospital and Community Psychiatry 37:481–484, 1986

Perlstadt H, Hembroff LA, Zonia SC: Changes in status, attitude and behavior toward alcohol and drugs on a university campus. Family and Community Health 14:44–62, 1991

Peterson JB, Rothfleisch J, Zelazo PD, et al: Acute alcohol intoxication and cognitive functioning. J Stud Alcohol 51:114–122, 1990

Pope HG Jr, Yurgelun-Tood D: The residual cognitive effective of heavy marijuana use in college students. JAMA 275:521–527, 1996

Pope HG Jr, Ionescu-Pioggia M, Aizley HG, et al: Drug use and lifestyle among college undergraduates in 1989: a comparison with 1969 and 1978. Am J Psychiatry 147:998–1001, 1990

Porjesz B, Begleiter H: Human evoked brain potentials and alcohol. Alcoholism 5:304–316, 1981

Racine A, Joyce T, Anderson R: The association between prenatal care and birth weight among women exposed to cocaine in New York City. JAMA 270:1581–1586, 1993

Raw M: Does nicotine chewing gum work? BMJ 290:1231–1232, 1985

Redmond DE, Krystal JH: Multiple mechanisms of withdrawal from opioid drugs. Annu Rev Neurosci 7:443–478, 1984

Reed BJ, May PA: Inhalant abuse and juvenile delinquency: a control study in Albuquerque, New Mexico. International Journal of Addictions 19:789–803, 1984

Regier Da, Farmer ME, Rae DS, et al: Comorbidity of mental disorders with alcohol and other drug abuse: results from the Epidemiologic Catchment Area (ECA) study. JAMA 264:2511–2518, 1990

Resnick RB, Schuyten-Resnick E, Washton AM: Assessment of narcotic antagonists in the treatment of opiate dependence. Annu Rev Pharmacol Toxicol 20:463–474, 1980

Reuler JB, Girard DE, Cooney TG: Wernicke's encephalopathy. N Engl J Med 312:1035–1039, 1985

Rice DP: The economic cost of alcohol abuse and alcohol dependence: 1990. Alcohol Health Res World 17:10–11, 1993

Rickels K, Case WG, Downing RW, et al: Long-term diazepam therapy and clinical outcome. JAMA 251:767–771, 1983

Rickels K, Schweizer E, Case WG: Long-term therapeutic use of benzodiazepines. Arch Gen Psychiatry 47:899–902, 1990

Rivera FP, Koepsell TD, Jurkovich GJ, et al: The effects of alcohol abuse on readmission for trauma. JAMA 270:1962–1964, 1993

Robins LN, Helzer JE, Weissman MM, et al: Lifetime prevalence of specific psychiatric disorders in three sites. Arch Gen Psychiatry 41:949–958, 1984

Roth D, Alarcon FJ, Fernandez JA: Acute rhabdomyolysis associated with cocaine intoxication. N Engl J Med 319:673–677, 1988

Rounsaville BJ, Carroll K: Interpersonal psychotherapy for patients who abuse drugs, in New Applications of Interpersonal Psychotherapy. Edited by Klerman GL, Weissman MM. Washington, DC, American Psychiatric Press, 1993, pp 319–352

Rounsaville BJ, Kleber HD: Psychotherapy counseling for opiate addicts: strategies for use in different treatment settings. International Journal of Addictions 20:869–896, 1985

Rounsaville BJ, Weissman MM, Kleber HD, et al: The heterogeneity of psychiatric diagnosis in treated opiate addicts. Arch Gen Psychiatry 39:161–166, 1982

Rounsaville BJ, Kosten TR, Weissman MM, et al: Prognostic significance of psychopathology in treated opiate addicts: a 2.5-year follow-up. Arch Gen Psychiatry 43:739–745, 1986

Rounsaville BJ, Anton SF, Carroll K, et al: Psychiatric diagnoses of treatment-seeking cocaine abusers. Arch Gen Psychiatry 48:43–51, 1991

Roy A, Lamparski D, DeJong J, et al: Characteristics of alcoholics who attempt suicide. Am J Psychiatry 147:761–765, 1990

Roy M, Roy A, Williams J, Weinberger L, et al: Reduced blue cone electroretinogram in cocaine-withdrawn patients. Arch Gen Psychiatry 54:153–156, 1997

Saitz R, Mayo-Smith MF, Roberts MS, et al: Individualized treatment for alcohol withdrawal: a randomized double-blind controlled trial. JAMA 272:519–523, 1994

Salloum IM, Moss HB, Daley DC: Substance abuse and schizophrenia: impediments to optimal care. Am J Drug Alcohol Abuse 3:321–336, 1991

Salloum IM, Cornelius JR, Daley DC, et al: The utility of diazepam loading in the treatment of alcohol withdrawal among psychiatric inpatients. Psychopharmacol Bull 31:305–310, 1995

Salmela KS, Laitinen K, Nystrom M, et al: Carbohydrate-deficient transferrin during 3 weeks' heavy alcohol consumption. Alcohol Clin Exp Res 18:228–230, 1994

Santos de Barona M, Simpson DD: Inhalant users in drug abuse prevention programs. Am J Drug Alcohol Abuse 10:503–518, 1984

Sass H, Soyka M, Mann K, et al: Relapse prevention by acamprosate. Arch Gen Psychiatry 53:673–680, 1996

Satel SL, Edell WS: Cocaine-induced paranoia and psychosis proneness. Am J Psychiatry 148:1708–1711, 1991

Saunders JB, Aasland OG, Babor TF, et al: Development of the alcohol use disorders identification test (AUDIT): WHO collaborative project on early detection of persons with harmful alcohol consumption—part II. Addiction 88:791–804, 1993

Schlaepfer TE, Pearlson GD, Wong DF, et al: PET study of competition between intravenous cocaine and [^{11}C] raclopride at dopamine receptors in human subjects. Am J Psychiatry 154:1209–1213, 1997

Schmauss C, Krieg JC: Enlargement of cerebrospinal fluid spaces in long-term benzodiazepine abusers. Psychol Med 17:869–873, 1987

Schmidt LG, Schmidt K, Dufeu P, et al: Superiority of carbohydrate-deficient transferrin to γ-glutamyltransferase in detecting relapse in alcoholism. Am J Psychiatry 154:75–80, 1997

Schneier FR, Siris SG: A review of psychoactive substance use and abuse in schizophrenia: patterns of drug choice. J Nerv Ment Dis 175:641–652, 1987

Schottenfeld RS, Pakes JR, Oliveto A, et al: Buprenorphine vs methadone maintenance treatment for concurrent opioid dependence and cocaine abuse. Arch Gen Psychiatry 54:713–720, 1997

Schuckit MA: The clinical implications of primary diagnostic groups among alcoholics. Arch Gen Psychiatry 42:1043–1049, 1985

Schuckit MA: Low level of response to alcohol as a predictor of future alcoholism. Am J Psychiatry February 151:184–189, 1994

Schuckit MA, Gold EO, Croot K, et al: P300 latency after ethanol ingestion in sons of alcoholics and in controls. Biol Psychiatry 24:310–315, 1988

Schuckit MA, Klein J, Twitchell G, et al: Personality test scores as predictors of alcoholism almost a decade later. Am J Psychiatry 151:1038–1042, 1994

Schwartz RH, Hawks RL: Laboratory detection of marijuana use. JAMA 254:788–792, 1986

Schweizer E, Rickels KV, Case WG, et al: Long-term therapeutic use of benzodiazepines. Arch Gen Psychiatry 47:908–915, 1990

Schweizer E, Rickels KV, Case WG, et al: Carbamazepine treatment in patients discontinuing long-term benzodiazepine therapy: effects on withdrawal severity and outcome. Arch Gen Psychiatry 48:448–452, 1991

Sellers EM, Naranjo CA, Harrison M, et al: Diazepam loading: simplified treatment of alcohol withdrawal. Clin Pharmacol Ther 34:822–826, 1983

Selzer ML: The Michigan Alcoholism Screening Test: the quest for a new diagnostic instrument. Am J Psychiatry 127:1653–1658, 1971

Serdula M, Williamson DF, Kendrick JS, et al: Trends in alcohol consumption by pregnant women 1985 through 1988. JAMA 265:876–879, 1991

Sevy S, Kay SR, Opler LA, et al: Significance of cocaine history in schizophrenia. J Nerv Ment Dis 178:642–648, 1990

Shaner A, Khalsa ME, Roberts L, et al: Unrecognized cocaine use among schizophrenic patients. Am J Psychiatry 150:758–762, 1993

Shaw GK, Waller S, Majumdar SK, et al: Tiapride in the prevention of relapse in recently detoxified alcoholics. Br J Psychiatry 165:515–523, 1994

Sherer MA, Kumor KM, Cone EJ, et al: Suspiciousness induced by four-hour intravenous infusions of cocaine: preliminary findings. Arch Gen Psychiatry 45:673–677, 1988

Silber A: Rationale for the technique of psychotherapy with alcoholics. International Journal of Psychoanalytic Psychotherapy 3:28–47, 1974

Simpson DD: Treatment for drug abuse: follow-up outcomes and length of time spent. Arch Gen Psychiatry 38:875–880, 1981

Singer L, Arendt R, Song LY, et al: Direct and indirect interactions of cocaine with childbirth outcomes. Arch Pediatr Adolesc Med 148:959–964, 1994

Smart RG: Crack cocaine use: a review of prevalence and adverse effects. Am J Drug Alcohol Abuse 17:13–26, 1991

Smart RG, Murray GF: Narcotic drug abuse in 152 countries: social and economic conditions as predictors. International Journal of Addictions 20:737–749, 1985

Smith SS, O'Hara BF, Persico AM, et al: Genetic vulnerability to drug abuse: the D_2 dopamine receptor Taq I B1 restriction fragment length polymorphism appears more frequently in polysubstance abusers. Arch Gen Psychiatry 49:723–727, 1992

Smoking Cessation Clinical Practice Guideline Panel and Staff: The Agency for Health Care Policy and Research Smoking Cessation Clinical Practice Guideline. JAMA 275:1270–1280, 1996

Soderstrom CA, Smith GA, Dischinger P, et al: Psychoactive substance use disorders among seriously injured trauma center patients. JAMA 277:1769–1774, 1997

Spencer DJ: Cannabis-induced psychosis. Br J Addict 65:369–372, 1970

Spiehler VR, Reed D: Brain concentrations of cocaine and benzoylecgonine in fatal cases. J Forensic Sci 30:1003–1011, 1985

Spohr HL, Willms J, Steinhausen HC: Prenatal alcohol exposure and long term developmental consequences. Lancet 341:907–910, 1993

Spotts JV, Shontz FC: Drug-induced ego states, 1: cocaine: phenomenology and implications. International Journal of Addictions 19:119–151, 1984

Spotts JV, Shontz FC: A new perspective on intervention in heavy, chronic drug use. International Journal of Addictions 20:1545–1565, 1985

Stimmel B, Goldberg J, Rotkopf E, et al: Ability to remain abstinent after methadone detoxification: a six-year study. JAMA 237:1216–1220, 1977

Stimmel B, Goldberg J, Reisman A, et al: Fetal outcome in narcotic-dependent women: the importance of the type of maternal narcotic used. Am J Drug Alcohol Abuse 9:383–385, 1982–1983

Stine SM, Burns B, Kosten T: Methadone dose for cocaine abuse (letter). Am J Psychiatry 148:1268, 1991

Strug DL, Hunt DE, Goldsmith DS, et al: Patterns of cocaine use among methadone clients. International Journal of Addictions 20:1163–1175, 1985

Stuppacek CH, Pycha R, Miller C, et al: Carbamazepine versus oxazpam in the treatment of alcohol withdrawal: a double-blind study. Alcohol Alcohol 27:153–158, 1992

Substance Abuse and Mental Health Services Administration: National Household Survey on Drug Abuse: population estimates (DHHS Publ No SMA-96-3095). Washington, DC, Substance Abuse and Mental Health Services Administration, 1995

Sullivan JT, Swift RM, Lewis DC: Benzodiazepine requirements during alcohol withdrawal syndrome: clinical implications of using a standardized withdrawal scale. J Clinical Psychopharmacol 11:291–295, 1991

Suwanwela: The History of Opium in Asia. Bangkok, Thailand, Institute of Health Research, 1979

Talbott JA, Teague JW: Marijuana psychosis. JAMA 210:299–302, 1969

Tardiff K, Marzuk PM, Leon AC, et al: Homicide in New York City. JAMA 272:43–46, 1994

Tarter RE: Psychosocial history, minimal brain dysfunction and differential drinking patterns of male alcoholics. J Clin Psychol 38:867–873, 1982

Thacore VR, Shukla SRP: Cannabis psychosis and paranoid schizophrenia. Arch Gen Psychiatry 33:383–386, 1976

Tiihonen J, Kuikka J, Hakola P, et al: Acute ethanol-induced changes in cerebral blood flow. Am J Psychiatry 151:1505–1508, 1994

Treffert DA: Marijuana use in schizophrenia: a clear hazard. Am J Psychiatry 135:1213–1215, 1978

Trell E, Kristenson H, Fex G: Alcohol-related problems in middle-aged men with elevated serum gamma-glutamyltransferase: a preventive medical investigation. J Stud Alcohol 45:302–309, 1984

Tsai G, Gastfriend DR, Coyle JT: The glutamatergic basis of human alcoholism. Am J Psychiatry 152:332–340, 1995

Tunstall CD, Ginsberg D, Hall SM: Quitting smoking. Int J Addict 20:1089–1112, 1985

Turner CE: Chemistry and metabolism, in Marijuana Research Findings (NIDA Res Monogr No 31; DHHS Publ No ADM-AD-1001). Edited by Petersen RL. Rockville, MD, National Institute on Drug Abuse, 1980

Turner RG, Lichstein PR, Peden JG, et al: Alcohol withdrawal syndromes: a review of pathophysiology, clinical presentations and treatment. J Gen Intern Med 4:432–444, 1989

Uhl GR, Persico AM, Smith SS: Current excitement with D2 dopamine receptor gene alleles in substance abuse. Arch Gen Psychiatry 49:157–160, 1992

U.S. Department of Health and Human Services: Fifth special report to the United States Congress on alcohol and health from the Secretary of Health and Human Services. Washington, DC, U.S. Department of Health and Human Services, 1993

Vaillant GE (preceptor): Alcohol abuse and dependence, in Psychiatry Update: American Psychiatric Association Annual Review, Vol 3. Edited by Grinspoon L. Washington, DC, American Psychiatric Press, 1984, pp 299–381

Vaillant GE: A long-term follow-up of male alcohol abuse. Arch Gen Psychiatry 53:243–249, 1996

Vardy MM, Kay SR: LSD psychosis or LSD-induced schizophrenia? A multimethod inquiry. Arch Gen Psychiatry 40:877–883, 1983

Victor M, Wolfe SM: Causation and treatment of the alcohol withdrawal syndrome, in Alcoholism: Progress in Research and Treatment. Edited by Bourne G, Fox R. New York, Academic, 1973, pp 137–166

Victor M, Adams RD, Collins GH: The Wernicke-Korsakoff Syndrome and Related Neurologic Disorders Due to Alcoholism and Malnutrition. Philadelphia, PA, FA Davis, 1989

Virkkunen M, Eggert M, Rawlings R, et al: A prospective follow-up study of alcoholic violent offenders and fire setters. Arch Gen Psychiatry 53:523–529, 1996

Virmani R, Robinowitz M, Smialek JE, et al: Cardiovascular effects of cocaine: an autopsy study of 40 patients. Am Heart J 115:1068–1076, 1988

Volavka J, Czobor P, Goodwin DW, et al: The electroencephalogram after alcohol administration in high-risk men and the development of alcohol use disorders 10 years later. Arch Gen Psychiatry 53:258–263, 1996

Volkow ND, Fowler JS, Wolf AP, et al: Effects of chronic cocaine abuse on postsynaptic dopamine receptors. Am J Psychiatry 147:719–724, 1990

Volkow ND, Hitzemann R, Wang G-J, et al: Decreased brain metabolism in neurologically intact healthy alcoholics. Am J Psychiatry 149:1016–1022, 1992

Volkow ND, Wang GJ, Hitzemann R, et al: Recovery of brain glucose metabolism in detoxified alcoholics. Am J Psychiatry 151:178–183, 1994

Volpicelli JR, Alterman AI, Hayashida M, et al: Naltrexone in the treatment of alcohol dependence. Arch Gen Psychiatry 49:876–880, 1992

Volpicelli JR, Rhines KC, Rhines JS, et al: Naltrexone and alcohol dependence: role of subject compliance. Arch Gen Psychiatry 54:737–742, 1997

Voltaire A, Beck O, Borg S, et al: Urinary 5-hydroxytryptophol: a possible marker of recent alcohol consumption. Alcohol Clin Exp Res 16:281–285, 1992

Walsh DC, Ringson RW, Merrigan DM, et al: A randomized trial of treatment options for alcohol-abusing workers. N Engl J Med 325:775–782, 1991

Walsh DC, Hingson RW, Merrigan DM, et al: The impact of a physician's warning on recovery after alcoholism treatment. JAMA 267:663–667, 1992

Washton AM: Structured outpatient treatment of alcohol vs drug dependencies. Recent Dev Alcohol 8:285–304, 1990

Washton AM, Resnick RG: Clonidine in opiate withdrawal: a review and appraisal of clinical findings. Pharmacotherapy 1:140–146, 1981

Washton AM, Gold MS, Pottash AC: Adolescent cocaine abusers (letter). Lancet 2:746, 1984

Watson JM: Solvent abuse by children and young adults: a review. Br J Addict 75:27–36, 1980

Watters JK, Estilo MJ, Clark GL, et al: Syringe and needle exchange as HIV/AIDS prevention for injection drug users. JAMA 271:115–120, 1994

Weddington WW, Brown BX, Haertzen CA, et al: Changes in mood, craving, and sleep during short-term abstinence reported by male cocaine addicts: a controlled, residential study. Arch Gen Psychiatry 47:861–868, 1990

Weddington WW, Brown BS, Haertzen CA, et al: Comparison of amantadine and desipramine combined with psychotherapy for treatment of cocaine dependence. Am J Drug Alcohol Abuse 2:137–152, 1991

Weil AJ: Adverse reactions to marijuana. N Engl J Med 282:997–1000, 1970

Weil AT, Zinberg NE, Nelsen JM: Clinical and psychological effects of marijuana in man. Science 162:1234–1242, 1968

Weiss RD, Mirin SM: Subtypes of cocaine abusers. Psychiatr Clin North Am 9:491–501, 1986

Weiss RD, Mirin SM, Griffin ML, et al: Psychopathology in cocaine abusers: changing trends. J Nerv Ment Dis 176: 719–725, 1988

Weller RA, Halikas JA: Marijuana use and psychiatric illness: a follow-up study. Am J Psychiatry 142:848–850, 1985

Williams JBW: DSM-III-R preview: a look at organic mental and substance use disorders. Hospital and Community Psychiatry 37:995–996, 1986

Winokur GA, Cadoret R, Dorzab JA, et al: The division of depressive illness into depression spectrum disease and pure depressive illness. International Pharmacopsychiatry 9:5–13, 1974

Winokur G, Coryell W, Akiskal HS, et al: Alcoholism in manic-depressive (bipolar) illness: familial illness, course of illness, and the primary-secondary distinction. Am J Psychiatry 152:365–372, 1995

Woody GE, Luborsky L, McLellan AT, et al: Psychotherapy for opiate addicts: does it help? Arch Gen Psychiatry 40:639–645, 1983

Woody GE, McLellan AT, Luborsky L, et al: Severity of psychiatric symptoms as a predictor of benefits from psychotherapy: the Veterans Administration–Penn Study. Am J Psychiatry 141:1172–1177, 1984

Woody GE, McLellan AT, Luborsky L, et al: Sociopathy and psychotherapy outcome. Arch Gen Psychiatry 42:1081–1086, 1985

World Health Organization: International Classification of Diseases, 10th Revision. Geneva, World Health Organization, 1992

Worner TM: Propranolol versus diazepam in the management of the alcohol withdrawal syndrome: double-blind controlled trial. Am J Drug Alcohol Abuse 20:115–124, 1994

Yamaguchi K, Kandel DB: Patterns of drug use from adolescence to young adulthood, III: predictors of progression. Am J Public Health 74:673–680, 1984

CHAPTER 12

SCHIZOPHRENIA, SCHIZOPHRENIFORM DISORDER, AND DELUSIONAL (PARANOID) DISORDERS

DONALD W. BLACK, M.D.
NANCY C. ANDREASEN, M.D., PH.D.

Schizophrenia is perhaps the most enigmatic and tragic disease that psychiatrists treat, and perhaps also the most devastating. It strikes at a young age so that, unlike patients with cancer or heart disease, patients with schizophrenia usually live many years after onset of the disease and continue to suffer its effects, which prevent them from leading fully normal lives—attending school, working, having a close network of friends, marrying, or having children.

Apart from its impact on individuals and families, schizophrenia creates a huge economic burden for society. A study at the National Institute of Mental Health calculated the total cost of schizophrenia in 1991 at $65 billion (Wyatt et al. 1995). Nearly two-thirds was attributed to the indirect cost of family caregiving, lost wages, and losses due to early death from suicide, and the remainder went for treatment, public assistance, and other direct costs. Not taken into account is the enormous social and psychological anguish schizophrenia causes to patients and their families. Despite its emotional and economic costs, schizophrenia has yet to receive sufficient recognition as a major

health concern or the necessary research support to investigate its causes, treatments, and prevention. Large private foundations (e.g., the Dana Foundation, the National Association for Research in Schizophrenia and Affective Disorder [NARSAD]) have been working to meet these needs, however, indicating a groundswell of public awareness of the importance of schizophrenia that parallels that surrounding Alzheimer's disease a decade earlier.

The decade of the 1980s was a period of reassessment. Earlier optimism about the treatment of schizophrenia had been prompted by the introduction of neuroleptics and the community mental health movement. Deinstitutionalization took hold, and large numbers of people suffering from schizophrenia were released from hospitals. Optimism gradually led to pessimism as it became clear that neuroleptics had a limited ability to control the symptoms of schizophrenia and also exposed patients to health risks with long-term exposure to the drugs. Moreover, although many patients were released from hospitals, it became apparent that many discharged patients could not function in the community and had to be returned to state hospitals or

425

residential care facilities. Others became homeless or were trapped by the "revolving door" of frequent, brief hospitalizations.

Having perhaps promised too much, during the early 1990s clinicians and researchers interested in schizophrenia initially found themselves embattled. This resulted in a period of regrouping and reassessment that has led to a more realistic, integrated, and multifaceted approach to understanding this complex disorder. In the late 1990s, a new era of guarded optimism has emerged. Clinicians have agreed that the best treatment approaches combine medication with various forms of psychosocial care, and researchers have pioneered methods to integrate genetics, neurochemistry, and neuropathology. Rapidly evolving techniques in brain imaging and histopathology have provided a major boost to work in schizophrenia, assisted by concomitant advances in descriptive phenomenology, methods of classification, and epidemiology. The neuroscience community has joined together to identify the neural mechanisms of this important disease, promising that it may ultimately be understood at the systems, cellular, and molecular levels. Finally, after many years of "me too" antipsychotics with similar pharmacologic profiles, "atypical" medications have been introduced that are more effective for some patients and better tolerated.

HISTORICAL OVERVIEW

Schizophrenia and related disorders have been recognized in almost all cultures and described throughout much of recorded time. "Mania" or "phrensy" were generic terms that referred to a broad range of psychotic illnesses beginning in classical times. Literary portrayals, such as the madness of Orestes in *The Oresteia of Aeschylus* or the mumblings of Poor Tom in *King Lear,* make it clear that serious psychoses have been recognized even by lay people for many years. More technical descriptions appear in books such as Reginald Scot's *Discoveries of Witchcraft* in the 16th century or the classic psychiatric writings of Pinel in the 18th century (Andreasen 1984).

Although others before him, such as Kahlbaum, had circled around the topic of distinct subtypes of psychosis, Emil Kraepelin (1856–1926) is usually credited with delineating schizophrenia, principally on the basis of course and outcome. He observed that, among the seriously mentally ill whom he treated in Dorpat and later in Heidelberg and Munich, some began to have symptoms such as delusions and emotional withdrawal at a relatively early age and that these patients were likely to have a chronic and deteriorat-

ing course. Kraepelin worked closely with his colleague Alzheimer, who also studied patients with serious cognitive impairment and deterioration beginning at a later age; this condition is now referred to as Alzheimer's disease. The patients whom Kraepelin (1919) studied, in contrast, developed their "dementia" at an early age, and Kraepelin therefore chose to distinguish these patients from the late-onset dementias by referring to them as having "dementia praecox." Kraepelin was also instrumental in separating dementia praecox not only from Alzheimer's disease, but also from a third group of illnesses, which he referred to as "manic-depressive illness." Manic-depressive illness differed from dementia praecox in that it had an age at onset distributed throughout life and a more episodic and less deteriorating course and outcome.

The importance of distinguishing between dementia praecox and manic-depressive illness quickly gained wide acceptance because of its prognostic utility and remains one of the most important distinctions in modern psychiatry. At the urging of Eugen Bleuler (1857–1939), dementia praecox was eventually renamed "schizophrenia." Bleuler, who also honed his clinical and diagnostic skills through the close observation of large numbers of patients over long periods of time, was convinced that cross-sectional symptoms were more important defining features of schizophrenia than were course and outcome. He stressed that the fundamental and unifying abnormality in schizophrenia was cognitive impairment, which he conceptualized as a "splitting" or "loosening" in the "fabric of thought." He believed that "thought disorder" was the essential and pathognomonic symptom of schizophrenia and named the illness after this symptom: *schizophrenia,* or the fragmenting of mental capacities. He also believed that affective blunting, peculiar and distorted thinking (autism), avolition, impaired attention, and conceptual indecisiveness (ambivalence) were nearly equally important. Bleuler referred to this group of symptoms as "fundamental," whereas other symptoms such as delusions and hallucinations were regarded as "accessory," since they could occur in other disorders such as manic-depressive illness. Further, he pointed out that some patients with schizophrenia have a full recovery (or *restitutio ad integrum),* whereas others have a relatively chronic course but do not deteriorate. Finally, he pointed out that some patients begin to experience symptoms of schizophrenia in their 20s, 30s, or 40s. For all these reasons, the term schizophrenia seems preferable to dementia praecox.

After the publication of his classic textbook, *Dementia Praecox, or the Group of Schizophrenias* in 1911, Bleuler's ideas enjoyed increasing acceptance and became an influential description of schizophrenia in most of Europe,

England, and the United States for decades. Several generations of psychiatrists were taught to recite the Bleulerian "Four A's" (occasionally expanded to five or six in order to reflect more accurately what Bleuler actually said): associations, affect, autism, and ambivalence. Thought disorder, or associative loosening, was considered to be the most important among these. Unlike delusions and hallucinations, Bleulerian fundamental symptoms are on a continuum with normality and can be present in relatively mild forms; some, such as ambivalence, are common in normal persons. Consequently, the influence of Bleuler led to an increasingly broad definition and conceptualization of schizophrenia as psychiatry gathered strength and momentum during the postwar years and through the 1950s and 1960s. This phenomenon was particularly apparent in the United States, where concepts such as "latent schizophrenia" and "pseudoneurotic schizophrenia" became popular (Black and Bofelli 1989). These concepts were reflected in the initial editions of the Diagnostic and Statistical Manual of Mental Disorders, published by the American Psychiatric Association. The first edition (American Psychiatric Association 1952) emphasized intrapsychic mechanisms rather than classes of disease, whereas the second edition (American Psychiatric Association 1968) shifted the emphasis to classification, but without listing specific criteria.

By the late 1960s, a number of factors intervened to introduce a climate of change. Studies of comparative diagnostic practices in the United States, England, and other nations alerted American psychiatrists to the fact that their diagnostic habits were out of step. For example, the United States/United Kingdom diagnostic project (Cooper et al. 1972) set out to determine why the prevalence of schizophrenia was greater in New York than London, while the reverse was true for manic-depressive illness. The investigators discovered that the same patients received different diagnoses in different countries due to conceptual and theoretical differences between their respective diagnostic systems. At about the same time, findings were reported from the International Pilot Study of Schizophrenia (World Health Organization 1975), in which schizophrenia was studied in nine countries. The major finding to emerge was that similar criteria were used in seven of the nine countries, but broader criteria were used in the United States and the Soviet Union.

In the context of these studies, an interest in reliable diagnosis emerged, leading to the development of structured interviews such as the Present State Examination (Wing et al. 1967), and operational diagnostic criteria such as the St. Louis Criteria (Feighner et al. 1972) developed at Washington University. Structured interviews required

the definition of a symptom in a way that would insure close agreement among clinicians and were accompanied by the development of operational diagnostic criteria in which definitions were spelled out in a clear and objective way. Bleulerian symptoms, with their breadth and imprecision, did not lend themselves well to such techniques. On the other hand, the use of delusions and hallucinations as defining features emphasized phenomena that are clearly abnormal and relatively easy to identify. The Present State Examination helped to introduce the concepts of the German psychiatrist Kurt Schneider (1887–1967) and his emphasis on "first-rank symptoms" to the English-speaking world. These forces helped reshape the concept of schizophrenia into one of a relatively severe psychotic disorder, bringing it closer to the original ideas of Kraepelin, but lacking Kraepelin's emphasis on a longitudinal definition that used course and outcome as a diagnostic guide.

Finally, and perhaps more importantly, the development of effective treatments such as neuroleptics, antidepressants, and, eventually, lithium carbonate made diagnosis an important clinical issue. If a patient with bipolar disorder or major depression were misdiagnosed with schizophrenia because of an excessively broad diagnostic concept, that patient might be deprived of the most appropriate treatment available, potentially condemned to an unnecessarily chronic course of illness, and perhaps condemned to needlessly suffer permanent and irreversible medication side effects.

As this brief historical overview indicates, the concept of schizophrenia has varied enormously over time and space. Kraepelin's definition was concise and narrow. For him, dementia praecox was an illness with a characteristic age at onset in the teens or early twenties that had a relatively poor outcome and led much of the time to relatively severe cognitive and emotional impairment. Kraepelin believed that the disorder would eventually be understood in terms of neuropathological mechanisms in the brain because of this clinical course. Although he emphasized the importance of cognitive impairment (i.e., "dementia"), he did not choose any single symptom as characteristic or pathognomonic; rather, his description of the clinical phenomenology stresses a mixture of delusions, hallucinations, motor signs and symptoms, emotional blunting, avolition, and social isolation. The introduction of Bleulerian ideas simultaneously broadened the concept and stressed the importance of symptoms that affected cognition, emotion, and volition. The emphasis on Schneiderian symptoms in the 1970s reintroduced yet another set of cross-sectional symptoms, specific delusions and hallucinations, which were quite different from the Bleulerian symptoms.

All of these developments led to a reassessment of how schizophrenia and other mental disorders were diagnosed, culminating in the third edition of the Diagnostic and Statistical Manual of Mental Disorders (DSM-III), which enumerated specific criteria for all recognized psychiatric disorders. DSM-III (American Psychiatric Association 1980) and its revision (DSM-III-R; American Psychiatric Association 1987) represented a convergence of these various points of view. The criteria included the Kraepelinian emphasis on course through the requirement that the illness be present for at least 6 months, the emphasis on specific delusions and hallucinations thought important by Schneider, and the emphasis on the importance of fundamental Bleulerian symptoms (thought disorder in the form of associative loosening or incoherence and affective blunting).

The DSM-III and DSM-III-R compromise stirred debate among investigators interested in understanding the pathophysiology and etiology of schizophrenia. New technologies, such as molecular genetics or brain imaging, re-emphasized the importance of careful and precise definition of the disease, as had occurred with the introduction of neuroleptics. Geneticists interested in familial patterns of transmission wondered whether the DSM-III and DSM-III-R definitions, with their requirement of florid psychotic symptoms, were too narrow to pick up subclinical cases in family pedigrees. They considered whether the concept of schizophrenia should be expanded to include nonpsychotic forms (e.g., simple and latent schizophrenia), much as Bleuler originally suggested. Studies of the neurobiology of schizophrenia, made possible by brain imaging and postmortem brain banks, blurred the distinction between schizophrenia and "organic" disorders. Nearly four decades of psychopharmacologic treatment of schizophrenia demonstrated that florid psychotic symptoms are probably not the core defining features after all, since crippling negative or deficit symptoms persist and seem fundamental, much as Bleuler observed. These observations have now been given more weight in DSM-IV (American Psychiatric Association 1994). Research conducted in the 1980s, as well as field trials conducted specifically for the Task Force on DSM-IV, showed that deficit symptoms can be reliably defined and should be considered as core features of the disorder.

diagnosis. The St. Louis criteria developed in 1972 include both longitudinal and cross-sectional criteria designed to identify schizophrenic patients with poor prognosis. The criteria require the exclusion of affective illness, drug abuse, or alcoholism and exclusion of cases of less than 6 months' duration. The Research Diagnostic Criteria (RDC) were introduced later and differ from the St. Louis criteria mainly in emphasis on course of illness (Spitzer et al. 1978). The St. Louis criteria require 6 months of continuous illness, whereas the RDC require only a 2-week history. These two sets of criteria were instrumental in the development of the DSM-III in 1980 and DSM-III-R in 1987 and include definitions of schizophrenia requiring both longitudinal and cross-sectional features.

The concept of including both cross-sectional and longitudinal features remains in DSM-IV, but more prominence is given to the Bleulerian concept of fundamental symptoms. According to DSM-IV, schizophrenia consists of the presence of characteristic positive or negative symptoms of at least 1 month in duration (unless successfully treated); deterioration in work, interpersonal relations, or self-care; continuous signs of the disturbance for at least 6 months; the ruling out of schizoaffective disorder and mood disorder with psychotic features; the determination that the disturbance is not due to a general medical condition or the direct physiological effects of a substance; and, finally, if autistic disorder or another pervasive developmental disorder is present, prominent hallucinations or delusions have also been present for at least 1 month. Schizophrenia is further classified according to course of illness as shown in Table 12–1.

If an illness otherwise meets the criteria, but has a duration of at least 1 month but less than 6 months, it is termed a *schizophreniform disorder*. If it has lasted less than 4 weeks, it may be classified as either a brief psychotic disorder or a psychotic disorder not otherwise specified, which is a residual category for psychotic disturbances that cannot be better classified.

Changes made in the diagnostic criteria of schizophrenia from DSM-III to DSM-IV are shown in Table 12–2. The major changes involve the description of and time requirement for active-phase symptoms, the deletion of the age at onset criterion, various exclusions, and the expansion of choices for classification of course.

DIAGNOSIS

Several sets of operational criteria were developed in the United States during the 1970s to increase the reliability of

DIFFERENTIAL DIAGNOSIS

The diagnosis of schizophrenia should be thought of as a diagnosis of exclusion, because none of its clinical features

TABLE 12–1.   DSM-IV criteria for schizophrenia

A. *Characteristic symptoms:* Two (or more) of the following, each present for a significant portion of time during a one-month period (or less if successfully treated):

(1) Delusions

(2) Hallucinations

(3) Disorganized speech (e.g., frequent derailment or incoherence)

(4) Grossly disorganized or catatonic behavior

(5) Negative symptoms (i.e., affective flattening, alogia, or avolition)

Note: Only one A symptom is required if delusions are bizarre or hallucinations consist of a voice keeping up a running commentary on the person's behavior or thoughts, or two or more voices conversing with each other.

B. *Social/occupational dysfunction:* For a significant portion of the time since the onset of the disturbance, one or more major areas of functioning such as work, interpersonal relations, or self-care are markedly below the level achieved prior to the onset (or when the onset is in childhood or adolescence, failure to achieve expected level of interpersonal, academic, or occupational achievement).

C. *Duration:* Continuous signs of the disturbance persist for at least 6 months. This 6-month period must include at least 1 month of symptoms (or less if successfully treated) that meet criterion A (i.e., active-phase symptoms) and may include periods of prodromal or residual symptoms. During these prodromal or residual periods, the signs of the disturbance may be manifested by only negative symptoms or two or more symptoms listed in criterion A present in an attenuated form (e.g., odd beliefs, unusual perceptual experiences).

D. *Schizoaffective and mood disorder exclusion:* Schizoaffective disorder and mood disorder with psychotic features have been ruled out because either 1) no major depressive, manic, or mixed episodes have occurred concurrently with the active-phase symptoms; or 2) if mood episodes have occurred during active-phase symptoms, their total duration has been brief relative to the duration of the active and residual periods.

E. *Substance/general medical condition exclusion:* The disturbance is not due to the direct physiological effects of a substance (e.g., a drug of abuse, a medication) or a general medical condition.

F. *Relationship to a pervasive developmental disorder:* If there is a history of autistic disorder or another pervasive developmental disorder, the additional diagnosis of schizophrenia is made only if prominent delusions or hallucinations are also present for at least 1 month (or less if successfully treated).

Classification of longitudinal course (can be applied only after at least 1 year has elapsed since the initial onset of active-phase symptoms):

Episodic with interepisode residual symptoms (episodes are defined by the reemergence of prominent psychotic symptoms); *also specify if:* **with prominent negative symptoms**

Episodic with no interepisode residual symptoms

Continuous (prominent psychotic symptoms are present throughout the period of observation); *also specify if:* **with prominent negative symptoms**

Single episode in partial remission; *also specify if:* **with prominent negative symptoms**

Single episode in full remission

Other or unspecified pattern

---

are pathognomonic. Schizophrenia remains a clinical diagnosis that rests on historical information and a careful mental status examination, and there are no predictable laboratory abnormalities that are diagnostic of the disorder. The first step in diagnosis is to take a careful history and perform a physical examination to exclude psychoses with known medical causes. Psychotic symptoms have been found to result from substance abuse (e.g., hallucinogens, phencyclidine, amphetamines, cocaine, alcohol); intoxication due to commonly prescribed medications (e.g., corticosteroids, anticholinergics, levodopa); infectious, metabolic, and endocrine disorders; tumors and mass lesions; and temporal lobe epilepsy. Atypical presentations such as a relatively acute onset, clouding of the sensorium, or onset occurring after age 30 years demand careful investigation.

Routine lab tests may be helpful in ruling out potential medical causes. Common screening tests include a complete blood count (CBC), urinalysis, liver enzymes, serum creatinine, blood urea nitrogen (BUN), thyroid function tests, and serologic tests for evidence of an infection with syphilis or the human immunodeficiency virus (HIV). Other tests will be indicated in selected patients, such as a serum ceruloplasmin to rule out Wilson's disease. Electroencephalography (EEG), computed tomography (CT), or magnetic resonance imaging (MRI) may be useful in selected cases to rule out alternate diagnoses, such as a tumor or mass lesion, or epilepsy.

The major task in differential diagnosis involves separating schizophrenia from schizoaffective disorder, mood disorder with psychotic features, delusional disorder, or a personality disorder. To rule out schizoaffective disorder

TABLE 12–2.   Differences among DSM-III, DSM-III-R, and DSM-IV criteria for schizophrenia

DSM-III	DSM-III-R	DSM-IV
Characteristic active-phase symptoms	Characteristic active-phase symptoms for 1 week or more	Characteristic active-phase symptoms 1 month or more (less if treated)
Deterioration in functioning	Impairment in functioning	Social/occupational dysfunction
Duration at least 6 months or more (including active phase)	Duration at least 6 months or more (including active phase)	Duration at least 6 months or more (including active phase)
Depression and mania ruled out	Schizoaffective disorder and psychotic mood disorder ruled out	Schizoaffective disorder and psychotic mood disorder ruled out
Organic mental disorder and mental retardation ruled out	Organic mental disorder ruled out Autistic disorder ruled out	Effects of substance or general medical condition ruled out
Onset before age 45		If there is a history of pervasive developmental disorder, prominent delusions, hallucinations must also be present for at least 1 month (or less if successfully treated)
Classification of course	**Classification of course**	**Classification of course**
Subchronic (> 6 months but < 2 yrs)	Subchronic (> 6 months but < 2 yrs)	Episodic with interepisode residual symptoms
Chronic (> 2 yrs)	Chronic (> 2 years)	Episodic with no interepisode residual symptoms
Subchronic with acute exacerbation	Subchronic with acute exacerbation	Continuous
Chronic with acute exacerbation	Chronic with acute exacerbation	Single episode in partial remission
In remission	In remission	Single episode in full remission
	Unspecified	Other or unspecified pattern

and psychotic mood disorders, major depressive or manic episodes should have been absent during the active phase, or the mood episode should have been brief relative to the total duration of the psychotic episode. Unlike delusional disorder, schizophrenia is characterized by bizarre delusions, and hallucinations are common. Patients with personality disorders, particularly those in the "eccentric" cluster (e.g., schizoid, schizotypal, and paranoid personality), may be indifferent to social relationships and display restricted affect, may have bizarre ideation and odd speech, or may be suspicious and hypervigilant, but they do not have delusions, hallucinations, or grossly disorganized behavior. Furthermore, patients with schizophrenia may develop other symptoms, such as a profound thought disorder, behavioral disturbances, and enduring personality deterioration. These symptoms are uncharacteristic of the mood disorders, delusional disorder, or the personality disorders.

Depersonalization disorder and sometimes panic disorder are accompanied by feelings of unreality, such as that one's mind and body are separate; however, insight is generally well preserved, and hallucinations and delusions are absent. The rituals occurring in a patient with obsessive-compulsive disorder may result in bizarre behavior, but they are performed to relieve anxiety, and not in response to delusional beliefs.

Other psychiatric disorders also must be ruled out, including schizophreniform disorder, brief psychotic disorder, factitious disorder with psychological symptoms, and malingering. If symptoms persist for more than 6 months, schizophreniform disorder can be ruled out. The history of how the illness presents will help to rule out an brief psychotic disorder, since schizophrenia generally has an insidious onset and there are usually no precipitating stressors. Factitious disorder may be difficult to delineate from schizophrenia, especially when the patient is knowledgeable about mental illness or is medically trained, but careful observation should enable the clinician to make the distinction between real or feigned psychosis. Likewise, a malingerer could attempt to simulate schizophrenia, but careful observation will help to distinguish the disorders. With the malingerer, there will be evidence of obvious secondary gain, such as avoiding incarceration, and the history may suggest antisocial personality disorder. The differential diagnosis for schizophrenia is summarized in Table 12–3.

TABLE 12–3. **Differential diagnosis of schizophrenia**

Psychiatric illness	General medical illness	Drugs of abuse
Psychotic mood disorders	Temporal lobe epilepsy	Stimulants (e.g., amphetamine, cocaine)
Schizoaffective disorder	Tumor, stroke, brain trauma	Hallucinogens (e.g., phencyclidine [PCP])
Brief reactive psychosis	Endocrine/metabolic disorders (e.g., porphyria)	Anticholinergics (e.g., belladonna alkaloids)
Schizophreniform disorder	Vitamin deficiency (e.g., B_{12})	Alcohol withdrawal delirium
Delusional disorder	Infectious (e.g., neurosyphilis)	Barbiturate withdrawal delirium
Induced psychotic disorder	Autoimmune (e.g., systemic lupus erythematous)	
Panic disorder	Toxic (e.g., heavy metal poisoning)	
Depersonalization disorder		
Obsessive-compulsive disorder		
Personality disorders (e.g., "eccentric" cluster)		
Factitious disorder with psychological symptoms		
Malingering		

CLINICAL FINDINGS

Clinical manifestations of schizophrenia and schizophreniform disorders are diverse and can change over time. Because of their variety, it has been said that to know schizophrenia is to know psychiatry. Whereas many symptoms are obvious, such as hallucinations, others such as affective blunting or incongruity are relatively subtle and can be easily missed by a casual observer.

A variety of methods have been developed to describe and classify the multiplicity of symptoms in schizophrenia. Traditionally, schizophrenia is considered to be a type of "psychosis," yet the definition of psychosis has been elusive. Older definitions stressed the subjective and internal psychological experience and defined psychosis as an "impairment in reality testing." More recently, psychosis has been defined objectively and operationally as the occurrence of hallucinations and delusions. Because schizophrenia is characterized by so many different types of symptoms, clinicians and scientists have tried to simplify the description of the clinical presentation by dividing the symptoms into subgroups. The most widely used subdivision classifies the symptoms as positive and negative.

POSITIVE AND NEGATIVE SYMPTOMS

The concept of positive and negative symptoms was originally formulated by the British neurologist John Hughlings Jackson (1931). Jackson believed that positive symptoms reflected release phenomena occurring in more phylogenetically advanced brain regions, due to injury to the brain at a more primitive level. Negative symptoms, on the other hand, simply represented a "dissolution," or a loss of brain function. Current definitions of positive and negative symptoms are an amplification of these earlier ideas.

Positive symptoms, including hallucinations, delusions, marked positive formal thought disorder (manifested by marked incoherence, derailment, tangentiality, or illogicality), and bizarre or disorganized behavior reflect a distortion or exaggeration of functions that are normally present. For example, hallucinations are a distortion or exaggeration of the function of the perceptual systems of the brain: the person experiences a perception in the absence of an external stimulus.

Negative symptoms reflect a deficiency of a mental function that is normally present. For example, some patients display *alogia* (i.e., marked poverty of speech, or poverty of content of speech). Others show *affective flattening*, *anhedonia/asociality* (i.e., inability to experience pleasure, few social contacts), *avolition/apathy* (i.e., anergia, impersistence at work or school), and *attentional impairment*. These negative or deficit symptoms are not only difficult to treat and respond less well to neuroleptics than positive symptoms, but they are also the most destructive because they render the patient inert and unmotivated. The schizophrenic patient with prominent negative symptoms may be able to raise his or her performance under supervision but cannot maintain it when supervision is withdrawn.

Recent research suggests that these symptoms reflect dimensions rather than discrete categories of psychopathology and that there are probably three dimensions rather than two (Andreasen et al. 1995; Arndt et al. 1995; Bilder et al. 1985; Liddle et al. 1989). Positive symptoms can be further divided into dimensions of psychoticism (i.e., delusions and hallucinations) and disorganization (i.e., disorganized speech and behavior and inappropriate affect). Negative (or deficit) symptoms represent a third dimension. The relationship between these three dimensions and their underlying pathophysiology continues to be studied and discussed (Andreasen et al. 1995).

Crow (1980) has proposed a method for classifying schizophrenic patients based on the presence of positive or negative symptoms. He has designated schizophrenic patients with mostly positive symptoms as Type I and those with mostly negative symptoms as Type II. However, in practice patients generally display a mixture of both positive and negative symptoms (Andreasen et al. 1990b).

The frequency of these and other common symptoms reported in 111 schizophrenic patients is presented in Table 12–4.

THE PSYCHOTIC DIMENSION

This symptom dimension refers to two classic "psychotic" symptoms that reflect a patient's confusion about the loss of boundaries between him- or herself and the external world: hallucinations and delusions. Both symptoms reflect a "loss of ego boundaries": the patient is unable to distinguish between his or her own thoughts and perceptions and those that he or she obtains by observing the external world.

Hallucinations have sometimes been considered the hallmark of schizophrenia. Although hallucinations may occur in a variety of other disorders, including mood and organic disorders, they remain important symptoms of schizophrenia and schizophreniform disorders. *Hallucinations* are perceptions experienced without an external stimulus to the sense organs that have qualities similar to a true perception (e.g., intensity, location). They are usually experienced as originating in the outside world, or within one's own body, but not within the mind as through imagination. Hallucinations vary in complexity and in sensory modality. Schizophrenic patients commonly have auditory, visual, tactile, gustatory, or olfactory hallucinations, or a combination of several types. Auditory hallucinations are the most frequent type observed in schizophrenia and may be experienced as noises, music, or more typically "voices." Voices may be mumbled or may sound clear and distinct,

and words, phrases, or sentences may be heard. Hallucinations may be inferred when the patient appears to be talking in response to the voices and may whisper, mutter incomprehensibly, talk normally, or shout out loud. Visual hallucinations may be simple or complex and include flashes of light or the image of persons, animals, or objects; they may be smaller or larger than a true perception. They may be experienced as being located outside the field of vision such as being behind the head and are usually reported in normal color. Olfactory and gustatory hallucinations are often experienced together, leading to unpleasant tastes and odors. Tactile hallucinations (or *haptic* hallucinations) may be experienced as sensations of being touched or pricked, electrical sensations, or even a sensation of insects crawling under the skin, which is called *formication*. Tactile hallucinations may occur as feelings of body organs being pulled upon and distended, and sexual stimulation may be experienced. Schizophrenic patients in all cultures experience hallucinations, although they may differ in frequency and type depending on the patient's experience and background (Ndetei and Vadher 1984).

Delusions involve a disturbance in inferential thinking rather than perception. Delusions are firmly held beliefs that are untrue; the judgment of "untrueness" must always be made within the context of the person's educational and cultural background. Delusions occurring in patients with schizophrenia may have somatic, grandiose, religious, nihilistic, or persecutory themes (see Table 12–5). None is specific to schizophrenia, and, like hallucinations, delusions tend to be culturally based. For example, a patient in the United States may worry about persecution by the CIA or FBI; a Bantu or Zulu might worry about persecution by spirits or demons.

Certain types of auditory hallucinations and delusions were considered symptoms of the first rank by Schneider. These symptoms share the common feature that all represent an intrusion of "personal space" by some outside influence: an extreme example of the loss of personal boundaries and the difficulty in distinguishing between internal experiences and the external world.

First-rank hallucinations were described by Schneider as prolonged, clearly audible voices, often commenting upon a person's actions or arguing with each other about the patient or repeating aloud the patient's thoughts. First-rank delusions were those of thought broadcasting, thought withdrawal, thought insertion, or delusions of passivity (i.e., being controlled as if a puppet). First-rank symptoms are present in up to three-quarters of schizophrenic patients but are also present in many patients with psychotic mood disorders (Andreasen and Akiskal 1983). These symptoms have not proven useful in predicting

TABLE 12–4. **Frequency of symptoms in 111 schizophrenic patients**

Symptom	%	Symptom	%
Negative symptoms		**Positive symptoms**	
Affective flattening		*Hallucinations*	
Unchanging facial expression	96	Auditory	75
Decreased spontaneous movements	66	Voices commenting	58
Paucity of expressive gestures	81	Voices conversing	57
Poor eye contact	71	Somatic-tactile	20
Affective nonresponsivity	64	Olfactory	6
Inappropriate affect	63	Visual	49
Lack of vocal inflections	73		
		Delusions	
Alogia		Persecutory	81
Poverty of speech	53	Jealous	4
Poverty of content of speech	51	Guilt, sin	26
Blocking	23	Grandiose	39
Increased response latency	31	Religious	31
		Somatic	28
Avolition-apathy		Delusions of reference	49
Impaired grooming and hygiene	87	Delusions of being controlled	46
Lack of persistence at work or school	95	Delusions of mind reading	48
Physical anergia	82	Thought broadcasting	23
		Thought insertion	31
Anhedonia-asociality		Thought withdrawal	27
Few recreational interests/activities	95		
Little sexual interest/activity	69	*Bizarre behavior*	
Impaired intimacy/closeness	84	Clothing, appearance	20
Few relationships with friends/peers	96	Social, sexual behavior	33
		Aggressive-agitated	27
Attention		Repetitive-stereotyped	28
Social inattentiveness	78		
Inattentiveness during testing	64	*Positive formal thought disorder*	
		Derailment	45
		Tangentiality	50
		Incoherence	23
		Illogicality	23
		Circumstantiality	35
		Pressure of speech	24
		Distractible speech	23
		Clanging	3

Source.   Adapted from Andreasen 1987.

treatment response or outcome in schizophrenia (see Table 12–6 for a list of common first-rank symptoms).

Several unusual delusions have been described that are often part of a schizophrenic illness. In the *Capgras syndrome*, a patient believes that a person closely related to him or her has been replaced by a double. (This belief was the theme of the 1950s "B" horror movie, *Invasion of the Body Snatchers*.) In the *Fregoli syndrome*, a patient identifies a familiar person in various other people he or she encounters. The patient may maintain that although there is no physi-

TABLE 12–5.   Varied content in delusions

Delusions	Foci of preoccupation
Grandiose	Possessing wealth, great beauty, or having a special ability (e.g., extrasensory perception); having influential friends; being an important figure (e.g., Napoleon, Hitler)
Nihilistic	Belief that one is dead or dying; belief that one does not exist or that the world does not exist
Persecutory	Being persecuted by friends, neighbors, or spouses; being followed , monitored, or spied on by the government (e.g., FBI, CIA) or other important organizations (e.g., the Catholic Church)
Somatic	Belief that one's organs have stopped functioning (e.g., that the heart is no longer beating) or are rotting away; belief that the nose or other body part is terribly misshapen or disfigured
Sexual	Belief that one's sexual behavior is commonly known; that one is a prostitute, a pedophile, or a rapist; that masturbation has led to illness or insanity
Religious	Belief that one has sinned against God; that one has a special relationship to God or some other deity; that one has a special religious mission; that one is the Devil or is condemned to burn in Hell

cal resemblance between the familiar person and others, they are nonetheless psychologically identical. *Cotard's syndrome* is characterized by the belief that one of the patient's bodily organs (e.g., brain, bowel) has changed in some impossible way, has stopped functioning, or has even disappeared.

THE DISORGANIZATION DIMENSION

The disorganization dimension includes disorganized speech, disorganized or bizarre behavior, and incongruous affect.

Disorganized speech, or *thought disorder*, was regarded as the most important symptom of schizophrenia by Bleuler. Historically, types of thought disorder have included associative loosening, illogical thinking, overinclusive thinking, and loss of ability to engage in abstract thinking. A standard set of definitions for various types of thought disorder has been developed (Andreasen 1979b) that stresses objective aspects of language and communication (which are empirical indicators of "thought"), such as derailment, poverty of speech, poverty of content of speech, or tangen-

TABLE 12–6.   Schneider's first-rank symptoms

Hallucination of one's thoughts being spoken aloud

Hallucination of voices in the form of a running commentary about the patient

Hallucination of voices conversing about the patient ("third person" hallucination) or arguing

Somatic hallucination attributed to outside forces (e.g., X rays, hypnosis)

Delusions of thoughts being withdrawn or inserted from patient's mind by an outside person or force

Delusions of thoughts being broadcast so that patient's private thoughts are known to others

Delusional perceptions in which highly personal meanings are attributed to perceptions

Delusions of being influenced or forced to do things or want things the patient does not wish to do and does not want

Delusions of being made to feel emotions or sensations (often sexual) that are not the patient's own

tial replies, and all have been found to occur frequently in both schizophrenia and mood disorders. Manic patients often have a thought disorder characterized by tangentiality, derailment (loose associations) and illogicality. Depressed patients manifest thought disorder less frequently than manic patients, but often display a poverty of speech, tangentiality, or circumstantiality. Other types of formal thought disorder include perseveration, distractibility, clanging, neologisms, echolalia, and blocking; with the possible exception of clanging in mania, none appears to be disorder specific. An example of speech from a patient with a prominent thought disorder (particularly derailment) follows:

> Let's see, there was one I would have liked if it wasn't for the instructor, well I go along with him, he was always wanting me to do the worse in class, it seemed like, and I'd always get bad, the grade, in my grading, and he tried to make other people like they were good enough to be in Hollywood or something, you know I'd be the last one down the ladder. That, that's the way they wanted the grading to be in the first place according to whose, theirs, they, they have all different reasons that I, I, I think that they use that they want one, won't come out. (Andreasen 1984, p. 61)

Because these various forms of thought disorder are inferred from listening to patients speak, the concept of disorganized speech has evolved and appears as such in the diagnostic criteria.

Disorganized or *catatonic motor behavior* is another aspect of this dimension. Many patients with schizophrenia display various motor disturbances and changes in social behavior. Abnormal motor behaviors range from catatonic stupor to excitement. In a catatonic stupor, the patient may be immobile, mute, and unresponsive, and yet remain fully conscious. A patient may exhibit uncontrolled and aimless motor activity while in a state of catatonic excitement. Some patients manifest *waxy flexibility* (flexibilitas cerea), in which they allow themselves to be placed in uncomfortable positions, which are maintained without apparent distress. Schizophrenic patients sometimes assume bizarre or awkward postures and maintain them for long periods, such as squatting for hours, which would cause obvious discomfort to most people.

Several disorders of movement that occur in schizophrenia need to be distinguished from drug-induced extrapyramidal side effects of antipsychotics and tardive dyskinesia (Manshreck et al. 1982). These include *stereotypies*, which are repeated movements that are not goal directed such as rocking; *mannerisms*, which are normal goal-directed activities that appear to have social significance but are either odd in appearance or out of context, such as grimacing or repeatedly running a hand through one's hair. *Mitgehen* is seen when the slightest pressure causes the patient's limbs to move in the direction of the push, despite being told to resist the pressure. Less common symptoms are *echopraxia*, which is imitating the movements and gestures of another person; *automatic obedience*, which is carrying out simple commands in a robotlike fashion; and *negativism*, which is refusing to cooperate with simple requests for no apparent reason. Many schizophrenic patients display ritualistic behaviors resembling those seen in obsessive-compulsive disorder, such as repetitive handwashing, checking, arranging, or counting (Fenton and McGlashan 1986). Some schizophrenic patients develop compulsive water drinking, which can lead to water intoxication necessitating careful attention to fluid and electrolyte balance (deLeon et al. 1994).

Antipsychotic medications are often responsible for inducing a variety of extrapyramidal side effects (EPS) as well as tardive dyskinesia, all of which are discussed in Chapter 27. Many schizophrenic patients were reported to display EPS or spontaneous involuntary movements before antipsychotics became available (Chatterjee et al. 1995). The presence of spontaneous EPS has been linked to poorer treatment response and negative symptoms. When tardive dyskinesia is present, schizophrenic patients are often unaware of their involuntary movements. Even when the abnormal movements are pointed out, the patient may remain unconcerned (Caracci et al. 1990).

Deterioration of social behavior often develops along with social withdrawal. Patients may neglect themselves and become messy or unkempt, wear dirty, unmended, or inap-

propriate clothing, and ignore or neglect their cluttered, untidy surroundings. Patients may develop other odd behaviors, breaking social conventions by exhibiting crude table manners, foraging through garbage bins, or shouting obscenities. It has been estimated that between one-third and one-half of today's "homeless" persons have schizophrenia (Susser et al. 1989).

Incongruity of affect is the third component of the disorganization dimension. Patients may smile inappropriately when speaking of neutral or sad topics, or giggle for no apparent reason. This symptom should not be confused with the nervous smiling or giggling that sometimes occurs in anxious patients. Affective incongruity should only be considered a symptom of schizophrenia when it occurs in the context of other characteristic symptoms.

THE NEGATIVE DIMENSION

DSM-IV lists three negative symptoms as characteristic of schizophrenia: alogia, affective blunting, and avolition. Other negative symptoms that are common in schizophrenia include anhedonia and attentional impairment (Andreasen 1982; Andreasen and Olson 1982).

Alogia is characterized by a diminution in the amount of spontaneous speech, a tendency to produce speech that is empty or impoverished in content when the amount is adequate. It is the external expression in language of the impoverishment of thought that occurs in many patients with schizophrenia. Patients may have great difficulty in producing fluent responses to questions. Instead, they tend to say little or reply concretely. For example, if asked "What brought you to the hospital?" the patient may reply "a car."

Affective flattening or blunting is a reduced intensity of emotional expression and response. It is manifested by unchanging facial expression, decreased spontaneous movements, poverty of expressive gestures, poor eye contact, lack of vocal inflections, and slowed speech.

Anhedonia, or the inability to experience pleasure, is also very common. Many patients describe themselves as feeling emotionally empty. They are no longer able to enjoy activities that previously gave them pleasure, such as playing sports or seeing family or friends. Their awareness that they have lost the capacity to enjoy themselves may be a source of great psychological pain.

Avolition is a loss of the ability to initiate goal-directed behavior and carry it through to completion. Patients seem to have lost their will or drive. They may initiate a project and then abandon it for no apparent reason. They may take a job, go to work for a few days or weeks, and then fail to appear or wander aimlessly away while at work. This symptom is sometimes interpreted as laziness, but in fact it represents the loss or diminution of basic drives and the capacity to formulate and pursue long-range plans.

Attentional impairment is reflected in the inability to concentrate or focus on a task or a question. Patients may complain of feeling bombarded by stimuli that they cannot process or filter; this in turn causes them to feel confused or to experience fragmented thoughts.

The negative symptoms of schizophrenia and the symptoms of depression are somewhat similar, making differential diagnosis of depression and schizophrenia difficult in some patients. Significant depressive symptoms occur in up to 60% of schizophrenic patients (Guze et al. 1983), leading to substantial distress, prompting suicidal behavior in some patients, and compromising what little energy and motivation the patient has. Antipsychotic medication itself may induce what appears to be depression, but is actually a drug-induced akinesia. This "depression" may go away when the dosage of antipsychotic is reduced or an anticholinergic medication is added (King et al. 1995). The International Classification of Diseases, 10th Edition (ICD-10) (World Health Organization 1992), recognizes a category called "post-psychotic depression," a full-blown depression occurring after the acute phase symptoms have fully resolved. In DSM-IV, a postpsychotic depression, or a major depression occurring in a patient with well-established schizophrenia, is diagnosed as a depressive disorder not otherwise specified.

The following case example (adapted from Andreasen 1984, pp. 57–58) illustrates many of the symptoms found in schizophrenia, and shows the profound impact of negative symptoms.

CASE EXAMPLE 1

Ronald, a 42-year-old unmarried man, had lived in a state hospital more or less continuously since the death of his last surviving parent 5 years earlier. As a youngster, his family noted that he was extremely shy and withdrawn. Although clearly attached to them, he did not enjoy hugging, kissing, or other expressions of affection. In school, he tended to be solitary, and although he functioned at an average level, his parents considered him bright and creative because he read a great deal, had a large vocabulary, and enjoyed various intellectual games. He was also preoccupied with inventing things. In high school, he invented a new alphabet that was supposed to be more phonetically functional than the one currently in use. Although he tried to explain its basic principles, no one seemed to understand it. Sometimes his parents were unable to determine whether he was difficult to understand because he was so much smarter than they or whether his thinking was simply disorganized.

During high school Ronald did not participate in any activities, had no friends, and never dated. He entered college, but dropped out with failing grades at the end of his first semester. He returned home to live with his parents, but despite repeated efforts to get him out of the house and into various types of jobs, he was never able to persist and perform any task dependably. He became increasingly absorbed in a fantasy world and spent much of his time involved in "intergalactic communication." He claimed to receive messages from an unknown galaxy in a special language that only he was able to understand. These messages, which he heard as if they were voices talking to him inside his head, would describe events in the distant galaxy of Atan. As he grew older, he seemed to lose interest in discussing this inner world and his inner voices with anyone. Never interested in appearance, he became disheveled. He had to be encouraged by his parents to wear clean clothing, to bathe, and to shave. He tended to select rather bizarre attire and hairstyles and preferred to wear long underwear, overalls, and a baseball cap placed backwards.

Ronald was briefly hospitalized after he returned home from college and placed on antipsychotic medication, which helped minimally. He was unable to follow through on tasks, developed extreme social withdrawal, and became fully preoccupied with his fantasy world. After the death of his mother when he was 32, he again required hospitalization. High doses of antipsychotic medication appeared to help temporarily, but had no lasting benefit. He was 36 when his father died. He lived at home alone for the next year, but was eventually rehospitalized after complaints from neighbors brought him to the attention of community agencies. He had been living in the house for the past year without ever having done laundry, taken out the garbage, or washed the dishes. The house gradually had filled with rotting food, debris, and old newspapers. He was placed in a chronic care facility because he was unable to function independently.

COGNITIVE IMPAIRMENT AS THE FUNDAMENTAL DEFICIT

Many thinkers, beginning with both Kraepelin and Bleuler, have considered schizophrenia to be a neurocognitive disorder, with the various signs and symptoms reflecting the downstream effects of a fundamental cognitive deficit. This fundamental cognitive deficit was highlighted in the original name *dementia praecox* and the later name *schizophrenia* ("fragmented mind"). Schizophrenia poses special challenges to the development of cognitive models because of its breadth and diversity of symptoms. The symptoms include nearly all domains of function: perception (hallucinations), inferential thinking (delusions), fluency of thought and speech (alogia), clarity and organization of thought and speech ("formal thought disorder"), motor activity (catatonia), emotional expression (affective blunting), ability to initiate and complete goal-directed behavior (avolition), and ability to seek out and experience emotional gratification (anhedonia). Not all these symptoms are present in any given patient, however, and none is pathognomonic of the illness. An initial survey of the diversity of symptoms might suggest that multiple brain regions are involved, in a spotty pattern much as once occurred in neurosyphilis. In the absence of visible lesions and known pathogens, however, investigators have turned to the exploration of models that could explain the diversity of symptoms by a single cognitive mechanism. Several leading cognitive neuroscientists and psychiatrists have developed models that can explain the symptoms based on a fundamental cognitive deficit. The convergent conclusions of these different models are striking.

Approaching schizophrenia from the background of cognitive psychology, Frith (1992) has divided the symptoms of schizophrenia into three broad groups or dimensions: 1) disorders of willed action (which lead to symptoms such as alogia and avolition), 2) disorders of self-monitoring (which lead to symptoms such as auditory hallucinations and delusions of alien control), and 3) disorders in monitoring the intentions of others ("mentalizing") (which lead to symptoms such as "formal thought disorder" and delusions of persecution). Frith believes that all these are special cases of a more general underlying mechanism: a disorder of consciousness or self-awareness that impairs the ability to think with "meta-representations" (higher order abstract concepts that are representations of mental states) (Frith 1992). Frith and colleagues are currently testing this conceptual framework using positron emission tomography (PET) (see functional imaging below).

Approaching schizophrenia from a background that blends lesion studies and single cell recordings in nonhuman primates to study cognition, Goldman-Rakic (1994) has proposed a model suggesting that the fundamental impairment in schizophrenia is an inability to guide behavior by representations, often referred to as a defect in working memory. *Working memory*, or the ability to hold a representation "online" and perform cognitive operations using it, permits individuals to respond in a flexible manner, to formulate and modify plans, and to base behavior on internally held ideas and thoughts rather than being driven by external stimuli (Goldman-Rakic 1987). A defect in this ability can explain a variety of symptoms of schizophrenia. For example, the inability to hold a discourse plan in mind and monitor speech output leads to disorganized speech and thought disorder; the inability to maintain a plan for behavioral activities could lead to negative symptoms such as avolition or alogia; the inability to reference a specific ex-

ternal or internal experience against associative memories (mediated by cortical and subcortical circuitry involving frontal/parietal/temporal regions and the thalamus) could lead to an altered consciousness of sensory experience that would be expressed as delusions or hallucinations. The model also explains the perseverative behavior observed in studies using the Wisconsin Card Sorting Test and is consistent with the compromised blood flow to the prefrontal cortex in these patients (Weinberger 1987). Overall, Goldman-Rakic's work supports a model that suggests a major role for prefrontal regions and their multiple distributed cortical, thalamic, and striatal connections in a fundamental cognitive function, representationally guided behavior, that permits organisms to adapt flexibly to a changing environment and to achieve temporal and spatial continuity between past experiences and present and future actions.

Using techniques originally derived from neurophysiology, Braff and colleagues have developed another complementary model. This model begins from the perspective of techniques used to measure brain electrical activity, particularly various types of evoked potentials, and hypothesizes that the core underlying deficit in schizophrenia involves information processing and attention (Braff 1993). This model derives from the empirical clinical observation that patients with schizophrenia frequently complain that they are bombarded with more stimuli than they can interpret (McGhie and Chapman 1961). Consequently, they misinterpret (i.e., have delusions), confuse internal with external stimuli (hallucinations), or retreat to safety ("negative symptoms" such as alogia, anhedonia, or avolition). Early interpretations of this observation drew on the Broadbent filter theory and postulated that patients had problems with early stages in serial order processing that led to downstream effects such as psychotic or negative symptoms (Broadbent 1958). As serial models have been supplanted by distributed models, the deficit may be better conceptualized in terms of resource allocation: Patients cannot mobilize attentional resources and allocate them to relevant tasks.

Andreasen and colleagues have used the clinical presentation of schizophrenia as a point of departure, postulating that the symptoms arise from "cognitive dysmetria." This refers to impaired connectivity between frontal, cerebellar, and thalamic regions as a consequence of a neurodevelopmental defect or perhaps a series of them (Andreasen et al. 1994a, 1994b; Nopoulos et al. 1997; Swayze et al. 1990). Motor dysmetria has been observed in schizophrenia since its original description by Kraepelin, and "soft signs" of poor coordination are reported in more contemporary studies (Gupta et al. 1995a; Kraepelin

1919). More injurious, however, is the related "cognitive dysmetria," which produces "poor coordination" of mental activities (Andreasen et al. 1996). The word *metron* literally means "measure": a person with schizophrenia has a fundamental deficit in taking measure of time and space, in making inferences about interrelationships between him- or herself and others, or between past, present, and future. He or she cannot accurately time input and output, and therefore cannot coordinate the perception, prioritization, retrieval, and expression of experiences and ideas. This model has received extensive support from work with MRI and PET (see below).

The common thread in these observations, gleaned from very different starting points, is that schizophrenia reflects a disruption in a fundamental cognitive process that affects a specific circuitry in the brain. Various research teams may use different terminology and somewhat different concepts—meta-representations, representationally guided behavior, information processing/attention, cognitive dysmetria—but they convey a common theme. The cognitive dysfunction in schizophrenia is an inefficient temporal and spatial referencing of information and experience as the person attempts to determine boundaries between self and not-self and to formulate effective decisions or plans that will guide him or her through the small scale (speaking a sentence) or large scale (finding a job) maneuvers of daily living. This capacity is sometimes referred to as *consciousness*.

Using diverse technologies and techniques—PET scanning, animal models, lesion methods, single-cell recordings, evoked potentials—the investigators also converge on similar conclusions about the neuroanatomic substrates of the cognitive dysfunction. All agree that it must involve distributed circuits rather that a single specific "localization," and all suggest a key role for interrelationships among prefrontal cortex, other interconnected cortical regions, and subcortical regions, particularly the thalamus and striatum. Animal models are being developed based on knowledge of this circuitry and the fundamental cognitive process, which can be applied to understanding the mechanism of drug actions and to the development of new medications.

CLINICAL VALIDITY OF COGNITIVE MODELS

The clinical validity of these cognitive models of schizophrenia is supported by a variety of studies using neuropsychological testing. One crucial question addressed by these studies is whether patients with schizophrenia experience cognitive deterioration over time, as occurs in Alzheimer's disease, or whether the cognitive impairment is stable. The bulk of the evidence supports the latter. Premorbidly, schizophrenic patients have subtle deficits in information processing tasks or on neuropsychological tests and have a slightly lower IQ than their siblings and peers (Aylward et al. 1984; Hyde et al. 1994). Following the onset of clinical disorder, mild deterioration occurs in cognitive functioning and neuropsychological test results (Hoff et al. 1991). There is little additional deterioration beyond that resulting from the normal aging process, even for patients who have been ill for more than 50 years. In a study of 74 schizophrenic patients in five age cohorts (i.e., 18–29, 30–39, 40–49, 50–59, 60–69 years), results from a battery of neuropsychological tests were abnormal across all age cohorts (Hyde et al. 1994). Research has also shown that both young and old schizophrenic patients exhibit a similar pattern of deficits (Bilder et al. 1991). This body of work suggests that there is little evidence of a progressive decline in cognitive function during the course of schizophrenia.

Neuropsychological impairment is not restricted to a small subset of patients; measurable impairment is present in 40%–60% of schizophrenic patients (Goldberg et al. 1988). Cognitive impairment tends to be generalized but is most pronounced for cognitive tasks involving attention, memory, and executive functions. Braff and colleagues (1991) found in a sample of 40 schizophrenic patients selective deficits in tests of complex reasoning, psychomotor speed, new learning, incidental memory, and both motor and sensory-perceptual abilities. Neuropsychological impairment has been linked with enlarged cerebral ventricles (Keilp et al. 1988), negative or deficit forms of schizophrenia (Buchanan et al. 1994), and the presence of neurologic soft signs (Flashman et al. 1996).

OTHER SYMPTOMS

Lack of Insight

Lack of insight is common in schizophrenia. Patients often deny they are ill or abnormal, and insist their hallucinations and delusions are real. Poor insight is one of the most difficult symptoms to treat and often persists even when other symptoms (e.g., hallucinations) respond to medication. Orientation and memory are generally preserved, unless impaired by the patient's psychotic symptoms, inattention, or distractibility.

Soft Signs

Nonlocalizing *soft signs* occur in a substantial proportion of schizophrenic patients and include abnormalities in stereognosis, graphesthesia, balance, and proprioception

(Gupta et al. 1995a). Although their clinical significance is unclear, their presence may reflect dysfunction in areas of motor coordination, integrative sensory function, and ordering complex motor tasks. In one study (Krakowski et al. 1989), violent schizophrenic patients were more likely to exhibit neurologic soft signs than were nonviolent patients.

Ocular Symptoms

Schizophrenic patients frequently display abnormal smooth pursuit eye movements (SPEM). This is a disorder of the visual tracking of smoothly moving targets and has been consistently observed in schizophrenic patients for nearly 90 years. Some experts believe that abnormal SPEM may represent a biologic marker for schizophrenia, because it has been observed in patients with remitted schizophrenia and schizotypal personality disorder and is more frequently found in relatives of schizophrenic patients than in the general population (Holzman et al. 1984; Thacker et al. 1996). Abnormal SPEM is more common in schizophrenic patients with predominantly negative or deficit symptoms (Ross et al. 1996). A similar abnormality in visual fixation that may have greater familial specificity than SPEM has also been reported (Amador et al. 1991).

Vegetative Functions

Some patients display disturbances of sleep, sexual interest, or other bodily functions. A variety of disrupted sleep measures have been reported in schizophrenia, but decreased delta sleep with diminished stage 4 is the most consistent finding (Neylan et al. 1992). Schizophrenic patients often have little interest in sexual activity and may derive little or no pleasure from sexual experiences (Lyketsos et al. 1983).

Immune System Function

Disturbed immune functioning has been reported in schizophrenia and includes abnormalities of circulating lymphocytes, peripheral and/or cerebrospinal fluid immunoglobulin and interferon levels, and the production of anti-brain antibodies. In one study (McAllister et al. 1989), schizophrenic patients were more likely than control subjects to show an increase in the subpopulation of CD5+ β-lymphocytes, cells that have been demonstrated to be increased in patients with certain autoimmune disorders such as rheumatoid arthritis. In another study (Ganguli et al. 1995), schizophrenic patients had decreased interleukin-2 production, which is also characteristic of autoimmune disease.

PREMORBID PERSONALITY

Several early writers including Kraepelin and Bleuler observed that patients with schizophrenia often had abnormal premorbid personalities. In a review of early studies of personality and schizophrenia, Cutting (1985) reported that premorbid schizoid traits were present in one-fourth of schizophrenic patients, but one-sixth had a range of other personality disturbances. Consistent with this review, a study of 52 chronic schizophrenic patients from the Iowa 500 sample (Pfohl and Winokur 1983) found 35% to meet criteria for a DSM-III personality disorder premorbidly; 44% of these personality disorders were schizoid, and the rest were a mixture of avoidant, paranoid, histrionic, compulsive, and other personality disorders. Poor premorbid adjustment has been shown to correlate with early disease onset, poor overall prognosis, negative symptoms, cognitive deficits, and poor social functioning (Gupta et al. 1995b).

SUBSTANCE ABUSE AND SMOKING

Comorbid alcohol and drug abuse is common in patients with schizophrenia and occurs at rates exceeding that found in the community (Dixon et al. 1991). Drug-taking schizophrenic patients tend to be younger and are more likely to be male than non–drug-taking schizophrenic patients. They also have poorer medication compliance, higher rates of rehospitalization, and poorer adjustment and treatment response than patients without such abuse or dependence (Drake et al. 1989). Some researchers believe that schizophrenic patients abuse drugs in an attempt to self-medicate, to treat their medication side effects (i.e., drug-induced akinesia), or to lessen their amotivation and avolition. Cigarette smoking is also very common, and in one study nearly three out of four schizophrenic patients smoke (Goff et al. 1992). Smoking increases neuroleptic metabolism and consequently may be associated with the need for higher neuroleptic dosages.

SUBTYPES OF SCHIZOPHRENIA AND SCHIZOPHRENIFORM DISORDER

DSM-IV recognizes five subtypes of schizophrenia: 1) paranoid, 2) disorganized, 3) catatonic, 4) undifferentiated, and 5) residual. The ICD-10 includes the simple, latent, and schizoaffective subtypes as well. The main purpose of subtyping is to improve predictive validity, to help the clinician to select treatments and predict outcome, and to help the researcher delineate homogeneous subtypes. These promises remain largely unfulfilled, and the reliability and validity of different schizophrenic subtypes are not fully established.

Data collected in the International Pilot Study of Schizophrenia failed to substantiate the usefulness of the classic subtypes of schizophrenia (Strauss and Carpenter 1981). Another effort to validate schizophrenic subtypes (Kendler et al. 1984) compared four diagnostic systems: DSM-III, RDC, ICD-9, and the Tsuang-Winokur criteria (Tsuang and Winokur 1974), which divide schizophrenia into paranoid and nonparanoid subtypes. The authors found that in all diagnostic systems, short- and long-term outcome were better for paranoid than hebephrenic or undifferentiated (or indeterminate) subtypes. No significant differences were found between hebephrenic or undifferentiated subtypes. These authors also reported (Kendler et al. 1985a) only moderate stability and reliability of subtype diagnosis in follow-up; the paranoid subtype was the most stable and reliable, but there was no evidence of subtypes breeding true within families (Kendler et al. 1988). While these studies provide some validation for the paranoid/nonparanoid subtyping, the usefulness of the other traditional subtypes remains uncertain. As a practical matter, many patients seem to fit several of these subtypes during the course of their illness. The DSM-IV subtypes are summarized in Table 12–7.

PARANOID SCHIZOPHRENIA

Kraepelin was the first to identify a paranoid subtype of schizophrenia, in which patients had bizarre and fragmented delusions and, ultimately, personality deterioration. The concept of a paranoid subtype was included in DSM-I (American Psychiatric Association 1952) and has continued to the present. The paranoid subtype is characterized by a preoccupation with one or more delusions and/or frequent auditory hallucinations; disorganized speech/behavior, catatonic behavior, and flat or inappropriate affect is not prominent.

In contrast to other subtypes, patients with paranoid schizophrenia have an older age at onset, better premorbid functioning, and a better outcome. They are more likely to marry and have better occupational functioning than patients with other subtypes (Fenton and McGlashan 1991; Winokur et al. 1974).

An example of a patient with the paranoid subtype of schizophrenia follows.

CASE EXAMPLE 2

Jane, a 55-year-old unmarried woman, was admitted to the hospital for evaluation of bizarre behavior. She had been pounding on her apartment ceiling and walls with a broom and yelling loudly in an attempt to stop her neighbors from harassing her.

A former schoolteacher, Jane had lived in a series of rooming houses and held temporary jobs in the past 10 years. She was socially isolated and interacted with others only at her church. Jane had been born with a cleft palate that was surgically corrected at age 4 years. She was teased unmercifully as a child due to her appearance, despite good cosmetic results from the surgery. Socially awkward and shy, Jane had few friends, but was an avid reader and model student. She showed little interest in boys, never dated, and briefly joined a convent after graduating from high school. She eventually obtained her teaching certificate after finishing college and lived with her mother.

Jane was briefly hospitalized at age 25 after developing the belief that her neighbors were harassing her. Over the next 20 years, her beliefs evolved into a complex delusion in which she believed that she was at the center of a cabal to change her identity. The judiciary, the Roman Catholic Church, and most of her neighbors were involved, she believed. She was convinced that her neighbors were recruited to spy on and harass her in order to make her life miserable. She would often overhear them plotting to assault or rape her.

As a result of her delusional beliefs, Jane moved about every 6 months, but discovered that wherever she went, her new neighbors were also part of the plot. Still, she continued working, but was gradually relegated to substitute teaching positions until these opportunities also dried up. A doctor had suggested that she obtain disability benefits from the government, but she denied having any mental illness and refused to apply. She obtained temporary jobs and, at admission, had been working several weeks in telemarketing schemes.

In the hospital Jane dressed modestly and was always neatly groomed. She cooperated well with her physicians and showed no evidence of depressed mood. Jane spoke in a clear, strong voice that one might expect after years of teaching, although she was markedly circumstantial. She was visibly upset about her hospitalization, which she felt unnecessary and inappropriate. She explained that yelling and screaming was her way of protesting the discomfort the landlord and neighbors had created by "zapping" her with electronic beams. She believed that electromagnetic waves were being used to control her actions and thoughts and described a bizarre sensation of electricity moving around her body when the landlord was near. It was learned that she had been hospitalized 6 years earlier under similar circumstances.

After 1 month of antipsychotic therapy, she remained delusional but was no longer as concerned about her perceived harassment. Due to her poor insight and history of medication noncompliance, Jane was placed on an intramuscular antipsychotic before discharge (adapted from Andreasen and Black 1991, pp. 162–163).

TABLE 12-7. DSM-IV subtypes of schizophrenia

Subtype	Criteria	Associated features
Paranoid	Preoccupation with one or more delusions or frequent auditory hallucinations.	Often associated with unfocused anger, anxiety, argumentativeness, or violence.
	None of the following is prominent: disorganized speech, disorganized or catatonic behavior, flat or inappropriate affect.	Stilted, formal quality or extreme intensity of interpersonal interactions may be seen.
Disorganized	All of the following are prominent:	Silly and childlike behavior is common; associated with extreme social impairment, poor premorbid functioning, and poor long-term functioning.
	Disorganized speech	
	Disorganized behavior	
	Flat or inappropriate affect	
	The criteria are not met for catatonic type.	
Catatonic	The clinical picture is dominated by at least two of the following:	Marked psychomotor disturbance present (stupor or agitation), and unusual motor disturbances may be present.
	Motoric immobility as evidenced by catalepsy (including waxy flexibility) or stupor	
	Excessive motor activity (that is apparently purposeless and not influenced by extreme stimuli)	May need medical supervision due to malnutrition, exhaustion, hyperpyrexia, or self-injury.
	Extreme negativism (an apparently motiveless resistance to all instructions or maintenance of a rigid posture against attempts to be moved) or mutism	
	Peculiarities of voluntary movement as evidenced by posturing (voluntary assumption of inappropriate or bizarre postures), stereotyped movements, prominent mannerisms, or prominent grimacing	Sodium amobarbital interview may be helpful diagnostically.
	Echolalic or echopraxia	
Undifferentiated	Symptoms meeting criterion A are present, but the criteria are not met for paranoid, disorganized, or catatonic types.	Probably the most common presentation in clinical practice.
Residual	The following criteria are met:	
	Absence of prominent delusions, hallucinations, disorganized speech, and grossly disorganized or catatonic behavior	Active phase symptoms (i.e., psychotic symptoms) are not present, but patient still exhibits emotional blunting, eccentric behavior, illogical thinking, and mild loosening of associations.
	Continuing evidence of the disturbance, as indicated by the presence of negative symptoms or two or more symptoms listed in criterion A for schizophrenia, present in an attenuated form (e.g., odd beliefs, unusual perceptual experiences)	

DISORGANIZED SCHIZOPHRENIA

Disorganized schizophrenia was first described in 1871 by Ewald Hecker, who used the term *hebephrenia*. This subtype is characterized by disorganized speech and behavior, and flat or inappropriate affect; it does not meet criteria for catatonic schizophrenia. Generally, delusions and halluci-nations, if present, are fragmentary, unlike the well-systematized delusions of the paranoid schizophrenic. Hebephrenia typically has an early onset that begins with the insidious development of avolition, affective flatten-ing, deterioration of habits, and cognitive impairment, as well as delusions and hallucinations (Winokur et al. 1974). Hebephrenic patients are also reported to have a greater family history of psychopathology, poorer premorbid functioning, and poorer long-term prognosis with continuous illness than patients with paranoid schizophrenia (Fenton and McGlashan 1991). Clinically, hebephrenic patients often seem silly and childlike. They sometimes grimace or giggle inappropriately or appear self-absorbed (Figure 12–1). Mirror gazing is commonly described in these patients.

CATATONIC SCHIZOPHRENIA

In 1874 Karl Kahlbaum used the term catatonia to describe a disorder with abnormal motor, sensory, and verbal symptoms including verbigeration, mutism, negativism, stereotyped movements, waxy flexibility, and decreased sensitivity to pain (Magrinat et al. 1983). Kraepelin, and later Bleuler, considered catatonia a subtype of schizophrenia. This tradition was continued to the present, and in

DSM-IV catatonic schizophrenia is defined as a type of schizophrenia dominated by at least two of the following: motoric immobility as evidenced by catalepsy or stupor, extreme agitation, extreme negativism or mutism, peculiarities of voluntary movement (e.g., stereotypies, mannerisms, grimacing), and echolalia or echopraxia (Figure 12–2). Compared with other subtypes, patients with catatonic schizophrenia tend to have the earliest age at onset, the most chronic course, and the poorest social and occupational functioning (Kendler et al. 1994a). This subtype of schizophrenia is reportedly less common than in the past, at least in developed countries (Sartorius et al. 1986).

Isolated catatonic symptoms are often found in other subtypes of schizophrenia, in other psychotic disorders, and in medical illnesses such as a viral encephalitis, frontal lobe tumors, metabolic disturbances (i.e., acute intermittent porphyria), and toxic reactions. Patients displaying catatonic features require careful evaluation and differential diagnosis (Stoudemire 1982). Intravenous sodium amobarbital may be helpful in the differential diagnosis of catatonia. Perry and Jacobs (1982) report that functional catatonia will clear temporarily during an "Amytal interview," and, for example, a mute patient may begin to speak. Patients in whom a catatonic syndrome has resulted from a medical disorder will become drowsy and less responsive.

UNDIFFERENTIATED AND RESIDUAL SUBTYPES

DSM-IV also includes the undifferentiated subtype, which is a residual category for patients meeting criteria

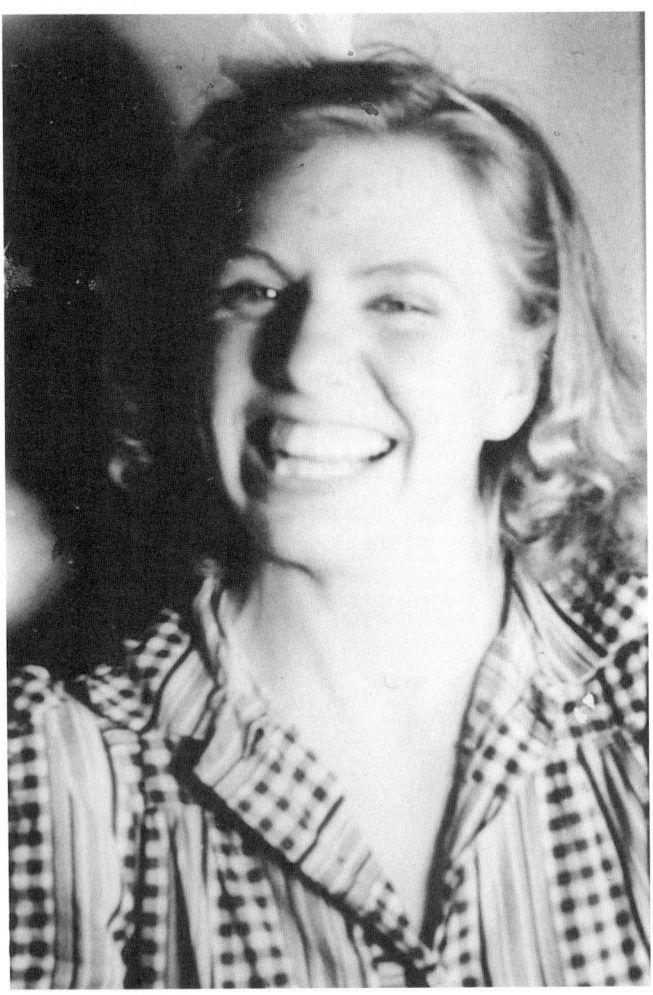

FIGURE 12–1. A young woman with disorganized schizophrenia (photo courtesy of D. W. Black, M.D.).

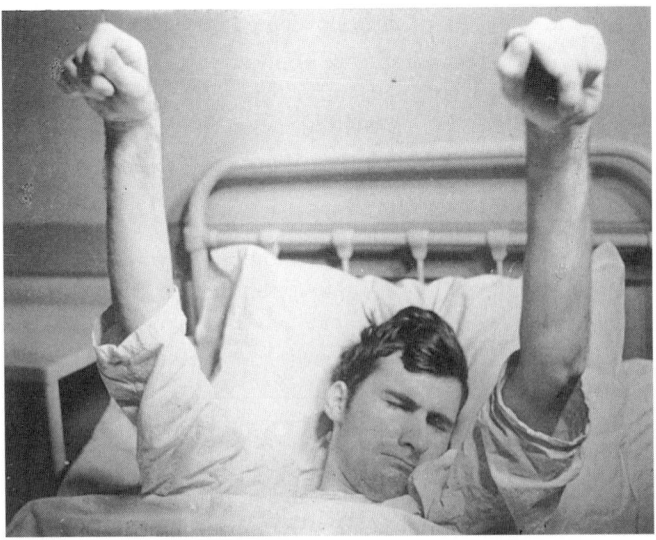

FIGURE 12–2. A young man with catatonic schizophrenia exhibiting waxy flexibility (flexibilitas cerea) (photo courtesy of D. W. Black, M.D.).

for schizophrenia but not meeting criteria for the paranoid, disorganized, or catatonic subtypes. This subtype is the most widely diagnosed.

The residual subtype as described in DSM-IV is applied to patients who no longer have prominent psychotic symptoms, but who once met criteria for schizophrenia and have continuing evidence of illness. Ongoing illness may be indicated by the presence of negative symptoms or of two or more symptoms listed in Criterion A for schizophrenia, present in an attenuated form (e.g., odd beliefs, unusual perceptual experiences).

OTHER SUBTYPES NOT IN DSM-IV

Simple schizophrenia was included in DSM-II (American Psychiatric Association 1968), is included in Appendix B of DSM-IV, and remains in ICD-10. The disorder is characterized by the insidious development of odd behavior, inability to meet societal demands, and decline in performance, but the absence of true delusions or hallucinations (Black and Boffeli 1989). In a recent epidemiologic study in Ireland, Kendler and colleagues (1994b) estimated the lifetime prevalence at 5.3 per 10,000. From a family perspective, the disorder appears related to typical schizophrenia.

Latent schizophrenia was also included in DSM-II and remains in ICD-10. This diagnosis is used to describe patients with eccentric behavior and odd affect who create the impression of having schizophrenia, but who do not have the syndrome's core features. *Pseudoneurotic schizophrenia* is a term peculiar to the United States but was never included in official nomenclature. It was used to describe patients with predominantly neurotic symptoms who on close examination were believed to exhibit mild abnormalities of thinking and emotion. A schizoaffective subtype was included in DSM-II and continues in ICD-10. This diagnosis is used with individuals who have pronounced manic or depressive features comingled with schizophrenic symptoms. DSM-IV recognizes schizoaffective disorder as a separate and distinct illness.

SCHIZOPHRENIFORM DISORDER

The term *schizophreniform psychosis* was introduced by Gabriel Langfeldt in 1939 to describe psychoses that were acute and reactive and occurred in persons with normal personalities. The term was reintroduced in 1980 in DSM-III to identify patients with a good prognosis, nonmood disorder distinct from schizophrenia. The current definition of schizophreniform disorder in DSM-IV requires active positive or negative symptoms and requires

that the disorder is not due to a schizoaffective disorder or a mood disorder with psychotic features, is not substance induced or due to a general medical condition, and lasts more than 1 month but less than 6 months (see Table 12–8). The diagnosis changes to schizophrenia if symptoms extend past 6 months, even if the symptoms are residual. The disorder can be further subdivided into cases with and without good prognostic features (e.g., acute onset).

Data collected since 1980 have not supported the validity of schizophreniform disorder as a distinct diagnosis. In a review, Strakowski (1994) reports that the diagnosis identifies a heterogeneous group of patients. Follow-up studies show that the majority of schizophreniform patients eventually develop other psychiatric syndromes, including schizophrenia, mood disorders, or schizoaffective disorder. Family study results have been contradictory, some finding an increased rate of schizophrenia in relatives, others finding an increased rate of mood disorders. Neurobiological studies have generally failed to show any difference between schizophreniform patients and control subjects. In one intriguing study (DeLisi et al. 1992), ventriculomegaly occurring in patients with schizophreniform disorder was associated with poor outcome and progression to schizophrenia. Perhaps in a subset of these patients, enlarged ventricles may provide useful prognostic information.

Neuroendocrine challenge studies suggest that some patients with schizophreniform disorder exhibit abnormalities similar to those shown in patients with mood disorders. For example, Targum (1983) concluded that patients with schizophreniform disorder can be separated

---

TABLE 12–8. DSM-IV criteria for schizophreniform disorder

A. Criteria A, D, and E of schizophrenia are met

B. An episode of the disorder (including prodromal, active, and residual phases) lasts at least 1 month but less than 6 months. (When the diagnosis must be made without waiting for recovery, it should be qualified as "provisional.")

Specify if:

Without good prognostic features

With good prognostic features as evidenced by two (or more) of the following:

(1) Onset of prominent psychotic symptoms within 4 weeks of first noticeable change in usual behavior or functioning

(2) Confusion or perplexity at the height of the psychotic episode

(3) Good premorbid social and occupational functioning

(4) Absence of blunted or flat affect

into those with atypical mood disorders and those with early schizophrenia by virtue of their neuroendocrine challenge test results including the dexamethasone suppression test. Outcome studies show that overall, patients with schizophreniform disorder have better outcomes than patients with schizophrenia (Coryell and Tsuang 1986), although outcome depends on whether or not the patient proceeded to develop schizophrenia or a mood disorder.

Clearly, the proper boundaries for schizophreniform disorder have not been established, so that the main use of the diagnosis is to guard against a premature diagnosis of schizophrenia. Treatment of schizophreniform disorder is similar to that of an acute episode of schizophrenia, which is described later in this chapter.

COURSE AND OUTCOME

The course of schizophrenia can follow various patterns, although it is typically viewed as a chronic disorder that begins in late adolescence and has a poor long-term outcome. Its onset may be insidious or abrupt, although generally begins with a *prodromal phase* characterized by social withdrawal and other subtle changes in behavior and emotional responsiveness. A patient may be seen as remote, aloof, emotionally detached, or even odd or eccentric. The onset of subtle thought disturbances and impaired attention may also occur at this stage. The prodrome varies in length, but typically lasts from months to years (Carpenter and Buchanan 1994).

The prodrome is followed by an *active phase* in which psychotic symptoms predominate. At this point, clinical disorder becomes evident, and a diagnosis of schizophrenia can usually be made. This phase is characterized by florid hallucinations and delusions, which alarm friends and family members and often lead to medical intervention. A *residual phase* follows the resolution of the active phase and is similar to the prodrome. Psychotic symptoms may persist during this phase, but at a lower level of intensity, and they may not be as troublesome to the patient. Active-phase symptoms may occur episodically ("acute exacerbations"), with variable levels of remission seen between episodes. The frequency and timing of these episodes is unpredictable, although stressful situations may precede these relapses or, in some instances, drug abuse (Linszen et al. 1994). Relapses are often preceded by changes in thought, feeling, or behavior noticed by the patient and family members. Symptoms preceding relapse include dysphoria, seclusiveness, sleep disturbance, anxiety, and ideas of reference (Herz 1985). Through this process patients accrue increased levels of morbidity in the form of residual or per-

sistent symptoms and decrements in function from their premorbid status. Relatively severe psychosis is continuous and unrelenting in some patients. The course of schizophrenia is shown in Figure 12–3.

There is a tendency for the symptoms of schizophrenia to evolve. Patients may show a preponderance of positive symptoms early in their illness, but gradually develop more negative or deficit symptoms. In a longitudinal study of 52 schizophrenic patients (Pfohl and Winokur 1983), 85% were reported to have persecutory delusions of some type at index hospitalization, but after 10 years of illness only 50% had such delusions; after 20 years of illness, only 40% had persecutory delusions. This trend was true for hallucinations and motor symptoms as well. On the other hand, these investigators found that negative symptoms such as avolition, asociality, and affective flattening increased in frequency during the same period of time. There is some evidence that schizophrenia may plateau at about 5 years without further deterioration (Carpenter and Strauss 1991).

OUTCOME

The clinical course and outcome in schizophrenia has been studied and debated since Kraepelin first described dementia praecox as chronic and progressive, leading inevitably to severe impairment. Recently, Hegarty and colleagues (1994) summarized the outcome of 51,800 schizophrenic patients from 320 studies reported in the psychiatric literature between 1895 and 1992. Followed an average of nearly 6 years, 40% of patients were considered improved. Improvement was essentially defined as recov-

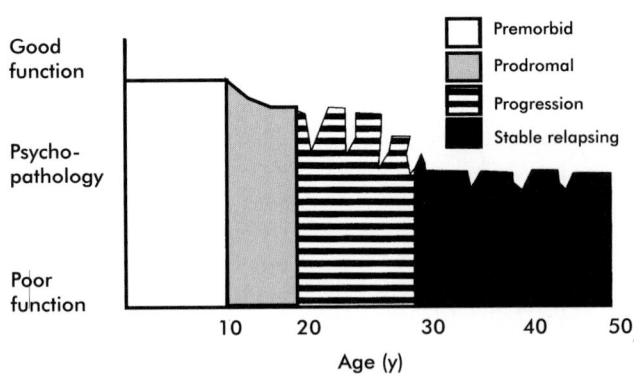

FIGURE 12–3.   The natural history of schizophrenia is portrayed.
Source.   Reprinted with permission from Lieberman JA: Atypical antipsychotic drugs as a first-line treatment of schizophrenia: a rationale end hypothesis. J Clin Psychiatry 57 (suppl 11):68–71, 1996.

ery, remission, or being well with minimal symptoms. They reported that outcome was much better when patients were diagnosed according to diagnostic symptoms with broad criteria (47% improved), rather than narrow criteria (27% improved). Further, the proportion of patients who improved was greater after the mid-century mark than before (49% versus 35%), perhaps reflecting a broadened concept of schizophrenia as well as improved treatment. Since 1975 the rate of favorable improvement has fallen to 36%, perhaps reflecting the impact of the reemergence of narrowed diagnostic criteria.

Several long-term follow-up studies have been published using contemporary American definitions of schizophrenia. The two best known are the "Iowa 500," which used the St. Louis criteria, and the "Chestnut Lodge" study, which used the DSM-III criteria. The findings of these studies are remarkably similar (McGlashan 1984; Tsuang et al. 1979). In the Iowa 500 study, 186 schizophrenic patients admitted to the University of Iowa Psychiatric Hospital between 1934 and 1944 were followed up in the early 1970s. Twenty percent of schizophrenic patients were reported to be psychiatrically well at follow-up, but 54% had incapacitating psychiatric symptoms; 21% were married or widowed, but 67% had never married; 34% lived in their own home or with a relative, but 18% were in mental institutions; 35% were economically productive, but 58% had never worked. The group experienced excess mortality from both natural and unnatural causes, and more than 10% committed suicide. In a recent reanalysis of this seminal study, Winokur and Tsuang (1996) report that only two of the schizophrenic patients followed up were completely free of symptoms (i.e., had "zero symptoms"). They conclude that whereas a patient may be considered improved and is able to work and to live independently, he or she is unlikely to be free of all symptoms.

In the Chestnut Lodge study, 163 schizophrenic patients discharged from the private hospital between 1950 and 1975 were followed up in the early 1980s. While 37% were living in a hospital or sheltered environment, only 28% were living independently; 26% had been employed 50% of the follow-up period or better; 41% were considered continuously incapacitated, and only 6% had recovered. McGlashan (1984) noted that roughly two-thirds of the schizophrenic patients were functioning marginally or worse at follow-up and that 7% had killed themselves during the interim.

In summary, outcome studies show that schizophrenia is a devastating illness that affects every aspect of a patient's life. Fortunately, many patients with schizophrenia will have a relatively good outcome and will avoid the severe deterioration considered by some a hallmark of the disorder.

PREDICTING OUTCOME

Although a variety of prognostic factors have been reported (Jonnson and Nyman 1984; McCabe et al. 1972; McGlashan 1986; Vaillant 1964), prediction of outcome remains a difficult task. Research has shown that definitions of schizophrenia that exclude patients with mood symptoms or those having a duration of illness under 6 months generally predict a poor prognosis. This is because these relatively restrictive definitions exclude patients with mood disorder, schizophreniform disorder, or schizoaffective disorders, who tend to have better outcomes. Perhaps the best study of outcome prediction was the International Pilot Study of Schizophrenia (World Health Organization 1975), in which psychiatrists in nine different countries participated. Regression analysis showed the five most powerful predictors of poor outcome to be social isolation, long duration of episode, history of past psychiatric treatment, being unmarried, and having a history of behavioral problems in childhood such as truancy and tantrums. The investigators also found that all 47 potential predictors accounted for only 38% of the variance. A summary of commonly reported prognostic factors is shown in Table 12–9.

OTHER FACTORS THAT AFFECT OUTCOME

Cultural Factors

Cross-cultural studies have shown that schizophrenic patients in less developed countries tend to have better outcomes than those in more developed countries. This unexpected finding was reported in the International Pilot Study of Schizophrenia (World Health Organization 1975), which demonstrated that the average outcome was considerably better in the developing countries (Colombia, India, and Nigeria) than in the industrialized countries (Czechoslovakia, Denmark, United Kingdom, United States, and the former Soviet Union). Despite extensive follow-up treatment available in industrialized countries, a high proportion of their patients had additional psychotic episodes not seen in the patients in developing countries. Although there were no important differences in the initial symptoms and other characteristics of the patients at the nine study sites, the possibility cannot be dismissed that these differences in outcome were due to unrecognized differences in the types of patients seeking treatment. One explanation is that the schizophrenic patient is better accepted in less developed countries, has fewer external demands, and is more likely to be taken care of by interested family members. The same finding

TABLE 12–9. Features associated with good and poor outcome in schizophrenia

Feature	Good outcome	Poor outcome
Onset	Acute	Insidious
Duration	Short	Chronic
Psychiatric history	Absent	Present
Affective symptoms	Present	Absent
Sensorium	Clouded	Clear
Obsessions/ compulsions	Absent	Present
Assaultiveness	Absent	Present
Premorbid functioning	Good	Poor
Marital history	Married	Never married
Psychosexual functioning	Good	Poor
Neurological functioning	Normal	Soft signs present
Neuropsychological test results	Normal	Abnormal
Structural brain abnormalities	None	Present
Social class	High	Low
Family history of schizophrenia	Negative	Positive

emerged from a comparison of outcome of schizophrenia in London and Mauritius (Murphy and Raman 1971).

Gender

Women with schizophrenia appear to have a more favorable outcome than men in treatment response, social functioning, and overall prognosis. A study of 121 schizophrenic patients in England (Watt et al. 1983) found that at a 5-year follow-up, 62% of women had a good outcome as compared with 35% of men. Women also had better housing, probably due to the fact that they were less likely than men to live alone or to be institutionalized. A similar study of 278 schizophrenic patients in Germany (Angermeyer et al. 1989), found women to have fewer rehospitalizations and shorter lengths of stay.

EPIDEMIOLOGY

Schizophrenia presents a challenge to the epidemiologist, due to disagreements about the definition of its core features and the breadth of its spectrum. The development of operational criteria, such as those in DSM-IV, has provided greater specificity for the diagnosis of schizophrenia and has resulted in a more cautious use of the concept. This has led to a reassessment of earlier epidemiologic studies that generated rates based on older conceptualizations of schizophrenia. Despite these advances, case identification remains an ongoing problem among epidemiologists. Efforts to standardize the diagnosis have met with some success, such as with the Present State Exam used in the International Pilot Study of Schizophrenia and the Composite Interview Diagnostic Instrument used in the recent National Comorbidity Study (Kessler et al. 1994).

PREVALENCE AND INCIDENCE

In a comprehensive review, Eaton and colleagues (1988) reported that the median point prevalence of schizophrenia was 3.2 per 1,000 (range 0.6–8.3). The median lifetime prevalence rate was 4.4 per 1,000 (range 1.7–7.0). *Point prevalence* includes all identified cases at a given point in time. *Lifetime prevalence*, or "disease expectancy," includes the proportion of persons studied who have ever experienced the disorder up to the time of assessment. The type of prevalence measure reported (i.e., point, lifetime) appears not to strongly influence the rate, presumably due to the chronic nature and low incidence of schizophrenia (Eaton 1985). In the National Comorbidity Study, in which lay-interviewed cases evidencing symptoms of psychosis were reinterviewed by a psychiatrist, the lifetime rate for schizophrenia was 0.14% (Bromet et al. 1995). This rate is much lower than that reported in the Epidemiologic Catchment Area survey (1.3% lifetime; Robins et al. 1984). That finding was based on results of the lay-administered Diagnostic Interview Schedule, an instrument with relatively poor reliability for the diagnosis of schizophrenia (Anthony et al. 1985).

A review of annual incidence rates of schizophrenia (Eaton et al. 1988) show a median rate of 0.20 per 1,000 (range 0.11–0.70). *Incidence* is the number of new cases that arise in a given time per unit of population. (A simple formula, prevalence = incidence × duration, shows the relationship between these two parameters.) Because incidence does not confound the rate of occurrence with duration, many investigators find it a more useful measure for etiologic studies, although both measures are helpful for planning health services. A World Health Organization study (Jablensky et al. 1992) involving 10 research sites showed that incidence rates were remarkably similar across the various sites. A reported decline in the incidence rate of schizophrenia has been debated, as some researchers believe that new cases are less frequent than many decades ago (Eaton 1991). It is likely that any apparent rate decline is tied to changing diagnostic practices that favor more restrictive definitions such as that in DSM-IV.

AGE AT ONSET AND SEX RATIO

Schizophrenia typically begins in early adulthood, but can develop at any age including early childhood (Beitchman 1985). Both Bleuler and Kraepelin reported an earlier onset for men than women, a finding confirmed by subsequent research. In one study (Loranger 1984), mean age at onset was 21.4 years for men and 26.8 years for women. Mean age at first treatment occurred 5 and 7 years later, respectively. A total of 9 of 10 males, but only 2 of 3 females, had developed schizophrenia by age 30. Onset after age 35 occurred in 17% of women, but in only 2% of men. The reason women develop schizophrenia later than men remains a mystery, but it is apparently not an artifact resulting from women having a more sheltered existence that conceals their illness. Kendler and colleagues (1996) recently concluded that environmental or developmental factors probably account for the variation seen in the age at onset in schizophrenia.

Early epidemiologic studies showed approximately equal rates of schizophrenia for men and women, but the broad concept of schizophrenia used in the past may have led to the inclusion of a disproportionate number of women with mood disorders. Lewine and colleagues (1984) analyzed the effect of using six different diagnostic systems on the male-to-female ratio of schizophrenia among 387 inpatients. Diagnostic criteria that present a broad concept of schizophrenia, such as the New Haven schizophrenia index, yielded equal rates of schizophrenia among men and women. Diagnostic systems with more stringent criteria, such as the Research Diagnostic Criteria, yielded a greater male-to-female ratio.

MARITAL STATUS AND REPRODUCTION

Patients with schizophrenia are more likely to remain single and unmarried than are patients in other diagnostic groups. This is particularly true in male patients (Eaton 1985) and can probably be explained by the fact that women tend to be younger than men when first married and are less likely to have experienced an initial psychotic episode. From a cultural perspective, women have traditionally been less active in initiating relationships, which may account for some of the difference.

Early researchers tended to find low rates of fertility and reproduction among schizophrenic patients (Kallman 1938). This finding can probably be explained by several factors including lack of interest in social relations, general apathy, low sex drive, and lack of opportunity for a sexual relationship due to hospitalization or institutionalization. Rates of reproduction in schizophrenic patients have probably increased since deinstitutionalization, although likely remain lower than those found in the general population (Erlenmeyer-Kimling 1978). The persistence of the disease in spite of low fertility rates is an intriguing fact that may suggest a contribution from environmental factors and/or a particular type of genetic transmission (e.g., recessive, low penetrance).

SOCIOECONOMIC STATUS

Patients with schizophrenia generally have low social status. Eaton (1985) reviewed 17 studies of incidence of treated schizophrenia that included indicators of social class. The highest rate of schizophrenia was found in the lowest social class in 15 of the studies. Earlier studies suggested that lower social class status seen in schizophrenic patients probably results from the "downward drift" in socioeconomic status they experience due to the debilitating effects of its symptoms, which impair social and occupational functioning.

ETHNICITY AND RACE

Jablensky and Sartorius (1975) concluded from a literature review that except for a high rate found by Böök in north Sweden (10.8 per 1,000) and a low rate reported by Eaton and Weil for the Hutterite sect in the United States (1.1 per 1,000), prevalence rates for schizophrenia are relatively similar worldwide. Pockets of high prevalence have been reported in areas of the Istrian peninsula in Croatia, on the western coast of Ireland, among Canadian Catholics, and among the Tamils of southern India. Low prevalence has been reported among American Old Order Amish, in the aboriginal tribes of Taiwan, and in the native population in Ghana. Although early studies in the United States suggested a higher rate of schizophrenia in African Americans than in whites, this finding was probably due to a systematic bias to overdiagnose schizophrenia in blacks (Mukherjee et al. 1983).

MORTALITY AND MORBIDITY

Research has long shown increased mortality in patients with schizophrenia (Simpson and Tsuang 1996). In the past, high death rates were attributed to both natural and unnatural causes. Before modern medical and psychiatric treatments were available, many patients suffered the ill effects of prolonged psychiatric symptoms leading to malnutrition or dehydration or were exposed to tuberculosis and other infectious diseases in large institutions. Because general medical and psychiatric care has improved, high death rates in schizophrenic patients are now due primarily to suicide and accidents. In one study (Black and Fisher 1992), schizophrenic patients showed a near three-fold increase over expected mortality. Those at risk for premature death were patients younger than 40 years and who were in their first few years of follow-up.

Based on early epidemiologic studies, schizophrenic patients were once thought to have some immunity from cancer. Recent research shows that while cancer death rates in general are not different than expected, there is evidence of lower risk for lung cancer despite high rates of smoking in those patients (Black and Winokur 1986; Gulbinat et al. 1992). There is evidence, too, that rheumatoid arthritis is less common in schizophrenic patients (Eaton et al. 1992) than among persons in the general population, although the reason for this association is unknown.

SUICIDE AND SUICIDAL BEHAVIOR

Patients with schizophrenia are at high risk for suicidal behavior. Nearly one-third will attempt suicide (Allebeck et al. 1987), and about 1 in 10 will complete suicide (Tsuang 1978). Between 2% and 3% of suicide completers have schizophrenia (Barraclough et al. 1974). Risk factors for suicide include male gender, age less than 30 years, living alone, unemployment, chronic relapsing course, prior depression, past treatment for depression, depression during the last episode of illness, history of substance abuse, and recent hospital discharge (Allebeck et al. 1987; Roy 1982). Schizophrenic patients with the paranoid subtype and those with a high level of education appear to be at greater risk for suicide (Fenton and McGlashan 1991), perhaps due to the patients' feelings of inadequacy and hopelessness, fear of disintegration, and a realization that desired expectations will never be met. Unlike other psychiatric patients who commit suicide, schizophrenic patients may fail to communicate their suicidal intentions and may act impulsively, complicating any effort at intervention (Breier and Astrachan 1984).

VIOLENCE AND CRIMINALITY

Until quite recently it was thought that mentally ill persons were not predisposed to violent behavior (Teplin 1985). Recent research shows that schizophrenic patients and other severe mental disorders exhibit relatively high rates of violent behavior and criminality. In the Epidemiologic Catchment Area study (Swanson et al. 1990), schizophrenic patients had rates of violent behavior five times higher than persons without mental illness, although the rate was about one-half that seen in persons with alcohol abuse or dependence. Schizophrenic patients with coexisting alcoholism are even more likely to commit violent acts, including homicide, than patients not abusing substances (Modestin and Ammann 1996). The severely mentally ill have high rates of conviction for criminal offenses and incarceration, although many of the offenses have been called "survival crimes," such as shoplifting and petty thievery thought due to homelessness or deinstitutionalization (Csillag 1993). To some extent violent behavior may be a function of the stage of a schizophrenic patient's illness (e.g., in response to persecutory delusions) and remains one of the primary reasons for hospitalization.

UTILIZATION OF HEALTH SERVICES

Patients with schizophrenia utilize a disproportionate share of general medical and psychiatric services. According to information from the Monroe County Psychiatric Case Register, schizophrenia accounted for 16.4% of the treatment population in 1975, but 47.6% of psychiatric inpatient days and 36.9% of new state hospital inpatient admissions (Babigian 1984). Schizophrenic patients 65 years and older utilized a disproportionate share of hospitalization days, especially at state facilities, whereas those aged 25–44 years had the highest rate of acute hospitalization episodes.

National Institute of Mental Health data show schizophrenia to be the first or second most frequent diagnosis for admissions to various types of psychiatric inpatient services, ranging from 21% for private hospitals to 38% for state and county hospitals, with a length of stay averaging 18–42 days, respectively. There were over 1.6 million admissions for schizophrenic patients to inpatient facilities in 1980 (Taube and Barrett 1985). Results from the Epidemiologic Catchment Area study (Shapiro et al. 1984) showed that nearly 78% of schizophrenic patients surveyed had health care visits during the previous 6 months; 45% of visits were for mental health care. Patients with schizophrenia tended to obtain mental health care from specialists rather than from general medical providers, which indicates the severity of the illness, since the opposite was true for most nonpsychotic disorders.

Most schizophrenic patients are brought to medical attention at some point during the course of their illness, but many will go untreated. A survey in Baltimore (Von Korff et al. 1985) found that approximately 50% of persons with schizophrenia were not receiving any form of mental health care. Nonetheless, all were deemed to be in need of these services, and only 14% had never received treatment.

PATHOPHYSIOLOGY AND ETIOLOGY

The development of multiple competing theories about the cause of schizophrenia parallels its history. Early theories were shaped by limited knowledge about the nature of mental illness and inadequate research methods. There is still disagreement about the relative contribution of genetic and environmental factors to the development of schizophrenia, despite advances in psychiatric nosology, epidemiology, and genetics. Recent work, however, has emphasized the importance of the interaction of both genetic and nongenetic factors in disease expression.

Consensus now exists among many investigators that schizophrenia is best conceptualized as a "multiple-hit" illness similar to cancer. Individuals may carry a genetic predisposition, but this vulnerabilty is not "released" unless other factors also intervene. Although the majority of these factors are considered environmental, in the sense that they are not encoded in DNA and could potentially produce mutations or influence gene expression, the majority are also biological rather than psychological and include factors such as birth injuries or nutrition. Current studies of the neurobiology of schizophrenia examine a multiplicity of factors, including genetics, anatomy (primarily through structural neuroimaging), functional circuitry (through functional neuroimaging), neuropatholgy, electrophysiology, neurochemistry and neuropharmacology, and neurodevelopment.

GENETICS

Evidence for a hereditary contribution to schizophrenia is based on family studies, twin studies, and studies of adoptees. As early as 1916, Rudin reported an increased prevalence of dementia praecox among the siblings of affected probands. Subsequent family studies have confirmed an increased prevalence of schizophrenia and related disorders in family members, with risk related to the number of shared genes of family members with the schizophrenic proband. Summaries of individual family studies have shown siblings of schizophrenic patients to have a near 10% lifetime risk of developing schizophrenia, while children who have one parent with schizophrenia have a 5%–6% lifetime risk (Gottesman and Shields 1982). The risk of a family member developing schizophrenia markedly increases when two or more family members

have the illness, with a lifetime expectancy of schizophrenia of 17% for siblings with one sib and one parent with schizophrenia and up to 46% in children of two parents with schizophrenia. These findings strongly support the familial nature of schizophrenia, but do not confirm a genetic over a familial environmental cause.

Twin studies and adoption studies allow a natural experimental paradigm to separate the genetic and environmental effects of familial associations. Despite varying methods, twin studies have been remarkably consistent in demonstrating high concordance rates for monozygotic twins (Farmer et al. 1987; Gottesman and Shields 1982). Rates have averaged 46% as compared with 14% in dizygotic twins across multiple studies, with only one negative twin study (Tienari 1963). However, the failure of monozygotic twins to be 100% concordant suggests that a hereditary component may be necessary but is insufficient to cause schizophrenia and that environmental factors are also important.

Adoption studies present another paradigm for evaluating genetic influences in familial illness. Heston (1966) examined grown children of mothers with schizophrenia who had been adopted and compared them with control adoptees whose mothers had no psychiatric disorder. He found a nearly 17% age-corrected morbidity risk of schizophrenia in the adoptees of schizophrenic mothers, figures similar to those reported family studies of children of mothers with schizophrenia not given up for adoption; no control adoptees had schizophrenia. The best-known adoption study was conducted in Denmark using a national psychiatric case register and a register of adoptions. Kety and colleagues (1975) reported that schizophrenia and *schizophrenia spectrum disorders* were more common in the biologic relatives of index adoptees who had schizophrenia than in the biologic relatives of mentally healthy control adoptees. Schizophrenia spectrum disorders include personality disorders that share certain characteristics with schizophrenia, such as paranoid ideas or eccentric behavior, without meeting full syndromal criteria. A blind reanalysis of the data (Kendler and Gruenberg 1984) using DSM-III criteria essentially replicated the original results. An ongoing adoption study in Finland (Tienari 1992) has shown similar results. Thus, adoption studies have demonstrated that having a schizophrenic parent increases the risk in offspring not only for schizophrenia, but also for spectrum disorders such as schizotypal personality.

Mode of inheritance of schizophrenia has also been studied mainly by using mathematical modeling of pedigrees and twin and adoption study data. Models currently proposed include a single-gene model and a polygenic model. A simple Mendelian model of transmission involving a single dominant or recessive gene is not clearly present in the pedigrees of most probands who suffer from schizophrenia, although a single gene is possible if one assumes incomplete penetrance and dominant transmission (Slater 1958), or if eye-tracking dysfunction (i.e., abnormal smooth pursuit eye movement) is considered an expression of schizophrenia (Holzman et al. 1988). However, polygenic models of inheritance are consistent with published family and twin data (Gottesman and Shields 1982); they are also consistent with genetic studies finding increased risk in families with more than one schizophrenic member and increased risk in first-degree relatives of more severely ill probands compared to less severely ill probands (Rice and McGuffin 1985). Polygenic models may provide a better explanation of the persistence of schizophrenia in light of the reduced fertility characteristic of the disorder. Sufficient data do not presently exist to definitively support or reject either single gene or polygenetic models.

The molecular genetic techniques described in Chapter 2 are now being used in attempts to pin down mode of inheritance and to locate a "schizophrenia gene" (or genes). The task is complicated by the lack of biological traits or vulnerability markers specific to schizophrenia, as well as clinical heterogeneity. Researchers have implicated several different gene regions (e.g., chromosome 6, chromosome 11); the short arm of chromosome 6 has been most consistently replicated (Crowe et al. 1991; Schwab et al. 1995; Wang et al. 1993). The nonreplications do not rule out involvement of a particular gene region in some families and may indicate only that schizophrenia is genetically heterogeneous. Efforts to link schizophrenia to particular gene regions will undoubtedly continue at a rapid pace (Vallada and Kunugi 1996).

Some evidence also suggests that schizophrenia may show the phenomenon of anticipation: increasingly severe onset at earlier ages within multigeneration affected families. Huntington's disease is a classic example of a severe genetically induced CNS disease characterized by anticipation. Because the mechanism causing anticipation is known (increasing proliferation of trinucleotide repeats in the DNA in successive generations), the occurrence of anticipation in schizophrenia may provide some clues as to its specific genetic loci and mechanisms (Petronis and Kennedy 1995).

NEUROANATOMY AND STRUCTURAL NEUROIMAGING

Since the early work of Kraepelin, Alzheimer, and Nissl in the late 19th and early 20th centuries, many psychiatrists have been convinced that patients with schizophrenia have some type of structural brain abnormality (Kraepelin 1919). Early pneumoencephalographic and neuropathological studies provided partial support for this hypothesis (Storey 1966), but in recent years new technology has been able to support it more fully. When Johnstone and colleagues (1976) first described the use of the technique to study brain abnormalities in chronic schizophrenia, their report elicited considerable controversy, but the finding of ventricular enlargement in schizophrenia has now been confirmed by numerous CT studies and is perhaps the best-replicated finding in psychiatry (Andreasen et al. 1982, 1990c; Weinberger et al. 1979, 1980). This early work with CT, conducted during the 1980s, firmly established that schizophrenia is a brain disorder with a measurable structural component that can be observed at the gross anatomic level when groups of patients are pooled together, averaged, and compared with normal volunteer control subjects.

Cerebral ventricular enlargement is the most consistently replicated finding, but sulcal enlargement or cerebellar atrophy are also reported. Although these findings cannot be explained on the basis of such factors as treatment with medications, they may be explained in part by gender, because it may be predominantly a male effect (Flaum et al. 1990). Examination of ventricular size in schizophrenia and normal subjects over a broad age range suggest that enlargement does not progress over time at a greater rate in schizophrenic patients than normally and that structural brain abnormalities are present from the outset (Andreasen et al. 1990b; Nopoulos et al. 1995a). Although not all studies show exactly the same correlates, there is substantial evidence to suggest that ventricular enlargement is associated with poor premorbid functioning, negative symptoms, poor response to treatment, and cognitive impairment. CT scan abnormalities may have some clinical significance, but they are not diagnostically specific; similar abnormalities are seen in other disorders such as Alzheimer's disease or alcoholism.

MRI has now largely supplanted CT as a clinical and research tool. Its particular advantage lies in its ability to distinguish gray and white matter, allowing the size of particular brain regions and structures to be measured. MRI has permitted investigators to move from asking "Is there a grossly measurable brain abnormality in schizophrenia?" to asking "Is a specific region or group of regions affected?" Many candidate regions have been explored but none has been conclusively confirmed. The conflicting reports appear to largely reflect the growing maturity of this method of study. Early reports used relatively primitive techniques such as area measurements on single slices and manual tracing. More recent studies apply automated volumetric measures that have greater power and sophistication.

The earliest MRI study reported a selective decrease in the frontal cortex, in addition to smaller cerebral and intracranial size, and it suggested that this combination of findings was consistent with a neurodevelopmental process in which the brain failed to grow normally, rather than with a neurodegenerative process (Andreasen et al. 1986). Many subsequent studies examined the issue of brain size; a recent meta-analysis examining all available studies of intracranial size (*N* = 18) and brain volume (*N* = 27) has confirmed a small but highly statistically significant difference between patients and control subjects in both brain and intracranial volume (Ward et al. 1996).

A decrease in frontal lobe size has been less consistently replicated, although hypotheses about a dysfunction of the frontal cortex continue to be widely discussed, particularly in functional imaging studies (see below). The prefrontal cortex performs a large array of higher cortical functions that are disrupted in schizophrenia (e.g., "executive functions," abstract thinking, working memory), making it an attractive candidate for study. Yet, it is also a large and functionally diverse brain region that was difficult to measure accurately prior to the recent development of 3-D acquisition procedures with MRI and volume-rendering techniques that permit visualization of cortical surface anatomy (see Figure 12–4). Three of the four recent studies that used relatively sophisticated measurement techniques have shown decreased frontal size in both chronic and first episode patients (Andreasen et al. 1994a; Breier et al. 1992; Nopoulos et al. 1995a; Wible et al. 1995). If all studies are pooled, however, negative studies are as frequent as positive ones (for a review, see Shenton et al. 1997).

MRI has also been used to explore possible abnormalities in other specific brain subregions, such as the thalamus, amygdala/hippocampus, temporal lobes, or basal ganglia. Several studies have indicated that the size of temporal regions is decreased in schizophrenia and that there may even be a relatively specific abnormality in the superior temporal gyrus or planum temporale that is correlated with the presence of hallucinations or formal thought disorder (Barta et al. 1990; Shenton et al. 1992).

The thalamus is relatively difficult to measure reliably using MRI, because it is composed of multiple nuclei, is a mixture of grey and white matter, and has relatively fuzzy borders as visualized on nearly all types of MRI sequences. Nonetheless, it has been noted to have a decreased size in several studies, and a novel application of image averaging and subtraction methods has indicated that this structure shows the greatest effect size difference when patients are compared to control subjects (Andreasen et al. 1994b). Like the prefrontal cortex, the thalamus is also an interest-ing candidate region for schizophrenia; although the precise functions of the various thalamic nuclei are still being mapped, it is clearly a major relay station that could serve functions such as gating or filtering or even generating input and output, because it receives afferent input and sends efferent output from and to widely distributed cortical and primary sensory and motor regions.

Sophisticated image analysis techniques have been developed to measure the total volume of grey matter, white matter, and cerebrospinal fluid (CSF), and these have also been applied to the study of schizophrenia (Cohen et al. 1992; Gur and Pearlson 1993; Harris et al. 1997; Lim et al. 1996). Figure 12–5 shows an image in which the MRI data have been reclassified in these three tissue types to permit quantitative measurement. Most studies consistently show a decrease in total brain tissue volume in schizophrenia as well as an increase in CSF in the ventricles and on the brain surface. Most studies that have evaluated the relative changes in gray and white matter have found a selective decrease in cortical gray matter, although some have also found white matter decreases as well (Breier et al. 1992; Flaum et al. 1997; Schlaepfer et al. 1994; Zipursky et al. 1994).

MRI studies have also provided some confirmation for neurodevelopmental theories of schizophrenia apart from the observation of decreased intracranical volume and decreased tissue discussed above. A variety of developmental anomalies are seen by MRI in some patients suffering from schizophrenia. The most consistently reported is an increased frequency of large cavum septi pellucidi, a midline anomaly reflecting a fusion failure of the septal leaflets (Lewis et al. 1985; Nopoulos et al. 1996; Nopoulos et al. 1997) In addition, partial callosal agenesis (a severe midline anomaly) appears to be modestly increased in schizophrenia (Swayze et al. 1990). Finally, findings that reflect abnormalities in neuronal migration (e.g., gray matter heterotopias) are also seen with increased incidence, although only in a small number of patients (Nopoulos et al. 1995b).

FUNCTIONAL CIRCUITRY AND FUNCTIONAL NEUROIMAGING

Beginning with the work of Ingvar and Franzen (1974), studies of regional cerebral blood flow (rCBF) have been used to explore the possibility of functional or metabolic abnormalities in schizophrenia. Their work suggested that schizophrenic patients had a relative "hypofrontality," which was associated with prominent negative symptoms. Since that early work, functional imaging studies have become more sophisticated, and it is now clear that PET can be used to explore the functional circuitry used by normal

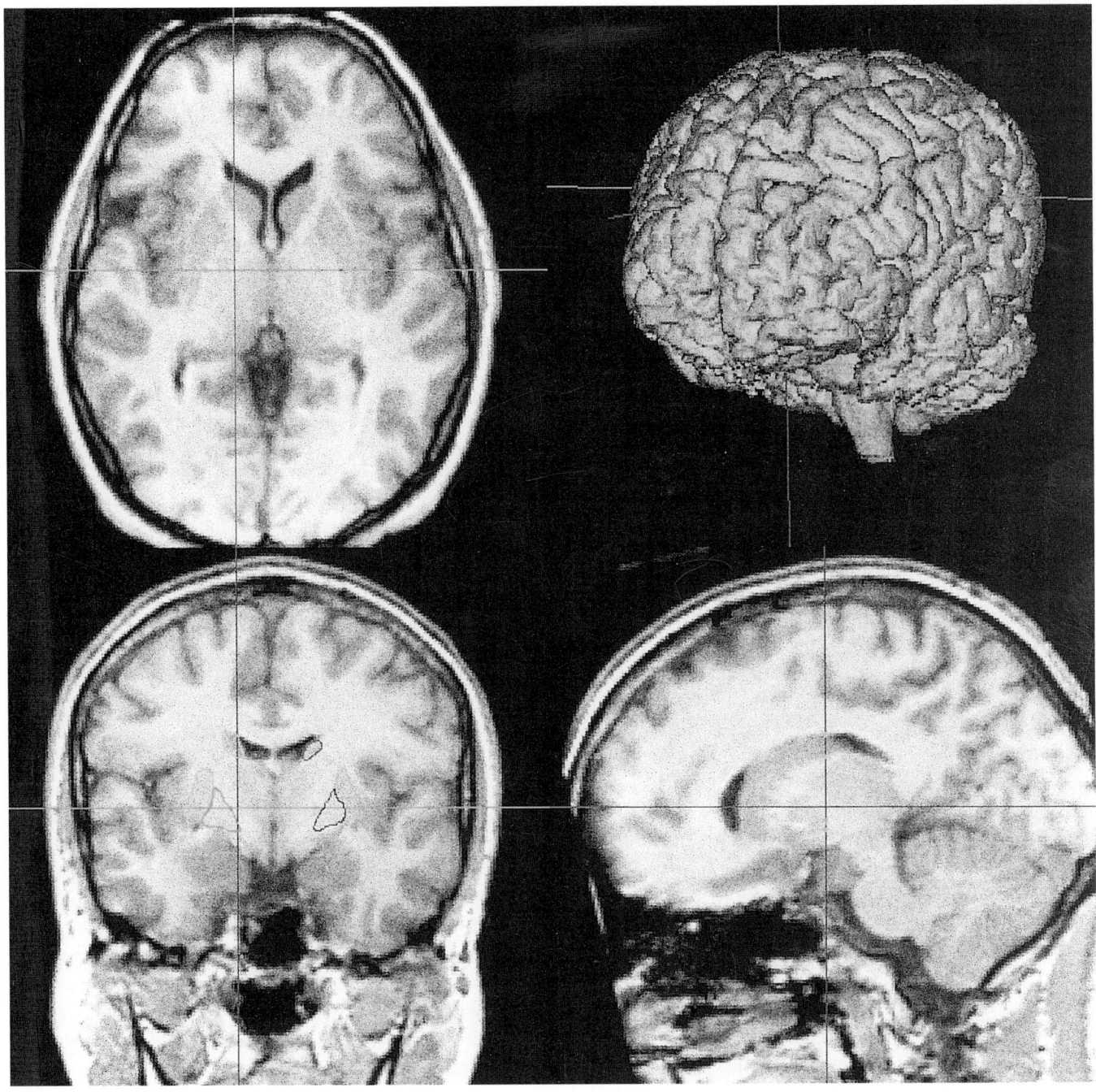

FIGURE 12-4.   This magnetic resonance image (MRI) scan shows how 3-D acquisition procedures and volume rendering techniques permit visualization of cortical surface anatomy (photo courtesy of N. C. Andreasen, M.D., Ph.D.).

individuals while they perform a variety of mental tasks and to identify circuits that are dysfunctional in schizophrenia. Much of this work has been facilitated by the maturation of the ^{15}O H$_2$O technique with PET. ^{15}O H$_2$O is a tracer with a very short half-life (around 2 minutes), which permits investigators to do multiple repeated scans (usually 6–12) with differing cognitive tasks during a short time period (around 2 hours). This permits the dissection of the

components of cognitive activities (e.g., memory encoding versus retrieval) and visualization of their associated circuitry.

Current thinking about the mechanisms of schizophrenia, based on functional imaging, postulates a disruption in distributed functional circuits rather than a single abnormality in a single brain region such as the prefrontal cortex or one of its specific subregions such as the

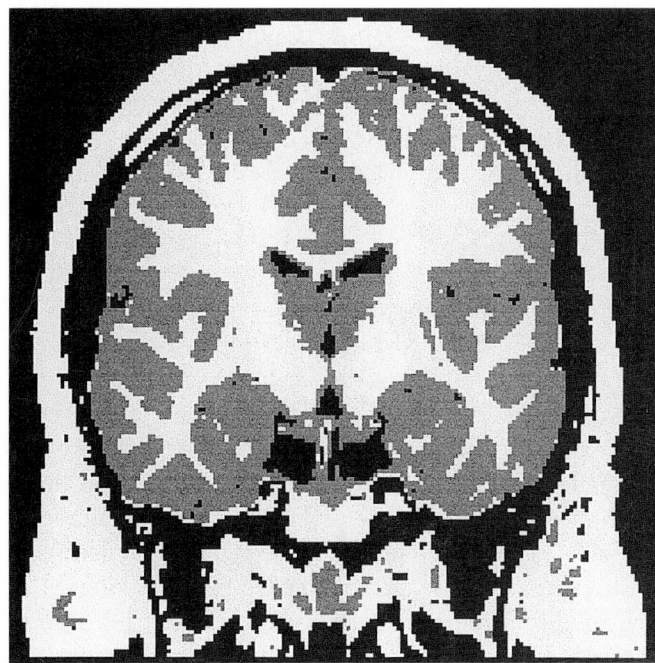

FIGURE 12–5. This magnetic resonance (MR) imaging scan shows how MR data can be reclassified to permit quantitative measurement of gray matter, white matter, and cerebrospinal fluid (photo courtesy of N. C. Andreasen, M.D.., Ph.D.).

dorsolateral prefrontal cortex. Although no single group of regions has definitely emerged as the "schizophrenia circuit," a consensus is developing concerning some of the nodes that may be involved. They include a variety of subregions within the frontal cortex (orbital, dorsolateral, medial), the anterior cingulate gyrus, the thalamus, several temporal lobe subregions, and the cerebellum.

For example, Frith and colleagues (1991) began their earliest work by studying *willed action* (their first symptom dimension and analogous to negative symptoms). They tested the neural substrates of willed action by giving subjects tasks for which the correct response is not evident from context, such as verbal fluency or choosing a finger movement. Normal subjects activate a frontal circuit during such tasks, whereas patients with schizophrenia show relative decreases in frontal regions and decreases in temporal regions in comparison with normal subjects (Liddle et al. 1992). If the pace of the verbal fluency task is slowed, however, frontal function is similar to normal subjects and only the temporal abnormality remains (Frith 1995). Examination of the correlations between flow in these regions suggests that the normal relationship between them has broken down and that there is abnormal functional connectivity (McGuire and Frith 1996).

More recently this research group completed a systematic study of hallucinations, their second dimension of psychopathology. They assume that hallucinations are caused by an erroneous attribution of the person's own inner speech to another person, reflecting a defect in self-monitoring. Starting first with normal subjects, they developed a task that could potentially mimic this mechanism of hallucinations; subjects were asked to perform a sentence completion task and imagine that the response was spoken in another person's voice. They found that this task led to activation of speech production and perception regions, such as Broca's area, the supplementary motor area, and the left superior and middle temporal regions (McGuire et al. 1996a). Applying the same task to people with schizophrenia and comparing hallucinators to nonhallucinators, they found the hallucinators to have decreased flow in the areas used to monitor speech, such as the left middle temporal gyrus and supplementary motor area (McGuire et al. 1996b). They have also examined flow in patients while they were experiencing auditory hallucinations and found activations primarily in subcortical regions (thalamus, striatum), limbic and paralimbic regions (anterior cingulate, parahippocampal gyrus), and cerebellum; they speculate that activity in subcortical regions may generate or moderate hallucinations, whereas the content (e.g., auditory, tactile) may be determined by the specific neocortical regions that are engaged (Silbersweig et al. 1995).

Other research groups have also used functional imaging in order to explore functional circuitry. Buchsbaum, who conducted the earliest PET studies suggesting hypofrontality (Buchsbaum et al. 1982), more recently measured glucose metabolism in a sample of 20 nevermedicated schizophrenic patients and also observed thalamic abnormalities using fluorodeoxyglucose (Buchsbaum et al. 1996). Interestingly, Buchsbaum and colleagues also reported a diminished metabolic rate in the cerebellum in this study.

Andreasen and colleagues have also provided support for abnormalities in multiple frontal subregions, the thalamus, and the cerebellum. In one study comparing schizophrenic patients to healthy volunteers during random episodic silent thought (REST), they observed blood flow abnormalities in medial, orbital, and dorsolateral frontal regions, as well as temporal, cingulate, thalamic, and cerebellar areas (Andreasen et al. 1994b). In another study of practiced and novel recall of complex narrative material, they also observed abnormalities in multiple brain regions, including frontal, thalamic, and cerebellar sites (Andreasen et al. 1996). These investigators have also observed similar abnormalities in schizophrenic patients during episodic memory and semantic/working memory tasks.

These findings are consistent with the theory that schizophrenia is a disease of multiple distributed circuits in the brain. The disease is characterized by a cognitive dysmetria caused by a disruption in pontine-cerebellar-thalamic-frontal feedback loops. The thalamus is a crucial waystation in the brain that has complex interconnections to many other regions. Various parts of the prefrontal cortex (i.e., dorsolateral, orbital, and medial) are connected to it, as are other regions such as the basal ganglia and anterior cingulate. Further, various thalamic nuclei have relay connections to virtually all other parts of the cerebral cortex, including sensory, motor, and association regions. Finally, the cerebellum also projects to multiple cortical regions via thalamic relay nuclei.

The concept of cognitive dysmetria postulates three key nodes in a feedback loop that involves frontal regions, the cerebellum, and the thalamus. Each of these nodes is assumed to have a particular function. The prefrontal node serves the classic "executive function": Prioritizing data, placing it within a broad context using information gleaned from other intercommunicating cortical regions, formulating decisions or responses, and initiating their action. The thalamus serves as the filter, receiving sensory information from multiple sources, simplifying it by excluding redundant or extraneous stimuli, and forwarding on the important or relevant information. The cerebellum, which contains half the neurons in the human brain and is composed of cells designed to handle massive amounts of information, may serve as the "metron." That is, it coordinates the information forwarded back to it from cortical regions and sent to it through subcortical and brain stem regions. As a metron, its primary role is to match data within the context of time and perhaps of space in order to make sure that the correct pieces of information are connected and coordinated with one another.

For example, a person carrying on a conversation must hear and "understand" the words of the other speaker, formulating an interpretation of the speaker's implicit and explicit meaning in order to generate an appropriate reply. In this simple model, the prefrontal cortex does most of the interpretation, whereas the thalamus permits the brain to focus on the conversation itself rather than on the multiple other people that may be nearby or ambient background noise in the room. The thalamus may damp down visual stimulation in order to focus on the auditory stimulation. The cerebellum, acting as the metron or coordinating organ, would be the site where information from the frontal executive and other sensory regions converges and would serve the responsibility of doing extremely rapid online processing, for which it appears to be well designed anatomically. A patient suffering from schizophrenia manifests impaired verbal and social responses in such situations because of a dysfunction in the circuitry that permits prioritizing information, excluding extraneous information, and performing these functions in a rapid, efficient, and well-coordinated manner.

Neuropathology

A better understanding of neurodevelopment has helped shape contemporary postmortem studies. During the second trimester neurons in the fetal brain must migrate to the appropriate layers of the cortex, then connect with other groups of neurons to form functional networks. Other developmental processes include excessive proliferation of cells and dendrites, which are subsequently followed by pruning and programmed cell death (apoptosis) of subplate neurons; surviving cells remain as interstitial neurons (or interneurons) of the white matter. The resulting network of neurons and cytoplasmic processes is called the *neuropil*. Recent work suggests that schizophrenia could be related to disturbances in any of these phases of brain maturation, ranging from migration to apoptosis. Failure of the cells to migrate to their proper position may show up as ectopic gray matter (Nopoulos et al. 1995b) or neuronal disarray in specific regions of the hippocampus (Conrad et al. 1991; Kovelman and Scheibel 1984). Arnold and colleagues (1991) reported displacement of neurons and a paucity of neurons in the superficial layers in the rostral and intermediate portions of the entorhinal cortex of the parahippocampal gyrus, which they attributed to faulty neuronal migration. Benes and colleagues (1991) reported a decreased density of interneurons in the prefrontal, anterior cingulate, and primary motor cortex of the brains of schizophrenic patients, findings that could indicate an accelerated process of neuronal cell death. More recently, Akbarian and colleagues (1996) found selective displacement of interneurons in the frontal lobe cortex, including decreased cell density in the superficial white matter, and increased cell density in the deeper white matter, findings also thought consistent with an alteration in the migration of subplate neurons or in the pattern of programmed cell death.

Neuropathology has also been used to explore whether abnormalities can be found in key candidate regions such as the thalamus or prefrontal cortex. Pakkenberg (1990) has noted decreased cell density in the medial dorsal nucleus of the thalamus, a crucial nucleus that projects to the prefrontal cortex. Thalamic abnormalities have also been noted in other neuropathologic studies (Bogerts 1993). Selemon et al. (1995) have also demonstrated increased cell packing density in prefrontal cortex in schizophrenic patients, consistent with a loss of the surrounding neuropil and consequent shrinkage of the interneuronal space. A convergence of findings is beginning to emerge from the variable perspectives of structural and functional neuroimaging and neuropathology. These perspectives are all consistent with neurodevelopmental mechanisms and with abnormalities in frontal, temporal, and thalamic regions.

Electrophysiologic Studies

Braff (1993) has developed a cognitive model of schizophrenia by using neurophysiological paradigms to examine sensory gating. Prepulse inhibition is a technique that measures gating of the startle response that can be triggered by a bright light or loud auditory stimulus; in normal subjects the startle response can be diminished (inhibited) if a weak prepulse stimulus is delivered in the same modality. Patients with schizophrenia have impaired prepulse inhibition, which occurs across a broad range of stimulus intensities (Grillon et al. 1992). A related paradigm, gating of the P50 evoked potential by a prepulse stimulus, has also been shown to be impaired in schizophrenic patients by this group and others (Judd et al. 1992). Waldo and colleagues (1994) have also shown impairment in P50 gating in unaffected family members of patients with schizophrenia, raising the possibility that this could be used as a trait or vulnerability measure.

Prepulse inhibition can be readily modeled in animals and used to study the effects of medications, because all mammals display the startle response. This group has demonstrated that cortical-striatal-pallidal-thalamic circuitry plays a key role in modulating the startle response in rats, using lesion methods and single-cell recordings. They have found that dopamine agonists such as apomorphine can also lead to loss of sensory gating and that both typical and atypical antipsychotic medications restore prepulse inhibition in apomorphine-treated rats in a profile that correlates with their clinical efficacy, suggesting that this model could serve as a screen for neuroleptic medications using a cognitive measure that may be related to the underlying neural defect in schizophrenia (Swerdlow and Geyer 1993).

Neurodevelopment

Several lines of evidence support speculation that schizophrenia is a neurodevelopmental disorder resulting from neuronal injury occurring early in life that interferes with normal brain maturation (Andreasen et al. 1986; Feinberg 1982; Weinberger 1987). As described above, MRI studies have shown an increased rate of neurodevelopmental brain anomalies in this illness. The observation that perinatal complications often precede the development of severe neurological and psychological disorders, such as cerebral palsy and mental retardation, have led investigators to explore the role of perinatal and obstetrical complications in the etiology of schizophrenia. Schizophrenic patients are more likely to have a history of obstetrical complications than other psychiatric patients or normal control subjects (Geddes and Lawrie 1995). Prematurity, oxygen deprivation, and long labor are especially common complications. McNeil and Kaij (1978) observed that among monozygotic twins discordant for schizophrenia, the co-twin with schizophrenia is more likely to have suffered an obstetrical complication. Schizophrenic patients with a history of obstetrical complications are also more likely to exhibit minor physical anomalies (O'Callaghan et al. 1991). Minor physical anomalies (slight anatomical defects of the head, hands, feet, and face) are relatively common in schizophrenia patients and are themselves believed to reflect abnormal neurodevelopment (Green et al. 1994).

Several groups of investigators have looked at the relationship between obstetrical complications and cerebral ventricular size. Turner and colleagues (1986) reported that ventricular size was positively correlated with obstetrical complications in a small sample of first episode schizophrenic patients. Pearlson et al. (1985) similarly found that perinatal complications were associated with larger ventricles and earlier age at onset. DeLisi and colleagues (1986) noted that schizophrenic patients had larger ventricles than their well siblings and that seven of eight schizophrenic patients with ventricles more than one standard deviation larger than the control mean had a history of obstetrical complications or head injury. These studies suggest that obstetrical complications may contribute to neuronal injury and perhaps predispose to the development of schizophrenia in genetically vulnerable persons.

Other lines of evidence supporting neurodevelopmental theories of schizophrenia are more circumstantial. Throughout the temperate northern latitudes, the birth dates of schizophrenic patients tend to cluster in the winter months, although the excess is minor (Hare et al. 1973). This finding suggests that a seasonally varying influence (a viral infection, for example) is acting in utero or in early life to cause neurologic injury. Thus, children born during the winter months would be more vulnerable to brain injury, due to the increased frequency of viral infections. This was the case in the study by Mednick and colleagues (1988), who reported that individuals who were in their second trimester of fetal development during a 1957 A_2 influenza epidemic in Finland were at a higher risk of hospitalization for schizophrenia than those born in the same months over the previous 6 years. The finding was replicated using data from influenza cases reported to the Ministry of Health in Denmark (Barr et al. 1990). Rh incompatibility, a form of obstetrical complication, could also be a risk factor for schizophrenia. Hollister and colleagues (1996) reported that the rate of schizophrenia was much higher in Rh incompatible men than in Rh compatible men. The authors suggest that hemolytic disease in the newborn resulting from Rh incompatibility may lead to fetal hypoxia, adversely affecting neurodevelopment. Tying maternal influenza, obstetrical complications, and schizophrenia together, Wright and colleagues (1995) reported that mothers of schizophrenic patients were more likely than control subjects to report both second-trimester influenza and at least one obstetrical complication.

Another interesting lead into the etiology of schizophrenia concerns nutritional factors during gestation. Susser and colleagues (1996) looked at the development of schizophrenia after prenatal exposure to the Dutch hunger winter of 1944–1945, when the Nazis imposed a complete food blockade against the populous northeastern section of the Netherlands. The average amount of food eaten was less than 1000 Kcals per day. The incidence of schizophrenia was increased twofold, suggesting the possibility that malnutrition has a detrimental effect on fetal neurodevelopment.

NEUROCHEMISTRY AND NEUROPHARMACOLOGY

For many years, the most widely accepted explanation for the biochemical pathophysiology of schizophrenia was the *dopamine hypothesis*, which suggests that the disorder is primarily caused by a functional hyperactivity in the dopamine system (Carlsson 1988; Davis et al. 1991). Much of the support for the dopamine hypothesis arose from the observation that the efficacy of many of the neuroleptic drugs used to treat schizophrenia were highly correlated with their ability to block dopamine D_2 receptors (Creese et al. 1976; Seeman et al. 1976). Conversely, drugs that enhance dopamine transmission, such as the amphetamines, tend to worsen the symptoms of schizophrenia (Snyder 1972). Therefore, the dopamine hypothesis also suggested that the abnormality in this illness might specifically lie in the D_2 receptors. For many years, the "ideal drug" was thought to be a highly specific D_2 blocker.

Recent work in neuropharmacology and chemical anatomy has demonstrated that there are five types of dopamine receptors, which differ in their cerebral distribution. The D_1 receptor is linked to adenylate cyclase and is located in the cortex and basal ganglia. The D_2 receptor is not linked to adenylate cyclase and is prominent in the striatum. The D_3 and D_4 receptors have a higher distribution in limbic regions. This distribution raises questions about the classic dopamine hypothesis, because limbic regions (or, alternately, frontal or temporal regions) have been the presumed target for neuroleptic drug action, yet D_2 receptors are not densely concentrated in these target regions.

Postmortem brain research has documented an increase in D_2 receptors in the caudate and nucleus accumbens in postmortem brains (Clardy et al. 1993). Other postmortem studies have documented increased dopamine or homovanillic acid in these regions as well as the left amygdala in schizophrenic patients (Davis et al. 1991). There is a concern, however, that these findings may be an artifact of treatment with antipsychotics. Animal work has shown that antipsychotics produce receptor supersensitivity in response to receptor blockade by increasing the number of D_2 receptors available. Consequently, an increase in D_2 receptors in postmortem brains could be a direct consequence of neuroleptic treatment itself.

Recently, PET has provided another way to assess neurochemical transmission in schizophrenia. This work has involved the use of labeled ligands known to bind to D_2 receptors. Two such ligands—^{3}H-labeled spiroperidol and ^{11}C-labeled raclopride—are currently used. Spiroperidol binds to both D_1 and D_2 receptors as well as serotonin sites, but raclopride is highly specific for D_2 receptors. Farde et al. (1985) used this technique to demonstrate D_2 receptor blockade in human beings in vivo, using both normal subjects and patients with schizophrenia. Early work (Wong et al. 1986) appeared to confirm the presence of increased D_2 receptors in schizophrenia, but the finding was not verified by subsequent research (Farde et al. 1990). These results have also lessened confidence that D_2 receptors alone could explain the symptoms of schizophrenia.

PET has also been used to measure receptor occupancy, providing an in vivo method for directly observing the mechanisms of pharmacologic action. This work, taken together with the development of the highly effective atypical antipsychotics, has shed further doubt on a simple D_2 theory of schizophrenia. As described later in the section on treatment, the new atypicals have a very broad pharmacologic profile, blocking $5HT_2$, D_1, and some subtypes of adrenergic receptors as well. One study showed that conventional antipsychotics have prominent D_2 occupancy (78%) and no obvious D_1 occupancy, whereas the atypical antipsychotics showed a 48% occupancy of D_2 receptors and a 38%–52% occupancy of D_1 receptors (Farde et al. 1992). This may help to explain why atypical antipsychotics are much less likely to induce extrapyramidal side effects, because patients with these effects have a higher D_2 receptor occupancy than do those without (Farde et al. 1992).

Alternative biochemical hypotheses have been advanced, in part because of the difficulty in confirming the dopamine hypothesis and in the realization that antidopaminergic agents are not always effective. More recent hypotheses also include the role of other neurotransmitter systems (e.g., norepinephrine, serotonin, glutamate, γ-aminobutyric acid [GABA]), neuropeptides, and neuromodulatory substances in the pathophysiology of schizophrenia (Meltzer 1987; VanKammen et al. 1990). The development of the new atypical neuroleptics, which have potent effects on serotonin, provides partial confirmation for the importance of additional neurotransmitter systems in schizophrenia, because they not only cause fewer extrapyramidal side effects than conventional antipsychotics but are more effective as well. The observation that phencyclidine intoxication leads to schizophrenia-like manifestations has also stimulated interest in the N-methyl-D-aspartic acid (NMDA) receptor complex and the possible role of glutamate in the pathophysiology of schizophrenia (Javitt and Zukin 1991; Olney and Farber 1995).

SOCIAL AND FAMILY FACTORS

Theories about the role of society, urbanization, and stress on the development of mental illness, including schizophrenia, were popular during the 1930s and 1940s. In an early study, Faris and Durham (1939) found higher rates for mental hospital admissions, including admissions for schizophrenia, in central slums rather than in the suburbs. This finding was replicated in other cities in both the United States and Europe. The conclusion was drawn that schizophrenia was caused by the ill effects of a slum environment, where people were faced with enormous stress from social disorganization, poverty, and the general adversity imposed by poor living conditions. These conditions were believed to produce or "breed" schizophrenia (Hare 1956).

Another explanation soon developed to explain the finding of geographic isolation of the severely mentally ill. The drift hypothesis stated that living in poor areas *resulted from* schizophrenia and was not causal (Wender et al. 1973). Rather, because schizophrenia leads to amotivation, cognitive impairment, poor hygiene, and other symptoms that make it impossible for the person with schizophrenia to maintain employment and survive in middle and upper class structures, persons with schizophrenia drift down in social class as their illness progresses. Subsequent research

has supported this view. Silverton and Mednick (1984) found, for example, that schizophrenic patients have lower social status on average than their parents.

The social isolation typically experienced by schizophrenic patients has also been suggested as a cause of schizophrenia. However, social isolation typically occurs before illness onset. For reasons of economics and personal choice, persons with schizophrenia tend to live alone, often segregated in certain areas. On the other hand, schizophrenic patients who live with their relatives are more evenly distributed among residential areas (Gerard and Houston 1953) and are less likely to experience downward drift in social class.

Studies of mental illness in immigrants have found a high rate of psychotic disorders (Malzberg 1964), including schizophrenia. Although it was originally believed that the stress of migration caused or contributed to the onset of mental illness, later studies showed that immigrants were more likely to come from low social classes and that immigrant populations were overrepresented with severe mental illness including schizophrenia (Murphy 1977).

CLINICAL MANAGEMENT

ANTIPSYCHOTIC MEDICATION

Antipsychotic medication has been the mainstay of treatment for schizophrenia since chlorpromazine was introduced in 1952. In fact, these agents are probably responsible in large measure for the deinstitutionalization that occurred in the 1950s and 1960s. Because these medications were so effective, large numbers of patients were able to leave psychiatric hospitals. In 1955, for instance, over one-half million hospital beds were filled by the chronic mentally ill, mainly schizophrenic patients; by the early 1990s the number of beds had been reduced to 103,000 (Lamb 1993).

Many conventional antipsychotic drugs are now available, each differing in potency and side effects, but similar in mode of action and efficacy. Their putative mechanism of action is their ability to block postsynaptic dopamine D_2 receptors in the limbic forebrain. This blockade is thought to initiate a series of events responsible for both acute and chronic therapeutic actions. Whereas these drugs block dopamine D_2 receptors almost immediately, onset of antipsychotic action takes weeks to develop. Antipsychotics also block the extrapyramidal motor system with equal affinity. Thus, their therapeutic effects are inseparable from their tendency to induce extrapyramidal side effects. Although many side effects of antipsychotics can be directly attributed to their dopamine-blocking properties, these drugs also block noradrenergic, cholinergic, and histaminic receptors to differing degrees, accounting for the unique side-effect profile of each agent.

All conventional antipsychotics are superior to placebo in the treatment of schizophrenia in the majority of drug trials. These drugs are used to control acute psychosis and to provide long-term maintenance, but they are not curative. They act by reducing positive symptoms like hallucinations and delusions, and gradually diminishing a patient's disturbed thought processes. Improvement is often dramatic, and medication effectiveness is generally sustained over years and decades. Nonetheless, from 10%–20% of patients respond poorly to traditional antipsychotic drugs, and the quality of response varies from patient to patient (Carpenter and Buchanan 1994). Further, the drugs seem to do little for negative symptoms such as apathy and avolition. Recently, several "atypical" antipsychotics have been introduced that represent the most important advance in the treatment of schizophrenia since the introduction of chlorpromazine. Clozapine, risperidone, and olanzapine are the first in this new generation of drugs and will soon be joined by other atypical antipsychotics. They appear more effective than conventional antipsychotics and are less likely to induce extrapyramidal side effects. They do not appear to increase prolactin levels, making them potentially useful for women who develop galactorrhea or irregular menses while taking conventional antipsychotics. In addition to their dopamine D_2 receptor blockade, these agents also block serotonin 5-HT_{2A} receptors in the frontal cortex and striatal system, which may help to mitigate against the development of extrapyramidal side effects. Clozapine was first used in the mid-1970s, but early reports of agranulocytosis in 1%–2% of patients delayed its introduction. A multicenter clinical trial (Kane et al. 1988) found that about 30% of inpatients with schizophrenia who had failed to respond to traditional antipsychotics responded to clozapine within 4–6 weeks; up to 60% may respond within 4–6 months (Schooler et al. 1995).

The major differences among the conventional antipsychotic agents lay in their chemical structure, rate of absorption, distribution, potency, and side effects. Rate of absorption is variable among agents, may be complicated by the presence of food, antacids, cigarette smoking, and anticholinergic agents, and may itself be under genetic control. Because smoking tends to stimulate hepatic enzymes, which increases drug metabolism, patients who smoke may require higher doses of antipsychotics (Goff et al. 1992). Once absorbed, distribution varies dramatically depending on the agent, dose used, and individual kinetics.

Intramuscular administration usually produces effects (e.g., sedation) within 10 minutes because injectable antipsychotic agents have much greater bioavailability than oral medication. Metabolism occurs almost entirely in the liver, largely by oxidation, and these highly lipid-soluble agents are converted to water-soluble metabolites and excreted through the kidneys. Excretion of antipsychotic agents tends to be slow as a result of drug accumulation in fatty tissue. Many antipsychotics, including the atypicals, have a half-life of 24 hours or longer; depot formulations have even longer elimination half-lives. This, and the fact that many of these drugs have active metabolites, have made it difficult to correlate plasma levels with therapeutic response. As a result, no definitive dose-response curve has been demonstrated for the antipsychotic agents (Kane and Marder 1993). Elimination half-life of these drugs from the brain is unknown. Animal studies show that behavioral effects persist even when brain levels are undetectable, suggesting slow dissociation from small pools in CNS tissue including receptor sites (Campbell et al. 1980). This finding could be responsible for the lag in the time from discontinuing a medication to clinical relapse.

With the exception of the new atypicals, no conventional antipsychotic has been shown to be superior to another. Controlled studies have not supported using a specific agent for a specific subtype of schizophrenia, nor is there any benefit from prescribing more than a single antipsychotic at a time.

TREATMENT OF ACUTE PSYCHOSIS

The majority of acutely psychotic schizophrenic patients will respond to a daily dose between 10 and 15 mg of haloperidol (or its equivalent) within several days or weeks (Kane and Marder 1993). Higher dosages of conventional antipsychotics may be needed in some patients, but controlled studies have not shown an advantage to either rapid loading or sustained high dosages. Further, higher dosages will increase the likelihood of adverse side effects. For example, in one study (McEvoy et al. 1991), acutely psychotic schizophrenic patients were given relatively low doses (generally from 2–6 mg) of haloperidol for 2 weeks, then randomly assigned to a dosage 2–10 times higher or to the same dosage for another 2 weeks. Higher dosages caused significantly more extrapyramidal side effects, but not greater improvement in measures of psychosis. In another study, Rifkin and colleagues (1991) found no difference in the response of newly admitted schizophrenic patients given 10 mg, 30 mg, or 80 mg of oral haloperidol for 6 weeks. High dosages of atypical antipsychotics also appear unnecessary. In a fixed-dose trial of risperidone

(Marder and Meibach 1994), doses of 2 mg, 6 mg, 10 mg, and 16 mg were compared with doses of 20 mg of haloperidol and placebo. All doses of risperidone were effective in relieving the symptoms of schizophrenia, but the 6-mg dose was the most effective and also proved superior to haloperidol.

Measuring plasma levels of antipsychotic drugs can be helpful in selected cases, but there is little to be gained by routine monitoring, because most patients will respond to moderate doses of antipsychotics. Plasma levels are most useful 1) in patients who have failed to respond to conventional doses, 2) when antipsychotic medications are combined with other drugs that can affect its pharmacokinetics (e.g., carbamazepine), and 3) to assess compliance. The very young, the elderly, or the medically compromised patient with schizophrenia may also benefit from plasma level monitoring. Because of the difficulties involved in correlating plasma levels and response, research results are not entirely consistent. Nonetheless, levels of haloperidol between 5–18 ng/mL appear to be effective for most patients (Perry and Smith 1993). Levels of fluphenazine between 0.6–1.5 ng/mL (Levinson et al. 1995) and levels of clozapine approaching 350 ng/mL (VanderZwaag et al. 1996) appear effective for most patients. Plasma levels of many other antipsychotic drugs can be reliably measured, but attempts to correlate responses with levels have not been successful.

A high-potency conventional antipsychotic (e.g., haloperidol), risperidone (i.e., 4–6 mg daily), or olanzapine (10–20 mg daily) have been recommended as an initial choice for treatment of acute psychosis (American Psychiatric Association 1997). If there is no response after 3–8 weeks, one of the other drugs should be tried. If a patient shows a partial response to the initial antipsychotic at 3 weeks, the trial should be extended another 2–9 weeks (Expert Consensus Guideline Series Steering Committee 1996). In this algorithm, clozapine is a second line choice because of its expense and propensity to cause agranulocytosis.

Highly agitated patients who are out of control require rapid control of their symptoms and should be given frequent, equally spaced doses of an antipsychotic drug. High potency antipsychotic medications (e.g., haloperidol) can be given every 30–120 minutes orally or intramuscularly until agitation is under control (Dubin et al. 1985). Rarely is more than 20–30 mg of haloperidol required in a 24-hour period. It is likely its effectiveness in subduing patients results from sedation, rather than from any specific antipsychotic effect. Since sedation is desired, a combination of antipsychotic medication and a benzodiazepine may work even better for the rapid control of agitated psychotic patients. In one study (Garza-Trevino et al. 1989), haloperidol (5 mg) and lorazepam (4 mg) were adminis-

tered and repeated every 30 minutes. Most patients achieved tranquilization after the initial dosage. The average time required to achieve a satisfactory response was 60 minutes. Once the patient has calmed down, the benzodiazepine can be gradually withdrawn. Rapid sedation may also be achieved through administration of droperidol (5–10 mg im) (Slaby and Moreines 1990).

A common practice is to prescribe "prn" or extra doses of antipsychotic medication to subdue acutely agitated patients (Cole 1985). This practice almost always occurs in hospitalized patients already receiving antipsychotic medications. It is likely that any benefit is due to nonspecific sedation, rather than antipsychotic action. As a rule prn dosing of antipsychotics is not recommended.

MAINTENANCE THERAPY

Patients benefiting from short-term treatment with antipsychotic medications are candidates for long-term prophylactic treatment, which has as its goal the sustained control of psychotic symptoms. To minimize the risk of side effects, particularly tardive dyskinesia, an often irreversible movement disorder, the lowest effective antipsychotic dose should be used. In a review of 35 well-designed studies of relapse rates, Davis and colleagues (1993) concluded that patients on placebo relapsed at a rate of 55%, whereas only 21% of schizophrenic patients relapsed when maintained on antipsychotic drugs. Further, they conclude that all patients not receiving antipsychotic medication will relapse within about 3 years, essentially guaranteeing multiple relapses and disrupted lives. Patients who experience a temporary worsening of psychotic symptoms in response to methylphenidate administration and those with tardive dyskinesia may be more likely to relapse when off medication (Lieberman et al. 1987).

Although duration of treatment for relapse prevention has not been established, the following guidelines were developed at an international consensus conference (Kissling 1991):

1. Prevention of relapse is more important than risk of side effects, since most side effects are reversible and the consequences of relapse may be irreversible.
2. At least 1–2 years of treatment are recommended after the initial episode due to the high risk of relapse and the possibility of social deterioration from further relapses.
3. At least 5 years of treatment for multi-episode patients, since high risk of relapse remains. Beyond this, data are incomplete, but indefinite, perhaps life-

long, treatment is recommended to patients who pose a danger to themselves or to others.

A reliable dose-response curve has not been established for maintenance medication, but recent literature supports the use of lower and more conservative doses. For example, Lehmann and colleagues (1983) evaluated 94 chronically ill patients who were shifted from their usual dose (equivalent of 452 mg of chlorpromazine) to a moderate or low dose (equivalent to 100 mg or 50 mg). After 1 year, 28% of those kept on the highest dose regimen had relapsed, and 42%–45% on the lower doses had relapsed. In a double-blind study (Kane 1985; Kane et al. 1983), 126 schizophrenic patients were assigned either to a standard dose (equivalent to 500–600 mg of chlorpromazine) or two lower dose groups (100–120 mg, or 50–60 mg). The full dosing was associated with a relapse rate of 7% after 1 year, compared with 20% for the intermediate dose and 50% for the low dose. Similarly, Hogarty (1984) compared a standard dose regimen (equivalent to 400–500 mg chlorpromazine) to low dose (equivalent to 80–100 mg chlorpromazine). The 1-year relapse rates were 25% and 23%, respectively. Baldessarini and colleagues (1988) reviewed these and other studies from the 1980s and concluded that doses between 50 mg and 150 mg of chlorpromazine daily or its equivalent are probably adequate for most patients. Atypical antipsychotic drugs also appear effective for long-term maintenance therapy but, as with the conventional antipsychotic medications, doses need to be individually adjusted.

Clinicians should periodically reassess whether the patient requires continued maintenance treatment. When it is time to reassess the need for medication, an attempt should be made to withdraw the drug slowly over weeks or months. Should symptoms reoccur, the drug should be immediately reinstituted and the dosage increased. Because many patients develop increased negative symptoms and decreased positive symptoms over time, they may have less need for antipsychotic medication (Carpenter 1996). Some research suggests that risk of relapse remains greater on oral rather than intramuscular antipsychotics, probably because of patient noncompliance (Davis et al. 1993). Drug holidays have been recommended by some investigators as a means of lowering the risk of tardive dyskinesia, but cannot be recommended. Targeted medication leads to more decompensation and rehospitalization than continuous medication, without lowering risk for tardive dyskinesia (Carpenter et al. 1990). For patients who are unable to take oral medication on a regular basis or are noncompliant, long-acting preparations are available, such as fluphenazine decanoate or haloperidol decanoate. There is no uni-

versally accepted method for converting a patient from oral to long-acting forms, and dosing with sustained-released preparations must be individualized. Further information about antipsychotic drugs and their rational use is found in Chapter 27.

NONCOMPLIANCE

Noncompliance with antipsychotic medication is a significant problem in the care of schizophrenic patients. There are many contributing factors, but denial of illness resulting from poor insight and discomfort from adverse medication side effects are among the most common. In a cohort of schizophrenic patients, between 30%–40% were noncompliant at any given time, and by 2 years after hospital discharge, three-quarters had stopped taking medication for at least 1 week (Weiden et al. 1991). Noncompliance needs to be carefully assessed with schizophrenic patients, in some cases involving alternative sources of information. Strategies to minimize drug side effects (e.g., lowering the dosage, prescribing adjunctive medication or switching to a better tolerated drug such as one of the atypical antipsychotics) may work to enhance compliance. In some cases, long-acting intramuscular antipsychotics may be necessary.

ADJUNCTIVE PHARMACOLOGIC TREATMENTS

Medications other than antipsychotics are occasionally useful in the schizophrenic patients, but their role has not been clearly defined. Conventional agents primarily used for the treatment of other psychiatric disorders such as benzodiazepines, propranolol, lithium carbonate, carbamazepine, sodium valproate, and antidepressants have been used with varying degrees of success.

Benzodiazepines have been used alone and in combination with antipsychotic medications (Christison et al. 1991). High doses have been used with the intent of relieving agitation, thought disorder, delusions, and hallucinations. The theoretical justification supporting the use of benzodiazepines is that they facilitate GABA neurotransmission, which may inhibit dopamine neurotransmission. Individual response to these agents is highly variable, and the greatest use for benzodiazepines may be as an adjunct to antipsychotic medications in the acute management of psychotic agitation (Wolkowitz and Pickar 1991). Benzodiazepines have also been used to relieve the akathisia associated with antipsychotic medications.

Propranolol, and other β-blockers, have been used to treat schizophrenia, alone and in conjunction with antipsychotic drugs (Christison et al. 1991). One of its actions may be to raise plasma antipsychotic levels, but it has been reported to reduce aggressive behaviors and temper outbursts (Peet et al. 1981). It has also been used to relieve neuroleptic-induced akathisia (Lipinsky et al. 1984).

Lithium carbonate, which has a clear role in bipolar affective disorder, has been used mainly in an attempt to reduce impulsive and aggressive behaviors, hyperactivity, or excitation, as well as to stabilize mood (Delva and Letemendia 1982). Carbamazepine and sodium valproate have also been used in schizophrenic patients. Their main benefit, too, has probably been to reduce aggressive behavior and to modulate mood (Johns and Thompson 1995). Nonetheless, the effectiveness of the mood stabilizers in schizophrenia has not been adequately determined and requires further study.

Antidepressants have also been used in the treatment of schizophrenic patients, primarily in those who have developed a serious depression. Although early research suggested that antidepressants could cause worsening of a thought disorder, more recent work suggest that they have a legitimate role in treating the depressed patient with schizophrenia. When used, antidepressants should be prescribed with an antipsychotic to prevent worsening of psychosis and should not be routinely used in floridly psychotic patients. A trial of an antiparkinsonian agent to rule out an antipsychotic induced akinesia should be tried initially. Continuation treatment appears to be safe and effective in patients who respond to adjunctive antidepressants (Siris et al. 1987, 1994).

PHYSICAL TREATMENTS

Electroconvulsive Therapy

Although electroconvulsive therapy (ECT) has been found primarily to benefit those with mood disorders, it is still widely used in the treatment of schizophrenia. Early uncontrolled studies were generally enthusiastic, but later studies failed to show a strong therapeutic effect of ECT in schizophrenia. It is now generally acknowledged that ECT is effective in acute and subacute forms of schizophrenia, but is rarely helpful in chronic cases (Johns and Thompson 1995). Its primary usefulness is in the treatment of a few specific syndromes and in patients not responding to antipsychotic medication. Catatonia and depression secondary to schizophrenia have both been recognized as indications for ECT. In these situations, ECT appears to be rapidly effective based on clinical reports, although neither its use in catatonia nor depression secondary to schizophrenia has been carefully studied.

Other Physical Treatments

Many physical treatments have been developed and later abandoned due to ineffectiveness. Insulin coma therapy was introduced in the 1930s as a treatment for schizophrenia, and despite initial enthusiasm and acceptance, it was abandoned after the introduction of ECT and, later, the antipsychotic medications. Psychosurgery, too, was developed enthusiastically, but currently has no role in the treatment of schizophrenia. Hemodialysis has also been tried, based on the theory that it cleared the blood of a toxin (or toxins) responsible for causing schizophrenia. A controlled study (Carpenter et al. 1983) failed to show any benefit from this treatment, and no such toxins have ever been identified.

PSYCHOSOCIAL AND PROGRAMMATIC INTERVENTION

Psychosocial interventions play an important role in the management of schizophrenic patients and should be integrated with pharmacotherapy. Like antipsychotic medication, psychosocial treatments should be tailored to fit the schizophrenic patient's needs. The fit will depend on the individual, the phase of illness, and the living situation. For example, patients living with their families might benefit from family therapy, whereas patients living alone might benefit from the social stimulation provided in a day hospital program or contact with a visiting home nurse. Some patients may be self-sufficient and employed, while others may require around-the-clock care for extended periods in the hospital. Further, patients may require one type of intervention early in the course of illness and different interventions in later stages, when clinical symptoms have changed. Clinicians must work actively to ensure that schizophrenic patients receive adequate mental health care and community benefits and are encouraged to develop a close working relationship with their local social service agencies. While optimal care necessitates the availability of a range of services to fit the needs of the patient, including social, vocational, and housing needs, these services are inadequate in many communities (Lamb 1986).

During the past 20 years significant changes have occurred in the way the treatment of schizophrenia is conceptualized. In the 1960s and 1970s much emphasis was given to repeated hospital stays for the pharmacologic treatment of psychotic episodes. As hospitalizations have become briefer and more restricted, the locus of treatment has shifted to outpatient settings and the community. At the same time, it became clear that insight-oriented psychotherapy was not only ineffective in treating schizophrenia, but had the potential to worsen its symptoms (Mueser and Berenbaum 1990). Newer psychosocial treatment models have been developed that emphasize the practical resolution of common social and psychological difficulties seen in schizophrenic patients. Meanwhile, older models involving family therapy have received greater prominence. The latter interventions are especially important since they have a direct impact on relapse rates. It is now clear that combining pharmacologic treatment with psychosocial interventions offers advantages beyond the power of any single approach. Most clinicians understand the importance of integrated treatment approaches. For example, common sense tells us that although medication will not teach patients social skills, or to budget and shop for themselves, it may facilitate learning by diminishing psychotic symptoms.

LOCUS OF CARE

Patients with schizophrenia are rarely placed in long-term custodial institutions today, as the locus of care has shifted to outpatient clinics and the community. Patients, their families, and society at large have benefited from this shift, as greater emphasis has been placed on outpatient management and brief hospital stays. Patients are able to achieve greater degrees of independence and have more opportunities to participate in community life. But many communities have been unable to provide the kind of integrated and coordinated system of care that patients need to reduce risk of relapse and enhance functioning.

Hospitalization

Hospitalization is reserved for schizophrenic patients who pose a danger to themselves or others; patients who refuse to properly care for themselves (e.g., refuse food or fluids); and patients requiring special medical observation, tests, or treatments (see Table 12–10). When the patient is a danger to himself or others and refuses to enter the hospital, it is usually necessary to obtain a court order for hospitalization. When hospitalized, schizophrenic patients stay briefly in special psychiatric hospitals or in psychiatric units found in general hospitals. Stays are short (e.g., days to weeks), and the patient is generally returned to the community.

An active ward milieu is superior to a custodial one in the hospital, especially if well structured and not overly stimulating (Maxmen 1984). The following characteristics have been found optimal: small units, short stays, high staff to patient ratio, low staff turnover, low percentage of psychotic patients, broad delegation of responsibility with

clear lines of authority, low perceived levels of anger and aggression, high levels of support, and a practical problem-solving approach (Ellsworth 1983). Token economies in which patients are provided a high degree of ward structure and are rewarded for desired behaviors seem to be effective in controlling behavior in the hospital, but this improvement often does not generalize to situations outside the hospital.

Group therapy is frequently used with schizophrenic patients in the hospital to provide emotional support in a setting where a patient can learn social skills, and where friendships can develop. Inpatient groups that are most successful are highly structured and set limited goals (Yalom 1983). Traditional group therapy approaches that encourage self-exploration and the seeking of insight are generally countertherapeutic (Kanas 1985). This is particularly true with psychotic or highly paranoid individuals who might misinterpret situations that arise in group therapy.

Partial Hospitalization/Day Treatment

Schizophrenic patients not needing to be hospitalized may still benefit from the structure provided in day treatment or partial hospital programs, especially patients with substantial symptoms who have not responded adequately to medication. The two programs are similar, although they differ in the intensity of services provided. These programs generally operate weekdays, with patients returning home on evenings and weekends. Psychopharmacologic management is provided along with psychosocial rehabilitation. With most programs, the services provided and frequency of attendance will be individualized to fit the needs of the patient (Gudeman et al. 1983).

TABLE 12–10.   Reasons to hospitalize the schizophrenic patient

When the illness is new, to rule out alternative diagnoses, and to stabilize the dose of antipsychotic medication

For special medical procedures such as electroconvulsive therapy (ECT)

When aggressive or assaultive behavior presents a danger to the patient or others

When the patient becomes suicidal

When the patient is unable to properly care for himself or herself (e.g., refuses to eat or take fluids).

When medication side effects become disabling or potentially life threatening (e.g., severe pseudoparkinsonism, severe tardive dyskinesia, neuroleptic malignant syndrome)

Outpatient Care

The outpatient clinic will be the locus of treatment for most schizophrenic patients and is the most appropriate setting in which to coordinate care. A well-equipped clinic should be able to provide close monitoring of patients for relapse detection and prevention through careful medication management, to provide both individual or group counseling and psychoeducation, to arrange family interventions, and to arrange special programmatic interventions such as social skills training or cognitive rehabilitation. Case managers should be available to help coordinate the patient's care and to help them access governmental programs to which they may be entitled.

Family Interventions

When combined with antipsychotic medication, family therapy has been demonstrated to reduce relapse rates in schizophrenia. Carpenter (1996) reviewed 14 controlled trials and reported relapse rates to range from 40% to 53% in the control condition compared with 6%–23% in the experimental condition (i.e., family therapy). While family therapy may gain some of its impact through enhanced medication compliance, it may also help to protect the schizophrenic patient from the demands of the "real world" by providing improved social support, structure, and guidance.

Although the exact mechanism of improvement in family therapy is unknown, and no specific approach is better than another (Penn and Mueser 1996), several recommendations can be made. First, families can benefit from education about schizophrenia itself. This should include information about the chronic nature of the disorder and the need for long-term care based on realistic expectations. Education will improve cooperation and compliance of both patient and family. However, education needs to be combined with other family interventions aimed at improving communication and, at the same time, learning to minimize criticism and emotional overinvolvement that will help to decrease the schizophrenic patient's level of stress. Gaining a more realistic appraisal of the patient's illness and future expectations will reduce expressed emotion, which, as discussed earlier in the chapter, has been shown to lead to schizophrenic relapse. Family therapy also benefits family members and can help to reduce their feelings of anger, frustration, and helplessness. Research shows that multiple-family groups may work even better than single-family interventions (McFarlane et al. 1995).

Self-Help Organizations

In addition to more formal family interventions, self-help organizations for family members can be enormously beneficial. They provide a forum for family members to learn about schizophrenia, to gain encouragement from others, and to learn how to cope with its manifestations. The best known group in the United States is the Alliance for the Mentally Ill (AMI), and local chapters can be found in many communities. Many other countries have similar national organizations (e.g., the Schizophrenia Fellowship of Canada or Great Britain) that emphasize education, advocacy, mutual support, and self-help.

COGNITIVE THERAPY TECHNIQUES

Cognitive Rehabilitation

Cognitive rehabilitation has as its goal the remediation of abnormal thought processes known to occur in schizophrenia (Penn and Mueser 1996) and uses techniques pioneered in the treatment of brain-injured persons. Work with schizophrenic patients is focused on improving information processing skills such as attention, memory, vigilance, and conceptual abilities. Early studies have had mixed results, but suggest that performance on specific tasks (e.g., Wisconsin Card Sort Test) can be improved. Whether improvement on specific tasks can generalize to other situations needs further study.

Cognitive Content

Content approaches focus on changing the schizophrenic patient's abnormal thoughts (e.g., delusions) or his responses to them or to his abnormal experiences (e.g., hallucinations) (Tarrier et al. 1993). Patients learn various coping strategies such as listening to music to mask auditory hallucinations or reality testing of delusional beliefs. While these techniques appear promising as a way to reduce residual psychotic symptoms, more research is needed to learn which techniques are most effective.

SOCIAL SKILLS TRAINING

Because social and interpersonal skills are generally deficient in schizophrenic patients, social skills training aims to help the patient develop more appropriate behavior. This is accomplished by using modeling and social reinforcement and by providing opportunities, both individual and group, to practice the new behaviors. This could be as simple as helping the patient learn to maintain eye contact or as complicated as helping him learn conversational skills. Research has shown that social skills training can significantly enhance social functioning, but probably has little effect on risk of relapse (Marder et al. 1996). The best results appear to occur in early onset schizophrenic patients whose social development would have been disrupted by the emergence of illness and in persons who persist in a training program for more than 1 year (Penn and Mueser 1996).

ALCOHOL/DRUG ABUSE

Alcohol and other drug abuse is a significant problem for many schizophrenic patients and needs to be a focus of concern. Substance abuse or dependence aggravates the symptoms of schizophrenia, leads to medication noncompliance, and undermines other treatment interventions. Abstinence should be encouraged in all patients, and some will need referral for drug detoxification and rehabilitation (Ziedonis and Fisher 1994). Although these services may not be helpful in acutely psychotic or agitated patients, they may be enormously beneficial once the patient has improved and the schizophrenic illness has stabilized. Disulfiram should be used with caution because it inhibits dopamine β hydroxylase, increasing the dopamine available to the CNS, and may exacerbate psychotic symptoms (Kingsbury and Salzman 1990).

PSYCHOSOCIAL REHABILITATION

Psychosocial rehabilitation is a term used to describe services that aim to restore the patient's ability to function in the community. This may involve the medical and psychosocial treatments described above, but may also involve ways to foster social interaction, to promote independent living, and to encourage vocational performance (Cook et al. 1996). Patients are encouraged to become involved in developing and implementing their rehabilitation plan, which has as its focus enhancing the patient's talents and skills. The goal of psychosocial rehabilitation is to integrate the patient back into his or her community, rather than segregating the patient in separate facilities as has occurred in the past. In many locations, patient clubhouses are available to promote psychosocial rehabilitation, such as Fountain House, a program in New York City that patients help to run. The organization serves a variety of functions including providing job training, social and leisure time activities, residential assistance, and skills training (Beard et al. 1982).

Appropriate and affordable housing is a major concern for many patients, and, depending on the community, options may range from supervised shelters and group homes ("halfway houses") to boarding homes to supervised apartment living. Group homes provide peer support and companionship, along with on-site staff supervision. Supervised apartments provide greater independence and offer the availability and back-up of trained staff. Clearly, not all schizophrenic patients will be able to take advantage of sheltered care residences. Persons with greater levels of impairment may need round-the-clock supervision in a nursing home (Lamberti and Tariot 1995).

Vocational training and support can also be of enormous benefit to schizophrenic patients in helping to mainstream them back into the community. Research shows that vocational interventions can be effective in helping patients find and maintain paid jobs (Lehman 1995). Vocational rehabilitation may involve supported employment, competitive work in integrated settings, and more formal job training programs. A simple, repetitive job environment offering both interpersonal distance and on-site supervision may be the best initial setting, such as that found in a "sheltered workshop." While some patients will not be employable in any setting because of apathy, amotivation, or chronic psychosis, employment should be encouraged in able patients. A job will serve to improve self-esteem, provide additional income, as well as provide a social outlet for the patient (Mackota and Lamb 1989). Gradually, a patient may move toward a more demanding work setting, although the clinician should help the patient develop appropriate goals. Failure will only diminish a patient's already shaky self-esteem and reinforce the "sick" role. Assessment by a vocational guidance counselor will be helpful in matching patients with appropriate jobs by gaining a better understanding of the patient's abilities, aptitudes, and interests.

In some areas assertive community treatment (ACT) is available (Stein 1993), which consists of the careful monitoring of patients, the availability of mobile mental health teams, and aggressive programming individually tailored to each patient. ACT programs operate 24 hours a day and have been shown to reduce hospital admission rates and to improve quality of life for many schizophrenic patients. ACT involves teaching patients basic living skills, helping patients work with community agencies, and helping patients develop a social support network. Voluntary job placement and supported work settings (i.e., sheltered workshops) are an important part of the program.

DELUSIONAL DISORDERS

Delusional disorders constitute a small but important group of conditions characterized by the presence of systematized, non-bizarre delusions accompanied by affect appropriate to the delusion. Personality is generally spared, but the delusion may preoccupy and dominate the patient's life.

HISTORICAL OVERVIEW

The term *paranoia* was used by the Greeks nearly two 2,000 years ago to describe insanity or "craziness" and can be literally translated as "a mind beside itself." The term was revived in the early nineteenth century by German psychiatrists who were interested in disorders characterized by delusions of persecution and grandeur (Lewis 1970; Tanna 1974). Karl Kahlbaum (1828–1899) first applied the term to a chronic delusional disorder. Kraepelin, like Kahlbaum, was concerned with longitudinal course and gradually altered his formulation of paranoia. By the eighth revision of his *Lehrbuch der Psychiatrie*, he had restricted the term to describe persons with systematized delusions, an absence of hallucinations, and a prolonged course without recovery but not leading to mental deterioration (Kendler 1988). Kraepelin also identified *paraphrenia* as an intermediate group of paranoid disorders between dementia praecox and paranoia characterized by unremitting systematized delusions and hallucinations without progression to dementia. The latter term is still used in Britain. Both Kraepelin and Bleuler believed that paranoia was a condition distinct from dementia praecox, although unlike Kraepelin, Bleuler maintained that hallucinations occurred in some patients. Ernst Kretschmer (1888–1964) regarded paranoia as a psychogenic reaction occurring in people with sensitive personalities rather than as an organic illness.

Delusional disorder, as represented in DSM-IV, resembles the definition put forth by Kraepelin in 1912 for paranoia. The original term for this condition, *paranoid disorder*, which was used in DSM-III, has been abandoned because the word paranoid is usually construed to mean "persecutory." Because the delusions found in patients with delusional disorders are not restricted to persecutory themes, the former term was no longer believed appropriate. Kendler (1980) has further proposed that in the absence of hallucinations the term *simple delusional disorder* be used, and that when hallucinations are present the term *hallucinatory delusional disorder* be used.

DIAGNOSIS

According to DSM-IV (Table 12–11), delusional disorders are characterized by nonbizarre delusions lasting at least 1 month, behavior that is not obviously odd or bizarre apart from the delusion or its ramifications, absence of active phase symptoms that may occur in schizophrenia (e.g., hallucinations, disorganized speech, negative symptoms), and the determination that the disorder is not due to a mood disorder with psychotic features, is not substance induced, and is not due to a medical condition. The core feature, however, is the presence of a well-systematized, often logical, nonbizarre delusion. The term *systematized* indicates that the delusion and its ramifications fit into an all-encompassing, complex scheme that makes sense to the patient. The term *nonbizarre* implies that the delusion involves situations that can occur in real life, such as being followed, and not implausible or impossible situations, such as having all of one's internal organs replaced by those of bug-eyed Martians. Auditory or visual hallucinations, if present, are not prominent. However, olfactory or tactile hallucinations may be present and prominent.

TABLE 12–11. **DSM-IV criteria for delusional disorder**

A. Nonbizarre delusions (i.e., involving situations that occur in real life, such as being followed, poisoned, infected, loved at a distance, deceived by one's spouse or lover, or having a disease) of at least 1 month's duration

B. Criterion A for schizophrenia has never been met
Note: Tactile and olfactory hallucinations may be present in delusional disorder if they are related to the delusional theme

C. Apart from the impact of the delusion(s) or its ramifications, functioning is not markedly impaired and behavior is not obviously odd or bizarre

D. If mood episodes have occurred concurrently with delusions, their total duration has been brief relative to the duration of the delusional periods

E. The disturbance is not due to the direct physiological effects of a substance (e.g., a drug of abuse, a medication) or a general medical condition

Specify type: (The following types are assigned based on the predominant delusional theme)

Erotomanic type: Delusions that another person, usually of higher status, is in love with the individual

Grandiose type: Delusions of inflated worth, power, knowledge, identity, or special relationship to a deity or famous person

Jealous type: Delusions that the individual's sexual partner is unfaithful

Persecutory type: Delusions that the person (or someone to whom the person is close) is being malevolently treated in some way

Somatic type: Delusions that the person has some physical defect or general medical condition

Mixed type: Delusions characteristic of more than one of the above types but no one theme predominates

Unspecified type

DIFFERENTIAL DIAGNOSIS

A careful assessment is necessary to rule out other functional or medical causes for the delusions. The workup should include a physical examination to rule out alcohol-, amphetamine-, cocaine-, and other drug-induced conditions; dementia; infectious; metabolic; and endocrine disorders (Manschreck 1996). Routine lab tests may be indicated depending on the results of the history and physical examination. CT or MRI may be helpful in selected cases, especially when mass lesions are suspected. Symptom onset, course, and associated features are also relevant. Abrupt changes in mood, mental state, personality, or ability to function strongly suggest a medical origin. Disturbed consciousness, perceptual disturbances, or physical signs (e.g., fever) may point to specific causes. Isolated paranoid symptoms are often an early sign of medical illness, and are especially common among elderly inpatients.

The major diagnostic task remains in separating delusional disorder from mood disorders, schizophrenia, and paranoid personality. The chief distinction is that in delusional disorder a full depressive or manic syndrome is absent, developed after the psychotic symptoms, or was brief in duration relative to the duration of the psychotic symptoms. Unlike schizophrenia, delusional disorder is characterized by nonbizarre delusions and generally either no hallucinations or hallucinations that are not prominent. Furthermore, patients with delusional disorder do not typically develop other schizophrenic symptoms such as incoherence or grossly disorganized behavior, and personality is generally preserved. Persons with paranoid personality are suspicious and hypervigilant, but are not delusional.

Associated features of delusional disorder include anger, social isolation and seclusiveness, eccentric behavior, suspiciousness, hostility, and sometimes violence prompted by the delusion (Kennedy et al. 1992). Winokur (1977) reported that patients with delusional disorders frequently develop sexual problems and depression, and described many as overtalkative and circumstantial. Clinical wisdom suggests that many patients become litigious and end up as lawyer's clients rather than as psychiatrists' patients.

Delusional disorder includes the following DSM-IV subtypes:

1. *Erotomanic type* (de Clerambault's syndrome), in which there is a belief that a person, usually of higher status, is in love with the patient
2. *Grandiose type*, in which there is a belief that one is of inflated worth, power, knowledge, or identity or has a special relation to a deity or famous person

3. *Jealous type*, in which the delusion is that one's sexual partner is unfaithful
4. *Persecutory type*, in which there is a belief that one is being malevolently treated in some way
5. *Somatic type*, in which the delusion is that a person has some physical defect, disorder or disease, such as acquired immunodeficiency syndrome (AIDS)

There is a residual category (*unspecified type*) for patients who do not fit the previous categories; for example, those who have been ill less than 1 month. Another category (*mixed type*) is for patients with delusions of more than one characteristic theme and in which no one theme predominates. The DSM-IV diagnosis of *shared psychotic disorder* is made when two or more persons share a delusion (*folie à deux*).

The following case example illustrates the jealous subtype of delusional disorder:

CASE EXAMPLE 3

Harvey, a 64-year-old electrician, lived with his wife of 43 years. He voluntarily presented for hospital admission, reporting that he was tired of his wife calling him "crazy." His wife reported that Harvey was chronically jealous, and she was unable to reassure him that she was faithful.

Harvey's family of origin was poor, and his father was alcoholic. Nonetheless, he had achieved good grades in school and participated in sport activities, even though he was considered aloof and distant by his peers. After graduating from high school, he married and joined the Army, serving honorably in World War II. He later worked as an electrician, eventually starting his own business. Although hardworking and honest, he had few friends and was viewed as excessively rigid and humorless by his family. Harvey and his wife had three children, all of whom were healthy and emotionally stable.

Several years after returning from the war, Harvey began to suspect his wife of infidelity. Over the following decades he continued to be convinced that his wife was involved with other men. Although he had never seen her with another man, he was convinced of her infidelity by trivial evidence such as frequently washed bed linen, spots on his wife's undergarments, or unfamiliar tire tracks in the driveway. He once accused his wife of placing sleeping pills in his coffee at night so that after he had fallen asleep she could leave the house for a sexual liaison with a lover. Incredibly, he maintained that several times his wife actually had sexual intercourse with another man in the same bed where he lay sleeping. One particular time, he reported awakening to find the bed sheets in disarray and his shorts pulled down to his knees in what he believed was his wife's lover's attempt to harass him. He also claimed that neighbors had commented to him about the large number of men who visited his wife when he was away on business.

His wife became aware of Harvey's suspiciousness and jealousy early in their marriage, and when confronted by him, she steadfastly maintained that there was no basis for the accusations. No amount of reassurance could alter her husband's convictions. She reported that her husband's jealous beliefs would wax and wane, alternating with periods of relative normalcy. While she continued to love and care for her husband, Harvey's wife admitted that the delusional beliefs had strained the marriage and had led to several trial separations.

In the hospital, Harvey was observed to be friendly with his peers and appropriate with the medical staff. He persisted with the belief that his wife had been unfaithful to him. There was no evidence of hallucinations. A trial of antipsychotic medication did not alter his delusion.

EPIDEMIOLOGY

Delusional disorder constitutes from 1% to 4% of psychiatric admissions, and from 2% to 7% of admissions for functional psychosis (Kendler 1982). The incidence of first admissions for paranoia was estimated to fall between 1–3/100,000/year and the prevalence to fall between 24–30/100,000 population. Delusional disorder occurs mainly in middle to late adult life, with a peak frequency of first admissions between 35 and 55 years of age. More women than men develop the disorder, and while 60%–75% of patients are married, up to one-third are widowed, divorced, or separated. Persons with delusional disorder are economically and educationally disadvantaged, and immigrants seem especially prone to develop the disorder. They are also more extroverted, dominant, and hypersensitive premorbidly than are schizophrenic patients, who, as discussed earlier in the chapter, are likely to be introverted and schizoid premorbidly. Once established, delusional disorder is generally chronic and lifelong. However, it appears to have a better long-term prognosis than schizophrenia (Opjordsmoen 1989; Winokur 1977). Remission is reported in one-third to one-half of cases (Jorgensen 1994).

ETIOLOGY

The cause of delusional disorder is unknown, although it is unlikely that delusional disorders are related to schizophrenia or the mood disorders. The relatives of probands with delusional disorder show increased rates of jealously, suspiciousness, paranoid personality, and delusional disorder over control relatives, but the families have no increase in schizophrenia or mood disorders (Kendler et al. 1982,

1985b; Watt 1985; Winokur 1985).

Other potentially relevant risk factors for delusional disorder include social isolation and immigration. *Prison psychosis* has been described in which persons placed in solitary confinement have developed a paranoid psychosis. *Migration psychoses*, which are often persecutory, have been described in persons migrating from one country to another (although it is reasonable to assume that persons in whom paranoia is prone to develop may be more likely to emigrate than others). *Querulent paranoia*, a special form of paranoia characterized by litigiousness, is believed by Scandinavian investigators to be a psychogenic disorder in which unlucky personal experiences precipitate paranoia in persons with deviant personalities (Astrup 1984).

CLINICAL MANAGEMENT

Clinical management of the patient with delusional disorder involves establishing the diagnosis, instituting appropriate interventions, and providing follow-up care. Because there are no systematic data comparing treatments in delusional disorder, recommendations are based on clinical observation, not empirical evidence. Treatment will most often include both psychotherapy and medication.

Most patients have little insight about their illness and refuse to acknowledge a problem, so an initial obstacle is getting the patient to the physician. This fact might account for the low percentage of cases reported by physicians. Most patients can be treated as outpatients, but hospitalization is necessary if threats of self-harm or harm to others are present. Suicide is uncommon, but may occur when the patient becomes depressed and despondent. The potential for violence may exist because some patients will act on their delusions, particularly jealous or erotomanic men. In these cases the target is not random, but specific to the delusional concern. Thus, a clinician caring for a patient with delusional disorder must carefully assess potential for harm to self or others.

Tact and skill are necessary to help persuade a delusional disorder patient to accept treatment. It may help to first convince the patient to receive treatment for depressive or anxiety symptoms and not the delusions. Once a therapeutic relationship is established, a clinician can begin to gently challenge the delusional beliefs by showing how they interfere with the patient's life, but must neither condemn nor collude in the beliefs. The patient should be assured of privacy, and the physician should take care not to discuss confidential matters with the patient's family without the patient's consent. Group therapy is usually not recommended; the patient's chronic suspiciousness and hypersensitivity may lead him or her to misinterpret situations that may arise in the context of group therapy.

Because delusional disorder is relatively uncommon, its treatment with antipsychotic medication has never been properly evaluated; anecdotal evidence suggests that response is poor (Winokur 1977). Antipsychotics may reduce the agitation, apprehension, and anxiety that accompany delusions, but leave the core delusion untouched. Any of the standard antipsychotics can be used. The selection of medication and dosage will depend on the patient's age and the drug's potential side effects. If the patient is helped by the antipsychotic, depot forms of several are available to ensure compliance (e.g., haloperidol decanoate, fluphenazine decanoate). Neuroleptics have been reported to specifically reduce the intensity of the delusions in erotomania and the associated ideas of reference (Segal 1989).

Monohypochondriacal paranoia (i.e., delusional disorder, somatic type) has been reported to respond to the antipsychotic pimozide at doses of 4–8 mg per day (Munro 1992). Selective serotonin reuptake inhibitors have also been reported helpful in reducing the delusional beliefs, as have the atypical antipsychotics clozapine and risperidone.

Antidepressants and anxiolytics may be indicated for accompanying depressive or anxiety syndromes, but have not been systematically evaluated in patients with delusional disorder. ECT has no role in the treatment of delusional disorder, unless it is used to treat a superimposed major depression.

CONCLUSIONS

Tremendous progress has been made during the past two decades to better our understanding of schizophrenia, schizophreniform disorder, and delusional disorder. While the introduction of DSM-III criteria in 1980 narrowed the definition for schizophrenia and created a more homogeneous group of subjects for research, some experts believed the narrowing went too far. A reemphasis on negative symptoms of schizophrenia (Bleuler's "fundamental" symptoms) in DSM-IV has added balance to the perhaps too-rigid emphasis on Schneiderian symptoms in the 1970s. Advances in classification and epidemiology have allowed us to reevaluate the distribution of schizophrenia and its risk factors.

The development of brain-imaging techniques such as CT, MRI, SPECT, and PET have enhanced our understanding of schizophrenia. This technology is allowing us to explore the nature and pattern of brain deficits and examine the possibility of symptom localization in schizophrenia. The development of "brain banks" as well as new techniques in histopathology have given renewed emphasis to postmortem research, permitting a more detailed investigation of abnormalities in neurotransmitter systems and in the neuropathology of schizophrenia. While the nosologists and neuroscientists have been clarifying the classification and pathologic mechanisms of schizophrenia, geneticists have been amassing large family data sets and applying new methods such as gene mapping that promise to enrich the study of genetic factors in schizophrenia.

Whereas technological advances are helping us to explore the etiology of schizophrenia, knowledge about course and outcome has been enhanced through long-term studies. We have learned that the best treatment approach to schizophrenia combines pharmacologic and psychosocial measures. The pharmacologic treatment of schizophrenia has been hampered by undue reliance on the well-worn dopamine theory, and investigators are now looking at other neurotransmitter systems that may yield a more complex interactive model of neurotransmission abnormalities that will result in new pharmacological approaches. Meanwhile, newer atypical antipsychotics have become available, helping many patients formerly thought to be treatment refractory to achieve better functioning in the community. New research has highlighted the importance of family interaction models in schizophrenia, leading to more specific psychosocial interventions in the treatment of this disorder.

During the 1990s, the "Decade of the Brain," the drive in psychiatry has been to develop a comprehensive understanding of brain function at levels that range from mind to molecule and to determine how aberrations in these normal functions lead to the development of symptoms of mental illness. Progress in the coming decade will be to build on the foundation of current research and enhance our understanding of the pathophysiology and etiology of schizophrenia. Our ultimate goal is to give physicians more powerful tools to treat those who suffer from schizophrenia and, if possible, prevent its development.

REFERENCES

Akbarian S, Kim JJ, Potkin SG, et al: Maldistribution of interstitial neurons in prefrontal white matter of the brains of schizophrenic patients. Arch Gen Psychiatry 53:428–436, 1996

Allebeck P, Varla A, Kristjansson E, et al: Risk factors for suicide among patients with schizophrenia. Acta Psychiatr Scand 76:414–419, 1987

Amador XF, Sackheim HA, Mukerjee S et al: Specificity of smooth pursuit eye movement and visual fixation abnormalities in schizophrenia: Comparison to mania and normal controls. Schizophr Res 5:135–144, 1991

American Psychiatric Association: Diagnostic and Statistical Manual of Mental Disorders. Washington, DC, American Psychiatric Press, 1952

American Psychiatric Association: Diagnostic and Statistical Manual of Mental Disorders, Second Edition. Washington, DC, American Psychiatric Press, 1968

American Psychiatric Association: Diagnostic and Statistical Manual of Mental Disorders, Third Edition. Washington, DC, American Psychiatric Press, 1980

American Psychiatric Association: Diagnostic and Statistical Manual of Mental Disorders, Third Edition, Revised. Washington, DC, American Psychiatric Press, 1987

American Psychiatric Association: Diagnostic and Statistical Manual of Mental Disorders, Fourth Edition. Washington, DC, American Psychiatric Press, 1994

American Psychiatric Association: Practice Guidelines for the Treatment of Patients With Schizophrenia. Am J Psychiatry 154:4:1–63, 1997

Andreasen NC: Affective flattening and the criteria for schizophrenia. Am J Psychiatry 136:944–947, 1979a

Andreasen NC: Thought, language, and communication disorders I; clinical assessment, definition of terms, and evaluation of their reliability. Arch Gen Psychiatry 36:1315–1321, 1979b

Andreasen NC: Negative symptoms in schizophrenia: definition and realiability. Arch Gen Psychiatry 39:784–788, 1982

Andreasen NC: The Broken Brain: The Biologic Revolution in Psychiatry. New York, Harper and Row, 1984

Andreasen NC: The diagnosis of schizophrenia. Schizophr Bull 13:9–22, 1987

Andreasen NC, Akiskal HS: The specificity of Bleulerian and Schneiderian symptoms: a critical reevaluation. Psychiatr Clin North Am 6:41–54, 1983

Andreasen NC, Black DW: Schizophrenia in The Introductory Textbook of Psychiatry. Washington, DC, American Psychiatric Press, 1991, pp 157–174

Andreasen NC, Olson S: Negative versus positive schizophrenia: definition and validation. Arch Gen Psychiatry 39:789–794, 1982

Andreasen NC, Smith MR, Jacoby CG, et al: Ventricular enlargement in schizophrenia: definition and prevalence. Am J Psychiatry 139:292–296, 1982

Andreasen NC, Nasrallah HA, Dunn V, et al: Structural abnormalities in the frontal system in schizophrenia: a magnetic resonance imaging study. Arch Gen Psychiatry 43:136–144, 1986

Andreasen NC, Ehrhardt JC, Swayze VW, et al: Magnetic resonance imaging of the brain in schizophrenia: the pathophysiologic significance of structural abnormalities. Arch Gen Psychiatry 47:35–44, 1990a

Andreasen NC, Flaum M, Swayze VW, et al: Positive and negative symptoms in schizophrenia: a critical reappraisal. Arch Gen Psychiatry 47:615–621, 1990b

Andreasen NC, Swayze VW, Flaum M, et al: Ventricular enlargement in schizophrenia: evaluation with computed tomographic scanning. Arch Gen Psychiatry 47:1008–1015, 1990c

Andreasen NC, Rezai K, Alliger R, et al: Hypofrontality in neuroleptic-naive patients and in patients with chronic schizophrenia: assessment with xenon 133 single-photon emission computed tomography and the Tower of London. Arch Gen Psychiatry 49:943–958, 1992

Andreasen NC, Flashman L, Flaum M, et al: Regional brain abnormalities in schizophrenia measured with magnetic resonance imaging. JAMA 272:1763–1769, 1994a

Andreasen NC, Arndt S, Swayze V, et al: Thalamic abnormalities in schizophrenia visualized through magnetic resonance image averaging. Science 266:294–298, 1994b

Andreasen NC, Arndt S, Alliger R, et al: Symptoms of schizophrenia: methods, meanings, and mechanisms. Arch Gen Psychiatry 52:341–351, 1995

Andreasen NC, O'Leary DS, Cizadlo T, et al: Schizophrenia and cognitive dysmetria: a positron-emission tomography study of dysfunctional prefrontal-thalamic-cerebellar circuitry. Proc Natl Acad Sci U S A 93:9985–9990, 1996

Angermeyer ML, Goldstein JM, Kuehn L: Gender differences in schizophrenia: rehospitalization and community survival. Psychol Med 19:365–382, 1989

Anthony JC, Folstein M, Romanoski AJ, et al: Comparison of the lay Diagnostic Interview Schedule and a standardized psychiatric diagnosis. Arch Gen Psychiatry 42:667–675, 1985

Arndt S, Andreasen NC, Flaum M, et al: A longitudinal study of symptom dimensions in schizophrenia: prediction and patterns of change. Arch Gen Psychiatry 52:352–360, 1995

Arnold SE, Hyman BT, VanHoesen GW, et al: Some cytoarchitectural abnormalities of the entorhinal cortex in schizophrenia. Arch Gen Psychiatry 48:625–632, 1991

Astrup C: Querulent paranoia: a follow-up. Neuropsychobiology 11:149–154, 1984

Aylward E, Walker E, Bettes B: Intelligence in schizophrenia: meta-analysis of the research. Schizophr Bull 10:430–459, 1984

Babigian HM: Schizophrenia: Epidemiology in Comprehensive Textbook of Psychiatry, Fourth Edition, Vol I. Edited by Kaplan HI, Sadock BJ. Baltimore, MD, Williams & Wilkins, 1984, pp 643–650

Baldessarini RJ, Cohen BM, Teicher MH: Significance of neuroleptic dose and plasma level in the pharmacologic treatment of psychosis. Arch Gen Psychiatry 45:79–91, 1988

Barr CE, Mednick SA, Munk-Jorgensen P: Exposure to influenza epidemics during gestation and adult schizophrenia—a 40-year study. Arch Gen Psychiatry 47:869–874, 1990

Barraclough B, Bunch J, Nelson B, et al: A hundred cases of suicide: clinical aspects. Br J Psychiatry 125:355–373, 1974

Barta PE, Pearlson GD, Powers RE, et al: Auditory hallucinations and smaller superior temporal gyral volume in schizophrenia. Am J Psychiatry 147:1457–1462, 1990

Beard JH, Propst RN, Malamud TJ: The Fountain House model of psychiatric rehabilitation. Psychosocial Rehabilitation J 5:47–54, 1982

Beitchman JH: Childhood schizophrenia—a review and comparison with adult onset schizophrenia. Pediatr Clin North Am 8:793–814, 1985

Benes FM, McSparren J, Bird ED, et al: Deficits in small interneurons in prefrontal and cingulate cortices of schizophrenic and schizoaffective patients. Arch Gen Psychiatry 48:996–1001, 1991

Bilder RM, Mukherjee S, Rieder RO, et al: Symptomatic and neuropsychological components of defect states. Schizophr Bull 11:409–491, 1985

Bilder RM, Lipschutz-Broch L, Reiter G, et al: Neuropsychological deficits in the early course of first-episode schizophrenia. Schizophr Res 5:198–199, 1991

Black DW, Boffeli TJ: Simple schizophrenia: past, present, and future. Am J Psychiatry 146:1267–1273, 1989

Black DW, Fisher R: Mortality in DSM-III-R schizophrenia. Schizophr Res 7:109–116, 1992

Black DW, Winokur G: Cancer mortality in psychiatric patients: the Iowa Record-Linkage Study. Int J Psychiatry Med 16:189–198, 1986

Bleuler E: Dementia Praecox, or the Group of Schizophrenias (1911). Translated by Zinken J. New York, International Universities Press, 1950

Bloom F: Advancing a neurodevelopmental origin for schizophrenia. Arch Gen Psychiatry 50: 224–227, 1993

Bogerts B: Recent advances in the neuropathology of schizophrenia. Schizophr Bull 19:431–445, 1993

Braff DL: Information processing and attention dysfunctions in schizophrenia. Schizophr Bull 192:233–259, 1993

Braff DL, Heaton R, Kuck J, et al: The generalized pattern of neuropsychological deficits in outpatients with chronic schizophrenia with heterogeneous Wisconsin Card Sorting Test results. Arch Gen Psychiatry 48:891–898, 1991

Breier A, Astrachan BM: Characterization of schizophrenic patients who commit suicide. Am J Psychiatry 141:206–209, 1984

Breier A, Buchanan RW, Elkashef A, et al: Brain morphology and schizophrenia: a magnetic resonance imaging study of limbic, prefrontal cortex, and caudate structures. Arch Gen Psychiatry 49:921–926, 1992

Broadbent DE: Perception and Communication. London, Pergamon Press, 1958

Bromet EJ, Dew MA, Eaton W: Epidemiology of psychosis with special reference to schizophrenia, in Textbook of Psychiatric Epidemiology. Edited by Tsuang MT, Tohen M, Zahner GEP. New York, Wiley-Liss, 1995, pp 283–300

Buchanan RW, Strauss ME, Kirkpatrick B, et al: Neuropsychological impairments in deficit versus non-deficit forms of schizophrenia. Arch Gen Psychiatry 51:804–811, 1994

Buchsbaum MS, Ingvar DH, Kessler R, et al: Cerebral glucography with positron tomography. Arch Gen Psychiatry 39:251–259, 1982

Buchsbaum MS, Someya T, Teng CY, et al: PET and MRI of the thalamus in never-medicated patients with schizophrenia. Am J Psychiatry 153:191–199, 1996

Campbell A, Herschel M, Cohen BM, et al: Tissue levels of haloperidol by radioreceptor assay and behavioral effects of haloperidol in the rat. Life Sci 27:633–640, 1980

Caracci G, Mukherjee S, Roth SD, et al: Subjective awareness of abnormal involuntary movements in chronic schizophrenic patients. Am J Psychiatry 147:295–298, 1990

Carlsson A: The current status of the dopamine hypothesis of schizophrenia. Neuropsychopharmacology 1:179–186, 1988

Carpenter WT: Maintenance therapy of persons with schizophrenia. J Clin Psychiatry 57 (suppl 19):10–18, 1996

Carpenter WT, Buchanan RW: Schizophrenia. N Engl J Med 330:681–690, 1994

Carpenter WT Jr, Strauss JS: The prediction of outcome in schizophrenia IV: eleven year follow-up of the Washington IPSS Cohort. J Nerv Ment Dis 179:517–525, 1991

Carpenter WT Jr, Hanlon TL, Heinrichs DW, et al: Continuous versus targeted medication in schizophrenic outpatients: outcome results. Am J Psychiatry 147:1138–1148, 1990

Carpenter WT Jr, Sadler JH, Light PD, et al: The therapeutic efficacy of hemodialysis in schizophrenia. N Engl J Med 308:669–675, 1983

Chatterjee A, Chako SM, Koreen A, et al: Prevalence and clinical correlates of extrapyramidal signs and spontaneous dyskinesia in never-medication schizophrenic patients. Am J Psychiatry 152:1724–1729, 1995

Christison GW, Kirch DG, Wyatt RJ: When symptoms persist: choosing among alternative somatic treatments for schizophrenia. Schizophr Bull 17:217–245, 1991

Clardy JA, Hyde TM, Kleinman JE: Post-mortem Neurochemical and Neuropathological Studies in Schizophrenia, in Schizophrenia: From Mind to Molecule. Edited by Andreasen NC. Washington, DC, American Psychiatric Press, 1993

Cohen G, Andreasen NC, Alliger R, et al: Segmentation techniques for the classification of brain tissue using magnetic resonance imaging. Psychiatry Res: Neuroimaging 45: 33–51, 1992

Cole JO: Psychopharmacology update: Medication and seclusion and restraint. McLean Hosp J 10:37–53, 1985

Conrad AJ, Abebe T, Austin R, et al: Hippocampal pyramidal cell disarray in schizophrenia as a bilateral phenomenon. Arch Gen Psychiatry 48:413–417, 1991

Cook JA, Pickett SA, Razzano L, et al: Rehabilitation services for persons with schizophrenia. Psychiatric Annals 26:97–104, 1996

Cooper JE, Kendall RE, Gurland BJ, et al: Psychiatric Diagnosis in New York and London: A Comparative Study of Mental Hospital Admissions. Institute of Psychiatry, Maudsley Monographs, No 20. London, UK, Oxford University Press, 1972

Coryell W, Tsuang MT: Outcome after 40 years in DSM-III schizophreniform disorder. Arch Gen Psychiatry 43:324–328, 1986

Creese R, Burt BR, Snyder SH: Dopamine receptor binding predicts clinical and pharmacologic potencies of antipsychotic drugs. Science 192:81–84, 1976

Crow TJ: Positive and negative schizophrenic symptoms and the role of dopamine. Br J Psychiatry 137:383–386, 1980

Crowe RR, Black DW, Wesner R, et al: Lack of linkage to chromosome 5q11-q13 markers in six schizophrenia pedigrees. Arch Gen Psychiatry 48:357–361, 1991

Csillag C: Denmark: psychiatric offenders. Lancet 341: 683–684, 1993

Cutting J: The Psychology of Schizophrenia. London, UK, Churchill Livingstone, 1985

Davis KL, Kahn RS, Ko G, et al: Dopamine in schizophrenia: a review and reconceptualization. Am J Psychiatry 148:1474–1486, 1991

Davis JM, Kane JM, Marder SR, et al: Dose response of prophylactic antipsychotics. J Clin Psychiatry 54 (suppl 3):24–30, 1993

deLeon J, Verghese C, Tracy JI, et al: Polydipsia and water intoxication in psychiatric patients: a review of the epidemiologic literature. Biol Psychiatry 35:519–530, 1994

DeLisi LE, Goldin LR, Hamovit VR, et al: A family study of the association of increased ventricular size with schizophrenia. Arch Gen Psychiatry 43:48–53, 1986

DeLisi LE, Hoff Al, Kushner M, et al: Left ventricular enlargement associated with diagnostic outcome of schizophreniform disorder. Biol Psychiatry 32:199–201, 1992

Delva NJ, Letemendia FJJ: Lithium treatment in schizophrenia and schizoaffective disorders. Br J Psychiatry 141:387–400, 1982

Dixon L, Haas G, Weiden PJ, et al: Drug abuse in schizophrenic patients: clinical correlates and reasons for use. Am J Psychiatry 148:224–230, 1991

Drake RE, Osher FC, Wallach MA: Alcohol use and abuse in schizophrenia: a prospective community study. J Nerv Ment Dis 177:408–414, 1989

Dubin WR, Waxman HM, Weiss KJ, et al: Rapid tranquilization: The efficacy of oral concentrate. J Clin Psychiatry 46:475–478, 1985

Eaton WW: Epidemiology of schizophrenia. Epidemiol Rev 7:105–126, 1985

Eaton WW: Update on epidemiology of schizophrenia. Epidemiol Rev 13:320–328, 1991

Eaton WW, Day R, Kramer M: The use of epidemiology for risk factor research in schizophrenia: an overview and methodologic critique, in Handbook of Schizophrenia, Vol 3—Nosology, Epidemiology, and Genetics. Edited by Tsuang MT, Simpson JC. Amsterdam, Elsevier Science Publishers, 1988, pp 169–204

Eaton WW, Hayward C, Ram R: Schizophrenia and rheumatoid arthritis: a review. Schizophr Res 6:181–192, 1992

Ellsworth RB: Characteristics of effective treatment milieu, in Principles and Practice of Milieu Therapy. Edited by Gunderson JG, Will OA, Mosher LF. New York, Jason Aronson, 1983, pp 87–123

Erlenmeyer-Kimling L: Fertility in psychotics, in Annual Review of the Schizophrenic Syndrome, Vol 5. Edited by Cancro R. New York, Brunner/Mazel, 1978, pp 298–325

Expert Consensus Guideline Series Steering Committee: Treatment of schizophrenia. J Clin Psychiatry 57 (suppl 12B):1–58, 1996

Farde L, Nordstrom AL: PET analysis indicates atypical central dopamine receptor occupancy in clozapine-treated patients. Br J Psychiatry 160:30–33, 1992

Farde L, Ehrin E, Eriksson E, et al: Substituted benzamides as ligands for visualization of dopamine receptor binding in the human brain by positron emission tomography. Proc Nat Acad Sci U S A 81:3863–3867, 1985

Farde L, Wiesel F-A, Stone-Elander S, et al: D_2 dopamine receptors in neuroleptic-naive schizophrenic patients: positron emission tomography study with [^{11}C]raclopride. Arch Gen Psychiatry 47:213–219, 1990

Faris REL, Durham HL: Mental Disorder in Urban Areas. Chicago, IL, University of Chicago Press, 1939

Farmer AE, McGuffin P, Gottesman II: Twin concordance for DSM-III schizophrenia: scrutinizing the validity of the definition. Arch Gen Psychiatry 44:634–641, 1987

Feighner JP, Robins F, Guze SB, et al: Diagnostic criteria for use in psychiatric research. Arch Gen Psychiatry 26:57–63, 1972

Feinberg I: Schizophrenia and late maturational brain changes in man. Psychopharmacol Bull 18:29–31, 1982

Fenton WS, McGlashan TH: The prognostic significance of obsessive-compulsive symptoms in schizophrenia. Am J Psychiatry 143:437–441, 1986

Fenton WS, McGlashan TH: Natural history of schizophrenia subtypes I: longitudinal study of paranoid, hebephrenic, and undifferentiated schizophrenia. Arch Gen Psychiatry 48:969–977, 1991

Flashman LA, Flaum M, Gupta S, Andreasen NC: Soft signs and neuropsychological performance in schizophrenia. Am J Psychiatry 153:526–532, 1996

Flaum M, Arndt S, Andreasen NC: The role of gender in studies of ventrical enlargement in schizophrenia: a predominantly male effect. Am J Psychiatry 147:1327–1332, 1990

Flaum M, Nopoulos P, Arndt S, et al: Improving tissue segmentation in magentic resonance imaging: multiple pulse sequences and automated training class selection. Third International Conference on Functional Mapping of the Human Brain, Copenhagen, 1997

Frith CD: The Cognitive Neuropsychology of Schizophrenia. East Sussix, Lawrence Erlbaum, 1992

Frith C: Functional imaging and cognitive abnormalities. Lancet 346:615–620, 1995

Frith CD, Friston K, Liddle PF, et al: Willed action and the prefrontal cortex in man: a study with PET. Proc R Soc Lond 244:241–246, 1991

Ganguli R, Brar JS, Chengappa KNR: Mitogen stimulated interleukin-2 production in never-medicated, first-episode schizophrenic patients. Arch Gen Psychiatry 52:668–672, 1995

Garza-Trevino ES, Hollister LE, Overall JE, et al: Efficacy of combinations of intramuscular antipsychotics and sedative-hypnotics for control of psychotic agitation. Am J Psychiatry 146:1598–1601, 1989

Geddes JR, Lawrie SM: Obstetrical complications and schizophrenia: a meta-analysis. Br J Psychiatry 167:786–793, 1995

Gerard DL, Houston LG: Family setting and social etiology of schizophrenia. Psychiatr Q 27:90–101, 1953

Goff DC, Henderson DC, Amico E: Cigarette smoking and schizophrenia: relationship to psychopathology and medication side effects. Am J Psychiatry 149:1189–1194, 1992

Goldberg TE, Kelsoe JR, Weinberger DR, et al: Performance of schizophrenic patients on putative neuropsychological tests of frontal lobe function. Int J Neurosci 42:51–58, 1988

Goldman-Rakic PS: Circuitry of primate prefrontal cortex and regulation of behavior by representational memory, in Handbook of Physiology. Edited by Plum F, Mountcastle V. Bethesda, MD, American Physiological Society, 1987, pp 373–417

Goldman-Rakic PS: Working memory dysfunction in schizophrenia. J Neuropsychiatry Clin Neurosci 64:348–357, 1994

Gottesman II, Shields J: Schizophrenia: The Epigenetic Puzzle. Cambridge, UK, Cambridge University Press, 1982

Green MF, Satz P, Christensen C: Minor physical remedies in schizophrenia patients, bipolar patients, and their siblings. Schizophr Bull 20:433–440, 1994

Grillon C, Ameli R, Charney DS, et al: Startle gating deficits occur across prepulse intensities in schizophrenic patients. Biol Psychiatry 32:939–943, 1992

Gudeman JE, Shore MF, Dickey B: Day hospitalization and an inn instead of inpatient care for psychiatric patients. N Eng J Med 308:749–753, 1983

Gulbinat W, Dupont A, Jablensky A, et al: Cancer incidence in schizophrenic patients: results of record linkage studies in three countries. Br J Psychiatry Suppl 18:75–83, 1992

Gupta S, Andreasen NC, Arndt S et al: Neurological soft signs in neuroleptic-naïve and neuroleptic treated schizophrenic patients and in normal comparison subjects. Am J Psychiatry 152:191–196, 1995a

Gupta S, Rajaprabhakaran R, Arndt S, et al: Premorbid adjustment as a predictor of phenomenological and neurobiological indices of schizophrenia. Schizophr Res 16:189–197, 1995b

Gur RC, Gur RE: Hypofrontality in schizophrenia: RIP. Lancet 345:1383–1384, 1995

Gur RE, Pearlson GD: Neuroimaging in schizophrenia research. Schizophren Bull 19:332–353, 1993

Guze SB, Cloninger CR, Martin RL, et al: A follow-up and family study of schizophrenia. Arch Gen Psychiatry 40:1273–1276, 1983

Hare EH: Mental illness and social conditions in Bristol. J Ment Sci 102:349–357, 1956

Hare EH, Price JS, Slater E: Mental disorder and season of birth. Nature 241:480, 1973

Harris G, Andreasen NC, Cizadlo T, et al: Improving tissue segmentation in magentic resonance imaging: multiple pulse sequences and automated training class selection. Third International Conference on Functional Mapping of the Human Brain, Copenhagen, 1997

Hegarty JD, Baldessarini RJ, Tohen M, et al: One hundred years of schizophrenia: a meta-analysis of the outcome literature. Am J Psychiatry 151:1409–1415, 1994

Herz M: Prodromal symptoms and prevention of relapse in schizophrenia. J Clin Psychiatry 46:22–25, 1985

Heston LL: Psychiatric disorders in foster home reared children of schizophrenic mothers. Br J Psychiatry 112:819–825, 1966

Hoff Al, Riordan H, O'Donnell DW, et al: Cross-sectional and longitudinal neuropsychological test findings in first-episode schizophrenic patients. Schizophr Res 5:197–198, 1991

Hogarty GE: Depot neuroleptics: the relevance of psychosocial factors—a United States perspective. J Clin Psychiatry 45:36–42, 1984

Hollister JM, Laing P, Mednick SA: Rhesus incompatibility as a risk factor for schizophrenia in male adults. Arch Gen Psychiatry 53:19–24, 1996

Holzman PS, Soloman CM, Levin S, et al: Pursuit eye movement dysfunctions in schizophrenia: family evidence for specificity. Arch Gen Psychiatry 41:136–139, 1984

Holzman PS, Kringlen E, Matthysse S, et al: A single dominant gene can account for eye tracking dysfunction and schizophrenia in offspring of discordant twins. Arch Gen Psychiatry 45:641–647, 1988

Hughlings-Jackson J: Selected Writings. London, UK, Hodder & Stoughton, 1931

Hyde TM, Nawroz S, Goldberg TE, et al: Is there a cognitive decline in schizophrenia? A cross-sectional study. Br J Psychiatry 164:494–500, 1994

Ingvar DH, Franzen G: Abnormalities of cerebral blood flow distribution in patients with chronic schizophrenia. Acta Psychiatr Scand 50:425–462, 1974

Jablensky A, Sartorius N: Culture and schizophrenia. Psychol Med 5:113–124, 1975

Jablensky A, Sartorius N, Ernberg G, et al: Schizophrenia: manifestation, incidence, and course, in Different Cultures: A World Health Organization Ten-Country Study—Psychological Medicine Monograph Supplement 20. Cambridge, UK, Cambridge University Press, 1992

Javitt DC, Zukin SR: Recent advances in the phencyclidine model of schizophrenia. Am J Psychiatry 148:1301–1308, 1991

Johns CA, Thompson JW: Adjunctive treatments in schizophrenia: pharmacotherapies and electroconvulsive therapy. Schizophr Bull 21:607–619, 1995

Johnstone EC, Crow TJ, Frith CD, et al: Cerebral ventricular size and cognitive impairment in chronic schizophrenia. Lancet 2:924–926, 1976

Jonsson H, Nyman AK: Prediction of outcome in schizophrenia. Acta Psychiatr Scand 69:274–291, 1984

Jorgensen P: Course and outcome in dimensional disorders. Psychopathology 27:79–88, 1994

Judd LL, McAdams LA, Budnick B, et al: Sensory gating deficits in schizophrenia: new results. Am J Psychiatry 149:448–493, 1992

Kallman FJ: The Genetics of Schizophrenia. New York, Augustin, 1938

Kanas N: Inpatient and outpatient group therapy for schizophrenic patients. Am J Psychother 39:431–439, 1985

Kane JM: Antipsychotic drug side effects: their relationship to dose. J Clin Psychiatry 46:16–21, 1985

Kane JM, Marder SR: Psychopharmacologic treatment of schizophrenia. Schizophr Bull 19:287–302, 1993

Kane JM, Honigfeld G, Singer J, et al: Clozapine for the treatment-resistant schizophrenic: a double-blind comparison with chlorpromazine. Arch Gen Psychiatry 45:789–796, 1988

Kane JM, Rifkin A, Woerner M, et al: Low-dose neuroleptic treatment of outpatient schizophrenics I: preliminary results for relapse rates. Arch Gen Psychiatry 40:893–896, 1983

Keilp TG, Sweeney JA, Jacobsen P, et al: Cognitive impairment in schizophrenia: specific relations to ventricular size and negative symptomatology. Biol Psychiatry 24:47–55, 1988

Kendler KS: The nosological validity of paranoia (simple delusional disorder): a review. Arch Gen Psychiatry 37:699–706, 1980

Kendler KS: Demography of paranoid psychosis (delusional disorder): a review and comparison with schizophrenia and affective illness. Arch Gen Psychiatry 39:890–902, 1982

Kendler KS: Kraepelin and the diagnostic concept of paranoia. Compr Psychiatry 29:4–11, 1988

Kendler KS, Gruenberg AM: An independent analysis of the Danish Adoption Study of Schizophrenia VI: the relationship between psychiatric disorders as defined by DSM-III in the relatives and adoptees. Arch Gen Psychiatry 41:555–564, 1984

Kendler KS, Gruenberg AM, Strauss JS: An independent analysis of the Copenhagen sample of the Danish Adoption Study of Schizophrenia III: the relationship between paranoid psychosis (delusional disorder) and the schizophrenia spectrum disorders. Arch Gen Psychiatry 38:985–987, 1982

Kendler KS, Gruenberg AM, Tsuang MT: Outcome of schizophrenic subtypes defined by four diagnostic systems. Arch Gen Psychiatry 41:149–154, 1984

Kendler KS, Gruenberg AM, Tsuang MT: Subtype stability in schizophrenia. Am J Psychiatry 142:827–832, 1985a

Kendler KS, Masterson CC, Davis KL: Psychiatric illness in first-degree relatives of patients with paranoid psychosis, schizophrenia, and medical illness. Br J Psychiatry 147:524–531, 1985b

Kendler KS, Gruenberg AM, Tsuang MT: A family study of the subtypes of schizophrenia. Am J Psychiatry 145:57–62, 1988

Kendler KS, McGuire M, Gruenberg AM, Walsh D: Outcome and family study of the subtypes of schizophrenia in the west of Ireland. Am J Psychiatry 151:849–856, 1994a

Kendler KS, McGuire M, Gruenberg AM, Walsh D: An epidemiologic, clinical, and family study of simple schizophrenia in County Roscommon, Ireland. Am J Psychiatry 151:27–34, 1994b

Kendler KS, Karkowski-Shuman L, Walsh D: Age at onset in schizophrenia and risk of illness in relatives—results from the Roscommon Family Study. Br J Psychiatry 169:213–218, 1996

Kennedy HG, Kemp LI, Dyer DE: Fear and anger in delusional (paranoid) disorder: the association with violence. Br J Psychiatry 160:488–492, 1992

Kessler R, McGonagle K, Zhao S, et al: Lifetime and 12-month prevalence of DSM-III-R psychiatric disorders in the United States: results from the National Comorbidity Study. Arch Gen Psychiatry 51:8–19, 1994

Kety SS, Rosenthal D, Wender PH, et al: Mental illness in the biologic and adoptive families of adopted individuals who have become schizophrenic: a preliminary report based on psychiatric interviews, in Genetic Research in Psychiatry. Edited by Fieve R, Rosenthal D, Brill H. Baltimore, MD, Johns Hopkins Press, 1975, pp 147–165

King DJ, Burke M, Lucas RA: Antipsychotic drug-induced dysphoria. Br J Psychiatry 167:480–482, 1995

Kingsbury SJ, Salzman C: Disulfiram in the treatment of alcoholic patients with schizophrenia. Hospital and Community Psychiatry 41:133–134, 1990

Kissling W (ed): Guidelines for Neuroleptic Relapse Prevention in Schizophrenia. Berlin, Springer-Verlag, 1991

Kovelman JA, Scheibel AB: A neurohistological correlate of schizophrenia. Biol Psychiatry 19:1601–1621, 1984

Kraepelin E: Dementia Praecox and Paraphrenia. Translated by Barkley RM. Edinburgh, E & S Livingstone, 1919

Krakowski MI, Convit A, Jaeger J, et al: Neurologic impairment in violent schizophrenic inpatients. Am J Psychiatry 146:849–853, 1989

Lamb HR: Some reflections on treating schizophrenics. Arch Gen Psychiatry 43:1007–1011, 1986

Lamb HR: Lessons learned from deinstitutionalization in the United States. Br J Psychiatry 162:587–592, 1993

Lamberti JS, Tariot PN: Schizophrenia in nursing home patients. Psychiatric Annals 25:441–448, 1995

Langfeldt G: Schizophreniform States. Copenhagen, E Munksguard, 1939

Lehman AF: Vocational rehabilitation in schizophrenia. Schizophr Bull 21:645–656, 1995

Lehmann HE, Wilson H, Deutsch M: Minimal maintenance medication: effect of three dose schedules on relapse rates and symptoms in chronic schizophrenic outpatients. Compr Psychiatry 24:293–303, 1983

Levinson DF, Simpson GM, Lo ES, et al: Fluphenazine plasma levels, dosage, efficacy, and side effects. Am J Psychiatry 152:765–771, 1995

Lewine R, Burbach D, Melzer HY: Effect of diagnostic criteria on the ratio of male to female schizophrenic patients. Am J Psychiatry 141:84–87, 1984

Lewis A: Paranoia and paranoid: a historical perspective. Psychol Med 1:2–12, 1970

Lewis SW, Mezey GC: Clinical correlates of septum pellucidum cavities: an unusual association with psychosis. Psychol Med 15:43–54, 1985

Liddle PF, Barnes TRE, Morris D, et al: Three symptoms in chronic schizophrenia. Br J Psychiatry 7:119–122, 1989

Liddle PF, Friston KJ, Frith CD, et al: Patterns of cerebral blood flow in schizophrenia. Br J Psychiatry 60:179–186, 1992

Lieberman JA, Kane JM, Sarantakos S, et al: Prediction of relapse in schizophrenia. Arch Gen Psychiatry 44:592–603, 1987

Lim KO, Tew W, Kushner M, et al: Cortical gray matter volume deficit in patients with first-episode schizophrenia. Am J Psychiatry 153:1548–1553, 1996

Linszen DH, Dingemans PM, Lenior ME: Cannabis abuse and the course of recent-onset schizophrenic disorders. Arch Gen Psychiatry 51:273–279, 1994

Lipinsky JF, Zubenko G, Cohen BM, et al: Propranolol in the treatment of neuroleptic-induced akathisia. Am J Psychiatry 141:412–415, 1984

Loranger AW: Sex difference in age at onset of schizophrenia. Arch Gen Psychiatry 41:157–161, 1984

Lyketsos GC, Sakka P, Mailis A: The sexual adjustment of chronic schizophrenics: a preliminary study. Br J Psychiatry 143:376–382, 1983

Mackota G, Lamb HR: Vocational rehabilitation. Psychiatric Annals 19:548–552, 1989

Magrinat G, Danziger JA, Lorenzo IC, et al: A reassessment of catatonia. Compr Psychiatry 24:218–228, 1983

Malzberg B: Mental disease among foreign-born in Canada, 1950–1952, in relation to period of immigration. Am J Psychiatry 120:971–973, 1964

Manschreck TC, Maher BA, Rucklos ME, et al: Disturbed voluntary motor activity in schizophrenic disorder. Psychol Med 12:73–84, 1982

Manschreck TC: Delusional disorder: the recognition and management of paranoia. J Clin Psychiatry 57 (suppl 3):32–38, 1996

Marder SR, Meibach RC: Risperidone in the treatment of schizophrenia. Am J Psychiatry 151:825–835, 1994

Marder SR, Wirshing WC, Mintz J, et al: Two-year outcome of social skills training and group psychotherapy for outpatients with schizophrenia. Am J Psychiatry 153:1585–1592, 1996

Maxmen JS: Delivery of After Care Services in Management of Chronic Schizophrenia. Edited by Caton CLM. New York, Oxford University Press, 1984

McAllister CG, Rapaport MH, Pickar D, et al: Increased number of CD5$^+$ B lymphocytes in schizophrenic patients. Arch Gen Psychiatry 46:890–894, 1989

McCabe MS, Fowler RC, Cadoret RJ, et al: Symptom differences in schizophrenics with good and poor prognosis. Am J Psychiatry 128:1239–1243, 1972

McEvoy JP, Hogarty GE, Steingard S: Optimal dose of neuroleptic in acute schizophrenia. Arch Gen Psychiatry 48:734–745, 1991

McFarlane WR, Lukens E, Link B, et al: Multiple family groups and psychoeducation in the treatment of schizophrenia. Arch Gen Psychiatry 52:679–687, 1995

McGhie A, Chapman J: Disorders of attention and perception in early schizophrenia. Br J Med Psychol 34:103–116, 1961

McGlashan TH: The Chestnut Lodge Follow-Up Study II: long-term outcome of schizophrenia and the affective disorders. Arch Gen Psychiatry 41:586–601, 1984

McGlashan TH: The prediction of outcome in chronic schizophrenia IV: the Chestnut Lodge Follow-Up Study. Arch Gen Psychiatry 43:167–176, 1986

McGuire PK, Frith CD: Disordered functional connectivity in schizophrenia. Psychol Med 26:663–667, 1996

McGuire PK, Silbersweig DA, Murray RM, et al: Functional anatomy of inner speech and auditory verbal imagery. Psychol Med 26:29–38, 1996a

McGuire PK, Silbersweig DA, Wright I, et al: The neural correlates of inner speech and auditory verbal imagery in schizophrenia: relationship to auditory verbal hallucinations. Br J Psychiatry 169:148–159, 1996b

McNeil T, Kaij L: Obstetric factors in the development of schizophrenia: complications in the births of three schizophrenics and in reproduction by schizophrenic patients, in The Nature of Schizophrenia: New Approaches to Research and Treatment. Edited by Wynn LC, Cromwell RL, Matthysse S. New York, Wiley, 1978, pp 401–429

Mednick SA, Machon RA, Hultunen MO, et al: Adult schizophrenia following prenatal exposure to an influenza epidemic. Arch Gen Psychiatry 45:189–192, 1988

Meltzer HY: Biological studies in schizophrenia. Schizophr Bull 13:77–100, 1987

Modestin T, Ammann R: Mental disorders and criminality: male schizophrenia. Schizophr Bull 22:69–82, 1996

Mueser KT, Berenbaum H: Psychodynamic treatment of schizophrenia: is there a future? Psychol Med 20:253–262, 1990

Mukherjee S, Shukla S, Woodle J, et al: Misdiagnosis of schizophrenia in bipolar patients: a multiethnic comparison. Am J Psychiatry 140:1571–1574, 1983

Munro A: Psychiatric disorders characterized by delusions: treatment in relation to specific types. Psychiatric Annals 22:232–240, 1992

Murphy HBM: Migration, culture and mental health. Psychol Med 7:677–684, 1977

Murphy HBM, Raman AC: The chronicity of schizophrenia in indigenous tropical people: results of a twelve-year follow-up survey in Mauritius. Br J Psychiatry 118:489–497, 1971

Ndetei DM, Vadher A: A comparative cross-cultural study of the frequencies of hallucinations in schizophrenia. Acta Psychiatr Scand 70:545–549, 1984

Neylan TC, van Kammen DP, Kelley ME, et al: Sleep in schizophrenic patients on and off haloperidol therapy: clinically stable versus relapsed patients. Arch Gen Psychiatry 49:643–649, 1992

Nopoulos P, Torres I, Flaum M, et al: Brain morphology in first-episode schizophrenia. Am J Psychiatry 152:1721–1723, 1995a

Nopoulos PC, Flaum M, Andreasen NC, et al: Gray matter heterotopias in schizophrenia. Psychiatry Res: Neuroimaging 61:11–14, 1995b

Nopoulos P, Swayze V, Andreasen NC: Pattern of brain morphology in patients with schizophrenia and large cavum septi pellucidi. J Neuropsychiatry Clin Neurosci 8:147–152, 1996

Nopoulos P, Swayze V, Flaum M: Cavum septi pellucidi in normals and patients with schizophrenia as detected by MRI. Biol Psychiatry 41:1102–1108, 1997

O'Callaghan E, Larkin C, Kinsella A, et al: Familial, obstetric, and other clinical correlates of minor physical anomalies in schizophrenia. Am J Psychiatry 148:479–483, 1991

Olney JW, Farber NB: Glutamate receptor dysfunction and schizophrenia. Arch Gen Psychiatry 52:998–1007, 1995

Opjordsmoen S: Delusional disorders I: comparative long-term outcome. Acta Psychiatr Scand 80:603–612, 1989

Pakkenberg B: Pronounced reduction of total neuron number in mediodorsal thalamic nucleus and nucleus accumens in schizophrenics. Arch Gen Psychiatry 47:1023–1028, 1990

Pearlson GD, Garbacz DJ, Moberg PJ, et al: Symptomatic, familial, perinatal, and social correlates of computerized axial tomography (CAT) changes in schizophrenics and bipolars. J Nerv Ment Dis 173:42–50, 1985

Peet M, Middlemiss DN, Yates RA: Propranolol in schizophrenia II: clinical and biochemical aspects of combining propranolol with chlorpromazine. Br J Psychiatry 139:112–117, 1981

Penn DL, Mueser KT: Research update on the psychosocial treatment of schizophrenia. Am J Psychiatry 153:607–617, 1996

Perry JC, Jacobs D: Overview: clinical applications of the Amytal interview in psychiatric emergency settings. Am J Psychiatry 139:552–559, 1982

Perry PJ, Smith DA: Neuroleptic plasma concentrations: an estimate of their sensitivity and specificity as predictors of response, in Clinical Use of Neuroleptic Plasma Levels. Edited by Marder SR, Davis JM, Janicak PG. Washington, DC, American Psychiatric Press, 1993, pp 113–135

Petronis A, Kennedy JL: Unstable genes—unstable mind? Am J Psychiatry 152:164–172, 1995

Pfohl B, Winokur G: The micropsychopathology of hebephrenic/catatonic schizophrenia. J Nerv Ment Dis 171:296–300, 1983

Rice JP, McGuffin P: Genetic Etiology of Schizophrenia and Affective Disorders in Psychiatry, Vol 1. Edited by Michels R, Cavenar JO. Philadelphia, PA, JB Lippincott, 1985

Rifkin A, Doddi S, Karajgi B, et al: Dosage of haloperidol for schizophrenia. Arch Gen Psychiatry 48:166–170, 1991

Robins LN, Helzer JE, Weissman MM, et al: Lifetime prevalence of specific psychiatric disorders in three sites. Arch Gen Psychiatry 41:949–958, 1984

Ross DE, Thaker GK, Buchanan RW, et al: Association of abnormal smooth pursuit eye movements with the deficit syndrome in schizophrenic patients. Am J Psychiatry 153:1158–1165, 1996

Roy A: Suicide in chronic schizophrenia. Br J Psychiatry 141:171–177, 1982

Rudin E: Studien uber Vererbung und Entstehung geistiger storungen I: Zur vererbung und Neuenstehung der Dementia Praecox. Berlin, Springer-Verlag, 1916

Sartorius N, Jablensky A, Korten A: Early manifestations and first contact incidence of schizophrenia in different cultures: a preliminary report on the evaluation of the WHO Collaborative Study in Determinants of Outcome of Severe Mental Disorders. Psychol Med 16:909–928, 1986

Schlaepfer TE, Harris GJ, Tien AY, et al: Diseased regional cortical gray matter volume in schiozphrenia. Am J Psychiatry 151:842–848, 1994

Schooler NR, Kane JM, Marder SR, et al: Efficacy of clozapine vs. haloperidol in a long-term clinical trial: preliminary findings (abstract). Schizophr Bull 15:165, 1995

Schwab SG, Albus M, Hallmayer J, et al: Evaluation of a susceptibility gene for schizophrenia on chromosome 6p by multipoint affected sib-pair linkage analysis. Nature Genetics 11:325–327, 1995

Seeman P, Lee T, Chau-Wong M, et al: Antipsychotic drug doses and neuroleptic-dopamine receptors. Nature 261:717–719, 1976

Segal JH: Erotomania revisited: from Kraepelin to DSM-III-R. Am J Psychiatry 146:1261–1266, 1989

Selemon LD, Rajkowska G, Goldman-Rakic S: Abnormally high neuronal density in the schizophrenic cortex. Arch Gen Psychiatry 52:805–818, 1995

Shapiro S, Skinner EA, Kessler LG, et al: Utilization of health and mental health services: three Epidemiologic Catchment Area sites. Arch Gen Psychiatry 41:971–978, 1984

Shenton ME, Kikinis R, Jolesz FA, et al: Abnormalities of the left temporal lobe and thought disorder in schizophrenia: a quantitative magnetic resonance imaging study. N Eng J Med 327:604–612, 1992

Shenton ME, Wible CG, McCarley RW: A review of magnetic resonance imaging studies of brain anomalies in schizophrenia, in Brain Imaging in Clinical Psychiatry. Edited by Krishnan KRR, Doraiswamy PM. New York, Marcel Dekker, 1997, pp 297–380

Silbersweig DA, Stern E, Frith C, et al: A functional neuroanatomy of hallucinations in schizophrenia. Nature 378:176–179, 1995

Silverton L, Mednick S: Class drift and schizophrenia. Acta Psychiatr Scand 70:304–309, 1984

Simpson JC, Tsuang MT: Mortality among patients with schizophrenia. Schizophr Bull 22:485–499, 1996

Siris SG, Morgan V, Fagerstrom R, et al: Adjunctive imipramine in the treatment of postpsychotic depression: a controlled trial. Arch Gen Psychiatry 44:533–539, 1987

Siris SG, Bermanzohn PC, Mason SE, et al: Maintenance imipramine therapy for secondary depression in schizophrenia: a controlled trial. Arch Gen Psychiatry 51:109–115, 1994

Slaby AE, Moreines R: Emergency room evaluation and management of schizophrenia, in Handbook of Schizophrenia, Vol 4: Psychosocial Treatment of Schizophrenia. Edited by Herz MI, Keith SJ, Docherty JP. New York, Elsevier, 1990, pp 247–268

Slater E: The monogenetic theory of schizophrenia. Acta Genet Med Gemellol 8:50–56, 1958

Snyder SH: Catecholamines in the brain as mediators of amphetamine psychosis. Arch Gen Psychiatry 27:169–179, 1972

Snyder SH: The dopamine hypothesis in schizophrenia: focus on the dopamine receptor. Am J Psychiatry 133:197–202, 1976

Spitzer RL, Endicott J, Robins E: Research diagnostic criteria: rationale and reliability. Arch Gen Psychiatry 35:773–782, 1978

Stein L: A system approach to reducing relapse in schizophrenia. J Clin Psychiatry 54 (suppl 3):7–12, 1993

Storey PB: Lumbar air encephalography in chronic schizophrenia: a controlled experiment. Br J Psychiatry 112:135–144, 1966

Stoudemire A: A differential diagnosis of catatonic states. Psychosomatics 23:245–251, 1982

Strakowski SM: Diagnostic validity of schizophreniform disorder. Am J Psychiatry 151:815–824, 1994

Strauss JS, Carpenter WJ: Schizophrenia. New York, Plenum Press, 1981

Suddath RC, Christison GW, Torrey EF, et al: Anatomical abnormalities in the brains of monozygotic twins discordant for schizophrenia. N Eng J Med 322:789–794, 1990

Susser E, Struening EL, Conover S: Psychiatric problems in homeless men: lifetime psychosis, substance use, and current disorders in new arrivals at New York City shelters. Arch Gen Psychiatry 46:845–850, 1989

Susser E, Neugebauer R, Hoek H, et al: Schizophrenia after premorbid famine: further evidence. Arch Gen Psychiatry 53:25–31, 1996

Swanson JW, Holtzer CE, Ganju VK, et al: Violence and psychiatric disorder in the community: evidence from the Epidemiology Catchment Area Surveys. Hospital and Community Psychiatry 41:761–770, 1990

Swayze VW, Andreasen NC, Ehrhardt JC, et al: Developmental abnormalities of the corpus callosum in schizophrenia. Arch Neurol 47:805–808, 1990

Swerdlow NR, Geyer MA: Clozapine and haloperidol in an animal model of sensorimotor gating deficits in schizophrenia. Pharmacol Biochem Behav 44:741–744, 1993

Tanna VL: Paranoid states: a selected review. Compr Psychiatry 15:453–470, 1974

Targum SD: Neuroendocrine dysfunction in schizophreniform disorder: correlation with 6-month clinical outcome. Am J Psychiatry 140:309–313, 1983

Tarrier N, Beckett R, Harwood S, et al: A trial of two cognitive-behavioral methods of treating drug-resistant residual psychotic symptoms in schizophrenic patients, I: outcome. Br J Psychiatry 162:524–532, 1993

Taube CA, Barrett SA (eds): Mental Health United States 1985 (DHHS Publ No ADM 85–1378). Rockville, MD, National Institute of Mental Health, 1985

Teplin LA: The criminality of the mentally ill: a dangerous misconception. Am J Psychiatry 142:593–599, 1985

Thacker GK, Cassady S, Adami H, et al: Eye movements in spectrum personality disorders: comparison of community subjects and relatives of schizophrenic patients. Am J Psychiatry 153:362–368, 1996

Thompson C: The use of high-dose antipsychotic medication. Br J Psychiatry 164:448–458, 1994

Tienari P: Psychiatric illness in identical twins. Acta Psychiatr Scand Suppl, No 171, 1963

Tienari P: Implications of adoption studies in schizophrenia. Br J Psychiatry 151 (suppl 18):52–58, 1992

Tsuang MT: Suicide in schizophrenics, manics, depressives, and surgical controls: a comparison with general population suicide mortality. Arch Gen Psychiatry 35:153–155, 1978

Tsuang MT, Winokur G: Criteria for subtyping schizophrenia: clinical differentiation of hebephrenic and paranoid schizophrenia. Arch Gen Psychiatry 31:43–47, 1974

Tsuang MT, Woolson RF, Fleming JA: Long-term outcome of major psychoses I: schizophrenia and affective disorders compared with psychiatrically symptom-free surgical conditions. Arch Gen Psychiatry 36:1295–1304, 1979

Turner SW, Toone BK, Brett-Jones JR: Computerized tomographic scan change in early schizophrenia. Psychol Med 16:209–225, 1986

Vaillant GE: Prospective prediction of schizophrenic remission. Arch Gen Psychiatry 11:509–518, 1964

Vallada HP, Kunugi H: An overview of schizophrenia genetic research presented at the 1995 World Congress on Psychiatric Genetics, Cardiff. Schizophr Res 19:87–92, 1996

VanderZwaag C, McGee M, McEvoy JP, et al: Response of patients with treatment-refractory schizophrenia to clozapine with three serum level ranges. Am J Psychiatry 153:1579–1584, 1996

VanKammen DP, Peters J, Yao J, et al: Norepinephrine in acute exacerbations of chronic schizophrenia: negative symptoms revisited. Arch Gen Psychiatry 47:161–168, 1990

Von Korff M, Nestadt G, Romanoski A, et al: Prevalence of treated and untreated DSM III schizophrenia: results of a two-stage community survey. J Nerv Ment Dis 173:577–581, 1985

Waldo M, Cawthra E, Adler L, et al: Auditory sensory gating, hippocampal volume, and catecholamine metabolism in schizophrenics and their siblings. Schizophr Res 12:93–106, 1994

Wang ZW, Black D, Andreasen N C, Crowe RR: A linkage study of chromosome 11q in schizophrenia. Arch Gen Psychiatry 50:212–216, 1993

Ward KE, Friedman L, Wise A, et al: Meta-analysis of brain and cranial size in schizophrenia. Schizophr Res 22:197–123, 1996

Watt DC, Katz K, Shepard M: The natural history of schizophrenia: a five-year prospective follow-up of a representative sample of schizophrenics by means of a standardized clinical and social assessment. Psychol Med 13:663–670, 1983

Watt JAG: The relationship of paranoid states to schizophrenia. Am J Psychiatry 142:1456–1458, 1985

Weiden PJ, Dixon L, Frances A, et al: Neuroleptic noncompliance in schizophrenia, in Advances in Neuropsychiatry and Psychopharmacology, Vol 1: Schizophrenia Research. Edited by Tamminga CA, Schulz SC. New York, Raven Press, 1991, pp 285–296

Weinberger DR: Implications of normal brain development for the pathogenesis of schizophrenia. Arch Gen Psychiatry 44:660–669, 1987

Weinberger DR, Torrey EF, Neophytides AN, et al: Lateral cerebral ventricle enlargement in chronic schizophrenia. Arch Gen Psychiatry 36:735–755, 1979

Weinberger DR, Bigelow LB, Kleinman JE, et al: Cerebral ventricular enlargement in chronic schizophrenia: an association with poor response to treatment. Arch Gen Psychiatry 37:11–13, 1980

Weinberger DR, Berman KF, Zec RF: Physiologic dysfunction of dorsolateral prefrontal cortex in schizophrenia I: regional cerebral blood flow evidence. Arch Gen Psychiatry 43:114–124, 1986

Wender PH, Rosenthal D, Kety SS, et al: Social class and psychopathology in adoptees: a natural experimental method for separating the roles of genetic and experimental factors. Arch Gen Psychiatry 28:318–325, 1973

Wible CG, Shenton ME, Hokama H: Prefrontal cortex and schizophrenia: a quantitative magnetic resonance imaging study. Arch Gen Psychiatry 52:279–288, 1995

Wing JK, Birley JLT, Cooper JE, et al: Reliability of a procedure for measuring and classifying "present psychiatric state." Br J Psychiatry 113:499–515, 1967

Winokur G: Delusional disorder (paranoia). Compr Psychiatry 18:511–521, 1977

Winokur G: Familial psychopathology in delusional disorder. Compr Psychiatry 26:241–248, 1985

Winokur G, Tsuang MT: The Natural History of Mania, Depression, and Schizophrenia. Washington, DC, American Psychiatric Press, 1996

Winokur G, Morrison J, Clancy J, et al: Iowa 500: the clinical and genetic distinction of hebephrenic and paranoid schizophrenia. J Nerv Ment Dis 159:12–19, 1974

Wolkowitz OM, Pickar D: Benzodiazepines in the treatment of schizophrenia: a review and reappraisal. Am J Psychiatry 148:714–726, 1991

Wong DF, Wagner HN, Tune LE, et al: Positron emission tomography reveals elevated D_2 dopamine receptors in drug-naive schizophrenics. Science 234:1558–1563, 1986

World Health Organization: International Statistical Classification of Diseases and Related Health Problems, 10th Revision (ICD-10). Geneva, World Health Organization, 1992

World Health Organization: Schizophrenia: The International Pilot Study of Schizophrenia, Vol 1. Geneva, World Health Organization, 1975

Wright P, Takai N, Rifkin L, et al: Maternal influenza, obstetrical complications, and schizophrenia. Am J Psychiatry 152:1714–1720, 1995

Wyatt RJ, Henter I, Leary MC, et al: An economic evaluation of schizophrenia 1991. Soc Psychiatry Psychiatr Epidemiol 30:196–205, 1995

Yalom ID: Inpatient Group Psychotherapy. New York, Basic Books, 1983

Ziedonis DM, Fisher W: Assessment and treatment of comorbid substance abuse in individuals with schizophrenia. Psychiatric Annals 24:477–483, 1994

Zipursky RB, Lim KO, DeMent S: Volumetric MRI assessment of temporal lobe structures in schizophrenia. Biol Psychiatry 35:501–516, 1994

CHAPTER 13

MOOD DISORDERS

STEVEN L. DUBOVSKY, M.D.
RANDALL BUZAN, M.D.

One knows not whether there can be human compassion for anemia of the soul. When the pitch of life is dropped and the spirit is so put over and reversed that only is horrible which before was sweet and worldly and of the day, the human relation disappears.

—Oliver Onions

Mood disorders can be relatively straightforward, or they can assume complex forms that can be difficult to treat. In this chapter, we review the epidemiology, diagnosis, comorbidity, and treatment of the wide variety of affective syndromes that are encountered in psychiatric practice.

EPIDEMIOLOGY

Estimates of the incidence and prevalence of mood disorders vary. In the United States, the lifetime risk of a major depressive episode is said to be around 6%, and the lifetime risk of any mood disorder is said to be around 8% (Cassem 1995; Kashani and Nair 1995). The prevalence of major depression ranges from 2.6% to 5.5% in men and from 6.0% to 11.8% in women (Fava and Davidson 1996). The prevalence of dysthymia is 3%–4% (Keller et al. 1996). Some reports suggest that as much as 48% of the United States population has had one or more lifetime mood episodes (Cassem 1995). Most studies have found unipolar depression in general to be twice as common in women as in men (Reynolds et al. 1990). The meaning of the gender difference remains to be clarified. Gender does not appear to affect the prevalence of bipolar disorder (Reynolds et al. 1990). The incidence of major depression is higher in separated or divorced people than in married individuals, especially men, and in medically ill patients (Lehtinen and Joukamaa 1994; Reiger et al. 1988), and depression is associated with greater use of general health services

(Weissman et al. 1988b). The prevalence of major depression in primary care practice is 4.8%–9.2%, and the prevalence of all depressive disorders is 9%–20%, which makes mood disorders the most common psychiatric problems in primary care (McDaniel et al. 1995).

The effects of culture and stress on the prevalence of depression were illustrated by the Cross-National Collaborative Group study of 10 countries, which used the Diagnostic Interview Schedule to make DSM-III (American Psychiatric Association 1980) diagnoses (Weissman et al. 1996). In this study, the lifetime rate for major depression varied from a low of 1.5 cases/100 adults in Taiwan to as many as 19.0/100 in Beirut, and the annual rate of depression was as low as 0.8 cases/100 in Taiwan and as high as 5.8/100 in New Zealand.

The prevalence of bipolar disorder is generally reported as being between 1% and 2.5% (Akiskal 1995b; Angst 1995; Bebbington 1995; Kashani and Nair 1995); however, some studies suggest rates for bipolar mood disorders of 3%–6.5% (Akiskal 1995b; Angst 1995). The frequency with which bipolar disorder is diagnosed probably depends on how it is defined; broader definitions produce significantly higher rates (Akiskal 1995b; Angst 1995). Most prevalence studies require the presence of mania for a bipolar diagnosis to be recorded, but the bipolar II variant, which is characterized by episodes of hypomania but not mania, is more common than the bipolar I variant (Cassano et al. 1989; Simpson et al. 1993). If bipolar spectrum disorders (Akiskal 1995b), or subsyndromal and complex forms of bipolar disorder (discussed later in this chapter), are also considered, the incidence of bipolar mood disorder is substantially higher. Roughly 10%–15% of patients with a diagnosis of unipolar depression will eventually receive a revised diagnosis of bipolar disorder (Olie et al. 1992).

When conservative criteria are used, between 5% and 15% of cases of adult depression are found to be bipolar (Bebbington 1995; Geller et al. 1996). Akiskal's group (Cassano et al. 1989) found that one-third of patients with primary depression met their criteria for bipolar spectrum disorders. The risk of bipolarity is higher in juvenile major depression—at least 20% in adolescents and 32% in children ages less than 11 years (Geller et al. 1996). The lifetime rate of bipolar disorder is relatively consistent across cultures, ranging from 0.3/100 in Taiwan to 1.5/100 in New Zealand (Weissman et al. 1996).

In all industrialized countries in the world, the incidence of depression, mania, suicide, and psychotic mood disorders has been increasing in every generation born after 1910 (Cross-National Collaborative Group 1992; Klerman 1988; Klerman et al. 1985). For unknown reasons, there was an abrupt jump in the rate of increase for people born after 1940—a true increase in the incidence of mood disorders (cohort effect) and not a function of better recognition (Cross-National Collaborative Group 1992; Klerman 1988; Klerman et al. 1985). Not only are mood disorders becoming more common, but they are appearing at an earlier age (especially bipolar mood disorders) (Lasch and Weissman 1990).

Suicide is an obvious public health problem that complicates mood disorders more frequently than other conditions. The lifetime risk of suicide in mood disorders is 10%–15% (Barklage 1991; Guze and Robbins 1970; Mueller and Leon 1996), and the risk of attempted suicide was increased 41-fold in depressed patients compared with those with other diagnoses in the Epidemiologic Catchment Area survey (Petronis et al. 1990). It is well known that women attempt suicide more frequently than men, but men are more likely to succeed. In one study, however, the excess risk of completed suicide in men was entirely accounted for by a higher prevalence of substance abuse in men and a greater likelihood that women have primary responsibility for children under age 18 (Young et al. 1994). The risk of suicide is high in mania as well as in depression. Patients with mixed bipolar states characterized by a combination of depression, rage, and grandiosity may be more likely to involve others in a suicide attempt—for example, through gunfights with the police. As many as 4% of people who commit suicide murder someone else first.

Although many clinicians agree on factors that increase the risk of suicide, formal attempts to predict suicide have been disappointing (Oxley and Van Meter 1996). This is not surprising; suicide is such a rare event (in the United States, the rate is about 11/100,000) that a prohibitively large number of patients would have to be followed prospectively to demonstrate that a constellation of features predicted an increased risk. In addition, no consensus exists about how long to follow a depressed patient before a conclusion can be made that suicide will not occur. There may be a statistically significant association between suicide and traditional risk factors such as older age, recent loss, male sex, bipolar depression, psychosis, comorbid substance abuse, history of a suicide attempt (especially if it was dangerous), and family history of suicide, but this association is not necessarily helpful in predicting suicide in an individual patient.

Despite the demonstrated inability of mental health professionals to predict (or prevent) suicide in any systematic manner (H. L. Miller et al. 1984), patients, families, and courts expect them to be able to do so. In an evaluation of immediate suicide risk, factors summarized in Table 13–1 can be considered (Oxley and Van Meter 1996; Pokorny 1993; Young et al. 1994). However, these factors

TABLE 13–1. **Factors suggesting an increased risk of suicide**

Demographic factors
    Male sex
    Recent loss
    Never married
    Older age
Symptoms
    Severe depression
    Anxiety
    Hopelessness
    Psychosis, especially with command hallucinations
History
    History of suicide attempts, especially if multiple or severe attempts
    Family history of suicide
    Active substance abuse
Suicidal thinking
    Presence of a specific plan
    Means available to carry out the plan
    Absence of factors that would keep the patient from completing the plan
    Rehearsal of the plan

at best suggest increased immediate risk. In addition, it is not known whether one risk factor is more important than another or how risk factors may interact with each other (Oxley and Van Meter 1996). Given the current state of knowledge, it is probably impossible for anyone to predict with any accuracy the long-term risk of completed suicide.

MOOD DISORDERS IN SPECIAL POPULATIONS

Postpartum depression occurs in about 10% of mothers; risk factors include a history of a mood disorder, unwanted pregnancy, unemployment of the mother, lack of breast-feeding, and the mother as head of the household (J. Hopkins et al. 1984; Warner et al. 1996). Postpartum depression increases the chance of alcohol and illicit drug use in teenage mothers (Barnet et al. 1995). There is some evidence that depression in a mother adversely affects temperament (C. T. Beck 1996) and cognitive development (Hay and Kumar 1995) in the infant. Depressed mothers of preschoolers have more negative perceptions of and interactions with their children (Lang et al. 1996).

Estimates of the prevalence of major depression in elderly people range from 2%–4% in community samples to 12% of medically hospitalized patients to 16% of geriatric patients in long-term care (Blazer and Koenig 1996). Geri-

atric depression is associated with an increased likelihood of cerebrovascular disease and enlarged ventricles and may be more likely than depression in younger patients to be accompanied by prominent cognitive complaints (Soares and Mann 1997).

Major depressive disorder (MDD) is said to occur in as many as 18% of preadolescents, with no gender differences (Kashani and Nair 1995). However, mood disorders are often underdiagnosed in this population because many clinicians still do not believe that depression occurs in children and because depression may be more difficult to recognize in children than in older patients. Among adolescents, the prevalence of MDD has been reported to be 4.7% in 14- to 16-year-olds (Kashani and Nair 1995). By this age, depression is more common in girls than in boys (Kashani and Nair 1995). In nonclinical samples, up to one-third of adolescents reported some depressive symptoms (Kashani and Nair 1995). Major depression in adolescents is associated with substance abuse and antisocial behavior, both of which sometimes obscure the affective diagnosis (Kashani and Nair 1995). The lifetime prevalence of bipolar disorder was 0.6% in 150 adolescents who were not psychiatrically referred (Kashani and Nair 1995). As discussed later in this chapter, many cases of bipolar disorder in younger patients may be overlooked because many depressed children and adolescents have not yet had time to exhibit mania and because manic symptoms, when present, may be confused with behavior disorders and attention-deficit disorder.

ECONOMICS OF MOOD DISORDERS

Depression produces more impairment of physical functioning, role functioning, social functioning, and perceived current health, is associated with more bodily pain, and causes patients to spend more days in bed due to poor health than hypertension, diabetes, arthritis, and chronic pulmonary disease (Wells et al. 1989). In a study of general medical patients in a health maintenance organization, patients with depressed mood or anhedonia of 2 weeks' duration but with an insufficient number of additional symptoms to meet full criteria for MDD still had 7.7 times as much impairment of social, family, and work functioning as did patients without any depressive symptoms (Olfson 1996). The total cost of depressive disorders in the United States is generally estimated at $44 billion (Hall and Wise 1995). This is equivalent to the total cost of coronary heart disease, a condition that is no more prevalent and less readily treatable than depression. The direct costs of treating depression are about $12 billion, only $890 million of which is accounted for by the price of antidepressants (Hall and Wise 1995). Yet, tremendous effort is being expended by third-party reviewers to get physicians to prescribe cheaper antidepressants. The morbidity cost of depressive disorders in the United States is around $24 billion, and the mortality costs are $8 billion; these costs can be attributed in part to increased accident rates, substance abuse, development of somatic illness, and increased use of medical hospitalization and outpatient treatment (Hall and Wise 1995).

DIAGNOSIS

Attempts to classify depression date back to at least the fourth century B.C., when Hippocrates coined the terms *melancholia* (black bile), and *mania* (to be mad). The independent descriptions in 1854 by two French physicians, Falret and Baillarger, of *folie circulaire* and *la folie à double forme* were the first formal diagnoses of alternating episodes of mania and depression as a single disorder (Sedler 1983). At the beginning of the current century, Emil Kraepelin differentiated schizophrenia (dementia praecox) from "manic-depressive insanity" on the basis of a deteriorating course of the former and an episodic course of the latter (Akiskal 1996). Kraepelin (1921) believed that manic-depressive insanity was a single illness that included "periodic and circular insanity," mania, and melancholia. Many of Kraepelin's observations of the symptoms and course of mood disorders remain accurate, but manic-depressive (bipolar) disorder is now known to be a complex group of disorders that share features such as a high rate of recurrence and alternations of mood states but differ in other important respects.

In the United States, the first edition of DSM, *Diagnostic and Statistical Manual: Mental Disorders* (American Psychiatric Association 1952), reflected the influence of Adolph Meyer. Meyer believed that psychiatric disorders were reactions to conflict or stress that were more specific to the individual than to the illness. Psychotic mood disorders (e.g., psychotic depressive reaction) were diagnosed on the basis not of hallucinations and delusions but of severity and lack of a precipitant (American Psychiatric Association 1952). In DSM-II (American Psychiatric Association 1968), *involutional melancholia* and *manic-depressive psychosis* were added. The concept of a depressive reaction was maintained as *depressive neurosis*, which was considered a neurotic reaction to an internal conflict or external event. In the absence of a precipitant, a diagnosis of psychotic depressive reaction was made for a single episode and manic-depressive psychosis for recurrent depressive episodes, whether or not the patient met traditional criteria

for psychosis in use by most clinicians. Alternating depression and elation was called *cyclothymia*, which was classified with the personality disorders on the grounds that it was chronic and was not caused by a specific circumstance. In subsequent editions of DSM (discussed later in this chapter), mood disorder diagnoses are based on symptom clusters rather than the presence or absence of an identifiable precipitant, since the presence of a precipitant does not demonstrably affect the course or treatment response of mood disorders.

ENDOGENOUS AND REACTIVE DEPRESSION

The differentiation of depression according to whether a precipitant is present is derived from an early distinction between endogenous (vital or melancholic) and reactive depression. In its original use by German descriptive psychiatrists, the term *reactive* referred to a depressed patient's ability to react positively to interactions and events and thus implied the presence of milder symptomatology. As the term was translated into English, however, it came to mean depression that developed in reaction to some external stress, thus implying an association between mild depression and depression in response to stress. In DSM-II, this concept was conserved as *neurotic depressive reaction*. In later informal diagnostic schemes, milder forms of depression that are more responsive to the environment evolved into the concept of *hysteroid dysphoria*, which is a type of depression with atypical symptoms that occurs in a patient with interpersonal sensitivity and a characterological tendency to dramatize (Shea and Hirschfeld 1996). In DSM-III-R (American Psychiatric Association 1987) and DSM-IV (American Psychiatric Association 1994a), the term *atypical depression* (a modifier of a major depressive episode) is more or less equivalent to *hysteroid dysphoria* and the modern derivative of neurotic depression.

Atypical depression is distinguished by mood reactivity (i.e., the capacity to be cheered up temporarily by positive interactions or events) as well as by severe fatigue (leaden paralysis), sensitivity to rejection, self-pity, a reverse diurnal mood swing (depression is worse later in the day), and reverse vegetative symptoms (e.g., increased instead of decreased appetite and sleep) (M. T. Tsuang and Faraone 1996). About 15% of depressive episodes have atypical features. Atypical symptoms are more common in bipolar depression. As is discussed later, atypical depression appears to respond better to monoamine oxidase inhibitor (MAOI) antidepressants than to other antidepressants.

In contrast to reactive depression, the term *endogenous depression* referred in the German literature to depression that was unresponsive to the environment and in the American literature to depression with greater severity, more considerable guilt and loss of interest, typical vegetative symptoms such as decreased appetite and sleep, and other physical symptoms such as difficulty concentrating, early morning awakening, and a diurnal mood swing (depression is worse in the morning) (M. T. Tsuang and Faraone 1996). In DSM-IV, the *melancholic features* specifier retains most of the features of endogenous depression; recent research suggests that "lack of reactivity" and "distinct quality of depressed mood" predict the full syndrome most consistently (K. S. Kendler 1997). However, melancholic depression can appear in response to an obvious precipitant. Endogenous depression has a better response to tricyclic antidepressants than does reactive depression and has a lower rate of response to psychotherapy and placebo (M. T. Tsuang and Faraone 1996).

Recent work has confirmed that the melancholic subtype of major depression is a more severe form of major depression that is associated with more depressive episodes, more symptoms, more impairment, more help-seeking, and more comorbidity with anxiety disorders and nicotine dependence but that is not qualitatively different from nonmelancholic major depression (K. S. Kendler 1997). In twins, the presence of MDD with melancholic features in one twin increased the risk of major depression but not necessarily melancholia in the other twin (K. S. Kendler 1997). Twin studies do not suggest an environmental influence on liability to melancholia in depressed patients (K. S. Kendler 1997). It is also now appreciated that melancholic and atypical depression are not necessarily mutually exclusive.

DIAGNOSIS AND DSM-IV

The term *affect* usually refers to the outward and changeable manifestation of a person's emotional tone, whereas *mood* is a more enduring emotional orientation that colors the person's psychology (American Psychiatric Association 1984a). However, the change from *affective disorders* in DSM-III to *mood disorders* in DSM-IV does not imply a reconceptualization of what these disorders primarily involve (i.e., dysregulation of mood or dysregulation of affect); the two terms are used interchangeably in DSM-IV.

DSM-IV distinguishes between mood episodes and mood disorders (Fava and Davidson 1996; First et al. 1996). An episode is a period lasting at least 2 weeks during which there are enough symptoms for full criteria to be met for the disorder. The criteria for a major depressive episode are summarized in Table 13–2. Patients with or without a history of mania may have a major depressive episode if

TABLE 13–2. DSM-IV criteria for a major depressive episode

A. Five (or more) of the following symptoms have been present during the same 2-week period and represent a change from previous functioning; at least one of the symptoms is either (1) depressed mood or (2) loss of interest or pleasure.

Note: Do not include symptoms that are clearly due to a general medical condition, or mood-incongruent delusions or hallucinations.

(1) depressed mood most of the day, nearly every day, as indicated by either subjective report (e.g., feels sad or empty) or observation made by others (e.g., appears tearful). **Note:** In children and adolescents, can be irritable mood.

(2) markedly diminished interest or pleasure in all, or almost all, activities most of the day, nearly every day (as indicated by either subjective account or observation made by others)

(3) significant weight loss when not dieting or weight gain (e.g., a change of more than 5% of body weight in a month), or decrease or increase in appetite nearly every day. **Note:** In children, consider failure to make expected weight gains.

(4) insomnia or hypersomnia nearly every day

(5) psychomotor agitation or retardation nearly every day (observable by others, not merely subjective feelings of restlessness or being slowed down)

(6) fatigue or loss of energy nearly every day

(7) feelings of worthlessness or excessive or inappropriate guilt (which may be delusional) nearly every day (not merely self-reproach or guilt about being sick)

(8) diminished ability to think or concentrate, or indecisiveness, nearly every day (either subjective account or as observed by others)

(9) recurrent thoughts of death (not just fear of dying), recurrent suicidal ideation without a specific plan, or a suicide attempt or a specific plan for committing suicide

B. The symptoms do not meet criteria for a mixed episode.

C. The symptoms cause clinically significant distress or impairment in social, occupational, or other important areas of functioning.

D. The symptoms are not due to the direct physiological effects of a substance (e.g., a drug of abuse, a medication) or a general medical condition (e.g., hypothyroidism).

E. The symptoms are not better accounted for by Bereavement, i.e., after the loss of a loved one, the symptoms persist for longer than 2 months or are characterized by marked functional impairment, morbid preoccupation with worthlessness, suicidal ideation, psychotic symptoms, or psychomotor retardation.

they fulfill these criteria, but *major depressive disorder* (MDD) refers to one or more episodes of major depression in the absence of mania or hypomania (i.e., unipolar depression). A major depressive episode may be modified by additional specifiers for melancholic features (Table 13–3) and/or atypical features (Table 13–4).

The interpretation of studies of mood disorders is facilitated by familiarity with several common terms (Fava and Davidson 1996; First et al. 1996). In most treatment studies, *response* is defined as at least 50% improvement, whereas *partial response* is 25%–50% improvement and *nonresponse* is < 25% improvement. According to this terminology, patients who are still half as symptomatic as at the beginning of treatment will be considered responders at the end of a treatment study. This is not a trivial point, given that most studies consider improvement rather than remission as the end point. *Remission* is defined as the state of having few or no symptoms of a mood disorder for at least 8 weeks. *Recovery*, the period after remission, is present if no symptoms have been present for more than 8 weeks, and the term implies that the disorder is quiescent. A *relapse* is a return of symptoms during the period of remission, and the term implies continuation of the original episode; whereas *recurrence* is a later return of symptoms (during recovery), and this term implies development of a new episode. These distinctions can be difficult to make in clinical practice. For example, mild residual symptoms of an initial episode may be overlooked or may be attributed to character pathology after improvement of the more dramatic manifestations of an episode; this may lead to the conclusion that a return of more severe symptoms represents a new episode rather than an exacerbation of the original episode.

TABLE 13–3. DSM-IV melancholic features specifier

With melancholic features (can be applied to the current or most recent major depressive episode in major depressive disorder and to a major depressive episode in bipolar I or bipolar II disorder only if it is the most recent type of mood episode)

A. Either of the following, occurring during the most severe period of the current episode:
   (1) loss of pleasure in all, or almost all, activities
   (2) lack of reactivity to usually pleasurable stimuli (does not feel much better, even temporarily, when something good happens)

B. Three (or more) of the following:
   (1) distinct quality of depressed mood (i.e., the depressed mood is experienced as distinctly different from the kind of feeling experienced after the death of a loved one)
   (2) depression regularly worse in the morning
   (3) early morning awakening (at least 2 hours before usual time of awakening)
   (4) marked psychomotor retardation or agitation
   (5) significant anorexia or weight loss
   (6) excessive or inappropriate guilt

TABLE 13–4. DSM-IV atypical features specifier

With atypical features (can be applied when these features predominate during the most recent 2 weeks of a major depressive episode in major depressive disorder or in bipolar I or bipolar II disorder when the major depressive episode is the most recent type of mood episode, or when these features predominate during the most recent 2 years of dysthymic disorder)

A. Mood reactivity (i.e., mood brightens in response to actual or potential positive events)

B. Two (or more) of the following features:
   (1) significant weight gain or increase in appetite
   (2) hypersomnia
   (3) leaden paralysis (i.e., heavy, leaden feelings in arms or legs)
   (4) long-standing pattern of interpersonal rejection sensitivity (not limited to episodes of mood disturbance) that results in significant social or occupational impairment

C. Criteria are not met for with melancholic features or with catatonic features during the same episode.

UNIPOLAR AND BIPOLAR MOOD DISORDERS

One of the most important distinctions between mood disorders is the distinction between unipolar and bipolar categories (Leonhard 1987a, 1987b). Unipolar mood disorders are characterized by depressive symptoms in the absence of a history of a pathologically elevated mood. In bipolar mood disorders, depression alternates or is mixed with mania or hypomania. Patients who have only had recurrent mania ("unipolar mania") are given the diagnosis of bipolar mood disorder on the assumption that they will eventually develop an episode of depression (M. T. Tsuang and Faraone 1996). DSM-IV criteria for a manic episode are summarized in Table 13–5. Hypomania, a milder form of pathologically elevated mood that can be present for a shorter period before it is diagnosed, is described in Table 13–6. Although most people think of elation as a defining characteristic of mania and hypomania, many patients experience only irritability, anxiety, or a dysphoric sense of

TABLE 13–5. **DSM-IV criteria for a manic episode**

A. A distinct period of abnormally and persistently elevated, expansive, or irritable mood, lasting at least 1 week (or any duration if hospitalization is necessary).

B. During the period of mood disturbance, three (or more) of the following symptoms have persisted (four if the mood is only irritable) and have been present to a significant degree:

    (1) inflated self-esteem or grandiosity

    (2) decreased need for sleep (e.g., feels rested after only 3 hours of sleep)

    (3) more talkative than usual or pressure to keep talking

    (4) flight of ideas or subjective experience that thoughts are racing

    (5) distractibility (i.e., attention too easily drawn to unimportant or irrelevant external stimuli)

    (6) increase in goal-directed activity (either socially, at work or school, or sexually) or psychomotor agitation

    (7) excessive involvement in pleasurable activities that have a high potential for painful consequences (e.g., engaging in unrestrained buying sprees, sexual indiscretions, or foolish business investments)

C. The symptoms do not meet criteria for a mixed episode.

D. The mood disturbance is sufficiently severe to cause marked impairment in occupational functioning or in usual social activities or relationships with others, or to necessitate hospitalization to prevent harm to self or others, or there are psychotic features.

E. The symptoms are not due to the direct physiological effects of a substance (e.g., a drug of abuse, a medication, or other treatment) or a general medical condition (e.g., hyperthyroidism).

TABLE 13–6. **DSM-IV criteria for a hypomanic episode**

A. A distinct period of persistently elevated, expansive, or irritable mood, lasting throughout at least 4 days, that is clearly different from the usual nondepressed mood.

B. During the period of mood disturbance, three (or more) of the following symptoms have persisted (four if the mood is only irritable) and have been present to a significant degree:

    (1) inflated self-esteem or grandiosity

    (2) decreased need for sleep (e.g., feels rested after only 3 hours of sleep)

    (3) more talkative than usual or pressure to keep talking

    (4) flight of ideas or subjective experience that thoughts are racing

    (5) distractibility (i.e., attention too easily drawn to unimportant or irrelevant external stimuli)

    (6) increase in goal-oriented activity (either socially, at work or school, or sexually) or psychomotor agitation

    (7) excessive involvement in pleasurable activities that have a high potential for painful consequences (e.g., the person engages in unrestrained buying sprees, sexual indiscretions, or foolish business investments)

C. The episode is associated with an unequivocal change in functioning that is uncharacteristic of the person when not symptomatic.

D. The disturbance in mood and the change in functioning are observable by others.

E. The episode is not severe enough to cause marked impairment in social or occupational functioning, or to necessitate hospitalization, and there are no psychotic features.

F. The symptoms are not due to the direct physiological effects of a substance (e.g., a drug of abuse, a medication, or other treatment) or a general medical condition (e.g., hyperthyroidism).

Note: Hypomanic-like episodes that are clearly caused by somatic antidepressant treatment (e.g., medication, electroconvulsive therapy, light therapy) should not count toward a diagnosis of bipolar II disorder.

increased energy, as if they were "crawling out of their skins." This kind of presentation may occur most frequently in women and younger patients with bipolar disorder and in antidepressant-induced hypomania. In DSM-IV, it is noted that mania is a state of increased goal-directed behavior that is pleasurable and has obvious potential for harm, whereas behavior in mania is often excessive, disorganized, and dysphoric but not clearly harmful or dangerous (American Psychiatric Association 1994a).

Most authorities agree that the bipolar-unipolar distinction is dichotomous: a patient either is or is not manic. In addition, the course of bipolar disorders differs from that of unipolar disorders (Dubovsky et al. 1989, 1991a; Faedda et al. 1995; Leibenluft et al. 1995; M. T. Tsuang and Faraone 1996; Weissman et al. 1996; Winokur 1995); the

differences are summarized in Table 13–7. On closer scrutiny, these distinctions may not be as obvious as they might seem at first. For example, unipolar depression can be psychotic with severe depressive symptoms, and depressive episodes may be highly recurrent without ever being associated with mania. Lithium can increase the effectiveness of antidepressants in unipolar depression, and electroconvulsive therapy (ECT) is effective in treating both mania and depression (Dubovsky and Buzan 1997). Patients

TABLE 13–7. Differences between unipolar and bipolar depression

Unipolar	Bipolar
Later onset	Earlier onset
Fewer episodes	More episodes
Female >> male	Female = male
More psychomotor agitation	More psychomotor retardation and lethargy
Typical symptoms	Atypical symptoms
Insomnia	Hypersomnia
Lower risk of suicide	Greater risk of suicide
Less frequently accompanied by psychotic symptoms in younger patients	Greater likelihood of psychotic symptoms in younger patients
Antidepressants more effective	Antidepressants less effective
Lithium less effective	Lithium more effective
Family history of depression	Family history of mania and depression
Normal $[Ca^{2+}]_i$	Increased $[Ca^{2+}]_i$

Note. $[Ca^{2+}]_i$ = increase in free intracellular concentration of calcium ions.

with unipolar depression may have symptoms generally associated with bipolar disorder such as agitation, racing thoughts, and overspending. Unipolar and bipolar disorders can aggregate in the same families, and some studies suggest there are no significant differences between unipolar and bipolar disorder with regard to familial rates of bipolar illness (E. S. Gershon et al. 1982; Weissman et al. 1984; Winokur 1995). Unipolar and bipolar illness may not be totally distinct, because they coaggregate in families.

Given that mania and depression are opposites of each other, one would think that only one of the two disorders could be present at a time. However, between 30% and 50% of manic episodes are accompanied by depressive symptoms (Bowden et al. 1995; McElroy et al. 1992). If the full criteria (except duration) are met for both mania and major depression, a mixed episode (dysphoric mania) should be diagnosed, according to DSM-IV. However, many more patients with one diagnosis have some symptoms of the other, as exemplified by exhibitionistic depression with outbursts of rage and decreased need for sleep or by hypomania with suicide attempts and fatigue (McElroy et al. 1992). Dysphoric mania is more common in females and is associated with a greater risk of suicide and a poorer response to lithium (McElroy et al. 1992).

SPECIFIC MOOD DISORDERS

The identification of an episode of mania and/or depression is the first step in making a comprehensive diagnosis. The next steps are to decide which modifiers in addition to melancholia and atypical features apply to the episode and then to consider specific subtypes of mood disorders. Some of these subtypes meet criteria for DSM-IV mood disorders with or without symptomatic or course specifiers, and some are commonly recognized syndromes that are not thought to meet formal diagnostic criteria.

MAJOR DEPRESSIVE DISORDER

MDD is characterized by one or more major depressive episodes in the absence of mania or hypomania. Depressive syndromes caused by medical illnesses (mood disorder due to a general medical condition) and by medications or psychoactive substances (substance-induced mood disorder) are not considered to be primary mood disorders and do not qualify for a diagnosis of MDD. In DSM-IV there are a number of course specifiers that can be applied to the current or most recent depressive episode. These course specifiers (severity, psychosis, degree of remission, chronicity, catatonic features, melancholic features, atypical features, and postpartum onset) are discussed throughout this chapter. DSM-IV provides two additional descriptors for patients with recurrent depressive episodes: with (or without) interepisode recovery and with seasonal pattern.

Although MDD can consist of a single episode, recurrence is the rule rather than the exception. After a single major depressive episode, the risk of a second episode is around 50%; after a third episode, the risk of a fourth is around 90% (Thase 1990). Each new episode tends to occur sooner and more abruptly, and new episodes often include the same symptoms that previous episodes included, along with new and more severe symptoms. The importance of this tendency of major depression to accelerate over time will be discussed later.

DSM-IV specifiers are used to indicate whether a major depressive episode has remitted fully (i.e., no symptoms for at least 2 months), partially (i.e., not enough ongoing depressive symptoms to qualify for a diagnosis of a major depressive episode or no symptoms for less than 2 months), or not at all (i.e., a chronic major depressive episode). Longitudinal course specifiers for MDD indicate whether recurrent major depressive episodes remit completely or partially in between episodes and whether major depressive episodes are superimposed on dysthymia. If one counts only the defining symptoms listed in Table 13–2, these kinds of distinctions may be relatively uncomplicated. However, recall of depressive symptoms may be greater when a patient feels more depressed than when depression is less severe (i.e., recall is state dependent). Because the severity of depression tends to fluctuate in all but the most profoundly depressed patients, a history obtained when a patient feels worse may suggest a more chronic illness than may a history obtained when the same patient feels better. One way to clarify whether the first instance represents retrospective amplification of past symptoms in the light of current mood or more accurate recall is to gather additional data from family members and others who have known the patient over time.

Another difficult judgment to make in assessing remission of a major depressive episode is the judgment of whether the psychology of depression represents residual depression. Patients who have one or two major depressive symptoms—insomnia and low energy, for example—along with the kind of pervasive negative thinking that is characteristic of depression may have a subsyndromal form of depression that might resolve completely with more aggressive treatment. Depression is associated with globally negative thinking such that negative events are attributed to inadequacies in the self and are seen as having pervasive and irreversible consequences (A. T. Beck et al. 1979; Thase 1996). Depressive thinking is derived from rigid, all-or-nothing assumptions such as "If everyone doesn't accept me all the time, no one cares about me at all" or "If I make a mistake, I'm totally incompetent" (Thase 1996). People who maintain these attitudes or who are chronically joyless, cranky, or hypersensitive may have partial depressive syndromes.

MASKED DEPRESSION

As many as 50% of major depressive episodes are unrecognized because a depressed mood is less obvious than other symptoms of the disorder. Alexithymia, or inability to express emotions in words, can focus a patient's attention on physical symptoms of depression, such as insomnia, low energy, and difficulty concentrating, without any awareness of feeling depressed. Minor physical dysfunction may be magnified by hypervigilance for anything that feels dangerous or bad, and therefore it may be difficult to distinguish chronic major depression from somatization disorder and hypochondriasis. Substance use as a form of self-treatment for depression can be more obvious than the underlying mood disorder. When pathological character traits are intensified in response to an underlying mood disorder, a personality disorder may seem to be the primary problem. Additional common masked presentations of major depression include marital and family conflicts, absenteeism from work, poor school performance, social withdrawal, and lack of motivation.

Many depressed patients have mild cognitive dysfunction that improves with encouragement. However, some depressed patients have a pattern of subcortical dementia that may be indistinguishable from primary dementia. The term *depressive pseudodementia* is often used to describe this presentation, but a more accurate term would be *dementia syndrome of depression* or *reversible dementia of depression*. There may be a neurological component to depressive dementia, as is suggested by an association of imaging evidence of global brain atrophy and white matter lesions with greater levels of cognitive impairment in depressed patients who do not have obvious neurological disease (Soares and Mann 1997).

In older patients and patients with preexisting mild dementia, depression may be expressed mainly as a disturbance of memory and concentration. The dementia syndrome of depression may be found on close questioning to be accompanied by changes in energy, appetite, and sleep but not necessarily changes in mood and by a family history of depression, but the only way to be confident that depression is not the cause of apparent dementia may be to observe the patient's response to an antidepressant. However, a majority of patients whose depressive dementias remit partially or completely with antidepressant treatment are found on follow-up to develop a primary dementia that no longer responds to antidepressants (Reynolds and Hoch 1987). One explanation for this outcome is that the effect of depression on subcortical structures causes a lowering of the threshold for the expression of coexisting early dementia that would otherwise be unrecognizable. With successful treatment of the depression, dementia is no longer apparent, but as dementia progresses it becomes severe enough to be identifiable in its own right. Even in these cases, treatment of depression can delay the onset of obvious irreversible primary dementia.

Another form of masked depression encountered in neurological settings occurs in patients with aprosodia (Ramasubbu and Kennedy 1994). Aprosodia, or loss of the capacity to convey emotional and other nuances of speech and behavior (prosody), is a manifestation of disease of the nondominant hemisphere. Patients with aprosodia, like those with aphasia, lose the capacity to understand, repeat, or communicate emotional meaning, even when speech remains intact (Ross 1981). If they become depressed, such patients may appear or feel sad or unhappy, but their thoughts and actions are derivatives of a depressive orientation (Dubovsky 1986). For example, affect may be irritable or blunted rather than depressed. Negativistic behavior (e.g., mutism, gross noncompliance with medical therapy, refusal to eat), withdrawal, catatonia, or violent outbursts may be much more obvious than a depressed mood. Vegetative symptoms such as disturbances of appetite, energy, and sleep may appear to be symptoms of the neurological illness. However, treatment with an antidepressant or with ECT can produce dramatic improvement (Dubovsky 1986).

CHRONIC DEPRESSION

Chronic forms of depression account for 12%–35% of depressive disorders (First et al. 1996; J. Scott 1988). Rates of chronicity in depression vary with the evaluation performed (J. Scott 1988). More patients meet criteria for chronicity when it is defined by the presence of any depressive symptoms than when it is defined as a level of symptomatology that is above some definite level, such as a Hamilton Rating Scale for Depression (HRSD) score of 10. Even after remission of specific depressive symptoms, many patients continue to experience family dysfunction, occupational impairment, and poor physical health (Keitner and Miller 1990; Thase 1992). If chronic depression is defined in part by impaired functioning, some of these patients may be considered chronically depressed even if specific depressive symptoms are not obvious.

DYSTHYMIC DISORDER

Dysthymic disorder (DD) (*dysthymia* means "ill-tempered") was introduced in DSM-III to indicate a nonepisodic chronic depression that was thought to be less severe than major depression (First et al. 1996). The cardinal feature of DD is a chronically depressed mood that is present most of the day, more days than not, for at least 2 years (First et al. 1996). The concept of DD as mild, chronic depression began with diagnoses in earlier versions of the DSM such as chronic depression and depressive personality (Klein et al. 1996), and this concept has continued to evolve. For example, in the change from DSM-III to DSM-III-R, eight symptoms were deleted, an appetite disturbance was added, and descriptions of some symptoms were reworded so that the number of associated symptoms was decreased from 13 to 6. In addition, the minimum number of symptoms required for a diagnosis of DD was reduced from three to two (Klein et al. 1996). However, the same patients with adult dysthymia appear to meet criteria of each DSM (Gwirtsman et al. 1997). It is not known whether this is also true of patients with adolescent- or geriatric-onset dysthymia (Gwirtsman et al. 1997).

DSM-IV criteria for DD (Table 13–8) are essentially the same as DSM-III-R criteria for DD, the primary changes being the addition of the impairment criterion and the elimination of a distinction between primary and secondary dysthymia. In an attempt to distinguish between chronic MDD and DD, DSM-IV stipulates that chronic depressive symptoms lasting less than 2 years after a major

---

TABLE 13–8. DSM-IV criteria for dysthymic disorder

A. Depressed mood for most of the day, for more days than not, as indicated either by subjective account or observation by others, for at least 2 years. **Note:** In children and adolescents, mood can be irritable and duration must be at least 1 year.

B. Presence, while depressed, of two (or more) of the following:
   (1) poor appetite or overeating
   (2) insomnia or hypersomnia
   (3) low energy or fatigue
   (4) low self-esteem
   (5) poor concentration or difficulty making decisions
   (6) feelings of hopelessness

C. During the 2-year period (1 year for children or adolescents) of the disturbance, the person has never been without the symptoms in Criteria A and B for more than 2 months at a time.

D. No major depressive episode has been present during the first 2 years of the disturbance (1 year for children and adolescents); i.e., the disturbance is not better accounted for by chronic major depressive disorder, or major depressive disorder, in partial remission.

Note: There may have been a previous major depressive episode provided there was a full remission (no significant signs or symptoms for 2 months) before development of the dysthymic disorder. In addition, after the initial 2 years (1 year in children or adolescents) of dysthymic disorder, there may be superimposed episodes of major depressive disorder, in which case both diagnoses may be given when the criteria are met for a major depressive episode.

E. There has never been a manic episode, a mixed episode, or a hypomanic episode, and criteria have never been met for cyclothymic disorder.

F. The disturbance does not occur exclusively during the course of a chronic psychotic disorder, such as schizophrenia or delusional disorder.

G. The symptoms are not due to the direct physiological effects of a substance (e.g., a drug of abuse, a medication) or a general medical condition (e.g., hypothyroidism).

H. The symptoms cause clinically significant distress or impairment in social, occupational, or other important areas of functioning.

depressive episode and otherwise meeting criteria for DD be diagnosed as major depressive episode in partial remission; if a full remission from a major depressive episode lasts at least 6 months and is then followed by dysthymia, a diagnosis of DD is justified (Keller et al. 1996).

What is the real difference between MDD and DD? Dysthymia begins insidiously and to be diagnosed must be present for at least 2 years, during which time criteria for a major depressive episode must not be met (First et al. 1996). However, retrospective accounts of the onset of a mood disorder years in the past are likely to be colored by patients' moods at the time of recall, making anything but prospective evaluation of patients who are at risk of depression unreliable in distinguishing between DD and chronic MDD. Another defining difference is that more depressive symptoms are required to diagnose MDD than DD (American Psychiatric Association 1994a). However, as Table 13–9 (First et al. 1996) shows, if a dysthymic patient reports only two more symptoms, the diagnosis is changed to MDD (Kocsis and Frances 1987). This commonly occurs because most patients who meet criteria for DD exceed the minimum number of symptoms required for the diagnosis, regardless of the diagnostic method used (e.g., DSM-III, DSM-III-R, DSM-IV, DSM-IV alternative criteria) (Klein et al. 1996). Indeed, 80% of patients with dysthymia also have a lifetime diagnosis of major depression (Keller et al. 1996; Klein et al. 1996), and most patients with DD seek treatment for superimposed major depression (Keller et al. 1996). Because a patient with depression meeting criteria for MDD may barely have the requisite number of symptoms, do the inevitable fluctuations in DD signify that a different disorder has developed? Does the advent of one particular additional symptom in a dysthymic patient have more significance than another for a new diagnosis of MDD? Is there any difference between severe dysthymia and mild major depression (First et al. 1996)?

When studied separately, MDD is associated with more vegetative symptoms; loss of interest or pleasure; loss of appetite and weight; trouble thinking, concentrating, or making decisions; reduced activity level; feelings of worthlessness; diurnal mood swing; fatigue or loss of energy; feelings of hopelessness; and social withdrawal than is DD, which suggests that major depression is a more severe condition, at least with regard to current symptoms (Keller et al. 1996; Klein et al. 1996). Cognitive and social-motivational symptoms have been reported to be more frequent in DD (Klein et al. 1996). However, even though patients with MDD usually have higher rates of most depressive symptoms than do patients with DD, there are no substantive qualitative differences in symptomatology between the two conditions (Klein et al. 1996). Patients with MDD usually have higher scores on the HRSD than do patients with DD, but the difference is not great (Kocsis 1993).

When severity is examined from the standpoint of functioning rather than of number of symptoms, the distinction between MDD and DD becomes less reliable (Angst and Wicki 1991). DD produces as much impairment as MDD in work, leisure activities, relationships, general health, and ability to perform social roles (Frances 1993). Even minor depression (a Research Diagnostic Criteria [RDC] condition in which the number of depressive symptoms is insufficient to meet criteria for DD or MDD) is associated with almost as much impairment as are DD and MDD (Broadhead et al. 1990). Comorbidity with other Axis I disorders and with personality disorders is about equally frequent in the two conditions (Howland 1993; Kocsis 1993; J. C. Perry 1985). Despite DD's being defined as a less severe condition, the prognosis of DD is not substantially different from that of MDD (Wells et al. 1992). Both disorders respond to the same antidepressant and psychotherapeutic regimens (Frances 1993; Kocsis et al. 1989; J. Scott 1992; Stewart et al. 1993).

Chronic MDD and DD may be related to each other in a number of ways. One possibility is that they are separate disorders with overlapping symptoms and with a high rate of comorbidity with each other, with a number of other conditions (such as anxiety, substance-related, eating, somatoform, and personality disorders), and with chronic medical illnesses (Conte and Karasu 1992; Howland 1993; Marin et al. 1993; J. C. Perry 1985). Another possibility is that DD is an early phase of MDD (Frances 1993), a theory that is suggested by the observation that childhood-onset DD does not persist into adulthood in its original form but is replaced by recurrent MDD and bipolar disorder (Kovacs et al. 1994). Or both disorders may be different presentations over time of the same disturbance of mood, personality traits, and psychosocial functioning, combining chronic low-grade or residual depression with recurrence of more severe depression.

TABLE 13–9. **Dysthymic disorder versus major depressive disorder**

Dysthymic disorder	Major depressive disorder
2 years	2 weeks
Depressed mood	Depressed mood
Two additional symptoms	Four additional symptoms
More cognitive symptoms	More vegetative symptoms
Mild onset may be followed after 2 years by major depression	Onset may begin with more severe symptoms

In the DSM-IV field trials, patients who met criteria for dysthymia on average also reported two-thirds of the symptoms listed in Table 13–10 (Keller et al. 1996). Some of these symptoms are attenuated versions of typical depressive symptoms, whereas others describe global ways of thinking about oneself that overlap with personality traits. A modified version of this symptom list (Table 13–11A) was placed in the Appendix to DSM-IV, the implication being that these symptoms might end up differentiating DD from MDD (Klein et al. 1996; Shea and Hirschfeld 1996). A recent consensus panel that considered this and five other proposed sets of research criteria for DD concluded that the core symptoms common to these sets of criteria and essential for a diagnosis of DD include dysphoria or gloominess for at least 2 years in adults and 1 year in children, along with at least three of the six symptoms listed in Table 13–11B (Gwirtsman et al. 1997) (as opposed to two of four symptoms in DSM-IV). However, more study is necessary before the value of alternative research criteria for DD is clarified (Keller et al. 1996). The overlap between chronic depressive symptoms and personality traits is discussed later in the chapter.

MINOR DEPRESSION

Minor depressive disorder is an RDC diagnosis in which the most prominent disturbance is a sustained depressed mood without the full depressive syndrome (Keller et al. 1996). The RDC for minor depression include feeling depressed or down in the dumps for 1 week (probable) or 2 weeks (definite) (Keller et al. 1996). At least two symptoms from a larger symptom list than the list of DSM-IV criteria for MDD that includes pessimistic attitude and self-pity are required for the diagnosis; impairment or seeking treatment are not required (M. T. Tsuang and

TABLE 13–10. **Symptoms endorsed by patients meeting DSM-IV criteria for dysthymic disorder**

Low self-esteem, feelings of inadequacy

Pessimism, despair, or hopelessness

Social withdrawal

Chronic fatigue or tiredness

Guilt, brooding about the past

Irritability, excessive anger

Decreased activity, effectiveness, or productivity

Difficulty thinking: poor concentration, poor memory, indecisiveness

Generalized loss of interest or pleasure (hypohedonia)

TABLE 13–11. **Research criteria for dysthymic disorder**

A.   DSM-IV criteria

Presence, while depressed, of three or more of the following:

    (1)   Low self-esteem or self confidence or feelings of inadequacy

    (2)   Feelings of pessimism, despair, or hopelessness

    (3)   Generalized loss of interest or pleasure

    (4)   Social withdrawal

    (5)   Chronic fatigue or tiredness

    (6)   Feelings of guilt, brooding about the past

    (7)   Subjective feeling of irritability or excessive anger

    (8)   Decreased activity, effectiveness, or productivity

    (9)   Difficulty thinking reflected by poor concentration, poor memory, or indecisiveness

B.   Consensus panel core symptom of dysthymia

    (1)   Low self-esteem

    (2)   Pessimism, hopelessness

    (3)   Social withdrawal

    (4)   Irritability, excessive anger

    (5)   Concentration or thinking problems

    (6)   Low energy, low initiative

Faraone 1996). Minor depression may be chronic, and, like DD, it may be complicated by superimposed major depressive episodes (Keller et al. 1996). In the DSM-IV mood disorders field trial, three of 524 subjects met criteria for a lifetime history of minor depression (Keller et al. 1996).

DOUBLE DEPRESSION

Although it is not a separate DSM-IV diagnosis, double depression, or DD with a superimposed major depressive episode, has been extensively discussed in the literature and the term is used widely by clinicians. The major depressive episode must appear 2 years or more (1 year in children and adolescents) after the onset of dysthymia for double depression to be diagnosed (First et al. 1996). Double depression is far from uncommon in dysthymic patients. Between 68% and 90% of dysthymic patients experience at least one major depressive episode (Thase 1992), and 25%–50% of patients with MDD have coexisting DD (Hirschfeld 1994; Levitt et al. 1991). It has been estimated that 22%–66% of all patients with unipolar depression have experienced a combination of dysthymia and major depression (Hirschfeld 1994; Keller 1994). A 9-year prospective study found DD with superimposed MDD or recurrent brief depression in 3% of the general population (Hirschfeld 1994).

Compared with major depressive episodes alternating with euthymia (episodic MDD), MDD superimposed on dysthymia has an earlier onset of major depression (Levitt et al. 1991), more severe depressive symptoms (Belsher and Costello 1988; Wells et al. 1992), more psychosocial impairment (Belsher and Costello 1988; Conte and Karasu 1992; Kovacs et al. 1994), a greater risk of suicide (Angst and Wicki 1991), more treatment resistance (Barrett 1984), and more comorbidity (Klein et al. 1988), especially with avoidant and dependent personality disorders (Sanderson et al. 1992). The major depressive episode in double depression is less likely to remit (I. W. Miller et al. 1986; Wells et al. 1992) than that in episodic MDD and is more likely to recur (Levitt et al. 1991). In one report (Belsher and Costello 1988), the relapse rate of major depression after 8 weeks of recovery was 30% for double depression and 4% for episodic MDD. In this study, major depression recurred in 50% of patients with double depression and 35% of patients with episodic MDD after 1 year and in 65% and 37%, respectively, after 2 years. The risk of a bipolar outcome also appears greater in double depression: 29% of patients with double depression in the NIMH-CS developed hypomania, compared with 9% of patients with episodic MDD (Keller 1994).

SUBSYNDROMAL DEPRESSION

Subsyndromal disorders are conditions that partially meet diagnostic criteria for a particular disorder (Jamison 1996). Some subsyndromal forms of unipolar depression such as RDC minor depressive disorder have formal diagnostic criteria, and even though impairment or seeking treatment is not required for the diagnosis, they are associated with clinically important functional impairment (Keller et al. 1996; M. T. Tsuang and Faraone 1996). In the Epidemiologic Catchment Area study, one-third of people using mental health services had subsyndromal mood disorders (Gwirtsman et al. 1997). There is less certainty about the degree to which some constellations of personality traits may also represent subsyndromal forms of chronic depression.

The concept of a depressive temperament or personality representing either a subsyndromal form of depression expressed through the personality, an inherited temperamental disposition, or a "fundamental state" from which more severe depressive episodes emerge later in life was proposed early in this century by Emil Kraepelin and again in the middle of the century by Kurt Schneider (Shea and Hirshfeld 1996). These and other investigators noted that depression is predictably associated with such personality

traits as persistent gloominess or despondency (Keller et al. 1996), seriousness (Shea and Hirshfeld 1996), guilt (Keller et al. 1996; Shea and Hirshfeld 1996), lack of self-confidence (Keller et al. 1996; Shea and Hirshfeld 1996), self-denial (Shea and Hirshfeld 1996), conscientiousness (Shea and Hirshfeld 1996), introversion, and neuroticism (Thase 1996). The question that remains to be formally answered is whether such traits are partial expressions of a depressive disorder, manifestations of mildly pathological personality traits mobilized in response to an underlying mood disorder that is less obvious than the overlying personality traits, or markers of a propensity to develop full syndromal mood disorders later in life.

Akiskal (1991, 1994a, 1994b) divided syndromes marked by depressive traits into *subaffective dysthymia*, in which depressive personality traits are caused by chronic subclinical depression, and *character spectrum disorder*, which he considered a type of personality disorder in which depressed mood is just one feature of a chronically unhappy and unfulfilled orientation of the personality. As a result of deliberations by the DSM-IV Personality Disorders Work Group, a version of character spectrum disorder is included in the Appendix to DSM-IV as *depressive personality disorder* (Keller et al. 1996). The DSM-IV field trials suggested that this condition "requiring further research" (Table 13–12) was associated with a passive, unassertive style, in the absence of current diagnosable dysthymia, in almost 50% of cases (Keller et al. 1996). Patients thought to have depressive personality disorder were noted to have a tendency to develop DD or MDD after the diagnosis of depressive personality disorder was made, which suggests

TABLE 13–12.   DSM-IV research criteria for depressive personality disorder

A. A pervasive pattern of depressive cognitions and behaviors beginning by early adulthood and present in a variety of contexts, as indicated by five (or more) of the following:

   (1) usual mood is dominated by dejection, gloominess, cheerlessness, joylessness, unhappiness

   (2) self-concept centers around beliefs of inadequacy, worthlessness, and low self-esteem

   (3) is critical, blaming, and derogatory toward self

   (4) is brooding and given to worry

   (5) is negativistic, critical, and judgmental toward others

   (6) is pessimistic

   (7) is prone to feeling guilty or remorseful

B. Does not occur exclusively during major depressive episodes and is not better accounted for by dysthymic disorder

that the apparent personality disorder might be an early-onset trait-like variant of other depressive disorders. This hypothesis is supported by the existence of a familial association between depressive personality disorder and other depressive disorders (American Psychiatric Association 1994a) and by earlier onset and more depressive episodes in patients with MDD and a premorbid depressive personality than in patients with major depression but without this premorbid temperament (Cassano et al. 1992).

From a clinical standpoint, defining a personality disorder that overlaps with but is distinct from primary mood disorders has the theoretical benefit of identifying a group of patients who would be expected to have a poor response to typical treatments for depression and a better response to specialized psychotherapeutic approaches. However, the overlap between abnormal mood and stable personality traits is often so extensive that it is indistinguishable (Shea and Hirschfeld 1996). Obviously, many people with diagnoses of MDD and/or dysthymia meet DSM-IV symptomatic criteria for depressive personality disorder. In one study, 41% of patients with a major depressive episode were found to meet all criteria for depressive personality disorder, including persistence of symptoms when the full mood disorder was not present (Shea and Hirschfeld 1996).

The impact of an abnormal mood on thinking and behavior is so profound that it can distort most assessments of personality, making it impossible to determine the degree to which a personality disorder is present when a primary mood disorder and a personality disorder appear to coexist. Chronically unstable or depressed mood can intensify pathological defenses and can skew the ways in which a person experiences the self and others (Deitz 1995). On personality inventories, depressed people resemble each other more than they resemble themselves when they are not depressed (Hirschfeld et al. 1989; Loranger et al. 1991). In several studies, more than 50% of patients (or their relatives) with a diagnosis of borderline personality disorder were found to develop major depression, mania, or hypomania or commit suicide (Akiskal 1984, 1991). This finding could indicate a high rate of comorbidity or an aggravation of pathological personality traits by subclinical mood disorders that are not obvious until they eventually become severe enough to be recognized. Because mild depressive symptoms as well as social impairment can persist after remission of a full depressive syndrome, persistent passivity, negative thinking, low self-esteem, cynicism, and related traits in the absence of a diagnosable mood disorder could represent residual symptoms of a previous episode or prodromal symptoms of another episode, rather than a true

personality disorder. In the absence of any validated method of distinguishing the two, the most prudent approach for the clinician is to treat depression as vigorously as possible before diagnosing a personality disorder. However, the fact that psychological issues that can interfere with the response of mood disorders to standard treatments—such as negative therapeutic reactions, attachment to a negative view of the self and others, self-destructive motivations, and treatment nonadherence—may not always be diagnostic of a personality disorder does not mean that it is possible to ignore these issues in treatment.

PSYCHOTIC DEPRESSION

The term *psychotic depression* (or *delusional depression*) refers to a major depressive episode accompanied by psychotic features (i.e., delusions and/or hallucinations). Some clinicians believe that psychotic depression is relatively uncommon. However, most studies continue to demonstrate that 16%–54% of depressed patients have psychotic symptoms (Dubovsky and Thomas 1992). Delusions occur without hallucinations in one-half to two-thirds of adults with psychotic depression, whereas hallucinations are unaccompanied by delusions in 3%–25% of patients (Dubovsky and Thomas 1992). Hallucinations occur more frequently than delusions in younger depressed patients and in patients with bipolar psychotic depression (Chambers et al. 1982; Goodwin and Jamison 1991). Half of all psychotically depressed patients experience more than one kind of delusion (Dubovsky and Thomas 1992). The common belief that visual and olfactory hallucinations are signs of neurological disease and do not occur commonly in mood disorders has been contradicted by clinical experience, which demonstrates that auditory and visual hallucinations are equally frequent and that olfactory hallucinations are not uncommon in psychotic depression (Dubovsky and Thomas 1992).

The classification of psychotic symptoms as mood congruent (i.e., consistent with a depressed or elated mood) or mood incongruent is complex. Prominent mood-incongruent psychotic symptoms in depressed patients such as delusions of control, along with poor adolescent adjustment, may be associated with a somewhat worse prognosis of psychotic depression (K. S. Kendler 1991; D. Tsuang and Coryell 1993). The RDC, which were used in many earlier studies of psychotic depression, indicate a diagnosis of schizoaffective disorder in depressed patients with concurrent mood-incongruent psychotic features. However, bipolar psychotic depression is frequently associated with mood-incongruent psychotic symptoms, some of which may be bizarre and easily mistaken for typical "schizophrenic" symptoms (Akiskal et al. 1983, 1985; McGlashan 1988); a formal thought disorder occurs in at least 20% of psychotically depressed patients (Goodwin and Jamison 1991). Because bipolar illness is over-represented in psychotic depression (Coryell 1996; Weissman et al. 1988a), it may be bipolar illness and not mood incongruence that contributes to a poorer treatment response in mood-incongruent psychotic depression. In recognition of the uncertain contribution of mood incongruence to the prognosis, DSM-IV requires the existence of psychotic symptoms for 2 or more weeks in the absence of prominent mood symptoms for a diagnosis of schizoaffective disorder, a feature that seems more consistently associated with a somewhat poorer prognosis of mixed affective and psychotic syndromes (Coryell 1996).

Recognizing psychotic symptoms in depressed patients is not always straightforward. If the patient does not seem severely depressed (this can occur in patients with bipolar psychotic depression who have a mixed element of elevated mood and energy that makes them appear less depressed than they feel), the clinician might not inquire about psychotic symptoms in the first place. Some patients do not consider hearing voices or ideas of reference to be abnormal and do not report such symptoms. Other patients conceal psychotic symptoms because they do not want to be considered "crazy." To be certain that psychotic symptoms are not present, it may be necessary to ask repeatedly about them, beginning with nonspecific questions such as "Does your mind ever play tricks on you?" and progressing gradually to more specific questions such as "Do you ever hear your name called when there's no one there?" and then "Do you ever hear a voice saying more than your name?"

Psychotic features tend to develop after several episodes of nonpsychotic depression. Once psychotic symptoms occur, they reappear with each subsequent episode, even if later episodes are not as severe. With each recurrence, psychotic symptoms take the same form that they did in previous episodes (e.g., patients with hallucinations have them in the same modality and with the same content from episode to episode) (Dubovsky and Thomas 1992). Relatives of psychotically depressed patients have an increased risk of psychotic depression themselves; and when psychotic depression is present, the content of the psychosis tends to be similar to that of the proband. The families of psychotically depressed patients also have an elevated risk of schizophrenia.

Whereas treatment with both an antipsychotic drug and an antidepressant is usually necessary for a remission of psychotic depression, antipsychotic drugs may improve the depression and the antidepressant may improve psychosis (Dubovsky and Thomas 1992). Further, coaggregation of severe mood disorders and schizophrenia exists in families of patients with psychotic depression. These two observations suggest that psychotic depression is not a simple combination of psychosis and depression but rather a complex interaction between the capacity to become psychotic and the capacity to become severely depressed (Dubovsky and Thomas 1992). Depression may have to reach a certain level of severity for psychosis to be expressed; but once psychosis develops, a unique disorder has evolved. Some features in addition to the unique treatment response that distinguish psychotic from nonpsychotic depression include a greater rate of recurrence; a higher suicide risk; more nonsuppression on the dexamethasone suppression test (DST), with higher post-dexamethasone cortisol levels; more prominent sleep abnormalities; and higher ventricle-to-brain ratios (Coryell 1996; Dubovsky and Thomas 1992). The extent to which the symptomatology, course, and treatment response of psychotic depression are a function of psychosis itself or the over-representation of bipolar disorder in psychotically depressed patients (Weissman et al. 1988a) has not been studied.

RECURRENT BRIEF DEPRESSION

Both the RDC (M. T. Tsuang and Faraone 1996) and DSM-IV criteria (First et al. 1996; M. T. Tsuang and Faraone 1996) require 2 weeks of continuous symptoms for a diagnosis of a major depressive episode to be made. Researcher Jules Angst and his colleagues elucidated a depressive disorder called *recurrent brief depression* in which depressive episodes meet DSM-IV symptomatic but not duration criteria for major depression. Depressive episodes in recurrent brief depression have the same number and severity of symptoms as DSM-IV major depressive episodes but last 1 day to 1 week (Keller et al. 1996). Depressive episodes must recur at least once per month over at least 12 months (not in association with the menstrual cycle) for recurrent brief depression to be diagnosed (Angst and Hochstrasser 1994). Although each acute depressive episode is short-lived, recurrent brief depression carries a high risk of suicide (Lepine et al. 1995), perhaps because of the inevitable return of depression and the repeated drastic contrast between the depressed and well states.

The appendix to DSM-IV lists recurrent brief depressive disorder defined by Angst's criteria as a condition requiring further study because it was thought that not enough data had accumulated to warrant its inclusion as an established diagnosis (American Psychiatric Association

1994a). In the DSM-IV mood disorders field trial, 1.5% of 524 subjects had a lifetime history of recurrent brief depression (Keller et al. 1996) and the 1-year prevalence of recurrent brief depressive disorder was 7% (American Psychiatric Association 1994a). Recurrent brief depression has been found to have high rates of comorbidity with panic disorder, generalized anxiety disorder, and substance abuse that are similar to comorbidity rates with MDD (Keller et al. 1996; Lepine et al. 1995). Recurrent brief depression has also been found often to have a seasonal pattern, with more recurrences in the winter (American Psychiatric Association 1994a; Keller et al. 1996).

One might assume that such a highly recurrent mood disorder likely would eventually have a bipolar outcome (Cassano et al. 1992), and in fact, prophylaxis of brief depressive recurrences is more successful with lithium than with antidepressants (Angst et al. 1990). However, extended follow-up of patients with this condition demonstrates that they never develop mania or hypomania (Angst and Hochstrasser 1994; Angst et al. 1990). This important observation suggests that recurrence may be a feature of mood disorders that is more common in, but not restricted to, bipolar subtypes and that lithium may be an antirecurrence as much as an antimanic treatment. The latter point is supported by the capacity of lithium to prevent recurrences of other cyclical disorders such as cluster headaches.

BIPOLAR SUBTYPES

Bipolar disorder is a mood disorder that is accompanied by episodes of mania and/or hypomania (DSM-IV criteria for manic, hypomanic, and mixed episodes are summarized in Tables 13–5, 13–6, and 13–7). DSM-IV includes three primary subtypes of bipolar disorder. Bipolar I disorder is characterized by manic episodes with or without episodes of hypomania. In bipolar II disorder, one or more hypomanic episodes occur but the patient never experiences mania; hypomanic episodes may be milder than depressive episodes (Akiskal 1995b). Evidence that bipolar II disorder is distinct from bipolar I disorder comes from several sources (Akiskal 1996; Bowden 1993; Bowden et al. 1995; Leibenluft 1996; Solomon et al. 1995). Patients with bipolar II disorder never become manic, despite multiple hypomanic episodes. In addition, the bipolar II diagnosis seems to "breed true" in that patients with this diagnosis have close relatives with hypomania but not mania, whereas patients with bipolar I disorder have some relatives who have had mania and some who have had only

hypomania. Rapid cycling, which is described later, seems to be more common in bipolar II disorder.

Although bipolar III disorder is not a DSM-IV diagnosis, the term has been used to describe patients with a history of depression who have at least one blood relative with a history of mania (M. T. Tsuang and Faraone 1996), on the grounds that such patients may have a bipolar diathesis that has not yet been expressed. In DSM-IV, mania or hypomania that appears in response to treatment with an antidepressant is not counted toward a diagnosis of a bipolar mood disorder, but many clinicians consider antidepressant-induced mania to be an indication of the capacity to develop mania or hypomania spontaneously and therefore a sign of a type of bipolar mood disorder (this seems very likely to be true of children and adolescents [Akiskal 1995a; Strober and Carlson 1982]). In some circles, *bipolar III* refers to patients with antidepressant-induced mania and *bipolar IV* is used to describe depressed patients with a family history of mania.

CYCLOTHYMIC DISORDER

Cyclothymic disorder (cyclothymia) was originally classified as a personality disorder with mood swings that were not clearly manic. Although many investigators now consider cyclothymic disorder to be a mood disorder, it is called *cyclothymic personality* in the RDC (M. T. Tsuang and Faraone 1996). As Table 13–13 indicates, cyclothymia can be diagnosed with DSM-IV in patients with recurrent hypomania and depressive symptoms that may not permit a diagnosis of major depression. In the RDC, cyclothymia is characterized by recurrent depressed mood lasting several days, alternating with elevated mood with at least two hypomanic symptoms. In both schemes, the patient rarely experiences a normal mood (M. T. Tsuang and Faraone 1996).

Patients with cyclothymia typically experience mood states that alternate between depression, irritability, cheerfulness, and relative normality that last days, weeks, or months (Jamison 1993, 1996). Many complain of unpredictable changes in energy, vague physical symptoms, and a seasonal pattern of mood swings (e.g., depression in the winter) (Jamison 1996). In some studies, 44% of cyclothymic patients develop hypomania while taking antidepressants, and about one-third develop full-blown hypomanic, manic, or depressive episodes during drug-free follow-up (Akiskal et al. 1977; Jamison 1996). In addition, at least one-third of the time the onset of clear bipolar I or bipolar II mood disorder is preceded by cyclothymia, which usually begins in adolescence or early adulthood (Jamison 1996).

TABLE 13-13. DSM-IV criteria for cyclothymic disorder

A. For at least 2 years, the presence of numerous periods with hypomanic symptoms and numerous periods with depressive symptoms that do not meet criteria for a major depressive episode. **Note:** In children and adolescents, the duration must be at least 1 year.

B. During the above 2-year period (1 year in children and adolescents), the person has not been without the symptoms in Criterion A for more than 2 months at a time.

C. No major depressive episode, manic episode, or mixed episode has been present during the first 2 years of the disturbance.

Note: After the initial 2 years (1 year in children and adolescents) of cyclothymic disorder, there may be superimposed manic or mixed episodes (in which case both bipolar I disorder and cyclothymic disorder may be diagnosed) or major depressive episodes (in which case both bipolar II disorder and cyclothymic disorder may be diagnosed).

D. The symptoms in Criterion A are not better accounted for by schizoaffective disorder, schizophreniform disorder, delusional disorder, or psychotic disorder not otherwise specified.

E. The symptoms are not due to the direct physiological effects of a substance (e.g., a drug of abuse, a medication) or a general medical condition (e.g., hyperthyroidism).

F. The symptoms cause clinically significant distress or impairment in social, occupation, or other important areas of functioning.

RAPID CYCLING

In DSM-IV, *rapid cycling* is a specifier that refers to a bipolar I or bipolar II mood disorder in which four or more episodes of depression and/or mania or hypomania occur per year, with either 2 weeks of normal mood between episodes or a shift directly from one pole to the other (e.g., from mania to depression) with no intervening period of normal mood (American Psychiatric Association 1994a). Rapid-cycling bipolar disorder is probably not a separate illness but a phase in the evolution of bipolar disorder that may last years but may not be permanent (Tomitaka and Sakamoto 1994). Rapid cycling appears to cause a decreased response to lithium (Roy-Byrne et al. 1984). Rapid cycling is more common in women and in patients with bipolar II disorder (Leibenluft 1996; Lish et al. 1993) and is more likely to occur after an episode of mania or hypomania than after depression (Altschuler et al. 1995; Post 1988). Additional risk factors for the development of rapid cycling include hypothyroidism, right cerebral hemisphere disease, mental retardation, and use of alcohol and stimulants (Ananth et al. 1993; Leibenluft 1996; Sachs 1996). As many as 60%–90% of patients with rapid cycling have been found to have hypothyroidism, and this condition often is too mild to produce medical morbidity but not too mild to contribute to mood instability (Bauer et al. 1990; Cowdry et al. 1983). Lithium itself may cause rapid cycling by inducing hypothyroidism (Terao 1993). Correcting subclinical forms of hypothyroidism therefore is an important intervention in rapid cycling (Extein et al. 1985).

A causal role of antidepressants in rapid cycling has been widely debated. A number of authorities argue that antidepressants can contribute to rapid cycling by inducing mania or by speeding up the inherent cyclicity of bipolar mood disorders (Altschuler et al. 1995; Goodwin et al. 1982; Post 1994; Sachs 1996; Wehr 1993). The majority of patients with rapid-cycling bipolar disorder are taking antidepressants, but it is difficult to prove that antidepressants are the cause of rapid cycling (Altschuler et al. 1995). Perhaps antidepressants are administered more frequently to patients with rapid-cycling and other forms of deteriorating bipolar disorder because depression is prominent or because nothing else is helping. The only way to prove a causal relationship would be to follow prospectively matched patients with bipolar mood disorder who were randomly assigned to take antidepressants or placebos, an experiment that is too difficult technically and ethically to likely be performed. If assessment of the association between starting antidepressants and developing rapid cycling is retrospective, the results are subject to being skewed by state-dependent recall and difficulty remembering the exact onset of complex mood swings. Even in a prospective study, it is difficult to be certain whether rapid cycling that develops after prolonged treatment with an antidepressant was caused by the medication or simply reflected the natural history of the condition.

These issues were recently addressed to some extent by Altschuler and associates (1995), who defined antidepressant-induced mania and rapid cycling as a change in order of episodes or a first episode of severe mania or cycling appearing within 8 weeks of starting antidepressants. In a literature review, the authors (Altschuler et al. 1995) identified 158 patients with bipolar depression in 15 placebo-controlled antidepressant trials in patients with mostly unipolar depression. Within this subgroup, 35% had likely antidepressant-induced mania by the stringent criteria used, the risk being more than 2.5 times as great (72% vs. 28%) for patients who were not also taking lithium. Among the limitations of the literature review were the relatively small number of patients with bipolar mood disorders, the lack of reliable data from trials of other antidepressants, and the lack of inclusion of hypomania as an antidepressant-induced event. In addition, patients in these studies were not identified as having bipolar mood disorders in the first place and might have had a different response to antidepressants than patients with more obvious bipolar disorder.

Altschuler and her colleagues (1995) then used a life-chart method to characterize affective episodes carefully in 51 patients with lithium-refractory bipolar mood disorders, 55% of whom had rapid cycling. Although 82% of the patients developed mania while taking an antidepressant, the investigators concluded that only one-third met their criteria for definite antidepressant-induced mania. One reason for this unexpectedly low rate may have been that their patients had such a high rate of spontaneous affective episodes that it was not possible to detect increases attributable to an antidepressant. The authors found that antidepressant-induced mania increased the risk of rapid cycling by 4.6-fold; 50% of the increase was directly attributable to the use of antidepressants and 50% was assumed to reflect the natural history of bipolar disorder. On the basis of their study and literature review, the authors suggested that continuing antidepressants aggravated rapid cycling, but withdrawing the antidepressant did not necessarily stop cycling. Most ominously, antimanic drugs did not predictably prevent or treat rapid cycling.

These results must be considered conservative for several reasons. First, hypomania and more subtle forms of pathologically elevated mood were not considered. Second, only classically defined rapid cycling was considered; other forms of mood cycling (described in a later section) may be even more common. Because there is no reason to think that antidepressants must take 8 weeks or fewer to induce hypomania or mood swings, using this arbitrary cutoff value may result in the overlooking of many patients for whom months or even years of antidepressants may be necessary to destabilize mood but who would not develop rapid cycling without antidepressants.

BRIEF HYPOMANIA

Angst (1995) defined a subtype of hypomania called *brief hypomania*. Brief hypomania consists of the same symptoms as hypomania, but the duration of symptoms is 1–3 days, rather than the 4 days or more required by DSM-IV for a diagnosis of hypomania. Angst found that despite the short duration of any episode, brief hypomania has a very high rate of recurrence and produces marked impairment. The prevalence of brief hypomania was 2.28% among pa-

tients with bipolar mood disorders in one study (Angst 1995), but further data are needed before diagnostic precision can be achieved for brief manic or hypomanic symptoms. Ultrarapid cycling, which is discussed in the next section, probably would qualify as a condition associated with manic or hypomanic symptoms lasting only a short time but recurring very frequently.

ULTRADIAN CYCLING

In a malignant form of rapid cycling called *ultradian cycling* (or *ultrarapid cycling*) (Pazzaglia et al. 1993; Roy-Byrne et al. 1984), patients appear chronically depressed. On close inspection, however, it is found that they experience multiple recurrences of mania and depression over the course of hours to days. For example, a patient wakes up feeling emotionally paralyzed and unable to get out of bed. A few hours later, the patient feels so energized that it is impossible to sit still and to refrain from acting impulsively; shortly thereafter, the patient sinks abruptly into suicidal despair. The patient briefly feels relatively well but then flies into a rage when criticized and hears voices saying the situation is hopeless. Racing thoughts keep the patient from falling asleep, but once the patient does fall asleep, sleep lasts 14 hours and the patient is exhausted the next day. Rather than having nonspecific "mood swings," the patient is experiencing distinct but very brief recurrences of bipolar depression, dysphoric hypomania, a mixture of depressive and hypomanic symptoms, and a psychotic energized state, with fleeting euthymia between episodes or an abrupt switch from one pole to the other. Akiskal (1991) called this a "protracted pseudo unipolar mixed state" (p. 161) that fluctuates considerably in intensity and with regard to the kinds of symptoms that predominate. The labile moods and behavior of the patient with ultradian cycling are often mistaken for evidence of borderline personality disorder (Akiskal 1996).

It is not clear whether ultradian cycling is a deteriorated form of rapid cycling or a different condition. However, there is no evidence that ultradian cycling is a separate bipolar subtype. The research that has been performed with patients with ultradian cycling suggests that it is even more refractory to treatment than traditionally diagnosed rapid cycling (Pazzaglia et al. 1993; Post 1988). There are no prospective studies to support the assertion that precipitating mania with antidepressants could be followed by ultradian cycling, but ultradian cycling, like rapid cycling, may be preceded by one or more hypomanic episodes (Post 1988, 1990b, 1994). Experience does suggest that the depression of ultradian cycling is aggravated rather than ameliorated by antidepressants (Akiskal 1991; J. Scott 1988).

MASKED AND SUBSYNDROMAL BIPOLAR DISORDER

When features listed in Tables 13–5 and 13–6 are obvious and sustained, the diagnosis of a bipolar mood disorder is straightforward. However, brief mood swings with mixed symptoms that wax and wane rather than clearly remit and recur can be more difficult to identify. Hypomania presenting not as elation but as anxiety attacks, insomnia, difficulty concentrating, irritability, dysphoria, agitation, impulsivity, or hypersexuality can easily be mistaken for an anxiety disorder or a personality disorder. Bipolar depression with mixed dysphoric hypomanic symptoms such as anxiety, restlessness, and agitation may be confused with agitated unipolar depression (Akiskal 1996). Because mania is often associated with a formal thought disorder and with bizarre hallucinations (Goodwin and Jamison 1991), some bipolar psychoses can be confused with excited schizophreniform psychoses.

Subclinical and masked forms of bipolar disorder range from agitated psychoses to temperamental dysregulation of mood (Akiskal 1995b). As with depressive disorders, the most subtle forms of subsyndromal bipolar disorders border personality disorders. Hyperthymia, which was originally described by J. Delay in 1946, is a chronic pattern of elevated mood that is less obvious than hypomania. Hyperthymic individuals are expansive, dynamic, joyful, and optimistic and have a robust sense of well-being, a decreased need for sleep, decreased appetite, increased energy, increased creativity, and a family history of bipolar disorder (Cassano et al. 1992; Hellekson 1989). Although there is no impairment of social or occupational functioning, hyperthymic people are prone to more blatant episodes of hypomania and depression (Hellekson 1989). Some investigators consider hyperthymia to be the premorbid personality style of bipolar disorder (Feline 1993).

Subaffective mania may mimic such personality traits as arrogance, pushiness, irritability, insensitivity, talkativeness, emotional intensity and hypersensitivity, temper tantrums, promiscuity, restlessness, and unpredictability. Never at a loss for a cutting repartee or an excuse, the person may be at the forefront of new movements and groups, only to lose interest after getting everyone else involved. Mixtures of subsyndromal mania and depression are frequently present, as exemplified by wild jokes with a dark or cynical edge, self-destructive thrill seeking, or suicidal humor (McElroy et al. 1992). Bipolar individuals who are chronically high-strung, moody, exhibitionistic, grandiose, hypersensitive, overreactive, and unstable often are thought to have dramatizing personality disorders such as borderline or narcissistic personality disorder. If they seek excitement through stealing or are habitually aggressive, they may appear to have an antisocial personality disorder. Indeed, a number of diagnostic criteria for borderline personality disorder—unstable, intense relationships; affective instability; inappropriate, intense anger; impulsivity; and recurrent suicidal behavior—are also typical of bipolar mood disorders. In one report, hysteria or sociopathy had previously been diagnosed in two-thirds of patients with cyclothymia (Akiskal et al. 1977). In another report, 22% of 23 patients with bipolar mood disorders met criteria for a personality disorder (Carpenter et al. 1995). High rates of narcissistic pathology have been noted in people with bipolar mood disorders (Grubb 1997), possibly reflecting subsyndromal grandiosity as well as a chronic attempt to bolster self-esteem that is undermined by feelings of helplessness to control an unpredictable mood. Patients may also attempt to achieve a sense of control over unstable mood and impulsivity by becoming purposefully self-destructive, impulsive, or thrill seeking, as if they wanted to behave in this manner and were not at the mercy of their mood swings. Making the distinction between borderline and narcissistic personality disorders and chronic bipolar disorders therefore can be challenging.

SEASONAL AFFECTIVE DISORDER

Many people living in climates in which there are marked seasonal differences in the length of the day have seasonal changes in mood and energy (Hellekson 1989; Kasper et al. 1989). There are also seasonal variations in most mood disorders. For example, unipolar depression is more likely to recur in the spring, whereas bipolar depression is more likely to recur in the fall and mania is more likely to recur during the summer (Barbini et al. 1995). Contrary to popular wisdom, the time of greatest risk of suicide is not during the Christmas holidays but during the months of May and June (Hellekson 1989). The time of the seasonal peak in the incidence of suicide is independent of latitude, but the amplitude of the peak is greatest where there is the greatest seasonal variation in light (Hellekson 1989). Hospital admissions for unipolar depression peak in the spring, whereas admissions for mania peak in the summer (Hellekson 1989). The observations that seasonal variations in mood disorders in the Southern hemisphere are the reverse of those in the Northern Hemisphere (e.g., more admissions for mania during the winter) and that the pattern of seasonal affective disorder (SAD) is the reverse in the Northern and Southern Hemispheres support the hypothesis that these changes are dependent on variations in available daylight (Hellekson 1989).

SAD was defined by Norman Rosenthal and associates (Hellekson 1989) as a condition that meets criteria for an RDC major affective disorder in which major depression occurs during the fall or winter for at least 2 consecutive years, with remission in the spring or summer. In SAD, depressive episodes cannot be associated with seasonal stressors, and no other Axis I diagnoses can be present. DSM-IV criteria (Table 13–14) are derived from the criteria of Rosenthal et al. (Hellekson 1989) and include additional provisos that hypomania as well as remission of depression may occur during the summer and that seasonal depressive episodes should substantially outnumber nonseasonal episodes (American Psychiatric Association 1994a). In DSM-IV, a seasonal pattern is considered to be not a separate diagnosis but an additional specifier of major depressive disorder (MDD) with recurrent depression, bipolar I disorder, or bipolar II disorder. As we noted in the previous paragraph, the well-described pattern of winter depression and summer euthymia or hypomania is reversed in the Southern Hemisphere (Hellekson 1989). In the Northern Hemisphere, a reverse SAD, in which patients become depressed in the summer, seems related to seasonal changes in temperature and humidity rather than changes in light (Hellekson 1989).

SAD occurs more frequently in women than in men; the female-to-male ratio is greater than it is in nonseasonal MDD (Hellekson 1989). SAD occurs in children as well as adults (Hellekson 1989). In a survey of centers specializing in the treatment of SAD (Hellekson 1989), the most common symptoms reported during depressive episodes were sadness, irritability, anxiety, decreased activity, increased appetite with carbohydrate craving, increased weight, increased sleep, daytime drowsiness, work and interpersonal problems, and menstrual difficulties. Symptoms began in November in Washington, D.C., and in late August in Alaska; this finding added to the data supporting the role of shortening of the day as the precipitant of seasonal depression. The mean duration of depressive symptoms across centers was about 5–6 months. More than half the patients had a family history of affective disorder, and many had a family history of SAD.

In some samples, the majority of patients with SAD have summer hypomania and therefore meet criteria for a diagnosis of bipolar II disorder; in other samples the incidence of hypomania is low (Hellekson 1989). Some of the discrepancy may be a function of the frequency with which increased energy, decreased sleep, and related experiences during the summer are viewed as hypomania or simply relief of depression. More data are needed to determine how frequently SAD is bipolar and how frequently it is unipolar. There is greater agreement about the presence of atypical depressive symptoms in the winter depressions of SAD (Hellekson 1989).

TABLE 13–14. DSM-IV seasonal pattern specifier

A. There has been a regular temporal relationship between the onset of major depressive episodes in bipolar I or bipolar II disorder or major depressive episode, recurrent, and a particular time of the year (e.g., regular appearance of the major depressive episode in the fall or winter).

Note: Do not include cases in which there is an obvious effect of seasonal-related psychosocial stressors (e.g., regularly being unemployed every winter).

B. Full remission (or a change from depression to mania or hypomania) also occurs at a characteristic time of the year (e.g., depression disappears in the spring).

C. In the last 2 years, two major depressive episodes have occurred that demonstrate the temporal seasonal relationships defined in Criteria A and B, and no nonseasonal major depressive episodes have occurred during that same period.

D. Seasonal major depressive episodes (as described above) substantially outnumber the nonseasonal major depressive episodes that may have occurred over the individual's lifetime.

SECONDARY MOOD DISORDERS

In some circles, the term *secondary mood disorder* is used to indicate a mood disorder having another cause—for example, a medical illness or use of a medication. To other experts, a secondary mood disorder is a mood disorder that occurs in the context of another disorder, such as schizophrenia or an anxiety disorder, with etiology not necessarily being implied (Knesper 1995; M. T. Tsuang and Faraone 1996). DSM-IV implies causality of secondary mood disorders with the phrases *mood disorder due to a general medical disorder* (mood disorder caused by a medical or surgical illness; see Table 13–15) and *substance-induced mood disorder* (mood disorder caused by a medication or a psychoactive substance; see Table 13–16) ("Drugs That Cause Psychiatric Symptoms" 1993; Long and Kathol 1993).

The other meaning of secondary mood disorder has been addressed in two ways in DSM-IV. Although it is permissible to make a diagnosis of a mood disorder in a patient with another Axis I disorder such as schizophrenia, chronic affective symptoms that occur exclusively during the course of a psychotic disorder such as schizophrenia are not given a separate diagnosis of a depressive disorder (First et

TABLE 13–15. Some medical conditions that can cause manic or depressive syndromes

Neurological disease: Parkinson's disease, Huntington's disease, traumatic brain injury, stroke, dementias, multiple sclerosis

Metabolic disease: Electrolyte disturbances, renal failure, vitamin deficiencies or excess, acute intermittent porphyria, Wilson's disease, environmental toxins, heavy metals

Gastrointestinal disease: Irritable bowel syndrome, chronic pancreatitis, Crohn's disease, cirrhosis, hepatic encephalopathy

Endocrine disorders: Hypo- and hyperthyroidism, Cushing's disease, Addison's disease, diabetes mellitus, parathyroid dysfunction

Cardiovascular disease: Myocardial infarction, angina, coronary artery bypass surgery, cardiomyopathies

Pulmonary disease: Chronic obstructive pulmonary disease, sleep apnea, reactive airway disease

Malignancies and hematologic disease: Pancreatic carcinoma, brain tumors, paraneoplastic effects of lung cancers, anemias

Autoimmune disease: Systemic lupus erythematosis, fibromyalgia, rheumatoid arthritis

---

al. 1996). The purpose of this approach is to avoid implying meaningless comorbidity. In addition, mood disorders that are truly secondary to another condition have a poorer treatment response than primary mood disorders (Knesper 1995). On the other hand, if affective symptoms are considered secondary to the psychotic (or other) Axis I illness, treatment may be directed only toward the "primary" disorder, and coexisting mood disorders that might respond to therapies directed specifically toward them could be overlooked. Differentiating between comorbidity of a mood disorder with another Axis I condition and affective symptoms that are manifestations of another disorder therefore has important clinical implications.

MOOD DISORDERS IN CHILDREN AND ADOLESCENTS

When it was thought that the child's superego was too immature to experience depression or mania (which was considered a defense against depression), childhood depression was thought to be very rare. As a result, DSM-I did not include psychiatric disorders of children, and DSM-II included only behavioral disorders of children. However, it is now known that depression can be diagnosed in children

as young as 3 years old. Consequently, DSM-III and DSM-III-R criteria for juvenile mood disorders were similar to those for adult mood disorders except that irritability could substitute for depressed mood, failure to maintain weight gain could substitute for weight loss, decreased school performance could substitute for decreased occupational function, and loss of interest in friends and play could substitute for loss of interest or pleasure. Symptom duration for a diagnosis of dysthymia in children and adolescents was established as 1 year; in adults, the required duration is 2 years (Kashani and Nair 1995). These criteria have not been changed substantially in DSM-IV.

Because of continued disagreement about the nature of juvenile mood disorders, estimates of prevalence and incidence vary. When the Schedule for Affective Disorders and Schizophrenia for School Age Children (K-SADS) was administered to 1,710 adolescents ages 14–18 years, almost 30% had at least one current depressive symptom, the most common symptoms being depressed mood, disturbed sleep, problems thinking, and anhedonia (Roberts et al. 1995). However, only 2.6% of the sample met full criteria for a current diagnosis of a mood disorder. In contrast to adults in other studies, adolescents in this study who had experienced two episodes of major depression had different symptoms during each episode. Other reports suggest that childhood mood disorders have more familial loading than adult mood disorders and that when children from depressed families become depressed, the depression occurs earlier than does depression in children of families that are not depressed (ages 12–13 years vs. ages 16–17 years) (Geller et al. 1996). These kinds of findings suggest that inherited factors may be more important in juvenile mood disorders. Mood disorders in younger patients, as in adults, present a definite risk of suicide, as does substance use (Marttunen et al. 1995; Shaffer et al. 1996).

One area of ongoing investigation is the presentation of bipolar disorder in children and adolescents. Compared with adult bipolar disorder, juvenile bipolar disorder is characterized by more irritability, dysphoria, psychosis, hyperactivity, mixed mania, rapid cycling, chronicity, and familial loading (Faedda et al. 1995; Geller et al. 1995). An important question is whether a first episode of major depression in a younger patient is more likely than a first episode in an adult to be the initial presentation of a bipolar mood disorder (i.e., to be followed by the later development of mania or hypomania) (Akiskal 1995a; Kashani and Nair 1995). When conservative criteria are used, it is found that between 5% and 15% of cases of major depression in adults are bipolar (Bebbington 1995; Geller et al. 1996), compared with at least 20% of cases among adolescents and 32% of cases among children ages less than 11 years (Geller

TABLE 13-16. Some medications that can cause mania or depression

Drug	Reaction	Comments
Acyclovir	Psychosis, depression	At high doses
Alcohol	Depression, withdrawal, mania	
Amantadine	Psychosis, mania	More frequent in elderly
Amphetamine-like drugs	Psychosis, mania, anxiety, withdrawal, depression	
Anabolic steroids	Mania, depression, psychosis	
Anticonvulsants	Depression, mania	Usually with high doses or blood levels
Antidepressants	Mania, anxiety; abulia with SSRIs	Mania to hypomania in 0.5%–10% of patients
Asparaginase	Depression, paranoia	May occur frequently
Baclofen	Psychosis, mania, depression	Sometimes with treatment and high doses, but usually with sudden withdrawal
Barbiturates	Depression, excitement	Especially in children and elderly
Benzodiazepines	Depression, psychosis, mania	During treatment and withdrawal
β-Adrenergic blockers	Depression, confusion, mania	With usual doses, including ophthalmologic use
Bromocriptine	Mania, psychosis, depression	Not dose related; may persist for weeks after drug is stopped
Bupropion	Mania, psychosis, agitation	Can aggravate schizophrenia
Buspirone	Mania, panic attack	In a few patients
Captopril	Mania, anxiety, psychosis	Especially in depressed patients
Carbamazepine	See Anticonvulsants	
Chloroquine	Psychosis, mania	Several reports
Clonidine	Depression	May resolve with continued use
Contraceptives, oral	Depression	In 15% in 1 study
Corticosteroids	Mania, depression, psychosis	Especially with high doses or withdrawal
Cyclobenzaprine	Mania, psychosis	Several reports
Cycloserine	Anxiety, depression, psychosis	Common
Cyclosporine	Psychosis, mania	Each in 1 patient
Dapsone	Psychosis, mania, depression	Several reports, even with low doses
DEET	Mania, psychosis	With excessive or prolonged use
Digitalis glycosides	Psychosis, depression	Especially with high doses or blood levels
Diltiazem	Depression, suicidal thoughts	Reported in 8 patients
Disopyramide	Psychosis, depression	Within 24–48 hours of starting
Disulfiram	Depression, psychosis	Not related to alcohol reactions
Enalapril	Depression, psychosis	2 reports
Ethionamide	Depression, psychosis	Multiple reports
Etretinate	Severe depression	
Fenfluramine	See Amphetamine-like drugs	
Histamine H_2-receptor antagonists	Psychosis, depression, mania	Usually with high doses, more often in elderly, and with renal dysfunction
HMG-CoA reductase inhibitors	Depression	In several patients, may be rare
Interferon-α	Delirium, psychosis, depression, suicidal thoughts	In 10 of 58 patients with viral hepatitis; depression may be treated with fluoxetine

(continued)

TABLE 13–16. Some medications that can cause mania or depression *(continued)*

Drug	Reaction	Comments
Isocarboxazid	See Monoamine oxidase inhibitors	Mania and psychosis in 2 patients during withdrawal
Isoniazid	Depression, psychosis	Several reports
Isosorbide	Psychosis, depression	In 1 elderly woman on 2 occasions
Isotretinoin	Depression	Several reports
Levodopa	Depression, hypomania, psychosis	More common in elderly or with prolonged use
L-Glutamine	Grandiosity, hyperactivity	In 2 men
Loxapine	Mania	In 1 man
Mefloquine	Psychosis, depression	Several reports
Methyldopa	Depression, psychosis	Several reports
Metoclopramide	Mania, severe depression, crying	Several reports
Metrizamide	Psychosis, depression	May be prolonged
Metronidazole	Depression, crying, psychosis	2 cases with oral use
Monoamine oxidase inhibitors	Mania, psychosis	
Nalidixic acid	Depression	Rare
Narcotics	Euphoria, dysphoria, depression, psychosis	Usually with high doses
Nifedipine	Irritability, depression	Several reports
Nonsteroidal anti-inflammatory drugs	Psychosis, depression	Not reported with all drugs in this class
Norfloxacin	Depression	
Ofloxacin	Depression, mania	Single reports of each
Penicillin G procaine	See Procaine derivatives	
Pergolide	Psychosis, depression	On withdrawal
Phenelzine	See Monoamine oxidase inhibitors	
Phentermine	See Amphetamine-like drugs	
Phenylephrine	Depression, psychosis	Overuse of nasal spray; single report with oral use
Phenylpropanolamine	See Amphetamine-like drugs	
Phenytoin	See Anticonvulsants	
Prazosin	Psychosis, depression	In 4 patients, 2 had renal failure
Procaine derivatives	Psychosis, depression, anxiety	Many reports, especially with penicillin G procaine
Procarbazine	Mania	In 2 children
Propafenone	Psychosis, mania	Several reports
Pseudoephedrine	Psychosis, mania	Reported with usual doses in children and with overuse in 1 adult
Quinacrine	Mania, psychosis	More common with high doses
Reserpine	Depression	Common with > 0.5 mg/day
Selegiline	See Monoamine oxidase inhibitors	
Sulfonamides	Depression, euphoria	Several reports
Theophylline	Mania, depression	Usually with high serum concentrations
Thiazides	Depression, suicidal ideation	In several patients after weeks to months of use

(continued)

TABLE 13–16. **Some medications that can cause mania or depression** (*continued*)

Drug	Reaction	Comments
Thyroid hormones	Mania, depression, psychosis	Initial doses in susceptible patients
Tranylcypromine	See Monoamine oxidase inhibitors	Hypomania or mania in up to 10% of depressed patients
Trimethoprim-sulfamethoxazole	Psychosis, depression	Several reports
Valproic acid	See Anticonvulsants	
Vinblastine	Depression	
Vincristine	Depression	
Zidovudine	Mania, psychosis	Reported in 2 patients

Note. DEET = diethyltoluamide; HMG-CoA = hepatic hydroxymethylglutaryl-coenzyme A; SSRI = selective serotonin reuptake inhibitor.

et al. 1996). Features that juvenile major depressive episodes share with bipolar disorder include an early age at onset, equal numbers of males and females affected, mood lability, a high rate of recurrence, prominent irritability and explosive anger suggestive of mixed bipolar episodes, and a relatively poor response to antidepressants (Akiskal 1995a). In addition, juvenile major depressive episodes are often associated with cyclothymic or hyperthymic temperaments (Akiskal 1995a).

The diagnostic challenge implied by these kinds of observations is to identify those juvenile patients with major depressive episodes who are at greater risk of a bipolar outcome and who might have a better ultimate response to mood-stabilizing treatments than to antidepressants. Features of major depressive episodes in younger patients listed in Table 13–17 have been found to be associated with the eventual occurrence of mania (Akiskal 1995a, 1995b; Strober and Carlson 1982). Although no predictive studies exist regarding the prognostic validity of these features, their regular occurrence in younger patients with bipolar disorder is reason for caution in treating juvenile major depression. One of these factors in particular warrants additional discussion. As we noted earlier, hypomania that occurs only when antidepressants are being taken is excluded in DSM-IV as a diagnostic criterion for bipolar disorder in

TABLE 13–17. **Features associated with a bipolar outcome in juvenile major depression**

Early onset

Acute onset

Psychotic symptoms, especially hallucinations

Significant psychomotor slowing

Family history of bipolar disorder

Any mood disorder in three consecutive generations

Antidepressant-induced hypomania

adults because not all patients with this experience will become manic spontaneously. However, several small studies of depressed adolescents and children indicate a very high rate of spontaneous mania or hypomania following antidepressant-induced hypomania (Akiskal 1995a, 1995b, 1996).

Difficulty recognizing juvenile bipolar disorder accounts for the recent finding that half of the children who fulfilled diagnostic criteria for mania had received a different diagnosis (Kashani and Nair 1995). A controversial area of diagnostic confusion concerns attention-deficit/hyperactivity disorder (ADHD). Some reports suggest a familial link between juvenile bipolar disorder and ADHD, and these conditions are frequently diagnosed together (Biederman 1995). For example, in a study in which 28% of 270 psychiatric inpatients ages 5–18 years given the K-SADS met criteria for ADHD, 36% of the patients with ADHD met criteria for nonpsychotic depression, 8% met criteria for an affective psychosis, and 22% met criteria for bipolar disorder (Butler et al. 1995); there was no follow-up to determine how many of the depressed patients developed mania.

Clinical experience also suggests that ADHD and bipolar disorder are often diagnosed in the same patient, but it is not clear whether this means that the two disorders are frequently comorbid or that the symptoms of the two disorders overlap, so that patients who meet criteria for one condition will regularly also meet criteria for the other (Butler et al. 1995). The latter point is illustrated in Table 13–18 (American Psychiatric Association 1994a; Kashani and Nair 1995).

Most patients with bipolar disorder meet criteria for ADHD, but patients with ADHD do not meet most criteria for bipolar disorder. For example, elation, depression, decreased need for sleep, hypersomnia, grandiosity, psychosis, and rapid, pressured speech are not characteristic of ADHD (Biederman 1995; Kashani and Nair 1995) except

TABLE 13–18. Common features of juvenile bipolar disorder and attention-deficit/hyperactivity disorder (ADHD)

ADHD	Bipolar disorder[a]
Mood lability, temper outbursts	Mood lability, temper outbursts
Fails to give close attention to detail	(Racing thoughts, impulsivity)
Difficulty sustaining attention	Racing thoughts
Does not listen when spoken to directly	Self-involvement
Does not follow through	(Impulsivity, distractibility, tangential thinking, changeable direction of effort driven by mood swings)
Difficulty organizing tasks and activities	(Disorganization, changeable focus of attention, impulsivity)
Loses things necessary for tasks	(Distractibility, impulsivity)
Easily distracted	Distractibility
Forgetful in daily activities	(Fluctuating interest and motivation)
Fidgets or squirms	(Increased levels of activity)
Leaves seat when remaining seated is expected	Increased energy
Runs about or climbs excessively	Increased activity
Difficulty playing quietly	Increased energy and activity
Often on the go or as if driven by a motor	Increased energy and activity
Talks excessively	Pressure of speech
Blurts out answers before questions have been completed	Racing thoughts
Difficulty awaiting turn	(Impulsivity, increased energy)
Interrupts or intrudes on others	(Impulsivity, grandiose self-centeredness)

[a]DSM-IV symptoms of bipolar disorder that could be mistaken for ADHD symptoms and features of bipolar disorder not formally listed as diagnostic criteria for bipolar disorder are noted in parentheses.

as manifestations of stimulant toxicity. Racing and tangential thinking may be difficult to differentiate from the kind of talkativeness that is encountered in patients with ADHD, but an increased content of thought, especially with multiple coexisting complex ideas and plans, is more suggestive of bipolar disorder than ADHD. Irritability, fighting, and thrill seeking can be encountered in both disorders, but attacks of rage that provoke prolonged organized attacks on others in response to threats to self-esteem and attempts to control the patient are more common in bipolar disorder, as is the kind of grandiosity that leads to fighting multiple opponents, fearlessness in the face of overwhelming odds, and jumping from extreme heights with the belief that one cannot be hurt and a response of hilarity on being injured. Historical elements listed in Table 13–17 are more common in bipolar disorder, although, as we noted earlier, bipolar disorder and ADHD may aggregate in the same families. Finally, bipolar disorder may be more common in tertiary care centers, given that uncomplicated ADHD is usually treated successfully in the offices of psychiatrists, pediatricians, and family physicians.

A study of 140 boys ages 6–17 years with diagnoses of ADHD attempted to address the question of symptomatic overlap by rediagnosing patients after specific symptoms of ADHD listed in Table 13–18 had been subtracted (Milberger et al. 1995). Seventy-nine percent of the patients still met criteria for MDD, 56% met criteria for bipolar disorder, and 75% met criteria for generalized anxiety disorder. One interpretation of these findings is that a number of other disorders may share characteristics sufficiently similar to those of ADHD (and each other) to result in diagnostic confusion between these conditions. A positive response to stimulants is often interpreted as evidence in favor of a diagnosis of ADHD, but the effect of stimulants in enhancing attention is not specific to ADHD. In addition, depressed patients with slowed thinking may show improvement of attention with stimulants, and some manic patients have been noted to experience calming and behavioral slowing in response to stimulants (Max et al. 1995). Although no controlled studies have addressed this issue, adolescent and young adult patients are encountered in practice who were apparently treated successfully with stimulants or antidepressants for ADHD, only to develop dysphoric manic symptoms such as increasing irritability, anxiety, impulsivity, thrill seeking, grandiose defiance, mood swings, and psychosis with continued treatment. It is impossible to know whether long-term treatment with stimulants eventually destabilized mood in patients with bipolar disorders misdiagnosed as ADHD or whether the adverse outcome represented the natural progression of bipolar disorder.

Deciding whether to institute treatment for bipolar disorder, ADHD, or both in situations in which a juvenile patient might qualify for either diagnosis is not easy. Stimulants probably have fewer adverse effects and are easier to monitor than mood-stabilizing medications. With the possible exception of clonidine, medications used to treat bipolar disorder have never been thought to be helpful for ADHD, but they do not have any special risks in patients with ADHD beyond physical adverse effects. Stimulants may temporarily improve mood in bipolar individuals, but there is a risk that they could induce mania and/or rapid cycling, which is more difficult to treat than less complicated forms of bipolar disorder. It would therefore seem prudent to initiate therapy with a mood-stabilizing medication in unclear cases. If the elevated rate of co-occurrence of bipolar disorder and ADHD is evidence of comorbidity as well as of symptom overlap, a distinct subpopulation will have both disorders. In this case, ADHD symptoms should persist after treatment of the mood disorder, at which time the need for additional treatment of ADHD can be assessed.

MOOD DISORDERS AND CREATIVITY

An association between mood disorders, especially bipolar mood disorders, and creativity has been noted for some time. Reviews of the histories of prominent artists and writers suggest that some, including Honoré de Balzac, F. Scott Fitzgerald (and his wife, Zelda), Ernest Hemingway, Randall Jarrell, Charles Lamb, Robert Lowell, Theodore Roethke, Delmore Schwartz, Anne Sexton, and Virginia Woolf, had bipolar disorder (Jamison 1996). Andreasen (1987) found that 80% of 30 writers at a creative writing workshop had at least one episode of affective illness and 43% had a history of hypomania or mania; the relatives of these writers also had elevated rates both of mood disorders and creativity. In a study of 20 award-winning European writers, painters, and sculptors, Akiskal found that two-thirds had recurrent cyclothymia or hypomania and half had depressive episodes (Jamison 1996).

Psychologist Kay Redfield Jamison, an influential researcher and writer who described her own experience with a bipolar mood disorder (Jamison 1995), found that 38% of distinguished British writers and visual artists had been treated for a mood disorder (Jamison 1996). In her book *Touched With Fire: Manic-Depressive Illness and the Artistic Temperament*, Jamison (1993) reviewed the personal histories of well-known artists and writers with mood disorders, many of them bipolar. Other biographical studies, as well as studies of living artists, demonstrate that compared with the general population, individuals who are successful in the arts are up to 18 times as likely to commit suicide, 8–10 times as likely to have major depressive episodes, and 10–20 times as likely to have a bipolar mood disorder (Jamison 1996).

The apparent link between mood disorders and creativity has yet to be examined systematically. One possibility is that elevated energy and expansive thinking of manic and hypomanic individuals may contribute to increased frequency of ideas and an increased rate and content of thought may result in unique ways of synthesizing ideas (Jamison 1996). High levels of energy and of mental and physical activity can enhance productivity, but productivity is usually uneven and at times impulsive, and periods of energetic hyperactivity are often interrupted by episodes of depressive inaction. Another possibility is that ordinary situations are experienced so intensely by people with mood disorders that they can be communicated more powerfully to others, although an active mood disorder is at least as likely to make the artist feel overwhelmed and disorganized by minor events. It is also conceivable that artistic people with mood disorders are more likely to put themselves in adverse situations that result in the kinds of experiences that can be successfully represented in their art, and it may be that some mood disorders are genetically linked to creative temperaments.

Lest mood disorders, and bipolar illness in particular, be romanticized as a condition that is necessary for artistic success, it is important to note that most people with mood disorders are not particularly creative (Jamison 1996) and many highly creative people do not have mood disorders. There is no evidence that an active mood disorder actually improves creativity or that successful treatment hinders an artist's career. If anything, treatment of mood disorders improves productivity (Jamison 1993) and can make an artist's work more comprehensible and organized.

CATEGORICAL VERSUS DIMENSIONAL DIAGNOSES

The DSM-III/DSM-IV approach to diagnosis has its limitations (M. T. Tsuang and Faraone 1996), but it has facilitated achieving a consensus about the number and kinds of symptoms that define a particular disorder so that more homogeneous populations can be defined and treatment outcomes can be better studied. Symptom specifiers such as *with atypical features* and course modifiers such as *seasonal pattern* represent a preliminary attempt to enhance the categorical approach to define subtypes of mood disorders. However, no categorical diagnosis in psychiatry is as uniform as is suggested in the diagnostic manual (S.-L. Brown et al. 1994). Some people with bipolar disorder have many manic episodes and some do not. Some depressed people who never experience a hint of mania have recurrences more frequently than do patients with bipolar depression.

Some patients with bipolar depression become psychotic, as do some unipolar patients. Some depressed people are very aggressive or suicidal, and some are not. Some people who are prone to depression have had traumatic experiences early in life, some have had families who misunderstood or did not care about them, and some have had highly supportive families. Some kinds of depression start early in life without any particular precipitant, some occur only after a stress, and some appear for the first time in later years. Some mood disorders are associated with substantial character pathology, and some are not. Some are accompanied by medical comorbidity, and some are not.

Mood disorders are diverse physiologically as well as phenomenologically. Within a given DSM-IV diagnosis (e.g., MDD), some subtypes are accompanied by one of the biological markers described later in this chapter, some by a different marker, and some by no known marker. Some patients have obvious familial transmission of a mood disorder that has similar manifestations in most family members, and some have sporadic illnesses. Some manic episodes respond to lithium, some to an anticonvulsant, and some to combinations of treatments. Even within the same individual, the presentation and treatment response of affective episodes may vary from one episode to the next.

Within categorical constraints, there are therefore many dimensions of abnormal mood, and the expression of a given type of mood disorder will depend on the net interaction between these factors (Figure 13–1). This is not to say that every depressed person is different from every other depressed person; rather, more categories of depression, and more treatment options, exist in real life than are listed in the textbooks. As more knowledge accumulates about the importance of specific dimensions of depression, it may become possible to make dimensional as well as categorical diagnoses that suggest more specific treatment options.

COMORBIDITY

Mood disorders are frequently comorbid with other psychiatric and medical conditions (Weissman et al. 1996), especially anxiety, substance-related, eating, somatoform, and personality disorders and chronic medical illnesses (Conte and Karasu 1992; Howland 1993; Marin et al. 1993; J. C. Perry 1985). In a recent study of this issue, 11,701 medically ill patients were compared with 9,039 psychiatric patients in the Department of Veterans Affairs database (Moos and Mertens 1996). As many as 60% of patients with mood disorders treated in mental health set-

tings had a comorbid psychiatric diagnosis, as did 30% of mood disorder patients treated in medical settings. Eighty percent of the psychiatric patients had comorbid medical conditions.

MEDICAL ILLNESS

The prevalence of major depressive episodes in patients with malignancies has been reported to be around 50% in those with pancreatic cancer, 22%–40% in those with cancer of the oropharynx, 10%–32% in patients with breast cancer, 13%–25% in those with colon cancer, and 23%, 17%, and 11%, respectively, in patients with gynecological cancer, lymphoma, and gastric carcinoma (McDaniel et al. 1995). Depression was found in 16% of bone marrow transplantation patients (Fann and Tucker 1995). Major depression occurs at increased rates in patients with myocardial infarction, ventricular arrhythmias, and congestive heart failure (Franco-Bronson 1996). Major depression has been found to increase the risk of developing coronary heart disease and to increase mortality after myocardial infarction (Barefoot and Schroll 1996). Hypothyroidism is very common in depressed patients, especially in those with treatment-refractory mood disorders and rapid-cycling bipolar disorder (Franco-Bronson 1996). Much of the hypothyroidism that occurs in depressed patients is caused by thyroiditis, which suggests a link between susceptibility loci for major depression and thyroiditis. There appears to be a similar link between migraine headaches and MDD. Additional medical conditions frequently associated with depression include irritable bowel syndrome, fibromyalgia, chronic fatigue

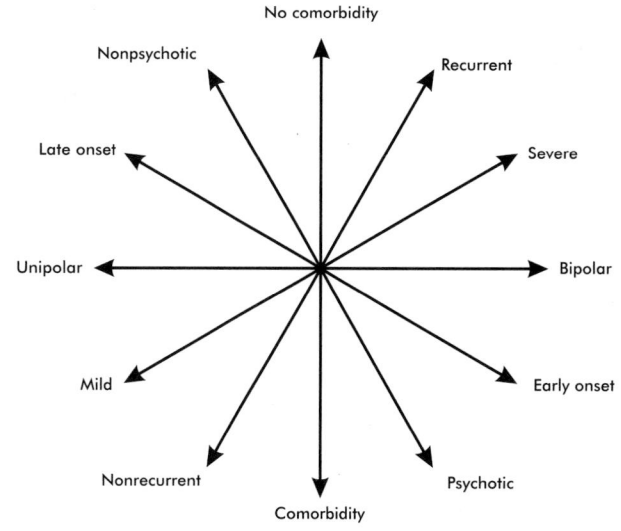

FIGURE 13–1. Dimensions of mood disorders.

syndrome, acquired immunodeficiency syndrome, renal failure, and autoimmune disease (Franco-Bronson 1996; Gruber et al. 1996).

A number of neurological illnesses are also associated with an increased risk of mood disorders (Fann and Tucker 1995). Between 8% and 75% of patients with cerebrovascular accidents develop major depression; in one study, depressed stroke patients had an eightfold risk of mortality compared with matched nondepressed stroke patients (P. L. P. Morris et al. 1993). Anatomic location of the stroke appears to have a marked effect on the prevalence of associated depression: left prefrontal and basal ganglia strokes more frequently result in depressive disorders than do right hemisphere lesions (P. L. P. Morris et al. 1993). Conversely, right hemisphere lesions are often associated with development of secondary mania (Berthier et al. 1996). Depression is the most frequent psychiatric complication of Parkinson's disease, possibly because of the participation of the basal ganglia in mood regulation (Klassen et al. 1995).

Depression is also frequently comorbid with Alzheimer's disease: about 50% of patients with Alzheimer's disease meet criteria for major depression or dysthymia (Petracca et al. 1996). Roughly 2%–3.8% of Alzheimer's disease patients develop mania (Fann and Tucker 1995). Despite the fact that the pattern of dementia is cortical in Alzheimer's disease and subcortical in the dementia syndrome of depression, it can be impossible to distinguish one from the other clinically, and depression can aggravate the dementia of Alzheimer's disease. The interaction of depression and dementia was discussed earlier in this chapter. The incidence of depression is also increased in temporal lobe epilepsy, AIDS, Huntington's disease, traumatic brain injury, spinal cord injury, and multiple sclerosis, and AIDS can also present as mania (Blumer et al. 1995; Fann and Tucker 1995; Kishi and Robinson 1996; T. F. Scott et al. 1996).

ANXIETY DISORDERS

Anxiety is a prominent symptom in as many as 70% of depressed outpatients (Rosenbaum et al. 1995). In addition, comorbidity of specific mood and anxiety disorders has been found consistently in large studies (Weissman et al. 1996). The NIMH Collaborative Program on the Psychobiology of Depression, a community survey, found that 32% of depressed patients had phobias, 31% had panic attacks, and 11% had obsessions or compulsions (Glass et al. 1989). Conversely, major depressive episodes have been reported in 8%–39% of patients with generalized anxiety disorder (Brawman-Mintzer and Lydiard

1996), 50%–90% of patients with panic disorder, 35%–70% of patients with social phobia, and 33% of patients with obsessive-compulsive disorder (OCD) (Gorman and Coplan 1996). Social phobia has been reported in more than 40% of patients with MDD (Bruder et al. 1997). Bipolar illness is also more common in patients with panic disorder and OCD (Strakowski et al. 1994).

There are a number of possible associations between mood and anxiety disorders. Many kinds of distress in depressed patients can be grouped by patients as well as independent raters under the rubric of *anxiety* (Bruder et al. 1997), and patients may describe arousal and dysphoria as anxiety at one point and depression at another. Some patients cannot tell the difference between anxiety and depression, and some of the items on mood rating scales such as the Hamilton Rating Scale for Depression are symptoms of anxiety. In other patients, anxiety may reflect a separate disorder that occurs at a higher-than-expected rate in depressed patients; this rate may be higher because one disorder lowers the threshold for the expression of the other or because susceptibility to one disorder is linked to susceptibility to the other. Manic overstimulation may be expressed as panic attacks, which can be distinguished from panic disorder by the presence of racing thoughts and a sense of having too much energy. Anxiety in patients with bipolar mood disorders is often an indication of mixed (dysphoric) states, which are more difficult to treat.

Anxiety and mood disorders may alternate with as well as accompany each other. A group of patients with depressive disorders followed prospectively are rediagnosed with anxiety disorders, and patients with initial diagnoses of anxiety disorders may receive a later diagnosis of a mood disorder (Kovacs et al. 1989). In some instances, the predominance of one or the other symptom may represent a prodromal phase of a mood disorder in which both anxiety and depression are important symptoms. The extent to which one disorder is emphasized over the other (e.g., depression with secondary anxiety or anxiety with secondary depression) may be more a matter of features that strike the examiner or the patient at a particular moment than of the nature of the illness.

In addition to their comorbidity, depression, mania, and anxiety as dimensions of affective experience have complex overlap and interactions with each other. Anxiety in depressed patients increases severity, chronicity, and impairment associated with depression and makes depression more refractory to treatment; anxiety also increases the risk of suicide in depressed patients, perhaps because it is a marker of higher levels of arousal (Keck et al. 1994; Rudd et al. 1993). Depressed people who are anxious have more anxious people in their families, and they also have more depressed relatives (Breier et al. 1985; Clayton et al. 1991). In these families, anxiety may be a marker of a risk factor for more severe, treatment-resistant, and/or familial depression (K. K. Kendler et al. 1987).

SUBSTANCE USE DISORDERS

Major mood disorders have high rates of comorbidity with use of many substances, especially alcohol (Maier et al. 1995b; Weissman et al. 1996). Alcohol abuse or dependence occurs in 50% of unipolar depression patients, 60% of bipolar I disorder patients, and 50% of bipolar II disorder patients (Feinman and Dunner 1996). Comorbid alcoholism worsens the course of both unipolar depression (Hasin et al. 1996) and bipolar disorder (Feinman and Dunner 1996). Conversely, abstinence improves the response of the mood disorder to treatment (Hasin et al. 1996).

Use of sedatives by manic patients to tone down dysphoric overstimulation is readily understandable. The reason some patients with bipolar mood disorders use stimulants to induce mania would be obvious if the mania were pleasurable, but substance-induced mania is frequently unpleasant. By purposely making themselves manic, some of these patients may be attempting to achieve a sense of mastery over fluctuations in mood that they otherwise feel helpless to control. Patients with mood disorders who are treated acutely with neuroleptics may note blunting of the rewarding properties of cocaine, but chronic neuroleptic therapy, which is common in patients who have been hospitalized for bipolar mood disorders (Sernyak and Woods 1993), may enhance the euphoric effects of cocaine.

SCHIZOPHRENIA

Major depressive episodes occur in 25%–50% of cases of schizophrenia (American Psychiatric Association 1993). The traditional belief that most of these episodes are "postpsychotic" and involve reactions to awareness of having a severe illness is contradicted by the finding that half of the depressive episodes occurring during the course of schizophrenia develop in the midst of an acute psychotic episode; the affective component, however, may become apparent only after the psychosis resolves (Dubovsky and Thomas 1992). Fears that administration of antidepressants may aggravate schizophrenia have been set aside by observations that in all but the most acute psychotic exacerbations, treatment of depression improves the prognosis of comorbid schizophrenia (Dubovsky and Thomas 1992).

PERSONALITY DISORDERS

Between 30% and 70% of depressed patients receive a concurrent diagnosis of a personality disorder (Thase 1996), usually in Cluster B (i.e., borderline, histrionic, and antisocial personality disorder) (Corruble et al. 1996). Similar diagnoses, along with narcissistic personality disorder, are often made in patients with bipolar mood disorders. At the same time, 95% of personality disorder patients who commit suicide have a comorbid Axis I diagnosis, usually depression (Isometsa et al. 1996). As we noted earlier, personality disorders may be diagnosed frequently in association with mood disorders because pathological defenses mobilized to deal with abnormal mood mimic character pathology. In support of this possibility, Thase's group (Thase 1996) found that when they reinterviewed depressed patients after successful treatment, the rate of personality disorder was half the rate before treatment.

There are a number of additional possible explanations for the association between mood and personality disorders (Riso et al. 1996; Thase 1996). One possibility is that certain personality traits or disorders may predispose to mood disorders. For example, an overly dependent patient might be more vulnerable to depression in response to loss of an important source of support. Or chronic mood disorders may skew experience in ways that lead to the development of personality disorders, as when grandiosity, impulsivity, and expansiveness associated with a bipolar mood disorder become integrated into a patient's habitual behavioral repertoire, leading to histrionic or narcissistic personality. Vulnerability to depression and to personality disorders may be inherited or acquired together, or common etiological factors may lead to both mood and personality disorders.

Patients with mood disorders who have comorbid personality disorders have more overall symptomatology and experience worse social adjustment than do mood disorder patients without personality disorders (Carpenter et al. 1995). Depressed patients with personality disorders are less responsive to antidepressants and electroconvulsive therapy (ECT) (Black et al. 1988; Thase 1996). The presence of a comorbid personality disorder has also been found to impair response to interpersonal therapy (Thase 1996). However, cognitive-behavior therapy has been reported to be equally effective in depressed patients with and without personality disorders (Shea et al. 1990; Stuart et al. 1992; Thase 1996).

In clinical practice, apparent comorbid personality disorders that actually reflect exaggeration of pathological character traits often are no longer problematic when the mood disorder responds to treatment. On the other hand, issues related to truly comorbid personality disorders such as self-destructive motivations, negative therapeutic reactions, and attachment to an identity as a depressed person can lead to noncompliance, turning of treatments against the clinician, and other behaviors that interfere with a positive response to treatment. The role of personality disorders is further complicated by a tendency of clinicians to attribute to a personality disorder the failure of depressed patients to respond as expected (Thase 1996). This kind of assessment may be premature if there is not a careful longitudinal assessment including an evaluation of the doctor-patient relationship.

STUDIES OF INHERITED FACTORS

Despite the progress made in DSM-IV and the Research Diagnostic Criteria toward defining homogeneous subtypes of mood disorders, there is enough remaining diversity of phenomenology and comorbidity to complicate studies of etiology. Research investigating causes of mood disorders is often contradictory and incomplete because all relevant features of the disorder are not included in each study.

When interpreting studies of etiological factors in mood disorders, it is important to be aware that it is not likely that there is a single cause of even the most rigidly defined mood disorder. There is no reason to think that any inborn factor causes mood disorders; such factors interact with experiential and other environmental influences to lead to illness. Etiologies considered in a single dimension are no less complex. One abnormal gene may produce an abnormal protein that produces a positive symptom, whereas another gene may fail to make a protein that regulates the emergence of the same symptom. A neurotransmitter may set in motion a chain of events that overlaps a second cascade initiated by another neurotransmitter, so that dysfunction of either transmitter can have the same end result. In the same manner, any one of a number of symptoms may be a cue for the entire symptom complex that is clinically called an *affective syndrome*. Bearing these limitations in mind, we will consider a number of areas of research and will then attempt to integrate the current state of knowledge about the causes of mood disorders.

FAMILY STUDIES

Family studies have repeatedly demonstrated that mood disorders are familial (M. T. Tsuang and Faraone 1996). Relatives of people with mood disorders are consistently two to three times as likely to have mood disorders than are relatives of controls (E. S. Gershon 1990). If one parent has a bipolar mood disorder, the risk that a child will have a unipolar or bipolar mood disorder is around 28%; if both parents have mood disorders, the risk is two to three times as great (Jamison 1996). Patients with mood disorders also have an elevated familial incidence of substance abuse (Geller et al. 1996), and patients who are depressed and anxious have more relatives who are depressed, anxious, or both (Breier et al. 1985; Gorman and Coplan 1996; K. K. Kendler et al. 1987).

Familial aggregation of mood disorders does not prove genetic transmission. Wealth and political affiliation also run in families, but they are not genetic. One way to begin to determine a genetic contribution is to compare the concordance of mood disorders in first- and second-degree relatives of probands with mood disorders. Because first-degree relatives (parents, children, and siblings) share 50% of their genomes, whereas only 25% of genes are identical in second-degree relatives (grandparents, uncles, aunts, nephews, and nieces), a greater rate of a mood disorder in first-degree relatives of individuals with the same disorder than in second-degree relatives of these individuals suggests a genetic influence (M. T. Tsuang and Faraone 1996). The expectation of a greater likelihood of mood disorders in first-degree relatives of patients with mood disorders than in second-degree relatives or control populations has usually been borne out (M. T. Tsuang and Faraone 1996).

Most studies suggest a more prominent familial transmission of bipolar than of unipolar mood disorders, often with affected relatives in consecutive generations. Family members of patients with bipolar disorder are more likely to have bipolar as well as unipolar mood disorders themselves than are family members of patients with unipolar disorders (Jamison 1996). However, the rate of bipolar disorder in the families of patients with unipolar depression is as much as three to four times the rate in controls (E. S. Gershon et al. 1982; Weissman et al. 1984). According to published family studies (E. S. Gershon et al. 1982; M. T. Tsuang and Faraone 1996; Weissman et al. 1984), first-degree relatives of patients with unipolar depression have a risk of unipolar depression of 5.5%–28.4% and a risk of bipolar disorder of 0.7%–8.1%; and first-degree relatives of probands with bipolar disorder have a 4.1%–14.6% likelihood of having a bipolar disorder themselves and a 5.4%–14% likelihood of having unipolar depression. As we noted earlier, bipolar II disorder "breeds true"; that is, bipolar II disorder patients have relatives who are hypomanic but not manic, whereas patients with bipolar I disorder have some relatives who are manic and some who are hypomanic (Jamison 1996).

TWIN STUDIES

Another approach to investigating genetic contributions to mood disorders is to study differences in concordance between monozygotic (MZ) (identical) and dizygotic (DZ) (fraternal) twins. MZ twins come from the same egg and have the same genes, whereas DZ twins come from different eggs and share 50% of their genes, like any other sibling. If the concordance rate for a disorder is greater in MZ twins than in DZ twins, it suggests a genetic influence because the role of intrauterine and postnatal environments is presumably similar for both kinds of twins (M. T. Tsuang and Faraone 1996). Concordance studies (Jamison 1996; M. T. Tsuang and Faraone 1996) reliably demonstrate that the overall risk of mood disorders is three times as great in MZ as in DZ twins of probands with mood disorders. For bipolar disorder, concordance rates average 0.67–1.0 for MZ and 0.20 for DZ twins. Concordance rates for unipolar depression are generally 0.50 in MZ twins and 0.20 in DZ twins. The greater difference in concordance rates between MZ and DZ twins in bipolar disorder may reflect a greater genetic influence in bipolar disorder.

The assumption that identical twins grow up in identical environments may not be entirely accurate. The phase of division of the egg at which two embryos begin to emerge differs in different MZ twin pairs, and this has potential implications for later development of the nervous system. Parents can usually tell MZ twins apart, and not all sets of MZ twins are exposed to the same interpersonal fields as they grow up. Concordance rates for mood disorders in MZ twins reared apart from infancy can help to differentiate genetic influences from potential differences in the postnatal environment. In one study, 8 of 12 MZ twins of probands with bipolar mood disorders had bipolar mood disorders themselves, a rate similar to the concordance rate of MZ twins of bipolar mood disorder patients reared with their ill twins (Jamison 1996).

Because concordance rates for mood disorders in twin studies are less than 100%, any genetic factors that are present must interact with environmental influences to create the risk for development of the actual disorder (M. T. Tsuang and Faraone 1996). Reviews of twin studies suggest that 21%–45% of the variance in the risk of depressive disorders can be attributed to genetic factors and 55%–75% of the variance can be attributed to environmental factors (K. K. Kendler et al. 1992b). A substantial amount (60%) of the effect of genetic factors appears to be direct, but 40% appears to reflect genetic factors that increase the likelihood that people will put themselves in situations that lead to depression (e.g., through heightened sensitivity to loss) (K. K. Kendler et al. 1993). Of the latter, stressful life events, especially losses, seem to be most influential (K. K. Kendler et al. 1993).

It was mentioned earlier that patients with major depression and comorbid anxiety have both anxiety and depression in their families. In support of this observation, K. K. Kendler et al. (1992a) reported that 1,033 pairs of female twins had increased concordance for both major depression and generalized anxiety disorder, agoraphobia, and social phobia. K. K. Kendler and his group (K. K. Kendler et al. 1987, 1992a, 1993) hypothesized that some common trait predisposing to anxiety and depression may be inherited and that which one predominates depends on experience.

ADOPTION STUDIES

The influence of the environment on the development of mood disorders can also be assessed by examining rates of mood disorders in adoptive and biological families of people who were adopted in infancy. Most of these studies report that adoptees with mood disorders are more likely to have biological than adoptive relatives with mood disorders (M. T. Tsuang and Faraone 1996). Because rates of bipolar disorder in adoptive families of probands with bipolar disorder are no greater than in the general population, whereas rates of bipolar disorder in the biological families of these adoptees are the same as those in bipolar individuals raised with bipolar family members, adoptive factors have little or no role in bipolar mood disorders (M. T. Tsuang and Faraone 1996). Adoptive studies suggest that genetic factors are most important in determining transmission of unipolar depression, but adoptive (i.e., environmental) mechanisms also play an important role; similar findings have emerged for transmission of suicide risk (M. T. Tsuang and Faraone 1996).

LINKAGE STUDIES

Less inferential studies of genetic factors examine linkage between biological phenotypes or genetic markers with mood disorders. Presumably, a gene or genes influencing development of the mood disorder would be close to the gene for the phenotype or the genetic marker that aggregates with the mood disorder. Linkage studies are most reliable for disorders that have a single dominant gene mode of transmission with complete penetrance, such as Huntington's disease. However, it is not clear whether the mode of transmission of most mood disorders involves one gene or is polygenic, and incomplete penetrance and variable expressivity are likely to be the rule (M. T. Tsuang and

Faraone 1996). Because the familial pattern of some bipolar mood disorders seems more consistent with a dominant mode of transmission, linkage studies of bipolar families have been most promising.

Red-green color blindness, a recessive X-linked trait, has been repeatedly linked to bipolar mood disorders in about one-third of cases studied (M. T. Tsuang and Faraone 1996). An X-linked factor near the gene for color blindness would be expected to demonstrate mother-to-son transmission, which is observed in some bipolar families. Of three linkage studies involving glucose-6-phosphate dehydrogenase (G6PD) deficiency, the gene for which is thought to be close to the gene for color blindness, findings of one supported and findings of another were highly suggestive of linkage of G6PD deficiency to bipolar disorder (M. T. Tsuang and Faraone 1996). A study of the F9 DNA marker on the X chromosome suggested linkage to bipolar disorder, but studies of other DNA markers from the same region did not reveal such linkage (M. T. Tsuang and Faraone 1996). Results of studies of linkage of bipolar mood disorder to different traits thought to be carried on the X chromosome may not have been more consistent because some bipolar subtypes in some families may have X-linkage, whereas others do not. Additional reasons for apparently contradictory findings in linkage studies are discussed later in this section.

Attempts to link human leukocyte antigen (HLA) phenotypes to bipolar mood disorders have generally been unsuccessful (M. T. Tsuang and Faraone 1996). The fact that bipolar disorder and thalassemia minor cosegregated in a family seemed to suggest linkage to a gene on the short arm of chromosome 11 close to the HRAS1 locus, because thalassemia minor is caused by a mutation at that locus (Joffe et al. 1986). This possibility was interesting because HRAS may be involved in the translation of experience into changes in neuronal functioning (Post 1992b). However, these results have not been replicated. An association between bipolar mood disorder and blood type O, the gene for which is on chromosome 9, was found in one report (Lavori et al. 1984). This finding was also of theoretical interest because the ABO blood type gene is close to the gene for dopamine β-hydroxylase; however, additional studies have rejected the concept of linkage of bipolar disorder to ABO markers (M. T. Tsuang and Faraone 1996).

A more specific type of linkage analysis involves restriction fragment length polymorphisms (RFLPs), which are DNA fragments prepared by digestion of chromosomes with restriction endonucleases that break DNA at known nucleotide sequences. Each RFLP contains more than one gene. In a widely publicized RFLP study of bipolar disorder in a large pedigree of old-order Amish

(Egeland et al. 1987), linkage was found to an RFLP on the short arm of chromosome 11 (11p15), another finding of theoretical interest because this locus is close to the gene for tyrosine hydroxylase, the rate-limiting step in the synthesis of norepinephrine. The model derived from this study suggested a penetrance of about 60%; that is, about 60% of subjects with a specific allele of the marker had a diagnosis of bipolar disorder. Unfortunately, additional data from patients who did not have the 11p15 marker but developed bipolar disorder appeared to refute the original findings and actually exclude linkage to chromosome 11p15 (Kelsoe et al. 1989). European studies of different pedigrees never showed linkage to 11p15 (Berrettini et al. 1997).

Studies of other loci have had equally confusing results. An investigation of one family suggested linkage of bipolar disorder to the long arm of chromosome 11, but other work rejected this hypothesis (M. T. Tsuang and Faraone 1996). Suggestions of linkage of bipolar disorder to markers on chromosome 21q22.3 in a few families were refuted in later research (Vallada et al. 1996). A study of 310 DNA markers covering about 50% of the genome excluded linkage of bipolar I disorder; bipolar II disorder; schizoaffective disorder, bipolar type; and recurrent unipolar depression to all markers except a marker on the centromeric region of chromosome 18 (Berrettini et al. 1997). However, linkage to chromosome 18 was not confirmed in another study of five families (Maier et al. 1995a).

There are a number of reasons genetic markers for bipolar disorder are reported in one study and refuted in another (Berrettini et al. 1997; M. T. Tsuang and Faraone 1996). Methodologies used differ substantially, as do diagnostic instruments. Even though bipolar and unipolar mood disorders can run in the same families, they probably have different patterns of familial aggregation, and bipolar II disorder has a different familial pattern than does bipolar I disorder. Yet linkage studies do not distinguish between bipolar I disorder and bipolar II disorder, and many studies group subjects with schizoaffective disorder and even recurrent unipolar depression with patients with bipolar disorder so that there will be enough patients to achieve statistically significant findings. If attempts are made to distinguish between unipolar disorder and bipolar disorder in a linkage study, patients with bipolar disorder who have not yet had a manic episode may be counted as unipolar disorder patients, as apparently happened in the Amish study (Egeland et al. 1987). If patients with subsyndromal bipolar mood disorders are counted as unipolar disorder patients, evidence of an association between a particular marker and bipolar disorder will be diluted. Positive associations that are found may reflect some dimension of the mood disorder such as recurrence or psychosis or a comorbid condition that is subject to genetic influences such as anxiety, substance use, or ADHD. Additional methodological issues include possible genetic differences between ethnic groups that are lumped together in genetic studies and flaws in statistical assumptions on which measures of significance are based.

Even if financial and technical barriers to large multicenter studies of homogeneous populations of patients with narrowly defined bipolar or unipolar mood disorders could be overcome and more discrete genetic markers could be employed, there are several reasons contradictory findings are likely to continue to emerge from linkage studies. First, there is no reason to believe that only one inherited factor predisposes to a given mood disorder, no matter how much patients with the disorder resemble each other clinically. Any one of a number of genes could produce abnormal proteins that alter a cascade of physiological events at different points to produce the same end result. Another gene might fail to produce a protein with sufficient activity to keep the abnormal cascade from having an effect. The same phenotype therefore could be associated with any one of a number of genotypes. In addition, because people with mood disorders tend to marry each other at a greater-than-random rate (assortative mating), members of the same family are likely to have clinically as well as genetically different mood disorders. Conversely, variable expressivity and penetrance can result in patients with the same gene having phenotypically distinct disorders. Finally, some cases of a mood disorder in a given family may clinically resemble a genetic form of the disorder without there being any genetic contribution at all (phenocopies), whereas spontaneous mutations can result in new cases of a genetic form of mood disorder in the absence of a prominent family history of the disorder.

The implication of these complexities is not that linkage and other genetic studies of mood disorders are invalid but that the genetic component of mood disorders is probably underestimated by the current methodology. Subsequent findings in the Amish study do not mean that there is no linkage between bipolar disorder and chromosome 11p15; rather, some cases of bipolar disorder in this population probably do have a genetic contribution at this locus, whereas others do not. Some bipolar disorders probably are X-linked, some are sporadic, and some may have no genetic influence. The degree to which a pathogenic gene is expressed as a mood disorder probably depends on interactions of the gene with experience and with other genes. The earlier the onset of the mood disorder, the less adverse experience is associated with its development; and the greater the incidence of similar mood disorders in consecu-

tive generations in the family, the more important the genetic influence is likely to be.

IMAGING FINDINGS

A variety of findings have emerged from structural and brain imaging studies of depressed patients. One of the most consistent generalized brain abnormalities in structural imaging studies of unipolar depression has been enlarged lateral ventricles, which are reported most frequently in late-onset major depressive disorder (MDD) (Soares and Mann 1997). Subcortical white matter and periventricular hyperintensities have been found on magnetic resonance imaging (MRI) in older but not younger depressed patients. Regional abnormalities most consistently reported in unipolar depression have included decreased size of the caudate, putamen, and possibly the cerebellum. The basal ganglia receive input from medial temporal lobe structures that regulate emotion, such as the amygdala and hippocampus, but there has not been any reliable evidence of abnormalities in the amygdala and hippocampus in mood disorders (Soares and Mann 1997). Reduced frontal lobe volume has been variably reported (Soares and Mann 1997).

Imaging studies in patients with bipolar mood disorders (Geller et al. 1996; Soares and Mann 1997; Woods et al. 1995) have noted enlarged third ventricles at all ages in adults (and in a small sample of children), as well as the same kinds of subcortical white matter and periventricular hyperintensities that are seen in older patients with unipolar depression. White matter hyperintensities on MRI increase with age in patients with bipolar mood disorders but not in controls, suggesting an interaction between age and diagnosis (Woods et al. 1995). Bipolar disorder is associated with more subcortical hyperintensities on MRI than are unipolar depression and no mood disorder (Dupont et al. 1995). Because the presence of psychotic symptoms may be correlated with enlarged lateral ventricles in depressed patients and because psychotic features are more frequent in bipolar depression than in unipolar depression, ventricular enlargement in bipolar patients at any age may reflect psychosis rather than bipolarity itself. However, although enlarged lateral ventricles are more common in major depression with psychotic features, white matter hyperintensities are not (Soares and Mann 1997). In contrast to unipolar depression, no consistent MRI changes in the frontal lobes have been reported in bipolar mood disorders (Soares and Mann 1997).

Subcortical white matter hyperintensities, which are

found in a number of disorders, may be better markers of cerebrovascular disease than of any particular mood disorder (Soares and Mann 1997). This could explain why a greater volume of abnormal white matter in bipolar mood disorder patients is correlated with more cognitive impairment (Dupont et al. 1995). A substrate of neurological dysfunction associated with white matter hyperintensities could also account for an increased risk of delirium with ECT, extrapyramidal side effects with neuroleptic medications, chronicity, and overall poor treatment response in patients with this MRI finding (Soares and Mann 1997).

CEREBRAL BLOOD FLOW FINDINGS

Functional brain imaging with positron emission tomography (PET) and single photon emission computed tomography (SPECT) measures regional cerebral blood flow, which is closely related to regional brain metabolism (Bonne et al. 1996; Gyulai et al. 1997). PET has demonstrated reduced metabolic activity in the frontal lobes (i.e., hypofrontality) in unipolar (Buchsbaum et al. 1997) and bipolar (Gyulai et al. 1997) depression. Antidepressants were found to normalize frontal metabolic activity (Buchsbaum et al. 1997). Asymmetries in cerebral blood flow have also been found in depression, but such findings have been variable (Bonne et al. 1996).

Most but not all SPECT studies using technetium Tc 99m hexamethyl propylenamine oxime (Tc99m HMPAO) have demonstrated reduced global cerebral blood flow in depressed patients compared with controls; frontal, prefrontal, cingulate, temporal, and sometimes parietal and subcortical regions have most commonly had specific perfusion deficits (Bonne et al. 1996). I-123 p-iodoamphetamine-SPECT in 12 rapid-cycling bipolar patients in manic, depressed, and euthymic states showed greater uptake in the right than in the left anterior temporal lobe in both the depressed and manic phase but not during euthymia, which suggests state-dependent metabolic asymmetry in both poles of abnormal mood (Gyulai et al. 1997).

ELECTROENCEPHALOGRAPHIC FINDINGS

The same direction of cerebral asymmetry has been found in electroencephalographic studies of major depression, with less left frontal activation and greater right frontal activation (as measured by alpha suppression) in major depression (Davidson 1992). Davidson (1992) suggested that reduced left frontal activation is associated with a deficit in approach-related behaviors and that right frontal activa-

tion is associated with an increase in withdrawal-related behaviors. The interpretation of electroencephalographic findings is complicated by the fact that depression and anxiety may have additive effects on anterior activation and contradictory effects on parietotemporal electroencephalographic activity (Bruder et al. 1997). Bruder et al. (1997) found less left than right anterior cortical activation in depressed patients with comorbid anxiety disorders but not in depressed patients without anxiety disorders. In contrast, nonanxious depressed patients had less activation at right posterior sites than at left posterior sites. These patterns could reflect differences in mobilization of the stress response in anxious arousal compared with that in pure anhedonia. They also illustrate the importance of controlling for specific dimensions of the mood disorder.

BIOLOGICAL MARKERS

Clear associations have been established between mood disorders and alterations in biological functioning measurable in the laboratory. Most biological markers are reported more frequently in severe, psychotic, and bipolar mood disorders and in inpatients, who are of course more severely ill. No marker has consistently shown any promise of distinguishing between bipolar and unipolar mood disorders. Although there has been extensive theorizing on the issue, it is not certain whether well-replicated biological markers reflect a cause or a result of mood disorders.

DEXAMETHASONE SUPPRESSION TEST

The dexamethasone suppression test (DST) was initially used to study adrenal cortical activity in mood disorders because hypercortisolemia has repeatedly been observed in depressed patients (S.-L. Brown et al. 1994). In the DST, 1 mg of dexamethasone (a synthetic adrenal steroid) is given in the afternoon to provide feedback inhibition of cortisol production by the adrenal cortex, and serum cortisol levels are measured one or more times the following day. Because the assay for cortisol does not read dexamethasone, the level of cortisol the day after dexamethasone administration is a measure of how readily the pituitary-adrenal-cortical axis can be suppressed. Normally, cortisol levels decrease to 5 µg/dL or less with dexamethasone suppression. Hyperactivity at any point between the hypothalamus and the adrenal cortex can be associated with failure of dexamethasone suppression, demonstrated by higher postdexamethasone cortisol levels (i.e., nonsuppression).

Melancholic major depression is associated with a 40%–50% rate of dexamethasone nonsuppression (S.-L. Brown et al. 1994). The frequency of nonsuppression is higher (80%–90%) in severe and psychotic unipolar depression, in major depression associated with more severe suicide attempts, in inpatients, and in those with a family history of affective disorder (Rush et al. 1997). Bipolar depression and mania have the same frequency of dexamethasone nonsuppression as melancholic unipolar depression (Rush et al. 1997). The DST has been found to be a state variable; DST results convert to normal 1–3 weeks before clinical remission and revert to nonsuppression within 1–3 weeks of clinical relapse (S.-L. Brown et al. 1994; Rao et al. 1997; Rush et al. 1997).

The proximate cause of dexamethasone nonsuppression associated with mood disorders may be hypersecretion of corticotropin-releasing factor (CRF) (S.-L. Brown et al. 1994), the hypothalamic hormone that stimulates the pituitary to release adrenocorticotropic hormone (ACTH), which in turn stimulates the adrenal cortex to release cortisol. Serotonergic input stimulates secretion both of CRF and ACTH and participates in inhibition by corticosteroids of CRF and ACTH (S.-L. Brown et al. 1994). Noradrenergic influences inhibit CRF production but can stimulate release of ACTH (S.-L. Brown et al. 1994). A functional deficiency of norepinephrine activity and/or an excess of serotonin (5-HT) transmission could contribute to dexamethasone nonsuppression (S.-L. Brown et al. 1994; Rush et al. 1997), the former possibility being supported by a significant correlation between postdexamethasone plasma cortisol and cerebrospinal fluid (CSF) levels of the norepinephrine metabolite 3-methoxy-4-hydroxyphenylglycol in depressed patients in many but not all studies (S.-L. Brown et al. 1994). An entirely different mechanism is suggested by findings of considerable variability in dexamethasone levels between patients taking the same dose of the steroid (Devanand et al. 1991b). This observation raises the possibility that in some patients, apparent dexamethasone nonsuppression may actually reflect faster metabolism of dexamethasone, with serum levels that are insufficient to provide feedback inhibition of CRF and cortisol production.

Although it may create a window into the physiology of arousal in mood disorders, the DST has not proved useful as a screening tool (Carroll 1986; Pitts 1984). Dexamethasone nonsuppression can be a response to hospitalization, acute illness, dementia, and recent weight loss. Smoking, alcohol use, and medications that accelerate dexamethasone metabolism can make it more difficult to achieve levels of dexamethasone necessary to suppress cortisol and can therefore increase the number of

false-positive results in actual clinical practice. Because the 50%–60% of endogenously depressed patients with normal DST results still have a depressive illness, without a clinical evaluation it is not possible to differentiate true-positive from false-positive results. On the other hand, persistent dexamethasone nonsuppression in a patient with remitted major depression may be a marker of increased risk of a relapse if treatment is stopped, and very high postdexamethasone cortisol levels (> 10 µg/dL) may be a marker of psychosis in depressed patients (Dubovsky and Thomas 1992). The DST has a specificity of 87% and a sensitivity of 48% for distinguishing between melancholic and nonmelancholic depression (Rush et al. 1997), but this is not of great practical importance, given that a positive DST result does not inform treatment of depression.

THYROTROPIN-RELEASING HORMONE STIMULATION TEST

There are important reasons for interest in the thyroid function in mood disorders. As we mentioned earlier, thyroiditis is more common in patients with mood disorders, and hypothyroidism occurs with increased frequency in rapid-cycling bipolar disorder. Thyroid hormones play an important role in the regulation of biological cycles (Cowdry et al. 1983) as well as neurotransmitter (Cowdry et al. 1983; Extein et al. 1982) and receptor function (Bernstein 1992; Cowdry et al. 1983; Stancer and Persad 1982). Thyroid dysfunction can induce abnormal fluctuations of monoaminergic systems involved in mood regulation (Cowdry et al. 1983; Extein et al. 1982), which may occur at normal circulating thyroid hormone levels if central nervous system delivery or processing of thyroid hormones is reduced, levels of thyroid-stimulating hormone (TSH) or thyrotropin-releasing hormone (TRH) are altered (Bauer and Whybrow 1990), or cycling of the thyroid axis is disrupted (Bauer and Whybrow 1986). TRH (protirelin), the hypothalamic hormone that stimulates release of TSH by the pituitary gland, has direct effects on the central nervous system, including modulation of the actions of 5-HT and dopamine, independent of stimulation of the thyroid or pituitary gland (Marangell et al. 1997).

The TRH stimulation test, an assay of the activity of the hypothalamic-pituitary-thyroid axis, involves measuring the increase in TSH ½–1½ hours after intravenous infusion of a standard dose (usually 500 IU) of protirelin. A TRH-induced increase in TSH greater than around 30 IU/mL is considered hyperactive, indicating reduced feedback inhibition of the pituitary by thyroid hormone, which often indicates hypothyroidism or primary hyperactivity at the level of the pituitary. If TSH increases by less than 5 IU/mL after TRH infusion, the TRH stimulation test result is blunted, in which case feedback inhibition of the pituitary by a hyperactive thyroid gland is excessive or primary pituitary failure has occurred.

About one-third of otherwise euthyroid melancholic depressed patients have been found to have a blunted TRH stimulation test result (Rush et al. 1997). In some studies this finding has been a state variable, reverting to normal with remission of depression (Rush et al. 1997), whereas in other studies it has been a trait variable, remaining abnormal after mood normalizes (S.-L. Brown et al. 1994). There is at most a modest likelihood that depressed patients with nonsuppressed DST result will also have a blunted TRH stimulation test result (S.-L. Brown et al. 1994; Rush et al. 1997). Conversely, in one study, 74% of patients with melancholic major depression or bipolar depression who had a blunted TRH stimulation test result also had nonsuppressed dexamethasone in the DST (Rush et al. 1997).

A blunted TRH stimulation test in melancholic depression is not associated with changes in circulating levels of thyroid hormones, and therefore it is unlikely that the test is a marker of true hyperthyroidism. However, delivery of thyroid hormone to feedback systems in the pituitary and hypothalamus may be excessive. It is also possible that TRH receptors in the pituitary are hypoactive. Chronic overstimulation of these receptors by endogenous TRH might lead to their downregulation but would also result in elevated thyroid hormone levels, so a primary defect in cellular signaling seems more likely. The input of serotonergic and noradrenergic tracts to the pituitary could permit a functional deficiency of norepinephrine activity or an excess of 5-HT transmission could contribute to a blunted TRH stimulation test result (Rush et al. 1997).

ABNORMAL SLEEP

Abnormal sleep is one of the most common symptoms of depression, and the most frequent cause of sleep disorders in patients evaluated at sleep centers is depression (Buysse et al. 1994). Well-replicated changes in sleep architecture in MDD include decreased sleep continuity, more awakenings, decreased rapid-eye-movement (REM) latency (i.e., decreased length of time between the onset of sleep to the first REM cycle), increased REM density (increased number of REMs per unit of time during REM sleep), increased length of time in REM sleep, and difficulty entering and remaining in slow-wave sleep (McDermott et al. 1997; Rush et al. 1997). Some of the decreased REM latency observed in melancholic depression is primary, and

some is secondary to reduced slow-wave sleep, which allows REM sleep to shift to the earlier part of the night (Kupfer 1995). Deficiencies in sleep efficiency and slow-wave sleep may explain why depressed patients sometimes feel tired even if they appear to sleep excessively.

Abnormalities of sleep architecture have been most notable in melancholic depression (Thase et al. 1997) and in bipolar and psychotic depression, the latter being accompanied by sleep-onset REMs, or a REM latency of less than 20 minutes (Dubovsky and Thomas 1992). However, reduced REM latency has not been found in seasonal affective disorder (SAD) (Hellekson 1989). Polysomnographic sleep measures were initially thought to be trait variables but more recently have been found to persist after clinical remission (Rao et al. 1997; Rush et al. 1997). Results may be contradictory because some findings—such as decreased slow-wave sleep—are trait variables, whereas others—such as decreased sleep continuity, decreased REM latency, and increased phasic REM activity—are state variables (Buysse et al. 1997).

Any single abnormality of sleep architecture is not strongly associated with major depression (Rush et al. 1997; Thase et al. 1997). For example, reduced REM latency has a false-positive rate of 20%–40% or more (Thase et al. 1997). On the other hand, the triad of reduced REM latency, increased REM density, and decreased sleep efficiency reliably discriminated between patients with MDD and controls in a recent carefully controlled study (Thase et al. 1997). Even in this study, however, 55% of depressed outpatients had no abnormalities on any of the three measures, which makes the sleep electroencephalogram a poor diagnostic test (Thase et al. 1997).

Attempts have been made to correlate polysomnographic findings with treatment outcome in MDD. Treatment with antidepressants delays REM onset, decreases total REM sleep, and shifts slow-wave sleep to earlier in the night (Buysse et al. 1997). When slow-wave sleep occupies a more normal position earlier in the night, patients feel more rested, whereas a shift of REM sleep to the latter part of the night and closer to the time of awakening can cause patients to remember more of their dreams. When suppression of REM sleep by antidepressants leads to REM rebound, however, dreams may become disturbingly vivid.

As presumed markers of a potent "biological" influence, sleep findings such as decreased REM latency have been said to predict a poorer response to psychotherapy, although this impression was not confirmed in later work (Thase et al. 1997). Thase's group (Thase et al. 1997) found that the triad mentioned earlier of reduced REM latency, increased REM density, and decreased sleep efficiency, but not any single measure, predicted a poorer response to interpersonal and cognitive-behavior psychotherapy for major depression. It has also been reported that failure of slow-wave sleep to increase or at least shift to earlier in the night in response to any kind of treatment predicts a higher risk of relapse or recurrence (Buysse et al. 1997).

Hypotheses about mechanisms of the complex changes in sleep architecture in major depression are incomplete. In cases of early morning awakening and decreased REM latency, there appears to be a phase advance of the sleep-wake cycle, which is driven by the "weak oscillator" that also drives activity-rest cycles, and of the REM sleep cycle, which is dependent on the "strong oscillator" that also controls body temperature. Because muscarinic cholinergic systems increase REM sleep (Poland et al. 1997), cholinergic excess could be one cause of increased REM density and increased time in REM sleep (Rush et al. 1997). However, decreased REM latency is more likely to be a function of noradrenergic deficiency (Poland et al. 1997). Changes in REM sleep may be secondary to a disturbance of non-REM sleep, which is regulated by corticothalamic circuits (Buysse et al. 1997).

CLINICAL USES OF BIOLOGICAL TESTS

Laboratory tests are useful for examining the pathophysiology of mood disorders, but the large numbers of false-positive and false-negative results make them relatively ineffective for diagnosing mood disorders. In addition, no laboratory test can outperform the gold-standard clinical interview to which it is referenced (Somoza and Mossman 1990), and no studies exist in which diagnosis was prospectively predicted by laboratory test alone. A single laboratory test such as the DST can occasionally be used to predict the risk of a relapse if an antidepressant is withdrawn or to increase the index of suspicion of psychosis in refractory depression. However, studies of correlations between multiple tests may create a better window into the complex phenomenology of mood disorders.

The DST, the TRH stimulation test, and sleep electroencephalography can distinguish between melancholic and nonmelancholic major depression but not between bipolar and unipolar depression (Rush et al. 1997). For identifying melancholic depression, a blunted TRH stimulation test result has the greatest specificity and the least sensitivity, whereas shortened REM latency has the greatest sensitivity and the least specificity (Rush et al. 1997). The sensitivity and specificity of any of these tests can be adjusted by altering the cutoff point for a positive test result. For example, using a postdexamethasone cortisol level

of 10 μg/dL as a positive result will increase the number of true-positive results as well as the number of false-negative results. However, at least one-fourth of patients with endogenous major depression demonstrate no abnormality on any of the three tests (Rush et al. 1997).

ETIOLOGY: BIOLOGICAL FACTORS AND THEORIES

Theories linking disordered physiology to disordered mood go back to at least the fourth century B.C., when Hippocrates hypothesized that mood depends on a balance among the four bodily humors—blood, phlegm, yellow bile, and black bile, found in the heart, brain, liver, and spleen, respectively (Whybrow et al. 1984). Hippocrates proposed that depression was caused by an excess of black bile in the spleen (Leonard 1994). Because the spleen occupied a position in the body analogous to the position of Saturn in the heavens, it was believed that those born under the sign of Saturn were prone to depression. These ideas are the basis of references to an attitude of depressive hostility as *spleen* and to morose people as *saturnine*.

The conviction that there must be some inherent biodynamic alteration in mood disorders has continued to be held over the years (Whybrow et al. 1984). Herman Boerhaave, a prominent Leiden physician of the eighteenth century, argued that depression was caused by "nervous and melancholy juice." The psychologist William James carried forth the argument that changes in mood must be accompanied by some form of "chemical action." In his "Project for a Scientific Psychology," Sigmund Freud (1895/1950) proposed a complex pathophysiological theory based on a hydraulic model of neuronal functioning, which he later abandonned. Modern technology has made it possible to study the "humors" and "melancholy juices" of the twentieth century—biological rhythms, neuroanatomy, neurotransmitters, receptors, and intracellular messengers. However, we will see that, as van Praag (1990) pointed out, "though a lot of biology has been uncovered in mental disorders, most of it seems to be devoid of nosological specificity" (p. 2).

BIOLOGICAL RHYTHMS

Depression has a diurnal variation, and episodes follow a monthly or seasonal pattern of recurrence (S.-L. Brown et al. 1994). Some mood disorders, such as SAD and rapid-cycling bipolar disorder, are defined by their periodicity. Phase advances (i.e., peaking earlier in the day) have been noted in sleep onset, REM sleep, temperature, and hormonal and neurotransmitter rhythms, including those of concentrations of cortisol, 5-HT, dopamine, and norepinephrine (S.-L. Brown et al. 1994).

This kind of cyclicity has led to hypotheses of chronobiological causes of mood disorders (S.-L. Brown et al. 1994; Goodwin et al. 1982; Teicher et al. 1997). One such hypothesis is that abnormalities of mood in MDD are related to a phase advance or at least desynchronization of the strong oscillator (which controls rhythms of body temperature, REM sleep, plasma cortisol, and melatonin) with respect to the weak oscillator (which controls the sleep-wake and rest-activity cycles). Loss of predictability of circadian rhythms—with reduced amplitude of rhythms of body temperature, norepinephrine, cortisol, and melatonin—could suggest impaired entrainment of these rhythms. Antidepressants restore normal organization of circadian rhythms and resynchronize the two oscillators, but it is not clear whether this is a therapeutic mechanism or one of a number of markers of overall improvement of psychobiology.

NEUROANATOMICAL FACTORS

Injury to the left frontal anterior cortical or subcortical areas causes secondary depression (Bonne et al. 1996; Soares and Mann 1997), whereas right-sided lesions in the limbic system, temporobasal areas, basal ganglia and thalamus induce secondary mania (Robinson et al. 1988; Soares and Mann 1997). It is possible that subtle alterations in the structure or function of brain areas that participate in mood regulation could contribute to primary mood disorders. Relevant areas of the brain for this kind of formulation include the prefrontal cortex; subcortical structures such as the basal ganglia, thalamus, and hypothalamus; the brain stem; and white matter structures connecting these structures to each other and the cerebral cortex (e.g., the limbic-thalamic-cortical circuit and the limbic-striatal-pallidal-thalamic-cortical circuit), and possibly the cerebellum (Soares and Mann 1997). Abnormalities in these areas that could contribute to affective symptoms might include abnormal brain development, vascular injury, aging, and degenerative disease (Soares and Mann 1997).

One finding that suggests a degenerative process in some of these areas is the global brain atrophy that occurs in older patients with unipolar depression and patients with bipolar disorder at all ages. Although some argue that enlarged ventricles and sulci are found more frequently (Elkis et al. 1995) and that the severity of structural brain changes is greater (Soares and Mann 1997) in mood disorders than in schizophrenia, others point out that such findings are found in many different psychiatric and medical illnesses

(Soares and Mann 1997). White matter hyperintensities in mood disorders seem to be a marker of vascular risk factors or perhaps of weight loss or alcohol use (Soares and Mann 1997). The most cogent explanation for apparent structural abnormalities in primary mood disorders is that they identify neuroanatomical substrates that can cause secondary mood disorders in older patients and that contribute to dementia syndromes in interaction with a primary mood disorder. Coexisting neurological factors may lead to treatment resistance, but there is no evidence that they are primary etiological factors in most cases.

BIOGENIC AMINES

Biologically active (biogenic) amines such as norepinephrine, 5-HT, dopamine, and acetylcholine (ACh) are neurotransmitters in brain systems that originate in the brain stem. These systems modulate background activity of multiple neuronal systems, and abnormal function of biogenic amines has been proposed in mood disorders (Salomon et al. 1997). The monoamine hypothesis, which was first proposed in 1965, holds that monoamines such as norepinephrine and 5-HT are deficient in depression and that the action of antidepressants depends on increasing synaptic availability of these monoamines (Schildkraut 1965). The monoamine hypothesis was based on observations that antidepressants block reuptake inhibition of norepinephrine, 5-HT, and/or dopamine. However, inferring neurotransmitter pathophysiology from an observed action of a class of medications on neurotransmitter availability is similar to concluding that because aspirin causes gastrointestinal bleeding, headaches are caused by too much blood and the therapeutic action of aspirin in headaches involves blood loss.

Additional experience has not confirmed the monoamine depletion hypothesis (S.-L. Brown et al. 1994; Salomon et al. 1997). Monoamine precursors such as tyrosine or tryptophan by themselves do not improve mood. Depletion of monoamines does not predictably cause depression, and when it does cause depression, the depression is not sustained. Some substances that are monoamine reuptake inhibitors, such as amphetamines and cocaine, do not have reliable antidepressant properties, and antidepressant medications exist (e.g., iprindole, mianserin, mirtazepine) that have no effect on monoamine reuptake. In the case of monoamine reuptake inhibitors that are antidepressants, reuptake inhibition is immediate, whereas the onset of antidepressant effect is delayed a month or more.

Neurotransmitter reuptake inhibition may not predict antidepressants' therapeutic effects, but it does predict side effects (S.-L. Brown et al. 1990, 1994). Norepinephrine is a neurotransmitter in arousal centers such as the locus coeruleus and in the sympathetic nervous system. Medications that increase noradrenergic activity can produce anxiety, tremor, tachycardia, diaphoresis, insomnia, and related symptoms of arousal. Because 5-HT influences gastrointestinal motility, cerebral vasomotor tone, appetitive functions, and arousal, 5-HT reuptake inhibitors can produce nausea, diarrhea, headaches, appetite loss, sexual dysfunction, sedation, and jitteriness. Dopamine is a neurotransmitter of activation, movement, and blood vessel tone, and dopamine reuptake inhibitors tend to be activating and may elevate blood pressure.

NOREPINEPHRINE

Relative deficiencies and excesses of central noradrenergic activity have both been postulated to exist in depression (S.-L. Brown et al. 1994). An early hypothesis was that decreased activity and motivation in depression was related to reduced noradrenergic tone and hyperactivity in mania was related to noradrenergic excess (Schildkraut 1965). However, reports of increased norepinephrine activity in depression have been more frequent than reports of reduced activity (S.-L. Brown et al. 1994). This is consistent with evidence of high levels of arousal such as the non-suppressed DST or phase advance of circadian rhythms, which are present even in behaviorally slowed depressed patients.

Unmedicated depressed patients do not show consistent changes in α_1-adrenergic receptor numbers (S.-L. Brown et al. 1994). However, downregulation and hyposensitivity of β and possibly α_2-adrenergic receptors have been reported (S.-L. Brown et al. 1994). In animal studies, chronic antidepressant treatment decreases the number of α_2 and β-adrenergic receptors and increases the density of α_1-adrenergic receptors (S.-L. Brown et al. 1994; Leonard 1994). The first change would increase norepinephrine release, whereas the second would be expected to reduce adrenergic transmission through postsynaptic receptors. However, although a number of antidepressants downregulate β-adrenergic receptors, ECT upregulates these receptors, and mianserin, an antidepressant in use in Europe, does not affect β-adrenergic receptor density at all (Leonard 1994). Actions on other adrenergic receptor subtypes may not be relevant to the therapeutic effect of antidepressants (S.-L. Brown et al. 1994).

Drawing on studies of responsiveness of noradrenergic measures such as plasma 3-methoxy-4-hydroxyphenylglycol (MHPG), a norepinephrine metabolite, to mild stresses, Siever and Davis (1985) suggested that depression is associated not with consistently elevated or reduced norepinephrine activity but with uneven responsiveness to stresses that activate noradrenergic stress response systems. Like the heat produced by a furnace that is controlled by a poorly regulated thermostat, baseline noradrenergic activity is excessive, but acute stresses that call for mobilization of the stress response result in inadequate mobilization of additional noradrenergic transmission.

SEROTONIN

Neurons utilizing serotonin, which is phylogenetically the oldest neurotransmitter, originate in raphe (midline) nuclei in the brain stem and project throughout the brain. These connections and interactions make it possible for 5-HT to interact with other biogenic amines and to contribute to the regulation of many core psychobiological functions that are disrupted in mood disorders, including mood, anxiety, arousal, vigilance, irritability, thinking, cognition, appetites, aggression, circadian and seasonal rhythms, nociception, and neuroendocrine functions (Coccaro 1989; Grahame-Smith 1992; Leonard 1992; Montgomery and Fineberg 1989; Murphy et al. 1989). 5-HT may serve as a "neurochemical brake" on certain innate behaviors that are normally suppressed, such as aggression, including aggression turned against the self (Benkelfat 1993). Therefore, it is not surprising that serotonergic dysfunction has been implicated in mood disorders and that medications that act on 5-HT are useful in the treatment of mood disorders.

A number of studies have found lower concentrations of 5-hydroxyindoleacetic acid (5-HIAA, the major 5-HT metabolite) in the CSF of depressed patients than in that of controls (S.-L. Brown et al. 1994). The finding of reduced platelet 5-HT uptake in unmedicated major depression (S.-L. Brown et al. 1994; Leonard 1994) could represent hypofunction of a cellular 5-HT transporter. If a similar malfunction existed in the brain, it could result in reduced 5-HT stores, or reduction of 5-HT uptake could be a means of compensating for increased 5-HT availability. Decreased binding of [3H]-imipramine, a marker of the 5-HT uptake site, has been found in platelets of unmedicated depressed patients, but not consistently (S.-L. Brown et al. 1994). Additionally, no change in platelet binding of [3H]-paroxetine, which may be a better marker of the 5-HT uptake site, has been found in major depression (S.-L. Brown et al. 1994). Many platelet 5-HT findings may be confounded by seasonal and circadian variations in platelet 5-HT uptake (S.-L. Brown et al. 1994). Reduced [3H]-imipramine binding has been found in the brains of depressed patients who died of suicide and of natural causes, but this finding has been inconsistent (S.-L. Brown et al. 1994). A more reliable finding has been increased numbers of platelet 5-HT$_2$ receptor sites, consistent with a reduction of systemic serotonergic activity (McBride et al. 1994).

Reduction of central 5-HT and its metabolites may not be a marker of depression so much as a feature that commonly accompanies depression. Of seven studies, five demonstrated modestly reduced brain stem 5-HT and 5-HIAA in persons who committed suicide, regardless of diagnosis (J. J. Mann et al. 1989). In 10 of 15 studies of CSF 5-HIAA, levels were lower in depressed patients who made a suicide attempt than in those who did not attempt suicide (J. J. Mann et al. 1989). Increased binding of labeled markers to 5-HT$_2$ and 5-HT$_{1A}$ receptors in the frontal cortex of individuals who committed suicide suggests that these receptors upregulated to compensate for decreased synaptic availability of 5-HT in suicide (Buchsbaum et al. 1997). A study of 22 drug-free depressed inpatients with a history of a suicide attempt found that current depressive episodes in patients whose past attempts caused more medical damage and were better planned were associated with lower CSF 5-HIAA (but no changes in other neurotransmitter metabolites) than were depressive episodes in patients who had made less lethal and less well planned suicide attempts, which suggests that reduced 5-HIAA may be a marker of seriousness of suicidal ideation (J. J. Mann and Malone 1997).

Reduced central 5-HT activity was originally thought to be specific for depression (Meltzer and Lowry 1987) and then for suicidal depression, but this finding appears to be correlated with violent and/or impulsive unpremeditated suicidal behavior, whether the descriptive diagnosis is depression, schizophrenia, behavior disorder, or personality disorder (Lopez-Ibor 1988; J. J. Mann et al. 1989; McBride et al. 1994; van Praag et al. 1987). Reduced serotonergic tone is not even restricted to suicidality per se but is also associated with loss of control over many forms of impulsivity and/or aggression, regardless of whether they are directed inward or outward (Coccaro 1989; Linnoila and Virkkunen 1992; J. J. Mann et al. 1989; Siever and Trestman 1993).

Serotonergic transmission is mediated through at least seven major 5-HT receptor subtypes, each with subtypes of its own, with overlapping functions and different signaling mechanisms (Dubovsky 1994a). We have already mentioned the association of depression with upregulation of the 5-HT$_2$ receptor—which mediates such functions as mood, anxiety, aggression, and vasomotor tone—in the brains of individuals who committed suicide. In animal studies, antidepressants downregulate 5-HT$_2$ receptors; however, electroconvulsive shock in animals increases

5-HT$_2$ receptor binding (S.-L. Brown et al. 1994; Leonard 1994; Mikuni and Meltzer 1984). No consistent changes have been reported in 5-HT$_1$ receptors in depression (S.-L. Brown et al. 1994; Leonard 1994).

One strategy to assess serotonergic function indirectly in mood disorders involves depletion of tryptophan, the amino acid precursor of 5-HT. Some studies have shown that tryptophan-depleting diets produce acute but brief relapses of depression in patients with remitted depression but no effect of tryptophan depletion in normal subjects (Salomon et al. 1997). Another indirect approach uses neuroendocrine probes of the 5-HT system. For example, the 5-HT precursors L-tryptophan and 5-hydroxytryptophan and the 5-HT releaser and reuptake inhibitor fenfluramine release hormones under serotonergic control such as cortisol, growth hormone, and prolactin (S.-L. Brown et al. 1994). Findings of blunted release of prolactin in response to tryptophan and fenfluramine in some patients with major depression have been interpreted as indicating primary subsensitivity of postsynaptic 5-HT receptors located on prolactin-releasing cells (S.-L. Brown et al. 1994). However, these kinds of neuroendocrine challenges are not selective for serotonergic systems, and variations in methodology limit generalizability of the findings. Studies of prolactin response to serotonergic provocation suggest postsynaptic 5-HT receptor subsensitivity in major depression, but cortisol release studies suggest the opposite (S.-L. Brown et al. 1994).

Considered together, studies of 5-HT in major depression suggest both hypofunction and hyperfunction (S.-L. Brown et al. 1994; Leonard 1994). Findings such as decreased 5-HT and 5-HIAA levels in postmortem brain and CSF studies, brief relapse of depression with diets that deplete 5-HT precursors, decreased postsynaptic 5-HT receptor sensitivity in depression, and the existence of antidepressant properties of some medications that enhance serotonergic transmission suggest underactivity of 5-HT systems. Conversely, decreased platelet 5-HT uptake in depression, increased 5-HT$_2$ receptor binding in the frontal cortex of individuals who committed suicide, and reduction of postsynaptic 5-HT$_2$ binding and CSF 5-HIAA by chronic antidepressant treatment suggest increased serotonergic transmission in major depression.

One reason for this uncertainty is that neurobiological and pharmacological studies generally emphasize isolated aspects of 5-HT function although in the intact organism the activity of this neurotransmitter cannot be separated from the action of other transmitters. For example, 5-HT is a cotransmitter with γ-aminobutyric acid (GABA) (Kahn et al. 1990) and norepinephrine (Jaim-Etcheverry and Zieher 1982). Serotonergic and noradrenergic neurons can take up each other's transmitter, altering the functioning of the parent neuron (Jaim-Etcheverry and Zieher 1982). Serotonergic raphe neurons inhibit noradrenergic neurons in the locus coeruleus (Kahn et al. 1990) and regulate β-adrenergic receptor number and function (Charney et al. 1990). Conversely, agonists of α and β-adrenergic receptors and GABA$_B$ receptors alter the function of several 5-HT receptors (Grahame-Smith 1992).

Many other 5-HT interactions have been identified. Raphe serotonergic neurons synapse with nigrostriatal and mesolimbic dopaminergic neurons (Bleich et al. 1990), and dopaminergic neurons have 5-HT receptors that permit tonic control of dopamine release in the midbrain, striatum, and nucleus accumbens (Meltzer 1992). Depending on the circumstances, 5-HT may facilitate dopamine release in the nucleus accumbens and inhibit dopaminergic activity in the striatum (Meltzer 1992). Serotonergic neurons have glucocorticoid receptors that alter gene transcription, perhaps providing a feedback loop between the stress response and resetting of 5-HT function (Leonard 1994).

In evaluating the effect of new serotonergic medications, it is important to bear in mind that there is usually no information about the functional subtypes of the disorders in which they are studied. For example, is it clear that the selective serotonin reuptake inhibitors (SSRIs) are specific treatments for MDD, or are they effective for any syndrome of depressed mood, self-destructive behavior, circadian rhythm disturbance, or appetitive dysfunction? Are drugs that antagonize the 5-HT$_2$ receptor such as clozapine specific for diagnoses such as schizophrenia and psychotic depression, or do they have applications in any disorder characterized by dysregulated thought and mood? Until validated rating scales for serotonergic functions are used along with measurements of categorical diagnosis in treatment outcome studies, such questions will remain incompletely answered.

DOPAMINE

Some investigations have found that CSF concentrations of the dopamine metabolite homovanillic acid (HVA) are lower in patients with major depression than in controls and that lower CSF HVA levels are found in more severely depressed patients, but results have not been consistent (S.-L. Brown et al. 1994). The dopamine reuptake inhibitors nomifensine (no longer available), amineptine (available in Europe), and bupropion are antidepressants. Dopaminergic agonists such as bromocriptine and piribedil and the dopamine-releasing stimulants methylphenidate and dextroamphetamine have antidepressant properties that make them useful adjuncts in the treatment of depression (S.-L. Brown et al. 1994).

As is true of 5-HT, any apparent dopaminergic hypofunction may have a greater impact on dimensions of mood disorders than on specific diagnoses. Because mobilization of goal-directed behavior is mediated by dopamine, underactivity of dopaminergic systems may be related to decreased drive and motivation in depression (S.-L. Brown et al. 1994). Hyperactivity of dopaminergic motivational and action systems could be related to manic or psychotic symptoms in mood disorders.

GABA

GABA is the major inhibitory neurotransmitter in the central nervous system. Inadequate GABAergic input to noradrenergic arousal systems could lead to the kind of unrestrained arousal that characterizes mood disorders. Decreased CSF GABA levels have been reported in major depression (Leonard 1994), and some antidepressants increase the number of GABA$_B$ receptor sites in rat brain (Leonard 1994). Benzodiazepines, which increase the affinity of GABA$_B$ receptors for endogenous GABA, are usually thought to aggravate depression, but this class of medications can reduce depressive symptoms in patients who are anxious and depressed. Reduction of depression could be secondary to decreased anxiety in these situations. Because GABA$_B$ receptors may act as heteroreceptors on serotonergic terminals in limbic regions (Leonard 1994), in addition to moderating noradrenergic output, any pathophysiological contribution of GABA and any therapeutic effect of GABAergic medications in mood disorders may ultimately be mediated by other neurotransmitter systems.

ACETYLCHOLINE

It has been hypothesized that cholinergic transmission, relative to noradrenergic transmission, is excessive in depression and inadequate in mania. Because acetylcholine (ACh) is a neurotransmitter in structures that mediate withdrawal and punishment such as the periventricular system, cholinergic hyperactivity could increase withdrawal behavior and contribute to depression (Poland et al. 1997). In support of this hypothesis are the findings that cholinergic input reduces REM latency (decreased REM latency is seen in depression); some antidepressants have anticholinergic properties; lecithin, an ACh precursor, reduces mania in some patients and can induce depression; and cholinergic rebound following abrupt withdrawal of anticholinergic medications can cause a relapse of depression (Dilsaver and Coffman 1989; Janowsky and Risch 1984; Keshavan 1985). Lithium was thought to induce upregulation of cholinergic receptors, but this finding has been contested (Lerer and Stanley 1985). In contrast to earlier suggestions of the existence of muscarinic receptor supersensitivity in depression, no change in muscarinic receptor number was found in the brains of persons who committed suicide (Kaufmann 1984). Additional objections raised against the cholinergic hypothesis include observations that not all anticholinergic medications are antidepressants; that none of the newer antidepressants is anticholinergic; and that muscarinic receptors were initially considered in testing the hypothesis, although most agents used to test the hypothesis act on nicotinic receptors (Dilsaver et al. 1989).

INTERACTIONS OF NEUROTRANSMITTER SYSTEMS

Early attempts to understand the role of neurotransmitters and their receptors involved the hypothesis that some depressions were characterized by functional norepinephrine deficiency, whereas others were associated with 5-HT abnormalities. According to this hypothesis, low norepinephrine depression would respond preferentially to noradrenergic antidepressants, and low 5-HT depressions respond better to treatments that enhance 5-HT availability. This prediction was never confirmed, and no evidence of differing "serotonergic" and "noradrenergic" depressive subtypes has emerged (S.-L. Brown et al. 1994). The hypothesis was then revised (termed the *permissive amine hypothesis*) to include the concept that serotonergic deficiency contributed to most cases of depression, some of which had additional noradrenergic dysfunction and others of which did not. This hypothesis would predict that treatments that enhance serotonergic transmission are antidepressants. However, tianeptine—an effective tricyclic antidepressant available in France—enhances 5-HT reuptake, reducing available synaptic 5-HT (Wilde and Benfield 1995).

These kinds of observations further amplify the importance of dimensional analyses of mood disorders (S.-L. Brown et al. 1990, 1994; Lopez-Ibor 1988; O'Keane et al. 1992). What appears to be comorbidity between mood disorders and other Axis I conditions may represent an overlap of dimensional malfunctions driven by dysfunction of one or more 5-HT systems in interaction with other neurotransmitter systems. For example, when arousal associated with noradrenergic excess is sufficient to overwhelm regulation of aggression and impulsivity that has been impaired by suboptimally active 5-HT systems, suicide, various forms of outwardly directed aggression, or generalized impulsivity

may be the predominant problem, whether the primary diagnosis is a mood disorder, an anxiety disorder, schizophrenia, or a personality disorder. If obsessiveness is the primary problem, a diagnosis of obsessive-compulsive disorder is made, but if it interacts with a marked disturbance of mood, ruminative depressive states may emerge; if the interaction is with the consequences of traumatic experiences, the intrusive recall of posttraumatic stress disorder may develop. Dysregulation of thought processes is a feature of schizophrenia, and when this interacts with the psychobiology of mood, the same malfunction may figure in psychotic depression, bipolar illness, and schizoaffective disorder.

Traditional neurotransmitter hypotheses ignore evidence of dysfunction of other neurotransmitters in mood disorders. In addition, none of these hypotheses is readily applicable to bipolar mood disorders. If mania is associated with neurotransmitter changes (e.g., increased norepinephrine and dopaminergic activity) that are the opposites of changes in depression, for example, why are 50% of manic patients depressed at the same time they are manic (i.e., mixed mania)? And how can mood shift so abruptly and rapidly from predominance of one neurotransmitter to predominance of another, as would be necessary if these shifts were driving rapid mood swings such as those in ultradian cycling?

It is impossible to understand reported neurotransmitter changes in mood disorders without appreciating that all neurotransmitters and receptors that have been studied interact with and influence each other (S.-L. Brown et al. 1994; Leonard 1994). Cotransmission using more than one neurotransmitter in the same neuron is the rule (Jaim-Etcheverry and Zieher 1982; McCormick and Williamson 1989). Most cerebral functions are the result of the converging action of many different neurotransmitters. For example, excitability in the human cortex is regulated by ACh, GABA, norepinephrine, histamine, and purines, in addition to 5-HT (McCormick and Williamson 1989). Each of these transmitters may produce more than one postsynaptic signal in the same neuron by activating interacting receptors, and more than one transmitter may induce the same change in postsynaptic neurons. This kind of overlap provides a mechanism for fine-tuning of complex adaptations to multiple kinds of input (McCormick and Williamson 1989).

Such interactions make it unlikely that the pathophysiology of mood disorders can be linked to any single neurotransmitter (S.-L. Brown et al. 1994). Instead, different aspects of the psychobiological malfunctions in mood disorders may be related to different kinds of neurotransmitter dysfunctions (S.-L. Brown et al. 1994; Leonard 1994). For example, disordered noradrenergic function may be related to anhedonia, anxiety, and excessive arousal, whereas loss of dopaminergic function could lead to deficits in mobilizing goal-directed behaviors and emotional incentives. Loss of serotonergic regulation of aggression would be best correlated with violent, dangerous and/or impulsive suicidal behavior, anxiety, rumination, and appetitive dysfunction, and excessive cholinergic tone could lead to withdrawal and an experience of events as punitive. It is likely that other neurotransmitters and neuromodulators such as neuropeptides and prostaglandins are also dysregulated, contributing to increased intensity of dysphoric affect (Leonard 1994; S.-L. Brown et al. 1994).

Rather than being related to any particular neurotransmitter disturbance, mood disorders may be disorders of the overall cohesiveness of multiple transmitter systems involved in responding to danger. Antidepressant therapies do not affect one of these systems but produce adaptational changes in multiple neurotransmitter systems (Leonard 1994). Greater coordination between affective, cognitive, and behavioral systems associated with these transmitters may be associated with normalization of mental state (S.-L. Brown et al. 1994).

SECOND MESSENGERS

Simultaneous loss of regulation of multiple neurotransmitter systems, or multiple downstream effects of loss of regulation of a single neurotransmitter system, do not on the surface represent compelling descriptions of the pathophysiology of mood disorders, especially if one must postulate opposing neurotransmitter changes at the same time in patients with mixed bipolar syndromes. Given that there are many neurotransmitters and neuromodulators and many more receptors, an alternative hypothesis is that one or more of the few second messengers that mediate diverse neurotransmitter and receptor actions are poorly regulated. The bidirectional actions of second messengers allow unitary changes in second messenger function to produce diverse changes in transmitter synthesis and release and in receptor activity, leading to complex neurotransmitter and receptor effects.

Three primary second messenger families (Dubovsky et al. 1992b) have been well studied. Cyclic adenosine monophosphate (cAMP) acts directly as an intracellular messenger by phosphorylating proteins and activating them. The phosphatidylinositol (PI) system is a self-recycling cascade of membrane events in which phosphatidylinositol 4,5-bisphosphate is hydrolyzed to inositol 1,4,5-trisphosphate (IP_3) and diacylglycerol (DG) by phospholipase C (PLC). IP_3 releases calcium ions (Ca^{2+}) from intracellular stores and contributes to influx of Ca^{2+} from the extracellular space, whereas DG activates a ubiquitous intracellular enzyme called protein kinase C (PKC). In the presence of Ca^{2+}, PKC phosphorylates many enzymes involved in processes implicated in mood disorders. Entry of positively charged ions such as Ca^{2+}, sodium, and potassium into neurons increases neuronal excitability, and influx of negatively charged chloride ions is hyperpolarizing. Different receptors may utilize different second messengers. For example, the α_1-adrenergic receptor primarily utilizes cAMP signaling and the dopamine D_2 receptor and 5-HT$_2$ receptor increase PI turnover, resulting in an increase in free intracellular Ca^{2+} concentration ($[Ca^{2+}]_i$). The 5-HT$_3$ and GABA$_A$ receptors are linked directly to ion channels.

Many second messenger effector systems are linked to their receptors through a guanyl-nucleotide-binding protein (G protein). Receptor occupation leads to hydrolysis of the G protein, which in turn produces the sequence of events that mobilizes second messengers. A single receptor may be associated with more than one G protein, permitting a neurotransmitter to activate more than one second messenger. The same G protein may be associated with more than one receptor, so that a single second messenger can be mobilized by more than one receptor.

The PI/Ca^{2+} second messenger system has been of interest to investigators of bipolar mood disorders because of the biphasic action of the intracellular calcium ion (Dubovsky et al. 1992b). Free intracellular Ca^{2+} concentration ($[Ca^{2+}]_i$) is normally regulated very tightly at around 100 nM, or $\frac{1}{10,000}$ the Ca^{2+} concentration in the extracellular fluid. Modest elevations of $[Ca^{2+}]_i$ accelerate many intracellular actions, whereas greater elevations can inhibit the same actions. In addition, the same $[Ca^{2+}]_i$ elevation can inhibit a function in one system and activate another function in some other location. Excessive signaling by this messenger, inhibiting some neuronal processes and activating others at the same time, could explain two aspects of bipolar mood disorders that have been difficult to understand—namely, mixtures of manic and depressive symptoms in the same patient and rapid alternations between mania and depression in rapid-cycling bipolar disorder.

In a number of studies, $[Ca^{2+}]_i$ was elevated in blood platelets (Dubovsky et al. 1989, 1991a, 1991b, 1992a; Tan et al. 1990) and lymphocytes (Dubovsky et al. 1992a) of affectively ill manic and bipolar depressed patients but not in platelets of unipolar depressed patients, controls, or bipolar patients who were euthymic after treatment with various medications or ECT. Serotonin-induced Ca2+ mobilization in platelets is increased in mania (Okamoto et al. 1995). In vitro incubation with lithium (Dubovsky et al. 1991b) and carbamazepine (Dubovsky et al. 1994; Walden et al. 1992) lowers platelet [Ca2+]i markedly in ill bipolar patients but not in controls or euthymic bipolar patients (Tan et al. 1990). Carbamazepine and lithium have calcium antagonist properties (Dubovsky 1995a; Walden et al. 1992), and lithium modulates PI turnover, in part by inhibiting a key but not rate-limiting enzyme called *inositol 1-monophosphatase* (Jope and Williams 1994; E. Friedman et al. 1993). Calcium channel blockers such as verapamil have antimanic properties (Dubovsky 1995a).

Excessive intracellular calcium signaling could be caused by increased mobilization of stored intracellular Ca^{2+} (which could result from increased IP_3 production) or by increased influx of calcium influx. Any of these processes could be caused by increased G protein activity. Hyperactivity of G proteins and of G protein–linked PLC has been found in mononuclear leukocytes and platelets of patients with bipolar disorder and in postmortem brain samples of bipolar patients who had been dying from various causes (Avissar and Schreiber 1992b; E. Friedman et al. 1993; Jope and Williams 1994; Mathews et al. 1997). The additional observation that lithium blunts the G protein response to stimulation in animal studies (Avissar et al. 1992a) suggests that increased Ca^{2+} signaling may be the effector arm of a cascade of intracellular events that begins with G protein hyperactivity and that is corrected with antimanic drugs. Antidepressants may have actions on G proteins and other aspects of the second messenger cascade (Avissar and Schreiber 1992b; Leonard 1994), but more work is needed to define these actions.

ETIOLOGY: PSYCHOLOGICAL FACTORS AND THEORIES

Mood disorders are psychological as well as physiological conditions. As with biological data, there is less disagreement about whether specific psychological dimensions of mood disorders exist than about whether they are etiological. And as is true of biological factors, proving that a particular psychological factor is causal would require prospectively following people at risk of depression to see whether those with the factor are more likely to develop a mood disorder. A finding that patients who have already had an affective episode and who exhibit the factor in question are more likely to have a recurrence could simply imply that the factor is a residual symptom of the index episode and not an independent risk factor. Even if expensive and difficult prospective studies of psychological risk factors were conducted, a positive finding would not guarantee that any factors identified were not markers of an underlying biological factor.

Most hypothesized psychological causes of mood dis-

orders have involved depression. Because none of the psychological theories of mania (e.g., that it is a defense against depression) has ever been tested empirically, we will focus on psychological hypotheses of depression.

ABNORMAL REACTIONS TO LOSS

Loss is one of the life events that has been most reliably linked to depression. Sigmund Freud (1917[1915]/1957) pointed out that both grief and depression are reactions to loss but depressive symptoms include guilt and low self-esteem. On the basis of psychoanalytic experience with depressed patients, Freud believed that grieving turned into depression when the bereaved felt ambivalent about the lost object (i.e., person) and could not tolerate the negative side of the ambivalence. An unconscious attack against an internalized image of the lost object that undermines self-esteem that depends in part on identification with the lost person is manifested as depression. Freud thought that early, unresolved losses made the patient more likely to have difficulty dealing with losses as an adult (Whybrow et al. 1984). Later theorists pointed out that loss of anything that represents a person and that is overvalued or ambivalently viewed—a group, a profession, a cherished belief, or an ideal, for example—can result in depression.

In a majority of studies comparing depressed patients with normal controls, childhood loss—especially loss of a parent—has had a positive association with adult depression, which has been temporally associated with a recent loss, separation, or disappointment (Bemporad 1988; Paykel 1982). In primate studies, separation from a peer reliably results in behavioral depression and in the physiology of human depression; separation depression can be prevented or reversed by use of antidepressants (Kaufman and Rosenblum 1967; Suomi et al. 1978). Separation during infancy from the mother or, in the case of animals raised with peers, from the peer group notably increases the risk of adult separation depression (Kaufman and Rosenblum 1967; McKinney 1988). Experience with human infants has also demonstrated that early separation can produce a depressive syndrome that predisposes to later depression (Bowlby 1980). Taken together, these kinds of findings suggest a role for loss in the etiology of depression, but the role may involve the physiology as much as the psychology of loss. In particular, disruption of an attachment bond in any primate leads first to distress, which, from an evolutionary standpoint, helps to attract back a parent from whom an infant has been separated. If reunion does not occur promptly, separation distress is replaced by withdrawal, which conserves energy and reduces the chance of attack by a predator (Dubovsky 1997). Early separations may sensitize arousal and withdrawal systems to react excessively to subsequent losses, whether real or symbolic.

Although the association between depression and loss seems reliable, it is not as strong as was originally thought. Not only does loss account for only a relatively small portion of the variance in the risk of depression (Paykel 1982), but losses of one kind or another precede many other medical and psychiatric illnesses (MagPhil and Thomas 1981). Loss, an event that is stressful in itself and that removes an important external source of regulation of disrupted psychology and physiology, may be a more severe instance of a range of stresses that predispose to mood disorders.

OTHER PSYCHODYNAMIC THEORIES

Psychoanalyst Karl Abraham postulated that depression is a manifestation of aggression turned against the self in a patient who is unable to express anger against loved ones (Whybrow et al. 1984). Attacks on the introjected other, who psychologically has become a part of the self, undermine adaptive capacities and produce negative affect. In support of this hypothesis is the fact that many depressed patients have difficulty expressing anger openly, either because they lack self-confidence or because they are afraid of being abandoned by a loved one on whom they are excessively dependent. However, it seems unlikely that anger is converted directly into depression in such individuals, because many depressed patients are openly irritable. A more likely explanation is that dependency, sensitivity to loss, and lack of assertiveness lead depressed people to conceal anger, or even differences of opinion with others, until it becomes overwhelming, at which point it intrudes into everyday interactions. This problem may be compounded by intensification of all emotional experience in depression.

A hypothesis first clearly articulated by Edward Bibring is that the central psychological fault in depression is loss of self-esteem (Whybrow et al. 1984). According to this hypothesis, the depression-prone person is an overambitious, conventional individual with unrealistically high ego ideals. Depression represents deflation of self-confidence and vitality within the self that results from failing to live up to internalized standards that are essential to the patient's self-concept. This concept was expanded in self theory (Kohut 1971), which emphasizes the central role of the self as an organizer and driving force of all mental functions. Without coherence, mental activities are fragmented and ineffective. Without a sense of vitality, there is inadequate psychic fuel for optimism and useful engagement with challenges and stress.

It is traditionally held that the premorbid personality of the depressed patient is perfectionistic, involving high expectations of the self and others. However, this opinion is based primarily on retrospective recall by patients, which is likely to be influenced by patients' current states. Low self-esteem is a symptom of depression, but it has not yet been demonstrated to be a cause. On the other hand, unrealistic expectations and perceptions of the self and others are also invoked in cognitive theories of depression, which employ more objective measures and more formal studies of this variable.

INTERPERSONAL THEORY

Interpersonal theory emphasizes four basic interpersonal issues: unresolved grief, disputes between partners and family members about roles and responsibilities in the relationship, transitions to new roles such as parent and retired person, and deficits in the social skills that are necessary to sustain a relationship (Klerman et al. 1984). As in other psychodynamic theories, depressed mood and altered biology are hypothesized to be responses to loss or the threat of loss. A psychotherapy derived from interpersonal theory (i.e., interpersonal therapy), which is described later in this chapter, has been found to be effective as a primary treatment for depression and an adjunct in the treatment of bipolar disorder, although this does not prove that the etiological concept behind the psychotherapy is accurate.

COGNITIVE THEORY

Cognitive theory, which is related to hypotheses derived from an earlier construct called *rational emotive therapy*, holds that negative thinking is a cause rather than a result of depression (A. T. Beck et al. 1979, 1985; Thase 1996; Whybrow et al. 1984). According to the cognitive model, early experience leads to the development of global negative assumptions called *schemata*. Depressive schemata involve such all-or-nothing assumptions as

- If I'm not completely happy, I'll be totally miserable.
- If something isn't done exactly right, it's worthless.
- If I'm not perfect, I'm a failure.
- If everyone doesn't love me unconditionally then no one loves me at all.
- If I'm not in complete control, I'm helpless.
- If I depend on anyone for anything, I'm totally needy.

As long as experience seems to support a schema—for example, if everything a person does seems to work out or if a person never leans on anyone else—mood remains unambivalently positive. However, if something happens to contradict an all-or-nothing assumption, the negative side of the patient's thinking predominates. Failure in one endeavor makes the patient feel like a complete failure, or becoming ill or otherwise requiring assistance results in the patient's thinking, "I'm totally needy" or "I can't do anything for myself." These negative beliefs, or negative cognitions, are supported by self-fulfilling prophecies that reinforce negative thinking. For instance, the patient who feels helpless as a result of not having been able to influence the outcome of a complex situation that nobody could have expected to control stops trying to do anything to deal with later stresses. When this lack of effort leads to subsequent failures, the patient's belief that nothing can be done to influence the environment seems to have been proven. Systematic errors in thinking lead to catastrophic thinking and generalization of single negative events to global negative expectations of the self, the environment, and the future (the "cognitive triad").

Much of the evidence in favor of the cognitive theory of depression comes from demonstrations that psychotherapy based on the theory (i.e., cognitive therapy, discussed in a later section) is an effective treatment for major depression. However, cognitive therapy is effective even when patients do not express negative cognitions, and any psychotherapy or antidepressant can reverse depression whether or not negative thinking is formally addressed. In addition, all-or-nothing thinking is characteristic of a number of conditions (e.g., personality disorders) in addition to depression.

LEARNED HELPLESSNESS

A concept related to cognitive theory is *learned helplessness*, which was first clearly demonstrated experimentally by psychologist Martin Seligman (Abramson et al. 1978; Seligman 1975). The classic learned helplessness paradigm involves exposing an animal to an inescapable noxious but harmless stimulus such as a mild electrical shock. At first, the animal attempts to flee from the shock, but when escape proves impossible it lies down and accepts the shock passively. If the situation is changed so that the animal can escape the stimulus (for example, if the investigator removes a barrier that was preventing the animal from leaving the portion of the cage where the shock is applied), the animal continues to act as though it cannot get away. The animal cannot be coaxed away from the shock; only forcibly dragging the animal to safety reverses the learned helpless behavior. A second instance of learned helplessness develops more readily than a first episode. Learned helplessness that develops in one situation may generalize to other situations.

Learned helplessness resembles the passive, withdrawn behavior of depression, and refusal to overcome a negative experience is reminiscent of the self-fulfilling negative expectations of depression. Learned helplessness can be demonstrated in humans—for example, by exposing normal subjects to an inescapable noxious sound—and subjects who score higher on depression rating scales develop learned helplessness more readily than do those without depressive symptoms (Abramson et al. 1978). In animals, pretreatment with an antidepressant prevents learned helplessness. Considering all these data, it has been postulated that previous experiences with uncontrollable situations create a predisposition to learned helplessness. In response to a new uncontrollable circumstance, more severe learned helplessness develops more rapidly than in the past, resulting in the behaviors and cognitions of depression.

Experimental evidence in favor of the learned helplessness theory of depression may not be as strong as it might seem. It is not clear that learned helplessness in animals is equivalent to human depression. Human subjects with elevated depression scores have not been clinically depressed and have not sought treatment for any reason. In addition, depression involves symptoms beyond those of learned helplessness.

BEHAVIORAL THEORIES

Behavioral theories of depression, which are related to learned helplessness, hold that depression is caused by loss of reinforcement for nondepressive behaviors, resulting in deficits in adaptive social behaviors such as assertiveness, responding positively to challenge, and otherwise seeking important reinforcers such as affection, caretaking, and attention (Whybrow et al. 1984). At the same time that environmental rewards are no longer forthcoming with positive behavior (this is known as *noncontingent reinforcement*), helplessness, expressions of distress, physical complaints, and other depressive behaviors may be rewarded, especially if significant others pay more attention to disability than to competence. Loss, in addition to rupturing an important attachment bond, removes a major social reinforcer and results in depressive behaviors if the patient has not developed an adequate repertoire of adaptive behaviors and does not have other sources of reinforcement. Like negative cognitions, depressive behaviors would be expected to drive a depressed mood.

There is little question that interpersonal rewards influence behavior. If important people pay more attention to expressions of helplessness and inadequacy than to expressions of competence, it may be more rewarding to be depressed than to be healthy. However, it remains to be demonstrated that behavioral factors by themselves can induce depression or that treatment of clinically important depression by behavioral techniques alone is effective.

COURSE OF MOOD DISORDERS

The mean age of onset of unipolar depression is 24.8–34.8 years (Weissman et al. 1996). About 25% of patients have low-grade chronic or intermittent depression before developing a major depressive episode (Keller et al. 1996). Extrapolation from early studies that showed an increasing number of patients remitting with extended follow-up led to the conclusion that most patients would eventually recover from a major depressive episode; however, more extensive studies have disproved this assumption (Mueller and Leon 1996). There is a 50% chance of remission of depression that has been present for 3–6 months, but there is only a 5% likelihood of remission within the next 6 months of a major depressive episode that has been present for 2 years (Keller et al. 1996). About 12% of patients with acute major depression do not recover after 5 years of illness; 7% have not recovered after 10 years (Keller et al. 1996; Mueller and Leon 1996).

Prospective follow-up studies lasting 2–20 years after an index major depressive episode suggest that 5%–27% (mean, 17%) of patients with MDD remain chronically ill (Fava and Davidson 1996; Keller et al. 1984; Mueller and Leon 1996; Piccinelli and Wilkinson 1994; Winokur and Morrison 1973). In longitudinal investigations, about one-third of depressed patients are ill at any time (Mueller and Leon 1996). Chronicity may occur after a relapse following initial improvement (Fava and Davidson 1996). The presentations of chronic and recurrent MDD are diagnosed in DSM-IV as recurrent major depression with full interepisode recovery and no dysthymia; recurrent major depressive episode without full interepisode recovery (i.e., residual major depression) but with no dysthymia; recurrent major depressive episode with full interepisode recovery but superimposed on dysthymia (double depression); and recurrent major depressive episode without full interepisode recovery, superimposed on dysthymia (First et al. 1996). However, as we noted earlier, these categories represent only some of the courses that unipolar mood disorders may follow.

In the National Institute of Mental Health Collaborative Study of the Psychobiology of Depression (NIMH-CS), 54% of patients with major unipolar depression recovered within the first 6 months of entry into the study, whereas only 18% of those who were still depressed after a year recovered between then and the fifth year of this naturalistic study (Keller 1994). In a sample selected for an episodic course of major depression, Coryell and associates (1994) found that patients who did not recover from an episode within 2 months had a one-in-three chance of recovery over the next 2 months. The odds of recovery in any 2 of the next 8 months declined to one in five to six. In the second year of depression, the likelihood of recovery in any 2-month period decreased to a little more than 7%. Such results indicate that the longer major depression has been present, the more likely it is to persist (Piccinelli and Wilkinson 1994). On the other hand, even chronically depressed patients may recover (Mueller and Leon 1996).

Major depressive episodes also have a tendency to recur, even with treatment (Thase 1992). In the NIMH-CS, 25% of patients who recovered during the first year relapsed within 3 months (Keller 1994). The rates of recurrence after recovery from an episode of major depression have been found to range from 50% within 2 years (Keller et al. 1996) to 90% in 6 years (Coryell et al. 1994). After having been depressed once, the average person has at least a 50% chance of becoming depressed again, but after two episodes the risk of a third episode is 70%, after the third episode the risk of a fourth is 80%, and after four episodes the risk of another one is 90%. Overall, between 75% and 95% of patients with a major depressive episode will have at least one more episode over the course of their lives. On average, major depressive episodes recur every 5 years, the latency between episodes shortening from an average of 6 years after two episodes to just 2 years after three episodes (Keller et al. 1996; Mueller and Leon 1996). Around 15% of unipolar patients have only one episode of major depression, whereas 13%–54% (mean, 27%) have three or more episodes (Mueller and Leon 1996). The average lifetime number of episodes of unipolar depression is four (Mueller and Leon 1996). The recurrence rates of both major depression and dysthymia are higher in double depression than in episodic MDD or dysthymic disorder without MDD (J. Scott 1988). In the NIMH-CS, 4% of patients with episodic MDD experienced a relapse of an index major depressive episode within the first month of recovery, compared with 30% of patients with double depression (Keller 1994).

A number of factors have been found to increase the risk of relapse and recurrence of unipolar depression (Belsher and Costello 1988; Boyce et al. 1991; Conte and Karasu 1992; Coryell et al. 1991; Dubovsky and Thomas 1992; Keitner and Miller 1990; Keitner et al. 1991; Keller 1994; Mueller and Leon 1996; J. Scott 1988; Thase 1992). One of the most important of these is inadequate treatment. Because residual depressive symptoms increase the risk of a relapse fourfold, any depressive episode should be treated as completely as possible. Discontinuation of effective treatment often leads to relapse, especially if medications are withdrawn rapidly. The greater the number of previous recurrences, the higher the risk of future recurrences. High expressed emotion in the family, marital problems, and psychosis also increase the risk of a relapse of unipolar depression. Secondary depression, whether associated with medical or nonaffective psychiatric illness, increases the risk of a relapse by 60% and reduces the length of time to relapse. Severity of a depressive episode does not affect the risk of relapse.

In two 16-year follow-up studies of hospitalized depressed patients (Paykel 1982), only 18%–20% recovered and were continuously well. Another 63% recovered, but these patients had subsequent episodes, and 17%–19% were continuously ill or committed suicide. Keller (1994) estimated that there is only a 22% chance of sustaining a recovery from major unipolar depression. In a review of published outcome studies, Piccinelli and Wilkinson (1994) noted that even though 90% of patients were found to have had remissions during 5 years of follow-up, only 24% of patients remained well during the 10 years after an index episode. Maj et al. (1992) reported that 25% of patients remained well 5 years after recovering from an index major depressive episode. Angst (1988) found over a 20-year investigation that patients with an index episode of major depression spent an average of 20% of their lives in depressive episodes. In the NIMH-CS, one-third of 495 patients who were followed for 10 years after an index major depressive episode were in an episode at any point during the follow-up (Mueller and Leon 1996).

The average age at first onset of bipolar disorder is 6 years less than that for unipolar depression (Weissman et al. 1996); the first onset of bipolar disorder usually occurs by the second or third decade of life. However, first episodes of mania have been reported after age 50 years (Sachs 1996). The median duration of a manic episode is 5–10 weeks and that of a bipolar depressive episode is 19 weeks. Mixed bipolar episodes have a median duration of 36 weeks. Kraepelin distinguished between manic-depressive insanity and dementia praecox on the grounds that the former was characterized by complete remission between episodes and lack of deterioration (Mueller and Leon 1996). However, fewer than one-third of patients with acute bipolar affective episodes remain euthymic for a year, and 20% of acute affective episodes in bipolar disorder become chronic, with the highest rate of chronicity occurring in mixed bipolar episodes (Sachs 1996).

In patients who experience discrete recurrent bipolar affective episodes, cycle length shortens during the first 3–6 episodes and then stabilizes at 1–2 episodes per year, the frequency of depressive and manic recurrences being about the same (Sachs 1996). The average patient with a bipolar mood disorder has an onset of symptoms in adolescence and has had 10 or more acute affective episodes before age 35 (Sachs 1996). Residual hypomanic symptoms increase the risk of depressive recurrences in bipolar mood disorder even more than do residual depressive symptoms (Thase 1992). As with unipolar depression, the risk of bipolar relapse or recurrence decreases the longer a patient remains completely well (Coryell et al. 1994; Keller 1994).

FUNCTIONAL OUTCOME

Functional outcome in depression is as poor as it is in chronic medical disorders such as diabetes mellitus and cardiovascular disease (Mueller and Leon 1996). In the prospective study of the Iowa 500, 17% of depressed patients were unable to work because of depression and 22% had incapacitating symptoms (Mueller and Leon 1996). The medical outcomes study of 22,462 outpatients in a health maintenance organization found that those with depressive disorders functioned more poorly in almost all areas measured than did patients with diabetes, cardiovascular disease, arthritis, or pulmonary disease (Mueller and Leon 1996). Similarly, in the NIMH-CS study, depressed patients were less likely to be employed; earned less money; were more likely never to have been married, had poorer spousal relationships when they were married, and were less satisfied with sexual activity compared with control subjects, even when the patients were not clinically ill (Mueller and Leon 1996).

Residual symptoms (Sotsky et al. 1991) and impairment of work, social, and parental roles (R. A. Friedman 1993; Hay and Kumar 1995; J. Scott 1988) often persist after improvement of depression, perhaps more frequently in double depression than in episodic MDD (R. A. Friedman 1993; Hellerstein et al. 1994). Stewart et al. (1993) found that only 28% of patients with double depression who showed marked symptomatic improvement with treatment rated themselves as well. Refractory major depression is associated with an increased risk of suicide, a 50% chance of work impairment, and a 65% risk of ongoing interpersonal distress (Fava and Davidson 1996). The risk of accidental death as well as of suicide is increased in all depressed patients (Mueller and Leon 1996). Compared with controls, depressed children are more impaired in mother-child interactions, peer relationships, and achievement and have more behavior problems (Geller et al. 1996); impaired relationships may persist after remission of depression (Geller et al. 1996).

PHYSICAL TREATMENTS

Given that psychological and behavioral therapies are effective for major depression that is accompanied by vegetative symptoms and antidepressants can reverse chronic depressive symptoms that mimic personality disorders, it seems arbitrary to dichotomize treatments into "biological" and "psychological" forms. In all but the least complicated mood disorders, both kinds of treatment are usually combined. It is therefore only a matter of convenience to discuss broad categories of treatment separately. More comprehensive discussions of pharmacological therapies can be found in standard texts (Schatzberg and Nemeroff 1995).

ANTIDEPRESSANT MEDICATION

Antidepressants are traditionally classified according to their structure (e.g., tricyclic, tetracyclic) or their effect on neurotransmitter dynamics (e.g., norepinephrine reuptake inhibitors, 5-HT reuptake inhibitors, monoamine oxidase inhibitors [MAOIs]). As we mentioned earlier, it seems unlikely that any particular neurotransmitter action can account for the therapeutic effect of antidepressants. However, neurotransmitter actions do predict side effects. For example, noradrenergic antidepressants can produce jitteriness, tremor, sweating, and insomnia; serotonergic antidepressants cause nausea, headaches, and sexual dysfunction; and dopaminergic antidepressants are activating.

All antidepressants produce about a 60% response rate in unipolar nonpsychotic depression, which is significantly higher than the 20%–40% rate of placebo response. Although antidepressants have been found to be effective for milder depression (Stewart et al. 1993), the difference between active antidepressant and placebo diminishes in the case of less severe depression (Elkin et al. 1989). A number of limitations of clinical trials make extrapolating to practice difficult. For example, the end point of most trials is response (i.e., 50% improvement) rather than remission, which occurs in 10%–20% fewer patients (Burke and Preskhorn 1995). Studies required for Food and Drug Administration approval need last only 4–6 weeks and do not provide information about long-term efficacy or adverse effects. The use in many trials of the method of analysis involving the last observation carried forward can also be problematic. In this method, the last measure obtained

from patients who drop out is considered to be the final value for those patients. Patients who withdraw early from a clinical trial because of adverse effects or some other reason may appear to be nonresponders because the antidepressant has not yet had a chance to become effective; the apparent efficacy of the drug is thus artificially reduced. This problem is common in comparisons with older antidepressants (e.g., imipramine), which have adverse effects that frequently lead patients to discontinue them prematurely. In actual clinical settings, more attention is paid to providing support for medication continuation than in a placebo-controlled study, and the response rate to active medication is often higher. The use of fixed doses and a lack of opportunities to treat adverse effects or change medications can also lead to an underestimation of antidepressant efficacy in clinical trials.

Premarketing studies involve, in addition to relatively brief trials, relatively small numbers of patients, typically 2,500 or fewer people, 90% of whom have been enrolled in phase I or phase II studies in which doses are different from those most commonly used in clinical practice (Burke and Preskhorn 1995). Patients selected for clinical trials usually are ages 18–65 years and have milder forms of depression without comorbidity, making them more similar to depressed patients treated by primary care physicians than to the more complex and severely ill patients treated by psychiatrists (Partonen et al. 1996). New antidepressants are usually compared with placebo and/or the reference antidepressants amitriptyline or imipramine, which makes it difficult to know whether one new antidepressant is better than another in a particular situation. Because the cost of putting a new antidepressant on the market exceeds $250 million (Burke and Preskhorn 1995), minor differences that are not clinically meaningful are exploited by pharmaceutical manufacturers to convince clinicians to prescribe their product.

Tricyclic and tetracyclic antidepressants (Table 13–19) have a three- or four-carbon ring structure (Bech 1993; Kasper et al. 1992; Osser 1993). All of these medications have similar properties. In most cases, either the parent drugs (e.g., desipramine) or their metabolites (e.g., desmethylclomipramine) block norepinephrine reuptake, and some parent drugs (e.g., chlorimipramine) block 5-HT reuptake. As was mentioned earlier, neurotransmitter reuptake inhibition mainly predicts adverse effects. For example, noradrenergic antidepressants are more likely to cause arousal, diaphoresis, tremor, and insomnia, and serotonergic antidepressants are more likely to produce headaches, gastrointestinal side effects, and sexual dysfunction (Leonard 1994). However, clomipramine (chlorimipramine) is the only tricyclic antidepressant

(TCA) that is effective in the treatment of obsessive-compulsive disorder (OCD), apparently because of its ability to block 5-HT reuptake.

All TCAs have similar side effect profiles (Glassman and Proud'homme 1993; Preskhorn 1991). A quinidine-like effect makes TCAs as effective as the type I antiarrhythmics in the treatment of ventricular tachyarrhythmias; on the other hand, these medications can aggravate heart block and have a negative inotropic effect. Tertiary amine TCAs such as imipramine and amitriptyline have more anticholinergic and sedative side effects. The tertiary amines also produce more α_1-adrenergic blockade, resulting in postural hypotension, and more histamine H_1 antagonism, which contributes to weight gain. These kinds of adverse effects, along with the potential negative impact on memory of anticholinergic side effects, make the tertiary amine TCAs poor choices for older patients and patients with dementia. Nortriptyline and desipramine are better tolerated by older patients. Nortriptyline definitely has a therapeutic window, and desipramine may have a therapeutic window (Preskhorn 1991). Aside from a sinusoidal correlation between serum level and clinical response for imipramine and possibly amitriptyline, no other correlations between antidepressant serum level and clinical response have been demonstrated (P. J. Perry et al. 1994). Measuring antidepressant levels (i.e., therapeutic drug monitoring) may be useful in determining whether nonresponse to a high antidepressant dose or adverse effects with a low dose may be due to unexpectedly low or high serum levels (Preskhorn 1991).

Second- and third-generation antidepressants (Table 13–20) are heterogeneous with respect to their structures and actions (Bech 1993; Danish University Antidepressant Group 1986, 1990; Kasper et al. 1992; Lader 1988; Montgomery 1995). Trazodone is primarily a 5-HT$_2$ receptor antagonist with prominent sedative properties. It is frequently used as a hypnotic because its short elimination half-life results in less daytime impairment than that caused by some traditional hypnotics. The same feature means that multiple doses of trazodone are necessary to achieve steady-state concentrations. However, daytime sedation may limit this schedule. In 1 in 6,000 patients taking trazodone, α_1-adrenergic blockade causes priapism. Bupropion is not sedating and does not have anticholinergic or cardiotoxic effects. Unlike the 5-HT reuptake inhibitors, bupropion does not have sexual side effects. However, divided doses are necessary and doses greater than 450 mg/day are associated with a 5% inci-

TABLE 13–19. Tricyclic and tetracyclic antidepressants

Generic name	Trade name	Usual daily dose (mg)	Comments
Amitriptyline	Elavil	150–300	Sedating, anticholinergic; metabolized to nortriptyline
Nortriptyline	Pamelor, Aventyl	75–150	Therapeutic window 50–150 ng/mL
Protriptyline	Vivactil	15–60	Used for sleep apnea
Trimipramine	Surmontil	150–300	As potent as cimetidine as histamine H_2 antagonist
Imipramine	Tofranil	150–300	Reference antidepressant; metabolized to desipramine
Desipramine	Norpramin, Pertofrane	150–300	Therapeutic window in some studies 125–200 ng/mL
Doxepin	Sinequan, Adapin	100–300	Like trimipramine; useful for treating allergies, esophagitis, peptic ulcer
Amoxapine	Asendin	150–600	A metabolite of loxapine, a neuroleptic; 7-OH metabolite of amoxapine has neuroleptic properties
Maprotiline	Ludiomil	150–225	A tetracyclic antidepressant between imipramine and desipramine in side effect profile; doses >225 mg/day associated with increased risk of seizures
Clomipramine	Anafranil	150–250	Only tricyclic effective for OCD; doses > 250 mg/day can cause seizures

Note. OCD = obsessive-compulsive disorder.

dence of seizures, which is a greater problem in bulimic patients.

Four 5-HT reuptake inhibitors (see Table 13–20) are available in the United States. Although these medications are called *selective serotonin reuptake inhibitors* (SSRIs), none is truly selective clinically or pharmacologically (Benkelfat 1993; Dubovsky 1994a; Grahame-Smith 1992; Jaim-Etcheverry and Zieher 1982; Lopez-Ibor 1988; McCormick and Williamson 1989; Meltzer 1989, 1992; van Praag et al. 1987; Wilde and Benfield 1995). In addition to being equally effective treatments for major depression, the SSRIs have applications in anxiety disorders, OCD, posttraumatic stress disorder, eating disorders, and any condition associated with dysregulation of functions that are moderated by serotonergic systems, such as unpredictable, unprovoked aggression; recurrent, intrusive thinking; and excessive sexual or appetitive behavior. Although SSRIs are more effective at blocking in vitro reuptake of 5-HT than are other neurotransmitters, effectiveness at 5-HT reuptake inhibition does not parallel antidepressant potency, and tianeptine, a TCA discussed earlier, enhances 5-HT reuptake (Wilde and Benfield 1995). Interactions of 5-HT with other neurotransmitters make an isolated action on 5-HT in the intact nervous system impossible. SSRIs all have similar side effects, including nausea, diarrhea, headache, activation, sedation, and sexual dysfunction. Fluoxetine and paroxetine inhibit the CYP 2D6 isoenzyme, whereas fluvoxamine inhibits the 3A4 isoenzyme. Some interactions that result are elevations of serum levels and elimination half-lives of TCAs, phenothiazines, warfarin, and many other medications by fluoxetine and paroxetine and of triazolobenzodiazepines, haloperidol, and astemizole by fluvoxamine. Additional P450 enzyme inhibitions occur with many of the SSRIs.

Several third-generation antidepressants act on various receptors, with or without 5-HT reuptake inhibition (Dubovsky 1994a; Montgomery and Fineberg 1989). Treatment with venlafaxine—which inhibits reuptake of 5-HT, norepinephrine, and, to a lesser extent, dopamine—has been found to be efficacious in refractory depression. Venlafaxine requires divided dosing and can have adverse effects related to all three neurotransmitters affected (e.g., headaches, jitteriness, activation). Mild elevation of diastolic blood pressure can occur; more severe hypertension develops rarely. Nefazodone has 5-HT reuptake inhibition and 5-HT$_2$ antagonist properties. Unlike most antidepressants, nefazodone does not suppress REM sleep, and therefore the drug is associated with a lower incidence of disturbing dreams caused by REM rebound. The sedative properties of nefazodone and possibly its effect on slow-wave sleep make nefazodone a useful drug for treating patients with insomnia, but because of its short half-life, divided dosing is required, which can be difficult when patients experience daytime sedation or dizziness. Mirtazepine, which is related to the antidepressant mianserin, is an antagonist of 5-HT$_2$ and 5-HT$_3$ receptors and norepinephrine presynaptic α_2-adrenergic receptors. Antagonism of 5-HT$_2$ receptors could prove useful for treating psychotic depression (as could also be true of nefazodone), whereas 5-HT$_3$ receptor blockade could have an antiemetic effect.

The MAOIs (Priest et al. 1995; Quitkin et al. 1991;

TABLE 13–20. Second- and third-generation antidepressants

Generic name	Trade name	Usual daily dose (mg)	Comments
Trazodone	Desyrel	200–600	Divided dose necessary for antidepressant effect
Bupropion	Wellbutrin	200–450	Sustained-release preparation still requires bid dosing; drug can be used to treat SSRI-induced sexual dysfunction
Fluoxetine	Prozac	10–60	Therapeutic window may develop over time, requiring reduction in dose; parent drug has half-life of 3 days; biologically active metabolite has half-life of 6–9 days; drug can be more activating than other SSRIs
Sertraline	Zoloft	50–200	One metabolite with minimal activity
Paroxetine	Paxil	10–40	Anticholinergic properties equivalent to those of nortriptyline
Fluvoxamine	Luvox	100–300	Shorter half-life may necessitate bid dosing for some patients
Venlafaxine	Effexor	75–375	Effective for refractory depression
Nefazodone	Serzone	200–600	Useful for sleep disorders
Mirtazepine	Remeron	15–45	Could have antiemetic properties; oversedation may occur

Note. SSRI = selective serotonin reuptake inhibitor.

Stewart et al. 1993) may be more frequently effective than TCAs for major depression with atypical features (SSRIs also appear to be more effective than the TCAs for atypical depression, although possibly less effective than the MAOIs). Three MAOIs are currently available in the United States. Phenelzine has more sedative and anticholinergic properties than do the other MAOIs but has probably been most widely studied. Reports of the use of tranylcypromine, a more activating MAOI, in bipolar depression have been more consistently positive than those of the use of other antidepressants. L-deprenyl (selegiline), which is used to treat Parkinson's disease in doses of 10 mg/day and may inhibit the progression of neurological damage as a result of an antioxidant effect, has antidepressant properties at doses of 30–50 mg/day.

The most important limitations to the use of MAOIs have been hypertensive reactions when foods high in content of the pressor monoamine tyramine or sympathomimetic medications are ingested and serotonin syndrome when serotonergic substances such as SSRIs and dextromethorphan are used concurrently. These problems arise because inhibition of the A form of monoamine oxidase (MAO-A) in the small intestine as well as the brain leads to absorption of excessive amounts of tyramine. Systemic inhibition of MAO leads to accumulation of toxic levels of 5-HT, another monoamine. Two approaches to minimizing this problem have emerged. The first involves developing medications that are selective for the B form of monoamine oxidase (MAO-B), which is present in high concentrations in the brain but not the gastrointestinal tract. Selegiline is an example of a selective MAOI, but at antidepressant doses it loses its selectivity and dietary restrictions must be followed. Moclobemide is a reversible inhibitor of MAO-A that is displaced from the enzyme by tyramine, allowing the tyramine to be metabolized normally. Moclobemide is available in a number of countries but not in the United States.

ANTIMANIC DRUG THERAPY

Medications that are used to treat mania (i.e., antimanic drugs) are also used to prevent or reduce the frequency of affective recurrences in bipolar disorder, in which case they are called *mood stabilizers*. Lithium, the best studied of the antimanic drugs, has established efficacy as an antimanic and is prophylactic against recurrences of mania and depression in bipolar disorder (Schou 1997). Lithium may reduce depressive recurrences in highly recurrent unipolar depression (Schou 1995, 1997). Lithium appears to be most effective in pure (i.e., not mixed) mania, infrequent episodes, the absence of rapid cycling, and situations

in which there is a lack of a requirement for neuroleptics (Bowden 1995; Gelenberg and Hopkins 1993; H. S. Hopkins and Gelenberg 1994; Schou 1997). On the other hand, more than 50% of lithium-treated patients have another affective episode within 2 years (Goldberg et al. 1995) and 20%–40% stop experiencing the prophylactic effect of the drug over time (Goldberg et al. 1995, 1996; Harrow et al. 1990; Post 1990b). Discontinuation of administration of lithium (and probably other mood stabilizers), especially if it is rapid, can result in rebound (i.e., worsening) of the mood disorder as well as refractoriness to the therapeutic effect of the medication (Hopkins and Gelenberg 1994; Post 1990a, 1990b).

Lithium doses are adjusted by serum level, levels greater than 0.8 mEq/L (0.8 mmol) being associated with greater efficacy but also more side effects (Gelenberg et al. 1989). Common adverse effects of lithium at therapeutic levels include polydipsia, polyuria, hypothyroidism, hyperparathyroidism, tremor, impaired cognitive function, nausea, and weight gain. The last-named side effect, along with interference with signaling of insulin receptors, makes lithium therapy problematic for diabetic patients. Lithium toxicity, which becomes more likely as serum levels exceed 1.5 mmol, causes a coarse tremor, ataxia, vertigo, dysarthria, vomiting, delirium, muscle fasciculations, cardiotoxicity, and death. Debate continues about whether chronic lithium therapy causes nephrotoxicity (Schou 1997), but permanent neurotoxicity after lithium intoxication has been reported (Saxena and Maltikarjuna 1988). The 24-hour elimination half-life of chronically administered lithium permits once-daily dosing, which may reduce the frequency of adverse effects.

The anticonvulsants carbamazepine and valproate (divalproex) have also been widely studied as antimanic drugs and mood stabilizers (Bowden 1995; Bowden et al. 1994; Chou 1991; Keck et al. 1992; McElroy et al. 1996b; Post 1988; Post et al. 1993; Simhandl et al. 1993). Alone or in combination with each other or with lithium, the anticonvulsants may be more frequently effective than lithium in mixed mania, rapid-cycling bipolar disorder, and refractory bipolar disorder. More-rapid dosage escalation may be possible with valproate than with lithium and carbamazepine, an effect that could result in faster achievement of therapeutic levels and possibly earlier discharge of hospitalized manic patients. However, studies with findings supporting briefer hospitalizations of patients treated primarily with valproate versus those treated with lithium have not been controlled for the fact that valproate became a common treatment for mania at the same time that inpatient length of stay began to decline substantially as a result of managed care, new therapeutic philosophies, and other changes in hospital treatment of mania.

The therapeutic level of valproate in the treatment of acute mania seems to be around 100 μg/mL, which is achieved with daily doses of 750–5,000 mg (Bowden et al. 1994). Therapeutic levels can be achieved quickly through rapid oral loading (Keck et al. 1993). The dose of carbamazepine (usually 400–1,200 mg/day) is frequently adjusted on the basis of serum level, but aside from findings that higher levels are more effective than lower ones, there is no scientific evidence of a specific therapeutic level for carbamazepine in epilepsy, let alone mood disorders (Chen 1931; Froscher 1992; Schoenenberger et al. 1995). On the other hand, higher serum levels are associated with more psychomotor impairment from the anticonvulsant (Thompson and Trimble 1983). Valproate can often be administered in one bedtime dose, which facilitates sleep, whereas carbamazepine is usually administered in a divided dose. The practice of obtaining periodic complete blood counts and of withdrawing carbamazepine if the white blood count drops below 3,000 will not prevent agranulocytosis because this extremely rare (2 cases in 525,000 patients) event occurs abruptly and is not correlated with the benign gradual decrease in white blood count that takes place during the first few months of carbamazepine treatment and then remits in one-third of patients. Routine liver function tests with anticonvulsants are not cost-effective because hepatotoxicity is rarely caused by these drugs and when it is, it can be better identified by clinical observation than by laboratory testing (Hoshino et al. 1995; Verma and Haidukewych 1993). Use of valproate and carbamazepine during pregnancy may be associated with neural tube defects and cognitive deficits (Lindhout and Omtzigt 1992).

Although no formal studies have been completed, two new anticonvulsants, lamotrigine and gabapentin, which have been approved in the United States only as adjuncts in the treatment of refractory epilepsy (Mattson 1995; M. J. McLean 1995; Messenheimer 1995), have been used recently in clinical settings to treat refractory bipolar illness (Calabrese et al. 1996a; Walden and Hesslinger 1995). In addition, the novel anticonvulsant zonisamide was found to have antimanic properties in an open trial (Kanba et al. 1994). Positive effects of lamotrigine and gabapentin on mood are suggested by reports that patients in continuation studies elect more often to keep taking these medications than would be expected on the basis of improved seizure control alone, apparently because of an improved sense of well-being (Messenheimer 1995; Smith et al. 1993).

The most frequent adverse effects of lamotrigine and gabapentin have been dizziness, headache, diplopia, ataxia, nausea, amblyopia, somnolence, fatigue, ataxia, rash, weight gain, and vomiting (Beydoun et al. 1995; Matsuo et al. 1996; M. J. McLean 1995; Messenheimer 1995; G. L. Morris 1995). The manufacturer recently raised concerns about dangerous allergic rashes with use of lamotrigine, but the precise risk is not clear. Gabapentin was thought to induce mania in one bipolar patient (Hauck and Bhaumik 1995) and was associated with aggressive behavior, hyperactivity, and tantrums in a number of children, most of whom had attention-deficit/hyperactivity disorder (Lee et al. 1996; Tallian et al. 1996).

Calcium Channel Blockers

Increasing experience with refractory bipolar syndromes has created pressure for the development of alternative treatments for patients who do not tolerate or respond to lithium and the anticonvulsants. Of the various innovative therapies that have been proposed, the best studied are the calcium channel blockers. Double-blind trials of verapamil in manic or hypomanic individuals (Dose et al. 1986; Dubovsky et al. 1986; Garza-Trevino et al. 1992; Giannini et al. 1984, 1985, 1987; Hoschl and Kozemy 1989; Pazzaglia et al. 1993) and a blinded trial of nimodipine in 11 rapidly cycling patients (Pazzaglia et al. 1993; Post et al. 1993) have been reported. In two 4- to 5-week double-blind trials (Garza-Trevino et al. 1992; Hoschl and Kozemy 1989), equivalent antimanic efficacy of verapamil and lithium was found. Verapamil and nimodipine have been noted to have mood-stabilizing properties in some manic and rapidly cycling patients (Barton and Gitlin 1987; Giannini et al. 1987; Goodnick 1995a; Manna 1991; Pazzaglia et al. 1993; Wehr et al. 1988). One trial has been reported in which verapamil appeared to be less effective than lithium in the treatment of acute mania (Walton et al. 1996), but the results were limited by small absolute numerical differences between groups in rating-scale scores, P values that would not usually be considered significant with the statistical measures used in the study, and the absence of any differences between mania rating-scale scores in the lithium and verapamil groups.

The dose of verapamil that has most frequently been found to be effective in bipolar mood disorders is 360–480 mg/day. A short elimination half-life requires dosing four times daily; the sustained-release formulation of verapamil is not predictably effective for mood disorders. The most common side effects are related to vasodilation and include dizziness, skin flushing, tachycardia, and nausea (Bigger and Hoffman 1991; Gerber and Nies 1991; Murad 1991). In randomized trials during pregnancy, the use of calcium channel blockers for the treatment of maternal hypertension, premature labor, and fetal arrhythmias was studied;

no evidence of teratogenicity was found, nor were there significant effects on uterine or placental blood flow (Byerly et al. 1991; Carbonne et al. 1993; Ulmsten et al. 1980; Wide-Swensson et al. 1996). In the single published report of the use of verapamil in pregnant patients, good control of mania in three manic women and uneventful delivery of normal infants occurred (Goodnick 1993).

Antipsychotic Drugs

Case reports, studies, and reviews have suggested that chlorpromazine, haloperidol, pimozide, thiothixene, and thioridazine have applications alone or as adjuncts to lithium in maintenance as well as acute treatment of bipolar disorder (Ahlfors et al. 1981; Bigelow et al. 1981; Chou 1991; Esparon et al. 1986; Hendrick et al. 1994; Littlejohn et al. 1994; Lowe 1985; McCabe and Norris 1977; McElroy et al. 1996a; Prien et al. 1972; Rifkin et al. 1994). Published reports suggest that clozapine, an atypical antipsychotic drug that acts on dopaminergic, serotonergic, and other receptors, may have an antimanic effect in nonpsychotic as well as psychotic patients with bipolar and schizoaffective disorders (Banov et al. 1994; Calabrese et al. 1991, 1996a; Frye et al. 1996; Klapheke 1991; McElroy et al. 1991; Privitera et al. 1993; Small et al. 1996a; Suppes et al. 1992, 1994; Zarate et al. 1995a). Clozapine has been found useful for treating nonrapid- as well as rapid-cycling bipolar disorder (Calabrese et al. 1991; 1996b). There is insufficient experience to ascertain whether observations of better prophylaxis against recurrent mania than depression (Banov et al. 1994) are isolated or whether they represent a common phenomenon. Impressions of a positive effect of risperidone in bipolar mood disorders (Madhusoodanan et al. 1995; Singh and Catalan 1994; Tohen et al. 1996a, 1996b) have involved low doses and trials that were probably too brief for any antidepressant properties of risperidone to predominate over the sedating and antipsychotic effects. Further, there have been a number of reports of increased manic symptoms with risperidone (Dwight et al. 1994; Koek and Kessler 1996; Schaffer and Schaffer 1996; Sajatovic 1996; Sajatovic et al. 1996); in contrast, clozapine has not been reported to induce mania or rapid cycling. There has been insufficient experience with olanzapine to determine whether this drug has mood-stabilizing or mood-destabilizing effects in bipolar mood disorder.

With neuroleptic therapy, there is the possibility of an increased risk of tardive dyskinesia and neuroleptic malignant syndrome in bipolar patients (Bowden et al. 1994; R. J. Miller and Chouinard 1993; Mukherjee et al. 1986; Sernyak and Woods 1993), as well as neurotoxic interactions with lithium (Small et al. 1996a). In addition, concern has been raised that neuroleptic use could be associated with withdrawal or supersensitivity (tardive) psychoses (appearing with reduction in neuroleptic dosages), presumably caused by supersensitivity of postsynaptic dopamine receptors (Chouinard 1991; Kirkpatrick et al. 1992). Most putative cases of tardive psychoses have been reported in schizophrenic patients in whom chronic neuroleptic use was thought to induce rather than prevent psychotic relapses (Chouinard 1991; Kirkpatrick et al. 1992; R. J. Miller and Chouinard 1993). Although this problem is rare, if it occurs at all, concerns have been raised that continuing neuroleptics for too long could make manic patients prone to more severe and prolonged depressive episodes and rapid cycling (Kukopulos et al. 1980; McElroy et al. 1996a). Naturalistic follow-up studies found that 34%–95% of patients continue to take neuroleptics alone or in combination with lithium 6–12 months after an index manic episode (Harrow et al. 1990; Sernyak and Woods 1993). In some of these cases, continued neuroleptic therapy may be necessary for prevention of affective recurrence even if psychosis has remitted (Aronson et al. 1988; Dubovsky and Thomas 1992). Such a possibility is supported by a finding that lithium alone ameliorated bipolar psychotic depression in 10 patients but 8 patients required the addition of a neuroleptic to prevent relapses (Aronson et al. 1988).

Benzodiazepines

In the treatment of acute mania, addition of benzodiazepines, especially lorazepam and clonazepam, appears to provide more rapid control of agitation than do neuroleptics alone (Chouinard et al. 1983; Garza-Trevino et al. 1989; Salzman et al. 1986)—as well as a reduction in neuroleptic requirement—but not always with fewer extrapyramidal side effects (Busch et al. 1989). The effectiveness of benzodiazepines as adjuncts in maintenance therapy with any goal other than that of normalizing sleep or reducing anxiety or agitation has not been demonstrated. Benzodiazepines can have neurotoxic interactions with lithium (Aronson et al. 1989; Colwell and Lopez 1987; Freinhar and Alvarez 1985; Santos and Morton 1987). Tolerance may develop to the psychotropic (Post 1990b) and antiepileptic (Colwell and Lopez 1987) effects of clonazepam.

Thyroid Hormone

In patients treated openly, L-thyroxine in doses of 0.025–0.5 mg/day added to lithium or taken alone appeared to reduce or totally eliminate rapid affective recurrences in patients with bipolar mood disorders (Bauer and Whybrow 1986; Bernstein 1992; Extein et al. 1982; Stancer and Persad 1982). Most of these patients had laboratory evidence of hypothyroidism (usually in the form of an elevated thyroid-stimulating hormone [TSH] level), whereas in some cases, results of thyroid testing, including a TRH stimulation test, were normal (Bernstein 1992). Bauer and Whybrow (Bauer et al. 1990) prospectively studied 11 patients with rapid-cycling bipolar I or bipolar II illness who were taking lithium (6 patients); lithium and carbamazepine (2 patients); antidepressants alone (2 patients); a benzodiazepine alone (1 patient); neuroleptics as needed, combined with other medications (4 patients); or thyroxine with other medications (3 patients). At the beginning of the study, only 3 patients had normal thyroid function, as demonstrated in part by normal results of a TRH stimulation test. In all patients, open addition of 0.15–0.4 mg/day of thyroxine (or increase of the existing thyroxine dose for patients already taking thyroxine) resulted in increases in serum thyroxine and decreases in TSH concentrations into the hyperthyroid range. Of the 11 patients, 10 demonstrated significant decreases in depression and mania ratings and increases in ratings of quality of life for 78–370 days of follow-up. Of 4 patients in whom a placebo was then substituted for thyroxine in a single-blind protocol, 3 experienced a return of cycling. Although these findings are provocative, the study is complicated by the open method in most patients, a single-blind discontinuation protocol in only 4 patients, a diverse group of patients likely to have had highly variable courses, and different lengths of thyroxine trials in different patients. To the extent that these high doses of thyroxine did in fact enhance the therapeutic effect of the thymoleptics, it is not clear whether this involved a primary action of the hormone or correction of peripheral or central hypothyroidism. There is no reason to think that thyroxine by itself has antimanic or mood-stabilizing properties in euthyroid patients. Risks of excessive thyroid replacement include anxiety, atrial fibrillation, and osteoporosis.

Psychosurgery

Stereotactic subcaudate tractotomy (SST), which involves precise localization of a lesion beneath the caudate nucleus, has been found on unstructured follow-up to benefit 50%–60% of the small number of patients with refractory bipolar disorder who have undergone this procedure (Bridges et al. 1994). In two cohorts of 9 patients each—all patients with continuous cycling refractory to all treatments—who were followed more carefully for 2–13 years after SST, 3 patients were essentially well and required no

further treatment, 1 patient had mild residual symptoms, 11 patients continued to have affective episodes but they were less severe, and 1 patient's condition was unchanged (Lovett and Shaw 1987; Poynton et al. 1988). SST was more effective in ameliorating hypomania than depression. Complications of surgery included cognitive deficits in a few patients, schizophreniform symptoms in 1 patient, and partial escape from the beneficial effects of surgery in several patients.

ELECTROCONVULSIVE THERAPY

Electroconvulsive therapy (ECT) is the oldest and most reliable of the modern somatic therapies for mood disorders (Abrams 1988; Dubovsky 1995b). In ECT, a bidirectional square wave lasting about 2 milliseconds is applied through right (nondominant) unilateral (RUL) or bilateral electrodes to produce a generalized electrical seizure in the brain lasting 20–150 seconds. Although it was initially introduced as a treatment for schizophrenia, ECT is now known to benefit only about 15% of patients with this diagnosis—generally those with an acute illness of relatively brief duration accompanied by affective symptoms, perplexity, catatonia, and a good premorbid adjustment. ECT is most clearly useful in the case of acute major depressive episodes, especially when they are characterized by rapid onset, brief duration, severity, psychosis, motor retardation, catatonia, severe pseudodementia, lack of insight, and inability to tolerate antidepressants (Dubovsky 1995b). ECT is also highly effective in mania and catatonia (Small et al. 1988, 1996b). At one time, it was thought that ECT would be inappropriate in the presence of delirium because ECT induces an acute confusional state, but more recent experience demonstrates that ECT can produce rapid improvement in delirium; motor symptoms of Parkinson's disease also improve with ECT, independent of ECT's effect on depressed mood (American Psychiatric Association 1990; Dubovsky 1986, 1995b; Folkerts 1995).

Evidence has emerged of a relationship between the dose of the electrical stimulus and response to ECT; stimulus intensities $1\frac{1}{2}$ to three times the seizure threshold appear to be more reliably effective in major depression (Devanand et al. 1991a; Dubovsky 1995b; Lamy et al. 1994). In routine use, RUL electroconvulsive therapy is usually used first in the treatment of a major depressive episode because it is associated with a lower risk of cognitive impairment. Bilateral ECT is used in cases of nonresponse to unilateral ECT and as an initial approach in severe depression, psychotic depression, catatonic stupor, Parkinson's disease, and depression in which a smaller number of ECT treatments is desirable (e.g., in cases of high anesthetic risk). Although 6–12 ECT treatments are usually sufficient for major depression, standard practice is to continue treatment until the patient responds; further treatment after this point is unnecessary and may produce intolerable cognitive impairment (Dubovsky 1995b). An early practice of estimating the "dose" in ECT by the number of seizure seconds was not supported by later research.

ECT is usually recommended for depressed patients who are refractory to antidepressants, because the expectation is that it will be effective when medications were not. Comparisons of patients who received adequate doses of antidepressants (or antidepressant-neuroleptic combinations for psychotic depression) with those who received inadequate medication doses demonstrated that about 90% of the latter respond to ECT, whereas the response rate was only about 50% for patients who received adequate antidepressant doses (Devanand et al. 1991a; Piper 1993; Sackeim 1994). The assumption that patients who were unresponsive to a particular antidepressant before ECT respond to that medication after ECT was also contradicted by the same research, which showed that antidepressants are no more effective after ECT than they were before it. However, a patient's ability to tolerate an antidepressant may be enhanced by ECT. Some form of maintenance therapy involving either adequate doses of antidepressants that have not been ineffective previously or continued periodic ECT treatments is necessary to prevent relapse and recurrence of depression (Sackeim 1994; Schwarz et al. 1995).

Mania is the third most common indication for ECT (Small et al. 1988), which appears to be the most rapidly effective treatment for mania (H. S. Hopkins and Gelenberg 1994; Small et al. 1996a) and the most effective treatment for bipolar depression (Bergsholm et al. 1992; H. S. Hopkins and Gelenberg 1994; Zornberg and Rose 1993). In a review of the published literature on the efficacy of ECT for acute mania, Mukherjee et al. (1994) found that the overall rate of "remission or marked clinical improvement" was 80% (470 of 589 patients). Interpretation of these composite figures is limited by differences in methodology and outcome measures in the studies reviewed and by the secondhand assessment of data using a nonstandard method. Although some studies found that unilateral ECT is as effective as bilateral ECT (Black et al. 1987), others found bilateral ECT to be more frequently and more rapidly effective (Milstein et al. 1987; Small et al. 1985, 1996a), possibly because of shunting of current through the scalp with the Lancaster RUL electrode placement, which was used in one study showing superiority of bilateral ECT (Mukherjee et al. 1994). In a prospective study (Schnur et al. 1992), five of eight manic patients had a complete remis-

sion with the d'Elia RUL electrode placement, which has a greater interelectrode distance, but the number of patients is too small for definitive conclusions to be drawn. Maintenance ECT was as effective as lithium in preventing manic relapse and recurrence in a prospective study and some case series (Avissar and Schreiber 1992b; Bigelow et al. 1981; Jaffe et al. 1991; Sachs 1989).

The most common side effects of ECT are confusion and memory loss, and these effects are more pronounced after bilateral ECT (Aperia 1985; Calev et al. 1989, 1995; Krueger et al. 1992; Pettinati and Rosenberg 1984). Anterograde amnesia is most obvious within 45 minutes of a treatment, but loss of memory of events occurring from a few days to as long as 2 years before ECT (i.e., retrograde amnesia) also occurs. In some cases, personally significant memories from the recent or distant past (i.e., autobiographical memory) may be lost permanently. Most of the time, however, cognitive functioning after recovery from the acute effects of ECT is better than it was before the treatment, probably because of recovery from the cognitive impairment of depression (Calev et al. 1995; Krueger et al. 1992; Sackeim et al. 1992). There is no evidence from studies of cerebral structure or function that ECT as it is currently administered causes brain damage (Coffey et al. 1991; Dubovsky 1995b; Weiner 1984).

PSYCHOTHERAPY

Antidepressants have become the predominant form of treatment for unipolar depression. One report (Roose and Stern 1995) stated that even 29% of 56 patients in psychoanalysis with analytic candidates were taking antidepressants. However, a number of psychotherapies have been found to be as effective as antidepressants (Antonuccio et al. 1995), especially in less severe cases of unipolar depression (Sotsky et al. 1991). Two psychotherapies designed specifically for major depression—cognitive therapy (and a variant, cognitive-behavior therapy) and interpersonal therapy (IPT)—have been subjected to controlled research and have been compared with reference antidepressants. However, these studies have several features that complicate interpretation of the results. For example, most studies have involved mildly to moderately depressed nonpsychotic, nonbipolar patients. In addition, comparisons of psychotherapy with medication utilize imipramine, the standard reference antidepressant, in a fixed-dose protocol. The dropout rate in such protocols is undoubtedly greater than it is for patients taking antidepressants in clinical practice because newer, better-tolerated antidepressants are used and because a component of pharmacotherapy includes increasing the dose in the case of nonresponse, treating side effects, and encouraging compliance. In addition, antidepressant medications and psychotherapies may not be directly comparable, because they act on different symptoms, psychotherapy working faster to improve social function and suicidal thinking and medications demonstrating a faster onset of improvement of disturbed mood, sleep, and appetite.

In the National Institute of Mental Health (NIMH) multicenter collaborative study of treatments for depression (Elkin et al. 1989), unipolar, nonpsychotically depressed patients received a 16-week course of placebo plus "clinical management" (i.e., nonspecific supportive psychotherapy), imipramine plus clinical management, IPT, or cognitive-behavior therapy. For mildly depressed patients, no active treatment was any more effective than placebo plus clinical management. As depression became more severe, imipramine plus clinical management was found to be consistently superior on the broadest range of outcome measures. IPT was better than a placebo but not as effective as imipramine. Cognitive-behavior therapy was only slightly less effective than IPT but it was not significantly better than a placebo (Hollon and Fawcett 1995; Hollon et al. 1992). The results suggested that support and no medication may be effective for mild acute depression, whereas more severely depressed patients do best with antidepressants. The efficacies of specific psychotherapies appeared to be intermediate between placebo and medication and these psychotherapies may work on different symptoms.

This conclusion is not as straightforward as it might seem. The method of analysis involving the last observation carried forward may have underestimated the efficacy of both psychotherapies, and other research suggests that cognitive-behavior psychotherapy and IPT are effective for severe depression (Antonuccio et al. 1995; Jarrett 1997; McLean and Taylor 1992). However, IPT and behavioral therapy may be less effective in melancholic than in nonmelancholic depression (Frank et al. 1992; McLean and Taylor 1992). Relapse of depression does not occur as rapidly after discontinuation of psychotherapy as it does after withdrawal of antidepressants, and continuation of psychotherapy after recovery reduces the relapse rate (Evans et al. 1992; Kupfer et al. 1992; Thase and Kupfer 1996; Weissman 1994), as is true of antidepressants.

COGNITIVE THERAPY

Cognitive therapy (CT) is based on the premise that the negative emotions of depression are reactions to negative thinking derived from global dysfunctional negative attitudes. Patient and therapist work together to identify automatic negative thoughts, correct the pervasive beliefs that generate these thoughts, and develop more realistic basic assumptions (A. T. Beck et al. 1979, 1985). Treatment involves systematically monitoring negative cognitions whenever the patient feels depressed; recognizing the association between cognition, affect, and behavior; generating data that support or refute the negative cognition; generating alternative hypotheses to explain the event that precipitated the negative cognition; and identifying the negative schemata predisposing to the emergence of global negative thinking when one side of an all-or-nothing assumption is disappointed. In the course of examining dysfunctional attitudes, the patient learns to label and counteract information processing errors such as overgeneralization, excessive personalization, all-or-nothing thinking, and generalizing from single negative events.

For example, after keeping track of what he was thinking at the moment he began to feel depressed, a man might realize that the feeling started after he began thinking "nobody loves me" when his wife did not greet him enthusiastically. This thought might be seen to follow logically from the assumption "If she isn't always happy to see me, she doesn't love me." Two kinds of alternative hypotheses could be generated in considering this cognition. First, the patient's wife may have been preoccupied with something else or may have been happy to see him but did not demonstrate it in exactly the way he expected. Second, lack of enthusiasm at one particular moment is not necessarily a sign of generalized lack of love. Eventually, the patient learns to correct the underlying all-or-nothing belief "People either are completely devoted to me or they don't care at all."

The best studied of the psychotherapies for major depression (Thase 1995), cognitive therapy has been compared with nonpharmacological-control conditions for the acute-phase treatment of depression in at least 21 randomized controlled clinical trials (Shea et al. 1988; Thase 1995). In a meta-analysis of 12 suitable studies, CT had an overall efficacy rate of 46.6% and was 30.1% more effective than no therapy in waiting-list control subjects (two studies) but was only 9.4% more effective than placebo plus clinical management in the collaborative study mentioned earlier. Although early studies demonstrated superiority of CT over pharmacotherapy provided by a primary care physician, comparisons with more rigorous pharmacological treatment provided by psychiatrists in recent studies suggest equivalence of the two treatments for depression of moderate severity (Hollon et al. 1992; Elkin et al. 1989). As we noted earlier, pharmacotherapy was more effective than

CT in more severely depressed patients in the NIMH collaborative study (Elkin et al. 1989). The onset of action of antidepressants has been found to be faster than the onset of action of CT (Watkins et al. 1993).

Although some studies suggest that adding CT to antidepressant medication therapy may improve efficacy more than adding antidepressants to CT (Bowers 1990; Hollon et al. 1992; Thase 1995), in clinical practice patients with a poor response to CT (or any psychotherapy) alone often respond to addition of antidepressants. Response rates to individual CT exceed those to group CT (50.1% vs. 39.2%). Modified cognitive therapy has been shown to be effective for hospitalized depressed patients (Stuart and Thase 1994). Depressed patients with personality disorders may be more likely to drop out of CT (Persons et al. 1996), but those who remain in treatment can improve as much as patients without Axis II disorders (Stuart et al. 1992).

Monthly CT achieved the same level of prophylaxis as continuation pharmacotherapy in one study (Blackburn et al. 1986). In a naturalistic follow-up study of CT responders compared with antidepressant responders who had been withdrawn from medication therapy and antidepressant responders treated with continuation pharmacotherapy, CT-treated patients relapsed significantly less often than did patients withdrawn from medication therapy (21% vs. 50% at 2 years) and at a rate comparable to that for patients who continued to take medication (15%) (Evans et al. 1992).

INTERPERSONAL THERAPY

Interpersonal therapy (IPT) is designed to improve depression by enhancing the quality of the patient's interpersonal world (Klerman et al. 1984). The treatment begins with an explanation of the diagnosis and treatment options, legitimizing depression as a medical illness. The acute course of treatment is conducted according to a manualized protocol over 12–16 weeks. A protocol for maintenance IPT has also been developed. Through structured assignments, IPT helps the patient to work toward explicit goals related to whichever of the four basic interpersonal problems (unresolved grief, role disputes, transitions to new roles, and social skills deficits) is believed to be present. Role-playing is used to help the patient acquire new interpersonal skills, and structured conjoint meetings are used to help partners to clarify their expectations of each other.

It is frequently claimed that IPT is no more than a specialized form of expressive (psychodynamic) psychotherapy, but there are important differences between the two treatments. Unlike expressive psychotherapy, IPT follows a structured approach outlined in a manual and uses explicit homework assignments. Its focus is exclusively on the present; there is no systematic attempt to explore conflicts related to early experience, to address transference, or to change underlying character structure. IPT may be a more acceptable treatment than medication or cognitive or behavioral therapies, at least to younger patients (Banken and Wilson 1992).

In initial randomized clinical trials involving outpatients with nonpsychotic major depression, IPT was superior to amitriptyline in producing improvement in mood, suicidal ideation, and interest, whereas the antidepressant was more effective for appetite and sleep disturbances (DiMascio et al. 1979; Elkin et al. 1989; Schneider et al. 1986; Thase 1995; Weissman et al. 1979). In a comparison with nortriptyline in older patients, IPT was found to be as effective in reducing depressive symptoms, and more IPT-treated patients than nortriptyline-treated patients remained in the study (Schneider et al. 1986). In the collaborative study mentioned earlier comparing IPT, CT, imipramine plus clinical management, and placebo plus clinical management, IPT was found to be equivalent to imipramine and CT by the end of 16 weeks, but imipramine was more rapidly effective (Elkin et al. 1989; Watkins et al. 1993).

Efficacy as a maintenance treatment as well as acute therapy has been demonstrated for IPT. In a prospective study of 128 patients, each of whom had had at least two previous episodes of recurrent unipolar depression, patients were randomized after remission with treatment with imipramine to one of five treatment conditions: continued monthly IPT with imipramine, monthly IPT with placebo, monthly IPT without medication, imipramine with supportive management, and placebo with supportive management (Frank et al. 1990). Both active-medication conditions were associated with roughly 80% relapse-free rates at 3-year follow-up. In addition, IPT with or without a placebo more than doubled relapse-free survival rates compared with placebo and supportive care at 3 years (30%–40% vs. 10%). Blind independent ratings of the quality of IPT demonstrated that patients treated with higher-quality IPT had 2-year relapse-free survival rates comparable to rates among patients treated with imipramine, and 3-year survival rates for patients in the former group were about 40%. Patients receiving IPT of below-average quality had survival rates that were no better than rates for patients receiving a placebo (Frank et al. 1991).

In a subsequent study, 20 patients who had been treated with imipramine and had remained in remission for the first 3 years of the first study (Frank et al. 1990) were randomized to an additional 2 years of placebo or continued medication therapy (Kupfer et al. 1992). Eighty-two percent of those treated with medication survived the next 2 years without a depressive recurrence, compared with 33% of those randomized to placebo. Of the latter group, only 11% of those receiving placebo alone survived, whereas 78% of those continuing with monthly IPT and placebo survived. The possibility remains that a "dose" of maintenance IPT that is greater than the monthly sessions used in these studies would have produced even better results. IPT was an effective adjunct to maintenance antidepressants in elderly patients (Reynolds et al. 1995).

A form of IPT called *interpersonal and social rhythm therapy* (IPSRT) is currently under study as an adjunct to thymoleptic medication therapy in the maintenance treatment of bipolar mood disorders (Frank et al. 1994). In addition to interpersonal techniques such as encouraging the expression of grief for the loss of the person the patient was before the illness began and resolving interpersonal conflicts, IPSRT includes a structured approach to normalizing circadian rhythms. The patient first keeps a log in which he or she notes the timing of 17 zeitgebers (e.g., getting out of bed, meals, first interaction with another person, exercising, and going to bed). Average times for each of these cues to circadian rhythms are computed, and the patient is helped to keep a regular schedule for each of them.

After 1 year of prospective comparison of IPSRT with supportive psychotherapy, using an education and medication compliance module (each psychotherapy added to standard pharmacotherapy protocols), in patients who had achieved a remission of mania or bipolar depression for at least 4 months, patients treated with IPSRT were significantly more likely to have normalized their schedules of the 17 circadian cues (i.e., their schedules were identical to those of control populations studied with the same instrument) (Frank et al. 1997). There were no significant clinical differences between the IPSRT and supportive psychotherapy groups after half of this planned 2-year study of a relatively small population had been completed. However, the effectiveness of IPSRT as an adjunctive maintenance treatment probably will not be apparent for several years.

BEHAVIOR THERAPY

Therapies for depression derived from principles of classic and operant conditioning, social learning theory, and learned helplessness include social learning approaches (Lewinsohn et al. 1984; P. D. McLean 1982), self-control therapy (Rehm 1977), social skills training (Hersen et al.

1984), and structured problem-solving therapy (Nezu 1986). Behavioral therapies utilize education, guided practice, homework assignments, and social reinforcement of successive approximations in a time-limited format, typically over 8–16 weeks. Depressive behaviors such as self-blame, passivity, and negativism are ignored, whereas behaviors that are inconsistent with depression, such as activity, experiencing pleasure, and solving problems, are rewarded. Rewards can include anything that the patient seems to seek out—from attention, to praise, to being permitted to withdraw or complain, to money. Learned helplessness is combated by the therapist's giving patients small, discrete tasks that very gradually become more demanding. For example, the person who feels hopeless about ever finding a job is first given the task of getting a newspaper. The next task is merely to look at the want ads, and only later is a list of possible jobs drawn up and one letter of application written. Each positive experience reinforces a feeling of accomplishment that makes the next task easier. Social skills training teaches self-reinforcement, assertive behavior, and the use of social reinforcers such as eye contact and compliments (Thase 1995).

In a meta-analysis of 10 suitable studies by the Agency for Health Care Policy and Services Research (1993), behavior therapy had an overall intention-to-treat efficacy rate of 55.3% and appeared to have a small advantage in relation to comparison psychotherapies in six studies and to pharmacotherapy in two studies. However, the adequacy of the treatments to which behavior therapy was compared has been questioned (Crits-Christoph 1992; Meterissian and Bradwejn 1989). Behavior therapy has had similar efficacy rates in depressed patients (R. A. Brown and Lewinsohn 1984) and in populations with a variety of psychiatric disorders (Budman et al. 1988). Group and individual behavioral therapies appear to have similar efficacy rates.

Support for the efficacy of maintenance behavior therapy in preventing depressive recurrence is not as well developed as support for its efficacy as an acute treatment (Thase 1995). Some studies comparing behavior therapy with no psychotherapy suggest that the benefits of behavior therapy persist after treatment is discontinued (P. McLean and Hakstian 1990; Nezu 1986), whereas other studies do not support this hypothesis (R. A. Brown and Lewinsohn 1984; Gallagher-Thompson et al. 1990). Adding antidepressants to behavior therapy did not enhance the outcome in three randomized outpatient trials of the combination (Hersen et al. 1984; Roth et al. 1982; Wilson 1982), but improvement was more rapid in two of the trials (Roth et al. 1982; Wilson 1982). Antidepressants may also have caused a greater number of more severely depressed patients to remain in trials of behavior therapy (Last et al. 1985; Thase 1995).

PSYCHODYNAMIC PSYCHOTHERAPY

At one time, extended and often unstructured psychodynamic psychotherapy was the standard psychotherapy for depression, and some case reports seemed to support its efficacy (Arieti and MacKenzie 1988; Gabbard 1995). With more experience, the utility of nondirective "traditional" psychodynamic approaches as a treatment for depression (as opposed to character pathology) was increasingly questioned (Thase 1995). There are no controlled studies of prolonged psychodynamic psychotherapy or psychoanalysis in mood disorders (Gabbard 1995). Brief dynamic psychotherapies have been applied to depressive disorders (Davenloo 1982; Luborsky 1984; J. Mann 1973; Strupp and Binder 1984), but they have not been studied as rigorously as have cognitive therapy and IPT (American Psychiatric Association 1993; Gabbard 1995). In eight randomized controlled trials, the utility of brief dynamic therapy has been studied, but methodological considerations limit the conclusions that can be drawn (Gabbard 1995). For example, low response rates (~35%) both to psychotherapy and treatment with antidepressants raise questions about the adequacy of either treatment. In addition, five of the six studies examined the treatments in a group format even though individual therapy is more widely practiced, and the therapy was usually performed by nonprofessional therapists who were not formally trained in brief dynamic therapy (Gabbard 1995).

CHARACTERISTICS OF AN EFFECTIVE PSYCHOTHERAPY FOR DEPRESSION

Even though data from controlled studies of psychotherapy of depression are limited, characteristics listed in Table 13–21 have repeatedly emerged as distinguishing effective treatments, regardless of the technical details of the therapy (Keller et al. 1996; Thase 1996). Extended, unstructured psychotherapies may be useful for treating associated problems such as personality disorders, but given the lack of data supporting the use of these therapies as primary treatments for depression, more focused, time- limited therapies seem appropriate, at least as initial approaches.

COMBINING MEDICATIONS AND PSYCHOTHERAPY

A recent review of two studies of dynamic psychodynamic therapy, three trials of behavior therapy, and nine studies of cognitive therapy, all of which included added antidepressants during the acute phase of treatment, found only a trend favoring a modest advantage for combined treatment, mainly because the studies reviewed had insufficient statistical power (Hollon and Fawcett 1995; Kazdin et al. 1989). Until more informative data become available about mild to moderate unipolar nonpsychotic depression, the recommendation that such depressive episodes be treated initially either with antidepressants or with one of the focused psychotherapies for depression (Klerman et al. 1974) seems reasonable. Some experts suggest that more severe major depressive episodes be treated first with antidepressants alone, so that time is not lost and the expense of psychotherapy is avoided for those patients who respond to a single treatment. These experts recommend combining medication and psychotherapy for patients with an inadequate response to either modality, with multiple symptom clusters that might respond differentially to psychotherapy and medication, or with a previously chronic course. Because addition of IPT to antidepressants reduced the attrition rate from 21% to 8% in the continuation therapy study of patients with recurrent unipolar depression (Frank et al. 1990), psychotherapy should be included in the maintenance treatment of recurrent unipolar depression, even if the index episode was not severe. Combining thymoleptic (mood-stabilizing) medications with IPSRT and behavioral techniques that reduce expressed emotion in the family shows promise of improving both medication compliance (Cochran 1984) and overall treatment response in bipolar mood disorders (Goodwin and Jamison 1991; Miklowitz 1992; Miklowitz and Goldstein 1990; Miklowitz et al. 1988).

INTEGRATED TREATMENT OF MOOD DISORDERS

Data from controlled studies are sufficiently limited and open to conflicting interpretations that practitioners must

TABLE 13–21. **Characteristics of an effective psychotherapy for depression**

Time limited

Explicit rationale for treatment shared by patient and therapist

Active and directive therapist

Focus on current problems

Emphasis on changing current behavior

Self-monitoring of progress

Involvement of significant others

Expression of cautious optimism

Problems divided into manageable units with short-term goals

Homework assignments

also consider in treatment planning the aggregate of anecdotal experience with patients with mood disorders, who often have complex syndromes with considerable comorbidity that do not resemble the purer mood disorders that are the subject of formal studies. Decisions about continuation therapy are made even more difficult by the lack of a sufficient number of prospective discontinuation studies.

The American Psychiatric Association's "Practice Guidelines for the Treatment of Major Depressive Disorder in Adults" (American Psychiatric Association 1993) state that successful treatment of mood disorders begins with a careful diagnostic, psychosocial, and medical evaluation and consideration of the patient's treatment preferences. The initial assessment of the patient with a mood disorder (and all subsequent treatment) occurs in the context of a relationship between doctor and patient. This interaction is crucial to the development of a therapeutic alliance (Sexton et al. 1996) in which the patient is engaged in a collaborative enterprise (A. T. Beck et al. 1979). In the National Institute of Mental Health Treatment of Depression Collaborative Research Program, the therapeutic alliance significantly affected outcomes of IPT, cognitive-behavior therapy, active pharmacotherapy, and placebo (Blatt et al. 1996; Krupnick et al. 1996). Treatment dropout rates are less than 10% when a collaborative alliance has been fostered (Frank et al. 1995). Informed consent is an essential component of a therapeutic alliance. Insofar as no treatment is clearly established as superior to other reasonable therapies for most mood disorders, the process of obtaining consent should involve a discussion of alternative therapies, the evidence in favor of and against the treatment course that is being recommended, and the likely outcome of no treatment. Like most aspects of the treatment of mood disorders, informed consent is a dynamic process that should periodically be reevaluated.

Evaluation of risk factors for suicide is essential in all patients with mood disorders (Buzan and Weissberg 1992). Because suicidal patients, especially those with psychotic or bipolar illness or both, may kill someone else before they kill themselves (Dubovsky and Thomas 1992), homicide risk should also be evaluated. Dangerousness is not a static issue but one that evolves with the mood disorder. It is therefore necessary to reevaluate dangerousness to self and others repeatedly throughout the treatment of a mood disorder. It is also important to inquire about nonsuicidal forms of self-destructive behavior, which are particular common in patients with comorbid mood and personality disorders.

Review of the patient's use of substances that can cause or aggravate depression and mania is another essential component of the evaluation of the patient with a mood disorder. Ongoing debate about the issue notwithstanding, it is much more difficult to treat a mood disorder in a patient who is actively using alcohol or illicit drugs. Because the presence of comorbid disorders in addition to substance-related disorders such as medical illness, panic disorder, eating disorders, obsessive-compulsive disorder, generalized anxiety, social phobia, posttraumatic stress disorder, and personality disorders can alter prognosis and call for a modification of the treatment, it is also important to diagnose these disorders in patients with mood disorders.

The next important step is to decide whether the mood disorder is unipolar or bipolar. Such a distinction is crucial, given the different treatment approaches in the two disorders. When a patient has a clear-cut history of mania, the diagnosis is straightforward; bipolar disorder may be more difficult to identify when a patient has had one or a few depressive episodes without obvious manic or hypomanic symptoms. Clues to bipolarity in a depressed patient are summarized in Table 13–22, although like all other aspects of mood disorders, the bipolar-unipolar distinction is one that may only be clarified with continued observation.

UNIPOLAR MAJOR DEPRESSIVE DISORDER

A mildly to moderately severe single major depressive episode without psychotic features can be treated with antidepressants or psychotherapy. However, the longer the duration of the episode or the greater its severity, the more likely an antidepressant is to be needed. Even if formal psychotherapy is not provided, antidepressant prescriptions should at least be accompanied by informed psychological management (Merriam and Karasu 1996). Because the presence of a comorbid personality disorder or perfectionism predicts a poorer response to antidepressants (Blatt 1995; Shea et al. 1990), as well as to briefer psycho-

TABLE 13–22. **Clues to bipolarity in depressed patients**

Highly recurrent depression

Intense anger

Racing thoughts

Mood-incongruent psychotic symptoms

Hallucinations

Thrill seeking

Increased libido with severe depression

Family history of bipolar disorder

Three consecutive generations with mood disorders

therapies (Shea and Hirschfeld 1996; Thase 1996), more intensive forms of psychodynamic psychotherapy may be appropriately added to antidepressants when these factors are present (Conte et al. 1986; Gabbard 1995; I. W. Miller and Keitner 1996), although empirical support for this approach has not yet emerged. Treatment of depression in a primary care setting is much less likely to include psychotherapy or counseling in any form than is treatment by mental health professionals, which produces better results (Meredith 1996; Schulberg 1996).

As was mentioned earlier, all of the currently available antidepressants are equally effective (Bech 1993; Hollon and Fawcett 1995; Kasper et al. 1992). This is not to say that all antidepressants are equally effective for all patients; many patients who do not respond to one agent will respond to another (Rush and Kupfer 1995). The initial choice of an antidepressant generally depends on history and current symptoms. For example, patients who have had a good response to a particular antidepressant may respond to the same medication again, although an antidepressant that was effective at one point may not be as effective on a second trial. Insomnia associated with depression often improves with remission of depression, but more sedating antidepressants such as doxepin, imipramine, trazodone, and nefazodone can produce more rapid relief of insomnia, whereas more activating antidepressants such as fluoxetine and tranylcypromine can aggravate insomnia (Neylan 1995). Because of their antihistamine properties, trimipramine and doxepin can be useful for treating allergies and peptic ulcer disease, and nefazodone may be useful for treating fibromyalgia. Newer antidepressants are safer than tricyclic antidepressants (TCAs) in patients with heart block and probably in patients with recent myocardial infarctions (Glassman and Proud'homme 1993). Patients with atypical depression appear to respond most frequently to monoamine oxidase inhibitors (MAOIs) and least frequently to TCAs (which are still more effective than placebos); selective serotonin reuptake inhibitors (SSRIs) are intermediate in efficacy (Quitkin et al. 1990, 1991; Rabkin et al. 1995).

An antidepressant overdose is the most common method of suicide in the United States (Buzan and Weissberg 1992). A large group of data contradicts a report of a small number of cases in which suicidal ideation was thought to be increased by SSRIs (Teicher et al. 1993) and indicates that the risk of suicide is reduced by all antidepressants, especially SSRIs, which decrease inwardly as well as outwardly directed aggression (Isacsson et al. 1996; Letizia et al. 1996; Warshaw and Keller 1996). Because SSRIs and other newer antidepressants are safer in overdose than TCAs (Glassman and Proud'homme

1993), SSRIs, venlafaxine, mirtazepine, and nefazodone may be the best initial choices for suicidal patients (Montgomery 1995). Prescribing small quantities of antidepressants to a suicidal patient in an attempt to prevent the patient from taking a lethal overdose causes the patient to make frequent trips to the pharmacy, which may encourage noncompliance and indirectly increase the risk of suicide. If the risk of suicide is so great that the physician cannot trust the patient with an antidepressant, the patient should be hospitalized.

Debate continues about the best antidepressant for severe depression. Well-publicized controlled studies found clomipramine to be superior to the SSRIs citalopram and paroxetine in severely depressed inpatients (Danish University Antidepressant Group 1986, 1990). However, not all controlled studies support the hypothesis that TCAs are more effective than SSRIs in more severe forms of unipolar depression (Nierenberg 1994). This issue remains unresolved because detecting a statistically significant difference in the efficacy of two active antidepressants requires the existence of more than 350 patients in each treatment group and is otherwise methodologically difficult (Lader 1988). ECT is a particularly appropriate option for patients who are too severely depressed or suicidal to wait for an antidepressant to take effect, patients who cannot tolerate an antidepressant, and patients with associated illnesses that might benefit from ECT, such as delirium or Parkinson's disease (Devanand et al. 1991a; Dubovsky 1995b).

A large body of data has accumulated about the treatment of major depression with psychotic features. Psychotic depression has a very low rate of spontaneous recovery (Kettering et al. 1987) and responds little or not at all to a placebo (Spiker and Kupfer 1988) or psychotherapy alone Dubovsky and Thomas 1992). Only 0%–46% (average, about 25%–35%) of patients with psychotic depression respond to TCAs (Avery and Lubano 1979; W. H. Nelson et al. 1984), even in high doses (Avery and Lubano 1979; W. H. Nelson et al. 1984; Spiker et al. 1986b); MAOIs do not produce better results (Janicak et al. 1988). Whereas 19%–48% of psychotically depressed patients recover with antipsychotic drugs therapy alone (Spiker et al. 1986a; 1986b), the combination of a neuroleptic and an antidepressant leads to improvement in an average of 70%–80% of patients (Anton and Burch 1986; Aronson et al. 1988; Spiker et al. 1986b)."Combination therapy" involves more than separate treatment of psychosis by the antipsychotic drug and depression by the antidepressant, because neuroleptic therapy alone ameliorates depression in some patients and antidepressants alone ameliorates psychosis in others (Dubovsky and Thomas 1992). Higher neuroleptic doses than those used for schizophrenia may be needed for psychotic depression (Aronson et al. 1987; J. C. Nelson et al. 1986; Spiker et al. 1985; Spiker et al. 1986b). Amoxapine, an antidepressant that is a metabolite of the neuroleptic amoxapine that also has neuroleptic properties, is almost as effective as traditional neuroleptic-antidepressant combinations in psychotic depression (Anton and Burch 1986). Preliminary experience suggests that clozapine may also be effective as monotherapy (McElroy et al. 1991). The response rate of psychotic depression is greatest with ECT (Solan et al. 1988).

DYSTHYMIC DISORDER

Placebo-controlled trials demonstrate that dysthymia responds as well as major depression does to TCAs, SSRIs, MAOIs, and atypical antidepressants such as tianeptine, although rates of noncompliance related to demoralization and intolerance of adverse effects are high (Conte and Karasu 1992; Harrison and Stewart 1993; Keller et al. 1996; Kocsis et al. 1988, 1989). In a comparison of the effect of ECT in 25 patients with double depression and 75 patients with MDD only, Prudic et al. (1993) found that both groups demonstrated the same level of improvement in depression rating-scale scores. However, patients with double depression had more residual symptoms and were more likely to relapse in the year following ECT, which suggests that the underlying dysthymia had been incompletely treated.

Psychotherapies that have been found useful for treating chronic depressive disorders, albeit creating a less robust response than in acute depression (Keller et al. 1996; Thase et al. 1994), include cognitive therapy, interpersonal therapy, behavior therapy, cognitive-behavior therapy, supportive therapy, psychoeducation, and family and marital therapy (Akiskal 1994; Conte and Karasu 1992; Frances 1993; Keitner and Miller 1990). Combining specific psychotherapies with antidepressants produces better results than medication therapy alone in dysthymic patients (Conte and Karasu 1992; Frances 1993; J. Scott 1988). Maintenance pharmacotherapy as well as psychotherapy is particularly important in reducing the risk of recurrence of dysthymia, as well as that of major depression in patients with double depression.

RECURRENT BRIEF DEPRESSION

There have been only a few studies of the treatment of recurrent brief depression. The data that have emerged suggest that antidepressants are not particularly effective in preventing acute depressive recurrences (Angst et al. 1990). Lithium may reduce acute recurrences, even though no evidence has emerged of a bipolar outcome in recurrent brief depression (Angst and Hochstrasser 1994). It is not known whether other mood-stabilizing medications might reduce the rate of recurrence of this form of depression, but insofar as all of these medications have antirecurrence as well as antimanic properties, it seems reasonable to consider using them. If recurrent brief depression is considered a mood disorder in which a bipolar trait (i.e., a high rate of recurrence) is combined with a type of depression that is unipolar in its form, the possibility must be considered that chronic use of antidepressants could have the potential to speed up the rate of recurrence of acute depressive episodes. This hypothesis awaits formal testing.

SEASONAL AFFECTIVE DISORDER

Artificial bright light is an effective treatment for seasonal affective disorder (SAD) (Rosenthal et al. 1989); rates of remission in published studies range from 36% to 75% (Rosenthal and Oren 1995; Tam et al. 1995). The minimal intensity of light that appears necessary for an antidepressant effect is 2,500 lux (1 lux = 10 foot candles) placed about 1 meter from the patient (Rosenthal et al. 1989). At greater intensities of light, a shorter duration of exposure to the light appears necessary. For example, remission rates with a 10,000-lux light unit for 30 minutes are similar to those with 2,500 lux for 2 hours (Tam et al. 1995). To be effective, light must enter the patient's eyes (Rosenthal et al. 1989), where it has been postulated that melatonin secretion is altered. However, this assumption has been questioned (Thalen et al. 1995), and resetting of the sleep-wake cycle could be a mechanism of action in some cases (Rosenthal et al. 1989). A light visor is available that has a lower intensity of light but is closer to the eyes than the standard light box, but the 35%–40% response rate to light-visor treatment is no better than to a placebo (Teicher et al. 1995). Use of an "artificial dawn," in which light of gradually increasing intensity is turned on before the patient wakes up, may be useful but is not as effective as standard light therapy (Tam et al. 1995).

Although some patients respond exclusively to morning light and some respond equally well to light administered at any time of the day, few patients respond preferentially to evening light (Rosenthal et al. 1989). Some authorities recommend that the patient start the treatment at whatever time of day is most convenient, so that compliance is increased, whereas others think that morning light should be tried first, especially in patients who tend to sleep late (Rosenthal and Oren 1995). Exposure to light too late in the day may make it difficult to fall asleep. There do not appear to be clinically significant differences in the effectiveness of any particular wavelength of light or of full-spectrum light versus cool-white fluorescent light (Tam et al. 1995).

Many patients respond to bright light within 3–5 days and relapse if they discontinue the light for treatment 3 days in a row during the winter. However, some patients who do not respond after 1 week of treatment will respond during the second week (Labbate et al. 1995). Patients with bipolar SAD may have a better response to artificial bright light than may patients with unipolar SAD (Deltito et al. 1991). Nonseasonally depressed patients may not respond as well as patients with SAD to light therapy, but chronically depressed patients with fall-winter exacerbations of depression may benefit from this treatment (Rosenthal et al. 1989). Artificial bright light may also be useful for treating seasonal lethargy without obvious depression, midwinter insomnia, jet lag, and adaptation to work shift changes (Rosenthal et al. 1989).

Artificial bright light appears to be safe if it does not contain light in the ultraviolet spectrum (Rosenthal et al. 1989). The most common side effects include headache and nausea; fatigue due to alteration of the sleep-wake cycle may occur acutely, but this often remits after about a week (Rosenthal et al. 1989). Concerns that lithium might sensitize the retina to damage from artificial bright light have not been borne out by recent research. Like anything with antidepressant properties, artificial bright light has the potential to induce mania or hypomania in bipolar patients (Rosenthal and Oren 1995).

A number of medications, including fluoxetine, moclobemide, tranylcypromine, bupropion, and alprazolam, appear to be at least as effective as bright light for treating SAD (Tam et al. 1995; Partonen et al. 1996). Whereas some patients prefer bright light because it is not a medication and has no real interactions, others find antidepressants more convenient, especially if they travel frequently. In patients with yearly recurrences of seasonal depression, bright light therapy is usually begun in the early fall and continued until the spring. It is not known whether seasonal administration of antidepressants is as effective in preventing winter recurrences of depression or whether chronic antidepressants would be more appropriate. Patients with bipolar SAD can be treated with seasonal use of bright light with or without a thymoleptic, depending on the response to the light and whether thymoleptics alone prevent seasonal recurrences. Prophylactic artificial bright light therapy from the fall through the spring prevents seasonal depressive recurrences.

UNIPOLAR DEPRESSION: MAINTENANCE TREATMENT

It is commonly recommended that antidepressants be continued for 6–9 months after a single episode of unipolar major depression (Consensus Development Panel 1985). However, this recommendation does not take into account the capacity of antidepressants to prevent recurrence, which occurs in 50% of patients within 2 years (Consensus Development Panel 1985). The decision to withdraw an antidepressant after the first major depressive episode therefore is more complex than it might appear at first glance. Obviously, patient preference is a crucial factor. Depressed patients often do not like taking antidepressants for extended periods. Cost and adverse effects are considerations, but many patients object even more to the idea of needing a medication because this appears to signify weakness or dependency. As is discussed below, patients may appreciate the benefit of an antidepressant while they are acutely ill, but when their mental state changes, they may no longer believe that they need the medication.

The risk-benefit ratio of continuing antidepressants is another factor to consider in deciding whether to continue treatment with an antidepressant after a first major depressive episode. If the episode was relatively mild and easy to treat, the risk of discontinuing antidepressants is low. Conversely, if the episode was severe or had major consequences such as a serious suicide attempt, inability to work, or disruption of the family, the risk of another episode may be substantially greater than the inconvenience of continuing antidepressant treatment. If depression only responded after multiple antidepressant trials, the benefit of continuing antidepressants may outweigh the risk of another long and difficult course of treatment. After improvement of depression with psychotherapy or pharmacotherapy, relapse and recurrence are up to five times more likely to occur after treatment withdrawal if residual symptoms are present (Blackburn et al. 1986; Thase et al. 1992). Slower antidepressant withdrawal may be less likely to be followed by relapse than rapid drug discontinuation.

There have been no prolonged antidepressant discontinuation studies after treatment of a first or second major depressive episode. However, after three or more episodes, withdrawal of the antidepressant within 5 years of remission has been found to be associated with an increased risk of recurrence (Frank et al. 1990; Kupfer et al. 1992). In view of reliable data indicating that relapse and recurrence of unipolar depression are reduced by continuation of the antidepressant (Devanand et al. 1991a; Fava and Kaji 1994; Frank et al. 1990, 1993b; Keller 1994; Kupfer et al. 1992), patients with recurrent unipolar depression should continue to take an effective antidepressant indefinitely. Of 23 prospective double-blind randomized studies of continuation and maintenance pharmacotherapy for depression, 22 found more recurrences in the placebo group, and the only study that detected no difference involved too small a sample to be reliable (Solomon and Bauer 1993). The same dose that produced a remission appears necessary to prevent recurrence (Blackburn 1994; Devanand et al. 1991a; Frank et al. 1993).

There have been at least 25 reports on the use of continuation/maintenance ECT since 1987 that suggest that such therapy can decrease rehospitalization rates by two-thirds or more (Petrides et al. 1994; Schwarz et al. 1995; Vanelle et al. 1994; Weiner 1995). Continuation/maintenance ECT is frequently administered on an outpatient basis, which increases patient acceptance (Association for Convulsive Therapy 1996). The frequency of maintenance treatments is based on symptom emergence as the time between ECT treatments is gradually increased.

Because cognitive therapy (Belsher and Costello 1988; Fava and Kaji 1994), cognitive-behavior therapy (J. Scott 1992), and interpersonal therapy (Frank et al. 1990; Frank et al. 1991; Kupfer et al. 1992) have an additive effect with antidepressants in reducing the risk of recurrence of unipolar depression, there is good reason to assume that continuation, possibly at a reduced frequency (Frank et al. 1990), of one of these psychotherapies—or any other psychotherapeutic approach that has proven useful in acute depression—along with the antidepressant will reduce the risk of relapse or recurrence of major depression or dysthymia (Weissman 1994). This is not an easy recommendation to implement in an era of cost containment that limits visits to the clinician after a patient is well. However, the cost of maintenance psychotherapy may be much less than the cost of treating another major episode, which could prove more difficult to treat than to prevent.

One problem that might be particularly responsive to maintenance psychotherapy is nonadherence with continuation of antidepressants. Between 33% and 68% of depressed patients have been found to be noncompliant with antidepressants (Burrows 1992; Jacob et al. 1984; Overall et al. 1987). Compliance with psychotherapy is usually better than with pharmacotherapy (Basco and Rush 1995), probably because psychotherapy has fewer adverse effects. When patients are acutely depressed, they may be more motivated to comply with pharmacotherapy, but when they feel better they are often less motivated to continue treatment (Last et al. 1985). The longer treatment must be continued, the more important addressing the meaning of the medication in psychotherapy may become to medication adherence.

MOOD DISORDERS IN CHILDREN AND ADOLESCENTS: USE OF ANTIDEPRESSANTS

Experience with antidepressants has not been as positive in younger patients as it has been in adults (Kashani and Nair 1995). In placebo-controlled trials, the efficacy of TCAs has consistently been found to be equivalent to that of placebo in children with major depression and less than that of placebo in adolescents with this disorder (Ambrosini et al. 1993; Geller et al. 1996). There are several possible explanations for these findings (Geller et al. 1996; Kashani and Nair 1995; Mandoki et al. 1997). The placebo response rate may be so high in juvenile patients with depression that it is impossible to demonstrate a differential effect of active treatment. Environmental factors may be more important in some younger patients, and antidepressants alone may be less effective in such patients. Fear of adverse effects and lack of knowledge about effective doses may result in underdosing, especially given the fact that antidepressants are metabolized more rapidly in younger than in older patients. For the same reason, once-a-day dosing may produce serum levels that are not as consistent in children and younger adolescents as they are in adults. In some cases, early-onset depression may be more severe and therefore more likely to be refractory to treatment. High rates of bipolarity and comorbidity could also contribute to lower antidepressant response rates in younger patients, whose illnesses may be biologically different from adult mood disorders. Finally, not all results of antidepressant trials in adults have been positive, and there may not have been a sufficient number of controlled trials in children and adolescents to yield positive results.

Childhood and adolescent depression is often accompanied by atypical features, and it has been suggested that treatment with MAOIs may be more effective than that with TCAs, but dietary noncompliance is often a problem with treatment with MAOIs (Kashani and Nair 1995). The SSRIs are safer and better tolerated in younger populations. One of two controlled studies of fluoxetine in children and adolescents demonstrated superiority of fluoxetine to placebo, and one study showed no difference between placebo and active drug (Geller et al. 1996). A controlled study of venlafaxine in 33 patients ages 8–17 years showed no differences between active drug and placebo, but doses were very low and patients given placebo as well as those given venlafaxine received psychotherapy in addition to medication (Mandoki et al. 1997). Ongoing studies suggest superiority to placebo of paroxetine and fluvoxamine in younger depressed patients. ECT is about as effective and safe in juvenile patients as it is in adults (Bertagnolli and Borchardt 1990; Fink 1993; Schneekloth et al. 1993; Walter and Rey 1997), but informed consent is more difficult and fears of the treatment are greater the younger the patient.

Given the current state of knowledge, children and adolescents should be treated first with individual and/or family psychotherapy (Emslie et al. 1995; Mandoki et al. 1997); more intensive psychotherapies may be more likely to achieve full recovery (Geller et al. 1996). Nonresponders to psychotherapy might receive an SSRI before any other class of antidepressant. The high rate of bipolar outcome and the lack of any prospective studies of antidepressant maintenance therapy warrant discontinuation of antidepressants at some point after remission, but the timing of this intervention remains to be studied.

MANIA

Lithium, carbamazepine, valproic acid (divalproex), and verapamil appear to be equally effective in the treatment of acute mania; response rates range from 60% to 78% (American Psychiatric Association 1994b; Bowden 1995; Bowden et al. 1994; Delgado and Gelenberg 1995; Dubovsky 1994b, 1995a; Dubovsky and Buzan 1997). Lithium is the best studied and most clearly established of these agents, whereas verapamil has not been subjected to multicenter studies. Treatment with lithium may be less effective than treatment with the anticonvulsants in mixed (dysphoric) mania and rapid cycling (McElroy et al. 1992); however, a direct comparison of carbamazepine and lithium in rapid-cycling bipolar disorder found both drugs to be equally effective (Okuma et al. 1990). Treatment with combinations of antimanic drugs may be more effective than that with a single medication (Keck et al. 1992).

Rapid oral loading with divalproex may produce a more rapid antimanic action (Keck et al. 1993). Most of the time, however, the antimanic effect of this and other antimanic drugs is delayed. Until recently neuroleptics, particularly haloperidol, were used routinely to control agitation until the antimanic drug took effect. However, not all manic patients are psychotic, and psychosis accompanying mania may remit with adequate treatment of the mania (Cohen and Lipinski 1986; Fennig et al. 1995; Goodwin and Jamison 1991; Prien et al. 1972). Supplementation of neuroleptics with the benzodiazepines lorazepam or clonazepam was introduced as a means of minimizing neuroleptic exposure with its attendant risks of side effects and adverse interactions with antimanic drugs (Sachs 1990; Salzman et al. 1986). More recently, benzodiazepines have been used without antipsychotic drugs in the initial treatment of mania (Bradwejn et al. 1990; Colwell and Lopez 1987; Lenox et al. 1986; Modell et al. 1985; Santos and Morton 1987). The benzodiazepine, with or without a neuroleptic, can be administered first to improve agitation and sleep. Once the patient's behavior is under better control, any neuroleptics that have been prescribed are withdrawn as an antimanic drug is gradually introduced. Minimizing neurotoxic medication interactions permits more rapid release from the hospital.

BIPOLAR DEPRESSION

There are fewer controlled studies of the treatment of bipolar depression than of that of other forms of depression (Brady et al. 1995). However, in view of the risk of antidepressant-induced mania and rapid cycling noted earlier, American Psychiatric Association practice guidelines for the treatment of bipolar disorder recommend that treatment of bipolar depression begin with an antimanic drug (American Psychiatric Association 1994b). Lithium has been noted to be an effective antidepressant in 30%–79% of bipolar depressed patients (Sachs et al. 1994b; Zornberg and Rose 1993). The finding that a full response to lithium took up to 8 weeks in nine controlled studies (Zornberg and Rose 1993) may imply that the treatment trial was inadequate in studies with a lower response rate. Valproate and carbamazepine have not been as well studied for treatment of bipolar depression, but experience suggests that they are not usually effective antidepressants as monotherapies (American Psychiatric Association 1994b). Divalproex may be effective for depressive symptoms occurring during a manic episode (Swann et al. 1997).

When bipolar depression does not remit with treatment with an antimanic drug, the psychiatrist must decide whether to add a second antimanic drug or an antidepressant. Antimanic drugs are not as effective as antidepressants for treating depression and have more adverse effects, but all antidepressants carry the risk of inducing mania and rapid cycling (Akiskal 1994; Peet and Peters 1995; Srisurapanont et al. 1995). In the absence of controlled data, there is only clinical experience and expert opinion to guide the choice between these two courses. Our experience has been that antidepressants do not produce a predictably positive response in bipolar depression with prominent mixed hypomanic symptoms such as profound irritability, decreased sleep without feeling tired during the day, racing thoughts, or increased libido. Instead, the antidepressant either provokes more dysphoric hypomania or produces initial improvement followed by more recurrences of mixed bipolar depression. Treatment with a combination of antimanic drugs may produce a remission, or it may at least convert a refractory mixed state to a more uncomplicated bipolar depression with hypersomnia, lethargy, slowed thinking, and lack of interpersonal sensitivity that may respond more predictably to addition of an antidepressant.

The combination of lithium and carbamazepine has been found to have antidepressant properties in some reported cases (Ketter et al. 1995; Post 1988). Verapamil has been used to treat bipolar depression in a few cases (Deicken 1990). Initial experience suggested that lamotrigine and gabapentin may have antidepressant as well as antimanic properties that could prove useful for treating mixed bipolar depression (Calabrese et al. 1996a), but no studies of this indication exist. If psychotic symptoms are present, it may be necessary to add neuroleptic therapy, but continuation of neuroleptic therapy may contribute to depressive recurrences in some cases (Dubovsky and Buzan 1997; Hendrick et al. 1994). As we pointed out earlier, clozapine appears to have both antidepressant and mood-stabilizing properties (Zarate et al. 1995a, 1996), but risperidone has been noted to destabilize mood in some patients with bipolar mood disorders (Dubovsky and Buzan 1997).

It seems clear that antidepressants should normally not be administered to patients with bipolar depression unless an antimanic drug is coadministered. However, the choice of a specific antidepressant in treating bipolar depression is limited by lack of replicated data. The TCAs seem more likely to induce mania and rapid cycling than bupropion, the MAOIs, and the SSRIs (Akiskal 1994; Rosenbaum et al. 1995; Sachs et al. 1994a; Stoll et al. 1994). Stimulants are generally not used as antidepressants in unipolar depression because tolerance to their antidepressant action develops, but the rapid onset and short duration of antidepressant effect of stimulants can be useful for treating bipolar depression. Artificial bright light can be a rapidly effective and safe antidepressant for bipolar depression with a seasonal component or with lethargy and oversleeping (Papatheodorou and Kutcher 1995a); as is true of stimulants, the short duration of action may make adverse effects on mood remit more rapidly. The most reliable class of antidepressant medication for bipolar depression is probably the MAOIs, particularly tranylcypromine (Ketter et al. 1995). ECT is the most effective treatment for bipolar depression (Dubovsky 1995b), which is unlike other antidepressant therapies in that it rarely induces mania, and when it does, further ECT usually normalizes mood.

There is no evidence that continuation of antidepressants after remission of bipolar depression prevents further depressive recurrences (Loo and Brochier 1995); this is in contrast to unipolar depression. In view of the risks of long-term antidepressants, it seems prudent to attempt to withdraw the antidepressant once mood normalizes, while continuing the mood-stabilizing regimen. Gradual discontinuation of antidepressants may reduce the risk of rebound of depression. If it becomes necessary to continue treatment with the antidepressant, lower doses may be less likely to destabilize mood. As described later in this chapter, maintenance ECT can prevent recurrences of bipolar depression as well as mania.

MIXED AND RAPID-CYCLING BIPOLAR DISORDER

Although the response rate of uncomplicated mania to lithium in three recent trials ranged from 59% to 91%, response rates in patients with mixed states were only 29%–43% (S. Gershon and Soares 1997); similar results have been obtained in patients with rapid cycling. Patients with either form of complex mood disorder may have a better response to valproate or carbamazepine (Freeman et al. 1992; Post 1992a; Swann et al. 1997). Valproic acid appears to be equally effective in rapidly and non–rapid-cycling bipolar disorder (Bowden et al. 1994). A recent consensus panel recommended valproate as the first choice for treating rapid cycling, followed by carbamazepine and then lithium (Expert Consensus Panel 1996). Additional treatments that have been reported to be useful for some patients with rapid-cycling bipolar disorder include ECT, antimanic combinations, nimodipine, clozapine, and supplementation with suprametabolic doses of thyroxine (Bauer and Whybrow 1990; Baumgartner et al. 1994; Calabrese et al. 1991, 1996b; Expert Consensus Panel 1996; Frye et al. 1996; Goodnick 1995b; Pazzaglia et al. 1993; Stancer and Persad 1982; Suppes et al. 1994; Swann 1995; Terao 1993; Wehr et al. 1988).

BIPOLAR DISORDER: MAINTENANCE TREATMENT

The high rates of affective recurrence, as well as the increasing severity and decreasing latency of each recurrence (Keller et al. 1993), are reasons to continue a mood-stabilizing regimen after remission of any acute episode of mania or bipolar depression. Treatment response can be assessed over time with the help of a structured mood chart. Post (1992a) and others (Altschuler et al. 1995; Pazzaglia et al. 1993; Roy-Byrne et al. 1984) developed a "life-charting" method that quantifies symptoms and important life events. However, life-charting is time-consuming and relies on observations by nursing staff. In everyday outpatient practice, it may be equally helpful to construct with the patient a graph on which specific symptoms are rated one or more times per day on whatever scale makes the most sense (e.g., mood can be rated from −5 for very depressed to +5 for manic, with 0 signifying euthymia). Different symptoms can be indicated by different line colors or styles, and changes in treatment and important events can be noted on the same graph.

At least 10 double-blind, placebo-controlled studies of more than 200 patients demonstrate that lithium substantially reduces the number of manic and depressive recurrences (0%–44% of patients taking lithium had recurrences, compared with 38%–93% of patients taking placebo) (Goodwin and Jamison 1991; Solomon and Bauer 1993). Serum lithium levels greater than 0.8 mM are associated with half the recurrence rate of levels less than 0.6 mM , although adverse effects are more common at higher levels (American Psychiatric Association 1994b; Gelenberg et al. 1989). The prophylactic effect of lithium results in a substantial decrease in suicide rates, resulting in turn in the addition of 7 years to life expectancy (National Institute of Mental Health 1995). More than 50% of patients experience an affective episode within 6 months of discontinuing lithium therapy, but the risk of recurrence is almost five times as great (median time in remission, 4 months) in patients who discontinue lithium therapy rapidly than in those who taper the drug (median time in remission, 20 months) (Baldessarini et al. 1996). There is no reason to expect different results with discontinuation of other thymoleptics.

Carbamazepine was effective as a maintenance treatment in bipolar illness in four published trials; however, lack of a placebo control in three of these trials and only a trend toward superiority of carbamazepine in the only placebo-controlled trial limit the strength of this conclusion (Solomon et al. 1995). Retrospective studies suggest that valproate prevents affective recurrences in bipolar disorder, but only one prospective placebo-controlled study of maintenance with valproate—in which patients were randomized to lithium monotherapy, divalproex monotherapy, or placebo—has been conducted, and the results have not yet been published (Solomon et al. 1995). Verapamil and nimodipine have had mood-stabilizing effects in small numbers of cases of bipolar mood disorder (Dubovsky 1995a; Dubovsky and Buzan 1997).

Case series suggest that combinations of two or three mood stabilizers may provide better affective prophylaxis than can be achieved with monotherapy (Bowden 1996; Expert Consensus Panel 1996). ECT is a highly effective maintenance therapy (Karliner and Wehrheim 1965;

Vanelle et al. 1994). Neuroleptics may be necessary adjuncts in the maintenance therapy of psychotic bipolar disorder, although as noted earlier these medications are thought to increase depressive recurrences in some cases. Clozapine seems more consistently effective as a mood stabilizer (Calabrese et al. 1991; Puri et al. 1995; Zarate et al. 1995b, 1996).

The efficacy of antimanic drugs in preventing recurrences (i.e., as mood stabilizers) has been noted to decline significantly from the first year to the fifth year of treatment (Peselow et al. 1994). Although the evolving physiology of bipolar disorder is probably one important factor in the increasing rate of recurrence with time, the fact that only one-third of outpatients are estimated to remain compliant is at least as important an issue (S. Gershon and Soares 1997). Noncompliance with mood stabilizers occurred in 64% of patients in the month preceding hospitalization for acute mania in a recent study (Keck et al. 1996). On follow-up of 140 patients recently hospitalized for bipolar disorder, 51% were partially or totally noncompliant with medications (Keck et al. 1997). Nonadherence, the most common cause of which is denial of illness and the need for treatment, is more common in patients with comorbid substance use disorders (Keck et al. 1996).

Obviously, one important goal of any form of maintenance psychotherapy is to improve medication compliance (Frank et al. 1995; Miklowitz 1992). Interpersonal and social rhythm therapy (IPSRT) has been shown to stabilize circadian rhythms, and preliminary evidence suggests that it can enhance the action of mood-stabilizing medications (Frank et al. 1997; Miklowitz and Goldstein 1990). Even if formal interpersonal therapy and logs of circadian cues are not utilized, helping the patient to keep regular hours, especially of going to sleep and waking up, and resolving interpersonal and family distress, including unrealistic expectations and high levels of expressed emotion, has an additive effect with mood-stabilizing medications (Frank et al. 1997; Miklowitz and Goldstein 1990; Miklowitz et al. 1988).

MOOD DISORDERS IN CHILDREN AND ADOLESCENTS: ANTIMANIC DRUGS

Lithium has not consistently been found to be effective in mania or bipolar depression in younger patients (Geller et al. 1996; Kafantaris 1995); the same is true of therapy with antidepressants in major depression. Although there is no reason to think that a high placebo response rate accounts for the apparent reduced rate of responsiveness to lithium in juvenile bipolar mood disorder, it is possible that this population requires more frequent dosing or higher serum levels than are required for a thymoleptic response in adults. Anticonvulsants have been the subject of open trials in childhood and adolescent bipolar disorder but not of placebo-controlled studies (Kafantaris 1995; Papatheodorou et al. 1995; Porter 1987). The results of these trials demonstrate that divalproex and carbamazepine are well tolerated and possibly effective. Verapamil, which is used regularly to treat childhood and adolescent cardiovascular disease, has been used successfully in a few cases of adolescent mania (Kastner and Friedman 1992). Case series and clinical experience indicate that ECT is as effective for treating mania in juvenile patients as it is in adults (Bertagnolli and Borchardt 1990; Carr et al. 1983; Kutcher and Robertson 1995). The course of juvenile bipolar disorder is more chronic than is that of adult bipolar disorder (Lewinsohn et al. 1995), but until empirical data are accumulated, decisions about the balance between potential positive and negative effects of maintenance medications on affective recurrence and intellectual and personality development are matters of opinion and personal experience.

CONCLUSIONS

Mood disorders are not unitary illnesses but complex syndromes with distinct etiologies, courses, and treatment responses that may ultimately be better understood through the addition of a more thorough dimensional analysis (e.g., early vs. late onset, comorbidity, disordered thinking, degree of intrusion into the personality) to existing categorical diagnoses. Even the most complete description of an affective episode at one point in time does not fully capture the picture of a mood disorder as it evolves over time. Mood disorders are not static but are dynamic conditions in which each new episode is a function of previous episodes (Post 1992b).

The evolving course of mood disorders is the result of an incompletely understood interaction of genetics, environmental factors, and cell biology (Consensus Development Panel 1985; Dubovsky 1997; Post 1990a, 1992b, 1994; Post et al. 1986, 1992; Thase 1990; Thase and Kupfer 1996). In many cases, initial episodes appear in response to an external stress, usually a loss or separation, or an event that evokes strong arousal or helplessness. The degree to which such events provoke an affective episode depends on their intrinsic severity and on predisposing and protective factors within the individual who experiences them. Mood in early episodes is often more reactive to the environment. Symptoms are less complex, and psychosocial disruption is

less complete. The neurobiology of an initial affective episode may be less complex, because a single treatment is often effective, and the physiology as well as the psychology of abnormal mood remits completely with treatment in the absence of substantial genetic loading or overwhelming early adverse experience. If they are not too severe, early depressive episodes respond equally well to environmental manipulation, psychotherapy, or medications. Early uncomplicated hypomanic episodes may respond fully to a single antimanic drug, and it is possible that normalization of circadian rhythms, IPSRT, reduction of expressed emotion in the family, and other psychosocial interventions could be equally effective.

With succeeding affective episodes, the psychobiology of mania or depression becomes more deeply ingrained by processes such as kindling, resetting of synaptic connections, and changes in gene expression induced by neurotransmitter, receptor, and second messenger responses to abnormal moods. At this stage, dysregulated affect becomes part of the normal repertoire of the synapse. At the same time, negative thinking, withdrawal, social ineptitude, irritability, and other depressive behaviors elicit negative input from others, which reinforces feelings of helplessness and solidifies the patient's identity as someone who is unfulfilled, overwhelmed, unpredictable, impulsive, incompetent, or unreliable. As more time is spent in the neurobiology and the psychology of abnormal mood, remissions are less complete and new recurrences develop with less provocation. These episodes are more likely to cause losses than to be caused by them.

Later affective recurrences are more abrupt, more severe, and more complex, as additional systems are recruited into an abnormal state. Environmental manipulations are not as successful at this point because the mood disorder is less responsive to external events. Psychological constellations are less amenable to structured psychotherapies and require more vigorous efforts to become reorganized. In cases in which single medications initially were effective, more complex interventions are necessary to address multiple interacting elements of abnormal cellular function. New medications aimed at second messengers or gene expression may prove useful for treating later-stage mood disorders involving multiple transmitter and receptor systems and more aggressive and extended forms of psychotherapy may be necessary for mood disorders that have become integrated into the personality.

One important implication of the accumulating data about the course of mood disorders is that it is easier to treat early episodes than it is to treat later episodes of unipolar or bipolar mood disorders. Another is that complete treatment of early episodes and continuation of effective therapy reduces the risk of later, more refractory episodes. Unfortunately, denial, reluctance to acknowledge needing help because being helped feels like a sign of weakness, and pressure from family members who themselves may have mood disorders make it difficult for people in the early stages of a mood disorder to recognize the seriousness of the illness, let alone treat it. Public education has reduced the stigma of seeking treatment for depression to some extent, but efforts to educate primary care physicians, who are more likely than mental health professionals to encounter patients with mood disorders for the first time, have not been successful in increasing rates of effective recognition, treatment, and, where necessary, referral of these patients for specialty care. Research into strategies for approaching mood disorders in primary care practice is therefore as important as research into new treatment technologies.

REFERENCES

Abrams RC: Electroconvulsive Therapy. New York, Oxford University Press, 1988

Abramson LY, Seligman MEP, Teasdale JD: Learned helplessness in humans: critique and reformulation. J Abnorm Psychol 87:49–74, 1978

Agency for Health Care Policy and Services Research: Clinical Practice Guideline: Depression in Primary Care, Vol 2: Treatment of Major Depression. Rockville, MD, U.S. Department of Health and Human Services, 1993

Ahlfors UG, Baastrup PC, Dencker SJ: Flupenthixol decanoate in recurrent manic-depressive illness: a comparison with lithium. Acta Psychiatr Scand 64:226–237, 1981

Akiskal HS: The interface of chronic depression with personality and anxiety disorders. Psychopharmacol Bull 20:393–398, 1984

Akiskal HS: Chronic depression. Bull Menninger Clin 240:349–354, 1991

Akiskal HS: Dysthymic and cyclothymic depressions: therapeutic considerations. Compr Psychiatry 55 (suppl 4):46–52, 1994

Akiskal HS: Developmental pathways to bipolarity: are juvenile-onset depressions pre-bipolar? J Am Acad Child Adolesc Psychiatry 34:754–763, 1995a

Akiskal HS: Le spectre bipolaire: acquisitions et perspectives cliniques. Encephale 21 (Spec No 6):3–11, 1995b

Akiskal HS: The prevalent clinical spectrum of bipolar disorders: beyond DSM-IV. J Clin Psychopharmacol 16 (2 suppl 1):4S–14S, 1996

Akiskal HS, Djenderedjian AM, Rosenthal RH, et al: Cyclothymic disorder: validating criteria for inclusion in the bipolar affective group. Am J Psychiatry 134: 1227–1233, 1977

Akiskal HS, Walker P, Puzantian VR, et al: Bipolar outcome in the course of depressive illness. J Affect Disord 5:115–128, 1983

Akiskal HS, Downs J, Jordan P, et al: Affective disorders in referred children and younger siblings of manic-depressives. Arch Gen Psychiatry 42:996–1003, 1985

Altschuler LL, Post RM, Leverich GS: Antidepressant-induced mania and cycle acceleration: a controversy revisited. Am J Psychiatry 152:1130–1138, 1995

Ambrosini PJ, Bianchi MD, Rabinovich H, et al: Antidepressant treatments in children and adolescents, I: affective disorders. J Am Acad Child Adolesc Psychiatry 32:1–5, 1993

American Psychiatric Association: Diagnostic and Statistical Manual: Mental Disorders. Washington, DC, American Psychiatric Association, 1952

American Psychiatric Association: Diagnostic and Statistical Manual of Mental Disorders, 2nd Edition. Washington, DC, American Psychiatric Association, 1968

American Psychiatric Association: Diagnostic and Statistical Manual of Mental Disorders, 3rd Edition. Washington, DC, American Psychiatric Association, 1980

American Psychiatric Association: American Psychiatric Glossary. Washington, DC, American Psychiatric Press, 1984

American Psychiatric Association: Diagnostic and Statistical Manual of Mental Disorders, 3rd Edition, Revised. Washington, DC, American Psychiatric Association, 1987

American Psychiatric Association: The Practice of Electroconvulsive Therapy: Recommendations for Treatment, Training and Privileging. Washington, DC, American Psychiatric Association, 1990

American Psychiatric Association: Practice guidelines for treatment of major depression in adults. Am J Psychiatry 150 (suppl 4):1–26, 1993

American Psychiatric Association: Diagnostic and Statistical Manual of Mental Disorders, 4th Edition. Washington, DC, American Psychiatric Association, 1994a

American Psychiatric Association: Practice guidelines for the treatment of patients with bipolar disorder. Am J Psychiatry 151 (suppl 12):1–36, 1994b

Ananth J, Wohl M, Ranganath V: Rapid cycling patients: conceptual and etiological factors. Neuropsychobiology 27:193–198, 1993

Andreasen NC: Creativity and mental illness: prevalence rates in writers and their first-degree relatives. Am J Psychiatry 144:1288–1292, 1987

Angst J: Clinical course of affective disorders, in Depressive Illness: Prediction of Course and Outcome. Edited by Hedgson T, Daly RJ. Berlin, Springer, 1988, pp 205–250

Angst J: Epidémiologie du spectre bipolaire. Encephale 21 (Spec No 6): 37–42, 1995

Angst J, Hochstrasser B: Recurrent brief depression: the Zurich Study. Compr Psychiatry 55 (suppl 4):3–9, 1994

Angst J, Wicki W: The Zurich Study, XI: is dysthymia a separate form of depression? Results of the Zurich Cohort Study. Eur Arch Psychiatry Clin Neurosci 240:349–354, 1991

Angst J, Merikangas K, Scheidegger P, et al: Recurrent brief depression: a new subtype of affective disorder. J Affect Disord 19:87–98, 1990

Anton RF, Burch EA: Amoxapine versus amitriptyline combined with perphenazine in the treatment of psychotic depression. Am J Psychiatry 147:1203–1208, 1986

Antonuccio DO, Danton WG, DeNelsky GY: Psychotherapy versus medication for depression: challenging the conventional wisdom with data. Professional Psychology—Research and Practice 26:574–585, 1995

Aperia B: Effects of electroconvulsive therapy on neuropsychological function and circulating levels of ACTH, cortisol, prolactin, and TSH in patients with major depressive illness. Acta Psychiatr Scand 72:536–541, 1985

Arieti S, MacKenzie KR: Psychotherapy of severe depression: recent developments in brief psychotherapy. Am J Psychiatry 39:852–864, 1988

Aronson TA, Shukla S, Hoff A: Continuation therapy after ECT for delusional depression: a naturalistic study of prophylactic treatments and relapse. Convuls Ther 3:251–259, 1987

Aronson TA, Shukla S, Hoff A, et al: Proposed delusional depression subtypes: preliminary evidence from a retrospective study of phenomenology and treatment course. J Affect Disord 14:69–74, 1988

Aronson TA, Shukla S, Hirschowitz J: Clonazepam treatment of five lithium-refractory patients with bipolar disorder. Am J Psychiatry 146:77–80, 1989

Association for Convulsive Therapy: Ambulatory electroconvulsive therapy: report of a task force of the Association for Convulsive Therapy. Convuls Ther 12:42–55, 1996

Avery D, Lubano A: Depression treated with imipramine and ECT: the DeCarolis study reconsidered. Am J Psychiatry 136:559–562, 1979

Avissar S, Schreiber G: Interaction of antibipolar and antidepressant treatments with receptor-coupled G proteins. Pharmacopsychiatry 25:44–50, 1992a

Avissar S, Schreiber G: The involvement of guanine nucleotide binding proteins in the pathogenesis and treatment of affective disorders. Biol Psychiatry 31:435–459, 1992b

Baldessarini RJ, Tondo L, Faedda GL, et al: Effects of the rate of discontinuing lithium maintenance treatment in bipolar disorders. Compr Psychiatry 57:441–448, 1996

Banken DM, Wilson GL: Treatment acceptability of alternative therapies for depression: a comparative analysis. Psychotherapy: Research, Theory, and Practice 29:610–619, 1992

Banov MD, Zarate CA, Tohen M, et al: Clozapine therapy in refractory affective disorders: polarity predicts response in long-term follow-up. Compr Psychiatry 55:295–300, 1994

Barbini B, Di Molfetta D, Gasperini M, et al: Seasonal concordance of recurrence in mood disorder patients. European Psychiatry 10:171–174, 1995

Barefoot JC, Schroll M: Symptoms of depression, acute myocardial infarction, and total mortality in a community sample. Circulation 93:1976–1980, 1996

Barklage NE: Evaluation and management of the suicidal patient. Emergency Care Quarterly 7:9–17, 1991

Barnet B, Duggan AK, Wilson MD, et al: Association between postpartum substance use and depressive symptoms, stress, and social support in adolescent mothers. Pediatrics 96:659–666, 1995

Barrett JE: Naturalistic change after 2 years in neurotic depressive disorders (RDC categories). Compr Psychiatry 25:404–418, 1984

Barton BM, Gitlin MJ: Verapamil in treatment-resistant mania: an open trial. J Clin Psychopharmacol 7:101–103, 1987

Basco MR, Rush AJ: Compliance with pharmacotherapy in mood disorders. Psychiatric Annals 25:269–279, 1995

Bauer MS, Whybrow PC: The effect of changing thyroid function on cyclic affective illness in a human subject. Am J Psychiatry 143:633–636, 1986

Bauer MS, Whybrow PC: Rapid cycling bipolar affective disorder. Arch Gen Psychiatry 47:435–440, 1990

Bauer MS, Whybrow PC, Winokur A: Rapid cycling bipolar affective disorder, I: association with grade I hypothyroidism. Arch Gen Psychiatry 47:427–432, 1990

Baumgartner A, Bauer M, Hellweg R: Treatment of intractable non-rapid cycling bipolar affective disorder with high-dose thyroxine: an open clinical trial. Neuropsychopharmacology 10:183–189, 1994

Bebbington R: The epidemiology of bipolar affective disorder. Soc Psychiatry Psychiatr Epidemiol 30:279–292, 1995

Bech P: Acute therapy of depression. Compr Psychiatry 54 (suppl 8):18–27, 1993

Beck AT, Rush AJ, Shaw BF: Cognitive Therapy of Depression. New York, Guilford, 1979

Beck AT, Jallon SD, Young JE: Treatment of depression with cognitive therapy and amitriptyline. Arch Gen Psychiatry 42:142–148, 1985

Beck CT: A meta-analysis of the relationship between postpartum depression and infant temperament. Nurs Res 45:225–230, 1996

Belsher G, Costello CG: Relapse after recovery from unipolar depression: a critical review. Psychol Bull 104:84–96, 1988

Bemporad JR: Psychodynamic models of depression and mania, in Depression and Mania. Edited by Georgotas A, Cancro R. New York, Elsevier, 1988, pp 167–180

Benkelfat C: Serotonergic mechanisms in psychiatric disorder: new research tools, new ideas. Int Clin Psychopharmacol 8 (suppl 2):53–56, 1993

Bergsholm P, Martinsen EW, Svoen N, et al: Affective disorders: drug treatment and electroconvulsive therapy. Tidsskr Nor Laegeforen 112:2651–2656, 1992

Bernstein L: Abrupt cessation of rapid-cycling bipolar disorder with the addition of low-dose L-tetraiodothyronine to lithium. J Clin Psychopharmacol 12:443–444, 1992

Berrettini WH, Ferraro TN, Goldin LR, et al: A linkage study of bipolar illness. Arch Gen Psychiatry 54:27–35, 1997

Bertagnolli MW, Borchardt CM: A review of ECT for children and adolescents. J Am Acad Child Adolesc Psychiatry 29:302–307, 1990

Berthier ML, Kulisevsky J, Gironell A: Poststroke bipolar affective disorder: clinical subtypes, concurrent movement disorders, and anatomical correlates. J Neuropsychiatry Clin Neurosci 8:160–167, 1996

Beydoun A, Uthman BM, Sackellares JC: Gabapentin: pharmacokinetics, efficacy, and safety. Clin Neuropharmacol 18:469–481, 1995

Biederman J: Developmental subtypes of juvenile bipolar disorder. Sexual and Marital Therapy 3:227–230, 1995

Bigelow LB, Weinberger DR, Wyatt RJ: Synergism of combined lithium-neuroleptic therapy: a double-blind, placebo-controlled case study. Am J Psychiatry 138:81–83, 1981

Bigger JT, Hoffman BF: Antiarrhythmic drugs, in Goodman and Gilman's The Pharmacological Basis of Therapeutics, 8th Edition. Edited by Gilman AG, Rall TW, Nies AS, et al. New York, Pergamon, 1991, pp 840–873

Black DW, Winokur G, Nasrallah A: Treatment of mania: a naturalistic study of electroconvulsive therapy versus lithium in 438 patients. Compr Psychiatry 48:132–139, 1987

Black DW, Bell S, Hulbert J: The importance of Axis II in patients with major depression. J Affect Disord 14:114–122, 1988

Blackburn I-M: Psychology and psychotherapy of depression. Current Opinion in Psychiatry 7:30–33, 1994

Blackburn I-M, Eunson KM, Bishop S: A two-year naturalistic follow-up of depressed patients treated with cognitive therapy, pharmacotherapy, and a combination of both. J Affect Disord 10:67–75, 1986

Blatt SJ: The destructiveness of perfectionism: implications for the treatment of depression. Am Psychol 50:1003–1020, 1995

Blatt SJ, Sanislow CA, Zuroff DC, et al: Characteristics of effective therapists: further analyses of data from the National Institute of Mental Health Treatment of Depression Collaborative Research Program. J Consult Clin Psychol 64:1276–1284, 1996

Blazer DG: Epidemiology of psychiatric disorders in late life, in Textbook of Geriatric Psychiatry. Edited by Busse EW, Blazer DG. Washington, DC, American Psychiatric Press, 1996, pp 155–174

Blazer DG, Koenig HG: Mood disorders, in Textbook of Geriatric Psychiatry. Edited by Busse EW, Blazer DG. Washington, DC, American Psychiatric Press, 1996, pp 235–264

Bleich A, Brown, S-L, van Praag HM: A serotonergic theory of schizophrenia, in The Role of Serotonin in Psychiatric Disorders. Edited by Brown S-L, van Praag HM. New York, Brunner/Mazel, 1990, pp 183–214

Blumer D, Montouris G, Hermann B: Psychiatric morbidity in seizure patients on a neurodiagnostic monitoring unit. J Neuropsychiatry Clin Neurosci 7:445–456, 1995

Bonne O, Krausz Y, Gorfine M, et al: Cerebral hypoperfusion in medication resistant, depressed patients assessed by Tc99m HMPAO SPECT. J Affect Disord 41:163–171, 1996

Bowden CL: The clinical approach to the differential diagnosis of bipolar disorder. Psychiatric Annals 23:57–63, 1993

Bowden CL: Predictors of response to divalproex and lithium (review). Compr Psychiatry 56 (suppl 3):25–30, 1995

Bowden CL: Dosing strategies and time course of response to antimanic agents. Compr Psychiatry 57 (suppl 13):4–9, 1996

Bowden CL, Brugger AM, Swann AC: Efficacy of divalproex vs lithium in the treatment of mania. JAMA 271:918–924, 1994

Bowden CL, Calabrese JR, Wallin BA, et al: Illness characteristics of patients in clinical drug studies of mania. Psychopharmacol Bull 31:103–109, 1995

Bowers WA: Treatment of depressed inpatients: cognitive therapy plus medication, relaxation plus medication, and medication alone. Br J Psychiatry 156:73–78, 1990

Bowlby J: Loss: Sadness and Depression. New York, Basic Books, 1980

Boyce P, Parker G, Barnett B, et al: Personality as a vulnerability factor to depression. Br J Psychiatry 159:106–114, 1991

Bradwejn J, Shriqui C, Koszycki D, et al: Double-blind comparison of the effects of clonazepam and lorazepam in acute mania. J Clin Psychopharmacol 10:403–408, 1990

Brady KT, Sonne SC, Anton R, et al: Valproate in the treatment of acute bipolar affective episodes complicated by substance abuse: a pilot study. Compr Psychiatry 56:118–121, 1995

Brawman-Mintzer O, Lydiard RB: Generalized anxiety disorder: issues in epidemiology. Compr Psychiatry 57 (suppl 7):3–8, 1996

Breier A, Charney DS, Heniger GR: The diagnostic validity of anxiety disorders and their relationship to depressive illness. Am J Psychiatry 142:787–797, 1985

Bridges PK, Bartlett JR, Hale AS, et al: Psychosurgery: stereotactic subcaudate tractotomy: an indispensable treatment. Br J Psychiatry 165:599–611, 1994

Broadhead WE, Blazer DG, George LK, et al: Depression, disability days, and days lost from work in a prospective epidemiologic survey. JAMA 264:2524–2528, 1990

Brown RA, Lewinsohn PM: A psychoeducational approach to the treatment of depression: comparison of group, individual, and minimal contact procedures. J Consult Clin Psychol 52:774–783, 1984

Brown S-L, Bleich A, van Praag HM: The monoamine hypothesis of depression: the case for serotonin, in The Role of Serotonin in Psychiatric Disorders. Edited by Brown S-L, van Praag HM. New York, Brunner/Mazel, 1990, pp 91–128

Brown S[-L], Steinberg RL, van Praag HM: The pathogenesis of depression: reconsideration of neurotransmitter data, in Handbook of Depression and Anxiety. Edited by den Boer JA, Sitsen JMA. New York, Marcel Dekker, 1994, pp 317–347

Bruder GE, Fong R, Tenke CE, et al: Regional brain asymmetries in major depression with or without an anxiety disorder: a quantitative electroencephalographic study. Biol Psychiatry 41:939–948, 1997

Buchsbaum MS, Wu J, Siegel BV, et al: Effect of sertraline on regional metabolic rate in patients with affective disorder. Biol Psychiatry 41:15–22, 1997

Budman SH, Demby A, Redondo JP, et al: Comparative outcome in time-limited individual and group psychotherapy. Int J Group Psychother 38:63–86, 1988

Burke MJ, Preskhorn SH: Short-term treatment of mood disorders with standard antidepressants, in Psychopharmacology: The Fourth Generation of Progress. Edited by Bloom FE, Kupfer DJ. New York, Raven, 1995, pp 1053–1065

Burrows GD: Long-term clinical management of depressive disorders. Compr Psychiatry 53 (suppl 3):32–35, 1992

Busch FN, Miller FT, Weiden PJ: A comparison of two adjunctive treatment strategies in acute mania. Compr Psychiatry 50:453–455, 1989

Butler SF, Arredondo DE, McCloskey V: Affective comorbidity in children and adolescents with attention deficit hyperactivity disorder. Ann Clin Psychiatry 7:51–55, 1995

Buysse DJ, Reynolds CF, Kupfer DJ, et al: Clinical diagnoses in 216 insomnia patients using the International Classification of Sleep Disorders (ICSD), DSM-IV and ICD-10 categories: a report from the APA/NIMH DSM-IV field trial. Sleep 17:630–637, 1994

Buysse DJ, Frank EF, Lowe KK, et al: Electroencephalographic sleep correlates of episode and vulnerability to recurrence in depression. Biol Psychiatry 41:406–418, 1997

Buzan RD, Weissberg M: Suicide: risk factors and prevention in medical practice. Annu Rev Med 43:37–46, 1992

Byerly WG, Hartmann A, Foster DE, et al: Verapamil in the treatment of maternal paroxysmal supraventricular tachycardia. Ann Emerg Med 20:552–554, 1991

Calabrese JR, Meltzer HY, Markovitz PJ: Clozapine prophylaxis in rapid cycling bipolar disorder. J Clin Psychopharmacol 11:396–397, 1991

Calabrese JR, Fatemi SH, Woyshville MJ: Antidepressant effects of lamotrigine in rapid cycling bipolar disorder (letter). Am J Psychiatry 153:1236, 1996a

Calabrese JR, Kimmel SE, Woyshville MJ, et al: Clozapine for treatment-refractory mania. Am J Psychiatry 153:759–764, 1996b

Calev A, Ben-Tzvi E, Shapira B, et al: Distinct memory impairments following electroconvulsive therapy and imipramine. Psychol Med 19:111–119, 1989

Calev A, Gaudino EA, Squires NK, et al: ECT and non-memory cognition: a review. Br J Clin Psychol 34 (part 4):505–515, 1995

Carbonne B, Jannet D, Touboul C, et al: Nicardipine treatment of hypertension during pregnancy. Obstet Gynecol 81:908–914, 1993

Carpenter D, Clarkin JF, Glick ID, et al: Personality pathology among married adults with bipolar disorder. J Affect Disord 34:269–274, 1995

Carr V, Dorrington C, Schrader G, et al: The use of ECT for mania in childhood bipolar disorder. Br J Psychiatry 143:411–415, 1983

Carroll BJ: Informed use of the dexamethasone suppression test. Compr Psychiatry 47 (suppl):10–12, 1986

Cassano GB, Akiskal HS, Musetti L, et al: Psychopathology, temperament, and past course in primary major depressions, 2: toward a redefinition of bipolarity with a new semistructured interview for depression. Psychopathology 22:278–288, 1989

Cassano GB, Akiskal HS, Perugi G, et al: The importance of measures of affective temperaments in genetic studies of mood disorders. Special issue: Genetics and gene expression in mental illness. J Psychiatr Res 26:257–268, 1992

Cassem EH: Depressive disorders in the medically ill: an overview. Psychosomatics 36:S2–S10, 1995

Chambers WJ, Puig-Antich J, Tabrizi MA, et al: Psychotic symptoms in prepubertal major depressive disorder. Arch Gen Psychiatry 39:921–927, 1982

Charney DS, Delgado PL, Price LH, et al: The receptor sensitivity hypothesis of antidepressant action: a review of antidepressant effects on serotonin function, in The Role of Serotonin in Psychiatric Disorders. Edited by Brown S-L, van Praag HM. New York, Brunner/Mazel, 1990, pp 27–56

Chen PJ: The efficacy and blood concentration monitoring of carbamazepine on mania [in Chinese]. Chung Hua Shen Ching Ching Shen Ko Tsa Chih 23:261–265, 1931

Chou JCY: Recent advances in treatment of acute mania. J Clin Psychopharmacol 11:3–21, 1991

Chouinard G: Severe cases of neuroleptic-induced supersensitivity psychosis: diagnostic criteria for the disorder and its treatment. Schizophr Res 5:21–33, 1991

Chouinard G, Young SN, Annable L: Antimanic effect of clonazepam. Biol Psychiatry 18:451–466, 1983

Clayton PJ, Grovw WM, Coryell W, et al: Follow-up and family study of anxious depression. Am J Psychiatry 148:1512–1517, 1991

Coccaro EF: Central serotonin and impulsive aggression. Br J Psychiatry 155 (suppl 8):52–62, 1989

Cochran SD: Preventing medical noncompliance in the outpatient treatment of bipolar affective disorder. J Consult Clin Psychol 52:873–878, 1984

Coffey CE, Weiner RD, Djang WT, et al: Brain anatomic effects of electroconvulsive therapy: a prospective magnetic resonance imaging study. Arch Gen Psychiatry 48:1013–1017, 1991

Cohen BM, Lipinski JF: Treatment of acute psychosis with non-neuroleptic agents. Psychosomatics 26 (suppl):7–16, 1986

Colwell BL, Lopez JR: Clonazepam in mania. Drug Intelligence and Clinical Pharmacy 21:794–795, 1987

Consensus Development Panel: NIMH/NIH Consensus Development Conference statement: mood disorders—pharmacologic prevention of recurrences. Am J Psychiatry 142:469–476, 1985

Conte HR, Karasu TB: A review of treatment studies of minor depression: 1980–1981. Am J Psychother 46:58–74, 1992

Conte HR, Plutchik R, Wild K, et al: Combined psychotherapy and pharmacotherapy for depression. Arch Gen Psychiatry 43:471–479, 1986

Corruble E, Ginestet D, Guelfi JD: Comorbidity of personality disorders and unipolar major depression: a review. J Affect Disord 37:157–170, 1996

Coryell W: Psychotic depression. Compr Psychiatry 57 (suppl 3):27–31, 1996

Coryell W, Endicott J, Keller MB: Predictors of relapse into major depressive disorder in a nonclinical population. Am J Psychiatry 148:1353–1358, 1991

Coryell W, Akiskal HS, Leon AC, et al: The time course of nonchronic major depressive disorder. Arch Gen Psychiatry 51:405–410, 1994

Cowdry RW, Wehr TA, Zis AP, et al: Thyroid abnormalities associated with rapid-cycling bipolar illness. Arch Gen Psychiatry 40:414–420, 1983

Crits-Christoph P: The efficacy of brief dynamic psychotherapy: a meta-analysis. Am J Psychiatry 149:151–158, 1992

Cross-National Collaborative Group: The changing rate of major depression: cross-national comparisons. JAMA 268:3098–3105, 1992

Danish University Antidepressant Group: Citalopram: clinical effect profile in comparison with clomipramine: a controlled multicenter study. Psychopharmacology 90:131–138, 1986

Danish University Antidepressant Group: Paroxetine: a selective serotonin reuptake inhibitor showing better tolerance, but weaker antidepressant effect than clomipramine in a controlled multicenter study. J Affect Disord 18:289–299, 1990

Davenloo H: Short-Term Dynamic Psychotherapy. New York, Jason Aronson, 1982

Davidson RJ: Anterior cerebral asymmetry and the nature of emotion. Brain Cogn 20:125–151, 1992

Deicken RF: Verapamil treatment of bipolar depression. J Clin Psychopharmacol 10:148–149, 1990

Deitz IJ: The self-psychological approach to the bipolar spectrum disorders. J Am Acad Psychoanal 23:475–492, 1995

Delgado PL, Gelenberg AJ: Antidepressant and antimanic medications, in Treatment of Psychiatric Disorders. Edited by Gabbard GO. Washington, DC, American Psychiatric Press, 1995, pp 1131–1168

Deltito JA, Moline M, Pollak C, et al: Effects of phototherapy on non-seasonal unipolar and bipolar depressive spectrum disorders. J Affect Disord 23:231–237, 1991

Devanand DP, Sackeim HA, Prudic J: Electroconvulsive therapy in the treatment-resistant patient. Psychiatr Clin North Am 14:905–923, 1991a

Devanand DP, Sackeim HA, Lo E-S, et al: Serial dexamethasone suppression tests and plasma dexamethasone levels. Arch Gen Psychiatry 48:525–533, 1991b

Dilsaver SC, Coffman JA: Cholinergic hypothesis of depression: a reappraisal. J Clin Psychopharmacol 9:173–179, 1989

DiMascio A, Weissman MM, Prusoff BA: Differential symptom reduction by drugs and psychotherapy in acute depression. Arch Gen Psychiatry 36:1450–1456, 1979

Dose M, Emrich HM, Cording-Tommel C: Use of calcium antagonists in mania. Psychoneuroendocrinology 11:241–243, 1986

Drugs that cause psychiatric symptoms. Medical Letter 35:65–70, 1993

Dubovsky SL: Using electroconvulsive therapy for patients with neurological disease. Hospital and Community Psychiatry 37:819–825, 1986

Dubovsky SL: Beyond the serotonin reuptake inhibitors: rationales for the development of new serotonergic agents. Compr Psychiatry 55 (suppl 2):34–44, 1994a

Dubovsky SL: Why don't we hear more about the calcium antagonists? An industry-academia interaction. Biol Psychiatry 35:149–150, 1994b

Dubovsky SL: Calcium channel antagonists as novel agents for manic-depressive disorder, in American Psychiatric Press Textbook of Psychopharmacology. Edited by Schatzberg AF, Nemeroff CB. Washington, DC, American Psychiatric Press, 1995a, pp 377–388

Dubovsky SL: Electroconvulsive therapy, in Comprehensive Textbook of Psychiatry/VI, 6th Edition, Vol 2. Edited by Kaplan HI, Sadock BJ. Baltimore, MD, Williams & Wilkins, 1995b, pp 2129–2140

Dubovsky SL: Mind-Body Deceptions. New York, WW Norton, 1997

Dubovsky SL, Buzan RD: Novel alternatives and supplements to lithium and anticonvulsants for bipolar affective disorder. J Clin Psychiatry 58:224–242, 1997

Dubovsky SL, Thomas M: Psychotic depression: advances in conceptualization and treatment. Hosp Community Psychiatry 43:1189–1198, 1992

Dubovsky SL, Franks RD, Allen S, et al: Calcium antagonists in mania: a double-blind study of verapamil. Psychiatry Res 18:309–320, 1986

Dubovsky SL, Christiano J, Daniell LC: Increased platelet intracellular calcium concentration in patients with bipolar affective disorders. Arch Gen Psychiatry 46:632–638, 1989

Dubovsky SL, Lee C, Christiano J: Elevated intracellular calcium ion concentration in bipolar depression. Biol Psychiatry 29:441–450, 1991a

Dubovsky SL, Lee C, Christiano J: Lithium decreases platelet intracellular calcium ion concentrations in bipolar patients. Lithium 2:167–174, 1991b

Dubovsky SL, Murphy J, Thomas M, et al: Abnormal intracellular calcium ion concentration in platelets and lymphocytes of bipolar patients. Am J Psychiatry 149:118–120, 1992a

Dubovsky SL, Murphy J, Christiano J, et al: The calcium second messenger system in bipolar disorders: data supporting new research directions. J Neuropsychiatry Clin Neurosci 4:3–14, 1992b

Dubovsky SL, Thomas M, Hijazi A, et al: Intracellular calcium signaling in peripheral cells of patients with bipolar affective disorder. Eur Arch Psychiatry Clin Neurosci 243:229–234, 1994

Dupont RM, Jernigan TL, Heindel W, et al: Magnetic resonance imaging and mood disorders: localization of white matter and other subcortical abnormalities. Arch Gen Psychiatry 52:747–755, 1995

Dwight MM, Keck PE, Stanton SP, et al: Antidepressant activity and mania associated with risperidone treatment of schizoaffective disorder. Lancet 344:554–555, 1994

Egeland JA, Gerhard DS, Pauls D, et al: Bipolar affective disorders linked to DNA markers on chromosome 11. Nature 325:783–787, 1987

Elkin I, Shea MT, Watkins JT, et al: National Institute of Mental Health Treatment of Depression Collaborative Research Program: general effectiveness of treatments. Arch Gen Psychiatry 46:971–982, 1989

Elkis H, Friedman L, Wise A, et al: Meta-analysis of studies of ventricular enlargement and cortical sulcal prominence in mood disorders: comparisons with controls or patients with schizophrenia. Arch Gen Psychiatry 52:735–746, 1995

Emslie GJ, Kennard BD, Kowatch RA: Affective disorders in children: diagnosis and management. J Child Neurol 10 (suppl 1):S42–S49, 1995

Esparon J, Kolloori J, Naylor GJ: Comparison of the prophylactic action of flupenthixol with placebo in lithium treated manic-depressive patients. Br J Psychiatry 148:723–725, 1986

Evans MD, Hollon SD, DeRubeis RJ, et al: Differential relapse following cognitive therapy and pharmacotherapy for depression. Arch Gen Psychiatry 49:802–808, 1992

Expert Consensus Panel: Treatment of bipolar disorder. Compr Psychiatry 57 (suppl 12A):1–88, 1996

Extein I, Pottash ALC, Gold MS: Does subclinical hypothyroidism predispose to tricyclic-induced rapid mood cycles? Compr Psychiatry 43:290–291, 1982

Extein I, Pottash ALC, Gold MS: Thyroid tests as predictors of treatment response and prognosis in psychiatry. Psychiatric Hospital 16:127–130, 1985

Faedda GL, Baldessarini RJ, Suppes T, et al: Pediatric-onset bipolar disorder: a neglected clinical and public health problem. Sexual and Marital Therapy 3:171–195, 1995

Fann JR, Tucker GJ: Mood disorders with general medical condition. Current Opinion in Psychiatry 8:13–18, 1995

Fava M, Davidson KG: Definition and epidemiology of treatment-resistant depression. Psychiatr Clin North Am 19:179–195, 1996

Fava M, Kaji J: Continuation and maintenance treatments of major depressive disorders. Psychiatric Annals 24:281–290, 1994

Feinman JA, Dunner DL: The effect of alcohol and substance abuse on the course of bipolar affective disorder. J Affect Disord 37:43–49, 1996

Feline A: Les hyperthymies. Encephale 19:103–107, 1993

Fennig S, Craig TJ, Tanenberg-Karant M, et al: Medication treatment in first-admission patients with psychotic affective disorders: preliminary findings on research-facility diagnostic agreement and rehospitalization. Ann Clin Psychiatry 7:87–90, 1995

Fink M: Electroconvulsive therapy in children and adolescents. Convuls Ther 9:155–157, 1993

First MB, Donovan S, Frances A: Nosology of chronic mood disorders. Psychiatr Clin North Am 19:29–39, 1996

Folkerts H: Electroconvulsive therapy in neurologic diseases. Nervenarzt 66:241–251, 1995

Frances AJ: An introduction to dysthymia. Psychiatric Annals 23:607–608, 1993

Franco-Bronson K: The management of treatment-resistant depression in the medically ill. Psychiatr Clin North Am 19:329–350, 1996

Frank E, Kupfer DJ, Perel JM, et al: Three-year outcomes for maintenance therapies in recurrent depression. Arch Gen Psychiatry 47:1093–1099, 1990

Frank E, Kupfer DJ, Wagner EF, et al: Efficacy of interpersonal psychotherapy as a maintenance treatment of recurrent depression: contributing factors. Arch Gen Psychiatry 48:1053–1059, 1991

Frank E, Kupfer DJ, Hamer T, et al: Maintenance treatment and psychobiologic correlates of endogenous subtypes. J Affect Disord 25:181–189, 1992

Frank E, Kupfer DJ, Perel JM, et al: Comparison of full-dose versus half-dose pharmacotherapy in the maintenance treatment of recurrent depression. J Affect Disord 27:139–145, 1993

Frank E, Kupfer DJ, Ehlers CL, et al: Interpersonal and social rhythm therapy for bipolar disorder: integrating interpersonal and behavioral approaches. Behavior Therapy 17:143–149, 1994

Frank E, Kupfer DJ, Siegel LR: Alliance not compliance: a philosophy of outpatient care. Compr Psychiatry 56 (suppl 1):11–17, 1995

Frank E, Hlastala S, Ritenour A, et al: Inducing lifestyle regularity in recovering bipolar disorder patients: results from the maintenance therapies in bipolar disorder protocol. Biol Psychiatry 41:1165–1173, 1997

Freeman TW, Clothier JL, Pazzaglia P, et al: A double-blind comparison of valproate and lithium in the treatment of acute mania. Am J Psychiatry 149:108–111, 1992

Freinhar JP, Alvarez WH: Use of clonazepam in two cases of acute mania. Compr Psychiatry 46:29–30, 1985

Freud S: Mourning and melancholia (1917[1915]), in Standard Edition of the Complete Psychological Works of Sigmund Freud, Vol 14. Translated and edited by Strachey J. London, Hogarth Press, 1957, pp 237–260

Freud S: Project for a scientific psychology (1950[1895]), in Standard Edition of the Complete Psychological Works of Sigmund Freud, Vol 1. Translated and edited by Strachey J. London, Hogarth Press, 1966, pp 281–397

Friedman E, Wang HY, Levinson D, et al: Altered platelet protein kinase C activity in bipolar affective disorder, manic episode. Biol Psychiatry 33:520–525, 1993

Friedman RA: Social impairment in dysthymia. Psychiatric Annals 23:632–637, 1993

Froscher W: Clinical relevance of the determination of antiepileptic drugs in serum. Wien Klin Wochenschr Suppl 191:15–18, 1992

Frye M, Altschuler LL, Bitran JE: Clozapine in rapid cycling bipolar disorder (letter). J Clin Psychopharmacol 16:87–90, 1996

Gabbard GO: Psychodynamic psychotherapies, in Treatment of Psychiatric Disorders. Edited by Gabbard GO. Washington, DC, American Psychiatric Press, 1995, pp 1205–1220

Gallagher-Thompson D, Hanley-Peterson P, Thompson LW: Maintenance of gains versus relapse following brief psychotherapy for depression. J Consult Clin Psychol 58:371–374, 1990

Garza-Trevino ES, Hollister LE, Overall JE, et al: Efficacy of combinations of intramuscular antipsychotics and sedative-hypnotics for control of psychotic agitation. Am J Psychiatry 146:1598–1601, 1989

Garza-Trevino ES, Overall JE, Hollister LE: Verapamil versus lithium in acute mania. Am J Psychiatry 149:121–122, 1992

Gelenberg AJ, Hopkins HS: Report on efficacy of treatments for bipolar disorder. Psychopharmacol Bull 29:447–456, 1993

Gelenberg AJ, Kane JM, Keller MB, et al: Comparison of standard and low serum levels of lithium for maintenance treatment of bipolar disorder. N Engl J Med 321:1489–1493, 1989

Geller B, Sun K, Zimerman B, et al: Complex and rapid-cycling in bipolar children and adolescents: a preliminary study. J Affect Disord 34:259–268, 1995

Geller B, Todd RD, Luby J, et al: Treatment-resistant depression in children and adolescents. Psychiatr Clin North Am 19:253–265, 1996

Gerber JS, Nies AS: Antihypertensive agents and the drug therapy of hypertension, in Goodman and Gilman's The Pharmacological Basis of Therapeutics, 8th Edition. Edited by Gilman AG, Rall TW, Nies AS, et al. New York, Pergamon, 1991, pp 784–813

Gershon ES: Genetics, in Manic-Depressive Illness. Edited by Goodwin FK, Jamison KR. New York, Oxford University Press, 1990, pp 373–401

Gershon ES, Hamovit J, Guroff I, et al: A family study of schizoaffective, bipolar I, bipolar II, unipolar and normal control probands. Arch Gen Psychiatry 39:1157–1167, 1982

Gershon S, Soares JC: Current therapeutic profile of lithium. Arch Gen Psychiatry 54:16–18, 1997

Giannini AJ, Houser WL, Loiselle RH: Antimanic effects of verapamil. Am J Psychiatry 141:1602–1603, 1984

Giannini AJ, Loiselle RH, Price WA: Comparison of antimanic efficacy of clonidine and verapamil. J Clin Pharmacol 25:307–308, 1985

Giannini AJ, Taraszewski R, Loiselle RH: Verapamil and lithium as maintenance therapy of manic patients. J Clin Pharmacol 27:980–982, 1987

Glass DR, Pilkonis PA, Leber WR, et al: National Institute of Mental Health Treatment of Depression Collaborative Research Program. Arch Gen Psychiatry 46:971–982, 1989

Glassman A, Proud'homme X: Review of the cardiovascular effects of heterocyclic antidepressants. Compr Psychiatry 54 (suppl 2):16–22, 1993

Goldberg JF, Harrow M, Grossman LS: Course and outcome in bipolar affective disorder: a longitudinal follow-up study. Am J Psychiatry 152:379–384, 1995

Goldberg JF, Harrow M, Leon AC: Lithium treatment of bipolar affective disorders under naturalistic followup conditions. Psychopharmacol Bull 32:47–54, 1996

Goodnick PJ: Verapamil prophylaxis in pregnant women with bipolar disorder (letter). Am J Psychiatry 150:1560, 1993

Goodnick PJ: Nimodipine treatment of rapid cycling bipolar disorder (letter). Compr Psychiatry 56:330, 1995a

Goodnick PJ: Nimodipine treatment of rapid cycling bipolar disorder. J Clin Psychiatry 56:330, 1995b

Goodwin FK, Jamison KR: Manic Depressive Illness. New York, Oxford University Press, 1991

Goodwin FK, Wirz-Justice A, Wehr TA: Evidence that the pathophysiology of depression and the mechanism of antidepressant drugs both involve alterations in circadian rhythms. Adv Biochem Psychopharmacol 32:1–11, 1982

Gorman JM, Coplan JD: Comorbidity of depression and panic disorder. Compr Psychiatry 57 (suppl 10):34–41, 1996

Grahame-Smith DG: Serotonin in affective disorders. Int Clin Psychopharmacol 6 (suppl 4):5–13, 1992

Grubb D: Three Bipolar Women: The Boundary Between Bipolar Disorders and Disorders of the Self. New York, Brunner/Mazel, 1997

Gruber AJ, Hudson JI, Pope HG: The management of treatment-resistant depression in disorders on the interface of psychiatry and medicine. Psychiatr Clin North Am 19:351–369, 1996

Guze SB, Robbins E: Suicide and primary affective disorders. Br J Psychiatry 117:437–438, 1970

Gwirtsman HE, Blehar MC, McCullough JP, et al: Standardized assessment of dysthymia: report of a National Institute of Mental Health conference. Psychopharmacol Bull 33:3–11, 1997

Gyulai L, Alavi A, Broich K, et al: I-123 iofetamine single-photon computed emission tomography in rapid cycling bipolar disorder: a clinical study. Biol Psychiatry 41:152–161, 1997

Hall RC, Wise MG: The clinical and financial burden of mood disorders: cost and outcome. Psychosomatics 36:S11–S18, 1995

Harrison WM, Stewart JW: Pharmacotherapy of dysthymia. Psychiatric Annals 23:638–648, 1993

Harrow M, Goldberg JF, Grossman LS, et al: Outcome in manic disorders: a naturalistic follow-up study. Arch Gen Psychiatry 47:665–671, 1990

Hasin DS, Tsai W-Y, Endicott J, et al: Five-year course of major depression: effects of comorbid alcoholism: the effect of alcohol and substance abuse on the course of bipolar affective disorder. J Affect Disord 37:43–49, 1996

Hauck A, Bhaumik S: Hypomania induced by gabapentin (letter). Br J Psychiatry 167:549, 1995

Hay DF, Kumar R: Interpreting the effects of mothers' postnatal depression on children's intelligence: a critique and re-analysis. Child Psychiatry Hum Dev 25:165–181, 1995

Hellekson C: Phenomenology of seasonal affective disorder: an Alaskan perspective, in Seasonal Affect Disorders and Phototherapy. Edited by Rosenthal NE, Blehar MC. New York, Guilford, 1989, pp 33–43

Hellerstein DJ, Yanowitch P, Rosenthal J, et al: Long-term treatment of double depression: a preliminary study with serotonergic antidepressants. Prog Neuropsychopharmacol Biol Psychiatry 18:139–147, 1994

Hendrick V, Altschuler LL, Szuba MP: Is there a role for neuroleptics in bipolar depression? Compr Psychiatry 55:533–535, 1994

Hersen M, Bellack AS, Himmelhoch JM, et al: Effects of social skills training, amitriptyline, and psychotherapy in unipolar depressed women. Behavior Therapy 15:21–40, 1984

Hirschfeld RMA: Guidelines for the long-term treatment of depression. Compr Psychiatry 55 (suppl 12):61–69, 1994

Hirschfeld RMA, Klerman GL, Lavori P: Premorbid personality assessments of first onset of major depression. Arch Gen Psychiatry 46:345–350, 1989

Hollon SD, Fawcett J: Combined medication and psychotherapy, in Treatment of Psychiatric Disorders. Edited by Gabbard GO. Washington, DC, American Psychiatric Press, 1995, pp 1221–1236

Hollon SD, DeRubeis RJ, Evans MD, et al: Cognitive therapy and pharmacotherapy for depression: singly and in combination. Arch Gen Psychiatry 49:774–781, 1992

Hopkins HS, Gelenberg AJ: Treatment of bipolar disorder: how far have we come? Psychopharmacol Bull 30:27–38, 1994

Hopkins J, Marcus M, Campbell SB: Postpartum depression: a critical review. Psychol Bull 95:498–515, 1984

Hoschl C, Kozemy J: Verapamil in affective disorders: a controlled, double-blind study. Biol Psychiatry 25:128–140, 1989

Hoshino M, Heise CO, Puglia P, et al: Hepatic enzymes' level during chronic use of anticonvulsant drugs. Arq Neuropsiquiatr 53:719–723, 1995

Howland RH: General health, health care utilization, and medical comorbidity in dysthymia. Int J Psychiatry Med 23:211–238, 1993

Isacsson G, Bergman U, Rich CL: Epidemiological data suggest antidepressants reduce suicide risk among depressives. J Affect Disord 41:1–8, 1996

Isometsa ET, Henriksson MM, Heikkinen ME: Suicide among subjects with personality disorders. Am J Psychiatry 153:667–673, 1996

Jacob M, Turner L, Kupfer DJ, et al: Attrition in maintenance therapy for recurrent depression. J Affect Disord 6:181–189, 1984

Jaffe RL, Rives W, Dubin WR, et al: Problems in maintenance ECT in bipolar disorder: replacement by lithium. Convuls Ther 7:288–294, 1991

Jaim-Etcheverry G, Zieher LM: Coexistence of monoamines in peripheral adrenergic neurones, in Co-Transmission. Edited by Cuello AC. London, Macmillan, 1982, pp 189–207

Jamison KR: Touched With Fire: Manic-Depressive Illness and the Artistic Temperament. New York, Free Press, 1993

Jamison KR: An Unquiet Mind. New York, Knopf, 1995

Jamison KR: Manic-depressive illness, genes, and creativity, in Genetics and Mental Illness: Evolving Issues for Research and Society. Edited by Hall LL. New York, Plenum, 1996, pp 111–132

Janicak PG, Pandey GN, Davis JM, et al: Response of psychotic and nonpsychotic depression to phenelzine. Am J Psychiatry 145:93–95, 1988

Janowsky DS, Risch SC: Adrenergic-cholinergic balance and affective disorders: a review of clinical evidence and therapeutic implications. Psychiatric Hospital 15:163–171, 1984

Jarrett RB: Comparing and combining short-term psychotherapy and pharmacotherapy for depression. New York, Guilford, 1997

Joffe RT, Horvath Z, Tarvydas I: Bipolar affective disorder and thalassemia minor (letter). Am J Psychiatry 143:933, 1986

Jope RS, Williams MB: Lithium and brain signal transduction systems. Biochem Pharmacol 47:429–441, 1994

Kafantaris V: Treatment of bipolar disorder in children and adolescents. J Am Acad Child Adolesc Psychiatry 34:732–741, 1995

Kahn RS, Kalus O, Wetzler S, et al: The role of serotonin in the regulation of anxiety, in The Role of Serotonin in Psychiatric Disorders. Edited by Brown S-L, van Praag HM. New York, Brunner/Mazel, 1990, pp 129–160

Kanba S, Yagi G, Kamijima K, et al: The first open study of zonisamide, a novel anticonvulsant, shows efficacy in mania. Prog Neuropsychopharmacol Biol Psychiatry 18:707–715, 1994

Karliner W, Wehrheim HK: Maintenance convulsive treatments. Am J Psychiatry 121:1113–1115, 1965

Kashani JH, Nair J: Affective/mood disorders, in Diagnosis and Psychopharmacology of Childhood and Adolescent Disorders, 2nd Edition. Edited by Weiner JM. New York, Wiley, 1995, pp 229–263

Kasper S, Wehr TA, Bartko JJ, et al: Epidemiological findings of seasonal changes in mood and behavior. Arch Gen Psychiatry 46:823–833, 1989

Kasper S, Fuger J, Moller H-J: Comparative efficacy of antidepressants. Drugs 43 (suppl 2):11–23, 1992

Kastner T, Friedman DL: Verapamil and valproic acid treatment of prolonged mania. J Am Acad Child Adolesc Psychiatry 31:271–275, 1992

Kaufman IC, Rosenblum LA: The reaction to separation in infant monkeys: anaclitic depression and conservation-withdrawal. Psychosom Med 29:648–675, 1967

Kaufmann CA: Muscarinic binding in suicides. Psychiatry Res 12:47–55, 1984

Kazdin A, Bass D: Power to detect differences between alternative treatments in comparative psychotherapy outcome research. J Consult Clin Psychol 57:138–147, 1989

Keck PE, McElroy SL, Vuckovic A, et al: Combined valproate and carbamazepine treatment of bipolar disorder. J Neuropsychiatry Clin Neurosci 4:319–322, 1992

Keck PE, McElroy SL, Tugrul KC, et al: Valproate oral loading in the treatment of acute mania. J Clin Psychiatry 54:305–308, 1993

Keck PE, Merikangas KR, McElroy SL, et al: Diagnostic and treatment implications of psychiatric comorbidity with migraine. Ann Clin Psychiatry 6:165–171, 1994

Keck PE, McElroy SL, Strakowski SM: Factors associated with pharmacologic noncompliance in patients with mania. J Clin Psychiatry 57:292–297, 1996

Keck PE, McElroy SL, Strakowski SM, et al: Compliance with maintenance treatment in bipolar disorder. Psychopharmacol Bull 33:87–91, 1997

Keitner GI, Miller IW: Family functioning and major depression: an overview. Am J Psychiatry 147:1128–1137, 1990

Keitner GI, Ryan CE, Miller IW, et al: 12-month outcome of patients with major depression and comorbid psychiatric or medical illness (compound depression). Am J Psychiatry 148:345–350, 1991

Keller MB: Dysthymia in clinical practice: course, outcome and impact on the community. Acta Psychiatr Scand 383 (suppl):24–34, 1994

Keller MB, Klerman G, Lavori PW: Long-term outcome of episodes of major depression. JAMA 252:788–792, 1984

Keller MB, Lavori PW, Coryell W, et al: Bipolar I: a five-year prospective follow-up. J Nerv Ment Dis 181:238–245, 1993

Keller MB, Hanks DL, Klein DN: Summary of the DSM-IV mood disorders field trial and issue overview. Psychiatr Clin North Am 19:1–27, 1996

Kelsoe JR, Ginns EI, Egeland JA, et al: Re-evaluation of the linkage relationship between chromosome 11p loci and the gene for bipolar affective disorder in the old order Amish. Nature 342:238–243, 1989

Kendler KS: Mood-incongruent psychotic affective illness. Arch Gen Psychiatry 48:362–369, 1991

Kendler KS: The diagnostic validity of melancholic major depression in a population-based sample of female twins. Arch Gen Psychiatry 54:299–304, 1997

Kendler KK, Heath AC, Martin NG, et al: Symptoms of anxiety and symptoms of depression: same genes, different environments? Arch Gen Psychiatry 44:451–457, 1987

Kendler KK, Neale MC, Kessler RC, et al: Major depression and generalized anxiety disorder: same genes, (partly) different environments? Arch Gen Psychiatry 49:716–722, 1992a

Kendler KK, Neale MC, Kessler CC, et al: A population-based twin study of major depression in women: the impact of varying definitions of illness. Arch Gen Psychiatry 49:257–266, 1992b

Kendler KK, Kessler CC, Neale MC, et al: The prediction of major depression in women: toward an integrated etiologic model. Am J Psychiatry 150:1139–1148, 1993

Keshavan MS: Benzhexol withdrawal and cholinergic mechanisms in depression. Br J Psychiatry 147:560–564, 1985

Ketter TA, Post RM, Parekh PI, et al: Addition of monoamine oxidase inhibitors to carbamazepine: preliminary evidence of safety and antidepressant efficacy in treatment-resistant depression. Compr Psychiatry 56:471–475, 1995

Kettering RL, Harrow M, Grossman L, et al: The prognostic relevance of delusions in depression: a follow-up study. Am J Psychiatry 144:1154–1160, 1987

Kirkpatrick B, Alphs L, Buchanan RW: The concept of supersensitivity psychosis. J Nerv Ment Dis 180:265–270, 1992

Kishi Y, Robinson RG: Suicidal plans following spinal cord injury: a six-month study. J Neuropsychiatry Clin Neurosci 8:442–445, 1996

Klapheke MM: Clozapine, ECT, and schizoaffective disorder, bipolar type. Convuls Ther 7:36–39, 1991

Klassen T, Verhey FRJ, Rozendaal N: Treatment of depression in Parkinson's disease: a meta-analysis. J Neuropsychiatry Clin Neurosci 7:281–286, 1995

Klein DN, Taylor EB, Harding K, et al: Double depression and episodic major depression: demographic, clinical, family, personality, and socioenvironmental characteristics and short-term outcome. Am J Psychiatry 145:1225–1231, 1988

Klein DN, Kocsis JH, McCullough JP, et al: Symptomatology in dysthymic and major depressive disorder. Psychiatr Clin North Am 19:41–53, 1996

Klerman GL: The current age of youthful melancholia: evidence for increase in depression among adolescents and young adults. Br J Psychiatry 152:4–14, 1988

Klerman GL, DiMascio A, Weissman MM, et al: Treatment of depression by drugs and psychotherapy. Am J Psychiatry 131:186–191, 1974

Klerman GL, Weissman MM, Rounsaville BJ, et al: Interpersonal Psychotherapy of Depression. New York, Basic Books, 1984

Klerman GL, Lavori PW, Rice J, et al: Birth-cohort trends in rates of major depressive disorder among relatives of patients with affective disorder. Arch Gen Psychiatry 42:689–693, 1985

Knesper DJ: The depressions of Alzheimer's disease: sorting, pharmacotherapy, and clinical advice. J Geriatr Psychiatry Neurol 8 (suppl 1):S40–S51, 1995

Kocsis JH: DSM-IV "major depression": are more stringent criteria needed? Depression 1:24–28, 1993

Kocsis JH, Frances AJ: A critical discussion of DSM-III dysthymic disorder. Am J Psychiatry 144:1534–1542, 1987

Kocsis JH, Frances AJ, Voss C, et al: Imipramine treatment for chronic depression. Arch Gen Psychiatry 45:253–257, 1988

Kocsis JH, Mason BJ, Frances AJ, et al: Prediction of response of chronic depression to imipramine. J Affect Disord 17:255–260, 1989

Koek RJ, Kessler CC: Possible induction of mania by risperidone (letter). Compr Psychiatry 57:174, 1996

Kohut H: The Analysis of the Self. New York, International Universities Press, 1971

Kovacs M, Gatsonis C, Paulauskas SL, et al: Depressive disorders in childhood, IV: a longitudinal study of comorbidity with and risk for anxiety disorders. Arch Gen Psychiatry 46:776–782, 1989

Kovacs M, Akiskal HS, Gatsonis C, et al: Childhood-onset dysthymic disorder: clinical features and prospective naturalistic outcome. Arch Gen Psychiatry 51:365–374, 1994

Kraepelin E: Manic-Depressive Insanity and Paranoia. Translated by Barclay RM. Edinburgh, Livingstone, 1921

Krueger RB, Sackeim HA, Gamzu ER: Pharmacological treatment of the cognitive side effects of ECT: a review. Psychopharmacol Bull 28:409–424, 1992

Krupnick JL, Sotsky SM, Simmens S, et al: The role of the therapeutic alliance in psychotherapy and pharmacotherapy outcome: findings in the National Institute of Mental Health Treatment of Depression Collaborative Research Program. J Consult Clin Psychol 64:532–539, 1996

Kukopulos A, Reginaldi D, Laddomada P: Course of the manic-depressive cycle and changes caused by treatment. Pharmakopsychiatry Neuropsychopharmakoly 13:156–167, 1980

Kupfer DJ: Sleep research in depressive illness: clinical implications—a tasting menu. Biol Psychiatry 36:391–403, 1995

Kupfer DJ, Frank E, Perel JM: Five-year outcome for maintenance therapies in recurrent depression. Arch Gen Psychiatry 49:769–773, 1992

Kutcher S, Robertson HA: Electroconvulsive therapy in treatment-resistant bipolar youth. J Child and Adolescent Psychopharmacology 5:167–175, 1995

Labbate LA, Lafer B, Thibault A, et al: Influence of phototherapy treatment duration for seasonal affective disorder: outcome at one vs. two weeks. Biol Psychiatry 38:747–750, 1995

Lader M: Fluoxetine efficacy vs. comparative drugs: an overview. Br J Psychiatry 153 (suppl 3):51–58, 1988

Lamy S, Bergsholm P, d'Elia G: The antidepressant efficacy of high-dose nondominant long-distance parietotemporal and bitemporal electroconvulsive therapy. Convuls Ther 10:43–52, 1994

Lang C, Field T, Pickens J, et al: Preschoolers of dysphoric mothers. Journal of Child Psychology and Psychiatry 37:221–224, 1996

Lasch K, Weissman MM: Birth cohort changes in the rate of mania. Psychiatry Res 33:31–37, 1990

Last CG, Thase ME, Hersen M, et al: Patterns of attrition for psychosocial and pharmacologic treatments of depression. Compr Psychiatry 46:361–366, 1985

Lavori P, Keller MB, Roth SL: Affective disorders and ABO blood groups: new data and a reanalysis of the literature using the logistic transformation of proportions. J Psychiatr Res 18:119–129, 1984

Lee DO, Steingard RJ, Cesena M, et al: Behavioral side effects of gabapentin in children. Epilepsia 37:87–90, 1996

Lehtinen V, Joukamaa M: Epidemiology of depression: prevalence, risk factors and treatment situation. Acta Psychiatr Scand 89 (suppl):7–10, 1994

Leibenluft E: Women with bipolar illness: clinical and research issues. Am J Psychiatry 153:163–173, 1996

Leibenluft E, Clark CH, Myers FS: The reproducibility of depressive and hypomanic symptoms across repeated episodes in patients with rapid-cycling bipolar disorder. J Affect Disord 33:83–88, 1995

Lenox RH, Modell JG, Weiner S: Acute treatment of manic agitation with lorazepam. Psychosomatics 27 (suppl):28–31, 1986

Leonard BE: Sub-types of serotonin receptors: biochemical changes and pharmacological consequences. Int Clin Psychopharmacol 7:13–21, 1992

Leonard BE: Effect of antidepressants on specific neurotransmitters: are such effects relevant to the therapeutic action? in Handbook of Depression and Anxiety. Edited by den Boer JA, Sitsen JMA. New York, Marcel Dekker, 1994, pp 379–404

Leonhard K: Differential diagnosis and different aetiology of monopolar and bipolar depressions. Psicopatologia 7:277–285, 1987a

Leonhard K: Differential diagnosis and different etiology of monopolar and bipolar phasic psychoses [in German]. Psychiatrie, Neurologie und Medizinische Psychologie 39:524–533, 1987b

Lepine J, Pelissolo A, Weiller E, et al: Recurrent brief depression: clinical and epidemiological issues. Psychopathology 28 (suppl 1):86–94, 1995

Lerer B, Stanley M: Does lithium stabilize muscarinic receptors? Biol Psychiatry 20:1247–1248, 1985

Letizia C, Kapik B, Flanders WD: Suicidal risk during controlled clinical investigations of fluvoxamine. Compr Psychiatry 57:415–421, 1996

Levitt AJ, Joffe RT, MacDonald C: Life course of depressive illness and characteristics of current episode in patients with double depression. J Nerv Ment Dis 179:678–682, 1991

Lewinsohn PM, Antonuccio DA, Steinmetz J, et al: The Coping With Depression Course: A Psychoeducational Intervention for Unipolar Depression. Eugene, OR, Castalia Press, 1984

Lewinsohn PM, Klein DN, Seeley JR: Bipolar disorders in a community sample of older adolescents: prevalence, phenomenology, comorbidity, and course. J Am Acad Child Adolesc Psychiatry 34:454–463, 1995

Lindhout D, Omtzigt JG: Pregnancy and the risk of teratogenicity. Epilepsia 33 (suppl 4):S41–S48, 1992

Linnoila M, Virkkunen M: Biologic correlates of suicidal risk and aggressive behavioral traits. J Clin Psychopharmacol 12:19S–20S, 1992

Lish JD, Gyulai L, Resnick SM, et al: A family history study of rapid-cycling bipolar disorder. Psychiatry Res 48:37–46, 1993

Littlejohn R, Leslie F, Cookson J: Depot antipsychotics in the prophylaxis of bipolar affective disorder. Br J Psychiatry 165:827–829, 1994

Long TD, Kathol RG: Critical review of data supporting affective disorder caused by nonpsychotropic medication. Ann Clin Psychiatry 5:259–270, 1993

Loo H, Brochier T: Long-term treatment with antidepressive drugs [in French]. Ann Med Psychol (Paris) 153:190–196, 1995

Lopez-Ibor JL: The involvement of serotonin in psychiatric disorders and behaviour. Br J Psychiatry 153 (suppl 3):26–39, 1988

Loranger AW, Lenzenweger MF, Gartner AF, et al: Trait-state artifacts and the diagnosis of personality disorders. Arch Gen Psychiatry 48:720–728, 1991

Lovett LM, Shaw DM: Outcome in bipolar affective disorder after stereotactic tractotomy. Br J Psychiatry 151:113–116, 1987

Lowe MR: Treatment of rapid cycling affective illness (letter). Br J Psychiatry 146:558, 1985

Luborsky L: Principles of Psychoanalytic Psychotherapy: A Manual for Supportive-Expressive Treatment. New York, Basic Books, 1984

Madhusoodanan S, Brenner R, Araujo L, et al: Efficacy of risperidone treatment for psychoses associated with schizophrenia, schizoaffective disorder, bipolar disorder, or senile dementia in 11 geriatric patients: a case series. Compr Psychiatry 56:514–518, 1995

MagPhil PLG, Thomas CB: Themes of interaction in medical students' Rorschach responses as predictors of midlife health or disease. Psychosom Med 43:215–225, 1981

Maier W, Hallmayer J, Zill P, et al: Linkage analysis between pericentrometric markers on chromosome 18 and bipolar disorder: a replication test. Psychiatry Res 59:7–15, 1995a

Maier W, Lichtermann D, Minges J, et al: The relationship between bipolar disorder and alcoholism: a controlled family study. Psychol Med 25:787–796, 1995b

Maj M, Veltro F, Pirozzi R, et al: Pattern of recurrence of illness after recovery from an episode of major depression: a prospective study. Am J Psychiatry 149:795–800, 1992

Mandoki MW, Tapia MR, Tapia MA, et al: Venlafaxine in the treatment of children and adolescents with major depression. Psychopharmacol Bull 33:149–154, 1997

Mann J: Time-Limited Psychotherapy. Cambridge, MA, Harvard University Press, 1973

Mann JJ, Malone KM: Cerebrospinal fluid amines and higher-lethality suicide attempts in depressed inpatients. Biol Psychiatry 41:162–171, 1997

Mann JJ, Arango V, Marzuk PM: Evidence for the 5-HT hypothesis of suicide: a review of post-mortem studies. Br J Psychiatry 155 (suppl 8):7–14, 1989

Manna V: Disturbi affettivi bipolari e ruolo del calcio intraneuronale: effetti terapeutici del trattamento con cali di litio e/o calcio antagonista in pazienti con rapida inversione di polarita. Minerva Med 82:757–763, 1991

Marangell LB, George MS, Callahan AM, et al: Effects of intrathecal thyrotropin-releasing hormone (protirelin) in refractory depressed patients. Arch Gen Psychiatry 54:214–222, 1997

Marin DB, Kocsis JH, Frances AJ, et al: Personality disorders in dysthymia. Journal of Personality Disorders 7:223–231, 1993

Marttunen MJ, Henriksson MM, Aro HM, et al: Suicide among female adolescents: characteristics and comparison with males in the age group 13 to 22 years. J Am Acad Child Adolesc Psychiatry 34:1297–1307, 1995

Mathews R, Li PP, Young T, et al: Increased $G\alpha_{q/11}$ immunoreactivity in postmortem occipital cortex from patients with bipolar affective disorder. Biol Psychiatry 41:649–656, 1997

Matsuo F, Madsen J, Tolman KG, et al: Lamotrigine high-dose tolerability and safety in patients with epilepsy: a double-blind, placebo-controlled, eleven-week study. Epilepsia 37:857–862, 1996

Mattson RH: Efficacy and adverse effects of established and new antiepileptic drugs. Epilepsia 36 (suppl 2):S13–S26, 1995

Max JE, Richards L, Hamdan-Allen G: Case study: antimanic effectiveness of dextroamphetamine in a brain-injured adolescent. J Am Acad Child Adolesc Psychiatry 34:472–476, 1995

McBride PA, Brown RP, DeMeo M: The relationship of platelet 5-HT2 receptor indices to major depressive disorder, personality traits, and suicidal behavior. Biol Psychiatry 35:295–308, 1994

McCabe MS, Norris B: ECT versus chlorpromazine in mania. Biol Psychiatry 12:245–254, 1977

McCormick DA, Williamson A: Convergence and divergence of neurotransmitter action in human cerebral cortex. Proc Natl Acad Sci U S A 86:8098–8102, 1989

McDaniel JS, Musselman DL, Proter MR: Depression in patients with cancer. Arch Gen Psychiatry 52:89–99, 1995

McDermott OD, Prigerson HG, Reynolds CF III, et al: Sleep in the wake of complicated grief symptoms: an exploratory study. Biol Psychiatry 41:710–716, 1997

McElroy SL, Dessain EC, Pope HG, et al: Clozapine in the treatment of psychotic mood disorders, schizoaffective disorder, and schizophrenia. Compr Psychiatry 52:411–414, 1991

McElroy SL, Keck PE, Pope HG, et al: Clinical and research implications of the diagnosis of dysphoric or mixed mania or hypomania. Am J Psychiatry 149:1633–1644, 1992

McElroy SL, Keck PE, Strakowski SM: Mania, psychosis, and antipsychotics. Compr Psychiatry 57 (suppl 3):14–26, 1996a

McElroy SL, Keck PE, Stanton SP, et al: A randomized comparison of divalproex oral loading versus haloperidol in the initial treatment of acute psychotic mania. Compr Psychiatry 57:142–146, 1996b

McGlashan TH: Adolescent versus adult onset of mania. Am J Psychiatry 145:221–223, 1988

McKinney WT: Animal models for depression and mania, in Depression and Mania. Edited by Georgotas A, Cancro R. New York, Elsevier, 1988, pp 181–196

McLean MJ: Gabapentin. Epilepsia 36 (suppl 2):S73–S86, 1995

McLean PD: Behavior therapy: theory and research, in Short-Term Psychotherapies for Depression. Edited by Rush AJ. New York, Guilford, 1982, pp 19–49

McLean PD, Hakstian AR: Relative endurance of unipolar depression treatment effects: a longitudinal follow-up. J Consult Clin Psychol 58:482–488, 1990

McLean P[D], Taylor S: Severity of unipolar depression and choice of treatment. Behav Res Ther 30:443–451, 1992

Meltzer HY: Serotonergic dysfunction in depression. Br J Psychiatry 155 (suppl 8):25–31, 1989

Meltzer HY: The importance of serotonin-dopamine interactions in the action of clozapine. Br J Psychiatry 160 (suppl 17):22–29, 1992

Meltzer HY, Lowy MT: The serotonin hypothesis of depression, in Psychopharmacology: The Third Generation of Progress. Edited by Meltzer HY. New York, Raven, 1987, pp 513–526

Meredith LS: Counseling typically provided for depression: role of clinician specialty and payment system. Arch Gen Psychiatry 53:905–912, 1996

Merriam AE, Karasu TB: The role of psychotherapy in the treatment of depression. Arch Gen Psychiatry 53:301–302, 1996

Messenheimer JA: Lamotrigine. Epilepsia 36 (suppl 2):S87–S94, 1995

Meterissian GB, Bradwejn J: Comparative studies on the efficacy of psychotherapy, pharmacotherapy, and their combination in depression: was adequate pharmacotherapy provided? J Clin Psychopharmacol 9:334–339, 1989

Miklowitz DJ: Longitudinal outcome and medication noncompliance among manic patients with and without mood-incongruent psychotic features. J Nerv Ment Dis 180:703–711, 1992

Miklowitz DJ, Goldstein MJ: Behavioral family treatment for patients with bipolar affective disorder. Behav Modif 14:457–489, 1990

Miklowitz DJ, Goldstein MJ, Nuechterlein KH, et al: Family factors and the course of bipolar disorder. Arch Gen Psychiatry 45:225–231, 1988

Mikuni M, Meltzer HY: Reduction of serotonin-2 receptors in rat cerebral cortex after incubation with imipramine and chlorpromazine. Life Sci 34:87–92, 1984

Milberger S, Biederman J, Faraone SV, et al: Attention deficit hyperactivity disorder and comorbid disorder: issues of overlapping symptoms. Am J Psychiatry 152:1793–1799, 1995

Miller HL, Coombs DW, Leeper JD, et al: An analysis of the effect of suicide prevention facilities on suicide rates in the United States. Am J Public Health 74:340–343, 1984

Miller IW, Keitner GI: Combined medication and psychotherapy in the treatment of chronic mood disorders. Psychiatr Clin North Am 19:151–171, 1996

Miller IW, Norman WH, Dow MG: Psychosocial characteristics of "double depression." Am J Psychiatry 153:1042–1044, 1986

Miller RJ, Chouinard G: Loss of striatal cholinergic neurons as a basis for tardive and L-dopa-induced dyskinesias, neuroleptic-induced supersensitivity psychosis and refractory schizophrenia. Biol Psychiatry 34:713–738, 1993

Milstein V, Small JG, Klapper MH: Uni- versus bilateral ECT in the treatment of mania. Convuls Ther 3:1–9, 1987

Modell JG, Lenox RH, Weiner S: Inpatient clinical trial of lorazepam for the management of manic agitation. J Clin Psychopharmacol 5:109–113, 1985

Montgomery SA: Selective serotonin reuptake inhibitors in the acute treatment of depression, in Psychopharmacology, The Fourth Generation of Progress. Edited by Bloom FE, Kupfer DJ. New York, Raven, 1995, pp 1043–1051

Montgomery SA, Fineberg N: Is there a relationship between serotonin receptor subtypes and selectivity of response in specific psychiatric illnesses? Br J Psychiatry 155 (suppl 8):63–70, 1989

Moos RH, Mertens JR: Patterns of diagnoses, comorbidities, and treatment in late-middle-aged and older affective disorder patients: comparison of mental health and medical sectors. J Am Geriatr Soc 44:682–688, 1996

Morris GL: Efficacy and tolerability of gabapentin in clinical practice. Clin Ther 17:891–900, 1995

Morris PLP, Robinson RG, Samuels J: Depression, introversion and mortality following stroke. Aust N Z J Psychiatry 27:443–449, 1993

Mueller TI, Leon AC: Recovery, chronicity, and levels of psychopathology in major depression. Psychiatr Clin North Am 19:85–102, 1996

Mukherjee S, Rosen AM, Caracci G, et al: Persistent tardive dyskinesia in bipolar patients. Arch Gen Psychiatry 43:342–346, 1986

Mukherjee S, Sackeim HA, Schnur DB: Electroconvulsive therapy of acute manic episodes: a review of 50 years' experience. Am J Psychiatry 151:169–176, 1994

Murad F: Drugs used for the treatment of angina: organic nitrates, calcium-channel blockers, and β-adrenergic agents, in Goodman and Gilman's The Pharmacological Basis of Therapeutics, 8th Edition. Edited by Gilman AG, Rall TW, Nies AS, et al. New York, Pergamon, 1991, pp 764–783

Murphy DL, Zohar J, Benkelfat C: Obsessive-compulsive disorder as a 5-HT subsystem-related behavioural disorder. Br J Psychiatry 155 (suppl 8):15–24, 1989

National Institute of Mental Health: Affective Disorders (Mood Disorders): Budget Estimate. Bethesda, MD, National Institute of Mental Health, 1995

Nelson JC, Price LH, Jatlow PI: Neuroleptic dose and desipramine concentrations during combined treatment of unipolar delusional depression. Am J Psychiatry 143:1151–1154, 1986

Nelson WH, Khan A, Orr WW: Delusional depression: phenomenology, neuroendocrine function and tricyclic antidepressant response. J Affect Disord 6:297–306, 1984

Neylan TC: Treatment of sleep disturbances in depressed patients. Compr Psychiatry 56 (suppl 2):56–61, 1995

Nezu AM: Efficacy of a social problem-solving therapy for unipolar depression. J Consult Clin Psychol 54:196–202, 1986

Nierenberg AA: The treatment of severe depression: is there an efficacy gap between SSRI and TCA antidepressant generations? Compr Psychiatry 55 (suppl A):55–59, 1994

Okamoto Y, Kagaya A, Shinno H, et al: Serotonin-induced platelet calcium mobilization is enhanced in mania. Life Sci 56:327–332, 1995

O'Keane V, Maloney E, O'Neill H, et al: Blunted prolactin responses to d-fenfluramine in sociotopathy: evidence for subsensitivity of central serotonergic function. Br J Psychiatry 160:643–646, 1992

Okuma T, Yamashita I, Takahashi R, et al: Comparison of the antimanic efficacy of carbamazepine and lithium carbonate by double-blind controlled study. Pharmacopsychiatry 23:143–150, 1990

Olfson M: Subthreshold psychiatric symptoms in a primary care group practice. Arch Gen Psychiatry 53:880–886, 1996

Olie JP, Brochier T, Bouvet O, et al: La conception actuelle des troubles de l'humeur: incidence sur la prise en charge thérapeutique. Encephale 18 (Spec No 1): 55–63, 1992

Osser DN: A systematic approach to the classification and pharmacotherapy of nonpsychotic major depression and dysthymia. J Clin Psychopharmacol 13:133–144, 1993

Overall JE, Donachie ND, Faillace LA: Implications of restrictive diagnosis for compliance to antidepressant drug therapy: alprazolam versus imipramine. Compr Psychiatry 48:51–54, 1987

Oxley SL, Van Meter S: The assessment and management of the suicidal patient. Journal of Practical Psychiatry and Behavioral Health 6:327–335, 1996

Papatheodorou G, Kutcher S: The effect of adjunctive light therapy on ameliorating breakthrough depressive symptoms in adolescent-onset bipolar disorder. J Psychiatry Neurosci 20:226–232, 1995

Papatheodorou G, Kutcher SP, Katic M, et al: The efficacy and safety of divalproex sodium in the treatment of acute mania in adolescents and young adults: an open clinical trial. J Clin Psychopharmacol 15:110–116, 1995

Partonen T, Sihvo S, Lonnqvist JK: Patients excluded from an antidepressant efficacy trial. Compr Psychiatry 57:572–575, 1996

Paykel ES: Handbook of Affective Disorders. New York, Guilford, 1982, pp xii, 699

Pazzaglia PJ, Post RM, Ketter TA, et al: Preliminary controlled trial of nimodipine in ultra-rapid cycling affective dysregulation. Psychiatry Res 49:257–272, 1993

Peet M, Peters S: Drug-induced mania. Drug Saf 12:146–153, 1995

Perry JC: Depression in borderline personality disorder: lifetime prevalence at interview and longitudinal course of symptoms. Am J Psychiatry 142:15–21, 1985

Perry PJ, Zeilmann C, Arndt S: Tricyclic antidepressant concentrations in plasma: an estimate of their sensitivity and specificity as a predictor of response. J Clin Psychopharmacol 14:230–235, 1994

Persons JB, Thase ME, Crits-Christoph P: The role of psychotherapy in the treatment of depression. Arch Gen Psychiatry 53:283–290, 1996

Peselow ED, Fieve RR, Difiglia C, et al: Lithium prophylaxis of bipolar illness. Br J Psychiatry 164:208–214, 1994

Petracca G, Teson A, Chemerinski E: A double-blind placebo-controlled study of clomipramine in depressed patients with Alzheimer's disease. J Neuropsychiatry Clin Neurosci 8:270–275, 1996

Petrides G, Dhossche D, Fink M, et al: Continuation ECT: relapse prevention in affective disorders. Convuls Ther 10:189–194, 1994

Petronis KR, Samuels JF, Moscicki EK, et al: An epidemiologic investigation of potential risk factors for suicide attempts. Soc Psychiatry Psychiatr Epidemiol 25:193–199, 1990

Pettinati HM, Rosenberg J: Memory self-ratings before and after electroconvulsive therapy: depression versus ECT induced. Biol Psychiatry 19:539–548, 1984

Piccinelli M, Wilkinson G: Outcome of depression in psychiatric settings. Br J Psychiatry 164:297–304, 1994

Piper AJ: Tricyclic antidepressants versus electroconvulsive therapy: a review of the evidence for efficacy in depression. Ann Clin Psychiatry 5:13–23, 1993

Pitts FN: Recent research on the DST. Compr Psychiatry 45:380–381, 1984

Pokorny AD: Suicide prevention revisited. Suicide Life Threat Behav 23:1–10, 1993

Poland RE, McCracken JT, Lutchmansingh P, et al: Differential response of rapid eye movement sleep to cholinergic blockade by scopolamine in currently depressed, remitted, and normal control subjects. Biol Psychiatry 41:929–938, 1997

Porter RJ: How to initiate and maintain carbamazepine therapy in children and adults. Epilepsia 28 (suppl 3):S59–S63, 1987

Post RM: Approaches to treatment-resistant bipolar affectively ill patients. Clin Neuropharmacol 11:93–104, 1988

Post RM: Non-lithium treatment for bipolar disorder. Compr Psychiatry 51 (suppl 8):9–16, 1990a

Post RM: Prophylaxis of bipolar affective disorders. International Review of Psychiatry 2:277–320, 1990b

Post RM: Anticonvulsants and novel drugs, in Handbook of Affective Disorders. Edited by Paykel ES. Edinburgh, Churchill Livingstone, 1992a, pp 387–417

Post RM: Transduction of psychosocial stress into the neurobiology of recurrent affective disorder. Am J Psychiatry 149:999–1010, 1992b

Post RM: Mechanisms underlying the evolution of affective disorders: implications for long-term treatment. Washington, DC, American Psychiatric Press, 1994, pp 23–65

Post RM, Rubinow DR, Ballenger JC: Conditioning and sensitisation in the longitudinal course of affective illness. Br J Psychiatry 149:191–201, 1986

Post RM, Weiss SR, Chuang DM: Mechanisms of action of anticonvulsants in affective disorders: comparisons with lithium. J Clin Psychopharmacol 12 (suppl 1):23S–35S, 1992

Post RM, Ketter TA, Pazzaglia PJ, et al: New developments in the use of anticonvulsants as mood stabilizers. Neuropsychobiology 27:132–137, 1993

Poynton A, Bridges PK, Bartlett JR, et al: Resistant bipolar affective disorder treated by stereotactic subcaudate tractotomy. Br J Psychiatry 152:354–358, 1988

Preskhorn SH: Pharmacokinetics of antidepressants: why and how they are relevant to treatment. Compr Psychiatry 52:4–8, 1991

Prien RF, Caffey EM, Klett CJ: Comparison of lithium carbonate and chlorpromazine in the treatment of mania. Arch Gen Psychiatry 26:146–153, 1972

Priest RG, Gimbrett R, Roberts M, et al: Reversible and selective inhibitors of monoamine oxidase A in mental and other disorders. Acta Psychiatr Scand Suppl 386:40–43, 1995

Privitera MR, Lamberti JS, Maharaj K: Clozapine in a bipolar depressed patient (letter). Am J Psychiatry 150:986, 1993

Prudic J, Sackeim HA, Devanand DP, et al: The efficacy of ECT in double depression. Depression 1:38–44, 1993

Puri BK, Taylor DG, Alcock ME: Low-dose maintenance clozapine treatment in the prophylaxis of bipolar affective disorder. Br J Clin Pract 49:333–334, 1995

Quitkin FM, McGrath PJ, Stewart JW, et al: Atypical depression, panic attacks, and response to imipramine and phenelzine: a replication. Arch Gen Psychiatry 47:935–941, 1990

Quitkin FM, Harrison W, Stewart JW, et al: Response to phenelzine and imipramine in placebo nonresponders with atypical depression: a new application of the crossover design. Arch Gen Psychiatry 48:319–323, 1991

Rabkin JG, Stewart JW, Quitkin F, et al: Should atypical depression be included as a separate entity in DSM-IV? A review of the research evidence, in DSM-IV Sourcebook. Edited by Widiger TA, Frances AJ, Pincus HA, et al. Washington, DC, American Psychiatric Press, 1995, pp 140–154

Ramasubbu R, Kennedy SH: Factors complicating the diagnosis of depression in cerebrovascular disease, II: neurological deficits and various assessment methods. Can J Psychiatry 39:601–607, 1994

Rao U, McCracken JT, Lutchmansingh P, et al: Electroencephalographic sleep and urinary free cortisol in adolescent depression: a preliminary report of changes from episode to recovery. Biol Psychiatry 41:369–373, 1997

Rehm LP: A self-control model of depression. Behavior Therapy 8:787–804, 1977

Reiger DA, Boyd JH, Burke JD: One-month prevalence of mental disorders in the United States. Arch Gen Psychiatry 45:977–986, 1988

Reynolds CF III, Hoch CC: Differential diagnosis of depressive pseudodementia and primary degenerative dementia. Psychiatric Annals 17:743–748, 1987

Reynolds CF III, Kupfer DJ, Thase ME, et al: Sleep, gender and depression: an analysis of gender effects on the electroencephalographic sleep of 302 depressed outpatients. Biol Psychiatry 28:673–684, 1990

Reynolds CF III, Frank E, Perel JM, et al: Maintenance therapies for late-life recurrent major depression: research and review circa 1995. Int Psychogeriatr 7 (suppl):27–39, 1995

Rifkin A, Doddi S, Karajgi B, et al: Dosage of haloperidol for mania. Br J Psychiatry 165:113–116, 1994

Riso LP, Klein DN, Ferro T: Understanding the comorbidity between early onset dysthymia and cluster B personality disorders: a family study. Am J Psychiatry 153:900–906, 1996

Roberts RE, Lewinsohn PM, Seeley JR: Symptoms of DSM-III-R major depression in adolescence: evidence from an epidemiological survey. J Am Acad Child Adolesc Psychiatry 34:1608–1617, 1995

Robinson RG, Bostan JD, Sarkstein SE, et al: Comparison of mania and depression after brain injury. Am J Psychiatry 145:172–175, 1988

Roose SP, Stern RH: Medication use in training cases: a survey. J Am Psychoanal Assoc 43:163–170, 1995

Rosenbaum JF, Fava M, Nierenberg AA, et al: Treatment-resistant mood disorders, in Treatment of Psychiatric Disorders. Edited by Gabbard GO. Washington, DC, American Psychiatric Press, 1995, pp 1275–1328

Rosenthal N[E], Sack DA, Skwerer RG, et al: Phototherapy for seasonal affective disorder, in Seasonal Affective Disorders and Phototherapy. Edited by Rosenthal NE, Blehar MC. New York, Guilford, 1989, pp 273–294

Rosenthal NE, Oren DA: Light therapy, in Treatment of Psychiatric Disorders. Edited by Gabbard GO. Washington, DC, American Psychiatric Press, 1995, pp 1263–1273

Ross ED: The aprosodias: functional anatomic organization of the affective components of language in the right hemisphere. Arch Neurol 38:561–569, 1981

Roth D, Bielsky R, Jones M, et al: A comparison of self-control therapy and combined self-control therapy and antidepressant medication in the treatment of depression. Behavior Therapy 13:133–144, 1982

Roy-Byrne PP, Joffe RT, Uhde TW, et al: Approaches to the evaluation and treatment of rapid-cycling affective illness. Br J Psychiatry 145:543–550, 1984

Rudd MD, Dahm PF, Rajab MH: Diagnostic comorbidity in persons with suicidal ideation and behavior. Am J Psychiatry 150:928–934, 1993

Rush AJ, Kupfer DJ: Strategies and tactics in the treatment of depression, in Treatment of Psychiatric Disorders. Edited by Gabbard GO. Washington, DC, American Psychiatric Press, 1995, pp 1349–1368

Rush AJ, Giles DE, Schlesser MA, et al: Dexamethasone response, thyrotropin-releasing hormone stimulation, rapid eye movement latency, and subtypes of depression. Biol Psychiatry 41:915–928, 1997

Sachs GS: Adjuncts and alternatives to lithium therapy for bipolar affective disorder. Compr Psychiatry 50 (suppl 12):31–39, 1989

Sachs GS: Use of clonazepam for bipolar disorder. Compr Psychiatry 51 (suppl 5):31–34, 1990

Sachs GS: Treatment-resistant bipolar depression. Psychiatr Clin North Am 19:215–235, 1996

Sachs GS, Lafer B, Stoll AL, et al: A double-blind trial of bupropion versus desipramine for bipolar depression. Compr Psychiatry 55:391–393, 1994a

Sachs GS, Lafer B, Truman CJ, et al: Lithium monotherapy: miracle, myth and misunderstanding. Psychiatric Annals 24:299–306, 1994b

Sackeim HA: Continuation therapy following ECT: directions for future research. Psychopharmacol Bull 30:501–521, 1994

Sackeim HA, Freeman J, McElhiney M, et al: Effects of major depression on estimates of intelligence. J Clin Exp Neuropsychol 14:268–288, 1992

Sajatovic M: A pilot study evaluating the efficacy of risperidone in treatment-refractory, acute bipolar, and schizoaffective mania (abstract). Psychopharmacol Bull 31:613, 1996

Sajatovic M, DiGiovanni SK, Bastani B, et al: Risperidone therapy in treatment refractory acute bipolar and schizoaffective mania. Psychopharmacol Bull 32:55–61, 1996

Salomon RM, Miller HL, Krystal JH, et al: Lack of behavioral effects of monoamine depletion in healthy subjects. Biol Psychiatry 41:58–64, 1997

Salzman C, Green AI, Rodriguez-Villa F, et al: Benzodiazepines combined with neuroleptics for management of severe disruptive behavior. Psychosomatics 27 (suppl):17–21, 1986

Sanderson WC, Wetzler S, Beck AT, et al: Prevalence of personality disorders in patients with major depression and dysthymia. Psychiatry Res 42:93–99, 1992

Santos AB, Morton WA: More on clonazepam in manic agitation. J Clin Psychopharmacol 7:439–440, 1987

Saxena S, Maltikarjuna P: Severe memory impairment with acute overdose lithium toxicity. Br J Psychiatry 152:853–854, 1988

Schaffer CB, Schaffer LC: The use of risperidone in the treatment of bipolar disorder (letter). Compr Psychiatry 57:136, 1996

Schatzberg AF, Nemeroff CB (eds): American Psychiatric Press Textbook of Psychopharmacology. Washington, DC, American Psychiatric Press, 1995a, pp 377–388

Schildkraut JJ: The catecholamine hypothesis of affective disorders: a review of supporting evidence. Am J Psychiatry 122:509–514, 1965

Schneekloth TB, Rummans TA, Logan KM: Electroconvulsive therapy in adolescents. Convuls Ther 9:158–166, 1993

Schneider LS, Sloane RB, Staples FR, et al: Pretreatment orthostatic hypotension as a predictor of response to nortriptyline in geriatric depression. J Clin Psychopharmacol 6:172–176, 1986

Schnur DB, Mukherjee S, Sackeim HA, et al: Symptomatic predictors of ECT response in medication-nonresponsive bipolar illness. Compr Psychiatry 53:63–66, 1992

Schoenenberger RA, Tanasijevic MJ, Jha A, et al: Appropriateness of antiepileptic drug level monitoring. JAMA 274:1622–1626, 1995

Schou M: Prophylactic lithium treatment of unipolar and bipolar manic-depressive illness. Psychopathology 28 (suppl 1):81–85, 1995

Schou M: Forty years of lithium treatment. Arch Gen Psychiatry 54:9–13, 1997

Schulberg HC: Treating major depression in primary care practice: eight-month clinical outcomes. Arch Gen Psychiatry 53:913–919, 1996

Schwarz T, Loewenstein J, Isenberg KE: Maintenance ECT: indications and outcome. Convuls Ther 11:14–23, 1995

Scott J: Chronic depression. Br J Psychiatry 153:287–297, 1988

Scott J: Chronic depression: can cognitive therapy succeed when other treatments fail? Behavioral Psychotherapy 20:25–36, 1992

Scott TF, Allen D, Price TRP: Characterization of major depression symptoms in multiple sclerosis patients. J Neuropsychiatry Clin Neurosci 8:318–323, 1996

Sedler MJ: Falret's discovery: the origin of the concept of bipolar affective illness. Am J Psychiatry 140:1127–1133, 1983

Seligman MEP: Helplessness: On Depression, Development and Death. San Francisco, CA, WH Freeman, 1975

Sernyak MJ, Woods SW: Chronic neuroleptic use in manic-depressive illness. Psychopharmacol Bull 29:375–381, 1993

Sexton HC, Hembre K, Kvarme G: The interaction of the alliance and therapy microprocess: a sequential analysis. J Consult Clin Psychol 64:471–480, 1996

Shaffer D, Gould MS, Fisher P, et al: Psychiatric diagnosis in child and adolescent suicide. Arch Gen Psychiatry 53:339–348, 1996

Shea MT, Hirschfeld RM: A chronic mood disorder and depressive personality. Psychiatr Clin North Am 19:103–120, 1996

Shea MT, Elkin I, Hirschfeld RMA, et al: Psychotherapeutic treatment of depression, in American Psychiatric Press Review of Psychiatry. Edited by Frances AJ, Hales RE. Washington, DC, American Psychiatric Press, 1988, pp 235–255

Shea MT, Pilkonis PA, Beckman E, et al: Personality disorders and treatment outcome in the NIMH Treatment of Depression Collaborative Research Program. Am J Psychiatry 147:711–718, 1990

Siever LJ, Davis KL: Overview: toward a dysregulation hypothesis of depression. Am J Psychiatry 142:1017–1025, 1985

Siever L[J], Trestman RL: The serotonin system and aggressive personality disorder. Int Clin Psychopharmacol 8 (suppl 2):33–39, 1993

Simhandl CA, Denk E, Thau K: The comparative efficacy of carbamazepine low and high serum level and lithium carbonate in the prophylaxis of affective disorders. J Affect Disord 28:221–231, 1993

Simpson SG, Folstein SE, Meyers DA, et al: Bipolar II: the most common bipolar phenotype? Am J Psychiatry 150:901–903, 1993

Singh AN, Catalan J: Risperidone in HIV-related manic psychosis. Lancet 344:1029–1030, 1994

Small JG, Small IF, Milstein V: Manic symptoms: an indication for bilateral ECT. Biol Psychiatry 20:125–134, 1985

Small JG, Klapper MH, Kellams JJ: Electroconvulsive treatment compared with lithium in the management of manic states. Arch Gen Psychiatry 45:727–732, 1988

Small JG, Klapper MH, Milstein V, et al: Comparison of therapeutic modalities for mania. Psychopharmacol Bull 32:623–627, 1996

Smith D, Baker G, Davies G, et al: Outcomes of add-on treatment with lamotrigine in partial epilepsy. Epilepsia 34:312–322, 1993

Soares JC, Mann JJ: The anatomy of mood disorders—review of structural neuroimaging studies. Biol Psychiatry 41:86–106, 1997

Solan WJ, Khan A, Avery DH, et al: Psychotic and nonpsychotic depression: comparison of response to ECT. Compr Psychiatry 49:97–99, 1988

Solomon DA, Bauer MS: Continuation and maintenance pharmacotherapy for unipolar and bipolar mood disorders. Psychiatr Clin North Am 16:515–540, 1993

Solomon DA, Keitner GI, Miller IW, et al: Course of illness and maintenance treatments for patients with bipolar disorder. Compr Psychiatry 56:5–13, 1995

Somoza E, Mossman D: Optimizing REM latency as a diagnostic test for depression using receiver operating characteristic analysis and information theory. Biol Psychiatry 27:990–1006, 1990

Sotsky SM, Glass DR, Shea MT, et al: Patient predictors of response to psychotherapy and pharmacotherapy: findings in the NIMH Treatment of Depression Collaborative Research Program. Am J Psychiatry 148:997–1008, 1991

Spiker DG, Kupfer DJ: Placebo response rates in psychotic and nonpsychotic depression. J Affect Disord 14:21–23, 1988

Spiker DG, Weiss JC, Dealy RS, et al: The pharmacological treatment of delusional depression. Am J Psychiatry 142:430–436, 1985

Spiker DG, Perel JM, Hanin I, et al: The pharmacological treatment of delusional depression: part II. J Clin Psychopharmacol 6:339–342, 1986a

Spiker DG, Dealy RS, Hanin I, et al: Treating delusional depressives with amitriptyline. Compr Psychiatry 47:243–246, 1986b

Srisurapanont M, Yatham LN, Zis AP: Treatment of acute bipolar depression: a review of the literature. Can J Psychiatry 40:533–544, 1995

Stancer HC, Persad E: Treatment of intractable rapid-cycling manic-depressive disorder with levothyroxine: clinical observations. Arch Gen Psychiatry 39:311–312, 1982

Stewart JW, McGrath PJ, Quitkin FM: Chronic depression: response to placebo, imipramine, and phenelzine. J Clin Psychopharmacol 13:391–396, 1993

Stoll AL, Mayer PV, Kolbrener M, et al: Antidepressant-associated mania: a controlled comparison with spontaneous mania. Am J Psychiatry 151:1642–1645, 1994

Strakowski S, McElroy SL, Keck PW Jr: The co-occurrence of mania with medical and other psychiatric disorders. Int J Psychiatry Med 24:305–328, 1994

Strober M, Carlson G: Bipolar illness in adolescents with major depression. Arch Gen Psychiatry 39:549–555, 1982

Strupp HH, Binder JL: Psychotherapy in a New Key: A Guide to Time-Limited Dynamic Psychotherapy. New York, Basic Books, 1984

Stuart S, Thase ME: Inpatient application of cognitive behavior therapy: a review of recent developments. Journal of Psychotherapy Practice and Research 3:284–299, 1994

Stuart S, Simons AD, Thase ME, et al: Are personality assessments valid in acute major depression? J Affect Disord 24:281–290, 1992

Suomi SJ, Seaman SF, Lewis JK: Effects of imipramine treatment of separation-induced social disorders in rhesus monkeys. Arch Gen Psychiatry 35:321–325, 1978

Suppes T, McElroy SL, Gilbert J, et al: Clozapine in the treatment of dysphoric mania. Biol Psychiatry 32:270–280, 1992

Suppes T, Phillips KA, Judd CR: Clozapine treatment of nonpsychotic rapid cycling bipolar disorder: a report of three cases. Biol Psychiatry 36:338–340, 1994

Swann AC: Mixed or dysphoric manic states: psychopathology and treatment. Compr Psychiatry 56 (suppl 3):6–10, 1995

Swann AC, Bowden CL, Morris D: Depression during mania. Arch Gen Psychiatry 54:37–42, 1997

Tallian KB, Nahata MC, Lo W, et al: Gabapentin associated with aggressive behavior in pediatric patients with seizures. Epilepsia 37:501–502, 1996

Tam EM, Lam RWA, Levitt AJ: Treatment of seasonal affective disorder: a review. Can J Psychiatry 40:457–466, 1995

Tan CH, Javors MA, Seleshi E: Effects of lithium on platelet ionic intracellular calcium concentration in patients with bipolar (manic-depressive) disorder and healthy controls. Life Sci 46:1175–1180, 1990

Teicher MH, Glod CA, Cole JO: Antidepressant drugs and the emergence of suicidal tendencies. Drug Saf 8:186–212, 1993

Teicher MH, Glod CA, Oren DA, et al: The phototherapy light visor: more to it than meets the eye. Am J Psychiatry 152:1197–2002, 1995

Teicher MH, Glod CA, Magnus E, et al: Circadian rest-activity disturbances in seasonal affective disorder. Arch Gen Psychiatry 54:124–130, 1997

Terao T: Subclinical hypothyroidism in recurrent mania. Biol Psychiatry 33:853–854, 1993

Thalen BE, Kjellman BF, Morkrid L, et al: Melatonin in light treatment of patients with seasonal and nonseasonal depression. Acta Psychiatr Scand 92:274–284, 1995

Thase ME: Relapse and recurrence in unipolar major depression: short-term and long-term approaches. Compr Psychiatry 51 (suppl 26):51–57, 1990

Thase ME: Long-term treatments of recurrent depressive disorders. Compr Psychiatry 53 (suppl 9):32–44, 1992

Thase ME: Reeducative psychotherapies, in Treatment of Psychiatric Disorders. Edited by Gabbard GO. Washington, DC, American Psychiatric Press, 1995, pp 1169–1204

Thase ME: The role of Axis II comorbidity in the management of patients with treatment-resistant depression. Psychiatr Clin North Am 19:287–309, 1996

Thase ME, Kupfer DJ: Recent developments in the pharmacotherapy of mood disorders. J Consult Clin Psychol 64:646–659, 1996

Thase ME, Simons AD, McGeary J, et al: Relapse after cognitive behavior therapy of depression: potential implications for longer courses of treatment. Am J Psychiatry 149:1046–1052, 1992

Thase ME, Reynolds CF, Frank E, et al: Response to cognitive-behavioral therapy in chronic depression. Journal of Psychotherapy Practice and Research Y1—1994 3:204–214, 1994

Thase ME, Kupfer DJ, Fasiczka AJ, et al: Identifying an abnormal electroencephalographic sleep profile to characterize major depressive disorder. Biol Psychiatry 41:964–973, 1997

Thompson PJ, Trimble MR: Anticonvulsant serum levels: relationship to impairments of cognitive functioning. J Neurol Neurosurg Psychiatry 46:227–233, 1983

Tohen M, Zarate CA, Centorrino F, et al: Risperidone in the treatment of mania. Compr Psychiatry 57:249–253, 1996a

Tohen M, Zarate CA, Centorrino F, et al: Risperidone in the treatment of mania (abstract). Psychopharmacol Bull 31:626, 1996b

Tomitaka S, Sakamoto K: Definition and prognosis of rapid cycling affective disorder (letter). Am J Psychiatry 151:1524, 1994

Tsuang D, Coryell W: An 8-year follow-up of patients with DSM-III-R psychotic depression, schizoaffective disorder and schizophrenia. Am J Psychiatry 150:1182–1188, 1993

Tsuang MT, Faraone SV: The inheritance of mood disorders, in Genetics and Mental Illness: Evolving Issues for Research and Society. Edited by Hall LL. New York, Plenum, 1996, pp 79–109

Ulmsten U, Anderson KE, Wingerup I: Treatment of premature labor with the calcium antagonist nifedipine. Arch Gynecol 229:1–5, 1980

Vallada H, Craddock N, Vasquez L, et al: Linkage studies in bipolar affective disorder with markers on chromosome 21. J Affect Disord 41:217–221, 1996

Vanelle J-M, Loo H, Galinowski MD, et al: Maintenance ECT in intractable manic-depressive disorders. Convuls Ther 10:195–205, 1994

van Praag HM: Two-tier diagnosing in psychiatry. Psychiatry Res 34:341–311, 1990

van Praag HM, Kahn RS, Asnis GM: Denosologization of biological psychiatry or the specificity of 5-HT disturbances in psychiatric disorders. J Affect Disord 13:1–8, 1987

Verma NP, Haidukewych D: Differential but infrequent alterations of hepatic enzyme levels and thyroid hormone levels by anticonvulsant drugs. Arch Neurol 2:319–323, 1993

Walden J, Hesslinger B: Value of old and new anticonvulsants in treatment of psychiatric diseases. Fortschr Neurol Psychiatr 63:320–335, 1995

Walden J, Grunze H, Bungmann D, et al: Calcium antagonistic effects of carbamazepine as a mechanism of action in neuropsychiatric disorders: studies in calcium dependent model epilepsies. Eur Neuropsychopharmacol 2:455–462, 1992

Walter G, Rey J: An epidemiological study of the use of ECT in adolescents. J Am Acad Child Adolesc Psychiatry 36:809–815, 1997

Walton SA, Berk M, Brook S: Superiority of lithium over verapamil in mania: a randomized, controlled, single-blind trial. Compr Psychiatry 57:543–546, 1996

Warner R, Appleby L, Whitton A, et al: Demographic and obstetric risk factors for postnatal psychiatric morbidity. Br J Psychiatry 168:607–611, 1996

Warshaw MG, Keller MB: The relationship between fluoxetine use and suicidal behavior in 654 subjects with anxiety disorders. Compr Psychiatry 57:158–166, 1996

Watkins JT, Leber WR, Imber SD, et al: Temporal course of change of depression. J Consult Clin Psychol 61:858–864, 1993

Wehr TA: Can antidepressants induce rapid cycling? Arch Gen Psychiatry 50:495–496, 1993

Wehr TA, Sack DA, Rosenthal NE, et al: Rapid cycling affective disorder: contributing factors and treatment responses in 51 patients. Am J Psychiatry 145:179–184, 1988

Weiner RD: Does electroconvulsive therapy cause brain damage? Behavioral and Brain Sciences 7:1–13, 1984

Weiner RD: Electroconvulsive therapy, in Treatment of Psychiatric Disorders. Edited by Gabbard GO. Washington, DC, American Psychiatric Press, 1995, pp 1237–1273

Weissman MM: Psychotherapy in the maintenance treatment of depression. Br J Psychiatry 165 (suppl 26):42–50, 1994

Weissman MM, Prusoff BA, DiMascio A, et al: The efficacy of drugs and psychotherapy in the treatment of acute depressive episodes. Am J Psychiatry 136:555–558, 1979

Weissman MM, Prusoff BA, Gammon GD, et al: Psychopathology in the children (ages 6–18) of depressed and normal parents. J Am Acad Child Adolesc Psychiatry 23:78–84, 1984

Weissman MM, Warner V, John K, et al: Delusional depression and bipolar spectrum: evidence for a possible association from a family study of children. Neuropsychopharmacology 1:257–264, 1988a

Weissman MM, Leaf PJ, Bruce ML: The epidemiology of dysthymia in five communities: rates, risks, comorbidity, and treatment. Am J Psychiatry 145:815–819, 1988b

Weissman MM, Bland RC, Canino GJ, et al: Cross-national epidemiology of major depression and bipolar disorder. JAMA 276:293–299, 1996

Wells KB, Stewart A, Hays RD: The functioning and well-being of depressed patients. JAMA 262:914–919, 1989

Wells KB, Burnnam A, Rogers WH, et al: The course of depression in adult outpatients: results from the medical outcomes study. Arch Gen Psychiatry 49:788–794, 1992

Whybrow PC, Akiskal HS, McKinney WT: Mood Disorders: Toward a New Psychobiology. New York, Plenum, 1984, pp 21–42

Wide-Swensson DG, Ingemarsson I, Lunell N, et al: Calcium channel blockade (isradipine) in treatment of hypertension in pregnancy: a randomized placebo-controlled study. Am J Obstet Gynecol 173:872–878, 1996

Wilde MI, Benfield P: Tianeptine: a review of its pharmacodynamic and pharmacokinetic properties, and therapeutic efficacy in depression and coexisting anxiety and depression. Drugs 49:411–439, 1995

Wilson PH: Combined pharmacological and behavioral treatment of depression. Behav Res Ther 20:173–184, 1982

Winokur G: Manic-depressive disease (bipolar): is it autonomous? Psychopathology 28 (suppl 1):51–58, 1995

Winokur G, Morrison J: The Iowa 500: follow-up of 225 depressives. Br J Psychiatry 123:543–548, 1973

Woods BT, Yurgelun-Todd D, Mikulis D, et al: Age-related MRI abnormalities in bipolar illness: a clinical study. Biol Psychiatry 38:846–847, 1995

Young MA, Fogg LF, Schefner WA, et al: Interaction of risk factors in predicting suicide. Am J Psychiatry 151:434–435, 1994

Zarate CA Jr, Tohen M, Baldessarini RJ: Clozapine in severe mood disorders. Compr Psychiatry 56:411–417, 1995a

Zarate CA Jr, Tohen M, Banov MD, et al: Is clozapine a mood stabilizer? Compr Psychiatry 56:108–112, 1995b

Zarate CA [Jr], Tohen M, Baldessarini RJ: Clozapine in severe mood disorders (abstract). Psychopharmacol Bull 31:636, 1996

Zornberg GL, Rose HG: Treatment of depression in bipolar disorder: new directions for research. J Clin Psychopharmacol 13:397–408, 1993

CHAPTER 14

ANXIETY DISORDERS

ERIC HOLLANDER, M.D.
DAPHNE SIMEON, M.D.
JACK M. GORMAN, M.D.

nxiety disorders are the most common of all psychiatric illnesses and result in considerable functional impairment and distress. Recent research developments have had a broad impact on our understanding of the underlying mechanisms of illness and treatment response. Working with patients who have an anxiety disorder can be highly gratifying for the informed psychiatrist, because these patients, who are in considerable distress, often respond to proper treatment and return to a high level of functioning.

In this chapter we have divided the anxiety disorders into four broad categories: panic and anxiety disorders (panic disorder and generalized anxiety disorder), phobic disorders (agoraphobia, social phobia, and specific phobia), obsessive-compulsive disorder, and posttraumatic stress disorder (PTSD). A diagnostic decision tree of the anxiety disorders is presented in Figure 14–1.

PANIC AND GENERALIZED ANXIETY DISORDERS

DEFINITIONS

The *Diagnostic and Statistical Manual of Mental Disorders*, 2nd Edition (DSM-II; American Psychiatric Association

1968) described an ill-defined condition of "anxiety neurosis," a term first coined by Freud in 1895 (Breuer and Freud 1893–1895/1955), which included any patient suffering from chronic tension, excessive worry, frequent headaches, or recurrent anxiety attacks. However, subsequent findings suggested that discrete spontaneous panic attacks may be qualitatively dissimilar to other chronic anxiety states. For example, patients with panic attacks were found to be unique in their panic-induction responsiveness to sodium lactate infusion, familial aggregation, development of agoraphobia, and treatment response to tricyclic antidepressants (TCAs). Thus, DSM-III (American Psychiatric Association 1980) and the subsequent DSM-III-R (American Psychiatric Association 1987) divided the category of anxiety neurosis into *panic disorder* and *generalized anxiety disorder*.

The DSM-IV (American Psychiatric Association 1994) definition of a panic attack is presented in Table 14–1. Panic disorder is subdivided into panic disorder with and panic disorder without agoraphobia, as in DSM-III-R, depending on whether there is any secondary phobic avoidance (see Tables 14–2 and 14–3). The DSM-IV definition of generalized anxiety disorder (GAD) is presented in Table 14–4.

In DSM-IV, several issues were clarified regarding the diagnosis and differential diagnosis of panic disorder.

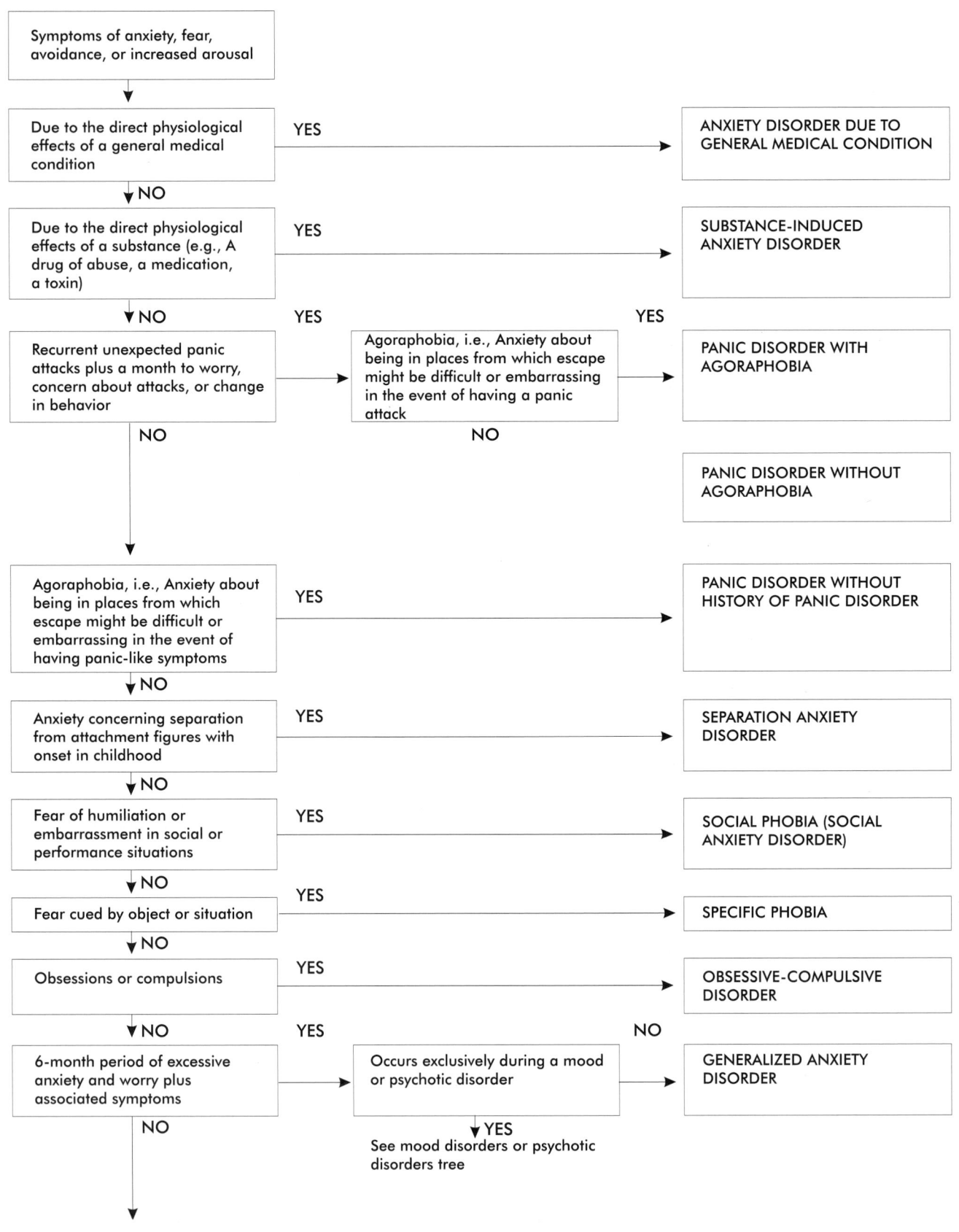

FIGURE 14–1.   Diagnostic decision tree for anxiety disorders.

Note.   Patients may have more than one disorder and thus must be evaluated for each disorder.

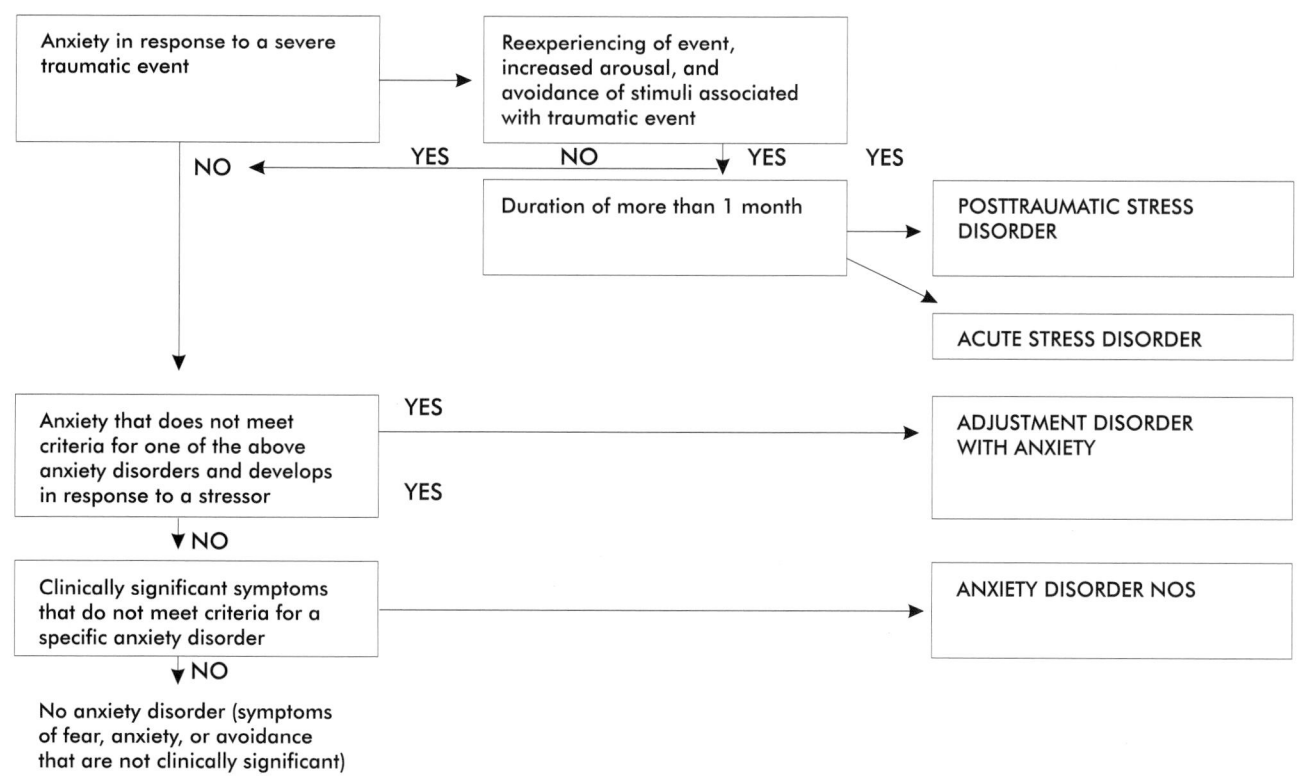

FIGURE 14–1.   Diagnostic decision tree for anxiety disorders *(continued)*.
Note.   Patients may have more than one disorder and thus must be evaluated for each disorder.

Panic attacks are known to occur not only in panic disorder but in other anxiety disorders as well (e.g., specific phobia, social phobia, and PTSD). In these other disorders, panic attacks are situationally bound or cued—that is, they occur exclusively within the context of the feared situation. DSM-IV explicitly presents the definition of panic attacks independently of panic disorder (Table 14–1) and specified that a panic attack can be unexpected (uncued), situationally bound (cued), or situationally predisposed.

The differential diagnosis can sometimes become complicated when, historically, one or several unexpected panic attacks had initially occurred in a specific situation, consistent with a diagnosis of panic disorder, but later evolved into a chronic condition in which the attacks are cued only by that situation or when avoidance of that situation develops because of fear of another attack. Is the diagnosis in such a case panic disorder with agoraphobia or social/specific phobia? DSM-IV retains the distinct diagnoses of panic disorder with agoraphobia, social phobia, and specific phobia and specifies that panic attacks can occur as a feature of all three of these disorders. Therefore, clinical judgment is called for in making the differential diagnosis in such cases.

DSM-IV also sharpened the distinction of GAD from "normal" anxiety by specifying that in GAD, the worry must be clearly excessive, pervasive, difficult to control, and associated with marked distress or impairment. DSM-IV also clarified that the diagnosis of GAD is excluded in the presence of other major Axis I disorders, and the cumbersome somatic symptom list from DSM-III-R was simplified.

Mixed Anxiety-Depressive Disorder

In primary care and community settings, a condition characterized by both anxious and depressive symptoms seems to be often encountered but does not meet the criteria for either an anxiety disorder or a depressive disorder. This entity underwent extensive critical consideration in the making of DSM-IV. On one hand, the condition is clinically identifiable and can cause notable distress and impairment, and a clinician would not want to miss or inconsistently treat such individuals (Zinbarg et al. 1994). On the other hand, there can be a risk of overdiagnosing psychiatric illness when it blends in with more universal human vicissitudes, of encouraging nonspecific diagnoses made in nonpsychiatric settings by nonexperts, and of overmedicating with drugs that may not necessarily be ef-

TABLE 14–1.   DSM-IV definition of panic attack

A discrete period of intense fear or discomfort, in which four (or more) of the following symptoms developed abruptly and reached a peak within 10 minutes:

> Palpitations, pounding heart, or accelerated heart rate
>
> Sweating
>
> Trembling or shaking
>
> Sensations of shortness of breath or smothering
>
> Feeling of choking
>
> Chest pain or discomfort
>
> Nausea or abdominal distress
>
> Feeling dizzy, unsteady, lightheaded, or faint
>
> Derealization (feelings of unreality) or depersonalization (being detached from oneself)
>
> Fear of losing control or "going crazy"
>
> Fear of dying
>
> Paresthesias (numbness or tingling sensations)
>
> Chills or hot flushes

The essential feature of a panic attack is a discrete period of intense fear or discomfort that is accompanied by at least 4 of 13 somatic or cognitive symptoms. The attack has a sudden onset and builds to a peak rapidly (usually in 10 minutes or less) and is often accompanied by a sense of imminent danger or impending doom and an urge to escape. The 13 somatic or cognitive symptoms are palpitations, sweating, trembling or shaking, sensations of shortness of breath or smothering, feeling of choking, chest pain or discomfort, nausea or abdominal distress, dizziness or lightheadedness, derealization or depersonalization, fear of losing control or "going crazy," fear of dying, paresthesias, and chills or hot flushes. Attacks that meet all other criteria but that have fewer than 4 somatic or cognitive symptoms are referred to as limited-symptom attacks.

Individuals seeking care for unexpected panic attacks will usually describe the fear as intense and report that they thought they were about to die, lose control, have a heart attack or stroke, or "go crazy." They also usually report an urgent desire to flee from wherever the attack is occurring. With recurrent attacks, some of the intense fearfulness may wane. Shortness of breath is a common symptom in panic attacks associated with panic disorder with and without agoraphobia. Blushing is common in situationally bound panic attacks related to social or performance anxiety. The anxiety that is characteristic of a panic attack can be differentiated from generalized anxiety by its intermittent, almost paroxysmal nature and its typically greater severity.

Panic attacks can occur in a variety of anxiety disorders (e.g., panic disorder, social phobia, specific phobia, posttraumatic stress disorder, acute stress disorder). In determining the differential diagnostic significance of a panic attack, it is important to consider the context in which the panic attack occurs. There are three characteristic types of panic attacks with different relationships between the onset of the attack and the presence or absence of situational triggers: **unexpected (uncued) panic attacks,** in which the onset of the panic attack is not associated with a situational trigger (i.e., occurring spontaneously "out of the blue"); **situationally bound (cued) panic attacks,** in which the panic attack almost invariably occurs immediately on exposure to, or in anticipation of, the situational cue or trigger (e.g., seeing a snake or dog always triggers an immediate panic attack); and **situationally predisposed panic attacks,** which are more likely to occur on exposure to the situational cue or trigger, but are not invariably associated with the cue and do not necessarily occur immediately after the exposure (e.g., attacks are more likely to occur while driving, but there are times when the individual drives and does not have a panic attack or times when the panic attack occurs after driving for a half hour).

The occurrence of unexpected panic attacks is required for a diagnosis of panic disorder (with or without agoraphobia). Situationally bound panic attacks are most characteristic of social and specific phobias. Situationally predisposed panic attacks are especially frequent in panic disorder but may at times occur in specific phobia or social phobia. The differential diagnosis of panic attacks is complicated by the fact that an exclusive relationship does not always exist between the diagnosis and the type of panic attack. For instance, although panic disorder definitionally requires that at least some of the panic attacks be unexpected, individuals with panic disorder frequently report having situationally bound attacks, particularly later in the course of the disorder.

TABLE 14–2. DSM-IV diagnostic criteria for panic disorder with agoraphobia

A. Both (1) and (2):

   (1) Recurrent unexpected panic attacks

   (2) At least one of the attacks has been followed by 1 month of one (or more) of the following:

      (a) persistent concern about having additional attacks;

      (b) worry about the implications of the attack or its consequences (e.g., losing control, having a heart attack, "going crazy");

      (c) a significant change in behavior related to the attacks

B. The presence of agoraphobia, i.e., anxiety about being in places or situations from which escape might be difficult (or embarrassing) or in which help may not be available in the event of having an unexpected or situationally predisposed panic attack or panic-like symptoms. Agoraphobic fears typically involve characteristic clusters of situations that include being outside the home alone; being in a crowd or standing in a line; being on a bridge; and traveling in a bus, train, or automobile.

   Note: Consider the diagnosis of specific phobia if limited to one or only a few specific situations, or social phobia if the avoidance is limited to social situations.

C. The panic attacks are not due to the direct physiological effects of a substance (e.g., a drug of abuse, a medication) or a general medical condition (e.g., hyperthyroidism).

D. The panic attacks are not better accounted for by another mental disorder, such as social phobia (e.g., occurring on exposure to feared social situations), specific phobia (e.g., on exposure to a specific phobic situation), obsessive-compulsive disorder (e.g., on exposure to dirt in someone with an obsession about contamination), posttraumatic stress disorder (e.g., in response to stimuli associated with a severe stressor), or separation anxiety disorder (e.g., in response to being away from home or close relatives).

---

fective on or specific to their target symptoms. As an interim solution, the diagnosis of mixed anxiety-depressive disorder has been included in an appendix to DSM-IV. It is a diagnosis of exclusion and stipulates a 1-month duration of symptoms; its institution may promote more conclusive research in this area.

Organic Etiologies

If pathological anxiety is induced by either psychoactive substance use or an Axis III physical illness, it is classified in DSM-IV under the anxiety disorders (substance-induced anxiety disorder or anxiety disorder due to a general medical condition, respectively). DSM-III-R had placed any psychopathology associated with organicity, regardless of

its form, under *organic mental disorders*. It is hoped that the new DSM-IV format will encourage greater specificity in the differential diagnosis of organic conditions. DSM-IV specifies the subtype of organic anxiety as *generalized anxiety*, *panic attacks*, or *obsessive-compulsive symptoms*.

CLINICAL DESCRIPTIONS

Panic Disorder

Onset.   In the typical onset of a case of panic disorder, subjects are engaged in some ordinary aspect of life when suddenly their heart begins to pound and they cannot catch their breath. They feel dizzy, light-headed, and faint and are convinced they are about to die. Panic disorder patients are usually young adults, most likely in the third decade. However, there have been cases in which the disorder began in the sixth decade.

Although the first attack generally strikes during some routine activity, several events are often associated with the early presentation of panic disorder. Not uncommonly, the first panic attack occurs in the context of a life-threatening illness or accident, the loss of a close interpersonal relationship, or during separation from family (e.g., after starting

TABLE 14–3. DSM-IV diagnostic criteria for panic disorder without agoraphobia

A. Both (1) and (2):

   (1) Recurrent unexpected panic attacks

   (2) At least one of the attacks has been followed by 1 month (or more) of one (or more) of the following:

      (a) persistent concern about having additional attacks;

      (b) worry about the implications of the attack or its consequences (e.g., losing control, having a heart attack, "going crazy");

      (c) a significant change in behavior related to the attacks

B. Absence of agoraphobia [defined in Table 14–2(B)].

C. The panic attacks are not due to the direct physiological effects of a substance (e.g., a drug of abuse, a medication) or a general medical condition (e.g., hyperthyroidism).

D. The panic attacks are not better accounted for by another mental disorder, such as social phobia (e.g., occurring on exposure to feared social situations), specific phobia (e.g., on exposure to a specific phobic situation), obsessive-compulsive disorder (e.g., on exposure to dirt in someone with an obsession about contamination), posttraumatic stress disorder (e.g., in response to stimuli associated with a severe stressor), or separation anxiety disorder (e.g., in response to being away from home or close relatives).

TABLE 14–4.   **DSM-IV diagnostic criteria for generalized anxiety disorder**

A. Excessive anxiety and worry (apprehensive expectation), occurring more days than not for at least 6 months, about a number of events or activities (such as work or school performance).

B. The person finds it difficult to control the worry.

C. The anxiety and worry are associated with three (or more) of the following six symptoms (with at least some symptoms present for more days than not for the past 6 months). **Note:** Only one item is required in children.

   (1) Restlessness or feeling keyed up or on edge

   (2) Being easily fatigued

   (3) Difficulty concentrating or mind going blank

   (4) Irritability

   (5) Muscle tension

   (6) Sleep disturbance (difficulty falling or staying asleep, or restless, unsatisfying sleep)

D. The focus of the anxiety and worry is not confined to features of an Axis I disorder, e.g., the anxiety or worry is not about having a panic attack (as in panic disorder), being embarrassed in public (as in social phobia), being contaminated (as in obsessive-compulsive disorder), being away from home or close relatives (as in separation anxiety disorder), gaining weight (as in anorexia nervosa), having multiple physical complaints (as in somatization disorder), or having a serious illness (as in hypochondriasis), and the anxiety and worry do not occur exclusively during posttraumatic stress disorder.

E. The anxiety, worry, or physical symptoms cause clinically significant distress or impairment in social, occupational, or other important areas of functioning.

F. The disturbance is not due to the direct physiological effects of a substance (e.g., a drug of abuse, a medication) or a general medical condition (e.g., hyperthyroidism) and does not occur exclusively during a mood disorder, a psychotic disorder, or a pervasive developmental disorder.

college or accepting a job out of town). Patients developing either hypothyroidism or hyperthyroidism may get the first flurry of attacks at this time. Attacks also begin in the immediate postpartum period. Finally, many patients have reported experiencing their first attacks while taking mind-altering drugs, especially marijuana, LSD, sedatives, cocaine, and amphetamines. However, even when these concomitant conditions are resolved, the attacks often continue unabated. This situation gives the impression that some stressors may act as triggers to provoke the beginning of panic attacks in patients who are already predisposed.

Patients experiencing their first panic attack generally fear they are having a heart attack or losing their mind.

Such patients often rush to the nearest emergency room, where routine laboratory tests, electrocardiography, and physical examination are performed. All that is found is an occasional case of sinus tachycardia, and the patients are reassured and sent home.

These patients may indeed feel reassured, and at this point the diagnosis of panic disorder would be premature. However, perhaps a few days or even weeks later they will again have the sudden onset of severe anxiety with all of the associated physical symptoms. Again, they seek emergency medical treatment. At this point, they may be told the problem is "psychological," be given a prescription for a benzodiazepine tranquilizer, or be referred for extensive medical workup.

Symptoms.   Typically, during a panic attack, a patient will be engaged in a routine activity—perhaps reading a book, eating in a restaurant, driving a car, or attending a concert—when he or she will experience the sudden onset of overwhelming fear, terror, apprehension, and a sense of impending doom. Several of a group of associated symptoms, mostly physical, are also experienced: dyspnea, palpitations, chest pain or discomfort, choking or smothering sensations, dizziness or feelings of unsteadiness, feelings of unreality (derealization and/or depersonalization), paresthesias, hot and cold flashes, sweating, faintness, trembling and shaking, and a fear of dying, going crazy, or losing control of oneself. It is clear that most of the physical sensations of a panic attack represent massive overstimulation of the autonomic nervous system.

Attacks usually last from 5 to 20 minutes and rarely last as long as an hour. Patients who claim they have attacks that last a whole day may fall into one of four categories. Some patients continue to feel agitated and fatigued for several hours after the main portion of the attack has subsided. At times, attacks occur, subside, and occur again in a wave-like manner. Alternatively, the patient with so-called long panic attacks is often suffering from some other form of pathological anxiety, such as severe generalized anxiety, agitated depression, or obsessional tension states. In some cases, such severe anticipatory anxiety may develop with time in expectation of future panic attacks so that the two may blend together in the patient's description and be difficult to distinguish.

Although many people experience an occasional unexpected attack of panic, the diagnosis of panic disorder is only made when the attacks occur with some regularity and frequency. However, patients with occasional unexpected panic attacks may be genetically similar to patients with panic disorder. A twin study found the best results for genetic linkage when patients with regular panic attacks were included with patients who had only occasional "panics" (Torgersen 1983).

Some patients do not progress in their illness beyond the point of continuing to have unexpected panic attacks. Most patients develop some degree of anticipatory anxiety consequent to the experience of repetitive panic attacks. The patient comes to dread experiencing an attack and starts worrying about doing so in the intervals between attacks. This can progress until the level of fearfulness and autonomic hyperactivity in the interval between panic attacks almost approximates the level during the actual attack itself. Such patients may be mistaken for GAD patients.

It is warranted to draw some further attention to what appears to be the cardinal symptom of panic. A number of lines of research evidence indicate that *hyperventilation* may be the central feature in the pathophysiology of panic attacks and panic disorder. Patients with panic disorder have been shown to be chronic hyperventilators who also acutely hyperventilate during spontaneous and induced panic. (The possible etiologies of this will be discussed later in this section.) This hyperventilation then induces hypocapnia and alkalosis, leading to decreased cerebral blood flow and to the dizziness, confusion, and derealization characteristic of panic attacks. Indeed, signs and symptoms of hyperventilation seem to disappear once a patient with panic disorder has been successfully treated with antipanic medication. Also, behavioral breathing retraining treatments aimed at teaching the patient not to hyperventilate are successful in decreasing the frequency of panic attacks (Clark et al. 1985; Lum 1981), presumably through dampening the ventilatory overreaction that may constitute the hallmark of panic.

Generalized Anxiety Disorder

Generalized anxiety disorder (GAD) is the main diagnostic category for prominent and chronic anxiety in the absence of panic disorder. The essential feature of this syndrome, according to DSM-IV, is persistent anxiety lasting at least 6 months. The symptoms of this type of anxiety fall within two broad categories: apprehensive expectation and physical symptoms.

Patients with GAD are constantly worried over trivial matters, fearful, and anticipating the worst. Muscle tension, restlessness, feeling keyed up (hypervigilance), difficulty concentrating, insomnia, irritability, and fatigue are typical signs of generalized anxiety and have become the symptom criteria for GAD in DSM-IV, a number of studies having been performed to single out the physical symptoms that are the most distinctive and characteristic of GAD. Motor tension and hypervigilance better differenti-

ate GAD from other anxiety states than does autonomic hyperactivity (Marten et al. 1993; Starcevic et al. 1994).

CHARACTER TRAITS

It has not been clearly established whether particular character types are correlated with panic disorder, and studies are further confounded because the presence of panic disorder may have secondary effects on personality. Noyes et al. (1991) conducted personality follow-up of panic disorder patients treated for panic over 3 years and found that the initial avoidant and dependent traits were to a large extent state related and waned with the treatment of panic. On the other hand, experience leads many clinicians to believe that patients with agoraphobia and panic more often show dependent character traits that antedate the onset of panic.

The personality types of patients with GAD are also not well characterized. One study reported that approximately one-third of patients with GAD also suffered from a DSM-III personality disorder, and the most common one was dependent personality disorder (Noyes et al. 1987).

EPIDEMIOLOGY

The National Institute of Mental Health Epidemiologic Catchment Area (ECA) study examined the population prevalence of DSM-III–diagnosed panic disorder using the Diagnostic Interview Schedule (DIS; Regier et al. 1988). The 1-month, 6-month, and lifetime prevalence rates for panic disorder at all five study sites combined were 0.5%, 0.8%, and 1.6%, respectively. Women had a 1-month prevalence rate of 0.7%, which was markedly higher than the 0.3% rate found among men; women also tended to have a greater increase in panic disorder in the age range of 25–44 years, and their attacks tended to continue longer into older age (Regier et al. 1988). The epidemiology of panic disorder appears to be similar in whites and blacks (Horwath et al. 1993).

The relationship between panic disorder and major depression has been questioned in numerous studies because the two are well known commonly to co-occur. A recent family study found that panic disorder and major depression are clearly distinct disorders, despite their frequent co-occurrence, and panic comorbid with major depression does not segregate in families as a distinct disorder (Weissman et al. 1993).

Findings on GAD from the ECA study must be interpreted more cautiously, because they were assessed only in the second wave of the study and only at three of the five sites. Also, the DIS criteria, in accordance with DSM-III, required only a total of three somatic symptoms and only a 1-month duration of illness. Therefore, according to the stricter DSM-III-R or DSM-IV criteria, the incidence of GAD would be lower. One-year prevalence rates for the three sites combined were 3.8% without any exclusions, 2.7% when concurrent panic or major depression was excluded, and 1.7% when any other DSM-III diagnoses were excluded. Lifetime prevalence when panic and major depression were excluded ranged from 4.1% to 6.6%, according to the site. Rates were higher overall in women (Blazer et al. 1991).

Another large epidemiologic study, the National Comorbidity Survey, assessed DSM-III-R–diagnosed GAD and found it to have a current (in the past year) prevalence of 3.1% and a lifetime prevalence of 5.1% in the age group of 15–45 years, to be as common in women, and to have a very high lifetime comorbidity of 90% with a wide spectrum of other psychiatric disorders. Even so, the prevalence and comorbidity patterns of current GAD supported its conceptualization as a distinct disorder (Wittchen et al. 1994).

ETIOLOGY

Biological Theories

A number of biological theories of both panic disorder and, to a much lesser extent, GAD are prominent in the psychiatric literature. We will summarize the evidence for or against some of the most promising of these. Certain agents have a powerful and specific capacity to induce panic, in contrast to other agents that produce prominent physiological changes but fail to induce panic. These findings argue strongly against the notion that panic is a reaction to nonspecific distressing stimuli and suggest a specific biological basis. The various theories described in this subsection, such as the carbon dioxide chemoreceptor and the locus coeruleus theories of panic, need not be viewed as mutually exclusive. For example, the relationship between central respiratory regulation and central neurotransmitter function in panic is very complex and still under investigation. Biological theories of panic are summarized in Table 14–5.

Catecholamine theory. Some investigators have found anxiety reactions associated with increases in levels of urinary catecholamines, especially epinephrine. Studies of normal subjects exposed to novel stress also demonstrate elevations in plasma catecholamine levels (Dimsdale and Moss 1980). However, elevated plasma levels of epinephrine are not a regular accompaniment of panic attacks

induced in the laboratory (Liebowitz et al. 1985a). It is not clear whether administration of catecholamines can actually provoke anxiety reactions and, if this is the case, whether the reaction is specific only to patients with anxiety disorder. Researchers in the 1930s and 1940s did show that epinephrine infusion caused the physical, but not necessarily the emotional, symptoms of anxiety in human subjects.

For many years the possibility that panic attacks are manifestations of massive discharge from the β-adrenergic nervous system has been considered. Frohlich and colleagues (1969) gave intravenous isoproterenol infusions to patients with a "hyper-dynamic beta-adrenergic circulatory state" and produced "hysterical outbursts" that in retrospect seem similar to panic attacks. Patients with spontaneous anxiety may be more sensitive to the effects of isoproterenol than are normal control subjects (Rainey et al. 1984). Gorman and colleagues (1989b) suggested that the putative panicogenic effect of isoproterenol may be indirect, because isoproterenol does not cross the blood-brain barrier. Peripheral mismatch may occur between induced metabolic demands and actual physiological state, is then conveyed to the brain stem, and elicits a panic reaction.

The β-adrenergic hypothesis received further support from studies claiming that β-adrenergic blocking drugs, such as propranolol, have an ameliorative effect on panic attacks and anxiety. When the properly designed and controlled studies of β-adrenergic blockers used in specific, well-diagnosed anxiety disorders are reviewed, however,

TABLE 14–5. Biological theories of panic

Catecholamine theory	Massive β-adrenergic nervous system discharge
Locus coeruleus theory	Increased discharge of central nervous system noradrenergic nuclei
Metabolic theory	Aberrant metabolic changes induced by lactate infusion
False suffocation alarm carbon theory	Hypersensitive brain-stem dioxide receptors
γ-Aminobutyric acid (GABA)-benzodiazepine theory	Abnormal receptor function leading to decreased inhibitory activity
Genetic theory	Attempts to isolate a panic gene from family pedigrees (without positive results to date)
Neuroethological theory	Biologically disrupted innate attachment mechanism

only modest antianxiety effects can actually be demonstrated. No study has ever shown that β-adrenergic blockers are specifically effective in blocking spontaneous panic attacks. For example, intravenously administered propranolol, in doses sufficient to achieve full peripheral β-adrenergic blockade, is not able to block a sodium lactate–induced panic attack in patients with panic disorder (Gorman et al. 1983). Examination of various autonomic variables seems to lead to the dispelling of the notion of simple autonomic dysregulation in panic (M. B. Stein and Asmundson 1994).

Locus coeruleus theory.   Another prominent hypothesis regarding the etiology of panic attacks involves the locus coeruleus. This nucleus is located in the pons and contains more than 50% of all noradrenergic neurons in the entire central nervous system. It sends afferent projections to a wide area of the brain, including the hippocampus, amygdala, limbic lobe, and cerebral cortex.

Support for this hypothesis comes from the fact that electrical stimulation of the animal locus coeruleus produces a marked fear and anxiety response, whereas ablation of the animal locus coeruleus renders an animal less susceptible to fear response in the face of threatening stimuli (Redmond 1979). In humans, drugs known to be capable of increasing locus coeruleus discharge in animals are anxiogenic, whereas many drugs that curtail locus coeruleus firing and decrease central noradrenergic turnover are antianxiety agents. Yohimbine, an α$_2$-adrenergic antagonist, is an example of a drug that increases locus coeruleus discharge and has been shown to provoke anxiety and panic attacks in humans. However, buspirone, which is also reported to increase locus coeruleus firing, is an anxiolytic medication and has not been reported to induce panic. Examples of medications that curtail locus coeruleus firing are clonidine, propranolol, benzodiazepines, morphine, endorphin, and TCAs. These drugs range from those clearly effective in blocking human panic attacks (e.g., TCAs) to those of more dubious efficacy (e.g., clonidine, propranolol, and standard benzodiazepines).

A controversy exists about the relevance of these animal models. Redmond (1979) and colleagues produced abundant evidence that situations that provoke fear and anxiety in laboratory animals are associated with increases in locus coeruleus discharge and in central noradrenergic turnover. This would, of course, support the idea that the locus coeruleus is a kind of generator for anxiety attacks. However, there is no consistent pattern of increased locus coeruleus discharge associated with anxiety in animals (S. T. Mason and Fibiger 1979). The locus coeruleus may

be involved in arousal and response to novel stimuli rather than in anxiety (Aston-Jones et al. 1984).

The refinement of neurochemical challenge techniques has provided us with an additional tool for investigating central neurotransmitter function in human subjects in a relatively noninvasive fashion. Yohimbine challenge was reported to induce greater anxiety and a greater increase in plasma 3-methoxy-4-hydroxyphenylglycol (MHPG), a major noradrenergic metabolite, in patients with frequent panic attacks, compared with patients who have panic attacks less frequently or with healthy control subjects. Such a finding is suggestive of heightened central noradrenergic activity in panic (Charney et al. 1984). The results from challenge tests with the α$_2$-adrenergic agonist clonidine, although difficult to interpret, have suggested noradrenergic dysregulation in panic, with hypersensitivity of some and subsensitivity of other brain α$_2$-adrenoreceptors. Compared with control subjects, panic disorder patients had heightened cardiovascular responses (Nutt 1989) but blunted growth hormone responses (Charney and Heninger 1986; Nutt 1989; Tancer et al. 1993) to clonidine. Similarly, in patients with GAD, Abelson et al. (1991) reported a blunted growth hormone response to clonidine compared with responses in normal control subjects. In summary, such findings continue to implicate a possible role of the central noradrenergic system in anxiety and panic but require further replication and elucidation.

Lactate panicogenic metabolic theory.   Although not without some controversy, sodium lactate provocation of panic attacks has captured much attention as an experimental model for understanding the pathogenesis of spontaneous panic attacks. Lactate-provoked panic is specific to patients with prior spontaneous attacks, closely resembles such attacks, and can be blocked by the same drugs that block natural attacks (Liebowitz et al. 1984a). Cohen and White (1950) first noted that patients with neurocirculatory asthenia, a condition closely related to anxiety disorder, developed higher levels of blood lactate while exercising than did normal control subjects. This finding stimulated Pitts and McClure (1967) to administer intravenous infusions of sodium lactate to patients with "anxiety disorder"; they found that most of the patients had an anxiety attack during the infusion. The subjects all believed that these attacks were quite typical of their naturally occurring attacks. Normal control subjects did not experience panic attacks during the infusion.

Having been replicated on numerous occasions under proper experimental conditions, the finding that 10 ml/kg of 0.5-M sodium lactate infused over 20 minutes will provoke a panic attack in most patients with panic disorder but not in normal control subjects is now a well-accepted fact. The mechanism, however, that may account for the observed biochemical and physiological changes (Liebowitz et al. 1985a) is surrounded by much uncertainty and controversy. Theories have included nonspecific arousal that cognitively triggers panic; induction of metabolic alkalosis; hypocalcemia; alteration of the nicotinamide adenine dinucleotide (NAD)–reduced form of NAD (NADH) ratio; and transient intracerebral hypercapnia. Of these, transient intracerebral hypercapnia has been the subject of considerable interest and received considerable validation in recent studies; it is discussed in the next subsection. Of interest, cortisol responses in lactate-induced panic have suggested hypothalamic-pituitary axis involvement in anticipatory anxiety, as is known to occur in other anxiety and stress states but not in the actual panic attack (Hollander et al. 1989).

Carbon dioxide hypersensitivity theory. Controlled hyperventilation and respiratory alkalosis do not routinely provoke panic attacks in most patients with panic disorder. Surprisingly, however, giving these patients a mixture of 5% carbon dioxide (CO_2) in room air to breathe causes panic almost as often as does a sodium lactate infusion (Gorman et al. 1984). This finding has been rather consistently replicated. Similarly, sodium bicarbonate infusion provokes panic attacks in patients with panic disorder at a rate comparable to that induced by CO_2 inhalation (Gorman et al. 1989a).

By what mechanism, then, does 5% CO_2 induce panic? Such a phenomenon may be partially explained by the findings of Svensson and colleagues, who showed that CO_2, when added to inspired air, causes a reliable dose-dependent increase in rat locus coeruleus firing (Elam et al. 1981). Alternatively, panic disorder patients may have hypersensitive brain-stem CO_2 chemoreceptors in the medulla. Indeed, during the CO_2 induction procedure, panic disorder patients who experience panic attacks while breathing 5% CO_2 demonstrate a much faster increase in inspiratory drive than do nonpanicking patients or normal control subjects; inspiratory drive is thought to reflect most directly the brain-stem component of respiratory regulation (Gorman et al. 1988).

Such a model is of interest because it could account for the generally well-established fact that hyperventilation does not cause panic, whereas CO_2, lactate, and bicarbonate do. Infused lactate is metabolized to bicarbonate, which is then converted in the periphery to CO_2. In other words, CO_2 constitutes the common metabolic product of both lactate and bicarbonate. This CO_2 then selectively crosses the blood-brain barrier and produces transient cerebral

hypercapnia. The hypercapnia then sets off the brain-stem CO_2 chemoreceptors, leading to hyperventilation and panic. Thus, a "false suffocation alarm" theory of panic has been formulated (D. F. Klein 1993) that proposes that patients with panic are hypersensitive to CO_2 because they have an overly sensitive brain-stem suffocation alarm system. This condition constitutes, in a sense, the opposite of the hyposensitive suffocation alarm seen in Ondine's curse, a rare illness in which there is a risk of suffocating in one's sleep. D. F. Klein (1993) proposed that such a theory of panic could explain, for example, the tendency of panic attacks to occur during high-CO_2 states such as deep non–rapid eye movement (REM) sleep, premenstrually, and sometimes with relaxation but not during childbirth, an event otherwise characterized by extreme hyperventilation and potentially catastrophic cognitions. This theory may be supported by the variety of subtle respiratory dysfunctions that appear to be associated with panic, such as preexisting pulmonary disease, panic disorder patients' tendency chronically to hyperventilate, their increased variance in tidal volume during steady-state respiration, and their greater irregularities in nocturnal breathing (Papp et al. 1993; M. B. Stein et al. 1995).

In contrast with panic, the response to inhaled CO_2 in GAD has received only limited attention, but results so far have not been remarkable.

GABA-benzodiazepine theory. Another subject of inquiry that may relate to the biological etiology of GAD and panic is the recently discovered brain benzodiazepine receptor. This receptor is linked to a receptor for the inhibitory neurotransmitter γ-aminobutyric acid (GABA). Binding of a benzodiazepine to the benzodiazepine receptor facilitates the action of GABA, effectively slowing neural transmission. The receptor is found in gray matter throughout the human brain.

One series of compounds, the β-carbolines, which are inverse agonists of this receptor complex, produce an acute anxiety syndrome when administered to laboratory animals or to normal human volunteers (Dorrow et al. 1983; Skolnick and Paul 1982). This raises the possibility that either aberrant production of an endogenous ligand or altered receptor sensitivity may occur in patients with GAD or panic, interfering with proper benzodiazepine receptor function and causing their symptoms.

There is some support for such a theory. One study found that panic disorder patients, compared with normal control subjects, demonstrated less reduced saccadic eye movement velocity in response to diazepam, suggesting hyposensitivity of the benzodiazepine receptor in panic (Roy-Byrne et al. 1990). Another study showed that the benzodiazepine antagonist flumazenil is panicogenic in panic patients but not in normal control subjects; this finding suggests a deficiency in an endogenous anxiolytic ligand or altered benzodiazepine receptor sensitivity in panic (Nutt et al. 1990). Clearly, the role of the benzodiazepine-GABA receptor complex in anxiety and panic merits further research.

Genetic basis of anxiety and panic.   The final line of evidence for a biological etiology of anxiety disorders is provided by studies that indicate the possible inherited nature of such disorders. Several family history studies of panic disorder found a higher rate in relatives of probands with panic disorder than in relatives of normal subjects. Crowe and colleagues (1983) found a morbidity risk for panic disorder of 24.7% among relatives of patients with panic disorder, compared with a risk of only 2.3% among normal control subjects. A 19.5% morbidity risk for GAD was found among relatives of GAD patients, compared with a 3.5% risk in normal control relatives; this may have been somewhat of an overestimate, because the GAD in the relatives was less chronic, less severe, or less likely to be treated than that in the probands (Noyes et al. 1987).

This kind of study cannot, of course, rule out the possibility that environmental rather than genetic influences are operant. Therefore, studies comparing rates of illness in monozygotic (MZ) and dizygotic (DZ) twins are best for distinguishing these two components of familial transmission of a psychiatric illness. Simple adoption studies can also serve this purpose but have not yet been reported for anxiety disorders.

Early twin studies involving patients with anxiety disorder included a mixed group of anxiety patients. These studies showed a higher concordance rate for anxiety disorder among MZ twins than among DZ twins, a finding indicating that genetic influence predominates over environmental influence. More recently, Torgersen (1983) completed a study of 32 MZ and 53 DZ twins. Panic attacks were five times more frequent in MZ than in DZ twins. However, the absolute concordance rate in MZ twins was 31%, which suggests that nongenetic factors play an important role in the development of the illness. For GAD, there was no MZ-DZ concordance rate difference in this study. However, Kendler et al. (1992a), also studying GAD in female twins, determined that the familial component of the disorder was almost entirely genetic; heritability was about 30%.

Even twin studies are open to question because they assume that parents treat identical twins in the same way that they treat fraternal twins. More definitive proof of a genetic component to a psychiatric illness can only come from studies comparing concordance rates in identical and fraternal twins who were separated at birth. No such studies have been reported for the anxiety disorders. Molecular genetic studies of panic in large, multigenerationally affected pedigrees initially appeared quite encouraging. However, several putative genetic markers and candidate genes for panic have been ruled out in the last several years, and no genetic linkage to panic disorder has yet been determined. Active research continues in this promising area, and in summary, to date, there seems to be a stronger case for inheritance in panic than in generalized anxiety.

Psychodynamic Theories

In this subsection we present the major landmarks in the evolution of psychodynamic theories of anxiety and panic, along with their relationship to recent biological advances. More lengthy expositions and critiques of the psychoanalytic theories can be referred to by interested readers (Cooper 1985; Michels et al. 1985; Nemiah 1988). Psychological theories of panic are summarized in Table 14–6.

Freud's first theory of anxiety neurosis (id or impulse anxiety).   In his earliest concept of anxiety formation, Freud (1895b[1894]/1962) postulated that anxiety stems from the direct physiological transformation of libidinal energy into the somatic symptoms of anxiety, without the mediation of psychic mechanisms. He found evidence for this process in the sexual practices and experiences of patients with anxiety, which were characterized by disturbed sexual arousal and continence and coitus interruptus. He termed such anxiety an "actual neurosis," as opposed to a psychoneurosis, because of the postulated absence of psychic processes. Such anxiety, originating from overwhelm-

TABLE 14–6.   **Psychological theories of panic**

Psychodynamic theory (qualitative distinction between anxiety and panic not made)

Freud's first theory of anxiety neurosis: direct physiological transformation of undischarged sexual energy

Freud's second theory of signal anxiety: anxiety as a signal to the ego of intrapsychic conflict

Separation anxiety: psychologically increased vulnerability to separation

Behavioral theory

Pairing of an unconditioned stimulus to a conditioned stimulus, leading to a conditioned response

Cognitive theory

Catastrophic cognitive misinterpretation of uncomfortable physical sensations and affects

ing instinctual urges, would today be referred to as *id* or *impulse anxiety.*

Over the next several years, Freud started to modify his theory. Although the basic tenet that anxiety stemmed from undischarged sexual energy remained the same, this was no longer posited to be due to external constraints such as sexual dysfunctions. In accordance with Freud's developing topographic theory of the mind, anxiety resulted from forbidden sexual drives in the unconscious being repressed by the preconscious.

Structural theory and intrapsychic conflict. By 1926, with the advent of the structural theory of the mind, Freud's theory of anxiety had undergone a major transformation (Freud 1926/1959). According to Freud, anxiety is an affect belonging to the ego and acts as a signal alerting the ego to internal danger. The danger stems from intrapsychic conflict between instinctual drives from the id, superego prohibitions, and external reality demands. Anxiety acts as a signal to the ego for the mobilization of repression and other defenses to counteract the threat to intrapsychic equilibrium. Inhibitions and neurotic symptoms develop as measures designed to avoid the dangerous situation and to allow only partial gratification of instinctual wishes, thus warding off signal anxiety. In the revised theory then, anxiety leads to repression, instead of the reverse.

The *intrapsychic conflict model of anxiety* continues to constitute a major tenet of contemporary psychoanalytic theory. Psychoanalytic theorists after Freud, such as Melanie Klein (1948) and Joachim Flescher (1955), also made important contributions to the understanding of the psychodynamic origins of anxiety. Whereas Freud concentrated on the role of sexual impulses and the oedipal conflict in the genesis of anxiety, these theorists drew attention to the role that aggressive impulses and preoedipal dynamics can also play in generating anxiety.

Although psychoanalytic theories are not universally accepted by psychiatrists today, they remain an invaluable tool in the understanding and treatment of at least some patients. Also, Freud's theory of anxiety formation is not incompatible with biological theories of anxiety. Although Freud's first model of anxiety was later overshadowed by the conflictual model, modern biological theories of panic are in many ways more reminiscent of his original physiological formulation. Furthermore, Freud maintained on numerous occasions that biological predispositions to psychiatric symptoms are undoubtedly operant in most conditions and that constitutional factors could play a role in the particular form that neurotic symptoms take in different patients.

Indeed, what psychoanalytic theory does not help us to do is better understand the determinants of the various specific forms in which anxiety symptoms manifest themselves. Some patients have anxiety attacks, others have more chronic forms of anxiety, and still others have phobias, obsessions, or compulsions. Freud himself attempted to address this problem of choice of neurosis and partly explained it on the basis of constitutional factors—a concept essentially similar to modern biological notions. In an attempt to reconcile this unpredictability with classic psychodynamic theory, it has been postulated that patients with unconscious conflict and a neural predisposition to panic may manifest their anxiety in the form of panic attacks, whereas individuals without this neural predisposition may manifest milder forms of signal anxiety (Nemiah 1981). A recent psychodynamic study of patients with panic disorder proposed that in patients who are neurophysiologically predisposed to early fearfulness, exposure to parental behaviors that augment this fearfulness may result in disturbances of object relations and persistence of conflicts surrounding dependence and catastrophic fears of helplessness that can be addressed in psychodynamic treatment (Shear et al. 1993).

With the broadening of psychodynamic theory over the decades, different forms of anxiety have been elaborated and have received increased attention: annihilation (i.e., fusion or persecutory) anxiety, separation anxiety, anxiety over the loss of others' love, castration anxiety, superego anxiety, and id anxiety. In particular, greater emphasis on preoedipal dynamics and research in child development has brought to the forefront attachment theories, the importance of negotiating the ubiquitous fear of object loss, and the central role of separation anxiety in the genesis of psychopathology.

Separation anxiety. In the mid-1960s, D. F. Klein (1964) advanced an etiological theory that agoraphobia with panic attacks represents an aberrant function of the biological substrate that underlies normal human separation anxiety. D. F. Klein (1981) advanced the notion, based on Bowlby's (1973) work on attachment and separation, that the attachment of an infant animal or human to its mother is not simply a learned response but is genetically programmed and biologically determined. Indeed, 20%–50% of adults with panic disorder and agoraphobia recall manifesting symptoms of pathological separation anxiety, often taking the form of school phobia, when they were children. Furthermore, the initial panic attack in the history of a patient who goes on to develop panic disorder is sometimes preceded by the real or threatened loss of a significant relationship. One systematic study showed the number and severity of recent life events—especially events related to loss—to be greater in new-onset panic patients than in control subjects (Faravelli and Pallanti 1989). A blinded psychodynamic study showed separation anxiety to be a significantly more prevalent theme in the dreams and screen memories of panic patients than in normal controls.

Infant animals demonstrate their anxiety when separated from the mother by a series of high-pitched cries, called *distress vocalizations*. Imipramine has been found to be effective in blocking distress vocalizations in dogs by Scott (1975) and in monkeys by Suomi and his co-workers (1978). Imipramine is a highly effective antipanic drug in adult humans (see later in this chapter). Hypothesizing a link between adult panic attacks and childhood separation anxiety, Gittelman-Klein and Klein (1971) conducted a study of imipramine treatment for children with school phobia. In these children, fear of separation from their mothers was usually the basis behind refusing to go to school. The drug proved successful in getting the children to return to school. In a related finding, Weissman et al. (1984) found a threefold increase in risk for separation anxiety in children of parents with panic disorder.

Thus, evidence suggests that the same drug that diminishes protest anxiety in higher mammals also reduces separation anxiety in children and blocks panic attacks in adults. This is further confirmation of the link between separation anxiety and panic attacks. Is early separation anxiety linked to agoraphobia or also to panic attacks per se? If imipramine affects panic attacks, and separation anxiety is linked to agoraphobia, then why is imipramine effective in the treatment of school phobia? On the other hand, children with school phobia do not have spontaneous panic attacks, but this could be related to their young age. Perhaps both panic disorder and panic disorder with agoraphobia are linked to a biologically disordered separation mechanism that is responsive to imipramine. This may occur if the retrospective histories of a lesser degree of separation anxiety in patients with panic attacks alone are misremembered.

Contemporary psychoanalysts, in response, have claimed that this neurophysiological and ethological model of a disrupted separation mechanism and panic may be unnecessarily reductionistic (Michels et al. 1985). They point out an inconsistency between the conceptualization of panic attacks as "spontaneous" and the frequently reported histories of childhood separation anxiety in patients with panic attacks and state that psychological difficulties with separation can also play a role in subsequent vulnerability to panic. On the other hand, contemporary psychoanalysts have also given more credence to the role of biological substrates in the genesis of anxiety symptoms in at

least some patients who "have developed their anxious personality structure secondary to a largely contentless biologic dysregulation," so that "while psychological triggers for anxiety may still be found, the anxiety threshold is so low in these patients that it is no longer useful to view the psychological event as etiologically significant" (Cooper 1985, p. 1398).

Learning Theories

Behavior or learning theorists hold that anxiety is conditioned by the fear of certain environmental stimuli. If every time a laboratory animal presses a bar it receives a noxious electric shock, the pressing of the lever becomes a conditioned stimulus that precedes the unconditioned stimulus (i.e., the shock). The conditioned stimulus releases a conditioned response in the animal, namely anxiety, which leads the animal to avoid contact with the lever, thereby avoiding the shock. Successful avoidance of the unconditioned stimulus, namely the shock, reinforces the avoidant behavior. This leads to a decrease in anxiety level.

By analogy with this animal model, we might say that anxiety attacks are conditioned responses to fearful situations. For example, an infant learns that if his or her mother is not present (i.e., the conditioned stimulus) he or she will experience hunger (i.e., the unconditioned stimulus) and learns to become anxious automatically whenever the mother is absent (i.e., the conditioned response). The anxiety may persist even after the child is old enough to feed himself or herself. Or, to give another example, a life-threatening situation in someone's life (e.g., skidding in a car during a snowstorm) is paired with the experience of rapid heartbeat (i.e., the conditioned stimulus) and tremendous anxiety. Long after the accident, rapid heartbeat alone, whether during vigorous exercise or minor emotional upset, becomes capable by itself of provoking the conditioned response of an anxiety attack.

Several problems are posed by such a theory. First, although we have pointed out some traumatic situations, such as thyroid disease, cocaine intoxication, or life-threatening event, that do seem to be paired with the onset of panic disorder, for many patients no such traumatic event can ever be located. In patients with GAD, attempting to find a precipitating event that makes sense as an unconditioned stimulus is even more difficult. It is also the case that most conditioned responses ultimately become extinguished in laboratory animals if they are not at least intermittently reinforced. Clinical experience does not support that patients with panic disorder or GAD undergo repeat traumatic events, and therefore they should be able to "unlearn" their anxiety and panic. Thus, even though learning theories have a powerful basis in experimental animal research, they do not seem to explain adequately, in and of their own, the pathogenesis of human anxiety disorders.

COURSE AND PROGNOSIS

The course of illness without treatment is highly variable. At present, there is no reliable way to know which patient will develop, for example, agoraphobia. The illness seems to have a waxing and waning course in which spontaneous recovery occurs, only to be followed months to years later by a new outburst. At the extreme, some patients become completely housebound for decades.

Treatment aimed at blocking the occurrence of the attacks, described in detail later in this chapter, is appropriate at any point in the course of the illness when such attacks are occurring. Results are often dramatic. Pharmacological blockade of panic attacks early in the illness, before phobic avoidance has become an ingrained way of life, often leads to complete remission. Even years into the illness, effective disruption of the attacks with medication can lead to resolution of anticipatory anxiety and phobias without other treatment.

However, a substantial number of patients with marked phobic avoidance remain anxious and frightened of confronting feared situations even after the attacks have been blocked. Such patients require other forms of intervention, described elsewhere in this text. A 7-year follow-up study examined prognostic factors in naturalistically treated patients with panic disorder. Although patients had generally good outcomes, there were several predictors of poorer outcome, including greater severity of initial attacks and agoraphobia, longer duration of illness, comorbid major depression, separation from a parent by death or divorce, high interpersonal sensitivity, low social class, and unmarried marital status (Noyes et al. 1990). Five-year findings of another long-term outcome study were also fairly optimistic: 34% of patients were recovered, 46% were minimally impaired, and 20% remained moderately to severely impaired. The most important predictor of poor outcome was an anxious-fearful personality type, followed by poor response to initial treatment (O'Rourke et al. 1996). Finally, another large outcome study over 4 years similarly showed that fewer than 20% of panic disorder patients remained seriously agoraphobic or disabled. Panic attack frequency at baseline, time of initial medication, and continuous use of medication were not related to outcome, whereas longer duration of illness and more severe initial avoidance were unfavorable predictors (Katschnig et al. 1995).

An earlier study had shown a higher incidence of premature death due to cardiovascular illness and suicide among patients with panic disorder compared with normal subjects (Coryell et al. 1982). However, the group of patients studied had all been hospitalized at one point and therefore may have constituted a more severely ill group of patients than is generally encountered in clinical practice.

The increased death rate from cardiovascular illness described in the clinical study of Coryell and colleagues (1982) was partly supported in an epidemiologic investigation by Weissman and her group (1990). In this study, panic disorder patients had a significantly higher risk for strokes than did patients with other psychiatric disorders, although several methodological limitations were identified. Of note, such medical risks are not routinely evident to clinicians in the usual status of patients undergoing treatment for panic disorder. Most such patients have normal medical workups. The one cardiovascular abnormality that has been found to occur at a higher rate in patients with panic disorder is mitral valve prolapse. This association could conceivably explain a higher incidence of cardiovascular-related death in patients with panic disorder; however, mitral valve prolapse itself is rarely a cause of premature death or major morbidity. One other possible explanation for increased cardiovascular/cerebrovascular risk in patients with panic disorder may be related to aspects of their lifestyle. Such patients tend to live relatively sedentary lives, and some report that vigorous physical exercise precipitates their panic attacks, leading them to avoid exertion of any kind. Heavy cigarette smoking, alcoholism, and poor diets could also contribute to an increased risk in panic patients. Alternatively, left ventricular enlargement and increased risk of thromboembolic events have also been contemplated as possibly accounting for the association (Weissman et al. 1990).

The putative association between panic disorder and increased suicide risk has received much attention in the past several years. It used to be thought that the association may have been due to the fact that patients with panic disorder are more prone than the normal population to major depressive disorder and to alcoholism at some point in their lives, and in part that probably remains valid. However, Allgulander and Lavori (1991) conducted a large retrospective survey in Sweden and found an increased suicide risk in panic disorder in the absence of comorbid diagnoses. Epidemiologic data further support this finding. In the Epidemiologic Catchment Area (ECA) study, the lifetime rate of suicide attempts in persons with uncomplicated panic disorder was found to be 7%, about the same as the 7.9% rate for persons with uncomplicated major depression (Johnson et al. 1990). However, in a reanalysis of the

ECA data, controlling for all comorbidity rather than one disorder at a time, an association between panic and suicide attempts could no longer be shown (Hornig and McNally 1995). In a clinical sample of panic disorder patients, a 17% incidence of suicide attempts was found for those without comorbid major depression or substance abuse, but these patients did have other comorbidity with some depressive symptomatology and/or personality disorder (Lepine et al. 1993). The ECA study also documented a variety of frequently neglected aspects of the marked morbidity associated with panic disorder (Markowitz et al. 1989). How exactly panic disorder could lead to suicide remains unclear and is not an established fact. One might speculate that impaired quality of life, marred by a subjective sense of poor health, financial dependency, and occupational and social dysfunction, could lead to demoralization and hopelessness and pose a suicide risk.

In contrast with panic disorder, no single, overwhelming event prompts the patient with GAD to seek help. Such patients seem only over time to develop the recognition that their experience of chronic tension, hyperactivity, worry, and anxiety is excessive. Often they will state that there has never been a time in their lives, as long as they can remember, that they were not anxious. In one study of a small number of patients, GAD appeared to be a more chronic condition than panic disorder (Raskin et al. 1982), involving fewer periods of spontaneous remission.

GAD is twice as common in women as in men. Age greater than 24 years; being separated, widowed, or divorced; unemployment; and being a homemaker are all strong correlates of GAD. Patients with GAD experience substantial interference with their lives, seek professional help to a high degree, and have a high use of medications (Wittchen et al. 1994). GAD patients with an earlier onset of anxiety symptoms in the first two decades of life appear to be more impaired overall, to have more severe anxiety that may not be precipitated by specific stressful events, and to have histories of more childhood fears, disturbed family environments, and greater social maladjustment; this finding could be due to constitutional and/or environmental influences (Hoehn-Saric et al. 1993b). In clinical samples, GAD is commonly comorbid with major depression and social phobia but still emerges as a distinct entity (Brawman et al. 1993). Abuse of alcohol, barbiturates, and antianxiety medications is said to be common in this group. GAD and chronic depression also overlap substantially. Breslau and Davis (1985) showed that if GAD is persistent for 6 months, as was required by the DSM-III-R definition and still is for DSM-IV, the comorbidity of depressive disorder is very high. Contrary to panic disorder, which declines in old age, GAD appears to account for many of the anxiety states in late life, often comorbidly with medical illnesses (Flint 1994). In these elderly patients, it is particularly important to differentiate generalized anxiety from other anxiety states that could be related to delirium, dementia, psychosis, and depression or that could be manifestations of underlying medical illnesses.

DIAGNOSIS

Physical Signs and Behavior

The diagnosis of panic disorder is made when a patient experiences recurrent panic attacks that are discrete and unexpected and followed by a month of persistent anticipatory anxiety or behavioral change. These panic attacks are characterized by a sudden crescendo of anxiety and fearfulness, in addition to the presence of at least four physical symptoms. Finally, these attacks are not secondary to a known organic factor or due to another mental disorder.

The diagnosis of GAD is made when a patient experiences at least 6 months of chronic anxiety and excessive worry. At least three of six physical symptoms must also be present. Finally, this chronic anxiety must not be secondary to another Axis I disorder or a specific organic factor.

However, these diagnoses are not always obvious, and a number of other psychiatric and medical disorders may mimic these conditions (see Table 14–7).

Differential Diagnosis

Other psychiatric illnesses. Although the medical conditions that mimic anxiety disorder are usually easily ruled out, psychiatric conditions that involve pathological anxiety can make the differential diagnosis of panic disorder and GAD difficult. By far the most problematic is the differentiation of primary anxiety disorder from depression.

TABLE 14–7. **Psychiatric and medical differential diagnosis of panic disorders**

Psychiatric	
Generalized anxiety disorder	Depersonalization disorder
Depressive disorders	Somatoform disorders
Schizophrenia	Character disorders
Medical	
Hyperthyroidism	Pheochromocytoma
Hypothyroidism	Hypoglycemia
Hyperparathyroidism	True vertigo
Mitral valve prolapse	Drug withdrawal
Cardiac arrhythmias	Alcohol withdrawal
Coronary insufficiency	

Patients experiencing depression often manifest signs of anxiety and agitation and may even have frank panic attacks. On the other hand, patients with GAD or panic disorder, if untreated for some time, routinely become demoralized as the illness causes progressive restriction of their ability to enjoy a normal life. Further complicating the picture is the fact that some, but not all, studies have shown that patients with anxiety disorder have increased family history of affective disorder.

Although the differentiation of anxiety from depression can at times strain even the most experienced clinician, several points are helpful. Patients with GAD or panic disorder generally do not demonstrate the full range of vegetative symptoms that are seen in depression. Thus, anxious patients usually have trouble falling asleep, rather than experiencing early morning awakening, and do not lose their appetite. Diurnal mood fluctuation is uncommon in anxiety disorder. Perhaps of greatest importance is the fact that most anxious patients do not lose the capacity to enjoy things or to be cheered up as endogenously depressed patients do.

The distinction between atypical depression and anxiety disorders is even more difficult because of the lack of typical endogenous features in the former. However, although patients with atypical depression can also be cheered up, they tend to slump faster than patients with anxiety disorder. Panic attacks and atypical depression frequently coexist, and coexisting panic attacks may increase the monoamine oxidase inhibitor (MAOI) responsivity of patients with atypical depression (Liebowitz et al. 1984b).

The order of developing symptoms also differentiates depression from anxiety. In cases of panic disorder or GAD, anxiety symptoms usually precede any seriously altered mood. Patients can generally recall having anxiety attacks first, then becoming gradually more disgusted with life, and then feeling depressed. In depression, patients usually experience dysphoria first and anxiety symptoms later. However, panic disorder can be complicated by secondary major depression or vice versa.

A few other psychiatric conditions often need to be differentiated from panic disorder and GAD. Patients with somatization disorder complain of a variety of physical ailments and discomforts, none of which are substantiated by physical or laboratory findings. They can present in a way that is similar to the way in which GAD patients present, because of their constant worry, but they are distinguished from GAD patients by their almost exclusive preoccupation with physical complaints. Unlike panic disorder patients, patients with somatization disorder present with physical problems that do not usually occur in episodic attacks but are virtually constant.

Patients with depersonalization disorder have episodes of derealization/depersonalization without the other symptoms of a panic attack. However, panic attacks not infrequently involve depersonalization and derealization as prominent symptoms.

Although patients with panic disorder often fear they will lose their minds or go crazy, psychotic illness is not an outcome of anxiety disorder. Reassuring the patient on this point is often the first step in a successful treatment.

Undoubtedly some patients with anxiety disorder abuse alcohol and illicit drugs such as sedatives in attempts at self-medication (Quitkin and Babkin 1982). In one study, after successful detoxification a group of alcoholic patients with a history of panic disorder were treated with medication to block spontaneous panic attacks (Quitkin and Babkin 1982). These patients did not resume alcohol consumption once their panic attacks were eliminated. Therefore, in evaluating any patient with substance abuse, the possibility that his or her illness began with spontaneous panic attacks or chronic anxiety should be considered. As discussed later, social phobia also is frequently associated with alcoholism and may contribute to its onset, continuation, or relapse.

Hyperthyroidism and hypothyroidism. Both hyperthyroidism and hypothyroidism can present with anxiety unaccompanied by other signs or symptoms. For this reason, it is imperative that all patients complaining of anxiety undergo routine thyroid function tests, including the evaluation of the level of thyroid-stimulating hormone. It should be remembered, however, that thyroid disease can act as one of the predisposing triggers to panic disorder, so that even when the apparently primary thyroid disease is corrected, panic attacks may continue until specifically treated.

Cardiac disease. The relationship of mitral valve prolapse to panic disorder has attracted a great deal of attention over the years. This usually benign condition has been shown by a number of investigators to occur more frequently in patients with panic disorder than in normal subjects. However, screening of patients known to have mitral valve prolapse reveals no greater frequency of panic disorder than that which is found in the overall population.

Although patients with mitral valve prolapse occasionally complain of palpitations, chest pain, light-headedness, and fatigue, symptoms of a full-blown panic attack are rare. A comparison of symptoms in mitral valve prolapse and panic disorder is provided in Table 14–8. Panic patients with and panic patients without mitral valve prolapse are similar in several important ways. Treatment for panic attacks works regardless of the presence of the prolapsed valve, and patients with both mitral valve prolapse and

TABLE 14-8. **Comparison of symptoms of mitral valve prolapse and panic disorder**

Symptoms	Mitral valve prolapse	Panic disorder
Fatigue	+	–
Dyspnea	+	++
Palpitations	++	++
Chest pain	++	+
Syncope	+	–
Choking	–	++
Dizziness	–	++
Derealization	–	++
Hot/cold flashes	–	++
Sweating	–	++
Fainting	–	++
Trembling	–	++
Fear of dying, going crazy, losing control	–	++

Note. + = occasionally; ++ = often present; – = rarely present.

panic disorder are just as sensitive to sodium lactate as are those with panic disorder alone. Some researchers have speculated that mitral valve prolapse and panic disorder may represent manifestations of the same underlying disorder of autonomic nervous system function (Gorman et al. 1981). Others have suggested that panic disorder actually causes mitral valve prolapse, by creating intermittent states of high circulating catecholamine levels and tachycardia (Mattes 1981). There are reports that mitral valve prolapse might disappear if the panic disorder is kept under control (Gorman et al. 1981). In a recent meta-analysis of 21 studies, it was found that there does appear to be a significant association between panic disorder and mitral valve prolapse, although the possibility of publication bias toward favorite positive reports cannot be ruled out (Katerndahl 1993).

In any event, it is clear that the presence of mitral valve prolapse in patients with panic disorder has little clinical or prognostic importance in the management of spontaneous panic attacks. What it may tell us about the underlying etiology of panic disorder is a question currently under vigorous investigation.

Other medical illnesses. Hyperparathyroidism occasionally presents as anxiety symptoms, warranting a serum calcium level determination before definitive diagnosis is made.

A variety of cardiac conditions can initially present as anxiety symptoms, although, in most cases, the patient's prominent complaints are of chest pain, skipped beats, or palpitations. Ischemic heart disease and arrhythmias, especially paroxysmal atrial tachycardia, should be ruled out by electrocardiography.

Pheochromocytoma is a rare, usually benign tumor of the adrenal medulla that secretes catecholamines in episodic bursts. During an active phase, the patient characteristically experiences flushing, tremulousness, and anxiety. Blood pressure is usually elevated during the active phase of catecholamine secretion but not at other times. Therefore, merely finding a normal blood pressure does not rule out a pheochromocytoma. If this condition is suspected, urine is collected for 24 hours so that a diagnosis can be attempted through determination of catecholamine metabolite concentration. In a study of patients with confirmed pheochromocytoma, about half met criteria for the physical symptoms of panic attacks, but none had panic disorder, because they did not experience terror during the attacks and did not develop anticipatory anxiety or agoraphobia (Starkman et al. 1990).

Disease of the vestibular nerve can cause episodic bouts of vertigo, light-headedness, nausea, and anxiety that mimic panic attacks. Rather than merely feeling dizzy, patients with disease of the vestibular nerve often experience true vertigo in which the room seems to spin in one direction during each attack. Otolaryngologic consultation is warranted when this condition is suspected. Some panic patients complain primarily of dizziness or unsteadiness. Whether they are a distinct subgroup with definite neurotological abnormalities is currently under study.

Although many patients believe that their anxiety disorder is caused by reactive hypoglycemia, there is no scientific proof at present that this condition is ever a cause of any psychiatric disturbance. Glucose tolerance tests are not helpful in establishing hypoglycemia as the cause of anxiety, because up to 40% of the normal population will have a random low blood-sugar level during a routine glucose tolerance test. The only convincing way to establish hypoglycemia as a cause of symptoms is to document a low blood-sugar level at the same time the patient is symptomatic. Studies with insulin tolerance tests in panic disorder have yielded negative results.

TREATMENT

Pharmacotherapy

Antidepressants. The central feature in the treatment of panic disorder is the pharmacological blockade of the spontaneous panic attacks. Several classes of medication have been shown to be effective in accomplishing this goal, and a summary of the pharmacological treatment of panic disorder is presented in Table 14–9. The most widely used and studied medications are the tricyclic antidepressants (TCAs), especially imipramine (D. F. Klein 1964; Mavissakalian and Michelson 1986a, 1986b; McNair and Kahn 1981; Sheehan et al. 1980; Zitrin et al. 1980, 1983). Other TCAs, such as desipramine, have also been found effective, although they have not been studied as extensively as imipramine. Nortriptyline has not been systematically studied, but in clinical experience it also tends to be efficacious and often better tolerated. The presence of de-

TABLE 14–9. **Pharmacological treatment of panic disorder**

Tricyclic antidepressants

General indications: First-line drugs; most established efficacy

Imipramine: Most studied

Desipramine: If low tolerance of anticholinergic side effects

Nortriptyline: If prone to orthostatic hypotension, elderly

Serotonin reuptake inhibitors

General indications: First-line drugs; inability to tolerate tricyclics; first choice with comorbid obsessive-compulsive symptoms or comorbid social phobia

Fluoxetine: Fewer anticholinergic side effects than tricyclics

Sertraline: Fewer anticholinergic side effects than tricyclics

Paroxetine: Fewer anticholinergic side effects than tricyclics

Fluvoxamine: Fewer anticholinergic side effects than tricyclics

Monoamine oxidase inhibitors

General indications: Poor response to or tolerance of other antidepressants; comorbid atypical depression or social phobia

Phenelzine: Most studied

Tranylcypromine: Less sedation

High-potency benzodiazepines

General indications: Poor response to or tolerance of antidepressants; prominent anticipatory anxiety or phobic avoidance; necessity for rapid initial effect

Alprazolam: Most studied

Clonazepam: Longer-acting, less frequent dosing, less withdrawal

Other medications

General indications: Patients who are refractory or intolerant of other options; not well tested to date

Venlaxafine

Nefazodone

Valproic acid

Inositol

Clonidine

pressed mood is not a predictor or requirement for these drugs to be effective in blocking panic attacks.

When a drug regimen is being initiated for a patient with panic disorder, it is crucial for the patient to understand that the drug will block the panic attacks but may not necessarily decrease the amount of intervening anticipatory anxiety. To reduce the level of anticipatory anxiety in patients with severe anxiety, it may be helpful for these patients initially to take a concomitant benzodiazepine; the dose can be gradually tapered and the drug discontinued after several weeks of antidepressant treatment.

Some patients with panic disorder display an initial hypersensitivity to TCAs, during which they complain of jitteriness, agitation, a "speedy" feeling, and insomnia. Although this is usually transient, such hypersensitivity is one of the main reasons why patients opt to discontinue medication early on. Therefore, it is recommended that patients with panic disorder be started on lower doses of tricyclics than would be given to depressed patients.

A standard regimen is to start the patient at a dosage of 10 mg qhs of imipramine and increase the dose by 10 mg every other night until 50 mg is reached. The dose can be given all at once. Because 50 mg is usually inadequate for full panic blockade, the dose can then be raised by 25-mg increments every 3 days or by 50-mg increments weekly to as high as 300 mg. Most patients need at least 150 mg of a TCA daily, and, unfortunately, underdosage commonly occurs. In some cases, a dose of more than 300 mg of imipramine is necessary. More than 80% of patients on "high" imipramine dosing of around 200 mg/day show a marked response in panic attacks (Mavissakalian and Perel 1989). Panic patients not responding to high doses of imipramine should have blood tricyclic levels measured. Often, blood levels will be disproportionately low for the dose, suggesting rapid metabolism or excretion, malabsorption, or noncompliance. It appears that patients do not show further antipanic responses at combined plasma levels of more than 140 ng/mL (Mavissakalian and Perel 1995). Patients who experience excessive anticholinergic side effects to imipramine can be given desipramine instead. Nortriptyline therapy can be tried in elderly patients or patients who are otherwise very sensitive to orthostatic hypotension.

Results of a number of open and controlled treatment trials have shown that the potent serotonin reuptake inhibitors (SSRIs) are also highly effective in the treatment of panic. Given their greater safety and ease of administration compared with tricyclics, they have recently started to be used as first-line therapy in the treatment of panic disorder and certainly would be the second choice in patients who do not respond to or cannot tolerate tricyclics. When comorbid obsessive-compulsive symptoms are present, they would be the first choice. In several controlled trials, the efficacy of fluvoxamine in dosages up to 150 mg/day has been documented (Den Boer 1988; Hoehn-Saric et al. 1993a). The efficacy of paroxetine in dosages of 20–60 mg/day has also been demonstrated in controlled studies (Oehrberg et al. 1995). One meta-analysis found that SSRIs were superior to imipramine and to alprazolam in treating panic, although lower doses of imipramine and alprazolam may have partly accounted for this difference (Boyer 1995). Like the tricyclics, fluoxetine can cause uncomfortable overstimulation in panic patients if started at the usual dosage of 20 mg/day. It is therefore suggested that treatment be started at 5 mg/day and that the dose be very gradually increased by 5 mg every week. A daily dose of 20 mg is adequate for most patients. Other SSRIs should be started at low doses as well. Clomipramine has been used in doses of 25–200 mg daily, titrated to patients' individual responses.

MAOIs are equally effective as the tricyclics and the SSRIs in treating panic. Both phenelzine and tranylcypromine successfully treat panic, although phenelzine has been studied more extensively. Phenelzine can be started at 15 mg daily in the morning. The dose is then increased by 15 mg every 4–7 days as tolerated, up to a maximum of 60–90 mg daily. If sedation or weight gain is of concern, tranylcypromine may be tried, starting at 10 mg in the morning and increasing by 10 mg every 4 days to a maximum of 80 mg daily. Tricyclics and SSRIs are typically preferred over MAOIs because they are better tolerated and they obviate the need for dietary restrictions and the risk of hypertensive crises. Furthermore, patients who do not respond to a tricyclic or an SSRI alone may respond to a combination of the two (Tiffon et al. 1994). However, MAOIs are an option to consider for patients who fail to tolerate or to respond well to other antidepressants. In patients with concomitant atypical depression or social phobia, MAOIs may be an appropriate earlier choice for treatment.

Full remission of panic attacks with antidepressants usually requires 4–12 weeks of treatment. Subsequently, the duration of required treatment to prevent relapse is a function of the natural course of panic disorder. The disorder can probably best be characterized as chronic, with an exacerbating and remitting course. Therefore, complete agreement has not been reached regarding the recommended course of treatment. In a naturalistic follow-up study, Noyes and his group (1989) found that the majority of panic patients initially treated with tricyclics had a relatively good prognosis when followed over a few years, whether they had continued (60% of the sample) or stopped (40% of the sample) taking medication. In a con-

trolled and prospective study with somewhat less optimistic results, a very high relapse rate for panic was found when imipramine therapy was discontinued after 6 months of acute treatment. However, half-dose imipramine at around 80 mg/day was successful in preventing relapse during 1 year of maintenance treatment (Mavissakalian and Perel 1992). Thus, a reasonable recommendation in treating panic patients is to keep them on full-dose medication for at least 6 months to prevent early relapse. Afterward, doses can be tapered to half-dose level and patients can be followed to ensure that clinical improvement is maintained. Subsequently, the clinician may attempt gradual dose decreases every few months as long as the improvement is maintained and reach a minimal dose at which the patient is relatively symptom free. Some patients may eventually be able to discontinue drug therapy. Other patients may require more chronic maintenance treatment, especially in light of the morbidity and mortality risk that may be associated with the disorder.

Newer antidepressants also appear to be beneficial in the treatment of panic disorder, although the data are fewer. The number of panic attacks diminished in four patients treated openly with venlafaxine in low dosages of 50–75 mg/day (Geracioti 1995). Nefazodone also appears promising for treating panic: 70% of 14 patients treated openly for 8 weeks with dosages of 200–600 mg/day were substantially improved (DeMartinis et al. 1996).

The pharmacological treatment of GAD is summarized in Table 14–10. With regard to GAD, a few studies have shown TCAs to be effective in treating chronically anxious patients independent of the presence of depressive

TABLE 14–10. Pharmacological treatment of generalized anxiety disorder

Benzodiazepines

General indications: Known efficacy; widely used; issues of dependence and withdrawal in certain patients

Buspirone

General indications: Proven efficacy; generally well tolerated; a trial is generally indicated; compared with benzodiazepines, delayed action and not associated with a "high"

Tricyclics

General indications: Shown efficacy in few trials; delayed action compared with benzodiazepines; may be more effective for cognitive rather than physical symptoms of anxiety

Imipramine: Shown efficacy; more side effects than benzodiazepines and buspirone

Trazodone: Shown efficacy; more side effects than benzodiazepines and buspirone

symptoms. In one controlled study comparing imipramine and alprazolam specifically in the treatment of GAD, similar efficacy was found for the two medications, with imipramine acting more on negative affects and cognitions and alprazolam acting more on somatic symptoms (Hoehn-Saric et al. 1988). In a more recent large study, therapy with up to 143 mg of imipramine per day, therapy with up to 255 mg of trazodone per day, and therapy with up to 26 mg of diazepam per day were found comparable after 8 weeks of treatment, and about two-thirds of GAD patients experienced moderate to marked improvement in anxiety. Not surprisingly, during the first 2 weeks of treatment somatic symptoms responded more rapidly to diazepam (Rickels et al. 1993a). In summary, the findings for tricyclics in the treatment of nonpanic anxiety are still preliminary but merit further attention.

Anxiolytics. Although benzodiazepines as a group have not been shown to be useful in blocking panic attacks, the high-potency benzodiazepines are highly effective antipanic drugs. In a large, multicenter, placebo-controlled study (Ballenger et al. 1988), 82% of patients treated acutely with alprazolam showed at least moderate improvement in panic, compared with 43% of patients taking placebo. Onset of response was rapid, in that significant improvement occurred in the first couple weeks of treatment, and the mean final dosage was 5.7 mg/day. After 8 weeks of acute treatment, medication therapy was gradually discontinued over 4 weeks; 27% of patients experienced rebound panic attacks and 35% had withdrawal symptoms. After discontinuation, panic outcome for the alprazolam-treated group was not significantly different from that for the placebo group (Pecknold et al. 1988). Although there are fewer data about the efficacy of clonazepam and lorazepam, these drugs appear equally promising for the acute treatment of panic. Long-term efficacy, possible tolerance and dependency, and difficulties in discontinuing medication therapy are the main areas of concern when benzodiazepine treatment is being chosen. Results of naturalistic follow-up studies of long-term benzodiazepine treatment appear generally optimistic, in that most patients maintain their therapeutic gains without an increase in benzodiazepine dose over time (Nagy et al. 1989; Schweizer et al. 1993).

These medications have fewer initial side effects than do tricyclics and SSRIs. However, the general treatment principle is that anxiolytics should be reserved until treatment with the different classes of antidepressants has failed, because anxiolytics do pose some risk for tolerance, dependence, and withdrawal. In the case of patients with severe acute distress and disability—patients who may re-

quire immediate relief—starting with a benzodiazepine and then replacing this drug with an antidepressant may be indicated. There is also some evidence that benzodiazepines may be more effective, at least initially, in ameliorating the associated anticipatory anxiety and phobic avoidance, and this may be another indication for their initial use. Systematic comparisons of antidepressants and benzodiazepines in the acute and maintenance treatment of panic disorder have shown that patients treated with alprazolam are notably more likely to stay in treatment and experience panic attack relief than are patients taking imipramine; the latter drug is associated with worse patient compliance (Schweizer et al. 1993).

Alprazolam therapy is usually started at a dosage of 0.5 mg qid and the dose is gradually increased to an average dosage of 4–6 mg/day and a range of 2–10 mg/day according to the individual patient. Clonazepam should generally be the first choice, because it is longer acting and thus has the advantage of less frequent bid dosing and less risk of withdrawal symptoms than does alprazolam. Treatment of at least 6 months is recommended, as with the antidepressants. Patients' moods must be followed, because alprazolam therapy may occasionally cause mania and clonazepam therapy can cause depression. Discontinuation must be gradual to prevent withdrawal: 0.5 mg every 3–4 days is generally a safe regimen, but a much slower rate may be required to prevent the recurrence of panic. In a controlled study, one-third of patients were unable to tolerate a gradual discontinuation of alprazolam over 4 weeks after 8 months of maintenance treatment; the strongest predictor of taper failure was initial severity of panic attacks, rather than alprazolam dose (Rickels et al. 1993b). How to distinguish between actual withdrawal and a simple recrudescence of the original anxiety symptom when the benzodiazepine is stopped remains controversial and the distinction can be difficult to make clinically. It has been convincingly shown that the introduction of cognitive-behavior therapy greatly increases the likelihood that panic patients will be able gradually to discontinue benzodiazepine treatment (Otto et al. 1993; D. A. Spiegel et al. 1994).

The pharmacological treatment of GAD involves more limited medication choices. Chronically anxious patients generally respond well to benzodiazepine therapy and are generally treated with benzodiazepines if a trial of buspirone (see later in this subsection) fails to ameliorate their symptoms. One study of GAD patients showed similar efficacy for alprazolam and imipramine, with alprazolam having a greater effect on somatic symptoms and imipramine on psychic symptoms (Hoehn-Saric et al. 1988). It has also been suggested that benzodiazepines such as chlordiazepoxide may peak in effectiveness after 4 weeks of treatment, whereas tricyclics such as imipramine may be more effective over the longer term for patients with anxiety (Kahn et al. 1986).

Although benzodiazepines are generally safe—side effects are limited mainly to sedation—there is a concern that some patients may develop tolerance or even become addicted to these medications. Available data indicate that most patients are able to stop taking them without serious sequelae and that the problem of frank addiction is overestimated and probably limited to an addiction-prone population or to patients with panic disorder who often increase benzodiazepine usage in unsuccessful attempts at self-medication.

Buspirone is a 5-hydroxytryptamine (5-HT$_{1a}$) agonist, nonbenzodiazepine antianxiety agent that appears to be as effective as the benzodiazepines in treating GAD. Its advantages are a better side-effect profile and the absence of tolerance and withdrawal. Its disadvantages include a slower rate of onset (Rickels et al. 1988), which can lead to early patient noncompliance. Rickels et al. (1988) compared the efficacy of the benzodiazepine clorazepate with that of the nonbenzodiazepine buspirone in the acute treatment and the maintenance of and the discontinuation of therapy in patients with GAD. The two medications were similarly effective by the fourth week of treatment, and benefits were maintained over a 6-month period, with an approximately 60% reduction of anxiety scores. There was no evidence of tolerance to either medication over the 6-month period. In the first 2 weeks of medication discontinuation, patients who had been taking clorazepate had a transient increase of anxiety consistent with withdrawal, whereas patients who had been taking buspirone did not. It has also been suggested that patients who have previously been treated with benzodiazepines may not respond as well to buspirone (Schweizer et al. 1986). However, one recent controlled study has refuted this hypothesis, showing that patients who gradually discontinued lorazepam therapy and then were treated with buspirone in a double-blind fashion did not exhibit benzodiazepine withdrawal or rebound anxiety and did as well with buspirone treatment as they had done with lorazepam therapy (Delle Chiaie et al. 1995). Treatment with buspirone is usually started at 5 mg tid, and the dose can be increased until a maximum dosage of 60 mg/day is reached. A bid regimen is probably as efficacious as a tid regimen and is an easier one with which to comply; because of ease of compliance, the dosage can be increased to 15–30 mg bid. Buspirone has not been found, to date, to be effective in treating panic attacks.

Other medications. β-Adrenergic blocking drugs, such as propranolol, are said by some to be useful in the treatment of a variety of anxiety disorders, but there is no convincing evidence that they are specifically effective in blocking spontaneous panic attacks. The same applies for GAD, in which propranolol may only be rarely indicated as an adjuvant in patients who experience notable palpitations or tremor.

Clonidine, which inhibits locus coeruleus discharge, would seem for theoretical reasons to be a good antipanic drug. Although two-thirds of patients in a small series responded initially, the therapeutic effect tends to be lost in a matter of weeks, despite continuation of dose (Liebowitz et al. 1981). A later study confirmed a similar pattern of loss of response during a 10-week trial (Uhde et al. 1989). This loss of response, plus a number of bothersome side effects, makes clonidine a poor initial choice for treatment of panic disorder. However, one controlled study found clonidine to be efficacious for both panic disorder and GAD (Hoehn-Saric et al. 1981).

Valproic acid may also have some beneficial effects in the treatment of panic attacks (Keck et al. 1993). In one open trial, all of 12 patients were moderately to markedly improved after 6 weeks of treatment, and 11 continued taking the medication and maintained their gains after 6 months (Woodman and Noyes 1994).

In a placebo-controlled 4-week trial, inositol, an intracellular second messenger precursor, was found to be effective in treating panic disorder at a dosage of 12 g/day (Benjamin et al. 1995).

Psychotherapy

Psychodynamic psychotherapy. Even after medication has blocked the actual panic attacks, a subgroup of panic patients remain wary of independence and assertiveness. In addition to supportive and behavioral treatment, traditional psychodynamic psychotherapy might be helpful for some of these patients. Considerable unconscious conflict over separations during childhood sometimes appears to operate in patients with panic disorder, leading to a reemergence of anxiety symptoms in adult life each time a new separation is imagined or threatened. Furthermore, it has been found that comorbid personality disorder is the major predictor of continued social maladjustment in patients otherwise treated for panic disorder (Noyes et al. 1990), which suggests that psychodynamic therapy may be an important additional treatment for at least some patients with panic disorder.

However, there are hardly any systematic studies documenting the efficacy of psychodynamic psychotherapy in panic disorder, and anecdotally it appears that this modality alone is often unsuccessful in treating panic attacks. Psychodynamically oriented clinicians tend to agree that psychological factors do not appear to be consequential in a proportion of patients with panic disorder, and they emphasize the importance of conducting a psychodynamic assessment to determine whether a particular patient may benefit from a psychodynamic treatment component (Gabbard 1990). Moreover, Cooper (1985) emphasized that in those patients with a predominant biological component to their illness, insistence on dynamic understanding and on responsibility for one's symptoms may be, in the long run, not only useless but potentially harmful, in that it may lead to further damage in self-esteem and strengthened masochistic defenses. However, there are case reports of patients who were successfully treated for panic with psychodynamic therapy or psychoanalysis. A recent controlled study showed that a 15-session course of brief dynamic psychotherapy combined with initial clomipramine treatment led to much lower relapse rates up to 9 months after the medication had been gradually discontinued (Wiborg and Dahl 1996).

Psychodynamic psychotherapy may also be helpful in some patients with GAD, particularly when unconscious conflict is believed by the clinician to be the cause of the patient's chronic anxiety. From a psychodynamic viewpoint, the more contained anxiety characteristic of GAD may be more akin to Freud's concept of signal anxiety and may thus be more amenable to psychodynamic exploration than panic is. Here, the emphasis is on anxiety not as an illness but as a ubiquitous affect hinting at underlying conflict. Thus, anxiety that appears generalized, free floating, or attached to a particular conscious and more acceptable fear might reveal a deeper conflict when explored (Gabbard 1990). Determining the capacity of individual patients for psychological-mindedness and exploration is a necessary prerequisite to embarking on a psychodynamic treatment. The specific nature of the patient's unconscious fear must be diagnosed, with the clinician's keeping in mind that symptoms are often multidetermined, and the ego's capacity to tolerate the anxiety associated with deeper exploration needs to be assessed. At present, no firm scientific data indicate which form of treatment—behavioral, psychodynamic, or pharmacological—is truly best for patients with GAD.

Pharmacotherapy is in no way incompatible with behavioral or psychodynamic treatment for patients with GAD or panic disorder. The notion that reducing the symptoms of anxiety disorder with medication will disturb a successful psychotherapy has never been convincingly demonstrated and is largely dogmatic. Indeed, successful psychotherapy often cannot take place until the more debilitating aspects of these syndromes have been eliminated pharmacologically.

Supportive psychotherapy.   Despite adequate treatment of panic attacks with medication, phobic avoidance may remain. Supportive psychotherapy and education about the illness are necessary in order for the patient to confront the phobic situation. Patients who fail to respond may then need additional psychotherapy, dynamic or behavioral. Encouragement from other patients with similar conditions is often quite helpful.

Cognitive-behavior therapy.   Behavioral treatments have long focused on phobic avoidance, but more recently, techniques have been developed and shown to be effective for panic attacks per se. In the last several years, interest in cognitive-behavior therapy (CBT) for panic has surged.

The major behavioral techniques for the treatment of panic attacks are breathing retraining, to control both acute and chronic hyperventilation; exposure to somatic cues, usually involving a hierarchy of exposure to feared sensations through imaginal and behavioral exercises; and relaxation training, achieved by the tensing and relaxing of different muscle groups. Cognitive treatment of panic involves cognitive restructuring, through which the uncomfortable affects and physical sensations associated with panic are given a more benign interpretation. These cognitive-behavioral techniques can be performed in various combinations. The extreme cognitive view is that panic attacks consist of normal physical sensations (e.g., palpitations, slight dizziness) to which panic disorder patients grossly overreact with catastrophic cognitions. A more moderate view is that panic patients do have extreme physical sensations such as bursts of tachycardia but can still help themselves substantially by changing their interpretation of the event from "I am going to die of a heart attack" to "There go my heart symptoms again." Such a theory has received experimental validation. Sanderson et al. (1989) provoked panic attacks in panic disorder patients with CO_2 inhalation; it was found that when patients had an illusion of control over the inhaled mixture, they experienced significantly fewer and less severe attacks and had less catastrophic cognitions.

Several studies have shown that these various cognitive-behavioral techniques are undoubtedly successful in the treatment of panic attacks (Barlow et al. 1989; Beck et al. 1992; Michelson et al. 1990; Salkovskis et al. 1986). Group-format cognitive-behavioral treatment for panic attacks has also been shown to be highly successful (Telch et al. 1993). Less is known about the relative or combined efficacy of medications versus that of CBT in the treatment of panic attacks without agoraphobia. In one controlled study, fluvoxamine was significantly beneficial in the acute treatment of panic disorder whereas cognitive therapy did not surpass placebo in efficacy (D. W. Black et al. 1993). Another controlled study found cognitive therapy, relaxation, and imipramine therapy to be similarly effective, and cognitive therapy had more lasting effects at 9-month follow-up after treatment was discontinued (Clark et al. 1994). After the initiation of medication treatment for initial symptom control, the introduction of CBT seems greatly to increase the likelihood that a patient will be able to gradually discontinue medication therapy (Otto et al. 1993). Preliminary findings on long-term outcome of panic with cognitive-behavioral treatment appear to be favorable, especially in the case of combined cognitive restructuring and exposure, whereas relaxation alone or added to the aforementioned does not appear to be helpful and may even be detrimental (Craske et al. 1991). Findings are inconsistent with regard to whether applied relaxation is equally efficacious or inferior to CBT for controlling panic attacks (Arntz and van den Hout 1996; Ost and Westling 1995).

Relaxation may also be a useful technique for generalized anxiety. In anxiety management training for generalized anxiety, relaxation training is specifically applied to both imagined and real-life anxiety-provoking situations. Relaxation helps reduce tension and other physical manifestations of anxiety and can be combined with cognitive restructuring to alleviate the cognitive component of negative anticipation and worrying. CBT is superior to general nondirective or supportive therapy in treating GAD (Chambless and Gillis 1993) and may be superior to applied relaxation therapy as well (Borkovec and Costello 1993).

Meditation and biofeedback.   The relaxation response is a physiological reaction brought about by stimulation of the hypothalamus that results in decreased sympathetic nervous system activity (Benson et al. 1974). The physiological changes of the relaxation response occur with Zen, yoga, and transcendental meditation. These techniques combine assuming a passive attitude and repetition of a word or a phrase. Meditation and the relaxation response may be a useful adjunct in the treatment of anxiety; there are, however, no systematic clinical data to support their efficacy. Biofeedback also appears promising for the treatment of GAD in controlled studies (Rice et al. 1993).

PHOBIC DISORDERS

DEFINITION

A *phobia* is defined as a persistent and irrational fear of a specific object, activity, or situation that results in a com-

pelling desire to avoid the dreaded object, activity, or situation (i.e., phobic stimulus). The fear is recognized by the individual as excessive or unreasonable in proportion to the actual dangerousness of the object, activity, or situation. Irrational fears and avoidance behavior are seen in a number of psychiatric disorders. However, in DSM-IV, phobic disorder is considered to be present only when single or multiple phobias are the predominant aspect of the clinical picture and a source of notable distress to the individual and are not the result of another mental disorder.

Phobias were classified in DSM-I under the rubric *phobic reaction* and in DSM-II as *phobic neurosis*. No subtypes were listed in either edition, reflecting the assumption of a qualitative unity implicit in the psychoanalytic model of phobias. DSM-III markedly differed from the previous editions in classifying distinct subtypes of phobias, suggesting a qualitative distinction between these subtypes. This distinction between agoraphobia, social phobia, and miscellaneous specific phobias stemmed from empirical findings, including findings of behavioral treatment studies by Marks (1969) and pharmacological treatment studies by D. F. Klein (1964). These three major categories of phobias were maintained in DSM-III-R and in DSM-IV. In DSM-III-R, agoraphobia was subdivided into *panic disorder with agoraphobia* and *agoraphobia without panic disorder*, which emphasizes the primacy of panic when the two conditions coexist. This classification is maintained in DSM-IV.

The major changes in the phobic disorders instituted in DSM-IV, in relation to DSM-III-R, were as follows. In agoraphobia without panic disorder, it is specified that the condition centers on the fear of developing incapacitating symptoms typically in characteristic situational clusters. It is also specified that agoraphobia related to embarrassment over a medical illness is a diagnosis that can be subject to clinical judgment. The two major changes in social phobia and in specific phobia in DSM-IV are similar for the two disorders. First, it is made explicit that panic attacks can occur as a feature of these phobias, and therefore clinical judgment is required to make the differential diagnosis between panic disorder with agoraphobia and social or specific phobia. Second, specific phobia is now divided into types, because new evidence has accumulated that phenomenology, natural history, and treatment response may differ according to type. The generalized type of social phobia was retained as in DSM-III-R.

DSM-IV diagnostic criteria for agoraphobia without history of panic disorder, social phobia, and specific phobia are presented in Tables 14–11, 14–12, and 14–13, respectively.

TABLE 14-11. DSM-IV diagnostic criteria for agoraphobia without history of panic disorder

A. The presence of agoraphobia related to fear of developing panic-like symptoms (e.g., dizziness or diarrhea). Agoraphobia: anxiety about being in places or situations from which escape might be difficult (or embarrassing) or in which help may not be available in the event of having an unexpected or situationally predisposed panic attack or panic-like symptoms. Agoraphobic fears typically involve characteristic clusters of situations that include being outside the home alone; being in a crowd or standing in a line; being on a bridge; and traveling in a bus, train, or automobile.

B. Criteria have never been met for panic disorder.

C. The disturbance is not due to the direct physiological effects of a substance (e.g., a drug of abuse, a medication) or a general medical condition.

D. If an associated general medical condition is present, the fear described in criterion A is clearly in excess of that usually associated with the condition.

CLINICAL DESCRIPTIONS

Agoraphobia

The clinical picture in agoraphobia consists of multiple and varied fears and avoidance behaviors that center around three main themes: 1) fear of leaving home, 2) fear of being alone, and 3) fear of being away from home in situations in which one can feel trapped, embarrassed, or helpless. According to DSM-IV, the fear is one of developing distressing symptoms in such situations in which escape is difficult or help is unavailable.

Typical agoraphobic fears are fears of using public transportation (buses, trains, subways, planes); of being in crowds, theaters, elevators, restaurants, supermarkets, or department stores; of waiting in line; and of traveling a distance from home. In severe cases patients may be completely housebound, fearful of leaving home without a companion, or may even be fearful of staying home alone.

Most cases of agoraphobia begin with a series of spontaneous panic attacks (see section on panic and generalized anxiety disorders earlier in this chapter). If the attacks continue, the patient usually develops a constant anticipatory anxiety characterized by continued apprehension about the possible occasion and consequences of the next attack. Agoraphobic symptoms represent a tertiary phase in the illness. Many patients will causally relate their panic attacks to the particular situation in which the attacks have oc-

curred. They then avoid these situations in an attempt to prevent further panic attacks (Figure 14–3). For example, a man who has had several attacks while taking the train to work may attribute the attacks to the train and, to avoid the train, start driving to work. If he still experiences panic at-

TABLE 14-12. DSM-IV diagnostic criteria for social phobia (social anxiety disorder)

A. A marked and persistent fear of one or more social or performance situations in which the person is exposed to unfamiliar people or to possible scrutiny by others. The individual fears that he or she will act in a way (or show anxiety symptoms) that will be humiliating or embarrassing. **Note:** In children, there must be evidence of the capacity for age-appropriate social relationships with familiar people and the anxiety must occur in peer settings, not just in interactions with adults.

B. Exposure to the feared situation almost invariably provokes anxiety, which may take the form of a situationally bound or situationally predisposed panic attack. **Note:** In children, the anxiety may be expressed by crying, tantrums, freezing, or shrinking from social situations with unfamiliar people.

C. The person recognizes that the fear is excessive or unreasonable. **Note:** In children, this feature may be absent.

D. The feared social or performance situations are avoided or else are endured with intense anxiety or distress.

E. The avoidance, anxious anticipation, or distress in the feared social or performance situation(s) interferes significantly with the person's normal routine, occupational (academic) functioning, or social activities or relationships, or there is marked distress about having the phobia.

F. In individuals under age 18 years, the duration is at least 6 months.

G. The fear or avoidance is not due to the direct physiological effects of a substance (e.g., a drug of abuse, a medication) or a general medical condition and is not better accounted for by another mental disorder (e.g., panic disorder with or without agoraphobia, separation anxiety disorder, body dysmorphic disorder, a pervasive developmental disorder, or schizoid personality disorder).

H. If a general medical condition or another mental disorder is present, the fear in criterion A is unrelated to it, e.g., the fear is not of stuttering, trembling in Parkinson's disease, or exhibiting abnormal eating behavior in anorexia nervosa or bulimia nervosa.

Specify if:

Generalized: if the fears include most social situations (also consider the additional diagnosis of avoidant personality disorder)

TABLE 14–13. **DSM-IV diagnostic criteria for specific phobia**

A. Marked and persistent fear that is excessive or unreasonable, cued by the presence or anticipation of a specific object or situation (e.g., flying, heights, animals, receiving an injection, seeing blood).

B. Exposure to the phobic stimulus almost invariably provokes an immediate anxiety response, which may take the form of a situationally bound or situationally predisposed panic attack. **Note:** In children, the anxiety may be expressed by crying, tantrums, freezing, or clinging.

C. The person recognizes that the fear is excessive or unreasonable. **Note:** In children, this feature may be absent.

D. The phobic situation(s) is avoided or else is endured with intense anxiety or distress.

E. The avoidance, anxious anticipation, or distress in the feared situation(s) interferes significantly with the person's normal routine, occupational (or academic) functioning, or social activities or relationships, or there is marked distress about having the phobia.

F. In individuals under age 18 years, the duration is at least 6 months.

G. The anxiety, panic attacks, or phobic avoidance associated with the specific object or situation are not better accounted for by another mental disorder, such as obsessive-compulsive disorder (e.g., fear of dirt in someone with an obsession about contamination), posttraumatic stress disorder (e.g., avoidance of stimuli associated with a severe stressor), separation anxiety disorder (e.g., avoidance of school), social phobia (e.g., avoidance of social situations because of fear of embarrassment), panic disorder with agoraphobia, or agoraphobia without history of panic disorder.

Specify type:

Animal type

Natural environment type (e.g., heights, storms, water)

Blood-injection-injury type

Situational type (e.g., airplanes, elevators, enclosed spaces)

Other type (e.g., phobic avoidance of situations that may lead to choking, vomiting, or contracting an illness; in children, avoidance of loud sounds or costumed characters)

tacks in the morning while driving to work rather than while taking the train, he interprets this as a sign that the attacks have spread to driving situations rather than as an indication that they were not caused by the train in the first place. Agoraphobic patients often fear situations that they believe they cannot leave abruptly if an attack occurs, such as crowded rooms, front-row seats, tunnels, bridges, and airplanes. Some individuals continue to have spontaneous panic attacks throughout the course of the illness. In other cases, after the initial phase of the illness, attacks may occur rarely or may occur exclusively when the patient ventures into the feared situation. The clinician must then decide whether the diagnosis is panic disorder with agoraphobia or social or specific phobia.

One interesting aspect of agoraphobia is the effect of a trusted companion on phobic behavior. Many patients who are unable to leave the house alone can travel long distances and partake in most activities if accompanied by a spouse, family member, or close friend. It is unclear whether vulnerability to panic attacks is actually decreased in this situation or whether the patient feels less helpless and isolated.

In addition to panic attacks, multiple phobias, and chronic anxiety, agoraphobic patients frequently exhibit symptoms of demoralization or secondary depression, multiple somatic complaints, and alcohol or sedative drug abuse.

According to most clinical studies and most clinicians, agoraphobia without any history of panic attacks is infrequently encountered in clinical settings. Indeed, some investigators believe that an initial panic attack, whether remote or forgotten, is a necessary prerequisite for the development of agoraphobia (see Figure 14–2). However, this conclusion is controversial. For example, in one clinical series of panic disorder with agoraphobia, 23% of patients reported that agoraphobia preceded the initial panic attack, although the existence of retrospective biases may cast some doubt on such a finding (Lelliott et al. 1989). Most striking is the high prevalence of agoraphobia without panic that has been reported in epidemiologic samples. According to the findings of the Epidemiologic Catchment Area (ECA) study, the majority of new-onset agoraphobia (about two-thirds) occurred without a history of panic attacks (Eaton and Keyl 1990). Such a discrepant finding may, at least in part, be accounted for by an excessively low severity threshold and weaknesses in differential diagnosis in epidemiologic assessments.

Social Phobia

In *social phobia*, the individuals' central fear is that they will act in such a way that they will humiliate or embarrass themselves in front of others. Socially phobic individuals fear and/or avoid a variety of situations in which they would be required to interact with others or to perform a task in front of other people. Typical social phobias are phobias of speaking, eating, or writing in public; of using public lavatories; and of attending parties or interviews. In addition, a common fear of socially phobic individuals is that other people will detect and ridicule their anxiety in

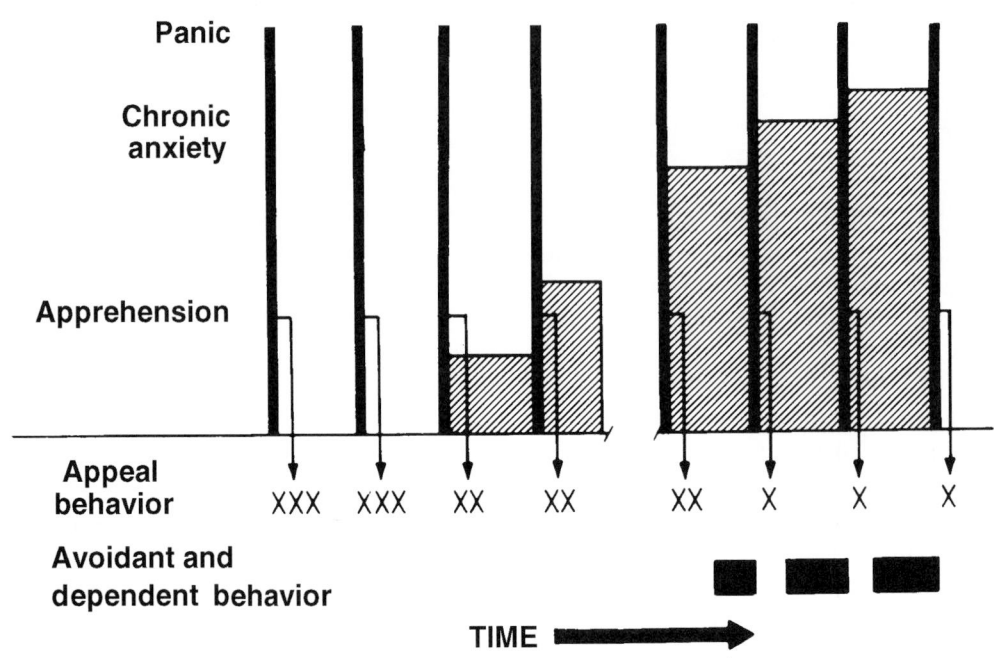

FIGURE 14-2.   Development of agoraphobia. After onset of unexpected panic attacks (solid bars), patient develops acute help-seeking behavior (**XX**), then apprehension culminating in chronic anxiety (shaded areas), and finally agoraphobic behavior (black blocks).

social situations. An individual may have a single social fear or limited or numerous social fears. Social phobia is described as *generalized* if the social fear encompasses most social situations as opposed to being present in circumscribed ones. Generalized social phobia is overall a more serious and impairing condition. This phobia can be reliably diagnosed as a subtype and involves an earlier age at onset than does limited social phobia; patients with generalized social phobia are more often single and have more interactional fears; and there is greater comorbidity with atypical depression and alcoholism (Manuzza et al. 1995).

As in specific phobia, the anxiety in social phobia is stimulus-bound. When forced or surprised into the phobic situation, the individual experiences profound anxiety accompanied by a variety of somatic symptoms. Interestingly, different anxiety disorders tend to be characterized by their own constellation of most-prominent somatic symptoms. For example, palpitations and chest pain or pressure are more common in panic attacks, whereas sweating, blushing, and dry mouth are more common in social anxiety (Amies et al. 1983; Reich et al. 1988). Actual panic attacks may also occur in individuals with social phobia in response to feared social situations. Blushing is the cardinal physical symptom characteristic of social phobia, whereas commonly encountered cognitive symptoms include tendencies toward self-focused attention, negative self-evaluation regarding social performance, difficulty gauging nonverbal aspects of one's behavior, discounting of social competence in positive interactions, and a positive bias towards appraising others' social performance (Alden and Wallace 1995).

Individuals who have only limited social fears may be functioning well overall and may be relatively asymptomatic unless confronted with the necessity of entering their phobic situation. When faced with this necessity, they are often subject to intense anticipatory anxiety. Multiple social fears, on the other hand, can lead to chronic demoralization, social isolation, and disabling vocational and interpersonal impairment. Alcohol and sedative drugs are often used to alleviate at least the anticipatory component of this anxiety disorder and substance abuse may result. In a study in which public-speaking–phobic individuals were systematically compared with individuals with generalized social phobia, the latter were found to be younger, less well educated, and less often employed and to have greater anxiety, depression, and fears of negative social evaluation (Heimberg et al. 1990b).

Specific Phobias

Specific phobias are circumscribed fears of specific objects, situations, or activities. This syndrome has three components: 1) an anticipatory anxiety that is brought on by the possibility of confrontation with the phobic stimulus, 2) the central fear itself, and 3) the avoidance behavior by which the patient minimizes anxiety.

In specific phobia, the fear is usually not of the object itself but of some dire outcome that the individuals believe may result from contact with that object. For example, persons with driving phobia are afraid of accidents; those with snake phobia are afraid that they will be bitten; and those who are claustrophobic are afraid that they will suffocate or be trapped in an enclosed space. These fears are excessive, unreasonable, and enduring; although most individuals with specific phobias will readily acknowledge that they know there is really nothing to be afraid of, reassuring them of this does not diminish their fear.

In DSM-IV, for the first time, types of specific phobias have been adopted: natural environment (e.g., storms); animal (e.g., insects); blood-injury-injection; situational (e.g., cars, elevators, bridges); and other (e.g., choking, vomiting). The validity of such distinctions is supported by data showing that these types tend to differ with respect to age at onset, mode of onset, familial aggregation, and physiological responses to the phobic stimulus (Curtis and Thyer 1983; Fyer et al. 1990; Himle et al. 1991; Ost 1987).

EPIDEMIOLOGY

In the ECA study, in which trained lay interviewers used the Diagnostic Interview Schedule to make DSM-III diagnoses of psychiatric disorders in five cities in the United States, phobias as a group were found to be the most common current psychiatric disorder: 1-month and 6-month prevalence rates were 6.2% and 7.7%, respectively, and the lifetime rate was 12.5% (Regier et al. 1988). Specific phobias were the most common (11.3%)—based on lifetime prevalence at four sites—followed by agoraphobia (5.6%) and social phobia (2.7%). Specific phobias were more common in women than in men (14.5% vs. 7.8%). Agoraphobia was also more common in women (7.9% vs. 3.2%). Social phobia was similar between the two genders (2.9% in women vs. 2.5% in men) (Eaton et al. 1991).

In the more recent National Comorbidity Survey (Kessler et al. 1994; Magee et al. 1996), which employed DSM-III-R criteria, specific phobias had the same lifetime prevalence (11.3%) as in the ECA study. However, social phobia appeared markedly more prevalent than in the ECA study (lifetime occurrence of 13.3%, 1-year incidence of 7.9%, and 1-month incidence of 4.5%) and was somewhat more common in women than in men (lifetime occurrence of 15.5% versus 11.1%). Findings concerning agoraphobia were similar to those in the ECA study; the lifetime prevalence was 6.7% and the 1-month prevalence was 2.3%. Median ages of illness onset were 15 years for specific phobias, 16 years for social phobia, and 29 years for agoraphobia. The phobias were highly comorbid with each other, and despite notable functional impairment, only a minority of the individuals interviewed had sought professional help.

ETIOLOGY

Psychodynamic Theory

Early on, Freud (1895a[1894]/1962) observed that in the analysis of phobias, "nothing is ever found but *the emotional state of anxiety.* . . . In the case of agoraphobia we often find *the recollection of an anxiety attack;* and what the patient actually fears is the occurrence of such an attack under the special conditions in which he believes he cannot escape it" (pp. 80–81). This is a succinct description, from more than one century ago, of the development of anticipatory anxiety and agoraphobia after a panic attack. At that time, Freud did not consider phobias to be psychologically mediated. Rather, he understood them, like anxiety neurosis, to be manifestations of a physiologically induced tension state. Undischarged libidinal energy was physiologically transformed into anxiety, which became attached to and partly discharged through objects that were, by their nature or in the patient's prior experience, dangerous.

However, with the 1909 publication of the case of Little Hans, Freud (1909/1955) started to develop a more psychological theory of phobic symptom formation. Little Hans was a 5-year-old boy who developed a phobia of horses. Through an analysis of the boy's conversations with his parents over a period of months, Freud hypothesized that Little Hans's unconscious and forbidden sexual feelings for his mother and aggressive, rivalrous feelings for his father, blocked from discharge because of repression, became physiologically transformed into anxiety, which was then displaced onto a symbolic object, in this case horses, the avoidance of which partly relieved Little Hans's anxiety.

Freud later reconceptualized the case of Little Hans in the context of his evolving structural theory. Freud hypothesized that phobic symptoms occur as part of the resolution of intrapsychic conflict between instinctual impulses, superego prohibitions, and external reality constraints. Signal anxiety is experienced by the ego when such unconscious impulses threaten to break through. Such anxiety serves to mobilize not only further repression but also, in the case of phobia formation, projection and displacement of the conflict onto a symbolic object, which can then be avoided as a neurotic solution to the original conflict. In the case of Little Hans, sexual feelings for his mother, aggressive feelings toward his father, and the guilty fear of retribution and castration by his father generated anxiety as a signal of oedipal conflict. The conflict became displaced and projected onto an avoidable object, horses, which Little Hans consequently feared would bite him. According to Freud, such a phobic symptom had two advantages. It allowed Little Hans to avoid the ambivalence inherent in his original conflict—Little Hans not only hated but also loved his father. It also allowed his ego to cease generating anxiety as long as he could avoid the sight of horses. The cost of this compromise was that Little Hans became housebound.

Since Freud, the psychodynamic literature has to a degree shifted away from formulations that primarily emphasize libidinal wishes and castration fears in understanding phobias (Michels et al. 1985). For example, the importance of a trustworthy and safe companion in the case of individuals with agoraphobia could be understood as a simultaneous expression of aggressive impulses toward the companion and a magical wish to protect the companion from such impulses by always being together. Alternatively, excessive fear of object loss and its concomitant separation anxiety could explain both the fear of being away from home alone and the alleviation of this fear when a companion is present.

Conditioned Reflex Theories

In learning theory, phobic anxiety is thought to be a conditioned response that is acquired through association of the phobic object (i.e., the conditioned stimulus) with a noxious experience (i.e., the unconditioned stimulus). Initially, the noxious experience (e.g., an electric shock) produces an unconditioned response of pain, discomfort, and fear. If the individual frequently receives an electric shock when in contact with the phobic object, then by contiguous conditioning the appearance of the phobic object alone may come to elicit an anxiety response (i.e., conditioned response). Avoidance of the phobic object prevents or reduces this conditioned anxiety and is therefore perpetuated through drive reduction.

This classic learning theory model of phobias received much reinforcement from the relative success of behavioral (i.e., deconditioning) techniques in the treatment of many patients with simple phobia. However, more recently the model has been criticized on the grounds that it is not consistent with a number of empirically observed aspects of phobic behavior in humans. Among the major criticisms are the following:

1. Many cases of phobia do not appear to have begun with a traumatic incident in which the phobic object is associated with an unpleasant unconditioned stimulus.
2. The learning theory model suggests that any object or situation that is regularly associated with noxious stimuli has an equal likelihood of becoming a phobic object. However, the range of phobic objects is actually relatively small and is neither random nor predominantly made up of those items that in a modern industrial society might be most likely to be frequently associated with noxious stimuli (e.g., electric switches, stoves, oncoming cars).
3. Learning theory does not account for the qualitative distinctions between panic and anticipatory anxiety delineated by pharmacological and sodium lactate infusion studies.

Conditioning theory may account for some cases of social and simple phobias (e.g., a traumatic early public speaking or social experience or being bitten by a dog). Prospective studies are needed to clarify this issue fully. Furthermore, even though learning theory could account for the initial emergence of certain phobic symptoms, it does not fully account for their maintenance; repeated exposure to the conditioned stimulus should extinguish the conditioned response. In this scenario, psychodynamic theory suggests that unconscious conflict may be the continuing driving force that maintains the phobic symptom (Nemiah 1981).

Findings of recent controlled studies examining the etiology of social phobia also do not favor conditioning theory as a putative explanation for the condition (Hofmann et al. 1995).

Biological Theories

Some interesting hypotheses about the origin of phobias have resulted from integration of ethological, biological, and learning theory approaches.

Seligman (1971) suggested that simple phobias are an example of evolutionarily prepared learning. The term *preparedness* refers to the observation that certain responses to stimuli are more easily learned than others and that the ease of learning in any one instance varies from species to species. Preparedness is a measure of the ease with which a particular stimulus becomes paired with a particular response. Most specific phobias involve stimuli that over the course of evolution might have been dangerous to humans and are still reacted to as though they were intrinsically dangerous. In support of a biological component in specific phobias,

Fyer et al. (1990) found high familial transmission for specific phobias; the risk for first-degree relatives of affected subjects was roughly threefold. Interestingly, there was no increased risk found for other phobic or anxiety disorders. Twin studies have not supported a genetic component to social and specific phobia, in contrast to panic disorder, generalized anxiety disorder, and posttraumatic stress disorder (PTSD); this finding suggests environmental causation (Skre et al. 1993).

Social phobia symptoms are accompanied in perhaps 50% of cases by a surge of plasma epinephrine. Such a surge distinguishes them from panic attacks, in which an adrenaline surge is not regularly seen. Patients with social phobia exhibit a blunted growth-hormone response to clonidine challenge, which suggests underlying noradrenergic dysfunction similar to that seen in panic disorder patients (Tancer et al. 1993). Cognitive features also play a role in social phobia, however, because rapid infusions of adrenaline in nonperformance situations do not fully reproduce the symptoms. Phenylethylamine or similar endogenous amines may be involved in mood response to social approval and disapproval. This system could be poorly regulated in patients with social phobia and those with atypical depression (Liebowitz et al. 1984b). Both of these groups overreact to criticism or rejection and greatly benefit from treatment with MAOIs, which reduce their sensitivity to rejection and also inhibit the metabolism of endogenous biogenic amines.

Agoraphobia is a response, in most cases, to spontaneous panic attacks, the etiology of which has already been discussed. Why only some individuals with panic attacks develop agoraphobia is uncertain and involves an interplay of environmental, gender, and genetic features. Individuals who must go out to earn a living are less likely to become housebound than those whose primary occupation is in the home. This may explain the greater female-to-male ratio for agoraphobia than for panic disorder. Agoraphobic individuals may also have more severe or chronic panic disorder. Family studies suggest genetic transmission for agoraphobia both related to and independent of panic disorder.

In a large study of phobias in twins, Kendler and his group (1992b) determined that the familial aggregation of phobias was mostly accounted for by genetic factors; heritability was 30%–40%, depending on the particular phobia. Environmental factors also played an important role in the development of phobic disorders.

Brain imaging studies of phobias are still in their infancy and have not yet yielded powerful or consistent findings. In one recent interesting study that examined simple phobia symptom provocation using positron-emission tomography, it appeared that the phobic anxiety is mediated by paralimbic structures; additionally, activation of the somatosensory cortex suggested that tactile imagery is one component of the phobic response (Rauch et al. 1995).

COURSE AND PROGNOSIS

There are very few systematically collected data on the natural history of agoraphobia. The usual age at onset of agoraphobia is between 18 and 35 years. Individuals whose panic episodes are characterized principally by feelings of unsteadiness and a fear of falling (leading to a fear of open spaces) typically have onset of the disorder in their 40s. Although in those patients who eventually seek treatment the overall course of the illness is thought to be chronic, the general impression of experienced clinicians is that the illness waxes and wanes and that many patients have at least brief periods of improvement or even remission. There are no follow-up studies of untreated agoraphobic individuals. Follow-up studies of treated patients are discussed in the subsection on treatment.

Onset of social phobia is mainly in adolescence and early adulthood, earlier than the onset of agoraphobia, and the course of illness is very chronic. Mean age at onset in two clinical series was 19 years (Amies et al. 1983; Marks and Gelder 1966). Onset of symptoms is sometimes acute after a humiliating social experience but is usually insidious over months or years and without a clear-cut precipitant. Interestingly, clinical studies have found men and women to be equally affected or have even found men to be more commonly affected than women, in distinction to other anxiety disorders. However, these findings may reflect the fact that men are more likely to seek treatment, because of societal role demands, rather than prevalence rates in the population at large. In a large epidemiologic survey of social phobia, Schneier et al. (1992) found that 70% of those with the disorder were women. Otherwise, findings were similar to those in clinical samples. Mean age at onset was 15 years, and there was substantial associated morbidity, including greater financial dependency and increased suicidal ideation. It has been found that more than half of social phobia patients report notable impairment in some area or areas of their lives, independent of the degree of social support (Schneier et al. 1994). Predictors of good outcome in social phobia are onset after age 11 years, absence of psychiatric comorbidity, and higher educational status (Davidson et al. 1993a).

Animal phobias usually begin in childhood, whereas situational phobias tend to start later in life. Marks (1969) found the mean age at onset for animal phobias to be 4.4 years, whereas patients with situational phobias had a mean age at onset of 22.7 years. Although systematic prospective studies are limited, it appears that specific phobias follow a chronic course unless treated.

DIAGNOSIS AND DIFFERENTIAL DIAGNOSIS

Before the diagnosis of phobic disorder can be made, the presence of other disorders that may cause irrational fears and avoidance behaviors must be ruled out. For a complete decision tree of the differential diagnosis of the anxiety disorders, see Figure 14–1.

Agoraphobia

Widespread fears and avoidance of being alone or of leaving home can be seen in paranoid and psychotic states, posttraumatic disorders, and major depressive disorders. Psychotic states can be differentiated from agoraphobia by the presence of delusions, hallucinations, and thought process disorder. Although agoraphobic patients are frequently afraid that they are going crazy, they do not exhibit psychotic symptomatology. Patients with PTSD have a typical history, such as a fear of being or of traveling alone after an assault.

Distinguishing between depressive disorders and agoraphobia is more difficult. Patients with depressive disorders and patients with agoraphobia commonly experience spontaneous panic attacks. Patients with agoraphobia are frequently demoralized and will state that they feel depressed. Close questioning, however, usually does not reveal further vegetative symptoms or a loss of pleasure or interest in activities. Early morning awakening and pervasive anhedonia, which are common symptoms in endogenous depression, are rare in agoraphobia. Agoraphobic individuals will usually say they would love to leave home and engage in a variety of activities if only they could be sure of not panicking. In contrast, depressed individuals usually see no point in going out because nothing gives them any pleasure and they believe that people will be better off without them.

Patients with atypical depression (i.e., depression characterized by hypersomnia, hyperphagia, extreme low energy, and depressed but reactive mood) frequently have panic attacks but rarely have agoraphobia as part of their life history or current symptomatology. Patients with atypical depression and a history of panic attacks may respond preferentially to MAOIs (Liebowitz et al. 1985b).

Social Phobia

Avoidance of social situations is seen as part of avoidant, schizoid, and paranoid personality disorders; agoraphobia; obsessive-compulsive disorder; depressive disorders; schizophrenia; and paranoid disorders.

Persons with paranoid disorders fear that something unpleasant will be done to them by others. In contrast, individuals with social phobia fear that they themselves will act inappropriately and cause their own embarrassment or humiliation.

In avoidant personality disorder, the central fear is also fear of rejection, ridicule, or humiliation by others. The distinction between this entity and generalized social phobia may be conceptual and semantic, and its validity is a subject of dispute. Automatically labeling such patients as having avoidant personalities may lead practitioners away from potentially useful pharmacotherapy and behavioral treatment efforts.

Some agoraphobic patients say that they are afraid they will embarrass themselves by losing control if they panic while in a social situation. These patients are distinguished from patients with social phobia by the presence of panic attacks that also occur in situations not involving scrutiny or evaluation by others.

Interpersonal anxiety or fears of humiliation leading to social avoidance are not diagnosed as social phobia when they occur in the context of schizophrenia, schizophreniform or brief reactive psychoses, and major depressive disorder. Patients with psychotic vulnerabilities and massive social isolation or poor interpersonal skills may occasionally be mistakenly considered as having social phobia if seen when they are in nonpsychotic or prepsychotic phases of illness.

Social withdrawal seen in depressive disorders is usually associated with a lack of interest or pleasure in the company of others rather than with a fear of scrutiny. In contrast, individuals with social phobia generally express the wish to be able to interact appropriately with others and they anticipate pleasure in this eventuality.

TREATMENT

Pharmacotherapy

Agoraphobia. There continues to be disagreement in the literature regarding the best method of treatment of agoraphobia with panic attacks. Antipanic medication is given to block the occurrence of panic attacks, and its efficacy in this regard is well documented. The pharmacological treatment of panic attacks has already been outlined in the section on panic and generalized anxiety. However, medication alone is often not adequate treatment in patients with significant agoraphobic avoidance. It is generally accepted that some means of exposing agoraphobic patients to the feared situations is necessary for overall improvement. Such exposure may be achieved by various nonspecific methods, such as psychoeducation, reassurance, and supportive therapy (D. F. Klein et al. 1983). However, it appears that focused cognitive-behavior therapy (CBT) is, on the whole, more successful than nonspecific techniques in reducing agoraphobic avoidance. Consequently, the relative and combined efficacy of treatment with medication and CBT for panic with agoraphobia has been the focus of a number of investigations.

Some studies have not found imipramine to have a significant effect on agoraphobia when given alone or with antiexposure instructions (Marks et al. 1983; Telch et al. 1985), whereas others have shown imipramine therapy alone to decrease phobic avoidance at combined plasma levels of 110–140 ng/mL (Mavissakalian and Perel 1995). Most studies concur that the combination of medication and behavioral treatment (exposure) is superior to medication or behavioral treatment alone for treating phobic avoidance (de Beurs et al. 1995; Mavissakalian and Michelson 1986a; Telch et al. 1985; Zitrin et al. 1980).

In summary, antipanic medication is indicated in the treatment of agoraphobia with panic, because one major goal of treatment is to block the occurrence of panic attacks. This approach should be applied even when panic attacks are sporadic or have limited symptoms. However, the efficacy of medication for phobic symptoms does not appear to be as great as that for panic symptoms, and if, as is often the case, psychoeducational and supportive measures are not adequate in encouraging the patient to enter feared situations, behavioral treatment should be instituted. Combination treatment in such patients appears to be superior to either treatment alone. In a large controlled study of alprazolam plus exposure in patients with panic disorder and agoraphobia, it emerged that the improvements in panic attacks, anticipatory anxiety, and phobic avoidance are largely independent of each other, and only early improvement in avoidance predicted global improvement after treatment (Basoglu et al. 1994). Cognitive therapy has been shown to decrease panic attacks but not agoraphobia, whereas exposure reduces agoraphobia but not panic (van den Hout et al. 1994).

Social phobia. The pharmacological treatment of social phobia is summarized in Table 14–14. Certain medication options are clearly efficacious in social phobia. In performance-type social phobia, several analog (i.e., involving nonclinical samples with performance or social anxiety) studies have shown β-blocker efficacy, particularly when these agents are used acutely before a performance (Brantigan et al. 1982; Hartley et al. 1983; I. M. James et al. 1977, 1983; Liden and Gottfries 1974; Neftel

TABLE 14–14. Pharmacological treatment of social phobia

Monoamine oxidase inhibitors

General indications: Demonstrated high effectiveness; may be difficult to tolerate and require dietary restrictions; effective for several comorbid conditions, including atypical depression, social phobia, panic

Phenelzine: Most studied

Tranylcypromine: Also effective

Reversible monoamine oxidase inhibitors

General indications: Demonstrated efficacy; no dietary restrictions or hypertensive crisis risk; not marketed in United States

Moclobemide

Brofaromine

Selective serotonin reuptake inhibitors

General indications: Recently shown efficacy; well tolerated; currently may be first choice in patients unwilling or unable to tolerate irreversible monoamine oxidase inhibitors; effective for comorbid depression, panic, obsessive-compulsive disorder

Fluvoxamine: Efficacy demonstrated in controlled trials

Sertraline: Efficacy demonstrated in controlled trials

Fluoxetine: Efficacy demonstrated in open trials

Paroxetine: Efficacy demonstrated in open trials

Benzodiazepines

General indications: Clinically widely used; reportedly efficacious in open trials; generally well tolerated

Clonazepam: Long-acting; efficacy demonstrated in controlled trial

Buspirone

General indications: Well tolerated; only open trials; comorbid generalized anxiety

β-Blockers

General indications: Highly effective for performance anxiety, taken as needed; generally not helpful in patients with generalized social phobia

Propranolol

Atenolol

et al. 1982). Many performing artists or public speakers find that β-blockers, taken orally a few hours before stage time, reduce palpitations, tremor, and the "butterfly feeling." Although a variety of β-blockers have been used in studies and are probably efficacious for performance anxiety, the most common ones used are propranolol (20 mg) or atenolol (50 mg). It also seems that β-blockers are more effective in controlling stage fright, with minimal or no side effects, than are benzodiazepines, which may decrease subjective anxiety but not optimize performance and may have an adverse effect on "sharpness."

To date, MAOIs have proved to be the most effective medications for treating generalized social phobia. Older studies had shown these drugs to be effective in mixed agoraphobic/social phobia samples (Mountjoy et al. 1977; C. Solyom et al. 1981; L. Solyom et al. 1973; Tyrer et al. 1973). More recently, Liebowitz et al. (1992) conducted a controlled study comparing phenelzine, atenolol, and placebo in the treatment of patients with DSM-III–diagnosed social phobia. About two-thirds of patients had a marked response to phenelzine, in dosages of 45–90 mg/day, whereas atenolol was not superior in efficacy to placebo. Tranylcypromine in dosages of 40–60 mg/day was also associated with notable improvement in about 80% of patients with DSM-III–diagnosed social phobia treated openly for 1 year (Versiani et al. 1988). The comparative and combined efficacy of medications and behavioral treatments for social phobia has also been investigated. One study (Gelernter et al. 1991) compared cognitive-behavioral group treatment with phenelzine, alprazolam, and placebo therapy. Although all groups improved markedly with treatment, phenelzine therapy tended to be superior with regard to absolute clinical response and decreased impairment. Further studies are expected to shed more light on relative efficacy and combined treatments.

Other medications have recently begun being tested and show some promise for the treatment of social phobia, although it is as yet uncertain whether they are as efficacious as the irreversible MAOIs. Results of several recent trials of selective serotonin reuptake inhibitors (SSRIs) have been positive. Treatment with 150 mg of fluvoxamine per day for 12 weeks resulted in substantial improvement in 46% of patients compared with 7% improvement in the placebo group (van Vliet et al. 1994). Of 20 patients treated openly with sertraline for at least 8 weeks, 80% showed some improvement of their social phobia (Van Ameringen et al. 1994), and the efficacy of sertraline was duplicated in one placebo-controlled study at dosages of 50–200 mg/day (Katzelnick et al. 1995). A similar response rate was found in an open trial of fluoxetine (Van Ameringen et al. 1993). The reversible MAOIs moclobemide and brofaromine also appear to be effective in social phobia and treatment involves no dietary restrictions or hypertensive risks, but the likelihood of their being marketed in the United States appears small (Den Boer et al. 1994; Fahlen et al. 1995). Treatment with benzodiazepines also appears promising for some patients with social phobia, but these drugs are used clinically more widely than supported by actual studies. Results of several open trials have been positive, and in one recent controlled study, clonazepam at dosages of

0.5–3 mg/day was found to be superior to placebo, with a response rate of 78% and improvement in social anxiety, avoidance, performance, and negative self-evaluation (Davidson et al. 1993b). Treatment with buspirone, a 5-hydroxytryptamine (5-HT_{1a}) agonist, may also hold some promise for social phobia; results of double-blind trials are needed before recommendations concerning such therapy can be made (Schneier et al. 1993).

Specific phobias.   No medication has been shown to be effective in treating specific phobias. Tricyclics, benzodiazepines, and β-blockers generally do not appear useful for treating specific phobias, based on the limited number of studies available to date.

Cognitive-Behavior Therapy

Agoraphobia.   The goal of psychotherapeutic intervention in agoraphobia is to encourage patients to reenter the phobic situation and demonstrate to themselves that they will not have panic attacks while taking medication and therefore may give up both the avoidance and the worry, or anticipatory anxiety, about having attacks.

At the start of treatment, the therapist explains to the patient the three-stage development of the illness and the fact that the medication will block the spontaneous panics but may not alleviate anticipatory anxiety or the desire to avoid. Once the frequency of spontaneous panics has abated, some patients will begin to try out previously avoided situations on their own. Others will need structured encouragement in the form of supportive psychotherapy. On the whole, focused behavioral therapies appear to be more effective for patients with more severe or resistant agoraphobia; exposure techniques have been used in conjunction with antipanic medication in the treatment of patients with agoraphobia with panic attacks. A popular form of behavior therapy is group in vivo exposure, in which groups of agoraphobic patients (initially accompanied by the therapist) travel together to restaurants, shopping malls, and other locations. Self-help groups are also helpful for raising morale and sharing information among agoraphobic individuals.

As already elaborated in the pharmacotherapy subsection, a persistent area of disagreement has been the sequence of applying medication and behavior therapy in the treatment of patients who have agoraphobia with panic attacks. Psychopharmacologically oriented clinicians recommend first blocking panics with medication and then using in vivo exposure for patients who cannot regain full mobility once their panics are blocked. Behavior therapists, on the other hand, advocate applying exposure treatment first and reserve medication for resistant cases. Behavior therapy that focuses principally on exposure often leaves panic attacks unblocked even if mobility is enhanced, a situation that argues for routine use of antipanic medication. However, newer behavioral techniques may be effective in ameliorating panic symptoms as well (see subsection on behavior therapy of panic). In all, it appears that combination treatments are clearly indicated, at least for those patients who are resistant to either form of treatment alone.

Social phobia. Three major cognitive-behavioral techniques are used in the treatment of social phobia: exposure, cognitive restructuring, and social skills training. Exposure treatment involves imaginal or in vivo exposure to specific feared performance and social situations. Although patients with very high levels of social anxiety may need to start out with imaginal exposure until a certain degree of habituation is attained, therapeutic results are not gained until in vivo exposure is done to the real-life feared situations. Social skills training employs modeling, rehearsal, role-playing, and assigned practice to help individuals learn appropriate behaviors and to decrease anxiety in social situations. This type of training is not necessary for all individuals with social phobia and is more applicable to those who have actual deficits in social interacting above and beyond their anxiety or avoidance of social situations. Cognitive restructuring focuses on poor self-concepts, the fear of negative evaluation by others, and the attribution of positive outcomes to chance or circumstance and negative outcomes to one's own shortcomings.

Results of older studies of behavioral treatments for social phobia were difficult to evaluate because of heterogeneous phobic patient samples, lack of operational definitions of disorder and improvement ratings, and the presentation of outcome data in terms of mean change scores rather than level of achieved functioning. However, over the past several years, the cognitive-behavioral treatment of social phobia has attracted great attention, detailed treatment strategies and approaches have been delineated, and more thorough systematic studies in well-defined clinical populations have emerged.

More recent studies have shown that exposure, cognitive restructuring, and social skills training may all be of substantial benefit to patients with social phobia. Attempts to correlate patient type (social skills deficits vs. phobic anxiety/avoidance) with preferred treatment modality (social skills training vs. exposure) have not always been fruitful (Wlazlo et al. 1990). Heimberg and his group (1990a) compared cognitive-behavioral group treatment with a credible psychoeducational-supportive control intervention in patients with DSM-III–diagnosed social phobia; both groups got better, but the cognitive-behavioral group showed more improvement, especially in patients' self-appraisal. Finally, it has been suggested that cognitive aspects may be of greater importance in social phobia than in other anxiety or phobic conditions, and therefore cognitive restructuring may be a necessary component to maximize treatment gains. Mattick et al. (1989) reported that combination treatment was superior to either exposure or cognitive restructuring alone in social phobia; cognitive restructuring was inferior to exposure in decreasing avoidant behavior, but exposure alone did not change self-perception and attitude.

Although long-term outcome is more difficult to assess, studies suggest that CBT leads to long-lasting gains (Turner et al. 1995) and therefore may be of particular importance in this disorder, which tends to have a chronic, often lifetime, course. At this point, it appears that in vivo exposure is a critical component of the treatment and that the introduction of cognitive restructuring at some point in the treatment contributes to further gains and to their long-term maintenance.

Specific phobias. The treatment of choice for specific phobias is exposure. The problem lies in persuading the patient that exposure is worth trying and will be beneficial.

Exposure treatments may be divided into two groups, depending on whether exposure to the phobic object is in vivo or imaginal. In vivo exposure involves the patient in real-life contact with the phobic stimulus. When imaginal techniques are used, the phobic stimulus is confronted through the therapist's descriptions and the patient's imagination.

The method of exposure in both the in vivo and imaginal techniques can be graded or ungraded. Graded exposure uses a hierarchy of anxiety-provoking events, varying from least to most stressful. The patient begins at the least stressful level and gradually progresses up the hierarchy. Ungraded exposure begins with the patients confronting the most stressful items in the hierarchy.

Most exposure techniques have been used in both individual and group settings. In a group setting, both the example and the encouragement of other members are often particularly helpful in persuading the patient to reenter the phobic situation. Techniques may include systematic desensitization, imaginal flooding, prolonged in vivo exposure, and participant modeling and reinforced practice.

Studies thus far have not conclusively shown any one exposure technique to be superior to other techniques or to be specifically indicated for particular phobic subtypes. In those patients whose phobic symptoms include panic attacks, antipanic medication may also be indicated.

Other Psychotherapy

All patients suffering from phobias require emotional support and confident guidance from the treating professional. For some phobic patients, the simple exhortation to face phobic objects or situations will suffice; for others, structured behavioral programs are more effective. Medication can facilitate confronting phobic fears in agoraphobia and social phobia.

In more recent years, the successful use of medication and/or behavioral treatments has resulted in psychodynamic therapy for phobias falling out of favor to some degree (Gabbard 1990). However, in those patients in whom underlying conflicts associated with phobic anxiety and avoidance can be identified by the clinician and lend themselves to insightful exploration, psychodynamic therapy may be of benefit. Furthermore, a psychodynamic approach may be valuable in understanding and resolving the secondary interpersonal ramifications in which phobic patients and their partners are often caught up and that could serve as resistances to the successful implementation of medication or behavioral treatments (Gabbard 1990).

OBSESSIVE-COMPULSIVE DISORDER

DEFINITION

The essential features of obsessive-compulsive disorder (OCD) are obsessions or compulsions. The definition and criteria for OCD in DSM-IV are presented in Table 14–15.

The terms *obsession* and *compulsion* are sometimes used to characterize conditions that are not true OCD. Although some activities—such as eating, sexual behavior, gambling, or drinking—when engaged in excessively may be referred to as "compulsive," these activities are distinguished from true compulsions in that they are experienced as pleasurable and ego-syntonic, although their consequences may become increasingly unpleasant and ego-dystonic over time. Obsessive brooding, ruminations, or preoccupations, typically characteristic of depression, may be unpleasant but are distinguished from true obsessions because they are not as senseless or intrusive and the individual regards them as meaningful although possibly excessive and painful.

The several presentations of OCD are based on symptom clusters. One group of OCD patients includes patients

with obsessions about dirt and contamination, patients whose rituals center around compulsive washing and avoidance of contaminated objects. A second group includes patients who engage in pathological counting and compulsive checking. A third group includes purely obsessional patients with no compulsions. Primary obsessional slowness is evident in another group of patients, in whom slowness is the predominant symptom. Patients may spend many hours every day getting washed, dressed, and eating breakfast, and life goes on at an extremely slow speed. Some OCD patients, called *hoarders*, are unable to throw anything out for fear they might someday need something they discarded.

In DSM-IV, OCD is classified among the anxiety disorders because 1) anxiety is often associated with obsessions and resistance to compulsions, 2) anxiety or tension is often immediately relieved by yielding to compulsions, and 3) OCD often occurs in association with other anxiety disorders. However, compulsions decrease anxiety only transiently, and the nature of the fears in OCD is distinct from that in other anxiety disorders.

Certain diagnostic disputes regarding OCD were investigated in the DSM-IV field trial and the findings led to some changes in criteria and clarifications in DSM-IV. Even though obsessions are typically experienced as ego-dystonic, there is a wide range of insight in patients with OCD. Although most patients have some degree of insight, about 5% are convinced that their obsessions and compulsions are reasonable (Foa et al. 1995). On the basis on this finding, DSM-IV specified a poor insight type, which describes a patient who, for most of the time during the current episode, does not recognize that the obsessions and compulsions are excessive or unreasonable. DSM-IV has also made explicit that compulsions can be either behavioral or mental. Mental rituals are encountered in the great majority of OCD patients and, like behavioral compulsions, are intended to reduce anxiety or prevent harm. Although more than 90% of patients have features of both obsessions and compulsions, 28% are bothered mainly by obsessions, 20% by compulsions, and 50% by both (Foa et al. 1995).

CLINICAL DESCRIPTION

Onset

Obsessive-compulsive disorder usually begins in adolescence or early adulthood but can begin before that time; 31% of first episodes occur between ages 10 and 15 years and 75% develop by age 30 years (A. Black 1974). In most cases, no particular stress or event precipitates the onset of

TABLE 14–15.   DSM-IV diagnostic criteria for obsessive-compulsive disorder

A. Either obsessions or compulsions:

Obsessions as defined by (1), (2), (3), and (4):

(1) Recurrent and persistent thoughts, impulses, or images that are experienced, at some time during the disturbance, as intrusive and inappropriate and that cause marked anxiety or distress.

(2) The thoughts, impulses, or images are not simply excessive worries about real-life problems.

(3) The person attempts to ignore or suppress such thoughts, impulses, or images or to neutralize them with some other thought or action.

(4) The person recognizes that the obsessional thoughts, impulses, or images are a product of his or her own mind (not imposed from without as in thought insertion).

Compulsions as defined by (1) and (2):

(1) Repetitive behaviors (e.g., handwashing, ordering, checking) or mental acts (e.g., praying, counting, repeating words silently) that the person feels driven to perform in response to an obsession or according to rules that must be applied rigidly.

(2) The behaviors or mental acts are aimed at preventing or reducing distress or preventing some dreaded event or situation; however, these behaviors or mental acts either are not connected in a realistic way with what they are designed to neutralize or prevent or are clearly excessive.

B. At some point during the course of the disorder, the person has recognized that the obsessions or compulsions are excessive or unreasonable. **Note:** This does not apply to children.

C. The obsessions or compulsions cause marked distress, are time consuming (take more than 1 hour a day), or significantly interfere with the person's normal routine, occupational (or academic) functioning, or usual social activities or relationships.

D. If another Axis I disorder is present, the content of the obsessions or compulsions is not restricted to it (e.g., preoccupation with food in the presence of an eating disorder; hair pulling in the presence of trichotillomania; concern with appearance in the presence of body dysmorphic disorder; preoccupation with drugs in the presence of a substance use disorder; preoccupation with having a serious illness in the presence of hypochondriasis; preoccupation with sexual urges or fantasies in the presence of a paraphilia; or guilty ruminations in the presence of major depressive disorder).

E. The disturbance is not due to the direct physiological effects of a substance (e.g., a drug of abuse, a medication) or a general medical condition.

Specify if:

With poor insight: if, for most of the time during the current episode, the person does not recognize that the obsessions and compulsions are excessive or unreasonable

---

OCD symptoms, and after an insidious onset there is a chronic and often progressive course. However, some patients describe a sudden onset of symptoms. This is particularly true of patients with a neurological basis for their illness. There is evidence of OCD onset associated with the 1920s encephalitis epidemic (Meyer-Gross and Steiner 1921), abnormal birth events (Capstick and Seldrup 1977), head injury (McKeon et al. 1984), and seizures (Kehl and Marks 1986). Of interest are reports of new onset of OCD during pregnancy (Neziroglu et al. 1992).

Symptoms

Obsessions.   Obsessive and compulsive symptoms have been recognized for centuries and were first described in the psychiatric literature by Esquirol in 1838 (Rachman and Hodgson 1980). Obsessional thoughts were defined by Karl Westphal in 1878 as "ideas that in an otherwise intact intelligence, and without being caused by an emotional or affect-like state, against the will of the person . . . come into the foreground of the consciousness" (Westphal 1878, p. 735).

An obsession is an intrusive, unwanted mental event

usually evoking anxiety or discomfort. Obsessions may be thoughts, ideas, images, ruminations, convictions, fears, or impulses and are often of an aggressive, sexual, religious, disgusting, or nonsensical nature. Obsessional ideas are repetitive thoughts that interrupt the normal train of thinking, whereas obsessional images are often vivid visual experiences. Much obsessive thinking involves horrific ideas. The person may think of doing the worst possible thing (e.g., blasphemy, rape, murder, child molestation). Obsessional convictions are often characterized by an element of magical thinking, such as "step on the crack, break your mother's back." Obsessional ruminations may involve prolonged, excessive, and inconclusive thinking about metaphysical questions. Obsessional fears often involve dirt or contamination and differ from phobias in that they are present in the absence of the phobic stimulus. Other common obsessional fears have to do with harm coming to oneself or to others as a consequence of the patient's misdoings, such as burning one's home because the stove was not checked or running over a pedestrian because of careless driving. Obsessional impulses may be aggressive or sexual, such as intrusive impulses of stabbing one's spouse or raping one's child.

Attributing these obsessions to an internal source, the patient resists or controls them to a variable degree, and substantial impairment in functioning can result. *Resistance* is the struggle against an impulse or intrusive thought, and *control* is the patient's ability to divert his or her thinking. Obsessions are usually accompanied by compulsions but may also occur as the main or only symptom. Approximately 10%–25% of OCD patients are purely obsessional or suffer predominantly from obsessions (Akhtar et al. 1975; Rachman and Hodgson 1980; Welner et al. 1976).

Another hallmark of obsessive thinking involves lack of certainty or persistent doubting. In contrast to manic or psychotic patients, who manifest premature certainty, OCD patients are unable to achieve a sense of certainty between incoming sensory information and internal beliefs. They ask themselves such questions as "Are my hands clean?" "Is the door locked?" and "Is the fertilizer poisoning the water supply?" Compulsive rituals such as excessive washing or checking appear to arise from this lack of certainty and are misguided attempts to increase certainty.

Compulsions.   A compulsive ritual is a behavior that usually reduces discomfort but is carried out in a pressured or rigid fashion. Such behavior may include rituals involving washing, checking, repeating, avoiding, striving for completeness, and being meticulous. *Washers* represent about 25%–50% of most OCD samples (Akhtar et al. 1975; Rachman and Hodgson 1980; Rasmussen and Tsuang 1986). These individuals are concerned with dirt, contaminants, or germs and may spend many hours a day washing their hands or showering. They may also attempt to avoid contaminating themselves with feces, urine, or vaginal secretions.

Checkers have pathological doubt and thus compulsively check to see whether they have, for example, run over someone with their car or left the door unlocked. Checking often fails to resolve the doubt and in some cases may actually exacerbate it. In the DSM-IV field trial, washing and checking were the two most common groups of compulsions.

Although slowness results from most rituals, it is the *major* feature of the rare and disabling syndrome of primary obsessional slowness. It may take several hours for the obsessionally slow individual to get dressed or get out of the house. This slowness may be a response to a lack of certainty as well. These patients may have little anxiety despite their obsessions and rituals.

Mental compulsions are also quite common and should be inquired about directly, because they could go undetected if the clinician asks only about behavioral rituals. Such patients, for example, may replay over and over in their minds past conversations with others to make sure they did not somehow incriminate themselves. In the DSM-IV OCD field trials, 80% of patients had both behavioral and mental compulsions, and mental compulsions were the third most common type after checking and washing.

Although distinct symptom clusters exist (washers, checkers, those who are purely obsessional, hoarders, and those with primary slowness), these symptoms may overlap or develop sequentially.

Character Traits

Psychoanalytic theorists have suggested that there is a continuum between compulsive personality and OCD. Janet (1908) stated that all obsessional patients have a premorbid personality that is causally related to the disorder. Freud (1913/1958) noted an association between obsessional neurosis (i.e., OCD) symptoms and personality traits such as obstinacy, parsimony, punctuality, and orderliness.

However, phenomenological and epidemiologic evidence suggests that OCD is frequently distinct from obsessive-compulsive personality disorder. OCD symptoms are ego-dystonic, whereas obsessive-compulsive personality traits are ego-systonic and do not involve a sense of compulsion that must be resisted against. Epidemiologic studies show that obsessive-compulsive character pathology is neither necessary nor sufficient for the development of OCD symptoms. When patients with obsessional traits decompensate, they often develop depression, paranoia, or somatization rather than OCD. Although the older literature suggested the presence of definite obsessional traits in as many as two-thirds of OCD patients, structured personality assessments were not used. In more recent, standardized evaluations, only a minority of OCD patients had DSM-III-R–diagnosed obsessive-compulsive personality disorder, whereas other personality disorders such as avoidant or dependent personality disorder were more common (Thomsen and Mikkelsen 1993). In addition, personality disorders may be more common in the presence of OCD of a longer duration, which suggests that they could be secondary to the Axis I disorder, and criteria for personality disorders may no longer be met after successful treatment of OCD (Baer and Jenike 1992; Baer et al. 1990).

EPIDEMIOLOGY

Obsessive-compulsive disorder was previously considered one of the rarest mental disorders. Early studies suggested a maximum incidence of 5 in 10,000 persons (Woodruff and Pitts 1964). This finding was probably due to clinicians' relative unfamiliarity with the disorder until the last decade, OCD patients' secretiveness about their symptoms, and the fact that the average wait before seeking psychiatric help was 7.5 years (Rasmussen and Tsuang 1986). Current data from the Epidemiologic Catchment Area (ECA) study (described earlier in this chapter) suggest that OCD is quite common; the 1-month prevalence is 1.3%, the 6-month prevalence is 1.5%, and the lifetime rate is 2.5% (Regier et al. 1988).

In clinical samples of adult OCD, there is a roughly equal ratio of men to women (A. Black 1974). In the ECA epidemiologic sample, a slightly higher 1-month prevalence was found for women (1.5%) compared with men (1.1%), which was accounted for in the age range of 25–64 years, but this difference was not significant (Karno et al. 1988; Regier et al. 1988). However, in childhood-onset OCD, about 70% of patients are male (Hollingsworth et al. 1980; Swedo et al. 1989c). This difference seems to be accounted for by the earlier age at onset in males, and it may suggest partly differing etiologies or vulnerabilities in the two genders.

Twin and family studies have found a greater degree of concordance for OCD (defined broadly to include obsessional features) among monozygotic (MZ) twins compared with dizygotic twins (Carey and Gottesman 1981), which suggests that some predisposition to obsessional behavior is inherited. There have been no studies of OCD in adopted children or MZ twins raised apart. Studies of first-degree relatives of OCD patients show a higher-than-expected incidence of a variety of psychiatric symptoms and disorders, including obsessive-compulsive symptoms, anxiety disorders, and depression (D. W. Black et al. 1992; Carey and Gottesman 1981; Rapoport et al. 1981). Findings of family studies suggest a genetic link between OCD and Tourette's syndrome (Nee et al. 1982).

There are reports demonstrating comorbidity of OCD with schizophrenia, depression, other anxiety disorders such as panic disorder and simple and social phobia, eating disorders, autism, and Tourette's syndrome. Epidemiologically, the OCD comorbidity risk for other major psychiatric disorders was found to be fairly high but nondistinctive (Karno et al. 1988).

ETIOLOGY

Psychodynamic Theory

Psychodynamic theory views OCD as residing on a continuum with obsessive-compulsive character pathology and suggests that OCD develops when defense mechanisms fail to contain the obsessional character's anxiety. In this model, obsessive-compulsive pathology involves fixation and subsequent regression from the oedipal to the earlier, anal developmental phase. The fixation is presumably due to excessive investment in anal eroticism, resulting from excessive frustrations or gratifications in the anal phase.

Obsessive-compulsive patients are thought to use the defense mechanisms of isolation, undoing, reaction formation, and displacement to control unacceptable sexual and aggressive impulses. The defense mechanisms are unconscious and thus not readily apparent to the patient.

Isolation. Isolation is an attempt to separate the feelings or affects from the thoughts, fantasies, or impulses that are associated with them. An example of isolation is seen in the patient who describes a particularly gruesome thought or fantasy but denies any feelings of anxiety or disgust associated with it.

Undoing. Undoing is an attempt to reverse a psychological event, such as a word, thought, or gesture. An act can be undone by performing or evoking its opposite. For example, a patient who believes he has spent too much money on an item for his own pleasure may attempt to undo this by returning the object or by punishing himself through some other deprivation.

Reaction formation. In the defense of reaction formation, an unacceptable unconscious impulse is substituted with its opposite. A patient who has sadistic impulses to hurt people might behave in a passive or masochistic manner or pronounce his love excessively at moments of heightened anger.

Regression. In OCD, regression is theorized to take place from the genital oedipal phase to the earlier pregenital anal-sadistic phase, which has not been fully relinquished. This regression helps the patient avoid genital conflicts and the anxiety associated with them. Themes characteristic of the anal phase typically reflect conflicts surrounding ambivalence, control, dirt, order, and parsimony.

Ambivalence. In normal development, aggressive impulses are neutralized and loving feelings predominate toward significant objects. In OCD, strong aggressive impulses are thought to reemerge toward love objects, resulting in displaced ambivalence and paralyzing doubts. In addition, magical ideation and lack of certainty may predominate, such that thoughts of harming someone may lead to uncertainty over actually having harmed someone.

Learning Theory

A prominent behavioral model of the acquisition and maintenance of obsessive-compulsive symptoms derives from the two-stage learning theory of Mowrer (1939). In stage 1, anxiety is classically conditioned to a specific environmental event (i.e., classical conditioning). The person then engages in compulsive rituals (escape/avoidance responses) to decrease anxiety. If the individual is successful in reducing anxiety, the compulsive behavior is more likely to occur in the future (stage 2: operant conditioning). Higher-order conditioning occurs when other neutral stimuli such as words, images, or thoughts are associated with the initial stimulus and the associated anxiety is diffused. Ritualized behavior preserves the fear response, because the person avoids the eliciting stimulus and thus avoids extinction. Likewise, anxiety reduction following the ritual preserves the compulsive behavior.

Biological Theories

Although OCD used to be viewed as having a psychological etiology, a wealth of biological findings that have emerged over the past 15 years have rendered OCD one of the most elegantly elaborated psychiatric disorders from a biological standpoint. The association of OCD with a variety of neurological conditions or more subtle neurological findings has been known for some time. Such findings include

- The onset of OCD following head trauma (McKeon et al. 1984) or von Economo's disease (Schilder 1938)
- A high incidence of neurological premorbid illnesses in OCD (Grimshaw 1964)
- An association of OCD with birth trauma (Capstick and Seldrup 1977)
- Abnormalities on the electroencephalogram (Pacella et al. 1944), auditory evoked potentials (Ciesielski et al. 1981; Towey et al. 1990), and ventricular brain ratio on computed tomography scan (Behar et al. 1984)
- An association with diabetes insipidus (Barton 1965)
- The presence of significantly more neurological soft signs in OCD patients compared with healthy control subjects (Hollander et al. 1990b)

Basal ganglia abnormalities were particularly suspected in the pathogenesis of OCD. The disorder is closely associated with Tourette's syndrome (Nee et al. 1982; Pauls et al. 1986), in which basal ganglia dysfunction results in abnormal involuntary movements. OCD is also associated with Sydenham's chorea, another disorder of the basal ganglia (Barton 1965; Swedo et al. 1989b). Neuropsychological findings in OCD, although not always consistent, have suggested abnormalities in memory, memory confidence, trial-and-error learning, and processing speed (Christensen et al. 1992; Galderisi et al. 1996; Hollander et al. 1991b; McNally and Kohlbeck 1993; Otto 1992; Rubenstein et al. 1993).

Neuroimaging techniques permit a more sophisticated and elaborate elucidation of the functional anatomy underpinning OCD. In particular, orbitofrontal-limbic–basal ganglia circuits have been implicated in numerous studies. Baxter et al. (1987) compared OCD patients and normal control subjects using positron-emission tomography and found higher metabolic rates in the orbitofrontal gyri and caudate nuclei in OCD. Similarly, Swedo and her group (1989a) showed higher metabolic activity in the orbitofrontal and cingulate regions in OCD. After treatment of the OCD with serotonin reuptake inhibitors or with behavior therapy, hyperactivity decreases in the caudate, orbitofrontal lobes, and cingulate cortex in patients with good treatment responses (Baxter et al. 1992; Benkelfat et al. 1990; Perani et al. 1995; Swedo et al. 1992a). Also after successful behavioral treatment, the correlations in brain activity between the orbital gyri and the caudate nucleus decrease significantly, which suggests a decoupling of malfunctioning brain circuits (Schwartz et al. 1996). Flor-Henry (1983) hypothesized that "the fundamental symptomatology of obsessions is due to a defect in neural inhibition of dominant frontal systems, leading to the inability to inhibit unwanted verbal-ideational mental representations and their corresponding motor sequences" (p. 309). It has been suggested that the severity of obsessive urges correlates with orbitofrontal and basal ganglia activity, whereas the accompanying anxiety is reflected by activity in the hippocampus and cingulate cortex (McGuire et al. 1994). With functional magnetic resonance imaging (MRI), it has been possible to demonstrate that during the behavioral provocation of symptoms in OCD patients, significant increases in relative blood flow occur in real time in the caudate, cingulate cortex, and orbitofrontal cortex relative to the resting state (Breiter et al. 1996; Rauch et al. 1994).

A neuroethological model of OCD was proposed by Rapoport, Swedo, and their group (Swedo 1989; Wise and Rapoport 1989), based on the hypothesized orbitofrontal–limbic–basal ganglia dysfunction. The basal ganglia act as a gating station, filtering input from the orbitofrontal lobes and the cingulate cortex and mediating the execution of motor patterns. Obsessions and compulsions are conceptualized as species-specific fixed action patterns that normally are adaptive but in OCD become inappropriately released, repetitive, and excessive. This could be due to a heightened internal drive state or an increased responsivity to external releasers. For example, OCD behaviors such as excessive washing or saving may be dysregulated manifestations of normal grooming or hoarding behaviors.

The neurochemistry of OCD has also been extensively elaborated. Serotonin (5-hydroxytryptamine) has been implicated in the mediation of impulsivity, suicidality, aggression, anxiety, social dominance, and learning. Dysregulation of this behaviorally inhibitory neurotransmitter possibly contributes to the repetitive obsessions and ritualistic behaviors seen in OCD patients. Despite some conflicting and nonreplicated data, extensive research has now clearly implicated the serotonergic system in the pathogenesis of OCD. Considerable indirect evidence supporting the role of serotonin in OCD stems from the well-documented antiobsessional effects of potent serotonin reuptake inhibitors such as clomipramine and SSRIs, in contrast to the ineffectiveness of noradrenergic antidepressants such as desipramine. Furthermore, reduction of OCD symptoms during clomipramine treatment was shown to correlate with a decrease in platelet serotonin level (Flament et al. 1987) and in cerebrospinal fluid (CSF) 5-hydroxyindoleacetic acid (5-HIAA) (Altemus et al. 1992; Swedo et al. 1992b; Thorén et al. 1980b). Although one study reported higher CSF 5-HIAA in untreated OCD patients than in normal control subjects (Insel et al. 1985), this finding has not been replicated (Thorén et al. 1980b).

The use of pharmacological challenge agents to stimulate or block serotonin receptors has also led to elucidation of the neurochemistry of OCD. Oral *m*-chlorophenylpiperazine (m-CPP), a partial serotonin agonist, has been found to exacerbate obsessive-compulsive symptoms transiently in a subgroup of OCD patients (Hollander et al. 1992; Zohar et al. 1987). Results of studies involving intravenous m-CPP have been mixed (Charney et al. 1988; Pigott et al. 1993). After treatment of the OCD with serotonin reuptake inhibitors such as clomipramine or fluoxetine, m-CPP challenge no longer induced symptom exacerbation (Hollander et al. 1991a; Zohar et al. 1988). A blunted prolactin response to m-CPP challenge has also been found in OCD patients by some investigators (Charney et al. 1988; Hollander et al. 1992) but not others (Zohar et al. 1987). Similarly blunted prolactin responses in OCD have been induced with the serotonin agonist MK-212 (Bastani et al. 1990). Other serotonin agonists, such as tryptophan, fenfluramine, and ipsapirone, or antagonists such as metergoline, have not been shown to induce consistent behavioral or neuroendocrine response abnormalities in patients with OCD (Benkelfat et al. 1989; Charney et al. 1988; Hewlett et al. 1992b; Hollander et al. 1992; Lesch et al. 1991; McBride et al. 1992; Zohar et al. 1987).

In summary, all studies taken together suggest that serotonergic dysregulation in OCD is complex and probably involves variations in receptor function according to brain region and receptor subtypes. Thus, global hyperactivity or hypoactivity of the serotonergic system in OCD is a simplistic formulation. The m-CPP findings may suggest not only hypersensitivity of the serotonin receptors mediating obsessive-compulsive behaviors but also hyporesponsivity of the hypothalamic serotonin receptors mediating prolactin secretion (Hollander et al. 1992).

It also does not appear that serotonergic dysregulation alone can fully explain the neurochemistry of OCD. It is possible that the serotonergic system may, in part, be modulating or compensating for other dysfunctional neurotransmitter systems or neuromodulators. Various neuropeptide abnormalities have begun to be elucidated. Abnormalities in CSF vasopressin (Altemus et al. 1992; Swedo et al. 1992b), CSF somatostatin (Altemus et al. 1993), and CSF oxytocin (Leckman et al. 1994) have been implicated in OCD. With clomipramine treatment, CSF levels of vasopressin and somatostatin tend to decrease whereas oxytocin levels increase (Altemus et al. 1994). All these neuropeptides may be implicated in arousal, memory, and the acquisition and maintenance of conditioned perseverative behaviors. The noradrenergic α_2-agonist clonidine has been reported to induce a transient improvement in OCD symptoms when administered to patients intravenously (Hollander et al. 1991c) or orally (Knesevich 1982), although other noradrenergic challenge findings have been negative (Lucey et al. 1992). Dopaminergic dysregulation has been variously implicated in OCD (Goodman et al. 1990a) through the association between OCD and Tourette's syndrome; reports of exacerbation of obsessive-compulsive symptoms with chronic stimulants; an association between higher pretreatment CSF homovanillic acid (HVA) and good treatment outcome (Swedo et al. 1992b); and use of dopamine blockers to augment partial treatment response with serotonin reuptake inhibitors (McDougle et al. 1990).

Future studies on the biology of OCD will need to examine the interplay of abnormalities in functional neuroanatomy and in neurochemistry and to determine whether pathophysiologically distinct subgroups exist. Presumably, structural abnormalities are intimately linked with chemical disruptions in the neurotransmitter systems that make these structures function.

COURSE AND PROGNOSIS

Recent studies of the natural course of the illness suggest that 24%–33% of patients have a fluctuating course,

11%–14% have a phasic course with periods of complete remission, and 54%–61% have a constant or progressive course (A. Black 1974). Although prognosis of OCD has traditionally been considered to be poor, developments in behavioral and pharmacological treatments have improved prognosis considerably.

The disorder usually has a major impact on daily functioning; some patients with OCD spend many waking hours consumed with their obsessions and rituals. Patients are often socially isolated, marry at an older age, and have high celibacy rates (this is particularly true of male patients) and low fertility rates. Depression and anxiety are common complications of OCD.

DIAGNOSIS

Although a variety of biological and neuropsychiatric markers have been associated with OCD, the diagnosis rests on the psychiatric examination and history. DSM-IV defines OCD as the presence of either obsessions or compulsions that cause marked distress, are time consuming, or interfere with social or occupational functioning. Although all other Axis I disorders are allowed to be comorbidly present, the OCD symptoms must not be merely secondary to another disorder; for example, thoughts about food in the presence of an eating disorder and guilty thoughts in the presence of major depression are not OCD symptoms. The diagnosis is usually clear-cut, but occasionally it can be more difficult to distinguish OCD from depression, psychosis, phobias, or severe obsessive-compulsive personality disorder.

DIFFERENTIAL DIAGNOSIS

Schizophrenia

The course of OCD may more closely resemble that of schizophrenia, in that there may be chronic debilitation, decline, and profound impairment in social and occupational functioning. Sometimes it is difficult to distinguish between an obsession (i.e., contamination) and a delusion (i.e., being poisoned). An obsession is typically egodystonic, resisted, and recognized as having an internal origin. A delusion is not resisted and is believed to be external. However, OCD patients may lack insight, and obsessions in 12% of cases may become delusions (Gittleson 1966). Yet longitudinal studies show that OCD patients are not at increased risk for developing schizophrenia (A. Black 1974). Both disorders may exist independently, and DSM-IV allows the diagnosis of both disorders. Thus, notable obsessive-compulsive symptoms in a schizophrenic patient warrant separate treatment.

Depression

Patients with OCD frequently have complicating depressions, and these patients may be difficult to distinguish from depressed patients who have complicating obsessive symptoms. Patients with psychotic depression, agitated depression, or premorbid obsessional features that occur before development of depression are particularly likely to develop obsessions (Gittleson 1966). These "secondary" obsessions often involve aggressive themes, but the distinction between primary and secondary obsessions rests on the order of occurrence. In addition, depressive ruminations, in contrast to pure obsessions, are often focused on a past incident rather than on a current or future event and are rarely resisted.

Phobic Disorders

A close connection exists between OCD and phobic and anxiety disorders. OCD patients who are compulsive cleaners appear very similar to phobic individuals and are often mislabeled "germ phobics." Both exhibit avoidant behavior, both show intense subjective and autonomic responses to focal stimuli, and both are said to respond to similar behavioral interventions (Rachman and Hodgson 1980). Both have excessive fear, although disgust is prominent in OCD patients and not in phobic patients. Also, OCD patients can never entirely avoid the obsession, whereas phobic patients have more focal, external stimuli that they can successfully avoid.

Patients with OCD who experience high levels of anxiety may describe panic-like episodes, but these episodes are secondary to obsessions and do not arise spontaneously. Unlike in panic disorder patients, there is no precipitation of anxiety attack with lactate infusions in OCD patients (Gorman et al. 1985). However, OCD does appear to have increased comorbidity with simple and social phobia and panic disorder (Rasmussen and Tsuang 1986).

TREATMENT

Pharmacotherapy

Advances of the past decade in the pharmacotherapy of OCD have been dramatic and have generated excitement in the study of this disorder. What was previously thought to be a rare, psychodynamically laden, and difficult-to-treat illness now appears to have a strong biological component and to respond well to potent serotonin reuptake inhibitors. The pharmacological treatment approach to OCD is summarized in Table 14–16.

The most extensively studied medication for the treat-

TABLE 14–16. Pharmacological treatment of obsessive-compulsive disorder

Serotonin reuptake inhibitors

General indication: First-choice treatment

Clomipramine: Most studied in efficacy

Fluvoxamine: Superior to desipramine and placebo, well studied

Fluoxetine: Effective

Sertraline: Effective, less well studied

Paroxetine: Effective, less well studied

Augmentation strategies

General indications: Partial response to serotonin reuptake inhibitors; presence of other target symptoms

Buspirone: Anxiety

Clonazepam: Anxiety, insomnia, panic attacks

Fenfluramine: Depression

Trazodone: Insomnia, depression

Lithium: Affective lability, bipolar features

Pimozide: Tics, schizotypal features, delusional symptoms

Haloperidol: Tics, schizotypal features, delusional symptoms

Combination treatments

General indications: Poor tolerance of clomipramine or selective serotonin reuptake inhibitor alone; partial response to clomipramine or selective serotonin reuptake inhibitor alone

Precautions: Use low doses of each medication; monitor clomipramine levels

Clomipramine + a selective serotonin reuptake inhibitor (i.e., fluoxetine, sertraline, fluvoxamine)

---

ment of OCD is clomipramine, a potent serotonin reuptake inhibitor with weak norepinephrine reuptake blockade. A series of well-controlled double-blind studies have undisputedly documented the efficacy of clomipramine in reducing OCD symptoms (Ananth et al. 1981; Flament et al. 1985; Insel et al. 1983; Thorén et al. 1980a). The largest of these studies was a multicenter trial in which clomipramine therapy was compared with placebo in more than 500 patients with OCD. At an average dosage of 200–250 mg/day of clomipramine, the average reduction in OCD symptoms was about 40%, and about 60% of all patients were clinically much or very much improved (Clomipramine Collaborative Study Group 1991). The very low placebo response rate of 2% documents that OCD is a chronic disorder with infrequent spontaneous remissions. Therapy should typically be begun at 25 mg of clomipramine at night, and the dose should then be gradually increased by 25 mg every 4 days or by 50 mg every week, until a maximum dose of 250 mg is reached. Some pa-

tients are unable to tolerate the highest dose and may be stabilized on 150 or 200 mg. Improvement with clomipramine therapy is relatively slow; maximal response occurs after 5–12 weeks of treatment. Some of the more common side effects reported by patients are dry mouth, tremor, sedation, nausea, and ejaculatory failure (in men). The seizure risk is comparable to that of other tricyclics and is acceptable in the absence of neurological history for dosages up to 250 mg/day. Clomipramine therapy is equally effective for OCD patients with pure obsessions and those with rituals; behavioral treatments, on the other hand, are less useful for patients suffering predominantly from obsessions. Although one study found a greater effect of clomipramine therapy compared with placebo only in the most depressed subgroup (Marks et al. 1980), the majority of studies found specific antiobsessional effects irrespective of depressive symptoms (Ananth et al. 1981; Clomipramine Collaborative Study Group 1991; Flament et al. 1985; Insel et al. 1983; Thorén et al. 1980a). Controlled studies have also demonstrated that clomipramine is effective in treating OCD when other antidepressants, such as amitriptyline, nortriptyline, desipramine, and the MAOI clorgyline, have no therapeutic effect (Ananth et al. 1981; Insel et al. 1983; Leonard et al. 1989; Thorén et al. 1980a; Zohar and Insel 1987). This finding strongly suggests that improvement in OCD symptoms is mediated through the blockade of serotonin reuptake.

Studies involving the more selective serotonin reuptake inhibitors, such as fluoxetine, fluvoxamine, sertraline, and paroxetine, have further supported this hypothesis. A controlled study comparing clomipramine and fluoxetine treatment in OCD did not find a significant difference in efficacy between the two drugs (Pigott et al. 1990), although the response with fluoxetine appeared somewhat less robust than did the response with clomipramine. Patients usually experience fewer anticholinergic side effects when taking fluoxetine than when taking clomipramine. Fluoxetine has been shown to be superior to placebo in treating OCD, in dosages of 20–60 mg/day, and there may be greater efficacy at higher doses (Montgomery et al. 1993; Tollefson et al. 1994). Similarly, fluoxetine has been shown to be safe and efficacious in treating OCD in children (Riddle et al. 1992).

Fluvoxamine was also found to have a significant antiobsessional effect in several controlled studies (Goodman et al. 1989, 1990b; Jenike et al. 1990a; Perse et al. 1987); efficacy was comparable to that of clomipramine (Freeman et al. 1994; Koran et al. 1996). Goodman and his group (1990b) showed that fluvoxamine is superior to desipramine in treating OCD. In their study, 52% of patients demonstrated marked clinical improvement independent of initial depression. The required daily dose is titrated up to a maximum of 300 mg. The efficacy of fluvoxamine in OCD has also been demonstrated in adolescent patients, at dosages of 100–300 mg/day (Apter et al. 1994).

Sertraline is another serotonin reuptake inhibitor whose efficacy in OCD has been established. Although an initial placebo-controlled study revealed no beneficial effect (Jenike et al. 1990b), subsequent studies showed sertraline to be superior to placebo, at daily doses ranging from 50 mg to 200 mg (Chouinard 1992; Greist et al. 1995a, 1995b).

Although clomipramine appears to have an edge in documented efficacy for treating OCD, satisfactory systematic comparisons of the various serotonin reuptake inhibitors, in which benefits and side effects are balanced, have not been conducted. Given the similar efficacy of these five medications in OCD, an extremely large prospective study would have to be undertaken to demonstrate small but significant differences between the various medications. Three meta-analyses addressed these questions by retrospective analysis of treatment data from past trials and showed clomipramine to be slightly but significantly more effective than the SSRIs (Greist et al. 1995b; Piccinelli et al. 1995; D. J. Stein et al. 1995). However, the clinical applicability of this finding may be limited, because in clinical practice actual or expected tolerability of different medications often takes precedence over small differences in efficacy.

The response to medication therapy in OCD is not as dramatic as in, for example, major depression; a considerable number of patients show a negligible or partial response to the aforementioned first-line medications. Approximately 50%–60% of OCD patients improve by about 50%–60% with a first-line drug. Thus, various combination and augmentation strategies are often needed to attain a satisfactory response. The most commonly used augmenting agents, aimed at further boosting the serotonergic system, are buspirone, lithium, tryptophan, fenfluramine, trazodone, and clonazepam (Hewlett et al. 1990; Hollander et al. 1990a; Jenike et al. 1991a; Rasmussen 1984). Although augmentation has been reported to be effective, negative reports on the subject are also common and thus general augmentation strategies for OCD have not been convincingly demonstrated. Still, given the often limited treatment options, such strategies are well worth undertaking sequentially on an individual-case basis.

Although a small study reported similar efficacy for clomipramine alone versus buspirone alone in treating OCD (Pato et al. 1991), three other studies failed to show that buspirone augmentation had a significant benefit in clomipramine-treated (Pigott et al. 1992b), fluoxetine-treated (Grady et al. 1993), or fluvoxamine-treated

(McDougle et al. 1993b) patients. A controlled study of lithium augmentation of clomipramine did not detect any additional benefit (Pigott et al. 1991). A controlled study of trazodone alone in OCD showed no benefit compared with placebo (Pigott et al. 1992a). A controlled crossover study showed clonazepam to be effective in 40% of OCD subjects failing to respond to clomipramine (Hewlett et al. 1992a). Neuroleptics are another class of medications that can be successfully used to augment partial response to serotonin reuptake inhibitors. McDougle et al. (1990) reported that about 50% of OCD patients improved noticeably when pimozide was added to fluvoxamine therapy; comorbid tic disorders or schizotypal personality predicted a good response, which is in support of the hypothesis that the dopaminergic system may be dysregulated in at least a subgroup of patients with OCD (Goodman et al. 1990a). OCD patients with comorbid tic disorders may actually be less responsive to SSRI monotherapy (McDougle et al. 1993a) and appear to respond well to haloperidol augmentation (McDougle et al. 1994). Risperidone has also been successfully used for augmentation; the drug has had good results in cases of horrific mental imagery rather than in comorbid tic disorders (Saxena et al. 1996). The atypical neuroleptic clozapine has been reported to worsen OCD, possibly because of its particular serotonergic properties, although reports are contradictory (Baker et al. 1992; Ghaemi et al. 1995). Clomipramine combined with an SSRI is also used to treat refractory patients and is generally well tolerated, although lower doses of clomipramine should be used and blood levels should be monitored so that toxicity is avoided, because clomipramine levels can become markedly elevated (Szegedi et al. 1996). Finally, intravenous clomipramine has met with success in some patients refractory to oral clomipramine therapy (Fallon et al. 1992; Warneke 1985). The next line of medications for refractory patients, although their use is supported by fewer data, are the MAOIs (Vallejo et al. 1992). Electroconvulsive therapy may also be considered in highly refractory patients, although its efficacy is debatable (Maletzky et al. 1994).

Although there are no definitive predictors of medication treatment response, several factors appear to be predictive of a poorer prognosis, including earlier age at onset, longer duration of illness, higher frequency of compulsions, washing rituals, a chronic course, previous hospitalizations, and the presence of avoidant, borderline, and schizotypal as well as multiple personality disorders (Ackerman et al. 1994; Baer and Jenike 1992; Baer et al. 1992; Ravizza et al. 1995).

In extreme cases, involving refractory, severely impaired OCD patients, neurosurgery can be considered. In a thorough retrospective analysis, Jenike and his group (1991b) estimated that in at least 25%–30% of patients, cingulotomy resulted in notable improvement. This response rate was confirmed in a 2-year prospective cingulotomy study (Baer et al. 1995). A comparable response rate of 38% was reported in another study in 10 years of follow-up after the stereotactic surgery (Hay et al. 1993). Guidelines for the use of neurosurgical techniques in the treatment of severe, refractory OCD—including selection, documented failed treatments, indications, contraindications, benefits, risks, and workup—have been thoroughly reviewed elsewhere (Mindus and Jenike 1992).

OCD tends to be a chronic illness, and many patients may require drug treatment for an indefinite length of time to stay well. Long-term continuation of medication treatment generally maintains a good treatment response; this statement is widely supported in clinical treatment and has been validated by a 1-year, double-blind sertraline maintenance study in dosages of 50–200 mg/day (Greist et al. 1995a). In a double-blind discontinuation study of OCD patients who had done well on clomipramine for about 1 year, 90% experienced substantial worsening within 7 weeks (Pato et al. 1988). The same relapse rate of 90% was found in an adolescent OCD group when chronic clomipramine was blindly substituted with 8 weeks of desipramine (Leonard et al. 1991). At follow-up after several years, most patients remain symptomatic and require continued pharmacotherapy; a substantial minority of 20% remain refractory to multiple treatment regimens (Leonard et al. 1993).

Behavior Therapy

Behavioral treatments of OCD involve two separate components: 1) exposure procedures that aim to decrease the anxiety associated with obsessions and 2) response prevention techniques that aim to decrease the frequency of rituals or obsessive thoughts. Exposure techniques range from systematic desensitization with brief imaginal exposure, to flooding, in which prolonged exposure to the real-life ritual-evoking stimuli causes profound discomfort. Exposure techniques aim to ultimately decrease the discomfort associated with the eliciting stimuli through habituation. In exposure therapy, the patient is assigned homework exercises that must be performed and the patient may require assistance in achieving exposure at home through therapists' home visits or from family members. Response prevention involves having patients face feared stimuli (e.g., dirt, chemicals) without excessive hand washing or having them tolerate doubt (e.g., doubt about whether the door is locked) without excessive checking. Initial work may in-

volve delaying performance of the ritual, but ultimately the patient attempts to resist the compulsions fully. The psychoeducation and support of family members can be pivotal to the success of the behavior therapy, because family dysfunction is prevalent and the majority of parents or spouses accommodate to or are involved in the patients' rituals, possibly as a way to reduce the anxiety or anger that patients may direct at their family members (Calvocoressi et al. 1995; Shafran et al. 1996).

It is generally agreed that combined behavioral techniques (i.e., exposure with response prevention) yield the greatest improvement. It is also generally reported that patients who primarily suffer from obsessions and have few rituals are the least responsive to behavioral treatment, although new behavioral techniques for obsessions may be more promising (Salkovskis and Westbrook 1989). When the combined techniques of in vivo exposure and response prevention were used, up to 75% of ritualizing patients willing and able to undergo the arduous treatment were reported to show substantial improvement (Marks et al. 1975). Marks et al. (1988) reported that self-exposure constitutes the most powerful treatment component; however, clomipramine doses in this study were rather low (i.e., 125–150 mg), and therapist-aided exposure was instituted late in the treatment and briefly. The addition of imaginal exposure to in vivo exposure/response prevention is reported to help maintain treatment gains, perhaps by moderating obsessive fears of future catastrophes (Steketee et al. 1982). Foa and her group (1984) systematically compared in vivo exposure, response prevention, and the two treatments combined. All study groups improved, but the combined treatment was superior in decreasing anxiety, rituals, and overall impairment. The proportion of clinical responders, defined as those patients who showed at least 30% improvement with treatment, was 33% in the response prevention group, 55% in the exposure group, and 90% in the group receiving combination treatment. This study also found that the majority of OCD patients successfully treated with behavior therapy had relapsed at follow-up, which suggests that, just as with medication, long-term behavioral maintenance treatment may be necessary. Predictors of poorer outcome for behavioral treatment of OCD include initial depression, initial OCD severity, longer duration, and lower motivation for treatment (Keijsers et al. 1994). It is not yet known how behavioral techniques compare with medications in treating OCD. Controlled studies, in which patients with comparable illness severity and symptomatology are randomized to the different treatments, are needed to determine the relative and combined efficacy of behavior therapy and pharmacotherapy. Such trials are currently under way.

Cognitive Therapy

Also more recently advocated for the treatment of OCD has been cognitive therapy, a form of therapy centering on cognitive reformulation of themes related to the perception of danger, estimation of catastrophe, expectations about anxiety and its consequences, excessive responsibility, thought-action fusion, and illogical inferences (Freeston et al. 1996; O'Connor and Robillard 1996; Rachman et al. 1995; vanOppen and Arntz 1994). A review of 15 open and controlled cognitive trials showed overall little evidence of improvement in OCD when cognitive therapy was added to the existing pharmacological and behavioral techniques (I. A. James and Blackburn 1995). However, one controlled study showed cognitive therapy, exposure, and response prevention to have similar effectiveness in treating OCD (vanOppen et al. 1995).

Other Psychotherapy

Patients with OCD frequently present with symptoms that appear laden with unconscious symbolism and dynamic meaning. However, OCD has generally proven refractory to psychoanalytically oriented, as well as to loosely structured, nondirective exploratory psychotherapies. In contrast to its lack of efficacy in treating chronic OCD, dynamic psychotherapy may be helpful for patients with acute and limited symptoms who are otherwise psychologically minded and motivated to explore their conflicts, as well as in dealing with obsessive character traits of perfectionism, doubting, procrastination, and indecisiveness (Salzman 1985). However, controlled clinical data are not available to support these clinical impressions.

OCD patients need supportive treatment even while pharmacotherapy or behavior therapy is being applied. Because of their tendency toward excessive doubt, these patients may require a great deal of reassurance during the early phase of treatment. More active supportive therapy that encourages risk taking helps OCD patients live with their anxiety, and a focus on the present has been reported to be helpful (Salzman 1985). In addition, psychoeducational support groups for OCD patients and their families have been described as being highly successful in helping treat these patients (D. W. Black and Blum 1992; Tynes et al. 1992).

POSTTRAUMATIC STRESS DISORDER

DEFINITION

Posttraumatic stress disorder (PTSD) was first introduced in DSM-III, its inclusion being spurred in part by the increasing recognition of posttraumatic conditions in veterans of the Vietnam War. The current DSM-IV criteria for PTSD are presented in Table 14–17. As in DSM-III-R, the disorder continues to be classified with the anxiety disorders, and the major criteria of an extreme precipitating stressor, intrusive recollections, emotional numbing, and hyperarousal have been maintained. The DSM-III-R descriptor of the traumatic event—one "outside the range of usual human experience"—was considered vague and unreliable and was eliminated. New duration criteria were also established, subdividing the disorder into acute or chronic.

Not all investigators agree that PTSD belongs with the anxiety disorders. Although anxiety is a prominent symptom, depression and dissociation are prominent symptoms as well. The diagnostic criterion of a precipitating stressor or trauma in PTSD makes this disorder different from other anxiety disorders and is more reminiscent of conditions such as brief reactive psychosis, acute stress disorder, pathological bereavement, and adjustment disorders. The International Classification of Diseases, 10th Revision (ICD-10; World Health Organization 1992), for example, classifies all such disorders as stress related. In acknowledgment of the spectrum of disorders stemming from severe stress, DSM-IV added acute stress disorder to the anxiety disorders. Acute stress disorder is similar to PTSD with regard to the precipitating traumatic event and to symptomatology but is time limited, occurring up to 1 month after the event.

Beyond the symptoms of PTSD per se, increasing attention has been drawn to an enduring constellation of traits that frequently develop in individuals subjected to chronic trauma as children or adults. Investigators such as Herman and van der Kolk have suggested that a discrete entity of complicated posttraumatic syndromes be recognized, otherwise designated as *DESNOS* (disorders of extreme stress not otherwise specified), characterized by lasting changes in identity, interpersonal relationships, and the sense of life's meaning (Herman et al. 1989; van der Kolk and Saporta 1991). Similar personality changes are recognized by ICD-10 and classified as "enduring personality change after catastrophic experience." Attention has been drawn to a concept of "trauma-spectrum" disorders, which result primarily from chronic childhood intrafamilial abuse and encompass diverse manifestations such as borderline personality disorder and multiple personality disorder (Herman and van der Kolk 1987; Herman et al. 1989; van der Kolk 1988).

CLINICAL DESCRIPTION

A soldier participates in the torture and murder of civilians. A passenger is the sole survivor of a commercial air-

TABLE 14-17. **DSM-IV diagnostic criteria for posttraumatic stress disorder**

A. The person has been exposed to a traumatic event in which both of the following were present:

   (1) The person experienced, witnessed, or was confronted with an event or events that involved actual or threatened death or serious injury or a threat to the physical integrity of self or others.

   (2) The person's response involved intense fear, helplessness, or horror. **Note:** In children, this may be expressed instead by disorganized or agitated behavior.

B. The traumatic event is persistently reexperienced in one (or more) of the following ways:

   (1) Recurrent and intrusive distressing recollections of the event, including images, thoughts, or perceptions. **Note:** In young children, repetitive play may occur in which themes or aspects of the trauma are expressed.

   (2) Recurrent distressing dreams of the event. **Note:** In children, there may be frightening dreams without recognizable content.

   (3) Acting or feeling as if the traumatic event were recurring (includes a sense of reliving the experience, illusions, hallucinations, and dissociative flashback episodes, including those that occur on awakening or when intoxicated). **Note:** In young children, trauma-specific reenactment may occur.

   (4) Intense psychological distress at exposure to internal and external cues that symbolize or resemble an aspect of the traumatic event.

   (5) Physiologic reactivity on exposure to internal or external cues that symbolize or resemble an aspect of the traumatic event.

C. Persistent avoidance of stimuli associated with the trauma and numbing of general responsiveness (not present before the trauma), as indicated by three (or more) of the following:

   (1) Efforts to avoid thoughts, feelings, or conversations associated with the trauma

   (2) Efforts to avoid activities, places, or people that arouse recollections of the trauma

   (3) Inability to recall an important aspect of the trauma

   (4) Markedly diminished interest or participation in significant activities

   (5) Feeling of detachment or estrangement from others

   (6) Restricted range of affect (e.g., unable to have loving feelings)

   (7) Sense of a foreshortened future (e.g., does not expect to have a career, marriage, children, or a normal life span)

D. Persistent symptoms of increased arousal (not present before the trauma), as indicated by two (or more) of the following:

   (1) Difficulty falling or staying asleep

   (2) Irritability or outbursts of anger

   (3) Difficulty concentrating

   (4) Hypervigilance

   (5) Exaggerated startle response

E. Duration of the disturbance (symptoms in criteria B, C, and D) is more than 1 month.

F. The disturbance causes clinically significant distress or impairment in social, occupational, or other important areas of functioning.

Specify if:

Acute: if duration of symptoms is less than 3 months

Chronic: if duration of symptoms is 3 months or more

Specify if:

With delayed onset: if onset of symptoms is at least 6 months after the stressor

---

liner. A woman is raped and severely beaten by an unknown assailant.

The characteristic features that may develop after a traumatic event such as those just described include psychic numbing, reexperiencing of the trauma, and increased autonomic arousal. The trauma is reexperienced in recurrent painful, intrusive recollections, daydreams, or nightmares. Dissociative states may occur, lasting from minutes to days, in which there is an actual reliving of the event. Psychic numbing or emotional anesthesia is manifested by diminished responsiveness to the external world, involving feelings of being detached from other people, loss of interest in usual activities, and inability to feel emotions such as intimacy, tenderness, or sexual interest. Symptoms of ex-

cessive autonomic arousal may include hyperactivity and irritability, an exaggerated startle response, difficulty concentrating, and sleep abnormalities. Rape or mugging victims sometimes become afraid to venture out alone for variable periods. Situations reminiscent of the original trauma may be systematically avoided.

Other symptoms may include guilt about having survived, guilt about not having prevented the traumatic experience, depression, anxiety, panic attacks, shame, and rage. There may be prolonged episodes of intense affect; increased irritability; explosive, hostile behavior; and impulsive behavior. Other accompanying or complicating symptoms associated with PTSD may include substance abuse, self-injurious behavior and suicide attempts, occupational impairment, and interference with interpersonal relationships.

EPIDEMIOLOGY

Although there are marked individual differences in how people react to stress, when stressors become extreme (such as in concentration camp situations or in extended combat) the rate of morbidity rapidly increases (Eitinger 1971; Krystal 1968). Posttraumatic syndromes may be found in up to 30% of victims of disasters (Chapman 1962). Long-term physical health effects have been noted in persons 30 years after their having survived concentration camps (Eitinger 1971).

Although this disorder has been more extensively studied in select groups, such as survivors of combat, concentration camps, and natural disasters, the Epidemiologic Catchment Area (ECA) study (described earlier in this chapter) investigated the occurrence of PTSD in the general population (Helzer et al. 1987). A 1% lifetime prevalence of PTSD was found (0.5% in men and 1.3% in women). The nature of the precipitating trauma differed between the two genders. Combat and witnessing someone's injury or death were the two traumas identified in men, whereas physical attack or threat accounted for almost half of the traumas in women. The presence of a few symptoms of PTSD (that is, too few to meet the full diagnostic criteria) was quite common in the general population. A high rate of comorbid disorders was found. The highest comorbidity was with affective disorders and OCD. Men with PTSD had no increased risk for panic disorder or phobias, whereas women with PTSD had a threefold to fourfold risk for these disorders.

In another large, random community survey of young adults, the lifetime prevalence of PTSD was 9.2%, higher than that found in the ECA study (Breslau et al. 1991). As in the ECA study, the prevalence was higher in women (11.3%) than in men (6%). A high comorbidity risk was found for OCD, agoraphobia, panic, and depression. The association with drug or alcohol abuse was weaker. In the more recent National Comorbidity Survey, the lifetime prevalence of PTSD was found to be 7.8%, much higher than in the ECA study, and was more common in women; the most common stressors were combat exposure in men and sexual assault in women (Kessler et al. 1995).

ETIOLOGY

The Role of the Stressor

The severity of the stressor in PTSD differs in magnitude from that in adjustment disorder; in adjustment disorder, the stressor is usually less severe and within the range of common life experience. However, this relationship between the severity of the stressor and the type of subsequent symptomatology is not always predictable. For example, studies of bereavement and divorce have found that stressors within the range of usual human experience can also produce a distinctive syndrome of reexperiencing the trauma (Horowitz et al. 1980).

Nevertheless, events such as rape and burglary, which are insults to personal integrity, self-esteem, and security, are particularly likely to lead to PTSD. When stressors become extreme (e.g., rape, extended combat, torture, or concentration camp experiences), the rate of morbidity increases markedly. For example, the ECA study found that among men who had served in Vietnam, 4% of those who had been in combat but had not been wounded had PTSD, whereas 20% of those who had been in combat and had been wounded developed PTSD. In a random community survey, approximately one-fourth of all individuals who experienced major trauma developed PTSD (Breslau et al. 1991). As described by McFarlane, a definite dose-response relationship exists between the impact of the trauma and PTSD. Still, it is rare even for overwhelming trauma to lead to PTSD in more than half of the exposed populations, which suggests that other etiological factors also play a role (McFarlane 1990).

In recent years, greater attention has been given to dissociative phenomena and to their relationship to posttraumatic symptoms. Such study has revealed that greater dissociation around the time of the traumatic event is a strong predictor of the later development of PTSD (Marmar et al. 1994; Shalev et al. 1996). It may be that early peritraumatic dissociation can serve as a "marker" to identify individuals who will be at high risk for developing future PTSD.

Premorbid Predictors

There is some disagreement in the literature concerning whether premorbid factors predispose to the development of PTSD. Although the disorder can develop in people who do not have much preexisting psychopathology, some studies suggest that predisposing psychological factors or adverse childhood experiences may render individuals more vulnerable to the development of PTSD. A number of confounding problems makes the study of the relationship of premorbid factors and PTSD difficult (Lindy et al. 1984):

- There may be a lack of reliable premorbid data.
- Retrospective self-reports may be unreliable.
- Character pathology may influence group selection

(such as volunteers vs. draftees, assignment to combat duty, survival).

■ Character pathology may be secondary to the trauma rather than precede it.

■ Indicators of character pathology may overlap with characteristics of PTSD.

In one study of a Vietnam veteran outreach center, a history of good adolescent friendships was predictive of PTSD, whereas a history of poor adolescent friendships was more likely in those who did not have PTSD (Lindy et al. 1984). In addition, this study reported that a number of patients with good premorbid adjustment, low level of childhood trauma, and good adolescent relationships experienced prolonged trauma in Vietnam and developed severe PTSD.

It has been suggested that the greater the amount of previous trauma experienced by an individual, the more likely he or she is to develop symptoms after a stressful life event (Horowitz et al. 1980). In addition, individuals with previous traumatic experiences may be more likely to become exposed to future traumas, because they can be prone to reenact the original trauma behaviorally (van der Kolk 1989). McFarlane (1989) found that the severity of exposure to disaster was the major determinant of early posttraumatic morbidity, whereas preexisting psychological disorders better predicted the persistence of posttraumatic symptoms after 29 months. In the ECA sample, a history of childhood conduct problems before age 15 years was predictive of PTSD. Patients with anxious premorbid states and family histories of anxiety may also respond to a trauma with pathological anxiety and develop PTSD (Scrignar 1984). An epidemiologic survey identified, albeit retrospectively, different risk factors for becoming exposed to trauma versus developing PTSD after traumatic exposure (Breslau et al. 1991). Risk factors for exposure to trauma were male gender, childhood conduct problems, extroversion, and family history of substance abuse or psychiatric problems. Risk factors for developing PTSD after traumatic exposure were disrupted parental attachments, anxiety, depression, and family history of anxiety. Compared with nonchronic PTSD, chronic PTSD of more than 1 year's duration has been specifically associated with female gender, higher rates of comorbid anxiety and depressive disorders, and a family history of antisocial behavior (Breslau and Davis 1992). In a study of Vietnam veterans, individuals with PTSD had higher rates of childhood physical abuse than veterans without PTSD, as well as a significantly higher rate of total traumatic events before entrance into the military (Bremner et al. 1993a).

Biological Theories

More than a century ago, Janet described the breakdown in normal adaptation, information processing, and action that can result from overwhelming trauma and noted the automatic emotional and physical overreaction that occurs with reexposure (van der Kolk and van der Hart 1989). Freud (1919/1955) implicated a biological basis to posttraumatic symptoms, in the form of a physical fixation to the trauma. Pavlov (1927/1960) demonstrated chronic change in autonomic nervous system activity level in response to repeated traumatic exposure. Kardiner (1959) comprehensively described the phenomenology of war traumatic neurosis, identifying five cardinal features: 1) persistence of startle response, 2) fixation on the trauma, 3) atypical dream life, 4) explosive outbursts, and 5) overall constriction of personality. He called this condition a "physioneurosis," a term implying an interaction of psychological and biological processes; the condition serves as a forerunner of current psychobiological models of PTSD.

Noradrenergic system. The neurobiological response to acute stress and trauma involves the release of various stress hormones that allow the organism to respond adaptively to stress. These releases include heightened secretion of catecholamines and cortisol. When PTSD develops under severe or repeated trauma, the stress response becomes dysregulated and chronic autonomic hyperactivity sets in, manifesting itself in the "positive" symptoms of PTSD—that is, hyperarousal and intrusive recollections. A wide range of data support this hypothesis. The noradrenergic system, originating in the locus coeruleus, regulates arousal. Animals exposed to inescapable shock initially show evidence of increased turnover of norepinephrine, with subsequent depletion of central norepinephrine (Anisman et al. 1980). Animals that have experienced previous inescapable shock are more sensitive to norepinephrine depletion. In patients with PTSD, heightened physiological responses to stressful stimuli, such as increased blood pressure, heart rate, respiration, galvanic skin response, and electromyographic activity, have been consistently documented (Kolb 1987; Pitman et al. 1987). Long-standing increases in the urinary catecholamines norepinephrine and epinephrine have been found in PTSD patients (Kosten et al. 1987). Agents that stimulate the arousal system, such as lactate (Rainey et al. 1987) and yohimbine (Southwick et al. 1993), induce flashbacks and increases in core PTSD symptoms. Clinical improvement in intrusive recollections and hyperarousal during open treatment with adrenergic blocking agents, such as clonidine or propranolol, also suggests adrenergic hyperactivity (Kolb et al. 1984).

A decrease in the number and sensitivity of α_2-adrenergic receptors, possibly as a consequence of chronic noradrenergic hyperactivity, has been reported in PTSD (Perry et al. 1987). Downregulation of the α_2-adrenergic receptor is also supported by one case report of a PTSD patient with a blunted growth hormone response to clonidine, which normalized after behavioral treatment (Hansenne et al. 1991). In addition, there is evidence that chronic hyperarousal blunts the adaptive steroid response to stress.

A kindling model has also been proposed to clarify the positive symptoms of PTSD (Lipper 1990). It posits that intrusive recollections, such as flashbacks or nightmares, are actual reexperiences of stored memories, triggered by oversensitization of the limbic system. Presumably, such kindling is a result of the repeated traumatic experiences and associated hyperarousal, which progressively sensitize the limbic neurons and lower their firing threshold. Indirect evidence for such a theory comes from results of an open treatment trial of carbamazepine in PTSD, which include the finding of substantial improvement in intrusive, but not in numbing, symptoms (Lipper et al. 1986). In rat models it has been shown that inescapable stress sensitizes the hippocampus to increase norepinephrine release in response to a subsequent smaller stressor (Petty et al. 1994).

Another neurophysiological model posits that the intrusive and hyperactive symptoms in PTSD are secondary symptoms of release that result from inadequate cortical inhibition of lower brain-stem structures, such as the hypothalamus and the locus coeruleus (Kolb 1987). Kolb (1987) proposed that the primary pathology is one of impaired perceptual discrimination and learning. Repeated, excessive stressful stimuli do not allow normal habituation of cortical neuronal synapses and their accompanying neurochemical changes to occur, as would happen in adaptive learning.

Endogenous opioid system. Whereas affective numbing was understood, in the past, primarily as a psychological defense against overwhelming emotional pain, more recent research has suggested a biological component to the "negative" symptoms of PTSD. Van der Kolk and his group (1984) proposed that animal models of inescapable shock may parallel the development of PTSD in humans. Animals prevented from escaping from severe stress develop a syndrome of learned helplessness (Maier and Seligman 1976) that resembles the symptoms of constricted affect, withdrawal, amotivation, and decline in functioning associated with PTSD.

Animals exposed to prolonged or repeated inescapable stress develop analgesia, which appears to be mediated by release of endogenous opiates and which is blocked by the opiate antagonist naloxone (Kelly 1982; Maier et al. 1980). Similarly, it is suggested that in humans who have experienced prolonged or repeated trauma, endogenous opiates are readily released with any stimulus that is reminiscent of the original trauma, leading to analgesia and psychic numbing (van der Kolk et al. 1984). Pitman and his group (1990) compared pain intensity with thermal stimuli in Vietnam veterans with PTSD and veterans without PTSD who were watching a war videotape. PTSD patients, but not control subjects, had on average a 30% analgesia when pretreated with a placebo injection; this analgesia was eliminated with naloxone pretreatment. On the basis of such findings, the concept of trauma addiction has been proposed (van der Kolk et al. 1984). After a transient opioid burst on reexposure to traumatic stimuli, accompanied by a subjective sense of calm and control, opiate withdrawal may set in. This withdrawal may then contribute to the hyperarousal symptoms of PTSD, leading the individual into a vicious cycle of traumatic reexposures to gain transient symptomatic relief.

The noradrenergic and opiatergic systems of the brain interact and may serve reciprocal functions. Clonidine, an α_2-adrenergic agonist, has been shown to suppress opiate withdrawal symptoms in opiate addiction (Gold et al. 1980). Open treatment with clonidine in Vietnam veterans with PTSD demonstrated substantial decreases in hyperreactivity (Kolb et al. 1984). Clonidine's opiate-enhancing effects may be mediated either through suppression of the noradrenergic system or by a direct morphine-like agonist effect.

The relationship of dissociation to PTSD is an area of particular interest that has received increased attention in the last few years. The emotional numbing encountered in PTSD is on a spectrum with a variety of other dissociative processes, such as depersonalization, amnesia, and identity alteration, that are known to occur in response to trauma (D. Spiegel and Cardeña 1990). Dissociative symptoms are commonly encountered, in varying degrees, in PTSD patients—amnesia in particular (Bremner et al. 1993c).

Parasympathetic system. Another pathophysiological model of PTSD involves abnormalities in parasympathetic tone in the development of symptoms (De la Pena 1984). Parasympathetic-dominant individuals are thought to experience a lower rate of information flow in the central nervous system at baseline and may be at a greater risk for developing PTSD after exposure to an information-rich combat environment. Although capable of handling well the increased sensory information load in combat with a rebound of excessive parasympathetic activity, on return home to a more normal sensory environment these individuals experience understimulation and sensory deprivation, accompanied by boredom and depression. Thus, information-augmenting and sensation-seeking responses develop as a compensatory response of the understimulated, bored brain. This development may be reflected in the high REM density, shortened REM latency, and impaired sleep efficiency seen in PTSD patients in the sleep laboratory.

Serotonergic system. The serotonergic system has also been implicated in the symptomatology of PTSD (van der Kolk and Saporta 1991), although such work is still in its infancy. The septohippocampal brain system contains serotonergic pathways and mediates behavioral inhibition and constraint. The role of serotonergic deficit in impulsive aggression has been studied extensively. In animals, repeated inescapable shock can lead to serotonin depletion. Thus, the irritability and outbursts seen in patients with PTSD may be related to serotonergic dysfunction. Results of open clinical trials have suggested that SSRIs may be the most effective medications for both the positive and negative symptoms of PTSD (Davidson et al. 1991; McDougle et al. 1991; Shay 1992).

Hypothalamic-pituitary-adrenal axis. A number of findings concerning PTSD have implicated a chronic dysregulation of hypothalamic-pituitary-adrenal (HPA) axis functioning that is highly characteristic of this disorder and distinct from that seen in other psychiatric disorders such as depression. The findings include low urinary cortisol concentrations (J. W. Mason et al. 1986) and an elevated urinary norepinephrine-cortisol ratio (J. W. Mason et al. 1988), a blunted adrenocorticotropic hormone response to corticotropin-releasing factor (Smith et al. 1989), enhanced suppression of cortisol, and a decrease in lymphocyte glucocorticoid receptor number after dexamethasone administration consistent with a model of enhanced negative feedback sensitivity of the HPA axis in PTSD (Yehuda et al. 1993, 1995a).

Neuroanatomic and neuropsychological findings. A number of studies have shown that subjects with PTSD, as well as subjects with childhood histories of physical or sexual abuse, have certain types of cognitive deficits related to memory functions, especially impairment of short-term verbal memory (Bremner et al. 1993b) and retroactive interference in short-term recall (Yehuda et al. 1995b). These functional deficits in verbal memory have been cor-related with a decreased right hippocampal volume on MRI (Bremner et al. 1995).

Positron-emission tomography with PTSD symptom provocation using audiotaped traumatic scripts showed activation of the right limbic and paralimbic systems and of the visual cortex (Rauch et al. 1996).

Genetic predisposition. A large study of Vietnam veteran twins found that genetic factors accounted for 13%–34% of the variance in liability to the various PTSD symptom clusters, whereas no etiological role was found for shared environment (True et al. 1993).

COURSE AND PROGNOSIS

Scrignar (1984) divided the clinical course of PTSD into three stages. Stage 1 involves the response to trauma. Nonsusceptible persons may experience an adrenergic surge of symptoms immediately after the trauma but do not dwell on the incident. Predisposed persons have higher levels of anxiety at baseline, an exaggerated response to the trauma, and an obsessive preoccupation with the trauma after the trauma has occurred. If symptoms persist beyond 4–6 weeks, the patient enters stage 2, or acute PTSD. Feelings of helplessness and loss of control, symptoms of increased autonomic arousal, reliving of the trauma, and somatic symptoms may occur. The patient's life becomes centered around the trauma and there are subsequent changes in lifestyle, personality, and social functioning. Phobic avoidance, startle responses, and angry outbursts may occur. In stage 3, chronic PTSD develops, in which the patient experiences disability, demoralization, and despondency. The patient's emphasis changes from preoccupation with the actual trauma to preoccupation with the physical disability resulting from the trauma. Somatic symptoms, chronic anxiety, and depression are common complications at this time, as are substance abuse, disturbed family relations, and unemployment. Some patients may focus on compensation and lawsuits.

DSM-IV states that delayed PTSD occurs when symptoms do not begin until 6 months after the trauma. Survivors of major catastrophes rather than ordinary accidents are more likely to have delayed-onset PTSD.

A retrospective study examined patterns of treatment length in PTSD and compared characteristics of short-term patients (i.e., those who were successfully treated within 3 months) with those of long-term patients (i.e., those who received treatment for more than 12 months) (Burstein 1986). All patients were treated with medication and psychotherapy. No difference was found between the two groups with regard to type of stressor, reported symptom distress, possible financial compensation factors, length of time from trauma to intervention, and various demographic features. In this study, the number of patients who were treated successfully in a brief period was almost equal to the number of patients who underwent a prolonged course of treatment. Compared with the patients who were treated over a short period, the patients who required long-term treatment needed higher daily doses of imipramine and may have been more depressed after the first 3 months of treatment. This study did not relate imipramine effects to presence of panic attacks.

DIAGNOSIS

The diagnosis of PTSD is usually not difficult if there is a clear history of exposure to a traumatic event, followed by symptoms of intense anxiety lasting at least 1 month, along with arousal and stimulation of the autonomic nervous system, numbing of responsiveness, and avoidance or reexperiencing of the traumatic event. However, a wide variety of anxiety, depressive, somatic, and behavioral symptoms for which the relationship between their onset and the traumatic event is less clear-cut may easily lead to misdiagnosis.

DIFFERENTIAL DIAGNOSIS

Organic Mental Disorders

Following acute physical traumas, head trauma, or concussion, an organic mental disorder must be ruled out, because this diagnosis has important treatment implications. Mild concussions may leave no immediate apparent neurological signs but may have residual long-term effects on mood and concentration. A careful evaluation of the nature of the head trauma, including a review of medical records and witnesses' observations, followed by mental status evaluation and neurological examination, and, if indicated, laboratory examinations, is essential in a diagnostic workup. Malnutrition may occur during prolonged stressful periods and may also lead to organic brain syndromes. Survivors of death camps may have symptoms of an organic mental disorder such as failing memory, difficulty concentrating, emotional lability, headaches, and vertigo. Other causes of organic mental disorder may occasionally mimic PTSD if anxiety, depression, personality changes, or abnormal behaviors are present. Abnormalities of cognition, memory, altered sensorium or level of consciousness, or focal neurological signs would suggest an organic mental disorder.

Organic mental disorders that could mimic PTSD include organic personality syndrome, delirium, amnestic syndrome, organic hallucinosis, and organic intoxication and withdrawal states.

In addition, patients with PTSD may cope with their disorder through excessive use of alcohol, drugs, caffeine, or tobacco and thus may present with a combination of organic and psychological factors. In this case, each concomitant disorder should be diagnosed.

Mood and Anxiety Disorders

Major depression.   There is much overlap between PTSD and major mood disorders. Symptoms such as psychic numbing, irritability, sleep disturbance, fatigue, anhedonia, impairments in family and social relationships, anger, concern with physical health, and pessimistic outlook may occur in both disorders. In some veteran outreach populations, 70%–80% of patients meet diagnostic criteria for both disorders. Major depression is a frequent complication of PTSD; when it occurs, major depression must be treated aggressively, because comorbidity carries an increased risk of suicide. If major depression develops secondary to PTSD, both disorders should be diagnosed. Dysthymic symptoms are frequently secondary to PTSD, but if they are of sufficient severity, the additional diagnosis of dysthymic disorder should be made.

Phobic disorders.   After a traumatic event, patients may be aversively conditioned to the surroundings of the trauma and may develop a phobia of objects, surroundings, or situations that remind them of the trauma itself. Phobic patients experience anxiety in the feared situation, whereas avoidance is accompanied by anxiety reduction that reinforces the avoidant behavior. In PTSD, the phobia may be symptomatically similar to specific phobia, but the nature of the precipitant and the symptom cluster of PTSD distinguish this condition from simple phobia.

Generalized anxiety disorder.   The symptoms of generalized anxiety disorder (GAD), such as motor tension, autonomic hyperactivity, apprehensive expectation, and vigilance and scanning, are also present in PTSD. However, the onset and course of the illness differ: GAD has an insidious or gradual onset and a course that fluctuates with environmental stressors, whereas PTSD has an acute onset often followed by a chronic course. Phobic symptoms, which are absent in GAD, are often present in PTSD. DSM-IV does not allow for the diagnosis of GAD if PTSD is present.

Panic disorder.   Patients with PTSD may also experience panic attacks. In some patients, panic attacks predate the PTSD or do not occur exclusively in the context of stimuli reminiscent of the traumatic event. In other patients, however, panic attacks may develop after the PTSD and are cued solely by traumatic stimuli.

Adjustment disorder. Adjustment disorders are maladaptive reactions to identifiable psychosocial pressures. Signs and symptoms may include a wide variety of disturbances and emerge within 3 months of the stressful event. If symptoms are of sufficient severity to meet other Axis I criteria, the diagnosis of adjustment disorder is not made. Adjustment disorder differs from PTSD in that the stressor in adjustment disorder is usually less severe and within the range of common experience and the characteristic symptoms of PTSD, such as reexperiencing the trauma, are absent. The prognosis of full recovery in adjustment disorder is usually excellent.

Compensation neurosis (factitious disorder and malingering). Both factitious disorder and malingering involve conscious deception and feigning of illness, although the motivation for each condition differs. Factitious disorder may present with physical or psychological symptoms, the feigning of symptoms is under voluntary control, and the motivation is to assume the "patient" role. Chronic factitious disorder with physical symptoms (i.e., Munchausen's syndrome) involves frequent doctor visits and surgical interventions. PTSD differs from this disorder by absence of fabricated symptoms, acute onset after a trauma, and absence of a bizarre pretraumatic medical history.

Malingering involves the conscious fabrication of an illness for the purpose of achieving a definite goal such as obtaining money or compensation. Malingerers often reveal an inconsistent history, unexpected symptom clusters, a history of antisocial behavior and substance abuse, and a chaotic lifestyle, and there is often a discrepancy between history, claimed distress, and objective data.

Postconcussion syndrome. Mental disorders secondary to head injury are influenced by physiological, psychological, and environmental factors. Psychological symptoms are extremely common after mild closed head injuries, even when the injuries do not involve loss of consciousness. The so-called postconcussion syndrome comprises the symptoms of headache, dizziness, irritability, and emotional lability after head injury with concussion. Depression and lethargy are the affective symptoms that occur most commonly. These symptoms bear no relation to the degree of physical injury.

TREATMENT

Pharmacotherapy

A variety of different psychopharmacological agents have been used in the treatment of PTSD by clinicians and reported in the literature as case reports, open clinical trials, and controlled studies.

Adrenergic blockers. Kolb et al. (1984) treated 12 Vietnam veterans with PTSD in an open trial of the β-blocker propranolol over a 6-month period. Dosage ranged from 120 to 160 mg/day. Eleven patients reported a positive change in self-assessment at the end of the 6-month period, claiming to experience less explosiveness, fewer nightmares, improved sleep, and a decrease in intrusive thoughts, hyperalertness, and startle response. Another open pilot study by this group (Kolb et al. 1984) was conducted in nine Vietnam veterans with PTSD. Daily doses of 0.2–0.4 mg of clonidine, a noradrenergic α_2-agonist, were administered over a 6-month period. Eight patients reported lessened explosiveness and improvements in their capacity to control their emotions, and a majority reported improvements in sleep and nightmares and lowered startle response, hyperalertness, and intrusive thinking, as well as psychosocial improvement. These findings support the role of noradrenergic hyperactivity in the maintenance of autonomic arousal symptoms in PTSD. In a retrospective treatment review of Cambodian patients with PTSD, Kinzie and Leung (1989) found that the majority of patients benefited from the combination of clonidine and a tricyclic, as opposed to either medication taken alone. Controlled studies of adrenergic blockers in PTSD are needed.

Tricyclics. Most reports thus far on the pharmacotherapy of PTSD involve the use of antidepressants. A retrospective study by Bleich et al. (1986) of 25 PTSD patients treated with a variety of different antidepressants, including tricyclics and MAOIs, reported good or moderate results in 67% of patients treated. Response was not clearly related to the presence of somatization symptoms, depression, or panic attacks. Antidepressants appeared to be more useful than major tranquilizers. Although antidepressants improved intrusion-type symptoms, the most prominent overall effects were overall sedation and alleviation of insomnia. Antidepressants also were found to have a positive impact on psychotherapy in 70% of cases.

Burstein (1984), in a report of a study involving 10 patients with PTSD of recent onset who received 50–350 mg of imipramine daily, observed marked improvement in intrusive recollections, sleep and dream disturbance, and flashbacks. Similar improvement in intrusive symptomatology was reported with an open trial of desipramine (Kauffman et al. 1987). A positive effect of imipramine therapy on posttraumatic night terrors was reported by Marshall (1975).

More recently, controlled studies of tricyclics in PTSD have been conducted but, overall, have not replicated the decreasing of posttraumatic symptoms reported in earlier trials. In a 4-week, double-blind, crossover study of desipramine and placebo in 18 veterans with PTSD, only depressive symptoms improved; anxiety, intrusive symptoms, and avoidance did not change with desipramine therapy (Reist et al. 1989). Davidson et al. (1990) conducted a 4- to 8-week double-blind comparison of amitriptyline and placebo in 46 veterans with PTSD. Although depression and anxiety decreased with amitriptyline therapy, decrease in intrusive and avoidant symptoms was apparent only in the subgroup of patients who completed 8 weeks of amitriptyline therapy and was modest and of marginal significance. At the end of the study, roughly two-thirds of patients in both treatment groups still met the criteria for PTSD.

Monoamine oxidase inhibitors. An early study of MAOIs described five cases of "traumatic war neurosis"; in these patients, phenelzine, in dosages of 45–75 mg/day, improved traumatic dreams, flashbacks, startle reactions, and violent outbursts (Hogben and Cornfield 1981). Panic attacks were also described in all of the patients in this study. Positive effects of phenelzine on intrusive posttraumatic symptoms have been reported in subsequent small open trials (Davidson et al. 1987; van der Kolk 1983).

More recently, an 8-week randomized double-blind trial compared treatment with phenelzine (71 mg), with imipramine (240 mg), and with placebo in 34 veterans with PTSD (Frank et al. 1988). Both antidepressant therapies resulted in some overall improvement in patients' posttraumatic symptoms, and phenelzine therapy tended to be superior to imipramine therapy. The most marked improvement was the decrease in intrusive symptoms in patients taking phenelzine; there was a 60% average reduction on the intrusion scale measure.

Lithium. In a small open trial of lithium in PTSD patients, van der Kolk (1983) reported improvement in intrusive recollections and irritability in more than half of the patients treated. However, there have been no controlled trials.

Anticonvulsants. In an open trial of carbamazepine in 10 patients with PTSD, Lipper and his group (1986)

reported moderate to great improvement in intrusive symptoms in 7 patients. Wolf et al. (1988) reported decreased impulsivity and angry outbursts in 10 veterans who were also treated with carbamazepine; all patients had normal electroencephalographic findings. Valproic acid was reported to decrease irritability and angry outbursts in two veterans with PTSD (Szymanski and Olympia 1991). Controlled trials, however, have not been conducted.

Serotonin reuptake inhibitors. Results of multiple open trials of SSRIs suggest that these medications have at least modest efficacy in the treatment of PTSD, and SSRIs appear to have become the medications of choice for this disorder. In a series of five patients with PTSD related to life-threatening accidents or sexual abuse, treatment with fluoxetine in dosages of 20–80 mg/day resulted in marked improvement of both intrusive and avoidant symptoms (Davidson et al. 1991). Reports of two larger trials involving war veterans with PTSD also documented benefits from fluoxetine treatment (McDougle et al. 1991; Shay 1992). Shay (1992) reported that two-thirds of patients experienced decreased anger, reduced explosive outbursts, and better mood with fluoxetine therapy. McDougle and colleagues (1991) treated 20 consecutive Vietnam veterans with fluoxetine for at least 4 weeks at a mean dosage of 35 mg/day. PTSD symptoms showed much improvement in two-thirds of patients in all three domains: re-experiencing, avoidance, and hyperarousal. Of particular interest, avoidance improved more than hyperarousal, independent of changes in depression. In a fairly large, double-blind trial comparing fluoxetine and placebo, fluoxetine treatment led to a significant reduction of PTSD symptomatology, especially arousal and numbing symptoms (van der Kolk et al. 1994). Open trials of other SSRIs, including fluvoxamine (De Boer et al. 1992) and sertraline (Brady et al. 1995), have also resulted in at least modest benefits with regard to PTSD symptoms.

Buspirone. In a small open trial of buspirone, seven of eight patients experienced a marked reduction in PTSD symptoms; no controlled studies have been undertaken (Duffy and Malloy 1994).

Psychotherapy

It is generally agreed that some form of psychotherapy is necessary in the treatment of posttraumatic pathology. Crisis intervention shortly after the traumatic event is effective in reducing immediate distress, possibly prevents chronic or delayed responses, and, if the pathological response is still tentative, may allow for briefer intervention.

Brief dynamic psychotherapy has been advocated both as an immediate treatment procedure and as a way of preventing chronic disorder. The therapist must establish a working alliance that allows the patient to work through his or her reactions.

The literature has suggested that persons with disrupted early attachments or abuse, who have been traumatized earlier in their lives, are more likely to develop PTSD than are those with stable backgrounds. The presence of psychic trauma in a person's past may psychologically and biologically predispose him or her to respond excessively and maladaptively to intense experiences and affects (Herman et al. 1989; Krystal 1968; van der Kolk 1987b). Therefore, attempting to modify preexisting conflicts, developmental difficulties, and defensive styles that render the person especially vulnerable to traumatization by particular experiences is central to the treatment of traumatic syndromes.

The "phase-oriented" treatment model suggested by Horowitz (1976) strikes a balance between initial supportive interventions to minimize the traumatic state and increasingly aggressive "working through" at later stages of treatment. Establishment of a safe and communicative relationship, reappraisal of the traumatic event, revision of the patient's inner model of self and world, and planning for termination with a reexperiencing of loss are all important therapeutic issues in the treatment of PTSD. Herman and her group (1989) emphasized the importance of validating the patient's traumatic experiences as a precondition for reparation of damaged self-identity.

Embry (1990) outlined seven major parameters for effective psychotherapy in war veterans with chronic PTSD: 1) initial rapport building, 2) limit setting and supportive confrontation, 3) affective modeling, 4) defocusing on stress and focusing on current life events, 5) sensitivity to transference-countertransference issues, 6) understanding of secondary gain, and 7) therapist's maintenance of a positive treatment attitude.

Group psychotherapy can also serve as an adjunctive treatment, or as the central treatment mode, in traumatized patients (van der Kolk 1987a). Because of past experiences, such patients are often mistrustful and reluctant to depend on authority figures, whereas the identification, support, and hopefulness of peer settings can facilitate therapeutic change.

Drug treatment has been impressionistically reported to have a positive impact on psychotherapy in 70% of cases, with improvements in symptom severity leading to a more positive and motivated approach to psychotherapy, and an enhanced accessibility to uncovering and working through traumatic memories (Bleich et al. 1986).

Behavior Therapy

A variety of behavioral techniques have been applied in the treatment of PTSD. People involved in traumatic events such as accidents frequently develop phobias or phobic anxiety related to or associated with these situations. Systematic desensitization or graded exposure has been found to be effective in cases of phobia or phobic anxiety associated with PTSD. This technique is based on the principle that when patients are gradually exposed to a phobic or anxiety-provoking stimulus, they will become habituated or deconditioned to the stimulus. Variations of this treatment include using imaginal techniques (i.e., imaginal desensitization) and exposure to real-life situations (i.e., in vivo desensitization). Prolonged exposure (i.e., flooding), if tolerated by patients, can be useful and has been reported to be successful in the treatment of Vietnam veterans (Fairbank and Keane 1982).

Relaxation techniques produce the beneficial physiological result of reducing motor tension and lowering the activity of the autonomic nervous system—effects that may be particularly efficacious in PTSD. Progressive muscle relaxation involves contracting and relaxing various muscle groups to induce the relaxation response. This technique is useful for symptoms of autonomic arousal such as somatic symptoms, anxiety, and insomnia. Hypnosis has also been used, with success, to induce the relaxation response in PTSD.

Cognitive therapy and thought stopping, in which a phrase and momentary pain are paired with thoughts or images of the trauma, have been used to treat unwanted mental activity in PTSD.

CONCLUSIONS

In this chapter we have presented a comprehensive discussion of panic disorder, generalized anxiety disorder, the phobic disorders, obsessive-compulsive disorder, and posttraumatic stress disorder. A review of history, differing theoretical models, and new developments in epidemiology, classification, pathophysiology, and treatment have been presented. For additional information, the reader is encouraged to consult the suggested readings that are listed at the end of this chapter. An explosion of research has led to dramatic developments in the understanding and alleviation of various forms of anxiety and has made the anxiety disorders an exciting field of modern psychiatry.

REFERENCES

Abelson JL, Glitz D, Cameron OG, et al: Blunted growth hormone response to clonidine in patients with generalized anxiety disorder. Arch Gen Psychiatry 48:157–162, 1991

Ackerman DL, Greenland S, Bystritsky A, et al: Predictors of treatment response in obsessive-compulsive disorder: multivariate analyses from a multicenter trial of clomipramine. J Clin Psychopharmacol 14:247–254, 1994

Akhtar S, Wig NN, Varma VK, et al: A phenomenological analysis of symptoms in obsessive-compulsive neurosis. Br J Psychiatry 127:342–348, 1975

Alden LE, Wallace ST: Social phobia and social appraisal in successful and unsuccessful social interactions. Behav Res Ther 33:497–505, 1995

Allgulander C, Lavori PW: Excess mortality among 3302 patients with "pure" anxiety neurosis. Arch Gen Psychiatry 48:599–602, 1991

Altemus M, Pigott T, Kalogeras KT, et al: Abnormalities in the regulation of vasopressin and corticotropin releasing factor secretion in obsessive-compulsive disorder. Arch Gen Psychiatry 49:9–20, 1992

Altemus M, Pigott T, L'Heureux F, et al: CSF somatostatin in obsessive-compulsive disorder. Am J Psychiatry 150:460–464, 1993

Altemus M, Swedo SE, Leonard HL, et al: Changes in cerebrospinal fluid neurochemistry during treatment of obsessive-compulsive disorder with clomipramine. Arch Gen Psychiatry 51:794–803, 1994

American Psychiatric Association: Diagnostic and Statistical Manual of Mental Disorders, 2nd Edition. Washington, DC, American Psychiatric Association, 1968

American Psychiatric Association: Diagnostic and Statistical Manual of Mental Disorders, 3rd Edition. Washington, DC, American Psychiatric Association, 1980

American Psychiatric Association: Diagnostic and Statistical Manual of Mental Disorders, 3rd Edition, Revised. Washington, DC, American Psychiatric Association, 1987

American Psychiatric Association: Diagnostic and Statistical Manual of Mental Disorders, 4th Edition. Washington, DC, American Psychiatric Association, 1994

Amies PL, Gelder MG, Shaw PM: Social phobia: a comparative clinical study. Br J Psychiatry 142:174–179, 1983

Ananth J, Pecknold JC, Van Den Steen N, et al: Double-blind comparative study of clomipramine and amitriptyline in obsessive neurosis. Prog Neuropsychopharmacol Biol Psychiatry 5:257–262, 1981

Anisman HL, Pizzino A, Sklar LS: Coping with stress, norepinephrine depletion and escape performance. Brain Res 191:583–588, 1980

Apter A, Ratzoni G, King RA, et al: Fluvoxamine open-label treatment of adolescent inpatients with obsessive-compulsive disorder or depression. J Am Acad Child Adolesc Psychiatry 33:342–348, 1994

Arntz A, van den Hout M: Psychological treatments of panic disorder without agoraphobia: cognitive therapy versus applied relaxation. Behav Res Ther 34:113–121, 1996

Aston-Jones SL, Foote FE, Bloom FE: Norepinephrine, in Frontiers of Clinical Neuroscience, Vol 2. Edited by Ziegler MG, Lake CR. Baltimore, MD, Williams & Wilkins, 1984, pp 92–116

Baer L, Jenike MA: Personality disorders in obsessive-compulsive disorder. Psychiatr Clin North Am 15:803–812, 1992

Baer L, Jenike MA, Ricciardi JN, et al: Standardized assessment of personality disorders in obsessive-compulsive disorder. Arch Gen Psychiatry 47:826–830, 1990

Baer L, Jenike MA, Black DW, et al: Effect of axis II diagnoses on treatment outcome with clomipramine in 55 patients with obsessive-compulsive disorder. Arch Gen Psychiatry 49:862–866, 1992

Baer L, Rauch SL, Ballantine HT, et al: Cingulotomy for intractable obsessive-compulsive disorder: prospective long-term follow-up of 18 patients. Arch Gen Psychiatry 52:384–392, 1995

Baker RW, Chengappa KN, Baird JW, et al: Emergence of obsessive compulsive symptoms during treatment with clozapine. J Clin Psychiatry 53:439–442, 1992

Ballenger JC, Burrows GD, DuPont RL Jr, et al: Alprazolam in panic disorder and agoraphobia: results from a multicenter trial, I: efficacy in short-term treatment. Arch Gen Psychiatry 45:413–422, 1988

Barlow DH, Craske MG, Cerny JA, et al: Behavioral treatment of panic disorder. Behavior Therapy 20:261–282, 1989

Barton R: Diabetes insipidus and obsessional neurosis: a syndrome. Lancet 1:133–135, 1965

Basoglu M, Marks IM, Kilic C, et al: Relationship of panic, anticipatory anxiety, agoraphobia and global improvement in panic disorder with agoraphobia treated with alprazolam and exposure. Br J Psychiatry 164:647–652, 1994

Bastani B, Nash JF, Meltzer HY: Prolactin and cortisol responses to MK-212, a serotonin agonist, in obsessive-compulsive disorder. Arch Gen Psychiatry 47:833–839, 1990

Baxter LR Jr, Phelps ME, Mazziotta JC, et al: Local cerebral glucose metabolic rates in obsessive-compulsive disorder: a comparison with rates in unipolar depression and in normal controls. Arch Gen Psychiatry 44:211–218, 1987

Baxter LR Jr, Schwartz JM, Bergman KS, et al: Caudate glucose metabolic rate changes with both drug and behavior therapy for obsessive-compulsive disorder. Arch Gen Psychiatry 49:681–689, 1992

Beck AT, Sokol L, Clark DA, et al: A crossover study of focused cognitive therapy for panic disorder. Am J Psychiatry 149:778–783, 1992

Behar D, Rapoport JL, Berg CJ, et al: Computerized tomography and neuropsychological test measures in adolescents with obsessive-compulsive disorder. Am J Psychiatry 141:363–369, 1984

Benjamin J, Levine J, Fux M, et al: Double-blind, placebo-controlled, crossover trial of inositol treatment for panic disorder. Am J Psychiatry 152:1084–1086, 1995

Benkelfat C, Murphy DL, Zohar J, et al: Clomipramine in obsessive-compulsive disorder: further evidence for a serotonergic mechanism of action. Arch Gen Psychiatry 46:23–28, 1989

Benkelfat C, Nordahl TE, Semple WE, et al: Local cerebral glucose metabolic rates in obsessive-compulsive disorder: patients treated with clomipramine. Arch Gen Psychiatry 47:840–848, 1990

Benson H, Beary JF, Carol MP: The relaxation response. Psychiatry 37:37–46, 1974

Black A: The natural history of obsessional neurosis, in Obsessional States. Edited by Beech HK. London, Methuen Press, 1974

Black DW, Blum NS: Obsessive-compulsive disorder support groups: the Iowa model. Compr Psychiatry 33:65–71, 1992

Black DW, Noyes R, Goldstein RB, et al: A family study of obsessive-compulsive disorder. Arch Gen Psychiatry 49:362–368, 1992

Black DW, Wesner R, Bowers W, et al: A comparison of fluvoxamine, cognitive therapy, and placebo in the treatment of panic disorder. Arch Gen Psychiatry 50:44–50, 1993

Blazer DG, Hughes D, George LK: Generalized anxiety disorder, in Psychiatric Disorders in America. Edited by Robins LN, Regier DA. New York, Free Press, 1991, pp 180–203

Bleich A, Siegel B, Garb R, et al: Post-traumatic stress disorder following combat exposure: clinical features and psychopharmacological treatment. Br J Psychiatry 149:365–369, 1986

Borkovec TD, Costello E: Efficacy of applied relaxation and cognitive-behavioral therapy in the treatment of generalized anxiety disorder. J Consult Clin Psychol 61:611–619, 1993

Bowlby J: Attachment and Loss, Vol 2: Separation: Anxiety and Anger. New York, Basic Books, 1973

Boyer W: Serotonin uptake inhibitors are superior to imipramine and alprazolam in alleviating panic attacks: a meta-analysis. Int Clin Psychopharmacol 10:45–49, 1995

Brady KT, Sonne SC, Roberts JM: Sertraline treatment of comorbid posttraumatic stress disorder and alcohol dependence. J Clin Psychiatry 56:502–505, 1995

Brantigan CO, Brantigan TA, Joseph N: Effect of beta blockade and beta stimulation on stage fright. Am J Med 72:88–94, 1982

Brawman MO, Lydiard RB, Emmanuel N, et al: Psychiatric comorbidity in patients with generalized anxiety disorder. Am J Psychiatry 150:1216–1218, 1993

Breiter HC, Rauch SL, Kwong KK, et al: Functional magnetic resonance imaging of symptom provocation in obsessive-compulsive disorder. Arch Gen Psychiatry 53:595–606, 1996

Bremner JD, Southwick SM, Johnson DR, et al: Childhood physical abuse and combat-related posttraumatic stress disorder in Vietnam veterans. Am J Psychiatry 150:235–239, 1993a

Bremner JD, Scott TM, Delaney RC, et al: Deficits in short-term memory in posttraumatic stress disorder. Am J Psychiatry 150:1015–1019, 1993b

Bremner JD, Steinberg M, Southwick SM, et al: Use of the Structured Clinical Interview for DSM-IV Dissociative Disorders for systematic assessment of dissociative symptoms in posttraumatic stress disorder. Am J Psychiatry 150:1011–1014, 1993c

Bremner JD, Randall P, Scott TM, et al: MRI-based measurement of hippocampal volume in patients with combat-related posttraumatic stress disorder. Am J Psychiatry 152:973–981, 1995

Breslau N, Davis GC: DSM-III generalized anxiety disorder: an empirical investigation of more stringent criteria. Psychiatry Res 15:231–238, 1985

Breslau N, Davis GC: Posttraumatic stress disorder in an urban population of young adults: risk factors for chronicity. Am J Psychiatry 149:671–675, 1992

Breslau N, Davis GC, Andreski P, et al: Traumatic events and posttraumatic stress disorder in an urban population of young adults. Arch Gen Psychiatry 48:216–222, 1991

Breuer T, Freud S: Studies on hysteria (1893–1895), in The Standard Edition of the Complete Psychological Works of Sigmund Freud, Vol 2. Translated and edited by Strachey J. London, Hogarth Press, 1955, pp 1–319

Burstein A: Treatment of post-traumatic stress disorder with imipramine. Psychosomatics 25:681–687, 1984

Burstein A: Treatment length in post-traumatic stress disorder. Psychosomatics 27:632–637, 1986

Calvocoressi L, Lewis B, Harris M, et al: Family accommodation in obsessive-compulsive disorder. Am J Psychiatry 152:441–443, 1995

Capstick N, Seldrup V: Obsessional states: a study in the relationship between abnormalities occurring at birth and subsequent development of obsessional symptoms. Acta Psychiatr Scand 56:427–439, 1977

Carey G, Gottesman II: Twin and family studies of anxiety, phobic, and obsessive disorders, in Anxiety: New Research and Changing Concepts. Edited by Klein DF, Rabkin J. New York, Raven, 1981, pp 117–136

Chambless DL, Gillis MM: Cognitive therapy of anxiety disorders. J Consult Clin Psychol 61:248–260, 1993

Chapman D: A brief introduction to contemporary disaster research, in Man and Society in Disaster. Edited by Boher G, Chapman D. New York, Basic Books, 1962

Charney DS, Heninger GR: Abnormal regulation of noradrenergic function in panic disorders: effects of clonidine in healthy subjects and patients with agoraphobia and panic disorder. Arch Gen Psychiatry 43:1042–1054, 1986

Charney DS, Heninger GR, Breier A: Noradrenergic function in panic anxiety: effects of yohimbine in healthy subjects and patients with agoraphobia and panic disorder. Arch Gen Psychiatry 41:751–763, 1984

Charney DS, Goodman WK, Price LH, et al: Serotonin function in obsessive-compulsive disorder: a comparison of the effects of tryptophan and *m*-chlorophenylpiperazine in patients and healthy subjects. Arch Gen Psychiatry 45:177–185, 1988

Chouinard G: Sertraline in the treatment of obsessive compulsive disorder: two double-blind, placebo-controlled studies. Int Clin Psychopharmacol 7 (suppl 2):37–41, 1992

Christensen KJ, Kim SW, Dysken MW, et al: Neuropsychological performance in obsessive-compulsive disorder. Biol Psychiatry 31:4–18, 1992

Ciesielski KT, Beech HR, Gordon PK: Some electrophysiological observations in obsessional states. Br J Psychiatry 138:479–484, 1981

Clark DM, Salkovskis PM, Chalkly AJ: Respiratory control as a treatment for panic attacks. J Behav Ther Exp Psychiatry 16:23–30, 1985

Clark DM, Salkovskis PM, Hackmann A, et al: A comparison of cognitive therapy, applied relaxation therapy and imipramine in the treatment of panic disorder. Br J Psychiatry 164:759–769, 1994

Clomipramine Collaborative Study Group: Clomipramine in the treatment of patients with obsessive-compulsive disorder. Arch Gen Psychiatry 48:730–738, 1991

Cohen ME, White ID: Life situation, emotions, and neurocirculatory asthenia. Research in Nervous and Mental Disease Proceedings 29:832–869, 1950

Cooper AM: Will neurobiology influence psychoanalysis? Am J Psychiatry 142:1395–1402, 1985

Coryell W, Noyes R, Clancy J: Excess mortality in panic disorder: a comparison with primary unipolar depression. Arch Gen Psychiatry 39:701–703, 1982

Craske MG, Brown TA, Barlow DH: Behavioral treatment of panic disorder: a two-year follow-up. Behavior Therapy 22:289–304, 1991

Crowe RR, Noyes R, Pauls DL, et al: A family study of panic disorder. Arch Gen Psychiatry 40:1065–1069, 1983

Curtis GC, Thyer B: Fainting on exposure to phobic stimuli. Am J Psychiatry 140:771–774, 1983

Davidson J, Walker JI, Kilts C: A pilot study of phenelzine in the treatment of post-traumatic stress disorder. Br J Psychiatry 150:252–255, 1987

Davidson J, Kudler H, Smith R, et al: Treatment of posttraumatic stress disorder with amitriptyline and placebo. Arch Gen Psychiatry 47:259–266, 1990

Davidson J, Roth S, Newman E: Fluoxetine in post-traumatic stress disorder. J Trauma Stress 4:419–423, 1991

Davidson JR, Hughes DL, George LK, et al: The epidemiology of social phobia: findings from the Duke Epidemiological Catchment Area Study. Psychol Med 23:709–718, 1993a

Davidson J, Potts N, Richichi E, et al: Treatment of social phobia with clonazepam and placebo. J Clin Psychopharmacol 13:423–428, 1993b

de Beurs E, van Balkom AJ, Lange A, et al: Treatment of panic disorder with agoraphobia: comparison of fluvoxamine, placebo and psychological panic management combined with exposure and of exposure in vivo alone. Am J Psychiatry 152:683–691, 1995

De Boer M, Op den Velde W, Falger PJ, et al: Fluvoxamine treatment for chronic PTSD: a pilot study. Psychother Psychosom 57:158–163, 1992

De la Pena A: Post-traumatic stress disorder in the Vietnam veteran: a brain modulated, compensatory in formation-augmenting response to information underload in the central nervous system? in Post-Traumatic Stress Disorder: Psychological and Biological Sequelae. Edited by van der Kolk BA. Washington, DC, American Psychiatric Press, 1984, pp 108–122

Delle Chiaie R, Pancheri P, Casacchia M, et al: Assessment of the efficacy of buspirone in patients affected by generalized anxiety disorder, shifting to buspirone from prior treatment with lorazepam: a placebo-controlled, double-blind study. J Clin Psychopharmacol 15:12–19, 1995

DeMartinis NA, Schweizer E, Rickels K: An open-label trial of nefazodone in high comorbidity panic disorder. J Clin Psychiatry 57:245–248, 1996

Den Boer JA: Serotonergic Mechanisms in Anxiety Disorders: An Inquiry Into Serotonin Function in Panic Disorder. The Hague, Cip-Gegevens Koninklijke Bibliotheek, 1988

Den Boer JA, Van Vlliet IM, Westenberg HG: Recent advances in the psychopharmacology of social phobia. Prog Neuropsychopharmacol Biol Psychiatry 18:625–645, 1994

Dimsdale JE, Moss J: Plasma catecholamines in stress and exercise. JAMA 243:340–342, 1980

Dorrow R, Horowski R, Paschelke G, et al: Severe anxiety induced by FG-7142, a beta-carboline ligand for benzodiazepine receptors. Lancet 1:98–99, 1983

Duffy JD, Malloy PF: Efficacy of buspirone in the treatment of posttraumatic stress disorder: an open trial. Ann Clin Psychiatry 6:33–37, 1994

Eaton WW, Keyl PM: Risk factors for the onset of Diagnostic Interview Schedule/DSM-III agoraphobia in a prospective, population-based study. Arch Gen Psychiatry 47:819–824, 1990

Eaton WW, Dryman A, Weissman MM: Panic and phobia, in Psychiatric Disorders in America. Edited by Robins LN, Regier DA. New York, Free Press, 1991, pp 155–179

Eitinger L: Organic and psychosomatic aftereffects of concentration camp imprisonment. International Psychiatry Clinics 8:205–215, 1971

Elam M, Yoat TP, Svensson TH: Hypercapnia and hypoxia: chemoreceptor-mediated control of locus ceruleus neurons and splanchnic, sympathetic nerves. Brain Res 222:373–381, 1981

Embry CK: Psychotherapeutic interventions in chronic posttraumatic stress disorder, in Posttraumatic Stress Disorder: Etiology, Phenomenology, and Treatment. Edited by Wolf ME, Mosnaim AD. Washington, DC, American Psychiatric Press, 1990, pp 226–236

Fahlen T, Nilsson HL, Borg K, et al: Social phobia: the clinical efficacy and tolerability of the monoamine oxidase-A and serotonin reuptake inhibitor brofaromine: a double-blind placebo-controlled study. Acta Psychiatr Scand 92: 351–358, 1995

Fairbank TA, Keane TM: Flooding for combat-related stress disorders: assessment of anxiety reduction across traumatic memories. Behavior Therapy 13:499–510, 1982

Fallon BA, Campeas R, Schneier FR, et al: Open trial of intravenous clomipramine in five treatment-refractory patients with obsessive-compulsive disorder. J Neuropsychiatry Clin Neurosci 4:70–75, 1992

Faravelli C, Pallanti S: Recent life events and panic disorder. Am J Psychiatry 146:622–626, 1989

Flament MF, Rapoport JL, Berg CJ, et al: Clomipramine treatment of childhood obsessive-compulsive disorder: a double-blind controlled study. Arch Gen Psychiatry 42:977–983, 1985

Flament MF, Rapoport JL, Murphy DL, et al: Biochemical changes during clomipramine treatment of childhood obsessive-compulsive disorder. Arch Gen Psychiatry 44:219–225, 1987

Flescher J: A dualistic viewpoint on anxiety. J Am Psychoanal Assoc 3:415–446, 1955

Flint AJ: Epidemiology and comorbidity of anxiety disorders in the elderly. Am J Psychiatry 151:640–649, 1994

Flor-Henry P: The obsessive-compulsive syndrome, in Cerebral Basis of Psychopathology. Edited by Flor-Henry P. Boston, John Coright, 1983, pp 301–311

Foa EB, Steketee G, Grayson JB, et al: Deliberate exposure and blocking of obsessive-compulsive rituals: immediate and long-term effects. Behavior Therapy 15:450–472, 1984

Foa EB, Kozak MJ, Goodman WK, et al: DSM-IV field trial: obsessive-compulsive disorder. Am J Psychiatry 152:90–96, 1995

Frank JB, Kosten TR, Giller EL Jr, et al: A randomized clinical trial of phenelzine and imipramine for posttraumatic stress disorder. Am J Psychiatry 145:1289–1291, 1988

Freeman CP, Trimble MR, Deakin JF, et al: Fluvoxamine versus clomipramine in the treatment of obsessive compulsive disorder: a multicenter, randomized, double-blinded, parallel group comparison. J Clin Psychiatry 55:301–305, 1994

Freeston MH, Rheaume J, Ladouceur R: Correcting faulty appraisals of obsessional thoughts. Behav Res Ther 34:433–446, 1996

Freud S: Obsessions and phobias (1895a[1894]), in The Standard Edition of the Complete Psychological Works of Sigmund Freud, Vol 3. Translated and edited by Strachey J. London, Hogarth Press, 1962, pp 69–84

Freud S: On the grounds for detaching a particular syndrome from neurasthenia under the description anxiety neurosis (1895b[1894]), in The Standard Edition of the Complete Psychological Works of Sigmund Freud, Vol 3. Translated and edited by Strachey J. London, Hogarth Press, 1962, pp 85–117

Freud S: Analysis of a phobia in a five-year-old boy (1909), in The Standard Edition of the Complete Psychological Works of Sigmund Freud, Vol 10. Translated and edited by Strachey J. London, Hogarth Press, 1955, pp 1–149

Freud S: The disposition to obsessional neurosis: a contribution to the problem of choice of neurosis (1913), in The Standard Edition of the Complete Psychological Works of Sigmund Freud, Vol 12. Translated and edited by Strachey J. London, Hogarth Press, 1958, pp 311–326

Freud S: Introduction to psychoanalysis and the war neuroses (1919), in The Standard Edition of the Complete Psychological Works of Sigmund Freud, Vol 17. Translated and edited by Strachey J. London, Hogarth Press, 1955, pp 205–215

Freud S: Inhibitions, symptoms and anxiety (1926), in The Standard Edition of the Complete Psychological Works of Sigmund Freud, Vol 20. Translated and edited by Strachey J. London, Hogarth Press, 1959, pp 75–175

Frohlich ED, Tarazi KC, Duston HP: Hyperdynamic beta-adrenergic circulatory state. Arch Intern Med 123:1–7, 1969

Fyer AJ, Mannuzza S, Gallops MS, et al: Familial transmission of simple phobias and fears: a preliminary report. Arch Gen Psychiatry 47:252–256, 1990

Gabbard GO: Psychodynamic Psychiatry in Clinical Practice. Washington, DC, American Psychiatric Press, 1990

Galderisi S, Mucci A, Catapano F, et al: Neuropsychological slowness in obsessive-compulsive patients: is it confined to tests involving the fronto-subcortical systems? Br J Psychiatry 167:394–398, 1996

Gelernter CS, Uhde TW, Cimbolic P, et al: Cognitive-behavioral and pharmacological treatments of social phobia: a controlled study. Arch Gen Psychiatry 48: 938–945, 1991

Geracioti TD: Venlafaxine treatment of panic disorder: a case series. J Clin Psychiatry 56:408–410, 1995

Ghaemi SN, Zarate CA, Popli AP, et al: Is there a relationship between clozapine and obsessive-compulsive disorder? A retrospective chart review. Compr Psychiatry 36:267–270, 1995

Gittelman-Klein R, Klein DF: Controlled imipramine treatment of school phobia. Arch Gen Psychiatry 25:204–207, 1971

Gittleson NL: The effect of obsessions on depressive psychosis. Br J Psychiatry 112:253–259, 1966

Gold M, Pottash AC, Sweeney DR, et al: Opiate withdrawal using clonidine. JAMA 243:343–346, 1980

Goodman WK, Price LH, Rasmussen SA, et al: Efficacy of fluvoxamine in obsessive-compulsive disorder: a double-blind comparison with placebo. Arch Gen Psychiatry 46:36–44, 1989

Goodman WK, McDougle CJ, Price LH, et al: Beyond the serotonin hypothesis: a role for dopamine in some forms of obsessive compulsive disorder? J Clin Psychiatry 51 (suppl):36–43, 1990a

Goodman WK, Price LH, Delgado PL, et al: Specificity of serotonin reuptake inhibitors in the treatment of obsessive-compulsive disorder: comparison of fluvoxamine and desipramine. Arch Gen Psychiatry 47:577–585, 1990b

Gorman JM, Fyer AF, Gliklich J, et al: Effect of imipramine on prolapsed mitral valves of patients with panic disorder. Am J Psychiatry 138:977–978, 1981

Gorman JM, Levy GF, Liebowitz MR, et al: Effect of acute β-adrenergic blockade on lactate-induced panic. Arch Gen Psychiatry 40:1079–1082, 1983

Gorman JM, Askanazi J, Liebowitz MR, et al: Response to hyperventilation in a group of patients with panic disorder. Am J Psychiatry 141:857–861, 1984

Gorman JM, Liebowitz MR, Fyer AJ, et al: Lactate infusions in obsessive-compulsive disorder. Am J Psychiatry 142:864–866, 1985

Gorman JM, Fyer MR, Goetz R, et al: Ventilatory physiology of patients with panic disorder. Arch Gen Psychiatry 45:31–39, 1988

Gorman JM, Battista D, Goetz RR, et al: A comparison of sodium bicarbonate and sodium lactate infusion in the induction of panic attacks. Arch Gen Psychiatry 46:145–150, 1989a

Gorman JM, Liebowitz MR, Fyer AJ, et al: A neuroanatomical hypothesis for panic disorder. Am J Psychiatry 146:148–161, 1989b

Grady TA, Pigott TA, L'Heureux F, et al: Double-blind study of adjuvant buspirone for fluoxetine-treated patients with obsessive-compulsive disorder. Am J Psychiatry 150:819–821, 1993

Greist JH, Jefferson JW, Kobak KA, et al: A 1 year double-blind placebo-controlled fixed dose study of sertraline in the treatment of obsessive-compulsive disorder. Int Clin Psychopharmacol 10:57–65, 1995a

Greist J[H], Chouinard G, DuBoff E, et al: Double-blind parallel comparison of three dosages of sertraline and placebo in outpatients with obsessive-compulsive disorder. Arch Gen Psychiatry 52:289–295, 1995b

Greist JH, Jefferson JW, Kobak KA, et al: Efficacy and tolerability of serotonin transport inhibitors in obsessive-compulsive disorder: a meta-analysis. Arch Gen Psychiatry 52:53–60, 1995c

Grimshaw L: Obsessional disorder and neurological illness. J Neurol Neurosurg Psychiatry 27:229–231, 1964

Hansenne M, Pitchot W, Ansseau M: The clonidine test in posttraumatic stress disorder (letter). Am J Psychiatry 148:810–811, 1991

Hartley LR, Ungapen S, Davie I, et al: The effect of beta adrenergic blocking drugs on speakers' performance and memory. Br J Psychiatry 142:512–517, 1983

Hay P, Sachdev P, Cumming S, et al: Treatment of obsessive-compulsive disorder by psychosurgery. Acta Psychiatr Scand 87:197–207, 1993

Heimberg RG, Dodge CS, Hope DA, et al: Cognitive behavioral group treatment for social phobia: comparison with a credible placebo control. Cognitive Therapy and Research 14:1–23, 1990a

Heimberg RG, Hope DA, Dodge CS, et al: DSM-III-R subtypes of social phobia: comparison of generalized social phobics and public speaking phobics. J Nerv Ment Dis 178:172–179, 1990b

Helzer JE, Robins LN, McEvoy L: Post-traumatic stress disorder in the general population: findings of the Epidemiologic Catchment Area survey. N Engl J Med 317:1630–1634, 1987

Herman JL, van der Kolk BA: Traumatic antecedents of borderline personality disorder, in Psychological Trauma. Edited by van der Kolk BA. Washington, DC, American Psychiatric Press, 1987, pp 111–126

Herman JL, Perry JC, van der Kolk BA: Childhood trauma in borderline personality disorder. Am J Psychiatry 146:490–495, 1989

Hewlett WA, Vinogradov S, Agras WS: Clonazepam treatment of obsessions and compulsions. J Clin Psychiatry 51:158–161, 1990

Hewlett WA, Vinogradov S, Agras WS: Clomipramine, clonazepam, and clonidine treatment of obsessive-compulsive disorder. J Clin Psychopharmacol 12:420–430, 1992a

Hewlett WA, Vinogradov S, Martin K, et al: Fenfluramine stimulation of prolactin in obsessive-compulsive disorder. Psychiatry Res 42:81–92, 1992b

Himle JA, Crystal D, Curtis GC, et al: Mode of onset of simple phobia subtypes: further evidence of heterogeneity. Psychiatry Res 36:37–43, 1991

Hoehn-Saric R, Merchant AF, Keyser ML, et al: Effects of clonidine on anxiety disorders. Arch Gen Psychiatry 38:1278–1282, 1981

Hoehn-Saric R, McLeod DR, Zimmerli WD: Differential effects of alprazolam and imipramine in generalized anxiety disorder: somatic versus psychic symptoms. J Clin Psychiatry 49:293–301, 1988

Hoehn-Saric R, McLeod DR, Hipsley PA: Effect of fluvoxamine on panic disorder. J Clin Psychopharmacol 13:321–326, 1993a

Hoehn-Saric R, Hazlett RL, McLeod DR: Generalized anxiety disorder with early and late onset of anxiety symptoms. Compr Psychiatry 34:291–298, 1993b

Hofmann SG, Ehlers A, Roth WT: Conditioning theory: a model for the etiology of public speaking anxiety? Behav Res Ther 33:567–571, 1995

Hogben GL, Cornfield RB: Treatment of traumatic war neurosis with phenelzine. Arch Gen Psychiatry 38:440–445, 1981

Hollander E, Liebowitz MR, Gorman JM, et al: Cortisol and sodium lactate–induced panic. Arch Gen Psychiatry 46:135–140, 1989

Hollander E, DeCaria CM, Schneier FR, et al: Fenfluramine augmentation of serotonin reuptake blockade antiobsessional treatment. J Clin Psychiatry 51:119–123, 1990a

Hollander E, Schiffman E, Cohen B, et al: Signs of central nervous system dysfunction in obsessive-compulsive disorder. Arch Gen Psychiatry 47:27–32, 1990b

Hollander E, DeCaria C, Gully R, et al: Effects of chronic fluoxetine treatment on behavioral and neuroendocrine responses to meta-chlorophenylpiperazine in obsessive-compulsive disorder. Psychiatry Res 36:1–17, 1991a

Hollander E, Liebowitz MR, Rosen WG: Neuropsychiatric and neuropsychological studies in obsessive-compulsive disorder, in The Psychobiology of Obsessive-Compulsive Disorder. Edited by Zohar J, Insel T, Rasmussen SA. New York, Springer, 1991b, pp 126–145

Hollander E, DeCaria C, Nitescu A, et al: Noradrenergic function in obsessive-compulsive disorder: behavioral and neuroendocrine responses to clonidine and comparison to healthy controls. Psychiatry Res 37:161–177, 1991c

Hollander E, DeCaria CM, Nitescu A, et al: Serotonergic function in obsessive-compulsive disorder: behavioral and neuroendocrine responses to oral m-chlorophenylpiperazine and fenfluramine in patients and healthy volunteers. Arch Gen Psychiatry 49:21–28, 1992

Hollingsworth CE, Tanguay PE, Grossman L, et al: Long-term outcome of obsessive-compulsive disorder in childhood. Journal of the American Academy of Child Psychiatry 19:134–144, 1980

Hornig CD, McNally RJ: Panic disorder and suicide attempt: a reanalysis of data from the Epidemiologic Catchment Area study. Br J Psychiatry 167:76–79, 1995

Horowitz MJ: Stress-Response Syndromes. New York, Jason Aronson, 1976

Horowitz MJ, Wilner N, Kaltreider N, et al: Signs and symptoms of posttraumatic stress disorders. Arch Gen Psychiatry 37:88–92, 1980

Horwath E, Johnson J, Hornig CD: Epidemiology of panic disorder in African-Americans. Am J Psychiatry 150:465–469, 1993

Insel TR, Murphy DL, Cohen RM, et al: Obsessive-compulsive disorder: a double-blind trial of clomipramine and clorgyline. Arch Gen Psychiatry 40:605–612, 1983

Insel TR, Mueller EA, Alterman I, et al: Obsessive-compulsive disorder and serotonin: is there a connection? Biol Psychiatry 20:1174–1188, 1985

James IA, Blackburn IM: Cognitive therapy with obsessive-compulsive disorder. Br J Psychiatry 166:444–450, 1995

James IM, Griffith DNW, Pearson RM, et al: Effect of oxprenolol on stage-fright in musicians. Lancet 2:952–954, 1977

James IM, Borgoyne W, Savage IT: Effect of pindolol on stress-related disturbances of musical performance: preliminary communication. J R Soc Med 76:194–196, 1983

Janet P: Les Obsessions et la psychasthénie, 2nd Edition. Paris, Bailliere, 1908

Jenike MA, Hyman S, Baer L, et al: A controlled trial of fluvoxamine in obsessive-compulsive disorder: implications for a serotonergic theory. Am J Psychiatry 147:1209–1215, 1990a

Jenike MA, Baer L, Summergrad P, et al: Sertraline in obsessive-compulsive disorder: a double-blind comparison with placebo. Am J Psychiatry 147:923–928, 1990b

Jenike MA, Baer L, Buttolph L, et al: Buspirone augmentation of fluoxetine in patients with obsessive-compulsive disorder. J Clin Psychiatry 52:13–14, 1991a

Jenike MA, Baer L, Ballantine HT, et al: Cingulotomy for refractory obsessive-compulsive disorder: a long-term follow-up of 33 patients. Arch Gen Psychiatry 48:548–555, 1991b

Johnson J, Weissman MM, Klerman GL: Panic disorder, comorbidity, and suicide attempts. Arch Gen Psychiatry 47:805–808, 1990

Kahn RJ, McNair DM, Lipman RS, et al: Imipramine and chlordiazepoxide in depressive and anxiety disorders, II: efficacy in anxious outpatients. Arch Gen Psychiatry 43:79–85, 1986

Kardiner A: Traumatic neurosis of war, in American Handbook of Psychiatry, Vol 1. Edited by Arieti S. New York, Basic Books, 1959, pp 245–257

Karno M, Golding JM, Sorenson SB, et al: The epidemiology of obsessive-compulsive disorder in five US communities. Arch Gen Psychiatry 45:1094–1099, 1988

Katschnig H, Amering M, Stolk JM, et al: Long-term follow-up after a drug trial for panic disorder. Br J Psychiatry 167:487–494, 1995

Katerndahl DA: Panic and prolapse: meta-analysis. J Nerv Ment Dis 181:539–544, 1993

Katzelnick DJ, Kobak KA, Greist JH, et al: Sertraline for social phobia: a double-blind, placebo-controlled crossover study. Am J Psychiatry 152:1368–1371, 1995

Kauffman CD, Reist C, Djenderedjian A, et al: Biological markers of affective disorders and posttraumatic stress disorder: a pilot study with desipramine. J Clin Psychiatry 48:366–367, 1987

Keck PE, Taylor VE, Tugrul KC, et al: Valproate treatment of panic disorder and lactate-induced panic attacks. Biol Psychiatry 33:542–546, 1993

Kehl PA, Marks IM: Neurological factors in obsessive-compulsive disorder: two case reports and a review of the literature. Br J Psychiatry 149:315–319, 1986

Keijsers GP, Hoogduin CA, Schaap CP: Predictors of treatment outcome in the behavioral treatment of obsessive-compulsive disorder. Br J Psychiatry 165:781–786, 1994

Kelly DD: The role of endorphins in stress-induced analgesia. Ann N Y Acad Sci 398:260–271, 1982

Kendler KS, Neale MC, Kessler RC, et al: Generalized anxiety disorder in women: a population-based twin study. Arch Gen Psychiatry 49:267–272, 1992a

Kendler KS, Neale MC, Kessler RC, et al: The genetic epidemiology of phobias in women: the interrelationship of agoraphobia, social phobia, situational phobia, and simple phobia. Arch Gen Psychiatry 49:273–281, 1992b

Kessler RC, McGonagle KA, Zhao S, et al: Lifetime and 12-month prevalence of DSM-III-R psychiatric disorders in the United States: results from the National Comorbidity Survey. Arch Gen Psychiatry 51:8–19, 1994

Kessler RC, Sonnega A, Bromet E, et al: Posttraumatic stress disorder in the National Comorbidity Survey. Arch Gen Psychiatry 52:1048–1060, 1995

Kinzie JD, Leung P: Clonidine in Cambodian patients with posttraumatic stress disorder. J Nerv Ment Dis 177:546–550, 1989

Klein DF: Delineation of two drug responsive anxiety syndromes. Psychopharmacologia 5:397–408, 1964

Klein DF: Anxiety reconceptualized, in Anxiety: New Research and Changing Concepts. Edited by Klein DF, Rabkin JG. New York, Raven, 1981, pp 235–263

Klein DF: False suffocation alarms, spontaneous panics, and related conditions: an integrative hypothesis. Arch Gen Psychiatry 50:306–317, 1993

Klein DF, Zitrin CM, Woerner MG, et al: Treatment of phobias, II: behavior therapy and supportive psychotherapy: are there any specific ingredients? Arch Gen Psychiatry 40:139–145, 1983

Klein M: A contribution to the theory of anxiety and guilt. Int J Psychoanal 29:114–123, 1948

Knesevich JW: Successful treatment of obsessive-compulsive disorder with clonidine hydrochloride. Am J Psychiatry 139:364–365, 1982

Kolb LC: A neuropsychological hypothesis explaining posttraumatic stress disorders. Am J Psychiatry 144:989–995, 1987

Kolb LC, Burris BC, Griffiths S: Propranolol and clonidine in treatment of the chronic post-traumatic stress disorders of war, in Post-Traumatic Stress Disorder: Psychological and Biological Sequelae. Edited by van der Kolk BA. Washington, DC, American Psychiatric Press, 1984, pp 97–105

Koran LM, McElroy SL, Davidson JR, et al: Fluvoxamine versus clomipramine for obsessive-compulsive disorder: a double-blind comparison. J Clin Psychopharmacol 16:121–129, 1996

Kosten TR, Mason JW, Giller EL, et al: Sustained urine norepinephrine and epinephrine elevation in PTSD. Psychoneuroendocrinology 12:13–20, 1987

Krystal H: Massive Psychic Trauma. New York, International Universities Press, 1968

Leckman JF, Goodman WK, North WG, et al: Elevated cerebrospinal fluid levels of oxytocin in obsessive-compulsive disorder: comparison with Tourette's syndrome and healthy controls. Arch Gen Psychiatry 51:782–792, 1994

Lelliott P, Marks I, McNamee G, et al: Onset of panic disorder with agoraphobia: toward an integrated model. Arch Gen Psychiatry 46:1000–1004, 1989

Leonard HL, Swedo SE, Rapoport JL, et al: Treatment of obsessive-compulsive disorder with clomipramine and desipramine in children and adolescents: a double-blind crossover comparison. Arch Gen Psychiatry 46:1088–1092, 1989

Leonard HL, Swedo SE, Lenane MC, et al: A double-blind desipramine substitution during long-term clomipramine treatment in children and adolescents with obsessive-compulsive disorder. Arch Gen Psychiatry 48:922–927, 1991

Leonard HL, Swedo SE, Lenane MC, et al: A 2- to 7-year follow-up study of 54 obsessive compulsive children and adolescents. Arch Gen Psychiatry 50:429–439, 1993

Lepine JP, Chignon JM, Teherani M: Suicide attempts in patients with panic disorder. Arch Gen Psychiatry 50:144–149, 1993

Lesch KP, Hoh A, Disselkamp-Tietze J, et al: 5-Hydroxytryptamine$_{1A}$ receptor responsivity in obsessive-compulsive disorder: comparison of patients and controls. Arch Gen Psychiatry 48:540–547, 1991

Liden S, Gottfries CG: Beta-blocking agents in the treatment of catecholamine-induced symptoms in musicians. Lancet 2:529, 1974

Liebowitz MR, Fyer AJ, McGrath P, et al: Clonidine treatment of panic disorder. Psychopharmacol Bull 17:122–123, 1981

Liebowitz MR, Fyer AJ, Gorman JM, et al: Lactate provocation of panic attacks, I: clinical and behavioral findings. Arch Gen Psychiatry 41:764–770, 1984a

Liebowitz MR, Quitkin FM, Stewart JW, et al: Phenelzine v imipramine in atypical depression: a preliminary report. Arch Gen Psychiatry 41:669–677, 1984b

Liebowitz MR, Gorman JM, Fyer AJ, et al: Lactate provocation of panic attacks, II: biochemical and physiological findings. Arch Gen Psychiatry 42:709–719, 1985a

Liebowitz MR, Gorman JM, Fyer AJ, et al: Social phobia: review of a neglected anxiety disorder. Arch Gen Psychiatry 42:729–736, 1985b

Liebowitz MR, Schneier F, Campeas R, et al: Phenelzine vs atenolol in social phobia: a placebo-controlled comparison. Arch Gen Psychiatry 49:290–300, 1992

Lindy JD, Grace MC, Green BL: Building a conceptual bridge between civilian trauma and war trauma: preliminary psychological findings from a clinical sample of Vietnam veterans, in Post-Traumatic Stress Disorder: Psychological and Biological Sequelae. Edited by van der Kolk BA. Washington, DC, American Psychiatric Press, 1984, pp 44–57

Lipper S: Carbamazepine in the treatment of posttraumatic stress disorder: implications for the kindling hypothesis, in Posttraumatic Stress Disorder: Etiology, Phenomenology, and Treatment. Edited by Wolf ME, Mosnaim AD. Washington, DC, American Psychiatric Press, 1990, pp 184–203

Lipper S, Davidson JRT, Grady TA, et al: Preliminary study of carbamazepine in post-traumatic stress disorder. Psychosomatics 27:849–854, 1986

Lucey JV, Barry S, Webb MG, et al: The desipramine-induced hormone response and the dexamethasone suppression test in obsessive-compulsive disorder. Acta Psychiatr Scand 86:367–370, 1992

Lum LC: Hyperventilation and anxiety states. J R Soc Med 74:1–4, 1981

Magee WJ, Eaton WW, Wittchen HU, et al: Agoraphobia, simple phobia, and social phobia in the National Comorbidity Survey. Arch Gen Psychiatry 53:159–168, 1996

Maier SF, Seligman ME: Learned helplessness: theory and evidence. J Exp Psychol 105:3–46, 1976

Maier SF, Dovies S, Gran JW: Opiate antagonists and long-term analgesic reaction induced by inescapable shock in rats. Journal of Comparative and Physiological Psychology 94:1172–1183, 1980

Maletzky B, McFarland B, Burt A: Refractory obsessive compulsive disorder and ECT. Convuls Ther 10:34–42, 1994

Manuzza S, Schneier FR, Chapman TF, et al: Generalized social phobia: reliability and validity. Arch Gen Psychiatry 52:230–237, 1995

Markowitz JS, Weissman MM, Ouellette R, et al: Quality of life in panic disorder. Arch Gen Psychiatry 46:984–992, 1989

Marks IM: Fears and Phobias. New York, Academic Press, 1969

Marks IM, Gelder MG: Different ages of onset in varieties of phobia. Am J Psychiatry 123:218–221, 1966

Marks IM, Hodgson R, Rachman S: Treatment of chronic obsessive-compulsive neurosis by in vivo exposure: a two-year follow-up and issues in treatment. Br J Psychiatry 127:349–364, 1975

Marks IM, Stern RS, Mawson D, et al: Clomipramine and exposure for obsessive-compulsive rituals, I. Br J Psychiatry 136:1–25, 1980

Marks IM, Gray S, Cohen D, et al: Imipramine and brief therapist-aided exposure in agoraphobics having self-exposure homework. Arch Gen Psychiatry 40:153–162, 1983

Marks IM, Lelliott P, Basoglu M, et al: Clomipramine, self-exposure and therapist-aided exposure for obsessive-compulsive rituals. Br J Psychiatry 152:522–534, 1988

Marmar CR, Weiss DS, Schlenger WE, et al: Peritraumatic dissociation and posttraumatic stress in male Vietnam theater veterans. Am J Psychiatry 151:902–907, 1994

Marshall JR: The treatment of night terrors associated with posttraumatic syndrome. Am J Psychiatry 132:293–295, 1975

Marten PA, Brown TA, Barlow DH, et al: Evaluation of the ratings comprising the associated symptom criterion of DSM-III-R generalized anxiety disorder. J Nerv Ment Dis 181:676–682, 1993

Mason JW, Giller EL, Kosten TR, et al: Urinary free-cortisol levels in posttraumatic stress disorder patients. J Nerv Ment Dis 174:145–149, 1986

Mason JW, Giller EL, Kosten TR, et al: Elevation of urinary norepinephrine/cortisol ratio in posttraumatic stress disorder. J Nerv Ment Dis 176:498–502, 1988

Mason ST, Fibiger HC: Anxiety: the locus ceruleus disconnection. Life Sci 25:2141–2147, 1979

Mattes J: More on panic disorder and mitral valve prolapse (letter). Am J Psychiatry 138:1130, 1981

Mattick RP, Peters L, Clarke JC: Exposure and cognitive restructuring for social phobia: a controlled study. Behavior Therapy 20:3–23, 1989

Mavissakalian M, Michelson L: Agoraphobia: relative and combined effectiveness of therapist-assisted in vivo exposure and imipramine. J Clin Psychiatry 47:117–122, 1986a

Mavissakalian M, Michelson L: Two-year follow-up of exposure and imipramine treatment of agoraphobia. Am J Psychiatry 143:1106–1112, 1986b

Mavissakalian M, Perel JM: Imipramine dose-response relationship in panic disorder with agoraphobia: preliminary findings. Arch Gen Psychiatry 46:127–131, 1989

Mavissakalian M, Perel JM: Clinical experiments in maintenance and discontinuation of imipramine therapy in panic disorder with agoraphobia. Arch Gen Psychiatry 49:318–323, 1992

Mavissakalian M, Perel JM: Imipramine treatment of panic disorder with agoraphobia: dose ranging and plasma level-response relationships. Am J Psychiatry 152:673–682, 1995

McBride PA, DeMeo MD, Sweeney JA, et al: Neuroendocrine and behavioral responses to challenge with the indirect serotonin agonist dl-fenfluramine in adults with obsessive-compulsive disorder. Biol Psychiatry 31:19–34, 1992

McDougle CJ, Goodman WK, Price LH, et al: Neuroleptic addition in fluvoxamine-refractory obsessive-compulsive disorder. Am J Psychiatry 147:652–654, 1990

McDougle CJ, Southwick SM, Charney DS, et al: An open trial of fluoxetine in the treatment of posttraumatic stress disorder. J Clin Psychopharmacol 11:325–327, 1991

McDougle CJ, Goodman WK, Leckman JF, et al: The efficacy of fluvoxamine in obsessive-compulsive disorder: effects of comorbid chronic tic disorder. J Clin Psychopharmacol 13:354–358, 1993a

McDougle CJ, Goodman WK, Leckman JF, et al: Limited therapeutic effect of addition of buspirone in fluvoxamine-refractory obsessive-compulsive disorder. Am J Psychiatry 150:647–649, 1993b

McDougle CJ, Goodman WK, Leckman JF, et al: Haloperidol addition in fluvoxamine-refractory obsessive-compulsive disorder: a double-blind, placebo-controlled study in patients with and without tics. Arch Gen Psychiatry 51:302–308, 1994

McFarlane AC: The aetiology of post-traumatic morbidity: predisposing, precipitating and perpetuating factors. Br J Psychiatry 154:221–228, 1989

McFarlane AC: Vulnerability to posttraumatic stress disorder, in Posttraumatic Stress Disorder: Etiology, Phenomenology, and Treatment. Edited by Wolf ME, Mosnaim AD. Washington, DC, American Psychiatric Press, 1990, pp 2–20

McGuire PK, Bench CJ, Frith CD, et al: Functional anatomy of obsessive-compulsive phenomena. Br J Psychiatry 164:459–468, 1994

McKeon J, McGuffin P, Robinson P: Obsessive-compulsive neurosis following head injury: a report of four cases. Br J Psychiatry 144:190–192, 1984

McNair DM, Kahn RJ: Imipramine compared with a benzodiazepine for agoraphobia, in Anxiety: New Research and Changing Concepts. Edited by Klein DF, Rabkin JG. New York, Raven, 1981, pp 69–80

McNally RJ, Kohlbeck PA: Reality monitoring in obsessive-compulsive disorder. Behav Res Ther 31:24–53, 1993

Michels R, Frances A, Shear MK: Psychodynamic models of anxiety, in Anxiety and the Anxiety Disorders. Edited by Tuma AH, Maser JD. Hillsdale, NJ, Erlbaum, 1985, pp 595–618

Michelson L, Marchione K, Greenwald M, et al: Panic disorder: cognitive-behavioral treatment. Behav Res Ther 28:141–151, 1990

Mindus, Jenike MA: Neurosurgical treatment of malignant obsessive-compulsive disorder. Psychiatr Clin North Am 15:921–938, 1992

Montgomery SA, McIntyre A, Osterheider M, et al: A double-blind, placebo-controlled study of fluoxetine in patients with DSM-III-R obsessive-compulsive disorder: the Lilly European OCD Study Group. Eur Neuropsychopharmacol 3:143–152, 1993

Mountjoy CQ, Roth M, Garside RF, et al: A clinical trial of phenelzine in anxiety depressive and phobic neuroses. Br J Psychiatry 131:486–492, 1977

Mowrer O: A stimulus response analysis of anxiety and its role as a reinforcing agent. Psychol Rev 46:553–565, 1939

Nagy LM, Krystal JH, Woods SW, et al: Clinical and medication outcome after short-term alprazolam and behavioral group treatment in panic disorder: 2.5-year naturalistic follow-up study. Arch Gen Psychiatry 46:993–999, 1989

Nee LE, Caine ED, Polinsky RJ, et al: Gilles de la Tourette syndrome: clinical and family study of 50 cases. Ann Neurol 7:41–49, 1982

Neftel KA, Adler RH, Kappell K, et al: Stage fright in musicians: a model illustrating the effect of beta blockers. Psychosom Med 44:461–469, 1982

Nemiah JC: A psychoanalytic view of phobias. Am J Psychoanal 41:115–120, 1981

Nemiah JC: The psychodynamic view of anxiety: an historical approach, in Handbook of Anxiety, Vol 1. Edited by Roth M, Noyes R, Burrows GD. Amsterdam, Elsevier, 1988, pp 277–303

Neziroglu F, Anemone R, Yaryura-Tobias JA: Onset of obsessive-compulsive disorder in pregnancy. Am J Psychiatry 149:947–950, 1992

Noyes R Jr, Clarkson C, Crow RR, et al: A family study of generalized anxiety disorder. Am J Psychiatry 144:1019–1024, 1987

Noyes R Jr, Garvey MJ, Cook BL: Follow-up study of patients with panic disorder and agoraphobia with panic attacks treated with tricyclic antidepressants. J Affect Disord 16:249–257, 1989

Noyes R Jr, Reich JH, Christiansen J, et al: Outcome of panic disorder: relationship to diagnostic subtypes and comorbidity. Arch Gen Psychiatry 47:809–818, 1990

Noyes R Jr, Reich JH, Suelzer M, et al: Personality traits associated with panic disorder: change associated with treatment. Compr Psychiatry 32:283–294, 1991

Nutt DJ: Altered central α_2-adrenoreceptor sensitivity in panic disorder. Arch Gen Psychiatry 46:165–169, 1989

Nutt DJ, Glue P, Lawson C, et al: Flumazenil provocation of panic attacks: evidence for altered benzodiazepine receptor sensitivity in panic disorder. Arch Gen Psychiatry 47:917–925, 1990

O'Connor K, Robillard S: Inference processes in obsessive-compulsive disorder: some clinical observations. Behav Res Ther 33:887–896, 1996

Oehrberg S, Christiansen PE, Behnke K, et al: Paroxetine in the treatment of panic disorder: a randomised, double-blind, placebo-controlled study. Br J Psychiatry 167:374–379, 1995

O'Rourke D, Fahy TJ, Brophy J, et al: The Galway study of panic disorder, III: outcome at 5 to 6 years. Br J Psychiatry 168:462–469, 1996

Ost LG: Age of onset of different phobias. J Abnorm Psychol 96:223–229, 1987

Ost LG, Westling BE: Applied relaxation vs cognitive behavior therapy in the treatment of panic disorder. Behav Res Ther 33:145–158, 1995

Otto MW: Normal and abnormal information processing: a neuropsychological perspective on obsessive-compulsive disorder. Psychiatr Clin North Am 15:825–848, 1992

Otto MW, Pollack MH, Sachs GS, et al: Discontinuation of benzodiazepine treatment: efficacy of cognitive-behavioral therapy for patients with panic disorder. Am J Psychiatry 150:1485–1490, 1993

Pacella BL, Polatin P, Nagler SH: Clinical and EEG studies in obsessive-compulsive states. Am J Psychiatry 100:830–838, 1944

Papp LA, Klein DF, Gorman JM: Carbon dioxide hypersensitivity, hyperventilation and panic disorder. Am J Psychiatry 150:1149–1157, 1993

Pato MT, Zohar-Kadouch R, Zohar J, et al: Return of symptoms after discontinuation of clomipramine in patients with obsessive-compulsive disorder. Am J Psychiatry 145:1521–1525, 1988

Pato MT, Pigott TA, Hill JL, et al: Controlled comparison of buspirone and clomipramine in obsessive-compulsive disorder. Am J Psychiatry 148:127–129, 1991

Pauls DL, Towbin KE, Leckman JF, et al: Gilles de la Tourette's and obsessive-compulsive disorder: evidence supporting a genetic relationship. Arch Gen Psychiatry 43:1180–1182, 1986

Pavlov IP: Conditional Reflexes: An Investigation of the Physiological Activity of the Cerebral Cortex (1927). Edited by Anrep GV. New York, Bover, 1960

Pecknold JC, Swinson RP, Kuch K, et al: Alprazolam in panic disorder and agoraphobia: results from a multicenter trial, III: discontinuation effects. Arch Gen Psychiatry 45:429–436, 1988

Perani D, Colombo C, Bressi S, et al: [18F]FDG PET study in obsessive-compulsive disorder: a clinical/metabolic correlation study after treatment. Br J Psychiatry 166:244–250, 1995

Perry BD, Giller EL Jr, Southwick SM: Altered plasma α_2-adrenergic binding sites in posttraumatic stress disorder (letter). Am J Psychiatry 144:1511–1512, 1987

Perse TL, Greist JH, Jefferson JW, et al: Fluvoxamine treatment of obsessive-compulsive disorder. Am J Psychiatry 144:1543–1548, 1987

Petty F, Chae Y, Kramer G, et al: Learned helplessness sensitizes hippocampal norepinephrine to mild restress. Biol Psychiatry 35:903–908, 1994

Piccinelli M, Pini S, Bellantuono C, et al: Efficacy of drug treatment in obsessive-compulsive disorder: a meta-analytic review. Br J Psychiatry 166:424–443, 1995

Pigott TA, Pato MT, Bernstein SE, et al: Controlled comparisons of clomipramine and fluoxetine in the treatment of obsessive-compulsive disorder: behavioral and biological results. Arch Gen Psychiatry 47:926–932, 1990

Pigott TA, Pato MT, L'Heureux F, et al: A controlled comparison of adjuvant lithium carbonate or thyroid hormone in clomipramine-treated patients with obsessive-compulsive disorder. J Clin Psychopharmacol 11:242–248, 1991

Pigott TA, L'Heureux F, Rubenstein CS, et al: A double-blind, placebo controlled study of trazodone in patients with obsessive-compulsive disorder. J Clin Psychopharmacol 12:156–162, 1992a

Pigott TA, L'Heureux F, Hill JL, et al: A double-blind study of adjuvant buspirone hydrochloride in clomipramine-treated patients with obsessive-compulsive disorder. J Clin Psychopharmacol 12:11–18, 1992b

Pigott TA, Hill JL, L'Heureux, et al: A comparison of the behavioral effects of oral versus intravenous m-CPP administration in OCD patients and the effect of metergoline prior to iv m-CPP. Biol Psychiatry 33:3–14, 1993

Pitman RK, Orr SP, Forgue DF, et al: Psychophysiologic assessment of post-traumatic stress disorder imagery in Vietnam combat veterans. Arch Gen Psychiatry 44:970–975, 1987

Pitman RK, van der Kolk BA, Orr SP, et al: Naloxone-reversible analgesic response to combat-related stimuli in posttraumatic stress disorder: a pilot study. Arch Gen Psychiatry 47:541–544, 1990

Pitts FN, McClure JN: Lactate metabolism in anxiety neurosis. N Engl J Med 277:1329–1336, 1967

Quitkin F, Babkin J: Hidden psychiatric diagnosis in the alcoholic, in Alcoholism and Clinical Psychiatry. Edited by Soloman J. New York, Plenum, 1982, pp 129–140

Rachman SJ, Hodgson RJ: Obsessions and Compulsions. Englewood Cliffs, NJ, Prentice-Hall, 1980

Rachman S, Thordarson DS, Shafran R, et al: Perceived responsibility: structure and significance. Behav Res Ther 33:779–784, 1995

Rainey JM Jr, Pohl RB, Williams M, et al: A comparison of lactate and isoproterenol anxiety states. Psychopathology 17 (suppl 1):74–82, 1984

Rainey JM Jr, Aleem A, Ortiz A, et al: Laboratory procedure for the inducement of flashbacks. Am J Psychiatry 144:1317–1319, 1987

Rapoport JL, Elkins R, Langer DH, et al: Childhood obsessive-compulsive disorder. Am J Psychiatry 138:1545–1554, 1981

Raskin M, Peeke HVS, Dickman W, et al: Panic and generalized anxiety disorders: developmental antecedents and precipitants. Arch Gen Psychiatry 39:687–689, 1982

Rasmussen SA: Lithium and tryptophan augmentation in clomipramine-resistant obsessive-compulsive disorder. Am J Psychiatry 141:1283–1285, 1984

Rasmussen SA, Tsuang MT: Clinical characteristics and family history in DSM-III obsessive compulsive disorder. Am J Psychiatry 143:317–322, 1986

Rauch SL, Jenike MA, Alpert NM, et al: Regional cerebral blood flow measured during symptom provocation in obsessive-compulsive disorder using oxygen 15–labeled carbon dioxide and positron emission tomography. Arch Gen Psychiatry 51:62–70, 1994

Rauch SL, Savage CR, Alpert NM, et al: A positron emission tomographic study of simple phobic symptom provocation. Arch Gen Psychiatry 52:20–28, 1995

Rauch SL, van der Kolk BA, Fisler RE, et al: A symptom provocation study of posttraumatic stress disorder using positron emission tomography and script-driven imagery. Arch Gen Psychiatry 53:380–387, 1996

Ravizza L, Barzega G, Bellino S, et al: Predictors of drug treatment response in obsessive-compulsive disorder. J Clin Psychiatry 56:368–373, 1995

Redmond DE Jr: New and old evidence for the involvement of a brain norepinephrine system in anxiety, in Phenomenology and Treatment of Anxiety. Edited by Fann WE, Karacan I, Pokorny AD, et al. New York, Spectrum, 1979, pp 153–203

Regier DA, Boyd JH, Burke JD Jr, et al: One-month prevalence of mental disorders in the United States, based on five Epidemiologic Catchment Area sites. Arch Gen Psychiatry 45:977–986, 1988

Reich J, Noyes R, Yates W: Anxiety symptoms distinguishing social phobia from panic and generalized anxiety disorders. J Nerv Ment Dis 176:510–513, 1988

Reist C, Kauffmann CD, Haier RJ, et al: A controlled trial of desipramine in 18 men with posttraumatic stress disorder. Am J Psychiatry 146:513–516, 1989

Rice KM, Blanchard EB, Purcell M: Biofeedback treatments of generalized anxiety disorder: preliminary results. Biofeedback Self Regul 18:93–105, 1993

Rickels K, Schweizer E, Csanalosi I, et al: Long-term treatment of anxiety and risk of withdrawal: prospective comparison of clorazepate and buspirone. Arch Gen Psychiatry 45:444–450, 1988

Rickels K, Downing R, Schweizer E, et al: Antidepressants for the treatment of generalized anxiety disorder: a placebo-controlled comparison of imipramine, trazodone, and diazepam. Arch Gen Psychiatry 50:884–895, 1993a

Rickels K, Schweizer E, Weiss S, et al: Maintenance drug treatment for panic disorder, II: short- and long-term outcome after drug taper. Arch Gen Psychiatry 50:61–68, 1993b

Riddle MA, Scahill L, King RA, et al: Double-blind, crossover trial of fluoxetine and placebo in children and adolescents with obsessive-compulsive disorder. J Am Acad Child Adolesc Psychiatry 31:1062–1069, 1992

Roy-Byrne PP, Cowley DS, Greenblatt DJ, et al: Reduced benzodiazepine sensitivity in panic disorder. Arch Gen Psychiatry 47:534–538, 1990

Rubenstein CS, Peynircioglu ZF, Chambless DL, et al: Memory in sub-clinical obsessive-compulsive checkers. Behav Res Ther 31:759–765, 1993

Salkovskis PM, Westbrook D: Behaviour therapy and obsessional ruminations: can failure be turned into success? Behav Res Ther 27:149–160, 1989

Salkovskis PM, Jones DRO, Clark DM: Respiratory control in the treatment of panic attacks: replication and extension with concurrent measurement of behaviour and pCO_2. Br J Psychiatry 148:526–532, 1986

Salzman L: Comments on the psychological treatment of obsessive-compulsive patients, in Obsessive-Compulsive Disorder: Psychological and Pharmacological Treatment. Edited by Mavissakalian M, Turner SM, Michelson L. New York, Plenum, 1985, pp 155–165

Sanderson WC, Rapee RM, Barlow DH: The influence of an illusion of control on panic attacks induced via inhalation of 5.5% carbon dioxide–enriched air. Arch Gen Psychiatry 46:157–162, 1989

Saxena S, Wang D, Bystritsky A, et al: Risperidone augmentation of SRI treatment for refractory obsessive-compulsive disorder. J Clin Psychiatry 57:303–306, 1996

Schilder P: The organic background of obsessions and compulsions. Am J Psychiatry 94:1397–1416, 1938

Schneier FR, Johnson J, Hornig CD, et al: Social phobia: comorbidity and morbidity in an epidemiologic sample. Arch Gen Psychiatry 49:282–288, 1992

Schneier FR, Saoud JB, Campeas R, et al: Buspirone in social phobia. J Clin Psychopharmacol 13:251–256, 1993

Schneier FR, Heckelman LR, Garfinkel R, et al: Functional impairment in social phobia. J Clin Psychiatry 55:322–331, 1994

Schwartz JM, Stoessel PW, Baxter LR, et al: Systematic changes in cerebral glucose metabolic rate after successful behavior modification treatment in obsessive-compulsive disorder. Arch Gen Psychiatry 53:109–113, 1996

Schweizer E, Rickels K, Lucki I: Resistance to the anti-anxiety effect of buspirone in patients with a history of benzodiazepine use. N Engl J Med 314:719–720, 1986

Schweizer E, Rickels K, Weiss S, et al: Maintenance drug treatment of panic disorder, I: results of a prospective, placebo-controlled comparison of alprazolam and imipramine. Arch Gen Psychiatry 50:51–60, 1993

Scott JP: Effects of psychotropic drugs on separation distress in dogs, in Proceedings of the IX Congress of Neuropsychopharmacology. Amsterdam, Excerpta Medica, 1975, pp 735–745

Scrignar CB: Post-Traumatic Stress Disorder: Diagnosis, Treatment, and Legal Issues. New York, Praeger, 1984

Seligman ME: Phobias and preparedness. Behavior Therapy 2:307–320, 1971

Shafran R, Ralph J, Tallis F: Obsessive-compulsive symptoms and the family. Bull Menninger Clin 59:472–479, 1996

Shalev AY, Peri T, Canetti L, et al: Predictors of PTSD in injured trauma survivors: a prospective study. Am J Psychiatry 153:2219–2225, 1996

Shay J: Fluoxetine reduces explosiveness and elevates mood of Vietnam combat vets with PTSD. J Trauma Stress 5:97–101, 1992

Shear MK, Cooper AM, Klerman GL, et al: A psychodynamic model of panic disorder. Am J Psychiatry 150:859–866, 1993

Sheehan DV, Ballenger J, Jacobsen G: Treatment of endogenous anxiety with phobic, hysterical, and hypochondriacal symptoms. Arch Gen Psychiatry 37:51–59, 1980

Skolnick P, Paul SM: Benzodiazepine receptors in the central nervous system. Int Rev Neurobiol 23:103–140, 1982

Skre I, Onstad S, Torgensen S, et al: A twin study of DSM-III-R anxiety disorders. Acta Psychiatr Scand 88:85–92, 1993

Smith MA, Davidson J, Ritchie JC, et al: The corticotropin releasing hormone test in patients with posttraumatic stress disorder. Biol Psychiatry 26:349–355, 1989

Solyom C, Solyom L, LaPierre Y, et al: Phenelzine and exposure in the treatment of phobias. Biol Psychiatry 16:239–247, 1981

Solyom L, Heseltine GFD, McClure DJ, et al: Behaviour therapy versus drug therapy in the treatment of phobic neurosis. Can J Psychiatry 18:25–32, 1973

Southwick SM, Krystal JH, Morgan CA, et al: Abnormal noradrenergic function in posttraumatic stress disorder. Arch Gen Psychiatry 50:266–274, 1993

Spiegel D, Cardeña E: Dissociative mechanisms in posttraumatic stress disorder, in Posttraumatic Stress Disorder: Etiology, Phenomenology, and Treatment. Edited by Wolf ME, Mosnaim AD. Washington, DC, American Psychiatric Press, 1990, pp 22–34

Spiegel DA, Bruce TJ, Gregg SF, et al: Does cognitive behavior therapy assist slow-taper alprazolam discontinuation in panic disorder? Am J Psychiatry 151:876–881, 1994

Starcevic V, Fallon S, Uhlenhuth EH: The frequency and severity of generalized anxiety disorder symptoms: toward a less cumbersome conceptualization. J Nerv Ment Dis 182: 80–84, 1994

Starkman MN, Cameron OG, Nesse RM, et al: Peripheral catecholamine levels and the symptoms of anxiety: studies in patients with and without pheochromocytoma. Psychosom Med 52:129–142, 1990

Stein DJ, Spadaccine E, Hollander E: Meta-analysis of pharmacotherapy trials for obsessive-compulsive disorder. Int Clin Psychopharmacol 10:11–18, 1995

Stein MB, Asmundson GJ: Autonomic function in panic disorder: cardiorespiratory and plasma catecholamine responsivity to multiple challenges of the autonomic nervous system. Biol Psychiatry 36:548–558, 1994

Stein MB, Millar TW, Larsen DK, et al: Irregular breathing during sleep in patients with panic disorder. Am J Psychiatry 152:1168–1173, 1995

Steketee GS, Foa EB, Grayson JB: Recent advances in the behavioral treatment of obsessive-compulsives. Arch Gen Psychiatry 39:1365–1371, 1982

Suomi SJ, Seaman SF, Lewis JK, et al: Effects of imipramine treatment of separation-induced social disorders in rhesus monkeys. Arch Gen Psychiatry 35:321–325, 1978

Swedo SE: Rituals and releasers: an ethological model of obsessive-compulsive disorder, in Obsessive-Compulsive Disorder in Children and Adolescents. Edited by Rapoport JL. Washington, DC, American Psychiatric Press, 1989, pp 269–288

Swedo SE, Schapiro MB, Grady CL, et al: Cerebral glucose metabolism in childhood-onset obsessive-compulsive disorder. Arch Gen Psychiatry 46:518–523, 1989a

Swedo SE, Rapoport JL, Cheslow DL, et al: Increased incidence of obsessive-compulsive symptoms in patients with Sydenham's chorea. Am J Psychiatry 146:246–249, 1989b

Swedo SE, Rapoport JL, Leonard H, et al: Obsessive-compulsive disorder in children and adolescents: clinical phenomenology of 70 consecutive cases. Arch Gen Psychiatry 46:335–341, 1989c

Swedo SE, Pietrini P, Leonard HL, et al: Cerebral glucose metabolism in childhood-onset obsessive-compulsive disorder: revisualization during pharmacotherapy. Arch Gen Psychiatry 49:690–694, 1992a

Swedo SE, Leonard HL, Kruesi MJP, et al: Cerebrospinal fluid neurochemistry in children and adolescents with obsessive-compulsive disorder. Arch Gen Psychiatry 49:29–36, 1992b

Szegedi A, Wetzel H, Leal M, et al: Combination treatment with clomipramine and fluvoxamine: drug monitoring, safety, and tolerability data. J Clin Psychiatry 57:257–264, 1996

Szymanski HV, Olympia J: Divalproex in posttraumatic stress disorder (letter). Am J Psychiatry 148:1086–1087, 1991

Tancer ME, Stein MB, Uhde TW: Growth hormone response to intravenous clonidine in social phobia: comparison to patients with panic disorder and healthy volunteers. Biol Psychiatry 34:591–595, 1993

Telch MJ, Agras WG, Taylor CM, et al: Combined pharmacological and behavioral treatment for agoraphobia. Behav Res Ther 23:325–335, 1985

Telch MJ, Lucas JA, Schmidt NB, et al: Group cognitive-behavioral treatment of panic disorder. Behav Res Ther 31:279–287, 1993

Thomsen PH, Mikkelsen HU: Development of personality disorders in children and adolescents with obsessive-compulsive disorder: a 6- to 22-year follow-up study. Acta Psychiatr Scand 87:456–462, 1993

Thorén P, Åsberg M, Cronholm B, et al: Clomipramine treatment of obsessive-compulsive disorder, I: a controlled clinical trial. Arch Gen Psychiatry 37:1281–1285, 1980a

Thorén P, Åsberg M, Bertilsson L, et al: Clomipramine treatment of obsessive-compulsive disorder, II: biochemical aspects. Arch Gen Psychiatry 37:1289–1294, 1980b

Tiffon L, Coplan JD, Papp LA, et al: Augmentation strategies with tricyclic or fluoxetine treatment in seven partially responsive panic disorder patients. J Clin Psychiatry 55:66–69, 1994

Tollefson GD, Rampey AH, Potvin JH, et al: A multicenter investigation of fixed-dose fluoxetine in the treatment of obsessive-compulsive disorder. Arch Gen Psychiatry 51:559–567, 1994

Torgersen S: Genetic factors in anxiety disorders. Arch Gen Psychiatry 40:1085–1089, 1983

Towey J, Bruder G, Hollander E, et al: Endogenous event-related potentials in obsessive-compulsive disorder. Biol Psychiatry 28:92–98, 1990

True WR, Rice J, Eisen SA, et al: A twin study of genetic and environmental contributions to liability for posttraumatic stress symptoms. Arch Gen Psychiatry 50:257–264, 1993

Turner SM, Beidel DC, Cooley-Quille MR: Two-year follow-up of social phobias treated with social effectiveness therapy. Behav Res Ther 33:553–555, 1995

Tynes LL, Salins C, Skiba W, et al: A psychoeducational and support group for obsessive-compulsive disorder patients and their significant others. Compr Psychiatry 33:197–201, 1992

Tyrer P, Candy J, Kelly D: A study of the clinical effects of phenelzine and placebo in the treatment of phobic anxiety. Psychopharmacology (Berl) 32:237–254, 1973

Uhde TW, Stein MB, Vittone BJ, et al: Behavioral and physiologic effects of short-term and long-term administration of clonidine in panic disorder. Arch Gen Psychiatry 46:170–177, 1989

Vallejo J, Olivares J, Marcos T, et al: Clomipramine versus phenelzine in obsessive-compulsive disorder: a controlled clinical trial. Br J Psychiatry 161:665–670, 1992

Van Ameringen M, Mancini C, Streiner DL: Fluoxetine efficacy in social phobia. J Clin Psychiatry 54:27–32, 1993

Van Ameringen M, Mancini C, Streiner D: Sertraline in social phobia. J Affect Disord 31:141–145, 1994

van den Hout M, Arntz A, Hoekstra R: Exposure reduced agoraphobia but not panic, and cognitive therapy reduced panic but not agoraphobia. Behav Res Ther 32:447–451, 1994

van der Kolk BA: Psychopharmacological issues in posttraumatic stress disorder. Hosp Community Psychiatry 34:683–691, 1983

van der Kolk BA: The role of the group in the origin and resolution of the trauma response, in Psychological Trauma. Edited by van der Kolk BA. Washington, DC, American Psychiatric Press, 1987a, pp 153–171

van der Kolk BA: The separation cry and the trauma response: developmental issues in the psychobiology of attachment and separation, in Psychological Trauma. Edited by van der Kolk BA. Washington, DC, American Psychiatric Press, 1987b, pp 31–62

van der Kolk BA: The trauma spectrum: the interaction of biological and social events in the genesis of the trauma response. J Trauma Stress 1:273–290, 1988

van der Kolk BA: The compulsion to repeat the trauma: reenactment, revictimization, and masochism. Psychiatr Clin North Am 12:389–411, 1989

van der Kolk BA, Saporta J: The biological response to psychic trauma: mechanisms and treatment of intrusion and numbing. Anxiety Research 4:199–212, 1991

van der Kolk BA, van der Hart O: Pierre Janet and the breakdown of adaptation in psychological trauma. Am J Psychiatry 146:1530–1540, 1989

van der Kolk BA, Boyd H, Krystal J, et al: Post-traumatic stress disorder as a biologically based disorder: implications of the animal model of inescapable shock, in Post-Traumatic Stress Disorder: Psychological and Biological Sequelae. Edited by van der Kolk BA. Washington, DC, American Psychiatric Press, 1984, pp 123–134

van der Kolk BA, Dreyfuss D, Michaels M, et al: Fluoxetine in posttraumatic stress disorder. J Clin Psychiatry 55:517–22, 1994

vanOppen P, Arntz A: Cognitive therapy for obsessive-compulsive disorder. Behav Res Ther 32:79–87, 1994

vanOppen P, deHaan E, vanBalkom AJ, et al: Cognitive therapy and exposure in vivo in the treatment of obsessive compulsive disorder. Behav Res Ther 33:379–390, 1995

van Vliet IM, den Boer JA, Westenberg HG: Psychopharmacological treatment of social phobia; a double blind placebo controlled study with fluvoxamine. Psychopharmacology (Berl) 115:128–134, 1994

Versiani M, Mundim FD, Nardi AE, et al: Tranylcypromine in social phobia. J Clin Psychopharmacol 8:279–283, 1988

Warneke LB: Intravenous chlorimipramine in the treatment of obsessional disorder in adolescence: case report. J Clin Psychiatry 46:100–103, 1985

Weissman MM, Leckman JF, Merikangas KR, et al: Depression and anxiety disorders in parents and children. Arch Gen Psychiatry 41:845–852, 1984

Weissman MM, Markowitz JS, Ouellette R, et al: Panic disorder and cardiovascular/cerebrovascular problems: results from a community survey. Am J Psychiatry 147:1504–1508, 1990

Weissman MM, Wickramaratne P, Adams PB, et al: The relationship between panic disorder and major depression: a new family study. Arch Gen Psychiatry 50:767–780, 1993

Welner A, Reich T, Robins E, et al: Obsessive-compulsive neurosis: record, family, and follow-up studies. Compr Psychiatry 17:527–539, 1976

Westphal K: Ueber Zwangsvorstellungen. Arch Psychiatr Neurol 8:734–750, 1878

Wiborg IM, Dahl AA: Does brief dynamic psychotherapy reduce the relapse rate of panic disorder? Arch Gen Psychiatry 53:689–694, 1996

Wise SP, Rapoport JL: Obsessive-compulsive disorder: is it a basal ganglia dysfunction? in Obsessive-Compulsive Disorder in Children and Adolescents. Edited by Rapoport JL. Washington, DC, American Psychiatric Press, 1989, pp 327–344

Wittchen HU, Zhao S, Kessler RC, et al: DSM-III-R generalized anxiety disorder in the National Comorbidity Survey. Arch Gen Psychiatry 51:355–364, 1994

Wlazlo Z, Schroeder-Hartwig K, Hand I, et al: Exposure in vivo vs social skills training for social phobia: long-term outcome and differential effects. Behav Res Ther 28:181–193, 1990

Wolf ME, Alavi A, Mosnaim AD: Posttraumatic stress disorder in Vietnam veterans, clinical and EEG findings: possible therapeutic effects of carbamazepine. Biol Psychiatry 23:642–644, 1988

Woodman CL, Noyes R: Panic disorder: treatment with valproate. J Clin Psychiatry 55:134–136, 1994

Woodruff R, Pitts FN Jr: Monozygotic twins with obsessional illness. Am J Psychiatry 120:1075–1080, 1964

World Health Organization: International Classification of Diseases, 10th Revision. Geneva, World Health Organization, 1992

Yehuda R, Southwick SM, Krystal JH, et al: Enhanced suppression of cortisol following dexamethasone administration in posttraumatic stress disorder. Am J Psychiatry 150:83–86, 1993

Yehuda R, Boisoneau D, Lowy MT, et al: Dose-response changes in plasma cortisol and lymphocyte glucocorticoid receptors following dexamethasone administration in combat veterans with and without posttraumatic stress disorder. Arch Gen Psychiatry 52:583–593, 1995a

Yehuda R, Keefe RS, Harvey PD, et al: Learning and memory in combat veterans with posttraumatic stress disorder. Am J Psychiatry 152:137–139, 1995b

Zinbarg RE, Barlow DH, Liebowitz M, et al: The DSM-IV trial for mixed anxiety-depression. Am J Psychiatry 151:1153–1162, 1994

Zitrin CM, Klein DF, Woerner MG: Treatment of agoraphobia with group exposure in vivo and imipramine. Arch Gen Psychiatry 37:63–72, 1980

Zitrin CM, Klein DF, Woerner MG, et al: Treatment of phobias, I: comparison of imipramine hydrochloride and placebo. Arch Gen Psychiatry 40:125–138, 1983

Zohar J, Insel TR: Obsessive-compulsive disorder: psychobiological approaches to diagnosis, treatment, and pathophysiology. Biol Psychiatry 22:667–687, 1987

Zohar J, Mueller EA, Insel TR, et al: Serotonergic responsivity in obsessive-compulsive disorder: comparison of patients and healthy controls. Arch Gen Psychiatry 44:946–951, 1987

Zohar J, Insel TR, Zohar-Kadouch RC, et al: Serotonergic responsivity in obsessive-compulsive disorder: effects of chronic clomipramine treatment. Arch Gen Psychiatry 45:167–172, 1988

SUGGESTED READINGS

Ballenger JC (ed): Neurobiology of Panic Disorder. New York, Wiley/Alan R Liss, 1990

Beck AT, Emery G, Greenberg RL: Anxiety Disorders and Phobias: A Cognitive Perspective. New York, Basic Books, 1985

Bowlby J: Attachment and Loss, Vol 2: Separation: Anxiety and Anger. New York, Basic Books, 1973

Gray J: The Neuropsychology of Anxiety. Oxford, Clarendon Press/Oxford University Press, 1982

Hollander E (ed): Obsessive-Compulsive Related Disorders. Washington, DC, American Psychiatric Press, 1993

Jenicke MA, Baer L, Minichiello WE: Obsessive-Compulsive Disorders: Theory and Management, 2nd Edition. Chicago, IL, Year Book Medical, 1990

Klein DF (ed): Anxiety. New York, Karger, 1987

Klein DF, Rabkin JG (eds): Anxiety: New Research and Changing Concepts. New York, Raven, 1981

Marks IM: Fears, Phobias, and Rituals: Panic, Anxiety, and Their Disorders. New York, Oxford University Press, 1987

Noyes R, Roth M, Burrows GD (eds): Handbook of Anxiety, Vol 4: The Treatment of Anxiety. New York, Elsevier, 1990

Pato MT, Zohar J (eds): Current Treatments of Obsessive-Compulsive Disorder. Washington, DC, American Psychiatric Press, 1991

Rapoport JL (ed): Obsessive-Compulsive Disorder in Children and Adolescents. Washington, DC, American Psychiatric Press, 1989

Roth M, Noyes R, Burrows GD (eds): Handbook of Anxiety, Vol 1: Biological, Clinical, and Cultural Perspectives. Amsterdam, Elsevier, 1988

Tuma AH, Mazer J (eds): Anxiety and Anxiety Disorders. Hillsdale, NJ, Erlbaum, 1985

van der Kolk BA (ed): Psychological Trauma. Washington, DC, American Psychiatric Press, 1987

Wolf ME, Mosnaim AD (eds): Posttraumatic Stress Disorder: Etiology, Phenomenology, and Treatment. Washington, DC, American Psychiatric Press, 1990

Zohar J, Insel TR, Rasmussen SA (eds): The Psychobiology of Obsessive-Compulsive Disorder. New York, Springer, 1991

CHAPTER 15

PSYCHOLOGICAL FACTORS AFFECTING MEDICAL CONDITIONS

JAMES L. LEVENSON, M.D.
J. STEPHEN MCDANIEL, M.D.
MICHAEL G. MORAN, M.D.
ALAN STOUDEMIRE, M.D.

The fact that psychological factors and psychiatric disorders may affect the clinical course of medical illness is incontrovertible and is no longer the topic of serious debate. For example, psychiatric disorders may adversely affect outcome and length of stay in general hospital patients (Levenson et al. 1990b; Marcantonio et al. 1994; Saravay and Lavin 1994), and the presence of major depression increases morbidity rates in patients with coronary artery disease (Carney et al. 1988; Frasure-Smith et al. 1993). In some situations, timely psychiatric intervention in medical patients can improve psychosocial adjustment (Evans et al. 1988) and even survival (Spiegel et al. 1989). It should be noted, however, that although most of the consultation-liaison literature has focused on interrelationships between comorbid psychiatric and medical disorders, a wealth of epidemiological research has identified behavioral risk factors for the development of medical illness. Research has documented that behavioral factors such as cigarette smoking, obesity, alcohol and substance dependency, and hazardous sexual practices are major causes of premature death and medical morbidity both in the United States and worldwide (Stoudemire et al. 1987a). For example, the total number of annual premature deaths due to behaviorally determined factors in the United States (excluding acquired immunodeficiency syndrome [AIDS]) is almost 2 million (Stoudemire et al. 1987b). A description of areas of investigation (Lipowski 1986) for classifying the psychological, behavioral, and social factors that may affect physical health is presented in Table 15–1.

This chapter consolidates the work of the committee that examined the DSM-III-R (American Psychiatric Association 1987) diagnostic category "Psychological Factors Affecting Physical Condition" (PFAPC) for revisions

The authors of this chapter would like to thank other members of the Work Group involved in revising the diagnostic criteria for this category in DSM-IV, whose background literature research contributed substantially to the information contained in this chapter. (The background papers are listed in the references to this chapter.) These individuals include Gale Beardsley, M.D., Claudia Bemis, M.D., Susan Glocheski, M.D., Michael Goldstein, M.D., F. Cleveland Kinney, M.D., David G. Folks, M.D., Robert E. Hales, M.D., M. Eileen McNamara, M.D., and Raymond Niaura, Ph.D.

TABLE 15–1. **Psychological and behavioral factors affecting medical conditions**

I. Psychophysiology
  A. Physiological reactions to psychological and behavioral variables
  B. Biological regulatory mechanisms associated with behavioral and psychological variables
    1. Psychoneurophysiology
    2. Psychoneuroendocrinology
    3. Psychoneuroimmunology
    4. Psychocardiology
II. Effects of concurrent psychiatric illness on the course and outcome of medical disorders
III. Behavioral risk factors for disease and injury
  A. Personality variables
  B. Cigarette smoking
  C. Dietary habits
  D. Alcohol and substance abuse
  E. Hazardous sexual behavior
  F. Risk-taking behaviors (accidents, injury)
  G. Noncompliance with medical treatment
  H. Violence, suicide, homicide
  I. Stressful or disruptive life change

Source. Reprinted with permission from Stoudemire A, Hales RE: "Psychological and Behavioral Factors Affecting Medical Conditions and DSM-IV: An Overview." *Psychosomatics* 32:5–13, 1991. Copyright 1991, Academy of Psychosomatic Medicine.

that are reflected in DSM-IV (American Psychiatric Association 1994) (see Table 15–2). Detailed literature reviews were conducted, with emphasis on studies employing systematic methodology examining the relationship among psychiatric, behavioral, and psychological factors and the onset, precipitation, and exacerbation of medical disorders. Expanded versions of those reviews—organized largely by organ system and medical specialty categories—have been published elsewhere (Beardsley and Goldstein 1993; Folks and Kinney 1992a, 1992b; Goldstein and Niaura 1992; Levenson and Bemis 1991; Levenson and Glocheski 1991; McNamara 1991; Moran 1991; Niaura and Goldstein 1992; Stoudemire 1993; Stoudemire and Hales 1991; Stoudemire et al. 1993). The essential findings of these reviews are summarized in this chapter, with special emphasis on their implications for clinical practice.

In this chapter, we focus on disorders of most interest to clinicians practicing in medical-psychiatric settings. We do not, for example, discuss relatively common nonspecific psychophysiological symptoms, such as diaphoresis, palpitations, gastric distress, diarrhea, urinary frequency, "tension" headaches, and vasovagal and other predominantly autonomically mediated reactions, as these are quite familiar to most clinicians. (Reviews of the traditional psychosomatic/psychophysiological theoretical and research literature may be found elsewhere [Stoudemire and McDaniel, in press].)

TABLE 15–2. **DSM-IV diagnostic criteria for psychological factors affecting general medical condition**

A. A general medical condition (coded on Axis III) is present.
B. Psychological factors adversely affect the general medical condition in one of the following ways:
  (1) The factors have influenced the course of the general medical condition as shown by a close temporal association between the psychological factors and the development or exacerbation of, or delayed recovery from, the general medical condition.
  (2) The factors interfere with treatment of the general medical condition.
  (3) The factors constitute additional health risks for the individual.
  (4) Stress-related physiological responses precipitate or exacerbate symptoms of the general medical condition.

Choose name based on the nature of the psychological factors (if more than one factor is present, indicate the most prominent):

Mental disorder affecting general medical condition (e.g., Axis I disorder such as major depressive disorder delaying recovery from a myocardial infarction)

Psychological symptoms affecting general medical condition (e.g., depressive symptoms delaying recovery from surgery; anxiety exacerbating asthma)

Personality traits or coping style affecting general medical condition (e.g., pathological denial of the need for surgery in a patient with cancer; hostile, pressured behavior contributing to cardiovascular disease)

Maladaptive health behaviors affecting general medical condition (e.g., overeating; lack of exercise; unsafe sex)

Stress-related physiological response affecting general medical condition (e.g., stress-related exacerbations of ulcer, hypertension, arrhythmia, or tension headache)

Other or unspecified psychological factors affecting general medical condition (e.g., interpersonal, cultural, or religious factors)

THE ROLE OF PSYCHOLOGICAL FACTORS IN CANCER ONSET AND PROGRESSION

The relationship between psychological factors and the onset and course of neoplastic disease serves as a prototype in examining the literature on this topic because many health care professionals and laypersons believe that psychological factors play a major role in cancer onset and progression. This belief has been strengthened, in part, by a rapidly growing literature, both scientific and popular, examining the role of psychological factors in cancer. Enthusiasm for therapeutic interventions based on "psychosomatic" relationships in oncology should be tempered by the recognition that the scientific evidence of such relationships is still in a relatively early stage of development and has many methodological limitations. In this section we critically summarize the literature on cancer and its potential connections to affective states, coping/defensive style and personality traits, interpersonal relationships, stressful life events, and psychosocial interventions.

AFFECTIVE STATES AND CANCER

The relationship between depression and cancer has been the focus of extensive study from several perspectives. The large epidemiological Western Electric study reported that depressive symptoms were associated with twice as high a risk of death from cancer 17 years later and with a higher-than-normal incidence of cancer for the first 10 years (Shekelle et al. 1981). This finding persisted at 20-year follow-up (Persky et al. 1987). The Western Electric study has been cited for many years as supporting the association between depressive symptoms and increased cancer risk. Other studies, however, have demonstrated negative findings (e.g., see Hahn and Petitti 1988). Dattore et al. (1980) found significantly *lower* depression scores in men who subsequently developed any type of cancer. A study by Zonderman et al. (1989) with a 10-year follow-up from the National Health and Nutrition Examination Survey found no significant depressive symptoms that could be seen as predictors of cancer morbidity or mortality, as did another study with a 15-year follow-up (Vogt et al. 1994).

Besides epidemiological studies, other studies have examined the effect of depression on outcome in cancer patients, most often those with breast cancer. Breast cancer patients who demonstrated a "fighting spirit" or who used denial had a higher survival rate than those with stoic acceptance or expressed hopelessness and helplessness (Greer et al. 1979). Although some clinical studies have not found a relationship between depression and cancer outcome (Cassileth et al. 1985), one study involving radiation therapy patients actually found high anxiety or depression to be predictive of lower mortality 3 years later (Leigh et al. 1987).

Bereavement has been recognized as a significant stressor and often has been assumed to be a risk factor in cancer onset and progression. An early retrospective study showed that the onset of hematological malignancy appeared to be preceded by significant losses in children and young adults (Greene et al. 1956). Other studies, however, have not shown bereavement to be a factor in the development or progression of cancer (Greer et al. 1979; Helsing and Szklo 1981; Klerman and Clayton 1984).

COPING STYLES, PERSONALITY TRAITS, AND CANCER

A large body of literature has described the cancer patient's degree of emotional expressiveness versus repressiveness and its purported effect on prognosis. Temoshok and Heller (1981) have described a Type C behavior pattern (in contrast to the Type A studied in coronary disease), typified as a cooperative, unassertive patient who suppresses negative emotions, particularly anger, and who accepts and complies with external authorities. Type C has been associated with increased melanoma tumor thickness (Temoshok et al. 1985), and its characteristics were found to be more common in melanoma patients than in control subjects (Kneier and Temoshok 1984). The Melbourne Colorectal Cancer Study found that cancer patients were more likely to have certain personality traits (similar to the Type C pattern) than were control subjects (G. A. Kune et al. 1991).

In contrast, Cassileth et al. (1985, 1988) found that none of the multiple psychosocial factors thought to be predictive of health predicted cancer survival (see also Holland 1989; Jamison et al. 1987). Other studies have demonstrated no differences in coping styles between breast cancer patients and control subjects (Buddeberg et al. 1991) or head and neck cancer patients and control subjects (Yamagiwa et al. 1991), and no relationship between coping style and breast cancer course (Edwards et al. 1990). Kreitler et al. (1993) found that repression and defensiveness increase in patients *after* the diagnosis of cancer is made. Epidemiological studies have not supported a relationship between "emotional repression" and cancer incidence or mortality (Shekelle et al. 1981).

Relatively less research has examined the effects of interpersonal variables on cancer. One prospective study of former medical students reported that lack of closeness with parents and less satisfactory relationships were associated with later development of cancer (Graves et al. 1991). A prospective study of breast cancer patients found several positive relationship variables that were predictive of increased survival (Waxler-Morrison et al. 1991).

A number of human studies have shown increased incidence of stressful life events preceding the onset of cervical, pancreatic, gastric, and lung cancer (Ernster et al. 1979; Fras et al. 1967; Horne and Picard 1979; Leherer 1980; Schmale and Iker 1965) and, as more recently noted, colorectal (S. Kune et al. 1991) and breast (Geyer 1991) cancer. Some work has linked stressful life events to progression or recurrence of cancer (Funch and Marshall 1983; Ramirez et al. 1989). Many other studies, however, have failed to find an association between preceding stressful life events and cancer onset (Barraclough et al. 1992; Edwards et al. 1990; Finn et al. 1974; Graham et al. 1971; Greer and Morris 1975). In a review of human and animal studies, Fox (1983) concluded that if stressful events and/or other psychological factors do have an effect on cancer incidence, it is small—a conclusion still appropriate today.

PSYCHOSOCIAL INTERVENTION AND CANCER OUTCOME

In contrast to studies lacking convincing support for an etiological relationship between psychological factors and cancer, some studies have shown improvement in the quality of life in cancer patients receiving group therapy (Fawzy et al. 1990a; Grossarth-Maticek et al. 1984; Spiegel et al. 1989). Relaxation training (Bindemann et al. 1991; Holland et al. 1991) and cognitive-behavior therapy (Greer et al. 1991) also have reduced anxiety and depression in cancer patients.

Spiegel and colleagues (Spiegel and Bloom 1983; Spiegel et al. 1981, 1989) performed a small randomized, controlled trial of supportive group therapy with training in self-hypnosis for pain control in women with metastatic breast cancer. At 1 year, the psychotherapy treatment group had less mood disturbance and fewer phobic responses (Spiegel et al. 1981) and complained of half as much pain (Spiegel and Bloom 1983). The treatment group also had increased survival compared with the control group (34.8 versus 18.9 months). Greater longevity was associated with less mood disturbance and greater vigor (Spiegel et al. 1989).

Fawzy et al. (1990a) evaluated the immediate and prolonged effects of a 6-week structured psychiatric group intervention for postsurgical patients with malignant melanoma. Patients who received the intervention had greater vigor than did control subjects at 6 weeks and less depression, fatigue, and total mood disturbance at 6-month follow-up. Experimental subjects demonstrated more active coping than control subjects both at the conclusion of the intervention and at follow-up. This study is the first to examine group psychiatric intervention in patients with early-stage cancer and good prognosis. The investigators also reported that patients who received group therapy had statistically significant increases in immunological function at 6-month follow-up (Fawzy et al. 1990b). Six years later, those who had received group therapy had significantly lower mortality and a trend for less recurrence of melanoma (Fawzy et al. 1993).

In controlled comparisons of women with metastatic breast cancer who did or did not receive psychotherapy, Grossarth-Maticek and colleagues also found psychotherapy to be associated with increased survival and higher lymphocyte counts (Grossarth-Maticek and Eysenck 1989; Grossarth-Maticek et al. 1984). Studies also have demonstrated no beneficial differences in cancer progression or mortality after psychotherapeutic intervention (Gellert et al. 1993). Larger, multisite studies are currently under way.

MECHANISMS

The question of *how* psychological factors might influence cancer onset and progression has many potential answers. The immune system is probably important for some, but not all, cancer surveillance, and much research has focused on the influence of psychological factors on immune function. Bereavement (Holland 1989), depression (Stein et al. 1991), stress (Kiecolt-Glaser et al. 1986), insomnia (Everson 1993), and level of social support (S. Levy et al. 1990) have all been shown to affect immune function, although the clinical significance of these effects is not clear. In the few studies to date, relationships between psychosocial factors, immune function, and cancer course have been complex (S. Levy et al. 1985, 1987, 1991).

Other mechanisms have been examined. The effect of some psychological factors (e.g., cynicism) on mortality may be mediated by smoking and alcohol (Almada et al. 1991), although these relationships may be interactive rather than simple (Grossarth-Maticek and Eysenck 1990). Psychological factors also affect whether and when patients seek medical attention for their initial cancer symptoms (Vracko-Tusevljak and Kambic 1989) and which treatment options they choose (Margolis et al. 1989). Some relationships may be cancer-type specific (e.g., sexual behavior and cervical cancer [Lambley 1993]).

In summary, a number of studies have lent some support to the relationship among a variety of psychological factors and the onset, exacerbation, or outcome of neoplastic disease. Currently, no clear associations (let alone causal relationships) have been proven, both because of methodological limitations in the positive studies and because of the failure of other studies of comparable methodology to find such relationships. Compared with other known risk factors, psychological factors alone (other than cigarette smoking and alcoholism) make a small contribution to cancer onset. However, more recent, methodologically sounder studies have suggested that cancer progression, rather than onset, may be influenced more by psychosocial factors.

CLINICAL IMPLICATIONS

Depression and anxiety remain common but relatively underdiagnosed and undertreated in cancer patients. Whether mood disorders affect the incidence, course, or clinical outcomes of cancer has not yet been definitively answered by systematic research. Nevertheless, depression and anxiety warrant clinical attention because of their clearly adverse effects on quality of life. Behaviors with obviously harmful effects on cancer patients (e.g., smoking, alcohol abuse, noncompliance with treatment) should also be targeted for intervention. The current literature on coping and personality style does not support the conclusions that any particular type of coping style is superior for all patients. Popular literature may lead some patients to feel responsible for their disease (or relapse) because they were unable to develop the "right attitude" or personality characteristics to "beat" cancer. Psychiatrists have a responsibility not only to avoid contributing to such simplistic, guilt-generating views, but also to help patients (and some other physicians) understand the value of a range of individualized approaches to adaptation.

Psychotherapeutic interventions may be of great benefit to cancer patients. If it is suggested, however, in an overly optimistic manner that psychological therapies will actually deliver cure or remission, there is a risk of deeply disappointing patients and their families and distracting from the direct benefits of psychiatric treatment for quality of life. Psychiatrists should keep in mind that psychosocial interventions are more likely to contribute to *quality* than to *quantity* of life in cancer patients. There is much enthusiasm among many professionals and laypersons for treatments promising to overcome cancer through "mind over body," but current scientific evidence supports a more cautious view. Psychiatric interventions are primarily justified if they reduce distress and dysfunction, such as when depressive or anxiety disorders are diagnosed in the context of oncological illness. Studies show that psychotherapy interventions can reduce anxiety and depression in cancer patients (Bindemann et al. 1991; Fawzy et al. 1990a; Greer et al. 1991; Grossarth-Maticek et al. 1984; Holland et al. 1991; Spiegel and Bloom 1983; Spiegel et al. 1981, 1989). A smaller number of studies have demonstrated the benefits of antianxiety and antidepressant medications in oncology (Costa et al. 1985; Holland et al. 1991). The diagnosis and treatment of psychiatric illness in cancer patients are discussed in detail elsewhere (Holland 1989; Lesko et al. 1993; McDaniel et al. 1995). Several of the most important findings in the relationship between psychological factors and cancer, including a number of sentinel outcome studies, are highlighted in Table 15–3.

PSYCHONEUROIMMUNOLOGY

The observation that psychosocial variables may affect outcome in cancer has focused attention on the immune system as a mediating mechanism, since the bidirectional interrelationship of the brain and the immune system has now been well documented (McDaniel 1995). This evidence ranges from anatomical confirmation of central nervous system (CNS) innervation of immune organs to reports documenting behavioral effects on immune response and tumor acquisition in experimental animals. Lymphocyte receptors have been identified for gonadal steroids, endorphins, enkephalins, corticotropin (adrenocorticotropic hormone [ACTH]), vasointestinal peptide, cholecystokinin, neurotensin, acetylcholine, and serotonin (Gorman and Kertzner 1990).

Just as cells of the peripheral immune system seem to be influenced by circulating factors of brain origin, a reciprocal relationship is demonstrated by the brain's susceptibility to certain lymphokines (i.e., substances produced by lymphocytes). The lymphokine interleukin-1 has been shown to directly stimulate the hypothalamus to produce corticotropin-releasing factor (CRF). This stimulation of CRF is believed to be a physiologically important part of an inhibitory feedback loop that functions to regulate the immune response. CRF increases secretion of ACTH, which in turn increases secretion of cortisol by the adrenal glands, thus serving to inhibit immune function. Glucocorticoids have a well-known immunosuppressive effect peripherally. This inhibitory feedback loop has been of particular interest to researchers studying immune aspects of mood disorders. Because of the overactivity of the hypothalamic-pituitary-adrenal (HPA) axis among some populations of depressed patients, the role of increased hypothalamic CRF production has now been documented and continues to be investigated with respect to more

TABLE 15–3. Illustrative studies supporting the effects of psychological factors on cancer

Psychological factor	Study type	Cancer type	Findings	Reference(s)
Depression	Epidemiological	Mixed	2× risk of death from cancer at 17-year follow-up	Shekelle et al. 1981
Personality traits	Case control	Colorectal	Cancer cases less likely to have expressive personality traits	G. A. Kune et al. 1991; S. Kune et al. 1991
Stressful life events	Case control	Breast	Increased stressful life events preceding cancer onset	Geyer 1991
Group therapy with training in self-hypnosis	Randomized controlled trial	Breast	Reductions in distress and pain, and increased survival in treatment group	Spiegel and Bloom 1983; Spiegel et al. 1981, 1989
Group therapy	Randomized controlled trial	Melanoma	Less distress, better coping, and increased immune function in treatment group	Fawzy et al. 1990a, 1990b

wide-ranging immunological implications.

The natural progression of study in psychoneuroimmunology has led investigators to focus on the role of psychological and psychosocial factors influencing physical health (Leonard and Miller 1995). For example, at least in the case of less serious infectious diseases (colds, influenza, herpes), convincing evidence links stress, negative affect, and disease onset and progression (Cohen and Herbert 1996). There is consistency in the literature describing the association between bereavement and immune function. Researchers have documented decreased mitogen stimulation in vitro in recently bereaved subjects, as well as decreased natural killer cell activity (NKA) in vitro in individuals with anticipatory bereavement.

A large amount of research has focused on a possible relationship between depression and the immune system. However, the studies have led to considerable confusion regarding conceptualizations, methods, experimental designs, and results. Stein et al. (1991) reviewed this literature and concluded that "alterations in the immune system in MD [major depression] do not appear to be a specific biological correlate of this disorder, but, rather, may occur in association with other variables that characterize depressed patients, including age and symptom severity" (p.175). These conclusions were drawn as a result of their study in which significant age-related differences between depressed subjects and control subjects were found. Specifically, the depressed patients did *not* show increases in lymphocyte function or number of CD_4 lymphocytes with advancing age as did the control subjects.

Literature examining psychosocial correlates and psychoneuroimmunology in cancer patients has increased. S. Levy et al. (1987, 1990) found that psychosocial variables such as lack of social support and depressive symptoms may be linked to reduced NKA in women with breast cancer and that more metastatic nodes and decreased NKA are associated with depressive symptoms in these patients, illuminating the need for more research in the area. Addressing psychoneuroimmunological aspects of depression with cancer may have important treatment implications, particularly regarding HPA axis hyperactivity associated with depression. In fact, HPA hyperactivity in depressed cancer patients may have important prognostic implications, particularly with regard to findings that in rats, HPA hyperactivity induced by exposure to stress is associated with increased tumor growth, especially in older rats (Sapolsky and Donnelly 1985). The possible role of psychological interventions affecting immune parameters has recently been studied in a group of postsurgical patients with malignant melanoma (Fawzy et al. 1990a). Those individuals randomized to the group intervention showed reduced psychological distress and enhanced longer-term effective coping. At 6-month follow-up, these patients also showed increases in the percentage of large granular lymphocytes and natural killer cells, as well as increased natural killer cytotoxic activity. These findings add to existing hypotheses regarding the earlier work of Spiegel et al. (1989), who reported significant increases in survival time in a group of patients with metastatic breast cancer who received 1 year of group psychotherapy, discussed earlier in this chapter.

While the field of psychoneuroimmunology continues to draw wide public interest, investigators must keep in mind how valid current methodological techniques are in evaluating the immune system. It has yet to be determined how accurate in vitro correlates are in reflecting actual in vivo immune responses. Therefore, each study must be critically examined within the context of the limitations of our current laboratory techniques.

CLINICAL IMPLICATIONS

The research literature suggests that immune modulation by psychosocial stressors and/or interventions may influence health status. Moreover, findings suggest that the impact of chronic stressors and psychosocial factors on sympathetic nervous system and endocrine function influences the immune system, thereby providing shared mechanisms that may impact on disease susceptibility and progression across a broad spectrum of disorders (Kiecolt-Glaser and Glaser 1995). Particularly in those patients experiencing bereavement and other significant psychosocial stress, as well as the spectrum of mood disorders, the possibility of coexisting immune changes should be considered. Similarly, in patients with some cancers (e.g., malignant melanoma and breast cancer), group psychotherapy both may decrease medical morbidity and may be associated with positive changes in immunity. Clearly, much more research is needed to correlate clinical presentations with in vitro immune measures. Nonetheless, as the literature continues to expand on this topic, clinicians must continue to respect the potential clinical effects of psychoneuroimmunology.

The most consistent findings in the study of psychoneuroimmunology are summarized in Table 15–4.

PSYCHOLOGICAL FACTORS AND ENDOCRINE DISEASE

Although there is a considerable amount of literature on psychoneuroendocrinology, particularly regarding the biology of mood disorders, there is little methodologically sound research regarding the clinical aspects of psychological factors and how these factors potentially influence endocrine diseases. Beardsley and Goldstein (1993, 1995) critically reviewed empirical findings on these factors and their influences. Of the existing literature, most research is focused primarily on three diseases: diabetes mellitus, Graves' disease, and Cushing's disease. The following discussions explore these three diseases and how psychological factors may influence them. The subject of psychiatric symptoms caused or exacerbated by endocrine disorders will not be reviewed.

DIABETES MELLITUS

Since the 17th century, there has been speculation about the role of psychological factors and the onset of diabetes mellitus. Although early studies aimed to show a relationship between stress and the onset of diabetes mellitus, these studies were significantly flawed, yielding inconclusive findings regarding the causal relationship between stress and disease onset (Beardsley and Goldstein 1995).

However, more current investigations have supported a relationship between stressful life events and diabetes mellitus. For example, Robinson and Fuller (1985) examined 13 newly diagnosed patients with insulin-dependent diabetes mellitus (IDDM) to ascertain the role of stressful life events as etiological triggering factors. By using siblings and neighborhood volunteers as control subjects, these investigators found a higher frequency of severe life events in the 3 years before diagnosis of IDDM in the patients compared with control subjects. In their study of 338 children with IDDM, Hagglof et al. (1991) found significant increases in events related to actual or threatened loss within the family of patients compared with nondiabetic control subjects. Because these investigators found no difference in the total frequency of life events between the two groups, their findings suggest that qualitative aspects of stress may be a more important cofactor than frequency of life events in understanding the relationship between stress and diabetes onset.

Other investigators have found no evidence of a causal relationship between stressful life events and the onset of diabetes mellitus (Gendel and Benjamin 1946). Studies utilizing retrospective design, as well as one large prospective study of air traffic controllers (Cobb and Rose 1973), failed to yield evidence of psychological factors such as stress being causally related to diabetes mellitus. In one recent review, Wales (1995) takes into account these conflicting data and suggests that in general, psychological stress may produce a deterioration in glycemic control in the as yet undiagnosed, asymptomatic patient, which in turn precipitates symptoms and makes the diagnosis evident.

Other investigators have speculated on the role of psychological factors in affecting the course of diabetes mellitus. Although early studies were flawed primarily because of difficulties in accurately measuring glucose control, more recent studies measuring glycosylated hemoglobin have proven this to be a reliable measure of metabolic control.

Two studies involving IDDM found significant associ-

TABLE 15-4.   Psychological factors associated with in vitro immune changes

Stressor	Effects	Reference(s)
Bereavement	↓ Lymphocyte mitogen response	Bartrop et al. 1977; Schleifer et al.1983
	↓ NKA	Irwin et al. 1987
Experimental stress paradigms		
Medical school final examination	↓ Lymphocyte mitogen response	Kiecolt-Glaser et al. 1984, 1986
	↓ Immunoglobulin A	
	↑ Antibody levels to EBV, HSV, CMV	
Work-related stress	↓ NKA	Dorian et al. 1985
Alzheimer's caregivers	↓ Percentage of T-lymphocytes	Kiecolt-Glaser et al. 1987a
	↓ CD$_4$/CD$_8$	
Divorce		
Women	↓ Lymphocyte mitogen response	Kiecolt-Glaser et al. 1987b, 1988
	↑ Antibody levels to EBV	
Men	↑ Antibody levels to EBV, HSV	Kiecolt-Glaser et al. 1987b, 1988
Depression	Some studies have shown normal lymphocyte mitogen responses and normal NKA, whereas others have shown reduced lymphocyte mitogen responses and reduced NKA. Other evidence suggests that patient age and illness severity may be important variables.	Schleifer et al. 1989; Stein et al.1991

Note.   NKA = natural killer cell activity; EBV = Epstein-Barr virus; HSV = herpes simplex virus; CMV = cytomegalovirus; CD$_4$ = helper cells; CD$_8$ = suppressor cells.

ations between psychological stress and blood glucose levels. Whereas one group of investigators monitored patients' self-perceptions of life stress over 8 weeks (Halford et al. 1990), Gonder-Frederick et al. (1990) monitored continuous blood glucose after exposing their cohort of patients to laboratory stress under controlled conditions. Similarly, Goetsch et al. (1993) found that laboratory stress yielded hyperglycemic effects in their cohort of patients with non–insulin-dependent diabetes mellitus (NIDDM). These experimental designs used the within-subject approach and, although based on relatively small numbers of subjects, suggest that some individuals are more vulnerable to the effects of stress than are others.

As with other medical illnesses, the role of personality characteristics and coping strategies also has been studied with relation to the course of diabetes mellitus. A number of these investigations have examined diabetic children. For example, Rovet and Ehrlich (1988) examined the effect of temperament on metabolic control in children with IDDM. Although no cause-effect relationship was concluded, these investigators found that diabetic children who were more active, better at following routines, less attentive, and more prone to negative moods, and who displayed milder responses to external stimuli, had improved metabolic control compared with the other diabetic children. Some of these findings are counterintuitive and require replication before accepting them as valid. Another investigation examined the relationship between specific personality traits and glucose regulation in diabetic children. Children with Type A behavior as identified by their responses to video games were found to have a hyperglycemic response to stress that was not exhibited by children with a Type B behavior pattern (Stabler et al. 1987). Other investigators have examined the relationship between low social competence and worsening of metabolic control (Hanson et al. 1987).

Although a number of studies have reported the effects of behavioral or psychosocial interventions on glucose control in diabetic patients, results have not been consistent. However, two groups of investigators have found that relaxation training can improve blood glucose control in NIDDM patients (Lammers et al. 1984; Surwit and Feinglos 1983).

Further studies evaluating the role of psychological factors in the onset and course of diabetes mellitus are needed to clarify the current conflicting data regarding stress and this disease. Clarifying this relationship will improve our understanding of the potential role of behavioral interventions as mediators in the effects of stress on diabetic patients.

GRAVES' DISEASE

Graves' disease, sometimes called *exophthalmic goiter*, has been in the differential diagnosis of psychosomatic illness used by clinicians for many years. To date, Weiner (1977) has provided the most extensive review of psychological factors in Graves' disease in his textbook *Psychobiology and Human Disease*. It is apparent from Weiner's review that numerous methodological flaws have made previous studies difficult to interpret. Complicating the studies of Graves' disease are the variable onset and course of the disease itself, making it difficult to measure changes in onset and course related to psychological factors. Furthermore, hyperthyroidism is often characterized by numerous psychological, behavioral, and neuropsychiatric signs and symptoms.

There appears to be minimal evidence to date suggesting that psychological characteristics of patients predispose them to develop Graves' disease or any thyroid disorder for that matter (Weiner 1977). However, one study has suggested that negative life events may be risk factors for Graves' disease (Winsa et al. 1991). These investigators studied patients with newly diagnosed Graves' disease and matched control subjects over a 2-year period. Patients and control subjects responded to a mailed questionnaire assessing demographic variables, life events, social support, and personality. Compared with control subjects, patients with Graves' disease had more negative life events in the 12 months preceding the diagnosis, and negative life events scores were significantly higher. These findings are of interest with regard to their psychosomatic implication; however, prospective studies are needed to confirm these results. There is currently insufficient evidence to suggest that psychological factors affect the course of Graves' disease.

CUSHING'S DISEASE

As is the case for Graves' disease, evidence that psychological factors affect Cushing's disease is lacking. Although Dr. Cushing himself argued that emotional stress contributed to the development of the disease that bears his name, methodologically sound prospective studies have yet to be conducted. Although it is clearly known that stressful stimuli may acutely lead to increased secretion of corticosteroids, hypercortisolism per se cannot be equated with illness and disease (Beardsley and Goldstein 1995). However, there is strong evidence that hypercortisolism of

several etiologies, including Cushing's disease, has been associated with the development of a wide range of neuropsychiatric phenomena (Hall et al. 1986). Nevertheless, anecdotal reports and descriptive analogies do not confirm a true relationship between psychological factors and the onset and/or course of Cushing's disease. Controlled human studies are needed to clarify these and other questions pertaining to psychological conditions and effects on endocrine disorders (see Table 15–5).

PSYCHOCARDIOLOGY

The effects of psychosocial and behavioral factors in cardiovascular disease have garnered considerable attention and have been a primary focus of epidemiological and psychosomatic medicine research for the past 20 years. This research has looked both at hypertension and coronary artery disease, including myocardial infarction and sudden cardiac death. Because approximately 85% of hypertension cases are classified as primary, or essential, hypertension in which the exact regulatory disruption leading to elevated blood pressure cannot be specified, psychological factors have been closely studied as part of the pathogenesis. These factors have been categorized as

---

TABLE 15–5. Psychological factors associated with endocrine disorders

Diabetes mellitus

Onset of illness: Some studies suggest a relationship between **stressful life events** and the onset of diabetes mellitus. These events in children have been categorized as experiences related to actual or threatened losses (Rovet and Ehrlich 1988).

Course of illness: Some studies have linked self-perceived **psychological stress** as well as experimental laboratory stress to changes in the course of the disease. One study found that Type A behavior in children is associated with a worse hyperglycemic response to stress than is a Type B behavior pattern (Stabler et al. 1987).

Graves' disease

Onset of illness: One study suggests that **negative life events** (e.g., death of loved one, divorce, loss of job) may be risk factors for onset of Graves' disease (Winsa et al. 1991).

Course of illness: There is no current evidence that psychological factors affect the course of illness.

Cushing's disease

There is little evidence of a causal relationship linked to psychological factors, but there is well-established evidence of neuropsychological manifestations of Cushing's disease.

"pressure reactivity" on the one hand and, on the other, as personality/behavioral factors. In the many reviews that have examined physiological hyperreactivity to environmental stimuli, there is relatively strong evidence that there exist subsets of individuals who have greater blood pressure reactivity to a variety of stressors than do others, ranging from experimental stress induced in the laboratory to stressful social conditions such as racism. However, the evidence linking reactivity in normotensive individuals with the eventual development of hypertension is equivocal. Perhaps most importantly, pressure reactivity in patients who have already developed hypertension may exacerbate and even accelerate their disease process.

Research examining personality traits in hypertension has been criticized because of the lack of prospective, longitudinal design. The most positive correlates have involved anger coping styles, but the relationship has not been a simple one; hypertension has positively correlated with both *inhibited* anger expression and *excessive* anger expression. Reviews of the epidemiological evidence of psychosocial precursors of hypertension have noted that individuals using an active coping style under environmental conditions that are not conducive to success may be predisposed to hypertension.

Some treatment interventions have been aimed specifically at affecting psychological factors related to hypertension. Various behavioral procedures (including biofeedback and relaxation training), as well as psychotherapy, have been used to treat hypertension. A number of investigators have reported clinically significant success in controlled studies, whereas other investigators have not found significant treatment effects when compared with the effects of interventions designed to act as a placebo or as attention control conditions.

Stress as a behavioral risk factor in coronary artery disease is another major focus of research in psychocardiology. Stress has been shown to cause a sympathetic-adrenomedullary alarm reaction characterized by excess catecholamine secretion. It is believed that catecholamine-mediated cardiac effects such as increased heart rate, contractility, and conduction velocity, as well as a shorter atrioventricular refractory period, may be pathogenically related to adverse cardiac events.

A host of studies have retrospectively examined temporally related stressful life experiences in patients who have experienced sudden death attributed to arrhythmias. In his study of patients who die suddenly, Engel (1971) found that uncertainty and fear of loss of control contributed to a giving-up state. This state, similar to depression, was thought to have possibly led to vasodepressor syncope, arrhythmias, and sudden death in patients predisposed to

myocardial disease. One study (Deanfield et al. 1984) has examined the use of positron-emission tomography (PET) to measure the diminished myocardial perfusion during mental stress in patients with typical angina and coronary heart disease. Seventy-five percent of the patients in this study showed perfusion abnormalities produced by a mental arithmetic stressor. Through the use of radionucleotide ventriculography and 48-hour Holter monitoring, Jiang et al. (1996) found mental stress-induced ischemia to be associated with significantly high rates of subsequent fatal and nonfatal cardiac events independent of age, baseline left ventricular ejection fraction, and previous myocardial infarction, and they predicted events over and above exercise-induced ischemia.

Another method of examining behavioral risks factors has resulted from investigations of psychosocial variables in coronary artery disease (Friedman and Rosenman 1959). These investigations led to the Type A versus Type B categorization first proposed in the 1950s. After a large number of studies, there remains disagreement regarding how important a risk factor the Type A behavior pattern is for the development and progression of coronary artery disease. Therefore, further studies have examined aspects of the Type A behavior pattern that are themselves more strongly associated with coronary artery disease, primarily hostility. A multidimensional item analysis from the Cook-Medley Hostility Scale (Cook and Medley 1954), derived from the Minnesota Multiphasic Personality Inventory (MMPI; Hathaway and McKinley 1943), has shown a significant relationship to mortality when specifically focusing on the items of cynicism, hostile affect, and aggressive responding in patients with a Type A behavior pattern (Goldstein and Niaura 1992).

The physiological correlates of Type A behavior patterns also have been studied with regard to cardiac morbidity. Type A behavior is believed to be a part of the stress paradigm. Individuals with Type A behavior patterns have been shown to display larger episodic increases in blood pressure, heart rate, and catecholamine levels when confronted by a stressful task. There is now evidence from primate studies that links the development of atherosclerosis in clinical coronary disease to the activation of the sympathetic nervous system. These findings suggest a link between psychological states, physiological reactivity, and subsequent cardiovascular morbidity (Manuck et al. 1989).

The role of mood states and cardiovascular morbidity and mortality also has been an important focus in cardiovascular research. One study showed that a major depression was the best predictor of major cardiac events during the 12 months after cardiac catheterization (Carney et al. 1988). Subsequent events were independent of variables such as severity of cardiac disease, left ventricular function, and smoking. In a recent progressive study of patients hospitalized following a myocardial infarction, major depressive disorder was found to be an independent risk factor for mortality at 6 months and 18 months (Frasure-Smith et al. 1993, 1995). The risk was at least equivalent to that of left ventricular dysfunction and previous myocardial infarction. When these patients were studied 18 months after their hospitalization for myocardial infarction, depression was a significant predictor of cardiac mortality, particularly among patients with ≥ 10 premature ventricular contractions per hour. Mood states associated with acute situational disturbances have been linked to sudden cardiac death. Reich et al. (1981) found that the onset of malignant ventricular arrhythmias was associated with identifiable psychologically stressful events in 21% of their patients referred for antiarrhythmic management.

Sociological factors such as work overload and life stress in addition to lack of social support have been shown to enhance coronary risk. Studies have specifically examined the role of social support in coronary disease in community samples. One community-based study of Japanese-American men living in Hawaii was designed to examine the influence of a variety of social network attributes on the incidence and prevalence of coronary heart disease. In this population, social networks tended to be significantly associated with the prevalence of coronary heart disease, but not with the incidence of coronary heart disease, between 1971 and 1977 (Welin et al. 1985). Other studies have found social connections to be negatively associated with the prevalence of coronary heart disease among men (Joseph 1980). A reduced level of socioeconomic resources enhances risk for cardiovascular death with coronary artery disease after all other risk factors are controlled (Williams et al. 1992). Nonmarried individuals with coronary artery disease are also at higher risk for death when compared with married individuals (Chandra et al. 1983). The role of social connections in the onset and course of coronary disease is an important focus of psychosomatic research, particularly as data continue to support the hypothesis that more socially isolated and/or less socially integrated individuals are overall less healthy psychologically and physically (Berkman 1995).

CLINICAL IMPLICATIONS

The role of psychological factors and cardiac morbidity is perhaps one of the most well-documented categories of psychosomatic medicine. Because of the role of pressure reactivity in patients with hypertension and its association with Type A behavior patterns, those patients who exhibit

manifestations of Type A behavior should be strongly considered for psychological interventions (Ketterer 1993). Particularly in view of existing evidence that Type A behavior patterns may be a risk factor for developing coronary artery disease, and evidence that mental stress is associated with decreased myocardial perfusion, patients who are at risk of developing, or those who currently have a diagnosis of, coronary artery disease are potentially excellent candidates for interventions such as stress management, biofeedback, and relaxation training. The work of Carney et al. (1988) and Frasure-Smith et al. (1995) clarifies the potential negative consequences of comorbid depression in patients following cardiac catheterization or myocardial infarction. Depression warrants aggressive treatment in this patient population. Further details regarding the diagnosis and treatment of specific psychiatric disorders in cardiology patients may be found elsewhere (Levenson 1993). The most consistent clinical findings between psychological factors and cardiovascular disease are summarized in Table 15–6.

LIFESTYLE RISK FACTORS

As emphasized in the introduction to this chapter, it is now well established that lifestyle behaviors are risk factors that

---

TABLE 15–6. **Psychological factors associated with cardiac disease**

Hypertension

Anger coping styles: Some research suggests that personality traits, particularly *anger coping styles* (both inhibited anger expression and excessive anger expression), may be precursors to hypertension.

Coronary artery disease (CAD)

Type A behavior pattern: A Type A behavior pattern is a risk factor for developing CAD. Studies suggest subsequent morbidity (i.e., related to cynicism, hostile affect, and aggressive responding) (Goldstein and Niaura 1992).

Stress: Primate studies have linked development of atherosclerosis to sympathetic nervous system activation (Manuck et al. 1989). Stressful life events have been linked to sudden cardiac death (Engel 1971).

Mood states: Major depression predicts cardiac morbidity up to 12 months postcardiac catheterization (Carney et al. 1988).

Social support: Nonmarried status, lack of social support, and reduced socioeconomic resources are linked to increased mortality in CAD (Chandra et al. 1983; Joseph 1980; Welin et al. 1985; Williams et al. 1992).

significantly contribute to the mortality rate in the United States. The most widely studied risk factors are cigarette smoking and obesity, both of which affect the development, perpetuation, and exacerbation of medical illnesses.

Cigarette smoking remains the single most important modifiable risk factor for illness and the greatest single cause of preventable premature deaths (Peto et al. 1992). Cigarette smoking is a powerful independent contributor to the occurrence of myocardial infarction, sudden death, peripheral vascular disease, and stroke. It has been shown to act synergistically with other traditional risk factors such as hypertension and high blood cholesterol to increase the risk of coronary artery disease. In 1985, smoking accounted for 87% of lung cancer deaths and 82% of deaths relating to chronic obstructive lung disease (U.S. Department of Health and Human Services 1989). In reviewing the behavioral risk factor literature, Goldstein found evidence that smoking cessation was effective in decreasing risk for the development of illness, as well as morbidity and mortality, once smoking-related illness develops (Stoudemire et al. 1993). Fifteen years after smoking cessation, the risk factor for coronary heart disease approaches the risk of individuals who never smoked. Rosenberg et al. (1985) have reported that the risk of myocardial infarction for cigarette smokers decreases within 2 years of quitting to a level similar to that in men who have never smoked.

Unfortunately, smoking cessation is a difficult intervention. The difficulty is compounded by the physical dependence on nicotine in chronic smokers, which has led to a separate category for nicotine dependence in DSM-IV. Such dependence can now be treated effectively, especially when behavioral and pharmacological approaches are combined.

After cigarette smoking, obesity is the second most widely studied risk factor associated with increased morbidity and mortality. There is a strong association between obesity and hypertension, hypercholesterolemia, and diabetes mellitus as risk factors for cardiovascular disease. Obesity also may increase the risk of prostate, colon, and rectal cancer in men and endometrial, cervical, ovarian, breast, and gallbladder cancer in women. For those individuals with morbid obesity (more than 100 pounds overweight), sudden death, pulmonary disorders, cardiomyopathy, congestive heart failure, liver dysfunction, and thromboembolic disease are common complications. Functional limitations and negative psychosocial sequelae also are well-documented outcomes in individuals with morbid obesity.

Because of the aforementioned associated medical complications, weight reduction for obese individuals has become an important medical intervention. However, recent evidence has shown that individuals who repeatedly diet are more likely to increase their weight over time when compared with obese individuals who do not repeatedly attempt to lose weight. This finding has led to speculation that repeated dieting may be associated with increases in morbidity.

The concept of weight reduction is complicated by psychological, social, and cultural differences. There is some evidence that psychological factors such as anxiety, depression, and stress contribute to overeating. Early learning and environmental reinforcement also play roles as mediators of behavior that can result in obesity. However, behavioral treatments for obesity have demonstrated efficacy, especially when they have focused on maintenance of behavior change. Strategies combining exercise, dietary restriction, longitudinal monitoring, and professionally led skills training have produced positive outcomes.

Other lifestyle factors that have been associated with negative health outcomes are as follows: 1) a sedentary lifestyle and diet high in cholesterol and fats and low in fiber; 2) sexual practices known to increase the risk of infection with human immunodeficiency virus (HIV), hepatitis B, and other transmissible organisms; 3) exposure to sun and other ultraviolet light; 4) lack of use of safety restraints when riding in motor vehicles; and 5) psychoactive substance use and abuse (Stoudemire et al. 1993).

CLINICAL IMPLICATIONS

With the currently established evidence of the morbidity and mortality associated with lifestyle risk factors, psychiatrists, perhaps more so than other clinicians, have an active role to play in assisting patients with behavioral changes. With cigarette smoking being the single most important modifiable risk factor for illness in this country, treatment of nicotine dependence should play a central role in the treatment plans of those patients who continue to abuse tobacco. Similarly, interventions for modifying obesity are paramount in preventing and treating conditions such as heart disease, diabetes mellitus, pulmonary disease, and certain cancers. At the very least, psychoeducation about these two risk behaviors, as well as about risk behaviors that include unsafe sexual practices, exposure to sun, psychoactive substance use and abuse, use of safety restraints in motor vehicles, and certain dietary habits, should be addressed with patients when considering their overall psychosomatic-psychophysiological profile. Clinicians are referred to practical reviews of the treatment interventions in cigarette smoking and obesity (Brown et al. 1993; Clark et al. 1993; Goldstein et al. 1991) (see also Table 15–7 and Figure 15–1).

TABLE 15–7. Lifestyle risk factors affecting health outcome

Cigarette smoking

Obesity

Sedentary lifestyle

Diet (high cholesterol, low fiber)

Unsafe sexual practices

Exposure to sun/ultraviolet light

Lack of use of safety restraints when riding in motor vehicles

Psychoactive substance abuse

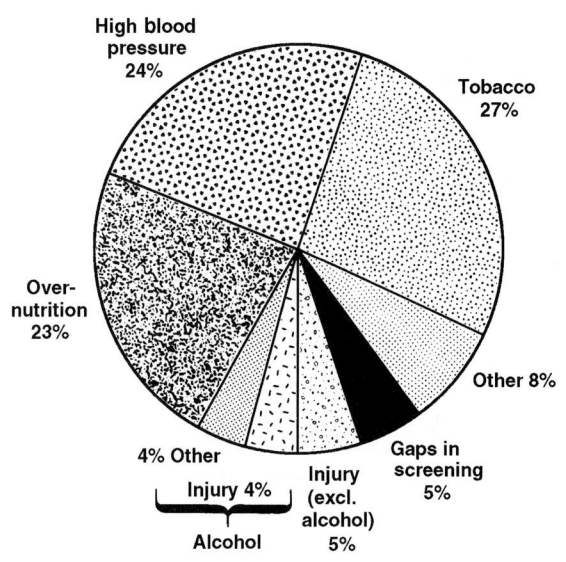

FIGURE 15–1. Premature deaths. Three precursors—tobacco, high blood pressure, and overnutrition—account for 73.5% of premature deaths in the United States.
Source. Reprinted with permission from Amler RW, Eddins DL: "Cross-Sectional Analysis: Precursors of Premature Death in the United States." *American Journal of Preventive Medicine* 3 (No 5, Suppl):181–187, 1987. Copyright 1987, Society for Neuroscience.

PULMONARY DISEASES

Asthma historically was considered to be a classic "psychosomatic" illness. Doctors and patients alike describe exacerbation of symptoms as a result of "stress." Classical psychoanalytic theories based on particular unconscious conflicts (Dunbar 1947) and models based on personality structure sought to demonstrate the vulnerability of certain character types to asthma, but there is no evidence that psychoanalytic therapy alone represents a comprehensive treatment for psychosomatic illnesses.

Most practitioners now embrace a multifactorial model in which a range of childhood trauma and predispositions (including genetic ones) set the stage for vulnerability to asthma in childhood or later in life (Knapp and Mathe 1985; Moran 1994). Current psychoanalytic models are more complex than Alexander's (1950) original formulations that implied specificity of childhood conflict, although Alexander himself regarded the so-called psychosomatic illnesses as multifactorially determined. More modern, analytically oriented models emphasize that optimal psychophysiological regulatory functions occur within a successful infant-mother attachment. Confirmation of these models is derived in part from observations that derangement or disruption of this attachment in monkeys may cause dysregulation of affect and physiological processes such as sleep-wake cycle, body temperature, and heart rate, among others (Hofer 1984; Reite and Short 1986). Some authors have proposed that adult asthma patients with a poor ability to manage loss and other stressors through verbal expression may be at increased risk for asthma attacks (Gaddini 1978; Rees 1956). Many researchers have investigated the role of personality traits and adaptive strategies in predisposing one to asthma or its relapses. Extreme inhibition, covert aggression, and marked dependency needs appear to be highly associated with asthma (Sharma and Nandkumar 1980). The lack of prospective studies and adequate animal models interferes with efforts to interpret these traits as predisposing individuals to asthma or as evidence of nonspecific adaptation to chronic illness.

From a more purely biological perspective, the usefulness of sympathomimetic agents in the treatment of asthma led to the formulation of asthma as a state of relative parasympathetic dominance (or β_2-receptor blockade). β_2-receptor blockade can produce bronchoconstriction in susceptible individuals, including most asthmatic persons. Stress and anxiety should produce functionally increased sympathetic outflow and should at least theoretically not worsen or provoke an attack. Asthmatic patients, however, may respond to stressful events with abnormally low epinephrine secretion (Mathe and Knapp 1969). Panic and anxiety disorders may worsen the course of asthma. Conversely, repeated episodes of respiratory distress probably predispose an asthma patient to panic and anxiety disorders (Smoller et al. 1996).

Through another route, sleep disruption caused by psychiatric disturbances such as depression or anxiety may cause impaired patient awareness of bronchoconstriction

(Ballard et al. 1990) and thus may delay appropriate self-medication in the early stages of an asthma attack. Psychosis and poor reality testing in schizophrenic or cognitively impaired individuals also could interfere with adherence to any prescribed medical regimen.

Studies of chronic obstructive pulmonary disease (COPD) have centered on personality types, ability to interpret symptoms such as dyspnea, and patient and family factors in ventilator dependence.

Although there is agreement that major personality disorders and mood disorders contribute to functional disability in COPD patients (Weiner 1985), no studies clearly designate these factors as specifically predisposing traits or maladaptive consequences of COPD. Dyspnea "out of proportion" to pertinent clinical measurements of airway resistance appears to be augmented or maintained by depressive and anxious mood, as well as by histrionic personality traits. Panic and anxiety in COPD patients may produce significant morbidity, through phobic avoidance of activity, excessive anxiolytic use, and more frequent hospitalizations (Smoller et al. 1996).

COPD itself, through adverse effects on arterial oxygen concentrations, can cause neuropsychiatric disturbances that impair compliance. Memory and concentration disturbances are especially common. Chronic ventilator patients present a number of diagnostic and therapeutic problems. Varying arterial oxygen tensions directly and negatively affect neuropsychiatric functioning in these patients, particularly elderly patients.

Anxiety within the family system of a ventilator patient can hinder progress in weaning. Adequate family ego strength (Sivak et al. 1986), especially the presence of defensive mechanisms that limit the effects of anxiety (Ford 1983), suggests the best prognosis. Educability, optimism, high motivation, and lack of preexisting psychopathology also improve the prospects for handling the on-again, off-again experience of ventilator dependence and marginal pulmonary functioning (Gilmartin 1986; Weisman 1987).

CLINICAL IMPLICATIONS

History that suggests a clear-cut connection between stressful events and aggravation of asthmatic symptoms should lead to psychiatric consultation. A specific aim of the consultation would include helping the patient develop heightened awareness of the typical stressors that appear to trigger breathing-related symptoms so that the patient can develop coping strategies for dealing with them. The psychiatrist also can evaluate the role of anxiolytics in those asthmatic patients who temporarily may need extra assistance with the burden of affect. Generally, asthmatic patients do not chronically retain CO_2 unless another lung condition, such as chronic obstructive disease, is present, and thus the judicious use of low-dose benzodiazepines is not necessarily contraindicated. Panic disorder may be indistinguishable from the expectable physiological reaction to severe dyspnea, and patients may inappropriately use bronchodilator medications for the treatment of such episodes. Careful history taking and education can reveal such situations, and the psychiatrist may then elect to use antidepressants for prophylactic management.

Personality profiles that include extreme inhibition and covert aggression often manifest themselves in the family setting as problematic dependency and undermine the asthmatic patient's potential for reasonable separation and individuation. Such a constellation should alert the psychiatrist to the potential need for family evaluation and treatment, directed at promoting more autonomous functioning for the patient.

If anxiety or depressive affect is severe enough, pulmonary outcome is eroded in at least two ways: through the patient's inability to adhere to the treatment regimen and, possibly, through autonomic pathways (Yellowlees and Kalucy 1990). In addition, nonspecific induction of stress may worsen the course of the asthma (Gorman 1990). The appropriate treatment of panic disorder or major depression thus forms an essential part of the medical management of pulmonary patients, especially asthmatic patients.

Certain pathological family dynamics, especially the presence of severe avoidance and denial of intense affect, suggest a poor prognosis for ventilator-dependent patients with COPD and require early and firm intervention by the psychiatrist. Family sessions focused on the family members' helplessness and anger are crucial in the overall approach. As for cardiac patients, the psychiatric issues that lead to or maintain smoking (such as masochistic traits, depression, or nicotine addiction) must be addressed in persons with COPD. Depression may be especially important in this regard: failure to treat a coexistent mood disorder seriously undermines the success of smoking-cessation treatments.

RHEUMATOLOGICAL DISEASE

Among patients and physicians there is widespread anecdotal agreement that emotional factors affect the clinical course of rheumatoid arthritis (RA). Since the work of Alexander and others, there has been interest in the personality profiles of RA patients, although the theory that certain neurotic conflicts were specific for RA has been disproven. Patients with RA were seen as self-sacrificing, masochistic, inhibited, and perfectionistic (Moos 1964). In turn, such persons also were considered to be at a higher-than-average risk for developing a new psychiatric disturbance (Cassileth et al. 1984). Depression, hypochondriacal symptoms, and endorsement of psychotic symptoms on psychological testing occur at an increased frequency among RA patients (Polley et al. 1970). The loss of mobility, jobs, and relationships contributes to depressive affect and withdrawal, eroding support systems that are so necessary in any chronically ill patient's struggle for rehabilitation. Certain "personality traits" and an increased incidence of psychiatric disturbance should be considered complications of RA and not causes of the disease.

Certain psychological factors appear to predict a poor course of RA, including poor motivation, low intelligence, depressed mood unassociated with pain, poor impulse control, and deficits in ego strength (Molodofsky and Chester 1970). These factors operate through mechanisms such as diminished energy for rehabilitation, decreased understanding of the treatment regimen, and impulsive, maladaptive acting out of anger and depressed mood as reactions to the chronic illness. Psychological strengths that constructively affect the course of RA include a positive attitude toward rehabilitation personnel and a flexible and adjustable view of the goals of the rehabilitation process (Vogel and Rosillo 1971).

Brief mention should be made of the so-called fibrositis or fibromyalgia syndrome (FMS). Emotional distress, such as depressive affect, is considered universal among patients with this condition. Symptoms include muscular trigger points, a characteristic sleep disorder, and widespread myalgias. The affective disturbances may be pathogenic (FMS as a depressive equivalent) or the result of having a chronic, poorly understood, and misdiagnosed disorder. First-degree relatives frequently demonstrate "depressive characteristics." Sedating, serotonergically active antidepressants such as doxepin or nortriptyline are the drugs of first choice (Goldenberg 1986).

CLINICAL IMPLICATIONS

Psychiatrists treating patients with rheumatological diseases should be especially alert to the existence of mood and cognitive impairment disorders. It has been estimated that *40%–50%* of RA patients appear depressed on psychological testing (Halliday 1942). The motoric retardation associated with depression can produce severe debili-

tation (Molodofsky and Chester 1970). Thus, clinicians should be alert to the development of anxiety and depression in these patients (Meenan 1981). Both anxiety and depression can erode patients' capacity and will for long-term adherence to medical treatment plans, essential components of therapeutic success for these patients.

Assessment of the support system is an early step in the total evaluation of a patient, and aggressive attempts should be made to maintain the involvement of the patient's family and friends. The frustration and self-criticism associated with depression undermine the patient's willingness and ability to continue physical therapy. This physical withdrawal can lead to severe debilitation, loss of important muscle mass, and resentment and functional abandonment by the patient's support system. Psychological withdrawal can produce enhanced experience of bodily symptoms such as pain and can increase the use of analgesics.

Psychological testing and a thorough history will be helpful in identifying a pattern of poor impulse control, low intelligence quotient, and depressed mood unassociated with pain, all of which reduce chances for adherence to the medical regimen. Family involvement and support, frequent rheumatology office visits, home visits by physician assistants or nurse specialists, and psychotherapy and pharmacotherapy directed at the depressed mood all play a role in ensuring maintenance of function and early detection of relapse.

FMS is frequently associated with depressive affect or major depression. The patient is often despondent over the repeated failures of previous treatments and may be angry about the long and seemingly wasteful lapse of time preceding actual diagnosis. Most FMS patients without major depression can benefit from antidepressant treatment. Selected FMS patients may obtain relief from a systematic program of meditation and yoga (Kaplan et al. 1993). Details regarding the treatment of psychiatric disorders in patients with arthritis and other connective tissue diseases may be found elsewhere (Moran and Dubester 1993).

GASTROINTESTINAL DISORDERS

Gastric and duodenal ulcers have long been recognized to differ in their etiologies. Understanding the pathogenesis of peptic ulcers has been revolutionized by discovery of the central role of the bacterium *Helicobacter pylori*. Early investigators of psychosomatic illnesses primarily focused on duodenal ulcer, for which psychological factors were thought to play a larger role. Alexander (1950) suggested that duodenal ulcer occurred after an increase in responsibility or frustration in individuals with unmet wishes to be cared for ("oral dependency"). In a classic study testing this hypothesis, Weiner et al. (1957) combined preexisting individual psychological characteristics and a biological trait (high pepsinogen secretion) to successfully predict when men undergoing the stress of army draft would develop duodenal ulcer. Recent studies continue to confirm that psychological stress is an independent risk factor for the development (Armstrong et al. 1994) and recurrence (Levenstein et al. 1995) of duodenal ulcer. Whether specific emotions or character traits are pathogenic for peptic disease remains controversial, and some "neurotic" traits may be the consequence rather than the cause of ulcer (Jess 1994; Jess and Eldrup 1994). There are several mechanisms by which psychological factors could impact ulcer disease, including pepsinogen secretion (P. Walker et al. 1988) or risk behaviors, including smoking, alcohol, and overuse of analgesics (Folks and Kinney 1992b).

Studies revealing the association between peptic ulcer and divorce, separation, and widowhood are intriguing (Gilligan et al. 1987). Such associations suggest that loss of attachment may be a precipitating factor. Attachment relationships may serve as a regulating influence for a number of physiological processes and for disturbing affects (Hofer 1984; Reite and Short 1986). Loss of these attachments could severely dysregulate susceptible individuals and lead to ulcer disease.

In irritable bowel syndrome (IBS), as in asthma, target organ hypersensitivity to mechanical and chemical stimuli, as well as to pathological stress, plays a major pathophysiological role. Increased vagal activity appears to have a mediating function in both disorders (Read 1987). Symptoms include abdominal pain and alterations in bowel habits, either constipation or diarrhea, in the absence of abnormalities on physical examination or traditional laboratory and radiological tests. Underlying motility disturbances appear to respond to psychological symptoms (Folks and Kinney 1992b) and produce a relapsing-remitting course. Morphology of the intestine does not appear to be altered in IBS, but electrical and motor activities are increased compared with such activities in control subjects.

Concomitant psychological symptoms appear to increase the chances that a patient with abdominal complaints will consult a physician, irrespective of the ultimate gastrointestinal diagnosis. When altered bowel habits are added to the symptom of abdominal pain, the patient also is more likely to complain of psychological distress (Whitehead et al. 1988).

Psychopathology is extremely common in patients with IBS, but there is no unique pattern of psychological

characteristics (E. A. Walker et al. 1990). IBS patients are more likely to have a history of childhood sexual abuse compared with patients who have other gastrointestinal disorders (E. A.Walker et al. 1993).

Developmental histories also reveal that control subjects had many *fewer* childhood doctor visits and less discomfort with bowel symptoms than did individuals with IBS (Lowman et al. 1987). Loss and separation are recurrent early developmental themes in patients with IBS. The early childhood of the patient may reflect an attempt by the child to find a regulatory relationship outside the family unit. Persistent or neurotic pursuit of such regulation by others may account for the frequently reported histories of conflicted, dependent marriages in IBS patients (Lowman et al. 1987). Ulcerative colitis was described in early literature as a psychosomatic disease, but no specific psychological factor has ever been demonstrated to contribute to the cause of ulcerative colitis or Crohn's disease. However, psychological stress does affect symptom complaints and aggravate mucosal disease activity in ulcerative colitis (Levenstein et al. 1994). The presence of a concurrent psychiatric disorder contributes substantially to disability and distress in patients with inflammatory bowel disease (E. A.Walker et al. 1996).

CLINICAL IMPLICATIONS

Patients with peptic ulcer of the duodenum whose condition is refractory to treatment should be screened for high state and trait anxiety characteristics. Psychotherapy focused on intellectualizing and problem-solving techniques can help patients feel a greater sense of mastery over feared calamities and less helpless and overwhelmed. The psychiatrist also can evaluate patients for appropriate use of anxiolytics. Conflict over aggression is also common among Type A patients and may be amenable to psychotherapy. Cognitive therapy may be useful, although one randomized trial found no benefits in preventing recurrence, but other benefits were found (Wilhelmsen et al. 1994). Hostility, irritability, and hypersensitivity are associated with high serum pepsinogen levels and may require more aggressive pharmacotherapy.

Patients with IBS frequently have had losses and significant separations as children and may as a result be more predisposed to depression as adults. Careful psychotherapeutic assessment and treatment of mood disorder and the propensity for conflicted adult relationships may help IBS patients avoid destructive repetitions of those losses. Cognitive therapy may be helpful in treatment of patients with IBS, as demonstrated in controlled trials (A. Payne and Blanchard 1995). The treatment of psychiatric complications of gastroenterological disease is examined in detail elsewhere (Epstein et al. 1993).

DERMATOLOGICAL DISORDERS

By way of its appearance and sensory capacities, the skin serves as a major conduit for emotional interchange in the interpersonal world. The range of normal emotions affect the appearance of the skin: flushing, sweating, and blanching. Psychopathological processes come into play—through neglect of normal skin care and reduced adherence to prescribed treatment of skin diseases, through overt self-inflicted lesions such as scratches and cuts, and through stress and anxiety—to produce a number of dermatoses by way of incompletely understood mechanisms. Because of the central social and psychological role played by the skin and its appearance, skin diseases in turn can produce a host of psychological reactions, including depressive affect, shame, social withdrawal, rage, and paradoxical aggravation of a primary skin condition (Folks and Kinney 1992a). Psychiatric consultation is thus an important part of the treatment approach with many dermatological patients.

Psoriasis produces hyperproliferative dry patches that require chronic treatment with topical preparations. It is a common illness, affecting up to 3 million individuals in the United States. The anxiety and shame associated with the disorder combine to exact a tremendous psychological toll on the individuals, with intense anticipation of rejection, a sense of defectiveness, and social withdrawal. Bleeding psoriatic lesions are strongly correlated with feelings of stigma. Despair and stigmatization have maladaptive effects and are highly associated with noncompliance of prescribed treatment (Gupta et al. 1989; Ramsay and O'Reagan 1988). Stress- and depression-related neuropeptides may have a role in the pathogenesis of psoriasis (Panconesi and Hautmann1996). More than half of all patients with the disease never enter remission and may be at greatest risk for social isolation. Defensive maneuvers such as social isolation contribute to the lack of potentially helpful relationships that could provide the regulation of painful effects (Hofer 1984; Reite and Short 1986). The presence of severe pruritus portends an unfortunate course for the disease (Faulstich et al. 1985). However, pruritus does not correlate with stressful life events, marital status, or use of alcohol (R. A. Payne et al. 1985).

Dermatitis was one of Alexander's (1950) "Holy Seven" psychosomatic illnesses, arising, he believed, from intense conflicts over cravings for physical closeness and exhibitionistic wishes. The coexistence of IBS and mi-

graine headaches with dermatitis kindled interest in a common neurophysiological mediator; serotonergic pathways have been implicated (Garvey and Tollefson 1988). Indexes of family stress correlate positively with severity of dermatitis symptoms (Gil et al. 1987).

Many psychological studies of patients with acne show a high prevalence of emotional symptoms, with poor self-esteem and negative self-image being the most common (Rubinow et al. 1987). Successful treatment of severe acne tends to reverse symptoms such as depressive affect and anxiety but produces little change in personality structure (Van der Meeren et al. 1985). Although adherence to treatment regimens constitutes an important variable in outcome, few studies have examined the psychological factors involved.

Urticaria is a common dermatological syndrome, producing wheal and flare "hives" that disappear within 24 hours. Lesions lasting longer should raise the suspicion of a vasculitic process and provoke a focus on etiologies other than the drugs and psychological causes common in urticaria. Neurophysiological mechanisms in anxiety-induced urticaria are similar to those in systemic anaphylaxis (Sell 1990). Treatment generally involves antihistamines and reassurance about the transience of the lesions.

Self-induced dermatoses occur frequently among psychiatric patients. Representing the effects of rage and narcissistic injury (borderline personality disorder), depression, psychosis (schizophrenia), malingering, and agitation and poor impulse control (mental retardation), the lesions can be wide ranging in their appearance and course (Levitz and Tan 1988). Serious lesions may result in tendon and nerve injury, as well as infection.

CLINICAL IMPLICATIONS

The psychological sequelae of dermatological illnesses may be as important as the antecedents, so destructive is the social withdrawal that occurs. The effect is particularly noticeable on the support system, which for the psoriasis patient plays an essential role in regulating dysphoria. In addition, noncompliance with medical treatment may result.

For many patients with chronic pruritus, psychosocial stressors have a direct exacerbating effect, and supportive psychotherapy, with or without careful use of anxiolytics, may help immensely in mitigating the adverse effects of such stressors. Patients with idiopathic urticaria commonly experience flares due to anxiety. Assessment of the severity of the attacks and their correlation with emotional triggers can direct the psychiatrist toward supportive psychotherapy in the less severe cases and toward use of prophylactic antidepressants in those more affected patients with panic disorder.

END-STAGE RENAL DISEASE

As treatment for end-stage renal disease (ESRD) has evolved, there has been extensive interest in the psychiatric and psychosocial aspects of dialysis and transplantation. In the following sections, the literature regarding quality of life and different treatment modalities, the effects of depression and noncompliance on outcome, and the case of patients who wish to withdraw from dialysis are discussed.

QUALITY OF LIFE AND TREATMENT MODALITY

A number of studies have compared psychosocial quality of life for patients who have dialysis versus renal transplantation. Including studies in the United States (Petrie 1989; Simmons and Abress 1990) and in other countries (Gudex 1995; Laupacis et al. 1996; Zimmermann 1989), most have found better psychosocial functioning in transplant patients. Similar results have been demonstrated in children with renal failure (Brownbridge and Fielding 1991; Reynolds et al. 1991). Other studies have shown no difference in the psychological adjustment of patients receiving either of the two treatment modalities (Kalman et al. 1983; Sayag et al. 1990). Investigators also have compared the quality of life among patients receiving different dialysis modalities. Some have found continuous ambulatory peritoneal dialysis (CAPD) to be associated with better psychological outcome (Brownbridge and Fielding 1991; Rydholm and Pauling 1991; Wolcott et al. 1988). Others have found mixed results or no differences in psychosocial outcomes (Griffin et al. 1994; Moreno et al. 1996). Home dialysis is preferred over center dialysis by those patients capable of handling it (Oberley and Schatell 1996). All of these quality-of-life studies must be interpreted cautiously because patients are never randomized to receive a particular form of dialysis or transplantation. Thus, outcome differences may be related to pretreatment differences in medical, psychosocial, or other variables.

EFFECTS OF DEPRESSION ON OUTCOME IN RENAL PATIENTS

A Canadian research group (Burton et al. 1986; Richmond et al. 1982; Wai et al. 1981) found that *depression* was a better predictor of shorter survival than was age or a composite physiological index of clinical variables (Burton et

al. 1986). Several other investigators have noted that depression in ESRD patients is associated with higher mortality and morbidity (Numan et al. 1981; Shulman et al. 1989). Other studies have found no effects of depression on survival (Devins et al. 1990; Kutner et al. 1994). A fundamental weakness of these earlier studies is that no attempt was made to measure and/or to control for disease severity, a major confounding factor in studies relating psychopathology to outcome in the medically ill (Levenson et al. 1990a).

EFFECTS OF COMPLIANCE ON OUTCOME

From a clinical standpoint, compliance is an important factor in the management of dialysis patients, but formal definition and measurement have been problematic. Psychosocial factors with demonstrated effects on compliance in ESRD include patients' beliefs about their health behaviors (Cummings et al. 1982), "locus of control" and self-efficacy (Schneider et al. 1991), family problems (Cummings et al. 1982), and social support (O'Brien 1990). The relationship between compliance and health outcomes in dialysis patients is not a simple one. More recent studies have controlled for illness severity and other potential confounds, and depression still predicts higher mortality (Peterson et al. 1991). Depressive symptoms predict overall quality of life more than does adequacy of biochemical dialysis, even after adjusting for other variables (Steele et al. 1996). In a study of the effects of family process variables on the survival of center hemodialysis patients, Reiss et al. (1986) examined 23 families in a laboratory setting. In contrast to the investigators' expectations, *better* family functioning predicted early death rather than survival. Patient noncompliance accounted for most of the associations between the family variables and survival. Although in this study the relationship found between noncompliance and survival is consistent with other work, the association between noncompliance and early death with indicators of *higher* family functioning is quite contrary to most clinical experience. O'Brien (1990) studied a cohort of 126 center hemodialysis patients at 3- and 6-year follow-up and found that patients who died earliest demonstrated the *highest* compliance, whereas those patients still surviving at the end of the study had reported the *lowest* compliance. Christensen et al. (1992) found social support predicted compliance with restriction of fluids but not dietary restrictions. Sensky et al. (1996) found that dietary and fluid compliance were not linked and had different psychosocial correlates. Other forms of noncompliance affected by psychological factors include skipping or shortening time on dialysis (Kimmel et al. 1995). Overall, although the effects of noncompliance on dialysis patients' outcomes are well recognized by clinicians, compliance should be regarded as a complex set of behaviors that remains insufficiently empirically characterized and classified.

Small studies of kidney transplant patients have shown that pretransplant noncompliance predicts posttransplant noncompliance and graft failure (Rodriguez et al. 1991). Noncompliant kidney transplant patients are more likely to be depressed and have other psychosocial problems than are compliant patients (Rodriguez et al. 1991).

WITHDRAWAL FROM DIALYSIS

Psychiatric consultation may be requested when long-term dialysis patients wish to discontinue treatment, raising clinical (Greene 1983), liaison (Slevin 1983), and ethical (Wright 1993) issues. In a large study of dialysis patients (Neu and Kjellstrand 1986), dialysis was discontinued in 9%, accounting for 22% of all deaths. Half of the patients withdrawn were incompetent and required surrogate decision making. Similar studies have been done in other countries (Catalano et al. 1996). Early studies that had pointed to a high rate of suicide in dialysis patients overestimated suicide prevalence by not distinguishing rational treatment withdrawal from suicide. A more recent study points to a suicide rate of 4% of those withdrawing from dialysis (Catalano et al. 1996). The true rate of suicide in dialysis has not been established systematically, nor has there been careful attention to the psychological factors that may affect the decision to withdraw from treatment.

Several of the major studies examining psychological factors and outcome in renal disease are summarized in Table 15–8.

MECHANISMS

The current state of research allows for informed speculation on how psychological factors such as depression might influence outcome in ESRD. Depression may adversely affect immune function (Stein et al. 1991). Clinical experience is that depressed ESRD patients are more likely to evidence poor self-care, noncompliance, and poor medical follow-up. Depression has been associated in other populations with increased use of analgesics, which in turn have been demonstrated to have a role in the etiology and exacerbation of chronic renal failure (Sandler et al. 1989; Schwarz et al. 1989). Depression is associated with smoking, alcoholism, and other forms of substance abuse that are themselves major causes of increased morbidity and mortality. Depression may adversely impact outcome in ESRD by serving as a risk factor for other medical comorbidity—for example, myocardial infarction (Booth-Kewley and Friedman 1987), reduced aerobic capacity (Carney et al. 1986), or malnutrition.

CLINICAL IMPLICATIONS

Psychiatrists are sometimes asked to participate in decision making about which ESRD treatment modality best suits a particular patient. Current research sheds some light on this question, but it still must be answered based on the preferences and needs of the particular patient. Which modality is most appealing to the patient (i.e., regarding lifestyle, body image, and demands of the treatment)? With which treatment will the patient be most successful in compliance?

Depression is the most common psychiatric disorder in ESRD patients, and the symptoms may be difficult to distinguish from uremia or other comorbid medical conditions (Hart and Kreutzer 1988; Levenson and Glocheski 1991). Careful differential diagnosis will identify those patients who should be treated for depression, with subsequent expectable improvement in quality of life and functional capacity. (Details of the treatment of psychiatric disorders in renal failure and dialysis patients may be found elsewhere [N. B. Levy 1993].)

Noncompliance remains the reason why psychiatrists

TABLE 15–8. Illustrative studies supporting the effects of psychological factors on end-stage renal disease

Psychological factor	Study type	Treatment modality	Findings	Reference(s)
Depression	Cohort	Home hemodialysis	Depression predicted shorter survival	Burton et al. 1986
Noncompliance	Family process	Center hemodialysis	Noncompliance associated with shorter survival	Reiss et al. 1986
Noncompliance	Cohort	Renal transplantation	Pretransplant noncompliance predicts posttransplant noncompliance and graft failure	Rodriguez et al. 1991

are most often consulted by nephrologists. The psychiatrist should help the ESRD treatment team avoid simplistic thinking about noncompliance and be aware of the risk of scapegoating the patient. *Noncompliance*, as previously noted, represents a complex set of behaviors and interpersonal relationships (patient, family, physician, nurse) with important cultural and ethical considerations. The most extreme form of noncompliance is refusal to accept, or withdrawal from, treatment for ESRD. Some clinicians err in regarding such patients as always depressed and suicidal, whereas others err in the opposite direction, too often accepting such a decision at face value as rational. Psychiatrists have a crucial role in what can be a difficult distinction between autonomous rational decision making versus irrational suicidal giving up, symptomatic of a treatable depression.

CONCLUSIONS

The revised diagnostic criteria for DSM-IV "Psychological Factors Affecting Medical Conditions" are shown in Table 15–2. These criteria emphasize the clinician's noting of relationships between psychological factors and medical conditions in regard to not only the onset but also the course and outcome of illness. As may be readily gathered from this overview of the literature, the fact that such relationships exist and that timely psychotherapeutic interventions can make a positive difference in many disorders has been well documented. These observations emphasize the importance of the detection of psychiatric factors in the context of medical illness and augur increased involvement of the psychiatrist in the clinical care of patients with medical disorders.

REFERENCES

Alexander F: Psychosomatic Medicine: Its Principles and Applications. New York, WW Norton, 1950

Almada SJ, Zonderman AB, Shekelle RB, et al: Neuroticism and cynicism and risk of death in middle-aged men: the Western Electric Study. Psychosom Med 53:165–175, 1991

American Psychiatric Association: Diagnostic and Statistical Manual of Mental Disorders, 3rd Edition, Revised. Washington, DC, American Psychiatric Association, 1987

American Psychiatric Association: Diagnostic and Statistical Manual of Mental Disorders, 4th Edition. Washington, DC, American Psychiatric Association, 1994

Amler RW, Eddins DL: Cross-sectional analysis: precursors of premature death in the United States. Am J Prev Med 3 (No 5, suppl):181–187, 1987

Armstrong D, Arnold R, Classen M, et al: RUDER—a prospective, two-year, multicenter study of risk factors for duodenal ulcer relapse during maintenance therapy with ranitidine. RUDER Study Group. Dig Dis Sci 39:1425–1433, 1994

Ballard RD, Tan WC, Kelly PL, et al: Effect of sleep and sleep deprivation on ventilatory response to bronchoconstriction. J Appl Physiol 69:490–497, 1990

Barraclough J, Pinder P, Cruddas M, et al: Life events and breast cancer prognosis. BMJ 304:1078–1081, 1992

Bartrop RW, Luckhurst E, Lazarus L, et al: Depressed lymphocyte function after bereavement. Lancet 1:834–836, 1977

Beardsley G, Goldstein MG: Psychological factors affecting physical condition: endocrine disease literature review. Psychosomatics 34:12–19, 1993

Beardsley G, Goldstein MG: Endocrine diseases, in Psychological Factors Affecting Medical Conditions. Edited by Stoudemire A. Washington, DC, American Psychiatric Press, 1995, pp 173–186

Berkman LF: The role of social relations in health promotion. Psychosom Med 57:245–54, 1995

Bindemann S, Soukop M, Kaye SB: Randomized controlled study of relaxation training. Eur J Cancer 27:170–174, 1991

Booth-Kewley S, Friedman HS: Psychological predictors of heart disease: a quantitative review. Psychol Bull 101:343–362, 1987

Brown RA, Goldstein MG, Niarua R, et al: Nicotine dependence: assessment and management, in Psychiatric Care of the Medical Patient. Edited by Stoudemire A, Fogel BS. New York, Oxford University Press, 1993, pp 877–901

Brownbridge G, Fielding DM: Psychosocial adjustment to end-stage renal failure: comparing hemodialysis, continuous ambulatory peritoneal dialysis and transplantation. Pediatr Nephrol 5:612–616, 1991

Buddeberg C, Wolf C, Sieber M, et al: Coping strategies and course of disease of breast cancer patients: results of a 3-year longitudinal study. Psychother Psychosom 55:151–157, 1991

Burton JJ, Kline SA, Lindsay RM, et al: Relationship of depression to survival in chronic renal failure. Psychosom Med 48:261–269, 1986

Carney RM, Wetzel RD, Hagberg J, et al: The relationship between depression and aerobic capacity in hemodialysis patients. Psychosom Med 48:143–147, 1986

Carney RM, Rich MW, Freedland KE, et al: Major depressive disorder predicts cardiac events in patients with coronary artery disease. Psychosom Med 50:627–633, 1988

Cassileth BR, Lusk EJ, Strouse TB, et al: Psychological status in chronic illness: a comparative analysis of six diagnostic groups. N Engl J Med 311:506–511, 1984

Cassileth BR, Lusk EJ, Miller DS, et al: Psychological correlates of survival in advanced malignant disease? N Engl J Med 312:1551–1555, 1985

Cassileth BR, Walsh WP, Lusk EJ: Psychosocial correlates of cancer survival: a subsequent report 3 to 8 years after cancer diagnosis. J Clin Oncol 6:1753–1759, 1988

Catalano C, Goodship TH, Graham KA, et al: Withdrawal of renal replacement therapy in Newcastle Upon Tyne. Nephrol Dial Transplant 11:133–139, 1996

Chandra V, Szklo M, Goldberg R, et al: The impact of marital status on survival after an acute myocardial infarction: a population-based study. Am J Epidemiol 117:320–325, 1983

Christensen AJ, Smith TW, Turner CW, et al: Family support, physical impairment, and adherence in hemodialysis: an investigation of main and buffering effects. J Behav Med 15:313–325, 1992

Clark MM, Ruggiero L, Pera V, et al: Assessment, classification, and treatment of obesity: a psychobiobehavioral perspective, in Psychiatric Care of the Medical Patient. Edited by Stoudemire A, Fogel BS. New York, Oxford University Press, 1993, pp 903–926

Cobb S, Rose RM: Hypertension, peptic ulcer, and diabetes in air traffic controllers. JAMA 224:489–492, 1973

Cohen S, Herbert TB: Health psychology: psychological factors and physical disease from the perspective of human psychoneuroimmunology. Ann Rev Psychol 47:113–142, 1996

Cook W, Medley D: Proposed hostility and pharisaic-virtue scales for the MMPI. J Appl Psychol 238:414–418, 1954

Costa D, Mogos I, Toma T: Efficacy and safety of mianserin in the treatment of depression of women with cancer. Acta Psychiatr Scand Suppl 72 (No 320):85–92, 1985

Cummings K, Becker M, Kirscht J, et al: Psychosocial factors affecting adherence to medical regimens in a group of hemodialysis patients. Med Care 20:567–580, 1982

Dattore PJ, Shontz FC, Coyne L: Premorbid personality differentiation of cancer and noncancer groups: a test of the hypothesis of cancer proneness. J Consult Clin Psychol 48:388–394, 1980

Deanfield JE, Kensett M, Wilson RA, et al: Silent myocardial ischemia due to mental stress. Lancet 2:1001–1005, 1984

Devins GM, Mann J, Mandin H, et al: Psychosocial predictors of survival in end-stage renal disease. J Nerv Ment Dis 178:127–133, 1990

Dorian B, Garfinkel P, Keystone E, et al: Occupational stress and immunity (abstract). Psychosom Med 47:77, 1985

Dunbar F: Mind and Body: Psychosomatic Medicine. New York, Random House, 1947

Edwards JR, Cooper CL, Pearl SS, et al: The relationship between psychosocial factors and breast cancer: some unexpected results. Behav Med 16:5–14, 1990

Engel GL: Sudden and rapid death during psychological stress. Ann Intern Med 74:771–782, 1971

Epstein SA, Wise TN, Goldberg RL: Gastroenterology, in Psychiatric Care of the Medical Patient. Edited by Stoudemire A, Fogel BS. New York, Oxford University Press, 1993, pp 611–625

Ernster VL, Sucks ST, Selvin S, et al: Cancer incidence by marital status: U.S. Third National Cancer Survey. J Natl Cancer Inst 63:567–585, 1979

Evans DL, McCartney CF, Haggerty JJ, et al: Treatment of depression in cancer patients is associated with better life adaptation: a pilot study. Psychosom Med 50:72–76, 1988

Everson CA: Sustained sleep deprivation impairs host defense. Am J Physiol 265:1148–1154, 1993

Faulstich ME, Williamson DA, Duchmann EG, et al: Psychophysiological analysis of atopic dermatitis. J Psychosom Res 29:415–417, 1985

Fawzy FI, Cousins N, Fawzy NW, et al: A structured psychiatric intervention for cancer patients, I: changes over time in methods of coping and affective disturbance. Arch Gen Psychiatry 47:720–725, 1990a

Fawzy FI, Kemeny ME, Fawzy NW, et al: A structured psychiatric intervention for cancer patients, II: changes over time in immunological measures. Arch Gen Psychiatry 47:729–735, 1990b

Fawzy FI, Fawzy NW, Hyun CS, et al: Malignant melanoma: effects of an early structured psychiatric intervention, coping, and affective state on recurrence and survival 6 years later. Arch Gen Psychiatry 50:681–9, 1993

Finn F, Mulcahy R, Hickey W: The psychological profiles of coronary and cancer patients, and of matched controls. Ir J Med Sci 143:176–178, 1974

Folks DG, Kinney FC: The role of psychological factors in dermatologic conditions. Psychosomatics 33:45–54, 1992a

Folks DG, Kinney FC: The role of psychological factors in gastrointestinal conditions: a review pertinent to DSM-IV. Psychosomatics 33:257–270, 1992b

Ford CV: The Somatizing Disorders: Illness as a Way of Life. New York, Elsevier, 1983

Fox BH: Current theory of psychogenic effects on cancer incidence and prognosis. Journal of Psychosocial Oncology 1:17–31, 1983

Fras I, Litin EM, Pearson JS: Comparison of psychiatric symptoms in carcinoma of the pancreas with those in some other intra-abdominal neoplasms. Am J Psychiatry 123:1553–1562, 1967

Frasure-Smith N, Lesperance F, Talajic M: Depression following myocardial infarction: impact on 6-month survival. JAMA 270:1819–1825, 1993

Frasure-Smith N, Lesperance F, Talajic M: Depression and 18-month prognosis after myocardial infarction. Circulation 91:999–1005, 1995

Friedman M, Rosenman RH: Association of specific overt behavior pattern with blood and cardiovascular findings. JAMA 169:1085–1096, 1959

Funch DP, Marshall J: The role of stress, social support and age in survival from breast cancer. J Psychosom Res 27:77–83, 1983

Gaddini R: Transitional object origins and the psychosomatic symptom, in Between Fantasy and Reality: Transitional Objects and Phenomena. Edited by Grolnick A, Barkin L. New York, Jason Aronson, 1978, pp 17–21

Garvey MJ, Tollefson GD: Association of affective disorder with migraine headaches and neurodermatitis. Gen Hosp Psychiatry 10:148–149, 1988

Gellert GA, Maxwell RM, Siegel BS: Survival of breast cancer patients receiving adjunctive psychosocial support therapy: a 10-year follow-up study. J Clin Oncol 11:66–69, 1993

Gendel BR, Benjamin JE: Psychogenic factors in the etiology of diabetes. N Engl J Med 234:556–562, 1946

Geyer S: Life events prior to manifestation of breast cancer: a limited prospective study covering eight years before diagnosis. J Psychosom Res 35:355–363, 1991

Gil KM, Keefe FJ, Sampson HA, et al: The relation of stress and family environment to atopic dermatitis symptoms in children. J Psychosom Res 31:673–684, 1987

Gilligan I, Fung L, Piper DW, et al: Life event stress and chronic difficulties in duodenal ulcer: a case control study. J Psychosom Res 31:117–123, 1987

Gilmartin ME: Patient and family education. Clin Chest Med 7:619–627, 1986

Goetsch VL, VanDorsten B, Pbert LA, et al: Acute effects of laboratory stress on blood glucose in non-insulin-dependent diabetes. Psychosom Med 55:492–496, 1993

Goldenberg DL: Psychological studies in fibrositis. Am J Med 81:67–70, 1986

Goldstein MG, Niaura R: Psychological factors affecting physical condition: cardiovascular disease literature review, I: coronary artery disease and sudden death. Psychosomatics 33:134–145, 1992

Goldstein MG, Niaura R, Abrams DB: Pharmacological and behavioral treatment of nicotine dependence: nicotine as a drug of abuse, in Medical Psychiatric Practice, Vol 1. Edited by Stoudemire A, Fogel BS. Washington, DC, American Psychiatric Press, 1991, pp 541–596

Gonder-Frederick LA, Carter WR, Cox DJ, et al: Environmental stress and blood glucose change in IDDM. Health Psychol 9:503–515, 1990

Gorman JM: Psychobiological aspects of asthma and the consequent research implications (editorial). Chest 97:514–515, 1990

Gorman JM, Kertzner R: Psychoneuroimmunology and HIV infection. J Neuropsychiatry Clin Neurosci 2:241–252, 1990

Graham S, Snell LM, Graham JB, et al: Social trauma in the epidemiology of cancer of the cervix. Journal of Chronic Diseases 24:711–735, 1971

Graves PL, Thomas CB, Mead LA: Familial and psychological predictors of cancer. Cancer Detect Prev 15:59–64, 1991

Greene WA: Problems in discontinuation of hemodialysis, in Psychonephrology 2: Psychological Problems in Kidney Failure and Their Treatment. Edited by Levy NB. New York, Plenum, 1983, pp 131–144

Greene WA, Young LE, Swisher SN: Psychological factors and reticuloendothelial disease. Psychosom Med 18:284–303, 1956

Greer S, Morris T: Psychological attributes of women who develop breast cancer: a controlled study. J Psychosom Res 19:147–153, 1975

Greer S, Morris T, Pettingale KW: Psychological response to breast cancer: effect on outcome. Lancet 2:785–787, 1979

Greer S, Moorey S, Baruch J: Evaluation of adjuvant psychological therapy for clinically referred cancer patients. Br J Cancer 63:257–260, 1991

Griffin KW, Wadhwa NK, Friend R, et al: Comparison of quality of life in hemodialysis and peritoneal dialysis patients. Adv Perit Dial 10:104–108, 1994

Grossarth-Maticek R, Eysenck HJ: Length of survival and lymphocyte percentage in women with mammary cancer as a function of psychotherapy. Psychol Rep 65:315–321, 1989

Grossarth-Maticek R, Eysenck HJ: Personality, smoking, and alcohol as synergistic risk factors for cancer of the mouth and pharynx. Psychol Rep 67:1024–1026, 1990

Grossarth-Maticek R, Schmidt P, Vetter H, et al: Psychotherapy research in oncology, in Health Care and Human Behaviour. Edited by Steptoe A, Mathews A. London, Academic Press, 1984, pp 325–341

Gudex CM: Health-related quality of life in end-stage renal failure. Qual Life Res 4:359–366, 1995

Gupta MA, Gupta AK, Kirkby S, et al: A psychocutaneous profile of psoriasis patients who are stress reactors: a study of 127 patients. Gen Hosp Psychiatry 11:166–173, 1989

Hagglof B, Dahlquist G, Lonnbert G, et al: The Swedish childhood diabetes study: indications of severe psychological stress as a risk factor for type 1 (insulin dependent) diabetes mellitus in childhood. Diabetologia 34:579–583, 1991

Hahn RC, Petitti DB: Minnesota Multiphasic Personality Inventory–rated depression and the incidence of breast cancer. Cancer 61:845–848, 1988

Halford WK, Cuddily S, Mortimer RH: Psychological stress and blood glucose regulation in type 1 diabetic patients. Health Psychol 9:516–528, 1990

Hall RCW, Stickney S, Beresford TP: Endocrine disease and behavior. Integrative Psychiatry 4:122–135, 1986

Halliday JL: Psychological aspects of rheumatoid arthritis. Proceedings of the Royal Society of Medicine 35:455–457, 1942

Hanson CL, Henggeler SW, Burghen GA: Social competence and parental support as mediators of the link between stress and metabolic control in adolescents with insulin-dependent diabetes mellitus. J Consult Clin Psychol 55:529–533, 1987

Hart RP, Kreutzer JS: Renal system, in Medical Neuropsychology: The Impact of Disease on Behavior. Edited by Tarter RE, Van Thiel DH, Edwards KL. New York, Plenum, 1988, pp 99–120

Hathaway SR, McKinley JC: Minnesota Multiphasic Personality Inventory. Minneapolis, MN, University of Minnesota, 1943

Helsing KJ, Szklo M: Mortality after bereavement. Am J Epidemiol 114:41–52, 1981

Hofer MA: Relationships as regulators: a psychobiological perspective on bereavement. Psychosom Med 46:183–197, 1984

Holland JC: Behavioral and psychosocial risk factors in cancer: human studies, in Handbook of Psychooncology. Edited by Holland JC, Rowland JH. New York, Oxford University Press, 1989, pp 705–726

Holland JC, Morrow GR, Schmale A, et al: A randomized clinical trial of alprazolam versus progressive muscle relaxation in cancer patients with anxiety and depressive symptoms. J Clin Oncol 9:1004–1011, 1991

Horne RL, Picard RS: Psychosocial risk factors for lung cancer. Psychosom Med 43:431–438, 1979

Irwin M, Daniel S, Smith TL, et al: Impaired natural killer cell activity during bereavement. Brain Behav Immun 1:98–104, 1987

Jamison RN, Burish TG, Wallston KA: Psychogenic factors in predicting survival of breast cancer patients. J Clin Oncol 5:768–772, 1987

Jess P: Gastric acid secretion in relation to personality, affect and coping ability in duodenal ulcer patients: a multivariate analysis—Hvidovre Ulcer Project Group. Dan Med Bull 41:100–103, 1994

Jess P, Eldrup J: The personality patterns inpatients with duodenal ulcer and ulcer-like dyspepsia and their relationship to the course of the diseases—Hvidovre Ulcer Project Group. J Intern Med 235:589–594, 1994

Jiang W, Babyak M, Krantz DS, et al: Mental stress-induced myocardial ischemia and cardiac events. JAMA 275:1651–1656, 1996

Joseph J: Social affiliation, risk factor status, and coronary heart disease: a cross-sectional study of Japanese-American men. Unpublished doctoral dissertation, University of California, Berkeley, 1980

Kalman TP, Wilson PG, Kalman CM: Psychiatric morbidity in long-term renal transplant recipients and patients undergoing hemodialysis. JAMA 250:55–58, 1983

Kaplan KH, Goldenberg DL, Galvin-Nadeau M: The impact of a meditation-based stress reduction program on fibromyalgia. Gen Hosp Psychiatry 15:284–289, 1993

Ketterer MW: Secondary prevention of ischemic heart disease: the case for aggressive behavioral monitoring and intervention. Psychosomatics 34:78–84, 1993

Kiecolt-Glaser JK, Garner W, Speicher C, et al: Psychosocial modifiers of immunocompetence in medical students. Psychosom Med 46:7–14, 1984

Kiecolt-Glaser JK, Glaser R: Psychoneuroimmunology and health consequences: data and shared mechanisms. Psychosom Med 57:269–274, 1995

Kiecolt-Glaser JK, Glaser R, Strain EC, et al: Modulation of cellular immunity in medical students. J Behav Med 9:5–21, 1986

Kiecolt-Glaser JK, Glaser R, Shuttleworth EC, et al: Chronic stress and immunity in family caregivers of Alzheimer's disease victims. Psychosom Med 49:523–535, 1987a

Kiecolt-Glaser JK, Fisher L, Ogrocki P, et al: Marital quality, marital disruption, and immune function. Psychosom Med 49:13–34, 1987b

Kiecolt-Glaser JK, Kennedy S, Malkoff S, et al: Marital discord and immunity in males. Psychosom Med 50:213–229, 1988

Kimmel PL, Peterson RA, Weihs KL, et al: Behavioral compliance with dialysis prescription in hemodialysis patients. J Am Soc Nephrol 5:1826–34, 1995

Klerman GL, Clayton P: Epidemiologic perspectives on the health consequences of bereavement, in Bereavement: Reactions, Consequences, and Care. Edited by Osterweis M, Solomon F, Green M. Washington, DC, National Academy Press, 1984, pp 15–44

Knapp PH, Mathe AA: Psychophysiologic aspects of bronchial asthma: a review, in Bronchial Asthma: Mechanisms and Therapeutics. Edited by Weiss EB, Segal MS, Stein M. Boston, Little, Brown, 1985, pp 914–931

Kneier AW, Temoshok L: Repressive coping reactions in patients with malignant melanoma as compared to cardiovascular patients. J Psychosom Res 28:145–155, 1984

Kreitler S, Chaitchik S, Kreitler H: Repressiveness: cause or result of cancer? Psychooncology 2:43–54, 1993

Kune GA, Kune S, Watson LF, et al: Personality as a risk factor in large bowel cancer: data from the Melbourne Colorectal Cancer Study. Psychol Med 21:29–41, 1991

Kune S, Kune GA, Watson LF, et al: Recent life change and large bowel cancer: data from the Melbourne Colorectal Cancer Study. J Clin Epidemiol 44:57–68, 1991

Kutner NG, Lin LS, Fielding B, et al: Continued survival of older hemodialysis patients: investigation of psychosocial predictors. Am J Kidney Dis 24:42–49, 1994

Lambley P: The role of psychological processes in the aetiology and treatment of cervical cancer: a biopsychological perspective. Br J Med Psychol 66:43–60, 1993

Lammers CA, Naliboff BD, Straatmeyer AJ: The effects of progressive relaxation on stress and diabetic control. Behav Res Ther 22:641–650, 1984

Laupacis A, Keown P, Pus N, et al: A study of the quality of life and cost-utility of renal transplantation. Kidney Int 50:235–242, 1996

Leherer S: Life change and gastric cancer. Psychosom Med 42:499–502, 1980

Leigh H, Percarpio B, Opsahl C, et al: Psychological predictors of survival in cancer patients undergoing radiation therapy. Psychother Psychosom 47:65–73, 1987

Leonard BE, Miller K: Stress, the immune system and psychiatry. Chichester, UK, John Wiley, 1995

Lesko LM, Massie MJ, Holland J: Oncology, in Psychiatric Care of the Medical Patient. Edited by Stoudemire A, Fogel BS. New York, Oxford University Press, 1993, pp 565–590

Levenson JL: Cardiovascular disease, in Psychiatric Care of the Medical Patient. Edited by Stoudemire A, Fogel BS. New York, Oxford University Press, 1993, pp 539–563

Levenson JL, Bemis C: The role of psychological factors in cancer onset and progression. Psychosomatics 32:124–132, 1991

Levenson JL, Glocheski S: Psychological factors affecting end-stage renal disease: a review. Psychosomatics 32:382–389, 1991

Levenson JL, Colenda C, Larson DB, et al: Methodology in consultation-liaison research: a classification of biases. Psychosomatics 31:367–376, 1990a

Levenson JL, Hamer RM, Rossiter LF: Relation of psychopathology in general medical inpatients to use and cost of services. Am J Psychiatry 147:1498–1503, 1990b

Levenstein S, Prantera C, Varvo V, et al: Psychological stress and distress activity in ulcerative colitis: a multidimensional cross-sectional study. Am J Gastroenterol 89: 1219–1225, 1994

Levenstein S, Kaplan GA, Smith M: Sociodemographic characteristics, life stressors, and peptic ulcer: a prospective study. J Clin Gastroenterol 21:185–192, 1995

Levitz SM, Tan OT: Factitious dermatosis masquerading as recurrent herpes zoster. Am J Med 84:781–783, 1988

Levy NB: Chronic renal failure and its treatment: dialysis and transplantation, in Psychiatric Care of the Medical Patient. Edited by Stoudemire A, Fogel BS. New York, Oxford University Press, 1993, pp 627–635

Levy S, Herberman RB, Maluish A, et al: Prognostic risk assessment in primary breast cancer by behavioral and immunological parameters. Health Psychol 4:99–113, 1985

Levy S, Herberman RB, Lippman M, et al: Correlation of stress factors with sustained depression of natural killer activity and predicted prognosis in patients with breast cancer. J Clin Oncol 5:348–353, 1987

Levy S, Herberman RB, Whiteside T, et al: Perceived social support and tumor estrogen/progesterone receptor status as predictors of natural killer cell activity in breast cancer patients. Psychosom Med 52:73–85, 1990

Levy S, Herberman RB, Lippman M, et al: Immunological and psychosocial predictors of disease recurrence in patients with early stage breast cancer. Behav Med 17:67–75, 1991

Lipowski ZJ: Psychosomatic medicine: past and present, III: current research. Can J Psychiatry 31:14–21, 1986

Lowman BC, Drossman DA, Cramer EM, et al: Recollection of childhood events in adults with irritable bowel syndrome. J Clin Gastroenterol 9:324–330, 1987

Manuck SB, Kaplan JR, Adams MR, et al: Behaviorally elicited heart rate reactivity and atherosclerosis in female cynomolgus monkeys (*Macaca fascicularis*). Psychosom Med 51:306–318, 1989

Marcantonio ER, Goldman L, Manigone CM, et al: A clinical prediction rule for delirium after elective non-cardiac surgery. JAMA 271:134–139, 1994

Margolis GJ, Goodman RL, Rubin A, et al: Psychological factors in the choice of treatment for breast cancer. Psychosomatics 30:192–197, 1989

Mathe AA, Knapp PH: Decreased plasma free fatty acids and urinary epinephrine in bronchial asthma. N Engl J Med 281:234–238, 1969

McDaniel JS, Musselman DL, Porter MR, et al: Depression in patients with cancer: diagnosis, biology, and treatment. Arch Gen Psychiatry 52:89–99, 1995

McNamara ME: Psychological factors affecting neurological conditions: depression and stroke, multiple sclerosis, Parkinson's disease, and epilepsy. Psychosomatics 32:255–267, 1991

Meenan RF: The impact of chronic disease: a sociomedical profile of rheumatoid arthritis. Arthritis Rheum 24:544–549, 1981

Molodofsky H, Chester WJ: Pain and mood patterns in patients with rheumatoid arthritis. Psychosom Med 32:309–317, 1970

Moos RH: Personality factors associated with rheumatoid arthritis: a review. Journal of Chronic Diseases 17:41–55, 1964

Moran MG: Psychological factors affecting pulmonary and rheumatologic diseases: a review. Psychosomatics 32:14–23, 1991

Moran MG: Psychiatric aspects of asthma. Seminars in Respiratory and Critical Care Medicine 15:168–174, 1994

Moran MG, Dubester SN: Connective tissue diseases, in Psychiatric Care of the Medical Patient. Edited by Stoudemire A, Fogel BS. New York, Oxford University Press, 1993, pp 739–756

Neu S, Kjellstrand CM: Stopping long-term dialysis: an empirical study of withdrawal of life-supporting treatment. N Engl J Med 314:14–20, 1986

Niaura R, Goldstein MG: Psychological factors affecting physical condition: cardiovascular disease literature review, II: coronary artery disease and sudden death and hypertension. Psychosomatics 33:146–155, 1992

Numan IM, Barklind KS, Lubin B: Correlates of depression in chronic dialysis patients: morbidity and mortality. Res Nurs Health 4:295–297, 1981

Oberley ET, Schatell DR: Home hemodialysis: survival, quality of life, and rehabilitation. Adv Ren Replace Ther 3: 147–153, 1996

O'Brien ME: Compliance behavior and long-term maintenance dialysis. Am J Kidney Dis 15:209–214, 1990

Panconesi E, Hautmann G: Psychophysiology of stress in dermatology: the psychobiologic pattern of psychosomatics. Dermatol Clin 14:399–421, 1996

Payne A, Blanchard EB: A controlled comparison of cognitive therapy and self-help support groups in the treatment of irritable bowel syndrome. J Consult Clin Psychol 63:779–786, 1995

Payne RA, Payne CME, Marks R: Stress does not worsen psoriasis? a controlled study of 32 patients. Clin Exp Dermatol 10:239–245, 1985

Persky VW, Kempthorne-Rawson J, Shekelle RB: Personality and risk of cancer: 20-year follow-up of the Western Electric Study. Psychosom Med 49:435–449, 1987

Peterson RA, Kimmel PL, Sacks CR, et al: Depression, perception of illness and mortality in patients with end-stage renal disease. Int J Psychiatry Med 21:343–354, 1991

Peto R, Lopez AD, Boreham J, et al: Mortality from tobacco in developed countries: indirect estimation from national vital statistics. Lancet 339:1268–1278, 1992

Petrie K: Psychological well-being and psychiatric disturbance in dialysis and renal transplant patients. Br J Med Psychol 62:91–96, 1989

Polley HF, Swenson WM, Steinhilber RM: Personality characteristics of patients with rheumatoid arthritis. Psychosomatics 11:45–49, 1970

Ramirez AJ, Craig TKJ, Watson JP, et al: Stress and relapse of breast cancer. BMJ 298:291–293, 1989

Ramsay B, O'Reagan M: A survey of the social and psychological effects of psoriasis. Br J Dermatol 118:195–201, 1988

Read NW: Irritable bowel syndrome (IBS): definition and pathophysiology. Scand J Gastroenterol Suppl 130:7–13, 1987

Rees L: Physical and emotional factors in bronchial asthma. J Psychosom Res 1:98–114, 1956

Reich P, DeSilva RA, Lown B, et al: Acute psychological disturbance preceding life-threatening ventricular arrhythmias. JAMA 246:233–235, 1981

Reiss D, Gonzalez S, Kramer N: Family process, chronic illness, and death: on the weakness of strong bonds. Arch Gen Psychiatry 43:795–804, 1986

Reite M, Short R: Behavior and physiology in young bonnet monkeys. Dev Psychobiol 19:567–579, 1986

Reynolds JM, Garralda ME, Postlethwaite RJ, et al: Changes in psychosocial adjustment after renal transplantation. Arch Dis Child 66:509–513, 1991

Richmond JM, Lindsay RM, Burton HJ, et al: Psychological and physiological factors predicting the outcome of home hemodialysis. Clin Nephrol 17:109–113, 1982

Robinson N, Fuller JH: Role of life events and difficulties in the onset of diabetes mellitus. J Psychosom Res 29:583–591, 1985

Rodriguez A, Diaz M, Colon A, et al: Psychosocial profile of noncompliant transplant patients. Transplant Proc 23:1807–1809, 1991

Rosenberg L, Kaufman DW, Helmrich SP, et al: The risk of myocardial infarction after quitting smoking in men under 55 years of age. N Engl J Med 313:1511–1514, 1985

Rovet J, Ehrlich RM: Effect of temperament on metabolic control in children with diabetes mellitus. Diabetes Care 11:77–82, 1988

Rubinow DR, Peck GL, Squillace KM, et al: Reduced anxiety and depression in cystic acne patients after successful treatment with oral isotretinoin. J Am Acad Dermatol 17:25–32, 1987

Rydholm L, Pauling J: Contrasting feelings of helplessness in peritoneal and hemodialysis patients: a pilot study. American Nephrological Nurses Association Journal 18:183–186, 187, 200, 1991

Sandler DP, Smith JC, Weinberg CR, et al: Analgesic use and chronic renal disease. N Engl J Med 320:1238–1243, 1989

Sapolsky RM, Donnelly TM: Vulnerability to stress-induced tumor growth increases with age: role of glucocorticoids. Endocrinology 117:662–666, 1985

Saravay SM, Lavin M: Psychiatric comorbidity and length of stay in the general hospital: a critical review of outcome studies. Psychosomatics 35:233–252, 1994

Sayag R, Kaplan De-Nour A, Shapire Z, et al: Comparison of psychosocial adjustment of male nondiabetic kidney transplant and hospital hemodialysis patients. Nephron 54:214–218, 1990

Schleifer SJ, Keller SE, Camerino M, et al: Suppression of lymphocyte stimulation following bereavement. JAMA 250:374–377, 1983

Schleifer SJ, Keller SE, Bond RN, et al: Major depressive disorder and immunity: role of age, sex, severity, and hospitalization. Arch Gen Psychiatry 46:81–87, 1989

Schmale AH, Iker HP: The psychological setting of uterine cervical cancer. Ann N Y Acad Sci 125:807–813, 1965

Schneider MS, Friend R, Whitaker P, et al: Fluid noncompliance and symptomatology in end-stage renal disease: cognitive and emotional variables. Health Psychol 10:209–215, 1991

Schwarz A, Kunzendorf U, Keller F, et al: Progression of renal failure in analgesic-associated nephropath. Nephron 53:244–249, 1989

Sell S: Immunopathology (hypersensitivity diseases), in Anderson's Pathology, 9th Edition. Edited by Kissane JE. St Louis, MO, CV Mosby, 1990, pp 487–545

Sensky T, Leger C, Gilmour S: Psychosocial and cognitive factors associated with adherence to dietary and fluid restriction regimens by people on chronic hemodialysis. Psychother Psychosom 65:36–42, 1996

Sharma S, Nandkumar VK: Personality structure and adjustment pattern in bronchial asthma. Acta Psychiatr Scand 61:81–88, 1980

Shekelle RB, Raynor WJ Jr, Ostfeld AM: Psychological depression and 17-year risk of death from cancer. Psychosom Med 43:117–125, 1981

Shulman R, Price JD, Spinelli J: Biopsychosocial aspects of long-term survival on end-stage renal failure therapy. Psychol Med 19:945–954, 1989

Simmons RG, Abress L: Quality of life issues for end-stage renal disease patients. Am J Kidney Dis 15:201–208, 1990

Sivak ED, Cordasco EM, Gipson GT, et al: Home care ventilation: the Cleveland Clinic experience from 1977 to 1985. Respiratory Care 31:294–301, 1986

Slevin SE: Termination of hemodialysis treatment: staff reactions, in Psychonephrology 2: Psychological Problems in Kidney Failure and Their Treatment. Edited by Levy NB. New York, Plenum, 1983, pp 117–130

Smoller JW, Pollack MH, Otto M, et al: Panic anxiety, dyspnea, and respiratory disease: theoretical and clinical considerations. Am J Respir Crit Care Med 154:6–17, 1996

Spiegel D, Bloom JR: Group therapy and hypnosis reduce metastatic breast carcinoma pain. Psychosom Med 45:333–339, 1983

Spiegel D, Bloom JR, Yalom I: Group support for patients with metastatic cancer: a randomized prospective outcome study. Arch Gen Psychiatry 38:527–533, 1981

Spiegel D, Bloom JR, Kraemer HC, et al: Effect of psychosocial treatment on survival of patients with metastatic breast cancer. Lancet 2:888–891, 1989

Stabler B, Surwit RS, Lane JD, et al: Type A behavior pattern and blood glucose control in diabetic children. Psychosom Med 49:313–316, 1987

Steele TE, Baltimore D, Finkelstein SH, et al: Quality of life in peritoneal dialysis patients. J Nerv Ment Dis 184:368–374, 1996

Stein M, Miller AH, Trestman RL: Depression, the immune system, and health and illness: findings in search of meaning. Arch Gen Psychiatry 48:171–177, 1991

Stoudemire A: Psychological factors affecting physical condition and DSM-IV. Psychosomatics 34:8–11, 1993

Stoudemire A, Hales RE: Psychological and behavioral factors affecting medical conditions and DSM-IV: an overview. Psychosomatics 32:5–13, 1991

Stoudemire A, McDaniel JS: History and current trends in psychosomatic medicine, in Comprehensive Textbook of Psychiatry, 7th Edition. Edited by Kaplan HI, Sadock BJ. Baltimore, MD, Williams & Wilkins (in press)

Stoudemire A, Wallack L, Hedemark N: Alcohol dependence and abuse. Am J Prev Med 3 (No 5, suppl):9–18, 1987a

Stoudemire A, Frank R, Kamlet M, et al: Depression. Am J Prev Med 3 (No 5, suppl):65–71, 1987b

Stoudemire A, Beardsley G, Folks DG, et al: Psychological factors affecting physical condition (PFAPC) 316.00: proposals for revisions in DSM-IV, in DSM-IV Sourcebook: Literature Reviews. Edited by Widiger TA, Frances A, Pincus H, et al. Washington, DC, American Psychiatric Press, 1993

Surwit RS, Feinglos MN: The effects of relaxation on glucose tolerance in non–insulin-dependent diabetes. Diabetes Care 6:176–179, 1983

Temoshok L, Heller BW: Stress and "type C" versus epidemiological risk factors in melanoma. Paper presented at the 89th annual convention of the American Psychological Association, Los Angeles, CA, August 1981

Temoshok L, Heller BW, Sageviel RW, et al: The relationship of psychological factors of prognostic indicators in cutaneous malignant melanoma. J Psychosom Res 29:139–153, 1985

U.S. Department of Health and Human Services: The Health Consequence of Smoking: Reducing the Health Consequences of Smoking: 25 Years of Progress: A Report of the Surgeon General. Rockville, MD, U.S. Department of Health and Human Services, Public Health Service, Office on Smoking and Health, 1989

Van der Meeren HLM, Van der Schaar WW, Van den Hurk CMAM: The psychological impact of severe acne. Cutis 36:84–86, 1985

Vogel ML, Rosillo RH: Correlation of psychological variables and progress in physical rehabilitation, III: ego functions and defensive and adaptive mechanisms. Arch Phys Med Rehabil 52:15–21, 1971

Vogt T, Pope C, Mullooly J, et al: Mental health status as a predictor of morbidity and mortality: a 15-year follow-up of members of a health maintenance organization. Am J Public Health 84:227–231, 1994

Vracko-Tusevljak M, Kambic V: The significance of psychological factors in the early diagnosis of laryngeal and hypopharyngeal tumors. Laryngorhinootologie 68:118–121, 1989

Wai L, Richmond J, Burton HJ, et al: Influence of psychosocial factors on survival of home-dialysis patients. Lancet 2:1155–1156, 1981

Wales JK: Does psychological distress cause diabetes? Diabet Med 12:109–112, 1995

Walker EA, Roy-Byrne RP, Katon WJ: Irritable bowel syndrome and psychiatric illness. Am J Psychiatry 174:565–572, 1990

Walker EA, Katon WJ, Roy-Byrne RP, et al: Histories of sexual victimization in patients with irritable bowel syndrome or inflammatory bowel disease. Am J Psychiatry 150:1502–1506, 1993

Walker EA, Gelfand MD, Gelfand AN, et al: The relationship of current psychiatric disorder to functional disability and distress in patients with inflammatory bowel disease. Gen Hosp Psychiatry 18:220–229, 1996

Walker P, Luther J, Samloff IM, et al: Life events stress and psychosocial factors in men with peptic ulcer disease, II: relationships with serum pepsinogen concentrations and behavioral risk factors. Gastroenterology 94:323–330, 1988

Waxler-Morrison N, Hislop TG, Mears B, et al: Effects of social relationships on survival for women with breast cancer: a prospective study. Soc Sci Med 33:177–183, 1991

Weiner H: Psychobiology and Human Disease. New York, Elsevier, 1977

Weiner H: Respiratory disorders, in Comprehensive Textbook of Psychiatry/IV, 4th Edition. Edited by Kaplan HI, Sadock BJ. Baltimore, MD, Williams & Wilkins, 1985, pp 1159–1167

Weiner H, Thaler M, Reiser MF, et al: Etiology of duodenal ulcer, I: relation of specific psychological characteristics to rate of gastric secretion (serum pepsinogen). Psychosom Med 19:1–10, 1957

Weisman AD: Coping with illness, in Massachusetts General Hospital Handbook of General Hospital Psychiatry. Edited by Hackett TP, Cassem NH. Littleton, MA, PSG Publishing, 1987, pp 297–308

Welin L, Svardsudd K, Ander-Perciva S, et al: Prospective study of social influences on mortality: the study of men born in 1913 and 1923. Lancet 1:915–918, 1985

Whitehead W, Bosmajian L, Zonderman A, et al: Symptoms of psychologic distress associated with irritable bowel syndrome: comparison of community and medical clinic samples. Gastroenterology 95:709–714, 1988

Wilhelmsen I, Haug TT, Ursin H, et al: Effect of short-term cognitive psychotherapy on recurrence of duodenal ulcer: a prospective randomized trial. Psychosom Med 56:440–448, 1994

Williams RB, Barefoot JC, Califf RM, et al: Prognostic importance of social and economic resources among medically treated patients with angiographically documented coronary artery disease. JAMA 267:520–524, 1992

Winsa B, Adami HO, Bergstrom R, et al: Stressful life events and Graves' disease. Lancet 338:1475–1479, 1991

Wolcott DL, Wellisch DK, Marsh JT, et al: Relationship of dialysis modality and other factors to cognitive function in chronic dialysis patients. Am J Kidney Dis 12:275–284, 1988

Wright J: On discontinuing dialysis. J Med Ethics 19:77–81, 1993

Yamagiwa M, Harada T, Kubo M, et al: Psychological states and personality as factors in the morbidity of head and neck malignant tumors. Nippon Jibiinkoka Gakkai Kaiho 94:67–73, 1991

Yellowlees PM, Kalucy RS: Psychobiological aspects of asthma and the consequent research implications. Chest 97:628–634, 1990

Zimmermann E: [Quality of life in artificial kidney therapy]. Wien Klin Wochenschr 101:780–784, 1989

Zonderman AB, Costa PT Jr, McCrae RR: Depression as a risk for cancer morbidity and mortality in a nationally representative sample. JAMA 262:1191–1195, 1989

CHAPTER 16

SOMATOFORM DISORDERS

RONALD L. MARTIN, M.D.[†]

SEAN H. YUTZY, M.D.

The somatoform disorders were first delineated as a class of psychiatric disorders in the third edition of the *Diagnostic and Statistical Manual of Mental Disorders* (DSM-III; American Psychiatric Association 1980). The class was created to facilitate the differential diagnosis of disorders characterized primarily by "physical symptoms suggesting physical disorder (hence, *somatoform*) for which there are no demonstrable organic findings or known physiological mechanisms and for which there is positive evidence, or a strong presumption, that the symptoms are linked to psychological factors or conflicts" (American Psychiatric Association 1980, p. 241). With minor modifications, this grouping and its underlying concept were retained in DSM-III-R (American Psychiatric Association 1987) and, after some debate (Martin 1995), in DSM-IV (American Psychiatric Association 1994). In contrast to factitious disorders and malingering, somatoform disorder symptoms are *not* under voluntary control. The stipulation in DSM-IV that symptoms are *not* fully accounted for by known physiological mechanisms distinguishes somatoform disorders from disorders formerly designated as psychophysiological disorders, some

of which are included in DSM-IV under "Psychological Factors Affecting Medical Condition." Beliefs or preoccupations with symptoms are not of delusional intensity, except for body dysmorphic disorder, wherein such a differentiation is difficult to make and does not generally determine management strategy. Symptoms are not better accounted for by other mental disorders.

In DSM-IV, the disorders included under the somatoform rubric are *somatization disorder, undifferentiated somatoform disorder, conversion disorder, pain disorder, hypochondriasis, body dysmorphic disorder,* and the residual category *somatoform disorder not otherwise specified (NOS).* DSM-IV criteria for these disorders are outlined in Table 16–1. The grouping is based on the clinical utility of a shared diagnostic concern rather than assumptions regarding shared etiology or mechanism: the exclusion of occult "physical" or "organic" pathology underlying the symptoms. In DSM-IV terminology, such etiologies are referred to as "general medical conditions" or the "direct effects of a substance." General medical conditions include all conditions not included in the mental disorders section of the tenth revision of the *International Classification of Diseases,* ICD-10 (World Health Organization 1992b). As

[†] Deceased.

TABLE 16–1. DSM-IV somatoform disorders: a comparison

DSM-IV somatoform disorder	General description	Temporal and other requirements	Exclusions by other psychiatric illness	Other exclusions
Somatization disorder	History of many physical complaints: pain in at least four different sites or functions, two nonpain gastrointestinal, one sexual or reproductive, one pseudoneurological (conversion or dissociative).	Onset before age 30. Occurs over a period of several years. Treatment sought or significant impairment in social, occupational, or other important areas of functioning.	Not specified.	Not fully explained by a known general medical condition or the direct effect of a substance.
Undifferentiated somatoform disorder	One or more physical complaints.	Duration of at least 6 months. Clinically significant distress or impairment in social, occupational, or other important areas of functioning.	Not better accounted for by another mental disorder.	Not fully explained by a known general medical condition or pathophysiological mechanism (i.e., the effects of injury, medication, drugs, alcohol).
Conversion disorder	Symptoms or deficits affecting voluntary motor or sensory function suggesting a neurological or other general medical condition.	Psychological factors associated. Clinically significant distress or impairment in social, occupational, or other important areas of functioning; or warrants medical evaluation.	Not limited to pain or sexual dysfunction. Not exclusively during course of somatization disorder. Not better accounted for by another mental disorder.	Not intentionally produced or feigned. Not fully explained by a neurological or other general medical condition, or by the direct effect of a substance, or as a culturally sanctioned behavior or experience.
Pain disorder	Pain as predominant focus of clinical presentation. Of sufficient severity to warrant clinical attention.	Clinically significant distress or impairment in social, occupational, or other important areas of functioning. Psychological factors have an important role.	Not better accounted for by a mood, anxiety, or psychotic disorder, and does not meet criteria for dyspareunia.	Not specified.
Hypochondriasis	Preoccupation with fears of having, or the idea that one has, a serious disease based on the misinterpretation of bodily symptoms. Persists despite appropriate medical evaluation and reassurance.	Duration of at least 6 months. Clinically significant distress or impairment in social, occupational, or other important areas of functioning.	Not exclusively during course of a generalized anxiety, obsessive-compulsive, or panic disorder; a major depressive episode; separation anxiety; or another somatoform disorder.	Not of delusional intensity. Not restricted to circumscribed concern about appearance.

(continued)

TABLE 16–1. DSM-IV somatoform disorders: a comparison *(continued)*

DSM-IV somatoform disorder	General description	Temporal and other requirements	Exclusions by other psychiatric illness	Other exclusions
Body dysmorphic disorder	Preoccupation (may be of delusional intensity) with imagined defect in appearance or markedly excessive concern with slight physical anomaly.	Clinically significant distress or impairment in social, occupational, or other important areas of functioning.	Not better accounted for by another mental disorder (e.g., dissatisfaction with body shape or size in anorexia nervosa).	Not specified.
Somatoform disorder not otherwise specified	Disorders with specified somatoform symptoms. Examples: pseudocyesis; disorders of less than 6 months' duration with fatigue or body weakness, nonpsychotic hypochondriacal symptoms, or other physical complaints.	Can be of less than 6 months' duration.	Does not meet criteria for any specific somatoform disorder.	Not specified.

Source.   Adapted with permission from Martin RL: "Somatoform Disorders in the General Hospital Setting," in *Handbook of Studies on General Psychiatry.* Edited by Judd FK, Burrows GD, Lipsitt DR. Amsterdam, Elsevier, 1991, pp 251–266. Copyright 1991, Elsevier Science Publishers.

examples, all infectious and parasitic, endocrine, nutritional, metabolic, immunity, and congenital disorders affecting virtually any organ system (including the nervous system) are considered general medical conditions. This terminology was adopted to avoid the implication that *mental* (i.e., psychiatric) conditions do not have *organic* causes and to underscore the view that psychiatric disorders are also *medical* conditions.

The utility of grouping disorders on the basis of a shared clinical concern was endorsed by the symptom-driven *Diagnostic and Statistical Manual of Mental Disorders, Fourth Edition, Primary Care Version* (DSM-IV–PC; American Psychiatric Association 1995), which includes "unexplained physical symptoms" as the basis of one of its 10 algorithms. Likewise, the ICD-10 *Diagnostic and Management Guidelines for Mental Disorders in Primary Care* (World Health Organization 1996) is organized similarly with a diagnostic category for "unexplained somatic complaint."

Criticisms of the somatoform disorders category were summarized by M. R. Murphy (1990), who contended that the category is "superficial" because it is delineated on the basis of presenting physical symptoms. Furthermore, the individual disorders are not qualitatively distinct, would be better described dimensionally than categorically, are derived from data on hospital- rather than community- or primary care–based populations, give the "spurious impression of understanding" leading to "naive assumptions about disease entities," and have diagnostic criteria that are either too restrictive for clinical use or are insufficiently

operationalized. Others (e.g., Cloninger 1987) maintain that the somatoform grouping represents a major advance over previous systems. Segregation of such disorders into a grouping has promoted clarification of concepts and greater consistency in terminology and descriptive distinctions between specific somatoform disorders. It is argued that such clarification and consistency will foster research that is more generalizable and therefore more clinically applicable. Indeed, comparison of post- versus pre-DSM-III literature on these disorders reveals greater consistency.

It is assumed that the specific disorders in the somatoform grouping are heterogeneous. In somatization, undifferentiated somatoform, conversion, and pain disorders, the focus is on the symptoms themselves. In hypochondriasis and body dysmorphic disorder, the emphasis is on preoccupations: in hypochondriasis, with the interpretation and possible implications of bodily symptoms; in body dysmorphic disorder, with an imagined or exaggerated defect in appearance. Because of their emphasis on preoccupations, hypochondriasis and body dysmorphic disorder more closely resemble obsessive-compulsive or even psychotic disorders than they do the symptom-centered somatoform disorders (Hollander et al. 1992; Phillips et al. 1995).

The *somatoform* concept, with a history dating only to the introduction of DSM-III in 1980, must not be equated with two concepts of long tradition: *psychosomatic illness* and *somatization.* Theoretically, in psychosomatic illnesses, structural or physiological changes result from psychological factors. In the somatoform disorders, however, such changes are generally not evident. The "classic" psychosomatic illnesses described by Alexander (1950) included bronchial asthma, ulcerative colitis, thyrotoxicosis, essential hypertension, rheumatoid arthritis, neurodermatitis, and peptic ulcer. In DSM-IV, these illnesses are considered general medical conditions, with additional mention under "Psychological Factors Affecting Medical Conditions" (see Chapter 15 in this volume).

The term *somatization* is attributed to Stekel (Lipowski 1988), who early in this century defined it as a bodily disorder that arises as the expression of a deep-seated neurosis. This conceptualization of somatization should not be confused with the descriptive use of the term in somatization disorder. Many elaborate hypotheses of somatization have been advocated (Kellner 1990; Lipowski 1988), with most postulating that somatic syndromes represent the expression of psychological distress somatically. However, others posit that "somatization is neither a discrete clinical entity, nor the result of a single pathological process" and that it "cuts across diagnostic categories" (Kellner 1990). The author goes on to argue that "empirical studies . . . suggest that there is no single theory that can adequately explain somatization, which is not only multifactorially determined but is an exceedingly complex phenomenon" (Kellner 1990, p. 157). Generally, somatization theories have been difficult to demonstrate. The effectiveness of treatment strategies derived from such theories, such as promoting verbal expression of emotions and psychological conflict in "alexithymic" patients (i.e., patients who are presumed deficient in such expression) so that expression of emotions somatically becomes unnecessary, has not been demonstrated (Bach et al. 1996).

Historically, many overlapping, conflicting, and even contradictory diagnostic conventions have been employed to identify and distinguish somatoform disorders. For the sake of consistency, this chapter uses DSM-IV criteria and terminology, with other systems reviewed and contrasted when appropriate. Table 16–2 lists the categories best corresponding to DSM-IV somatoform disorders in DSM (American Psychiatric Association 1952), DSM-II (American Psychiatric Association 1968), DSM-III, and DSM-III-R, as well as ICD-9 (World Health Organization 1977) and ICD-10.

No general heading corresponding to "somatoform" existed in DSM and DSM-II. In DSM, with only "Conversion Reaction" specifically listed, conditions corresponding to the DSM-IV somatoform disorders would have been diagnosed under "psychoneurotic disorders." DSM-II

included "Hysterical Neurosis, Conversion Type" under "Neuroses." Both DSM and DSM-II included a "psychophysiologic" category, encompassing syndromes involving organ systems under autonomic nervous system control. A somatoform grouping was not incorporated into the international system until ICD-10. In ICD-9, disorders corresponding to DSM-IV somatoform disorders were included under "Neurotic Disorders." The ICD-10 somatoform category is conceptualized in a manner similar to what was introduced with DSM-III, emphasizing as the main feature "physical symptoms" that are not adequately explained by physical disorders. In addition, ICD-10 includes a medical utilization specification requiring a "repeated presentation" of symptoms, "persistent requests for medical investigations," and resistance to consideration of "psychological causation" despite "repeated negative findings and reassurances by doctors that the symptoms have no physical basis" (World Health Organization 1992a, p. 161). ICD-10 somatoform disorders include somatization disorder, undifferentiated somatoform disorder, hypochondriacal disorder (which also subsumes DSM-IV body dysmorphic disorder), somatoform autonomic dysfunction (a category not included in DSM-IV that corresponds, in part, to the DSM and DSM-II psychophysiological disorders), persistent somatoform pain disorder, other somatoform disorders, and somatoform disorder, unspecified. Conversion disorder is not included as a somatoform disorder but is subsumed under a fused dissociative (conversion) disorder. As will be discussed in the section on conversion disorder in this chapter, this option was considered carefully in the preparation of DSM-IV, but it was decided to leave conversion disorder in the somatoform grouping on the basis that it met the essential requirement of presentation with physical symptoms suggesting a general medical condition but for which there is no adequate medical or physiological explanation (Martin 1996).

Despite inconsistencies between DSM-IV and ICD-10, sufficient overlap exists to permit generalizations regarding specific somatoform disorders, as long as the differences are kept in mind. The comparability and, by design, compatibility of DSM-IV and ICD-10 provide evidence of expanding international cooperation in developing a common language to foster better communication among clinicians and researchers worldwide.

Given the heterogeneity of the somatoform disorder class, extensive discussion of the class, in general, is not particularly useful. The specific somatoform disorders are best discussed individually. Thus, with the exception of pain disorder, which is reviewed in a separate chapter of this textbook (see Chapter 26), we review the somatoform disorders included in DSM-IV. For convenience, the disor-

TABLE 16-2. **DSM-IV somatoform disorders and corresponding categories in previous DSM and ICD diagnostic systems**

DSM-IV (1994)	DSM (1952)	DSM-II (1968)	ICD-9 (1977)	DSM-III (1980)	DSM-III-R (1987)	ICD-10 (1992)
Somatoform disorders	—	—	—	Somatoform disorders	Somatoform disorders	Somatoform disorders; also dissociative (conversion) disorders
Somatization disorder	—	—	Other neurotic disorders: somatization disorder, Briquet's disorder.	Somatization disorder	Somatization disorder	Somatization disorder
Undifferentiated somatoform disorder	—	—	—	Atypical somatoform disorder	Undifferentiated somatoform disorder	Undifferentiated somatoform disorder
Conversion disorder	Conversion reaction	Hysterical neurosis: conversion type	Conversion disorder	Conversion disorder	Conversion disorder	Dissociative (conversion) disorders
Pain disorder	—	Hysterical neurosis: conversion type	Psychalgia, psychogenic pain	Psychogenic pain disorder	Somatoform pain disorder	Persistent pain disorder
Hypochondriasis	Psycho-neurotic reaction: other	Hypochon-driacal neurosis	Hypochon-driasis	Hypochon-driasis	Hypochondriasis	Hypochondriasis
Body dysmorphic disorder	—	—	—	Atypical somatoform disorder: dys-morphophobia	Body dysmorphic disorder	Included under hypochondriacal disorder
Somatoform disorder not otherwise specified	—	—	—	Atypical somatoform disorder	Somatoform disorder not otherwise specified	Other somatoform disorders

Source. Adapted with permission from Martin RL: "Somatoform Disorders in the General Hospital Setting," in *Handbook of Studies on General Psychiatry.* Edited by Judd FK, Burrows GD, Lipsitt DR. Amsterdam, Elsevier, 1991, pp 251–266. Copyright 1991, Elsevier Science Publishers.

ders are discussed in the order in which they appear in DSM-IV.

SOMATIZATION DISORDER

DEFINITION AND CLINICAL DESCRIPTION

The core features of somatization disorder are recurrent multiple physical complaints that are not fully explained by physical factors and that result in medical attention or significant impairment.

A patient with somatization disorder is typified by the following example:

A married woman in her 30s was referred to a psychiatrist by her internist, who had become frustrated after several unsuccessful attempts to establish a clear longitudinal history for her numerous physical complaints and failure to demonstrate any plausible general medical explanation for the symptoms through physical examination and laboratory testing. In addition, the patient had been treated by the internist for depressive and anxiety complaints with a number of different antidepressants and anxiolytics. Some of these agents had shown promise of effectiveness initially, only to fail later, and they were associated with a number of subjective adverse effects.

On her initial visit to the psychiatrist, the patient focused on a number of physical complaints that had mystified the primary care physician. The psychiatrist noted the vague and dramatic presentation of a long and complicated medical history. At times, the patient focused not on somatic symptoms but on an elaborate and dramatic discussion of marital, social, and occupational problems. As the medical history was more completely elicited, a chronic pattern emerged of many physical complaints that had never been adequately explained medically. Furthermore, there seemed to be a temporal association between the medical complaints and periods of psychosocial stress.

Somatization disorder is the most pervasive somatoform disorder. By definition, somatization disorder is a polysymptomatic disorder affecting multiple body systems. Symptoms of other specific somatoform disorders (e.g., *conversion disorder* and *pain disorder*) are included in the diagnostic criteria for somatization disorder. Undifferentiated somatoform disorder, in essence, represents a syndrome similar to somatization disorder but with a less extensive symptomatology. From a hierarchical perspective, none of these disorders is diagnosed if symptoms occur exclusively during the course of somatization disorder.

Somatization disorder has been the most rigorously studied somatoform disorder and is the best validated in terms of diagnostic reliability, stability over time, prediction of medical utilization, and even heritability. Yet its validity as a discrete syndrome has been challenged (Bass and Murphy 1990). Vaillant (1984), noting that the majority of the research on this disorder has emanated from four academic centers in the midwestern United States, went so far as to state that the diagnosis "lies in the eyes of the beholder" (p. 543).

DIAGNOSIS

History

The DSM-IV criteria for somatization disorder are the product of a long and inconsistent approach to a syndrome characterized by multiple unexplained physical complaints (Martin 1988). Originally designated as *hysteria*, the syndrome was first described at least 4,000 years ago, with its conceptualization probably originating in Egypt

(Goodwin and Guze 1996). In Egyptian medicine, it was believed that physical displacement of the uterus precipitated symptoms (Veith 1965); treatment consisted of attempting to attract the "wandering womb" back to its proper site.

Freud devoted a great deal of attention to the concept of hysteria (Breuer and Freud 1893–1895/1955). In fact, many of the principles of psychoanalysis were engendered by observations of hysteria. Dynamic theorists postulated the operation of the ego defense mechanism of conversion in hysteria. This mechanism was conceptualized as the converting of "psychic energy" into physical symptoms. Later, Stekel (1943) coined the term *somatization*, which he regarded as similar to Freud's concept of conversion.

Paul Briquet (1859) described in a monograph, *Traité, Clinique et Thérapeutique Y l'Hystérie*, a syndrome corresponding to somatization disorder as it is conceptualized today, describing hysteria as characterized by multiple dramatic and excessive medical complaints in the absence of demonstrable organic pathology. Purtell et al. (1951) resurrected Briquet's concept, adding a quantitative perspective by providing a list of associated symptoms, which was further refined by Perley and Guze (1962).

Hysteria was included as one of the 14 "canonized" psychiatric disorders in the influential criteria described by Feighner et al. (1972). The disorders included were those considered by the authors to have been validated sufficiently. For hysteria, the Feighner criteria required a chronic or recurrent illness beginning before age 30 years that includes a dramatic, vague, or complicated medical history. The diagnosis required 25 "positive" medically unexplained symptoms (from a list of 59) in 9 of 10 groups (Table 16–3); 20 symptoms in the same number of groups were necessary for a probable diagnosis. In order to be counted as positive, a symptom 1) caused the patient to see a physician or other health care provider, 2) was disabling enough to interfere with the patient's life, 3) led the patient to take medicine on more than one occasion, or 4) was of "clinical significance" despite not fulfilling one of the other three previously mentioned criteria. An example of this fourth criterion would be a brief spell of blindness that the patient minimizes.

As is discussed in this chapter, the syndrome as defined by Feighner et al. (1972) remains the gold standard because it has been the best validated. In particular, clinical, epidemiological, and follow-up studies using Feighner criteria support its validity, reliability, and internal consistency (Barsky 1989). The stability of the disorder is supported by the finding that in the 6–8 years after initial diagnosis there is a 90% probability that the clinical picture will remain essentially unchanged and that no general medical or new mental disorder will de-

TABLE 16–3. Feighner symptom list for hysteria (somatization disorder)

Group 1	Group 6
Headaches	Abdominal pain
Sickly most of life	Vomiting
Group 2	**Group 7**
Blindness	Dysmenorrhea
Paralysis	Menstrual irregularity
Anesthesia	Amenorrhea
Aphonia	Excessive bleeding
Fits or convulsions	**Group 8**
Unconsciousness	Sexual indifference
Amnesia	Frigidity
Deafness	Dyspareunia
Hallucinations	Other sexual difficulties
Urinary retention	Vomiting all 9 months of
Trouble walking	pregnancy at least once,
Other unexplained	or hospitalization for
"neurological" symptoms	hyperemesis gravidarum
Group 3	**Group 9**
Fatigue	Back pain
Lump in throat	Joint pain
Fainting spells	Extremity pain
Visual blurring	Burning pains of the sexual
Weakness	organs, mouth, or rectum
Dysuria	Other bodily pains
Group 4	**Group 10**
Breathing difficulty	Nervousness
Palpitation	Fears
Anxiety attacks	Depressed feelings
Chest pain	Need to quit working, or
Dizziness	inability to carry on
Group 5	regular duties because of
Anorexia	feeling sick
Weight loss	Crying easily
Marked fluctuations in weight	Feeling life is hopeless
Nausea	Thinking a good deal
Abdominal bloating	about dying
Food intolerances	Wanting to die
Diarrhea	Thinking of suicide
Constipation	Suicide attempts

Note. Twenty-five positive symptoms in nine groups required for a diagnosis of definite hysteria; 20 positive symptoms in nine groups required for a diagnosis of probable hysteria.
Source. Adapted from Perley and Guze 1962. Reprinted with permission from Cloninger CR: "Somatoform and Dissociative Disorders," in *The Medical Basis of Psychiatry, Second Edition.* Edited by Winokur G, Clayton P. Philadelphia, PA, WB Saunders, 1994, pp 169–192. Copyright 1994, WB Saunders.

velop to explain the original symptoms (Barsky 1989).

Despite such validation, the construct was underused by clinicians (Cloninger 1994). This underuse has been at-tributed to two sources: the pejorative connotation of the term *hysteria* and the complexity of remembering the numerous symptoms divided into various groups not organized according to any obvious logic. The criteria were intended principally for a research setting where the investigator followed a checklist to systematically evaluate for the presence of the syndrome.

In addition to its definition as a syndrome characterized by many somatic complaints, hysteria was frequently confused with the dramatic and volatile hysterical personality characteristics as described by Chodoff and Lyons (1958). Guze (1970) suggested the more neutral Briquet's syndrome. In DSM-III, the syndrome was descriptively renamed somatization disorder.

In DSM-III, the criteria were simplified as follows:

1. The required number of symptoms was lowered to 14 for women and 12 for men, from a list of 37 commonly identified somatic complaints. The 37 symptoms listed were those that best discriminated somatization disorder from other disorders. The number of symptoms required of men was lowered in an attempt to reduce a possible sex bias because of the impossibility of menstrual and pregnancy symptoms in men.

2. The group requirement was dropped as it seemed to add little information.

3. Depressive and panic attack symptoms were eliminated to avoid overlap with depressive and panic disorders.

Because DSM-III, DSM-III-R, and DSM-IV criteria for somatization disorder have the same conceptual base as Briquet's syndrome and identify a similar population as that identified by the well-studied Feighner hysteria syndrome, in subsequent discussions in this chapter—except when specifically noted—the term *somatization disorder* is used even when findings are reviewed from studies in which the term *hysteria* or *Briquet's syndrome* was used.

The diagnostic criteria for somatization disorder in DSM-III required a history of physical symptoms of several years' duration beginning before the patient was age 30 years. Conditions similar to those defined by the Feighner criteria were necessary to consider a symptom positive. Exclusion of a medical explanation was determined if the symptoms were not adequately explained by a "physical disorder or physical injury" and were "not side effects of medication, drugs or alcohol" (American Psychiatric Association 1980, p. 243). The clinician did not need to be convinced that the symptom had actually occurred; a patient's report was sufficient.

The criteria for somatization disorder were modified slightly for DSM-III-R. The changes included shortening the symptom list to 35 and requiring 13 symptoms for the diagnosis in both sexes. A symptom was not counted if it occurred only during a panic attack. Symptoms were to be counted as present if there was no specific pathology or pathophysiological mechanism. In addition, if organic pathology was identified, the complaint or resulting social or occupational impairment must have grossly exceeded what would be expected from the physical findings.

Unfortunately, diagnostic concordance between the simplified DSM-III somatization disorder criteria and the Feighner criteria was less than optimal. As a result, the question was raised as to whether the types of cases identified by DSM-III criteria constituted a valid disease entity (Cloninger et al. 1986; Guze et al. 1986). The adequacy of the criteria also was questioned when the National Institute of Mental Health (NIMH) Epidemiologic Catchment Area (ECA) studies (L. N. Robins et al. 1984), using DSM-III criteria, found a much lower lifetime prevalence rate (0.2%–0.3%) of somatization disorder for women in the general population than the 2% estimated by Woodruff et al. (1971), using Feighner criteria. In addition, many psychiatrists considered both the DSM-III and DSM-III-R criteria too lengthy and complex for routine clinical use.

DSM-IV Criteria

In an attempt to address these issues for DSM-IV, a comprehensive reassessment of the extant literature and preexisting data sets was coordinated by the American Psychiatric Association. On the basis of this review, Cloninger and Yutzy (1993) suggested a diagnostic strategy that simplified the criteria for somatization disorder and appeared usable in routine practice. Data from a sample of 500 psychiatric outpatients were reanalyzed, leading to the development of an empirically derived algorithm to diagnose somatization disorder. This algorithm required four pain symptoms, two nonpain gastrointestinal symptoms, one nonpain sexual or reproductive symptom, and one pseudoneurological (conversion or dissociative) symptom. This approach was adopted for DSM-IV (Table 16–4). The data reanalysis criteria identified nearly the same patients as did both the original Feighner criteria for hysteria and the DSM-III-R criteria for somatization disorder ($\kappa = .79$; sensitivity = 81%; specificity = 96%) (Yutzy et al. 1992).

The new criteria were tested in a multicenter field trial designed to examine their concordance with previous diagnostic criteria. This study (Yutzy et al. 1995) found excellent agreement with the newly proposed diagnostic strategy and the following earlier criteria: DSM-III-R ($\kappa = .84$;

TABLE 16–4. DSM-IV diagnostic criteria for somatization disorder

A. A history of many physical complaints beginning before age 30 years that occur over a period of several years and result in treatment being sought or significant impairment in social, occupational, or other important areas of functioning.

B. Each of the following criteria must have been met, with individual symptoms occurring at any time during the course of the disturbance.

  (1) *Four pain symptoms:* a history of pain related to at least four different sites or functions (e.g., head, abdomen, back, joints, extremities, chest, rectum, during menstruation, during sexual intercourse, or during urination)

  (2) *Two gastrointestinal symptoms:* a history of at least two gastrointestinal symptoms other than pain (e.g., nausea, bloating, vomiting other than during pregnancy, diarrhea, or intolerance of several different foods)

  (3) *One sexual symptom:* a history of at least one sexual or reproductive symptom other than pain (e.g., sexual indifference, erectile or ejaculatory dysfunction, irregular menses, excessive menstrual bleeding, vomiting throughout pregnancy)

  (4) *One pseudoneurological symptom:* a history of at least one symptom or deficit suggesting a neurological disorder not limited to pain (conversion symptoms such as impaired coordination or balance, paralysis or localized weakness, difficulty swallowing or lump in throat, aphonia, urinary retention, hallucinations, loss of touch or pain sensation, double vision, blindness, deafness, seizures, dissociative symptoms such as amnesia, or loss of consciousness other than fainting)

C. Either (1) or (2):

  (1) After appropriate investigation, each of the symptoms in criterion B cannot be fully explained by a known general medical condition or the direct effects of a substance (e.g., a drug of abuse, a medication).

  (2) When there is a related general medical condition, the physical complaints or resulting social or occupational impairment is in excess of what would be expected from the history, physical examination, or laboratory findings.

D. The symptoms are not intentionally produced or feigned (as in factitious disorder or malingering).

sensitivity = 84%; specificity = 98%), DSM-III (κ = .82; sensitivity = 82%; specificity = 98%), and the original Feighner criteria for hysteria (κ = .79; sensitivity = 80%; specificity = 97%). These findings supported the DSM-IV diagnostic strategy for somatization disorder.

Differential Diagnosis

The symptom picture encountered in somatization disorder is frequently nonspecific and can overlap with a multitude of medical disorders. According to Cloninger (1994), three features are useful in discriminating between somatization disorder and physical illness: 1) involvement of multiple organ systems, 2) early onset and chronic course without development of physical signs of structural abnormalities, and 3) absence of characteristic laboratory abnormalities of the suggested physical disorder (Table 16–5). These features should be considered in cases for which careful analysis leaves the etiology unclear. The clinician also should be aware that several medical disorders may be confused with somatization disorder (Table 16–6). Patients with multiple sclerosis (MS) and systemic lupus erythematosus (SLE) may have vague functional and sensory disturbances with unclear physical signs. Patients with acute intermittent porphyria (AIP) may have a history of episodic pain and various neurological disturbances, and patients with hemochromatosis associated with vague pains may be confused with patients who have somatization disorder.

According to Cloninger (1994), three psychiatric disorders must be carefully considered in the differential diagnosis of somatization disorder: anxiety disorders (in particular, panic disorder), mood disorders, and schizophrenia. The most troublesome distinction is between anxiety disorders and somatization disorder. Individuals with generalized anxiety disorder may have a multitude of physical complaints that also frequently are found in patients with somatization disorder. Individuals with anxiety disorders also may have disease concerns and hypochondriacal complaints common to somatization disorder. Similarly, patients with somatization disorder often report panic attacks. Although the usual parameters of age at onset and course may be helpful in differentiating between an anxiety disorder and somatization disorder, the presence of certain traits, symptoms, and factors can be of assistance. In particular, the presence of histrionic personality traits, conversion and dissociative symptoms, sexual and menstrual problems, and social impairment supports a diagnosis of somatization disorder (Cloninger 1994). In addition, gender should be considered because men are much more likely to suffer from anxiety disorders than from somatization disorder. Precise diagnosis, although difficult, is clinically important because the medical management of somatization disorder differs from that of anxiety disorders.

Patients with mood disorders, especially depression, may have somatic complaints. Commonly, the chief complaint is headache, gastrointestinal disturbance, or unexplained pain. However, such symptoms resolve with successful treatment of the mood disorder, whereas in somatization disorder the physical complaints continue. From the other perspective, patients with somatization disorder often complain of depression, often fulfilling criteria for major depression (DeSouza et al. 1988). It is not clear, however, whether these complaints truly reflect the clinical state or are simply a reflection of overreporting.

Patients with schizophrenia may have unexplained somatic complaints. Careful evaluation will reveal delusions, hallucinations, and/or a formal thought disorder. Rarely will the somatic symptoms be extensive enough to meet the criteria for somatization disorder. It should be noted that occasionally a patient with extensive somatic symptomatology and no evidence of psychosis subsequently will develop clinical symptoms of schizophrenia (Goodwin and Guze 1996). As described in the section on conversion disorder later in this chapter, reports of hallucinations are common among women with somatization disorder (R. L. Martin, unpublished observations, 1998). Caution must be taken not to equate such reports with a psychotic diagnosis, which can lead to unnecessary long-term treatment with neuroleptics.

Individuals with antisocial, borderline, and/or histrionic personality disorder may have an associated somatiza-

TABLE 16–5. Features useful in discriminating between somatization disorder and general medical conditions

Involvement of multiple organ systems

Early onset and chronic course without development of physical signs of structural abnormalities

Absence of characteristic laboratories of the suggested physical disorder

TABLE 16–6. General medical conditions that may be confused with somatization disorder

Multiple sclerosis (MS)

Systemic lupus erythematosus (SLE)

Acute intermittent porphyria (AIP)

Hemochromatosis

tion disorder (Cloninger et al. 1997; Hudziak et al. 1996; Stern et al. 1993). Antisocial personality disorder has been shown to cluster both within individuals and within families (Cloninger and Guze 1970; Cloninger et al. 1975) and may have a common etiology in many cases.

Patients with somatization disorder often complain of psychological or interpersonal problems, in addition to somatic symptoms. Wetzel et al. (1994) summarized these as "psychoform symptoms." In this study, Minnesota Multiphasic Personality Inventory (MMPI; Hathaway and McKinley 1943) profiles of somatization disorder patients mimicked multiple psychiatric disorders.

NATURAL HISTORY

E. Robins and O'Neal (1953) found somatization disorder to be unusual in children younger than age 9 years. In the majority of cases, characteristic symptoms begin during adolescence, and the criteria were satisfied by the mid-20s (Guze and Perley 1963; Purtell et al. 1951).

Somatization disorder is a chronic illness with fluctuations in the frequency and diversity of symptoms, but it rarely, if ever, remits totally (Guze and Perley 1963; Guze et al. 1986). The most active symptomatic phase is usually early adulthood, but aging does not lead to total remission (Goodwin and Guze 1996). Pribor et al. (1994) found that somatization disorder patients age 55 years and older did not differ from younger patients in terms of the number of somatization symptoms or the use of health care services. Longitudinal prospective studies have confirmed that 80%–90% of patients diagnosed with somatization disorder maintain consistent clinical syndrome and retain the same diagnosis over many years (Cloninger et al. 1986; Guze et al. 1986; Perley and Guze 1962).

According to Goodwin and Guze (1996), the most frequent and important complications of somatization disorder are repeated surgical operations, drug dependence, marital separation or divorce, and suicide attempts. These authors suggest that the first two complications are preventable if the disorder is recognized and the patient is managed appropriately. Generally, because awareness that somatization disorder is an alternative explanation for various pains and other symptoms, invasive techniques can be withheld or postponed when objective indications are absent or equivocal. There is no evidence of excess mortality in patients with somatization disorder. Suicide attempts are common, but completed suicide is not (Martin et al. 1985; G. E. Murphy and Wetzel 1982). Avoidance of prescribing habit-forming or addictive substances for persistent or recurrent complaints of pain should be paramount in the mind of the treating physician. It is unclear whether marital or occupational dysfunction can be minimized through psychotherapy.

EPIDEMIOLOGY

The lifetime risk, prevalence, and incidence of somatization disorder are unclear. The lifetime risk for somatization disorder was estimated at about 2% in women when age at onset and method of assessment were taken into account (Cloninger et al. 1975). This risk is similar to the previously noted 2% prevalence rate identified by Woodruff et al. (1971). Cloninger et al. (1984), using complete lifetime medical records, found a 3% frequency of somatization disorder in 859 Swedish women in the general population. However, the ECA study (L. N. Robins et al. 1984), using nonphysician interviewers, found a lifetime risk of somatization disorder of only 0.2%–0.3% of women. However, the prevalence of somatization disorder may be underestimated in studies relying on interviews by nonphysicians. In a study by L. N. Robins et al. (1981), nonphysicians, when compared with psychiatrists, showed high (i.e., 97%–99%) diagnostic specificity for somatization disorder. However, diagnostic sensitivity for nonphysicians was low (55% for Feighner-defined hysteria and 41% for DSM-III-defined somatization disorder). The diagnostic criteria for somatization disorder require judgments as to whether or not symptoms are fully explained medically. Patients with somatization disorder often attribute symptoms to various physical disorders. Nonphysicians rarely have the expertise to evaluate such statements critically and may tend to accept them. To properly assess somatic complaints relative to objective findings and the known course of disease may require that the interviewer have an adequate medical background (Cloninger 1994). Additionally, patients may be less inclined to describe physical complaints to nonphysicians. All of these factors may lead to the underdiagnosis of somatization disorder, which may account for the low prevalence of somatization disorder in large-scale population surveys that use nonphysician interviewers.

Somatization disorder is diagnosed predominantly in women and rarely in men. Some have suggested that this sex difference may be artifactual, since somatization disorder criteria are biased against making the diagnosis in men because of the inapplicability of pregnancy and menstrual complaints. Also, men tend to report fewer symptoms than do women. Some investigators have suggested an adjustment for this discrepancy (Temoshok and Attkisson 1977). DSM-III reduced the number of symptoms required to diagnose somatization disorder from 14 in women to 12 in men, compensating for the inapplicable gynecological symptoms but not for the response bias in the number of somatic complaints. Diagnosis of somatization disorder remains much less frequent in men than in women unless the number of somatic complaints required for diagnosis in men is reduced to half (i.e., 7) of the 14 required in women (Cloninger 1994). The symptoms of somatization disorder were counted in a study of psychiatric outpatients and their relatives (Cloninger et al. 1986). The frequency counts were identified for probands and for the relatives of nonsomatizing subjects. The prevalence of somatization disorder was 22% in outpatient women when DSM-III criteria of 14 unexplained symptoms in women were used, compared with 2.9% in the female relatives of nonsomatizing subjects. When the DSM-III criterion of 12 unexplained symptoms in men was applied, the prevalence of somatization disorder in the male relatives of nonsomatizing subjects was only 0.3%, making the disorder more than 10 times as prevalent in women as in men. When the symptom count for men was reduced to 7 or 8 symptoms, the prevalences in men and women were about the same. However, according to Cloninger (1994), men who had from 7 to 11 somatic complaints had a mixed picture of anxiety and personality disorders and did not cluster in families with somatizing subjects of either sex.

ETIOLOGY

The etiology of somatization disorder is unknown, but it is clearly a familial disorder. In a number of studies, approximately 20% of the female first-degree relatives of patients with somatization disorder also met criteria (Cloninger and Guze 1970; Guze et al. 1986; Woerner and Guze 1968). Guze et al. (1986) further demonstrated the familial nature of somatization disorder in a "blind" family study and documented an association between somatization disorder and antisocial personality in male and female relatives. In addition, several studies have suggested that male relatives of female patients with somatization disorder have an increased risk of antisocial personality disorder and alcoholism (Cloninger et al. 1975; Woerner and Guze 1968). As noted previously, Cloninger et al. (1986) found men with multiple somatic complaints to be clinically heterogeneous and not to aggregate in families with either male or female somatizing subjects. Overall, these findings suggest that somatization disorder in women shares a common etiology with antisocial personality disorder, whereas somatization disorder in men may be related more to anxiety disorders (Cloninger et al. 1984, 1986).

A relationship between somatization disorder and certain personality disorders has been posited. Hudziak et al.

(1996) and Cloninger et al. (1997) identified similarities and even overlap between somatization disorder and borderline personality disorder, as did Stern et al. (1993) with personality disorders broadly. These studies support interpretations that somatization disorder is more of a personality (Axis II) disorder than an Axis I disorder, considering its early onset, nonremitting nature, and pervasiveness, which in some cases results in chronic dysfunctional states.

Familial aggregation in somatization disorder could result from genetic factors, environmental influences, or both. Using comprehensive lifetime medical records, Bohman et al. (1984), in an adoption study in Sweden, identified two discrete types of somatoform disorders in women. One form, described as "high-frequency somatization," was characterized by frequent headaches, backaches, gastrointestinal disturbances, and gynecological complaints associated with psychiatric disability (Figure 16–1). Review of the psychiatric evaluations revealed overlap with somatization disorder. Women who were adopted before age 3 years had a fivefold increase in high-frequency somatization disorder if their biological parents had alcoholism or were antisocial. Risk of somatization disorder in the adopted children varied according to the social status of

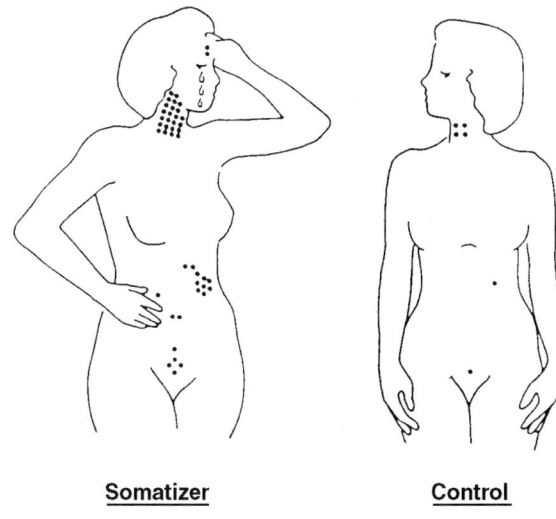

Somatizer   **Control**

• 1 Somatic sick leave/10 person years

⏚ 1 Psychiatric sick leave/10 person years

FIGURE 16–1. Distribution and number of sick leave occasions in Swedish frequently ("high frequency") somatizing subjects and control nonsomatizing subjects. Reprinted with permission from Cloninger CR: "Somatoform and Dissociative Disorders," in *The Medical Basis of Psychiatry, Second Edition.* Edited by Winokur G, Clayton P. Philadelphia, PA, WB Saunders, 1994, pp 169–192. Copyright 1994, WB Saunders.

the adoptive parents. In a cross-fostering analysis that considered the possible combinations of genetic background and postnatal influences, both factors contributed independently to the risk of somatization.

Experimental neuropsychological testing indicates that individuals with somatization disorder demonstrate difficulty with information processing related to problems with attention and memory (Almgren et al. 1978; Bendefeldt et al. 1976; Ludwig 1972). Flor-Henry et al. (1981) investigated the neuropsychological functioning of patients with somatization disorder and compared them with control subjects, psychotic depressive patients, and schizophrenic patients. All comparison groups were matched to the patients with somatization disorder for sex, age, handedness, and Wechsler Adult Intelligence Scale–Revised (WAIS-R; Wechsler 1981) full-scale IQ. Compared with the control subjects, patients with somatization disorder had bilateral, symmetrical patterns of frontal lobe dysfunction. The authors also noted non-dominant hemisphere dysfunction, with impairment greater in the anterior as opposed to the posterior regions. Patients with somatization disorder had greater dominant hemisphere impairment than did control subjects and psychotic depressive patients, a finding also reported for persons with antisocial personality disorder. Patients with somatization disorder had less nondominant hemisphere disorganization than did schizophrenic patients. This pattern of neuropsychological impairment permitted identification of patients with somatization disorder from control subjects and patients in the comparison groups.

There are other theories that attempt to explain the characteristics of patients with somatization disorder. In particular, Shapiro (1965) and Horowitz (1977) suggested that "hysterical" information processing may be responsible for many of the clinical features. The information-processing deficit may be the basis for the somatic complaints, mental status findings of vagueness and circumstantiality, and many social, interpersonal, and occupational problems prominent in these patients and their biological relatives (Cloninger 1978; Flor-Henry et al. 1981; Horowitz 1977). Ford (1983) and Quill (1985) postulated a social communication model based on the theory that individuals with somatization disorder learn to somatize as a means of expressing emotion (i.e., distress) in their family constellation, evoking support and care from significant individuals. Further work needs to be done to evaluate these theories.

TREATMENT

Somatization disorder is difficult to treat, and there appears to be no single superior treatment approach (G. E. Murphy 1982). Although primary care physicians can generally manage patients with somatization disorder adequately, the expertise of a psychiatrist, at least as a consultant to provide management suggestions, has been shown to be useful. In a prospective, randomized controlled study, Smith et al. (1986) found a reduction in health care costs for patients with somatization disorder receiving a psychiatric consultation relative to the time before the consultation, as well as in comparison to costs for patients who did not receive such consultation. Reduced expenditures were largely the result of decreased rates of hospitalization. These gains were accomplished with no decrement in medical status or in patient satisfaction, suggesting that many of the evaluations and treatments otherwise provided to somatization disorder patients are unnecessary. Smith et al. (1986) suggest that treatment include regularly scheduled visits with an appropriate physician. The frequency of visits should be determined on the basis of needed support for the patient, not in response to the frequency or severity of complaints.

Scallet et al. (1976), reviewing the earlier literature on hysteria, reported the success rates of various treatment modalities. Although most of the studies were uncontrolled and otherwise methodologically flawed, one study by Luff and Garrod (1935) noted a 51% improvement rate at 3-year follow-up in patients treated with an "eclectic approach." As summarized by Scallet et al. (1976), this treatment involved "reeducation, reassurance and suggestion" (p. 348). These techniques also were described by Carter (1949) as being effective in the treatment of acute conversion.

An eclectic approach comports well with the general principles of treatment recommended by Quill (1985), Cloninger (1994), and Smith et al. (1986). Three important suggestions emerge from review of these reports: 1) establish a firm therapeutic alliance with the patient, 2) educate the patient regarding the manifestations of somatization disorder, and 3) provide consistent reassurance. Implementation of these principles, as described in more detail below, may greatly facilitate clinical management of somatization disorder and prevent potentially serious complications, including the effects of unnecessary diagnostic and therapeutic procedures. The superiority of any more specific treatment approaches has not been documented by controlled trials (Kellner 1989).

First, a firm therapeutic alliance must be established. The basis of any satisfactory treatment relationship is a firm therapeutic alliance; it is particularly important in the treatment of patients with somatization disorder but often is difficult to attain. Generally, multiple physicians already have been consulted in an attempt to uncover physical explanations for the symptoms that a somatization disorder patient has. Also, the patient probably has received the message (overtly or covertly) that the difficulty is "mental," "psychological," or "psychiatric" and that the physician is not particularly interested in continuing to provide care to him or her. This message promotes a pattern of "doctor shopping," which may lead to unnecessary diagnostic procedures and treatments. To prevent these unnecessary procedures and treatments, a therapeutic alliance is essential. The first step in establishing such an alliance is for the physician to acknowledge the patient's pain and suffering. This acknowledgment communicates to the patient that the physician is caring, compassionate, and interested in providing help. The physician then should conduct an exhaustive review of the patient's medical history, including careful examination of medical records. Such a review generally will strengthen the incipient therapeutic bond, demonstrating the physician's willingness to take the time and effort to gain an understanding of the patient. In addition, this step is crucial in ruling out medical disorders that can include nonspecific motor and sensory abnormalities or transient or equivocal signs (e.g., MS, SLE, AIP, hemochromatosis) (Table 16–6). Also, a thorough medical knowledge of the patient initially will allow better ongoing assessment of symptoms. After the diagnosis of somatization disorder is firmly established, elaborate diagnostic evaluations should be conducted based on objective evidence, not just on subjective complaints. However, the clinician must always remain cognizant that patients with somatization disorder are not immune to developing physical illnesses.

Education is the second general principle. Cloninger (1994) favors informing the patient of the diagnosis and describing the various facets of somatization disorder in a positive light. Advising the patient that he or she is not "crazy" but is suffering from a medically recognized illness and that the condition will not lead to chronic mental or physical deterioration or death may bring some comfort. However, the clinician should be careful to strike a balance between painting a positive picture of the disorder, on the one hand, and, on the other, realistically discussing prognosis, goals, and treatment plans.

The third principle is consistent reassurance. A patient with somatization disorder often becomes concerned that the physician is not performing a sufficiently thorough evaluation and may threaten to seek care from a different physician. Such challenges should be directly addressed with reassurance that the possibility of an undiscovered physical illness is being appropriately assessed on a continuing basis and that changing physicians would place decisions in the hands of someone unaware of the complexities of the patient's case. The patient should be reassured that there is no evidence of a physical cause for the complaint but that there may be a link with "stress." A thorough review of complaints commonly identifies a temporal association of symptoms with interpersonal, social, or occupational problems. Discussion of such associations may help the patient gain insight that the problems may precipitate somatic or psychological symptoms. In patients for whom introspection is difficult, modification of behavior by using simple behavioral management techniques may be useful.

In addition to these general principles, several other issues merit consideration in the treatment of somatization disorder. Because patients with somatization disorder also frequently complain of anxiety and depressive symptoms, prescription medications for these complaints should be held to a minimum and carefully monitored. Wheatley (1962, 1964, 1965) found that low doses of anxiolytic drugs provided some improvement in symptoms in a series of double-blind clinical trials. Although chlordiazepoxide was recommended for reasons of safety, patient preference, and effectiveness in symptom relief, the best results were obtained by optimistic physicians using low doses of anxiolytic medications, regardless of which drug was given (Wheatley 1965). Pharmacotherapy in the management of patients with somatization disorder must be tempered with the knowledge that these patients may take medicines inconsistently and unpredictably, may develop drug dependence, and may overdose in suicide attempts or gestures.

The clinician should develop a relationship with the patient's family. This facilitates attaining a better appreciation of the patient's social structure, which may be crucial to understanding and managing the somatization disorder patient's often chaotic personal lifestyle. When appropriate, the clinician must place firm limits on excessive demands, manipulations, and attention seeking (G. E. Murphy 1982; G. E. Murphy and Guze 1960).

UNDIFFERENTIATED SOMATOFORM DISORDER

DEFINITION AND CLINICAL DESCRIPTION

The essential aspect of undifferentiated somatoform disorder is the presence of one or more clinically significant medically unexplained somatic symptoms with a duration of 6 months or more that are not better accounted for by another mental disorder (Table 16–7; see also Table 16–1 for comparison with other somatoform disorders). In ef-

TABLE 16–7. DSM-IV diagnostic criteria for undifferentiated somatoform disorder

A. One or more physical complaints (e.g., fatigue, loss of appetite, gastrointestinal or urinary complaints).

B. Either (1) or (2):

(1) After appropriate investigation, the symptoms cannot be explained by a known general medical condition or the direct effects of a substance (e.g., a drug of abuse, a medication).

(2) When there is a related general medical condition, the physical complaints or resulting social or occupational impairment is in excess of what would be expected from the history, physical examination, or laboratory findings.

C. The symptoms cause clinically significant distress or impairment in social, occupational, or other important areas of functioning.

D. The duration of the disturbance is at least 6 months.

E. The disturbance is not better accounted for by another mental disorder (e.g., another somatoform disorder, sexual dysfunction, mood disorder, anxiety disorder, sleep disorder, or psychotic disorder).

F. The symptom is not intentionally produced or feigned (as in factitious disorder or malingering).

fect, this category serves to capture syndromes that resemble somatization disorder but do not meet the full criteria. Symptoms that may be seen include the same as those that are considered for somatization disorder.

DIAGNOSIS

History

The category of undifferentiated somatoform disorder did not exist prior to DSM-III-R. At that time it was added to cover those syndromes that in DSM-III simply would have been included under "Atypical Somatoform Disorder." It is not clear whether the category undifferentiated somatoform disorder has been well adopted by clinicians, but a number of studies support its existence. Alternative terms that have been proposed include *subsyndromal, forme fruste,* or *abridged* somatization disorder (Kirmayer and Robbins 1991) and more recently *multisomatoform disorder* (Kroenke et al. 1997).

DSM-IV

After some debate, minor changes in the category undifferentiated somatoform disorder were made in DSM-IV.

Because of perceived low use of the diagnosis undifferentiated somatoform disorder by clinicians, which was attributed to ambiguity of the term *undifferentiated disorder,* the term *multisomatoform disorder* was suggested. However, because the few empirical data available seemed to indicate a variable course, with unclear boundaries with normality and other mental disorders (especially anxiety and depressive disorders), this term was not adopted. As a result, the only changes involved substituting the standard "general medical condition" for DSM-III-R's "organic pathology." A threshold for diagnosis also was added, requiring clinically significant distress or impairment. Instead of excluding the diagnosis on the basis of "occurrence exclusively during the course of another mental disorder," exclusion in DSM-IV is on the basis of "not better accounted for by another mental disorder."

Kroenke et al. (1997), using improved diagnostic criteria with inclusion and exclusion criteria, found that the proposed multisomatoform disorder had a large and independent effect on impairment in a study of 1,000 patients from four primary care sites. Still lacking in terms of validity of the proposed disorder is evidence of temporal stability.

Differential Diagnosis

Principal considerations in the differential diagnosis include the question of whether or not, with follow-up, criteria for somatization disorder will be met. Patients with somatization disorder are typically inconsistent historians. During one evaluation, they may report a large number of symptoms and fulfill criteria for the full syndrome, whereas during another, they may report fewer symptoms, perhaps only fulfilling criteria for an abridged syndrome (Martin et al. 1979). Another consideration is whether the somatic symptoms qualifying a patient for a diagnosis of undifferentiated somatoform disorder are the manifestation of a depressive or an anxiety disorder. Indeed, high rates of major depression and anxiety disorders have been found in somatizing patients attending family medicine clinics (Kirmayer et al. 1993).

EPIDEMIOLOGY

Some investigators have argued that undifferentiated somatoform disorder is the most common somatoform disorder. Escobar et al. (1991), using a construct requiring six somatic symptoms for women and four for men, reported that in the United States 11% of non-Hispanic whites and Hispanics and 15% of blacks, and in Puerto Rico 20% of Puerto Ricans fulfilled the criteria. A preponderance of women was evident in all groups except the Puerto Rican sample.

ETIOLOGY

If undifferentiated somatoform disorder is simply an abridged form of somatization disorder, etiological theories reviewed under that diagnosis also should apply to undifferentiated somatoform disorder. Of theoretical interest would be the question of why the syndrome is fully expressed in some and only partially in others. Some investigators postulate theories of etiology involving primarily the concept of somatization, for which there are a large number of explanations. As reviewed by Kirmayer and Robbins (1991), somatization can be viewed as a pattern of illness behavior by which bodily idioms of distress may serve as symbolic means of social regulation as well as protest or contestation. As yet, there is little, if any, empirical evidence for such theories.

TREATMENT

Existing data have been derived from studies fraught with methodological problems, including the use of diverse groups with only a certain number of chronic somatic complaints in common. A number of studies suggest that improvement is accelerated with psychotherapy of a supportive, rather than a nondirective, type. However, a substantial proportion of patients improve or recover with no formal psychotherapy. Judicious use of pharmacotherapy also appears to be beneficial, with trials of antidepressant medications indicated for patients with depressive symptoms and trials of buspirone, benzodiazepines, and propranolol for patients with anxiety symptoms. Again, definitive recommendations await a more extensive empirical data base.

CONVERSION DISORDER

DEFINITION AND CLINICAL DESCRIPTION

The essential features of conversion disorder are the nonintentionally produced symptoms or deficits affecting voluntary motor or sensory function that suggest but are not fully explained by a neurological or general medical condition, by the direct effects of a substance, or by a culturally sanctioned behavior or experience. Specific symptoms mentioned as examples in DSM-IV include motor symptoms such as impaired coordination or balance, paralysis or localized weakness, tremor, difficulty swallowing or lump in throat (e.g., "globus hystericus"), aphonia, and

urinary retention; sensory symptoms, including hallucinations, loss of touch or pain sensation, double vision, blindness, and deafness; and seizures or convulsions with voluntary motor or sensory components. Single episodes usually involve one symptom, but longitudinally, other conversion symptoms will be evident as well. Psychological factors generally appear to be involved in that symptoms often occur in the context of a conflictual situation that may in some way be resolved with the development of the symptom.

An example of a typical patient with conversion disorder follows:

A woman in her early 20s was brought to the emergency room by female relatives after an argument with her husband, leading to his leaving the household. She showed variable impairment in gait, at times appearing quite unstable and needing the support of another person, a piece of furniture, or the walls to ambulate. At other times her gait was only mildly unsteady. A psychiatry consultation was requested, but before it occurred, the woman was observed to have a "seizure" during which she showed generalized shaking that seemed to wax and wane. No incontinence was noted. Following the episode, she had a questionable Babinski sign on the left side. Her eyes remained closed, and she was variously unresponsive to questions, sometimes answering incoherently and at other times not attending to conversations at all. When unresponsive, she showed no spontaneous voluntary movement, but she resisted passive movement, such as when attempts were made to open her eyelids to evaluate her pupils.

Internal medicine consultation resulted in routine laboratory work, lumbar puncture, and magnetic resonance imaging (MRI). The patient was admitted to the medical intensive care unit. No abnormalities were noted in any of the laboratory or imaging procedures.

The next day, the patient was fully responsive, showed no impairment in gait, and had no episodes of "seizures." When questioned, she had hazy recall of the preceding day but did remember the argument with her husband. She reported unhappiness about her marital difficulties, but she did not report enough symptoms to warrant diagnosis of a depressive episode. She was not particularly interested in exploring psychological issues. She denied prior psychiatric problems or treatment, although relatives reported a similar episode 4 years previously, after a disagreement with a boyfriend. The patient had a normal neurological examination except for a questionable Babinski sign on the left side. It was concluded that her apparent neurological presentation was attributable to a mixture of conversion and dissociative symptoms. The patient and her family were cautioned to be vigilant for any symptoms suggesting neurological dysfunction.

She was transferred to the psychiatry service, from which she was discharged 2 days later with a follow-up plan that included marital counseling.

This case illustrates several typical aspects of the presentation and course of conversion disorder to be discussed later in this section.

DIAGNOSIS

History

Some of the major early contributions to the study of conversion disorder were by neurologists, including Charcot (Torack 1978) and Breuer and Freud (1893–1895/1955) in the late 19th century and early 20th century. As shown in Table 16–2, conversion disorder was called "conversion reaction" in DSM and "hysterical neurosis, conversion type" in DSM-II. In both DSM and DSM-II, the conversion process was restricted to the production of symptoms affecting the voluntary motor and sensory nervous system. Symptoms for which there was a physiological understanding (generally involving the autonomic nervous system) were subsumed under the psychophysiological disorders.

Other terms such as *acute hysteria* also have been used. Unfortunately, conversion disorder or *conversion hysteria* was used by some clinicians synonymously with *hysteria*, a term replaced by somatization disorder in DSM-III. Generally, hysteria was used to describe a more pervasive, chronic, and polysymptomatic disorder. Although conversion symptoms are perhaps the most dramatic symptoms of somatization disorder, the disorder is characterized by multiple unexplained symptoms in many organ systems. In conversion disorder, a single symptom, traditionally of a pseudoneurological type (i.e., suggesting neurological disease), suffices. Such inconsistency in the use of terms has resulted in a great deal of confusion, both in research and in clinical practice.

Adding to this confusion was a change introduced in DSM-III and retained in DSM-III-R, whereby the concept of conversion was expanded to include disorders characterized by symptoms involving any "loss of, or alteration in, physical functioning suggesting a physical disorder" (American Psychiatric Association 1987, p. 259) as long as the mechanism of conversion was evident; that is, the symptom was "an expression of a psychological conflict or need" (American Psychiatric Association 1987, p. 257). Thus, symptoms involving the autonomic or endocrine systems, such as vomiting (supposedly representing revulsion and disgust) and pseudocyesis (as a manifestation of unconscious conflict about, or the need for, pregnancy), were included as examples of conversion symptoms.

DSM-IV Criteria

Several questions about modifications of conversion disorder criteria for DSM-IV were carefully considered, including where in the nosology conversion disorder should be included (i.e., should it remain with the somatoform disorders or be grouped with the dissociative disorders?) and what the syndrome boundaries should be (i.e., what types of symptoms are to be included?) (Martin 1992, 1996). Although the symptomatic, epidemiological, and perhaps pathogenetic similarities of conversion and dissociative symptoms were acknowledged, the review argued for the retention of conversion disorder with the somatoform disorders because of the advantages of facilitating the critical differential diagnosis of patients who have physical symptoms that suggest physical disorders. Review of the literature supported the utility of again restricting conversion disorder to symptoms affecting voluntary motor and sensory functions.

As defined in DSM-IV, nonintentional "symptoms or deficits affecting voluntary motor or sensory function"

TABLE 16–8. DSM-IV diagnostic criteria for conversion disorder

A. One or more symptoms or deficits affecting voluntary motor or sensory function that suggest a neurological or other general medical condition.

B. Psychological factors are judged to be associated with the symptom or deficit because the initiation or exacerbation of the symptom or deficit is preceded by conflicts or other stressors.

C. The symptom or deficit is not intentionally produced or feigned (as in factitious disorder or malingering).

D. The symptom or deficit cannot, after appropriate investigation, be fully explained by a general medical condition, or by the direct effects of a substance, or as a culturally sanctioned behavior or experience.

E. The symptom or deficit causes clinically significant distress or impairment in social, occupational, or other important areas of functioning or warrants medical evaluation.

F. The symptom or deficit is not limited to pain or sexual dysfunction, does not occur exclusively during the course of somatization disorder, and is not better accounted for by another mental disorder.

Specify type of symptom or deficit:

With motor symptom or deficit

With sensory symptom or deficit

With seizures or convulsions

With mixed presentation

(American Psychiatric Association 1994, p. 457) are central to conversion disorder (see Table 16–8). The majority of such symptoms will suggest a neurological condition (i.e., are pseudoneurological), but other general medical conditions may be suggested as well. However, pseudoneurological symptoms remain the classic symptoms. By definition, symptoms limited to pain or disturbance in sexual functioning are not included.

In conversion disorder, as in the other somatoform disorders, the symptom cannot be fully explained by a known physical disorder. This criterion is perhaps the most imperative diagnostic consideration. In addition, the symptom is defined as not fully explained by a culturally sanctioned behavior or experience. Symptoms such as seizure-like episodes, occurring in conjunction with certain religious ceremonies, and culturally expected responses, in times past, such as women swooning in response to excitement would qualify as examples.

DSM-IV specifies that the symptoms in conversion disorder are not intentionally produced, thus distinguishing conversion symptoms from those of malingering or a factitious disorder. Although this judgment is difficult to make, it is an important one because the recommended management and expected outcome of malingering and factitious disorder are markedly different.

Clinical judgment also is required in determining whether psychological factors are etiologically related to the symptom. Inclusion of this criterion is perhaps a holdover from the initial conceptualization of conversion symptoms as representing the conversion of unconscious psychic conflict into a physical symptom. As reviewed by Cloninger (1987), such determination is virtually impossible except in cases in which there is a temporal relationship between a psychosocial stressor and the symptom or in cases in which similar situations led to conversion symptoms in the past.

Differential Diagnosis

Because conversion symptoms suggest physical illness, nonpsychiatrists are generally seen at least initially. Neurologists are probably most consulted by primary physicians for such symptoms, since the majority suggest neurological disease. It has been estimated that 1% of patients admitted to the hospital for neurological problems exhibit conversion symptoms (Marsden 1986).

A diagnostic problem is not simply that conversion symptoms suggest neurological or general medical conditions but that symptoms of such illness are misdiagnosed as conversion. A number of studies have found that significant proportions of patients initially diagnosed with con-

version symptoms have neurological illnesses on follow-up. Slater and Glithero (1965) found a misdiagnosis rate of 50% during a 7- to 11-year follow-up; Gatfield and Guze (1962) reported 21%; and more recently, Mace and Trimble (1996) observed a rate of 15%. The trend toward less misdiagnosis may reflect increasing sophistication in neurological diagnosis. Although Slater and Glithero's study often has been used to challenge the validity of hysteria (now called somatization disorder), its importance lies in underscoring the need to remain tentative in making a diagnosis of conversion disorder.

Symptoms of a variety of neurological illnesses may seem to be inconsistent with known neurophysiology or neuropathology and may suggest conversion. Diseases to be considered include MS (consider blindness secondary to optic neuritis with initially normal fundi), myasthenia gravis, periodic paralysis, myoglobinuric myopathy, polymyositis, other acquired myopathies (all of which may include marked weakness in the presence of normal deep tendon reflexes), and Guillain-Barré syndrome, in which early weakness of the arms and legs may be inconsistent (Cloninger 1994). As reviewed by Ford and Folks (1985), more than 13% of actual neurological cases are diagnosed as "functional" prior to the elucidation of a neurological illness. Initial evidence of some neurological disease is predictive of a subsequent neurological explanation (Mace and Trimble 1996).

Complicating diagnosis is the fact that physical illness and conversion (or other apparent psychiatric overlay) are not mutually exclusive. Patients with incapacitating and frightening physical illnesses may appear to be exaggerating their symptoms. Patients with actual neurological illness also may have "pseudosymptoms." For example, patients with actual seizures often have pseudoseizures (Desai et al. 1982).

Considering these observations, physicians should resist an incautious diagnosis of conversion disorder when faced with difficult-to-interpret symptoms. The occurrence of apparent conversion symptoms mandates a thorough evaluation for possible underlying physical explanation. This evaluation may include physical and psychiatric examination, X rays, and blood and urine tests as the symptoms and signs would indicate.

Longitudinal studies indicate that the most reliable predictor that a patient with apparent conversion symptoms will not later be shown to have a physical disorder is a history of previous conversion or other unexplained symptoms (Cloninger 1994). Patients with somatization disorder will manifest multiple symptoms in multiple organ systems, including the voluntary motor and sensory nervous systems. Thus, apparent conversion symptoms in the context of somatization disorder should indicate that an underlying physical disorder is unlikely. Although conversion symptoms may occur at any age, vulnerability for conversion symptoms is first manifest most often in late adolescence or early adulthood (Cloninger 1994). Conversion symptoms first occurring in middle age or later should increase suspicion of an occult physical illness.

The DSM-IV lists hallucinations among the sensory nervous system examples. Reports of hallucinations suggest psychosis, especially schizophrenia, or a mood disorder with psychotic features. In fact, DSM-III and DSM-III-R virtually forced this interpretation in that the only contexts in which hallucinations were mentioned in conjunction with a nonpsychotic disorder were with the reexperiencing of the traumatic event in posttraumatic stress disorder and with the hearing, by one personality, the voice(s) of one or more of the other personalities in multiple personality disorder (dissociative identity disorder in DSM-IV). Hallucinations as conversion symptoms have long been reported (Andrade and Srinath 1986; Fitzgerald and Wells 1977; Goodwin et al. 1971; Modai and Cygielman 1986). In DSM-IV's somatization disorder field trial, one-third of a large sample of nonpsychotic women with evidence of unexplained somatic complaints reported a history of hallucinations. Among the 40% who met criteria for somatization disorder, more than one-half reported hallucinations (R. L. Martin, unpublished observations, 1998). Women with other conversion symptoms were more likely to report hallucinations than were those women with no other conversion symptoms, giving further support for including hallucinations as conversion symptoms.

Generally, conversion disorder hallucinations differ in several ways from hallucinations in psychotic conditions and are referred to by some as *pseudohallucinations*. Conversion disorder hallucinations typically occur in the absence of other psychotic symptoms. Insight that the hallucinations are not "real" is generally retained. Whereas hallucinations in psychoses generally involve a single sensory modality (especially auditory; secondarily, tactile), conversion hallucinations often involve more than one modality. They may have a naive, fantastic, or childish content, as in a fairy tale, and are described eagerly as an interesting story (e.g., "A big green frog came in, sat down next to me, and began talking to me"). Conversion hallucinations are often psychologically meaningful (e.g., "I heard my ex-boyfriend's voice telling me that he had made a big mistake"). Because hallucinations as part of psychoses also may share some of these features, vigilance must be maintained for the emergence of other signs of psychosis. A diagnosis of conversion disorder should not be made if the hallucinations are better accounted for by posttraumatic stress disorder or

dissociative identity disorder (multiple personality disorder).

An association between conversion symptoms affecting voluntary motor and sensory functioning and dissociative symptoms affecting memory and identity should be noted. Traditionally, such symptoms have been attributed to similar psychological mechanisms. The two types of symptoms often occur in the same individual, sometimes during the same episode of illness (consider the example of the patient with conversion disorder discussed at the beginning of this section). Thus, patients with conversion disorder should be screened for dissociative symptoms, and patients with a dissociative disorder should be evaluated for conversion symptoms.

NATURAL HISTORY

Onset is generally from late childhood to early adulthood. Conversion disorder is rare before age 10 years (Maloney 1980) and seldom first presents after age 35 years, but it has been reported to begin as late as the ninth decade (Weddington 1979). When onset is in middle or late age, the possibility of a neurological or other medical condition is increased. Onset is generally acute but may be characterized by gradually increasing symptomatology. The course of individual conversion symptoms is generally short; half (Folks et al. 1984) to nearly all (Carter 1949) patients show a disappearance of symptoms by the time of hospital discharge. However, 20%–25% will relapse within 1 year. Factors traditionally associated with good prognosis include acute onset, presence of clearly identifiable stress at the time of onset, a short interval between onset and institution of treatment, and good intelligence (Toone 1990). A recent study notes better outcome for patients with affective illnesses and a poor prognosis for those with personality disorders (Mace and Trimble 1996). In the Mace and Trimble study, a diagnosis of somatization disorder at follow-up was especially associated with chronicity. Symptoms of blindness, aphonia, and paralysis have been noted to have a relatively good prognosis, whereas seizures and tremor were said to be more persistent (Toone 1990). However, these findings were not supported in the Mace and Trimble study. When followed longitudinally, some patients initially diagnosed only with conversion disorder will subsequently meet the criteria for somatization disorder (Kent et al. 1995; Mace and Trimble 1996).

Generally, individual conversion symptoms are self-limited and do not lead to physical changes or disabilities. Occasionally, physical sequelae such as atrophy may occur, but this is rare. Morbidity in terms of marital and occupational impairment appears to be less than that in somatization disorder (Kent et al. 1995; Tomasson et al. 1991). In a long-term follow-up study (up to 44 years) of a small number ($N = 28$) of individuals with conversion disorder, excess mortality by unnatural causes was observed (Coryell and House 1984). None of the deaths in this study was by suicide.

EPIDEMIOLOGY

Conclusions regarding the epidemiology of conversion disorder are compromised by methodological differences in diagnostic boundaries as well as by ascertainment procedures from study to study. Vastly different estimates have been reported. Lifetime prevalence rates of treated conversion symptoms in general populations have ranged from 11/100,000 to 300/100,000 (Ford and Folks 1985; Toone 1990). A marked excess of women compared with men develop conversion symptoms. More than 25% of healthy postpartum and medically ill women report having had conversion symptoms sometime during their life (Cloninger 1994).

Under 5%–24% of psychiatric outpatients, 5%–14% of general hospital patients, and 1%–3% of outpatient psychiatric referrals have a history of conversion symptoms (Cloninger 1994; Ford 1983; Toone 1990). There is an association with lower socioeconomic status, with less educated and less psychologically sophisticated and/or rural populations overrepresented (Folks et al. 1984; Guze and Perley 1963; Lazare 1981; Stefansson et al. 1976; Weinstein et al. 1969). Consistent with this finding, much higher rates (nearly 10%) of outpatient psychiatric referrals in developing countries are for conversion symptoms. As countries develop, there may be a declining incidence over time, which may relate to increasing levels of education and sophistication (Stefanis et al. 1976).

Conversion disorder appears to be diagnosed more often in women than in men, with ratios varying from 2:1 (Ljundberg 1957; Stefansson et al. 1976) to 10:1 (Raskin et al. 1966). In part, this variance may relate to referral patterns, but it also appears that indeed a predominance of women compared with men develop conversion symptoms.

ETIOLOGY

An etiological hypothesis is implicit in the term *conversion*. The term conversion, in fact, is derived from the hypothesized conversion of psychological conflict into a somatic symptom. A number of psychological factors have been implicated in the pathogenesis, or at least pathophysiology, of conversion disorder. However, as the following discussion will show, such etiological relationships are difficult to demonstrate.

In *primary gain*, anxiety is theoretically reduced by keeping an internal conflict or need out of awareness by symbolic expression of an unconscious wish as a conversion symptom. However, individuals with active conversion symptoms often continue to show marked anxiety, especially on psychological tests (Lader and Sartorious 1968; Meares and Horvath 1972). Symbolism is infrequently evident, and its evaluation involves highly inferential and unreliable judgments (Raskin et al. 1966). Interpretation of symbolism in persons with occult medical disorder has been noted to contribute to misdiagnosis. *Secondary gain*, whereby conversion symptoms allow avoidance of noxious activities or the obtaining of otherwise unavailable support, also may occur in persons who have medical conditions, who often take advantage of such benefits (Raskin et al. 1966; Watson and Buranen 1979).

Individuals with conversion disorder may show a lack of concern, in keeping with the nature or implications of the symptom (the so-called *la belle indifférence*). However, such indifference to symptoms is not invariably present in conversion disorder (Lewis and Berman 1965; Sharma and Chaturvedi 1995), and it also can be seen in individuals with general medical conditions (Raskin et al. 1966), sometimes as denial or stoicism (Pincus 1982). Conversion symptoms may be revealed in a dramatic or histrionic fashion and may be highly suggestible. A minority of individuals with conversion disorder fulfill criteria for histrionic personality disorder. A dramatic presentation of conversion disorder also is seen in distressed individuals with medical conditions. Even symptoms based on underlying medical conditions often respond to suggestion, at least temporarily (Gatfield and Guze 1962). Persons with conversion disorder often may have a history of disturbed sexuality (Lewis 1974), with many (one-third) reporting a history of sexual abuse, especially incestuous. (Thus, two-thirds do *not* report such a history.) Individuals with conversion disorder often are reported to be the youngest, or else the youngest of a sex, in sibling order, but these are not consistent findings (Stephens and Kamp 1962; F. J. Ziegler et al. 1960).

Limited data suggest that conversion symptoms are more frequent in relatives of individuals with conversion disorder (Toone 1990). Rates that were 10 times greater than similarly derived general-population estimates in female relatives and approximately five times the corresponding rate in male relatives were reported in a nonblind study (Ljundberg 1957). Accumulated data from available twin studies show 9 concordant and 33 discordant monozygotic pairs, and 0 concordant and 43 discordant dizygotic pairs (Inouye 1972). Nongenetic familial factors, particularly incestuous childhood sexual abuse, also may be frequent. Nearly one-third of individuals with medically unexplained seizures reported childhood sexual abuse, as compared with less than 10% of those with complex partial epilepsy (Alper et al. 1993). High rates also have been noted in overlapping dissociative conditions. Rates of reported childhood sexual abuse as high as 85% have been noted in individuals with dissociative identity disorder, of whom approximately half will have conversion symptoms, and in as many as 50% of individuals with somatization disorder, of whom all will have either conversion or dissociative symptoms (Martin 1996).

If not directly etiological, many factors have been suggested as predisposing individuals to conversion disorder. In many instances, preexisting personality disorders are diagnosable and may predispose some individuals to conversion disorder. A number of psychosocial factors in addition to a history of abuse may be involved. Individuals from rural backgrounds and those who are psychologically and medically unsophisticated appear to be predisposed to conversion disorder, as are those with existing neurological disorders. In the latter case, a tendency to conversion symptoms has been attributed to "modeling"; that is, patients with neurological disorders are likely to observe in others, as well as in themselves, various neurological symptoms that they at other times simulate as conversion symptoms.

TREATMENT

Generally, the initial aim in treating patients with conversion disorder is the removal of the symptom. The pressure behind accomplishing this goal depends on the distress and disability associated with the symptom (Merskey 1989). If the patient is not in particular discomfort and the need to regain function is not great, direct attention may not be necessary. In any situation, direct confrontation is not recommended. Such a communication may cause a patient to feel even more isolated. A conservative approach of reassurance and relaxation is effective. Reassurance need not come from a psychiatrist but can be performed effectively by the primary physician. Once physical illness is excluded, prognosis for conversion symptoms is good. Folks et al. (1984), for example, found that half of 50 general hospital patients with conversion symptoms showed complete remission by the time of discharge.

If symptoms do not resolve with a conservative approach and there is an immediate need for symptom resolution, a number of techniques, including narcoanalysis (e.g., amobarbital interview), hypnosis, and behavior therapy, may be tried (Merskey 1989). It does appear that

prompt resolution of conversion symptoms is important in that the duration of conversion symptoms is associated with greater risk of recurrence and chronic disability (Cloninger 1994).

In narcoanalysis, amobarbital or another sedative-hypnotic medication such as lorazepam is given to the patient intravenously to the point of drowsiness. Sometimes this is followed by administration of a stimulant medication such as methamphetamine. The patient is then encouraged to discuss stressors and conflicts. This technique may be effective in the short term, leading to at least temporary symptom relief and expansion of the information known about the patient. This technique has not been shown to be especially effective with more chronic conversion symptoms. In hypnotic therapy, symptoms may be removed during a hypnotic state, with the suggestion that the symptoms will gradually improve posthypnotically. Information regarding stressors and conflicts may be explored as well. Behavior therapy, including relaxation training and even aversion therapy, has been proposed and reported by some investigators to be effective.

It should be evident that it may not be the particular technique that is associated with symptom relief but the influence of suggestion. Various rituals such as exorcism and other religious ceremonies undoubtedly have led to immediate "cures." Suggestion seems to play a big part in cases of mass hysteria, in which individuals exposed to a "toxin" develop similar symptoms that do not appear to have any organic basis. Often, the epidemic can be contained if affected individuals are segregated. Simple announcements that no toxin is present and that symptoms have been linked to mass hysteria have been effective.

Anecdotal reports exist of positive response to somatic treatments such as phenothiazines, lithium, and even electroconvulsive therapy (ECT). Of course, in some cases such a response again may be attributable to suggestion. In others, it may be that symptom removal occurred because of resolution of another psychiatric disorder, especially a mood disorder.

Thus far, the discussion on treatment of conversion disorder has centered on acute treatment primarily for symptom removal. Longer-term approaches include strategies that were previously discussed for somatization disorder. These involve a pragmatic, conservative approach that entails support for and exploration of various areas of conflict, particularly interpersonal relationships. Ford (1995) suggests a treatment strategy based on "three Ps," whereby predisposing factors, precipitating stressors, and perpetuating factors are identified and addressed. A certain degree of insight may be attained, at least in terms of appreciating relationships between various conflicts and stressors and the development of symptoms. More ambitious goals have been adopted by some in terms of long-term, intensive insight-oriented psychotherapy, especially of a psychodynamic nature. Reports of such approaches date from Freud's work with Anna O. Three studies involving a series of patients treated with psychoanalytic psychotherapy have reported success (Merskey 1989).

HYPOCHONDRIASIS

DEFINITION AND CLINICAL DESCRIPTION

The essential feature in hypochondriasis is not preoccupation with symptoms themselves but rather with the fear or idea of having a serious disease, based on the misinterpretation of bodily signs and sensations (Table 16–1). The preoccupation persists despite evidence to the contrary and reassurance from physicians. Some degree of preoccupation with disease is apparently quite common. As reviewed by Kellner (1987), 10%–20% of "normal" and 45% of "neurotic" persons have intermittent, unfounded worries about illness, with 9% of patients doubting reassurances given by physicians. In another review, Kellner (1985) estimates that 50% of all patients attending physicians' offices "suffer either from primary hypochondriacal syndromes or have 'minor somatic disorders with hypochondriacal overlay' " (p. 822). How these estimates relate to hypochondriasis as a disorder is difficult to assess because they do not appear to distinguish between preoccupation with symptoms (as is present in somatization disorder) and preoccupation with the implications of the symptoms (as is the case with hypochondriasis).

DIAGNOSIS

History

Clinical descriptions of a syndrome designated *hypochondriasis* and characterized by preoccupation with bodily function can be found in the writings of the Hippocratic era (Stoudemire 1988). The Greeks attributed the syndrome to disturbances of viscera below the xiphoid cartilage, hence the term *hypochondria*. Even into the 19th century, the term hypochondriasis, unlike the topographically nonspecific concept of more recent usage, was used specifically for somatic complaints below the diaphragm (Cloninger et al. 1984). As reviewed by M. R. Murphy (1990), Gillespie, in 1928, encapsulated a concept of hypochondriasis that is essentially identical with modern concepts, emphasizing preoccupation with a disease con-

viction "far in excess of what is justified," implying "an indifference to the opinion of the environment, including irresponsiveness to persuasion" (p. 28). Gillespie considered hypochondriasis a discrete disease entity. DSM did not include hypochondriasis as a separate illness, only mentioning "hypochondriacal preoccupation" as one of the malignant symptoms observed in psychotic but not reactive depression. As shown in Table 16–2, the syndrome was included in DSM-II as hypochondriacal neurosis and in ICD-9, DSM-III, DSM-III-R, and ICD-10 as hypochondriasis.

Throughout the modern period, there has been controversy as to whether or not hypochondriasis represents an independent, discrete disease entity, as was proposed by Gillespie. Kenyon (1976), in an often quoted but perhaps methodologically flawed study (see M. R. Murphy 1990), concluded that hypochondriasis was virtually always secondary to another psychiatric disorder, usually depression. Barsky and various colleagues (Barsky and Klerman 1983; Barsky et al. 1986, 1993) extensively have studied patients with hypochondriacal complaints, using a set of operational criteria derived from DSM-III. These authors conclude that of the many patients with such complaints, few will meet criteria for the full diagnosis. However, they note no bimodality, suggesting that hypochondriasis represents a continuum rather than a discrete entity.

DSM-IV Criteria

Specific criteria for the diagnosis of hypochondriasis are included in Table 16–9. As mentioned previously, in hypochondriasis, emphasis is on the patient's preoccupation with the implication that a serious illness is present based on the misinterpretation of bodily symptoms. There was some debate in the development of DSM-IV that it was not necessary that a symptom be present. However, on the basis of empirical data, it was determined that this symptom requirement was a valid one and helped to distinguish the "disease conviction" of hypochondriasis from "disease fear" as in a phobic disorder (Cote et al. 1996). "Bodily symptoms" may be interpreted broadly to include misinterpretation of normal bodily functions. The requirement that the preoccupation persist despite medical evaluation and reassurance was included to emphasize the disease conviction aspect of the syndrome. The exclusionary criterion of delusion was debated. Although this criterion was maintained for the purpose of discriminating hypochondriasis from delusional disorders, somatic type, a specifier "with poor insight" was added. To distinguish hypochondriasis from clinically insignificant states, the requirement for distress or impairment is as in

TABLE 16–9.   DSM-IV diagnostic criteria for hypochondriasis

A. Preoccupation with fears of having, or the idea that one has, a serious disease based on the person's misinterpretation of bodily symptoms.

B. The preoccupation persists despite appropriate medical evaluation and reassurance.

C. The belief in criterion A is not of delusional intensity (as in delusional disorder, somatic type) and is not restricted to a circumscribed concern about appearance (as in body dysmorphic disorder).

D. The preoccupation causes clinically significant distress or impairment in social, occupational, or other important areas of functioning.

E. The duration of the disturbance is at least 6 months.

F. The preoccupation is not better accounted for by generalized anxiety disorder, obsessive-compulsive disorder, panic disorder, a major depressive episode, separation anxiety, or another somatoform disorder.

Specify if:

With poor insight: if, for most of the time during the current episode, the person does not recognize that the concern about having a serious illness is excessive or unreasonable

---

the other somatoform disorders. A requirement of 6 months' duration was maintained to distinguish hypochondriasis from transient syndromes that have been shown to have a more variable longitudinal course, suggesting heterogeneity (Barsky et al. 1993).

As is explained in the following discussion, hypochondriasis is not diagnosed if symptoms occur exclusively during the course of generalized anxiety disorder, anxiety disorder, obsessive-compulsive disorder, panic disorder, a major depressive episode, separation anxiety, or another somatoform disorder.

Differential Diagnosis

The first step in evaluating patients with hypochondriasis is to assess the possibility of physical disease. The list of serious diseases associated with the type of complaints seen in hypochondriacal patients is extensive, yet certain general categories emerge (Kellner 1985; 1987). These include neurological diseases, such as myasthenia gravis and MS; endocrine diseases; systemic diseases, such as SLE, that affect several organ systems; and occult malignancies.

If after appropriate assessment the probability of physical illness appears low, the condition should be considered relative to other psychiatric disorders (i.e., whether the hypochondriacal symptoms represent a primary disorder

or are secondary to another psychiatric illness). As previously mentioned, one useful criterion is whether the belief is of delusional proportions. Patients with hypochondriasis as a primary disorder, although extremely preoccupied, are generally able to acknowledge the possibility that their concerns are unfounded. Delusional patients, on the other hand, are not. Hypochondriasis with poor insight would lie somewhere in between, with the patient not recognizing the concern is unwarranted for most of the episode. Somatic delusions of serious illness are seen in some cases of major depressive disorder and with schizophrenia. A useful discriminator is the presence of other psychiatric symptoms. A patient with hypochondriacal concerns secondary to depression should show other symptoms of depression such as sleep and appetite disturbance, feelings of worthlessness, self-reproach, and so forth, although elderly patients particularly may deny sadness or other expressions of depressed mood. Generally, schizophrenic patients will have bizarre delusions of illness (e.g., "I have congenital Hodgkin's caused by a snail hormone imbalance") and will show other signs of schizophrenia such as looseness of associations, peculiarities of thought and behavior, hallucinations, and other delusions. A confounding feature is the fact that hypochondriacal patients often will develop anxiety or depression in association with their hypochondriacal concerns. In general, characterizing the chronology of the episode will separate such patients from those with hypochondriasis.

Treatment trials also may have diagnostic significance. Depressed patients who are hypochondriacal may respond to antidepressant medication or ECT (often necessary in reversing a depressive state of sufficient severity to lead to such profound symptoms), with resolution of the hypochondriacal as well as the depressive symptoms. In schizophrenic patients a disease-related delusion may show improvement with neuroleptic treatment. Although, if questioned carefully, a patient still may report a somatic delusion, preoccupation with the delusion will have diminished.

NATURAL HISTORY

Traditionally, limited data suggested that approximately one-fourth of patients with a diagnosis of hypochondriasis do poorly, two-thirds show a chronic but fluctuating course, and one-tenth recover. However, such predictions may not reflect advances in psychopharmacology. It also must be remembered that such findings pertain to the full syndrome. A much more variable course is seen in patients with some hypochondriacal concerns.

EPIDEMIOLOGY

Estimates of the frequency of hypochondriacal symptoms warranting a diagnosis are somewhat compromised in that DSM-III-R did not provide threshold criteria, other than requiring a duration of more than 6 months. The ECA study (L. N. Robins et al. 1984) did not assess for hypochondriasis. One study reported prevalence figures ranging from 3% to 13% in different cultures (Kenyon 1965), but it is not clear whether this range represented the full syndrome or just hypochondriacal symptoms. As previously mentioned, many patients have such symptoms as part of other psychiatric disorders, particularly depressive and anxiety disorders, whereas others develop transient hypochondriacal symptoms in response to stress, particularly serious physical illness.

ETIOLOGY

In considering hypochondriasis as an aspect of depression or anxiety disorders, it has been posited that these conditions create a state of hypervigilance to insult, including overperception of physical problems (Barsky and Klerman 1983). Hypochondriasis has been discussed extensively in the psychoanalytic literature. Freud hypothesized that it represented "the return of object libido onto the ego with cathexis to the body" (Viederman 1985, p. 10). This theory has formed the basis for a number of psychoanalytic interpretations, including disturbed object relations and repressed hostility displaced to the body so that anger can be communicated indirectly to others, as well as dynamics involving masochism, guilt, conflicted dependency needs, and a need to suffer and be loved at the same time (Stoudemire 1988). Such "narcissistic" mechanisms have been thought to make patients unanalyzable. Other psychological theories involve defenses against feelings of low self-esteem and inadequacy, perceptual and cognitive abnormalities, and reinforcement for assuming the sick role.

More recently, hypochondriasis has been included by some in a posited "obsessive-compulsive spectrum disorder," which includes, in addition to obsessive-compulsive disorder, body dysmorphic disorder, anorexia nervosa, Tourette's disorder, and certain impulsive disorders, including trichotillomania and pathological gambling (Hollander et al. 1992). This clustering is based, in part, on the phenomenological similarity of repetitive thoughts and behaviors that are difficult or impossible to delay or inhibit (Martin and Yutzy 1997).

TREATMENT

Patients referred early for psychiatric evaluation and treatment of hyphochondriasis appear to have a better progno-

sis than those continuing with only medical evaluations and treatments (Kellner 1983). Psychiatric referral should be performed with sensitivity. Perhaps the best guideline to follow is for the referring physician to stress that the patient's distress is serious and that psychiatric evaluation will be a supplement to, not a replacement for, continued medical care.

Hypochondriacal symptoms secondary to depressive and anxiety disorders may improve with successful treatment of the primary disorder. However, until recently, hypochondriasis as a primary condition was not seen to be responsive to known psychopharmacological drugs. Now, although results of placebo-controlled, double-blind studies are pending, anecdotal case reports, open-label trials, and review of preliminary data show promise for the selective serotonin reuptake inhibitors (SSRIs; Fallon 1996). Interestingly, these drugs have been shown to be effective in obsessive-compulsive disorder, and at least anecdotal or preliminary data are promising for their use in other obsessive-compulsive spectrum disorders such as body dysmorphic disorder and anorexia nervosa.

Investigators have tried a large number of psychotherapeutic approaches in treating patients with hypochondriasis. These may be summarized as supportive, rational, ventilative, and educative (Kellner 1987). However, there is no evidence demonstrating the superiority of any one of these methods over the others. An approach suggested by Stoudemire (1988)—one that includes consistent treatment, generally by the same primary physician, with supportive, regularly scheduled office visits, not based on the evaluation of symptoms—should be considered. Hospitalization, medical tests, and medications with addictive potential are to be avoided if possible. Focus during the office visits gradually should be shifted from symptoms to social or interpersonal problems. Psychotherapeutic approaches may be enhanced greatly by the promising potential of effective pharmacotherapy. Thus, there is increasing hope for attaining the overriding goal in treating hypochondriacal patients: preventing adoption of the sick role and chronic invalidism (Kellner 1987).

BODY DYSMORPHIC DISORDER

DEFINITION AND CLINICAL DESCRIPTION

The essential feature of body dysmorphic disorder is a preoccupation with some imagined defect in appearance or markedly excessive concern with a minor physical anomaly (Table 16–10). Such preoccupation persists even after reassurance. Common complaints include a diversity of

TABLE 16–10. DSM-IV diagnostic criteria for body dysmorphic disorder

A. Preoccupation with an imagined defect in appearance. If a slight physical anomaly is present, the person's concern is markedly excessive.

B. The preoccupation causes clinically significant distress or impairment in social, occupational, or other important areas of functioning.

C. The preoccupation is not better accounted for by another mental disorder (e.g., dissatisfaction with body shape and size in anorexia nervosa).

imagined flaws of the face or head, including various defects in the hair (too much or too little), skin, shape of the face, or facial features. However, any body part may be the focus, including genitals, breasts, buttocks, extremities, shoulders, and even overall body size. De Leon et al. (1989) stated that the nose, ears, face, or sexual organs are most often involved. It is not surprising, then, that patients with body dysmorphic disorder are found most commonly among persons seeking cosmetic surgery.

The following case example illustrates some of the diagnostic and therapeutic uncertainties involving body dysmorphic disorder, especially regarding overlap with depressive and obsessive-compulsive disorders.

The patient, a male in his mid-20s, received outpatient psychiatric care after 4 years of preoccupation with facial asymmetry and a blemish, defects not evident to others. He had been treated previously with unsuccessful trials of imipramine, phenelzine, perphenazine, and haloperidol. Seeing his reflection in a mirror or shiny surface resulted in a compulsion (accompanied by "a sick, anxious feeling") to inspect the blemish; thus, the patient avoided viewing all such surfaces. He also experienced what he described as a "sinking feeling" in his chest if he touched his face, particularly in the area of the blemish. He grew a beard so that he would not have to shave himself and went to a barber weekly for a shave and a haircut that required nothing more than drying with a towel after showering. He retained insight that there was no actual defect but had once made an appointment with a plastic surgeon. He was embarrassed about his preoccupation and concealed it from others. Although diligent in his work and studies and somewhat perfectionistic in general, he had no other evident obsessions or compulsions.

From the start of his current treatment, an educative approach was taken. He did extensive reading on body dysmorphic and obsessive-compulsive disorders and their therapies.

The SSRIs fluoxetine, sertraline, paroxetine, and fluvoxamine were not available at the time the patient was

treated. With clomipramine, 100 mg daily (he was not able to tolerate larger doses because of extreme dry mouth), he showed some improvement in that he was less dysphoric when ruminating about the blemish, but the preoccupation remained. Similarly, alprazolam "only took the edge off."

The patient became markedly dysphoric and developed suicidal ideation after a breakup with a girlfriend. He received six ECTs, and his depressive and body dysmorphic symptoms improved dramatically. Although the "idea" of the blemish remained, he was no longer preoccupied with it. For the first time in several years he could actually look at himself in the mirror and touch his face without discomfort. Although the benefit from ECT was transient, it gave him hope that he could be free of his preoccupation. He continued taking clomipramine.

On his own initiative he obtained bromazepam (Lexotanil), a benzodiazepine available in Europe but not the United States. He reported that with this drug, his preoccupation was "more under control." This drug has been found in some, but not all, studies to be effective in treating obsessive-compulsive disorder (Hewlett 1993). After fluvoxamine was introduced, he began taking this drug. He tolerated it much better than clomipramine, and the dose was increased to 300 mg daily. Buspirone was added, and the bromazepam was discontinued. On this regimen he still has concerns about his face, but "it doesn't rule me the way it used to." He maintains a successful professional practice. He has never married but has had a succession of girlfriends.

DIAGNOSIS

History

As is evident in Table 16–2, body dysmorphic disorder was not even mentioned in the official nomenclatures until DSM-III and then only parenthetically as *dysmorphophobia*. The syndrome, generally under the rubric of dysmorphophobia, has a long history in the European and Japanese literature, with much less attention in the United States literature (Phillips and Hollander 1996). Because the symptoms are not really of a typical phobic nature with avoidance behavior, the condition was renamed *body dysmorphic disorder* in DSM-III-R. There is a continuous debate as to whether body dysmorphic disorder is a discrete disorder. It is variously argued that it represents a variant of a social phobia, a mood disorder, an obsessive-compulsive disorder, hypochondriasis, a psychotic disorder (particularly delusional disorder), or just the extreme of the continuum of normal concern with appearance. ICD-9 did not include mention of any such disorder. ICD-10 lists it as a type of hypochondriacal disorder. Since inclusion of body dysmorphic disorder in DSM-III, increased study has occurred so that the disorder is now more clearly characterized.

DSM-IV

In DSM-IV, the essential feature of body dysmorphic disorder is preoccupation with an imagined defect in appearance or markedly excessive concern for a slight anomaly (Table 16–10). This criterion represents a slight change from that in DSM-III-R, in which the phrase "in a normal-appearing person" was included. Because a person with some defect may have a preoccupation with a different imagined or exaggerated defect, this phrase was dropped.

As in other somatoform disorders, diagnosis requires that the preoccupation causes clinically significant distress or impairment to exclude those individuals with trivial symptoms. As is explained in the following discussion, body dysmorphic disorder is not diagnosed if the preoccupation is better accounted for by another mental disorder. On the other hand, DSM-IV dropped exclusion on the basis of the preoccupation being delusional, which was included in DSM-III-R and in ICD-10.

Differential Diagnosis

By definition, body dysmorphic disorder is not diagnosed when the body preoccupation is better accounted for by another mental disorder. Anorexia nervosa, in which there is dissatisfaction with body shape and size, is specifically mentioned in the criteria as an example of such an exclusion. In DSM-III-R, transsexualism (gender identity disorder in DSM-IV) also was mentioned as such a disorder. Although not specifically mentioned in DSM-IV, if a preoccupation is limited to discomfort or a sense of inappropriateness of one's primary and secondary sex characteristics, coupled with a strong and persistent cross-gender identification, body dysmorphic disorder would not be diagnosed. Diagnostic problems may develop when a patient has the mood-congruent ruminations of major depression (e.g., preoccupation with a perceived unattractive appearance in association with poor self-esteem). However, such concerns generally lack the focus on a particular body part that is seen in body dysmorphic disorder. Somatic obsessions and even grooming or cleaning rituals in obsessive-compulsive disorder may suggest body dysmorphic disorder; however, in such cases, other obsessions and compulsions are seen as well. In body dysmorphic disorder, the preoccupations are limited to concerns with appearance. Preoccupations in body dysmorphic disorder may reach delusional proportions, and patients with this disorder may show ideas of reference regarding defects in their appearance, which may lead to consideration of the

diagnosis schizophrenia. However, bizarre delusions and hallucinations are not seen in patients with body dysmorphic disorder. From the other perspective, schizophrenic patients with somatic delusions generally do not focus on a specific defect in appearance.

Unlike the diagnostic guideline for hypochondriasis, if the preoccupation is of psychotic proportions, a diagnosis of body dysmorphic disorder still can be made. De Leon et al. (1989) point out the difficulties in determining whether a dysmorphophobic concern is delusional or not. They suggest that cases be classified as "primary dysmorphophobia" without attempting to distinguish between delusional and nondelusional concerns, as long as schizophrenia, major depression, and organic mental disorders are excluded. This point of view was adopted in DSM-IV (Phillips and Hollander 1996). In body dysmorphic disorder, it appears that a continuum exists between preoccupations and delusions, and thus it is difficult, if not impossible, to draw a discrete boundary between body dysmorphic disorder and delusional disorder, somatic type. Furthermore, individual patients seem to move along this continuum. Thus, it was decided to allow both diagnoses if a dysmorphic preoccupation was delusional.

Because patients with body dysmorphic disorder often isolate themselves, social phobia may be suspected. Indeed, the two conditions may coexist. In social phobia alone, however, the person may feel self-conscious but will not focus on a specific imagined defect. Persons with histrionic personality disorder may be vain and excessively concerned with appearance. However, in this disorder, the focus is on maintaining a good or even exceptional appearance rather than preoccupation with a defect.

NATURAL HISTORY

Onset of body dysmorphic disorder peaks in adolescence or early adulthood (Phillips 1991). The disorder is generally a chronic condition, with a waxing and waning of intensity but rarely full remission (Phillips et al. 1993). Over a lifetime, multiple preoccupations are typical. (In their study, Phillips et al. [1993] found an average of four.) In some persons, the same preoccupation remains unchanged; in others, preoccupations with newly perceived defects are added to the original ones. In some individuals, symptoms remit only to be replaced by others.

Body dysmorphic disorder is highly incapacitating. Almost all persons with this disorder show marked impairment in social and occupational activities. About 75% will never marry and among those who do, most will divorce (Phillips 1995). Perhaps a third become housebound. Most attribute their limitations to embarrassment concerning their "defect." The extent to which patients with body dysmorphic disorder receive surgery or medical treatments is unknown. Superimposed depressive episodes are common, as are suicidal ideation and suicide attempts. The actual suicide risk is unknown.

EPIDEMIOLOGY

The lifetime risk of body dysmorphic disorder in the general population is unknown. Although body dysmorphic disorder is seldom seen in psychiatric settings, Andreasen and Bardach (1977) estimate that 2% of patients seeking corrective cosmetic surgery have this disorder. Generally, patients with body dysmorphic disorder are seen psychiatrically only after referral from plastic surgery, dermatology, and otorhinolaryngology clinics (De Leon et al. 1989). The male to female ratio is about 1:1 (Phillips 1995).

ETIOLOGY

Traditionally, little emphasis was devoted to etiological possibilities other than suggested relationships to underlying mood disorders, schizophrenia, obsessive-compulsive disorder, or social phobia. More recently, body dysmorphic disorder has been included with a posited obsessive-compulsive spectrum disorder and with delusional disorders for which a variety of biological pathologies have been posited (Phillips et al. 1995). The latter association is reflected in DSM-IV's allowing both disorders to be diagnosed in the same patient for the same symptoms.

TREATMENT

Simply recognizing that a complaint derives from body dysmorphic disorder may have therapeutic benefit by interrupting an unending procession of repeated evaluations by physicians and the possibility of needless surgery. Surgery actually has been recommended as a treatment for this disorder, but there is no clear evidence that it is helpful. There is a long history of anecdotal reports suggesting the value of diverse treatments, including behavior therapy, dynamic psychotherapy, and pharmacotherapy, the last of which involves neuroleptics and antidepressants, particularly monoamine oxidase inhibitors (De Leon et al. 1989). Response to neuroleptic treatment has been suggested as a diagnostic test to distinguish body dysmorphic disorder from delusional disorder, somatic type (Riding and Munro 1975). Delusional syndromes, in general, may respond to neuroleptics, whereas in body dysmorphic disorder, even when the bodily preoccupations are psychotic, there is less likelihood of success. Pimozide has been sin-

gled out as a neuroleptic having specific effectiveness for somatic delusions, but this drug does not appear to be any more effective than other neuroleptics in treating body dysmorphic disorder.

In earlier reports it was not clear if reported response to antidepressant drugs or ECT was due to amelioration of dysmorphic symptoms per se or to improvement in depressive symptoms. Recently, promising results have been noted with SSRIs at higher dosage levels as in obsessive-compulsive disorder (Phillips 1995). Patients showing a partial response to the SSRI may benefit further from augmentation with buspirone. Improvement with SSRIs seems to be a primary effect in that response was not predicted on the basis of coexisting major depression or obsessive-compulsive disorder. Also of note are observations that patients with somatic delusions may respond to SSRIs.

SOMATOFORM DISORDER NOT OTHERWISE SPECIFIED

DEFINITION AND CLINICAL DESCRIPTION

Somatoform disorder NOS is the true residual category for the somatoform disorders. By definition, conditions included under this category are characterized by somatoform symptoms criteria that are not met for any of the specified somatoform disorders. DSM-IV gives several examples, but syndromes potentially included under this category are not limited to those examples. Unlike undifferentiated somatoform disorder, no minimum duration is required. In fact, some disorders may be relegated to NOS because they do not meet the time requirements for a specified somatoform disorder.

DIAGNOSIS

History

DSM-III included atypical somatoform disorder, a minimally defined residual category requiring only that the predominant disturbance of a disorder be characterized by organically or pathophysiologically unexplained physical symptoms or complaints that are apparently linked to psychological factors. The only example given was dysmorphophobia. In DSM-III-R, the atypical category was renamed and redefined, requiring only the presence of "somatoform symptoms" (implying that no organic or pathophysiological mechanism was present) and that criteria for any specific somatoform or other psychiatric disorder with physical symptoms were not present. Examples given included nonpsychotic hypochondriacal symptoms or physical complaints of less than 6 months' duration that are not related to stress.

DSM-IV

The basic DSM-IV requirement for a diagnosis of somatoform disorder NOS is that a disorder with somatoform symptoms does not meet criteria for a specified somatoform disorder. The first example listed in DSM-IV is pseudocyesis. In DSM-III and DSM-III-R, pseudocyesis was included as a conversion disorder under criteria broadened to include any alteration or loss of physical functioning, suggesting a physical disorder that was an expression of psychological conflict or need. With the contraction of conversion disorder to voluntary motor and sensory dysfunction in DSM-IV, pseudocyesis was excluded and relegated to the NOS category. Oddly enough, pseudocyesis lends itself to a quite specific definition (see Table 16–11). The criteria for pseudocyesis were derived from a review of the existing literature (Martin 1994). However, given its rarity, pseudocyesis is not listed as a specified somatoform disorder.

Two other examples given are syndromes that resemble specified somatoform syndromes, somatization disorder, undifferentiated somatoform disorder, or hypochondriasis but have a duration less than the required 6 months. An additional example is a condition described as involving complaints such as fatigue or body weakness not

TABLE 16–11. DSM-IV diagnostic criteria for somatoform disorder not otherwise specified

This category includes disorders with somatoform symptoms that do not meet the criteria for any specific somatoform disorder. Examples include

1. *Pseudocyesis:* a false belief of being pregnant that is associated with objective signs of pregnancy, which may include abdominal enlargement (although the umbilicus does not become everted), reduced menstrual flow, amenorrhea, subjective sensation of fetal movement, nausea, breast engorgement and secretions, and labor pains at the expected date of delivery. Endocrine changes may be present, but the syndrome cannot be explained by a general medical condition that causes endocrine changes (e.g., a hormone-secreting tumor).

2. A disorder involving nonpsychotic hypochondriacal symptoms of less than 6 months' duration.

3. A disorder involving unexplained physical complaints (e.g., fatigue or body weakness) of less than 6 months' duration that are not due to another mental disorder.

due to another mental disorder, again with a duration of less than 6 months. Such a syndrome would resemble neurasthenia, a syndrome with a long historical tradition. Included in DSM-II, ICD-9, and ICD-10, neurasthenia was considered for inclusion as a specified DSM-IV somatoform disorder. After careful review, neurasthenia was not adopted because it was difficult to delineate it from depressive, anxiety, and other somatoform disorders, and there was a lack of systematic study supporting it. Finally, there was concern that neurasthenia would become a wastebasket category, the availability of which might promote premature closure of the diagnostic process so that other mental disorders, as well as other general medical disorders, would be overlooked.

DIFFERENTIAL DIAGNOSIS

As mentioned in the preceding discussion, DSM-IV lists several syndromes that, if not for their short duration, would qualify for a diagnosis as the specified somatoform disorder that they resemble.

Pseudocyesis deserves special attention. Although not mentioned in DSM-II, it probably would have fit best as a psychophysiological endocrine disorder. In DSM-III and DSM-III-R, pseudocyesis was specifically listed as a conversion symptom. Its presumed mechanism was ambivalence about pregnancy, with the resulting conflict expressed somatically, leading to resolution (primary gain) and unconsciously needed environmental support (secondary gain). Pseudocyesis could have been subsumed under the heading "Psychological Factors Affecting Medical Condition." An argument can be made for its inclusion as a medical condition because, based on a literature review (Martin 1996), in most if not all cases it appears that a neuroendocrine change accompanies, and at times may antedate, the false belief of pregnancy. However, in most instances a discrete general medical condition (such as a hormone-secreting tumor) cannot be identified. It might have been included as a specified somatoform disorder except for its rarity; Whelan and Stewart (1990) reported six cases in 20 years of consulting to a unit delivering 2,500 women per year. Yet, pseudocyesis appears as a reasonably discrete syndrome such that specific criteria derived from the literature are included in its listing as a somatoform disorder NOS (see Table 16–11).

EPIDEMIOLOGY, ETIOLOGY, AND TREATMENT

Discussion of epidemiology, etiology, and treatment for a residual category such as somatoform disorder NOS would not be meaningful, since it represents a grouping of diverse disorders. Conditions that would warrant diagnosis of a specified somatoform disorder except for their insufficient duration (less than 6 months) are probably best considered to be in the spectrum of the resembled disorder. Thus, the epidemiological, etiological, and treatment considerations pertaining to the specified disorder should be reviewed because these may apply, at least in part, to the shorter-duration syndromes.

In a comprehensive review of pseudocyesis, Small (1986) states: "Of all that has been written on the subject [pseudocyesis], therapy is least discussed. What has been written is reviewed by Ford." In another report, Whelan and Stewart (1990) emphasize two principles in treating patients with pseudocyesis. First, the patient is to be clearly, yet "empathically" advised that she (or the rare he) is not pregnant. If such simple advice is not effective, objective procedures such as ultrasound are recommended to demonstrate to the patient that there is no visible evidence of a fetus. Alternatively, menses are to be induced. Remarkably, such straightforward approaches are often effective (Cohen 1982). According to Whelan and Stewart (1990), the second principle, which goes hand in hand with the first, is that the patient's expectations, fears, and fantasies be explored to discover the reason why the false pregnancy was "needed." Also advised is providing a face-saving resolution to the patient's lack of pregnancy, such as allowing the patient to take the position that a "miscarriage" has occurred. However, systematic data on the effectiveness of these and other approaches are lacking. Whatever the therapy, relapses are common. According to Ford (1995) there is limited data on the prognosis for women with pseudocyesis. Concomitant disorders such as major depression should be treated in the usual manner.

CONCLUSIONS

Syndromes now subsumed under the rubric "Somatoform Disorders" have had a tortuous course in the evolution of psychiatric nosology and therapy. Yet, they are extremely important because they are disorders that must be differentiated from conditions with identifiable, and often treatable, physical bases.

Developments in the last decade are encouraging. Coordinated effort has been made to establish a common, globally used nomenclature. Somatoform disorders as delineated in DSM-IV are compatible with, although not identical to, counterparts in ICD-10. A common and more explicitly defined nosology is conducive to empirical research that is truly comparable from one investigation to the next. Initial observations on the pharmacological treatment of several of the disorders, namely hypochondriasis and body dysmorphic disorder, are promising and not only may add to our therapeutic armamentarium, but also may suggest avenues for improved pathophysiological and even etiological understanding these two somatoform disorders.

Ultimately, it may prove possible to obtain a better understanding of the somatoform disorders, a group of complex, incapacitating disorders. Better understanding should facilitate more effective treatments for them. Already, there has been some preliminary discussion of the development of practice guidelines for somatoform disorders. Consideration of practice guidelines would have been highly unlikely even a few years ago.

REFERENCES

Alexander F: Psychosomatic Medicine: Its Principles and Applications. New York, WW Norton, 1950

Almgren P-E, Nordgren L, Skantze H: A retrospective study of operationally defined hysterics. Br J Psychiatry 132:67–73, 1978

Alper K, Devinsky O, Vasquez B, et al: Nonepileptic seizures and childhood sexual and physical abuse. Neurology 43:1950–1953, 1993

American Psychiatric Association: Diagnostic and Statistical Manual: Mental Disorders. Washington, DC, American Psychiatric Association, 1952

American Psychiatric Association: Diagnostic and Statistical Manual of Mental Disorders, 2nd Edition. Washington, DC, American Psychiatric Association, 1968

American Psychiatric Association: Diagnostic and Statistical Manual of Mental Disorders, 3rd Edition. Washington, DC, American Psychiatric Association, 1980

American Psychiatric Association: Diagnostic and Statistical Manual of Mental Disorders, 3rd Edition, Revised. Washington, DC, American Psychiatric Association, 1987

American Psychiatric Association: Diagnostic and Statistical Manual of Mental Disorders, 4th Edition. Washington, DC, American Psychiatric Association, 1994

American Psychiatric Association: Diagnostic and Statistical Manual of Mental Disorders, 4th Edition, Primary Care Version. Washington, DC, American Psychiatric Association, 1995

Andrade C, Srinath S: True auditory hallucinations as a conversion symptom. Br J Psychiatry 148:100–102, 1986

Andreasen NC, Bardach J: Dysmorphophobia: symptom or disease? Am J Psychiatry 134:673–676, 1977

Bach M, Bach D, de Zwaan M: Independency of alexithymia and somatization. Psychosomatics 37:451–458, 1996

Barsky AJ: Somatoform disorders, in Comprehensive Textbook of Psychiatry/V, 5th Edition, Vol 1. Edited by Kaplan HI, Sadock BJ. Baltimore, MD, Williams & Wilkins, 1989, pp 1009–1027

Barsky AJ, Klerman GL: Overview: hypochondriasis, bodily complaints, and somatic styles. Am J Psychiatry 140:273–283, 1983

Barsky AJ, Wyshak G, Klerman GL: Hypochondriasis: an evaluation of the DSM-III criteria in medical outpatients. Arch Gen Psychiatry 43:493–500, 1986

Barsky AJ, Cleary PD, Sarnie MK, et al: The course of transient hypochondriasis. Am J Psychiatry 150:484–488, 1993

Bass CM, Murphy MR: Somatization disorder: critique of the concept and suggestions for future research, in Somatization: Physical Symptoms and Psychological Illness. Edited by Bass C. Oxford, UK, Blackwell Scientific, 1990, pp 301–332

Bendefeldt F, Miller LL, Ludwig AM: Cognitive performance in conversion hysteria. Arch Gen Psychiatry 33:1250–1254, 1976

Bohman M, Cloninger CR, von Knorring A-L, et al: An adoption study of somatoform disorders, III: cross-fostering analysis and genetic relationship to alcoholism and criminality. Arch Gen Psychiatry 41:872–878, 1984

Breuer J, Freud S: Studies on hysteria (1893–1895), in the Standard Edition of the Complete Psychological Works of Sigmund Freud, Vol 2. Translated and edited by Strachey J. London, Hogarth, 1955, pp 1–311

Briquet P: Traité Clinique et Thérapeutique Y l'Hystérie. Paris, J-B Balliere & Fils, 1859

Carter AB: The prognosis of certain hysterical symptoms. BMJ 1:1076–1079, 1949

Chodoff P, Lyons H: Hysteria, the hysterical personality and "hysterical" conversion. Am J Psychiatry 114:734–740, 1958

Cloninger CR: The link between hysteria and sociopathy: an integrative model based on clinical, genetic, and neurophysiological observations, in Psychiatric Diagnosis: Explorations of Biological Predictors. Edited by Akiskal HS, Webb WL. New York, Spectrum, 1978, pp 189–218

Cloninger CR: Diagnosis of somatoform disorders: a critique of DSM-III, in Diagnosis and Classification in Psychiatry: A Critical Appraisal of DSM-III. Edited by Tischler GL. New York, Cambridge University Press, 1987, pp 243–259

Cloninger CR: Somatoform and dissociative disorders, in The Medical Basis of Psychiatry, 2nd Edition. Edited by Winokur G, Clayton P. Philadelphia, WB Saunders, 1994, pp 169–192

Cloninger CR, Guze SB: Psychiatric illness and female criminality: the role of sociopathy and hysteria in the antisocial woman. Am J Psychiatry 127:303–311, 1970

Cloninger CR, Yutzy S: Somatoform and dissociative disorders: a summary of changes for DSM-IV, in Current Psychiatric Therapy. Edited by Dunner DL. Philadelphia, WB Saunders, 1993, pp 310–313

Cloninger CR, Reich T, Guze SB: The multifactorial model of disease transmission, III: familial relationship between sociopathy and hysteria (Briquet's syndrome). Br J Psychiatry 127:23–32, 1975

Cloninger CR, Sigvardsson S, von Knorring A-L, et al: An adoption study of somatoform disorders, II: identification of two discrete somatoform disorders. Arch Gen Psychiatry 41:863–871, 1984

Cloninger CR, Martin RL, Guze SB, et al: A prospective follow-up and family study of somatization in men and women. Am J Psychiatry 143:873–878, 1986

Cloninger CR, Bayon C, Przybeck TR: Epidemiology and axis I comorbidity of antisocial personality, in Handbook of Antisocial Behavior. Edited by Stoff DM, Breiling J, Maser JD. New York, John Wiley, 1997, pp 12–21

Cohen LM: A current perspective of pseudocyesis. Am J Psychiatry 139:1140–1144, 1982

Coryell W, House D: The validity of broadly defined hysteria and DSM-III conversion disorder: outcome, family history, and mortality. J Clin Psychiatry 45:252–256, 1984

Cote G, O'Leary T, Barlow DM, et al: Hypochondriasis: integrative review for DSM-IV, in DSM-IV Sourcebook, Vol 2. Edited by Widiger TA, Frances AJ, Pincus HA, et al. Washington, DC, American Psychiatric Press, 1996, pp 933–947

De Leon J, Bott A, Simpson GM: Dysmorphophobia: body dysmorphic disorder or delusional disorder, somatic subtype? Compr Psychiatry 30:457–472, 1989

Desai BT, Porter RJ, Penry K: Psychogenic seizures: a study of 42 attacks in six patients, with intensive monitoring. Arch Neurol 39:202–209, 1982

DeSouza C, Othmer E, Gabrielli W Jr, et al: Major depression and somatization disorder: the overlooked differential diagnosis. Psychiatric Annals 18:340–348, 1988

Escobar JI, Swartz M, Rubio-Stipec M, et al: Medically unexplained symptoms: distribution, risk factors, and comorbidity, in Current Concepts of Somatization: Research and Clinical Perspectives. Edited by Kirmayer LJ, Robbins JM. Washington, DC, American Psychiatric Press, 1991, pp 63–78

Fallon BA, Schneir FR, Narshall R, et al: The pharmacotherapy of hypochondriasis. Psychopharmacol Bull 32:607–611, 1996

Feighner JP, Robins E, Guze SB, et al: Diagnostic criteria for use in psychiatric research. Arch Gen Psychiatry 26:57–63, 1972

Fitzgerald BA, Wells CE: Hallucinations as a conversion reaction. Diseases of the Nervous System 38:381–383, 1977

Flor-Henry P, Fromm-Auch D, Tapper M, et al: A neuropsychological study of the stable syndrome of hysteria. Biol Psychiatry 16:601–626, 1981

Folks DG, Ford CV, Regan WM: Conversion symptoms in a general hospital. Psychosomatics 25:285–295, 1984

Ford CV: The Somatizing Disorders: Illness as a Way of Life. New York, Elsevier, 1983

Ford CV: Conversion disorder and somatoform disorder not otherwise specified, in Treatment of Psychiatric Disorders, 2nd Edition. Edited by Gabbard GO. Washington, DC, American Psychiatric Press, 1995, pp 1737–1753

Ford CV, Folks DG: Conversion disorders: an overview. Psychosomatics 26:371–383, 1985

Gatfield PD, Guze SB: Prognosis and differential diagnosis of conversion reactions (a follow-up study). Diseases of the Nervous System 23:623–631, 1962

Goodwin DW, Guze SB: Psychiatric Diagnosis, 5th Edition. New York, Oxford University Press, 1996

Goodwin DW, Alderson P, Rosenthal R: Clinical significance of hallucinations in psychiatric disorders. Arch Gen Psychiatry 24:76–80, 1971

Guze SB: The role of follow-up studies: Their contribution to diagnostic classification as applied to hysteria. Seminars in Psychiatry 2:392–402, 1970

Guze SB, Perley MJ: Observations on the natural history of hysteria. Am J Psychiatry 119:960–965, 1963

Guze SB, Cloninger CR, Martin RL, et al: A follow-up and family study of Briquet's syndrome. Br J Psychiatry 149:17–23, 1986

Hathaway SR, McKinley JC: Minnesota Multiphasic Personality Schedule. Minneapolis, MN, University of Minnesota Press, 1943

Hewlett HA: The use of benzodiazepines in obsessive-compulsive disorder and Tourette's syndrome. Psychiatric Annals 23:309–316, 1993

Hollander E, Neville D, Frenkel M, et al: Body dysmorphic disorder: diagnostic issues and related disorders. Psychosomatics 33:156–165, 1992

Horowitz MJ: Hysterical Personality. New York, Jason Aronson, 1977

Hudziak JJ, Boffeli TJ, Kreisman JJ, et al: Clinical study of the relation of borderline personality disorder to Briquet's syndrome (hysteria), somatization disorder, antisocial personality disorder, and substance abuse disorders. Am J Psychiatry 153:1598–1606, 1996

Inouye E: Genetic aspects of neurosis. International Journal of Mental Health 1:176–189, 1972

Kellner R: The prognosis of treated hypochondriasis: a clinical study. Acta Psychiatr Scand 67:69–79, 1983

Kellner R: Functional somatic symptoms and hypochondriasis: a survey of empirical studies. Arch Gen Psychiatry 42:821–833, 1985

Kellner R: Hypochondriasis and somatization. JAMA 258:2718–2722, 1987

Kellner R: Somatization disorder, in Treatments of Psychiatric Disorders: A Task Force Report of the American Psychiatric Association, Vol 3. Washington, DC, American Psychiatric Association, 1989, pp 2166–2171

Kellner R: Somatization: theories and research. J Nerv Ment Dis 178:150–160, 1990

Kent D, Tomasson K, Coryell W: Course and outcome of conversion and somatization disorders: a four-year follow-up. Psychosomatics 36:138–144, 1995

Kenyon FE: Hypochondriasis: a survey of some historical, clinical, and social aspects. Br J Psychiatry 138:117–133, 1965

Kenyon FE: Hypochondriacal states. Br J Psychiatry 129:1–14, 1976

Kirmayer LJ, Robbins JM: Introduction: concepts of somatization, in Current Concepts of Somatization: Research and Clinical Perspectives. Edited by Kirmayer LJ, Robbins JM. Washington, DC, American Psychiatric Press, 1991, pp 1–19

Kirmayer LJ, Robbins JM, Dworkind M, et al: Somatization and the recognition of depression and anxiety in primary care. Am J Psychiatry 150:734–741, 1993

Kroenke K, Spitzer RL, de Gruy FV, et al: Multisomatoform disorder: an alternative to undifferentiated somatoform disorder for the somatizing patient in primary care. Arch Gen Psychiatry 54:352–358, 1997

Lader M, Sartorious N: Anxiety in patients with hysterical conversion symptoms. J Neurol Neurosurg Psychiatry 31:490–495, 1968

Lazare A: Conversion symptoms. N Engl J Med 305:745–748, 1981

Lewis WC: Hysteria: the consultant's dilemma: twentieth century demonology, pejorative epithet, or useful diagnosis? Arch Gen Psychiatry 30:145–151, 1974

Lewis WC, Berman M: Studies of conversion hysteria, I: operational study of diagnosis. Arch Gen Psychiatry 13:275–282, 1965

Lipowski ZJ: Somatization: the concept and its clinical application. Am J Psychiatry 145:1358–1368, 1988

Ljundberg L: Hysteria: clinical, prognostic and genetic study. Acta Psychiatr Scand Suppl 32:1–162, 1957

Ludwig AM: Hysteria: a neurobiological theory. Arch Gen Psychiatry 27:771–777, 1972

Luff MC, Garrod M: The after-results of psychotherapy in 500 adult cases. BMJ 2:54–59, 1935

Mace CJ, Trimble MR: Ten-year prognosis of conversion disorder. Br J Psychiatry 169:282–288, 1996

Maloney MJ: Diagnosing hysterical conversion disorders in children. J Pediatr 97:1016–1020, 1980

Marsden CD: Hysteria: a neurologist's view. Psychol Med 16:277–288, 1986

Martin RL: Problems in the diagnosis of somatization disorder: effects on research and clinical practice. Psychiatric Annals 18:357–362, 1988

Martin RL: Somatoform disorders in the general hospital setting, in Handbook of Studies on General Hospital Psychiatry. Edited by Judd FK, Burrows GD, Lipsitt DR. Amsterdam, Elsevier, 1991, pp 251–266

Martin RL: DSM-IV in progress: diagnostic issues for conversion disorder. Hospital and Community Psychiatry 43:771–773, 1992

Martin RL: DSM-IV changes in the somatoform disorders. Psychiatric Annals 25:29–39, 1995

Martin RL: DSM-IV diagnostic options for conversion disorder: proposed autonomic arousal disorder and pseudocyesis, in DSM-IV Sourcebook, Vol 2. Edited by Widiger TA, Frances AJ, Pincus HA, et al. Washington, DC, American Psychiatric Press, 1996, pp 893–914

Martin RL, Yutzy SH: Somatoform disorders, in Psychiatry. Edited by Tasman A, Kay J, Lieberman JA. Philadelphia, WB Saunders, 1997, pp 1119–1155

Martin RL, Cloninger CR, Guze SB: The evaluation of diagnostic concordance in follow-up studies, II: a blind prospective follow-up of female criminals. J Psychiatr Res 15:107–125, 1979

Martin RL, Cloninger CR, Guze SB, et al: Mortality in a follow-up of 500 psychiatric outpatients, II: cause-specific mortality. Arch Gen Psychiatry 42:58–66, 1985

Meares R, Horvath T: "Acute" and "chronic" hysteria. Br J Psychiatry 121:653–657, 1972

Merskey H: Conversion disorder, in Treatments of Psychiatric Disorders: A Task Force Report of the American Psychiatric Association, Vol 3. Washington, DC, American Psychiatric Association, 1989, pp 2152–2159

Modai I, Cygielman G: Conversion hallucinations: a possible mental mechanism. Psychopathology 19:324–326, 1986

Murphy GE: The clinical management of hysteria. JAMA 247:2559–2564, 1982

Murphy GE, Guze SB: Setting limits. Am J Psychother 14:30–47, 1960

Murphy GE, Wetzel RD: Family history of suicidal behavior among suicide attempters. J Nerv Ment Dis 170:86–90, 1982

Murphy MR: Classification of the somatoform disorders, in Somatization: Physical Symptoms and Psychological Illness. Edited by Bass C. Oxford, UK, Blackwell Scientific, 1990, pp 10–39

Perley M, Guze SB: Hysteria: the stability and usefulness of clinical criteria: a quantitative study based upon a 6–8 year follow-up of 39 patients. N Engl J Med 266:421–426, 1962

Phillips KA: Body dysmorphic disorder: the distress of imagined ugliness. Am J Psychiatry 148:1138–1149, 1991

Phillips KA: Body dysmorphic disorder: clinical features and drug treatment. CNS Drugs 3:30–40, 1995

Phillips KA, Hollander E: Body dysmorphic disorder, in DSM-IV Sourcebook, Vol 2. Edited by Widiger TA, Frances AJ, Pincus HA, et al. Washington, DC, American Psychiatric Press, 1996, pp 949–960

Phillips KA, McElroy SL, Keck PE Jr, et al: Body dysmorphic disorder: 30 cases of imagined ugliness. Am J Psychiatry 150:302–308, 1993

Phillips KA, Kim JM, Hudson JI: Body image disturbance in body dysmorphic disorder and eating disorders: obsessions or delusions? Psychiatr Clin North Am 18:317–334, 1995

Pincus J: Hysteria presenting to a neurologist, in Hysteria. Edited by Roy A. London, Wiley, 1982, pp 131–144

Pribor EF, Smith DS, Yutzy SH: Somatization disorder in the elderly. Am J Geriatr Psychiatry 2:109–117, 1994

Purtell J, Robins E, Cohen M: Observations on clinical aspects of hysteria: a quantitative study of 50 hysteria patients and 156 control subjects. JAMA 146:902–909, 1951

Quill TE: Somatization disorder: one of medicine's blind spots. JAMA 254:3075–3079, 1985

Raskin M, Talbott JA, Meyerson AT: Diagnosis of conversion reactions: predictive value of psychiatric criteria. JAMA 197:530–534, 1966

Riding J, Munro A: Pimozide in the treatment of monosymptomatic hypochondriacal psychosis. Acta Psychiatr Scand 52:23–30, 1975

Robins E, O'Neal P: Clinical features of hysteria in children. The Nervous Child 10:246–271, 1953

Robins LN, Helzer JE, Croughan J, et al: National Institute of Mental Health Diagnostic Interview Schedule: its history, characteristics, and validity. Arch Gen Psychiatry 38:381–389, 1981

Robins LN, Helzer JE, Weissman MM, et al: Lifetime prevalence of specific psychiatric disorders in three sites. Arch Gen Psychiatry 41:949–958, 1984

Scallet A, Cloninger CR, Othmer E: The management of chronic hysteria: a review and double-blind trial of electrosleep and other relaxation methods. Diseases of the Nervous System 37:347–353, 1976

Shapiro D: Neurotic Styles. New York, Basic Books, 1965

Sharma P, Chaturvedi SK: Conversion disorder revisited. Acta Pschiatr Scand 92:301–304, 1995

Slater ETO, Glithero C: A follow-up of patients diagnosed as suffering from "hysteria." J Psychosom Res 9:9–13, 1965

Small GW: Pseudocyesis: an overview. Can J Psychiatry 31:452–457, 1986

Smith GR Jr, Monson RA, Ray DC: Psychiatric consultation in somatization disorder: a randomized controlled study. N Engl J Med 314:1407–1413, 1986

Stefanis C, Markidis M, Christodoulou G: Observations on the evolution of the hysterical symptomatology. Br J Psychiatry 128:269–275, 1976

Stefansson JH, Messina JA, Meyerowitz S: Hysterical neurosis, conversion type: clinical and epidemiological considerations. Acta Psychiatr Scand 59:119–138, 1976

Stekel W: The Interpretation of Dreams: New Developments and Technique, Vols 1 and 2. Translated by Paul E, Paul C. New York, Liveright, 1943

Stephens JH, Kamp M: On some aspects of hysteria: a clinical study. J Nerv Ment Dis 134:305–315, 1962

Stern J, Murphy M, Bass C: Personality disorders in patients with somatization disorder: a controlled study. Br J Psychiatry 163:785–789, 1993

Stoudemire GA: Somatoform disorders, factitious disorders, and malingering, in American Psychiatric Press Textbook of Psychiatry. Edited by Talbott JA, Hales RE, Yudofsky SC. Washington, DC, American Psychiatric Press, 1988, pp 533–556

Temoshok L, Attkisson CC: Epidemiology of hysterical phenomena: evidence for a psychosocial theory, in Hysterical Personality. Edited by Horowitz MJ. New York, Jason Aronson, 1977, pp 143–222

Tomasson K, Kent D, Coryell W: Somatization and conversion disorders: comorbidity and demographics at presentation. Acta Psychiatr Scand 84:288–293, 1991

Toone BK: Disorders of hysterical conversion, in Physical Symptoms and Psychological Illness. Edited by Bass C. London, Blackwell Scientific, 1990, pp 207–234

Torack RM: Historical overview of dementia, in The Pathologic Physiology of Dementia. Edited by Torack RA. New York, Springer-Verlag, 1978, pp 1–16

Vaillant GE: The disadvantages of DSM-III outweigh its advantages. Am J Psychiatry 141:542–545, 1984

Veith I: Hysteria: The History of a Disease. Chicago, University of Chicago Press, 1965

Viederman M: Somatoform and factitious disorders, in Psychiatry, Vol 1. Edited by Cavenar JO. Philadelphia, JB Lippincott, 1985, pp 1–20

Watson CG, Buranen C: The frequency and identification of false positive conversion reactions. J Nerv Ment Dis 167:243–247, 1979

Wechsler D: Wechsler Adult Intelligence Scale–Revised. New York, Psychological Corporation, 1981

Weddington WW: Conversion reaction in an 82-year-old man. J Nerv Ment Dis 167:368–369, 1979

Weinstein EA, Eck RA, Lyerly OG: Conversion hysteria in Appalachia. Psychiatry 32:334–341, 1969

Wetzel RD, Guze SB, Cloninger CR, et al: Briquet's syndrome (hysteria) is both a somatoform and a "psychoform" illness: an MMPI study. Psychosom Med 56:564–569, 1994

Wheatley D: Evaluation of psychotherapeutic drugs in general practice. Psychopharmacol Bull 2:25–32, 1962

Wheatley D: General practitioner clinical trials: phenobarbitone compared with an inactive placebo in anxiety states. Practitioner 192:147–151, 1964

Wheatley D: General practitioner clinical trials: chlordiazepoxide in anxiety states, II: long-term study. Practitioner 195:692–695, 1965

Whelan CI, Stewart DE: Pseudocyesis: a review and report of six cases. International Journal of Psychiatry in Medicine 20:97–108, 1990

Woerner PI, Guze SB: A family and marital study of hysteria. Br J Psychiatry 114:161–168, 1968

Woodruff RA, Clayton PJ, Guze SB: Hysteria: studies of diagnosis, outcome, and prevalence. JAMA 215:425–428, 1971

World Health Organization: The ICD-9 Classification of Mental and Behavioural Disorders, 9th Revision: Clinical Descriptions and Diagnostic Guidelines. Geneva, World Health Organization, 1977

World Health Organization: The ICD-10 Classification of Mental and Behavioural Disorders, 10th Revision: Clinical Descriptions and Diagnostic Guidelines. Geneva, World Health Organization, 1992a

World Health Organization: International Statistical Classification of Diseases and Related Health Problems, 10th Revision. Geneva, World Health Organization, 1992b

World Health Organization: Diagnostic and Management Guidelines for Mental Disorders in Primary Care: ICD-10 Chapter V Primary Care Version. Gottingen, Germany, Hogrefe & Huber, 1996

Yutzy SH, Pribor EF, Cloninger CR, et al: Reconsidering the criteria for somatization disorder. Hospital and Community Psychiatry 43:1075–1076, 1149, 1992

Yutzy SH, Cloninger CR, Guze SB, et al: The DSM-IV field trial: somatization disorder: testing a new proposal. Am J Psychiatry 152:97–101, 1995

Ziegler FJ, Imboden JB, Meyer E: Contemporary conversion reactions: a clinical study. Am J Psychiatry 116:901–910, 1960

CHAPTER 17

FACTITIOUS DISORDERS AND MALINGERING

MARTIN H. LEAMON, M.D.
JOHN PLEWES, M.D.

FACTITIOUS DISORDER

Factitious disorder is characterized by a person intentionally fabricating signs or symptoms of other illnesses solely to become identified as "ill" or as a "patient." Such patients have been described in medical writing throughout history (Feldman and Ford 1994) and throughout the world (Lim et al. 1991; Linde 1996; Seersholm et al. 1991; Seguel et al. 1990). The concept became firmly established in modern medical thinking in 1951 when Asher (1951) described what has since been classified a subtype of factitious disorders: Munchausen syndrome. Many patients with factitious disorders remain undiagnosed, and even when recognized, they often go untreated (Toth and Baggaley 1991). Yet, factitious disorders cause significant morbidity and mortality (Baker and Major 1994; Folks 1995; Higgins 1990), cause an astonishing amount of medical resources to be consumed (Feldman 1994a; Frumkin and Victoroff 1990; Higgins 1990; Powell and Boast 1993a; Schwarz et al. 1993), and cause significant emotional distress in the patients, their caregivers, and in their close relationships (Feldman and Smith 1996). Since the last edition of this textbook, there has been a continued expansion of the medical literature about factitious disorders, with the publication of lay and professional books on the topic

(Feldman and Eisendrath 1996; Feldman and Ford 1994) and the establishment of a factitious disorders site on the World Wide Web (Feldman 1997).

CLASSIFICATION

DSM-IV (American Psychiatric Association 1994) requires three criteria for the diagnosis of factitious disorder (Table 17–1). The first, the intentional production or feigning of physical or psychological signs or symptoms, distinguishes factitious disorder from the somatoform disorders, in which physical symptoms are viewed as unconsciously produced. The second and third criteria, that the motivation for the behavior is to assume the sick role and that external incentives for the behavior are absent, distinguish factitious disorder from malingering. The tenth revision of *International Classification of Diseases*, (ICD-10; World Health Organization 1992), although slightly different, uses similarly defined operational criteria (Freyberger and Schneider 1994).

DSM-IV (Table 17–1) classifies the disorder based on the predominant type of factitious symptom presented—physical or psychological. Individual case histories (Bauer and Boegner 1996; Craddock and Brown 1993; Zimmerman et al. 1991) suggest that this categorization

TABLE 17-1. **DSM-IV diagnostic criteria for factitious disorder**

A. Intentional production or feigning of physical or psychological signs or symptoms.

B. The motivation for the behavior is to assume the sick role.

C. External incentives for the behavior (such as economic gain, avoiding legal responsibility, or improving physical well-being, as in malingering) are absent.

Code based on type:

300.16 **With predominantly psychological signs and symptoms:** if psychological signs and symptoms predominate in the clinical presentation

300.19 **With predominantly physical signs and symptoms:** if physical signs and symptoms predominate in the clinical presentation

300.19 **With combined psychological and physical signs and symptoms:** if both psychological and physical signs and symptoms are present but neither predominates in the clinical presentation

may be somewhat arbitrary, as the same patient may have different presentations across time. Predominantly physical symptoms may be feigned at one episode and predominantly psychological or a mixed picture at another. Rogers et al. (1989) also have raised epistemological objections to this subtyping, arguing in part that factitious disorder with predominantly psychological signs and symptoms confers a psychiatric disorder to someone who by definition is merely pretending to have one. The fourth subtype is factitious disorder not otherwise specified (NOS) (Table 17–2). The code for factitious disorder NOS should be used for disorders with factitious symptoms that do not meet criteria for one of the other subtypes. An example is factitious disorder by proxy, discussed later in this chapter.

Other authors have used different typologies. Nadelson (1979) distinguished between "prototypical" and "nonprototypical" factitious disorders. This typology may have prognostic and treatment implications.

TABLE 17-2. **DSM-IV diagnostic criteria for factitious disorder not otherwise specified**

300.19 This category includes disorders with factitious symptoms that do not meet the criteria for factitious disorder. An example is factitious disorder by proxy: the intentional production or feigning of physical or psychological signs or symptoms in another person who is under the individual's care for the purpose of indirectly assuming the sick role.

Prototypical factitious disorder refers to Munchausen syndrome, the term coined by Asher (1951), and actually comprises only about 10% of patients with factitious disorders (Eisendrath 1996). The eponym remains in wide use and describes a variant of DSM-IV's factitious disorder with predominantly physical signs and symptoms. In this special type of factitious disorder, multiple hospitalizations with dramatic and often life-threatening presentations, wandering from hospital to hospital (peregrination), and pathological lying (*pseudologia fantastica,* the telling of tall tales that the listener initially finds intriguing and fascinating) are prominent. The patient shows a pattern of feigning illness at numerous hospital emergency rooms, often in different cities; gaining admission and sometimes receiving invasive procedures; becoming quarrelsome with the staff; and being discharged against medical advice when the ruse is discovered. Asher, using the anglicized spelling, drew the term from Rudolf Erich Raspe's 1784 book, *Baron Münchhausen's Narrative of His Marvelous Travels and Campaigns in Russia,* which detailed the exaggerated accounts of the sporting and military adventures, as well as the peregrinations, of a German cavalry officer in the Russian army, Baron Karl Friedrich Hieronymous von Münchhausen (Encarta Multimedia Encyclopedia 1993).

Other expressions concerning patients of this type have been quite colorful: "hospital hobos" (Clark and Melnich 1958), "hospital addicts" (J. P. Barker 1962), and "metabolic malingerers" (C. A. Gorman et al. 1970). Additional terms for the disorder have included "chronic factitious illness" (Spiro 1968) and "Kopenickades syndrome" and "Ahasuerus syndrome" ("Clinical Case Conference" 1984).

Nonprototypical Munchausen patients comprise the vast majority of patients with factitious disorders. Characterized by several authors (Carney 1980; Ford 1986; Freyberger et al. 1994; Guziec et al. 1994; Plassmann 1994b; Reich and Gottfried 1983), these patients are mostly young women with conforming lifestyles and more family support and involvement. The patients have been described as passive, immature, and hypochondriacal, and a significant proportion have health-related jobs. Most are not wanderers, have single-system complaints, and generate fewer hospitalizations than do the prototypical Munchausen patients, but the overall severity and morbidity of their illness may be just as great (Sutherland and Rodin 1990).

Others (Eisendrath 1996; Overholser 1990) have classified patients with factitious disorders according to the manner in which illness is simulated and by the type of simulated illness. Patients may simply report invented symptoms and false medical histories, as in the case example in the following discussion. Or they may manipulate diagnostic instruments to give false readings, such as manipulating electrocardiogram (ECG) leads to simulate arrhythmia (Ludwigs et al. 1994) or rubbing thermometers to fake fevers (Aduan et al. 1979). They also may tamper with laboratory specimens, adding blood to urine or sputum. Finally, they purposefully may cause actual tissue damage or biochemical abnormalities in their bodies by methods such as intentionally traumatic self-catheterization, self-induced infection of wounds or skin with bacteria, injection of insulin, and ingestion of thyroid hormones or anticoagulants.

Classification by type of simulated illness is most useful to the clinician who begins to suspect factitious illness and who then looks for evidence to support the suspicion. Wallach (1994) and Nordmeyer (1994) give thorough descriptions of presentations of factitious illness in the different organ systems and some suggestions for their detection. Patients with this disorder can simulate almost any conceivable condition, depending on their knowledge and covert skill.

DIAGNOSIS

John was a middle-aged, middle-ranking United States military officer stationed at what was widely held to be a desirable post in Europe. He was married with no children, by mutual decision with his attentive wife. His superiors described his military career performance as slightly better than average. He was hospitalized for evaluation when a sentry discovered him one evening walking around outside, disorganized and talking disjointedly about Vietnam.

He was hospitalized at one of the United States military psychiatric wards in Europe, where he described long-standing symptoms of posttraumatic stress disorder (PTSD) from his experiences as part of an elite covert operations team functioning behind enemy lines. He readily engaged in ward activities and in his treatment program. The historical details he provided were accurate, although some details he said he could not reveal, due to their classified nature. He was evaluated by experienced psychiatrists, psychologists, and nursing staff. His cognitive and affective presentations, in ward activities, group psychotherapy, and individual psychotherapy, were all consistent with delayed-onset PTSD. When he showed no improvement after 2 weeks of intensive treatment, he was transferred to a military medical center in the United States for further treatment.

His presentation remained unchanged, although he seemed to show some improvement. He received much support from the other military patients and was regarded as tragically courageous. The psychiatric resident responsible for John's direct care (one of the authors of this chapter [M. L.]) spent time reading the literature on the treatment of PTSD, and John received extra individual psychotherapy, a valued commodity on a busy inpatient service. A search of his military records revealed no history of Vietnam service, and John carefully explained that his record had been officially manipulated, again because of the classified nature of his activities. Knowledgeable military sources confirmed that although John's explanation was unusual, it could be correct. In couples psychotherapy sessions, John gently explained to his wife that he had withheld this important part of his premarital history from her because of the pain it caused him to recall these experiences, as well as the classified nature of his activities. She continued to be emotionally supportive after gradually accepting that her husband had been so secretive. As time went on, it became clear that John was facing discharge from military service, which neither he nor his wife wanted. For a number of reasons, it also seemed unlikely that John would receive any disability payments once discharged.

After John was hospitalized for several months, his mother was contacted (with his consent). She seemed to be a reliable source and expressed complete bewilderment at her son's predicament. She explained that John had not been in Vietnam or even in the military during the time he claimed but had been living with her, working in a store.

When John was presented with his mother's information, he seemed nonplussed, confirmed that his mother was correct, and acknowledged that he had fabricated the Vietnam and PTSD history. He would not engage in further discussion of his hospitalization or his story. The other patients on the ward continued to support John and were indignant that his doctors questioned the veracity of his story (despite John's public admission of its invention). His wife was confused. He continued to be superficially pleasant and cooperative on the ward until he was released from the hospital and the military. He received no disability, returned to his wife's hometown, and was lost to follow-up at that time.

Many factors can suggest a diagnosis of factitious disorder (Freyberger et al. 1994; Popli et al. 1992). There can be discrepancies between objective findings, such as differences between oral and rectal temperatures. Objective findings might be inconsistent with clinical history or symptoms, as in the preceding case example or when mixed bowel flora is isolated from "spontaneous" skin lesions. Illness course could be markedly atypical, or the condition can fail to respond as expected to usual therapies, as demonstrated by erratic blood sugars or failure of wounds to heal. A patient may be unusually acquiescent to invasive diagnostic studies or may be unusually quarrelsome and argumentative with staff, particularly when it comes to trying to obtain old records to confirm history. A patient who describes a flamboyant, fascinating life with connections to well-known people may have no visitors or callers.

Verification of the diagnostic criteria, however, can be problematic. The patient must be feigning illness. The physician becomes a detective, working against the patient's overt desires, trying to discover the ruse. This role shift destabilizes the relationship (Duffy 1993; Paar 1994). Some patients may have combinations of feigned and actual illness (Nordmeyer 1994; Sutherland and Rodin 1990). The patient may develop an actual illness in the attempt to simulate one. An example is the ambulance attendant who repeatedly infected her surgical incision with fecal material; with worsening infections and continued antibiotic treatment, she developed kidney failure (Feldman and Ford 1994). Similarly, the patient who has had multiple abdominal surgeries for factitious causes may develop adhesions that require surgical intervention.

The feigning must be intentional. Psychoses (Gielder 1994), mood disorders (Roy and Roy 1995), and dissociative disorders (Goodwin 1988; Toth and Baggaley 1991) need to be ruled out as alternative etiologies. In an adversarial physician-patient relationship, the hunt for intentionality raises ethical and legal issues of informed consent, right to privacy, and malpractice (Frumkin and Victoroff 1990; Houck 1992; Markantonakis and Lee 1988; Powell and Boast 1993a). Almost by definition, patients with factitious disorders deny their simulations, and intention is often inferred rather than proved (Dixon and Abbey 1995).

The patients' motivation must be "to assume the sick role" (American Psychiatric Association 1994). Yet such patients are usually unaware of their motivations, despite being aware of their role in producing their illness (Bhugra 1988; Eisendrath 1996). Patients can be extremely resistant to psychological inquiry or prematurely may leave the hospital (Bauer and Boegner 1996), rendering psychological motivational assessment incomplete (Baker and Major 1994; Churchill et al. 1994; Harrington et al. 1990; Topazian and Binder 1994). Motivations may be multiple and mixed (Rogers et al. 1989), with clear secondary gains coexisting with less conscious ones (Lawrie et al. 1993). Nonetheless, thorough attempts must be made to investigate and clarify the motivational factors operative in the patients (e.g., Feldman and Russell 1991; Feldman et al. 1994).

The notion of the sick role is complex. Some authors see it as a psychological position in which the patient receives overt empathic support and is subject to overtly reduced expectations; that is, the sick role is a nonpathological mode of functioning that the factitious disorder patient adopts for pathological reasons. Others see the sick role of the factitious disorder patient as inherently

pathological. Plassmann (1994b) sees it in terms of the patient's "disturbed relationship to his or her own body" combined with a "seriously disturbed doctor-patient relationship." Spivak et al. (1994) similarly describe "disturbances in the sense of self and in the sense of reality."

Another factor complicating the diagnosis is the high prevalence of comorbid disorders (Sutherland and Rodin 1990). Substance use disorders (Bauer and Boegner 1996; Burge and Lacey 1993; Harrington et al. 1990; Kent 1994; McDaniel et al. 1992; Parker 1993; Popli et al. 1992), personality disorders (particularly borderline and antisocial) (Bauer and Boegner 1996; Nadelson 1979; Overholser 1990; Parker 1993), malingering (W. F. Gorman and Winograd 1988; Harrington et al. 1990), dissociative disorders (Goodwin 1988; Toth and Baggaley 1991), eating disorders (Burge and Lacey 1993; McDaniel et al. 1992), and suicidality and mood disorders (Earle and Folkes 1986; Gielder 1994; Paar 1994; Roy and Roy 1995; Sutherland and Rodin 1990) may coexist. The comorbidities can overwhelm the diagnostic picture, and the diagnosis can be ignored altogether (Roy and Roy 1995; Toth and Baggaley 1991).

There are no diagnostic tests for factitious disorders. Psychological testing may reflect comorbid conditions (Babe et al. 1992) or in cases of factitious disorder with predominantly psychological signs and symptoms may give "fake bad" or invalid results (Zimmerman et al. 1991). Such results are not pathognomonic but of the same order as spurious thermometer readings in cases of factitious fever. Neuroimaging studies are explained in the following discussion.

EPIDEMIOLOGY

Data on incidence and prevalence rates for the factitious disorders are difficult to gather, vary considerably, and must be viewed with a critical eye. The covert nature of the disorder can lead to missed diagnosis and underestimation of rates or, conversely, to the same case being counted twice (Duffy 1992, 1993; Ifudu and Friedman 1993; Ifudu et al. 1992) and inflating apparent rates. There even has been one "case," humorously invented and reported by its physician authors, that was accepted and cited in the literature as genuine (Feldman 1992; Gurwith and Langston 1992). Most studies have used the form of simulated illness typology. Sutherland and Rodin (1990) diagnosed factitious disorder in 0.8% of all psychiatric consultation-liaison service referrals of medical or surgical inpatients. Bhugra (1988) found 0.5% of psychiatric admissions to have Munchausen syndrome. Ballas (1996) found that

0.9% of patients in a sickle-cell program could have factitious disorder, type unspecified. Bauer and Boegner (1996) diagnosed 0.3% of neurological admissions with factitious disorders. Others (Eisendrath 1996) have reported rates between approximately 2% and 10%, with the higher rates in case series of fevers of unknown origin.

ETIOLOGY

Psychodynamic explanations for these paradoxical disorders have been provided by several authors. Many have noted the apparent prevalence of histories of early childhood physical or sexual abuse, with disturbed parental relationships and emotional deprivation. Histories of early illness or extended hospitalizations also have been noted. Nadelson (1985) conceptualizes factitious disorder as a manifestation of borderline character pathology rather than as an isolated clinical syndrome. The patient becomes both the "victim and victimizer" by garnering medical attention from physicians and other health care workers while defying and devaluing them. Projection of hostility and worthlessness onto the caretaker occurs as he or she is both desired and rejected. Plassmann (1994b, 1994c) views the disorders as a "symptom of a psychic problem complex." Early traumas are dealt with narcissistically and through dissociation, denial, and a type of projection. The patient's body, or part of the body, becomes perceived as an external object or as a fused, symbiotic combination of self and object, which then comes to represent negative affects (hate, fear, pain), the associated negative object concepts, and negative self-concepts. In the face of early deprivation and assaults, the "body-self" is split off to preserve the "psychic self" (Hirsch 1994). When subsequent life events activate these affects or concepts, the result is extreme anxiety and growing derealization. Eventually, the patient acts out or involves the medical system in a type of countertransference identification, which results in manipulations of the body of the patient. The manipulation results in emotional relief, albeit transient and incomplete, in the manner of most repetitious compromises.

Neuropathological bases for the disorders also have been suggested, based on abnormal single photon emission computed tomography (SPECT) scans (Lawrie et al. 1993; Mountz et al. 1996), computed tomography (CT) abnormalities (Babe et al. 1992), and magnetic resonance imaging (MRI) abnormalities (Fenelon et al. 1991). No consistent findings have yet been reported. Intriguing, however, is the suggestion that pseudologia fantastica may be a syndrome related to, but distinct from, factitious disorders with its own associated pathology (Abed 1995; Mountz et al. 1996)

Many cases of factitious disorder are chronic (Sutherland and Rodin 1990; Zimmerman et al. 1991); the stressor of recurrent object loss, or fear of loss, occurs over and over in the literature as an antecedent of a factitious episode (Ballard and Stoudemire 1992; Linde 1996; Rothchild 1994; Songer 1995). For example, Carney (1980) found that 74% of his factitious disorder patients experienced severe sexual or marital stress prior to the development of factitious signs or symptoms.

TREATMENT

Once the diagnosis is suspected, it is essential to examine the treatment team for countertransference reactions. Plassmann (1994b) sees the patient's ability to induce a countertransference identification in the physician as a core of the disorder, and several authors (Amirault 1995; Freyberger et al. 1994; Kalivas 1996) see the physician's countertransference feelings as partially diagnostic for the disorder. In general medical settings, examining countertransference reactions usually means obtaining psychiatric consultation (Stotland 1989) involving the entire treatment team of physicians, nurses, ethics and risk management committees, and others (Eisendrath and Feder 1996). In psychiatric settings, the examination may call for some additional reflection on the case, a treatment planning conference if on an inpatient unit, or a discussion with a clinical consultant or with colleagues. As Feldman and Feldman (1995) describe, countertransference can lead to a number of adverse consequences. "Therapeutic nihilism" on the part of the treatment system may lead to an unexamined assumption that the patient cannot or should not be treated, with subsequent failure to diagnose or refer (Bhugra 1988; Toth and Baggaley 1991). "Anger and aversion" can rupture any therapeutic alliance, undermine the unity of a treatment team, or lead to punitive acting out against the patient. Genuine comorbid or concomitant illness may be ignored (Lewis 1993; Powell and Boast 1993a). Breaches of confidentiality may ensue in the diagnostic hunt or in the supposed effort to "warn" colleagues (see Markantonakis and Lee 1988; Powell and Boast 1993a). Overidentification with the patient or activation of rescue fantasies can sabotage treatment efforts and as Willenberg (1994) warns can reinforce the patient's internal splitting and actually support continued factitious behaviors.

As discussed previously, the diagnosis must be confirmed. Erroneous diagnosis of a factitious disorder can result in its own trauma and may be perpetuated in medical records (Feldman and Ford 1994; Guziec et al. 1994). However, Teasell and Shapiro (1994) argue against the necessity of accurate diagnosis once the contribution of general medical illness has been factored out. The patient then must be informed generally of a change in treatment plan, and an attempt must be made to enlist him or her in that plan. The literature generally refers to this process (perhaps alluding to its countertransference aspects) as containing an element of "confrontation." There is now general agreement that treatment begins at this point, and that it is best done indirectly, with minimal expectation that the patient "confess" or acknowledge the deception. It is a delicate process, with patients frequently leaving the hospital against medical advice or otherwise leaving treatment (Baile et al. 1992; Baker and Major 1994; Ballas 1996; Songer 1995). Guziec et al. (1994) aptly liken this process to making a psychodynamic interpretation. Eisendrath (1989) describes techniques for reducing confrontation, including the use of inexact interpretations, therapeutic double binds, and face-saving techniques to engage the patient in treatment.

Some authors recommend inpatient psychiatric hospitalization, often involuntary (Aduan et al. 1979; Plassmann 1994a; Powell and Boast 1993b). However, many (Ballard and Stoudemire 1992; Guziec et al. 1994; Parker 1993; Rothchild 1994; Spivak et al. 1994; Teasell and Shapiro 1994, among others) describe treatment being initiated in the general medical inpatient setting where the factitious disorder has been diagnosed and continuing in the psychiatric outpatient setting. Whereas the patient with Munchausen syndrome is regarded as less likely to engage in treatment (Eisendrath 1989; Stotland 1989), and the nonprototypical factitious disorder patient is seen as generally more available for intervention, there are case reports of Munchausen syndrome patients responding favorably to treatment (Parker 1993; Rothchild 1994; Spivak et al. 1994).

There have been no comparative studies of different therapeutic approaches, but several different techniques have been described. Regardless of modality, treatment must be collaborative and must involve some level of communication among all of the patient's treatment providers (Eisendrath and Feder 1996; Feldman and Duval 1997; Higgins 1990). The psychodynamic approach to treatment (Plassmann 1994a; Spivak et al. 1994) generally focuses not on the factitious behaviors themselves but on the underlying dynamic issues, with the therapist taking a neutral stance toward the factitious nature of the behaviors. Strategic-behavioral approaches also have been used (Solyom and Solyom 1990; Teasell and Shapiro 1994), implementing standard behavioral techniques as well as the therapeutic double bind, which requires the patient to abandon the target factitious behaviors. In one particularly intractable

case, Schwarz et al. (1993) used a unique combination strategy involving weekly psychotherapy provided by the primary care physician and a carefully designed paradoxical unrestricted hospital admission policy to control factitious behavior. When used, pharmacotherapy targets specific symptoms, such as depression or transient psychosis, or comorbid disorders.

The treatment of factitious disorders is not without its pitfalls. In addition to the challenges of diagnosis and countertransference, there are significant medicolegal issues to be considered, both in the malpractice and workers' compensation arenas. Houck (1992) provides a thorough review, and Janofsky (1994) discusses several forensic cases.

There have been insufficient studies to address conclusively the prognostic factors in factitious disorder, but the case literature is certainly ample and implies that the factitious disorder patient, although requiring considerable therapeutic skill, may be approached with a cautious hope for improvement (Feldman 1992; Mayo and Haggerty 1984).

FACTITIOUS DISORDER BY PROXY

Meadow (1977), the British pediatrician, described another scenario involving factitious illness. He presented his observations on a number of cases in each of which a mother had fabricated illness in her infant child, not in herself. Concealing the fabrication, the mother then presented the child for medical care, resulting in extensive, often invasive, evaluations and examinations of the child. The mother seemed to be concerned and caring, perhaps overly so. Despite the outward appearance of being concerned and caring, the mother continued to fabricate illness in her child. Meadow coined the term "Munchausen syndrome by proxy" (MSBP) to describe such scenarios. The children in these situations may be subject to considerable and prolonged morbidity, with a mortality of approximately 10% (Rosenberg 1987; Schreier and Libow 1993b). As Schreier and Libow (1993a) write, "With the exception perhaps of incest, this simultaneously long-term, close-yet-destructive relationship between perpetrator and victim has no parallel in human psychology" (p. 53). Since the last edition of this textbook, there has been a continued expansion of the medical literature about this type of fabricated illness, with the publication of lay and professional books on the topic (Brownlee 1996; Feldman and Eisendrath 1996; Levin and Sheridan 1995; Schreier and Libow 1993a; Schreier and Libow 1996).

CLASSIFICATION

DSM-IV provides research criteria for factitious disorder by proxy (FBP) in the appendix "Criteria Sets and Axes Provided for Further Study" (American Psychiatric Association 1994). The criteria are similar to those for factitious disorder, with the addition of the "by proxy" specification (see Table 17–3). However, much of the literature retains the use of the eponym Munchausen syndrome by proxy, and there is considerable debate about the notion of proxy-fabricated illness (see Fisher and Mitchell 1995; Meadow 1995b; Morley 1995).

The debate revolves around four questions:

1. Does the syndrome require child abuse to have occurred?
2. Does the syndrome pertain to the diagnosis of an individual (implying some degree of homogeneous individual psychopathology), or does it pertain to a situation (without homogeneous psychopathology in the fabricator)?
3. Does the syndrome require an attribution or determination of the fabricator's primary motivation, and if so, what is the nature of that motivation?
4. Does the conferring of a psychiatric diagnosis mitigate the fabricator's responsibility for egregious behavior?

In DSM-IV, FBP describes a mental disorder in an individual who is specifically motivated to attain the sick role through someone else who is under that individual's care. Technically, since FBP is a research diagnosis, an individual meeting FBP criteria would actually be diagnosed with factitious disorder NOS. The proxy, if psychiatrically diagnosed, could receive different diagnoses, depending on the circumstances and the proxy's psychiatric symptomatology (American Psychiatric Association 1994).

Meadow (1995b) uses MSBP to refer to a particular

TABLE 17–3.   **DSM-IV research criteria for factitious disorder by proxy**

A. Intentional production or feigning of physical or psychological signs or symptoms in another person who is under the individual's care.

B. The motivation for the perpetrator's behavior is to assume the sick role by proxy.

C. External incentives for the behavior (such as economic gain) are absent.

D. The behavior is not better accounted for by another mental disorder.

form of child abuse characterized by a particular behavior and attitude on the part of the mother and would reserve FBP as an individual diagnosis were one needed. MSBP is something a mother commits, not a disorder she has (Meadow 1995a). Bools (1996) sees the attempt to label the perpetrator of child abuse with any new diagnosis as "(pseudo) psychiatric" and reserves either term to describe a situation of child abuse. Other authors similarly use the terms to refer to situations of abuse (Blix and Brack 1988; Donald and Jureidini 1996; Fisher and Mitchell 1995; Rosenberg 1996).

Schreier and Libow (1993a) do not insist that statutory child abuse be present, although they acknowledge that it usually is. They apply the term MSBP to describe a disorder in the fabricator who has a specific and particular primary motivation, which is "the mother's intense need to be in a relationship with doctors and/or hospitals. The child is used to gain and maintain this contact" (p. 13). This motivation is a true perversion in the analytical sense of the term (Schreier 1992). Schreier's more recent writing (1996) agrees with the broadened DSM-IV criteria that include perpetrators who fabricate with a proxy in order to build "a highly manipulative relationship with a powerful transferential figure," specifically "professionals who occupy positions of power in society," not just physicians.

Ford (1996) argues that the fabricator should receive no syndrome-related diagnosis for the factitious behavior out of concern that diagnosis may provide a legal defense for behavior he views as predominantly criminal. Uniquely, however, he would use the diagnosis factitious disorder NOS to apply to the proxy-victim.

DSM-IV criteria allow the proxy to be other than a child and the caregiver other than the mother. Although the overwhelming majority of cases involve mother and child (McClure et al. 1996), instances have been described wherein the proxies are able-bodied adults or hospital and nursing home patients and wherein the perpetrators are fathers, other relatives, baby-sitters, partners, and health care professionals or paraprofessionals (Chantada et al. 1994; Makar and Squier 1990; Repper 1995; Sigal et al. 1986; Yorker 1996a).

In the following discussions, we use the term FBP, as equivalent to MSBP, rely primarily on the DSM-IV research criteria, and use the paradigm of the mother perpetrator and the child proxy-victim.

DIAGNOSIS

Certain clusters of warning signs can suggest a diagnosis of FBP (see Table 17–4). Another diagnostic indicator, described by Szajnberg et al. (1996), is a particular type of

TABLE 17–4. Warning signs of factitious disorder by proxy

- The parent has taken the child to numerous caregivers, resulting in multiple diagnostic evaluations but neither cure nor definitive diagnosis.
- The parent seems overly attentive to or overly involved in the child's medical care or with the medical staff.
- The other parent (usually the father) is notably uninvolved.
- The parent seems less concerned than the physicians or medical staff about painful or risky diagnostic tests for the child.
- The child persistently fails to tolerate or respond to usual medical therapies.
- Signs and symptoms abate or do not occur when the child is separated from the parent.
- Another child in the family has had unexplained illness or childhood death.
- The parent has a history of factitious disorder or unusual obstetrical complications.

Source. Adapted from Bools et al. 1992; Jani et al. 1992; Jureidini 1993; Libow 1995; R. Meadow 1982; Schreier and Libow 1996.

countertransference that the clinician experiences, even in cases in which the illness fabrication has been proven: "the clinician has a recurrent, uncanny, ego-dystonic, and uncomfortable sense of *disbelief* that this parent has perpetrated his or her child's symptoms and illness" (p. 230). They recommend that two clinicians be present during a diagnostic FBP interview: one to conduct the interview and the other to observe the interpersonal process.

Verification of the DSM-IV diagnosis is a process fraught with the same type of difficulties mentioned in the discussion of factitious disorder earlier in this chapter. The mother's motivation must be determined (Kahan and Yorker 1991; Morley 1995; Schreier 1996), and any motivation other than attaining the sick role by proxy must be ruled out (Bools 1996; Meadow 1995b). Also required is the determination that the mother is intentionally fabricating the child's illness. Because child abuse is a crime, proving the fabrication becomes a forensic process rather than a clinical medical investigation (Yorker 1996b). Various techniques have been used, including covert video surveillance in the hospital (Byard and Burnell 1994; Lacey et al. 1993; Samuels et al. 1992), searching rooms and belongings (Ford 1996; Ostfeld and Feldman 1996), and special handling of laboratory specimens (Kahan and Yorker 1991). Some of these techniques raise obvious legal and ethical issues that must be resolved before their implementation (Evans 1995; Ford 1996; Samuels et al. 1992). Once the fabrication is identified, the intentionality usually

readily is inferred, given the amount of premeditation that is required, for example, to suffocate repeatedly (Samuels et al. 1992), poison (McClure et al. 1996), or inject (Sigal et al. 1990) the proxy-victim.

The ability of the mother with FBP to deceive and to appear to be a caring, concerned parent can be astounding. In one case, the mother confessed to poisoning repeatedly two of her children with salt but was "so convincing in her performance that local authorities were reported as digging up pipes in the street looking for contamination" (Coombe 1995, p. 195), presumably of the water supply. Video surveillance has shown clearly how the "caring" is a performance; when the mother thinks she is unobserved, she gives the child minimal attention (Samuels et al. 1992).

The cautions against making a false-positive diagnosis of factitious disorder apply to FBP as well (Barker and Howell 1994; Meadow 1995b; Schreier and Libow 1994). Added to these risks is that of making false criminal accusations with adverse results for the involved family (Schreier and Libow 1993a). There is even an organization that has been formed to "stop the assault on innocent mothers (or fathers) from MSBP accusations" (Mothers Against Munchausen Syndrome by Proxy Allegations 1997).

Once FBP has been diagnosed, it is important to assess the entire family, including the proxy. Other children also may be proxies, other family members may be participating in the factitious behavior, and the proxy himself or herself may be actively cooperating with the fabrications (Alexander et al. 1990; Rand 1996; Sanders 1995; Smith and Ardern 1989).

EPIDEMIOLOGY

The prevalence of FBP is unknown, but one study estimates 2.8 cases per 100,000 children age 1 year or younger or 0.5 cases per 100,000 children age 16 years or younger (McClure et al. 1996). Among select populations, such as in cases of fevers of unknown origin (Chantada et al. 1994), against medical advice discharges (Jani et al. 1992), or pediatric specialty registers (Schreier and Libow 1993b), the rates may be higher. The child typically is age 2 or 3 years at diagnosis (Donald and Jureidini 1996; Yorker and Kahan 1990). Length of time from onset of symptoms in the child to diagnosis can vary widely, averaging 15 months (± 14 months) in one series (Rosenberg 1987) to undetected in another (Libow 1995). Methods are legion, but smothering, poisoning, and fabricated history of seizures are most commonly reported (McClure et al. 1996). In the majority of cases, however, multiple methods have been employed to fabricate a variety of illnesses in the child (Bools et al. 1992). In 25%–45% of cases, another sibling has been a proxy-victim as well (Alexander et al. 1990).

A substantial minority (i.e., greater than would be expected in a general population sample but still the minority) of the mothers have connections to the health professions (Ostfeld and Feldman 1996), have received prior psychiatric attention (Alexander et al. 1990; Samuels et al. 1992), or have indications of preexisting factitious disorder themselves (Meadow 1982). Actual psychosis is rare (Bools 1996). No consistent profile on psychological testing has been shown (Rand 1996). In contrast to factitious disorder, the most common comorbid psychiatric disorder in FBP is narcissistic personality disorder (Schreier 1992), and substance use disorders are less commonly reported.

ETIOLOGY

Most authors see the maternal pathology arising from childhood roots, characterized by "quietly traumatic" emotional neglect and abandonment. Some descriptions of the hypothesized childhood deficits suggest that they occur later than those hypothesized to result in factitious disorder, whereas other authors see the dynamics as more similar (Schreier and Libow 1993a; Sigal et al. 1988). Others have emphasized the role of modern medicine, with its predilection for invasive and aggressive diagnostic testing, in the etiology of the syndrome (Donald and Jureidini 1996). Schreier and Libow (1993a) have written extensively on the etiological hypotheses.

TREATMENT

Mothers diagnosed with FBP are universally regarded as very resistant and difficult to treat (Schreier and Libow 1994). Some of the difficulty stems from the mothers' massive use of denial and projective identification (Coombe 1995; Feldman 1994b; Schreier 1992). Another source stems from the process by which treatment is usually initiated. Experience with treatment of factitious disorder patients has shown that an indirect, nonconfrontational approach is most effective and that some continuing of the factitious behavior is to be expected during the course of treatment. In treating FBP patients, because of the necessity to protect the proxy, an indirect approach permitting continued factitious behavior is not possible. The first stage of treatment in FBP usually begins with the involvement of child protection authorities, the initiation of legal proceedings against the parent, and the removal of the child from the home.

The few cases of continued treatment of FBP that have been described note the necessity of coordinating multidisciplinary, multiagency involvement (Coombe 1995; Lyons-Ruth et al. 1991; Smith and Ardern 1989). Individual treatment is long-term psychotherapy (group, individual, or combined), and focuses on helping the mother express feelings and needs for support and recognition more directly, with less use of projection and a development of empathic capacity (Coombe 1995; Lyons-Ruth et al. 1991). As with the treatment of factitious disorder patients, the factitious behavior is rarely the primary focus. Pharmacotherapy is used only to treat comorbid conditions.

In the absence of effective treatment, prognosis is poor, with a high likelihood of continued FBP behavior (Bools et al. 1993, 1994; Libow 1995; Meadow 1993). Management of FBP patients is usually coordinated and directed through the legal system, and protection of the child is priority (Brady 1994; Kahan and Yorker 1991; Ostfeld and Feldman 1996).

MALINGERING

CLASSIFICATION

Malingering is usually considered to occur infrequently. Experienced clinicians report rates of an estimated 16% in forensic examinations and of an estimated 7% in nonforensic clinical settings (Rogers et al. 1994). However, nonclinical examples abound. Almost everyone has malingered an illness at some time in his or her life: as children, most have feigned a headache or stomachache to avoid going to school. In DSM-IV, malingering is classified under "Other Conditions That May Be a Focus of Clinical Attention," the V codes, and is not considered to be a mental disorder or a psychiatric illness (American Psychiatric Association 1994). It is defined as

> the intentional production of false or grossly exaggerated physical or psychological symptoms, motivated by external incentives such as avoiding military duty, avoiding work, obtaining financial compensation, evading criminal prosecution, or obtaining drugs. Under some circumstances, Malingering may represent adaptive behavior—for example, feigning illness while a captive of the enemy during wartime. (American Psychiatric Association 1994, p. 683)

In malingering, as differentiated from factitious disorders, the motivation for the symptom production is an external incentive; the goal is something *other* than attaining the sick role. In contrast to somatoform disorders and conversion disorder, malingering involves the awareness of intentional feigning of symptoms. The term *malingering by proxy* also has been suggested (Bools 1996) for those cases in which illness is fabricated in a child for secondary gain (e.g., for the purpose of obtaining social assistance benefits).

Diagnostic confusion between malingering and other mental disorders, particularly factitious disorders, can be traced to Asher's (1951) original description of Munchausen syndrome. He attributed several possible motives for Munchausen syndrome, including "a desire to escape from the police" and "a desire to get free board and lodgings for the night" (Asher 1951, p. 339), motives that would now clearly classify feigned illness behavior as malingering. The tendency to include malingering within the factitious disorders spectrum was further reinforced by Spiro (1968), who recommended that in individuals with Munchausen syndrome, "malingering should only be diagnosed in the absence of psychiatric illness and the presence of behavior appropriately adaptive to a clear-cut long-term goal" (p. 569). There are, however, many examples of patients with factitious disorder who also malinger (see Diagnosis section of Factitious Disorder section earlier in this chapter).

The term *malingering* describes or attributes motivation to someone's behavior or set of behaviors in a particular environmental context. In this necessary linkage to circumstances and life events, it is most akin to the adjustment disorders. Whether it is deemed adaptive or dysfunctional often depends on the observer's perspective. The prisoner of war feigning illness to avoid torture or to effect an escape may be regarded as clever and courageous, whereas the conscientious objector feigning illness to avoid military duty may be regarded as a maladaptive coward (for more examples, see Cappucci and Flemming 1994; Sung et al. 1995; Witztum et al. 1996).

DIAGNOSIS

Essentially all authors note the potential difficulty of detecting malingering. As in the factitious disorders, the first task of the physician is to ensure that a true medical or psychiatric cause for the symptoms is not overlooked. A thorough, unbiased, and well-planned evaluation must be performed. Witztum et al. (1996) describe a number of military inductees, erroneously diagnosed as malingerers, in whom diagnoses of severe psychiatric disorders were missed because of assessment problems. They also note, as do DuAlba and Scott (1993), the important role of cross-cultural issues in the assessment of malingering.

Nonetheless, there are clinical warning signs for malingering (see Table 17–5). Yudofsky (1991) emphasizes that these signs are not *diagnostic*, as they may be present in

other situations as well. Rogers (1990) also cautions against the uncritical application of such indicators, noting, for example, that psychotic patients are more frequently uncooperative than malingerers and that there is limited evidence for the association between antisocial personality disorder and malingering. Many strategies have been proposed to attempt clinical detection of deception (Annon 1988; Nordmeyer 1994; Wallach 1994). Resnick (1993) gives some clinical clues and interview techniques for the detection of malingered psychosis and other disorders. Table 17–6 lists guidelines on how to approach possible malingerers.

Should specific testing be desired to diagnose malingering, such testing should generally include "multiple measures and methodologies" (Nies and Sweet 1994) to enhance diagnostic reliability. Testing may include structured interviewing (Rogers et al. 1991), symptom validity testing or other forced-choice techniques (Fautek 1995; Pankratz and Erickson 1990), physiological techniques (Annon 1988), and specific neuropsychological testing performed by a knowledgeable neuropsychologist (Annon 1988; Fauteck 1995; Lees-Haley and Fox 1990; Nies and Sweet 1994).

TABLE 17–5.   Warning signs of malingering

- Symptoms are vague, ill defined, and do not conform to discrete diagnostic entities.
- Complaints, signs, or symptoms seem excessive or overdramatized.
- Injuries appear to be self-inflicted.
- Unexplained toxic substances or unprescribed medications are detected in drug screens.
- Medical records or diagnostic data appear to have been altered or tampered with.
- There is a history of recurrent injuries or accidents.
- History, physical examination, and diagnostic data do not support complaints.
- The patient is uncooperative in the diagnostic evaluation or treatment.
- The patient is reluctant to accept a favorable prognosis.
- The patient requests addicting or commonly abused drugs to treat the disorder.
- The patient derives financial compensation or other gain as a result of the disorder.
- The patient is able to avoid painful, dangerous, anxiety-producing, or otherwise unpleasant situations as a result of the disorder.
- The patient is able to avoid legal or social responsibilities or to evade legal penalties as a result of the disorder.
- There is a concomitant diagnosis of antisocial personality disorder.

Source.   Adapted from Yudofsky 1991.

TABLE 17–6. **Tips on evaluating suspected malingering**

- Do not let your subjective confidence in your diagnostic acumen be your guide.
- Consider the strength of the examinee's motive to deceive.
- Do not depend on interview results and the physical examination alone to exclude malingering.
- Obtain collateral and corroborative information.
- Consider specific testing designed to detect malingering.

Source. Adapted from Faust 1995.

TREATMENT

Although "treatment" for a nondisorder seems odd, several authors describe the potential usefulness of helping malingerers develop alternate coping skills (Rabinowitz et al. 1990; Yudofsky 1991). Pankratz and Erickson (1990) stress the importance of allowing the malingerer to save face, and it seems likely that some of the techniques employed in the treatment of the factitious disorder patient (discussed earlier in this chapter) also could be used with the malingerer. Finally, many of Houck's (1992) warnings about the medicolegal pitfalls in the assessment and treatment of the patient with a factitious disorder also apply to the assessment, treatment, and disposition of the malingerer.

REFERENCES

Abed RT: Voluntary false confessions in a Munchausen patient: a new variant of the syndrome? Irish Journal of Psychological Medicine 12:24–26, 1995

Aduan RP, Fauci AS, Dale DC, et al: Factitious fever and self-induced infection: a report of 32 cases and review of the literature. Ann Intern Med 90:230–242, 1979

Alexander R, Smith W, Stevenson R: Serial Munchausen syndrome by proxy. Pediatrics 86:581–585, 1990

American Psychiatric Association: Diagnostic and Statistical Manual of Mental Disorders, 4th Edition. Washington, DC, American Psychiatric Association, 1994

Amirault C: Pseudologica fantastica and other tall tales: the contagious literature of Munchausen syndrome. Lit Med 14:169–190, 1995

Annon JS: Detection of deception and search for truth: a proposed model with particular reference to the witness, the victim, and the defendant. Forensic Reports 1:303–360, 1988

Asher R: Munchausen's syndrome. Lancet 1:339–341, 1951

Babe KS Jr, Peterson AM, Loosen PT, et al: The pathogenesis of Munchausen syndrome: a review and case report. Gen Hosp Psychiatry 14:273–276, 1992

Baile WF, Kuehn CV, Straker D: Factitious cancer. Psychosomatics 33:100–105, 1992

Baker CE, Major E: Munchausen's syndrome: a case presenting as asthma requiring ventilation. Anaesthesia 49:1050–1051, 1994

Ballard RS, Stoudemire A: Factitious apraxia. Int J Psychiatry Med 22:275–280, 1992

Ballas SK: Factitious sickle-cell acute painful episodes: a secondary type of Munchausen-syndrome. Am J Hematol 53:254–258, 1996

Barker JP: The syndrome of hospital addiction (Munchausen syndrome): a report on the investigation of seven cases. Journal of Mental Sciences 108:107–182, 1962

Barker LH, Howell RJ: Munchausen syndrome by proxy in false allegations of child sexual abuse: legal implications. Bulletin of the American Academy of Psychiatry and the Law 22:499–510, 1994

Bauer M, Boegner F: Neurological syndromes in factitious disorder. J Nerv Ment Dis 184:281–288, 1996

Bhugra D: Psychiatric Munchausen's syndrome: literature review with case reports. Acta Psychiatr Scand 77:497–503, 1988

Blix S, Brack G: The effects of a suspected case of Munchausen's syndrome by proxy on a pediatric nursing staff. Gen Hosp Psychiatry 10:402–409, 1988

Bools C: Factitious illness by proxy; Munchausen syndrome by proxy. Br J Psychiatry 169:268–275, 1996

Bools CN, Neale BA, Meadow SR: Co-morbidity associated with fabricated illness (Munchausen syndrome by proxy). Arch Dis Child 67:77–79, 1992

Bools CN, Neale BA, Meadow SR: Follow up of victims of fabricated illness (Munchausen syndrome by proxy). Arch Dis Child 69:625–630, 1993

Bools C, Neale B, Meadow R: Munchausen syndrome by proxy: a study of psychopathology. Child Abuse Negl 18:773–788, 1994

Brady MM: Munchausen syndrome by proxy: how should we weigh our options? Law and Psychology Review 18:361–375, 1994

Brownlee S: Mother love betrayed: a rare psychiatric disorder turns parents into tormenters (http://www.usnews.com/usnews/issue/munch.htm). U.S. News and World Report, April 29, 1996

Burge CK, Lacey JH: A case of Munchausen's syndrome in anorexia nervosa. Int J Eat Disord 14:379–381, 1993

Byard RW, Burnell RH: Covert video surveillance in Munchausen syndrome by proxy: ethical compromise or essential technique? Med J Aust 160:352–356, 1994

Cappucci DT Jr, Flemming SL: Medical observations of malingering in Iraqi enemy prisoners of war during Operation Desert Storm. Mil Med 159:462–464, 1994

Carney MWP: Artefactual illness to attract medical attention. Br J Psychiatry 136:542–547, 1980

Chantada G, Casak S, Plata JD, et al: Children with fever of unknown origin in Argentina: an analysis of 113 cases. Pediatr Infect Dis J 13:260–263, 1994

Churchill DR, De Cock KM, Miller RF: Feigned HIV infection/AIDS: malingering and Munchausen's syndrome. Genitourin Med 70:314–316, 1994

Clark EJ, Melnich SC: Munchausen's syndrome or the problem of hospital hoboes. Am J Med 25:6–12, 1958

Clinical Case Conference. N Engl J Med 311:108–115, 1984

Coombe P: The inpatient psychotherapy of a mother and child at the Cassel hospital: a case of Munchausen's syndrome by proxy. British Journal of Psychotherapy 12:195–207, 1995

Craddock N, Brown N: Munchausen syndrome presenting as mental handicap. Mental Handicap Research 6:184–190, 1993

Dixon D, Abbey S: Cupid's arrow: an unusual presentation of factitious disorder. Psychosomatics 36:502–504, 1995

Donald T, Jureidini J: Munchausen syndrome by proxy: child abuse in the medical system. Arch Pediatr Adolesc Med 150:753–758, 1996

DuAlba L, Scott RL: Somatization and malingering for workers' compensation applicants: a cross-cultural MMPI study. J Clin Psychol 49:913–917, 1993

Duffy TP: The red baron. N Engl J Med 327:408–411, 1992

Duffy TP: Kidney-related Munchausens-syndrome and the red baron. N Engl J Med 328:61–62, 1993

Earle JR Jr, Folks DG: Factitious disorder and coexisting depression: a report of successful psychiatric consultation and case management. Gen Hosp Psychiatry 8:448–450, 1986

Eisendrath SJ: Factitious physical disorders: treatment without confrontation. Psychosomatics 30:383–387, 1989

Eisendrath SJ: Current overview of factitious physical disorders, in The Spectrum of Factitious Disorders. Edited by Feldman MD, Eisendrath SJ. Washington, DC, American Psychiatric Press, 1996, pp 21–36

Eisendrath SJ, Feder A: Management of factitious disorders, in The Spectrum of Factitious Disorders. Edited by Feldman MD, Eisendrath SJ. Washington, DC, American Psychiatric Press, 1996, pp 195–214

Encarta Multimedia Encyclopedia, 1994 Edition. Redmond, WA, Microsoft Corporation, 1993

Evans D: The investigation of life-threatening child abuse and Munchausen syndrome by proxy. J Med Ethics 21:9–13, 1995

Faust D: The detection of deception. Neurol Clin 13:255–265, 1995

Fauteck PK: Detecting the malingering of psychosis in offenders: no easy solutions. Criminal Justice and Behavior 22:3–18, 1995

Feldman MD: Factitious Munchausen's syndrome: a confession. N Engl J Med 327:438–439, 1992

Feldman MD: The costs of factitious disorders. Psychosomatics 35:506–507, 1994a

Feldman MD: Denial in Munchausen syndrome by proxy: the consulting psychiatrist's dilemma. Int J Psychiatry Med 24:121–128, 1994b

Feldman MD: Dr. Marc Feldman's Munchausen syndrome and factitious disorders page (http://ourworld. compuserve.com/homepages/Marc_Feldman_2/). June 8, 1997

Feldman MD, Duval NJ: Factitious quadriplegia: a rare new case and literature review. Psychosomatics 38:76–80, 1997

Feldman MD, Feldman JM: Tangled in the web: countertransference in the therapy of factitious disorders. Int J Psychiatry Med 25:389–399, 1995

Feldman MD, Ford CV: Patient or Pretender: Inside the Strange World of Factitious Disorders. New York, John Wiley & Sons, 1994

Feldman MD, Russell JL: Factitious cyclic hypersomnia: a new variant of factitious disorder. South Med J 84:379–381, 1991

Feldman MD, Smith R: Personal and interpersonal toll of factitious disorders, in The Spectrum of Factitious Disorders. Edited by Feldman MD, Eisendrath SJ. Washington, DC, American Psychiatric Press 1996, pp 175–194

Feldman MD, Ford CV, Stone T: Deceiving others/deceiving oneself: four cases of factitious rape. South Med J 87: 736–738, 1994

Feldman MD, Eisendrath SJ (eds): The Spectrum of Factitious Disorders. Washington, DC, American Psychiatric Press, 1996

Fenelon G, Mahieux F, Roullet E, et al: Munchausen's syndrome and abnormalities on magnetic resonance imaging of the brain. BMJ 302:996–997, 1991

Fisher GC, Mitchell I: Is Munchausen syndrome by proxy really a syndrome? Arch Dis Child 72:530–534, 1995

Folks DG: Munchausen's syndrome and other factitious disorders. Neurol Clin 13:267–281, 1995

Ford CV: The somatizing disorders. Psychosomatics 27:327–337, 1986

Ford CV: Ethical and legal issues in factitious disorders: an overview, in The Spectrum of Factitious Disorders. Edited by Feldman MD, Eisendrath SJ. Washington, DC, American Psychiatric Press, 1996, pp 51–64

Freyberger H, Nordmeyer JP, Freyberger HJ, et al: Patients suffering from factitious disorders in the clinico-psychosomatic consultation liaison service: psychodynamic processes, psychotherapeutic initial care and clinicointerdisciplinary cooperation. Psychother Psychosom 62:108–122, 1994

Freyberger H, Schneider W: Diagnosis and classification of factitious disorder with operational diagnostic systems. Psychother Psychosom 62:327–337, 1986

Frumkin LR, Victoroff JI: Chronic factitious disorder with symptoms of AIDS. Am J Med 88:694–696, 1990

Gielder U: Factitious disease in the field of dermatology. Psychother Psychosom 62:48–55, 1994

Goodwin J: Munchausen's Syndrome as a dissociative disorder. Dissociation: Progress in the Dissociative Disorders 1:54–60, 1988

Gorman CA, Wahner HW, Tauxe WN: Metabolic malingerers: patients who deliberately induce or perpetuate a hypermetabolic or hypometabolic state. Am J Med 48:708–714, 1970

Gorman WF, Winograd M: Crossing the border from Munchausen to malingering. J Fla Med Assoc 75:147–150, 1988

Gurwith M, Langston C: Factitious Munchausen-syndrome: a confession: reply (letter). N Engl J Med 327:439, 1992

Guziec J, Lazarus A, Harding JJ: Case of a 29-year-old nurse with factitious disorder: the utility of psychiatric intervention on a general medical floor. Gen Hosp Psychiatry 16:47–53, 1994

Harrington WZ, Jackimczyk KC, Seligson RA: Thiopental-facilitated interview in respiratory Munchausen's syndrome. Ann Emerg Med 19:941–942, 1990

Higgins PM: Temporary Munchausen syndrome. Br J Psychiatry 157:613–616, 1990

Hirsch M: The body as a transitional object. Psychother Psychosom 62:78–81, 1994

Houck CA: Medicolegal aspects of factitious disorder. Psychiatric Medicine 10:105–116, 1992

Ifudu O, Friedman EA: Kidney-related Munchausens-syndrome and the red baron (letter). N Engl J Med 328:61, 1993

Ifudu O, Kolasinski SL, Friedman EA: Brief report: kidney-related Munchausen's syndrome. N Engl J Med 327:388–389, 1992

Jani S, White M, Rosenberg LA, et al: Munchausen syndrome by proxy. Int J Psychiatry Med 22:343–349, 1992

Janofsky JS: The Munchausen syndrome in civil forensic psychiatry. Bulletin of the American Academy of Psychiatry and the Law 22:489–497, 1994

Jureidini J: Obstetric factitious disorder and Munchausen syndrome by proxy. J Nerv Ment Dis 181:135–137, 1993

Kahan B, Yorker BC: Munchausen syndrome by proxy: clinical review and legal issues. Behav Sci Law 9:73–83, 1991

Kalivas J: Malingering versus factitious disorder (letter). Am J Psychiatry 153:1108, 1996

Kent JD: Munchausen's syndrome and substance abuse. J Subst Abuse Treat 11:247–251, 1994

Lacey SR, Cooper C, Runyan DK, et al: Munchausen syndrome by proxy: patterns of presentation to pediatric surgeons. J Pediatr Surg 28:827–832, 1993

Lawrie SM, Goodwin G, Masterton G: Munchausen's syndrome and organic brain disorder. Br J Psychiatry 162:545–549, 1993

Lees-Haley PR, Fox DD: MMPI subtle-obvious scales and malingering: clinical versus simulated scores. Psychol Rep 66:907–911, 1990

Levin AV, Sheridan MS (eds): Munchausen Syndrome by Proxy: Issues in Diagnosis and Treatment. New York, Lexington Books, 1995

Lewis EJ: Kidney-related Munchausen's syndrome and the red baron. N Engl J Med 328:60–61, 1993

Libow JA: Munchausen by proxy victims in adulthood: a first look. Child Abuse Negl 19:1131–1142, 1995

Lim LC, Yap HK, Lim JW: Munchausen syndrome by proxy. Journal of the Singapore Paediatric Society 33:59–62, 1991

Linde PR: A bewitching case of factitious disorder in Zimbabwe. Gen Hosp Psychiatry 18:440–443, 1996

Ludwigs U, Ruiz H, Isaksson H, et al: Factitious disorder presenting with acute cardiovascular symptoms. J Intern Med 236:685–690, 1994

Lyons-Ruth K, Kaufman M, Masters N, et al: Issues in the identification and long-term management of Munchausen by proxy syndrome within a clinical infant service. Infant Mental Health Journal 12:309–320, 1991

Makar AF, Squier PJ: Munchausen syndrome by proxy: father as a perpetrator. Pediatrics 85:370–373, 1990

Markantonakis A, Lee AS: Psychiatric Munchausen's syndrome: a college register (letter). Br J Psychiatry 152:867, 1988

Mayo JP Jr, Haggerty J Jr: Long-term psychotherapy of Munchausen syndrome. Am J Psychother 38:571–578, 1984

McClure RJ, Davis PM, Meadow SR, et al: Epidemiology of Munchausen syndrome by proxy, non-accidental poisoning, and non-accidental suffocation. Arch Dis Child 75:57–61, 1996

McDaniel JS, Desoutter L, Firestone S, et al: Factitious disorder resulting in bilateral mastectomies. Gen Hosp Psychiatry 14:355–356, 1992

Meadow R: Munchausen by proxy: the hinterland of child abuse. Lancet 2:343–345, 1977

Meadow R: Munchausen syndrome by proxy. Arch Dis Child 57:92–98, 1982

Meadow R: False allegations of abuse and Munchausen syndrome by proxy. Arch Dis Child 68:444–447, 1993

Meadow R: Munchausen syndrome by proxy. Med Leg J 63:89–104, 1995a

Meadow R: What is, and what is not, 'Munchausen syndrome by proxy'? Arch Dis Child 72:534–538, 1995b

Morley CJ: Practical concerns about the diagnosis of Munchausen syndrome by proxy. Arch Dis Child 72:528–529, 1995

Mothers Against Munchausen Syndrome by Proxy Allegations (MAMA; http://www.mbsp.com/). July 7, 1997

Mountz JM, Parker PE, Liu HG, et al: Tc-99m HMPAO brain SPECT scanning in Munchausen syndrome. J Psychiatry Neurosci 21:49–52, 1996

Nadelson T: The Munchausen spectrum: borderline character features. Gen Hosp Psychiatry 1:11–17, 1979

Nadelson T: The false patient: chronic factitious disease, Munchausen syndrome, and malingering, in Psychiatry, Vol 2. Edited by Cavenar JO, Jr. Philadelphia, PA, JB Lippincott, 1985

Nies KJ, Sweet JJ: Neuropsychological assessment and malingering: a critical review of past and present strategies. Archives of Clinical Neuropsychology 9:501–552, 1994

Nordmeyer JP: An internist's view of patients with factitious disorders and factitious clinical symptomatology. Psychother Psychosom 62:30–40, 1994

Ostfeld BM, Feldman MD: Factitious disorder by proxy: clinical features, detection, and management, in The Spectrum of Factitious Disorders. Edited by Feldman MD, Eisendrath SJ. Washington, DC, American Psychiatric Press, 1996, pp 83–108

Overholser JC: Differential diagnosis of malingering and factitious disorder with physical symptoms. Behav Sci Law 8:55–65, 1990

Paar GH: Factitious disorders in the field of surgery. Psychother Psychosom 62:41–47, 1994

Pankratz L, Erickson RC: Two views of malingering. Clinical Neuropsychologist 4:379–389, 1990

Parker PE: A case report of Munchausen syndrome with mixed psychological features. Psychosomatics 34:360–364, 1993

Plassmann R: Inpatient and outpatient long-term psychotherapy of patients suffering from factitious disorder. Psychother Psychosom 62:96–107, 1994a

Plassmann R: Munchhausen syndromes and factitious diseases. Psychother Psychosom 62:7–26, 1994b

Plassmann R: Structural disturbances in the body self. Psychother Psychosom 62:91–95, 1994c

Popli AP, Masand PS, Dewan MJ: Factitious disorders with psychological symptoms. J Clin Psychiatry 53:315–318, 1992

Powell R, Boast N: The million dollar man: resource implications for chronic Munchausen's syndrome. Br J Psychiatry 162:253–256, 1993a

Powell R, Boast N: Resource implications of Munchausen's syndrome (letter). Br J Psychiatry 162:848, 1993b

Rabinowitz S, Mark M, Modai I, et al: Malingering in the clinical setting: practical suggestions for intervention. Psychol Rep 67:1315–1318, 1990

Rand DC: Comprehensive psychosocial assessment in factitious disorder by proxy, in The Spectrum of Factitious Disorders. Edited by Feldman MD, Eisendrath SJ. Washington, DC, American Psychiatric Press, 1996, pp 109–134

Reich P, Gottfried LA: Factitious disorders in a teaching hospital. Ann Intern Med 99:240–247, 1983

Repper J: Munchausen syndrome by proxy in health care workers. J Adv Nurs 21:299–304, 1995

Resnick PJ: Defrocking the fraud: the detection of malingering. Isr J Psychiatry Relat Sci 30:93–101, 1993

Rogers R: Development of a new classificatory model of malingering. Bulletin of the American Academy of Psychiatry and the Law 18:323–333, 1990

Rogers R, Bagby RM, Rector N: Diagnostic legitimacy of factitious disorder with psychological symptoms. Am J Psychiatry 146:1312–1314, 1989

Rogers R, Gillis JR, Bagby RM, et al: Detection of malingering on the Structured Interview of Reported Symptoms (SIRS): a study of coached and uncoached simulators. Psychological Assessment 3:673–677, 1991

Rogers R, Sewell KW, Goldstein AM: Explanatory models of malingering: a prototypical analysis. Law Hum Behav 18:543–552, 1994

Rosenberg DA: Web of deceit: a literature review of Munchausen syndrome by proxy. Child Abuse Negl 11:547–563, 1987

Rosenberg DA: Portable guides to investigating child abuse: child neglect and Munchausen syndrome by proxy (http://www.ncjrs.org/txtfiles/chnegmun.txt). United States Department of Justice, Office of Juvenile Justice and Delinquency Prevention, September 1996

Rothchild E: Fictitious twins, factitious illness. Psychiatry 57:326–332, 1994

Roy M, Roy A: Factitious hypoglycemia: an 11-year follow-up. Psychosomatics 36:64–65, 1995

Samuels MP, McClaughlin W, Jacobson RR, et al: Fourteen cases of upper airway obstruction. Arch Dis Child 67:162–170 1992

Sanders MJ: Symptom coaching: factitious disorder by proxy with older children. Clin Psychol Rev 15:423–442, 1995

Schreier HA: The perversion of mothering: Munchausen syndrome by proxy. Bull Menninger Clin 56:421–437, 1992

Schreier HA: Repeated false allegations of sexual abuse presenting to sheriffs: when is it Munchausen by proxy? Child Abuse Negl 20:985–991, 1996

Schreier HA, Libow JA: Hurting for Love: The Munchausen by Proxy Syndrome. New York, Guilford, 1993a

Schreier HA, Libow JA: Munchausen syndrome by proxy: diagnosis and prevalence. Am J Orthopsychiatry 63:318–321, 1993b

Schreier HA, Libow JA: Munchausen by proxy syndrome: a clinical fable for our times. J Am Acad Child Adolesc Psychiatry 33:904–905, 1994

Schreier HA, Libow JA: Munchausen by proxy: the deadly game. Saturday Evening Post 22(4):40–46, 1996

Schwarz K, Harding R, Harrington D, et al: Hospital management of a patient with intractable factitious disorder. Psychosomatics 34:265–267, 1993

Seersholm NJ, Frolich S, Jensen NH, et al: Uaegte sygdom: en iatrogen lidelse? (Factitious disorder: an iatrogenic disease?). Ugeskr Laeger 153:2133–2135, 1991

Seguel M, Arrese M, Perez C, et al: Sindrome de Munchausen: estudio de 6 casos (Munchausen syndrome: study of 6 cases). Rev Med Chil 118:1090–1097, 1990

Sigal MD, Altmark D, Carmel I: Munchausen syndrome by adult proxy: a perpetrator abusing two adults. J Nerv Ment Dis 174:696–698, 1986

Sigal MD, Carmel I, Altmark D, et al: Munchausen syndrome by proxy: a psychodynamic analysis. Med Law 7:49–56, 1988

Sigal MD, Gelkopf M, Levertov G: Medical and legal aspects of the Munchausen by proxy perpetrator. Med Law 9:739–749, 1990

Smith NJ, Ardern MH: More in sickness than in health: a case study of Munchausen by proxy in the elderly. Journal of Family Therapy 11:321–334, 1989

Solyom C, Solyom L: A treatment program for functional paraplegia/Munchausen syndrome. J Behav Ther Exp Psychiatry 21:225–230, 1990

Songer DA: Factitious AIDS: a case report and literature review. Psychosomatics 36:406–411, 1995

Spiro HR: Chronic factitious illness: Munchausen's syndrome. Arch Gen Psychiatry 18:569–579, 1968

Spivak H, Rodin G, Sutherland A: The psychology of factitious disorders: a reconsideration. Psychosomatics 35:25–34, 1994

Stotland NL: Munchausen syndrome. JAMA 261:447, 1989

Sung JJ, Tam LS, Ko GT, et al: Deception and self-harm in the quest for freedom: an audit of Vietnamese boat people admitted to a regional hospital in Hong Kong. Med J Aust 163:524–526, 1995

Sutherland AJ, Rodin GM: Factitious disorders in a general hospital setting: clinical features and a review of the literature. Psychosomatics 31:392–399, 1990

Szajnberg NM, Moilanen I, Kanerva A, et al: Munchausen-by-proxy syndrome: countertransference as a diagnostic tool. Bull Menninger Clin 60:229–237, 1996

Teasell RW, Shapiro AP: Strategic-behavioral intervention in the treatment of chronic nonorganic motor disorders. Am J Phys Med Rehabil 73:44–50, 1994

Topazian M, Binder HJ: Factitious diarrhea detected by measurement of stool osmolality. N Engl J Med 330:1418–1419, 1994

Toth EL, Baggaley A: Coexistence of Munchausen's syndrome and multiple personality disorder: detailed report of a case and theoretical discussion. Psychiatry 54:176–183, 1991

Wallach J: Laboratory diagnosis of factitious disorders. Arch Intern Med 154:1690–1696, 1994

Willenberg H: Countertransference in factitious disorder. Psychother Psychosom 62:129–134, 1994

Witztum E, Grinshpoon A, Margolin J, et al: The erroneous diagnosis of malingering in a military setting. Mil Med 161:225–229, 1996

World Health Organization: International Statistical Classification of Diseases and Related Health Problems, 10th Revision. Geneva, World Health Organization, 1992

Yorker BC: Hospital epidemics of factitious disorder by proxy, in The Spectrum of Factitious Disorders. Edited by Feldman MD, Eisendrath SJ. Washington, DC, American Psychiatric Press, 1996a, pp 157–174

Yorker BC: Legal issues in factitious disorder by proxy, in The Spectrum of Factitious Disorders. Edited by Feldman MD, Eisendrath SJ. Washington, DC, American Psychiatric Press, 1996b, pp 135–156

Yorker BC, Kahan BB: Munchausen's syndrome by proxy as a form of child abuse. Arch Psychiatr Nurs 4:313–318, 1990

Yudofsky SC: Malingering: reply. J Clin Psychiatry 52:281–282, 1991

Zimmerman JG, Hussian RA, Tintner R, et al: Factitious disorder in a geriatric patient. Clinical Gerontologist 11:3–11, 1991

CHAPTER 18

DISSOCIATIVE DISORDERS

DAVID SPIEGEL, M.D.
JOSE R. MALDONADO, M.D.

The dissociative disorders involve a disturbance in the integrated organization of identity, memory, perception, or consciousness. Events normally experienced on a smooth continuum are isolated from the other mental processes with which they would ordinarily be associated. This isolation results in a variety of dissociative disorders depending on the primary cognitive process affected. When memories are poorly integrated, the resulting disorder is *dissociative amnesia*. Fragmentation of identity results in *dissociative fugue* or *dissociative identity disorder* (DID; formerly known as multiple personality disorder or MPD). Disordered perception yields *depersonalization disorder*. Dissociation of aspects of consciousness produces *acute stress disorder* and various dissociative trance and possession states (see Table 18–1).

These dissociative disorders are more a disturbance in the organization or structure of mental contents than in the contents themselves. Memories in dissociative amnesia are not so much distorted or bizarre as they are segregated from one another. The identity temporarily lost in dissociative fugue, or the aspects of the self that are fragmented in DID, are two-dimensional aspects of an overall personality structure. In this sense, it has been said that patients with DID suffer not from having more than one personality, but rather from having less than one personality. The problem is the failure of integration rather than the contents of the fragments. In summary, all types of dissociative disorders have in common a lack of immediate access to the entire personality structure or mental content in one form or another.

The dissociative disorders have a long history in classical psychopathology but until recently have been largely ignored. Nonetheless, the phenomena are sufficiently persistent and interesting that they have elicited growing attention from both professionals and the public. The dissociative disorders remain an area of psychopathology for which the best treatment is psychotherapy (Maldonado et al. 1997). As mental disorders, they have much to teach us about the way humans adapt to traumatic stress and about information processing in the brain.

The dissociative disorders were included in DSM-III (American Psychiatric Association 1980) and its revised edition, DSM-III-R (American Psychiatric Association 1987), and have been retained with some changes in nomenclature and diagnostic criteria in DSM-IV (American Psychiatric Association 1994). The discussion of each disorder later in this chapter will follow the DSM-IV structure.

TABLE 18–1. DSM-IV dissociative disorders

Dissociative amnesia (300.12)

Dissociative fugue (300.13)

Dissociative identity disorder (300.14; multiple personality disorder)

Depersonalization disorder (300.6)

Dissociative disorder not otherwise specified (300.15)

Others:

Dissociative trance disorder

Acute stress disorder (308.3)

DEVELOPMENT OF THE CONCEPT

Jean Martin Charcot (1890), a well-known French neurologist, became interested in the dissociated-like features experienced by some of his patients who had unusual neurological-like symptoms. He discovered that hypnosis could reproduce and reverse some of the deficits manifested by his patients. Charcot believed that even a normal process such as hypnosis, which could be used to access desegregated mental contents, was itself evidence of pathology (*un etat nerveux artificiel ou experimentale,* "an artificial or experimental nervous state"). He thought, for example, that once patients were cured of hysteria, they would no longer be hypnotizable. We now know this not to be the case because many "normal" individuals are highly hypnotizable (Hilgard 1965; H. Spiegel and Spiegel 1978/1987).

Nevertheless, the French physician and psychologist Pierre Janet (1920) is credited with the initial description of dissociation as a disorder, a *desagregation mentale.* The term *desagregation* carries with it a slightly different nuance than does the English translation (i.e., dissociation) because it implies a separation of certain mental contents from their general tendency to aggregate or be processed together. Janet (1920) described hysteria as "a malady of the *personal synthesis*" (p. 332). He viewed dissociation as a purely pathological process.

The dissociative disorders might have been studied more intensively during this century had not Janet's and Charcot's work been so thoroughly eclipsed by the psychoanalytic approach pioneered by Freud. Freud learned the use of hypnotic techniques from Charcot and applied them in the treatment of some of his first cases. In his early writings with Breuer, Freud began an exploration of dissociative phenomena, similar to those that Janet had described earlier. Cases in the *Studies on Hysteria* (Breuer and Freud 1893–1895/1955), such as that of Anna O., clearly involved dissociative phenomena. Indeed, Anna O. had many symptoms suggestive of DID (Nakdimen 1988).

However, Breuer and Freud reformulated the role of the capacity to dissociate through the concept of "hypnoid states, rather than the mechanism of dissociation." Indeed, they thought that dissociative symptoms should be attributed to the capacity to enter these hypnoid states rather than the reverse (Breuer and Freud 1893–1895/1955). However, in an effort to develop a more general theory of human psychopathology, Freud went on to study other kinds of patients, such as those with "obsessive compulsive neurosis" (i.e., obsessive-compulsive disorder) (Freud 1909/1955) and schizophrenia (Freud 1911/1958). This shift in the patient population studied may well account for much of Freud's waning interest in dissociation as a defense and his increasing interest in repression as a more general model for motivated forgetting in unconscious processes. Much has recently been made of the fact that Freud abandoned the seduction theory of the etiology of the neuroses. What may have happened is that he abandoned the study of individuals for whom trauma plausibly could be applied as an etiological factor in their psychiatric disorder.

Hilgard (1977) developed a neodissociation theory designed to revive interest in Janetian psychology and psychopathology. He postulated a mental structure with divisions that were horizontal rather than vertical, as in Freud's (1923/1961) archaeological model. Unlike Freud's system, Hilgard's model would allow for immediate access to consciousness of any of a variety of warded-off memories. In the dynamic unconscious model, repressed memories must first go through a process of transformation as they are accessed and lifted from the depths of the unconscious. In Hilgard's model, amnesia is a crucial mediating mechanism that provides the barriers that divide one set of mental contents from another. Thus, the flexible and reversible use of amnesia is a key defensive tool, whereas the reversal of amnesia is an important therapeutic tool.

Repression as a general model for keeping information out of conscious awareness differs from dissociation in six important ways (see Table 18–2):

1. The organizational structure of mental contents in dissociation is horizontal, with subunits of information divided from one another but equally available to consciousness (Hilgard 1977). Repressed information, on the other hand, is presumed to be stored in an archeological manner, at various depths, and therefore different parts are not equally accessible (Freud 1923/1961).

2. Subunits of information are presumed to be divided by amnesic barriers in dissociation, whereas dynamic conflict, motivated forgetting, is the mechanism underlying repression.

TABLE 18–2. Differences between dissociation and repression

	Dissociation	Repression
Organizational structure	Horizontal	Vertical
Barriers	Amnesia	Dynamic conflict
Etiology	Trauma	Developmental conflict over unacceptable wishes
Contents	Untransformed: traumatic memories	Disguised, primary process: dreams, slips
Means of access	Hypnosis	Interpretation
Psychotherapy	Access, control, and working through traumatic memories	Interpretation, transference

3. The information kept out of awareness in dissociation is often for a discrete and sharply delimited period of time, usually for a traumatic experience, whereas repressed information may be for a variety of experiences, fears, or wishes scattered across time. Dissociation seems to be elicited as a defense especially after episodes of physical trauma, whereas repression is a response to warded-off fears and wishes or in response to other dynamic conflicts.

4. Dissociated information is stored in a discrete and untransformed manner, whereas repressed information is usually disguised and fragmented. Even when repressed information becomes available to consciousness, its meaning is hidden (e.g., in dreams, slips of the tongue).

5. Retrieval of dissociated information often can be direct. Techniques such as hypnosis can be used to access warded-off memories. In contrast, uncovering of repressed information often requires repeated recall trials through intense questioning, psychotherapy, or psychoanalysis with subsequent interpretation (i.e., of dreams).

6. The focus of psychotherapy for dissociation is integration, via control of access to dissociated states and working through of traumatic memories. The classical psychotherapy for repression involves interpretation, including working through of the transference.

There is debate about whether dissociation is a subtype of repression or vice versa. Such a dispute is probably not resolvable, but what has become clear in recent years is

that given the complexity of human information processing, the accomplishment of a sense of mental unity is an achievement, not a given (Kihlstrom and Hoyt 1990; D. Spiegel 1990a). What is remarkable is not that dissociative disorders occur but rather that they do not occur more often, given the fact that information processing comprises a variety of reasonably autonomous subsystems involving perception, memory storage and retrieval, intention, and action (Baars 1988; Cohen and Servan-Schreiber 1992a, 1992b; Rumelhart and McClelland 1986; D. Spiegel 1991c).

MODELS AND MECHANISMS OF DISSOCIATION

DISSOCIATION AND INFORMATION PROCESSING

Modern information processing–based theories, including connectionist and parallel distributed processing (PDP) models (Rumelhart and McClelland 1986), take a bottom-up rather than a top-down approach to cognitive organization. Traditional models emphasize a superordinate organization in which broad categories of information structure the processing of specific examples. In the more Aristotelian PDP models, subunits or neural nets process information through computation of co-occurrence of input stimuli. The activation patterns in these neural nets allow for category recognition. For example, the category "kitchen" is built up from the frequent co-occurrence of "appliances of a certain type" rather than being the basis for recognizing its components. The output of one set of nets becomes the input to another, thereby gradually building up integrated and complex patterns of activation and inhibition. Such bottom-up processing models have the advantage of accounting for the processing of vast amounts of information and for the human ability to recognize patterns on the basis of approximate information. However, such models make the classification and integration of information problematic. In PDP models, it is theoretically likely that failures in integration of mental contents will occur. Indeed, attempts have been made to model psychopathology based on difficulties in neural net information processing, for example, in schizophrenia and bipolar disorder (Hoffman 1987), as well as in dissociative disorders (D. Li and Spiegel 1992). The idea is that when a net runs into difficulty in balancing the processing of input information (a model for traumatic input), it is more likely to have difficulty achieving a unified and balanced output. Such neural nets tend to fall into a "dissociated" situation in which they move in one direction or another but cannot reach an optimal balanced solution, and therefore they are unable to process smoothly all of the incoming information.

Such bottom-up information processing systems have more the problems of a democracy than a monarchy. The difficulty is achieving unity of representation and action. In such models, consciousness is viewed as analogous to the rostrum in a legislature where competing subunits vie for attention and the ability to broadcast their input to the system as a whole (Baars 1988). Indeed, such information processing models have now become of considerable interest in cognitive psychology (Kihlstrom 1987), and modern memory research, as mentioned earlier in this chapter, provides other examples of structural dissociation of mental elements (Schacter 1996).

DISSOCIATION AND MEMORY SYSTEMS

Modern research on memory demonstrates that there are at least two broad categories of memory, variously described as explicit and implicit (Schacter 1992; Squire 1992) or episodic and semantic (Tulving 1983). These two memory systems serve different functions. *Explicit (or episodic) memory* involves recall of personal experience identified with the self (e.g., "I was at the ball game last week"). The other type, *implicit (or semantic) memory*, involves the execution of routine operations, such as riding a bicycle or typing. Such operations may be carried out with a high degree of proficiency with little conscious awareness of either their current execution or the learning episodes on which the skill is based. Indeed, these two types of memory may well have different anatomical localizations: the limbic system, especially the hippocampal formation, and mamillary bodies for episodic memory, and the basal ganglia and cortex for procedural (or semantic) memory (Mishkin 1991; Squire 1992).

Indeed, the distinction between these two types of memory may account for certain dissociative phenomena (D. Spiegel et al. 1993). The automaticity observed in certain dissociative disorders may be a reflection of the separation of self-identification in certain kinds of explicit memory from routine activity in implicit or semantic memory. It is thus not at all foreign to our mental processing to act in an automatic way devoid of explicit self-identification. Were it necessary for us to retrieve explicit memories of how and when we learned all of the activities we are required to perform, it is highly unlikely that we would be able to function with anything like the degree of efficiency we have. Many athletes report focusing on some detail of the event and allowing their bodies to do what they need to, when in fact they are performing extremely well. There is thus a fundamental model in memory research for the dissociation between identity and performance that may well find its pathological reflection in disorders such as dissociative amnesia, fugue, and identity disorder.

DISSOCIATION AND TRAUMA

An important development in the modern understanding of dissociative disorders is the exploration of the link between trauma and dissociation (D. Spiegel and Cardeña 1991). Trauma can be understood as the experience of being made into an object or a thing, the victim of someone else's rage or of nature's indifference. It is the ultimate experience of helplessness and loss of control over one's own body. There is growing clinical and some empirical evidence that dissociation may occur especially as a defense during trauma—an attempt to maintain mental control at the very moment when physical control has been lost (Bremner and Brett 1997; Butler et al. 1996; Eriksson and Lundin 1996; Kluft 1984a, 1984c; Koopman et al. 1995, 1996; Putnam 1985; D. Spiegel 1984; D. Spiegel et al. 1988). One DID patient reported "going to a mountain meadow full of wildflowers" when she was being sexually assaulted by her drunken father. She would concentrate on how pleasant and beautiful this imaginary scene was as a way of detaching herself from the immediate experience of terror, pain, and helplessness. Such individuals often report seeking comfort from imaginary playmates or imagined protectors or absorbing themselves in some perceptual distraction, such as the pattern of the wallpaper. Many rape victims report floating above their bodies, feeling sorry for the persons being assaulted beneath them. There is recent evidence (Putnam 1993; Terr 1991) that children exposed to multiple traumas are more likely to use dissociative defense mechanisms, which include spontaneous trance episodes and amnesia.

As is noted in the discussion on dissociative identity disorder later in this chapter, an accumulating literature suggests a connection between a history of physical and sexual abuse in childhood and the development of dissociative symptoms (Anderson et al. 1993; Coons 1994; Coons and Milstein 1986; Ellason et al. 1996; Kaplan et al. 1995; Kluft 1984c, 1985a; Roesler and McKenzie 1994; Sar et al. 1996; Saxe et al. 1993; D. Spiegel 1984). Similarly, evidence is accumulating that dissociative symptoms are more prevalent in patients with Axis II disorders such as borderline personality disorder when there has been a history of childhood abuse (Brenner 1996a, 1996b; Brodsky et al. 1995; Chu and Dill 1990; Darves-Bornoz 1997; Herman et al. 1989; Zweig-Frank et al. 1994). However, another way to examine the connection between dissociation and trauma is to look at the link between recent trauma and dissociative symptoms (Carlier et al. 1996; Darves-Bornoz 1997; Eriksson and Lundin 1996; Koopman et al. 1994, 1995, 1996; Marmar et al. 1996; D. Spiegel 1991a, 1991b; D. Spiegel and Cardeña 1991; van der Kolk et al. 1994). If it is indeed the case that trauma seems to elicit dissociation, this should be observable in the immediate aftermath of natural disasters, combat, and physical assault.

The early literature examining responses to trauma provides hints of dissociative symptoms, but these symptoms often were not systematically assessed. In a classic article on the symptomatology and management of acute grief in the aftermath of the Coconut Grove fire, Lindemann (1944) noted that those individuals who had been injured or had lost loved ones but who acted as though little or nothing had happened had an extremely poor prognosis. Indeed, it was the absence of posttraumatic symptoms in this group compared with the agitation, dysphoria, and restlessness that typified the majority of survivors that led Lindemann to formulate the normal process of acute grief.

More recently researchers have observed that numbing (i.e., loss of responsiveness in the wake of trauma) is a predictor of later posttraumatic stress disorder (PTSD) symptomatology. For example, Z. Solomon et al. (1988, 1989) observed that psychic numbing accounted for 20% of the variance in later PTSD among Israeli combat soldiers. McFarlane (1986) found that numbing in response to the Ash Wednesday Bush Fires in Australia was a strong predictor of later posttraumatic symptomatology. Similarly, research on hostages and survivors of other life-threatening events indicates that more than half have experienced feelings of unreality, automatic movements, lack of emotion, and a sense of detachment (Madakasira and O'Brien 1987; Noyes and Kletti 1977; Sloan 1988). Symptoms of depersonalization and hyperalertness also frequently occur (Noyes and Slymen 1978–1979). Numbing, loss of interest, and an inability to feel deeply about anything were reported in about a third of the survivors of the Hyatt Regency skywalk collapse (Wilkinson 1983) and in a similar proportion of survivors of the North Sea oil rig collapse (Holen 1993). This finding is consistent with studies of survivors of the Loma Prieta earthquake (Cardeña and Spiegel 1993), in which a quarter of a sample of healthy students reported marked depersonalization during and immediately after the earthquake.

Such dissociative experiences, especially numbing, have been found to be rather strong predictors of later PTSD (McFarlane 1986). In fact, Z. Solomon et al. (1989) found numbing to be the single best predictor of a later diagnosis of PTSD. After the Loma Prieta earthquake in 1989, Weiss et al. (1995) found a strong correlation be-

tween peritraumatic dissociation and later PTSD among earthquake rescue workers. McFarlane (1992) found that high levels of intrusion, measured 4 months after the trauma, strongly predict the development of PTSD. Koopman et al. (1994) discovered that a combination of acute dissociative and anxiety symptoms was a significant predictor of PTSD 7 months after the Oakland-Berkeley fires. Shalev et al. (1993, 1996) have found that symptoms of intrusion as measured by the Impact of Event Scale (IES; Horowitz et al. 1979) remained elevated in PTSD subjects, whereas they decreased in subjects who did not develop PTSD. They also found that avoidance symptoms dramatically increased between the first week and the 6-month follow-up examination, although they remained low in subjects without PTSD (Shalev et al. 1996). S. Perry et al. (1992) found similar results following burn trauma. Thus, physical trauma seems to elicit dissociation or compartmentalization of experience and may often become the matrix for later posttraumatic symptomatology, such as dissociative amnesia for the traumatic episode. Indeed, more extreme dissociative disorders, such as DID, have been conceptualized as chronic PTSDs (Kluft 1984b, 1991; D. Spiegel 1984, 1986a). Recollection of trauma tends to have an off-on quality involving either intrusion or avoidance (Horowitz 1976) in which victims either intensively relive the trauma as though it were recurring or have difficulty remembering it (Cardeña and Spiegel 1993; Christianson and Loftus 1987; Madakasira and O'Brien 1987).

ACUTE STRESS DISORDER

Although acute stress disorder is classified among the anxiety disorders in DSM-IV, mention is made of it in this chapter because half of the symptoms of this disorder are dissociative in nature (Table 18–3). The diagnostic criteria for this disorder would designate as symptomatic in approximately one-fourth to one-third of individuals exposed to serious trauma. These symptoms are strongly predictive of later development of PTSD (Butler et al. 1996; Koopman et al. 1994). Similarly, the occurrence of PTSD is predicted by intrusion, avoidance, and hyperarousal symptoms in the immediate aftermath of rape (Rothbaum and Foa 1993) and combat trauma (Blank 1993; Z. Solomon and Mikulincer 1988). Although most individuals experiencing serious trauma are initially symptomatic, the majority will recover without developing PTSD. Most studies demonstrate that 25% or less of those who experience serious trauma later become symptomatic.

TABLE 18–3.   DSM-IV diagnostic criteria for acute stress disorder

A.   The person has been exposed to a traumatic event in which both of the following were present:

   (1)   the person experienced, witnessed, or was confronted with an event or events that involved actual or threatened death or serious injury, or a threat to the physical integrity of self or others

   (2)   the person's response involved intense fear, helplessness, or horror

B.   Either while experiencing or after experiencing the distressing event, the individual has three (or more) of the following dissociative symptoms:

   (1)   a subjective sense of numbing, detachment, or absence of emotional responsiveness

   (2)   a reduction in awareness of his or her surroundings (e.g., "being in a daze")

   (3)   derealization

   (4)   depersonalization

   (5)   dissociative amnesia (i.e., inability to recall an important aspect of the trauma)

C.   The traumatic event is persistently reexperienced in at least one of the following ways: recurrent images, thoughts, dreams, illusions, flashback episodes, or a sense of reliving the experience; or distress on exposure to reminders of the traumatic event.

D.   Marked avoidance of stimuli that arouse recollections of the trauma (e.g., thoughts, feelings, conversations, activities, places, people).

E.   Marked symptoms of anxiety or increased arousal (e.g., difficulty sleeping, irritability, poor concentration, hypervigilance, exaggerated startle response, motor restlessness).

F.   The disturbance causes clinically significant distress or impairment in social, occupational, or other important areas of functioning or impairs the individual's ability to pursue some necessary task, such as obtaining necessary assistance or mobilizing personal resources by telling family members about the traumatic experience.

G.   The disturbance lasts for a minimum of 2 days and a maximum of 4 weeks and occurs within 4 weeks of the traumatic event.

H.   The disturbance is not due to the direct physiological effects of a substance (e.g., a drug of abuse, a medication) or a general medical condition, is not better accounted for by brief psychotic disorder, and is not merely an exacerbation of a preexisting Axis I or Axis II disorder.

This new diagnostic category should be useful not only for research on the normal and abnormal processes of adjusting to trauma, but also as a means of providing an im-

portant opportunity for early preventive intervention. It may be that dissociation works well at the time of trauma, but if the defense persists too long, it interferes with the working through (in Lindemann's term, the "grief work") necessary to put traumatic experience into perspective and reduce the likelihood of later PTSD or other symptomatology. Therefore, psychotherapy aimed at helping individuals acknowledge, bear, and put into perspective traumatic experience shortly after the trauma should be helpful in reducing the incidence of later PTSD.

In the following discussions, we review the diagnosis and treatment of the dissociative disorders as defined in DSM-IV.

DISSOCIATIVE AMNESIA

The hallmark of this disorder is the inability to recall important personal information, usually of a traumatic or stressful nature, which cannot be explained by ordinary forgetfulness (American Psychiatric Association 1994) (Table 18–4). Dissociative amnesia is considered the most common of all dissociative disorders (Putnam 1985). Amnesia is a symptom commonly found in a number of other dissociative and anxiety disorders, including acute stress disorder, PTSD, somatization disorder, dissociative fugue, and DID (American Psychiatric Association 1994). A higher incidence of dissociative amnesia has been described in the context of war and other natural and man-made disasters (Maldonado et al. 1997). There appears to be a direct relationship between the severity of the exposure to trauma and the incidence of amnesia (G. R. Brown and Anderson 1991; Chu and Dill 1990; Kirshner 1973; Putnam 1985, 1993; Sargant and Slater 1941).

Dissociative amnesia is the classical functional disorder of memory and involves difficulty in retrieving discrete components of episodic memory (Table 18–2). It does not, however, involve a difficulty in memory storage, as in Wernicke-Korsakoff syndrome. Because the amnesia involves primarily difficulties in retrieval rather than encoding or storage, the memory deficits exhibited are usually reversible. Once the amnesia has cleared, normal memory function is resumed (Schacter et al. 1982). Dissociative amnesia has three primary characteristics:

1.   The memory loss is episodic. The first-person recollection of certain events is lost rather than knowledge of procedures.

2.   The memory loss is for a discrete period of time, ranging from minutes to years. It is not vagueness or inefficient retrieval of memories but rather a dense

TABLE 18–4.   **DSM-IV diagnostic criteria for dissociative amnesia**

A.   The predominant disturbance is one or more episodes of inability to recall important personal information, usually of a traumatic or stressful nature, that is too extensive to be explained by ordinary forgetfulness.

B.   The disturbance does not occur exclusively during the course of dissociative identity disorder, dissociative fugue, posttraumatic stress disorder, acute stress disorder, or somatization disorder and is not due to the direct physiological effects of a substance (e.g., a drug of abuse, a medication) or a neurological or other general medical condition (e.g., amnestic disorder due to head trauma).

C.   The symptoms cause clinically significant distress or impairment in social, occupational, or other important areas of functioning.

unavailability of memories that had been clearly available. Unlike in the amnestic disorders, for example, from damage to the medial temporal lobe in surgery (Squire and Zola-Morgan 1991) or in Wernicke-Korsakoff syndrome, there is usually no difficulty in learning *new* episodic information. Thus, the amnesia is typically retrograde rather than anterograde (Loewenstein 1991a), with one or more discrete periods of past information becoming unavailable. However, Kluft (1988) has observed a syndrome of continuous difficulty in incorporating new information that mimics organic amnestic syndromes.

3.   The memory loss is generally for events of a traumatic or stressful nature. In one study (Coons and Milstein 1986), the majority of cases involved child abuse (60%), but disavowed behaviors such as marital problems, sexual activity, suicide attempts, criminal behavior, and the death of a relative were also precipitants.

Dissociative amnesia is most frequent in the third and fourth decades of life (Abeles and Schilder 1935; Coons and Milstein 1986). It usually involves one episode, but multiple periods of lost memory are not uncommon (Coons and Milstein 1986). Comorbidity with conversion disorder, bulimia, alcohol abuse, and depression is common, and Axis II diagnoses of histrionic, dependent, and borderline personality disorders occur in a substantial minority of such patients (Coons and Milstein 1986). Legal difficulties, such as driving under the influence of alcohol, also accompany dissociative amnesia in a minority of cases. Occasionally, there may be a history of head trauma. If that is the case, usually the

trauma is too slight to have physiological consequences.

The typical course of dissociative amnesia is described in the following case:

A 54-year-old man was involved in a motorcycle accident. He was wearing a helmet, which was damaged but did protect him during the accident. He was determined to have suffered no significant head trauma. The patient did not lose consciousness, and he talked with a friend after the accident about it. However, he had no memory of the accident, nor of the 12 hours afterward. His first recollection was of a friend telling him, "You crashed my motorcycle." When he returned the next day to the hospital where he had been treated, he recognized a nurse as someone familiar, and she told him he had been yelling when they treated his injured left knee. Yet this visit did not stimulate any direct recollection of his time in the hospital. The man had recovered no memory of the accident a month later.

Dissociative amnesia usually involves discrete boundaries around the period of time unavailable to consciousness. Individuals with such a disorder lose the ability to recall what happened during a specific period of time. They demonstrate not vagueness or spotty memory but rather a loss of any episodic memory for a finite period of time. Such individuals initially may not be aware of the memory loss—that is, they may not remember that they do not remember. However, they may find, for example, new purchases in their homes but have no memory of having obtained them. They report being told that they have done or said things that they cannot remember.

Dissociative amnesia most frequently occurs after an episode of trauma, and the onset may be sudden or gradual.

A 30-year-old woman was beaten and raped by a man who drove her home from a party. She had refused to let him enter her apartment, but he returned a few minutes later claiming that he had to make a telephone call. He then sexually assaulted her. She screamed and struggled and called the police immediately afterward. The man was arrested when he returned to retrieve some jewelry she had pulled off his neck during the struggle. Although she had not suffered a concussion, she began to lose memory of the rape in the ensuing week. By the end of the week, she had no memory of the rape but became listless and depressed. In psychotherapy, she used hypnosis to help retrieve her memory, which she was gradually able to do.

Some individuals do suffer from episodes of selective amnesia, usually for specific traumatic incidents, which may be more interwoven with periods of intact memory. In these cases, the amnesia is for a type of material remembered rather than for a discrete period of time.

Despite the fact that certain information is kept out of consciousness in dissociative amnesia, such information may exert an influence on consciousness. For example, a rape victim with no conscious recollection of the assault will nonetheless behave like someone who has been sexually victimized. Such individuals often suffer detachment and demoralization, are unable to enjoy intimate relationships, and show hyperarousal to stimuli reminiscent of the trauma. This phenomenon is similar to priming in memory research. Individuals who have read a word in a list will complete a word stem for such a word (e.g., a partial word such as *pre* for *prepare*) minutes or hours later more quickly than they would for a word they have not recently seen. This phenomenon occurs despite the fact that they cannot consciously recall having read the word. Similarly, individuals instructed in hypnosis to forget having seen a list of words will nonetheless demonstrate priming effects from the hypnotically suppressed list. It is the essence of dissociative amnesia that material being kept out of conscious awareness is nonetheless active and may influence consciousness indirectly: out of sight does not mean out of mind.

Individuals with dissociative amnesia generally do not suffer disturbances of identity, except to the extent that their identity is influenced by the warded-off memory. It is not uncommon for such individuals to develop depressive symptoms as well, especially when the amnesia is in the wake of a traumatic episode.

TREATMENT

To date there are no controlled studies addressing the treatment of dissociative amnesia. There are no established pharmacological treatments except for the use of benzodiazepines or barbiturates for drug-assisted interviews (Maldonado et al. 1997). Most cases of dissociative amnesia revert spontaneously, especially when the individuals are removed from stressful or threatening situations, when they feel physically and psychologically safe, and/or when they are exposed to cues from the past (i.e., family members) (W. Brown 1918; Kardiner and Spiegel 1947; Loewenstein 1991b; Maldonado et al. 1997; Reither and Stoudemire 1988). When a safe environment is not enough to restore normal memory functioning, the amnesia can sometimes be breached by using techniques such as pharmacological-mediated interviews (i.e., barbiturates and benzodiazepines) (Baron and Nagy 1988; Naples and Hackett 1978; J. C. Perry and Jacobs 1982; Wettstein and Fauman 1979).

On the other hand, most dissociative disorder patients are highly hypnotizable on formal testing and therefore are easily able to make use of hypnotic techniques such as age regression (H. Spiegel and Spiegel 1978/1987). Patients are hypnotized and instructed to experience a time before the onset of the amnesia as though it were the present. Then the patients are reoriented in hypnosis to experience events during the amnesic time period. Hypnosis can enable such patients to reorient temporally and therefore to achieve access to otherwise dissociated memories.

If there is traumatic content to the warded-off memory, patients may abreact (i.e., express strong emotion) as these memories are elicited, and they will need psychotherapeutic help in integrating these memories and the associated affect into consciousness.

One technique that can help bring such memories into consciousness while modulating the affective response to them is the screen technique (D. Spiegel 1981). In this approach, patients are taught, by using hypnosis, to relive the traumatic event as if they were watching it on an imaginary movie or television screen. This technique is often helpful for individuals who are unable to relive the event as if it were occurring in the present tense, either because that process is too emotionally taxing or because they are not sufficiently hypnotizable to be able to engage in hypnotic age regression. The screen technique also can be used to provide dissociation between the psychological and somatic aspects of the memory retrieval. Individuals can be put into self-hypnosis and instructed to get their bodies into a state of floating comfort and safety. They are reminded that no matter what they see on the screen their bodies will be safe and comfortable.

A victim of a violent attempted rape had developed a selective amnesia for much of the physical struggle itself. She had suffered a basilar skull fracture, although she had not been rendered unconscious. She also had a generalized seizure shortly after the assault. She initially sought help with hypnosis in an attempt to improve her recollection of the assailant's face.

The woman was instructed in the screen technique and used it to relive the assault. She remembered two things she had not previously recalled: 1) the assailant was surprised at how hard she was fighting with him, and 2) she recognized that he intended not merely to rape her but to kill her. She became convinced that had she let him drag her into her apartment, she likely would not have survived. She was tearful and frightened as she recalled this aspect of the assault that had been previously unavailable to consciousness.

She was then instructed to divide the imaginary screen in half, picturing on the left side an image of the viciousness and intensity of the assault on her and on the other to recognize what she had done to protect herself. She was instructed to concentrate on these two aspects of the assault and then, when she was ready, to bring herself out of the state of self-hypnosis. She was told that she could use this as a self-hypnosis exercise to be employed several times a day if she wished, as a means of putting her memories of the rape into perspective. This cognitive and emotional restructuring of the traumatic memories made them more bearable in consciousness.

Before this psychotherapy, she had blamed herself for having fought so hard that she was seriously injured. Afterward, she recognized that she may have saved her life by fighting off the assailant so vigorously. This positive therapeutic outcome occurred despite the fact that she was unable to recall any new details about the assailant's physical appearance.

The psychotherapy of dissociative amnesia involves accessing the dissociated memories, working through affectively loaded aspects of these memories, and supporting the patient through the process of integrating these memories into consciousness.

DISSOCIATIVE FUGUE

Dissociative fugue combines failure of integration of certain aspects of personal memory with loss of customary identity and automatisms of motor behavior (Table 18–5). Patients appear "normal," usually exhibiting no signs of psychopathology or cognitive deficit. Fugue involves one or more episodes of sudden, unexpected, purposeful travel away from home, coupled with an inability to recall portions or all of one's past, and a loss of identity or the assumption of a new identity. In contrast to patients who have DID, if patients with dissociative fugue develop a new identity, the old and new identities do not alternate. The onset is usually sudden, and it frequently occurs after a traumatic experience or bereavement. A single episode is not uncommon, and spontaneous remission of symptoms can occur without treatment.

It was thought that the assumption of a new identity, as in the classical case of the Reverend Ansel Bourne (James 1890/1950), was typical of dissociative fugue. However, Reither and Stoudemire (1988), in their review of the literature, document that in the majority of

TABLE 18–5. DSM-IV diagnostic criteria for dissociative fugue

A. The predominant disturbance is sudden, unexpected travel away from home or one's customary place of work, with inability to recall one's past.

B. Confusion about personal identity or assumption of a new identity (partial or complete).

C. The disturbance does not occur exclusively during the course of dissociative identity disorder and is not due to the direct physiological effects of a substance (e.g., a drug of abuse, a medication) or a general medical condition (e.g., temporal lobe epilepsy).

D. The symptoms cause clinically significant distress or impairment in social, occupational, or other important areas of functioning.

cases there is loss of personal identity but no clear assumption of a new identity.

Many cases of dissociative fugue remit spontaneously. But again, hypnosis can be useful in accessing dissociated material. The following case was reported by H. Spiegel and Spiegel (1978/1987):

A woman who appeared dazed but physically unharmed was brought into an army hospital emergency room by the base guards because she had been found wandering near the army base. She reported that she did not know who she was, where she lived, or how she happened to be there. Initially, plans were made to admit her to the hospital for a full neurological and psychiatric evaluation. She proved to be highly hypnotizable, and in hypnosis, age regression was used to take her back to an earlier year. She then reported her name and that she lived some 500 miles away. The time was changed again in hypnosis to a period just before this apparent fugue episode. She then reported having received unsigned letters from someone at the army base where her husband was stationed, reporting that her husband was having an affair. This had deeply upset her, and it turned out that her husband was indeed a soldier on the base near which she had been found wandering. They were reunited and reconciled, and the fugue episode ended.

Not infrequently, fugue episodes represent dissociated but purposeful activity, as in the following case:

A businessman found himself on several occasions on transatlantic flights from California to London without recollecting who he was or how he had gotten on the airplane. In psychotherapy exploring these fugue episodes, it was determined that he had had an extremely conflicted relationship with a successful but neglectful father. The father had recently died, leaving the patient financially well off but emotionally ambivalent, with a sense of incompleteness about his relationship with his father. The patient had spent his boyhood years in London, and he recognized in therapy that the travel to London seemed to represent an unconscious attempt to revisit his childhood years and "set his father straight"—something he had never been able to do while his father was alive.

In this case, the dissociative fugue was a form of pathological grief reaction.

Hypnosis can be helpful in accessing otherwise unavailable components of memory and identity. The approach used is similar to that for dissociative amnesia. Hypnotic age regression can be used as the framework for accessing information available at a previous time. Demonstrating to patients that such information can be made available to consciousness enhances their sense of control over the material and facilitates the therapeutic working through of emotionally laden aspects of it.

A woman in a Veterans Administration hospital had lost all memory of the preceding 10 months and insisted that she was in another hospital where she had been during the previous December. She proved on testing with the Hypnotic Induction Profile (H. Spiegel and Spiegel 1978/1987) to be highly hypnotizable. She was then put into hypnosis with a simple, rapid induction technique involving the following instruction: On 1, do one thing, look up. On 2, do two things, slowly close your eyes, and take a deep breath. On 3, do three things, let the breath out, let your eyes relax, but keep them closed, and let your body float. Then let one hand or the other float up into the air like a balloon, and that is your signal to yourself that you are ready to concentrate.

When she did this, she was told that we would be changing times, that we would count backward in years, and that when her eyes opened she would be at an earlier time in her life. We agreed that when I touched her forehead, she would close her eyes and we would change times again. We then began counting several years back. When she opened her eyes, she spoke as though she were in some different place earlier in her life. She was reoriented to the time

when she really was in another psychiatric hospital in a different city, and she talked about that experience. She was then instructed to close her eyes again and count forward in months to the present month. She opened her eyes and was then properly oriented and had episodic memory for what had transpired in her life in recent months.

Once reorientation is established and the overt aspects of the fugue have been resolved, it is important to work through interpersonal or intrapsychic issues that underlie the dissociative defenses. Individuals with dissociative fugue are often relatively unaware of their reactions to stress because they so effectively can dissociate them (H. Spiegel 1974). Thus, effective psychotherapy is also anticipatory, helping patients to recognize and modify their tendency to set aside their own feelings in favor of those of others.

Patients with dissociative fugue may be helped with a psychotherapeutic approach that facilitates conscious integration of dissociated memories and motivations for behavior previously experienced as automatic and unwilled. It is often helpful to address current psychosocial stressors, such as marital conflict, with the involved individuals, as in the previously discussed case of the woman found on the army base. To the extent that current psychosocial stress triggers fugue, resolution of that stress can help resolve the fugue state and reduce the likelihood of recurrence. Highly hypnotizable individuals prone to these extreme dissociative symptoms (D. Spiegel et al. 1988; H. Spiegel 1974; H. Spiegel and Spiegel 1978/1987) often have great difficulty in asserting their own point of view in a personal relationship. Rather, they interact with others as though they were undergoing a spontaneous trance experience. One individual described herself as a "disciple in search of a teacher." Psychotherapy can be effective in helping such individuals recognize and modify their tendency toward unthinking compliance with others and toward extreme sensitivity to rejection and disapproval.

In the past, sodium amobarbital or other short-acting sedatives were used to reverse dissociative amnesia or fugue. However, such techniques offer no advantage over hypnosis and are not especially effective (J. C. Perry and Jacobs 1982). Not infrequently, the ceremony of injecting the drug elicits spontaneous hypnotic phenomena before the pharmacological effect is felt, and sedation and other side effects can be troublesome.

DEPERSONALIZATION DISORDER

The essential feature of depersonalization disorder is the occurrence of persistent feelings of unreality, detachment, or estrangement from oneself or one's body, usually with the feeling that one is an outside observer of one's own mental processes (Steinberg 1991). Thus, depersonalization disorder is primarily a disturbance in the integration of perceptual experience (Table 18–6). Individuals who have depersonalization disorder are distressed by it. Different from those with delusional disorders and other psychotic processes, those with depersonalization disorder have intact reality testing. Patients are aware of some distortion in their perceptual experience and therefore are not delusional. The symptom is not infrequently transient and may co-occur with a variety of other symptoms, especially anxiety, panic, or phobic symptoms. Indeed, the content of the anxiety may involve fears of "going crazy." Derealization frequently co-occurs, in which affected individuals notice an altered perception of their surroundings, resulting in the world seeming unreal or dreamlike. Affected individuals often will ruminate about this alteration and be preoccupied with their own somatic and mental functioning.

Depersonalization as a symptom is seen in a number of psychiatric and neurological disorders (Pies 1991; Putnam 1985). Unlike other dissociative disorders, the presence of which excludes other mental disorders such as schizophrenia and substance abuse, depersonalization disorder frequently co-occurs with such disorders. It is often a symptom of anxiety disorder and PTSD, and it also occurs as a symptom of alcohol and drug abuse, as a side-effect of prescription medication, and during stress and sensory deprivation. Depersonalization is considered a disorder when it is a persistent and predominant symptom. The phenomenology of the disorder involves both the initial symptoms themselves and the reactive anxiety caused by them.

TABLE 18–6. **DSM-IV diagnostic criteria for depersonalization disorder**

A. Persistent or recurrent experiences of feeling detached from, and as if one is an outside observer of, one's mental processes or body (e.g., feeling like one is in a dream).

B. During the depersonalization experience, reality testing remains intact.

C. The depersonalization causes clinically significant distress or impairment in social, occupational, or other important areas of functioning.

D. The depersonalization experience does not occur exclusively during the course of another mental disorder, such as schizophrenia, panic disorder, acute stress disorder, or another dissociative disorder and is not due to the direct physiological effects of a substance (e.g., a drug of abuse, a medication) or a general medical condition (e.g., temporal lobe epilepsy).

TREATMENT

Depersonalization is most often transient and may remit without formal treatment. Recurrent or persistent depersonalization should be thought of both as a symptom in and of itself and as a component of other syndromes requiring treatment, such as anxiety disorders and schizophrenia.

The symptom itself may respond to self-hypnosis training. Often, hypnotic induction will induce transient depersonalization symptoms in patients. This is a useful exercise because by having a structure for inducing the symptoms, one provides patients with a context for understanding and controlling them. The symptoms are presented as a spontaneous form of hypnotic dissociation that can be modified. Individuals for whom this approach is effective can be taught to induce a pleasant sense of floating lightness or heaviness in place of the anxiety-related somatic detachment. Often, the use of an imaginary screen to picture problems in a way that detaches them from the typical somatic response is also helpful (H. Spiegel and Spiegel 1978/1987).

Other treatment modalities employed (Maldonado et al. 1997) include behavioral techniques, such as paradoxical intention (Blue 1979), record keeping, and positive reward (Dollinger 1983); flooding (Sookman and Solyom 1978); psychotherapy, especially psychodynamic (Noyes and Kletti 1971; Schilder 1939; Shilony and Grossman 1993; Torch 1987); and psychoeducation (Fewtrell 1986; Torch 1987). Some have suggested the use of psychotropic medications, including psychostimulants (Cattell and Cattell 1974; Davison 1964; Shorvon 1946), antidepressants (Fichtner et al. 1992; Hollander et al. 1989, 1990; Noyes et al. 1987; Walsh 1975), antipsychotics (Ambrosino 1973; Nuller 1982), anticonvulsants (Stein and Uhde 1989), and benzodiazepines (Ballenger et al. 1988; Nuller 1982; Spier et al. 1986; Stein and Uhde 1989). Finally, others have suggested the use of electroconvulsive therapy (ECT; Ambrosino 1973; Davison 1964; Roth 1959; Shorvon 1946). Appropriate treatment for comorbid disorders is an important part of treatment. Use of antianxiety medications for generalized anxiety or phobic disorders and antipsychotic medications for schizophrenia should help in these conditions.

DISSOCIATIVE IDENTITY DISORDER (MULTIPLE PERSONALITY DISORDER)

PREVALENCE

There are no convincing studies of the absolute prevalence of DID. The initial systematic report on the epidemiology of DID estimated a prevalence in the general population of 0.01% (Coons 1984). The estimated prevalence is approximately 3% of psychiatric inpatients (Ross 1991; Ross et al. 1991b). Studies conducted in the general population suggest a higher prevalence than initially reported by Coons (1984) but lower (about 1%) than the one described in psychiatric settings and specialized treatment units (Ross 1991; Vanderlinden et al. 1991). Loewenstein (1994) reported that the prevalence in North America is about 1%, compared with a prevalence of 10% for all dissociative disorders as a group.

There has been a considerable rise in the number of reported DID cases in recent years. Factors that account for this increase include a more general awareness of the diagnosis among mental health professionals; the availability, starting with DSM-III, of specific diagnostic criteria (Table 18–7); and reduced misdiagnosis of DID as schizophrenia or borderline personality disorder. Whereas the increase in reported cases is best documented in North America, a recent study shows similar phenomenology and link to trauma history in Europe (Boon and Draijer 1993a, 1993b). In fact, there are reports of DID in almost all societies and races, making it a true cross-cultural diagnosis (Coons et al. 1991). Indeed, case reports have described DID or related disorders among Asians (Putnam 1989; Yap 1960), blacks (Coons et al. 1986; R. Solomon 1983; Stern 1984), Europeans (van der Hart 1993), Hispanics (Allison 1974; Ronquillo 1991; R. Solomon 1983), and inhabitants of Australia and New Zealand (Gelb 1993; Price and Hess 1979), Canada (Horen et al. 1995; Ross et al. 1989, 1991a, 1991b; Vincent and Pickering 1988), the Caribbean (Wittkower 1970), India (Adityanjee et al. 1989; Varma et

al. 1981), Japan (Berger et al. 1994), the Netherlands (Boon and Draijer 1993b; van der Hart and Nijenhuis 1993; Vanderlinden et al. 1991; van Dyck 1993), Norway (Boe et al. 1993), Sweden (Eriksson and Lundin 1996), and Turkey (Sar et al. 1996).

Other authors attribute the increase in reported cases to hypnotic suggestion and misdiagnosis (Brenner 1994, 1996a; Frankel 1990; Ganaway 1989, 1995; Mayer-Gross et al. 1969; McHugh 1995a, 1995b; Spanos et al. 1985, 1986). Proponents of this point of view argue that individuals with DID are as a group highly hypnotizable and therefore quite suggestible and that not infrequently a few specialist clinicians make the vast majority of diagnoses. However, it has been observed that the symptomatology of patients diagnosed by specialists in dissociation does not differ from that assessed by psychiatrists, psychologists, and physicians in more general practice, who diagnose one or two cases a year. Furthermore, were such patients so suggestible and subject to directive influence by diagnosticians, it is surprising that their presenting symptoms persist for an average of 6.5 years before attaining the diagnosis (Putnam et al. 1986). Rather, it would seem likely that such patients would accept a suggestion that they have another disorder, such as schizophrenia or borderline personality disorder, because they encounter many clinicians who are unaware of or not familiar with DID, especially if it is suggested that the patients have something else. Because these patients are indeed highly hypnotizable and therefore suggestible (Frischholz 1985), care must be taken in the manner in which the illness is presented to them. However, it is unlikely that the increased number of cases currently reported is accounted for by suggestion alone. Rather, a reduction in previous misdiagnoses and an increase in recognition of the prevalence and sequelae of physical and sexual abuse in childhood (Braun 1990; Bryer et al. 1987; Coons et al. 1988; Finkelhor 1984; Frischholz 1985; Goodwin 1982; Herman et al. 1989; Kluft 1984b, 1991; Pribor and Dinwiddie 1992; Putnam 1988; Putnam et al. 1986; Ross 1989; Russell 1986; D. Spiegel 1984; Terr 1991) are also likely explanations. Recently, there have been reports of "definite independent confirmation of the histories of abuse" (Coons 1994; Martinez-Taboas 1996) confirming not only the association between dissociative disorders and trauma, but also the occurrence of amnesia in response to traumatic experiences.

COURSE

DID is diagnosed in childhood with increasing frequency (Kluft 1984b) but typically emerges between adolescence and the third decade of life; it rarely presents as a new dis-

---

TABLE 18–7.   DSM-IV diagnostic criteria for dissociative identity disorder (multiple personality disorder)

A. The presence of two or more distinct identities or personality states (each with its own relatively enduring pattern of perceiving, relating to, and thinking about the environment and self).

B. At least two of these identities or personality states recurrently take control of the person's behavior.

C. Inability to recall important personal information that is too extensive to be explained by ordinary forgetfulness.

D. The disturbance is not due to the direct physiological effects of a substance (e.g., blackouts or chaotic behavior during alcohol intoxication) or a general medical condition (e.g., complex partial seizures). **Note:** In children, the symptoms are not attributable to imaginary playmates or other fantasy play.

order after an individual reaches age 40 years, but there is often considerable delay between initial symptom presentation and diagnosis (American Psychiatric Association 1994; Putnam et al. 1986).

Untreated, it is a chronic and recurrent disorder. It rarely remits spontaneously, but the symptoms may not be evident for some time (Kluft 1985b). DID has been called "a pathology of hiddenness" (Gutheil, as quoted in Kluft 1988, p. 575). The dissociation itself hampers self-monitoring and accurate reporting of symptoms. Many patients with the disorder are not fully aware of the extent of the dissociative symptomatology. They may be reluctant to bring up symptoms because of having encountered frequent skepticism. Furthermore, because the majority of DID patients report histories of sexual and physical abuse (Braun and Sachs 1985; Coons and Milstein 1992; Coons et al. 1988; Kluft 1985, 1988, 1991; Putnam 1988; Putnam et al. 1986; Ross 1989; Ross et al. 1990; Schultz et al. 1989; D. Spiegel 1984), the shame associated with that experience, as well as fear of retribution, may inhibit reporting of symptoms.

COMORBIDITY

The major comorbid psychiatric illnesses of DID are the depressive disorders (Putnam et al. 1986; Ross and Norton 1989; Ross et al. 1989), substance use disorders (Anderson et al. 1993; Coons 1984; Dunn et al. 1995; Ellason et al. 1996; Putnam et al. 1986; Rivera 1991), and borderline personality disorder (Anderson et al. 1993; Brodsky et al. 1995; Horevitz and Braun 1984; Shearer 1994). Sexual (Brenner 1996b; van der Kolk et al. 1994), eating (Berger et al. 1994; Valdiserri and Kihlstrom 1995; van der Kolk et al. 1994), and sleep disorders (Putnam et al. 1986) occur less commonly. Patients with DID frequently display self-mutilative behavior (Bliss 1980, 1984; Coons 1984; Gainer and Torem 1993; Greaves 1980; Putnam et al. 1986; Ross and Norton 1989; Zweig-Frank et al. 1994), impulsiveness, and overvaluing and devaluing of relationships that make approximately a third of DID patients fit the criteria for borderline personality disorder as well. Such individuals also show higher levels of depression (Horevitz and Braun 1984). Conversely, recent research shows dissociative symptoms in many patients with borderline personality disorder, especially those who report histories of physical and sexual abuse (Chu and Dill 1990; Ogata et al. 1990). Indeed, the impulsiveness, splitting, and hostility frequently seen in some older personality states are similar to the presentations seen in many patients with borderline personality disorder.

Comorbidity is complex in that patients with concur-rent diagnoses of DID and borderline personality disorder (approximately one-third) are also more likely to meet the criteria for major depressive disorder. In addition, they frequently meet the criteria for PTSD, with intrusive flashbacks, recurring dreams of physical and sexual abuse, avoidance and loss of pleasure of usually pleasurable activities, and symptoms of hyperarousal, especially when exposed to reminders of childhood trauma (Kluft 1985, 1991; Putnam 1993; D. Spiegel 1990b; van der Kolk and Fisler 1995; van der Kolk et al. 1994, 1996).

In addition, these patients are not infrequently misdiagnosed as having schizophrenia (Coons 1984; Ellason and Ross 1995; Kluft 1987; Putnam et al. 1986; Ross and Norton 1988, Ross et al. 1990; Steinberg et al. 1994). This diagnostic confusion is understandable given that the first-rank criterion for schizophrenia is that the patient has an apparent delusion (i.e., that his or her body is occupied by more than one person). These patients frequently have auditory hallucinations in which one personality state speaks to or comments on the activities of another (Bliss 1986; Bliss et al. 1983; Coons 1984; Kluft 1987; Peterson 1995; Putnam et al. 1986; Ross et al. 1990). When misdiagnosed as having schizophrenia, these patients are frequently put on neuroleptics, with poor therapeutic response.

Individuals with DID report an average of 15 somatic or conversion symptoms (Anderson et al. 1993; Bowman 1993; Bowman and Markand 1996; Kaplan et al. 1995; Ross et al. 1989, 1990) and other psychosomatic symptoms such as migraine headaches (D. Spiegel 1987). Studies show that approximately one-third of these patients have complex partial seizures (Schenk and Bear 1981), although more recent studies have not found seizure rates to be that high and do not show substantial elevations in Dissociative Experiences Scale scores of patients with complex partial seizures compared with those of other neurological patients (Loewenstein and Putnam 1988). There is sufficient comorbidity that patients recently diagnosed with DID should be evaluated for the possibility of a seizure disorder.

PSYCHOLOGICAL TESTING

The diagnosis of DID can be facilitated by psychological testing. Form level on the Rorschach is usually within the normal range, but there are frequent emotionally dramatic responses, often involving mutilation, especially on the color cards (such responses are often seen in patients with histrionic personality disorder as well). Good form level is useful in distinguishing DID patients from schizophrenic patients, who have poor form level. Also, unlike individuals with schizophrenia, those with DID score far higher than healthy individuals on standard measures of hypnotizability, whereas schizophrenic patients tend to show lower than normal or the absence of high hypnotizability (Lavoie and Sabourin 1980; Pettinati 1982; Pettinati et al. 1990; D. Spiegel and Fink 1979; D. Spiegel et al. 1982; van der Hart and Spiegel 1993). Thus, there is comparatively little overlap in the hypnotizability scores of schizophrenic patients versus those of DID patients.

More recently, scales of trait dissociation have been developed (Bernstein and Putnam 1986; Ross 1989), and patients with DID score extremely high on these scales in contrast to healthy populations and other patient groups (Ross et al. 1990; Steinberg et al. 1990).

TREATMENT

Psychotherapy

Therapeutic direction. It is possible to help DID patients gain control in several ways over the dissociative process underlying their symptoms. The fundamental psychotherapeutic stance should involve meeting patients halfway in the sense of acknowledging that they experience themselves as fragmented, yet the reality is that the fundamental problem is a failure of integration of disparate memories and aspects of the self. Therefore, the goal in therapy is to facilitate integration of disparate elements. This can be done in a variety of ways.

Secrets are frequently a problem with DID patients, who attempt to use the therapist to reinforce a dissociative strategy that withholds relevant information from certain personality states. Such patients often like to confide plans or stories in the therapist with the idea that the information is to be kept from other parts of the self, for example, traumatic memories or plans for self-destructive activities. Clear limit setting and commitment on the part of the therapist to helping all portions of a patient's personality structure learn about warded-off information is important. It is wise to clarify explicitly that the therapist will not become involved in secret collusion. Furthermore, when important agreements are negotiated, such as a commitment on the part of the patient to seek medical help before acting on a thought to harm self or others, it is useful to discuss with the patient that this is an "all-points bulletin," that is, one that requires attention from all the relevant personality states. The excuse that certain personality states were "not aware" of the agreement should not be accepted.

For example, a patient with DID who had been in treatment for many years demonstrated a new alter who threatened to arrange for an apparently accidental death. The therapist told the alter that he, the therapist, would have to share this information with the other personalities. "You can't do that," the alter replied. "That would violate doctor-patient confidentiality." Suppressing a smile, the therapist explained that confidentiality did not apply between identities.

Hypnosis. Hypnosis can be helpful in therapy as well as in diagnosis (Braun 1984; Kluft 1982; Maldonado and Spiegel 1995, 1998; Maldonado et al. 1997; Smith 1993; H. Spiegel and Spiegel 1978/1987).

First, the simple structure of hypnotic induction may elicit dissociative phenomena. For example, the Hypnotic Induction Profile (H. Spiegel and Spiegel 1978/1987) was administered to a woman who had suffered hysterical pseudoseizures. In the middle of a routine induction, her head suddenly turned to the side and she relived, with considerable affect, as if it were happening in present tense, an episode in which she had been abducted and sexually assaulted. This enabled her and the clinician to reanalyze her symptoms as spontaneous dissociation, similar to the hypnotic state she had been in. The capacity to elicit such symptoms on command provides the first hint of the ability to control these symptoms. Most of these patients have the experience of being unable to stop dissociative symptoms but are often intrigued by the possibility of starting them. This carries with it the potential for changing or stopping the symptoms as well.

Hypnosis can be helpful in facilitating access to dissociated personalities. The personalities may simply occur spontaneously during hypnotic induction. An alternative strategy is to hypnotize the patient and use age regression to help the patient reorient to a time when a different personality state was manifest. An instruction later to change times back to the present tense usually elicits a return to the other personality state. This then becomes an alternative means of teaching the patient control over the dissociation.

Alternatively, entering the state of hypnosis may make it possible to simply "call up" different identities or personality states. Patients can be taught a simple self-hypnosis exercise (as noted earlier in this chapter and covered in more detail in Chapter 32). For example, the patient can be told to count to herself from one to three: On 1, do one thing: look up. On 2, do two things: slowly close your eyes and take a deep breath. On 3, do three things: let the breath out, let your eyes relax but keep them closed, and let your body float. Then let one hand float up in the air like a balloon. Develop a pleasant sense of floating throughout your body. After some formal exercises such as this, it is often possible to simply ask to speak with a given alter personality, without the formal use of hypnosis. Merely asking to talk with a given identity usually suffices after a while.

Memory retrieval. Because loss of memory in DID is complex and chronic, its retrieval is likewise a more extended and integral part of the psychotherapeutic process. The therapy becomes an integrating experience of information sharing among disparate personality elements. In conceptualizing DID as a chronic PTSD, the psychotherapeutic strategy involves a focus on working through traumatic memories in addition to controlling the dissociation.

Controlled access to memories greatly facilitates psychotherapy. As in the treatment of patients with dissociative amnesia, a variety of strategies can be employed to help DID patients break down amnesic barriers. Using hypnosis to go to that place in imagination and ask one or more such parts of the self to interact can be helpful.

Once these memories of earlier traumatic experience have been brought into consciousness, it is crucial to help the patient work through the painful affect, inappropriate self-blame, and other reactions to these memories. A model of grief work is helpful, enabling the patient to acknowledge and bear the import of such memories (Lindemann 1944; D. Spiegel 1981). It may be useful to have the patient visualize the memories rather than relive them as a way of making their intensity more manageable. It also can be useful to have the patient divide the memories onto two sides of an imaginary screen; for example, on one side, picturing something an abuser did to him or her and on the other side, picturing how the patient tried to protect himself or herself from the abuse.

> A young woman with DID remembered a particularly painful episode in hypnosis. When she was 12 years old, her stepfather smoked a good deal of marijuana and then forced her to have oral sex with him. She recalled being repelled by what he was forcing her to do and then remembered that she had gagged and vomited all over him. "I spoiled his fun. He threw me up against a wall, but it did not bother me a bit because I knew I ruined it for him." She was instructed to picture on one side of the screen what he had done to her and on the other, what she had done to him.

Such techniques can help make the traumatic memories more bearable by placing them in a broader perspective, one in which the trauma victim also can identify adaptive aspects of his or her response to the trauma.

This technique and similar approaches can help these individuals work through traumatic memories, enabling them to bear the memories in consciousness and therefore reducing the need for dissociation as a means of keeping such memories out of consciousness. Although these techniques can be helpful and often result in reduced fragmentation and integration (Kluft 1986; Maldonado and Spiegel 1995, 1998; D. Spiegel 1984, 1986a), there are a number of complications that can occur in the psychotherapy of these patients as well.

The information retrieved from memory in these ways should be reviewed, traumatic memories put into perspective, and emotional expression encouraged and worked through, with the goal of sharing the information as widely as possible among various parts of the patient's personality structure. Instructions to other alter personalities to "listen" while a given alter is talking, and reviewing previously dissociated material uncovered, can be helpful. The therapist conveys his or her desire to disseminate the information, without accepting responsibility for transmitting it across all personality boundaries.

The "rule of thirds." Psychotherapy with a DID patient can be a time-consuming and emotionally taxing process. The "rule of thirds" (Kluft 1988, 1991) is a helpful guideline. Spend the first third of the psychotherapy session assessing the patient's current mental state and life problems and defining a problem area that might benefit from retrieval into conscious memory and working through. Spend the second third of the session accessing and working through this memory. Allow a final third for helping the patient assimilate the information, regulate and modulate emotional responses, and discuss any responses to the therapist and plans for the immediate future.

It is wise to use this final third of the session for debriefing and helping the patient to reorient, to attempt to integrate the new material, to transmit information across personalities, and to prepare to terminate the session. There may be resistance on the part of the therapist to doing this because the intense abreactive materials are often so compelling and interesting. There also may be resistance on the part of the patient to sharing of information across personalities.

Given the intensity of the material that often emerges involving memories of sexual and physical abuse, and the sudden shifts in mental state accompanied by amnesia, the therapist is called upon to take a clear and structured role in managing the psychotherapy. Appropriate limits must be set about self-destructive or threatening behavior and agreements made regarding physical safety and treatment compliance, and other matters must be presented to the patient in such a way that dissociative ignorance is not an acceptable explanation for failure to live up to agreements.

Traumatic transference. Transference applies with special meaning in patients who have been physically and sexually abused. These patients have experienced presumed caretakers who acted instead in an exploitative and sometimes sadistic fashion. These patients thus expect the same from their therapists. Although their reality testing is good enough that they can perceive genuine caring, they expect therapists either to exploit them, with the patients viewing the working through of traumatic memories as a reinflicting of the trauma and the therapists' taking sadistic pleasure in the patients' suffering, or to be excessively passive, with the patients identifying the therapist with some uncaring family figure who knew abuse was occurring but did little or nothing to stop it. It is important in managing the therapy to keep these issues in mind and make them frequent topics of discussion. Attention to these issues can diffuse, but not eliminate, such traumatic transference distortions of the therapeutic relationship (Maldonado and Spiegel 1995, 1998; D. Spiegel 1988).

Integration. The ultimate goal of psychotherapy for DID patients is integration of the disparate states. There can be considerable resistance to this process. Early in therapy, the patient views the dissociation as tremendous protection: "I knew my father could get some of me, but he couldn't get all of me." Indeed, he or she may experience efforts of integration as an attempt on the part of the therapist to "kill" personalities. These fears must be worked through and the patient shown how to control the degree of integration, giving the patient a sense of gradually being able to control his or her dissociative processes in the service of working through traumatic memories. The process of the psychotherapy, in emphasizing control, must alter rather than reinforce the content, which involves reexperiencing of helplessness, a symbolic reenactment of trauma (D. Spiegel 1986b).

As previously mentioned, a patient with DID often fears integration as an attempt to kill alter personalities and make the patient more vulnerable to mistreatment by depriving him or her of the dissociative defense. At the same time, this defense represents an internalization of the abusive person or persons in the patient's memory. Setting aside the defense also means acknowledging and bearing the discomfort of helplessness at having been victimized and working through the irrational self-blame that gave the patient a fantasy of control over events that he or she was in fact helpless to control. Yet difficult as it is, ultimately, the goal of psychotherapy is mastery over the dissociative process, controlled access to dissociative states, integration of warded-off painful memories and material, and a more integrated continuum of identity, memory, and consciousness (Maldonado and Spiegel 1995, 1998; D. Spiegel 1988). Although there have been no controlled trials of

psychotherapy outcome in patients with this disorder, case series reports indicate a positive outcome in a majority of cases (Kluft 1984c, 1986, 1991).

Psychopharmacology

To this day, there is no good evidence that medication of any type has a direct therapeutic effect on the dissociative process manifested by DID patients (Loewenstein 1991b; Markowitz and Gill 1996; Putnam 1989). In fact, most dissociative symptoms seem relatively resistant to pharmacological intervention (Loewenstein 1991a, 1991b). Thus, pharmacological treatment has been limited to the control of signs and symptoms afflicting DID patients or comorbid conditions rather than the treatment of dissociation per se.

Whereas in the past, short-acting barbiturates such as sodium amobarbital were used intravenously to reverse functional amnesias, this technique is no longer employed, largely because of poor results (J. C. Perry and Jacobs 1982).

Benzodiazepines have at times been employed to facilitate recall through controlling secondary anxiety associated with retrieval of traumatic memories. However, these effects may be nonspecific at best. Furthermore, sudden mental state transitions induced by medications may increase rather than decrease amnesic barriers, as the recent concern about triazolam, a short-acting benzodiazepine hypnotic, indicates. Thus, inducing state changes pharmacologically could in theory add to difficulty in retrieval. The only systematic study on the use of benzodiazepines in DID patients was conducted by Loewenstein et al. (1988). In his study, he used clonazepam successfully to control PTSD-like symptoms in a small sample ($n = 5$) of DID patients, achieving improvement in sleep continuity and a decrease in frequency of flashbacks and nightmares.

Antidepressants are the most useful class of psychotropic agents for patients with DID. Such patients frequently have dysthymic disorder or major depression as well, and when these disorders are present, especially with somatic signs and suicidal ideation, antidepressant medication can be helpful. At least two studies report on the successful use of antidepressant medications (Barkin et al. 1986; Kluft 1984a, 1985). The use of antidepressants should be limited to the treatment of DID patients who experience symptoms of major depression (Barkin et al. 1986). The newer selective serotonin reuptake inhibitors (SSRIs) are effective at reducing comorbid depressive symptoms and have the advantage of far less lethality in overdose compared with tricyclics and monoamine oxidase inhibitors (MAOIs). Medication compliance is a problem with such patients because dissociated personality states may interfere with the taking of medication by the patients' "hiding" or hoarding of pills, or patients may overdose.

Antipsychotics are rarely useful in reducing dissociative symptoms. They are used occasionally for containing impulsive behavior, with varying effect. More often, they are employed with little benefit when DID patients have been misdiagnosed as being schizophrenic (Kluft 1987). In addition to the risks of side effects such as tardive dyskinesia, there is a risk that the neuroleptics will reduce the range of affect, thereby making patients with DID look spuriously as though they were schizophrenic. In fact, most DID researchers have reported an extremely high incidence of adverse side effects to the use of neuroleptic medications (Barkin et al. 1986; Kluft 1984a, 1988; Putnam 1989; Ross 1989).

Anticonvulsants have been used to treat seizure disorders (Mesulam 1981; Schenk and Bear 1981), which have a high rate of comorbidity with DID, comorbid mood disorders (Fichtner et al. 1990), and the impulsiveness associated with personality disorders. These agents are rarely definitively helpful and should be avoided due to the high incidence of serious side effects (Devinsky et al. 1989).

There have been case reports suggesting that β-blockers may be useful in the treatment of hyperarousal, anxiety, poor impulse control, disorganized thinking, and rapid or uncontrolled switching in DID patients (Braun 1990). But little information is available regarding the actual success rate, comorbid diagnoses, or prevalence of adverse drug reactions.

DISSOCIATIVE TRANCE DISORDER

CULTURAL CONTEXT

Dissociative phenomena are ubiquitous around the world, occurring in virtually every culture (Castillo 1994a, 1994b; Kirmayer 1993; Lewis-Fernandez 1993). These phenomena seem to be more prevalent in the less heavily industrialized second- and third-world countries, although they can be found everywhere. For this reason, a number of scholars have argued against the inclusion of possession or trance disorder as a DSM diagnostic category (Noll 1993). There are descriptions of mediums or possession episodes in different cultures, but they may all serve a similar purpose. There are shamans among Hispanics (Alonso 1988) and in Brazil (Shapiro 1992), China (Kua et al. 1993), India (Moore 1993; Nuckolls 1991), Iran (Safa 1988), Israel (Bilu and Beit-Hallahmi 1989; Shirali and Bharti 1986), Japan (Eguchi 1991; Etsuko 1991), Madagascar (Lambek

1988; Sharp 1990, 1994), Malaysia (McLellan 1991; Ong 1988), New Guinea (Schieffelin 1996), Samoa (Mageo 1996), Singapore (Kua et al. 1986), South Africa (Heap and Ramphele 1991), South Asia (Castillo 1994a, 1994b), Thailand (Trangkasombat et al. 1995), Zambia (Pullela 1986), and Zanzibar (Tantam 1993). Other dissociative syndromes include demonic possession in Brazil (Heap and Ramphele 1991), Chilopa ritual sacrifices in Malawi (Machleidt and Peltzer 1991), and Zar possession in Northen Sudan (Boddy 1988) and Ethiopia (Witztum et al. 1996).

Most scholars agree that the most common clinical features of trance states are amnesia, emotional disturbances, and loss of identity (D. Li and Spiegel 1992). In a study comparing the characteristic features of the possession-trance in three different ethnic groups in Chinese, Malayans, and Indians, Kua et al. (1986) found a set of similarities, including alteration in the level of consciousness, amnesia for the period of the trance, stereotyped behavior characteristic of a deity, duration of less than 1 hour, fatigue at the termination of the trance, normal behavior in the interval between trances, onset before age 25 years, low social class status, poor educational level, and prior witnessing of a trance.

Dissociative symptoms are widely understood as an idiom of distress. The major purposes served by possession and trance states include the need to gain power, prestige, and status and the desire to express aggressive and sexual impulses (Shirali and Bharti 1986), especially given the cultural overdetermination of women's selfhood (Boddy 1988). Spirit-possession rituals may mystify the source of women's suppression and absolve women of any responsibility for an otherwise unacceptable challenge to patriarchal control (Sered 1994). They also may provide the subject with a sense of social association and ultimately attempt to make something socially useful from feelings such as aggression that were previously socially disintegrative (Tantam 1993), may provide a release from normative structural constraints, and may facilitate role reversal and role enhancement (McLellan 1991).

Some even suggest that possession can be interpreted as historical discourse, usually containing tales of tradition (Mageo 1996), or even as an alternative method of healing—not too different from Western psychotherapy (Machleidt and Peltzer 1991; Mulhern 1991; Tantam 1993)—thus performing a wider social function. In fact, "when the embodiment of an alternative identity is exercised in the cross-cultural complex of spirit possession, it provides a conduit through which subjective suffering can be transcended and through which the past, present, and future can be expressed" (Mulhern 1991).

The trance and possession categories of dissociative trance disorder constitute by far the most common kind of dissociative disorder around the world. Several studies of dissociative disorders in India, for example, demonstrate that dissociative trance and possession are the most prevalent dissociative disorders (i.e., approximately 3.5% of psychiatric admissions (Adityanjee et al. 1989; Saxena and Prasad 1989). On the other hand, DID, which is relatively more common in the United States, is virtually never diagnosed in India. Cultural as well as biological factors may account for the different content and form of dissociative symptoms. Nonetheless, the underlying dissociative mechanism inhibiting integration of perception, memory, and identity makes these syndromes an important class of dissociative disorders.

Differences in culture clearly influence almost all mental disorders, and therefore the contents of religious delusions will be different in a Hindu or Muslim person with schizophrenia than in a Christian person with the same disorder. Depression takes a very different form in China, resembling what used to be called *neurasthenia*, with a variety of somatic symptoms predominating more so than the guilty ruminations seen in the West (Kleinman 1977). Likewise, the variations in form of the dissociative disorders only serve to underscore the ubiquity of the dissociative mechanism. Nonetheless, the variety of mental contents is worthy of attention. The DSM-IV Task Force voted to include dissociative trance disorder in an appendix of DSM-IV to stimulate further research on the question of whether or not it should be a separate Axis I disorder rather than an example in the category of dissociative disorders not otherwise specified, in which it was placed in DSM-III-R (Table 18–8). Some suggest, and we agree, that the inclusion of trance and possession disorder in DSM-IV intends to develop a sense of cultural sensitivity and internationalization of DSM. On the other hand, designating trance and possession disorder as a formal diagnostic disorder carries with it the risks in attempting to craft a global nosological system, an impossible task. Furthermore, the composite category "dissociative trance disorder," encompassing both trance and possession phenomena, may be misinterpreted as "a single, uniform diagnostic construct and may suggest a greater degree of phenomenological uniformity than exists among indigenous syndromes, creating a hybrid nosological entity without validity" (Lewis-Fernandez 1992, p. 123–167).

These dissociative episodes are usually understood as an idiom of distress, and yet they are not viewed as normal. That is, they are not a generally accepted part of cultural and religious practice that may often involve normal trance phenomena, such as trance dancing in the Balinese Hindu

TABLE 18–8. DSM-IV (appendix) diagnostic criteria for dissociative trance disorder

A. Either (1) or (2):

    (1) Trance, i.e., temporary marked alteration in the state of consciousness or loss of customary sense of personal identity without replacement by an alternate identity, associated with at least one of the following:

        (a) Narrowing of awareness of immediate surroundings or unusually narrow and selective focusing on environmental stimuli

        (b) Stereotyped behaviors or movements that are experienced as being beyond one's control

    (2) Possession trance, i.e., a single or episodic alteration in the state of consciousness characterized by the replacement of customary sense of personal identity by a new identity. This is attributed to the influence of a spirit, power, deity, or other person, as evidenced by one (or more) of the following:

        (a) Stereotyped and culturally determined behaviors or movements that are experienced as being controlled by the possessing agent

        (b) Full or partial amnesia for the event

B. The trance or possession trance state is not accepted as a normal part of a collective cultural or religious practice.

C. The trance or possession trance state causes clinically significant distress or impairment in social, occupational, or other important areas of functioning.

D. The trance or possession trance state does not occur exclusively during the course of a psychotic disorder (including mood disorder with psychotic features and brief psychotic disorder) or dissociative identity disorder and is not due to the direct physiological effects of a substance or a general medical condition.

Note. The diagnostic criteria for DSM-IV dissociative trance disorder appear in Appendix B: "Criteria Sets and Axes Provided for Further Study."

culture. Trance dancers in that culture are remarkable for being the only portion of this socially stable society able to elevate their social status. This elevation of social status is done through developing an ability to enter trance states. They are able within the social ceremony to induce an altered state of consciousness in which they dance over hot coals, hold a sword at their throat, or in other ways exhibit exceptional powers of concentration and physical prowess. They are frequently watched by other dancers to make sure that they retain control and do not hurt themselves. This form of trance is considered socially normal and even exalted. By contrast, trance and possession disorder is viewed by the local community as a common but aberrant form of behavior that requires intervention. Although trance and possession disorder is clearly an idiom of distress (e.g., discomfort in a new family environment), there is an array of alternative strategies that the majority of individuals use for coping with such distress. Thus, cultural informants make it clear that persons with trance and possession trance disorders are acting abnormally, if recognizably.

It is interesting that the most common form of dissociative disorder in the West is DID—that is, the experience of fragmentation of individual identity—whereas in the East this disorder involves possession by an outside spirit, deity, or other entity. Given the greater sociocentric organization of culture in the East, it makes sense that the dissociative problem would take the form of an intruding outside identity, whereas in the West the disorder takes the form of competing internal identities. Nevertheless, some have proposed that possession trance and multiple personality disorders arose on the basis of similar histories of child abuse and the use of dissociation as a defense mechanism (Bourguignon 1989). Still, different cultures apply their own idiosyncratic etiological theories. The therapeutic approaches and subjects responses may be rather similar or radically different, depending on the traditional beliefs of the culture in question.

CLASSIFICATION

Dissociative trance disorder has been divided into two broad categories: dissociative trance and possession trance (Table 18–9).

Dissociative Trance

Dissociative trance phenomena are characterized by a sudden alteration in consciousness not accompanied by distinct alternative identities. In this form, the dissociative symptom involves consciousness rather than identity. Also, in dissociative trance, the activities performed are rather simple, usually involving sudden collapse, immobilization, dizziness, shrieking, screaming, or crying. Memory is rarely affected, and amnesia, if any, is fragmented.

Dissociative trance phenomena frequently involve sudden, extreme changes in sensory and motor control. Classic examples include *ataque de nervios*, which is prevalent throughout Latin America. This condition, for example, is estimated to have a 12% lifetime prevalence rate in Puerto Rico (Lewis-Fernandez 1993). Typically, the individual suddenly starts to shake convulsively, hyperventilate, scream, and exhibit agitation and aggressive movements. These behaviors may be followed by collapse and loss of consciousness. Afterward, such individuals report

TABLE 18–9. Comparison of Western and Eastern types of dissociative syndromes

Dissociative phenomenon	Western	Eastern
Identity	DID (MPD): multiple internal identities	Possession trance: control by external identities
	Dissociative fugue	
Memory	Dissociative amnesia	Secondary in dissociative trance, more common in possession trance
Perception	Depersonalization disorder	Dissociative trance (e.g., *latah*, *ataque de nervios*)
Consciousness	Acute stress disorder	Dissociative trance

DID = dissociative identity disorder; MPD = multiple personality disorder.

being exhausted and may have some amnesia for the event (Lewis-Fernandez 1993).

Falling out occurs frequently among African Americans in the southern United States. Affected individuals may collapse suddenly, unable to see or speak even though they are conscious. These persons may be confused afterward but usually are not amnesic to the episode (Lewis-Fernandez 1993).

In the Malay version of trance disorder, *latah*, affected individuals may have a sudden vision of a spirit that is threatening them. These persons scream or cry, strike out physically, and may need restraints. They may report amnesia, but they do not clearly take on the identity of the offending spirit (Lewis-Fernandez 1993).

Possession Trance

In contrast to dissociative trance, possession trance involves the assumption of a distinct alternate identity, usually that of a deity, ancestor, or spirit. The person in this trance often engages in rather complex activities, which may take the form of expressing otherwise forbidden thoughts or needs, negotiating for change in family or social status, or engaging in aggressive behavior. Possession usually involves amnesia for a large portion of the episode during which the alternate identity was in control of the person's behavior.

In Indian possession syndrome, the affected individual suddenly begins speaking in an altered voice with an altered identity, usually that of a deity recognizable to others. Through this voice, a person may refer to himself or herself in the third person. The affected person's "spirit" may negotiate for changes in the family environment or become agitated or aggressive. Possession syndrome typically occurs in a recently married woman who finds herself uncomfortable or unwelcome in her mother-in-law's home. Such individuals are usually unable to directly express their discomfort.

TREATMENT

Treatment of these disorders varies from culture to culture. Most syndromes occur within the context of acute social stress and thus serve the purpose of recruiting help from the family and other support systems or removing the subject from the immediate danger or threat. Ceremonies to remove or appease the invading spirit are commonly used. The role of psychiatry should be focused on ruling out any possible organic cause for the symptoms displayed, treating comorbid psychiatric conditions (if any are present), avoiding excess medication, understanding the social context and role of the syndrome, and facilitating a favorable outcome.

CONCLUSIONS

The dissociative disorders constitute a challenging component of psychiatric illness. The failure of integration of memory, identity, perception, and consciousness seen in these disorders results in symptomatology that illustrates fundamental problems in the organization of mental processes. Dissociative phenomena often occur during and after physical trauma but also may represent transient or chronic defensive patterns. Dissociative disorders are generally treatable and constitute a domain in which psychotherapy is a primary modality, although pharmacological treatment of comorbid conditions such as depression can be quite helpful. The dissociative disorders are ubiquitous around the world, although they take a variety of forms. They represent a fascinating window into the processing of identity, memory, perception, and consciousness, and they pose a variety of diagnostic, therapeutic, and research challenges.

REFERENCES

Abeles M, Schilder P: Psychogenic loss of personal identity: amnesia. Archives of Neurology and Psychiatry 34:587–604, 1935

Adityanjee, Raju GSP, Khandelwal SK: Current status of multiple personality disorder in India. Am J Psychiatry 146:1607–1610, 1989

Allison RB: A new treatment approach for multiple personalities. Am J Clin Hypn 17:15–32, 1974

Alonso L: Mental illness complicated by the santeria belief in spirit possession. Hospital and Community Psychiatry 39:1188–1191, 1988

Ambrosino SV: Phobic anxiety-depersonalization syndrome. New York State Journal of Medicine 73: 419–425, 1973

American Psychiatric Association: Diagnostic and Statistical Manual of Mental Disorders, 3rd Edition. Washington, DC, American Psychiatric Association, 1980

American Psychiatric Association: Diagnostic and Statistical Manual of Mental Disorders, 3rd Edition, Revised. Washington, DC, American Psychiatric Association, 1987

American Psychiatric Association: Diagnostic and Statistical Manual of Mental Disorders, 4th Edition. Washington, DC, American Psychiatric Association, 1994

Anderson G, Yasenik L, Ross CA: Dissociative experiences and disorders among women who identify themselves as sexual abuse survivors. Child Abuse Negl 17:677–686, 1993

Baars BJ: A Cognitive Theory of Consciousness. New York, Cambridge University Press, 1988

Ballenger JC, Burrows GD, Dupont RL, et al: Alprazolam in panic disorder and agoraphobia: results from a multicenter trial, I: efficacy in short term treatment. Arch Gen Psychiatry 45:413–422, 1988

Barkin R, Braun BG, Kluft RP: The dilemma of drug therapy for multiple personality disorder, in Treatment of Multiple Personality Disorder. Edited by Braun BG. Washington, DC, American Psychiatric Press, 1986, pp 107–132

Baron DA, Nagy R: The amobarbital interview in a general hospital setting, friend or foe: a case report. Gen Hosp Psychiatry 10:220–222, 1988

Berger D, Saito S, Ono Y, et al: Dissociation and child abuse histories in an eating disorder cohort in Japan. Acta Psychiatr Scand 90:274–280, 1994

Bernstein EM, Putnam FW: Development, reliability, and validity of a dissociation scale. J Nerv Ment Dis 174:727–735, 1986

Bilu Y, Beit-Hallahmi B: Dybbuk-possession as a hysterical symptom: psychodynamic and socio-cultural factors. Isr J Psychiatry Relat Sci 26:138–149, 1989

Blank AS Jr: The longitudinal course of posttraumatic stress disorder, in Posttraumatic Stress Disorder: DSM-IV and Beyond. Edited by Davidson JRT, Foa EB. Washington, DC, American Psychiatric Press, 1993, pp 3–22

Bliss EL: Multiple personalities: a report of 14 cases with implications for schizophrenia and hysteria. Arch Gen Psychiatry 37:1388–1397, 1980

Bliss EL: A symptom profile of patients with multiple personalities, including MMPI results. J Nerv Ment Dis 172: 197–202, 1984

Bliss EL: Multiple Personality, Allied Disorders, and Hypnosis. New York, Oxford University Press, 1986

Bliss EL, Larson EM, Nakashima SR: Auditory hallucinations and schizophrenia. J Nerv Ment Dis 171:30–33, 1983

Blue FR: Use of directive therapy in the treatment of depersonalization neurosis. Psychol Rep 49:904–906, 1979

Boddy J: Spirits and selves in Northern Sudan: the cultural therapeutics of possession and trance. American Ethnologist 15:4–27, 1988

Boe T, Haslerud J, Knudsen H: Multiple personality: a phenomenon also in Norway? Tidsskr Nor Laegeforen 113: 3230–3232, 1993

Boon S, Draijer N: Multiple personality disorder in the Netherlands: a clinical investigation of 71 patients. Am J Psychiatry 150:489–494, 1993a

Boon S, Draijer N: Multiple Personality Disorder in the Netherlands: A Study on Reliability and Validity of the Diagnosis. Amsterdam, Swets & Zeitlinger, 1993b

Bourguignon E: Multiple personality, possession trance, and the psychic unity of mankind. Ethos 17:371–384, 1989

Bowman ES: Etiology and clinical course of pseudoseizures: relationship to trauma, depression, and dissociation. Psychosomatics 34:333–342, 1993

Bowman ES, Markand ON: Psychodynamics and psychiatric diagnoses of pseudoseizure subjects. Am J Psychiatry 153:57–63, 1996

Braun BG: Uses of hypnosis with multiple personality. Psychiatric Annals 14:34–36; 39–40, 1984

Braun BG: Multiple personality disorder: an overview. Am J Occup Ther 44:971–976, 1990

Braun BG, Sachs RG: The development of multiple personality disorder: predisposing, precipitating, and perpetuating factors, in Childhood Antecedents of Multiple Personality Disorder. Edited by Kluft RP. Washington, DC, American Psychiatric Press, 1985, pp 37–64

Bremner JD, Brett E: Trauma-related dissociative states and long-term psychopathology in posttraumatic stress disorder. J Trauma Stress 10:37–49, 1997

Brenner I: The dissociative character: a reconsideration of "multiple personality." J Am Psychoanal Assoc 42:819–846, 1994

Brenner I: The characterological basis of multiple personality. Am J Psychother 50:154–166, 1996a

Brenner I: On trauma, perversion, and "multiple personality." J Am Psychoanal Assoc 44:785–814, 1996b

Breuer J, Freud S: Studies on hysteria (1893–1895), in The Standard Edition of the Complete Psychological Works of Sigmund Freud, Vol 2. Translated and edited by Strachey J. London, Hogarth Press, 1955, pp 201–319

Brodsky BS, Cloitre M, Dulit RA: Relationship of dissociation to self-mutilation and childhood abuse in borderline personality disorder. Am J Psychiatry 152:1788–1792, 1995

Brown GR, Anderson B: Psychiatric morbidity in adult inpatients with childhood histories of sexual and physical abuse. Am J Psychiatry 148:55–61, 1991

Brown W: The treatment of cases of shell shock in an advanced neurological centre. Lancet 2:197–200, 1918

Bryer JB, Nelson BA, Miller JB, et al: Childhood sexual and physical abuse as factors in adult psychiatric illness. Am J Psychiatry 144:1426–1430, 1987

Butler LD, Duran EFD, Jasiukatis P, et al: Hypnotizability and traumatic experience: a diathesis-stress model of dissociative symptomatology. Am J Psychiatry 153:42–63, 1996

Cardeña E, Spiegel D: Dissociative reactions to the San Francisco Bay Area earthquake of 1989. Am J Psychiatry 150:474–478, 1993

Carlier IV, Lamberts RD, Fouwels AJ, et al: PTSD in relation to dissociation in traumatized police officers. Am J Psychiatry 153:1325–1328, 1996

Castillo RJ: Spirit possession in South Asia, dissociation or hysteria? I: theoretical background. Cult Med Psychiatry 18:1–21, 1994a

Castillo RJ: Spirit possession in South Asia, dissociation or hysteria? II: case histories. Cult Med Psychiatry 18:141–162, 1994b

Cattell JP, Cattell JS: Depersonalization: psychological and social perspectives, in American Handbook of Psychiatry. Edited by Arieti S. New York, Basic Books, 1994, pp 767–799

Charcot JM: Oeuvres Completes de J M Charcot, Tome XI. Paris, Lecrosnier et Babe, 1890

Christianson SA, Loftus EF: Memory for traumatic events. Applied Cognitive Psychology 1:225–239, 1987

Chu JA, Dill DL: Dissociative symptoms in relation to childhood physical and sexual abuse. Am J Psychiatry 147:887–892, 1990

Cohen JD, Servan-Schreiber D: Introduction to neural network models in psychiatry. Psychiatric Annals 22:113–118, 1992a

Cohen JD, Servan-Schreiber D: A neural network model of disturbances in the processing of context in schizophrenia. Psychiatric Annals 22:131–136, 1992b

Coons PM: The differential diagnosis of multiple personality: a comprehensive review. Psychiatr Clin North Am 7:51–65, 1984

Coons PM: Confirmation of childhood abuse in child and adolescent cases of multiple personality disorder and dissociative disorder not otherwise specified. J Nerv Ment Dis 182:461–464, 1994

Coons PM, Milstein V: Psychosexual disturbances in multiple personality: characteristics, etiology, and treatment. J Clin Psychiatry 47:106–110, 1986

Coons PM, Milstein V: Psychogenic amnesia: a clinical investigation of 25 cases. Dissociation 5:73–79, 1992

Coons PM, Bowman ES, Milstein V: Multiple personality disorder: a clinical investigation of 50 cases. J Nerv Ment Dis 17:519–527, 1988

Darves-Bornoz JM: Rape-related psychotraumatic syndromes. Eur J Obstet Gynecol Reprod Biol 71:59–65, 1997

Davison K: Episodic depersonalization: observations on 7 patients. Br J Psychiatry 110:505–513, 1964

Devinsky O, Putnam F, Grafman J, et al: Dissociative states and epilepsy. Neurology 39:835–840, 1989

Dollinger S: A case report of dissociative neurosis (depersonalization disorder) in an adolescent treated with family therapy and behavior modification. J Consult Clin Psychol 51:479–484, 1983

Dunn GE, Ryan JJ, Paolo AM, et al: Comorbidity of dissociative disorders among patients with substance use disorders. Psychiatr Serv 46:153–156, 1995

Eguchi S: Between folk concepts of illness and psychiatric diagnosis: kitsune-tsuki (fox possession) in a mountain village of western Japan. Cult Med Psychiatry 15:421–451, 1991

Ellason JW, Ross CA: Positive and negative symptoms in dissociative identity disorder and schizophrenia: a comparative analysis. J Nerv Ment Dis 183:236–241, 1995

Ellason JW, Ross CA, Sainton K, et al: Axis I and II comorbidity and childhood trauma history in chemical dependency. Bull Menninger Clin 60:39–51, 1996

Eriksson NG, Lundin T: Early traumatic stress reactions among Swedish survivors of the Estonia disaster. Br J Psychiatry 169:713–716, 1996

Etsuko M: The interpretations of fox possession: illness as metaphor. Cult Med Psychiatry 15:453–477, 1991

Fewtrell W: Depersonalization: a description and suggested strategies. British Journal of Guidance and Counseling 14:263–269, 1986

Fichtner CG, Kuhlman DT, Gruenfeld MJ, et al: Decreased episodic violence and increased control of dissociation in a carbamazepine-treated case of multiple personality. Biol Psychiatry 27:1045–1052, 1990

Fichtner CG, Horevitz RP, Braun BG: Fluoxetine in depersonalization disorder. Am J Psychiatry 149:1750–1751, 1992

Finkelhor D: Child Sexual Abuse: New Theory and Research. New York, Free Press, 1984

Frankel FH: Hypnotizability and dissociation. Am J Psychiatry 147:823–829, 1990

Freud S: Notes upon a case of obsessional neurosis (1909), in The Standard Edition of the Complete Psychological Works of Sigmund Freud, Vol 10. Translated and edited by Strachey J. London, Hogarth Press, 1955, pp 151–320

Freud S: Psycho-analytic notes on an autobiographical account of a case of paranoia (dementia paranoides) (1911), in The Standard Edition of the Complete Psychological Works of Sigmund Freud, Vol 12. Translated and edited by Strachey J. London, Hogarth Press, 1958, pp 1–82

Freud S: The ego and the id (1923), in The Standard Edition of the Complete Psychological Works of Sigmund Freud, Vol 19. Translated and edited by Strachey J. London, Hogarth Press, 1961, pp 3–66

Frischholz EJ: The relationship among dissociation, hypnosis, and child abuse in the development of multiple personality disorder, in Childhood Antecedents of Multiple Personality Disorder. Edited by Kluft RP. Washington, DC, American Psychiatric Press, 1985, pp 99–126

Gainer MJ, Torem MS: Ego-state therapy for self-injurious behavior. Am J Clin Hypn 35:257–266, 1993

Ganaway GK: Historical versus narrative truth: clarifying the role of exogenous trauma in the etiology of MPD and its variants. Dissociation 2:205–220, 1989

Ganaway GK: Hypnosis, childhood trauma, and dissociative identity disorder: toward an integrative theory. Int J Clin Exp Hypn 43:127–144, 1995

Gelb JL: Multiple personality disorder and satanic ritual abuse. Aust N Z J Psychiatry 27:701–708, 1993

Goodwin J: Sexual Abuse: Incest Victims and Their Families. Boston, Wright/PSG, 1982

Greaves GB: Multiple personality: 165 years after Mary Reynolds. J Nerv Ment Dis 168:577–596, 1980

Heap M, Ramphele M: The quest for wholeness: health care strategies among the residents of council-built hostels in Cape Town. Soc Sci Med 32:117–126, 1991

Herman JL, Perry JC, van der Kolk BA: Childhood trauma in borderline personality disorder. Am J Psychiatry 146:490–495, 1989

Hilgard ER: Hypnotic Susceptibility. New York, Harcourt, Brace & World, 1965

Hilgard ER: Divided Consciousness: Multiple Controls in Human Thought and Action. New York, Wiley-Interscience, 1977

Hoffman RE: Computer simulations of neural information processing and the schizophrenia-mania dichotomy. Arch Gen Psychiatry 44:178–188, 1987

Holen A: Normal and pathological grief: recent views. Tidsskr Nor Laegeforen 113:2089–2091, 1993

Hollander E, Fairbanks J, Decaria C, et al: Pharmacological dissection of panic and depersonalization (letter). Am J Psychiatry 146:402, 1989

Hollander E, Liebowitz MR, Decaria C, et al: Treatment of depersonalization with serotonin reuptake blockers. J Clin Psychopharmacol 10:200–203, 1990

Horen SA, Leichner PP, Lawson JS: Prevalence of dissociative symptoms and disorders in an adult psychiatric inpatient population in Canada. Can J Psychiatry 40:185–191, 1995

Horevitz RP, Braun BG: Are multiple personalities borderline? An analysis of 33 cases. Psychiatr Clin North Am 7:69–87, 1984

Horowitz MJ: Stress Response Syndromes. New York, Jason Aronson, 1976

Horowitz MJ, Wilner NR, Alvarez W: Impact of Event Scale: a measure of objective distress. Psychosom Med 41:208–218, 1979

James W: The Principles of Psychology (1890). New York, Dover, 1950

Janet P: The Major Symptoms of Hysteria: Fifteen Lectures Given in the Medical School of Harvard University, 2nd Edition. New York, Macmillan, 1920

Kaplan ML, Asnis GM, Lipschitz DS, et al: Suicidal behavior and abuse in psychiatric outpatients. Compr Psychiatry 36:229–235, 1995

Kardiner A, Spiegel H: War, Stress and Neurotic Illness. New York, Hoeber, 1947

Kihlstrom JF: The cognitive unconscious. Science 237:1445–1452, 1987

Kihlstrom JF, Hoyt IP: Repression, dissociation, and hypnosis, in Repression and Dissociation: Implications for Personality Theory, Psychopathology, and Health. Edited by Singer JL. Chicago, University of Chicago Press, 1990, pp 181–208

Kirmayer LJ: Pacing the void: social and cultural dimensions of dissociation, in Dissociation: Culture, Mind, and Body. Edited by Spiegel D. Washington, DC, American Psychiatric Press, 1993, pp 91–122

Kirshner LA: Dissociative reactions: an historical review and clinical study. Acta Psychiatr Scand 49:698–711, 1973

Kleinman A: Depression, somatization and the "new cross-cultural psychiatry." Soc Sci Med 11:3–10, 1977

Kluft RP: Varieties of hypnotic intervention in the treatment of multiple personality. Am J Clin Hypn 24:230–240, 1982

Kluft RP: An introduction to multiple personality disorder. Psychiatric Annals 14:19–24, 1984a

Kluft RP: Multiple personality in childhood. Psychiatr Clin North Am 7:121–134, 1984b

Kluft RP: Treatment of multiple personality disorder: a study of 33 cases. Psychiatr Clin North Am 7:9–29, 1984c

Kluft RP: The natural history of multiple personality disorder, in Childhood Antecedents of Multiple Personality. Edited by Kluft RP. Washington, DC, American Psychiatric Press, 1985a, pp 197–238

Kluft RP: Using hypnotic inquiry protocols to monitor treatment progress and stability in multiple personality disorder. Am J Clin Hypn 28:63–75, 1985b

Kluft RP: Hypnotherapy of chilandood multiple personality disorder. Am J Clin Hypn 27:201–210, 1985c

Kluft RP: Personality unification in multiple personality disorder: a follow-up study, in Treatment of Multiple Personality Disorder. Edited by Braun BG. Washington, DC, American Psychiatric Press, 1986, pp 29–60

Kluft RP: First-rank symptoms as a diagnostic clue to multiple personality disorder. Am J Psychiatry 144:293–298, 1987

Kluft RP: The dissociative disorders, in American Psychiatric Press Textbook of Psychiatry. Edited by Talbott JA, Hales RE, Yudofsky SC. Washington, DC, American Psychiatric Press, 1988, pp 557–585

Kluft RP: Using hypnotic inquiry protocols to monitor treatment progress and stability in multiple personality disorder. Am J Clin Hypn 28:63–75, 1985b

Kluft RP: Hypnotherapy of chilandood multiple personality disorder. Am J Clin Hypn 27:201–210, 1985c

Kluft RP: Multiple personality disorder, in American Psychiatric Press Review of Psychiatry, Vol 10. Edited by Tasman A, Goldfinger SM. Washington, DC, American Psychiatric Press, 1991, pp 161–188

Kluft RP: The use of hypnosis with dissociative disorders. Psychiatr Med 10:31–46, 1992

Koopman C, Classen C, Spiegel D: Predictors of posttraumatic stress symptoms among survivors of the Oakland/Berkeley, Calif., firestorm. Am J Psychiatry 151:888–894, 1994

Koopman C, Classen C, Cardeña E, et al: When disaster strikes, acute stress disorder may follow. J Trauma Stress 8:29–46, 1995

Koopman C, Classen C, Spiegel D: Dissociative responses in the immediate aftermath of the Oakland/Berkeley firestorm. J Trauma Stress 9:521–540, 1996

Kua EH, Sim LP, Chee KT: A cross-cultural study of the possession-trance in Singapore. Aust N Z J Psychiatry 20:361–364, 1986

Kua EH, Chew PH, Ko SM: Spirit possession and healing among Chinese psychiatric patients. Acta Psychiatr Scand 88:447–450, 1993

Lambek M: Spirit possession/spirit succession: aspects of social continuity among Malagasy speakers in Mayotte. American Ethnologist 15:710–731, 1988

Lavoie G, Sabourin M, Langlois J: Hypnotic susceptibility, amnesia, and IQ in chronic schizophrenia. Int J Clin Exp Hypn 21:157–168, 1973

Lavoie G, Sabourin M: Hypnosis and schizophrenia: a review of experimental and clinical studies, in Handbook of Hypnosis and Psychosomatic Medicine. Edited by Burrows GD, Dennerstein L. New York, Elsevier, 1980

Lewis-Fernandez R: Culture and dissociation: a comparison of ataque de nervios among Puerto Ricans and "possession syndrome" in India, in Dissociation: Culture, Mind, and Body. Edited by Spiegel D. Washington, DC, American Psychiatric Press, 1993, pp 123–167

Li C, Sun Y, Fang M: Trance states, altered states of consciousness, and related issues. Chinese Mental Health Journal 6:167–170, 1992

Li D, Spiegel D: A neural network model of dissociative disorders. Psychiatric Annals 22:144–147, 1992

Lindemann E: Symptomatology and management of acute grief. Am J Psychiatry 101:141–148, 1944

Loewenstein RJ: An official mental status examination for complex chronic dissociative symptoms and multiple personality disorder. Psychiatr Clin North Am 14:567–604, 1991a

Loewenstein RJ: Psychogenic amnesia and psychogenic fugue: a comprehensive review, in American Psychiatric Press Review of Psychiatry, Vol 10. Edited by Tasman A, Goldfinger SM. Washington, DC, American Psychiatric Press, 1991b, pp 189–222

Loewenstein RJ: Diagnosis, epidemiology, clinical course, treatment, and cost effectiveness of treatment of dissociative disorders and MPD: report submitted to the Clinton Administration Task Force on Health Care Financing Reform. Dissociation 7:3–11, 1994

Loewenstein RJ, Putnam FW: A comparative study of dissociative symptoms in patients with complex partial seizures, multiple personality disorder and posttraumatic stress disorder. Dissociation 1:17–23, 1988

Loewenstein RJ, Hornstein N, Farber B: Open trial of clonazepam in the treatment of posttraumatic stress symptoms in MPD. Dissociation 1:3–12, 1988

Machleidt W, Peltzer K: The Chilopa ceremony: a sacrificial ritual for mentally (spiritually) ill patients in a traditional healing centre in Malawi. Psychiatria Danubina 3:205–227, 1991

Madakasira S, O'Brien KF: Acute posttraumatic stress disorder in victims of a natural disaster. J Nerv Ment Dis 175:286–290, 1987

Mageo JM: Spirit girls and marines: possession and ethnopsychiatry as historical discourse in Samoa. American Ethnologist 23:61–82, 1996

Maldonado JR, Spiegel D: Using hypnosis, in Treating Women Molested in Childhood. Edited by Classen C. San Francisco, Jossey-Bass, 1995, pp 163–186

Maldonado JR, Spiegel D: Trauma, dissociation, and hypnotizability, in Trauma, Memory, and Dissociation. Edited by Marmar CR, Bremmer JD. Washington, DC, American Psychiatric Press, 1998, pp 57–106

Maldonado JR, Butler LD, Spiegel D: Treatment of dissociative disorders, in Treatments That Work. Edited by Nathan P, Gorman JM. New York, Oxford University Press, 1997, pp 423–446

Markowitz JS, Gill HS: Pharmacotherapy of dissociative identity disorder. Ann Pharmacother 30:1498–1499, 1996

Marmar CR, Weiss DS, Metzler TJ, et al: Characteristics of emergency services personnel related to peritraumatic dissociation during critical incident exposure. Am J Psychiatry 153(suppl 7):94–102, 1996

Martinez-Taboas A: Repressed memories: some clinical data contributing toward its elucidation. Am J Psychother 50:217–230, 1996

Mayer-Gross W, Slater E, Roth M: Clinical Psychiatry, 3rd Edition. London, Bailliere, Tindal & Cassell, 1969

McConkey KM: Memory, repression, and abuse: recovered memory and confident reporting of the personal past, in American Psychiatric Press Review of Psychiatry, Vol 16. Edited by Dickstein LJ, Riba MB, Oldham JM. Washington, DC, American Psychiatric Press, 1997, pp II55—II78

McFarlane AC: Posttraumatic morbidity of a disaster: a study of cases presenting for psychiatric treatment. J Nerv Ment Dis 174:4–14, 1986

McFarlane AC: Avoidance and intrusion in posttraumatic stress disorder. J Nerv Ment Dis 180:439–445, 1992

McHugh PR: Dissociative identity disorder as a socially constructed artifact. Journal of Practical Psychiatry and Behavioral Health 1:158–166, 1995a

McHugh PR: Witches, multiple personalities, and other psychiatric artifacts. Nature Medicine 1:110–114, 1995b

McLellan S: Deviant spirits in West Malaysian factories. Anthropologica 33:145–160, 1991

Mesulam MM: Dissociative states with abnormal temporal lobe EEG: Multiple personality and the illusion of possession. Arch Neurol 38:178–181, 1981

Mishkin M, Appenzeller T: The anatomy of memory. Sci Am 256:80–89, 1987

Moore EP: Gender, power, and legal pluralism: Rajasthan, India. American Ethnologist 20:522–542, 1993

Mulhern S: Patients reporting ritual abuse in childhood (letter and comment). Child Abuse Negl 15:609–613, 1991

Nakdimen KA: Psychoanalysis and multiple personality. Am J Psychiatry 145:896–897, 1988

Naples M, Hackett T: The Amytal interview: history and current uses. Psychosomatics 19:98–105, 1978

Noll R: Exorcism and possession: the clash of worldviews and the hubris of psychiatry. Dissociation 6 (special issue):250–253, 1993

Noyes R, Kletti R: Depersonalization in response to life-threatening danger. Compr Psychiatry 18:375–384, 1977

Noyes R, Slymen DJ: The subjective response to life-threatening danger. Omega 9:313–321, 1978–1979

Noyes R, Kupperman S, Olson SB: Desipramine: a possible treatment for depersonalization. Can J Psychiatry 32:782–784, 1987

Nuckolls CW: Deciding how to decide: possession-mediumship in Jalari divination. Med Anthropol 13 (special issue):57–82, 1991

Nuller YL: Depersonalization: symptoms, meaning, therapy. Acta Psychiatr Scand 66:451–458, 1982

Ogata SN, Silk KR, Goodrich S, et al: Childhood sexual and physical abuse in adult patients with borderline personality disorder. Am J Psychiatry 147:1008–1013, 1990

Ong A: The production of possession: spirits and the multinational corporation in Malaysia. American Ethnologist 15:28–42, 1988

Perry JC, Jacobs D: Overview: clinical applications of the Amytal interview in psychiatric emergency settings. Am J Psychiatry 139:552–559, 1982

Perry S, Difede J, Musngi G, et al: Predictors of posttraumatic stress disorder after burn injury. Am J Psychiatry 149:931–935, 1992

Peterson G: Auditory hallucinations and dissociative identity disorder. Am J Psychiatry 152:1403–1404, 1995

Pettinati HM: Measuring hypnotizability in psychotic patients. Int J Clin Exp Hypn 30:404–416, 1982

Pettinati HM, Kogan LG, Evans FJ, et al: Hypnotizability of psychiatric inpatients according to two different scales. Am J Psychiatry 147:69–75, 1990

Pies R: Depersonalization's many faces. Psychiatric Times 8(4):27–28, 1991

Pribor EF, Dinwiddie SH: Psychiatric correlates of incest in childhood. Am J Psychiatry 149:52–56, 1992

Pullela S: An outbreak of epidemic hysteria: an illustrative case study. Irish Journal of Psychiatry 7:9–11, 1986

Putnam FW: Dissociation as a response to extreme trauma, in Childhood Antecedents of Multiple Personality. Edited by Kluft RP. Washington, DC, American Psychiatric Press, 1985, pp 65–97

Putnam FW: The disturbance of "self" in victims of childhood sexual abuse, in Incest-Related Syndromes of Adult Psychopathology. Edited by Kluft RP. Washington, DC, American Psychiatric Press, 1988, pp 113–132

Putnam FW: Diagnosis and Treatment of Multiple Personality Disorder. New York, Guilford, 1989

Putnam FW: Dissociative disorders in children: behavioral profiles and problems. Child Abuse Negl 17:39–45, 1993

Putnam FW, Guroff JJ, Silberman EK, et al: The clinical phenomenology of multiple personality disorder: review of 100 recent cases. J Clin Psychiatry 47:285–293, 1986

Reither AM, Stoudemire A: Psychogenic fugue states: a review. South Med J 81:568–571, 1988

Rivera M: Multiple personality disorder and the social systems: 185 cases. Dissociation 4:79–82, 1991

Roesler TA, McKenzie N: Effects of childhood trauma on psychological functioning in adults sexually abused as children. J Nerv Ment Dis 182:145–150, 1994

Ronquillo EB: The influence of "espiritismo" on a case of multiple personality disorder. Dissociation 4:39–45, 1991

Ross CA: Multiple Personality Disorder: Diagnosis, Clinical Features, and Treatment. New York, Wiley, 1989

Ross CA: Epidemiology of multiple personality disorder and dissociation. Psychiatr Clin North Am 14:503–518, 1991

Ross CA, Norton GR: Multiple personality disorder patients with a prior diagnosis of schizophrenia. Dissociation 1:39–42, 1988

Ross CA, Norton GR: Suicide and parasuicide in multiple personality disorder. Psychiatry 52:365–371, 1989

Ross CA, Norton GR, Wozney K: Multiple personality disorder: an analysis of 236 cases. Can J Psychiatry 34:413–418, 1989

Ross CA, Miller SD, Reagor P, et al: Structured interview data on 102 cases of multiple personality disorder from four centers. Am J Psychiatry 147:596–601, 1990

Ross CA, Joshi S, Currie R: Dissociative experiences in the general population: a factor analysis. Hospital and Community Psychiatry 42:297–301, 1991a

Ross CA, Anderson G, Fleischer WP, et al: The frequency of multiple personality disorder among psychiatric inpatients. Am J Psychiatry 148:1717–1720, 1991b

Roth M: The phobic-anxiety-depersonalization syndrome. Proceedings of the Royal Society of Medicine 52:587–595, 1959

Rothbaum BO, Foa EB: Subtypes of posttraumatic stress disorder and duration of symptoms, in Posttraumatic Stress Disorder: DSM-IV and Beyond. Edited by Davidson JRT, Foa EB. Washington, DC, American Psychiatric Press, 1993, pp 23–35

Rumelhart DE, McClelland JL: Parallel Distributed Processing: Explorations in the Microstructure of Cognition, Vols 1 and 2. Cambridge, MA, MIT Press, 1986

Russell DEH: The Secret Trauma: Incest in the Lives of Girls and Women. New York, Basic Books, 1986

Safa K: Reading Saedi's Ahl-e Hava: pattern and significance in spirit possession beliefs on the southern coasts of Iran. Cult Med Psychiatry 12:85–111, 1988

Sar V, Yargic LI, Tutkun H: Structured interview data on 35 cases of dissociative identity disorder in turkey. Am J Psychiatry 153:1329–1333, 1996

Sargant W, Slater E: Amnestic syndromes in war. Proceedings of the Royal Society of Medicine 34:757–764, 1941

Saxe GN, van der Kolk BA, Berkowitz R, et al: Dissociative disorders in psychiatric inpatients. Am J Psychiatry 150:1037–1042, 1993

Saxena S, Prasad KVSR: DSM-III subclassification of dissociative disorders applied to psychiatric outpatients in India. Am J Psychiatry 146:261–262, 1989

Schacter DL: Understanding implicit memory: a cognitive neuroscience approach. Am Psychol 47:559–569, 1992

Schacter DL: In Search of Memory. Cambridge, MA, Harvard University Press, 1996

Schacter DL, Wang PL, Tulving E, et al: Functional retrograde amnesia: a quantitative case study. Neuropsychologia 20:523–532, 1982

Schenk L, Bear D: Multiple personality and related dissociative phenomena in patients with temporal lobe epilepsy. Am J Psychiatry 138:1311–1316, 1981

Schieffelin EL: Evil spirit sickness, the Christian disease: the innovation of a new syndrome of mental derangement and redemption in Papua, New Guinea. Cult Med Psychiatry 20:1–39, 1996

Schilder P: The treatment of depersonalization. Bulletin of the New York Academy of Science 15:258–272, 1939

Schultz R, Braun BG, Kluft RP: Multiple personality disorder: phenomenology of selected variables in comparison to major depression. Dissociation 2:45–51, 1989

Sered SS: Ideology, autonomy, and sisterhood: an analysis of the secular consequences of women's religions. Gender and Society 8:486–506, 1994

Shalev AY, Schreiber S, Galai T: Early psychiatric responses to traumatic injury. J Trauma Stress 6:441–450, 1993

Shalev AY, Peri T, Canetti L, et al: Predictors of PTSD in injured trauma survivors: a prospective study. Am J Psychiatry 153:219–225, 1996

Shapiro DJ: Symbolic fluids: the world of spirit mediums in Brazilian possession groups. Dissertation Abstracts International 53:867–868, 1992

Sharp LA: Possessed and dispossessed youth: spirit possession of school children in northwest Madagascar. Cult Med Psychiatry 14:339–364, 1990

Sharp LA: Exorcists, psychiatrists, and the problems of possession in northwest Madagascar. Soc Sci Med 38:525–542, 1994

Shearer SL: Dissociative phenomena in women with borderline personality disorder. Am J Psychiatry 151:1324–1328, 1994

Shilony E, Grossman FK: Depersonalization as a defense mechanism in survivors of trauma. J Trauma Stress 6:119–128, 1993

Shirali P, Kishwar A, Bharti SP: Life stress, demographic variables and personality (TAT) in eleven cases of possession (trance-medium) in Shimla Tehsil. Personality Study and Group Behaviour 6:73–81, 1986

Shorvon HJ: The depersonalization syndrome. Proceedings of the Royal Society of Medicine 39:779–785, 1946

Sloan P: Posttraumatic stress in survivors of an airplane crash landing: a clinical and exploratory research intervention. J Trauma Stress 1:211–229, 1988

Smith WH: Incorporating hypnosis into the psychotherapy of patients with multiple personality disorder. Bull Menninger Clin 57:344–354, 1993

Solomon R: The use of the MMPI with multiple personality patients. Psychol Rep 53:1004–1006, 1983

Solomon Z, Mikulincer M: Psychological sequelae of war: a 2-year follow-up study of Israeli combat stress reaction casualties. J Nerv Ment Dis 176:264–269, 1988

Solomon Z, Mikulincer M, Bleich A: Characteristic expressions of combat-related posttraumatic stress disorder among Israeli soldiers in the 1982 Lebanon war. Behav Med 14:171–178, 1988

Solomon Z, Mikulincer M, Benbenisty R: Combat stress reaction: clinical manifestations and correlates. Military Psychology 1:17–33, 1989

Sookman D, Solyom L: Severe depersonalization treated with behavior therapy. Am J Psychiatry 135:1543–1545, 1978

Spanos NP, Weekes JR, Bertrand LD: Multiple personality: a social psychological perspective. J Abnorm Psychol 94:362–376, 1985

Spanos NP, Weekes JR, Menary E, et al: Hypnotic interview and age regression procedures in elicitation of multiple personality symptoms: a simulation study. Psychiatry 49:298–311, 1986

Spiegel D: Vietnam grief work using hypnosis. Am J Clin Hypn 24:33–40, 1981

Spiegel D: Multiple personality as a post-traumatic stress disorder. Psychiatr Clin North Am 7:101–110, 1984

Spiegel D: Dissociating damage. Am J Clin Hypn 29:123–131, 1986a

Spiegel D: Dissociation, double binds, and posttraumatic stress in multiple personality disorder, in Treatment of Multiple Personality Disorder. Edited by Braun BG. Washington, DC, American Psychiatric Press, 1986b, pp 61–77

Spiegel D: Chronic pain masks depression, multiple personality disorder. Hospital and Community Psychiatry 38:933–935, 1987

Spiegel D: Dissociation and hypnosis in posttraumatic stress disorders. J Trauma Stress 1:17–33, 1988

Spiegel D: Hypnosis, dissociation, and trauma: hidden and overt observers, in Repression and Dissociation: Implications for Personality Theory, Psychopathology, and Health. Edited by Singer JL. Chicago, University of Chicago Press, 1990a, pp 121–142

Spiegel D: Trauma, dissociation, and hypnosis, in Incest-Related Syndromes of Adult Psychopathology. Edited by Kluft RL. Washington, DC, American Psychiatric Press, 1990b, pp 247–261

Spiegel D: Dissociation and trauma, in American Psychiatric Press Review of Psychiatry, Vol 10. Edited by Tasman A, Goldfinger SM. Washington, DC, American Psychiatric Press, 1991a, pp 261–275

Spiegel D: Dissociative disorders: afterword, in American Psychiatric Press Review of Psychiatry, Vol 10. Edited by Tasman A, Goldfinger SM. Washington, DC, American Psychiatric Press, 1991b, p 276

Spiegel D: Dissociative disorders: foreword, in American Psychiatric Press Review of Psychiatry, Vol 10. Edited by Tasman A, Goldfinger SM. Washington, DC, American Psychiatric Press, 1991c, pp 143–144

Spiegel D, Cardeña E: Disintegrated experience: the dissociative disorders revisited. J Abnorm Psychol 100:366–378, 1991

Spiegel D, Fink R: Hysterical psychosis and hypnotizability. Am J Psychiatry 136:777–781, 1979

Spiegel D, Detrick D, Frischholz E: Hypnotizability and psychopathology. Am J Psychiatry 139:431–437, 1982

Spiegel D, Hunt T, Dondershine HE: Dissociation and hypnotizability in posttraumatic stress disorder. Am J Psychiatry 145:301–305, 1988

Spiegel D, Frischholz EJ, Spira J: Functional disorders of memory, in American Psychiatric Press Review of Psychiatry, Vol 12. Edited by Oldham JM, Riba MB, Tasman A. Washington, DC, American Psychiatric Press, 1993, pp 747–782

Spiegel H: The grade 5 syndrome: the highly hypnotizable person. Int J Clin Exp Hypn 22:303–319, 1974

Spiegel H, Spiegel D: Trance and Treatment: Clinical Uses of Hypnosis (1978). Washington, DC, American Psychiatric Press, 1987

Spier SA, Tesar GE, Rosenbaum JF, et al: Treatment of panic disorder and agoraphobia with clonazepam. J Clin Psychiatry 47:238–242, 1986

Squire LR: Memory and the hippocampus: a synthesis from findings with rats, monkeys, and humans. Psychol Rev 99:195–231, 1992

Squire LR, Zola-Morgan S: The medial temporal lobe memory system. Science 253:1380–1386, 1991

Stein MB, Uhde TW: Depersonalization disorder: effects of caffeine and response to pharmacotherapy. Biol Psychiatry 26:315–320, 1989

Steinberg M: The spectrum of depersonalization: assessment and treatment, in American Psychiatric Press Review of Psychiatry, Vol 10. Edited by Tasman A, Goldfinger SM. Washington, DC, American Psychiatric Press, 1991, pp 223–247

Steinberg M, Rounsaville B, Cicchetti DV: The Structured Clinical Interview for DSM-III-R Dissociative Disorders: preliminary report on a new diagnostic instrument. Am J Psychiatry 147:76–82, 1990

Steinberg M, Cicchetti D, Buchanan J, et al: Distinguishing between multiple personality disorder (dissociative identity disorder) and schizophrenia using the Structured Clinical Interview for DSM-IV Dissociative Disorders. J Nerv Ment Dis 182:495–502, 1994

Stern CR: The etiology of multiple personalities. Psychiatr Clin North Am 7:149–160, 1984

Tantam D: An exorcism in Zanzibar: insights into groups from another culture. Group Analysis 26:251–260, 1993

Terr LC: Childhood traumas: an outline and overview. Am J Psychiatry 148:10–20, 1991

Trangkasombat U, Su-umpan U, Churujikul V, et al: Epidemic dissociation among school children in southern Thailand. Dissociation 8:130–141, 1995

Torch EM: The psychotherapeutic treatment of depersonalization disorder. Hillside Journal of Clinical Psychiatry 9:133–143, 1987

Tulving E: Elements of Episodic Memory. Oxford, UK, Clarendon Press, 1983

Valdiserri S, Kihlstrom JF: Abnormal eating and dissociative experiences. Int J Eat Disord 17:373–380, 1995

van der Hart O: Multiple personality disorder in Europe: impressions. Dissociation 6:102–118, 1993

van der Hart O, Nijenhuis E: Dissociative disorders, especially multiple personality disorder. Ned Tijdschr Geneeskd 137:1865–1868, 1993

van der Hart O, Spiegel D: Hypnotic assessment and treatment of trauma-induced psychoses: the early psychotherapy of Breukink and modern views. Int J Clin Exp Hypn 41:191–209, 1993

van der Kolk BA, Fisler R: Dissociation and the fragmentary nature of traumatic memories: overview and exploratory study. J Trauma Stress 8:505–525, 1995

van der Kolk BA, Hostetler A, Herron N, et al: Trauma and the development of borderline personality disorder. Psychiatr Clin North Am 17:715–730, 1994

van der Kolk BA, Pelcovitz D, Roth S, et al: Dissociation, somatization, and affect dysregulation: the complexity of adaptation of trauma. Am J Psychiatry 153 (suppl 7):83–93, 1996

Vanderlinden J, Van Dyck R, Vandereycken W, et al: Dissociative experiences in the general population of the Netherlands and Belgium: a study with the Dissociative Questionnaire (DIS-Q). Dissociation 4:180–184, 1991

van Dyck R: Dissociation, hypnosis and multiple personality disorders. Ned Tijdschr Geneeskd 137:1863–1864, 1993

Varma VK, Bouri M, Wig NN: Multiple personality in India: comparison with hysterical possession state. Am J Psychother 35:113–120, 1981

Vincent M, Pickering MR: Multiple personality disorder in childhood. Can J Psychiatry 33:524–529, 1988

Walsh RN: Depersonalization: definition and treatment (letter). Am J Psychiatry 132:873–874, 1975

Weiss DS, Marmar CR, Metzler TJ, et al: Predicting symptomatic distress in emergency services personnel. J Consult Clin Psychol 63:361–368, 1995

Wettstein RM, Fauman BJ: The amobarbital interview. JACEP 8:272–274, 1979

Wilkinson CB: Aftermath of a disaster: the collapse of the Hyatt Regency hotel skywalks. Am J Psychiatry 140:1134–1139, 1983

Wittkower ED: Transcultural psychiatry in the Caribbean: past, present and future. Am J Psychiatry 127:162–166, 1970

Witztum E, Grisaru N, Budowski D: The "Zar" possession syndrome among Ethiopian immigrants to Israel: cultural and clinical aspects. Br J Med Psychol 69:207–225, 1996

Yap PM: The possession syndrome: a comparison of Hong Kong and French findings. Journal of Mental Science 106:114–137, 1960

Zweig-Frank H, Paris J, Guzder J: Psychological risk factors for dissociation and self-mutilation in female patients with borderline personality disorder. Can J Psychiatry 39:259–264, 1994

CHAPTER 19

SEXUAL AND GENDER IDENTITY DISORDERS

JUDITH V. BECKER, PH.D.
BRADLEY R. JOHNSON, M.D.
RICHARD J. KAVOUSSI, M.D.

Clinicians see patients who have a variety of sexual disorders or dysfunctions. A woman who is sexually assaulted may no longer experience sexual desire. A man who is recently widowed may experience difficulty in achieving erections when he begins to date. A woman with multiple sclerosis may no longer have orgasms. Recent postmenopausal women may find intercourse painful. Patients placed on antidepressants or antipsychotic medication may report impairment in sexual functioning. An adolescent may request a consultation because he is troubled by his cross-dressing. An adult male who has been fantasizing sex with prepubertal children may seek treatment because he is fearful that he will act on his fantasies. Consequently, it is important for clinicians to become educated about the categories of sexual disorders, become adept at taking sexual histories, and become adept in the various modalities and interventions.

GENDER IDENTITY DISORDERS

GENDER AND SEXUAL DIFFERENTIATION

The genetic sex of an individual is determined at conception, but development from that point on is influenced by many factors. For the first few weeks of gestation, the gonads are undifferentiated. If the Y chromosome is present in the embryo, the gonads will differentiate into testes. A substance referred to as the H-Y antigen is responsible for this transformation. If the Y chromosome or H-Y antigen is not present in the developing embryo, the gonads will develop into ovaries.

Like the gonads, the internal and external genital structures are initially undifferentiated in the fetus. If the gonads differentiate into testes, fetal androgen (i.e., testosterone) is secreted, and these structures develop into male genitalia (epididymis, vas deferens, ejaculatory ducts, penis, and scrotum). In the absence of fetal androgen, these structures develop into female genitalia (fallopian tubes, uterus, clitoris, and vagina). It is important to note that the development of genitalia in utero depends on the presence or absence of fetal androgen, from whatever source. Thus, if fetal androgen is present in a genetically determined female (e.g., adrenal hyperplasia), male genitalia will develop, even in the presence of ovaries, and the child will be born with either ambiguous or male genitals. Likewise, if fetal androgen is missing (e.g., enzyme deficiency) or androgen receptors are defective (e.g., testicular feminization), female genitalia will develop even though the individual has the Y chromosome and testes.

Psychosexual development also is thought to be influenced by a complex interaction of factors, both pre- and postnatal. Before discussing these factors, however, it is important to break down psychosexual behavior into several components. *Gender identity* is an individual's perception and self-awareness of being male or female. *Gender role* is the behavior that an individual engages in that identifies him or her to others as being male or female (e.g., wearing dresses and makeup). *Sexual orientation* is the erotic attraction that an individual feels (e.g., arousal to men, women, children, nonsexual objects, and so on).

Prenatal hormones play a role in the differentiation of the mammalian brain. However, their exact effect on psychosexual development in humans has not been established. Although they may contribute to the development of gender role behaviors, their effect on the development is still debated. In fact, some have proposed that hormones have little or no effect on sexual orientation (Bancroft 1994; Byne and Parsons 1993). All in all, they do not appear to play a major part in gender identity differentiation (Ehrhardt and Meyer-Bahlburg 1981).

Gender identity appears to develop in the early years of life and is generally established by age 3 years. Gender identity seems to depend on the sex in which an individual is reared, regardless of biological factors. The evidence for this comes from studies of children born with genitalia that are ambiguous or opposite from their genetic sex (Money and Ehrhardt 1974). These children have been found to develop gender identity consistent with the gender assigned to them at birth as long as their parents are unambiguous about the child's sex and surgical and hormonal corrections are made. Thus, a child with testicular feminization will grow up with a female gender identity, even though "she" has testes, if assigned and raised as a girl and the aforementioned conditions are met. Similarly, a genetic female with ambiguous genitalia due to congenital adrenal hyperplasia, if reared as a boy, will develop a male gender identity; if reared as a girl, the individual will develop a female gender identity.

Gender identity, once firmly established, is extremely resistant to change. For example, if a genetic female is reared as a boy (e.g., due to exposure to fetal androgens) but suddenly develops breasts and other female secondary sex characteristics during puberty, his gender identity will remain male, and he will want to correct the changes. However, if a child's physical appearance is ambiguous or if the caregivers are inconsistent in their view of the child as male or female, gender identity may not develop strongly, leading to possible "change" or confusion regarding gender identity at a later time in life.

If gender identity develops between birth and age 3 years and depends on sex of rearing, what are the factors that contribute to its development? Several theories attempt to answer this question. There may be biological factors that influence the development of gender identity that have not yet been discovered, and there are instances in which it has been suggested that biological factors may override sex assignment at birth (Ehrhardt and Meyer-Bahlburg 1981). According to a learning theory model, gender identity begins to develop when the child imitates or identifies with same-sexed models. The child is then reinforced for this identification and for engaging in "appropriate" sex-role behaviors. In psychoanalytic theory, gender identity develops as part of overall identity formation in the phase of separation and individuation and is very much dependent on the quality of the mother-infant dyad. Later, during the oedipal phase, gender role and sexual orientation are shaped.

CRITERIA FOR DIAGNOSING GENDER IDENTITY DISORDERS

Gender identity disorders are characterized by strong and persistent cross-gender identification (not merely a desire for any perceived cultural advantages of being the other sex), as well as a persistent discomfort with one's sex or sense of inappropriateness in the gender role of that sex.

In children, the disorder is manifested by at least four of the five following criteria:

1. A repeatedly stated desire to be, or insistence that he or she is, a member of the opposite sex
2. In boys, a preference for cross-dressing or simulating female attire; in girls, insistence on wearing stereotypically masculine clothing
3. A strong or persistent preference for cross-sex roles in make-believe play or persistent fantasies of being the other sex
4. An intense desire to participate in the stereotypical games and pastimes of the opposite sex
5. A strong preference for playmates of the opposite sex

In adolescents or adults, the symptoms include

- A stated desire to be the opposite sex
- Frequently "passing" as the opposite sex
- A desire to live or be treated as a member of the opposite sex
- Having the conviction that one experiences the typical feelings and reactions of the opposite sex

The diagnosis is made if there are no concurrent physical intersex conditions. Finally, the disturbance could clinically cause significant distress or impairment in social, occupational, or other important areas of functioning. In DSM-IV (American Psychiatric Association 1994), gender identity disorder is grouped in one single broad category (Table 19–1). In this chapter, however, gender identity disorder of adulthood and of childhood are reviewed.

GENDER IDENTITY DISORDER OF ADULTHOOD

Gender identity disorders were first introduced in DSM-III (American Psychiatric Association 1980) and were included in the section on psychosexual disorders. In DSM-III-R (American Psychiatric Association 1987), the gender identity disorders were moved to the section "Disorders Usually First Evident in Infancy, Childhood, or Adolescence." Additionally, in DSM-III-R, gender identity disorder of adulthood, nontranssexual type, was added. Up to this point, the essential features of the principle diagnostic categories in the subclass *transsexualism* were a persistent sense of discomfort and inappropriateness about one's anatomical sense and a persistent wish to be rid of one's genitals and to live as a member of the other sex.

The term *transsexualism* was eliminated in DSM-IV. A single diagnostic term, *gender identity disorder*, exists for the childhood form and for the adult and adolescent form. The elimination of the term transsexualism alters the sense that it exists as a single disorder and presents it conceptually, as a spectrum of disorders. However, the term transsexualism still appears to describe appropriately what is now referred to as gender identity disorder of adulthood.

Gender identity disorder of adulthood is rare, with estimates of 30,000 cases worldwide (Lothstein 1980). There have been cases described throughout history, but only in the past 25 years scientific and media attention has focused on this phenomenon, and specialized gender identity clinics have been developed. Transsexual individuals most commonly request *sex reassignment*; that is, change in their physical appearance (usually by hormonal and surgical means) to correspond with their self-perceived gender. However, it is important to remember that not all those who seek sex reassignment are transsexual; cross-gender wishes may occur in transvestism (i.e., wearing opposite-gender clothes for erotic purposes) or effeminate homosexuality. Therefore, it is important to conduct a thorough evaluation before recommending sex reassignment.

Three to four times as many males as females apply for sex reassignment, but approximately equal numbers of males and females are reassigned (J. K. Meyer 1982). Vir-

TABLE 19–1.   DSM-IV diagnostic criteria for gender identity disorder

A. A strong and persistent cross-gender identification (not merely a desire for any perceived cultural advantages of being the other sex).

In children, the disturbance is manifested by four (or more) of the following:

(1) Repeatedly stated desire to be, or insistence that he or she is, the other sex

(2) In boys, preference for cross-dressing or simulating female attire; in girls, insistence on wearing only stereotypical masculine clothing

(3) Strong and persistent preferences for cross-sex roles in make-believe play or persistent fantasies of being the other sex

(4) Intense desire to participate in the stereotypical games and pastimes of the other sex

(5) Strong preference for playmates of the other sex

In adolescents and adults, the disturbance is manifested by symptoms such as a stated desire to be the other sex, frequent passing as the other sex, desire to live or be treated as the other sex, or the conviction that he or she has the typical feelings and reactions of the other sex.

B. Persistent discomfort with his or her sex or sense of inappropriateness in the gender role of that sex.

In children, the disturbance is manifested by any of the following: in boys, assertion that his penis or testes are disgusting or will disappear or assertion that it would be better not to have a penis, or aversion toward rough-and-tumble play and rejection of male stereotypical toys, games, and activities; in girls, rejection of urinating in a sitting position, assertion that she has or will grow a penis, or assertion that she does not want to grow breasts or menstruate, or marked aversion toward normative feminine clothing.

In adolescents and adults, the disturbance is manifested by symptoms such as preoccupation with getting rid of primary and secondary sex characteristics (e.g., request for hormones, surgery, or other procedures to physically alter sexual characteristics to simulate the other sex) or belief that he or she was born the wrong sex.

C. The disturbance is not concurrent with a physical intersex condition.

D. The disturbance causes clinically significant distress or impairment in social, occupational, or other important areas of functioning.

Code based on current age:

Gender identity disorder in children

Gender identity disorder in adolescents or adults

(continued)

TABLE 19–1.   DSM-IV diagnostic criteria for gender identity disorder (continued)

Specify if (for sexually mature individuals):

Sexually attracted to males

Sexually attracted to females

Sexually attracted to both

Sexually attracted to neither

Gender identity disorder not otherwise specified

This category is included for coding disorders in gender identity that are not classifiable as a specific gender identity disorder. Examples include

(1)   Intersex conditions (e.g., androgen insensitivity syndrome or congenital adrenal hyperplasia) and accompanying gender dysphoria

(2)   Transient, stress-related cross-dressing behavior

(3)   Persistent preoccupation with castration or penectomy without a desire to acquire the sex characteristics of the other sex

---

tually all of the women who apply have a sexual orientation toward women. Male transsexuals are predominately homosexual in orientation, but approximately 25% are sexually attracted to women. Some of these "heterosexual" transsexuals enter into "lesbian" relationships after they are reassigned as females. These findings provide further evidence of the separateness of gender identity and sexual orientation. Many male and female transsexuals also have been described as being hyposexual or asexual. However, both male and female patients often have a fear of homosexual attraction and thus choose to remain asexual rather than acknowledge their homosexual orientation.

Among those adults who are diagnosed as having gender identity disorder, there is a high degree of concomitant psychiatric disorder, most commonly borderline, antisocial, or narcissistic personality disorder; substance abuse; and suicidal or self-destructive behavior (J. K. Meyer 1982). These individuals can be demanding and manipulative and often resist interventions other than sex reassignment.

The term *gender dysphoria* has been used to characterize a person's sense of discomfort or unease about his or her status as male or female (Zucker and Green 1997). Gender dysphoria has been classified as primary or secondary as it relates to transsexualism (Person and Ovesey 1974). *Primary transsexuals* have a lifelong, profound disturbance of core gender identity. They have histories of cross-dressing as children but never were aroused by wearing opposite-sex clothes. They usually have a clear history of engaging in opposite-sex gender-role behaviors. *Secondary transsexuals*

also can have a long history of gender identity confusion; however, in these individuals the identity disturbance follows other cross-gender behavior such as transvestism or effeminate homosexuality.

ETIOLOGY

There are no well-established or exhaustive explanations for the development of gender identity disorder. As noted earlier in this chapter, gender identity appears to be established and influenced by psychosocial factors during the first few years of life. However, many authors have argued that biological factors, if not causative, may predispose an individual to a gender identity disorder. It is important to realize, however, that researchers still have been unable to identify a biological anomaly or variant associated specifically with gender identity disorder.

As previously mentioned, prenatal sex hormones probably have little causal effect on gender identity and possibly sexual orientation. However, studies of females with congenital adrenal hyperplasia that is due to high levels of androgens prenatally (Collaer and Hines 1995) suggest there may be a relation in such disorders and gender identity problems. This type of example leads us to realize that further research in this area needs to be done.

Some researchers have found decreased levels of testosterone in male transsexuals and abnormally high levels of testosterone in female transsexuals, but the findings have been inconsistent and the studies from which they were obtained were not well controlled. Tests for H-Y antigen have been found to be negative in male transsexuals and positive in female transsexuals in a high percentage of cases; however, there has been a consistent failure to replicate these findings (Hoenig 1985).

Although no correlation has been made with specific temporal lobe abnormalities, there have been case reports of individuals who developed gender identity disorder following onset of temporal lobe seizures, which reverted with the use of anticonvulsive medication. Studies of electroencephalograms (EEGs) in male and female transsexuals have revealed abnormalities in 30%–70%; however, only one of the studies used control groups, and the effect of medications, especially estrogen, was not taken into account (Hoenig 1985).

Family studies have been difficult to carry out given the low incidence of gender identity disorders. To date, no clear increase in familial incidence has been demonstrated.

Learning theory models suggest that gender dysphoria arises from absent or inconsistent reinforcement for identification with same-sexed models. Cross-gender identification and behaviors take place, and these are reinforced with either overt or covert approval from the child's caregivers.

Psychoanalytic theory argues that early deprivation of the male child by his mother leads to a symbiotic merger with the mother and lack of full individuation as a separate person. In the case of borderline personality disorder, this process leads to general identity confusion and loss of ego boundaries when the individual is under stress. In gender dysphoria, the defect is isolated to gender. However, the same ego impairment, disordered object relations, and primitive defense mechanisms (i.e., denial and splitting) are present (J. K. Meyer 1982).

Clinical studies (Green 1987; Stoller 1968, 1975a, 1975b, 1979) described that boys with gender identity disorder often have an overly close relationship with their mother and a distant, ambivalent relationship with their father. Stoller argues that the boy who is excessively close to his mother, in absence of the father, may have difficulty in separating himself from the female body and feminine behavior.

DIAGNOSIS AND EVALUATION

Individuals who request sex reassignment require careful and patient evaluation by a psychiatrist or psychologist with experience in the management of gender identity disorders. Patients with other primary psychiatric diagnoses may present as transsexuals. Psychotic patients may have delusions centered around their genitalia (e.g., that someone has substituted the incorrect genitals, that God is telling them to change their sex). When the psychosis is treated, the cross-gender wishes usually resolve. Individuals with severe personality disorders, especially borderline, can have transient wishes to change gender as part of their overall identity diffusion during times of stress. Effeminate homosexuals may desire to change sex in order to be more attractive to men; usually this desire fluctuates with time. Transvestites (described later in this chapter) are aroused by wearing female garments, although these individuals may be of a homosexual or heterosexual orientation. To increase their arousal, they may progress to actually wishing to become a woman; again, however, this wish is usually not continuous over a long period, and their gender identity is male. Adolescents sometimes become gender dysphoric because of developing homosexual feelings that need to be resolved. In each of these cases, psychotherapy is indicated to deal with the appropriate issues leading to their request for sex reassignment.

Unfortunately, individuals requesting sex reassignment often hide the truth in an effort to obtain hormonal and surgical change. Therefore, it is imperative to contact significant others in the patient's life (e.g., family members, spouse, sexual partners) to confirm the pervasive and nonremitting nature of the gender identity disturbance.

TREATMENT

Because most gender dysphoric individuals have adamant requests for sex reassignment (many often already taking opposite-sex hormones supplied by other physicians), it is extremely difficult to engage these patients in treatment with anything other than surgical sex reassignment as the goal. These patients see psychotherapy as a means of discouraging them from surgery. However, because surgery is irreversible, it is important to engage these patients in psychotherapy, even if surgery is indicated. The therapist should be careful to base the goals of therapy on what is desired by the patient. These goals should be identified at the beginning of therapy, including a discussion on informed consent as to the possible outcomes and complications that could arise secondary to the use of psychotherapy.

Supportive psychotherapy can serve various purposes in transsexual individuals. First, there have been reports, albeit few, of reversal of patients' gender identity disorders. Second, a trial of psychotherapy is often useful in cases in which the diagnosis is not clear. Third, dealing with patients' fears of homosexuality may sometimes change their wishes for surgical reassignments. Fourth, psychotherapy plays an important role in patients' adjustment to the process of sex reassignment. Finally, therapy is often helpful in the postsurgical adjustment of patients with gender identity disorder.

The therapist must be comfortable in treating patients who have gender identity disorders. Furthermore, the therapist must be comfortable with his or her sexual identity and sexual issues so that countertransference does not adversely affect the treatment. Psychoanalysis generally is not indicated in the treatment of transsexuals secondary to occasional poor ego functioning (J. K. Meyer 1982). Dynamic psychotherapy may be used but must involve parameters applied to borderline patients (i.e., structured therapy, limit setting, ego support, and short-term goals).

Behavior therapy has been used with success in ego-dystonic male transsexuals in several cases (Barlow et al. 1979). The treatment can be helpful to those who wish to alter their effeminate behaviors, including female patterns of behavior (e.g., sitting, walking, social behavior, and vocal characteristics). These behaviors are then changed using videotapes and modeling of masculine behaviors in which the patients are trained to engage. Attempts also can be made to change the patients' arousal pattern from homosexual to heterosexual; however, this attempt was successful in only one of three cases. Again, it is important to attempt therapy to change an arousal pattern only if it is the wish or goal of the patient, not the therapist.

Sexual reassignment to the opposite gender has been the most widely used and studied treatment modality for adults with gender identity disorder. Early reports of outcome were extremely positive, with dramatic changes in social functioning and satisfaction. Hormonal treatment and surgery have become more readily available for adults with gender identity disorder, often with little preparation other than a brief consultation with a psychiatrist. This approach led to an increase in the reports of poor results and realization that sex reassignment was not a panacea.

Green and Fleming (1990) reviewed the literature written during 1979 through 1989 on both male-to-female and female-to-male postoperative transsexuals. Only 11 follow-up studies were located in the literature. These authors concluded that preoperative factors that were indicative of a favorable outcome included an absence of psychosis, as well as mental and emotional stability shown prior to the surgery; a successful adaptation to the desired gender for at least 1 year; an understanding of the consequences and limitations of the surgery; and the seeking of preoperative psychotherapy. These authors reported that there was some evidence that outcome was somewhat less favorable for secondary transsexuals, even when these individuals were denied surgery. Data from this report indicated that outcomes were considered satisfactory for 97% of the female-to-male transsexuals and for 87% of the male-to-female transsexuals.

Sex reassignment is a long process that must be carefully monitored. Patients with other primary psychiatric diagnoses and secondary transsexuals should be screened out and given other appropriate treatment. If the patient is considered appropriate for sex reassignment, psychotherapy should be started to prepare the patient for the cross-gender role. The patient should then go out into the world and live in the cross-gender role before surgical reassignment. Males should cross-dress, have electrolysis, and practice female behaviors. They can even change their identity to female on official documents and at work. Females should cut their hair, bind or conceal their breasts, and similarly take on the identity of a man. After 1–2 years, if these measures have been successful and the patient still wishes reassignment, hormone treatment is begun. Estrogens are given to the male patient, resulting in redistribution of body fat in a more "feminine" pattern and enlargement of the breasts. This treatment is not without possible medical complications, and patients should be followed closely by a physician. Side effects of estrogen treatment may include deep vein thrombosis, thromboembolic disorders, increased blood pressure, weight gain, impaired glucose tolerance, liver abnormalities, and depression. Testosterone given to the female patient causes redistribution of fat, growth of facial and body hair, enlargement of the clitoris, and deepening of the voice. Unwanted side effects of testosterone treatment include acne, edema secondary to sodium retention, and impairment of liver function. After 1–2 years of hormone therapy, the patient may be considered for surgical reassignment if such a procedure is still desired. In the male-to-female patient this consists of bilateral orchiectomy, penile amputation, and creation of an artificial vagina. Female-to-male patients undergo bilateral mastectomy and optional hysterectomy with removal of ovaries. Efforts to create an artificial penis have met with mixed results thus far; at this point, it is better to counsel the patient to downplay the role of the penis in sexual activity. Overall cosmetic and functional results from surgery have been variable in both male and female transsexuals. Psychotherapy after surgery is indicated to help the patient adjust to the surgical changes and discuss sexual functioning and satisfaction.

GENDER IDENTITY DISORDER OF CHILDHOOD

DESCRIPTION

Because of the difficulty and turmoil involved in treating late-adolescent and adult patients who have gender identity disorder, researchers and clinicians began to evaluate and treat children with gender identity problems. Strictly speaking, this disorder is seen in a child who perceives himself or herself as being of the opposite sex.

However, it is often difficult to separate gender identity from gender role behavior in children. Boys with normal gender identity may play with "girl" dolls. Many girls in our culture are "tomboys" and like rough and contact games. However, in this gender identity syndrome there is a repeated pattern of opposite-gender role behavior accompanied by a disturbance in the child's perception of "being" a boy or a girl. The exact incidence of gender identity disorder in children is not known, but, like adult gender dysphoria, it is a rare disorder.

Children with gender identity problems express a desire to become a member of the opposite sex. Boys wish to have a vagina and may play at breast-feeding. Girls wish to have a penis and may simulate a penis with various objects or stand to urinate. Boys cross-dress with dresses, makeup, and jewelry, whereas girls may resist wearing dresses at any cost and wear short hair. Both sexes identify with role models of the opposite sex (e.g., a boy insists that he is Supergirl in a game). In evaluating a child, it is important not to look solely at behavior; there must be a disturbance in the child's sexual identity. As in the evaluation of adults, the child should be evaluated for other psychiatric disorders such as psychosis or adjustment disorder.

ETIOLOGY

As with adult gender dysphoria, the etiology of childhood gender identity disorder is unclear. The theories outlined earlier in this chapter for adults who have gender identity disorder also apply to children. Additional factors that have been suggested are parents' indifference to or encouragement of opposite-sex behavior; regular cross-dressing as a young boy by a female; lack of male playmates during a boy's first years of socialization; excessive maternal protection, with inhibition of rough-and-tumble play; or absence of or rejection by an older male early in life (Green 1974).

PHYSICAL APPEARANCE

It is interesting to note that a number of studies have associated gender identity disorder with greater physical attractiveness in boys when compared with the physical attractiveness of clinical control subjects who did not have the disorder (Green 1987; Zucker et al. 1993). Fridell et al. (1996) concluded that girls with gender identity disorder were often seen as less attractive than those in a control group.

COURSE

Retrospective studies of transsexuals (Green 1974) have shown a high incidence of childhood cross-gender behavior. Follow-up studies of children with gender identity disorder have found a high incidence of continued manifestations in adulthood, with a higher incidence of homosexual or bisexual behavior and fantasies than those in a control group (Green 1985).

TREATMENT

Treatment of the child with gender identity disorder is offered in an attempt to help the child avoid peer ostracism and humiliation, be comfortable with his or her own sex, and avoid the possible development of adult gender dysphoria. Behavior therapy has been used to modify specific cross-gender behaviors in a manner similar to that described for adults, as well as to enhance contingency management (e.g., reinforcing appropriate behaviors with tokens). Analytically oriented treatment deals with the family dynamics (e.g., a powerful, masculine-devaluing mother; an ineffective, emotionally absent father) and individual dynamics (e.g., castration anxiety following surgery) of the child. An eclectic approach to treatment has been advocated that involves the development of a close, trusting relationship between a male therapist and the boy; stopping parental encouragement of feminine behaviors; interrupting the excessively close relationship between mother and son; enhancing the role of father and son; and reinforcing male behaviors (Green 1974).

SEXUAL DYSFUNCTIONS

MALE AND FEMALE PHYSIOLOGY

Human sexual functioning requires a complex interaction of the nervous, vascular, and endocrine systems to produce arousal and orgasm. Sexual arousal in men occurs in the presence of visual stimuli (e.g., a naked partner), fantasies, or physical stimulation of the genitals or other areas of the body (e.g., the nipples). This stimulation leads to involuntary discharge in the parasympathetic nerves that control the diameter and valves of the penile blood vessels. There is then increased blood flow into the corpora cavernosa, two cylinders of specialized tissue in the penis that distend with blood to produce an erection. Continued stimulation leads to emission of semen and ejaculation, which are controlled through sympathetic fibers and the pudendal nerve. Dopaminergic systems in the central nervous system facilitate arousal and ejaculation, whereas serotonergic systems inhibit these functions. In addition, androgens must be present to expedite sexual arousal (and to some extent erection and ejaculation).

In women, as in men, arousal depends on fantasies, visual stimuli, and physical stimulation; in general, the latter is more important for women, whereas visual cues are more important for men. Again, this stimulation leads to parasympathetic nervous discharge that increases blood flow to the female genitalia, resulting in lubrication of the vagina and some enlargement of the clitoris. Continued stimulation of the clitoris either directly or through intercourse results in orgasm. Estrogens and progestins play a role in female sexual functioning; however, androgens are important in the maintenance of sexual arousal in women. As in men, dopaminergic systems facilitate female sexual arousal and orgasm, whereas serotonergic systems inhibit these functions.

It is readily apparent that normal sexual functioning and processes require intact neural and vascular connections to the genitals along with normal endocrine functioning. Any illness that interferes with these systems can lead to sexual dysfunction: neurological diseases (e.g., multiple sclerosis, lumbar or sacral spinal cord trauma, herniated disks), thrombosis of the arteries or veins of the penis, diabetes mellitus (which causes both neurological and vascular damage), endocrine disorders (e.g., hyperprolactinemia), liver disease (which leads to a buildup of estrogens), and so forth.

Similarly, drugs that affect these systems also can impair sexual functioning (Table 19–2). Thus, antihypertensives, because of their antiadrenergic effects, can impair erectile function in men and lubrication in women. Antipsychotics, tricyclic antidepressants, and monoamine oxidase inhibitors can inhibit these same functions through their anticholinergic effects. Antipsychotics can impair

TABLE 19–2.   Some commonly used medications that may interfere with sexual functioning

Abused drugs
  Alcohol
  Opiates
  Cocaine

Antihypertensives
  Diuretics (thiazides, spironolactone)
  Methyldopa
  Clonidine
  β-Blockers
  Reserpine
  Guanethidine

Antipsychotics
  Thioridazine (retarded ejaculation)
  Thiothixine
  Chlorpromazine
  Perphenazine
  Fluphenazine
  Risperidone
  Olanzapine

Antidepressants
  Tricyclics
  Monoamine oxidase inhibitors
  Serotonin reuptake inhibitors
  Trazodone (priapism)
  Nefazodone
  Venlafaxine
  Mirtazapine

Others
  Cimetidine
  Steroids
  Estrogens

arousal and orgasm because of their dopamine-blocking effects, whereas serotonin reuptake inhibitors (e.g., fluoxetine, sertraline, paroxetine, and fluvoxamine) can inhibit arousal and orgasm through their serotonergic effects. Spironolactone, steroids, and estrogens can decrease sexual desire through their antiandrogenic effects.

The sexual response cycle of men and women consists of four stages: appetitive, excitement, orgasm, and resolution (Masters and Johnson 1970). The *appetitive stage* is characterized by sexual fantasies or a desire to be sexual. The *excitement stage* in both men and women is characterized by erotic feelings that lead to vaginal lubrication in women and penile erection in men. There also is an increase in both heart rate and blood pressure. During the male *orgasmic stage*, semen is ejaculated from the penis in spurts. Orgasm for women consists of reflex rhythmic contractions of the circumvaginal muscles. During *resolution*, the final stage, the sex-specific physiological responses return to a resting state. In men, there is a refractory period after orgasm during which it is not possible to have another erection (the length of this period varies between individuals and increases with age). Women are variable: some have a refractory period after orgasm, whereas others do not and can have multiple sequential orgasms.

Sexual dysfunctions (Table 19–3) occur when there are disruptions of any of the four stages of sexual response because of anatomical, physiological, or psychological factors. Sexual orientation is not a determining factor; consequently, heterosexual, homosexual, or bisexual individuals may experience a sexual dysfunction at some point in their lives. Sexual dysfunctions may be lifelong or may develop after a period of normal sexual functioning. For example, a woman who has never achieved an orgasm would be classified as having a primary female orgasmic disorder, whereas a woman who has been orgasmic at one point in her life but is presently unable to achieve orgasm is experiencing a secondary orgasmic disorder. Sexual dysfunctions may be further characterized as to whether they are present in all sexual activities or are situational. For example, a man who has an erection during masturbation but not during sexual interaction with a partner has a situational erectile disorder.

When a sexual dysfunction is diagnosed, the following types should be specified: dysfunction due to psychological factors or dysfunction due to combined psychological factors and a general medical condition. The dysfunction may be recent or lifelong.

EPIDEMIOLOGY

The exact prevalence of sexual dysfunctions is difficult to determine (Table 19–4). Frank et al. (1978) surveyed 100

TABLE 19-3. Sexual dysfunctions

- Hypoactive sexual desire disorder
- Sexual aversion disorder
- Female sexual arousal disorder
- Male erectile disorder
- Female orgasmic disorder (i.e., inhibited female orgasm)
- Male orgasmic disorder (i.e., inhibited male orgasm)
- Premature ejaculation
- Dyspareunia (not due to a general medical condition)
- Vaginismus (not due to a general medical condition)
- Sexual dysfunction due to a general medical condition
- Substance-induced sexual dysfunction
- Sexual dysfunction not otherwise specified

well-educated, happily married couples. Forty percent of the men reported erectile or ejaculatory dysfunctions at some point during their lives. Sixty-three percent of the women reported arousal or orgasmic dysfunctions at some point. In addition, 50% of the men and 77% of the women reported other sexual difficulties, including lack of interest or inability to relax. Nathan (1986) analyzed the findings of 22 sex surveys of the general population to estimate prevalence rates for various sexual dysfunctions; Spector and Carey (1990) evaluated 23 community samples to estimate prevalence rates. These studies found a wide range in prevalence estimates (Table 19–4) for sexual dysfunctions. Studies of clinical samples suggest an increase in the frequency of hypoactive sexual desire disorder, male and female orgasmic disorder, and male erectile disorder as presenting problems and a decrease in premature ejaculation as a presenting problem (Spector and Carey 1990). Clearly, a significant percentage of men and women in our society experience sexual problems at some time in their lives.

ETIOLOGY

Kaplan (1974) argues for a multicausal theory of sexual dysfunctions on several levels (intrapsychic, interpersonal, and behavioral) and lists four factors as playing a role in the development of these disorders (Table 19–5).

Other factors that may lead to the development of a sexual dysfunction include an unacknowledged homosex-

TABLE 19-4. Prevalence of sexual dysfunctions

Disorder	Prevalence (%)
Female orgasmic disorder	5–30
Male orgasmic disorder	4–10
Premature ejaculation	35–38
Male erectile disorder	4–20

ual orientation and attempts to function sexually with a person of the opposite sex. Some sexual dysfunctions lead to secondary sexual problems; for example, an individual who does not have erections or cannot achieve orgasm may develop a lack of sexual desire secondary to not experiencing any positive gratification from the sexual interaction.

Many sexual problems are related to sexual trauma. For example, a history of incest, child sexual abuse, or rape may place an individual at risk for developing sexual problems (Becker et al. 1986).

Many sexual dysfunctions occur secondary to major psychiatric disorders such as schizophrenia, depression, and severe personality disorders (Fagan et al. 1988).

As previously discussed, physical, neurological, and physiological problems can lead to sexual dysfunction. The use of a single medication, or multiple medications, is one of the most common causes of sexual dysfunction.

Finally, many cases of dysfunction involve both organic and psychogenic factors, especially in the case of an erectile disorder. A man may have a mild degree of organic impairment (e.g., due to diabetes or vascular insufficiency), fail several times at obtaining an erection, and become vulnerable to performance anxiety. In this case, treatment aimed at reducing the psychogenic factors may be sufficient to improve sexual functioning. Conversely, even if a man has evidence of psychological factors contributing to erectile disorder, it is still necessary to evaluate him for organic abnormalities (LoPiccolo and Stock 1986).

DIFFERENTIAL DIAGNOSIS

Patients with a sexual dysfunction should be medically evaluated by a gynecologist or urologist to rule out treatable organic etiologies. These organic factors may be local diseases of the genitals, vascular illnesses, neurological diseases, endocrine disorders, or systemic illnesses. Patients always should be asked about medications, including over-the-counter medicines and illegal drugs.

Psychophysiological procedures have been developed

TABLE 19-5. Multicausal theory of sexual dysfunctions

1. Misinformation or ignorance regarding sexual and social interaction
2. Unconscious guilt and anxiety concerning sex
3. Performance anxiety, as the most common cause of erectile and orgasmic dysfunctions
4. Partners' failure to communicate to each other their sexual feelings and those behaviors in which they want to engage

to assess patients' erections. During rapid eye movement (REM) sleep, men experience penile erections defined as nocturnal penile tumescence (NPT). Although NPT measures can be equivocal, they help in evaluating a patient with erectile problems for organic factors (e.g., a man with "psychogenic" impotence should have erections while sleeping, whereas a man with "organic" impotence should not have an erection at any time). However, many men have both organic and psychological causes for erectile problems, and thus the results of NPT testing must be interpreted cautiously. Men with a predominance of psychogenic factors may not have nocturnal tumescence, whereas men with an organically based dysfunction actually may have nocturnal erections.

Researchers also have demonstrated the occurrence of vaginal vascular changes in women during REM sleep, and assessment techniques are being explored to evaluate these changes in women who have sexual dysfunctions. Other assessment procedures include Doppler flow studies and penile blood pressure measurement, arteriography and papaverine injections of the corpora cavernosa to assess vascular competence, and nerve root stimulation to assess neurological impairment.

DESCRIPTIONS AND TREATMENTS OF SEXUAL DYSFUNCTIONS

Sexual Desire Disorders

Hypoactive sexual desire disorder. Hypoactive sexual desire disorder (also known as inhibited sexual desire or ISD) is characterized by persistent or recurrent deficient sexual fantasies and desire for sexual activity. The disturbance also causes marked distress or interpersonal difficulty. The diagnosis is made if the dysfunction does not occur exclusively during the course of another Axis I disorder (e.g., major depression) and is not due to the direct effects of a substance (alcohol or illegal drugs or prescription drugs) or a general medical condition.

It is also important to determine whether hypoactive sexual desire is the primary problem or rather the consequence of another underlying sexual problem. Frequently, a male or female who is experiencing either inhibited sexual excitement or an orgasmic problem may develop hypoactive sexual desire because sexual activity is not found to be reinforcing. It is also important to differentiate this disorder, in which there is an absence of sexual desire and fantasies, from sexual aversion, in which there is avoidance of sexual activity due to extreme anxiety. As with the other dysfunctions, this disorder may be lifelong, may occur after

a period of good sexual appetite, or may occur only in a certain context (e.g., with the individual's current partner). It is important to assess whether the desire disorder is substance induced (i.e., drugs or medications). Assessment of individuals with hypoactive sexual desire disorder requires medical workup, psychological evaluation, and assessment of the relationship.

Hypoactive sexual desire disorder has been the most difficult of all the dysfunctions to treat. Testosterone has been used (in both men and women) to treat ISD; however, masculinizing side effects make its use problematic in women. There is no consistent evidence that it is useful in raising sexual interest in men, even when serum testosterone levels are low (O'Carroll and Bancroft 1984). In addition, a placebo-controlled study in women found no advantage of testosterone over therapy (Dow and Gallagher 1989). The most effective treatments involve a combination of cognitive therapy to deal with maladaptive beliefs (e.g., that partners must always want sex at the same time), behavioral treatment (e.g., exercises to enhance sexual pleasure and communication), and marital therapy (e.g., to deal with the individual's use of sex to control the relationship).

Sexual aversion disorder. Sexual aversion disorder is characterized by a persistent or recurrent extreme aversion to and avoidance of all (or almost all) genital sexual contact with a partner. The disturbance causes marked distress or interpersonal difficulties and does not occur exclusively during the course of another Axis I disorder. It is important to differentiate this disorder from hypoactive sexual desire disorder (Ponticas 1992).

The major goal of treatment is to reduce the patient's fear and avoidance of sex. This goal can be accomplished via systematic desensitization in which the patient is gradually exposed in imagination and then in vivo to the actual sexual situations that generate anxiety. Kaplan et al. (1982) have reported successful treatment of sexual phobias with tricyclic medications and sex therapy.

Sexual Arousal Disorders

Male erectile disorder. Male erectile disorder is characterized by persistent or recurrent inability to attain or maintain an adequate erection until completion of the sexual activity. Another criterion is that the disturbance causes marked distress or interpersonal difficulty.

The treatment of erectile problems is generally easier if the patient has a willing sexual partner to participate in therapy. However, treatment is possible without a partner's attendance.

Initially, the clinician should inform the patient with male erectile dysfunction that he is not alone in this problem and that, in fact, most men are unable to generate an erection at some time in their lives. The most successful treatment for arousal and erectile disorders in patients with partners has been the use of behavioral assignments to gradually decrease performance anxiety. Sensate focus exercises (Masters and Johnson 1970) are examples of such techniques in which the patient engages in nongenital, nondemand caressing with a partner and concentrates on pleasurable feelings. Gradually, the patient engages in pleasurable, genital sexual activities (e.g., touch, oral contact) with no penetration permitted until anxiety has been decreased sufficiently to permit full erectile function.

Group therapy, hypnotherapy, and systematic desensitization also have been used successfully in cases of erectile difficulties. Again, these treatments act to reduce anxiety associated with being sexual. Although psychoanalysis is not indicated in the treatment of simple erectile dysfunction, psychodynamic interventions may be helpful in alleviating intrapsychic conflicts contributing to performance anxiety. Couples therapy also is often helpful in treating these patients (Leiblum and Rosen 1991).

Various somatic treatments also can be used for erectile disorders, even when these disorders are primarily due to nonorganic factors. Testosterone is often used by nonpsychiatric physicians to treat impotence; however, there is no indication for its use except when erectile problems are due to hypogonadism (O'Carroll and Bancroft 1984).

Vasoactive injections into the corpora cavernosa can be used to treat erectile disorders. These injections can produce erections that last up to several hours. Most injections consist of a combination of papaverine (a smooth-muscle relaxant) and phentolamine (an α-adrenergic blocker), although other agents (e.g., prostaglandin E_1) also can be used (Mahmoud et al. 1992). Side effects of the injections include priapism (i.e., a prolonged, painful erection), fibrotic nodules in the penis, and mild alteration in liver function tests (Levine et al. 1989). Success rates for this treatment are high (about 85%), with improvements in erectile capacity, sexual satisfaction, and frequency of intercourse (Althof et al. 1991). However, there is a high dropout rate (about 55%) due to pain of the injection, side effects, and the fact that the injections should not be used more than twice a week (Cooper 1991). The combination of traditional sex therapy techniques and these injections may be helpful even in those men with purely psychogenic erectile dysfunction (Weiss et al. 1991).

Topical medications also may play a role in the treatment of erectile dysfunction by directly relaxing arterial smooth muscle in the penis. Nitroglycerin patches have been found to improve erectile function in about 40% of patients (Meyhoff et al. 1992); the most common side effect is headache. Topical minoxidil also has been found to be helpful in some patients (Cavallini 1991); however, further evaluation of this treatment is required.

Oral medications such as yohimbine, an α-adrenergic antagonist, also have been used to treat erectile dysfunction. Full or partial improvement has been reported in about 34%–38% of patients when compared with those taking a placebo, although the benefits can take several weeks to develop (Sonda et al. 1990; Susset et al. 1989). Dopamine agonists such as bromocriptine also have been found to be effective in preliminary trials (Lal et al. 1991).

A major noninvasive, nonpharmacological treatment for erectile dysfunction is an external vacuum device. The device consists of a plastic cylinder with one end open and the other end connected to a vacuum pump. A vacuum is created that draws blood into the penis. A tension ring is then slipped from the cylinder to the base of the penis for up to 30 minutes. This treatment has a high success rate (about 85%) and a low dropout rate (about 20% per year) (Turner et al. 1991). The external vacuum device has the advantages of being noninvasive, being relatively inexpensive, and having few side effects (bruising, physical discomfort, and blocked ejaculation are the most common). Disadvantages are that erections last only 30 minutes and the patient must interrupt sexual activity to use the device (Turner et al. 1992).

For men with pure organic or combination organic-psychogenic impotence who do not respond to other treatment measures, penile prostheses can be implanted. There are two types currently available: a bendable silicone implant and an inflatable implant. However, these only should be used after careful psychiatric, sexual, and urological evaluations. There are several drawbacks that must be taken into account when considering patients for this form of treatment: the risk of surgery and postoperative infection, the destruction of natural erectile capacity, and mechanical breakdown (about 20%). However, follow-up studies have suggested high patient and partner satisfaction in carefully screened candidates (Pedersen et al. 1988).

Female sexual arousal disorder. Female sexual arousal disorder is characterized by persistent or recurrent inability to attain or maintain an adequate lubrication-swelling response of sexual excitement until completion of the sexual activity. Diagnosis is made if the disorder does not occur exclusively during the course of another Axis I disorder and is not due to the direct effects of a substance (illegal or prescription drugs) or a general medical condition.

Treatment of impairment of sexual arousal in women often involves the reduction of anxiety associated with sexual activity. Thus, behavioral techniques such as those involving sensate focus are most often effective (Kaplan 1974).

Orgasmic Disorders

Female orgasmic disorder. Female orgasmic disorder (also known as inhibited female orgasm) is characterized by persistent or recurrent delay in, or absence of, orgasm following a normal sexual excitement phase. Clinicians should take into consideration that females exhibit great variability in both the type and the intensity of stimulation required to trigger an orgasm. Other factors to be evaluated include the woman's age and sexual experience and the adequacy of sexual stimulation she receives. As with the other dysfunctions, the diagnosis is made if the disorder causes marked distress or interpersonal difficulty, if it does not occur exclusively during the course of another Axis I disorder, and if it is not due to the direct effects of a substance or a general medical condition.

The most likely way for a woman with general anorgasmia (i.e., never having had an orgasm) to become orgasmic is through a program of directed masturbation (LoPiccolo and Stock 1986). Any discomfort the patient may feel about exploring her own body should be discussed. Next, the patient should be instructed in a systematic program for exercising the pubococcygeus muscle, a muscle involved in orgasms. Once the patient has mastered these exercises, she is placed on a masturbatory program that begins with a gradual visual and tactile exploration of her body and moves toward focused genital touching. Use of sexual fantasies combined with stimulation is also taught. The clinician may recommend use of a vibrator if the woman is unable to have an orgasm when engaging in focused genital touching. Once the woman is able to have an orgasm through self-stimulation, she then teaches her sexual partner (using sensate focus exercises) the type of genital stimulation she requires to have an orgasm.

For a woman with situational anorgasmia, it is imperative to explore the relationship and involve her partner in treatment. Couples therapy, if indicated, and graduated exposure exercises also can be used in treatment. Treatments that focus on communication and relationship skills have been found to have high success rates (Milan et al. 1988).

The most frequent complaint of women experiencing an orgasmic problem is that they are not orgasmic through penile-vaginal intercourse. When becoming orgasmic through intercourse is a patient's treatment goal, the clinician should ensure that she and her partner are aware that adequate stimulation both before and during intercourse is necessary. In addition, the clinician may suggest various sexual positions that allow stimulation of the clitoris by the patient or her partner during intercourse. For women who are fearful of "letting go" during intercourse, systematic desensitization is often helpful. The therapist may wish to explore with the patient psychodynamic reasons, religious concerns, or personal beliefs regarding intercourse and sexual pleasure. Appropriate therapy can be offered to deal with these issues while still working within the parameters of the patient's personal beliefs and morals. Finally, the patient should be told not to expect to have an orgasm every time she has intercourse, as only a minority of women are orgasmic regularly during intercourse.

Male orgasmic disorder. Male orgasmic disorder (also known as inhibited male orgasm or retarded ejaculation) is characterized by persistent or recurrent delay in or absence of orgasm following a normal sexual excitement phase during sexual activity. The patient's age as well as the focus, intensity, and duration of sexual stimulation must be considered. As with the other disorders, the disturbance must cause marked distress.

The treatment for this disorder is similar to that used for inhibited orgasm in females. The patient should be told that when he masturbates, he should masturbate as quickly as possible to ejaculation while fantasizing that his penis is inside his partner's vagina and ejaculating. A second technique is to teach the patient and his partner sensate focus exercises. If the patient is able to masturbate in the presence of his partner, he is instructed to place his partner's hand over his so that she can see how much touching he requires. He should then place his hand over hers while she masturbates him to ejaculation. Finally, she should sit astride him and stimulate him, eventually putting his penis in her vagina when he reaches the point of ejaculatory inevitability. If a man is uncomfortable ejaculating in the presence of his partner, systematic desensitization is used to help him become more comfortable in her presence.

Premature ejaculation. Premature ejaculation is characterized by persistent or recurrent ejaculation with minimal sexual stimulation before, on, or shortly after penetration and before the person wishes. The patient's age, novelty of situation, sexual partner, and frequency of sexual activity must be taken into consideration in making this diagnosis.

The treatment of premature ejaculation involves training the individual to tolerate high levels of excitement without ejaculating and reducing anxiety associated with sexual arousal. One successful intervention is the start-stop technique (Semans 1956). This procedure involves having the patient lie on his back while his partner strokes his penis. The patient focuses on the pleasurable feelings resulting from the penile stimulation and the sensations that precede his urge to ejaculate. When he feels that he is about to ejaculate, he signals his partner to stop stimulation. The patient should start and stop at least four times before he allows himself to ejaculate.

A second procedure, the "squeeze" technique (Masters and Johnson 1970), can be done in conjunction with the start-stop technique. In the squeeze technique, the patient's partner is taught to place her thumb on the frenulum of the penis and her first and second fingers on the opposite sides of the head of the penis. When the patient feels that he is going to ejaculate, the partner squeezes for up to 5 seconds and then releases the penis for up to 30 seconds. This technique is continued until the individual is no longer on the verge of ejaculating, then the patient's partner resumes penile stimulation.

Somatic treatments for premature ejaculation include intracavernous injection of papaverine and phentolamine (Fein 1990) and oral medications such as clomipramine (Colpi et al. 1991).

Sexual Pain Disorders

Dyspareunia. Dyspareunia is characterized by recurrent or persistent genital pain in either a male or female before, during, or after sexual intercourse. A substance-induced disorder and other Axis I disorders or general medical conditions should be ruled out. It is imperative that a comprehensive physical and gynecological or urological examination be conducted. In the absence of organic pathology, the patient's fear and anxiety underlying sexual functioning should be investigated. Systematic desensitization has been found to be successful in the treatment of this disorder in some women.

Vaginismus. Vaginismus is characterized by recurrent or persistent involuntary spasm of the musculature of the outer one-third of the vagina that interferes with sexual intercourse. This problem can be diagnosed with certainty only through a gynecological examination. Some women who are anxious about sex may experience muscular tightening and some pain during penetration, but these women do not have vaginismus. It is important to rule out other Axis I disorders (e.g., somatization disorder), substance-induced disorders, or a general medical condition.

Systematic desensitization has been the most effective treatment method for vaginismus. A useful procedure involves the systematic insertion of dilators of graduated

sizes, either in the physician's office or in the privacy of the patient's home. Some clinicians have the patient or her partner gradually insert a tampon or fingers until penile penetration can be effected (Kaplan 1974). The clinician may suggest that the patient gently stroke her genitals and clitoris during the insertion procedure. Additionally, penile penetration should be effected with the partner lying on his back and the patient controlling the actual insertion and subsequent movement during intercourse. Follow-up studies have demonstrated maintenance of treatment gains over time for most women (Scholl 1988).

Sexual Dysfunction Due to a General Medical Condition

The diagnosis of sexual dysfunction due to a general medical condition is made if there is evidence from the history, physical examination, or laboratory findings of a general medical condition judged to be etiologically related to the sexual dysfunction (e.g., male erectile disorder due to a general medical condition, dyspareunia due to a general medical condition).

Substance-Induced Sexual Dysfunction

The diagnosis of substance-induced sexual dysfunction is made if the patient has been using either medications or drugs that result in the impairment of sexual functioning, and the symptoms of the dysfunction are manifested either during use of the substance or within 6 weeks of cessation of the substance. Individuals who abuse drugs have a high rate (up to 60%) of sexual dysfunctions (Cocores et al. 1988; Schiavi 1990). Drugs of abuse can impair sexual functioning through various mechanisms. Cocaine may impair sexual functioning because of its ability to deplete dopamine stores with chronic use. Chronic opiate and alcohol use also may interfere with endogenous dopamine and serotonin functioning, leading to impaired sexual functioning.

PARAPHILIAS

The paraphilias (Table 19–6) are characterized by experiencing, over a period of at least 6 months, recurrent intense sexual urges and sexually arousing fantasies that involve nonhuman objects or nonconsenting partners. Examples are fetishism (i.e., sexual arousal to nonliving objects, female undergarments), transvestic fetishism (i.e., sexual urges and fantasies involving cross-dressing), and pedophilia (i.e., sexual urges and fantasies involving pre-

TABLE 19–6.   Paraphilias

- Exhibitionism
- Fetishism
- Frotteurism
- Pedophilia
- Sexual masochism
- Sexual sadism
- Transvestic fetishism
- Voyeurism
- Paraphilia not otherwise specified
- Sexual disorder not otherwise specified

pubescent children). Sexual sadism involves urges toward, and sexually arousing fantasies of, acts (real, not simulated) in which the psychological and/or physical suffering (including humiliation) of the victim is sexually exciting to the perpetrator. In sexual masochism, an individual derives sexual excitement from being humiliated, beaten, bound, or otherwise made to suffer.

Other paraphilias that involve nonconsenting partners are exhibitionism (i.e., exposure of genitals to an unsuspecting stranger), voyeurism (i.e., observing an unsuspecting person naked, in the process of disrobing, or engaging in sexual activity), and frottage (i.e., sexual arousal caused by rubbing up against a stranger). Some individuals are aroused by sexual contact with corpses (necrophilia), urine (urophilia), feces (coprophilia), or enemas (klismaphilia).

In diagnosing all of the paraphilias, a further criterion is that the person has acted on the urges or is markedly distressed by them.

EPIDEMIOLOGY

The paraphilias rarely cause personal distress, and individuals with these disorders usually come for treatment because of pressure from their partners or the authorities. Thus, there are few data on the prevalence or course of many of these disorders. Historically, information on those paraphilias involving victims (pedophilia, exhibitionism) has been obtained from studies of incarcerated sex offenders. However, these data are limited in that many sex offenders are not arrested and those who are tend to underreport their deviant behavior for fear of further prosecution. For example, two large studies of incarcerated sex offenders found that the offenders had committed only a small number of sexually deviant acts (Gebhard et al. 1965). In contrast, studies of nonincarcerated pedophiles have demonstrated a high number of paraphilic acts: 23.2–281.7 acts per offender (Abel et al. 1985).

The vast majority of individuals with these disorders are men. For example, among reported cases of sexual abuse, over 90% of offenders are men (Finkelhor 1986). However, it is interesting to note that one study (Risin and Koss 1988) reported that 42.7% of college males who reported they had been sexually victimized were abused by women. Fallen (1989) reported that 5%–15% of perpetrators were females. It also has been traditionally held that persons with paraphilias engage in only one type of deviant sexual behavior. However, studies have suggested that these individuals often have multiple paraphilias (Abel et al. 1985). It is important to note that more than 50% of these individuals develop the onset of their paraphilic arousal before age 18 years.

ETIOLOGY

Various theories have been put forth to explain the development of paraphilias. As with the gender identity disorders, biological factors have been postulated. Destruction of parts of the limbic system in animals causes hypersexual behavior (Klüver-Bucy syndrome), and temporal lobe diseases such as psychomotor seizures or temporal lobe tumors have been implicated in some persons with paraphilias. It also has been suggested that abnormal levels of androgens may contribute to inappropriate sexual arousal. The majority of studies, however, have dealt only with violent sex offenders and have yielded inconclusive results (Bradford and McLean 1984).

Psychoanalytic theories have postulated that severe castration anxiety during the oedipal phase of development leads to the substitution of a symbolic object (inanimate or an anatomical part) for the mother, as in fetishism and transvestism. Similarly, anxiety over arousal to the mother can lead to the choice of "safe," inappropriate sexual partners, as in pedophilia or zoophilia, or safe sexual behaviors in which there is no sexual contact, as in exhibitionism and voyeurism. Some psychoanalytic theories have suggested that a paraphilia represents an attempt by an individual to recreate and master early childhood punishment or humiliation (Stoller 1975a, 1975b). Some view deviant sexual behavior as an alternative to neurotic development, attributing it to ego acceptance of unrepressed infantile sexual fantasies (Abel et al. 1993).

According to learning theory, sexual arousal develops when an individual engages in a sexual behavior that is subsequently reinforced through sexual fantasies and masturbation. It is thought that there are certain vulnerable periods (e.g., puberty) when the development of sexual arousal can occur. For example, if an adolescent boy is sexual with a 7-year-old boy and there are no negative consequences, the adolescent may continue to fantasize about having sex with the boy and masturbate to those fantasies, developing arousal to young boys (i.e., pedophilia). Similarly, if a young boy is experimenting and puts on his sister's panties or is cross-dressed by a relative and he becomes aroused, he may develop arousal to wearing women's clothes (i.e., transvestism).

Another theoretical model of the development of paraphilias is based on cognitive distortions. Distortions in thinking, or thinking errors, provide a way for an individual to give himself or herself permission to engage in inappropriate or deviant sexual behaviors. Examples of such faulty beliefs include the following: it's all right to have sex with a child as long as the child agrees; watching a woman through a window as she undresses does not cause her any harm; and if a child stares at my penis, he or she likes what he or she is seeing and wants to be sexual (Abel et al. 1984).

Other factors also play a role in the development of paraphilias. For instance, it has been shown that many pedophiles have impaired social and adult heterosexual relationships (Araji and Finkelhor 1985).

While theory and model development continues, it is important that developing theories are comprehensive and include evolutionary, neuroendocrine, and social learning factors.

DIAGNOSIS

It is important to distinguish paraphilias such as fetishism and transvestism from normal variations of sexual behavior. Some couples occasionally augment their usual sexual activities with activities such as bondage or cross-dressing. Transvestism, however, would be diagnosed only if a heterosexual male, over a period of at least 6 months, had recurrent intense sexual urges and sexually arousing fantasies involving cross-dressing and if the person is distressed by the urges or has acted on them. It is only when these activities are the exclusive or preferred means of achieving sexual excitement and orgasm, or when the sexual behavior is not consensual, that the diagnosis of paraphilia is made. Obviously, nonconsensual sexual activities such as sexual contact with children or exhibitionism never can be appropriate; children never can give consent for sexual activity with an adult.

Inappropriate sexual behavior is not always the result of a paraphilia. A psychotic patient may cross-dress due to a delusional belief that God wishes him or her to hide his or her true sex. A manic patient may expose himself to women due to his hypersexuality and belief that he will be able to "pick them up." A patient with dementia can behave in a sexually inappropriate manner (e.g., masturbate in a room full of people) because of cognitive impairment. An individual with mental retardation may engage in a sexually inappropriate behavior because of cognitive impairment,

poor impulse control, and lack of sexual knowledge. Individuals with antisocial personality disorder also can commit deviant sexual acts; such behaviors are usually part of their overall disregard for societal norms and sanctions.

In evaluating an individual for paraphilic behavior, a careful psychiatric evaluation must be done to exclude the aforementioned possible causes of this behavior. A detailed sexual history should be taken, noting the onset and course of paraphilic and appropriate sexual fantasies and behavior and the present degree of control over the deviant behavior. In addition, the individual should be evaluated for faulty beliefs about his or her sexual behavior (i.e., cognitive distortions), social and assertive skills with appropriate adult partners, sexual dysfunctions, and sexual knowledge.

Phallometric assessments (i.e., measurements of penile erection) have been used to objectively assess sexual arousal in individuals who have engaged in paraphilic behavior. This finding is important because persons with paraphilias, especially those in trouble with the law, are reluctant to disclose the full extent of their deviant behavior and fantasies. A transducer (either a thin metal ring or mercury-in-rubber strain gauge) is placed around the penis, and the degree of erection is recorded while the individual is exposed to various sexual stimuli (audiotapes, slides, videotapes) depicting paraphilic and appropriate sexual scenes. This information is then recorded on a polygraph or computer, and the degree of arousal to deviant sexual scenes is compared with arousal to nonparaphilic scenes.

Phallometric assessments of sexual age and gender preferences have excellent discriminant validity with extrafamilial child molesters (Freund and Blanchard 1989). However, exclusively incestuous offenders are less likely to show inappropriate sexual age preferences in phallometric assessment as compared with extrafamilial child molesters (Barbaree and Marshall 1989). Although phallometric assessments attempt to measure the degree of sexual preference among stimulus categories, they do not detail whether someone has engaged in paraphilic behavior or has committed a sexual offense. Furthermore, some individuals are able to influence their responses in order to appear to have nonparaphilic preferences (Freund et al. 1988). Further research is indicated to standardize this form of assessment and to establish the psychometric properties.

As with the interpretation of most physiological procedures, many urge caution in interpreting plethysmograph outcomes; that is, the setting in which the data is obtained is quite different from the real world. There can be variation within subjects over time, and therefore the interpretation must be made within the context of the offender's history, available records, and psychological characteristics (Dougher 1995).

TREATMENT

Biological treatments traditionally have been reserved for individuals with pedophilia or exhibitionism, although occasionally, individuals with other paraphilias receive treatment with medications. In view of the important role androgens play in maintaining sexual arousal, treatments have focused on blocking or decreasing the level of circulating androgens. Surgical castration has been used widely in Europe with incarcerated sex offenders. However, studies have suggested that surgical castration is not an effective means of eliminating deviant sexual behavior and that almost one-third of castrated men can still engage in intercourse. Many view surgical castration not only as highly intrusive, but also as cruel and unusual punishment. The results from this procedure are variable, unpredictable, and irreversible (Heim 1981).

Antiandrogenic medications have been used widely throughout the world since the late 1960s to treat sex offenders. The most extensively used and studied are the progestin derivatives medroxyprogesterone acetate (MPA) and cyproterone acetate (CPA). They have been used less extensively in this country due to ethical and legal considerations involving the ability of an individual facing a prison term to give informed consent. MPA appears to act by blocking testosterone synthesis, whereas CPA acts primarily by blocking central and peripheral androgen receptors. These medications may be given orally or via long-acting intramuscular depot injection (to improve compliance). They do not appear to influence the direction of sexual drive toward appropriate adult partners; rather, they act to decrease libido and thus break the individual's pattern of compulsive deviant sexual behavior. MPA and CPA thus work best in those paraphilic persons with a high sexual drive and less well in those with a low sexual drive or an antisocial personality (Cooper 1986).

Some researchers have examined the effect that CPA has on sleeping and waking penile erections in pedophiles. Cooper and Cernovovsky (1992) reported that all measures of NPT decreased while the patients were taking CPA. Results of arousal assessment while patients were awake were somewhat more variable. While the subjects were taking CPA, levels of serum testosterone, follicle-stimulating hormone (FSH), and luteinizing hormone (LH) also decreased, but prolactin levels did not show consistent changes. These medications never should be used as the only form of treatment; the patient must acknowledge his or her responsibility for his or her sexual behavior and participate in individual or group psychotherapy. The most significant long-term side effects are weight gain, increased blood pressure, impaired glucose tolerance, and

gallbladder disease (W. J. Meyer et al. 1985). The use of antiandrogenic medications often is referred to as *chemical castration*. Although the legal issues raised concerning surgical castration are similar to those concerning chemical castration, the use of these medications is at least reversible and less invasive.

Another promising focus of research has been on the use of other forms of pharmacological treatment. Fluoxetine has been used successfully in the treatment of patients with voyeurism (Emmanuel et al. 1991), exhibitionism, pedophilia, and frottage (Perilstein et al. 1991) and in persons who have committed rape (Kafka 1991).

Stein et al. (1992) reported on the use of serotonergic medications (i.e., fluoxetine, clomipramine, fluvoxamine, or fenfluramine) in the treatment of patients who had sexual obsessions, addictions, and paraphilias. In contrast to authors of the previously mentioned studies, these authors found that serotonergic medications were ineffective in treating the paraphilias. Stein et al. (1992) hypothesized that compulsivity and impulsivity may occur on a neurobiological spectrum on which obsessions and compulsions are at the compulsive end of the spectrum and paraphilias at the impulsive end. Clearly, further controlled research is needed to evaluate the efficacy of serotonergic medications in treating patients with these disorders.

Psychoanalysis and psychodynamic therapy have been used in treating paraphilias. Identification and resolution of early conflicts, trauma, and humiliation are thought to remove the individual's anxiety toward appropriate partners and enable him or her to give up the paraphilic fantasies. Although psychodynamic psychotherapy has been useful in the treatment of some individuals, there has been disappointment with the results of this therapy as the sole form of treatment in cases of deviant sexual arousal (Crawford 1981).

A variety of behavior therapies have been used to treat paraphilias. Various aversive conditioning methods (e.g., noxious odors) and covert sensitization have been used to decrease deviant sexual behavior. (In the latter approach, the individual pairs his or her inappropriate sexual fantasies with aversive, anxiety-provoking scenes, under the guidance of a therapist.) Satiation is a technique in which the individual uses his or her deviant fantasies postorgasm in a repetitive manner to the point of satiating himself or herself with the deviant stimuli, in essence making the fantasies and behavior boring (Marshall and Barbaree 1978).

Skills training and cognitive restructuring to change the individual's maladaptive beliefs are also used in behavioral treatments. Marshall et al. (1991), in an extremely comprehensive review of the literature of treatment outcome studies for a variety of sex offenders, concluded that treatment programs that use comprehensive cognitive-behavioral interventions, as well as those that use antiandrogens in combination with psychological treatment, are the most effective. Recent outcome studies of sex offender programs have yielded generally optimistic results regarding recidivism outcome (Freeman-Longo and Knopp 1992; Marshall and Pithers 1994).

SEXUAL DISORDER NOT OTHERWISE SPECIFIED

There are several sexual disturbances that are neither dysfunctions nor paraphilias but are still considered sexual disturbances. These include marked feelings of inadequacy concerning sexual performance or other traits related to self-imposed standards of masculinity or femininity, distress about a pattern of repeated sexual relationships involving a succession of lovers who are experienced by the person only as things to be used, or persistent and marked distress about one's sexual orientation.

REFERENCES

Abel GG, Becker JV, Cunningham-Rathner J: Complications, consent, and cognitions in sex between children and adults. Int J Law Psychiatry 7:89–103, 1984

Abel GG, Mittelman MS, Becker JV: Sexual offenders: results of assessment and recommendations for treatment, in Clinical Criminology. Edited by Ben-Aron HH, Hucker SI, Webster CD. Toronto, Ontario, MM Graphics, 1985, pp 191–205

Abel GG, Osborn CA, Twigg DA: Sexual assault through the life span: adult offenders with juvenile histories, in The Juvenile Sex Offender. Edited by Barbaree HE, Marshall WL, Hudson SM. New York, Guilford, 1993

Althof SE, Turner LA, Levine SB, et al: Sexual, psychological, and marital impact of self-injection of papaverine and phentolamine: a long-term prospective study. J Sex Marital Ther 17:101–112, 1991

American Psychiatric Association: Diagnostic and Statistical Manual of Mental Disorders, 3rd Edition. Washington, DC, American Psychiatric Association, 1980

American Psychiatric Association: Diagnostic and Statistical Manual of Mental Disorders, 3rd Edition, Revised. Washington, DC, American Psychiatric Association, 1987

American Psychiatric Association: Diagnostic and Statistical Manual of Mental Disorders, 4th Edition. Washington, DC, American Psychiatric Association, 1994

Araji S, Finkelhor D: Explanations of pedophilia: review of empirical research. Bulletin of the American Academy of Psychiatry and the Law 13:17–37, 1985

Bancroft J: Homosexual orientation: the search for a biological basis. Br J Psychiatry 164:437–440, 1994

Barbaree HE, Marshall WL: Erectile responses among heterosexual child molesters, father-daughter incest offenders, and matched non-offenders: five distinct age preference profiles. Canadian Journal of Behavioral Sciences 21:70–82, 1989

Barlow DH, Abel GG, Blanchard EB: Gender identity change in transsexuals: follow-up and replications. Arch Gen Psychiatry 36:1001–1007, 1979

Becker JV, Skinner LJ, Abel GG, et al: Level of postassault sexual functioning in rape and incest victims. Arch Sex Behav 15:37–49, 1986

Bradford JMW, McLean D: Sexual offenders, violence, and testosterone: a clinical study. Can J Psychiatry 29:335–343, 1984

Byne W, Parsons B: Human sexual orientation: the biological theories reappraised. Arch Gen Psychiatry 50:228–239, 1993

Cavallini G: Minoxidil versus nitroglycerin: a prospective double-blind controlled trial in transcutaneous erection facilitation for organic impotence. J Urol 146:50–53, 1991

Cocores JA, Miller NS, Pottash AC, et al: Sexual dysfunction in abusers of cocaine and alcohol. Am J Drug Alcohol Abuse 14:169–173, 1988

Collaer ML, Hines M: Human behavioral sex differences: a role for gonadal hormones during early development? Psychol Bull 118:55–107, 1995

Colpi GM, Fanciullacci F, Aydos K, et al: Effectiveness mechanism of clomipramine by neurophysiological tests in subjects with true premature ejaculation. Andrologia 23:45–47, 1991

Cooper AJ: Progestogens in the treatment of male sex offenders: a review. Can J Psychiatry 31:73–79, 1986

Cooper AJ: Evaluation of I-C papaverine in patients with psychogenic and organic impotence. Can J Psychiatry 36:574–578, 1991

Cooper AJ, Cernovovsky Z: The effects of cyproterone acetate on sleeping and waking penile erections in pedophiles: possible implications for treatment. Can J Psychiatry 37:33–39, 1992

Crawford D: Treatment approaches with pedophiles, in Adult Sexual Interest in Children. Edited by Cook M, Howells K. New York, Academic, 1981, pp 181–217

Dougher MJ: Clinical assessment of sex offenders, in The Sex Offender: Corrections, Treatment and Legal Practice. Edited by Schwartz BK, Cellini HR. Kingston, NJ, Civic Research Institute, 1995

Dow MGT, Gallagher J: A controlled study of combined hormonal and psychological treatment for sexual unresponsiveness in women. Br J Clin Psychol 28:201–212, 1989

Ehrhardt AA, Meyer-Bahlburg HFL: Effects of prenatal sex hormones on gender-related behavior. Science 211: 1312–1318, 1981

Emmanuel NP, Lydiard RB, Ballenger JC: Fluoxetine treatment of voyeurism (letter). Am J Psychiatry 148:950, 1991

Fagan PJ, Schmidt CW Jr, Wise TN, et al: Sexual dysfunction and dual psychiatric diagnoses. Compr Psychiatry 29:278–284, 1988

Fallen KC: Characteristics of a clinical sample of sexually abused children: how boy and girl victims differ. Child Abuse Negl 13:281–291, 1989

Fein RL: Intracavernous medication for treatment of premature ejaculation. Urology 35:301–303, 1990

Finkelhor D: Source Book on Child Sex Abuse. Beverly Hills, CA, Sage, 1986

Frank E, Anderson C, Rubenstein D: Frequency of sexual dysfunctions in normal couples. N Engl J Med 299: 111–115, 1978

Freeman-Longo RE, Knopp FH: State-of-the-art sex offender treatment: outcome and issues. Annals of Sex Research 5:1992

Freund K, Blanchard R: Phallometric diagnosis of pedophilia. J Consult Clin Psychol 57:100–105, 1989

Freund K, Watson R, Rienzo D: Signs of feigning in the phallometric test. Behav Res Ther 26:105–112, 1988

Fridell SR, Zucker KJ, Bradley SJ, et al: Physical attractiveness of girls with gender identity disorder. Arch Sex Behav 25:17–31, 1996

Gebhard PH, Gagnon JH, Pomeroy WB, et al: Sex Offenders. New York, Harper & Row, 1965

Green R: Sexual Identity Conflict in Children and Adults. New York, Basic Books, 1974

Green R: Gender identity in childhood and later sexual orientation: follow-up of 78 males. Am J Psychiatry 142:339–341, 1985

Green R: "The Sissy Boys Syndrome" and the Development of Homosexuality. New Haven, CT, Yale University Press, 1987

Green R, Fleming DT: Transsexual surgery follow-up: status in the 1990s, in Annual Review of Sex Research, Vol 1. Edited by Bancroft J, Davis CM, Weinstein D. Lake Mills, IA, Society for the Scientific Study of Sex, 1990, pp 163–174

Heim N: Sexual behavior of castrated sex offenders. Arch Sex Behav 10:11–19, 1981

Hoenig J: Etiology of transsexualism, in Gender Dysphoria: Development, Research, Management. Edited by Steiner BW. New York, Plenum, 1985, pp 33–73

Kafka MP: Successful treatment of paraphilic coercive disorder (a rapist) with fluoxetine hydrochloride. Br J Psychiatry 158:844–847, 1991

Kaplan HS: The New Sex Therapy: Active Treatment of Sexual Dysfunctions. New York, Brunner/Mazel, 1974

Kaplan HS, Fyer AJ, Novick A: Sexual phobia. J Sex Marital Ther 8:3–28, 1982

Lal S, Kiely ME, Thavundayil JX, et al: Effect of bromocriptine in patients with apomorphine-responsive erectile impotence: an open study. J Psychiatry Neurosci 16:262–266, 1991

Leiblum SR, Rosen RC: Couples therapy for erectile disorders: conceptual and clinical considerations. J Sex Marital Ther 17:147–59, 1991

Levine SB, Althof SE, Turner LA, et al: Side effects of self-administration of intracavernous papaverine and phentolamine for the treatment of impotence. J Urol 141: 54–57, 1989

LoPiccolo J, Stock WE: Treatment of sexual dysfunction. J Consult Clin Psychol 54:158–167, 1986

Lothstein L: The postsurgical transsexual: empirical and theoretical considerations. Arch Sex Behav 9:547–564, 1980

Mahmoud KZ, el Dakhli MR, Fahmi IM, et al: Comparative value of prostaglandin E_1 and papaverine in treatment of erectile failure: double-blind crossover study among Egyptian patients. J Urol 147:623–626, 1992

Marshall WL, Barbaree HE: The reduction of deviant arousal: satiation treatment for sexual aggressors. Criminal Justice and Behavior 5:294–303, 1978

Marshall WL, Pithers W: A reconsideration of treatment outcome with sex offenders. Criminal Justice and Behavior 21:6–27, 1994

Marshall WL, Jones R, Ward T, et al: Treatment outcome with sex offenders. Clin Psychol Rev 11:465–485, 1991

Masters WH, Johnson VE: Human Sexual Inadequacy. Boston, MA, Little, Brown, 1970

Meyer JK: The theory of gender identity disorders. J Am Psychoanal Assoc 30:381–418, 1982

Meyer WJ, Walker PA, Emory LE, et al: Physical, metabolic, and hormonal effects on men of long-term therapy with medroxyprogesterone acetate. Fertil Steril 43:102–109, 1985

Meyhoff HH, Rosenkilde P, Bodker A: Non-invasive management of impotence with transcutaneous nitroglycerin. Br J Urol 69:88–90, 1992

Milan RJ, Kilmann PR, Boland JP: Treatment outcome of secondary orgasmic dysfunction: a two- to six-year follow-up. Arch Sex Behav 17:463–480, 1988

Money J, Ehrhardt AA: Man and Woman, Boy and Girl: The Differentiation and Dimorphism of Gender Identity From Conception to Maturity. Baltimore, MD, Johns Hopkins University Press, 1974

Nathan SG: The epidemiology of the DSM-III psychosexual dysfunctions. J Sex Marital Ther 12:267–281, 1986

O'Carroll R, Bancroft J: Testosterone therapy for low sexual interest and erectile dysfunctions in men: a controlled study. Br J Psychiatry 145:146–151, 1984

Pedersen B, Tiefer L, Ruiz M, et al: Evaluation of patients and partners 1 to 4 years after penile prosthesis surgery. J Urol 139:956–958, 1988

Perilstein RD, Lipper S, Friedman LJ: Three cases of paraphilias responsive to fluoxetine treatment. J Clin Psychiatry 52:169–170, 1991

Person E, Ovesey L: The transsexual syndrome in males, II: secondary transsexualism. Am J Psychother 28:174–193, 1974

Ponticas Y: Sexual aversion versus hypoactive sexual desire: a diagnostic challenge. Psychiatric Medicine 10:273–281, 1992

Risin LI, Koss MP: The sexual abuse of boys: childhood victimizations reported by a national survey, in Rape and Sexual Assault II. Edited by Burgess AW. New York, Garland, 1988, pp 91–104

Schiavi RC: Chronic alcoholism and male sexual dysfunction. J Sex Marital Ther 16:23–33, 1990

Scholl GM: Prognostic variables in treating vaginismus. Obstet Gynecol 72:231–235, 1988

Semans JH: Premature ejaculation: a new approach. South Med J 9:353–357, 1956

Sonda LP, Mazo R, Chancellor MB: The role of yohimbine for the treatment of erectile impotence. J Sex Marital Ther 16:15–21, 1990

Spector IP, Carey MP: Incidence and prevalence of the sexual dysfunctions: a critical review of the empirical literature. Arch Sex Behav 19:389–408, 1990

Stein DJ, Hollander E, Anthony DT, et al: Serotonergic medications for sexual obsessions, sexual addictions and paraphilias. J Clin Psychiatry 53:267–271, 1992

Stoller RJ: Sex and Gender, Vol 1: The Development of Masculinity and Femininity. New York, Science House, 1968

Stoller RJ: Perversion: The Erotic Form of Hatred. New York, Pantheon, 1975a

Stoller RJ: Sex and Gender, Vol 2: The Transsexual Experiment. London, Hogarth Press, 1975b

Stoller RJ: Fathers of transsexual children. J Am Psychoanal Assoc 27:837–866, 1979

Susset JG, Tessier CD, Wincze J, et al: Effect of yohimbine hydrochloride on erectile impotence: a double-blind study. J Urol 141:1360–1363, 1989

Turner LA, Althof SE, Levine SB, et al: External vacuum devices in the treatment of erectile dysfunction: a one-year study of sexual and psychosocial impact. J Sex Marital Ther 17:81–93, 1991

Turner LA, Althof SE, Levine SB, et al: Twelve-month comparison of two treatments for erectile dysfunction: self-injection versus external vacuum devices. Urology 39:139–144, 1992

Weiss JN, Ravalli R, Badlani GH: Intracavernous pharmacotherapy in psychogenic impotence. Urology 37:441–443, 1991

Zucker KJ, Bradley SJ, Lowry Sullivan CB, et al: A gender identity interview for children. J Pers Assess 61:443–456, 1993

Zucker KJ, Green R: Gender identity and psychosexual disorders, in Textbook of Child and Adolescent Psychiatry, 2nd Edition. Edited by Wiener JM. Washington, DC, American Psychiatric Press, 1997, pp 657–676

CHAPTER 20

ADJUSTMENT DISORDER

JAMES J. STRAIN, M.D.
JEFFREY NEWCORN, M.D.
GEORGE FULOP, M.D.
MIRIAM SOKOLYANSKAYA, B.A.

Adjustment disorder is a subthreshold diagnosis that has undergone a major evolution since 1952 (Table 20–1). As with all subthreshold diagnoses, it presents major taxonomical and diagnostic dilemmas. In the gray area of diagnoses that lie between normal behavior and major disorders reside the subthreshold disorders, which are often poorly defined, overlap with other diagnostic groupings, have indefinite symptomatology, and present problems of reliability and validity. These disorders are also juxtaposed between problem-level diagnoses and more clearly defined disorders. At the same time, the indefiniteness of these subthreshold disorders permits the classification of early or temporary states when the clinical picture is vague and indiscrete, and yet the morbid state is more than that expected in a normal reaction. Therefore, adjustment disorder occupies an important place in the psychiatric lexicon spectrum: normal, problem-level diagnoses (V codes), adjustment disorder, disorders not otherwise specified (NOS), and major disorders. As such, adjustment disorder would "trump" problem-level disorders but be trumped by a specific diagnosis, even if it were in the NOS category.

In the previous edition of this textbook, numerous questions regarding the diagnosis of adjustment disorder were raised in this chapter but never answered because of the absence of research in pertinent areas at that time. These questions included those about the role of stressors and the value of specific stressors in the adjustment disorders, the importance of age and medical conditions, the clarity of the diagnostic criteria, and the lack of a symptoms checklist, as well as issues of treatment and prognosis. These questions will be discussed in relationship to the new research findings, which support or refute some of the points cited in the previous edition and clarify or expand others.

Adjustment disorder is a stress-related phenomenon in which the stressor has resulted in maladaptation and symptoms that are time limited until the stressor is removed or a new state of adaptation has occurred (Table 20–2). At the same time that the diagnosis of adjustment disorder has evolved, so has the recognition of other stress-related disorders, such as posttraumatic stress disorder (PTSD). Other acute stress disorders were described as possible options during the development of the fourth edition of the *Diagnostic and Statistical Manual of Mental Disor-*

TABLE 20–1. **Diagnostic categories of adjustment disorder**

DSM-I (1952): Transient situational personality disorder
Gross stress reaction
Adult situational reaction
Adjustment reaction of infancy
Adjustment reaction of childhood
Adjustment reaction of adolescence
Adjustment reaction of late life
Other transient situational personality disturbance

DSM-II (1968): Transient situational disturbance
Adjustment reaction of infancy
Adjustment reaction of childhood
Adjustment reaction of adolescence
Adjustment reaction of adult life
Adjustment reaction of late life

DSM-III (1980): Adjustment disorder
Adjustment disorder with depressed mood
Adjustment disorder with anxious mood
Adjustment disorder with mixed emotional features
Adjustment disorder with disturbance of conduct
Adjustment disorder with mixed disturbance of emotions
    and conduct
Adjustment disorder with work (or academic) inhibition
Adjustment disorder with withdrawal
Adjustment disorder with atypical features

DSM-III-R (1987): Adjustment disorder
Adjustment disorder with depressed mood
Adjustment disorder with anxious mood
Adjustment disorder with mixed emotional features
Adjustment disorder with disturbance of conduct
Adjustment disorder with mixed disturbance of emotions
    and conduct
Adjustment disorder with work (or academic) inhibition
Adjustment disorder with withdrawal
Adjustment disorder with physical complaints
Adjustment disorder not otherwise specified (NOS)

DSM-IV (1994): Adjustment disorder
Adjustment disorder with depressed mood
Adjustment disorder with anxiety
Adjustment disorder with mixed anxiety and depressed mood
Adjustment disorder with disturbance of conduct
Adjustment disorder with mixed disturbance of emotions and
    conduct
Adjustment disorder unspecified

TABLE 20–2. **DSM-IV diagnostic criteria for adjustment disorders**

A. The development of emotional or behavioral symptoms in response to an identifiable stressor(s) occurring within 3 months of the onset of the stressor(s).

B. These symptoms or behaviors are clinically significant as evidenced by either of the following:
1. Marked distress that is in excess of what would be expected from exposure to the stressor
2. Significant impairment in social or occupational (academic) functioning

C. The stress-related disturbance does not meet the criteria for another specific Axis I disorder and is not merely an exacerbation of a preexisting Axis I or Axis II disorder.

D. The symptoms do not represent bereavement.

E. Once the stressor (or its consequences) has terminated, the symptoms do not persist for more than an additional 6 months.

Specify if:

Acute: if the disturbance lasts less than 6 months

Chronic: if the disturbance lasts for 6 months or longer

Adjustment disorders are coded based on the subtype, which is selected according to the predominant symptoms. The specific stressor(s) can be specified on Axis IV.

309.0   **With depressed mood**

309.24   **With anxiety**

309.28   **With mixed anxiety and depressed mood**

309.3   **With disturbance of conduct**

309.4   **With mixed disturbance of emotions and conduct**

309.9   **Unspecified**

ders, DSM-IV (American Psychiatric Association 1994)—for example, those stress reactions that follow a disaster or cataclysmic personal event (e.g., acute distress disorder) (Spiegel 1994). The stress disorders are also unique in the psychiatric DSM lexicon in that they are diagnoses with a known etiology and in which the etiological agent is central to the diagnosis. DSM by design was intended to have an atheoretical and phenomenological base as the cornerstone of its conceptual framework for diagnostic assignment. The deviance of the stress-induced disorders requires the diagnostician to impute etiological significance to a life event—a stressor—and relate its effect in clinical terms to the patient. The diagnosis of adjustment disorder also requires a careful assessment of the timing of the stressor to the adverse psychological sequelae that ensue, and until DSM-IV, a time limit was imposed on how long this diagnosis could be employed after the stressor had ceased. Until DSM-IV directives, adjustment disorder was a transitory diagnosis that could not exceed 6 months.

The etiological and dynamic attributes of the diagnosis of adjustment disorder make it a fascinating diagnostic category that constitutes a linchpin between normality and pathology.

DEFINITION AND HISTORY

Wise (1988) has summarized the history of adjustment disorder since 1945. Historically, the concept included the notion of a transient situational disturbance, initially codified by developmental epochs (Table 20–1); and then evolved to embody a disorder of adjustment characterized by mood, behavior, or work (or academic) inhibition (DSM-III [American Psychiatric Association 1980]); and finally evolved to include physical complaints as well (DSM-III-R [American Psychiatric Association 1987]).

With the opportunity to develop another evolutionary step of DSM-IV, the authors were asked to reexamine the subthreshold diagnostic category of adjustment disorder. From a review of the literature, reanalysis of existing data sets, and observations of the other pertinent diagnoses (e.g., minor depression, PTSD, minor anxiety), modifications for DSM-IV and their rationale were formulated.

As a result of the review of the literature and the Western Psychiatric Institute and Clinic data reanalysis, the American Psychiatric Association (APA) Task Force on Psychological System Interface Disorders supported that the following changes be included in DSM-IV:

1. Enhance the language.
2. Describe the time of the reaction to reflect duration: acute (less than 6 months) or chronic (6 months or longer).
3. Allow for the continuation of the stressor for an indefinite period.
4. Eliminate the subtypes of mixed emotional features, work (or academic) inhibition, withdrawal, and physical complaints.

Although it might be argued that adjustment disorder could be placed in a new category of "stress response syndromes," the literature does not offer any data to support such a grouping. In the extreme, adjustment disorder could be eliminated altogether, with the advantage of maintaining the atheoretical approach of DSM-III-R. This solution, however, does not seem beneficial in view of the recent findings that show adjustment disorder to be a valid diagnosis (Kovacs and Pollock 1995). In following the guidelines for recommending changes for DSM-IV—based on scientifically derived data—no clear evidence exists for selecting a placement alternative to this disorder's independent listing. The MacArthur field trials on the minor depressive and anxiety disorders that have collected data on the presence of stressors immediately preceding the occurrence of symptoms have become important data

bases to establish whether stress per se is a distinguishing characteristic between adjustment disorder and the other minor mood disorders. These studies include diagnosis of adjustment disorder in more than 1) 60% of burned inpatients (Perez-Jimenez et al. 1994), 2) 20% of patients in early stages of multiple sclerosis (Sullivan et al. 1995), and 3) 40% of poststroke patients (Shima et al. 1994).

In reviewing the diagnosis of adjustment disorder for DSM-IV, two issues emerge as fundamental. First, the effect of the imprecision of this diagnosis on reliability and validity, because of the lack of behavioral or operational criteria, must be determined. One study (Aoki et al. 1995), however, found three psychological tests, Zung's Self-Rating Anxiety Scale (Zung 1971), Zung's Self-Rating Depression Scale (Zung 1965), and Profile of Mood States (McNair et al. 1971), to be useful tools for adjustment disorder diagnosis among physical rehabilitation patients. Although Aoki et al. (1995) succeeded in reliably differentiating patients with adjustment disorder from healthy patients, they did not distinguish them from patients with major depression or PTSD. Second, the classification of syndromes that do not fulfill the criteria for a major mental illness but indicate serious (or incipient) symptomatology that requires intervention and/or treatment, by default, may be viewed as "subthreshold" and afforded a subthreshold interest by health care workers and third-party payers. Thus, the construct of adjustment disorder is designed as a means for classifying psychiatric conditions having a symptom profile that is as yet insufficient to meet the more specifically operationalized criteria for the major syndromes but that is 1) clinically significant and deemed to be in excess of a normal reaction to the stressor in question, 2) associated with impaired vocational or interpersonal functioning, and 3) not solely the result of a psychosocial problem (V code) requiring medical attention (e.g., noncompliance, phase-of-life problem).

Attention to minor mental symptomatology (and psychiatric morbidity) may forestall the evolution to more serious disorders and allow remediation before relationships, work, and functioning have been so impaired that they are disrupted or permanently sundered. Yet, in the gray area in which early diagnosis may take place and has enormous value with modest therapeutic investment, guidelines are the most tenuous. It is the professionals at the "front door"—those involved in primary care, triage, and emergency room treatment—who must be assisted to make this most difficult call: Is there sufficient psychiatric morbidity to warrant mental health assessment and/or intervention? Another problem that is shown in a number of studies is that due to the subthreshold nature of the adjustment disorder diagnosis and an absence of the symptoms checklist, nonpsychiatric physicians and nurses find adjustment disorder more difficult to diagnose than a major psychiatric disorder (Fincannon 1995; Margolis 1994; Perez-Jimenez et al. 1994; Silverstone 1996). The positive side of this issue, however, is that the presence of medical illness, which is a frequent comorbidity of adjustment disorder, does not confound this gray-area diagnosis. Without a symptoms checklist, the presence of medical symptoms does not intrude on the diagnosis. In major affective disorder, if seminal symptoms key to the diagnosis (e.g., appetite, sleep, energy, libido) are attributable to a medical diagnosis, they cannot be used to support a psychiatric diagnosis. Of course, at times the attribution of the symptoms is unclear.

In contrast to other DSM-IV disorders, adjustment disorder includes no clear and specific profile (or checklist) of symptoms that collectively constitutes a psychiatric (medical) syndrome or disorder. Field studies, however, are being performed (i.e., *DSM-IV Sourcebook*, Volume 4) to create a reliable checklist from an elaborate list of symptoms associated with adjustment disorder (Table 20–3). (The V codes, a problem level of diagnoses outside the realm of a medical disorder, understandably are devoid of a symptom-based diagnostic schema.) The imprecision of the diagnostic criteria for adjustment disorder is immediately apparent in DSM-IV's description of this disorder as a maladaptive reaction to an identifiable psychosocial

TABLE 20–3.   **Symptomatological comparisons among subtypes of adjustment disorder in 2,224 adult (19–64 years of age) psychiatric patients**

Differential symptoms	AD AII	ADD	ADA	ADE	ADC	ADM
1. Hyposomnia	1.19	1.33[a]	0.99	1.03	0.63	0.98
3. Appetite decreased	0.76	0.89[a]	0.41	0.58	0.35	0.66
5. Weight decreased	0.47	0.53[a]	0.22	0.33	0.23	0.40
12. Alcohol use	0.60	0.67	0.20	0.35	0.70	1.03[a]
14. Non-CNS depressant	0.45	0.51	0.10	0.28	0.40	0.66[a]
15. Violent behavior	0.437	0.30	0.19	0.33	1.14[a]	0.95
16. Impulsivity	0.72	0.69	0.41	0.57	1.67[a]	1.35
17. Other antisocial behavior	0.24	0.25	0.09	0.16	0.35	0.46[a]
22. Self-centered	0.12	0.08	0.15	0.17	0.09	0.28[a]
25. Undue perfectionism	0.15	0.11	0.31[a]	0.26	0.00	0.04
27. Decreased motor activity	0.39	0.48[a]	0.09	0.30	0.12	0.28
28. Increased motor activity	0.44	0.32	0.68[a]	0.58	0.58	0.65
29. Social withdrawal	0.58	0.67[a]	0.29	0.52	0.16	0.36
31. Bizarre behavior	0.03	0.03	0.01	0.02	0.21[a]	0.09
32. Hostility	0.28	0.23	0.11	0.26	0.60	0.71[a]
38. Generalized anxiety	0.63	0.49	1.52[a]	0.85	0.37	0.55
39. Panic attacks	0.11	0.08	0.32[a]	0.16	0.00	0.04
40. Situational anxiety	0.13	0.09	0.37[a]	0.20	0.00	0.09
41. Depressed mood	1.52	1.78[a]	0.70	1.27	0.65	1.16
42. Low self-esteem	0.98	1.10[a]	0.82	0.84	0.51	0.77
44. Elated mood	0.04	0.02	0.03	0.05	0.00	0.13[a]
46. Suspiciousness	0.21	0.19	0.16	0.22	0.14	0.37[a]
47. Somatic preoccupation	0.09	0.07	0.24[a]	0.13	0.05	0.05
48. Suicidal indicators	0.87	1.04[a]	0.14	0.56	0.77	1.04
49. Homicidal ideation	0.21	0.19	0.02	0.18	0.42	0.48[a]
50. Homicidal behavior	0.07	0.05	0.02	0.05	0.40[a]	0.23
62. Developmental intellectual deficit	0.06	0.04	0.07	0.07	0.26[a]	0.11
64. Lack of insight	0.60	0.56	0.37	0.57	1.42[a]	0.97

AD AII = Adjustment disorder Axis II; ADD = AD with depression; ADA = AD with anxiety; ADE = AD with emotional features; ADC = AD with conduct disorder; ADM = AD with mixed features; CNS = central nervous system.
[a]Group with the highest score, significantly higher than at least one other AD subtype at *P* < .01.

stressor, or stressors, that occurs within 3 months after on-set of the stressor. It is assumed that the disturbance will re-mit soon after the stressor ceases or, if the stressor persists, when a new level of adaptation is achieved (American Psychiatric Association 1994). Difficulties are inherent within these diagnostic constructional elements.

First, with regard to the "maladaptive reaction," it is unclear how this concept can or should be operationalized. The social, vocational, and relationship dysfunctions that are qualitatively or quantitatively unspecified lend them-selves neither to reliability nor to validity—or even to agreement when this clinical situation obtains. The con-cept of maladaptive reaction is further confounded by the elements of culture—that is, the expectable reactions within a specific cultural environment, gender responses, developmental level differences, and the "meaning" of events to an individual and his or her reactions to them. "Average expectable environment" and "patient's explana-tory belief model" are examples of concepts for which there is an attempt to weigh cultural and subjective differences in the assessment of an individual's mental state and reaction (Kleinman 1980). Such considerations are not part of the decision-making algorithm of DSM-IV, which strives for a phenomenological, atheoretical orientation to enhance re-liability and validity by describing what can be seen and heard. Another question is whether the assessment of maladaptation is subjective or objective—by a third party, by a mental health professional, or by an admixture of these. When does an individual cross the threshold into "patienthood," and who will make the decision? As men-tioned previously, detection of early states with poorly de-veloped psychiatric prodromi—leading to early warning or prevention—is desired but presents a quandary, and no-where is this more apparent than in the measurement of "maladaptation."

The patient's functional status evaluation (Axis V) is not linked via an algorithm to the adjustment disorder con-struct in DSM-IV. Fabrega et al. (1987) contend that both subjective symptoms and decrement in social function can be considered maladaptive and that the severity of either of these is subject to great individual variation. Using data from Axis V and their "Axis VI"—an additional and more specific functional status axis on their Initial Evaluation Form (Mezzich et al. 1981)[1]—these authors could not con-clude that the level of psychopathology correlates with im-paired functioning. However, Bodlund et al. (1994) found that, according to Axis V, the Global Assessment of Func-tioning Scale self-report was a poor predictor for an adjust-ment disorder with depressive symptoms because patients who have this illness tended more so than others to score themselves lower.

Second, no criteria or "guidelines" are offered in DSM-IV to quantify stressors for adjustment disorder or to assess their effect or meaning for a particular individual at a given time. Many of the statements regarding maladapta-tion described previously apply to the assessment of stress-ors as well (Cohen 1981; Perris et al. 1984; Zilberg et al. 1982). Mezzich et al. (1981) attempted to classify and quan-tify the psychosocial stressors in 13 domains: health, be-reavement, love and marriage, parental, family stressors for children and adolescents, other familial relationships, other relationships outside the family, work, school, finan-cial, legal, housing, and miscellaneous. Another study (Despland et al. 1995), showed that type of stressor may in-deed be of help in diagnosing adjustment disorder. The study demonstrated that adjustment disorder with de-pressed mood and mixed mood was associated with more marital problems than were depressive disorders, whereas adjustment disorder with anxiety could be distinguished from anxiety disorder by the quantity of family and marital problems. The measurement of the severity of the stressor, however, and its temporal and causal relationship to de-monstrable symptoms are often uncertain and at times im-possible. Furthermore, the assessment of stress is not linked by an algorithm to Axis IV—a statement of stress during the previous year—so internal consistency or rein-forcement within the diagnostic lexicon is not required (D. Schafer, personal communication, April 1990).

The time course and chronicity of both stressors and symptoms need further exploration. The modifications in-troduced in DSM-IV, which differentiate between acute and chronic forms of adjustment disorder, solved the prob-lem of a 6-month limitation in DSM-III-R's criteria. This change was validated by Despland et al. (1995), who found that 16% of patients with adjustment disorder required treatment for longer than 1 year, with the mean length ex-ceeding the prior limitation of 6 months.

Although the diagnosis of adjustment disorder is not scientifically rigorous, this imprecision makes the diagno-sis useful to psychiatry. It is difficult to identify an emerging illness in its early stages, and in such instances the diagnosis of adjustment disorder serves as a temporary diagnosis that can be modified with information from longitudinal evalu-ation and treatment. It is a way to "tag" an individual for

---

[1] The functional status measure, involving seven levels of impairment, is used to assess "current functioning" of patients in three dimensions: "at work or at school, with family, and with other persons or groups" (Fabrega et al. 1987, p. 569)

possible difficulty before the morbidity becomes more apparent.

Even serious symptomatology (e.g., suicidal behavior) that is not regarded as part of a major mental disorder needs treatment and a "diagnosis" under which it can be placed. De Leo et al. (1986a, 1986b) reported on adjustment disorder and suicidality. Recent life events, which would constitute an acute stress, were commonly found to correlate with suicidal behavior in a group that included those with adjustment disorder (Isometsa et al. 1996). Spalletta et al. (1996) found assessment of suicidal behavior an important tool in differentiating major depression, dysthymia, and adjustment disorder. Furthermore, adjustment disorder patients were found to be among the most common recipients of a deliberate self-harm (DSH) diagnosis, with the majority involving self-poisoning (Vlachos et al. 1994). Thus, DSH is more common in adjustment disorder patients (Vlachos et al. 1994), whereas the percentage of suicidal behavior was found to be higher in depressed patients (Spalletta et al. 1996). It had been suggested by the DSM-IV Adjustment Disorder Work Group that suicide and DSH could be subtypes of adjustment disorder, but the problem of suicidal symptomatology without another psychiatric diagnosis is placed in the F-code section in DSM-IV, "Other Conditions That May Be a Focus of Clinical Attention." Clearly, what is regarded as a subthreshold diagnosis—adjustment disorder—does not necessarily imply the presence of subthreshold symptomatology within its domain.

Finally, the issue of boundaries between depression NOS, anxiety NOS, and adjustment disorder remains problematic. How often are the major syndromes associated with a stressor? How different are the symptom profiles of depression and anxiety NOS from those of adjustment disorder? Studies have been performed to examine these issues in an attempt to further the understanding of the specificity of the diagnosis and the construct of the stressor-related disorders and of those disorders not related to stressors. Although some of the findings seem to shed light on these issues, other data are still controversial. The diagnosis of adjustment disorder was consistently associated with shorter length of stay compared with that for major psychiatric diagnoses (Despland et al. 1995; Greenberg et al. 1995). Whereas Despland et al. (1995) found a significantly greater number of Axis II comorbidities in adjustment disorder patients compared with patients who have other psychiatric diagnosis, Spalletta et al. (1996) found the prevalence of Axis II personality disorder to occur the least among patients with adjustment disorder with depressed mood relative to patients with major depression or dysthymia.

Mixed anxiety-depressive disorder is another subthreshold diagnosis that has only recently been included in DSM-IV. The disorder is similar to adjustment disorder with mixed mood, thus making it difficult to draw a boundary between the two disorders. Furthermore, until DSM-IV had been implemented, the main difference between the two diagnoses was the chronicity of the mixed anxiety-depressive disorder, as was noted in the mixed anxiety-depression field trial (Zinbarg et al. 1994). In DSM-III-R, chronic adjustment disorder was not yet described. Now, with the change in criterion C for adjustment disorder, chronic or recurrent disturbance does not eliminate adjustment disorder, and the problem of differentiating the two subthreshold diagnoses remains a gray area. This uncertainty is further complicated by the question of treatment. Is this an anxiety accompanied by depression that should be treated with anxiolytics, such as benzodiazepines, or is this a depression accompanied by anxiety that should be treated with an antidepressant, such as a selective serotonin reuptake inhibitor (SSRI)?

A potential mood disorder, subsyndromal symptomatic depression (SSD), has been recently described (Judd et al. 1994). It also joined adjustment disorder in the gray area of subthreshold diagnoses. However, there are two critical differences between SSD and adjustment disorder: 1) SSD has a symptom checklist, and 2) SSD is not associated with a stressor. Nevertheless, our earlier definitions become blurred. Earlier in this chapter, we defined adjustment disorder as a diagnosis that will trump a problem-level diagnosis but that will be trumped by a specific psychiatric diagnosis, even if it is in the NOS category. By definition, "SSD is the simultaneous presence of any two or more symptoms of depression, present for most or all of the time, at least 2 weeks in duration, associated with evidence of social dysfunction, occurring in individuals who do not meet criteria for diagnosis of minor depression, major depression, and/or dysthymia" (Judd et al. 1994, p. 27). In some cases, the SSD diagnosis is the same as DSM-IV diagnosis for minor depression, termed by Judd et al. (1994) "SSD with mood disturbance," and has to be documented as such. In other cases, the disorder is SSD "without mood disturbance." Now, SSD with mood disturbance (i.e., minor depression) would trump adjustment disorder by definition. But should SSD without mood disturbance trump adjustment disorder or should adjustment disorder trump SSD? Research is needed to demarcate more carefully the boundaries among the problem-level, subthreshold, minor, and major disorders and, in particular, demarcate with regard to the role of stressors as etiological precipitants, concomitants, or essentially unrelated factors.

DSM-III-R has been described as "medical illness and

age unfair" (i.e., it does not sufficiently take into account the issues of age and/or medical illness) (L. George, personal communication, June 1981; Strain 1981), and eventually, to enhance reliability and validity, there needs to be a psychiatric taxonomy that considers developmental epochs (e.g., children and youth, adults, young elderly, and "old" elderly) and medical illness with its symptomatology. For example, with regard to the latter issue, Endicott (1984) has described replacing vegetative with ideational symptoms when evaluating depressed patients with medical illness. Rapp and Vrana (1989) confirmed Endicott's proposed changes in the diagnostic criteria for depression in medically ill elderly persons and observed a maintenance of specificity and sensitivity, respectively, when substituting for vegetative symptoms. Recent studies found adjustment disorder patients to be significantly younger compared with patients who have a major psychiatric diagnosis (Despland et al. 1995; Mok and Walter 1995). Zarb's (1996) study suggests that cognitively impaired elderly, when evaluated using individual items of the Geriatric Depression Scale (Yesavage et al. 1982–1983), exhibited adjustment disorder rather than major depression. In addition, Despland et al. (1995) showed that the patients' group with adjustment disorder with depressive or mixed symptoms included more women, thus exhibiting a sex ratio resembling that for major depression or dysthymia. Therefore, future editions of DSM may be able to take into account the differences encountered in symptom profiles for gender, various developmental epochs, and medical and psychiatric comorbidity. (See Table 20–2 for DSM-IV diagnostic criteria for adjustment disorders.)

EPIDEMIOLOGY

Andreasen and Wasek (1980) reported that 5% of an inpatient and outpatient sample were labeled as having adjustment disorder. Fabrega et al. (1987) observed that 2.3% of a sample of patients at a walk-in clinic (diagnostic and evaluation center) met criteria for adjustment disorder, with no other diagnoses on Axis I or Axis II; 20% had the diagnosis of adjustment disorder when patients with other Axis I diagnoses (i.e., Axis I comorbidities) also were included. In general hospital psychiatric consultation populations, adjustment disorder was diagnosed as 21.5% (Popkin et al. 1990), 18.5% (Foster and Oxman 1994), and 11.5% (Snyder and Strain 1989). D. Schafer (personal communication, April 1990) noted that up to 70% of children in the psychiatric setting may be given the diagnosis of adjustment disorder in a variety of mental health care settings. Faulstich et al. (1986) reported the prevalence of DSM-III

conduct and adjustment disorders for adolescent psychiatric inpatients. Andreasen and Wasek (1980), using a chart review, reported that more adolescents than adults experienced acting out and behavioral symptoms, but adults had significantly more depressive symptomatology (87.2% vs. 63.8%). Anxiety symptoms were frequent at all ages.

Fabrega et al. (1987) and Mezzich et al. (1981) evaluated 64 symptoms present in three cohorts: subjects with specific diagnoses, those with adjustment disorder, and those who were not ill. Vegetative, substance use, and characterological symptoms were greatest in the specific-diagnosis group, intermediate in the adjustment disorder group, and least in the group with no illness. The symptoms of mood and affect, general appearance, behavior, disturbance in speech and thought pattern, and cognitive functioning had a similar distribution. The adjustment disorder group was significantly different from the no-illness group with regard to more "depressed mood" and "low self-esteem" ($P = < .0001$). The adjustment disorder and no-illness groups both had minimal pathology of thought content and perception. Twenty-nine percent of the adjustment disorder group versus 9% of the no-illness group had a positive response on the suicide indicators. The three cohorts did not differ on the frequency of Axis III disorders.

An example of associated features in adjustment disorder is provided by Andreasen and Wasek (1980), who observed that in their adjustment disorder cohorts 21.6% of the adolescents' and 11.8% of the adults' fathers had problems with alcohol. Greenberg et al. (1995) report more substance abuse in adults with diagnosed adjustment disorder compared with all those with other diagnoses. Breslow et al. (1996), comparing patients with adjustment disorder and patients with other psychiatric diagnoses, showed that alcohol or substance use/abuse did not help to differentiate between diagnostic groups. Thus, higher rate of substance use at this time does not serve as an incontrovertible prediction factor for the diagnosis of an adjustment disorder.

ETIOLOGY

Stress has been described as the etiological agent for adjustment disorder. However, diverse variables and modifiers are involved regarding who will experience an adjustment disorder following stress. Cohen (1981) argues that 1) acute stresses are different from chronic ones in both psychological and physiological terms, 2) the meaning of the stress is affected by "modifiers" (i.e., ego strengths, support systems, prior mastery), and 3) one must differentiate the manifest and latent meanings of the stressor(s) (e.g., loss of job may be a relief or a catastrophe). Adjustment disorder with maladaptive denial of pregnancy, for example, can be a consequence of a stressor such as separation from a partner (Brezinka et al. 1994). An objectively overwhelming stress may have little impact on one individual, whereas a minor one could be regarded as cataclysmic by another. A recent minor stress superimposed on a previous underlying (major) stress that has no observable effect on its own may have a significant additive impact (i.e., concatenation of events) (B. Hamburg, personal communication, April 1990).

The chronological relationship between the stressor and symptoms has been examined less extensively. Depue and Monroe (1986) and Skodol et al. (1990) identified significant methodological problems in evaluating the quality, quantity, and timing of both stressors and symptoms. Depue and Monroe (1986) and Rahe (1990) state that the model of a single stressor impinging on an undisturbed individual to cause symptoms at a single point in time is insufficient to account for the many presentations of stress and illness in the clinical situation. Limitations of the current construct of stress for research have been described (Cohen 1981). Holmes and Rahe (1967) assigned relative values to specific stressors, but there has been much concern about the methodology used and the results obtained (Cohen 1981). Other life event scales (Dohrenwend et al. 1978; Paykel and Tanner 1976; Paykel et al. 1971; Tennant 1983) also have been shown to be inconsistent in their ability to link stress and illness. Many authors have cautioned that the vulnerability of the individual (e.g., ego strengths, support system, underlying personality disorders, timing and concatenation of the stressors, control over the stressors, and desirability of the event) needs to be assessed to ascertain the import of the situation on the individual. Axis IV of DSM-III was included to allow the clinician to assess the presence of stress in the multiaxial diagnoses of psychiatric disorders, but it has been confounded by low reliability (Rey et al. 1988; Spitzer and Forman 1979; Zimmerman et al. 1987). Almost 100% presence of stressors on Axis IV was reported by Despland et al. (1995) for adjustment disorder with depressed mood, whereas 83% was reported for major depression, 80% for dysthymia, and only 67% for nonspecific depression, supporting importance of stressors in the adjustment disorder diagnosis.

Hirschfeld (1981) and Winokur (1985) discussed both sides of the controversy regarding *neurotic* (i.e., related to a stressor) and *endogenous* (i.e., not related to a stressor) depression. From the examination of several studies, it has been difficult to demonstrate a significant temporal link between the onset of an identified stressor and the occurrence of depressive illness (Akiskal et al. 1978; Andreasen and Winokur 1979; Benjaminsen 1981; Garvey et al. 1984; Hirschfeld 1981; Paykel and Tanner 1976; Winokur 1985).

Andreasen and Wasek (1980) described the differences between the types of stressors found in adolescents versus those in adults: respectively, 59% and 35% of the precipitants had been present for a year or more and 9% and 39% for 3 months or less. Fabrega et al. (1987) reported that their adjustment disorder group had greater registration of stressors compared with the specific-diagnosis and the non-illness cohorts. There was a significant difference in the amount of stressors reported relevant to the clinical request for evaluation: the group with adjustment disorder, compared with the specific-diagnosis and the non-illness patients, was overrepresented in the "higher stress category." Popkin et al. (1990) reported that in 68.6% of the cases in their consultation cohort, the medical illness itself was judged to be the primary psychosocial stressor. Snyder and Strain (1989) observed that stressors as assessed on Axis IV were significantly higher ($P = .0001$) for consultation patients with adjustment disorder than for patients with other diagnostic disorders.

CLINICAL FEATURES

Nine different types of adjustment disorder are listed in DSM-III-R. As in DSM-III, DSM-III-R adjustment disorder is classified according to the predominant symptoms. In DSM-IV, adjustment disorder has been reduced to six types that again are classified according to their clinical features: adjustment disorder with depressed mood, adjustment disorder with anxious mood, adjustment disorder with mixed anxiety and depressed mood, adjustment disorder with disturbance of conduct, adjustment disorder with mixed disturbance of emotions and conduct, and adjustment disorder NOS (Table 20–4). In their study, Despland et al. (1995) suggested to reduce the subtypes even further, demonstrating identical profiles for adjustment disorder with depressed mood and adjustment disorder with mixed mood and proposing assimilation of mixed mood into the depressed mood category. Fifty-seven percent of their adjustment disorder sample were represented by these two groups; the rest of the sample was accounted for by adjustment disorder with anxiety and other categories.

TREATMENT

Treatment of adjustment disorder rests primarily on psychotherapeutic measures that enable reduction of the stressor, enhanced coping with the stressor that cannot be

TABLE 20–4. Types of DSM-IV adjustment disorder

Adjustment disorder with depressed mood: The predominant symptoms are those of a minor depression. For example, the symptoms might be depressed mood, tearfulness, and hopelessness.

Adjustment disorder with anxious mood: This type of adjustment disorder is diagnosed when anxiety symptoms are predominant, such as nervousness, worry, and jitteriness. The differential diagnosis would include anxiety disorders.

Adjustment disorder with mixed anxiety and depressed mood: This category should be used when the predominant symptoms are a combination of depression and anxiety or other emotions. An example would be an adolescent who, after moving away from home and parental supervision, reacts with ambivalence, depression, anger, and signs of increased dependence.

Adjustment disorder with disturbance of conduct: The symptomatic manifestations are those of behavioral misconduct that violated societal norms or the rights of others. Examples are fighting, truancy, vandalism, and reckless driving.

Adjustment disorder with mixed disturbance of emotions and conduct: This diagnosis is made when the disturbance combines affective and behavioral features of adjustment disorder with mixed emotional features and adjustment disorder with disturbance of conduct.

Adjustment disorder not otherwise specified (NOS): This is a residual diagnosis within the diagnostic category. This diagnosis can be used when a maladaptive reaction that is not classified under other adjustment disorders occurs in response to stress. An example would be a patient who, when diagnosed as having cancer, denies the diagnosis of malignancy and is noncompliant with treatment recommendations.

reduced or removed, and establishment of a support system to maximize adaptation. The first goal is to note significant dysfunction secondary to a stressor and help the patient to moderate this imbalance. Many stressors may be avoided or minimized (e.g., taking on more responsibility than can be managed by the individual or putting oneself at risk by having unprotected sex with an unknown partner). Other stressors may elicit an overreaction on the part of the patient (e.g., abandonment by a lover). The patient may attempt suicide or become reclusive, damaging his or her source of income. In this situation, the therapist would attempt to help the patient put his or her feelings and rage into words rather than into destructive actions and assist more optimal adaptation and mastery of the trauma-stressor. The role of verbalization cannot be overestimated in an attempt to reduce the pressure of the stressor and enhance coping. The therapist also needs to clarify

and interpret the meaning of the stressor for the patient. For example, a mastectomy may have devastated a patient's feelings about her body and herself. It is necessary to clarify that the patient is still a woman, capable of having a fulfilling relationship, including a sexual one, and that the patient can have the cancer removed/treated and not have a recurrence. Otherwise, the patient's pernicious fantasies—"all is lost"—may take over in response to the stressor (i.e., the mastectomy) and make her dysfunctional in work and/or sex and precipitate a painful disturbance of, or typhoidal, mood that is incapacitating.

Counseling, psychotherapy, crisis intervention, family therapy, and group treatment may be employed to encourage the verbalization of fears, anxiety, rage, helplessness, and hopelessness to the stressors imposed upon a patient. The goals of treatment in each case are to expose the concerns and conflicts that the patient is experiencing, identify means to reduce the stressors, enhance the patient's coping skills, and help the patient gain perspective on the adversity and establish relationships (i.e., a support network) to assist in the management of the stressors and the self. The primary treatment for adjustment disorder is talking. However, in some patients, as in the following case example, small doses of antidepressants and anxiolytics may be appropriate.

> A 35-year-old married woman, mother of three children, was desperate when she learned she had cancer and would need a mastectomy followed by chemotherapy and radiation. She was convinced that she would not recover, that her body would be forever distorted and ugly, that her husband would no longer find her attractive, and that her children would be ashamed of her baldness and the fact she had cancer. She wondered if anyone would ever want to touch her again. Because her mother and sister also had experienced breast cancer, the patient felt she was fated to an empty future. Despite several sessions to deal with her feelings, the patient's dysphoria remained quite profound. It was decided to add antidepressant chemotherapy (fluoxetine, 20 mg qd) in addition to her psychotherapy sessions to decrease the patient's continuing unpleasant symptoms. Two weeks later, the patient reported that she was feeling less despondent and less concerned about the future and that she had a desire to start resuming her former activities with her family.

Few data are available on pharmacological treatment of adjustment disorder. It seems that formal psychotherapy is presently the treatment of choice (Uhlenhuth et al. 1995), although psychotherapy combined with benzodiazepines also is used, especially for patients with severe life stress and a significant anxious component (Uhlenhuth et al. 1995). Tricyclic antidepressants or buspirone were recommended in place of benzodiazepines for patients with current or past heavy alcohol use because of the greater risk of dependence in these patients (Uhlenhuth et al. 1995).

As mentioned earlier in this chapter, the diagnosis of an adjustment disorder may be applied to a patient who is in the early phase of a disorder that has not yet developed to the extent that full-blown symptoms are evident. Therefore, if a patient continues to worsen, becomes more symptomatic, and does not respond to treatment, it is critical to review the diagnosis for the presence of a major disorder. The patient in the case example could have been in the early phases of a major depressive disorder, but at the time of assessment, she was still subthreshold.

COURSE AND PROGNOSIS

With regard to the long-term outcome of adjustment disorder, Andreasen and Hoenk (1982) suggest that the prognosis is good for adults but that in adolescents many major psychiatric illnesses eventually occur. At 5-year follow-up, 71% of adults were completely well, 8% had an intervening problem, and 21% developed a major depressive disorder or alcoholism. In adolescents at 5-year follow-up, only 44% were without a psychiatric diagnosis, 13% had an intervening psychiatric illness, and 43% went on to develop major psychiatric morbidity (i.e., schizophrenia, schizoaffective disorders, major depression, bipolar disorder, substance abuse, and personality disorders). In contrast to the predictors for major pathology in adults, the chronicity of the illness and the presence of behavioral symptoms in the adolescents were the strongest predictors for major pathology at the 5-year follow-up. The number and type of symptoms were less useful than the length of treatment and chronicity of symptoms as predictors of future outcome. Mezzich et al. (1981) and J. J. Strain et al. (1998) found that many of the subtypes of adjustment disorder were infrequently used (e.g., "with mixed emotional features"), whereas "with physical complaints," a DSM-III-R category, has had insufficient time to be observed.

As Chess and Thomas (1984) have reported, it is important to note that adjustment disorder with disturbance of conduct, regardless of age, has a more guarded outcome. Just as Andreasen and Wasek (1980) reported, Chess and Thomas (1984) underscored that "a significant number [of adjustment disorder patients] did not improve or even grew worse in adolescence and early adult life, and it was not always possible to predict the developmental course of

the disorder in the early period after its identification. Hence, we would suggest active appropriate therapeutic intervention in all cases" (p. 58).

Although there was considerable discussion regarding the inclusion of a subtype of adjustment disorder for use with patients with suicidal thoughts, behaviors, and attempts or DSH, who did not qualify for another psychiatric diagnosis, this proposed subtyping was believed to raise other conflicts. None of the other diagnoses has a code for suicidal or DSH behavior, although it is a common behavior in major depression, substance abuse, and borderline personality disorder. In fact, suicidal behavior or DSH can accompany any psychiatric diagnosis. Suicidal behavior and DSH are important predictors in diagnosis of adjustment disorder (Spalletta et al. 1996). They are symptoms that can lead to the most distressing consequence—death. This outcome, when reached, neither can be corrected nor resolved. If the new subtyping were to be implemented, the patient might then be given the diagnosis of adjustment disorder with suicidal ideation, behavior, or attempt or DSH, rather than the more exact diagnosis, and the assessors might tag suicide or DSH to trump the specificity of the diagnosis. In effect, a behavior would trump the syndromal diagnosis of a disorder. Consequently, the behavior of suicide or self-mutilation is coded in DSM-IV under an F code: "Other Conditions That May Be a Focus of Clinical Attention." Therefore, there would be two Axis I designations: the primary disorder and the condition indicated by the F code.

CONCLUSIONS

The issues of diagnostic rigor and clinical utility seem at odds for adjustment disorder, and field studies that would employ reliable and valid instruments (e.g., depression or anxiety rating scales, stress assessments, length of disability, treatment outcome, family patterns) would allow more exact specification of the parameters of the diagnosis. Identification of the time course, remission or evolution to another diagnosis, and evaluation of stressors (characteristics, duration, and nature of adaptation to stress) would enhance understanding of the concept of a stress-response illness.

Studies with adequate symptom checklists rated independently from the establishment of the diagnosis would help clarify the threshold between major and minor depression and anxiety, as well as help guide an entry cutoff point for adjustment disorder. Although the upper threshold is established by the criteria for the major syndromes, the lower threshold between an adjustment disorder and problem/normality is undesignated with operational criteria and illustrates the difficulty of the "boundary issue" described earlier in this chapter. The careful examination of associated demographic and treatment outcome variables also would enable clinicians to describe more specifically the boundaries between diagnoses. Associated features such as family history, biological correlates, treatment response, and long-term course are all critical to establishing the authenticity of a diagnosis and do not just represent a current symptom checklist and profile. The theory and practice of medicine have demonstrated the need for a comprehensive multidimensional formulation of all these physiological and functional variables to describe an illness.

Regardless of their position on the diagnostic tree, subthreshold syndromes can encompass significant psychopathology that not only must be recognized but also treated (e.g., suicidal ideation/behavior). Cross-sectionally, adjustment disorder may appear to be the incipient phase of an emerging major syndrome. Consequently, adjustment disorder, despite the problems of reliability and validity associated with such a category, could serve an important diagnostic function in the practice of psychiatry, especially when the typology is more fully developed. Problem- and subthreshold-level diagnoses are critical to the function of any medical discipline. Because this disorder may be the initial phase, or a mild form, of a dysfunction that is not yet fully developed, there is a need to describe the relationship between the incipient and the developed and between the subthreshold and the defined. This apparent chaos, lack of specificity, and questionable reliability and validity are the hallmark of interface disorders and subthreshold phenomena, whether they be in diabetes mellitus, hypertension, or depression.

Combined with the remaining problem of the certainty of the diagnosis, the question prevails: Should drugs be used in the treatment of adjustment disorders? The solution to this dilemma is an extreme caution with drug use. The pharmacological studies are currently inconclusive. The diagnostic uncertainty of adjustment disorder presents sufficient difficulty in and of itself, with its mixed features, great amount of medical comorbidity, and placement in the gray area (Hosaka et al. 1994; Hugo et al. 1996; Oxman et al. 1994). It is better to be cautious and delay psychotropic drug administration rather than subject the patient to the risk of unfavorable drug–psychotropic drug interaction. The condition may resolve or evolve into a major psychiatric illness and then be treated accordingly. This treatment may include pharmacological agents.

The characteristics of a mental disorder vary over the life cycle, and this variation is clearly illustrated by adjustment disorder. Certain developmental epochs may be associated with a particular symptom profile, as seen with acute myocardial infarction or appendicitis. The effect of the stressor may vary, and the assessment of functioning must be "measured" according to the demands of the developmental stage (i.e., school [youth], work [adults], self-care and maintenance [elderly]). The symptom characteristics and functional assessment of other diagnoses also may vary along the developmental schema from birth to senescence; illnesses such as major depressive disorders, organic mental disorders, sexual dysfunctions, and eating disorders need to be recast in another hierarchy to incorporate the stage of the life cycle extant at the time of the assessment. Considering normal variations across developmental epochs would make adjustment disorder and other DSM disorders much more applicable and less vulnerable to being characterized as "unfair" in regard to the aged, the child/youth, or the medically ill (L. George, personal communication, May 1981; Strain 1981). The result would be a taxonomy tempered by the vicissitudes of development and medical illness.

Such an effort also may make adjustment disorder, and DSM in general, more useful to child psychiatrists, pediatricians, geriatricians, geriatric psychiatrists, and primary care specialists, who currently feel that too often their patients' problems do not conform with psychiatry's lexicon. In fact, a significant number of their patients remain at the problem level of diagnoses with their somatic complaints as well. It is common for a fever of unknown origin not to be diagnosed or for a chest pain to remain unspecified. It is the *art* of medicine that makes it a profession, and it is a most difficult one at the interface of medicine and psychiatry or at the interface of normality and pathology. Anna Freud (1968) has emphasized the difficulty of understanding normality and pathology in her assessments of childhood. This important advice would obtain across the life cycle and be an important challenge to the developers of the subthreshold diagnoses (e.g., adjustment disorder) and future editions of DSM.

REFERENCES

Akiskal HS, Bitar AH, Puzantian VR, et al: The nosological status of neurotic depression: a prospective three- to four-year follow-up examination in light of the primary-secondary and unipolar-bipolar dichotomies. Arch Gen Psychiatry 35:756–766, 1978

American Psychiatric Association: Diagnostic and Statistical Manual of Mental Disorders, 3rd Edition. Washington, DC, American Psychiatric Association, 1980

American Psychiatric Association: Diagnostic and Statistical Manual of Mental Disorders, 3rd Edition, Revised. Washington, DC, American Psychiatric Association, 1987

American Psychiatric Association: Diagnostic and Statistical Manual of Mental Disorders, 4th Edition. Washington, DC, American Psychiatric Association, 1994

Andreasen NC, Hoenk PR: The predictive value of adjustment disorders: a follow-up study. Am J Psychiatry 139:584–590, 1982

Andreasen NC, Wasek P: Adjustment disorders in adolescents and adults. Arch Gen Psychiatry 37:1166–1170, 1980

Andreasen NC, Winokur G: Secondary depression: familial, clinical, and research perspectives. Am J Psychiatry 136:62–66, 1979

Aoki T, Hosaka T, Ishida A: Psychiatric evaluation of physical rehabilitation patients. Gen Hosp Psychiatry 17:440–443, 1995

Benjaminsen S: Stressful life events preceding the onset of neurotic depression. Psychol Med 11:369–378, 1981

Bodlund O, Kullgren G, Ekselius L, et al: Axis V—Global Assessment of Functioning Scale: evaluation of a self-report version. Acta Psychiatr Scand 90:342–347, 1994

Breslow RE, Klinger BI, Erickson BJ: Acute intoxication and substance abuse among patients presenting to a psychiatric emergency service. Gen Hosp Psychiatry 18:183–191, 1996

Brezinka C, Huter O, Biebl W, et al: Denial of pregnancy: obstetrical aspects. J Psychosom Obstet Gynaecol 15:1–8, 1994

Chess S, Thomas A: Origins and Evolution of Behavior Disorders: From Infancy to Early Adult Life. New York, Brunner/Mazel, 1984

Cohen F: Stress and bodily illness. Psychiatr Clin North Am 4:269–286, 1981

De Leo D, Pellegrini C, Serraiotto L: Adjustment disorders and suicidality. Psychol Rep 59:355–358, 1986a

De Leo D, Pellegrini C, Serraiotto L, et al: Assessment of severity of suicide attempts: a trial with the dexamethasone suppression test and two rating scales. Psychopathology 19:186–191, 1986b

Depue RA, Monroe SM: Conceptualization and measurement of human disorder in life stress research: the problem of chronic disturbance. Psychol Bull 99:36–51, 1986

Despland JN, Monod L, Ferrero F: Clinical relevance of adjustment disorder in DSM-III-R and DSM-IV. Compr Psychiatry 36:456–460, 1995

Dohrenwend BS, Krasnoff L, Askenasy AR, et al: Exemplification of a method for scaling life events: the PERI Life Event Scale. J Health Soc Behav 19:205–229, 1978

Endicott J: Measurement of depression in patients with cancer. Cancer 53:2243–2249, 1984

Fabrega H Jr, Mezzich JE, Mezzich AC: Adjustment disorder as a marginal or transitional illness category in DSM-III. Arch Gen Psychiatry 44:567–572, 1987

Faulstich ME, Moore JR, Carey MP, et al: Prevalence of DSM-III conduct and adjustment disorders for adolescent psychiatric inpatients, in Adolescence, Vol 21, No 82. San Diego, CA, Libra Publishers, 1986, pp 333–337

Fincannon JL: Analysis of psychiatric referrals and interventions in an oncology population. Oncol Nurs Forum 22:87–92, 1995

Foster P, Oxman T: A descriptive study of adjustment disorder diagnoses in general hospital patients. Irish Journal of Psychological Medicine 11:153–157, 1994

Freud A: Normality and Pathology: Assessment of Childhood. New York, International Universities Press, 1968

Garvey MJ, Tollefson GD, Mungas D, et al: Is the distinction between situational and nonsituational primary depression valid? Compr Psychiatry 25:372–375, 1984

Greenberg WM, Rosenfeld DN, Ortega EA: Adjustment disorder as an admission diagnosis. Am J Psychiatry 152:459–461, 1995

Hirschfeld RMA: Situational depression: validity of the concept. Br J Psychiatry 139:297–305, 1981

Holmes TH, Rahe RH: The Social Readjustment Rating Scale. J Psychosom Res 11:213–218, 1967

Hosaka T, Aoki T, Ichikawa Y: Emotional states of patients with hematological malignancies: preliminary study. Jpn J Clin Oncol 24:186–190, 1994

Hugo FJ, Halland AM, Spangenberg JJ, et al: DSM-III-R classification of psychiatric symptoms in systemic lupus erythematosus. Psychosomatics 37:262–269, 1996

Isometsa E, Heikkinen M, Henriksson M, et al: Suicide in non-major depressions. J Affect Disord 36:117–127, 1996

Judd LL, Rapaport MH, Paulus MP, et al: Subsyndromal symptomatic depression: a new mood disorder? J Clin Psychiatry 55 (suppl):18–28, 1994

Kleinman A: Patients and Healers in the Context of Culture: An Exploration of the Borderland Between Anthropology, Medicine, and Psychiatry. Berkeley, CA, University of California Press, 1980

Kovacs M, Ho V, Pollock MH: Criterion and predictive validity of the diagnosis of adjustment disorder: a prospective study of youths with new-onset insulin-dependent diabetes mellitus. Am J Psychiatry 152:523–528, 1995

Margolis RL: Nonpsychiatrist house staff frequently misdiagnose psychiatric disorders in general hospital inpatients. Psychosomatics 35:485–491, 1994

McNair DM, Lorr M, Doppelman LF (eds): Manual for the Profile of Mood States. San Diego, CA, Educational and Industrial Testing Service, 1971

Mezzich JE, Dow JT, Rich CL, et al: Developing an efficient clinical information system for a comprehensive psychiatric institute, II: initial evaluation form. Behavioral Research Methods and Instrumentation 13:464–478, 1981

Mok H, Walter C: Brief psychiatric hospitalization: preliminary experience with an urban sort-stay unit. Can J Psychiatry 40:415–417, 1995

Oxman TE, Barrett JE, Freeman DH, et al: Frequency and correlates of adjustment disorder relates to cardiac surgery in older patients. Psychosomatics 35:557–568, 1994

Paykel ES, Tanner J: Life events, depressive relapse and maintenance treatment. Psychol Med 6:481–485, 1976

Paykel ES, Prusoff BA, Uhlenhuth EH: Scaling of life events. Arch Gen Psychiatry 25:340–347, 1971

Perez-Jimenez JP, Gomez-Bajo GJ, Lopez-Catillo JJ, et al: Psychiatric consultation and post-traumatic stress disorder in burned patients. Burns 20:532–536, 1994

Perris H, von Knorring L, Oreland L, et al: Life events and biological vulnerability: a study of life events and platelet MAO activity in depressed patients. Psychiatry Res 12:111–120, 1984

Popkin MK, Callies AL, Colón EA, et al: Adjustment disorders in medically ill patients referred for consultation in a university hospital. Psychosomatics 31:410–414, 1990

Rahe RH: Psychosocial stressors and adjustment disorder: Van Gogh's life chart illustrates stress and disease. J Clin Psychiatry 51 (suppl):13–19, 1990

Rapp SR, Vrana S: Substituting nonsomatic for somatic symptoms in the diagnosis of depression in elderly male medical patients. Am J Psychiatry 146:1197–1200, 1989

Rey JM, Stewart GW, Plapp JM, et al: DSM-III Axis IV revisited. Am J Psychiatry 145:286–292, 1988

Shima S, Kitagawa Y, Kitamura T, et al: Poststroke depression. Gen Hosp Psychiatry 16:286–289, 1994

Silverstone PH: Prevalence of psychiatric disorders in medical inpatients. J Nerv Ment Dis 184:43–51, 1996

Skodol AE, Dohrenwend BP, Line BG, et al: The nature of stress: problems of measurement, in Stressors and the Adjustment Disorders. Edited by Noshpitz JD, Coddington RD. New York, Wiley, 1990, pp 3–20

Snyder S, Strain JJ: Differentiation of major depression and adjustment disorder with depressed mood in the medical setting. Gen Hosp Psychiatry 12:159–165, 1989

Spalletta G, Troisi A, Saracco M, et al: Symptom profile: axis II comorbidity and suicidal behaviour in young males with DSM-III-R depressive illnesses. J Affect Disord 39:141–148, 1996

Spiegel D: DSM-IV Options Book. Washington, DC, American Psychiatric Association, 1994

Spitzer RL, Forman JBW: DSM-III field trials, II: initial experience with the multiaxial system. Am J Psychiatry 136:818–820, 1979

Strain JJ: Diagnostic considerations in the medical setting. Psychiatr Clin North Am 4:287–300, 1981

Strain JJ, Newcorn JH, Mezzich JE, et al: Adjustment Disorder: the MacArthur Reanalysis, in DSM-IV Sourcebook, Vol 4. Washington, DC, American Psychiatric Association, 1998, pp 403–424

Sullivan MJ, Winshenker B, Mikail S: Screening for major depression in the early stages of multiple sclerosis. Can J Neurol Sci 22:228–231, 1995

Tennant C: Life events and psychological morbidity: the evidence from prospective studies. Psychol Med 13:483–486, 1983

Uhlenhuth EH, Balter MB, Ban TA, et al: International study of expert judgment on therapeutic use of benzodiazepines and other psychotherapeutic medications, III: clinical features affecting experts' therapeutic recommendations in anxiety disorders. Psychopharmacol Bull 31:289–296, 1995

Vlachos IO, Bouras N, Watson JP, et al: Deliberate self-harm referrals. European Journal of Psychiatry 8:25–28, 1994

Winokur G: The validity of neurotic-reactive depression: new data and reappraisal. Arch Gen Psychiatry 42:1116–1122, 1985

Wise MG: Adjustment disorders and impulse disorders not otherwise classified, in American Psychiatric Press Textbook of Psychiatry. Edited by Talbot JA, Hales RE, Yudofsky SC. Washington, DC, American Psychiatric Press, 1988, pp 605–620

Yesavage JA, Brink TL, Rose TL, et al: Development and validation of geriatric depression screening scale: a preliminary report. J Psychiatry Res 17:37–49, 1983–1983

Zarb J: Correlates of depression in cognitively impaired hospitalized elderly referred for neuropsychological assessment. J Clin Exp Neuropsychol 18:713–723, 1996

Zilberg NJ, Weiss DS, Horowitz MJ: Impact of Event Scale: a cross-validation study and some empirical evidence supporting a conceptual model of stress response syndromes. J Consult Clin Psychol 50:407–414, 1982

Zimmerman M, Pfohl B, Coryell W, et al: The prognostic validity of DSM-III Axis IV in depressed inpatients. Am J Psychiatry 144:102–106, 1987

Zinbarg RE, Barlow DH, Liebowitz M, et al: The DSM-IV field trial for mixed anxiety-depression. Am J Psychiatry 151:1153–1162, 1994

Zung W: A self-rating depression scale. Arch Gen Psychiatry 12:63–70, 1965

Zung W: A rating instrument for anxiety disorders. Psychosomatics 12:371–379, 1971

CHAPTER 21

IMPULSE CONTROL DISORDERS NOT ELSEWHERE CLASSIFIED

MICHAEL G. WISE, M.D.
JOHN G. TIERNEY, M.D.

The DSM-IV (American Psychiatric Association 1994a) diagnostic category called "Impulse Control Disorders Not Elsewhere Classified" is a "residual" diagnostic category, even though there is no other distinct group of disorders in DSM-IV classified as impulse disorders. The diagnoses found in this category are intermittent explosive disorder, kleptomania, pyromania, pathological gambling, trichotillomania, and impulse control disorder not otherwise specified (ICDNOS). The features common to all these impulse disorders are listed in Table 21–1.

In the nineteenth century, Pinel and Esquirol introduced the concept of *instinctive impulse* and the term *instinctive monomania*. The original monomanias included alcoholism, fire setting, and homicide. Kleptomania, a disorder first described by Marc in 1838, was later added to the monomanias by Mathey (Gibbens and Prince 1962). Many changes in the nomenclature of monomanias have occurred since the nineteenth century. Kleptomania, pyromania, pathological gambling, and trichotillomania were not listed as mental disorders in either DSM-I (American Psychiatric Association 1952) or DSM-II (American Psychiatric Association 1968). In 1980, kleptomania, pyroma-

nia, and pathological gambling were all added to the official DSM nomenclature in DSM-III (American Psychiatric Association 1980), along with two new disorders, intermittent explosive disorder and isolated explosive disorder. Seven years later, in DSM-III-R (American Psychiatric Association 1987), *isolated* explosive disorder was deleted "because of the high potential for misdiagnosis based on a single episode of aggressive behavior" (p. 427). *Intermittent* explosive disorder was retained, even though it was noted that "serious questions have been raised about its validity" (p. 427), and trichotillomania was added.

As more research on impulse disorders is conducted, other changes in this category will occur. Research indicates that there is a relationship between low cerebrospinal fluid (CSF) 5-hydroxyindoleacetic acid (5-HIAA; a metabolite of serotonin) and impulsivity (Virkkunen et al. 1987, 1989, 1994), as well as between low CSF 5-HIAA and recidivist violent crimes (Virkkunen et al. 1996). In addition, antidepressants, especially those antidepressants with the ability to block the reuptake of serotonin in a selective fashion, are often effective in the treatment of these disorders (McElroy et al. 1991c). This new research has stimulated discussion concerning whether the impulse control disor-

TABLE 21–1.   Essential features of impulse control disorders not elsewhere classified

Failure to resist an impulse, drive, or temptation to perform some act that is harmful to the person or others

An increasing sense of tension or arousal before committing the act

A sense of pleasure, gratification, or release at the time of committing the act, or shortly thereafter

ders are "affective spectrum disorders" (McElroy et al. 1992), are related to obsessive-compulsive disorder (OCD) (Hollander et al. 1996; Swedo et al. 1989), or are a convergence of mood, impulse, and compulsive disorders (Kafka and Coleman 1991).

INTERMITTENT EXPLOSIVE DISORDER

DEFINITION AND DIAGNOSTIC CRITERIA

The classification of individuals who exhibit episodic violent behavior has undergone considerable change in the literature (Table 21–2). DSM-I described an aggressive type of person who manifested "a persistent reaction to frustration with irritability, temper tantrums and destructive behavior" (American Psychiatric Association 1952, p. 37) as a "Passive Aggressive Personality." In 1956, Menninger and Mayman introduced the term *episodic dyscontrol*, and Menninger, in his 1963 book *The Vital Balance*, subdivided dyscontrol into three distinct types: 1) chronic, repetitive aggressive behavior (antisocial personality); 2) episodic, impulsive violence (homicidal assaultiveness, shell shock, hypomania, and delirious syndromes); and 3) disorganized episodic violence (seizure disorders and brain-damage syndromes).

In 1968, DSM-II introduced a new diagnostic category: "Explosive Personality (Epileptoid Personality Disorder)." The diagnostic criteria for this category seem contradictory in that the intermittent violent behavior needed to occur in an aggressive person who has "gross outbursts of rage or of verbal or physical aggressiveness" that are "strikingly different from the patient's usual behavior." Nonetheless, as DSM-II noted, "these patients are generally considered excitable, aggressive and over-responsive to environmental pressures" (p. 42).

In 1970, Mark and Ervin described a "dyscontrol syndrome," characterized by 1) a history of physical assault, especially spouse and child abuse; 2) the symptom of pathological intoxication; 3) a history of impulsive sexual behavior, at times including sexual assaults; and 4) a history of many traffic violations and serious automobile acci-

dents. This syndrome was thought to represent behavioral manifestations of disordered brain physiology, particularly in the limbic system. That same year, Monroe (1970) reinforced the idea that subtle brain dysfunction could cause episodic violent behavior and also used the term *episodic dyscontrol*. Despite a lack of diagnostic specificity, the label *episodic dyscontrol* has persisted, primarily in the neurological literature (Elliott 1990).

The diagnostic term *intermittent explosive disorder* first appeared in the *International Classification of Diseases, 9th Revision, Clinical Modification* (ICD-9-CM) (World Health Organization 1978). This was the first time that an official diagnostic nomenclature had categorized episodic violence as a disorder separate from personality. Intermittent explosive disorder with different diagnostic criteria appeared in DSM-III, and then in DSM-III-R, but with this disclaimer:

> This category has been retained in DSM-III-R despite the fact that many doubt the existence of a clinical syndrome characterized by episodic loss of control that is not symptomatic of one of the disorders that must be ruled out before the diagnosis of intermittent explosive disorder can be made. (American Psychiatric Association 1987, p. 321)

Despite reservations, intermittent explosive disorder was retained in DSM-IV. In the DSM-IV diagnostic criteria for intermittent explosive disorder (Table 21–3), the requirement that impulsivity be absent between episodes has been eliminated and additional exclusionary diagnoses have been added.

Two DSM-IV diagnoses are currently available to the clinician who wishes to diagnose a patient who primarily manifests episodic violent behavior: *intermittent explosive disorder* and *personality change due to a general medical condition, aggressive type*. Intermittent explosive disorder has numerous exclusion criteria, whereas personality change due to a general medical condition requires the presence of a specific organic factor that is judged to be causally related to the violence. The majority of individuals with episodic violent behavior do not meet the diagnostic criteria for either disorder but have another psychiatric disorder such as schizophrenia, paranoid disorder, mania, substance abuse, drug withdrawal, delirium, a personality disorder (especially borderline or antisocial), mental retardation, a conduct disorder, or organic brain disease (Tardiff 1992).

EPIDEMIOLOGY

Monopolis and Lion (1983) call attention to the tendency of clinicians to diagnose intermittent explosive disorder

TABLE 21–2. **Diagnosis of episodic violent behavior: historical perspective**

1952	DSM-I	Passive-aggressive personality (aggressive type)
1955	ICD-7	Immature personality (aggressiveness subtype)
1956	Menninger and Mayman	"Episodic dyscontrol"
1963	Menninger	Dyscontrol: chronic, repetitive; episodic, impulsive; disorganized
1968	DSM-II	Explosive personality
1970	Monroe	Episodic behavioral disorders
1970	Mark and Ervin	"Dyscontrol syndrome"
1977	ICD-9	Explosive personality (exclude: dyssocial, hysterical)
1979	ICD-9-CM	Intermittent explosive disorder 　Recurrent, significant outbursts 　Not due to other mental disorder 　Aggression disproportionate to stressors 　Regret, self-reproach (remorse) present
1980	DSM-III	Intermittent explosive disorder 　Several discrete, serious episodes 　Aggression disproportionate to stressors 　No other impulsivity, aggression 　Exclude: schizophrenia, antisocial personality disorder, 　　conduct disorder
1987	DSM-III-R	Intermittent explosive disorder 　Several discrete, serious episodes 　Aggression disproportionate to stressors 　No other impulsivity, aggression 　Exclude: psychosis, organic personality syndrome, antisocial 　　personality disorder, borderline personality disorder, conduct 　　disorder, intoxication
1994	DSM-IV	Intermittent explosive disorder 　Several discrete, serious episodes 　Aggression disproportionate to stressors 　Exclude: antisocial personality disorder, borderline personality 　　disorder, a psychotic disorder, a manic episode, conduct disorder, 　　attention-deficit/hyperactivity disorder, substance intoxication, 　　and a general medical condition that caused the aggression

without using any diagnostic criteria. A literature review prepared for the sourcebook for DSM-IV (American Psychiatric Association 1994b) reaffirms this impression and notes that authors typically consider the occurrence of one or more explosive outbursts sufficient for the diagnosis of intermittent explosive disorder. This means that the information published about intermittent explosive disorder, a relatively rare disorder, is actually information about individuals who are violent, an all too common phenomenon. Males account for 80% of persons who display episodic violence (American Psychiatric Association 1994b). In the

introduction to a recent volume titled *Anger, Aggression, and Violence in the Psychiatric Clinics of North America*, Fava (1997) stated: "Intermittent Explosive Disorder seems to create the illusion of the existence of a relatively homogenous group of individuals displaying pathological aggressive behavior. In reality, any rigorous approach to the study and the classification of pathological anger and violence has to take into account both the complexity and the heterogeneity of these behaviors" (p. xi).

The characteristics of 842 individuals who were reported to display episodic violent behavior[1] are summa-

---

[1] In this chapter, the authors use the general term *episodic violent behavior* to describe individuals who display recurrent violent behavior. Intermittent explosive disorder, as defined in DSM-IV, if it exists as a diagnostic entity, is quite rare.

TABLE 21–3. **DSM-IV diagnostic criteria for intermittent explosive disorder**

A. Several discrete episodes of failure to resist aggressive impulses that result in serious assaultive acts or destruction of property.

B. The degree of aggressiveness expressed during the episodes is grossly out of proportion to any precipitating psychosocial stressors.

C. The aggressive episodes are not better accounted for by another mental disorder (e.g., antisocial personality disorder, borderline personality disorder, a psychotic disorder, a manic episode, conduct disorder, or attention-deficit/hyperactivity disorder) and are not due to the direct physiological effects of a substance (e.g., a drug of abuse, a medication) or a general medical condition (e.g., head trauma, Alzheimer's disease).

rized in Table 21–4 (American Psychiatric Association 1994b). When all 842 cases were carefully reviewed and compared against DSM-III-R criteria for intermittent explosive disorder, only 17 patients were found to have possible intermittent explosive disorder. Mattes (1990) reported 4 (8%) of 51 patients diagnosed with intermittent explosive disorder who were free of any evidence of organicity. No systematic personality analysis was done, although the authors stated that the patients did not have borderline or antisocial personality disorders. In the only study that used DSM-III-R criteria for the diagnosis of intermittent explosive disorder, Felthous et al. (1991), after an extensive evaluation process, reported 13 patients with intermittent explosive disorder, although no neuropsychological testing or systematic personality assessment was performed.

Despite the knowledge that individuals who exhibit episodic violence often have personality disorders, no investigator of intermittent explosive disorder has evaluated personality in a systematic fashion. This is a critical factor, because antisocial personality disorder and borderline personality disorder are part of the exclusion criteria for the intermittent explosive disorder diagnosis.

ETIOLOGY

Monroe (1970) originally noted that episodic violent behavior occurs in patients because of excessive neuronal discharges or purely motivational causes. He described a continuum between "faulty learning" and "faulty equipment." Patients with episodic violent behavior frequently have neurological abnormalities. A significant percentage of patients have abnormal neurological examination results (65%), abnormal neuropsychological test results (58%), abnormal electroencephalogram (EEG) results (55%), a history of attention-deficit/hyperactivity disorder (45%), or a history of learning disability (38%) (Table 21–4). Despite evidence of central nervous system (CNS) dysfunction, it is often impossible to establish a clear cause-and-effect relationship between the CNS dysfunction and episodic violent behavior. Occasionally, special diagnostic techniques, such as EEG activation with α-chloralose (Monroe 1970) may prove useful in evaluation of these patients.

Research has implicated abnormalities in noradrenergic and serotonergic function (Eichelman 1992; Kruesi et al. 1992; Tardiff 1992; Virkkunen 1996), as well as high testosterone levels, increased dopamine levels, and increased arginine vasopressin levels (Kavoussi et al. 1997), in individuals who display episodic violence. This research is promising, and further investigation into the relationship between biological factors and behavioral disorders is warranted. McElroy et al. (1998), in a recent report of 27 cases of individuals with intermittent explosive disorder (IED) as defined in DSM-IV, stated that IED "appears to be a bona fide impulse-control disorder that may be related to mood disorder and may represent another form of affective spectrum disorder."

TREATMENT/COURSE AND PROGNOSIS

According to a review of the literature published between 1937 and 1991, episodic violent behavior is quite common in the general population, but strictly diagnosed intermittent explosive disorder is quite rare (American Psychiatric Association 1994b). Consequently, although information on the management and treatment of aggressive behavior is available, no information exists on the treatment, course, or prognosis of rigorously diagnosed intermittent explosive disorder. In addition, studies of aggressive behavior consist primarily of anecdotal case reports or open drug trials; few studies are placebo controlled. Research in this area is also complicated by the ethical dilemma of randomizing potentially violent patients to placebo treatment.

The development of a treatment plan for a patient who has long-standing, episodic aggressive behavior is complicated and involves the assessment and amelioration (when possible) of multiple factors, such as temperament, sensory cues, neuroanatomy, neurochemistry, neuroendocrine function, stress, and social conditions (Eichelman 1992). Presently, there is no drug specifically approved by the Food and Drug Administration (FDA) for the treatment of aggression. However, numerous pharmacological

TABLE 21-4. Characteristics of 842 patients with episodic violent behavior

	Percentage of patients examined out of total sample (N = 842)	Number positive/ total examined (%)
History of seizures	87	215/733 (29)
Legal problems	74	216/621 (35)
Head trauma	73	182/617 (30)
History of attention deficit	69	262/582 (45)
Drugs involved	65	82/547 (15)
Neurological abnormality	64	350/539 (65)
History of psychosis	62	33/527 (6)
Antisocial personality	53	15/445 (3)
Alcohol abuse/pathological intoxication	50	238/417 (57)
Electroencephalogram (EEG)	44	202/368 (55)
Family history of violence	31	109/264 (41)
Prodromal symptoms	24	77/202 (38)
Other personality disorder	20	39/168 (23)
Neuropsychological tests	20	97/167 (58)
Presence of remorse	18	96/153 (63)
Genetic abnormality	18	4/151 (3)
Learning disability	12	38/99 (38)
Computed tomography scan	12	16/98 (16)

agents—including neuroleptics, benzodiazepines, lithium, β-blockers (especially propranolol), anticonvulsants (especially carbamazepine), serotonin-modulating drugs (tryptophan, trazodone, buspirone, clomipramine, fluoxetine), polycyclic antidepressants, monoamine oxidase inhibitors (MAOIs), and psychostimulants—and long-term psychotherapy are effective in diminishing violent behavior in some individuals (Eichelman 1992; Tardiff 1992). The task for the clinician is to select the most effective and safest intervention for an individual patient who either is acutely violent or has chronic difficulty controlling violent impulses.

The treatment of a patient who becomes acutely violent, regardless of the underlying etiology, commonly involves physical restraint, seclusion, and sedation. Neuroleptics and benzodiazepines, such as haloperidol and lorazepam (or a combination of the two), are often appropriate and effective interventions to control an acutely violent individual. It is more difficult to decide how to treat a patient who has long-standing bouts of aggressive behavior.

Because there are no universally effective anti-aggression medications, selection of a pharmacological agent is based on the clinical diagnosis of the patient. For example, when aggressive behavior is the result of psychotic ideation or mania, treatment with a neuroleptic or a mood stabilizer will likely decrease aggressivity. In the absence of a treatable psychiatric condition, lithium, carbamazepine, propranolol, and more recently serotonin-selective agents are increasingly being used in the management of chronic aggressive behavior.

There is a small body of literature on the efficacy of lithium in the treatment of aggression not associated with a manic episode. Campbell et al. (1984) treated children who had conduct disorder with lithium and reported decreases in aggressive behavior, especially when the behavior contained strong affective components. In a double-blind, placebo-controlled study, Sheard et al. (1976) demonstrated that lithium reduced aggression in prisoners who did not have affective disorders. Fava (1997) noted that lithium appears to be effective in the treatment of aggression in prison inmates without epilepsy, mentally retarded and disabled patients, children with conduct disorder, and patients with bipolar disorder.

On the basis of the hypothetical relationship between seizures and aggressive behavior, carbamazepine was used in the early 1970s to treat patients with rage outbursts, especially patients who had seizure foci located in the temporal lobe or limbic structures (Mattes 1986). Several additional studies reported that carbamazepine reduces aggressive behavior in patients without overt epilepsy (Mattes 1990; Mattes et al. 1984; Stone et al. 1986).

Elliott (1977) was among the first to use propranolol to treat the aggressive behavior seen in brain-injured patients. Numerous other studies demonstrate the relative benefit of β-blockers in patients with and without overt brain injury (Mattes 1990; Mattes et al. 1984; Sheard 1988; Williams et al. 1982; Yudofsky et al. 1981). More recent research has suggested that compounds that modulate serotonin transmission, such as buspirone, serotonin-reuptake-inhibiting antidepressants, trazodone, and clomipramine, may benefit some patients. In disorders of pathological aggression, "the most promising agents overall are those affecting the serotonin system" (Fava 1997, p. 444).

KLEPTOMANIA

DEFINITION AND DIAGNOSTIC CRITERIA

There is no systematic research on kleptomania to establish or refute the validity of the existing DSM criteria (American Psychiatric Association 1994b). The DSM-IV diagnostic criteria for kleptomania are given in Table 21–5. The only modification in these criteria from those in DSM-III-R is the addition of mania as an exclusionary diagnosis.

The reader must exercise caution when reading literature about "kleptomania." Much of the literature presents information about shoplifters and thieves and does not discuss the rare subgroup of those individuals who meet the diagnostic criteria for kleptomania. Shoplifters and thieves are different from persons with kleptomania in that thieves steal for financial gain or to use the stolen object for personal use (and are excluded by criterion A of the DSM-IV diagnostic criteria for kleptomania).

EPIDEMIOLOGY

Little is known about the epidemiology of kleptomania, because it is a relatively rare disorder and is seldom the subject of research. According to McElroy et al. (1991a, 1991b), most of the information on kleptomania is derived from three sources: studies of "legally referred" shoplifters, case reports or small series of psychiatric patients, and cases of kleptomanic patients with eating disorders. Consequently, estimates on the incidence and sex ratios of

TABLE 21–5. DSM-IV diagnostic criteria for kleptomania

A. Recurrent failure to resist impulses to steal objects that are not needed for personal use or for their monetary value.

B. Increasing sense of tension immediately before committing the theft.

C. Pleasure, gratification, or relief at the time of committing the theft.

D. The stealing is not committed to express anger or vengeance and is not in response to a delusion or a hallucination.

E. The stealing is not better accounted for by conduct disorder, a manic episode, or antisocial personality disorder.

kleptomania vary widely. Among shoplifters (Table 21–6), the incidence of kleptomania has been estimated as "no clear entity exists" (Gibbens and Prince 1962), 3.8% (Arieff and Bowie 1947), 8% (Medlicott 1968), and less than 5% (American Psychiatric Association 1994b). In a review, Goldman (1991), noting that "kleptomania may account for a substantial portion of the staggering $40 billion in business losses attributed to shoplifting each year" (p. 986), estimated that the rate of kleptomania is at least 6 per 1,000 persons. Cupchik (1992), however, questioned the validity of Goldman 's statements.

Goldman (1991), on the basis of his review, concluded that the typical individual with kleptomania is a 35-year-old woman who began to steal when she was 20 years old. In a study by Bradford and Balmaceda (1983), a 1:1 male-to-female ratio among shoplifters was found; however, more females (62%) than males (38%) were sent for pretrial psychiatric evaluation, which would skew the data. In a study by McElroy et al. (1991a), 15 (75%) of 20 individuals who met DSM-III-R criteria for kleptomania were female. The peak frequency of stealing was 27 episodes per month (range, 0.3–120 episodes), the mean age was 36 years (range, 21–48 years), and the mean duration of illness was 16 years (range, 3–38 years).

ETIOLOGY

Hypotheses about the cause of kleptomania are legion and little agreement exists.[2] In a detailed discussion of the anal-

---

[2] Hypotheses to explain the stealing behavior in kleptomania are that such behavior is an antidepressant, compensation for an actual or anticipated loss, an act for intrapsychic profit, a fetishistic behavior, a sexual act, a symptom of an underlying conflict, a behavior related to depression, a defense, a neurotic conflict, a form of psychopathy, or an OCD-related disorder (Goldman 1991). Kleptomanic behavior can also result from brain disease, mania, or medications.

TABLE 21-6. Frequency of kleptomania among shoplifters

Study	N	Clinical features
Arieff and Bowie (1947)	338	93% female; 70% some psychiatric disorder; sample 1.8% of total group of shoplifters arrested during the time period of study; kleptomania only in 3.8% of total sample
Gibbens and Prince (1962)	776	69% female; depression common; higher than average psychiatric hospital admission; 0% kleptomanic
Ordway (1964)	85	43% depressed (DSM-I); unknown % kleptomanic
Cameron (1964)	873	Only females in the study; 1.4% depressed; < 1% kleptomanic
Medlicott (1968)	50	52% female; 28% depressed (all female); all had some psychiatric disorder; 8% kleptomanic
Gillen (1976)	48	100% females; 100% psychiatric disorder; < 5% kleptomanic
Bradford and Balmaceda (1983)	50	62% female; 42% depressed; 4% kleptomanic
Cupchik and Atcheson (1983)	24	71% female; unknown % kleptomanic
Silverman and Brener (1988)	34	100% female; unknown % kleptomanic; shoplifters were compared with agoraphobic, depressive subjects; shoplifters had high levels of psychosocial stress (e.g., marital discord)

yses of three males with kleptomania, Wilhelm Stekel (1924) noted: "All three are dominated by the Oedipus complex—which is certainly far from an accident. All presented a tremendous sexual energy which may be released, as kinetic energy, temporarily, in cleptomaniac deeds" (p. 122). Fenichel (1945) pointed out that the unconscious formula for kleptomania is "If you don't give it to me, I'll take it" (p. 370).

Bradford and Balmaceda (1983) found an association between shoplifting (not kleptomania) and psychosocial stress: 78% of shoplifters had a mild to moderate psychosocial stressor on DSM-III Axis IV, and an additional 14% had a severe level of stress. McElroy et al. (1991a) found that none of the 20 persons with kleptomania whom they studied developed stealing behavior as a result of stressful or traumatic events.

Gibbens (1981) commented on the motivation behind kleptomanic behavior:

The motive is often obscure, and the objects stolen useless or very trivial, but most often it seems to be a sudden impulse to give themselves a treat, like a child stealing for lack of love; to punish others by punishing themselves; hysterical secondary gain; or, in the newly poor, to keep up appearances. (p. 347)

Stealing is occasionally a presenting feature of brain disease (Wood and Garralda 1990) or a response to medications. McIntyre and Emsley (1990) described the case of an individual who "impulsively" stole inexpensive cosmetics and who was found to have normal-pressure hydrocephalus. Khan and Martin (1977) described a man who stole as a presenting feature of presenile dementia, and Mendez (1988) discussed the case of a 66-year-old man who compulsively stole as a presenting feature of multi-infarct dementia. Coid (1984) reported on the case of a 54-year-old woman who apparently sought relief of her withdrawal symptoms from diazepam through stealing.

McElroy et al. (1991a) found that all 20 of her patients who met the DSM-III-R diagnostic criteria for kleptomania had either a current diagnosis (65%) or a lifetime history (100%) of depression. Also, a particularly high association with bipolar disorder was noted (35%). In addition, 17 (85%) met criteria during their lifetime for at least four or more other psychiatric disorders, including psychoactive substance use disorders (50%), anxiety disorders (80%), eating disorders (60%), and other impulse control disorders (60%). First-degree relatives of these 20 patients were found to have major mood disorders (22 of 103, or 21%), substance abuse (21 of 103, or 20%), or anxiety disorders (13 of 103, or 13%), such as OCD (7 of 103, or 7%) (McElroy et al. 1995).

TREATMENT/COURSE AND PROGNOSIS

Literature reviews of kleptomania report no systematic studies of individuals with rigorously diagnosed kleptomania (American Psychiatric Association 1994b; Goldman 1991; McElroy et al. 1991a, 1995). The secretive nature of the disorder also complicates systematic study. In addition, as noted in the foregoing discussion, many case reports and studies fail to distinguish adequately between shoplifting and kleptomania. Without systematic studies and careful differentiation of kleptomania from shoplifting, little useful information exists about treatment, course, or prognosis of individuals with kleptomania. Available information on treatment is limited to a number of case reports that use a broad range of therapeutic interventions.

The psychoanalytic view suggests that kleptomania is a symptom of an underlying conflict (Goldman 1991). Unfortunately, because systematic studies are lacking, the success of psychoanalytic treatment of kleptomania is unknown. In one example, Fishbain (1987) reported the cure of a patient with kleptomania using a combination of insight-oriented and supportive psychotherapy, as well as antidepressant medication.

There are a number of reports of the use of behavior therapy to treat kleptomania. Glover (1985) described the successful use of covert sensitization in the treatment of this disorder. Guidry (1975) and Wetzel (1966) described single case reports using covert punishing contingency and behavioral modification, respectively. Also, Marzagao (1972) reported success using systematic desensitization to reduce the anxiety that had prompted the stealing behavior of a patient with kleptomania.

Somatic therapies are credited with partial or full remission of kleptomanic symptoms. For example, McElroy et al. (1991a) cited several reports of electroconvulsive therapy (ECT) alone, or ECT in combination with antidepressants, decreasing kleptomanic behavior. Burstein (1992) reported remission of kleptomanic behavior in one patient treated with a combination of fluoxetine and lithium. Kmetz et al. (1997) reported the case of a 36-year-old woman whose mixed mania and stealing behavior markedly worsened when she was taking fluoxetine and completely resolved with valproate.

McElroy's group is responsible for much of the recent work on pharmacotherapeutic interventions in kleptomania. McElroy and associates suggested that kleptomania is part of a group of disorders called *affective spectrum disorders*. Included in this category are OCD, eating disorders, and major mood disorders. These disorders are hypothesized to represent a spectrum of behaviors that occur secondary to abnormalities in the serotonergic system. Consequently, much of the research on affective spectrum disorders focuses on treatment using antidepressants that modulate serotonergic activity. For example, McElroy et al. (1989) reported a complete or partial decrease in kleptomania in three patients with bulimia treated with a serotonergic antidepressant (either trazodone or fluoxetine). In another study, McElroy et al. (1991c), reported that 10 (56%) of 18 patients with kleptomania had a partial or complete remission of stealing behavior as a result of treatment with antidepressants.

Future research on kleptomania must differentiate individuals who shoplift from patients who have kleptomania. It must also focus on associated clinical characteristics, such as OCD, eating disorders, and major mood disorders. This will allow for the scientific evaluation of various treatments and help delineate the course and prognosis of kleptomania (American Psychiatric Association 1994b).

PYROMANIA

DEFINITION AND DIAGNOSTIC CRITERIA

Pyromania has been described as "motiveless arson" (Koson and Dvoskin 1982). This description would imply that if no motivation can be determined, pyromania exists. The problem with this diagnostic approach is that arsonists often do not admit motivation, or even the crime itself. To do so would be to admit guilt. This has led to misclassification of arsonists as persons with pyromania and contaminates much of the data on pyromania. Geller (1987) cautioned that "pathologic fire setting needs to be viewed not as pathognomonic of pyromania but as a symptom, present in a range of psychiatric disorders, that must be addressed clinically" (p. 501).

In a literature review on pyromania written by Geller for the DSM-IV Sourcebook (American Psychiatric Association 1994b), there was found to be "a small frequency of pyromania in reported cases of fire setting since 1970 and no cases reported in the literature from the United States since 1970" (Table 21–7). Because there is little new literature on pyromania, few changes were made in DSM-IV to the DSM-III-R diagnostic criteria for pyromania. The additions to DSM-IV state that pyromania is not diagnosed if fire setting occurs only during a manic episode or if fire setting is better accounted for by a conduct disorder or an antisocial personality disorder (Table 21–8).

Geller noted that the individual with pyromania may make considerable advanced preparation before setting the fire, be an avid fire watcher, set off false fire alarms, be interested in fire-fighting paraphernalia, and even seek work as a firefighter (American Psychiatric Association 1994b).

TABLE 21-7. Frequency of pyromania in adult fire setters

Dates	Cases of fire setting	Cases of pyromania	Percentage of fire setters diagnosed with pyromania
1840–1919	22	3–4	14–18%
1920–1959	1,496	781	52
1960–1969	169	42	25
1970–1979	161	0	0
1980–1989	932	27[a]	3

[a]Contains 2 cases from Canada and 25 cases from Finland. The number of cases from Finland (Virkkunen) may be less if individuals were reported in more than one article.

TABLE 21-8. DSM-IV diagnostic criteria for pyromania

A. Deliberate and purposeful fire setting on more than one occasion.

B. Tension or affective arousal before the act.

C. Fascination with, interest in, curiosity about, or attraction to fire and its situational contexts (e.g., paraphernalia, uses, consequences).

D. Pleasure, gratification, or relief when setting fires or when witnessing or participating in their aftermath.

E. The fire setting is not done for monetary gain, as an expression of sociopolitical ideology, to conceal criminal activity, to express anger or vengeance, to improve one's living circumstances, in response to a delusion or hallucination, or as a result of impaired judgment (e.g., in dementia, mental retardation, substance intoxication).

F. The fire setting is not better accounted for by *conduct disorder*, a *manic episode*, or *antisocial personality disorder*.

Note. Italics indicate changes from DSM-III-R criteria.

EPIDEMIOLOGY

The diagnosis of pyromania is rarely made when DSM-III or DSM-III-R criteria are applied; the diagnosis is much more readily given in studies of arsonists in which no clear diagnostic criteria are used. Therefore, one cannot be sure whether individuals with pyromania are adequately differentiated in the literature from persons who exhibit other types of fire-setting behavior or arson behavior. This flaw brings into question the characteristics often associated with pyromania.

The classic monograph *Pathological Fire Setting (Pyromania)* by Lewis and Yarnell (1951) is the largest study of this topic. Lewis and Yarnell collected cases from a wide variety of sources, including approximately 2,000 records from the National Board of Fire Underwriters. Additional cases were provided through fire departments, psychiatric clinics and institutions, and police departments in the vicinity of New York City. A detailed survey of 1,145 adult male cases was made. (Even with intense efforts, these authors were able to find only 120 records of adult female fire setters.) The peak incidence of fire setting occurred at age 17. Table 21–9 contains a summary of motivations found in the 1,145 cases of fire setting. Concerning the individuals with pyromania (39% of the selected sample), Lewis and Yarnell noted: "Many of them offered the excuse of finding themselves controlled by the 'irresistible impulse' and, though their stories implied a mixture of all the above motives, they more often denied such motives, and for this reason we have allowed them to remain loosely classified as pyromaniacs" (p. 32). Of the 1,145 cases, 48% were classified as "morons" or "imbeciles," 22% as having borderline to dull normal intelligence, and 13% as having between dull and low average intelligence. Only 17% of the entire group were rated as having average to superior intelligence.

Other studies indicate that the clinical phenomenon of pyromania is more rare than was found in Lewis and Yarnell's samples. Robbins and Robbins (1967) reported that 23% of 239 convicted arsonists were identified as persons with pyromania; Koson and Dvoskin (1982) reported that no cases (0%) of pyromania were found during the pretrial evaluation of 26 arsonists. Bradford (1982) found only 1 individual (3% of sample) who "had some features of this phenomenon" in 34 pretrial arson evaluations. In two studies of fire setting among psychiatric patients at Northampton State Hospital (Geller 1984; Geller and Bertsch 1985), only 1 patient with pyromania (2%) was found among a total of 45 fire setters.

Whereas pyromania is a rare disorder, fire-setting behavior among adults and children with other psychiatric disorders is not (Kolko and Kazdin 1992). In a study of psychiatric patients in a state hospital, 26% had a history of fire-setting behaviors and 16% had actually set fires

TABLE 21–9. Survey of motivation in 1,145 fire setters

Motivation	% of sample
Pyromania	39
Revenge/jealous resentment	23
Psychosis	13
Volunteer firefighters or fire "buffs"	9
Tramps/migrant workers	7
"Would-be heroes"	6
Associated with burglary	3

Source. Data derived from Lewis and Yarnell (1951).

(Geller and Bertsch 1985). Preliminary data on another chronic mentally ill population showed a lifetime prevalence rate of 30% in fire-setting behaviors.

In DSM-III, a number of features are associated with pyromania. These include alcohol intoxication, psychosexual dysfunction, lower-than-average IQ, chronic personal frustrations, resentment of authority figures, and the occurrence of sexual arousal secondary to fires. Whether these features are associated with pyromania per se or represent a general characteristic of arsonists/fire setters remains a question for further study. Neither DSM-III-R nor DSM-IV lists any features associated with pyromania.

ETIOLOGY

Fire symbolizes many things, from the "fires of Hell" to "fiery passion." The diverse symbolism of fire is represented in the psychoanalytic interpretations of pyromania. Wilhelm Stekel (1924), in his discussion of 95 cases and a case report of an analysis of a patient with pyromania, emphasized that "awakening and ungratified sexuality impels the individual to seek a symbolic solution to his conflict between instinct and reality" (p. 126). Sigmund Freud (1932[1931]/1964) considered fire setting a masturbatory equivalent with homosexual features. He noted that "in order to gain control over fire, men had to renounce the homosexually tinged desire to put it out with a stream of urine" (p. 187). He further noted that "the warmth that is radiated by fire calls up the same sensation that accompanies a state of sexual excitation, and the shape and movement of a flame suggest a phallus in activity" (p. 190). Fenichel (1945) discussed pyromania as a specific form of urethral-erotic fixation and emphasized the sadistic and destructive symbolism of fire. Later writers, such as Lewis and Yarnell (1951), stressed that revenge is an important underlying motive for pyromania. Geller (1987) suggested that fire setting as a symptom can best be understood as a

communication from an individual with few social skills.

Research (Virkkunen 1984; Virkkunen et al. 1987, 1994) raises questions about whether the behavior of arson is associated with reactive hypoglycemia and/or lower concentration of 3-methoxy-4-hydroxyphenylglycol (MHPG) and 5-HIAA in CSF. Virkkunen et al. (1987) noted that their results "support the hypothesis that poor impulse control in criminal offenders is associated with low levels of certain CSF monoamine metabolites and with a hypoglycemic tendency" (p. 241). A small subgroup of subjects with pyromania in this study (3 of 20 arsonists) had the lowest blood glucose nadirs among the arsonists. In addition, impulse fire setters who are violent offenders are often alcoholic and have a father who is alcoholic (Linnoila et al. 1989).

TREATMENT

Most writers on the treatment of pyromania approach the patients from a psychoanalytic perspective (Macht and Mack 1968; Stekel 1924). Mavromatis and Lion (1977) pointed out that "treatment for fire setters has been traditionally problematic due to the frequent refusal to take responsibility for the act, the use of denial, the existence of alcoholism, and the lack of insight" (p. 955).

Most behavioral researchers have used aversive therapy to treat fire setters (McGrath and Marshall 1979), although others have used positive reinforcement with threats of punishment, stimulus satiation, and operant structured fantasies with positive reinforcement (Bumpass et al. 1983). Bumpass et al. (1983) treated 29 child fire setters and used a graphing technique that sequentially correlated external stress, behavior, and feeling on graph paper. These authors reported that after treatment (average follow-up of 2.5 years), only 2 of the 29 children subsequently set fires. Milrod and Urion (1992) reported the cases of three boys with abnormal EEG results who were fire setters; the patients improved with anticonvulsant therapy.

COURSE AND PROGNOSIS

The pyromanic impulse to set fires is episodic and often self-limited and frequently appears during a developmental or situational crisis. Fire setting associated with mental retardation, alcoholism, or a ritualistic pattern indicates a poor prognosis. A better prognosis exists if the patient can verbalize and work through frustrations in therapy. Studies indicate that the recidivism rate for fire setters ranges from 4.5% (Mavromatis and Lion 1977) to 28% (Lewis and Yarnell 1951).

PATHOLOGICAL GAMBLING

DEFINITION AND DIAGNOSTIC CRITERIA

Gambling is now legal in some form in 48 of 50 states and in more than 90 countries. The amount of money spent gambling legally has increased from $17 billion in 1974 to $482 billion in 1995, and consequently the likelihood that clinicians will encounter individuals who have this disorder has increased (Lesieur and Rosenthal 1990; Westphal and Rush 1996).

The diagnostic criteria for pathological gambling in DSM-IV (Table 21–10) incorporate features from the criteria found in DSM-III and DSM-III-R. In general, the criteria for pathological gambling are similar to the criteria for psychoactive substance abuse disorders. Freud was one of the first to recognize this similarity, which prompted him to categorize pathological gambling as an addiction along with alcoholism and drug dependence (Lesieur and Rosenthal 1990).

TABLE 21–10. DSM-IV diagnostic criteria for pathological gambling

A. Persistent and recurrent maladaptive gambling behavior as indicated by five (or more) of the following:

(1) is preoccupied with gambling (e.g., preoccupied with reliving past gambling experiences, handicapping or planning the next venture, or thinking of ways to get money with which to gamble)

(2) needs to gamble with increasing amounts of money in order to achieve the desired excitement

(3) has repeated unsuccessful efforts to control, cut back, or stop gambling

(4) is restless or irritable when attempting to cut down or stop gambling

(5) gambles as a way of escaping from problems or of relieving a dysphoric mood (e.g., feelings of helplessness, guilt, anxiety, depression)

(6) after losing money gambling, often returns another day to get even ("chasing" one's losses)

(7) lies to family members, therapist, or others to conceal the extent of involvement with gambling

(8) has committed illegal acts such as forgery, fraud, theft, or embezzlement to finance gambling

(9) has jeopardized or lost a significant relationship, job, or educational or career opportunity because of gambling

(10) relies on others to provide money to relieve a desperate financial situation caused by gambling

B. The gambling behavior is not better accounted for by a manic episode.

CLINICAL FEATURES

Edmond Bergler (1957), a psychoanalyst who treated more than 60 compulsive gamblers, characterized the compulsive gambler as a risk taker who fails to profit from his gambling misadventures. The compulsive gambler is often described as fiercely competitive, highly independent, individualistic, overconfident, and profoundly optimistic. He resents the intrusion of authority figures into his life, just as he resented his parents' intrusions during his childhood. The compulsive gambler is likely to marry and provide reasonably well for his family before his gambling losses precipitate a financial crisis. Contrary to what one might suspect, the compulsive gambler is extremely knowledgeable about the technical aspects of gambling and his skills are impressive, particularly when he is winning. It is when he is "chasing" his losses by larger and larger wagers that he disregards his technical knowledge. The compulsive gambler rarely seeks psychiatric help on his own but is generally forced into consultation.

Speculation about the personality structure of a pathological gambler deserves comment. Comparison of the pathological gambler's premorbid personality with the "premorbid" personality of an individual with alcoholism seems appropriate, especially because the two disorders are so often linked. George Vaillant's (1980) prospective research on the personality of the alcoholic individual showed that this person does not have a premorbid oral, passive, dependent personality. Rather, when the person with alcoholism drinks excessively and continuously, these traits emerge as a secondary rather than a primary phenomenon. The same may be true of the pathological gambler.

The clinical features of a pathological gambler are listed in Table 21–11. The individual is progressively preoccupied with gambling, spends more time gambling and needs higher bets to experience excitement, experiences

---

TABLE 21–11. Clinical features of pathological gambling

Progressive gambling

Development of *tolerance*

Symptoms on discontinuation (*withdrawal*)

Gambling as *escape* from dysphoria

Chasing of losses

Lies/deception

Illegal acts

Family/job disruption

Financial *bailout*

Inability to stop (*loss of control*)

withdrawal symptoms if gambling is abruptly discontinued, may use gambling to forget or avoid dysphoric mood states, wagers larger and larger amounts to win back losses (called *chasing*), creates family and job disruption by telling lies to sustain gambling and performing illegal acts to pay debts, requests and often receives financial help (a bailout) from family and/or friends to pay off debts and to sustain gambling, and attempts unsuccessfully to cut back on or stop gambling. Westphal and Rush (1996) found that pathological gamblers wagered from 14% to 45% of their monthly income.

EPIDEMIOLOGY

Dickerson (1984) estimated that 1% of men are pathological gamblers, an estimate that is consistent with data obtained by Volberg and Steadman (1988); in DSM-IV, the prevalence is estimated as being 2%–3% of the adult population. States that provide increased opportunity for legal gambling have higher rates (DeCaria et al. 1996). The rate among psychiatric inpatients is higher and goes largely unrecognized. Lesieur and Blume (1990) found that 6.7% of patients admitted to an adult general psychiatry ward were pathological gamblers. Prevalence rates among alcohol- and substance-abusing individuals are estimated to be from 8% to 33% (Daghestani et al. 1996; Lesieur and Rosenthal 1990). It is likely that equal numbers of men and women gamble, but the vast majority of compulsive gamblers are men. The membership of Gamblers Anonymous ranges from 1% to 2% women in the United Kingdom to 5% to 10% women in Australia. Pathological gambling and alcoholism are more common in the fathers of males with the disorder and in the mothers of females with the disorder.

ETIOLOGY

Numerous theories have been invoked to explain the origin of pathological gambling, including unconscious motivations, behavioral anomalies, the presence of an affective disorder, addiction, and biological abnormalities. Hollander et al. (1992, 1995) reiterated the idea that pathological gambling might be an obsessive-compulsive spectrum disorder. Lesieur and Blume (1993) conceptualized pathological gambling as an addictive disease comparable to alcoholism, McElroy et al. (1996) hypothesized that impulsivity and bipolarity (or mania) are related, and Sharpe and Tarrier (1993) advanced a cognitive-behavioral theory of problem gambling. Any one explanation seems insufficient to explain the heterogeneous nature of this patient population.

Bergler (1957) believed that the compulsive gambler's illogical, senseless certainty that he will win stems from a childhood sense of omnipotence. His unconscious aggression against the reality principle leads to an unconscious need for punishment. The punishment, achieved through losing, becomes essential for psychic equilibrium. H. R. Greenberg (1980) reviewed the psychodynamic formulations of other analysts, including the analogies between gambling, childhood play, and masturbation; the classification of compulsive gamblers as compulsive neurotic individuals with latent homosexual tendencies; and a variant of *Schicksal* (fate) neurosis in which the person surrenders responsibility for his actions to an omnipotent force, such as Lady Luck.

Gambling is also an activity that is reinforced by both the cash that one may win and the many exciting stimuli associated with the process. The validity of this hypothesis to explain pathological gambling is challenged by the observation that individuals have losing streaks that last for months. The compulsive gambler will continue gambling regardless of the losses. He appears desperate and oblivious to the rest of the world as he "chases" his losses.

Platelet monoamine oxidase (MAO) activity is a peripheral index of serotonin function; low platelet MAO activity has been linked to impulsivity (Blanco et al. 1996; Carrasco et al. 1994). Pathological gamblers have been found to have low platelet MAO activity (Blanco et al. 1996; Carrasco et al. 1994). Many studies (Lesieur and Rosenthal 1990; Linden et al. 1986; McCormick et al. 1984) have reported an extremely high incidence of affective disorders among pathological gamblers. McCormick et al. (1984) examined 25 compulsive gamblers and found a 72% incidence of major depression around the time they stopped gambling. Linden et al. (1986) reported that 76% of 50 compulsive gamblers had a major depressive disorder. These authors also found that 32% of the subjects had first-degree relatives with major affective disorders, and 36% had at least one first-degree relative who abused alcohol or had alcohol dependence. Gambling may also be an antidepressant, protecting the gambler from dysphoria and depression. The analogy can be drawn between the manic and depressive cycles of a patient with bipolar disorder and the frenetic, high-energy mood of a winning gambler versus the desperate low of the losing gambler.

There are many interesting similarities between substance abuse, particularly alcoholism, and compulsive gambling. In both disorders, dependencies are developed that exclude basic human needs such as sleep, food, and sex. The insidious downward trajectory of both disorders leads to loss of family, friends, and position. Custer (1982) noted that compulsive gamblers who abruptly stop gambling during a hospital admission are frequently tremulous and experience headaches, abdominal pain, diarrhea, nightmares, and cold sweats. Blaszczynski et al. (1986) found that a subgroup of gamblers had lower baseline β-endorphin levels. Roy and co-workers (1988) found evidence of elevated noradrenergic function in pathological gamblers and, in a later study (Roy et al. 1989), noted that elevation in noradrenergic function was correlated with personality extraversion. The pathological gambler's EEG activation patterns to right and left brain tasks are similar to patterns found in alcoholic adults and unmedicated children diagnosed as having attention-deficit disorder (ADD). Goldstein et al. (1985) noted that "both pathological gambling and alcoholism may be related to dysfunctional attention mechanisms and, more to the point, to the deficits in impulse control that characterize ADD" (p. 1233). The course of a recovering substance abuser and that of a compulsive gambler are very much alike in that relapses are common and occur at times of increased stress. Abstinence is thought by many to be an essential part in the recovery from both disorders. The mainstay of treatment, Gamblers Anonymous, is patterned after Alcoholics Anonymous.

TREATMENT

A number of diverse treatments for compulsive gambling have been reported (Legg England and Götestam 1991). These include psychoanalysis, behavior therapy, cognitive therapy, medications, and ECT. There are no controlled studies that compare these treatment modalities. Regardless of the choice of therapy, the pathway to recovery is likely to be fraught with difficulties. Relapses are common, as are missed sessions. During treatment, financial crises may occur (some clinicians experienced in treating compulsive gamblers recommend collecting the fee before each session!), and legal sequelae of gambling may arise.

The high incidence of major affective disorders among pathological gamblers leads one to question the relationship between these disorders. The dearth of articles on somatic treatments of compulsive gamblers leaves this question unanswered. Moskowitz (1980) did report improvement in three compulsive gamblers who were taking lithium carbonate. Hollander et al. (1992), in a double-blind, placebo-controlled trial with clomipramine, reported a successful response in one treatment-resistant case. Wong and Hollander (1996), in a preliminary report, stated that four (66%) of six patients were much or very much improved when taking fluvoxamine at doses between 100 and 300 mg/day. In some gamblers the affective disorder may promote the gambling, whereas in other gamblers it seems likely that the depletion of resources (e.g., emo-

tional, family, friends, financial) is responsible for the affective state of the gambler when he enters treatment. There may be a subgroup of compulsive gamblers who remain depressed in spite of abstinence. In a follow-up study of gamblers who continued abstinence 6 months after inpatient treatment, 18% reported "significant improvement in work and family life . . . but still were significantly depressed" (Taber et al. 1987, p. 761).

Behavioral treatments, particularly aversive therapy, have been used to treat compulsive gamblers. However, review of the literature on aversive treatments reveals disappointing results. McConaghy et al. (1983) compared aversive therapy with imaginal desensitization and found the latter more effective. Dickerson (1984) noted that there is "a trend away from the use of single limited procedures such as aversion therapy toward a multimodal approach" (p. 113). Greenberg and Rankin (1982) reported on the behavioral treatment of 25 compulsive gamblers. After treatment, 5 (20%) had their gambling "well under control," 7 (28%) alternated between periods of control and periods of gambling, and 14 (56%) were gambling when last followed up. Bujold et al. (1994) reported successful treatment of three pathological gamblers using a combination of cognitive interventions, problem solving, and relapse prevention.

Bolen and Boyd (1968) stated that psychoanalysis was the treatment of choice for the compulsive gambler. In Bergler's (1957) collection of 60 individual case reports, 15 patients (25%) discontinued treatment in the first 6 weeks; of those who underwent treatment, 33 (55%) received an analysis of their neurosis, and 30 (50%) were judged to be cured.

Custer (1982) recommended that the compulsive gambler be admitted to an inpatient psychiatric treatment center, particularly when there is a risk of suicide, emotional decompensation, or exhaustion. The initial assessment must include the compulsive gambler's areas of high risk: marital problems, large debts, demands or threats from creditors, loss of employment, legal problems, and isolation from friends and relatives. The treatment plan is then designed to treat problems identified during the intake process. In addition, Custer recommended group therapy with other compulsive gamblers and involvement of the compulsive gambler with Gamblers Anonymous.

Gamblers Anonymous and its sister groups Gam-Anon (for families and spouses of compulsive gamblers) and Gam-a-Teen (for adolescent children of compulsive gamblers) are important resources for treatment. The only requirement for membership in Gamblers Anonymous is an expressed desire to stop gambling. Unfortunately, retrospective studies have found that overall dropout rates range from 75% to 90% and the abstinence rate at 1-year follow-up was 8% (DeCaria et al. 1996).

COURSE AND PROGNOSIS

The clinical course of compulsive gambling is outlined in Figure 21–1. The compulsive gambler's early history often involves winning and periods of considerable profits. Once the gambler falls behind, he is unable to cut his losses. Instead, he increases his wagers and begins to chase his losses on long shots. This leads to a tightening spiral of involvements and fewer options (Lesieur 1979). In a study of 50 compulsive gamblers, Lesieur (1979) noted that all 50 participated in some activity such as pool, golf, and bowling hustling; bookmaking; obtaining loans from friends, loan sharks, or loan companies; "borrowing" from personal checking accounts and from work; and committing petty larceny. Seventeen (34%) participated in check forgery, burglary, fencing stolen goods, stealing company checks, or swindling.

The prognosis of the untreated compulsive gambler is unknown. Few creditable data exist about the prognosis of the treated pathological gambler. The follow-up study by Taber et al. (1987) of 66 male veterans 6 months after the completion of a 28-day inpatient program indicated that 56% were totally abstinent. Outcome in this study was found to correlate with attendance at Gamblers Anonymous meetings. It does seem clear that keeping the compulsive gambler engaged in any form of therapy is very difficult. In our opinion, data currently available on the long-term prognosis of alcoholism might come close to predicting the outcome of pathological gambling.

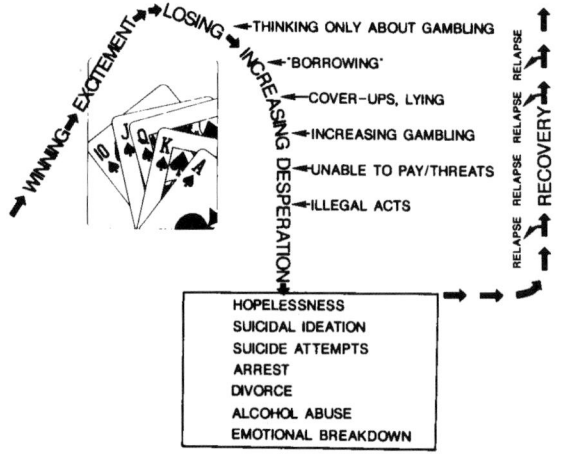

FIGURE 21–1.   The clinical course of a pathological gambler.

TRICHOTILLOMANIA

DEFINITION AND DIAGNOSTIC CRITERIA

Trichotillomania is a term created by Hallopeau in 1889 (Krishnan et al. 1985) to describe a compulsion to pull out one's own hair. Trichotillomania was not listed in DSM-III but was added to DSM-III-R because "this well- recognized disorder involving the pulling out of hair fulfills the general criteria for the Impulse Control Disorders" (American Psychiatric Association 1987, p. 427). Although there has been more recent research on trichotillomania than on most of the other disorders in this chapter, insufficient information was available at the time DSM-IV was developed to warrant significant changes to the DSM-III-R diagnostic criteria (Table 21–12). A significant number of individuals do not fulfill Criterion B, increased tension immediately before hair pulling (Christenson and Crow 1996), and gratification or relief after pulling the hair (Criterion C) is not always present.

Trichotillomania produces irregular, nonscarring focal patches of hair loss that are linear, rectangular, or oval (Figure 21–2). Hair loss usually occurs in the scalp region but can involve eyebrows, eyelashes, or pubic hair. These areas of hair loss are more likely to be found on the opposite side of the body from the dominant hand. Within the area of hair loss, broken hairs of varying lengths are found, and the scalp may have a slight brownish discoloration secondary to rubbing the area. Two clinical findings can help with the diagnosis. In trichotillomania, the patient should not have changes in fingernails or toenails (except possibly signs of nail biting) usually associated with dermatological conditions. Second, hair regrowth follows the application of collodion to the area of hair loss for 1 week.

TABLE 21–12.   DSM-IV diagnostic criteria for trichotillomania

A. Recurrent pulling out of one's hair resulting in noticeable hair loss.

B. An increasing sense of tension immediately before pulling out the hair or when attempting to resist the behavior.

C. Pleasure, gratification, or relief when pulling out the hair.

D. The disturbance is not better accounted for by another mental disorder and is not due to a general medical condition (e.g., a dermatological condition).

E. The disturbance causes clinically significant distress or impairment in social, occupational, or other important areas of functioning.

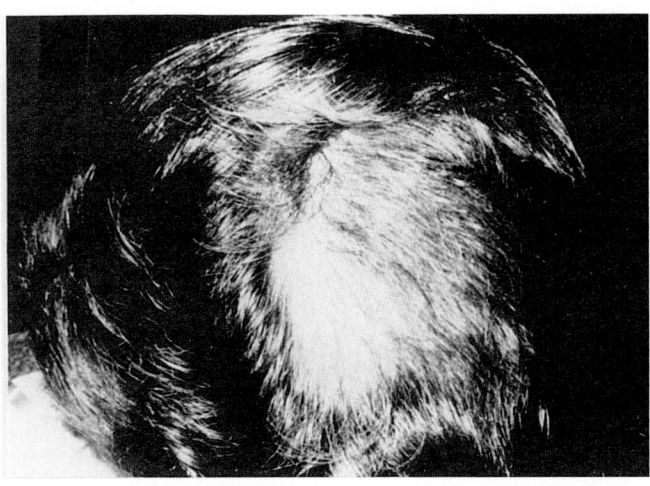

Figure 21-2. Trichotillomania. Note the irregular pattern of hair loss, the hair of varying lengths within the patch of hair loss, and the scalp, which has no evidence of scarring.

Parents may resist the suggestion that a child is pulling out his or her own hair. In these cases, a biopsy is diagnostic and provides evidence for the doubting parents. Careful parental observation of the child, which includes looking for hair among the child's playthings, is often helpful in making the diagnosis. The child may also practice onychophagy (i.e., nail biting). If the child complains of gastrointestinal symptoms such as abdominal pain, diarrhea and/or constipation, or decreased appetite, examination of the oral cavity for evidence of trichophagy (i.e., hair biting) and X-ray examination of the stomach for a trichobezoar (i.e., hairball) are warranted.

EPIDEMIOLOGY

The frequency of trichotillomania in the adult population is unknown, but most literature suggests that it is rare. The literature also suggests that females have the disorder much more frequently than do males. However, Christenson et al. (1991b), in a questionnaire survey of 2,579 first-year college students, concluded that trichotillomania may not be as rare as previously suspected and that males may be affected as frequently as females. Prevalence ranged between 0.6% and 1.5% for males and between 0.6% and 3.4% for females.

Christenson et al. (1991a) reported on the characteristics of 60 adult hair pullers. The mean age at onset was 13 years, and 93% of the subjects were female. Hair was pulled primarily from the scalp (67%); however, subjects also pulled eyelashes (22%), eyebrows (8%), facial hair (2%), and pubic hair (2%). Subjects in this study were just as likely to use the nondominant as the dominant hand for

hair pulling. All subjects believed that their hair pulling was an excessive or unusual behavior, and 95% reported a diurnal variation, with the worst hair pulling in the evening. The comorbidity with other psychiatric disorders was striking (Table 21–13).

The dermatological literature most commonly reports pathological hair pulling in preadolescent children. For example, Stroud (1983), a dermatologist, reviewed diagnoses of all patients who came to his office with hair loss. During 1982, 59 children under the age of 13 came to his office with hair loss. Of these 59 children, 31 (53%) had tinea capitis (i.e., a fungal infection), 12 (20%) had alopecia areata (i.e., a suspected autoimmune phenomenon), 7 (11%) had traction alopecia (i.e., a disorder associated with hairstyles that apply excessive prolonged tension to the hair), and 6 (10%) had trichotillomania. In another report of trichotillomania in children, Oranje et al. (1986) found that the female-to-male ratio was 2.5:1 and also that 25% of the children with trichotillomania had associated onychophagy, trichophagy, or automutilation. A small sample of 10 children with trichotillomania was systematically evaluated by Reeve et al. (1992), who found that hair pulling was not always a benign habit and was frequently associated with anxiety and affective disorders.

ETIOLOGY

From a psychoanalytic perspective, hair may have many possible symbolic meanings. According to Krishnan et al. (1985), hair can represent beauty, virility, sexual conflicts, physical prowess, and sexuality; haircutting or plucking

Table 21–13. Lifetime prevalence of psychiatric disorders in a population of 60 chronic hair pullers

Diagnosis	% of sample
Trichotillomania	83[a]
Mood disorders	65
Psychotic disorders	2
Anxiety disorders	57
Eating	20
Substance abuse	22
No disorder (except trichotillomania)	18

[a]Not all individuals had both an increasing sense of tension before pulling the hair and gratification, or a relief after pulling out the hair (both are required in DSM-IV).
Source. Modified and reprinted with permission from Christenson GA, Mackenzie TB, Mitchell JE: "Characteristics of 60 Adult Chronic Hair Pullers." *American Journal of Psychiatry* 158:365–370, 1991a. Copyright 1991, American Psychiatric Association.

can signify castration. Oguchi and Miura (1977) believed that when trichotillomania occurs in a child, the hair pulling is a manifestation of mild frustration and is analogous to nail biting. In children, the syndrome usually develops at a time of psychosocial stress (Oranje et al. 1986), such as when there is a disturbed mother-child relationship, hospitalization, or family stress associated with raising a mentally retarded child. These authors believed that the hair pulling can develop into a habit even though the stressor(s) may no longer be present.

Stroud (1983) pointed out that "trichotillomania in adolescents and adults may indicate a more serious psychological problem and require psychiatric help" (p. 648). Krishnan et al. (1985) noted that trichotillomania can be present as a major symptom in OCD, mental retardation, schizophrenia, borderline personality disorder, and depression. Some authors have even questioned the validity of trichotillomania as a unique diagnostic entity (Dean et al. 1992; Werry 1990).

Some literature suggests that trichotillomania may be a type of OCD (Jenike 1989; Swedo et al. 1989). Stanley et al. (1992, 1993), however, reported a number of differences between OCD and trichotillomania, including the facts that hair pulling is usually associated with pleasure, patients with trichotillomania have few associated obsessive-compulsive symptoms, and patients with OCD differ from patients with trichotillomania in terms of anxiety, depression, and personality characteristics. In addition, findings from regional cerebral blood flow studies of women with trichotillomania appear different from those of women with OCD (Christenson and Crow 1996; Swedo et al. 1991). Blunting of neuroendocrine response to meta-chlorophenylpiperazine (m-CPP), a measure of serotonin responsivity sometimes present in patients with OCD, was not found in 10 patients with trichotillomania (Stein et al. 1995). In addition, Ninan et al. (1992) did not find abnormalities in CSF cortisol, 5-HIAA, homovanillic acid (HVA), or MHPG levels in patients with trichotillomania but did find that baseline CSF 5-HIAA levels correlated with response to treatment with SSRI-type antidepressants. In a single case report (Graae et al. 1992), a 13-year-old girl's OCD responded to fluoxetine and to clomipramine, but her trichotillomania responded minimally to each medication.

TREATMENT

According to Dean et al. (1992), "treatment modalities reported to be successful in ameliorating pathologic hair-pulling include a large part of the armamentarium of psychiatry and clinical psychology" (p. 89). Consequently, there is no specific treatment for trichotillomania; rather, psychoanalytic, behavioral, or pharmacological treatment may each potentially decrease hair pulling.

Swedo et al. (1989) found that clomipramine was significantly more effective than desipramine in a double-blind crossover treatment of trichotillomania. This study has been criticized for selection bias toward OCD patients, because 9 of 20 subjects were self-referred to the study after a television advertisement on OCD (Dean et al. 1992). Christenson et al. (1991d), in another placebo-controlled, double-blind crossover study, reported the response of 21 patients with chronic hair pulling to fluoxetine. In this 6-week trial, fluoxetine was no better than placebo. In a 16-week open-label trial of fluoxetine, Winchel et al. (1992) reported that 8 of 12 patients treated had a meaningful decrease in hair pulling. Streichenwein and Thornby (1995), in a placebo-controlled, double-blind crossover trial, found that fluoxetine was not effective in the 23 chronic hair pullers. Christenson et al. (1991c) reported success in an open trial using lithium carbonate; 8 of 10 patients taking lithium had mild to moderate improvement. Stein and Hollander (1992) found that augmentation of serotonergic agents with pimozide (a dopamine blocker) led to improvement in 6 of 7 patients, and Stein et al. (1997) found that 4 of 5 patients with trichotillomania improved when risperidone (1 mg/day) was added to a serotonin reuptake inhibitor. Keuthen et al. (1998), in a retrospective review of 63 patients with trichotillomania, found that "state-of-the-art behavioral and pharmacological treatments offer substantial clinical benefits" (p. 560).

Isolated case reports of successful treatment of trichotillomania have been published discussing the use of medications (paroxetine [Reid 1994]; buspirone [Reid 1992]; chlorpromazine, in a schizophrenic individual; amitriptyline; a monoamine oxidase inhibitor [MAOI]), hypnosis (with and without other treatments), and numerous behavior modification techniques (Krishnan et al. 1985). Behavior therapy for trichotillomania is different from that for OCD; a technique called *habit reversal* is reportedly the most effective (Baer 1992). Occasional cases of successful treatment with hypnosis have been reported (Christenson and Crow 1996).

COURSE AND PROGNOSIS

According to Stroud (1983), most cases of trichotillomania in young children resolve spontaneously. In younger children, trichotillomania usually represents a transient behavior in response to a psychosocial stressor, or it may represent a habit, without the presence of an obvious precipitant. However, if hair loss persists, psychiatric consultation is indicated, and inquiry into areas of parent- child relationships or other areas of potential conflict may illuminate the problem. Oranje et al. (1986), in their study of 21 children under the age of 15, found that psychiatric consultation was necessary in 11 cases (52%); 4 of these consultees (19%) required psychiatric intervention. Sullivan (1989) raised two issues with regard to patients with trichotillomania: the possibility of trichophagia (i.e., hair eating) leading to the complication of a trichobezoar, and the rare possibility that iron deficiency may cause the hair pulling/eating behavior.

Psychiatric evaluation is indicated when trichotillomania occurs in adolescents and adults. Trichotillomania in adults, as Christenson et al. (1991a) noted, "follows a chronic course, frequently involves multiple hair sites, and is associated with high rates of psychiatric comorbidity" (p. 370).

IMPULSE CONTROL DISORDER NOT OTHERWISE SPECIFIED

The DSM-IV criteria for ICDNOS are essentially unchanged from those for DSM-III-R; therefore, the diagnosis of ICDNOS remains a residual category for impulse control disorders that do not meet the criteria for other impulse control disorders discussed in this chapter.

The Impulse Control Disorders Committee of the DSM-IV Task Force reviewed diagnoses such as amok, pathological spending, pathological shopping, and self-mutilation disorder for listings as examples of impulse control disorders in DSM-IV. The Task Force determined that insufficient scientific data existed to support including any of these conditions as examples of an ICDNOS diagnosis. Since the publication of DSM-IV, the terms *compulsive buying* (Black 1996; Christenson et al. 1994; McElroy et al. 1994) and *uncontrolled buying* (Lejoyeux et al. 1996) have appeared in the literature and diagnostic criteria for this disorder have been proposed (McElroy et al. 1994).

CONCLUSIONS

The disorders that are considered impulse control disorders not elsewhere classified represent a diverse array, including intermittent explosive disorder, kleptomania, pathological gambling, pyromania, trichotillomania, and impulse control disorder not otherwise specified. The disorders in this diagnostic category, when diagnosed using DSM criteria, are rare, with the exception of pathological gambling. For example, in the United States literature during the last 20 years, no new cases of pyromania were reported. The limited number of available cases hampers research and gathering of information on the epidemiology, treatment, course, and prognosis of these disorders, as well as refinement of diagnostic criteria.

Promising research is under way, especially on the relationship between serotonin, selective serotonin reuptake inhibitors, and impulsivity. This research may help clarify this diagnostic category, as well as answer questions regarding whether the impulse control disorders not elsewhere classified are part of an affective spectrum that includes disorders such as OCD, eating disorders, and major mood disorders.

REFERENCES

American Psychiatric Association: Diagnostic and Statistical Manual: Mental Disorders. Washington, DC, American Psychiatric Association, 1952

American Psychiatric Association: Diagnostic and Statistical Manual of Mental Disorders, 2nd Edition. Washington, DC, American Psychiatric Association, 1968

American Psychiatric Association: Diagnostic and Statistical Manual of Mental Disorders, 3rd Edition. Washington, DC, American Psychiatric Association, 1980

American Psychiatric Association: Diagnostic and Statistical Manual of Mental Disorders, 3rd Edition, Revised. Washington, DC, American Psychiatric Association, 1987

American Psychiatric Association: Diagnostic and Statistical Manual of Mental Disorders, 4th Edition. Washington, DC, American Psychiatric Association, 1994a

American Psychiatric Association: DSM-IV Sourcebook, Vol 2. Washington, DC, American Psychiatric Association, 1994b

Arieff AJ, Bowie CG: Some psychiatric aspects of shoplifting. Journal of Clinical Psychopathology 8:565–576, 1947

Baer L: Behavior therapy for obsessive-compulsive disorder and trichotillomania, in Advances in Neurology. Edited by Chase TN, Friedhoff AJ, Cohen DJ. New York, Raven, 1992, pp 333–340

Bergler E: The Psychology of Gambling. New York, International Universities Press, 1957

Black DW: Compulsive buying: a review. J Clin Psychiatry 57:50–55, 1996

Blanco C, Orensanz-Munoz L, Blanco-Jerez C, et al: Pathological gambling and platelet MAO activity: a psychobiological study. Am J Psychiatry 153:119–121, 1996

Blaszczynski AP, Winter SW, McConaghy N: Plasma endorphin levels in pathologic gambling. Journal of Gambling Behavior 2:3–14, 1986

Bolen DW, Boyd WG: Gambling and the gambler: a review and preliminary findings. Arch Gen Psychiatry 18:617–630, 1968

Bradford J: Arson: a clinical study. Can J Psychiatry 27:188–193, 1982

Bradford J, Balmaceda R: Shoplifting: is there a specific psychiatric syndrome? Can J Psychiatry 28:248–254, 1983

Bujold A, Ladouceur R, Sylvain C, et al: Treatment of pathological gamblers: an experimental study. J Behav Ther Exp Psychiatry 25:275–282, 1994

Bumpass ER, Fagelman FD, Brix RJ: Intervention with children who set fires. Am J Psychother 37:328–345, 1983

Burstein A: Fluoxetine-lithium treatment for kleptomania (letter). J Clin Psychiatry 53:28–29, 1992

Cameron MB: Department Store Shoplifting: The Booster and the Snitch. London, Free Press of Glencoe/Collier-Macmillan, 1964

Campbell M, Perry R, Green WH, et al: Use of lithium in children and adolescents. Psychosomatics 25:95–101, 105–106, 1984

Carrasco JL, Sai-Ruiz J, Hollander E, et al: Low platelet monoamine oxidase activity in pathological gambling. Acta Psychiatr Scand 90:427–431, 1994

Christenson GA, Crow SJ: The characterization and treatment of trichotillomania. J Clin Psychiatry 57:42–49, 1996

Christenson GA, Mackenzie TB, Mitchell JE: Characteristics of 60 adult chronic hair pullers. Am J Psychiatry 148:365–370, 1991a

Christenson GA, Pyle RL, Mitchell JE: Estimated lifetime prevalence of trichotillomania in college students. J Clin Psychiatry 52:415–417, 1991b

Christenson GA, Popkin MK, Mackenzie TB, et al: Lithium treatment of chronic hair pulling. J Clin Psychiatry 52:116–120, 1991c

Christenson GA, Mackenzie TB, Mitchell JE, et al: A placebo-controlled, double-blind crossover study of fluoxetine in trichotillomania. Am J Psychiatry 148:1566–1571, 1991d

Christenson GA, Faber RJ, deZwann M, et al: Compulsive buying: descriptive characteristics and psychiatric comorbidity. J Clin Psychiatry 55:5–11, 1994

Coid J: Relief of diazepam-withdrawal syndrome by shoplifting. Br J Psychiatry 145:552–554, 1984

Cupchik W: Kleptomania and shoplifting (letter). Am J Psychiatry 149:1119, 1992

Cupchik W, Atcheson JD: Shoplifting: an occasional crime of the moral majority. Bull Am Acad Psychiatry Law 11:343–354, 1983

Custer RL: An overview of compulsive gambling, in Addictive Disorders Update: Alcoholism, Drug Abuse, Gambling. Edited by Carone PA, Yolles SF, Kieffer SN, et al. New York, Human Sciences Press, 1982, pp 107–124

Daghestani AN, Elenz E, Crayton JW: Pathological gambling in hospitalized substance abusing veterans. J Clin Psychiatry 57:360–363, 1996

Dean JT, Nelson E, Moss L: Pathologic hair-pulling: a review of the literature and case reports. Compr Psychiatry 33:84–91, 1992

DeCaria CM, Hollander E, Grossman R, et al: Diagnosis, neurobiology, and treatment of pathological gambling. J Clin Psychiatry 57:80–84, 1996

Dickerson MG: Compulsive Gambling. New York, Longman Group Ltd, 1984

Eichelman B: Aggressive behavior: from laboratory to clinic. Quo vadit? Arch Gen Psychiatry 49:488–492, 1992

Elliott FA: Propranolol for the control of belligerent behavior following acute brain damage. Ann Neurol 1:489–491, 1977

Elliott FA: Neurology of aggression and episodic dyscontrol. Semin Neurol 10:303–311, 1990

Fava M: Psychopharmacologic treatment of pathologic aggression, in The Psychiatric Clinics of North America. Edited by Fava M. Philadelphia, WB Saunders, 1997

Felthous AR, Bryant SG, Wingerter CB, et al: The diagnosis of intermittent explosive disorder in violent men. Bull Am Acad Psychiatry Law 19:71–79, 1991

Fenichel O: The Psychoanalytic Theory of Neurosis. New York, WW Norton, 1945

Fishbain DA: Kleptomania as risk-taking behavior in response to depression. Am J Psychother 41:598–603, 1987

Freud S: The acquisition and control of fire (1932[1931]), in Standard Edition of the Complete Psychological Works of Sigmund Freud, Figure 22. Translated and edited by Strachey J. London, Hogarth Press, 1964, pp 181–193

Geller J[L]: Arson: an unforeseen sequela of deinstitutionalization. Am J Psychiatry 141:504–508, 1984

Geller JL: Firesetting in the adult psychiatric population. Hospital and Community Psychiatry 38:501–506, 1987

Geller JL, Bertsch G: Fire-setting behavior in the histories of a state hospital population. Am J Psychiatry 142:464–468, 1985

Gibbens TCN: Shoplifting. Br J Psychiatry 138:346–347, 1981

Gibbens TCN, Prince J: Shoplifting. London, Institute for the Study and Treatment of Delinquency, 1962

Gillen RS: A study of woman shoplifters. South Australian Clinics 11:173–176, 1976

Glover JH: A case of kleptomania treated by covert sensitization. Br J Clin Psychol 24:213–214, 1985

Goldman MJ: Kleptomania: making sense of the nonsensical. Am J Psychiatry 148:986–996, 1991

Goldstein L, Manowitz P, Nora R, et al: Differential EEG activation and pathological gambling. Biol Psychiatry 20:1232–1234, 1985

Graae F, Gitow A, Piacentini J, et al: Response of obsessive-compulsive disorder and trichotillomania to serotonin reuptake blockers (letter). Am J Psychiatry 149:149–150, 1992

Greenberg D, Rankin H: Compulsive gamblers in treatment. Br J Psychiatry 140:364–366, 1982

Greenberg HR: Psychology of gambling, in Comprehensive Textbook of Psychiatry/III, 3rd Edition, Figure 3. Edited by Kaplan HI, Freedman AM, Sadock BJ. Baltimore, MD, Williams & Wilkins, 1980, pp 3274–3283

Guidry LS: Use of a covert punishing contingency in compulsive stealing. J Behav Ther Exp Psychiatry 6:169, 1975

Hollander E, Wong CM: Body dysmorphic disorder, pathological gambling, and sexual compulsions. J Clin Psychiatry 56:7–12, 1995

Hollander E, Frenkel M, DeCaria C, et al: Treatment of pathological gambling with clomipramine (letter). Am J Psychiatry 149:710–711, 1992

Hollander E, Kwon JH, Stein DJ, et al: Obsessive-compulsive and spectrum disorders: overview and quality of life issues. J Clin Psychiatry 57:3–6, 1996

Jenike MA: Obsessive-compulsive and related disorders (editorial). N Engl J Med 321:539–541, 1989

Kafka MP, Coleman E: Serotonin and paraphilias: the convergence of mood, impulse, and compulsive disorders (editorial). J Clin Psychopharmacol 11:223–224, 1991

Kavoussi R, Armstead P, Coccaro E: The neurobiology of impulsive aggression, in The Psychiatric Clinics of North America. Edited by Fava M. Philadelphia, WB Saunders, 1997

Keuthen NJ, O'Sullivan RL, Goodchild P, et al: Retrospective review of treatment outcome for 63 patients with trichotillomania. Am J Psychiatry 155:560–561, 1998

Khan K, Martin ICA: Kleptomania as a presenting feature of cortical atrophy. Acta Psychiatr Scand 56:168–172, 1977

Kmetz GF, McElroy SL, Collins DJ: Response of kleptomania and mixed mania to valproate (letter). Am J Psychiatry 154:580–581, 1997

Kolko DJ, Kazdin AE: The emergence and recurrence of child firesetting: a one-year prospective study. J Abnorm Child Psychol 20:17–37, 1992

Koson DF, Dvoskin J: Arson: a diagnostic study. Bull Am Acad Psychiatry Law 10:39–49, 1982

Krishnan KRR, Davidson JRT, Guajardo C: Trichotillomania—a review. Compr Psychiatry 26: 123–128, 1985

Kruesi MJP, Hibbs ED, Zahn TP, et al: A 2-year prospective follow-up study of children and adolescents with disruptive behavior disorders: prediction by cerebrospinal fluid 5-hydroxyindoleacetic acid, homovanillic acid, and autonomic measures? Arch Gen Psychiatry 49:429–435, 1992

Legg England S, Götestam KG: The nature and treatment of excessive gambling. Acta Psychiatr Scand 84:113–120, 1991

Lejoyeux M, Ades J, Tassain V, et al: Phenomenology and psychopathology of uncontrolled buying. Am J Psychiatry 153:1524–1529, 1996

Lesieur HR: The compulsive gambler's spiral of options and involvement. Psychiatry 42:79–87, 1979

Lesieur HR, Blume SB: Characteristics of pathological gamblers identified among patients on a psychiatric admissions service. Hospital and Community Psychiatry 41: 1009–1012, 1990

Lesieur HR, Blume SB: Pathological gambling, eating disorders, and the psychoactive substance use disorder, in Comorbidity of Addictive and Psychiatric Disorders. Edited by Miller NS, Stimmel B. Binghamton, NY, Haworth, 1993

Lesieur HR, Rosenthal RJ: Pathological gambling, a review of the literature prepared for DSM-IV Work Group on Disorders of Impulse Control Not Elsewhere Classified. Washington, DC, American Psychiatric Association, 1990

Lewis NDC, Yarnell H: Pathological Firesetting (Pyromania) (Nervous and Mental Disease Monogr 82). New York, Coolidge Foundation, 1951

Linden RD, Pope HG Jr, Jonas JM: Pathological gambling and major affective disorder: preliminary findings. J Clin Psychiatry 47:201–203, 1986

Linnoila M, De Jong J, Virkkunen M: Family history of alcoholism in violent offenders and impulsive fire setters. Arch Gen Psychiatry 46:613–616, 1989

Macht LB, Mack JE: The firesetter syndrome. Psychiatry 31:277–288, 1968

Mark V, Ervin F: Violence and the Brain. New York, Harper & Row, 1970

Marzagao LR: Systematic desensitization treatment of kleptomania. J Behav Ther Exp Psychiatry 3:327–328, 1972

Mattes JA: Psychopharmacology of temper outbursts: a review. J Nerv Ment Dis 174:464–470, 1986

Mattes JA: Comparative effectiveness of carbamazepine and propranolol for rage outbursts. J Neuropsychiatry Clin Neurosci 2:159–164, 1990

Mattes JA, Rosenberg J, Mays D: Carbamazepine versus propranolol in patients with uncontrolled rage outbursts: a random assignment study. Psychopharmacol Bull 20: 98–100, 1984

Mavromatis M, Lion JR: A primer on pyromania. Diseases of the Nervous System 38:954–955, 1977

McConaghy N, Armstrong MS, Blaszczynski A, et al: Controlled comparison of aversive therapy and imaginal desensitization in compulsive gambling. Br J Psychiatry 142: 366–372, 1983

McCormick RA, Russo AM, Ramirez LF, et al: Affective disorders among pathological gamblers seeking treatment. Am J Psychiatry 141:215–218, 1984

McElroy SL, Keck PE Jr, Pope HG Jr, et al: Pharmacological treatment of kleptomania and bulimia nervosa. J Clin Psychopharmacol 9:358–360, 1989

McElroy SL, Pope HG Jr, Hudson JI, et al: Kleptomania: a report of 20 cases. Am J Psychiatry 148:652–657, 1991a

McElroy SL, Hudson JI, Pope HG Jr, et al: Kleptomania: clinical characteristics and associated psychopathology. Psychol Med 21:93–108, 1991b

McElroy SL, Satlin A, Pope HG Jr, et al: Treatment of compulsive shopping with antidepressants: a report of three cases. Ann Clin Psychiatry 3:199–204, 1991c

McElroy SL, Hudson JI, Pope HG Jr, et al: The DSM-III-R impulse control disorders not elsewhere classified: clinical characteristics and relationship to other psychiatric disorders. Am J Psychiatry 149:318–327, 1992

McElroy SL, Keck PE, Pope HG, et al: Compulsive buying: a report of 20 cases. J Clin Psychiatry 55:242–248, 1994

McElroy SL, Keck PE, Phillips KA: Kleptomania, compulsive buying, and binge-eating disorder. J Clin Psychiatry 56:14–26, 1995

McElroy SL, Pope HG Jr, Keck PE, et al: Are impulse-control disorders related to bipolar disorder? Compr Psychiatry 37:229–240, 1996

McElroy SL, Soutullo CA, Beckman DA, et al: DSM-IV Intermittent Explosive Disorder: a report of 27 cases. J Clin Psychiatry 59:203–210, 1998

McGrath P, Marshall PG: A comprehensive treatment program for a fire setting child. J Behav Ther Exp Psychiatry 10:69–72, 1979

McIntyre AW, Emsley RA: Shoplifting associated with normal-pressure hydrocephalus: report of a case. J Geriatr Psychiatry Neurol 3:229–230, 1990

Medlicott RW: Fifty thieves. N Z Med J 67:183–188, 1968

Mendez MJ: Pathological stealing in dementia. J Am Geriatr Soc 36:825–826, 1988

Menninger KA: The Vital Balance. New York, Viking, 1963

Menninger KA, Mayman M: Episodic dyscontrol: a third order of stress adaptation. Bull Menninger Clin 20:153–165, 1956

Milrod LW, Urion DK: Juvenile fire setting and the photoparoxysmal response. Ann Neurol 32:222–223, 1992

Monopolis S, Lion JR: Problems in the diagnosis of intermittent explosive disorder. Am J Psychiatry 140:1200–1202, 1983

Monroe RR: Episodic Behavioral Disorders. Cambridge, MA, Harvard University Press, 1970

Moskowitz JA: Lithium and Lady Luck. New York State Journal of Medicine 80:785–788, 1980

Ninan PT, Rothbaum BO, Stipetic M, et al: Assessment update: trichotillomania. CSF 5-HIAA as a predictor of treatment response in trichotillomania. Psychopharmacol Bull 28:451–455, 1992

Oguchi T, Miura S: Trichotillomania: its psychopathological aspect. Compr Psychiatry 18:177–182, 1977

Oranje AP, Pureboom-Wynia JDR, De Raeymaechec CMJ: Trichotillomania in childhood. J Am Acad Dermatol 16:614–619, 1986

Ordway JA: "Successful" court treatment of shoplifters. Journal of Criminal Law, Criminology and Political Science 53:344–347, 1964

Reeve EA, Bernstein GA, Christenson GA: Clinical characteristics and psychiatric comorbidity in children with trichotillomania. J Am Acad Child Adolesc Psychiatry 31:132–138, 1992

Reid TL: Treatment of generalized anxiety disorder and trichotillomania with buspirone (letter). Am J Psychiatry 149:573–574, 1992

Reid TL: Treatment of resistant trichotillomania with paroxetine (letter). Am J Psychiatry 151:290, 1994

Robbins E, Robbins L: Arson, with special reference to pyromania. New York State Journal of Medicine 67:795–798, 1967

Roy A, Adinoff B, Roehrich L, et al: Pathological gambling: a psychobiological study. Arch Gen Psychiatry 45:369–373, 1988

Roy A, De Jong J, Linnoila M: Extraversion in pathological gamblers correlates with indexes of noradrenergic function. Arch Gen Psychiatry 46:679–681, 1989

Sharpe L, Tarrier N: Towards a cognitive-behavioural theory of problem gambling. Br J Psychiatry 162:407–412, 1993

Sheard MH: Clinical pharmacology of aggressive behavior. Clin Neuropharmacol 11:483–492, 1988

Sheard MH, Marini JL, Bridges CI, et al: The effect of lithium on impulsive aggressive behavior in man. Am J Psychiatry 133:1409–1413, 1976

Silverman G, Brener N: Psychiatric profile of shoplifters (letter). Lancet 2:157, 1988

Stanley MA, Swann AC, Bowers TC, et al: A comparison of clinical features in trichotillomania and obsessive-compulsive disorder. Behav Res Ther 30:39–44, 1992

Stanley MA, Prather RC, Wagner AL, et al: Can the Yale-Brown obsessive compulsive scale be used to assess trichotillomania? A preliminary report. Behav Res Ther 31:171–177, 1993

Stein DJ, Hollander E: Low-dose pimozide augmentation of serotonin reuptake blockers in the treatment of trichotillomania. J Clin Psychiatry 53:123–126, 1992

Stein DJ, Hollander E, Cohen L, et al: Serotonergic responsivity in trichotillomania: neuroendocrine effects of m-chlorophenylpiperazine. Biol Psychiatry 37:414–416, 1995

Stein DJ, Bouwer C, Hawkridge S, et al: Risperidone augmentation of serotonin reuptake inhibitors in obsessive-compulsive and related disorders. J Clin Psychiatry 58:119–122, 1997

Stekel W: Peculiarities of Behavior: Wandering Mania, Dipsomania, Cleptomania, Pyromania and Allied Impulsive Acts, Figure 2. New York, Liveright, 1924

Stone JL, McDaniel KD, Hughes JR, et al: Episodic dyscontrol disorder and paroxysmal EEG abnormalities: successful treatment with carbamazepine. Biol Psychiatry 21:208–212, 1986

Streichenwein SM, Thornby JI: A long-term, double-blind, placebo-controlled crossover trial of the efficacy of fluoxetine for trichotillomania. Am J Psychiatry 152:1192–1196, 1995

Stroud JD: Hair loss in children. Pediatr Clin North Am 30: 641–657, 1983

Sullivan C: Trichotillomania (letter). Br J Psychiatry 155:869, 1989

Swedo SE, Leonard HL, Rapoport JL, et al: A double-blind comparison of clomipramine and desipramine in the treatment of trichotillomania (hair pulling). N Engl J Med 321: 497–501, 1989

Swedo SE, Rapoport JL, Leonard HL, et al: Regional cerebral glucose metabolism of women with trichotillomania. Arch Gen Psychiatry 48:828–833, 1991

Taber JI, McCormick RA, Russo AM, et al: Follow-up of pathological gamblers after treatment. Am J Psychiatry 144: 757–761, 1987

Tardiff K: The current state of psychiatry in the treatment of violent patients. Arch Gen Psychiatry 49:493–499, 1992

Vaillant GE: Natural history of male psychological health, VIII: antecedents of alcoholism and "orality." Am J Psychiatry 137:181–186, 1980

Virkkunen M: Reactive hypoglycemia tendency among arsonists. Acta Psychiatr Scand 69:445–452, 1984

Virkkunen M, Nuutila A, Goodwin FK, et al: Cerebrospinal fluid monoamine metabolite levels in male arsonists. Arch Gen Psychiatry 44:241–247, 1987

Virkkunen M, De Jong J, Bartko J, et al: Psychobiological concomitants of history of suicide attempts among violent offenders and impulsive fire setters. Arch Gen Psychiatry 46:604–606, 1989

Virkkunen M, Rawlings R, Takola R, et al: CSF biochemistries, glucose metabolism, and diurnal activity rhythms in alcoholic, violent offenders, fire setters, and healthy volunteers. Arch Gen Psychiatry 51:20–27, 1994

Virkkunen M, Eggert M, Rawlings R, et al: A prospective follow-up study of alcoholic violent offenders and fire setters. Arch Gen Psychiatry 53:523–529, 1996

Volberg RA, Steadman HJ: Refining prevalence estimates of pathological gambling. Am J Psychiatry 145:502–505, 1988

Werry JS: Trichotillomania—taxonomic issues. Literature review prepared for the DSM-IV Task Force Childhood Disorders Committee. Washington, DC, American Psychiatric Association, 1990

Westphal JR, Rush J: Pathological gambling in Louisiana: an epidemiological perspective. J La State Med Soc 148: 353–358, 1996

Wetzel R: Use of behavior techniques in a case of compulsive stealing. J Consult Psychol 30:367–374, 1966

Williams DT, Mehl R, Yudofsky S, et al: The effect of propranolol on uncontrolled rage outbursts in children and adolescents with organic brain dysfunction. J Am Acad Child Psychiatry 21:129–135, 1982

Winchel RM, Jones JS, Stanley B, et al: Clinical characteristics of trichotillomania and its response to fluoxetine. J Clin Psychiatry 53:304–308, 1992

Wong CM, Hollander E: New dimensions in the OCD spectrum: autism, pathological gambling, and compulsive buying. CNS Spectrums 1:44–53, 1996

Wood A, Garralda ME: Kleptomania in a 13-year old boy: a sequel of a 'lethargic' encephalitic/depressive process? Br J Psychiatry 157:770–772, 1990

World Health Organization: International Classification of Diseases, 9th Revision, Clinical Modification. Ann Arbor, MI, Commission on Professional and Hospital Activities, 1978

Yudofsky SC, Williams D, Gorman J: Propranolol in the treatment of rage and violent behavior in patients with chronic brain syndromes. Am J Psychiatry 138:218–220, 1981

CHAPTER 22

PERSONALITY DISORDERS

KATHARINE A. PHILLIPS, M.D.
JOHN G. GUNDERSON, M.D.

All clinicians frequently encounter patients with personality disorders. These patients are commonly seen in a variety of treatment settings, both inpatient and outpatient. Studies indicate that 30%–50% of outpatients have a personality disorder (Koenigsberg et al. 1985) and that 15% of inpatients are hospitalized primarily for problems caused by a personality disorder; as many as half of the remaining inpatients have a comorbid personality disorder (Loranger 1990) that significantly affects their response to treatment. It has also been estimated that personality disorders are relatively common in the general population, the prevalence being between 10% and 13% (Lenzenweger et al. 1997; Weissman 1993).

Patients with personality disorders present with problems that are among the most complex and challenging that clinicians encounter. Some patients intensely desire relationships but fearfully avoid them because they anticipate rejection; others seek endless admiration and are engrossed with grandiose fantasies of limitless power, brilliance, or ideal love. Still others have a self-concept so disturbed that they feel they embody evil or do not exist. This complexity is amplified by the fact that these and other personality disorder characteristics are not simply a problem the person has but are in fact central to who the person is.

Personality disorders, according to DSM-IV (American Psychiatric Association 1994), are patterns of inflexible and maladaptive personality traits that cause subjective distress, significant impairment in social or occupational functioning, or both. These traits must also deviate markedly from the culturally expected and accepted range, or *norm*, and this deviation must be manifested in more than one of the following areas: cognition, affectivity, control over impulses and need gratification, and ways of relating to others. In addition, the deviation must have been stably present and enduring since adolescence or early adulthood, and it must be pervasive—that is, it must manifest itself across a broad range of situations, rather than in only one specific triggering situation or in response to a particular stimulus.

Although useful, this definition has its ambiguities and limitations. It can be difficult, for example, to determine whether personality traits are inflexible or to differentiate deviance from the norm or sickness from health. Whether dependence on others, compulsive work habits, or passive resistance to demands is considered excessive or problematic depends to some extent on the personal, social, and cultural context in which each occurs.

Nonetheless, it is important that clinicians attempt to recognize personality disorders in their patients. First, personality disorders do, by definition, cause significant problems for those who have them. Persons with these disorders often suffer, and their relationships with others are problematic. They have difficulty responding flexibly and adaptively to the environment and to the changes and demands of life, and they lack resilience when under stress. Instead, their usual ways of responding tend to perpetuate and intensify their difficulties. However, these individuals are often oblivious to the fact that their personality causes them problems, and they may instead blame others for their difficulties or even deny that they have any problems at all.

Personality disorders also often cause problems for others and are costly to society. Individuals with personality disorders frequently have considerable difficulty in their family, academic, occupational, and other roles. They have elevated rates of separation, divorce, child custody proceedings, unemployment, homelessness (Caton et al. 1994), and perpetration of child abuse (Dinwiddie and Bucholz 1993). They also have increased rates of accidents (McDonald and Davey 1996); emergency department visits; medical hospitalization (J. [H.] Reich et al. 1989); violence, including homicide (Miller et al. 1993; Raine 1993); self-injurious behavior (Hillbrand et al. 1994); attempted suicide; and completed suicide (Brent et al. 1994; Hawton et al. 1993). A high percentage of criminals (70%–85% in some studies) (Jordan et al. 1996), 60%–70% of alcoholic individuals, and 70%–90% of persons who abuse drugs have a personality disorder.

Finally, personality disorders need to be identified because of their treatment implications. These disorders often need to be a focus of treatment or, at the very least, need to be taken into account when comorbid Axis I disorders are treated, because their presence often affects an Axis I disorder's prognosis and treatment response. For example, patients with depressive disorders (Black et al. 1988; Nelson et al. 1994), bipolar disorder (Calabrese et al. 1993), panic disorder (J. H. Reich 1988), obsessive-compulsive disorder (Jenike et al. 1986), and substance abuse (Fals-Stewart 1992) often respond less well to pharmacotherapy when they have a comorbid personality disorder. In addition, as most clinicians are well aware, the characteristics of patients with personality disorders are likely to be manifested in the treatment relationship, whether or not the personality disorder is the focus of treatment. For example, some patients may be overly dependent on the clinician, others may not follow treatment recommendations, and still others may experience significant conflict about getting well. Although individuals with personality disorders tend to use psychiatric services extensively, they are more likely to be dissatisfied with the treatment they receive (Kelstrup et al. 1993; Kent et al. 1995).

What follows is a clinically oriented overview of the personality disorders and a description of each disorder. These descriptions, although based on clinical tradition, have also been informed by the recent explosion of empirical research on the personality disorders—a development that was facilitated by the placement of these disorders on a separate axis in DSM-III (American Psychiatric Association 1980). This research has focused on many different aspects of these disorders. Their descriptive features, family history, course, and treatment response have been addressed, as has their etiology, including their psychodynamic, biogenetic, and sociocultural roots. This research, which continues, is greatly enhancing our understanding of these complex disorders.

GENERAL CONSIDERATIONS

HISTORY OF PERSONALITY DISORDERS

Personality types and disorders have been described for thousands of years, as evidenced by Hippocrates' description of four temperaments: the pessimistic melancholic, the overly optimistic sanguine, the irritable choleric, and the apathetic phlegmatic. It is interesting that the early Greeks' theory that these temperaments were determined by the relative proportion of the four bodily humors (black bile, blood, yellow bile, and phlegm, respectively) is reflected in current attempts to discover biogenetic bases of personality.

In the early 1800s, psychiatrists such as Pinel, Esquirol, Rush, and Pritchard described socially maladaptive personality types seen in clinical settings. More specific personality types were then described at the turn of the century, when, for example, Janet (1901) and Freud (Breuer and Freud 1893–1895/1957) described the psychological traits associated with hysteria, the forerunner of histrionic personality disorder. Subsequently, within the framework of early psychoanalytic instinct theory, Abraham proposed that arrests at the three psychosexual stages of childhood development—the oral, anal, and phallic phases—led to the development of the dependent, obsessive-compulsive, and hysterical character types, respectively. However, this view changed as early instinct theory and the subsequent ego-psychological model of psychoanalytic theory were gradually supplanted by object relations theory, which proposes that personality is shaped largely by the child's early parental relationships. In this framework, dependent personality traits derive from parental deprivation, obsessive-compulsive traits from control struggles with parental figures, and hysterical traits, in part, from parental seduction and competition. The borderline and narcissistic personality disorder concepts also developed out of the object relations framework.

From a quite different perspective, in the 1920s the German phenomenologists Kraepelin (1921) and Kretschmer (1925) described personality types in terms of the spectrum concept—the theory that personality types are biogenetically related variants of the paranoid and affective psychoses (which would now be considered Axis I disorders). These early spectrum personality types were forerunners of the current paranoid, schizotypal, cyclothymic, and depressive personality disorders. In contrast, Schneider (1958), another German phenomenologist, did not subscribe to the spectrum concept but considered personality disorders to represent socially deviant and extreme variants of normally occurring personality traits. He developed the first comprehensive system of personality disorder categories, which provided the template for many of those contained in the *International Statistical Classification of Diseases and Related Health Problems, 10th Revision* (ICD-10) (World Health Organization 1992) and DSM-IV.

Personality disorders have been included in every version of DSM, but only paranoid, obsessive-compulsive, and antisocial personality disorders have been consistent DSM "members." Some current categories (e.g., borderline) were added to later editions, whereas others (e.g., inadequate) were dropped. The theoretical underpinnings of the DSM personality disorder categories have also changed over the years (Gunderson 1992).

DSM-I, published in 1952 by the American Psychiatric Association, defined personality disorders not as stable and enduring patterns but as traits that malfunction under stressful circumstances, which leads to inflexible and maladaptive behavior. DSM-II (American Psychiatric Association 1968) emphasized that personality disorders involve distress and impairment in functioning, not merely socially deviant behavior.

In DSM-III, several major changes in personality disorder conceptualization and classification were made. There was a shift away from a psychoanalytic orientation and toward an atheoretical, descriptive approach. Specific diagnostic criteria were added, and the personality disorders were placed on a separate axis, which highlighted the importance of their diagnosis.

The changes made in DSM-III-R (American Psychiatric Association 1987) and DSM-IV attempted to increase the validity of the personality disorder categories by incorporating findings from the growing empirical literature. Although current DSM descriptions attempt to represent an optimal synthesis of clinical tradition and research findings, such descriptions are likely to continue to evolve over time as our understanding of these disorders increases.

CLASSIFICATION ISSUES

Since DSM-III, the personality disorders have been grouped into three clusters: the *odd or eccentric cluster* (schizotypal, schizoid, and paranoid); the *dramatic, emotional, or erratic cluster* (borderline, histrionic, narcissistic, and antisocial); and the *anxious or fearful cluster* (avoidant, dependent, and obsessive-compulsive) (Table 22–1). Although these clusters were originally based on face validity alone, they have since received some empirical support (Kass et al. 1985; Zimmerman and Coryell 1989). Nonetheless, these clusters are limited because they are based on descriptive similarities rather than on similarities in etiology or external validators such as family history or treatment response.

TABLE 22–1. **Summary of personality disorder features**

Cluster	Model	Key clinical features	Treatment	Course/prognosis
A				
Odd, eccentric	Spectrum disorders	Social deficits, absence of close relationships	Structure, rehabilitation, support, medication	Stable/poor
B				
Dramatic, emotional, erratic	Self disorders	Social and interpersonal instability	Support, exploration, sociotherapy, individual therapy, medication	Unstable/some remission with age
C				
Anxious, fearful	Dimensional disorders	Interpersonal and intrapsychic conflicts	Exploration, individual therapy, group therapy	Modifiable/good

Another classification issue is whether the personality disorders are best classified as dimensions or categories (Frances 1982; Gunderson et al. 1991b). Do personality disorders exist along dimensions that reflect extreme variants of normal personality, or are they distinct categories that are qualitatively different, and clearly demarcated, from normal personality traits and one another? Each model has its advantages and disadvantages. For example, the *dimensional model*, with its potential use of many personality descriptors and its ability to assess the degree to which traits are present, may more comprehensively cover problematic traits. It does not confine clinicians to the use of a limited number of categories. In addition, most of the traits embodied by Axis II criteria can be found in less extreme form in psychiatrically healthy people. Indeed, one of the frontiers in personality disorder research is the development of types that relate to personality dimensions found in populations that are psychiatrically healthy (Widiger 1991). Of special significance are the widely heralded "Big Five" dimensions of neuroticism, extroversion, openness, agreeableness, and conscientiousness (Costa and McCrae 1990). Cloninger's seven-dimension psychobiological model of temperament and character, which is theoretically linked to abnormalities in specific neurotransmitter systems, is also of great interest and is receiving increasing investigation (Cloninger et al. 1993).

The *categorical model*, however, better reflects how clinicians think—that is, in terms of pathological syndromes that a person either has or does not have. The use of categories also makes it possible for clinicians succinctly to summarize patients' difficulties and facilitates communication about them. Although DSM-IV is based primarily on the categorical model, it also incorporates a dimensional approach to some extent, in that it encourages clinicians to identify problematic personality traits that are subthreshold for any particular diagnosis. Classification models that incorporate both a dimensional and a categorical approach may ultimately prove most useful to clinicians, and several such models have been proposed (Gunderson 1992).

These and other classification issues are currently being debated and researched, and such action may change the future classification of personality disorders. Whatever system is used, it is important that it be useful to clinicians and, ultimately, reflect what is known about the etiology of these disorders.

ASSESSMENT ISSUES AND METHODS

The assessment of Axis II disorders is in some ways more complex than that of Axis I disorders. It can be difficult to assess multiple domains of experience and behavior (i.e.,

cognition, affect, intrapsychic experience, and interpersonal interactions) and to determine that traits are not only distressing, impairing, and of early onset, but also pervasive and enduring. Nonetheless, a personality disorder assessment is essential to the comprehensive evaluation and adequate treatment of all patients. What follows is a discussion of such an assessment and steps that can be taken to avoid commonly encountered problems.

Comprehensiveness of Evaluation

A skilled, psychodynamically informed clinical interview is the mainstay of personality disorder diagnosis and is particularly useful if the clinician is familiar with DSM criteria, takes a longitudinal view, and uses multiple sources of information. However, because an open-ended approach may inadequately cover all Axis II disorders, the additional use of a self-report or semistructured (i.e., interviewer-administered) personality disorder assessment instrument can be useful (Table 22–2). Such instruments systematically assess each personality disorder criterion with the use of standard questions or probes. Although self-report instruments have the advantage of saving interviewer time, they often yield false-positive diagnoses and allow contamination of Axis II traits by Axis I states (Widiger and Frances 1987). Semistructured interviews—which require the interviewer to use certain questions but allow further probing—facilitate accurate diagnosis in several ways: they allow the interviewer to attempt to differentiate Axis II traits from Axis I states, clarify contradictions or ambiguities in the patient's response, and determine that traits are pervasive rather than limited to a specific situation.

Nonetheless, even with the use of a structured interview, the interviewer must often use his or her judgment. For example, is a given trait present in enough situations to be considered pervasive? How much distress or impairment is necessary to consider the criterion present? Is a given characteristic a personality trait or a symptom of an Axis I disorder (i.e., a state)? Another limitation is that agreement among existing instruments is fairly low, and the instruments do not indicate which disorder in any given patient is most severe or should be the focus of treatment.

Syntonicity of Traits

As was noted earlier, because personality disorders to some extent reflect who the person is—and not simply what he or she has—some patients are unaware of the traits that reflect their disorder or may not perceive them as problematic. This limited self-awareness can interfere with personality disorder assessment, especially if the questions

TABLE 22–2. Features of interviews and self-report instruments for the assessment of personality disorders

Interview or instrument	Author	Type	Special features
Structured Interview for DSM-III-R Personality Disorders (SIDP)	Pfohl et al. 1989	Interview	Patient and informant questions
Personality Disorders Examination (PDE)	Loranger 1988	Interview	Detailed instruction manual
Structured Clinical Interview for DSM-III-R Personality Disorders (SCID-II)	Spitzer et al. 1990	Interview	Axis I section; Axis II screening questionnaire
Diagnostic Interview for Personality Disorders (DIPD)	Zanarini et al. 1987	Interview	Good test-retest reliability
Personality Interview Questions–II (PIQ-II)	Widiger 1987	Interview	Nine-point scale for traits and behaviors
Personality Diagnostic Questionnaire— Revised (PDQ-R)	Hyler et al. 1987	Self-report	Face-valid items
Millon Clinical Multiaxial Inventory–II (MCMI-II)	Millon 1987	Self-report	Dimensions of Axis I and Axis II psychopathology
Wisconsin Personality Inventory (Revised) (WPI-R)	M. Klein 1990	Self-report	Integrates structural analysis of social behavior model[a]
Schedule for Normal and Abnormal Personality (SNAP)	Clark 1990	Self-report	Normal and abnormal personality measures
Minnesota Multiphasic Personality Inventory (MMPI) scales for DSM-III personality disorders	Morey et al. 1985	Self-report	Constructed from MMPI item pool

Note. All instruments listed assess the full range of personality disorders. Other instruments are available to assess certain individual personality disorders.
[a]See Benjamin 1974.
Source. Modified from Skodol and Oldham 1991.

asked have negative or unflattering implications. This problem can be minimized by the use of a skilled psychodynamic interview, comprehensive coverage of all personality disorder criteria with a semistructured assessment instrument, and the use of multiple sources of information (e.g., medical records and informants who know the patient well).

State Versus Trait

Another potential problem in personality disorder assessment is that the presence of an Axis I disorder can complicate the assessment of Axis II traits. For example, a person with social withdrawal, low self-esteem, and lack of motivation or energy due to major depression might appear to have avoidant or dependent personality disorder, when in fact these features reflect the Axis I condition. Or a hypomanic person with symptoms of grandiosity or hypersexuality might appear narcissistic or histrionic. In some cases, assessment of Axis II disorders may need to wait until the Axis I condition, such as florid psychosis or mania, has subsided. However, the clinician can often differentiate personality traits from Axis I states during an Axis I episode by asking the patient to describe his or her usual personal-

ity outside Axis I episodes; the use of informants who have observed the patient over time and without an Axis I disorder can be helpful. Prior systematic assessment of Axis I conditions is invaluable in terms of alerting the clinician to which Axis II traits will need particularly careful assessment. This task can be very difficult, however, in patients with certain Axis I conditions that are chronic and of early onset.

Medical Illness Versus Trait

Similarly, the interviewer must ascertain that what appear to be personality traits are not symptoms of a medical illness. For example, aggressive outbursts caused by a seizure disorder should not be attributed to borderline or antisocial personality disorder; nor should the unusual perceptual experiences that can accompany temporal lobe epilepsy be attributed to schizotypal personality disorder. A medical evaluation should be included in a thorough patient assessment.

Situation Versus Trait

The interviewer should also ascertain that personality disorder features are pervasive—that is, not limited to only one situation or occurring in response to only one specific trigger. Similarly, these features should be enduring rather than transient. Asking the patient for behavioral examples of traits can help determine that the trait is indeed present in a wide variety of situations and is expressed in many relationships.

Sex and Cultural Bias

Although most research suggests that existing personality disorder criteria are relatively free of sex bias, interviewers can unknowingly allow such bias to affect their assessments. It is important, for example, that histrionic, borderline, and dependent personality disorders be assessed as carefully in men as in women and that obsessive-compulsive, antisocial, and narcissistic personality disorders be assessed as carefully in women as in men. Interviewers should also be careful to avoid cultural bias when diagnosing personality disorders, especially when evaluating such traits as promiscuity, suspiciousness, or recklessness, which may have different norms in different cultures.

Diagnosing Disorders in Children and Adolescents

Because the personality of children and adolescents is still developing, personality disorders should be diagnosed with care in this age group. It is in fact often preferable to defer these diagnoses until late adolescence or early adulthood, at which time a personality disorder diagnosis may be appropriate if the features appear to be pervasive, stable, and likely to be enduring. The diagnosis, however, may prove to be wrong as any stage-specific difficulties of adolescence resolve and as the person further matures.

ETIOLOGY AND PATHOGENESIS

What causes personality disorders is the most enigmatic and challenging question pertaining to this complex group of disorders. As was described in the section on the history of personality disorders, various hypotheses have been formulated over the years. Although earlier views tended to emphasize the contribution of developmental and environmental factors, such as pathological or inadequate parenting, constitutional or biological factors have also long been postulated to play an important role in the etiology of personality disorders.

As is the case with other psychiatric disorders, the answer is not likely to be simple. It is unlikely that any personality disorder has a single cause, whether environmental (e.g., childhood abuse) or biological (e.g., a gene). Rather, available data suggest that personality disorders (as well as

normal personality traits) result from a complex combination of, and interaction between, temperament (genetic and other biological factors) and psychological (developmental or environmental) factors (Paris 1993). Although the degree to which genetic and environmental factors contribute to etiology appears to vary for different personality disorders, these factors appear to be important to all of these disorders. For example, family, twin, and adoption studies provide compelling evidence that antisocial personality disorder has a significant genetic component and that schizotypal personality disorder also has a substantial degree of heritability and is genetically linked to schizophrenia. On the other hand, although there is some evidence for a genetic component to borderline personality disorder, the impact of environment (i.e., developmental experiences) appears to be more important. The etiology and pathophysiology of the cluster C disorders have undergone little investigation. Of relevance, however, are studies indicating that approximately half the observed variance in personality traits such as neuroticism, introversion, and submissiveness can be traced to genetic variation (Carey and DiLalla 1994).

Investigation of the underlying neurobiology of these disorders is rapidly increasing. A growing body of evidence supports the importance of various neurobiological abnormalities in persons with schizotypal personality disorder; alterations in brain structure and function have been shown to be related to deficitlike symptoms and increased dopaminergic function to psychoticlike symptoms. Abnormalities in the serotonin system, which appears to mediate behavioral inhibition, have been found in individuals with borderline and antisocial personality disorders. The recent finding, which requires replication, that the amount of neuroticism is influenced by two alleles of a gene encoding a transporter for serotonin (Lesch et al. 1996) is an example of the groundbreaking work being done in this important area.

Increasing numbers of studies of environmental antecedents of personality disorders, such as family environment and sexual and physical abuse, are substantiating a likely role for such factors in the development of certain disorders (e.g., borderline personality disorder). In addition, defense mechanisms appear to play an important role in the expression of personality disorders, which are characterized by less mature defense mechanisms such as projection and acting out (Vaillant 1994). Research in these areas is expected to continue to increase rapidly; in addition to providing information about the origins of the personality disorders, such findings are also expected to open new avenues for treating these often difficult-to-treat patients.

TREATMENT

Because personality disorders consist of deeply ingrained attitudes and behavior patterns that consolidate during development and have endured since adulthood, they cannot be readily changed. As previously noted, treatment efforts are further confounded by the degree to which patients view their personality disorder traits as constituting who they are and not as what they have. Often, the personality characteristics that others find offensive or that impair the social adjustment of the individual with the personality disorder are not experienced by the person as undesirable or related to his or her problems. For all of these reasons, there has been a general wariness about the treatability of patients with personality disorders.

Psychoanalysts pioneered the hope that persons with personality disorders could respond to treatment. The original conception of neurosis as a discrete set of symptoms related to a discrete developmental phase or to discrete conflicts was gradually replaced by the idea that more enduring defensive styles and identification processes were the building blocks of character traits. From this perspective, Wilhelm Reich (1949) and others developed the concept of character analysis and defense analysis. These processes refer to an analyst's efforts to address the ways in which a person resists learning or the confrontations by which the analyst draws attention to the maladaptive effects of the patient's character traits (i.e., his or her usual interpersonal and behavioral style). A parallel development in technique evolved from group therapy experience. Maxwell Jones (1953) identified the value of confrontations delivered within group settings in which peer pressure made it difficult for patients to ignore feedback or to leave the group. Here, too, a primary goal of treatment was to render more dystonic the ego-syntonic but maladaptive aspects of the patient's interpersonal and behavioral style. This general principle was subsequently adopted by other forms of sociotherapies, notably those within hospital milieus and family therapies.

Families or couples may present other complications insofar as the designated patient's disordered interpersonal and behavioral patterns may serve functions for, or be complementary to, the disordered patterns of persons with whom the patient is closely associated. For example, a dependent person is apt to bond with an overly authoritarian partner, or an emotionally constricted obsessional person may find an emotionally expressive, hysterical person particularly compatible. Under these circumstances, treatment is primarily directed not at confronting the maladaptive aspects of one person's character traits but rather at identifying the way in which these aspects may be welcomed and reinforced in one setting but maladaptive and impairing in others.

In the past decade, the use of pharmacotherapy for personality disorders has begun to be explored. To the prospect of using specific medications for specific disorders has been added that of identifying biological dimensions of personality psychopathology that may respond to different medication classes (Cloninger 1987; Coccaro and Kavoussi 1997; Siever and Davis 1991). For example, research has increasingly suggested that impulsivity and aggression may respond to serotonergic medications, mood instability and lability may respond to serotonergic medications and to other antidepressants, and psychoticlike experiences may respond to neuroleptics (Coccaro and Kavoussi 1997; Cornelius et al. 1993; Soloff et al. 1993).

The most recent development in the treatment of personality disorders involves cognitive-behavioral strategies. These strategies generally are more focused and structured than psychodynamic therapies and offer the hope of more discrete, time-limited forms of intervention. Behavioral strategies typically involve efforts to diminish impulsivity or increase assertiveness by using relaxation techniques or role-playing exercises. Cognitive strategies involve first identifying specific internal mental schemes by which patients typically misunderstand certain situations or misrepresent themselves, and then learning how to modify those internal schemes.

The overall development of treatment strategies for personality disorders has involved a movement away from therapeutic nihilism to the present widespread but inconsistent use of a full spectrum of treatment modalities. An overview of our knowledge about the potential usefulness of the three major types of psychiatric treatment—psychotherapies, sociotherapies, and pharmacotherapies—is provided in Table 22–3. It is expected that use of these therapies will increasingly be guided by more specific and empirically based information on which modalities, in what sequence, are most effective for treatment of each personality disorder.

SPECIFIC PERSONALITY DISORDERS

PARANOID PERSONALITY DISORDER

History

Paranoid personality disorder has been richly and consistently represented in this century's descriptive psychiatric literature. It was described by Mayer, Koch, Kraepelin, Bleuler, Kretschmer, and Schneider under such rubrics as

TABLE 22–3.   Evidence of treatment effectiveness for personality disorders

	ST	SZ	P	B	AS	H	N	OC	D	AV
Psychotherapies	–	+	–	+	–	++	++	++	++	++
Sociotherapies	±	+	–	++	+	–	–	–	+	+
Pharmacotherapies	+	–	±	+	–	–	–	–	–	±

Note.   – = no support; ± = uncertain support; + = modestly helpful; ++ = significantly helpful. ST = schizotypal; SZ = schizoid; P = paranoid; B = borderline; AS = antisocial; H = histrionic; N = narcissistic; OC = obsessive-compulsive; D = dependent; AV = avoidant.

the "pseudoquerulent type" and the "fanatic psychopath" (Millon 1981). This disorder has, however, received less attention in the psychoanalytic literature than have many other personality disorders.

Paranoid personality disorder is one of the few personality disorders to have been included in every version of DSM, and its description has consistently focused on the disorder's central feature of a pervasive and unwarranted mistrust of others (Bernstein et al. 1993).

Clinical Features

Persons with paranoid personality disorder have a pervasive, persistent, and inappropriate mistrust of others (Table 22–4). They are suspicious of others' motives and assume that others intend to harm, exploit, or trick them. Thus, they may question, without justification, the loyalty or trustworthiness of friends or sexual partners, and they are reluctant to confide in others for fear the information will be used against them. Persons with paranoid personality disorder appear guarded, tense, and hypervigilant, and they constantly scan their environment for clues of possible attack, deception, or betrayal. They often find "evidence" of such malevolence by misinterpreting benign events (such as a glance in their direction) as demeaning or threatening. In response to perceived or actual insults or betrayals, these individuals overreact, quickly becoming excessively angry and responding with counterattacking behavior. They are unable to forgive or forget such incidents and instead bear long-term grudges against their supposed betrayers; some persons with paranoid personality disorder are litigious. Whereas some individuals with this disorder appear quietly and tensely aloof and hostile, others are overtly angry and combative. Persons with this disorder are usually socially isolated and, because of their paranoia, often have difficulties with co-workers.

Differential Diagnosis

Unlike paranoid personality disorder, the Axis I disorders paranoid schizophrenia and delusional disorder, paranoid type, are both characterized by prominent and persistent paranoid delusions of psychotic proportions; paranoid

TABLE 22–4.   DSM-IV diagnostic criteria for paranoid personality disorder

A.   A pervasive distrust and suspiciousness of others such that their motives are interpreted as malevolent, beginning by early adulthood and present in a variety of contexts, as indicated by four (or more) of the following:

(1)   Suspects, without sufficient basis, that others are exploiting, harming, or deceiving him or her

(2)   Is preoccupied with unjustified doubts about the loyalty or trustworthiness of friends or associates

(3)   Is reluctant to confide in others because of unwarranted fear that the information will be used maliciously against him or her

(4)   Reads hidden demeaning or threatening meanings into benign remarks or events

(5)   Persistently bears grudges, i.e., is unforgiving of insults, injuries, or slights

(6)   Perceives attacks on his or her character or reputation that are not apparent to others and is quick to react angrily or to counterattack

(7)   Has recurrent suspicions, without justification, regarding fidelity of spouse or sexual partner

B.   Does not occur exclusively during the course of schizophrenia, a mood disorder with psychotic features, or another psychotic disorder and is not due to the direct physiological effects of a general medical condition.

Note: If criteria are met prior to the onset of schizophrenia, add "premorbid," e.g., "paranoid personality disorder (premorbid)."

schizophrenia is also accompanied by hallucinations and other core symptoms of schizophrenia. Although paranoid and schizotypal personality disorders both involve suspiciousness, paranoid personality disorder does not entail perceptual distortions and eccentric behavior.

Etiology

Early psychoanalytic speculation suggested that this personality type derived from reaction formation against and projection onto others of homosexual impulses, a theory that is no longer widely accepted. However, the defense mechanism of projection is generally assumed to be involved in the expression of this disorder's features (Vaillant 1992). Some theories suggest that persons with this disorder have been the object of excessive parental rage, whereas others suggest that these persons have been humiliated by others, perhaps, in particular, by members of the same sex. Either type of experience could in theory lead to feelings of inadequacy and vulnerability followed by projection onto others of hostility and rage as well as a tendency to blame others for one's shortcomings and problems.

It seems likely that paranoid personality disorder has biogenetic contributions. Early in this century, Kraepelin (1921) theorized that this personality disorder was the premorbid character type of persons predisposed to paranoia (now known as Axis I delusional disorder). The existence of an association between these two disorders has received some support from family history studies that found a greater morbid risk of paranoid personality disorder in the first-degree relatives of delusional disorder probands than in the relatives of probands with schizophrenia or medical illness (Kendler and Gruenberg 1982). Such a link implicates the involvement of both environmental and constitutional factors in the etiology of paranoid personality disorder.

Treatment

Because they mistrust others, persons with paranoid personality disorder usually avoid psychiatric treatment. If they do seek treatment, the therapist immediately encounters the challenge of engaging them and keeping them in treatment. This can best be accomplished by maintaining an unusually respectful, straightforward, and unintrusive style aimed at building trust. If a problem develops in the treatment relationship—for example, the patient accuses the therapist of some fault—it is best simply to offer a straightforward apology, if warranted, rather than to respond evasively or defensively. It is also best to avoid an overly warm style, because excessive warmth and expression of interest can exacerbate the patient's paranoid tendencies. A supportive psychotherapy that incorporates such an approach may be the best treatment for these patients.

Although group treatment or cognitive-behavioral treatment (Turkat and Maisto 1985) aimed at anxiety management and the development of social skills might be of benefit, these patients, because of their suspiciousness and fears of losing control and being criticized, tend to resist such approaches.

Antipsychotic medications are sometimes useful in the treatment of this disorder. Patients may view such treatment with mistrust; however, these medications are particularly indicated in the treatment of the overtly psychotic decompensations that these patients sometimes experience.

SCHIZOID PERSONALITY DISORDER

History

Schizoid personality disorder was originally conceptualized as the personality type associated with schizophrenia—a role that is now largely assumed by schizotypal personality disorder. As such, during the early part of this century, schizoid personality disorder as a traitlike variant of schizophrenia was described by Hoch (1910) as the "shut-in personality," by Bleuler (1922) as "schizoidie," and by Kraepelin (1919) as "autistic personality." A similar personality type was also described in the psychoanalytic literature by the object relations theorists Fairbairn (1940/1952) and Guntrip (1971), who used the term in a broader fashion to describe socially withdrawn patients who had difficulties with intimacy and some of those behavioral peculiarities now subsumed by schizotypal personality disorder.

Schizoid personality disorder has been included in every version of DSM, but its meaning has varied significantly in the different DSM editions (Kalus et al. 1993). Broadly defined in DSM-I and DSM-II, the category was later divided into the schizoid, avoidant, and schizotypal types of personality disorder.

Clinical Features

Schizoid personality disorder is characterized by a profound defect in the ability to relate to others in a meaningful way (Table 22–5). Persons with this disorder have little or no desire for relationships with others and, as a result, are extremely socially isolated. They prefer to engage in solitary, often intellectual, activities, such as computer games or puzzles, and they often create an elaborate fantasy world into which they retreat and which substitutes for relationships with others. As a result of their lack of interest in relationships, they have few or no close friends or confidants. They date infrequently and seldom marry, and they often work at jobs requiring little interpersonal interaction (e.g., in a laboratory). These individuals are also notable for their lack of affect. They usually appear cold, detached, aloof, and constricted, and they have particular discomfort when experiencing warm feelings. Few, if any, activities or experiences give them pleasure, which is reflected in their chronic anhedonia.

TABLE 22–5. DSM-IV diagnostic criteria for schizoid personality disorder

A. A pervasive pattern of detachment from social relationships and a restricted range of expression of emotions in interpersonal settings, beginning by early adulthood and present in a variety of contexts, as indicated by four (or more) of the following:

   (1) Neither desires nor enjoys close relationships, including being part of a family

   (2) Almost always chooses solitary activities

   (3) Has little, if any, interest in having sexual experiences with another person

   (4) Takes pleasure in few, if any, activities

   (5) Lacks close friends or confidants other than first-degree relatives

   (6) Appears indifferent to the praise or criticism of others

   (7) Shows emotional coldness, detachment, or flattened affectivity

B. Does not occur exclusively during the course of schizophrenia, a mood disorder with psychotic features, another psychotic disorder, or a pervasive developmental disorder and is not due to the direct physiological effects of a general medical condition.

Note: If criteria are met prior to the onset of schizophrenia, add "premorbid," e.g., "schizoid personality disorder (premorbid)."

Differential Diagnosis

Schizoid personality disorder shares the features of social isolation and restricted emotional expression with schizotypal personality disorder, but it lacks the latter disorder's cognitive and perceptual distortion characteristics. Unlike individuals with avoidant personality disorder, who intensely desire relationships but avoid them because of exaggerated fears of rejection, persons with schizoid personality disorder have little or no interest in developing relationships with others.

Etiology

Clinicians have noted that schizoid personality disorder occurs in adults who experienced cold, neglectful, and ungratifying relationships in early childhood, which leads these persons to assume that relationships are not valuable or worth pursuing. There is reason to believe that constitutional factors contribute to the childhood pattern of shyness that often precedes the disorder. Introversion, which characterizes schizoid (as well as avoidant and schizotypal)

personality disorder, appears to be highly heritable. Although family history studies give stronger support to a link between schizophrenia and schizotypal personality disorder, some studies suggest an association of schizophrenia with schizoid personality disorder, which would implicate the importance of genetic factors in the latter disorder's etiology.

Treatment

Persons with schizoid personality disorder, like those with schizotypal personality disorder, rarely seek treatment. They do not perceive the formation of any relationship—including a therapeutic relationship—as potentially valuable or beneficial. They may, however, occasionally seek treatment for an associated problem, such as depression, or they may be brought for treatment by others. Whereas some patients can tolerate only a supportive therapy or treatment aimed at the resolution of a crisis or associated Axis I disorder, others do well with insight-oriented psychotherapy aimed at effecting a basic shift in their comfort with intimacy and affects.

Development of an alliance may be difficult and can be facilitated by an interested and caring attitude and an avoidance of early interpretation or confrontation. Some authors have suggested the use of so-called inanimate bridges, such as writing and artistic productions, to ease the patient into the therapy relationship. Incorporation of cognitive-behavioral approaches that encourage gradually increasing social involvement may be of value (Liebowitz et al. 1986). Although many patients may be unwilling to participate in a group, group therapy may also facilitate the development of social skills and relationships.

SCHIZOTYPAL PERSONALITY DISORDER

History

Early concepts, like current concepts, of schizotypal personality disorder were linked to schizophrenia. Bleuler's (1922) concept of latent schizophrenia, which consisted of mild or attenuated schizophrenia symptoms without deterioration into psychosis, was one of the major clinical forerunners of schizotypal personality disorder. The term *schizotype*, coined by Rado (1956), denoted a nonpsychotic phenotypic variant of the schizophrenia genome. This term was later used as an alternative label for the "borderline schizophrenia" syndrome identified in the Danish adoption studies, which was a milder schizophrenialike disorder present in the biological relatives of schizophrenic probands (Kety et al. 1968).

Schizotypal personality disorder was new to DSM-III and was based on the characteristics of the relatives (i.e., the "schizotypes") identified in the Danish adoption studies. An additional impetus for its addition to DSM-III was the concern that the schizoid and borderline personality disorder constructs were too broadly defined (Siever et al. 1991).

Clinical Features

Persons with schizotypal personality disorder experience cognitive or perceptual distortions, behave in an eccentric manner, and are socially inept and anxious (Table 22–6). Their cognitive and perceptual distortions include ideas of reference, bodily illusions, and unusual telepathic and clairvoyant experiences. These distortions, which are inconsistent with subcultural norms, occur frequently and are an important and pervasive component of the person's experience. They are in keeping with the odd and eccentric behavior characteristic of this disorder. These individuals may, for example, talk to themselves in public, gesture for no apparent reason, or dress in a peculiar or unkempt fashion. Their speech is often odd and idiosyncratic—unusually circumstantial, metaphorical, or vague, for instance—and their affect is constricted or inappropriate. Such a person may, for example, laugh in a silly manner when discussing his or her problems.

Persons with schizotypal personality disorder are also socially uncomfortable and isolated, and they have few friends. This isolation is often due to their eccentric cognitions and behavior as well as to their lack of desire for relationships, which stems in part from their suspiciousness of others. If they develop a relationship, they tend to remain distant or may even terminate it because of their persistent social anxiety and paranoia.

Differential Diagnosis

Schizotypal personality disorder shares the feature of suspiciousness with paranoid personality disorder and that of social isolation with schizoid personality disorder, but these latter two disorders lack the markedly peculiar behavior and significant cognitive and perceptual distortions typically present in schizotypal personality disorder. Schizotypal personality disorder, although on a spectrum with Axis I schizophrenia, lacks enduring overt psychosis.

Etiology

Schizotypal personality disorder is a schizophrenia-spectrum disorder—that is, it is related to Axis I schizophrenia. Phenomenological, biological, genetic, treatment response, and outcome data support this link.

TABLE 22-6. **DSM-IV diagnostic criteria for schizotypal personality disorder**

A. A pervasive pattern of social and interpersonal deficits marked by acute discomfort with, and reduced capacity for, close relationships as well as by cognitive or perceptual distortions and eccentricities of behavior, beginning by early adulthood and present in a variety of contexts, as indicated by five (or more) of the following:

(1) Ideas of reference (excluding delusions of reference)

(2) Odd beliefs or magical thinking that influences behavior and is inconsistent with subcultural norms (e.g., superstitiousness, belief in clairvoyance, telepathy, or "sixth sense"; in children and adolescents, bizarre fantasies or preoccupations)

(3) Unusual perceptual experiences, including bodily illusions

(4) Odd thinking and speech (e.g., vague, circumstantial, metaphorical, overelaborate, or stereotyped)

(5) Suspiciousness or paranoid ideation

(6) Inappropriate or constricted affect

(7) Behavior or appearance that is odd, eccentric, or peculiar

(8) Lack of close friends or confidants other than first-degree relatives

(9) Excessive social anxiety that does not diminish with familiarity and tends to be associated with paranoid fears rather than negative judgments about self

B. Does not occur exclusively during the course of schizophrenia, a mood disorder with psychotic features, another psychotic disorder, or a pervasive developmental disorder.

Note: If criteria are met prior to the onset of schizophrenia, add "premorbid," e.g., "schizotypal personality disorder (premorbid)."

For example, family history studies show an increased risk for schizophrenia-related disorders in the relatives of schizotypal probands and, conversely, an increased risk for schizotypal personality disorder in the relatives of schizophrenia probands (Kendler et al. 1993; Torgersen et al. 1993). In addition, at least some forms of schizotypal personality disorder involve biological abnormalities characteristic of schizophrenia—for example, an increased ventricular-brain ratio on computed tomography scan; higher cerebrospinal fluid homovanillic acid concentrations (Siever et al. 1993); impaired smooth pursuit eye movements; and impaired performance on tests of executive function and other tests of visual or auditory attention, such as the Wisconsin Card Sorting Test, the backward masking task, the continuous performance task, and sensory gating tests, suggesting altered precortical functioning (Siever et al. 1991; Trestman et al. 1995).

Because of this evidence, schizotypal personality disorder is classified in ICD-10 with schizophrenia rather than with the personality disorders. However, it may be that certain subtypes of this personality disorder are not related to schizophrenia—a reflection of the fact that schizotypal personality disorder's DSM definition has been modified over time to better reflect clinical impressions of a syndrome characterized by cognitive, perceptual, and behavioral eccentricities and to better differentiate it from near-neighbor personality disorders. It is not clear whether those variants of schizotypal personality disorder that are related to schizophrenia represent a milder, traitlike, nonpsychotic variant of schizophrenia or whether they in fact constitute schizophrenia's core features, on which the more florid psychotic episodes of schizophrenia can be superimposed.

Treatment

Because they are socially anxious and somewhat paranoid, persons with schizotypal personality disorder usually avoid psychiatric treatment. They may, however, seek such treatment—or be brought for treatment by concerned family members—when they become depressed or overtly psychotic. As with patients with paranoid personality disorder, it is difficult to establish an alliance with schizotypal patients, and they are unlikely to tolerate exploratory techniques that emphasize interpretation or confrontation. A supportive relationship that counters cognitive distortions and ego-boundary problems may be useful (Stone 1985). This may involve an educational approach that fosters the development of social skills or encourages risk-taking behavior in social situations, or, if these efforts fail, encourages the development of activities with less social involvement. If the patient is willing to participate, cognitive-behavioral therapy and highly structured educational groups with a social skills focus may also be helpful.

Several case series support the usefulness of low-dose antipsychotic medications in the treatment of schizotypal personality disorder (Goldberg et al. 1986; Serban and Siegel 1984). These medications may ameliorate the anxiety and psychoticlike features associated with this disorder, and they are particularly indicated in the treatment of the more overt psychotic decompensations that these patients can experience. In addition, results of an open-label trial suggested that fluoxetine may also diminish features of schizotypal personality disorder (Markovitz et al. 1991).

ANTISOCIAL PERSONALITY DISORDER

History

Pritchard (1835) used the term *moral insanity* to describe people with a pattern of repeated immoral behaviors for which they were not fully responsible. The disorder he characterized has been described by many other psychiatric luminaries under a variety of labels (Millon 1981). Even as psychiatry has decried the use of this diagnosis for excusing antisocial acts, it has been steadfast in recognizing that such persons have significant psychological impairment.

By the late nineteenth century, the term *psychopathic personality* had become a broadly applicable category for persons with socially undesirable character traits. Harvey Cleckley's 1941 definition of the psychopath (Cleckley 1964) heavily influenced the DSM-I and DSM-II definitions of antisocial personality, whereas the definitions of antisocial personality in DSM-III and DSM-III-R rested on the empirical work of L. N. Robins (1966). The DSM-III and DSM-III-R definitions consisted of an established pattern of conduct disorder in childhood as well as a set of socially noxious behaviors (e.g., arrests, truancy, and assaultiveness) occurring in adulthood. These definitions had the assets of being explicitly behavioral and of permitting reliable assessment but had the liabilities of being cumbersome and too specific to Western culture. On the basis of empirical evidence, in DSM-IV the Robins' behaviorally based version is combined with Cleckley's personologic traits to bring the disorder's definition back in line with clinical observations and with personality trait–based descriptions.

Clinical Features

The central characteristic of antisocial personality disorder is a long-standing pattern of socially irresponsible behaviors that reflects a disregard for the rights of others (Table 22–7). Many persons with this disorder engage in repetitive unlawful acts. The more prevailing personality characteristics include a lack of interest in or concern for the feelings of others, deceitfulness, and, most notably, a lack of remorse over the harm they may cause others. These characteristics generally make these individuals fail in roles requiring fidelity (e.g., as a spouse or a parent), honesty (e.g., as an employee), or reliability in any social role. Some antisocial persons possess a glibness and charm that can be used to seduce, outwit, and exploit others. Although most antisocial persons are indifferent to their effects on others, a notable subgroup takes sadistic pleasure in being harmful. Antisocial personality disorder is associated with high rates of substance abuse (Dinwiddie et al. 1992).

TABLE 22-7. DSM-IV diagnostic criteria for antisocial personality disorder

A. There is a pervasive pattern of disregard for and violation of the rights of others occurring since age 15 years, as indicated by three (or more) of the following:

    (1) Failure to conform to social norms with respect to lawful behaviors as indicated by repeatedly performing acts that are grounds for arrest

    (2) Deceitfulness, as indicated by repeated lying, use of aliases, or conning others for personal profit or pleasure

    (3) Impulsivity or failure to plan ahead

    (4) Irritability and aggressiveness, as indicated by repeated physical fights or assaults

    (5) Reckless disregard for safety of self or others

    (6) Consistent irresponsibility, as indicated by repeated failure to sustain consistent work behavior or honor financial obligations

    (7) Lack of remorse, as indicated by being indifferent to or rationalizing having hurt, mistreated, or stolen from another

B. The individual is at least age 18 years.

C. There is evidence of conduct disorder with onset before age 15 years.

D. The occurrence of antisocial behavior is not exclusively during the course of schizophrenia or a manic episode.

Differential Diagnosis

The primary differential diagnostic issue involves narcissistic personality disorder. Indeed, these two disorders may be variants of the same basic type of psychopathology (Hare et al. 1991). However, the antisocial person, unlike the narcissistic person, is likely to be reckless and impulsive. In addition, narcissistic individuals' exploitativeness and disregard for others are attributable to their sense of uniqueness and superiority rather than to a desire for materialistic gains.

Etiology

Findings of twin and adoptive studies indicate that genetic factors predispose to the development of antisocial personality disorder (Grove et al. 1990; Lyons et al. 1995). Nonetheless, it is unclear how much variance is accounted for by genetic factors and whether the nature of the predisposition is relatively specific or is best conceptualized in terms of relatively nonspecific traits such as impulsivity, excitability, or hostility (Widiger et al. 1992). Growing evidence indicates that the impulsive and aggressive behav-

iors may be mediated by abnormal serotonin transporter functioning in the brain (Coccaro et al. 1996). It is clear that even in the absence of genetic vulnerability, the early family life of these persons often poses severe environmental handicaps in the form of absent, assaultive, or inconsistent parenting. Indeed, many family members also have significant action-oriented psychopathology such as substance abuse or antisocial personality disorder itself. Notably, children who have seen a sibling treated harshly (in ways that might render the sibling likely to engage in antisocial behavior) may learn inhibitions and civility, and thus the exposure may have protective effects on them (Reiss et al. 1995).

Treatment

It is clinically important to recognize antisocial personality disorder because an uncritical acceptance of these individuals' glib or shallow statements of good intentions and collaboration can permit them to have a disruptive influence on treatment teams and other patients. However, there is little evidence to suggest that this disorder can be successfully treated by usual psychiatric interventions. Of interest, nonetheless, are reports suggesting that in confined settings, such as the military or prisons, depressive and introspective concerns may surface (Vaillant 1975). Under these circumstances, confrontation by peers may bring about changes in the antisocial person's social behaviors. It is also notable that some antisocial patients demonstrate an ability to form a therapeutic alliance with psychotherapists, which augurs well for these patients' future course (Woody et al. 1985). These findings contrast with the clinical tradition that emphasizes such persons' inability to learn from harmful consequences. Yet longitudinal follow-up studies have shown that the prevalence of this disorder diminishes with age as these individuals become more aware of the social and interpersonal maladaptiveness of their most noxious social behaviors.

BORDERLINE PERSONALITY DISORDER

History

The borderline personality disorder construct originated from the observations of psychoanalytic psychotherapists who were impressed by these patients' demanding search for nurturance, their disregard for the usual boundaries of therapy, and their tendency to regress in unstructured situations. Impelled by the clinical importance of foreseeing such problems and by a new wave of psychotherapeutic optimism, empirical work was done to better define this disorder. This work raised the question of whether such patients had an atypical form of mood disorder rather than an atypical form of schizophrenia, as had been previously thought, and, more importantly, led to this disorder's inclusion in DSM-III.

The development of operationalized diagnostic criteria provoked an effusion of further empirical research that has led to revisions of this disorder's construct and informed its treatment (Gunderson et al. 1991a). Borderline personality disorder is the most widely studied personality disorder. It is also common, occurring in approximately 2%–3% of the population and in every culture. Evidence for its validity is growing, and the disorder is now recognized as the most prevalent Axis II disorder in all kinds of clinical settings, cases of the disorder making up 12%–15% of cases of Axis II disorders (Gunderson 1992).

Clinical Features

Central to this disorder's psychopathology are a severely impaired capacity for attachment and predictably maladaptive behavior patterns related to separation (Gunderson 1984). When borderline patients feel cared for, held on to, and supported, depressive features (notably loneliness and emptiness) are most evident (Table 22–8). When the loss of such a sustaining relationship is threatened, the lovingly idealized image of a beneficent caregiver is replaced by a hatefully devalued image of a cruel persecutor. This shift is called *splitting*. An impending separation also evokes intense abandonment fears. To minimize these fears and to prevent the separation, rageful accusations of mistreatment and cruelty and angry self-destructive behaviors frequently occur. These behaviors often elicit a guilty or fearful protective response from others. When patients experience an absence of a sustaining, holding, or caring relationship, dissociative experiences, ideas of reference, or desperate impulsive acts (including substance abuse and promiscuity) predictably occur.

Differential Diagnosis

Borderline patients' intense feelings of being bad or evil are distinctly different from the idealized self-image of narcissistic persons. Although borderline patients, like persons with antisocial personality disorder, may be reckless and impulsive, their behaviors are primarily interpersonally oriented and aimed toward obtaining support rather than materialistic gains.

Etiology

Psychoanalytic theories have emphasized the importance of early parent-child relationships in the etiology of bor-

derline personality disorder. Such reports have emphasized maternal mismanagement of the 2- to 3-year-old child's efforts to become autonomous (Masterson 1972), exaggerated maternal frustration that aggravates the child's anger (Kernberg 1975), and inattention to the child's emotions and attitudes (Adler 1985). A considerable body of empirical research has embellished these theories by documenting a high frequency of traumatic early abandonment, physical abuse, and sexual abuse (Table 22–9). It is clear that these traumatic experiences occur within a context of sustained neglect from which the preborderline child develops an enduring rage and self-hatred. The lack of stably involved attachment during development is a source of the inability of borderline patients to maintain a stable sense of themselves or of others without ongoing contact (i.e., their defects of object constancy or stable introjects) (Gunderson 1996). This combination of factors may be more specific than any one factor to the pathogenesis of this disorder.

TABLE 22–8. **DSM-IV diagnostic criteria for borderline personality disorder**

A pervasive pattern of instability of interpersonal relationships, self-image and affects, and marked impulsivity beginning by early adulthood and present in a variety of contexts, as indicated by five (or more) of the following:

(1) Frantic efforts to avoid real or imagined abandonment. **Note:** Do not include suicidal or self-mutilating behavior covered in criterion 5.

(2) A pattern of unstable and intense interpersonal relationships characterized by alternating between extremes of idealization and devaluation

(3) Identity disturbance: markedly and persistently unstable self-image or sense of self

(4) Impulsivity in at least two areas that are potentially self-damaging (e.g., spending, sex, substance abuse, reckless driving, binge eating). **Note:** Do not include suicidal or self-mutilating behavior covered in criterion 5.

(5) Recurrent suicidal behavior, gestures, or threats, or self-mutilating behavior

(6) Affective instability due to a marked reactivity of mood (e.g., intense episodic dysphoria, irritability, or anxiety usually lasting a few hours and only rarely more than a few days)

(7) Chronic feelings of emptiness

(8) Inappropriate, intense anger or difficulty controlling anger (e.g., frequent displays of temper, constant anger, recurrent physical fights)

(9) Transient, stress-related paranoid ideation or severe dissociative symptoms

TABLE 22–9. Studies of childhood trauma in borderline personality disorder

Study	BPD (N)	Controls	Separation/Loss	Physical abuse	Sexual abuse	No trauma
Soloff and Millward (1983)	45	SZ, DEP	56%–62%[a]			
Akiskal et al. (1985)	100	OPD, Bi, DEP	37%[a]			
Links et al. (1988)	88	BL traits	25%[a]	29%[a]	26%[a]	44%[a]
Zanarini et al. (1989)	50	OPD, ASPD	46%[a]	46%	26%[a]	26%
Herman et al. (1989)	24	OPD		71%[a]	67%[a]	19%[a]
Johnson et al. (1989)	43	OPD, NL	40%			
Ogata et al. (1990)	24	DEP		42%	71%[a]	21%[a]
Shearer et al. (1990)	40	—		25%	40%	
Stone (NYPI) (1990)	29	—		28%	35%	
	206	SZ, SZ aff	37%	11%	17%	45%
Westen et al. (1990)	23	"Other"		52%	52%[a]	
Paris (1992)	78	OPD		70%[a]	70%[a]	27%[a]

Note. SZ = schizophrenia; DEP = depressed; OPD = other personality disorder; Bi = bipolar; BL traits = subthreshold borderline criteria; ASPD = antisocial personality disorder; NL = normal; SZ aff = schizoaffective; "other" = undefined.
[a]Prevalence significantly greater in BPD sample.
Source. Reprinted from Gunderson JG, Sabo AS: "The Phenomenological and Conceptual Interface of Borderline Personality Disorder and Posttraumatic Stress Disorder." *American Journal of Psychiatry* 150:19–27, 1993. Copyright 1993, American Psychiatric Association. Used with permission.

Various efforts to identify inherited temperamental predispositions to borderline personality disorder have yielded support for the presence of nonspecific problems with regulation of affects, aggression, and impulses.

Treatment

The extensive literature on the treatment of borderline personality disorder universally notes the extreme difficulties that clinicians encounter with these patients. These problems derive from the patients' appeal to their treaters' nurturing qualities and their rageful accusations in response to their treaters' perceived failures. Often therapists develop intense countertransference reactions that lead them to attempt to re-parent or reject borderline patients. As a consequence, regardless of the treatment approach used, personal maturity and considerable clinical experience are important assets.

As a result of the work of Kernberg (1968) and Masterson (1972), much of the treatment literature has focused on the value of intensive exploratory psychotherapies directed at modifying borderline patients' basic character structure. However, this literature has increasingly suggested that improvement may be related not to the acquisition of insight but to the corrective experience of developing a stable, trusting relationship with a therapist who fails to retaliate in response to these patients' angry and disruptive behaviors. Paralleling this development has been the suggestion that supportive psychotherapies or group therapies

may bring about similar changes.

Treatment of borderline patients has now expanded to include pharmacological and cognitive-behavioral interventions. Although no one medication has been found to have dramatic or predictable effects, results of short-term studies indicate that many medications may diminish specific problems such as impulsivity, affective lability, or intermittent cognitive and perceptual disturbances (Table 22–10), as well as irritability and aggressive behavior (Cornelius et al. 1993; Cowdry and Gardner 1988; Salzman et al. 1995; Soloff 1989; Soloff et al. 1993). Linehan et al. (1991) showed that behavioral treatment consisting of a once-weekly individual and twice-weekly group regimen can effectively diminish the self-destructive behaviors and hospitalization of borderline patients. The success and cost benefits of this treatment, called *dialectical behavior therapy*, have led to a rapid expansion of its usage. In general, the profusion of treatment modalities and the introduction of empiricism point toward the increasing use of more time-limited and focused treatment strategies.

HISTRIONIC PERSONALITY DISORDER

History

The forerunner of histrionic personality disorder can be found in turn-of-the-century accounts of hysteria by Pierre Janet and Sigmund Freud. Janet was impressed with the role of actual seduction (or other trauma) in childhood,

TABLE 22–10.　Medication efficacy in borderline personality disorder

Medication	Mood	Suicidality/ Self-destructiveness	Impulsivity	Psychoticlike features
Monoamine oxidase inhibitors	+	++	+	?
Serotonin reuptake inhibitors	++	++	++	++
Tricyclic antidepressants	+	±	±	±
Antipsychotics	±	++	+	+
Carbamazepine	+	++	++	+
Benzodiazepines	±	–	–	?

Note. The information in this table should be considered tentative, because most medication trials in borderline personality disorder have been small and open, and few of the medications listed have been directly compared with one another. ++ = clear improvement; + = modest improvement; ± = variable improvement or worsening; – = some worsening. Most published studies of serotonin reuptake inhibitors have used fluoxetine.

whereas Freud focused on the unconscious elaboration of the child's sexual drive (i.e., libido). Subsequent psychoanalytic observers noted that hysterical symptoms were often associated with a particular set of character traits. This finding led to the designation of a hysterical type of personality disorder in DSM-II.

The initial empirical examination of hysterical personality traits used factor-analytic methods, which helped consolidate this syndrome's components but also led to a broad definition (Lazare et al. 1970). Indeed, this disorder's early definitions were so broad that they rendered the diagnosis "meaningless" (Easser and Lesser 1965).

The label *hysterical* was changed to the label *histrionic* in DSM-III in an effort to use a term that was more theoretically neutral and more in line with psychiatry's descriptive tradition. Whereas the term *hysterical personality* still connotes the conflicted eroticization of parental figures, the term "histrionic" that replaced it in DSM-III reflects the diagnostician's concern with the observable features of emotional instability and attention seeking. The DSM-III version of the operationalized criteria of this disorder largely captured its more severe "oral" and manipulative variants and thereby unintentionally magnified its overlap with other categories, such as borderline personality disorder (Pfohl 1991).

The modifications of DSM-III-R and DSM-IV helped distinguish this category from others and placed it within the range of less severe personality disorders that can be conceptualized as maladaptive variants of normally occurring traits. This view was reflected by Chodoff's (1982) suggestion that this disorder represents a caricature of stereotypic femininity.

Clinical Features

Central to histrionic personality disorder is an over-concern with attention and appearance (Table 22–11).

Persons with this disorder spend an excessive amount of time seeking attention and making themselves attractive. The desire to be found attractive may lead to inappropriately seductive or provocative dress and flirtatious behavior, and the desire for attention may lead to other flamboyant acts or self-dramatizing behavior. All of these features reflect these persons' underlying insecurity about their value as anything other than a fetching companion. Persons with histrionic personality disorder also display an effusive but labile and suspiciously shallow range of feelings. They are often overly impressionistic and given to hyperbolic descriptions of others (e.g., "She's wonderful" or "She's horrible"). More generally, these persons do not attend to detail or facts, and they are reluctant or unable to

TABLE 22–11.　DSM-IV diagnostic criteria for histrionic personality disorder

A pervasive pattern of excessive emotionality and attention seeking, beginning by early adulthood and present in a variety of contexts, as indicated by five (or more) of the following:

(1) Is uncomfortable in situations in which he or she is not the center of attention

(2) Interaction with others is often characterized by inappropriate sexually seductive or provocative behavior

(3) Displays rapidly shifting and shallow expression of emotions

(4) Consistently uses physical appearance to draw attention to self

(5) Has a style of speech that is excessively impressionistic and lacking in detail

(6) Shows self-dramatization, theatricality, and exaggerated expression of emotion

(7) Is suggestible, i.e., easily influenced by others or circumstances

(8) Considers relationships to be more intimate than they actually are

make reasoned critical analyses of problems or situations. Persons with this disorder often present with complaints of depression, somatic problems of unclear origin, and a history of disappointing romantic relationships.

Differential Diagnosis

This disorder can be confused with dependent, borderline, and narcissistic personality disorders. Histrionic individuals are often willing, even eager, to have others make decisions and organize their activities for them. However, unlike persons with dependent personality disorder, histrionic persons are uninhibited and lively companions who willfully forgo appearing autonomous because they believe this is desired by others. Unlike persons with borderline personality disorder, they do not perceive themselves as bad, and they lack ongoing problems with rage or willful self-destructiveness. Persons with narcissistic personality disorder also seek attention to sustain their self-esteem but differ in that their self-esteem is characterized by grandiosity, and the attention they crave must be admiring—for example, unlike the histrionic person, they would be crushed to be described as "cute" or "silly."

Etiology

Psychoanalytic theory proposes that histrionic personality disorder originates in the oedipal phase of development (i.e., 3–5 years of age) when an overly eroticized relationship with the opposite-sex parent is unduly encouraged and the child fears that the consequences of this excitement will be the loss of, or retaliation by, the same-sex parent. This conflict results in lasting character formations of exaggerated fantasy and exhibitionistic promise with inhibited factual analysis and diminished actual productivity. More recently, research suggests that qualities such as emotional expressiveness and attention seeking may be characteristics of biogenetically determined temperament. From this perspective, histrionic personality disorder would be considered an extreme variant of a temperamental disposition, the environmental contributions of which may be less specific than those of the aforementioned theories.

Treatment

Individual psychodynamic psychotherapy, including psychoanalysis, remains the cornerstone of most treatment for persons with histrionic personality disorder. This treatment is directed at increasing patients' awareness of 1) how their self-esteem is maladaptively tied to their ability to attract attention at the expense of developing other skills and 2) how their shallow relationships and emotional experience reflect unconscious fears of real commitments. Most of this increase in awareness occurs through analysis of the here-and-now doctor-patient relationship rather than through the reconstruction of childhood experiences. Therapists should be aware that the typical idealization and eroticization that such patients bring into treatment are the material for exploration, and thus therapists should be aware of countertransferential gratification.

NARCISSISTIC PERSONALITY DISORDER

History

Havelock Ellis (1898) introduced the term *narcissism* in 1898 to describe a type of sexual perversion involving treating oneself as a sexual object. Freud then adopted the term to describe a more general attitude of self-absorption and self-love. Later, analysts moved the concept toward excessive self-love and grandiosity that develop in response to injured self-esteem (Morrison 1989; Pulver 1970). The concept of a narcissistic type of personality disorder developed only during the 1980s and was inspired largely by the enormous attention given to pathological narcissism in the psychoanalytic community (Gunderson et al. 1991c). Ironically, this attention was largely an outgrowth of Heinz Kohut's (1971, 1977) theoretical and clinical contributions, many of which focused on nonpathological narcissism.

Clinical Features

Because persons with narcissistic personality disorder have grandiose self-esteem, they are vulnerable to intense reactions when their self-image is damaged (Table 22–12). They respond with strong feelings of hurt or anger to even small slights, rejections, defeats, or criticisms. As a result, persons with narcissistic personality disorder usually go to great lengths to avoid exposure to such experiences and, when that fails, react by becoming devaluative or rageful. Serious depression can ensue, which is the usual precipitant for their seeking clinical help. In relationships, narcissistic persons are often quite distant, try to sustain "an illusion of self-sufficiency" (Modell 1975), and may exploit others for self-serving ends. They are likely to feel that those with whom they associate need to be special and unique because they see themselves in these terms; thus, they usually wish to be associated only with persons, institutions, or possessions that will confirm their sense of superiority. The DSM-IV criteria are most accurate in identifying the arrogant, socially conspicuous forms of

TABLE 22–12.   DSM-IV diagnostic criteria for narcissistic personality disorder

A pervasive pattern of grandiosity (in fantasy or behavior), need for admiration, and lack of empathy, beginning by early adulthood and present in a variety of contexts, as indicated by five (or more) of the following:

(1) Has a grandiose sense of self-importance (e.g., exaggerates achievements and talents, expects to be recognized as superior without commensurate achievements)

(2) Is preoccupied with fantasies of unlimited success, power, brilliance, beauty, or ideal love

(3) Believes that he or she is "special" and unique and can only be understood by, or should associate with, other special or high-status people (or institutions)

(4) Requires excessive admiration

(5) Has a sense of entitlement, i.e., unreasonable expectations of especially favorable treatment or automatic compliance with his or her expectations

(6) Is interpersonally exploitative, i.e., takes advantage of others to achieve his or her own ends

(7) Lacks empathy: is unwilling to recognize or identify with the feelings and needs of others

(8) Is often envious of others or believes that others are envious of him or her

(9) Shows arrogant, haughty behaviors or attitudes

---

narcissistic personality disorder; however, there are other forms in which a conviction of personal superiority is hidden behind social withdrawal and a facade of self-sacrifice and even humility (Cooper and Ronningstam 1992).

Differential Diagnosis

Narcissistic personality disorder can be most readily confused with histrionic and antisocial personality disorders. Like persons with antisocial personality disorder, those with narcissistic personality disorder are capable of exploiting others but usually rationalize their behavior on the basis of the specialness of their goals or their personal virtue. In contrast, antisocial persons' goals are materialistic, and their rationalizations, if offered, are based on a view that others would do the same to them. The narcissistic person's excessive pride in achievements, relative constraint in expression of feelings, and disregard for other people's rights and sensitivities help distinguish him or her from persons with histrionic personality disorder. Perhaps the most difficult differential diagnostic problem is whether a person who meets criteria for narcissistic personality disorder has a stable personality disorder or an

adjustment reaction. When the emergence of narcissistic traits has been defensively triggered by experiences of failure or rejection, these traits may diminish radically and self-esteem may be restored when new relationships or successes occur.

Etiology

Little scientific evidence is available about the pathogenesis of narcissistic personality disorder. Reconstructions based on developmental history and observations in psychoanalytic treatment indicate that this disorder develops in persons who have had their fears, failures, or dependency responded to with criticism, disdain, or neglect during their childhood years. Such experiences leave them contemptuous of such reactions in themselves and others and inexperienced in viewing others as sources of comfort and support. They develop a veneer of invulnerability and self-sufficiency that masks their underlying emptiness and constricts their capacity to feel deeply.

Treatment

Individual psychodynamic psychotherapy, including psychoanalysis, is the cornerstone of treatment for persons with narcissistic personality disorder. Following Kohut's lead, some therapists believe that the vulnerability to narcissistic injury indicates that intervention should be directed at conveying empathy for the patient's sensitivities and disappointments. This approach, in theory, allows a positive idealized transference to develop that will then be gradually disillusioned by the inevitable frustrations encountered in therapy—disillusionment that will clarify the excessive nature of the patient's reactions to frustrations and disappointments. An alternative view, explicated by Kernberg (1974, 1975), is that the vulnerability should be addressed earlier and more directly by interpretations and confrontations by which these persons will come to recognize their grandiosity and its maladaptive consequences. With either approach, the psychotherapeutic process usually requires a relatively intensive schedule over a period of years in which the narcissistic patient's hypersensitivity to slights is foremost in the therapist's mind and interventions.

AVOIDANT PERSONALITY DISORDER

History

Avoidant personality disorder, which was new to DSM-III, was theoretically derived from Millon's (1981) typology of personality disorders (corresponding to his active-detached pattern). Despite its theoretical basis, the disorder does have some historical clinical antecedents, including Kretschmer's (1925) hyperaesthetic type, Schneider's (1959) sensitive type, Horney's (1945) detached type, and Fenichel's (1945) phobic character. In DSM-III-R, in fact, the avoidant personality disorder construct was brought closer to the psychoanalytic construct of the phobic character. The changes of DSM-IV focused on better differentiating this disorder from the Axis I condition of generalized social phobia (Millon 1991).

Clinical Features

Persons with avoidant personality disorder experience excessive and pervasive anxiety and discomfort in social situations and in intimate relationships (Table 22–13). Although strongly desiring relationships, they avoid them because they fear being ridiculed, criticized, rejected, or humiliated. These fears reflect their low self-esteem and hypersensitivity to negative evaluation by others. When they do enter into social situations or relationships, they feel inept and are self-conscious, shy, awkward, and preoccupied with being criticized or rejected. Their lives are constricted in that they tend to avoid not only relationships but also new activities because they fear that they will embarrass or humiliate themselves.

TABLE 22–13. DSM-IV diagnostic criteria for avoidant personality disorder

A pervasive pattern of social inhibition. feelings of inadequacy, and hypersensitivity to negative evaluation, beginning by early adulthood and present in a variety of contexts, as indicated by four (or more) of the following:

(1) Avoids occupational activities that involve significant interpersonal contact, because of fears of criticism, disapproval, or rejection

(2) Is unwilling to get involved with people unless certain of being liked

(3) Shows restraint within intimate relationships because of the fear of being shamed or ridiculed

(4) Is preoccupied with being criticized or rejected in social situations

(5) Is inhibited in new interpersonal situations because of feelings of inadequacy

(6) Views self as socially inept, personally unappealing, or inferior to others

(7) Is unusually reluctant to take personal risks or to engage in any new activities because they may prove embarrassing

---

Differential Diagnosis

Schizoid personality disorder also involves social isolation, but the schizoid person does not desire relationships, whereas the avoidant person desires them but avoids them because of anxiety and fears of humiliation and rejection. And whereas avoidant personality disorder is characterized by avoidance of all situations and relationships involving possible rejection or disappointment, Axis I social phobia usually consists of specific fears related to social performance (e.g., a fear of saying something inappropriate or of being unable to answer questions in social situations).

Etiology

Millon (1981), from whose work DSM avoidant personality disorder was derived, suggested that the disorder develops from parental rejection and censure, which may be reinforced by rejecting peers. Psychodynamic theory suggests that avoidant behavior may derive from early life experiences that lead to an exaggerated desire for acceptance or an intolerance of criticism. Research in the biological sphere has implicated the importance of inborn temperament in the development of avoidant behavior. Kagan (1989) found that some children as young as 21 months of age manifest increased physiological arousal and avoidant traits in social situations (e.g., retreat from the unfamiliar and avoidance of interaction with strangers) and that this social inhibition tends to persist for many years.

Treatment

Because of their excessive fear of rejection and criticism and their reluctance to form relationships, persons with avoidant personality disorder may be difficult to engage in treatment. Engagement in psychotherapy may be facilitated by the therapist's use of supportive techniques, sensitivity to the patient's hypersensitivity, and gentle interpretation of the defensive use of avoidance. Although early in treatment these patients may tolerate only supportive techniques, they may eventually respond well to all kinds of psychotherapy, including short-term, long-term, and psychoanalytic approaches. Clinicians should be aware of the potential for countertransference reactions such as overprotectiveness, hesitancy to adequately challenge the patient, or excessive expectations for change.

Although few data exist, it seems likely that assertiveness and social skills training may increase patients' confidence and willingness to take risks in social situations. Cognitive techniques that gently challenge patients' pathological assumptions about their sense of ineptness may also be useful. Group experiences—perhaps, in particular, homogeneous supportive groups that emphasize the development of social skills—may prove useful for avoidant patients.

Promising preliminary data suggest that avoidant personality disorder may improve with treatment with monoamine oxidase inhibitors or serotonin reuptake inhibitors (Deltito and Stam 1989; Versiani et al. 1992). Anxiolytics sometimes help patients better manage anxiety (especially severe anxiety) caused by facing previously avoided situations or trying new behaviors.

DEPENDENT PERSONALITY DISORDER

History

Abraham's (1927) "oral" character was the major clinical forerunner of dependent personality disorder. This character type was thought to result from fixation at the first, or oral, stage of psychosexual development—a theory that was reflected in Fenichel's (1945) observation that "certain persons act as nursing mothers in all their object relationships" (p. 489). This personality type was similar to Horney's "compliant" type (Millon 1981).

Dependent personality disorder was a subtype of passive-aggressive personality disorder in DSM-I and did not become a separate disorder until DSM-III. The changes of DSM-IV put greater emphasis on the disorder's central features and attempted to diminish its overlap with other personality disorders (Hirschfeld et al. 1991).

Clinical Features

Dependent personality disorder is characterized by an excessive need to be cared for by others, which leads to submissive and clinging behavior and excessive fears of separation from others (Table 22–14). Although these individuals are able to care for themselves, they so doubt their abilities and judgment, and they view others as so much stronger and more capable than they, that they can be quite disabled. These persons excessively rely on "powerful" others to initiate and do things for them, make their decisions, assume responsibility for their actions, and guide them through life. Low self-esteem and doubt about their effectiveness lead them to avoid positions of responsibility. Because they feel unable to function without excessive guidance, they go to great lengths to maintain the dependent relationship. They may, for example, always agree with those on whom they depend, and they tend to be excessively clinging, submissive, passive, and self-

sacrificing. If the dependent relationship ends, these individuals feel helpless and fearful, because they feel incapable of caring for themselves, and they often then indiscriminately find another person with whom to have a relationship, so that they can be provided with direction and nurturance—an unfulfilling or even an abusive relationship may seem better than being on their own.

Differential Diagnosis

Although persons with borderline personality disorder also dread being alone and need ongoing support, dependent persons want others to assume a controlling function that would frighten the borderline patient. Moreover, persons with dependent personality disorder become appeasing rather than rageful or self-destructive when threatened with separation. Although both avoidant and dependent personality disorders are characterized by low self-esteem, rejection sensitivity, and an excessive need for reassurance, persons with dependent personality disorder seek out rather than avoid relationships, and they quickly and indiscriminately replace ended relationships instead of further withdrawing from others.

TABLE 22–14. **DSM-IV diagnostic criteria for dependent personality disorder**

A pervasive and excessive need to be taken care of that leads to submissive and clinging behavior and fears of separation, beginning by early adulthood and present in a variety of contexts, as indicated by five (or more) of the following:

(1) Has difficulty making everyday decisions without an excessive amount of advice and reassurance from others

(2) Needs others to assume responsibility for most major areas of his or her life

(3) Has difficulty expressing disagreement with others because of fear of loss of support or approval
   Note: Do not include realistic fears of retribution.

(4) Has difficulty initiating projects or doing things on his or her own (because of a lack of self-confidence in judgment or abilities rather than a lack of motivation or energy)

(5) Goes to excessive lengths to obtain nurturance and support from others, to the point of volunteering to do things that are unpleasant

(6) Feels uncomfortable or helpless when alone because of exaggerated fears of being unable to care for himself or herself

(7) Urgently seeks another relationship as a source of care and support when a close relationship ends

(8) Is unrealistically preoccupied with fears of being left to take care of himself or herself

Etiology

Abraham suggested that the dependent character derives from either overindulgence or underindulgence during the oral phase of development (i.e., birth to age 2). Subsequent empirical data have given more support to the underindulgence hypothesis. However, studies of adults have not supported a specific association between feeding or other oral habits in childhood and dependency in adulthood. It may be that ongoing patterns unrelated to the oral phase per se—for example, chronic physical illness, or underindulgent parenting that also prohibits independent behavior—are more important to this disorder's development. Genetic or constitutional factors, such as innate submissiveness, may also be a factor in this disorder's etiology; twin studies have found that monozygotic twins score more similarly on scales measuring submissiveness than do dizygotic twins.

Cultural and social factors may also play a role in the development of dependent personality disorder. Dependency is considered not only normative but desirable in certain cultures, and Gilligan (1982) argued that it is encouraged in women in our own culture. Thus, dependent personality disorder may represent an exaggerated and maladaptive variant of normal dependency; that is, it may—along with histrionic, obsessive-compulsive, and avoidant personality disorders—best be conceptualized as a "trait" disorder (i.e., occurring on a continuum with normal personality traits). It is important to recognize that to qualify as dependent personality disorder, the dependent traits should be so extreme that they cause significant distress or impairment in functioning.

Treatment

Patients with dependent personality disorder often enter therapy with complaints of depression or anxiety that may be precipitated by the threatened or actual loss of a dependent relationship. They often respond well to various types of individual psychotherapy. Treatment may be particularly helpful if it explores patients' fears of independence; uses the transference to explore their dependency; and is directed toward increasing patients' self-esteem, sense of effectiveness, assertiveness, and independent functioning. These patients often seek an excessively dependent relationship with the therapist, which can lead to countertransference problems that may actually reinforce their dependence. The therapist may, for example, overprotect or be overly directive with the patient, give inappropriate reassurance and support, or prolong the treatment unnecessarily. He or she may also have excessive expectations for change or withdraw

from a patient who is perceived as too needy.

Group therapy and cognitive-behavioral therapy aimed at increasing independent functioning, including assertiveness and social skills training, may be useful for some patients. If the patient is in a relationship that is maintaining and reinforcing his or her excessive dependence, couples or family therapy may be helpful.

OBSESSIVE-COMPULSIVE PERSONALITY DISORDER

History

In the early 1900s, Freud (1908/1924) made his often-cited observation that persons with obsessive-compulsive personality disorder were characterized by the three "peculiarities" of orderliness (which included cleanliness and conscientiousness), parsimoniousness, and obstinacy. Similarly, in 1918, Ernest Jones (1918/1938) described these individuals as being preoccupied with cleanliness, money, and time. These observations were repeatedly cited and amplified in the subsequent psychoanalytic literature—the disorder often being referred to as *anal character*—and in the descriptive literature (Millon 1981).

This disorder's DSM description has closely mirrored these earlier clinical observations (Pfohl and Blum 1991). In addition, in keeping with its consistent representation in the clinical literature, obsessive-compulsive personality disorder is one of the few personality disorders that has been included in every version of DSM. In European psychiatry, this disorder has been referred to as *anancastic personality disorder*, a term used by Kretschmer and Schneider in the 1920s and still used in ICD-10.

Clinical Features

As Freud noted, and as DSM-IV criteria reflect, persons with obsessive-compulsive personality disorder are excessively orderly (Table 22–15). They are neat, punctual, overly organized, and overconscientious. Although these traits might be considered virtues, especially in cultures that subscribe to the Puritan work ethic, to qualify as obsessive-compulsive personality disorder the traits must be so extreme that they cause significant distress or impairment in functioning. As Abraham (1923) noted, these individuals' perseverance is unproductive. For example, attention to detail is so excessive or time consuming that the point of the activity is lost, conscientiousness is so extreme that it causes rigidity and inflexibility, and perfectionism interferes with task completion. And although these individuals tend to work extremely hard, they do so at the expense of leisure activities and relationships. As Shapiro

TABLE 22-15. **DSM-IV diagnostic criteria for obsessive-compulsive personality disorder**

A pervasive pattern of preoccupation with orderliness, perfectionism, and mental and interpersonal control, at the expense of flexibility, openness, and efficiency, beginning by early adulthood and present in a variety of contexts, as indicated by four (or more) of the following:

(1) Is preoccupied with details, rules, lists, order, organization, or schedules to the extent that the major point of the activity is lost

(2) Shows perfectionism that interferes with task completion (e.g., is unable to complete a project because his or her own overly strict standards are not met)

(3) Is excessively devoted to work and productivity to the exclusion of leisure activities and friendships (not accounted for by obvious economic necessity)

(4) Is overconscientious, scrupulous, and inflexible about matters of morality, ethics, or values (not accounted for by cultural or religious identification)

(5) Is unable to discard worn-out or worthless objects even when they have no sentimental value

(6) Is reluctant to delegate tasks or to work with others unless they submit to exactly his or her way of doing things

(7) Adopts a miserly spending style toward both self and others; money is viewed as something to be hoarded for future catastrophes

(8) Shows rigidity and stubbornness

(1965) pointed out, the most characteristic thought of obsessive-compulsive persons is "I should"—a phrase that aptly reflects their severe superego and captures their overly high standards, drivenness, and excessive conscientiousness, perfectionism, rigidity, and devotion to work and duties.

These individuals also tend to be overly concerned with control—not only over the details of their own lives but over their emotions and other people. They have difficulty expressing warm and tender feelings, often using stilted, distant phrasing that reveals little of their inner experience. And they may be obstinate and reluctant to delegate tasks or to work with others unless others submit exactly to their way of doing things, which reflects their need for interpersonal control as well as their fear of making mistakes. Their tendency to doubt and worry also manifests itself in their inability to discard worn-out or worthless objects that might be needed for future catastrophes, and, as Freud and Jones noted, persons with obsessive-compulsive personality are miserly toward themselves and others. A

caricatured description of such persons is Rado's (1959) "living machines."

Differential Diagnosis

Obsessive-compulsive personality disorder differs from Axis I obsessive-compulsive disorder in that the latter disorder consists of specific repetitive thoughts and ritualistic behaviors rather than personality traits. In addition, obsessive-compulsive disorder has traditionally been considered ego-dystonic whereas obsessive-compulsive personality disorder has been considered ego-syntonic. These two disorders are sometimes, but not necessarily, comorbid.

Etiology

Freud's view that obsessive-compulsive personality disorder derives from difficulties occurring during the anal stage of psychosexual development (age 2–4 years) was echoed and elaborated on by subsequent psychoanalytic thinkers, such as Karl Abraham and Wilhelm Reich (1933). According to this theory, children's infantile anal-erotic libidinal impulses conflict with parental attempts to socialize them—in particular, to toilet train them. Although these theories emphasize the importance of children's perception of parental disapproval during toilet training, and of ensuing parent-child control struggles—what Rado (1959) referred to as "the battle of the chamber pot"—these factors are not currently considered central to this disorder's etiology. It may be, however, that conflicts arising during toilet training—such as those characteristic of Erikson's (1950) stage of autonomy versus shame—and continuing during other developmental stages do play a role in this disorder's etiology (Perry and Vaillant 1989). In particular, excessive parental control, criticism, and shaming may result in an insecurity that is defended against with perfectionism, orderliness, and an attempt to maintain excessive control.

Freud believed that constitutional factors also play an important role in the formation of this personality type; similarly, Rado postulated the etiological importance of constitutionally excessive rage that leads to power struggles with others. As is the case with other personality disorders, empirical studies are needed to clarify this disorder's sources.

Treatment

Persons with obsessive-compulsive personality disorder may seem difficult to treat because of their excessive intellectualization and difficulty expressing emotion. However, these patients often respond well to psychoanalytic psychotherapy or psychoanalysis. Therapists usually need to be relatively active in treatment. They should also avoid being drawn into interesting but affectless discussions that are unlikely to have therapeutic benefit; in other words, rather than intellectualizing with the patient, therapists should focus on the feelings these patients usually avoid. Other defenses common in this disorder, such as rationalization, isolation, undoing, and reaction formation, should also be identified and clarified. Power struggles that may occur in treatment offer opportunities to address the patient's excessive need for control.

Cognitive techniques may also be used to diminish the patient's excessive need for control and perfection. Although patients may resist group treatment because of their need for control, dynamically oriented groups that focus on feelings may provide insight and increase their comfort with exploring and expressing new affects.

OTHER PERSONALITY DISORDERS

The following three personality disorders were considered for inclusion on DSM-IV Axis II on the basis of their historical tradition, clinical utility, and/or empirical support. However, for various reasons they were thought to require further study. Of note, all three disorders involve chronically morose people who have problems with direct expression of their aggression.

DEPRESSIVE PERSONALITY DISORDER

Of all the personality disorders, depressive personality disorder may have the longest clinical tradition, having been recognized 2,000 years ago by Hippocrates in his description of the "black gall," or melancholic, temperament (Phillips et al. 1990). Kraepelin (1921) also described this temperament and, like Hippocrates, considered it a depressive-spectrum disorder—a constitutional traitlike variant of the more severe depressive disorders and one predisposing to their occurrence. Schneider's (1959) description of this personality type led to its inclusion in ICD-9 as an affective personality disorder. Kernberg (1988), who drew from the writings of Laughlin, emphasized this personality type's psychodynamic features, which include a severe superego, the inhibited expression of aggression, and an excessive dependence that is defended against with counterdependence. Because of the strength of this disorder's historical tradition, its inclusion in ICD-9, and some empirical evidence in its support, depressive personality disorder was added to the appendix in DSM-IV.

Persons with this disorder are persistently gloomy, burdened, worried, serious, pessimistic, and incapable of enjoyment or relaxation (Table 22–16). They also tend to be guilty, moralistic, self-denying, passive, nonassertive, and introverted. They have low self-esteem and are excessively sensitive to criticism and rejection. Although they may be critical of others, they have difficulty directing criticism or any form of aggression toward others and find it easier to criticize themselves. They are also overly dependent on the love and acceptance of others, but they inhibit the expression of this dependency and may instead appear counterdependent.

Although concern has been expressed that this personality disorder may overlap excessively with Axis I depressive disorders—in particular, dysthymia—available data suggest that its overlap with dysthymia, major depression, and other personality disorders is far from complete and that depressive personality disorder appears be a separate construct (D. N. Klein 1990; Phillips et al. 1988). This disorder should not be diagnosed, however, if it occurs only during major depressive episodes. Although depressive personality disorder appears distinct from Axis I depressive disorders, family history and other data suggest that it may be related to these disorders, giving support to Kraepelin's spectrum concept.

Depressive personality disorder has been noted to respond well to psychoanalytic psychotherapy and psychoanalysis. Although it has been proposed that the major depressive episodes that can co-occur with this personality type may be particularly responsive to antidepressant med-

---

TABLE 22–16. Research criteria for depressive personality disorder

A. A pervasive pattern of depressive cognitions and behaviors beginning by early adulthood and present in a variety of contexts, as indicated by five (or more) of the following:

 (1) Usual mood is dominated by dejection, gloominess, cheerlessness, joylessness, unhappiness

 (2) Self-concept centers around beliefs of inadequacy, worthlessness, and low self-esteem

 (3) Is critical, blaming, and derogatory toward self

 (4) Is brooding and given to worry

 (5) Is negativistic, critical, and judgmental toward others

 (6) Is pessimistic

 (7) Is prone to feeling guilty or remorseful

B. Does not occur exclusively during major depressive episodes and is not better accounted for by dysthymic disorder.

ications (Akiskal 1983), this assertion awaits further empirical validation.

NEGATIVISTIC PERSONALITY DISORDER

Negativistic personality disorder entered the appendix in DSM-IV as a replacement for the excessively narrow category of passive-aggressive personality disorder, which was thought to represent a single defense mechanism rather than a personality disorder. Other limitations of passive-aggressive personality disorder were its limited empirical support and the fact that passive-aggressive behavior can be normative, even laudable, in certain situations. Negativistic personality disorder is a broader construct that has some historical precedents, including Schneider's (1923) "ill-tempered depressives."

Negativistic personality disorder, like passive-aggressive personality disorder, describes a pervasive pattern of passive resistance to demands for social and occupational performance (Table 22–17). But it also encompasses a wide range of negativistic attitudes and behaviors, such as anger, pessimism, and cynicism; sullenness and argumentativeness; criticism of others; and envy of those who are perceived as more fortunate. In addition, these individuals tend to alternate between hostile self-assertion and contrite submission. The clinical features of this disorder and its differentiation from other personality disorders remain to be empirically confirmed.

TABLE 22–17. Research criteria for passive-aggressive personality disorder

A. A pervasive pattern of negativistic attitudes and passive resistance to demands for adequate performance, beginning by early adulthood and present in a variety of contexts, as indicated by four (or more) of the following:

   (1) Passively resists fulfilling routine social and occupational tasks

   (2) Complains of being misunderstood and unappreciated by others

   (3) Is sullen and argumentative

   (4) Unreasonably criticizes and scorns authority

   (5) Expresses envy and resentment toward those apparently more fortunate

   (6) Voices exaggerated and persistent complaints of personal misfortune

   (7) Alternates between hostile defiance and contrition

B. Does not occur exclusively during major depressive episodes and is not better accounted for by dysthymic disorder.

SELF-DEFEATING PERSONALITY DISORDER

Self-defeating personality disorder has been the subject of much controversy. This personality type has a significant historical and clinical tradition, beginning with Kraft-Ebbing's nineteenth-century description of sexual masochism (which is classified as a paraphilia in DSM) and Freud's subsequent description of moral masochism, a pattern of nonsexual submissive behavior that leads to psychological pain and mistreatment. Nonetheless, concerns have been raised about the misuse of the diagnosis of this disorder—in particular, that it may be misapplied to women who are actually being abused and thereby be used to blame the victim. In part as a reflection of these concerns, self-defeating personality disorder has never been an official psychiatric diagnosis. It was included in the DSM-III-R appendix (Fiester 1991) and is not included in DSM-IV. However, this disorder's proponents argue that it applies to men as well as to women and that it is a clinically useful concept with important treatment implications.

Self-defeating personality disorder applies to persons who exhibit a pervasive pattern of self-defeating behavior that does not occur only in response to, or in anticipation of, physical, sexual, or psychological abuse. Persons with this disorder feel unworthy of being treated well and, as a result, treat themselves poorly and unwittingly encourage others to make them suffer. They may, for example, reject opportunities for pleasure, choose people or situations that lead to mistreatment or failure, and incite others to become angry with them or reject them. If things do go well for them, they attempt to undermine themselves by, for example, becoming depressed or causing themselves pain.

This disorder's treatment is complicated by the patient's self-defeating tendencies; patients may unknowingly undermine the treatment and their progress because they feel undeserving of improvement or happiness. Exploring the patient's need to be victimized and making their investment in suffering ego-dystonic may allow a successful outcome with insight-oriented psychotherapy or psychoanalysis.

CONCLUSIONS

Clinical interest and research in the personality disorders have grown enormously since 1980, when these disorders were put on a separate axis in DSM-III. The ensuing period has brought to light more specific treatment strategies and a better understanding of the prognosis and etiology of these disorders. Even more dramatic than the knowledge gained are the heightened awareness of these disorders and the new and more informed questions that this awareness has generated. Remaining challenges include an explication of the boundaries between personality disorders and both normalcy and Axis I conditions, as well as the discovery of biogenetic bases for personality disorder classification. There is good reason to believe that with continued inquiry by clinical and basic-science investigators, the classification system will continue to change so that it becomes even more tightly linked to these disorders' etiology and treatment.

REFERENCES

Abraham K: Contributions to the theory of the anal character. Int J Psychoanal 4:400–418, 1923

Abraham K: The influence of oral eroticism on character formation, in Selected Papers on Psychoanalysis. Edited by Jones E. London, Hogarth Press, 1927, pp 393–406

Adler G: Borderline Psychopathology and Its Treatment. New York, Jason Aronson, 1985

Akiskal HS: Dysthymic disorder: psychopathology of proposed chronic depressive subtypes. Am J Psychiatry 140:11–20, 1983

Akiskal HS, Chen SE, Davis GC, et al: Borderline: an adjective in search of a noun. J Clin Psychiatry 46:41–48, 1985

American Psychiatric Association: Diagnostic and Statistical Manual: Mental Disorders. Washington, DC, American Psychiatric Association, 1952

American Psychiatric Association: Diagnostic and Statistical Manual of Mental Disorders, 2nd Edition. Washington, DC, American Psychiatric Association, 1968

American Psychiatric Association: Diagnostic and Statistical Manual of Mental Disorders, 3rd Edition. Washington, DC, American Psychiatric Association, 1980

American Psychiatric Association: Diagnostic and Statistical Manual of Mental Disorders, 3rd Edition, Revised. Washington, DC, American Psychiatric Association, 1987

American Psychiatric Association: Diagnostic and Statistical Manual of Mental Disorders, 4th Edition. Washington, DC, American Psychiatric Association, 1994

Benjamin LS: Structural analysis of social behavior. Psychol Rev 81:392–425, 1974

Bernstein DP, Useda D, Siever LJ: Paranoid personality disorder: a review of its current status. Journal of Personality Disorders 7:53–62, 1993

Black DW, Bell S, Hulbert J, et al: The importance of Axis II in patients with major depression: a controlled study. J Affect Disord 14:115–122, 1988

Bleuler E: Die Probleme der Schizoidie und der Syntonie. Zeitschrift für die gesamte Neurologie und Psychiatrie 78: 373–388, 1922

Brent DA, Johnson BA, Perper J, et al: Personality disorder, personality traits, impulsive violence, and completed suicide in adolescents. J Am Acad Child Adolesc Psychiatry 33:1080–1086, 1994

Breuer J, Freud S: Studies on Hysteria (1893–1895). Translated and edited by Strachey J. New York, Basic Books, 1957

Calabrese JR, Woyshville MJ, Kimmel SE, et al: Predictors of valproate response in bipolar rapid cycling. J Clin Psychopharmacol 13:280–283, 1993

Carey G, DiLalla DL: Personality and psychopathology: genetic perspectives. J Abnorm Psychol 103:32–43, 1994

Caton CL, Shrout PE, Eagle PF, et al: Risk factors for homelessness among schizophrenic men: a case-control study. Am J Public Health 84:265–270, 1994

Chodoff P: Hysteria and women. Am J Psychiatry 139:545–551, 1982

Clark LA: Schedule for Normal and Abnormal Personality (SNAP). Dallas, TX, Southern Methodist University, 1990

Cleckley H: The Mask of Sanity, 4th Edition. St Louis, CV Mosby, 1964

Cloninger CR: A systematic method for clinical description and classification of personality variants. Arch Gen Psychiatry 44:573–588, 1987

Cloninger CR, Svrakic DM, Przybeck TR: A psychobiological model of temperament and character. Arch Gen Psychiatry 50:975–990, 1993

Coccaro EF, Kavoussi RJ: Fluoxetine and impulsive aggressive behavior in personality-disordered subjects. Arch Gen Psychiatry 54:1081–1088, 1997

Coccaro EF, Kavoussi RJ, Sheline YI, et al: Impulsive aggression in personality disorder correlates with tritiated paroxetine binding in the platelet. Arch Gen Psychiatry 53:531–536, 1996

Cooper AM, Ronningstam E: Narcissistic personality disorder, in American Psychiatric Press Review of Psychiatry, Vol 11. Edited by Tasman A, Riba ME. Washington, DC, American Psychiatric Press, 1992, pp 80–97

Cornelius JR, Soloff PH, Perel JM, et al: Continuation pharmacotherapy of borderline personality disorder with haloperidol and phenelzine. Am J Psychiatry 150: 1843–1848, 1993

Costa P, McCrae R: Personality disorders and the five-factor model of personality. Journal of Personality Disorders 4:3 62–371, 1990

Cowdry RW, Gardner DL: Pharmacotherapy of borderline personality disorder: alprazolam, carbamazepine, trifluoperazine, and tranylcypromine. Arch Gen Psychiatry 45:111–119, 1988

Deltito JA, Stam M: Psychopharmacological treatment of avoidant personality disorder. Compr Psychiatry 30: 498–504, 1989

Dinwiddie SH, Bucholz KK: Psychiatric diagnoses of self-reported child abusers. Child Abuse Negl 17:465–476, 1993

Dinwiddie SH, Reich T, Cloninger CR: Psychiatric comorbidity and suicidality among intravenous drug users. J Clin Psychiatry 53:364–369, 1992

Easser BR, Lesser SR: Hysterical personality: a re-evaluation. Psychoanal Q 34:390–405, 1965

Ellis H: Auto-erotism: a psychological study. Alienist and Neurologist 19:260–299, 1898

Erikson EH: Childhood and Society. New York, WW Norton, 1950

Fairbairn WRD: Schizoid factors in the personality (1940), in Psychoanalytic Studies of the Personality. London, Tavistock, 1952, pp 3–27

Fals-Stewart W: Personality characteristics of substance abusers: an MCMI cluster typology of recreational drug users treated in a therapeutic community and its relationship to length of stay and outcome. J Pers Assess 59:515–527, 1992

Fenichel O: The Psychoanalytic Theory of the Neurosis. New York, WW Norton, 1945

Fiester SJ: Self-defeating personality disorder: a review of data and recommendations for DSM-IV. Journal of Personality Disorders 5:194–209, 1991

Frances A: Categorical and dimensional systems of personality diagnosis: a comparison. Compr Psychiatry 23:516–527, 1982

Freud S: Character and anal erotism (1908), in Collected Papers, Vol 2. London, Hogarth Press, 1924, pp 45–50

Gilligan C: In a Different Voice: Psychological Theory and Women's Development. Cambridge, MA, Harvard University Press, 1982

Goldberg SC, Schulz C, Schulz PM, et al: Borderline and schizotypal personality disorders treated with low-dose thiothixene vs placebo. Arch Gen Psychiatry 43:680–686, 1986

Grove WM, Eckert ED, Heston L, et al: Heritability of substance abuse and antisocial behavior: a study of monozygotic twins reared apart. Biol Psychiatry 27:1293–1304, 1990

Gunderson JG: Borderline Personality Disorder. Washington, DC, American Psychiatric Press, 1984

Gunderson JG: Diagnostic controversies, in American Psychiatric Press Review of Psychiatry, Vol 11. Edited by Tasman A, Riba M. Washington, DC, American Psychiatric Press, 1992, pp 9–24

Gunderson JG: The borderline patient's intolerance of aloneness: insecure attachment and therapist availability. Am J Psychiatry 153:752–758, 1996

Gunderson JG, Zanarini MC, Kissiel C: Borderline personality disorder: a review of data on DSM-III-R descriptions. Journal of Personality Disorders 5:340–352, 1991a

Gunderson JG, Links PS, Reich JH: Competing models of personality disorders. Journal of Personality Disorders 5:60–68, 1991b

Gunderson JG, Ronningstam E, Smith LE: Narcissistic personality disorder: a review of data on DSM-III-R descriptions. Journal of Personality Disorders 5:167–177, 1991c

Guntrip HJ: The schizoid problem, in Psychoanalytic Theory, Therapy, and the Self. New York, Basic Books, 1971, pp 145–174

Hare RD, Hart SD, Harpur TJ: Psychopathy and the DSM-IV criteria for antisocial personality disorder. J Abnorm Psychol 100:391–398, 1991

Hawton K, Fagg J, Platt S, et al: Factors associated with suicide after parasuicide in young people. BMJ 306:1641–1644, 1993

Herman JL, Perry JC, van der Kolk BA: Childhood trauma in borderline personality disorder. Am J Psychiatry 146:490–495, 1989

Hillbrand M, Krystal JH, Sharpe KS, et al: Clinical predictors of self-mutilation in hospitalized forensic patients. J Nerv Ment Dis 182:9–13, 1994

Hirschfeld RMA, Shea MT, Weise R: Dependent personality disorder: perspectives for DSM-IV. Journal of Personality Disorders 5:135–149, 1991

Hoch A: Constitutional factors in the dementia praecox group. Review of Neurology and Psychiatry 8:463–475, 1910

Horney K: Our Inner Conflicts: A Constructive Theory of Neurosis. New York, WW Norton, 1945

Hyler SE, Rieder RO, Williams JBW, et al: Personality Diagnostic Questionnaire—Revised (PDQ-R). New York, New York State Psychiatric Institute, 1987

Janet P: The Mental State of Hystericals: A Study of Mental Stigmata and Mental Accidents. Translated by Corson CR. New York, Putnam, 1901

Jenike MA, Baer L, Minichiello WE, et al: Coexistent obsessive-compulsive disorder and schizotypal personality disorder: a poor prognostic indicator (letter). Arch Gen Psychiatry 43:296, 1986

Johnson C, Tobin D, Enright A: Prevalence and clinical characteristics of borderline patients in an eating-disordered population. J Clin Psychiatry 50:9–15, 1989

Jones E: Anal-erotic character traits (1918), in Papers on Psychoanalysis. London, Balliere, Tindall and Cox, 1938, pp 531–555

Jones M: The Therapeutic Community—A New Treatment in Psychiatry. New York, Basic Books, 1953

Jordan BK, Schlenger WE, Fairbank JA, et al: Prevalence of psychiatric disorders among incarcerated women. Arch Gen Psychiatry 53:513–519, 1996

Kagan J: Temperamental influences on the preservation of styles of social behavior. McLean Hospital Journal 14:23–34, 1989

Kalus O, Bernstein DP, Siever LJ: Schizoid personality disorder: a review of its current status. Journal of Personality Disorders 7:43–52, 1993

Kass F, Skodol AE, Charles E, et al: Scaled ratings of DSM-III personality disorders. Am J Psychiatry 142:627–630, 1985

Kelstrup A, Lund K, Lauritsen B, et al: Satisfaction with care reported by psychiatric inpatients. Relationship to diagnosis and medical treatment. Acta Psychiatr Scand 87:374–379, 1993

Kendler KS, Gruenberg AM: Genetic relationship between paranoid personality disorder and the "schizophrenic spectrum" disorders. Am J Psychiatry 139:1185–1186, 1982

Kendler KS, McGuire M, Gruenberg AM, et al: The Roscommon family study, III: schizophrenia-related personality disorders in relatives. Arch Gen Psychiatry 50:781–788, 1993

Kent S, Fogarty M, Yellowlees P: A review of studies of heavy users of psychiatric services. Psychiatr Serv 46:1247–1253, 1995

Kernberg OF: Treatment of patients with borderline personality organization. Int J Psychoanal 49:600–619, 1968

Kernberg OF: Further contributions to the treatment of narcissistic personalities. Int J Psychoanal 55:215–240, 1974

Kernberg OF: Borderline Conditions and Pathological Narcissism. New York, Jason Aronson, 1975

Kernberg OF: Clinical dimensions of masochism. J Am Psychoanal Assoc 36:1005–1029, 1988

Kety SS, Rosenthal D, Wender PH, et al: The types and prevalence of mental illness in the biological and adoptive families of adopted schizophrenics, in The Transmission of Schizophrenia. Edited by Rosenthal D, Kety SS. Oxford, UK, Pergamon, 1968, pp 345–362

Klein DN: Depressive personality: reliability, validity, and relation to dysthymia. J Abnorm Psychol 99:412–421, 1990

Klein M: Wisconsin Personality Inventory—Revised. Madison, WI, University of Wisconsin, 1990

Koenigsberg HW, Kaplan RD, Gilmore MM, et al: The relationship between syndrome and personality disorder in DSM-III: experience with 2,462 patients. Am J Psychiatry 142:207–212, 1985

Kohut H: The Analysis of the Self: A Systematic Approach to the Psychoanalytic Treatment of Narcissistic Personality Disorders. New York, International Universities Press, 1971

Kohut H: The Restoration of the Self. New York, International Universities Press, 1977

Kraepelin E: Dementia Praecox and Paraphrenia. Edinburgh, E and S Livingstone, 1919

Kraepelin E: Manic-Depressive Insanity and Paranoia. Translated by Barclay RM. Edited by Robertson GM. Edinburgh, E and S Livingstone, 1921

Kretschmer E: Physique and Character. New York, Harcourt, Brace, 1925

Lazare A, Klerman G, Armor D: Oral, obsessive and hysterical personality patterns: replication of factor analysis in an independent sample. J Psychiatr Res 7:275–279, 1970

Lenzenweger MF, Loranger AW, Korfine L, et al: Detecting personality disorders in a nonclinical population. Arch Gen Psychiatry 54:345–351, 1997

Lesch KP, Bengel D, Heils A: Association of anxiety-related traits with a polymorphism in the serotonin transporter gene regulatory region. Science 274:1527–1531, 1996

Liebowitz MR, Stone MH, Turkat ID: Treatment of personality disorders, in Psychiatry Update: American Psychiatric Association Annual Review, Vol 5. Edited by Frances AJ, Hales RE. Washington, DC, American Psychiatric Press, 1986, pp 356–393

Linehan MM, Armstrong HE, Suarez A, et al: Cognitive behavioral treatment of chronically parasuicidal borderline patients. Arch Gen Psychiatry 48:1060–1064, 1991

Links PS, Steiner M, Offord DR, et al: Characteristics of borderline personality disorder: a Canadian study. Can J Psychiatry 33:336–340, 1988

Loranger AW: Personality Disorders Examination (PDE) Manual. Yonkers, NY, DV Communications, 1988

Loranger AW: The impact of DSM-III on diagnostic practice in a university hospital. Arch Gen Psychiatry 47:672–675, 1990

Lyons MJ, True WR, Eisen SA, et al: Differential heritability of adult and juvenile antisocial traits. Arch Gen Psychiatry 52:906–915, 1995

Markovitz PJ, Calabrese JR, Schulz SC, et al: Fluoxetine in the treatment of borderline and schizotypal personality disorders. Am J Psychiatry 148:1064–1067, 1991

Masterson JF: Treatment of the Borderline Adolescent: A Developmental Approach. New York, Wiley-Interscience, 1972

McDonald AS, Davey GCL: Psychiatric disorders and accidental injury. Clinical Psychology Review 16:105–127, 1996

Miller RJ, Zadolinnyj K, Hafner RJ: Profiles and predictors of assaultiveness for different psychiatric ward populations. Am J Psychiatry 150:1368–1373, 1993

Millon T: Disorders of Personality—DSM-III: Axis II. New York, Wiley, 1981

Millon T: Millon Clinical Multiaxial Inventory–II Manual. Minnetonka, MN, National Computer Systems, 1987

Millon T: Avoidant personality disorder: a brief review of issues and data. Journal of Personality Disorders 5:353–362, 1991

Modell AH: A narcissistic defense against affects and the illusion of self-sufficiency. Int J Psychoanal 56:275–282, 1975

Morey LC, Waugh MH, Blashfield RK: MMPI scales for DSM-III personality disorders: their derivation and correlates. J Pers Assess 49:245–251, 1985

Morrison AP: Introduction, in Essential Papers on Narcissism. Edited by Morrison AP. New York, University Press, 1989, pp 1–11

Nelson JC, Mazure CM, Jatlow PI: Characteristics of desipramine-refractory depression. J Clin Psychiatry 55: 12–19, 1994

Ogata SN, Silk KR, Goodrich S, et al: Childhood sexual and physical abuse in adult patients with borderline personality disorder. Am J Psychiatry 147:1008–1013, 1990

Paris J: Social risk factors for borderline personality disorder: a review and hypothesis. Can J Psychiatry 37:510–515, 1992

Paris J: Personality disorders: a biopsychosocial model. Journal of Personality Disorders 7:255–264, 1993

Perry JC, Vaillant GE: Personality disorders, in Comprehensive Textbook of Psychiatry/V, 5th Edition, Vol 2. Edited by Kaplan HI, Sadock BJ. Baltimore, MD, Williams & Wilkins, 1989, pp 1352–1387

Pfohl B: Histrionic personality disorder: a review of available data and recommendations for DSM-IV. Journal of Personality Disorders 5:150–166, 1991

Pfohl B, Blum N: Obsessive-compulsive personality disorder: a review of available data and recommendations for DSM-IV. Journal of Personality Disorders 5:363–375, 1991

Pfohl B, Blum N, Zimmerman M, et al: The Structured Interview for DSM-III-R Personality Disorders. Iowa City, IA, University of Iowa Press, 1989

Phillips KA, Gunderson JG, Hirschfeld RMA, et al: A review of the depressive personality. Am J Psychiatry 147:830–837, 1990

Phillips KA, Gunderson JG, Triebwasser J, et al: Reliability and validity of depressive personality disorders. Am J Psychiatry 155:1044–1048, 1988

Pritchard JC: A Treatise on Insanity. London, Sherwood, Gilbert and Piper, 1835

Pulver SE: Narcissism: the term and the concept. J Am Psychoanal Assoc 18:319–341, 1970

Rado S: Schizotypal organization: preliminary report on a clinical study of schizophrenia, in Psychoanalysis and Behavior. New York, Grune & Stratton, 1956, pp 1–10

Rado S: Obsessive behavior, in American Handbook of Psychiatry, Vol 1. Edited by Arieti S. New York, Basic Books, 1959, pp 324–344

Raine A: Features of borderline personality and violence. J Clin Psychology 49:277–281, 1993

Reich JH: DSM-III personality disorders and the outcome of treated panic disorder. Am J Psychiatry 145:1149–1152, 1988

Reich J[H], Boerstler H, Yates W, et al: Utilization of medical resources in persons with DSM-III personality disorders in a community sample. Int J Psychiatry Med 19:1–9, 1989

Reich W: Charakteranalyse: Technik und Grundlagen für studierende und praktizierende Analytiker. Leipzig, IM Selbstverlage des Verfassers, 1933

Reich W: On the technique of character analysis, in Character Analysis, 3rd Edition. New York, Simon & Schuster, 1949, pp 39–113

Reiss D, Hetherington EM, Plomin R, et al: Genetic questions for environmental studies: differential parenting and psychopathology in adolescence. Arch Gen Psychiatry 52:925–936, 1995

Robins LN: Deviant Children Grown Up: A Sociological and Psychiatric Study of Sociopathic Personality. Baltimore, MD, Williams & Wilkins, 1966

Salzman C, Wolfson AN, Schatzberg A, et al: Effect of fluoxetine on anger in symptomatic volunteers with borderline personality disorder. J Clin Psychopharmacol 15:23–29, 1995

Schneider K: Die psychopathischen Personlichkeiten. Vienna, Deuticke, 1923

Schneider K: Psychopathic Personalities. Springfield, IL, Charles C Thomas, 1958

Schneider K: Clinical Psychopathology. Translated by Hamilton MW. London, Grune & Stratton, 1959

Serban G, Siegel S: Response of borderline and schizotypal patients to small doses of thiothixene and haloperidol. Am J Psychiatry 141:1455–1458, 1984

Shapiro D: Neurotic Styles. New York, Basic Books, 1965

Shearer SL, Peters CP, Quaytman MS, et al: Frequency and correlates of childhood sexual and physical abuse histories in adult female borderline inpatients. Am J Psychiatry 147:214–216, 1990

Siever LJ, Davis KL: A psychobiological perspective on the personality disorders. Am J Psychiatry 148:1647–1658, 1991

Siever LJ, Bernstein DP, Silverman JM: Schizotypal personality disorder: a review of its current status. Journal of Personality Disorders 5:178–193, 1991

Siever LJ, Amin F, Coccaro EF, et al: CSF homovanillic acid in schizotypal personality disorder. Am J Psychiatry 150:149–151, 1993

Skodol AE, Oldham JM: Assessment and diagnosis of borderline personality disorder. Hospital and Community Psychiatry 42:1021–1028, 1991

Soloff PH: Psychopharmacologic therapies in borderline personality disorder, in American Psychiatric Press Review of Psychiatry, Vol 8. Edited by Tasman A, Hales RE, Frances AJ. Washington, DC, American Psychiatric Press, 1989, pp 65–83

Soloff PH, Millward JW: Developmental histories of borderline patients. Compr Psychiatry 24:574–588, 1983

Soloff PH, Cornelius J, George A, et al: Efficacy of phenelzine and haloperidol in borderline personality disorder. Arch Gen Psychiatry 50:377–385, 1993

Spitzer RL, Williams JBW, Gibbon M, et al: Structured Clinical Interview for DSM-III-R (SCID). Washington, DC, American Psychiatric Press, 1990

Stone M: Schizotypal personality: psychotherapeutic aspects. Schizophr Bull 11:576–589, 1985

Stone M: Abuse and abusiveness in borderline personality disorder, in Family Environment and Borderline Personality Disorder. Edited by Links PS. Washington, DC, American Psychiatric Press, 1990

Torgersen S, Onstad S, Skre I, et al: "True" schizotypal personality disorder: a study of co-twins and relatives of schizophrenic probands. Am J Psychiatry 150:1661–1667, 1993

Trestman RL, Keefe RSE, Mitropoulou V, et al: Cognitive function and biological correlates of cognitive performance in schizotypal personality disorder. Psychiatry Res 59:127–136, 1995

Turkat I, Maisto S: Application of the experimental method to the formulation and modification of personality disorders, in Clinical Handbook of Psychological Disorders. Edited by Barlow D. New York, Guilford, 1985, pp 502–570

Vaillant GE: Sociopathy as a human process: a viewpoint. Arch Gen Psychiatry 32:178–183, 1975

Vaillant GE: Ego Mechanisms of Defense: A Guide for Clinicians and Researchers. Washington, DC, American Psychiatric Press, 1992

Vaillant GE: Ego mechanisms of defense and personality psychopathology. J Abnorm Psychol 103:44–50, 1994

Versiani M, Nardi AE, Mundim FD, et al: Pharmacotherapy of social phobia. A controlled study with moclobemide and phenelzine. Br J Psychiatry 161:353–360, 1992

Weissman MM: The epidemiology of personality disorders: a 1990 update. Journal of Personality Disorders 7:44–62, 1993

Westen D, Ludolph P, Misle B, et al: Physical and sexual abuse in adolescent girls with borderline personality disorder. Am J Orthopsychiatry 60:55–66, 1990

Widiger TA: Personality Interview Questions–II. Lexington, KY, University of Kentucky, 1987

Widiger TA: Personality disorder dimensional models proposal for DSM-IV. Journal of Personality Disorders 5:386–398, 1991

Widiger TA, Frances AJ: Interviews and inventories for the measurement of personality disorders. Clinical Psychology Review 7:49–75, 1987

Widiger TA, Corbitt EM, Millon T: Antisocial personality disorder, in American Psychiatric Press Review of Psychiatry, Vol 11. Edited by Tasman A, Riba ME. Washington, DC, American Psychiatric Press, 1992, pp 63–79

Woody GE, McLellan AT, Luborsky L, et al: Sociopathy and psychotherapy outcome. Arch Gen Psychiatry 42:1081–1086, 1985

World Health Organization: International Statistical Classification of Diseases and Related Health Problems, 10th Revision. Geneva, World Health Organization, 1992

Zanarini MC, Frankenburg FR, Chauncey DL, et al: The Diagnostic Interview for Personality Disorders: interrater and test-retest reliability. Compr Psychiatry 28:467–480, 1987

Zanarini MC, Gunderson JG, Marino MF, et al: Childhood experiences of borderline patients. Compr Psychiatry 30:18–25, 1989

Zimmerman M, Coryell W: DSM-III personality disorder diagnoses in a nonpatient sample: demographic correlates and comorbidity. Arch Gen Psychiatry 46:682–689, 1989

CHAPTER 23

DISORDERS USUALLY FIRST DIAGNOSED IN INFANCY, CHILDHOOD, OR ADOLESCENCE

CHARLES POPPER, M.D.
SCOTT A. WEST, M.D.

Childhood is recognized in psychiatry as a period of vulnerability and progressive development toward adult personality and character. The psychiatric disorders in children and adolescents are increasingly coming into focus as serious treatable conditions and as precursors of adult psychopathology.

In this chapter, the discrete psychopathological entities that are usually first diagnosed in youth are discussed. These disorders often emerge in combinations, change in presentation during maturation, interact with each other over time, and can be obscured or amplified by intervening developmental events. As in DSM-IV (American Psychiatric Association 1994), these childhood-onset disorders are described here as crystalline abstract entities, a presentation that does not respect the individuality of their appearance in each child, cradled in a particular family and society, and undergoing continual change.

The primary "work" of children is to change and grow, a task that reflects their push to interact and modify in multiple dimensions. Rigid crystallized descriptions of their disorders do not convey the liveliness and energy of children who are coping and growing in ways that are characteristic of these disorders and in ways quite independent of psychiatric states.

The main message of this chapter concerns the dynamic undercurrent: not the rigidity of diagnostic categories, but the flux and change that these abstract entities produce in the lives of children—and of the adults they become.

Multiple psychiatric disorders are typical in a single child psychiatric patient. Each primary psychiatric disorder in childhood can lead to secondary developmental complications, such as conduct disorder or school failure, and more persistently to low self-esteem and disorders of social assertiveness. Primary syndromes quickly expand with secondary complications during development, blurring the boundaries of the "original" psychopathology. Certain disorders move in clusters through families and individuals, and interact with each other to produce more virulent forms of the disorders. These interactive effects of multiple concurrent disorders are particularly evident in children and adolescents. Even though personality diagnoses are usually withheld before age 18, the average child psychiatric outpatient carries two separate DSM diagnoses, and the average inpatient carries four.

This developmental expansion of childhood psychopathology may generate a lifetime of "associated features." In dyslexia, the ectopic neurons and cytoarchitectonic anomalies in the cerebral cortex commonly lead to low frustration tolerance in childhood, rigidity in learning in adolescence, and underachievement in adulthood. The adult outcome of childhood psychopathology depends partly on the ways in which the psychopathology is amplified or contained by individual, family, cultural, and therapeutic forces.

Where were adult psychiatric patients during their childhoods? Part of the answer rests in the ability to see disease in children. Not long ago, it was believed that mood disorders did not begin until mid or late adolescence. Now it is known that all "adult" psychiatric disorders in DSM-IV can begin during childhood. Any diagnosis can be used as a primary diagnostic label in a child. Even personality disorders (except for antisocial personality disorder) may be diagnosed in children if the characteristics of the personality disorder appear pervasive and unusually persistent. It also is now known that all childhood-onset disorders can have major sequelae in adults or develop into adult disorders.

Medical conditions in children are crucial in evaluating their behavior; even mild or transient Axis III medical problems can cause flagrant behavioral symptoms, especially in young children (Cantwell and Baker 1988). There is a doubling of the prevalence of psychiatric disorders in children with non–central nervous system (CNS) physical handicaps and diseases (Rutter and Yule 1970). On Axis IV, DSM-IV provides a modified version of the Severity of Psychosocial Stressors Scale for children and adolescents. Parental absence or neglect, physical and sexual abuse, psychiatric disorders among caregivers, and even puberty exert age-specific effects on children. The Axis V Global Assessment of Functioning Scale incorporates features of the Children's Global Assessment Scale (Shaffer et al. 1983).

Developmental stage can influence the presentation, significance, and course of a psychiatric disorder. Coping functions and adaptive strengths change with development and are not related in a simple way to chronological age. Under the current DSM system, such developmental characteristics are not classified, and the clinician is left to personal judgment to assess the developmental stage of the individual and the developmental significance of presenting symptoms.

The DSM-IV category "Disorders Usually First Diagnosed in Infancy, Childhood, or Adolescence" includes conditions that not only begin in childhood but also are typically *diagnosed* during childhood (Table 23–1). Some behavioral patterns are normal at certain developmental stages but become pathological at later developmental stages (e.g., separation anxiety disorder, enuresis, encopresis, and oppositional defiant disorder). Most of the

TABLE 23–1. DSM-IV disorders usually first diagnosed in infancy, childhood, or adolescence

Mental retardation
Mild mental retardation
Moderate mental retardation
Severe mental retardation
Profound mental retardation
Mental retardation, severity unspecified

Learning disorders (academic skills disorders)
Reading disorder
Mathematics disorder
Disorder of written expression
Learning disorder not otherwise specified

Motor skills disorder
Developmental coordination disorder

Pervasive developmental disorders
Autistic disorder
Rett's disorder
Childhood disintegrative disorder
Asperger's disorder
Pervasive developmental disorder not otherwise specified

Disruptive behavior and attention-deficit disorders
Attention-deficit/hyperactivity disorder
    Predominantly inattentive type
    Predominantly hyperactive-impulsive type
    Combined type
    Not otherwise specified
Conduct disorder
Oppositional defiant disorder
Disruptive behavior disorder not otherwise specified

Feeding and eating disorders of infancy or early childhood
Pica
Rumination disorder of infancy
Feeding disorder of infancy or early childhood

Tic disorders
Tourette's disorder
Chronic motor or vocal tic disorder
Transient tic disorder
Tic disorder not otherwise specified

Communication disorders
Expressive language disorder
Mixed receptive-expressive language disorder
Phonological disorder
Stuttering
Communication disorder not otherwise specified

Elimination disorders
Encopresis
Enuresis

Other disorders of infancy, childhood, or adolescence
Separation anxiety disorder
Selective mutism
Reactive attachment disorder of infancy or early childhood
Stereotypic movement disorder
Disorder of infancy, childhood, or adolescence not otherwise specified

behaviors exhibited in these disorders, however, are not "normal" at any age.

In this chapter, we do not discuss adjustment disorders in children (Newcorn and Strain 1992) or problems of parent-child relationships. Child development and child psychiatric treatment are discussed in Chapters 4 and 35, respectively. Important psychiatric disorders in youth, including mood and anxiety disorders, substance use disorders, eating disorders, and schizophrenia, also are described elsewhere in this volume. Although these conditions generally present with symptoms during childhood, they are not usually diagnosed until the individual reaches maturity.

Just as psychopathological influences can undergo developmental expansion during early life, so can early therapeutic interventions. In knowing and treating childhood psychopathology, professionals serve children and the adults they become (parents, caregivers) as well as adults and the children they once were.

ATTENTION-DEFICIT/ HYPERACTIVITY DISORDER

Children or adults with attention-deficit/hyperactivity disorder (ADHD) show the behavioral characteristics of impulsivity (or motor hyperactivity), the cognitive characteristics of inattention (e.g., short attention span and distractibility), or both. The DSM-IV criteria (Table 23–2) no longer suggest that ADHD is a child's disorder, a loose mix of scattered attention and annoying behaviors, or a problem that is confined to one setting. Although ADHD is now understood to affect people of all ages, most of the available research has concentrated on children and adolescents. Many documented findings about ADHD in children and adolescents point to working hypotheses and speculations about ADHD in adults. So far, most findings concerning ADHD in adults have been consistent with previous findings in youths with ADHD.

Originally described in antiquity and documented anecdotally throughout the world literature, ADHD was first identified on a large scale in the early 20th century, when children with von Economo's encephalitis developed symptoms of hyperactivity, impulsivity, and inattention. Impulsive children such as these have been labeled as having "minimal brain damage" (even though there is no direct evidence of brain damage), "minimal brain dysfunction" (although overt neurological damage can produce similar dysfunctions), "hyperkinetic syndrome" (although more is involved than motor systems alone), and "hyperactivity

syndrome" (although 50% of all "normal" boys are rated as "hyperactive" by their parents and teachers).

Psychostimulant therapy of behavior disorders is one the oldest and most established psychopharmacological treatments. Although there have been more than 200 double-blind demonstrations of its clinical effectiveness in children, some aspects of its clinical use remain open to question. Despite 60 years of identification of ADHD and its treatment with psychostimulants, the disorder is often "diagnosed" in clinical practice after a beneficial response to an empirical trial of psychostimulant medication. However, therapeutic responsiveness to a drug (or drug category) cannot be taken as a biological marker of a single disorder, because many psychiatric conditions respond to psychostimulants. Similarly, behavioral predictors of stimulant response are quite nonspecific. In children particularly, it is unsatisfying that this drug-treatable disorder is defined purely by the co-occurrence of common behaviors. Unfortunately, in adults and children, this diagnostic label is not clinically meaningful and is often functionally equivalent to "stimulant-responsive impulsivity."

More generally, there remains considerable uncertainty about the validity of ADHD as a diagnostic entity. For example, there is ongoing debate about whether ADHD should be conceptualized in "dimensional" terms (i.e., the disorder is best described by a set of numbers quantitating its various symptoms, each of which may be present in greater or lesser amounts—a multispectrum disorder) or in categorical terms (i.e., the disorder is best described as present or absent, because its features distinguish it from other disorders—with no in-between disorders). These two models support different concepts of the illness: ADHD may be viewed as a diverse group of behavior-management problems or as a disorder with a final common physiological pathway. Clinically, both models are useful.

CLINICAL DESCRIPTION

Major symptoms include motoric hyperactivity, impulsivity, and inattention. These symptoms are emphasized in DSM-IV and often viewed as the "core" symptoms of ADHD. Because measures of activity and attention in ADHD generally are only weakly correlated, the two symptoms appear to reflect independent dimensions of psychopathology. These two dimensions are also independent in children without psychiatric disorders. In factor analyses of behavioral ratings on Conners' Hyperactivity Scale and the Achenbach Child Behavioral Checklist (CBCL; Achenbach and Ruffle 1998), the "hyperactivity" factor emerges robustly as a distinct component of

TABLE 23–2.   DSM-IV diagnostic criteria for attention-deficit/hyperactivity disorder

A. Either (1) or (2):

(1) Six (or more) of the following symptoms of **inattention** have persisted for at least 6 months to a degree that is maladaptive and inconsistent with developmental level:

Inattention

(a) Often fails to give close attention to details or makes careless mistakes in schoolwork, work, or other activities

(b) Often has difficulty sustaining attention in tasks or play activities

(c) Often does not seem to listen when spoken to directly

(d) Often does not follow through on instructions and fails to finish schoolwork, chores, or duties in the workplace (not due to oppositional behavior or failure to understand instructions)

(e) Often has difficulty organizing tasks and activities

(f) Often avoids, dislikes, or is reluctant to engage in tasks that require sustained mental effort (such as schoolwork or homework)

(g) Often loses things necessary for tasks or activities (e.g., toys, school assignments, pencils, books, or tools)

(h) Is often easily distracted by extraneous stimuli

(i) Is often forgetful in daily activities

(2) Six (or more) of the following symptoms of **hyperactivity-impulsivity** have persisted for at least 6 months to a degree that is maladaptive and inconsistent with developmental level:

Hyperactivity

(a) Often fidgets with hands or feet or squirms in seat

(b) Often leaves seat in classroom or in other situations in which remaining seated is expected

(c) Often runs about or climbs excessively in situations in which it is inappropriate (in adolescents or adults, may be limited to subjective feelings of restlessness)

(d) Often has difficulty playing or engaging in leisure activities quietly

(e) Is often "on the go" or often acts as if "driven by a motor"

(f) Often talks excessively

Impulsivity

(g) Often blurts out answers before questions have been completed

(h) Often has difficulty awaiting turn

(i) Often interrupts or intrudes on others (e.g., butts into conversations or games)

B. Some hyperactive-impulsive or inattentive symptoms that caused impairment were present before age 7 years.

C. Some impairment from the symptoms is present in two or more settings (e.g., at school [or work] and at home).

D. There must be clear evidence of clinically significant impairment in social, academic, or occupational functioning.

E. The symptoms do not occur exclusively during the course of a pervasive developmental disorder, schizophrenia, or other psychotic disorder and are not better accounted for by another mental disorder (e.g., mood disorder, anxiety disorder, dissociative disorder, or personality disorder).

Code based on type:

314.01   Attention-deficit/hyperactivity   disorder, combined type: if both Criteria A1 and A2 are met for the past 6 months.
314.00   Attention-deficit/hyperactivity disorder, predominantly inattentive type: if criterion A1 is met but criterion A2 is not met for the past 6 months.
314.01   Attention-deficit/hyperactivity disorder, predominantly hyperactive-impulsive type: if criterion A2 is met but criterion A1 is not met for the past 6 months.

Coding note: For individuals (especially adolescents and adults) who currently have symptoms that no longer meet full criteria, "in partial remission" should be specified.

---

general childhood behavior, and "inattention" emerges as a separate factor less powerfully but consistently in clinical and community samples of children.

This separation between the cognitive and the behavioral factors is clinically useful. The DSM-IV subtyping of ADHD into "predominantly inattentive," "predominantly hyperactive-impulsive," and "combined" types allows the diagnostic label of ADHD to designate three of the most pronounced symptom complexes. Each of these three

DSM-IV ADHD "subtypes" appears to have a distinct prognosis and response to psychosocial treatment; therefore, the separate clinical assessment of inattention and hyperactivity/impulsivity is necessary.

The DSM-IV diagnosis of ADHD Not Otherwise Specified (NOS) subsumes conditions similar to ADHD that do not fulfill diagnostic criteria. Although this might be expected to be a diagnosis of convenience (useful for paperwork) rather than a biologically distinct disorder, researchers using quantitative electroencephalography (EEG) and evoked response potentials have found electrophysiological characteristics that distinguish ADHD-NOS from the three main forms of ADHD (Kuperman et al. 1996). This finding suggests that an additional form of ADHD may exist, that it is currently hidden within the group of patients with ADHD-NOS, and that focused research on individuals with ADHD-NOS is warranted.

Naturalistic measurements of children with ADHD generally show that their motor activity is high across various environmental settings (Porrino et al. 1983). In situations in which motor activity in all children is expected to be high (in the cafeteria, at recess, and in the gym), activity levels are quantitatively similar in both children with and children without ADHD. In contrast, children with ADHD are most different from "normal" children during structured classroom activities. Even at their quietest, children with ADHD show excessive activity. Motor activity remains elevated during sleep, suggesting that "attention" is not the central or primary area of deficit.

Although people with ADHD tend to be symptomatic in many if not all settings, the intensity of symptoms varies across settings. Symptoms can vary with environmental structure, sensory stimulation, and emotional state, as well as with physiological factors such as general alertness, hunger, and sleep deprivation. Many children experience more environmental stimulation and affective "pressure" at school than at home, and the "overflow" into hyperactivity and impulsivity is particularly clear in classrooms and job sites, where people are expected to inhibit their physical and mental impulses. Hyperactivity/impulsivity and inattention are also readily viewed in noisy places and group settings that require some physical stillness, such as fast-food restaurants or movie theaters. Depending on whether home or hospital unit is more stimulating or disruptive, a child with ADHD can become more symptomatic or can "improve" when hospitalized (such hospitalizations are usually due to the comorbid disorders, because ADHD itself rarely justifies hospitalization). ADHD patients may appear quite different to observers in different environments, such as the home, school or job, hospital, or supermarket. Symptoms are often more apparent in the "real world" (crowded waiting rooms or clinic hallways) than to a physician in a quiet office.

Although DSM-IV emphasizes the three core symptoms, pathological functioning is also seen in motivation, emotionality, anger control, and aggressivity. Noncompliance with instructions or plans, "forgetting" to bring required work or study materials, losing track of goals and of conversation flow, lessened ability to formulate a plan in-

volving sequential actions, problems in multitasking, and other symptoms of "disorganization" are common in ADHD.

Motivational problems in ADHD can include variability, unpredictability, difficulty in sustaining interest and completing projects, and simple frustration and discouragement. Although these characteristics are considered in DSM-IV to be "associated features" of ADHD, lack of motivation and difficulty in self-organization produce more functional interference than do the "core" symptoms of ADHD in many cases.

Emotional impulsivity is most obvious in anger and aggressive behavior. These symptoms can be regularly triggered in response to minor provocation. Once started, anger or aggression can stimulate a further increase in impulsivity; that is, anger can stimulate itself.

Exploratory behavior can seem "aggressive," involving an energetic foraging into new places and things. On entering a room, a child with ADHD may immediately begin to touch and climb. These "exploratory" inclinations can lead to rough handling of objects, accidental breakage, intrusive entry into unsafe areas, physical injuries including bone fractures, and accidental ingestions. Property damage may result without malicious intent (i.e., nonangry destructiveness).

Not all children with ADHD have behavior problems, hyperactivity, or excessive aggressivity. The predominantly inattentive type of ADHD is relatively less common in psychiatric populations (inpatients) and more common in other settings, such as learning disorder clinics, where the threshold for entry does not require high levels of aggressivity. In contrast to children with the predominantly hyperactive type of ADHD, predominantly inattentive children show more manageable behavior, mild anxiety and shyness, more sluggishness and drowsiness, less impulsivity, less conduct disorder and problem behavior, and more mood and anxiety disorders (Gaub and Carlson 1997; Lahey et al. 1987). Like the predominantly hyperactive children with ADHD, their inattention can be psychostimulant-responsive (Famularo and Fenton 1987).

Girls and women with ADHD have received little study. Nearly all ADHD research has been concerned with preadolescent boys. Generally, girls have been reported to have less impulsivity and conduct disorder than boys; therefore, it may be appropriate to use a lower cutoff score for girls on rating scales of hyperactivity and conduct disorder (Berry et al. 1985). However, factor analysis of behavioral data in adults with ADHD suggests that certain inattention and impulsivity items load on different factors in men than in women; that is, gender affects factor composition. Therefore, the core behaviors of ADHD may have more distinctive mechanisms in men versus women than is currently believed (Stein et al. 1995). Girls with ADHD have been reported to show more fear, depression, mood swings, cognitive difficulties, and language problems than boys with ADHD.

The sense of time has been proposed to be a common feature of ADHD, although this feature has received relatively little attention. Impairments in time sense, along with other characteristics of ADHD, might contribute (although independently of mathematics disorder or sequencing problems) to poor planning, lateness, difficulty in correcting self-regulation, gross mistaken sense of past or recent events, and genuine surprise at unexpected outcomes.

The affective and cognitive experiences of a person with ADHD may be heuristically likened to perceptions under a strobe light. Sudden attentional shifts and brief flashes of experience lead to a constantly changing and disjointed view of the world. Disconnected experiences might impair the ability to form complex cognitions, respond emotionally, and learn social norms. In some cases, attention shifting appears to complicate learning about human emotions and complex thinking.

Although inattention and impulsivity/hyperactivity are currently the two defining dimensions of ADHD in DSM-IV, the organizational deficits, motivational problems, and impaired time sense in ADHD deserve considerably more clinical attention. These features might constitute three additional dimensions of ADHD. If the impulsivity and hyperactivity dimensions were eventually parsed into components, ADHD could then be identified with six independent dimensions. Although the current two-dimensional concept of ADHD has some degree of clinical usefulness and scientific validity, it is likely that our construct of ADHD will become much more differentiated and multidimensional.

EPIDEMIOLOGY

In the United States, approximately 10% of boys and 2% of girls have ADHD, and the general prevalence in the school-age population has been estimated at 6% (range 3%–10%). ADHD is present in 30%–50% of child psychiatric outpatients and in 40%–70% of child psychiatric inpatients. The strong male predominance ranges from 3 to 10 boys for each girl. Although girls are generally reported to constitute 10%–25% of children with ADHD, this may be an underestimate resulting from the expectations of diagnosticians. Women may constitute a higher proportion of the adult ADHD population than men, and, compared to men, present for treatment more frequently (Wender

1987). About 17% of children with ADHD are extrafamilial adoptees, compared to 4% of child psychiatric patients and 1% of the general population (Deutsch et al. 1982).

The prevalence of childhood ADHD has been consistently reported to be higher in the United States than in other countries. This difference has been hypothesized to result from exposure to products of advanced technologies (such as lead-containing gasoline, paints, and synthetic food additives), but it is more likely due to diagnostic practices. Traditionally, about 2% of child psychiatric outpatients in Great Britain have a diagnosis of ADHD versus 40% in the United States. DSM-IV criteria require that there be symptoms of ADHD in two or more settings but not necessarily all. In England, the diagnostic label has usually been restricted to children with "pervasive" presentations (symptoms occurring in all settings, including home and school or job). Those with "situational" symptoms (occurring only in certain settings, such as home or school) have not been designated as having ADHD in Great Britain. Also, comorbid ADHD with conduct disorder has traditionally been diagnosed as conduct disorder in England but as ADHD in the United States. These differences reflect the emphasis in the United States on biological causes and drug treatment of ADHD and the British emphasis on social causes and psychological treatment of conduct disorder.

Pharmacoepidemiological studies have estimated that 2%–4% of the United States school population were being treated with psychostimulant medications in the mid-1980s. Family physicians treated about 60% of these children (vs. 98% in the early 1970s). Psychostimulants were prescribed for 20% of special education students. Public campaigns by the Church of Scientology in the late 1980s appear to have contributed to a temporary reduction in the clinical use of psychostimulants (Safer and Krager 1992). Between 1990 and 1995, however, there has been a 2.5-fold rise in the use of stimulants in the United States (Safer et al. 1996), and significant increases have also been noted in Australia (Valentine et al. 1997). Factors that have been proposed to explain this sudden increase in stimulant use include the growing recognition and treatment of ADHD in adolescents and adults, increasing drug treatment of predominantly inattentive ADHD, more extensive treatment of young females, lengthier treatments, physician familiarity and comfort in prescribing psychostimulants for ADHD, increased visibility of ADHD and its treatment in the public media, and the growth of national organizations such as Children and Adults with ADD (ChADD) that provide grassroots support and information to individuals and families affected by ADHD.

ETIOLOGY AND MECHANISMS

There is no evidence that there is only one attention deficit or that a single brain mechanism is responsible for all manifestations of ADHD. Similarly, there is no evidence of a single gene defect or a specific mechanism of genetic transmission in ADHD, and the hereditary component will probably be explained as polygenic (Vandenberg et al. 1986). Different etiologies and different sites of psychostimulant action may be relevant for different individuals with ADHD.

Genetics

Although family studies have suggested strong genetic and nongenetic contributions (Pauls 1991), the genetic ones appear to predominate (Sherman et al. 1997). The prevalence of psychopathology is two to three times higher in the relatives of children with ADHD, even after controlling for socioeconomic class and family intactness. In adopted children with ADHD, biological parents have been found to have more psychopathology than adopting parents (Deutsch et al. 1982). Family members of children with ADHD show an increased prevalence of ADHD, conduct disorder and antisocial personality disorder, mood disorders, anxiety disorders, and substance abuse.

The family transmission of ADHD is particularly prominent in males. It is common in clinical practice to find families in which ADHD is present in numerous males across generations. Girls with ADHD are diagnosed less commonly and appear to have less gender-specific transmission of ADHD than boys. However, girls with ADHD generally have a stronger family history of ADHD than boys with ADHD, suggesting a higher genetic loading for ADHD in girls (Vandenberg et al. 1986) and a higher "gene load" threshold. This "gender threshold effect" might be explained by a variety of biological, psychodynamic, and cultural factors, such as reduced penetrance for the expression of the genetic form of ADHD in girls, gender-related differences in the profile of ADHD etiologies or symptoms, gender-based differences in cognitive processing and processing mechanisms in the central nervous system, or cultural differences in the frequency or recognition of aggressivity and impulsivity in boys and girls. In any case, it seems that genetic loading can interact with gender-related factors in modulating the phenomenology of ADHD.

A strong genetic influence is consistent with findings that ADHD appears in particular families that comorbidly transmit other psychiatric disorders, so that ADHD appears to form clusters with certain psychiatric conditions that are transmitted together in particular families. Such findings suggest that genetic factors related to comorbidity might be relevant to an etiologically based subtyping of ADHD; for example, ADHD may present with (or as) bipolar disorder in some families and with (or as) anxiety disorders in other families. Such familial patterns of ADHD comorbidity have been frequently described; however, the literature is full of inconsistencies regarding ADHD comorbidity, and contrary to common belief, one cannot yet conclude that patients with ADHD have an increased prevalence of comorbid anxiety disorders (Perrin and Last 1996), substance abuse (Hazell 1997), or mood disorders in adulthood (Murphy and Barkley 1996). Furthermore, separate genetic factors may be involved in the etiology of different features of ADHD (Sherman et al. 1997) or of associated features of ADHD.

Specific genetic mechanisms are beginning to be described. Although the extent of genetic influence appears to vary, there seem to be individuals who have a primarily genetic version of the disorder. A single-gene (20p11–p12 region), autosomal dominant, sex-influenced pattern has been identified in some families (Hess et al. 1995).

Another genetic mechanism that appears relevant in ADHD is the D_4 dopamine receptor. The D_4 receptor, distributed in cortical and limbic regions, has been associated with novelty-seeking behavior. The gene for D_4 dopamine receptor has a region with a 48-bp repeat sequence that has been found to have the sevenfold repetition more frequently in children with ADHD than in children without ADHD. This receptor form mediates a diminished intracellular response to dopamine, effectively functioning as an underresponsive receptor (LaHoste et al. 1996). These findings suggest a specific link between D_4 receptor pathology and a decreased postreceptor response to postsynaptic dopamine in ADHD.

The genetics of the dopamine transporter is another potential clue to understanding ADHD. The dopamine transporter is carrier protein involved in presynaptic reuptake of dopamine, and the gene for the dopamine transporter (480-bp DAT1) has also been associated with ADHD. Linkage has been established between ADHD and the gene for the dopamine D_2 receptor, which has been associated with central reward mechanisms (Blum et al. 1996). Also, a chromosome containing two separate specific alleles (the null allele of the C4B gene and the β-1 allele of the DR gene) located within the major histocompatibility complex that appears to produce immunological substances has been identified in 55% of individuals with ADHD and in only 8% of control subjects (Odell et al. 1997).

Variations in the dopamine transporter, the dopamine D_4 receptor, and the D_2 receptor suggest that several variants in dopaminergic structures may be helpful in exploring the mechanisms underlying ADHD and that immune functions associated with the major histocompatibility complex may be involved in the etiology of some common forms of ADHD.

Together, these genetic findings suggest that immune functions encoded within the major histocompatibility complex may be involved in the etiology of some common forms of ADHD; in addition, variations in the dopamine transporter, the dopamine D_4 receptor, and the D_2 receptor suggest that variants in several dopaminergic structures may be helpful in exploring the mechanisms underlying ADHD.

General Medical Factors

A variety of medical factors can lead to the appearance of ADHD or ADHD-like symptoms, including streptococcal infection, (generalized) resistance to thyroid hormone, hyperthyroidism, ordinary hunger, and occasionally constipation. Certain psychiatric medications may mimic ADHD by inducing anxiety, agitation, manic switch, behavioral activation, or disinhibition. These medications include psychostimulants, antidepressants, carbamazepine, valproate, benzodiazepines, and phenobarbital, as well as substances such as caffeine or theophylline.

Pediatric autoimmune neuropsychiatric disorders associated with streptococcal infections (PANDAS), such as obsessive-compulsive disorder and Tourette's disorder, present with ADHD symptoms (see the section "Tic Disorders" later in the chapter). About half of the preadolescent children with PANDAS have symptoms of ADHD (Swedo et al. 1998).

Generalized resistance to thyroid hormone (GRTH) results from an autosomal dominant mutation in the human thyroid receptor (chromosome 3) that makes target sites underresponsive to the action of thyroid hormone, and 50% of the cases present with ADHD (Hauser et al. 1993). It is interesting that GRTH in males is associated with brain abnormalities accrued during early fetal development, including multiple appearances of Heschl's gyrus bilaterally and Sylvian fissure anomalies in the left hemisphere (Leonard et al. 1995). Although GRTH is often associated with ADHD, the reverse is not true: the prevalence of GRTH among ADHD patients is too low to warrant routine thyroid screening. Apart from the uncommon disorder of GRTH, thyroid disorders are diagnosed in about 2%–3% of children with ADHD, which is within the 1%–4% prevalence rate for a general pediatric population (Valentine et al. 1997). However, the association of GRTH with low intelligence might be stronger than its association with ADHD (Weiss et al. 1994), and the apparent association of GRTH and ADHD might be mediated by intelligence.

Nutrition is a critical factor in the development of the central nervous system. Severe early malnutrition is probably the most common cause of ADHD worldwide. In children who experience severe malnutrition during the first year of life, 60% show inattention, impulsivity, and hyperactivity persisting at least into adolescence (Galler et al. 1983). In addition, pyloric stenosis is associated with the subsequent appearance of ADHD, even when corrected by age 2 months. The specific nutritional deficiencies that contribute to the etiology of ADHD are unknown.

Hyperthyroidism only rarely underlies ADHD. Very rarely, hunger (without malnutrition) and constipation are causes of acute transient but repeated episodes of ADHD symptoms.

Neuromedical Factors

Neuromedical etiologies of ADHD include brain damage (often frontal cortex), neurological disorders, low birth weight, perinatal anoxia of extreme severity, and exposure to neurotoxins (pre- and postnatal).

Intrauterine exposure to toxic substances, including alcohol, lead, cigarette smoke, and probably cocaine, can produce teratogenic effects on behavior. For example, fetal alcohol syndrome includes hyperactivity, impulsivity, and inattention as well as physical anomalies and diminished intelligence.

Lead can produce a broad range of toxic effects, especially during development, and these effects are more common and more persistent than generally realized. Both prenatal and postnatal toxic lead exposure can precede ADHD and other cognitive deficits (Bellinger et al. 1987). Transient lead exposure during childhood produces neurocognitive and neurobehavioral abnormalities that may persist for 10 or more years. Although its physical toxicity rises in a dose-dependent manner, there appears to be no minimal level below which lead ceases to have toxic effects on the development of cognition. A doubling of blood lead levels (from 100 to 200 µg/L) has been associated with an estimated mean reduction of 1–3 IQ points (Winneke and Krämer 1997).

Children with ADHD have higher mean blood lead levels than their siblings. In first-grade students, a dose-response relationship has been found between lead concentrations in hair and teachers' ratings of disruptive behavior, regardless of socioeconomic class. A large-scale study in Ottawa showed a topological distribution of children with ADHD living in public housing, perhaps reflecting the lead-containing paints in residential buildings

(Trites 1979). However, far higher Connors scores were observed in children living near a major roadway, apparently demonstrating the strong effect of lead-containing gasolines (Figure 23–1).

Intrauterine exposure to cigarette smoke appears to be associated with ADHD. In one study, 22% of the mothers of children with ADHD smoked during pregnancy, compared to 8% of the mothers of children without ADHD (Milberger et al. 1996).

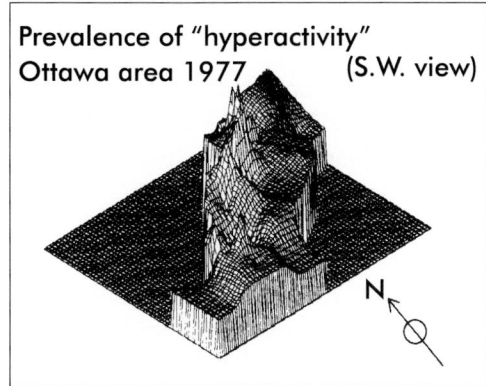

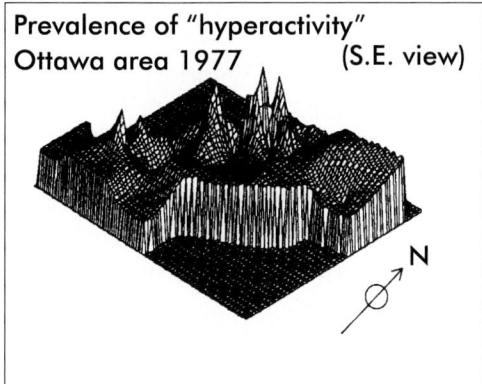

FIGURE 23–1. Map of Ottawa showing topographic distribution of hyperactivity scores on the Conners Teaching Rating Scale administered to 14,000 elementary school children in Ottawa, Canada. The scores are topographically exhibited on a map of the city. The peaks and valleys are population-corrected. A river runs along the low side of the plot. About one-half of the peak areas appear in low socioeconomic regions. Some peaks clearly coincide with high-density public housing, perhaps reflecting the effects of lead paint in the dwellings. The main peaks follow the course of the Queen Mary Highway, a major source of lead-containing gas emissions in the 1970s.
Source. Reprinted with permission from Trites RL: "Prevalence of Hyperactivity in Ottawa, Canada," in *Hyperactivity in Children.* Edited by Trites RL. Baltimore, MD, University Park Press, 1979. Copyright 1979, University Park Press.

Obstetrical complications during late pregnancy or delivery may result in ADHD, but only occasionally. Contrary to earlier belief, only the most severe perinatal problems increase the risk of enduring changes in brain function. Generally, obstetrical difficulties and perinatal asphyxia are not tightly correlated with the appearance of neurological disorders such as cerebral palsy (Nelson and Ellenberg 1986), and such events probably do not account for more than a small percentage of cases of ADHD (Nichols and Chen 1981). Instead, prenatal predisposing factors seem more important than birth or perinatal complications in the etiology of ADHD and probably of other neuropsychiatric disorders. Prenatal predisposing factors appear to increase the risk both for both ADHD and for birth complications. For example, low birth weight is predictive of subsequent ADHD, regardless of whether there were obstetrical complications. Correlations between two characteristics (e.g., perinatal distress and neuropsychiatric disorder) might not reflect a causal link, because a remote causal factor (e.g., maternal behavior, pica, prenatal care, socioeconomic factors, lead exposure) may contribute to the appearance of both characteristics.

Overt neurological disorders, most commonly seizures and cerebral palsy, are present in 5% of children with ADHD, but they do not correlate with the severity of ADHD symptoms. Like other children with learning and behavior disorders, children with ADHD may have multiple minor physical and neurological anomalies. Nonlocalizing neurological "soft signs" (e.g., clumsiness, left-right confusion, perceptual-motor dyscoordination, and dysgraphia) are commonly seen in children with ADHD; however, 15% of normal children exhibit up to five neurological soft signs, so the clinical relevance is usually presumed to be insignificant. ADHD is associated with a mild decrement in IQ, but it is so small that it is measurable only in comparison to sibling controls, and it might be due only to attention-related test behaviors.

ADHD with onset after toddlerhood suggests the presence of "acquired" neuropathological changes, such as traumatic brain injury, encephalitis, or CNS infection. Frontal lobe injury is often involved in ADHD, but brain lesions in a variety of locations can lead to a clinical picture that resembles ADHD and responds to medication in a similar manner. Brain localization may be crucial to specific ADHD symptoms and might be related to variations in clinical presentation, prognosis, and treatment outcome.

Right Hemisphere Syndrome

ADHD-like symptoms are present in 93% of people with right hemisphere syndrome (Voeller 1986). Right hemisphere syndrome is not a medical disorder, a result of injury or disease, or a learning disorder in the usual sense (involving a particular skill, such as reading or arithmetic). Instead, it consists of a series of right cortical deficits that can appear in healthy individuals who have difficulties in learning, memory, concentration, and organization. The entire right hemisphere appears to be involved, and no more specific localization is assignable. Typically from birth, children with right hemisphere syndrome grow up with nonverbal learning problems; often familial transmission is evident.

Right hemisphere syndrome is readily identifiable in routine intelligence testing by a verbal IQ score that is significantly higher than the performance IQ score. Usually, a 20-point IQ difference can generate noticeable characteristics, and 20- to 50-point differences account for most cases. Extreme cases can involve differences of 100 points or more. The level of intelligence in individuals with right hemisphere syndrome ranges from retarded to brilliant.

The crucial feature in right hemisphere syndrome is not poor right hemisphere functioning but a marked mismatch between the "intelligence" of each hemisphere. Because neither hemisphere is usually defective, right hemisphere syndrome is typically conceptualized as a "difference" in functioning rather than as a "medical disorder." In addition to the expected right-sided characteristics classically seen in patients with right hemisphere neurological damage, individuals with right hemisphere syndrome have what might be called "social dyslexia": difficulty in perceiving and reacting to social cues, bafflement at or incomplete comprehension of other people's sense of humor (although they may be quite witty themselves), generally slow acquisition of social skills, the disadvantage of being viewed by others as different or a bit strange (but not at all bizarre), and a tendency to become angry or aggressive because of social misunderstandings. Depressive disorders seem to be overrepresented, perhaps because depressive symptoms are often associated with relatively weak right-sided functioning as well as with diminished social functioning and demoralization. As children and adults, individuals with right hemisphere syndrome are far more verbally gifted than their other achievements might suggest.

The ADHD characteristics in right hemisphere syndrome typically respond poorly to medications, but cognitive-behavioral treatment (including interventions at school or on the job) appears helpful. A more ambitious approach is a developmentally guided cognitive therapy, similar in some ways to the neuropsychological rehabilitative treatments offered to people who have sustained major brain trauma. This constructional treatment involves step-by-step learning, starting with simple mental tasks, progressively building on newly acquired skills, with the progression of specific steps determined by cognitive and developmental principles.

Among adolescents with right hemisphere disorder and ADHD, patients without hyperactivity have been found to have more cognitive difficulty on right hemisphere tasks than do patients with hyperactivity (García-Sánchez et al. 1997). More generally, patients with ADHD have been shown to have widespread anatomical abnormalities in the right hemisphere (Castellanos et al. 1996).

Misdiagnosis

Misidentification does not normally function as an etiological factor, but ADHD can be viewed as a special case because many psychiatric disorders look somewhat similar to ADHD in clinical presentation (Table 23–3). Disorders that look like ADHD ("ADHD look-alikes") include oppositional defiant disorder, conduct disorder, bipolar disorder, Tourette's disorder, posttraumatic stress disorder (PTSD), abuse or neglect (without PTSD), and even major depressive disorder. For example, about 25% of patients who traditionally might have been diagnosed as having ADHD are now diagnosed with bipolar disorder. The high prevalence of ADHD look-alike disorders poses a variety of problems for both diagnostic practice and the understanding of the etiology of ADHD.

TABLE 23–3. **Psychiatric disorders often associated with attention-deficit/hyperactivity disorder**

Conduct disorder

Oppositional defiant disorder

Bipolar disorder

Learning disorders

Motor skills disorder

Substance use disorders

Communication disorders

Major depression

Posttraumatic stress disorder

Obsessive-compulsive disorder

Tourette's disorder

Schizophrenia

Mental retardation

Pervasive developmental disorders, including autistic disorder

Note. Various psychiatric states should be assessed clinically in individuals with ADHD, even though strong statistical associations have not been demonstrated for each of these conditions.

ADHD look-alike disorders pose two problems for diagnosis. First, some patients diagnosed with ADHD in fact have a different psychiatric disorder, so that the ADHD look-alike might be considered to be a form of "counterfeit ADHD" or "pseudo-ADHD." Such patients might receive stimulant treatment that exacerbates their disorder (e.g., psychosis, tics) and fail to receive appropriate treatment for their medical problem (e.g., neuroleptics). Second, some patients who have ADHD are diagnosed with and treated for an irrelevant disorder; they can be considered to have a form of "masked ADHD" or "hidden ADHD." Such patients might inappropriately receive benzodiazepines or lithium, because they were misdiagnosed as having an anxiety disorder or bipolar disorder. In cases of both masked ADHD and counterfeit ADHD, misdiagnosis may delay appropriate treatment or produce iatrogenic complications.

Such misdiagnosis leads to faulty or confusing research findings on etiology. In studies of patient samples with counterfeit ADHD, irrelevant etiological factors may be attributed to ADHD (e.g., aggression attributed to ADHD rather than conduct disorder, provocative behavior overattributed to ADHD rather than oppositional defiant disorder or bipolar disorder). Similarly, in studies focused on other disorders, the presence of subjects who have hidden ADHD may lead to a false association of ADHD characteristics with the other disorder (e.g., impulsivity attributed to conduct disorder rather than ADHD). Such misdiagnosis can influence the understanding of the etiology of ADHD, as well as of ADHD look-alikes, by distorting scientific findings.

This problem is more severe and pervasive with ADHD than with other disorders because groups of persons with ADHD often are flooded with diagnostic contamination. ADHD is unique, at least in psychiatry, in being a highly prevalent disorder that is misdiagnosed in a large proportion (and perhaps even the majority) of cases. Although misdiagnosis can distort the understanding and treatment of any medical condition, ADHD is a special case because of the high frequency of diagnostic error. This situation goes beyond the common problem of diagnostic contamination reducing the "purity" of a patient group (patient caseload or study sample); the results may be extensive damage to the diagnosis, treatment, and understanding of ADHD.

Because of the advances afforded by the major diagnostic systems, misdiagnosis of ADHD is probably declining. Recent studies have suggested that about 90% of patients treated for ADHD in community settings appear to have valid diagnoses, at least as judged by symptoms documented in the medical records. Nonetheless, the impact of ADHD look-alikes on etiological understanding and clinical practice remains to be adequately assessed and controlled. As recognition of the ADHD look-alike conditions grows, the process of diagnosing ADHD has become more complex and sophisticated. To diagnose ADHD, all ADHD look-alike conditions need to be considered and ruled out (Table 23–3).

COMORBIDITY

Although ADHD can mimic or be mimicked by other disorders, it can also present concurrently with other DSM-IV disorders, and it often does. For example, ADHD is associated with a high prevalence of all learning, motor, and communication disorders. Similarly, ADHD has a relatively high prevalence in samples of individuals with mental retardation. These common comorbidities may result from shared neurodevelopmental etiologies (learning or communication disorders) or shared related prenatal pathology (mental retardation). In general, the possibility of comorbid learning disorders or mental retardation needs to considered whenever ADHD is diagnosed.

As previously discussed, there is continuing debate about the possible clustering of ADHD with other diagnoses such as major depressive disorder and certain anxiety disorders. When such clustering occurs, the usual diagnostic question ("Is this ADHD or something else?") is further complicated by the possibility of comorbid presentation ("It could be ADHD or something else, but it could also be ADHD and something else presenting concurrently"). The possibility of a comorbid presentation of ADHD and another psychiatric disorder (including an ADHD look-alike) must be considered whenever a diagnosis of ADHD is evaluated. The possibility of comorbidity can generate complications in differential diagnosis (bipolar disorder vs. ADHD) and also in choices regarding target symptoms, symptom control, and safety.

ADHD can divert the clinician's attention away from concurrent psychopathologies, and vice versa. The comorbid conditions might not be treated adequately if the treatment is overfocused on the disruptive behavior, and ADHD might not be adequately addressed if a patient has a prominent anxiety disorder or bipolar disorder. A diagnosis of ADHD is not excluded by the presence of learning and communication disorders, mental retardation, or any other psychopathology. In fact, there are no disorders whose presence excludes a diagnosis of ADHD.

Conduct Disorder

Conduct disorder (not merely conduct problems or symptoms) is seen in 40%–70% of children with ADHD, and about the same percentage of children with conduct disorder have ADHD (Soussignan and Tremblay 1996). This high comorbidity rate of ADHD and conduct disorder implies that most of the available ADHD literature is based on studies of children who did not simply have ADHD but instead had conduct disorder with comorbid ADHD. That is, the current concept of ADHD is likely to consist of some characteristics that are true of conduct disorder and not of ADHD.

For example, there is some question whether excessively aggressive behavior is more of a component of ADHD or of conduct disorder. Similarly, are language disorders associated with ADHD or with conduct disorder? Is antisocial personality disorder, long viewed as a major developmental risk for children with ADHD, merely a reflection of the more expectable adult outcome of conduct disorder in children? Only occasionally do children with the predominantly inattentive type of ADHD have conduct disorder or aggressive behavior. Several studies have suggested that conduct disorder is not closely linked to the presence of attention deficit but that aggressivity may be associated more closely with conduct disorder than with ADHD.

The reattribution of aggressive behavior to conduct disorder (or oppositional defiant disorder) rather than ADHD has important treatment implications for the management of aggressivity. Steps toward separating the symptoms of conduct disorder from the symptoms of ADHD allow a more accurate understanding of ADHD. Children with "predominantly hyperactive/impulsive ADHD plus conduct disorder" have been found to have high levels of family psychopathology, whereas the predominantly inattentive type of ADHD is linked to neurological disorders, lower IQ, and additional cognitive deficits (August et al. 1983).

Tic Disorders

Tourette's disorder is overrepresented in patients with ADHD, and at least 25% of males with Tourette's disorder have ADHD. Obsessive-compulsive disorder (OCD) in children also appears to be linked to ADHD, often in association with Tourette's disorder. One of the earliest signals of this association was the unexpected finding (Achenbach and Edelbrock 1983) that, as a group, children with ADHD have high ratings for obsessive-compulsive features on the Achenbach and Edelbrock Child Behavior Checklist than do children without ADHD (Figure 23–2). More recently, children who have comorbid tic disorder with ADHD as well as those who have comorbid OCD with ADHD have been found to have antistrepto-

coccal/antineuronal antibodies. About half of these PANDAS fulfill criteria for ADHD (Swedo et al. 1998). This association is described more fully in the section "Tic Disorders" later in the chapter.

The comorbid appearance of ADHD, Tourette's disorder, and OCD has emerged as a clinically significant cluster of diagnoses, with each of these three disorders apparently sharing a common genetic etiology. Their shared genetic characteristics suggest that ADHD associated with Tourette's disorder and/or OCD might be different from other forms of ADHD in terms of physiological, phenomenological, or pharmacological features. For example, such genes might increase vulnerability to streptococcal infections, leading to the autoimmune forms of ADHD syptoms (see the section "Tic Disorders" later in the chapter). Alternatively, aggressive behavior in some patients with ADHD may result partially from the anxiety associated with OCD or from the complex tics associated with Tourette's disorder. Children with concurrent ADHD, Tourette's disorder, and OCD can be appropriately treated with serotonin reuptake inhibitors and concurrently with either stimulants or low doses of neuroleptic agents. These medication regimens are not usually considered first-line treatments of ADHD, but they can reduce inattention, hyperactivity, and impulsivity in patients with ADHD, OCD, and Tourette's disorder.

Pervasive Developmental Disorders

Autistic disorder presents so commonly with ADHD that the DSM-III-R criteria (American Psychiatric Association 1987) for ADHD excluded its diagnosis in the presence of autism. In DSM-IV that exclusion has been removed, so patients with autistic disorder and ADHD can legitimately be treated with psychostimulants without the necessity of declaring autism to be a new indication for stimulants.

Psychotic Agitation

Accurate differential diagnosis of psychotic agitation is particularly crucial, because psychostimulant or antidepressant treatment can exacerbate psychotic symptoms. The differentiation can be based on several features. Typically, people with ADHD have absolutely no hallucinations, delusional thinking, or breakthroughs of primary process thinking. However, similar to patients with psychotic disorders, ADHD patients may exhibit "loose" thought patterns, self-endangering behavior, and underawareness of environmental events. The motoric activity in ADHD appears continuous and endless, and the tempo of the impulsivity is roughly constant, in contrast to the irregular and less predictable body and affective tempo of

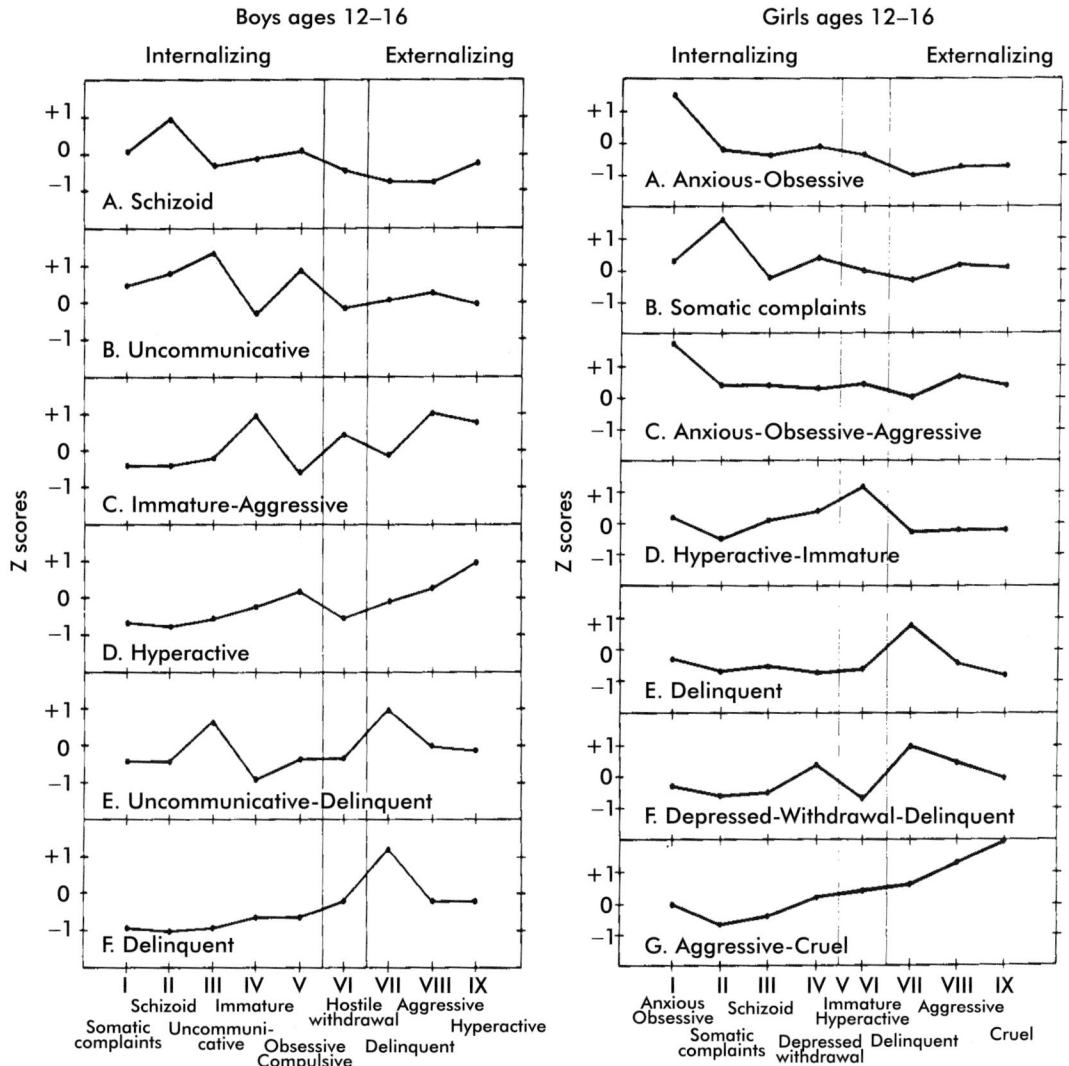

FIGURE 23–2. Behavior profile for attention-deficit/hyperactivity disorder. An early version of the Child Behavior Checklist of Achenbach and Edelbrock (Rapoport 1985; Achenbach and McConaughy 1987) was administered to children with ADHD and analyzed for specific behavioral features. A small peak in obsessive-compulsive behaviors is seen for boys, but not for girls, who have ADHD. A symptom profile may be used for quantitative descriptions of psychopathology in childhood. The updated version of the Child Behavior Checklist includes a new set of symptom groupings that have been identified across reports from parents, teachers, and children. The newer groupings (syndrome constructs) are titled Withdrawn, Somatic Complaints, Anxious/Depressed, Social Problems, Thought Problems, Attention Problems, Delinquent Behavior, and Aggressive Behavior (Achenbach and Ruffle 1998)

Source. Reprinted with permission from Achenbach TM, Edelbrock C: *Manual for the Child Behavioral Checklist and Revised Child Behavioral Profile.* Burlington, VT, University of Vermont Psychology Department, 1983.

psychotic children. Psychotic children may show anger and emotional overreactions that are primarily derived from cognitive (or paranoid) distortions and can have a long duration (30 minutes to 5 hours). In contrast, emotional overreactions in ADHD patients usually are based on misunderstandings and accidents, and tantrums in these patients usually resolve within 30 minutes. Generally, the long-term course of ADHD is gradual improvement. Behavioral worsening, apart from periods of overt

environmental stress, suggests the emergence of a different psychiatric disorder.

Mood and Thought Disorders

Children with ADHD may have an increased prevalence of major depressive disorder, but the findings concerning this association have been mixed. If there is a link, whether minimal or robust, the connection might be in part biological, because both ADHD and major depressive disorder are associated with decreased rapid eye movement (REM) latency, responsiveness to tricyclic antidepressants, genetic interrelationships, anxiety disorders, and bipolar disorder. About 50%–100% of bipolar children are also hyperactive or fulfill ADHD criteria (Butler et al. 1995; West et al. 1996), and about 20%–25% of children with ADHD also fulfill criteria for bipolar disorder (Biederman et al. 1996; Butler et al. 1995). Also, some children of mothers with schizophrenia have motor and attention deficits and, according to follow-up studies, often grow up to become adults with schizophrenia; their non-ADHD siblings have a low incidence of adult schizophrenia (Marcus et al. 1985). Thus, certain children with ADHD may have "precursor conditions" of adult mood or psychotic disorders.

Psychosocial Factors

Psychosocial factors such as situational anxiety, child abuse and neglect, and simple boredom can clinically manifest in symptoms that mimic ADHD. Examination of the course of illness distinguishes these conditions from ADHD.

PATHOPHYSIOLOGY

The large array of etiological factors, mechanisms, symptom overlap, look-alike disorders, comorbid disorders, and complications of illness—and especially their interactions—demonstrates why each individual with ADHD can present with a genuinely unique set of symptoms. This maze also demonstrates why it is so difficult to identify the essential attributes of ADHD as distinct from those of other disorders. Professionals are left wondering, even in individual cases, how to sort through this cloud of causality and identify the "edges" of ADHD itself.

With unclear diagnostic boundaries, it is difficult to define or even conceptualize a unitary concept of ADHD or of its etiology. One generally cannot even specify the sequence of mechanisms involved, because biological findings that might play a role in the etiology might reflect effects of ADHD. One can say with reasonable certainty that both biological and psychosocial factors are involved in shaping the appearance of ADHD in individuals. It remains beyond reach to identify specific etiological events, the balance of etiological factors, or various influences that modify ADHD in a patient. However, it appears that most cases of ADHD, at least in the United States, have their origins somewhere in the biological realm.

Clinical research has yielded a wide variety of biological findings concerning ADHD (and ADHD look-alikes)

that can contribute to the descriptive and etiological understanding of this disorder (Table 23–4). These biological findings reflect the diversity of etiologies that lead to ADHD and, to a lesser degree, the characteristics that are common across the numerous etiologically and phenomenologically similar types of ADHD.

Neurochemical and Pharmacological Studies

Neurochemical studies of ADHD were initially organized around the catecholamine hypothesis, beginning with norepinephrine as the crucial neurotransmitter (Wender 1971). Despite unreplicated and inconsistent neuropharmacological findings, the neurochemical model has undergone numerous revisions over the years. Currently, particular emphasis is placed on the roles of dopamine, serotonin, glutamate, and γ-aminobutyric acid (GABA) in the frontal (especially prefrontal) cortex and the caudate, with less involvement of norepinephrine and acetylcholine. This model has been supported by autoradiographic studies showing the binding of stimulants to the striatal structures and pharmacological studies showing altered stimulant effects when the striatum or frontal cortex is chemically lesioned.

A dopamine hypothesis of ADHD is supported by findings that 1) psychostimulants, still the most effective treatment, have prominent (although not exclusively) dopaminergic effects and that their therapeutic effects are reduced when dopamine receptors are blocked; 2) experimental rats with neonatal lesions of their dopamine neuronal systems have motoric hyperactivity and learning deficits, which are reversed by psychostimulants; 3) children with von Economo's encephalitis acquired an ADHD-like clinical picture (and years later, as adults, Parkinson's disease); 4) low levels of the dopamine metabolite (homovanillic acid) appear in the cerebrospinal fluid of children with ADHD; and 5) children with ADHD have a low spontaneous blink rate (Caplan et al. 1996), which is an observable correlate of dopamine function.

However, the dopamine hypothesis is not supported by findings that 1) dopamine receptor blockers can also exert therapeutic effects, 2) not all dopamine agonists are therapeutic for ADHD, and 3) clinical studies of dopamine concentrations in blood and cerebrospinal fluid have, taken together, yielded quite contradictory findings. The seeming paradoxes concerning the effects of dopamine agonists will probably be resolved when more receptor-specific and subreceptor-specific dopamine agonists and antagonists become available. These differences may also reflect the diverse etiologies of various subtypes of ADHD or perhaps simply reflect different symptoms of ADHD. At

TABLE 23–4. Physical and laboratory findings in attention-deficit/hyperactivity disorder

Motor activity meters

Increased locomotion during daytime (especially during quiet activities) and sleep.

Increased head and body motion during mental concentration.

Increased body motion during sleep.

Upward flattening of the daytime biological rhythm of motor activity (high activity with relatively little diurnal change).

Clinical laboratory

Lead levels increased.

(Thyroid abnormalities—questionable.)

Neuromedical examination

Multiple minor physical anomalies, including neurological "soft signs."

Seizure disorders, with slight increase in electroencephalographic abnormalities.

Low spontaneous blink rate.

Psychological testing

Various signs of distractibility and attentional pathology, variable motivational state, and various localized cortical deficits (often associated with comorbid learning disorders).

Autonomic responsiveness

Mixed findings of increased or decreased autonomic and central "tone."

Sleep physiology

Decreased latency of rapid eye movements.

Increased sleep latency (initial insomnia).

Increased motor activity (restlessness during sleep).

Neuroanatomy

Small right frontal cortex.

Small right-greater-than-left asymmetry of caudate (suggestive that left caudate had less developmental reduction in size).

Small right globus pallidus.

Small right corpus callosum.

Small cerebellum.

Neurotransmitter metabolites

Mixed findings on neurochemical assays of biogenic amines and metabolites in cerebrospinal fluid, but tendency toward low levels of dopamine, norepinephrine, and phenylethylamine, and elevations of serotonin and possibly epinephrine.

Regional metabolism in brain

High blood flow in primary sensory regions of temporal and occipital cortex, and low blood flow in frontal cortex (and usually in caudate nuclei).

Cerebral glucose metabolism reduced by 8%, with decreases in many brain regions, with the largest reductions in the premotor cortex and superior prefrontal cortex.

Clinical pharmacology

Therapeutic responsiveness to psychostimulants, tricyclic antidepressants, and monoamine oxidase inhibitors.

Possibly, responsiveness to α_2-adrenergic agonists (clonidine, guanfacine) and selective serotonin reuptake inhibitors.

Stimulant responders have a smaller left anterior frontal cortex and a smaller and more symmetrical caudate, especially head of caudate, in comparison to both nonresponders and normal controls.

Stimulant nonresponders have reversed caudate asymmetry (left is larger than right) and a smaller parietal-occipital cortex (especially retrocallosal white matter), in comparison to nonresponders and normal controls.

Stimulant nonresponders also have lower α_2-receptor binding (in platelet model).

Note. Many of these findings appear only in certain individuals or subgroups rather than throughout the entire ADHD population.

present, it appears that the eventual availability of receptor-specific dopamine D_4 agonists may provide an important advance in the treatment of ADHD.

A norepinephrine hypothesis of ADHD is supported by 1) reports of low levels of 3-methoxy-4-hydroxyphenylglycol (MHPG) in ADHD, although this finding is complicated by the finding that MHPG levels are lowered even further by psychostimulant treatment; 2) the therapeutic efficacy of tricyclic antidepressants and monoamine oxidase inhibitors (MAOIs), although these agents can also modify serotonin transmission; 3) the therapeutic effectiveness of the α_2 (autoreceptor) agonists clonidine and guanfacine, although their effectiveness has been seriously challenged by recent data; and 4) the diminished platelet α_2-receptor binding in boys with ADHD who do not respond therapeutically to D-amphetamine treatment, compared to normal binding in boys with ADHD who do respond.

Studies of serotonin generally have been inconsistent, but often they have shown elevations of plasma serotonin in children with ADHD. These findings may be contaminated by the low serotonin levels that are commonly found in highly aggressive children, but the serotonin levels appear to be normally distributed and so do not support a subtyping of children with ADHD. In adults with ADHD as well (Ernst et al. 1997), plasma levels of serotonin and its metabolite have been found to correlate with the clinical effects of treatment with L-deprenyl (selegiline), a selective inhibitor of MAO-B.

The proposed explanations of ADHD involving links between specific brain functions and neurotransmitters have been somewhat contradictory. Studies of laboratory rats, involving selective neonatal depletion of catecholamine systems during early development (B. A. Shaywitz et al. 1976), suggested a role of dopamine in behavioral hyperactivity (Teicher and Baldessarini 1987). In a study of circulating bioamines in humans, dopamine measures were found to correlate with the severity of the behavioral symptoms, and norepinephrine measures correlated with performance on tests of attention (Ernst et al. 1997). It has been suggested that norepinephrine is involved in alerting (i.e., signaling) the posterior attention system of the cortex to receive incoming stimuli and that dopamine might influence the cortical anterior attention system, subserving executive functions that are linked to behavioral responses (Pliszka et al. 1996). These findings are consistent with a norepinephrine/attention and dopamine/behavior model of ADHD, with "behavior" encompassing hyperactivity, impulsivity, and self-control. Another study in humans provided evidence for a model of norepinephrine/hyperactivity, dopamine/impulsivity, and serotonin/aggression (Castellanos et al. 1994). In addition, in the same study it was found that increased cerebrospinal fluid (CSF) levels of serotonin were correlated with increased aggression, rather than lowered levels as predicted by prevailing theory, and that CSF levels of dopamine correlated with hyperactivity.

Taken together, the findings of the available neurotransmitter studies in humans are not fully consistent. Nonetheless, they might be interpreted as pointing toward a model linking norepinephrine with attention, dopamine with impulsive behavior (and self-control), serotonin with aggression, and hyperactivity with both norepinephrine and dopamine.

Neuronal circuitry models of ADHD now routinely synthesize findings concerning multiple neurotransmitter systems, including epinephrine and GABA (Pliszka et al. 1996). In addition to dopamine and norepinephrine, peripheral and possibly central epinephrine might be involved in the mechanism of psychostimulant action on attention and impulsivity (Pliszka et al. 1996). Therefore, the early "monotransmitter theories" of ADHD have been replaced by more sophisticated models that reflect the heterogeneous neurochemical mechanisms or etiologies of ADHD (Zametkin and Rapoport 1987). Also, conceptualizations linking specific brain functions with neurotransmitter systems in ADHD are being synthesized with emerging findings in human neurochemical anatomy and cognitive neuroscience.

Neuroimaging and Anatomical Studies

EEG findings are abnormal in only 20% of children with ADHD (vs. 15% generally), and computed tomography (CT) scans are typically normal. However, the results of other types of cerebral imaging and of numerous neuropsychological studies are consistent with impaired functioning of the frontal cortex in at least some children with ADHD. ADHD-like symptoms are typically observed in humans with lesions and disorders of certain regions of the frontal cortex. These frontal regions are believed to inhibit subcortically guided automatic ("impulsive") responses to sensory stimulation from external sources and to prepare the brain for voluntary movements based on external stimuli.

In an imaging study of cerebral blood flow, children with ADHD showed high blood flow in the primary sensory regions of the occipital and temporal cortices. All 11 children with ADHD had hypoperfusion of the frontal lobes (especially white matter), and 7 out of 11 had hypoperfusion of the caudate nuclei. Psychostimulant medication increased blood flow in the basal ganglia (consistent with activation of dopamine neurons) and decreased flow in primary sensory and motor cortices (Lou 1996; Lou et al. 1989).

In contrast, a PET scan study of adults with ADHD demonstrated an overall reduction in global cerebral glucose metabolism of 8% (Zametkin et al. 1990). Significant reductions were found in 30 of the 60 brain regions examined, and the largest decreases were in the premotor cortex and superior prefrontal cortex (Figure 23–3; also see Zametkin et al. 1990). In another study, chronic stimulant treatment resulted in no PET scan evidence of change in global brain metabolism in response to methylphenidate or dextroamphetamine; significant changes were observed in only 2 of 60 brain regions during chronic methylphenidate treatment and in none of the regions during chronic methylphenidate treatment (Matochik et al. 1994). These findings are consistent with the hypothesis of hypofrontality in children and adults with ADHD, but they also support the notion that abnormalities in other brain regions may be relevant to the pathophysiology of ADHD.

Quantitative magnetic resonance imaging (MRI) studies have demonstrated several anatomical characteristics of ADHD. Boys with ADHD are reported to have small volumes of their anterior frontal cortex and left caudate structures (Filipek et al. 1997). The caudate region shows less of its usual right-larger-than-left asymmetrical structure, suggesting that the caudate does not have its normal extent of developmental reduction in size. In contrast, the anterior frontal cortex and globus pallidus are smaller on the right side. Cerebellar volume is also reduced (Castellanos et al. 1996). These findings are consistent with other lines of evidence that suggest predominant abnormalities in the striatum and right frontal cortex in ADHD.

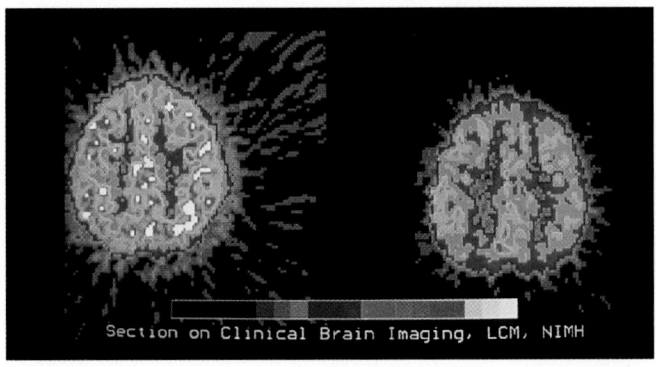

FIGURE 23–3. Positron-emission tomography (PET) scan of an adult with attention-deficit/hyperactivity disorder (ADHD) and an adult control subject. The two subjects were selected as representative of the ADHD and control groups. The study was conducted while each subject was engaged in a continuous performance task based on auditory discrimination. Frontal regions are at the top, and the left side of the image represents the right side of the brain. The occiput is at the bottom. Colors indicate high (white, red, orange) and low (blue, green, purple) levels of glucose metabolism. The purple halo is an artifact. This scan demonstrates significant reductions in 30 of the 60 brain regions examined, with the largest decreases in the premotor and somatosensory cortex. These data are consistent with neuropsychological findings of decreased frontal lobe functioning in children and adults with ADHD.
Source. Adapted with permission from information appearing in Zametkin AJ, Nordahl TE, Gross M, et al: "Cerebral Glucose Metabolism in Adults With Hyperactivity of Childhood Onset." *New England Journal of Medicine* 323:1361–1366, 1990.

Structure-function correlations in ADHD are reportedly strongest in the right prefrontal and caudate areas. Performance on neuropsychological tasks that require response inhibition correlates with anatomical differences in the prefrontal cortex, caudate, and globus pallidus. These studies of structure-function relationships suggest that, in children with ADHD, anatomical changes in the right frontostriatal neuronal systems correlate specifically with the deficits in response inhibition (Casey et al. 1997).

Responders to psychostimulant treatment have been reported to have anatomical characteristics that distinguish them from nonresponders. Stimulant responders appeared to have smaller (and more symmetrical) caudate heads and smaller left anterior frontal cortical regions than nonresponders and normal control subjects, whereas stimulant nonresponders had reversed caudate asymmetry (i.e., left was larger than right) and smaller parietal-occipital cortex, particularly retrocallosal white matter (Filipek et al. 1997), than did stimulant responders and normal controls.

MRI findings on the corpus callosum in ADHD are less consistent. A small anterior corpus callosum has been reported (Giedd et al. 1994), but a normal anterior corpus callosum and a smaller splenium in the posterior corpus callosum have also been described (Semrud-Clikeman et al. 1994). The corpus callosum, presumably involved in the transfer of information between hemispheres, may be relevant to understanding the symptoms reflecting the imbalance in hemispheric functioning observed in right hemisphere syndrome.

Together, these studies concerning children with ADHD suggest that hemispheric differences in the frontal cortex and caudate might be associated with deficits in response inhibition, the presence of ADHD, and responsiveness to stimulants. Right hemisphere syndrome may represent an anatomical and functional variant involving the right frontostriatal pathology of ADHD.

Neuropsychological Studies

Deficits in response inhibition have been long recognized as a component of ADHD, but this feature has been increasingly recognized as the most central element in the disorder (Barkley 1990; Quay 1997). Response inhibition can be assessed on simple, well-established neuropsychological tasks that assess the capacity for withholding or suppressing a physical or mental response that might otherwise be expected (e.g., because of impulsive force due to drive, instinct, automatic response, or reflexive reaction). The effect of response inhibition is to hold in check impulsive reactions. These reactions might be improved adaptively if allowed to rein in semiautomatic responses and if allowed more time (thought) before acting. For example, an individual's adaptive interests are generally served by the capacity to minimize or avoid distractions by irrelevant stimuli, to delay tempting but counterproductive responses, and to minimize pointless motion.

Another neuropsychological mechanism that appears to constitute a basic defect in ADHD is encoding, the processes associated with "translation" of information into changes in the nervous system that can be mapped into a language-like system. Encoding into working memory (a type of "short-term" 30-second memory) appears to be especially disrupted in ADHD.

A third realm of basic neuropsychological deficit in ADHD is a defect in higher order, "executive" cortical functions (Denckla and Reader 1993). For example, patients have difficulty in organization, such as structuring a narrative, multitasking, and self-monitoring. In young children, the difficulty of organizing can be demonstrated clinically when a child is telling a story (Purvis and Tannock 1997).

Clinicians use the term *attention* in a manner different

from that of cognitive scientists. In the language of clinicians, children with ADHD show distractibility (especially when bored), other abnormalities in attention regulation (including attention span), stimulus seeking, and motivational variability.

In short, cognitive studies have demonstrated that clinical manifestations of ADHD are tied to problems in response inhibition, encoding, intention, and other elements of executive functioning. An impairment is observed in sustaining focus on a specific task of a continuous performance test in ADHD, but it is also seen in learning disorders and mental retardation. An increase in the number of shifts of attention has been viewed as a nonspecific neuropsychological marker for ADHD. Other cognitive findings in ADHD include state-dependent learning while taking psychostimulants (learning that is not maintained when medication is discontinued), which has been reported in laboratory studies of children with ADHD, but not clinically.

Neurophysiological Studies

Neurophysiological studies show that children with ADHD differ in autonomic responsiveness from children without ADHD by exhibiting either more or less reactivity, both in the tonic resting state and in response to novel situations. Again, because similar findings are observed in children with learning disorders or mental retardation, autonomic responsiveness is not a distinguishing feature of ADHD.

Although routine clinical EEGs are interpreted as normal in the majority of patients with ADHD, quantitative EEG data have shown that 93% of children with ADHD could be categorized as exhibiting either hyperarousal (increased activity, especially frontal) or hypoarousal (slowing, especially frontal) relative to normal (Chabot and Serfontein 1996). This finding suggests that ADHD involves both hyper- and hypoarousal (in different individuals) and supports ADHD as a disorder (deviation) rather than as a developmental delay.

Evoked potentials (event-related electrical waves in the brain) in ADHD show a smaller P3 amplitude and longer P3 latency than normal. Earlier responses are inconsistent (between studies) but generally normal in ADHD, suggesting that mental priming (readiness) for incoming information is normal. P1 amplitude seems generally smaller, except for visually evoked potentials. ADHD individuals have more slow wave negativity (700–900 msec) at midline occipital than normal. Compared to non-aggressive individuals with ADHD, aggressive individuals with ADHD have more frontocentral negativity (640–900 msec slow wave); they also have more right-sided than left-sided negativity in the parietal regions.

When stimulants are taken, evoked potentials show a normalizing increase in the small P3 amplitude, which is accompanied by better accuracy and reaction times in performing a task. There is a further slowing of the P3b response latency in response to increasing memory load. Among the early peaks, there is probably no change in the earliest peaks (N1 and P1), but N2 increases in amplitude, especially in the frontal region.

Some characteristics have been proposed to distinguish stimulant responders from nonresponders. Although stimulant nonresponders and responders have similar P3b amplitudes before medication, P3b amplitude appears to show a larger increase in stimulant *nonresponders*. P300, a later wave related to attention and processing, appears normal in pemoline responders, but poor responders have a small P300 amplitude in the right frontal (center) cortex (1).

These diverse and partially inconsistent neurophysiological findings do not lend themselves to easy summation, but it appears that ADHD involves a disorder of arousal in addition to a defect in response inhibition. Two main forms of arousal can be distinguished in different patients. Hyperarousal and hypoarousal, both in comparison to normal arousal, presumably linked to high and low autonomic reactivity, might represent two subtypes of ADHD. Both forms of ADHD appear to be associated with particularly prominent abnormalities in the frontal regions. An abnormality in the right frontal cortex, associated with impaired attention and information processing (small P300 amplitude), correlates with diminished effectiveness of stimulants in some patients. However, stimulant nonresponders may have a paradoxically smaller normalization of the ADHD-related small P3 amplitude than do responders. The mechanisms involved in preparing (or priming) for incoming information (corresponding to the nearly normal form of the earliest evoked response potentials) seem intact in ADHD and are not changed by stimulants.

Sleep Studies

Children with ADHD show increased motoric activity during sleep ("restless sleep"), increased sleep latency (time required to fall asleep), and decreased REM latency (similar to adults with major depressive disorder), but no other consistent EEG architectural changes.

COURSE AND PROGNOSIS

Most cases of ADHD are congenital and lifelong. Clinical anecdotal lore suggests that some mothers of children with

ADHD recall excessive intrauterine "kicking" or report that "when he began to walk, he ran." Even when parents view the young child as troublesomely active, they are usually more concerned about ongoing behavior management than about any long-term liability of the hyperactivity.

ADHD can be diagnosed by age 36 months, but it is usually difficult to recognize the disorder before age 5 years because there is a normal developmental stage of hyperactivity beginning at about age 24 months. Identification is often delayed until elementary school, where demands for physical stillness are greater, comparison to peers is easier, and there is more group stimulation.

Onset of ADHD after toddlerhood suggests the possibility of acute onset or a new episode of a concomitant biopsychiatric illness, situational anxiety, physical or sexual abuse, neglect, adverse effects of medications, acute neurological trauma, or other "acquired" neuropathology.

Individuals with ADHD are said to experience their strongest lifetime barriers to adjustment during the regimented school years, in part because they are not yet free to select areas of learning and work that are least affected by their cognitive and behavioral symptoms. In addition to academic challenges and behavioral infractions, school-age children with ADHD may be significantly compromised in social skills and self-esteem.

The ADHD component of motoric hyperactivity often improves during childhood and early adolescence. In general, the symptoms of hyperactivity improve notably, impulsivity improves to a lesser degree, but the inattention does not improve (Hart et al. 1995). The age-related reduction in hyperactivity appears to be concentrated mainly in children with demonstrable developmental disorders and delays only; apparently it is not a significant feature of most other forms of ADHD (Pearson and Aman 1994). In addition, social skills and general adaptive abilities appear to fall progressively further behind over time (Roizen et al. 1994).

The prevalence of ADHD is estimated to decline by 50% about every 5 years until the mid-20s (Hill and Schoener 1996), regardless of the type and duration of treatment (Hart et al. 1995). Features of impulsivity persist into adolescence in 70% and into adulthood in 30%–50% of cases of childhood ADHD (Barkley 1990; Gittelman et al. 1985; Weiss and Hechtman 1986).

Clearly, ADHD is not a benign or self-limited childhood disorder. By young adulthood, ADHD is associated with fewer completed years of schooling, more changes of residence, more (and earlier) cigarette smoking, more marijuana use, more alcohol use, more traffic violations, more speeding, more car accidents and crashes, more court appearances, and more felony convictions. In terms of psychiatric symptoms, young adults with ADHD have more

suicide attempts, phobic anxiety, somatization symptoms, and psychosexual traumas, but no general excess of schizophrenia.

As adults, many individuals with ADHD continue to show inattention, impulsivity, and emotional changeability long after the motoric hyperactivity is no longer clinically prominent. In some cases, the symptoms continue to interfere with functioning, and treatment for ADHD is extended into adolescence or adulthood. In other cases, adults with ADHD have a good adjustment and outcome but persistently experience mild residual ADHD symptoms, such as restlessness or fidgeting.

Certain of the associated features of ADHD also tend to resolve over time. For example, although substance use disorders emerge in children with ADHD earlier and more often than in children without ADHD (Pomerleau et al. 1995), substantial evidence shows that there may be no general excess of substance use disorders in adults with ADHD. Furthermore, in the absence of conduct disorder, ADHD does not appear to be associated with subsequent substance abuse (Lynskey and Fergusson 1995). If there is a link between ADHD and substance abuse, therefore, it can probably be explained by comorbidity such as conduct disorder in children and antisocial personality or personality disorder in adults. Other forms of comorbidity that might mediate a link of ADHD and substance abuse include risk-taking behavior, difficulty in anticipating or planning for consequences, aggressive behavior, or bipolar disorder. Owing to inconsistent research findings, the comorbidity links between ADHD and substance-related disorders (and most other psychopathology) remain unsettled.

Overall, the most frequent outcome of childhood ADHD is clinical normalcy. However, major and enduring psychopathology is dramatically overrepresented in ADHD patients examined as an entire population. Antisocial personality disorder in adulthood is the most common serious outcome of ADHD in adulthood. It has been confirmed in several follow-up studies that 25%–30% of children with ADHD eventually develop antisocial personality disorder.

The high risk of antisocial outcome is likely to be concentrated in children with ADHD who have comorbid conduct disorder. Although 40%–70% of ADHD in children is associated with conduct problems, and about the same percentage of children with conduct disorder also have ADHD (Soussignan and Tremblay 1996), ADHD without aggressiveness does not appear to lead to conduct problems, aggressivity, or antisocial behavior in adulthood (August et al. 1983).

An adult with pronounced inattention, impulsivity, and hyperactivity does not necessarily have ADHD. The

DSM-IV diagnosis of ADHD in adults requires a history of ADHD during childhood. For children whose symptoms continue into adulthood, the adult course tends to be stable or to improve gradually over the years. Their residual symptoms remain responsive to psychostimulants, tricyclic antidepressants, bupropion, venlafaxine, and possibly selective serotonin reuptake inhibitors.

As an individual with ADHD enters parenthood, problems of impulsivity in caregiving, inattentiveness to child-rearing details, disorganization, identification with the child's ADHD, projection of the parent's ADHD tendencies, and guilt (regarding genetic transmission to the child) may become evident. It is not reasonable to assume that parents with ADHD know how to manage a child with ADHD because of their familiarity with the symptoms of ADHD. The parent's ability to overcome the obstacles of his or her disorder, and sometimes to start pharmacological treatment if not previously initiated, can have a major impact on the child's treatment, course of illness, and prognosis.

The actual course and prognosis of ADHD in an individual patient depend on the etiology of the ADHD as well as other individual factors, including the presence of comorbid psychiatric disorders. ADHD symptoms tend to improve gradually over time if they are not complicated by other factors. Comorbid psychiatric disorders that present episodically tend to yield periodic exacerbations of the ADHD symptoms. More chronic or deteriorative psychiatric disorders, such as bipolar disorder or schizophrenia, tend to intensify ADHD symptoms over time.

Generalizations about the prognosis of ADHD are difficult because both ADHD and other psychiatric disorders, especially in children and adolescents, may be aggravated in a nonsupportive environment, mitigated by the availability of supportive people and opportunities, altered in ways that cannot easily be predicted by intercurrent situational events, and influenced by the patients' (and families') ability to face problems, seek help, and make use of the help.

Effective help-seeking behavior is a crucial determinant of the management, course, and prognosis of ADHD. This characteristic, an ego function that modifies the course of all psychiatric disorders, is itself subject to learning, especially during childhood when adaptive skills are initially developing.

Distinguishing the natural course of ADHD from its secondary complications and comorbid disorders can be clinically difficult. Low self-esteem, compromised social skills, major conduct problems, aggressivity, antisocial personality, and criminality are probable complications (or features of comorbid disorders) rather than "core" symptoms of ADHD.

Complications in family functioning are virtually inevitable (Hechtman 1996). A child's ADHD is likely to influence parental satisfaction, marital harmony, and sibling development. Behavioral observation studies indicate that parents tend to have more anxious, controlling, directive, structure-setting, and negative responses to their children with ADHD, but at least part of the parents' behavior is elicited by the difficult behavior of the child (Barkley et al. 1990). Similar effects on peer relations and behavior are also worthy of clinical monitoring.

Completing the circle, parent and sibling responses to the behavior of children with ADHD can readily aggravate or improve the course of the child's illness. Owing to genetic transmission, parents of children with ADHD often have ADHD themselves. A parent's ADHD can be a psychosocial modulator of the severity of a child's symptoms. Stimulant treatment of a parent with ADHD can produce clinically significant improvement in the child's ADHD symptoms. When both parent and child have ADHD, treatment of either the parent or child can improve the condition of the other. Alternatively, failure to treat parent or child can be a rate-limiting step in the clinical improvement of both. As in many disorders, the concurrent treatment of child and family is usually a major advantage in managing ADHD in a child. In general, the interpersonal and social complications of ADHD can be complex, even in relatively mild cases (Hechtman 1996; Whalen et al. 1989).

EVALUATION AND DIFFERENTIAL DIAGNOSIS

Clinical evaluation entails assessing etiologies of ADHD, considering similarly presenting disorders, and delineating concomitant psychiatric and neurological disorders (Table 23–5).

A psychodynamic, psychosocial, and developmental evaluation of the individual and family is basic. Special emphasis is placed on school reports of grades and behavior (including behavior on the bus and in the cafeteria) or work history, concomitant learning disorders (or disorders of motor skills or communication) and major psychiatric disorders, social functioning and social skills, obstetrical history (maternal alcohol use, fetal overactivity, prenatal or perinatal injury), family residence (lead exposure in paints and car exhaust fumes), family psychiatric history (including ADHD in males), family medical history (thyroid disorder), medication use (barbiturates, benzodiazepines, stimulants, carbamazepine), history of child abuse or neglect, and potential risks of medication abuse by the patient or family members. A full psychiatric evaluation is certainly appropriate if there is conduct disorder, aggressivity, or a

TABLE 23–5.   Differential diagnosis of attention-deficit/hyperactivity disorder

Psychiatric

Conduct disorder

Oppositional defiant disorder

Major depression

Anxiety (situational, developmental)

Separation anxiety disorder

Posttraumatic stress disorder

Panic disorder

Phobic disorder

Dissociative disorders

Bipolar disorder

Early schizophrenia

Psychotic agitation

Substance use disorders (intoxication or withdrawal)

Attention-seeking or manipulative behavior

Psychosocial

Physical or sexual abuse

Neglect

Boredom

Overstimulation

Sociocultural deprivation

Medical

Thyroid disorders

Drug-induced agitation

   Recreational stimulants

   Medical stimulants: pseudoephedrine

   Barbiturates, benzodiazepines

   Carbamazepine

   Theophylline

Extreme prenatal or perinatal problem (rare)

Brain damage (following trauma or infection)

Lead poisoning (postnatal toxicity)

Teratogenic effect of exposure to alcohol, cocaine, lead, probably cigarette smoke

Dietary

Excessive caffeine

Hunger

Constipation

Minor persistent pain

Normal behavior

Note.   A variety of etiological factors give rise to ADHD or to conditions that look like ADHD. ADHD look-alike disorders may be more clinically appropriate diagnoses for individual patients than ADHD, and some look-alikes may be better diagnosed as comorbid conditions along with ADHD. Owing to the common co-occurrence of ADHD and ADHD look-alike conditions, all these disorders and some etiological conditions that give rise to them must be considered in the differential diagnosis of ADHD. In clinical practice, all the factors listed in the table (disorders, symptoms, situations, and states) should be considered—either identified or ruled out —before a firm diagnosis of ADHD is made. In effect, ADHD is a "diagnosis of exclusion"—a diagnosis that is made by the exclusion of other factors.

family psychiatric history of mood disorder or psychosis. Essential sources of information include the patient, parents, teachers, and pediatrician.

Physical examination and laboratory testing can identify physical anomalies and thyroid disorders. Neurological evaluation can uncover possible localizing symptoms, neuromaturational signs (choreiform movements, overflow and mirror movements, tremor, gross and fine motor function, cerebral laterality), and baseline (premedication) frequency of tics or dystonias. Lead screening is appropriate when excessive lead exposure is suspected, and possibly even if not suspected. The screening test is a plasma level of zinc protoporphyrin (ZPP), which has replaced the free erythrocyte protoporphyrin because it has fewer false positives and is an indicator of long-term lead exposure. A plasma lead level is optional at initial screening, because it reflects lead exposure over the previous 4 weeks only. A baseline sample of handwriting permits visual documentation of clinical change in the medical record. In the absence of suggestive symptoms, baseline (premedication) electroencephalogram, electrocardiogram, and thyroid evaluation are not essential and probably not cost-effective. Diagnostic blood tests might not be necessary in routine cases.

Educational testing and, often, neuropsychological evaluation are useful to assess academic achievement, intelligence, cortical functioning, attention, impulsivity, and developmental skills (including symptoms of learning, motor skills, and communication disorders).

Comorbidity rates are sufficiently high that evaluations of ADHD should be initially based on the expectation that concurrent psychiatric disorders will be identified. ADHD is often diagnosed in association with conduct disorder, oppositional defiant disorder, bipolar disorder, and learning disorders (Table 23–3). The differential diagnosis of ADHD is also challenging because of a high rate of comorbidity of neurological disorders and the extensive phenomenological similarity to other psychiatric disorders and to normal behavior.

Many of the defining criteria of ADHD are shared with numerous psychiatric disorders. Notable progress has been made in eliminating diagnostic criteria of ADHD that are common behaviors of "normal" people, but several of the 18 symptoms of ADHD listed in DSM-IV are still problematic. Fidgeting, acting driven or on-the-go, talking excessively, interrupting or intruding, making careless mistakes, glossing over errors, and engaging reluctantly in effortful thinking are hardly overt signs of significant psychopathology. However, these symptoms are helpful diagnostically in distinguishing ADHD from conduct disorder and oppositional defiant disorder when they present in the context of disruptive behavioral symptoms.

At present, however, the main clinical problem is no longer differentiating ADHD from normal behavior but differentiating ADHD from other psychopathology, including conduct disorder and oppositional defiant disorder. Some of the earlier diagnostic criteria for ADHD were discarded after the field trials for DSM-IV because they lacked the power to differentiate DSM-IV ADHD from other DSM-IV disorders, including anxiety and bipolar disorder. For example, the symptoms of excessive talking, intruding and interrupting, and thoughtless self-endangering behavior were found to be too nonspecific to warrant their continued use.

With such extensive symptom overlap, several neuropsychiatric disorders can readily be misdiagnosed as ADHD, and ADHD can readily be mistaken for a variety of psychiatric disorders. For example, bipolar disorder and ADHD have several symptoms in common, or perhaps it is more accurate to say that bipolar disorder has ADHD-like symptoms and ADHD has bipolarlike symptoms. These two disorders can mimic each other sufficiently to lead to diagnostic error. As discussed earlier, ADHD look-alikes are often misdiagnosed as ADHD ("counterfeit ADHD"), and ADHD is at times treated as if it were one (or more) of its look-alikes. All ADHD look-alike conditions need to be considered in the evaluation of ADHD and viewed as part of the differential diagnosis of ADHD to reduce the risk of overdiagnosis of ADHD.

The comorbidity of similarly appearing disorders presents additional problems that complicate the differential diagnosis. Although they resemble and mimic each other, both ADHD and bipolar disorder can appear comorbidly as distinct disorders, presenting simultaneously in one individual, even if their symptom overlap can make them difficult to differentiate. As previously noted, about 20%–25% of youths with ADHD also have bipolar disorder by DSM-IV criteria (Butler et al. 1995), and between 50% and 100% of youths with bipolar disorder fulfill criteria for ADHD (Butler et al. 1995; West et al. 1996). Therefore, caution must be taken to avoid oversimplifying by diagnosing a single diagnosis, because this can significantly impair treatment and prognosis.

In addition to the comorbidity, ADHD is typically accompanied by "associated features," as described in DSM-IV. For instance, when compared to adolescents with bipolar disorder, adolescents who have both bipolar disorder and ADHD are more likely to have mixed mania, irritability, higher scores on mania rating scales, and lower serum thyroxine concentrations (West et al. 1996). Such findings highlight the fact that clinically relevant features of ADHD are difficult to conceptualize but nonetheless

can be helpful in clinical diagnosis.

Often in psychiatry, diagnostic confidence cannot be achieved, and a "working diagnosis" is used as a basis for treatment. With ADHD, this approach can lead (often automatically and inappropriately) to an empirical trial of psychostimulants and to a common diagnostic error. A positive treatment response to a stimulant does not imply a diagnosis of ADHD; patients with several other disorders can show a therapeutic response to stimulants. On the other hand, a negative response to a stimulant does not rule out ADHD, because patients with ADHD may respond only to certain stimulants or to no stimulant at all. In general, it is helpful to keep the diagnostic process "open-ended" and to expect that emerging clinical data will probably shift diagnostic impressions, if only because of developmental changes.

The eventual identification of specific and sensitive criteria for ADHD will create a major advantage in diagnosing ADHD and differentiating it from other conditions and from normalcy. An easy and objective method to assess both attention and hyperactivity/impulsivity is solely needed, and some progress is being made in this direction (Teicher et al. 1996).

At present, clinical diagnosis of ADHD rests to a large degree on clinical judgment. The looseness of this approach is unsatisfactory for the diagnosis of a significant psychiatric disorder in children. Furthermore, the use of purely behavioral features, cognitive performance, and affective symptoms is particularly frustrating in distinguishing ADHD from the many ADHD look-alike conditions.

Currently, making a diagnosis of ADHD is much more complicated than in past decades. It is no longer possible to make a firm diagnosis of ADHD without assessing the presence or absence of many disorders (Table 23–3). It is no longer easy to make this diagnosis in a single office visit, because the accumulation of adequate clinical data to address each of these possibilities requires careful evaluation and observation over time. In effect, ADHD has become a "diagnosis of exclusion."

TREATMENT

A variety of treatment methods are useful; both multimodal and sequential approaches are generally needed. Certain interventions are specific to particular etiologies, but some treatments are helpful regardless of etiology.

Environmental management of sensory stimulation can reduce overstimulation from external sources, keep impulsivity and aggressivity in better control, and provide a sense of control and basis for self-esteem. Environmental measures can involve arranging the patient's home and job or school setting to reduce stimuli and distractions. For children at home, parents can be advised to establish quiet spaces, decorate with simple furniture and subdued colors, keep toys put away in the closet, permit only one friend to visit at a time, avoid supermarkets and parties, and encourage fine motor exercises (e.g., jigsaw puzzles). At work, adolescents and adults should be encouraged to make arrangements to use a quiet, small office space with no officemates, to have a minimum of visitors (or visiting), to avoid chatting or visual contact with passersby, and to have few telephone interruptions. The work environment should be uncluttered and undistracting, containing few windows and no nearby refrigerator, radio or television, or sound-making machinery. These recommendations have not been evaluated in controlled studies, but they are commonly offered and appear clinically valuable.

Special education is generally required, because children with ADHD are typically below achievement levels expected for school grade, even after accounting for IQ (Cantwell and Baker 1988). At school, beneficial accommodations include a small and self-contained classroom, small-group activities, thoughtful selection of seating location to minimize distractions, high teacher-to-student ratio, quiet ambience, routine and predictable structure, one-to-one tutoring, and use of a resource room. Arrangements for supervision or modifications at recess, in gym class, on the bus, and in the cafeteria are sometimes helpful. Careful management of transitions to new schools and between programs requires administrative foresight and detail-oriented planning. It is essential to inform school officials about the child's strengths and problems, self-esteem, social skills, and useful environmental measures as well as to receive regular reports from school personnel regarding behavior and academic performance. An individualized educational plan (IEP) can be developed with the school to facilitate classroom arrangements, perhaps with concomitant interventions to accommodate specific learning disorders.

For children and adolescents, psychostimulant treatment of ADHD has well-documented efficacy and effectiveness, and tricyclic antidepressants have been shown to be effective in double-blind placebo-controlled studies conducted by 11 separate research groups during the past 30 years. Drug studies in adults are less plentiful, but the same medications seem to be successful in treating adults. Dosage ranges in adults and children are approximately comparable because of the faster hepatic biotransformation of drugs in youths.

It is usually reported that approximately 75% of children with ADHD respond therapeutically to psycho-

stimulants; however, the response rate to psychostimulants has been reported to be as high as 93% when careful dosing and monitoring are provided. Similarly high rates of response have been reported in preschool children (Mayes et al. 1994). It is common practice to initiate treatment with a short-acting psychostimulant (D-amphetamine 5–40 mg or methylphenidate 10–60 mg daily). If one stimulant fails, there is a 25% chance that another will be helpful. These psychostimulants have therapeutic effects that last about 4–6 hours. A "rebound" period can then ensue, during which behavioral symptoms may become more severe than at baseline and, in addition, tics may transiently emerge. A commercially available product containing a mixture of four salts of D- and L-amphetamine (Adderall) appears to have a more prolonged duration of clinical effect, perhaps lasting for 6–10 hours, which is helpful for patients who are reluctant to take midday doses at work or school. Methamphetamine is another commercially available alternative with a long duration of clinical action (8–12 hours) at dosages of 5–40 mg daily. The long-acting formulations of D-amphetamine and methylphenidate appear to be less effective than standard formulations. Magnesium pemoline (Cylert) is another longer acting psychostimulant that can be successfully administered once daily, but 3% of patients form hepatotoxic metabolites that cause chemical hepatitis with increased liver transaminase levels; recently, the U.S. Food and Drug Administration (FDA) discouraged the use of pemoline as a first-line treatment of ADHD in view of 11 deaths owing to acute fulminant hepatitis in the past 25 years.

Some patients do not experience therapeutic effects from psychostimulants. Several factors can be considered in these cases. Some comorbid psychiatric disorders are aggravated by stimulants, including anxiety disorders or symptoms, bipolar disorder, and schizophrenia. Most psychotic disorders or symptoms can be aggravated by stimulants. Any neurological condition or neurodevelopmental idiosyncrasy that occurs concomitantly with ADHD might lead to drug-induced neurotoxic symptoms, often at unexpectedly low doses of psychotropic medications. The presence of anxiety (and perhaps other internalizing symptoms) has been reported by numerous research groups to be associated with a weaker and less prevalent therapeutic effect of psychostimulants. Patients with internalizing disorders tend to be overly inhibited, whereas ADHD patients typically have deficits in inhibitory self-control (Oosterlaan and Sergeant 1996). It may be hypothesized that the changing balance between these characteristics and the intermittent nature of anxiety contribute to the unevenness of stimulant effects in patients with ADHD and anxiety. In some cases, the dosage of the stimulant may need to be altered when ADHD with comorbid anxiety is treated in order to obtain stable therapeutic effects (Livingston et al. 1992).

The effect of stimulants in treating core symptoms of ADHD has been shown to persist for at least 15 months (Gillberg et al. 1997), but the effectiveness of these drugs in clinical use appears to endure for many years. However, some clinicians have described a small percentage of patients who appear to develop tolerance to stimulants after several months of treatment; that is, the stimulants become ineffective despite dose increases. If a therapeutic effect diminishes over time and is not due to intercurrent illness (including psychiatric illness) or stress, it might be due to a form of tolerance. This problem can generally be clinically managed by alternating between two different stimulants, switching every few weeks or months.

The cognitive deficits in response inhibition appear to improve with low doses (0.3–0.6 mg/kg) of methylphenidate but improve to a lesser degree at 0.9 mg/kg; the dose-response curve is ∪-shaped. In contrast, the behavioral effects of stimulants appear to be linearly dose-dependent. These findings suggest that various symptoms of ADHD do not respond in unison to stimulants and that stimulant effects on behavior and attention involve separate pharmacological mechanisms. Identification of a single "optimal" stimulant dose for an individual may not be possible; clinicians instead must make judgments in dose selection that are aimed at optimizing or balancing control among different ADHD behaviors.

Current concepts of the mechanism or mechanisms of psychostimulant action in ADHD are undergoing continual revision. The largely dopaminergic, lesser adrenergic, still lesser serotonergic, and probably other pharmacological effects of the stimulants are consistent with many different (and conflicting) models of ADHD. Simple single-neurotransmitter explanations are viewed as unlikely. Newer theories, incorporating nonpharmacological and neurophysiological findings, can become quite elaborate and interesting. For instance, the unexpected finding that methylphenidate slows right hemisphere processing (i.e., slower reaction time on neuropsychological tasks without a change in accuracy) seems to imply that the therapeutic effects of stimulants must be strong enough to outweigh their seemingly negative effects on right-sided functioning (Campbell et al. 1996).

In healthy individuals, the most serious risks of stimulants include tics and psychosis. Seizures are not induced by stimulants, and cardiac and cardiovascular effects are generally not clinically significant. Common side effects include delayed sleep onset, minor increase in blood pressure and heart rate, decreased appetite, reduced (or slowed)

height and weight gain, tremor or adventitious movements, cognitive overfocusing, anxiety, dysphoria, irritability, nightmares, and social withdrawal.

In general, nonstimulant medications are notably less effective in treating ADHD, especially in treating symptoms of inattention. Low dosages of tricyclic antidepressants (e.g., nortriptyline 0.3–2.0 mg/kg daily) provide therapeutic effects that last more than 24 hours, and once-daily use does not elicit rebound symptoms. The tricyclics are not as effective as psychostimulants in treating the attention deficits and cognitive symptoms of ADHD, although they do provide comparable effectiveness in treating the behavioral symptoms.

Reports of sudden death during routine desipramine treatment in five children and adolescents (Popper and Elliott 1990; Riddle et al. 1991, 1995) have led to general concern about the use of tricyclic antidepressants in youths, particularly for treating nonlethal disorders such as ADHD. The problem appears to be specific to desipramine; even imipramine has not been implicated, probably because its anticholinergic side effects are cardioprotective. Most of these cases of sudden death involved treatments for ADHD rather than enuresis (the most common pediatric use of tricyclic antidepressants) or mood disorders. Some of the patients who died had significant preexisting cardiovascular risks, including one patient whose coronary artery anomaly could not have been identified before death unless invasive arteriography had been obtained.

Desipramine treatment of ADHD is easy to avoid because so many other tricyclic antidepressants are readily available, and all appear to be equally effective in treating ADHD. Therefore, tricyclic antidepressants other than desipramine can be reasonably considered if rebound effects of psychostimulants are disruptive, if tics emerge specifically during rebound, if once-a-day administration is needed for treatment adherence, if the child or family is potentially drug-abusing, if mood disorder is a codiagnosis, if diurnal sleep or arousal symptoms are prominent, and perhaps if the family psychiatric history of mood disorder is strong.

MAOI antidepressants are usually clinically effective, but they are not typically used for treating ADHD because of the dietary restrictions and potential risks. The newer MAOIs, such as L-deprenyl (selegiline) and moclobemide (available in Canada), are more isoenzyme-specific than traditional MAOIs. Early findings suggest that moclobemide is effective in ADHD (Trott et al. 1992) and that L-deprenyl is not (Ernst et al. 1996; Feigin et al. 1996).

Clonidine is a frequently used treatment for ADHD (Hunt et al. 1990), but more extensive documentation of its therapeutic effectiveness is needed. Its effectiveness in ADHD has been seriously questioned, and its safety when used in combination with stimulants is unclear. If clonidine is effective for ADHD, it may be similar to tricyclic antidepressants in being helpful for behavioral symptoms (impulsivity, hyperactivity) but less helpful for cognitive symptoms (inattention). If these medications fail, magnesium pemoline might be considered, although it carries a 1%–3% risk of chemical hepatitis from hepatotoxic metabolite formation. The risk of fatality from fulminant hepatitis is small, but recent warnings from the FDA advise caution.

Bupropion has demonstrated efficacy in ADHD, but its effects are weaker than those of stimulants, and skin rash has appeared in 17% of treated children (Conners et al. 1996). Carbamazepine has been commonly used in England for many years, but formal demonstration of its efficacy has only recently been obtained (Silva et al. 1996). Pindolol has been shown in a well-designed study to treat behavioral symptoms in children with ADHD (Buitelaar et al. 1996), although other β-adrenergic blocking agents would be expected to have fewer adverse effects.

Major tranquilizers in low doses (e.g., chlorpromazine 10–50 mg four times a day) might also be considered, but their therapeutic effects are nonspecific, and side effects make them unsuitable for long-term treatment. Both olanzapine (5 mg daily at most) and risperidone (0.25–2 mg twice daily) have been reported to be effective in open-label trials, but more information about these agents is needed.

Other pharmacological treatments might be proposed. L-Thyronine (L-T_3), when used in supraphysiological doses, was found to reduce impulsivity and hyperactivity in children with comorbid ADHD and generalized resistance to thyroid hormone; in a small, well-controlled study, it appeared ineffective or worse in children with ADHD with generalized resistance to thyroid hormone (Weiss et al. 1994). Nicotine has been found to produce a beneficial effect on attention and concentration in a well-controlled 1-week study of adults with ADHD, using administration by patch. Because this effect was seen in nonsmokers but not in smokers, it cannot be attributed to withdrawal effects (Levin et al. 1996). With the use of a patch that released about 67 mg daily, few side effects were observed (Conners et al. 1996).

The pharmacology of hypericum (St. John's wort) suggests that it might be therapeutic for ADHD, but it has not been evaluated, and anxiety can emerge in some patients with ADHD.

Lithium is generally not effective for ADHD and can aggravate its symptoms (Greenhill et al. 1973; McKnew et al. 1981; Whitehead and Clark 1970). However, lithium can be helpful if the disorder is not in fact ADHD but bipolar disorder presenting with impulsivity, inattention, and hyperactivity (Butler et al. 1995). It is also strongly advisable to avoid benzodiazepines and barbiturates, which induce excitation and agitation, perhaps more so in patients with ADHD or neurodevelopmental disorders. Diphenhydramine (Benadryl) and chloral hydrate can induce sleep and are less likely to cause paradoxical excitation in children with ADHD, but bedtime administration of trazodone, melatonin, or nortriptyline is usually preferable.

Overall, psychostimulants remain the preferred treatment for ADHD, primarily because their ability to improve inattention and other cognitive symptoms is not matched by antidepressants, clonidine, or any of the other proposed drug treatments.

Dose optimization in ADHD patients is complicated by the variations in the level of ambient environmental stimulation, changes in emotionality and excitement, and diurnal patterns of hunger and arousal. These factors produce shifts in attentional and neurophysiological reactivity, as well as shifts in stimulant-induced effects. Clinically significant differences often exist between home and job (or school) environments. Dose selection becomes an artful task in which one attempts to optimize the balance of behaviors in different settings.

Drug treatment may continue for several years, with periodic dose adjustments needed for changes in body weight, varying environmental or developmental stress, or metabolic (including drug-induced autometabolic) changes in drug biotransformation rate. In 30%–50% of cases, treatment is no longer required by adolescence, but another 30%–50% of individuals with ADHD continue to need treatment into adulthood (Barkley 1990; Gittelman et al. 1985; Weiss and Hechtman 1986).

Psychostimulant effects in ADHD include a clinical improvement in impulsivity, hyperactivity, inattention, and emotional lability. This quieting is distinct from caffeine-induced focusing of attention, the antianxiety effect of benzodiazepines, or the tranquilization of antipsychotic agents. These agents act by different neurochemical and neurophysiological mechanisms, and they produce chemically different forms of "sedation." Children with ADHD can show a calming response to other medical stimulants (pseudoephedrine) and behavioral excitation to sedatives (benzodiazepines and barbiturates). Such "paradoxical" clinical effects may not be specific to hyperactive children. Under laboratory conditions, normal boys and adult men show a qualitatively similar stimulant-induced reduction of motor behavior, but the quantitative effect in hyperactive boys is significantly larger (Rapoport et al. 1980). The explanation of this apparent difference in the human laboratory, and of the clinical finding that not all people with ADHD respond "therapeutically" to psychostimulants, is uncertain. It appears that psychostimulant-responsiveness is not specifically tied to diagnostic state but reflects more basic biological mechanisms.

Treatment outcome studies of ADHD have led to some striking findings. In addition to helping reduce inattention, impulsivity, and hyperactivity, treatment with psychostimulants can lead to enduring improvement in social skills and attitudes toward self. However, psychostimulant treatment alone has not been found routinely to lead to improved academic performance or school grades, even in children whose attention and classroom behavior improve (Barkley and Cunningham 1978). Similarly, stimulants do not appear to produce lasting improvements in aggressivity, conduct disorder, criminality, educational achievement, job functioning, marital relationships, or long-term adjustment.

Although psychostimulants alone can treat the core symptoms of ADHD, they are not sufficient to affect ego-developmental and cognitive deficits incurred before drug treatment, concomitant biopsychiatric disorders, or ongoing environmental influences that can disrupt learning and adaptive functioning. Multiple treatment methods involving special educational and psychological help are likely to be needed for establishing a normal developmental outcome.

The clear value of psychostimulants in treating the defining behavioral and cognitive symptoms of ADHD contrasts with their ineffectiveness—when used alone—for treating more complex, integrated aspects of psychological functioning and for future development. The experience with psychostimulants may serve as a reminder that the value of an effective treatment can easily be overestimated and that empirical studies are required to define the value and scope of medical interventions.

In other dimensions of the management of ADHD, a variety of psychosocial interventions appear helpful in supporting the patient and family and in relieving some of the predictable problems associated with ADHD. Education of the family members about ADHD, its treatment, and its management is necessary as well. Family members can usually be "coached" in behavior-management techniques that can be applied at home. For children, the psychological impact of the parents can be pivotal in exacerbating or diminishing symptoms; therefore, parent counseling or therapy is sensible in most cases.

Environmental manipulation and drug treatment can be sufficient when behavior problems are not prominent, adaptive functioning is good, and study habits and interest in school have not been disrupted. However, additional treatment approaches are useful in most cases, particularly if medication and environmental interventions do not lead to improved behavior, academic or job performance, or social adjustment.

Contingent rewards, response-cost management, and time-outs can help build impulse control in children. Behavioral methods can be as effective as psychostimulants in modifying classroom behavior, but generalization beyond the treatment setting may be limited. Cognitive-behavioral therapy is used for teaching problem-solving strategies, self-monitoring, verbal mediation (using internal speech) for self-praise and self-instruction, and seeing rather than glossing over errors.

Group treatments can be helpful for children with ADHD and adolescents who need training in social skills. Deficits in the development of social skills are commonly found in individuals with ADHD, including those without aggressive behavior, oppositional behavior, impulsivity, or hyperactivity. Other areas of adaptive functioning are also compromised, even in patients with predominantly inattentive ADHD. Children with ADHD of normal intelligence (full-scale IQ of 101±14) may have low-to-borderline scores on the Vineland Adaptive Behavior Scale (73±14), and this discrepancy increases with age (Roizen et al. 1994). Social and adaptive dysfunctions have only recently been viewed as standard components of ADHD, and they may justify incorporation into the routine management of ADHD (Stein et al. 1995).

For nonsmoking youths, it is advisable to reinforce smoking prevention attitudes and to foster the acquisition of alternative means of dealing with peer pressure, self-image, anxiety, and peers' opinions. Early intervention is particularly valuable for youths with ADHD, who generally start smoking earlier than their peers who do not have ADHD. Their tendency to be less concerned about future health problems (and other delayed risks) and their novelty-seeking behavior may also interfere with subsequent smoking cessation efforts (Downey et al. 1997). Moreover, the therapeutic effects of nicotine on ADHD symptoms (Levin et al. 1996) may lead to exacerbation during smoking cessation, making it difficult for persons with ADHD to stop smoking. In a similar manner, preventive measures to stem alcohol and other substance use disorders are useful.

Education and support for parents and family members are crucial, and they can be provided through programmed group training sessions (Barkley 1990). In addition, national organizations for parents, such as ChADD, have many local chapters throughout the United States that can provide crucial support, education, and advocacy for families and patients.

If a patient's conflicts or resistances interfere with general adjustment, development, or treatment, or if comorbid disorders require more intensive treatment, individual and family psychotherapy can become a component of ADHD treatment. Although no studies support the effectiveness of psychotherapy alone in treating ADHD, it can be a critical part of multimodal treatment for some individuals.

Nutritional therapy of ADHD has a murky history, involving a string of cures too good to be true and "new" treatments that have been used for years. Perhaps frustrated by behavioral methods and frightened by "mind drugs," parents are often interested in hearing physicians' views on nutritional and other unproven treatments of ADHD. Some of these parents seem willing to accept that their child has a "physical problem" but are not ready to acknowledge a "medical disorder." It is also striking that ADHD has attracted more medical and professional advocates of nutritional treatment than any other psychiatric and most other medical disorders. Possibly reflecting acute clinical intuition, numerous forms of elimination diets have been enthusiastically promulgated and enforced for years on the basis of anecdotes and repeated assertions, without the benefit of adequate testing or even attempts at controlled trials.

Although no dietary treatment of ADHD has been consistently demonstrated to have clinical value, some studies cannot be readily dismissed. Several reasonable reports are consistent with a possible role of dietary factors in the etiology and treatment of ADHD. In a controlled trial employing dye washout periods and high-dose dye challenges, specific restriction of a set of food dyes (with no other restrictions) was found to be effective for treating a subgroup (5%–10%) of children with ADHD. In another controlled rechallenge study, a diet that minimized the intake of certain "reactive" foods, preservatives, and artificial food dyes was found to produce a clinically and statistically significant improvement in children with ADHD (Boris and Mandel 1994); in this study, atopic children with ADHD appeared to be more likely to respond than other children with ADHD. In an EEG study examining children whose ADHD appeared to be aggravated by specific foods (as determined by previous deprivation and challenge), an increase was found in beta activity in the frontotemporal cortex during rechallenge with the sensitizing food (Uhlig et al. 1997). A controlled study of a low-antigen diet found no changes on attention or activity measures, but the children with ADHD reported significant subjective improvement (Schulte-Körne et al. 1996).

Other dietary treatments of ADHD have been examined but without convincing evidence of clinical value. The well-publicized Feingold diet, involving reduced dietary intake of salicylates and food dyes, has yielded contradictory findings in controlled trials. Data on salicylate elimination and challenge have demonstrated minimal effects (Perry et al. 1996). Sugar toxicity, sugar withdrawal, and reactive hypoglycemia have been reported to induce ADHD symptoms, but these claims do not appear to be valid (unless perhaps there were preexisting nutritional deficiencies). It has been well documented that aspartame has no clinical effects on ADHD. Dietary treatments based on trace mineral content in hair analysis (particularly zinc deficiency and cadmium excess) have not been rigorously evaluated. Megavitamin treatments appear ineffective and can cause toxic effects.

Despite prevailing skepticism of dietary treatments of ADHD, some studies of dietary treatments of ADHD have produced enough suggestive evidence to warrant a measure of respect and to justify further disciplined research. There is reasonably good evidence that some foods or food dyes induce hyperactive behavior or other ADHD symptoms in a small percentage of children; perhaps atopic children are more vulnerable to this effect. Although the clinical significance of these findings remains to be determined, new data have confirmed the folklore that mood and sleep are influenced by a broad range of foods in children (Breakey 1997); therefore, it should not be implausible or surprising that diet may significantly influence ADHD and other behavioral conditions.

In another interesting area of ADHD research, investigators have examined the effects of iron because of the involvement of iron in mechanisms affecting dopaminergic activity. Confirming preliminary reports, in a well-conducted open-label study boys with ADHD seemed to respond to 30-day iron supplementation with improvements in ADHD symptoms that were concomitant with the increasing serum ferritin levels (Sever et al. 1997).

To monitor treatment effects in research and clinical practice, a variety of standardized scales have been developed. The best available instrument for adults is the Wender Utah Rating Scale, which is also useful in assessing ADHD symptoms in children (Stein et al. 1995). Other options are available for children as well. The Child Attention/Activity Profile (CAP) assesses both the inattention and hyperactivity/impulsivity factors (Figure 23–4) and is sensitive to stimulant effects (Edelbrock 1987). Early versions of Conners's parents' rating scales and teachers' rating scales (Rapoport et al. 1985) were widely employed, but they functioned as nonspecific measures of "misbehavior" and conduct problems; they were not as useful for monitoring specific ADHD symptoms or for the predominantly inattentive type of ADHD. However, Conners updated these scales to keep pace, and the current versions appear to function quite well (Conners et al. 1996). The Home Situations Questionnaire (HSQ) can be used by parents or residential caregivers (Barkley 1990); it assesses behaviors in a variety of different settings and can also measure drug effects. All these instruments, although developed for drug research, can be applied to outcome assessment of ADHD for any treatment method. An additional method assessment, which is one of the best (although not as systematic or reproducible as the scales), is an arrangement for clinicians to receive reports on behavior and cognition from teachers as well as parents.

Peer ratings by children have been used clinically

(Glow and Glow 1980), but a standardized scale has not yet been devised. Peers perceive children with ADHD as different from others, and their perception of "hyperactive" children is clearer than their perceptions of "popular" and "bully" children. Ratings by classroom peers show a closer correlation to teachers' than to parents' ratings, presumably because ADHD symptoms are modified by situation.

Self-rating scales have been developed for adolescents but not yet for children. Children may be aware of their ADHD and of "getting into trouble," but they are less effective than parents as observers of their ADHD behavior.

Certain laboratory tests, mostly variations on the continuous performance test (CPT), have been used clinically

---

Child Attention/Activity Profile (CAP)

Child's Name: _____   Child's Age: _____

Today's Date: _____   Child's Sex: [ ]M   [ ]F

Filled out by: _____

Directions: Below is a list of items that describe pupils. For each item that describes the pupil *now* or *within the past week,* check whether the item is Not True, Somewhat or Sometimes True, or Very or Often True. Please check all items as well as you can, even if some do not seem to apply to this pupil.

	Not true	Somewhat or sometimes true	Very or often true
1. Fails to finish things he/she starts	[ ]	[ ]	[ ]
2. Can't concentrate, can't pay attention for long	[ ]	[ ]	[ ]
3. Can't sit still, restless, or hyperactive	[ ]	[ ]	[ ]
4. Fidgets	[ ]	[ ]	[ ]
5. Daydreams or gets lost in his/her thoughts	[ ]	[ ]	[ ]
6. Impulsive or acts without thinking	[ ]	[ ]	[ ]
7. Difficulty following directions	[ ]	[ ]	[ ]
8. Talks out of turn	[ ]	[ ]	[ ]
9. Messy work	[ ]	[ ]	[ ]
10. Inattentive, easily distracted	[ ]	[ ]	[ ]
11. Talks too much	[ ]	[ ]	[ ]
12. Fails to carry out assigned tasks	[ ]	[ ]	[ ]

Please feel free to write any comments about the pupil's work or behavior in the last week.

FIGURE 23–4.   Child Attention/Activity Profile (CAP). Entries are raw scale scores that fall at or below the designated percentile rank.
Source.   C. Edelbrock, Ph.D., S-211 Henderson, Pennsylvania State University, University Park, Pennsylvania 16802. In the public domain.

to measure attentiveness and responsiveness to changing sensory cues. Although these tests (computerized or otherwise) have been used to monitor treatment and to adjust medication dosages, their usefulness is open to question: attentional performance in a laboratory is not related in a simple manner to naturalistic behavior or cognitive functioning in different life spaces.

It is unlikely that any rating scale or protocol has the clinical usefulness of reports from a variety of observers in a variety of settings. Treatment outcome is best evaluated by speaking to parents, teachers, and observers in different environments. Rather than relying on clinical interviews in a quiet office (where ADHD behaviors may be least evident) or on laboratory tests (which may not reflect usual functioning), the clinician should consider the primary assessment instrument for evaluating treatment of ADHD to be the telephone.

Multimodal treatment of ADHD is currently the standard of care for children with ADHD, especially those with major psychiatric or neurological comorbidity, behavior disorders, aggressivity, disruptiveness, learning disorders, developmental disorders, or poor prognosis. In a major study of multimodal treatment, substantial clinical value was suggested. A combination of medication, special edu-

---

Child Attention/Activity Profile (CAP) Rating Scale Scoring

Normative cutoff points for inattention, overactivity, and total score:

Inattention: Sum of items 1, 2, 5, 7, 9, 10, 12; each scored 0, 1, or 2. Range 0–14.

	Boys		Girls	
Age	6–11	12–16	6–11	12–16
Median	2	2	0	0
69%ile	4	4	1	3
84%ile	6	7	5	5
93%ile	9	9	8	7
98%ile	12	12	11	10

Overactivity: Sum of items 3, 4, 6, 8, 11; each scored 0, 1, or 2. Range 0–10

	Boys		Girls	
Age	6–11	12–16	6–11	12–16
Median	1	0	0	0
69%ile	3	2	1	1
84%ile	3	4	3	2
93%ile	6	7	5	4
98%ile	8	9	7	7

Total Score: Sum of all items 1–12; each scored 0, 1, or 2. Range 0–24.

	Boys		Girls	
Age	6–11	12–16	6–11	12–16
Median	4	4	1	1
69%ile	8	7	3	5
84%ile	11	12	8	8
93%ile	15	16	12	11
98%ile	20	20	16	15

FIGURE 23–4. Child Attention/Activity Profile (CAP). Entries are raw scale scores that fall at or below the designated percentile rank. *(continued)*
Source. C. Edelbrock, Ph.D., S-211 Henderson, Pennsylvania State University, University Park, Pennsylvania 16802. In the public domain.

cation, and psychotherapy resulted in improved education, increased attentional functioning, better psychosocial adjustment, and reduced antisocial activity (Satterfield et al. 1981). However, 50% of the patients had dropped out of treatment within 3 years, limiting the generalizability to the full ADHD population.

In contrast, other reports have been less favorable. Two studies of children with ADHD found surprisingly small benefits of multimodal treatment in comparison to medication treatment alone. A well-controlled study of 96 children with ADHD found little evidence that the effects of treatment with methylphenidate alone were enhanced by the addition of psychosocial treatments. The nondrug treatments were a combination of behavioral training for the parents and self-control instruction for the child, which included both cognitive-behavioral and social learning interventions (Ialongo et al. 1993). Similarly, in an independent study of 31 children, researchers examined the effects of another psychostimulant and multimodal psychosocial treatment. The combined treatment included a well-structured program of behavior modification that targeted both classroom behavior and academic performance. The multimodal treatment was found to produce more clinical improvement than stimulants alone in only 41% of cases. Furthermore, the improvements afforded by the nondrug treatments were viewed as having minor clinical significance. Also, the medications resulted in improved academic performance, whereas the behavioral program did not (Pelham et al. 1993).

More studies are needed to examine the multimodal and interactive effects of various treatments of ADHD in both children and adults. It seems surprising, however, that despite its common use in treating children with ADHD, the multimodal approach may not be significantly more effective than psychostimulant monotherapy, even before cost-effectiveness is considered.

CLINICAL COMMENT

ADHD provides an example of a congenital or early-onset disorder, often with a genetic or neurological etiology, that can be modified by life experiences. Untoward genetic and biological processes that are prominent during early childhood can be "washed over" in time by social and environmental factors. Socioeconomic opportunities, family variables, education, and the ability to seek and use medical treatment exert prominent influences on the development of behavior and behavior disorders, regardless of cause. In this way, ADHD characteristics can be amplified into psychopathology or channeled into useful energetic activity, depending on a series of psychosocial factors.

A large variety of etiologies, environmental circumstances, developmental processes, and psychiatric disorders can result in behavioral hyperactivity, impulsivity, and inattention. Whether there is a final common pathway, similar among all "varieties" of ADHD, remains to be determined. Although genetic and some toxin-induced forms of ADHD appear to share virtually identical clinical features and possibly common pathways, a single physiological explanation of ADHD is doubtful in view of the apparent differences in medication responsiveness of ADHD of different etiologies; for example, genetic ADHD versus right hemisphere syndrome versus ADHD with anxiety.

Psychostimulants continue to be employed to treat the mixed population of patients with ADHD, and ADHD continues to be defined by use of nonspecific criteria consisting of relatively common behaviors. Attempts to subtype this complex population on the basis of behavioral criteria alone remain elusive, probably in part because of the confounding effects of genetics; psychiatric and neurological comorbidity; somatic, affective, and cognitive features; and a vast array of family and social variables.

Because it appears that nearly all cases of ADHD have comorbidity, there has been relatively little study of "pure" ADHD in the absence of comorbidity. After subtracting out children with ADHD who also have learning disorders, conduct disorder, mood and anxiety disorders, Tourette's disorder, and the like, one might even wonder whether ADHD exists in "pure" form at all. Estimates suggest that up to 5% of children with ADHD may present without neurological or psychiatric comorbidity. Nonetheless, the hypothesis has been advanced that comorbidity rather than ADHD may be responsible for the severity of presenting symptoms and the likelihood of referral, and that children with the "pure" forms of ADHD may be seen simply as energetic personalities and not referred for treatment.

In view of the large number of "ADHD look-alike" conditions, it is no longer sufficient to identify a child who is hyperactive (e.g., by broken furniture in a physician's office) and proceed with a stimulant trial. Instead, a thorough evaluation is essential to rule out a host of other psychiatric diagnoses. In effect, ADHD has become a "diagnosis of exclusion," requiring a large number of alternative disorders to be considered before the decision is made.

Although the clinical concept of ADHD is largely based on nongenetic factors, the "gene revolution" in medicine may hold some promise for identifying the different subtypes of ADHD. Gene markers might provide a system for identifying and classifying psychiatric disorders. If the comorbidity associated with ADHD turns out to be inheritable, a subtyping of ADHD based on its comorbidity could be solidified. In this way, the gene revolution may offer new ways to recognize different "ADHD" subtypes that are in fact the presentation of different disorders (the comorbid disorders) that happen to "look like" ADHD.

Owing to the extensive comorbidity of ADHD, psychiatrists are still trying to sort out characteristics ascribed to ADHD that should be viewed as features of other disorders. Furthermore, contemporary knowledge about ADHD is limited by the historical use of patient samples that were composed mainly of prepubertal boys from white, middle-class America who mostly had both ADHD and conduct disorder. From such research, it is difficult to distinguish ADHD symptoms from symptoms of conduct disorder, even within the select population. It is perilous to draw inferences about ADHD in patients who were not represented in this large but limited sample.

For example, the understanding of ADHD in adults is still based mainly on inferences from studies of children and partially on clinical drug trials that have faithfully replicated well-established findings in children. In a reversal of the common pattern in which knowledge of adult psychopathology informs and distorts the initial approach to the psychiatric treatment of children, studies of ADHD in children are now expanding the treatment opportunities for adults with ADHD. The usual provisos about the perils of generalizing across age groups now are used to temper the overconfidence engendered by impatient clinical speculation.

Although stimulant treatments are well established in medicine, these agents are not viewed favorably by some members of the public. Despite the sometimes overstated objections, there is considerable substance in the concern that psychostimulant treatments present a major public policy problem. Amphetamines and methylphenidate are highly abusable and, in fact, were highly abused into the late 1980s. During much of the 1980s, more than 95% of prescriptions for amphetamines were estimated to be used for "diet control" or recreational abuse, and responsible critics recommended their withdrawal from the commercial market. Public education regarding these treatments has provided some relief, but the potential for abuse is undiminished and poses a threat to the patient, family members, or peers.

ADHD has provided some unexpected findings, challenging the ability to rethink concepts and procedures. The few longitudinal studies have provided convincing evidence that many children with ADHD grow up to have significant adult psychopathology. The traditional view of ADHD as a benign and perhaps amusing childhood condition has been rejected. The assumption that effective stimulant treatment predictably leads to improved school grades has turned out to be debatable. Although

multimodal treatment is the long-established norm in the psychiatric treatment of ADHD, even this approach is questioned by findings that the addition of psychosocial treatment may provide little benefit over the use of stimulants alone. If simple stimulant treatment is the best treatment option, and if additional psychosocial interventions do not yield as much as generally believed, it is conceivable that long-term developmentally oriented early intervention might be less powerful than assumed. The advantage of early intervention is a bedrock concept in child psychiatric treatment, but recent findings concerning ADHD suggest that even bedrock should be examined and tested. The experience with ADHD serves as a reminder that, even with the oldest and most established diseases and treatments, empirical study is needed to define the scope and limits of knowledge.

CONDUCT DISORDER

Conduct disorder is the most common diagnosis of child and adolescent patients in both clinic and hospital settings. This disorder entails repeated violations of personal rights or societal rules, including violent and nonviolent behaviors. The syndrome is not a single medical entity but consists of various forms of "major misbehavior." The diagnostic criteria include offenses ranging from frequent lying, cheating, and truancy to vandalism, running away, car theft, arson, and rape (Table 23–6). The validity of a single categorical grouping has been questioned by proponents of a more symptomatic or dimensional approach to conduct problems. Conduct disorders can present with or derive from biopsychiatric disease (mood disorders, psychosis, ADHD), organic impairment, and mental retardation or psychodevelopmental (or personality) disorders. However, in most cases, family, socioeconomic, and environmental factors contribute heavily to the genesis of conduct disorder.

Conduct disorder encompasses some of the most severe behavior disorders of childhood. Only a fraction of children with this disorder are treated. Many can be rehabilitated or habilitated, but some lead lives of delinquency or undergo long-term incarceration. Early onset has been found to be the strongest predictor of poor outcome in a variety of studies (Tolan 1987), forming the basis for the DSM-IV subtyping of conduct disorder into early and late onset.

CLINICAL DESCRIPTION

Conduct disorder accounts for 50% of convicted juvenile delinquents and a higher proportion of incarcerated

TABLE 23-6.   DSM-IV diagnostic criteria for conduct disorder

A. A repetitive and persistent pattern of behavior in which the basic rights of others or major age-appropriate societal norms or rules are violated, as manifested by the presence of three (or more) of the following criteria in the past 12 months, with at least one criterion present in the past 6 months:

Aggression to people and animals

(1) Often bullies, threatens, or intimidates others.
(2) Often initiates physical fights.
(3) Has used a weapon that can cause serious physical harm to others (e.g., a bat, brick, broken bottle, knife, gun).
(4) Has been physically cruel to people.
(5) Has been physically cruel to animals.
(6) Has stolen while confronting a victim (e.g., mugging, purse snatching, extortion, armed robbery).
(7) Has forced someone into sexual activity.

Destruction of property

(8) Has deliberately engaged in fire setting with the intention of causing serious damage.
(9) Has deliberately destroyed others' property (other than by fire setting).

Deceitfulness or theft

(10) Has broken into someone else's house, building, or car.
(11) Often lies to obtain goods or favors or to avoid obligations (i.e., "cons" others).
(12) Has stolen items of nontrivial value without confronting a victim (e.g., shoplifting, but without breaking and entering; forgery).

Serious violations of rules

(13) Often stays out at night despite parental prohibitions, beginning before age 13 years.
(14) Has run away from home overnight at least twice while living in parental or parental surrogate home (or once without returning for a lengthy period).
(15) Is often truant from school, beginning before age 13 years.

B. The disturbance in behavior causes clinically significant impairment in social, academic, or occupational functioning.

C. If the individual is age 18 years or older, criteria are not met for antisocial personality disorder.

Code based on type:

312.81   Conduct disorder, childhood-onset type: onset of at least one criterion characteristic of conduct disorder prior to age 10 years.
312.82   Conduct disorder, adolescent-onset type: absence of any criteria characteristic of conduct disorder prior to age 10 years.
312.89   Conduct disorder, unspecified onset: age at onset is not known.

Specify severity:

Mild: Few if any conduct problems in excess of those required to make the diagnosis **and** conduct problems cause only minor harm to others.
Moderate: Number of conduct problems and effect on others intermediate between "mild" and "severe."
Severe: Many conduct problems in excess of those required to make the diagnosis **or** conduct problems cause considerable harm to others.

---

youths. These youths are often products of low socioeconomic status, unstable homes with family discord, maternal rejection, and absent or alcoholic fathers. Other youths with conduct disorder come from more favorable environments. As a group, youths with conduct disorder have measurably lower cognitive and moral development, more behavioral impulsivity, greater susceptibility to boredom and stimulus-seeking behavior, and lower nutritional status. There is an overrepresentation of homicidal behavior, particularly directed against the parents, in youths with conduct disorder as compared to those without it. Outcome and course depend partially on involvement in a delinquency group, the nature of the delinquency group, the availability of alternative social supports, the comorbidity, and the age of onset.

Not all delinquent behavior is conduct disorder. Youths with *adaptive delinquency* or *subcultural delinquency*

are conceptualized to have made an "adaptive" response to social and cultural disadvantage, parental neglect, and delinquent peers. Viewed as social victims rather than as mentally ill, these youths are commonly seen in juvenile delinquency centers and inner-city clinics, and less commonly in prisons. There is a wide range of severity in adaptive delinquency, and the condition is not always apparent. The diagnosis of conduct disorder was developed to identify more serious cases that may have psychiatric dimensions. Misconduct (especially severe delinquency) is more frequent in boys, but the symptom profile is similar in both genders (Table 23–7).

A crucial feature of conduct disorder is the absence of impulsivity (Halperin et al. 1995). Impulsive anger in patients with conduct disorder typically derives from comorbid disorders, especially ADHD. Both impulsive and nonimpulsive anger (and actions) can play a role in the conduct of illegal behavior. Drug dealing (selling) requires much more thoughtful planning and effective action than does abusing drugs. The strong association between conduct disorder and impulsivity is an artifact of the frequent comorbid presentation of ADHD and conduct disorder. These disorders appear to be separate conditions or dimensions. Impulsive and nonimpulsive subtypes might turn out to be useful subdivisions of conduct disorder. In fact, many of the characteristics attributed to conduct disorder result from comorbid psychiatric disorders. The high rate of comorbidity has complicated delineation of the features specific to conduct disorder, of which impulsivity is just one example.

Across a diversity of presentations, children and adolescents with conduct disorder show alterations of mood (sullenness, anger), attention (and learning disorders), and

TABLE 23-7. Common misbehaviors of adolescents

Misbehaviors	Self-reported misconduct (%)		
	Male	Female	Total
Skipping school	82	81	82
Drinking alcohol	83	73	78
Disturbing the peace	72	69	71
Having sex with opposite sex	78	62	70
Smoking marijuana	67	59	63
Committing theft (less than $2)	67	58	62
Defying parents' authority	41	42	42
Attacking someone with fists	48	25	37
Driving car without permission	42	25	34
Using fake ID	35	27	31
Driving while intoxicated on marijuana	40	22	31
Driving while intoxicated on alcohol	39	22	30
Theft ($2–$50)	34	26	30
School problem, suspension, expulsion	32	27	29
Selling marijuana	35	19	27
Gang fighting	39	15	27
Property destruction (less than $10)	37	16	26
Carrying weapon	34	17	25
Using hard drugs	15	19	17
Running away from home	16	16	16
Property destruction (over $10)	20	6	13
Joyriding	18	6	12
Theft of car parts	20	3	12
Extortion	14	8	11
Burglary—unoccupied	17	4	10
Selling hard drugs	12	9	10
Driving while intoxicated on hard drugs	12	7	10
Using weapon to attack someone	12	7	9
Theft (over $50)	13	5	9
Burglary—occupied	10	2	6
Robbery	5	1	3
Car theft	5	1	3
Sex for money	5	1	3

Note.   Self-reports obtained by anonymous questionnaires distributed to 822 high school students in two midwestern cities in 1977.
Source.   Data from Cernkovich and Giordano 1979.

other aspects of cognition. Cognitive problems in these youths include a faulty sense of size and time, distorted view of the consequences of previous events, difficulty in imagining the expectable outcome of current events, underestimation of risks, disrupted awareness of causal connections (particularly regarding their own behavior), reduced problem-solving ability, blocks in logical thinking, and impaired moral reasoning. Pathological defenses include minimizing, avoiding, lying, externalizing, unconscious manipulation, and denial. Interpersonal impairments appear as suspiciousness or paranoia (with cognitive distortions sometimes triggering fights and resentments), a minimum of guilt and empathy, and difficulty in relating to professionals.

Although symptoms such as driving recklessly, carrying weapons, or demonstrating impulsive and non-impulsive violence may be observed, wanton dangerousness to the public is not typical of all youths with conduct disorder. However, dangerousness may be significant in the small subgroup of children whose aggressive or suicidal behavior is a direct response to hallucinations.

Typically, concomitant psychiatric or neurological pathology is observed in association with severe conduct disorder. Adolescents in prisons, especially those slated for execution, show an exceedingly high prevalence of conduct disorder, comorbid neuropsychiatric disorders, and brain injury (Lewis et al. 1982). Substance use disorders are known to contribute to both the severity and duration of symptoms. Low self-esteem and passivity are common but might be covered by an exterior of bravado, or "toughness." Academic underachievement is typical and may be related to the commonly comorbid learning and communication disorders, especially reading disorder and expressive language disorders. If behavioral impulsivity and hyperactivity are present, they can be due to ADHD. Alcohol and substance use for self-stimulation or self-medication (of anxiety, depression, boredom, pathological excitement, temper, or psychosis) can become a complicating (and mediating) factor that aggravates the impulsivity, rage, and passivity associated with comorbid disorders. In general, concomitant psychopathology is often present and can contribute to the chronicity, severity, and social spread of conduct disorder.

Embedded within the concept of conduct disorder is the stereotype of the young "hardened criminal" who is dangerous and sociopathic but has not yet been imprisoned. DSM-IV makes no attempt to designate such youths. In attempts at a more precise description of such youths, researchers have considered a variety of attributes hypothesized to be specific to these individuals, including callousness, low emotional responsiveness (reactivity), and family

history (of antisocial personality disorder, illegal behavior, and career criminality).

EPIDEMIOLOGY

More epidemiological information is available about crime than about conduct disorder. The prevalence of delinquency in the general child and adolescent population in the United States is approximately 10% (range 5%–15%). There is a male predominance for property crimes (4:1) and violent crimes (8:1).

The distribution of violent crimes in the United States among urban, suburban, and rural areas is 10:2:1. After adjustment for population density, however, violent crime is found to be highest in rural areas. Minors (younger than 18 years) are responsible for 40% of arrests for property crimes and 20% of arrests for violent crimes (Figure 23–5). Children under 15 years old account for 5% of all arrests for violent crimes. These statistics probably overestimate the general worldwide problem, because violent crime appears to be more prevalent in the United States than in other countries. Conduct disorder itself has been found to be more prevalent in youths residing in large cities (Wichstrøm et al. 1996). The prevalence of conduct disorders has been increasing in females in recent years, so that the traditional male predominance is decreasing over time.

These epidemiological estimates are based on government crime data and clinical records, which are not fully reliable sources regarding prevalence. When self-report data are used instead of official statistics, the prevalence of misconduct and delinquent behaviors becomes much greater, and the male predominance lowers to about 2:1. The prev-

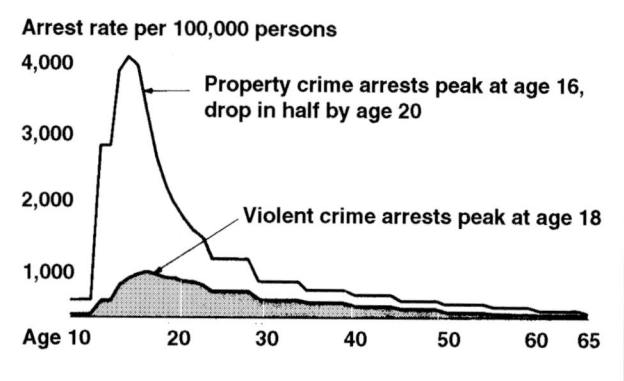

FIGURE 23–5. Age-related incidence of serious crime arrests. Arrests for serious crimes are highest in adolescents and young adults.
Source. FBI Uniform Crime Reports, 3-year average, 1978–1980.

alence of nondestructive behavioral components of conduct disorder is not well documented. The epidemiology of conduct disorder will continue to vary, depending on changes in population size and distribution, family and community structure, and socioeconomic conditions.

ETIOLOGY

A wide variety of etiological factors have been described, reflecting the full range of explanatory models of behavioral causation and the importance of delinquency as a central societal problem. Early speculation centered on intrapsychic structures, such as "superego defects" (Aichhorn 1925/1955), and on parental influences on unconscious motivation (Johnson et al. 1941), such as "superego lacunae" and the "acting out" of parents' unverbalized antisocial wishes or impulses. These inferences were never subjected to large-scale or epidemiological studies in children or adults.

Sociological theories focused on the effects of social deprivation (poverty and cultural disadvantage), substance use (cigarettes, alcohol, recreational drugs), local variations in behavioral norms (street-corner gangs), status seeking, escape from social entrapment, early rejection by peers, and school failure. Researchers in the field of sociology have been using sophisticated mathematical modeling to determine the role of specific socialization experiences in the path that leads to delinquent behavior and drug use (Elliott et al. 1985).

Family history studies show an overrepresentation of antisocial personality, substance abuse, addictive behaviors, mood disorders, ADHD, learning disorders, and schizophrenia. There is an increased incidence of antisocial behavior and conduct disorder in fathers and male relatives of children with conduct disorder. These findings can be explained by familial or genetic transmission.

Genetic studies suggest some inheritable predisposing factors. Elevated rates of conduct disorder in adopted-away children complicate the use of adoption studies, but both adoption and twin studies suggest that genetic and environmental factors are operational. For example, one twin study found that a family history of antisocial personality disorder increased a child's risk of having aggressive behavior and conduct disorder in youth and antisocial features in adulthood. An adverse home environment was found to predispose a child to the development of conduct disorder, but only if there was antisocial personality disorder in the biological family history. That is, a problematic home in the absence of the genetic loading does not lead to conduct disorder (Cadoret et al. 1995). It is likely that the conduct disorders will be shown to have polygenic transmission that

interacts etiologically with environmental and other biological mechanisms.

Follow-up studies of early childhood "personality" suggest that both aggressive and overinhibited personalities can predispose to subsequent conduct disorder in later childhood. Overall, "externalizing" behaviors present a higher risk for conduct disorder than "internalizing" tendencies.

Neurological factors appear significant in some individuals with conduct disorder, especially in more aggressive and violent children. Conduct disorder is associated with an increased prevalence of neurological symptoms (both "hard" and "nonlocalizing"), neuropsychological deficits (especially inattention), and seizures. The degree of aggressivity correlates with a history of physical abuse, head and face injuries, neurological findings, ADHD, and possibly perinatal problems. In extremely violent youths, severe learning and communication problems are common. Psychomotor seizures occur in 20% of these individuals, compared to below 1% in a general population of youths (Lewis et al. 1982). Furthermore, psychotic symptoms appear in up to 60% of severely violent youths with conduct disorder (Lewis et al. 1988).

Biological markers of conduct disorder might be reflective of biological etiologies. Decreased resting heart rate has been reported in numerous studies. The combination of decreased heart rate, lowered skin conductance, and increased slow wave activity on EEG at age 15 was found to correlate with the presence of criminality at age 24 (independently of some demographic and academic factors); this suggests that autonomic underarousal (presumably associated with low levels of anxiety) may be a biological mediator of the tendency toward the development of conduct disorder (Raine et al. 1990). Comorbid conduct disorder and substance use disorder have been associated (during abstinence) with reduced secretion of dense granules from platelets; this might be related to the altered signal transduction associated with the (agonist-nonspecific) underresponsiveness of platelet aggregation in these patients (Moss and Yao 1996). A large and somewhat inconsistent literature supports the hypotheses that changes in serotonin, norepinephrine, or dopamine metabolism may be involved in at least some cases of conduct disorder, but these observations may be a consequence of the high comorbidity of ADHD with conduct disorder. More fruitful findings may come from studies that take the more dimensional approach of seeking biological markers for individual symptoms of conduct disorder (impulsivity, aggressivity, callousness, sullenness, cognitive impairments) rather than for the entire diagnostic category of conduct disorder (Zubieta and Alessi 1993).

Concomitant psychopathology can operate as a pathogenic factor: substance use disorders, ADHD, bipolar disorder, learning and communication disorders, individual psychodynamic features such as counterphobic behavior and avoidance, identification with the aggressor, and stimulus seeking (including novelty seeking and risk taking) may predispose to conduct disorder. The pathogenic mechanisms involved in the interrelationships among conduct disorder, ADHD, and oppositional defiant disorder are not well understood.

Parent, caregiver, and home "microenvironment" characteristics are believed to be particularly important in the presentation of conduct disorder. Proposed factors in the etiology of conduct disorder include fathers with antisocial personality disorder, absent or alcoholic fathers, large families, shifting caregivers, parental rejection, parental abandonment, parental role modeling of impulsive or injurious behaviors, inadequate limit setting, harsh discipline, inconsistent or unpredictable discipline, parental overstimulation or understimulation, parental manipulative behavior, difficult temperament at age 2, separation from parents, institutional care, early onset of unsanctioned use of alcohol, proximity of a delinquent peer group, and chronic poverty. Empirical evidence for the validity of these factors (and their interactions) varies in strength. It is most likely that each factor contributes significantly in some cases.

The macroenvironment also influences the development and outcome of conduct disorder. Geography appears to be a significant factor once a threshold level of urbanization is reached. Living in a city—whether a small city or a metropolitan area—is associated with an increased prevalence of conduct disorder. This finding may reflect the availability of "soft drugs" and the proximity of peers with antisocial characteristics. Involvement in religion was not found to be associated with the increased prevalence in cities (Wichstrøm et al. 1996).

Some counterintuitive findings are clinically helpful. Coming from a single-parent home appears not to be a major risk factor. Family discord rather than separation appears to mediate the risk for conduct disorder (Rutter and Giller 1984), and other factors associated with single-parent homes also appear to be mediating factors (Lahey et al. 1988). Keeping some families together can have disastrous developmental consequences.

Certain microenvironmental factors can also "statistically protect" a child. Intelligence and small family size repeatedly have been found to be protective factors against both the development and persistence of conduct disorder. Adequate supervision at home, especially when parents are away, has been shown to reduce the risk of conduct disor-

der. After-school activities, involvement of neighbors and relatives, community centers, and extended school hours can provide this type of supervision.

One might conclude that all these etiological factors for conduct disorder could be predicted with the use of common sense alone. Indeed, there are few surprises: only an observer without psychiatric knowledge would be surprised by the clinical correlates with family psychiatric history, concomitant individual psychopathology, neurological factors, home microenvironment, intrapsychic dynamics, sociocultural and economic factors, and temperament. These factors are relevant to the production of any abnormal (and normal) behavior. However, as noted, there are counterintuitive findings and interactions among factors, and these easily overload any rigorous etiological explanation about the individuality of each case. Although common sense and basic psychiatric knowledge can make a large proportion of these cases understandable in a general way, the appearance of conduct disorder is not readily predictable. No single factor mentioned is able to account for more than 50% of the variance in the occurrence of childhood disorders. When factors are grouped together, no combination of factors can account for more than 70% of the variance in the occurrence of conduct disorder (Elliott et al. 1985). Given this variety of factors operating at the "population" level, it is a daunting (if not impossible) task to accumulate predictive knowledge about the development of individual cases of conduct disorder.

COURSE AND PROGNOSIS

The major outcome risk of conduct disorder in childhood is antisocial personality disorder in adulthood. In a 30-year follow-up study of 500 child guidance clinic patients (Robins 1966), antisocial behavior in childhood was found to predict maladjustment and a high prevalence (37%) of severe psychopathology in adulthood: antisocial behavior, alcohol abuse, psychiatric hospitalization, child neglect, nonsupport, financial dependency, and poor employment and military records. The children of these patients showed a high prevalence of truancy, running away, theft, and dropping out of high school.

Of particular interest is the finding by Robins (1966) that the natural course of conduct disorder did not appear to be influenced by psychiatric treatment, lengthy incarceration, job or military experiences, or degree of religious involvement. In contrast, marriage to a stable spouse, support from siblings and parents, and brief incarceration were found to be helpful in promoting stability.

In a separate follow-up study of 9,945 Philadelphia boys with conduct disorder, 35% were arrested by their

18th birthday, and 6% became chronic offenders accounting for more than 50% of delinquencies. Recidivists in this sample were more likely to have early onset, poor school grades, and low socioeconomic status (Wolfgang et al. 1972). In another study it was found that about 50% of youths (median age 15) with conduct disorder had no Axis I diagnosis at follow-up 18–21 months later, but 33% had antisocial personality disorder; about 25% of these adults had anxiety disorders, and 25% had substance use disorders (Storm-Mathisen and Vaglum 1994).

Among youths with conduct disorder, childhood predictors of chronicity and unfavorable outcome in adulthood include antisocial behavior, substance abuse, family history of antisocial personality disorder, early onset, low socioeconomic status, school failure, attentional problems, anxiety disorders (two or more in childhood), arson, socialization deficits, nonsupportive family life, family discord, and family deviance. Family risk factors appear to be more prognostically significant for the development of conduct disorder than for any other child psychiatric diagnosis (Fendrich et al. 1990).

Better socialization, positive social experiences, and adequate social skills (especially assertiveness and problem solving) are useful in predicting a better long-term outcome (Jenkins 1973; Rutter and Giller 1984). The nature of involvement with peers is also a predictor of course and severity. Peer ratings of misbehavior and low popularity in first grade were found to predict delinquent behavior during adolescence (Tremblay et al. 1988). Furthermore, ratings of aggressivity made by a child's peers at age 8 may predict certain features of the psychiatric, marital, and legal status at age 28–30 (Huesmann et al. 1984).

Beyond the further development of problem behaviors listed in the definition of conduct disorder, complications of conduct disorder are numerous: school failure, school suspension, legal problems, injuries due to fighting or retaliation, accidents, sexually transmitted disease, teenage pregnancy, prostitution, being raped or murdered, criminal activity, imprisonment, fugitive status, abandonment of family, drug addiction, suicide, and homicide. Consequences of comorbid attention deficits and learning disorders can include low frustration tolerance, educational failure, loss of interest in school, underdevelopment of verbal skills, school dropout, and subsequent unemployment. Children with conduct disorder have a high rate of physical injuries, accidents, and illnesses, as well as emergency room visits and hospitalizations. At follow-up, the most common causes of mortality in conduct disorder were found to be suicide, motor vehicle accidents, and death from uncertain causes (Rydelius 1988).

When compared to children with conduct disorder alone, children with comorbid ADHD and conduct disorder tend to have an earlier onset of symptoms, more aggressive behavior, more severe and diverse conduct problems, and a more troubled course and outcome. The fathers of children presenting with comorbid ADHD and conduct disorder tend to be more aggressive and to be imprisoned more often (Walker et al. 1987). Both conduct disorder and ADHD contribute, separately, to the development of illegal behavior (Foley et al. 1996).

As age increases (up to about 26 years old), there is a tendency toward progressively more serious crime and a higher incidence of incarceration (Figure 23–6) or, alternatively, toward general improvement in overall self-management. Over time, interactions among etiological factors become accumulative. The "spiraling down" and "spiraling up" are viewed as the result of interactions among disadvantages or advantages.

Among incarcerated youths, there is an 85% prevalence of conduct disorder. About 20% have ADHD or a learning disorder; and about 50% have an IQ below 85. Therefore, although conduct disorder is highly linked to family factors, incarceration status is more strongly associated with psychiatric diagnosis (or intelligence) than with family or economic variables (Hollander and Turner 1985).

Despite the extremely high incidence of major psychopathology, maladjustment, and incarceration, about half of children with conduct disorder achieve a favorable adult adjustment (Loeber 1982; Rutter and Giller 1984). There is a tendency toward a reduction in antisocial symptoms after age 40 (Hare et al. 1988; Robins 1966). Although later onset, adequate supervision at home, and good socialization skills are predictors of better course and adult outcome, it is unknown to what degree the good outcomes are associated with the natural course of illness, life experiences, therapeutic intervention, comorbidity, or preexisting characteristics.

EVALUATION AND DIFFERENTIAL DIAGNOSIS

For youths with conduct disorder who have impaired verbal skills, use manipulative defenses, or become uncomfortable when talking with professionals, interactive diagnostic interviews can be difficult. Specific verbal inquiries or repetitive questioning can elicit inconsistent or hostile responses. For these individuals, standard interviews can be ineffective or even counterproductive. Assessments based on highly verbal and structured interviews may overestimate psychopathology and underestimate the interpersonal or intellectual strengths of these individuals.

Child self-reports of conduct symptoms are not fully reliable. Although parents' reports are often viewed by cli-

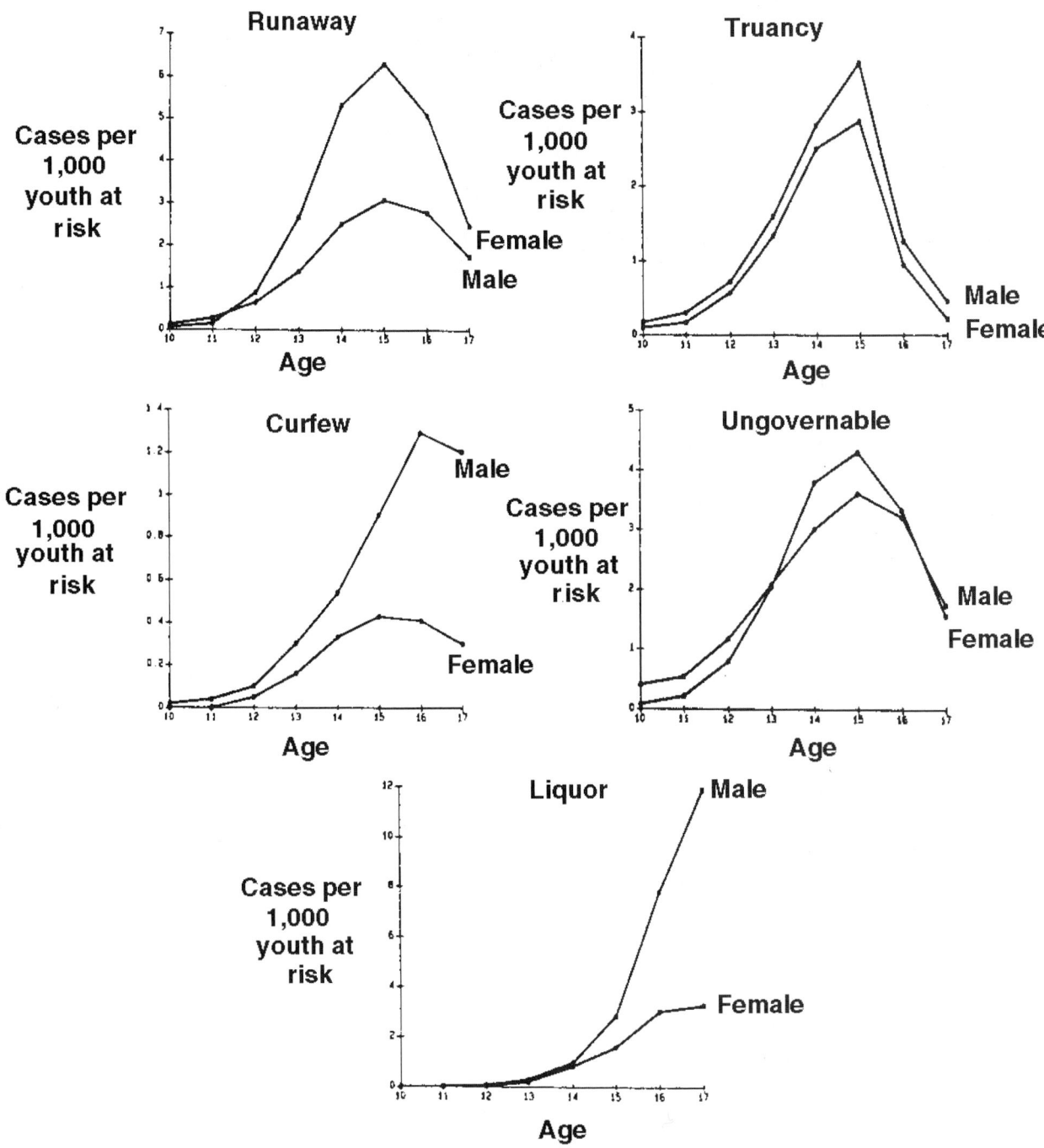

FIGURE 23–6. Age-related incidence of legal violations by youths for certain behavioral symptoms. Official statistics on juvenile court cases disposed in 1983 regarding children charged with a "status offense" (the legal term for an act that would not be considered criminal if committed by an adult). Shown are rates in the general population, not in a clinical population or a conduct-disordered population. Runaway, truancy, and curfew violations are diagnostic criteria for conduct disorder, but liquor violations are nondiagnostic legal offenses. These behaviors generally peak in mid-adolescence, but liquor law violations continue to increase into adulthood (especially in males). The chronicity of alcohol-related problems contrasts with other features of major adolescent misbehavior.

Source. Reprinted with permission from Snyder HN, Finnegan TA: *Delinquency in the United States, 1983*. Pittsburgh, PA, National Center for Juvenile Justice, 1987.

nicians as more trustworthy, there are good reasons to question the accuracy of these data. Because some of the behaviors of conduct disorder appear infrequently, historical rather than observational data are often preferred. However, the secrecy of the behaviors, the fears or wishes for punishment, and the amplifying or diminishing influences of extraneous feelings and biases confound the reliability of all reporters (child, parents, teachers, police). Correlations between the behavioral reports of different types of reporters are quite low (Achenbach and McConaughy 1997), leading to unresolved clinical dilemmas concerning how to combine the data derived from different informants.

Virtually any child psychiatric disorder can present with behavior problems or with comorbid conduct disorder. In assessing an individual with conduct disorder, it is essential to evaluate the full range of psychiatric diagnoses, neurological status, intelligence and neuropsychological features, educational skills and deficits, social adaptiveness and assertiveness, and family functioning.

A search for comorbid psychiatric diagnoses is critical, especially for bipolar disorder (McGee and Williams 1988). It appears that about 25% of adolescents with conduct disorder also have bipolar disorder (Arredondo and Butler 1994), and much higher lifetime rates have been reported. However, conduct disorder does not have a high rate of comorbidity with other mood disorders such as major depressive disorder or dysthymic disorder (Arredondo and Butler 1994; Rey 1994). Adolescents with conduct disorder have major depressive disorder at the rate that would be expected if there were no association between the two disorders. Anxiety tends to be present in children with comorbid conduct and major depressive disorders, but not in children with conduct disorder only (Meller and Borchardt 1996).

In the other direction, most studies have suggested that 10%–20% of youths with major depressive disorder also have conduct disorder, although rates as high as 30% have been reported in preadolescent children (Puig-Antich 1982). These figures are probably underestimates, because some youths with conduct disorder are later rediagnosed as having bipolar disorder.

The finding that 25% of children with conduct disorder also have bipolar disorder, but that there is no overrepresentation of conduct disorder with major depressive disorder, challenges the common clinical belief that a diagnosis of conduct disorder is a signal that the child might be depressed. Instead, conduct disorder can be interpreted as a signal that the child might have bipolar disorder. Conduct disorder can appear before or after the apparent onset of bipolar disorder, and the conduct disorder may persist or remit after the resolution of the bipolar symptoms (Kovacs et al. 1988).

Bipolar disorder is not the only major disorder that often presents with conduct disorder. Learning and communication disorders are common concomitants of conduct disorder and can contribute to the chronicity. Developmental deficits in social skills and other adaptive functions are often apparent, even in individuals who have predominantly inattentive ADHD. Mild mental retardation is often overlooked. Prepsychotic children and intermittently psychotic children may have or appear to have conduct disorder. Substance use is often present in association with conduct disorder. However, even among adolescents with conduct disorder, substance use disorders are commonly underdiagnosed.

The understanding of conduct disorder has progressed dramatically from the days, not long ago, when delinquency was viewed largely in terms of personality development or family functioning. At present, it would be a significant error to assume that a child with conduct disorder should be first conceptualized as having merely a "personality disorder" or a "prepersonality disorder." The differential diagnosis of conduct disorder has become more complex, responding to increasing awareness of the multiple paths that lead to conduct disorder.

The biopsychosocial evaluation of conduct disorder typically involves a multidisciplinary team including a psychiatrist, psychologist, pediatrician, neurologist, educational consultant, speech and language specialist, occupational and recreational supervisor, social worker, legal advisor, parole officer, school liaison person, and case manager. Children with conduct disorders challenge the capacity to think and respond in a multidimensional manner.

TREATMENT

Psychiatric treatment of conduct disorder depends more on individual variables than on diagnosis. Given the diversity of presentations and severities of conduct disorder, it is unsurprising that treatment can move in several directions: legal sanctions, family interventions, social support, psychotherapeutic treatment of individual or family psychopathology, or neuromedical treatment (Kazdin 1987). The treatment site can be a home, school, hospital, residential school, or specialized delinquency program.

From the very start and to the end of treatment, the quick establishment of a containment structure and an expectation of effective limit setting—to provide both safety and a holding environment for treatment—are essential. Limit setting at home may be compromised by parental conflict, parental absence, inconsistent discipline, vague or low behavioral expectations, or parental depression or other psychiatric illness. Creating or reinforcing limits can involve parent counseling, psychiatric treatment of parents, increased supervision at home, surveillance at school, or use of legal mechanisms. Guardianship, hearings before judges, counseling by parole officers, and brief incarceration may be essential for effective limit setting and for communicating the significance of behavioral violations. Treatment of conduct disorder typically requires the involved management of multiple systems (Kazdin 1997).

The possible primary and sustaining roles of comorbid mental disorders in most cases of conduct disorder require that mental health professionals evaluate and follow psychiatric factors in essentially all cases. The minimum required would be a consultative role in a multimodal treatment program. A single treatment method can be decisive for some individuals with conduct disorder, but the vast majority of patients require multimodal treatment.

Cognitive-behavioral therapy can help in the development of skills for managing anger, controlling impulsivity, and communicating (Faulstich et al. 1988). Training in problem-solving skills may be more effective than individual psychotherapy (Kazdin et al. 1989), but specific psychotherapeutic methods can also be used to treat conduct disorder (Kernberg and Chazan 1991).

Parental guidance can help in decision making and management of difficult behaviors as well as promote effective limit setting on impulsive behavior. Functional family therapy can be useful in some cases for reducing interpersonal manipulativeness (Patterson 1982) and for limiting projective identification between family members (Tolan et al. 1986). Psychiatric treatment of the parents or siblings is often needed to treat their biopsychiatric disorders. Group therapy, particularly in residential treatment or group-oriented facilities, often permits the "gang orientation" of these youths to be used in promoting positive change and improving socialization skills.

School interventions can include informing teachers about the nature of this condition, training teachers in management techniques for enhancing learning and behavioral control, and encouraging individualized educational programming, vocational training, and remediation of language and learning disorders. There is evidence that the early treatment of learning disorders may help prevent the development of conduct disorder.

Owing to the complexity of individual cases, most youths with conduct disorder need lengthy therapeutic interventions. Because treatment may "terminate" by graduation into another treatment or facility, a therapist may not see the long-term effects of a particular intervention. Man-

agement of a case often entails repeated setbacks that can frustrate caregivers.

For treatment-resistant patients, effortful attention and purposeful persistence may be needed to establish empathic understanding of the child's view of life and to develop a motivation for change. Failure to diagnose additional concomitant psychiatric disorders (in child or family) is a common source of poor outcome in conduct disorder. When necessary, parent counseling involves helping parents learn to secure psychiatric hospitalization, use the legal system, avoid inappropriate attempts at defending or excusing the child's actions, or, in extreme cases, accept the "loss" of the child to a life of imprisonment, crime, or fugitive status.

Pharmacological research on conduct disorder is quite limited, and most therapeutic effects have appeared to be more closely related to the comorbidity than to the conduct disorder itself. That is, the range of medications used in treatment reflects the range of comorbidity presenting with conduct disorder, and it appears to have little to do with specific treatment of conduct disorder. Pharmacotherapy can involve virtually any psychotropic drug, depending on the concomitant neuropsychiatric findings in the individual: psychostimulants for ADHD, lithium or antidepressants for mood disorders or aggressivity, neuroleptics for psychotic features (or, in low dose, for impulsive behavior), β-adrenergic blocking agents for aggressivity, or anticonvulsants. Lithium treatment has been examined in several controlled trials, but the exclusive focus has been on conduct disorder with prominent aggressive features. Findings have been mixed. When used to treat an entire group of aggressive patients with conduct disorder as a whole (rather than treating only patients with bipolar disorder), lithium appears to have small or clinically insignificant effects (Campbell et al. 1995a, 1995b; Rifkin et al. 1997). Alternatively, lithium might be exerting a substantial effect in a subgroup of these patients. Despite the mixed showing of lithium in controlled trials, clinicians widely report that it appears to be effective in many cases, perhaps because about 25% of youths with conduct disorder have bipolar disorder. Carbamazepine is believed not effective in treating conduct disorder with aggressivity.

For treating comorbid ADHD and conduct disorder, open trials of pemoline (Shah et al. 1994) have indicated some therapeutic effects, but there is no evidence of the value of this drug in treating conduct disorder in the absence of ADHD. In using pemoline, the risks of substance abuse (although less than with short-acting stimulants such as dextroamphetamine), drug dealing, and chemical hepatitis (potentially fulminant) must be clinically considered. Open-label clonidine has also been reported helpful in treating comorbid conduct disorder and ADHD (Schvehla et al. 1994).

In clinical settings, when medication appears useful in treating conduct and comorbid disorders, therapeutic drug effects may not be evident because they are masked by numerous concurrent behavioral symptoms and other problems. However, even if the medication treatment has minimal impact on the overall complex of symptoms and circumstances, continuation of the drug treatment can provide at least a limited degree of symptom reduction. For example, adolescents with comorbid ADHD and conduct disorder may show little reduction of illegal behavior during treatment for ADHD, but the diminished level of impulsivity and inattention may be crucial to their learning alternative methods for social coping.

The value of nonpharmacological treatments can often be seen when pharmacological therapies are not initiated immediately in treatment. Especially with psychiatric hospitalization, the cost-cutting method of starting pharmacotherapy on admission increases the risk of misattributing clinical stabilization to medications rather than to hospitalization, the milieu, and other treatments (Malone et al. 1997). Unnecessary drug treatments and excessive dosing can potentially be avoided by delaying pharmacotherapy long enough to make a specific diagnosis of a comorbid drug-treatable disorder rather than quickly starting a nonspecific drug treatment.

Conduct disorder is based on family factors as fully as is any psychiatric disorder. Individuals with conduct disorder (and perhaps psychiatric comorbidity) and family members with externalizing psychiatric disorders have ways of disrupting the people and environment around them. Maintaining effective limits and a focused orientation toward treatment (rather than punishment) may challenge not only other family members but mental health professionals and legal systems as well. Clearly, the combination of medications, religion, community supports, and psychotherapy does not substitute for family. The treatment of conduct disorder, with or without concurrent psychiatric disorders, with or without "family deprivation," can be quite taxing.

CLINICAL COMMENT

There has been a debate regarding whether the diagnosis of conduct disorder should be "constructed" to be independent of gender and social class: should criteria be selected to remove gender and class bias so that all children are viewed democratically as equally likely to have conduct disorder? Or should the definition of conduct disorder be constructed by using criteria that make no attempt to diminish or hide differences in the prevalence of conduct disorder that might appear among cultural, socioeconomic, ethnic, or gender subgroups? Even if the definitional criteria for conduct disorder were selected to be class-independent, it is unsurprising that patterns of referral, availability of treatments, and course of illness remain class-dependent.

Governmental planning for a full and balanced range of treatment services for delinquency requires a mandated sense of priority at the national and state levels. Outpatient clinics, hospital units, residential treatment facilities, aftercare (posthospitalization) services, emergency and short-term facilities, specialized delinquency programs and correctional services, and juvenile courts are essential services to permit a child with conduct disorder to move through an appropriate sequence of treatments.

Controlled comparisons of the psychiatric and legal models for the management of the conduct disorders are not currently available, despite the widespread use of both models. In practice, both models are blended in many treatments. The evaluation of such complicated multimodal treatments would be an exceedingly costly, large-scale, multicenter, and multiyear project. In the meantime, the treatment of these children continues to remain subject to judgments made in a diversity of locales and based on a variety of child-rearing and psychiatric treatment philosophies.

Conduct disorder is an umbrella term that unifies under a single name tremendously diverse forms of misbehavior that derive from biological, psychodynamic, familial, and social factors. Attempts to subcategorize conduct disorder need to become more sophisticated, allowing for multiple dimensions and their interactions (e.g., aggressive vs. nonaggressive, socialized vs. unsocialized, impulsive vs. nonimpulsive, early vs. late onset, with vs. without family history of antisocial personality disorder). Until psychiatry can delineate specific criteria for clinically useful subgroups, treatment will continue to be offered in individualized but nonspecific psychiatric plans for this mixture of children with "major misbehavior."

OPPOSITIONAL DEFIANT DISORDER

Children with oppositional defiant disorder show argumentative and disobedient behavior but, unlike children with conduct disorder, respect the personal "rights" of other people. Similar provocative and antiauthority behavior is common in children with conduct disorders and ADHD, but oppositional defiant disorder is a separate diagnosis in its own right. In addition, children may show oppositional or defiant behavior during major affective episodes (depression or hypomania) or more enduringly in chronic mood disorder. However, the term *oppositional defiant disorder* describes children whose provocative, antiauthority, or angry behavior occurs apart from psychosis or symptomatic periods of mood disorders. Oppositional defiant disorder often presents in association with ADHD, conduct disorder, or other psychiatric diagnoses (Table 23–8).

This diagnostic designation permits the study and treatment of "difficult" behavior that is not as severe as conduct disorder and that presumably does not have the same genetic transmission, psychodynamics, family features, or drug responsiveness as the psychotic and mood disorders.

CLINICAL DESCRIPTION

Oppositional and defiant features can be normal for young children at 18–36 months and for adolescents; the 6-month minimum duration criterion for oppositional defiant disorder is used to exclude ordinary developmental phenomena.

TABLE 23–8.   DSM-IV diagnostic criteria for oppositional defiant disorder

A. A pattern of negativistic, hostile, and defiant behavior lasting at least 6 months, during which four (or more) of the following are present:

   (1) Often loses temper.
   (2) Often argues with adults.
   (3) Often actively defies or refuses to comply with adults' requests or rules.
   (4) Often deliberately annoys people.
   (5) Often blames others for his or her mistakes or misbehavior.
   (6) Is often touchy or easily annoyed by others.
   (7) Is often angry and resentful.
   (8) Is often spiteful or vindictive.

   Note: Consider a criterion met only if the behavior occurs more frequently than is typically observed in individuals of comparable age and developmental level.

B. The disturbance in behavior causes clinically significant impairment in social, academic, or occupational functioning.

C. The behaviors do not occur exclusively during the course of a psychotic or mood disorder.

D. Criteria are not met for conduct disorder, and, if the individual is age 18 years or older, criteria are not met for antisocial personality disorder.

Anger-related symptoms are the presenting behavior problems, but management of anger appears to be a circumscribed problem. Unlike children with ADHD, the oppositional and angry behavior demonstrated by these children does not lead to impulsivity throughout their behavior, affect, and cognition (Halperin et al. 1995). The anger is typically directed at parents and teachers, and a lesser degree of anger dyscontrol may be seen in peer relationships. Temper tantrums typically subside in minutes, at most in 30 minutes. Children with mood disorders can require considerably longer to reorganize after an angry outburst.

A crucial feature of oppositional struggling is the self-defeating stand that these children take in arguments. They may be willing to lose something they want (a privilege or toy) rather than lose a struggle. The oppositional struggle takes on a life of its own in the child's mind and becomes more important than the reality of the situation. This "holding onto" or "winning" the struggle may feel paramount to the child. "Rational" objections voiced to the child become counterproductive, and the child may experience these interventions as the adult continuing the argument.

Passive-aggressive and "sneaky" behavior can also be seen, but it does not have the self-centered manipulative quality or the persistent continuity of the coping style seen in children with conduct disorder. Alternatively, oppositional children can also display excessive compliance, passivity, and "goody-goody" or perfectionistic behavior. At times, these children seem to live by their own sense of justice, without regard for the realities or circumstances of other people.

The oppositional and defiant symptoms are generally reported by parents and caregivers; the children typically are not able to provide reliable information pertaining to this diagnosis. The children do not view themselves as oppositional or argumentative, and they externalize blame onto parents, authority figures, and peers. In addition to the symptoms of oppositional behavior, intentional defiance is a hallmark of this disorder. Behavior problems may include verbal fighting and bullying.

In a follow-up study of children with oppositional defiant disorder and conduct disorder, there was little crossover between these two diagnostic categories in the course of 18 months. The distinction between the disruptive behavior disorders, on the basis of the criterion of "violation of personal rights and societal rules," appears to be useful and stable. This lack of crossover may explain the finding that youths with oppositional defiant disorder have a lower than normal prevalence of substance-related disorders.

EPIDEMIOLOGY

It has been estimated that 6% of children have oppositional defiant disorder. Along with ADHD, it is the most prevalent psychiatric disorder in 5- to 9-year-old children (August et al. 1996). A male predominance of 2–3:1 was reported in a nonreferred epidemiological sample (Anderson et al. 1987). Oppositional defiant disorder is commonly seen in classrooms for emotionally disturbed and learning-disabled children. The majority of children with ADHD also have oppositional defiant disorder.

ETIOLOGY

Oppositional defiant disorder often appears to be a characteristic of a family rather than of a child (Fletcher et al. 1996). In the absence of direct studies of the etiology of oppositional defiant disorder, several psychosocial mechanisms have been hypothesized: 1) parental problems (too harsh or inadequate) in disciplining, structuring, and limit setting; 2) identification by the child with an impulse-disordered parent, who sets a role model for oppositional and defiant interactions with other people; and 3) attachment deficits due to parents' emotional or physical unavailability (e.g., depression, separation, evening work hours). However, neurobiological influences and temperamental factors may also contribute. Preliminary results suggest a familial aggregation of oppositional defiant disorder. Mechanisms of transmission are undetermined.

COURSE AND PROGNOSIS

Oppositional defiant disorder can be diagnosed after age 3 but usually appears in late childhood. Follow-up studies suggest that 40% of children with oppositional defiant disorder retain the diagnosis for at least 4 years and 93% retain psychiatric symptoms (Cantwell and Baker 1989). There is a developmental progression for certain individuals from oppositional defiant disorder (with or without ADHD) to conduct disorder as well as to other psychiatric disorders.

DIAGNOSTIC EVALUATION

Behavioral evidence of oppositional defiant disorder can often be obtained within 30 minutes by observing peer interactions (Matthys et al. 1995). Psychiatric evaluation of the child and family is needed to investigate family and psychosocial factors as well as to identify comorbid presentations with conduct disorder, ADHD, mood disorders, or psychotic disorders. It is also worthwhile to evaluate for a learning disorder, language disorder, or low

intelligence; the persistence of these conditions can contribute to a child's oppositional behavior.

TREATMENT

Several studies in the psychology literature have demonstrated that behavioral techniques can modify oppositional behavior. There are virtually no other reports of specifically psychiatric treatments of children with oppositional defiant disorder. In one large-scale study, it was reported that psychoanalytic psychotherapy has greater effectiveness in treating oppositional defiant disorder (56%) than in treating conduct disorder (23%), especially if the patient and family do not drop out during the first year of treatment (Fonagy and Target 1994). There are no controlled studies to support the typical practice of treating these children with individual or family psychotherapy.

CLINICAL COMMENT

Although oppositional defiant disorder is a distinct disruptive behavior disorder, considerable research is needed to define its clinical characteristics, epidemiology, etiology, course, and relationship to other disorders. At present, there is little psychiatric research concerning treatment.

Although the oppositional behavior and defiance are distressing to families, these symptoms are not necessarily more pathological than excessive compliance in a child. Pathological compliance can be a significant developmental liability and reason for treatment, but it is not recognized as a psychopathological entity in a culture that places a high social value on harmonious conformity.

LEARNING, MOTOR SKILLS, AND COMMUNICATION DISORDERS

Developmental problems and barriers to the acquisition or performance of specific skills are usually first diagnosed in childhood and can have major consequences for lifetime functioning. Three major domains of skills are addressed by DSM-IV. The "learning disorders" involve a series of impairments in the learning of academic skills, particularly reading, arithmetic, and expressive writing. "Motor skills disorder" entails difficulty with physical coordination. The "communication disorders" involve developmental problems with language and speech, specifically deficits of expressive language, receptive (plus expressive) language, stuttering, and articulation.

These disorders often occur in combination and often

with other psychiatric comorbidity in individuals and families. In practice, these children commonly present with psychiatric or behavioral problems, and the learning and communication disorders are uncovered secondarily.

Most of these disorders are defined by a particular skill or area of functioning that is impaired relative to general intelligence. DSM-IV criteria specify that these diagnoses should be based on more than simple clinical observation: when possible, standardized test protocols are important for documenting the presence of a specific deficit. Depending on the disorder, formal measurements of both intelligence and specific skills may be required for diagnosis.

As a group, these disorders are present in 10%–15% of the school-age population. There is a male predominance of 3–4:1 for most of these disorders. Equal gender ratios are reported for reading disorder, mathematics disorder, and mixed receptive/expressive language disorder. All of these disorders run in families.

The etiology is unknown but is generally believed to be related to slow maturation, dysfunction, or damage of the cerebral cortex or other brain areas related to these specific processing functions. The strength of the direct evidence for genetic or biological abnormalities varies with each disorder, and nonbiological factors are clearly also involved. There is no reason to assume that each disorder is due to a single pathological mechanism, and subtyping may become possible as the brain mechanisms involved become better understood. The clustering of these disorders in the same individuals suggests that these neuropsychological impairments reflect an early disruption in developmental processes, can involve wide-ranging but potentially related cerebral dysfunctions, and are likely to require multimodal educational remediation.

These learning, language, and coordination disorders are commonly associated with high rates of comorbid psychiatric disorders as well as a variety of psychological complications, including low self-esteem ("feeling stupid"), poor frustration tolerance, passivity, rigidity in new learning situations, truancy, and dropping out of school. Disruptive behavior disorder can be a complication of these disorders, but signs of developmental dysfunction may appear before school failure, in the preschool years. Although there has been considerable emphasis on the "emotional overlay" resulting from learning and communication disorders, there is an increasing awareness of the neuropsychiatric and sociofamilial antecedents of these disorders.

Over time, mild cases may "resolve" through persistent education and practice. Certain individuals may compensate by "overlearning," but others retain specific deficits in adulthood. Often, the associated behavioral symptoms and intrapsychic complications persist beyond the duration of the developmental deficits, and they may remain problematic during adult life (J. Cohen 1985).

Evaluation includes intelligence testing, a battery of specific achievement tests (of the full range of academic skills, language, speech, and motor coordination), and observation of the child's behavior in the classroom. A general determination of the quality of teaching available at the school is needed before a diagnosis is made. It is also essential to evaluate for possible mental retardation, ADHD, mood disorder (causing low motivation), and other psychiatric and neurological disorders. Sensory perception tests are obtained to assess possible impairments of vision or hearing, which can aggravate or mimic features of these disorders.

Treatment for these disorders in public schools is guaranteed (in principle) by law. The Education for Handicapped Children Act of 1978 (federal law P.L. 94-142) mandates "special education" of all learning-disabled children in the "least restrictive environment." P.L. 94-142 is usually interpreted to include at most the learning disorders, communication disorders, and ADHD, although other psychiatric disorders that entail symptoms of inattention are sometimes considered. In practice, remediation of only the more basic skills in the most severe cases is funded. An "individual educational plan" (IEP) is designed for each child, but the quality of initial evaluation and treatment services is variable. Part-time "resource rooms," full-time "self-contained classrooms," and "mainstream" classrooms (with special education consultants) provide the major part of special education services. Sometimes, specialized schools and residential treatment programs are employed.

Multidisciplinary communication is essential, because many specialists and teachers may be involved in the education of a single child. Careful communication, particularly during transitions, is vital to maintain developmental and educational progress.

Parents of children with learning and communication disorders often fear the irreversibility of these conditions and may contribute to a climate of negativity and criticism. These parents may be responsive to supportive interventions such as involvement in educational planning and adjustment of expectations to anticipate slower-than-standard learning with no clear "ceiling" on educational outcome.

Since the enactment of PL 94-142, children with these underdiagnosed and undertreated disorders have begun to receive remediation during childhood. Despite the use of many types of psychoeducational and educational techniques nationwide, these methods are rarely evaluated in comparative studies. Psychopharmacological therapy is not helpful in treating learning, communication, or motor skills disorders. Aggressive management is required for psychological effects on self-esteem, patience, assertiveness, and flexibility. The evaluation and treatment of concurrent psychiatric disorders, as well as the management of secondary psychological complications, require more than a purely educational or neuropsychiatric perspective.

These neurodevelopmental disorders appear to be predominantly genetic or neuromaturational in origin; however, socioenvironmental factors are critical in the appearance of the complications of these disorders, so that psychosocial and interpersonal factors are central in treatment and prognosis.

LEARNING DISORDERS

The learning disorders involve deficits in the acquisition and performance of reading, writing (not handwriting but expressive writing), or arithmetic. These conditions are meant to designate individuals who have specific deficits in acquiring skills and neurointegrative processing, and so are qualitatively different from other slow learners.

Learning disorders are defined to exclude individuals whose slow learning is explainable by weak educational opportunities, low intelligence, motor or sensory (visual or auditory) handicaps, or neurological problems. In understanding the impact of these disorders, it is helpful to hold a broad psychiatric and neurological view of development in childhood and functioning in adulthood, because the estimated 5%–10% of the population with learning disorders is at increased risk for other psychiatric disorders. People with learning disorders commonly have a comorbid communication or motor skills disorder, low self-esteem, motivational problems, and symptoms of anxiety.

The diagnosis of a learning disorder is often made initially during grade school. During the early school years, basic skills, attention, and motivation are building blocks for subsequent learning. Major impairments in these fundamental abilities require identification and remediation to avoid developmental derailment in multiple spheres of functioning. In later school years, organizational skills become increasingly significant: problems with note taking, time management, and book and paper arrangements may be signs of cortical deficits, even for individuals whose basic skills are well remedied. In high school and college, these students may have difficulty in learning foreign languages, writing efficiently, reading for fun, enjoying sports, pursuing scientific studies, setting high personal goals, and striving to achieve their goals (J. Cohen 1985).

Depending on the type of disorder, a child can be encouraged to make use of a calculator or word processor, take "time-extended" tests, receive tutoring individually or in a small group, or use self-paced programmed texts or computerized self-instruction. Cognitive-behavioral techniques are employed to emphasize success, develop pride and self-esteem, foster enjoyment of mastering a skill, give opportunities to experiment with less defensive rigidity, enhance learning by confronting established patterns ("do something new"), and promote interests in new situations and new experiences.

Reading Disorder

Learning to read can be compromised in many ways, but reading disorder is a specific neuropsychiatric form of reading disability. Reading disorder can be a severe impairment, even in the presence of normal intelligence, educational opportunity, motivation, and emotional control. Commonly called *dyslexia*, this learning disorder is characterized by a slow acquisition of reading skills resulting from demonstrable cognitive deficits, primarily in cortical function. Slow reading speed, impaired comprehension, word omissions or distortions, and letter reversals result in functioning below the expected performance levels based on age and intelligence (Table 23–9).

Reading disorder is different from simple learning slowness, just as small body size induced by an endocrinological disorder is different from simple short stature. The distinctiveness of reading disorder has been questioned by findings indicating that it may simply represent the low end of the spectrum (a normal distribution) of reading abilities (Shaywitz et al. 1990). However, there appears to be a hump at the "slow" end of the curve for reading acquisition and no analog of "fast" learners at the high end

TABLE 23–9. DSM-IV diagnostic criteria for reading disorder

A. Reading achievement, as measured by individually administered standardized tests of reading accuracy or comprehension, is substantially below that expected given the person's chronological age, measured intelligence, and age-appropriate education.

B. The disturbance in criterion A significantly interferes with academic achievement or activities of daily living that require reading skills.

C. If a sensory deficit is present, the reading difficulties are in excess of those usually associated with it.

Coding note: If a general medical (e.g., neurological) condition or sensory deficit is present, code the condition on Axis III.

of the curve (Rutter and Yule 1975). This distribution implies that pathogenic processes are associated with reading disorder and can be identified amid the numerous possible sources of slowness in reading acquisition. It appears that reading disorder does not merely reflect a developmental lag, therefore, but is a specific abnormality. Reading disorder (a specific disorder that is defined relative to intelligence) is distinct from reading acquisition slowness (a temporary developmental lag that may be present or absent regardless of intelligence).

For reading acquisition to develop in the normal way, a wide variety of neurological and psychiatric functions must be intact. Eye control (not slipping off letters or lines), spatial orientation (attacking letters and words from the left, retaining a memory trace of letter forms), verbal sequencing, grasping the structural sense of a sentence, and abstraction and categorization require intact eye and brain functions as well as cortical integration. Reading also involves the simultaneous use of visual and spatial perception (shape discrimination), sequencing (spatial and temporal), cross-modal visual-auditory processing, phonemic processing (linguistic sound units), syntactic (grammatical) and semantic (meaning) analysis, and the pursuit of understanding. Attention, motivation, and effort must be reasonably intact. In addition, "reading readiness" skills are necessary, including the ability to take instruction, remain seated, and avoid disrupting other individuals in the classroom.

Both reading disorder and reading acquisition slowness can result from processes that interfere with any of these functions. Processes that interfere with these functions include psychiatric disorders (especially if associated with symptoms of anxiety, agitation, or inattention), sensory deficits, cultural deprivation, inadequate schooling, brain damage, and mental retardation. Although reading ability generally correlates with IQ (especially verbal coding and sequencing), these forms of interference can break the correlation.

The focus of cognitive research on reading disorder has shifted away from an emphasis on visual-perceptual and visuospatial (decoding) problems. There is a newer focus on the language (and symbol-processing) characteristics of children with reading disorder that is consistent with the structuralist trends in language analysis and neuroscience.

Clinical description. Individuals with reading disorder typically show difficulty in the "paired-associate task" of translating verbal symbols (letters) into auditory-based sounded words. In addition, left-right orientation, sound discrimination, and perceptual-motor skills are often impaired. Signs of visual and perceptual-motor skill impairment include letter reversals (e.g., b, d), word transposition (e.g., saw, was), omissions (e.g., truck, tuck), and substitution (e.g., truck, trick).

Virtually all individuals with reading disorder have spelling problems, which may be more severe and long lasting than the reading problem. About 80% have other verbal language deficits. Many have DSM-IV disorder of written expression, phonological disorder, motor skills disorder, or poor handwriting. Some have seizures or symptoms of nondominant hemisphere injury. Attentional difficulties are common and are noted also on tasks unrelated to reading and language. About 25% have conduct disorder, usually beginning before adolescence and sometimes before the school years. About one-third of children with conduct disorder have reading disorder.

Epidemiology. Reading disorder is by far the most prevalent of the learning disorders, involving 80% of all individuals with learning disorders. Prevalence estimates for reading disorder vary widely but usually range from 5% to 15% of the general population. Reading disorder was believed to show the 3:1–4:1 male predominance observed in most learning disorders, but more recent data suggest an equal prevalence in males and females (S. E. Shaywitz et al. 1990; Wadsworth et al. 1992). These children often have a parent with reading disorder, perhaps in the majority of cases. Increased prevalence of reading disorder is associated with low socioeconomic class, large family size, and social disadvantage. Prevalence varies considerably with geographic region. The nature and prevalence of reading disorder may differ in other countries, where demands for high-quality reading may vary and where reading may involve different linguistic structures or pictographic symbols.

Etiology. The main etiological factors appear to be neurological, but symptom severity and duration are affected by learning and experience. When neuropsychological testing of a patient identifies patterns similar to the cognitive characteristics of individuals with localizable brain disorders, brain defects in similar cortical regions are postulated.

Anomalous cerebral morphology in the bilateral frontal and left temporoparietal regions have been described in numerous imaging studies of reading disorder. These structures are hypothesized to play a role in reading, and the anomalies are postulated to contribute to the etiology of reading disorder. Magnetic resonance imaging data demonstrate subtle variations in the morphology of the corpus callosum. The reduction in the anterior (genu) volume of the corpus callosum suggests potential difficulties with interhemispheric transfer (Hynd et al. 1995). These studies also found a significant correlation between corpus callosum volume and reading achievement. Together, these findings suggest that reading disorder might be a result of structural changes in the anterior corpus callosum that interfere with interhemispheric transfer or coordination of information.

Developmental abnormalities of the cerebral cortex in reading disorder are suggested by neuroanatomical anomalies (Figure 23–7) that have been demonstrated in neuropathological studies (Galaburda et al. 1985). These neuronal ectopias and dysplasias are widespread through-

out the cortex but are primarily concentrated in the left hemisphere, especially in the perisylvian region. In the inferior frontal and superior temporal regions, these neuronal anomalies include micropolygyria, neuronal ectopia in layer 1, nodules (brain warts), and architectonic dysplasias.

There is also an absence of the usual cerebral pattern of a larger language-dominant region (Broca's area) in the left hemisphere (Haslam et al. 1981). Instead, the planum temporale is symmetrical in these brains, indicating that the usual asymmetry in this part of the brain is absent and suggesting that the normal development of a differentiated language center does not occur in reading disorder.

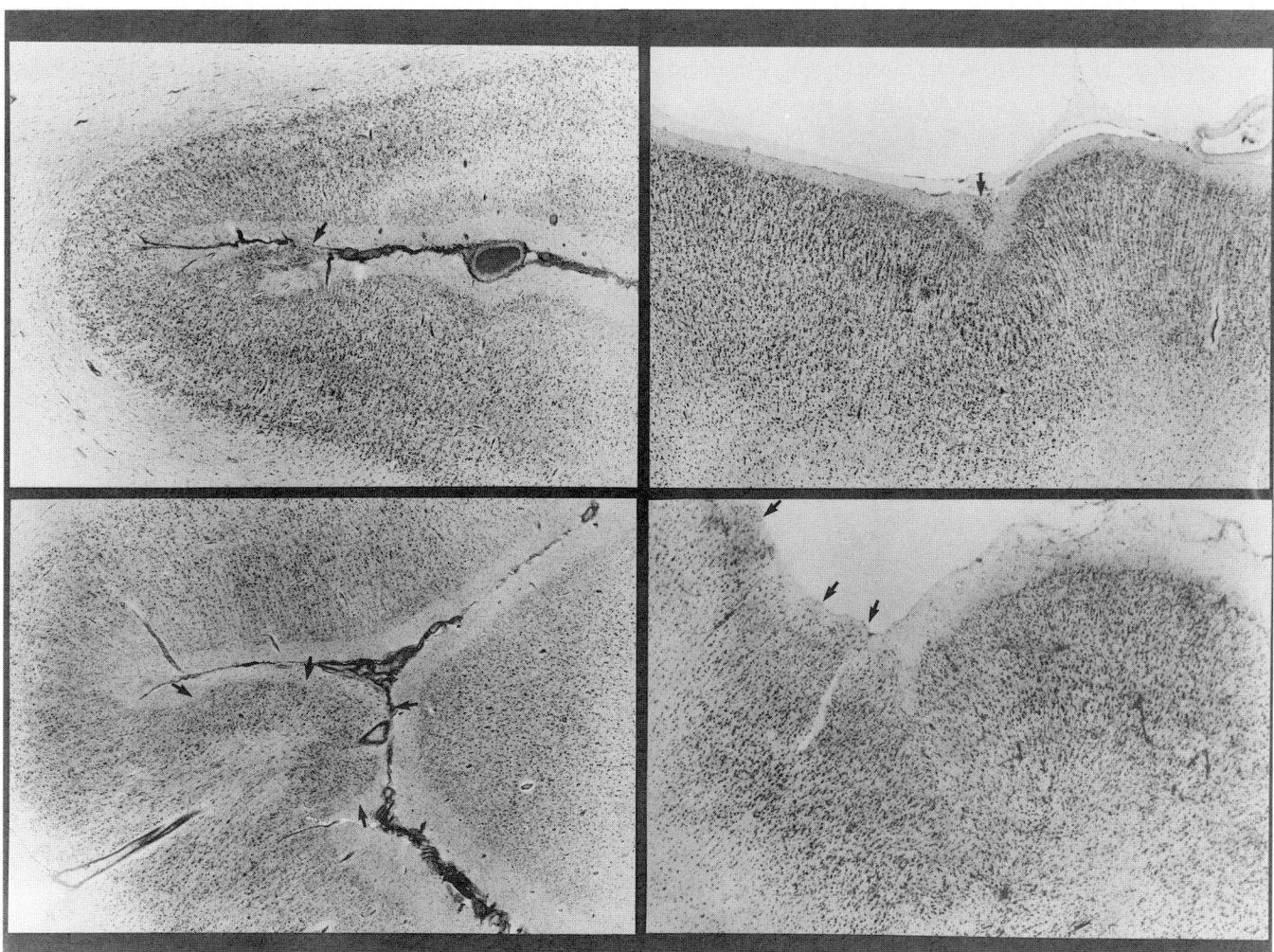

FIGURE 23–7. Neuroanatomical abnormalities of the cerebral cortex in reading disorder. Examples of neuronal ectopias and architectonic dysplasias (arrows) in the cerebral cortex of four patients with reading disorder. These neuroanatomical anomalies imply abnormal structural development of the cerebral cortex. In Patient C (lower left), an artery and a cell-free area appear near a brain wart (about 500 microns).

Source. Reprinted with permission from Galaburda AM, Sherman GF, Rosen GD, et al: "Developmental Dyslexia: Four Consecutive Patients With Cortical Anomalies." *Annals of Neurology* 18:222–233, 1985. Copyright 1985, Little, Brown.

These studies provide evidence of a relatively underdeveloped Broca's area (left planum temporale) as well as more widespread cortical anomalies. The neuronal ectopias and anomalous symmetry imply a relative failure in brain development that is not restricted to language-dominant regions. More generalized dysfunction is implied by findings that cerebral blood flow is more left-asymmetrical (i.e., predominates on the left side of the brain) during a semantics task in individuals with reading disorder (Rumsey et al. 1985a). These anomalous brain structures are associated with a broad range of cerebral functions, including spatial and verbal abilities, motor dominance (i.e., handedness), and left-right sense. The wide distribution of anomalous structures and function may be consistent with the variety of other learning disorders that frequently accompany reading disorder, underscoring again that reading disorder is not merely a localized defect in this cortical language center.

The cytoarchitectonic anomalies were probably acquired during the midgestational period of massive neuronal migration in the topographic formation of the cerebral cortex. Because early acquired lesions can cause a reorganization of the structure and interconnections of the cortex (even at distant points, remote from the original lesions), it is possible to speculate that brain architectonic and connectional features may lead to a "cerebral reorganization" and deliver unusual functioning in people with reading disorder. Such alterations in organization suggest that older theories based on "loss-of-function" models of reading disorder significantly underestimate these individuals' potentials and special talents. None of these abnormalities can be assumed to be causes of reading disorder, because educational and environmental factors interact to alter the expression of these neuronal lesions.

Numerous findings and theories regarding hemisphere function and specialization during development have been proposed. A study comparing strongly left-handed and strongly right-handed people demonstrated that left-handers (and their relatives) have more reading disorder, stuttering, and immune disorders (Geschwind and Behan 1982). Geschwind and Galaburda (1985) speculated that a prenatal testosterone spurt may lead to slowed cortical lateralization (reduced left hemisphere function), reading disorder, left-handedness, and autoimmune disease (thymus suppression). Although many of the predictions based on this hypothesis have been shown to be incorrect, there are some biological interconnections among these conditions (Galaburda 1993) that underscore the medical basis of reading disorder.

Various neuropsychological formulations of reading disorders have been proposed, mainly regarding differences in language-related functions and symbolic processing deficits. The disability appears to involve both word recognition and phonological perception.

For example, people with reading disorder have been shown to process phonemes slowly (Fletcher et al. 1994; Stanovich and Siegel 1994); that is, they have difficulty in breaking words down into small sound segments. This difficulty in associating words with sounds involves problems in two directions: a difficulty in decoding and a difficulty in identification. Phonological processing ability appears to be genetically transmitted, and impairments generally persist into adulthood unless remediated (Bruck 1992; Felton et al. 1990). The phonological processing problem can be diminished when the rate of verbal input is slowed, thereby providing more processing time for phonemic analysis (Tallal and Stark 1982). Cognitive exercises have been developed that are targeted to improve phonemic processing speed. In patients with reading disorder, treatment of the impaired phonological processing leads to enhanced reading ability (Bradley and Bryant 1983; Wise and Olson 1995).

Visual acuity is generally normal, but some dyslexic patients have nonprocessing visual deficits (Geiger and Lettvin 1987). Eye-training methods are numerous, have been tested, and are not helpful.

Family psychiatric histories show an overrepresentation of reading, speech, and language disorders in siblings and parents. A concordance rate approaching 100% in identical twins has been found in several studies of reading disorder (Vandenberg et al. 1986). The lower concordance in fraternal twins supports a genetic factor. Family pedigrees are generally not consistent with a single mode of transmission, suggesting that the disorder is genetically heterogeneous. Gene linkage analysis has implicated chromosome 15 in the autosomal dominant transmission of certain cases of reading disorder (Smith et al. 1983). Chromosome 6 is also involved in some cases (Cardon et al. 1994; Grigorenko et al. 1997), and other linkages have been established as well.

The extent to which neurological comorbidity influences the etiology of reading disorder is unclear. EEG abnormalities appear to be associated with the presence of reading disorder, but this association can be explained by a variety of mechanisms.

Despite the neurogenetic factors in the etiology of reading disorder, environmental factors exert a strong influence on its expression and clinical presentation. Reading disorder can be negatively influenced by maternal smoking, low birth weight, and prenatal and perinatal mishaps. In the positive direction, reading disorder can be beneficially influenced by educational opportunities; family support; and individual personality, drive, and ambition.

In surveying this diversity of findings, it may be inferred that reading disorder is not a unitary disorder and that multiple etiological factors could operate in the same individual. The numerous neurological, physiological, attentional, behavioral, family, educational, and cultural factors are best understood as correlates or risk factors rather than as causes. This implies that correction of any one of these deficits may contribute only marginally to the general remediation of reading disorder and that the opportunity to maximize the potential anomalous strengths and special talents of these individuals would be missed.

Course and prognosis. For reading disorder and slow reading acquisition, adequate reading skills may eventually be acquired with sufficient time and effort. Educational interventions appear to accelerate this process, especially if family support and personal motivation are strong. The extent of residual symptoms in reading disorder and its associated features is quite variable.

Delayed acquisition of reading skills is usually identified in grade school. Typically, by third grade the child with reading disorder is 1–2 years behind expectations and may fall further behind unless remediation is received. Adolescents may become frustrated with learning, lose interest in school, and drop out of school; in addition, there may be an exacerbation (or clinical recognition) of conduct disorder or other concomitant psychiatric disorders. Although reading usually improves over time, spelling problems and delinquency may persist. In adulthood, there is an elevated rate of unemployment and placement in unskilled jobs.

Some adults never attain substantial reading skills and may adapt by hiding the disability from their children, friends, and employers. They may not seek remedial education or may continue to resist remediation in adulthood, either because of embarrassment, pride, or the required effort. The associated feature of rejection of help may be both a cause and a complication of persistent reading problems. Mismanagement of this major problem in early learning can become a model for the child's subsequent approach to problem solving. Alternatively, proper management can teach the child how to persevere in the face of a seemingly hopeless personal problem.

Evaluation and differential diagnosis. It can be useful to obtain neurological and psychiatric assessment (especially regarding disruptive behavior, ADHD, other learning and communication disorders, and social deprivation), hearing and vision tests, as well as IQ, psychological, neuropsychological, and educational measurements (including reading speed, comprehension, and spelling).

The new neuroimaging techniques are expected to contribute significantly to diagnostic assessment in the future.

Reading disorder is clinically distinguishable from simple slowness in reading acquisition in several characteristics. Compared to reading disorder, slow reading acquisition is more closely associated with slow arithmetic learning, constructional apraxia, physical clumsiness, cerebral palsy, and other neurological conditions. In contrast, unlike slow reading acquisition, reading disorder is often associated with the other DSM-IV learning disorders. Similarly, the mean IQ in reading disorder is quite normal (Rutter and Yule 1975), whereas slow reading acquisition is associated with a lower IQ.

Treatment. Early educational intervention may involve one of the many remedial systems; comparative studies of the different educational approaches to reading disorder are lacking. There is little evidence supporting the use of any particular teaching method, including the usual perceptual training based on an individual's "strong" learning modality (e.g., auditory vs. visual). Self-esteem may need to be bolstered to help the child (or adult) tolerate the remedial efforts. Treatment should be directed at the reading disorder and any associated learning and communication disorders, conduct disorder, or ADHD.

Parental involvement is crucial in providing support for the educational program and for the child's persistent efforts in a criticism-free learning environment. Some parents may advocate alternative vitamin or dietary approaches, but no data support these options for treating learning disorders. Parents can be advised that it is more beneficial for them to listen to their children read at home daily (Tizard et al. 1982).

The standard psychotropic medications are not useful in treating reading disorder. Somewhat unexpectedly, piracetam has been found in numerous double-blind placebo-controlled studies, with standardized reading tests among the outcome measures, to improve reading in children with developmental reading disorder. Most studies show that the improvements in children are modest but consistent and statistically significant. The longer studies (5–9 months) showed more pronounced improvements in reading. Furthermore, five double-blind placebo-controlled studies in adults with reading disorder have confirmed the findings in children. Piracetam, a derivative of γ-aminobutyric acid (GABA), has been used outside the United States to treat cognitive changes in the elderly. It is not a psychostimulant and does not alter levels of alertness or arousal. With strong accumulated evidence that piracetam can improve reading in children and adults with reading disorder, this noötropic agent (memory or learning enhancer) may open the door to important new directions in treatment and research.

Mathematics Disorder

The capacity for making simple mathematical calculations is critical in a consumer economy and high-technology culture. Arithmetic, calculation (fractions, decimals, percentages), measurement (space, time, weight), and logical reasoning are basic skills.

Mathematics disorder can present with circumscribed deficits associated with fact retrieval or with more globalized deficits associated with problem conceptualization. Arithmetic facts may be deficient despite preserved mathematical conceptual knowledge (Hittmair-Delazer et al. 1995). Individuals with mathematics disorder (Table 23–10) have difficulty in learning to count, doing simple mathematical calculations, conceptualizing sets of objects, and thinking spatially (right-left, up-down, east-west). Deficits may be seen in copying shapes, mathematical memory, number and procedure sequencing, and the naming of mathematical concepts and operations. Also, reading and spelling problems may be seen in association with mathematics disorder.

Factors that produce slow academic development of mathematical abilities include neurological, genetic, psychological, and socioeconomic conditions as well as learning experiences. Typically, arithmetic ability correlates with IQ and classroom training. However, mathematics disorder is not defined to designate individuals who are merely slow learners or who have poor educational opportunities; instead, it labels individuals whose mathematical abilities are low for their IQ. In addition, these individuals often have comorbid psychiatric disorders or symptoms,

TABLE 23–10. **DSM-IV diagnostic criteria for mathematics disorder**

A. Mathematical ability, as measured by individually administered standardized tests, is substantially below that expected given the person's chronological age, measured intelligence, and age-appropriate education.

B. The disturbance in criterion A significantly interferes with academic achievement or activities of daily living that require mathematical ability.

C. If a sensory deficit is present, the difficulties in mathematical ability are in excess of those usually associated with it.

   Coding note: If a general medical (e.g., neurological) condition or sensory deficit is present, code the condition on Axis III.

although descriptions of the psychiatric aspects of this disorder are limited.

Approximately 6% of the population is affected by mathematics disorder, and the gender distribution appears to be equal (Gross-Tsur et al. 1996). As in other learning disabilities, psychiatric comorbidities are common, especially conduct disorder. Also, ADHD occurs in about 25% of children with mathematics disorder (Shalev et al. 1995a). Attentional problems may lead to arithmetic difficulties (Ehlers et al. 1997) in children who do not have mathematics disorder, but children with such difficulties need to be evaluated for this disorder. Lower socioeconomic classes show an overrepresentation of mathematics disorder as well as other learning disorders. Although genetic contributions are largely unknown, in a large sample of patients with developmental dyscalculia, it was reported that 42% of the first-degree relatives also had learning disabilities (Gross-Tsur et al. 1996).

Etiological factors are not well defined. Individuals with mathematics disorder appear to have a type of neurocortical abnormality that is linked to a deficit in processing speed in some areas of mathematics (Bull and Johnston 1997). Neuropsychological deficits may be demonstrated in number manipulation, spatial relationships, and mathematical reasoning. Both verbal (sequencing) and visuospatial deficits can contribute to mathematics disorder, suggesting that bilateral hemisphere dysfunction may be involved (Rourke and Strang 1983), although neurological damage in the language-dominant hemisphere is not typically demonstrable. Nonetheless, there is evidence that the left hemisphere may play a relatively more important role, at least in certain functional deficits (Shalev et al. 1995b). For example, the left prefrontal region has been implicated in mathematics disorder (Tohgi et al. 1995). Subcortical mechanisms have also been proposed.

During the school years, the course of mathematics disorder usually entails a progressive increase in disability, because the learning of mathematical skills is based on the developmental completion of earlier steps. Some children perform well on rote arithmetic and fail later in trigonometry and geometry, which require more abstract and spatial thinking. Over time, most individuals show gradual improvement. As in other learning disorders, complications include low self-esteem, truancy, dropping out of school, symptoms of disruptive behavior disorders, and avoidance (or poor performance) of jobs that require mathematical skills.

Evaluation for mathematics disorder includes psychiatric (i.e., disruptive behavior disorders, other learning disorders, and mental retardation), neurological, cognitive (i.e., intelligence, psychological, neuropsychological, and educational achievement testing), and social assessments. Standardized tests of arithmetic skills may need to be individually adjusted for the child's educational experience with an older (rote calculation) or newer (logical concept) mathematics curriculum.

Treatment of mathematics disorder involves special education, with initial evaluation and subsequent monitoring of the possible need for psychiatric and neurological intervention. It is interesting that when mathematics disorder is accompanied by ADHD, salient auditory stimulation has been found to improve mathematical performance (Abikoff et al. 1996).

The mathematical skills of a normal fifth- or sixth-grader are quite sufficient for the practical requirements of most adults, although concomitant social and nonverbal deficits that accompany mathematics disorder may be more significant as well as enduring (Semrud-Clikeman and Hynd 1990). After the school years (and even during them), weakness in arithmetic skills is not socially stigmatic and may not be a direct source of personal distress. It is likely that this disorder is quietly present in many adults, who make accommodations in their lives and choice of work to manage a residue of dysfunctions that were more evident during school years.

Disorder of Written Expression

Disorder of written expression is not well characterized in the psychiatric literature, and its assessment and treatment are not well developed. Spelling, grammar, sentence and paragraph formation, organizational structure, and punctuation are the areas of difficulty (Table 23–11).

Symptoms include slow writing speed, low written yield, illegibility, letter reversals, word-finding and syntax errors, erasures, rewritings, spacing errors, and punctuation and spelling problems. A more generalized "developmental output failure" may be suggested by low productivity, refusal to complete work or submit assignments, and chronic underachievement (Levine et al. 1981). Ideational content and intellectual abstraction may be limited, although not necessarily. The "sense of audience," a social cognition of the interests and needs of the reader, may be impaired (Gregg and McAlexander 1989).

These deficits in written expression may result from underlying problems with graphomotor (hand and pencil control), fine motor, and visuomotor function; attention; memory; concept formation and organization (prioritizing and flow); and expressive language function. Other motor dysfunctions may be present. Like other learning disorders, disorder of written expression is presumed to result from neurocortical dysfunctions, which may be modified by environmental experiences. The prevalence of disorder of written expression is not well delineated. There is a standard 3:1–4:1 male predominance.

Formal methods for assessment and measurement of expressive writing have been developed, but adequate clinical screening can be obtained from samples of copied, dictated, and spontaneous writing. In evaluating disorder of written expression, it is worthwhile to screen for developmental coordination disorders and other motor abnormalities.

Genuine remedial therapy is possible. Educational interventions have traditionally consisted of alternative writing formats and skill building. The wide availability of computers has promoted new methods in remediation. Pending more specific research, the psychiatric evaluation and intervention for the disorder of written expression resemble the approach to the other learning disorders.

MOTOR SKILLS DISORDER: DEVELOPMENTAL COORDINATION DISORDER

Developmental coordination disorder, the only motor skills disorder recognized in DSM-IV, involves deficits in the learning and performance of motor skills (Table 23–12). Integration of motor functions and memory of motor tasks are also impaired. Overall, about 5% of children have significant impairments of gross or fine motor functions, which are apparent in running, throwing a ball, buttoning, holding a pencil, and moving with grace; the disorder also may manifest as generalized physical awkwardness. None of the motor impairments in developmental coordination disorder can be explained by fixed or

---

TABLE 23–11. DSM-IV diagnostic criteria for disorder of written expression

A. Writing skills, as measured by individually administered standardized tests (or functional assessments of writing skills), are substantially below those expected given the person's chronological age, measured intelligence, and age-appropriate education.

B. The disturbance in criterion A significantly interferes with academic achievement or activities of daily living that require the composition of written texts (e.g., writing grammatically correct sentences and organized paragraphs).

C. If a sensory deficit is present, the difficulties in writing skills are in excess of those usually associated with it.

Coding note: If a general medical (e.g., neurological) condition or sensory deficit is present, code the condition on Axis III.

localizable neurological abnormalities or by mechanical interference.

Although this disorder is rarely the primary complaint leading to psychiatric evaluation, it is commonly found in association with many psychiatric disorders, especially learning disorders. The psychiatric literature contains little other information on developmental coordination disorder, except for some continuing debate regarding its classification and descriptive criteria (Miyahara and Mobs 1995).

Three main areas of motor deficits have been defined: clumsiness, adventitious movements, and dyspraxia. *Clumsiness*, technically defined as a slowness or awkwardness in the movement of single joints, involves disruption of the integration of agonist and antagonist muscle groups. Although it is defined in terms of dysfunction at the basic level of single-joint movements, clumsiness can reduce the capacity to perform more complex motor tasks, such as riding a bike or drawing. Clinically, clumsiness is easily observed in finger tapping or in picking up very small objects. Clumsiness may present alone or associated with ADHD, learning disorders, or mental retardation (especially trisomy 21/Down's syndrome), and it sometimes is aggravated by anticonvulsants. Although it was previously assumed that these children would "outgrow" their clumsiness, long-term data suggest that these symptoms commonly persist into adulthood (Fox and Lent 1996).

Adventitious movements are involuntary movements that occur during voluntary movements. Overflow move-

ments (i.e., synkinesias) may include mirror movements (which occur in symmetrically active muscles) or motions seen in unrelated muscle groups (e.g., opening the mouth while reaching). Other adventitious movements include tics, tremor, and chorea. Clinically, adventitious movements can be observed while the child is performing specific tasks that emphasize voluntary control.

Dyspraxia, the impaired learning or performance of sequential voluntary movements (relative to age or verbal intelligence) that cannot be attributed to sensory or mechanical limitations, does not improve when specific tasks are executed without time limits or hurry. Its expression may involve a range of muscle movements, from localized (face, tongue, or hands) to global, and may depend partially on cerebral dominance (both in spatial vs. linguistic functions and in left- vs. right-sided tasks). This symptom is also seen in mental retardation, especially fragile X syndrome. Dyspraxia may be screened clinically by asking the child to imitate some unusual hand or finger positions and by pantomiming sequential tasks (e.g., taking a bottle out of a refrigerator, opening it, pouring the contents, and having a drink from the glass).

Common concomitants of developmental coordination disorder include ADHD, and common complications include being scapegoated, impaired self-esteem, and sports avoidance.

Research into the mechanisms underlying clinical decrements in motor performance and integration is scarce. Both the database and theoretical knowledge in this area are limited, but simple concepts of control by fixed motor pathways do not seem able to explain these motor decrements. The emerging view of motor integration deficits is based on a model of interactive failures between different autonomic and functional units of motor systems, which are composed of neurons that themselves have flexible functions in different neural networks (Getting 1989). This model is consistent with magnetic resonance imaging data suggesting that damage to the ventral part of the posterior end of the body of the corpus callosum is correlated with the dyspraxia (Tanaka et al. 1996). These findings also suggest that developmental coordination disorder is associated with a disconnection between the right and left superior parietal lobe. In most right-handed subjects, the left superior parietal lobe is dominant for volitional control of movement.

Treatment may seem questionable in clinical settings, especially for mild presentations. However, because "good hands" and athletic ability are crucial building blocks of self-esteem for children and adolescents, and may be economically vital for some adults, remediation is warranted to promote general development, even if special education

TABLE 23–12.   DSM-IV diagnostic criteria for developmental coordination disorder

A. Performance in daily activities that require motor coordination is substantially below that expected given the person's chronological age and measured intelligence. This may be manifested by marked delays in achieving motor milestones (e.g., walking, crawling, sitting), dropping things, "clumsiness," poor performance in sports, or poor handwriting.

B. The disturbance in criterion A significantly interferes with academic achievement or activities of daily living.

C. The disturbance is not due to a general medical condition (e.g., cerebral palsy, hemiplegia, or muscular dystrophy) and does not meet criteria for a pervasive developmental disorder.

D. If mental retardation is present, the motor difficulties are in excess of those usually associated with it.

   Coding note: If a general medical (e.g., neurological) condition or sensory deficit is present, code the condition on Axis III.

funding is limited. It is unclear whether developmental co-ordination disorder, apart from identifiable neurological disorders or more focal findings, has prognostic significance in psychiatry beyond the factors related to its comorbidity (Deuel and Robinson 1987).

COMMUNICATION DISORDERS

Speech problems (regarding sound production) are seen in about 15% of the general school-age population, and language problems (involving the communicative use of speech as well as other communicative modes) are seen in about 6%. The frequent association of communication disorders, including disorders of speech or language, with the learning disorders highlights the general cerebral dysfunctions that characterize both groups of disorders. There is some evidence to suggest that language disorders may be developmental precursors of learning disorders rather than merely comorbid disorders of independent etiology (Tallal 1988). Language disorders in young children may not become clinically evident until the appearance of learning disorders during the school years.

About 25%–50% of child psychiatric patients have a communication disorder. About 50% of children with communication disorders have concomitant psychiatric disorders, most notably ADHD, and in an additional 20%, learning disorders eventually appear (Beitchman et al. 1986; Cantwell and Baker 1987). Children with developmental language disorders (and speech disorders) also tend to have motor deficits, and these deficits also may require treatment (Owen and McKinlay 1997). Language deficiencies observed in children with ADHD are typically higher order executive deficiencies and not deficits in basic language processing (Purvis and Tannock 1997).

As in the learning disorders, recent research in communication disorders is moving away from an emphasis on deficits in audioperceptual processing and toward a conceptualization based on language and symbolic functions. Sensory, perceptual, motor, and cognitive processes are closely connected in cerebral development. During the course of early development of the cerebral cortex, there is a progressive leftward lateralization of language functions, including speech (sound production), phonetic and syntactic analysis, and verbal (as well as nonverbal) sequence analysis. The right hemisphere appears to be more involved in sound recognition than the left. Lesion data and neurobiological theory have implicated the left perisylvian regions in the processing of phonemes and auditory information. These findings have been confirmed by magnetic resonance imaging, single photon emission spectroscopy, and PET. The areas of the planum temporale and angular

gyrus appear compromised in both children and adults with language impairments (Semrud-Clikeman 1997). There is also emerging evidence of familial transmission of these precise deficits.

The usual development of language and speech skills occurs over many years, and there is a wide range of normal functioning. By age 5 years, children are expected to speak fluently, comprehend, and express themselves. Gender differences in cortical maturation may relate to girls' developmental advantage in verbal skills (which lasts until adolescence), which is comparable to boys' advantage in spatial processing. Speech and language may interact with other environmental factors in influencing development and adult skills. In social interactions, nonverbal (gestures of eye, face, and hand; vocal qualities) and verbal communication includes word finding (access and retrieval of verbal information), word relationships (semantics), sentence formation (syntax), giving and receiving feedback, following of conversational structure and flow, responding to the context, adapting to meanings and external events, responding to one's own internal sense of events, and monitoring one's own communicative productions (metalinguistic skills). The development of these skills is a formidable task to complete in 5 years.

In speech and language disorders, deficits in articulation (diction or speech sound production), expression (oral language production and use), and reception (comprehension) may be evident by age 2–3 years. Early speech and language problems frequently improve during development, and these early delays are not strongly predictive of subsequent learning disorders. However, children with early genuine speech and language problems are at high risk for later learning disorders as well as persistent communication disorders. Most preschool children with communication disorders (70%) are placed in special education or repeat a grade within the first 10 years of schooling (Aram et al. 1984).

Hearing loss plays a significant role in the etiology of the communication disorders. Hearing is crucial in the development of speech and language, and impairments of hearing operate etiologically alongside genetic, neurological, environmental, and educational factors. Deafness is associated with clear reduction in communication skills, but milder hearing decrements may also be developmentally significant. A mild hearing loss (25–40 decibels) resulting from chronic otitis media or perforation of the tympanic membrane may delay development of articulation, expressive and receptive language, and spelling. During the formative period for language development, fluctuating hearing capacity can diminish verbal intelligence and academic performance in a persistent way (Howie 1980).

Early middle-ear pathology may cause language or

speech symptoms, particularly if the hearing impairment is chronic. Otitis media, a common infectious disease in children, may leave a residual hearing decrement in 20% of the American population. The degree of language and speech delay may correlate to the number of otitis episodes. Determinants of otitis media include socioeconomic class, allergies, and oropharyngeal (palate) or craniofacial malformations. Hearing loss may also result from genetic and metabolic disorders, chromosomal anomalies, low birth weight, perinatal anoxic damage, CNS infections, ototoxic medications (e.g., antibiotics, diuretics), and toxin exposures (e.g., alcohol, anticonvulsants). Sociofamilial as well as medical factors can contribute, via otitis media, to the appearance of communication disorders.

It appears that impairment in cognitive and educational development may occur at levels of hearing loss that are considered medically insignificant (Howie 1980). It may be speculated that early fluctuations in conductive hearing lead to anomalies in brain development, perhaps leading to enduring changes in auditory attention or signal/noise discrimination. However, not all children who have had episodes of otitis media have developmental delays. Sensory stimulation is crucial in organizing the visual cortex (Wiesel 1982), but there is less clarity regarding the effect of early auditory experience on the acquisition of language, speech, and central auditory-processing mechanisms.

An interesting line of research has led to the proposal that the neurophysiological problem in language disorders may be a deficit in processing rapidly presented stimuli (Tallal 1988). This problem in the perception and memory of rapidly appearing stimuli may involve not only linguistic tasks but a variety of sensory and motor functions as well as integrative processing. Laboratory tests to identify these neuropsychological deficits might be helpful in the direct diagnosis of language disorders, without the use of standard neuropsychological testing batteries, at least in certain children. These sensory and motor deficits in response to rapid stimuli are also found in children with reading disorder (although not phonological disorder), again supporting the notion of a continuity between language and learning disorders.

Although it is only speculative, the mechanisms involved in early influences on the development of the cerebral cortex may be useful in understanding the pathogenesis of learning disorders as well as communication disorders, and they may apply to a broader range of mental functions.

Speech and language skills are eventually acquired in virtually all children with communication disorders, but lower IQ and concomitant psychopathology appear to predict less favorable outcome. Complications include progressive academic impairments, psychological distress, low self-esteem, rigidity regarding learning, and dropping out of school.

Evaluation includes a medical, psychiatric, social, and developmental workup as well as language and speech assessment (Cantwell and Baker 1987). Because 20% of children have hearing deficits due to otitis media, it is helpful to test for hearing acuity, using methods such as audiometry or auditory evoked response (which does not require a young child's cooperation). Parents may give a history of few startle reactions, lack of sound imitation (at 6 months) or reactiveness (at 12 months), unintelligibility (at 2.5 years), loud speech, frequent misunderstandings ("Huh?"), speech avoidance, or communication-associated embarrassment or tension (e.g., blinking). Assessing family characteristics (e.g., family size, birth order, socioeconomic status, parental verbal skills, familial speech patterns, interpersonal stimulation), as well as observing free speech between parents and child, may be useful. The child's speech may be studied for language comprehension (linguistic structures), expression (structure and length of utterances), and logical reasoning. Auditory attention (e.g., keeping up with the flow of conversation, ability to hear in a crowd, lack of distractibility), discrimination (e.g., distinguishing similar sounds), and memory (e.g., the ability to repeat sequences of words or digits) can be assessed informally or formally. In neuropsychological tests, nonverbal measures of IQ (e.g., Leiter International Performance Scale, Columbia Scale of Mental Maturity) are employed. Also, a neurological evaluation may be indicated for children with a communication disorder in whom a motor abnormality is suspected.

Treatment of communication disorders includes educational and behavioral interventions, as well as treatment of concomitant medical (e.g., hearing), neurological (e.g., seizures), and psychiatric problems. Aggressive treatment of otitis media is particularly indicated in these children, despite the uncertainty about the relation of this disease to language and speech development. It is particularly helpful to encourage social involvement, imitation, and imaginative play as a means of increasing verbal, communicative, and symbolic exercise. There is no evidence that use of nonverbal communication by child or parents inhibits the development of language skills, and it might even enhance such skills.

Expressive Language Disorder

In this linguistic "encoding" problem, the symbolic production and communicative use of language are impaired. The individual cannot put the idea into words ("I can't get the words out") and also has problems in nonverbal expression. There are similar difficulties with repeating, imitating, pointing to named objects, or acting on commands. Unlike autistic and pervasive developmental disorders, there is typically normal comprehension in verbal and nonverbal communication. In verbal language, both semantic and syntactic errors occur so that word selection and sentence construction may be impaired; paraphrasing, narrating, and explaining are unintelligible or incoherent. The child with expressive language disorder may use developmentally earlier forms of language expression and may rely more on nonverbal communication for requests and comments. Short sentences and simple verbal structures may be employed, even with nonverbal communications such as sign language (Paul et al. 1994). This feature implies a problem in symbolic development across language modalities, leading to a diverse group of delays in articulation, vocabulary, and grammar (Table 23–13).

Individuals with expressive language disorder generally learn language in a normal sequence, but slowly. These children can adjust their speech to talk appropriately to young children (Fey et al. 1981), suggesting some facility and flexibility in the use of their language skills. There may be associated learning disorders, phonological disorder, inattentiveness, impulsivity, or aggressivity.

When frustrated, the child may have tantrums during

TABLE 23–13. DSM-IV diagnostic criteria for expressive language disorder

A. The scores obtained from standardized individually administered measures of expressive language development are substantially below those obtained from standardized measures of both nonverbal intellectual capacity and receptive language development. The disturbance may be manifest clinically by symptoms that include having a markedly limited vocabulary, making errors in tense, or having difficulty recalling words or producing sentences with developmentally appropriate length or complexity.

B. The difficulties with expressive language interfere with academic or occupational achievement or with social communication.

C. Criteria are not met for mixed receptive-expressive language disorder or a pervasive developmental disorder.

D. If mental retardation, a speech-motor or sensory deficit, or environmental deprivation is present, the language difficulties are in excess of those usually associated with these problems.

   Coding note: If a speech-motor or sensory deficit or a neurological condition is present, code the condition on Axis III.

the early years or may briefly refuse to speak when older. Problems in social interactions may lead to peer problems and overdependence on family members.

Approximately 1 in 1,000 children have a severe form of expressive language disorder, but mild forms may be 10 times more common. The standard 3:1–4:1 male predominance of some of the other developmental disorders is seen in this disorder.

Diverse etiologies involving neurological, genetic, environmental, and familial factors have been described. Teratogenic, perinatal, toxic, and metabolic influences are linked to certain cases. When hearing loss is present, the degree to which hearing is lost strongly correlates with the amount of language impairment (Martin 1980). Children with expressive language disorder are reported to have low cerebral blood flow to the left hemisphere (Raynaud et al. 1989).

Although expressive language disorder is often associated with seemingly secondary behavioral and attentional problems, a high incidence of various psychiatric problems is also observed in relatives, suggesting that concomitant psychiatric disorders may be present in children with difficulties in expressive language.

This condition usually causes parental concern by the time the child reaches age 2–3 years, when the child may appear to be bright but is not yet talking, has acquired only a small vocabulary, or is difficult to comprehend. The period from age 4 to age 7 years is crucial. By age 8, one of two developmental courses is usually established. The child may be progressing toward nearly normal speech, retaining only subtle defects and perhaps symptoms of other learning disorders. Alternatively, the child may remain disabled, show slow progress, and subsequently lose some previously achieved capacities. There appears to be a decrease in nonverbal IQ, possibly owing to the failure of development of sequencing, categorization, and related higher cortical functions. The child may lose some of his or her earlier brightness and come to resemble a mentally retarded adolescent. In both courses, complications of expressive language disorder include shyness, withdrawal, and emotional lability.

Evaluation includes psychiatric (attentional and behavior problems), neurological, cognitive, and educational assessments. Intelligence is determined by a nonverbal measure of IQ. A test of hearing acuity is sensible, and workup for concomitant learning disorders is essential.

Mixed Receptive-Expressive Language Disorder

Mixed receptive-expressive language disorder is the impaired development of language comprehension that entails impairments in both decoding (i.e., comprehension) and encoding (i.e., expression). Multiple cortical deficits are usually observed, including sensory, integrative, recall, and sequencing functions (Table 23–14). Because it involves both receptive and expressive language deficits, mixed receptive-expressive language disorder is considerably more severe and socially disruptive than expressive language disorder (D. Cohen et al. 1976).

Although receptive aphasia in adults leaves expression intact, a similar condition during development leaves a child impaired in the learning of a first verbal language. Depending on the nature of the deficits, nonverbal comprehension may be preserved or disrupted.

In mild cases, there may be slow "processing" of certain linguistic forms (e.g., unusual, uncommon, or abstract words; spatial or visual language) or slow comprehension of complicated sentences. There may also be difficulty in understanding humor and idioms and in "reading" situational cues. In severe cases, these difficulties may extend to simpler phrases or words, reflecting slow auditory processing. Muteness, echolalia, or neologisms may be observed. During the developmental period, the learning of expressive language skills becomes impaired by the slowness in receptive language processing.

Mixed receptive-expressive language disorder is distinguished from aphasia (which is not a developmental disorder but a loss of preexisting language functions), other acquired deficits (usually caused by neurological trauma or

---

TABLE 23–14. DSM-IV diagnostic criteria for mixed receptive-expressive language disorder

A. The scores obtained from a battery of standardized individually administered measures of both receptive and expressive language development are substantially below those obtained from standardized measures of nonverbal intellectual capacity. Symptoms include those for expressive language disorder as well as difficulty understanding words, sentences, or specific types of words, such as spatial terms.

B. The difficulties with receptive and expressive language significantly interfere with academic or occupational achievement or with social communication.

C. Criteria are not met for a pervasive developmental disorder.

D. If mental retardation, a speech-motor or sensory deficit, or environmental deprivation is present, the language difficulties are in excess of those usually associated with these problems.

　　Coding note: If a speech-motor or sensory deficit or a neurological condition is present, code the condition on Axis III.

---

disease), or the absence of language (a rare condition usually associated with profound mental retardation).

Mixed receptive-expressive language disorder may approach the severity of autistic disorder during adolescence because of social awkwardness, stereotypies, resistance to change, and low frustration tolerance (D. Cohen et al. 1976). However, these individuals typically demonstrate better social skills, environmental awareness, abstraction, and nonverbal communication than do those with autism.

About 3%–10% of school-age children have mixed receptive-expressive language disorder, but severe cases have a prevalence of 1 in 2,000. Unlike the male predominance of expressive language disorder and many of the learning disorders, there is an equal gender ratio in mixed receptive/expressive language disorder.

The main etiology of mixed receptive-expressive language disorder appears to be neurobiological, usually genetic factors or cortical damage. Neurological examination reveals abnormalities in about two-thirds of cases. Electroencephalographic findings include a slight increase in nondiagnostic abnormalities, especially in the language-dominant hemisphere. CT scans may show abnormalities, but these are not uniform or diagnostic. Similarly, dichotic listening may be abnormal but without specific or lateralizing findings.

Evaluation includes assessment of nonverbal IQ, social skills, hearing acuity, articulation, receptive skills (understanding single words, word combinations, and sentences), nonverbal communication (vocalizations, gestures, and gazes), and expressive language skills. Expressive language skills can be measured in terms of the mean length of utterances (MLU), which is compared with developmental norms. Syntactic structures should be assessed and also compared with developmental norms. There are standardized instruments to assess comprehension, with norms starting at age 18 months. Concomitant medical, neurological, and psychiatric (e.g., learning disorders, mood disorders, autistic disorder and other pervasive developmental disorders, mental retardation, and selective mutism) diagnoses should be considered.

For treatment of expressive and receptive language problems, special education should be maintained until the symptoms improve. After a child is "mainstreamed," supplemental academic and language supports may be helpful. Psychiatric treatment for attention deficits, behavior problems, and other comorbidity, as well as speech therapy for phonological disorder, may be needed.

Phonological Disorder

Diction problems, especially for late-acquired sounds, may be seen in children who have normal vocabulary and grammar. This impairment in articulation and in learning sound production for speech includes substitutions ("wery" for "very"), omissions ("cayon" for "crayon"), additions ("blook" for "book"), and distortions (Table 23–15). Speech may be slightly or largely unintelligible, or it may sound like "baby talk." The understandability of speech may be further compromised by problems that are not part of phonological disorder: accent, intonation (e.g., neurologically induced), stuttering, cluttering, physical conditions (orofacial disorders such as cleft palate), neurological disease, or psychotropic medication (especially neuroleptics).

Early in development, infant sounds are similar cross-culturally, apparently because they are based on biologically directed processes. As an infant learns the sounds of the local language and environment, sound productions change and become culture-specific. Subsequent speech sound production depends on the development of speech motor control (tongue, lips, palate, larynx, jaw, breathing muscles), auditory perception (vowel and consonant phonemes, rhythm, intensity, intonation), and the ability to make sounds, contrasts, combinations, plural formations, and emphases. By age 8 years, a child has typically acquired all speech sounds.

Age at diagnosis of phonological disorder is generally about 3 years, but the disorder may appear earlier or later depending on its severity. Approximately 6% of boys and 3% of girls have phonological disorder, but problems with articulation become less prevalent with age. The etiology of phonological disorder is often unknown; contributing factors may include faulty speech models within the family,

mild hearing impairment, or neurocortical deficits.

In addition to an evaluation of intelligence, these children should receive a full language assessment, because many have an associated disorder of grammatical (syntactic) expression.

Spontaneous recovery usually occurs by age 8, but individual or group speech therapy may help the speed and completeness of speech development. "Communicative low self-esteem" is a potential complication.

Stuttering

Stuttering, the disruption of normal speech flow, is characterized by involuntary and irregular hesitations, prolongations, repetitions, or blocks on sounds, syllables, or words (Table 23–16). Unlike the case of cluttering or other dysfluencies in children, anxiety produces a noticeable aggravation of speech rhythm and rate in people who stutter. There may be a transient worsening during periods of performance anxiety or "communicative stress" (e.g., during public speaking or a job interview). In laboratory studies, abnormalities of speech behavior and body movement are seen even during periods of apparently fluent speech.

Approximately 2%–4% of children have this speech disorder. Stuttering improves spontaneously in 50%–80%

TABLE 23–15. DSM-IV diagnostic criteria for phonological disorder

A. Failure to use developmentally expected speech sounds that are appropriate for age and dialect (e.g., errors in sound production, use, representation, or organization such as, but not limited to, substitutions of one sound for another [use of /t/ for target /k/ sound] or omissions of sounds such as final consonants).

B. The difficulties in speech sound production interfere with academic or occupational achievement or with social communication.

C. If mental retardation, a speech-motor or sensory deficit, or environmental deprivation is present, the speech difficulties are in excess of those usually associated with these problems.

Coding note: If a speech-motor or sensory deficit or a neurological condition is present, code the condition on Axis III.

TABLE 23–16. DSM-IV diagnostic criteria for stuttering

A. Disturbance in the normal fluency and time patterning of speech (inappropriate for the individual's age), characterized by frequent occurrences of one or more of the following:

(1) Sound and syllable repetitions
(2) Sound prolongations
(3) Interjections
(4) Broken words (e.g., pauses within a word)
(5) Audible or silent blocking (filled or unfilled pauses in speech)
(6) Circumlocutions (word substitutions to avoid problematic words)
(7) Words produced with an excess of physical tension
(8) Monosyllabic whole-word repetitions (e.g., "I-I-I-I see him.")

B. The disturbance in fluency interferes with academic or occupational achievement or with social communication.

C. If a speech-motor or sensory deficit is present, the speech difficulties are in excess of those usually associated with these problems.

Coding note: If a speech-motor or sensory deficit or a neurological condition is present, code the condition on Axis III.

of cases, and 1% of adolescents and adults continue to fulfill criteria for the disorder. In young children, poor phonological ability contributes to the appearance of stuttering, and developmental improvement in phonological performance appears to contribute to resolution (Paden and Yairi 1996). A male predominance of 3:1–4:1 is found in stuttering.

Etiological theories of stuttering are based on genetic, neurological, and behavioral concepts. There may be several etiological subgroups of stuttering. A strikingly higher concordance in monozygotic than dizygotic twins suggests a large genetic etiological factor (Vandenberg et al. 1986). For 60% of persons who stutter, the disorder runs in families, appearing in about 20%–40% of first-degree relatives (especially in males). Because the prevalence is lower in females but the familial prevalence is higher in the relatives of female stutterers, a gender threshold effect on penetrance (gender-specific difference in penetrance or in the genetic loading required for penetrance) is apparent.

Current data are not consistent with a single-gene mode of transmission but can fit a polygenic model with a gender-influenced differential threshold of phenotypic expression. When a multifactorial model was used, 86% of the variance in the pedigree data could be explained by genetic factors (Kidd 1980).

Certain forms of acquired stuttering are clearly neurological in origin, such as stuttering that begins after stroke (presumably owing to damage to fluency centers) or secondary to degenerative brain disease. These acquired forms may be transient, but they can persist, particularly if there is bilateral and multifocal brain disease. These neurologically based forms of stuttering have clinical characteristics that differ from the developmental form of stuttering: blocks and prolongations occur but are not primarily at initial syllables and substantive words, and associated grimacing and hand movements are unusual.

Several investigators have found that non-right-handedness (mixed or left-handedness) is overrepresented in stutterers (and in their first- and second-degree relatives), suggesting that stuttering may be associated with anomalous cortical organization (Geschwind and Galaburda 1985). Also, some stuttering is associated with mental retardation, specifically trisomy 21 (Down's syndrome) and Hunter-Hurler's syndrome (a mucopolysaccharide disorder). In rare cases, stutterlike dysfluency can be caused by psychotropic medications (tricyclic antidepressants, neuroleptics, lithium, alprazolam).

Stuttering often starts at age 2–4 years or, less commonly, at age 5–7 years. For toddlers, stuttering is usually a transient developmental symptom lasting less than 6 months, but 25% of early-onset cases have persistent stuttering beyond age 12 years. For onset during latency, symptoms are usually stress-related, and there is typically a benign course of 6 months' to 6 years' duration.

At the onset, the child is usually unaware of the symptom. The disorder typically waxes and wanes during childhood, either gradually improving during childhood or worsening and leading to a chronic course. Males tend to have more chronic forms of the disorder. If the condition progresses, word blocking and involuntary tension of the jaw and face muscles may become conspicuous. In persistent cases, people who stutter become painfully aware of the problem. These individuals find that anxiety further aggravates their dysfluency and that they cannot improve their speech by slowing their speech rate or by focusing attention on their speech.

Neurological and acquired stuttering tend to be more constant and fixed, in contrast to a greater variability of the genetic, constitutional, and psychodynamic forms. For nonneurogenic stuttering, the symptoms are often absent during singing, reading aloud, talking in unison, or talking to pets or inanimate objects.

Complications include fearful anticipation, eye blinking, tics, and avoidance of problematic words and situations. The child may experience negative emotional reactions of family and peers (embarrassment, guilt, anger), teasing, and social ostracism. Speech avoidance and poor self-image may affect language and social development, and may lead to academic and occupational problems.

Evaluation of stuttering includes a workup for possible neurological causes (cortical, basal ganglial, cerebellar). A full developmental history and general evaluation of speech, language, and hearing are needed. Behavioral assessment includes delineating any restrictions in social interactions and activities. Referral for evaluation to a speech and language pathologist is indicated in all cases of stuttering. It is helpful to assess the dysfluency in monologue, conversation, play, and anxiety; to test the effects of slowed speech and focused attention on the dysfluency; and to observe parent-child interactions for communicative stress placed on the child (e.g., rapid questioning, interruptions, repeated corrections, frequent topic shifts).

Speech therapy involves some elements of behavioral therapy, including modifying environmental and conversational factors that trigger stuttering, relaxation, rhythm control, feedback, and dealing with accessory body movements, as well as fostering self-esteem and social assertiveness. Specific therapies for stuttering include intensive smooth speech, intensive electromyography feedback, and home-based smooth speech; all have been reported to reduce stuttering frequency by 85%–90%, and these gains have persisted 1 year after treatment (Craig et al. 1996). Other methods include imitation, role-playing, practice in speaking (while reading, choral reading, conversing), and talking in different settings (alone, in a group, in front of a classroom, on a telephone) and with different people (parents, relatives, friends, strangers).

Education and counseling of family members are advised. Psychotherapy is generally not indicated, but it might be considered if stuttering persists or begins in adolescence. Antianxiety drugs are generally of minimal value. Neuroleptics may be useful in some cases, but there are no controlled studies. Some studies have suggested the possible effectiveness of serotonin reuptake inhibitors for stuttering. A controlled trial found that clonidine did not improve stuttering (Althaus et al. 1995). Therefore, the role of pharmacotherapy seems limited at best, especially in view of the effectiveness of speech therapy.

CLINICAL COMMENT

The preceding neurodevelopmental disorders highlight the potential for underachievement in specific domains. Despite educational opportunities, adequate intelligence, and emotional stability, they emerge in both clinical populations and "normal" samples.

Anomalous strengths and special talents can be associated with these "disorders." Mental age and IQ do not set an upper level for achievement for individuals with any of these disorders. In theory and in practice (Rutter and Yule 1975), many children and adults attain personal goals that are far beyond predicted capacity.

For learning and language disorders that are defined as a weakness relative to general intelligence, there are no formal standards yet for choosing which instruments should be used to assess the specific developmental skills or for determining what degree of test score discrepancies should count for diagnosis. Clinically, it is also difficult to be precise about distinguishing "ordinary statistical slowness" (i.e., at the low end of the normal curve for learning rate) from genuine neurodevelopmental slowness, especially in individuals who have other signs of delays.

This is an arena in which psychiatric and neuropsychological findings are quite thin, especially in view of the broad impact of these disorders on the education of children and opportunities for adults. Wide-reaching recommendations have been made for educational programs and legally mandated treatments on the basis of little rigorous research and relatively simple theories of cognitive functioning.

Although spelling problems are commonly seen in association with these disorders, they are not classified as a separate disorder. In the general population, spelling problems are typically a result of weak instruction or concentration problems rather than cognitive processing deficits. In some cases, however, a "spelling disorder" can be labeled as a "learning disorder not otherwise specified," as can certain types of spatial processing difficulties, handwriting problems, social skills deficits, or (in a slightly different world) lack of musicality. The focus on learning, motor skills, and communication is based on culturally defined notions of essential skills as well as the psychiatric comorbidity that accompanies deficits in these functions.

In view of suggestions that learning problems may be increased through prenatal exposure by maternal use of cigarettes (Nichols and Chen 1981) or alcohol (S. E. Shaywitz et al. 1980), some cases of these disorders may be preventable.

MENTAL RETARDATION

Intelligence (e.g., as measured by IQ) might be considered an independent dimension that deserves its own separate DSM-IV axis. However, the diagnosis of mental retardation encompasses more than low intelligence; it also requires deficits in adaptive functioning. The diagnostic concept of mental retardation as constituting low-IQ-plus-adaptive-deficits was developed by the American Association on Mental Retardation (1992) and essentially adopted as the DSM-IV alternative. It emphasizes that mental retardation is not an innate characteristic of an individual but the result of an interaction between personal intellectual capacities and the environment.

At least 90% of individuals with low intelligence are identified by age 18, but the diagnosis of mental retardation requires onset during the developmental period. Furthermore, developmental understanding is basic to the treatment of mental retardation, although psychiatric treatment of people with mental retardation is typically provided by general as well as child psychiatrists.

The definition of mental retardation encompasses three features: 1) subaverage intelligence (e.g., IQ of 70 or below), 2) impaired adaptive functioning, and 3) childhood onset (Table 23–17). The system for subclassifying the severity of mental retardation in DSM-IV is based on IQ scores, but the American Association on Mental Retardation (1992) instead subclassifies by the required "intensity and pattern of support systems" (intermittent, limited, extensive, and pervasive).

Intelligence is routinely measured by standardized tests, such as the Wechsler Adult Intelligence Scale

TABLE 23–17. **DSM-IV diagnostic criteria for mental retardation**

A. Significantly subaverage intellectual functioning: an IQ of approximately 70 or below on an individually administered IQ test (for infants, a clinical judgment of significantly subaverage intellectual functioning).

B. Concurrent deficits or impairments in present adaptive functioning (i.e., the person's effectiveness in meeting the standards expected for his or her age by his or her cultural group) in at least two of the following areas: communication, self-care, home living, social/interpersonal skills, use of community resources, self-direction, functional academic skills, work, leisure, health, and safety.

C. The onset is before age 18 years.

Code based on degree of severity reflecting level of intellectual impairment:

317	Mild mental retardation:	IQ level 50–55 to approximately 70
318.0	Moderate mental retardation:	IQ level 35–40 to 50–55
318.1	Severe mental retardation:	IQ level 20–25 to 35–40
318.2	Profound mental retardation:	IQ level below 20 or 25

| 319 | **Mental retardation, severity unspecified:** when there is strong presumption of mental retardation but the person's intelligence is untestable by standard tests |

(WAIS), the Wechsler Intelligence Scale for Children—Revised (WISC-R) for 6- to 16-year-olds, the Stanford-Binet IQ—Revised for 2- to 18-year-olds, or sections of the Bayley Scales of Mental Development for children from 2 months to 2.5 years of age. Specialized test protocols are being developed for infants. Major limitations of these standardized methods include cultural variations in question meaning and test performance, language and communicational differences among individuals, the unresponsiveness of standardized tests to "creative" responses, the dangers of employing a rigid construct of intelligence that masks individual strengths, and over-reliance on test findings in planning education. Even the concept of intelligence may be questioned, in view of the wide varieties of cognition (verbal and nonverbal, conscious and unconscious, emotional and "other"). However, these standardized IQ tests (Figure 23–8) are able to provide a global assessment that is of clinical value,

particularly when combined with an evaluation of adaptive behavior.

Adaptive capacities may be judged by many means, including standardized instruments for assessing social maturity and adaptive skills. For example, the Vineland Adaptive Behavior Scale is a multidimensional measure of adaptive behaviors in five "domains": communication, daily living skills, socialization, motor skills, and maladaptive behaviors. Data are provided by a semistructured interview of a parent or caregiver. Age-dependent expected competency scores of adaptive skills are established for children up to 18 years of age with different levels of mental retardation. Adaptive competence may be above or below the level of general intelligence (Figure 23–9).

The Vineland Adaptive Behavior Scale assesses typical performance (not optimal ability) of the "daily activities required for personal and social sufficiency" (Sparrow et al. 1984). For instance, in the socialization domain, there is an assessment of coping skills, including manners, following rules, apologizing, keeping secrets, and controlling impulses (Table 23–18).

Multidimensional scoring in different domains permits assessment of specific skills and deficits for an individual, facilitates the targeting of goals in different areas of adaptive functioning, helps in planning (for school, job, and residential placements), and allows measurement of changes in adaptive functioning over time. It is possible for scores in each domain to show more "scatter" than is shown by the intelligence subtests.

Because adaptive behavioral functioning may vary in different environments, a single measurement may be an oversimplification. In practice, it is rare that a single observer sees a patient in all settings or at all times of the day. This complicates the assessment of adaptive behavior in both standardized and global clinical methods. Clinicians typically use data from multiple sources to draw a composite picture of life functioning.

Because the diagnosis of mental retardation requires onset during childhood, an adult who experiences severe neurological damage is not classified as mentally retarded, even if both intelligence and adaptive skills are impaired. The adult-onset condition is diagnosed as dementia, which is an organic mental disorder (although certain dementias can also be designated as occurring in children). Disruption of the developmental process is required, by definition, for the diagnosis of mental retardation.

Minimal forms of mental retardation, present in individuals with an IQ below 71 who do not meet criteria for diagnosis, may receive a V code for borderline intellectual functioning.

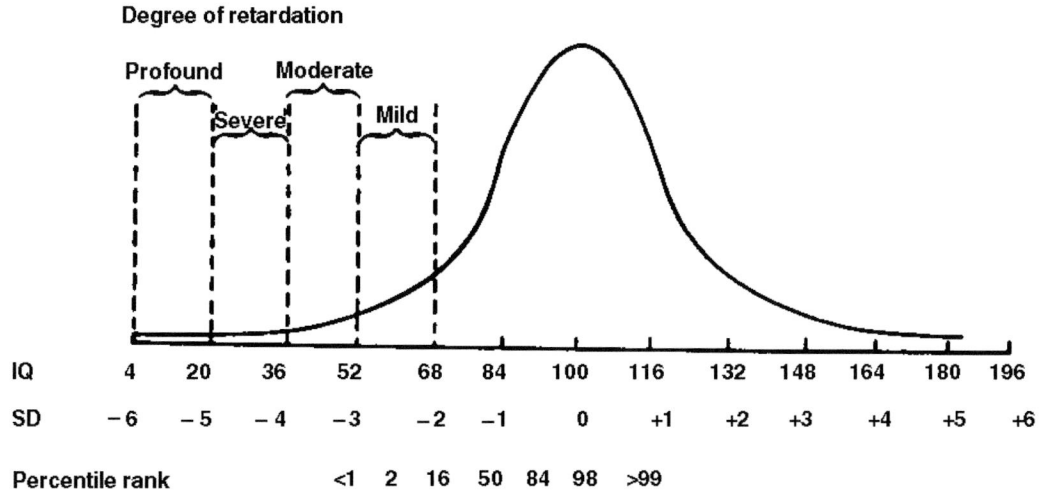

FIGURE 23-8.   The normal distribution of Stanford-Binet IQ. The theoretical distribution of IQ scores is symmetrical. Criteria for mental retardation (and its degrees of severity) are defined by arbitrary boundaries, typically statistical parameters such as standard deviation from the mean. In practice, the bell curve is skewed by a raised tail to the left, representing neuromedical disorders and socioenvironmental barriers.
Source.   Reprinted with permission from Baroff GS: *Mental Retardation: Nature, Cause and Management.* New York, Hemisphere Publishers, 1986. Copyright 1986, Hemisphere Publishers.

Measured intellectual functioning

	Retarded	Not retarded
Adaptive behavior — Retarded	Mentally retarded	NOT mentally retarded
Adaptive behavior — Not retarded	NOT mentally retarded	NOT mentally retarded

FIGURE 23-9.   Possible combinations of measured intellectual functioning and adaptive behavior. Mental retardation is diagnosed only if low intelligence is accompanied by impaired adaptive functioning. Low intelligence alone, or deficits in adaptive behavior alone, do not result in a diagnosis of mental retardation.
Source.   Reprinted with permission from Grossman HJ (ed): *Classification in Mental Retardation.* Washington, DC, American Association on Mental Deficiency [American Association on Mental Retardation], 1983. Copyright 1983, American Association on Mental Deficiency.

CLINICAL DESCRIPTION

Developmental slowness may appear in mental retardation across all areas of functioning, but it is primarily evident in cognition and intellectual functioning. Certain clinical features depend on the degree of intellectual functioning in mental retardation (Table 23–19). Neurobiological, motor, sensory, and integrative features; parent-child attachment; self-other differentiation; and subsequent emotional development are commonly affected. Although other aspects of psychological development are often impaired secondarily, there can be a remarkable degree of preservation of psychological growth. There may be wide "scatter" among various subtests of intellectual and adaptive functions, reflecting significant strengths in particular areas.

Because there is a two- to fourfold increase in psychopathology among mentally retarded persons, many of these individuals have "dual diagnoses." Fully half or more of persons with mental retardation have an additional psychiatric diagnosis (Gillberg et al. 1986; Gostason 1985). The frequency appears to be the same in both children and adults with severe or profound mental retardation (Cherry et al. 1997), which suggests that the comorbid diagnoses are distinct clinical entities and do not represent age-related manifestations of mental retardation.

TABLE 23–18.   Vineland Adaptive Behavior Scales: daily living skills domain, community subdomain

Safety skills

Demonstrates understanding that hot things are dangerous.

Looks both ways before crossing street or road alone.

Demonstrates understanding that it is unsafe to accept rides, food, or money from strangers.

Obeys traffic lights and Walk and Don't Walk signs.

Fastens seatbelt in automobile independently.

Telephone skills

Answers the telephone appropriately.

Summons to the telephone the person receiving a call, or indicates that the person is not available.

Initiates telephone calls to others.

Uses emergency telephone number in emergency.

Uses the telephone for all kinds of calls without assistance.

Uses a pay telephone.

Money skills

Demonstrates understanding of the function of money.

States value of penny, nickel, dime, and quarter.

Correctly counts change from a purchase costing more than a dollar.

Saves for and has purchased one major recreational item.

Earns spending money on a regular basis.

Budgets for weekly expenses.

Manages own money without assistance.

Budgets for monthly expenses.

Has checking account and uses it responsibly.

Time and dates

Demonstrates understanding of the function of a clock, either standard or digital.

States current day of the week when asked.

States current date when asked.

Tells time by five-minute segments.

Left-right orientation

Identifies left and right on others.

Restaurant skills

Orders own complete meal in restaurant.

Job skills

Arrives at work on time.

Notifies supervisor if arrival at work will be delayed.

Notifies supervisor when absent because of illness.

Obeys time limits for coffee breaks and lunch at work.

Holds full-time job responsibly.

Adapted with permission from Sparrow SS, Balla DA, Cicchetti DV: *Vineland Adaptive Behavior Scales.* Circle Pines, MN, American Guidance Service, 1984.

Any psychiatric diagnosis may occur in combination with mental retardation: DSM-IV criteria list no psychiatric disorder excluding the diagnosis of mental retardation. Several disorders occur at higher rates in association with mental retardation: impulse control disorders, anxiety disorders, mood disorders, ADHD, communication disorders, pervasive developmental disorders (including autistic disorder), stereotypic movement disorder (including self-injurious behavior), pica, and seizures (King et al. 1994). Posttraumatic stress disorder and adjustment disorders may certainly be seen, and the full array of personality types and all personality disorders may appear. The same DSM-IV criteria for defining these disorders may be applied without modification for the population with mental retardation, and some psychiatric ratings scales have been formally tested (Aman 1991). However, some clinicians are less inclined to diagnose or evaluate psychiatric comorbidity in individuals with mental retardation. Mentally retarded people also receive less treatment for their concomitant psychopathology, in part because of their low self-expectations (derived from family and clinician attitudes), economic limitations, and difficulties in managing complex organizational systems.

Distinguishing primary elements of mental retardation from its complications can be difficult. People commonly expect these individuals to be dull and lifeless. It is clear that depression can be a concomitant disorder or a complication; for example, it may be in response to extra burdens, low self-image, and stigma. Many apparent characteristics of mental retardation are not essential to the syndrome, may "disappear" during the course of effective treatment, and are merely associated findings or developmental complications. These features should be distinguished from true comorbid diagnoses, although both may warrant treatment.

Some clinical findings are primary cognitive and neurobiological features of mental retardation. Cognitively, there may be concreteness, egocentricity, distractibility, and short attention span. Sensory hyperreactivity may lead to "overflow" behaviors, stimulus avoidance, and the need to process stimuli at low levels of intensity.

Emotional features may include difficulty in expressing feelings and perceiving affect in self and others. Slow development of self-other differentiation may be clinically evident in affect management. The affective expressivity may be modified by physical disabilities (hypertonia, hypotonia). There may be cognitively based difficulty in "reading" facial expressions. With delays in speech and language development, limitations in communication may inhibit expression of negative affect, leading to instances of apparent affective hyperreactivity including impulsive an-

TABLE 23–19. **Clinical features of mental retardation**

	Mild	Moderate	Severe	Profound
IQ	50–55 to approximately 70	35–40 to 50–55	20–25 to 35–40	Below 20–25
Age of death (years)	50s	50s	40s	About 20
Percentage of mentally retarded population	89	7	3	1
Socioeconomic class	Low	Less low	No skew	No skew
Academic level achieved by adulthood	6th grade	2nd grade	Below 1st grade level in general	Below 1st grade level in general
Education	Educable	Trainable (self-care)	Untrainable	Untrainable
Residence	Community	Sheltered	Mostly living in highly structured and closely supervised settings	Mostly living in highly structured and closely supervised settings
Economic	Makes change; manages a job; budgets money with effort or assistance	Makes small change; usually able to manage change well	Can use coin machines; can take notes to shop owner	Dependent on others for money management

ger, low frustration tolerance, and reactive agitation. In extreme cases, impulse dyscontrol may lead to violence and destructiveness. These behavioral manifestations may show only modest improvement over time, especially in patients with severe or profound mental retardation (Reid and Ballinger 1995) and may justify chronic treatment with a β-adrenergic blocking agent (such as nadolol) or an α_2-adrenergic agonist (such as clonidine).

The ordinary complexities of daily human interactions may test an individual's cognitive limits (Sigman 1985). Cognitive capacities may be taxed in the parallel processing of speech production; thought communication; listening; and the understanding of situational context, social cues, and emotional signals. Changes in daily situation may stretch cognitive capacities and coping abilities, sometimes leading to frustration. Resistance to novelty and environmental change may be viewed as an associated finding or developmental consequence of mental retardation.

Defensive style can include rigidity or withdrawal. Primitive reactions to frustration and tension may involve not only aggressive responses but also self-injurious, self-stimulatory, or habitual behaviors. Self-injurious behavior is commonly observed in this population, although visual and auditory deficits can induce or aggravate such behavior (Davidson et al. 1996; Wieseler et al. 1995).

Rehabilitation may be inhibited by the individual's difficulty in recognizing the historical and interpersonal dimensions of his or her behavioral and affective problems, limitations in memory, cognitive processing, abstract thinking, sense of time, and perspective taking.

Medical problems (including associated neurological or metabolic disorders, physical disabilities, and sensory deficits) often are undertreated. When motor deficits are present, their specific characteristics should be identified and targeted for treatment. However, receiving adequate medical care may require organizational and social skills that exceed the easy grasp of mentally retarded people.

Generalizations about mental retardation are increasingly coming into question as research permits the understanding and differentiation of specific mental retardation syndromes. Contrasting with the old notion that mental retardation is a nonspecific form of slow development, newer phenomenological data indicate that these syndromes share many commonalities but are not the same. Persons with trisomy 21 (Down's syndrome) and fragile X syndrome tend to have quite different characteristics of language, cognition, social behavior, and adaptive skills (Bregman and Hodapp 1991; Lachiewicz et al. 1994) as well as different psychiatric comorbidity (Bregman 1991). Such findings suggest that individuals with mental retardation of different etiologies, not just of different severities, have distinct profiles of strengths and weaknesses that may be expected to influence their development.

EPIDEMIOLOGY

Prevalence figures in the United States are 1%–3%, depending mainly on the definition of adaptive functioning. Approximately 90% of cases are mildly retarded (IQ 55–70). There appears to be a male predominance at all levels of mental retardation (overall, about 1.5:1–6:1), although there may be a female predominance in severe mental retardation (Katusic et al. 1996).

Diagnostic labeling is low before age 5, rises sharply in the early school years, peaks in the later school years (about age 15), and then declines during adulthood toward 1%. High prevalence rates during the school years are usually attributed to the adaptive and intellectual demands of school (especially social and abstract thinking) and the high degree of supervision in classrooms (increased recognition of the child's difficulties). The decline during adulthood is usually attributed to improving social and economic skills, less supervision at work, and possibly (in some cases) delayed intellectual development. Typically, there is an earlier age of diagnosis for more severe levels of mental retardation.

Socioeconomic class is a crucial variable. Severe and profound mental retardation are distributed uniformly across all socioeconomic classes, but mild mental retardation is more common in low socioeconomic classes (Figure 23–10).

In the lowest socioeconomic class, there is a 10%–30% prevalence of mental retardation in the American school-age population. This "multiply disadvantaged" poverty class consists of inhabitants of city slums and poor rural areas, migrant workers, and economically oppressed groups. This fact highlights the etiological role of genetic-environmental interactions in mental retardation, especially in cases for which there is no obvious cause (Thapar et al. 1994).

In underdeveloped countries, the quality of nutrition, hygiene, sanitation, prenatal care, and mass immunization influences the incidence of mental retardation, but prevalence is reduced by infant mortality. In technologically advanced countries, medical and social supports enhance survival and longevity, although the impact on quality of life is less clear.

ETIOLOGY

The etiology is partially dependent on the level of mental retardation. Mild retardation is generally idiopathic and familial, but severe and profound retardation are typically genetic or related to brain damage.

The most common form is idiopathic mental retardation, which is associated with sociocultural or psychosocial disadvantage and is typically seen in the offspring of retarded parents ("familial"). The degree of retardation in this form is generally mild and sometimes moderate. Intellectual and adaptive deficits are presumed to be determined by a polygenic mechanism, although emphasis is currently placed on the intervening social factors. These individuals

live in low socioeconomic circumstances, and their functioning is influenced by poverty, disease, deficiencies in health care, and impaired help seeking. Family size may exceed parental capacities for attention and positive stimulation of the children, inducing marked effects on several dimensions of development. Social disadvantage contributes heavily to the etiology of some forms of mild mental retardation (Table 23–20). Nonetheless, the overrepresentation of various genetic, physical, and neurological abnormalities in people with mild mental retardation is a reminder that social forces may not be the predominant etiological factors.

Both inherited (presumably polygenic) factors and environmental mechanisms may contribute to the familial transmission of mild mental retardation across generations. This common form of mental retardation is associated with a high prevalence of conduct, attention, and language disorders.

Moderate and severe forms of mental retardation are less likely to be idiopathic. Specific biomedical etiologies may be identified in 25% of all cases of mental retardation and in 60%–80% of cases of severe or profound mental retardation. These moderate and severe cases are usually first diagnosed in infancy or early childhood, and 90% have prenatal causes. Major mechanisms include genetic and neurodevelopmental damage (Table 23–21). When biological causes are identifiable, there are more severe disabilities, physical limitations, and dependency.

In cases of idiopathic mental retardation, there is sub-

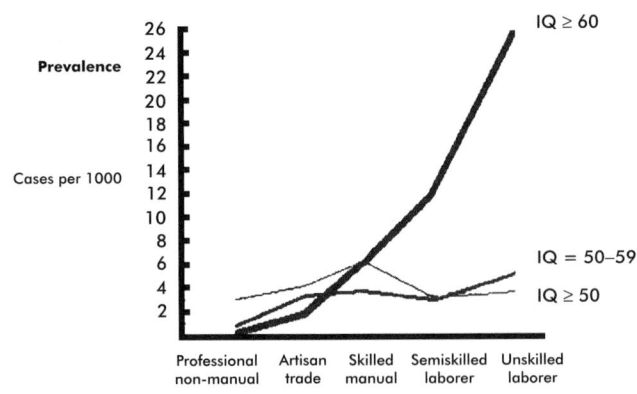

FIGURE 23–10. Prevalence of mental retardation in children from various socioeconomic classes. The more serious forms of mental retardation show an even distribution across socioeconomic class, but mild mental retardation is more prevalent in lower socioeconomic groups. Social class is indicated by occupation of the child's father.
Source. Adapted from Birch et al. 1970.

TABLE 23-20.   Psychosocial etiologies and determinants of mental retardation

Poverty

Inadequate housing

Weak hygiene

Malnutrition

Disease and infection

Inadequate medical treatment

Insufficient preventive medical care (prenatal, postnatal)

Sociocultural deprivation

Parental factors

IQ (can lead to impaired use of personal resources, help, and agencies)

Age (e.g., unplanned teenage pregnancies)

Education (regarding parenting skills)

Income and employment record

Psychiatric disorders

Help-seeking behavior (e.g., regarding medical care)

Child care

   Supervision and caretaking (can lead to risk of accidents and ingestions)

   Limit setting and discipline (quality, predictability)

   Psychosocial stimulation

Child abuse and neglect

Family variables

Family size (may exceed parental resources)

Family organization

Planning for future needs and opportunities

Intrapsychic dimensions

Self-esteem

Personal assertiveness

Mastery of challenges and management of failures

Exploration and novelty seeking

Concomitant psychiatric disorder

Community

Housing

Medical care

Safety of neighborhood

Specialized facilities for mental retardation

Funding resources

   Political attitudes

   Economic stability of nation

   Advocacy on behalf of individuals with mental retardation

stantial evidence for a biological basis of brain abnormalities. Enlarged ventricles, similar to findings in schizophrenia, have been reported in 75% of children with mental retardation of unknown cause (Prassopoulos et al. 1996). Infants with mental retardation show an abnormal thickening of the corpus callosum during development in the first year of life (Fujii et al. 1994).

There are more than 200 recognized biological syndromes involving mental retardation (Grossman 1983), entailing disruptions in virtually any sector of brain biochemical or physiological functioning.

Neurodevelopmental damage may be produced by a variety of mechanisms. Physical insults that are typically damaging to the brain are catastrophic in early development. Because the fetus has no demonstrable immunological response in early gestation, maternal infections (e.g., congenital AIDS or toxoplasmosis) may cause major damage. If rubella is contracted during the first month of pregnancy, there is a 50% rate of fetal abnormalities. Intrauterine exposure to toxins (e.g., lead), medications, and radiation may result in intrauterine growth retardation and other toxic effects on brain development (Herskowitz 1987). Similarly, intrauterine exposures to nicotine, alcohol, and cocaine are preventable causes of mental retardation (Drews et al. 1996). Intrauterine seizures can be a prenatal cause of brain damage and impaired brain development (Volpe 1987). Certain forms of maternal illness (toxemia or diabetes) may also be dangerous to the developing nervous system in utero.

At birth, obstetrical trauma and Rh isoimmunization may cause brain injury. Birth asphyxia is probably not a significant source of mental retardation; there has recently been a deemphasis on the role of perinatal hypoxia in the etiology of neuropsychiatric problems (Nelson 1991). Hypoxic changes typically result in maturational delays that are no longer diagnosed by age 7 years, except perhaps in severe and profound mental retardation. Prematurity (or low birth weight) is not typically causal, but it may be in extreme cases (less than 28 weeks of gestation or birth weight less than 1,500 g).

Several forms of neurodevelopmental damage may occur postnatally. Environmental factors are particularly crucial in underdeveloped countries, where distribution of medical care may be limited. Neurological infections and disease, including seizures, may contribute. Neurological trauma may result from falls, accidents, athletic injury, extreme fever, child abuse, and severe malnutrition.

Chromosomal factors can be identified in 10% of institutionalized individuals with mental retardation. Apart from polygenetic inheritance, the major chromosomal mechanisms include dominantly inherited single-gene

TABLE 23–21. Selected biological mechanisms causing mental retardation and pervasive developmental disorders

Hereditary

Single gene defects; dominant (e.g., tuberous sclerosis)

Inborn errors of metabolism; recessive (e.g., phenylketonuria)

Chromosome aberrations (e.g., fragile X chromosome syndrome)

Polygenic inheritance (postulated for familial retardation associated with sociocultural or psychosocial disadvantage)

Prenatal

Early (embryonic) developmental alterations

Gene-related defects, but not inherited (e.g., trisomy 21/Down's syndrome)

Maternal infection (e.g., sexually transmitted diseases, rubella, toxoplasmosis, cytomegalovirus)

Toxic exposures (e.g., alcohol, crack or cocaine, lead)

Medical exposures (e.g., anticonvulsants, warfarin, radiation)

Later (fetal) developmental alterations

Brain malformations

Extreme prematurity or low birth weight

Small for gestational age (e.g., SGA babies)

Extreme malnutrition

Neurological abnormalities (as a result of trauma, disease)

Intrauterine seizures [questionable]

Gestational disorders

Maternal illness (e.g., toxemia, diabetes, hypoglycemia)

Perinatal

Rh or ABO isoimmunization

Birth-related brain trauma

Birth-related asphyxia [questionable]

Respiratory distress [questionable]

Postnatal (acquired) neurological conditions

Brain infection (e.g., encephalitis, meningitis)

Head trauma (as a result of child abuse or neglect; accidents, including falls, athletic injury, car accidents)

Neurological damage or disease

Metabolic or endocrinological disorder (e.g., hypothyroidism)

Toxic exposure (e.g,. to lead, irradiation)

Extreme malnutrition

---

defects, recessively inherited inborn errors of metabolism, recessive chromosomal aberrations, and early developmental (embryonic) gene alterations.

Trisomy 21 (Down's syndrome) is the most common and well-described form of mental retardation. Patients with trisomy 21 have neurochemical pathology including major loss of acetylcholine (nucleus basalis) and somatostatin (cerebral cortex) neurons, as well as loss in serotonin and norepinephrine pathways. Patients with Down's syndrome show progressive neuropathological changes similar to those in Alzheimer's disease, including neurofibrillary tangles and neuritic plaques, which are seen in 100% of individuals with Down's syndrome who survive beyond age 30 (Figure 23–11). Chromosome 21 contains the gene for β-amyloid, the brain protein that accumulates in the neuritic plaques of patients with Down's syndrome or Alzheimer's disease. The effectiveness of centrally acting cholinesterase inhibitors, such as tacrine (Cognex) and donepezil (Aricept), in the treatment of Alzheimer's disease raises the question of whether these anticholinesterases might also be effective in treating Down's syndrome, at least during its later stages. However, the prevalence of dementia in adults with trisomy 21 is well below the prevalence of the anatomical changes (Zigman et al. 1996), suggesting that other mechanisms may be involved in Down's dementia. For example, cerebral glucose metabolism appears to decrease with age (Bregman and Hodapp 1991), which is consistent with the wide variety of neurological symptoms.

Fragile X chromosome syndrome is the second most common genetic cause of moderate and severe mental re-

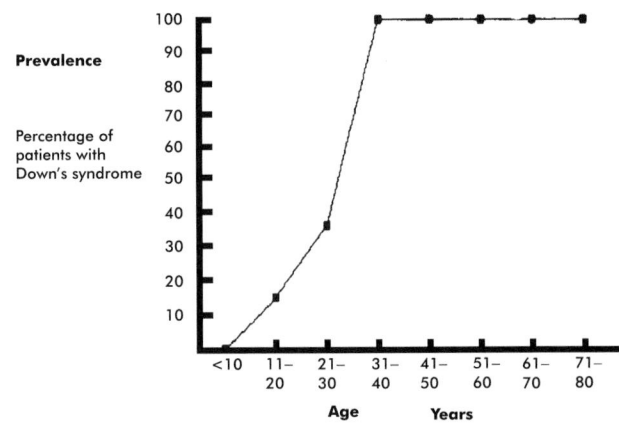

FIGURE 23–11. Development of Alzheimer's neuropathology in patients with Down's syndrome. In all individuals with Down's syndrome who survive past age 30 years, the neuropathological changes that are characteristic of Alzheimer's disease are observed at autopsy. Neurofibrillary tangles and senile plaques are seen in 100% of these people.
Source. Data from Wisniewski KE, Wisniewski HM, Wen GY: "Occurrence of Neuropathological Changes and Dementia of Alzheimer's Disease in Down's Syndrome." *Annals of Neurology* 17:278–282, 1985.

tardation, affecting about 1 in 1,000 males (Bregman et al. 1987). About 80% of males with fragile X syndrome have moderate-to-severe mental retardation, which accounts for 40% of the male predominance in moderate and severe mental retardation. Affected males have large testes in 25% of cases before puberty and in 85% after puberty. Macro-orchidism is an unusual symptom in medicine, and its high frequency in this syndrome makes it useful as a screening question. Most symptomatic males have an elongated dysmorphic face (large jaw, forehead, and ears), large head circumference, mitral valve prolapse (80%), hyper-extensible joints, and a highly arched palate. Behavioral abnormalities are present in 80% of males, including hy-peractivity, violence, stereotypies, resistance to environ-mental changes, and self-mutilating behaviors. Language and speech deficits include immature syntax, poor abstrac-tion, expressive and receptive language deficits, and articu-lation problems. Frontal lobe symptoms may include perseverative language and behavior, attention deficits, and impaired shifting between mental sets (Mazzocco et al. 1992). Approximately 20%–40% of fragile X males have features of autistic disorder, but less than 10% of autistic males have fragile X chromosome syndrome. About one-third of fragile X males have neuroendocrine abnormali-ties: increased baseline leutinizing hormone (LH) and fol-licle-stimulating hormone (FSH), decreased testosterone, and blunted thyroid-stimulating hormone (TSH) follow-ing thyroid-releasing hormone (TRH) infusion. Females have elevated rates of fertility and twinning. In females, a "carrier" state may be asymptomatic or associated with learning disorders or mild mental retardation (females are partially protected by having two X chromosomes).

The proposed gene abnormality involves a nucleotide sequence (CGG, cytosine-guanine-guanine) that is redun-dantly repeated to variable degrees and becomes quite lengthy in patients with fragile X chromosome syndrome (Verkerk et al. 1991). These patients show an increased number of "fragile sites" at q27.3 at the end of the long arm of the X chromosome, corresponding to the location of the abnormal gene sequence, when their cells are incubated in a low folate and thymidine medium. Clinical severity ap-pears to correlate with the degree of cytogenetic expres-sion. Oral folate reduces the frequency of fragile sites in vivo and improves behavior and attention; however, this therapeutic effect is mainly seen in preadolescent children, and postpubertally the effect is minimal (Aman and Kern 1991). In males, intelligence scores plateau and then de-cline after age 10–15, although adaptive functions may be maintained (Dykens et al. 1989). Genetic, diet, drug, gen-der, and age factors appear to interact in modifying the penetrance of fragile X chromosome syndrome.

As mental retardation in general and the specific disor-ders are more intensively studied, there is an emerging pic-ture of the extraordinary complexity of genetic and neuro-developmental processes, as well as of sociodevelopmental processes, that contribute to the different presentations. Specific genetic mechanisms, molecular events, develop-mental courses, cognitive features, language abilities, and adaptive strengths and weaknesses are being identified for the various mental retardation syndromes (Bregman and Hodapp 1991).

COURSE AND PROGNOSIS

Although biological factors of each mental retardation syndrome in each individual may determine certain as-pects of development, the course and outcome of mental retardation depend largely on social, economic, health/medical, educational, and developmental circumstances. Whether the disorder is a mild familial form or the result of a severe inborn metabolic error, the course of mental re-tardation is influenced by interactions with environmental opportunities and barriers. Parental characteristics may entail advantages that are compensatory or disadvantages that are compounding. Such features of the micro-environment operate as intervening factors and may have a stronger influence on adult psychiatric outcome than the causative factors, except in extreme cases. The course and prognosis of mental retardation is much less predictable than originally believed (Figure 23–12).

Neurodevelopmental evaluation during the first year can predict intellectual outcome and neurological status in later childhood in nearly 90% of premature children (Largo et al. 1990). Premature infants with intracranial hemorrhage (demonstrated on ultrasound) are especially likely to demonstrate impaired cognitive and motor abili-ties later, especially if there are persistent signs of periventricular abnormalities (Williams et al. 1987).

Current data on the course of mental retardation re-flect varying degrees of aggressivity in rehabilitative ef-forts. The prognosis in mental retardation may be expected to improve as therapeutic interventions become available to more members of the general public and as adaptive be-havior improves over the course of a lifetime.

At present, about two-thirds of mentally retarded indi-viduals shed their diagnoses in adulthood, as adaptive skills increase (Grossman 1983). Typically, the global level of adaptive functioning is found to change over the course of months or years in response to changes in economic and so-cial supports, living arrangements, work opportunities, and parental support.

For mental retardation at all levels of severity, and for

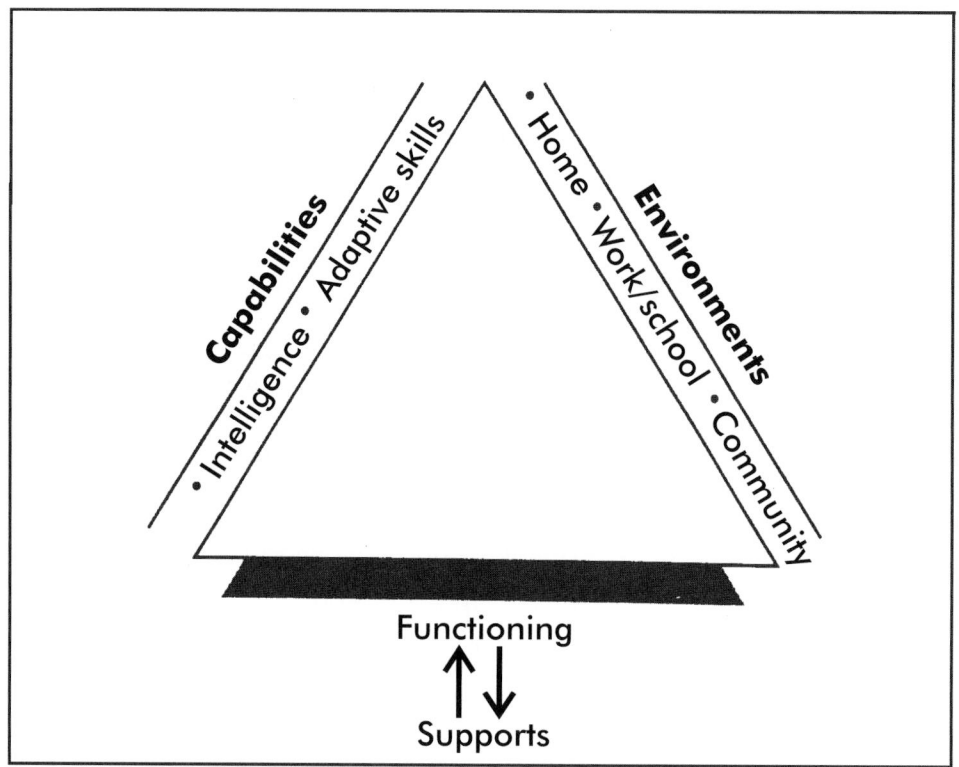

FIGURE 23–12. Opportunities for growth and change in mental retardation. The general structure of the current definition of mental retardation emphasizes the balance of strengths and weaknesses in multiple domains. It highlights the potential for change based on growing adaptive skills, changing environments, and shifting supports for functioning. An individual's innate capacities and learnable skills interact with different types of ecological opportunities. External support, which may be available from a variety of sources, can also influence functioning. Improvements in functioning can promote the individual's capacity to seek and use external supports, whether they be social, financial, educational, cultural, or medical.
Source.   Reprinted with permission from American Association on Mental Retardation: *Mental Retardation: Definition, Classification, and Systems of Supports*, 9th Edition. Washington, DC, American Association on Mental Retardation, 1992. Copyright 1992, American Association on Mental Retardation.

cases of both idiopathic and known etiologies, the developmental course is slow but not "deviant." The normal sequence of cognitive developmental stages is observed. The speed of developmental change is slow, and there appears to be a "ceiling" on ultimate achievement. In addition, secondary emotional and social "complications" may influence the clinical presentation and outcome.

Too low or too high expectations maintained by family, therapeutic team, or patient constitute significant obstacles to therapeutic improvement. The habitual resignation to low expectation of achievement has a chilling effect on self-esteem, hope, and outcome.

Common psychological complications include frequent experiencing of failure, low self-esteem, frustration in fulfillment of dependency needs and wishes for love, wavering parental support, regressive wishes for institutionalization, anticipation of failure (leading to avoidance of problem solving and challenges, reduced curiosity and exploration, and impaired mastery seeking and pride), defensive rigidity, and excessive caution (e.g., resistance to dealing with new people and places, including helping professionals). Additional psychosocial complications are impaired interactions and communications, inappropriate social assertiveness, and vulnerability to being exploited.

Financial complications (poverty) entail further medical complications, including impaired care seeking (delayed treatment, excessive use of emergency facilities), rarity of preventive treatment (prenatal and well-baby care, periodic checkups), accidents and trauma, malnutrition, lead exposure, child abuse, prematurity, and teenage pregnancy. Complications of mental retardation are numerous. A lack of aggressivity, integration, or continuity in the provision of care can hinder basic medical treatment. Institutionalization may promote passivity and excessive compliance. Societal ignorance and stigmatization may lead to avoidance by potential social companions and professionals.

Family complications may include parental disappointment, anger, guilt, overprotectiveness, infantilization, overinvolvement, or detachment. Siblings may experience annoyance at sharing in sibling care, loss of parents' attention, parents' compensatory overexpectations, and realistic fears concerning genetic risks for their own children. It is interesting, however, that the impact on parents of having a child with mental retardation is in fact positive in many cases (Taanila et al. 1996).

A major part of the care of mentally retarded individuals includes prevention and management of the numerous medical, psychological, and family complications. Another major component of care is the monitoring of overall speed of progress: a lack of developmental improvement raises the possibility of concomitant psychiatric diagnoses.

EVALUATION AND DIFFERENTIAL DIAGNOSIS

It cannot be overemphasized that all psychiatric diagnoses may co-occur with mental retardation and that all personality types may occur in mental retardation. Approximately one-third to one-half of these patients have ADHD. Mentally retarded individuals may also have unipolar and bipolar mood disorders, anxiety disorders, psychotic reactions, autistic disorder, and learning disorders (Menolascino et al. 1986).

Sadness, lack of enthusiasm, excessive anxiety, and "primary process" associations are not primary features of mental retardation; these symptoms should be evaluated as complications or as signs of concomitant disorders.

Medical evaluation should include physical examination (seeking physical stigmata) and laboratory tests, including chromosomal analysis, amino and organic acids studies, thyroid function, lead testing, and a mucopolysaccharide screen. X-ray studies of long bones and wrists should be obtained. Neurological evaluation, including EEG and CT scan, should be performed to discover possible treatable causes of mental retardation, seizure disor-

ders, and possibly deafness and blindness. Head and face size and symmetries, head shape (including hair patterns), eye and ear position, and asymmetries of motor and sensory function should be checked. A history of maternal miscarriage, toxic exposures, infections, and fetal size and activity should be elicited. Psychological testing, including neuropsychological evaluation, is commonly required. Social adaptive skills of the individual should be measured (e.g., the Vineland Scale) to target areas of remediation and strength.

Families of people with mental retardation experience considerable challenge. The burden of management can tax the efforts of any family (Cooper 1981), especially the parents (Figure 23–13). Because intensive intervention is required to minimize developmental complications, this burden can continue for many years. The growth-promoting characteristics of the family can be assessed (through interviews and home visit) by investigating the level of stimulation, emotional support, help seeking, decision making, future orientation, and financial planning for the mentally retarded individual.

TREATMENT

Treatment of the multiple handicaps and complications commonly associated with mental retardation is typically multimodal, with a developmental orientation (Sigman 1985; Szymanski 1987; Szymanski and Tanguay 1980). Long-term rehabilitative programs involve many specialists and agencies working collaboratively over time and across agency boundaries.

The specifically psychiatric component includes the

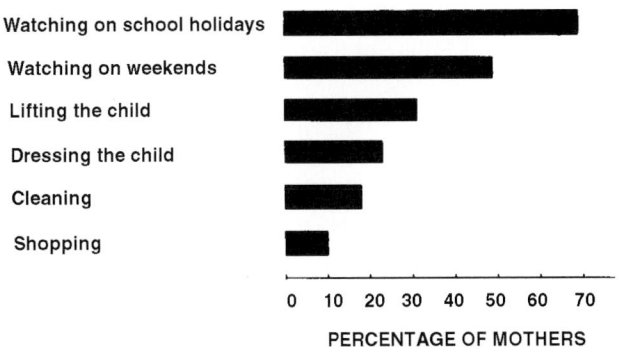

FIGURE 23–13. Caregiving burdens described by mothers of children with mental retardation. The care of a child with mental retardation places practical responsibilities as well as emotional strains on the families.
Source. Adapted from Birch et al. 1970.

coordination of the primary diagnostic evaluation of medical and psychiatric conditions, parental guidance (behavior management, educational and environmental planning, long-term monitoring, and advocacy), and the usual variety of psychiatric therapies for specific concomitant psychiatric disorders (Szymanski and Tanguay 1980).

Although treatments based on abstract thinking may not be helpful, developmentally oriented psychotherapeutic interventions may be effective for crisis management or for achieving long-term psychosocial goals. For some adolescent or adult patients with mild mental retardation, verbal psychotherapy may be used to promote self-other differentiation, self-esteem, identity formation, interpersonal development, emotional and behavioral control, management of power, and expression of love and sexuality. Technical modifications include the use of briefer and clearer verbalizations, focus on current events and feelings, reinforcement of reality-fantasy differentiations, management of projections, teaching about the nature of emotional life, and free use of positive reinforcement. Brief, frequent sessions may be more useful than standard formats. For children, play therapy may be used. Behavior modification can be useful for treating symptoms of aggressivity, defiance, overactivity, asocial behavior, self-injury, stereotypies, and pica; in some cases, toilet training, dressing and grooming, and eating skills may be taught. Educational and developmental training to enhance speech and language, motor, cognitive, occupational, social, recreational, sexual, and adaptive skills are commonly provided by specialized professionals. The individual may be trained to initiate task simplifications, request communicational clarifications, and perform environmental improvements. Parent counseling and education, as well as family support, are standard. Special attention is needed for managing the conflicts regarding standard of living (economic) and behavioral expectations between home and treatment settings.

Pharmacotherapy may be helpful in the management of some symptoms associated with mental retardation as well as in the treatment of comorbid psychiatric disorders. Although controlled studies are still relatively few, certain symptoms associated with mental retardation have been amply shown to respond to conventional neuroleptics. Less well-established treatments include use of atypical neuroleptics, β-adrenergic blockers, clonidine (or guanfacine) for agitation, psychostimulants for hyperactivity, tricyclic antidepressants for mood disorders, serotonin reuptake inhibitors for mood and perseverative symptoms, anticonvulsants for seizures, mood stabilizers for comorbid psychiatric disorders, and naltrexone for self-injurious behaviors.

CLINICAL COMMENT

The development of treatment resources for mentally retarded individuals requires the collaboration of professionals in the fields of medicine, psychology, education, law, and ethics, as well as representatives of private agencies and government. The ethical issues involved in the treatment of mentally retarded patients may inhibit some physicians and other professionals from taking an aggressively therapeutic stance. The tremendous dependency needs and the lifelong duration of treatment may also operate to scare physicians away.

In schools, the ongoing controversy about the merits of "mainstream" classroom versus specialized "resource room" placements remains to be resolved by psychological and educational outcome assessment; the debate will interact with public and political processes.

In underdeveloped countries, improved nutrition, hygiene, sanitation, and prenatal care, as well as mass immunizations, are crucial to the prevention and treatment of mental retardation. Within the United States, large variations in the regional distribution of mental retardation treatment programs, in addition to the high needs of inner cities and some rural areas, limit the effectiveness of governmental service and planning.

Advances in medicine are fostering the survival of very premature and low-weight infants, whose persistent neurological and intellectual deficits are a new source of mental retardation. There is also an increasing number of known causes of mental retardation and an expanding awareness of the effectiveness of aggressive treatment. In research, mental retardation offers the opportunity for investigating the interrelationships of intellectual and emotional functioning in human development. The revolution in molecular medicine and neuroscience will undoubtedly lead to further identification of genetic, morphogenetic, and physiological (including neuronal plasticity and brain "reorganization") processes that underlie or remediate many presentations of mental retardation.

This ancient disorder, described in classical Thebes, has been viewed with tolerance and respect in many historical cultures, although the Christian concept of the "feeble-minded" established a curious mix of sensitivities. In the 18th century, John Locke made the pivotal distinction between mental retardation and emotional disorders. In the 19th century, a period of rehabilitative optimism was followed by subsequent disillusionment at slow therapeutic progress. In the 20th century, some states enacted laws that required sterilization of mentally retarded individuals. By midcentury, medical research had challenged the ancient notion of untreatability. In 1975, federal law P.L. 94-142 mandated special educational services for all mentally retarded children. There remain some legal anachronisms and funding limitations that obstruct opportunities for contributory work, dignified living, and personal growth. Interest in this disorder is unfashionable in this age, which is oriented toward productivity and efficiency. However, within professional circles, it is believed that aggressive treatment works and that the implementation of a humane public policy entails funding of the required services.

Medical professionals will continue to investigate causes, psychiatric concomitants, psychological complications, and psychosocial treatment interventions. The ongoing revolutions in molecular medicine and neuroscience will undoubtedly lead to further identification of genetic, morphogenetic, and physiological processes that underlie many presentations of mental retardation. Management of the family's "postdiagnosis crisis," the siblings' psychological burdens, and the family's financial planning remain the most immediate ways of improving the mentally retarded child's microenvironment. Family support can also be provided by local chapters of the Association for Retarded Citizens. Research on adaptive skills, education, and development remain the focus of long-term efforts. A particular contribution of psychiatrists is in aiding patients with "dual diagnoses."

There are numerous aspects of prevention, including public education, destigmatization, alleviation of poverty, wider medical care, genetic counseling, and advocacy in law and government for the development of treatment resources and special education.

Aggressive treatment can improve the quality of life and longevity of mentally retarded persons. At least some future cases of mental retardation may be prevented or treated through genetic alteration.

PERVASIVE DEVELOPMENTAL DISORDERS

The pervasive developmental disorders make up a neurobiologically diverse group of conditions characterized by deficits across many areas of functioning that lead to a remarkably pervasive but diffuse disruption of developmental processes. These multiply handicapped individuals typically have a developmental process that is not merely slow or limited but is "atypical" or "deviant." Anomalous strengths can emerge from this developmental process in some cases, but many of these individuals have mental retardation. Comorbidity may include any of the psychiatric disorders, and there may be an increased prevalence of obsessive-compulsive disorder (often identified as

"perseveration"), stereotypic movement disorder, tic disorders, ADHD, and mood disorders among individuals with a pervasive developmental disorder.

DSM-IV recognizes several pervasive developmental disorders that differ in course of illness, symptoms, and severity. *Autistic disorder* involves an early onset of impairments in social interaction, communication deficits, and restricted activities and interests; there is some tendency toward partial improvement over time, but unpredictable periods of rapid improvement appear between extended periods of minimal change. *Childhood disintegrative disorder* entails symptoms that are largely similar, but the symptoms follow at least 2 years of seemingly normal development; the child then loses early developmental gains and reaches a stable level of autistic-like functioning. *Rett's disorder*, an early-onset progressive disorder of females, is associated with mental retardation, generalized growth retardation, and multiple neurological symptoms (including stereotyped movements of the hands); this disorder appears similar to autistic disorder during early childhood, but it progressively takes on characteristics of a neurodegenerative or neurodevelopmental disorder. *Asperger's disorder* is largely similar to "high-functioning" autistic disorder in its relative preservation of language skills and intellect; despite some remaining skepticism about its validity as a distinct DSM-IV disorder, several features of Asperger's disorder have been found that distinguish it from autism and other developmental disorders.

Early intervention and multiyear treatment of the pervasive developmental disorders emphasize communication and occupational functions. The treatment can be effective, although the benefits accrue slowly and its value has not been well documented in controlled studies. General management requires a long-term multimodal developmentally oriented clinical program. Medical treatments are aimed at symptom relief and management of any comorbid neurological or psychiatric disorders.

AUTISTIC DISORDER

This early-onset pervasive developmental disorder entails disabilities in virtually all psychological and behavioral sectors. In view of the severity of extreme cases of autistic disorder, it is remarkable that this condition was not documented until the late 19th century and not described until the mid 20th century. However, most individuals with autistic disorder do not have the massive, severe developmental impairments seen in the classically described cases. Although it was initially conceptualized as a deprivation syndrome, later evidence of neuropsychiatric dysfunction led to a more biological construct of the affective, cogni tive, social, communicative, motor, neurovegetative, integrative, and adaptive abnormalities of autistic disorder. The current view of the phenomenology is remarkably similar to the early description, but there have been major shifts in the understanding of prevalence, severity, etiology, and especially treatment (D. Cohen et al. 1987).

Clinical Description

The DSM-IV definition of autistic disorder puts particular emphasis on the impairments in social interaction and reciprocity, the difficulties with verbal and nonverbal communication (and related capacities such as symbolization), and the stereotyped pattern of behaviors and interests (Table 23–22).

Autistic disorder presents in a wide spectrum of severities. The classic form of "early infantile autism," described by Kanner (1943), was a severe infancy-onset disorder with profoundly disturbed social relations (e.g., detachment, aloofness), communication disruption, motor abnormalities, affective atypicality, massive cognitive impairments, multiple behavioral oddities, distorted perception, and bizarre thoughts. These symptoms led to conceptualizations based on failed ego development or severe regression, and the bizarre thoughts and behaviors were viewed as suggestive of psychotic development. The notion of autistic disorder as a variant of schizophrenia or of any psychotic disorder is no longer considered heuristically useful.

Despite the extremely disrupted integration of brain functions, an almost chaotic form of disorganization, and cognitive and emotional confusion, autistic disorder is not associated with delusions, hallucinations, or loose associations. It is no longer viewed as a psychotic disorder, and emphasis is placed on the neurointegrative features of the disorganization and the idiosyncratic traits of the individual. There are relatively mild forms of autistic disorder in which the social, communicative, and behavioral abnormalities are so subtle that they merge into the range of character pathology.

Children with autistic disorder may show limited social interactiveness, a seeming indifference to human warmth, little imitation or sharing, and rare smiling. Socially, these children appear passive and aloof, initially avoiding social contact, but they can come to enjoy and seek interpersonal experiences. Autistic children often have difficulty in comprehending verbal and nonverbal language and are often misinterpreted; typically these issues need to be a focus of treatment. They often show persistent deficits in sensing or appreciating the feelings of other people and in understanding the process and nuances

TABLE 23–22.   DSM-IV diagnostic criteria for autistic disorder

A. A total of six (or more) items from (1), (2), and (3), with at least two from (1), and one each from (2) and (3):

  (1) qualitative impairment in social interaction, as manifested by at least two of the following:

   (a) marked impairment in the use of multiple nonverbal behaviors such as eye-to-eye gaze, facial expression, body postures, and gestures to regulate social interaction

   (b) failure to develop peer relationships appropriate to developmental level

   (c) a lack of spontaneous seeking to share enjoyment, interests, or achievements with other people (e.g., by a lack of showing, bringing, or pointing out objects of interest)

   (d) lack of social or emotional reciprocity

  (2) qualitative impairments in communication as manifested by at least one of the following:

   (a) delay in, or total lack of, the development of spoken language (not accompanied by an attempt to compensate through alternative modes of communication such as gesture or mime)

   (b) in individuals with adequate speech, marked impairment in the ability to initiate or sustain a conversation with others

   (c) stereotyped and repetitive use of language or idiosyncratic language

   (d) lack of varied, spontaneous make-believe play or social imitative play appropriate to developmental level

  (3) restricted repetitive and stereotyped patterns of behavior, interests, and activities, as manifested by at least one of the following:

   (a) encompassing preoccupation with one or more stereotyped and restricted patterns of interest that is abnormal either in intensity or focus

   (b) apparently inflexible adherence to specific, nonfunctional routines or rituals

   (c) stereotyped and repetitive motor mannerisms (e.g., hand or finger flapping or twisting, or complex whole-body movements)

   (d) persistent preoccupation with parts of objects

B. Delays or abnormal functioning in at least one of the following areas, with onset prior to age 3 years: (1) social interaction, (2) language as used in social communication, or (3) symbolic or imaginative play.

C. The disturbance is not better accounted for by Rett's disorder or childhood disintegrative disorder.

of social communication. Communicative speech and gesturing are limited and may be difficult to understand because of echolalia, pronoun reversals, and idiosyncratic meanings. Speech is typically late and unusual, and it sometimes fails to develop altogether. Phonological (i.e., sound production) and syntactic (i.e., grammar) functions may be relatively spared, with more significant impairments of semantics (i.e., sociocultural meanings) and pragmatics (i.e., rules of interpersonal exchange), as well as other aspects of communication. Imaginative and symbolic functions (e.g., use of toys in play) may be deeply affected. Rituals, stereotypies (e.g., rocking, whirling), self-stimulation, self-mutilation, and unusual mannerisms are common. There is often an obsessive attachment to certain people or objects (resistance to change) and a lack of ordinary spontaneity. Affect may be "shallow," overly responsive to small changes, oblivious to large changes in the environment, and unpredictably labile and odd. Cognitive deficits include impairments in abstraction, sequencing, and integration. There may be distorted perception for smell, taste, or touch and underdevelopment of visual and auditory processing.

The majority of individuals with autistic disorder show subnormal intelligence, but some show significant "increases" in measured IQ during the course of treatment or development. There are often dramatic inconsistencies, with extraordinary "scatter" of capabilities among different IQ subtests and over time. Unusual or special capacities ("savant" skills) may be present in particular areas such as music, drawing, arithmetic, or calendar calculation.

Epidemiology

The available prevalence estimates for autistic disorder are based on criteria that emphasize the more severe forms of this disorder. When these criteria are used, prevalence is estimated at approximately 30 to 50 per 100,000. The less severe forms are more common. There is a male predominance of approximately 3:1–4:1, but females often have more severe symptoms. Contrary to early belief, increased prevalence is not associated with higher socioeconomic class or higher intelligence.

Etiology

Genetic and biological factors appear to play a significant role in autistic disorder (Folstein and Piven 1991). However, because individuals with autistic disorder rarely marry, genetic studies remain limited. The higher concordance in monozygotic than dizygotic twins (36% vs. 0%) suggests a genetic factor. The probable overrepresentation of ADHD, obsessive-compulsive symptoms, and

Tourette's disorder may also suggest that autistic disorder involves genetic factors that are related to the transmission of these disorders and, perhaps, the transmission of the syndrome entailing all three conditions (Stern and Robertson 1997). Siblings of autistic children show a prevalence of autistic disorder of 2% (50 times the expected prevalence), and about 5%–25% of siblings have delays in learning (usually language or speech disorder), mental retardation, or physical defects. In family studies, there have been suggestions of autosomal recessive inheritance for certain cases of autistic disorder. Neuropathological studies have suggested that neurodevelopmental changes begin early in gestation, probably in the second trimester (Bauman 1991). There is no evidence that psychosocial factors or parenting abnormalities cause autistic disorder.

Studies of evoked response potentials often yield abnormalities that are nonspecific, nondiagnostic, or suggestive of neuromaturational delays. CT scans also show inconsistent, diverse, and nonspecific findings, typically including suggestions of ventricular enlargement, left temporal abnormalities, and abnormal symmetry. MRI studies have also yielded mixed findings, but they most commonly show hippocampal dysfunction secondary to sclerosis (DeLong and Heinz 1997) and reduced posterior corpus callosum volumes (Rimland and Baker 1996). Cell loss in the vermis of the cerebellum (Courchesne et al. 1988; Peterson 1995) is a finding that has not been replicated in several other studies (Schaefer et al. 1996). An early PET study showed a modest and generalized increase in glucose metabolism in some brain regions (Rumsey et al. 1985a). More recent PET studies have shown decreased volume and metabolic activity in the anterior cingulate gyrus as well as bitemporal glucose hypometabolism (Haznedar et al. 1997). High-resolution single photon emission computed tomography (SPECT) scanning has also revealed abnormalities in the temporal and parietal lobes (Mountz et al. 1995). The most consistent neuroimaging findings implicate abnormalities in the temporal and parietal lobes of patients with autistic disorder.

A specific medical cause may be identified in some individuals. An elevated prevalence of early developmental problems, such as postnatal neurological infections, congenital rubella, and phenylketonuria, has been reported. About 2%–5% of autistic individuals appear to have fragile X syndrome. Seizure disorders are also common in autism, including both major motor seizures and partial complex seizures. Seizure onset is typically either during early childhood or during adolescence, and clinical seizures can be observed in up to 50% of autistic persons by age 20. Children with an early onset of seizures may show an increase in seizure symptoms during adolescence. Adolescence-onset seizures are observed more commonly in autistic disorder than in mental retardation.

Neurochemical assays suggest a decrease in urinary catecholamines (and related metabolites) and perhaps an increase in the dopamine metabolite homovanillic acid (HVA) in CSF. Elevated blood serotonin concentration appears to be a stable trait that remains for decades in one-third of patients with autism, but it does not appear to correlate with specific clinical features. Regional studies have suggested asymmetries of serotonin synthesis in the frontal cortex, thalamus, and dentate nucleus of the cerebellum (Chugani et al. 1997). Acute tryptophan depletion markedly exacerbated symptoms of autism, again suggesting a role for serotonin (McDougle et al. 1996). Elevated plasma levels of the excitatory amino acids glutamine and asparagine have been found (Moreno-Fuenmayor et al. 1996). Oxytocin and vasopressin may be involved in social attachment, which might be relevant to the symptoms of autistic disorder (Insel 1997). Other studies support the possible involvement of opiate peptides in autistic disorder (Sandman 1991; Willemsen-Swinkels et al. 1996).

A variety of immunological abnormalities have been proposed to contribute to the development of autism. Several reports have suggested an overrepresentation of several different autoimmune disorders in autistic patients. Preliminary reports have suggested the possible role of various autoantibodies and of interleukin.

Neuropsychological testing typically reveals global dysfunctions, but no discrete pathways or regions are consistently identified. Low IQ is associated with a higher prevalence of seizures, social impairment, bizarre behavior, self-mutilation, and poor prognosis. The increase in seizures during adolescence is observed particularly often in autistic individuals with low IQ. There is delayed development of cerebral dominance and an excess of non-right-handedness, primitive neurological reflexes, soft neurological signs, and physical anomalies.

Together, these findings suggest that autistic disorder entails 1) neuromaturational abnormalities that affect the development of brain structure and cerebral asymmetry, 2) pervasive and diffuse changes in widely disparate parts of the brain, 3) diffuse but pervasive symptoms in a variety of dimensions, and 4) serotonergic abnormalities in at least a subgroup of patients. The etiology of the neuromaturational problem is unknown, but such atypical brain development might be induced by genetic predisposition, infection or immunological reaction in the second trimester, or possibly a metabolic disturbance in brain chemistry during early or mid gestation. It may be speculated that the serotonergic abnormalities are related to comorbid obses-

sive-compulsive features, mood or anxiety disorder, or immunological changes. In sum, the neurobiological dysfunction appears to be quite diffuse, and there is no clear "primary" deficit in the majority of autistic individuals.

Course and Prognosis

Autistic disorder is often apparent at birth or early infancy, and parents may seek a medical evaluation during the child's first year (often for deafness). The DSM-IV definition of autistic disorder requires an apparent onset before age 3 years.

The general course of autistic disorder is gradual improvement, but there is a high degree of irregularity and unpredictability in the speed of improvement. Periods of rapid developmental growth alternate with periods of slow, stable growth. The changes in maturational tempo occur abruptly or gradually. Developmental progress can be slow or rapid in pace, and the periods of improvement may last for a couple of weeks or many months. Developmental change may be made in particular skills without improvement in other areas of functioning, or it may occur pervasively across many areas of functioning. Episodes of overt regression may occur during concurrent medical illness, situational stress, or puberty, and even during periods of otherwise rapid developmental progress unexplained by environmental factors. Overall, predictors of good adaptive outcome include later onset, higher IQ, better language skills (especially vocabulary), and greater social and communicative skills.

The availability of educational and supportive services has a marked beneficial impact, just as in mental retardation. In the severe, classic forms, some adaptive skills can be learned. In the less severe forms, the acquired social skills and adaptations may eventually permit performance in an ordinary occupation. Even a relatively interactive and pleasant social life can be attained.

Over the years, the time course of change remains unpredictable. As adults, autistic individuals continue to show a gradual clearing of symptoms but retain clinical evidence of residual deficits (Rumsey et al. 1985b). Depending on the severity of the autistic disorder, perhaps 2%–15% achieve a nonretarded level of cognitive and adaptive functioning. "Obsessive-compulsive" features remain predominant in adulthood and may include stereotyped pacing, rocking, perseveration, and stuttering. Adults with autistic disorder remain socially aloof and often retain an oppositional streak. Expressive and receptive language often become normal, although speech may continue to have a singsong, or monotonous, sound. No delusions or hallucinations are evident. Adults may achieve employment (generally in simple rote jobs) and the capacity for independent residence, but they rarely marry. The few outcome studies currently available describe the follow-up of severe and largely untreated cases; adult outcome may be better in less severe and more aggressively treated cases. It is unclear whether the features that persist into adulthood are "core" symptoms or developmental complications of autistic disorder, but these persistent features are not typically shared by individuals with mental retardation. There are many other complications of autistic disorder, even in the nonretarded subgroup, that are similar to the complications typically seen in mental retardation.

Evaluation and Differential Diagnosis

In addition to the standard psychiatric and behavioral evaluation, a workup of autistic disorder includes assessment of language skills, cognition, social skills, and adaptive functioning. Neurological examination includes consideration of possible inborn metabolic and degenerative diseases. Screening for phenylketonuria is probably cost-effective. MRI studies may be helpful in some cases as a part of the general neurological evaluation, but they cannot be used for diagnosis of autistic disorder at this time. It is typically worthwhile to obtain an EEG in view of the high prevalence of seizure disorders in this population. Chromosomal analysis should also be considered to evaluate for relatively frequent genetic abnormalities, such as fragile X syndrome. In some cases, audiological examination for possible deafness and examinations for other sensory deficits may be considered. Psychological and neuropsychological testing for mental retardation, juvenile-onset psychotic disorders, and mixed receptive/expressive language disorder is valuable but can be difficult. Evaluation for communication disorders may be particularly difficult if the child's nonverbal skills are also impaired. An assessment of the home environment and emotional supportiveness of the family is needed. Standardized evaluation checklists can be used to collect and organize information based on clinical observations and parental recall of early behavior (Parks 1983).

It is also important to evaluate patients with autistic disorder for comorbidity, especially obsessive-compulsive disorder, ADHD, tic disorders, and mood disorders (particularly major depressive or dysthymic disorder). Although ADHD may be functionally present and fulfill diagnostic criteria, it is not designated as a separate DSM-IV disorder when it occurs in the context of a pervasive developmental disorder.

Differential diagnosis includes congenital deafness (although deaf children typically learn an alternate lip or sign language, lose their isolative behaviors, and develop sensitive expressive communication), congenital blindness (although blind children relate more socially), mental retardation (although mentally retarded children do not show the islands of special capacity that autistic children sometimes have), expressive and mixed receptive-expressive language disorder (although children with these disorders are typically more interactive and can communicate well in gestures), schizophreniform disorder, schizotypal personality disorder, and juvenile-onset schizophrenia (although children with schizophrenia typically have hallucinations, delusions, or thought disorder).

In many cases, particularly those involving less severe forms, it is difficult to make a definitive diagnosis of autistic disorder. The appearance of hallucinations, delusions, or clear thought disorder should lead to the consideration of a primary psychotic disorder rather than autism. However, children and adults with autistic disorder may have concomitant psychotic disorders, comorbid mood disorders, or anxiety disorders.

Treatment

Historically, treatment neglect resulted in a generation of individuals with autistic disorders who had a relatively poor outcome. More recently, several studies have shown that rigorous multimodal treatment may be useful and sometimes has dramatic effects, although controlled and systematic studies are needed.

Behavioral therapy has been demonstrated to be helpful in controlling unwanted symptoms, promoting social interactions, increasing self-reliance, and facilitating exploration (i.e., novelty-seeking behavior). Specialized assertiveness training may be helpful in enhancing adaptive skills. Special education, vocational training, teaching of adaptive skills, and support in managing major life events are basic. Environmental management, especially predictable or programmed structure, has a particularly powerful effect.

Providing guidance to parents is critical, especially for those who are making the chronically afflicted child the emotional center of their lives. Although this attentiveness may have beneficial effects for the child, it is often driven by unjustified guilt, unrealistic pessimism, or narcissism. Parents can contribute to the child's learning of self-care and adaptive skills, arrange for special education and management with schools and other public agencies, and make long-term plans for the child's future. Because long-term treatment is essential, periodic medical reassessment is needed to monitor for the possible appearance of seizures or concomitant psychiatric disorders that may be masked by the autistic disorder.

A long-term program involving high levels of supervision and structure is generally required. Specialized day care and group settings, incorporating elements of behavioral treatment in a naturalistic setting with a stable interpersonal network, are helpful in some cases (Landesman and Vietze 1987). At times, residential care is needed to provide a more enveloping structure of protection and supervision.

Most of the pharmacological studies of autistic disorder have been conducted in children, with little research concerning adults. There is no drug treatment of autistic disorder itself, but psychotropic medications can be used to target particular symptoms, symptom clusters, and comorbid disorders in individual patients. There are still no psychotropic medications that provide generally useful treatment for the majority of patients with autistic disorder.

The symptoms most amenable to pharmacotherapy include perseverative behaviors (comparable to obsessive-compulsive symptoms), depressive disorders, aggressivity, impulsivity, destructiveness, bipolar disorder, anxiety, hyperactivity, hypoactivity, pica, and self-injurious behavior. Management of seizures is also approached medically. In general, the risk of overmedication requires continual attentiveness.

Although no single medication is generally indicated, a variety of different agents can provide symptomatic benefit. Low doses of nonsedating conventional neuroleptics (such as haloperidol) have been found helpful for promoting learning, controlling behavioral symptoms, reducing excessive activity levels, controlling aggressive and disruptive behavior, and enhancing the effects of behavioral therapy and other interventions. The newer atypical antipsychotics, such as risperidone, appear to be more beneficial in some patients (McDougle et al. 1997), better tolerated, and less risky. Olanzapine is generally less satisfactory because of its tendency to aggravate obsessive-compulsive symptoms. Psychostimulants, anticonvulsants, and neuroleptics may be useful for symptoms of impulsivity. Psychostimulants are employed for children who either are underactive or have concurrent ADHD. β-Blocking agents and perhaps clonidine might have some value in managing symptoms of impulsivity and aggression. Early reports on naltrexone, an opiate receptor blocking agent, suggested that this drug could improve affective availability, promote social reciprocity, and reduce stereotyped motor and self-injurious behaviors; however, more recent data suggest that it has little or no clinically significant effects. Several preliminary reports have suggested that fluoxetine can be helpful in treating obsessional and depressive symptoms in patients with autistic disorder. Serotonin reuptake inhibitors have also been found to reduce anxiety symptoms in some children (Steingard et al. 1997). A controlled study of fluvoxamine in adults with autism found that drug to be significantly more beneficial than placebo (McDougle et al. 1997), and lithium has been found to be helpful as an adjunctive treatment, particularly when supplementing serotonin reuptake inhibitors. Other researchers have suggested possible benefits of H_2 blockers (famotidine), adrenocorticotropic hormone (ACTH) analogs, and inositol.

Controlled clinical studies of intervention in autistic disorder have been almost exclusively restricted to behavioral and pharmacological treatments. Reports on family, individual, group, and program interventions are generally based on impressionistic evaluations.

Working closely with autistic children may present a challenge to a therapist's empathic capacities. These individuals learn about reality in slow steps and may take considerable time to learn about human beings and the nature of feelings. Children with less severe cases of autistic disorder may present more subtle empathic challenges. Over time, many of these children are capable of deeply joyous and genuine interpersonal interactions, albeit unusual ones that may be lacking in the more transcendental aspects of human interaction.

CHILDHOOD DISINTEGRATIVE DISORDER

Childhood disintegrative disorder differs from autistic disorder in time of onset, clinical course, and prevalence. In contrast to autistic disorder, in this disorder there is an early period of normal development until age 3–4 years. This is followed by a period of marked deterioration of capacities (Table 23–23), usually occurring rapidly over the course of 6–9 months. Childhood disintegrative disorder may begin with behavioral symptoms, such as anxiety, anger, or outbursts, but the general loss of functions becomes pervasive and severe. The deterioration leads to a syndrome that is symptomatically similar to autistic disorder, except that mental retardation (typically in the moderate-to-profound range) tends to be more frequent and pronounced. Over time, the deterioration remains stable, although some capacities may be regained to a limited degree. About 20% regain the ability to speak in sentences, but their communication skills remain impaired (Hill and Rosenbloom 1986). Most adults are completely dependent and require institutional care, and some have a shortened life span.

No specific neurobiological deficit or cause of childhood disintegrative disorder has been identified (Volkmar and Cohen 1989). Significant psychosocial or medical stressors have been reported in association with the onset or worsening of the disorder, but their etiological significance is unclear.

Childhood disintegrative disorder appears to be less prevalent than autistic disorder, with estimates ranging from 1 to 4 in 100,000. There appears to be a male predominance of greater than 4:1.

The evaluation and treatment of childhood disintegrative disorder are essentially comparable to the approach to autistic disorder, although much more active support, behavioral treatment, neurological care, and medical monitoring are needed. A change in the disease label is also needed, because of the crudity of the term "disintegrative," especially when used in speaking with parents about their child.

RETT'S DISORDER

Rett's disorder is a progressive neuropsychiatric disorder in girls, who typically present with autistic features. The disorder classically unfolds in four stages: relative nor-

---

TABLE 23–23. DSM-IV diagnostic criteria for childhood disintegrative disorder

A. Apparently normal development for at least the first 2 years after birth as manifested by the presence of age-appropriate verbal and nonverbal communication, social relationships, play, and adaptive behavior.

B. Clinically significant loss of previously acquired skills (before age 10 years) in at least two of the following areas:

   (1) Expressive or receptive language
   (2) Social skills or adaptive behavior
   (3) Bowel or bladder control
   (4) Play
   (5) Motor skills

C. Abnormalities of functioning in at least two of the following areas:

   (1) Qualitative impairment in social interaction (e.g., impairment in nonverbal behaviors, failure to develop peer relationships, lack of social or emotional reciprocity)
   (2) Qualitative impairments in communication (e.g., delay or lack of spoken language, inability to initiate or sustain a conversation, stereotyped and repetitive use of language, lack of varied make-believe play)
   (3) Restricted, repetitive, and stereotyped patterns of behavior, interests, and activities, including motor stereotypies and mannerisms

D. The disturbance is not better accounted for by another specific pervasive developmental disorder or by schizophrenia.

---

malcy, developmental arrest, plateau, and significant motor decline (Hagberg and Witt-Engerstrom 1986). Recent epidemiological and neurological data suggest that the deviance from normal development often begins in the perinatal period and becomes more prominent with age.

Once considered a clearly neurodegenerative process, serial neurodevelopmental evaluations have indicated that there may not be any actual loss of developmental gains, but rather an arrest of developmental functions at various stages, particularly during periods of rapid neuronal growth, pruning, and maturation (Naidu et al. 1995). Debate continues about the neurodevelopmental versus neurodegenerative nature of the disease process and course, but it is clear that the onset of Rett's disorder can be observed in very young girls and that progressive clinical decline is the hallmark.

The estimated prevalence of Rett's disorder ranges from 5 to 15 in 100,000 girls. All the documented cases have been girls, although some undocumented cases are rumored to have been boys. Etiological factors remain unclear. A strong genetic component is suggested by the finding of 100% concordance for Rett's disorder in eight sets of monozygotic twins and 0% in six sets of zygotic twins (Hagberg 1989). Data are suggestive of a dominant X-linked inheritance with full or nearly full penetrance, and with early death of the males (and perhaps some females) in spontaneous abortion.

The progressive clinical decline is not initially apparent. Typically, after 6–18 months of relatively normal development, the first social, language, neurological, and motor deficiencies become apparent. Initially, the clinical decline is gradual, but it becomes quite evident by 4 years of age (Table 23–24). Head and body growth retardation, along with other developmental delays, can be seen during this phase. Then, starting during the early school years, there is a period of more rapid functional deterioration in which intellectual and communicative capacities diminish, and purposeful control of hand movements is replaced with apraxia, wringing, and washing motions. Following this rapid deterioration, these girls appear to have a pervasive developmental disorder, which is usually identified as autistic disorder or childhood disintegrative disorder (Moeschler et al. 1988). This rapid decline in functioning usually reaches an apparent plateau that may last for months or years. However, this plateau is eventually seen to be a gradual decline that is much slower than that of the previous stage. Gait and truncal ataxia, respiratory symptoms involving dysregulation of breathing functions, and scoliosis typically begin to emerge during this slow decline.

By age 3–5 years, girls with Rett's disorder are less likely to be viewed as having either autistic or childhood disintegrative disorder because of the progressive appearance of increasingly severe neurological symptoms. Mental retardation is generally apparent, and most patients have intelligence scores in the severely retarded range. Seizures, decreasing physical mobility, spasticity, muscle weakness, severe scoliosis, wasting, dystonia, and choreoathetosis may emerge. Typically, these girls are eventually confined to wheelchairs, often before adolescence. Feeding can become quite difficult because of compromised motor functioning (swallowing). Caretakers need to be aware of the high risk of aspiration, which may be compounded by the dysregulation of breathing. Seizures occur in 80% of patients and add to the management problems. Although some girls with Rett's disorder die suddenly of unexplained causes, most patients have a normal life span despite the severe symptoms and disabilities.

The etiology of Rett's disorder remains obscure. An atypical glycolipid has been described in the majority of these patients. Investigators evaluating the CSF of patients with Rett's disorder have reported reduced concentrations of substance P (Matsuishi et al. 1997) and nerve growth factor, and elevated concentrations of β-endorphin and glutamate. Abnormalities of monoamine levels have been reported. Two studies show underpigmentation in the zona compacta. Neuropathological studies have demonstrated a generalized atrophy involving both the cerebrum and the cerebellum, a generalized decrease in neuronal cell size and increased cell density, a reduction in the number of basal

TABLE 23-24.   **DSM-IV diagnostic criteria for Rett's disorder**

A. All of the following:

  (1) Apparently normal prenatal and perinatal development
  (2) Apparently normal psychomotor development through the first 5 months after birth
  (3) Normal head circumference at birth

B. Onset of all of the following after the period of normal development:

  (1) Deceleration of head growth between ages 5 and 48 months
  (2) Loss of previously acquired purposeful hand skills between ages 5 and 30 months with the subsequent development of stereotyped hand movements (e.g., hand wringing or hand washing)
  (3) Loss of social engagement early in the course (although often social interaction develops later)
  (4) Appearance of poorly coordinated gait or trunk movements
  (5) Severely impaired expressive and receptive language development with severe psychomotor retardation

forebrain cholinergic neurons, and reduced melanin-containing neurons in the substantia nigra (Wong et al. 1998).

Data from neuroimaging studies are preliminary, but SPECT studies have suggested that bifrontal hypoperfusion correlates with severity of Rett's disorder. Diffuse atrophy (most notably in the prefrontal, posterior frontal, and anterior temporal regions) was noted in an MRI study. Abnormal EEGs are typically found after 2 years of age; despite the high prevalence of seizures, the EEG findings are typically nonspecific. Taken together, the neurobiological abnormalities suggest an X-linked generalized atrophy with global dysfunction that correlates with severity of the symptoms.

Treatment of Rett's disorder is supportive. Generally, these multiply handicapped patients require intensive care (Lindberg 1992). The role of psychopharmacotherapy is limited, but several reports found have carbamazepine to be more effective than other anticonvulsants for seizure control in girls with Rett's disorder.

ASPERGER'S DISORDER

Asperger's disorder is another pervasive developmental disorder that is similar to autistic disorder except that language skills and cognition are partially preserved (Table 23–25). Because of its similarities to autism, the status of Asperger's disorder as a distinct form of pervasive developmental disorder is often questioned, and many specialists believe that it is a mild version of autistic disorder (i.e., high-functioning autism) rather than a separate and distinct disorder (Gillberg 1989; Rapin 1991).

Recently researchers have focused on discriminating between Asperger's and autistic disorders by analysis of speech and communication patterns, cognitive batteries, and the WISC alone (Ehlers et al. 1997). Generally, the newer studies have suggested that the two entities are distinct, which is consistent with the current DSM-IV categorization. On the other hand, categorization does not preclude a "spectrum" of illness, so that Asperger's disorder might be considered, at least heuristically, a "right-hemisphere-only version of autistic disorder."

There tends to be a relative sparing of intelligence, language, and cognition, as well as a lower prevalence of mental retardation, in Asperger's disorder. Only 12% of children with this disorder have IQ scores below 70. It is characteristic of these patients to misread nonverbal cues, have marked difficulties with peer interactions (especially in groups), focus repetitively in conversation on topics of interest only to themselves, appear not particularly empathic, and speak without normal inflection and tone varia-

TABLE 23–25. DSM-IV diagnostic criteria for Asperger's disorder

A. Qualitative impairment in social interaction, as manifested by at least two of the following:

   (1) Marked impairment in the use of multiple nonverbal behaviors such as eye-to-eye gaze, facial expression, body postures, and gestures to regulate social interaction

   (2) Failure to develop peer relationships appropriate to developmental level

   (3) A lack of spontaneous seeking to share enjoyment, interests, or achievements with other people (e.g., by a lack of showing, bringing, or pointing out objects of interest to other people)

   (4) Lack of social or emotional reciprocity

B. Restricted repetitive and stereotyped patterns of behavior, interests, and activities, as manifested by at least one of the following:

   (1) Encompassing preoccupation with one or more stereotyped and restricted patterns of interest that is abnormal either in intensity or focus

   (2) Apparently inflexible adherence to specific, nonfunctional routines or rituals

   (3) Stereotyped and repetitive motor mannerisms (e.g., hand or finger flapping or twisting, or complex whole-body movements)

   (4) Persistent preoccupation with parts of objects

C. The disturbance causes clinically significant impairment in social, occupational, or other important areas of functioning.

D. There is no clinically significant general delay in language (e.g., single words used by age 2 years, communicative phrases used by age 3 years).

E. There is no clinically significant delay in cognitive development or in the development of age-appropriate self-help skills, adaptive behavior (other than in social interaction), and curiosity about the environment in childhood.

F. Criteria are not met for another specific pervasive developmental disorder or schizophrenia.

---

tion; they may be relatively unexpressive affectively, and they tend to have few friends (Wing 1981). Even with these limitations, persons with Asperger's disorder are often quite sociable and talkative, and they may form affectionate bonds with family members (Frith 1991). The course tends to be stable over time, often with some gradual gains (Szatmari et al. 1989).

Epidemiological data are limited, but the prevalence of Asperger's disorder is estimated at 5 to 15 in 100,000. The male predominance is 3:1–4:1.

The etiology of Asperger's disorder remains unknown. In some cases, it follows a familial pattern, consistent with genetic, psychosocial, or environmental transmission. A possible role of fetal exposure to alcohol has been raised (Aronson et al. 1997).

Neurobiological studies are extremely limited. About 30% of patients with Asperger's disorder have nonspecific EEG abnormalities, and 15% show evidence of brain atrophy. In a recent SPECT study, abnormal right hemisphere metabolism was reported; although the significance of this finding is not entirely known, it lends some support to the concept of "right-hemisphere-only autistic disorder" (Szatmari et al. 1995).

Treatment includes social and motor skills training, remedial educational interventions when indicated, and vocational training. The relative sparing of language and intelligence allows individuals with Asperger's disorder to have a better outcome than do most persons with autistic disorder. Temple Grandin is a productive member of society with good verbal skills who has Asperger's disorder (formerly diagnosed as autism). Her self-report (Grandin and Scariano 1986) demonstrates that a high-functioning individual with a pervasive developmental disorder can vividly describe personal experiences and complex cognitions. Persons with Asperger's disorder, despite their relative handicaps in social functioning, can become quite expert and effective in their chosen activities, and perhaps they are even helped in these accomplishments by the highly focused nature of their interests.

CLINICAL COMMENT

A sensible subtyping of pervasive developmental disorders has long been awaited (Table 23–26), and recent research and the clinical awareness of the diversity of pervasive developmental disorders can be expected to lead to improved understanding and eventually to improved treatments. At this time, however, treatments remain largely supportive and symptomatic.

These disorders, relatively rare and still of unknown etiology, are receiving intensive study. Because maternal factors are no longer considered primary or in any way etiological, research has focused on biological description and evaluation of psychosocial treatment interventions. The critical role of aggressive treatment and the need for a variety of community resources have been generally accepted, although the development of appropriate community supports is limited by funding. Effective public advocacy has provided some genuine opportunities for individuals with pervasive developmental disorders. With improving treatment, increasingly more adults with pervasive developmental disorder have overcome the disease label.

TIC DISORDERS

Tic disorders are stereotyped abnormalities of semi-involuntary movement presumably related to dysfunction in the basal ganglia, which are situated at a midway position among higher and lower centers within the brain. Symptoms of these disorders are subject to moment-to-moment influences from environmental and internal stimuli and thus permit study of interacting biopsychosocial influences (Chase et al. 1992; D. Cohen et al. 1988; Kurlan 1993).

Although tics are experienced as involuntary (Table 23–27), patients may consciously (although only temporarily) suppress tic movements, in contrast to choreiform (i.e., disruptions of normal synergistic movement by coordinated muscle groups, such as blinks or grimaces) and athetoid (i.e., slow writhing) movements. Tics are distinct from dyskinesias (i.e., disruptions of voluntary and involuntary motions), dystonias (i.e., abnormal muscle tone), and other neurological movement disorders. Instead, tics are brief and repetitive—but not rhythmic—motor (muscular) or vocal (phonic) responses that are purposeless but may resemble purposeful acts. They involve recurrent movements of the same muscle groups, but their location can change gradually over time. Their form may be simple (motor: jerking movements, shrugging, eye blinking; vocal: grunting, sniffing, throat clearing) or complex (motor: grimacing, bending, banging; vocal: echolalia, odd inflections and accents).

Individual tics may be seen occasionally in normal children and adults, but such "twitches" (e.g., blinks, grimaces) and habits are not diagnosed unless they persist for at least 2 weeks.

Tic disorders are subtyped into transient tic, chronic tic, and Tourette's disorders. These conditions appear to be closely related in descriptive, genetic, and developmental characteristics. They vary in intensity over time, usually increasing during times of psychosocial stress (including teasing and social ostracism), intrapsychic conflict, and positive or negative emotional excitement. Psychosocial stress may be particularly symptom inducing at the start of

TABLE 23–26. Characteristics and differential diagnosis of the pervasive developmental disorders

Characteristics	Autistic disorder	Childhood disintegrative disorder	Rett's disorder	Asperger's disorder	PDD-NOS
Feature	Standard autism	Delayed onset but severe autism	"Midchildhood" autism	High functioning autism	Atypical and subthreshold
Intelligence	Severe MR to normal	Severe MR	Severe MR	Mild MR to normal	Mild MR to normal
Age at recognition	0–3 years	>2 years	0.5–2.5 years	Usually >2 years	Variable
Communication skills	Usually limited	Poor	Poor	Limited to fair	Limited to fair
Social skills	Very limited	Very limited	Varies with age	Limited	Variable
Loss of skills	Usually not	Marked	Marked	Usually not	Usually not
Restricted interests	Variable	Not applicable	Not applicable	Marked	Variable
Seizure disorder	Uncommon	Frequent	Uncommon	Common	Common
Head growth deceleration	No	No	Yes	No	No
Prevalence per 100,000 estimated	30–50	1–4	5–15	5–100	>15
Family history of similar problems	Uncommon	No	No	Frequent	Unknown
Gender ratio	M > F	M > F	F	M > F	M > F
Course in adulthood	Stable	Declining	Declining	Stable	Usually stable
Outcome	Poor	Very poor	Very poor	Fair to poor	Fair to good

Note. PDD-NOS = pervasive developmental disorder not otherwise specified; MR = mental retardation.
Source. Modified with permission from Volkmar FR, Cohen DJ: "Nonautistic Pervasive Developmental Disorders" (Chapter 27.2), in *Psychiatry*. Edited by Michels R, Cooper AM, Guze SB, et al. Philadelphia, PA, JB Lippincott, 1991. Copyright 1991, JB Lippincott.

TABLE 23–27.   DSM-IV diagnostic criteria for tic disorders

Diagnostic criteria for Tourette's disorder

A. Both multiple motor and one or more vocal tics have been present at some time during the illness, although not necessarily concurrently. (A *tic* is a sudden, rapid, recurrent, nonrhythmic, stereotyped motor movement or vocalization.)

B. The tics occur many times a day (usually in bouts) nearly every day or intermittently throughout a period of more than 1 year, and during this period there was never a tic-free period of more than 3 consecutive months.

C. The disturbance causes marked distress or significant impairment in social, occupational, or other important areas of functioning.

D. The onset is before age 18 years.

E. The disturbance is not due to the direct physiological effects of a substance (e.g., stimulants) or a general medical condition (e.g., Huntington's disease or postviral encephalitis).

Diagnostic criteria for chronic motor or vocal tic disorder

A. Single or multiple motor or vocal tics (i.e., sudden, rapid, recurrent, nonrhythmic, stereotyped motor movements or vocalizations), but not both, have been present at some time during the illness.

B. The tics occur many times a day nearly every day or intermittently throughout a period of more than 1 year, and during this period there was never a tic-free period of more than 3 consecutive months.

C. The disturbance causes marked distress or significant impairment in social, occupational, or other important areas of functioning.

D. The onset is before age 18 years.

E. The disturbance is not due to the direct physiological effects of a substance (e.g., stimulants) or a general medical condition (e.g., Huntington's disease or postviral encephalitis).

F. Criteria have never been met for Tourette's disorder.

Diagnostic criteria for transient tic disorder

A. Single or multiple motor and/or vocal tics (i.e., sudden, rapid, recurrent, nonrhythmic, stereotyped motor movements or vocalizations).

B. The tics occur many times a day nearly every day for at least 4 weeks, but for no longer than 12 consecutive months.

C. The disturbance causes marked distress or significant impairment in social, occupational, or other important areas of functioning.

D. The onset is before age 18 years.

E. The disturbance is not due to the direct physiological effects of a substance (e.g., stimulants) or a general medical condition (e.g., Huntington's disease or postviral encephalitis).

F. Criteria have never been met for Tourette's disorder or chronic motor or vocal tic disorder.

Specify if:

Single episode or recurrent
tic disorder not otherwise specified
This category is for disorders characterized by tics that do not meet criteria for a specific tic disorder. Examples include tics lasting less than 4 weeks or tics with an onset after age 18 years.

---

the school year, at times of parental separation and divorce, and during physical fatigue. Tics typically decrease in frequency and severity during focused mental activity, concentration, or sudden alerting (e.g., by a distraction), but they may not fully disappear during sleep.

Family genetic studies show that first-degree relatives of patients with Tourette's disorder (50% of males and 30% of females) have an overrepresentation of transient tic disorder, chronic tic disorders, and OCD, suggesting a genetic interrelationship among all three tic disorders as well as OCD. Because the etiologies of the three tic disorders seem closely interrelated, it is appropriate that tic disorders are subtyped by clinical description and course rather than by etiology.

TRANSIENT TIC DISORDER

Transient tic disorder is diagnosed if daily tics persist for 2 weeks to 1 year (the threshold for the label of chronic tic disorder). Although a single symptomatic period may be observed, recurrent episodes may come and go for years.

Transient tics are usually motoric, but they are otherwise similar in appearance to chronic and Tourette's tics. Transient tic disorder may be relabeled later in its course if tics persist. These tics do not appear to be consistently associated with other symptoms, but situational or developmental anxiety may be prominent during episodes.

Up to 12% of children have tic symptoms, but the prevalence of transient tic disorder is undetermined. There is a male-to-female predominance of 3:1.

Both genetic and psychosocial factors influence the appearance of transient tic disorder. Episodes are typically seen during periods of increased stress or excitement, which contribute to the transient presentation and the variability of symptom intensity. When tics present in apparent response to physical or emotional trauma, the individual generally has an underlying genetic vulnerability (Alegre et al. 1996).

The onset of single or recurrent episodes of transient tic disorder is usually during midchildhood (age 5–10 years) or early adolescence. If episodes recur, there is typically a reduction in the frequency and severity of symptoms over the course of years. The symptoms do not usually interfere with functioning, although tics may interact with anxiety and social stressors to produce interpersonal and self-esteem complications.

Neuromedical and psychiatric evaluations of these children are needed to assess possible concomitant disorders, including other neurological movement disorders, virus-induced tics (typically herpes), and posttraumatic tics from head trauma. Children should also be carefully screened for anxiety disorders (e.g., PTSD, OCD) because of their exacerbating effect on tics.

Individuals with transient tic disorder typically do not require treatment. It is usually helpful to advise the family to reduce attention to the symptom and criticism of the child. Behavioral techniques (e.g., relaxation), medications (e.g., minor tranquilizers, low dosages of major tranquilizers), or brief psychotherapy may be helpful in certain cases for anxiety management and tic control. The patient and family may be provided with education and reassurance, and they may be encouraged to return for reevaluation if symptoms persist.

CHRONIC MOTOR OR VOCAL TIC DISORDER

The diagnosis of chronic motor or vocal tic disorder is made if either motor or vocal tics persist for more than 1 year. Tourette's disorder is diagnosed if both motor and vocal tics are chronic.

Chronic tics are typically motoric and similar in form to those in other motor tic disorders. Chronic vocal tics are rare, usually mild, and generally consist of grunts (e.g., diaphragmatic contractions) rather than true vocal or verbal tics. The persistence of chronic tics can be associated with anxiety or depressive disorders, both of which may aggravate tic disorders.

Prevalence data are not available for chronic tic disorders, because the durational characteristics of tics have not been studied epidemiologically. Chronic tic disorder is probably less common than Tourette's disorder in clinical populations, but it is unclear whether this reflects general prevalence or referral bias (e.g., help seeking).

There is typically little variation in the intensity of chronic tics over the course of weeks, although changes may be noted over the course of months or years. The onset is usually during early childhood (ages 5–10 years). In about two-thirds of cases the disorder ends during adolescence, but some cases may persist in mild form for years or even decades. A subtype of chronic tic disorder can also appear in adulthood, typically after age 40.

Neuromedical and psychiatric evaluations, similar to the workup for transient tic disorder, are indicated. Specific evaluation for anxiety and depressive disorders, as possible sustaining factors of chronic tics, is helpful.

Behavioral and pharmacological treatments are effective, and psychosocial interventions (including individual and family psychotherapy) are used to target the symptoms of anxiety. Minor tranquilizers and low dosages of major tranquilizers should be considered. Although systematic data are lacking, anecdotal information suggests that these medications are quite useful. The use of stimulants and tricyclic antidepressants in treating chronic tic disorder is discussed in the section on Tourette's disorder.

TOURETTE'S DISORDER

Tourette's disorder is a lifelong disease entailing vocal tics and multiple motor tics. During the first 12 months that both motor and verbal tics are observed, transient tic disorder is diagnosed. Beyond 1 year, the diagnosis is converted to Tourette's disorder. The DSM-IV definition of Tourette's disorder is considerably looser than the classic criteria and permits inclusion of a wider range of patients.

Clinical Description

Both the motor and vocal tics of Tourette's disorder may be simple or complex. The behavioral component can be suppressed voluntarily, but then a premonitory sensory urge (usually with a subjective sense of tension) builds. This sensation of craving before a tic is relieved temporarily when patients allow themselves to express their tics in action. Many patients experience their tics as a voluntary response to these premonitory urges, and they may feel more troubled by the continual pre-tic tension than by the tics themselves (Leckman et al. 1993).

Some patients find that they can control their tics during the daytime at school or work, and then "let off the tension" later, when alone in their bedrooms. For these individuals, the use of the home as a haven for the release of symptoms can be an effective way to reduce the impact of their symptoms on their social and occupational life. However, some patients with severe Tourette's disorder feel that "saving" their tics in this manner is even more problematic because it interferes with the comfort of family members.

Tourette's disorder involves a typical pattern of waxing and waning over time. Severity varies widely. Mild cases may go undiagnosed even in television personalities, and severe cases may be disabling and socially disfiguring. As in other tic disorders, anxiety and excitement lead to increased symptoms, relaxation and focused attention can reduce symptoms, and symptoms are typically minimal or absent during sleep. Increased symptom severity may be evident for several minutes during stressful situations, may last for months during periods of developmental anxiety and stress, or may last for years (particularly when associated with concomitant anxiety or mood disorders).

The clinical presentation of Tourette's disorder may change during the course of development. Onset is usually between ages 2 and 13 years. Symptoms begin as a single tic in 50% of patients. At about age 7 years (mean age at onset), motor tics become evident and show a rostral-caudal progression over time (i.e., head before trunk and limbs). At about age 11 years (on average), phonic and vocal tics may appear, followed by obsessive-compulsive behaviors. Vocal tics may start as a single syllable, progress to longer exclamations, and occasionally progress to complex verbal structures and gestures. Classic coprolalia is observed in 60% of patients with Tourette's disorder, with an initial appearance typically in early adolescence. Copropraxia (i.e., complex obscene gestures) may appear later, as coprolalia resolves. Complex motor tics may appear to be purposeless, or they may be camouflaged by being blended into other purposeful movements. Sometimes these complex motor tics are self-destructive (e.g., scratching or cutting oneself) or violent (e.g., temper tantrums, assaults). Sensory tics are present in up to 30% of patients with Tourette's disorder and typically present in a rostral-caudal distribution (Chee and Sachdev 1997). Obsessive-compulsive symptoms usually begin about 5–10 years after the first appearance of simple tics (Bruun 1988) and may elaborate extensively.

Early in development, before the appearance of tics, 25%–50% of children with Tourette's disorder show impulsivity, hyperactivity, and inattention similar to the symptoms of ADHD. Conduct disorder is also common. Obsessive-compulsive symptoms appear in about 20%–40% of cases, and full obsessive-compulsive disorder presents in 7%–10%.

Structured diagnostic assessments in adults with Tourette's disorder have revealed a significantly elevated rate of personality disorders in comparison to the general population (64% vs. 6%). In adulthood, it is common for patients with Tourette's disorder to meet criteria for more than one personality disorder. Moreover, depressive and anxiety disorders are significantly more prevalent in patients with Tourette's disorder than in control samples (Robertson et al. 1997).

Neurological symptoms are typically observed in patients with Tourette's disorder. Neurological soft signs (50% of patients) and choreiform movements (30% of patients) are common. Approximately 50% of patients show abnormal EEG findings, particularly immature patterns (excess slow waves and posterior sharp waves). CT scans are usually normal. Disordered sleep and enuresis may be overrepresented.

Some patients have a form of Tourette's disorder that is an autoimmune reaction to a streptococcal infection; that is, a pediatric autoimmune neuropsychiatric disorder associated with streptococcal infections (PANDAS). Choreiform "piano-playing" movements are present in essentially all of these cases. About 80% of patients with PANDAS also have OCD, and about 50% have ADHD. Other neuropsychiatric symptoms associated with PANDAS include emotional lability, oppositional behavior, separation anxiety, (such as nighttime fears), bedtime rituals, and deterioration in math skills and handwriting (Swedo et al. 1998).

There is no evidence of psychosis, impaired reality sense, or intellectual deterioration, but Tourette's disorder can appear in combination with other psychiatric disorders. Increased aggressive (Stefl 1983) or sexual (Jagger et al. 1982) behavior each may be seen in about one-third of patients with Tourette's disorder.

Although the diagnostic criteria are clearly defined, the clinical boundaries between Tourette's disorder, ADHD, and OCD are blurred in many patients who exhibit combined features of these three disorders.

Epidemiology

Up to 12% of children may have tic symptoms. The general prevalence of tic disorders is currently estimated at 1%–2%, but it is probably higher in children and adolescents. Prevalence estimates for Tourette's disorder itself are about 1 in 1,500. There is a male predominance of at least 3:1 (perhaps as high as 10:1). There is no apparent socioeconomic skewing. Cross-cultural studies have suggested that Tourette's disorder displays strong similarities across cultures in its clinical features, comorbidity, family history, and treatment outcomes, further suggesting an underlying genetic and neurobiological basis (Staley et al. 1997).

Etiology

Genetic, biological, and psychosocial factors appear operative in Tourette's disorder, as in other tic disorders. Tics are noted in two-thirds of relatives of patients with Tourette's disorder. Family studies of patients with tic disorders and OCD show that both groups are associated with a similar prevalence of tics and compulsive behaviors in family members. The higher concordance of Tourette's disorder in monozygotic than dizygotic twins suggests an inheritable component. Genetic studies show a link between Tourette's disorder, chronic tics, and OCD. There may also be a link between Tourette's disorder and ADHD in the absence of OCD. The familial predisposition to tic disorders and OCD appears to be governed by a single gene with autosomal dominant transmission (Pauls and Leckman 1986).

About one-third of preadolescent children with Tourette's disorder appear to have a genuine autoimmune disorder. Their episodes are caused or triggered by group A β-hemolytic streptococcal infections, such as pharyngitis, upper respiratory infections, or subclinical streptococcal infections (i.e., exposure). The mechanism involves the production of antistreptococcal antibodies that also have antineuronal properties and that attack the basal ganglia (Swedo et al. 1994). This mechanism also underlies other PANDAS, including OCD and Sydenham's chorea (St. Vitus dance). Separation anxiety disorder and anorexia nervosa have also been proposed to be PANDAS.

A "gender threshold effect" is observed for Tourette's disorder (as well as for ADHD). Tourette's disorder is more common in boys, but there is a higher prevalence of chronic tic and Tourette's disorders in the relatives of girls than with boys with Tourette's. Both the apparent 3:1 male predominance and the more common appearance of Tourette's disorder in boys at a given level of genetic loading could reflect a lower penetrance for the genetic form of Tourette's disorder in girls.

When all forms of the disorder are considered, the penetrance is 100% for males and 71% for females. Within affected families, males are more likely to have tic disorders, and females are more likely to have OCD (Pauls and Leckman 1986). There is a gender-related difference in the phenomenology (or phenotype) or in the penetrance of single genetically transmitted disorders (i.e., a gender threshold effect). No mechanistic explanation has been provided for the gender threshold effect in Tourette's disorder, OCD, or ADHD. For these disorders, gender may be considered a predisposing factor that contributes to the presentation or emergence of symptoms.

About 10% of individuals with Tourette's disorder have a nonfamilial version, which is a phenocopy similar in appearance to the genetic form of Tourette's disorder. In the nonfamilial cases, family psychiatric history is negative for these disorders (Pauls and Leckman 1986).

Additional etiological factors are suggested by retrospective findings of increased prenatal complications, lower birth weight (in affected monozygotic than dizygotic twins), greater emotional stress during pregnancy, and more nausea/vomiting during the first trimester (Leckman et al. 1990). It may be speculated that such environmental factors modulate the expression of the genetic predisposition to Tourette's disorder, perhaps operating through stress- or gender-related hormonal mechanisms.

The usual absence of motor developmental delays in Tourette's disorder (Bruun 1988) suggests that a relatively specific effect is exerted on the involved neural pathways rather than a generalized neurodevelopmental effect on neuromotor functions.

A leading hypothesis suggests that Tourette's disorder is associated with a supersensitivity of postsynaptic dopaminergic D_2 receptors in the basal ganglia; however, abnormalities of serotonin, dynorphin, γ-aminobutyric acid (GABA), acetylcholine, and norepinephrine have also been described. The metabolites of dopamine and sometimes serotonin are reduced in the CSF of patients with Tourette's disorder. Decreased levels of the endogenous opiate dynorphin Al-17 have been found in striatal pathways projecting to the globus pallidus (Haber and Wolfer 1992), and dynorphin Al-8 is increased in the CSF of Tourette's patients (Leckman et al. 1988), which is consistent with the involvement of opioid mechanisms. Autopsy studies have described abnormalities of dopamine in the striatum, of serotonin in the basal ganglia, of dynorphin in the globus pallidus, and of glutamic acid in the subthalamic region. Genetic studies of serotonin receptors suggest that this neurotransmitter system plays a minor role, if any (Brett et al. 1995).

Imaging studies are generally consistent in finding involvement of the basal ganglia, although specific findings vary. The globus pallidus is reported to be small and the caudate enlarged, perhaps with greater changes on the left side (Peterson et al. 1993). A recent quantitative MRI study of monozygotic twins concordant for tics found significantly reduced right caudate volumes in the more severely affected twins (Hyde et al. 1995). Also, the more severely affected twins did not have the normal asymmetry of the lateral ventricles observed in the less affected twins and in control groups of previous studies. SPECT studies have shown decreased cerebral blood flow in the left lenticular nucleus (Riddle et al. 1992) and a significant decrease in right basal ganglia activity; these findings are suggestive of functional asymmetry (Klieger et al. 1997). A PET study quantifying dopamine receptors in Tourette's disorder found an elevated number of D_2 receptors in a small subgroup of patients (Wong et al. 1997). Taken together, these data implicate the basal ganglia, both anatomically and functionally, in the pathophysiology of Tourette's disorder.

Motor tics may be related to abnormalities in the nigrostriatal neurons, and the other symptoms of Tourette's disorder may be related to limbic and cortical neurons, although these links appear to be overly simplistic. Interactions between the basal ganglia and the limbic system are quite complex and may play a direct role (Haber and Lynd-Balta 1993). Relevant pathways may include dopaminergic nuclei in the substantia nigra (projecting to the striatum), their neighboring midbrain nuclei in the ventral tegmental area (projecting to various cortical and limbic areas), and their descending pathways into the pons. In addition, corticothalamic pathways, which are involved in motor and sensorimotor functions, use the basal ganglia as a relay site. Therefore, the tics observed in Tourette's disorder may originate from a primary subcortical disorder affecting the motor cortex through disinhibited afferent signals or from impaired inhibition directly at the level of the motor cortex, or from both (Ziemann et al. 1997).

Course and Prognosis

The onset of illness is typically during childhood (ages 2–13 years) and is rarely postpubertal. This lifelong disease shows characteristic waxing and waning in frequency and severity, corresponding in part to periods of increased stress or anxiety. Presentation varies during development (see the section Clinical Description). Maximal tic symptoms may be seen in the early adolescent years, although obsessive-compulsive symptoms may become more prominent and troubling.

In the autoimmune forms of Tourette's disorder (PANDAS), the course is characterized by a periodic worsening of symptoms (waxing and waning). These exacerbations typically present days to months after the onset of the streptococcal infection; the interval is initially about 6–9 months and then decreases with recurrent infections. A worsening of tic symptoms can result from a so-called strep throat or from a respiratory cold and can even be triggered by simple exposure to other people with streptococcal infections. The tic symptoms in PANDAS usually begin at around 6 years (Swedo et al. 1998).

Complications of Tourette's disorder generally include major effects on self-esteem and social performance. Teasing, shame, self-consciousness, and social ostracism are standard features of these patients' lives. These individuals show a reluctance to involve themselves in socially demanding situations. Particularly if their symptoms are severely socially disfiguring, these patients may avoid entering intimate relationships, marriage, and other interpersonally gratifying activities. The rate of unemployment is reportedly as high as 50% in adults with Tourette's disorder.

Evaluation and Differential Diagnosis

A complete psychiatric evaluation of the child and parents is indicated, including assessment of possible ADHD, conduct disorder, OCD, learning disorders, pervasive developmental disorders, and mental retardation. Neurological examination is appropriate to rule out other movement disorders, including Wilson's disease. An assessment of baseline dyskinesias is needed before the start of neuroleptic drug treatments. An EEG is helpful in ruling out myoclonic seizures and other neurological disorders. All children with tic disorders should be evaluated for antistreptococcal antibodies, because this may expand the treatment options. School reports, including those addressing academic performance, general behavior, severity of tics, and social skills, are useful. The child's self-consciousness, management of teasing and social ostracism, and assertiveness may be assessed. The possibility of concurrent mood or anxiety disorder should be evaluated. Evaluation of tic disorders in relatives may be considered.

Following patients with Tourette's disorder is complicated by the variability in types of tics, which reduces the usefulness of a strictly quantitative approach to estimates of tic severity. Symptom lists are idiosyncratic to individuals, so it is helpful to obtain periodic individual evaluations of symptom severity, symptom shifting, and functional interference (i.e., disruptiveness of the symptoms).

Treatment

Pharmacotherapy, behavioral therapy, and sometimes psychotherapy and special education may be employed. Although medications play a vital role in the management of Tourette's disorder, a child's adaptive capacities, comorbid diagnoses, coping mechanisms, interpersonal skills, and social support play a significant role in outcome. Subsequently, treatment must employ strategies for developing and maintaining these factors.

Conventional neuroleptic drugs are the cornerstone of pharmacotherapy, but recent findings have suggested that the newer atypical neuroleptics (e.g., risperidone and olanzapine) are highly effective as well. Approximately 60%–80% of Tourette's patients demonstrate improvement with conventional neuroleptics. Low dosages of high-potency neuroleptics (haloperidol and pimozide) have been prescribed most commonly, but low-potency neuroleptics appear to be approximately as effective. Pimozide has shown better therapeutic effects than haloperidol in a controlled comparison. The atypical neuroleptics have the major advantage of a markedly reduced incidence of adverse short-term and long-term motor effects, but all neuroleptics carry a risk of inducing neuroleptic malignant syndrome (Latz and McCracken 1992; Steingard et al. 1992) and tardive tourettism (Bharucha and Sethi 1995). Neuroleptic dosages may require gradual elevation over time, but decreases in dosage may be possible depending on life circumstances and waxing and waning of symptoms.

Clonidine is an alternative treatment that has been reported to be helpful in about 50% of patients with Tourette's disorder, particularly for children with behavior disorders whose ADHD might be improved by clonidine. At low dosages, clonidine stimulates α_2-adrenergic presynaptic receptors, leading acutely to decreased norepinephrine neurotransmission and, with chronic treatment, to increased dopamine utilization (via an unknown indirect mechanism, possibly involving serotonin). The clinical effect of clonidine might increase over the course of 2–3 months of treatment. Similar to clonidine, the α_2-adrenergic receptor agonist guanfacine may also be effective in this population (Chappell et al. 1995). The effects of long-term clonidine and guanfacine treatment are not well defined.

The use of stimulants and tricyclic antidepressants in treating Tourette's disorder remains controversial because of past findings that these agents may exacerbate or trigger tic disorders. Although some controlled findings suggest that these agents exacerbate tics in many children (Gadow et al. 1995; Riddle et al. 1995), many physicians have returned to using these agents with only occasional complaints of tic induction. With or without the use of stimulants and tricyclic antidepressants, continued vigilance regarding tic induction is advisable if over-the-counter sympathomimetic drugs are used by patients with Tourette's disorder. Similarly, special warnings are needed concerning the recreational use of cocaine and related drugs. At this time, it is acceptable practice to prescribe psychostimulants in treating chronic tic disorders with comorbid ADHD, and tricyclic antidepressants may be considered for patients with comorbid anxiety or depressive disorders.

Preliminary data support the use of various other agents in Tourette's disorder, such as desipramine, pergolide, propoxyphene, nicotine, and selegiline (L-deprenyl). There is some evidence that androgens or the opiate receptor antagonist naltrexone may worsen tics (and obsessive-compulsive symptoms).

If comorbid psychiatric disorders are present in patients with Tourette's disorder, treatment of the comorbidity may improve the symptoms of Tourette's disorder. This parallel improvement can be seen with most comorbid psychiatric disorders, including mood and anxiety disorders, ADHD, and other behavior disorders.

For children with tic disorders associated with streptococcal infection, several immunologic treatments are under investigation, including plasmapheresis, intravenous immunoglobulins, chronic antibiotic treatments, and prednisone (Allen et al. 1995; Matarrazo 1992).

Neuropsychologically based educational interventions can be helpful in dealing with some of the "frontal" symptoms of ADHD (Denckla and Reader 1993). A variety of behavioral techniques have been used, but they are not uniformly effective. Standard procedures have not been established.

Although it is not a specific treatment of Tourette's disorder, psychotherapy may be useful to help an individual deal with the stigma of illness and with self-esteem problems, promote interpersonal comfort and social skills, improve the opportunities for and the odds of successful marriage, and enhance functioning and satisfaction at work. In addition to enhancing adaptive skills, psychotherapy may reduce the anxiety that aggravates symptom severity.

The family response to this disfiguring disorder is often significant, and its management is important for the welfare of both the family and the patient (D. Cohen et al. 1988). The Tourette Syndrome Association is a national organization that provides support and education to families and patients, funds and helps locate subjects for research, and advocates with public agencies.

Clinical Comment

The high incidence of social ostracism and self-consciousness, as well as the high rates of adult unemployment, among patients with Tourette's disorder requires special attention to the psychosocial consequences of this disorder. Control of the tics does not constitute the end point of treatment. This classic "neurological" disorder is no longer considered rare, is found to present comorbidly with other classic psychiatric disorders, and has a firm place in the psychiatric nosology.

FEEDING AND EATING DISORDERS OF INFANCY OR EARLY CHILDHOOD

Anorexia nervosa and bulimia nervosa, usually first diagnosed in adolescence, are discussed in Chapter 25. Three additional eating disorders usually first diagnosed in childhood are pica, rumination disorder of infancy, and feeding disorder of infancy or early childhood.

Pica and rumination disorder are rarely treated as isolated entities by psychiatrists, but these disorders are significant medical conditions with definite psychiatric dimensions. Feeding disorder of infancy or early childhood corresponds to a subcategory of the pediatric diagnosis of nonorganic failure to thrive (NFTT).

PICA

A pattern of eating nonfood materials can be seen in young children, individuals with severe or profound mental retardation, and pregnant women. Pica has been extensively documented in the pediatric literature but minimally documented in the psychiatric literature—despite its presumed biopsychosocial etiology and its potential for major behavioral, cognitive, neurological, and developmental complications.

Pica appears to be quite common in children, particularly young children, but it is infrequently diagnosed. When pica occurs in mentally retarded persons or in pregnant women, it can require a physician's vigilant inquiry to uncover. The psychiatric significance of pica is very different in these different populations.

Geophagia (the eating of clay or soil) is a similar phenomenon that is an ordinary and sanctioned activity in many cultures worldwide. Such culturally determined forms of pica are not considered a mental disorder (Table 23–28). Whatever the basis for the pica, the risk of accidental poisoning is significant.

Clinical Description

Children and people with mental retardation may eat paper, paint, coins, string, rags, hair, feces, vomitus, leaves, bugs, worms, and cloth. Pica in children is typically observed in association with behavioral and other medical problems, but such children are rarely brought for psychiatric treatment for the isolated problem of pica.

Pregnant women, apart from their common craving for fruit and sharp-tasting foods, have been reported at times to seek and eat starchy materials, refrigerator frost, or substances containing minerals. Cultural geophagia commonly involves the eating of earth, clay, sand, and pebbles. Geophagia is also common in children and in pregnant women.

Epidemiology

About 10%–20% of children in the United States exhibit pica at some point in their lives, and up to 50%–70% of children living in the inner cities exhibit picalike behaviors between ages 1 and 6 years. Boys and girls are equally involved. Epidemiological studies show that children with pica typically come from a low socioeconomic class, have pets at home, and display various behavioral abnormalities. Typically, they are not referred for treatment unless complications, such as lead poisoning, or concomitant disorders are identified. More than 50% of children hospitalized for accidental ingestions have been found to exhibit pica (Millican et al. 1968).

Mental retardation is associated with a high prevalence of pica. Approximately 20%–40% of institutionalized people with severe or profound mental retardation have pica. Gender prevalence is equal.

The prevalence of pica among pregnant women has been reported to vary geographically from 0% to 70%. In the lower socioeconomic classes of the United States, persistent nonnutritive eating is seen in about 60% of pregnant women. The specific eating of ice and freezer frost was reported by 8% of pregnant women in the inner city of Washington, D.C. (Edwards et al. 1994). Most children with pica have mothers or siblings who also have pica.

Pica increases the risk of exposure to environmental toxins. Lead poisoning has been reported in as many as 92% of children living near a lead smelter in Brazil (Silvany-Neto et al. 1996). Households may become contaminated by toxins inadvertently brought home from job sites despite precautions to avoid occupational exposure and transportation of potentially toxic materials (Chiaradia et al. 1997). Even in affluent locations, pica is a major route of exposure to lead, pesticides, and organic toxins through the ingestion of house dust in carpets, mattresses, and sofas (Roberts and Dickey 1995).

Culturally based pica is seen in some families of Third World origins (Vermeer and Frate 1979). For example, geophagia is observed in the general population

---

TABLE 23–28.　**DSM-IV diagnostic criteria for pica**

A. Persistent eating of nonnutritive substances for a period of at least 1 month.

B. The eating of nonnutritive substances is inappropriate to the developmental level.

C. The eating behavior is not part of a culturally sanctioned practice.

D. If the eating behavior occurs exclusively during the course of another mental disorder (e.g., mental retardation, pervasive developmental disorder, schizophrenia), it is sufficiently severe to warrant independent clinical attention.

(nonclinical samples) in many parts of Africa, South America, Asia, and aboriginal Australia. In different regions, earth eating is used as a simple "pacifier" for infants, a routine pastime (like smoking), or a culturally based method for respecting or incorporating magical spirits; it also is used for presumed medicinal value (e.g., to suppress nausea). The practice is not indiscriminate but involves careful selection of certain types of clay and specific preparations (such as cooking). When culturally proper soil or clay is not available to Americans of African descent in inner cities, laundry starch is used as a common substitute because of its claylike texture and consistency. The risks of pica remain potentially serious, even when culturally sanctioned. Among children, the prevalence of lead intoxication has been reported as high as 73% in Kenya and 90% in Pakistan (Hafeez and Malik 1996).

Etiology

Childhood pica is sometimes interpreted as an ordinary part of exploratory learning or as a reflection of a young child's inability to differentiate food from inedible objects. The findings of increased childhood pica in households with pets and of the eating of pet food by children suggest that imitation can be an etiological factor. Most children with pica have parents with a history of pica; the disorder may be passed along by a variety of mechanisms, including cultural ones. Psychoanalytic hypotheses have emphasized impairments in aggressivity or orality. Disorders of parent-child nurturance and of psychosocial deprivation (disruptive feeding, traumatic weaning, unmet "oral" needs) may contribute in certain cases. The overrepresentation of pica in lower socioeconomic classes may be a partial marker for psychosocial stress or family pathology, which may be involved in the etiology. Parental depression, neglect, and inadequate supervision are clearly related to the risk of toxic ingestions in children (Bithoney et al. 1985) and are presumed to be tangible behavioral factors that contribute to the appearance of pica. Mothers of children with pica have been described as immature, emotionally unavailable, and overwhelmed by parenting tasks. In general, the cultural and environmental origins of pica need to be considered, because they may explain some aspects of the family transmission of pica.

In individuals with severe or profound mental retardation, the primary mechanism is believed to be self-stimulation rather than impaired judgment. Children and adults with mental retardation and pica tend to engage in pica with a favorite object.

A nutritional etiology has been proposed for some adults, who are believed to have an instinctive craving for vitamins and minerals, especially iron and perhaps zinc or calcium. The eating is hypothesized to be an attempt to correct a nutritional deficiency. There is evidence that this mechanism operates in animals, but few data support this notion in humans. Eating of ice (or refrigerator frost) has been reported in pregnant women in association with iron deficiency, and prescription of iron supplements has been found to improve the anemia and reduce the ice eating (Danford 1982). Pica can instead be a cause of malnutrition, because the consumed objects or substances may interfere with the absorption of nutrients. Because anemia does not regularly induce pica in adults, it is more likely that pica causes nutritional imbalances in adults. The relevance of the nutritional deficiency theory of pica to children is undetermined.

Certain medical factors can also contribute to the appearance of pica in adults, including brain disorders, gastrointestinal disease, parasitic infestations, and inflammations. Family psychiatric history, biological concomitants, and transference manifestations of pica have not been systematically studied. However, some data have suggested that mood disorders may be overrepresented in families with pica.

Course and Prognosis

In children, pica usually starts at 12–24 months and resolves by age 6. However, in mentally retarded persons, pica can endure and persist in adulthood. In pregnant women, geophagia usually resolves at the end of pregnancy, although it may recur in subsequent pregnancies.

Complications of pica are numerous and potentially severe. Constipation and gastrointestinal malabsorption are common. Fecal impaction may occur repetitively. Ingestion of foreign bodies or hair balls can lead to intestinal obstruction, potentially leading to intestinal perforation or biliary obstruction, which sometimes requires colostomy. Anemias can be produced by nutritional deficiencies and sometimes traumatic intestinal bleeding. Salt imbalances, parasitic infections, vomiting, poisoning, and dental injury may be seen.

Ingestion of lead-containing paint, plaster, and earth can lead to toxic encephalopathy in severe cases, fatigue and weight loss (with constipation) in moderate cases, and learning impairments in mild cases. Approximately 80% of severely lead-poisoned children have pica, and at least 30% of children with pica show lead-related symptoms.

Lead intake by pregnant women can cause congenital plumbism. However, pica has developmental significance even without toxin ingestions: ice-eating pregnant women give birth to infants with smaller head circumferences than women without pica (Edwards et al. 1994). Children with pica can have slow motor and mental development, growth retardation, seizures, and neurological deficits, as well as behavioral abnormalities both before and after the period of pica.

Evaluation and Differential Diagnosis

Evaluation of children with pica involves behavioral and psychiatric evaluation of the child and parents, psychosocial evaluation of the home (including caregiver availability and presence of pets), nutritional status, feeding history, lead exposure, and cultural values. The possibility of inadequate supervision of children or parental neglect needs assessment.

The diagnosis is often missed, because children are typically brought for evaluation of other problems. Adults may not have directly observed the pica behavior in children or may volunteer such observations about their family only reluctantly.

Pica should be actively considered in children and adults (not only persons with mental retardation) with anemia, chronic constipation, fecal impaction, or accidental ingestions. Lead poisoning may be present in children with ADHD, unexplained fatigue or weight loss, learning impairments, mental retardation, or gingival "lead-lines."

In view of the high risk of lead intoxication, it is reasonable to assess children with pica by obtaining both a zinc protoporphyrin (ZPP) and a plasma lead level. Although there remains debate about whether there is a developmentally "safe" minimal blood level of lead, there is general agreement about the upper limits of acceptable plasma levels of lead (10 $\mu g/dL$) and zinc protoporphyrin (30 $\mu g/100$ mL). When identifying a child with pica, it is advisable to examine siblings and parents for pica as well.

Treatment

Behavioral therapy has been employed for children and mentally retarded individuals with pica. Rewarding appropriate eating, teaching the differentiation of edible foods, overcorrection (immediate enforcement of oral hygiene), and negative reinforcement (time-outs, physical restraint) have been successfully employed, especially for mentally retarded people. Psychosocial interventions include promotion of maternal supervision and stimulation, improvement of play opportunities (new toys), and placement in day care.

Concomitant medical treatments may be required. Management of lead poisoning may be handled in the routine manner. It has been suggested that nutritional iron and zinc treatments produce short-term improvements in some individuals.

Psychosocial and nutritional interventions have not been systematically evaluated. Improvements in personal and household hygiene can be beneficial. Removal of old or synthetic carpets and furniture, elimination of sources of dust and particulates, or even a family move away from a problematic home may be required in some cases.

Public health measures for reducing environmental lead levels have been shown to be dramatically effective in reducing plasma lead levels of children on a national level, including outside the United States. Despite these large gains, clinical caution continues to be required.

Effective correction of lead intoxication may not induce lasting improvements. For example, even after comprehensive management of lead poisoning in children with pervasive developmental disorder, 75% became reexposed to lead during the course of their medical management. In many cases of childhood pica, ongoing reassessments of lead and ZPP levels are advisable beyond the course of acute medical treatment.

Clinical Comment

Pica in children and mentally retarded individuals is a significant disorder that generally has not received systematic psychiatric attention. Nonnutritive eating in pregnant women and among some socioeconomic groups may represent a related or dissimilar condition. Increased clinical surveillance and research studies are needed to delineate possible differences in the forms of pica that appear in different populations, including the normative forms of pica that are prevalent in certain regions of the world.

The basic psychiatric dimensions of childhood pica are yet to be described, but the routine evaluation of the siblings and parents of American children with pica is clinically advisable. Beyond studies on lead exposure, there are no long-term follow-up studies of pica or its treatment.

RUMINATION DISORDER

Certain infants show a pleasurable relaxation as they regurgitate, rechew, drool, and reswallow their food, usually in the absence of caregivers and other sources of stimulation. Their continuing self-stimulation, apparent satisfaction, and languorous obliviousness highlight their full engrossment in rumination. Their obvious enjoyment and enthusiasm occurs despite malnourishment and diminished weight gain, and it stands in marked contrast to their parents' disgust at this activity.

This potentially fatal disorder of infants appears to reflect abnormal development of early self-stimulation and physiological regulation, and it is particularly apparent when infants are alone (Table 23–29). Rumination (merycism) may be a cause or result of disrupted parent-child attachments, and it can be associated with major developmental delays and mental retardation.

The symptom of rumination is relatively common in adults with mental retardation, and patients with anorexia or bulimia are occasionally observed to ruminate. Rumination may also present in developmentally normal children (Reis 1994) or adults (Parry-Jones 1994), seemingly as a transient response to situational stressors. The relationship of these forms of rumination to the pathological condition of rumination disorder in infants is unclear.

Clinical Description

Rumination involves the continued eating of partially digested stomach contents that are regurgitated into the esophagus or mouth. It is different from vomiting, in which the stomach contents are expelled through the mouth.

Rumination may start with the infant's placing fingers or clothes in the mouth to induce regurgitation, with rhythmic body or neck motions, or it may begin without any apparent initiating action. During rumination, the infant generally lies quietly, may look happy or "spacey," and may hold body and head in a characteristic arching position while sucking. There is no apparent nausea, discomfort, or disgust. If observed, the infant usually stops and fixes visual attention on the intruder; when the infant is no longer aware of being observed, sucking and tongue movements restart in seconds. When he or she is not ruminating, the infant may appear apathetic and withdrawn, irritable and fussy, or seemingly normal.

Self-stimulatory behaviors are commonly seen in association with rumination disorder. Often, thumb sucking,

---

TABLE 23–29. DSM-IV diagnostic criteria for rumination disorder

A. Repeated regurgitation and rechewing of food for a period of at least 1 month following a period of normal functioning.

B. The behavior is not due to an associated gastrointestinal or other general medical condition (e.g., esophageal reflux).

C. The behavior does not occur exclusively during the course of anorexia nervosa or bulimia nervosa. If the symptoms occur exclusively during the course of mental retardation or a pervasive developmental disorder, they are sufficiently severe to warrant independent clinical attention.

---

cloth sucking, head banging, and body rocking are observed, lending support to the hypothesis that rumination can be an infantile form of self-stimulation.

Epidemiology

There are no available prevalence figures, but rumination disorder is rare and decreasing in prevalence in the general population, perhaps owing to improving infant and child care. The disorder has almost disappeared in some countries (Guedeney 1995). However, rumination disorder is not rare in infants with mental retardation. About 10% of institutionalized mentally retarded adults show similar medically unexplained symptoms. About 93% of adults with rumination have severe or profound mental retardation. The few available studies consist of small samples and report contradictory findings on gender ratio. Both male predominance and equal gender prevalence have been reported.

Etiology

There is strong evidence of both organic and environmental contributions to the etiology of rumination disorder. Rumination in infants can result from gastroesophageal reflux due to esophageal sphincter disorder, such as hiatal hernia; such medical conditions are considered exclusion criteria for the diagnosis of rumination disorder of infancy. In these cases, the rumination can be viewed as an attempt to clear the esophagus of refluxed material or as a reflexive response triggered by esophageal dilation. Medical or surgical intervention reduces the rumination behavior.

The majority of infants with rumination disorder are not developmentally delayed. However, about 25% of infants with rumination disorder have a low developmental quotient score, as seen in mental retardation and pervasive developmental disorder. Obstetrical complications are seen in one-third of these infants, suggesting that perinatal brain damage can contribute to the appearance of rumination disorder. Alternatively, and more likely, prenatal pathology, such as impaired psychomotor or visceromotor capacities, can contribute to subsequent perinatal and postnatal difficulties. However, the majority of infants with rumination disorder achieve milestones normally and show no obvious developmental problems.

An understimulating environment might contribute to the appearance of rumination disorder. These infants are often from underprivileged families, in which sensory and interpersonal stimulation may be low. Primary caregivers for infants with rumination disorder are believed to provide inappropriate stimulation owing to inadequate time spent with the infant; preexisting parental anxiety or avoidance; or parental psychiatric impairment, absence, or harsh handling. Excessive parental stimulation can also lead to rumination disorder.

There is no specific psychopathology identified as characteristic of the primary caregiver, although depression, anxiety disorder, personality disorder, substance abuse, and schizophrenia have been reported (Mayes et al. 1988). Studies have typically centered on maternal stimulation, and there is little information regarding the father's role.

An etiology cannot be identified in all cases of rumination disorder of infancy. Predisposing impairments in the parent-infant relationship are not invariably seen. Some infants with rumination disorder appear happy and have parents who are emotionally supportive and interactive. These infants may be particularly likely to respond to simple behavioral interventions (Lavigne et al. 1981). The usual developmental psychodynamic (orality), organic, and genetic models might be more relevant for understanding rumination associated with mental retardation; however, the etiology of rumination in mentally retarded infants is usually ascribed to a need for self-stimulation.

It is presumed that infants who lack external sources of gratification use rumination for self-stimulation or tension discharge. There is speculation that the infant may gain a degree of "voluntary" control over regurgitation, shaping this physiological response into pleasurable self-stimulation.

Course and Prognosis

Regurgitation or vomiting (with reflux on barium fluoroscopy) is generally seen during the first 3 months of life, but rumination does not typically appear until 3–12 months of age. It usually resolves by the end of the second year but may persist until the third or fourth year. In more persistent cases, the patient generally has mental retardation. People with mental retardation can also show a later onset of rumination disorder; however, the disorder typically emerges during childhood or adolescence.

Dehydration, electrolyte imbalance, slow weight gain, growth retardation, malnutrition, and tooth decay can be seen in some individuals. Spontaneous remissions are common, but there is also a high risk of developmental delay and death. Reports in the literature from the 1950s indicate a 10%–25% mortality rate, with death from malnutrition. However, the risk of fatality depends on the availability of intervention, and the modern availability of parenteral hyperalimentation has probably led to a substantial reduction in deaths.

A major complication of rumination disorder of infancy is the parents' reaction to the symptoms. A parent's immediate response to observing rumination is typically acute anxiety and distress, which can lead to ongoing affective and cognitive responses that impair the formation of parental attachment to the child. The parents' frustration and disgust, particularly at the odor, may lead to further avoidance and understimulation of the child. This disruption of attachment can constitute a major complication in the child's development (Mayes et al. 1988).

The only available follow-up study of infants with rumination disorder indicates that about 50% have normal behavioral development and that 20% have severe developmental or medical pathology at age 5 years (Sauvage et al. 1985). Both mental retardation and pervasive developmental disorders are commonly associated with rumination disorder; they may be cause, effect, or concomitant disorders. Chronic malnutrition typically is not seen in rumination disorder. The course of rumination in adults with mental retardation has not been well described.

Evaluation and Differential Diagnosis

Evaluation includes behavioral and psychiatric evaluation of child and parents, with an emphasis on developmental history and psychosocial assessment, as well as eating history, nutritional status, and observation of parent-child interactions during feeding. Gastrointestinal disease needs to be considered, including gastroesophageal reflux, hiatus hernia, pyloric stenosis, other congenital anomalies, and infections. Gastrointestinal structural abnormalities (and other abnormalities) may be particularly common in individuals with cerebral palsy, physical anomalies, and developmental disorders.

The symptom of regurgitation in infants can also be due to anxiety; some children appear openly distressed during rumination. Usually, however, children with rumination disorder appear happy and enjoy the regurgitation, whereas children with gastrointestinal disorders vomit with discomfort and experience pain. Although this sounds like a simple distinction, the literature on rumination and reflux esophagitis is confounded by difficulties in this differential diagnosis. It is usually unclear whether reflux or rumination initiated the esophageal pathology. Clinically, it is advisable to obtain careful evaluation of esophageal function in parallel with the psychiatric evaluation. In addition, diagnosticians should keep in mind that rumination occasionally presents in developmentally normal children (Reis 1994) and adults (Parry-Jones 1994).

Treatment

There is no established treatment of rumination disorder of infancy, although various forms of behavioral therapy, parental guidance, and medication (antispasmodics and tranquilizers) have been tried. Psychotherapy for the caregiver, dietary changes, and hand restraints have not been found to be particularly effective.

Behavioral techniques include cuddling and playing with the child before, during, and after mealtime to reduce social deprivation and behavioral withdrawal. Aversive conditioning (e.g., putting hot pepper sauce or lemon on the infant's tongue, electroshock) produces the most rapid symptom suppression, but it generally elicits strong caregiver resistance and cannot usually be applied immediately or consistently. Negative attention, such as shouting or slapping the child, can serve to reinforce the behavior, especially if other forms of reinforcement and attention are lacking or ineffective. A combination of a negative reinforcement (a scolding and putting the child down for 2 minutes) with a reward for nonrumination (parental attention and social interaction, such as being cleaned and played with) has been successfully used in outpatient treatment (Lavigne et al. 1981).

Temporary hospitalization is commonly used to provide a separation of the child from the primary caregiver, an alternative feeding environment for the child (to "decondition" the symptoms), and a period of relaxation for the parent (to permit anxiety reduction). Reassurance, education, and support of the parents help reduce their preexisting anxiety and avoidance, diminish their acute stress at times of the infant's rumination, and reestablish the parents' comfort in the feeding process. Psychiatric and psychosocial evaluation of the parents may be valuable. Ongoing clinical follow-up is useful to facilitate attachment between infant and mother, monitor the psychosocial environment at home, and provide support in the event of emerging mental retardation. There has been limited systematic assessment of the treatment interventions used in rumination disorder (Chatoor et al. 1984).

Clinical Comment

Preexisting anxiety in the primary caregiver and impaired infant-handling methods are subject to preventive treatment. Early identification and preventive intervention might be helpful, but their efficacy has not been evaluated. It may be speculated that effective treatment of rumination disorder could reduce the incidence or severity of certain forms of mental retardation and other developmental abnormalities.

The relationship of this childhood eating disorder to adult psychiatric disorders is unknown. However, esophageal motility abnormalities are present in 84% of adult psychiatric patients, especially in those with mood and anxiety disorders; only 31% of nonpsychiatric patients show similar abnormalities in distal esophageal contraction (Clouse and Lustman 1983).

The establishment of physiological and affective regulation may be viewed as a precondition and a consequence of a deepening parent-child attachment; therefore, this rare disorder of infancy provides an unusual opportunity for child development research.

FEEDING DISORDER OF INFANCY OR EARLY CHILDHOOD

In pediatrics, the diagnosis of failure to thrive (FTT) indicates retardation of body growth or milestone attainment resulting from inadequate nutritional intake. The "organic" forms of FTT can result from chronic physical illness (congenital AIDS), neurological disease, sensory deficit, or virtually any serious pediatric disease. The "nonorganic" forms, constituting at least 80% of cases of FTT, encompass 1) homeostatic disorders of infancy (sleep and feeding dysregulation), 2) pathological food refusal, 3) protein-calorie malnutrition, and 4) social and emotional factors interfering with adequate nutritional care (including reactive attachment disorder, which is discussed later in the chapter).

The DSM-IV diagnosis of feeding disorder of infancy or early childhood does not include all forms of nonorganic failure to thrive (NFTT), but only the types of eating failure that occur in the context of adequate provision of food (Table 23–30). This disorder does not include cases of child neglect or cases of inadequate eating due to obviously defective parenting or feeding.

Clinical Description

Infants may gag when fed or refuse to open their mouths. Young children might decline to eat, or they may eat so slowly that their intake is drastically reduced. In infants, the retardation in weight gain is typically accompanied by motor, social, and linguistic delays as well as a problematic relationship with the feeder or caregiver (as a result if not a cause of the disorder). In early childhood, symptoms may include impaired interpersonal relationships and interactions, mood symptoms, behavior problems, developmental delays, unusual food preferences, excessively rigid or narrow food choices, and perhaps bizarre eating and foraging behaviors.

Epidemiology

Approximately 1%–5% of pediatric hospital admissions are due to NFTT. Epidemiological data concerning the

DSM-IV diagnosis of feeding disorder of infancy or early childhood are not available.

Etiology

The relative loss of weight is due to malnutrition, but the malnutrition may be due to various causes (Woolston 1983). Both physical and psychosocial etiologies may be involved, although the definition of the disorder excludes cases that clearly result from overt medical problems or other psychiatric disorders.

Various mechanisms (and potential subtypes) include difficulties with physiological homeostasis, attachment to the caregiver, and autonomy from the caregiver, as well as posttraumatic responses (Chatoor et al. 1985).

Homeostatic control of sleep and feeding is an early developmental accomplishment that is generally easy to achieve. The lability of the autonomic nervous system, presumably seen in "colicky" infants, needs the calming and soothing responses of the caregiver to promote the development of self-regulation. Even the physical requirements of eating may induce fatigue and interfere with feeding in some infants, especially those with medical conditions unrelated to feeding.

Attachment problems, reflected in impaired relatedness and reciprocal interactions with the caregiver, may operate to inhibit adequate feeding. The ordinary signals, including eye contact, smiling, vocal contact, visual stimulation, and physical touching, may not be provided (or responded to) by child or parent, undermining the reciprocal signaling that underlies effective feeding. Apathy might replace the enjoyment of feeding experienced by child and caregiver.

TABLE 23–30. **DSM-IV diagnostic criteria for feeding disorder of infancy or early childhood**

Diagnostic criteria for feeding disorder of infancy or early childhood

A. Feeding disturbance as manifested by persistent failure to eat adequately with significant failure to gain weight or significant loss of weight over at least 1 month.

B. The disturbance is not due to an associated gastrointestinal or other general medical condition (e.g., esophageal reflux).

C. The disturbance is not better accounted for by another mental disorder (e.g., rumination disorder) or by lack of available food.

D. The onset is before age 6 years.

Autonomy struggles, reflecting the negotiation of separation from the feeder, may be manifest by the child's food refusal, "pickiness" about food choices, or undereating. Between the ages of 6 months and 3 years, the child's agenda may effectively become "I will decide who puts food in my mouth." If the parent interprets the child's actions as rebellion or personal insult, a power struggle may become evident in feeding (before it becomes clear in other developmental arenas). Food refusal is often accompanied by other displays of autonomy and power, including temper tantrums and aggressivity (Chatoor 1989).

Additional socioemotional factors that might reduce nutritional intake and body growth include posttraumatic responses to medical procedures involving the mouth, child abuse, emotional deprivation, or family pathology.

Another type of feeding disorder is the pediatric syndrome called *psychosocial dwarfism*. This disorder has a later age of onset (or later age of recognition) and is usually based on a failure to gain height (whereas weight is the criterion in the DSM-IV definition of feeding disorder). This form of NFTT involves developmental and behavioral features similar to those of feeding disorder, as well as enuresis or encopresis, irritability, or apathy. These children typically also have a clinically apparent sleep problem and a reduced secretion of growth hormone at night. The reduced growth hormone secretion may result from the disturbed sleep and may serve as a biological marker for psychosocial dwarfism. Other forms of NFTT and reactive attachment disorder (discussed later in the chapter) do not appear to have the sleep or growth hormone abnormality of psychosocial dwarfism.

Course and Prognosis

The untreated course of these disorders may depend on the specific subtype or mechanisms involved, but the expected outcome ranges from spontaneous remission to malnutrition, infection, or death. Both nutritional and psychosocial deprivation may result in long-term behavioral changes, hyperactivity, short stature, and lowered IQ. The relationship of these feeding disorders to other psychiatric disorders, including the eating disorders of adulthood, is undetermined.

Evaluation and Treatment

It is not clear from the DSM-IV definition whether feeding disorder of infancy or early childhood includes cases in which food is available but the caregiver is simply an inept feeder. It is also unclear whether the reversal of the symptoms with appropriate care is characteristic. The services of a multidisciplinary team, preferably in a hospital setting, are helpful for evaluating and initiating treatment. Evaluation includes assessment of body growth as well as observations of the mother-child interactions in general and in feeding in particular. (A more detailed description of the multidisciplinary treatment is found in the section Reactive Attachment Disorder.)

ELIMINATION DISORDERS

ENCOPRESIS

This elimination disorder includes fecal soiling of clothes, voiding in bed, and excretion onto the floor, occurring after age 4 years when full bowel control is developmentally expected. Because "organic" causes of encopresis need to be excluded, medical evaluation for structural and other nonfunctional abnormalities must be obtained before the diagnosis is made (Table 23–31). Although the term *encopresis* is used loosely to denote both types of soiling, the medically explained cases are technically *fecal incontinence*, and the idiopathic ones are *encopresis* (Loening-Baucke 1996). Both biopsychiatric and psychodynamic theories have been proposed to explain the "etiology" of encopresis. However, if a specific neurobiological explanation were identified, the condition would no longer be idiopathic. *Idiopathic encopresis* would be a clearer term for this psychiatric disorder.

Behavior problems are found in one-third of children with encopresis (van der Plas et al. 1996). Some of the psychological and behavioral difficulties appear to resolve when the encopresis improves. In such cases, encopresis

---

TABLE 23–31. **DSM-IV diagnostic criteria for encopresis**

A. Repeated passage of feces into inappropriate places (e.g., clothing or floor) whether involuntary or intentional.

B. At least one such event a month for at least 3 months.

C. Chronological age is at least 4 years (or equivalent developmental level).

D. The behavior is not due exclusively to the direct physiological effects of a substance (e.g., laxatives) or a general medical condition except through a mechanism involving constipation.

Code as follows:

    With constipation and overflow incontinence
    Without constipation and overflow incontinence

---

appears to function as an etiological factor for the development of behavioral symptoms. In other cases, major psychiatric disorders appear comorbidly with encopresis and require concurrent treatment.

Most cases of encopresis result from chronic constipation that leads to overflow. The stool may be formed, semiformed, or liquid. At least some children have encopresis without constipation. Children who have encopresis with constipation were found to have a longer colonic transit time (slower movement) than encopretic children without constipation (Benninga et al. 1994), suggesting that some additional mechanisms might be involved. Children with soiling showed a general increase in behavioral symptoms, as measured on the Child Behavior Checklist, which were comparable in magnitude for both the constipated and nonconstipated children (Benninga et al. 1994).

Clinical Description

Encopresis is usually a result of chronic constipation and is generally accompanied by pain during defecation, smell, and embarrassment. Parents usually repeatedly ask the child to try to relieve the symptoms in the toilet. Encopresis during the daytime is much more common than nocturnal encopresis. In half of these patients, bowel control is not yet learned, so the symptom may be viewed as reflecting slow development or an early developmental fixation (primary encopresis). In the other half, the children initially learned bowel control, were continent for at least 1 year, and then regressed, typically by age 8 years (secondary encopresis).

Primary encopresis, in which the child has never learned control, appears to be the result of a developmental delay or fixation. It has been associated, in boys, with a high rate of developmental delays and enuresis compared with secondary enuresis. Secondary enuresis, in which control was learned and then lost, is associated more strongly with conduct disorder and psychosocial stressors than is primary enuresis (Foreman and Thambirajah 1996).

About 75%–90% of children with encopresis have the DSM-IV subtype designated as "constipation with overflow incontinence." These "retentive" cases involve a low frequency of bowel movements, impaction, overflow of liquid around a partially hardened stool, and leakage of liquid into the clothing. The cause may be chronic constipation, inadequate bowel training (e.g., overly coercive), pain (e.g., from an anal fissure), or phobic avoidance of toilets. These retentive episodes usually extend for several days and are followed by painful defecation.

Encopresis without constipation and overflow can involve a variety of causes, including a lack of sphincter awareness or weak sphincter control. In cases of postbath soiling, physical stimulation may be causative. If soiling is deliberate and the child is typically impulsive or hostile, antisocial or major psychiatric disorders may be associated. Smearing may be accidental (the child who tries to hide the accident) or purposeful (defiant or vindictive).

Behavior problems such as conduct disorder are common in the psychiatrically referred population of youths with encopresis (Friman et al. 1988), but there is comparatively little behavioral disturbance in samples seen by pediatricians (Gabel et al. 1988). In the psychiatric population, 25% of children with encopresis also have functional enuresis; in the pediatric population, this diagnostic overlap is less common. Some children withhold both urine and feces; they may develop megabladder and megacolon.

Chronic constipation, even without overflow incontinence, tends to be severe and is commonly associated with large stools and pain. In girls, urinary tract infection and chronic pyelonephritis are frequent.

Typically, children with encopresis experience shame and embarrassment, feel dirty, and have low self-esteem. They may suffer accusations from parents and sibs, fear discovery by peers, and hide physically and emotionally.

Epidemiology

Encopresis is less common than enuresis. Prevalence is approximately 1.5% after age 5; the disorder diminishes with age and is rare in adolescents. There is a 4:1 male predominance. Slightly higher prevalence rates are associated with the lower socioeconomic classes and with mental retardation, particularly in moderate and severe cases. However, most cases of encopresis are not associated with low intelligence. Overall, neither social class nor intelligence appears to correlate with the presence of encopresis.

Etiology

Medical causes of fecal incontinence include hypothyroidism, hypercalcemia, anal fissure or malformation, rectal stenosis, lactase deficiency, overeating of fried and fatty foods, trauma or surgery, congenital aganglionic megacolon (although Hirschsprung's disease is usually associated with large feces rather than incontinence), meningomyelocele (tissue protrusion through a defect in the vertebral column), and other neuromedical disorders. Pathophysiological mechanisms include altered colon motility and contraction patterns, stretching and thinning of colon walls (megacolon), and decreased sensation or perception (usually appearing early in development). During infancy, fecal soiling may result from severe diaper

rash: fecal withholding might help the infant avoid rectal pain. These medical causes of fecal soiling exclude the diagnosis of encopresis.

Abnormal secretion of gastrointestinal hormones or altered motility in the gastrointestinal tract could lead to constipation and overflow incontinence. Children with encopresis were reported to have normal secretion of gastrin and cholecystokinin; however, their levels of pancreatic polypeptide were found to reach their peak and remain abnormally high following meals, whereas postprandial motilin levels were diminished (Stern et al. 1995). These differences in hormone secretion and motility might explain the unusually chronic constipation associated with fecal overflow, although their association with encopresis might also be a result of the constipation.

Some encopretic children show neurodevelopmental symptoms, such as inattention, hyperactivity, impulsivity, low frustration tolerance, and dyscoordination. Neurodevelopmental theories of encopresis have been proposed, although most children with neurodevelopmental delays or disorders do not have encopresis, and most children with encopresis do not appear to have significant neurodevelopmental symptoms. Children with primary encopresis appear to have comorbid developmental delays and enuresis, whereas secondary enuresis is more likely to present with conduct disorder and psychosocial stressors (Foreman and Thambirajah 1996). This clustering supports a neurodevelopmental factor in the etiology of primary encopresis.

A familial occurrence of encopresis is well documented. About 15% of children with encopresis have fathers who had encopresis during childhood. Unlike the findings in enuresis, psychosocial factors appear to be stronger than genetic factors in the familial transmission of encopresis.

Psychosocial stressors (suggestive of adverse circumstances) and conduct disorder (suggestive of family psychopathology) are associated with encopresis, specifically secondary enuresis (Foreman and Thambirajah 1996). Presumably, the loss of previously established sphincter control is secondary to intercurrent life events, such as disorder in the family and environment. In general, family psychopathology is overrepresented in encopresis and, in some cases, intrudes on the development of self-control and disrupts its consolidation.

Inadequate or punitive toilet training appears to be a cause of encopresis in some cases. Pathogenic approaches are those that are usually considered coercive, aggressive, perfectionistic, inconsistent, or neglectful. Some cases of encopresis reflect developmental complications. For example, encopresis can result from toilet-related fears that are not properly managed or from physical discomfort associated with inadequate physical support during toilet training (e.g., feet do not touch the ground). Stress-related factors appear causative in one-half of cases of secondary encopresis, for example, frenetic rushing before school or during television commercials.

Course and Prognosis

Prevalence typically decreases over time throughout childhood, both for medically untreated and treated children. In children with chronic constipation and encopresis who also have psychopathology or concurrent medical disorders (unrelated to the encopresis), the disorder appearing comorbidly with encopresis can be the primary determinant of prognosis. For example, a more protracted course of encopresis is associated with the presence of conduct disorder, the use of soiling as a direct expression of anger, and parental disinterest in dealing with the problem.

Evaluation and Differential Diagnosis

Initial medical evaluation is required to evaluate possible structural abnormalities (e.g., anal fissure) and may involve barium enema. Psychiatric evaluation includes assessment of comorbid psychopathology, which is found in 35% of children with encopresis. Typical comorbidity with encopresis includes conduct disorder, oppositional defiant disorder, psychotic disorders, mood disorders, and mental retardation.

Treatment

Many cases can be treated in a pediatric model by decompaction and behavioral treatment, but resistant cases may require psychiatric intervention. Pediatric management of cases may include bowel cleansing (laxatives, enemas), daily maintenance on mineral oil, counseling (education, reducing interpersonal struggles and negative affects, and rewards), and follow-up.

Anal sphincter biofeedback also appears effective for children when used in combination with conventional treatment (Cox et al. 1996), although its value may be time-limited. When used in association with conventional pediatric management, biofeedback can increase the response rate after 6 weeks of treatment from 20% to about 40% of children. However, both types of treatment produced improvement in about 50% of the children after 1 year of treatment (van der Plas et al. 1996).

In pediatric practice, approximately 50%–75% of cases improve during the initial months of treatment (Levine 1982). Only 7% of children with pediatrically treated encopresis and chronic constipation were found to remain encopretic at 7-year follow-up, and those patients had significant behavioral symptoms. In contrast, children whose chronic constipation (without encopresis) was pediatrically treated usually become asymptomatic. At 7-year follow-up, 70% of such children had a complete resolution of symptoms, and 25% had mild constipation occasionally; only 5% required occasional laxatives (Sutphen et al. 1995). Thus, a small but significant fraction of children with encopresis remain encopretic despite extended medical treatment (Rockney et al. 1996). In adults with encopresis, the effectiveness of medical treatment is not well delineated. Generally, residual encopresis in adolescence and adulthood is associated with psychopathology.

In resistant cases, or if aggressive pediatric treatment becomes counterproductive, individual and family psychiatric interventions are indicated. The focus of treatment then shifts from the encopresis to a more general treatment of associated psychopathological disorders.

Clinical Comment

Encopresis may be successfully approached using a pediatric model in most cases, but treatment-resistant cases may need psychiatric intervention. Even if major psychopathology can be immediately identified, medical evaluation is required in all cases to rule out possible organic causes.

Encopresis is commonly experienced by clinicians as "unattractive," due to both personal meanings and odor. This symptom and the patients who carry it may be unconsciously but systematically avoided, and this avoidance constitutes a complication in psychiatric treatment as well as in the child's development.

ENURESIS (NOT DUE TO A GENERAL MEDICAL CONDITION)

Urinary incontinence in young children, and occasionally in older children after the completion of toilet training, is a normal developmental phenomenon. Enuresis (not due to a general medical condition) is diagnosed when medically unexplained urinary incontinence is frequent, distressing, or interfering with activities (Table 23–32). Urinary bladder control is typically attained by age 3 or 4; therefore, DSM-IV diagnosis requires a minimal age of 5. Before these presentations are designated as psychiatric disorders, a medical assessment of physical causes of enuresis (such as bladder infection or seizures) is required.

The DSM-IV term *enuresis (not due to a general medical condition)* is inconvenient for efficient communication, but it avoids the problems connected with the DSM-III-R

TABLE 23–32. DSM-IV diagnostic criteria for enuresis

A. Repeated voiding of urine into bed or clothes (whether involuntary or intentional).

B. The behavior is clinically significant as manifested by either a frequency of twice a week for at least 3 consecutive months or the presence of clinically significant distress or impairment in social, academic (occupational), or other important areas of functioning.

C. Chronological age is at least 5 years (or equivalent developmental level).

D. The behavior is not due exclusively to the direct physiological effect of a substance (e.g., a diuretic) or a general medical condition (e.g., diabetes, spina bifida, a seizure disorder).

Specify type:

Nocturnal only
Diurnal only
Nocturnal and diurnal

term *functional enuresis*. "Functional" disorders were originally distinguished from "organic" disorders to refer separately to the physical/medical and the mental/psychiatric realms. As the concepts of those realms have progressively merged, the terms have become outdated. Because the terms are convenient, however, they are used in the following discussion: *functional enuresis* refers here to enuresis (not due to a general medical condition), and *enuresis* refers to enuresis regardless of cause.

Once medical and anatomical etiologies are ruled out, enuresis can be due to neurodevelopmental or sleep disorders as well as psychodynamic and biopsychiatric disorders; this is not the case in the classification of encopresis.

Clinical Description

Bedwetting is more common than daytime urinary incontinence. In the large majority of school-age children, nocturnal enuresis is monosymptomatic (Varan et al. 1996), that is, not accompanied by daytime wetting or other urological conditions. Bedwetting typically occurs 30 minutes to 3 hours after sleep onset, with the child either sleeping through the episode or awakened by the moisture. For some children, however, enuresis may occur at any time during the night. Children with daytime (diurnal) enuresis usually have nocturnal enuresis too. About 30% of children with nocturnal enuresis also have enuresis during the daytime (Kalo and Bella 1996).

In 80% of enuretic children, bladder control has not yet been attained, and the enuresis is "primary" (caused either by a uromedical disorder or by delayed learning of bladder control). In 20%, urinary incontinence is "secondary," reappearing after competent functioning is attained (apparently caused by an intercurrent process). Several studies have suggested that primary (dysfunctional) enuresis is associated with less emotional disturbance or with mental retardation and that secondary (regressive) enuresis implies more serious psychopathology or stress (von Gontard et al. 1997). However, the distinction between primary and secondary enuresis has not been supported by other empirical studies. Most studies have demonstrated that stressors (concerning family stability, stressful life events before age 6 years, current psychosocial difficulties) are significant in both primary and second enuresis. Stronger evidence is available in youths to associate more comorbid psychopathology with older age of onset. Thus, the labels of *primary* and *secondary* enuresis may be used for descriptive rather than explanatory or mechanistic purposes. A more useful categorization is based on the distinction between patients with enuresis at night only, in the daytime only (rare), and in both the night and the day.

Epidemiology

Enuresis is common, but prevalence figures vary widely, depending partially on quantitative aspects of the definitional criteria. Nocturnal enuresis may occur occasionally in 25% of boys, but more problematic enuresis persists beyond age 5 in 7%–10% of boys and 3% of girls. The male predominance persists but decreases with age. At age 10, 3% of boys and 2% of girls are still diagnosable. In adulthood, general prevalence is 1%. A correlation with socioeconomic status has been suggested but not established.

Etiology

The mechanisms involved in developing and maintaining bladder control are not well described, and multiple etiologies are believed to produce enuresis. Nocturnal polyuria has become recognized as a major factor in the etiology of many cases of "functional" enuresis. In fact, nocturnal bed-wetting can be induced in healthy children with ingestion of a water load at bedtime. In these cases, the wetting is elicited by a threshold volume that is specific to each individual and bears no correlation to bladder filling rate (Kirk et al. 1996).

Enuresis can also be caused by urological (urinary tract infection, especially in secondary enuresis in girls, or obstruction), anatomical (spinal disease, weak bladder or supporting musculature), physiological (abnormally low bladder pressure threshold, leading to early emptying), metabolic (diabetes), and neurological (seizure disorder) mechanisms.

Some forms of functional enuresis may run in families, particularly in males. Approximately 65%–70% of children with this disorder have a first-degree relative with functional enuresis. The chances of a child having enuresis are 77% if both parents have history of enuresis and 44% if one parent has such a history (Bakwin 1973). Three studies of monozygotic and dizygotic twins demonstrated a strong genetic factor, but the mechanism of transmission has not yet been described.

Some children with nocturnal enuresis do not have a normal nighttime release of vasopressin (antidiuretic hormone) and so may not have the usual nocturnal reduction in urine production (Rittig et al. 1989). The low overnight plasma levels of vasopressin (that persist into the morning) are associated with increased urination volume and decreased osmolality. No pituitary abnormalities were found on magnetic resonance imaging to explain the defective control of the circadian rhythm of vasopressin (Hunsballe et al. 1996). Decreased nocturnal vasopressin secretion is the basis for pharmacological treatment with desmopressin, an analog of vasopressin.

Disorders of sleep or diurnal rhythm may be etiological in a minority of cases of functional enuresis. The EEG findings are still debated; enuretic episodes can occur during any EEG stage, but there seems to be a concentration of episodes during delta (stages 3 and 4, non-REM) sleep or postdelta arousal (transition from delta into REM sleep). One subtyping of enuresis involves the coupling of sleep EEG with sleep cystometry (Watanabe and Azuma 1989). In addition, some children with enuresis are described by their parents as "deep" sleepers, and "at-home" studies have confirmed that they were more difficult to awaken (arouse) in the morning.

A "maturational" disorder is suggested in certain cases by findings of short stature, low mean bone age for chronological age, delayed sexual maturation, and small volume of voidings (suggestive of small bladder capacity); however, bladder capacity is typically normal. More generally, enuresis is associated with an overrepresentation of developmental delays (Steinhausen and Gobel 1989). Also, children who have behavior problems and enuresis have more developmental delays and smaller voiding volumes than enuretic children who do not have behavior problems; this finding suggests that at least some forms of enuresis with behavior problems are reflections of a developmental delay (Shaffer et al. 1984).

Approximately 50% of children with functional enuresis have emotional or behavioral symptoms, but it is unclear whether this result represents cause, effect, or an associated finding (e.g., poor parental limit setting).

Functional enuresis may also be related to stress, trauma, or psychosocial crisis, such as the birth of a sibling, start of school, a move, hospitalization, a loss, parental absence, or developmental crisis. In contrast to other types of enuresis, stress-induced cases are equally prevalent in boys and girls. However, the roles of environmental stress, family support, and socioeconomic status have been questioned (Fergusson et al. 1986).

There is a higher prevalence of functional enuresis associated with moderate and severe mental retardation. Voluntary enuresis may imply psychopathology, but it is often difficult to identify such psychopathology in individual cases or events, particularly if voluntary episodes are used to camouflage or cover for unintentional events.

Genetic mechanisms appear to be heterogeneous, but linkage studies have demonstrated involvement of chromosomes 8, 12q, and 13g in different families with multiple cases of functional enuresis (von Gontard et al. 1997). Chromosome 13 was linked to dominant transmission of primary nocturnal enuresis in 43% of families with primary nocturnal enuresis; penetrance was greater than 90%. A recessive mode of inheritance was observed in 9% of the families (Arnell et al. 1997; Eiberg et al. 1995).

Course and Prognosis

Enuresis remits spontaneously at a rate of approximately 15% per year (Forsythe and Butler 1989). Approximately 1% of boys (and fewer girls) still have this condition at age 18, generally with little associated psychopathology. The adolescent-onset form of enuresis, however, appears to have more associated psychopathology and a less favorable outcome.

The symptoms of functional enuresis, at any age, can lead to embarrassment, anger and punishment from caregivers, teasing by peers, avoidance of overnight visiting and camp, social withdrawal, and angry outbursts. These complications, if not properly managed, can have more impact on long-term outcome than the enuresis itself.

Evaluation and Differential Diagnosis

An initial medical assessment is required to rule out the various nonfunctional forms of enuresis. With extensive urological evaluation, about 20% of patients with nocturnal enuresis are found to have a urological abnormality. In certain cases, a sleep evaluation may be useful, but an EEG is not routinely required. Measurement of certain maturational indices may be useful for identifying simple developmental variance.

A specific form of enuresis, *giggle incontinence*, appears to result from altered muscle tone during laughter or emotionally intense moments. Although this form was traditionally resistant to treatment, psychostimulants appear to be effective. Giggle incontinence should be routinely considered during diagnostic evaluation because of its distinctive treatment.

Psychiatric evaluation of the child and parents includes assessment of associated psychopathology, recent psychosocial stressors, family concern about the symptom, and previous management of the symptoms. Inquiry about possible enuresis in the siblings is appropriate in view of their threefold increased risk. The proposed specific association of enuresis and depressive disorders has not been consistently supported in well-designed studies, but a stronger link has been found with ADHD. Children with ADHD are three times more likely to have nocturnal enuresis and five times more likely to have daytime enuresis than children without ADHD (Robson et al. 1997); therefore, evaluation for ADHD is advisable in children with enuresis.

Treatment

Most cases of functional enuresis are treated by pediatricians, who strongly prefer behavioral to pharmacological interventions for enuresis (Skoog et al. 1997). Behavioral methods for treating nocturnal enuresis include restriction of pre-bedtime fluid intake, planned midsleep awakenings for voiding in toilet, and rewards for successful nights.

Since the 1930s, nocturnal enuresis has been commonly treated by a simple device: a moisture-sensitive blanket that, during an enuretic episode, sounds a bell whose ringing arouses the patient from sleep. The "bell and pad" method has a high success rate (80%–90%) but also a high relapse rate (up to 15%–40%). A lower relapse rate can usually be achieved if the bell is set up to awaken the parents, who themselves then awaken the child. If relapse occurs, reinitiation of the bell system is often effective (Forsythe and Butler 1989). There is sometimes considerable resistance to the consistent use of the alarm system, by either parent and child. A variety of other behavioral methods are in widespread use, but they have not been as systematically tested.

Desmopressin, an analog of the antidiuretic hormone vasopressin, has been successful in several double-blind trials in treating nocturnal enuresis and is now popularly prescribed by family practitioners and pediatricians. Its efficacy in 50%–80% of cases (Bonde et al. 1994; Caione et al. 1997; Wille 1986) is not as high as that of bell alarms, and

the extent of improvement appears more limited. Only 60%–65% of patients with primary nocturnal enuresis have a marked reduction in wet nights (Skoog et al. 1997; Uygur et al. 1997). There is some evidence that desmopressin might be more effective in older children. Desmopressin also appears to be more effective for patients with a demonstrable excess of nocturnal vasopressin release (Rittig et al. 1997). Relapse is common when treatment is discontinued. Adverse effects are usually minimal, with only 4% of patients experiencing any side effects; however, 0.8% of patients had hyponatremic seizures resulting from desmopressin-induced water intoxication. Because the seizures usually appear following excessive fluid intake, they might be significantly reduced if patients avoid excessive fluid ingestion, especially in the evening. Another major disadvantage is cost: a daily dosage of desmopressin costs more than $4.50 (average wholesale price in 1997), which is considerably higher than treatment with tricyclic antidepressants or the bell system.

Generally, desmopressin produces a more rapid therapeutic effect than the alarm system, but the alarm bell has a higher rate of improvement and is slightly more likely to elicit persistent symptom control after treatment discontinuation. Overall, use of the alarm and use of desmopressin are similarly effective, at least for treating primary nocturnal enuresis. However, on the basis of a cost-effectiveness analysis, researchers in Denmark concluded that the use of the alarm system would produce substantial net savings to society, whereas use of desmopressin would produce net losses (Ankjaer-Jensen and Sejr 1994).

Tricyclic antidepressants can be helpful if a patient does not respond well to behavioral interventions, if there is daytime as well as nighttime enuresis, or if there is associated mood or anxiety disorder. Tricyclic antidepressants have been shown to be effective in many double-blind studies, typically in low dosages (e.g., imipramine 25–125 mg or about 2 mg/kg nightly; EEG monitoring is absolutely mandatory; a daily dosage of 5 mg/kg is not to be exceeded). Some reports have suggested that the success rate is only 15% after discontinuation of antidepressants, but the success rate is probably higher if the dosage is tapered gradually. In view of the high rate of remission with placebo, it is sensible to attempt to lower the medication dosage every 4–6 months. In view of the high lethality of tricyclic antidepressants in overdose (particularly desipramine) and the reported sudden deaths during desipramine treatment (see earlier section concerning ADHD), treatment of enuresis with desipramine should be avoided. Imipramine is much safer and is effective in treating enuresis. Also, access to pill bottles at home should be carefully controlled to minimize risks of overdose, which might result from the child's attempt to make treatment go faster, a suicide attempt, or accidental ingestion by younger siblings.

The mechanism for the effect of tricyclics on enuresis is unknown, but it is not the anticholinergic properties (anticholinergic agents are not effective); it may be related to the antidepressant property (MAOIs are also effective). Consistent with a catecholamine/alertness hypothesis, pseudoephedrine was reported to provide statistically significant improvement in primary nocturnal enuresis (Varan et al. 1996). Selective serotonin reuptake inhibitors have not been examined for antienuretic properties. In patients with nocturnal polyuria (without enuresis), imipramine may produce reductions in urine osmolality as well as volume, suggesting that imipramine may have an antidiuretic effect that is independent of its antienuretic effect (Hunsballe et al. 1997).

In a provocative study, imipramine in combination with an inhibitor of prostaglandin synthesis, diclofenac, and was reported to have a 60% response rate (and only a 13% relapse rate) in primary nocturnal enuresis. The clinical significance of this finding will remain unclear until it is replicated.

Perhaps the most effective treatment for nocturnal enuresis is the bell alarm combined with desmopressin (Sukhai et al. 1989), although imipramine might be used instead of desmopressin if cost is a concern and immediate symptom control is not essential.

For daytime enuresis, oxybutynin (Ditropan) has been reported to produce significant improvement in 54% of cases; when combined with desmopressin, its success rate rises to 71% (Caione et al. 1997). Oxybutynin treats enuresis mainly by acting as a smooth muscle relaxant, and it also has anticholinergic effects. By diminishing bladder muscle contraction, oxybutynin increases bladder capacity, allows delay of the need to urinate, and thereby reduces the urgency and frequency of involuntary voiding (and voluntary urination). Another alternative is acupuncture, which is reported to be helpful in 40% of cases (Caione et al. 1997).

Other interventions are usually not necessary in most cases of functional enuresis, although the presence of secondary enuresis might suggest possible benefits from counseling. Psychotherapy may be useful for the uncommon case in which the symptom of enuresis is interpersonally cathected (e.g., into an oppositional struggle or into expression of rage) or for patients with significant comorbid psychopathology.

Management of the embarrassment, low self-esteem, and behavioral avoidance that often accompany this disorder is usually a critical part of the treatment for children and adults in the United States. In contrast, enuresis does not cause as much concern in Australia, either for the child or the family (Bower et al. 1996). When dealing with the emotional complications of enuresis, it is usually helpful to deemphasize the conscious or unconscious explanations that might engender shame or guilt, and instead to focus more specifically on the symptom alleviation.

CLINICAL COMMENT

Like encopresis, enuresis (not due to a general medical condition) may be managed successfully in most cases by pediatricians. Despite the multiple etiologies of this elimination disorder, behavioral interventions are effective in the majority of cases. Even when secondary functional enuresis appears to signal significant psychosocial or developmental stress, behavioral interventions may be sufficient to restore adequate developmental progress. Possible medical causes of enuresis (including neurodevelopmental and sleep disorders) require pediatric evaluation. Psychiatric intervention is crucial in a minority of cases of functional enuresis, particularly when there is late-onset enuresis without medical explanation, interpersonal cathexis of the symptoms, or associated psychopathology. The high success rate in treating nocturnal enuresis with a vasopressin analog, coupled with findings of diminished nocturnal release of the antidiuretic hormone, has added a new dimension to the understanding of this medical disorder that often responds to behavioral approaches.

OTHER DISORDERS OF INFANCY, CHILDHOOD, OR ADOLESCENCE

SEPARATION ANXIETY DISORDER

In addition to normal situational and developmental anxiety, children can show genuine anxiety disorders. These pathological states are common, but they are frequently dismissed by parents, pediatricians, and psychiatrists as mere "anxiety." Children are commonly imagined to be innately fearful, and adolescence is seen as naturally anxiety provoking. Anxiety is viewed as so ordinary in children that often due consideration is not given to the possibility of an anxiety disorder.

Separation anxiety disorder is the only anxiety disorder listed in DSM-IV as a disorder usually first diagnosed in children or adolescents. Like other anxiety disorders in children, separation anxiety disorder can lead to social problems, academic underachievement, and interference with developing assertiveness skills and personal autonomy, often resulting in social awkwardness (or "immaturity") and sometimes a reluctance to date. Unlike many childhood disorders, the anxiety disorders often cause more distress to the children than to the parents (although the parents may themselves be quite anxious owing to their own anxiety disorders). As in adults, anxiety disorders tend to present in clusters, and most children with separation anxiety disorder have other anxiety disorders comorbidly.

Separation anxiety, a normal developmental phenomenon at age 18–30 months, has been traditionally described in terms of attachment and separation theory (see Chapter 4). A nonpathological form of separation anxiety is sometimes observed in adults or children who have been geographically displaced and are feeling homesick; examples include students, soldiers, immigrants, refugees, and hospitalized patients (Van Tilburg et al. 1996).

In separation anxiety disorder, cognitive, affective, somatic, and behavioral symptoms appear in response to genuine or fantasied separation from attachment figures (Table 23–33). Separation anxiety disorder can present clinically in a variety of ways, including difficulty in falling asleep (pre-bedtime agitation) and school absenteeism (Bernstein and Borchardt 1991).

Clinical Description

The major attachment object is usually a parent or caregiver, but it can be a favorite toy or familiar place. Typically, even a young child can specify the attachment object that gives a sense of protection or safety (from anxiety). Common presentations include preoccupying or morbid fear of parents' death, clinging to parents, school avoidance, sleep refusal, resistance to being alone, nightmares, anticipatory worrying, cognitive disruption, or somatization. Although the anxiety is usually centered around separation from a parent, the fear can instead manifest as an anticipatory fear of being injured, kidnapped, or killed. Interference with autonomous functioning can extend to inability to sleep in one's own bed, visit friends, go on errands, or stay at camp. Homesickness may be freely described by young children ("I want my mommy") but can be hard to admit for adolescents, especially boys.

More than 92% of children with separation anxiety disorder have other DSM-IV disorders, typically anxiety or mood disorders (Table 23–34). Many children with major depressive disorder also fulfill criteria for separation anxiety disorder.

Children with separation anxiety may sense a clear "line of demarcation" that separates safe from unsafe: they may be able to enter the school hallways but not the classroom, or they may be able to play in the school yard but not

be able to walk into the school building; they may be able to leave the house but not cross a particular street.

These children typically display internalizing behaviors and psychological mechanisms. Pathological compliance, perfectionism, and "nicey-nice" presentation of self may be seen. The children can show somatizations (stomachaches, headaches) in the morning on school days, a fear of teachers ("They're mean"), or passive-aggressive traits. In some cases, anxiety disorders in children can become the basis for disruptive behavioral symptoms.

TABLE 23-33. DSM-IV diagnostic criteria for separation anxiety disorder

A. Developmentally inappropriate and excessive anxiety concerning separation from home or from those to whom the individual is attached, as evidenced by three (or more) of the following:

(1) Recurrent excessive distress when separation from home or major attachment figures occurs or is anticipated

(2) Persistent and excessive worry about losing, or about possible harm befalling, major attachment figures

(3) Persistent and excessive worry that an untoward event will lead to separation from a major attachment figure (e.g., getting lost or being kidnapped)

(4) Persistent reluctance or refusal to go to school or elsewhere because of fear of separation

(5) Persistently and excessively fearful or reluctant to be alone or without major attachment figures at home or without significant adults in other settings

(6) Persistent reluctance or refusal to go to sleep without being near a major attachment figure or to sleep away from home

(7) Repeated nightmares involving the theme of separation

(8) Repeated complaints of physical symptoms (such as headaches, stomachaches, nausea, or vomiting) when separation from major attachment figures occurs or is anticipated

B. The duration of the disturbance is at least 4 weeks.

C. The onset is before age 18 years.

D. The disturbance causes clinically significant distress or impairment in social, academic (occupational), or other important areas of functioning.

E. The disturbance does not occur exclusively during the course of a pervasive developmental disorder, schizophrenia, or other psychotic disorder and, in adolescents and adults, is not better accounted for by panic disorder with agoraphobia.

Specify if:

Early onset: if onset occurs before age 6 years

TABLE 23–34.   Comparison of children with separation anxiety disorder and children with school-related phobic disorders

	Children with separation anxiety disorder	Children with phobic disorders
Age at referral (mean)	9 years	14 years
Gender ratio (M:F)	1:2	2:1
Low socioeconomic class (Hollingshead IV or V)	32%	68%
Concurrent DSM-III disorder	92%	63%
Concurrent anxiety disorder	50%	53%
Concurrent mood disorder	33%	32%
Maternal anxiety disorder	83%	57%
Maternal mood disorder	63%	14%

Note.   These children were referred to an outpatient psychiatric clinic and were diagnosed with separation anxiety disorder or a phobic disorder (simple or social) regarding school. Although concomitant mood and anxiety disorders are common in both disorders, the children and mothers showed more psychopathology associated with separation anxiety disorder than with phobic disorders.
Source.   Data from Last et al. 1987.

The prominence of somatization with separation anxiety is similar to that of panic, phobic, generalized anxiety, and depressive disorders of adulthood. Children with separation anxiety disorder commonly experience stomachaches and palpitations, and they generally have more somatic complaints than children with any other psychiatric disorder (Livingston et al. 1988). Separation anxiety disorder has many characteristics of phobic disorders. Separation anxiety disorder differs from other anxiety disorders in its focus on separation and its early appearance (usually first diagnosed in childhood). It differs from phobic disorders in that the latter may be directed toward a myriad of potential sources of fear.

School absenteeism is reported in about 75% of children with separation anxiety disorder, and separation anxiety disorder is reported in up to 50%–80% of school absentees (Klein and Last 1989); however, these conditions are quite distinct. The terms *school phobia, school avoidance,* and *school refusal* are misnomers: most school "phobics" are not in fact phobic, and the terms *avoidance* and *refusal* imply psychological mechanisms that may not apply. A more descriptively neutral and accurate label is *school absenteeism,* a term that has the advantage of highlighting a possible connection with job absenteeism. School absenteeism has a variety of etiologies (Table 23–35). Not all children with

school absenteeism have separation anxiety, and not all children with separation anxiety disorder have school absenteeism (Last et al. 1987).

In some cases of school absenteeism, the parent and child are bound to each other by psychodynamically based fears of separation. The classical psychoanalytic description (Johnson et al. 1941) is consistent with recent findings of mood disorders and separation anxiety in both parent and child associated with school absenteeism.

Epidemiology

Separation anxiety disorder is common and tends to run in families. Epidemiological studies report a prevalence of 0.6%–6%. The gender ratio is equal or female predominant (2:1).

School absenteeism is common, with 75% of adults admitting to this behavior during childhood. At some inner-city schools, absenteeism may be observed in more than 90% of students. Large-scale studies of school absenteeism have not been pursued from a psychiatric point of view. The extent of school absenteeism that is specifically due to separation anxiety disorder, and not to comorbidity, is undetermined.

TABLE 23–35.   Sources of school absenteeism

Separation anxiety disorder

Truancy (often associated with conduct disorder)

Psychiatric disorders usually first diagnosed in adulthood

    Mood disorders

        Major depressive disorder

        Bipolar disorder

    Anxiety disorders

        Overanxious disorder

        Phobic disorder

        Panic disorder

        Obsessive-compulsive disorder

    Overt psychotic disorders (rare)

Sociocultural conformity

    Permission granted by family (e.g., overt or covert support to stay at home to take care of sibs, to earn money, or to avoid tests)

    Normative peer behavior in certain locales (spending time with peers rather than going to school)

Realistic fear of bodily harm in dangerous school setting

Drug-induced absenteeism (e.g., propranolol, haloperidol)

Etiology

Developmental theorists have speculated about mechanisms contributing to separation anxiety disorder. Unconscious internal conflicts regarding aggressive and sexual impulses, uncertainty regarding the location of caregivers after the toddler's initial ambulatory movements, and parent-induced anxious attachment are standard psychodynamic formulations. Learning theorists have emphasized the maintenance of symptoms by conditioned fear through stimulus generalization and reinforcement. Biological theorists focus on temperament factors, pharmacological features, and the relationship to childhood mood and adult anxiety disorders. Child psychiatrists and pediatricians might emphasize the roles of illness, helplessness, fear, and dependency.

More than half the children with separation anxiety disorder have parents with mood or anxiety disorders (Table 23–34). Similarly, many children with school absenteeism have mood disorders or one of several anxiety disorders, and their parents may also have these disorders (Figure 23–14).

Separation anxiety disorder is commonly seen in association with major depressive disorder in children and developmentally can precede the appearance of major depressive disorder. A study of dexamethasone suppression testing in children with separation anxiety disorder suggested that positive tests (nonsuppression) are seen nearly as often as in children with major depressive disorder, possibly reflecting a high rate of comorbidity or physiological similarity between separation anxiety disorder and major depressive disorder. There remains some debate about whether separation anxiety disorder in children exists entirely independently of associated major depressive disorder or other anxiety disorders.

Separation anxiety disorder may also occur at higher frequency in children whose family histories include alcoholism or panic disorder with agoraphobia. Agoraphobic mothers report a high incidence of stomachaches during their own childhoods, and their reports indicate that their children have a high incidence of school absenteeism (14%) and stomachaches (Berg 1976). Children who are shy, fearful, or "behaviorally inhibited" before age 3 (Kagan et al. 1987) show increased prevalence of anxiety disorders at follow-up (Biederman et al. 1990).

Another proposed etiological factor for separation anxiety disorder is posttraumatic stress disorder (PTSD). Separation anxiety disorder was found to be the most common cormorbid diagnosis in the 50% of sexually and/or physically abused boys who developed PTSD (Dykman et al. 1997). It is unclear whether the appearance of separation anxiety disorder in this group is due to traumatic abuse, PTSD, psychological grief, or concurrent depressive disorders, or whether it is a marker for family chaos and abuse.

Little research has been conducted on genetic factors in separation anxiety disorder. A twin study suggested a significant genetic influence toward the development of separation anxiety disorder, but only in females; environmental factors were demonstrated for both genders (Silove et al. 1995a).

Course and Prognosis

Separation anxiety disorder may be diagnosed after the normative period of separation anxiety, but it is typically not observed before age 4. It is usually first recognized in early or mid childhood. Separation anxiety disorder is typically a chronic disorder, but there can be exacerbations at times of actual separations, deaths, illness, family moves, or natural disasters. Symptoms might be aggravated during episodes of comorbid psychiatric disorders. Symptoms may also worsen during or after medical illness, particularly chronic medical conditions with acute exacerbations. Multiple medical evaluations are commonly sought by the child or parents.

A follow-up study of children with separation anxiety disorder (who also had a communication disorder) found that, after 4 years, 11% still had separation anxiety disorder, 33% had a different diagnosis (typically another anxiety disorder), and 44% no longer had an anxiety disorder (Cantwell and Baker 1989). Long-term follow-up studies

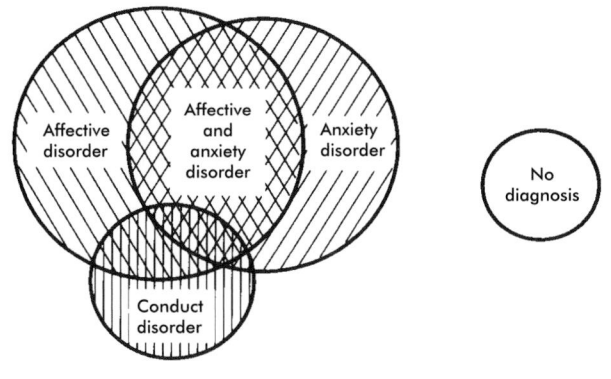

FIGURE 23-14. School absenteeism: overlap with affective, anxiety, and conduct disorders.
Source. Reprinted with permission from Bernstein GA, Garfinkel BD: "School Phobia: The Overlap of Affective and Anxiety Disorders." *Journal of the American Academy of Child Psychiatry* 25:235–241, 1986. Copyright 1986, American Academy of Child Psychiatry.

have suggested an increased risk for the development of other anxiety disorders (especially panic disorder with agoraphobia) and possibly depressive disorder (Klein and Last 1989). Furthermore, independently of depressive disorders, separation anxiety can be strongly associated with suicidality in adolescents (Feldman and Wilson 1997).

Separation anxiety disorder in childhood may be developmentally connected to panic disorder in adults. Separation anxiety disorder in childhood is associated with early-onset panic disorder (Battaglia et al. 1995). Adults with panic disorder, especially those with agoraphobia, reported childhood symptoms of separation anxiety disorder even more often than did adults with generalized anxiety disorder or phobic disorder (Silove et al. 1995b). In addition, adults with panic disorder reported family histories in which panic disorder (with and without agoraphobia) and alcohol use disorders were overrepresented (Battaglia et al. 1995). A developmental link with childhood separation anxiety disorder may not be specific to adult panic disorder, because separation anxiety disorder appears to function as a risk factor for the comorbid appearance of multiple anxiety disorders in adults (Lipsitz et al. 1994).

Conversely, the majority (68%) of children of adults with agoraphobia were found to have diagnosable psychiatric disorders, especially anxiety disorders in general and separation anxiety disorder in particular (Capps et al. 1996). One-half of children of parents with social phobia were found to have an anxiety disorder, and 19% of the total had separation anxiety disorder (Mancini et al. 1996). It may be speculated that childhood separation anxiety develops into adult panic disorder or, at least, that childhood separation anxiety is one of several possible antecedents of panic disorder in adults (Ollendick et al. 1994). A follow-up study is needed that reexamines children with separation anxiety once they become adults. At present, there remains considerable debate about whether separation anxiety disorder exists as a distinct disorder in adults and whether panic disorder exists in children.

School absentees often show academic underachievement and social avoidance, and they can be at risk for chronic unemployment in adulthood. Just as they have difficulty getting to school, they have difficulty getting to their jobs.

Diagnostic Evaluation

The workup includes assessment of possible mood disorder or anxiety (phobic, panic) disorder. These disorders, as well as separation anxiety disorder, should also be evaluated in the parents.

Clinically, it is sometimes difficult to distinguish the presenting symptoms of separation anxiety disorder from ordinary acute anxiety. Both conditions can involve distractibility, distorted cognition, depersonalization, transient impairment in reality sense, motoric overactivity, and angry outbursts. However, the presence of separation anxiety disorder implies that separation-related psychodynamics are a primary trigger of the acute anxiety.

Some severe disorders may present with separation anxiety and exclude a separate diagnosis of separation anxiety disorder. Children with autistic disorder or other PDDs often have separation anxiety, but evidence of neurological dysfunction can usually be identified across a wide area of functions. Schizophrenia can initially present in children as separation anxiety, with impaired early object relations (e.g., being viewed as "weird" by peers, living as a "loner") appearing before more overt psychotic symptoms emerge.

Occasionally, separation anxiety disorder, school absenteeism, and panic attacks are drug-induced. Propranolol (used for treating headache) or haloperidol (for associated Tourette's disorder or psychosis) may induce transient periods of separation anxiety disorder or school absenteeism that resolve on discontinuation of medication (Popper 1993); therefore, it is worth evaluating current medication regimens for agents that might aggravate "depression."

Differential diagnosis may be complicated by an unexpected form of separation anxiety. Developmentally normal children who had low birth weights and neonatal ultrasound evidence of ventricular enlargement or brain parenchymal lesions were found to have an increased likelihood of separation anxiety when 6 years old (Whitaker et al. 1997). In contrast, separation anxiety was not identified in similar children with neonatal intraventricular hemorrhage or brain matrix disorders, suggesting some degree of neuropathological specificity. This finding implies that early brain injury could be an etiology of some forms of separation anxiety in children.

Treatment

The traditional treatment of separation anxiety disorder entails psychosocial interventions (individual psychotherapy combined with family therapy or parental guidance), often with antianxiety or antidepressant medication.

Antidepressants are commonly used for treating separation anxiety disorder, despite the meager literature supporting their effectiveness and a substantial literature that questions its usefulness (Popper 1993). Tricyclic antidepressants have been studied mainly in children with school absenteeism and separation anxiety disorder rather than in children with separation anxiety disorder per se. Antidepressant treatment (e.g., fluoxetine, imipramine) may be considered for children whose school absenteeism exceeds 2 weeks and is not explained by a medical problem, truancy, overt psychosis, sociocultural conformity, or realistic fear of physical danger. An open-label study of fluoxetine reported clinical improvement in all 10 children and adolescents with separation anxiety disorder, 8 of 10 youths with social phobia, but only 1 of 7 with generalized anxiety disorder (Fairbanks et al. 1997). The value of these treatments remains in question, however, because the available studies are small; there have been no large-scale investigations of antidepressants for treating either separation anxiety disorder or school absenteeism. However, antidepressants are probably effective in the many cases of school absenteeism in which the underlying etiology is separation anxiety disorder, mood disorder, phobic disorder, or panic disorder.

If a parent has an anxiety or mood disorder causing difficulty in separating from the child, the parent should receive direct psychiatric treatment as well as behavioral guidance for parenting. Treatment of a parent with antidepressant medication for mood or anxiety disorders is commonly a part of the treatment of a child with separation anxiety disorder.

Benzodiazepines, mainly alprazolam and clonazepam, have also been employed for children and parents with separation anxiety disorder. Clinically, these agents appear to be particularly helpful for the "anticipatory" anxiety that can develop secondarily around "primary" anxiety symptoms. Buspirone might also be considered.

Separation anxiety disorder can also be partially alleviated by the use of a "high-tech" method: the attachment figure is given an electronic beeper, and the child is given a coin, allowing a telephone call to the parent in the event of a surge of anxiety. Typically, the child will use the beeper to contact the parent once or twice and then uses the coin as a symbol of the capacity to reach the attachment figure if needed. This technique can also be useful in facilitating school attendance.

Cognitive-behavioral therapy and family management appear to be useful in treating separation anxiety disorder (Barrett et al. 1996). Individual and family psychotherapies have more regularly appearing characteristics for this disorder than for most childhood disorders.

For children with separation anxiety disorder, the child's experience of psychotherapy is organized around the actual "separations within the therapy." It is advisable to pay special attention to planned and unplanned absences (vacations by the patient or therapist, school transitions, therapist or teacher pregnancy, parental unavailability, therapist illness, deaths) and to the termination of treatment. It is often useful to give the child a concrete object or souvenir, or a clearly verbalized image of the therapist's future activity, at the time of interruption or termination. Preventive verbal anticipation, preparation of the parents as well as the child, and active discussion of the practicalities surrounding expected separations are useful in the management of these cases.

It is advised that strong emphasis be placed on termination work with the parents as well as with the child. The parents' own separation issues and psychopathology may lead them to be intolerant of the "loss" affects, to push for an abrupt finish, or to undervalue the importance of psychodynamic issues elicited at termination. Both child and parents may be observed to "rehearse" different aspects of the treatment termination before its completion. Much like their children, parents with separation anxiety disorder may have distorted cognitions regarding terminations ("I was not sure that you would allow us to come back"); therefore, explicit articulation of this point before termination is useful. Particularly for parents with mood or anxiety disorders, who may themselves be vulnerable at times of psychological loss or stress, it is useful to be specific about the mechanism for return to treatment.

More generally, there is extensive dynamic interaction between the separation anxiety of the child and the anxiety of the parent or parents, even if the family conceals the more overt instances of parental encouragement of the child's dependency and parental worry about the child's independent action. The treatments of the child and the parent will interact extensively as well, giving a clinician opportunities to intervene at two points in the self-stimulating system. If hospitalization of the child is needed, the parent's own separation fears might make it difficult for him or her to tolerate having the child away from home. This may appear to be a lack of cooperation with treatment, but it is more helpful to understand that the parent can only view the measure as too extreme. Management of the parent's separation anxiety at this juncture is crucial and a major part of the treatment, because it allows the successful initiation of genuine psychotherapy of the separation anxiety disorder in the child. Occasionally, this situation can lead to joint hospitalization of the child and the parent (Chabrol et al. 1995).

A common pitfall in the treatment of this disorder is an overemphasis by the parents and professionals on the presenting symptoms (e.g., poor school attendance) rather than on the child's long-term development. A child's ability to attend school consistently or to manage anxiety quietly signifies behavioral improvement, but the child may be left with psychodevelopmental liabilities. It is essential to maintain a broad perspective on the psychopathology and the risk for adult impairment to prevent premature closure of therapeutic work.

Another pitfall in the treatment of children and parents with this disorder involves pathological compliance. Some parents and children have an overly "good" or "nice" presentation of self, and their perfectionistic manner of managing themselves can prevent them from exposing their deeper thoughts and feelings. "Pathological pleasantness" in child or parents needs to be monitored during the course of treatment and not mistaken for substantial understanding, support, or change.

Limit setting in the treatment of separation anxiety disorder can be useful or disruptive. If the child has a panic disorder or major depressive episode, limit setting can be counterproductive and aggravate the symptoms. Forcing a child with panic disorder to attend school can result in a temper tantrum or physical assault. However, "therapeutic coercion," sensitively applied, can be helpful in some cases of true separation anxiety disorder, particularly if the intervention is appropriately timed after drug treatment. For treating truancy (a far more common cause of school absenteeism), limit setting is certainly a useful and often necessary measure for establishing a routine daily structure in the child's life.

Psychosocial measures are also appropriate for managing school absenteeism based on fear of physical danger, family "permission," or subcultural "hanging out" with peers.

Clinical Comment

Research is needed regarding the relationship of separation anxiety disorder to other child and adult psychiatric disorders, especially in view of the high prevalence of school absenteeism and adult unemployment. Treatment of these children requires a serious focus beyond their prominent presenting symptoms. The high prevalence of concurrent psychopathology and long-term developmental liabilities requires anticipatory clinical attention. Helping parents and school personnel to recognize the broader psychopathology and psychodevelopmental risks of separation anxiety disorder requires ongoing collaborative work, consultation, and advocacy at schools.

SELECTIVE MUTISM

Children with selective mutism do not use speech in specific settings and show abnormalities of interpersonal behavior and social assertiveness. This uncommon disorder was initially described more than 100 years ago, but the medical literature on selective mutism still consists mainly of individual case reports. The paucity of large-scale controlled studies has impeded the accumulation of systematic and statistical descriptions.

Clinical Description

In selective mutism, children do not speak in one or several of the major environments in which they live. Even though they can talk without difficulty in certain places (usually at home), partial or total muteness appears selectively in unfamiliar places or particular social situations (Table 23–36). Typically, speech is normal at home when the child is alone with parents and siblings, and communication is constricted in the presence of teachers, peers, and strangers. When separated from a familiar or comfortable environment, these children might freely or hesitantly use gestural speech, nods, monosyllabic responses, written notes, or whispers, but they avoid full vocalization and verbal speech.

Although many children with selective mutism have normal language capabilities, approximately one-third of these children have a language disorder, and about one-half have a speech disorder or delayed speech development (Hayden 1980; Kolvin and Fundudis 1981). In addition, children with selective mutism have an increased prevalence of neurological disorders and mental retardation. The traditional assumption that children with selective mutism have normal speech, language, and biological development is not true in the majority of these children.

Many children with selective mutism also exhibit school absenteeism, problems with separation, anxiety, and

TABLE 23-36. DSM-IV diagnostic criteria for selective mutism

A. Consistent failure to speak in specific social situations (in which there is an expectation for speaking, e.g., at school) despite speaking in other situations.

B. The disturbance interferes with educational or occupational achievement or with social communication.

C. The duration of the disturbance is at least 1 month (not limited to the first month of school).

D. The failure to speak is not due to a lack of knowledge of, or comfort with, the spoken language required in the social situation.

E. The disturbance is not better accounted for by a communication disorder (e.g., stuttering) and does not occur exclusively during the course of a pervasive developmental disorder, schizophrenia, or other psychotic disorder.

obsessive-compulsive features. Most children had behavioral abnormalities that were observed before age 6 years.

There are usually widespread impairments of social behavior and sometimes behavioral control. Many of these children show early and persistent shyness, submissiveness, excessive dependency, timidity in activities involving personal assertiveness, clinging to parents, sulky behavior with strangers, temper tantrums, and regressive behaviors. At times, these children may show streaks of oppositionality, demanding and controlling behavior, passive-aggressiveness, and defiance.

In many of the published case reports, overly strong emotional ties to the mother and maternal overprotectiveness were emphasized. There were frequent descriptions of parental fear, anxiety, agoraphobia, and shyness, but also of parental aggressivity and violence. The parents' use of silence as a weapon of anger and a means of coercion is also repeatedly highlighted.

Early facial injury, mouth trauma (dental surgery), or oral punishment (washing out the mouth, slapping the face) are commonly described, especially during the period of speech development. Children with selective mutism are sometimes compared to children who, after the developmental period of normal stranger anxiety, are hesitant to speak in new situations. Many psychiatrically normal children have major difficulty in speaking on initially entering kindergarten, but this hesitancy resolves as the people and environment become familiar.

In a large study of 68 children with selective mutism (Hayden 1980), four subtypes of this disorder were distinguished on the basis of psychodynamic and behavioral features (Table 23–37). The *symbiotic* form of selective mutism involves a dominant mother who is openly jealous of the child's relationships with other people, a father who is passive or speaks minimally, and a child who seems submissive but can be intensely manipulative. This subgroup is the largest, and its description closely parallels the usual clinical descriptions. The *passive-aggressive* group of children with selective mutism use silence in a defiant and hostile manner, display antisocial and often aggressive behaviors, and generally have parents with overt antisocial features. The *reactive* (or perhaps depressed) children commonly

TABLE 23–37. A classification of selective mutism

	Symbiotic (*n* = 31) (% of children showing trait)	Passive-aggressive (*n* = 16) (% of children showing trait)	Reactive (*n* = 14) (% of children showing trait)	Speech-phobic (*n* = 7) (% of children showing trait)
Dominant mother, plus passive or absent father	97	0	7	0
School achievement above average	45	0	0	0
Mouthing words or whispering	13	0	0	0
Aggressive behavior	0	56	0	0
Antisocial behavior	10	82	14	0
Parental incarceration	3	75	36	0
Onset after age 5 years	6	50	14	0
Depressive features	6	50	100	14
Severe withdrawal, catatonic-like	6	37	100	0
Parental depression	3	0	43	0
Familial shyness	10	6	71	29
Shyness	3	0	32	86
Rituals and compulsions	10	6	7	100
Physical abuse (documented)	65	100	71	10
Sexual abuse (documented)	26	50	36	43

Source. Subtyping and data from a study of 68 children, Hayden 1980.

show depressive features and social withdrawal, have a parent with a mood disorder, and often have a family history of shyness. The *speech-phobic* children appear literally afraid to hear their own voices, show autonomic excitatory reactions in response to hearing themselves talk (even on audiotape), exhibit obvious ritualistic and compulsive behaviors, and show a strong motivation to overcome their symptoms.

In the same study, Hayden (1980) also reported a high prevalence of physical and sexual abuse in children with all forms of selective mutism (Table 23–37); the cases of physical and sexual abuse were documented by independent social welfare agencies. A similarly high rate of child abuse was found in an independent study (MacGregor et al. 1994). These findings suggest that, in some cases, selective mutism might be a posttraumatic phenomenon, which would have implications for the clinical management of these children and their families.

Epidemiology

An estimated prevalence of 180 per 100,000 children has recently been reported (Kopp and Gillberg 1997), indicating a higher prevalence than generally was reported in the past (when more stringent definitional criteria were used). There is a slight female predominance, with a gender ratio of 1:1–2. An increased prevalence of selective mutism in children from immigrant families is also reported.

Etiology

Mainly on the basis of the case studies, psychodynamic models of explanation have predominated. Psychoanalytic theorists have emphasized mechanisms involving oral inhibition, anal control, separation anxiety, and abandonment fears. The mutism is often conceptualized as a coping behavior and as a reflection of primitively asserted autonomy. Muteness can also be interpreted as a defense against emotional distress, pain, fear of punishment, and interpersonal interaction, occurring in families in which there is a tendency toward family enmeshment and overprotectiveness.

A variety of descriptive observations are consistent with these psychodynamic formulations. The selective appearance of symptoms in specific environments implies the operation of psychodynamic factors. A posttraumatic etiology is supported by the data suggesting a high prevalence of physical and sexual abuse, parental violence, and early mouth trauma. An etiology related to separation anxiety is consistent with some overt behavioral symptoms, as well as the strong maternal ties, family history of mood disorder, and history of loss (e.g., through geographic move or sociopolitical change). A lack of confidence and personal autonomy in managing the external world appears to be a contributing factor.

Several findings suggest biological etiological factors. Although the association of selective mutism with a history of early-onset shyness or a family history of shyness is consistent with a psychodynamic model, it is also consistent with a constitutional or temperamental contribution to childhood shyness (Kagan et al. 1987), anxiety disorders, or mood disorders. Although there are no controlled family history studies, numerous reports have suggested an increased prevalence of anxiety, mood, and personality disorders in the parents. The association of selective mutism with communication disorders, mental retardation, and neurological disorder suggests a neurodevelopmental etiological factor. These conditions can potentially aggravate the speech of a child with selective mutism.

Although it is difficult to provide more than speculation regarding the etiology, there is clear evidence of numerous and multidimensional etiological factors.

Course and Prognosis

Selective mutism typically starts at age 3–5, when developmentally normal children may still show brief periods of mutism on meeting strangers or in new settings. Although the gradual emergence of early "shyness" may be identified retrospectively (Kolvin and Fundudis 1981), selective mutism is typically diagnosed at ages 5–8, when symptoms become obvious at school. If school attendance is adequate and social behavior is compliant, recognition and referral for treatment may be delayed or avoided.

Symptoms may last for several weeks, months, or years. Some children improve without therapy. About 50% of children are no longer selectively mute by age 10, but the prognosis appears less encouraging if speech behaviors do not improve by then (Kolvin and Fundudis 1981).

Certain cases of selective mutism do not emerge until adolescence. These individuals typically do not speak to family members or outsiders, often show prominent passive-aggressive or antisocial features, and tend to have a less favorable prognosis (Hayden 1980).

Complications include academic underachievement, scapegoating, and satisfaction with the secondary gains of illness. The disadvantages of inappropriate special class and school placements are incurred, as teachers become helpless in dealing with the socially disruptive silence. Many children experience teasing and humiliation, but some children are apparently protected by peers, who may speak in their behalf or who bestow special services and personal attention. Excessive protection and tolerance by peers or parents usually reinforces the mute behavior.

The long-term outcome is not known. The abnormal social behavior, interpersonal manipulations, shyness, and aggressivity appear to persist beyond the period of symptomatic muteness. Further information about the natural course of illness may be derived from studies on co-morbidity. The relationship of selective mutism to mood, separation anxiety, and phobic disorders, as well as psychosis of childhood and adulthood, is only now being examined. The finding that 97% of children with selective mutism fulfill criteria for social phobia has led to the proposal that selective mutism may be a symptom of social anxiety disorder, a disorder commonly seen in adults (Black and Uhde 1992).

Evaluation

A full psychiatric evaluation of the child and parents is warranted. Neurological assessment is helpful to consider possible brain damage and mental retardation. Speech and language evaluation is needed, including examination of familial patterns of communication, silence, and anger. The child and family should be assessed for physical and sexual abuse, depression, antisocial behavior, shyness, and mental retardation. At times, a home visit is helpful. Differential diagnosis includes anxiety disorders such as social phobia, disuse of speech in schizophrenia (alogia) or schizotypal personality, deafness, aphasia, and hysteria.

Treatment

Selective mutism was notoriously difficult to treat until fluoxetine was demonstrated to produce substantial improvement in both mutism and global functioning of these children, as rated by parents (Black and Uhde 1992). This finding was particularly striking in view of the inability of tricyclic antidepressants to treat this condition. However, most of the children were still quite symptomatic after 12 weeks of treatment (Black and Uhde 1992), and the therapeutic effect appeared to drop with increasing age (Dummit et al. 1996); therefore, the use of other methods remains necessary.

Behavior therapy appears to have the next best outcome (Krohn et al. 1992; Labbe and Williamson 1984). Contingency management, positive reinforcement, desensitization, and assertiveness training have generally been employed. At present, behavior therapy should probably be used in combination with a selective serotonin reuptake inhibitor. Speech and language therapy are often indicated for children with selective mutism, especially in view of their communication disorders and neurodevelopmental problems.

Parent counseling can be effective. Accommodations to the child's muteness are often made by parents and teachers; however, it is generally useful to maintain a clear expectation that the child talk and communicate, at least for a structured period each day at home, at each school period, and at each treatment session. It is important for the parents, especially the symbiotic parent, to be explicit with the child about the expectation of talking at school and in therapy. Most parents and teachers need to be supported and repeatedly reminded to refrain from reinforcing the child's passivity or contributing to the secondary gain.

Therapists have anecdotally described a variety of practical techniques aimed at reducing the child's muteness. Minimizing the "directness" of verbal interaction can reduce the subjective feelings of threat or aggressivity that the child may experience in communicating. Clinicians have employed approaches such as covering their own mouths during speech, reducing eye contact with the child, using averted body positions, speaking in gestures (pantomime), and silent mouthing of words. Often, simple questions to the child are asked that require writing a response, tapping of the therapist's hand, or a one-word utterance. For children whose anxiety results from speech phobia, the production of a single word may be preceded by increased tension and rigidity, and followed by a sense of relief and pride, which a therapist can positively reinforce. It is unclear whether such methods are therapeutic or counterproductive.

Once the mute speech is improving, it may be anticipated that the child and parents will continue to require treatment for associated psychiatric disorders. Initial symptomatic improvement may be followed by resistance to investigating the causes and origins of the problem, by both child and parents. Both individual and family psychotherapy aimed at reducing the mutism are usually found to be slow, difficult, and disappointing. It may be helpful to focus the psychotherapies on issues related to fear, including self-esteem, separation and autonomy, and assertiveness. During the course of treatment, particularly of children with significant separation issues, missed appointments and illness may be followed by regressive behavior and speech.

Use of short-term therapy (Wright et al. 1985), phenelzine, and hospitalization have been suggested but not pursued. However, the treatment options and outlook for this disorder are beginning to expand (Dow et al. 1995).

Clinical Comment

There remains a clear need for systematic studies of virtually all aspects of selective mutism, including the essentially uncharted territory of its natural course, epidemiology, genetics and biological features, etiological role of abuse and neglect, and treatment outcomes. Investigation of this disorder, which has been dormant for years, has now been enlivened by the suggestion that selective mutism may be a childhood symptom of social phobia (Black and Uhde 1992) and the growing interest in its comorbidity and developmental relationships to other psychiatric disorders (especially anxiety and mood disorders), the effects of abuse and neglect, the possible etiological role of (developmental) stranger anxiety, and the "serotonergic view" of the disorder. At the level of clinical care, however, each case of this uncommon disorder teaches its own lessons.

REACTIVE ATTACHMENT DISORDER OF INFANCY OR EARLY CHILDHOOD

Following physical or emotional abuse by a caregiver, young children and even infants may display abnormal interpersonal behavior, altered emotional excitability, and cognitive changes. It is inferred that the abnormal behavior results from disordered development of early interpersonal attachment (Table 23–38). Reactive attachment disorder encompasses both increased and decreased social interactiveness after trauma in infancy or early childhood.

A variety of abusive conditions during childhood may lead to this posttraumatic syndrome. According to DSM-IV, reactive attachment disorder can be the consequence of physical or sexual abuse, caregiving by emotionally disturbed individuals, inappropriate parental emotional involvement, neglect, enduring posttraumatic reactions, instability of home environments, and impaired attachment or bonding (Tibbits-Kleber and Howell 1985). However, any failure of normal development may be labeled as reactive attachment disorder if preceded by clear failures in child care.

The hallmark of reactive attachment disorder is the appearance of grossly disturbed interpersonal relations following grossly inadequate early care in childhood, with or without evidence of their linkage. The pediatric label of nonorganic failure to thrive (NFTT) is a broader diagnostic category that encompasses 1) cases of reactive attachment disorder that involve physical growth retardation, 2) the DSM-IV category of feeding and eating disorders of infancy or early childhood, and 3) some cases of retarded physical growth without prominent social abnormalities.

Clinical Description

In normal development, an infant is expected to show overt behavioral signs of attachment and bonding to a parent by age 8 months. A variety of behavioral, cognitive, and

TABLE 23–38. **DSM-IV diagnostic criteria for reactive attachment disorder of infancy or early childhood**

A. Markedly disturbed and developmentally inappropriate social relatedness in most contexts, beginning before age 5 years, as evidenced by either (1) or (2):

  (1) Persistent failure to initiate or respond in a developmentally appropriate fashion to most social interactions, as manifest by excessively inhibited, hypervigilant, or highly ambivalent and contradictory responses (e.g., the child may respond to caregivers with a mixture of approach, avoidance, and resistance to comforting, or may exhibit frozen watchfulness).

  (2) Diffuse attachments as manifest by indiscriminate sociability with marked inability to exhibit appropriate selective attachments (e.g., excessive familiarity with relative strangers or lack of selectivity in choice of attachment figures).

B. The disturbance in criterion A is not accounted for solely by developmental delay (as in mental retardation) and does not meet criteria for a pervasive developmental disorder.

C. Pathogenic care as evidenced by at least one of the following:

  (1) Persistent disregard of the child's basic emotional needs for comfort, stimulation, and affection.

  (2) Persistent disregard of the child's basic physical needs.

  (3) Repeated changes of primary caregiver that prevent formation of stable attachments (e.g., frequent changes in foster care).

D. There is a presumption that the care in criterion C is responsible for the disturbed behavior in criterion A (e.g., the disturbances in criterion A began following the pathogenic care in criterion C).

Specify type:

Inhibited type: if criterion A1 predominates in the clinical presentation
Disinhibited type: if criterion A2 predominates in the clinical presentation

---

affective presentations may be seen at different ages. In children, odd social responsiveness, weak interpersonal attachment, apathy or inappropriate excitability, and mood abnormalities are common. In early infancy, diagnosis is based on the failure to achieve developmental expectations: lack of eye tracking or responsive smiling by age 2 months and failure to play simple games or reach out to be picked up by 5 months.

Children with reactive attachment disorder may present with the "inhibited" or "disinhibited" subtypes.

"Inhibited" infants with reactive attachment disorder may appear lethargic or show little activity. Their body movements are weak. Sleep is excessive and disrupted, and weight gain is slow. They may seem spacey and unengaged or, alternately, hypervigilant and avoidant. The infants have little interactive interest in the environment and often resist being held. As young children, individuals with reactive attachment disorder may appear withdrawn, passive, or disinterested in people, or they may respond to interpersonal stimuli in odd or inconsistent ways. Children who have the "inhibited" subtype of reactive attachment disorder seem to have closed down on incoming stimulation, interpersonal and otherwise, as if their general responsiveness were diminished and their reactivity were inhibited.

Children with the "disinhibited" form of reactive attachment disorder may show overly rapid familiarity; they may display inappropriate touching or clinging, excessive interest, and a sort of unmodulated "enthusiasm" with people, even in a first-time meeting. They readily switch their intense "attachment" from one person to another, acting as though people are interchangeable parts and repetitively reenacting a few rigid "scripts" in their interactions. Their behavior appears to convey the message "You can take care of me forever." Their immediate emotional involvement may seem initially gratifying to a stranger, but it is also experienced as weird or unusual.

In older children, reactive attachment disorder typically presents with socialization defects. In the absence of socialization problems, such a child might be labeled with a V code (parent-child relational problem) or diagnosed as having PTSD. At present, the DSM designation of this disorder has led to little further research on reactive attachment disorder, either biological or psychosocial.

Epidemiology

Approximately 1%–5% of pediatric hospital admissions are due to *nonorganic failure to thrive*, and the prevalence in the relevant age range is roughly estimated at 1% (Zeanah and Embe 1995).

Etiology

The etiology of this disorder is written into its definition, which is a unique occurrence in DSM-IV. Previous abuse, neglect, or impaired caregiving is definitionally required, and the disease label suggests that a disruption of parent-child bonding is the crucial mechanism. Although it emphasizes the interpersonal or social effects on the child, the definition implies that the parenting (i.e., the parent) is the cause of the child's problem.

The failure to offer normal instinctive parenting, or even minimally adequate parenting, is typically the result of an overt emotional or psychiatric problem afflicting parent or caregiver. The obstacles to parenting may include major depressive disorder, psychosis, substance abuse, or mental retardation; child phobia or fear of committing infanticide; frustration with a "difficult" child, active hostility, or indifference; parental isolation, poverty, or poor education; or grossly disturbed family life. These factors are presumed to have a disruptive effect on child-caregiver attachment that is expressed in the child's impaired social behavior (Call 1984).

A specific suppression of growth hormone release has been described in infants with reactive attachment disorder, and it has been interpreted as closely resembling the growth hormone hyposecretion in rat pups during maternal separation (Katz et al. 1996). It is unclear whether growth hormone suppression is a cause, a result, or an unrelated phenomenon (perhaps related instead to separation anxiety or hyperexploratory behavior). As is always the case, the relevance of this putative animal model to clinical matters is speculative. More extensive research has been conducted on pediatric failure to thrive, but that disorder is sufficiently different from reactive attachment disorder to prevent meaningful comparison. Nonetheless, these studies might suggest directions for further research on reactive attachment disorder.

Course and Prognosis

If this disorder is untreated, the course may vary from spontaneous remission to malnutrition, infection, or death. Both nutritional and psychosocial deprivation may result in long-term behavioral changes, hyperactivity, short stature, and lowered IQ. If emotional deprivation continues but enforced feeding is provided, children may show improved weight gain. However, even when body growth is preserved, ongoing emotional deprivation can cause depressive-type changes and developmental delays in infants. This consequence appears to be illustrated in the historical entity of *hospitalism* (Provence and Lipton 1962). Improved body growth does not guarantee a normal developmental outcome. Specific predictors of behavioral, cognitive, and physical sequelae have not been identified.

As longitudinal studies of reactive attachment disorder become available, more specific phenomenological and developmental detail will be known about this disorder, which has a clearly specified cause but no clearly defined outcome. The relationship of reactive attachment disorder to the subsequent appearance of mood disorders, anxiety disorders, eating disorders, and personality disorders has not been determined.

Evaluation and Differential Diagnosis

A diagnosis of reactive attachment disorder generally requires professional observation of mother-child interactions in the medical setting and at home. A home visit is central to evaluation and diagnosis. Psychiatric evaluation of the parents is essential. When possible, siblings should be assessed regarding their psychosocial experiences, social functioning, and possible psychiatric disorders. Medical assessment of the child patient is required to rule out chronic physical illness (organic FTT), homeostatic sleep and feeding disorders, food refusal, malnutrition, neurological disease, and sensory deficit.

The diagnosis is essentially confirmed by the child's symptomatic improvement following the provision of adequate care. The evaluation of the child's response can be most readily conducted in a hospital, which permits direct evaluation of the child and the parent-child interactions. Hospitalization also allows a multidisciplinary team to make the observations necessary for diagnosis. An alternative to hospitalization is a planned parent-child separation, which involves removal of the child to a different environment in which the caregiver has the capacity for care and observation.

Assessment of caregiver-child interactions can involve a high degree of sophistication and technical skill. Minimally, it involves observation of the caregiver's simple capacity for physical holding, physical and interpersonal stimulation, empathy, attentiveness to the child's behavior, fear of the child, anger, or indifference.

With or without hospitalization, home visits are generally indicated for evaluation of the adequacy of housing, safety, nutrition, stability, regularity of actions during the day and over time, use of space, supervision, other home dwellers, behavioral standards, and parental involvement with the child. Multiple shifts of routine, caregiver, home, and environment may undermine the consistency of the child's life and contribute to the development of reactive attachment disorder.

Although home visits can contribute to the evaluation of any psychiatric patient (including adults), this is the only psychiatric disorder for which a home visit is virtually required. In practice, however, parents may be reluctant to allow even one home visit. Parents may be defensive, angry, and ashamed concerning the professional's interest in home visits. The handling of privacy and personal concerns presents a challenge to the clinician to maintain empathy for the caregivers, especially if a child's suffering is at stake. Issues of privacy often generate sharp limitations on the evaluation of these children.

Many parents of children with this disorder are aware that their child is not receiving what is needed. They may wish to give care but find themselves incapable of providing it. It is a clinical error to presume that parents of children with reactive attachment disorder are not interested in what is best for the child. Parents often are gratified to receive outside assistance, help for the child (despite the sense of humiliation at "failing" to provide), and support and treatment for themselves.

Psychiatric evaluation of the parents is an essential component of the overall assessment. Particularly for the primary caregiver, the evaluation needs to be thorough, including the full range of debilitating psychiatric disorders and psychosocial stressors. Assessment must be made of the extent or lack of supports, the onset of the psychiatric disorder in relation to the period of neglect, the possibility of physical or sexual abuse, and the causes of any previous treatment failures. Child abuse and, at times, neglect may not be readily identifiable during the initial weeks or months of the treatment; they may not be revealed until months later, when the parents become more comfortable and trusting.

Treatment

Basic medical care, provision of adequate caregiving, parental education, and parental psychiatric treatment are generally needed to treat reactive attachment disorder of infancy or early childhood. Medical hospitalization, which is useful in evaluation, is generally justified also for performing this massive intervention.

The use of hospitalization is much preferable to parent-child separation for infants or very young children, but it can be useful for children at any age. Both removal from the home environment and hospitalization permit the establishment of normal feeding and physiological patterns as well as the opportunity for evaluating and expanding the parents' caregiving capacities.

Given the complexity of medical and psychiatric problems, the need for proficiency in baby care and nurturance, the required sensitivity in managing the parents, and the frequent need for social services and legal procedures, it is a major advantage for treatment to be delivered by a specialized team working in a hospital. This multidisciplinary team typically provides care on a pediatric inpatient unit and in an outpatient clinic, with a determined emphasis on coordination and continuity.

Hospitalization or treatment intervention typically leads to a major improvement in the clinical status of the child. This improvement in response to treatment is considered confirmation of the diagnosis of reactive attachment disorder. Clinical nonresponsiveness implies the presence of a different disorder, an additional disorder, or persistent physical damage resulting from extreme medical complications that occurred before treatment was begun.

If treatment is initiated long after the period of abuse and neglect, when early attachment problems are already a part of the past history and abnormal social behavior is prominent, standard psychiatric evaluation and treatment of child and parents are indicated. Hospitalization is not crucial if the child is no longer in the abusive phase. Although there are no controlled studies of treatment outcome, current medical and psychiatric practice involves multimodal therapy with child and parents.

Clinical Comment

The creation of a diagnostic category that entails a reasonable but hypothetical mechanism is an unusual occurrence in the DSM-IV system. Confusion may arise in individual cases if socialization defects are not preceded by clear antecedent abuse or neglect or if demonstrably disordered early attachment results in behavioral or affective symptoms without sociability deficits. The linkage between an early traumatic experience and subsequent symptoms may be speculative in individual cases, but repeated clinical observations of this coupling in many children allows the diagnosis to be defined by its apparent etiology.

In individual cases of reactive attachment disorder, the value of an etiology-based definition can appear questionable (Richters et al. 1994). The limitations often placed on the availability of accurate historical and social information may preclude fulfillment of the etiological criterion, forcing clinicians to improvise. The etiological criterion is also questionable because of the possibility, for example, that this condition is a developmental disorder such as atypical development (pervasive developmental disorder) and that the attachment deficits are not essential to this disorder.

On the other hand, it is a valuable experience for psychiatrists to be able to treat a neuropsychiatric disorder with a clear-cut etiology. Furthermore, the treatment of disorders of infancy, with major medical and psychophysiological complications as well as psychiatric liabilities, constitutes an important expansion of the clinical interests and activities of psychiatric practitioners.

STEREOTYPIC MOVEMENT DISORDER

Certain repetitive and purposeless motor behaviors may be seen in young children, sensory-deprived (deaf or blind) people, or individuals with mental retardation, pervasive developmental disorders, and some psychotic disorders (e.g., schizophrenia, mood disorders with psychomotor

changes). Many stereotypies appear to have a self-stimulatory component, but the diagnosis of stereotypic movement disorder is made only if these repetitive behaviors cause functional interference or physical injury (Table 23–39). Self-injurious behavior is a common and clinically important form of stereotypic behavior.

Clinical Description

Examples of stereotypies include head banging, body rocking, hand flapping, whirling, stereotyped laughter, thumb sucking, hair fingering, facial touching, eye poking, object biting, self-biting, self-scratching, self-hitting, teeth grinding, and breath holding. Although one behavioral stereotypy may predominate, it is typical for several stereotypies to co-occur. Different stereotypies may become prominent at different times. The rhythm of the repetitive behavior may be slow and gentle, fast and energetic, or even violently energized. Sometimes waves of increasing and decreasing energy may be seen over the course of several minutes. Frequency may increase during periods of tension, frustration, boredom, and isolation, as well as just before bedtime.

Two of the most common presentations are head bang-

TABLE 23-39. **DSM-IV diagnostic criteria for stereotypic movement disorder**

A. Repetitive, seemingly driven, and nonfunctional motor behavior (e.g., hand shaking or waving, body rocking, head banging, mouthing of objects, self-biting, picking at skin or bodily orifices, hitting own body).

B. The behavior markedly interferes with normal activities or results in self-inflicted bodily injury that requires medical treatment (or would result in an injury if preventive measures were not used).

C. If mental retardation is present, the stereotypic or self-injurious behavior is of sufficient severity to become a focus of treatment.

D. The behavior is not better accounted for by compulsion (as in obsessive-compulsive disorder), a tic (as in tic disorder), a stereotypy that is part of a pervasive developmental disorder, or hair pulling (as in trichotillomania).

E. The behavior is not due to the direct physiological effects of a substance or a general medical condition.

F. The behavior persists for 4 weeks or longer.

Specify if:

With self-injurious behavior: if the behavior results in bodily damage that requires specific treatment (or that would result in bodily damage if protective measures were not used)

ing and body rocking. Head banging may last for hours, particularly at bedtime or on morning awakening. The head banging can be soft and quiet, occurring during periods of isolation or boredom, and appear to have a self-stimulatory and pleasurable quality. Alternatively, head banging may occur during a clearly unpleasurable state. During a temper tantrum, a child may thrash on the floor, with limbs flailing and head banging vigorously against the floor or wall.

Body rocking may be slow swaying, with quiet murmuring or singing, or it may be violent enough to move a child's bed across the room. Whether pleasurable or unpleasurable, there is typically a self-absorbed quality of mentation.

Epidemiology

Approximately 15%–20% of a normal pediatric population may have a history of transient stereotypies, but there are no available data regarding the prevalence of stereotypic movement disorder with physical injury or functional interference. Stereotypic behaviors show equal gender prevalence. There are no data regarding socioeconomic influences. There is a higher prevalence in individuals with mental retardation. Among institutionalized people with severe and profound mental retardation, about 60% have stereotypic movement disorder, and 15% engage in self-injurious behaviors (Schroeder et al. 1979).

Etiology

There is no clear etiology, but several theories have been advanced, and multiple contributing or interacting factors are probably involved.

Organic influences are supported by the increased incidence of stereotypic movement disorder in individuals with abnormal brain structure or function, such as mental retardation, auditory or visual sensory deficit (blindness, deafness), brain disease (seizures, postinfection, metabolic abnormality), psychotic disorder, and drug-induced psychosis (amphetamines).

An etiological role of self-stimulation (or autoerotic stimulation) is suggested by the characteristic self-absorbed and apparently pleasurable appearance, and by the occurrence of this behavior during periods of boredom or physical isolation. Self-stimulation through repetitive physical activity may be satisfying if normal forms of stimulation are unavailable or ineffective. For example, patients with extreme impairments in cognition may body-rock if the ordinary array of sights and sounds is not as interpretable or pleasurable as the physical activity. Alternatively, a tension-relieving purpose is plausible, because these be-

haviors increase during periods of anxiety, tension, and frustration. An arousal factor has also been proposed, because the behaviors sometimes are more evident at bedtime or on arising in the morning. Thus, head banging during temper tantrums may be viewed in terms of self-stimulation, tension discharge, or arousal.

Self-injurious behaviors are particularly difficult to explain etiologically. Theories are easy to generate, but they are often shaped by counterintuitive clinical observations. For example, protective physical restraints that inhibit self-injurious behavior are welcomed and found to be relaxing by some people, yet removal of the restraints may lead promptly to a marked return or increase in stereotyped behavior. These patients can experience pain (in response to a pinch or electric shock) and, at times, seem to try to protect themselves from self-injury. These observations are difficult to integrate in terms of a general capacity to feel or avoid discomfort. It has been theorized that such observations concerning self-injurious behavior suggest a form of pain sensitivity that can be drastically altered by emotion, situation, or physiology in some unusual manner in patients with specific psychiatric disorders (e.g., autistic disorder).

Although there is an overrepresentation of stereotypic movement disorder among individuals with a history of neglect, understimulation, and mental retardation, these behaviors can be seen in patients with normal intelligence and normal caregiving experiences.

Certain types of stereotypies occur in normal development, particularly during the period of learning of motor patterns and rhythms (Kravitz and Boehm 1971). These behaviors appear to function as motoric exercises, aiding the child in feeling and acting within their neuromuscular/motoric system. Family history studies, biological markers, and physiological studies of stereotypic movement disorder are unavailable.

Course and Prognosis

Certain stereotypies begin as early as 6–12 months, such as head banging and body rocking. These behaviors typically resolve in 80% of normal children by age 4, although more subtle habits may persist, such as finger tapping or teeth grinding (DeLissovoy 1962). In people with mental retardation or pervasive developmental disorders, such early-onset stereotypies may persist for years. Later onset stereotypies may be descriptively similar, but they appear episodically and only during periods of anxiety or stress.

A complication of stereotypic movement disorder results from the attention that the behaviors (especially self-injurious behaviors) invoke from caregivers. These various forms of attention and care may unwittingly become sustaining behavioral reinforcers, leading to more intense or enduring symptoms.

Evaluation and Differential Diagnosis

When the disorder begins during infancy or very early childhood, evaluation for concurrent mental retardation and other developmental disabilities is appropriate. For later onset disorder, it is necessary to evaluate for agitation associated with psychosis or mood disorders as well as for mental retardation and pervasive developmental disorders. In some cases, the use of psychostimulant medications and other dopamine agonists may aggravate or produce stereotypic behaviors; therefore, evaluation of current medication use is appropriate.

Stereotypic movement disorder is not diagnosed if the symptoms can be explained by concomitant tic disorder or obsessive-compulsive disorder. Stereotypies may be distinguished from tics or compulsions when there is a self-stimulatory or pleasurable component. Although tics or compulsions may carry a tension-discharging function, they are not experienced as pleasurable.

Treatment

The symptoms of stereotypic movement disorder are often treatment resistant. Behavioral techniques, especially overcorrection, have been found most effective. Interventions involving anxiety reduction, sensory stimulation, and the offering of alternatives to self-stimulation are also helpful.

Although behavioral methods usually rely on reward systems when possible, positive reinforcement in treating stereotypic movement disorder is generally not effective when used alone. Overcorrection has the best empirical support, but it is a coercive treatment that may invoke anger, oppositionalism, and symptom substitution.

Blocking pleasurable feedback from self-stimulation can be useful. The particular technique depends on the sensory mode of predominant self-stimulation. For self-stimulation based on sound, a white noise or tape-recorded music may be considered. For rocking, a vibrator taped to the hand may distract from other kinesthetic self-stimulation. For finger waving, beads on a string may provide alternative proprioceptive stimulation. For visual stimulation, ambient lighting may be altered or a bubble-blower may be provided. Such distraction from self-stimulation and use of stimuli substitution can be helpful in some individuals (Baroff 1986).

In case of noninjurious behaviors, extinction (ignoring the symptom rather than giving attention) is sometimes suggested. In treating significant self-injurious behavior, mildly aversive stimuli might need to be employed, for example, facial puffs of air, sharp (tabasco) or sour (lemon) tastes, or scratchy skin contact (burlap). Physical restraints may also be used protectively or as a reward for increasing periods of abstaining from self-injury.

Neuroleptics or diphenhydramine may be helpful in some cases. Psychostimulants and other dopamine agonists may aggravate or induce the appearance of stereotypic behaviors. Because seizure disorders are commonly present in patients with self-injurious behaviors, anticonvulsants may be considered for some of these individuals. The opiate blocker naltrexone has been effective in reducing self-injurious behaviors, particularly in patients with mental retardation, presumably by blocking endorphin-mediated pleasure sensations (Sandman 1991).

Increased parental attention and involvement during performance of the stereotypies may be therapeutic, similar to treatment of apparent self-stimulation in rumination disorder. For example, during head banging, parents are advised to hold or sit with the child, holding and protecting the head until banging stops. Although this process can reduce the overall duration, it may take a long time, and parents often have difficulty in following through on suggestions to provide additional time with or attention to a child.

When stereotypies originate from a psychotic disorder, increased attention may be unhelpful or counterproductive. Treatment with antipsychotic or other sedative medications may be needed.

Some clinicians employ simple and practical management techniques, such as directing a child to head-bang on a soft surface, combined with interventions for stress reduction. Controlled studies of most treatments of stereotypic movement disorder are lacking.

Clinical Comment

This disorder, encompassing a variety of behavioral stereotypies, allows the diagnostic labeling of certain behavioral problems at any age. Although it may be found to represent a distinct diagnostic category in its own right, it is advisable at present to evaluate aggressively for possible concurrent mental retardation, developmental disorders, psychotic disorders, and agitation associated with mood or anxiety disorders (or related incipient or precursor conditions) in all patients with stereotypic movement disorder.

STANDARDIZED ASSESSMENT INSTRUMENTS FOR CHILDREN AND ADOLESCENTS

Structured and semistructured interview protocols, checklists, questionnaires, and rating scales have been developed for the evaluation and follow-up of many child psychiatric disorders (Rapoport et al. 1985). Similar to instruments developed for evaluating the major diagnoses in adults, these instruments are useful in clinical practice as well as research protocols (Achenbach and Ruffle 1988). Available instruments can provide a systematic review of general behaviors, psychiatric symptoms, and all DSM-IV diagnoses of childhood, as well as a global assessment of general functioning (Rutter et al. 1987).

Standardized instruments can yield findings that differ from those of clinical evaluations. The sources of these differences are probably numerous, and neither approach can be rigidly interpreted as correct. It is helpful to use standardized assessment procedures as a supplement to the clinical evaluation of children.

The standardized instruments are more systematic and complete than is scanning for disorders by clinicians. Clinicians tend to underreport substance abuse and related disorders in adolescents and to miss bipolar disorders in adolescents and children.

Children and parents each contribute useful but different observations. In general, children are more effective in reporting mood symptoms, and parents are more effective in reporting behavioral symptoms. However, features of conduct disorder may be reported at higher rates either by children or by parents, depending on the clinical situation. It is likely that children report more when the information will not be self-indicting, but less if punishment or treatment is being considered.

It is clear that no single informant can give a full description of a child. Children, teachers, parents, relatives, community members, and clinicians all view the child from different settings and with different biases. The gender, age, and psychiatric diagnosis of the child and the parents might influence the nature of observations. However, the differences between parents' and teachers' observations, and between two parents' observations, often relate to genuine variations in the behavior of children in different settings and with different people. Studies comparing the data of different reporters, evaluation techniques, and diagnostic subgroups are clarifying the sources of complexity that have long been inherent in the clinical process.

The standardized diagnostic instruments will facilitate epidemiological studies of the major psychiatric disorders in the general child and adolescent population. The classic work of Rutter, on the Isle of Wight and in inner-city London, has provided the first major comprehensive set of epidemiological data on psychiatric disorders in children (Rutter 1989; Rutter et al. 1970, 1976). Current estimates for prevalence and gender ratio for many childhood-onset disorders are still preliminary and sometimes vague (Table 23–40). These data are expected to improve as more information becomes available using current diagnostic criteria and standardized assessments of childhood psychopathology.

SUMMARY

Multiple comorbid diagnoses are typical in children and adolescents, and all psychiatric disorders in youth can induce developmental complications. Moreover, all the etiologic factors that give rise to psychiatric disorders (biogenetic, familial, intrapsychic, interpersonal, socioeconomic, and sociocultural) can also distort, delay, or strengthen a child's development independently of the psychiatric disorders. Developmental effects may manifest in multiple symptoms and realms of functioning, often cumulatively and enduringly.

The multidimensional interactions of comorbid conditions, etiologic factors, and developmental complications are immensely complicated. This complexity is barely reduced by its tendency to organize and snowball into final common pathways of child psychopathology. Final common nonspecific developmental complications include progressive learning lags, declining school grades, school failure, low self-esteem, being scapegoated, disorders of social assertiveness, demoralization, and societal dropout.

Psychiatric treatment too interacts with all these factors, adding another dimension to the system of intermeshing forces that create and surround a child.

This vast complexity can lead to murky theory and overreliance on impressionism in the clinical process. This impressionism demands more discipline rather than less in thinking about individual psychopathology.

REFERENCES

Abikoff H, Courtney ME, Szeibel PJ et al: The effects of auditory stimulation on the arithmetic performance of children with ADHD and nondisabled children. Journal of Learning Disabilities 29:238–246, 1996

Achenbach TM, Edelbrock C: Manual for the Child Behavioral Checklist and Revised Child Behavioral Profile. Burlington, University of Vermont Psychology Department, 1983

Achenbach TM, McConaughy SH: Empirically Based Assessment of Child and Adolescent Psychopathology. Newbury Park, CA, Sage, 1997

TABLE 23–40. Estimates of epidemiological characteristics of disorders usually first diagnosed in infancy, childhood, or adolescence

Diagnosis	Gender ratio (male:female)	Lifetime prevalence (per 100,000)
Conduct disorder	3:1–5:1	3,000–15,000
Reading disorder	3:1–4:1	3,000–15,000
Oppositional defiant disorder	2:1–3:1	2,000–15,000
Attention-deficit/hyperactivity disorder	3:1–10:1	3,000–10,000
Phonological disorder		3,000–10,000
Expressive language disorder	3:1–4:1	3,000–10,000 (1,000 for severe cases)
Mathematics disorder	2:1	3,000–10,000
Motor skills disorder		4,000–8,000
Mixed receptive/expressive language disorder	1:1	1,000–10,000 (500 for severe cases)
Separation anxiety disorder	1:1–2:1	600–6,000
Stuttering	3:1–4:1	1,000–4,000
Mental retardation	1:1–3:1	1,000–3,000
Tic disorders	3:1–9:1	1,000–2,000
Enuresis	2:1–3:1	1,000 (males at age 18)
Encopresis	4:1	1,000–1,500 (at age 5)
Selective mutism	1:1–2:1	180
Pervasive developmental disorder not otherwise specified	3:1–4:1	100–200
Tourette's disorder	3:1–9:1	40–80
Autistic disorder	3:1–4:1	30–50
Asperger's disorder	3:1–4:1	5–100
Rett's disorder	All female	5–15
Childhood disintegrative disorder	> 4:1	1–4
Disorder of written expression	3:1–4:1	?
Pica		?
Rumination disorder	1:1	?
Stereotypy/habit disorder	?	?
Reactive attachment disorder	?	?

Note. These estimates are based on current and often preliminary data from a variety of sources using different methods and diagnostic criteria. Thus, they are likely to be revised substantially as more studies become available. It is particularly important to note that the order of descending prevalence listed here is only approximate (and in some places arbitrary) because of the wide range of uncertainty and unknowns in the current prevalence estimates.

Achenbach TM, McConaughy SH: Empirically Based Assessment of Child and Adolescent Psychopathology: Practical Applications, 2nd Edition. Thousand Oaks, CA, Sage, 1997

Achenbach TM, Ruffle T: Medical Practitioners' Guide for the Child Behavior Checklist and Related Forms. Burlington, VT, University of Vermont College of Medicine, Department of Psychiatry, 1998

Aichhorn A: Wayward Youth (1925). New York, Meridian Books, 1955

Alegre S, Chacon J, Redondo L, et al: Post-traumatic tics. Rev Neurol 24:1280–1282, 1996

Allen AJ, Leonard HL, Swedo SE: Case study: A new infection-triggered, autoimmune subtype of pediatric OCD and Tourette's syndrome. J Am Acad Child Adolesc Psychiatry 34:307–311, 1995

Althaus M, Vink HJ, Minderaa RB, et al: Lack of effect of clonidine on stuttering in children. Am J Psychiatry 152:1087–1089, 1995

Aman MG: Assessing Psychopathology and Behavior Problems in Persons with Mental Retardation: A Review of Available Instruments (DHHS Publ No ADM-91-1712). Rockville, MD, U.S. Department of Health and Human Services, 1991

Aman MG, Kern RA: The efficacy of folic acid in fragile X syndrome and other developmental disabilities. J Child Adolesc Psychopharmacol 1:285–295, 1991

American Association on Mental Retardation: Mental Retardation: Definition, Classification, and Systems of Supports, 9th Edition. Washington, DC, American Association on Mental Retardation, 1992

American Psychiatric Association: Diagnostic and Statistical Manual of Mental Disorders, 3rd Edition, Revised. Washington, DC, American Psychiatric Association, 1987

American Psychiatric Association: Diagnostic and Statistical Manual of Mental Disorders, 4th Edition. Washington, DC, American Psychiatric Association, 1994

Anderson JC, Williams S, McGee R, et al: DSM-III disorders in preadolescent children. Prevalence in a large sample from the general population. Arch Gen Psychiatry 44:69–76, 1987

Ankjaer-Jensen A, Sejr TE: Costs of the treatment of enuresis nocturna. Health economic consequences of alternative methods in the treatment of enuresis nocturna. Ugeskr Laeger 156:4355–4360, 1994

Aram DM, Ekelman BL, Nation JE: Preschoolers with language disorder: 10 years later. J Speech Hear Res 27:232–244, 1984

Arnell H, Hjälmas K, Jägervall M, et al: The genetics of primary nocturnal enuresis: inheritance and suggestion of a second major gene on chromosome 12q. J Med Genet 34:360–365, 1997

Aronson M, Hagberg B, Gillberg C: Attention deficits and autistic spectrum problems in children exposed to alcohol during gestation: a follow-up study. Dev Med Child Neurol 39:583–587, 1997

Arredondo DE, Butler SF: Affective comorbidity in psychiatrically hospitalized adolescents with conduct disorder or oppositional defiant disorder: should conduct disorder be treated with mood stabilizers? J Child Adolesc Psychopharmacol 4:151–158, 1994

Attwood T: Asperger's Syndrome: A Guide for Parents and Professionals. Bristol, PA, Jessica Kingsley Publishers, 1997

August GJ, Stewart MA, Holmes CS: A four-year follow-up of boys with and without conduct disorder. Br J Psychiatry 143:192–198, 1983

August GJ, Realmuto GM, MacDonald AW III et al: Prevalence of ADHD and comorbid disorders among elementary school children screened for disruptive behavior. J Abnorm Child Psychol 24:571–595, 1996

Bakwin H: The genetics of enuresis, in Bladder Control and Enuresis. Edited by Kolvin RC, MacKeith RC, Meadow SR. London, W. Heinemann Medical Books, 1973

Barkley RA (ed): Attention Deficit Hyperactivity Disorder: A Handbook for Diagnosis and Treatment. New York, Guilford, 1990

Barkley RA, Cunningham CE: Do stimulant drugs improve the academic performance of hyperkinetic children? A review of outcome studies. Clin Pediatr 17:85–92, 1978

Baroff GS: Mental Retardation: Nature, Cause and Management. New York, Hemisphere, 1986

Barrett PM, Dadds MR, Rapee RM: Family treatment of childhood anxiety: a controlled trial. J Consult Clin Psychol 64:3333–3342, 1996

Battaglia M, Bertella S, Politi E, et al: Age at onset of panic disorder: influence of familial liability to the disease and of childhood separation anxiety disorder. Am J Psychiatry 152(9):1362–1364, 1995

Bauman ML: Microscopic neuroanatomical abnormalities in autism. Pediatrics 87 (suppl):791–796, 1991

Baumgardner TL, Singer HS, Denckla MB, et al: Corpus callosum morphology in children with Tourette syndrome and attention deficit hyperactivity disorder. Neurology 47:477–842, 1996

Beitchman JH, Nair R, Clegg M, et al: Prevalence of psychiatric disorders in children with speech and language disorders. J Am Acad Child Psychiatry 25:528–535, 1986

Bellinger D, Leviton A, Waternaux C, et al: Longitudinal analyses of prenatal and postnatal lead exposure and early cognitive development. N Engl J Med 316:1037–1043, 1987

Benninga MA, Buller HA, Heymans HS, et al: Is encopresis always the result of constipation? Arch Dis Child 71:186–193, 1994

Berg I: School phobia in the children of agoraphobic women. Br J Psychiatry 128:86–89, 1976

Bernstein GA, Borchardt CM: Anxiety disorders of childhood and adolescence: a critical review. J Am Acad Child Adolesc Psychiatry 30:519–532, 1991

Berry CA, Shaywitz SE, Shaywitz BA: Girls with attention deficit disorder: a silent minority? A report on behavioral and cognitive characteristics. Pediatrics 76:801–809, 1985

Bharucha KJ, Sethi KD: Tardive tourettism after exposure to neuroleptic therapy. Mov Disord 10:791–793, 1995

Biederman J, Rosenbaum JF, Hirschfeld DR, et al: Psychiatric correlates of behavioral inhibition in young children of parents with and without psychiatric disorders. Arch Gen Psychiatry 47:21–26, 1990

Biederman J, Faraone SV, Keenan K, et al: Further evidence for family genetic risk factors in attention deficit hyperactivity disorder: patterns of comorbidity in probands and relatives in psychiatrically and pediatrically referred samples. Arch Gen Psychiatry 49:728–738, 1992

Biederman J, Faraone S, Mick E, et al: Attention-deficit hyperactivity disorder and juvenile mania: an overlooked comorbidity? J Am Acad Child Adolesc Psychiatry 35:997–1008, 1996

Birch HG, Richardson SA, Baird D, et al: Mental Subnormality in the Community: A Clinical and Epidemiological Study. Baltimore, MD, Williams & Wilkins, 1970

Bithoney WG, Snyder J, Michalek J, et al: Childhood ingestions as symptoms of family distress. Am J Dis Child 139:456–459, 1985

Black B, Uhde TW: Elective mutism as a variant of social phobia. J Am Acad Child Adolesc Psychiatry 31:1090–1094, 1992

Blum K, Sheridan PJ, Wood RC, et al: The D$_2$ dopamine receptor gene as a determinant of reward deficiency syndrome. J R Soc Med 89:396–400, 1996

Bonde HV, Andersen JP, Rosenkilde P: Nocturnal enuresis: change of nocturnal voiding pattern during alarm treatment. Scand J Urol Nephrol 28:349–352, 1994

Boris M, Mandel FS: Foods and additives are common causes of the attention deficit hyperactive disorder in children. Ann Allergy 72:462–468, 1994

Bower WF, Moore KH, Shepherd RB, et al: The epidemiology of childhood enuresis in Australia. Br J Urol 78:602–606, 1996

Bradley L, Bryant PE: Categorizing sounds and learning to read: a causal connection. Nature 301:419–421, 1983

Breakey J: The role of diet and behaviour in childhood. J Paediatr Child Health 33:190–194, 1997

Bregman JD: Current developments in the understanding of mental retardation, Part 2: psychopathology. J Am Acad Child Adolesc Psychiatry 30:861–872, 1991

Bregman JD, Hodapp RM: Current developments in the understanding of mental retardation, Part 1: biological and phenomenological perspectives. J Am Acad Child Adolesc Psychiatry 30:707–719, 1991

Bregman JD, Dykens E, Watson M, et al: Fragile-X syndrome: variability of phenotypic expression. J Am Acad Child Psychiatry 26:463–471, 1987

Brett PM, Curtis D, Robertson MM, et al: Exclusion of the 5-HT1A serotonin neuroreceptor and tryptophan oxygenase genes in a large British kindred multiply affected with Tourette's syndrome, chronic motor tics, and obsessive-compulsive behavior. Am J Psychiatry 152:437–440, 1995

Bruck M: Persistence of dyslexics' phonological awareness deficits. Dev Psychol 28:874–886, 1992

Bruun RD: The natural history of Tourette's syndrome, in Tourette's Syndrome and Tic Disorders: Clinical Understanding and Treatment. Edited by Cohen D, Bruun R, Leckman J. New York, Wiley, 1988

Buitelaar JK, van der Gaag RJ, Swaab-Barneveld H, et al: Pindolol and methylphenidate in children with attention-deficit hyperactivity disorder. Clinical efficacy and side-effects. J Child Psychol Psychiatry 37:587–595, 1996

Bull R, Johnston RS: J Exp Child Psychol 65:1–24, 1997

Butler SF, Arredondo DE, McCloskey V: Affective comorbidity in children and adolescents with attention deficit hyperactivity disorder. Ann Clin Psychiatry 7:51–55, 1995

Cadoret RJ, Yates WR, Troughton E, et al: Genetic-environmental interaction in the genesis of aggressivity and conduct disorders. Arch Gen Psychiatry 52:916–924, 1995

Caione P, Arena F, Biraghi M, et al: Nocturnal enuresis and daytime wetting: a multicentric trial with oxybutynin and desmopressin. Eur Urol 31:459–463, 1997

Call JD: Child abuse and neglect in infancy: sources of hostility within the parent-infant dyad and disorders of attachment in infancy. Child Abuse Negl 8:185–202, 1984

Campbell M, Adams PB, Small AM, et al: Lithium in hospitalized aggressive children with conduct disorder: A double-blind and placebo-controlled study. J Am Acad Child Adolesc Psychiatry 34:445–453, 1995a

Campbell M, Kafantaris V, Cueva JE: An update on the use of lithium carbonate in aggressive children and adolescents with conduct disorder. Psychopharmacol Bull 31:93–102, 1995b

Campbell L, Malone MA, Kershner JR, et al: Methylphenidate slows right hemisphere processing in children with attention-deficit/hyperactivity disorder. J Child Adolesc Psychopharmacol 6:229–239, 1996

Cantwell DP, Baker L: Developmental Speech and Language Disorders. New York, Guilford, 1987

Cantwell DP, Baker L: Issues in classification of child and adolescent psychopathology. J Am Acad Child Adolesc Psychiatry 27:521–533, 1988

Cantwell DP, Baker L: Stability and natural history of DSM-III childhood diagnoses. J Am Acad Child Adolesc Psychiatry 28:691–700, 1989

Caplan R, Guthrie D, Komo S: Blink rate in children with attention-deficit-hyperactivity disorder. Biol Psychiatry 39:1032–1038, 1996

Capps L, Sigman M, Sena R, et al: Fear, anxiety and perceived control in children of agoraphobic parents. J Child Psychol Psychiatry 37:445–452, 1996

Cardon LR, Smith SD, Fulker DW, et al: Quantitative trait locus for reading disability on chromosome 6. Science 266:276–279, 1994

Casey BJ, Castellanos FX, Giedd JN, et al: Implication of right frontostriatal circuitry in response inhibition and attention-deficit/hyperactivity disorder. J Am Acad Child Adolesc Psychiatry 36:374–383, 1997

Castellanos FX, Elia J, Kruesi MJ, et al: Cerebrospinal fluid monoamine metabolites in boys with attention-deficit hyperactivity disorder. Psychiatry Res 52:305–316, 1994

Castellanos FX, Giedd JN, Marsh WL, et al: Quantitative brain magnetic resonance imaging in attention-deficit hyperactivity disorder. Arch Gen Psychiatry 53:607–616, 1996

Chabot RJ, Serfontein G: Quantitative electroencephalographic profiles of children with attention deficit disorder. Biol Psychiatry 40:951–963, 1996

Chabrol H, Fouraste R, Morón P, et al: Father-child hospitalization in separation anxiety [in Spanish]. Actas Luso Esp Neurol Psiquiatr Cienc Afines 23:223–226, 1995

Chappell PB, Riddle MA, Scahill L, et al: Guanfacine treatment of comorbid attention deficit hyperactivity disorder and Tourette's syndrome: preliminary clinical experience. J Am Acad Child Adolesc Psychiatry 34:1140–1146, 1995

Chase TN, Friedhoff AJ, Cohen DJ (eds): Tourette Syndrome: Genetics, Neurobiology, and Treatment (Advances in Neurology Series, Vol. 58). New York, Raven, 1992

Chatoor I: Infantile anorexia nervosa: a developmental disorder of separation or individuation. J Am Acad Psychoanal 17:43–64, 1989

Chatoor I, Dickson L, Einhorn A: Rumination: etiology and treatment. Pediatr Ann 13:924–929, 1984

Chatoor I, Dickson L, Schaefer S, et al: A developmental classification of feeding disorders associated with failure to thrive: diagnosis and treatment, in New Directions in Failure to Thrive: Research and Clinical Practice. Edited by Drotar D. New York, Plenum, 1985

Chee KY, Sachdev P: A controlled study of sensory tics in Gilles de la Tourette syndrome and obsessive compulsive disorder using a structured interview. J Neurol Neurosurg Psychiatry 62:188–192, 1997

Cherry KE, Matson JL, Paclawskyj TR: Psychopathology in older adults with severe and profound mental retardation. Am J Ment Retard 101:445–458, 1997

Chiaradia M, Gulson BL, MacDonald K: Contamination of houses by workers occupationally exposed in a lead-zinc-copper mine and impact on blood lead concentrations in the families. Occup Environ Med 54:117–124, 1997

Chugani DC, Muzik O, Rothermel R, et al: Altered serotonin synthesis in the dentatothalamocortical pathway in autistic boys. Ann Neurol 42:666–669, 1997

Clouse RE, Lustman PJ: Psychiatric illness and contraction abnormalities of the esophagus. N Engl J Med 309:1337–1342, 1983

Cohen D, Caparulo B, Shaywitz B: Primary childhood aphasia and childhood autism: clinical, biological and conceptual observations. Journal of the American Academy of Child Psychiatry 15:604–645, 1976

Cohen D, Caparulo B, Shaywitz B: Primary childhood aphasia and childhood autism: clinical, biological and conceptual observations. J Am Acad Child Psychiatry 4:604–645, 1979

Cohen D, Donnellan A, Rhea P (eds): Handbook of Autism and Pervasive Developmental Disorders. New York, Wiley, 1987

Cohen D, Bruun R, Leckman J: Tourette's Syndrome and Tic Disorders: Clinical Understanding and Treatment. New York, Wiley, 1988

Cohen J: Learning disabilities and adolescence: developmental considerations, in Adolescent Psychiatry, Vol 12. Edited by Feinstein SC, Sugar M, Esman AH, et al. Chicago, University of Chicago Press, 1985

Conners CK, Levin ED, Sparrow E, et al: Nicotine and attention in adult attention deficit hyperactivity disorder (ADHD). Psychopharmacol Bull 32:67–73, 1996

Cooper B (ed): Assessing the Handicaps and Needs of Mentally Retarded Children. New York, Academic Press, 1981

Courchesne E, Yeung-Courchesne R, Press GA, et al: Hypoplasia of cerebellar vermal lobules VI and VII in autism. N Engl J Med 318:1349–1354, 1988

Cox DJ, Sutphen J, Ling W, et al: Additive benefits of laxative, toilet training, and biofeedback therapies in the treatment of pediatric encopresis. J Pediatr Psychol 21:659–670, 1996

Craig A, Hancock K, Chang E, et al: A controlled trial for stuttering in persons aged 9 to 14 years. J Speech Hear Res 39:808–826, 1996

Danford DE: Pica and nutrition. Annu Rev Nutr 2:303–322, 1982

Davidson PW, Jacobson J, Cain NN, et al: Characteristics of children and adolescents with mental retardation and frequent outwardly directed aggressive behavior. Am J Ment Retard 101:244–255, 1996

DeLissovoy V: Head banging in early childhood. Child Dev 33:43–56, 1962

DeLong GR, Heinz ER: The clinical syndrome of early life bilateral hippocampal sclerosis. Ann Neurol 42:11–17, 1997

Denckla MB, Reader MJ: Education and psychosocial interventions: executive dysfunction and its consequences, in Handbook of Tourette's Syndrome and Related Tic and Behavioral Disorders. Edited by Kurlan R. New York, Marcel Dekker, 1993

Deuel RK, Robinson D: Developmental motor signs, in Soft Neurological Signs. Edited by Tupper D. New York, Grune & Stratton, 1987

Deutsch CK, Swanson JM, Bruell JH, et al: Overrepresentation of adoptees in children with the attention deficit disorder. Behav Genet 12:231–238, 1982

Dow SP, Sonies BC, Scheib D, et al: Practical guidelines for the assessment and treatment of selective mutism. J Am Acad Child Adolesc Psychiatry 34:836–846, 1995

Downey KK, Stelson FW, Pomerleau OF, et al: Adult attention deficit hyperactivity disorder: psychological test profiles in a clinical population. J Nerv Ment Dis 185:32–38, 1997

Drews CD, Murphy CC, Yeargin-Allsopp M, et al: The relationship between idiopathic mental retardation and maternal smoking during pregnancy. Pediatrics 97:547–553, 1996

Dummit ES III, Klein RG, Tancer NK, et al: Fluoxetine treatment of children with selective mutism: an open trial. J Am Acad Child Adolesc Psychiatry 35(5):615–621, 1996

Dykens EM, Hodapp RM, Ort S, et al: The trajectory of cognitive development in males with fragile X syndrome. J Am Acad Child Adolesc Psychiatry 28:422–426, 1989

Dykman RA, McPherson B, Ackerman PT, et al: Internalizing and externalizing characteristics of sexually and/or physically abused children. Integr Physiol Behav Sci 32:62–74, 1997

Edelbrock C: Behavioral checklists and rating scales, in Basic Handbook of Child Psychiatry, Vol 5. Edited by Noshpitz JD, Call JD, Cohen RL, et al. New York, Basic Books, 1987

Edwards CH, Johnson AA, Knight EM, et al: Pica in an urban environment. J Nutr 124(suppl 6):954S–962S, 1994

Ehlers S, Nyden A, Gillberg C, et al: Asperger syndrome, autism and attentional disorders: a comparative study of the cognitive profiles of 120 children. J Child Psychol Psychiatry 38:207–217, 1997

Eiberg H, Berendt I, Mohr J: Assignment of dominant inherited nocturnal enuresis (ENUR1) to chromosome 13q. Nat Genet 10:354–356, 1995

Elliott DS, Huizinga D, Ageton SS: Explaining Delinquency and Drug Use. Beverly Hills, CA, Sage, 1985

Ernst M, Liebenauer LL, Jons PH, et al: Selegiline in adults with attention deficit hyperactivity disorder: clinical efficacy and safety. Psychopharmacol Bull 32:327–334, 1996

Ernst M, Liebenauer LL, Tebeka D, et al: Selegiline in ADHD adults: plasma monoamines and monoamine metabolites. Neuropsychopharmacology 16:276–284, 1997

Fairbanks JM, Pine DS, Tancer NK, et al: Open fluoxetine treatment of mixed anxiety disorders in children and adolescents. J Child Adolesc Psychopharmacol 7:17–29, 1997

Famularo R, Fenton T: The effect of methylphenidate on school grades in children with attention deficit disorder without hyperactivity: a preliminary report. J Clin Psychiatry 48:112–114, 1987

Faulstich ME, Moore JR, Roberts RW, et al: A behavioral perspective on conduct disorders. Psychiatry 51:116–130, 1988

Feigin A, Kurlan R, McDermott MP, et al: A controlled trial of deprenyl in children with Tourette's syndrome and attention deficit hyperactivity disorder. Neurology 46:965–968, 1996

Feldman M, Wilson A: Adolescent suicidality in urban minorities and its relationship to conduct disorders, depression, and separation anxiety. J Am Acad Child Adolesc Psychiatry 36:75–84, 1997

Felton RH, Naylor CE, Wood FB: Neuropsychological profile of adult dyslexics. Brain Lang 39:485–497, 1990

Fendrich M, Warner V, Weissman MM: Family risk factors, parental depression, and psychopathology in offspring. Dev Psychol 26:40–50, 1990

Fergusson DM, Horwood LJ, Shannon FT: Factors related to the age of attainment of nocturnal bladder control. Pediatrics 78:884–890, 1986

Fey M, Leonard L, Wilcox K: Speech style modification in language-impaired children. J Speech Hear Disord 46:91–96, 1981

Filipek PA, Semrud-Clikeman M, Steingard RJ, et al: Volumetric MRI analysis comparing subjects having attention-deficit hyperactivity disorder with normal controls. Neurology 48:589–601, 1997

Fletcher JM, Shaywitz SE, Shankweiler DP, et al: Cognitive profiles of reading disability: comparisons of discrepancy and low achievement definitions. J Educ Psychol 86:6–23, 1994

Fletcher KE, Fischer M, Barkley RA, et al: A sequential analysis of the mother-adolescent interactions of ADHD, ADHD+ODD, and normal teenagers during neutral and conflict discussions. J Abnorm Child Psychol 24:271–297, 1996

Foley HA, Carlton CO, Howell RJ: The relationship of attention deficit hyperactivity disorder and conduct disorder to juvenile delinquency: legal implications. Bull Am Acad Psychiatry Law 24:333–345, 1996

Folstein SE, Piven J: Etiology of autism: Genetic influences. Pediatrics 87 (suppl):767–773, 1991

Fonagy P, Target M: The efficacy of psychoanalysis for children with disruptive disorders. J Am Acad Child Adolesc Psychiatry 33:45–55, 1994

Foreman DM, Thambirajah MS: Conduct disorder, enuresis and specific developmental delays in two types of encopresis: a case-note study of 63 boys. Eur Child Adolesc Psychiatry 5:33–37, 1996

Forsythe WI, Butler RJ: Fifty years of enuretic alarms. Arch Dis Child 64:879–885, 1989

Fox AM, Lent B: Clumsy children: primer on developmental coordination disorder. Can Fam Physician 42:1965–1971, 1996

Friman PC, Mathew JR, Finney JW, et al: Do encopretic children have clinically significant behavior problems? Pediatrics 82:407–409, 1988

Frith U (ed): Autism and Asperger Syndrome. Cambridge, UK, University of Cambridge, 1991

Fujii Y, Konishi Y, Kuriyama M, et al: Corpus callosum in developmentally retarded infants. Pediatr Neurol 11:219–223, 1994

Gabel S, Chandra R, Shindledecker R: Behavior ratings and outcome of medical treatment for encopresis. J Dev Behav Pediatr 9:129–133, 1988

Gadow KD, Sverd J, Sprafkin J, et al: Efficacy of methylphenidate for attention deficit hyperactivity disorder in children with tic disorder. Arch Gen Psychiatry 52:444–455, 1995

Galaburda AM (ed): Dyslexia and Development: Neurobiological Aspects of Extra-Ordinary Brains. Cambridge, MA, Harvard University Press, 1993

Galaburda AM, Sherman GF, Rosen GD, et al: Developmental dyslexia: four consecutive patients with cortical anomalies. Ann Neurol 18:222–233, 1985

Galler JR, Ramsey F, Solimano G, et al: The influence of early malnutrition on subsequent behavioral development, II. classroom behavior. Journal of the American Academy of Child Psychiatry 22:16–22, 1983

García-Sánchez C, Estévez-González A, Suárez-Romero E, et al: Right hemisphere dysfunction in subjects with attention-deficit disorder with and without hyperactivity. J Child Neurol 12:107–115, 1997

Gaub M, Carlson CL: Behavioral characteristics of DSM-IV ADHD subtypes in a school-based population. J Abnorm Child Psychol 25:103–111, 1997

Geiger G, Lettvin JY: Peripheral vision in persons with dyslexia. N Engl J Med 316:1238–1243, 1987

Geschwind N, Behan P: Left-handedness: association with immune disease, migraine, and developmental learning disorder. Proc Natl Acad Sci USA 79:5097–5100, 1982

Geschwind N, Galaburda AM: Cerebral lateralization: biological mechanisms, associations, and pathology. Arch Neurol 42:428–459, 521–552, 634–654, 1985

Getting P: Emerging principles governing the operations of neural networks. Ann Rev Neursci 12:185–204, 1989

Giedd JN, Castellanos FX, Casey BJ, et al: Quantitative morphology of the corpus callosum in attention deficit hyperactivity disorder. Am J Psychiatry 151:665–669, 1994

Gillberg C: Asperger syndrome in 23 Swedish children. Dev Med Child Neurol 31:520–531, 1989

Gillberg C, Persson E, Grufman M, et al: Psychiatric disorders in mildly and severely mentally retarded urban children and adolescents. Epidemiological aspects. Br J Psychiatry 149:68–74, 1986

Gillberg C, Melander H, von Knorring AL, et al: Long-term stimulant treatment of children with attention-deficit hyperactivity disorder symptoms. A randomized, double-blind, placebo-controlled trial. Arch Gen Psychiatry 54:857–864, 1997

Gittelman R, Mannuzza S, Shenker R, et al: Hyperactive boys almost grown up, I. Psychiatric status. Arch Gen Psychiatry 42:937–947, 1985

Glow RA, Glow PH: Peer and self-rating: children's perception of behavior relevant to hyperkinetic impulse disorder. J Abnorm Child Psychol 8:471–490, 1980

Gostason R: Psychiatric illness among the mentally retarded: a Swedish population study. Acta Psychiatr Scan 318 (suppl):1–117, 1985

Grandin T, Scariano MM: Emergence Labeled Autistic. Novato, CA, Arena Press, 1986

Greenhill LL, Rieder RO, Wender PH, et al: Lithium carbonate in the treatment of hyperactive children. Arch Gen Psychiatry 28:636–640, 1973

Gregg N, McAlexander PA: The relation between sense of audience and specific learning disabilities: an exploration. Annals of Dyslexia 39:206–226, 1989

Grigorenko EL, Wood FB, Meyer MS, et al: Susceptibility loci for distinct components of developmental dyslexia on chromosomes 6 and 15. Am J Hum Genet 60:27–39, 1997

Gross-Tsur V, Manor O, Shalev RS: Developmental dyscalculia: prevalence and demographic features. Dev Med Child Neurol 38:25–33, 1996

Grossman HJ (ed): Classification in Mental Retardation. Washington DC, American Association on Mental Deficiency, 1983

Guedeney A: An update on merycism and early depression: a critical review of the literature and a psychopathological hypothesis [in French]. Psychiatr Enfant (Paris) 38:345–363, 1995

Haber SN, Lynd-Balta E: Basal ganglia-limbic system interactions, in Handbook of Tourette's Syndrome and Related Tic and Behavioral Disorders. Edited by Kurlan R. New York, Marcel Dekker, 1993

Haber SN, Wolfer D: Basal ganglia peptidergic staining in Tourette syndrome, in Tourette Syndrome: Genetics, Neurobiology, and Treatment (Advances in Neurology Series, Vol. 58). Edited by Chase TN, Friedhoff AJ, Cohen DJ. New York, Raven, 1992

Hafeez A, Malik QU: Blood lead levels in preschool children in Rawalpindi. J Pak Med Assoc 46:272–274, 1996

Hagberg BA: Rett syndrome: clinical peculiarities, diagnostic approach, and possible cause. Pediatr Neurol 5:75–83, 1989

Hagberg BA, Witt-Engerstrom I: Rett's syndrome: a suggested staging system for describing the impairment profile with increasing age toward adolescence. Am J Med Genet 24:47–59, 1986

Halperin JM, Newcorn JH, Matier K, et al: Impulsivity and the initiation of fights in children with disruptive behavior disorders. J Child Psychol Psychiatry 36:1199–1211, 1995

Hare RD, McPherson LM, Forth AE: Male psychopaths and their criminal careers. J Consult Clin Psychol 56:710–714, 1988

Hart EL, Lahey BB, Loeber R, et al: Developmental change in attention-deficit hyperactivity disorder in boys: a four-year longitudinal study. J Abnorm Child Psychol 23:729–749, 1995

Haslam RH, Dalby JT, Johns RD, et al: Cerebral asymmetry in developmental dyslexia. Arch Neurol 38:679–682, 1981

Hauser P, Zametkin AJ, Martinez P, et al: Attention deficit-hyperactivity disorder in people with generalized resistance to thyroid hormone. N Engl J Med 328:997–1001, 1993

Hayden TL: Classification of elective mutism. Journal of the American Academy of Child Psychiatry 19:118–133, 1980

Hazell P: The overlap of attention deficit hyperactivity disorder with other common mental disorders. J Paediatr Child Health 33:131–137, 1997

Haznedar MM, Buchsbaum MS, Metzger M, et al: Anterior cingulate gyrus volume and glucose metabolism in autistic disorder. Am J Psychiatry 154:1047–1050, 1997

Hechtman L: Families of children with attention deficit hyperactivity disorder: a review. Can J Psychiatry 41:350–360, 1996

Herskowitz J: Developmental neurotoxicology, in Psychiatric Pharmacosciences of Adolescents and Children. Edited by Popper C. Washington, DC, American Psychiatric Press, 1987

Hess EJ, Rogan PK, Domoto M, et al: Absence of linkage of apparently single gene mediated ADHD with the human syntenic region of the mouse mutant Coloboma. Am J Med Genet 60:573–579, 1995

Hill AE, Rosenbloom L: Disintegrative psychosis of childhood: teenage follow-up. Dev Med Child Neurol 28:34–40, 1986

Hill JC, Schoener EP: Age-dependent decline of attention deficit hyperactivity disorder. Am J Psychiatry 153:1143–1146, 1996

Hittmair-Delazer M, Sailer U, Benke T: Impaired arithmetic facts but intact conceptual knowledge: a single case study of dyscalculia. Cortex 31:139–147, 1995

Hollander HE, Turner FD: Characteristics of incarcerated delinquents: relationship between development disorders, environmental and family factors, and patterns of offense and recidivism. J Am Acad Child Psychiatry 24:221–226, 1985

Howie VM: Developmental sequelae of chronic otitis media: a review. J Dev Behav Pediatr 1:34–38, 1980

Huesmann LR, Eron LD, Lefkowitz MM, et al: The stability of aggression over time and generations. Dev Psychol 20:1120–1134, 1984

Hunsballe JM, Lundorf E, Norgaard JP: The pituitary gland in nocturnal enuresis: MR findings. Scand J Urol Nephrol 30:85–87, 1996

Hunsballe JM, Rittig S, Pedersen EB, et al: Single dose imipramine reduces nocturnal urine output in patients with nocturnal enuresis and nocturnal polyuria. J Urol 158:830–836, 1997

Hunt RD, Capper L, O'Connell P: Clonidine in child and adolescent psychiatry. J Child Adolesc Psychopharmacol 1:87–102, 1990

Hyde TM, Stacey ME, Coppola R, et al: Cerebral morphometric abnormalities in Tourette's syndrome: a quantitative MRI study of monozygotic twins. Neurology 45:1176–1182, 1995

Hynd GW, Hall J, Novey ES: Dyslexia and corpus callosum morphology. Arch Neurol 52:32–38, 1995

Ialongo NS, Horn WF, Pascoe JM, et al: The effects of multimodal intervention with ADHD children: a 9-month follow-up. J Am Acad Child Adolesc Psychiatry 32:182–189, 1993

Insel TR: A neurobiological base of social attachment. Am J Psychiatry 154:726–735, 1997

Jagger J, Proshoff BA, Cohen DJ, et al: The epidemiology of Tourette syndrome: a pilot study. Schizophr Bull 8:267–279, 1982

Jenkins RL: Behavior Disorders of Childhood and Adolescence. Springfield, IL, Charles C Thomas, 1973

Johnson AM, Falstein EI, Szurek SA, et al: School phobia. Am J Orthopsychiatry 11:702–711, 1941

Kagan J, Reznick JS, Snidman N: The physiology and psychology of behavioral inhibition in children. Child Dev 58:1459–1473, 1987

Kalo BB, Bella H: Enuresis: prevalence and associated factors among primary school children in Saudi Arabia. Acta Paediatr 85:1217–1222, 1996

Kanner L: Autistic disturbances of affective contact. Nerv Child 2:217–250, 1943

Katusic SJ, Colligan RC, Beard CM, et al: Mental retardation in a birth cohort, 1976–1980, Rochester, Minnesota. Am J Ment Retard 100:335–344, 1996

Katz LM, Nathan L, Kuhn CM, et al: Inhibition of GH in maternal separation may be mediated through altered serotonergic activity at 5-HT2A and 5-HT2C receptors. Psychoneuroendocrinology 21:219–235, 1996

Kazdin AE: Conduct Disorders in Childhood and Adolescence. Newbury Park, CA, Sage, 1987

Kazdin AE: Practitioner review: psychosocial treatments for conduct disorder in children. J Child Psychol Psychiatry 38:161–178, 1997

Kazdin AE, Bass D, Siegel T, et al: Cognitive-behavioral therapy and relationship therapy in the treatment of children referred for antisocial behavior. J Consult Clin Psychol 57:522–535, 1989

Kernberg PF, Chazan SE: Children with Conduct Disorders: A Psychotherapy Manual. New York, Basic Books, 1991

Kidd KK: Genetic models of stuttering. Journal of Fluency Disorders 5:187–201, 1980

King BH, DeAntonio C, McCracken JT, et al: Psychiatric consultation in severe and profound mental retardation. Am J Psychiatry 151:1802–1808, 1994

Kirk J, Rasmussen PV, Rittig S, et al: Provoked enuresis-like episodes in healthy children 7 to 12 years old. J Urol 156:210–213, 1996

Klein RG, Last CG: Anxiety Disorders in Children. Newbury Park, CA, Sage, 1989

Klieger PS, Fett KA, Dimitsopulos T, et al: Asymmetry of basal ganglia perfusion in Tourette's syndrome shown by Technitium-99m-HMPAO SPECT. J Nucl Med 38:2188–2191, 1997

Kolvin I, Fundudis T: Elective mute children: psychological development and background factors. J Child Psychol Psychiatry 22:219–232, 1981

Kopp S, Gillberg C: Selective mutism: a population-based study: a research note. J Child Psychol Psychiatry 38(2):257–262, 1997

Kovacs M, Paulauskas S, Gatsonis C, et al: Depressive disorders in childhood, III. A longitudinal study of comorbidity with and risk for conduct disorders. J Affect Disord 15:205–217, 1988

Kravitz H, Boehm JJ: Rhythmic habit patterns in infancy: their sequence, age of onset, and frequency. Child Dev 42:399–413, 1971

Krohn DD, Weckstein SM, Wright HL: A study of the effectiveness of a specific treatment for elective mutism. J Am Acad Child Adolesc Psychiatry 31:711–718, 1992

Kuperman S, Johnson B, Arndt S, et al: Quantitative EEG differences in a nonclinical sample of children with ADHD and undifferentiated ADD. J Am Acad Child Adolesc Psychiatry 35:1009–1017, 1996

Kurlan R (ed): Handbook of Tourette's Syndrome and Related Tic and Behavioral Disorders. New York, Marcel Dekker, 1993

Labbe EE, Williamson DA: Behavioral treatment of elective mutism: a review of the literature. Clin Psychol Rev 4:273–294, 1984

Lachiewicz AM, Spiridigliozzi GA, Gullion CM, et al: Aberrant behaviors of young boys with fragile X syndrome. Am J Ment Retard 98:567–579, 1994

Lahey BB, Schaughency EA, Hynd GW, et al: Attention deficit disorder with and without hyperactivity: comparison of behavioral characteristics of clinic-referred children. J Am Acad Child Adolesc Psychiatry 26:718–723, 1987

Lahey BB, Hartdagen S, Frick PJ, et al: Conduct disorder: parsing the confounded relation to parental divorce and antisocial personality. J Abnorm Psychol 97:334–337, 1988

LaHoste GJ, Swanson JM, Wigal SB, et al: Dopamine D4 receptor gene polymorphism is associated with attention deficit hyperactivity disorder. Mol Psychiatry 1(2):121–124, 1996

Landesman S, Vietze P: Living Environments and Mental Retardation. Washington, DC, American Association on Mental Deficiency, 1987

Largo RH, Graf S, Kundu S, et al: Predicting developmental outcome at school age from infant tests of normal, at-risk, and retarded infants. Dev Med Child Neurol 32:30–45, 1990

Last CG, Francis G, Hersen M, et al: Separation anxiety and school phobia: a comparison using DSM-III criteria. Am J Psychiatry 144:653–657, 1987

Latz SR, McCracken JT: Neuroleptic malignant syndrome in children and adolescents: two case reports and a warning. J Child Adolesc Psychopharmacol 2:123–129, 1992

Lavigne JV, Burns WJ, Cotter PD: Rumination in infancy: recent behavioral approaches. Int J Eat Disord 1:70–82, 1981

Leckman JF, Riddle MA, Berrettini WH, et al: Elevated CSF dynorphin A [1–8] in Tourette's syndrome. Life Sci 43:2015–2023, 1988

Leckman JF, Dolnansky ES, Hardin MT, et al: Perinatal factors in the expression of Tourette's syndrome: an exploratory study. J Am Acad Child Adolesc Psychiatry 29:220–226, 1990

Leckman JF, Walker DE, Cohen DJ: Premonitory urges in Tourette's syndrome. Am J Psychiatry 150:98–102, 1993

Leonard CM, Martinez P, Weintraub BD, et al: Magnetic resonance imaging of cerebral anomalies in subjects with resistance to thyroid hormone. Am J Med Genet 60:238–243, 1995

Levin ED, Conners CK, Sparrow E, et al: Nicotine effects on adults with attention-deficit/hyperactivity disorder. Psychopharmacology (Berl) 123:55–63, 1996

Levine MD: Encopresis: its potentiation, evaluation, and alleviation. Pediatr Clin North Am 29:315–330, 1982

Levine MD, Oberklaid F, Meltzer LJ: Developmental output failure: a study of low productivity in school-aged children. Pediatrics 67:18–25, 1981

Lewis DO, Pincus JH, Shanok SS, et al: Psychomotor epilepsy and violence in a group of incarcerated adolescent boys. Am J Psychiatry 139:882–887, 1982

Lewis DO, Pincus JH, Bard B, et al: Neuropsychiatric, psychoeducational and family characteristics of 14 juveniles condemned to death in the United States. Am J Psychiatry 145:584–589, 1988

Lindberg B: Understanding Rett Syndrome: A Practical Guide for Parents, Teachers,. and Therapists. Göttingen, Germany, Hogrefe & Huber, 1992

Lipsitz JD, Martin LY, Mannuzza S, et al: Childhood separation anxiety disorder in patients with adult anxiety disorders. Am J Psychiatry 151:927–929, 1994

Livingston R, Taylor JL, Crawford SL: A study of somatic complaints and psychiatric diagnosis in children. J Am Acad Child Adolesc Psychiatry 27:185–187, 1988

Livingston RL, Dykman RA, Ackerman PT: Psychiatric comorbidity and response to two doses of methylphenidate in children with attention deficit disorder. J Child Adolesc Psychopharmacol 2:115–122, 1992

Loeber R: The stability of antisocial and delinquent childhood behavior. Child Dev 53:1431–1446, 1982

Loening-Baucke V: Encopresis and soiling. Pediatr Clin North Am 43:279–298, 1996

Lou HC: Etiology and pathogenesis of attention-deficit hyperactivity disorder (ADHD): significance of prematurity and perinatal hypoxic-haemodynamic encephalopathy. Acta Paediatr 85(11):1266–1271, 1996

Lou HC, Henriksen L, Bruhn P, et al: Striatal dysfunction in attention deficit and hyperkinetic disorder. Arch Neurol 46:48–52, 1989

Lynskey MT, Fergusson DM: Childhood conduct problems, attention deficit behaviors, and adolescent alcohol, tobacco, and illicit drug use. J Abnorm Child Psychol 23:281–302, 1995

MacGregor R, Pullar A, Cundall D: Silent at school: elective mutism and abuse. Arch Dis Child 70(6):540–541, 1994

Malone RP, Luebbert JF, Delaney MA, et al: Nonpharmacological response in hospitalized children with conduct disorder. J Am Acad Child Adolesc Psychiatry 36:242–247, 1997

Mancini C, van Ameringen M, Szatmari P, et al: A high-risk pilot study of the children of adults with social phobia. J Am Acad Child Adolesc Psychiatry 35:1511–1517, 1996

Marcus J, Hans SL, Mednick SA, et al: Neurological dysfunctioning in offspring of schizophrenics in Israel and Denmark. Arch Gen Psychiatry 42:753–761, 1985

Martin JAM: Syndrome delineation in communication disorders, in Language and Language Disorders in Children. Edited by Hersov LA, Berger M. Oxford, UK, Pergamon, 1980

Matarazzo EB: Tourette's syndrome treated with ACTH and prednisone: reports of two cases. J Child Adolesc Psychopharmacol 2:215–226, 1992

Matochik JA, Liebenauer LL, King AC, et al: Cerebral glucose metabolism in adults with attention deficit hyperactivity disorder after chronic stimulant treatment. Am J Psychiatry 151:658–664, 1994

Matsuishi T, Nagamitsu S, Yamashita Y, et al: Decreased cerebrospinal fluid levels of substance P in patients with Rett syndrome. Ann Neurol 42:978–981, 1997

Matthys W, Van Loo P, Pachen V, et al: Behavior of conduct disordered children in interaction with each other and with normal peers. Child Psychiatry Hum Dev 25:183–195, 1995

Mayes SD, Humphrey FJ 2d, Handford HA, et al: Rumination disorder: differential diagnosis. J Am Acad Child Adolesc Psychiatry 27:300–302, 1988

Mayes SD, Crites DL, Bixler EO, et al: Methylphenidate and ADHD: influence of age, IQ and neurodevelopmental status. Dev Med Child Neurol 36:1099–1107, 1994

Mazzocco MMM, Hagerman RJ, Cronister-Silverman A, et al: Specific frontal lobe deficits among women with the fragile X gene. J Am Acad Child Adolesc Psychiatry 31:1141–1148, 1992

McDougle CJ, Naylor ST, Cohen DJ, et al: Effects of tryptophan depletion in drug-free adults with autistic disorder. Arch Gen Psychiatry 53:980–983, 1996

McDougle CJ, Holmes JP, Bronson MR, et al: Risperidone treatment of children and adolescents with pervasive developmental disorders: a prospective open-label study. J Am Acad Child Adolesc Psychiatry 36:685–693, 1997

McGee R, Williams S: A longitudinal study of depression in nine-year-old children. J Am Acad Child Adolesc Psychiatry 27:342–348, 1988

McKnew DH, Cytryn L, Buchsbaum MS, et al: Lithium in children of lithium-responding parents. Psychiatry Res 4:171–180, 1981

Meller WH, Borchardt CM: Comorbidity of major depression and conduct disorder. J Affect Disord 39:123–126, 1996

Menolascino FJ, Levitas A, Greiner C: The nature and types of mental illness in the mentally retarded. Psychopharmacol Bull 22:1060–1071, 1986

Milberger S, Biederman J, Faraone SV, et al: Is maternal smoking during pregnancy a risk factor for attention deficit hyperactivity disorder in children? Am J Psychiatry 153:1138–1142, 1996

Millican FK, Layman EM, Lourie RS, et al: Study of an oral fixation: pica. J Am Acad Child Psychiatry 7:79–107, 1968

Miyahara M, Mobs I: Developmental dyspraxia and developmental coordination disorder. Neuropsychol Rev 5:245–268, 1995

Moeschler JB, Charman CD, Berg SZ, et al: Rett syndrome: natural history and management. Pediatrics 82:1–10, 1988

Moreno-Fuenmayor H, Borjas L, Arrieta A, et al: Plasma excitatory amino acids in autism. Invest Clin 37:113–128, 1996

Moss HB, Yao JK: Platelet dense granule secretion in adolescents with conduct disorder and substance abuse: preliminary evidence for variation in signal transduction. Biol Psychiatry 40:892–898, 1996

Mountz JM, Tolbert LC, Lill DW, et al: Functional deficits in autistic disorder: characterization by technetium-99m-HMPAO and SPECT. J Nucl Med 36:1156–1162, 1995

Murphy K, Barkley RA: Attention deficit hyperactivity disorder in adults: comorbidities and adaptive impairments. Compr Psychiatry 37:393–401, 1996

Naidu S, Hyman S, Harris EL, et al: Rett syndrome studies of natural history and search for a genetic marker. Neuropediatrics 26:63–66, 1995

Nelson KB: Prenatal and perinatal factors in the etiology of autism. Pediatrics 87 (suppl):761–766, 1991

Nelson KB, Ellenberg JH: Antecedents of cerebral palsy: multivariate analysis of risk. N Engl J Med 315:81–86, 1986

New York, Hemisphere, 1986

Newcorn JH, Strain J: Adjustment disorder in children and adolescents. J Am Acad Child Adolesc Psychiatry 31:318–327, 1992

Nichols PL, Chen T-C: Minimal Brain Dysfunction: A Prospective Study. Hillsdale, NJ, Lawrence Erlbaum, 1981

Odell JD, Warren RP, Warren WL, et al: Association of genes within the major histocompatibility complex with attention deficit hyperactivity disorder. Neuropsychobiology 35:181–186, 1997

Ollendick TH, Mattis SG, King NJ: Panic in children and adolescents: a review. J Child Psychol Psychiatry 35:113–134, 1994

Oosterlaan J, Sergeant JA: Inhibition in ADHD, aggressive, and anxious children: a biologically based model of child psychopathology. J Abnorm Child Psychol 24:19–36, 1996

Owen SE, McKinlay IA: Motor difficulties in children with developmental disorders of speech and language. Child Care Health Dev 23:315–325, 1997

Paden EP, Yairi E: Phonological characteristics of children whose stuttering persisted or recovered. J Speech Hear Res 39:981–990, 1996

Parks SL: The assessment of autistic children: a selective review of available instruments. J Autism Dev Disord 13:255–267, 1983

Parry-Jones B: Merycism or rumination disorder: a historical investigation and current assessment. Br J Psychiatry 165:303–314, 1994

Patterson GR: Coercive Family Processes. Eugene, OR, Castalia, 1982

Paul R, Cohen D, Caparulo B: A longitudinal study of patients with severe, specific developmental language disorders. J Am Acad Child Psychiatry 22:525–534, 1994

Pauls DL: Genetic factors in the expression of attention-deficit hyperactivity disorder. J Child Adolesc Psychopharmacol 1:353–360, 1991

Pauls DL, Leckman JF: The inheritance of Gilles de la Tourette's syndrome and associated behaviors. N Engl J Med 315:993–997, 1986

Pearson DA, Aman MG: Ratings of hyperactivity and developmental indices: should clinicians correct for developmental level? J Autism Dev Disord 24:395–411, 1994

Pelham WE, Carlson C, Sams SE, et al: Separate and combined effects of methylphenidate and behavior modification of boys with attention deficit hyperactivity disorder in the classroom. J Consult Clin Psychol 61:506–515, 1993

Perrin S, Last CG: Relationship between ADHD and anxiety in boys: results from a family study. J Am Acad Child Adolesc Psychiatry 35:988–996, 1996

Perry CA, Dwyer J, Gelfand JA, et al: Health effects of salicylates in foods and drugs. Nutr Rev 54:225–240, 1996

Peterson BS: Neuroimaging in child and adolescent neuropsychiatric disorders. J Am Acad Child Adolesc Psychiatry 12:1560–1576, 1995

Peterson B, Riddle MA, Cohen DJ, et al: Reduced basal ganglia volumes in Tourette's syndrome using three-dimensional reconstruction techniques from magnetic resonance images. Neurology 43:941–949, 1993

Pliszka SR, McCracken JT, Maas JW: Catecholamines in attention-deficit hyperactivity disorder: current perspectives. J Am Acad Child Adolesc Psychiatry 35:264–272, 1996

Pomerleau OF, Downey KK, Stelson FW, et al: Cigarette smoking in adult patients diagnosed with attention deficit hyperactivity disorder. J Subst Abuse 7:373–378, 1995

Popper C: Psychopharmacological treatment of anxiety disorders in adolescents and children. J Clin Psychiatry 54 (5 suppl):52–63, 1993

Popper CW, Elliott GR: Sudden death and tricyclic antidepressants: clinical considerations for children. Journal of Child and Adolescent Psychopharmacology 1:125–132, 1990

Porrino LJ, Rapoport JL, Behar D, et al: A naturalistic assessment of the motor activity of hyperactive boys, 1. comparison with normal controls. Arch Gen Psychiatry 40:681–687, 1983

Prassopoulos P, Cavouras D, Ioannidou M, et al: Study of subarachnoid spaces in children with idiopathic mental retardation. J Child Neurol 11:197–200, 1996

Provence S, Lipton RC: Infants and Institutions. New York, International Universities Press, 1962

Puig-Antich J: Major depression and conduct disorder in prepuberty. J Am Acad Child Psychiatry 21:118–128, 1982

Purvis KL, Tannock R: Language abilities in children with attention deficit hyperactivity disorder, reading abilities, and normal controls. J Abnorm Child Psychol 25:133–144, 1997

Quay HC: Inhibition and attention deficit hyperactivity disorder. J Abnorm Child Psychol 25:7–13, 1997

Raine A, Venables PH, Williams M: Relationships between central and autonomic measures of arousal at age 15 years and criminality at age 24 years. Arch Gen Psychiatry 47:1003–1007, 1990

Rapin I: Autistic children: diagnosis and clinical features. Pediatrics 87 (suppl):751–760, 1991

Rapoport JL, Buchsbaum MS, Weingartner H, et al: Dextroamphetamine: its cognitive and behavioral effects in normal and hyperactive boys and normal men. Arch Gen Psychiatry 37:933–943, 1980

Rapoport JL, Conners CK, Reatig N: Rating scales and assessment instruments for use in pediatric psychopharmacology research. Psychopharmacol Bull 21:713–1125, 1985

Raynaud C, Billard C Tzongrig H, et al: Study of rCBF developmental dysphasia children at rest and during verbal stimulation. Cerebral Blood Flow Metabolism 1 (suppl):S323, 1989

Reid AH, Ballinger BR: Behaviour symptoms among severely and profoundly mentally retarded patients. A 16–18 year follow-up study. Br J Psychiatry 167:452–455, 1995

Reis S: Rumination in two developmentally normal children: case report and review of the literature. J Fam Pract 38:521–523, 1994

Rey JM: Comorbidity between disruptive disorders and depression in referred adolescents. Aust NZ J Psychiatry 28:106–113, 1994

Richters MM, Volkmar FR: Reactive attachment disorder of infancy or early childhood. J Am Acad Child Adolesc Psychiatry 33:328–332, 1994

Riddle MA, Nelson JC, Kleinman CS, et al: Sudden death in children receiving Norpramin: a review of three reported cases and commentary. J Am Acad Child Adolesc Psychiatry 30:104–108, 1991

Riddle MA, Rasmussen AM, Woods SW, et al: SPECT imaging of cerebral blood flow in Tourette syndrome, in Tourette Syndrome: Genetics, Neurobiology, and Treatment (Advances in Neurology Series, Vol. 58). Edited by Chase TN, Friedhoff AJ, Cohen DJ. New York, Raven, 1992

Riddle MA, Lynch KA, Scahill L, et al: Methylphenidate discontinuation and reinitiation during long-term treatment of children with Tourette's disorder and attention-deficit/hyperactivity disorder: a pilot study. J Child Adolesc Psychopharmacol 5:205–214, 1995

Rifkin A, Karajgi B, Dicker R, et al: Lithium treatment of conduct disorders in adolescents. Am J Psychiatry 154:554–555, 1997

Rimland B, Baker SM: Brief report: alternative approaches to the development of effective treatments for autism. J Autism Dev Disord 26:237–241, 1996

Rittig S, Knudsen UB, Norgaard JP, et al: Abnormal diurnal rhythm of plasma vasopressin and urinary output in patients with enuresis. Am J Physiol 256:F664–F671, 1989

Rittig S, Schaumburg H, Schmidt F, et al: Long-term home studies of water balance in patients with nocturnal enuresis. Scand J Urol Nephrol [Suppl] 183:25–56, discussion 26–27, 1997

Roberts JW, Dickey P: Exposure of children to pollutants in house dust and indoor air. Rev Environ Contam Toxicol 143:59–78, 1995

Robertson MM, Banerjee S, Hiley PJ, et al: Personality disorder and psychopathology in Tourette's syndrome: a controlled study. Br J Psychiatry 171:283–286, 1997

Robins LN: Deviant Children Grown Up. Baltimore, MD, Williams & Wilkins, 1966

Robson WL, Jackson HP, Blackhurst D, et al: Enuresis in children with attention-deficit hyperactivity disorder. South Med J 90:503–505, 1997

Rockney RM, McQuade WH, Days AL, et al: Encopresis treatment outcome: long-term follow-up of 45 cases. J Dev Behav Pediatr 17:380–385, 1996

Roizen NJ, Blondis TA, Irwin M, et al: Adaptive functioning in children with attention-deficit hyperactivity disorder. Arch Pediatr Adolesc Med 148:1137–1142, 1994

Rourke BP, Strang JD: Subtypes of reading and arithmetic disabilities: a neuropsychological analysis, in Developmental Neuropsychiatry. Edited by Rutter M. New York, Guilford, 1983

Rumsey JM, Duara R, Grady C, et al: Brain metabolism in autism: resting cerebral glucose utilization rates as measured with positron emission tomography. Arch Gen Psychiatry 42:448–455, 1985a

Rumsey JM, Rapoport JL, Sceery WR: Autistic children as adults: psychiatric, social, and behavioral outcomes. Journal of the American Academy of Child Psychiatry 24:465–473, 1985b

Rutter M: Isle of Wight revisited: twenty-five years of child psychiatric epidemiology. J Am Acad Child Adolesc Psychiatry 28:633–653, 1989

Rutter M, Giller H: Juvenile Delinquency: Trends and Perspectives. New York, Guilford, 1984

Rutter M, Yule W: A Neuropsychiatric Study in Childhood. Suffolk, UK, Lavenhan Press, 1970

Rutter M, Yule W: The concept of specific reading retardation. J Child Psychol Psychiatry 16:181–197, 1975

Rutter M, Tizard J, Whitmore K: Education, Health and Behaviour: Psychological and Medical Study of Childhood Development. Harlow, UK, Longman, 1970

Rutter M, Tizard J, Yule W, et al: Isle of Wight studies, 1964–1974. Psychol Med 6:313–332, 1976

Rutter M, Tuma A, Lann I: Assessment and diagnosis in child psychopathology. New York, Guilford, 1987

Rydelius A: The development of antisocial behavior and sudden violent death. Acta Psychiatr Scand 77:398–403, 1988

Safer DJ, Krager JM: Effect of a media blitz on a threatened lawsuit on stimulant treatment. JAMA 268:1004–1007, 1992

Safer DJ, Zito JM, Fine EM: Increased methylphenidate usage for attention deficit disorder in the 1990s. Pediatrics 98:1084–1088, 1996

Sandman CA: The opiate hypothesis in autism and self-injury. J Child Adolesc Psychopharmacol 1:237–248, 1991

Satterfield JH, Satterfield BT, Cantwell DP: Three-year multimodality treatment study of 100 hyperactive boys. J Pediatrics 98:650–655, 1981

Sauvage D, Leddet I, Hameury L, et al: Infantile rumination: diagnosis and follow-up of twenty cases. J Am Acad Child Psychiatry 24:197–203, 1985

Schaefer GB, Thompson JN, Bodensteiner JB, et al: Hypoplasia of the cerebellar vermis in neurogenetic syndromes. Ann Neurol 39:382–385, 1996

Schroeder S, Schroeder C, Smith B, et al: Prevalence of self-injurious behaviors in a large state facility for the retarded: a three-year follow-up study. Journal of Autism and Childhood Schizophrenia 8:261–269, 1979

Schulte-Körne G, Deimel W, Gutenbrunner C, et al: Effect of an oligo-antigen diet on the behavior of hyperkinetic children [in German]. Z Kinder Jugenpsychiatr 24:176–183, 1996

Schvehla TJ, Mandoki MW, Sumner GS: Clonidine therapy for comorbid attention deficit hyperactivity disorder and conduct disorder: preliminary findings in a children's inpatient unit. South Med J 87:692–695, 1994

Semrud-Clikeman M: Evidence from imaging on the relationship between brain structure and developmental language disorders. Semin Pediatr Neurol 4:117–124, 1997

Semrud-Clikeman M, Hynd GW: Right hemispheric dysfunction in nonverbal learning disabilities: social, academic, and adaptive functioning in adults and children. Psychol Bull 107:196–209, 1990

Sever Y, Ashkenazi A, Tyano S, et al: Iron treatment in children with attention deficit hyperactivity disorder: a preliminary report. Neuropsychobiology 35:178–180, 1997

Shaffer D, Gould MS, Brasic J, et al: A children's global assessment scale (CGAS). Arch Gen Psychiatry 40:1228–1231, 1983

Shaffer D, Gardner A, Hedge B: Behavior and bladder disturbance of enuretic children: a common disorder. Dev Med Child Neurol 26:781–792, 1984

Shah MR, Seese LM, Abikoff H, et al: Pemoline for children and adolescents with conduct disorder: a pilot investigation. J Child Adolesc Psychopharmacol 4:255–261, 1994

Shalev RS, Auerbach J, Gross-Tsur V: Developmental dyscalculia behavioral and attentional aspects: a research note. J Child Psychol Psychiatry 36:1261–1268, 1995a

Shalev RS, Manor O, Amir N, et al: Developmental dyscalculia and brain laterality. Cortex 31:357–365, 1995b

Shaywitz BA, Yager RD, Klopper JH: Selective brain dopamine depletion in developing rats: an experimental model of minimal brain dysfunction. Science 191:305–308, 1976

Shaywitz SE, Cohen DJ, Shaywitz BA: Behavior and learning difficulties in children of normal intelligence born to alcoholic mothers. J Pediatr 96:978–982, 1980

Shaywitz SE, Shaywitz BA, Fletcher JM, et al: Prevalence of reading disability in boys and girls: results of the Connecticut Longitudinal Study. JAMA 264:998–1002, 1990

Sherman DK, Iacono WG, McGue MK: Attention-deficit hyperactivity disorder dimensions: a twin study of inattention and impulsivity-hyperactivity. J Am Acad Child Adolesc Psychiatry 36:745–753, 1997

Sigman M (ed): Children with Emotional Disorders and Developmental Disabilities: Assessment and Treatment. Orlando, FL, Grune & Stratton, 1985

Silove D, Manicavasagar V, O'Connell D, et al: Genetic factors in early separation anxiety: implications for the genesis of adult anxiety disorders. Acta Psychiatr Scand 92:17–24, 1995a

Silove D, Harris M, Morgan A, et al: Is early separation anxiety a specific precursor of panic disorder-agoraphobia? A community study. Psychol Med 25:405–411 1995b

Silva RR, Munoz DM, Alpert M: Carbamazepine use in children and adolescents with features of attention-deficit hyperactivity disorder: a meta-analysis. J Am Acad Child Adolesc Psychiatry 35:352–358, 1996

Silvany-Neto AM, Carvalho FM, Tavares TM, et al: Lead poisoning among children of Santo Amaro, Bahia, Brazil in 1980, 1985, and 1992. Bull Pan Am Health Organ 30:51–62, 1996

Skoog SJ, Stokes A, Turner KL: Oral desmopressin: a randomized double-blind placebo controlled study of effectiveness in children with primary nocturnal enuresis. J Urol 158:1035–1040, 1997

Smith S, Kimberling W, Pennington B, et al: Specific reading disability: identification of an inherited form through linkage analysis. Science 219:1345–1347, 1983

Soussignan R, Tremblay R: Other disorders of conduct, in Hyperactivity Disorders of Childhood. Edited by Sandberg S. Cambridge, UK, Cambridge University Press, 1996

Sparrow SS, Balla DA, Cicchetti DV: Vineland Adaptive Behavior Scales. Circle Pines, MN, American Guidance Service, 1984

Staley D, Wand R, Shady G: Tourette disorder: a cross-cultural review. Compr Psychiatry 38:6–19, 1997

Stanovich KE, Siegel LS: Phenotypic performance profile of children with reading disabilities: a regression-based test of the phonological-core-variable-difference model. J Educ Psychol 86:24–53, 1994

Stefl ME: The Ohio Tourette's Study. Cincinnati, OH, University of Cincinnati School of Planning, 1983

Stein MA, Sandoval R, Szumowski E, et al: Psychometric characteristics of the Wender Utah Rating Scale (WURS): reliability and factor structure for men and women. Psychopharmacol Bull 31:425–433, 1995

Steingard R, Khan A, Gonzalez A, et al: Neuroleptic malignant syndrome: review of experience with children and adolescents. J Child Adolesc Psychopharmacol 2:183–198, 1992

Steingard RJ, Zimnitzky B, DeMaso DR, et al: Sertraline treatment of transition-associated anxiety and agitation in children with autistic disorder. J Child Adolesc Psychopharmacol 7:9–15, 1997

Steinhausen HC, Gobel D: Enuresis in child psychiatric clinic patients. J Am Acad Child Adolesc Psychiatry 28:279–281, 1989

Stern JS, Robertson MM: Tics associated with autistic and pervasive developmental disorders. Neurol Clin 15:345–355, 1997

Stern HP, Stroh SE, Fiedorek SC, et al: Increased plasma levels of pancreatic polypeptide and decreased plasma levels of motilin in encopretic children. Pediatrics 96(Pt 1):111–117, 1995

Storm-Mathisen A, Vaglum P: Conduct disorder patients 20 years later: a personal follow-up study. Acta Psychiatr Scand 89:416–420, 1994

Sukhai RN, Mol J, Harris AS: Combined therapy of enuresis alarm and desmopressin in the treatment of nocturnal enuresis. Eur J Pediatr 148:465–467, 1989

Sutphen JL, Borowitz SM, Hutchison RL, et al: Long-term follow-up of medically treated childhood constipation. Clin Pediatr (Phila) 34:576–580, 1995

Swedo SE: Sydenham's chorea: A model for childhood autoimmune neuropsychiatric disorders. JAMA 272:1788–1791, 1994

Swedo SE, Leonard HL, Garvey M, et al: Pediatric autoimmune neuropsychiatric disorders associated with streptococcal infections: clinical description of the first 50 cases. Am J Psychiatry 154:264–271, 1998

Szatmari P, Bremner R, Nagy J: Asperger's syndrome: a review of clinical features. Can J Psychiatry 34:554–560, 1989

Szatmari P, Archer L, Fisman S, et al: Asperger's syndrome and autism: differences in behavior, cognition, and adaptive functioning. J Am Acad Child Adolesc Psychiatry 34:1662–1671, 1995

Szymanski LS: Prevention of psychosocial dysfunction in persons with mental retardation. Ment Retard 25:215–218, 1987

Szymanski LS, Tanguay LS (eds): Emotional Disorders of Mentally Retarded Persons. Baltimore, MD, University Park Press, 1980

Taanila A, Kokkonen J, Järvelin MR: The long-term effects of children's early onset disability on marital relationships. Dev Med Child Neurol 38:567–577, 1996

Tallal P: Developmental language disorders, in Learning Disabilities: Proceedings of the National Conference. Edited by Kavanagh JF, Truss TJ. Parkton, MD, York, 1988, pp 181–272

Tallal P, Stark PE: Perceptual/motor profiles of reading impaired children with or without concomitant oral language deficits. Annals of Dyslexia 32:163–176, 1982

Tanaka Y, Yoshida A, Kawahata N, et al: Diagnostic dyspraxia: clinical characteristics, responsible lesion and possible underlying mechanism. Brain 119:859–873, 1996

Teicher MH, Baldessarini RJ: Developmental pharmacodynamics, in Psychiatric Pharmacosciences of Adolescents and Children. Edited by Popper C. Washington, DC, American Psychiatric Press, 1987

Teicher MH, Ito Y, Glod CA, et al: Objective measurement of hyperactivity and attentional problems in ADHD. J Am Acad Child Adolesc Psychiatry 35:334–342, 1996

Thapar A, Gottesman II, Owen MJ, et al: The genetics of mental retardation. Br J Psychiatry 164:747–758, 1994

Tibbits-Kleber AL, Howell RJ: Reactive attachment disorder of infancy (RAD). Journal of Clinical Child Psychology 14:304–310, 1985

Tizard J, Schofield WN, Hewison J: Collaboration between teachers and parents in assisting children's reading. Br J Educ Psychol 52:1–15, 1982

Tohgi H, Saitoh K, Takahashi S, et al: Agraphia and acalculia after a left prefrontal (F1, F2) infarction. J Neurol Neurosurg Psychiatry 58:629–632, 1995

Tolan PH: Implications of age of onset for delinquency risk. J Abnorm Child Psychol 15:47–63, 1987

Tolan PH, Cromwell RE, Brasswell M: Family therapy with delinquents: a critical review of the literature. Fam Process 25:619–650, 1986

Tremblay RE, LeBlanc M, Schwartzman AE: The pediatric power of first-grade peer and teacher ratings of behavior: sex differences in antisocial behavior and personality at adolescence. J Abnorm Child Psychol 16:571–583, 1988

Trites RL: Prevalence of hyperactivity in Ottawa, Canada, in Hyperactivity in Children. Edited by Trites RL. Baltimore, MD, University Park Press, 1979

Trott GE, Friese HJ, Menzel M, et al: Use of moclobemide in children with attention deficit hyperactivity disorder. Psychopharmacology 106:S134–S136, 1992

Uhlig T, Merkenschlager A, Brandmaier R, et al: Topographic mapping of brain electrical activity in children with food-induced attention deficit hyperkinetic disorder. Eur J Pediatr 156:557–561, 1997

Uygur MC, Ozgü IH, Ozen H, et al: Long-term treatment of nocturnal enuresis with desmopressin intranasal spray. Clin Pediatr (Phila) 36:455–459, 1997

Valentine J, Rossi E, O'Leary P, et al: Thyroid function in a population of children with attention deficit hyperactivity disorder. J Paediatr Child Health 33:117–120, 1997

van der Plas RN, Benninga MA, Redekop WK, et al: Randomised trial of biofeedback training for encopresis. Arch Dis Child 75:367–374, 1996

Van Tilburg MA, Vingerhoets AJ, Van Heck GL: Homesickness: a review of the literature. Psychol Med 26:899–912, 1996

Vandenberg SG, Singer SM, Pauls DL: The Heredity of Behavior Disorders in Adults and Children. New York, Plenum, 1986

Varan B, Saatçi U, Ozen S, et al: Efficacy of oxybutynin, pseudoephedrine and indomethacin in the treatment of primary nocturnal enuresis. Turk J Pediatr 38:155–159, 1996

Verkerk AJMH, Piereti M, Sutcliffe JS, et al: Identification of a gene (FMR-1) containing a CGG repeat coincident with a breakpoint cluster region exhibiting length variation in fragile X syndrome. Cell 65:396–399, 1991

Vermeer DE, Frate DA: Geophagia in rural Mississippi: environmental and cultural contexts and nutritional implications. Am J Clin Nutr 32:2129–2135, 1979

Voeller K: Right-hemisphere deficit syndrome in children. Am J Psychiatry 143:1004–1009, 1986

Volkmar FR, Cohen DJ: Disintegrative disorder or "late onset" autism. J Child Psychol Psychiatry 30:717, 1989

Volkmar FR, Cohen DJ: Nonautistic pervasive developmental disorders, in Psychiatry. Edited by Michels R, Cooper AM, Guze SB, et al. Philadelphia, PA, JB Lippincott, 1991

Volpe JJ: Neurology of the Newborn. Philadelphia, PA, WB Saunders, 1987

von Gontard A, Hollmann E, Eiberg H, et al: Clinical enuresis phenotypes in familial nocturnal enuresis. Scand J Urol Nephrol [Suppl] 183:11–16, 1997

Wadsworth SJ, DeFries JC, Stevenson J, et al: Gender ratios among reading-disabled children and their siblings as a function of parent impairment. J Child Psychol Psychiatry 33:1229–1239, 1992

Walker JL, Lahey BB, Hynd GW, et al: Comparison of specific patterns of antisocial behavior in children with conduct disorder with or without coexisting hyperactivity. J Consult Clin Psychol 55:910–913, 1987

Watanabe H, Azuma Y: A proposal for a classification system of enuresis based on overnight simultaneous monitoring of electroencephalography and cystometry. Sleep 12:257–264, 1989

Weiss G, Hechtman LT: Hyperactive Children Grown Up. New York, Guilford, 1986

Weiss RE, Stein MA, Duck SC, et al: Low intelligence but not attention deficit hyperactivity disorder is associated with resistance to thyroid hormone caused by mutation R316H in the thyroid hormone receptor beta gene. J Clin Endocrinol Metab 78:1525–1528, 1994

Wender PH: Minimal Brain Dysfunction in Children. New York, Wiley, 1971

Wender PH: The Hyperactive Child, Adolescent, and Adult: Attention Deficit Disorder Through the Lifespan. New York, Oxford University Press, 1987

West SA, Sax KW, Stanton SP, et al: Differences in thyroid function studies in acutely manic adolescents with and without attention deficit hyperactivity disorder (ADHD). Psychopharmacol Bull 32:63–66, 1996

Whalen C, Henker B, Buhrmester D, et al: Does stimulant medication improve the peer status of hyperactive children? J Consult Clin Psychol 57:545–549, 1989

Whitaker AH, Van Rossem R, Feldman JF, et al: Psychiatric outcomes in low-birth-weight children at age 6 years: relation to neonatal cranial ultrasound abnormalities. Arch Gen Psychiatry 54:847–856, 1997

Whitehead PL, Clark LD: Effect of lithium carbonate, placebo, and thioridazine on hyperactive children. Am J Psychiatry 127:824–825, 1970

Wichstrøm L, Skogen K, Oia T: Increased rate of conduct problems in urban areas: what is the mechanism? J Am Acad Child Adolesc Psychiatry 35:471–479, 1996

Wiesel TN: Postnatal development of the visual cortex and the influence of environment. Nature 299:583–592, 1982

Wieseler NA, Hanson RH, Nord G: Investigation of mortality and morbidity associated with severe self-injurious behavior. Am J Ment Retard 100:1–5, 1995

Wille S: Comparison of desmopressin and enuresis alarm for nocturnal enuresis. Arch Dis Child 61:30–33, 1986

Wille S: Primary nocturnal enuresis in children. Background and treatment. Scand J Urol Nephrol [Suppl] 156:1–48, 1994

Willemsen-Swinkels SH, Buitelaar JK, Weijnen FG, et al: Plasma beta-endorphin concentrations in people with learning disability and self-injurious and/or autistic behavior. Br J Psychiatry 168:105–109, 1996

Williams ML, Lewandowski LJ, Coplan J, et al: Neurodevelopmental outcome of preschool children both preterm with and without intracranial hemorrhage. Dev Med Child Neurol 29:243–249, 1987

Wing L: Asperger's syndrome: a clinical account. Psychol Med 11:115–130, 1981

Winneke G, Krämer U: Neurobehavioral aspects of lead neurotoxicity in children. Cent Eur J Public Health 5:65–69, 1997

Wise BW, Olson RK: Computer-based phonological awareness and reading instruction. Annals of Dyslexia 45:99–122, 1995

Wolfgang ME, Figlio RM, Cellin T: Delinquency in a Birth Cohort. Chicago, IL, University of Chicago Press, 1972

Wong DF, Singer HS, Brandt J, et al: D_2-like dopamine receptor density in Tourette syndrome measured by PET. J Nucl Med 38:1243–1247, 1997

Wong DF, Ricaurte G, Grunder G, et al: Dopamine transporter changes in neuropsychiatric disorders. Adv Pharmacol 42:219–223, 1998

Woolston JL: Eating disorders in infancy and early childhood. J Am Acad Child Psychiatry 22:114–121, 1983

Wright HH, Miller MD, Cook MA, et al: Early identification and intervention with children who refuse to speak. J Am Acad Child Psychiatry 24:739–746, 1985

Zametkin AJ, Rapoport JL: Neurobiology of attention deficit disorder with hyperactivity: where have we come in 50 years? J Am Acad Child Adolesc Psychiatry 26:676–686, 1987

Zametkin AJ, Nordahl TE, Gross M, et al: Cerebral glucose metabolism in adults with hyperactivity of childhood onset. N Engl J Med 323:1361–1366, 1990

Zeanah CH, Embe RN: Attachment disorders in infancy and childhood, in Child and Adolescent Psychiatry, 3rd Edition. Edited by Rutter M, Hersov L, Taylor E. London, UK, Blackwell, 1995

Ziemann U, Paulus W, Rothenberger A: Decreased motor inhibition in Tourette's disorder: evidence from transcranial magnetic stimulation. Am J Psychiatry 154:1277–1284, 1997

Zigman WB, Schupf N, Sersen E, et al: Prevalence of dementia in adults with and without Down syndrome. Am J Ment Retard 100:403–412, 1996

Zubieta JK, Alessi NE: Is there a role of serotonin in the disruptive behavior disorders? A literature review. J Child Adolesc Psychopharmacol 3:11–35, 1993

CHAPTER 24

SLEEP DISORDERS

THOMAS C. NEYLAN, M.D.
CHARLES F. REYNOLDS III, M.D.
DAVID J. KUPFER, M.D.

This chapter is intended to provide a comprehensive overview of sleep disorders. Despite the extreme scientific and public interest in the function of sleep, its essential purposes remain unknown. There are many theories concerning its function, which include, among others, 1) homeostatic restoration of tissues, particularly the central nervous system (CNS); 2) energy conservation; 3) thermoregulation (Rechtschaffen et al. 1989); 4) discarding of irrelevant memories from the sensory-overloaded brain (Crick and Mitchison 1983); 5) consolidation of perceptual and implicit memory (Karni et al. 1994; Skaggs and McNaughton 1996; Wilson and McNaughton 1994); and 6) protection against predation by remaining aloof from predators.

Clearly a vital function is served by sleep, given the extraordinary adaptations many species have evolved to preserve sleep. For example, zebras on the savanna require the vigilance of awake members of the herd in order to sleep safely in the presence of predators (Moss 1975; Zepelin 1994). Dolphins and other cetaceans sleep one hemisphere at a time, which allows the animals to remain in motion and to continue with respiration (Mukhametov 1984). Yet whatever function is being served, some species have adapted to survive on very little sleep. For example, the giraffe sleeps an average of 2 hours per 24 hours (Zepelin 1994).

NORMAL HUMAN SLEEP

The brain has three major states of activity and function: wakefulness, rapid eye movement (REM) sleep, and non-REM sleep. The neuroanatomic substrate and neurophysiological activity of the brain are different in each major brain state (Hobson and Steriade 1986). For example, the responsiveness of the brain to auditory stim-

Supported in part by the National Alliance for Research in Schizophrenia and Affective Disorders Young Investigator Award (TCN), Veterans Affairs Merit Review (TCN), and National Institute of Mental Health Grants MH 00295 (CFR:RSA), MH37869 (CFR), MH30915 (DJK), and MH52247 (CFR).

uli, thermal stimuli, and hypoxia varies with each state.

REM sleep, identified in 1953 by Aserinsky and Kleitman, is a dramatic physiologic state in that the brain becomes electrically and metabolically activated with frequencies approaching those of wakefulness, accompanied by a 62%–173% increase in cerebral blood flow (Reivich et al. 1968). Perhaps as a defense to preserve sleep, there is a generalized muscle atonia that is detected polysomnographically by the disappearance of electromyographic activity. REMs occur in phasic bursts and are accompanied by fluctuations in respiratory and cardiac rate. There is penile and clitoral engorgement, which is presumed to be mediated by the increase in cholinergic tone associated with the REM state. There is also a suspension of normal temperature regulation; humans become transiently poikilothermic as a result (Parmeggiani 1980). Finally, dreaming in REM sleep is frequently vivid and affectively charged and is associated with activation of the amygdaloid complexes, which is thought to regulate emotionally influenced memory (Macquet et al. 1996).

Healthy sleep in humans consists of recurring 70- to 120-minute cycles of non-REM and REM sleep characterized polysomnographically by the electroencephalogram (EEG), the electrooculogram (EOG), and the electromyogram (EMG) (Rechtschaffen and Kales 1968). The conventional EEG lead used for sleep staging is either C3 or C4 (Jasper 1958). Eye movements are detected by the EOG because of the presence of an electrical dipole between the cornea and retina. Typically, sleep progresses from wakefulness through the four stages of non-REM sleep until the onset of the first REM period. In the healthy adult, the deepest stages of sleep, non-REM stages 3 and 4 (collectively referred to as *slow-wave sleep*), occur in the first two non-REM periods. In contrast, the REM periods in the first half of the sleep period are brief and lengthen in successive cycles.

During wakefulness, the EEG is characterized by low-voltage fast activity consisting of a mix of alpha (8–13 Hz) and beta (>13 Hz) frequencies. *Stage 1* of non-REM sleep is a transitional stage between wakefulness and sleep during which the predominant alpha rhythm disappears, giving way to the slower theta (4–7 Hz) frequencies. Tonic electromyographic activity decreases, and the eyes move in a slow, rolling pattern. *Stage 2* is characterized by a background theta rhythm and the episodic appearance of sleep spindles (i.e., brief bursts of 12- to 14-Hz activity) and K complexes (i.e., a high-amplitude, slow-frequency electronegative wave followed by an electropositive wave). Muscle tone remains diminished, and eye movements are rare. *Stages 3 and 4* are defined as epochs of sleep consisting of greater than 20% and 50%, respectively, of high-

amplitude activity in the delta band (0.5–3.0 Hz). Muscle tone is nearly atonic, and eye movements are absent.

Sleep cannot be localized to a single neurotransmitter system or anatomic location within the brain. The sleep-promoting and wake-promoting systems interact antagonistically and appear to be controlled by several neurotransmitters. Non-REM sleep appears to be driven by the basal forebrain, the area around the solitary tract in the medulla, and the dorsal raphe nucleus (serotonergic cells). Other areas of the brain, primarily the ascending reticular activating system and the posterior hypothalamus, facilitate waking and arousal. The suprachiasmatic nucleus functions as a pacemaker for most circadian rhythms and is involved in the sleep-wake cycle (Rusak and Zucker 1979). REM sleep may be under the control of a system of neurons and neurotransmitters that play antagonistic roles. Cells in the dorsal raphe nucleus (serotonergic), locus coeruleus (noradrenergic), and nucleus peribrachialis lateralis (noradrenergic) may be REM "off" cells. Cholinergic cells in the mesencephalic, medullary, and pontine gigantocellular regions may be REM "on" cells. These two antagonistic systems may interact to produce the alternations between non-REM and REM sleep (Siegel 1994). Sleep-promoting peptides have been found to accumulate in the cerebrospinal fluid (CSF) of sleep-deprived animals. For example, fatty acid primary amides have recently been found to have sleep-promoting properties (Cravatt et al. 1995).

ONTOGENY OF SLEEP STAGES

Infants at birth spend up to 20 hours per day asleep. REM and non-REM stages are not fully differentiated until 3–6 months of age, because of the relative immaturity of neural structures governing sleep. During the first 3 years, the sleep-wake rhythm develops from an ultradian to a circadian pattern, with the principal sleep phase occurring at night. Sleep in prepubertal children is characterized by large percentages of REM and high-amplitude slow-wave sleep. During adolescence, a precipitous decrease in slow-wave sleep (Feinberg 1974) occurs during a period of rapid neuronal senescence and synaptic pruning (Feinberg 1982; Huttenlocher 1979). In the third through sixth decades, there is a gradual and slight decline in sleep efficiency and total sleep time. With advancing age, sleep becomes more fragmented and lighter in depth (Ancoli-Israel 1997; Bliwise 1993; Monk et al. 1992; Neylan et al. 1996). There are more transient arousals, as well as sleep stage shifts, and there is also a gradual disappearance of slow-wave sleep (Gillin and Ancoli-Israel 1992). In addition, the diurnal sleep-wake pattern decays as sleep is redistributed into the light phase in the form of frequent naps (Buysse et al. 1992; Tune 1968).

CLINICAL MANIFESTATIONS AND EVALUATION OF SLEEP DISORDERS

In community and clinical studies, disorders of sleep and wakefulness have been found to be associated with poor job performance, accidents, impaired physical well-being, and increased use of alcohol (Ford and Kamerow 1989; Gallup Organization 1995; Kales et al. 1984; Mellinger et al. 1985; National Commission on Sleep Disorders Research 1993). By conservative estimate, the total annual cost of insomnia in the United States is between $92.5 billion and $107.5 billion (Stoller 1994). The chief complaint usually is related to disrupted or too little sleep, excessive sleepiness, or adverse events associated with the sleep period.

A thorough medical and psychiatric history is essential for diagnosing conditions that have an impact on sleep-wake function. The entire 24-hour period should be explored with respect to sleep-wake habits. Patients with insomnia should be questioned about their views on what constitutes healthy sleep. Very often patients who by virtue of their constitution are short sleepers are subjectively distressed by their inability to sleep for the popular standard of 8 hours. The severity of insomnia can be understood only in terms of its impact on daytime function such as mood, fatigue, muscle aches, attention, and concentration. Asking patients about the total number of hours of sleep typically obtained has limited value, given the overlap between good and poor sleepers (Figure 24–1). Self-rating instruments such as the Pittsburgh Sleep Quality Index (Buysse et al. 1989) are useful for measuring subjective sleep quality. A 2-week sleep-wake log is invaluable for obtaining a history of irregular sleep-wake patterns; napping; use of stimulants, hypnotics, or alcohol; diet; activity during the day; number of arousals; and perceived length of sleep time and its relationship to daytime mood and alertness.

Approximately 4%–5% of the general population complain of excessive sleepiness (Bixler et al. 1979). Sleepiness relates to the propensity to sleep, such as after sleep deprivation. Clinically, it is more alarming than insomnia because of the higher degree of psychosocial impairment as well as the high rate of automobile and occupational accidents (Guilleminault and Carskadon 1977; Mitler et al. 1988; T. Roth et al. 1994). The severity of sleepiness can be considered mild if sleep episodes occur during sedentary activity such as watching television; moderate if sleep occurs during mild physical activity such as driving; and severe if sleep occurs during physical activity that requires

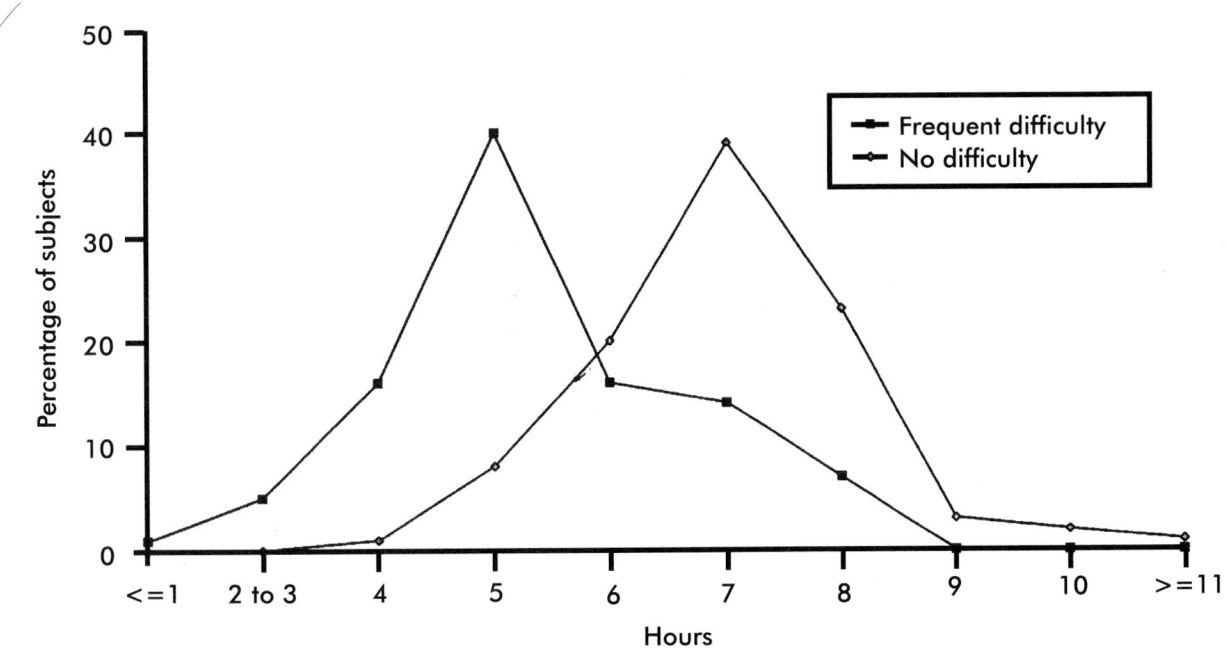

FIGURE 24–1. Average number of hours of sleep each night in good and poor sleepers. Adapted from Gallup Organization 1995.

moderate attention such as talking or eating (American Sleep Disorders Association Diagnostic Classification Steering Committee 1990). Patients should be asked about symptoms of morning headaches, cataplexy, hypnagogic or hypnopompic hallucinations, sleep paralysis, automatic behavior, or sleep drunkenness (Table 24–1). In addition, they should be questioned carefully about falling asleep while driving or while performing any other potentially dangerous activity. Additional history should be obtained from bed partners for events usually not perceived by the patients, such as snoring, respiratory pauses longer than 10 seconds, unusual body movements, or somnambulism.

Patients who complain of disturbances associated with

the sleep period should be questioned about nocturnal incontinence or polyuria, orthopnea, paroxysmal nocturnal dyspnea, headaches that interrupt sleep, jaw clenching or bruxism, sleeptalking, somnambulism, and, in the case of males, painful nocturnal erections (Aldrich 1994).

Polysomnography remains the principal diagnostic tool in the field of sleep medicine. A thorough polysomnographic study provides data on sleep continuity, sleep architecture, REM physiology, sleep-related respiratory impairment, oxygen desaturation, cardiac arrhythmias, and periodic movements. Additional measures may include nocturnal penile tumescence, temperature, and infrared video monitoring. The routine use of polysomnography in the evaluation of hypersomnolent patients is well justified given the high incidence of sleep apnea and narcolepsy in this group (Coleman et al. 1982). Polysomnography should be used in any patient with a parasomnia in which there is clinical suspicion of sleep apnea or nocturnal seizure disorder. Practice guidelines for the use of polysomnography in the evaluation of chronic insomnia have been recommended by the American Sleep Disorders Association (Table 24–2).

The Multiple Sleep Latency Test (MSLT) (Carskadon et al. 1986) is the most objective and valid measure of excessive sleepiness. Other measures such as the Stanford Sleepiness Scale (Hoddes et al. 1973) and the Maintenance of Wakefulness Test (Mitler et al. 1982) are less reliable, although they are easy and inexpensive to use. The Epworth Sleepiness Scale measures daytime sleepiness in eight common real-life situations (Johns 1991). In the MSLT, the patient is given the opportunity to fall asleep in a darkened room for five 20-minute periods in 2-hour intervals across

TABLE 24–1. Sleep definitions

Apnea	Cessation of airflow for at least 10 seconds.
Cataplexy	Sudden loss in muscle tone, usually precipitated by a sudden emotional response such as fear or laughter.
Chronobiology	The study of natural physiological rhythms.
Circadian rhythm	A regular pattern of fluctuation in physiology or behavior that is usually linked to the 24-hour light-dark cycle.
Diurnal	A behavior or physiological variable that is tied to daytime.
Hypersomnia	Excessive sleepiness. Pertains to the propensity to fall asleep.
Hypnagogic or hypnopompic hallucinations	Hallucinations occurring at the beginning or end of sleep that are usually a manifestation of REM sleep.
Hypopnea	Reduction in airflow by at least 50% for at least 10 seconds.
Insomnia	Difficulty with initiating or maintaining sleep.
Myoclonus	Abrupt contraction of a group of muscles, usually in the lower extremity.
Paradoxical sleep	Synonym for REM sleep.
Parasomnia	Adverse physiological or behavioral event occurring during sleep.
Phase advance or delay	Shift of the sleep or wake cycle to an earlier or later position in the 24-hour day.
Polysomnogram	The electrophysiological recording of multiple biological parameters during sleep.
Zeitgeber	An environmental factor, such as the light-dark cycle, that helps entrain biological rhythms to a 24-hour time period.

Note.   REM = rapid eye movement.
Source.   Adapted from American Sleep Disorders Association Diagnostic Classification Steering Committee 1990.

TABLE 24–2. Practice guidelines for the use of polysomnography in the evaluation of insomnia

Polysomnography is not routinely indicated for transient or chronic insomnia.

Polysomnography is indicated when sleep apnea or myoclonus is suspected, particularly in older patients.

Polysomnography should be considered if the diagnosis is uncertain *and* behavior or drug therapy is ineffective.

Polysomnography is indicated for patients with confusional or violent arousals, particularly if the clinical diagnosis is uncertain.

Polysomnography should be considered for circadian rhythm disorders if the clinical diagnosis is uncertain.

Source.   Adapted from American Sleep Disorders Association Standards of Practice Committee 1995.

the patient's usual period of wakefulness. The average latency to sleep onset, measured polysomnographically, is a direct measure of the propensity to fall asleep. Multiple studies have shown that an average sleep latency of less than 5 minutes indicates a pathological degree of sleepiness associated with a high rate of intrusive sleep episodes during the wake period and decrements in work performance (Carskadon et al. 1981; Dement et al. 1978; Nicholson and Stone 1986). The detection of sleep-onset REM periods in the MSLT has become a cornerstone in the diagnosis of narcolepsy (Mitler 1982).

CLASSIFICATION OF SLEEP DISORDERS

DSM-IV (American Psychiatric Association 1994) divides sleep disorders into four major categories: primary sleep disorders, sleep disorders related to another mental disorder, sleep disorder due to a general medical condition, and substance-induced sleep disorder (Table 24–3).

PRIMARY SLEEP DISORDERS

DYSSOMNIAS

Primary Insomnia

Primary insomnia is the term used to describe difficulty initiating or maintaining sleep, or nonrestorative sleep, lasting at least a month in duration. By definition, primary insomnia results in significant daytime impairment and is not secondary to another sleep disorder. It encompasses several terms, notably *idiopathic insomnia* and *psychophysiologic insomnia*. The degree of sleep fragmentation can be externally validated by polysomnography, which shows prolonged sleep latencies, decreased sleep efficiency, and a predominance of the lighter stages of non-REM sleep (Hauri and Fisher 1986; Hauri and Olmstead 1980). An overview of the evaluation of chronic insomnia is provided in Table 24–4.

For some patients, primary insomnia represents a lifetime disorder or trait characteristic in which the patient has a constitutional predisposition for fragmented sleep (Hauri and Olmstead 1980). The pathophysiology, although unknown, is presumed to be secondary to a neurochemical or structural disorder involving neural networks governing sleep-wake states. Patients with this pattern of primary insomnia are extremely light sleepers and are easily perturbed by environmental noise, temperature fluctuations, and situational anxiety. Several studies sug-

TABLE 24–3. DSM–IV classification of sleep disorders

Primary sleep disorders

Dyssomnias

    Primary insomnia

    Primary hypersomnia

    Narcolepsy

    Breathing-related sleep disorder

    Circadian rhythm sleep disorder (sleep-wake schedule disorder)

        Delayed sleep phase type

        Jet lag type

        Shift work type

        Unspecified

    Dyssomnia not otherwise specified

Parasomnias

    Nightmare disorder (dream anxiety disorder)

    Sleep terror disorder

    Sleepwalking disorder

    Parasomnia not otherwise specified

Sleep disorders related to another mental disorder

Insomnia related to another [Axis I or Axis II] disorder

Hypersomnia related to [Axis I or Axis II] disorder

Other sleep disorders

Sleep disorder due to a general medical condition

    Insomnia type

    Hypersomnia type

    Parasomnia type

    Mixed type

Substance-induced sleep disorder

    Insomnia type

    Hypersomnia type

    Parasomnia type

    Mixed type

gest that primary insomnia can be conceptualized as a disorder of hyperarousal (Regestein et al. 1993). For example, patients with insomnia have a greater 24-hour metabolic rate than age- and weight-matched normal sleepers (Bonnet and Arand 1995). Patients with insomnia have longer average sleep latencies on the MSLT (Stepanski et al. 1988).

Other patients develop primary insomnia following a period of severe stress. In these patients, the symptoms of insomnia do not remit with the resolution of the stressful event, because new behaviors that disrupt sleep have been adapted. For example, some patients develop a form of per-

TABLE 24–4.   Evaluation of chronic insomnia

Step 1	Evaluate for a general medical condition that may adversely affect sleep.
Step 2	Evalute whether medications or substance use is disrupting sleep.
Step 3	Evaluate whether another mental disorder such as depression, schizophrenia, or anxiety disorder is causing sleep disruption.
Step 4	Consider a breathing-related sleep disorder, particularly if the patient snores or is obese.
Step 5	Consider a sleep-wake schedule disorder if the patient has an irregular schedule or is involved in shift work.
Step 6	Consider a parasomnia diagnosis if the patient complains of behavioral or mental events that occur during sleep.
Step 7	If insomnia has persisted for more than a month and is not related to the above disorders, then the diagnosis is primary insomnia.
Step 8	If insomnia is not described by the above criteria, then the diagnosis of dyssomnia not otherwise specified is used.

Source.   Adapted from Reynolds et al. 1995.

formance anxiety associated with going to sleep. Their struggles to fall asleep and their anxiety about possible daytime fatigue set up a conditioned association between bedtime behavior and anxious arousal. Often environmental cues in the sleeping environment, such as clocks, become associated and paired with arousal, thus further reinforcing the sleep disturbance. Patients with this pattern of primary insomnia are often able to sleep better when they are away from home because of the removal of these environmental cues. The disorder can become chronic, persisting over many years, and can cause chronic fatigue, muscle aches, and mood disturbance (Hauri and Fisher 1986).

There are several effective treatment approaches to chronic insomnia that do not involve the use of hypnotics. Education about normal sleep and counseling around habits for promoting good sleep hygiene are a good but not sufficient intervention when used alone (Hauri 1989; Morin et al. 1994). Various relaxation therapies such as hypnosis, meditation, deep breathing, and progressive muscle relaxation can be helpful. These techniques, in contrast to the use of hypnotics, are not immediately beneficial but require several weeks of practice to improve sleep (McClusky et al. 1991). Success is dependent on a high degree of motivation in patients, who must devote considerable time to practicing these techniques. Those who succeed in learning these techniques have a greater satisfaction with main-

tenance treatment than do patients chronically using hypnotics (Bootzin and Perlis 1992; Morin et al. 1992). Further, responders to behavioral interventions have sustained benefits after 6 months (Jacobs et al. 1996). Biofeedback can be helpful in those patients who are not sensitive to their internal state of arousal (Hauri and Esther 1990). Patients are provided an external measure of a biological variable such as an EMG or EEG that allows them a means to influence their own level of arousal.

Stimulus control behavior modification focuses on eliminating environmental cues associated with arousal (Bootzin 1972). This technique is similar to implementing rules for sleep hygiene in that patients are instructed to use their bed only for sleep and intimacy, to go to bed only when sleepy, to remove clocks from sight, and to adhere to a stable sleep-wake schedule. The goal is to limit the amount of wake time spent in bed, thereby reestablishing the association between the bed and sleep.

Sleep restriction therapy is similarly aimed at reducing the amount of wake time spent in bed (Spielman et al. 1987). Patients are asked to record in a sleep diary the amount of time they estimate they are asleep. They are then instructed to restrict their time in bed to a degree commensurate to their estimate of their total sleep time. Patients often have their usual difficulties with sleep fragmentation during the first few nights and become sleep deprived. Sleep deprivation helps consolidate sleep on subsequent nights, thereby improving sleep efficiency. Increases in length of time in bed can subsequently be titrated to the presence of daytime fatigue.

Hypnotic medications.   Very few clinicians dispute that the use of benzodiazepines of short and intermediate half-life in appropriate doses is safe and effective in treating transient insomnia in non–substance-abusing young and middle-aged adults. However, a recent epidemiologic study in France showed that 82% of subjects who reported occasional use of hypnotics had used them for more than 6 months (Ohayon 1996). Elderly patients have reduced clearance of hypnotics and hence experience more sedation and cognitive side effects than do younger patients (Greenblatt et al. 1991). The use of hypnotics in treating chronic insomnia remains controversial, particularly in elderly patients, and is a subject of considerable debate. In this subsection we focus on treating the elderly, because they receive a disproportionate amount of prescribed sedatives (Wooten 1992). Concerns raised in the debate about hypnotic use are applicable to all patient groups.

The field of sleep medicine remains divided in this area, and at present there is no consensus on the long-term use of hypnotics in any patient population. Historically, there have always been concerns about hypnotics, many of which were realistic concerns about the potential for overdose and addiction with barbiturates. The introduction of long–half-life benzodiazepines brought about concerns of daytime impairment and memory disturbance (Gillin 1991). In particular, long–half-life benzodiazepines increase both the risk of falls in elderly persons (Mendelson 1996a; Ray et al. 1989) and the number of errors made while driving an automobile (Betts and Birtle 1982). Short–half-life benzodiazepines have fewer "hangover" effects (Johnson and Chernik 1982), but there are concerns about daytime anxiety, confusion, hyperexcitability (Oswald 1989), global amnesia (Morris and Estes 1987), and next-day memory impairment (Bixler et al. 1991). Rebound insomnia after drug withdrawal, particularly with short–half-life benzodiazepines, is well described and represents an abstinence syndrome (Roehrs et al. 1986).

All benzodiazepines, particularly those with short half-lives, have some potential for addiction. Abrupt withdrawal of any benzodiazepine will cause some degree of rebound anxiety and insomnia (Mendelson 1990); short-half-life compounds have the greatest effect. However, most patient groups who chronically use benzodiazepines do not escalate the dosages over time (American Psychiatric Association 1990). Further, careful tapering of benzodiazepines, including short–half-life compounds, is effective in eliminating the abstinence syndrome (Greenblatt et al. 1987).

Any discussion of safety must include a consideration of the alternative drugs used for insomnia. To date, there is no hypnotic available that can be used in elderly patients without risk. For example, over-the-counter hypnotics also cause amnesia and daytime sedation at a rate similar to that of prescription hypnotics (Balter and Uhlenhuth 1991). Since 1989, New York State has required the use of triplicate prescriptions for benzodiazepines. The result, predictably, has been a dramatic decline in the use of these drugs. During this time, there has been a reemergence of the use of more dangerous sedative-hypnotics, as evidenced by the increase in reported overdoses of meprobamate and methaqualone (Hoffman et al. 1991; Weintraub et al. 1991). Trazodone has several advantages as a hypnotic, with its sustained efficacy and its lack of anticholinergic effects (Ware and Pittard 1990). Trazodone has been found to be effective as an adjunctive medication for patients with depression who are being treated with other antidepressants (Nierenberg et al. 1994). However, it can cause hypotension and increase the risk of falls and fractures. Melatonin, which will be discussed in more detail in a subsequent section, has been found to be a modestly effective hypnotic in some but not all studies (Brzezinski 1997). Zolpidem is a short–half-life nonbenzodiazepine drug that binds selectively to the type-1 benzodiazepine receptor subtype (Langer et al. 1987). It has no effect on nocturnal respiratory function in patients with obstructive lung disease (Girault et al. 1996). In therapeutic doses, it has minimal effects on sleep architecture and does not cause rebound insomnia after discontinuation (Kryger et al. 1991; Merlotti et al. 1989). Like triazolam, zolpidem causes short-term impairment of memory that is reversible by flumazenil (Wesensten et al. 1995).

The pros and cons of various hypnotics are overviewed in Table 24–5. The guidelines of the National Institutes of Health Consensus Development Conference Statement on the Treatment of Sleep Disorders of Older People (1991) are pertinent. Hypnotics should be considered only after a thorough diagnostic assessment of secondary causes of insomnia, after sleep hygiene has been improved, and after behavioral treatments have been attempted. If these approaches are unsuccessful, then hypnotics can be used, starting with very low doses and limiting use to short periods. Long-term efficacy studies of behavior and pharmacological interventions in insomnia are clearly needed (Kupfer and Reynolds 1997).

Primary Hypersomnia

The diagnosis of primary hypersomnia subsumes two International Classification of Sleep Disorders categories: idiopathic hypersomnia and recurrent hypersomnia (Kleine-Levin syndrome). Both variants are characterized by prolonged nocturnal sleep and severe daytime sleepiness that can be objectively documented by a short mean sleep latency on the MSLT. Primary hypersomnia is a diagnosis of exclusion, made when other disorders causing excessive sleepiness have been ruled out. A recurrent form of primary hypersomnia is characterized by intermittent attacks of hypersomnolence and hyperphagia, often associated with indiscrete hypersexuality, poor social judgment, mood disturbance, and hallucinations. Between episodes there can be a complete remission of symptoms. This pattern of primary hypersomnia occurs most frequently in males in their late adolescence and early twenties, after which time there is a gradual decline in the frequency and duration of the episodes (Critchley 1962). The pathophysiology of primary hypersomnia is postulated to involve an underlying disturbance of limbic and hypothalamic function. Several abnormal laboratory findings have been documented, including slowing of background rhythm on the EEG, altered secretory pattern of growth hormone and thyroid-stimulating hormone, and elevated

TABLE 24-5.　Overview of the use of hypnotics in the treatment of elderly patients

Hypnotic	Advantages	Disadvantages
Antidepressants		
Amitriptyline	No tolerance	Anticholinergic delirium, increased risk of falls, daytime sedation
Doxepin	No tolerance	Increased risk of falls, daytime sedation
Trazodone	No tolerance, no anticholinergic effects	Increased risk of falls, daytime sedation
Antipsychotics		
Haloperidol	No tolerance, few anticholinergic effects	Extrapyramidal effects, increased risk of falls, not very sedating
Thioridazine	No tolerance	Extrapyramidal effects, increased risk of falls, anticholinergic delirium
Barbiturates	No pertinent advantages over benzodiazepines	High risk of addiction, dangerous withdrawal syndrome, overdose potential, daytime sedation
Benzodiazepines		
Estazolam	Intermediate half-life	Some daytime sedation and performance decrements
Flurazepam	Delayed rebound insomnia	Daytime sedation, high risk of falls, driving errors
Temazepam	Intermediate half-life	Some daytime sedation and performance decrements
Triazolam	No daytime sedation	Rebound insomnia
Miscellaneous		
Chloral hydrate	Less addictive than benzodiazepines	Overdose potential, tolerance to hypnotic effects over time, nausea
Diphenhydramine	No tolerance	Anticholinergic delirium, increased risk of falls, daytime sedation and memory impairment
Zolpidem	No disruption to sleep architecture, no tolerance	Memory impairment and sensory distortions immediately after usage

CSF serotonin and dopamine metabolites (Billiard 1989; Chesson et al. 1991). Polysomnographic studies have shown diminished delta sleep, increased number of awakenings, and reduced REM latency (Reynolds et al. 1980). In one report (Reynolds et al. 1984), the MSLT revealed the presence of sleep-onset REM periods during the acute attack but not during recovery. Treatment usually involves the use of stimulants for both the hypersomnolence and the increased appetite.

Narcolepsy

Narcolepsy is a common cause of daytime hypersomnolence in which REM sleep repeatedly and suddenly intrudes into wakefulness. It represents an impairment in the ability to maintain a stable neural state; REM is no longer segregated in its usual ultradian rhythm during sleep. The clinical phenomenology of narcolepsy is best understood through a consideration of normal REM physiology (e.g., activated EEG, generalized atonia, dream cognition). Both cataplexy and sleep paralysis involve muscle atonia occurring at a time when the patient is cognizant of

the environment and subjectively feels awake. Hypnagogic hallucinations are not well understood but are thought to be related to the dreamlike perceptual phenomenon of REM sleep. Nocturnal sleep is characterized by short REM latency and frequent arousals and shifts from non-REM sleep to REM sleep to wakefulness (Rechtschaffen et al. 1963).

Although the term *narcolepsy* (literally, *sleep seizure*), as coined by Gelineau (1880), suggests an ictal disorder, the pathophysiology remains unknown. There is convincing evidence of a heritable transmission of the disorder. A canine form of narcolepsy shows an autosomal recessive mode of transmission (Foutz et al. 1979). In humans, there is a close association of the disorder with the human leukocyte antigen (HLA) DR2 and DQw1 haplotypes genetically encoded on chromosome 6. Although the DR2 antigen is found in 10%–35% of the general population, it has been found in some ethnic groups to be 100% associated with narcolepsy (Juji et al. 1984; Langdon et al. 1986). The risk for narcolepsy in first-degree relatives of affected probands is 41 times that in the general population (Billiard et al. 1994).

Studies have shown that narcolepsy affects psychological state as well as cognition. Patients have been found to have more job-related injuries, problems with occupational or academic performance, and a higher prevalence of anxiety and mood disorders (Richardson et al. 1990). Several studies of patients with narcolepsy have shown impaired performance in tasks requiring sustained attention, as a result of intrusive microsleeps. However, not all performance decrements can be attributed to impaired arousal, because attention deficits have been found in narcoleptic patients during EEG-verified wakefulness (for review, see Mendelson 1987). In one study (Reynolds et al. 1983b), 20% of 25 patients with narcolepsy met criteria for major depression, 8% for generalized anxiety disorder, and 12% for alcohol abuse. An unresolved issue is whether the higher prevalence of psychiatric symptomatology is a response to the psychosocial consequences of having a chronic disorder in which existing treatments are often inadequate or whether the mood and affective disturbance are driven by a common pathophysiology.

Therapeutic approaches include the use of stimulants such as methylphenidate, amphetamine, pemoline, and modafinil to treat daytime somnolence. Modafinil, an atypical psychostimulant that affects postsynaptic α_1-adrenergic receptors, promotes wakefulness and is rarely associated with substance dependence (Besset et al. 1996). Modafinil is less effective than amphetamine in controlling cataplexy (Shelton et al. 1995). REM-suppressing agents such as tricyclic antidepressants and γ-hydroxybutyrate have been found to control cataplexy. Numerous other medications have been tried and found to have modest benefit, including codeine, propranolol, bromocriptine, L-tyrosine, selegiline, and methysergide (Aldrich 1992; Boivin et al. 1993; Laffont et al. 1994; Reinish et al. 1995). An important nonpharmacological approach is the use of scheduled naps throughout the wake period. Practice guidelines for the use of stimulants in the treatment of narcolepsy have been recommended by the American Sleep Disorders Association (Table 24–6). Patients with narcolepsy who are taking high doses of stimulants still have a greater degree of daytime somnolence compared with control subjects (Mitler 1994).

Breathing-Related Sleep Disorder

If evolution had led to the development of a stiff upper airway, the problems of snoring and obstructive apnea would never have occurred. Because it must be flexible for purposes of swallowing and production of speech, the upper airway has an inherent potential for collapse during respiration. To compensate for this vulnerability, there is a

TABLE 24–6. Practice guidelines for the use of stimulants in the treatment of narcolepsy

The diagnosis of narcolepsy should be established by a polysomnogram and the Multiple Sleep Latency Test.

Stimulants should be used to alleviate daytime sleepiness, not to maximize performance.

Pemoline, methylphenidate, dextroamphetamine, methamphetamine, and modafinil have proven efficacy.

The recommended maximum daily doses for some of the stimulants used to treat narcolepsy are as follows:

Pemoline	150 mg
Methylphenidate	100 mg
Dextroamphetamine	100 mg
Methamphetamine	80 mg

Combining short- and long-acting stimulants may be indicated in some patients.

Tolerance is most likely to occur in treatment with high-dose amphetamines.

Amphetamines have the highest potential for illicit use.

Most female patients should discontinue taking stimulants during pregnancy if this does not present intolerable risk to the woman.

Caution is urged in prescribing stimulants to nursing mothers.

Source. Adapted from American Sleep Disorders Association Standards of Practice Committee 1995.

complex set of muscles that dilate the upper airway during inspiration. The neurological regulation of these muscles differs in each of the major brain states: wakefulness, non-REM sleep, and REM sleep. For example, in REM sleep the phasic activity of these muscles with each breath is diminished, leading to an increased potential for collapse (Sauerland and Harper 1976). In addition, anatomic factors that affect lumen size (e.g., obesity) and exogenous factors that reduce phasic muscle activity of the upper airway (e.g., sedative-hypnotics [Bonora et al. 1984]) can independently lead to an increased potential for airway collapse. Genetic factors, independent of obesity, contribute to the heritability of sleep apnea, through the influence of craniofacial traits (Mathur and Douglas 1995; Nelson and Hans 1997).

Sleep-disordered breathing is an age-related disorder affecting approximately 24% of community-dwelling individuals over age 65 (Ancoli-Israel et al. 1991) and 42% of elderly persons living in nursing homes (Ancoli-Israel 1989). The estimated prevalence of apnea in a random sample of employed middle-aged subjects is 9% for women and 24% for men (Young et al. 1993). On the basis of findings of a multicenter study of polysomnographic diagnoses made in sleep centers nationwide, it was found that 43% of all patients with excessive daytime somnolence had a sleep apnea syndrome (Coleman et al. 1982). Although occasionally causing insomnia, sleep apnea is typically an occult disorder that causes daytime somnolence, impaired concentration and intellectual functioning, and morning headaches. It is associated with obesity, loud snoring, systemic and pulmonary hypertension, cardiac arrhythmias, nocturnal cardiac ischemia, myocardial infarction, and excessive mortality (Shafer et al. 1997; Strollo and Rogers 1996; Yamashiro and Kryger 1994). It can be caused by an impairment in central respiratory drive (central apnea), intermittent upper airway obstruction (obstructive apnea), or a combination of the two (mixed apnea). Patients with this disorder experience frequent respiratory pauses during sleep that are associated with oxygen desaturation. The apneic events are terminated by loud gasping, thrashing movements, as well as arousal on EEG. Patients, who usually have no awareness of these events, are often brought to clinical attention by alarmed bed partners (Guilleminault 1982).

Sleep apnea is quantified polysomnographically by measuring oral and nasal airflow with thermistors, which are warmed by exhaled air; respiratory effort with either thoracic and abdominal strain gauges, diaphragmatic or intercostal EMG, or an esophageal pressure gauge; oxygen saturation with an oximeter; and sleep architecture with a standard sleep montage (i.e., EEG, EOG, EMG). Patients with severe sleep apnea typically have evidence of pathological sleepiness as measured by latencies to sleep onset of less than 5 minutes on the MSLT. Ball et al. (1997) found that an effort by sleep specialists to increase awareness of obstructive sleep apnea among primary care physicians succeeded in dramatically increasing case recognition and treatment of the disorder.

The clinical impact of sleep apnea is related to two phenomena: hypoxia and sleep fragmentation. Cerebral hypoxia can lead to intellectual deterioration, impaired attention and memory, and personality changes. Successful treatment improves neurocognitive performance on most, but not all, measures, which suggests that permanent anoxic injury occurs in some patients (Bedard et al. 1993). Several investigators have attempted to discern whether hypersomnolence is related to sleep hypoxia or to sleep fragmentation. Roehrs et al. (1989) reported a study of 466 patients with obstructive sleep apnea in which multiple polysomnographic variables, including arousals on EEG and oxygen desaturations, were independently analyzed for prediction of excessive daytime somnolence. Although the number of arousals and hypoxic events covaried significantly, it was the arousal index that best predicted short

latencies on the MSLT. This finding suggests that hypersomnolence is secondary to the disruption in quantity and quality of sleep. A study of older insomnia patients with and without mild to moderate sleep apnea showed that when sleep fragmentation is controlled, apneas and hypoxic events do not predict additional psychomotor impairment (Stone et al. 1994).

There are a variety of behavioral, medical, pharmacological, and surgical treatments for sleep apnea. Behavioral approaches include weight loss, abstinence from sedative-hypnotics, and sleep-position training (which helps the patient avoid the supine position during sleep) (Cartwright et al. 1991a). Mechanical approaches include use of tongue-retaining devices, orthodontic appliances that advance the mandible (Loube and Strauss 1997; Nakazawa et al. 1992), and nasal continuous positive airway pressure (CPAP). Antidepressant medications, such as protriptyline and fluoxetine, play a limited role in the treatment of milder cases of obstructive sleep apnea (Hanzel et al. 1991). Surgical techniques aim to increase the lumen size of the oropharynx and include uvulopalatopharyngoplasty (UPPP), maxillomandibular and hyoid advancement, and chronic tracheostomy (Powell et al. 1994). Follow-up studies of patients who have undergone UPPP show that approximately half of the subjects benefit from surgery, and some who do benefit relapse after several years (Janson et al. 1997). Preliminary data suggest that laser-assisted UPPP is inferior to conventional UPPP in enhancing oropharyngeal air space; however, the clinical significance of this finding has not been established (Finkelstein et al. 1997).

To date, nasal CPAP remains the initial treatment of choice for moderate to severe sleep apnea. CPAP acts as a pneumatic splint that maintains the patency of the oropharynx during respiration (Sullivan and Grunstein 1994). The air pressure required to maintain airway patency should be directly titrated in the sleep laboratory. Reports of long-term compliance are variable, ranging from 25% to 70% (Guilleminault et al. 1992). Nightly compliance is required for optimal benefit. One night of discontinuation of nasal CPAP results in complete reversal of the gains made in daytime alertness (Kribbs et al. 1993).

Circadian Rhythm Sleep Disorder (Sleep-Wake Schedule Disorder)

The sleep-wake cycle, under the circadian control of endogenous regulators or oscillators, can be disrupted by a misalignment between biological rhythms and external demands on waking behavior. In mammals the circadian cycle is under the principal control of the suprachiasmatic nucleus, the destruction of which eliminates any circadian rhythmicity (Moore and Eichler 1972; Rusak and Zucker 1979). Circadian rhythm sleep disorders, the vast majority of which do not involve any known structural damage to neural oscillators, present with either insomnia or hypersomnolence, depending on the juxtaposition of performance demands and the underlying circadian cycle.

Circadian rhythm sleep disorders are associated with significant medical comorbidity and impairment in psychosocial functioning. Rotating-shift workers have been found to have an injury rate of two to three times that of their co-workers who work stable day, evening, or night shifts (M. Smith and Colligan 1982). *Shift work type disorder* is associated with high rates of gastrointestinal, cardiac, and reproductive disorders (Czeisler and Allan 1988). Several, but not all, studies show an increase in motor vehicle accidents after the switch to daylight savings time, in which the day is shortened by 1 hour (Coren 1996; Ferguson et al. 1995; Monk 1980).

Rapid shifts in the sleep-wake schedule cause an acute circadian dysrhythmia. The *jet lag type* is one of the most common of these disorders. Travelers flying across multiple time zones are met with a radical change in the cues, called *Zeitgebers*, that help entrain circadian rhythms with respect to both social schedule and the light-dark cycle. Similarly, workers who rotate onto different shifts experience an acute misalignment in their underlying biological rhythms: 65% of workers on rotating shifts complain of poor sleep as compared with 20% of workers on stable shifts (Czeisler et al. 1982). Night shift workers are usually in a state of permanent circadian misalignment because of their tendency to revert to conventional schedules on their days off. Air traffic controllers and attending emergency physicians make more cognitive errors while working night shifts (Luna et al. 1997; Smith-Coggins et al. 1994). Monk (1994) pointed out that the ability to cope with shift work is related to tolerance for circadian desynchrony and decreased sleep, as well as for domestic pressures often experienced by those who work unconventional hours. Although it has been argued that sleep-wake difficulties secondary to shift work are not pathological per se, it is true that, as a group, shift workers have higher rates of divorce, on-the-job sleepiness, and drug use (Regestein and Monk 1991). Patients with irregular sleep-wake patterns may have little to no circadian rhythmicity to their sleep cycle. For example, some institutionalized patients with dementia have a polyphasic sleep-wake cycle in which brief periods of wakefulness followed by napping persist throughout the 24-hour day.

All of these disorders give rise to sleep-wake complaints, mood disturbance, decreased work performance, and general physical malaise. The general treatment approach is to promote good sleep hygiene, with the goal of properly aligning the patients' circadian system with their sleep-wake schedule. Treatment of these disorders also requires an improved approach to shift work by industry and government (Czeisler et al. 1982; Regestein and Monk 1991).

Some circadian sleep-wake disorders are related to a diminished capacity to respond to external Zeitgebers. Congenitally blind subjects, for whom light is ineffective as a Zeitgeber, have been described as having a sleep-wake pattern longer than 24 hours (Miles et al. 1977). Of interest is a report that shows that melatonin administration can entrain a free-running blind subject to a conventional sleep-wake schedule (Sack et al. 1990). Patients with the *delayed sleep phase type* disorder are described as night owls, with an innate preference for beginning sleeping in the late hours of night and sleeping until the late morning or early afternoon. They experience sleep-onset insomnia and morning hypersomnolence when forced to comply with a conventional sleep-wake schedule. There are reports of patients with a phase advance in their sleep-wake schedule who experience hypersomnolence in the early evening hours, as well as midnight arousal. Typically these are older patients, because with age there is a tendency for the sleep-wake cycle to advance relative to clock time. The treatment for many of these disorders involves the realignment of the sleep-wake schedule with manipulation or augmentation of external Zeitgebers, such as with the use of bright light therapy.

Photiotherapy. Multiple studies have shown that exposure to light at 2,000 lux or more can shift circadian rhythms (Terman 1994). Bright light entrains multiple biological rhythms by means of a direct retinohypothalamic tract and excitatory amino acids transducing information to the suprachiasmatic nuclei (Dijk et al. 1995). Much of the literature examining the clinical utility of bright light has focused on seasonal affective disorder (Lewy et al. 1984; Rosenthal et al. 1984). Several investigators have suggested that seasonal affective disorder is a chronobiological disturbance in which the sleep-wake rhythm, as well as other circadian factors, is phase delayed. One hypothesis concerning the therapeutic value of morning bright light is related to its ability to phase-advance or realign these rhythms to a healthy baseline (Lewy et al. 1987; Terman et al. 1988). However, some studies have shown light therapy to be effective independent of circadian phase or time of day (Wirz-Justice et al. 1993). Recent studies have shown that rapid tryptophan depletion under double-blind conditions reverses the therapeutic gains of bright light, which suggests that serotonergic mechanisms are involved in phototherapy (Lam et al. 1996; Neumeister et al. 1997).

With respect to sleep disorders, bright light has been found to be effective in treating delayed sleep phase disorder (Rosenthal et al. 1990) and jet lag (Daan and Lewy 1984). Further, it has been found to improve alertness and cognitive performance in night shift workers (Campbell et al. 1995a). Bright light therapy improves sleep-wake patterns in institutionalized elderly persons. For example, evening light exposure improves sleep maintenance insomnia in the elderly (Campbell et al. 1995b; Mishima et al. 1994). Bright light exposure in the evening reduces sundowning behavior in hospitalized patients with Alzheimer's disease (Satlin et al. 1992).

In one method of therapy, patients are instructed to sit 3 feet in front of a bright light source of at least 2,500 lux intensity (Terman 1994). Typically, patients require between 30 minutes and 2 hours of exposure, depending on therapeutic response. Side effects include eyestrain, headache, and mild psychomotor agitation. At present, there is no evidence that long-term use of bright light therapy results in any ocular damage (Gallin et al. 1995). The timing of exposure depends on the direction in which patients wish to shift their sleep-wake schedule. Morning or evening exposure will phase-advance or phase-delay the sleep-wake schedule, respectively.

Melatonin. The popularity of use of melatonin as a sleep-promoting agent has persisted despite multiple warnings from sleep specialists. Melatonin increases after the onset of the dark cycle and is inhibited by photic stimuli transduced by the retinohypothalamic tract to the suprachiasmatic nucleus to the pineal gland. Currently, melatonin is used clinically primarily for its apparent ability to phase-shift the endogenous circadian rhythm. For example, ingestion of melatonin in the early evening causes the endogenous melatonin release to occur earlier and produces an enhanced propensity for an earlier sleep onset (Lewy et al. 1995). Hence, exogenous melatonin is a potential alternative to bright light therapy for manipulating sleep-wake rhythms to manage jet lag, delayed sleep phase syndrome, and adaptation to rotating work shifts.

Dyssomnia Not Otherwise Specified

The category of dyssomnia not otherwise specified (NOS) includes the phenomenon of *nocturnal myoclonus*, which is characterized by periodic leg movements of sufficient severity to cause sleep continuity disturbance, leading to complaints of either insomnia or daytime sleepiness.

Nocturnal myoclonus consists of repetitive, brief leg jerks that occur in regular 20- to 40-second intervals. These movements are frequently associated with transient arousals that lead to sleep fragmentation and a predominance of the lighter stages of non-REM sleep. Patients are usually unaware of this disorder, except that they may have the experience of morning leg cramps and a sense of insufficient sleep. Periodic leg movements are frequently found on polysomnographic record and are not correlated with subjective measures of sleep quality (Mendelson 1996b).

Nocturnal myoclonus is seen frequently in association with sleep apnea, narcolepsy, uremia, diabetes, and a variety of disorders affecting the cortex, brain stem, and spinal cord (Coleman et al. 1980). Typically, nocturnal myoclonus is idiopathic, with no evidence of gross CNS pathology. It is a normal phenomenon at birth, disappears in childhood, and frequently reemerges in old age. The emergence of myoclonus is thought to be secondary to the loss of inhibition of a naturally occurring pacemaker operating at the level of the spinal cord (Lugaresi et al. 1972; R. C. Smith 1985). The most common treatments involve the use of benzodiazepines, L-dopa/carbidopa, and cognitive-behavior therapy (Becker et al. 1993; Edinger et al. 1996).

Restless legs syndrome is a syndrome that causes sleep-onset insomnia. It is typically characterized by deep paresthesias in the calf muscles, prompting the urge to keep the legs in motion. However, it also can involve the arms in approximately half of those with the syndrome (Montplaisir et al. 1997). Restless legs syndrome can be extremely distressing and has been linked to suicide. It is associated with anemia, pregnancy, and nocturnal myoclonus. It is also associated with uremia and has diagnosed in 20% of patients with end-stage renal disease (Winkelman et al. 1996). There is a familial form of this disorder with an autosomal dominant pattern of transmission with complete penetrance (Trenkwalder et al. 1996). The main treatment involves the use of either benzodiazepines or dopaminomimetics such as L-dopa or bromocriptine (Montplaisir et al. 1992; Trenkwalder et al. 1995). Other agents currently under investigation for use in treatment of restless legs syndrome include opioids, carbamazepine, clonidine, and baclofen (Wagner et al. 1996).

PARASOMNIAS

Parasomnias are adverse events that occur during sleep. Many of these disorders have been described as disorders of partial arousal from various sleep stages (Karacan 1988). There has been much debate regarding whether these disorders emerge from specific sleep stages such as delta and

REM. Mahowald and Schenck (1992) argued that parasomnias and narcolepsy represent dissociated states with mixed features of REM sleep, non-REM sleep, and wakefulness. *Sleepwalking disorder* and *sleep terror disorder* involve intrusions of wake behavior into non-REM sleep. Similarly, *REM sleep behavior disorder*, in which patients are motorically active during dreams, represents an intrusion of wake behavior into a sleep state. This model is also helpful in understanding how some antidepressant medications cause sleep dissociation, as in the case of intrusion of REMs during non-REM sleep with fluoxetine treatment (Schenck et al. 1992).

Sleepwalking and *night terrors* are found normally in young children and are associated with psychopathology only if persisting into adulthood. Typically, they involve a partial arousal from sleep during the first third of the night, a period characterized by a predominance of slow-wave sleep. In sleepwalking, subjects become partially aroused and ambulatory; they are typically difficult to awaken and have amnesia for the events. Data from the Finnish Twin Cohort show that concordance for sleepwalking in childhood is 0.55 in monozygotic and 0.35 in dizygotic pairs (Hublin et al. 1997). Nocturnal violent behavior, seen predominantly in men, can be associated with sleepwalking (Moldofsky et al. 1995). Several forensic cases have involved the argument that sleep-related violence was defensible on the basis of its being a noninsane automatism (Broughton et al. 1994; Schenck and Mahowald 1995). In one survey of 170 adults with injurious parasomnias, long-term nightly use of benzodiazepines was found to be safe and effective (Schenck and Mahowald 1996). Night terrors involve an emergence of intense fear associated with autonomic arousal in which patients are inconsolable, difficult to awaken fully, and unable to assign specific cognitions associated with the anxiety. Treatment is directed toward reducing stress, anxiety, and sleep deprivation, all of which are known to exacerbate these disorders. In extreme cases, low-dose benzodiazepines are indicated and effective.

Nightmare disorder, formerly known as *dream anxiety disorder*, occurs in 10%–50% of children (American Psychiatric Association 1994). The incidence of the disorder peaks between the ages of 3 and 6 (Leung and Robson 1993) and declines with age (Hartmann 1984). According to survey results, 10%–29% of college students have one or more nightmares per month (Belicky and Belicky 1982; Feldman and Hersen 1967). In a survey of 1,006 adults (ages 18–80 years) in Los Angeles, 5.3% of respondents reported that "frightening dreams" were a current problem (Bixler et al. 1979). Results of this survey and others (Coren 1994) have indicated that there is a higher prevalence of

frightening dreams in women. Unfortunately, there is no reliable information about nightmare disorder in adults because nightmares are rarely captured in the sleep laboratory and because subjects are often confused about the difference between night terrors and nightmares, which can obscure survey data (Hartmann 1984). Individuals with nightmare disorder, unlike those with night terrors, have anxiety-provoking dreams characterized by vivid, detailed imagery that is associated with good recall. Further, in none of the aforementioned studies were attempts made to adjust or control for exposure to traumatic stress.

Historically, nightmares have been postulated to be a hallmark of traumatic stress responses (Brett and Ostroff 1985; Freud 1920/1955; Horowitz 1976; Kardiner and Spiegel 1947; Ross et al. 1989). Hartmann (1984), in his studies of patients with frequent nightmares, found that adult exposure to violent assault increased nightmare frequency; however, he was not able to obtain a history of early childhood trauma in his subjects. He and others obtained data from individuals with frequent nightmares and suggested that such persons were distrustful, schizoid, and alienated but were not psychotic (Hartmann et al. 1981; Kales et al. 1980). Kales et al. (1980) also found that the onset of nightmares was preceded by "major life events." The National Comorbidity Survey found a lifetime prevalence of posttraumatic stress disorder (PTSD) of 10.4% in women and 5.0% in men (Kessler et al. 1995), which is similar to the gender ratio reported for individuals who experience frequent nightmares. DSM-IV acknowledges that the prevalence of nightmare disorder is unknown. Given that this diagnosis is excluded when PTSD is present, the validity of nightmare disorder as a separate nosologic entity has not been well established.

REM sleep behavior disorder, which is listed as a parasomnia NOS in DSM-IV, occurs when there is incomplete or absent muscle atonia during REM sleep. The disorder is characterized by prominent motor activity during dreaming. Several dramatic cases have involved patients who suddenly assaulted their bed partners in response to frightening dreams. REM sleep behavior disorder can emerge transiently during drug intoxication or withdrawal or exist as a chronic condition, most typically in patients with demonstrable neurological disease (Mahowald and Schenck 1992; Nofzinger and Reynolds 1994). Benzodiazepines, particularly clonazepam, and carbamazepine have been found to be useful in reducing these events (Bamford 1993; Mahowald and Schenck 1994).

Nocturnal paroxysmal dystonia, another disorder subsumed under parasomnia NOS in DSM-IV, is characterized by stereotypical and violent movements of the trunk and limbs of short duration. These movements can resemble seizure activity and respond to treatment with carbamazepine (Lugaresi et al. 1986). They can occur multiple times during the night and are associated with non-REM sleep. A variant of this disorder involves similar movements, but longer in duration, that do not appear to be epileptic in origin and are not effectively treated with anticonvulsants (Lugaresi and Cirignotta 1984).

Some parasomnias occur during sleep-wake transitions. Head banging, formerly known as *jactatio capitis nocturnus*, is a rhythmic movement disorder that is thought to be a self-soothing behavior in children during the transition from wakefulness to sleep. Sleep starts, or hypnic jerks, are sudden muscle contractions that often occur during sleep onset and are thought to be clinically insignificant.

SLEEP DISORDERS RELATED TO ANOTHER MENTAL DISORDER

MOOD DISORDERS

The theory that disordered sleep physiology precedes the development of depression (Reynolds and Kupfer 1987) is supported by two prospective epidemiological studies that show that persons with insomnia have a higher risk of developing depression at follow-up (Breslau et al. 1996; Ford and Kamerow 1989). Other evidence supports an integral relationship between sleep and depression. For example, sleep deprivation has been shown to improve mood in more than 50% of patients with endogenous depression (Wu and Bunney 1990). The latency to the first REM period (i.e., REM latency) is frequently decreased in patients after clinical remission of their depressive episode (Cartwright et al. 1991b; Hauri et al. 1974; Rush et al. 1986), which suggests that some aspects of sleep physiology may serve as a trait marker for major depression. Several studies with pharmacological probes that affect sleep physiology have shown that patients with depression respond differently to such probes than do patients with other psychiatric disorders or psychiatrically healthy control subjects. For example, patients with depression who are administered a cholinergic agonist in the second non-REM period will enter REM sleep significantly faster than patients with other psychiatric disorders or control subjects without such disorders (Gillin et al. 1991; Sitaram et al. 1980). In contrast, patients with depression have less REM sleep suppression when administered clonidine than do psychiatric and psychiatrically healthy control subjects (Schittecatte et al. 1992). These data suggest that both depression and sleep are regulated in part by aminergic and cholinergic pathways.

Sleep disturbance is verifiable in 90% of patients with major depression and is characterized by sleep fragmentation, decreased quantity and altered distribution of delta sleep, reduced duration of the first non-REM period (i.e., REM latency), redistribution of REM sleep into the first half of the night, and increased number of REMs per minute of REM sleep (Kupfer and Foster 1972; Kupfer and Reynolds 1992; Reynolds and Kupfer 1987). Patients with bipolar disorder, in contrast, typically become hypersomnolent during depressive episodes and have comparatively increased sleep efficiency and total sleep time (Detre et al. 1972). They also report feeling hypersomnolent despite an absence of objective evidence of excessive sleepiness on the MSLT (Nofzinger et al. 1991). Patients with mania have polysomnographic abnormalities that are very similar to those of patients with unipolar depression (Hudson et al. 1992).

A review of sleep data from psychiatric patients leads to the conclusion that no single variable, such as REM latency, has diagnostic specificity (Benca et al. 1992). However, REM latency has been found to be a reliable marker for particular state and trait variables and to have value in predicting clinical course and treatment outcome. For example, first-degree relatives of depressed patients with short REM latency have been found to be at increased risk for major depression (Giles et al. 1988). In addition, first-degree relatives concordant for depression have been found also to be concordant for REM latency (Giles et al. 1987b). Kupfer et al. (1976) showed that the degree of REM latency prolongation and total REM suppression seen during initiation of treatment with amitriptyline predicted clinical response. Similarly, REM suppression by clomipramine has been found to predict response to treatment (Höchli et al. 1986). Short REM latency during an index episode of depression confers a higher risk of relapse after clinical remission (Giles et al. 1987a).

Multiple studies have shown that REM latency is related to state-dependent factors in major depression. For example, Giles et al. (1986) found that REM latency helped distinguish endogenous depression from nonendogenous depression. Short REM latency was related to appetite loss, terminal insomnia, anhedonia, and unreactive mood. In contrast, sleep electroencephalography does not support the biological validity of the diagnoses of primary versus secondary depression, in that the polysomnographic characteristics of each are similar (Thase et al. 1984). Reynolds et al. (1992) showed that subjects with bereavement-related depression had more sleep continuity disturbance and shorter REM latencies than did bereaved subjects without depression. Kupfer et al. (1988) showed, in one of the few longitudinal studies of sleep in depression, that

REM latency is shorter during the earlier phases of relapse in recurrent major depression. This finding was replicated in a study of elderly patients with depression (Dew et al. 1996). Short REM latency is more prevalent among inpatients with depression than among outpatients with depression, suggesting a relationship with the severity of the index episode (Spiker et al. 1978). Disturbed sleep, as measured by REM latency, REM density, and sleep efficiency, predicts a poorer response to cognitive-behavior therapy (Thase et al. 1996). Delusional depression is distinguishable from the nondelusional subtype because the former is associated with a higher frequency of sleep-onset REM periods and decreased total REM time (Thase et al. 1986). It is interesting to note that cerebral glucose metabolism during the first non-REM period has been found to be elevated in subjects with depression compared with controls; this supports the hypothesis that subjects with depression are hyperaroused (Ho et al. 1996).

There have been several attempts to integrate the aforementioned findings into a model that explains the association of sleep physiology with both state and trait characteristics in depression. Kupfer and Ehlers (1989) suggested that a subgroup of patients may have as a heritable characteristic an inherently weak slow-wave sleep process that allows REM to be expressed earlier. Patients with short REM latency may have a lifelong vulnerability for major depression. For example, Lauer et al. (1995) showed that subjects with no lifetime psychiatric disorder and a family history of depression have reduced slow-wave sleep and increased REM density in the first sleep cycle. In other patients, state-dependent phenomena such as arousal or stress temporarily affect sleep architecture. In this group, a short REM sleep measure serves as a state marker that is related to the severity of the episode. For example, unmedicated subjects with depression who are successfully treated with cognitive or interpersonal psychotherapy show a reduction in REM density (Buysse et al. 1997; Thase et al. 1994). Similarly, depressed patients with CNS hyperarousal, as indicated by decreased sleep efficiency, and increased REM density are less likely to respond well to interpersonal or cognitive-behavior therapy (Thase et al. 1996, 1997). Current research in sleep and depression is aimed at clarifying the influence of age, gender, and family history on sleep physiology.

Antidepressant medications vary in their effects on sleep continuity and architecture. Tricyclic antidepressants have different effects on sleep latency and stage 1 and stage 2 sleep, but all increase slow-wave sleep, suppress REM sleep, and prolong REM latency. Most tricyclics produce daytime sedation, which limits their tolerability; this is particularly true of amitriptyline and doxepin. The seda-

tive effect may explain why tricyclics enhance sleep continuity (Benca 1994; Kupfer et al. 1991; Shipley et al. 1985). Monoamine oxidase inhibitors prolong sleep latency, decrease sleep continuity, greatly suppress REM sleep, and prolong REM latency (Benca 1994; Minot et al. 1993). Selective serotonin reuptake inhibitors decrease sleep continuity, increase REM latency, and usually decrease REM time (Hendrickse et al. 1994; Mahowald and Schenck 1992; Nicholson and Pascoe 1988; Saletu et al. 1991). Trazodone increases slow-wave sleep, increases REM latency, decreases REM time, and improves sleep continuity (Muratorio et al. 1974; Scharf and Sachais 1990). Nefazodone produces no change in slow-wave sleep and improves sleep continuity but, in contrast to most other antidepressants, modestly increases REM sleep (Armitage et al. 1994; Rickels et al. 1994; Sharpley et al. 1992; Ware et al. 1994). Bupropion decreases sleep continuity and slow-wave sleep and, like nefazodone, increases REM sleep (Nofzinger et al. 1995). No data are available about the effects of venlafaxine on polysomnographic measures of sleep.

SCHIZOPHRENIA

Two years after the discovery of REM sleep, the first of many reports on REM sleep and schizophrenia was published (Dement 1955). The early studies were driven, in part, by the exciting prospect of finding a link between dream cognition and perception, and psychosis. In the latter half of the 1960s, approximately 50% of all studies of sleep and psychiatric disorders involved patients with schizophrenia (Nofzinger et al. 1993b). Although a specific link between REM sleep and psychosis was never found, most studies clearly show that patients with schizophrenia have disrupted sleep. Many studies are difficult to interpret because of the lack of suitable control subjects for confounding variables such as age, presence of centrally active medication, proximity to drug withdrawal, clinical features (e.g., negative and positive symptoms), and state-dependent characteristics such as acute relapse. Nevertheless, patients with schizophrenia have been found to have prolonged sleep latencies, sleep fragmentation with multiple arousals, decreased slow-wave sleep, variability in REM latency, and decreased REM rebound after REM sleep deprivation (Benson and Zarcone 1993; Ganguli et al. 1987; Keshavan et al. 1990b; Zarcone et al. 1987).

Several investigators have attempted to find correlations between clinical features of schizophrenia and specific sleep variables. For example, the variability in REM latency in schizophrenia has been found to be linked to family history of affective disorder (Keshavan et al. 1990a), presence of negative symptoms (Maggini et al. 1987; Tandon et al. 1989), tardive dyskinesia (Thaker et al. 1989), neuroleptic withdrawal (Neylan et al. 1992; Nofzinger et al. 1993a; Tandon et al. 1992), and non-suppression of cortisol by dexamethasone (Tandon et al. 1996). Increased REM sleep time and increased REM activity in subjects with schizophrenia are associated with suicidal behavior (Lewis et al. 1996). Diminished slow-wave sleep is one of the most replicated and stable findings in schizophrenia (Feinberg and Hiatt 1978; Keshavan et al. 1996), although it has not been observed in all studies (Lauer et al. 1997). It has been found to be associated with poor performance on neuropsychological tests of attention (Orzack et al. 1977) and with negative symptoms (Ganguli et al. 1987; Keshavan et al. 1995a; Tandon et al. 1992; van Kammen et al. 1988). Three studies have shown an inverse relationship between slow-wave sleep and cerebral atrophy as measured by the ventricular brain ratio on computed tomography scans (Benson and Zarcone 1992; Benson et al. 1996; van Kammen et al. 1988). A recent study of 31-P magnetic resonance spectroscopy found an inverse relationship between slow-wave sleep and brain anabolic processes (Keshavan et al. 1995b). Slow-wave sleep has also been found to be correlated with the serotonin metabolite 5-hydroxyindoleacetic acid (5-HIAA) (Benson et al. 1991) and delta sleep–inducing peptide-like immunoreactivity (van Kammen et al.1992) in CSF of volunteers with schizophrenia.

ANXIETY DISORDERS

Sleep in patients with generalized anxiety disorder is similar to that in patients with primary insomnia in that there are prolonged sleep latencies and increased sleep fragmentation. Subjective sleep quality is significantly impaired in subjects with social phobia (Stein et al. 1993). Sleep in patients with anxiety disorders differs from that seen in patients with major depression: patients with anxiety disorders exhibit normal REM latencies and decreased REM percentage (Reynolds et al. 1983a). It has been suggested that patients with symptoms of both depression and anxiety may be segregated with respect to sleep variables on the basis of the presence or absence of a family history of depression (Sitaram et al. 1984).

A study on sleep and panic disorder by Mellman and Uhde (1989) confirmed that panic attacks can arise during sleep. Six of 13 patients with panic disorder were observed to have panic symptoms during sleep when they were being studied electrographically. Of interest, all panic attacks occurred during non-REM sleep, particularly during transitions from stage 2 to delta sleep. This finding adds further data to support the theory that panic attacks can be physiologically provoked. The mild hypercapnia normally found in sleep may predispose patients to sleep panic, although this hypothesis needs further testing (Mellman and Uhde 1989). Patients with panic disorder who are experiencing sleep panic do have more irregularities in tidal volume and increased numbers of microapneas than do control subjects (Stein et al. 1995). Patients with sleep panic attacks have an earlier onset of illness and greater occurrence of comorbid mood and other anxiety disorders (Labbate et al. 1994).

Multiple studies have demonstrated that patients with PTSD have significant sleep continuity disturbance and increased REM phasic activity such as eye movements (Mellman et al. 1995a, 1995b; Ross et al. 1994; Woodward et al. 1996); these symptoms are directly correlated with PTSD symptom severity. Several studies suggest that nightmares may be uniquely related to exposure to traumatic stress. A survey of Holocaust survivors by Rosen et al. (1991) showed that the number of complaints of nightmares was higher in survivors with longer periods of imprisonment in the concentration camps. True et al. (1993) obtained self-report data about sleep in 4,042 monozygotic and dizygotic Vietnam era–veteran twins with varying degrees of combat exposure. Combat exposure was highly correlated with reports of dreams and nightmares but was only weakly associated with sleep-onset and sleep-maintenance insomnia. Neylan and colleagues (1998) conducted a secondary data analysis of the questionnaire items that address complaints about sleep from the National Vietnam Veterans Readjustment Study (NVVRS) (Kulka et al. 1990). The NVVRS was a major population-based study that sampled to represent the entire group of 3.1 million men and women who served in the Vietnam War. The results show that complaints of frequent nightmares are relatively rare and are found exclusively in subjects with PTSD (Neylan et al. 1998). These results support the hypothesis published by Ross and colleagues (1989), who stated that nightmares and disturbances of REM sleep are a hallmark of PTSD.

DEMENTIA

Patients with dementia of the Alzheimer's type (DAT) have more sleep fragmentation, less delta and REM sleep (Vitiello and Prinz 1988), and little to no spindle and K-complex activity (Reynolds et al. 1985a; Smirne et al. 1977) in comparison with age-matched control subjects. Vitiello et al. (1992) suggested that the poor sleep of these patients results from the loss of neurons from areas that participate in the regulation of sleep such as the nucleus basalis of Meynert (McKinney et al. 1982; Sterman and Clemente 1974) and the brain-stem reticular formation (Hirano and Zimmerman 1962). Patients with dementia have more sleep-related phenomena, such as sundowning and nocturnal wanderings, that provoke attempts to consolidate nocturnal sleep with hypnotics as well as prompt families to institutionalize their elderly relatives (Sanford 1975). Patients with DAT spend as much as half of the 24-hour day in bed, often experiencing a polyphasic sleep-wake pattern (Jacobs et al. 1989; Witting et al. 1990). Perhaps aggravating this pattern is the fact that institutionalized elderly patients spend less than 2 minutes per day exposed to bright light (Ancoli-Israel and Kripke 1989).

Studies examining the relationship between sleep, aging, and dementia suggest an important relationship between normal sleep-wake function and cognition. The severity of dementia has been found to correlate with severity of sleep disturbances (Bliwise et al. 1995). Feinberg et al. (1967) suggested that the sleep EEG is an indicator of the functional integrity of the cerebral cortex. An important unanswered question is whether sleep loss in aging is related to cognitive impairment or whether the two emerge secondary to some underlying, independent biological process.

There is evidence that the prevalence of sleep apnea is higher in patients with probable Alzheimer's dementia than in age- and sex-matched control subjects. Further, the severity of dementia is correlated with the severity of apnea (Hoch et al. 1986; Reynolds et al. 1985b). One study has shown that demented patients with sleep apnea have a higher rate of mortality at 2-year follow-up (Hoch et al. 1989).

SLEEP DISORDER DUE TO A GENERAL MEDICAL CONDITION

Sleep can be adversely affected by multiple medical disorders, particularly those that compromise cardiopulmonary function or cause chronic pain. Endocrine disorders such as diabetes and hyperthyroidism can cause significant sleep continuity disturbance. Hot flashes associated with normal menopause can occur in sleep and cause arousals. Patients may complain of insomnia, hypersomnia, parasomnia, or a combination of symptoms.

SLEEP AND SEIZURES

Non-REM sleep has a well-known activating effect on seizure activity. This is in contrast to REM sleep, during which epileptic discharges usually are suppressed. EEG synchronization may explain the higher prevalence of seizures and interictal discharges seen in non-REM sleep (Shouse 1994). Many patients with epilepsy have their seizures predominantly during sleep or on arousal from sleep (Janz 1962). The clinical course depends on the type and severity of the seizure disorder. Although complaints of insomnia are unusual, sleep can be sufficiently fragmented to cause daytime hypersomnolence.

Unusual nocturnal motor behavior, sleep-related incontinence, or nocturnal tongue biting warrants an evaluation for sleep seizures. Often seizure-related behavior is difficult to distinguish from parasomnias such as enuresis and somnambulism. Family history of either parasomnias or seizure disorder is useful collaborative evidence. Persons who exhibit somnambulism usually have more purposeful motor behavior and are easier to redirect. Finally, an all-night EEG may be needed to screen for epileptiform activity.

SLEEP AND PARKINSON'S DISEASE

Sleep disturbance is reported in approximately 75% of patients with Parkinson's disease. These patients' sleep is characterized by an increased number of awakenings, decreased delta and REM sleep, and a scarcity of sleep spindles. The resting tremor usually subsides with the onset of stage 1 sleep, but, depending on the severity of the disorder, it can persist into stage 2 or reemerge during sleep stage changes (April 1966). The pathophysiology of the sleep disturbance is unclear. Patients with Parkinson's disease have been shown to have a higher prevalence of sleep-disordered breathing (Hardie et al. 1986). Nigrostriatal degeneration may have a direct or indirect impact on the neural substrate regulating sleep. Dopaminomimetic drugs such as L-dopa have dose-dependent effects on sleep; lower doses improve sleep quality and higher doses cause decreased sleep efficiency (Bergonzi et al. 1974).

SUBSTANCE-INDUCED SLEEP DISORDER

Substance-induced sleep disorder is related to both direct and indirect toxic effects on sleep. Both alcohol- and hypnotic-induced sleep disorders involve the development of tolerance to the sleep-inducing effects of the agent, as well as increased arousals during withdrawal periods. Many studies have shown that acute alcohol administration causes REM sleep suppression in the first half of the night followed by a rebound increase of REM sleep and arousals in the second half (Mendelson 1987). Acute alcohol use in high doses suppresses REM sleep for the entire night (Knowles et al. 1968). During acute withdrawal, there is marked sleep continuity disturbance and prominent REM sleep rebound (Johnson et al. 1970). Alcoholic individuals admitted to a treatment unit who have evidence of increased REM pressure have a higher rate of relapse at 3 months (Gillin et al. 1994). Abstinent alcoholic subjects have been shown to have decreased slow-wave sleep and increased sleep stage changes for many months after alcohol withdrawal (Adamson and Burdick 1973).

Stimulants cause sleep-onset insomnia during usage and rebound hypersomnia during withdrawal. Food allergy– and toxin-induced sleep disorders presumably involve indirect toxic effects on the physiological substrate regulating sleep. In all of these disorders, careful removal of the offending agent either eliminates the problem or exposes an additional sleep disorder.

CONCLUSIONS

Careful assessment and treatment of sleep disorders can dramatically improve the quality of psychiatric care. Disordered sleep has protean effects on mood, attention, memory, and general sense of vigor. Further, disturbance in sleep has clear prognostic value and must be addressed to optimize clinical care. The search for the core function of sleep remains an exciting area for scientific research, with clear implications for our understanding of basic brain homeostatic mechanisms.

REFERENCES

Adamson J, Burdick JA: Sleep of dry alcoholics. Arch Gen Psychiatry 28:146–149, 1973

Aldrich MS: Narcolepsy. Neurology 42 (suppl 6):34–43, 1992

Aldrich MS: Cardinal manifestations of sleep disorders, in Principles and Practice of Sleep Medicine, 2nd Edition. Edited by Kryger MH, Roth T, Dement WC. Philadelphia, WB Saunders, 1994, pp 413–425

American Psychiatric Association: Benzodiazepine Dependence, Toxicity, and Abuse: A Task Force Report of the American Psychiatric Association. Washington, DC, American Psychiatric Association, 1990

American Psychiatric Association: Diagnostic and Statistical Manual of Mental Disorders, 4th Edition. Washington, DC, American Psychiatric Association, 1994

American Sleep Disorders Association Diagnostic Classification Steering Committee: International Classification of Sleep Disorders: Diagnostic and Coding Manual. Rochester, MN, American Sleep Disorders Association, 1990

American Sleep Disorders Association Standards of Practice Committee: Practice parameters for the use of stimulants in the treatment of narcolepsy. Sleep 17:348–351, 1994

American Sleep Disorders Association Standards of Practice Committee: Practice parameters for the use of polysomnography in the evaluation of insomnia. Sleep 18:55–57, 1995

Ancoli-Israel S: Epidemiology of sleep disorders. Clin Geriatr Med 5:347–362, 1989

Ancoli-Israel S: Sleep problems in older adults: putting myths to bed. Geriatrics 52:20–30, 1997

Ancoli-Israel S, Kripke DF: Now I lay me down to sleep: the problem of sleep fragmentation in elderly and demented residents of nursing homes. Bulletin of Clinical Neurosciences 54:127–132, 1989

Ancoli-Israel S, Kripke DF, Klauber MR, et al: Sleep disordered breathing in community dwelling elderly. Sleep 14:486–495, 1991

April RS: Observations on parkinsonian tremor in all-night sleep. Neurology (New York) 16:720–724, 1966

Armitage R, Rush AJ, Trivedi M, et al: The effects of nefazodone on sleep architecture in depression. Neuropsychopharmacology 10:123–127, 1994

Aserinsky E, Kleitman N: Regularly occurring periods of eye motility and concomitant phenomena during sleep. Science 118:273–274, 1953

Ball EM, Simon RD Jr, Tall AA, et al: Diagnosis and treatment of sleep apnea within the community. The Walla Walla Project. Arch Intern Med 157:419–424, 1997

Balter MB, Uhlenhuth EH: The beneficial and adverse effects of hypnotics. J Clin Psychiatry 52 (suppl):16–23, 1991

Bamford CR: Carbamazepine in REM sleep behavior disorder. Sleep 16:33–34, 1993

Becker PM, Jamieson AO, Brown WD: Dopaminergic agents in restless legs syndrome and periodic limb movements of sleep: response and complications of extended treatment in 49 cases. Sleep 16:713–716, 1993

Bedard MA, Montplaisir J, Malo J, et al: Persistent neuropsychological deficits and vigilance impairment in sleep apnea syndrome after treatment with continuous positive airway pressure (CPAP). J Clin Exp Neuropsychol 15:330–341, 1993

Belicky D, Belicky K: Nightmares in a university population. Sleep Research 11:116, 1982

Benca RM: Mood disorders, in Principles and Practice of Sleep Medicine, 2nd Edition. Edited by Kryger MH, Roth T, Dement WC. Philadelphia, WB Saunders, 1994, pp 899–913

Benca RM, Obermeyer WH, Thisted RA, et al: Sleep and psychiatric disorders: a meta-analysis. Arch Gen Psychiatry 49:651–668, 1992

Benson KL, Zarcone VP: Slow wave sleep and brain structural imaging in schizophrenia. Sleep Research 21:250, 1992

Benson KL, Zarcone VP Jr: Rapid eye movement sleep eye movements in schizophrenia and depression. Arch Gen Psychiatry 50:474–482, 1993

Benson KL, Faull KF, Zarcone VP: Evidence for the role of serotonin in the regulation of slow wave sleep in schizophrenia. Sleep 14:133–139, 1991

Benson KL, Sullivan EV, Lim KO, et al: Slow wave sleep and computed tomographic measures of brain morphology in schizophrenia. Psychiatry Res 60:125–134, 1996

Bergonzi P, Chiurulla C, Cianchetti C, et al: Clinical pharmacology as an approach to the study of biochemical sleep mechanisms: the action of L-dopa. Confinia Neurologica 36:5–22, 1974

Besset A, Chetrit M, Carlander B, et al: Use of modafinil in the treatment of narcolepsy: a long term follow-up study. Neurophysiol Clin 26:60–66, 1996

Betts TA, Birtle J: Effect of two hypnotic drugs on actual driving performance next morning. BMJ 285:852, 1982

Billiard M: The Kleine-Levin syndrome, in Principles and Practice of Sleep Medicine. Edited by Kryger MH, Roth T, Dement WC. Philadelphia, WB Saunders, 1989, pp 377–378

Billiard M, Pasquie-Magnetto V, Heckman M, et al: Family studies in narcolepsy. Sleep 17 (suppl 8):S54–S59, 1994

Bixler EO, Kales A, Soldatos CR, et al: Prevalence of sleep disorders in the Los Angeles metropolitan area. Am J Psychiatry 136:1257–1262, 1979

Bixler EO, Kales A, Manfredi RL, et al: Next-day memory impairment with triazolam use. Lancet 337:827–831, 1991

Bliwise DL: Sleep in normal aging and dementia. Sleep 16:40–81, 1993

Bliwise DL, Hughes M, McMahon PM, et al: Observed sleep/wakefulness and severity of dementia in an Alzheimer's disease special care unit. J Gerontol A Biol Sci Med Sci 50:M303–M306, 1995

Boivin DB, Montplaisir J, Lambert C: Effects of bromocriptine in human narcolepsy. Clin Neuropharmacol 16:120–126, 1993

Bonnet MH, Arand DL: 24-hour metabolic rate in insomniacs and matched normal sleepers. Sleep 18:581–588, 1995

Bonora M, Shields G, Knuths S, et al: Selective depression by ethanol of upper airway respiratory motor activity in cats. American Review of Respiratory Disease 130:156–161, 1984

Bootzin RR: A stimulus control treatment for insomnia (abstract), in Proceedings of the Annual Meeting of the American Psychological Association. Washington, DC, American Psychological Association, 1972, pp 395–396

Bootzin RR, Perlis ML: Nonpharmacologic treatments of insomnia. J Clin Psychiatry 53 (suppl):37–41, 1992

Breslau N, Roth T, Rosenthal L, et al: Sleep disturbance and psychiatric disorders: a longitudinal epidemiological study of young adults. Biol Psychiatry 39:411–418, 1996

Brett EA, Ostroff R: Imagery and posttraumatic stress disorder: an overview. Am J Psychiatry 142:417–424, 1985

Brzezinski A: Melatonin in humans. N Engl J Med 336: 186–195, 1997

Broughton R, Billings R, Cartwright R, et al: Homicidal somnambulism: a case report. Sleep 17:253–264, 1994

Buysse DJ, Reynolds CF, Monk TH, et al: The Pittsburgh Sleep Quality Index: a new instrument for psychiatric practice and research. Psychiatry Res 28:193–213, 1989

Buysse DJ, Browman KE, Monk TH, et al: Napping and 24-hour sleep/wake patterns in healthy elderly and young adults. J Am Geriatr Soc 40:779–786, 1992

Buysse DJ, Frank E, Lowe KK, et al: Electroencephalographic sleep correlates of episode and vulnerability to recurrence in depression. Biol Psychiatry 41:406–418, 1997

Campbell SS, Dijk DJ, Boulos Z, et al: Light treatment for sleep disorders: consensus report, III: alerting and activating effects. J Biol Rhythms 10:129–132, 1995a

Campbell SS, Terman M, Lewy AJ, et al: Light treatment for sleep disorders: consensus report, V: age-related disturbances. J Biol Rhythms 10:151–154, 1995b

Carskadon MA, Harvey K, Dement WC: Sleep loss in young adolescents. Sleep 4:299–312, 1981

Carskadon MA, Dement WC, Mitler MM, et al: Guidelines for the Multiple Sleep Latency Test (MSLT): a standard measure of sleepiness. Sleep 9:519–524, 1986

Cartwright RD, Ristanovic R, Diaz F, et al: A comparative study of treatments for positional sleep apnea. Sleep 14:546–552, 1991a

Cartwright RD, Kravitz HM, Eastman CI, et al: REM latency and the recovery from depression: getting over divorce. Am J Psychiatry 148:1530–1535, 1991b

Chesson AL, Levine SN, Kong LS, et al: Neuroendocrine evaluation in Kleine-Levin syndrome: evidence of reduced dopaminergic tone during periods of hypersomnolence. Sleep 14:226–232, 1991

Coleman RM, Pollack CP, Weitzman ED: Periodic movements in sleep (nocturnal myoclonus): relationship to sleep disorders. Ann Neurol 8:416–421, 1980

Coleman RM, Roffwarg HP, Kennedy SJ, et al: Sleep-wake disorders based on a polysomnographic diagnosis: a national cooperative study. JAMA 247:997–1003, 1982

Coren S: The prevalence of self-reported sleep disturbances in young adults. Int J Neurosci 79:67–73, 1994

Coren S: Daylight savings time and traffic accidents (letter). N Engl J Med 334:924, 1996

Cravatt BF, Prospero-Garcia O, Siuzdak G, et al: Chemical characterization of a family of brain lipids that induce sleep. Science 268:1506–1509, 1995

Crick F, Mitchison G: The function of dream sleep. Nature 304:111–113, 1983

Critchley M: Periodic hypersomnia and megaphagia in adolescent males. Brain 59:494–515, 1962

Czeisler CA, Allan JS: Pathologies of the sleep-wake schedule, in Sleep Disorders: Diagnosis and Treatment, 2nd Edition. Edited by Williams RL, Karacan I, Moore CA. New York, Wiley, 1988, pp 109–129

Czeisler CA, Moore-Ede MC, Coleman RM: Rotating shift work schedules that disrupt sleep are improved by applying circadian principles. Science 217:460–463, 1982

Daan S, Lewy AJ: Scheduled exposure to daylight: a potential strategy to reduce "jet lag" following transmeridian flight. Psychopharmacol Bull 20:566–568, 1984

Dement W[C]: Dream recall and eye movements during sleep in schizophrenics and normals. J Nerv Ment Dis 122: 263–269, 1955

Dement WC, Carskadon MA, Richardson GS: Excessive daytime sleepiness in the sleep apnea syndrome, in Sleep Apnea Syndromes. Edited by Guilleminault C, Dement WC. New York, Alan R Liss, 1978, pp 23–46

Detre T, Himmelhoch J, Swartzburg M, et al: Hypersomnia and manic-depressive disease. Am J Psychiatry 128:1303–1305, 1972

Dew MA, Reynolds CF, Buysse DJ, et al: Electroencephalographic sleep profiles during depression: effects of episode duration and other clinical and psychosocial factors in older adults. Arch Gen Psychiatry 53:148–156, 1996

Dijk DJ, Boulos Z, Eastman CI, et al: Light treatment for sleep disorders: consensus report, II: basic properties of circadian physiology and sleep regulation. J Biol Rhythms 10: 113–125, 1995

Edinger JD, Fins AI, Sullivan RJ, et al: Comparison of cognitive-behavioral therapy and clonazepam for treating periodic limb movement disorder. Sleep 19:442–444, 1996

Feinberg I: Changes in sleep cycle patterns with age. J Psychiatr Res 10:283–306, 1974

Feinberg I: Schizophrenia: caused by a fault in programmed synaptic elimination during adolescence? J Psychiatr Res 17:319–334, 1982

Feinberg I, Hiatt JF: Sleep patterns in schizophrenia: a selective review, in Sleep Disorders: Diagnosis and Treatment, 1st Edition. Edited by Williams RC, Karacan I. New York, Wiley, 1978, pp 205–231

Feinberg I, Koresko RL, Heller N: EEG sleep patterns as a function of normal and pathological aging in man. J Psychiatr Res 5:107–144, 1967

Feldman MJ, Hersen M: Attitudes toward death in nightmare subjects. J Abnorm Psychol 72:421–425, 1967

Ferguson SA, Preusser DF, Lund AK, et al: Daylight saving time and motor vehicle crashes: the reduction in pedestrian and vehicle occupant fatalities. Am J Public Health 85:92–95, 1995

Finkelstein Y, Shapiro-Feinberg M, Stein G, et al: Uvulopalatopharyngoplasty vs laser-assisted uvulopalatoplasty/Anatomical considerations. Arch Otolaryngol Head Neck Surg 123:265–276, 1997

Ford DE, Kamerow DB: Epidemiologic study of sleep disturbances and psychiatric disorders: an opportunity for prevention? JAMA 262:1479–1484, 1989

Foutz AS, Mitler MM, Cavalli-Sforza LL, et al: Genetic factors in canine narcolepsy. Sleep 1:413–422, 1979

Freud S: Beyond the pleasure principle (1920), in Standard Edition of the Complete Psychological Works of Sigmund Freud, Vol 18. Translated and edited by Strachey J. London, Hogarth Press, 1955, pp 1–64

Gallin PF, Terman M, Reme CE, et al: Ophthalmologic examination of patients with seasonal affective disorder, before and after bright light therapy. Am J Ophthalmol 119:202–210, 1995

Gallup Organization: Sleep in America. Princeton, NJ, Gallup, 1995

Ganguli R, Reynolds CF, Kupfer DJ: Electroencephalographic sleep in young, never-medicated schizophrenics: a comparison with delusional and nondelusional depressives and with healthy controls. Arch Gen Psychiatry 44:36–44, 1987

Gelineau JBE: De la narcolepsie. Gazette des Hôpitals (Paris) 53:626–628, 1880

Giles DE, Roffwarg HP, Schlesser MA, et al: Which endogenous depressive symptoms relate to REM latency reduction? Biol Psychiatry 21:473–482, 1986

Giles DE, Jarrett RB, Roffwarg HP, et al: Reduced rapid eye movement latency: a predictor of recurrence in depression. Neuropsychopharmacology 1:33–39, 1987a

Giles DE, Roffwarg HP, Rush AJ: REM latency concordance in depressed family members. Biol Psychiatry 22:910–914, 1987b

Giles DE, Biggs MM, Rush AJ, et al: Risk factors in families of unipolar depression, I: psychiatric illness and reduced REM latency. J Affect Disord 14:51–59, 1988

Gillin JC: The long and the short of sleeping pills. N Engl J Med 324:1735–1737, 1991

Gillin JC, Ancoli-Israel S: The impact of age on sleep and sleep disorders, in Clinical Geriatric Psychopharmacology, 2nd Edition. Edited by Salzman C. Baltimore, MD, Williams & Wilkins, 1992, pp 213–234

Gillin JC, Sutton L, Ruiz C, et al: The cholinergic rapid eye movement induction test with arecoline in depression. Arch Gen Psychiatry 48:264–270, 1991

Gillin JC, Smith TL, Irwin M, et al: Increased pressure of REM sleep at admission predicts relapse in non-depressed patients with primary alcoholism at 3 month follow-up. Arch Gen Psychiatry 51:189–197, 1994

Girault C, Muir JF, Mihaltan F, et al: Effects of repeated administration of zolpidem on sleep, diurnal and nocturnal respiratory function, vigilance, and physical performance in patients with COPD. Chest 110:1203–1211, 1996

Greenblatt DJ, Harmatz JS, Zinny MA, et al: Effect of gradual withdrawal on the rebound sleep disorder after discontinuation of triazolam. N Engl J Med 317:722–728, 1987

Greenblatt DJ, Harmatz JS, Shapiro L, et al: Sensitivity to triazolam in the elderly. N Engl J Med 324:1691–1698, 1991

Guilleminault C: Sleep and breathing, in Sleep and Waking Disorders: Indications and Techniques. Edited by Guilleminault C. Menlo Park, CA, Addison-Wesley, 1982, pp 155–182

Guilleminault C, Carskadon M: Relationship between sleep disorders and daytime complaints, in Sleep 1976. Edited by Koeller WP, Oevin PW. Basel, S Karger, 1977, pp 95–100

Guilleminault C, Stoohs R, Quera-Salva MA: Sleep-related obstructive and nonobstructive apneas and neurologic disorders. Neurology 42 (suppl 6):53–60, 1992

Hanzel DA, Proia NG, Hudgel DW: Response of obstructive sleep apnea to fluoxetine and protriptyline. Chest 100:416–421, 1991

Hardie RJ, Efthimiou J, Stern GM: Respiration and sleep in Parkinson's disease. J Neurol Neurosurg Psychiatry 49:1326, 1986

Hartmann E: The Nightmare: The Psychology and Biology of Terrifying Dreams. New York, Basic Books, 1984

Hartmann E, Russ D, van der Kolk B, et al: A preliminary study of the personality of the nightmare sufferer: relationship to schizophrenia and creativity? Am J Psychiatry 138:794–797, 1981

Hauri P: Primary insomnia, in Treatment of Psychiatric Disorders, Vol 3. Washington, DC, American Psychiatric Association, 1989, pp 2424–2433

Hauri PJ, Esther MS: Insomnia. Mayo Clin Proc 65:869–882, 1990

Hauri P, Fisher J: Persistent psychophysiologic (learned) insomnia. Sleep 9:38–53, 1986

Hauri P, Olmstead P: Childhood-onset insomnia. Sleep 3:59–65, 1980

Hauri P, Chernik D, Hawkins D, et al: Sleep of depressed patients in remission. Arch Gen Psychiatry 31:386–391, 1974

Hendrickse WA, Roffwarg HP, Grannemann BD, et al: The effects of fluoxetine on the polysomnogram of depressed outpatients: a pilot study. Neuropsychopharmacology 10:85–91, 1994

Hirano A, Zimmerman H: Alzheimer's neurofibrillary changes: a topographic study. Arch Neurol 7:227, 1962

Ho AP, Gillin JC, Buchsbaum MS, et al: Brain glucose metabolism during non-rapid eye movement sleep in major depression. A positron emission tomography study. Arch Gen Psychiatry 53:645–652, 1996

Hobson JA, Steriade M: Neuronal basis of behavioral state control, in Handbook of Physiology, Sec 1, Vol 4: The Nervous System. Edited by Bloom FE. Bethesda, MD, American Physiologic Society, 1986, pp 701–823

Hoch CC, Reynolds CF, Kupfer DJ, et al: Sleep-disordered breathing in normal and pathologic aging. J Clin Psychiatry 47:499–503, 1986

Hoch CC, Reynolds CF, Houck PR, et al: Predicting mortality in mixed depression and dementia using EEG sleep variables. J Neuropsychiatry Clin Neurosci 1:366–371, 1989

Höchli D, Riemann D, Zulley J, et al: Initial REM sleep suppression by clomipramine: a prognostic tool for treatment response in patients with a major depressive disorder. Biol Psychiatry 21:1217–1220, 1986

Hoddes E, Zarcone VP, Smythe H, et al: Quantification of sleepiness: a new approach. Psychophysiology 10:431–436, 1973

Hoffman RS, Wipfler MG, Maddaloni MA, et al: How the New York State triplicate benzodiazepine prescription regulation influenced sedative-hypnotic overdoses. New York State Journal of Medicine 91:436–439, 1991

Horowitz MJ: Stress Response Syndromes. New York, Jason Aronson, 1976

Hublin C, Kaprio J, Partinen M, et al: Prevalence and genetics of sleepwalking: a population-based twin study. Neurology 48:177–181, 1997

Hudson JI, Lipinski JF, Keck PE Jr, et al: Polysomnographic characteristics of young manic patients: comparison with unipolar depressed patients and normal control subjects. Arch Gen Psychiatry 49:378–383, 1992

Huttenlocher PR: Synaptic density in human frontal cortex: developmental changes and effects of aging. Brain Res 163:195–205, 1979

Jacobs D, Ancoli-Israel S, Parker L, et al: 24-hour sleep/wake patterns in a nursing home population. Psychol Aging 4:352–356, 1989

Jacobs GD, Benson H, Friedman R: Perceived benefits in a behavioral-medicine insomnia program: a clinical report. Am J Med 100:212–216, 1996

Janson C, Gislason T, Bengtsson H, et al: Long-term follow-up of patients with obstructive sleep apnea treated with uvulopalatopharyngoplasty. Arch Otolaryngol Head Neck Surg 123:257–262, 1997

Janz D: The grand mal epilepsies and the sleeping-waking cycle. Epilepsia 3:69–109, 1962

Jasper NH: The ten-twenty electrode system of the International Federation. Electroencephalogr Clin Neurophysiol 10:371–375, 1958

Johns MW: A new method for measuring daytime sleepiness: the Epworth sleepiness scale. Sleep 14:540–555, 1991

Johnson LC, Chernik DA: Sedative-hypnotics and human performance. Psychopharmacology (Berl) 76:101–113, 1982

Johnson LC, Burdick JA, Smith J: Sleep during alcohol intake and withdrawal in the chronic alcoholic. Arch Gen Psychiatry 22:406–418, 1970

Juji T, Satake M, Honda Y, et al: HLA antigens in Japanese patients with narcolepsy. Tissue Antigens 24:316–319, 1984

Kales A, Soldatos CR, Caldwell AB, et al: Nightmares: clinical characteristics and personality patterns. Am J Psychiatry 137:1197–1201, 1980

Kales JD, Kales A, Bixler EO, et al: Biopsychobehavioral correlates of insomnia, V: clinical characteristics and behavioral correlates. Am J Psychiatry 141:1371–1376, 1984

Karacan I: Parasomnias, in Sleep Disorder: Diagnosis and Treatment, 2nd Edition. Edited by Williams RL, Karacan I, Moore CA. New York, Wiley, 1988, pp 131–144

Kardiner A, Spiegel H: War Stress and Neurotic Illness. New York, Paul B Hoeber, 1947

Karni A, Tanne D, Rubenstein BS, et al: Dependence on REM sleep of overnight improvement of a perceptual skill. Science 265:679–682, 1994

Keshavan MS, Reynolds CF, Ganguli R, et al: EEG sleep in familial subgroups of schizophrenia. Sleep Research 19:330, 1990a

Keshavan MS, Reynolds CF, Kupfer KJ: Electroencephalographic sleep in schizophrenia: a critical review. Compr Psychiatry 31:34–47, 1990b

Keshavan MS, Miewald J, Haas G, et al: Slow-wave sleep and symptomatology in schizophrenia and related psychotic disorders. J Psychiatr Res 29:303–314, 1995a

Keshavan MS, Pettegrew JW, Reynolds CF III, et al: Biological correlates of slow wave sleep deficits in functional psychoses: 31P-magnetic resonance spectroscopy. Psychiatry Res 57:91–100, 1995b

Keshavan MS, Reynolds CF III, Miewald JM, et al: A longitudinal study of EEG sleep in schizophrenia. Psychiatry Res 59:203–211, 1996

Kessler RC, Sonnega A, Bromet E, et al: Posttraumatic stress disorder in the National Comorbidity Survey. Arch Gen Psychiatry 52:1048–1060, 1995

Knowles JB, Laverty SG, Kuechler HA: The effects of alcohol on REM sleep. Quarterly Journal Study Alcohol 29:342–349, 1968

Kribbs NB, Pack AI, Kline LR, et al: Effects of one night without nasal CPAP treatment on sleep and sleepiness in patients with obstructive sleep apnea. American Review of Respiratory Disease 147:1162–1168, 1993

Kryger MH, Steljes D, Pouliot Z, et al: Subjective versus objective evaluation of hypnotic efficacy: experience with zolpidem. Sleep 14:399–407, 1991

Kulka RA, Schlenger WE, Fairbank JA, et al: The National Vietnam Veterans Readjustment Study: Tables and Findings and Technical Appendices. New York, Brunner/Mazel, 1990

Kupfer DJ, Ehlers CL: Two roads to rapid eye movement latency. Arch Gen Psychiatry 46:945–948, 1989

Kupfer DJ, Foster FG: Interval between onset of sleep and rapid-eye-movement sleep as an indicator of depression. Lancet 2:684–686, 1972

Kupfer DJ, Reynolds CF: Sleep and affective disorders, in Handbook of Affective Disorders, 2nd Edition. Edited by Paykel ES. New York, Guilford, 1992, pp 311–323

Kupfer DJ, Reynolds CF III: Management of insomnia. N Engl J Med 336:341–346, 1997

Kupfer DJ, Foster FG, Reich L, et al: EEG sleep changes as predictors in depression. Am J Psychiatry 133:622–626, 1976

Kupfer DJ, Frank E, Grochocinski VJ, et al: Electroencephalographic sleep profiles in recurrent depression: a longitudinal investigation. Arch Gen Psychiatry 45:678–681, 1988

Kupfer DJ, Perel JM, Pollock BG, et al: Fluvoxamine versus desipramine: comparative polysomnographic effects. Biol Psychiatry 29:23–40, 1991

Labbate LA, Pollack MH, Otto MW, et al: Sleep panic attacks: an association with childhood anxiety and adult psychopathology. Biol Psychiatry 36:57–60, 1994

Laffont F, Mayer G, Minz M: Modafinil in diurnal sleepiness. A study of 123 patients. Sleep 17 (suppl 8):S113–S115, 1994

Lam RW, Zis AP, Grewal A, et al: Effects of rapid tryptophan depletion in patients with seasonal affective disorder in remission after light therapy. Arch Gen Psychiatry 53:41–44, 1996

Langdon N, Lock C, Welsh K, et al: Immune factors in narcolepsy. Sleep 9:143–148, 1986

Langer SZ, Arbilla S, Scatton B, et al: Receptors involved in the mechanism of action of zolpidem, in Imidazopyridines in Sleep Disorders: A Novel Experimental and Therapeutic Approach. Edited by Sauvanet JP, Langer SZ, Morselli PL. New York, Raven, 1987, pp 55–72

Lauer CJ, Schreiber W, Holsboer F, et al: In quest of identifying vulnerability markers for psychiatric disorders by all-night polysomnography. Arch Gen Psychiatry 52:145–153, 1995

Lauer CJ, Schreiber W, Pollmacher T, et al: Sleep in schizophrenia: a polysomnographic study on drug-naive patients. Neuropsychopharmacology 16:51–60, 1997

Leung AK, Robson WL: Nightmares. J Natl Med Assoc 85:233–235, 1993

Lewis CF, Tandon R, Shipley JE, et al: Biological predictors of suicidality in schizophrenia. Acta Psychiatr Scand 94:416–420, 1996

Lewy AJ, Sack RA, Singer CL: Assessment and treatment of chronobiologic disorders using plasma melatonin levels and bright light exposure: the clock-gate model and the phase response curve. Psychopharmacol Bull 20:561–565, 1984

Lewy AJ, Sack RA, Miller S, et al: Antidepressant and circadian phase-shifting effects of light. Science 235:352–354, 1987

Lewy AJ, Sack RL, Blood ML, et al: Melatonin marks circadian phase position and resets the endogenous circadian pacemaker in humans. Ciba Found Symp 183:303–317, 1995

Loube MD, Strauss AM: Survey of oral appliance practice among dentists treating obstructive sleep apnea patients. Chest 111:382–386, 1997

Lugaresi E, Cirignotta F: Two variants of nocturnal paroxysmal dystonia with attacks of short and long duration, in Epilepsy, Sleep and Sleep Deprivation. Edited by Degen R, Niedermeyer E. Amsterdam, Elsevier, 1984, pp 169–173

Lugaresi E, Coccagna G, Mantovani M, et al: Some periodic phenomenon arising during drowsiness and sleep in man. Electroencephalogr Clin Neurophysiol 32:701–705, 1972

Lugaresi E, Cirignotta F, Montagna P: Nocturnal paroxysmal dystonia. J Neurol Neurosurg Psychiatry 49:375–380, 1986

Luna TD, French J, Mitcha JL: A study of USAF air traffic controller shiftwork: sleep, fatigue, activity, and mood analyses. Aviat Space Environ Med 68:18–23, 1997

Macquet P, Peters J, Aerts J, et al: Functional neuroanatomy of human rapid-eye-movement sleep and dreaming. Nature 383:163–166, 1996

Maggini C, Guazzeli M, Ciapparelli A: All-night sleep abnormalities in schizophrenia, in Schizophrenia: A Psychobiological View. Edited by Casacchia M, Rossi A. Dordrecht, The Netherlands, Kluwer Academic Publishers, 1987, pp 125–136

Mahowald MW, Schenck CH: Dissociated states of wakefulness and sleep. Neurology 42 (suppl 6):44–52, 1992

Mahowald MW, Schenck CH: REM sleep behavior disorder, in Principles and Practice of Sleep Medicine, 2nd Edition. Edited by Kryger MH, Roth T, Dement WC. Philadelphia, WB Saunders, 1994, pp 574–588

Mathur R, Douglas NJ: Family studies in patients with sleep apnea-hypopnea syndrome. Ann Intern Med 122:174–178, 1995

McClusky HY, Milby JB, Switzer PK, et al: Efficacy of behavioral versus triazolam treatment in persistent sleep-onset insomnia. Am J Psychiatry 148:121–126, 1991

McKinney M, Hedreen C, Coyle JT: Cortical cholinergic innervation: implications for the pathophysiology and treatment of Alzheimer's disease, in Alzheimer's Disease: A Report of Progress in Research. Edited by Corkin S, Davis K, Crowden J, et al. New York, Raven, 1982, pp 259–265

Mellinger GD, Balter MB, Uhlenhuth EH: Insomnia and its treatment. Prevalence and correlates. Arch Gen Psychiatry 42:225–232, 1985

Mellman TA, Uhde TW: Electroencephalographic sleep in panic disorder: a focus on sleep-related panic attacks. Arch Gen Psychiatry 46:178–184, 1989

Mellman TA, David D, Kulick-Bell R, et al: Sleep disturbance and its relationship to psychiatric morbidity after Hurricane Andrew. Am J Psychiatry 152:1659–1663, 1995a

Mellman TA, Kulick-Bell R, Ashlock LE, et al: Sleep events among veterans with combat-related posttraumatic stress disorder. Am J Psychiatry 152:110–115, 1995b

Mendelson WB: Human Sleep: Research and Clinical Care. New York, Plenum, 1987

Mendelson WB: Hypnotics in the treatment of chronic insomnia, in Handbook of Sleep Disorders. Edited by Thorpy MJ. New York, Marcel Dekker, 1990, pp 737–753

Mendelson WB: The use of sedative/hypnotic medication and its correlation with falling down in the hospital. Sleep 19:698–701, 1996a

Mendelson WB: Are periodic leg movements associated with clinical sleep disturbance? Sleep 19:219–223, 1996b

Merlotti L, Roehrs T, Koshorek G, et al: The dose effects of zolpidem on the sleep of healthy normals. J Clin Psychopharmacol 9:9–14, 1989

Miles LM, Raynal DM, Wilson MA: Blind man living in normal society has circadian rhythms of 24.9 hours. Science 198:421–423, 1977

Minot R, Luthringer R, Macher JP: Effect of moclobemide on the psychophysiology of sleep/wake cycles: a neuroelectrophysiological study of depressed patients administered moclobemide. Int Clin Psychopharmacol 7:181–189, 1993

Mishima K, Okawa M, Hishikawa Y, et al: Morning bright light therapy for sleep and behavior disorders in elderly patients with dementia. Acta Psychiatr Scand 89:1–7, 1994

Mitler MM: The Multiple Sleep Latency Test as an evaluation for excessive somnolence, in Disorders of Sleeping and Waking: Indications and Techniques. Edited by Guilleminault C. Menlo Park, CA, Addison-Wesley, 1982, pp 145–153

Mitler MM: Evaluation of treatment with stimulants in narcolepsy. Sleep 17 (suppl 8):S103–S106, 1994

Mitler MM, Gujavarty KS, Browman CP: Maintenance of wakefulness test: a polysomnographic technique for evaluating treatment efficacy in patients with excessive somnolence. Electroencephalogr Clin Neurophysiol 53:658–661, 1982

Mitler MM, Carskadon MA, Czeisler CA, et al: Catastrophes, sleep, and public policy: consensus report. Sleep 11:100–109, 1988

Moldofsky H, Gilbert R, Lue FA, et al: Sleep-related violence. Sleep Nov, 18:731–739, 1995

Monk TH: Traffic accident increases as a possible indicant of desynchronosis. Chronobiologica 7:527–529, 1980

Monk TH: Shift work, in Principles and Practice of Sleep Medicine, 2nd Edition. Edited by Kryger MH, Roth T, Dement WC. Philadelphia, WB Saunders, 1994, pp 471–476

Monk TH, Reynolds CF, Machen MA, et al: Daily social rhythms in the elderly and their relation to objectively recorded sleep. Sleep 15:322–329, 1992

Montplaisir J, Lapierre O, Warnes H, et al: The treatment of the restless leg syndrome with or without periodic leg movements in sleep. Sleep 15:391–395, 1992

Montplaisir J, Boucher S, Poirier G, et al: Clinical, polysomnographic, and genetic characteristics of restless legs syndrome: a study of 133 patients diagnosed with new standard criteria. Mov Disord 12:61–65, 1997

Moore RY, Eichler VB: Loss of a circadian adrenal corticosterone rhythm following suprachiasmatic lesions in the rat. Brain Res 42:210–216, 1972

Morin CM, Gaulier B, Barry T, et al: Patients' acceptance of psychological and pharmacological therapies for insomnia. Sleep 15:302–305, 1992

Morin CM, Culbert JP, Schwartz SM: Nonpharmacological interventions for insomnia: a meta-analysis of treatment efficacy. Am J Psychiatry 151:1172–1180, 1994

Morris HH, Estes ML: Traveler's amnesia: transient global amnesia secondary to triazolam. JAMA 258:945–946, 1987

Moss C: Portraits in the Wild. Boston, Houghton Mifflin, 1975

Mukhametov LM: Sleep in marine mammals, in Sleep Mechanisms. Edited by Borbely AA, Valatx JL. Heidelberg, Springer, 1984, pp 227–236

Muratorio A, Maggini C, Coccagna G, et al: Polygraphic study of the all-night sleep pattern in neurotic and depressed patients treated with trazodone. Mod Probl Pharmacopsychiatry 9:182–189, 1974

Nakazawa Y, Sakamoto T, Yasutake R, et al: Treatment of sleep apnea with prosthetic mandibular advancement (PMA). Sleep 15:499–504, 1992

National Commission on Sleep Disorders Research: Wake Up, America: A National Sleep Alert. Submitted to the United States Congress, January 1993

National Institutes of Health Consensus Development Conference Statement: the treatment of sleep disorders of older people (March 26–28, 1990). Sleep 14:169–177, 1991

Nelson S, Hans M: Contribution of craniofacial risk factors in increasing apneic activity among obese and nonobese habitual snorers. Chest 111:154–162, 1997

Neumeister A, Praschak-Rieder N, Besselmann B, et al: Effects of tryptophan depletion on drug-free patients with seasonal affective disorder during a stable response to bright light therapy. Arch Gen Psychiatry 54:133–138, 1997

Neylan TC, van Kammen DP, Kelley ME, et al: Sleep in schizophrenic patients on and off haloperidol therapy: clinically stable vs relapsed patients. Arch Gen Psychiatry 49:643–649, 1992

Neylan TC, De May M, Reynolds CF: Sleep and Chronobiologic Disturbances in Late Life, in Geriatric Psychiatry, 2nd Edition. Edited by Busse EW, Blazer DG. Washington, DC, American Psychiatric Press, 1996, pp 329–339

Neylan TC, Marmar CR, Metzler TJ, et al: Sleep disturbances in the Vietnam generation: an analysis of sleep measures from the National Vietnam Veteran Readjustment Study. Am J Psychiatry 155:929–933, 1998

Nicholson AN, Pascoe PA: Studies on the modulation of the sleep-wakefulness continuum in man by fluoxetine, a 5-HT uptake inhibitor. Neuropharmacology 27:597–602, 1988

Nicholson AN, Stone BM: Impaired performance and the tendency to sleep. Eur J Clin Pharmacol 30:27–32, 1986

Nierenberg AA, Adler LA, Peselow E, et al: Trazodone for antidepressant-associated insomnia. Am J Psychiatry 151:1069–1072, 1994

Nofzinger EA, Reynolds CF III: REM sleep behavior disorder. JAMA 271:820, 1994

Nofzinger EA, Thase ME, Reynolds CF, et al: Hypersomnia in bipolar depression: a comparison with narcolepsy using the Multiple Sleep Latency Test. Am J Psychiatry 148:1177–1181, 1991

Nofzinger EA, van Kammen DP, Gilbertson MW, et al: Electroencephalographic sleep in clinically stable schizophrenic patients: two-weeks versus six-weeks neuroleptic-free. Biol Psychiatry 33:829–835, 1993a

Nofzinger EA, Buysse DJ, Reynolds CF, et al: Sleep disorders related to another mental disorder (nonsubstance/primary): a DSM-IV literature review. J Clin Psychiatry 54:244–255, 1993b

Nofzinger EA, Reynolds CF III, Thase ME, et al: REM sleep enhancement by bupropion in depressed men. Am J Psychiatry 152:274–276, 1995

Ohayon M: Epidemiological study on insomnia in the general population. Sleep 19 (suppl 3):S7–S15, 1996

Orzack MH, Hartmann EL, Kornetsky C: The relationship between attention and slow-wave sleep in chronic schizophrenia. Psychopharmacol Bull 13:59–61, 1977

Oswald I: Triazolam syndrome 10 years on. Lancet 2:451–452, 1989

Parmeggiani PL: Temperature regulation during sleep: a study in homeostasis, in Physiology in Sleep. Edited by Orem J, Barnes CD. New York, Academic Press, 1980, pp 98–143

Powell NB, Guilleminault C, Riley RW: Surgical therapy for obstructive sleep apnea, in Principles and Practice of Sleep Medicine, 2nd Edition. Edited by Kryger MH, Roth T, Dement WC. Philadelphia, WB Saunders, 1994, pp 706–771

Ray WA, Griffin MR, Downey W: Benzodiazepines of long and short elimination half-life and the risk of hip fracture. JAMA 262:3303–3307, 1989

Rechtschaffen A, Kales A: A Manual of Standardized Terminology, Techniques, and Scoring System for Sleep Stages of Human Subjects. Bethesda, MD, U.S. Department of Health, Education and Welfare, Public Health Service, 1968, pp 1–60

Rechtschaffen A, Wolpert EA, Dement WC, et al: Nocturnal sleep of narcoleptics. Electroencephalogr Clin Neurophysiol 15:599–609, 1963

Rechtschaffen A, Bergmann BM, Everson CA, et al: Sleep deprivation in the rat, X: integration and discussion of the findings. Sleep 12:68–87, 1989

Regestein QR, Monk TH: Is the poor sleep of shift workers a disorder? Am J Psychiatry 148:1487–1493, 1991

Regestein QR, Dambrosia J, Hallett M, et al: Daytime alertness in patients with primary insomnia. Am J Psychiatry 150:1529–1534, 1993

Reinish LW, MacFarlane JG, Sandor P, et al: REM changes in narcolepsy with selegiline. Sleep 18:362–367, 1995

Reivich M, Isaacs G, Evarts E, et al: The effect of slow wave sleep and REM sleep on regional cerebral blood flow in cats. J Neurochem 15:301–306, 1968

Reynolds CF, Kupfer DJ: Sleep research in affective illness: state of the art circa 1987. Sleep 10:199–215, 1987

Reynolds CF, Black RS, Coble P, et al: Similarities in EEG sleep findings for Kleine-Levin syndrome and unipolar depression. Am J Psychiatry 137:116–118, 1980

Reynolds CF, Christiansen CL, Taska LS, et al: Sleep in narcolepsy and depression: does it all look alike? J Nerv Ment Dis 171:290–295, 1983a

Reynolds CF, Shaw DH, Newton TF, et al: EEG sleep in outpatients with generalized anxiety: a preliminary comparison with depressed outpatients. Psychiatry Res 8:81–89, 1983b

Reynolds CF, Kupfer DJ, Christiansen CL, et al: Multiple Sleep Latency Test findings in Kleine-Levin syndrome. J Nerv Ment Dis 172:41–44, 1984

Reynolds CF, Kupfer DJ, Taska LS, et al: EEG sleep in elderly depressed, demented, and healthy subjects. Biol Psychiatry 20:431–442, 1985a

Reynolds CF, Kupfer DJ, Taska LS, et al: Sleep apnea in Alzheimer's dementia: correlation with mental deterioration. J Clin Psychiatry 46:257–261, 1985b

Reynolds CF, Hoch CC, Buysse DJ, et al: Electroencephalographic sleep in spousal bereavement and bereavement-related depression of late life. Biol Psychiatry 31:69–82, 1992

Reynolds CF III, Buysse DJ, Kupfer DJ: Disordered sleep: developmental and biopsychosocial perspectives on the diagnosis and treatment of persistent insomnia, in Psychopharmacology: The Fourth Generation of Progress. Edited by Bloom FE, Kupfer DJ. New York, Raven, 1995, pp 1617–1629

Richardson JW, Fredrickson PA, Siong-Chi L: Narcolepsy update. Mayo Clin Proc 65:991–998, 1990

Rickels K, Schweizer E, Clary C, et al: Nefazodone and imipramine in major depression: a placebo-controlled trial. Br J Psychiatry 164:802–805, 1994

Roehrs T, Jorick NJ, Wittig RM, et al: Dose determinants of rebound insomnia. Br J Clin Pharmacol 22:143–147, 1986

Roehrs T, Zorick F, Wittig R, et al: Predictors of objective level of daytime sleepiness in patients with sleep-related breathing disorders. Chest 95:1202–1206, 1989

Rosen J, Reynolds CF, Yeager AL, et al: Sleep disturbances in survivors of the Nazi Holocaust. Am J Psychiatry 148:62–66, 1991

Rosenthal NE, Sack DA, Gillin JC, et al: Seasonal affective disorder: a description of the syndrome and preliminary findings with light therapy. Arch Gen Psychiatry 41:72–80, 1984

Rosenthal NE, Joseph-Vanderpool JR, Levendosky AA, et al: Phase-shifting effects of bright morning light as treatment for delayed sleep phase syndrome. Sleep 13:354–361, 1990

Ross RJ, Ball WA, Sullivan KA, et al: Sleep disturbance as the hallmark of posttraumatic stress disorder. Am J Psychiatry 146:697–707, 1989

Ross RJ, Ball WA, Dinges DF, et al: Rapid eye movement sleep disturbance in posttraumatic stress disorder. Biol Psychiatry 35:195–202, 1994

Roth T, Roehrs T, Carskadon M, et al: Daytime sleepiness and alertness, in Principles and Practice of Sleep Medicine, 2nd Edition. Edited by Kryger MH, Roth T, Dement WC. Philadelphia, WB Saunders, 1994, pp 40–49

Rusak B, Zucker I: Neural regulation of circadian rhythms. Physiol Rev 59:449–526, 1979

Rush AJ, Erman MK, Giles DE, et al: Polysomnographic findings in recently drug-free and clinically remitted depressed patients. Arch Gen Psychiatry 43:878–884, 1986

Sack RL, Stevenson J, Lewy AJ: Entrainment of a previously free-running blind human with melatonin administration (abstract). Sleep Research 19:80, 1990

Saletu B, Frey R, Krupka M, et al: Sleep laboratory studies on the single-dose effects of serotonin reuptake inhibitors paroxetine and fluoxetine on human sleep and awakening qualities. Sleep 14:439–447, 1991

Sanford JRA: Tolerance of debility in elderly dependants by supporters at home: its significance for hospital practice. BMJ 3:471–473, 1975

Satlin A, Volicer L, Ross V, et al: Bright light treatment of behavioral and sleep disturbances in patients with Alzheimer's disease. Am J Psychiatry 149:1028–1032, 1992

Sauerland EK, Harper RM: The human tongue during sleep: electromyographic activity of the genioglossus muscle. Exp Neurol 51:160–170, 1976

Schafer H, Koehler U, Ploch T, et al: Sleep-related myocardial ischemia and sleep structure in patients with obstructive sleep apnea and coronary heart disease. Chest 111: 387–393, 1997

Scharf MB, Sachais BA: Sleep laboratory evaluation of the effects and efficacy of trazodone in depressed insomniac patients. J Clin Psychiatry 51:13–17, 1990

Schenck CH, Mahowald MW: A polysomnographically documented case of adult somnambulism with long-distance automobile driving and frequent nocturnal violence: parasomnia with continuing danger as a noninsane automatism? Sleep 18:765–772, 1995

Schenck CH, Mahowald MW: Long-term, nightly benzodiazepine treatment of injurious parasomnias and other disorders of disrupted nocturnal sleep in 170 adults. Am J Med 100:333–337, 1996

Schenck C, Mahowald M, Won Kim S, et al: Prominent eye movements during non-REM sleep and REM sleep behavior disorder associated with fluoxetine treatment of depression and obsessive-compulsive disorder. Sleep 15:226–235, 1992

Schittecatte M, Charles G, Machowski R, et al: Reduced clonidine rapid eye movement sleep suppression in patients with primary major affective illness. Arch Gen Psychiatry 49:637–642, 1992

Sharpley AL, Walsh AES, Cowen PJ: Nefazodone—a novel antidepressant—may increase REM sleep. Biol Psychiatry 31:1070–1073, 1992

Shelton J, Nishino S, Vaught J, et al: Comparative effects of modafinil and amphetamine on daytime sleepiness and cataplexy of narcoleptic dogs. Sleep 18:817–826, 1995

Shipley JE, Kupfer DJ, Griffin SJ, et al: Comparison of effects of desipramine and amitriptyline on EEG sleep of depressed patients. Psychopharmacology 85:14–22, 1985

Shouse MN: Epileptic seizure manifestations during sleep, in Principles and Practice of Sleep Medicine, 2nd Edition. Edited by Kryger MH, Roth T, Dement WC. Philadelphia, WB Saunders, 1994, pp 801–814

Siegel JM: Brainstem mechanisms generating REM sleep, in Principles and Practice of Sleep Medicine, 2nd Edition. Edited by Kryger MH, Roth T, Dement WC. Philadelphia, WB Saunders, 1994, pp 125–144

Sitaram N, Nurnberger JI Jr, Gershon ES, et al: Faster cholinergic REM induction in euthymic patients with primary affective illness. Science 208:200–202, 1980

Sitaram N, Gillin JC, Bunney WE Jr: Cholinergic and catecholaminergic receptor sensitivity in affective illness: strategy and theory, in Neurobiology of Mood Disorders. Edited by Post RM, Ballenger JC. Baltimore, Williams & Wilkins, 1984, pp 629–651

Skaggs WE, McNaughton BL: Replay of neuronal firing sequences in rat hippocampus during sleep following spatial experience. Science 271:1870–1873, 1996

Smirne S, Come G, Franceschi M, et al: Sleep in presenile dementia, in Communications in EEG. International Federation of Societies for Electroencephalography and Clinical Neurophysiology, 9th Congress. 1977, pp 521–522

Smith M, Colligan M: Health and safety consequences of shift work in the food processing industry. Ergonomics 25:133–144, 1982

Smith RC: Relationship of periodic movements in sleep (nocturnal myoclonus) and the Babinski sign. Sleep 8:239–243, 1985

Smith-Coggins R, Rosekind MR, Hurd S, et al: Relationship of day versus night sleep to physician performance and mood. Ann Emerg Med 24:928–934, 1994

Spielman A, Saskin P, Thorpy M: Treatment of chronic insomnia by restriction of time in bed. Sleep 10:45–56, 1987

Spiker DG, Coble P, Cofsky J, et al: EEG sleep and severity of depression. Biol Psychiatry 13:485–488, 1978

Stein MB, Kroft CD, Walker JR: Sleep impairment in patients with social phobia. Psychiatry Res 49:251–256, 1993

Stein MB, Millar TW, Larsen DK, et al: Irregular breathing during sleep in patients with panic disorder. Am J Psychiatry 152:1168–1173, 1995

Stepanski E, Zorick F, Roehrs T, et al: Daytime alertness in patients with chronic insomnia compared with asymptomatic control subjects. Sleep 11:54–60, 1988

Sterman MB, Clemente CD: Forebrain mechanisms for the onset of sleep, in Basic Sleep Mechanisms. Edited by Petre-Quadens O, Schlag JD. New York, Academic Press, 1974, pp 83–97

Stoller MK: Economic effects of insomnia. Clin Ther 16:873–897, 1994

Stone J, Morin CM, Hart RP, et al: Neuropsychological functioning in older insomniacs with or without obstructive sleep apnea. Psychol Aging 9:231–236, 1994

Strollo PJ Jr, Rogers RM: Obstructive sleep apnea. N Engl J Med 334:99–104, 1996

Sullivan CE, Grunstein RR: Continuous positive airway pressure in sleep-disordered breathing, in Principles and Practice of Sleep Medicine, 2nd Edition. Edited by Kryger MH, Roth T, Dement WC. Philadelphia, WB Saunders, 1994, pp 694–705

Tandon R, Shipley JE, Eiser AS, et al: Association between abnormal REM sleep and negative symptoms in schizophrenia. Psychiatry Res 27:359–361, 1989

Tandon R, Shipley JE, Taylor S, et al: Electroencephalographic sleep abnormalities in schizophrenia: relationship to positive/negative symptoms and prior neuroleptic treatment. Arch Gen Psychiatry 49:185–194, 1992

Tandon R, Lewis C, Taylor SF, et al: Relationship between DST nonsuppression and shortened REM latency in schizophrenia. Biol Psychiatry 40:660–663, 1996

Terman M: Light therapy, in Principles and Practice of Sleep Medicine, 2nd Edition. Edited by Kryger MH, Roth T, Dement WC. Philadelphia, WB Saunders, 1994, pp 1012–1029

Terman M, Terman JS, Quitkin FM, et al: Response of the melatonin cycle to phototherapy for seasonal affective disorder. J Neural Transm 72:147–165, 1988

Thaker GK, Wagman AM, Kirkpatrick B, et al: Alterations in sleep polygraphy after neuroleptic withdrawal: a putative supersensitive dopaminergic mechanism. Biol Psychiatry 25:75–86, 1989

Thase ME, Kupfer DJ, Spiker DG: Electroencephalographic sleep in secondary depression: a revisit. Biol Psychiatry 19:805–814, 1984

Thase ME, Kupfer DJ, Ulrich RF: Electroencephalographic sleep in psychotic depression: a valid subtype? Arch Gen Psychiatry 43:886–893, 1986

Thase ME, Reynolds CF III, Frank E, et al: Polysomnographic studies of unmedicated depressed men before and after cognitive behavioral therapy. Am J Psychiatry 1994 151:1615–1622, 1994

Thase ME, Simons AD, Reynolds CF: Abnormal electroencephalographic sleep profiles in major depression: association with response to cognitive behavior therapy. Arch Gen Psychiatry 53:99–108, 1996

Thase ME, Buysse DJ, Frank E, et al: Which depressed patients will respond to interpersonal psychotherapy? The role of abnormal EEG sleep profiles. Am J Psychiatry 154:502–509, 1997

Trenkwalder C, Stiasny K, Pollmacher T, et al: L-dopa therapy of uremic and idiopathic restless legs syndrome: a double-blind, crossover trial. Sleep 18:681–688, 1995

Trenkwalder C, Seidel VC, Gasser T, et al: Clinical symptoms and possible anticipation in a large kindred of familial restless legs syndrome. Mov Disord 11:389–394, 1996

True WR, Rice J, Eisen SA, et al: A twin study of genetic and environmental contributions to liability for posttraumatic stress symptoms. Arch Gen Psychiatry 50:257–264, 1993

Tune GS: Sleep and wakefulness in normal human adults. BMJ 2:269–271, 1968

van Kammen DP, van Kammen WB, Peters J, et al: Decreased slow-wave sleep and enlarged lateral ventricles in schizophrenia. Neuropsychopharmacology 1:265–271, 1988

van Kammen DP, Widerlov E, Neylan TC, et al: Delta sleep-inducing-peptide–like immunoreactivity (DSIP-LI) and delta sleep in schizophrenic volunteers. Sleep 15:519–525, 1992

Vitiello MV, Prinz PN: Aging and sleep disorders, in Sleep Disorders: Diagnosis and Treatment, 2nd Edition. Edited by Williams RL, Karacan I, Moore CA. New York, Wiley, 1988, pp 293–312

Vitiello MV, Bliwise DL, Prinz PN: Sleep in Alzheimer's disease and the sundown syndrome. Neurology 42 (suppl 6):83–94, 1992

Wagner ML, Walters AS, Coleman RG, et al: Randomized, double-blind, placebo-controlled study of clonidine in restless legs syndrome. Sleep 19:52–58, 1996

Ware JC, Pittard JT: Increased deep sleep after trazodone use: a double-blind placebo-controlled study in healthy young adults. J Clin Psychiatry 51 (suppl):18–22, 1990

Ware JC, Rose FV, McBrayer RH: The acute effects of nefazodone, trazodone and buspirone on sleep and sleep-related penile tumescence in normal subjects. Sleep 17:544–550, 1994

Weintraub M, Singh S, Byrne L, et al: Consequences of the 1989 New York State triplicate benzodiazepine regulations. JAMA 266:2392–2397, 1991

Wesensten NJ, Balkin TJ, Davis HQ, et al: Reversal of triazolam- and zolpidem-induced memory impairment by flumazenil. Psychopharmacology 121:242–249, 1995

Wilson MA, McNaughton BL: Reactivation of hippocampal ensemble memories during sleep. Science 265:676–679, 1994

Winkelman JW, Chertow GM, Lazarus JM: Restless legs syndrome in end-stage renal disease. Am J Kidney Dis 28:372–378, 1996

Wirz-Justice A, Graw P, Kräuchi K, et al: Light therapy in seasonal affective disorder is independent of time of day or circadian phase. Arch Gen Psychiatry 50:929–937, 1993

Witting W, Kwa IH, Eikelenboom P, et al: Alterations in the circadian rest-activity rhythm in aging and Alzheimer's disease. Biol Psychiatry 27:563–572, 1990

Woodward SH, Friedman MJ, Bliwise DL: Sleep and depression in combat-related PTSD inpatients. Biol Psychiatry 39:182–192, 1996

Wooten V: Sleep disorders in geriatric patients. Clin Geriatr Med 8:427–439, 1992

Wu JC, Bunney WE: The biological basis of an antidepressant response to sleep deprivation and relapse: review and hypothesis. Am J Psychiatry 147:14–21, 1990

Yamashiro Y, Kryger MH: Why should sleep apnea be diagnosed and treated? Clinical Pulmonary Medicine 1:250–259, 1994

Young T, Palta M, Dempsey J, et al: The occurrence of sleep-disordered breathing among middle-aged adults. N Engl J Med 328:1230–1235, 1993

Zarcone VP Jr, Benson KL, Berger PA: Abnormal rapid eye movement latencies in schizophrenia. Arch Gen Psychiatry 44:45–48, 1987

Zepelin H: Mammalian sleep, in Principles and Practice of Sleep Medicine, 2nd Edition. Edited by Kryger MH, Roth T, Dement WC. Philadelphia, WB Saunders, 1994, pp 69–80

CHAPTER 25

EATING DISORDERS: ANOREXIA NERVOSA, BULIMIA NERVOSA, AND OBESITY

KATHERINE A. HALMI, M.D.

The eating disorders *anorexia nervosa* and *bulimia nervosa* and the condition of *obesity* have been known since earliest times in Western civilization. Well-documented case reports of anorexia nervosa are found in literature describing early Christian saints. Bell (1985) reported the severe starving behavior and bingeing episodes of Saint Catherine of Siena, described the kind of reed she employed to induce vomiting, and listed the herbal cathartics that she used for purging. Although binge eating and purging behavior are certainly described in Roman civilization, the disorder bulimia nervosa as we define it today has not been so well documented.

The eating disorders are entities or syndromes and not specific diseases with a common cause, common course, and common pathology. They are best conceptualized as syndromes and are therefore classified on the basis of the clusters of symptoms they present.

Because there is an important interaction between psychology and physiology in the eating disorders, this chapter begins with a brief section on the physiology of eating. Following this, the characteristics of anorexia nervosa, bulimia nervosa, and obesity are reviewed, with emphasis on the distinctive clinical features, medical complications, epidemiology, course, prognosis, pathogenic development, treatment, and theories of etiology.

PHYSIOLOGY AND BEHAVIORAL PHARMACOLOGY OF EATING

A SYSTEMS CONCEPTUALIZATION

A major conceptual revision for understanding the physiology and behavior of eating has expanded the dual-center theory of hypothalamic facilitatory and inhibitory centers for eating. The sensitive hypothalamic eating centers are part of a broad complex of neuroregulator interactions that includes a peripheral satiety system (gastrointestinal and pancreatic hormones released by food passing through the gastrointestinal tract) and a broad neural network affecting feeding, within the brain. Eating behavior is now known to reflect an interaction between an organism's physiological state and environmental conditions. Salient physiological variables include the balance of various neuropeptides and neurotransmitters, metabolic state, metabolic rate, condition of the gastrointestinal tract, amount of storage tissue, and sensory receptors for taste and smell. Environmental conditions include features of the food such as taste, texture, novelty, accessibility, and nutritional composition, as well as other external conditions such as ambient temperature, presence of other people, and stress (Blundell and Hill 1986).

To understand eating behavior, it is also important to recognize the role of conditioned (learned) components in the initiation and termination of nutrient ingestion. Because of methodological complexities, this is an area that has received little study. Booth (1985) provided the best discussion of conditioned appetites and satieties because he focused attention on the interaction between psychological and physiological phenomena.

It is important to remember that when an exogenous agent such as a drug or peptide is given to an animal or a human, it does not simply activate a specific set of receptors that induce specific responses; it intervenes into a complex transactional fabric as well (Blundell and Hill 1986).

EXPERIMENTAL METHODS

Early test models for eating behavior in animals either used food deprivation to induce eating or involved observations of the effects of hypothalamic lesions. Several recently developed techniques have used pharmacological agents to probe the complex structure of feeding. A microstructural analysis of feeding behavior has been used that involves the simultaneous recording of many behaviors, such as drinking, grooming, locomotor activity, and resting, besides the eating behavior of animals, within a short time frame. The macroanalysis of feeding patterns is a measurement of long-term feeding patterns in free-feeding animals never subjected to food deprivation. This continuous monitoring procedure has improved the precision of measuring parameters of meal patterns such as meal size, meal duration, meal frequency, intermeal intervals, and ratios of meal size to meal interval. It allows assessments to be made under normal physiological conditions. Experimental obesity in animals can be produced by the technique of using varied and palatable diets. The dietary self-selection model allows the study of pharmacological agents and exogenously administered hormones on macronutrient (i.e., fat, protein, and carbohydrate) consumption.

These models developed to study feeding have been used successfully with humans. With the microanalysis technique, amphetamine was found to inhibit the onset of eating and increase eating rate, whereas fenfluramine shortened the duration of the meal and markedly slowed the rate of eating. Silverstone and Kyriades (1982) used an automated food dispenser to study the action of various anorectic drugs on eating profiles. For a more extensive discussion of these models, see Blundell and Hill (1986).

The effect of stress on eating has been studied in animals with the mild tail-pinching technique, immobilization, or exposure to a novel environment (Morley et al. 1986). To determine whether satiety signals arise from oral, gastric, or intestinal sites, a sham feeding model has been used in animals (Young et al. 1974). In this technique, cannulas are placed in the esophagus or stomach so that they can be temporarily opened during a test to allow drainage and recovery of an ingested food. When these cannulas are open (sham feeding), all species overeat, which demonstrates that food stimuli in the mouth are not sufficient to exert a normal satiety reaction. Food infused directly into the intestine produces a dose-related suppression of sham feeding.

All of these experimental models have been used to study the role of neurotransmitters, peptides, and opioids on feeding behavior.

NEUROTRANSMITTERS—BIOGENIC AMINES

The study of catecholaminergic pathways in the hypothalamus by Leibowitz (1980) led to the discovery of the role of α_2 adrenergic receptors in the paraventricular nucleus (PVN) and the β_2 adrenergic receptors in the perifornical hypothalamus (PFH) in feeding. Microinjection of α_2 agonists to the PVN produces hyperphagia and causes a preferential ingestion of carbohydrate. This adrenergic β_2-responsive circuit in the PFH inhibits feeding.

Serotonin, an indoleamine, has been demonstrated to facilitate satiety (Hoebel 1977) and may at least in part control the intake of carbohydrate (Wurtman and Wurtman 1979). Serotonin injected peripherally and centrally into the PVN suppresses deprivation-induced and norepinephrine-induced eating (Leibowitz 1980).

Dopamine seems to play a more complicated role in eating behavior. Low doses of dopamine and dopamine agonist stimulate feeding, whereas higher doses inhibit feeding (Leibowitz 1980). Glucose administration suppressed firing in substantia nigra dopamine neurons. There is evidence of increased hypothalamic dopamine turnover during feeding. This finding suggests that central dopamine mechanisms mediate the rewarding effects of food as they mediate rewarding effects of intracranial self-stimulation and the self-stimulation of psychoactive drugs. The dopamine antagonist pimozide suppressed sham feeding intake of sucrose. This may be due to the inhibition of the rewarding effect of glucose (Gibbs and Smith 1984). In free-feeding rats, however, pimozide causes an increase in meal size.

PEPTIDES AND OPIOIDS

Corticotropin-releasing factor (CRF) acts within the PVN to inhibit feeding. Norepinephrine seems to inhibit the CRF inhibitory feeding effect. The pancreatic polypeptide neuropeptide Y increases both food and water intake when injected into the PVN. Another pancreatic polypeptide, peptide YY, is a more potent stimulator of feeding than neuropeptide Y (Morley and Levine 1985).

Opioid antagonism decreases feeding in many species but has no effect in reducing food intake in other species. Under some physiological conditions, such as starving or insulin-induced hypoglycemia, naloxone fails to inhibit feeding. Stress-induced eating is probably driven by activation of the opioid system. Dynorphin, an endogenous κ opioid receptor ligand, enhances feeding. Again the major site of action for dynorphin appears to be the PVN (Morley and Levine 1985).

PERIPHERAL SATIETY NETWORK

Several peptides are released by ingested food from the gastrointestinal tract. Some of these inhibit feeding by activating ascending vagal fibers. Cholecystokinin (CCK) is the most extensively studied of these peptides. Its effects, mediated by vagal fibers, have been traced to the PVN of the hypothalamus, where lesions will abolish CCK's effect on feeding. Low doses of CCK infused into the PVN attenuate feeding, and central infusions of CCK antibodies enhance feeding. The potency of the satiety effect of CCK varies across animal species. Other peptides that appear to inhibit feeding via vagal fibers are glucagon, somatostatin, and thyrotropin-releasing hormone.

Bombesin is a gastric peptide that inhibits feeding, independent of vagus fibers. Gastrin-releasing peptide and calcitonin also inhibit feeding (Gibbs and Smith 1984). Some of these peptides, such as CCK, bombesin, and glucagon, when administered parenterally to humans, have produced satiety. However, their usefulness as therapeutic agents at present is limited because of their restricted absorption from the gut and because the high doses required induce adverse effects such as nausea.

The basic physiological information on eating obtained from animal research serves as the foundation for testable hypotheses relevant to anorexia nervosa, bulimia nervosa, and obesity.

ANOREXIA NERVOSA

DEFINITION

Anorexia nervosa is a disorder characterized by preoccupation with body weight and food, behavior directed toward losing weight, peculiar patterns of handling food, weight loss, intense fear of gaining weight, disturbance of body image, and amenorrhea. Criteria from DSM-IV (American Psychiatric Association 1994) for anorexia nervosa are contained in Table 25-1.

CLINICAL FEATURES

Anorexic individuals typically express an intense fear of gaining weight, tend to be preoccupied with thoughts of food, and worry irrationally about fatness. Denial of their own clearly observable symptoms is characteristic of anorectic patients. They frequently look in mirrors to make sure they are thin and they incessantly express concern about looking fat and feeling flabby. Collecting recipes and preparing elaborate meals for their families are other behaviors that reflect their preoccupation with food. Peculiar handling of food is frequent in anorectic individuals. They will hide carbohydrate-rich foods and hoard large quantities of candies, carrying them in their pockets and purses. Often they will try to dispose of their food sur-

TABLE 25-1. Diagnostic criteria for anorexia nervosa

A. Refusal to maintain body weight at or above a minimally normal weight for age and height (e.g., weight loss leading to maintenance of body weight less than 85% of that expected; or failure to make expected weight gain during period of growth, leading to body weight less than 85% of that expected).

B. Intense fear of gaining weight or becoming fat, even though underweight.

C. Disturbance in the way in which one's body weight or shape is experienced, undue influence of body weight or shape on self-evaluation, or denial of the seriousness of the current low body weight.

D. In postmenarcheal females, amenorrhea, i.e., the absence of at least three consecutive menstrual cycles. (A woman is considered to have amenorrhea if her periods occur only following hormone, e.g., estrogen, administration.)

Specify type:

Restricting type: during the current episode of anorexia nervosa, the person has not regularly engaged in binge-eating or purging behavior (i.e., self-induced vomiting or the misuse of laxatives, diuretics, or enemas)

Binge-eating/purging type: during the current episode of anorexia nervosa, the person has regularly engaged in binge-eating or purging behavior (i.e., self-induced vomiting or the misuse of laxatives, diuretics, or enemas)

reptitiously to avoid eating. Anorexic persons will spend a great deal of time cutting food into small pieces and rearranging the food on their plates.

Anorexic patients' fear that they are gaining weight exists even in the face of increasing cachexia, and they characteristically display disinterest in and even resistance to treatment. Persons with this disorder lose weight by drastically reducing their total food intake and disproportionately decreasing the intake of high-carbohydrate and fatty foods. Some anorectic individuals will develop rigorous exercise programs, and others will simply be as active as possible at all times. Self-induced vomiting, laxatives, and diuretic abuse are other purging behaviors by which anorectic persons attempt to lose weight. Weight loss and a refusal to maintain body weight over a minimal normal weight for age and height are the most characteristic features of this disorder. Anorexic individuals have a disturbance in the way in which they experience their body weight and shape. They often fail to recognize that their degree of emaciation is dangerous. Their cognition is so distorted that they judge their self-worth predominantly by body shape and weight.

Obsessive-compulsive behavior often develops after the onset of anorexia nervosa. An obsession with cleanliness, an increase in housecleaning activities, and a more compulsive approach to studying are not uncommonly observed in these patients.

Amenorrhea can appear before noticeable weight loss has occurred. Poor sexual adjustment is frequently present in anorectic patients. Many adolescent anorectic patients have delayed psychosocial sexual development, and adults often have a markedly decreased interest in sex with the onset of anorexia nervosa.

Patients with anorexia nervosa can be divided into two groups: those who binge and purge and those who merely restrict food intake to lose weight. There is a relatively frequent association with impulsive behavior such as suicide attempts, self-mutilation, stealing, and substance abuse (including alcohol abuse) among bulimic anorectic individuals, who are also less likely to be regressed in their sexual activity and may in fact be promiscuous. Bulimic anorectic patients are more likely to have discrete personality disorder diagnoses (Halmi 1987).

MEDICAL COMPLICATIONS

Most of the physiological and metabolic changes in anorexia nervosa are secondary to the starvation state or purging behavior and are reversed with nutritional rehabilitation. We often find abnormalities in hematopoiesis, such as leukopenia and relative lymphocytosis, in acutely emaciated anorectic patients. Individuals with anorexia nervosa who engage in self-induced vomiting or who abuse laxatives and diuretics are liable to develop hypokalemic alkalosis. These patients often have elevated serum bicarbonate levels, hypochloremia, and hypokalemia. Patients with electrolyte disturbances have physical symptoms of weakness and lethargy and, at times, have cardiac arrhythmias. The latter condition may threaten sudden cardiac arrest, a not infrequent cause of death in patients who purge. Other complications of bingeing and purging are discussed in the section on bulimia nervosa.

Elevation of serum enzymes reflects fatty degeneration of the liver and is observed both in the emaciated anorectic phase and during refeeding. Elevated serum cholesterol levels tend to occur more frequently in younger patients. Carotenemia is often observed in malnourished anorectic patients. All of these physiological changes reverse themselves with nutritional rehabilitation (Halmi and Falk 1981). Amenorrhea, which is a major diagnostic criterion for anorexia nervosa, is not related simply to weight loss and is discussed in the section on etiology and pathogenesis.

EPIDEMIOLOGY, COURSE, AND PROGNOSIS

The incidence of anorexia nervosa has increased in the past 30 years both in the United States and in Western Europe. In Monroe County, New York, the average annual incidence rate of 0.35 per 100,000 population in the 1960s increased to 0.64 per 100,000 in the 1970s (Jones et al. 1980). In London, the prevalence of anorexia nervosa was one severe case in approximately 200 girls ages 12–18 years in the 1970s (Crisp et al. 1976). An incidence study in northeastern Scotland in the 1980s found four cases of anorexia nervosa per 100,000 population per annum (Szmukler 1985). The most recent incidence study, also conducted in northeastern Scotland (Eagles et al. 1995), revealed that between 1965 and 1991, the incidence of anorexia nervosa increased nearly sixfold (from 3 per 100,000 to 17 per 100,000 cases). These studies probably underestimate the true incidence because not all cases come to the attention of health care providers. Hoek (1991) found the incidence of anorexia nervosa at the primary care level in Holland to be 6.3 per 100,000 population per year during the period 1985–1986 and 8.1 during the period 1987–1989. Rooney et al. (1995) surveyed patients recruited for study from the level of primary care in England. The prevalence of anorexia nervosa was 20.2 cases per 100,000 population (0.02% of the total population). The prevalence among female patients ages 15–29 years was 115.4 cases per 100,000 (0.1%). In Rochester, Minnesota, Lucas et al. (1991)

recorded a point prevalence of anorexia nervosa of 0.2% for females and 0.02% for males on January 1, 1980. Five years later, his survey showed that the point prevalence of anorexia nervosa had increased to 0.48% among female adolescents ages 15–19 years. Only 4%–6% of the anorectic population are males (Halmi 1974).

The course of anorexia nervosa varies from a single episode with weight and psychological recovery, to nutritional rehabilitation with relapses, to an unremitting course resulting in death. Two of the most methodologically satisfying long-term follow-up studies have shown a mortality rate of 6.6% at 10 years after a well-defined treatment program (Halmi et al. 1991) and a mortality rate of 18% at 30 years' follow-up (Theander 1985).

These studies, in addition to a follow-up study by Hsu et al. (1979), found that many anorectic patients may show considerable improvement their medical condition, but the majority still suffered from the characteristic psychological set of the illness. Less than one-fourth of these patients could be considered to have made a good psychological adjustment when they were followed to ages 20 through 50 years. In his 30-year follow-up study, Theander (1985) found that 75% of his patients could be classified as being in a psychologically stable state. This was not true at the time of earlier follow-up examinations. Generally speaking, poor outcome in the studies mentioned earlier was associated with longer duration of illness, older age at onset, previous admissions to psychiatric hospitals, poor childhood social adjustment, premorbid personality difficulties, and disturbed relationships between patients and other family members.

ETIOLOGY AND PATHOGENESIS

A specific etiology and pathogenesis leading to the development of anorexia nervosa are unknown. Anorexia nervosa begins after a period of severe food deprivation, which may be due to any of the following:

- Willful dieting for the purpose of being more attractive
- Willful dieting for the purpose of being more professionally competent (e.g., ballet dancers, gymnasts, jockeys)
- Food restriction secondary to severe stress
- Food restriction secondary to severe illness and/or surgery
- Involuntary starvation

Previous periods of severe food restriction are often reported, and a history of earlier dieting is not unusual. The question is, what is unique about the individual who goes on to develop anorexia nervosa?

The psychological theories concerning the causes of anorexia have centered mostly on phobic mechanisms and psychodynamic formulations. Crisp (1976) postulated that anorexia nervosa constitutes a phobic avoidance response to food resulting from the sexual and social tension generated by the physical changes associated with puberty.

Psychodynamic theories have focused on fantasies of oral impregnation and dependent seductive relationships with warm, passive fathers and guilt over aggression toward ambivalently regarded mothers.

A cognitive and perceptual developmental defect was postulated by Bruch (1962) as the cause of anorexia nervosa. She described the disturbances of body image (denial of emaciation), disturbances in perception (lack of recognition or denial of fatigue, weakness, hunger), and a sense of ineffectiveness as being caused by untoward learning experiences.

Russell (1969) suggested that the amenorrhea may be caused by a primary disturbance of hypothalamic function and that the full expression of this disturbance is induced by psychological stress. He thought that the malnutrition of anorexia nervosa perpetuates the amenorrhea but is not primarily responsible for the endocrine disorder. This hypothesis is supported by the fact that the return of normal menstrual cycles lags behind the return to a normal body weight; the resumption of menses in anorexia nervosa is associated with marked psychological improvement (Falk and Halmi 1982).

Further support for the theory of disturbed hypothalamic function in anorexia nervosa comes from recent neurotransmitter studies. The increased cortisol production present in anorexia nervosa has been traced to the hypothalamus. Two groups of investigators (Gold et al. 1986; Hotta et al. 1986) have shown that anorectic patients have increased CRF in their cerebrospinal fluid (CSF), which probably means that increased CRF production from the hypothalamus is causing the cortisol changes observed in anorexia. Because central neurotransmitters such as dopamine, serotonin, and norepinephrine all influence appetite, satiety, and eating behavior, it is reasonable to study these neurotransmitters in anorectic patients.

Although there are serious methodological problems in assessing neurotransmitter function in the brain in humans, preliminary indirect studies indicate that there is probably a dysregulation of all three of these neurotransmitters. Kaye et al. (1984b) showed a decreased serotonin turnover in bulimic anorectic patients compared with restricting anorectic patients. In addition, Kaye et al. (1984a) showed low CSF norepinephrine levels in long-term anorectic patients who have attained a weight within at least 15% of their normal weight range. Owen et al. (1983) showed that anorectic individuals have a blunted growth hormone response to L-dopa, indicating a defect at the postsynaptic dopamine receptor sites. Neuropeptide Y, a powerful endogenous stimulant of eating behavior in the central nervous system, was found to be significantly elevated in the CSF of emaciated anorectic patients (Kaye et al. 1990). The neuropeptide Y levels generally returned to a normal range with long-term weight restoration. A reduction of food intake may produce a homeostatic increase in neuropeptide Y secretion that should serve to stimulate feeding, but this mechanism seems to be ineffective in the anorectic patient. The relationship between neuropeptide Y and CRF and luteinizing hormone secretion in anorexia nervosa is an area that needs further investigation (see Table 25–2).

Family studies of anorexia nervosa have shown a tendency to familial occurrence of this disorder and a high association with affective disorder. Theander (1970) calculated the morbidity risk for a sister of an anorectic patient to be 6.6%, much higher than would be expected. In 30 female twin pair studies in London, 9 of 16 of the monozygotic and 1 of 14 of the dizygotic pairs were concordant for anorexia nervosa (Holland et al. 1984). In a later expansion of this study, Holland et al. (1988) concluded that their data indicated a genetic predisposition that could become manifest under adverse conditions, such as inappropriate dieting or emotional stress. The authors proposed that this genetic vulnerability might implicate a particular personality type or a general susceptibility to psychiatric instability (in particular, affective disorder) or might directly involve a hypothalamic dysfunction. A monozygotic twin carrying one or more vulnerability factors would have both the potential for developing anorexia nervosa under conditions of stress and some less specific genetic loading for this disorder. Family studies of anorexia nervosa have shown an increased frequency of affective disorder in the first-degree relatives of the anorectic probands compared with the first-degree relatives of subjects without anorexia. In two controlled studies, there was no higher prevalence of eating disorder in the first-degree relatives of affective disorder probands. This suggests that an independent predisposition to anorexia must be superimposed on a predisposition to affective disorder for anorexia nervosa to be manifest. Strober (1985) found increased rates of anorexia nervosa, bulimia nervosa, and subclinical anorexia nervosa in first- and second-degree relatives of anorectic probands compared with the relatives of nonanorectic psychiatrically ill control probands. He proposed that the pattern of familial clustering of these disorders represents variable expressions of a common underlying psychopathology.

In a study comparing mothers of 57 anorectic patients with mothers of age- and sex-matched controls, Halmi et al. (1991) found a significantly greater prevalence of obsessive-compulsive disorder (OCD) in the mothers of the anorectic patients. Serotonin dysregulation may be a link between the OCD of the mothers and the anorexia nervosa in their daughters.

TREATMENT

A multifaceted treatment endeavor with medical management and behavioral, individual, cognitive, and family therapy is necessary to treat anorexia nervosa (Table 25–3). The first step in treatment is to obtain the anorectic patient's cooperation in a treatment program. Most patients with anorexia nervosa are disinterested and even resistant

TABLE 25–2. Neurotransmitters and neuropeptides in anorexia nervosa

Hormone	Effect on eating behavior	Functional status in anorexia nervosa	Clinical manifestations
Norepinephrine	Inhibits the CRF-inhibiting feeding effect	↓	Decreased food intake
Serotonin	Facilitates satiety	↑	Feeling full after a minimal intake of food
Dopamine	Mediates rewarding effects of food	↓	?
Corticotropin-releasing factor (CRF)	Inhibits feeding; stimulates motor activity	↑	Decreased food intake; increased motor activity
Neuropeptide Y (NPY)	Increases food intake	↑	Should stimulate feeding, but ineffective in anorexia nervosa
Cholecystokinin (CCK)	Attenuates feeding	↑	Decreased meal size

Note. This table is, of course, oversimplified; actual phenomena are more complex.

TABLE 25–3.   Treatment of anorexia nervosa

Type of treatment	Key elements	Measurements	Indications
Medical management	Weight restoration	Weight (outpatient—weekly; inpatient—daily)	Below normal weight for age and height by ≥10%
	Rehydration and correction of serum electrolytes	Serum electrolytes	History of vomiting, laxative abuse, severe restriction of food and fluids
Behavior therapy	Positive reinforcements for weight gain	Weight (outpatient—weekly; inpatient—daily)	Underweight
	Response prevention for binge eating and purging	Serum electrolytes and serum amylase	Weakness, puffy cheeks–parotid enlargement, scars on dorsum of hands, fainting spells
Cognitive therapy	Operationalizing beliefs, evaluating automatic thoughts, prospective hypothesis testing, examination of underlying assumptions	Assessment of distorted cognitions (e.g., all-or-none/black-or-white thinking), feeling fat, self-worth measured solely by body image, pervasive sense of ineffectiveness except in losing weight	Disturbance in way one's body weight or shape is experienced; denial of seriousness of low body weight; relentless pursuit of thinness for control of environment
Family therapy	Family counseling or therapy format based on needs of specific family	Analysis of family functioning, roles, and interactions	If patient is living with family, some type of family counseling or therapy is essential
Pharmacotherapy			
Chlorpromazine	Liquid form, start low doses, such as 10 mg tid, and gradually increase	Complete blood count, lying and standing blood pressure	Severely delusional, overactive, hospitalized patients
Cyproheptadine	Liquid form, start 4 mg bid and increase to 8 mg tid if necessary	Complete blood count with platelets	Severely overactive anorexic patient who does not binge and purge
Fluoxetine	Preferable to use after weight restoration because of tendency to induce arousal	Complete blood count, observation of total sleep and activity	Severely obsessive-compulsive behaviors related or unrelated to eating disorders, severe depression
Clomipramine	Necessary to start in very low doses because of hypotension side effects; preferable to use after weight restoration	Complete blood count, lying and standing blood pressure, electrocardiogram	Severely obsessive-compulsive behaviors
Tricyclic antidepressants	Necessary to start in very low doses because of hypotension side effects; preferable to use after weight restoration	Complete blood count, lying and standing blood pressure, electrocardiogram	Severe depression

to treatment and are brought to the therapist's office unwillingly by relatives or friends. For these patients, it is important to emphasize the benefits of treatment and to reassure them that treatment can bring about a relief of insomnia and depressive symptoms, a decrease in the obsessive thoughts about food and body weight that interfere with the ability to concentrate on other matters, an increase in physical well-being and energy, and an improvement in peer relationships.

The immediate aim of treatment should be to restore the patient's nutritional state to normal. Mere emaciation or the state of being mildly underweight (15%–25%) can cause irritability, depression, preoccupation with food, and sleep disturbance. It is exceedingly difficult to achieve behavioral change with psychotherapy in a patient who is suffering the psychological effects of emaciation. Outpatient therapy as an initial approach has the best chance for success in anorectic patients who 1) have had the illness for less than 6 months, 2) are not bingeing and vomiting, and 3) have parents who are likely to cooperate and effectively participate in family therapy.

The more severely ill anorectic patient may present an extremely difficult medical-management challenge and should be hospitalized and undergo daily monitoring of weight, food, and calorie intake and urine output. In the patient who is vomiting, frequent assessment of serum electrolytes is necessary. Behavior therapy is most effective in the medical management and nutritional rehabilitation of the anorectic patient, although there are times when other target behaviors can be changed with this approach. Behavior therapy can be used in both outpatient and inpatient settings.

The operant conditioning paradigm has been the most effective form of behavioral therapy for the treatment of anorexia nervosa. This can be used both in the context of a structured ward setting and in an individualized treatment program set up after a behavioral analysis of the patient has been completed. Positive reinforcements are used and consist of increased physical activity, visiting privileges, and social activities contingent on weight gain. An individual behavioral analysis may show other positive reinforcements to be more clinically relevant in the particular cases. The timing of reinforcement is important in behavior therapy. An adolescent patient needs at least a daily reinforcement for weight increase, which should be approximately ¼ lb or 0.1 kg per day. Making positive reinforcements contingent only on weight gain is helpful in reducing the staff-patient arguments and stressful interactions concerning how and what the patient is eating, because weight is an objective measure. In addition to being used to induce weight gain, behavior therapy can be used to stop vomiting. A response-prevention technique is used when bingeing and purging patients are required to stay in an observed dayroom area for 2–3 hours after every meal. Very few patients vomit in front of other people, and thus the emesis response is prevented and, eventually, stopped completely.

Cognitive therapy techniques for treating anorexia nervosa were developed by Garner and Bemis (1982). The assessment of cognition is a first step in cognitive therapy. Patients are asked to write down their thoughts on an assessment form so that cognitions can be examined for systematic distortions in the processing and interpretation of events. Cognitive techniques include operationalizing beliefs, decentering, using the "what if" technique, evaluating autonomic thoughts, testing prospective hypotheses, reinterpreting body image misperception, examining underlying assumptions, and modifying basic assumptions.

Cognitive-behavioral treatment for prevention of relapse of anorexia nervosa was further developed by Kleifield et al. (1996), who created an easy-to-use treatment manual. The cognitive-behavioral treatment is based on two core assumptions about the disorder. The first assumption is that anorexia nervosa has a significant positive functioning in the patient's life and develops as a way of coping with adverse experiences often associated with developmental transitions and distressing life events. The anorectic patient's deficient coping abilities produce anxiety and fear, and the patient is distracted from these anxieties by an overwhelming preoccupation with food and weight. The anorectic condition is also a reinforcing one, in that the patient experiences a surge of confidence and a sense of competence and control after being successful in dieting. The second assumption is that food restriction and ritualistic food avoidance behaviors become independent of the events or issues provoking them. The anorectic patient's extreme anxiety about gaining weight and becoming fat is alleviated by not eating. The relief of anxiety about gaining weight—the anxiety being alleviated through avoidance of food—is another strong reinforcement and thus a key factor in the persistence with which these patients pursue food restriction.

On the basis of the aforementioned assumptions, two separate pathways are taken in treatment. First, the dietary restriction is regarded as a food phobia and change eating behavioral is a primary objective. Behavioral methods such as monitoring food intake and the details surrounding food intake, along with techniques such as increasing exposure, are used to increase the patient's food intake gradually. Cognitive-behavioral methods are employed to reduce the anxiety associated with behavioral change. Cognitive techniques such as cognitive restructuring and problem solving help the patient deal with distorted and overvalued beliefs about food and thinness and cope with life's stresses.

A family analysis should be done on all anorectic patients who are living with their families. On the basis of this analysis, a clinical judgment should be made regarding what type of family therapy or counseling is clinically advisable. There will be some cases in which family therapy is not possible. However, in those cases, issues of family relationships must be dealt with in individual therapy and, in some cases, in brief counseling sessions with immediate family members. A controlled family therapy study by Russell et al. (1987) showed that anorectic patients under age 18 benefited from family therapy and patients over age 18 did worse in family therapy compared with the control therapy. There are no controlled studies of the combination of individual and family therapy. In actual practice, many clinicians provide individual therapy and some sort of family counseling in managing anorexia nervosa.

Drugs can be useful adjuncts in the treatment of anorexia nervosa. The first drug used in treating anorectic patients was chlorpromazine. This medication is especially effective in anorectic patients who are severely obsessive-compulsive. There has been no controlled double-blind study to prove definitely the efficacy of chlorpromazine in inducing weight gain in persons with anorexia. This is surprising, given that it was the first drug used and that it is the preferred drug for most severely ill anorectic patients. Another category of drugs frequently used in the treatment of anorexia nervosa is the antidepressants. A double-blind study in which 72 anorectic patients were randomly assigned to amitriptyline, cyproheptadine (an antihistaminic drug), and placebo therapy showed that both cyproheptadine and amitriptyline had a marginal effect in decreasing the number of days necessary to achieve a normal weight. Cyproheptadine had an unexpected antidepressant effect, demonstrated by a significant decrease on the Hamilton Depression Rating Scale (Halmi et al. 1986). In the bulimic subgroups of anorectic patients, cyproheptadine had a negative effect compared with both placebo and amitriptyline. This differential effect within the bulimic anorectic subgroups indicates a real medical distinction and appears to justify this subgrouping. Cyproheptadine has the advantage of not having the tricyclic antidepressant side effects of reducing blood pressure and increasing heart rate. This makes it especially attractive for use in emaciated anorectic individuals.

Other drugs have been tested in anorectic patients but have not had much of an effect. The results of small studies exploring the efficacy of fluoxetine and clomipramine suggest that both these medications warrant further study (Crisp et al. 1987; Gwirtsman et al. 1990). Both fluoxetine and clomipramine are potent inhibitors of serotonin reuptake, and both have proven effective in OCD as well as depression. These medications may be effective in preventing relapse in anorexia nervosa. Because of certain side effects (anorexia and hyperactivity in fluoxetine therapy; hypotension and tachycardia in clomipramine therapy), special caution is necessary when these medications are given to underweight anorectic patients. At a 6- to 18-month follow-up of 31 patients who had been taking fluoxetine after inpatient weight restoration, 29 patients were found to have maintained their weight at or above 85% of average body weight (Kaye et al. 1991). In this study, restricting anorectic patients responded significantly better than did bulimic and purging-type anorectic patients. The authors judged the overall responses to be good in 10 patients, partial in 17, and poor in 4 patients.

A multifaceted treatment approach is necessary for effective care of patients with anorexia nervosa. As medical rehabilitation proceeds, there is an associated improvement in psychological state. Behavioral contingencies are useful for inducing weight gain and changing the medical condition of the patient. If an anorectic patient has a predominance of depressive symptomatology, a trial with amitriptyline (or cyproheptadine, in the case of restricting anorectic individuals) is warranted.

Severely obsessive-compulsive, anxious, and agitated anorectic patients are likely to require chlorpromazine. All patients need cognitive individual psychotherapy. The more severely ill patients need hospitalization initially, followed by a well-planned continued outpatient treatment program (Garner and Garfinkel 1985). Prevention of relapse is a major part of the treatment of anorexia nervosa. Multicenter controlled treatment studies are being conducted to test the efficacy of a specific cognitive-behavior therapy and serotonin reuptake inhibitors in the prevention of relapse in this disorder.

BULIMIA

DEFINITION

Bulimia is a term that means "binge eating." This behavior has become a common practice among female students in universities and, more recently, in high schools. Not all persons who engage in binge eating require a psychiatric diagnosis. Bulimia can occur in anorexia nervosa; when this happens, the patient, under DSM-IV system, should have a diagnosis of *anorexia nervosa—binge eating/purging type*. Bulimia can also occur in a normal weight condition associated with psychological symptomatology. In that case, a diagnosis of bulimia nervosa applies (Table 25–4). Normal-weight bingeing and purging patients can fall into two categories: 1) normal-weight bulimic patients who have never had a previous history of anorexia nervosa and 2) those who have had a previous history of anorexia nervosa. Unfortunately, DSM-IV classification system does not separate these two subgroups of bulimic patients. The term *bulimia nervosa* implies a psychiatric impairment and therefore is a better label than simply *bulimia*.

Bulimia nervosa is a disorder in which the behavior of bulimia or binge eating is the predominant behavior. Binge eating is defined as an episodic, uncontrolled, rapid ingestion of large quantities of food over a short period. Abdominal pain or discomfort, self-induced vomiting, sleep, or social interruption terminates the bulimic episode. Feelings of guilt, depression, or self-disgust follow. Bulimic patients often use cathartics for weight control and have an eating

TABLE 25-4. DSM-IV diagnostic criteria for bulimia nervosa

A. Recurrent episodes of binge eating. An episode of binge eating is characterized by both of the following:

   (1) Eating, in a discrete period of time (e.g., within any 2-hour period), an amount of food that is definitely larger than most people would eat during a similar period of time and under similar circumstances

   (2) A sense of lack of control over eating during the episode (e.g., a feeling that one cannot stop eating or control what or how much one is eating)

B. Recurrent inappropriate compensatory behavior in order to prevent weight gain, such as self-induced vomiting; misuse of laxatives, diuretics, enemas, or other medications; fasting; or excessive exercise.

C. The binge eating and inappropriate compensatory behaviors both occur, on average, at least twice a week for 3 months.

D. Self-evaluation is unduly influenced by body shape and weight.

E. The disturbance does not occur exclusively during episodes of anorexia nervosa.

Specify type:

Purging type: during the current episode of bulimia nervosa, the person has regularly engaged in self-induced vomiting or the misuse of laxatives, diuretics, or enemas.

Nonpurging type: during the current episode of bulimia nervosa, the person has used other inappropriate compensatory behaviors, such as fasting or excessive exercise, but has not regularly engaged in self-induced vomiting or the misuse of laxatives, diuretics, or enemas.

---

pattern of alternate binges and fasts. Bulimic patients have a fear of not being able to stop eating voluntarily. The food consumed during a binge usually has a highly dense calorie content and a texture that facilitates rapid eating. Frequent weight fluctuations occur but without the severity of weight loss present in anorexia nervosa.

Bulimia is also encountered in DSM-IV *binge-eating disorder* (BED), which did not exist in DSM-III-R (American Psychiatric Association 1987). This disorder is listed as an example under the category "eating disorders not otherwise specified" (Tables 25–5 and 25–6). There are not enough data currently available to make BED a distinct Axis I diagnosis. Preliminary field studies show that the majority of persons who meet criteria for BED are obese. In the next 5 years, epidemiological studies will determine whether BED is a distinct disorder or merely the nonpurging type of bulimia.

CLINICAL FEATURES

Bulimia nervosa usually begins after a period of dieting of a few weeks to a year or longer. The dieting may or may not have been successful in achieving weight loss. Most binge eating episodes are followed by self-induced vomiting. Episodes are less frequently followed by use of laxatives. A minority of bulimic patients use diuretics for weight control. The average length of a bingeing episode is about 1 hour. Most patients learn to vomit by sticking their fingers down their throat, and after a short time they learn to vomit on a reflex basis. Some patients have abrasions and scars on the backs of their hands (called *Russell's sign*) from their persistent efforts to induce vomiting. Most bulimic patients do not eat regular meals and have difficulty feeling satiety at the end of a normal meal. Bulimic patients usually prefer to eat alone and at their homes. Approximately one-third to one-fifth of bulimic patients will choose a weight within a normal weight range as their ideal body weight. About one-fourth to one-third of patients with bulimia nervosa have had a previous history of anorexia nervosa.

The majority of bulimic patients have depressive signs and symptoms. They have problems with interpersonal relationships, self-concept, and impulsive behaviors and show high levels of anxiety and compulsivity. Chemical

TABLE 25-5. DSM-IV diagnostic criteria for eating disorder not otherwise specified

This category is for disorders of eating that do not meet the criteria for any specific eating disorder. Examples include

(1) For females, all of the criteria for anorexia nervosa are met except that the individual has regular menses.

(2) All of the criteria for anorexia nervosa are met except that, despite significant weight loss, the individual's current weight is in the normal range.

(3) All of the criteria for bulimia nervosa are met except that the binge eating and inappropriate compensatory mechanisms occur at a frequency of less than twice a week or for a duration of less than 3 months.

(4) The regular use of inappropriate compensatory behavior by an individual of normal body weight after eating small amounts of food (e.g., self-induced vomiting after the consumption of two cookies).

(5) Repeatedly chewing and spitting out, but not swallowing, large amounts of food.

(6) Binge-eating disorder: recurrent episodes of binge eating in the absence of the regular use of inappropriate compensatory behaviors characteristic of bulimia nervosa [see Table 25–6].

TABLE 25–6. DSM-IV (appendix) research criteria for binge-eating disorder

A. Recurrent episodes of binge eating. An episode of binge eating is characterized by both of the following:

   (1) Eating, in a discrete period of time (e.g., within any 2-hour period), an amount of food that is definitely larger than most people would eat in a similar period of time under similar circumstances.

   (2) A sense of lack of control over eating during the episode (e.g., a feeling that one cannot stop eating or control what or how much one is eating).

B. The binge-eating episodes are associated with three (or more) of the following:

   (1) Eating much more rapidly than normal

   (2) Eating until feeling uncomfortably full

   (3) Eating large amounts when not feeling physically hungry

   (4) Eating alone because of being embarrassed by how much one is eating

   (5) Feeling disgusted with oneself, depressed, or very guilty after overeating

C. Marked distress regarding binge eating is present.

D. The binge eating occurs, on average, at least 2 days a week for 6 months.

   Note: The method of determining frequency differs from that used for bulimia nervosa; future research should address whether the preferred method of setting a frequency threshold is counting the number of days on which binges occur or counting the number of episodes of binge eating.

E. The binge eating is not associated with the regular use of inappropriate compensatory behaviors (e.g., purging, fasting, excessive exercise) and does not occur exclusively during the course of anorexia nervosa or bulimia nervosa.

dependency is not unusual in this disorder, alcohol abuse being the most common. Bulimic persons will abuse amphetamines to reduce their appetite and to lose weight. Impulsive stealing usually occurs after the onset of binge eating; however, about one-fourth of patients actually begin stealing before the onset of bulimia. Food, clothing, and jewelry are the items most commonly stolen.

MEDICAL COMPLICATIONS

Patients with bulimia nervosa who engage in self-induced vomiting and abuse purgatives or diuretics are susceptible to hypokalemic alkalosis. These patients have electrolyte abnormalities including elevated serum bicarbonate levels, hypochloremia, hypokalemia, and, in a few cases, low serum bicarbonate levels, indicating a metabolic acidosis. The latter is particularly true among individuals who abuse laxatives. It is important to remember that fasting can promote dehydration, which results in volume depletion. This in turn can promote generation of aldosterone, which promotes further potassium excretion from the kidneys. Thus there can be an indirect renal loss of potassium as well as a direct loss through self-induced vomiting. Patients with electrolyte disturbances have physical symptoms of weakness and lethargy and at times have cardiac arrhythmias. The latter, of course, can lead to a sudden cardiac arrest. Patients with bulimia nervosa can have severe attrition and erosion of the teeth, causing an irritating sensitivity, pathological pulp exposures, loss of integrity of the dental arches, diminished masticatory ability, and an unaesthetic appearance.

Parotid gland enlargement associated with elevated serum amylase levels is commonly observed in patients who binge and vomit. In fact, the serum amylase level is an excellent way to follow reduction of vomiting in patients with eating disorders who deny purging episodes. Acute dilatation of the stomach is a rare emergency condition for patients who binge. Esophageal tears can also occur through the process of self-induced vomiting. A complication of shock can result subsequent to the esophageal tear and should be treated by experienced medical and surgical personnel. Severe abdominal pain in the patient with bulimia nervosa should alert the physician to a diagnosis of gastric dilatation and the need for nasogastric suction, X rays, and surgical consultation.

Cardiac failure caused by cardiomyopathy from ipecac intoxication is a medical emergency that is being reported more frequently and that usually results in death. Symptoms of precardial pain, dyspnea, and generalized muscle weakness associated with hypotension, tachycardia, and abnormalities on the electrocardiogram should alert one to possible ipecac intoxication. Other laboratory findings may include elevated liver enzymes and an increased erythrocyte sedimentation rate. Obviously, at this point the patient should be under a cardiologist's care. An echocardiogram will show a cardiomyopathy contraction pattern associated with congestive heart failure.

There are probably other mechanisms for cardiac arrhythmias and sudden death in bulimic patients. The arrhythmias noted here are associated with electrolyte disturbances and ipecac intoxication. More recent studies have shown arrhythmias associated with bingeing behavior even when serum electrolytes are within normal limits.

A summary of medical complications is presented in Table 25–7.

EPIDEMIOLOGY, COURSE, AND PROGNOSIS

No satisfactory incidence studies on bulimia nervosa have been reported. This is not surprising, given the fact that this disorder emerged only in 1980 as the distinct diagnostic entity presented in DSM-III (American Psychiatric Association 1980). In DSM-III, bulimia nervosa was referred to as "bulimia," and the criteria did not allow one to distinguish between occasional binge eating episodes and the truly incapacitating disorder of bulimia nervosa. The bulimia nervosa diagnostic criteria have been revised every few years, and this may account for the disparity in reported prevalence rates for this disorder. Studies that used strict criteria found prevalence rates between 1 and 3.8 per 100 females (Hart and Ollendick 1985; Schotte and Stunkard 1987; Whitaker et al. 1989). In a recent study combining surveys and interviews of women in the first year of college, Kurth et al. (1995) found the prevalence of bulimia nervosa to be 2%. In a Canadian community sample, in a study in which a structured interview was used, prevalence rates of this disorder were 1% (Garfinkel et al. 1995). Hoek (1991) found a 1-year prevalence rate of bulimia nervosa of 0.17% among adolescent girls and young women ages 15–29 years in a primary care health delivery system. The prevalence of males in the bulimia nervosa population varies between 10% and 15%. In most studies, the average age at onset of bulimia nervosa is

18 years (range, 12–35 years). These studies have shown a much higher representation of the higher social classes IV and V in the patients with bulimia nervosa compared with the patients with anorexia nervosa.

There are virtually no long-term follow-up studies on patients with bulimia nervosa. Thus, little information is available on the natural course of this disorder and on outcome predictors.

ETIOLOGY AND PATHOGENESIS

Fairborn and Cooper (1984) found that a rigid diet was the most commonly reported precipitant of binge eating behavior and a gross bingeing bout was the most common precipitant for vomiting behavior. This finding may shed some light on the physiological mechanisms involved in binge eating and purging. For example, the period of strict dieting may influence peptide and neurotransmitter secretion, which may in turn affect appetite and satiety mechanisms. Studies of satiety responses in patients with eating disorders have shown that the perceptions of hunger and of satiety are disturbed in patients who binge and purge (Halmi and Sunday 1991). Another study has shown distinct differences in taste preferences for sweetness and "fattiness" in restricting anorectic patients, bulimic anorectic patients, normal-weight bulimic patients, and control subjects (Sunday and Halmi 1990). Further identification of disturbances in the psychological processes of hunger, satiety, and taste could provide important clues concerning impaired central mechanisms. In another study of clinical features, Hatsukami et al. (1984) found that 43.5% of a sample of 108 women with bulimia nervosa had an affective disorder at some time in their lives and 18.5% had a history of alcohol or drug abuse. Although there is a high association of affective disorder with bulimia nervosa, at present not enough evidence is available to support describing bulimia nervosa as a mere forme fruste of affective disorder. Bulimia nervosa theoretically fits well into an addictive model (Szmukler and Tantam 1984).

A study that used the Minnesota Multiphasic Personality Inventory to compare women with bulimia nervosa with women who abused alcohol and drugs found that the two groups had similar profiles. They had elevations on the scales denoting depression, impulsivity, anger, rebelliousness, anxiety, rumination, social withdrawal, and idiosyncratic thinking (Hatsukami et al. 1982). Two studies using the Social Adjustment Scale found that women with bulimia nervosa were significantly worse in all areas of adjustment (work, social, and leisure activities; relationship with extended family;

TABLE 25–7. Medical complications of bulimia nervosa

Behavioral and physical aberrations	Physiological disturbances
Binge eating	Acute dilatation of stomach–shock
Self-induced vomiting	Esophageal tears–shock; dehydration; metabolic alkalosis-hypochloremia, hypokalemia, weakness, lethargy; cardiac arrhythmias–cardiac arrest; erosion of dental enamel–caries, exposure of pulp
Parotid gland enlargement (self-induced vomiting or excessive gum chewing)	Elevated serum amylase
Ipecac use	Hypotension, tachycardia, electrocardiographic abnormalities, elevated liver enzymes

role as spouse; role as parent, and membership in a family unit) than were women in a control sample (Johnson and Berndt 1983; Norman and Herzog 1984). These findings remained stable after a year. These latter studies indicate one might expect to find a higher prevalence of Axis II DSM-IV diagnoses in the patients with bulimia nervosa than in a normal population.

The percentage of individuals with DSM-III-R bulimia (including anorectic bulimic individuals) who have at least one personality disorder has been reported to be 77% (Powers et al. 1988), 69% (Wonderlich et al. 1990), 62% (Gartner et al. 1989), 61% (Schmidt and Telch 1990), 33% (Ames-Frankel et al. 1992), and 23% (Herzog et al. 1992). All of these studies used established diagnostic interviews, but the findings are not in agreement. This is probably due to several factors: 1) some of the studies with very small numbers of patients may represent a biased sample; 2) studies used different criteria, ranging from DSM-III to DSM-III-R, for both eating disorders and personality disorders; and 3) some of the Axis II interviewers lacked information about the patients' Axis I diagnosis, which may have led to false-positive personality disorder diagnoses. Nonetheless, there is substantial evidence that personality disorders are commonly associated with bulimia nervosa.

TREATMENT

Treatment studies of bulimia nervosa have proliferated in the past 15 years, in contrast to the relatively few treatment studies of anorexia nervosa. This is probably due to the greater prevalence of bulimia nervosa and the fact that this disorder can usually be treated on an outpatient basis. Specific therapy techniques such as behavior therapy, cognitive therapy, psychodynamic therapy, and "psychoeducation therapy" have been conducted both in individual and group therapies (Table 25–8). There are no controlled studies in which patients were randomly assigned to individual or group therapy for any of these techniques. Multiple controlled drug treatment studies have also been conducted in the past decade. Often a variety of therapy techniques such as cognitive therapy, behavior therapy, and drug treatment may be used together in either individual or group therapy. Unfortunately, there is no way to predict at present what bulimic patient will respond to what type of therapy or treatment.

TABLE 25–8. Treatment of bulimia nervosa

Type of treatment	Indications	Measurements	Key elements
Cognitive-behavior therapy (CBT)			
Group	Outpatients—young adults	Psychiatric and medical evaluations before entering therapy	Psychoeducational component on all aspects of the bulimic disorder
Individual	Inpatients; outpatients—adolescents and adults with severe character disorders	Self-recording of medical consultations available throughout treatment	Self-monitoring, cognitive restructuring
Behavior therapy	Usually used in conjunction with computed tomography	Same as for CBT	Restricting exposure to cues, developing alternative behaviors, response prevention to stop vomiting
Interpersonal therapy	Outpatients—young adults	Psychiatric and medical evaluations before entering therapy and consultation available during treatment	Focuses on interpersonal relationships
Pharmacotherapy *Antidepressants* Desipramine Imipramine Nortriptyline Phenelzine Fluoxetine	Binge-eating behavior, depression, unwillingness to enter CBT	Initial evaluation: complete blood count, serum electrolytes and amylase electrocardiogram, blood pressure. Repeat above after 1 week and as often as clinically indicated	The antidepressant drugs affect catecholamine and indoleamine function, which in turn modulates eating behavior

Psychodynamic Therapy

Lacey (1983) described the use of psychodynamic therapy with cognitive and behavioral techniques in both the individual and group therapy format. Common themes that need to be dealt with are poor self-esteem, dependency problems, and a sense of ineffectiveness.

Cognitive-Behavior Therapy

Fourteen published controlled studies have examined the efficacy of cognitive-behavior therapy (CBT) in bulimia nervosa. One of the first and best descriptions of CBT was by Fairburn (1981). All of the subjects in these 14 studies were outpatients, with the exception of one study of the effectiveness of CBT in individual therapy, involving inpatients. Nearly all of the studies used a psychoeducational component that included information on the social-cultural emphasis on thinness; set point theory; the physical effects and medical complications of bingeing, purging, and abuse of laxatives and diuretics; and how dieting and fasting precipitate binge-purge cycles. Self-monitoring was an important part of all of these studies and usually consists of a daily record of the times and durations of meals and a record of binge eating and purging episodes, as well as descriptions of moods and circumstances surrounding binge-purge episodes. The studies stressed the importance of eating regular meals.

Cognitive restructuring is the basis of all the CBT programs. The first step in cognitive therapy is the assessment of cognition. Patients are asked to write their thoughts on an assessment form so that cognitions can be examined for systematic distortions in the processing and interpretation of events. Two reviews of controlled studies of CBT for bulimia nervosa concluded that CBT benefits the majority of patients (Fairburn et al. 1992a; Gotestam and Agras 1989). CBT was found to be more effective than treatment with antidepressants alone, self-monitoring plus supportive psychotherapy, and behavioral treatment without the cognitive treatment component. One-year follow-up studies with CBT have shown a good maintenance of change, superior to that following treatment with antidepressants.

Behavior therapy is used specifically to stop the binge-eating/purging behaviors. Behavioral approaches include restricting exposure to cues that trigger a binge-purge episode, developing a strategy of alternate behaviors, and delaying the vomiting response to eating. Response prevention is a technique used specifically to prevent vomiting. After eating, a patient is placed in a situation in which it is very difficult for him or her comfortably to vomit. Adding exposure (i.e., requiring the patient to binge) did not seem to enhance the effects of response pre-vention (Rosen 1982).

The combined effects of CBT and antidepressant medication for bulimia nervosa were examined in two studies. Mitchell et al. (1990) found that group CBT was superior to imipramine therapy for decreasing binge eating and purging and the combined treatment demonstrated no additive effects for those treated with group CBT alone. Agras et al. (1992) had similar results comparing individual CBT, desipramine therapy, or the combination at 16 weeks. However, at 32 weeks, only the combined treatment given for 24 weeks was superior to medication given for 16 weeks. A study of interpersonal therapy (IPT), which targets interpersonal functioning, showed that IPT was equivalent to CBT in reducing bulimic symptoms and psychopathology; at follow-up it was actually superior to CBT (Fairburn et al. 1992b). This is the first study to show that bulimia nervosa may be treated successfully without focusing directly on the patient's eating habits and attitudes toward shape and weight. This study should be replicated before definitive statements can be made concerning the effectiveness of IPT in the treatment of bulimia nervosa.

Currently, multicenter treatment studies are under way that use a sequential design, which more realistically represents the practice of treating bulimia nervosa patients by primary care physicians. In these studies, usually one form of treatment such as CBT or a serotonin reuptake inhibitor is administered for a period of 4 months. If the patients have not completely ceased bingeing and purging behavior at the end of that time, they are then assigned to another treatment modality. In the next 3–4 years, these studies will yield some very useful data to aid in the decisions concerning what kind of therapy should be given to which patients.

Drug Therapy

Studies of antidepressant medications have consistently shown some efficacy in the treatment of bulimia nervosa. These studies were prompted by observations that patients with bulimia nervosa also had significant mood disturbances. Since 1980, more than a dozen double-blind, placebo-controlled trials of various antidepressants were conducted in normal-weight outpatients with bulimia nervosa. (For a review of these studies, see Fairburn et al. 1992a.) All of these trials demonstrated a significantly greater reduction in binge eating when antidepressant medication was administered than when placebo was given. Antidepressants improved mood and reduced psychopathological symptoms such as preoccupation with shape and weight. These studies provide evidence for the short-term efficacy of antidepressant medication, but long-term efficacy remains unknown. The average rate of abstinence from bingeing and purging in these studies was 22%, indicating that the majority of patients remain symptomatic at the end of treatment with antidepressants. Both of the systematic studies conducted to evaluate maintenance of change in bulimic symptomatology yielded disappointing results: most subjects did not maintain improvement (Pyle et al. 1990; Walsh et al. 1991). The dosage of antidepressant medication to treat bulimia nervosa was similar to that used in the treatment of depression. The antidepressants used in the controlled treatment studies for bulimia nervosa included desipramine, imipramine, amitriptyline, nortriptyline, phenelzine, and fluoxetine.

The current data suggest that the treatment of choice for bulimia nervosa should be CBT and that a single antidepressant administered in the absence of psychotherapy cannot be considered an adequate treatment.

OBESITY

DEFINITION

In contrast to anorexia nervosa and bulimia nervosa, obesity is classified not as a psychiatric disorder but as a medical disorder. Obesity is an excessive accumulation of body fat and operationally is defined as being overweight. The body mass index (BMI), which is weight (kg)/height (m²), has the highest correlation, 0.8, with body fat measured by other more precise laboratory methods. *Mildly overweight* is defined as having a BMI of 25–30, or body weight between the upper limit of normal and 20% above that limit on standard height-weight charts. *Obesity* is defined as a BMI above 30, or body weight greater than 20% above the upper limit for height (Bray 1978).

CLINICAL FEATURES

The most obvious clinical features of obesity are physical; these features are discussed in the section on medical complications. The psychological and behavioral aspects of obesity are best considered grouped in two categories: *eating behavior* and *emotional disturbance*. There is considerable heterogeneity in eating patterns. Most commonly, obese persons complain that they cannot restrain their eating and that they have difficulty achieving satiety. Some obese persons cannot distinguish hunger from other dysphoric states and will eat when they are emotionally upset.

The most methodologically satisfying studies have shown that there is no distinct or excess psychopathology in obesity. In one study of severely obese patients who had gastric bypass surgery, the most prevalent psychiatric diag-

nosis was major depressive disorder. However, this diagnosis was no more prevalent in the obese patients than in the general population. Self-disparagement of body image is especially present in those who have been obese since childhood. This may be due to the continual bombardment of social prejudice against obese people. The stigmatization and prejudice against obese types is well documented in studies of educational disadvantages and of employment prejudices against obese persons. Many obese individuals develop anxiety and depression when they attempt to diet (Halmi et al. 1980). Because health risks and mortality vary with degree of adiposity, Bray (1986) proposed a classification into low-risk (BMI 25–30), moderate-risk (BMI 31–40), and high-risk (BMI greater than 40) individuals.

MEDICAL COMPLICATIONS

Obesity affects a great variety of physiological functions. Blood circulation may be overtaxed as body weight increases, and congestive heart failure may occur in grossly obese individuals. There is a high association of hypertension with obesity, and the prevalence of carbohydrate intolerance in grossly obese subjects is approximately 50%. Increased body fat in the upper region of the body as opposed to the lower region is more likely to be associated with the onset of diabetes mellitus. The impairment of pulmonary function becomes extreme in severe obesity and involves hypoventilation, hypercapnia, hypoxia, and somnolence (i.e., the pickwickian syndrome). The latter has a high mortality rate. Obesity may accelerate the development of osteoarthritis and of dermatological problems from stretching of the skin, intertrigo, and acanthosis nigricans. Obese women are an obstetrical risk, being susceptible to toxemia and hypertension.

Obesity has been associated with several types of cancer. Obese males have a higher rate of prostate and colorectal cancer, and obese females have increased incidences of gallbladder, breast, cervical, endometrial, uterine, and ovarian cancer. Most studies on the topic suggest that obesity influences the development and progression of both endometrial and breast cancer through influences on estrogen production. Low-density lipoprotein levels are increased in obesity and levels of high-density lipoproteins (HDL cholesterol) are reduced. The low levels of HDL may be one mechanism by which obesity is associated with an increased risk for cardiovascular disease.

EPIDEMIOLOGY, COURSE, AND PROGNOSIS

If obesity is defined as the state of being 20% above ideal weight, then nearly a quarter of the United States population would be considered obese (VanItallie 1985). Socioeconomic status is highly correlated with obesity: the condition is much more common among women (less so among men) of low status. This relationship is also present in obese children. Increasing age and obesity are associated until age 50. There is a higher prevalence of obesity in women compared with men; over age 50 years, this may be due to the increased mortality rate among obese men with advancing age.

Unfortunately, life expectancy and obesity studies are restricted to life insurance studies and therefore do not represent a random American population. Despite these limitations, studies have shown a progressive increase in "excess mortality" as BMI increased (Society of Actuaries 1992). Another study of grossly obese persons showed that excess mortality was greatly increased in younger men (ages 25–34 years) and gradually declined with age (Stevens et al. 1998).

ETIOLOGY AND PATHOGENESIS

It is unlikely that there is a single etiology for obesity. In the first section of this chapter, the complex neural mechanisms involved in the control of feeding behavior were discussed. Lipid, amino acid, and glucose metabolism all seem to affect, in some way, central neural regulatory mechanisms that influence eating behavior. Obesity is regarded today by most investigators as a disorder of energy balance, a disorder with a strong genetic component that is modulated by cultural and environmental influences.

There is a definite familial aspect to obesity. Eighty percent of the offspring of two obese parents are obese, compared with 40% of the offspring of one obese parent and only 10% of the offspring of lean parents. Findings of twin studies and adoption studies suggest that genetic factors play a strong role in the development of obesity.

The cloning and sequencing of the mouse obese (OB) gene and its human homologue in 1994 (Zhang et al. 1994) provided the basis for further research into the pathways that regulate adiposity and body weight. Leptin, the gene product of the OB gene, was shown to be a 16-kilodalton protein that is present in mouse and human plasma (Halaas et al. 1995). Intraperitoneal injections of recombinant leptin decrease food intake and increase energy expenditure in wild-type mice. Leptin reduces body fat in mice, and its absence in mice with the OB gene leads to a massive increase in body fat. In both humans and rodents, leptin is highly correlated with BMI and amount of body fat (Maffei et al. 1995). Weight loss due to food restriction was associated with a decrease in plasma leptin concentrations in mice and obese humans. These data suggest that leptin

serves an endocrine function, regulating body weight and stores of body fat.

Obese persons have larger and more numerous fat cells. Cellular proliferation tends to occur early in life but will also occur in adult life when the existing fat cells are greatly enlarged. The regulation of fat cell proliferation and size is not well understood. The relation of physical activity to obesity is complex. It is known that obese people are less active than people of normal weight. The increase in caloric expenditure by physical activity is small. Animal studies show that physical activity actually decreases food intake and may actually prevent the fall in metabolic rate that usually accompanies dieting.

TREATMENT

For mild obesity (20%–40% overweight), the most efficient treatment to date is behavior modification in groups, a balanced diet, and exercise. This is usually done by both commercial and nonprofit large organizations. For moderate obesity (41%–100% overweight), a medically supervised protein-sparing modified fast (400–700 calories per day) is often necessary. This diet may or may not be combined with behavior modification techniques. A behavior analysis is necessary to set up a sensible behavioral modification program. Antecedents of eating behavior, the eating behavior itself, the consequences of the behavior, and the acceptable rewards for carrying out various prescribed behaviors are all analyzed. Behavior treatment programs include self-monitoring, nutrition education, physical activity, and cognitive restructuring.

The use of medication such as phenylpropanolamine or fenfluramine was popular in the past. The problem with these drugs is that on withdrawal, there is a rebound ballooning up of weight and, in some patients, concomitant lethargy and depression. In 1997, fenfluramine was removed by the Food and Drug Administration from the market and for approved use for treatment of obesity because of the adverse effects of pulmonary hypertension and mitral valve impairment.

There is only one long-term (5 years) controlled study that has documented the safety and efficacy of the fenfluramine-phentermine combination (Weintraub 1992). The National Task Force on the Prevention and Treatment of Obesity (1996) reviewed all English-language reports of studies in which human obesity was treated with medication that was given for at least 24 weeks. The task force found that the net weight loss attributable to medication use is modest, ranging from 2 kg to 10 kg. The weight loss tends to reach a plateau by 6 months. Most adverse effects are mild and self-limited, but rare serious outcomes such as pulmonary hypertension have been reported. The task force's conclusion was that pharmacotherapy for obesity, when combined with appropriate behavioral approaches to change diet and amount of physical activity, helps some obese patients lose weight and maintain weight loss for at least 1 year (National Task Force on the Prevention and Treatment of Obesity 1996). The task force also stated that until more data are available, pharmacotherapy cannot be recommended for routine use in obese individuals. They did acknowledge that it may be helpful in carefully selected patients.

Severe obesity (greater than 100% over a normal weight) is the least common form of obesity and is most effectively treated by surgical procedures that reduce the size of the stomach. These procedures produce a large weight loss and show a good record of weight loss maintenance.

Behavior modification is the treatment of choice for overweight children and should include involvement of the parents and the schools. Psychotherapy is not recommended as a treatment per se for obesity, although it is possible that some patients may have particular problems that may be effectively treated or helped with psychotherapy. For excellent discussions on the treatment of obesity, see Stunkard (1984), Brownell (1984), and Lasagna (1987).

CONCLUSIONS

The eating disorders are complex syndromes in which the interactions among environmental, psychological, and physiological factors both create and maintain the disturbed eating behavior. The more precise an understanding we obtain of the connectedness of basic physiological changes, psychological changes, and eating behavior, the better we will be able to design effective treatment interventions.

Many questions remain to be asked about our current treatment interventions. For example, how long should the bulimic patient be treated with antidepressants? Would periodic follow-up behavioral sessions prevent relapse in bulimic patients treated with behavior therapy? How can we identify the most likely effective treatment for a patient?

Continued prospective longitudinal studies are necessary for bulimia nervosa because there is no information on what happens to this addictive-like bingeing-purging behavior over the course of a lifetime. Although disturbed eating behavior has been present throughout the history of humankind, it has been systematically studied with scientific methodology only in the past few decades. There is a continued need for further study of eating disorders.

REFERENCES

Agras WS, Rossiter EM, Arnow B, et al.: Pharmacologic and cognitive-behavioral treatment for bulimia nervosa: a controlled comparison. Am J Psychiatry 149:82–87, 1992

American Psychiatric Association: Diagnostic and Statistical Manual of Mental Disorders, 3rd Edition. Washington, DC, American Psychiatric Association, 1980

American Psychiatric Association: Diagnostic and Statistical Manual of Mental Disorders, 3rd Edition, Revised. Washington, DC, American Psychiatric Association, 1987

American Psychiatric Association: Diagnostic and Statistical Manual of Mental Disorders, 4th Edition. Washington, DC, American Psychiatric Association, 1994

Ames-Frankel J, Devlin MJ, Walsh BT, et al: Personality disorders and eating disorders. J Clin Psychiatry 53:90–96, 1992

Bell RM: Holy Anorexia. Chicago, University of Chicago Press, 1985

Blundell JE, Hill A: Behavioral pharmacology of feeding: relevance of animal experiments for studies in man, in Pharmacology of Eating Disorders. Edited by Carruba M, Blundell J. New York, Raven, 1986, pp 51–70

Booth DA: Food-conditioned eating preferences and aversions with interceptive elements: conditioned appetite and satieties. Ann N Y Acad Sci 443:22–41, 1985

Bray GA: Definitions, measurements and classification of the syndromes of obesity. Int J Obesity 2:99–112, 1978

Bray GA: Effects of obesity on health and happiness, in Handbook of Eating Disorders: Physiology, Psychology, and Treatment. Edited by Brownell KD, Foreyt JP. New York, Basic Books, 1986, pp 3–44

Brownell KD: New developments in the treatment of obese children and adolescents, in Eating and Its Disorders. Edited by Stunkard AJ, Stellar E. New York, Raven, 1984, pp 175–184

Bruch H: Perceptual and conceptual disturbance in anorexia nervosa. Psychosom Med 24:187–195, 1962

Crisp AH: The possible significance of some behavioral correlates of weight and carbohydrate intake. J Psychosom Res 11:117–123, 1976

Crisp AH, Palmer RL, Kalucy RS, et al: How common is anorexia nervosa? A prevalence study. Br J Psychiatry 128:549–552, 1976

Crisp AH, Lacey JH, Crutchfield M: Clomipramine and 'drive' in people with anorexia nervosa: an inpatient study. Br J Psychiatry 150:355–358, 1987

Eagles T, Johnston M, Hunter D, et al: Increasing incidence of anorexia nervosa in the female population of northeast Scotland. Am J Psychiatry 152:1266–1271, 1995

Eckert E, Halmi KA, Marchi M: Ten year outcome in anorexia nervosa. Paper presented at the annual meeting of the American Psychiatric Association, Washington, DC, May 1986

Fairburn C: A cognitive behavioral approach to the treatment of bulimia. Psychol Med 11:707–711, 1981

Fairburn CG, Cooper PJ: The clinical features of bulimia nervosa. Br J Psychiatry 144:238–246, 1984

Fairburn CG, Agra WS, Wilson GT: The research on the treatment of bulimia nervosa: practical and theoretical implications, in Biology of Feast and Famine: Relevance to Eating Disorders. Edited by GH Anderson, SH Kennedy. New York: Academic Press, 1992a, pp 318–340

Fairburn CG, Jones R, Pevelar RC et al: Three psychological treatments for bulimia nervosa: a comparative trial. Arch Gen Psychiatry 48:463–469, 1992b

Falk JR, Halmi KA: Amenorrhea in anorexia nervosa: examination of the critical body hypothesis. Biol Psychiatry 17:799–806,1982

Garfinkel P, Goering L, Spegg C, et al: Bulimia nervosa in a Canadian community sample: prevalence and comparison of subgroups. Am J Psychiatry 52:1052–1058, 1995

Garner DM, Bemis KM: A cognitive-behavioral approach to anorexia nervosa. Cognitive Therapy and Research 6: 1223–1250, 1982

Garner DM, Garfinkel PE: Handbook of Psychotherapy for Anorexia Nervosa. New York, Guilford, 1985

Gartner AF, Marcus RN, Halmi KA, et al: DSM-III-R personality disorders in patients with eating disorders. Am J Psychiatry 146:1585–1591, 1989

Gibbs J, Smith GP: Satiety hormones, in Frontiers in Neuroendocrinology, Vol 8. Edited by Martini L, Gonong W. New York, Raven, 1984, pp 98–132

Gold PW, Gwirtsman H, Kaye W, et al: Pathophysiologic mechanisms in underweight and weight corrected patients. N Engl J Med 314:335–342, 1986

Gotestam KA, Agras WS: Bulimia nervosa: pharmacologic and psychologic approaches to treatment. Nordisk Psykiatrisk Tidsskrift 43:543–551, 1989

Gwirtsman HE, Guze BH, Yager J, et al: Fluoxetine treatment of anorexia nervosa: an open trial. J Clin Psychiatry 51:378–382, 1990

Halaas J, Gajiwala K, Maffei M, et al: Weight-reducing effects of the protein encoded by the obese gene. Science 269:543–546, 1995

Halmi KA: Anorexia nervosa: demographic and clinical features in 94 cases. Psychosom Med 36:18–26, 1974

Halmi KA: Anorexia nervosa and bulimia, in Handbook of Adolescent Psychology. Edited by Hersen M, Van Hasselt T. New York, Pergamon, 1987, pp 265–287

Halmi KA, Falk JR: Common physiological changes in anorexia nervosa. Int J Eat Disord 1:16–27, 1981

Halmi KA, Sunday SR: Temporal patterns of hunger and satiety ratings and related cognitions in anorexia and bulimia. Appetite 16:219–237, 1991

Halmi KA, Stunkard AJ, Mason EE: Emotional responses to weight reduction by three methods: gastric bypass, jejunoileal bypass, diet. Am J Clin Nutr 33:446–451, 1980

Halmi KA, Eckert E, LaDu T, et al: Anorexia nervosa: treatment efficacy of cyproheptadine and amitriptyline. Arch Gen Psychiatry 43:177–181, 1986

Halmi KA, Eckert E, Marchi P, et al: Comorbidity of psychiatric diagnoses in anorexia nervosa. Arch Gen Psychiatry 48: 712–718, 1991

Hart K, Ollendick TH: Prevalence of bulimia in working and university women. Am J Psychiatry 142:851–854, 1985

Hatsukami J, Mitchell J, Eckert E: Similarities and differences on the MMPI between women with bulimia and women with alcohol and drug abuse problems. Addict Behav 7:435–439, 1982

Hatsukami J, Mitchell J, Eckert E, et al: Affective disorder and substance abuse in women with bulimia. Psychol Med 14:704–710, 1984

Herzog DB, Keller MB, Lavori PW, et al: The prevalence of personality disorders in 210 women with eating disorders. J Clin Psychiatry 53:147–152, 1992

Hoebel BG: Pharmacological control of feeding. Annu Rev Pharmacol Toxicol 17:605–621, 1977

Hoek H: The incidence and prevalence of anorexia nervosa and bulimia nervosa in primary care. Psychol Med 21:455–460, 1991

Holland AJ, Crisp A, Russell GFM, et al: Anorexia nervosa: a study of 34 twin pairs and one set of triplets. Br J Psychiatry 145:414–419, 1984

Holland AJ, Sicotte N, Tresure J: Anorexia nervosa: evidence for a genetic basis. J Psychosom Res 32:561–571, 1988

Hotta M, Chibasaki T, Masuda A, et al: The responses of plasma adrenal corticotropin and cortisol to corticotropin-releasing hormone and cerebral spinal fluid immunoreactive CRH in anorexia nervosa patients. J Clin Endocrinol Metab 62:319–321, 1986

Hsu G, Crisp A: Outcome of anorexia nervosa. Lancet 1:61–65, 1979

Johnson C, Berndt DJ: Preliminary investigation of bulimia and life adjustment. Am J Psychiatry 140:774–777, 1983

Jones D, Fox MM, Babigian HM, et al: Epidemiology of anorexia nervosa in Monroe County, N.Y., 1960–1976. Psychosom Med 42:551–558, 1980

Kaye WH, Ebert MH, Raleigh M, et al: Abnormalities in CNS monoamine metabolism in anorexia nervosa. Arch Gen Psychiatry 41:350–355, 1984a

Kaye WH, Ebert M, Gwirtsman H, et al: Differences in brain serotonergic metabolism between nonbulimic and bulimic patients with anorexia nervosa. Am J Psychiatry 141: 1598–1601, 1984b

Kaye WH, Berrettini W, Gwirtsman HE, et al: Altered cerebral spinal fluid neuropeptide Y and peptide YY immunoreactivity in anorexia and bulimia nervosa. Arch Gen Psychiatry 47:548–556, 1990

Kaye WH, Welzin T, Hsu J: An open trial of fluoxetine in patients with anorexia nervosa. J Clin Psychiatry 52:464–471, 1991

Kleifield E, Wagner S, Halmi K: Cognitive-behavioral treatment of anorexia nervosa. Psychiatr Clin North Am 19:715–734, 1996

Kurth C, Krahn D, Nairn K, et al: The severity of dieting and bingeing behaviors in college women: interview validation of survey data. J Psychiatry Res 29:211–225, 1995

Lacey JH: An outpatient treatment program for bulimia nervosa. Int J Eat Disord 2:209–241, 1983

Lasagna L: The pharmacotherapy of obesity, in Psychopharmacology: The Third Generation of Progress. Edited by Meltzer HY. New York, Raven, 1987, pp 1281–1284

Leibowitz SF: Neurochemical systems of the hypothalamus: control of feeding and drinking behavior and water electrolyte excretion, in Handbook of the Hypothalamus, Vol 3. Edited by Morgane PJ, Panksepp J. New York, Raven, 1980, pp 299–347

Lucas A, Beard C, O'Fallon W, et al: Fifty year trends in the incidence of anorexia nervosa in Rochester, Minnesota: a population-based study. Am J Psychiatry 148:917–922, 1991

Maffei M, Halaas J, Ravussin E, et al: Leptin levels in human and rodent: measurement of plasma leptin and OB RNA in obese and weight-reduced subjects. Nat Med 1:1155–1161, 1995

Mitchell JE, Pyle RL, Eckert ED, et al: A comparison study of antidepressants and structured intensive group therapy in the treatment of bulimia nervosa. Arch Gen Psychiatry 47:149–157, 1990

Morgan HG, Russell GFM: Values of family background and clinical features as predictors of long-term outcome in anorexia nervosa. Psychol Med 5:355–371, 1975

Morley J, Levine AS: Pharmacology of eating behavior. Annu Rev Pharmacol Toxicol 25:127–146, 1985

Morley J, Levine AS, Willenbring ML: Stress-induced feeding disorder, in Pharmacology of Eating Disorders. Edited by Carruba M, Blundell JE. New York, Raven, 1986, pp 71–100

National Task Force on the Prevention and Treatment of Obesity: Long-term pharmacotherapy in the management of obesity. JAMA 276:1907–1915, 1996

Norman KA, Herzog DB: Persistent social maladjustment in bulimia: one year follow-up. Am J Psychiatry 141:355–340, 1984

Owen WP, Halmi KA, Lasley E, et al: Dopamine regulation in anorexia nervosa. Psychopharm Bull 19:578–580, 1983

Pope H, Hudson JI, Jonas JM, et al: Bulimia treated with imipramine: a placebo-controlled double-blind study. Am J Psychiatry 140:554–560, 1983

Powers PS, Covert DL, Brightwell DR, et al: Other psychiatric disorders among bulimic patients. Compr Psychiatry 29:503–508, 1988

Pyle RL, Mitchell JE, Eckert ED, et al: Maintenance treatment and 6 month outcome for bulimia patients who respond to initial treatment. Am J Psychiatry 147:871–875, 1990

Rooney B, McClelland L, Crisp AH, et al: The incidence and prevalence of anorexia nervosa in three suburban health districts in southwest London, UK. Int J Eat Disord 18:299–307, 1995

Rosen J: Bulimia nervosa: treatment with exposure and response prevention. Behavior Therapy 13:117–124, 1982

Russell GFM: Metabolic, endocrine and psychiatric aspects of anorexia nervosa. Scientific Basis of Medicine Annual Review 14:236–255, 1969

Russell GFM, Szmukler JI, Dare C, et al: An evaluation of family therapy in anorexia nervosa and bulimia nervosa. Arch Gen Psychiatry 44:1047–1056, 1987

Schotte D, Stunkard A: Bulimia vs. bulimic behaviors on a college campus. JAMA 9:1213–1215, 1987

Schmidt ND, Telch MJ: Prevalence of personality disorders among bulimics, non-bulimic binge eaters and normal controls. Journal of Psychopathology and Behavioral Assessment 12:170–185, 1990

Silverstone T, Kyriades M: Clinical pharmacology of appetite, in Drugs and Appetite. Edited by Silverstone T. New York, Academic Press, 1982, pp 93–124

Society of Actuaries: Life tables for the United States Social Security Area 1900–2080: Actuarial Study No 107, August 1992 (SSA Publ No 11-11536). Washington, DC, U.S. Department of Health and Human Services, 1992

Stevens J, Ooi J, Pamuk E, et al: The effect of age on the association between body mass index and mortality. N Engl J Med 338:1–7, 1998

Strober M, Morell W, Burroughs J, et al: A controlled family study of anorexia nervosa. Psychiatry Res 19:329–346, 1985

Stunkard AJ: The current status of treatment for obesity in adults, in Eating and Its Disorders. Edited by AJ Stunkard, Stellar E. New York, Raven, 1984, pp 157–174

Sunday SR, Halmi KA: Taste perceptions and hedonics in eating disorders. Physiol Behav 48:587–594, 1990

Szmukler JI: The epidemiology of anorexia nervosa and bulimia. J Psychiatry Res 19:1243–1253, 1985

Szmukler JI, Tantam D: Anorexia nervosa: starvation dependence. Br J Med Psychol 57:305–310, 1984

Theander S: Anorexia nervosa. Acta Psychiatr Scand 214:1–300, 1970

Theander S: Outcome and prognosis in anorexia nervosa and bulimia, in Anorexia Nervosa and Bulimic Disorders. Edited by Szmukler GI, Slade PD, Harris P, et al: London, Pergamon, 1985, pp 493–508

VanItallie TB: Health implications of overweight and obesity in the United States. Ann Intern Med 103:983–988, 1985

Walsh BT, Hadigan CM, Devlin MJ, et al: Long-term outcome of antidepressant treatment for bulimia nervosa. Am J Psychiatry 148:1206–1212, 1991

Weintraub M: Long-term weight control: The National Heart, Lung and Blood Institute funded multi-modal intervention study. Clin Pharmacol Ther 51:581–585, 1992

Wonderlich SA, Swift WJ, Slotnick HB, et al: DSM-III-R personality disorders and eating disorder subtypes. Int J Eat Disord 9:607–616, 1990

Wurtman JJ, Wurtman RJ: Drugs that enhance central serotonergic transmission diminished elective carbohydrate consumption by rats. Life Sci 24:895–904, 1979

Young RC, Gibbs J, Antin J, et al: Sham-feeding. Journal of Comparative and Physiological Psychology 87:795–800, 1974

Zhang Y, Prenca R, Maffei M, et al: Positional cloning of the mouse obese gene and its human homologue. Nature 372:425–432, 1994

CHAPTER 26

PAIN DISORDERS

STEVEN A. KING, M.D.

Of all the problems faced by physicians, pain is among the most pervasive and difficult to diagnose and treat. It is not only one of the most frequently encountered complaints in medicine in general but also a common symptom of other mental disorders. The scope of the problem is reflected by the fact that in any given year, 10%–15% of adults in the United States have some form of work disability due to back pain alone (Osterweis et al. 1987). Unfortunately, psychiatry's involvement in the field of pain has been markedly limited by misconceptions and misunderstandings about the nature of pain, its assessment, and its management.

This chapter provides an overview of current concepts regarding the diagnosis and treatment of pain, with special emphasis on the role of the psychiatrist.

DEFINITION OF PAIN

One of the difficulties encountered by clinicians and researchers is defining pain. Although pain has not traditionally been considered a mental disorder, the current defini-

tions of pain accept the primacy of psychological factors in the pain experience. The most commonly accepted definition is that presented by the Committee on Taxonomy of the International Association for the Study of Pain: "An unpleasant sensory and emotional experience associated with actual or potential tissue damage, or described in terms of such damage. . . . Activity induced in the nociceptor and nociceptive pathways by a noxious stimulus is not pain, *which is always a psychological state*, even though we may well appreciate that pain most often has a proximate physical cause" (Merskey and Bogduk 1994, p. 210; emphasis added). The Institute of Medicine Committee on Pain, Disability, and Chronic Illness Behavior reported that "the experience of pain is more than a simple sensory process. It is a complex perception involving higher levels of the central nervous system, emotional states, and higher order mental processes" (Osterweis et al. 1987, p. 13).

These definitions indicate the necessity of terminating the dualistic concept that pain should be divided into that associated with identifiable organic pathology and that considered secondary to psychological factors. This outdated view has many drawbacks, most notably its often leading to the belief that the former is "real pain," whereas the latter is "imaginary," even though when the etiological factors involved in the pain are psychological, the patient's perception of the pain is the same and his or her suffering is just as real.

DIAGNOSTIC CLASSIFICATION OF PAIN

Problems were encountered in employing the pain-related diagnoses included in the previous editions of the *Diagnostic and Statistical Manual of Mental Disorders* (DSM) (King and Strain 1996). Therefore, a new pain-related category—*pain disorder* was introduced in the fourth edition, DSM-IV (American Psychiatric Association 1994) (Table 26–1). This is the first DSM category to provide for diagnosis in patients with acute pain and in patients in whom both psychological factors and general medical conditions are involved in the development or maintenance of the pain.

As yet, the extent of the use of this new diagnostic category has been the subject of limited research. King (1996) reported that 51% of patients with pain who were evaluated by a psychiatric consultation or liaison service fulfilled the diagnostic criteria for pain disorder, whereas less than 2% met the criteria for *somatoform pain disorder*, its predecessor in DSM-III-R (American Psychiatric Association 1987).

Other diagnostic classification systems for pain have been proposed, but none has yet been widely employed. The most extensive of these was developed by the Task Force on Taxonomy of the International Association for the Study of Pain (Merskey and Bogduk 1994). This five-axis classification system for categorizing pain is displayed in Table 26–2. The schema provides for comments on psychological factors on both the second axis, where psychiatric illness can be coded under the nervous system, and on the fifth axis, where possible etiologies include "psychophysiological" and "psychological." However, the diagnosis of the psychiatric illness is based on other classification systems for mental disorders, such as DSM.

Although it is not contained in any formal diagnostic classification systems for pain, the term *chronic pain syndrome* is frequently applied to extended pain. There are different views concerning what should be subsumed under this syndrome, but most clinicians employ Black's (1975) criteria: "intractable, often multiple pain complaints, which are usually inappropriate to existing somatogenic problems; multiple physician contacts and many nonproductive diagnostic procedures; excessive preoccupation with the pain problem; [and] an altered behavior pattern with some of the features of depression,

anxiety, and neuroticism." (p. 1000)

Because of the extremely subjective nature of many of the criteria, the validity of this diagnosis is questionable. Furthermore, some of the factors described, such as the overuse of diagnostic procedures, may be related as much to limitations in training and knowledge about pain among medical professionals as to patient behavior. Because of

---

TABLE 26–1. **DSM-IV criteria for pain disorder**

A. Pain in one or more anatomical sites is the predominant focus of the clinical presentation and is of sufficient severity to warrant clinical attention.

B. The pain causes clinically significant distress or impairment in social, occupational, or other important areas of functioning.

C. Psychological factors are judged to have an important role in the onset, severity, exacerbation, or maintenance of the pain.

D. The symptom or deficit is not intentionally produced or feigned (as in factitious disorder or malingering).

E. The pain is not better accounted for by a mood, anxiety, or psychotic disorder and does not meet criteria for dyspareunia.

Code as follows:

307.80 Pain disorder associated with psychological factors: Psychological factors are judged to have the major role in the onset, severity, exacerbation, or maintenance of the pain. (If a general medical condition is present, it does not have a major role in the onset, severity, exacerbation, or maintenance of the pain.) This type of pain disorder is not diagnosed if criteria are also met for somatization disorder.

Specify if:

Acute: duration of less than 6 months

Chronic: duration of 6 months or longer

307.89 Pain disorder associated with both psychological factors and a general medical condition: Both psychological factors and a general medical condition are judged to have important roles in the onset, severity, exacerbation, or maintenance of the pain. The associated general medical condition or anatomical site of the pain (see below) is coded on Axis III.

Specify if:

Acute: duration of less than 6 months

Chronic: duration of 6 months or longer

Note: The following is not considered to be a mental disorder and is included here to facilitate differential diagnosis and should be coded on Axis III.

Pain disorder associated with a general medical condition: A general medical condition has a major role in the onset, severity, exacerbation, or maintenance of the pain. (If psychological factors are present, they are not judged to have a major role in the onset, severity, exacerbation, or maintenance of the pain.)

TABLE 26–2. International Association for the Study of Pain classification of chronic pain

Axis I:	**Regions** (head, face, and mouth; abdominal region; lower back, etc.)
Axis II:	**Systems** (musculoskeletal system and connective tissue; nervous system; gastrointestinal system, etc.)
Axis III:	**Temporal characteristics of pain: pattern of occurrence** (single episode, limited duration; continuous or nearly continuous, non-fluctuating; recurring irregularly, etc.)
Axis IV:	**Patient's statement of intensity: time since onset of pain** (mild, medium, or severe with appropriate duration)
Axis V:	**Etiology** (inflammatory; neoplasm; degenerative; dysfunctional, including psychophysiological; psychological origin, etc.)

Source. Adapted from Merskey and Bogduk 1994.

these limitations and the pejorative connotations that have surrounded its use, the diagnostic category *chronic pain syndrome* is best avoided.

GATE CONTROL THEORY OF PAIN

Over the years, a variety of theories have been promulgated to explain pain. Although there is no universal acceptance of any one concept, the *gate control theory* developed by Melzack and Wall (1965) has received much attention. These authors believe that the transmission of nerve impulses from the periphery to the spinal cord is modified by a gate-like mechanism in the dorsal horn. The position of the gate and the amount of information subsequently conveyed to the brain are determined by several factors. Large A-beta fibers as well as small A-delta and C fibers carry impulses from the periphery to the substantia gelatinosa and spinal cord transmission (T) cells. Activation of the large fibers inhibits transmission to the T cells, thus closing the gate, whereas activation of the small fibers increases transmissions, thus opening the gate. The impact of the large and small fibers on the T cells is mediated by the substantia gelatinosa.

In addition to the impulses from the periphery, the gating mechanism is also influenced by descending messages from the brain and by a "central control" mechanism that is activated by the large-diameter fibers and involves certain cognitive processes. Thus, according to this theory,

pain is determined not only by peripheral stimulation, but also by information traveling from the brain to the spinal cord. This reaffirms the role of the mind-body interaction.

Although more recent research indicates that the gating system is more complicated than first conceived and that there may be more than one such mechanism involved, the basic concept remains intact (Melzack 1996; Wall 1996).

PAIN DISORDERS AND OTHER MENTAL DISORDERS

Although there is unquestionably a relationship between pain and other mental disorders, the exact nature of this relationship is unclear. Most research on this issue has focused on the frequency of psychiatric disorders among patients whose primary complaint is pain, but the few studies that addressed pain among psychiatric patients reported it to be a common problem. Delaplaine et al. (1978) found that 38% of 227 patients admitted to a psychiatric hospital complained of pain. Chaturvedi (1987a) identified pain in 18% of patients attending a psychiatric clinic. In both studies, pain was noted to be much more frequent among the patients whose diagnosis was neurosis than among those with schizophrenia or other psychoses.

Chronic pain appears to be most frequently associated with various forms of depressive disorders, including major depression, dysthymic disorder, and adjustment disorder with depressed mood. In the current literature, the range of prevalence of depression in patients with chronic pain is 10%–100% (King and Strain 1996; Romano and Turner 1985). Although the variability of these results may reflect difficulties in applying these diagnoses in patients with pain, it may also be due to differences in the patient populations studied. These disorders have been identified both in patients in whom there is clear evidence of an organic etiology for the pain and in patients in whom there is not, although it appears that the depressive disorders may be more common among the latter group (Magni 1987).

Although much research on pain has focused on the importance of psychological factors in the development and perpetuation of chronic pain, there is substantial evidence to support the role of these factors in acute pain and the role of psychologically based treatment modalities in its management. The decision to include a diagnostic category for acute pain in DSM-IV reflects this. Research demonstrates that pain ranging from traumatic to postoperative is strongly influenced by the mental state of the patient (Acute Pain Management Guideline Panel 1992; Chapman and Turner 1986).

It is often conceived that patients develop depression as a response to pain, but other opinions regarding this have been voiced. Blumer and Heilbronn (1982) suggested that the associated mental disorder may precede the pain and possibly predispose one to it, and they described the pain-prone individual whose pain is a form of masked depression. Research indicates that depressive disorders and alcohol dependence may be more common in the first-degree relatives of people with chronic pain, which suggests a possible environmental or genetic predisposition for developing pain (Chaturvedi 1987b; Hudson et al. 1985; Katon et al. 1985; Magni 1987; Violon and Giurgea 1984). Other studies suggest that depression is secondary to the pain (Atkinson et al. 1991; Brown 1990) or that these two problems may coexist either independently or as the result of a common psychological or neurochemical pathway (Feinmann 1985; Gamsa 1990; Magni 1987; von Knorring and Ekselius 1994). The relationship between pain and depression may be affected by variables such as age (Turk et al. 1995). As Magni et al. (1994) noted, all of the theories appear to have some validity, and currently the best conclusion seems to be that "depression promotes pain and pain promotes depression" (Magni et al. 1994, p. 289).

Certain forms of acute pain also appear to be frequently associated with other mental disorders. Beitman et al. (1988, 1989) observed that more than 30% of patients with chest pain and normal coronary arteries by cardiac catheterization met the criteria for panic disorder.

ASSESSMENT OF PAIN

Although physicians and health care professionals often seek to obtain evidence of the presence and severity of pain, in fact pain is a subjective experience for which there are no objective measures. The literature indicates that there is little correlation between the level of pain and physical findings. For example, Gore et al. (1987) reported that there was no relationship between radiological findings and the severity of neck pain experienced. In a study in which magnetic resonance imaging (MRI) of the lumbar spine was performed on asymptomatic subjects, Jensen et al. (1994) found that 64% had at least one abnormal lumbar disk and 38% had two or more.

To determine how much pain an individual patient should have requires the evaluation of multiple psychosocial factors that appear to influence the pain experience, including past pain, cultural factors, and family history of pain and mental disorders. Studies also suggest that the failure to identify underlying physical conditions etiologically related to the pain may result from these conditions' not having reached the threshold of clinical detection or may reflect deficiencies in the training of physicians in the diagnosis of pain-related conditions (Gunn and Sola 1989; Hendler et al. 1982; Rosomoff et al. 1989). Furthermore, many of the therapies used for pain—for example, medications, surgery, and extended periods of inactivity—can themselves cause or exacerbate pain, further obscuring the original etiology of the pain. Because mental health professionals usually do not evaluate patients with pain until long after its onset, if they evaluate such patients at all, these professionals are further handicapped in their attempts to assess the factors involved in the development of the pain.

Because pain is a complex, subjective experience, many different methods for assessing and measuring it have been promulgated (Acute Pain Management Guideline Panel 1992; Chapman et al. 1985; Jacox et al. 1994; Williams 1988). Although no single method has been found to be universally valid or reliable, those described in the following paragraphs are among the most commonly employed.

The simplest pain measurement is the Numerical Rating Scale (Scott and Huskisson 1976), in which the patient is asked to assign a numerical score to the pain. A typical scale ranges from 0 to 10, where "0" represents no pain and "10" represents the worst pain imaginable. A similar scale, the Visual Analog Scale (Scott and Huskisson 1976) requires the patient to mark a place on a 10-cm line, the ends of which are similarly labeled.

The McGill Pain Questionnaire permits a more in-depth analysis of the pain the patient is experiencing (Melzack 1975). The test lists 20 sets of words describing pain. These words are assigned to sensory, affective, and evaluative scales. The test can be scored based on the total number of words chosen or by the rank order of the words. Research indicates that patterns of response vary according to the type of pain experienced (Reading et al. 1982). The McGill Pain Questionnaire has been criticized for its reliance on language skills; results may reflect the patient's intelligence level, education, or cultural background.

A commonly employed alternative is the West Haven–Yale Multidimensional Pain Inventory, a 52-question instrument that measures the patient's perception of how others respond to his or her pain; participation in daily activities; and the effect of pain on the patient's overall lifestyle (Kerns et al. 1985).

Other, more traditional psychological testing instruments have also been used with pain patients, most notably the Minnesota Multiphasic Personality Inventory (MMPI) (Hathaway and McKinley 1989). However, the validity of this and similar psychological instruments is controversial when these tests are applied to patients with physical ailments such as pain. For example, it was reported more than 40 years ago that patients whose back pain did not have an organic etiology were more likely to demonstrate a certain configuration on the MMPI, the so-called Conversion V or neurotic triad, in which elevations on the hypochondriasis and hysteria scales were believed to reflect the patient's concerns about his or her health (Hanvik 1951). A lower depression score suggested that the patient was indifferent to these concerns. Although some support for this view still remains, other research indicates that this configuration may actually reflect adjustment to chronic illness and can be found among patients with chronic health problems, whether or not there is an identifiable organic etiology (Naliboff et al. 1982; Watson 1982). Similarly, instruments to detect depression, such as the Beck Depression Inventory, may be overinclusive, because many items such as problems with sleep, appetite, and health are as likely to be related to the pain as to depression (Novy et al. 1995). The MMPI and other psychological instruments have at times also been used to determine whether patients who develop chronic pain are characterologically prone to this problem, but studies have failed to reveal any marked evidence for this (Main et al. 1991).

To assist physicians in determining whether a patient's pain is of organic or psychological origin, Waddell et al. (1980) described five signs that they believed indicated that low back pain was of nonorganic origin:

- Tenderness that is superficial or nonanatomic in distribution
- Pain brought on by movements that should not cause pain but are simulations of those that do
- The disappearance of positive physical findings when the patient is distracted
- Regional disturbances involving weakness or sensory deficits that are nonanatomic in origin
- Overreaction by the patient during the examination

However, the authors noted that these signs are subject to a range of interpretation on the part of the clinicians and may be invalid for certain connective tissue disorders.

Because pain can be influenced by such a wide variety of factors, the concept *illness behavior* has been found by some to be useful (Mechanic 1962; Pilowsky 1968). Criteria included in illness behavior are

- Pain perception
- Decision making regarding whether to seek treatment and from whom to seek such treatment
- The meaning of the pain to the patient

- The manner in which the patient communicates about pain
- The effect pain has on the patient's functioning

Among the factors that affect illness behavior are cultural background, socioeconomic status, psychological functioning, experiences, memory, and learning.

Although the concept of illness behavior has been more frequently applied to chronic pain, extensive evidence indicates that some of these factors also play a major role in acute pain. In a pioneering study, Beecher (1946) observed that soldiers severely wounded in battle often did not complain of pain or described pain of a level far below that which would be expected. He postulated that this may have reflected the relief felt by the soldiers, who realized that they would be removed from the battlefield and their lives would no longer be endangered. Conversely, stressful life events may contribute to the development of chronic pain (Atkinson et al. 1988).

A person's knowledge of and expectations regarding a potentially painful insult to the body has also been demonstrated to alter patient response. Egbert et al. (1964) found that preoperative psychological preparation of the patient can have a profound influence on postsurgical recovery, including the degree of pain experienced.

Other work has indicated that there are significant differences between cultures and ethnic groups in the level of pain reported and the response to pain. What is considered to be acceptable illness behavior varies from culture to culture. Zborowski (1969) compared pain experiences among "Old Americans" (individuals of Anglo-Saxon ancestry), Italian Americans, and Jewish Americans and reported that the Old Americans were more stoic and had a greater tendency to withdraw from social contact when in pain than did the other two groups. Sternbach and Tursky (1965) similarly compared several ethnic groups and found that there were differences in pain tolerance. Greenwald (1991), Moore (1990), and Pilowsky and Spence (1977) also reported ethnic differences in responses to pain and pain-coping perceptions.

THE PROBLEM OF PAIN IN SPECIAL POPULATIONS

Because pain is a subjective problem, physicians must rely on patient self-report. However, in groups in which verbal skills may be diminished, most notably very young and elderly populations, this does not suffice. Unfortunately, failure to recognize this has resulted in the undertreatment of pain for both these groups. Furthermore, because these patients are often unable to complain of pain, myths have developed that they feel less pain than do nongeriatric adults (Acute Pain Management Guideline Panel 1992). Physicians who are caring for these patients must be especially vigilant for signs that the patients are in pain and they must use their experience to identify conditions and procedures that are likely to cause pain and treat it appropriately (Cummings et al. 1996; Sengstaken and King 1993). Assessment of pain may at times require the use of different tools—for example, the substitution of nonverbal scales of pain measurement, such as one employing faces ranging from happy to sad, developed for small children in place of the Numerical Rating and Visual Analog Scales. The recommendations for pain management in these two groups are similar to those for nongeriatric adults, although extra caution must be taken when providing medications to children and geriatric patients.

The care of the terminally ill is an issue that has received increasing attention as a result of the recent ongoing debate over physician-assisted suicide. Although there is a tendency for psychiatrists to focus on depression experienced by many terminally ill patients, it is important to remember that a large number of these patients also experience severe pain, which is often poorly managed (Jacox et al. 1994). The presence of depression and pain appear to increase the likelihood that a patient will request physician-assisted suicide, and both problems need to be addressed (Foley 1997). Unfortunately, although psychiatrists accept the importance of their role in evaluating and treating depression among the terminally ill, they may consider pain management to be better handled by other physicians, who they believe undergo more extensive training in this field. However, it is important to note that physicians in general, including those in primary care, also tend to receive limited training in pain during their postgraduate education (Sengstaken and King 1994).

EFFECT OF LITIGATION

Because many patients with chronic pain have developed the problem as the result of an injury, and because we live in an increasingly litigious society, psychiatrists who evaluate and treat such patients must be aware of the potential effects that involvement in the judicial system may have on the patient and his or her pain. When there is financial gain from having pain, the possibility of malingering is often paramount; however, concerns about this possibility are overstated. Patients may exaggerate symptoms and the ex-

tent of disability to attain secondary gains, but such exaggerations usually occur after the presence of the illness that initiated the pain is established. Actual falsification of pain and injury appears to be infrequent. The Report of the Commission on the Evaluation of Pain (1987) found that malingering was a rare problem in the Social Security Administration's disability system. Leavitt and Sweet (1986) similarly found malingering to be rare in individuals complaining of low back pain.

Studies have both supported and rejected the detrimental effects of litigation and involvement in worker's compensation systems on chronic pain. In their review, Osterweis et al. (1987) reported that the only consistent finding among these patients was that those who were employed at the outset of treatment appeared to do better. Unfortunately, involvement in the legal system may promote inactivity, which in turn can exacerbate pain and make it even more difficult for patients to return to their preinjury lifestyles. For example, in some situations, patients may find it more financially lucrative not to return to work. Even when patients desire to increase their activity levels, they may be fearful that this will demonstrate that they are not in pain and they will therefore lose benefits that are needed and are due. Patients in this situation often feel torn with regard to which of the possibly conflicting recommendations of physicians, friends, relatives, and lawyers to accept. Physicians who treat patients with chronic pain must be cognizant of this potential conflict and must make their patients aware that it is the individual's well-being that is of utmost importance.

MANAGEMENT OF PAIN

Although acute and chronic pain are often managed with similar therapeutic modalities, there are important differences in how these two types are approached and in the goals that the treating clinician should try to accomplish.

No method of differentiating acute pain from chronic pain has yet received universal acceptance. In its classification system, the Task Force on Taxonomy of the International Association for the Study of Pain recommends a criterion of 3 months' duration (Merskey and Bogduk 1994). Others suggest that the term *chronic pain* not be defined by any specific time limit but rather be used when the pain lasts beyond the expected period for its resolution (Brena et al. 1984). However, in the literature, the criterion most frequently employed is pain of 6 months' or longer duration, and this is the criterion included in DSM-IV.

APPROACHES TO MANAGEMENT

Acute Pain

The goal of treatment for acute pain is primarily to relieve the pain. Although the methods for effectively treating most cases of this form of pain appear to available, it is often undertreated. Marks and Sachar (1973) found that of 37 medical inpatients being treated for pain with narcotic analgesics, 32% were continuing to experience severe distress and another 41% experienced moderate distress, despite the medication regimen. The authors observed that misconceptions among physicians about the pharmacokinetics of these medications and concern about the potential for addiction were major factors in the physicians' failing to address adequately their patients' pain. Other more recent studies indicate that problems with undertreatment continue (Abbott et al. 1992; Choiniere et al. 1990; Melzack et al. 1987; Owen et al. 1990). In contrast to physicians' concern about starting the patient on the road to addiction by treating acute pain with opioid analgesics, the potential for developing opioid dependence after receiving one of these medications iatrogenically for acute pain is uncommon. Porter and Jick (1980) reported that among almost 12,000 patients, only four who had no previous history of dependence developed this problem.

Although the management of postoperative and other forms of acute pain will usually be provided by surgeons, anesthesiologists, and other physicians directly involved in the care of the patient, psychiatrists should be aware that there is much they can contribute to the care of patients with pain. The Acute Pain Management Guideline Panel (1992) highlighted the importance of employing cognitive and behaviorally based interventions such as relaxation, imagery, biofeedback, and education and instruction in the management of postoperative and other acute pain. However, many nonpsychiatric physicians involved in caring for patients with these forms of pain may lack the training and experience psychiatrists have that are needed to provide these therapeutic modalities.

Guidelines for the psychiatric approach to acute pain are presented in Table 26–3.

Chronic Pain

In treating chronic pain, it is important to address functioning as well as the pain. The goal of treatment should be to manage the pain as opposed to curing it. In many cases, this requires refocusing the patient away from the pain. In essence, patients with chronic pain must wrest control of their lives back from the pain. Much of the benefit from the use of the psychologically based treatment modalities may

relate more to their effect on the patient as a whole than to directly reducing the pain itself. In a meta-analysis of 109 studies of psychological treatments for pain, Malone and Strube (1988) found that these therapies had a greater effect on mood and the number of subjective symptoms than on the frequency, intensity, and duration of pain.

Although only a small percentage of patients with acute pain develop chronic pain, it is still unclear who these individuals are and whether there is any way to predict long-term disability. The literature supports the importance of psychosocial factors rather than organic variables in determining whether a person will recover from his or her pain (Dworkin et al. 1985; Osterweis et al. 1987).

In approaching the patient with chronic pain, the psychiatrist faces a number of obstacles. Unfortunately, many patients with this problem tend to view referrals to psychiatrists and other mental health practitioners negatively. They fear that such referrals may indicate that their treating physicians do not believe that the pain is "real." Furthermore, many patients with this problem believe that the physicians, in making such referrals, are giving up and that acceptance of the referrals forces patients to acquiesce in this condition. As Blumer and Heilbronn (1987) noted, "The chronic pain sufferer argues that he or she has no mental problem and needs no psychiatric intervention, that the only real problem is the pain and that the doctors

TABLE 26–3. **Guidelines for the psychiatric approach to acute pain**

1. In acute pain, the primary goal is to alleviate the pain as much as possible.

2. Although the appropriate use of analgesic medications is the mainstay of the effective management of acute pain, psychologically based interventions are also efficacious and should be employed.

3. The pain and the effectiveness of the therapeutic modalities being used to treat it should be frequently assessed.

4. Problems for which psychiatric consultations are often obtained on patients with acute pain, such as anxiety, depression, and problems coping with the illness, may reflect poor pain management.

5. When acute pain is accompanied by other mental disorders, relief of the pain may improve the mental state of the pain.

6. Be aware of the special issues that may be encountered in the management of acute pain. For example, patients with cancer pain may develop suicidal ideation.

7. Opioid analgesics may be safely used for the management of acute pain with minimal risk of abuse or dependence.

better find out what is wrong where it hurts" (p. 216). To help these patients, psychiatrists must recognize and address these concerns.

Many colleagues of psychiatrists may also mistakenly assume that psychiatrists have a role to play only when there is no organic pathology and may ask them to help determine whether the pain is real. Psychiatrists who are called on to settle this question might consider the following reply: "Pain occurring in unicorns, griffins and jabberwockies is always imaginary pain, since these are imaginary animals; patients, on the other hand are real, and so they always have real pain" (Sapira 1976, p. 116).

By the time they are referred to psychiatrists, patients with chronic pain often feel frustrated and abused by the health care system. Furthermore, if the pain is the result of an accident involving litigation, the patient has the additional problem of coping with the judicial system. In many cases, the specific form of therapy chosen may be less important than the therapist's willingness to display empathy and understanding and to set realistic goals for treatment. Unfortunately, modern Western medicine has, to a great degree, emphasized therapies that are performed on patients—rather than recognized that for many problems it is what patients do for themselves, not what is done to them, that is the most effective. This is especially true for chronic pain.

One of the obstacles that must frequently be overcome in cases of chronic pain is the common fears that the pain indicates the presence of a severe underlying condition that must be detected and that an increase in activity will exacerbate rather than improve the pain. Patients who manage to avoid or conquer these concerns tend to do better than those who retain them (Jensen et al. 1991).

Guidelines for the psychiatric approach to chronic pain are presented in Table 26–4.

PSYCHOLOGICALLY BASED MODALITIES

Psychologically based treatment approaches are considered to be a vital part of pain management programs (Fordyce et al. 1985). A wide variety of psychotherapies have been reported to be beneficial for pain, including many forms of individual, group, and family therapy. The most commonly used approaches fall into two major categories: 1) operant conditioning and 2) cognitive-behavior therapies, including biofeedback, relaxation training, and hypnosis. Each of these is more fully described elsewhere in this book; the following is a brief overview of their specific application to pain.

Operant conditioning is based on the concept that certain operant or learned behaviors develop in response to

TABLE 26–4. Guidelines for the psychiatric approach to chronic pain

1. The focus of the management of chronic pain should be on improving function rather than on alleviating pain.

2. Unless there is clear evidence that the patient is malingering, accept that the reported pain is present.

3. When evaluating patients with chronic pain, explain that psychiatrists' involvement in their care in no way suggests that they do not have "real" pain or that the pain is "all in their head."

4. To determine an appropriate treatment plan, attempt to discern the roles that psychological factors and a general medical condition are playing in the onset and maintenance of the pain. Be aware that even when a general medical condition is playing a major role in the pain, psychologically based therapeutic approaches are often efficacious.

5. Because psychosocial factors often determine the responses of patients with chronic pain to many therapeutic modalities, psychiatrists should endeavor to assist their nonpsychiatric physician colleagues in evaluating these patients before treatment plans are created.

6. Recognize that pain is often comorbid with other mental disorders. The pain may be a symptom of these mental disorders, lead to them, or coexist with them.

7. Be aware that the effective management of chronic pain often depends on the willingness and ability of patients with this problem to learn and practice strategies that will assist them in coping with their pain.

8. Be supportive. Patients with chronic pain often feel angry and frustrated about many issues, including interactions with the health care and legal systems.

9. Avoid therapeutic modalities such as the extended use of benzodiazepines or opioid analgesics that may worsen the patient's problems.

environmental cues. Common examples among pain patients include complaints of pain and reluctance to indulge in certain activities. The anticipated response to pain is often receipt of medication and being excused from work or normal daily tasks. The goal of operant conditioning is to reinforce the positive or "healthy" behaviors and to diminish the destructive behaviors that maintain the patient's pain.

Cognitive-behavior therapy involves identifying and correcting the patient's distorted attitudes, beliefs, and expectations. The goal of this therapy is, first, to make the patient more aware of factors that exacerbate and diminish the pain and, second, to cause the patient therefore to modify behavior accordingly. A variety of therapeutic modalities may be used to achieve this. In biofeedback, electronic equipment is employed to measure certain physiological functions of which the patient is usually unaware and to convey this information to the patient. One example of such physiological parameters is muscle tension. The patient may be instructed in specific relaxation techniques or be encouraged to achieve certain goals involving the biofeedback equipment, such as lowering the pitch of a tone.

A wide variety of relaxation techniques can be taught to patients. Among the most common methods is progressive muscle relaxation, in which the patient learns to relax different muscle groups by contracting and then relaxing each one (Jacobson 1970).

Although the exact nature of hypnosis and the associated trance remains the subject of debate, a British Medical Association (1955) report offered the following apt description:

> A temporary condition of altered attention in the subject which may be induced by another person and in which a variety of phenomena may appear spontaneously or in response to verbal or other stimuli. These phenomena included alterations in consciousness and memory, increased susceptibility to suggestion, and the production in the subject of responses and ideas unfamiliar to him in his usual state of mind. Further, phenomena such as anesthesia, paralysis and rigidity of muscles, and vasomotor changes can be produced and removed in the hypnotic state. (p. 191)

Although hypnosis involves relaxation, its efficacy in the treatment of pain extends beyond this. Patients can be taught to reduce pain through hypnotic suggestions such as forming a visual image of the pain and changing it or dissociating the painful part from the rest of the body. The benefits of hypnosis for acute pain are well documented, but, unfortunately, support for its efficacy in chronic pain is based primarily on anecdotal evidence (Hilgard and Hilgard 1983).

The application of each of these techniques to the management of pain has been studied to varying degrees, and controversy still remains concerning which approach is most efficacious. However, research suggests certain general guidelines regarding how each is best used. Through reviews of the literature, Turner and Chapman (1982a, 1982b) and Linton (1986) found that operant therapy is especially useful in decreasing patients' medication use and increasing their activity levels. In contrast, cognitive-behavior therapy was observed to be helpful in reducing pain complaints. Biofeedback was found to be of benefit in certain pain conditions, especially tension and migraine headaches, but was discovered overall to be inferior or at

best equal to relaxation therapy, which appears to be efficacious in the treatment of a wide variety of both acute and chronic pain conditions.

Each of these therapies may be employed when pain is the primary problem. However, when pain is the symptom of a mental disorder, that disorder should be addressed: appropriate treatment with psychotherapy and/or psychotropic medications must be initiated.

One additional method of treatment, the efficacy and actions of which are controversial, is the use of placebo. Research indicates that placebos can have a definite analgesic effect on a variety of painful conditions, including those in which there is an identifiable organic etiology (Turner et al. 1994).

PHARMACOLOGICAL MANAGEMENT OF PAIN

Opioid Analgesics

Although opioid analgesics play a primary role in the management of acute pain and the pain associated with cancer, the prescribing of opioid analgesics for patients with chronic noncancer pain continues to be the subject of controversy. Studies have shown that these medications can be safely prescribed and are effective for this form of pain (Portenoy 1994; Zenz et al. 1992). Furthermore, there is evidence that many painful conditions are undertreated and mismanaged because of physicians' concerns about the use of these drugs. However, physicians must also be aware that these medications are subject to abuse and can have potentially life-shattering side effects, the most notable being the development of dependence. Other potential problems must also be considered. Because patients can obtain medications from multiple sources, it may be difficult to determine whether they are being honest about their drug use. Furthermore, the issue of deciding what constitutes abuse and dependence for drugs that are prescribed is complex. The best recommendation is to consider the prescription of opioid analgesics for chronic noncancer pain on a case-by-case basis, with close monitoring of patients and continuous scrutiny for signs of abuse. Clearly the use of these medications for this problem should be limited to patients for whom objective benefits of treatment, such as an increase in activity levels or a return to or continuation of employment, can be observed. Physicians should be hesitant to prescribe these medications when the only sign of improvement is a reduction in pain without any other concurrent changes that would support the validity of this self-report. Those who fear that providing opioids to patients with chronic pain may result in legal sanctions should note that this result is unlikely to occur if the care provided conforms to published guidelines on pain management.

When opioid analgesics are being considered, the following guidelines should be employed (Table 26–5).

Guideline 1. In the case of mild to moderate postoperative and other acute pain, a nonsteroidal anti-inflammatory drug (NSAID) or acetaminophen should be used. More severe acute pain should be treated with an opioid analgesic. Treatment for cancer-related and chronic noncancer pain should begin with nonopioid analgesics, such as the NSAIDs and tricyclic antidepressants, and other forms of pain management. The World Health Organization Expert Committee (1990) recommends a stepwise approach starting with nonopioid analgesics, with the addition of opioid analgesics if pain is not controlled. Even if the nonopioid analgesics are insufficient for pain relief, they should be continued after the introduction of an opioid if they are providing some benefit. They may enable analgesia to be attained at a lower dosage of the opioid than would be required if it were used alone, and administration of a lower dosage will result in a reduction in frequency and severity of opioid-related side effects.

Guideline 2. Acute pain may require initial treatment with a stronger opioid analgesic such as morphine or hydromorphone. When treatment with opioid analgesics

TABLE 26–5. Guidelines for the use of opioid analgesics

1. Opioid analgesics may be used as the initial treatment for more severe acute pain conditions. In the case of cancer-related and chronic noncancer pain, initiate treatment with nonopioid analgesics (e.g., nonsteroidal anti-inflammatory drugs and tricyclic antidepressants) and other forms of pain management before employing opioid analgesics. Even if the addition of opioids is required, these other therapeutic modalities should be continued if they are providing analgesia.

2. In the case of acute pain, a stronger opioid may be initially required. Treatment for cancer-related and chronic noncancer pain should begin with the milder opioid analgesics such as codeine, oxycodone, and hydrocodone rather than the more potent ones.

3. Prescribe on a fixed schedule rather than on an "as needed" (prn) basis.

4. Unless a patient is unable to take medications in oral form, administer medications orally rather than parenterally.

5. Be aware of the available routes of administration and the potential side effects associated with these medications.

is initiated for cancer-related and chronic noncancer pain, the milder medications, such as codeine, oxycodone, and hydrocodone, should be tried first. If these are insufficient, the stronger narcotics, including morphine, methadone, and hydromorphone, should be considered. All the opioids just discussed are μ opioid receptor agonists. The other basic class of opioid analgesics consists of the mixed agonist-antagonists and partial agonist, which either bind at the κ opioid receptors and block the μ receptors or partially bind at the μ receptors. Although it has been reported that this second group of medications may have less potential for abuse than the μ receptor agonists, they do not appear to offer any marked benefit and they have the potential for creating additional problems. At least one study has suggested that treatment with mixed agonist-antagonists may be more efficacious in women, but further research is required to confirm this finding (Gear et al. 1996). Patients who take a mixed agonist-antagonist after receiving pure agonists may go into withdrawal. Furthermore, pentazocine, a commonly used mixed agonist-antagonist, can cause psychotomimetic effects including hallucinations. The use of the mixed agonist-antagonist is therefore not generally recommended. However, the mixed agonist-antagonist butorphanol is available in a nasal spray and is therefore suitable for patients who require an opioid but are temporarily unable to take one by mouth because of nausea and vomiting.

μ Opioid analgesics also have individual properties that affect their efficacy. Propoxyphene is a mild opioid that appears to possess a lesser analgesic effect than do similar opioids such as codeine. At one time, it appeared that propoxyphene offered a lower abuse potential than did these other medications. However, this has not been borne out in practice, and the use of this medication is not recommended. In the case of a patient who is prescribed a selective serotonin reuptake inhibitor antidepressant for depression and who is also receiving codeine, it is important to remember that codeine is metabolized to morphine by the hepatic cytochrome P450 2D6 enzyme system and that inhibition of this system results in a reduction in the analgesic effect of codeine.

When methadone is used, it must be given qid to be effective, because its duration of analgesia is shorter than its half-life. Also because of its long half-life, methadone may take 2–3 days before it provides effective analgesia. Therefore, another opioid analgesic should be provided for breakthrough pain during this period. The clinician should also be aware that because in the United States methadone is strongly associated with drug addiction, it is imperative that when the drug is prescribed for pain, the patient be made aware that it is being employed for its analgesic effects.

Meperidine is a strong opioid analgesic that is used in a variety of pain settings. Although the drug is an effective treatment for acute pain, the Acute Pain Management Guideline Panel (1992) stated that it is overused even for this indication and that other opioid analgesics are more effective. The extended use of meperidine (i.e., for more than 2–3 days) is contraindicated because repeated dosing may result in the accumulation of the toxic metabolite normeperidine, a cerebral irritant that can cause problems ranging from marked anxiety to convulsions. The oral bioavailability of meperidine is also poor, necessitating the switch to an alternative analgesic when parenteral administration is no longer required. Psychiatrists should know that, apparently alone among the opioid analgesics, meperidine can have a lethal interaction with monoamine oxidase inhibitors (MAOIs) (Browne and Lintner 1987) and increase the risk of postoperative delirium (Marcantonio et al. 1994).

Tramadol (Ultram) is a unique medication that combines a weak μ opioid receptor agonist ($\frac{1}{6000}$ the potency of morphine) with a weak inhibitor of norepinephrine and serotonin (5-HT) reuptake ("Tramadol" 1995). It has been reported to be beneficial for both acute and chronic pain, although in the United States it is currently available only in oral form, which somewhat limits its usefulness in certain cases of acute pain. Because of its weak μ opioid receptor affinity, it has been suggested that tolerance for, dependence on, and abuse of tramadol are less likely than for other opioids. The recommended oral dose is 50–100 mg every 4–6 hours up to 200 mg/day.

Recommended starting and equianalgesic doses of the opioid analgesics are listed in Table 26–6. The table is a general guide; the exact dosages administered should be determined on a case-by-case basis according to the status of the individual patient.

Guideline 3. The medications should be given on a fixed schedule rather than as needed (prn). When a fixed schedule is employed, better analgesia is often provided. Also, the patient is freed from the multitude of decisions that prn dosing engenders. The patient does not have to decide whether the pain is sufficient to warrant taking the medication, whether to take it as the pain is beginning or to wait until it becomes unbearable, or whether to delay taking it so that it will remain available. Unfortunately, these decisions tend to focus the patient's mind on the pain rather than away from it—the opposite of what is desired in the management of most cases of pain.

Patient-controlled analgesic (PCA) devices commonly combine a baseline fixed-schedule infusion of opioids with prn dosing. These devices have received widespread acceptance for the management of postoperative pain. However, there is currently no substantial evidence that this method provides better analgesia than fixed-schedule dosing alone, which is usually far less expensive.

Guideline 4. Physicians who prescribe opioid analgesics should be aware of the various ways they can be administered and of the potential side effects associated with them. Routes of administration for these medications include orally; intramuscularly; intravenously, either by bolus, continuous infusion, or pumps such as PCA devices; rectally; by epidural or intrathecal infusion; transdermally; and by nasal spray.

Fentanyl administered by a transdermal patch may provide a useful alternative to other forms of parenteral administration in patients who are unable to ingest oral medications. Because the patches need be changed only at 48- or 72-hour intervals and are easily applied, this method of opioid use may be especially beneficial for outpatients. However, in general, because oral administration is the simplest and usually the least expensive, this form is preferred unless the patient is unable to tolerate it or this method of administration has ceased to be effective. A major advantage of parenteral administration is more rapid onset of peak analgesia. For most of the opioids, the peak is reached at $\frac{1}{2}$ to 1 hour when the medication is given parenterally, compared with $1\frac{1}{2}$ to 2 hours when provided orally. However, this becomes a less important factor when the medication is provided on a fixed schedule. Furthermore, parenteral administration often results in a 1- to 2-hour reduction in the duration of analgesia when compared with oral administration (4–6 hours vs. 4–7 hours).

The side effects most commonly associated with the opioid analgesics are constipation, nausea and vomiting, and sedation. Treatment with stool softeners (e.g., docusate) and a large-bowel stimulant laxative (e.g., senna) should be initiated prophylactically to prevent constipation. Nausea and vomiting can be treated with hydroxyzine or a phenothiazine antiemetic. In patients with cancer who require high doses of opioids to control their pain, excessive sedation may be managed with a psychostimulant medication. Respiratory depression may develop with the administration of opioids and is the most frequent cause of mortality associated with this class of drugs. It may occur acutely as the result of an overdose, but in clinical situations it more commonly results from the gradual accumulation of the opioid. Psychiatrists at times may be asked by their physician colleagues to help in assessing whether a patient is abusing an opioid analgesic and in withdrawing a patient from such a medication. Because most physicians receive scant training in the problems of drug abuse and depend-

TABLE 26–6.   Opioid analgesics: recommended starting and equianalgesic doses

Drug	Approximate equianalgesic oral dose	Approximate equianalgesic parenteral dose	Recommended starting dose	
			Oral	Parenteral
μ opioid agonist				
Morphine	30 mg q 3–4 hr (around-the-clock dosing) 60 mg q 3–4 hr (single dose or intermittent dosing)	10 mg q 3–4 hr	30 mg q 3–4 hr	10 mg q 3–4 hr
Sustained-release morphine (MS Contin, Oramorph, Kadian)	60 mg q 12 hr	Not available	30 mg q 12 hr	Not available
Methadone	20 mg q 6–8 hr	10 mg q 6–8 hr	20 mg q 6–8 hr	10 mg q 6–8 hr
Transdermal fentanyl (Duragesic)		25 μg q hr		25 μg q hr (via transdermal patch)
Hydromorphone (Dilaudid)	7.5 mg q 3–4 hr	1.5 mg q 3–4 hr	6 mg q 3–4 hr	1.5 mg q 3–4 hr
Meperidine (Demerol)	300 mg q 2–3 hr	100 mg q 3 hr	Not recommended	100 mg q 3 hr
Codeine	130 mg q 3–4 hr	75 mg q 3–4 hr	60 mg q 3–4 hr	60 mg q 2 hr (intramuscular/ subcutaneous)
Oxycodone (Percodan, Percocet, Tylox) and hydrocodone (Vicodin, Lortab)	30 mg q 3–4 hr	Not available	10 mg q 3–4 hr	Not available
Sustained-release oxycodone (OxyContin)	30 mg q 12 hr	Not available	10 mg q 12 hr	Not available
Propoxyphene (Darvon-N, Darvocet-N)	250 mg 3–4 hr	Not available	200 mg q 3–4 hr	Not available
Opioid agonist-antagonist and partial agonist				
Buprenorphine (Buprenex)	Not available	0.3–0.4 mg q 6–8 hr	Not available	0.4 mg q 6–8 hr
Butorphanol (Stadol)	Not available	2 mg q 3–4 hr	Not available	2 mg q 3–4 hr
Nalbuphine (Nubaine)	Not available	10 mg q 3–4 hr	Not available	10 mg q 3–4 hr
Pentazocine (Talwin)	150 mg q 3–4 hr	60 mg q 3–4 hr	50 mg q 3–4 hr	Not recommended

Source.   Adapted from Jacox et al. 1994.

ence and their management, it falls to psychiatrists to possess the appropriate knowledge. Perhaps of most importance is understanding what is meant by *dependence* and *addiction* and knowing that they differ from physiological tolerance. Unfortunately, failure to understand these terms may result in unnecessary suffering. Patients who are undertreated for their pain and express desire for more effective pain management may be mislabeled as being

drug dependent, a problem that has been termed "pseudo-addiction" (Weissman and Haddox 1989). For further discussion of drug abuse and dependence, see Chapter 11 in this book.

In the treatment of patients who are receiving opioid analgesics, the recognition of withdrawal syndromes is vital. The DSM-IV criteria for opioid withdrawal disorder are presented in Table 26–7.

Multiple protocols for detoxifying patients from opioid analgesics are available. The simplest method is a gradual tapering of the opioid being used. This is usually accomplished by placing the patient on a fixed schedule and then reducing the dose. Several factors should be considered in determining the appropriate schedule: the length of time the patient has been using the medication, the dose, the patient's desire for detoxification and willingness to cooperate with the process, and the degree of pain still being experienced. Generally, the dose of the opioids can be safely reduced by 10%–20% each day with minimal risk of withdrawal.

An alternative schedule, one that is especially useful when the patient is taking large doses of an opioid, is a substitution/detoxification schedule employing methadone. In this case, the equianalgesic dose of methadone is determined (see Table 26–6). The methadone is then provided on a qid schedule. To avoid the necessity of waking the patient during the night, a schedule of 8:00 A.M., 12:00 noon, 5:00 P.M., and 9:00 P.M. is often followed. The methadone dose is then reduced by 10%–20% each day. Patient compliance may be improved by providing the methadone in a "pain cocktail" so that the patient is unaware of the amount of medication being taken. This method is commonly pro-vided by inpatient pain management programs and, with the help of cooperative pharmacies, in outpatient settings. The methadone withdrawal protocol should not be employed for patients using mixed agonist-antagonist opioids.

Although detoxification can be performed quickly and safely, most patients with chronic pain require the institution of other forms of pain management to prevent relapse. Simply detoxifying such patients without addressing the reasons why they required an opioid analgesic in the first place may make physicians feel they have accomplished something but offers little long-term benefit for the patients.

Nonsteroidal Anti-Inflammatory Drugs

The nonsteroidal anti-inflammatory drugs (NSAIDs) and acetaminophen (Table 26–8) are effective analgesics for a wide range of pain conditions. The NSAIDs are especially effective for the pain associated with bone metastases, one of the most common cancer-related pains.

The NSAIDs appear to exert their analgesic actions primarily through the inhibition of cyclooxygenase and, in turn, the synthesis of prostaglandins, although recent research indicates that they may have also have a central nervous system effect. The mechanism by which acetaminophen provides analgesia is still unknown. As others have noted, the selection of an NSAID appears to be more an art than a science (Gottlieb 1985). Aspirin is one of the most widely used, but it appears to be tolerated less well than other NSAIDs (Brooks and Day 1991). Acetaminophen has not classically been considered an NSAID, but it is an effective analgesic, and there is evidence to suggest that it may have a greater anti-inflammatory effect than was previously thought (Bradley et al. 1991). Although the newer NSAIDS such as nabumetone, oxaprozin, and piroxicam carry the benefit of having a longer half-life, allowing for once-per-day dosing, they are also more expensive than the older NSAIDs. Several NSAIDS, including ibuprofen, ketoprofen, and naproxen, are now available in over-the-counter preparations; because of the lower expense, it is recommended that these medications be tried first. If one NSAID is not beneficial after a 1- to 2-week period at a sufficient dose, an alternative should be considered.

Although NSAIDs are very effective analgesics, a large number of patients are unable to tolerate the associated side effects, primarily gastrointestinal (GI) distress, which is related to the inhibition of prostaglandin synthesis. At this time, there does not appear to be any substantial difference between the various NSAIDs in their potential for

---

TABLE 26–7. **DSM-IV criteria for opioid withdrawal**

A. Either of the following:
   (1) Cessation of (or reduction in) opioid use that has been heavy and prolonged (several weeks or longer)
   (2) Administration of an opioid antagonist after a period of opioid use

B. Three (or more) of the following, developing within minutes to several days after criterion A:
   (1) Dysphoric mood
   (2) Nausea or vomiting
   (3) Muscle aches
   (4) Lacrimation or rhinorrhea
   (5) Pupillary dilation, piloerection, or sweating
   (6) Diarrhea
   (7) Yawning
   (8) Fever
   (9) Insomnia

C. The symptoms in criterion B cause clinically significant distress or impairment in social, occupational, or other important areas of functioning

D. The symptoms are not due to a general medical condition and are not better accounted for by another mental disorder.

TABLE 26–8. Nonsteroidal anti-inflammatory drugs and acetaminophen

Drug	Usual adult dose (po)
Acetaminophen	650–975 mg q 4 hr
Oral	
Aspirin	650–975 mg q 4 hr
Choline magnesium trisalicylate (Trilisate)	1,000–1,500 mg bid
Diflunisal (Dolobid)	500 mg q 12 hr
Diclofenac sodium (Voltaren)	50 mg tid
Etodolac (Lodine)	200–400 mg q 4–6 hr
Fenoprofen calcium (Nalfon)	200 mg q 4–6 hr
Fluriprofen (Ansaid)	50 mg q 4–6 hr
Ibuprofen (Motrin, Advil)	400 mg q 4–6 hr
Indomethacin (Indocin)	25–50 mg q 8 hr
Ketoprofen (Orudis)	25–75 mg q 6–8 hr
Magnesium salicylate	650 mg q 4 hr
Meclofenamate sodium (Meclomen)	50 mg q 4–6 hr
Mefenamic acid (Ponstel)	250 mg q 6 hr
Nabumetone (Relafen)	1,000 mg q 24 hr
Naproxen (Naprosyn)	250 mg q 6–8 hr
Naproxen sodium (Anaprox, Naprelan)	275 mg q 6–8 hr
Oxaprozin (Daypro)	1200 mg q 24 hr
Piroxicam (Feldene)	20 mg q 24 hr
Salsalate (Disalcid)	500 mg q 4 hr
Sodium salicylate	325–650 mg q 3–4 hr
Sulindac (Clinoril)	200 mg q 12 hr
Parenteral	
Ketorolac (Toradol)	30 or 60 mg im initial dose followed by 15 or 30 mg q 6 hr / Oral dose following im dosage: 10 mg q 6–8 hr

Source. Adapted from Jacox et al. 1994.

causing GI problems. Certainly patients with a previous history of peptic or duodenal ulcers should be carefully monitored for signs of GI bleeding. The prescription of a histamine H_2-receptor antagonist, such as cimetidine, famotidine, or ranitidine, or a prostaglandin analog (misoprostol) should also be considered for these patients. If the NSAID is being used primarily for analgesia, a switch to acetaminophen should be considered for patients who complain of GI distress. Because NSAIDs inhibit prostaglandin synthesis, these drugs must be prescribed carefully to patients with impaired renal function. NSAIDS can cause renal toxicity due to papillary necrosis and a decrease in renal perfusion related to the reduction of prostaglandins. Although certain NSAIDs such as sulindac have been reported to be less likely to affect renal function, no clear evidence of this exists. Because the NSAIDs may interfere with renal function, the physician who is prescribing one of the drugs for a patient who is taking lithium must be aware that there may be a resultant increase in plasma lithium concentration. Although acetaminophen usually carries a much smaller risk of side effects than do the NSAIDs, long-term administration of this medication can result in impairment in hepatic function.

Ketorolac, the first NSAID to be available in parenteral form in the United States, can be prescribed to patients unable to tolerate oral medications. It also provides an effective alternative to opioid analgesics for the management of many cases of postoperative pain. However, because of its possible GI side effects and its cost, ketorolac should be used for no more than 5 days parenterally and 14 days orally, and the oral form should be used only in patients being converted from the parenteral form.

Antidepressants

During the past 30 years, there has been an increase in evidence supporting the analgesic properties of antidepressant medications, most notably the tricyclics, for both cancer pain and chronic nonmalignant pain. Although this effect was initially thought to be related to the antidepressant properties of these medications, substantial research indicates that they have separate analgesic effects unrelated to the emotional state of the patient.

The antidepressants appear to be efficacious for a wide range of painful conditions, including neuropathic pain, tension and migraine headaches (for which the drugs are used prophylactically), fibromyalgia, osteoarthritis and rheumatoid arthritis, and irritable bowel syndrome (Clouse 1994; King 1995; Magni 1991; McQuay et al. 1996; Saper 1997). The tricyclic antidepressants (TCAs) are now considered first-line drugs for the treatment of pain related to neuropathies, including postherpetic neuralgia and diabetic neuropathy. It should be noted that although many physicians still consider opioids the most potent analgesics available, painful conditions directly involving the nerves often respond poorly to these drugs. Even when the antidepressants themselves are not sufficient to control pain, as in many cases of cancer pain, they may enable reduction in the dose of opioids required, with a concomitant decrease in opioid side effects.

How antidepressants exert their analgesic effect is unclear. The primary focus has been on their effects on serotonin and norepinephrine reuptake; and it appears that the medications that act on both neurotransmitters, such as the TCAs, are more effective than those that act only on serotonin (Max 1994). Other mechanisms of action that have been suggested include enhanced endorphin secretion and the effect of antidepressants on calcium and sodium channels.

Which tricyclic has the most analgesic effects is a matter of controversy. Amitriptyline appears to be the TCA most widely used for pain. However, it is unclear whether this fact reflects a pharmacological advantage or is simply a result of its being the one most studied in the literature. Among the other tricyclics reported to have analgesic effects are nortriptyline, imipramine, desipramine, clomipramine, and doxepin. A major advantage of amitriptyline is its sedative effect. Amitriptyline may be especially beneficial for patients with chronic pain, given that problems with sleep often accompany chronic pain and these problems may be treated with benzodiazepines, which may exacerbate the pain.

Of the selective serotonin reuptake inhibitors, both fluoxetine and paroxetine have been studied as treatments for diabetic neuropathy but have been found to be less efficacious than the TCAs with which they were compared (Max et al. 1992; Sindrup et al. 1990). These medications, along with sertraline and fluvoxamine, have also been studied with regard to their efficacy in treatment for a variety of headache conditions, and the results have been mixed. Findings of several recent case studies and animal research indicate that venlafaxine provides analgesia. Currently, there are no reports in the literature on the analgesic effects of nefazodone or mirtazepine.

Although the TCAs appear to exert their analgesic effects at lower dosage levels than are required for their antidepressant actions, analgesia appears to be dose related. A commonly repeated myth is that the ceiling dose for analgesia is 75 mg/day of amitriptyline or the equivalent. In fact, the literature indicates that the optimal analgesic dose is usually in the 100- to 200-mg range. The best way to initiate treatment for analgesia with a TCA is to start at a dose smaller than the usual initial dose for depression and then to increase the dose gradually until side effects, most commonly daytime sedation, develop. For example, for analgesia the initial dose of amitriptyline is 25 mg 1–2 hours before bedtime or 10 mg in a debilitated patient. The dose can be increased by 10–25 mg every second to third day until side effects develop. Because the duration of analgesia appears to be similar to that of the antidepressant effect, once-a-day dosing is often sufficient. However, some patients may obtain a better analgesic effect with divided doses. Although patients often show improvement after treatment for several days, as in the case of depression, the analgesic effects of the tricyclics may take several weeks to develop.

As in the treatment of depression, the recommended length of maintenance therapy with antidepressants for chronic pain varies from patient to patient. These medications carry a lower risk of side effects than other medications that are commonly used for chronic pain, most notably the NSAIDs. Therefore, if a patient is doing well, these should be the last medications that are discontinued. Physicians should reassess the continuing need for an antidepressant every few months and should consider tapering and discontinuing the medication after the patient's condition has stabilized.

Benzodiazepines

As with the narcotics, the use of benzodiazepines for patients with chronic noncancer pain is controversial. Benzodiazepines appear to provide little benefit in most cases of cancer pain. There is evidence to support the efficacy of clonazepam and alprazolam for neuropathic pain, but there is little to indicate that these two are more effective than the TCAs for these conditions. Apart from these two medications, it is generally recommended that benzodiazepines be avoided when chronic pain is a problem. It has been noted that because of their gamma- aminobutyric acid (GABA)ergic effects, benzodiazepines may actually exacerbate pain rather than reduce it (Dellemijn and Fields 1994). Despite this, King and Strain (1990) found that these medications are often employed in the management of chronic pain. They also observed that the most frequently given reason that patients were taking these medications was that they improve sleep. Because of the additional analgesic effects provided by the TCAs, it is recommended that they be used to treat the insomnia that may accompany pain. When pain is accompanied by anxiety, the use of a benzodiazepine alternative such as buspirone should be considered.

Selected Other Medications Used as Analgesics

Because so many different medications have been employed for pain, it is impossible to provide a comprehensive list here. The following selected medications are included because of their special interest to psychiatrists.

In addition to the antidepressants, other psychotropic medications also appear to have analgesic effects. Several of the neuroleptics, including haloperidol and chlorpromazine, have been reported to provide analgesia, most notably for neuropathic pain. However, methotrimeprazine, a phenothiazine, is the only neuroleptic that has been found in controlled studies to have analgesic effects (Monks 1990).

Anticonvulsants, including phenytoin, carbamazepine, and sodium valproate, have also been found to be beneficial in pain that is due to peripheral nerve syndromes, including postherpetic neuralgia and diabetic neuropathy. However, because the TCAs are also efficacious for treating these syndromes and are less likely to result in major side effects, it is recommended that they be tried first. With regard to other specific pain syndromes, carbamazepine appears to be effective in treating trigeminal neuralgia, and sodium valproate is beneficial in prophylactic treatment of migraine headaches (McQuay et al. 1995). Currently, there is limited information on the use of the newer anticonvulsants as analgesics; of these, on the basis of case reports in the literature, gabapentin appears to be the most promising.

Lithium has been shown to be beneficial in cases of acute and cluster headaches. Therapeutic dosage is usually similar to that required when this medication is used to treat bipolar disorder.

Sumatriptan, a 5-HT_{1D}-receptor agonist, and zolmitriptan, a $5\text{-HT}_{1B,1D}$ agonist, are useful for abortive treatment of migraine headaches.

OTHER TREATMENT MODALITIES

It is beyond the scope of this chapter to present a comprehensive review of the many therapies available for the treatment of acute and chronic pain. Readers who are interested in a more detailed discussion are referred to textbooks on pain (Bonica 1990; Wall and Melzack 1994).

Among the other therapies found to be beneficial are various surgical interventions, nerve blocks, trigger point injections, acupuncture, physical therapy, and transcutaneous electrical nerve stimulation (TENS). The provision of each of these therapies requires clinicians with specific training and experience. As with the psychologically based modalities, support in the literature for the efficacy of each of these therapies is variable. The best recommendation is that, in the absence of a medical emergency, conservative therapies be tried before more invasive ones such as nerve blocks and surgery. Therapeutic interventions such as physical therapy, acupuncture, and TENS carry little risk of side effects or of worsening the patient's pain. It has often been noted that there is a dearth of well-performed research supporting the efficacy of these treatments. However, this statement can be applied to most of the therapies used for chronic pain, including surgery.

When any of the organic therapies are employed, they should be used in addition to, not in place of, the interventions that address the psychosocial aspects of the pain.

As the interest in pain has grown during the past quarter century, various forms of pain services, clinics, and treatment centers have been created. These vary from true multidisciplinary establishments to those offering single forms of treatment provided by one or more clinicians. Unfortunately, the type of therapy provided often is based less on what the patient needs than on what the clinician offers. Even when a truly multidisciplinary treatment team is present, the team may fail to recognize the differences between patients, and the clinicians may attempt a "one size fits all" treatment approach (Turk 1990). Patients appear to be much better served when a variety of treatment modalities are available.

Because of the importance of improving the functioning of patients with chronic pain, the best multidisciplinary pain programs offer services that focus on this goal. Central to such programs are physical therapy, occupational therapy, and behaviorally oriented therapies. Although patients may prefer programs in which treatment is done *on* them, lasting improvement appears to depend on health care professionals' teaching patients how to cope with and manage their pain and patients' willingness to do this.

CONCLUSIONS

Both acute and chronic pain are major health problems. Although the methods for effectively treating most cases of pain are currently available, misconceptions about pain and ignorance of the principles of its management have resulted in needless suffering. Psychiatrists have much to contribute to the care of patients with pain, and it is hoped that they will take a leading role in this important field.

REFERENCES

Abbott FV, Gray-Donald K, Sewitch MJ, et al: The prevalence of pain in hospitalized patients and resolution over six months. Pain 50:15–28, 1992

Acute Pain Management Guideline Panel: Acute Pain Management: Operative or Medical Procedures and Trauma. Clinical Practice Guideline, AHCPR Publ No 92–0032. Rockville, MD, Agency for Health Care Policy and Research, Public Health Service, U.S. Department of Health and Human Services, February 1992

American Psychiatric Association: Diagnostic and Statistical Manual of Mental Disorders, 3rd Edition, Revised. Washington, DC, American Psychiatric Association, 1987

American Psychiatric Association: Diagnostic and Statistical Manual of Mental Disorders, 4th Edition. Washington, DC, American Psychiatric Association, 1994

Atkinson JH, Slater MA, Grant I, et al: Depressed mood in chronic low back pain: relationship with stressful life events. Pain 35:47–55, 1988

Atkinson JH, Slater MA, Patterson TL, et al: Prevalence, onset and risk of psychiatric disorders in men with chronic low back pain: a controlled study. Pain 45:111–122, 1991

Beecher HK: Pain in men wounded in battle. Ann Surg 123:98–105, 1946

Beitman BD, Mukerji V, Flaker G, et al: Panic disorder, cardiology patients, and atypical chest pain. Psychiatr Clin North Am 11:387–397, 1988

Beitman BD, Mukerji V, Lamberti JW, et al: Panic disorder in patients with chest pain and angiographically normal coronary arteries. Am J Cardiology 63:1399–1403, 1989

Black RG: The chronic pain syndrome. Surg Clin North Am 55:999–1011, 1975

Blumer D, Heilbronn M: Chronic pain as a variant of depressive disease: the pain-prone disorder. J Nerv Ment Dis 170:381–394, 1982

Blumer D, Heilbronn M: Depression and chronic pain, in Presentations of Depression. Edited by Cameron OG. New York, Wiley, 1987, pp 215–235

Bonica JJ: The Management of Pain. Philadelphia, Lea & Febiger, 1990

Bradley JD, Brandt KD, Katz BP, et al: Comparison of an anti-inflammatory dose of ibuprofen and acetaminophen in the treatment of patients with osteoarthritis of the knee. N Engl J Med 325:87–91, 1991

Brena SF, Crue BL, Stieg RL: Comments on the classification of chronic pain: its clinical significance. Bulletin of the Clinical Neurosciences 49:67–81, 1984

British Medical Association: Report: medical use of hypnotism. BMJ I (suppl):190–193, 1955

Brooks PM, Day RO: Nonsteroidal anti-inflammatory drugs—differences and similarities. N Engl J Med 324:1716–1725, 1991

Brown GK: A causal analysis of chronic pain and depression. J Abnorm Psychol 99:127–137, 1990

Browne B, Lintner S: Monoamine oxidase inhibitors and narcotic analgesics: a critical review of the implications for treatment. Br J Psychiatry 151:210–212, 1987

Chapman CR, Turner JA: Psychological control of acute pain in medical settings. J Pain Symptom Manage 1:9–20, 1986

Chapman CR, Casey KL, Dubner R, et al: Pain measurement: an overview. Pain 22:1–31, 1985

Chaturvedi SK: Prevalence of chronic pain in psychiatric patients. Pain 19:231–237, 1987a

Chaturvedi SK: A comparison of depressed and anxious chronic pain patients. Gen Hosp Psychiatry 9:383–386, 1987b

Choiniere M, Melzack R, Giarard N, et al: Comparisons between patients' and nurses' assessment of pain and medication efficacy in severe burn injuries. Pain 40:143–152, 1990

Clouse RE: Antidepressants for functional gastrointestinal syndromes. Dig Dis Sci 39:2352–2363, 1994

Cummings EA, Reid GJ, Finley GA, et al: Prevalence and source of pain in pediatric inpatients. Pain 68:25–31, 1996

Delaplaine R, Ifabumuyi OI, Merskey H, et al: Significance of pain in psychiatric hospital patients. Pain 4:361–366, 1978

Dellemijn PLI, Fields HL: Do benzodiazepines have a role in chronic pain management? Pain 57:137–152, 1994

Dworkin RH, Handlin DS, Richlin DM, et al: Unraveling the effects of compensation, litigation, and employment on treatment response in chronic pain. Pain 23:49–59, 1985

Egbert LD, Battit GE, Welch CD, et al: Reduction of postoperative pain by encouragement and instruction of patients. N Engl J Med 270:825–827, 1964

Feinmann C: Pain relief by antidepressants: possible modes of action. Pain 23:1–8, 1985

Foley KM: Competent care for the dying instead of physician-assisted suicide. N Engl J Med 336:54–57, 1997

Fordyce WE, Roberts AH, Sternbach RA: The behavioral management of chronic pain: a response to critics. Pain 22:113–125, 1985

Gamsa A: Is emotional disturbance a precipitator or a consequence of chronic pain? Pain 42:183–195, 1990

Gear RW, Miaskowski C, Gordon NC, et al: Kappa-opioids produce significantly greater analgesia in women than in men. Nat Med 2:1248–1250, 1996

Gore DR, Sepic SB, Gardner GM, et al: Neck pain: a long-term follow-up of 205 patients. Spine 12:1–5, 1987

Gottlieb NL: The art and science of non-steroidal anti-inflammatory drug selection. Semin Arthritis Rheum 15 (suppl 2):1–3, 1985

Greenwald HP: Interethnic differences in pain perception. Pain 44:157–163, 1991

Gunn CC, Sola AE: Chronic intractable benign pain (CIBP) (letter). Pain 39:364–365, 1989

Hanvik LJ: MMPI profiles in patients with low-back pain. J Consult Clin Psychol 5:350–353, 1951

Hathaway SR, McKinley JC: Minnesota Multiphasic Personality Inventory—2. Minneapolis, MN, University of Minnesota, 1989

Hendler N, Uematsu S, Long D: Thermographic validation of physical complaints in "psychogenic pain" patients. Psychosomatics 23:283–287, 1982

Hilgard ER, Hilgard JR: Hypnosis in the Relief of Pain, Revised Edition. Los Altos, CA, William Kaufman, 1983

Hudson JI, Hudson MS, Pliner LF, et al: Fibromyalgia and major affective disorder: a controlled phenomenology and family history study. Am J Psychiatry 142:441–446, 1985

Jacobson E: Modern treatment of tense patients. Springfield, IL, Charles C Thomas, 1970

Jacox A, Carr DB, Payne R, et al: Management of Cancer Pain. Clinical Practice Guideline, AHCPR Publ No 94–0592. Rockville, MD, Agency for Health Care Policy and Research, Public Health Service, U.S. Department of Health and Human Services, March 1994

Jensen MP, Turner JA, Romano JM, et al: Coping with chronic pain: a critical review. Pain 47:249–283, 1991

Jensen MC, Bran-Zawadzki MN, Obuchowski N, et al: Magnetic resonance imaging of the lumbar spine in people without back pain. N Engl J Med 331:69–73, 1994

Katon W, Egan K, Miller D: Chronic pain: lifetime psychiatric diagnoses and family history. Am J Psychiatry 142:1156–1160, 1985

Kerns RD, Turk DC, Rudy TE: The West Haven–Yale Multidimensional Pain Inventory (WHYMPI). Pain 23:345–356, 1985

King SA: Antidepressants: a valuable adjunct for musculoskeletal pain. Journal of Musculoskeletal Medicine 12:51–57, 1995

King SA: The clinical application of DSM-IV for patients with pain, in Proceedings of the 8th World Congress on Pain. Vancouver, BC, IASP Press, 1996

King SA, Strain JJ: Benzodiazepine use by chronic pain patients. Clin J Pain 6:143–147, 1990

King SA, Strain JJ: Somatoform pain disorder, in DSM-IV Sourcebook, Vol 2. Edited by Widiger TA, Frances AJ, Pincus HA, et al. Washington, DC, American Psychiatric Press, 1996, pp 915–931

Leavitt F, Sweet JJ: Characteristics and frequency of malingering among patients with low back pain. Pain 25:357–374, 1986

Linton SJ: Behavioral remediation of chronic pain: a status report. Pain 24:125–141, 1986

Magni G: On the relationship between chronic pain and depression when there is no organic lesion. Pain 31:1–21, 1987

Magni G: The use of antidepressants in the treatment of chronic pain: a review of the current evidence. Drugs 42:730–748, 1991

Magni G, Moreschi C, Rigatti-Luchini S, et al: Prospective study on the relationship between depressive symptoms and chronic musculoskeletal pain. Pain 56:289–297, 1994

Main CJ, Evans PJD, Whitehead RC: An investigation of personality structure and other psychological features in patients presenting with low-back pain: a critique of the MMPI, in Proceedings of the VIth World Congress on Pain. Edited by Bond MR, Charlton JE, Woolf CJ. Amsterdam, Elsevier, 1991, pp 207–218

Malone MD, Strube MJ: Meta-analysis of non-medical treatments for chronic pain. Pain 34:231–244, 1988

Marcantonio ER, Juarez G, Goldman L, et al: The relationship of postoperative delirium with psychoactive medications. JAMA 272:1518–1522, 1994

Marks RM, Sachar EJ: Undertreatment of medical inpatients with narcotic analgesics. Ann Intern Med 78:173–181, 1973

Max MB: Antidepressants as analgesics, in Progress in Pain Research and Management, Vol 1. Edited by Fields HL, Liebeskind JC. Seattle, WA, IASP Press, 1994, pp 229–246

Max MB, Lynch SA, Muir J, et al: Effects of desipramine, amitriptyline, and fluoxetine on pain in diabetic neuropathy. N Engl J Med 326:1250–1256, 1992

McQuay H, Carroll D, Jadad AR, et al: Anticonvulsant drugs for management of pain: a systematic review. BMJ 311:1047–1052, 1995

McQuay H, Tanner M, Nye BA, et al: A systematic review of antidepressants for neuropathic pain. Pain 63:217–227, 1996

Mechanic D: The concept of illness behavior. Journal of Chronic Disease 15:189–194, 1962

Melzack R: The McGill Pain Questionnaire: major properties and scoring methods. Pain 1:277–299, 1975

Melzack R: Gate control theory. Pain Forum 5:128–138, 1996

Melzack R, Wall PD: Pain mechanisms: a new theory. Science 150:971–979, 1965

Melzack R, Abbott FV, Zackon W, et al: Pain on a surgical ward: a survey of the duration and intensity of pain and the effectiveness of medication. Pain 29:67–72, 1987

Merskey H, Bogduk N (eds): International Association for the Study of Pain Classification of Chronic Pain, 2nd Edition. Seattle, WA, IASP Press, 1994

Monks R: Psychotropic drugs, in The Management of Pain. Edited by Bonica JJ. Philadelphia, Lea & Febiger, 1990, pp 1676–1689

Moore R: Ethnographic assessment of pain coping perceptions. Psychosom Med 52:171–181, 1990

Naliboff BD, Cohen MJ, Yellen AN: Does the MMPI differentiate chronic illness from chronic pain? Pain 13:333–341, 1982

Novy DM, Nelson DV, Berry LA: What does the Beck Depression Inventory measure in chronic pain? A reappraisal. Pain 61:261–270, 1995

Osterweis M, Kleinman A, Mechanic D (eds): Pain and Disability. Washington, DC, National Academy Press, 1987

Owen H, McMillan V, Rogowski D: Postoperative pain therapy: a survey of patients' expectations and their experiences. Pain 41:303–307, 1990

Pilowsky I: Abnormal illness behavior. Br J Med Psychol 42:347–351, 1968

Pilowky I, Spence ND: Ethnicity and illness behavior. Psychol Med 7:447–452, 1977

Portenoy RK: Opioid therapy for chronic nonmalignant pain: current status, in Progress in Pain Research and Management, Vol 1. Edited by Fields HL, Liebeskind JC. Seattle, WA, IASP Press, 1994, pp 247–264

Porter J, Jick H: Addiction rare in patients treated with narcotics (letter). N Engl J Med 302:123, 1980

Reading AE, Everitt BS, Sledmere CM: The McGill Pain Questionnaire: a replication of its construction. Br J Clin Psychol 21:339–349, 1982

Report of the Commission on the Evaluation of Pain. U.S. Department of Health and Human Services, Social Security Administration, Office of Disability, Publ No 64-031, 1987

Romano JM, Turner JA: Chronic pain and depression: does the literature support a relationship? Psychol Bull 97:18–34, 1985

Rosomoff HL, Fishbain DA, Goldberg M, et al: Physical findings in patients with chronic intractable benign pain of the neck and/or back. Pain 37:279–287, 1989

Saper JR: Diagnosis and symptomatic treatment of migraine. Headache 37 (suppl 1):S1–S14, 1997

Sapira J: Real pain (letter). N Engl J Med 295:116, 1976

Scott J, Huskisson EC: Graphic representation of pain. Pain 2:175–184, 1976

Sengstaken EA, King SA: The problems of pain and its detection among geriatric nursing home residents. J Am Geriatr Soc 41:541–544, 1993

Sengstaken EA, King SA: Primary care physicians and pain: education during residency. Clin J Pain 10:303–309, 1994

Sindrup SH, Gram LF, Brosen K, et al: The selective serotonin reuptake inhibitor paroxetine is effective in the treatment of diabetic neuropathy symptoms. Pain 42:135–144, 1990

Sternbach RA, Tursky B: Ethnic differences among housewives in psychophysical and skin potential response to electric shock. Psychophysiology 1:241–246, 1965

Tramadol—a new oral analgesic. Med Lett Drugs Ther 37:59–60, 1995

Turk DC: Customizing treatment for chronic pain patients: who, what, and why. Clin J Pain 6:255–270, 1990

Turk DC, Okifuji A, Scharff L: Chronic pain and depression: role of perceived impact and perceived control in different age cohorts. Pain 61:93–101, 1995

Turner JA, Chapman CR: Psychological interventions for chronic pain: a critical review, I: relaxation training and biofeedback. Pain 12:1–21, 1982a

Turner JA, Chapman CR: Psychological interventions for chronic pain: a critical review, II: operant conditioning, hypnosis, and cognitive-behavioral therapy. Pain 12:23–46, 1982b

Turner JA, Deyo RA, Loeser JD, et al: The importance of placebo effects in pain treatment and research. JAMA 271:1609–1614, 1994

Violon A, Giurgea D: Familial models for chronic pain. Pain 18:199–203, 1984

von Knorring L, Ekselius L: Idiopathic pain and depression. Qual Life Res 3 (suppl 1):S57–S68, 1994

Waddell G, McCulloch JA, Kummel E, et al: Nonorganic physical signs in low back pain. Spine 5:117–125, 1980

Wall PD: Comments after 30 years of the gate control theory. Pain Forum 5:12–22, 1996

Wall PD, Melzack R: Textbook of Pain, 3rd Edition. Edinburgh, Churchill Livingstone, 1994

Watson D: Neurotic tendencies among chronic pain patients: an MMPI item analysis. Pain 14:365–385, 1982

Weissman DE, Haddox JD: Opioid pseudoaddiction: an iatrogenic syndrome. Pain 36:363–366, 1989

Williams RC: Toward a set of reliable and valid measures for chronic pain assessment and outcome research. Pain 35:239–251, 1988

World Health Organization Expert Committee on Cancer Pain Relief and Active Supportive Care: Cancer Pain Relief and Palliative Care: Report of a WHO Expert Committee (WHO Technical Series 804). Geneva, World Health Organization, 1990

Zborowski M: People in Pain. San Francisco, Jossey-Bass, 1969

Zenz M, Strumpf M, Tryba M: Long-term oral opioid therapy in patients with chronic nonmalignant pain. J Pain Symptom Manage 7:69–77, 1992

PSYCHIATRIC TREATMENTS

CHAPTER 27

PSYCHOPHARMACOLOGY AND ELECTROCONVULSIVE THERAPY

LAUREN B. MARANGELL, M.D.
STUART C. YUDOFSKY, M.D.
JONATHAN M. SILVER, M.D.

The skillful practice of psychopharmacology requires a broad knowledge of psychiatry, pharmacology, and medicine. We begin this chapter with an overview of general principles relevant to the safe and effective use of psychotropic medications. Subsequent sections cover the major classes of psychotropic medications—antidepressants, antipsychotics, anxiolytics, and mood stabilizers—and the disorders for which they are prescribed. The reader should be aware that this nomenclature is somewhat artificial; for example, many antidepressant medications are also used to treat anxiety disorders.

GENERAL PRINCIPLES

INITIAL EVALUATION

Like all areas of medicine, the art of psychopharmacology rests on proper diagnosis and delineation of medication responses. Before prescribing a psychotropic medication or ECT, a thorough evaluation must be performed with the goals of 1) establishing the diagnosis, course of illness, and target symptoms; 2) deciding whether the diagnosis and target symptoms are likely to respond to medication (for example, dysphoria related to a family problem gener-

The authors would like to thank Holly Zboyan, Becky Stager, and Kimberly Cress, M.D., for their invaluable assistance in the preparation of this chapter.

The Drug Interactions section contains material developed over many years for other purposes in collaboration with Ann Callahan, M.D., and Terence Ketter, M.D.

This work was supported in part by a Young Investigator's Award to Dr. Marangell by the National Alliance for Research on Schizophrenia and Depression.

ally should not be treated with medication, unless another medication-responsive condition, such as major depression, is also present); 3) ruling out nonpsychiatric causes, such as endocrine or neurological disorders and substance abuse; 4) noting the presence of other medical problems that will influence drug selection, such as cardiac or hepatic disease; 5) evaluating other medications that the patient is taking that might cause a drug-drug interaction; and 6) evaluating personal and family history of medication responses.

TARGET SYMPTOMS

A key component of a well-considered decision to use a medication is the delineation of target symptoms. The physician should determine and list the specific symptoms that are designated for treatment and monitor the response of these symptoms to treatment. Standard semistructured psychiatric interviews, such as the Schedule for Affective Disorders and Schizophrenia (SADS; Endicott and Spitzer 1978) and the Structured Clinical Interview for DSM-III (SCID; Spitzer et al. 1990), and rating scales, such as the Hamilton Depression Rating Scale (HDRS; Hamilton 1960) and the Overt Aggression Scale (OAS; Silver and Yudofsky 1991; Yudofsky et al. 1986), provide specific methods and structures for assessing symptoms and target behaviors and are also useful for monitoring change with treatment. In the absence of formal rating scales, target symptoms can be rated on a 1–10 scale.

MULTIPLE MEDICATIONS

A frequent and dangerous clinical error is the treatment of specific symptoms of a disorder with multiple drugs, rather than treating, more specifically, the underlying disorder. For example, it is not uncommon for a psychiatrist to receive a referral for a patient who is taking one type of benzodiazepine for anxiety, a different type of benzodiazepine for insomnia, an analgesic for nonspecific somatic complaints, and a subtherapeutic dosage of an antidepressant (for example, 50 mg/day of imipramine) for feelings of sadness. Often, the somatic complaints, insomnia, and anxiety are components of an underlying depression, which may be aggravated by the polypharmaceutical approach inherent in symptomatic treatment.

On the other hand, there are many patients whose psychiatric conditions require the concomitant use of several psychotropic agents. The carefully considered, rational use of several psychiatric medications must be distinguished from ill-considered polypharmacy. An example of useful combined treatment is augmentation of an antidepressant agent with lithium for patients who have experienced only a partial therapeutic response to an antidepressant alone.

CHOICE OF DRUG

Selection of a drug for a given diagnosis or symptom is made on the basis of both patient-specific and drug-specific considerations. Patient-specific factors include comorbid medical and psychiatric disorders, other medications being taken, previous history of response to medication, family history of medication responses, and life circumstances that will likely be affected by the specific side effects of the chosen agent. For example, for an elderly man with depression and prostatic hypertrophy, an antidepressant drug with minimal anticholinergic properties should be chosen to avoid urinary retention. For a patient with both panic disorder and major depression, an antidepressant medication that also treats panic disorder should be chosen. For an architect with bipolar disorder, medications that cause a hand tremor might be problematic. For a woman taking oral birth control pills, carbamazepine may increase the hepatic metabolism of the contraceptive agent, thereby lowering the contraceptive efficacy. Patients often, but not always (Post et al. 1992), respond positively to medications that were helpful in the past. For example, a patient with severe depression that was previously responsive to phenelzine but is now unresponsive to a variety of newer antidepressants might respond again to phenelzine.

The clinician must also consider the physical, intellectual, and psychological capacities of the patient and of his or her caregivers when selecting a new medication. For example, in patients with dementia it may not be safe to use a monoamine oxidase inhibitor (MAOI), for which it is important to remember dietary restrictions and potential drug interactions. An elderly patient with mild memory impairment may have difficulty following instructions about increasing the dosage of an antidepressant medication. In general, the more complicated the instructions or the more medications that are prescribed, the more difficulty the patient will have in complying with the therapeutic regimen.

Drug-specific factors include available preparations and cost. In most cases, once-a-day dosing is preferred for patient convenience and compliance. The choice of a particular medication may also depend on whether that drug is available in injectable and liquid forms in addition to tablet, pill, or capsule forms.

GENERIC SUBSTITUTION

Generic substitution, when available, may provide a less expensive alternative to the original proprietary (brand-name) formulation; however, some caution is warranted because generic "equivalents" may not be truly equivalent in all circumstances. After patent expiration, information relevant to producing a medication is in the public domain. At that point, the medication may be produced by other pharmaceutical companies, without the brand name, provided the drug is formulated according to U.S. Food and Drug Administration (FDA) requirements. The current FDA requirements center around the concept of *bioequivalence;* products are bioequivalent if there is no significant difference in the rate at which or extent to which the active ingredient becomes available to the site of action, given the same dose and conditions (FDA 1992). However, in some cases even small differences in bioavailability, or other differences in preparations such as type of preservatives or excipients, may become clinically meaningful. For example, a patient may have allergic reactions to one generic preparation but not another of the same drug because of differences in the dye used to color the pill.

Initial generic product selection is of less clinical significance than is switching between formulations. For example, if a patient is in remission and without side effects while taking one formulation of generic amitriptyline, pharmacy substitution risks both loss of efficacy and toxicity if the new preparation has a slightly lower or higher bioavailability. This type of substitution generally occurs when the patient changes pharmacies or when the pharmacy buys a different, often less expensive, generic preparation. This risk of an adverse clinical outcome is highest when switching between two generic preparations (Hauck and Anderson 1992). In many circumstances, generic substitution is a safe and effective cost-saving tool, but the clinician should be aware of potential problems and, in the event of an unexpected reaction, should ask the patient if the medication has changed in appearance. The change in appearance, such as in size, shape, or color, should alert the clinician to a probable change in generic formulations.

PATIENT INFORMATION AND PATIENT-PHYSICIAN COMMUNICATION

A general principle is that the more the patient and his or her family understand about the illness and the reason that medications have been chosen to treat the illness, the more compliant the patient and the more supportive the family will be. Failure to devote adequate time to discussion and instruction before recommending a medication may result in poor therapeutic response, poor compliance by the patient, areas of mistrust and miscommunication, and the requirement at a later time of extensive professional time and effort. We believe that excellent communication among the physician, the patient, and the family before the selection of a medication will increase the likelihood that the most therapeutically effective agent with the safest side-effect profile will be chosen.

Therapeutic skill and creativity on the part of a clinician are essential for effective treatment with medications. For example, the clinician must expect a patient with major depression associated with significant anxiety and somatic complaints to be concerned about and fearful of drug side effects. The way in which the clinician discusses such side effects with the patient will ultimately affect the patient's confidence in the treatment plan and his or her compliance. To an anxious and suspicious patient with major depression who is being given imipramine, the clinician may say the following:

> I expect that in the early stages of treatment you will experience dryness of your tongue and mouth. This is usually not a dangerous side effect—in fact, when you experience dryness of your mouth, it's an indication that the medication is acting within your system and that the time in which the therapeutic benefit is expected is drawing closer. The dryness will likely improve with time. Keeping your mouth moist by swallowing small amounts of water or sucking on dietetic hard candy may help reduce the discomfort of your dry mouth. If you do *not* experience dryness of your mouth after 1 week on this medication, please notify my office, as I will be concerned about whether or not we are achieving adequate treatment doses of the medication.

In this manner, the clinician alerts the patient to anticipate a side effect by emphasizing its positive implications rather than sharing the patient's anxious and pessimistic perspective.

COMPLIANCE

Less than 50% of patients who require subacute or chronic treatment continue to take their medications as prescribed (Sackett 1979). As discussed earlier, we believe that communication and patient education are the most important interventions to improve patient compliance. In addition to oral communication, written instructions are often helpful, particularly if the patient is to remember more complicated information, such as dose titration or instructions for multiple medications. Whenever possible, medication regimens should be simplified. For example, once-a-day dosing should be used when possible, and any medication that requires more than twice-a-day dosing should usually be avoided if a suitable alternative exists. To assist patients who have difficulty remembering to take their medication, the physician should help to identify cues from the daily routine that can be used as reminders (Cramer 1995). Often it is easiest to incorporate medication times with morning or evening toiletry routines; patients may be instructed to leave their medication by their toothbrush or razor. Midday doses are the most difficult to incorporate reliably into most people's daily activities and should be avoided if possible, unless the patient is extremely well motivated.

Patients value medication not only in terms of absolute efficacy, but with regard to how the medication affects all areas of their lives (Morris and Shulz 1993). As such, it is essential that the patient be an active part of the treatment and that the medication decisions be tailored to conform to the patient's lifestyle and values. For example, a benzodiazepine may be an appropriate medication for a patient with acute anxiety, but if the patient believes it to be a dangerous and addictive medication, despite physician reassurance, noncompliance is more likely. When multiple medications cannot be avoided, a pillbox with sections for each day of the week can be purchased at most pharmacies. Use of a pillbox is also helpful for patients who do not remember whether or they have taken their medication each day. When applicable, blood levels of medications can be used to monitor compliance.

EVALUATION OF RESPONSE

The treatment plan should include a predetermined dose and duration that will provide an adequate trial of the medication. Far too frequently, medications are discontinued with the assumption of failure of response without the benefit of an adequate drug trial (e.g., inadequate dosage or duration of treatment). A patient's treatment plan should be revised if the patient has an unusual sensitivity to the medication, if dangerous or disabling side effects emerge, or if the patient does not respond to an adequate drug trial. In such cases, a diagnostic reevaluation of the patient may be indicated, with further tests to detect any underlying nonpsychiatric physical illness that did not appear during the initial assessment but that may be related to the persistence of the symptoms. Different treatment approaches range from a second trial with a related class of medication to the use of complementary or different treatment methods. For example, a patient whose delusional depression does not respond to combined treatment with antipsychotic agents and antidepressant agents and for whom careful evaluation does not reveal an underlying physical etiology may be a candidate for ECT.

Finally, for patients who do respond, an end point for treatment must be determined. Far too frequently, medication regimens are continued beyond the point at which therapeutic benefit is derived. A common example is the use of benzodiazepines for the treatment of anxiety in which patients may be maintained for years without the assessment of the therapeutic benefit of the drug by gradual discontinuation.

ANTIDEPRESSANT DRUGS

OVERVIEW

The modern era of the treatment of depression with medication began in the 1950s when iproniazid, an MAOI used for the treatment of tuberculosis, was noted to elevate mood (Selikoff et al. 1952). Its efficacy in the treatment of depressed patients was subsequently shown in studies by Crane (1957) and Kline (1958). Unfortunately, hepatic necrosis was a side effect of iproniazid, and this led to its withdrawal from clinical use. In addition, dangerous hypertensive reactions associated with the MAOIs initially were poorly understood, and most psychiatrists were reluctant to use these drugs. Imipramine, the first of the tricyclic antidepressants (TCAs), was developed as a derivative of chlorpromazine; it was hoped that imipramine would be more effective than chlorpromazine as an antipsychotic agent. Although imipramine did not exhibit antipsychotic efficacy, it was shown to be effective in the treatment of depression (Kuhn 1958). Subsequently, many other antidepressants have been approved for use in the United States. All are equally effective for treating major depression, but individual patients may respond preferentially to one agent or another. In addition, these medications are significantly different from one another with regard to side effects, lethality in overdose, pharmacokinetics, and the ability to treat comorbid psychiatric disorders.

MECHANISMS OF ACTION

To date, all antidepressant drugs affect the serotonergic and/or catecholaminergic systems in the central nervous system (CNS), either by presynaptic reuptake inhibition, blocking catabolism, or by receptor agonist or antagonist effects, all of which have the end result of enhancing monoaminergic transmission. (For a review of antidepressant mechanisms, see Goodman and Charney 1985; Frazer 1997.)

The early observation of these effects of antidepressants led to the catecholamine hypothesis of depression (Schildkraut 1965). This theory postulates that depression is caused by a relative deficiency of catecholamine neurotransmitters that is corrected by antidepressant drugs; the theory further hypothesizes that some depressions are "serotonergic" whereas others are "noradrenergic." We now know that these two neurotransmitter systems—serotonin ascends from the raphe nucleus and norepinephrine from the locus coeruleus—are interconnected in a feedforward system, such that the induction of one serves to induce the other (Meltzer and Lowy 1987). In addition, the effects on reuptake inhibition are immediate, but the clinical response is delayed for several weeks. More closely paralleling the time course of clinical response, presynaptic autoreceptors, α- and β-noradrenergic receptors, and the $5\text{-}HT_1$ serotonergic receptors downregulate. This downregulation can be conceptualized as a marker of antidepressant-induced neuronal adaptation.

Many of these receptors are linked to G proteins. A defective linkage between the receptor and the G protein may result in abnormal intracellular transduction mechanisms (Bourin and Baker 1996). In patients with major depression, there may be alteration of G-protein-induced activation of the phosphoinositide signal transduction system (Pacheco et al. 1996). Antidepressants most likely act via modulating G proteins, second messenger systems, and gene expression.

INDICATIONS

Although the antidepressants have many potential therapeutic uses, the primary approved indication for these drugs is the treatment of major depression, as defined by DSM-IV (American Psychiatric Association 1994). Overall, approximately 70% of patients with depression respond to an adequate trial of antidepressant medication. In addition, antidepressants are effective for patients with obsessive-compulsive disorder (selective serotonin reuptake inhibitors [SSRIs] and clomipramine), panic disorder (TCAs and SSRIs), bulimia (TCAs, SSRIs, and MAOIs), dysthymia (SSRIs), bipolar depression (after treatment with a mood stabilizer), social phobia (MAOIs and SSRIs), posttraumatic stress disorder (SSRIs), irritable bowel syndrome (TCAs), enuresis (TCAs), neuropathic pain (TCAs), migraine headache (TCAs and SSRIs), attention-deficit/hyperactivity disorder (desipramine, bupropion), smoking cessation (bupropion), autism (SSRIs), and late luteal phase dysphoric disorder (SSRIs); however, the FDA has not evaluated or approved the use of antidepressants to treat many of these conditions.

CLINICAL USE

Each of the commonly used classes of antidepressants is discussed in the following sections and summarized in Table 27–1. The antidepressant classes are based on similarity of receptor effects and side effects. All are effective for depression when administered in therapeutic doses. The choice of antidepressant medication is based on the patient's psychiatric symptoms, his or her history of previous treatment response, family members' history of previous response, medication side-effect profile, comorbid psychiatric or medical disorders, and risk of suicide by overdose (Tables 27–2 and 27–3). In general, the SSRIs and the other newer antidepressants are better tolerated and safer than either the TCAs or the MAOIs, although there are still many patients who benefit from these older drugs. In the following sections, clinically relevant information is presented for each of the antidepressant medication classes individually, followed by a discussion of the pharmacological treatment of depression. Principles germane to the use of antidepressants to treat anxiety disorders can be found at the end of the section on anxiety later in this chapter.

TRICYCLIC AND HETEROCYCLIC ANTIDEPRESSANTS

Receptor Effects

Most TCAs inhibit the reuptake of norepinephrine, serotonin, and, to a lesser extent, dopamine. These mechanisms are thought to be responsible for the therapeutic action of TCAs. In addition, TCAs block muscarinic cholinergic receptors, H_1 histamine receptors, and α_1-adrenergic receptors. These mechanisms are thought to account for the side effects of the TCAs.

Background

Tricyclic antidepressants were first developed in the 1950s, and they are often considered the classic antidepressant drugs. The name *tricyclic* is based on the chemical structure; all tricyclics have a three-ring nucleus. (The chemical structure of selected psychotropic medications is illustrated in the appendix to this chapter.) Currently, most clinicians are moving away from use of TCAs as first-line drugs; relative to the newer antidepressants, they tend to have more side effects, to require gradual titration to achieve an adequate antidepressant dose, and to be lethal in overdose. Some data suggest that TCAs may be more effective than SSRIs in the treatment of major depression with melancholic features (Danish University Antidepres-

TABLE 27-1. Commonly used antidepressant drugs

Generic (trade) name	Starting dosage (mg)[a]	Usual daily dosage (mg)	Available oral dosages (mg)	Mean drug [active metabolite] half-life (hours)
Tricyclics and tetracyclics				
Tertiary amine tricyclics				
Amitriptyline (Elavil, Endep)	25–50	100–300	10, 25, 50, 75, 100, 150	15.6 [26.6]
Clomipramine (Anafranil)	25	100–250	25, 50, 75	32 [69]
Doxepin (Sinequan)	25–50	100–300	10, 25, 50, 75, 100, 150	16.8
Imipramine (Tofranil, Tofranil PM)	25–50	100–300	10, 25, 50, 75, 100, 125, 150	7.6 [17.1]
Trimipramine (Surmontil)	25–50	100–300	25, 50, 100	24
Secondary amine tricyclics				
Desipramine (Norpramin)	25–50	100–300	25, 50, 75, 100, 150	17.1
Nortriptyline (Pamelor, Aventyl)	25	50–200	10, 25, 50, 75	26.6
Protriptyline (Vivactil)	10	15–60	5, 10	78.4
Tetracyclics				
Amoxapine (Asendin)	50	100–400	25, 50, 100, 150	8
Maprotiline (Ludiomil)	50	100–225	25, 50, 75	43
Selective serotonin reuptake inhibitors				
Citalopram (Celexa)	20	20–60[b]	20, 40	35
Fluoxetine (Prozac)	20	20–60[b]	10, 20, liq	72 [144]
Fluvoxamine (Luvox)	50	50–300[b]	50, 100	15
Paroxetine (Paxil)	20	20–60[b]	10, 20, 30, 40	20
Sertraline (Zoloft)	50	50–200[b]	50, 100	26 [66]
Dopamine-norepinephrine reuptake inhibitors				
Bupropion (Wellbutrin)	150	300	75, 100	14
Bupropion SR (Wellbutrin SR, Zyban)	150	300	100, 150	21
Serotonin-norepinephrine reuptake inhibitors				
Venlafaxine (Effexor)	37.5	75–225	25, 37.5, 50, 75, 100	5[11]
Venlafaxine (XR) (Effexor XR)	37.5	75–225	37.5, 75, 150	5[11]
Serotonin modulators				
Nefazodone (Serzone)	50	150–300	100, 150, 200, 250	4
Trazodone (Desyrel)	50	75–300	50, 100, 150, 300	7
Norepinephrine-serotonin modulator				
Mirtazapine (Remeron)	15	15–45	15, 30	20
Monoamine oxidase inhibitors				
Irreversible, nonselective				
Phenelzine (Nardil)	15	15–90	15	2
Tranylcypromine (Parnate)	10	30–60	10	2
Reversible MAOI-A				
Moclobemide (Aurorix, Manerix)	150	300–600	100, 150	2

[a]Lower starting dosages are recommended for elderly patients and for those with panic disorder, significant anxiety, or hepatic disease. [b]Dosage varies with diagnosis. See text for specific guidelines.

Source. Dosing information is from American Psychiatric Association Practice Guidelines for Depression 1993. Half-life information is compiled from Amsterdam 1980 and *Physicians' Desk Reference* 1997, with added information on maprotiline, trimipramine, and moclobemide from Wells and Gelenberg 1981, Abernethy et al. 1984, and Freeman 1993, respectively.

TABLE 27–2. Guidelines for choosing an antidepressant medication

Unipolar depression	All antidepressants are equally effective. Choose on the basis of previous response, side effects, comorbid medical and psychotic disorders.
Depression with melancholia features	TCA[a]
Depression with atypical features	SSRI, MAOI[b]
Depression with psychotic features	Antidepressant + antipsychotic, or ECT; avoid bupropion
Bipolar depression	Lithium[c]
Depression + OCD	SSRI, clomipramine
Depression + panic disorder	SSRI, TCA, MAOI[b]
Depression + cardiovascular disease	SSRI, bupropion SR
Depression + seizures	Avoid bupropion and TCAs
Depression + Parkinson's disease	Bupropion
Depression + migraine	TCA, SSRI
Depression + sexual dysfunction	Bupropion, nefazodone, mirtazapine

Note. ECT = electroconvulsive therapy; MAOI = monoamine oxidase inhibitor; OCD = obsessive-compulsive disorder; SR = sustained release; SSRI = selective serotonin reuptake inhibitor; TCA = tricyclic antidepressant.
[a]Although some data suggest that TCAs are superior in melancholic depression, many clinicians choose the newer agents, even in melancholia, on the basis of improved tolerability and safety.
[b]Although MAOIs are highly effective, they are not used as first-line agents because of their increased risk relative to the newer agents.
[c]Mood stabilizers are first-line treatment for all phases of bipolar disorder. To date, lithium appears to be most the effective (see text section on mood stabilizers).

sant Group 1990; Perry 1996); however, many skilled clinicians and researchers continue to prefer the newer antidepressants, even in melancholia, for the aforementioned reasons.

Imipramine, amitriptyline, clomipramine, trimipramine, and doxepin are tertiary amines. Desipramine, nortriptyline, and protriptyline are secondary amines. The tertiary amines have more potent serotonin reuptake inhibition, and the secondary amines have more potent noradrenergic reuptake inhibition. The tertiary amines tend to have more side effects than the secondary amines; in our opinion, the tertiary amines do not usually offer any additional therapeutic benefits. Desipramine and protriptyline tend to be activating. Among the TCAs, nortriptyline is the least likely to produce orthostatic hypotension. Amoxapine has an active metabolite that antagonizes D_2 receptors and can therefore cause treatment-emergent extrapyramidal side effects (EPS; Coupet et al. 1979; see section on antipsychotic drugs later in this chapter). Maprotiline is characterized as a heterocyclic agent. The receptor effects of maprotiline are most similar to those of protriptyline.

Clinical Use

Before initiation of treatment with TCAs, the physician must obtain a comprehensive cardiovascular history and review of symptoms. Because TCAs often cause orthostasis, other potential risk factors for hypotension should

be considered, and patients should be instructed to change from sitting or lying to the standing position slowly. For patients with preexisting heart disease and for all patients older than 40, an electrocardiogram (ECG) should be obtained before the initiation of TCA treatment. If the initial ECG reveals clinically significant abnormalities, another ECG must be taken after the patient's medication has reached a steady-state level. For patients with bundle branch block, TCAs should not be used unless all other options have failed.

The following dosage guidelines are for healthy adults with minimal anxiety. Patients with significant anxiety, panic, or a tendency to be sensitive to side effects should receive initial dosages that are 50% lower. Similarly, elderly patients and those with cardiovascular or hepatic disease should receive lower initial dosages.

Imipramine, amitriptyline, doxepin, desipramine, clomipramine, and trimipramine can be initiated at 25–50 mg/day. Divided dosing may be used initially to minimize side effects, but eventually the entire dosage can be given at bedtime. The dosage can be increased to 150 mg/day the second week, 225 mg/day the third week, and 300 mg/day the fourth week. The dosage of clomipramine should not exceed 250 mg/day because of an increased risk of seizures at higher dosages.

Nortriptyline should be initiated at 25 mg/day and increased to 75 mg/day over 1–2 weeks depending on tolerability and clinical response. Some patients require

TABLE 27–3. Summary of key features and side effects of antidepressant medications

Medication	Proposed mechanism	Dosing	Key features				Other key side effects
			Titration required	Sedation	Weight gain	Sexual dysfunction	
TCAs	5-HT + NE reuptake inhibition	Once daily	Yes	Most, yes	Yes	Yes	Anticholinergic[a], orthostasis, quinidine-like effects on cardiac condition, lethal in overdose
SSRIs	5-HT reuptake inhibition	Once daily	Minimal	Minimal	Rare	Yes	Initial: nausea, loose bowel movements, headache, insomnia
Bupropion SR	DA + NE reuptake inhibition	Multiple if dose > 150 mg	Some	Rare	Rare	Rare	Initial: nausea, headache, insomnia, anxiety/ agitation; seizure risk
Venlafaxine XR	5-HT + NE >DA reuptake inhibition	Once daily	Some	Minimal	Rare	Yes	Similar to SSRIs; dose-dependent hypertension
Nefazodone	5-HT$_2$ antagonist + weak 5HT reuptake inhibition	bid	Yes	Yes	Rare	Rare	Initial: nausea, dizziness, confusion, visual changes, sedation
Trazodone	5-HT$_2$ antagonist + weak 5-HT$_2$ reuptake inhibition	bid	Yes	Yes	Rare	Rare	Initial sedation, priapism, dizziness, orthostasis
Mirtazapine	a$_2$-adrenergic + 5-HT$_2$ antagonism	Once daily	Minimal	Yes	Yes	Rare	Anticholinergic[a]; may increase serum lipids; rare: orthostasis, hypertension, peripheral edema, agranulocytosis
MAOIs	Inhibit MAO	bid–tid	Yes	Rare	Yes	Yes	Orthostatic hypotension, insomnia, peripheral edema; avoid in patients with CHF, avoid phenelzine in patients with hepatic impairment; potentially life-threatening drug interactions; dietary restrictions

Note. 5-HT = serotonin; CHF = congestive heart failure. DA = dopamine; MAO = monoamine oxidase; MAOI = MAO inhibitor; NE = norepinephrine.
[a]Anticholinergic side effects include dry mouth, blurred vision, constipation, urinary retention, tachycardia, and possible confusion.

dosages up to 150 mg/day. Amoxapine should be started at 50 mg/day and titrated up to 400 mg/day; it has a short half-life and should be given in divided doses. Protriptyline can be started at 10 mg/day and increased up to 60 mg/day. Maprotiline should be started at 50 mg/day and maintained at that dosage for 2 weeks because of an increased risk of seizure if the dosage is raised too quickly. The dosage can be increased over 4 weeks to 225 mg/day.

Plasma Levels and Therapeutic Monitoring

Clinically meaningful plasma levels are available for imipramine, desipramine, and nortriptyline. For imipramine, the combined sum of the plasma levels of imipramine and the desmethyl metabolite (desipramine) should be greater than 200–250 ng/mL. Desipramine levels should be greater than 125 ng/mL. A therapeutic window has been observed for nortriptyline, with optimal response between 50 and 150 ng/mL. These therapeutic levels are based on steady-state concentrations, which are reached after 5–7 days for these medications. Blood should be drawn approximately 10–14 hours after the last dose of medication.

Most patients respond to usual dosages of antidepressants and do not require monitoring of plasma levels. For example, in two-thirds of physically healthy adult patients with depression, a dosage of 75 mg/day of nortriptyline results in an optimal therapeutic plasma level of this drug (Åsberg 1974). Therefore, this dosage is used as a general guideline for initiating treatment and, in most cases, will lead to a satisfactory treatment response. Nonetheless, there are times when a plasma level determination can be useful (Table 27–4).

TABLE 27–4. **Indications for use of antidepressant levels**

1. Patient has not responded to an adequate trial of nortriptyline, desipramine, or imipramine.
2. Patient is at high risk because of age or medical illness and requires treatment with the lowest possible effective dose.
3. Patient requires rapid increases in dosage because of extraordinary suicide risk.
4. Concern about patient compliance with medication regimen.
5. Documentation is needed of plasma level to which the patient responded for use in future treatment.
6. Potential of drug interactions that may lead to an increase or decrease in plasma levels.

Source. Adapted from American Psychiatric Association 1985.

Risks, Side Effects, and Their Management

Anticholinergic effects. Anticholinergic side effects result from antagonism of muscarinic receptors. The most common anticholinergic side effects are dry mouth, constipation, urinary retention, blurred vision, and tachycardia. In predisposed patients, such as elderly persons, anticholinergic medications may cause cognitive impairment and confusion. Because the tertiary amines and protriptyline have a particularly high affinity for the muscarinic receptors, these medications are more likely than others to cause anticholinergic side effects.

Cholinergic medications have been reported to relieve some of the anticholinergic side effects (Everett 1976; Yager 1986). Bethanechol chloride may alleviate dry mouth, constipation, urinary hesitancy and retention, and erectile and ejaculatory dysfunction. The addition of a medication to treat side effects should be considered only after dosage reduction and alternative antidepressants with fewer anticholinergic side effects have been attempted. One must proceed with great caution when using antidepressants with anticholinergic side effects in treating patients with prostatic hypertrophy, narrow-angle glaucoma, or cognitive impairment. The newer antidepressant drugs may be preferable for patients with these disorders.

Sedation. The relative sedating properties of the tricyclic antidepressant drugs appear to parallel their respective histamine receptor binding affinities. Trimipramine, amitriptyline, and doxepin are the most sedating tricyclic antidepressants. Desipramine and protriptyline are less sedating.

Cardiac effects. Many of the TCAs have cardiovascular effects, including orthostatic hypotension and cardiac conduction delays. For many patients, especially those with preexisting heart disease, tricyclic antidepressants have clinically relevant effects on blood pressure, heart rate, cardiac conduction, and cardiac rhythm (Glassman 1984; Goodman et al. 1986; Roose 1992).

Orthostatic hypotension is the cardiovascular side effect that most commonly results in serious morbidity, especially in elderly patients and in patients with congestive heart failure (Glassman and Bigger 1981; Glassman et al. 1983). Glassman et al. (1979) reported an injury rate of 4% for patients with an average age of 60 years who were treated with imipramine. These injuries included fractures and lacerations requiring sutures. Although orthostatic hypotension may occur with any TCA, nortriptyline is the TCA least likely to cause this side effect (Roose et al. 1981). Orthostatic hypotension from TCAs may not be dose dependent; therefore, lowering the dosage of the antidepressant may not lessen the dizziness or the changes in blood pressure.

Increases in heart rate that occur with TCAs rarely result in morbidity or mortality (Glassman and Bigger 1981); however, patients often find tachycardia frightening or distracting. Antidepressants with greater anticholinergic properties are associated with a higher incidence of this side effect, which may be quite troublesome to patients with panic disorder.

Because TCAs at toxic levels (as occur in overdose) can cause life-threatening arrhythmias, many clinicians believe that these drugs can cause dangerous arrhythmias at treatment doses. In fact, TCAs are potent antiarrhythmic agents, possessing quinidine-like properties (Glassman and Bigger 1981). Because prolongation of the PR and QRS intervals can occur with TCA use, these drugs should not be used in patients with preexisting heart block (especially right bundle branch block and left bundle branch block). In such patients TCAs often lead to second- or third-degree heart block, both of which are life-threatening conditions (Roose et al. 1987).

Weight gain. Patients treated with TCAs may experience undesirable weight gain. This side effect appears to be unrelated to improvement in the patient's mood (Fernstrom et al. 1986; Kupfer et al. 1979).

Neurological effects. Tremor is a common side effect. Dose reduction or a change to a different type of antidepressant may ultimately be required to alleviate the tremor. However, treatment with a β-adrenergic blocking drug (e.g., propranolol) often provides symptomatic relief (Kronfol et al. 1983).

A dose-related risk of seizures has been found with clomipramine, which has led to the recommendation that the daily dosage of this drug should not exceed 250 mg (Clomipramine Collaborative Study Group 1991; see also Anafranil package insert). Overdoses of TCAs are associated with seizures, particularly amoxapine and desipramine (Wedin et al. 1986). Whether or not therapeutic dosages of TCAs lower the seizure threshold is controversial (Dailey and Naritoku 1996). Nonetheless, other classes may be safer options for individuals with epilepsy (Rosenstein et al. 1993).

Amoxapine, which has a mild neuroleptic effect, can cause extrapyramidal side effects, akathisia, and even tardive dyskinesia (Gammon and Hansen 1984; Ross et al. 1983; Thornton and Stahl 1984). For this reason, we do not recommend that amoxapine be prescribed as a first-line treatment for depression.

Overdose. The major complications from overdose with TCAs include those that arise from neuropsychiatric impairment, hypotension, cardiac arrhythmias, and seizures. Because the TCAs have significant anticholinergic activity, anticholinergic delirium may occur. This is particularly true for elderly patients and for patients with neuropsychiatric conditions. Other complications of anticholinergic overdose include agitation, supraventricular arrhythmias, hallucinations, severe hypertension, and seizures (Goldfrank et al. 1986). Patients with anticholinergic delirium manifest hot dry skin, dry mucous membranes, dilated pupils, absent bowel sounds, and tachycardia. Anticholinergic delirium constitutes a medical emergency and requires full supportive medical care. Physostigmine, a centrally and peripherally acting reversible anticholinesterase, may be used as a diagnostic agent in cases of suspected anticholinergic toxicity. This agent is administered at a dose of 1–2 mg intramuscularly or intravenously at a slow, controlled rate of no more than 1 mg/minute. Physostigmine should not be used to maintain reversal of the toxicity, however, because a cholinergic crisis may result. A cholinergic crisis is characterized by nausea, vomiting, bradycardia, and seizures. This reaction can be reversed by the administration of a potent anticholinergic drug such as atropine. A more detailed explanation of the treatment of these complications can be found elsewhere (Goldfrank et al. 1986).

Hypotension, which may result from norepinephrine depletion, as well as from other causes related to the peripheral and central effects of TCAs, should be treated with vigorous fluid replacement. Seizures and cardiac complications may also occur with antidepressant overdose (Boehnert and Lovejoy 1985). When the QRS interval is below 0.10, the likelihood of seizures or ventricular arrhythmias decreases (Boehnert and Lovejoy 1985). Ventricular arrhythmias that occur secondary to overdose are typical of the arrhythmias that occur with high doses of quinidine-like agents, and these begin within the first 24 hours after hospital admission (Goldberg et al. 1985). Ventricular arrhythmias should be treated with lidocaine, propranolol, or phenytoin. Prophylactic treatment with phenytoin and insertion of a temporary pacemaker should be considered in patients with prolonged QRS intervals (i.e., greater than 120 msec; Goldfrank et al. 1986).

Seizures associated with TCA overdose should be managed with standard emergency procedures (i.e., airway maintenance, proper ventilation, and treatment of the seizures with agents such as intravenous diazepam). Because many overdose situations involve combinations of drugs, the clinician should be alert to the possibility that alcohol or benzodiazepines may also have been ingested.

Allergic reactions. Allergic and hypersensitivity reactions may occur with TCAs, as they may with most drugs. If a mild rash develops, the drug may be continued and symptomatic treatment instituted. For more serious skin eruptions, the drug should be discontinued, preferably over several days to reduce the possibility of cholinergic rebound symptoms. If further antidepressant treatment is necessary, it is preferable to avoid drugs that are metabolites of the offending drug (i.e., one should not use nortriptyline if a reaction develops to amitriptyline or desipramine if a reaction develops to imipramine). Elevated temperature or signs of infection associated with the rash necessitate a complete medical evaluation, including complete blood count and liver function tests.

Drug interactions. Because the TCAs are metabolized by the liver, drugs that inhibit or induce hepatic microsomal enzymes may alter plasma tricyclic levels. This is particularly true for 2D6 inhibitors. In some individuals this interaction may cause dangerously high levels of the TCA (Vaughan 1988; see section on drug interactions later in this chapter).

Although tricyclic levels are affected by several agents, the effect is usually not reciprocal: the TCAs rarely affect the metabolism of other drugs. A notable exception to this general rule is the drug sodium valproate, levels of which may drop when a TCA is administered concurrently (Preskorn and Burke 1992). By a different mode of action, the TCAs may also interfere with the mechanism of action of two antihypertensive drugs. Both guanethidine and clonidine lose effectiveness if administered concomitantly with drugs, such as TCAs, that block reuptake of catecholamines into adrenergic neurons.

SELECTIVE SEROTONIN REUPTAKE INHIBITORS

Mechanism of Action

SSRIs inhibit the presynaptic serotonin reuptake pump. This reuptake inhibition initially increases serotonin in the synaptic cleft, which then causes presynaptic autoreceptors to downregulate and ultimately increases net 5-HT transmission (De Montigny et al. 1981).

Background

Selective serotonin reuptake inhibitors were developed in an attempt to formulate reuptake-blocking drugs that lacked the troublesome side effects of the TCAs. SSRIs largely lack four of the five pharmacological properties characteristic of TCAs—blockade of muscarinic receptors, of H_1-histaminergic receptors, and of α_1-adrenergic receptors, and norepinephrine reuptake blocking properties—leaving only the serotonin reuptake inhibitor property intact. This selectivity has several advantages, including a reduction in dangerous side effects. Other advantages are the ability to treat a variety of comorbid psychiatric disorders and ease of dosing. The SSRIs are much safer in overdose than the TCAs, because they do not have life-threatening effects at high plasma concentrations. A 15-day supply of TCAs is lethal in most patients. In addition, SSRIs are unlikely to affect the seizure threshold or cardiac conduction, making these drugs an excellent choice for patients for who have epilepsy or cardiac disease.

Because of the more tolerable side effects and once-a-day dosing, patients are more likely to comply with SSRI than with TCA treatment. Compliance is particularly important when considering first-line treatment and overall health care costs. In addition, SSRIs have an unusually broad spectrum of action. They are efficacious in the treatment not only of depression, but also of many other psychiatric disorders, as listed earlier in this chapter. This broad spectrum of efficacy is advantageous when treating patients who have more than one disorder. Only the SSRIs and clomipramine are effective for the treatment of obsessive-compulsive disorder (OCD).

The SSRIs are started at or near their therapeutic antidepressant doses, without the long titration period required with most TCAs. The most significant disadvantage of these medications is a high incidence of treatment-emergent sexual dysfunction (discussed later), which often persists for as long as the patient continues taking the medication.

All the SSRIs have a similar spectrum of efficacy and a similar side-effect profile. However, they are structurally and, in some instances, clinically distinct. For example, allergy to one SSRI does not predict allergy to another. Similarly, response or nonresponse to one does not ensure a similar reaction to another medication in the class. They also have different pharmacokinetic properties, the most important of which are half-life and inhibition of cytochrome P450 enzymes.

Fluvoxamine has an average half-life of 12–15 hours after a single oral dose, but this is prolonged by 30%–50% at steady state (van Harten 1995). Fluvoxamine requires bid administration at dosages above 50 mg/day. Sertraline and paroxetine both have an elimination half-life of approximately 24 hours. Sertraline has an active metabolite, desmethysertraline, that has a half-life of 62–104 hours. Citalopram has a half-life of 35 hours and no clinically significant metabolites. The moderate half-life of these drugs warrants once-daily dosing and allows for washout within about a week. Fluoxetine has a half-life of 2–4 days, and its active metabolite, norfluoxetine, has a half-life of 7–15 days. Although this long half-life results in a longer time to reach steady-state concentrations, the onset of therapeutic effects is not delayed beyond the 2–4 weeks required of all current antidepressant medications. A long half-life may be advantageous for patients who forget to take their medication.

Although drug-drug interactions are significantly less common with SSRIs than with either TCAs or MAOIs, most SSRIs inhibit various hepatic cytochrome P450 (CYP) enzymes, which may increase levels of other drugs. The individual drugs in the class have different profiles of CYP inhibition, as discussed later in this chapter.

Clinical Use

Although all patients with depression should receive a thorough medical evaluation, no specific tests are required before treatment is initiated with an SSRI. The usual starting dosages for the SSRIs are summarized in Table 27–1. These standard dosages should be decreased by 50% for patients with hepatic disease and for elderly persons. In addition, patients with panic disorder or significant anxiety symptoms are often intolerant of the initial stimulating side effects that commonly occur with SSRIs. In these cases also the initial dosage should be decreased by 50% (or more) and then increased as tolerated to the usual therapeutic dosage. It is often advantageous to apply this approach to patients who generally tend to be sensitive to side effects. A liquid preparation of fluoxetine is available for patients who require doses of less than 10 mg or who have difficulty swallowing pills. The other SSRIs are available in scored tablets.

The usual therapeutic dosages for the treatment of depression are citalopram 20 mg, fluoxetine 20 mg, paroxetine 20 mg, and sertraline 50–150 mg. Although the manufacturer of fluvoxamine has not pursued FDA approval for the treatment of depression in the United States (fluvoxamine is approved only for the treatment of OCD), this medication is an effective antidepressant at 50–150 mg/day (Claghorn et al. 1996; Walczak et al. 1996). For the treatment of depression, the SSRIs have a flat dose-response curve, meaning that higher dosages tend not to be more effective than standard dosages, although isolated patients respond better to higher dosages. Premature escalation of the SSRI dosage when treating a patient with depression is most likely to add side effects without improved antidepressant efficacy. Therefore, we recommend maintaining the usual therapeutic dosage for 4 weeks. If there is

no improvement at that time, a trial of a higher dose may be warranted. If a partial response is evident at 4 weeks, the dosage should remain constant for an additional 2 weeks because improvement to the initial dosage may continue.

The treatment of OCD requires a longer duration to assess efficacy and often higher dosages. A therapeutic trial for OCD is 8–12 weeks. In fixed-dose studies, fluoxetine and sertraline have appeared to be effective at dosages similar to those used to treat depression (Greist et al. 1995; Tollefson et al. 1994). However, some patients clearly benefit from higher doses. To avoid unnecessary side effects, the best course of action often is to treat first with modest dosages of medication and then increase the dosage if needed. The most common reason for nonresponse in patients with OCD is failure to increase the dose adequately.

In the treatment of panic disorder, data indicate that 40–60 mg/day of paroxetine is more efficacious than lower dosages (Oehrberg et al. 1995; Ballenger et al. 1998). However, available data indicate that the other SSRIs are effective for the treatment of panic disorder at their typical antidepressant dosages (van Vliet et al. 1996). Use of fluoxetine in panic disorder has been studied only in small, open studies, but the drug appears to exhibit antipanic effects at low dosages (Louie et al. 1993). Fluoxetine should be initiated at 5 mg/day and gradually increased to 20 mg/day because patients with panic disorder tend to be exquisitely sensitive to side effects (see subsection on the treatment of panic disorder in the section on anxiolytics in this chapter).

Late luteal phase dysphoric disorder appears to respond to doses similar to those used to treat depression. Gelenberg (1997) noted the successful treatment of late luteal phase dysphoric disorder even when medication was administered only in the 5–7 days of each month immediately before menses. Fluoxetine is effective in the treatment of bulimia at a dosage of 60 mg/day (Mitchell et al. 1993). Although the other SSRIs are probably also effective, data are limited and clear dosing guidelines are not available. The use of SSRIs to attenuate symptoms associated with borderline personality disorder and posttraumatic stress disorder (PTSD) typically requires relatively higher dosages.

Risks, Side Effects, and Their Management

Common side effects. Mild nausea, loose bowel movements, anxiety, headache, insomnia, and increased sweating are frequent initial side effects of SSRI treatment. They are usually dosage related and may be minimized with low initial dosing and gradual titration. These early adverse effects almost always attenuate after the first few weeks of treatment. Sexual dysfunction, discussed later, is the most common longer term side effect of the SSRIs.

Neurological effects.

Tension headaches are common early in treatment. These can usually be managed with over-the-counter pain relief preparations. SSRIs may initially worsen migraine headaches, but if the patient can tolerate the first few weeks of treatment with symptomatic relief, SSRIs are often effective in reducing the severity and frequency of migraines (Doughty and Lyle 1995; Hamilton and Halbreich 1993; Manna et al. 1994).

Tremor and akathisia are less common and can be managed with dosage reduction or the addition of a β-blocker. There are isolated case reports of SSRI-related dystonia and increasing reports of SSRI-related exacerbation of Parkinson's disease (Leo 1996; Lipinski et al. 1989; Tate 1989). However, in a review of case reports of movement disorders associated with SSRIs, Leo (1996) found that over half were confounded by the concomitant use of other medications that can contribute to EPS. The advisability of SSRI use in depressed patients with Parkinson's disease remains to be determined. Bupropion and ECT may be reasonable alternatives for patients with both Parkinson's disease and depression.

Stimulation/insomnia.

Some patients complain of jitteriness, restlessness, muscle tension, and disturbed sleep. These side effects typically occur early in treatment, before the antidepressant effect. All patients should be informed of the possibility of these side effects and reassured that if they develop, they will be transient. Patients with preexisting anxiety should be started at low dosages with subsequent titration as tolerated. In this way, if overstimulation occurs, it will not be so severe and persistent that it will discourage compliance with medication. The short-term use of a benzodiazepine may also help the patient cope with overstimulation in the early stages of treatment, until tolerance to this side effect occurs. Despite these common transient stimulating effects, SSRIs are clearly effective for patients with anxiety or agitated depression. Similarly, insomnia that commonly occurs early in treatment may be tolerable if the patient is reassured that the side effect will be transient. Symptomatic treatment with short-term use of benzodiazepines or low-dose trazodone (e.g., 50–150 mg) at bedtime is reasonable (Jacobsen 1990; Nierenberg and Keck 1989).

Sedation.

Despite occasional stimulating effects, SSRIs may induce sedation in some patients. In our experience, patients who experience significant treatment-emergent sedation with these medications often require lower doses.

Weight gain or loss.

Treatment with fluoxetine has been associated with weight loss (Ferguson 1986), and as a consequence, the drug has been studied as a possible treatment for obesity. However, it now appears that any weight reduction associated with fluoxetine may be transient (Marcus et al. 1990). Furthermore, all the SSRIs have the potential to cause weight gain in some individuals (Bouwer and Harvey 1996; Fisher et al. 1995). However, in most patients, SSRIs are not associated with either weight gain or weight loss.

Gastrointestinal symptoms.

Nausea and diarrhea may occur following treatment with an SSRI. This side effect is dose dependent and often transient.

Sexual dysfunction.

Decreased libido, anorgasmia, and delayed ejaculation are common side effects of SSRIs. When possible, the management of sexual side effects should be postponed until the patient has completed an adequate trial of the antidepressant. In some cases, tolerance to sexual side effects develops.

When significant sexual dysfunction persists for more than 1 month despite a positive response to treatment, a reduction in the dosage should be considered. In many cases, this results in a diminution of the symptoms without loss of therapeutic benefit. Unfortunately, in other instances there is no therapeutic dosage that does not cause the sexual side effect. In such cases, two strategies are available: the antidepressant can be replaced with an alternative, or other drugs may be prescribed to counteract the side effect. The decision to try a different antidepressant is potentially problematic because an equivalent therapeutic response is not guaranteed. In our experience, switching from one SSRI to another does not tend to decrease sexual side effects. Antidepressants that do not commonly cause sexual dysfunction are bupropion, nefazodone, and mirtazapine.

Several medications have been suggested as antidotes for the sexual side effects associated with antidepressants. Bupropion, 75 or 150 mg/day, has been added to an SSRI regimen with some success in minimizing sexual side effects (Labbate and Pollack 1994). Cyproheptadine, an antihistamine with antiserotonergic properties, has been successful in reversing anorgasmia, in doses of 4–12 mg, taken 1–2 hours before sexual activity (Steele and Howell 1987; Zajecka et al. 1991). Similarly, yohimbine, an inhibitor of the α_2-noradrenaline autoreceptor, has been successful in treating impotence, taken in a 10-mg dose 1 hour before sexual activity (Price and Grunhaus 1990). Because the sexual side effects of SSRIs reverse rapidly when the medication is stopped, it is sometimes feasible for patients to skip 1 or 2 days of medication each week and experience unimpaired sexual function the next day (Rothschild 1995). This "drug holiday," or "sex holiday," as it is sometimes referred to, is most easily accomplished with the shorter half-life agents. However, there is some concern regarding relapse and of fostering noncompliance with this strategy.

The syndrome of inappropriate secretion of antidiuretic hormone. Case reports have identified an association between SSRIs and the development of the syndrome of inappropriate secretion of antidiuretic hormone (SIADH). However, the actual incidence remains unclear, and a causative relationship has yet to be established (Woo and Smythe 1997). Published reports have indicated that elderly persons may be at a higher risk (Liu et al. 1996). Symptoms include lethargy, headache, hyponatremia, elevated urinary sodium excretion, and hyperosmolar urine. Acute treatment of SIADH should consist of discontinuation of the drug as well as restriction of fluid intake. Patients experiencing severe confusion, convulsions, or coma should receive intravenous sodium chloride. Physicians should be aware of this potentially serious but reversible side effect, especially when treating elderly patients.

Vivid dreams. Reports of vivid dreams, distinct from nightmares, are common with SSRIs. The mechanism is unknown; in fact, SSRIs tend to decrease rapid eye movement (REM) sleep.

Rash. If a mild rash develops, the drug may be continued and symptomatic treatment instituted. Severe rashes require discontinuation of medication. Because the SSRIs share a similar mechanism but not similar structures, an allergy to one agent does not predict an allergy to another.

The serotonin syndrome. There have been several reports of a medication-induced syndrome that has been attributed to excessive stimulation of the serotonergic system. This condition arises more commonly among patients treated concurrently with two or more serotonergic drugs (e.g., fluoxetine and an MAOI). However, it may occur also in patients treated with SSRI monotherapy. Affected individuals suffer from the constellation of lethargy, restlessness, confusion, flushing, diaphoresis, tremor, and myoclonic jerks. As the condition progresses, hyperthermia, hypertonicity, rhabdomyolysis, renal failure, and death may occur (Metz and Shader 1990). The syndrome must be identified as rapidly as possible, because discontinuation of the serotonergic medications is the first step in treatment, followed by emergency medical treatment, as required.

Discontinuation syndromes. A number of case reports have described transient dizziness, lethargy, paresthesia, nausea, vivid dreams, and irritability following the discontinuation or dose reduction of serotonergic antidepressant medications. This topic is addressed in greater detail at the end of this section under the heading "Antidepressant Discontinuation."

Apathy syndromes. We and others have noted an apathy syndrome in some patients after months or years of successful treatment with SSRIs. Patients often confuse this syndrome with a recurrence of depression, but the two conditions are quite distinct. The syndrome is characterized by a loss of motivation, increased passivity, and often feelings of lethargy and "flatness." However, there is no associated sadness, tearfulness, emotional angst, decreased concentration, or thoughts of hopelessness, worthlessness, or suicide. If specifically asked, patients often remark that the symptoms are not experientially similar to their original depressive symptoms. This syndrome has, to date, not been adequately studied, and the pathophysiology is not known. However, there is speculation that subchronic stimulation of central serotonin may attenuate dopamine functioning in several areas of the brain, including the frontal cortex. In this respect it is notable that the clinical presentation mirrors that of a frontal lobe syndrome.

The syndrome appears to be dose dependent and reversible. Mistakenly interpreting the apathy and lethargy for a relapse of depression, and hence increasing the dose of medication, will worsen the symptoms. If dosage reduction is not effective, patients may benefit from the addition of a stimulant. In our experience very low doses are effective, such as 18.75–37.5 mg of pimoline, with only rare development of tolerance. Other agents that increase dopamine may also be effective.

Risk of suicide. Teicher and colleagues (1990) reported that six depressed patients taking fluoxetine became intensely preoccupied with suicidal ideation. Subsequently, the question of fluoxetine-induced suicidality has received a great deal of attention in the media. Teicher's report emphasized the unusual, obsessive quality to the patients' suicidal ideation. Fluoxetine-induced akathisia has been implicated in several cases, on the basis of both the phenomenology of the symptom and a positive response to antiakathisia treatments (Hamilton and Opler 1992). Other cases of increased suicidality with SSRIs have been attributed to a well-known condition among severely depressed patients initiating treatment with antidepressants: relief from dysphoria may lag behind while energy levels begin to increase, with the result that the patient's motivation to complete suicide is greater than it was before treatment. Whatever the final explanation for the reports, studies of suicide rates among fluoxetine users to date have not indicated an increased risk of suicide attempts or completions relative to users of other antidepressants (Fava and Rosenbaum 1992; Mann and Kapur 1991). Larger controlled studies have confirmed that suicide rates among depressed patients treated with fluoxetine (and all other antidepressants) are markedly reduced from those of depressed patients who do not receive antidepressants.

Drug interactions. Several deaths have been reported in patients taking a combination of SSRIs and MAOIs, presumably owing to the serotonin syndrome (Francois et al. 1997; Hodgman et al. 1997; Kolecki 1997). Because of the potential lethality of this interaction, when it is necessary to switch from an SSRI to an MAOI, the patient must remain off the SSRI for a long enough time to ensure that it has been fully eliminated from the body. This time frame is the equivalent of five times the half-life of the SSRI. Therefore, 5 weeks are required between the discontinuation of fluoxetine and the institution of an MAOI (Beasley 1993) and about 1 week between other SSRIs and an MAOI. A 2-week waiting period is required when switching from an MAOI to an SSRI.

SSRIs should not be given to patients who are taking fenfluramine or dexfenfluramine because of the risk of precipitating the serotonin syndrome. These medications act synergistically: fenfluramine and dexfenfluramine cause the release of serotonin from the presynaptic neuron, whereas SSRIs decrease reuptake.

SSRIs vary with regard to inhibition of cytochrome P450 isozymes. Enzyme inhibition may result in increased blood levels of concomitantly administered medications (see section on drug interactions later in this chapter).

BUPROPION

Mechanism of Action

Bupropion's mechanism of antidepressant activity still remains unclear. Bupropion (Wellbutrin) is metabolized to hydroxybupropion, which appears to be the active entity. Hydroxybupropion inhibits the reuptake of norepinephrine and dopamine, hence the designation dopamine-norepinephrine reuptake inhibitor (DNRI).

Background

Bupropion's unique spectrum of putative receptor effects provides a useful addition to the therapeutic armamentarium. The most significant advantage of bupropion is its relative lack of sexual side effects. Indeed, the addition of low doses of bupropion may attenuate the sexual dysfunction caused by other medications. There has been some suggestion, on the basis of small clinical trials and case reports, that bupropion may be less likely than other antidepressants to precipitate mania or rapid cycling in patients with bipolar disorder (Ketter et al. 1995; Sachs et al. 1994; Stoll et al. 1994; Zarate et al. 1995). Because bupropion facilitates dopamine transmission, many clinicians preferentially use this agent for patients with Parkinson's disease. The fact that dopamine is integrally related to the brain's reward mechanisms, which are stimulated by nicotine and other addictive substances, has provided the theoretical underpinning for recent research demonstrating that bupropion is an effective aid to smoking cessation. Two placebo-controlled trials with nondepressed chronic cigarette smokers revealed a dose-dependent increase in the percentage of patients able to achieve abstinence. Individuals receiving 300 mg/day were able to sustain abstinence longer than those receiving 150 mg/day, and both groups were superior to placebo groups (Zyban package insert). Bupropion is being marketed under the name Zyban for smoking cessation.

Several small clinical trials have indicated that bupropion may be beneficial in the treatment of attention-deficit/hyperactivity disorder (Conners et al. 1996; Cook et al. 1995; Greenhill 1992). Unfortunately, bupropion does not treat panic disorder or obsessive-compulsive disorder, and clinical experience suggests that it has less ability than the SSRIs to attenuate symptoms of general anxiety.

Overall, bupropion has a favorable side-effect profile with little or no weight gain, few effects on cardiac conduction (Roose et al. 1991), and minimal sexual side effects (Kiev et al. 1994). Disadvantages include an increased risk of medication-induced seizures and the requirement for multiple daily doses.

Clinical Use

We recommend the use of the sustained-release preparation rather than the original preparation because of increased tolerability and decreased seizure risk. The sustained-release preparation is initiated at 150 mg, preferably taken in the morning. After 4 days the dosage may be increased to 150 mg bid. For the short-acting preparation, bupropion is initiated at 75 mg bid and increased as tolerated to a total daily dosage of 300 mg. Patients who do not respond after 4 weeks may warrant a trial of 450 mg/day. No single dose should exceed 150 mg. Gradual dose titration helps to minimize initial anxiety and insomnia. The temporary use of anxiolytic or hypnotic agents is reasonable in some patients but generally should be limited to the first few weeks of treatment.

Contraindications

Patients with seizure disorders should not use bupropion. Similarly, consideration of an alternative treatment is advised for patients with a history of head trauma, central nervous system tumor, or eating disorders.

Risks, Side Effects, and Their Management

The most common side effects of bupropion are initial headache, anxiety, insomnia, increased sweating, and gastrointestinal upset. Tremor and akathisia may also occur. Management is the same as previously discussed concerning the SSRIs. Bupropion is not associated with anticholinergic side effects, orthostatic hypotension, weight gain, or cardiac conduction changes.

The incidence of seizures is 0.4% with dosages less than 450 mg/day, provided no single dose of the short-acting preparation exceeds 150 mg. The incidence increases to 5% with dosages between 450 and 600 mg/day. The sustained-release preparation has a seizure incidence of 0.1% in dosages less than 300 mg/day and 0.4% in dosages between 300 and 400 mg/day. Higher dosages of the sustained-release preparation have not been evaluated. Patients with a history of seizure or who are taking concomitant medications that lower seizure threshold (e.g., antipsychotics, other antidepressants) should be given bupropion only with extreme caution.

Psychosis. Reports of delusions, hallucinations, and paranoia are consistent with bupropion-mediated increases in central dopamine. Bupropion should be used with caution in patients with psychotic disorder.

Overdose. Much more is known about overdose with the immediate-release formulation of bupropion than with the newer, sustained-release formulation. Reported reactions with the immediate-release form include seizures, hallucinations, loss of consciousness, and sinus tachycardia. Treatment of overdose should include induction of vomiting, administration of activated charcoal, and ECG and electroencephalographic (EEG) monitoring. For seizures, an intravenous benzodiazepine preparation is recommended.

The danger of bupropion overdose is, for the most part, limited to the risk of seizures. However, seizures are seldom a life-threatening event, unless they result in motor vehicle accidents, falls, or other trauma-related events. On the other hand, bupropion's lack of significant cardiovascular or respiratory toxicity means that it is rarely lethal in overdose.

Drug interactions. Combination with an MAOI is potentially dangerous, but less so than the combination of serotonergic drugs and MAOIs. Although the practice is not recommended, there are reports of combining MAOIs and bupropion in patients with refractory depression.

In vitro data suggest that bupropion is metabolized by CYP 2B6. Bupropion does not appear to inhibit cytochrome P450 enzymes. Because of the risk of dose-dependent seizures, caution is warranted when bupropion is combined with other medications that might inhibit its metabolism.

VENLAFAXINE

Mechanism of Action

Venlafaxine hydrochloride (Effexor) is a potent inhibitor of norepinephrine and serotonin reuptake, as well as a less potent dopamine reuptake inhibitor. At lower dosages, serotonin reuptake inhibition is prominent. At higher dosages, inhibition of norepinephrine reuptake becomes more significant. Inhibition of dopamine reuptake is manifest at the higher end of the dosage range (Ellingrod and Perry 1994).

Background

Venlafaxine is a phenylethylamine antidepressant released in the United States in 1994. Although it is indicated for the treatment of major depression, preliminary data suggest that it might also have a role in the treatment of chronic pain conditions and perhaps other disorders for which SSRIs are effective. Venlafaxine may be effective for patients who have not responded to other antidepressants; a 33% response rate to venlafaxine was reported in patients who failed to improve during adequate trials of other antidepressant treatments, including MAOIs and ECT (Nierenberg et al. 1994). Venlafaxine is 27% protein bound, which is substantially lower than all the other antidepressants. This property is advantageous when it is necessary to minimize the likelihood of protein-binding interactions. Venlafaxine is unlikely to inhibit cytochrome P450 enzymes, which further decreases the likelihood of drug interactions. Venlafaxine extended-release (XR) allows for once-a-day dosing. Blood pressure elevation may occur at higher doses, as discussed in the section on side effects.

Clinical Use

The recommended dosage range of venlafaxine is 75–225 mg/day. The extended-release (XR) preparation, which allows for once-daily dosing, is preferred. The usual starting dosage is 37.5–75 mg/day. Doses up to 375 mg/day have been used for patients who are otherwise nonresponsive to treatment. Blood pressure monitoring is required because of dose-dependent increases in mean diastolic blood pressure in some patients.

Recent data (Kelsey 1996) indicate a significant dose-response relationship for venlafaxine; patients with mild depression may respond to lower doses, whereas patients with more severe or recurrent depression may respond better to higher doses. Kelsey (1996) hypothesized that this difference exists because the mechanism of action involves mixed reuptake, with differential effects at higher dosages.

Risks, Side Effects, and Their Management

The side-effect profile of venlafaxine is similar to that of the SSRIs, including possible early stimulation, gastrointestinal symptoms, sexual dysfunction, and transient discontinuation symptoms. Like the SSRIs, venlafaxine does not affect cardiac conduction or lower the seizure threshold. For most patients venlafaxine is not associated with sedation or weight gain. Side effects that differ from those of the SSRIs are hypothesized to be related to the increased noradrenergic activity of this drug at higher doses, specifically dose-dependent anxiety and hypertension.

Hypertension.   Modest dose-dependent increases in blood pressure may occur with venlafaxine treatment. The incidence of elevated blood pressure is 3.0% with dosages less than 300 mg/day. For clinically significant treatment-emergent hypertension, dosage reduction or treatment discontinuation should be considered.

Overdose.   Few data are available regarding venlafaxine in overdose, but its pharmacological profile suggests it is safer than the tricyclic antidepressants. Of the reported cases to date, most patients did not have symptoms. For others, somnolence, mild sinus tachycardia, and generalized convulsions were reported. Recommended treatment includes general supportive and symptomatic measures; in severe cases, dialysis should be considered.

Drug interactions.   Venlafaxine does not appear to inhibit significantly cytochrome P450 enzymes, and it is the antidepressant least likely to contribute to protein-binding interactions. Venlafaxine should not be combined with MAOIs, fenfluramine, or dexfenfluramine because of the risk of serotonin syndrome.

NEFAZODONE

Mechanism of Action

Nefazodone (Serzone) is a 5-HT$_2$-receptor antagonist and a weak inhibitor of neuronal 5-HT reuptake. Together these properties are believed to enhance 5-HT$_{1A}$–mediated neuronal transmission.

Background

Nefazodone entered the United States market in 1995. The advantages of nefazodone are a low incidence of sexual dysfunction (Goldberg 1995) and early attenuation of symptoms of anxiety and insomnia (Armitage et al. 1994; Fawcett et al. 1995). The disadvantages are prominent early sedation, bid dosing, slow dosage titration, and inhibition of CYP 3A3/4.

Clinical Use

The clinically effective dosage range has been determined to be between 300 and 600 mg/day. Because of prominent early side effects, we recommend an initial dosage of 50 mg bid or qhs, with subsequent increases every 5–7 days, as tolerated, until the total daily dosage reaches 600 mg/day in divided doses or a therapeutic response emerges. The therapeutic range for elderly patients is slightly lower (i.e., between 200 and 400 mg/day in divided doses). As with other antidepressants, an adequate trial of at least 4 weeks is necessary to evaluate efficacy.

Risks, Side Effects, and Their Management

Common side effects are sedation, nausea, dizziness, confusion, and blurred vision. Nefazodone does not appear to cause weight gain or sexual dysfunction.

Visual effects.   Visual symptoms, such as blurred or abnormal vision, may accompany nefazodone treatment. Nefazodone does not have significant anticholinergic effects, and the mechanism for visual changes is not known. Treatment-emergent visual symptoms are generally mild and transient.

Effects on sleep.   Although it has been reported that nefazodone does not suppress REM sleep (Armitage et al. 1994), the clinical significance of this finding is unclear. Indeed, the ability of antidepressants to suppress REM sleep early in treatment may be predictive of therapeutic efficacy (Kupfer et al. 1981).

Overdose. Few data on nefazodone overdose exist. No deaths have been reported. Treatment should consist of supportive measures with specific attention to hypotension and excessive sedation. Gastric lavage is encouraged.

Contraindications and drug interactions. Nefazodone should not be used in combination with terfenadine (Seldane), astemizole (Hismanal), or cisapride (Propulsid) because of the potential for severe adverse cardiovascular events. This reaction is mediated by inhibition of the cytochrome P450 3A3/4 enzyme by nefazodone.

Coadministration with other medications that are metabolized by CYP 3A3/4 is not contraindicated, but the dosages of the other medications that are 3A3/4 substrates should be reduced (see the section on drug interactions later in this chapter). The interaction of nefazodone with MAOIs has not yet been evaluated, but it may be as dangerous as that of the SSRIs. Therefore, this combination should be avoided.

TRAZODONE

Mechanism of Action

Trazodone (Desyrel), like nefazodone, is a postsynaptic 5-HT$_2$ antagonist and a weak inhibitor of 5-HT reuptake.

Background

Trazodone is an older antidepressant that is associated with significant sedative activity. Currently, trazodone is not recommended as a first-line antidepressant because of an increased risk of orthostatic hypotension, arrhythmias, and priapism. Also, when compared with other available antidepressants, trazodone does not offer an advantage in terms of therapeutic efficacy (Haria et al. 1994). However, trazodone may be useful in patients with insomnia. It is currently common practice to use low dosages of trazodone, such as 50–100 mg, to assist with initial insomnia while starting one of the newer antidepressants to treat the underlying depression. If this strategy is used, we recommend tapering the dosage and discontinuing treatment with trazodone after 4–6 weeks.

Clinical Use

Trazodone is prescribed in much the same manner as the TCAs, although there is less danger of toxicity at higher doses. The recommended therapeutic dosage range for the treatment of depression is 200–400 mg/day in divided doses. Initial dosing should begin with 50 mg/day, with

subsequent increases as tolerated. Most of the daily dosage should be administered in the evening to minimize daytime sedation.

Risks, Side Effects, and Their Management

Excessive sedation is the most commonly encountered side effect of trazodone. Although trazodone has virtually no anticholinergic effects, dry mouth and blurred vision occur more frequently with trazodone treatment than with placebo.

Priapism. Trazodone is the only antidepressant that has been associated with priapism (Scher et al. 1983), which may be irreversible and require surgical intervention (Mitchell and Popkin 1983). This risk must always be considered before trazodone is chosen to treat male patients.

Cardiovascular effects. Trazodone can cause orthostatic hypotension and dizziness (Glassman 1984; Spivak et al. 1987), although these side effects do not appear to correlate with trazodone's binding to the α_2-adrenergic receptor. Because trazodone does not cause a significant change in cardiac conduction, for some time it was felt to be the antidepressant of choice among patients with cardiac conduction defects. However, there are now several reports of increased ventricular irritability among patients with conduction defects and preexisting ventricular arrhythmias (Aronson and Hafez 1986; Jankowsky et al. 1983; Vitullo et al. 1990), and multiple newer agents exist that do not appear to affect cardiac conduction.

Overdose. There is a risk in overdose of myocardial irritation in patients with preexisting ventricular conduction abnormalities.

MIRTAZAPINE

Mechanism of Action and Receptor Effects

Mirtazapine (Remeron) facilitates central serotonergic and noradrenergic transmission by antagonizing α_2-noradrenergic autoreceptors and heteroreceptors (De Boer 1996). In addition, mirtazapine antagonizes postsynaptic 5-HT$_{2A}$, 5-HT$_3$, and H$_1$ receptors. 5-HT$_{2A}$ antagonism may be related to the antidepressant properties of this drug and is likely to account for the low rate of occurrence of drug-induced sexual dysfunction. 5-HT$_3$ antagonism is thought to prevent nausea. Antagonism of H$_1$ receptors may account for the side effects of sedation and weight gain. Mirtazapine has moderate activity at α_1 receptors and muscarinic receptors.

Background

Mirtazapine entered the United States market in 1996. It has been shown to reduce anxiety symptoms and sleep disturbances associated with depression as early as 1 week after the start of treatment (Bremmer 1995; Smith et al. 1990). Other advantages are minimal sexual dysfunction, minimal nausea, and once-daily dosing. In addition, mirtazapine is unlikely to be associated with cytochrome-P450-mediated drug interactions. The disadvantages of mirtazapine are weight gain, prominent early sedation, and possible elevation of serum lipid levels.

Clinical Use

Mirtazapine treatment is initiated with 15 mg at bedtime. Depending on clinical response and side effects, the dosage can be increased to a maximum of 45 mg qhs. Elderly patients and those with renal or hepatic disease may require lower dosages.

Risks, Side Effects, and Their Management

As noted previously, sexual dysfunction and nausea are not commonly associated with mirtazapine treatment. The most common side effects are sedation, weight gain, and dizziness. Rare but potentially serious adverse events are agranulocytosis and increases in serum cholesterol and triglyceride levels.

Somnolence. Somnolence occurs in more than 50% of patients treated with mirtazapine (Bremmer 1995; Smith et al. 1990). Tolerance to this side effect develops after the first few weeks of treatment.

Weight gain. The weight gain associated with mirtazapine use may be partially due to an increased appetite. A mean increase of 8.2 lb over the first 28 weeks of treatment has been reported in several controlled studies (Bremmer 1995; Smith et al. 1990).

Agranulocytosis. In preliminary clinical trials, 2 of 2,796 mirtazapine-treated patients developed agranulocytosis, and 1 developed severe neutropenia. All three patients recovered after medication discontinuation. Thirteen patients with pretreatment neutropenia did not progress to more severe neutropenia or agranulocytosis. On the basis of this limited population, the risk of developing agranulocytosis with mirtazapine is estimated at 1.1/1,000 patients. The potential risk of agranulocytosis should be discussed with patients. Routine laboratory monitoring is not currently recommended. The development of fever, chills, sore throat, or other signs of infection in association with a low white blood cell (WBC) count warrants close monitoring and the discontinuation of mirtazapine.

Anticholinergic effects. Mirtazapine is associated with modest anticholinergic side effects, including dry mouth and constipation. Anticholinergic side effects and their management are discussed in the section of this chapter concerning TCAs.

Increased serum lipid levels. Nonfasting serum cholesterol levels increased by 20% or more in 15% of patients and to levels greater than or equal to 500 mg/dL in 6% of patients who participated in the United States clinical trials. These rates are twice those of patients taking either placebo or an active comparison drug. The clinical significance of mirtazapine-induced increases in serum lipid levels is not known.

Cardiac effects. Hypertension, orthostatic hypotension, dizziness, and vasodilation with peripheral edema may occur with mirtazapine treatment.

Overdose. Little is known about mirtazapine overdose. To date, patients who have overdosed have fully recovered. Warning signs include drowsiness, impaired memory, and tachycardia. Recommended treatment includes gastric lavage, cardiac monitoring, and supportive measures.

Drug interactions. Mirtazapine does not significantly inhibit hepatic cytochrome P450 enzymes. Additive effects may occur when mirtazapine is combined with other drugs with sedative or vascular effects. Mirtazapine should not be used in combination with an MAOI or within 14 days of discontinuing therapy with an MAOI.

MONOAMINE OXIDASE INHIBITORS

Mechanism of Action

The enzyme monoamine oxidase (MAO) inactivates biogenic amines such as norepinephrine, serotonin, dopamine, and tyramine through oxidative deamination. MAOIs block this inactivation and thereby increase the amount of these transmitters available for synaptic release. There are two types of MAO: A and B. Type A (MAO-A) acts selectively on the substrates norepinephrine and serotonin, whereas type B (MAO-B) preferentially affects phenylethylamine. Both MAO types oxidize dopamine and tyramine. MAO-A inhibition appears to be most relevant to the antidepressant effects of these drugs. Drugs that contain both MAO-A and MAO-B are called *nonselective*. The two MAOI antidepressants currently available in the United States, phenelzine (Nardil) and tranylcypromine (Parnate), are both nonselective inhibitors. Because tyramine can be metabolized by either MAO-A or MAO-B, drugs that selectively inhibit either one of these enzymes, but not the other, do not require dietary restrictions. MAO-A-selective drugs, such as moclobemide, are available in other countries for the treatment of depression. MAO-B-selective drugs, such as pargyline and L-deprenyl, are marketed for other indications and do not appear to treat depression in their usual dosages. At higher dosages both of these drugs become nonselective.

Another important characteristic of MAOIs is the production of reversible versus irreversible enzyme inhibition. An irreversible inhibitor permanently disables the enzyme. This means that MAO must be resynthesized, in the absence of the drug, before the activity of the enzyme can be reestablished. Resynthesis of the enzyme may take up to 2 weeks. For this reason, 10–14 days are required after discontinuation of irreversible inhibitors before instituting other antidepressants or before permitting the use of the drugs or foods that are known to be contraindicated (see section on clinical use of MAOIs later in this chapter). On the other hand, a reversible inhibitor can move away from the active site of the enzyme, enabling the enzyme to be available to metabolize other substances. The reversibility and selectivity of the currently available MAOIs are summarized in Table 27–5.

Clinical Use

The MAOIs are not currently used as first-line agents because of the improved tolerability and safety of the newer antidepressants. Because of this decline in use, isocarboxazid (Marplan) is no longer being manufactured. However, the MAOIs continue to be excellent medications for a subset of patients who do not respond to the newer antidepressants. Patients with a depressive syndrome that is characterized by mood reactivity (i.e., mood that is responsive acutely to favorable and unfavorable life experiences), oversleeping, overeating, extreme lethargy, and extreme sensitivity to rejection—the so-called atypical subtype—may show a preferential response to MAOI therapy (Liebowitz et al. 1984; Quitkin et al. 1979; Ravaris et al. 1980; Zisook 1985). These atypical symptoms may, in fact, provide a marker for patients who are likely to respond to MAOIs.

More so than with other medications, it is imperative to review the patient's medical status and current medications before prescribing an MAOI. The importance of following the dietary and medication restrictions, as outlined later, should be discussed with the patient; the discussion should be supplemented with written instructions, as presented in Table 27–6. Patients should also be warned against gaining a false sense of confidence if dietary guidelines are broken without consequences. We often recommend that our patients who take MAOIs read chapters on antidepressants in books written specifically for patients and their families (e.g., Gorman 1990; Kass et al. 1992; Yudofsky et al. 1991). Because the current use of MAOIs is predominantly in patients with refractory depression—patients who are often suicidal—too often clinicians are hesitant to use these medications for fear that patients will intentionally not comply with dietary restrictions in order to harm themselves. This is a difficult paradox: if the medication is effective, the patient will no longer want to commit suicide. Furthermore, withholding of effective treatment, with the likely continuation of the

TABLE 27–5.   Summary of MAOI reversibility and selectivity

Drug	Reversible inhibition	Enzyme selectivity	Indication
Phenelzine	No	MAO-A + B	Depression
Tranylcypromine	No	MAO-A + B	Depression
Isocarboxazid[a]	No	MAOI-A + B	Depression
Deprenyl	No	MAO-B[b]	Parkinson's disease
Pargyline	No	MAO-B[b]	Hypertension
Moclobemide[c]	Yes	MAO-A	Depression

Note.   MAOI = monoamine oxidase inhibitor.
[a]No longer manufactured.
[b]MAOI-B is selective at lower doses, nonselective at higher doses.
[c]Not available in the United States.

TABLE 27–6.   Instructions for patients taking monoamine oxidase inhibitors

While taking this medication:

1. Avoid all the foods and drugs indicated on the list (see Table 27–7).

2. In general, all the foods you should avoid are decayed, fermented, or aged in some way. Avoid any spoiled food even if it is not on the list.

3. If you get a cold or flu, you may use aspirin or Tylenol. For a cough, glycerin cough drops or cough syrup without dextromethorphan may be used.

4. All laxatives or stool softeners for constipation may be used.

5. For infections, all antibiotics may be safely prescribed, such as penicillin, tetracycline, or erythromycin.

6. Do not take any other medications without first checking with me. These include any over-the-counter medicines bought without prescription, such as cold tablets, nose drops, cough medicine, and diet pills.

7. Eating one of the restricted foods may cause a sudden elevation of your blood pressure. If this occurs, you will get an explosive headache, particularly in the back of your head and in your temples. Your head and face will feel flushed and full, your heart may pound, and you may perspire heavily and feel nauseated. If this rare reaction occurs, do not lie down because this elevates your blood pressure further. If your blood pressure is high, go to the nearest emergency center for evaluation and treatment. Do not wait for a phone call from our office.

8. If you need medical or dental care while taking this medication, show these restrictions and instructions to the doctor or dentist. Have the doctor or dentist call my office if he or she has any questions or needs further clarification or information.

9. Side effects such as postural lightheadedness, constipation, delay in urination, delay in ejaculation and orgasm, muscle twitching, sedation, fluid retention, insomnia, and excess sweating are quite common. Many of these side effects lessen after the third week.

10. Lightheadedness may occur after sudden changes in position. This can be avoided by getting up slowly. If tablets are taken with meals, this and the other side effects are lessened.

11. The medication is rarely effective in less than 3 weeks.

12. Care should be taken while operating any machinery or driving; some patients have episodes of sleepiness in the early phase of treatment.

13. Take the medication precisely as directed. Do not regulate the number of pills without first consulting me.

14. In spite of the side effects and special dietary restrictions, your medication (an MAO inhibitor) is safe and effective when taken as directed.

15. If any special problems arise, call me at my office.

Source.   Adapted from Jenike 1987.

---

depressed state, is associated with a higher risk for suicide. In these cases we often emphasize to the patient that failure to adhere to the instructions is more likely to cause cerebral hemorrhage and disability than to cause death.

Phenelzine is initiated with 15 mg in the morning and increased by 15 mg every other day until a total daily dosage of 60 mg is reached. If no response occurs within 2 weeks, the dosage may be increased in 15-mg increments to a usual maximum of 90 mg/day. Higher dosages are sometimes used, if tolerated, in patients with severe and refractory depression. Tranylcypromine is initiated at 10 mg and then increased every other day to 30 mg/day. As with phenelzine, higher doses may be necessary when the condition is refractory to treatment (Amsterdam and Berwish 1989). After tolerance to the hypotensive side effects has developed, usually after 1 or 2 weeks, the patient may take the medication as a single daily dose in the morning. Morning dosing is preferred because these medications tend to be activating, especially tranylcypromine, which is related to amphetamine. Some data suggest that once-a-day dosing of the MAOIs may be therapeutically superior to multiple dosing (Weise et al. 1980).

Risks, Side Effects, and Their Management

The following risks and side effects apply to the irreversible, nonselective MAOI antidepressants (phenelzine and tranylcypromine). The most common side effects are orthostatic hypotension, headache, insomnia, weight gain, sexual dysfunction, peripheral edema, and afternoon somnolence. Although the MAOIs do not have significant affinity for muscarinic receptors, anticholinergic-like side effects are present at the beginning of treatment. Dry mouth is common but not as marked as with the TCAs. Fortunately, the more serious risks, such as hypertensive crisis and serotonin syndrome, are not common.

Hypertensive crisis.   The inactivation of intestinal monoamine oxidase impairs the metabolism of tyramine. Tyramine can act as a false transmitter and displace norepinephrine from presynaptic storage granules. Therefore, large amounts of dietary tyramine can result in a hypertensive crisis in patients taking MAOIs because increased amounts of norepinephrine result in profound α-adrenergic activation. This reaction has also been called the "cheese reaction," because tyramine is present in relatively high concentrations in aged cheese.

Tyramine is formed in foods by the decarboxylation of tyrosine during the aging, ripening, or decay process of foods. Patients receiving MAOI treatment should be instructed to avoid eating the foods listed in Table 27–7. The

TABLE 27–7.   Dietary and medication restrictions for patients taking monoamine oxidase inhibitors

Foods that must be avoided while taking an MAOI and for 2 weeks after stopping the medication:[a]

Aged cheeses (fresh cheese such as cream cheese, cottage cheese, ricotta cheese, American cheese, and moderate amounts of mozzarella are currently considered safe)

Aged or fermented meats, such as sausages, salami and pepperoni (smoked salmon and whitefish are currently considered safe)

Sauerkraut

Soy sauce

Fava beans and broad bean pods

All food that may be spoiled

Alcohol may be consumed in moderation but tap beer should be avoided, including nonalcoholic tap beer

Yeast or meat extracts, such as Marmite and Bovril (yeast and baked goods containing yeast are safe)

Yogurt, if fresh, is safe

Drugs that must be avoided while taking MAOI, and for 2 weeks after stopping the medication[b]

All sympathomimetics and stimulant drugs, including:

Amphetamines	Local anesthetic drugs containing ephedrine or cocaine
Diet medications	Demerol
Ephedrine	Levodopa and dopamine
Isoproterenol	Flenfluramine and dexfenfluramine
Methylphenidate	Other antidepressant medications
Phenylpropanolamine	Buspirone
Phenylephrine	

Over-the-counter nasal decongestants and cold, sinus, and allergy medication containing pseudoephedrine, phenylephrine, or phenylpropanolamine:

Actifed	CoTylenol	Sine-Off
Alka-Seltzer Plus	Dristan	Sinex
Allerest	Neo-Synephrine	Triaminic
Contact	Robitussin PE, DM, CF, Night Relief	Tylenol
Coricidin D	Sine-Aid	Vicks Formula 44M, 44D, Nyquil

Safe cold/allergy medications:

Tylenol (plain), Robitussin (plain), Alka-Seltzer (plain), Chlor-Trimeton Allergy (without decongestant), steroid inhalers

Other safe medications:

Nonsteroidal anti-inflammatory drugs, codeine, morphine

Antibiotics

Laxatives and stool softeners

Local anesthetics without epinephrine or cocaine

[a]Food restrictions are based on tyramine contact data from Walker et al. 1996. [b]It is advisable to check the current *Physicians' Desk Reference* for any drug that is not known to be safe before prescribing it in combination with an MAOI.

key foods to avoid are aged cheeses, fermented sausage, sauerkraut, soy sauce, yeast extracts such as Marmite, fava beans and broad beans (which contain dopamine), and any food that is overripe or spoiled. Fresh, unaged cheeses, such as cottage cheese, ricotta, and cream cheese, are safe. Several foods that were formerly considered dangerous are no longer included on the list of prohibited substances. For example, domestic bottled or canned beer is now considered safe when consumed in moderation (Gardner et al. 1996). Most wines and liquors are also considered safe when taken in moderation. Liver, if fresh, is also probably safe, and caffeine and chocolate are of concern only when consumed in large amounts.

Some drugs with sympathomimetic activity, including certain decongestants and cough syrups, should be avoided because of the risk of precipitating a hypertensive crisis (Table 27–7). However, pure antihistamine drugs, such as diphenhydramine (Benadryl), and pure expectorants without dextromethorphan (e.g., guaifenesin) are permissible.

Unfortunately, even perfect compliance with the dietary and other restrictions does not guarantee complete protection from MAOI-induced hypertensive crises. Rare reports of spontaneous hypertension associated with MAOI use have come from several independent sources. Most of these reports involve the use of tranylcypromine, but phenelzine has also been implicated (da Motta and Cordas 1990; Fallon et al. 1988; Kahn 1988; Krause 1989; Linet 1986).

These reactions can range from mild to severe. In the mildest form, the patient may complain of sweating, palpitations, and a mild headache. The most severe form manifests as a hypertensive crisis, with severe headache, increased blood pressure, and possible intracerebral hemorrhage. If a patient experiences a severely painful or unremitting occipital headache when taking an MAOI, he or she should immediately seek medical assessment and monitoring.

If the blood pressure is severely elevated, pharmacological treatment should be instituted. We often recommend that patients purchase a home blood pressure cuff to help distinguish a true hypertensive crisis from more common, and benign, headaches of other etiologies. Currently, the most common treatment for MAOI-induced hypertension is the calcium channel blocker nifedipine. An oral dose of 10 mg of nifedipine often normalizes blood pressure in 1–5 minutes with little risk of overshoot hypotension (Schenk and Remick 1989). If patients are supplied with a prescription for nifedipine in advance, they may administer the medication immediately and then proceed to a hospital for further monitoring and treatment. A drug with α-adrenergic-blocking properties, such as intravenous phentolamine (Regitine) 5 mg or intramuscular chlorpro-

mazine 25–50 mg, may also be administered. Because treatment with phentolamine may be associated with cardiac arrhythmias or severe hypotension, this approach should be carried out only in an emergency room setting (Tollefson 1983).

It is advisable to have patients taking MAOIs carry an identification card as notification to emergency medical personnel that they are currently taking an MAOI. Patients should always carry the list of prohibited foods and medications, and they should be told to notify physicians that they are taking an MAOI before accepting any medication or anesthetic (Tables 27–6 and 27–7). When patients have dental procedures performed, local anesthetics without vasoconstrictors (e.g., epinephrine) must be used.

Serotonin syndrome. The combination of serotonergic drugs, such as the SSRIs, with MAOIs can result in a potentially fatal hypermetabolic reaction, which is often referred to as the *serotonin syndrome*. Affected individuals suffer from the constellation of lethargy, restlessness, confusion, flushing, diaphoresis, tremor, and myoclonic jerks. As the condition progresses, hyperthermia, hypertonicity, myoclonus, and death may occur. The syndrome must be identified as rapidly as possible. Discontinuation of the serotonergic medications is the first step in treatment, followed by emergency medical treatment, as required.

The combination of MAOIs with meperidine (Demerol), and perhaps with other phenylpiperidine analgesics, has also been implicated in fatal reactions that were attributed to the serotonin syndrome. Aspirin, nonsteroidal anti-inflammatory drugs, and acetaminophen should be used for mild-to-moderate pain. Among narcotic agents, codeine and morphine are safe in combination with MAOIs, although doses may need to be lower than usual.

Cardiovascular effects. The MAOIs cause significant hypotension, which is often the dosage-limiting side effect of these drugs. Expansion of the intravascular volume by using salt tablets or fludrocortisone may be an effective treatment. However, some patients manifest peripheral edema, which may mandate a reduction in salt intake. The addition in low dosage of a psychostimulant medication has been shown to alleviate this side effect as well.

Weight gain. MAOIs are associated with a risk of significant weight gain during treatment. It appears that this side effect occurs less frequently with tranylcypromine than it does with phenelzine (Rabkin et al. 1985).

Sexual dysfunction. MAOIs are commonly associated with treatment-emergent sexual dysfunction, including decreased libido, delayed ejaculation, anorgasmia, and impotence. Some patients become tolerant to this side effect over time, but more often the problem persists unless the dose is reduced or another medication is used to counter the sexual side effects. The treatment of sexual side effects is discussed in the section on SSRIs.

Central nervous system effects.   Headache and insomnia are common initial side effects that usually dissipate after the first few weeks of treatment. Patients taking MAOIs commonly experience somnolence in the afternoon, which is often described as an irresistible urge to take a nap. Even a brief nap, for example 20 minutes, will effectively restore alertness. This interesting effect is not related to insomnia or the timing of medication administration, but rather is a more direct chronobiological effect.

Overdose.   The MAOIs fall between the TCAs and the SSRIs in terms of lethality in overdose. Most complications related to MAOI overdose arise from its stimulation of the sympathetic nervous system. MAOIs are most dangerous when patients suffer from hypertensive crises as the result of ingesting foods with high tyramine content.

Drug interactions.   The inhibition of MAO can cause severe interactions with other drugs, as detailed in the earlier sections on hypertensive crisis and the serotonin syndrome. A list of MAOI drug interactions is provided in Table 27–7. In addition, MAOIs may prolong and amplify the sedative effects of medications and alcohol.

MOCLOBEMIDE

Moclobemide (Manerix, Aurorix) is a reversible inhibitor of MAO-A (RIMA). This drug is not available in the United States, but it is available in many other countries, including Mexico and Canada. As discussed earlier in this section, because the RIMAs are reversible and selective, dietary restrictions are not necessary. Controlled trials have indicated that moclobemide is effective in the treatment of depressive disorders and may have a role in refractory depression and social phobia (Fulton and Benfield 1996). When compared with SSRIs, moclobemide has similar tolerability, but it lacks the sexual dysfunction and gastrointestinal side effects.

Moclobemide is initiated at 150 mg bid. Although the suggested therapeutic range is 300–600 mg/day, we and others have found that dosages of 900 mg/day are often required to obtain optimal antidepressant effects.

OTHER ANTIDEPRESSANT TREATMENTS

Several investigators have examined the antidepressant effects of alprazolam (Fawcett et al. 1987; Feighner et al. 1983; Remick et al. 1988; Rickels et al. 1985). These researchers reported positive results when alprazolam was used in high dosages (i.e., in the range of 4.5–6.0 mg/day); however, they were skeptical as to whether a true antidepressant effect can be distinguished from alprazolam's anxiolytic and sedative effects. We share this skepticism. Because dependency and withdrawal effects occur with all benzodiazepines, using alprazolam for the treatment of a chronic illness such as depression should be carefully considered by the clinician and patient and only for highly specific and unusual indications.

Several nondrug methods have been investigated for the treatment of depression. ECT is a highly effective treatment that is fully reviewed later in this chapter. Some patients with mood disorder have recurrent annual depressions, a condition termed *seasonal affective disorder* (SAD). The most common form of this condition involves regularly occurring winter depressions, characterized by the reverse neurovegetative pattern found in atypical depressions (e.g., hypersomnia, hyperphagia with carbohydrate craving, weight gain; Wehr and Rosenthal 1989). Summer depressions have also been reported; these seem to present with a clinical picture consistent with typical depression. Although many patients with SAD have bipolar disorder (usually type II or cyclothymic), there remains some debate among investigators as to whether patients with SAD have exclusively bipolar disorders (Blehar and Rosenthal 1989). There is now strong evidence that patients with SAD who suffer from winter depressions respond to phototherapy. Morning exposure to bright light appears to be the most efficacious (Terman et al. 1989), with current recommendations for a minimum of 2,500 lux for 2 hours each day for 1 week. Doses as high as 10,000 lux for briefer daily periods of exposure may be even more effective. Patients with milder depressions respond best to this form of treatment (Terman et al. 1989).

Partial sleep deprivation may also induce remission in depressed patients (Post et al. 1976). This antidepressant effect is usually transient, but it may be prolonged by concomitant administration of lithium (Baxter et al. 1986).

ISSUES OF TREATMENT

Treatment of Acute Major Depression

The choice of an antidepressant medication is based on factors discussed earlier in this section and outlined in Table 27–2. The initial therapeutic response of the depressed patient to medications may be detected as early as the first week, but it is often delayed by several weeks. Neurovegetative symptoms usually improve before mood improves. The clinician must inform the patient of this latency in therapeutic response, because many patients expect antidepressants to be effective with the first dose. For patients with severe anxiety or insomnia, the concurrent use of a benzodiazepine may be considered. However, we restrict this practice solely to the treatment of depressed patients with marked anxiety, and we discontinue it by tapering the benzodiazepine dosage as the antidepressant begins to exert its therapeutic effect. A patient may experience a return of energy and motivation while still experiencing the subjective symptoms of hopelessness and excessive guilt. For such patients, there may be an increased risk of suicide, because a return of energy in an extremely dysphoric individual may provide the impetus and wherewithal for an act of self-destruction.

A clinical challenge in the evaluation of side effects of antidepressant drugs is to distinguish symptoms of the illness from complaints that are secondary to side effects. Nelson et al. (1984) carefully studied patient complaints before and during treatment with desipramine. Many symptoms that the patients attributed to antidepressant treatment, such as constipation, poor memory or concentration, nausea or vomiting, diarrhea, difficulty sitting still, drowsiness, difficulty with urination, palpitations, urinary frequency, and tremors, were attributable to the illness rather than medication side effects. A great deal of the skill required to treat patients with major depression involves encouraging them to continue treatment despite their perception of early medication side effects. It is important to inform patients that more serious antidepressant side effects subside after the first 2 weeks of treatment.

An adequate trial of antidepressant medication traditionally has been defined as treatment with therapeutic dosages of a drug for a total of 6–8 weeks. On the basis of more recent data, Quitkin et al. (1996) suggested that 4 weeks may be a more clinically meaningful point for reevaluation of treatment. After 4 weeks of antidepressant treatment, the patient can be conceptualized as falling into one of three groups, depending on whether there has been 1) a full response, 2) a partial response, or 3) no response at all. For the fortunate patients who achieve full remission, treatment should continue for a minimum of 4–6 months, or longer when there is a history of a recurrent course (see the subsection on maintenance therapy). If a partial response has been achieved by 4 weeks, a full response may be evident within an additional 2 weeks without further intervention. If there is no response at all, the dosage should be increased, the medication should be changed to another antidepressant, or the therapy should be augmented with another medication (see the subsection on refractory depression). These guidelines are summarized in Figure 27–1.

Treatment of Depression With Psychotic Features

Patients with psychotic depression have been reported to respond to combined treatment with antidepressants and antipsychotics (Nelson and Bowers 1978); they also show a dramatic response to ECT, which is often the treatment of choice in this disorder (Yudofsky 1981). Long-term antipsychotic medications are generally not warranted, but prophylactic antidepressant medication must be continued as in nonpsychotic depression.

Treatment of Bipolar Depression

A history of previous episodes of mania or hypomania should alert the clinician to the diagnosis of bipolar disorder. Because antidepressants can precipitate manic episodes and increase cycling in bipolar patients (Wehr and Goodwin 1979), mood stabilizers (e.g., lithium, valproate) are the appropriate first step in the treatment of a patient with bipolar depression (see the section on mood stabilizers later in this chapter).

Maintenance Treatment of Major Depression

Results from the National Institute of Mental Health (NIMH) collaborative study indicate that antidepressant therapy should not be discontinued before there have been 4–5 symptom-free months (Prien and Kupfer 1986). Most clinicians treat single episodes of depression for a minimum of 6 months. Antidepressants should be continued at the same dosage that resulted in remission of the acute episode. There is strong evidence that relapse is more likely when the antidepressant dosage is lowered from acute treatment levels (Frank et al. 1990).

Unfortunately, depression is often a recurrent disorder. After one episode of depression, there is a 50% chance that the patient will have a second episode; after three episodes, there is a 90% chance of recurrence (Angst 1990). Therefore, longer periods of antidepressant treatment, often called *maintenance treatment*, are warranted to protect against recurrence (NIMH 1985). The value of maintenance antidepressant treatment, with and without psychotherapy, for patients with recurrent depression has been demonstrated by Frank et al. (1990) in an elegant four-arm double-blind placebo-controlled trial (Figure 27–2). Cur-

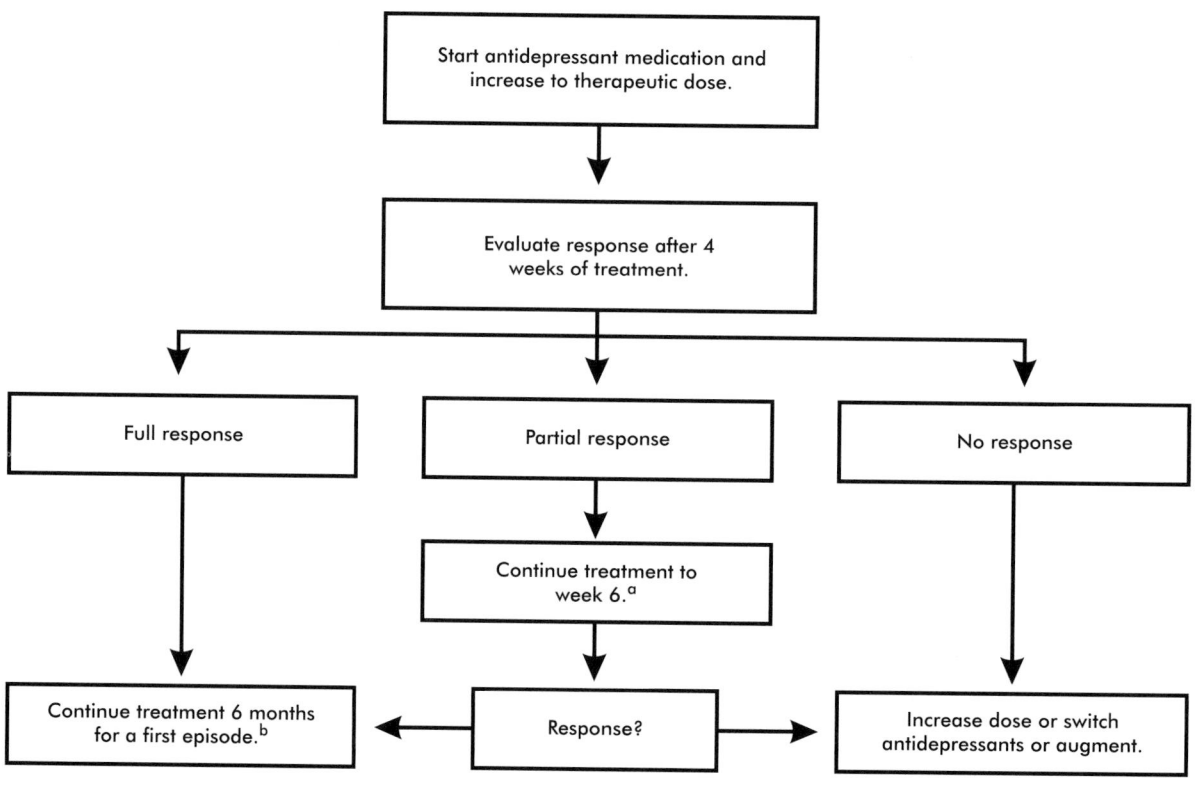

FIGURE 27-1.   Algorithm for the acute treatment of major depression.
[a]If no further response is seen at week 5, it is not necessary to wait until week 6. [b]See text for maintenance treatment guidelines for patients with recurrent depression.

rent World Health Organization guidelines recommend maintenance treatment for patients who have had two or more episodes of major depression within a 5-year period (Coppen et al. 1986). In patients with more than three episodes of depression, long-term prophylaxis is strongly recommended. The duration of treatment is individualized on the basis of the severity and impact of past episodes, and the time between episodes. Some patients may require lifelong antidepressant maintenance treatment. There is no evidence of increased risk associated with long term use of antidepressants.

Antidepressant Discontinuation

Discontinuation of antidepressant medication should be concordant with the guidelines for treatment duration, as outlined earlier. It is advisable to taper the medication while monitoring for signs and symptoms of relapse. Abrupt discontinuation is also more likely to lead to antidepressant discontinuation symptoms, which are often referred to as "withdrawal" symptoms. The occurrence of these symptoms following medication discontinuation does not imply that antidepressants are "addictive."

Abrupt discontinuation of TCAs commonly results in

diarrhea, increased sweating, anxiety, and dizziness—symptoms previously attributed to cholinergic rebound. However, the occurrence of similar symptoms following the discontinuation of many of the newer serotonergic antidepressants suggests that the pathophysiology may be more closely related to changes in serotonin. Among the newer antidepressants, withdrawal symptoms appear to occur most commonly following the discontinuation of short half-life serotonergic drugs (Coupland et al. 1996), such as fluvoxamine, paroxetine, and venlafaxine. Symptoms are discussed by patients as "flulike," including nausea, diarrhea, insomnia, malaise, muscle aches, anxiety, irritability, dizziness, vertigo, and vivid dreams (Coupland et al. 1996). Often and for unknown reasons, patients who experience this constellation of symptoms have transient "electric shock" sensations. This unique symptom is diagnostically useful and strongly suggests to the clinician that the patient is in fact experiencing withdrawal, because the symptom rarely occurs in other conditions such as viral infections or as a side effect of a new medication.

Symptoms usually occur for 1–2 days following the abrupt discontinuation of the medication and subside within 2–3 days. However, in some instances symptoms

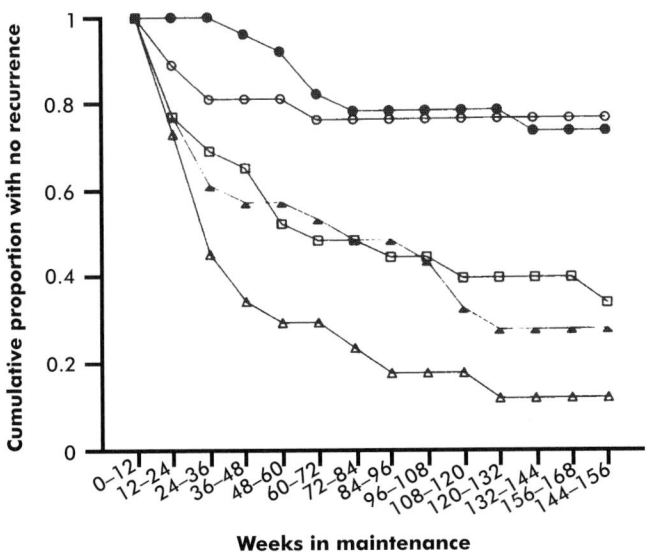

Weeks in maintenance

FIGURE 27–2. Outcome of the maintenance therapies in recurrent depression. 128 patients with a mean of 4 prior episodes participated in the study. Open circles represent group that underwent medication clinic and active imipramine; solid circles, interpersonal psychotherapy and active imipramine; squares, interpersonal psychotherapy alone; solid triangles, interpersonal psychotherapy and placebo; and open triangles, medication clinic and placebo.
Source. Reprinted with permission from Frank E, Kupfer DJ, Perel JM, et al.: "Three-Year Outcomes for Maintenance Therapies in Recurrent Depression." *Arch Gen Psychiatry* 47:1093–1099, 1990.

may also occur during tapering and dose reduction, and they may persist for up to 3 weeks. Restarting the medication with a slower taper may be necessary, although it is often possible to attenuate withdrawal symptoms produced by short-half-life SSRIs by administering one dose of fluoxetine (which has a more prolonged half-life). In our experience, the short-term addition of a benzodiazepine is often helpful.

Treatment of Refractory Depression

Careful review of the clinical history and response to previous treatment often reveals that patients in whom depression has been refractory to standard antidepressant treatment have had an inadequate therapeutic trial with the antidepressant (Lydiard 1985) or have been noncompliant with the medication. Failure to complete an adequate therapeutic trial with an antidepressant drug does not constitute a depression that is resistant to pharmacotherapy. In another pseudorefractory presentation, pa-

tients report a history of robust but short-lived responses to several antidepressants. This patient may be manifesting a medication-induced rapid-cycling course. Mild episodes of hypomania during the course of treatment may be overlooked, especially in a high-functioning, productive patient with a premorbid history of hyperthymic personality, which is defined as a chronic state of mild hypomania. Kukopoulos et al. (1983) and Akiskal (1992) claimed that hyperthymia and mild cyclothymia may be predictors of a medication-induced rapid-cycling course and suggested that these patients are at the milder end of a bipolar spectrum. Mixed mood states may ultimately develop if the patient continues taking antidepressants, and the diagnosis of a refractory, agitated depression may be made erroneously. In these cases, treatment with a mood stabilizer (discussed later in this chapter) is indicated.

For patients with true nonresponse and for those who achieve only partial response, treatment options include switching to another antidepressant and using an augmentation strategy. Augmentation involves the concurrent use of two antidepressants or the use of a single antidepressant in combination with another agent, such as lithium, thyroid hormone, or a psychostimulant. Whether to switch antidepressants or augment depends on the severity of illness, side effects of the current medication, and the patient's willingness to take more than one medication. For example, if a patient's illness is significantly interfering with his or her ability to function such that employment is compromised, and he or she has minimal medication side effects, augmentation should be considered because this often results in a quicker response. On the other hand, a patient with a milder illness, significant side effects of the current medication, and a general uneasiness about taking medication will probably be better off if the medication is switched to a different, single antidepressant.

Of the augmentation strategies, lithium augmentation has received the most attention. Since De Montigny and colleagues first reported successful antidepressant treatment with adjunctive lithium in 1981, there have been many reports of patients who failed to respond to TCA or SSRI treatment alone but whose depressions improved when the antidepressant was combined with lithium (Dinan and Barry 1989; Ontiveros et al. 1991; Thase et al. 1989). Although some of these patients manifested a rapid and dramatic response when lithium was added to their antidepressant regimen, improvement may require several weeks. Patients often respond to dosages of lithium lower than are used for the treatment of bipolar disorder. We typically start with 600 mg at bedtime. If there is no response after 2 weeks, the dosage should be increased as tolerated.

Thyroid supplementation has received a more mixed

endorsement in the scientific literature. Goodwin et al. (1982) performed the first double-blind study that found triiodothyronine (T_3) to be a useful adjunct in former nonresponders. However, Gitlin et al. (1987), in a follow-up study, found no benefit to this approach. A study by Joffe (1988) reported that patients who did respond to the addition of T_3 were less likely to benefit from adjunctive lithium, and vice versa. This double-blind, placebo-controlled trial found a 50% response rate for both lithium and T_3 augmentation. For unclear reasons, it appears that T_3 is more effective than T_4 as an augmenting agent in unipolar depression (Joffe and Singer 1990).

The use of more than one antidepressant for patients with refractory depression is potentially beneficial. SSRI-TCA combinations have been reported to be effective for patients who fail to respond to monotherapy and, perhaps, to cause a more rapid antidepressant effect (Nelson et al. 1991; Weilburg et al. 1989). Some SSRIs can cause tricyclic levels in the blood to rise (Aranow et al. 1989; Downs et al. 1989), but this effect is not likely to account for the synergism between the two antidepressants. However, because of this pharmacokinetic interaction, augmentation of the TCA dose should be reduced to achieve the same blood levels. Although there are few systematic data, other antidepressant combinations are commonly used in clinical practice to treat refractory depression. The principle of combining two antidepressants is to choose agents that have different mechanisms of action. For example, it makes little sense to combine two different SSRIs. However, the combination of an SSRI with mirtazapine or bupropion may provide mechanistic synergy. When combining antidepressants, it is important first to ensure that the patient has had an adequate trial of a single agent and to be aware of possible drug interactions or additive side effects.

Despite concerns about severe reactions that may occur with concomitant treatment with tricyclic antidepressants and MAOIs, the combination may be safely prescribed provided specific precautions are taken. It has been firmly established that it is hazardous to add a TCA to ongoing MAOI therapy. However, there are now many reports of the safe addition of an MAOI to ongoing treatment with a TCA (Kahn et al. 1989; for a review, see Pande et al. 1991). There is some evidence that such a combination may prove effective in depressed patients who have failed monotherapy with a TCA and an SSRI (Schmauss et al. 1988; White and Simpson 1981). There are two general strategies for combined therapy with MAOIs: 1) the MAOI is added to the TCA, or 2) the two drugs are begun concurrently. If the MAOI is to be added, the TCA should be raised, as usual, to a therapeutic level. The MAOI should be

added in small increments over protracted periods of time until a therapeutic response occurs or until side effects intervene. When the MAOIs and TCAs are initiated concurrently, we also recommend that gradual adjustments in small increments be made until an effect is obtained. If the patient responds, the clinician eventually may wish to determine whether it is the combined therapy or the MAOI alone that is responsible for the improvement. This can be accomplished by gradually reducing the TCA dose; if the depressive symptoms reappear, the combined treatment is, indeed, necessary. However, because of the risk of the serotonin syndrome, TCAs with strong serotonin reuptake inhibition, especially clomipramine, should be avoided in combination with MAOIs (Marley and Wozniak 1984). This caveat must be extended to the entire class of SSRIs and venlafaxine, all of which must never be administered together with an MAOI.

Stimulants such as amphetamine and methylphenidate have been used to treat depression for many years. Stimulants should not be used as monotherapy, except perhaps in geriatric patients with prominent apathy, medically ill patients with depression, or patients with poststroke depression (Lingam et al. 1988). However, psychostimulants are useful for augmentation of antidepressants in the treatment of refractory depression and they are generally safe, even for most patients with cardiac disorders. Fawcett et al. (1991) reported the successful use of stimulant-MAOI combinations among a group of patients who were nonresponders to various other treatments, including ECT. Only 1 of their 32 patients could not tolerate the combination because of hypertensive side effects.

Switching Antidepressants

Particular care must be exercised in switching patients from an MAOI to other antidepressant classes. For patients who have completed an MAOI trial without therapeutic response, other antidepressants should not be started until 14 days after the original MAOI has been discontinued. Equal care is required when switching from most other antidepressant to an MAOI. A time period equal to five times the half-life of the drug, including active metabolites, is required between stopping other antidepressant medications and starting an MAOI. However, as noted previously, MAOIs may be safely begun, with the appropriate precautions, while a patient continues taking certain of the TCAs (Kahn et al. 1989).

Switching between other antidepressants is less problematic. Current practice is to discontinue the first medication before starting the second one. There is no need for a medication-free period if neither medication is a MAOI.

However, some patients report increased side effects and anxiety when switching from fluoxetine to nefazodone. This reaction is most likely because fluoxetine and its active metabolite norfluoxetine inhibit cytochrome P450 2D6, which metabolizes a metabolite of nefazodone, which is known to be anxiogenic. Therefore, it may be prudent to wait 1–2 weeks between the discontinuation of fluoxetine and the start of nefazodone.

A 2-week interval is also recommended when switching from phenelzine to tranylcypromine because tranylcypromine is an amphetamine derivative. Theoretically, switching from tranylcypromine, which has a short half-life, to phenelzine should not require as prolonged a waiting period. A recent case series published by Szuba et al. (1997) suggested that some patients can be switched from one MAOI to another without a 14-day washout. The authors emphasized that this strategy should be used only when clinically essential and with close monitoring.

ANXIOLYTICS, SEDATIVES, AND HYPNOTICS

OVERVIEW

Anxiety and insomnia are prevalent symptoms with multiple etiologies. Effective treatments are available, but they vary by diagnosis; in most instances, the best course of action is to treat the underlying disorder rather than reflexively instituting a nonspecific anxiolytic. For example, a patient who has anxiety symptoms related to paranoid delusions should be treated with an antipsychotic medication, not with an anxiolytic. Likewise, patients with panic disorder, obsessive-compulsive disorder, or major depression should receive medications indicated for those disorders. In these cases, anxiety may be a target symptom, one of the group of target symptoms of the underlying disorder.

In some cases, anxiolytics serve a transitional purpose. Consider a patient with acute-onset panic disorder, severe anticipatory anxiety, and a family history of depression. An antidepressant medication that also has antipanic effects may be the optimal treatment, but it will not help the patient for several weeks, during which time there is a risk of progression to agoraphobia. For this patient we recommend starting the antidepressant and also targeting acute symptom relief with a benzodiazepine. After 4 weeks, the benzodiazepine should be slowly tapered so that the patient is controlled with the antidepressant alone.

In this section we discuss the pharmacology of medications that are classified as anxiolytic, sedative, or hypnotic,

primarily the benzodiazepines, buspirone, and zolpidem; subsequently, we present diagnosis-specific treatment guidelines as outlined in Table 27–8. The commonly used anxiolytics and hypnotics, together with their usual dosages, are shown in Table 27–9. In addition, many antidepressant medications are effective in the treatment of anxiety disorders. The pharmacology of the antidepressants was discussed in the previous section; their clinical use in anxiety disorders is included in the diagnosis-specific subsections that follow.

BENZODIAZEPINES

Mechanisms of Action

Benzodiazepines facilitate the inhibitory properties of γ-aminobutyric acid (GABA), the major inhibitory neurotransmitter in the brain (reviewed by Tallman et al. 1980). The benzodiazepine receptor is a subtype of the $GABA_A$ receptor. Activation of the benzodiazepine receptor facilitates the action of endogenous GABA, which results in the opening of chloride ion channels and a decrease in neuronal excitability. Benzodiazepines act rapidly because ion channels can open and close relatively quickly, in contrast to the slower onset of action that occurs when a drug acts via a metabotropic receptor and the resultant cascade of G proteins, second messengers, and subsequent indirect effects.

Indications and Efficacy

Benzodiazepines are highly effective anxiolytics and sedatives; they also possess muscle relaxant and anticonvulsant properties. Benzodiazepines effectively treat both acute

TABLE 27–8. **Medications of choice for specific anxiety disorders**

Diagnosis	Medication
Generalized anxiety disorder	Buspirone, benzodiazepines, antidepressants
Obsessive-compulsive disorder	Clomipramine, SSRIs
Panic disorder	SSRIs, TCAs, MAOIs, benzodiazepines, alprazolam, clonazepam
Performance anxiety	β-Blockers, benzodiazepines
Social phobia	SSRIs, MAOIs, benzodiazepines, buspirone

Note. MAOI = monoamine oxidase inhibitor; SSRI = selective serotonin reuptake inhibitor; TCA = tricyclic antidepressant.

TABLE 27-9. Commonly used anxiolytic and hypnotic medications

Generic (trade) name	Single dosage (mg)	Usual therapeutic dosage (mg/day)	Approximate dose equivalent (mg)	Methods of administration and supplied form	Approximate elimination half-life, including metabolites[a]	Lipophilicity
Benzodiazepines						
Alprazolam (Xanax and generics)	0.25–1	1–4	0.5	po: 0.25/0.5 mg	12 hours	0.54
Chlordiazepoxide (Librium and generics)	5–25	15–100	10	po: 5/10/25 mg; iv, im[b]	1–4 days	?
Clonazepam (Klonopin)	0.5–2	1–4	0.25	po: 0.5/2 mg	1–2 days	0.28
Clorazepate (Tranxene and generics)	3.75–22.5	15–60	7.5	po: 3.75/7.5/30 mg	2–4 days	0.79
Diazepam (Valium and generics)	2–10	4–40	5	po: 2/5/10 mg; iv, im[b]	2–4 days	1.00
Lorazepam (Ativan and generics)	0.5–2	1–6	1	po, s/l: 0.5/1/2 mg; iv, im[b]	12 hours	0.48
Oxazepam (Serax and generics)	10–30	30–120	15	po: 10/15/30 mg	12 hours	0.45
Nonbenzodiazepines						
Buspirone (BuSpar)	10–30	30–60	N/A	po: 5/10/15 mg	2–3 hours	N/A

[a]The clinical duration of action for the benzodiazepines does not correlate with the elimination half-life. See text for discussion. [b]Lorazepam im is well absorbed. We do not recommend chlordiazepoxide or diazepam im.

Source. Adapted with permission from Teboul and Chouinard 1990.

and chronic generalized anxiety (Elie and Lamontagne 1985; Greenblatt et al. 1983; Rickels et al. 1983, 1986) and panic disorder. The high-potency benzodiazepines alprazolam and clonazepam have received more attention as antipanic agents (Tesar 1990; Tesar et al. 1991), but double-bind studies have also confirmed the efficacy of diazepam (Dunner et al. 1986) and lorazepam (Charney and Woods 1989) in the treatment of panic disorder. Although only a few benzodiazepines have specific, FDA-approved indications for the treatment of insomnia, almost all benzodiazepines may be used for this purpose. Benzodiazepines are most clearly valuable as hypnotics in the general hospital setting, where high levels of sensory stimulation, pain, and acute stress may interfere with sleep. The safe, effective, and time-limited use of benzodiazepine hypnotics may, in fact, prevent chronic sleep difficulties from taking hold (NIMH Consensus Development Conference 1984). Benzodiazepines are also used to treat akathisia and catatonia and as an adjunct in the treatment of acute mania.

Because alcohol and barbiturates also act, in part, via the $GABA_A$- receptor-mediated chloride ion channel, benzodiazepines exhibit cross-tolerance with these substances. As such, benzodiazepines are used frequently for the treatment of alcohol or barbiturate withdrawal and detoxification. Alcohol and barbiturates are more dangerous than benzodiazepines because at high doses they can act directly at the chloride ion channel. In contrast, benzodiazepines have no direct effect on the ion channel; the effects of benzodiazepines are limited by the amount of endogenous GABA.

Three of the benzodiazepines are indicated for use in the control of seizure disorders. Diazepam is rapidly effective in the control of status epilepticus when administered intravenously. Clonazepam, either alone or in addition to other anticonvulsants, is indicated for control of absence, myoclonic, and atonic seizures. Clorazepate is indicated as adjunctive therapy for the control of grand mal and other seizure disorders. Intravenous lorazepam has gained acceptance as the treatment of choice for status epilepticus; its pharmacokinetic and pharmacodynamic properties result in a more prolonged anticonvulsant effect than is found with intravenous diazepam, which was formerly the standard treatment (Leppik et al. 1983).

Choice of Benzodiazepine

In equipotent doses, all benzodiazepines have similar effects. The choice among benzodiazepines is generally based on differences in half-life, rapidity of onset, metabolism, and potency. One frequently misunderstood issue is the relationship between pharmacokinetic half-life and pharmacodynamic effect. The pharmacodynamics (i.e., the effects of the drug on the CNS) depend on several factors, including pharmacokinetic half-life, affinity of the drug for the benzodiazepine receptor, and lipid solubility of the drug. For example, lorazepam has a higher binding affinity for the benzodiazepine receptor than does diazepam (Jack et al. 1982); therefore, lorazepam binds to the receptor for a longer time. Lipid solubility is another important factor in determining pharmacodynamic effects of benzodiazepines. A drug that is highly lipid soluble will rapidly distribute to fat tissues, including those within the brain, whereas a drug with a lower lipid solubility will reach the brain more slowly but maintain brain levels longer. Therefore, although diazepam (with high lipid solubility) has a more rapid onset of action than lorazepam (with moderate lipid solubility), the acute therapeutic effects will not last as long as those of lorazepam. When compared with diazepam, a single dose of lorazepam takes longer to produce sedation, but this sedation persists longer (Ellinwood et al. 1985). This occurs despite the fact that lorazepam has a markedly briefer pharmacokinetic half-life than does diazepam and its metabolites (8 hours vs. 48 hours, respectively).

The metabolism of benzodiazepines also is important in the choice of the specific therapeutic agent. For example, diazepam is metabolized in the liver to desmethyldiazepam, a metabolite with a long half-life. Lorazepam and oxazepam are not converted to active metabolites by the liver. Therefore, for patients with hepatic dysfunction, lorazepam and oxazepam are clinically indicated for relief of anxiety because their elimination from the body will not be significantly affected (Abernethy et al. 1984).

Sedative effects of diazepam have been demonstrated to persist for up to 2 weeks following discontinuation, after only 14 days of administration of diazepam 3 mg tid (Salzman et al. 1983). For patients with brain disorders and for elderly patients, benzodiazepines that are brief acting and devoid of active metabolites are usually indicated. As in all psychotropic medications, the most critical issue is that the lowest effective doses should be used in elderly patients, with careful and continuous monitoring of side effects.

Risks, Side Effects, and Their Management

Sedation and impairment of performance. Benzodiazepine-induced sedation may be considered either a therapeutic action or a side effect. Residual daytime somnolence is a function of two variables: drug half-life and dosage (Roth and Roehrs 1992). With longer acting agents, such as flurazepam and quazepam, a morning-after hang-

over is common, although some tolerance to this effect may develop with time. On the other hand, any benzodiazepine, short or long acting, can cause daytime drowsiness if the nighttime dose is too great. In general, it is clinically unclear and theoretically uncertain whether or not sedation is a desirable component of anxiolytic activity. Many patients both expect and desire some degree of sedation when they are intensely anxious. Anxious patients who have been treated chronically with benzodiazepines rarely complain about daytime sedation, even when compared with drug-free anxious subjects (Lucki et al. 1986).

Impairment of performance in sensitive psychomotor tests has been well documented after the administration of benzodiazepines. Diazepam, administered in a dosage of 10 mg tid, impaired driving skills in anxious patients during the first weeks of treatment (Linnoila et al. 1983). Lucki et al. (1986) found no impairment in a series of cognitive tasks in a group of anxious patients who had been taking benzodiazepines for an average of 5 years. Whether or not sedation is desired, patients must be warned that driving, engaging in dangerous physical activities, and using hazardous machinery should be avoided during the acute stages, and possibly during the later stages, of treatment with benzodiazepines.

Dependence, withdrawal, and rebound effects. Concerns about physical and psychological dependence on benzodiazepines are frequently raised by patients and often affect a clinician's choice of treatment. On the basis of the criterion of self-reinforcement, however, most of the benzodiazepines, with the possible exception of diazepam, have low abuse potential when properly prescribed and supervised (American Psychiatric Association 1990; Sellers et al. 1992). Illicit street traffic in such potent agents as alprazolam and triazolam has remained low, possibly because the rapidly developing sedation produced by these drugs interferes with the desired euphoriant effects (Mendelson 1992). Physical dependence often occurs when benzodiazepines are taken in higher than usual dosages or for prolonged periods of time (Busto et al. 1986; Schopf 1983; Tyrer et al. 1983).

If benzodiazepines are discontinued precipitously, withdrawal effects that include hyperpyrexia, seizures, psychosis, and even death may occur. Despite various methodological shortcomings, several studies also suggest that physical dependence may occur even when benzodiazepines are taken in usual clinical doses for prolonged periods beyond several weeks and that the symptoms of withdrawal may arise even when drug discontinuation is not abrupt (Ashton 1991; Noyes et al. 1988). Signs and symptoms of withdrawal may include tachycardia, increased blood pressure, muscle cramps, anxiety, insomnia, panic attacks, impairment of memory and concentration, and perceptual disturbances. In addition, withdrawal-related derealization, hallucinations, and other psychotic symptoms have been reported. These withdrawal symptoms may begin as soon as the day after discontinuation of benzodiazepines and may continue for weeks to months. There is evidence that withdrawal reactions peak more rapidly and more intensely with the benzodiazepines that have a briefer half-life (Busto et al. 1986). These withdrawal effects are rapidly reversed with the readministration of benzodiazepines. Although it is generally believed that there is cross-tolerance for all benzodiazepines, there has been a report of withdrawal symptoms from alprazolam that were not reversed with diazepam (Zipursky et al. 1985).

Rebound anxiety is defined as the return, on discontinuation of a benzodiazepine, of the anxiety signs and symptoms with greater intensity than existed before treatment. For this diagnosis, accurate documentation of specific symptoms and operationalized measures of the severity of preexisting anxiety are required. Fontaine et al. (1984) treated patients with generalized anxiety disorder for 4 weeks either with diazepam (a benzodiazepine with a long half-life) in a dosage of 15 mg/day or with placebo. After this time, both the drug and the placebo were withdrawn either abruptly or gradually. The patients who experienced abrupt withdrawal from diazepam had a 10% increase in anxiety, whereas no patient on the gradual withdrawal schedule or with placebo treatment had increased anxiety. Muscle spasms, insomnia, gastric symptoms, and agitation were documented in the benzodiazepine withdrawal group compared with the placebo group. Fewer cases of rebound anxiety were seen with diazepam than with bromazepam (which has a briefer half-life than diazepam).

Kales and Kales (1983) described rebound insomnia occurring after abrupt withdrawal of benzodiazepine drugs with relatively rapid elimination rates, such as triazolam. For patients with panic disorder treated with alprazolam, tapering and discontinuation of the medication may be associated with significant rebound anxiety and panic (Pecknold and Swinson 1986). Fyer et al. (1987) showed that significant withdrawal effects may occur when alprazolam, administered in a dosage of 2.5–8.0 mg/day for 12–47 weeks, is tapered at a rate of 10% every 3 days. In addition, there have been several reports of seizures occurring after the sudden discontinuation of alprazolam (Breier et al. 1984; Levy 1984). Kales et al. (1986) found no rebound effects with the discontinuation of the long-acting benzodiazepines flurazepam and quazepam. However, the patients were observed for only 15 days, which may be an insufficient length of time. In another study, the discontinuation of flurazepam led to rebound insomnia that occurred only during the second week of observation, whereas the rebound after triazolam discontinuation came within 2 days (Mitler et al. 1984).

A general principle for most psychoactive medications is that discontinuation should be accomplished gradually. For patients treated with benzodiazepines for longer than 2–3 months, we suggest that the dosage be decreased by approximately 10% per week. Therefore, for a patient receiving 4 mg/day of alprazolam, the dosage should be tapered by 0.5 mg/week for 8 weeks. The last few dosage levels may be the most difficult to discontinue, and the patient will require increased attention and support from the physician during this time.

Memory impairment.   Intravenous use of the benzodiazepines is associated with significant anterograde amnesia (Dixon et al. 1984; Reitan et al. 1986). For midazolam, diazepam, and lorazepam, this phenomenon may have clinical benefits, because amnesia for surgical or other invasive therapeutic procedures is often desired. Amnesia appears to be mediated through the central benzodiazepine receptor; therefore, it may occur with any benzodiazepine (Lister 1985). In contrast to use in anesthesia, when benzodiazepines are used to treat insomnia or anxiety, amnesia may be a serious liability. Several studies have documented the deleterious effects on memory of oral benzodiazepines (Angus and Romney 1984; Mac et al. 1985). Tolerance to these amnestic effects may not develop. The degree of anterograde amnesia appears to be related to dosage, and the amnesia may occur in the first several hours after each dose of benzodiazepine is taken, even after repeated use (Lucki et al. 1986). There is some evidence, however, that the disruption of memory may be, at least in part, a retrograde effect produced by the onset of sleep itself (Roth et al. 1980); for example, benzodiazepine doses too low to induce sleep are less likely to cause amnestic effects (Roth et al. 1984).

The newer, briefer acting benzodiazepines have been associated in some reports with a greater tendency to produce memory impairments (Roth et al. 1980), although a review of controlled studies does not seem to bear this out (Rothschild 1992). Following a 0.5-mg dose of triazolam, several individuals found themselves unable to recall a whole series of complex, though routine, daily activities (Ewing et al. 1988; Morris and Estes 1987).

Disinhibition and dyscontrol.   An area of controversy is the allegation that benzodiazepines may, in some instances, cause behavior disinhibition, leading to acts of aggression (Medawarn and Rassaby 1991; Regestein and Reich 1985). Greenblatt et al. (1984), in their review of double-blind, controlled studies of triazolam and flurazepam that included more than 5,400 patients, found no reports of bizarre, disinhibitory reactions. However, there is a long history of anecdotal reports suggesting that many of the benzodiazepines can cause paradoxical anger and behavioral disinhibition that is dose related (see review by Rothschild 1992). A history of hostility, impulsivity, or borderline or antisocial personality disorder has been implicated as a potential predictor of this reaction. In light of the heightened attention focused on triazolam and the resulting potential for a significant reporting bias, the increase in anecdotal reports citing this particular agent is difficult to interpret. At the present time, some caution should be exercised when benzodiazepines are prescribed to patients with a history of poor impulse control and aggression (see section on the treatment of aggression later in this chapter); this possibility should be communicated to patients and documented in the medical record.

Overdose. Benzodiazepines are remarkably safe when taken in overdose. Dangerous effects occur when the overdose includes several sedative drugs, especially when alcohol is included, because of synergistic effects at the chloride ion site and resultant membrane hyperpolarization. In an extensive review by Greenblatt et al. (1977a), no patient who suffered an overdose of benzodiazepines alone became seriously ill or had serious complications. When the overdose occurred in combination with other drugs, however, the complications depended on the type and quantity of the nonbenzodiazepines. Finkle and colleagues (1979) essentially confirmed these results by finding that in only 2 of 1,239 overdoses with benzodiazepines were the deaths associated with the benzodiazepine alone.

The diagnosis of benzodiazepine overdose is usually made on the basis of questioning by the clinician of the patient, family, or friends concerning what drugs were ingested. The result is confirmed by physical examination revealing signs and symptoms of toxicity with a CNS depressant (e.g., sedation, mental confusion, reduced respiration) and by either urine or blood drug screens. Because the standard urine drug screen assay may not detect the presence of many commonly prescribed benzodiazepines, including lorazepam, alprazolam, clonazepam, temazepam, and triazolam, the clinician should actively research the presence and accuracy of these tests in the laboratory that he or she uses. There now exists a safe and effective benzodiazepine antagonist, flumazenil, which may be used via intravenous injection in an emergency setting to reverse the effects of any potential overdose with a benzodiazepine (Votey et al. 1991). However, medical management of a patient who has had an overdose often still requires physical supportive measures, such as ensuring proper respiratory function.

Drug interactions. Most sedative drugs, including narcotics and alcohol, potentiate the sedative effects of benzodiazepines. In addition, medications that inhibit hepatic cytochrome P450 3A3/4, as discussed later in this chapter, increase blood levels and hence side effects of clonazepam, alprazolam, midazolam, and triazolam. Lorazepam, oxazepam, and temazepam are not dependent on hepatic enzymes for metabolism and therefore are not affected by hepatic disease or the inhibition of hepatic enzymes.

Use in pregnancy. Anxiolytics, like most medications, should be avoided during pregnancy or breast-feeding when possible. Although there have been concerns that benzodiazepines, when ingested during the first trimester of pregnancy, may increase the risk of the development of cleft palate, this has not been substantiated in controlled studies (Rosenberg et al. 1983; Shiono and Mills 1983).

BUSPIRONE

The azapirones are agonists at the 5-HT$_{1A}$ receptors. Unlike benzodiazepines and barbiturates, they do not interact with the GABA receptor or directly with chloride ion channels. As such, these medications do not produce sedation, interact with alcohol, impair psychomotor performance, or pose a risk of abuse. There is no cross-tolerance between benzodiazepines and azapirones; it is important to bear in mind that these classes of medication are not interchangeable. Like the antidepressants, azapirones have a relatively slow onset of action. Buspirone (BuSpar) is the only azapirone currently available in the United States.

Mechanism of Action

The anxiolytic effect of the azapirones is the result of a selective stimulation of the 5-HT$_{1A}$ receptor. Acute administration suppresses neuronal firing in the dorsal raphe through autoreceptor stimulation. Chronic administration desensitizes presynaptic, but not postsynaptic, 5-HT$_{1A}$ receptors (Suranyi-Cadotte et al. 1990).

Indications and Efficacy

Buspirone is effective in the treatment of generalized anxiety; although it has a longer onset of action, its efficacy is not statistically different from that of the benzodiazepines

(Cohn and Wilcox 1986; Goldberg and Finnerty 1979). Despite its successes in the treatment of generalized anxiety disorder, however, buspirone does not appear to be effective in the treatment of panic attacks (Sheehan et al. 1990), except perhaps in an auxiliary role for the treatment of anticipatory anxiety (Gastfried and Rosenbaum 1989). Buspirone is also used as an augmenting agent in the treatment of obsessive-compulsive disorder (Harvey and Balon 1995; Laird 1996) and depression (Rickels et al. 1988; Sramek et al. 1996), and there is some evidence that buspirone may be an effective treatment for social phobia (Munjack et al. 1991; Schneier et al. 1992).

Buspirone is available for oral administration in 5-, 10-, or 15-mg tablets. The 15-mg tablets are scored for division into bisections or trisections. We recommend an initial dosage of 15 mg bid. The dosage may be increased by 5 mg every 2–3 days as needed to achieve optimal therapeutic response. The usual recommended maximum daily dosage is 60 mg, but many patients safely tolerate and benefit from 90 mg/day. Because buspirone is metabolized by the liver and excreted by the kidneys, it should not be administered to patients with severe hepatic or renal impairment.

Side Effects

The side effects that are more common with buspirone than with the benzodiazepines are nausea, headache, nervousness, insomnia, dizziness, and lightheadedness (Rakel 1990). Restlessness has also been reported, which theoretically may be related to the activity of this drug at the dopamine receptor. Buspirone does not appear to interact with alcohol or other CNS depressants to increase sedation and motor impairment (Moskowitz and Smiley 1982). When administered to subjects who had histories of recreational sedative abuse, buspirone showed no abuse potential (Cole et al. 1982), a finding confirmed by subsequent studies (Sellers et al. 1992). As mentioned previously, buspirone is not sedating and does not impair mechanical performance, such as driving (Moskowitz and Smiley 1982). However, because side effects in any individual patient cannot be predicted, these activities should be avoided during the initial stages of buspirone therapy.

Drug Interactions

Buspirone should not be administered in combination with an MAOI.

Overdose

No fatal outcomes of buspirone overdose have been reported. However, overdose of buspirone with other drugs may result in more serious outcomes.

ZOLPIDEM

Mechanism of Action

Zolpidem (Ambien) is an imidazopyridine hypnotic. Although it is not a benzodiazepine, it acts selectively at the omega-1 subtype of the central benzodiazepine receptor. This selectivity is hypothesized to be associated with a lower risk of dependence (as reviewed by Schoch et al. 1993).

Indications

Zolpidem is a short-acting hypnotic with established efficacy in inducing and maintaining sleep. Unlike the benzodiazepines, zolpidem does not appear to have significant anxiolytic, muscle relaxant, or anticonvulsant properties. Owing to the short half-life of this drug, most patients report minimal daytime sedation.

Clinical Use

Zolpidem is available in 5- and 10-mg tablets for oral administration. The maximum recommended dosage for adults is 10 mg/day, administered at night. The initial dosage for elderly persons should not exceed 5 mg. With a half-life of 2.5 hours, daytime sedation is minimal. Sedative effects generally occur after 20–30 minutes. Zolpidem should be administered immediately before retiring. Caution is advised in patients with hepatic dysfunction. In general, hypnotics should be limited to short-term use, with reevaluation for more extended therapy (see discussion of the treatment of insomnia later in this section).

Risks, Side Effects, and Their Management

In general the side effects of zolpidem are similar to those of the short-acting benzodiazepines. In several controlled studies, no difference was reported between triazolam and zolpidem regarding amnestic effects and performance impairment (Berlin et al. 1993; Roehrs et al. 1994; Rush and Griffiths 1996; Wesensten et al. 1995). However, when it was compared to triazolam in a double-blind placebo-controlled study, zolpidem was found to be less likely to produce rebound insomnia when discontinued after 27 days of use (Monti et al. 1994). Although they are rare, there are reports of new-onset psychotic symptoms that resolved following discontinuation of zolpidem (Markowitz and Brewerton 1996; van Puijenbroek et al. 1996). In general, side effects of zolpidem, most commonly CNS and gastrointestinal symptoms, are dose dependent. Zolpidem should not be considered free of abuse potential.

Overdose.   Zolpidem appears to be nonfatal in overdose. However, overdoses involving zolpidem in combination with other CNS-depressant agents pose a greater risk. Recommended treatment consists of general symptomatic and supportive measures including gastric lavage. Use of flumazenil may be helpful.

Drug interactions.   Research is limited in this area, but any drug with CNS-depressant effects could potentially enhance the CNS-depressant effects of zolpidem via pharmacodynamic interactions. In addition, zolpidem is primarily metabolized by cytochrome P450 3A3/4 (Pichard et al. 1995), and inhibitors of this enzyme (discussed later in this chapter) may increase zolpidem blood levels and toxicity.

PHARMACOTHERAPY OF GENERALIZED ANXIETY DISORDER

Generalized anxiety disorder can be treated with benzodiazepines, buspirone, and certain of the antidepressants. Some of these agents are compared in Table 27–10.

Benzodiazepines have the advantage of being rapidly effective but the obvious disadvantages of abuse potential and sedation. Although benzodiazepines are indicated for relatively short-term use only (i.e., 1–2 months), they are, in general, safe and effective for long-term use for the minority of patients who require such medication (Greenblatt et al. 1983; Rickels et al. 1983). Whereas tolerance to sedation often develops, the same is not true of the anxiolytic effects of these agents. All benzodiazepines indicated for the treatment of anxiety are equally efficacious. The choice of a specific agent usually depends on the pharmacokinetics and pharmacodynamics of the drug. Some patients respond to extremely low dosages, such as 0.125 mg

of alprazolam bid, although mean dosages are higher. When using benzodiazepines to treat anxiety, we advocate starting with 0.25 mg bid or tid of alprazolam or an equivalent dosage of another benzodiazepine (Table 27–9) and then titrating according to anxiolysis versus sedation. Benzodiazepines should be avoided in patients with a history of recent and/or significant substance abuse, and all patients should be advised to take their first dose at home in a situation that would not be dangerous in the event of greater than expected sedation.

Buspirone does not cause the sedative or abuse problems of the benzodiazepines, but some clinicians have observed that the anxiolytic properties do not appear to be as potent as those of the benzodiazepines, particularly in patients who have previously received a benzodiazepine (Schweizer et al. 1986). Because buspirone is not sedating (Seidel et al. 1985) and has no psychomotor effects, it has a distinct advantage over the benzodiazepines when optimal alertness and motor performance are necessary. Buspirone has been assessed in subjects with histories of recreational sedative abuse (Cole et al. 1982) and in recently detoxified alcoholic patients (Griffith et al. 1986); in these groups, it demonstrated no abuse potential. Response to buspirone occurs in approximately 2–4 weeks. There is also evidence that the azapirones have modest antidepressant effects, perhaps at high doses (Jenkins et al. 1990; Lucki 1991). Buspirone does not exhibit cross-tolerance with benzodiazepines and other sedative/hypnotic drugs such as alcohol, barbiturates, and chloral hydrate. Therefore, buspirone does not suppress benzodiazepine withdrawal symptoms (Lader and Olajide 1987). For anxious patients treated with a benzodiazepine who require a switch to buspirone, the benzodiazepine must be tapered gradually to avoid withdrawal symptoms, despite the fact that the patient is receiving buspirone.

TABLE 27–10. **Comparison of benzodiazepines, buspirone, and SSRIs**

Characteristic	BZDs	Buspirone	SSRIs
Therapeutic effect of single dose	Yes	No	No
Time to full therapeutic action	Days	Weeks	Weeks
Sedation	Yes	No	No
Dependence liability	Yes	No	No
Impairs performance	Yes	No	No
Suppresses sedative withdrawal symptoms	Yes	No	No
Once-a-day dosing	No	No	Yes
Treats comorbid depression	No	No	Yes
Side effects	Sedation, memory impairment	Restlessness, nervousness	Gastrointestinal, sexual dysfunction

Note. BZD = benzodiazepines; SSRI = selective serotonin reuptake inhibitors.

Patients with generalized anxiety disorder also respond to antidepressant treatment (Hoehn-Saric et al. 1988; Kahn et al. 1986). In studies comparing benzodiazepines, MAOIs, SSRIs, and TCAs in the treatment of concurrent anxiety and depression, all have had some measure of success depending on the degree of depression and the type of anxiety disorder (Keller and Hanks 1995). Kahn et al. (1986) reported success comparable to that found with chlordiazepoxide in treating patients with generalized anxiety disorder with 75–150 mg/day of imipramine. Like the effect reported with buspirone, this anxiolytic effect was noted to have a delayed onset of approximately 2–3 weeks. Another research group, comparing imipramine with alprazolam in patients with generalized anxiety disorder, found imipramine to be more effective in treating the psychic symptoms, such as dysphoria and negative anticipatory thinking, and alprazolam more effective in treating the somatic symptoms (Hoehn-Saric et al. 1988). In a controlled study comparing imipramine, trazodone, diazepam, and placebo in 230 patients with generalized anxiety disorder not complicated by depression or panic disorder, moderate-to-marked improvement was reported by 73% of those treated with imipramine, 69% of those treated with trazodone, 66% of those treated with diazepam, and only 47% of those treated with placebo (Rickels et al. 1993). SSRIs also appear to be effective, but controlled studies are lacking.

The duration of pharmacotherapy for generalized anxiety disorder is controversial. Psychotherapy is recommended for most patients with this disorder, and it may facilitate the tapering of medication. However, generalized anxiety is often a chronic condition, and some patients require long-term pharmacotherapy. As in other anxiety disorders, the need for ongoing treatment should be reassessed every 6–12 months.

PHARMACOTHERAPY OF PANIC DISORDER

Benzodiazepines, tricyclic antidepressants, MAOIs, and SSRIs are all effective in the treatment of panic disorder. Among the benzodiazepines, the higher potency agents, alprazolam and clonazepam, are preferred because they are well tolerated in the higher dose ranges often required to treat panic disorder (Spier et al. 1986; Tesar 1990). Clonazepam has the advantage of a longer elimination half-life, which provides more stable plasma drug levels and allows twice-a-day dosing, whereas the shorter half-life of alprazolam is better suited for acute dosage titration. For the treatment of panic disorder, clonazepam is started at 0.5 mg bid and increased to a total of 1–2 mg/day in two divided doses. Higher dosage levels may be neces-sary for complete relief of symptoms. The starting dosage of alprazolam is usually 0.25 or 0.5 mg tid (Tesar 1990).

Because long-term exposure to high-dosage benzodiazepines may place some patients at risk of physical and/or psychological dependence, we recommend the use of antidepressants for the treatment of panic disorder. Many antidepressants have been demonstrated to be effective in this setting, including TCAs (Klein et al. 1987; Zitrin et al. 1983), MAOIs (Sheehan et al. 1980; van Vliet et al. 1993), and SSRIs (den Boer et al. 1995; Oehrberg et al. 1995; Schneier et al. 1990; Westenberg and den Boer 1988). For most patients, the SSRIs, imipramine, desipramine, and nortriptyline should be considered first-line agents. The choice should be based on the same factors discussed in the section on antidepressant drugs. MAOIs are usually reserved for patients who have not responded to SSRIs and TCAs. A major caveat is that patients with panic disorder initially may be highly sensitive to the stimulant effects of small doses of antidepressants, especially desipramine and fluoxetine. For highly anxious patients with panic disorder, we often initiate treatment with clonazepam or alprazolam and add a low-dose antidepressant, which is then increased slowly. The rapid onset of action of the benzodiazepine is helpful to the patient until the antidepressant becomes effective. In addition, the benzodiazepine will treat any stimulating effects of the antidepressant until tolerance to this side effect develops (which may require several weeks). When panic symptoms have not been present for several weeks, the benzodiazepine is slowly tapered. In patients with marked residual anticipatory anxiety, longer term use of a benzodiazepine or buspirone should be considered as an adjunct to the antidepressant. Although some patients respond to lower doses, standard-to-high-standard antidepressant doses generally are used for the treatment of panic disorder.

For most patients, pharmacotherapy combined with time-limited cognitive-behavioral therapy is highly effective in reducing panic attacks but possibly less effective in attenuating avoidance behavior. Unfortunately, there are no guidelines for the duration of pharmacotherapy. We recommend attempting to taper medication every 6–12 months if the patient has been relatively symptom-free. However, many patients require longer term pharmacotherapy.

PHARMACOTHERAPY OF SOCIAL PHOBIA

Social phobia responds to a variety of medications, including SSRIs (Black et al. 1992; den Boer et al. 1995; Van Ameringen et al. 1993; Westenberg and den Boer 1993), MAOIs (Liebowitz et al. 1988; Marshall et al. 1994), benzodiazepines (Davidson et al. 1991; Gelernter et al. 1991; Jefferson 1995), and buspirone (Munjack et al. 1991; Schneier et al. 1992). TCAs, although highly effective in the treatment of panic disorder, appear to be ineffective for most patients with social phobia. Similarly, β-blockers, although effective in treating performance anxiety, are not effective in treating generalized social phobia (Jefferson 1995).

The risks and side effects of the SSRIs, MAOIs, and benzodiazepines are discussed extensively elsewhere in the chapter. Dosages for the treatment of social phobia are similar to dosages of these medications for other disorders.

The high-potency agents alprazolam (Gelernter et al. 1991) and clonazepam (Davidson et al. 1991; Jefferson 1995) appear to be the most effective benzodiazepines for treating social phobia. Preliminary studies have shown that patients with generalized and specific social phobia benefited from treatment with the reversible MAOIs (moclobemide), but the irreversible MAOI phenelzine remains the best studied (Jefferson 1995). Although the MAOIs are highly effective in reducing both social anxiety and social avoidance, these drugs are not first-line agents, as they are not in the treatment of depression, because of their increased risks compared to other available agents.

PHARMACOTHERAPY OF PERFORMANCE ANXIETY

Several studies have demonstrated the efficacy of β-blockers in the treatment of performance anxiety. Taken within 2 hours of the stressor, propranolol, in doses ranging from 20 to 80 mg, may improve performance on examinations (Drew et al. 1985), in public speaking (Hertley et al. 1983), and in musical performances (Brantigan et al. 1982). A trial dose of 40 mg of propranolol (e.g., during a vacation day) should be administered before the specific performance situation in which the patient anticipates anxiety. This initial dose should not be taken in a high-risk or critical situation in which any unexpected side effect could result in serious consequences. Subsequently, doses of propranolol should be administered approximately 2 hours before the situation in which disabling performance anxiety is expected. The dose may be increased gradually by 20-mg increments during successive performances until adequate relief of performance distress is achieved (Yudofsky and Silver 1987). The risks and side effects of β-blockers are discussed extensively later in this chapter, in the section on antiaggression drugs.

PHARMACOTHERAPY OF OBSESSIVE-COMPULSIVE DISORDER

The discovery of the SSRIs has brought about a revolution in psychopharmacology, similar to the effect of the discovery of the neuroleptics and antidepressants a generation ago. As a consequence of the development of these drugs, the understanding of obsessive-compulsive disorder and related conditions has multiplied manyfold. Clomipramine, a tricyclic with potent serotonin reuptake inhibition, was the first medication with established efficacy for treatment of OCD (Clomipramine Collaborative Study Group 1991). Currently, clomipramine and the SSRIs provide the foundation of pharmacological treatment for OCD. In contrast to the experience of patients treated with pharmacotherapy for many other Axis I disorders, most patients with OCD experience only a 35%–60% improvement in symptoms (Jenike 1990). In addition, medication responses may not be apparent until treatment has been given for 10 weeks. Cognitive-behavioral therapy should be combined with pharmacological approaches.

Before initiating clomipramine treatment, the clinician must heed all the precautions associated with the use of any TCA (see discussion of TCAs earlier in this chapter). Initial dosing and titration of clomipramine must also follow the guidelines for TCAs, with the additional caveat that 250 mg is the maximum recommended dosage because of an increased risk of seizures above this level. Plasma levels are available but are only weakly correlated with therapeutic effect (Mavissakalian et al. 1990). Most patients with OCD respond to dosages of clomipramine between 150 and 200 mg/day. Because side effects associated with the anticholinergic, antihistaminic, and α_2-adrenergic actions of clomipramine may occur, patients must be monitored for and made aware of the potential for symptoms such as constipation, dry mouth, urinary hesitancy, sedation, and orthostatic hypotension.

As in the treatment of depression, the SSRIs tend to be better tolerated than the TCAs. Fluoxetine has been compared with clomipramine under double-blind conditions and found to have an approximately equivalent antiobsessional effect (Pigott et al. 1990). It has been suggested that an effective antiobsessional dosage of fluoxetine may be higher than its usual antidepressant dosage. Many clinicians seek to establish a daily dosage of 60–80 mg in treating patients with OCD. No systematic study of this issue has confirmed this common impression and widely used practice. In fact, a preliminary report by Wheadon (1991) found no greater antiobsessional effect of fluoxetine 40 or 60 mg/day compared with 20 mg/day. Nonetheless, on the basis of the current knowledge of the treatment of OCD, a trial of fluoxetine should not be considered complete until the patient has failed to respond to 80 mg/day after 8 weeks (Jenike 1990). In an open-label study, 198 patients with OCD who were previously nonresponsive to fixed doses of fluoxetine benefited from dosage titration up to 80 mg, with two-thirds achieving an optimal response within 24 weeks (Tollefson et al. 1994).

The other SSRIs are also effective treatments for OCD. Therapeutic dosages of fluvoxamine range from 100 to 300 mg/day in divided doses (Freeman et al. 1994; Goodman et al. 1990, 1996; Perse et al. 1988). In a double-blind comparison of flexible doses of paroxetine, clomipramine, and placebo, paroxetine was found to be as effective as clomipramine and significantly more effective than placebo in the treatment of patients with OCD (Zohar and Judge 1996). The recommended dosage range for paroxetine in the treatment of OCD is 40–60 mg/day. In a double-blind comparison of three dosages of sertraline (50, 100, and 200 mg/day) and placebo in patients with OCD, all three sertraline groups showed significantly greater improvement than the placebo group after 12 weeks (Greist et al. 1995).

A number of augmentation strategies have been suggested, none with uniformly positive results in controlled trials but with possible effectiveness in selected patients. OCD augmentation strategies include use of fenfluramine (Hollander et al. 1990), lithium (Feder 1988), antipsychotics (McDougle et al. 1990, 1995), clonazepam (Hewlett et al. 1990), and buspirone (Jenike et al. 1991; Markovitz et al. 1990).

As in the other anxiety disorders, there are relatively few data available to address longer term treatment. OCD is often a lifelong disorder with a waxing and waning course, for which many patients require prolonged pharmacotherapy. Although relatively high dosages of SSRIs are recommended for the acute treatment, lower dosages may be effective for maintenance treatment (Mundo et al. 1997). In a 2-year follow-up study comparing 130 obsessive-compulsive patients who were responders to treatment with clomipramine (150 mg/day), fluoxetine (40 mg/day), or fluvoxamine (300 mg/day) for 6 months, those who continued treatment with the same daily dosage or half dosage had significantly superior outcomes when compared to those who discontinued treatment. No differences in efficacy between the full and half doses were found (Ravizza et al. 1996).

PHARMACOTHERAPY OF INSOMNIA

Although the benzodiazepines and zolpidem are the mainstay of pharmacotherapy for insomnia, other sedating drugs, such trazodone or chloral hydrate, may also be used. As discussed previously, insomnia should first be addressed diagnostically, and in most cases nonpharmacological interventions should be attempted before treatment with a hypnotic is instituted. Hypnotic agents should be administered in the lowest effective dose. Medications commonly prescribed to treat insomnia, their recommended dosages, time of onset, and half-life are shown in Table 27–11. General principles for using medications to treat insomnia are outlined in Table 27–12.

Each hypnotic benzodiazepine has a distinct pharmacodynamic and pharmacokinetic profile that has an important influence on its use in clinical practice. Whereas all the currently available benzodiazepine hypnotics are absorbed relatively rapidly from the gastrointestinal tract and achieve peak plasma levels in approximately 1.5 hours (Greenblatt 1992), affinity for the benzodiazepine receptor and elimination half-life both affect the clinical use of these agents. For example, flurazepam and quazepam are both ultimately metabolized into a clinically active compound, desalkylflurazepam, which has an elimination half-life of 40–50 hours (Greenblatt 1992; Greenblatt et al. 1981). With successive days of treatment, the accumulation of this compound in the body may adversely affect motor performance and cause daytime drowsiness, a so-called hangover effect. Although tolerance to the daytime sedation may develop with time (Greenblatt et al. 1977b), we believe that for elderly patients and many others the risks of CNS side effects are too great with flurazepam and quazepam. On the other hand, a long elimination half-life reduces the risk of early-morning awakening and rebound insomnia after drug discontinuation, so that these agents may be appropriate for brief treatment. With a half-life of just 1.5–5 hours, triazolam is at the opposite end of the spectrum among the benzodiazepines (Greenblatt et al. 1983). The risks of accumulation of triazolam in the body are avoided in healthy patients, but the risk of rebound insomnia makes triazolam less useful for patients with early-morning awakening. Temazepam and estazolam have intermediate half-life values (Greenblatt 1992), and, as a result, day-after and rebound insomnia are less likely with these agents. Quazepam is unique among the benzodiazepines in that it is selective for the type 1 benzodiazepine receptor (Wamsley and Hunt 1991); however, desalkylflurazepam, a metabolite of quazepam, is a long-acting and nonselective benzodiazepine receptor agonist, which accounts for at least some of the clinical effects of this drug.

The nonbenzodiazepine hypnotic agent zolpidem also acts selectively at the type 1 benzodiazepine receptor, although, unlike quazepam, it has no nonselective metabo-

TABLE 27–11. **Medications commonly prescribed to treat insomnia**

Medication (trade name)	Usual therapeutic dosage (mg/day)		Time until onset of action (min)	Half-life (including metabolites; hr)
	Adult	Geriatric		
Clonazepam (Klonopin)[a]	0.5–2	0.25–1	20–60	19–60
Clorazepate (Tranxene)	3.75–15	3.75–7.5	30–60	48–96
Estazolam (ProSom)	1–2	0.5–1	15–30	8–24
Lorazepam (Ativan)[a]	1–4	0.25–1	30–60	8–24
Oxazepam (Serax)	15–30	10–15	30–60	2.8–5.7
Quazepam (Doral)	7.5–15	7.5	20–45	39–120
Temazepam (Restoril)	15–30	7.5–15	45–60	3–25
Triazolam (Halcion)	0.125–0.25	0.125	15–30	1.5–5
Chloral hydrate[b]	500–2000	500–2000	30–60	4–8
Haloperidol (Haldol)[a,b]	0.5–5	0.25–2	60	20
Trazodone (Desyrel)[a,b]	50–150	25–100	30–60	5–9
Zolpidem (Ambien)[b]	5–10	5	30	1.5–4.5

[a]Use of this drug as a hypnotic agent is not an indication approved by the Food and Drug Administration. [b]These drugs are not benzodiazepines.
Source. Adapted with permission from Kupfer and Reynolds 1997.

TABLE 27–12. **Guidelines for pharmacotherapy of insomnia**

1. Use the lowest effective dose.
2. Use agents with short or intermediate half-lives to avoid daytime sedation.
3. Use intermittent dosing (two to four times a week).
4. Use for no more than 3–4 weeks.
5. Discontinue medication gradually.
6. Be alert for rebound insomnia.

Source. Adapted with permission from Kupfer and Reynolds 1997.

lites. As discussed previously, the clinical characteristics of zolpidem are similar to those of triazolam, but zolpidem appears to be less likely to produce rebound insomnia. Sedating antidepressants such as trazodone are often effective and do not carry the risk of abuse associated with more traditional hypnotics.

ALCOHOL WITHDRAWAL

A relatively simple procedure for treating alcohol withdrawal is the benzodiazepine loading dose technique (Sellers et al. 1983). This technique takes advantage of the long half-lives of benzodiazepines such as diazepam and chlordiazepoxide. Doses of 20 mg of diazepam (or 100 mg of chlordiazepoxide) are administered hourly to patients until they exhibit no signs or symptoms of alcohol withdrawal. This state is usually accompanied by mild-to-moderate sedation. Thereafter, no further doses of benzodiazepine are administered. Because of the long half-life of diazepam and other long-acting benzodiazepines, the therapeutic plasma level of the benzodiazepine is maintained during the period of risk for alcohol withdrawal symptoms. Sullivan and Sellers (1986) recommended that healthy patients receive at least 60 mg of diazepam or 300 mg of chlordiazepoxide in the initial loading dose regimen. This technique has advantages over the method of repeat dosing with benzodiazepines in that the accumulation of benzodiazepines may lead to prolonged sedation and the development of benzodiazepine dependence in a population at high risk for chemical dependence.

ANTIPSYCHOTIC DRUGS

Antipsychotic medications, previously referred to as *major tranquilizers* or *neuroleptics*, are effective agents for the treatment of a variety of psychotic symptoms, such as hallucinations, delusions, and thought disorders, regardless of etiology (other indications are discussed later). The term *major tranquilizer* is a misnomer because sedation is generally a side effect, not the principal treatment effect. Similarly, the term *neuroleptic* is based on the neurological side effects characteristic of the older antipsychotic drugs, such as catalepsy in animals and predictable extrapyramidal side effects in humans.

There are a number of ways to classify antipsychotic drugs. One classification is based on chemical structure, for example, phenothiazines and butyrophenones. This classification is important to note primarily when switching from one conventional antipsychotic to another, such as in the case of allergy. We use the term *conventional* to signify the older antipsychotic drugs, to differentiate them from the newer, *atypical* antipsychotics. All conventional antipsychotics are equally effective when given in equivalent doses (Table 27–13). Although the term *atypical antipsychotic* lacks a single consistent definition, it generally implies fewer extrapyramidal side effects and superior efficacy, particularly for attenuating the negative symptoms of schizophrenia. Atypical antipsychotics (AAP) are also less likely to produce hyperprolactinemia. Currently, the AAPs include clozapine, risperidone, olanzapine, and quetiapine.

The favorable efficacy and safety profile of AAPs has led some authorities to recommend that, with the exception of clozapine because of the increased risk of agranulocytosis, they be used uniformly as first-line agents (Lieberman 1996). On the other hand, there are limited long-term data for the AAPs, which are markedly more expensive. Therefore, other experts recommend using conventional antipsychotics as first-line agents, reserving AAPs for nonresponders or individuals with preexisting movement disorders or tardive dyskinesia.

MECHANISMS OF ACTION

For many years the prevailing theory regarding the mechanism of action of antipsychotic drugs was based on the observation that all the available antipsychotics antagonize dopamine (D_2) receptors in vitro and that the relative affinities of the typical antipsychotic drugs for striatal D_2 re-

TABLE 27–13. Commonly used antipsychotic drugs

Generic (trade) name	Usual daily dosage (mg)	Methods of administration	Available oral doses (mg)	Approximate oral dose equivalents (mg)[a]
Conventional antipsychotics				
Phenothiazines				
Chlorpromazine (Thorazine)	300–600	po, im	10, 25, 50, 100, 200	100
Piperidines				
Thioridazine (Mellaril)	300–600	po, im	10, 15, 25, 50, 100, 150, 200	100
Mesoridazine (Serentil)	150–300	po	10, 25, 50, 100	50
Pimozide (Orap)	2–6	po	2	1–2
Piperazines				
Trifluoperazine (Stelazine)	15–30	po	1, 2, 5, 10	5
Fluphenazine (Prolixin)	5–15	po, L, im, D	1, 2.5, 5, 10	2
Perphenazine (Trilafon)	32–64	po	2, 4, 8, 16	10
Thioxanthenes				
Thiothixene (Navane)	15–30	po, L, im	1, 2, 5, 10, 20	5
Butyrophenones				
Haloperidol (Haldol)	5–15	po, im, D	0.5, 1, 2, 5, 10, 20	2
Dibenzoxazepines				
Loxapine (Loxitane)	45–90	po	5, 10, 25, 50	15
Molindone (Moban)	30–60	po	5, 10, 25, 50, 100	10
Atypical antipsychotics				
Clozapine (Clozaril)	250–500	po	25, 100	50
Risperidone (Risperdal)	4–6	po	1, 2, 3, 4	1
Olanzapine (Zyprexa)	10–15	po	2.5, 5, 7.5, 10	2–3
Quetiapine (Seroquel)	300–400	po	25, 100, 200	100

Note. D = long-acting decanoate preparation; im = short-acting intramuscular; L = liquid; po = oral tablets or capsules.
[a]Equivalent doses from American Psychiatric Association 1997.

ceptors correlate with the dosage required to treat psychotic symptoms (Creese et al. 1976; Seeman et al. 1976). Yet the theory that psychosis is a result simply of hyperdopaminergia is overly simplistic. Underactivity of dopamine in mesocortical pathways, specifically those projecting to the frontal lobes, may account for the negative symptoms of schizophrenia (e.g., anergia, apathy, aspontaneity; Crow 1995; Meltzer 1995). At the same time, this underactivity in the frontal lobe serves to disinhibit mesolimbic dopamine activity via a cortico-limbic feedback loop (Pycock et al. 1980). An overactivity of mesolimbic dopamine is the result, manifested by the positive symptoms of schizophrenia (e.g., hallucinations, delusions; Davis et al. 1991). This revised dopamine hypothesis is concordant with the clinical observation that conventional antipsychotic drugs are more effective in treating positive symptoms than negative symptoms.

As a result of functional interactions between the dopamine and serotonin systems, antagonism of the serotonin$_2$ (5-HT$_2$) receptor may regionally modify D$_2$. This dual 5-HT$_2$/D$_2$ antagonism is believed to account, at least in part, for the superior efficacy and side-effect profile of the AAPs (Meltzer et al. 1989). Also on the basis of this dual antagonism, atypical antipsychotics are often referred to as *serotonin-dopamine antagonists*, or SDAs. Other investigators have suggested that manipulation of the noradrenergic (Litman et al. 1993), glutaminergic-N-methyl-D-aspartate (NMDA) (Wachtel and Turski 1990), or GABAergic (Reynolds and Stroud 1993) system may be of therapeutic benefit in schizophrenia.

In addition, the more recently discovered D$_4$ receptor, which is found in frontal cortex and limbic areas, and not in striatal areas (Civelli et al. 1991), may be relevant to the distinctly different side-effect profiles and efficacy of the atypical antipsychotics, which tend to have a much greater affinity for this receptor (Meltzer 1990; Sokoloff et al. 1990; Van Tol et al. 1991).

Finally, neuropeptides, specifically cholecystokinin (Garver et al. 1990), neurotensin (Bisette and Nemeroff 1988; Garver et al. 1991), and vasopressin (Beckman et al. 1985; Sorensen et al. 1985), have each been implicated in either the pathophysiology or the treatment of psychotic disorders.

INDICATIONS AND EFFICACY

The most common indications for the use of antipsychotic drugs are in the treatment of acute psychosis and the maintenance of a remission of psychotic symptoms in patients with schizophrenia. All conventional antipsychotics (Table 27–13) have comparable efficacy but differing side-effect profiles. The atypical antipsychotics—

clozapine, risperidone, and olanzapine—appear to be at least as effective as the older medications for the treatment of positive symptoms and more efficacious for the treatment of negative symptoms of schizophrenia. Clozapine is effective in approximately 30% of patients who were nonresponsive to several trials of conventional antipsychotics (Kane 1996). Risperidone and olanzapine may also be advantageous for this difficult patient population, but to date adequate controlled trials are lacking.

Antipsychotic drugs are also effective in ameliorating psychotic symptoms that result from many diverse etiologies, such as mood disorders with psychotic features, drug toxicities, psychosis secondary to other brain disorders, and delusional disorders. Low dosages of antipsychotics may be effective in some patients with borderline or schizotypal personality disorders, particularly when used to target psychotic ideation (Gunderson 1986). In the treatment of severe obsessive-compulsive disorder, antipsychotics have been used to augment antiobsessional agents (McDougle et al. 1990). Antipsychotics and other drugs with dopamine-receptor-blocking action (e.g., metoclopramide) are also used for their antimimetic effect. Gilles de la Tourette's syndrome may be controlled with antipsychotic agents; haloperidol and pimozide are the most frequently used drugs for this disorder.

The sedative side effect of antipsychotic medications may lead to the misuse of these drugs in several clinical situations. Antipsychotics frequently are improperly prescribed as hypnotic or anxiolytic agents. In addition, antipsychotic drugs are administered to patients who are chronically agitated and violent. Because of the potential long-term risks of these drugs (see subsection on tardive dyskinesia), antipsychotics are not recommended for the treatment of anxiety or insomnia. Although they are sometimes valuable for acute episodes of agitation and aggression, these drugs should not be used for the treatment of chronic aggression and agitation.

CLINICAL USE

Medication Selection

The choice of medication is determined, in large part, by the side effects that either are desired or must be avoided in any individual patient. In most circumstances, the AAPs (except for clozapine) are preferred as first-line agents, if cost formulary constraints do not dictate otherwise. Clozapine is generally reserved for refractory patients because of the risk of agranulocytosis. For the conventional antipsychotic drugs, a useful construct for conceptualizing differences in side-effect profiles is the concept of "high-potency" versus "low-potency" drugs. Drug potency refers to the milligram equivalence of drugs, not to the relative efficacy. For example, although haloperidol is more potent than chlorpromazine (haloperidol 2 mg = chlorpromazine 100 mg), therapeutically equivalent doses are equally effective (haloperidol 12 mg = chlorpromazine 600 mg).

Potency of the antipsychotic drugs has generally been determined in two ways: 1) by ascertaining dosages that are efficacious in clinical trials and clinical practice and 2) by noting affinities of the drug for the D_2 receptor. Typically, the potency of antipsychotic drugs is compared to a standard 100-mg dose of chlorpromazine. As a rule, for conventional antipsychotics only, the high-potency antipsychotic drugs have an equivalent dose of less than 5 mg (Table 27–13). These medications have a high degree of extrapyramidal side effects (EPS) but less sedation, fewer anticholinergic side effects, and less hypotension. Low-potency antipsychotic drugs have an equivalent dose of greater than 40 mg. These drugs have a high level of sedation, anticholinergic side effects, and hypotension, but a lower degree of acute EPS. Tardive dyskinesia rates do not differ between high- and low-potency conventional antipsychotics. Antipsychotic drugs with intermediate potency (i.e., equivalent dose between 5 and 40 mg) have a side-effect profile that lies between the profiles of these two groups. In most circumstances, high-potency drugs are preferred among the conventional antipsychotics, because EPS can usually be minimized by using the lowest effective dosage or by symptomatic treatment, whereas anticholinergic and autonomic side effects are potentially more dangerous and difficult to manage.

Intermediate-potency drugs are used for patients who cannot tolerate either high- or low-potency drugs. The AAPs produce less EPS than even the low-potency conventional antipsychotics, and they may be preferred agents for patients with Parkinson's disease or prominent negative symptoms, and perhaps for patients with chronic schizophrenia, who require long-term treatment. Certain circumstances may call for a drug that has a low incidence of other particular side effects. Drugs with significant anticholinergic properties exacerbate cognitive impairment and constipation. Molindone and fluphenazine appear to have the least effect on seizure threshold. Although a preliminary report suggested that molindone produced less weight gain, clinical observation has not substantiated this finding.

Optimal Dosages

Despite years of use, there is no universally agreed-on optimal dosage for most of the antipsychotics. Older high-dosage strategies and "rapid tranquilization," which

often employed dosages of haloperidol of 60–100 mg or the equivalent of another antipsychotic, are no longer recommended. Antipsychotic drugs, with the exception of clozapine, have a high therapeutic index, and they can be administered at dosages substantially above the optimal therapeutic dosage without immediate and obvious adverse events. However, carefully controlled studies have confirmed that more modest dosages of antipsychotic drugs have equal efficacy and are more tolerable. Several reviewers of published studies have concluded that the optimal dosage for most patients is between 300 and 600 mg/day chlorpromazine-equivalents, with some patients responding to lower dosages and with little benefit above 700 mg/day (Appleton and Davis 1980; Baldessarini et al. 1988; Davis 1985).

In a randomized but not double-blind study of haloperidol, van Putten et al. (1990) found 20 mg initially superior to both 5 and 10 mg; after 2 weeks, however, patients in the 20-mg group experienced more social withdrawal, akinesia, and akathisia, culminating in 35% leaving the study against medical advice, compared to only 4% of patients who were taking the lower dosages. McEvoy et al. (1986) advocated using the "neuroleptic threshold," as initially suggested by Haase (1961). The neuroleptic threshold is defined as the lowest dosage that produces slight rigidity on clinical examination. For an individual patient, it is suggested that this threshold dosage is also the dosage at which optimal therapeutic benefit will occur after several weeks. In an open study designed to test this hypothesis, a mean haloperidol dosage of 4.2±2.4 mg/day resulted in significant therapeutic improvement in two-thirds of the patients (McEvoy et al. 1986).

In the initial stages of treatment with antipsychotic medication, sedation caused by the drug may predominate over the specific antipsychotic effects. Although it is widely recognized that antidepressant drugs may take 3–4 weeks before the patient shows clinical improvement, many psychiatrists incorrectly believe that if psychosis does not rapidly respond with the use of antipsychotics, higher dosages are necessary. In fact, as in antidepressant therapy, reversal of psychosis is often gradual and may occur over several weeks to several months. Unless this fact is recognized, a patient may be exposed to dosages of antipsychotic medication that are higher than required. Guidelines for the acute use of antipsychotic drugs are summarized in Table 27–14; usual dosages for each of the commonly used antipsychotic drugs are summarized in Table 27–13.

Long-Acting Injectable Antipsychotics

For patients with chronic psychotic symptoms who do not comply with a daily medication regimen, a long-acting de-

TABLE 27–14. Guidelines for the acute use of antipsychotic drugs

1. Before the initiation of treatment, obtain a medical history and perform a complete physical and neurological examination. The history and physical examination are necessary not only to ensure accurate diagnosis of the etiology of the psychosis, but also to ensure safe administration of the antipsychotic drugs. Because each antipsychotic drug has a slightly different side-effect profile, the examination may be tailored as appropriate. Among the elements of the examination that have particular importance are pulse rate and blood pressure, ophthalmological examination, and neurological examination with emphasis on extrapyramidal signs and symptoms and tardive dyskinesia.

2. After discussion with the patient and family about the risks and benefits of treatment, select the appropriate antipsychotic agent on the basis of the patient's physical status, the side-effect profile of the drug, and the history of previous response to medication, if available.

3. Inform and educate the patient and family about the risks of development of tardive dyskinesia. Document this discussion in the patient's chart.

4. Initiate antipsychotic medications in moderate dosages (e.g., 4–10 mg haloperidol, 4–6 mg risperidone [titrate from lower dose], or 10 mg olanzapine for healthy adults).

5. Consider anticholinergic medication for the prophylaxis of extrapyramidal symptoms when prescribing high-potency conventional antipsychotic drugs to patients at high risk for dystonia. Avoid anticholinergic medication in patients with confusion or urinary retention and in patients who are at low risk for dystonia, such as the elderly.

6. Maintain the treatment dosage for 2–4 weeks, because the response to antipsychotics is gradual.

7. When medication is necessary to control acute agitation, a sedative such as lorazepam 2 mg may be effective.

8. If possible, give all the antipsychotic medication at bedtime to increase compliance and minimize daytime side effects.

9. If there is no response, side effects are minimal, and you believe poor compliance is not the reason, increase the dosage gradually until mild side effects are seen (e.g., sedation, hypotension, extrapyramidal effects).

10. If no further improvement is seen after an additional 2–4 weeks at this dosage, substitute another antipsychotic drug from another class. Consider the use of another atypical antipsychotic drug.

pot preparation should be considered following stabilization with oral medication. Fluphenazine decanoate and haloperidol decanoate are the only long-acting injectables currently available in the United States.

Conversion to a decanoate preparation is complicated by the highly variable individual pharmacokinetics of the oral and long-term depot agents. Most patients respond to a fluphenazine decanoate dose of between 10 and 30 mg every 2 weeks (Baldessarini et al. 1988). A loading dose strategy has been established for haloperidol decanoate, in which patients receive an initial dose that is 20 times the oral maintenance dosage (Ereshefsky et al. 1993). The maximum volume per injection of haloperidol decanoate should not exceed 3 cc, and the maximum dose per injection should not exceed 100 mg. If 20 times the oral dose is greater than 100 mg, the dose is given in divided injections spaced 3–7 days apart. Subsequent doses are decreased monthly to about 10 times the oral dosage by the third or fourth month. For patients who are elderly or debilitated, the initial dose is 10–15 times the previous oral daily dosage.

Breakthrough psychotic symptoms are treated with supplemental oral medication, and the dose of the next scheduled depot injection is increased accordingly. Note that depot medications continue to be active for weeks to months after administration, and side effects that occur from such treatment may take months to subside. In addition, withdrawal dyskinesia may not appear for months after discontinuation of the decanoate formulation.

Risks, Side Effects, and Their Management

Many of the side effects of antipsychotic drugs can be understood on the basis of their receptor-blocking properties. When antipsychotics reduce dopamine activity in the nigrostriatum (via dopamine receptor blockade), extrapyramidal signs and symptoms result, similar to those of Parkinson's disease. Another locus of dopamine receptors resides in the pituitary and hypothalamus (the tuberoinfundibular system), where dopamine is synonymous with prolactin-inhibiting factor. As such, blocking dopamine in this system results in hyperprolactinemia. Similarly, antagonism of acetylcholine receptors produces symptoms such as dry mouth, blurred vision, and constipation. Antagonism of α_1-adrenergic receptors results in hypotension, and antagonism of histamine receptors is associated with sedation.

Extrapyramidal effects. Extrapyramidal symptoms include acute dystonic reactions, parkinsonian syndrome, akathisia, neuroleptic malignant syndrome, and tardive dyskinesia. Although high-potency antipsychotics are more likely to produce extrapyramidal symptoms, all conventional antipsychotic drugs are equally likely to produce tardive dyskinesia. Clozapine appears to be the only agent to date that does not cause tardive dyskinesia.

Acute dystonic reactions are among the most disturbing and acutely disabling adverse drug reactions that can occur with the administration of antipsychotic drugs. This reaction most frequently occurs within hours or days of the initiation of a high-potency conventional antipsychotic medication. The most common feature of this syndrome is uncontrollable tightening of the face and neck with spasm and distortions of the head and/or back (i.e., opisthotonos). If the extraocular muscles are involved, an oculogyric crisis may occur, wherein the eyes are locked up in an elevated position. Laryngeal involvement may lead to respiratory and ventilatory difficulties. These reactions are often terrifying to the patient and may result in deteriorating compliance with medications. Intravenous or intramuscular administration of anticholinergic medication is a rapid and effective treatment of acute dystonia, so rapid, in fact, that the dystonia may disappear before the injection is completed. The drugs and dosages used to treat dystonic reactions are listed in Table 27–15. The anticholinergic drug given to reverse the dystonia will wear off after several hours. Because antipsychotic drugs have long half-lives and durations of action, additional oral anticholinergic drugs should be prescribed for several days after an acute dystonic reaction or longer if the antipsychotic drug is continued unchanged. Patients for whom anticholinergic drugs are contraindicated require careful assessment of risk-benefit ratios before initiation of medications. Amantadine should be considered for such patients if extrapyramidal side effects occur.

Acute dystonic reactions may be treated prophylactically with anticholinergic medications; for example, benztropine 1–2 mg bid may be initiated at the same time as the antipsychotic agent haloperidol. Some patients, such as muscular young male African American or Hispanic patients, are at particularly high risk for the development of acute dystonia when treated with high-potency antipsychotic drugs. We suggest that prophylactic treatment is indicated for patients for whom the risk of developing extrapyramidal reactions is high, especially if these reactions are likely to diminish compliance (e.g., in angry, paranoid patients).

Parkinsonian syndrome (or pseudoparkinsonism) has many of the features of classic idiopathic Parkinson's disease: diminished range of facial expression (masked facies), cogwheel rigidity, slowed movements (bradykinesia), drooling, small handwriting (micrographia), and pill-rolling tremor. As in Parkinson's disease, the pathophysiology involves disproportionally less dopamine than acetylcholine in the basal ganglia. The onset of this side effect is gradual, and it may not appear for weeks after antipsychotics have been administered. The most common treatments for idiopathic Parkinson's disease restore the dopamine:acetylcholine (DA:ACH) balance by increasing dopamine. Because dopamine antagonism is putatively involved in the therapeutic effects of antipsychotics, treatment of parkinsonism most often involves decreasing the level of acetylcholine (although amantadine, a dopaminergic drug, often effectively attenuates parkinsonian side effects without exacerbating the underlying psychotic illness). Drugs used in the treatment of the parkinsonian side effects of antipsychotic agents are listed in Table 27–15.

The *rabbit syndrome*, consisting of fine, rapid movements of the lips that resemble the chewing movements of a rabbit, is often considered a subset of parkinsonian side

TABLE 27–15.   **Drugs commonly used for the treatment of acute extrapyramidal side effects**

Generic (trade) name	Mechanism	Usual dosage	Indications
Benztropine (Cogentin)	Anticholinergic	1–2 mg po bid	D, P
		2 mg iv[a]	Acute dystonia
Diphenhydramine (Benadryl)	Anticholinergic	25–50 mg po tid	D, P
		25 mg im/iv[a]	Acute dystonia
Trihexyphenidyl (Artane)	Anticholinergic	5–10 mg po bid	D, P
Amantadine (Symmetrel)	Dopaminergic	100 mg po bid	P
Propranolol (Inderal)	β-Blocker	20 mg po tid	A
		1 mg iv	

Note.   A = akathisia; D = dystonia; P = parkinsonian syndrome. Rabbit syndrome and akinesia respond to the medications used to treat parkinsonian syndrome.
[a]Follow with po medication.

effects. This side effect occurs after more prolonged treatment and may be confused with buccolingual tardive dyskinesia (Baldessarini 1988; Deshmukh et al. 1990). It has been found to be present in approximately 4% of patients receiving antipsychotics without concomitant anticholinergics (Yassa and Lal 1986). Like parkinsonian side effects, the rabbit syndrome is treated effectively with anticholinergic drugs.

Akinesia is defined as a behavioral state of diminished spontaneity characterized by decreased gestures, unspontaneous speech, and, particularly, apathy and difficulty with initiating usual activities (Rifkin et al. 1975). Akinesia may appear after several weeks of therapy and is often a subset of the parkinsonism syndrome. Among patients treated with antipsychotic agents, this syndrome may be mistaken for depression. The drugs suggested in Table 27–15 provide effective treatment. Akinesia may also be a manifestation of negative symptoms in a patient with schizophrenia. In this circumstance, use of atypical antipsychotics to improve the negative symptoms should be considered.

Akathisia is an extrapyramidal disorder consisting of a subjective feeling of needing to move, often manifested in an inability to sit still. It is a common reaction that most often occurs shortly after the initiation of antipsychotic medication. After a single oral dose of 5 mg of haloperidol, 40% of patients in one study experienced akathisia; after 1 week of receiving a 10-mg nighttime dose, this rate increased to 75% (van Putten et al. 1984). Unfortunately, akathisia is frequently mistaken for an exacerbation of psychotic symptoms, anxiety, and/or depression. If the dosage of antipsychotic medication is increased, the restlessness continues and eventually worsens. Lowering the dosage may improve the symptoms. Unfortunately, akathisia is among the most treatment resistant of the acute extrapyramidal side effects. In the past, anticholinergic drugs were suggested as the first line of therapy, but they are often ineffective, helping only occasionally when akathisia occurs in combination with other extrapyramidal symptoms, such as rigidity. Benzodiazepines are helpful in some cases.

The treatments of choice for akathisia are the β-adrenergic-blocking drugs, particularly propranolol. Several well-controlled studies have documented that propranolol, in dosages up to 120 mg/day, is an effective treatment for akathisia (Adler et al. 1985, 1989; Lipinski et al. 1984). In general, the lipophilic β-blockers are more effective in treating akathisia than the hydrophilic ones (Dupuis et al. 1987; Reiter et al. 1987; Zubenko et al. 1984). At present there remains a controversy as to whether β-selective drugs effectively treat akathisia, with some negative findings (Zubenko et al. 1984) and some positive reports

(Dumon et al. 1992; Dupuis et al. 1987). These drugs avoid the risk of bronchospasm in susceptible patients and, therefore, would be a welcome treatment alternative (Adler et al. 1991; Dumon et al. 1992; Lewis and Lofthouse 1993).

Tardive disorders. Tardive dyskinesia (TD) is a disorder characterized by involuntary choreoathetoid movements of the face, trunk, or extremities. The syndrome is usually associated with prolonged exposure to dopamine-receptor-blocking agents, most frequently, antipsychotic drugs. However, use of the drugs such as the antidepressant amoxapine, the antiemetic agents metoclopramide and prochlorperazine, and other drugs with dopamine-receptor-blocking properties also can result in TD. The American Psychiatric Association (APA) Task Force on TD estimated an incidence of 5% per year of exposure among young adults and 30% after 1 year of treatment among elderly patients (American Psychiatric Association 1992). Clozapine seems to carry little or no risk of inducing TD. The incidence of TD in association with the other AAPs has not yet been adequately determined. Preliminary evidence suggests a level of risk for olanzapine between the conventional antipsychotics and clozapine (Tollefson et al. 1997).

The diagnostic features of TD are listed in Table 27–16. These features have been adapted from one of the specific scales developed for the documentation of TD: the Abnormal Involuntary Movement Scale (AIMS). Although this scale is primarily for research use, physicians who prescribe antipsychotic drugs should be familiar with its contents in order to be able to perform a thorough examination for the presence of TD. A procedure for examining a patient for TD can be found in Table 27–17.

An evaluation for abnormal movements should be conducted before treatment begins and every 12 months thereafter. In the mildest stages, the patient may not be aware of the involuntary movements. As the movements become more severe, the patient may become dysfunctional to the point of experiencing difficulty eating or resting. Although the most common form of tardive disorder is the dyskinetic variety, other types have been observed. These include tardive akathisia, tardive dystonia, and tardive tics (Fahn 1985). Tardive dystonia is characterized by frequent contractions of the neck and shoulder muscles, such as seen in torticollis, which emerge with treatment with antipsychotic agents. The patient with tardive akathisia may experience continuous feelings of restlessness.

The most commonly accepted hypothesis of the mechanism for the development of TD is that postsynaptic dopamine receptors develop supersensitivity to dopamine

TABLE 27-16. Clinical features of tardive dyskinesia

1. Facial and oral movements
   a. Muscles of facial expression: involuntary movement of forehead, eyebrows, periorbital area, cheeks; involuntary frowning, blinking, smiling, grimacing.
   b. Lips and perioral area: involuntary puckering, pouting, smacking.
   c. Jaw: involuntary biting, clenching, chewing, mouth opening, lateral movements.
   d. Tongue: involuntary protrusion, tremor, choreo-athetoid movements (i.e., rolling, wormlike movement without displacement from the mouth).

2. Extremity movements
   a. Involuntary movement of upper arms, wrists, hands, fingers: choreic movements (i.e., rapid, objectively purposeless, irregular, spontaneous), athetoid movements (i.e., slow, irregular, complex, serpentine), tremor (i.e., repetitive, regular, rhythmic).
   b. Involuntary movement of lower legs, knees, ankles, toes: lateral knee movement, foot tapping, foot squirming, inversion and eversion of foot.

3. Trunk movements: Involuntary movement of neck, shoulders, hips: rocking, twisting, squirming, pelvic gyrations.

Source. Adapted from the Abnormal Involuntary Movement Scales (AIMS), National Institute of Mental Health 1988 ("AIMS: Abnormal Involuntary Movement Scale" 1988).

after prolonged dopamine receptor blockade. Other hypotheses have also been proposed, however. Noradrenergic hyperactivity may be an important factor in the development of TD (Jeste et al. 1982), and antipsychotic treatment may produce free radicals that can damage terminals of catecholaminergic systems (Cadet et al. 1986) or the system involving GABA (Fibinger and Lloyd 1986), or that can promote cerebral deterioration in general (Waddington et al. 1986).

The most significant and consistently documented risk factor for the development of TD is increasing age of the patient (Branchey and Branchey 1984; Jeste and Wyatt 1982; Kane and Smith 1982). Women have been found to be at a greater risk for severe TD, although the evidence to date suggests that this finding is limited to geriatric populations (Kennedy et al. 1971; Seide and Muller 1967). Other risk factors may include the dosage of the drug, total time taking the drug, EPS early in the course of treatment, a history of drug holidays (a greater number of drug-free periods is associated with an increased risk), the time since the first exposure to antipsychotic drugs (including drug holi-

TABLE 27-17. Examination procedure for tardive dyskinesia

Either before or after completing the examination procedure, unobtrusively observe the patient at rest (e.g., in the waiting room). The chair to be used in this examination should be a hard, firm one without arms.

Examination procedure:

1. Ask patient whether there is anything in his or her mouth (e.g., gum, candy), and if there is, ask him or her to remove it.
2. Ask patient about the current condition of his or her teeth. Ask patient if he or she wears dentures. Do teeth or dentures bother patient now?
3. Ask patient whether he or she notices any movements in mouth, face, hands, or feet. If yes, ask him or her to describe them and to assess to what extent they currently bother the patient or interfere with his or her activities.
4. Have patient sit in chair with hands on knees, legs slightly apart, and feet flat on floor. (Look at entire body for movements while patient is in this position.)
5. Ask patient to sit with hands hanging unsupported (if male) between legs or (if female and wearing a dress) hanging over knees. (Observe hands and other body areas.)
6. Ask patient to open mouth. (Observe tongue at rest within mouth.) Do this twice.
7. Ask patient to protrude tongue. (Observe abnormalities of tongue movement.) Do this twice.
8. Ask patient to tap thumb, with each finger, as rapidly as possible for 10–15 seconds, separately with right hand, then with left hand. (Observe facial and leg movements.)
9. Flex and extend patient's left and right arms one at a time. (Note any rigidity.)
10. Ask patient to stand up. (Observe in profile. Observe all body areas again, hips included.)
11. Ask patient to extend both arms outstretched in front with palms down. (Observe trunk, legs, and mouth.)
12. Have patient walk a few paces, turn, and walk back to chair. (Observe hands and gait.) Do this twice.

Source. Adapted from the Abnormal Involuntary Movement Scales (AIMS), National Institute of Mental Health 1988 ("AIMS: Abnormal Involuntary Movement Scale" 1988).

days), the presence of brain damage, and the diagnosis (especially the presence of affective disorder).

The issue of informed consent with respect to antipsychotic medications and the risk of TD has been extensively reviewed (Munetz and Roth 1985; Roth 1983). It is usually difficult, if not impossible, to obtain informed consent from a patient with acute psychosis. A general guideline is to inform and educate the family of the patient about the risks of TD before starting the antipsychotic and to educate the patient gradually about this disorder as soon as possible after agitation and psychosis remit. In many circumstances, true informed consent may not be obtainable from a patient with acute psychosis for several weeks. The psychiatrist also needs to be aware that some states (e.g., California and New Jersey) legally mandate that informed consent be obtained from patients before the initiation of antipsychotic treatment. All such discussions with patients and their families should be documented in the patients' records. Informed consent that is exclusively in the written form has been shown to be less effective in communicating information to the patient than verbal communication combined with written information (Munetz and Roth 1985). The psychiatrist must allocate adequate time to the provision of informed consent consistent with the confusional state and cognitive capabilities of the patient. Further discussion of this area may be found in Chapter 41 of this textbook.

Because antipsychotic medications remain the most effective treatment for most patients with schizophrenia, the case often arises in which a patient develops TD but still requires the medication to function. If discontinuation of the antipsychotic drug is clinically possible, improvement in the TD may be gradual. Worsening of the involuntary movements often occurs initially with tapering of the antipsychotic, a phenomenon referred to as *withdrawal dyskinesia*. These movements also may be masked temporarily by increasing the dosage of the antipsychotic medication, but the symptoms eventually reemerge, often in a more severe form. However, a 50% reduction in dyskinetic movement is documented in most patients by 18 months after discontinuation of antipsychotic agents (Glazer et al. 1984).

Anticholinergic drugs, often used for the control of EPS in patients taking neuroleptics, have been shown to worsen some forms of TD. Reunanen et al. (1982) and Yassa (1985) reported that TD improved for 9 of 15 patients whose anticholinergic medications had been discontinued. Paradoxically, anticholinergic drugs in high doses have been shown to be of value in the treatment of tardive dystonia (Burke et al. 1982; Fahn 1985).

There is no definitive treatment for TD. Alpha tocopherol (vitamin E) has been shown to be of some benefit, most often for patients who have had TD for less than 5 years (Adler et al. 1993; Akhtar et al. 1993; Dabiri et al. 1994; Egan et al. 1992; Elkashef et al. 1990; Lohr and Caligiuri 1996; Lohr et al. 1987). Vitamin E is a relatively nontoxic antioxidant that may protect neurons from the damaging effects of free radicals, which have been implicated in the etiology of TD. The typical dosage of vitamin

E is 1,600 IU/day. In addition to the treatment of existing TD, prophylaxis with vitamin E has been recommended. The most promising treatment for TD is clozapine. In an open trial, Lieberman et al. (1991) found at least 50% improvement in TD among 43% of patients switched from another antipsychotic to clozapine. Severe TD, and especially tardive dystonia, seem to respond best. In view of the risks of agranulocytosis with clozapine treatment (discussed later), this strategy is reserved for patients with severe TD or who are also poorly responsive to other agents. The efficacy of the other AAPs has not been systematically evaluated in this regard, but it is reasonable to attempt to use these agents prior to a clozapine trial. Other medications that have been used with limited benefit include dopamine-depleting agents, GABAergic drugs, low-dose dopamine agonists, and calcium channel blockers.

Neuroleptic malignant syndrome. In rare instances, patients taking antipsychotic medications may develop a potentially life-threatening disorder known as *neuroleptic malignant syndrome* (NMS). Although it occurs most frequently with the use of high-potency conventional antipsychotic drugs, this condition may accompany treatment with any antipsychotic agent, including the AAPs. Patients with NMS typically exhibit marked muscle rigidity, although this feature may be absent with the AAPs. Other salient features include fever, autonomic instability, elevated WBC count (above 15,000/mm^3), elevated creatinine phosphokinase (CPK) levels (above 300 U/mL), and delirium. The elevated CPK is due to muscle breakdown, which can lead to myoglobinuria and acute renal failure.

In a large prospective study, Rosebush and Stewart (1989) found that NMS was associated most often with the initiation or increase of antipsychotic medication, and in every case it occurred within 1 month of admission to a psychiatric unit. Episodes that occurred in patients taking stable dosages of antipsychotic medications were almost always associated with antecedent dehydration. Lithium use increases the risk appreciably, as does the presence of a mood disorder. Higher dosages, rapid escalation of dosage, and intramuscular injections of antipsychotics are all associated with the development of NMS (Keck et al. 1989). The keys to treatment after recognition of the syndrome are discontinuation of all medications, thorough medical evaluation, intravenous fluids, antipyretic agents, and cooling blankets. Several medications have been suggested to control NMS. Dantrolene and bromocriptine have received the most attention and are apparently the most successful agents. However, their efficacy over supportive care has not been proved (Guze and Baxter 1985; Levenson

1985). Because these two agents may treat different symptoms of NMS and act through distinct mechanisms, they may also be useful in combination. The most rational approach at present is to begin with supportive treatment and to initiate a trial of either dantrolene or bromocriptine only if supportive treatment proves inadequate.

Bromocriptine is a centrally active dopamine agonist that has been used successfully in some cases of NMS (Guze and Baxter 1985). The symptoms of rigidity may respond rapidly, although the temperature elevation, blood pressure instability, and creatinine kinase level may normalize only after several days. This drug should be administered in an initial dosage of 1.25–2.5 mg twice a day, and it may be increased to 10 mg three times a day (Guze and Baxter 1985).

Dantrolene sodium, also used in the treatment of malignant hyperthermia (a rare reaction to anesthetic drugs), is a direct-acting muscle relaxant that may reduce the thermogenesis of NMS caused by the tonic contraction of skeletal muscles (Guze and Baxter 1985). The manufacturer's recommendation for administration of dantrolene for acute malignant hyperthermia is 1 mg/kg by rapid intravenous push. The drug should be continued until the symptoms are reversed or until a maximum dose of 10 mg/kg is given. The oral dosage of dantrolene after a malignant hyperthermic crisis is 4–8 mg/kg/day in four divided doses. This regimen should be continued until all symptoms resolve. The clinician should be aware that dantrolene has a significant potential for hepatotoxicity and thus should not be administered to patients with liver dysfunction. For patients who have recovered from NMS but still require treatment with antipsychotic medication, rechallenge with neuroleptics is usually successful, although lower doses and low-potency neuroleptics should be used.

Anticholinergic side effects.	In general, the anticholinergic potency of the antipsychotic drugs is less than that of the anticholinergic drugs. However, when low-potency antipsychotic drugs are given in high dosages, anticholinergic side effects often become pronounced. Anticholinergic effects are categorized as peripheral or central. The most common peripheral side effects are dry mouth, decreased sweating, decreased bronchial secretions, blurred vision (owing to inhibition of accommodation), difficulty in urination, constipation, and tachycardia. Bethanechol chloride, a cholinergic drug that does not cross the blood-brain barrier, may effectively treat these side effects at a dosage of 25–50 mg tid; it may be required for the duration of therapy with the antipsychotic medication.

Central side effects of anticholinergic drugs include impairment in concentration, attention, and memory, and these side effects must be differentiated from symptoms caused by the patient's psychosis. Some patients are subject to these symptoms at relatively low dosages of medication. In cases of toxicity, anticholinergic delirium, which includes hot dry skin, dry mucous membranes, dilated pupils, absent bowel sounds, and tachycardia, may appear. Anticholinergic delirium constitutes a medical emergency and requires full supportive medical care. Physostigmine, a centrally and peripherally acting reversible anticholinesterase, may be used as a diagnostic agent in cases of suspected anticholinergic toxicity. This agent is administered intramuscularly at a dose of 1.0–to 2.0 mg or intravenously at a slow controlled rate of no more than 1 mg/minute. Physostigmine should not be used to maintain reversal of the toxicity, however, because a cholinergic crisis may result, which is characterized by nausea, vomiting, bradycardia, and seizures. This reaction can be reversed by the administration of a potent anticholinergic drug such as atropine.

Adrenergic side effects.	Antipsychotics also block α-adrenergic receptors, which can result in orthostatic hypotension and dizziness. The administration of epinephrine, which stimulates both α- and β-adrenergic receptors, will result in a paradoxical drop in blood pressure. This lowering of blood pressure is explained by the stimulation of β receptors in the presence of α-receptor blockade. In asthmatic patients who require treatment with antipsychotics as well as episodic treatment with α-adrenergic drugs, specific warnings are necessary regarding the dangers inherent in the use of epinephrine in the treatment of an acute asthmatic attack.

Endocrine and sexual side effects.	All the conventional antipsychotic medications and risperidone may produce hyperprolactinemia. Other side effects mediated, at least in part, by hyperprolactinemia include gynecomastia, galactorrhea, amenorrhea, and decreased libido. Amantadine may be an effective treatment for these side effects.

A combination of anticholinergic effects, α-adrenergic-receptor blockade, and hormonal effects may lead to several types of sexual difficulty. In men, inability to achieve or maintain erections, decreased ability to achieve orgasm, and changes in the pleasurable quality of orgasm have been reported (Ghadirian et al. 1982). Thioridazine may cause painful retrograde ejaculation, in which semen is ejected into the bladder (Shader 1964). Priapism, which necessitates immediate urological consultation, has been reported, especially with thioridazine and chlorpromazine (Mitchell and Popkin 1982). Women may experience changes in the quality of orgasm as well as decreased ability to achieve orgasm with use of antipsychotics. Sexual side effects are usually highly troubling to patients and often interfere with treatment compliance. Therefore, regular assessment by the clinician of sexual side effects is mandatory. Reducing the dosage or changing the type of agent usually reverses these symptoms. (Other treatment strategies are discussed in the subsection on sexual side effects of antidepressant drugs earlier in this chapter.)

Weight gain. Many patients experience weight gain while taking antipsychotic medication. Although one report suggested that molindone may be less likely than other drugs to cause weight gain (Gardos and Cole 1977), clinical experience has not confirmed this observation.

Ocular effects. Antipsychotics may cause pigmentary changes in the lens and retina, especially with long-term treatment. Pigment deposition in the lens of the eye does not affect vision; however, pigmentary retinopathy, which can lead to irreversible blindness, has been associated specifically with the use of thioridazine. Although pigmentary retinopathy has most often been reported with dosages above the recommended ceiling (i.e., 800 mg/day) of thioridazine, this condition has also occurred at usual clinical doses (Ball and Caroff 1986; Hamilton 1985). The clinician should be aware that drug interactions may increase plasma levels of thioridazine, which may increase the risk of development of this dangerous side effect (Silver et al. 1986).

Dermatological effects. Almost all patients taking antipsychotics, especially the aliphatic phenothiazines (e.g., chlorpromazine), become more sensitive to the effects of sunlight, which can lead to severe sunburn. Especially in the summer months, patients should avoid excessive sun exposure and use ultraviolet-blocking agents such as sunscreens that contain fully protective levels of para-aminobenzoic acid (PABA). As with many other medications, allergic maculopapular skin eruptions may occur. These are best treated by discontinuation of the agent, accompanied by symptomatic treatment with an antihistamines such as diphenhydramine. For subsequent treatment of psychosis, the patient should be given a drug from another family of antipsychotics.

Cardiac effects. Several of the antipsychotic medications have cardiac effects that can be detected both clinically and by ECG. Thioridazine is associated with prolonged QT intervals, related to plasma level concentration (Axelsson and Aspenstrom 1982). The pathophysiological significance of this change is not certain (Alvarez-Mena and Frank 1973); however, there have been reports of other arrhythmias and sudden death with antipsychotic agents. In our clinical experience, the most significant cardiovascular risks with antipsychotic use are associated with high or toxic doses. For example, using a 50-mg intramuscular dose of chlorpromazine to treat an acute psychotic event in a patient without a history of such treatment may cause sudden central suppression of the respiratory system, leading to cardiac arrest. We therefore recommend beginning treatment of patients who have no history of safely tolerating higher doses with frequent low doses of antipsychotic drugs, especially if intramuscular preparations are viable (e.g., chlorpromazine, 10 mg im every hour); this should be combined with careful monitoring of blood pressure and other vital signs.

Hepatic effects. Increased levels on liver function tests have been associated with antipsychotic treatment. Many cases of this reaction were linked to impurities in the original formulation of chlorpromazine, and the incidence has decreased over the years. These abnormalities usually suggest obstructive liver disease, with increases in bilirubin and alkaline phosphatase. In such circumstances the drug must be immediately discontinued and a different antipsychotic drug initiated. This reaction appears to be more common with low-potency conventional antipsychotics.

Hematological effects. Transient leukopenia and, in rare cases, agranulocytosis have been associated with neuroleptic treatment (Balon and Berchou 1986). Although agranulocytosis is strictly defined as a complete absence of all granulocytes in the blood, it may also refer to severe neutropenia, with a neutrophil count of less than 500/mL. This is an idiosyncratic reaction that usually occurs within the first 3–4 weeks after the initiation of treatment with an antipsychotic drug. However, the period of risk for agranulocytosis and leukopenia continues for 2–3 months of treatment. A higher risk for agranulocytosis is associated with low-potency conventional antipsychotic drugs, and most significantly, clozapine (Balon and Berchou 1986). (For discussion of clozapine-induced agranulocytosis, see subsection on the side effects of clozapine later in the chapter.)

Signs and symptoms of this reaction include high fever, stomatitis, severe pharyngitis, lymphadenopathy, and malaise. Treatment of this reaction requires immediate discontinuation of all medications and immediate medical evaluation and treatment. Agranulocytosis usually resolves after discontinuation of the causative agent. There must be vigorous treatment of any infections that develop. Further treatment of psychosis must be with an agent of a completely different chemical class.

Effects on seizure threshold. The antipsychotic drugs have been shown to lower seizure threshold, a phenomenon that has been confirmed in animal models. Of all the conventional antipsychotics, molindone and fluphenazine have most consistently been shown to have the lowest potential for this side effect (Itil and Soldatos 1980; Oliver et al. 1982). Clozapine is associated with a significant dose-dependent increase in seizures, an effect that is discussed more fully later. Special precautions must be taken with the use of antipsychotic agents for patients with a history of seizure disorder and for patients with other risk factors that decrease the seizure threshold.

Effects on temperature regulation. Antipsychotic drugs directly affect the hypothalamus and suppress temperature regulation. In combination with the α-adrenergic receptor- and cholinergic-receptor- blocking effects of antipsychotics, this effect becomes particularly serious in hot, humid weather. Severe hyperthermia, rhabdomyolysis, renal failure, and death may result. This potentially life-threatening condition requires immediate medical intervention and supportive treatment. It is mandatory that a cool environment and adequate amounts of fluids be provided for patients taking antipsychotic agents. Also, care must be taken that patients do not overexert themselves in warm weather or hot environments. Special monitoring is also required for acutely agitated or manic patients and for patients in restraints, because they are prone to this dangerous condition.

Use in pregnancy. Like most other drugs, antipsychotic agents should be avoided, if possible, during pregnancy and during lactation periods for mothers who breast-feed their infants. There is a possible increase in birth defects among infants born to mothers who were first exposed to antipsychotic drugs during the sixth to tenth week of gestation (Edlund and Craig 1984). Edlund and Craig (1984) pointed out that because there is an increased risk of fetal death in psychotic mothers, the small risk of neuroleptic-induced teratogenesis must be assessed carefully and balanced against the risks involved in withholding treatment. These important issues are reviewed in detail elsewhere (Cohen et al. 1989; Nurnberg and Prudic 1984; Robinson et al. 1986).

In addition, antipsychotic agents should be prescribed with great caution in the peripartum period. Extra-

pyramidal symptoms (Hill et al. 1966; Levy and Wisniewski 1974; Tamer et al. 1969) and neonatal jaundice (Scokel and Jones 1962) have been reported in infants following in utero exposure to these drugs. Also, neonates may be exposed to small amounts of antipsychotics in breast milk (Stewart et al. 1980). It is therefore necessary to reassess the potential risks and benefits of antipsychotic treatment as the pregnancy comes to term. As a general guideline, antipsychotic drugs should be used in pregnant patients only if absolutely necessary, at the minimal dose required, and for the briefest possible time. Documentation of informed consent from both the mother and the father is necessary. Use of ECT to treat acute psychosis in pregnant mothers should be considered.

Drug interactions. Antipsychotic drugs have profound effects on multiple CNS receptors, and these effects are compounded when other medications are added. For example, the α-adrenergic-receptor blockade of antipsychotics may interfere with the efficacy of the antihypertensive drug guanethidine. The sedative and anticholinergic effects of antipsychotic drugs are increased with the addition of other sedating or anticholinergic drugs. As mentioned previously, patients taking drugs with potentially serious adverse effects (such as the risk of retinopathy with thioridazine) should be monitored through plasma level determinations when other medications are used concurrently.

ATYPICAL ANTIPSYCHOTIC DRUGS

The first of the class of atypical antipsychotic drugs was clozapine (Clozaril). Clozapine is a landmark drug in the treatment of schizophrenia for several reasons. It was the first medication shown to be efficacious in otherwise nonresponsive patients, many of whom seemed destined to live out their lives in state psychiatric hospitals. Although it was not uniformly effective, clozapine was a "miracle" for many of these individuals. In addition, clozapine was the first agent to attenuate significantly the negative symptoms of schizophrenia, such as marked social withdrawal and apathy, thereby helping many patients return to meaningful and productive lives. Also, clozapine rarely produces EPS, and to date it is the only antipsychotic drug that is not associated with treatment-emergent tardive dyskinesia. This important clinical property is concordant with the observation that chronic administration of clozapine results in selective inhibition of dopamine neurons in the mesolimbic pathways, with little functional effect on striatal dopamine tracts. Finally, clozapine has minimal effects on the tuboinfundibular system, and therefore it does not cause hyperprolactinemia.

Clozapine has a wide range of physiological actions, and although there are a number of hypotheses to explain its unique spectrum of effects, the definitive answer awaits further research. A great deal of research has focused on clozapine's relatively greater 5-HT$_2$ than D$_2$ antagonism, and this property has been the predominant focus of new drug development in the class of drugs currently referred to as atypical antipsychotics. Risperidone (Risperdal), olanzapine (Zyprexa), and quetiapine (Seroquel) have subsequently been approved for use in the United States. In general, the atypical antipsychotics drugs appear to provide superior efficacy, most significantly in the treatment of negative symptoms, the reduction of acute motor side effects, and the possibility of a reduced risk of tardive dyskinesia compared to conventional antipsychotic drugs. These drugs may also improve cognitive function in patients with schizophrenia (Green et al. 1997; Hagger et al. 1993; Rossi et al. 1997). Although the use of these agents, as opposed to the less expensive, conventional drugs, is currently the subject of debate, the AAPs may dramatically improve the treatment of chronic psychotic disorders.

Clozapine

Clozapine, a dibenzodiazepine, is the prototype AAP. Because of a 1%–2% risk of producing a potentially fatal agranulocytosis, the use of clozapine is restricted to patients who have not responded to or cannot tolerate other antipsychotic drugs. Kane et al. (1988) studied patients with chronic schizophrenia who had failed to improve after at least three adequate trials of conventional antipsychotics. Data from this large, multicenter, double-blind prospective study demonstrated a significant improvement in 30% of the patients taking clozapine, compared to only 4% of those taking chlorpromazine. Less rigorous data suggest that clozapine may also be effective in refractory schizoaffective disorder, psychotic mood disorders, and rapid-cycling bipolar disorder, even in the absence of psychosis (Calabrese et al. 1996; Keck et al. 1996; McElroy et al. 1991; Suppes et al. 1992; Zarate et al. 1995). Because clozapine appears to be devoid of parkinsonian side effects, it is also useful in low dosages (25 mg/day) for patients with Parkinson's disease and psychosis induced by dopamine agonists (Ostergaard and Dupont 1988). Other indications require higher dosages, as discussed later, and an extended period of titration to achieve therapeutic dosages and clinical response.

Clozapine is a difficult drug for both patient and physician, but when other treatments have failed, there is no doubt that the potential benefits of this remarkable medication are worth the risks for many patients with severe psychotic illnesses.

Mechanism of action. Clozapine exhibits high in vitro receptor affinities for the D$_4$, 5-HT$_2$, α_1-adrenergic, muscarinic, and histamine H$_1$ receptors, and a relatively weak affinity for D$_1$, D$_2$, and D$_3$ receptors (Brunello et al. 1995; Meltzer et al. 1989). The high 5-HT$_2$:D$_2$ ratio is hypothesized to be responsible for many of clozapine's advantages over typical antipsychotic drugs, either directly or indirectly (Meltzer 1991). Other investigators have suggested that clozapine's superior efficacy may be related to the drug's ability to increase norepinephrine outflow (Breier et al. 1994). It is also of interest that clozapine appears to be able to block the behavioral effects of the NMDA-receptor antagonists PCP and MK801 (D. C. Hoffman 1992; Verma and Kulkarni 1992).

Clinical use. Because of prominent sedation and orthostatic hypotension, clozapine is initiated at a dosage of 12.5 mg/day and quickly increased to 12.5 mg bid. The dosage is then increased as tolerated in 25-mg increments every other day. The typical target dosage is 300–500 mg/day in divided doses, with a greater amount given in the evening to minimize daytime sedation. Although routine blood level monitoring is not recommended, it should be noted that a serum level of greater than 350 ng/mL is associated with a higher response rate (Perry et al. 1991). Serum levels should be ascertained in nonresponders. The duration of treatment required to assess the medication response adequately is longer than for most medications—typically, 3–6 months (Meltzer 1994). It is important that both the patient and the family understand this time frame before initiating treatment with clozapine. If patients are nonresponsive after 6 months of continuous clozapine treatment, the dosage may be gradually increased to a maximum of 900 mg/day.

Commonly, clozapine is initially combined with the antipsychotic medication presently being taken and then cross-tapered after 2–3 weeks to avoid a period of time when the patient is not taking an adequate amount of antipsychotic medication. This strategy should be used with caution if the existing medication is a low-potency conventional antipsychotic because of additive α-adrenergic and anticholinergic side effects.

Risks, Side Effects, and Their Management

Agranulocytosis. Agranulocytosis occurs in 0.8% of patients treated with clozapine during the first year of treatment, with a peak incidence at 3 months (Alvir and Lieberman 1994, Alvir et al. 1993). The institution of weekly WBC monitoring in most cases allows time for withdrawal of the drug. The dispensing of clozapine in the United States is linked to weekly WBC monitoring. On the basis of the patient's WBC and absolute neutrophil count, strict guidelines have been set (Table 27–18). Until recently, weekly WBC count monitoring was required throughout clozapine treatment. Recently, the Neuropsychopharmacology Advisory Committee to the US Food and Drug Administration unanimously recommended a reduction in frequency of WBC count monitoring after 6 months of continuous treatment to every 14 days (Honigfeld et al. 1998).

There may be a genetic susceptibility to clozapine-induced agranulocytosis. Although it was first reported in patients of Ashkenazi Jewish descent (Lieberman et al. 1990), the finding has been extended to non-Jewish populations and appears to be related to genetic variations in the major histocompatibility complex (Corzo et al. 1995; Turbay et al. 1997; Yunis et al. 1995). Although there are some promising leads for genetic markers, at this time genetic testing is not of clinical benefit and these findings do not preclude the use of clozapine in any ethnic group. For unknown reasons, women and elderly persons may also be at greater risk for clozapine-induced agranulocytosis.

If agranulocytosis develops, prompt consultation with a hematologist is indicated. Reverse isolation and prophy-

TABLE 27–18. Guidelines for hematological monitoring of patients taking clozapine

1. Initial white blood cell count (WBC) must be greater than 3,500/mm³.

2. A weekly WBC is required throughout treatment and for 4 weeks after discontinuation of clozapine.[a]

3. If WBC is 2,000–3,000/mm³ *or* granulocyte count is 1,000–1,500/mm³, interrupt therapy and monitor for signs of infection. Check WBC and differential daily. If there are no symptoms of infection, WBC returns to greater than 3,000/mm³, and granulocyte level is greater than 1,500/mm³, resume clozapine with twice-weekly WBC and differential counts until the total WBC returns to above 3,500/mm³.

4. If WBC is less than 2,000/mm³ *or* granulocyte count is less than 1,000/mm³, discontinue clozapine and do not rechallenge. Check WBC and differential daily. Treat infection with antibiotics. Consider bone marrow aspiration to ascertain granulopoietic status. If granulopoiesis is deficient, consider protective isolation.

[a]Monitoring every 14 days has recently been recommended for patients who have been taking clozapine for ≥ 6 months.

lactic antibiotics may be used to prevent infection. Granulocyte-stimulating factors may be used to shorten the duration and reduce the morbidity of agranulocytosis (Barnas et al. 1992; Chengappa et al. 1996; Gerson et al. 1992; Nielsen 1993). Although lithium often causes leukocytosis, it does not appear to treat or prevent clozapine-induced agranulocytosis. Once a patient has developed agranulocytosis while taking clozapine, he or she should not be rechallenged with this medication.

Clozapine is contraindicated in patients with myeloproliferative disorders or who are immunocompromised owing to diseases such as tuberculosis or human immunodeficiency virus (HIV) infection because of their increased risk of developing agranulocytosis. Concomitant medications that are associated with bone marrow suppression, such as carbamazepine, are also contraindicated.

Extrapyramidal effects. Extrapyramidal side effects are uncommon with clozapine at any dosage, although some patients experience akathisia or hand tremors. The incidence of akathisia is about 7% (Chengappa et al.1994).

Neuroleptic malignant syndrome. Despite the absence of EPS in clozapine-treated patients, there have been reports of NMS in patients medicated with clozapine alone (Anderson and Powers 1991; Das Gupta and Young 1991; Miller et al. 1991).

Sedation. Sedation is the most common side effect of clozapine, and it is particularly prominent early in treatment. Sedation generally attenuates with dosage reduction, when tolerance to this side effect develops, or when a disproportionate amount is given at bedtime.

Cardiovascular effects. Hypotension and tachycardia occur in the majority of patients treated with clozapine.

Weight gain. Weight gain occurs in most patients; in many cases patients gain 10% or more of their original body weight (Umbricht et al. 1994). Patients should receive nutritional counseling at the initiation of treatment with clozapine.

Hypersalivation. Hypersalivation occurs in one-third of patients taking clozapine, particularly at night. Although the basis for this side effect is unknown, the symptom is not related to drug-induced parkinsonism. Treatment with anticholinergic medications or an α_2 antagonist may be helpful.

Fever. For unclear reasons, clozapine treatment is associated with benign, transient temperature elevations, generally within the first 3 weeks of treatment. Patients taking clozapine who develop fevers must be evaluated for infectious etiologies and for agranulocytosis and NMS.

Seizures. Clozapine treatment is associated with a dose-dependent risk of seizures. The vast majority of clozapine-induced seizures are tonic-clonic, but myoclonic seizures also occur. Dosages of less than 300 mg/day are associated with a 1%–3% seizure risk. Dosages of 300–600 mg/day carry a 3%–4% risk, and dosages greater than 600 mg/day are associated with a 5% risk of seizures. Because of this risk, clozapine dosages greater than 600 mg/day are not recommended unless the patient has failed to respond at lower dosages. Many clinicians avoid using clozapine for patients with abnormal EEGs. Our clinical impression is that EEG abnormalities associated with clozapine use are much more common than clozapine-induced seizures. Once a seizure has occurred, the question of whether or not to continue using clozapine requires clinical judgment, including an assessment of the risk-benefit ratio. Because only patients with fairly serious and otherwise refractory illnesses receive clozapine, the medication is usually continued, with the addition of an anticonvulsant. Carbamazepine must be avoided because of the additive risk of bone marrow suppression. At the present time, valproate appears to be the safest anticonvulsant for patients taking clozapine.

Anticholinergic effects. Anticholinergic side effects, such as dry mouth, blurred vision, constipation, and urinary retention, are common early side effects.

Obsessive-compulsive disorder. Treatment with clozapine has been reported to exacerbate symptoms of obsessive-compulsive disorder, probably owing to 5-HT$_2$ antagonism (Ghaemi et al. 1995). If this effect occurs, symptoms are usually controlled with the addition of an SSRI.

Drug interactions. Clozapine should not be combined with any drugs that have the potential to suppress bone marrow function, such as carbamazepine. Clozapine should not be used in conjunction with bupropion because of the additive risk of seizures. There have been isolated reports of respiratory arrest in patients who were taking both clozapine and a high-potency benzodiazepine. Because of these reports, benzodiazepines should be avoided, but are not absolutely contraindicated, in patients who are taking clozapine.

Clozapine is metabolized by hepatic cytochrome P450 1A2 and, to a lesser degree, 3A3/4; therefore it is subject to changes in serum concentration when combined with medications that inhibit or induce these enzymes (see section on drug interactions later in this chapter). These pharmacokinetic interactions are particularly important regarding clozapine because of the dose-dependent risk of seizures.

RISPERIDONE

Risperidone (Risperdal), a novel benzisoxazole derivative, is an atypical antipsychotic medication that combines D$_2$-receptor antagonism with potent serotonin 5-HT$_2$-receptor antagonism. Risperidone has a higher affinity for D$_2$ receptors than does clozapine. Risperidone also antagonizes D$_1$, D$_4$, α_1, α_2, and H$_1$ histaminic receptors. Risperidone is effective against both the positive and the negative symptoms of chronic schizophrenia (Chouinard et al. 1993; Marder and Meibach 1994). In these controlled, fixed-dose studies, the optimal dosage of risperidone was 6 mg/day. Higher dosages (i.e., 10–16 mg/day), produced greater EPS and less robust antipsychotic effects. Risperidone is unlikely to cause acute EPS at lower dosages.

Risperidone (and the other AAPs except for clozapine) does not cause higher than expected rates of agranulocytosis and does not require routine hematological monitoring. The long-term risk of TD is not known, but it appears to be higher than for clozapine and lower than for conventional antipsychotic drugs. Unlike clozapine, risperidone is associated with elevated serum prolactin levels.

Bondolfi et al. (1996) reported that risperidone is comparable to clozapine in treatment-refractory schizophrenia; however, the patients in their study were not as highly refractory as were the patients in the earlier studies of clozapine in refractory schizophrenia (Kane et al. 1988). Clinical experience suggests that clozapine is superior to risperidone in highly refractory cases (i.e., patients who have not responded to risperidone may respond to clozapine). However, given the more benign side-effect profiles of risperidone and olanzapine, we recommend a trial of one of these drugs before beginning a trial of clozapine. We do not recommend switching patients who are stable while taking clozapine to risperidone because of the high frequency of severe relapses when this has been attempted.

Clinical Use

Risperidone is most effective in the 4- to 6-mg range. For initial treatment, we recommend using divided doses, starting at 1 mg bid and quickly increasing to 2 mg bid. For elderly persons, the initial dosage should be lower. After the first week of treatment, it may be useful to give the entire dosage at bedtime. This usually helps the patient to sleep and reduces daytime side effects. However, we do not suggest this practice for elderly persons because of an increased risk of falling. In addition, some patients feel an activating effect from risperidone; in these individuals the medication should be administered in the morning.

Risks, Side Effects, and Their Management

Insomnia, hypotension, agitation, headache, and rhinitis are the most common side effects of risperidone. These tend to lessen with time. Overall, the drug tends to be well tolerated. Overall, risperidone is not associated with significant anticholinergic side effects.

Extrapyramidal effects.   In comparison to haloperidol, risperidone is associated with a lower prevalence of acute extrapyramidal effects and akathisia (Owens 1996). EPS occurs in a dose-dependent manner, with more frequent occurrence when the dosage is above 6 mg/day.

Cardiovascular effects.   Brief hypotension may occur, as expected with α blockade (Owens 1994). Tachycardia is also common.

Tardive dyskinesia.   Risperidone at low doses produces few parkinsonian side effects, but it can cause tardive dyskinesia (Gwinn and Caviness 1997; Umbricht and Kane 1996). The incidence of risperidone-induced TD is not known, but it is assumed to be between that of clozapine and the conventional antipsychotics.

Weight gain.   Weight gain has been associated with risperidone treatment (Owens 1994; Umbricht and Kane 1996).

Drug interactions.   Risperidone is metabolized primarily by the cytochrome P450 2D6 enzyme. Medications that inhibit this enzyme, such as many of the SSRIs, cause increased risperidone plasma levels for any dosage. If such medications are being taken, it is important to monitor the patient for the development of EPS, because this side effect is dose dependent. If such a pharmacokinetic interaction is suspected, the dosage of risperidone is decreased on the basis of clinical observation; serum levels are not clinically meaningful with risperidone. Pharmacodynamic interactions may occur when risperidone is combined with other medications that share a similar physiological effect. Caution is particularly warranted when risperidone is combined with other medications that can cause hypotension.

OLANZAPINE

Olanzapine (Zyprexa), a thienobenzodiazapine, is the most recently released AAP. Compared to clozapine, olanzapine has greater D_2 and weaker D_4 and α-adrenergic affinity. Despite the structural similarity of these two drugs, olanzapine is not associated with higher than expected rates of agranulocytosis. Although in vitro binding studies have indicated a high affinity for M_1 receptors, anticholinergic side effects are clinically not as prominent as these data would predict.

Olanzapine has dose-dependent therapeutic effects on both positive and negative symptoms and a favorable side-effect profile (Beasley et al. 1996). Acute dystonia is distinctly uncommon. Akathisia is more common but significantly less common than with the conventional antipsychotic drugs. In prospective double-blind studies, treatment-emergent tardive dyskinesia has been reported to occur in 1% of the olanzapine group compared to 4.6% of the haloperidol group (Tollefson et al. 1997). Olanzapine is associated with modest dose-dependent elevations in serum prolactin levels, but most often these elevations are transient and within the normal reference range (Tollefson et al. 1997).

Although the effect of olanzapine on patients with primary mood disorders has not been systematically studied, this is an area of active interest. The results of an international collaborative trial of olanzapine versus haloperidol in the treatment of schizophrenia and schizoaffective disorders indicated that olanzapine is superior to haloperidol in treating comorbid depression (Tollefson et al. 1997). Olanzapine has not been directly compared to clozapine in patients with refractory schizophrenia. Olanzapine, like clozapine, prevents MK801 neurotoxicity in animal models (Farber et al. 1996).

Clinical Use

The recommended starting dosage of olanzapine is 5–10 mg at bedtime, subsequently titrated on the basis of tolerability and therapeutic effect. The clinically effective range is 7.5–20 mg/day, administered as a single daily dose at bedtime. Higher dosages are more effective but result in increased side effects. Dosages of 12.5–17.5 mg/day are superior to haloperidol in the treatment of negative symptoms (Borison 1995). Clinically meaningful improvement may not be evident for the first several weeks after initiating treatment, but improvement usually continues through week 6 and perhaps longer.

Although there are no systematic data regarding switching from other antipsychotic drugs to olanzapine, early clinical experience favors a gradual cross-titration.

Commonly, olanzapine is added to the existing antipsychotic medication, which is then tapered after 1–2 weeks. This strategy is applicable when switching from clozapine to olanzapine, but a word of caution is warranted. For patients who are stable taking clozapine, it is tempting to consider substituting olanzapine to avoid the risk of clozapine-induced agranulocytosis; however, it cannot be assumed that patients will do equally well on another AAP. There have been many instances of poor patient outcomes after attempts to switch from clozapine to another AAP, and we currently do not recommend this change despite the problems with clozapine. However, before initiating a trial of clozapine, it is reasonable to try olanzapine or risperidone in patients whose illness is refractory to conventional antipsychotic drugs.

Risks, Side Effects, and Their Management

Somnolence.   As one would predict on the basis of the histamine H_1 antagonism, somnolence is the most common side effect of olanzapine. Somnolence and psychomotor slowing are dose dependent, and patients often become tolerant to this side effect over time.

Anticholinergic side effects.   Anticholinergic side effects are clinically less significant than would be predicted on the basis of in vitro muscarinic receptor-binding affinity. However, dry mouth has been reported in association with olanzapine treatment (Beasley 1996).

Seizures.   Premarketing studies revealed a 0.9% incidence of seizures, some of which were attributed to concomitant medical disorders. Olanzapine should be used with caution in elderly patients, in patients with a history of seizures, and in those with conditions that may lower the seizure threshold, such as dementia.

Hepatic effects.   Increased transaminase levels were reported in 2% of patients taking olanzapine in premarketing evaluation. In many cases these levels normalized without medication discontinuation, and all cases to date have been clinically benign. Routine laboratory monitoring is not recommended, but olanzapine should be used with caution in patients with hepatic disease or with additional risk factors for hepatic toxicity. In this group of patients, serum transaminase levels must be monitored.

Weight gain.   Treatment-emergent weight gain has been observed in association with olanzapine treatment. Patients should be advised to monitor their caloric intake and increase their exercise levels whenever possible

Drug interactions.   Olanzapine is metabolized by several pathways and is therefore less likely to be affected by concurrent administration with other medications. Because olanzapine does not appear to inhibit any of the cytochrome P450 enzymes, it should not increase the availability of other medications through this mechanism. Additive pharmacodynamic effects are expected if olanzapine is combined with medications that also have anticholinergic, antihistaminic, or α-adrenergic side effects.

QUETIAPINE

Quetiapine (Seroquel), the newest of the AAPs to enter the U.S. market, is indicated for the treatment of psychotic disorders. Quetiapine is a dibenzothiazapine derivative with weak affinity for 5-HT_{1A}, 5-HT_2, D_1, D_2, H_1, α_1, and α_2 receptors. In a fixed-dose comparison of quetiapine to haloperidol (12 mg/day) and placebo, quetiapine was superior to placebo at doses of 150 mg–750 mg on most measures, but superior to placebo for the treatment of negative symptoms only at the 300-mg dose (Arvanitis et al. 1997). Quetiapine was not statistically superior to haloperidol in efficacy measures, but was comparable to placebo with regards to treatment-emergent extrapyramidal side effects (Arvanitis et al. 1997). The relatively high 5-HT_2-to-D_2 ratio is consistent with the hypothesized advantageous properties of the AAPs, antagonism of H_1 receptors is associated with sedative side effects, and α_1 antagonism is associated with orthostatic hypotension.

Clinical Use

Quetiapine is initiated at a dose of 25 mg bid, and then increased on day 2 to 50 mg bid, on day 3 to 100 mg bid, and on day 4 to 100 mg in the morning and 200 mg in the evening. The optimal dose for most patients appears to be 300 mg, although the drug appears to be safe and possibly efficacious within a dose range of 150–750 mg. A slower titration and lower daily doses may be warranted for patients with hepatic disease and for elderly patients.

Risks, Side Effects, and Their Management

Quetiapine was no different from placebo in doses to 750 mg/day regarding extrapyramidal side effects and changes in serum prolactin levels (Arvanitis et al. 1997).

Somnolence.   Somnolence is one of the most common side effects of quetiapine. Somnolence and psychomotor slowing are dose dependent, and patients often become tolerant to this side effect over time.

Ocular changes. The development of cataracts was observed in association with quetiapine treatment in studies of dogs and long-term studies of dogs and humans, but a causal relationship has not been established. Because of the possible risk of ocular changes, it is currently recommended that patients receive an ocular examination of sufficient sensitivity to detect cataract formation, such as a slit-lamp examination, at the initiation of treatment and at 6-month intervals. Because this is not an acute change, if the clinical situation dictates, quetiapine may be begun shortly before the ocular examination.

Cardiovascular effects. As predicted with α_1 antagonism, quetiapine may induce orthostatic hypotension and concomitant symptoms of dizziness, tachycardia, and syncope. The risk of symptomatic hypotension is particularly pronounced during initial dose titration. Quetiapine should be used with precaution in patients with cardiovascular disease, cerebral vascular disease, or other illnesses predisposing to hypotension.

Hepatic effects. Increased transaminase levels were reported in 6% of patients taking quetiapine in premarketing evaluation. These changes usually occur in the first weeks of treatment and to date have been benign. Routine laboratory monitoring is not recommended, but quetiapine should be used with caution in patients with hepatic disease or with additional risk factors for hepatic toxicity.

Weight gain. Quetiapine may induce weight gain. In premarketing placebo-controlled studies, a weight gain of $\geq 7\%$ of body weight was observed in 23% of quetiapine-treated patients, compared to 6% of placebo control subjects. Early clinical experience suggests that weight gain associated with quetiapine treatment is not generally as marked as has been observed with olanzapine.

Drug interactions. Quetiapine is metabolized by the hepatic cytochrome P450 3A3/4 enzyme. Concurrent administration of cytochrome P450–inducing drugs, such as carbamazepine, decreases quetiapine blood levels. In such circumstances, increased doses of quetiapine are appropriate. Quetiapine does not appreciably affect the pharmacokinetics of other medications. Pharmacodynamic effects are expected if quetiapine is combined with medications that also have antihistaminic or α-adrenergic side effects. Because of its potential for producing hypotension, quetiapine may also enhance the effects of certain antihypertensive agents.

PHARMACOLOGICAL TREATMENT OF SCHIZOPHRENIA

General Principles

There is evidence that the long-term outcome for a patient with schizophrenia is better when treatment of the acute episode is initiated rapidly. After a patient's first episode of schizophrenia, the antipsychotic medication should be continued for approximately 1 year after a full remission of psychotic symptoms (Johnson 1985). After that time, a trial period without medication may be considered, except for patients with a history of serious suicide attempts or violent aggressive behavior (American Psychiatric Association 1997). The patient and his or her family should be informed of the early signs and symptoms of relapse, such as suspiciousness, difficulty sleeping, and argumentativeness. The patient should be carefully monitored during this period.

When antipsychotic drugs are discontinued (especially when done precipitously) in patients who have been treated with these drugs for a year or longer, a withdrawal supersensitivity psychosis may appear (Chouinard et al. 1978). This psychosis may be due to the anticholinergic actions of antipsychotics, rather than to the dopamine-blocking activity (Luchins et al. 1980). If left untreated, the psychotic symptoms most often abate over several weeks. All too often, however, the clinician views the condition as the reemergence of the underlying psychosis and treats this psychosis with additional antipsychotic drugs. However, a relapse of the psychosis may take weeks to months to occur after discontinuation of antipsychotic drugs. The withdrawal psychosis usually resolves within days.

For patients with a chronic, relapsing form of schizophrenia, antipsychotic medication should be continued for up to 5 symptom-free years before discontinuation (Johnson 1985). Kane et al. (1983) performed careful studies of patients maintained with high-dose (12.5–50.0 mg every 2 weeks) and low-dose (1.25–5.0 mg every 2 weeks) treatment with fluphenazine decanoate. Although the high-dose medication prevented relapse better than the low-dose treatment, patients treated with low-dose medication had fewer extrapyramidal side effects. In addition, the mild exacerbations of the psychoses were successfully treated with periodic increases in medication, without the necessity of hospitalization. Marder et al. (1984) compared the clinical course in patients with schizophrenia treated with 5 or 25 mg of fluphenazine decanoate administered every 2 weeks. They found no difference in relapse rates between the two groups, although the higher dose group had evidence of more side effects.

Subsequent studies have further documented the advantage of dose reduction in the maintenance of schizophrenia (Johnson et al. 1987; Marder et al. 1987; Schooler et al. 1997); however, intermittent treatment is associated with a greater relapse rate and is not recommended (Herz et al. 1991; Schooler et al. 1997).

In light of these important studies, we recommend that patients be maintained on the lowest dosage of antipsychotic drugs possible. In addition, patients should be monitored closely for symptoms of relapse. If the patient is compliant with treatment, oral medications are usually sufficient. However, if there is concern, on the basis of the previous treatment history, that the patient may not reliably take daily oral medication, a long-acting depot preparation may be indicated.

Refractory Schizophrenia

If there is no response to the indicated treatment, minimal side effects are seen (e.g., EPS, hypotension, sedation), and poor compliance is not the cause, one can gradually increase the dosage until mild side effects are seen. If no further improvement is seen after an additional 2–4 weeks at this dosage, another antipsychotic drug from another class should be substituted. Atypical antipsychotics should be considered in patients who have not responded to conventional antipsychotic medication. At this time adequate data do not exist to suggest greater efficacy of one AAP, other than clozapine, over the others in patients with refractory illness. A trial of clozapine should be considered for patients who continue to have positive symptoms or violent behavior despite an adequate trial of at least one other antipsychotic medication and for patients with intolerable side effects to at least two different antipsychotic medications from different classes (American Psychiatric Association 1997). At least one of these drugs should be an AAP.

An additional strategy to use with nonresponsive patients is to add another medication to augment the therapeutic effects of the antipsychotic. The most common agents used to augment antipsychotic medications in the treatment of schizophrenia are lithium (Cole et al. 1984; Delva and Letemednia 1982), valproate (Linnoila et al. 1976), carbamazepine (Hakola and Loulumaa 1984; Klein et al. 1984; Luchins 1984; Neppe 1982), and benzodiazepines (Csernansky et al. 1988; Douyon et al. 1989; Nestoros et al. 1982). These medications are often quite helpful when there is a need to target specific symptoms, such as affective lability, aggression, or anxiety, in a patient with schizophrenia. However, with the current availability of the AAPs, particularly clozapine, the use of these aug-

menting strategies in patients with antipsychotic-resistant schizophrenia should be reserved for patients who cannot take clozapine or who have not fully responded to clozapine (American Psychiatric Association 1997). Although there are no systematic data to guide the treatment of patients who have not responded to clozapine, some patients are benefiting from the combination of clozapine and one of the other AAPs.

MOOD STABILIZERS

OVERVIEW

After an initial observation by Cade (1949) that the calming effect of lithium in animals could be extended to humans with manic-depressive illness, Baastrup and Schou (1967) conclusively demonstrated that lithium was effective in the prophylaxis of recurrence of affective disorders. Although lithium continues to be an invaluable primary treatment for acute mania and maintenance therapy in bipolar disorder, it is ineffective or suboptimal for many patients. More recently, the anticonvulsant medications valproate (Depakote) and carbamazepine (Tegretol) have been shown to be effective and, in some cases, superior to lithium. Although they are most often used to treat bipolar disorder, these medications are collectively referred to as *mood stabilizers* because of their ability to stabilize mood oscillations regardless of etiology. Other drugs that have been reported to be effective in the treatment of bipolar disorder include thyroxine (T_4) and the calcium channel blockers. In this section, we review the clinical use of these drugs and the treatment of bipolar disorder.

LITHIUM

Indications and Efficacy

Lithium has been proved effective for acute and prophylactic treatment of both manic and depressive episodes in patients with bipolar illness (Consensus Development Panel 1985; Prien et al. 1984) and cyclothymia (Akiskal et al. 1979). However, patients with rapid-cycling bipolar disorder (i.e., four or more mood disorder episodes per year) have been reported to respond less well to lithium treatment (Dunner and Fieve 1974; Prien et al. 1984; Wehr et al. 1988). Lithium is also effective in the prevention of future depressive episodes in patients with recurrent unipolar depressive disorder (Consensus Development Panel 1985) and as an adjunct to antidepressants in depressed patients whose illness is partially refractory to treatment with antidepressants alone (discussed earlier in this chapter in the section on antidepressant drugs). Furthermore, lithium may be useful in the maintenance of remission of depressive disorder after ECT (Coopen et al. 1981) and in the maintenance of the antidepressant effect of sleep deprivation (Baxter et al. 1986). Lithium has also been used effectively in some cases of aggression and behavioral dyscontrol (see section on the treatment of aggression later in this chapter).

Mechanism of Action

Lithium is a monovalent cation that is believed to affect intracellular second-messenger systems. According to a review by Jope and Williams (1994), lithium inhibits several steps in phosphoinositide metabolism as well as G-protein functioning (Manji et al. 1995). Lithium has been reported to inhibit the stimulation of adenylate cyclase by a number of different neurotransmitters without suppressing basal adenylate cyclase activity (Belmaker et al. 1983; Ebstein et al. 1980; Zohar et al. 1982). These effects on signal transduction have broad effects on neuronal function and gene expression.

Clinical Use

Before they begin treatment with lithium, patients should be told that they might experience nausea, diarrhea, polyuria, increased thirst, and fine hand tremor. These are often transient, but in some patients they persist with therapeutic lithium levels. Because of a narrow range between the therapeutic and toxic doses of lithium and the wide variability of lithium pharmacokinetics among different individuals, the optimal dosage for an individual patient cannot be based on the dosage administered. Rather, lithium dosing should be based on the concentration of lithium in the plasma. Lithium carbonate is completely absorbed by the gastrointestinal tract and reaches peak plasma levels in 1–2 hours. The elimination half-life is approximately 24 hours. Steady-state lithium levels are obtained in approximately 5 days.

Therapeutic plasma levels for patients undergoing lithium therapy range from 0.5 to 1.5 mEq/L. Although lower plasma levels are associated with less troubling side effects, most clinicians seek to establish levels of at least 0.8 mEq/L in treating acute manic episodes. Therefore, when intolerable side effects have not intervened, treatment of acute mania with lithium should not be considered a failure until plasma levels of 1.2–1.5 mEq/L have been reached and maintained for 2 weeks. However, when levels this high are necessary for acute treatment, the dosage often may be reduced to the range of 0.8–1.0 mEq/L for mainte-

nance therapy. Although Gelenberg et al. (1989) initially reported that levels in the range of 0.8–1.0 mEq/L provide better prophylaxis against relapse, this finding may be applicable only to patients who require relatively high levels for initial stabilization. Patients who are stabilized with blood levels in the range of 0.4–0.8 mEq/L may do well remaining at these relatively low levels, often with a reduced side-effect burden. It now appears that rapid decreases in lithium may be more strongly correlated with relapse than is the absolute blood level. Therapeutic lithium levels have not been established for other disorders.

There are several methods for initiating lithium treatment. Some investigators have suggested a test-dose method: a small dose of lithium is given, and the level is ascertained either 24 hours later (Cooper et al. 1973) or 12 and 36 hours later (Perry et al. 1986). From these levels, the required maintenance dosage can be calculated. Dose prediction tests require precise patient compliance and timing with respect to both the dose ingested and obtaining the blood test. A simple titration method we suggest is to start healthy adult patients on a dosage of lithium carbonate of 300 mg bid, increasing this dosage by 300 mg every 3–4 days. For healthy patients with no impairment in renal function, plasma level determinations should be obtained biweekly. Because steady-state plasma levels should not be taken until the patient has been on a constant dosage regimen for at least 5 days, this method may slightly underestimate the steady-state level. Lithium levels must be obtained 12 hours after the last lithium dose. After therapeutic lithium levels have been established, levels should be monitored every month for the first 3 months and every 3 months thereafter. For patients who have remained stable and who are aware of early signs of both relapse and lithium toxicity, lithium levels may be obtained less frequently.

Because lithium has a serum half-life of approximately 24 hours, it may be administered as a single daily dose. The results of several investigations favor such a dosing schedule. Divided daily doses with the usual carbonate salt result in several peak levels throughout the day, with a relatively rapid decrease between doses. The multiple-dose regimen exposes the kidney to multiple peak levels of intermediate concentration, whereas single daily dosing exposes the kidney to a single peak of higher absolute concentration. It has been suggested that nephrotoxicity is related to the duration of exposure to peak lithium levels and not to the absolute level of any particular peak (Bowen et al. 1991; Hetmar et al. 1987; Plenge et al. 1982). It is for this reason that single daily dosing is recommended. Although slow-release preparations of lithium are available, these are not necessary for obtaining adequate 24-hour levels. The main advantage of sustained release is that less lithium ion is released in the stomach, where it can act as an irritant, and more is released in the small intestines (Schatzberg and Cole 1991). For patients who experience nausea and gastric irritation, the slow-release formulations may provide protection from this unpleasant side effect. Patients with diarrhea may prefer the standard-release formulations. The patient and appropriate family members must be informed of the potential acute side effects and long-term consequences of lithium therapy. Side effects are described in detail in the following subsection. General guidelines for lithium treatment are listed in Table 27–19.

Contraindications and Pretreatment Medical Evaluation

Lithium should not be administered to patients with fluctuating or unstable renal function. In patients with statically impaired renal function, another mood stabilizer, such as valproate, is preferred. For patients who are unresponsive to alternate treatments, lithium may be administered if the dosage and dose frequency are suitably reduced to avoid toxic blood levels. Because lithium may affect functioning of the cardiac sinus node, patients with sinus node dysfunction (e.g., sick sinus syndrome) should not receive lithium. Although lithium also has acute and chronic

TABLE 27–19. Guidelines for lithium treatment

1. Review medical history and review of systems with particular attention to renal, thyroid, and cardiac status.

2. Order pretreatment pregnancy test and levels of BUN, creatinine, electrolytes, and TSH. If the patient is older than 40 years or has evidence of cardiac disease, order ECG.

3. Inform patient and family of proper use of lithium. Include a discussion of common side effects, the importance of monitoring of lithium levels, early signs and symptoms of toxicity, and potential long-term side effects. If patient is female, include warnings regarding pregnancy during treatment.

4. Initiate therapy at 300 mg bid, and increase by 300 mg every 3–4 days.

5. Obtain lithium levels (12 hours after last dose) twice a week, until there is a clinical response or the lithium level reaches approximately 1.0 mEq/L.

6. Monitor BUN/creatinine.

7. Monitor TSH every 6–12 months if symptoms of hypothyroidism develop.

Note. BUN = blood urea nitrogen; ECG = electrocardiography; TSH = thyroid-stimulating hormone.

effects on the thyroid, patients with hypothyroidism may receive lithium if the thyroid disease is adequately treated and monitored. Laboratory tests that should be performed before the initiation of lithium, valproate, and carbamazepine are outlined in Table 27–20.

Although initial uncontrolled reports have suggested a markedly increased risk of Ebstein's anomaly of the heart in infants who were exposed to lithium in utero (Nora et al. 1974), more recent controlled data predict a 0.1%–0.7% absolute risk (Edmonds and Oakley 1990; Jacobson et al. 1992; Kallen and Tandberg 1983; Zalzstein et al. 1990) compared to 0.01% in the general population. The overall risk of major congenital anomalies in association with lithium exposure is 4%–12%, compared with 2%–4% in comparison groups (Cohen et al. 1994). The increased risk of malformations must be weighed against the risk for both mother and fetus if lithium discontinuation results in a manic relapse. Guidelines for lithium use in pregnancy are outlined in Table 27–21.

Risks, Side Effects, and Their Management

Renal effects. For all patients taking lithium, a measure of serum blood urea nitrogen (BUN) and creatinine should be obtained at baseline and every 3–6 months after lithium therapy has commenced, with more frequent testing if there are specific complaints or signs of renal dysfunction. Most of the effects of lithium on the kidney are reversible after discontinuation of the drug. Although permanent morphological changes in renal structure have been reported, the clinical implications of these changes have yet to be established, and to date there have been no published reports of irreversible renal failure as a result of chronic, nontoxic lithium therapy (Hetmar et al. 1991).

However, lithium inhibits vasopressin with resultant impairment in renal concentrating ability. Termed *nephrogenic diabetes insipidus* (NDI), this condition results in polyuria for up to 60% of patients taking lithium (Lokkegaard et al. 1985). This side effect is associated with higher plasma lithium levels, a longer duration of treatment (DePaulo et al. 1986), and a multiple daily dosing schedule (Hetmar et al. 1991). NDI may result in serious complications, including dehydration, lithium toxicity, and electrolyte imbalance. Although clinically significant polyuria usually reverses itself after discontinuation of lithium therapy, it may persist for many months (Ramsey and Cox 1982; Simon et al. 1977). However, less serious increases in urine volume may persist indefinitely, an effect that some investigators believe is a consequence of renal tubular atrophy (Hetmar et al. 1991).

Preventive and management strategies for NDI

TABLE 27–20. Characteristics of commonly used mood stabilizers

	Lithium	Valproate	Carbamazepine
Available preparations	Lithium carbonate (Eskalith, Lithonate, Lithotabs, generics; 300-mg tabs, caps) Lithium citrate liquid (8 mEq/5 mL) Extended release (Eskalith CR 450 mg; Lithobid 300 mg)	Divalproex sodium (Depakote 125-, 250-, 500-mg tabs, 125-mg sprinkle caps) Depacon iv Valproic acid (Depakene, generics, 250-mg caps; Depakene 250 mg/5-mL syrup)	Tegretol, generics (200-mg tablets, 100-mg chewable tablets, 100-mg/5-mL suspension) Tegretol XR sustained release (100-, 200-, 400-mg tabs)
Half-life	24 hours	12–16 hours	24/12 hours[c]
Starting dosage	300 mg bid	250 mg tid or 20 mg/kg	200 mg bid
Blood level	0.8–1.2 mEq/L	45–125 µg/mL	4–12[d] µg/mL
Metabolism	Renal	Hepatic	Hepatic
Contraindications[a]	Unstable renal function	Hepatic dysfunction	Hepatic dysfunction
Pretreatment laboratory evaluation	Chem 20[b], CBC, TSH, ECG if ≥ 40 years old or cardiac disease; pregnancy test	SGOT, SGPT, pregnancy test	CBC, SGOT, SGPT, pregnancy test

Note. CBC = complete blood count; ECG = electrocardiography; SGOT = serum glutamic-oxaloacetic transaminase; SGPT = serum glutamate pyruvate transaminase; TSH = thyroid-stimulating hormone.
[a]All current mood stabilizers should be avoided in pregnancy. See text for discussion. [b]Especially BUN, creatinine, sodium, and calcium. [c]24 hours before hepatic autoinduction; 12 hours after autoinduction. [d]Not correlated with clinical response.

include increasing the patient's fluid intake and decreasing the amount of lithium given to the lowest effective dosage. Once-a-day dosing also results in lower urinary output than the multiple dosing schedule (Hetmar et al. 1991; Plenge et al. 1982). If these simpler management strategies fail to correct the polyuria, potassium supplementation, 10–20 mEq/day, may be effective (Klemfuss 1992; Martin 1993). Diuretics may also be used in the treatment of lithium-induced NDI. By causing sodium depletion, diuretics ultimately create in the kidney a compensatory conservation of sodium. The osmotic effect of this sodium conservation constrains the kidney's ability to dilute urine, thereby alleviating the polyuria. However, thiazide diuretics can raise lithium levels into the toxic range, an effect that is particularly dangerous in a patient already at risk for dehydration from polyuria. For this reason, the nonthiazide diuretic amiloride is now the preferred treatment for lithium-induced NDI, because it does not appear to increase plasma lithium levels (Battle et al. 1985). Amiloride apparently acts by blocking the absorption of lithium in the renal tubules, where the lithium would otherwise interfere with the action of vasopressin (Billings 1985). For lithium-induced NDI, amiloride is prescribed in a dosage of 5 mg bid and increased to 10 mg bid if necessary. Despite the claim that amiloride does not raise lithium levels, we believe it is prudent to continue to monitor serum lithium levels with greater frequency (at least every 2 months) when amiloride is combined with lithium.

Interstitial nephritis has been reported to be a consequence of long-term lithium therapy. Hetmar et al. (1987) performed renal biopsies on 46 bipolar patients with a mean of 8 years of lithium therapy and found that the proportion of sclerotic glomeruli, atrophic tubules, and interstitial fibrosis was significantly greater in patients who had received a multiple daily dosing schedule, compared with patients with a history of once-daily dosing and with a control group with no history of lithium exposure. Lokkegaard et al. (1985) reported that decreases in the glomerular filtration rate (GFR) are detectable only after many years of lithium therapy; however, most investigators have found no clinically significant effect on the GFR (Hetmar et al. 1991; Schou 1989; Waller and Edwards 1989). Proteinuria has been reported as a rare side effect and is thought to be the consequence of either glomerular leakage or the inhibition of tubular resorption (Waller and Edwards 1989; Wood et al. 1989).

Thyroid dysfunction. Reversible hypothyroidism may occur in as many as 20% of patients treated with lithium (Lindstedt et al. 1977; Myers et al. 1985). Although

TABLE 27-21. Treatment recommendations for lithium use in women with bipolar disorder

I. Encourage careful contraceptive practices for all women of childbearing age.

II. Evaluate the need for lithium prophylaxis.

    A. In women with single episodes of affective instability and long intervening periods of well-being:

        1. Attempt gradual tapering and discontinuation of lithium prophylaxis before pregnancy.

        2. Maintain lithium-free well-being for the entire pregnancy if possible; reintroduce lithium during the second and third trimesters if necessary.

    B. In women with severe bipolar disorder in whom discontinuation of lithium prophylaxis poses a *substantial* risk of increased morbidity:

        1. Temporarily discontinue lithium therapy for a period coinciding as closely as possible with that of embryogenesis.

        2. Consider reintroduction of lithium and/or treatment with antipsychotic agents if clinical deterioration occurs.

    C. In women with severe bipolar disorder in whom discontinuation of lithium prophylaxis poses an *unacceptable* risk of increased morbidity, maintain lithium therapy throughout pregnancy.

III. Other considerations for women who take lithium during all or part of the first trimester of pregnancy:

    A. Provide reproductive risk counseling as early in pregnancy as possible.

    B. Offer prenatal diagnosis by fetal echocardiography and high-resolution ultrasound examination at 16–18 weeks of gestation.

Source. Reprinted with permission from Cohen LS, Friedman JM, Jefferson JW, et al: A reevaluation of risk of in utero exposure to lithium. *JAMA* 271(2):146–150, 1994. Copyright 1994, American Medical Association.

this occurrence is hypothesized to be related to the effect of lithium on thyroid-stimulating hormone (TSH) adenylate cyclase, lithium may have important effects on other key areas of thyroid function (Waller 1985). Lithium-induced hypothyroidism occurs more frequently in women, in patients with thyroid antibodies, and in patients with an exaggerated TSH response to thyrotropin-releasing hormone (TRH; Calabrese et al. 1985; Myers et al. 1985). Because the development of hypothyroidism in bipolar patients is associated with intractable depression (Yassa et al. 1988) and with the development of a rapid-cycling course (Bauer and Whybrow 1989), thyroid function must be monitored every 6–12 months during lithium treatment or if symptoms develop that might be attributable to thyroid dysfunction. The TSH level is the most sensitive test for detecting hypothyroidism, especially with recent refinements in the assay. If laboratory tests reveal the development of hypothyroidism, the patient should be evaluated clinically for signs and symptoms of hypothyroidism and be referred to an endocrinologist for any further tests. In collaboration with the endocrinologist, the psychiatrist should decide on the appropriate treatment—in most cases, thyroid hormone replacement and continuation of lithium therapy.

Parathyroid dysfunction. The effects of lithium on calcium metabolism may be related to lithium-induced hyperparathyroidism (Anath and Dubin 1983; Mallette and Eichhorn 1986). Clinically significant effects of hypercalcemia associated with lithium have been reported, including back pain, kyphoscoliosis, osteoporosis, hypertension, cardiomegaly, and impaired renal function (Clur 1989). Potential neuropsychiatric sequelae include affective changes, anxiety, aggressiveness, sleep disturbance, apathy, psychosis, delirium, dementia, and seizures (Borer and Bhanot 1985). Although they are rare, symptoms of hyperparathyroidism may be misdiagnosed as lithium toxicity or the effects of the underlying affective disorder. When signs or symptoms that might be related to hyperparathyroidism develop, serum calcium ion levels should be checked, and if they are abnormal, parathyroid hormone levels should be obtained and an endocrinologist consulted.

Neurotoxicity. Lithium therapy may be associated with several types of neurological dysfunction. Fine resting tremor is a neurological side effect that may be detected in as many as one-half of patients taking lithium (Vestergaard et al. 1980). β-Adrenergic-blocking drugs, such as propranolol in divided daily doses below 80 mg/day, are effective in treating this tremor (Zubenko et al. 1984). Subjective memory impairment occurs in approximately 28% of patients taking lithium and is among the most frequent reasons for noncompliance (Goodwin and Jamison 1990). ECT-induced confusion is likely to be worsened by concurrent lithium administration; therefore, lithium is relatively contraindicated for patients who are receiving a course of ECT (Consensus Conference 1985; Penney et al. 1990).

Cardiac effects. Mitchell and Mackenzie (1982) reported changes in T-wave morphology on the ECG (flattening or inversion) in 20%–30% of patients taking lithium, changes that are most likely benign. Lithium also may suppress the function of the sinus node and result in sinoatrial block. Patients with sinus disease or conduction defects, therefore, should not be treated with lithium. Cases have also been reported of aggravation of preexisting ventricular arrhythmias with lithium therapy. An ECG should be checked before treatment with lithium is started in patients older than 40 years or in those with a history or symptoms of cardiac disease.

Weight gain.   Weight gain is a frequent side effect of lithium treatment (Peselow et al. 1980; Vendsborg et al. 1976; Vestergaard et al. 1980). Vendsborg et al. (1976) found a correlation between liquid intake and weight gain. Patients with polydipsia may drink fluids with a high caloric content, such as carbonated soft drinks, and thereby gain weight. These patients should be instructed to drink low-calorie liquids. Peselow et al. (1980) reviewed several hypotheses indicating that weight gain may also be a direct effect of lithium therapy. Possible mechanisms include influences on carbohydrate metabolism, changes in glucose tolerance, or changes in lipid metabolism. Diet and exercise should be recommended early in treatment.

Dermatological reactions.   Dermatological reactions to lithium include acne, follicular eruptions, and psoriasis (Bakris et al. 1980–1981; Deandrea et al. 1982). The most frequent of these reactions is skin rash, which is reported in up to 7% of lithium-treated patients (Bone et al. 1980). Changes in hair, including hair loss, hair thinning, and loss of wave, have also been reported. Except for cases of exacerbation of psoriasis, these reactions are usually benign and may not warrant discontinuation of lithium treatment. Lithium-induced acne responds to topical treatment with steroidal agents, such as tretinoin (Retin-A).

Gastrointestinal side effects.   Gastrointestinal difficulties occur frequently with lithium treatment, especially nausea and diarrhea. Although these side effects may be manifestations of toxicity, they also occur at lithium levels within the therapeutic range. Gastrointestinal symptoms may improve with reduction of dosage or ingestion of lithium with meals. Slow-release formulations are more often associated with nausea, whereas sustained-release preparations are more commonly associated with diarrhea.

Hematological side effects.   The most frequent hematological change detected in patients taking lithium is leukocytosis (approximately 15,000 white blood cells/mm^3). As reviewed by Brewerton (1986), this change is generally benign; lithium may, in fact, be used to treat several conditions associated with granulocytopenia. (The use of lithium to treat carbamazepine-induced granulocytopenia is discussed later in this section.) Lithium-induced leukocytosis is readily reversible with discontinuation of lithium therapy.

Overdose and toxicity.   Because of the narrow range between therapeutic and toxic plasma lithium levels, the physician must devote sufficient time to informing the patient and the family about the signs and symptoms of early lithium toxicity and the circumstances that may increase the chances of toxicity, such as drinking insufficient amounts of fluids, becoming overheated with increased perspiration, or ingesting too much medication. The physician must emphasize the prevention of lithium toxicity through the maintenance of adequate salt and water intake, especially during hot weather and exercise. Toxic lithium levels can produce severe neurotoxic reactions, with symptoms such as dysarthria, ataxia, and intention tremor. The signs and symptoms of lithium toxicity may be divided into those that usually occur at lithium levels between 1.5 and 2.0 mEq/L, those that occur between 2.0 and 2.5 mEq/L, and those that occur above 2.5 mEq/L (Table 27–22), although some patients may become clinically toxic with lithium levels in the standard therapeutic range. The recommended management of lithium toxicity is reviewed in Table 27–23.

Drug interactions.   Because of the narrow therapeutic range of lithium, knowledge of its drug-drug interactions is of paramount importance. Drugs that may potentially interact with lithium are outlined in Table 27–24. Concerns about increased risk of delirium, neuroleptic malignant syndrome, and irreversible brain damage have been raised for the combination of lithium and neuroleptic drugs on the basis of case reports (Cohen and Cohen 1974). However, a controlled investigation found no difference in side effects or complications between a group of patients with mania treated with antipsychotic medications alone and a group of patients with mania treated with antipsychotic drugs and lithium (Goldney and Spence 1986); this result is concordant with clinical experience. The preponderance of evidence indicates that lithium and antipsychotic medications, including haloperidol, can be safely and effectively combined, with appropriate monitoring.

VALPROATE

Lambert et al. (1966) were the first to report success in treating bipolar disorder with valproate (VPA). Since that time there have been numerous uncontrolled studies sup-

TABLE 27–22. Signs and symptoms of lithium toxicity

Mild-to-moderate intoxication
(lithium level = 1.5–2.0 mEq/L)

Gastrointestinal	Vomiting
	Abdominal pain
	Dryness of mouth
Neurological	Ataxia
	Dizziness
	Slurred speech
	Nystagmus
	Lethargy or excitement
	Muscle weakness

Moderate-to-severe intoxication
(lithium level = 2.0–2.5 mEq/L)

Gastrointestinal	Anorexia
	Persistent nausea and vomiting
Neurological	Blurred vision
	Muscle fasciculations
	Clonic limb movements
	Hyperactive deep tendon reflexes
	Choreoathetoid movements
	Convulsions
	Delirium
	Syncope
	Electroencephalographic changes
	Stupor
	Coma
	Circulatory failure (lowered blood pressure, cardiac arrhythmias, and conduction abnormalities)

Severe lithium intoxication
(lithium level = > 2.5 mEq/L)

Generalized convulsions
Oliguria and renal failure
Death

TABLE 27–23. Management of lithium toxicity

1. The patient should immediately contact his or her personal physician or go to a hospital emergency room.
2. Lithium should be discontinued and the patient instructed to ingest fluids, if possible.
3. Physical examination should be completed, including vital signs and a neurological examination with complete formal mental status examination.
4. Lithium level, serum electrolytes, renal function tests, and electrocardiogram should be obtained as soon as possible.
5. For significant acute ingestion, residual gastric contents should be removed by induction of emesis, gastric lavage, and absorption with activated charcoal.[a]
6. Vigorous hydration and maintenance of electrolyte balance are essential.
7. For any patient with a serum lithium level greater than 4.0 mEq/L or with serious manifestations of lithium toxicity, hemodialysis should be initiated.[a]
8. Repeat dialysis may be required every 6–10 hours, until the lithium level is within nontoxic range and the patient has no signs or symptoms of lithium toxicity.

[a]Information from Goldfrank et al. 1986.

tive as lithium in patients with euphoric mania. It is concordant with previous observations (Calabrese et al. 1992; McElroy et al. 1992; Post et al. 1987) that valproate was found to be more effective than lithium in patients with rapid-cycling and dysphoric mania. Valproate has also been reported to be especially effective for mania occurring in patients with a history of closed-head trauma (McElroy et al. 1989) and in patients with EEG abnormalities (Pope et al. 1988). Although several open-trial studies have suggested that valproate is also effective for prophylaxis in bipolar disorder, no controlled studies have confirmed this finding to date (Keck et al. 1992). The efficacy of valproate in the treatment of acute bipolar depression has yet to be studied systematically.

Mechanism of Action

Although many putative mechanisms have been proposed, the basis for the mood-stabilizing effects of valproate is largely unknown; it may involve enhanced GABAergic tone and sodium-channel-mediated membrane stabilization (Davies 1995; Macdonald and Kelly 1995; Post et al. 1992).

Clinical Use

Before beginning treatment with valproate, patients should be told that they might experience nausea, seda-

porting this initial claim. After the early 1980s, several controlled studies have established that valproate is effective in acute mania (Gerner and Stanton 1992; Keck et al. 1992; Pope et al. 1991). More recently, a collaborative study by Bowden et al. (1994) directly compared valproate with lithium and placebo in patients with mania. This study, which represents the largest controlled trial of these drugs used in mania to date, found valproate to be effec-

TABLE 27–24. Clinically important drug interactions with lithium

Drug	Interaction
Diuretics	
Thiazides	Reduce lithium clearance by effect on distal tubular function.
Loop diuretics (furosemide)	No effect on lithium clearance.
Potassium-sparing diuretics (amiloride)	Can be used to treat lithium-induced polyuria.
Nonsteroidal anti-inflammatory drugs	
Indomethacin, phenylbutazone, naproxen, ibuprofen (and others)	May increase lithium level by interfering with clearance.
Sulindac	No effect on serum lithium levels and lithium clearance.
Antibiotics[a]	
Metronidazole	Probable renal effect; may increase lithium level; may also induce diarrhea.
Antihypertensives	
Methyldopa	May increase lithium level, may cause neurotoxic symptoms; mechanism uncertain; lithium may decrease antihypertensive effect.
Cardiac medications	In combination with elevated lithium levels may cause serious prolonged dysrhythmias.
Calcium channel blockers	May increase rate of lithium excretion.
Bronchodilators (aminophylline, theophylline)	Cause significantly increased lithium excretion; possibly increased risk of mortality in those with certain cardiovascular abnormalities.
Insulin and oral hypoglycemics	Careful monitoring of glucose levels is necessary, because lithium can increase glucose tolerance; mechanism is unclear.
Digoxin, quinidine	Effects on cardiac condition may be potentiated by lithium; digoxin may reduce effect of lithium.
Neuroleptics	May increase the risk of neurotoxicity; tardive dyskinesia.
Anticonvulsants	
Carbamazepine	Additive CNS effects can produce neurotoxicity unless dosage is modified.
Valproate	May decrease lithium level.

[a] In 1978, a case report suggested that tetracycline might cause an increase in lithium levels (McGennis 1978). This report caused some concern, because tetracycline is commonly used to treat skin eruptions secondary to lithium; however, no other such cases have been reported. In normal volunteers, tetracycline has in fact been shown to decrease lithium levels (Fankhauser et al. 1988).

Source.   Reprinted with permission from Goodwin FK, Jamison R: *Manic-Depressive Illness.* New York, Oxford University Press, 1990.

tion, and a fine hand tremor. These are often transient, but in some patients they persist. There are several valproate preparations available in the United States, including valproic acid, sodium valproate, and divalproex sodium (Depakote). Divalproex sodium is a dimer of sodium valproate and valproic acid with an enteric coating, and it is much better tolerated than other oral valproate preparations. An intravenous preparation has also become available, but it has not yet been studied in psychiatric disorders. The half-life of valproate is 10 hours.

Valproate may be initiated gradually with subsequent dosage titration or with a more rapid "loading" strategy. Most commonly, valproate is initiated at a dosage of 250 mg tid and subsequently increased by 250 mg every 3 days.

Most patients require a daily dosage of 1,250–2,500 mg/day. Although valproate has a relatively short half-life, moderate doses may be given once a day at bedtime to reduce daytime sedation, often without compromising clinical efficacy. This strategy should not be employed when valproate is used to treat seizure disorders, for which more constant serum levels are required.

In situations for which rapid stabilization is of paramount importance, valproate treatment can be initiated at a dose of 20 mg per kilogram of body weight (Keck et al. 1993). There are patients who require relatively high dosages of valproate, sometimes greater than 4,000 mg/day, to achieve a sufficient plasma level and clinical response, and some patients do not respond until plasma valproate levels are greater than 100 mg/mL. Like that of all psychotropic medications, the final dosage is more dependent on the balance between clinical response and side effects than on absolute blood level. However, plasma levels of 45–100 mg/mL are recommended for the treatment of acute mania (Bowden et al. 1996). Patients with less severe symptoms, such as bipolar II disorder or cyclothymia, often respond at lower dosages and blood levels (Jacobsen 1993). Blood levels in other phases of bipolar disorder, such as bipolar depression, or in other indications, such as aggression, have not been established.

Contraindications

Valproate is relatively contraindicated for patients with hepatitis or liver disease; it may be pursued as treatment for such patients only as a last resort and with the approval and continuous involvement of a gastroenterologist. Valproate has been linked to spina bifida and other neural tube defects in the offspring of patients exposed to this medication in the first trimester of pregnancy (Lammer et al. 1987; Robert and Guibaud 1982); therefore, this agent should be avoided during pregnancy.

Risks, Side Effects, and Their Management

Hepatic toxicity. Although there have been reports of rare, non-dose-related hepatic failure with fatalities—estimated to occur in 1 in 118,000 patients—no cases have occurred in patients older than 10 years of age who were receiving valproate monotherapy (Dreifuss et al. 1987, 1989). Nonetheless, baseline liver function tests are indicated. If baseline tests are normal, monitoring for clinical signs of hepatotoxicity is more important than routine monitoring of liver enzymes, which has little predictive value and may be less effective than clinical monitoring (Pellock and Willmore 1991).

Transient, mild elevations in the liver enzymes, up to three times the upper limit of normal, do not require the discontinuation of valproate. Although γ-glutamyl transferase (GGT) levels are often checked by clinicians, this test is often elevated without clinical significance in patients receiving valproate and carbamazepine (Dean and Penry 1992). Likewise, plasma ammonia levels are often elevated transiently with valproate treatment, but this finding does not require that the treatment be interrupted (Jaeken et al. 1980). Because increases in transaminase levels are often dose dependent, if there is not a suitable alternative treatment, dosage reduction and careful monitoring may be attempted.

Hematological effects. Valproate has been associated with changes in platelet count, but clinically significant thrombocytopenia has rarely been documented (Dean and Penry 1992). Coagulation defects have also been reported. Overall, the risk of inducing a coagulation disturbance in an otherwise healthy adult is extremely low. However, in patients for whom anticoagulation is strictly contraindicated and in patients who already are receiving anticoagulation therapy, monitoring of the coagulation profile is required at baseline, at 1 month, and then every 3 months.

Gastrointestinal side effects. Indigestion, heartburn, and nausea are common side effects of valproate therapy. We recommend the divalproex sodium preparation to help mitigate these effects. Patients may also be encouraged to take their doses with food. The symptomatic use of histamine$_2$ blockers or famotidine is sometimes warranted. In most cases, however, dyspepsia is transient and not severe. Pancreatitis has been reported as a rare occurrence among some patients receiving relatively high doses of valproate (Murphy et al. 1981). If vomiting and severe abdominal pain develop in the context of valproate therapy, a serum amylase level should be obtained immediately.

Weight gain. Weight gain is a common side effect of valproate treatment. Isojarvi et al. (1996) reported significant weight gain with associated hyperinsulinemia in approximately 50% of a cohort of women taking valproate. This side effect does not appear to be dose dependent. Diet and exercise should be recommended early in treatment.

Neurological effects. One of the most common side effects associated with valproate use is benign essential tremor. This tremor is apparently not dose related and may first occur as late as 1 year after the initiation of therapy (Hyman et al. 1979). Drowsiness is another common side effect of valproate treatment, but tolerance often develops once a steady-state level of the drug is reached. A more gradual initial titration of valproate may be indicated for patients who complain of marked daytime sleepiness. In addition, once-a-day bedtime dosing often achieves symptomatic remission with less daytime sedation. Rarely, persistent somnolence, ataxia, or even delirium may occur, but these effects are more likely when other potentially sedating medications are being prescribed concurrently.

Alopecia. Both transient and persistent hair loss have been associated with valproate use. When hair loss occurs, it often begins 3 months or longer after the initiation of treatment and is probably not dose related. Regrowth may result in hair that is wavier or curlier than before (Jeavons et al. 1977). It is our observation that patients with thyroid abnormalities who receive valproate are more likely to suffer hair loss, even when ongoing thyroid replacement treatment has normalized their thyroid function. Patients with valproate-induced alopecia may benefit from zinc supplementation, at a dosage of 22.5 mg/day (Hurd et al. 1984). We routinely recommend supplementation with a multivitamin preparation containing zinc and selenium at the onset of valproate treatment.

Overdose. Valproate overdose results in increasing sedation, confusion, and ultimately coma. The patient may also manifest hyperreflexia or hyporeflexia, seizures, respiratory suppression, and superventricular tachycardia (Labar 1992). Treatment should include gastric lavage, ECG monitoring, treatment of emergent seizures, and respiratory support as indicated.

Drug interactions. Because valproate may inhibit hepatic enzymes, there is the potential for increases in the levels of other medications (Dean and Penry 1992). Valproate is also highly bound to plasma proteins and may displace other highly bound drugs from protein-binding sites. Therefore, coadministered drugs that are either highly protein bound or reliant on hepatic metabolism may require dose adjustment.

CARBAMAZEPINE

Takezaki and Hanaoka (1971) reported that carbamazepine was effective in controlling manic behavior; the first report from the United States of its efficacy for mania was by Ballenger and Post (1980). Subsequently, evidence from controlled studies has indicated that carbamazepine is effective in both the acute and the prophylactic treatment of mania, with overall response rates comparable to those of lithium treatment (Gerner and Stanton 1992; Keck et al. 1992). There is less evidence, however, to support the efficacy of carbamazepine in the acute treatment of depression and in the prophylactic treatment of unipolar depression. In two controlled studies, carbamazepine treatment was found to be effective in a subgroup of patients with refractory depression, with response rates greater among the patients with bipolar depression than among those with unipolar depression (Post et al. 1986; Small 1990). A systematic, controlled study of the antidepressant effects of carbamazepine in a more typical group of patients with depression remains to be conducted.

Clinical Use

Carbamazepine should be initiated at a dosage of 200 mg bid with increments of 200 mg/day every 3–5 days. Plasma levels of 8–12 µg/mL are based on clinical use in patients with seizure disorders and do not correlate with clinical response in psychiatric disorders. We recommend dosage titration to clinical response and side effects, rather than targeting of a particular dosage or blood level. During the titration phase, patients may be particularly prone to side effects such as sedation, dizziness, and ataxia, which indicates that a more gradual titration, such as 100 mg bid, should be instituted. Although the maximum recommended dosage of carbamazepine by the manufacturer is 1,200 mg/day, higher dosages are frequently required on the basis of plasma level determinations and clinical response (Placidi et al. 1986; Post et al. 1984). Tegretol XR is a sustained-release preparation that is less likely to cause gastrointestinal side effects. Generic preparations of carbamazepine are often poorly tolerated. Because carbamazepine induces its own metabolism (autoinduction), dose adjustments may be required for weeks or months after the initiation of treatment to maintain therapeutic plasma levels (Eichelbaum et al. 1985). Some investigators have suggested that the carbamazepine metabolite carbamazepine-10,11-epoxide has a major role in the therapeutic activity of carbamazepine in affective illness, especially in the treatment of depression (Post et al. 1983).

Contraindications

Because of the potential for hematological and hepatic toxicity, carbamazepine should not be administered to patients with liver disease or thrombocytopenia or those who are at risk for agranulocytosis. For this reason, carbamazepine is strictly contraindicated in patients receiving clozapine. Because of reports of teratogenicity, including increased risks of spina bifida (Rosa 1991), microcephaly (Bertollini et al. 1987), and craniofacial defects (Jones et al. 1989), carbamazepine is relatively contraindicated for use in pregnant women. Pretreatment evaluation should include a complete blood count (CBC), a serum glutamic-oxaloacetic transaminase (SGOT) level, and a serum glutamate pyruvate transaminase (SGPT) level. Because carbamazepine has a tricyclic structure, theoretical concerns have been raised about coadministration with monoamine oxidase inhibitors, but more recently Ketter et al. (1995a) suggested that this combination is well tolerated.

Risks, Side Effects, and Their Management

Hematological disorders. The most serious toxic hematological side effects of carbamazepine are agranulocytosis and aplastic anemia, which can be fatal. Whereas carbamazepine-induced agranulocytosis or aplastic anemia is extremely rare, now estimated to occur at the rate of 1 in 125,000 patients (Pellock 1987), leukopenia (total WBC count of less than 3000 cells/mm^3) is more common, with a prevalence of approximately 10%. Persistent leukopenia with thrombocytopenia occurs in approximately 2% of patients, and mild anemia occurs in fewer than 5% of patients. Although it is important to assess hematological function and risk factors before initiating treatment, there appears to be no benefit to ongoing monitoring in the absence of clinical indicators. When carbamazepine-induced agranulocytosis occurs, the onset is rapid, so that a normal CBC one day does not provide reassurance that agranulocytosis will not develop the next day. Therefore, as opposed to routine monitoring, we advise patients to call if they develop fever, sore throat, infection, petechiae, or extreme weakness and pallor.

Carbamazepine should be discontinued if the absolute neutrophil count is less than 1,000. Consultation with a hematologist is also required at this point. It is interesting that the use of lithium to counteract leukopenia induced by carbamazepine has been suggested (Brewerton 1986). However, lithium does not reverse the underlying pathophysiological effects of carbamazepine; therefore, the clinician should monitor patients taking carbamazepine as they are being withdrawn from lithium, because clinically significant leukopenia may be unmasked.

Hepatic toxicity. Carbamazepine occasionally causes hepatic toxicity (Gram and Bentsen 1983), usually a hypersensitivity hepatitis that appears after a latency period of several weeks and is associated with elevations in SGOT, SGPT, and lactic dehydrogenase (LDH). Cholestasis is also possible, with increases in bilirubin and alkaline phosphatase. Mild, transient elevations in transaminase levels can generally be monitored without discontinuation of carbamazepine. If SGOT or SGPT levels increase above three times the upper limit of normal, carbamazepine should be discontinued.

Dermatological conditions. An exanthematous rash is one of the more common side effects associated with carbamazepine, occurring in 3%–17% of patients (Warnock and Knesevich 1988). This reaction typically begins within 2–20 weeks after the start of treatment. Carbamazepine is generally discontinued if a rash develops because of the risk of progression to an exfoliative dermatitis or Stevens-Johnson syndrome, a severe bullous form of erythema multiforme (Patterson 1985). In patients who are nonresponsive to all other mood stabilizers,

carbamazepine may be reinstituted along with initial prednisone coverage (Murphy et al. 1991; Vick 1983).

Endocrinological disorders. Carbamazepine may cause a reduction in the circulating levels of T$_3$ and T$_4$, possibly by inducing their hepatic metabolism (Bentsen et al. 1983; Yeo et al. 1978); this effect rarely has clinical significance. However, when carbamazepine is used in combination with other agents that antagonize thyroid function, such as lithium, a clinically significant synergistic effect may emerge (Kramlinger and Post 1990). Carbamazepine may simultaneously reduce TSH levels, because it appears to diminish the pituitary response to TRH (Joffe et al. 1984).

The syndrome of inappropriate antidiuretic hormone (SIADH) with resultant hyponatremia may be induced by carbamazepine treatment. Alcoholic patients may be at greater risk for developing hyponatremia. If a patient taking carbamazepine develops confusion, the serum sodium level should be checked. When hyponatremia develops, it is often transient; however, even more severe cases of this condition can often be managed by fluid restriction, the addition of lithium, or use of the antibiotic demeclocycline (Brewerton and Jackson 1994).

Weight gain does not appear to be a side effect of carbamazepine therapy (Joffe et al. 1986).

Gastrointestinal disorders. Nausea and occasional vomiting are common side effects of carbamazepine, as they are with other mood stabilizers. Dosage reduction and institution of a slower titration rate help to minimize these effects.

Neurological effects. Patients may develop dizziness, drowsiness, and ataxia. These symptoms often occur at therapeutic plasma levels, especially in the early phases of treatment, and in such cases the dosage should be reduced and a slower titration schedule implemented.

Drug interactions. Carbamazepine induces hepatic cytochrome P450 enzymes, which may reduce the levels of other medications. Through the mechanism of hepatic enzyme induction, carbamazepine has been implicated in oral contraceptive failure (Coulam and Annegers 1979); therefore, women should be advised to consider alternative forms of birth control while taking carbamazepine. Similarly, medications or substances that inhibit cytochrome P450 3A3/4 (discussed in the section of this chapter on drug interactions) may result in significant elevations of plasma carbamazepine levels (Brodie and MacPhee 1986; Ketter et al. 1995b).

Overdose. Carbamazepine overdose is first manifested by neuromuscular disturbances, such as nystagmus, myoclonus, and hyperreflexia, with later progression to seizures and coma. Cardiac conduction changes may manifest at dosages higher than 60 g. Nausea, vomiting, and urinary retention may also occur. Treatment should include induction of vomiting, gastric lavage, and supportive care. Monitoring of blood pressure and respiratory and kidney functioning should follow for several days after a serious overdose.

LEVOTHYROXINE

There is evidence that high dosages of levothyroxine (T_4), as high as 400 µg/day, added to lithium or other mood stabilizers may convert partial responders or nonresponders to responders (Bauer and Whybrow 1990). Bauer and Whybrow (1989) recommended as a guideline that the T_4 dosage be increased until the patient's free thyroid index reaches 150% of the normal value. Alternatively, the T_4 dosage may be increased until the TSH level is suppressed to slightly below the low-normal value. Patients receiving high dosages of T_4 must be monitored for signs of thyroid toxicity.

CALCIUM CHANNEL BLOCKERS

Several investigators have studied the use of calcium channel blockers on the basis of the hypothesis that intracellular calcium signaling might be dysregulated in patients with bipolar disorder. Verapamil has been reported to be effective in the treatment of mania in several controlled studies (Brotman et al. 1986; Dubovsky et al. 1982, 1986; Gitlin and Weiss 1984; Hoschl and Kozeny 1989), although a recent study did not show significant improvement (Janicak et al. 1998). There also are preliminary data indicating that other calcium channel blockers—diltiazem (Caillard 1985), nifedipine (DeBeaurepair 1992), and nimodipine (Brunet et al. 1990)—may also be effective in treating mania or rapid cycling (Pazzaglia et al. 1993). The doses of verapamil used are in the range of 360–480 mg/day, taken tid in a divided regimen. Once patients are stabilized, they may be switched to the slow-release verapamil preparation, which allows for once-daily dosing. Nimodipine dosages are in the range of 120–720 mg/day.

LAMOTRIGINE

Lamotrigine (Lamictal) is a recently approved anticonvulsant medication that decreases sustained high-frequency repetitive firing of the voltage-dependent sodium channel, which may then decrease glutamate release (Leach et al. 1991; MacDonald and Kelly 1995). An initial report by Calabrese et al. (1995) suggested that lamotrigine may be effective in treating both the manic and depressive phases of bipolar disorder. In addition, there is some suggestion that this compound may have especially strong antidepressant effects (Calabrese et al. 1996). If further studies confirm these preliminary results, lamotrigine will be a valuable addition to the current therapeutic armamentarium because it is well tolerated and to date is not associated with hepatotoxicity, weight gain, or significant sedation. However, given the limited experience with lamotrigine in psychiatric patients, particularly regarding long-term use, lamotrigine currently should be reserved for patients who either do not benefit from or cannot tolerate lithium or valproate.

Lamotrigine treatment is usually initiated at 25 mg once a day and increased in 25-mg increments every week. This dosage should be reduced by half for patients who are also taking valproate and increased for those taking carbamazepine because of hepatic enzyme inhibition and induction, respectively. Lamotrigine requires slow dosage titration to minimize the risk to the patient of developing a skin rash. A maculopapular rash develops in 5% of patients treated with lamotrigine, usually in the first 4 weeks of treatment. Stevens-Johnson syndrome may occur, with an estimated risk of 1 in 1,000 patient years (Richens 1994). Stevens-Johnson syndrome is potentially fatal. It is essential to advise patients of this risk and to emphasize that they should call the office immediately if they develop a rash. A particular concern is a rash with concomitant systemic symptoms.

Although the drug is generally well tolerated, common early side effects include headache, dizziness, gastrointestinal distress, and blurred or double vision.

TREATMENT OF MANIA

The first step in treating mania is to initiate treatment with a mood stabilizer. Currently lithium, valproate, and to a lesser extent carbamazepine are all used as primary antimanic medications (Steering Committee, American Psychiatric Association 1996). Although the most extensive clinical experience is with lithium, recent controlled studies have found an overall similar response rate to lithium and divalproex (Bowden et al. 1994). Valproate appears to be particularly effective for patients with mixed mania and depression (Swann et al. 1997).

Other factors to consider in selecting a mood stabilizer include previous response to treatment, family history of response to a particular agent, side effects, concomitant medical problems, and concurrent medications. All mood stabilizers cause gastrointestinal side effects, especially initially, although some preparations do so more than others. Lithium and valproate both cause weight gain and tremor. Carbamazepine is more often associated with complex drug interactions. Starting dosages and rapidity of titration depend on balancing the clinical need for rapid control of symptoms, which dictates faster titration, with the improved tolerability of slower dose escalations. For example, after the clinician diagnoses acute mania and decides to use valproate as the primary mood stabilizer, the initial dose depends on the urgency of the clinical situation. If the patient is highly agitated on an inpatient hospital unit, use of the "loading" strategy may be indicated, in which case the patient is started with 20 mg/kg of divalproex. On the other hand, a patient with hypomania may do well at a substantially lower dose. Often patients with bipolar II disorder do well taking small doses of mood stabilizers, such as lithium 300–600 mg qhs, valproate 250–500 mg qhs, or carbamazepine 200–400 mg qhs.

When patients fail to respond to a single agent, the next step is to add a second mood stabilizer. Adding a second agent is preferred to substituting one mood stabilizer for another, unless there was a toxic or allergic reaction to the first drug. This strategy provides synergy and avoids the risk of exacerbating the patient's symptoms by withdrawing the first agent, which although seemingly ineffective may have been providing some therapeutic benefit. After the patient is stabilized, it may be reasonable to consider tapering the first agent, although it is not unusual for patients with bipolar disorder to require long-term treatment with a combination of medications. Lithium in combination with carbamazepine (Lipinski and Pope 1982; Moss and James 1983) or with valproate (McElroy et al. 1989) has produced remission for some patients who were unresponsive to lithium alone. In addition, some patients respond to a combination of two mood stabilizers even if they have previously failed to respond to each agent individually (Ketter et al. 1992).

Lithium with valproate is the most common and least complicated combination. Valproate and carbamazepine can be combined, but the pharmacokinetics are complicated. To compensate for the bimodal pharmacokinetic interactions, valproate dosages need to be higher and carbamazepine dosages lower than when these agents are used singly. Valproate shifts the metabolism of carbamazepine toward its active metabolite, which is not reflected in the serum carbamazepine levels. Therefore, carbamazepine levels appear artificially low.

If these combinations prove ineffective, preliminary data suggest that clozapine is an effective mood stabilizer, even in nonpsychotic patients (Suppes et al. 1992). In addition, levothyroxine (T_4, Synthroid) can be an effective augmentation, particularly in rapid-cycling bipolar disorder (Bauer and Whybrow 1990; Stancer and Persad 1982). For levothyroxine to be effective, serum T_4 levels should be 10%–50% above the upper limit of normal. This strategy generally does not cause clinical hyperthyroidism and is well tolerated by most patients. Finally, ECT is an effective treatment for acute mania and is especially useful for patients who cannot safely wait until medication becomes effective (Hirschfeld et al. 1994).

Although the mood stabilizers provide definitive treatment, they often require 1–2 weeks, and occasionally longer, before their efficacy is apparent. Because agitation and behavioral dyscontrol are often prominent in mania, additional agents are frequently used in the acute setting. The benzodiazepines lorazepam (Lenox et al. 1992) and clonazepam (Chouinard et al. 1983, 1993), even in high doses, can be safely used to treat agitation and insomnia until the mood stabilizer takes effect. High-potency benzodiazepines are preferred to conventional antipsychotics because of the more benign side-effect profile, specifically the avoidance of extrapyramidal side effects and tardive dyskinesia. Alprazolam is not recommended for patients with mania because, like all agents with antidepressant effects, it may precipitate mania (Arana et al. 1988). Patients who are psychotic can be acutely treated with medium doses of antipsychotics, such as 10–15 mg/day of haloperidol. In general, antipsychotic medication should be tapered after the acute episode, with continuation of the mood stabilizer as prophylaxis against recurrent episodes.

Occasionally patients require antipsychotic medications for longer periods of time, but this should not be assumed before attempting to taper the medication after an acute episode. Studies are currently under way to assess the antimanic and mood-stabilizing effects of the AAPs.

BIPOLAR DEPRESSION

Treatment

A common mistake is to treat bipolar depression in the same manner as unipolar depression, overlooking the need for a mood stabilizer. In bipolar depression, the first pharmacological intervention should be to start or optimize treatment with a mood stabilizer, rather than to start an antidepressant medication. In addition, thyroid function should be evaluated, particularly if the patient is taking lithium. Subclinical hypothyroidism, diagnosed by an elevated TSH level and normal T_3 and T_4 levels, may present as depression in affectively predisposed individuals. In such cases the addition of thyroid hormones may be beneficial, even if there is no other evidence of hypothyroidism.

Unless previous treatment history or comorbid medical problems dictate otherwise, lithium remains the first-line treatment for bipolar depression. The response rate to lithium in bipolar depression is 79% (Zornberg and Pope 1993), compared to approximately 30% for each of the anticonvulsants. For all the mood stabilizers, antidepressant efficacy is of slower onset than antimanic efficacy, and it may not become evident for 4–6 weeks, although some patients respond within days. If treatment with a single mood stabilizer is ineffective, many experts recommend adding a second mood stabilizer, particularly lithium if an anticonvulsant has been the primary mood stabilizer.

If the mood stabilizers prove to be insufficient in the treatment of bipolar depression, an antidepressant can then be carefully added. Although the switch rate into mania or induction of rapid cycling by antidepressants is controversial (Peet 1994; Wehr and Goodwin 1987), these agents do appear to present a risk for some patients, often with devastating consequences. Controlled comparative data on the use of specific antidepressant drugs in the treatment of bipolar depression are sparse. Current treatment guidelines extrapolate from these few studies and rely heavily on anecdotal clinical experience. Monoamine oxidase inhibitors appear to be more effective than tricyclic antidepressants in bipolar depression (Himmelhoch et al. 1991). Some data suggest that bupropion (Wellbutrin) may also be less likely to induce mania or cycle acceleration (Sachs et al. 1994; Shopsin 1983) compared to the tricyclic antidepressants. The serotonin reuptake inhibitors also appear to be relatively safe for many patients (Cohn et al. 1989). Overall, tricyclic antidepressants should be avoided when other viable treatment options exist. ECT, as discussed later in this chapter, should be considered in severe cases.

Prophylaxis

Patients with bipolar disorder require lifelong prophylaxis with a mood stabilizer, both to prevent new episodes and to decrease the likelihood that the illness will progress to a more malignant course. Ninety percent of bipolar patients relapse on stopping lithium, most within 6 months (Suppes et al. 1991). In addition to the single episode that may occur, each episode may further kindle the illness, thereby inducing a more malignant course of illness with decreased treatment responsiveness. The more episodes a patient has had, the less likely he or she is to respond to treatment (Gelenberg et al. 1989).

An additional rationale for continuing effective prophylactic treatment is the phenomenon of discontinuation-induced refractoriness (Post et al. 1992). It appears that some patients who were previously successfully treated with lithium, who then have another episode after lithium has been discontinued, fail to respond to the reinstitution of lithium. Moreover, these individuals tend to be poorly responsive to other treatments, such as the anticonvulsants. Although to date discontinuation-induced refractoriness has been reported only with lithium, it is feasible that the phenomenon may occur with other agents. However, if tolerance develops, a period of time off the ineffective medication, possibly combined with the institution of a different agent, is indicated. In other situations in which it is necessary to discontinue a mood stabilizer, it should be done with as slow a taper as possible. Abruptly stopping lithium is associated with a substantially higher rate of relapse than is tapering the drug (Faedda et al. 1994). Again, although most currently available data are for lithium, there is no reason to suspect that the principles differ for other mood stabilizers.

Finally, prophylaxis is best achieved when patients understand their illness, including the importance of treatment and the consequences of discontinuing medication. Referral to local support groups, such as the National Depressive and Manic-Depressive Association, can be invaluable. It is also helpful to simplify medication schedules, for example using qhs lithium dosing as opposed to divided doses. Minimizing side effects is also important. Although in a seminal study Gelenberg et al. (1989) concluded that relapse was more likely with serum lithium levels of 0.4–0.6 mEq/L compared to levels of 0.8–1.0 mEq/L, a recent reanalysis of these data suggested that the relapses that occurred in the group taking 0.4–0.6 mEg/L could be almost entirely accounted for by a rapid change from a previously higher blood level (J. F. Rosenbaum, personal communication, 1994). Patients who were previously stable at the lower blood level were as likely to remain stable as were patients in the group taking 0.8–1.0 mEq/L. Therefore, it may be possible to maintain patients on relatively lower levels, with a reduced side-effect burden, as long as dosage changes are not made abruptly.

DRUG INTERACTIONS

A drug interaction occurs when the pharmacological action of a medication is altered by a concurrently administered drug (or exogenous substance). With the increased use of psychotropic medications, the importance of drug interactions in psychopharmacology is increasingly apparent. Simultaneously, the characterization of specific cytochrome P450 isozymes facilitates the use of a more clinically meaningful and simpler conceptual framework to understand and predict many of the drug-drug interactions.

There are three types of drug interactions. *Pharmacokinetic interactions* involve an alteration by a second agent in the absorption, distribution, metabolism, or excretion of a drug, which changes the plasma concentration of the drug. *Pharmacodynamic interactions* involve a change in the action of a drug at a receptor or biologically active site, which alters the pharmacological effect of a given plasma concentration of the drug. Figure 27–3 illustrates potential sites and types of drug-drug interactions. *Idiosyncratic interactions* occur unpredictably in a small number of patients; they are unexpected, given the known pharmacological actions of the individual drugs.

PHARMACOKINETIC INTERACTIONS

Cytochrome P450 Enzymes

Clinically significant drug interactions are most commonly caused by changes in drug metabolism. All psychotropic drugs, except lithium, are metabolized by cytochrome P450 (CYP) enzymes. These enzymes are a heterogeneous group of mixed-function oxidases found predominantly in the liver and, to varying degrees, in the gut and brain. These enzymes catalyze the oxidative metabolism of a large number of drugs as well as many other endogenous and exogenous substances. The CYP enzymes are classified by families and subfamilies on the basis of similarities in amino acid sequence (Nelson et al. 1993). Enzymes within subfamilies have relatively specific affinities for various drugs and other substances. The enzymes that are primarily involved in drug metabolism are CYP 1A2, 2C, 2D6, and 3A3/4.

If one of these enzymes is inhibited by another drug, the result is an increase in the plasma level of concurrently administered drugs that rely on the enzyme for metabolism. A common analogy is blocking a drain, which results in a buildup of water. The drain is the metabolic pathway, the block is the enzyme inhibitor, and the water is the medications that are substrates for the enzyme. For example, the 2D6 enzyme is essential for the usual metabolism of TCAs (they are substrates for this enzyme). Fluoxetine inhibits the 2D6 enzyme. If a patient is taking a TCA and fluoxetine is added, or vice versa, TCA plasma levels increase, which may result in increased side effects or toxicity. Anticipating the potential for this reaction, the clinician can use a lower dosage of the TCA. This example illustrates the key clinical principle of prescribing enzyme inhibitors: in most cases, the combination of an enzyme inhibitor and a medication that is a substrate for that enzyme is not contraindicated, but the patient should be monitored for signs and symptoms related to increased substrate levels, with appropriate lowering of the substrate dose if necessary. The specific P450 enzymes that metabolize most drugs in clinical practice are not yet known, but information regarding the role of the cytochrome P450 enzymes in drug metabolism is rapidly evolving. Table 27–25 provides a list of the better recognized and clinically important substrates and inhibitors for the each of the CYP enzymes.

In most cases enzyme inhibitors and substrates can be safely combined, provided the dosage of the substrate is lowered if needed. However, there are a few important exceptions. Three medications—terfenadine, astemizole, and cisapride—are reliant on the 3A3/4 enzyme for conversion from a potentially cardiotoxic compound. When the 3A3/4 enzyme is not significantly inhibited, this is not clinically relevant because the heart is not exposed to the parent compound to any appreciable degree. However, if the 3A3/4 enzyme is significantly inhibited, clinically relevant QT prolongation and torsades de pointes may result (Honig et al. 1992; Monahan et al. 1990).

In general, enzyme inhibition is competitive and depends on both the relative concentration of the inhibitor and its affinity for the enzyme. The effects of inhibitors are relatively rapid (minutes to hours) and are reversible within a time frame that depends on the half-life of the inhibitor. There is a large amount of interindividual variation in drug metabolism and the propensity for enzyme inhibition to

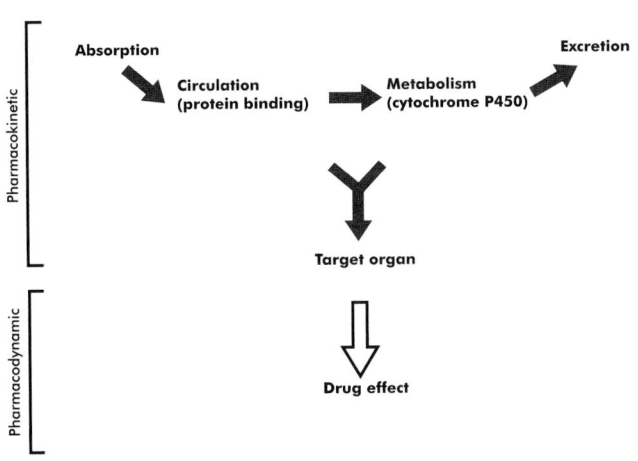

FIGURE 27–3. Potential sites and types of drug-drug interactions.

TABLE 27–25. Partial list of clinically relevant cytochrome P450 substrates and inhibitors

Enzyme	CYP 1A2	CYP 2C9/10	CYP 2D6	CYP 3A3/4

Substrates (medications metabolized by this enzyme)	Clozapine
	Tacrine
	Theophylline
	Caffeine
		Warfarin
		Phenytoin
			TCAs
			Trazodone, MCPP
			Type IC antiarrhythmics
			  Encainide
			  Flecainide
			  Mexiletine
			Lipophilic β-Blockers
			Most antipsychotics
			Codeine to morphine
			Dexfenfluramine
				Anticonvulsants
				  Carbamazepine
				  Ethosuximide
				Steroids
				Protease inhibitors
				Simvastin
				Pimozide[a] (Orap)
				Cyclosporine
				Lovastatin
				Cisapride[a] (Propulsid)
				Antihistamines
				  Terfenadine[a] (Seldane)
				  Astemizole[a] (Hismanal)
				Calcium channel blockers
				Benzodiazepines
				  Alprazolam
				  Midazolam
				  Triazolam
				Antiarrhythmics
				  Amiodarone
				  Quinidine
				  Lidocaine
				  Propafenone

Inhibitors (may increase levels of substrates)	Fluvoxamine (Luvox)
	Fluoroquinolones
	  Ciprofloxacin
	  Enoxacin
	  Norfloxacin
	Grapefruit juice
		Ritonavir
		?Antidepressants
		  Fluoxetine[b] (Prozac)
		  Sertraline[b] (Zoloft)
		  Fluvoxamine[b] (Luvox)
			Quinidine
			Antidepressants
			  Fluoxetine (Prozac)
			  Paroxetine (Paxil)
			  Sertraline (Zoloft)
			  Fluvoxamine[b] (Luvox)
			Ritonavir
			Phenothiazines
				Imidazole antifungal agents (e.g., ketoconazole)
				Some macrolide antibiotics (EES, clarithromycin, azithromycin)
				Protease inhibitors
				Verapamil, diltiazem
				Antidepressants
				  Nefazodone (Serzone)
				  Fluvoxamine (Luvox)
				  Fluoxetine[b] (Prozac)
				Grapefruit juice

CYP = cytochrome P450. [a]Do not use with 3A3/4 inhibitors. [b]Possible weak inhibition.
Source. Adapted from Callahan et al. 1996.

alter metabolism. Part of this variation is the result of genetic polymorphism (Shimada et al. 1994), which is a heritable alteration in the enzyme. The 2C19 and 2D6 enzymes are known to exhibit polymorphism. Persons who exhibit a genetic polymorphism causing a large reduction in the amount of active enzyme are referred to as "poor metabolizers" and are at risk for increased drug levels, which may lead to toxicity. Approximately 15%–20% of Asians and 1% of Caucasians have reduced amounts of the CYP 2C19 enzyme (Nakamura et al. 1985; Xie et al. 1996), whereas 7%–10% of Caucasians lack the CYP 2D6 enzyme (Dahl et al. 1995). In contrast, some persons have increased amounts of the CYP 2D6 enzyme (Johansson et al. 1993). These individuals are referred to as "ultrarapid metabolizers" and may have reduced levels of drugs that are metabolized by this enzyme, resulting in decreased efficacy. Polymorphism accounts for much of the well-known interindividual differences in drug metabolism and the occurrence of drug-drug interactions mediated by CYP 450.

In addition, the CYP enzymes can be induced (Watkins et al. 1985). CYP enzyme induction causes the liver to produce a greater amount of the enzyme, which can increase elimination and reduce plasma levels of a second drug or its metabolites. When clinically relevant, the drug dosage should be increased to achieve the same serum concentration. The effects of inducers tend to be delayed days to weeks because this process involves enzyme synthesis. Barbiturates, carbamazepine, phenytoin, rifampin, dexamethasone, smoking, and chronic alcohol use induce CYP enzymes.

Protein Binding

Medications are distributed to their sites of action through the circulatory system. In the bloodstream, all the psychotropic medications except lithium are bound to plasma proteins to varying degrees. A drug is considered highly protein bound if more than 90% is bound to plasma proteins. A reversible equilibrium exists between the bound and unbound drug; the unbound fraction is pharmacologically active, whereas the bound fraction is inactive and therefore cannot be metabolized or excreted. When two drugs exist simultaneously in the plasma, competition for protein-binding sites occurs. This can cause displacement of the previously protein-bound drug, which in the free state becomes pharmacologically active. Interactions that occur by this mechanism are called *protein-binding interactions*. They are transient because, although the plasma concentration of free drug initially increases, the drug then becomes subject to redistribution, metabolism, and excretion, producing a new steady-state concentration. This

type of interaction is generally not clinically significant unless the drugs involved are highly protein bound (which results in a large change in plasma concentration of free drug from a small amount of drug displacement) and have a low therapeutic index or narrow therapeutic window (in which case small changes in plasma levels can result in toxicity or loss of efficacy; Callahan et al. 1996).

Absorption and Excretion

Changes in plasma level as a result of alterations in absorption or excretion are less common with psychiatric medications. Drugs with anticholinergic effects, such as tricyclic antidepressants, tend to decrease gastrointestinal motility, which allows for longer periods of absorption of other medications (Greiff and Rowbotham 1994). Prolonged absorption may result in increased plasma levels of concomitantly administered medications. Changes in drug plasma concentration as a result of changes in excretion are most germane to lithium, which is dependent on renal excretion. Any medication that alters the kidney's excretion of lithium may result in clinically significant changes in the serum lithium level (as reviewed by Goodwin and Jamison 1990). These medications are listed in Table 27–24.

PHARMACODYNAMIC INTERACTIONS

Pharmacodynamic interactions involve a change in the pharmacological effect of a drug resulting from the action of a second drug at a common receptor or bioactive site. These interactions can be mediated directly or indirectly. Direct pharmacodynamic interactions involve agonist or antagonist actions of two drugs at a common site, which produces increased (additive) or decreased pharmacological effects. Such interactions generally result from known pharmacological actions of a drug, and for this reason agents with a multiplicity of pharmacological effects are more likely to be involved. For example, low-potency antipsychotics and tertiary amine tricyclic antidepressants have anticholinergic, antihistaminic, α-adrenergic-antagonist, and quinidine-like effects. In light of this, it can be predicted that the concurrent administration of chlorpromazine and imipramine will result in additive sedation, constipation, postural hypotension, and depression of cardiac conduction.

Indirect interactions involve changes in physiological functions owing to the combined action of two drugs at a common site. These interactions cannot be predicted on the basis of known pharmacological effects, and their mechanisms are poorly understood. Many indirect pharmacodynamic interactions have clinically significant consequences. For example, the adjunctive use of lithium with various antidepressant agents can potentiate antidepressant effects (synergism). On the other hand, the concurrent administration of a serotonin-reuptake inhibitor or meperidine with a monoamine oxidase inhibitor can produce a potentially lethal hypermetabolic reaction.

SUMMARY

Remembering the myriad of psychotropic drug interactions is extremely difficult. Nevertheless, by applying a systematic approach, the clinician can often predict the occurrence and time course of such interactions. Several factors must be considered when assessing the potential consequences of drug interactions. Drug-related factors that increase the risk for clinically significant interactions include a low therapeutic index or narrow therapeutic window, a multiplicity of pharmacological actions, and inhibition or inducement of cytochrome P450 enzymes. Next, patient-related factors that can increase the risk for significant drug interactions should be considered. These include genetically based variations in drug-metabolizing capacity, as well as advanced age, underlying medical illness, and comorbid substance abuse. Finally, the literature should be carefully reviewed to ascertain the potential clinical relevance of available data. If a clinically significant drug interaction appears likely to occur, the patient's clinical status should be followed closely; therapeutic drug monitoring should be used, if applicable, and dosage adjustments should be made accordingly. Rational polypharmacy requires an understanding of the pharmacological principles governing drug interactions and a knowledge of the factors that increase the likelihood of clinically significant variations in drug action. This understanding will allow the clinician to maximize beneficial effects while minimizing the risk of adverse events.

ANTIAGGRESSION DRUGS

OVERVIEW

Aggressive and violent behaviors are frequently encountered in patients with underlying disorders as diverse as traumatic brain injury; brain tumor; hereditary or metabolic brain disease; mental retardation; dementia; seizure disorders; sequelae of CNS infections; sequelae of substance abuse; DSM-IV Axis I psychiatric disorders such as schizophrenia, bipolar disorder, and conduct disorder; and Axis II personality disorders such as antisocial and border-

line personality disorders (Silver and Yudofsky 1987). Dyscontrol of aggression in many of these conditions is often the most significant source of disability and dysfunction among all the symptoms and signs associated with the underlying illness. These episodes range in severity from irritability to outbursts that result in damage to property or assaults on others. In severe cases, affected individuals cannot remain in the community or with their families and often are referred to the most restrictive long-term psychiatric or neurobehavioral facilities.

In establishing a treatment plan for patients with agitation or aggression, the overarching principle is that diagnosis comes before treatment. The history of the development of symptoms in a biopsychosocial context is usually the most critical part of the evaluation. It is essential to determine the mental status of the patient before the agitated or aggressive event, the nature of the precipitant, the physical and social environment in which the behavior occurs, the ways in which the event is mitigated, and the primary and secondary gains related to agitation and aggression. Evaluation and documentation of aggressive behaviors with objective measures such as the Overt Aggression Scale (Silver and Yudofsky 1991; Yudofsky et al. 1986) are often helpful.

Although no medication has been approved by the FDA specifically for the treatment of aggression, medications are widely used (and commonly misused) in the management of patients with acute or chronic aggression. The use of pharmacological interventions for aggression can be considered in two categories: 1) the use of the sedating effects of medications, as required in acute situations, so that the patient does not harm him- or herself or others, and 2) the use of nonsedating antiaggression medications for the treatment of chronic aggression (Corrigan et al. 1993; Silver and Yudofsky 1994; Yudofsky et al. 1990).

ACUTE AGGRESSION AND AGITATION

Medications that are sedating may be indicated for the treatment of agitation and for treating acute episodes of aggressive behavior. Because these drugs are not specific in their ability to inhibit aggressive behaviors, however, there may be detrimental effects on arousal and cognitive function. Therefore, the use of sedation-producing medications must be time-limited to avoid the emergence of seriously disabling side effects ranging from oversedation to tardive dyskinesia. Unless aggressive behavior is clearly related to psychotic ideation that is responding to treatment with antipsychotic agents, we limit the use of both antipsychotic agents and benzodiazepines for "sedating" aggression to a maximum time period of 4 weeks. Beyond this time, the clinician must consider whether or not the aggression is chronic and alter the treatment plan accordingly to use medications recommended to treat chronic behaviors (see the following section).

Antipsychotic Drugs

Antipsychotics are the most commonly used medications in the treatment of aggression. Although these agents are appropriate and effective when aggression is derivative of active psychosis, the use of neuroleptic agents to treat chronic aggression, especially when secondary to organic brain injury, is often ineffective and entails significant risk of serious complications. Usually, it is the sedative side effects rather than the antipsychotic properties of antipsychotics that are used (i.e., misused) to treat (i.e., mask) the aggression, and patients often develop tolerance to these sedative effects, requiring increasing doses. As a result, extrapyramidal and anticholinergic side effects occur. Paradoxically (and frequently), because of the development of akathisia, the patient may become more agitated and restless as the dosage of the neuroleptic is increased, especially when a high-potency antipsychotic such as haloperidol (Haldol) is administered. The akathisia is often mistaken for increased irritability and agitation, and a vicious cycle of increased dosages of neuroleptics and worsening akathisia develops. Herrera et al. (1988) demonstrated that there was a marked increase in violent behavior when patients with schizophrenia were treated with haloperidol (in dosages up to 60 mg/day) compared with the behaviors that occurred during treatment with chlorpromazine (1,800 mg/day) or clozapine (900 mg/day), two drugs that are associated with less akathisia than is haloperidol. Similarly, risperidone and olanzapine may have a role in the treatment of agitation and aggression, although this has not yet been demonstrated in controlled clinical trials.

There is some evidence from studies of injury to motor neurons in animals that haloperidol retards recovery. This effect was seen only when animals actively participated in a behavioral task and not when the animals were restrained after drug administration (Feeney et al. 1982). It is possible that the effect of haloperidol of decreasing dopamine levels and inhibiting neuronal function, which may be the mechanism of action in treating aggression, has other detrimental effects on recovery. Whether this finding is generalizable to recovery in brain injury remains unclear; however, it raises important potential risk-benefit issues that must be considered before antipsychotic drugs are used to treat aggressive behavior in patients with neuronal damage.

In patients with brain injury and acute aggression, we recommend starting a neuroleptic such as haloperidol at low doses: 1 mg orally or 0.5 mg intramuscularly, with repeated administration every hour until control of aggression is achieved (Yudofsky et al. 1990). If after several administrations of haloperidol, the patient's aggressive behavior does not improve, the hourly dose may be increased until the patient is sedated sufficiently that he or she no longer exhibits agitation or violence. Once the patient is not aggressive for 48 hours, the daily dosage should be decreased gradually (i.e., by 25% each day) to ascertain whether aggressive behavior reemerges. If it does, consideration should be given to increasing the dosage of haloperidol and then initiating treatment with a more specific antiaggression drug. Preliminary data suggest that risperidone may also be effective in the reduction of hostility and aggression in patients with mental retardation and behavioral disturbance (Lott et al. 1996), schizophrenia (Czobor et al. 1995; McCreadie 1996), and dementia (Jeanblanc and Davis 1995).

Benzodiazepines

The literature is inconsistent concerning the effects of the benzodiazepines in the treatment of aggression. The sedative properties of benzodiazepines are especially helpful in the management of acute agitation and aggression (Yudofsky et al. 1987); most likely, this is due to the effect of the benzodiazepines in facilitating the inhibitory neurotransmitter GABA. Paradoxically, several researchers have reported increased hostility and aggression, as well as the induction of rage, in patients treated with benzodiazepines (Yudofsky et al. 1987). However, these reports are balanced by the observation that this phenomenon is rare (Dietch and Jennings 1988). Benzodiazepines can produce amnesia (Angus and Romney 1984; Lucki et al. 1986; Roth et al. 1980) and can exacerbate preexisting memory dysfunction. Patients with brain injury may also experience increased problems with coordination and balance with benzodiazepine use.

For treatment of acute aggression, lorazepam, 1–2 mg, may be administered every hour by either the oral or the intramuscular route until sedation is achieved (Yudofsky et al. 1990). Intramuscular lorazepam has been suggested as an effective medication in the emergency treatment of violent patients (Bick and Hannah 1986). Intravenous lorazepam is also effective, although the onset of action is similar when administered intramuscularly. Caution must be taken with intravenous administration of lorazepam; it should be injected in doses of less than 1 cc (1 mg) per minute to avoid laryngospasm. As is done with neuroleptics, gradual tapering of lorazepam may be attempted when the patient has demonstrated control for 48 hours. If aggressive behavior recurs, medications for the treatment of chronic aggression may be initiated. Lorazepam in 1- or 2-mg doses, either orally or by injection, may be administered, if necessary, in combination with a neuroleptic medication (e.g., haloperidol, 2–5 mg). Other sedating medications such as valproate, chloral hydrate, or diphenhydramine may be preferable to sedative antipsychotic agents.

CHRONIC AGGRESSION

If a patient continues to have periods of agitation or aggression for longer than several weeks, maintenance approaches should be considered. We advocate that the choice of the specific psychopharmacological agent be guided by the determination of the underlying illness that leads to the chronic behavior; the co-occurrence of other psychiatric symptoms such as anxiety, mania, or depression; and the underlying hypothesized mechanism of action of the drug (e.g., effects on the serotonergic system, the adrenergic system, or kindling). Because no medication has been approved by the FDA for treatment of aggression, the clinician must use medications that may have an antiaggressive effect but have been approved for other uses (e.g., seizure disorders, depression, hypertension).

Antipsychotic Medications

It is generally clinically indicated to restrict the use of antipsychotic medications to the treatment of agitation or aggression that is the direct response to psychotic ideation or perception such as paranoid delusions or command hallucinations. When treating such patients, the clinician should attempt, at regular intervals, to taper the medication to gauge the efficacy of the antipsychotic agent in treating both the psychosis and the attendant aggression. The clinician should choose antipsychotics and dosages in the same manner as recommended for the treatment of psychosis.

Buspirone

As discussed earlier, serotonin appears to be a key neurotransmitter in the modulation of aggressive behavior. In preliminary reports, buspirone, a 5-HT$_1$A agonist, has been reported to be effective in the management of aggression and agitation for patients with head injury (Gualtieri 1991a, 1991b; Levine 1988; Ratey et al. 1992a), dementia (Colenda 1988; Tiller et al. 1988), and developmental disabilities and autism (Ratey et al. 1989; Realmuto et al. 1989). We have also noted that some patients become more aggressive when treated with buspirone; therefore,

buspirone should be initiated at low dosages (i.e., 5 mg bid) and increased by 5 mg every 3–5 days. Dosages of 45–60 mg/day may be required before there is improvement in aggressive behavior. A latency of 3–6 weeks before therapeutic effects are observed is not uncommon.

Anticonvulsants

The anticonvulsants carbamazepine and valproate have proved effective for the treatment of bipolar disorders and have been advocated for the control of aggression in both epileptic and nonepileptic patients (Yudofsky et al. 1987). The mechanism of action of the anticonvulsants in the treatment of aggression may be through their inhibition of kindling. Although a specific antiaggressive response to these agents has not yet been demonstrated according to the strictest scientific criteria, a vast amount of clinical experience strongly suggests the efficacy of carbamazepine and valproate. Several open studies have indicated that carbamazepine may be effective in decreasing aggressive behavior associated with dementia (Gleason and Schneider 1990; Leibovici and Tariot 1988), developmental disabilities (Folks et al. 1982; Tunks and Dermer 1973; Yatham and McHale 1988), and schizophrenia (Hakoloa and Loulumaa 1982; Luchins 1983), as well as in a variety of other organic brain disorders (Mattes 1988). Reports also have indicated that the antiaggressive response of carbamazepine can be found in patients with EEG abnormalities (Hakoloa and Loulumaa 1982; Stone et al. 1986; Tunks and Dermer 1973; Yatham and McHale 1988) and without EEG abnormalities (Luchins 1983; Mattes 1988). Similarly, valproate has been found to reduce agitation and aggression in patients with a wide variety of psychiatric and medical disorders (Giakas et al. 1990; Mazure et al. 1992; Mellow et al. 1993; Wilcox 1994).

Carbamazepine and valproate can be highly effective medications for treating aggression in patients with brain injury, and we believe these are the drugs of choice for patients who have aggressive episodes with concomitant seizures or epileptic foci.

Lithium

Lithium is known to be effective in controlling aggression related to manic excitement, and researchers have suggested that it may also have a role in the treatment of aggression in selected patients who do not have bipolar disorder (Yudofsky et al. 1987). Included have been patients with traumatic brain injury (Haas and Cope 1985), patients with mental retardation who exhibit self-injurious (Luchins and Dojka 1989) or aggressive behavior (Craft et al. 1987; Dale 1980; Dostal and Zvolsky 1970; Worrall et al. 1975), children and adolescents with behavioral disorders (Campbell et al. 1972; Vetro et al. 1985), prison inmates (Sheard et al. 1976; Tupin et al. 1973), and patients with other organic brain syndromes (Williams and Goldstein 1979). Primary antiaggressive effects may be due to the effect of lithium on the serotonergic system, although lithium also affects other important neuronal systems, such as inositol phosphate metabolism and kindling (Berridge et al. 1989).

Patients with brain injury have increased sensitivity to the neurotoxic effects of lithium (Hornstein and Seliger 1989; Moskowitz and Altshuler 1991). Because of its potential for neurotoxicity and its relative lack of efficacy in many patients with aggression secondary to brain injury, we limit the use of lithium in patients whose aggression is related to manic effects or recurrent irritability associated with cyclic mood disorders.

Antidepressant Medications

Antidepressants may have effects on the serotonergic, noradrenergic, and other neurotransmitter systems. The antidepressants that have been reported to control aggressive behavior are those that act preferentially or specifically on serotonin. In open studies, Mysiw et al. (1988) and Jackson et al. (1985) reported that amitriptyline (maximum dosage 150 mg/day) was effective in the treatment of patients with recent severe brain injury whose agitation had not responded to behavioral techniques. Szlabowicz and Stewart (1990) successfully treated a 43-year-old man with aggressive behavior subsequent to anoxic encephalopathy with amitriptyline 75 mg at bedtime. Trazodone has also been reported to be effective in treating the aggression that occurs with organic mental disorders (Greenwald et al. 1986; Pinner and Rich 1988; Simpson and Foster 1986). Gedye (1991) reported that a 17-year-old mentally disabled and autistic boy with aggressive and self-injurious behavior had a favorable response after treatment with trazodone. Fluoxetine, a potent serotonergic antidepressant, was reported to be effective in the treatment of aggressive behavior in a patient who had brain injury (Sorbin et al. 1989), as well as in patients with personality disorders (Coccaro et al. 1990) and depression (Fava et al. 1993). There have also been reports of the therapeutic effect of fluoxetine for adolescents with mental retardation and self-injurious behavior (Bass and Beltis 1991; King 1991). We have used fluoxetine with considerable success in aggressive patients with brain lesions. The drug may be started at a dosage of 10 mg/day and increased to 20 mg/day after 1 week. For some patients with aggression related to brain disorders, response to treatment with fluoxetine occurs in the range of 60–80 mg/day.

We have evaluated and treated many patients with emotional lability that is characterized by frequent episodes of tearfulness and irritability as well as the full symptomatic picture of organic aggressive syndrome (Silver and Yudofsky 1994). The patients, who would be diagnosed according to DSM-IV criteria as having personality change due to a general medical condition, labile type, have responded well to antidepressants. These therapeutic results are consistent with the reports of Schiffer et al. (1985), who used amitriptyline for patients with multiple sclerosis (MS), and of Seliger et al. (1992) and Sloan et al. (1992), who used fluoxetine to treat patients after brain injury, stroke, or MS. In addition, it appears that the other SSRIs are also effective in these disorders. It is usually necessary to administer these medications at standard antidepressant dosages to achieve full therapeutic effects.

Antihypertensive Medications (β-Blockers)

Since the first report of the use of β-adrenergic-receptor blockers in the treatment of acute aggression in 1977, more than 25 articles have appeared in the neurological and psychiatric literature reporting experience in using β-blockers with more than 200 patients with aggression (Yudofsky et al. 1987). Most of these patients had been unsuccessfully treated with antipsychotics, minor tranquilizers, lithium, and/or anticonvulsants before treatment with β-blockers was begun. The β-blockers that have been investigated in controlled prospective studies include propranolol (a lipid-soluble, nonselective receptor antagonist; Greendyke et al. 1986; Mattes 1988), nadolol (a water-soluble, nonselective receptor antagonist; Alpert et al. 1990; Ratey et al. 1992b), and pindolol (a lipid-soluble, nonselective receptor antagonist with partial sympathomimetic activity; Greendyke et al. 1986, 1989). A growing body of preliminary evidence suggests that β-adrenergic-receptor blockers are effective agents for the treatment of aggressive and violent behaviors, particularly those related to organic brain syndrome. Because of our own extensive clinical experience using β-blockers to treat aggressive patients with neuropsychiatric disorders, this approach has become our first line of treatment of organically induced agitation and aggression.

Guidelines for the use of propranolol are listed in Table 27–26. When a patient requires the use of a once-a-day medication because of compliance difficulties, long-acting propranolol (i.e., Inderal LA) or nadolol (Corgard) can be used. When patients develop bradycardia that prevents prescribing of therapeutic dosages of propranolol, pindolol (Visken) can be substituted, using one-tenth the dosage of propranolol. Pindolol's intrinsic sympathomimetic activity stimulates the β receptor and restricts the

TABLE 27–26.   Clinical use of propranolol

1. Conduct a thorough medical evaluation.

2. Exclude patients with the following disorders: bronchial asthma, chronic obstructive pulmonary disease, insulin-dependent diabetes mellitus, congestive heart failure, persistent angina, significant peripheral vascular disease, hyperthyroidism.

3. Avoid sudden discontinuation of propranolol (particularly in patients with hypertension).

4. Begin with a single test dose of 20 mg/day in patients for whom there are clinical concerns with hypotension or bradycardia. Increase dosage of propranolol by 20 mg/day every 3 days.

5. Initiate propranolol on a schedule of 20 mg tid for patients without cardiovascular or cardiopulmonary disorder.

6. Increase the dosage of propranolol by 60 mg/day every 3 days.

7. Increase medication unless the pulse rate is reduced to below 50 beats/minute or the systolic blood pressure is less than 90 mmHg.

8. Do not administer medication if severe dizziness, ataxia, or wheezing occurs. Reduce or discontinue propranolol if such symptoms persist.

9. Increase dosage to 12 mg/kg or until aggressive behavior is under control.

10. Dosages of greater than 800 mg are usually not required to control aggressive behavior.

11. Maintain the patient on the highest dosage of propranolol for at least 8 weeks before concluding that the patient is not responding to the medication. Some patients, however, respond rapidly to propranolol.

12. Use concurrent medications with caution. Monitor plasma levels of all antipsychotic and anticonvulsive medications.

Source. Reprinted with permission from Yudofsky SC, Silver JM, Schneider SE: "Pharmacologic treatment of aggression." *Psychiatric Annals* 17:397–407, 1987. Copyright Slack, Inc., 1987.

development of bradycardia.

The mechanism of action of β-blockers in the treatment of aggression is not known. Although some investigators have hypothesized a peripheral (e.g., nonbrain) site of action secondary to decreased afferent input to the brain (Ratey et al. 1992b), even nonlipid soluble β-adrenergic antagonists, when used for several days, gain access to the CNS (Gengo et al. 1988). On the basis of the presence of β receptors in the CNS (Alexander et al. 1979), and the fact that these agents have antiaggressive effects when administered intraventricularly to animals (Leavitt et al. 1989), we believe that there is a central site of action.

The major side effects of β-blockers when used to treat aggression are a lowering of blood pressure and a lowering of pulse rate. If orthostatic hypotension occurs, the physician should ensure that the patient's salt intake is adequate. Because peripheral β receptors are fully blocked with dosages of 300–400 mg/day, further decreases in these vital signs usually do not occur even when dosages are increased to much higher levels. Thereafter, increasing the dosage of a β-blocker is not typically associated with cardiovascular side effects. Therapeutic response may not be apparent for 6–8 weeks. Despite reports of depression with the use of β-blockers, controlled trials and our experience indicate that this rarely occurs (Yudofsky 1992). Because the use of propranolol is associated with significant increases in plasma levels of thioridazine, which has an absolute dosage ceiling of 800 mg/day, the combination of these two medications should be avoided whenever possible (Silver et al. 1986).

RECOMMENDATIONS FOR TREATMENT

In treating aggression, clinicians should, when possible, diagnose and treat underlying disorders and use agents that are specific for those disorders. For example, if aggression is related to active psychosis, antipsychotic agents should be used. In patients with aggression related to mania, valproate or lithium should be used. When aggression is related to seizure disorder, carbamazepine or valproate is indicated. Patients with mood lability or depression with concomitant irritability or rage attacks should be treated with serotonergic antidepressants or mood stabilizers. Finally, for patients in whom aggression is secondary to neurological syndromes, such as traumatic brain injury, Alzheimer's disease, or Huntington's disease, we recommend the use of β-blockers. β-blockers should also be considered for agitation and aggression in patients with schizophrenia whose aggression is not directly related to psychotic ideation. For example, if a patient is defensively violent because he delusionally believes a therapy aide is attempting to perpetrate an act of sexual violence against him, an antipsychotic agent would be indicated. However, if a patient with schizophrenia is chronically agitated, and the level of psychosis is independent of the dosage of antipsychotic agents, we recommend that β-blockers be considered.

ELECTROCONVULSIVE THERAPY

OVERVIEW

Electroconvulsive therapy (ECT) is the use of electrically induced repetitive firings of the neurons in the CNS (i.e., grand mal seizures) to treat psychiatric illnesses such as depression or mania and psychiatric symptoms such as psychosis or catatonia. Although ECT was first used in the late 1930s, before the era of potent psychopharmacological treatment of major affective disorders, the treatment today remains clinically relevant because of its high degree of efficacy, safety, and usefulness. Despite the extraordinary practical difficulties involved, scientific efforts to define its clinical efficacy and diagnostic indications have resulted in six published controlled trials since 1968 in which ECT has been shown to be superior to simulated treatment (Lerer and Belmaker 1986). For many patients, ECT is the safest and most effective form of treatment (American Psychiatric Association 1990). Many years ago ECT was used primarily in large state hospitals for the treatment of patients with chronic psychiatric disorders, including schizophrenia. Currently, in the United States, ECT is used primarily in the private sector for patients who do not receive prolonged inpatient care (Asnis et al. 1978).

MECHANISMS OF ACTION

The mechanisms of action of ECT, like those of other treatments in psychiatry, are complex and not completely understood. Nevertheless, ECT has been found to affect many of the neurotransmitters and receptors that have been implicated in depression and its treatment. In studies involving both humans and animals, ECT has been found to affect serotonin, GABA, endogenous opiates and their receptors, and catecholamines (including dopamine, norepinephrine, and epinephrine and their receptors). It also affects a wide variety of other neurotransmitters, neuropeptides, and neuroendocrine pathways (Kapur and Mann 1993; Nutt and Glue 1993). In addition, neurophysiological hypotheses regarding a range of effects of ECT (e.g., on kindling and on regional cerebral blood flow) increasingly are being advanced and studied (Silfverskiold et al. 1986).

INDICATIONS

The principal diagnostic indications for ECT are listed in Table 27–27 (American Psychiatric Association 1990). The APA Task Force on Electroconvulsive Therapy has recommended specific primary and secondary clinical indications for the use of ECT (Tables 27–28 and 27–29). Depressed patients adequately treated with either drugs or ECT have significantly lower mortality rates, not only related to suicide but also from natural causes, than patients with depression who are not treated with one of these

methods (Avery and Winokur 1976). According to an analysis of rigorously controlled studies that compared the efficacy of ECT with that of simulated ECT, placebo, and antidepressants, ECT was clearly superior to all the other forms of treatment for severe depression (Janicak et al. 1985). Although ECT and antidepressant agents are effective in similar patient populations with depression (except for patients with delusional depression, in whom ECT is superior), a number of comparative studies have shown that ECT is significantly more effective, with marked improvement generally occurring in 80%–90% of patients (Weiner 1979). ECT may also be of benefit in the treatment of manic excitement that is not responsive to medications (Small et al. 1986), as well as in the treatment of acute psychotic and affective symptoms of schizophrenia. In a review of the use of ECT in the treatment of schizophrenia, Salzman (1980) found that the few acceptable published studies showed that the clinical response to ECT was inversely proportional to the duration of the schizophrenic symptoms. In general, patients with schizophrenia who have affective and catatonic symptoms respond best to ECT. There is no indication that ECT alters the fundamental psychopathology of schizophrenia (Small et al. 1986).

Yudofsky (1981) outlined special clinical situations in which ECT may be advantageous over other treatment approaches. Among these situations, which are by no means all-inclusive, are the following:

1. Patients whose severe affective disorders have not responded to adequate psychopharmacological treatment (i.e., with appropriate dosage and duration of treatment).
2. Patients with delusional depression (Avery and

TABLE 27-27. **Diagnostic indications for electroconvulsive therapy**

I. Major depression

II. Mania

III. Schizophrenia and other functional psychoses

    1. Schizophrenic exacerbations:

        a. With catatonia

        b. When affective symptoms are prominent

        c. When there is a history of favorable response

    2. Schizophreniform and schizoaffective disorder

Source. Reprinted with permission from American Psychiatric Association: *The Practice of Electroconvulsive Therapy: Recommendations for Treatment, Training, and Privileging.* A Task Force Report of the American Psychiatric Association. Copyright 1990, American Psychiatric Association.

TABLE 27–28. **Primary clinical indications for the use of electroconvulsive therapy**

1. When there is a need for a rapid, definitive response on either medical or psychiatric grounds
2. When the risks of other treatments outweigh the risks of electroconvulsive therapy (ECT)
3. When there is a history of poor drug response and/or good response to ECT during previous episodes of the illness
4. Patient preference

Source. Adapted with permission from American Psychiatric Association 1990.

TABLE 27–29. **Secondary clinical indications for the use of electroconvulsive therapy**

1. When there has been treatment failure (taking into account issues such as choice of agent, dosage, and duration of trial)
2. When there are adverse effects that are unavoidable and that are deemed less likely and/or less severe with electroconvulsive therapy than with medication
3. When there is deterioration of the patient's condition such that rapid, definitive response is necessary on either psychiatric or medical grounds

Source. Adapted with permission from American Psychiatric Association 1990.

Lubrano 1979; Glassman and Roose 1981; Paul et al. 1977).

3. Patients—particularly elderly patients—who cannot tolerate the cardiovascular, genitourinary, or CNS side effects of antidepressant or antipsychotic agents.
4. Patients whose acute symptoms are so severe (i.e., manic excitement, active suicidal behavior, psychomotor retardation, or catatonia) that a rapid and dramatic response is required.
5. Patients with histories of depressive episodes that have responded successfully to previous electroconvulsive treatments.

CONTRAINDICATIONS

There are relatively few contraindications to ECT (American Psychiatric Association 1990). First, patients with clinically significant space-occupying cerebral lesions or conditions with increased intracranial pressure must not receive this treatment because of the risk of brain stem herniation (Maltbie et al. 1980). Second, patients with

significant cardiovascular problems, such as recent myocardial infarction, severe cardiac ischemia, and moderate-to-severe hypertension (including pheochromocytoma), are more prone to the transient fluctuations in the cardiovascular system that occur during and shortly after ECT. Such patients may or may not safely be given ECT, and they must be evaluated before treatment by a cardiologist familiar with the potential side effects of ECT. Patients with recent intracerebral hemorrhage are at increased risk, as are those with bleeding or unstable vascular aneurysm or abnormalities, or with retinal detachment. Before the use of muscle relaxants in ECT, degenerative diseases of the spine and other bones constituted a significant risk from ECT. Today, however, adequate anesthetic and muscle relaxant techniques render ECT generally safe in patients with these disorders. Although it has been suggested that patients should discontinue taking MAOIs at least 2 weeks before the initiation of ECT to prevent dangerous increases in blood pressure during treatment, ECT has been administered to patients currently treated with MAOIs without adverse effects (Wells and Bjorkstein 1989).

MEDICAL EVALUATION BEFORE TREATMENT

Before receiving ECT, patients should have a complete medical and neurological examination, complete blood count, serum electrolyte analysis, and ECG. An X ray of the lumbosacral region should be obtained if spinal orthopedic problems are suspected. A chest X ray must be obtained because of the use of positive pressure respiration during general anesthesia. Evaluation by an anesthesiologist to determine risk of anesthesia is recommended. In specific clinical situations, such as when there is clinical evidence of a brain tumor or intracerebral bleeding or if there are CNS symptoms of uncertain etiology, electroencephalography and brain computed tomography or magnetic resonance imaging are also required.

Informed consent of a competent patient is essential. Because of the high degree of fear and misinformation related to ECT, we encourage that ample time be devoted to the discussion of the risks, benefits, and techniques of ECT and of all treatment alternatives with patients and their families. This includes meeting with patients and family members to provide an ample opportunity for the exchange of ideas, feelings, and information related to electroconvulsive treatment. We consider this process an integral part of the overall ECT procedure. The clinician may wish to have the patient and his or her family read specially prepared information about the risks and benefits of ECT (Yudofsky et al. 1991).

TECHNIQUE

Anesthesia and Muscle Relaxation

Electroconvulsive therapy is used primarily for psychiatric inpatients, and it is becoming more common for an anesthetist or anesthesiologist to assist the psychiatrist in administering the treatment. The APA Task Force on ECT (American Psychiatric Association 1990) recommended pretreatment with an anticholinergic drug such as atropine (0.4–1.0 mg iv) or glycopyrrolate (0.2–0.4 mg iv) to decrease the morbidity of cardiac bradyarrhythmias and aspiration. General anesthesia is induced only to the degree that a light coma is produced, using a fast-acting anesthetic such as methohexital, which has fewer cardiac side effects than slower acting barbiturates such as thiopental. A starting dose of approximately 0.75–1.0 mg/kg of intravenous methohexital is recommended, but the amount required to induce safe and brief anesthesia may vary from considerably lower to considerably higher amounts depending on the patient's metabolism of the drug. Once the patient is anesthetized, intravenous succinylcholine is used for muscular relaxation. In general, approximately 0.5–1 mg/kg of intravenous succinylcholine is administered rapidly, immediately after the onset of general anesthesia. If there are preexisting skeletal problems or other orthopedic problems, a higher dose of succinylcholine may be required, whereas a history or evidence of pseudocholinesterase deficiency would call for a lower dose. Once the succinylcholine is administered, the patient is ventilated with 100% oxygen until muscle fasciculations occur and motoric relaxation of the patient is accomplished. Modern ECT devices allow for simultaneous monitoring of the EEG and ECG before, during, and after the ECT procedure. In addition, there should be frequent monitoring of blood pressure, pulse rate, and blood oxygen saturation (with pulse oximetry).

Devices

The electrical stimulation of ECT devices is classified on the basis of waveform. Mechanisms using sine wave stimuli historically were the most commonly used to initiate grand mal seizures, whereas newer devices using brief pulse stimulation are increasingly being used. With the latter technique, grand mal seizures usually can be initiated with an amount of electrical energy that is significantly lower than that required with devices using sine wave stimuli (Malitz and Sackeim 1986).

Parameters

Two major issues in the administration of the electrical stimulus include the stimulus dose and the electrode placement (i.e., placement may be nondominant unilateral or bilateral). It has been documented that seizure threshold, which is defined as the minimal electrical intensity needed to produce a generalized seizure, increases with age and is greater in men than in women. However, the threshold can vary by 40-fold among patients (Sackeim et al. 1991). Electrodes may be placed unilaterally on the nondominant hemisphere (i.e., the electrodes over the right hemisphere for a right-handed individual) or bilaterally. Although there have been observations that unilateral electrode placement is related to fewer cognitive side effects compared with bilateral stimulus, studies also have suggested that unilateral placement is less efficacious (Abrams 1986; American Psychiatric Association 1990; Malitz and Sackeim 1986).

In a recent study Sackeim and co-workers (1993) compared low-dose (i.e., just above threshold) unilateral ECT, high-dose (i.e., 2.5 times the threshold) unilateral ECT, low-dose bilateral ECT, and high-dose bilateral ECT for efficacy and cognitive effects. The response rates for the differing treatments are listed in Table 27–30. Whereas high-dose unilateral treatment is more efficacious than low-dose unilateral stimulation, bilateral treatment is superior. In measures of time to recover orientation, unilateral stimulation was associated with fewer deleterious effects than bilateral stimulation, regardless of dosage.

The decision to initiate treatment with unilateral or bilateral electrode placement may be influenced by a variety of factors, including preexisting cognitive impairment and the clinical requirement for rapid improvement. In our practice, we determine seizure threshold during the first treatment session, and we increase subsequent treatment doses to ensure that stimulation is above threshold (American Psychiatric Association 1990).

TABLE 27–30. Efficacy and cognitive effects of electroconvulsive therapy stimuli

Stimulus	Response rate (%)	Time to orientation (minutes)
Low-dose unilateral	17	11 ± 7
High-dose unilateral	43 ($P = .054$)	21 ± 11
Low-dose bilateral	65 ($P = .001$)	38 ± 21
High-dose bilateral	63 ($P = .001$)	41 ± 17

Source. Data from Sackeim et al. 1993.

Course of Treatment

In the United States, ECT treatments are generally given on an every-other-day basis for 2–3 weeks, usually Monday, Wednesday, and Friday. Twice-weekly treatments may be equally effective with less cognitive side effects but with a slower onset of action (Lerer et al. 1995). Duration of seizure for longer than 20 seconds per treatment (as assessed by motor activity, not EEG seizure activity) is considered adequate for therapeutic purposes. The number of treatments administered is generally determined by a patient's clinical response; the therapy is discontinued when successive treatments do not elicit further beneficial effects (Weiner 1979). With depressed patients, a typical course of ECT consists of 6–10 treatments, but sometimes more are required. We do not recommend more than 20 treatments in a single course of ECT.

After a course of treatment, ample time and permission must be given for the patient to discuss with the professional his or her feelings about having been depressed and having received ECT. Occasionally, a patient will erroneously attribute his or her inability to recall a name to permanent side effects of the procedure. In this situation, the normal forgetting process to which most people are subject can become a frightening and unwarranted symbol of depression and ECT. In addition, there must be the recognition that ECT is a specific therapeutic tool that should be used as a component of a larger therapeutic strategy (Yudofsky 1982; Yudofsky et al. 1991). Because the beneficial response to ECT is often so rapid and dramatic, insufficient emphasis may be placed on sociological and intrapsychic stresses that have contributed to the initial depression. It is only after the patient's affective illness has been improved by ECT that he or she is able to use psychotherapy, family therapy, and behavior therapy effectively to address the conditions that contributed to the depression.

RISKS AND SIDE EFFECTS

In general, ECT is an unusually safe procedure, with morbidity and mortality not significantly greater than that associated with general anesthesia. The mortality rate of patients with ECT is 2 per 100,000 treatments (Fink 1978). The most frequent complaints of patients are memory impairment, headaches, and muscle aches (Gomez 1975); the most significant risks associated with ECT are cardiovascular and intracerebral (Abrams 1992).

Medical Risks

Ictal and postictal fluctuations in autonomic tone can elicit cardiac arrhythmias of many varieties, including prema-

ture ventricular contractions during the immediate postictal period. Increase in vagal tone may result in sinus bradycardia or sinus arrest, whereas increases in sympathetic tone can elicit ventricular ectopy and increases in blood pressure and heart rate (Abrams 1992). To evaluate the safety of ECT in the cardiovascular realm, Dec et al. (1985) assessed serial ECGs and serum cardiac enzyme values of 29 patients who received a course of this therapy. The investigators could not find persistent electrocardiographic changes, elevations in creatinine phosphokinase, or elevations in SGOT levels after 85 treatments in these patients. It is important to note that 24% of these patients had stable, preexisting cardiovascular disease, which included conduction system disease, recent myocardial infarction, and depressed ventricular function. The authors concluded that with careful cardiac monitoring before and after the procedure, with frequent checks of electrolyte values, and with careful tailoring of the anesthetic regimen to the individual patient, cardiovascular morbidity and mortality can be minimized, even for patients with known cardiovascular disease. As we noted earlier, patients who have preexisting disorders that increase intracranial pressure (e.g., space-occupying brain lesions), other CNS dysfunctions, hypertension, degenerative bone disease, or severe cardiac disease are at increased risk for serious side effects related to ECT. Such patients may receive ECT only after thorough evaluation and carefully documented approval by the relevant nonpsychiatric medical specialists.

Memory Impairment

The initial confusion and cognitive deficits associated with ECT treatment are usually temporary, lasting approximately 30 minutes. Whereas many patients report no problems with their memory, aside from the time immediately surrounding the ECT treatments, others report that their memory is not as good as it was before receiving ECT (Squire and Slater 1983). However, the controversy surrounding the effect of ECT on memory results primarily from public misinformation (Reid 1993).

To date, no reliable data have shown permanent memory loss caused by modern ECT. Prospective computed tomography and magnetic resonance imaging studies of the brain show no evidence of ECT-induced structural changes (Coffey et al. 1991; Devanand et al. 1994). A comparison of eight patients who received more than 100 ECT treatments with matched controls who had never received ECT found no significant differences in cognitive function (Devanand et al. 1991). Ninety-two depressed patients receiving either unilateral or bilateral ECT were interviewed regarding side effects both before and after the course of treatment. There was no change in cognitive complaints from pre-ECT to immediately after the ECT course (Devanand et al. 1995). In considering the possible effects of ECT on memory and cognition, it is important to keep in mind that depression itself commonly results in both memory and cognitive deficits. For patients with cognitive impairment secondary to depression, the therapeutic effect of ECT may contribute to improved cognitive functioning over time (Stoudemire et al. 1995).

The use of brief pulse stimulation instead of sine wave stimulation can reduce the memory impairment (Squire et al. 1975). Unilateral stimulation results in fewer cognitive problems, although its efficacy may be inferior (Sackeim et al. 1993). Other cognitive deficits include memory deficits for nonverbal information and transient disorientation. Patients with pretreatment global cognitive impairment and prolonged disorientation in the acute postictal periods were the most vulnerable to persistent retrograde amnesia (Sobin et al. 1995).

POST-ECT PROPHYLACTIC TREATMENT

Despite the acute efficacy of ECT, appropriate prophylactic treatment must be instituted after ECT to prevent relapse. Most commonly, antidepressant medications are used for this purpose. Unfortunately, many patients who receive ECT have been previously nonresponsive to standard antidepressant medications, and the efficacy of these treatments post-ECT is not clear (Sackeim et al. 1990). In such patients, lithium carbonate may be a useful agent for continuation therapy (Coppen et al. 1991; Perry and Tsuang 1979; Shapira et al. 1995). Although continuation therapy for patients with delusional depression has not been systematically studied, it is our impression that some patients require combined antipsychotic and antidepressant continuation drug therapy after ECT. It is our practice to maintain patients on therapeutic levels of antidepressants for at least 6 months of euthymia following a course of ECT; after that time, we gradually taper the antidepressants over a period of 4–8 weeks. For patients who fail to respond to other prophylactic therapies, maintenance ECT (i.e., an outpatient treatment every week to every several weeks) may be effective (Schwarz et al. 1995).

CONCLUSIONS

After more than 50 years of use, electroconvulsive therapy remains a safe, specific, and effective treatment regimen in psychiatry. The treatment is particularly effective in patients with severe depressions, including those that have delusional, suicidal, or psychomotor components. New technologies involving varying electrode placement as well as a reduced energy requirement to initiate seizures have led to fewer side effects while maintaining the therapeutic advantage of this procedure. It is important, as it is concerning all somatic interventions in psychiatry, that ECT be recognized as a specific therapeutic tool that is only one component of a larger treatment plan and that includes psychosocial and other biological interventions. Adequate time must be allocated to discuss the risks, benefits, side effects, and overall experience of the procedure with patients and their families and to answer their questions.

REFERENCES

General Principles

Amsterdam JD, Brunswick DJ, Mendels J: Reliability of commercially available tricyclic antidepressant levels.

Bourin M, Baker GB: The future of antidepressants. Biomed Pharmacother 50 (1):7–12, 1996

Cramer JA: Optimizing long-term patient compliance. Neurology 45:S25–S28, 1995

Endicott J, Spitzer RL: A diagnostic interview: the Schedule for Affective Disorders and Schizophrenia. Arch Gen Psychiatry 35:837–844, 1978

Food and Drug Administration: Bioavailability and bioequivalence requirements. Federal Register 57: 17997–18001, 1992

Hamilton M: Rating depressive patients. J Clin Psychiatry 41:21–24, 1960

Hauck WW, Anderson S: Types of bioequivalence and related statistical considerations. International Journal of Clinical Pharmacology, Therapy, and Toxicology 30 (51):181–187, 1992

MacKinnon R, Yudofsky SC: Principles of Psychiatric Evaluation. Philadelphia, PA, JB Lippincott, 1991

Morris LS, Schulz RM: Medication compliance: the patient's perspective. Clin Ther 15 (3):593–606, 1993

Physicians Desk Reference, 51st Edition. Oradell, NJ, Medical Economics Co, 1997

Post RM, Leverich GS, Altshuler L, Mikalauskas K: Lithium-discontinuation-induced refractoriness: preliminary observations. Am J Psychiatry 149:1727–1729, 1992

Sackett DL, Snow JS: The magnitude and measurement of compliance, in Compliance in Health Care. John Hopkins University Press, 1979, p 11

Silver JM, Yudofsky SC: The Overt Aggression Scale: overview and clinical guidelines. J Neuropsychiatry Clin Neurosci 3:S22–S29, 1991

Spitzer RL, Williams JBW, Gibbon M, et al: Structured Clinical Interview for DSM-III-R. Washington, DC, American Psychiatric Press, 1990

Yudofsky SC, Silver JM, Jackson W, et al: The Overt Aggression Scale for the objective rating of verbal and physical aggression. Am J Psychiatry 143:35–39, 1986

Antidepressant Drugs

Abernethy DR, Greenblatt DJ, Shader RI: Trimipramine kinetics and absolute bioavailability: use of gas-liquid chromatography with nitrogen-phosphorus detection. Clin Pharmacol Ther 35:348–353, 1984

Akiskal HS: Depression in cyclothymic and related temperaments: clinical and pharmacologic considerations. J Clin Psychiatry Monogr 10[1]:37–43, 1992

American Psychiatric Association: Diagnostic and Statistical Manual of Mental Disorders, 4th Edition. Washington, DC, American Psychiatric Association, 1994

American Psychiatric Association: Practice guidelines for major depressive disorder in adults. Washington DC, American Psychiatric Association, 1993

Amsterdam J, Berwish NJ: High dose tranylcypromine therapy for refractory depression. Pharmacopsychiatry 22 (1):21–25, 1989

Angst J: Natural history and epidemiology of depression, in Results of Community Studies in Prediction and Treatment of Recurrent Depression. Edited by Cobb J, Goeting N. Southampton, England, Duphar Medical Relations, 1990

Aranow A, Hudson J, Pope HG Jr, et al: Elevated antidepressant plasma levels after addition of fluoxetine. Am J Psychiatry 148:911–913, 1989

Armitage R, Rush AJ, Trivedi M, et al: The effects of nefazodone on sleep architecture in depression. Neuropsychopharmacology 10:123–127, 1994

Aronson MD, Hafez H: A case of trazodone-induced ventricular tachycardia. J Clin Psychiatry 47:388–389, 1986

Åsberg M: Individualization of treatment with tricyclic compounds. Med Clin North Am 58:1084–1091, 1974

Ballenger JC, Wheadon DE, Steiner M, et al: Double-blind, fixed-dose, placebo-controlled study of paroxetine in the treatment of panic disorder. Am J Psychiatry 155 (1):36–42, 1998

Baxter LR Jr, Liston EH, Schwartz JM, et al: Prolongation of the antidepressant response to partial sleep deprivation by lithium. Psychiatry Res 19:17–23, 1986

Beasley CM Jr., Masica DN, Heiligenstein JH, et al: Possible monoamine oxidase inhibitor-serotonin uptake inhibitor interaction: fluoxetine clinical data and preclinical findings. J Clin Psychopharmacology 13 (5):312–320, 1993

Blehar MC, Rosenthal NE: Seasonal affective disorders and phototherapy: report of a National Institute of Mental Health–sponsored workshop. Arch Gen Psychiatry 46:469–474, 1989

Boehnert MT, Lovejoy FH: Value of the QRS duration versus the serum drug level in predicting seizures and ventricular arrhythmias after an acute overdose of tricyclic antidepressants. N Engl J Med 313:474–479, 1985

Bouwer CD, Harvey BH: Phasic craving for carbohydrate observed with citalopram. Int Clin Psychopharmacol 11:273–278, 1996

Bremmer JD: A double blind comparison of mirtazapine, amitriptyline, and placebo in major depression. J Clin Psychiatry 56:519–525, 1995

Claghorn JL, Earl CQ, Walczak DD, Stoner KA, Wong LF, Kanter D, Houser VP: Fluvoxamine maleate in the treatment of depression: a single-center, double-blind, placebo-controlled comparison with imipramine in outpatients. J Clin Psychopharmacol 16:113–120, 1996

Clomipramine Collaborative Study Group: Clomipramine in the treatment of patients with obsessive-compulsive disorder. Arch Gen Psychiatry 48:730–738, 1991

Conners CK, Casat CD, Gualtieri CT, et al: Bupropion hydrochloride in attention deficit disorder with hyperactivity. J Am Acad Child Adolesc Psychiatry 35:1314–1321, 1996

Cook EH Jr, Stein MA, Krasowski MD, et al: Association of attention-deficit disorder and the dopamine transporter gene. Am J Hum Genet 56: 993–998, 1995

Coppen A, Mendelwicz J, Kielholz P: Pharmacotherapy of depressive disorders: a consensus statement. Geneva: World Health Organization, 1986

Coupet J, Rauh CE, Szues-Myers VA, et al: 2-Chloro-11-(1-piperazinyl) dibenz [b, f] [1, 4] oxazepine (amoxapine), an antidepressant with antipsychotic properties: a possible role for 7-hydroxyamoxapine. Biochemical Pharmacology 28:2514–2515, 1979

Coupland NJ, Bell CJ, Potokar JP: Serotonin reuptake inhibitor withdrawal. J Clin Psychopharmacol 16:356–362, 1996

Crane GE: Iproniazid (Marsilid) phosphate, a therapeutic agent for mental disorders and debilitating disease. J Psychiatr Res 8:142–152, 1957

Dailey JW, Naritoku DK: Antidepressants and seizures: clinical anecdotes overshadow neuroscience. Biochem Pharmacol 52:1323–1329, 1996

Danish University Antidepressant Group: Paroxetine: a selective serotonin reuptake inhibitor showing better tolerance, but weaker antidepressant effect than clomipramine in a controlled multicenter study. J Affect Disord 18:289–299, 1990

De Boer T: The pharmacologic profile of mirtazapine. J Clin Psychiatry 57 (suppl 4):19–25, 1996

De Montigny C, Gunberg S, Mayer A, et al: Lithium induces rapid relief of depression in tricyclic antidepressant nonresponders. Br J Psychiatry 138:252–256, 1981

Dinan TG, Barry S: A comparison of electroconvulsive therapy with a combined lithium and tricyclic combination among depressed tricyclic nonresponders. Acta Psychiatr Scand 80:97–100, 1989

Doughty MJ, Lyle WM: Medications used to prevent migraine headaches and their potential ocular adverse effects. Optometry and Vision Science 72: 879–891, 1995

Downs JM, Downs AD, Rosenthal TL, et al: Increased plasma tricyclic antidepressant concentrations in two patients currently treated with fluoxetine. J Clin Psychiatry 50: 226–227, 1989

Ellingrod VL, Perry PJ: Venlafaxine: a heterocyclic antidepressant. Am J Hosp Pharm 51:3033–3046, 1994

Everett HC: The use of bethanechol chloride with tricyclic antidepressants. Am J Psychiatry 132:1202–1204, 1976

Fallon B, Foote B, Walsh T, et al: Spontaneous hypertensive episodes with monoamine oxidase inhibitors. J Clin Psychiatry 49:163–165, 1988

Fava M, Rosenbaum JF: Suicidality and fluoxetine: is there a relationship? J Clin Psychiatry 52:108–111, 1992

Fawcett J, Edwards JH, Kravitz HM, et al: Alprazolam an antidepressant? Alprazolam, desipramine, and an alprazolam-desipramine combination in the treatment of adult depressed outpatients. J Clin Psychopharmacol 7:295–310, 1987

Fawcett J, Kravitz HM, Zajecka JM, et al: CNS stimulant potentiation of monoamine oxidase inhibitors in treatment-refractory depression. J Clin Psychopharmacol 11:127–132, 1991

Fawcett J, Marcus RN, Anton SF, et al: Response of anxiety and agitation symptoms during nefazodone treatment of major depression. J Clin Psychiatry 56 (suppl 6):37–42, 1995

Feighner JP, Aden GC, Fabre LF, et al: Comparison of alprazolam, imipramine, and placebo in the treatment of depression. JAMA 249:3057–3064, 1983

Ferguson JM: Fluoxetine-induced weight loss in overweight, nondepressed subjects (letter). Am J Psychiatry 143:1496, 1986

Fernstrom MH, Krowinski RL, Kupfer DJ: Chronic imipramine treatment and weight gain. Psychiatry Res 17:269–273, 1986

Fisher S, Kent TA, Bryant SG: Postmarketing surveillance by patient self-monitoring: preliminary data for sertraline versus fluoxetine. J Clin Psychiatry 56:288–296, 1995

Francois B, Marquet P, Roustan J, et al: Serotonin syndrome due to an overdose of moclobemide and clomipramine: a potentially life-threatening association. Intensive Care Med 23 (1):122–124, 1997

Frank E, Kupfer DJ, Perel JM, et al: Three-year outcomes for maintenance therapies in recurrent depression. Arch Gen Psychiatry 47:1093–1099, 1990

Frazer A: Antidepressants. J Clin Psychiatry 58 (suppl 6):9–25, 1997

Freeman H: Moclobemide. Drug profile. Lancet 342: 1528–1532, 1993

Fulton B, Benfield P: Moclobemide: an update of its pharmacological properties and therapeutic use. Drugs 52: 450–474, 1996

Gammon GD, Hansen C: A case of akinesia induced by amoxapine. Am J Psychiatry 141:283–284, 1984

Gardner DM, Shulman KI, Walker SE, et al: The making of a user friendly MAOI diet. J Clin Psychiatry 57 (3):99–104, 1996

Gelenberg AJ: Treating PMS. Biological Therapies in Psychiatry Newsletter 20 (1):1, 1997

Gitlin MJ, Weiner H, Fairbanks L: Failure of T_3 to potentiate tricyclic antidepressant response. J Affect Disord 13: 267–272, 1987

Glassman AH: The newer antidepressant drugs and their cardiovascular effects. Psychopharmacol Bull 20:272–279, 1984

Glassman AH, Bigger JT: Cardiovascular effects of therapeutic doses of tricyclic antidepressants: a review. Arch Gen Psychiatry 39:815–820, 1981

Glassman AH, Roose SP: Delusional depression: a distinct clinical entity? Arch Gen Psychiatry 38:424–427, 1981

Glassman AH, Bigger JT, Giardina EGV, et al: Clinical characteristics of imipramine-induced orthostatic hypotension. Lancet 1:468–472, 1979

Glassman AH, Johnson LL, Giardina EGV, et al: Psychotropic drug use in depressed patients with congestive heart failure. JAMA 250:1997–2001, 1983

Goldberg RJ: Nefazodone and venlafaxine: two new agents for the treatment of depression. J Fam Pract 41:591–594, 1995

Goldberg RJ, Capone RJ, Hunt JD: Cardiac complications following tricyclic antidepressant overdose: issues for monitoring policy. JAMA 254:1772–1775, 1985

Goldfrank LR, Lewin NA, Flomenbaum NE, et al: Antidepressants: tricyclics, tetracyclics, monoamine oxidase inhibitors, and others, in Goldfrank's Toxicologic Emergencies, 3rd Edition. Edited by Goldfrank LR, Flomenbaum ME, Lewis NA, et al. Norwalk, CT, Appleton-Century-Crofts, 1986, pp 351–363

Goodman LS, Alexander RD, Laciness DJ: Monoamine oxidase inhibitors and tricyclic antidepressants: comparison of their cardiovascular effects. J Clin Psychiatry 47:225–229, 1986

Goodman WK, Charney DS: Therapeutic applications and mechanisms of action of monoamine oxidase inhibitor and heterocyclic antidepressant drugs. J Clin Psychiatry 46 (No 10, suppl 12):6–22, 1985

Goodwin FK, Prange AJ, Post RM, et al: Potentiation of antidepressant effects by L-triiodothyronine in tricyclic nonresponders. Am J Psychiatry 139:34–38, 1982

Gorman JM: The Essential Guide to Psychiatric Drugs. New York, St Martin's Press, 1990

Greenhill LL: Pharmacologic treatment of attention deficit hyperactivity disorder. Psychiatr Clin North Am 15:1–27, 1992

Greist JH, Jefferson JW, Kobak KA, et al: A 1 year double-blind placebo-controlled fixed dose study of sertraline in the treatment of obsessive-compulsive disorder. Int Clin Psychopharmacol 10 (2):57–65, 1995

Hamilton JA, Halbreich U: Special aspects of neuropsychiatric illness in women: with a focus on depression. Annu Rev Med 44:355–364, 1993

Hamilton MS, Opler LA: Akathisia, suicidality, and fluoxetine. J Clin Psychiatry 53:401–406, 1992

Haria M, Fitton A, McTavish D: Trazodone: a review of its pharmacology, therapeutic use in depression and therapeutic potential in other disorders. Drugs Aging 4:331–355, 1994

Hodgman MJ, Martin TG, Krenzelok EP: Serotonin syndrome due to venlafaxine and maintenance tranylcypromine therapy. Hum Exp Toxicol 16 (1):14–17, 1997

Jacobsen FM: Low-dose trazodone as a hypnotic in patients treated with MAOIs and other psychotropics: a pilot study. J Clin Psychiatry 51:298–302, 1990

Jankowsky D, Curtis G, Zisook S, et al: Trazodone-aggravated ventricular arrhythmias. J Clin Psychopharmacol 3:372–376, 1983

Jenike MA: Affective illness in elderly patients, part 2. Psychiatric Times 4 (3):1, 1987

Joffe RT: T$_3$ and lithium potentiation of tricyclic antidepressants. Am J Psychiatry 145:1317–1318, 1988

Joffe RT, Singer W: A comparison of triiodothyronine and thyroxine in the potentiation of tricyclic antidepressants. Psychiatry Res 32:241–251, 1990

Kahn D: Mysterious MAOI hypertensive episodes (letter). J Clin Psychiatry 49:38–39, 1988

Kahn D, Silver JM, Opler LA: The safety of switching rapidly from tricyclic antidepressants to monoamine oxidase inhibitors. J Clin Psychopharmacol 9:198–202, 1989

Kass FI, Oldham JM, Pardes H: The Columbia University College of Physicians and Surgeons Complete Home Guide to Mental Health. New York, Henry Holt, 1992

Kelsey JE: Dose-response relationship with venlafaxine. J Clin Psychopharmacol 16 (3 suppl 2):21S–28S, 1996

Ketter TA, Jenkins JB, Schroeder DH, et al: Carbamazepine but not valproate induces bupropion metabolism. J Clin Psychopharmacol 15:327–333, 1995

Kiev A, Masco HL, Wenger TL, et al: The cardiovascular effects of bupropion and nortriptyline in depressed outpatients. Ann Clin Psychiatry 6 (2):107–115, 1994

Kline NS: Clinical experience with iproniazid (Marsilid). Journal of Clinical and Experimental Psychopathology 19 (suppl 1):72–78, 1958

Kolecki P: Venlafaxine induced serotonin syndrome occurring after abstinence from phenelzine for more than two weeks (letter). J Toxicol Clin Toxicol 35:211–212, 1997

Krause R: Hypertensive episodes with tranylcypromine treatment. J Clin Psychopharmacol 9:232–233, 1989

Kronfol Z, Greden JF, Zis AP: Imipramine-induced tremor: effects of a beta-adrenergic blocking agent. J Clin Psychiatry 44:225–226, 1983

Kuhn R: The treatment of depressive states with G 22355 (imipramine hydrochloride). Am J Psychiatry 115:459–464, 1958

Kukopoulos A, Caliari B, Tundo A, et al: Rapid cyclers, temperament, and antidepressants. Compr Psychiatry 24:249–258, 1983

Kupfer DJ, Frank E: Relapse in recurrent unipolar depression. Am J Psychiatry 144:86–88, 1987

Kupfer DJ, Coble PA, Rubinstein MS: Changes in weight during treatment for depression. Psychosom Med 41:535–544, 1979

Kupfer DJ, Spiker DG, Coble PA, et al: Sleep and treatment prediction in endogenous depression. Am J Psychiatry 138:429–434, 1981

Labbate LA, Pollack MH: Treatment of fluoxetine-induced sexual dysfunction with bupropion: a case report. Ann Clin Psychiatry 6 (1):13–15, 1994

Liebowitz MR, Quitkin FM, Stewart JW, et al: Phenelzine vs imipramine in atypical depression: a preliminary report. Arch Gen Psychiatry 41:669–677, 1984

Linet LS: Mysterious MAOI hypertensive episodes. J Clin Psychiatry 47:563–565, 1986

Lingam VR, Lazarus LW, Groves L, et al: Methylphenidate in treating post-stroke depression. J Clin Psychiatry 49:151–153, 1988

Lipinski JF, Cohen BM, Frankenburg F, et al: An open trial of S-adenosyl methionine for treatment of depression. Am J Psychiatry 141:448–450, 1984

Lipinski JF, Mallya G, Zimmerman P, et al: Fluoxetine-induced akathisia: clinical and theoretical implications. J Clin Psychiatry 50:339–342, 1989

Liu BA, Mittmann N, Knowles SR, et al: Hyponatremia and the syndrome of inappropriate secretion of antidiuretic hormone associated with the use of selective serotonin reuptake inhibitors: a review of spontaneous reports. Can Med Assoc J 155:519–527, 1996

Louie AK, Lewis TB, Lannon RA: Use of low-dose fluoxetine in major depression and panic disorder. J Clin Psychiatry 54:435–438, 1993

Lydiard RB: Tricyclic-resistant depression: treatment resistance or inadequate treatment? J Clin Psychiatry 46:412–417, 1985

Mann J, Kapur S: The emergence of suicidal ideation and behavior during antidepressant pharmacotherapy. Arch Gen Psychiatry 48:1027–1033, 1991

Manna V, Bolino F, Di Cicco L: Chronic tension-type headache, mood depression and serotonin: therapeutic effects of fluvoxamine and mianserine. Headache 34 (1):44–49, 1994

Marcus MD, Wing RR, Ewing L, et al: A double-blind, placebo-controlled trial of fluoxetine plus behavior modification in the treatment of obese binge-eaters and non-binge-eaters. Am J Psychiatry 147:876–881, 1990

Marley E, Wozniak KM: Interactions of non-selective monoamine oxidase inhibitor, phenelzine, with inhibitors of 5-hydroxytryptamine, dopamine, or noradrenaline re-uptake inhibitors. J Psychiatr Res 18:191–203, 1984

Meltzer HY, Lowy MT: The serotonin hypothesis of depression, in Psychopharmacology: The Third Generation of Progress. Edited by Meltzer HY. New York, Raven, 1987, pp 513–526

Metz A, Shader RI: Adverse interactions encountered when using trazodone to treat insomnia associated with fluoxetine. Int Clin Psychopharmacol 5:191–194, 1990

Mitchell JE, Popkin JE: Antidepressant drug therapy and sexual dysfunction in men: a review. J Clin Psychopharmacol 3:76–79, 1983

Mitchell JE, Raymond N, Specker S: A review of the controlled trials of pharmacotherapy and psychotherapy in the treatment of bulimia nervosa. Int J Eat Disord 14:229–247, 1993

NIMH Consensus Development Conference Statement. Mood disorders: pharmacologic prevention of recurrences. Am J Psychiatry 142:469–476, 1985

Nelson JC, Bowers MB: Delusional unipolar depression: description and drug response. Arch Gen Psychiatry 35:1321–1328, 1978

Nelson JC, Jatlow PI, Quinlan DM: Subjective complaints during desipramine treatment: relative importance of plasma drug concentrations and the severity of depression. Arch Gen Psychiatry 41:55–59, 1984

Nelson JC, Mazure CM, Bowers MB: A preliminary, open study of the combination of fluoxetine and desipramine. Arch Gen Psychiatry 48:303–307, 1991

Nierenberg AA, Keck PE Jr: Management of monoamine oxidase inhibitor-associated insomnia with trazodone. J Clin Psychopharmacol 9:42–45, 1989

Nierenberg AA, Feighner JP, Rudolph R, et al: Venlafaxine for treatment resistant unipolar depression. J Clin Psychopharmacology 14:419–423, 1994

Oehrberg S, Christiansen PE, Behnke K, et al: Paroxetine in the treatment of panic disorder: a randomized, double-blind, placebo-controlled study. Br J Psychiatry 167 (3):374–379, 1995

Ontiveros A, Fontaine R, Elie PL, et al: Refractory depression: the addition of lithium to fluoxetine or desipramine. Acta Psychiatr Scand 83:188–192, 1991

Pacheco MA, Stockmeier C, Meltzer HY, et al: Alterations in phosphoinositide signaling and G-protein levels in depressed suicide brain. Brain Research 723 (1–2):37–45, 1996

Pande AC, Calarco MM, Grunhaus LJ: Combined MAOI-TCA treatment in refractory depression, in Refractory Depression. Edited by Amsterdam J. New York, Raven, 1991, pp 115–121

Perry PJ: Pharmacotherapy for major depression with melancholic features: relative efficacy of tricyclic versus selective serotonin reuptake inhibitor antidepressants. J Affect Disord 39:1–6, 1996

Post RM, Kopin IJ, Goodwin FK: Effects of sleep deprivation on mood and central amine metabolism in depressed patients. Arch Gen Psychiatry 33:627–632, 1976

Preskorn SH, Burke M: Somatic therapy for major depressive disorder: selection of an antidepressant. J Clin Psychiatry 53 (No 9, suppl):5–18, 1992

Price J, Grunhaus LJ: Treatment of clomipramine-induced anorgasmia with yohimbine: a case report. J Clin Psychiatry 51:32–33, 1990

Prien RF, Kupfer DJ: Continuation drug therapy for major depression episodes: how long should it be maintained? Am J Psychiatry 143:18–23, 1986

Quitkin F, Rifkin A, Klein DF: Monoamine oxidase inhibitors: a review of antidepressant effectiveness. Arch Gen Psychiatry 35:749–760, 1979

Quitkin FM, McGrath PJ, Stewart JW, et al: Chronological milestones to guide drug change. When should clinicians switch antidepressants? Arch Gen Psychiatry 53:785–792, 1996

Rabkin JG, Quitkin FM, McGrath P, et al: Adverse reactions to monoamine oxidase inhibitors, Part II: treatment correlates and clinical management. J Clin Psychopharmacol 5:2–9, 1985

Ravaris CL, Robinson DS, Ives JO, et al: Phenelzine and amitriptyline in the treatment of depression: a comparison of present and past studies. Arch Gen Psychiatry 37:1075–1080, 1980

Remick RA, Keller FD, Buchanan RA, et al: A comparison of the efficacy and safety of alprazolam and desipramine in depressed outpatients. Can J Psychiatry 33:590–594, 1988

Rickels K, Feighner JP, Smith WT: Alprazolam, amitriptyline, doxepin, and placebo in the treatment of depression. Arch Gen Psychiatry 42:134–141, 1985

Roose SP: Modern cardiovascular standards for psychotropic drugs. Psychopharmacol Bull 28:35–43, 1992

Roose SP, Glassman AH, Siris SG, et al: Comparison of imipramine- and nortriptyline-induced orthostatic hypotension: a meaningful difference. J Clin Psychopharmacol 1:316–319, 1981

Roose SP, Glassman AH, Giardina EGV, et al: Tricyclic antidepressants in depressed patients with cardiac conduction disease. Arch Gen Psychiatry 44:273–275, 1987

Roose SP, Dalack GW, Glassman AH, et al: Cardiovascular effects of bupropion in depressed patients with heart disease. Am J Psychiatry 148:512–516, 1991

Rosenstein DL, Nelson JC, Jacobs SC: Seizures associated with antidepressants: a review. J Clin Psychiatry 54:289–299, 1993

Ross DR, Walker JI, Paterson J: Akathisia induced by amoxapine. Am J Psychiatry 140:115–116, 1983

Rothschild AJ: Selective serotonin reuptake inhibitor-induced sexual dysfunction: efficacy of a drug holiday. Am J Psychiatry 152:1514–1516, 1995

Sachs GS, Later B, Stol AL, et al: A double-blind trial of bupropion versus desipramine for bipolar depression. J Clin Psychiatry 55:391–393, 1994

Schenk CH, Remick RA: Sublingual nifedipine in the treatment of hypertensive crisis associated with monoamine oxidase inhibitors (letter). Ann Emerg Med 18:114–115, 1989

Scher M, Krieger JN, Juergens S: Trazodone and priapism. Am J Psychiatry 140:1362–1363, 1983

Schildkraut JJ: The catecholamine hypothesis of affective disorders: a review of supporting evidence. Am J Psychiatry 122:509–522, 1965

Schmauss M, Kapfhammer HP, Meyr P, et al: Combined MAO-inhibitor and tri-(tetra)cyclic antidepressant treatment in therapy resistant depression. Prog Neuropsychopharmacol Biol Psychiatry 12:523–532, 1988

Selikoff IJ, Robitzek EH, Ornstein GG: Toxicity of hydrazine derivatives of isonicotinic acid in the chemotherapy of human tuberculosis. Quarterly Bulletin of SeaView Hospital 13 (1):17–26, 1952

Smith WT, Glaudin V, Panagides J, et al: Mirtazapine versus amitriptyline versus placebo in the treatment of major depressive disorder. Psychopharmacol Bull 20:191-196, 1990

Spiker DG, Cofsky Weiss J, Dealy RS, et al: The pharmacologic treatment of delusional depression. Am J Psychiatry 142:430–436, 1985

Spivak B, Ravdan M, Shine M: Postural hypotension with syncope possibly precipitated by trazodone. Am J Psychiatry 144:1512–1513, 1987

Steele TE, Howell EF: Cyproheptadine for imipramine-induced anorgasmia (letter). Am J Psychiatry 144:1243–1244, 1987

Stoll AL, Mayer PV, Kolbrener M, et al: Antidepressant-associated mania: a controlled comparison with spontaneous mania. Am J Psychiatry 151:1642–1645, 1994

Szuba MP, Hornig-Rohan M, Amsterdam J: Rapid conversion from one monoamine oxidase inhibitor to another. J Clin Psychiatry 58:307–310, 1997

Tate JL: Extrapyramidal symptoms in a patient taking haloperidol and fluoxetine (letter). Am J Psychiatry 148:339–340, 1989

Teicher MH, Glod C, Cole J: Emergence of intense suicidal preoccupation during fluoxetine treatment. Am J Psychiatry 52:294–299, 1990

Terman M, Terman JS, Quitkin FM, et al: Light therapy for seasonal affective disorder: a review of efficacy. Neuropsychopharmacology 2:1–22, 1989

Thase ME, Kupfer DJ, Frank E, et al: Treatment of imipramine-resistant depressant, II: an open clinical trial of lithium augmentation. J Clin Psychiatry 50:413–417, 1989

Thornton JE, Stahl SM: Case report of tardive dyskinesia and parkinsonism associated with amoxapine therapy. Am J Psychiatry 141:704–705, 1984

Tollefson GD: Monoamine oxidase inhibitors: a review. J Clin Psychiatry 44:280–288, 1983

Tollefson GD, Birkett M, Koran L, Genduso L: Continuation treatment of OCD: double-blind and open-label experience with fluoxetine. J Clin Psychiatry 55 (S):69–76, 1994

van Harten J: Overview of the pharmacokinetics of fluvoxamine. Clin Pharmacokinetics 29 (suppl 1):1–9, 1995

van Vliet IM, den Boer JA, Westenberg HG, et al: A double-blind comparative study of brofaromine and fluvoxamine in outpatients with panic disorder. J Clin Psychopharmacol 16:299–306, 1996

Vaughan DA: Interaction of fluoxetine with tricyclic antidepressants (letter). Am J Psychiatry 145:1478, 1988

Vitullo RN, Wharton JM, Allen NB, et al: Trazodone-related exercise-induced nonsustained ventricular tachycardia. Chest 98:247–248, 1990

Walczak DD, Apter JT, Halikas JA, et al: The oral dose-effect relationship for fluvoxamine: a fixed-dose comparison against placebo in depressed outpatients. Ann Clin Psychiatry 8 (3):139–151, 1996

Walker SE, Shulman KI, Tailor SA, Gardner D: Tyramine content of previously restricted foods in monoamine oxidase inhibitor diets. J Clin Psychopharmacol 16 (5):383–388, 1996

Wedin GP, Oderda GM, Klein-Schwartz W, et al: Relative toxicity of cyclic antidepressants. Ann Emerg Med 15:797–804, 1986

Wehr TA, Goodwin FK: Rapid cycling in manic-depressives induced by tricyclic antidepressants. Arch Gen Psychiatry 36:555–559, 1979

Wehr TA, Rosenthal NE: Seasonality and affective illness. Am J Psychiatry 146:829–839, 1989

Wehr TA, Sack DA, Rosenthal NE, et al: Rapid-cycling affective disorder: contributing factors and treatment responses in 51 patients. Am J Psychiatry 145:179–184, 1988

Weilburg JB, Rosenbaum JF, Biederman J, et al: Fluoxetine added to non-MAOI antidepressant converts non-responders to responders: a preliminary report. J Clin Psychiatry 50:447–449, 1989

Weise CC, Stein MK, Pereira-Ogan J, et al: Amitriptyline once daily versus three times daily in depressed outpatients. Arch Gen Psychiatry 37:555–560, 1980

Wells BG, Gelenberg AJ: Chemistry, pharmacology, pharmacokinetics, adverse effects, and efficacy of the antidepressant maprotiline hydrochloride. Pharmacotherapy 1 (2):121–139, 1981

White K, Simpson G: Combined MAOI-tricyclic antidepressant treatment: a reevaluation. J Clin Psychopharmacol 1:264–282, 1981

Woo MH, Smythe MA: Association of SIADH with selective serotonin reuptake inhibitors. Ann Pharmacotherapy 31 (1):108–110, 1997

Yager J: Bethanecol chloride can reverse erectile and ejaculatory dysfunction induced by tricyclic antidepressants and mazindol: case report. J Clin Psychiatry 47:210–211, 1986

Yudofsky SC: Electroconvulsive therapy in general hospital psychiatry: a focus of new indications and technologies. Gen Hosp Psychiatry 3:292–296, 1981

Yudofsky SC, Hales RE, Ferguson T: What You Need to Know About Psychiatric Drugs. New York, Grove Weidenfeld, 1991

Zajecka J, Fawcett J, Schaff M, et al: The role of serotonin in sexual dysfunction. J Clin Psychiatry 52:66–68, 1991

Zarate CA Jr, Tohen M, Baraibar G, et al: Prescribing trends of antidepressants in bipolar depression. J Clin Psychiatry 56:260–264, 1995

Zisook S: A clinical overview of monoamine oxidase inhibitors. Psychosomatics 26:240–246, 1985

Anxiolytics, Sedatives, and Hypnotics

Abernethy DR, Greenblatt DJ, Ochs HR, et al: Benzodiazepine drug-drug interactions commonly occurring in clinical practice. Curr Med Res Opin 8 (suppl 4):80–93, 1984

American Psychiatric Association: Benzodiazepine Dependence, Toxicity, and Abuse: A Task Force Report of the American Psychiatric Association. Washington, DC, American Psychiatric Association, 1990

Angus WR, Romney DM: The effect of diazepam on patients' memory. J Clin Psychopharmacol 4:203–206, 1984

Ashton H: Protracted withdrawal syndromes from benzodiazepines. J Subst Abuse Treat 8:19–28, 1991

Berlin I, Warot D, Hergueta T, et al: Comparison of the effects of zolpidem and triazolam on memory functions, psychomotor performances, and postural sway in healthy subjects. J Clin Psychopharmacol 13:100–106, 1993

Black B, Uhde TW, Tancer ME: Fluoxetine for the treatment of social phobia (letter). J Clin Psychopharmacol 12:293–295, 1992

Brantigan CO, Brantigan TA, Joseph N: Effect of beta blockade and beta stimulation on stage fright. Am J Med 72:88–94, 1982

Breier A, Charney DS, Nelson JC: Seizures induced by abrupt discontinuation of alprazolam. Am J Psychiatry 141: 1606–1607, 1984

Busto U, Sellers EM, Naranjo CA, et al: Withdrawal reactions after long-term therapeutic use of benzodiazepines. N Engl J Med 315:854–857, 1986

Charney DS, Woods SW: Benzodiazepine treatment of panic disorder: a comparison of alprazolam and lorazepam. J Clin Psychiatry 50:418–423, 1989

Clomipramine Collaborative Study Group: Clomipramine in the treatment of patients with obsessive-compulsive disorder. Arch Gen Psychiatry 48:730–738, 1991

Cohn J, Wilcox CS: Low-sedation potential of buspirone compared with alprazolam and lorazepam in the treatment of anxious patients: a double-blind study. J Clin Psychiatry 47:409–412, 1986

Cole JO, Orzak MG, Beake B, et al: Assessment of the abuse liability of buspirone in recreational sedative users. J Clin Psychiatry 43:69–74, 1982

Davidson JRT, Ford SM, Smith RD, et al: Long-term treatment of social phobia with clonazepam. J Clin Psychiatry 52 (No 11, suppl):16–20, 1991

den Boer JA, van Vliet IM, Westenberg HG: Recent developments in the psychopharmacology of social phobia. Eur Arch Psychiatry Clin Neurosci 244:309–316, 1995

Dixon J, Power SJ, Grundy EM, et al: Sedation for local anaesthesia: comparison of intravenous midazolam and diazepam. Anaesthesia 39:372–378, 1984

Drew PJ, Barnes JN, Evans SJ: The effect of acute beta-adrenoceptor blockade on examination performance. Br J Clin Pharmacol 19:783–786, 1985

Dunner DL, Ishiki D, Avery DH, et al: Effect of alprazolam and diazepam on anxiety and panic attacks in panic disorder: a controlled study. J Clin Psychiatry 47:458–460, 1986

Elie R, Lamontagne Y: Alprazolam and diazepam in the treatment of generalized anxiety. J Clin Psychopharmacol 4:125–129, 1985

Ellinwood EH Jr, Heatherly DG, Nikaido MA, et al: Comparative pharmacokinetics and pharmacodynamics of lorazepam, alprazolam and diazepam. Psychopharmacology (Berl) 86:393–451, 1985

Ewing JA, Elliot WJ, Maio LD, et al: You don't have to be a neuroscientist to forget everything with triazolam but it helps. JAMA 259:350–352, 1988

Feder R: Lithium augmentation of clomipramine (letter). J Clin Psychiatry 49:458, 1988

Finkle BS, McCloskey KL, Goodman LS: Diazepam and drug-associated deaths: a survey in the United States and Canada. JAMA 242:429–434, 1979

Fontaine R, Chouinard G, Annable L: Rebound anxiety in anxious patients after abrupt withdrawal of benzodiazepine treatment. Am J Psychiatry 141:848–852, 1984

Freeman CP, Trimble MR, Deakin JF, et al: Fluvoxamine versus clomipramine in the treatment of obsessive-compulsive disorder: a multicenter, randomized, double-blind parallel group. J Clin Psychiatry 55:301–305, 1994

Fyer AJ, Liebowitz JR, Gorman JM, et al: Discontinuation of alprazolam treatment in panic patients. Am J Psychiatry 144:303–308, 1987

Gastfried DR, Rosenbaum JF: Adjunctive buspirone in benzodiazepine treatment of four patient with panic disorder. Am J Psychiatry 146:914–916, 1989

Gelernter CS, Uhde TW, Cimbolic P, et al: Cognitive-behavioral and pharmacologic treatments for social phobia: a preliminary study. Arch Gen Psychiatry 48:938–945, 1991

Goldberg HL, Finnerty RJ: The comparative efficacy of buspirone and diazepam in the treatment of anxiety. Am J Psychiatry 136:1184–1187, 1979

Goodman WK, Price LH, Delgado PL, et al: Specificity of serotonin reuptake inhibitors in the treatment of obsessive-compulsive disorder: comparison of fluvoxamine and desipramine. Arch Gen Psychiatry 47:577–585, 1990

Goodman WK, Kozak MJ, Liebowitz M, White KL: Treatment of obsessive-compulsive disorder with fluvoxamine: a multicentre, double-blind, placebo-controlled trial. Int Clin Psychopharmacol 11:21–29, 1996

Greenblatt DJ: Pharmacology of benzodiazepine hypnotics. J Clin Psychiatry 53 (No 6, suppl):7–13, 1992

Greenblatt DJ, Allen MD, Noel BJ, et al: Acute overdosage with benzodiazepine derivatives. Clin Pharmacol Ther 21:497–514, 1977a

Greenblatt DJ, Allen MD, Shader RI: Toxicity of high dose flurazepam in the elderly. Clin Pharmacol Ther 21:355–361, 1977b

Greenblatt DJ, Divoll M, Harmatz JS, et al: Kinetics and clinical effects of flurazepam in young and elderly noninsomniacs. Clin Pharmacol Ther 30:475–486, 1981

Greenblatt DJ, Shader RI, Abernethy DR: Drug therapy. Current status of benzodiazepines. N Engl J Med 309 (7): 410–16, 1983

Greenblatt DJ, Shader RI, Divol M, et al: Adverse reactions to triazolam, flurazepam, and placebo in controlled clinical trials. J Clin Psychiatry 45:192–195, 1984

Greist J, Chouinard G, DuBoff E, et al: Double-blind parallel comparison of three dosages of sertraline and placebo in outpatients with obsessive-compulsive disorder. Arch Gen Psychiatry 52:289–295, 1995

Griffith JD, Jasinski DR, Casten GP, et al: Investigation of the abuse liability of buspirone in alcohol-dependent patients. Am J Med 80 (suppl 3B):30–35, 1986

Harvey KV, Balon R: Augmentation with buspirone: a review. Ann Clin Psychiatry 7 (3):143–147, 1995

Hertley LR, Ungapen S, Davie I, et al: The effect of beta-adrenergic blocking drugs on speakers' performance and memory. Br J Psychiatry 142:512–517, 1983

Hewlett WA, Vinogradov S, Agras WS: Clonazepam treatment of obsessions and compulsions. J Clin Psychiatry 51: 158–161, 1990

Hoehn-Saric R, McLeod DR, Zimmerli WD: Differential effects of alprazolam and imipramine in generalized anxiety disorder: somatic vs psychic symptoms. J Clin Psychiatry 49:293–301, 1988

Hollander E, DeCaria CM, Schneier FR, et al: Fenfluramine augmentation of serotonin reuptake blockade antiobsessional treatment. J Clin Psychiatry 51:119–123, 1990

Jack ML, Colburn WA, Spirt NM, et al: A pharmacokinetic/pharmacodynamic/receptor binding model to predict the onset and duration of pharmacological activity of the benzodiazepines. Prog Neuropsychopharmacol Biol Psychiatry 7:629–635, 1982

Jefferson JW: Social phobia: a pharmacologic treatment overview. 56 (No 5, suppl):18–24, 1995

Jenike MA: Approaches to the patient with treatment-refractory obsessive-compulsive disorder. J Clin Psychiatry 51 (No 2, suppl):15–21, 1990

Jenike MA, Baer L, Buttolph L: Buspirone augmentation of fluoxetine in patients with obsessive-compulsive disorder. J Clin Psychopharmacol 12:13–14, 1991

Jenkins SW, Ruegg R, Moeller FG: Gepirone in the treatment of major depression. J Clin Psychopharmacol 10 (suppl):77S–85S, 1990

Kahn RJ, Menair D, Lipman RS, et al: Imipramine and chlordiazepoxide in depressive and anxiety disorders: efficacy in anxious outpatients. Arch Gen Psychiatry 43:79–85, 1986

Kales A, Kales JD: Sleep laboratory studies of hypnotic drugs: efficacy and withdrawal effects. J Clin Psychopharmacol 3:140–150, 1983

Kales A, Bixler EO, Vela-Bueno A, et al: Comparison of short and long half-life benzodiazepine hypnotics: triazolam and guazepam. Clin Pharmacol Ther 40:378–386, 1986

Keller MB, Hanks DL: Anxiety symptom relief in depression treatment outcomes. J Clin Psychiatry 56 (No 6, suppl):22–29, 1995

Klein DF, Ross DC, Cohen P: Panic and avoidance in agoraphobia; application of path analysis to treatment studies. Arch Gen Psychiatry 44 (4):377–385, 1987

Kupfer KJ, Reynolds CF: Management of insomnia. N Engl J Med 336:341–346, 1997

Lader M, Olajide D: A comparison of buspirone and placebo in relieving benzodiazepine withdrawal symptoms. J Clin Psychopharmacol 7:11–15, 1987

Laird LK: Issues in the monopharmacotherapy and polypharmacotherapy of obsessive-compulsive disorder. Psychopharmacol Bull 32:569–578, 1996

Leppik IE, Derivan AT, Homan RW, et al: Double-blind study of lorazepam and diazepam in status epilepticus. JAMA 249:1452–1454, 1983

Levy AB: Delirium and seizures due to abrupt alprazolam withdrawal: case report. J Clin Psychiatry 45:38–39, 1984

Liebowitz MA, Gorman JM, Fyer AJ, et al: Pharmacotherapy of social phobia: an interim report of a placebo-controlled comparison of phenelzine and atenolol. J Clin Psychiatry 49:252–257, 1988

Linnoila M, Erwin CW, Brendle A, et al: Psychomotor effects of diazepam in anxious patients and healthy volunteers. J Clin Psychopharmacol 3:88–96, 1983

Lister RG: The amnestic action of benzodiazepines in man. Neurosci Biobehav Rev 9:87–94, 1985

Lucki I: Behavioral studies of serotonin receptor antagonists as antidepressant drugs. J Clin Psychiatry 52 (No 12, suppl):24–31, 1991

Lucki I, Rickels K, Geller AM: Chronic use of benzodiazepines and psychomotor and cognitive test performance. Psychopharmacology (Berl) 88:426–433, 1986

Mac DS, Kumar R, Goodwin DW: Anterograde amnesia with oral lorazepam. J Clin Psychiatry 46:137–138, 1985

Markovitz PJ, Stagro SJ, Calabrese JR: Buspirone augmentation of fluoxetine in obsessive-compulsive disorder. Am J Psychiatry 147:798–800, 1990

Markowitz JS, Brewerton TD: Zolpidem-induced psychosis. Ann Clin Psychiatry 8 (2):89–91, 1996

Marshall RD, Schneier FR, Fallon BA, et al: Medication therapy for social phobia. J Clin Psychiatry 55 (S):33–37, 1994

Mavissakalian MR, Jones B, Olson S, et al: Clomipramine in obsessive-compulsive disorder: clinical response and plasma levels. J Clin Psychopharmacol 10:261–268, 1990

McDougle CJ, Goodman WK, Price LH, et al: Neuroleptic addition in fluvoxamine-refractory obsessive-compulsive disorder. Am J Psychiatry 147:652–654, 1990

McDougle CJ, Fleischmann RL, Epperson CN, et al: Risperidone addition in fluvoxamine-refractory obsessive-compulsive disorder: three cases. J Clin Psychiatry 56:526–528, 1995

Medawarn C, Rassaby E: Triazolam overdose, alcohol, and manslaughter. Lancet 338:1515–1516, 1991

Mendelson WB: Clinical distinction between long-acting and short-acting benzodiazepines. J Clin Psychiatry 53 (No 12, suppl):4–7, 1992

Mitler MM, Seidel WF, Van Den Hoel J, et al: Comparative hypnotic effects of flurazepam, triazolam, and placebo: a long-term simultaneous nighttime and daytime study. J Clin Psychopharmacol 4:2–13, 1984

Monti JM, Attali P, Monti D, et al: Zolpidem and rebound insomnia: a double-blind, controlled polysomnographic study in chronic insomniac patients. Pharmacopsychiatry 27166–175, 1994

Morris HH, Estes ML: Traveler's amnesia: transient global amnesia secondary to triazolam. JAMA 258:945–946, 1987

Moskowitz H, Smiley A: Effects of chronically administered buspirone and diazepam on driving-related skills and performance. J Clin Psychiatry 43:45–55, 1982

Mundo E, Bareggi SR, Pirola R, et al: Long-term pharmacotherapy of obsessive-compulsive disorder: a double-blind controlled study. J Clin Psychopharmacol 17:4–10, 1997

Munjack DJ, Bruns J, Baltazar PL, et al: A pilot study of buspirone in the treatment of social phobia. Journal of Anxiety Disorders 5:87–98, 1991

NIMH [National Institute of Mental Health] Consensus Development Conference: Drugs and insomnia: the use of medication to promote sleep. JAMA 251:2410–2414, 1984

Noyes R Jr, Garvey MJ, Cook BL, et al: Benzodiazepine withdrawal: a review of evidence. J Clin Psychiatry 49:382–389, 1988

Oehrberg S, Christiansen PE, Behnke K, et al: Paroxetine in the treatment of panic disorder. A randomised, double-blind, placebo-controlled study. Br J Psychiatry 167:374–379, 1995

Pecknold JC, Swinson RP: Taper withdrawal studies with alprazolam in patients with panic disorder and agoraphobia. Psychopharmacol Bull 22:173–176, 1986

Perse TL, Greist JH, Jefferson JW, et al: Fluvoxamine treatment of obsessive-compulsive disorder. Am J Psychiatry 144:1543–1548, 1988

Pichard L, Gilbert G, Bonfils C, et al: Oxidative metabolism of zolpidem by human liver cytochrome P450S. Drug Metab Dispos 23:1253–1262, 1995

Pigott TA, Pato MT, Bernstein SE, et al: Controlled comparisons of clomipramine and fluoxetine in the treatment of obsessive-compulsive disorders: behavioral and biological results. Arch Gen Psychiatry 47:926–932, 1990

Rakel RE: Long-term buspirone therapy for chronic anxiety: a multicenter international study to determine safety. South Med J 83:194–198, 1990

Ravizza L, Barzega G, Bellino S, et al: Drug treatment of obsessive-compulsive disorder (OCD): long-term trial with clomipramine and selective serotonin reuptake inhibitors (SSRIs). Psychopharmacol Bull 32 (1):167–173, 1996

Regestein QR, Reich P: Agitation observed during treatment with newer hypnotic drugs. J Clin Psychiatry 46:280–283, 1985

Reitan JA, Porter W, Braunstein M: Comparison of psychomotor skills and amnesia after induction of anesthesia with midazolam or thiopental. Anesth Analg 65:933–937, 1986

Rickels K: The clinical use of hypnotics: indications for use and the need for a variety of hypnotics. Acta Psychiatr 332 (suppl):132–141, 1986

Rickels K, Case WG, Downing RW, et al: Long-term diazepam therapy and clinical outcome. JAMA 250:767–771, 1983

Rickels K, Schweizer E, Csanelosi I, et al: Long-term treatment of anxiety and risk of withdrawal: prospective comparison of clonazepam and buspirone. Arch Gen Psychiatry 45:444–450, 1988

Rickels K, Downing R, Schweizer E, et al: Antidepressants for the treatment of generalized anxiety disorder. A placebo-controlled comparison of imipramine, trazodone, and diazepam. Arch Gen Psychiatry 50:884–895, 1993

Roehrs T, Merlotti L, Zorick F, et al: Sedative, memory, and performance effects of hypnotics. Psychopharmacology 116:130–134, 1994

Rosenberg L, Mitchell AA, Parsells JL, et al: Lack of relation of oral clefts to diazepam use during pregnancy. N Engl J Med 309:1282–1285, 1983

Roth T, Roehrs TA: Issues in the use of benzodiazepine therapy. J Clin Psychiatry 53 (No 6, suppl):14–18, 1992

Roth T, Hartse KM, Saab PG, et al: The effects of flurazepam, lorazepam, and triazolam on sleep and memory. Psychopharmacology (Berl) 70:231–237, 1980

Roth T, Roehr T, Wittig R, et al: Benzodiazepines and memory. Br J Clin Pharmacol 18 (suppl):45S–49S, 1984

Rothschild AJ: Disinhibition, amnestic reactions, and other adverse reactions secondary to triazolam: a review of the literature. J Clin Psychiatry 53 (No 12, suppl):69–79, 1992

Rush CR, Griffiths RR: Zolpidem, triazolam, and temazepam: behavioral and subject-rated effects in normal volunteers. J Clin Psychopharmacol 16:146–157, 1996

Salzman C, Shader RI, Greenblatt DJ, et al: Long vs short half-life benzodiazepines in the elderly: kinetics and clinical effects of diazepam and oxazepam. Arch Gen Psychiatry 40:293–297, 1983

Schneier FR, Liebowitz MR, Davies SO, et al: Fluoxetine in panic disorder. J Clin Psychopharmacol 10:119–121, 1990

Schneier FR, Saoud JB, Campeas RC, et al: Buspirone in social phobia. J Clin Psychopharmacol 13:251–256, 1992

Schoch P, Moreau JL, Martin JR, et al: Aspects of benzodiazepine receptor structure and function with relevance to drug tolerance and dependence. Biochem Soc Symp 59:121–134, 1993

Schopf J: Withdrawal phenomena after long-term administration of benzodiazepines: a review of recent investigations. Pharmacopsychiatrie Neuro-Psychopharmakologie 16:1–8, 1983

Schweizer E, Rickels K, Lucki I: Resistance to anti-anxiety effects of buspirone in patients with a history of benzodiazepine use. N Engl J Med 314:719–720, 1986

Seidel WF, Cohen SA, Bliwise NG, et al: Buspirone: an anxiolytic without sedative effect. Psychopharmacology (Berl) 87:371–373, 1985

Sellers EM, Naranjo CA, Harrison M, et al: Oral diazepam loading: simplified treatment of alcohol withdrawal. Clin Pharmacol Ther 34:822–826, 1983

Sellers EM, Schneiderman JF, Romach MK, et al: Comparative drug effects and abuse liability of lorazepam, buspirone, and secobarbital in nondependent subjects. J Clin Psychopharmacol 12:79–85, 1992

Sheehan DV, Ballenger J, Jacobsen G: Treatment of endogenous anxiety with phobic, hysterical, and hypochondriacal symptoms. Arch Gen Psychiatry 39:51–59, 1980

Sheehan DV, Raj AB, Sheehan KH, et al: Is buspirone effective for panic disorder? J Clin Psychopharmacol 10:3–11, 1990

Shiono PH, Mills JL: Oral clefts and diazepam use during pregnancy (letter). N Engl J Med 311:919–920, 1983

Spier SA, Tesar GE, Rosenbaum JF, et al: Treatment of panic disorder and agoraphobia with clonazepam. J Clin Psychiatry 47:238–242, 1986

Sramek JJ, Tansman M, Suri A, et al: Efficacy of buspirone in generalized anxiety disorder with coexisting mild depressive symptoms. J Clin Psychiatry 57:287–291, 1996

Sullivan JT, Sellers EM: Treating alcohol, barbiturate, and benzodiazepine withdrawal. Ration Drug Ther 20:1–8, 1986

Suranyi-Cadotte BE, Bodnoff SR, Welner SA: Antidepressant-anxiolytic interactions: involvement of the benzodiazepine-GABA and serotonin systems. Prog Neuropsychopharmacol Biol Psychiatry 14:633–654, 1990

Tallman JF, Paul SM, Skolnick P, et al: Receptors for the age of anxiety: pharmacology of the benzodiazepines. Science 207:274–281, 1980

Teboul E, Chouinard G: A guide to benzodiazepine selection, Part 1: Pharmacological aspects. Can J Psychiatry 35:700–710, 1990

Tesar GE: High-potency benzodiazepines for short-term management of panic disorder: the U.S. evidence. J Clin Psychiatry 15 (No 5, suppl):4–10, 1990

Tesar GE, Rosenbaum JF, Pollack MH, et al: Double-blind, placebo-controlled comparison of clonazepam and alprazolam for panic disorder. J Clin Psychiatry 52:69–76, 1991

Tollefson GD, Birkett M, Koran L, et al: Continuation treatment of OCD: double-blind and open-label experience with fluoxetine. J Clin Psychiatry 55 (suppl):69–76, 1994

Tyrer PJ, Owen R, Dawling S: Gradual withdrawal of diazepam after long-term therapy. Lancet 1:1402–1406, 1983

Van Ameringen M, Mancini C, Streiner DL: Fluoxetine efficacy in social phobia. J Clin Psychiatry 54:27–32, 1993

van Puijenbroek EP, Egberts AC, Krom HJ: Visual hallucinations and amnesia associated with the use of zolpidem. Int J Clin Pharmacol Ther 34:318, 1996

van Vliet IM, Westenberg HG, Den Boer JA: MAO inhibitors in panic disorder: clinical effects of treatment with brofaromine. A double blind placebo controlled study. Psychopharmacology 112:483–489, 1993

Votey SR, Bosse GM, Bayer MJ, et al: Flumazenil: a new benzodiazepine antagonist. Ann Emerg Med 20:181–188, 1991

Wamsley JK, Hunt MA: Relative affinity of quazepam for type-1 benzodiazepine receptors in brain. J Clin Psychiatry 52 (No 9, suppl):15–20, 1991

Wesensten NJ, Balkin TJ, Belenky GL: Effects of daytime administration of zolpidem versus triazolam on memory. Eur J Clin Pharmacol 48:115–122, 1995

Westenberg HGM, den Boer JA: Clinical and biochemical effects of selective serotonin-uptake inhibitors in anxiety disorders, in Selective Serotonin Reuptake Inhibitors: Novel or Commonplace Agents? Edited by Gastpar M, Wakelin JS. Basel, Switzerland, S. Karger, 1988, pp 84–99

Westenberg HG, den Boer JA: New findings in the treatment of panic disorder. Pharmacopsychiatry 26 (No 1, suppl):30–33, 1993

Wheadon DE: Placebo controlled multi-center trial of fluoxetine in OCD. Paper presented at the Fifth World Congress of Biological Psychiatry, Florence, Italy, June 1991

Yudofsky SC, Silver JM: Beta-blockers in the treatment of performance anxiety. Harvard Mental Health Letter 4 (5):8, 1987

Zipursky RB, Baker RW, Zimmer B: Alprazolam withdrawal delirium unresponsive to diazepam: case report. J Clin Psychiatry 46:344–345, 1985

Zitrin CM, Klein DF, Woerner MG, et al: Treatment of phobias: comparison of imipramine and placebo. Arch Gen Psychiatry 40:125–138, 1983

Zohar J, Judge R: Paroxetine versus clomipramine in the treatment of obsessive-compulsive disorder. Br J Psychiatry 169:468–474, 1996

Antipsychotic Drugs

Adler LA, Angrist B, Peselow E, et al: Efficacy of propranolol in neuroleptic-induced akathisia. J Clin Psychopharmacol 5:164–166, 1985

Adler LA, Angrist B, Reiter S, et al: Neuroleptic-induced akathisia: a review. Psychopharmacology (Berl) 97:1–11, 1989

Adler LA, Angrist B, Weinreb H, et al: Studies on the time course and efficacy of β-blockers in neuroleptic-induced akathisia and the akathisia of idiopathic Parkinson's disease. Psychopharmacol Bull 27:107–111, 1991

Adler LA, Peselow E, Rotrosen J, et al: Vitamin E in the treatment of tardive dyskinesia. Am J Psychiatry 150:1405–1407, 1993

AIMS: Abnormal involuntary movement scale. Psychopharmacol Bull 24:781–783, 1988

Akhtar S, Jajor TR, Kumar S: Vitamin E in the treatment of tardive dyskinesia. J Postgrad Med 39 (3):124–126, 1993

Alvarez-Mena SC, Frank MJ: Phenothiazine-induced T-wave abnormalities: effects of overnight fasting. JAMA 224:1730–1733, 1973

Alvir JMJ, Lieberman JA: Agranulocytosis: incidence and risk factors. J Clin Psychiatry 55 (suppl B):137–138, 1994

Alvir JMJ, Lieberman JA, Safferman AZ: Clozapine-induced agranulocytosis: incidence and risk factors in the United States. N Engl J Med 329:162–167, 1993

American Psychiatric Association: Tardive Dyskinesia: A Task Force Report of the American Psychiatric Association. Washington, DC, American Psychiatric Association, 1992

American Psychiatric Association: Practice guideline for the treatment of patients with schizophrenia. Am J Psychiatry 154 (4, suppl):1–63, 1997

Anderson ES, Powers PS: Neuroleptic malignant syndrome associated with clozapine use. J Clin Psychiatry 52:102–104, 1991

Appleton WS, Davis JM: Practical Clinical Psychopharmacology, 2nd Edition. Baltimore, MD, Williams & Wilkins, 1980

Arvinitis LA, Miller BG: Multiple fixed doses of "Seroquel" (quetiapine) in patients with acute exacerbation of schizophrenia: a comparison with haloperidol and placebo. (The Seroquel Trial 13 Study Group.) Biol Psychiatry 42 (4):233–246, 1997

Axelsson R, Aspenstrom G: Electrocardiographic changes and serum concentrations in thioridazine-treated patients. J Clin Psychiatry 43:332–335, 1982

Baldessarini RJ: Drugs and the treatment of psychiatric disorders, in Goodman and Gilman's The Pharmacological Basis of Therapeutics, 7th Edition. Edited by Gilman AG, Goodman LS, Mured F. New York, Macmillan, 1985, pp 385–445

Baldessarini RJ: A summary of current knowledge of tardive dyskinesia. Encephale 14 (special no):263–268, 1988

Baldessarini RJ, Katz B, Cotton P: Dissimilar dosing with high-potency and low-potency neuroleptics. Am J Psychiatry 141:748–752, 1984

Baldessarini RJ, Cohen BM, Teicher MH: Significance of neuroleptic dose and plasma level in the pharmacological treatment of psychoses. Arch Gen Psychiatry 45:79–91, 1988

Ball WA, Caroff SN: Retinopathy, tardive dyskinesia, and low-dose thioridazine (letter). Am J Psychiatry 143:256–257, 1986

Balon R, Berchou R: Hematologic side effects of psychotropic drugs. Psychosomatics 27:119–127, 1986

Barnas C, Zwierzina H, Hummer M, et al: Granulocyte-macrophage colony-stimulating factor (GM-CSF) treatment of clozapine-induced agranulocytosis: a case report. J Clin Psychiatry 53:245–247, 1992

Beasley CM, Tollefson G, Tran P, et al: Olanzapine versus placebo and haloperidol: acute phase results of the Northern American double-blind olanzapine trial. Neuropsychopharmacology 14:111–123, 1996

Beckman H, Lang R, Gattoz WF: Vasopressin-oxytocin in cerebrospinal fluid of schizophrenic patients and normal controls. Psychoneuroendocrinology 10:187–191, 1985

Bisette G, Nemeroff CB: Neurotensin and the mesocortico-limbic dopamine system. Ann NY Acad Sci 537:397–404, 1988

Bondolfi G, Baumann P, Dufour H: Treatment-resistant schizophrenia: clinical experience with new antipsychotics. Eur Neuropsychopharmacol (6 suppl):S21–S25, 1996

Borison RL: Clinical efficacy of serotonin-dopamine antagonists relative to classic neuroleptics. J Clin Psychopharmacol 15 (suppl 1):24S–29S, 1995

Branchey M, Branchey L: Patterns of psychotropic drug use and tardive dyskinesia. J Clin Psychopharmacol 4:41–45, 1984

Breier A, Buchanan RW, Waltrip RW II, et al: The effect of clozapine on plasma norepinephrine: relationship to clinical efficacy. Neuropsychopharmacology 10:1–7, 1994

Brunello N, Masotto C, Steardo L, et al: New insights into the biology of schizophrenia through the mechanism of action of clozapine. Neuropsychopharmacology 13:177–213, 1995

Burke RE, Fahn S, Jankovic J, et al: Tardive dyskinesia: late-onset and persistent dystonia caused by antipsychotic drugs. Neurology 32:1335–1346, 1982

Cadet JL, Lohr JB, Jeste DV: Free radicals and tardive dyskinesia (letter). Trends Neurosci 9:107–108, 1986

Calabrese JR, Kimmel SE, Woyshville MJ, et al: Clozapine for treatment-refractory mania. Am J Psychiatry 153:759–764, 1996

Chengappa KN, Shelton MD, Baker RW, et al: The prevalence of akathisia in patients receiving stable doses of clozapine. J Clin Psychiatry 55:142–145, 1994

Chengappa KN, Gopalani A, Haught MK, et al: The treatment of clozapine-associated agranulocytosis with granulocyte colony-stimulating factor (G-CSF). Psychopharmacol Bull 32:111–121, 1996

Chouinard G, Jones BD, Annable L: Neuroleptic-induced supersensitivity psychosis. Am J Psychiatry 135:1409–1410, 1978

Chouinard G, Jones BD, Remington G, et al: A Canadian multicenter, placebo-controlled study of fixed doses of resperidone and haloperidol in the treatment of chronic schizophrenic patients. J Clin Psychopharmacol 13:25–40, 1993

Civelli O, Bunzow JR, Grandy DK, et al: Molecular biology of the dopamine receptors. Eur J Pharmacol 207:277–286, 1991

Cohen LS, Heller VL, Rosenbaum JF: Treatment guidelines for psychotropic drug use in pregnancy. Psychosomatics 30:25–33, 1989

Cole JO, Gardos G, Rapkin R, et al: Lithium carbonate in tardive dyskinesia and schizophrenia, in Tardive Dyskinesia and Affective Disorders. Edited by Gardos G, Casey D. Washington, DC, American Psychiatric Press, 1984, pp 50–73

Corzo D, Yunis JJ, Salazar M, et al: The major histocompatibility complex region marked by HSP70-1 and HSP70-2 variants is associated with clozapine-induced agranulocytosis in two different ethnic groups. Blood 86:3835–3840, 1995

Creese I, Burt DR, Snyder SH: Dopamine receptor binding predicts clinical and pharmacological potencies of antischizophrenic drugs. Science 192:481–483, 1976

Crow TJ: Brain changes and negative symptoms in schizophrenia. Psychopathology 28 (1):18–21, 1995

Csernansky JC, Riney SJ, Lombrozo L: Double-blind comparison of alprazolam, diazepam, and placebo for the treatment of negative schizophrenic symptoms. Arch Gen Psychiatry 45:655–659, 1988

Dabiri LM, Pasta D, Darby JK, et al: Effectiveness of vitamin E for the treatment of long-term tardive dyskinesia. Am J Psychiatry 151:925–926, 1994

Das Gupta K, Young A: Clozapine-induced neuroleptic malignant syndrome. J Clin Psychiatry 52:105–107, 1991

Davis JM: Maintenance therapy and the natural course of schizophrenia. J Clin Psychiatry 46 (No 11, Sec 2):18–21, 1985

Davis KL, Kahn RS, Ko G, et al: Dopamine in schizophrenia: a review and reconceptualization. Am J Psychiatry 148:1474–1486, 1991

Delva NJ, Letemednia FJJ: Lithium treatment in schizophrenia and schizo-affective disorders. Br J Psychiatry 141:387–400, 1982

Deshmukh DK, Joshi VS, Agarwal MR: Rabbit syndrome: a rare complication of long-term neuroleptic medication. Br J Psychiatry 157:293, 1990

Douyon R, Angrist B, Peselow E, et al: Neuroleptic augmentation with alprazolam: clinical effects and pharmacokinetic correlates (comment). Am J Psychiatry 146:1087–1088, 1989

Dumon J-P, Catteau J, Lanvin F, et al: Randomized, double-blind, crossover, placebo-controlled comparison of propranolol and betaxolol in the treatment of neuroleptic-induced akathisia. Am J Psychiatry 149:647–650, 1992

Dupuis B, Catteau J, Dumon J-P, et al: Comparison of propranolol, sotalol, and betaxolol in the treatment of neuroleptic-induced akathisia. Am J Psychiatry 144:802–805, 1987

Edlund MJ, Craig TJ: Antipsychotic drug use and birth defects: an epidemiologic reassessment. Compr Psychiatry 25:32–37, 1984

Egan MF, Hyde TM, Albers GW, et al: Treatment of tardive dyskinesia with vitamin E. Am J Psychiatry 149 (6):773–777, 1992

Elkashef AM, Ruskin PE, Bacher N, et al: Vitamin E in the treatment of tardive dyskinesia. Am J Psychiatry 147:505–506, 1990

Ereshefsky L, Toney G, Saklad SR, et al: A loading-dose strategy for converting from oral to depot haloperidol. Hosp Community Psychiatry 44:1155–1161, 1993

Fahn S: A therapeutic approach to tardive dyskinesia. J Clin Psychiatry 46 (No 4, Sec 2):19–24, 1985

Farber NB, Foster J, Duhan NL, et al: Olanzapine and fluperlapine mimic clozapine in preventing MK-801 neurotoxicity. Schizophr Res 21 (1):33–37, 1996

Fibinger HC, Lloyd KG: Is the dopamine hypothesis of tardive dyskinesia completely wrong? (reply to letter) Trends Neurosci 9:259–260, 1986

Gardos G, Cole JO: Weight reduction in schizophrenia by molindone. Am J Psychiatry 134:302–304, 1977

Garver DL, Beinfeld MC, Yao JK: Cholecystokinin, dopamine and schizophrenia. Psychopharmacol Bull 26:377–380, 1990

Garver DL, Bisette G, Yao JK, et al: Relation of CSF neurotensin concentrations to symptoms and drug response of psychotic patients. Am J Psychiatry 148:484–488, 1991

Gerson SL, Gullion G, Yeh HS, et al: Granulocyte colony-stimulating factor for clozapine-induced agranulocytosis (letter). Lancet 340 (8827): 1097, 1992

Ghadirian AM, Chouinard G, Annable L: Sexual dysfunction and plasma prolactin levels in neuroleptic-treated schizophrenic outpatients. J Nerv Ment Dis 170:463–467, 1982

Ghaemi SN, Zarate CA Jr, Popli AP, et al: Is there a relationship between clozapine and obsessive-compulsive disorder? A retrospective chart review. Compr Psychiatry 36:267–270, 1995

Glazer WM, Moore DC, Schooler NR, et al: Tardive dyskinesia: a discontinuation study. Arch Gen Psychiatry 41:623–627, 1984

Green MF, Marshall BD Jr., Wirshing WC, et al: Does risperidone improve verbal working memory in treatment-resistant schizophrenia? Am J Psychiatry 154: 799–804, 1997

Gunderson JG: Pharmacotherapy for patients with borderline personality disorder. Arch Gen Psychiatry 43:698–700, 1986

Guze BH, Baxter LR: Current concepts: neuroleptic malignant syndrome. N Engl J Med 313:163–166, 1985

Gwinn KA, Caviness JN: Risperidone-induced tardive dyskinesia and parkinsonism. Mov Disord 12 (1):119–121, 1997

Haase HJ: Extrapyramidal modification of fine movements: a "conditio sine qua non" of the fundamental therapeutic action of neuroleptic drugs, in Systeme Extrapyramidal et Neuroleptiques. Edited by Bordeleeau JM. Montreal, Quebec, Canada, Editions Psychiatriques, 1961

Hagger C, Buckley P, Kenny JT, et al: Improvement in cognitive functions and psychiatric symptoms in treatment-refractory schizophrenic patients receiving clozapine. Biol Psychiatry 34:702–712, 1993

Hakola H, Loulumaa V: Carbamazepine in violent schizophrenics, in Anticonvulsants in Affective Disorders. Edited by Emrich H, Okuma T, Muller A. Amsterdam, Excerpta Medica, 1984, pp 204–207

Hamilton JD: Thioridazine retinopathy within the upper dosage limit. Psychosomatics 26:823–824, 1985

Herz MI, Glazer WM, Mostert MA, et al: Intermittent versus maintenance medication in schizophrenia: two-year results. Arch Gen Psychiatry 48:333–339, 1991

Hill RM, Desmond NM, Kay JL: Extrapyramidal dysfunction in an infant of a schizophrenic mother. J Pediatr 69: 589–595, 1966

Hoffman DC: Typical and atypical neuroleptics antagonize MK-801-induced locomotion and stereotypy in rats. J Neural Transm 89 (1–2):1–10, 1992

Honigfeld G, Arellano F, Sethi J, et al: Reducing clozapine-related morbidity and mortality: 5 years of experience with the Clozaril National Registry. J Clin Psychiatry 59 (suppl 3):3–7, 1998

Itil TM, Soldatos CL: Epileptogenic side effects of psychotropic drugs: practical recommendations. JAMA 244:1460–1463, 1980

Jeste DV, Wyatt RJ: Understanding and Treating Tardive Dyskinesia. New York, Guilford, 1982

Jeste DV, Linnoila M, Fordis CM, et al: Enzyme studies in tardive dyskinesia, III: noradrenergic hyperactivity in a subgroup of dyskinetic patients. J Clin Psychopharmacol 2:318–320, 1982

Johnson DAW: Antipsychotic medication: clinical guidelines for maintenance therapy. J Clin Psychiatry 46 (No 205, Sec 2):6–15, 1985

Johnson DA, Ludlow JM, Street K, et al: Double-blind comparison of half-dose and standard-dose flupenthixol decanoate in the maintenance treatment of stabilized out-patients with schizophrenia. Br J Psychiatry 151:634–638, 1987

Kane JM: Treatment-resistant schizophrenic patients. J Clin Psychiatry 57:35–40, 1996

Kane JM, Smith JM: Tardive dyskinesia: prevalence and risk factors, 1959 to 1979. Arch Gen Psychiatry 39:473–481, 1982

Kane JM, Rifkin A, Woerner M, et al: Low-dose neuroleptic treatment of outpatient schizophrenics, I: preliminary results for relapse rates. Arch Gen Psychiatry 40:893–896, 1983

Kane JM, Honigfeld G, Singer J, et al: Clozapine for the treatment-resistant schizophrenic: a double-blind comparison vs chlorpromazine/benztropine. Arch Gen Psychiatry 45:789–796, 1988

Keck PE Jr, Pope HG Jr, Cohen BM, et al: Risk factor for neuroleptic malignant syndrome. Arch Gen Psychiatry 46:914–918, 1989

Keck PE Jr, McElroy SL, Strakowski SM: New developments in the pharmacologic treatment of schizoaffective disorder. J Clin Psychiatry 57 (suppl 9):41–48, 1996

Kennedy PF, Hershon HI, McGuire RJ: Extrapyramidal disorders after prolonged phenothiazine therapy. Br J Psychiatry 118:509–518, 1971

Klein E, Bental E, Lerer B, et al: Carbamazepine and haloperidol vs placebo and haloperidol in excited psychosis. Arch Gen Psychiatry 41:165–170, 1984

Levenson JL: Neuroleptic malignant syndrome. Am J Psychiatry 142:1137–1145, 1985

Levy W, Wisniewski K: Chlorpromazine causing extrapyramidal dysfunction in newborn infants of psychotic mothers. NY State J Med 74:684–685, 1974

Lewis RV, Lofthouse C: Adverse reactions with β-adrenoceptor blocking drugs: an update. Drug Saf 9:272–279, 1993

Lieberman JA: Atypical antipsychotic drugs as a first-line treatment of schizophrenia: a rationale and hypothesis. J Clin Psychiatry 57 (suppl 11): 68–71, 1996

Lieberman JA, Yunis J, Egea E, et al: HLA-B38, DR4, DQw3 and clozapine induced agranulocytosis in Jewish patients with schizophrenia. Arch Gen Psychiatry 47:945–948, 1990

Lieberman JA, Saltz BL, Johns CA, et al: The effects of clozapine on tardive dyskinesia. Br J Psychiatry 158: 503–510, 1991

Linnoila M, Vinkar M, Hiertala O: Effect of sodium valproate on tardive dyskinesia. Br J Psychiatry 129:114–119, 1976

Lipinski JF, Zubenko GS, Cohen BM, et al: Propranolol in the treatment of neuroleptic induced akathisia. Am J Psychiatry 141:412–415, 1984

Litman RE, Hong WW, Weismman EM, Su TP, et al: Idazoxan, an α-2 antagonist, augments fluphenazine in schizophrenic patients: a pilot study. J Clin Psychopharmacol 13: 264–267, 1993

Lohr JB, Caligiuri MP: A double-blind placebo-controlled study of vitamin E treatment of tardive dyskinesia. J Clin Psychiatry 57:167–173, 1996

Lohr JB, Cadet JL, Lohr MA, et al: L-Alpha-tocopherol in tardive dyskinesia. Lancet 1:913–914, 1987

Luchins DJ: Carbamazepine in violent non-epileptic schizophrenics. Psychopharmacol Bull 20:569–571, 1984

Luchins DJ, Freed WJ, Wyatt RJ: The role of cholinergic supersensitivity in the medical symptoms associated with withdrawal of antipsychotic drugs. Am J Psychiatry 137:1395–1398, 1980

Marder SR, Meibach RC: Risperidone in the treatment of schizophrenia. Am J Psychiatry 151: 825–835, 1994

Marder SR, van Putten T, Mintz J, et al: Costs and benefits of two doses of fluphenazine. Arch Gen Psychiatry 41:1025–1029, 1984

Marder SR, van Putten T, Mintz J, et al: Low and conventional dose maintenance therapy with fluphenazine decanoate: two-year outcome. Arch Gen Psychiatry 44:518–521, 1987

McDougle CJ, Goodman WK, Price LH, et al: Neuroleptic addition in fluvoxamine-refractory obsessive-compulsive disorder. Am J Psychiatry 147:652–654, 1990

McElroy SL, Dessain EC, Pope HG Jr, et al: Clozapine in the treatment of psychotic mood disorders, schizoaffective disorder, and schizophrenia. J Clin Psychiatry 52:411–414, 1991

McEvoy JP, Stiller RL, Farr R: Plasma haloperidol levels drawn at neuroleptic threshold doses: a pilot study. J Clin Psychopharmacol 6:133–138, 1986

Meltzer HY: The role of serotonin in the action of atypical antipsychotic drugs. Psychiatric Annals 20:571–579, 1990

Meltzer HY: The mechanism of action of novel antipsychotic drugs. Schizophr Bull 17:265–287, 1991

Meltzer HY: An overview of the mechanism of action of clozapine. J Clin Psychiatry 55 (suppl B): 47–52, 1994

Meltzer HY: Role of serotonin in the action of atypical antipsychotic drugs. Clin Neurosci 3 (2):64–75, 1995

Meltzer HY, Matsubara S, Lee J-C: Classification of typical and atypical antipsychotic drugs on the basis of dopamine D_1, D_2, and serotonin$_2$ pKi values. J Pharmacol Exp Ther 251:238–246, 1989

Miller DD, Sharafuddin MJA, Kathol RG: A case of clozapine-induced neuroleptic malignant syndrome. J Clin Psychiatry 52:99–101, 1991

Mitchell JE, Popkin MK: Antipsychotic drug therapy and sexual dysfunction in men. Am J Psychiatry 139:633–637, 1982

Munetz MR, Roth LH: Informing patients about tardive dyskinesia. Arch Gen Psychiatry 42:866–871, 1985

Neppe V: Carbamazepine in the psychiatric patient (letter). Lancet 2:334, 1982

Nielsen H: Recombinant human granulocyte colony-stimulating factor (rhG-CSF; filgrastim) treatment of clozapine-induced agranulocytosis. Journal of Internal Medicine 34 (5):529–531, 1993

Nestoros J, Suranyi B, Spees R, et al: Diazepam in high doses is effective in schizophrenia. Prog Neuropsychopharmacol Biol Psychiatry 6:513–518, 1982

Nurnberg HG, Prudic J: Guidelines for treatment of psychosis during pregnancy. Hosp Community Psychiatry 35:67–71, 1984

Oliver AP, Luchins DJ, Wyatt RJ: Neuroleptic-induced seizures: an in vitro technique for assessing relative risk. Arch Gen Psychiatry 39:206–209, 1982

Ostergaard K, Dupont E: Clozapine treatment of drug-induced psychotic symptoms in late stages of Parkinson's disease (letter). Acta Neurol Scand 78:349–350, 1988

Owens DG: Extrapyramidal side effects and tolerability of risperidone: a review. J Clin Psychiatry 55 (suppl):29–35, 1994

Owens DG: Adverse effects of antipsychotic agents. Do newer agents offer advantages? Drugs 51:895–930, 1996

Perry PJ, Miller DD, Arndt SV, et al: Clozapine and norclozapine plasma concentrations and clinical response of treatment-refractory schizophrenic patients. Am J Psychiatry 148:231–235, 1991

Pycock CJ, Carter CJ, Kerwin RW: Effect of 6-hydroxy-dopamine lesions of the medial prefrontal cortex on neurotransmitter systems in subcortical sites in the rat. J Neurochem 34 (1):91–99, 1980

Reiter S, Adler L, Angrist B, et al: Atenolol and propranolol in neuroleptic-induced akathisia (letter). J Clin Psychopharmacol 7:279–280, 1987

Reunanen M, Kaarnen P, Vaisanen E: The influence of anticholinergic treatment on tardive dyskinesia caused by neuroleptic drugs. Acta Neurol Scand 65 (Suppl 90): 278–279, 1982

Reynolds GP, Stroud D: Hippocampal benzodiazepine receptors in schizophrenia. J Neural Transm 93:151–155, 1993

Rifkin A, Quitkin F, Klein DF: Akinesia: a poorly recognized drug-induced extrapyramidal behavioral disorder. Arch Gen Psychiatry 32:672–674, 1975

Robinson GE, Stewart DE, Flak E: The rational use of psychotropic drugs in pregnancy and postpartum. Can J Psychiatry 31:1983–1990, 1986

Rosebush P, Stewart T: A prospective analysis of 24 episodes of neuroleptic malignant syndrome. Am J Psychiatry 146:717–725, 1989

Rossi A, Mancini F, Stratta P, et al: Risperidone, negative symptoms, and cognitive deficit in schizophrenia: an open study. Acta Psychiatr Scand 95:40–43, 1997

Roth LH: Question the experts. J Clin Psychopharmacol 3:206–207, 1983

Schooler NR: The efficacy of antipsychotic drugs and family therapies in the maintenance treatment of schizophrenia. J Clin Psychopharmacol 6:11S–19S, 1986

Schooler NR, Keith SJ, Severe JB, et al: Relapse and rehospitalization during maintenance treatment of schizophrenia. The effects of dose reduction and family treatment. Arch Gen Psychiatry 54:453–463, 1997

Scokel PW, Jones WD: Infant jaundice after phenothiazine drugs for labour: an enigma. Obstet Gynecol 20:124–127, 1962

Seeman P, Lee T, Chau-Wong M, et al: Antipsychotic drug doses and neuroleptic/dopamine receptors. Nature 261:717–719, 1976

Seide H, Muller HR: Choreiform movements as side effects of phenothiazine medication in elderly patients. J Am Geriatr Soc 15:517–522, 1967

Shader RI: Sexual dysfunction associated with thioridazine hydrochloride. JAMA 188:1007–1009, 1964

Silver JM, Yudofsky SC, Kogan M, et al: Elevation of thioridazine plasma levels by propranolol. Am J Psychiatry 143:1290–1292, 1986

Sokoloff P, Giros B, Martres M-P, et al: Molecular cloning and characterization of a novel dopamine receptor (D₃) as a target for neuroleptics. Nature 347:146–151, 1990

Sorensen SC, Gjerris A, Hammer M: Cerebrospinal fluid vasopressin in neurological and psychiatric disorders. J Neurol Neurosurg Psychiatry 48:50–57, 1985

Stewart RB, Karas B, Springer PK: Haloperidol excretion in human milk. Am J Psychiatry 137:849–850, 1980

Suppes T, McElroy SL, Gilbert J, et al: Clozapine in the treatment of dysphoric mania. Biol Psychiatry 32:270–280, 1992

Tamer A, McKay R, Arias D, et al: Phenothiazine-induced extrapyramidal dysfunction in the neonate. J Pediatr 75:479–480, 1969

Tollefson GD, Beasley CM Jr, Tamura RN: Blind, controlled, long-term study of the comparative incidence of treatment-emergent tardive dyskinesia with olanzapine or haloperidol. Am J Psychiatry 154 (9):1248–1254, 1997

Turbay D, Lieberman J, Alper CA, et al: Tumor necrosis factor constellation polymorphism and clozapine-induced agranulocytosis in two different ethnic groups. Blood 89:4167–4174, 1997

Umbricht D, Kane JM: Medical complications of new antipsychotic drugs. Schizophr Bull 22:475–483, 1996

Umbricht D, Pollack S, Kane JM: Clozapine and weight gain. J Clin Psychiatry 55 (suppl B):157–160, 1994

van Putten T, May PRA, Marder SR: Akathisia with haloperidol and thiothixene. Arch Gen Psychiatry 31:67–72, 1984

van Putten T, Marder SR, Mintz J: A controlled dose comparison of haloperidol in newly admitted schizophrenic patients. Arch Gen Psychiatry 47:754–758, 1990

Van Tol HHM, Bunzow JR, Hong-Chang G, et al: Cloning of the gene for a human dopamine D₄ receptor with high affinity for the antipsychotic clozapine. Nature 350:610–614, 1991

Verma A, Kulkarni SK: Modulation of MK-801 response by dopaminergic agents in mice. Psychopharmacology 107:431–436, 1992

Wachtel H, Turski L: Glutamate: a new target in schizophrenia? Trends Pharmacol Sci 11:219–220, 1990

Waddington JL, Molloy AG, O'Boyle KM, et al: Motor consequences of D-1 dopamine receptor stimulation and blockade. Clin Neuropharmacol 9 (suppl 4):20–22, 1986

Yassa R: Antiparkinsonian medication withdrawal in the treatment of tardive dyskinesia: a report of three cases. Can J Psychiatry 30:440–442, 1985

Yassa R, Lal S: Prevalence of the rabbit syndrome. Am J Psychiatry 143:656–657, 1986

Yunis JJ, Corzo D, Salazar M, et al: HLA associations in clozapine-induced agranulocytosis. Blood 86:1177–1183, 1995

Zarate CA Jr, Tohen M, Baldessarini RJ: Clozapine in severe mood disorders. J Clin Psychiatry 56:411–417, 1995

Zubenko GS, Lipinski JF, Cohen M, et al: Comparison of metoprolol and propranolol in the treatment of akathisia. Psychiatry Res 11:143–149, 1984

Mood Stabilizers

Akiskal HS, Khani MK, Scott-Strauss A: Cyclothymic temperamental disorders. Psychiatr Clin North Am 2:527–554, 1979

Anath J, Dubin SE: Lithium and symptomatic hyperparathyroidism. J R Soc Med 96:1026–1029, 1983

Arana GW, Epstein S, Molloy M, et al: Carbamazepine-induced reduction of plasma alprazolam concentrations: a clinical case report. J Clin Psychiatry 49:448–449, 1988

Baastrup PC, Schou M: Lithium as a prophylactic agent: its effect against recurrent depressions and manic-depressive psychosis. Arch Gen Psychiatry 16:162–172, 1967

Bakris GL, Smith DW, Tiwari S: Dermatologic manifestations of lithium: a review. Int J Psychiatry Med 10:327–331, 1980–1981

Ballenger JC, Post RM: Carbamazepine in manic-depressive illness: a new treatment. Am J Psychiatry 137:782–790, 1980

Battle DC, von Riotte AB, Gaviria M, et al: Amelioration of polyuria by amiloride in patients receiving long-term lithium therapy. N Engl J Med 312:408–414, 1985

Bauer MS, Whybrow PC: Rapid cycling bipolar affective disorder, II: Treatment of refractory rapid cycling with high dose levothyroxine. Arch Gen Psychiatry 47:435–440, 1990

Bauer MS, Whybrow PC, Winokur A: Rapid cycling bipolar affective disorder, I: association with grade I hypothyroidism. Arch Gen Psychiatry 47:427–432, 1989

Baxter LR Jr, Liston EH, Schwartz JM, et al: Prolongation of the antidepressant response to partial sleep deprivation by lithium. Psychiatry Res 19:17–23, 1986

Belmaker RH, Lerer B, Klein E, et al: Clinical implications of research on the mechanism of action of lithium. Prog Neuropsychopharmacol Biol Psychiatry 7:287–296, 1983

Bentsen KD, Gram L, Veje A: Serum thyroid hormones and blood folic acid during monotherapy with carbamazepine or valproate: a controlled study. Acta Neurol Scand 67:235–241, 1983

Bertollini R, Kallen B, Mastroiacovo P, et al: Anticonvulsant drugs in monotherapy: effect on the fetus. Eur J Epidemiol 3:164–171, 1987

Billings PR: Amiloride in the treatment of lithium-induced diabetes insipidus (letter). N Engl J Med 312:1575–1576, 1985

Bone S, Roose SP, Dunner DL, et al: Incidence of side effects in patients on long-term lithium therapy. Am J Psychiatry 137:103–104, 1980

Borer MS, Bhanot VK: Hyperparathyroidism: neuropsychiatric manifestations. Psychosomatics 26:597–601, 1985

Bowden CL, Brugger AM, Swann AC, et al: Efficacy of divalprox vs lithium and placebo in the treatment of mania. The Depakote Mania Study Group. JAMA 271:918–924, 1994

Bowden CL, Janicak PG, Orsulak P, et al: Relation of serum valproate concentration to response in mania. Am J Psychiatry 153:765–770, 1996

Bowen RC, Grof P, Grof E: Less frequent lithium administration and lower urine volume. Am J Psychiatry 148:189–192, 1991

Brewerton TD: Lithium counteracts carbamazepine-induced leukopenia while increasing its therapeutic effect. Biol Psychiatry 21:677–685, 1986

Brewerton TD, Jackson CW: Prophylaxis of carbamazepine-induced hyponatremia by demeclocycline in six patients. J Clin Psychiatry 55:249–251, 1994

Brodie MJ, MacPhee GJ: Carbamazepine neurotoxicity precipitated by diltiazem. BMJ 292:1170–1171, 1986

Brotman AW, Fahardi AM, Gelenberg AJ: Verapamil treatment of acute mania. J Clin Psychiatry 47:136–138, 1986

Brunet G, Cerlich B, Robert P, et al: Open trial of a calcium antagonist, nimodipine, in acute mania. Clin Neuropharmacol 13:224–228, 1990

Cade JFJ: Lithium salts in the treatment of psychotic excitement. Med J Aust 36:349–352, 1949

Caillard V: Treatment of mania using a calcium antagonist-preliminary trial. Neuropsychobiology 14:23–26, 1985

Calabrese JR, Gulledge AD, Hahn K, et al: Autoimmune thyroiditis in manic-depressive patients treated with lithium. Am J Psychiatry 142:1318–1321, 1985

Calabrese JR, Markowitz PJ, Kimmel SE, et al: Spectrum of efficacy of valproate in 78 rapid-cycling bipolar patients. J Clin Psychopharmacol 12:53S–56S, 1992

Calabrese JR, Fatemi SH, Woyshville MJ: Antidepressant effects of lamotrigine in rapid cycling bipolar disorder. Am J Psychiatry 153(9):1236, 1996

Chouinard G, Young SN, Annable L: Antimanic effect of clonazepam. Biol Psychiatry 18:451–466, 1983

Chouinard G, Annable L, Turnier L, et al: A double-blind randomized clinical trial of rapid tranquilization with I.M. clonazepam and I.M. haloperidol in agitated psychotic patients with manic symptoms. Can J Psychiatry 38 S4:S114–S121, 1993

Clur AWB: Hypothyroidism and hyperparathyroidism associated with lithium toxicity. S Afr Med J 76:124, 1989

Cohen LS, Friedman JM, Jefferson MD, et al: A reevaluation of risk of in utero exposure to lithium. JAMA 271:146–150, 1994

Cohen WJ, Cohen NH: Lithium carbonate, haloperidol and irreversible brain damage. JAMA 230:1283–1287, 1974

Cohn JB, Collins G, Ashbrook E, et al: A comparison of fluoxetine, imipramine, and placebo in patients with bipolar depressive disorder. Int Clin Psychopharmacol 4:313–322, 1989

Consensus Conference: Electroconvulsant therapy. JAMA 254:2103–2108, 1985

Consensus Development Panel: Mood disorders: pharmacologic prevention of recurrences. Am J Psychiatry 142:469–476, 1985

Coopen A, Abou-Saleh MT, Miller P, et al: Lithium continuation therapy following electroconvulsive therapy. Br J Psychiatry 139:284–287, 1981

Cooper TB, Bergner PEE, Simpson GM: The 24-hour serum lithium level as a prognosticator of dosage requirements. Am J Psychiatry 130:601–603, 1973

Coulam CB, Annegers JF: Do anticonvulsants reduce the efficacy of oral contraceptives? Epilepsia 20:519–525, 1979

Davies JA: Mechanisms of action of antiepileptic drugs (review). Seizure 4:267–271, 1995

Dean JC, Penry JK: Valproate, in The Medical Treatment of Epilepsy. Edited by Resor SR, Kutt H. New York, Marcel Dekker, 1992, pp 265–278

Deandrea D, Walker N, Mehlmauer M, et al: Dermatologic reactions to lithium: a critical review of the literature. J Clin Psychopharmacol 2:199–204, 1982

DeBeaurepair R: Treatment of neuroleptic-resistant mania and schizoaffective disorders (letter). Am J Psychiatry 149:1614–1615, 1992

DePaulo JR, Correa EI, Sapir DG: Renal function and lithium: a longitudinal study. Am J Psychiatry 143:892–895, 1986

Dreifuss FE, Santilli N, Langer DH, et al: Valproic acid hepatic fatalities: a retrospective review. Neurology 37:379–385, 1987

Dreifuss FE, Langer DH, Moline KA, et al: Valproic acid hepatic fatalities, II: US experience since 1994. Neurology 39:201–207, 1989

Dubovsky SL, Franks RD, Lifschitz M, et al: Effectiveness of verapamil in the treatment of manic patients. Am J Psychiatry 139:502–504, 1982

Dubovsky SL, Franks RD, Allen S, et al: Calcium antagonism in mania: a double-blind study of verapamil. Psychiatry Res 18:309–320, 1986

Dunner DL, Fieve RR: Clinical factors in lithium carbonate prophylaxis failure. Arch Gen Psychiatry 30:229–233, 1974

Ebstein RP, Hermoni M, Belmaker RH: The effect of lithium on noradrenaline-induced cyclic AMP accumulation in rat brain: inhibition after chronic treatment and absence of supersensitivity. J Pharmacol Exp Ther 213:161–167, 1980

Edmonds LD, Oakley GP: Ebstein's anomaly and maternal lithium exposure during pregnancy. Teratology 41:551– 552, 1990

Eichelbaum M, Tomson T, Tybring G, et al: Carbamazepine metabolism in man: induction and pharmacogenetic aspects. Clin Pharmacokinet 10:80–90, 1985

Faedda GL, Tondo L, Baldessarini RJ, et al: Outcome after rapid vs. gradual discontinuation of lithium treatment in bipolar disorders. Arch Gen Psychiatry 50: 448–455, 1994

Fankhauser MP, Lindon JL, Connolly B, et al: Evaluation of lithium-tetracycline interaction. Clin Pharm 7 (4): 314–317, 1988

Gelenberg AJ, Kane JM, Keller MB, et al: Comparison of standard and low blood levels of lithium for maintenance treatment of bipolar disorder. N Engl J Med 321:1489–1493, 1989

Gerner RH, Stanton A: Algorithm for patient management of acute manic states: lithium, valproate, or carbamazepine? J Clin Psychopharmacol 12 (No 1, suppl):57S–63S, 1992

Gitlin MJ, Weiss J: Verapamil as maintenance treatment in bipolar illness: a case report. J Clin Psychopharmacol 4: 341–343, 1984

Goldney RD, Spence ND: Safety of the combination of lithium and neuroleptic drugs. Am J Psychiatry 143:882–884, 1986

Goodwin FK, Jamison R: Manic-Depressive Illness. New York, Oxford University Press, 1990

Gram LM, Bentsen KD: Hepatic toxicity of antiepileptic drugs: a review. Acta Neurol Scand (Suppl) 97:81–90, 1983

Hetmar O, Bren C, Clemmesen L, et al: Lithium: long-term effects on the kidney, II: structural changes. J Psychiatr Res 21:279–288, 1987

Hetmar O, Poulsen UJ, Ladefoged J, et al: Lithium: long-term effects on the kidney: a prospective follow-up study ten years after kidney biopsy. Br J Psychiatry 158:53–58, 1991

Himmelhoch JM, Thase ME, Mallinger AG, et al: Tranylcypromine versus imipramine in anergic bipolar depression. Am J Psychiatry 148:910–916, 1991

Hirschfeld RMA, Clayton P, Cohen I, et al: Practice guideline for the treatment of patients with bipolar disorder. Am J Psychiatry 151:12, 1994

Hoschl C, Kozeny J: Verapamil in affective disorders: a controlled, double-blind study. Biol Psychiatry 25:128–140, 1989

Hurd RW, Rinsvelt V, Karas WB, et al: Selenium, zinc, and copper changes with valproic acid: possible relation to drug side effects. Neurology 34:1393–1395, 1984

Hyman NM, Dennis PD, Sinclair KG: Tremor due to sodium valproate. Neurology 29:1172–1180, 1979

Isojarvi JI, Laatikainen TJ, Knip M, et al: Obesity and endocrine disorders in women taking valproate for epilepsy. Ann Neurol 39:579–584, 1996

Jacobsen FM: Low-dose valproate: a new treatment for cyclothymia, mild rapid cycling disorders, and premenstrual syndrome. J Clin Psychiatry 54:229–234, 1993

Jacobson SJ, Jones K, Johnson K, et al: Prospective multicentre study of pregnancy outcome after lithium exposure during first trimester. Lancet 339:530–533, 1992

Jaeken J, Casaer P, Corbeel L: Valproate, hyperammonaemia and hyperglycinaemia (letter). Lancet 2:260, 1980

Janicak PG, Sharma RP, Pandey G, et al: Verapamil for the treatment of acute mania: a double-blind, placebo-controlled trial. Am J Psychiatry 155 (7):972–973, 1998

Jeavons PM, Clark JE, Harding GFA: Valproate and curly hair. Lancet 1:359, 1977

Joffe RT, Gold PW, Uhde TW, et al: The effects of carbamazepine on the thyrotropin response to thyrotropin releasing hormone. Psychiatry Res 12:161–166, 1984

Joffe RT, Post RM, Uhde TW: Effect of carbamazepine on body weight in affectively ill patients. J Clin Psychiatry 47:313–314, 1986

Jones KL, Lacro RV, Johnson KA, et al: Pattern of malformations in the children of women treated with carbamazepine during pregnancy. N Engl J Med 320:1661–1666, 1989

Jope RS, Williams MB: Lithium and brain signal transduction systems. Biochem Pharmacol 47:429–441, 1994

Kallen B, Tandberg A: Lithium and pregnancy: a cohort study in manic-depressive women. Acta Psychiatr Scand 68: 134–139, 1983

Keck PE Jr, McElroy SL, Nemeroff CB: Anticonvulsants in the treatment of bipolar disorder. J Neuropsychiatry Clin Neurosci 4:395–405, 1992

Keck PE Jr, McElroy SL, Tugrul KC, et al: Valproate oral loading in the treatment of acute mania. J Clin Psychiatry 54:305–308, 1993

Ketter TA, Pazzaglia PJ, Post RM: Synergy of carbamazepine and valproic acid in affective disorders. J Clin Psychopharmacol 12: 276–281, 1992

Ketter TA, Post RM, Parekh PI, et al: Addition of monoamine oxidase inhibitors to carbamazepine: preliminary evidence of safety and antidepressant efficacy in treatment- resistant depression. J Clin Psychiatry. 56:471–475, 1995a

Ketter TA, Flockhart DA, Post RM, et al: The emerging role of cytochrome P450 3A in psychopharmacology. J Clin Psychopharmacol 15:387–398, 1995b

Klemfuss H: Diminishing toxic effects of lithium administration (letter). Am J Psychiatry 149:846, 1992

Kramingler KG, Post RM: Addition of lithium carbonate to carbamazepine: hematological and thyroid effects. Am J Psychiatry 147:615–620, 1990

Labar DR: Antiepileptic drug toxic emergencies, in The Medical Treatment of Epilepsy. Edited by Resor SR, Kutt H. New York, Marcel Dekker, 1992, pp 573–588

Lambert P-A, Cavaz G, Borselli S, et al: Action neuropsychotrop diun nouvel anti-epileptique: le Depamide. Ann Med Psychol (Paris) 1:707–710, 1966

Lammer EJ, Sever LE, Oakley GP: Teratogen update: valproic acid. Teratology 35:465–473, 1987

Leach MJ, Baxter MG, Critchley MA: Neurochemical and behavioral aspects of lamotrigine. Epilepsia 32:S4–S8, 1991

Lenox RH, Newhouse PA, Creelman WL, et al: Adjunctive treatment of manic agitation with lorazepam versus haloperidol: a double blind study. J Clin Psychiatry 53:47–52, 1992

Lindstedt G, Nilsson L, Walinder J, et al: On the prevalence, diagnosis and management of lithium-induced hypothyroidism in psychiatric patients. Br J Psychiatry 130:452–458, 1977

Lipinski JF, Pope HG: Possible synergistic action between carbamazepine and lithium carbonate in the treatment of three acutely manic patients. Am J Psychiatry 139:948–949, 1982

Lokkegaard H, Andersen NF, Henriksen E: Renal function in 153 manic-depressive patients treated with lithium for more than five years. Acta Psychiatr Scand 71:347–355, 1985

MacDonald RL, Kelly KM: Antiepileptic drug mechanisms of action (review). Epilepsia 36 (2):S2–S12, 1995

Mallette LE, Eichhorn E: Effects of lithium carbonate on human calcium metabolism. Arch Intern Med 146:770–776, 1986

Manji HK, Chen G, Shimon H, et al: Guanine nucleotide-binding proteins in bipolar affective disorder: effects of long-term lithium treatment. Arch Gen Psychiatry 52:135–144, 1995

Martin A: Clinical management of lithium-induced polyuria. Hosp Community Psychiatry 44:427–428, 1993

McElroy SL, Keck PE Jr, Pope HG Jr, et al: Valproate in psychiatric disorders: literature review and clinical guidelines. J Clin Psychiatry 50 (No 20, suppl):23–29, 1989

McElroy SL, Keck PE Jr, Pope HG Jr, et al: Valproate in the treatment of bipolar disorder: literature review and clinical guidelines. J Clin Psychopharmacol 12 (No 1, suppl):42S–52S, 1992

McGennis AJ: Lithium carbonate and tetracycline interaction. BMJ 1 (6121):1183, 1978

Mitchell JE, Mackenzie TB: Cardiac effects of lithium therapy in man: a review. J Clin Psychiatry 43:47–51, 1982

Moss GR, James CR: Carbamazepine and lithium synergism in mania. Arch Gen Psychiatry 40:588–589, 1983

Murphy MJ, Lyon IW, Taylor JW, et al: Valproic acid associated with pancreatitis in an adult (letter). Lancet 1:41–42, 1981

Murphy JM, Mashman J, Miller JD, et al: Suppression of carbamazepine-induced rash with prednisone. Neurology 41:144–145, 1991

Myers DH, Carter RA, Burns BH, et al: A prospective study of the effects of lithium on thyroid function and on the prevalence of antithyroid antibodies. Psychol Med 15:55–61, 1985

Nora JJ, Nora AH, Toews WH: Lithium, Ebstein's anomaly and other congenital heart defects. Lancet 1:594–595, 1974

Patterson JF: Stevens-Johnson syndrome associated with carbamazepine therapy. J Clin Psychopharmacol 5:185, 1985

Pazzaglia PJ, Post RM, Ketter TA, et al: Preliminary controlled trial of nimodipine in ultra-rapid cycling affective dysregulation. Psychiatry Res 49:257–272, 1993

Peet M: Induction of mania with selective serotonin re-uptake inhibitors and tricyclic antidepressants. Br J Psychiatry 164:549–550, 1994

Pellock JM: Carbamazepine side effects in children and adults. Epilepsia 28 (3):S64–S70, 1987

Pellock JM, Willmore LJ: A rational guide to routine blood monitoring in patients receiving antiepileptic drugs. Neurology 41 (7):961–964, 1991

Penney JF, Dimwiddie SH, Zarumski CF, et al: Concurrent and close temporal administration of lithium and ECT. Convulsive Therapy 6:139–145, 1990

Perry PJ, Alexander B, Prince RA, et al: The utility of a single-point dosing protocol for predicting steady-state lithium levels. Br J Psychiatry 148:401–405, 1986

Peselow ED, Dunner DL, Fieve RR, et al: Lithium carbonate and weight gain. J Affect Disord 2:303–310, 1980

Placidi GF, Lenzi A, Lazzerini F, et al: The comparative efficacy and safety of carbamazepine versus lithium: a randomized double-blind 3-year trial in 83 patients. J Clin Psychiatry 47:490–494, 1986

Plenge P, Mellerup ET, Bolwig C, et al: Lithium treatment: does the kidney prefer one daily dose instead of two? Acta Psychiatr Scand 66:121–128, 1982

Pope HG Jr, McElroy SL, Sathin A, et al: Head injury, bipolar disorder, and response to valproate. Compr Psychiatry 29:34–38, 1988

Pope HG Jr, McElroy SL, Keck PE Jr, et al: Valproate in the treatment of acute mania: a placebo-controlled study. Arch Gen Psychiatry 48:62–68, 1991

Post RM, Uhde TW, Ballenger JC, et al: Carbamazepine and its 10-11-epoxide metabolite in plasma and CSF: relationship to antidepressant response. Arch Gen Psychiatry 40:673–676, 1983

Post RM, Uhde TW, Ballenger JC: Efficacy of carbamazepine in affective disorders: implications for underlying physiological and biochemical substrates, in Anticonvulsants in Affective Disorders. Edited by Emrich HM, Okuma T, Muller AS. Amsterdam, Elsevier, 1984, pp 93–115

Post RM, Uhde TW, Roy-Byrne PP, et al: Antidepressant effects of carbamazepine. Am J Psychiatry 143:29–34, 1986

Post RM, Uhde TW, Roy-Byrne PP, et al: Correlates of antimanic response to carbamazepine. Psychiatry Res 21:71–83, 1987

Post RM, Weiss SRB, Chuang D-M: Mechanisms of action of anticonvulsants in affective disorder: comparisons with lithium. J Clin Psychopharmacol 12 (No 1, suppl):23S–35S, 1992

Prien RF, Kupfer DJ, Mansky PA, et al: Drug therapy in the prevention of recurrences in unipolar and bipolar affective disorders: report of the NIMH Collaborative Study Group comparing lithium carbonate, imipramine, and a lithium carbonate-imipramine combination. Arch Gen Psychiatry 41:1096–1104, 1984

Ramsey TA, Cox M: Lithium and the kidney: a review. Am J Psychiatry 139:443–449, 1982

Richens A: Safety of lamotrigine. Epilepsia 35 (suppl 5):S37–S40, 1994

Robert E, Guibaud P: Maternal valproic acid and congenital neural tube defects (letter). Lancet 2:937, 1982

Rosa FW: Spina bifida in infants of women treated with carbamazepine during pregnancy. N Engl J Med 324:674–677, 1991

Sachs GS, Lafer B, Stoll AL, et al: A double-blind trial of bupropion versus desipramine for bipolar depression. J Clin Psychiatry 55:391–393, 1994

Schatzberg AF, Cole JO: Manual of Clinical Psychopharmacology, 2nd Edition. Washington, DC, American Psychiatric Press, 1991

Schou M: Lithium prophylaxis: myths and realities. Am J Psychiatry 146:573–576, 1989

Shopsin B: Bupropion's prophylactic efficacy in bipolar affective illness. J Clin Psychiatry 44:163–169, 1983

Simon MN, Garber E, Arieff AJ: Persistent nephrogenic diabetes insipidus after lithium carbonate. Ann Intern Med 86:446–447, 1977

Small JG: Anticonvulsants in affective disorders. Psychopharmacol Bull 26:25–36, 1990

Stancer HC, Persad E: Treatment of intractable rapid-cycling manic-depressive disorder with levothyroxine: clinical observations. Arch Gen Psychiatry 47:435–440, 1982

Steering Committee, American Psychiatric Association: The expert consensus guideline series: treatment of bipolar disorder. J Clin Psychiatry 57 (suppl 12a):3–88, 1996

Suppes T, Baldessarini RJ, Faedda GI, et al: Risk of recurrence following discontinuation of lithium treatment in bipolar disorder. Arch Gen Psychiatry 48:1082–1088, 1991

Suppes T, McElroy SL, Gilbert J, et al: Clozapine in the treatment of dysphoric mania. Biol Psychiatry 32:270–280, 1992

Swann AC, Bowden CL, Morris D, et al: Depression during mania: treatment response to lithium or divalproex. Arch Gen Psychiatry 54:37–42, 1997

Takezaki H, Hanaoka M: The use of carbamazepine (Tegretol) in the control of manic-depressive psychosis and other manic-depressive states. J Clin Psychiatry 13:173–183, 1971

Vendsborg PB, Bech P, Rafaelson OJ: Lithium treatment and weight gain. Acta Psychiatr Scand 53:139–147, 1976

Vestergaard P, Amdisen A, Schou M: Clinically significant side effects of lithium treatment. Acta Psychiatr Scand 62:193–200, 1980

Vick NA: Suppression of carbamazepine-induced skin rash with prednisone. New Engl J Med 309:1193–1194, 1983

Waller DG: Thyroid function and urine-concentrating ability during lithium treatment. J Psychiatr Res 19:569–571, 1985

Waller DG, Edwards JG: Lithium and the kidney: an update. Psychol Med 19:825–831, 1989

Warnock JK, Knesevich J: Adverse cutaneous reactions to antidepressants. Am J Psychiatry 145:425–430, 1988

Wehr TA, Goodwin FK: Do antidepressants cause mania? Psychopharmacol Bull 23:61–65, 1987

Wehr TA, Sack DA, Rosenthal NE, et al: Rapid cycling affective disorder: contributing factors and treatment responses in 51 patients. Am J Psychiatry 145:179–184, 1988

Wood IK, Parmalee DX, Foreman JW: Lithium-induced nephrotic syndrome. Am J Psychiatry 146:84–87, 1989

Yassa R, Saunders A, Nastase C, et al: Lithium-induced thyroid disorders: a prevalence study. J Clin Psychiatry 48:14–16, 1988

Yeo PP, Bates D, Howe JG, et al: Anticonvulsants and thyroid function. BMJ 1:1581–1583, 1978

Zalzstein E, Koren G, Einarson T, Freedom RM: A case-control study on the association between first trimester exposure to lithium and Ebstein's anomaly. Am J Cardiol 41:551–552, 1990

Zohar J, Ebstein RP, Belmaker RH: Adenylate cyclase as the therapeutic target site of lithium, in Basic Mechanisms in the Action of Lithium. Edited by Emrich HM, Aldenhoff JB, Lux HD. Amsterdam, Elsevier, 1982, pp 154–166

Zornberg GL, Pope HGJ: Treatment of depression in bipolar disorder: new directions for research. J Clin Psychopharmacol 13:397–408, 1993

Zubenko GS, Cohen BM, Lipinski JF: Comparison of metoprolol and propranolol in the treatment of lithium tremor. Psychiatry Res 11:163–164, 1984

Drug Interactions

Callahan AM, Marangell LB, Ketter TA: Evaluating the clinical significance of drug interaction: a systematic approach. Harvard Rev Psychiatry 4:153–158, 1996

Dahl ML, Johansson I, Bertilsson L, et al: Ultrarapid hydroxylation of debrisoquine in a Swedish population: Analysis of the molecular genetic basis. J Pharmacol Exp Ther 274:516–520, 1995

Goodwin FK, Jamison R: Manic-Depressive Illness. New York, Oxford University Press, 1990

Greiff JM, Rowbotham D: Pharmacokinetic drug interactions with gastrointestinal motility modifying agents. Clin Pharmacokinet 27:447–461, 1994

Honig PK, Woosley RL, Zamani K, et al: Changes in the pharmacokinetics and electrocardiographic pharmacodynamics of terfenadine with concomitant administration of erythromycin. Clin Pharmacol Ther 52:231–238, 1992

Johansson I, Lundqvist E, Bertilsson L, et al: Inherited amplification of an active gene in the cytochrome P450 CYP2D locus as a cause of ultrarapid metabolism of debrisoquine. Proc Nat Acad Sci USA 90:11825–11829, 1993

Monohan BP, Ferguson CL, Killeavy ES, et al: Torsades de pointes occurring in association with terfenadine use. JAMA 264:2788–2790, 1990

Nakamura K, Goto F, Ray WA, et al: Interethnic differences in genetic polymorphism of debrisoquine and mephenytoin hydroxylation between Japanese and Caucasian populations. Clin Pharmacol Ther 38:402–408, 1985

Nelson DR, Kamataki T, Waxman DJ, et al: The P450 superfamily: update on new sequences, gene mapping, accession numbers, early trivial names of enzymes, and nomenclature. DNA Cell Biol 12:1–51, 1993

Shimada T, Yamazaki H, Mimura M, et al: Interindividual variations in human liver cytochrome P-450 enzymes involved in the oxidation of drugs, carcinogens and toxic chemicals: studies with liver microsomes of 30 Japanese and 30 Caucasians. J Pharmacol Exp Ther 270:414–423, 1994

Watkins PB, Wrighton SA, Maurel P, et al: Identification of an inducible form of cytochrome P-450 in human liver. Proc Natl Acad Sci USA 82:6310–6314, 1985

Xie HG, Xu ZH, Luo X, et al: Genetic polymorphism of debrisoquine and S-mephenytoin oxidation metabolism in Chinese populations: a meta-analysis. Pharmacogenetics 6:235–238, 1996

Antiaggression Drugs

Alexander RW, Davis JN, Lefkowitz RJ: Direct identification and characterization of β-adrenergic receptors in rat brain. Nature 258:437–440, 1979

Alpert M, Allan ER, Citrome L, et al: A double-blind, placebo-controlled study of adjunctive nadolol in the management of violent psychiatric patients. Psychopharmacol Bull 28:367–371, 1990

Angus WR, Romney DM: The effect of diazepam on patients' memory. J Clin Psychopharmacol 4:203–206, 1984

Bass JN, Beltis J: Therapeutic effect of fluoxetine on naltrexone-resistant self-injurious behavior in an adolescent with mental retardation. J Child Adolesc Psychopharmacol 1:331–340, 1991

Berridge MJ, Downes CP, Hanley MR: Neural and developmental actions of lithium: a unifying hypothesis. Cell 59:411–419, 1989

Bick PA, Hannah AL: Intramuscular lorazepam to restrain violent patients. Lancet 1:206, 1986

Campbell M, Fish B, Korein J, et al: Lithium and chlorpromazine: a controlled crossover study of hyperactive severely disturbed young children. J Autism Child Schizophr 2:234–263, 1972

Coccaro EF, Astill JL, Herbert JL, et al: Fluoxetine treatment of impulsive aggression in DSM-III-R personality disorder patients. J Clin Psychopharmacol 10:373–375, 1990

Colenda CC: Buspirone in treatment of agitated demented patient. Lancet 1:1169, 1988

Corrigan PW, Yudofsky SC, Silver JM: Pharmacological and behavioral treatments for aggressive psychiatric inpatients. Hosp Community Psychiatry 44:125–133, 1993

Craft M, Ismail IA, Krishnamurti D, et al: Lithium in the treatment of aggression in mentally handicapped patients: a double-blind trial. Br J Psychiatry 150:685–689, 1987

Czobor P, Volavka J, Meibach RC: Effect of risperidone on hostility in schizophrenia. J Clin Psychopharmacol 15:243–249, 1995

Dale PG: Lithium therapy in aggressive mentally subnormal patients. Br J Psychiatry 137:469–474, 1980

Dietch JT, Jennings RK: Aggressive dyscontrol in patients treated with benzodiazepines. J Clin Psychiatry 49:184–189, 1988

Dostal T, Zvolsky P: Antiaggressive effects of lithium salts in severe mentally retarded adolescents. Int Pharmacopsychiatry 5:203–207, 1970

Fava M, Rosenbaum JF, Pava JA, et al: Anger attacks in unipolar depression, Part 1: clinical correlates and response to fluoxetine treatment. Am J Psychiatry 150:1158–1163, 1993

Feeney DM, Gonzalez A, Lewin A: Amphetamine, haloperidol, and experience interact to affect rate of recovery after motor cortex injury. Science 217:855–857, 1982

Folks DG, King LD, Dowdy SB, et al: Carbamazepine treatment of selective affectively disordered inpatients. Am J Psychiatry 139:115–117, 1982

Gedye A: Trazodone reduced aggressive and self-injurious movements in a mentally handicapped male patient with autism. J Clin Psychopharmacol 11:275–276, 1991

Gengo FM, Fagan SC, de Padova A, et al: The effect of beta-blockers on mental performance in older hypertensive patients. Arch Intern Med 148:779–784, 1988

Giakas WJ, Seibyl JP, Mazure CM: Valproate in the treatment of temper outbursts. J Clin Psychiatry 51:525, 1990

Gleason RP, Schneider LS: Carbamazepine treatment of agitation in Alzheimer's outpatients refractory to neuroleptics. J Clin Psychiatry 51:115–118, 1990

Greendyke RM, Kanter DR, Schuster DB, et al: Propranolol treatment of assaultive patients with organic brain disease: a double-blind crossover, placebo-controlled study. J Nerv Ment Dis 174:290–294, 1986

Greendyke RM, Berkner JP, Webster JC, et al: Treatment of behavioral problems with pindolol. Psychosomatics 30:161–165, 1989

Greenwald BS, Marin DB, Silverman SM: Serotonergic treatment of screaming and banging in dementia. Lancet 2:1464–1465, 1986

Gualtieri CT: Buspirone for the behavior problems of patients with organic brain disorders. J Clin Psychopharmacol 11:280–281, 1991a

Gualtieri CT: Buspirone: neuropsychiatric effects. Journal of Head Trauma and Rehabilitation 6:90–92, 1991b

Haas JF, Cope N: Neuropharmacologic management of behavior sequelae in head injury: a case report. Arch Phys Med Rehabil 66:472–474, 1985

Hakoloa HP, Loulumaa VA: Carbamazepine in treatment of violent schizophrenics. Lancet 1:1358, 1982

Herrera JN, Sramek JJ, Costa JF, et al: High potency neuroleptics and violence in schizophrenics. J Nerv Ment Dis 176:558–561, 1988

Hornstein A, Seliger G: Cognitive side effects of lithium in closed head injury (letter). J Neuropsychiatry Clin Neurosci 1:446–447, 1989

Jackson RD, Corrigan JD, Arnett JA: Amitriptyline for agitation in head injury. Arch Phys Med Rehabil 66:180–181, 1985

Jeanblanc W, Davis YB: Risperidone for treating dementia-associated aggression. Am J Psychiatry 152:1239, 1995

King BH: Fluoxetine reduced self-injurious behavior in an adolescent with mental retardation. J Child Adolesc Psychopharmacol 1:321–329, 1991

Leavitt ML, Yudofsky SC, Maroon JC, et al: Effect of intraventricular nadolol infusion on shock-induced aggression in 6-OHDA lesioned rats. J Neuropsychiatry Clin Neurosci 1:167–172, 1989

Leibovici A, Tariot PN: Carbamazepine treatment of agitation associated with dementia. J Geriatr Psychiatry Neurol 1:110–112, 1988

Levine AM: Buspirone and agitation in head injury. Brain Inj 2:165–167, 1988

Lott RS, Kerrick JM, Cohen SA: Clinical and economic aspects of risperidone treatment in adults with mental retardation and behavioral disturbance. Psychopharmacol Bull 32:721–729, 1996

Luchins DJ: Carbamazepine for the violent psychiatric patient. Lancet 2:755, 1983

Luchins DJ, Dojka D: Lithium and propranolol in aggression and self-injurious behavior in the mentally retarded. Psychopharmacol Bull 25:372–375, 1989

Lucki I, Rickels K, Geller AM: Chronic use of benzodiazepines and psychomotor and cognitive test performance. Psychopharmacology 88:426–433, 1986

Mattes JA: Carbamazepine vs propranolol for rage outbursts. Psychopharmacol Bull 24:179–182, 1988

Mazure CM, Druss BG, Cellar JS: Valproate treatment of older psychotic patients with organic mental syndromes and behavioral dyscontrol. J Am Geriatr Soc 40:914–916, 1992

McCreadie RG: Managing the first episode of schizophrenia: the new role of therapies. Eur Neuropsychopharmacol 6:S3–S5, 1996

Mellow AM, Solano-Lopez C, Davis S: Sodium valproate in the treatment of behavioral disturbance in dementia. J Geriatr Psychiatry Neurol 6:205–209, 1993

Moskowitz AS, Altshuler L: Increased sensitivity to lithium-induced neurotoxicity after stroke: a case report. J Clin Psychopharmacol 11:272–273, 1991

Mysiw WJ, Jackson RD, Corrigan JD: Amitriptyline for post-traumatic agitation. Am J Phys Med Rehabil 67:29–30, 1988

Pinner E, Rich CL: Effects of trazodone on aggressive behavior in seven patients with organic mental disorders. Am J Psychiatry 145:1295–1296, 1988

Ratey JJ, Sovner R, Mikkelsen E, et al: Buspirone therapy for maladaptive behavior and anxiety in developmentally disabled persons. J Clin Psychiatry 50:382–384, 1989

Ratey JJ, Leveroni CL, Miller AC, et al: Low-dose buspirone to treat agitation and maladaptive behavior in brain-injured patients: two case reports. J Clin Psychopharmacol 12:362–364, 1992a

Ratey JJ, Sorgi P, O'Driscoll GA, et al: Nadolol to treat aggression and psychiatric symptomatology in chronic psychiatric inpatients: a double-blind, placebo-controlled study. J Clin Psychiatry 53:41–46, 1992b

Realmuto FM, August GJ, Garfinkel BD: Clinical effect of buspirone in autistic children. J Clin Psychopharmacol 9:122–124, 1989

Roth T, Hartse KM, Saab PG, et al: The effects of flurazepam, lorazepam, and triazolam on sleep and memory. Psychopharmacology (Berl) 70:231–237, 1980

Schiffer RB, Herndon RM, Rudick RA: Treatment of pathologic laughing and weeping with amitriptyline. N Engl J Med 312:1480–1482, 1985

Seliger GM, Hornstein A, Flax J, et al: Fluoxetine improves emotional incontinence. Brain Inj 6:267–270, 1992

Sheard MH, Marini JL, Bridges C, et al: The effects of lithium in impulsive aggressive behavior in man. Am J Psychiatry 133:1409–1413, 1976

Silver JM, Yudofsky SC: Aggressive behavior in patients with neuropsychiatric disorders. Psychiatric Ann 17:367–370, 1987

Silver JM, Yudofsky SC: The Overt Aggression Scale: overview and clinical guidelines. J Neuropsychiatry Clin Neurosci 3:S22–S29, 1991

Silver JM, Yudofsky SC: Aggressive disorders, in Neuropsychiatry of Traumatic Brain Injury. Edited by Silver JM, Yudofsky SC, Hales RE. Washington, DC, American Psychiatric Press, 1994

Silver JM, Yudofsky SC, Kogan M, et al: Elevation of thioridazine plasma levels by propranolol. Am J Psychiatry 143:1290–1292, 1986

Simpson DM, Foster D: Improvement in organically disturbed behavior with trazodone treatment. J Clin Psychiatry 47:191–193, 1986

Sloan RL, Brown KW, Pentland B: Fluoxetine as a treatment for emotional lability after brain injury. Brain Inj 6:315–319, 1992

Sorbin P, Schneider L, McDermott H: Fluoxetine in the treatment of agitated dementia. Am J Psychiatry 146:1636, 1989

Stone JL, McDaniel KD, Hughes JR, et al: Episodic dyscontrol disorder and paroxysmal EEG abnormalities: successful treatment with carbamazepine. Biol Psychiatry 21: 208–212, 1986

Szlabowicz JW, Stewart JT: Amitriptyline treatment of agitation associated with anoxic encephalopathy. Arch Phys Med Rehabil 71:612–613, 1990

Tiller JWG, Dakis JA, Shaw JM: Short-term buspirone treatment in disinhibition with dementia. Lancet 2:510, 1988

Tunks ER, Dermer SW: Carbamazepine in the dyscontrol syndrome associated with limbic dysfunction. J Nerv Ment Dis 14:311–317, 1973

Tupin JP, Smith DB, Clanon TL, et al: Long-term use of lithium in aggressive prisoners. Compr Psychiatry 14: 311–317, 1973

Vetro A, Szentistvanyi L, Pallag M, et al: Therapeutic experience with lithium in childhood aggressivity. Pharmacopsychiatry 14:121–127, 1985

Wilcox J: Divalproex sodium in the treatment of aggressive behavior. Ann Clin Psychiatry 6 (1):17–20, 1994

Williams KH, Goldstein G: Cognitive and affective responses to lithium in patients with organic brain syndrome. Am J Psychiatry 136:800–803, 1979

Worrall EP, Moody JP, Naylor GT: Lithium in non-manic depressives: antiaggressive effect and red blood cell lithium values. Br J Psychiatry 126:464–468, 1975

Yatham LN, McHale PA: Carbamazepine in the treatment of aggression: a case report and a review of the literature. Acta Psychiatr Scand 78:188–190, 1988

Yudofsky SC: Beta-blockers and depression: the clinicians's dilemma. JAMA 267:1826–1827, 1992

Yudofsky SC, Silver JM, Jackson W, et al: The Overt Aggression Scale for the objective rating of verbal and physical aggression. Am J Psychiatry 143:35–39, 1986

Yudofsky SC, Silver JM, Schneider SE: Pharmacologic treatment of aggression. Psychiatric Annals 17:397–407, 1987

Yudofsky SC, Silver JM, Hales RE: Pharmacologic management of aggression in the elderly. J Clin Psychiatry 51 (No 10, suppl):22–28, 1990

Electroconvulsive Therapy

Abrams R: Is unilateral electroconvulsive therapy really the treatment of choice in endogenous depression? Ann NY Acad Sci 462:50–55, 1986

Abrams R: Electroconvulsive Therapy, 2nd Edition. New York, Oxford University Press, 1992

American Psychiatric Association: The Practice of Electroconvulsive Therapy: Recommendations for Treatment, Training, and Privileging. A Task Force Report of the American Psychiatric Association. Washington, DC, American Psychiatric Association, 1990

Asnis GM, Fink M, Saferstein S: ECT in metropolitan New York hospitals: a survey of practice, 1975–76. Am J Psychiatry 135:479–482, 1978

Avery D, Lubrano A: Depressions treated with imipramine and ECT: the DeCarolis study reconsidered. Am J Psychiatry 136:559–569, 1979

Avery D, Winokur G: Mortality in depressed patients treated with ECT and antidepressants. Arch Gen Psychiatry 33:1029–1037, 1976

Coffey CE, Weiner RD, Djang WT, et al: Brain anatomic effects of electroconvulsive therapy. A prospective magnetic resonance imaging study. Arch Gen Psychiatry 48:1013–1021, 1991

Coppen A, Abou-Saleb MT, Miller P, et al: Lithium continuation therapy following electroconvulsive therapy. Br J Psychiatry 139:284–287, 1981

Dec GW, Stern TA, Welsch C: The effects of electroconvulsive therapy on serial electrocardiograms and serum cardiac enzyme values: a prospective study of depressed hospitalized inpatients. JAMA 253:2525–2529, 1985

Devanand DP, Verma AK, Tirumalasetti F, et al: Absence of cognitive impairment after more than 100 lifetime ECT treatments. Am J Psychiatry 148:929–932, 1991

Devanand DP, Dwork AJ, Hutchinson ER, et al: Does ECT alter brain structure? Am J Psychiatry 151:957–970, 1994

Devanand DP, Fitzsimons L, Prudic J, et al: Subjective side effects during electroconvulsive therapy. Convulsive Therapy 11:232–240, 1995

Fink M: Efficacy and safety of induced seizures (ECT) in man. Compr Psychiatry 19:1–18, 1978

Glassman AH, Roose SP: Delusional depression: a distinct clinical entity. Arch Gen Psychiatry 38:424–427, 1981

Gomez J: Subjective side effects of ECT. Br J Psychiatry 127:609–611, 1975

Janicak PG, Davis JM, Gibbons RD, et al: Efficacy of ECT: a meta-analysis. Am J Psychiatry 132:297–302, 1985

Kapur S, Mann JJ: Antidepressant action and the neurobiologic effects of ECT: human studies, in The Clinical Science of Electroconvulsive Therapy. Edited by Coffey CE. Washington, DC, American Psychiatric Press, 1993, pp 236–250

Lerer B, Belmaker RH: ECT and lithium: basic mechanisms, parallels, and controls in receptor mechanisms, in ECT: Basic Mechanisms. Edited by Lerer B, Weiner D, Belmaker R. Washington, DC, American Psychiatric Press, 1986

Lerer B, Shapira B, Calev A, et al: Antidepressant and cognitive effects of twice- versus three-times-weekly ECT. Am J Psychiatry 152:4, 564–570, 1995

Malitz S, Sackeim HA: Preface. Ann NY Acad Sci 462, 1986

Maltbie AA, Wingfield MS, Volow MR, et al: Electroconvulsive therapy in the presence of brain tumor: case reports and an evaluation of risk. J Nerv Ment Dis 168:400–405, 1980

Nutt DJ, Glue P: The neurobiology of ECT: animal studies. in The Clinical Science of Electroconvulsive Therapy. Edited by Coffey CE. Washington, DC, American Psychiatric Press, 1993, pp 213–235

Paul SM, Extein I, Calih H, et al: The use of ECT with treatment resistant depressed patients at the National Institute of Mental Health. Am J Psychiatry 138:486–489, 1977

Perry P, Tsuang MT: Treatment of unipolar depression following electroconvulsive therapy: relapse rate comparison between lithium and tricyclic therapies following ECT. J Affect Disord 1:123–129, 1979

Reid WH: Electroconvulsive therapy. Tex Med 89 (5):58–62, 1993

Sackeim HA, Prudic J, Devanand DP, et al: The impact of medication resistance and continuation pharmacotherapy on relapse following response to electroconvulsive therapy in major depression. J Clin Psychopharmacol 10:96–104, 1990

Sackeim HA, Devanand DP, Prudic J: Stimulus intensity, seizure threshold, and seizure duration: impact on the efficacy and safety of electroconvulsive therapy. Psychiatr Clin North Am 14:803–843, 1991

Sackeim HA, Prudic J, Devanand DP, et al: Effects of stimulus intensity and electrode placement on the efficacy and cognitive effects of electroconvulsive therapy. N Engl J Med 328:839–846, 1993

Salzman C: The use of ECT in the treatment of schizophrenia. Am J Psychiatry 137:1031–1041, 1980

Schwarz T, Loenwenstein J, Isenberg KE: Maintenance ECT: indications and outcome. Convulsive Therapy 11:14–23, 1995

Shapira B, Gorfine M, Lerer B: A prospective study of lithium continuation therapy in depressed patients who have responded to electroconvulsive therapy. Convulsive Therapy 11:80–85, 1995

Silfverskiold P, Gustafon L, Risberg J: Changes in regional cerebral blood flow during ECT, in ECT: Basic Mechanisms. Edited by Lerer B, Weiner R, Belmaker R. Washington, DC, American Psychiatric Press, 1986

Small JG, Milstein V, Klapper MH, et al: Electroconvulsive therapy in the treatment of manic episodes. Ann NY Acad Sci 462:37–49, 1986

Sobin C, Sackeim HA, Prudic J, et al: Predictors of retrograde amnesia following ECT. Am J Psychiatry 152:995–1001, 1995

Squire LR, Slater PC: Electroconvulsive therapy and complaints of memory dysfunction: a prospective three-year follow-up study. Br J Psychiatry 142:1–8, 1983

Squire LR, Slater PC, Chance PM: Retrograde amnesia: temporal gradient in very long-term memory following electroconvulsive therapy. Science 187:77–79, 1975

Stoudemire A, Hill CD, Morris R, et al: Improvement in depression-related cognitive dysfunction following ECT. J Neuropsychiatry Clin Neurosci 7:31–34, 1995

Weiner RD: The psychiatric use of electrically induced seizures. Am J Psychiatry 136:1507–1516, 1979

Wells DG, Bjorkstein AR: Monoamine oxidase inhibitors revisited. Can J Anaesth 36:64–74, 1989

Yudofsky SC: ECT in general hospital psychiatry: focus on new indications and technologies. Gen Hosp Psychiatry 3:292–296, 1981

Yudofsky SC: Electroconvulsive therapy in the eighties: technique and technologies. Am J Psychother 36:391–398, 1982

Yudofsky SC, Hales RE, Ferguson T: What You Need to Know About Psychiatric Drugs. New York, Grove Weidenfeld, 1991

APPENDIX: CHEMICAL STRUCTURES OF SELECTED PSYCHOTROPIC MEDICATIONS

 Antidepressants

TCAs

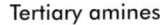

Tertiary amines

Amitriptyline

Imipramine

Secondary amines

Desipramine

Nortriptyline

SSRIs

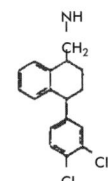

Fluoxetine

Paroxetine

Sertraline

Other 2nd-generation antidepressants

Bupropion

Mirtazapine

Nefazodone

Venlafaxine

MAOIs

Isocarboxazid

Phenelzine

Tranylcypromine

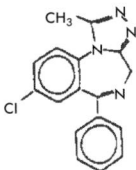 **Anxiolytics**

Alprazolam

Buspirone

Clonazepam

Lorazepam

C   Antipsychotics

Conventional

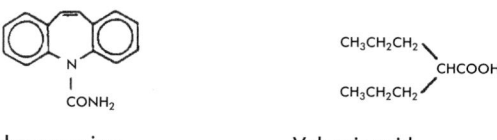

Fluphenazine

Haloperidol

Atypical

Clozapine

Olanapine

Risperidone

D   Mood stabilizers

Carbamazepine

Valproic acid

CHAPTER 28

BRIEF DYNAMIC INDIVIDUAL PSYCHOTHERAPY

HANNA LEVENSON, PH.D.
STEPHEN F. BUTLER, PH.D.

It has now been established in a number of studies with a variety of patients—across a range of settings with diverse agendas—that regardless of the type of outpatient treatment patients begin (e.g., long-term psychotherapy, short-term therapy), the great majority are seen only for 6 to 12 sessions (Garfield 1986; Goldman and Taube 1988; Olfson and Pincus 1994; Phillips 1987). In fact, it has been estimated that 50% of all outpatients drop out of treatment before the eighth session (Phillips 1987). These findings hold even when the treatments are specifically psychodynamic in nature.

Although there is evidence that the majority of therapy is brief, most of these therapies have been unplanned brief treatments (e.g., premature terminations, dropouts, no-shows). Levenson and colleagues, however, attempted to assess the prevalence of intentional short-term treatments. In a comprehensive national survey of 3,600 psychologists, psychiatrists, and social workers (response rate = 57%), almost all respondents in the three disciplines

(89% of psychologists, 77% of psychiatrists, and 84% of social workers) reported conducting some planned brief therapy (i.e., therapy designed to be limited in duration and/or focus) (Davidovitz and Levenson 1995). Overall, the psychodynamically oriented psychiatrists, psychologists, and social workers were responsible for one-quarter of all brief therapy conducted nationally. The type of location in which the therapy was conducted (rural, nonmetropolitan, or metropolitan) had no effect on the proportion of therapists conducting brief therapy or the amount of time spent conducting such therapy. In a random survey of 1,500 psychologists licensed in California or Massachusetts (response rate = 58%), Levenson et al. (1995) found that 80% of respondents were conducting some form of brief therapy and 40% of their clinical time was spent on this type of therapy. As expected, cognitive-behavior therapists conducted brief therapy for the greatest number of hours per week, and psychodynamic therapists spent the least amount of time conducting brief

The authors gratefully acknowledge the contributions of Drs. Joanna S. Burg, Robert Weisman, and David Overstreet to various sections.

therapy. Therefore, most mental health professionals are conducting treatments that are short-term, whether by default or by design.

In our first section we examine the past and present practice of short-term dynamic psychotherapy. We then elucidate those qualities that we believe describe contemporary, brief dynamic psychotherapy. In subsequent sections we examine clinically relevant research and factors influencing the practice of brief dynamic psychotherapy, such as training and therapist reluctance to use briefer treatment modes. We conclude with our best guesses regarding the future of brief dynamic psychotherapy.

HISTORICAL PERSPECTIVE

We provide a history of short-term therapy to emphasize the fact that brief therapy is not new. As pointed out by Miller (1996), "to a large extent, the implementation of brief therapy innovations occurred before managed care came to dominate mental health services" (p. 355). From a historical and conceptual viewpoint, short-term dynamic psychotherapies may be conveniently grouped into "generations" (Crits-Christoph et al. 1991). We will briefly mention four such generations as a way of tracing the evolution in the thinking and practice of brief dynamic psychotherapy. For further information on the history of brief dynamic psychotherapy, the reader is referred to Marmor's (1979) overview as well as to the original works.

FIRST GENERATION: FREUD AND PSYCHOANALYSIS

Contemporary brief dynamic psychotherapy is anchored in the work of Freud. Several of Freud's early treatments were short-term therapies. As described by Marmor (1979), Bruno Walter, the conductor, was treated successfully by Freud in six sessions in 1906, and in 1908 Freud cured Gustav Mahler, the composer, of impotency problems in one single 4-hour session. Even training analyses were conducted in less than 1 year. As psychoanalytic theory became more complex and elaborate, and the goals of analysis became more ambitious, the length of treatments increased. Freud's focus on free association was what Davanloo (1986) called a "fateful step," from which the early advocates of brief psychotherapy began to diverge. Davanloo noted: "Almost all attempts to reverse this trend and develop an effective technique of short-term psychotherapy have been based on taking back some of the control and putting more of the motive power [for the treatment] into the hands of the therapist" (p. 108).

In 1925, Sandor Ferenczi and Otto Rank published *The Development of Psychoanalysis*, in which were advocated time limits, a focus for the treatment, and a frequently active stance for the therapist. Even by today's standards, these authors' contributions to brief dynamic psychotherapy remain innovative and central to modern dynamic approaches. Ferenczi and Rank wished to increase the therapist's activity to counter the patient's passivity. Presaging many aspects both of object relations and of the interpersonal brief therapies was Ferenczi's stress on the frankness, empathy, and democracy of the patient-therapist relationship (Rachman 1988). Rank introduced precursors of two additional tenets of modern brief psychotherapy: 1) the issue of separation activated by setting a time limit in advance (Rank's concept of the *birth trauma*) and 2) assessment of the patient's motivation to change (Rank's concept of the *will*). For these reasons, Marmor (1979) wrote that Rank "may well be the most important historical forerunner of the brief dynamic psychotherapy movement" (p. 150).

Several years after Freud's death in 1939, another serious challenge to classical psychoanalysis unfolded. In their seminal book *Psychoanalytic Therapy: Principles and Applications*, Alexander and French (1946) questioned the presumed relationship between therapeutic outcome and length of therapy. Their book has been recognized by some current practitioners as the first brief therapy manual. Alexander and French's best-known recommendation is that psychotherapists should actively adjust their conduct or manner so that patients are provided with a "corrective emotional experience." Alexander and French advocated therapist flexibility and adjustment of the length and frequency of sessions. These maneuvers were intended to prevent the patient's passive dependency and the development of a transference neurosis. Intense controversy occurred within the psychoanalytic community in reaction to the ideas of Ferenczi, Rank, and Alexander and French, and, thus, the contributions of these investigators were ignored for many years.

SECOND GENERATION: SHORT-TERM DYNAMIC PSYCHOTHERAPIES

In this phase, from 1960 to 1980, brief dynamic therapy began to emerge as a legitimate therapeutic method. David Malan of the Tavistock Clinic in London, James Mann of Boston University School of Medicine, Peter Sifneos of Massachusetts General Hospital in Boston, and Habib Davanloo of Montreal General Hospital in Canada are usually seen as the main representatives of this generation.

Malan's brief therapy techniques derive from psychoanalytic principles—an "applied psychoanalysis" (Ursano and Hales 1986). Malan believed that "far reaching changes could be brought about in relatively severe and chronic illnesses by a technique of active interpretation containing all the essential elements of full scale analysis" (Malan 1976, p. 20). Malan concentrated on identification of a focal problem—a "nuclear" or childhood conflict that is manifested in some form in the current presenting problem. He emphasized making interpretations linking recurrent, maladaptive patterns apparent in the therapist-patient relationship (i.e., transference) with patterns evidenced in present and past relationships (i.e., triangle of insight). For example, the therapist might point out that a patient's deferential and dependent manner toward the therapist seems characteristic of childhood interactions that the patient had with his or her parents. Malan would also be interested in understanding the pattern of the patient's impulses, defenses, and anxieties concerning the focus (i.e., triangle of conflict). For example, the therapist would explore why the aforementioned patient needed to adopt an acquiescent attitude with the parents.

Mann is credited with deriving a generic theoretical orientation that focuses on the difficulties in dealing with separation and loss (Levenson and Butler 1997; Mann 1973). His *time-limited treatment* consists of 12 sessions. It is asserted that the fixed duration forces the patient to face unconscious issues related to the passage of time. In the relationship with the therapist, the patient is thought to relive (in a healthier way) reunion with and separation from that parent who has failed the patient and who is regarded with ambivalence and guilt.

Sifneos developed techniques and a rationale for his *short-term anxiety-provoking psychotherapy* (STAPP; Sifneos 1987). He contributed greater specificity to selection and exclusion criteria, focus of inquiry, and anxiety-provoking intervention techniques. His work focuses on the efficacy of brief dynamic therapy with relatively high-functioning patients experiencing conflicts associated with oedipal issues. No number of sessions is agreed on at the outset, but a length between 6 and 20 sessions is determined as the therapy proceeds. Sifneos assumes a role that is part therapist and part teacher (Bloom 1992). Burke et al. (1979) more descriptively noted that Sifneos "is like a schoolmaster seeing through the excuses and alibis of his recalcitrant pupils" (p. 178).

Davanloo, after training under Malan, developed his *intensive short-term dynamic psychotherapy* (ISTDP) approach. ISTDP was designed to break through the patient's defensive barrier using confrontive techniques similar to those of Sifneos. Vagueness, tentativeness, detachment, evasiveness, diversionary tactics, intellectualization, rationalization, rumination, projection, introjec-

tion, and weepiness are dramatically pointed out to patients to intensify feelings and crystallize the patients' resistance. The crisis of being confronted by the therapist "produces intense affects which tap into a reservoir of unconscious thoughts, memories and feelings, and activate the unconscious therapeutic alliance. This dynamic flow speeds and compresses the psychoanalytic process" (Laiken et al. 1991, p. 93). Davanloo (1978) sees himself as "the relentless healer." He is particularly interested in working with patients who have chronic, serious psychopathology; consequently, he offers treatment to a wider range of patients than do many other brief dynamic therapists.

THIRD GENERATION: RESEARCH-BASED INTERPERSONAL THERAPIES

The approaches of the second generation furthered the practice of brief dynamic psychotherapy, but empirical support was sparse. Selection criteria and interventions were formulated primarily by ideology, clinical judgment, and theoretical inference, rather than by systematic application of research findings (Perry et al. 1983).

The third generation of brief therapies has done much to provide empirical support for the efficacy of brief dynamic therapy, as well as to elucidate its active therapeutic ingredients. However, these therapies have tended to exclude particularly difficult patients from their research for methodological reasons. In addition to an empirical emphasis, the third-generation therapies herald a move away from *intra*psychic models of theory and practice to more *inter*personal ones. Representatives of this wave are *time-limited dynamic psychotherapy* (TLDP), developed by Hans Strupp and Jeffrey Binder at Vanderbilt University (Strupp and Binder 1984); *supportive-expressive psychotherapy*, formulated by Lester Luborsky at the University of Pennsylvania (Luborsky et al. 1990); and *control mastery theory*, created by Joseph Weiss and Harold Sampson at Mount Zion Hospital in San Francisco (Weiss et al. 1986).

As an example of this research-based interpersonal approach, Strupp and Binder's TLDP will be briefly reviewed. A manual for the practice of TLDP, *Psychotherapy in a New Key* (Strupp and Binder 1984), was developed as part of efforts of the Vanderbilt Psychotherapy Research Team. This manual, which was designed to standardize the application of TLDP technique, represents an attempt to make the model more learnable. (Some of the drawbacks of "manualized" therapies will be discussed later.)

TLDP has a psychoanalytic foundation; however, personality development and functioning are viewed from an interpersonal and object relations perspective. The major objective of TLDP is to examine recurrent, maladaptive themes from the patient's range of object relations that are activated in relation to the therapist. Consistent focus is directed to the patient's manner of construing and relating to the therapist both as a significant person in the present and as the personification of past relationships. The patient-therapist relationship is conceived of as a dyadic system in which the behavior of both participants is continually scrutinized and modified (Strupp and Binder 1984). The rationale for this approach stems from the view that regardless of the severity of psychopathology, interpersonal relations are the arena in which intrapsychic conflict is expressed. Very much in the tradition of Alexander and French, the goal of TLDP is to provide the patient with a new (i.e., healthier) experience of himself or herself and the other person (i.e., corrective interpersonal experience). In addition, the therapist, as Strupp and Binder (1984) noted, "helps patients discover, identify, and understand the meanings of the beliefs, feelings, and action patterns that interfere with their current living, built on erroneous and obsolescent assumptions carried forward automatically from earlier phases" (p. 137). The duration of treatment is approximately 25 sessions and is established very early in treatment.

FOURTH GENERATION: MANAGED HEALTH CARE

The fourth wave, which coexists with the second and third generations of brief dynamic psychotherapies, reflects the powerful major economic and market demands that are affecting the provision of mental health care. Numerous writers have discussed the current state of crisis in the health care industry, the urgent need for cost containment, and the impact and implications of this situation on mental health care providers and their clients (see, for example, Austad et al. 1988; Barron and Sands 1996; Fraser 1996; Koss et al. 1986). Predictions that from 45% (Austad et al. 1988) to 79% (Berkman et al. 1988) of the population will receive their health care, including mental health services, through a managed care system have come true. As a result, the nature of clinical work is being dramatically altered.

The current emphasis on briefer formats to meet the expectations for service delivery has led researchers and practitioners to address issues such as the ongoing need for more research and training in brief therapy, the necessity for clinicians to rethink their role in the health care field, and the need for mental health care providers to become more flexible in their treatment approaches. Increasing emphasis has been placed on the idea that the psychotherapist should function similarly to the old-fashioned family

doctor, who provides "brief, intermittent therapy through the life cycle," treating not only the problems of the individual client but, when indicated, those of other family members as well (Cummings 1987, p. 357).

Psychological health care that is provided by health maintenance organizations (HMOs) or financed by third-party payers tends to be severely limited in duration by either required practice styles, utilization review, or capitation (absolute dollar limits). The maximum number of sessions covered by HMOs or third-party payers is almost always 20 or fewer and in practice is considerably lower; an average of 2.5, 4.7, or 6.6 sessions is not uncommon (Miller 1996). Some authors have distinguished between brief therapy and that practiced in managed care settings by giving the latter a different label (e.g., "HMO-therapy" [Austad and Berman 1991] or "ultrabrief therapy" [Miller 1996]). Most of the models for short-term dynamic psychotherapy specify a treatment longer than an HMO would find desirable. Thus, there can be critical differences between brief therapy as practiced traditionally and brief therapy as practiced in many managed care settings. For an elucidation on how brief therapies are relevant for managed care, the reader is referred to the *Concise Guide to Brief Dynamic Psychotherapy* (Levenson and Butler 1997).

QUALITIES THAT DEFINE BRIEF DYNAMIC PSYCHOTHERAPY

What are the essential features that distinguish brief dynamic psychotherapy from other types of therapy? A review of the literature of the past 20 years reveals numerous publications addressing this topic (e.g., Bauer and Kobos 1987; Burlingame and Fuhriman 1987; Crits-Christoph and Barber 1991; Flegenheimer 1982; Gustafson 1984; Koss and Shiang 1994; Koss et al. 1986; Levenson 1995; Levenson and Hales 1993; MacKenzie 1991; Magnavita 1993; Marmor 1979; Mendelsohn 1978; Messer and Warren 1995; Small 1979; Wolberg 1980). A content analysis of these papers reveals a number of fundamental qualities. Some of these qualities have been mentioned repeatedly in the literature and, therefore, appear to be quite essential in defining brief dynamic psychotherapy; others are less frequently reported and seem more peripheral.

The qualities of brief dynamic psychotherapy can, in general, be organized into two main categories: those qualities pertaining to the *brief features* per se and those germane to the *psychodynamic aspects* (Table 28–1). Within each category the qualities are rank-ordered in terms of the number of times they are mentioned in these various publi-

TABLE 28–1. Qualities that define brief psychodynamic psychotherapy

Brief qualities

Limited focus (and limited goals)

Limited time

Selection criteria

Therapist activity

Therapeutic alliance

Rapid assessment/prompt intervention

Termination

Optimism

Contract

Psychodynamic qualities

Analytic concepts

Analytic techniques

Note. Qualities based on the frequency with which they are mentioned in the literature.

cations. These characteristics may be conceptualized as a consensual, operational definition of short-term dynamic psychotherapy. The first four brief qualities—limited focus and goals, limited time, selection criteria, and increased therapist activity—will be examined in some detail, followed by a discussion of brief therapy modifications in psychoanalytic concepts and techniques.

LIMITED THERAPEUTIC FOCUS

A major concept distinguishing the brief dynamic psychotherapy approaches from long-term psychotherapy or psychoanalysis is the idea of a limited focus of treatment. Probably the earliest attempt to provide a focus for analytically oriented treatment was when Rank (1929/1936) set a predetermined termination date and concentrated on the separation issues stimulated by this date. Ferenczi and Rank (1925) argued against attempting a complete analysis for every patient when they noted that "in the correctly executed analysis the whole development of the individual is not repeated, but only those phases of development of the infantile libido on which the ego . . . has remained fixed" (p. 19). Alexander and French (1946), likewise, argued that it is not necessary to analyze all aspects of every patient's mental life. Rather, the analysis need extend back only to the point at which the trauma causing the patient difficulty occurred (Flegenheimer 1982). Furthermore, Alexander and French (1946) advocated limiting the patient's regression by using such modifications as reducing the frequency of sessions and using a chair instead of a couch.

Brief therapists need a central theme, topic, or problem to serve as a guide so that they will be able to stay on target—a necessity when time is of the essence. Brief therapists cannot pay attention to all clinical data; even fascinating material must sometimes be ignored. Practitioners working with short-term models must learn to use *selective attention* (Malan 1963) and *benign neglect* (Pumpian-Mindlin 1953) or they run the risk of being overwhelmed by the patient's rich intrapsychic and interpersonal life.

A detailed presentation of the different foci represented by the various brief dynamic theorists is beyond the scope of this chapter. However, in Table 28–2 we summarize the focus of treatment for several of the main brief dynamic theorists. The reader is referred to the original sources or to the excellent volume edited by Crits-Christoph and Barber (1991) for more information.

Examination of the different brief dynamic psychotherapies reveals some general trends in the development of focal methods. As previously stated, the theoretical emphasis of brief dynamic therapy has shifted from an intrapsychic to an interpersonal focus, deemphasizing wishes and impulses in favor of efforts to define recurrent interpersonal patterns that create and maintain dysfunctional relationships in the patient's life. This interpersonal focus is typically identified early in the treatment and communicated to the patient, and digressions away from the focus are discouraged. In general, vignettes of interpersonal interactions with significant others are scrutinized by the therapist to extract repetitive maladaptive efforts to deal with interpersonal conflict. The patient's transference reaction to the therapist is presumed to be an expression of the same basic relationship problems that create difficulty for the patient in his or her daily life. The different theorists proffer different explanations for the link between the patient's core conflicts and the presenting symptomatology, but all agree that these relationship themes must be addressed in the therapy.

A particularly important development in the field is reflected in the efforts of Luborsky and colleagues (1990), Strupp and Binder (1984; Levenson 1995), the Mount Zion Psychotherapy Research Group (Weiss et al. 1986), and Horowitz and colleagues (1984), who offered explicit methodologies for generating a therapeutic focus. Prior to these efforts, a focal theme was left to be intuited based on clinical experience. The development of formalized, systematic methods for defining the focal theme promises more effective means of training therapists (Strupp et al. 1988) and greater accessibility to research protocols for investigating the role actually played by the dynamic focus.

Early research on therapeutic focus was conducted by Malan (1976), who reported that undirected interpretations (i.e., interpretations not associated with a central

TABLE 28–2.   Focus of treatment

Theorist(s)	Focus
Malan	Wish (impulse)–threat–defense (triangle of conflict)
	Therapist–current (parent) relationships–past (parent) relationships (triangle of insight)
Sifneos Short-term anxiety-provoking psychotherapy	Unresolved conflict defined during evaluation—typically oedipal issues
Mann Time-limited psychotherapy	Conflict over time limits and loss—especially the pain and limitations imposed by dealing with loss defensively
Davanloo Intensive short-term dynamic psychotherapy	Triangle of insight Triangle of conflict
Luborsky and Mark Supportive-expressive psychotherapy	Core conflictual relationship theme (CCRT)—wish-response from other-response from self
Strupp and Binder Time-limited dynamic psychotherapy	Cyclical maladaptive patterns/ dynamic focus—acts of self-expectations of others–acts of others–introject
Horowitz Treatment for stress response syndrome	Evaluate impact of stress on state of mind; work through trauma and reactions; integration of traumatic event
Sampson and Weiss Mt. Zion Group	Unconscious pathogenic beliefs that underlie the patient's "plan"

Source.   Adapted from Barber and Crits-Christoph 1991, p. 337.

issue) were negatively associated with outcome. This work, however, has been criticized for its methodology (e.g., no control group, use of case notes rather than audio- or videotapes). Malan's pioneering effort, however, was followed by a study conducted by the Mount Zion group (Silberschatz et al. 1986), which demonstrated that interpretations compatible with the patient's "plan" were more effective than other types of interpretations, including transference interpretations. Similarly, accuracy of interpretations has been found to be predictive of positive outcome (Crits-Christoph et al. 1988; Joyce et al. 1995). A convergence of findings appears to support the efficacy of establishing a focus and maintaining that focus throughout the treatment. However, a caveat is warranted here—namely, that the meager evidence available also supports the notion that the therapist should be *flexible*. Rounsaville et al. (1988) investigated therapists trained to adhere to an interpersonal focus with depressed patients and found that therapists were judged by supervisors to be more skillful when they deviated from the prescribed protocol with difficult patients. Clearly, rigid efforts to adhere to a focus and discourage deviations are likely to damage the therapeutic alliance and result in poor outcome.

Thus, paying attention to material directly related to the focus does not mean coercing patients or ignoring what is important to them. Schacht et al. (1984) emphasized that disregard for what a patient says or does could weaken the therapeutic alliance and be perceived as unempathic by the patient. Rather, the therapist should repeatedly attempt to enable the patient to work on the focal issue: "The therapist's patterning of questions, the timing and shaping of the context for questions, the choices of what to name and what to leave nameless, should all create an associative atmosphere in which focally relevant material predominates because it seems most narratively natural" (Schacht et al. 1984, p. 108). Some general guidelines for developing a psychodynamic focus are given in Table 28–3. These guidelines underscore the importance of sensitive and simultaneous attention to patterns of past and present functioning. As Wolberg (1980) stated,

TABLE 28–3.   General principles for developing a psychodynamic focus

1. Gather historical material and other data, but let the patient tell his or her own story.

2. Study the patient's characteristic defensive pattern.

3. Be sensitive to how present patterns have roots in the past.

4. Watch for transference patterns; deal with negative transference reactions rapidly and supportively.

5. Examine possible countertransference feelings and behavior for clues as to repetitive dysfunctional patterns.

6. Constantly look for resistances that threaten to block progress.

Source.   Adapted from Wolberg 1980.

Little time is available in short-term therapy to explore the past. Much better use can be made of the treatment hour by dealing with pertinent elements in the here and now. However, where the therapist can determine important past events and contingencies that have molded the personality organization, this will facilitate a better understanding of the patient's illness and help select an appropriate dynamic focus. (p. 101)

Bauer and Kobos (1987) contend that "the focus of treatment should be clear, specific, and manageable" (p. 157). Related to, but separate from, therapeutic focus is "manageability" of the focus within the allotted time, sometimes referred to as having "limited goals." The aim of brief dynamic psychotherapy is not "cure" once and for all. Rather, the therapy should provide an opportunity to foster some changes in behavior and thinking, permitting more adaptive coping and a better sense of one's self. Brief dynamic therapy is seen as an opportunity to begin a process of change that continues long after the therapy is over. Additionally, brief therapy is also viewed as rendering appropriate help for brief periods throughout the life cycle. This outlook has resulted in a more general-practice framework for brief psychotherapy (Budman and Gurman 1988) in which therapists (like internists or family practitioners) have discontinuous but enduring relationships with patients as the patients deal with developmental stresses and the intermittent strains of life.

TIME LIMITS AND TIME MANAGEMENT

Naturally, time is the critical variable that defines an approach as *short-term*, *brief*, or *time-limited*. The issue of time is the second most frequently mentioned brief therapy criterion. Although most clinicians set 25 sessions as the upper limit of brief therapy (Koss and Shiang 1994), the number of sessions may range from one session (e.g., Bloom 1992; Hoyt et al. 1992) to as many as 40 (Sifneos 1979).

Time, like focus, can be conceptualized in a variety of ways. Burlingame and Fuhriman (1987) divided considerations of duration into three categories: *specific time limits*, *variable time limits*, and *time attentive considerations* (MacKenzie 1991). Usually the *limiting* or *rationing* of time is used conceptually to accelerate the therapeutic work, either by raising the patient's awareness of the existential issues of finite time and mortality (e.g., Mann 1973) or by encouraging therapist activity and adherence to a focus (e.g., Horowitz et al. 1984).

Although it is most customary for psychodynamically oriented short-term therapists to use the traditional weekly 50-minute "hour," many are experimenting with the fre-

quency of sessions (e.g., frequent initial sessions with more intermittent later sessions), the duration of each therapy session (e.g., the 20-minute "hour"), and even the number of consecutive brief therapies (e.g., intermittent brief therapy throughout the life cycle). Marmor (1979) pointed out that setting time limits has three clinical consequences. First, it emphasizes individuation-separation issues, which commonly underlie presenting problems. Second, it acknowledges the autonomy of the patient. Third, it encourages the patient's independence and self-confidence.

Unfortunately, time limits are being used increasingly for administrative and economic reasons instead of therapeutic ones. In the worst of situations, there may be no therapeutic basis for the number of sessions patients receive, such decisions being determined only by the financial bottom line. In the best of situations, managed care programs monitor the quality of care and promote patients' resourcefulness.

The brief dynamic psychotherapies have been developed for and researched with highly selected, and usually highly functioning, patients (see following subsection on patient selection). It may be dangerous to make the assumption that brief (especially very brief) courses of treatment can be readily extended to severely disturbed patients with chaotic lifestyles. The amount of therapy that is appropriate for the treatment of severe conditions remains an important empirical question. *Variable time limits* are used by some therapeutic models that propose altering the time allotted based on various factors such as therapist experience (Malan 1976) or type and severity of presenting complaint (Davanloo 1978). Strupp and Binder (1984) suggested using 25-session "blocks" of therapy, with sharply defined goals for each block.

More recently, however, brief dynamic therapists are moving away from conceptualizing therapy merely in terms of a specific amount of time and are instead addressing ways to make every session count regardless of length of treatment. These models are categorized as *time attentive*. Examples of this approach include the idea of the therapist's *time-limited attitude* (regardless of the actual length of therapy) (Binder et al. 1987) and the notion of brief therapy as a "state of mind of the therapist and of the patient" (Budman and Gurman 1988, p. 10).

SELECTION CRITERIA

The importance of selection criteria is a controversial subject in the brief dynamic psychotherapy field. Early in the history of psychoanalysis, as psychoanalytic treatments became progressively longer, Freud (1904/1953) put forth the possibility that treatment might be shortened with healthier patients. Largely based on this comment, rigorous patient selection to identify the healthiest patients became an early and integral part of virtually all brief dynamic psychotherapies.

The problem then arose of how to determine which patients were the "healthiest" and which ones would respond well to a brief course of treatment. Rank (1929/1936) introduced the role of the patient's "will" or motivation for therapeutic change. That patients motivated for change are more likely than others to benefit from brief psychotherapy remains an important idea for modern short-term psychodynamic theorists. Later, Alexander and French (1946) proposed that brief treatment was suitable for patients with mild, chronic, and acute neurosis (Flegenheimer 1982). Good motivation, ego strength, and response to trial interpretations were also mentioned, along with the patient's willingness and ability to take an active role in the treatment. Although Alexander held that severity of symptoms bore no relationship to length of treatment, he reserved standard psychoanalysis for severe chronic neurosis.

Following these early pioneers, modern short-term theorists extended the applications of traditional psychoanalytic concepts to patient selection. In their reviews of the psychoanalytic literature on analyzability, Bachrach and Leaff (1978) noted that a patient's suitability for treatment is typically judged from reports of the patient's history and general level of functioning. Such concepts as high ego strength and a history of good object relations are considered prognostic indicators of significant therapeutic gains. Thus, those credited with bringing brief dynamic psychotherapy into the modern therapeutic arena (Malan 1963, 1976, 1979; Mann 1973; Sifneos 1972, 1979; Davanloo 1978, 1980) specified fairly stringent suitability characteristics:

1. Appropriate ego strength
2. Ability to become rapidly involved in and contribute to treatment
3. Adequate motivation
4. A history of meaningful relationships
5. Adequate intelligence or psychological sophistication
6. A relatively circumscribed problem or symptom presentation (as opposed to wide-ranging difficulties in many aspects of the patient's life)

In addition, these authors specified relatively consistent exclusion criteria, such as psychosis, major affective disorders (especially bipolar disorder), drug use, suicidal tendencies (and other acting out) or impulsive tendencies,

organic disorders, and some personality disorders (borderline personality disorder, especially in those patients with histories of acting out, and schizoid personality disorder, when interpersonal unresponsiveness on the part of the patient is noted). Finally, following Malan's (1976) notion of a "trial interpretation," short-term theorists generally suggest an interview or trial session to evaluate the patient's ability to engage in the therapeutic tasks. The inclusion and exclusion criteria for the major short-term dynamic approaches are given in Table 28–4.

How do these selection criteria hold up? Attempts to evaluate patients' suitability for brief dynamic psychotherapy generally recognize that there are two basic approaches. One involves an assessment of the patient's general state of psychological health and tends to focus on psychoanalytic formulations of *patient characteristics* antedating the psychotherapy (such as ego functioning and quality of object relations). However, such concepts are typically highly abstract and difficult to translate into specific clinical and empirical observations. Binder et al. (1987) pointed out that "it is much easier to agree about the importance of 'ego strength' than to specify its manifestations" (p. 156). Similarly, it has proven to be difficult to establish clear, concrete evidence of Sifneos' (1979) requirement of one "meaningful" relationship in the patient's history.

The other approach to evaluate patients' suitability for brief dynamic psychotherapy involves using *performance criteria*, that is, a patient's performance during early interviews. This approach echoes early attempts to gauge the willingness and ability of patients to become actively involved in treatment and their response to trial interpretations. Such trial interpretations were hoped to provide a stimulus from which to assess the patient's insightfulness and manner of dealing with psychological issues, sometimes referred to as *psychological mindedness*. Thus, this in vivo evaluation was thought to provide a direct assessment of the patient's ability to engage in the actual behavior demanded in the therapeutic situation.

Despite its promise, however, performance-based assessment has only minimally enhanced the ability to forecast outcome in brief dynamic psychotherapy. Thackrey and colleagues (1993; Butler et al. 1987) tested a scale that was intended to assess a patient's willingness and ability to engage in psychotherapy and that used low inference judgments made by independent raters and interviewing clinicians. These ratings yielded significant but modest correlations with outcome ($r = .30–.52$), accounting for 9%–25% of the variance in process and outcome measures. Thus, 75%–91% of the variance was *not accounted for* by ratings of the patient's performance in an early interview.

TABLE 28-4. Criteria for patient selection for brief dynamic psychotherapy

Theorist(s)	Inclusion criteria	Exclusion criteria
Malan	Capacity to form good relationships Good response to trial interpretations	Addictions, serious suicide attempts, ECT Severe major depression, acting out

Sifneos
Short-term anxiety-provoking
  psychotherapy
	Intelligence, psychological mindedness
	History of meaningful relationships
	Motivation for change beyond symptom
	  relief
	Appropriate affect during interview
	One major and specific complaint
		Psychosis, major affective syndrome,
		  addiction
		Suicidal tendencies and acting out
		Severe personality disorder

Mann
Time-limited psychotherapy
	Good ego strength, capacity for
	  rapid affective connection
	Definable focus
	Mild neurosis and personality disorders
		Psychosis, schizoid, and severe obsessional
		  personality disorders
		Severe psychosomatic disorders

Davanloo
Intensive short-term dynamic
  psychotherapy
	Wide range
	Pass trial therapy
		Psychosis, severe major depression, brain
		  damage, suicidal tendencies and acting
		  out, addictions
		"Decompensation" during or following
		  trial therapy

Luborsky and Mark
Supportive-expressive psychotherapy
		Psychotics, borderline personality disorder,
		  suicidal acting out, antisocial personality
		  without depression

Strupp and Binder
Time-limited dynamic psychotherapy
	Coherent, identifiable interpersonal
	  theme
	Distinction between self and others
	Capacity for human relationships
	Ability to form collaborative relationship
	  with therapist	

Horowitz
Treatment for stress response syndrome
	One or few recent traumatic events	Lack of capacity to be collaborative
		Unwillingness to enhance strength
		  (e.g., addiction)
		Value conflict with therapist
		Normative life crisis
		Inability to keep acting-out behavior under
		  control
		Active psychosis, brain damage

Sampson and Weiss **Mt. Zion Group** Plan formulation method	History of positive interpersonal relationships	Psychosis Organic brain syndrome Mental deficiency Serious substance abuse Suicide potential

Note. ECT = electroconvulsive therapy.
Source. Adapted from Barber and Crits-Christoph 1991, pp. 328–330.

Several possibilities might explain these disappointing results. First, as in most controlled psychotherapy studies, this study's inclusion criteria eliminated the most severe psychopathology. Thus, patients with psychosis, patients currently requiring hospitalization, actively suicidal or homicidal patients, and patients with active, severe comorbid substance abuse were excluded. Restricting the range of studied patients in this way would be expected to reduce the chances of obtaining strong correlations. The correlations observed in this study would undoubtedly have been higher had a broader range of patients been included.

Patients with severe personality disorder, for example, would seem less likely to benefit from brief psychodynamic therapy. Horowitz et al. (1986) reported that brief (i.e., 12-session) focused dynamic therapy was insufficient to improve the functioning of patients with more severe personality disorders. Likewise, Shea et al. (1990) found that depressed patients with personality disorders had worse outcomes than did patients without personality disorders after 16 sessions of treatment. On the other hand, Levenson and Overstreet (1993) found significant changes in some patients with personality disorders after 15 sessions of dynamic therapy. Also, some patients with personality disorders in the study by Thackrey and colleagues (Butler et al. 1987; Thackrey et al. 1993) were deemed suitable for outpatient brief therapy.

Kopta et al. (1994) found that it took half of the patients with acute distress symptoms (e.g., crying easily) an average of 5 sessions to return to normal functioning, whereas it took the same proportion of patients with chronic distress symptoms (e.g., feelings of guilt) an average of 14 sessions to achieve the same result. Patients with character symptoms (e.g., inability to trust others) required more than 52 sessions.

Hoglend (1993) found that patients with personality disorders did more poorly 2 years after brief dynamic therapy (9 to 53 sessions) than did patients without personality disorders. These groups, however, were not significantly different at the 4-year follow-up. Furthermore, there was some evidence that patients with personality disorders who received more therapy were the ones who did better in the long run. Perhaps the most interesting point made by this study is a methodological one—namely, that the effects of additional sessions on patients with personality disorders may not be evident at termination or even at the 1-year follow-up, the time point typically used in psychotherapy research designs.

One compounding problem in using such constructs in personality diagnosis to determine suitability was highlighted by Binder et al. (1987). These authors pointed to the fact that certain patients appeared bright, articulate, and seemingly insightful during the trial therapy interview, yet their "insights" tended to be superficial. The intellectual formulations of these patients camouflaged subtle, automatic maneuvers aimed at resisting true collaboration with the therapist. Furthermore, some patients who evidenced verbal fluency and intelligence in an initial interview appeared to use these qualities in therapy to divert attention away from painful emotional concerns. Finally, these evaluations did not take into account the contribution of the therapist. In several cases, the patient's problems in relating interpersonally were exacerbated in therapy by the therapist's counterresponse (i.e., countertransference) to the patient's style.

All of this suggests that prediction of a given patient's response to brief psychotherapy is risky. The kinds of scientific investigations just described are important in terms of identifying and defining explicitly relevant therapist and patient variables and for generating research hypotheses regarding how these variables interact. Clinically, however, such selection criteria can be used only to make very qualified predictions of how an individual patient will respond to therapy. As clinicians, we must also recognize that patients are not mere passive vessels whose conditions we diagnose and offer prognoses for. Rather, patients are responsive to our predictions and may respond to a judgment that they are "too sick" for brief therapy or "not sick enough" for long-term therapy in ways that confound our notions of how psychotherapy is supposed to work.

The present authors' position on the use of selection criteria is that, given the present state of knowledge, virtually any psychotherapy with virtually any patient can benefit from a time-limited attitude on the part of the therapist. This involves the promotion of a consistent, active engagement of both patient and therapist in the therapeutic relationship. Impediments on the part of the patient to becoming so engaged become an important issue to be addressed in the therapy.

THERAPIST ACTIVITY

Flegenheimer (1982) noted that

> it is striking to compare pages of written transcripts of long-term and brief therapy. While the former will show long productions by the patient interspersed with brief comments by the therapist, the brief therapy transcripts show almost equal productions by patient and therapist. . . .
>
> The activity of the therapist also brings a special tone to the therapeutic situation. By his or her activity the therapist shows an interest in the work at hand, and the properly selected patient will respond to this by an increase in motivation and interest in the treatment. (pp. 7–8)

Brief dynamic psychotherapy emphasizes the need for increased amounts of therapist activity. However, *activity* is only necessary to the extent that one needs to maintain the *focus* and make progress within a certain amount of *time*. Thus, activity is integrally related to the aforementioned aspects of focus and time. It is only through the interventions of the therapist that the focus can be achieved within a specified period. Mendelsohn (1978), writing on critical factors in short-term psychotherapy, viewed focusing as a type of therapist activity.

Many clinicians, when learning brief therapy techniques, become confused that therapist activity means confrontation, advice giving, or directive support. What it more appropriately entails is an awareness of the goals of the work and a plan of how to get there while being sensitive to the patient's presentation and the context of the clinical material. Therapist activity should aid the patient in increasing focally relevant thoughts and behaviors. As Schacht et al. (1984) noted, "If [therapy is] carried out in a crude, mechanical, or unempathic manner the patient may reject the therapist's efforts as tedious carping and the therapy may reach an impasse" (p. 108). Similarly, MacKenzie (1991) acknowledged that "clinical skill is required to be active, yet not controlling; stimulating, but not taking over" (p. 403).

That there can be detrimental results from therapist activity has been empirically demonstrated. Henry et al. (1993a) found that training therapists to become more active as they learn how to do time-limited dynamic psychotherapy may actually give them more opportunities to make clinical errors (see subsection on training later in this section). As Strupp (1982) poetically observed, "Therapy without guidance results in chaos; forcible therapy has its own built-in defeats; the therapist's task is to find the optimum balance. The therapist, like the good parent, needs to know how to love without spoiling and to discipline without hurting..." (p. 68). Several writers (e.g., Flegenheimer 1982; MacKenzie 1991) elaborated on how the focusing activity of the therapist not only keeps the therapy on target but also lessens patient regression and the development of a transference neurosis (i.e., the acting out of the patient's conflicts in the therapy), both of which could inhibit therapeutic progress in the abbreviated length of time. Typically the activity of the psychodynamic brief therapist refers to an increase in and earlier timing of interpretations, usually involving transference issues. This brings us to a discussion of brief therapy modifications of analytic concepts and techniques.

MODIFICATIONS OF PSYCHOANALYTIC CONCEPTS AND TECHNIQUES

Brief psychodynamic therapists adhere to many of the psychoanalytically inspired concepts familiar to the various forms of psychotherapy such as Freudian, ego analytic, object relations, interpersonal, and self psychology therapy. Specifically, brief dynamic therapeutic work relies on major psychoanalytic and psychodynamic concepts such as the importance of childhood experiences and developmental history, unconscious determinants of behavior, the role of conflicts, the transference relationship between therapist and patient, the patient's resistance to the therapeutic work, and repetitive behavior. Many brief therapists, however, do not feel obliged to adopt elaborate metapsychological models that incorporate highly infer-

ential constructs. Instead, they prefer to stick close to the observable data. Such an inclination may stem from the need to do pragmatic clinical work and from the interest many brief theorists have in conducting research, for which variables must be precisely defined.

Similarly, the techniques used in brief dynamic psychotherapy have been inspired by those used in psychoanalysis and long-term dynamic therapy:

> That is, the therapist makes use of clarifications and interpretations, pays attention to the transference and countertransference, and addresses other repetitive, often maladaptive, patterns of behavior, especially in the interpersonal domain. In general, no direct advice is given. Unlike formal psychoanalysis, brief dynamic psychotherapies use free association for specific issues and not as a general rule of treatment. (Crits-Christoph and Barber 1991, pp. 2–3)

As Crits-Christoph and Barber's description suggests, some classical techniques have been modified to be more compatible with a limited focus and limited time. Perhaps the most notable of these modifications is that of the *early transference interpretation*. Flegenheimer (1982) saw early interpretation of transference as preventing the occurrence of a transference neurosis: "The early interpretation of transference manifestations brings these phenomena under the scrutiny of the observing portion of the patient's ego, putting the patient on guard, so to speak, against the dangers of dependency and regression which lie ahead" (p. 9). Still others see value in demonstrating to the patient his or her characteristic style of relating. An example from a second hour of a brief psychotherapy will illustrate:

> A 45-year-old patient had been talking about how her parents always found fault with her and tried to make her feel inferior. The therapist pursued a series of questions in an attempt to understand the patient's parental experiences and dynamics better. The patient responded in an angry tone, "Your questions! I just don't know what you want or how to answer." To which the therapist replied, "Do you get the feeling that I want to make you feel stupid like your parents did?"

This early transference interpretation highlighted for the patient how the same interpersonal dynamic evident with her parents might also be occurring with her therapist. In addition, it also served to bring into awareness the negative feelings the patient was having in this early phase of treatment. Making such negative feelings obvious serves to limit their being acted on by the patient (e.g., prematurely ending therapy), a situation that often cannot be dealt with effectively within the brief format.

Another major modification of psychoanalytic technique involves the gathering of psychosocial and historical information. Clearly, in a brief therapy, the amount of time devoted to obtaining background material must be curtailed. Many brief therapists employ the concept of a *focused history*, in which the patient begins to tell his or her own story and the therapist asks clarifying questions designed to obtain information relevant to a particular theme that is emerging in the therapy. For example, a patient might enter therapy saying he is afraid his girlfriend might leave him. The therapist could ask whether he has had similar fears with other persons in the past. Or the therapist could pursue losses the patient has experienced in his life. Both of these lines of inquiry would be different from having a fixed set of intake questions covering such topics as family history and school history.

Also with regard to acquiring information, many brief dynamic therapists put less emphasis on knowing factual genetic material. They are more likely to base their focus and interventions on an assessment of patients in the here and now. How are the patients presenting themselves? Why now? What is the nature of the interaction between patient and therapist? What seem to be the characteristic defenses used? What is the therapist's own countertransference?

In summary, short-term psychodynamic psychotherapies can be described as treatments of limited duration in which therapists are active in maintaining a circumscribed focus with limited goals using a framework of psychoanalytically derived concepts and techniques.

FACTORS RELATED TO THE PRACTICE OF BRIEF DYNAMIC PSYCHOTHERAPY

MANAGED CARE, CONSUMERISM, AND THE ZEITGEIST

Managed care takes various forms, such as HMOs, preferred provider organizations (PPOs), independent practice associations, employee assistance programs (EAPs), and utilization review. Such systems have been established for the ostensible purpose of controlling costs while promoting efficient and effective (but usually limited-access) treatments. However, Bennett (1988) summarized that "over the past 15 years the health maintenance organization . . . movement has abandoned its social objectives in favor of economic ones" (p. 1544). Some writers (e.g.,

Ackley 1993) have suggested that the managed care industry, now so monetarily driven, be renamed the "managed cost industry."

More than one-half of the respondents to the national survey (Davidovitz and Levenson 1995) and the state survey (Levenson et al. 1995) were providing services for a PPO or an HMO. Another survey of therapists from several disciplines revealed that two-thirds had adopted time-limited therapy techniques or shortened the length of the therapy because of the restraints of managed care. Sixty percent of respondents reported that their incomes had declined (Fee, Practice and Managed Care Survey 1995). In a 1989 national survey of psychiatrists conducted by the American Psychiatric Association, 60% of those surveyed said they had received pressure from outside organizations to shorten inpatient hospitalizations and to deny treatment (Dorwart 1990).

It is no accident that much of the interest in brief approaches has occurred at a time when short-term interventions are being mandated by organizations needing to accommodate consumer needs within fiscal constraints. In a book on the subject of psychotherapy in managed health care, published by the American Psychological Association, Austad and Berman (1991) discussed what they call "HMO psychotherapy, . . . in which the parameters of treatment have been modified both consciously and unconsciously, to be compatible with the philosophy, theory, and economic and pragmatic conditions of a managed care system" (p. 8).

Recently, there has been a heated debate concerning the clinical, ethical, and practical effects of managed care practices on the delivery of mental health services (e.g., Austad 1996; Chipman 1995; Cummings 1995; Karon 1995; Stern 1993). (See Chapter 47 in the current volume.) Each side in this "psychobattle" (Hymowitz and Pollock 1995) has accused the other of bad practices, as is evident in the titles of some of the two sides' publications (e.g., "Is Long-Term Psychotherapy Unethical?" [Austad 1996] and "Managed Care Is Harmful to Outpatient Mental Health Services" [Miller 1996]). Iglehart (1996) made the point that at present little is known about the efficacy and effectiveness of these ultrabrief treatments.

The push for briefer treatments, however, is not based solely on economic considerations. Professionals in the mental health care system are concerned about providing more rapid relief of suffering and making services available to more people. Those persons seeking help are demanding the most for their time and money in an age of consumer awareness. Potential patients (more likely called *clients* or *consumers*) are questioning therapists (*providers*) regarding what results can be expected in what amount of time. Messer and Warren (1995) commented on other factors leading to an increase in short-term interventions: improved access to treatment by the Community Mental Health Centers Act of 1963; increased attention to the benefits of therapy through the popular media; decreased length of hospitalization; and development of brief, empirically based treatments.

Some commentators have also considered that the push toward brief therapies stems from American society's fascination with quick solutions. Cartoons in the popular press depict therapy drive-up windows ("Brief Therapy 1990"), and an article in *U.S. News and World Report* ("Therapy for the '90s" 1992) noted the following:

> Fast food, it is now clear, was only the beginning. Society has moved on to express checkout lines and automated teller machines, to plain-paper faxes and microwaved dinners. Value, in the 1990s, cleaves to what is quick. So it was perhaps inevitable that someone would come up with the idea of "single-session psychotherapy," an expedited approach to dealing with the ills of the psyche. If an hour is too long to wait for baked chicken, who can spend months or years on the analytic couch? (p. 55)

TRAINING

Another major factor influencing the practice of brief dynamic psychotherapy is training:

> Practice and systematic attention to detail are fundamental to learning any new skill. Short-term therapy based on psychoanalysis seems so familiar that there is a tendency to rush off equipped with one's comfortable therapeutic style and find, with dismay, [that] "there's nothing really new here." This is erroneous. The techniques are similar, but the differences are critical. (Goldin 1985, p. 55)

From the growing mass of clinical and empirical work, it can be stated emphatically that brief dynamic psychotherapy is not simply a shorter version of long-term therapy. The research literature is clear that brief therapy is a different treatment modality requiring specialized training in its own theories and techniques (e.g., Bauer and Kobos 1987; Budman and Stone 1983; Ursano and Hales 1986). However,

> students are instructed in the long-term model (usually psychoanalysis) whereas most patients are, in fact, seen on a short-term basis. The result is that most therapists struggle to develop bootstrap forms of the knowledge they have acquired in formal training to the realities of practice. (Strupp and Binder 1984, p. 6)

Despite its importance, training in brief therapy is far less researched and understood than brief therapy techniques and outcome. In one of the few studies to document the extent and type of training in brief dynamic psychotherapy, Levenson et al. (1995) found that of those clinicians who regularly offered brief therapy, more than one-third reported having little or no training in it. This is a distressing statistic, particularly because it is now widely accepted that brief therapy is not "dehydrated" long-term therapy (Cummings 1986) or "just less of the same" (Peake et al. 1988). However, the survey data also revealed that professionals with extensive training were conducting considerably more brief therapy than were those who received no training. Also, there is a significant positive relationship between the amount of training and attitudes about and skill in conducting brief therapy. The most common type of brief therapy training experience for the practicing professional is reading, followed by workshops, conferences, and supervision. Supervision, not unexpectedly, was considered to be the most useful experience. Psychiatrists (90% of whom identified themselves as having a psychodynamic or eclectic orientation) reported taking significantly more academic courses than psychologists or social workers. Furthermore, over time there appears to have been an increase in the psychiatric brief therapy course offerings, with 90% of current psychiatrists in practice less than 6 years reporting taking a brief therapy course (compared with 64% of new psychiatrists 20 years ago). However, after residency training, psychiatrists are less likely to take continuing education courses in time-limited therapy than are psychologists and social workers (26% of psychiatrists, 53% of psychologists, and 65% of social workers) (Fee, Practice and Managed Care Survey 1995).

Evans and Levenson (1997) conducted a survey of psychology graduate schools and internships. They found that 60% of institutions with a psychodynamic orientation offered some form of brief therapy training. When the teachers and supervisors in these settings were asked to identify the topics that were most difficult for trainees to grasp, they indicated the following: setting of limited goals, adherence to a focus, making a paradigm shift, rapid development of an alliance, and attitudinal bias toward long-term therapy.

The parallel processes of supervision and treatment have been observed for years (e.g., Ekstein and Wallerstein 1972). Frances and Clarkin (1981) noted that the brief therapy "treatment context requires a relatively high level of therapist activity and planning, the setting of clear and limited goals, the focus on a single problem or dynamic conflict, and a quick attachment to and then separation from the therapist. These same conditions are characteristic of the work of brief therapy supervision" (p. 244).

Dasberg and Winokur (1984) also discussed parallels between short-term dynamic treatment and training. Specifically, they mentioned similarities in structure and experiences (e.g., changing attitudes over time) and in attributes and actions (e.g., high motivation, commitment to change) between the learner and the patient in brief therapy. Hoyt (1991) pointed out congruences in phase-specific behaviors between supervisor and trainee. For example, early on, problems of focusing and establishing a working alliance may affect both therapy and supervision. Similarly, the supervisor may unrealistically try to "cram unassimilable amounts of clinical lore and wisdom into the last supervision meetings. The trainee, not feeling 'totally educated' and competent, may invite and welcome these eleventh-hour desperations" (Hoyt 1991, p. 105). This is a process that may be paralleled in the ending trainee-patient relationship. Levenson has detailed 10 similarities between supervision in time-limited dynamic psychotherapy (TLDP) and TLDP itself (Table 28–5).

Burlingame et al. (1989) randomly exposed trainee and senior staff of a counseling center to one of three training conditions: no training, self-instructional training, and intensive training (i.e., 10 hours of instruction, demonstration, role-playing, and discussion). All therapists then con-

TABLE 28–5. Parallels between brief therapy supervision and brief therapy treatment

1. Almost same number of meetings (21 vs. 20).
2. Generate hypotheses on relatively little information.
3. Model desirable therapist qualities in supervision (e.g., patience, activity, staying focused, awareness of time constraints, supportive yet confrontive and collaborative).
4. Work actively with trainee resistance.
5. Trainees not only have an educative, intellectual learning experience but also have a new affective experience (e.g., sense of competency).
6. Trainees take responsibility for choosing what they bring up in supervision.
7. Emphasize collaboration between supervisee and supervisor (e.g., supervisor shows own work and is open to feedback from trainees).
8. Create a safe environment in supervision.
9. Concerning termination, trainees are simultaneously dealing with issues about leaving supervision (e.g., have they learned enough) and leaving their patients (e.g., will they be okay).
10. Expectation that trainees will continue to incorporate and integrate what they have learned after the conclusion of the training rotation.

ducted an eight-session time-limited therapy. Although the more experienced therapists had superior outcomes in general, there were indications that greater amounts of training for *both* the inexperienced and experienced therapists led to greater patient improvements. In other words, even experienced therapists gained significantly from the brief therapy training program. The investigators concluded that "if a mental health agency is moving to a time-limited treatment policy in an attempt to be more cost effective, minimal training of [even experienced] therapists may be a more effective way to proceed than merely putting a limit on the number of sessions" (Burlingame et al. 1989, p. 312).

Training manuals have been one approach to provide more specific descriptions of treatment techniques. Butler and Strupp (1993) reviewed some of the best-known "manualized" psychodynamic/interpersonal therapies. One of these is TLDP (Strupp and Binder 1984; Levenson 1995). At the Vanderbilt Center for Psychotherapy Research, Strupp and colleagues completed a study on the effects of specialized training in TLDP (Vanderbilt II study). This 5-year Vanderbilt II study examined the effect of manualized training in TLDP on 16 experienced therapists (8 psychiatrists and 8 psychologists) and 80 patients. For the first phase of the study, therapists were assigned two patients and asked to treat them in up to 25 weekly sessions, as "they ordinarily would treat such patients" (Strupp 1990). In the second year of the study, therapists went through a training program to learn TLDP. The training program consisted of didactic presentations on TLDP principles and techniques, illustrated with clinical examples, and small-group supervision, including discussion of audio- and videotaped sessions of training cases.

In the third phase, therapists again treated two patients, this time according to the tenets of TLDP. The main Vanderbilt II results indicated that the training program was successful in changing therapists' interventions to be congruent with the manual (Henry et al. 1993a). Furthermore, at the 1-year follow-up, patients receiving TLDP (vs. the therapists' usual treatment) showed significant changes on TLDP-relevant interpersonal variables. This significant difference did not occur, however, at termination and was not apparent for less suitable patients.

The Vanderbilt II findings pertinent to the changes in therapists' behavior and their responses to training, however, are quite complex. Although there were positive changes in *general* therapist skills after training (this was not the focus of the training, however), there were also indications of negative changes. For example, the greater activity level of therapists after training resulted in the therapists' having more opportunities to make "mistakes." In addition, after training, therapists appeared less approving and less supportive in their therapies. The investigators speculated that there may be a post-training phase in which there is a decrement in therapists' performance as they attempt to adapt their customary style to accommodate new strategies. Suggestions on how to maximize manualized training effects, based on the Vanderbilt II findings, are presented in Table 28–6.

In addition to manuals, training in brief psychotherapy has emphasized the use of clinical material obtained directly from therapy sessions, including live supervision and use of audio- and videotaping (Evans and Levenson 1997). Goldin (1985) made a special plea for the inclusion of videotape recordings in brief dynamic therapy supervision:

> They enable one to check on the working alliance, find clues to the early development of transference outcroppings, and note physical clues that may indicate resistances of all kinds and harbingers of incipient acting out. They also are useful as a check on the therapist's ability to clarify and confront, and they assist in unearthing hidden countertransferential difficulties. (p. 72)

Students have found watching videotaped sessions of their teachers treating patients invaluable. Most brief dynamic therapy training programs routinely use videotape recordings for supervision and research purposes (e.g., Davanloo 1980; Gustafson 1984; Sifneos 1987) and usually will not accept patients for treatment who, for whatever reason, cannot consent to videotaping. In addition, videotaping has been widely used in workshops on short-term dynamic psychotherapy given by experts in the field (e.g., Budman, Hoyt, Levenson). Supervisors have found few negative effects from such procedures but have encountered resistance from therapists in training who either consciously or unconsciously fear exposing their work to such close scrutiny. Sifneos (1987) called videotape technology the "microscope" of psychiatry, which underscores both its usefulness and its feared inhibiting effect.

Budman and Armstrong (1992) discussed the lack of training in brief therapy even in such settings as PPOs, HMOs, and EAPs, which have promoted themselves as providing efficient and effective psychotherapeutic services. These authors noted that supervisors and teachers of psychotherapy rarely apply adult education principles, which hold that adults 1) have a wealth of previous experience to draw on when they are confronted with problems, 2) are autonomous learners who decide what, why, and whether to learn, and 3) want to use their new learning pragmatically and immediately. Budman has trainees apply the skills they are learning in brief psychotherapy in videotaped practice sessions with actors trained to play the roles of patients. Budman and Armstrong (1992) concluded their article with the caveat "High quality staff training in brief therapy is needed. It is dangerous to assume that the job of being an effective brief therapist can be learned without informed and well-designed input" (p. 420).

EXPERIENCE

Experience appears to be another factor that greatly influences the practice of brief dynamic psychotherapy. But how it exerts such influence is somewhat of a paradox. It is widely accepted that brief therapy is a very demanding endeavor—one best suited to be learned after one has already become facile with the basics. As Mann (1973) notes,

> Knowledge of the psychoanalytic theories of mental functioning heavily buttressed by experience in the long-term treatment of patients is the best preparation for this [brief] treatment plan. *Short treatment in no way suggests easy treatment.* In many ways, short treatment is more difficult than longer treatment, even for the experienced therapist. (p. 82; emphasis added)

As Mario Andolphi, an Italian family therapist and trainer, is quoted as saying: "To make shorter the therapy, make longer the training" (Ecker and Hulley 1996, p. ix).

However, the paradox is that although knowledge and skills gained over the years in conducting long-term therapy seem to be a prerequisite for learning brief therapy, one may need to set aside many of the assumptions of long-term therapy to make full use of brief therapy techniques and rationale (Flegenheimer 1982). Sifneos (1987), writing on learning to use STAPP, stated the following:

> From my own observations of the supervision of 70 therapists representing such disciplines as psychiatry, psychology, social work, and nursing during the last 25 years, I can

---

TABLE 28–6. Guidelines for maximizing manualized training

1. Choose competent but relatively less experienced therapists.
2. Select therapists who are less vulnerable to negative training effects (e.g., less hostile and controlling).
3. Assume that even experienced therapists are novices in the approach to be learned.
4. Provide close, directive, and specific feedback to therapists and focus on therapists' own thought processes.

Source. Adapted from Henry et al. 1993b.

state categorically that the main difficulty in learning to use STAPP has more to do with certain misconceptions about the superiority of long-term psychotherapy which were rigidly embedded in the minds of our trainees, and which they were reluctant to give up, than with anything else, including their relative inexperience. This problem was resolved when we decided . . . to offer [instruction in STAPP] early so as to avoid their being thoroughly indoctrinated in dogmatic points of view and in preconceived and narrow-minded ideas which tended to obscure their ability to make meaningful observations which interfered with their learning. (p. 189)

Because these inexperienced therapists were presumably open-minded (i.e., not indoctrinated), Sifneos found them easier to train than experienced therapists, and these therapists-in-training, therefore, "more often obtained successful results than did their more experienced counterparts" (Sifneos 1978, p. 493).

The issue of when to train in brief dynamic psychotherapy remains somewhat controversial. However, it seems that the enthusiasm and positive expectation of the neophyte learner may be as valuable as the knowledge and skill of the seasoned clinician. Winokur and Dasberg (1983) found that experienced therapists may suffer from a sense of loss of competence as they experiment with shorter-term treatments. These authors suggested allowing seasoned therapists time to work through negative attitudes they might have toward briefer methods. The diminished self-esteem or narcissistic injury that may occur while therapists are practicing new skills may, in part, account for the post-training decrements in performance evidenced by the experienced therapists in the Vanderbilt II study described earlier in this section.

Regardless of when brief therapy skills are learned, experience in brief therapy seems to be reliably related to greater skill and confidence in brief therapy techniques. Ursano and Dressler (1974, 1977) found that clinicians who were more experienced in brief therapy tended to refer patients to brief therapy more frequently than those who were less familiar. Also, those clinicians who had more brief therapy experience rated themselves as more skilled. Similarly, Levenson et al. (1995) found that the best predictor of self-assessed skill in all types of brief therapy was experience conducting brief therapy. For those therapists who were conducting brief therapy but who had little experience in that modality, formal training and the amount of brief therapy they were presently conducting were the most potent predictors of skill. For more experienced brief therapists, attitude toward brief therapy played a greater role in predicting skill. Levenson et al. (1995) concluded that novice therapists would do well to continue to increase their experience while receiving more training; experienced clinicians, however, might require training that focuses on values and attitudes as well as techniques. Experience alone does not appear to be a sufficient teacher.

RESISTANCES, ATTITUDES, EXPECTATIONS

Despite advances in the theory and technique of brief dynamic psychotherapy, as well as the existence of a number of research studies demonstrating its overall effectiveness, many therapists are still reluctant to learn these methods and apply them in their clinical practice (e.g., Bolter et al. 1990; Budman and Gurman 1983, 1988; Evans and Levenson 1997; Hoyt 1985; Levenson et al. 1995; Winokur and Dasberg 1983). Important variables in understanding this reluctance are therapists' values and assumptions regarding the nature and practice of brief psychotherapy.

Budman and Gurman (1983) proposed that the value systems of the long-term therapist are different from those of the short-term therapist. These authors identified eight dominant values pertaining to the ideal manner in which long-term therapy is practiced and contrasted these with the corresponding ideal values pertinent to the practice of short-term therapy. For example, Budman and Gurman postulated that one of the ideal value differences between long-term and short-term therapists involves the idea of "cure." Whereas the long-term therapist seeks a change in basic character or "therapeutic perfectionism" (Malan 1963), the short-term therapist does not believe in the notion of "cure" and prefers pragmatism, parsimony, and the least radical intervention.

Bolter et al. (1990) sought to assess empirically whether there were such value differences between short-term and long-term practicing therapists. Two hundred twenty-two psychologists were sent a questionnaire in order that relevant values and preferred therapeutic approaches (short-term vs. long-term) might be measured. The study provided partial support for Budman and Gurman's (1983) proposal: in two of the eight areas, long-term and short-term therapists' responses differed significantly. Short-term therapists believed more strongly that psychological change could occur outside therapy and that setting time limits would intensify the therapeutic work. Furthermore, results indicated that clinicians with a psychodynamic orientation, in contrast to those having a cognitive-behavioral orientation, were more likely to believe that therapy was necessary for change, that the focus of therapy should be on pathology, that therapy should be open-ended, and that ambitious goals were desirable. Thus, although the findings from the study by Bolter et al.

(1990) suggest that a short-term orientation is related to therapeutic values, it is important to note that the theoretical orientation of the therapist also plays a significant role in determining values.

The majority of the literature addressing therapists' reluctance to use brief therapy focuses on psychoanalytic or psychodynamic therapists. Bolter (1987) found that 91% of the psychodynamic therapists who responded to an attitude questionnaire favored long-term approaches. Speed (1992) similarly found that 87% of those therapists most comfortable with very long-term therapy were psychodynamic in orientation. In the psychologist survey (Levenson et al. 1995), psychodynamic brief therapists reported less skill, experience, and training in, and less of a positive attitude concerning the effectiveness of, brief therapy than did their cognitive-behavior therapy colleagues. Yet, these dynamically trained practitioners were conducting a large amount of brief therapy. This fact has tremendous implications for training. Are graduate school curricula, residency training programs, and continuing education experiences geared toward meeting the needs of these dynamic clinicians? The data from the national survey (Davidovitz and Levenson 1995) indicate that residency training programs may be doing an excellent job in providing brief therapy courses; 90% of recent graduates have taken at least one such course.

Hoyt (1985) proposed that dynamically trained therapists have resistances toward short-term psychotherapy. In trying to determine why many therapists are not learning and applying short-term dynamic methods as a treatment of choice, Hoyt rejected the idea that the situation is due chiefly to lack of awareness regarding recent clinical and research developments: "Rather, I would suggest, there are a number of myths, erroneous beliefs, and (perhaps unconscious) 'problems about learning' (Ekstein and Wallerstein 1972) that may make clinicians reluctant or resistant to using short-term dynamic methods" (Hoyt 1985, p. 95). Hoyt organized these resistances into six broad categories, as shown in Table 28–7.

Similarly, Budman and Armstrong (1992) addressed the topic of resistance, but from the perspective of mental health administrators who are against instituting brief therapy training in their agencies. Specifically, the authors mentioned the administrators' perceptions 1) that because someone has a psychotherapy license, he or she is qualified to provide any type of therapy; 2) that money should be used to hire new staff, with training seen as a luxury; and 3) that one must force staff to do brief therapy, without recognizing that staff members may have a poor attitude because of lack of training.

Negative attitudes toward briefer modes of intervention could adversely affect therapists' willingness and ability to use brief therapy methods effectively. Flegenheimer (1982) warned that problems could arise during a brief psychotherapy if the therapist's values are "inconsistent with the optimism and confidence that the brief therapist must have in the method and which must be brought to the treatment situation" (p. 13).

Similarly, Winokur and Dasberg (1983) suggested that

> when teaching professionals a new approach, it is not enough to rely on lectures, reading materials, or even live demonstrations and individual supervision. . . . In order to integrate a new approach into their professional identity, particularly if this identity is molded already, they need also to work through the intellectual, quasi-intellectual, and emotional difficulties encountered in the learning process. (p. 51)

Ursano and Dressler (1977) made the point that

> clinicians' attitudes toward various therapeutic approaches strongly influence the use of a particular treatment modality and the effectiveness with which it is conducted. These values are determined by the type of professional training, the amount of clinical experience, and the particular work setting of the clinician, as well as by individual personality characteristics. *A positive attitude toward brief psychotherapy* and a skill in practicing it are extremely important if the trend toward shorter term treatment continues. (p. 55 [emphasis added])

As early as 1969, it was found that therapists who were initially biased toward time-unlimited treatment later judged time-limited therapies to be more effective (Reid and Shyne 1969), suggesting that attitudes can be changed

TABLE 28–7. Sources of resistance against short-term dynamic psychotherapy

The belief that more is better (e.g., treatment must take a long time to be effective)

Myth of the "pure gold" of analysis

Confusion of patient's interests (in the most efficient, effective help) with the therapist's interests (in uncovering all aspects of the patient's personality)

Demanding hard work (to be active and intensely alert)

Economic and other pressures (desire to hold on to that which is profitable and dependable)

Countertransference and related therapist reactions to termination

Source. Adapted from Hoyt 1985.

with increased experience. Levenson and Bolter (1988) examined the values and attitudes of psychiatry residents and psychology interns before and after a 6-month seminar/supervision in brief dynamic psychotherapy. Findings revealed that after training, trainees were more willing to consider brief therapy for more than minor disorders, more positive about achieving significant insight, more expectant that the benefits would be long-lasting, and less likely to think that an extended "working through" was necessary. Also, they were more willing to be active, more likely to see that a time limit was helpful, and more prepared to believe that patients would change significantly after the therapy was over. An extension of this study (Neff et al. 1996), involving three experienced trainers with three different brief therapy models, indicated that intensive 1-day workshops can lead to more positive and optimistic attitudes toward brief therapy. These studies support the view that attending to values and attitudes associated with short-term versus long-term therapy may be a necessary component for the success of any teaching or training program in brief psychotherapy.

Similarly, other investigators (e.g., Johnson and Gelso 1980) have concluded that it is not feasible for agencies to institute time-limited policies without considering the staff's personal feelings and experiences. Ursano and Dressler (1977) found that therapists' attitudes were influenced by type of professional training, clinical experience, the institutional setting, and the clinic's team structure. They concluded that a multidisciplinary team with professionals of varying experience offered the best organizational structure to promote unbiased attitudes toward brief psychotherapy, provided there was openness and mutual respect.

In sum, the prevailing evidence suggests that those clinicians who may be naturally drawn to brief treatment models may express values and attitudes different from those whose preference is to conduct long-term therapy. This is not surprising; nor is it surprising that an individual's training greatly influences those values and attitudes. It is crucial, however, to ensure that the current economic climate is not used politically to elevate one set of values and attitudes at the expense of another. Indeed, earlier in this century, those therapists who sought to shorten therapy regularly found these efforts devalued by their peers. Clearly, brief treatment is not a panacea and should not be oversold. Neither should the important observations made by long-term therapists of patients over time be summarily rejected. There is much yet to be learned about the treatment of psychopathology, and it is unlikely that one set of values and attitudes is unquestionably superior.

CLINICALLY RELEVANT RESEARCH ON BRIEF DYNAMIC PSYCHOTHERAPY

THE THERAPEUTIC ALLIANCE

Several times in this chapter we have made reference to the importance of the therapeutic alliance and its relationship to the success or failure of therapy. The term *therapeutic alliance* typically refers to "the emotional bond and reciprocal involvement that develops between patient and therapist during the course of therapy" (Koss and Shiang 1994). The significance of at least an adequate alliance between patient and therapist extends to long-term therapy (Frank 1991), but such an alliance may be particularly important in brief therapy, in which time constraints may preclude extended efforts to correct alliance problems.

In correlational investigations the state of the alliance has consistently been found to be a predictor of therapeutic success (e.g., Eaton et al. 1988; Gaston et al. 1994; Marmar et al. 1989; Orlinsky et al. 1994). Findings of some studies (e.g., Strupp and Hadley 1979) suggest that the quality of the alliance tends to be established (as good or poor) early in therapy (i.e., by the third session). The "helping alliance" is positively correlated with initial, accurate therapeutic interventions (Crits-Christoph et al. 1993), and premature terminations are related to early misalliances (Magnavita 1993). Luborsky et al. (1985) reported that a helping alliance contributes far more than other factors, such as theoretical approach or use of techniques. For many brief dynamic therapies, the patient's ability to form a collaborative stance with the therapist is listed as a selection criterion (see Table 28–4). Such findings raise the question of what happens in cases of poor alliance.

Consistent with the general trend of findings, Marziali et al. (1981) found that patients rated as making a strong positive contribution to the alliance had good outcomes. However, in cases of poor outcome, patients with a "negative disposition to the treatment situation that persisted across the hours of the brief psychotherapy . . . [were] relatively intransigent to the therapist's efforts to shore up the alliance" (Marziali et al. 1981, p. 363). In a series of comparisons of good and poor outcome cases conducted by the same therapists, Strupp (1980b, 1980c, 1980d, 1980e) observed: "we failed to encounter a single instance in which a difficult patient's hostility and negativism were successfully confronted or resolved" (Strupp 1980d, p. 954). Further analyses of these cases by Henry et al. (1986) revealed that patient communications defined as hostile, withdrawn, or otherwise provocative tended to be met with complementary responses by the therapist. In other words, patient negativity tended to be met with subtly negative responses from the therapist, yielding a negative interaction sequence almost always associated with poor outcome. Rather than concluding that the therapist is helpless in the face of patient negativity or hostility, some authors (e.g., Butler and Strupp 1986; Levenson 1995; Safran et al. 1994) have proposed training therapists to rapidly detect and address such alliance problems. Although this appears to be a promising direction for research and training, an initial effort to train experienced therapists along these lines was only partially successful (Henry et al. 1993a). Obviously, further research into the therapist's contribution to the alliance is essential if brief forms of therapy are to be extended to difficult patients.

RESEARCH ON THE EFFICACY, EFFECTIVENESS, AND LONG-TERM OUTCOME OF SHORT-TERM THERAPY

To evaluate whether brief dynamic psychotherapy is efficacious (i.e., works under experimental conditions), Crits-Christoph (1992) combined the results of a number of outcome studies using the statistical procedure called *meta-analysis*. He found that brief dynamic psychotherapy is as effective as other forms of therapy. Review of the empirical literature in brief therapy indicates that empirical studies have failed to demonstrate that long-term (or open-ended) approaches achieve better outcomes than short-term (or time-limited) therapies (Barber 1994; Koss and Shiang 1994). Findings of some studies even indicate that briefer interventions are more effective. For example, Piper et al. (1984) found that short-term (6 months) individual dynamic psychotherapy and long-term (24 months) group therapy produced better outcomes than long-term individual therapy or short-term group therapy.

Howard et al. (1986) plotted improvement rates for a large number of studies as a function of time and concluded that 50% of patients show significant improvement by the 8th session and 75% by the 26th session. These improvement rates occur within the 10- to 25-session limit typical of many brief dynamic therapies. Moreover, these 50% and 75% effectiveness marks were derived almost exclusively from studies of long-term or open-ended therapies, rather than of ones that were specifically intended to be brief or time-limited (Hoyt and Austad 1992). However, one must be cautious in interpolating these empirical data. As pointed out by Barber and Ellman (1996), "The lack of studies comparing brief with long-term therapy has led to the unfounded 'verdict' that long-term dynamic psychotherapy is not effective or not worthwhile" (p. 189). When evaluating such findings, one must consider the inherent limitations of research with long-term psychotherapies.

For pragmatic reasons, research on long-term therapies usually involves observations of therapies in naturalistic studies, resulting in a loss of the experimental control that is possible in studies of shorter duration.

In trying to assess brief dynamic therapy's effectiveness (i.e., whether it works in clinical practice), *Consumer Reports* ("Mental Health 1995") surveyed its readership. Responses indicated that the longer people were in therapy, the more likely they were to say they had improved, although those staying in therapy a shorter time (6 months or less) also felt helped. Although there was no clear difference in outcome between people with fee-for-service coverage and those in HMOs or PPOs, respondents who thought that their choice of therapist or the duration of their care was limited by their insurance coverage did worse (Seligman 1995).

In assessing long-term outcome, research indicates that patients in brief dynamic therapy tend to maintain their therapeutic gains (Messer and Warren 1995), but there is some indication that treatments of less than 16 sessions may not be as effective for depressed patients (Shapiro et al. 1995).

CONCLUSIONS

Although there are now many types of brief dynamic individual psychotherapies, these therapies have several qualities in common. We have defined brief psychodynamic psychotherapy as treatment of limited duration in which therapists are active in maintaining a circumscribed focus with limited goals using a framework of psychoanalytically derived concepts and techniques. Much remains to be learned about who is an "appropriate" brief therapy patient. Using patient characteristics and performance criteria to identify such patients has not been as successful as had once been hoped. One of the most disturbing trends is that with the economically based, increased demand for briefer treatments, therapists are being required to do shorter-term interventions without adequate training. We strongly encourage universities, training programs, clinics, HMOs, and continuing education programs to offer and facilitate training in brief dynamic psychotherapy. If such training is absent, we fear that brief psychotherapy will be poorly conceptualized and executed. If this occurs, brief psychodynamic therapy could become synonymous with poor therapy.

We strongly believe that there is an important and major role for short-term *dynamically informed* therapy in the future. The dynamic brief therapist of the twenty-first century will need to be trained to be able to use appropriately and flexibly a variety of intervention techniques and to work collaboratively with other health care providers. What we envision is an emphasis on a psychodynamic understanding of the patient to provide a guide for these appropriate interventions. As stated by Gabbard (1990) in his book on psychodynamic psychiatry in clinical practice, "Dynamic psychiatry simply provides a coherent conceptual framework within which all treatments are prescribed. Regardless of whether the treatment is dynamic psychotherapy or pharmacotherapy, it is *dynamically informed*" (p. 204). If brief dynamic therapists of the future emphasize the psychodynamic understanding of patients and their situations, they will have a basis for using any one of a number of specialized techniques, such as cognitive restructuring, hypnosis, psychopharmacology, or more traditionally recognizable psychodynamic interventions. As part of this approach, there has been a liberating movement away from more elaborate metapsychological models, along with an increased focus on clinical phenomena and descriptive formulations to guide effective and efficient treatment (Levenson and Hales 1993).

We close with our admonition that brief treatments (psychodynamic or otherwise) must not be oversold. Clearly, brief treatment is not a panacea. There is a danger in this age of limited resources, consumerism, and quick fixes that brief therapy (and especially the ultrabrief treatments) will be touted and then expected to do the impossible. However, brief dynamic psychotherapy that is used in a realistic and informed fashion should continue to help many of our patients.

REFERENCES

Ackley DC: Employee health insurance benefits: a comparison of managed care in traditional mental health care: costs and results. The Independent Practitioner 13:49–53, 1993

Alexander F, French T: Psychoanalytic Therapy: Principles and Applications. New York, Ronald Press, 1946

Austad CS: Is Long-Term Psychotherapy Unethical? Toward a Social Ethic in an Era of Managed Care. San Francisco, CA, Jossey-Bass, 1996

Austad CS, Berman WH: Managed health care and the evolution of psychotherapy, in Psychotherapy in Managed Health Care: The Optimal Use of Time and Resources. Edited by Austad CS, Berman WH. Washington, DC, American Psychological Association, 1991, pp 3–18

Austad CS, DeStefano L, Kisch J: The health maintenance organization, II: implications for psychotherapy. Psychotherapy: Theory, Research and Practice 25:449–454, 1988

Bachrach HM, Leaff LA: "Analyzability": a systematic review of the clinical and quantitative literature. J Am Psychoanal Assoc 26:881–920, 1978

Barber JP: Efficacy of short-term dynamic psychotherapy: past, present, and future. Journal of Psychotherapy Practice and Research 3:108–121, 1994

Barber JP, Crits-Christoph P: Comparison of the brief dynamic therapies, in Handbook of Short-Term Dynamic Psychotherapy. Edited by Crits-Christoph P, Barber JP. New York, Basic Books, 1991, pp 323–356

Barber JP, Ellman J: Advances in short-term dynamic psychotherapy. Current Opinion in Psychiatry 9:188–192, 1996

Barron JW, Sands H (eds): Impact of Managed Care on Psychodynamic Treatment. Madison, CT, Universities Press, 1996

Bauer GP, Kobos JC: Brief Therapy: Short-Term Psychodynamic Intervention. Northdale, NJ, Jason Aronson, 1987

Bennett MJ: The greening of the HMO: implications for prepaid psychiatry. Am J Psychiatry 145:1544–1549, 1988

Berkman AS, Bassos CA, Post L: Managed mental health care and independent practice: a challenge to psychology. Psychotherapy: Theory, Research and Practice 25:434–440, 1988

Binder JL, Henry WP, Strupp HH: An appraisal of selection criteria for dynamic psychotherapies and implications for setting time limits. Psychiatry 50:154–166, 1987

Bloom BL: Planned Short-Term Psychotherapy. Boston, Allyn and Bacon, 1992

Bolter K: Differences in therapy-related values and attitudes between short-term and long-term therapists. Unpublished doctoral dissertation, California School of Professional Psychology, Berkeley, CA, 1987

Bolter K, Levenson H, Alvarez W: Differences in values between short-term and long-term therapists. Professional Psychology: Research and Practice 21:285–290, 1990

Brief therapy: fast relief for troubled people. Better Homes and Gardens, September 1990, pp 53–54

Budman SH, Armstrong E: Training for managed care settings: how to make it happen. Psychotherapy: Theory, Research and Practice 29:416–421, 1992

Budman SH, Gurman AS: The practice of brief therapy. Professional Psychology: Research and Practice 14:277–289, 1983

Budman SH, Gurman AS: Theory and Practice of Brief Psychotherapy. New York, Guilford, 1988

Budman SH, Stone J: Advances in brief psychotherapy: a review of recent literature. Hospital and Community Psychiatry 34:939–946, 1983

Burke JD Jr, White HS, Havens LL: Which short-term therapy? Matching patient and method. Arch Gen Psychiatry 36:177–186, 1979

Burlingame GM, Fuhriman JA: Clinician attitudes toward time-limited and time-unlimited therapy. Professional Psychology: Research and Practice 18:61–65, 1987

Burlingame GM, Fuhriman A, Paul S, et al: Implementing a time-limited therapy program: differential effects of training and experience. Psychotherapy: Theory, Research and Practice 26:303–312, 1989

Butler SF, Strupp HH: "Specific" and "nonspecific" factors in psychotherapy: a problematic paradigm for psychotherapy research. Psychotherapy: Theory, Research and Practice 23:30–40, 1986

Butler SF, Strupp HH: Effects of training psychoanalytically oriented therapists to use a manual, in Psychodynamic Treatment Research: A Handbook for Clinical Practice. Edited by Miller NE, Luborsky L, Barber JP, et al. New York, Basic Books, 1993, pp 191–210

Butler SF, Thackrey M, Strupp HH: Capacity for Dynamic Process Scale (CDPS): relation to patient variables, process and outcome. Paper presented at the annual meeting of Society for Psychotherapy Research, Ulm, West Germany, June 1987

Chipman A: Meeting managed care: an identity and value crisis for therapists. Am J Psychother 49:550–567, 1995

Crits-Christoph P: The efficacy of brief dynamic psychotherapy: a meta-analysis. Am J Psychiatry 149:151–158, 1992

Crits-Christoph P, Barber JP (eds): Handbook of Short-Term Dynamic Psychotherapy. New York, Basic Books, 1991

Crits-Christoph P, Cooper A, Luborsky L: The accuracy of therapists' interpretations and the outcome of dynamic psychotherapy. J Consult Clin Psychol 56:490–495, 1988

Crits-Christoph P, Barber JP, Kurcias JS: Introduction and historical background, in Handbook of Short-Term Dynamic Psychotherapy. Edited by Crits-Christoph P, Barber JP. New York, Basic Books, 1991, pp 1–12

Crits-Christoph P, Barber JP, Kurcias JS: The accuracy of therapist's interpretations and the development of the therapeutic alliance. Psychotherapy Research 3:25–35, 1993

Cummings NA: The dismantling of our health system: strategies for the survival of psychological practice. Am Psychol 41:426–431, 1986

Cummings NA: The future of psychotherapy: one psychologist's perspective. Am J Psychother 41:349–360, 1987

Cummings NA: Unconscious fiscal convenience. Psychotherapy in Private Practice 14:23–28, 1995

Dasberg H, Winokur M: Teaching and learning short-term dynamic psychotherapy: parallel processes. Psychotherapy: Theory, Research and Practice 21:184–188, 1984

Davanloo H (ed): Basic Principles and Techniques in Short-Term Dynamic Psychotherapy. New York, Spectrum, 1978

Davanloo H: A method of short-term dynamic psychotherapy, in Short-Term Dynamic Psychotherapy, Vol 1. Edited by Davanloo H. New York, Jason Aronson, 1980, pp 43–71

Davanloo H: Intensive short-term psychotherapy with highly resistant patients, I: handling resistance. International Journal of Short-Term Psychotherapy 1:107–133, 1986

Davidovitz D, Levenson H: A national survey on practice and training in brief therapy. Paper presented at the annual meeting of the American Psychological Association, New York, August 1995

Dorwart RA: Managed mental health care: myths and realities in the 1990s. Hospital and Community Psychiatry 41:1087–1091, 1990

Eaton TT, Abeles N, Gutfreund MJ: Therapeutic alliance and outcome: impact of treatment length and pretreatment symptomatology. Psychotherapy: Theory, Research and Practice 25:536–542, 1988

Ecker B, Hulley L: Depth-Oriented Brief Therapy. San Francisco, CA, Jossey-Bass, 1996

Ekstein R, Wallerstein RS: The Teaching and Learning of Psychotherapy. New York, International Universities Press, 1972

Evans S, Levenson H: Brief therapy training in APA-approved graduate programs and internships. Symposium presented at the annual meeting of the American Psychological Association, Chicago, August 1997

Fee, practice and managed care survey. Psychotherapy Finances 21:1–8, 1995

Ferenczi S, Rank O: The Development of Psychoanalysis. New York, Nervous and Mental Disease Publication Company, 1925

Flegenheimer WV: Techniques of Brief Psychotherapy. New York, Jason Aronson, 1982

Frances A, Clarkin J: Parallel techniques in supervision and treatment. Psychiatr Q 53:242–248, 1981

Frank A: The therapeutic alliances of borderline patients, in Borderline Personality Diagnoses. Edited by Clarkin JF, Marziali E, Moore H. New York, Guilford, 1991, pp 220–247

Fraser JS: All that glitters is not gold: medical offset effects and managed behavioral health care. Professional Psychology: Research and Practice 27:335–344, 1996

Freud S: Psycho-analytic method (1904), in Collected Papers: Early Papers, Vol 1. Translated by Riviere J. Edited by Jones E. London, Hogarth Press, 1953, pp 264–271

Gabbard GO: Psychodynamic Psychiatry in Clinical Practice. Washington, DC, American Psychiatric Press, 1990

Garfield SL: Research on client variables in psychotherapy, in Handbook of Psychotherapy and Behavior Change, 3rd Edition. Edited by Garfield SL, Bergin AE. New York, Wiley, 1986, pp 213–256

Gaston L, Piper WE, Debbane EG, et al: Alliance and technique for predicting outcome in short- and long-term analytic psychotherapy. Psychotherapy Research 4:121–135, 1994

Goldin V: Problems of technique, in Treating the Oedipal Patient in Brief Psychotherapy. Edited by Horner AJ. New York, Jason Aronson, 1985, pp 55–74

Goldman HH, Taube CA: High users of outpatient mental health services, II: implications for practice and policy. Am J Psychiatry 145:24–28, 1988

Gustafson JP: An integration of brief dynamic psychotherapy. Am J Psychiatry 141:935–944, 1984

Henry WP, Schacht TE, Strupp HH: Structural analysis of social behavior: application to a study of interpersonal process in differential therapeutic outcome. J Consult Clin Psychol 54:27–31, 1986

Henry WP, Strupp HH, Butler SF, et al: Effects of training in time-limited dynamic psychotherapy: changes in therapist behavior. J Consult Clin Psychol 61:434–440, 1993a

Henry WP, Schacht TE, Strupp HH, et al: Effects of training in time-limited dynamic psychotherapy: mediators of therapists' responses to training. J Consult Clin Psychol 61:441–447, 1993b

Hoglend P: Personality disorders and long-term outcome after brief dynamic psychotherapy. Journal of Personality Disorders 7:168–181, 1993

Horowitz M[J], Marmar CR, Krupnick J, et al: Personality Styles and Brief Psychotherapy. New York, Basic Books, 1984

Horowitz MJ, Marmar CR, Weiss DS, et al: Comprehensive analysis of change after brief dynamic psychotherapy. Am J Psychiatry 143:582–589, 1986

Howard KI, Kopta SM, Krause MS, et al: The dose-effect relationship in psychotherapy. Am Psychol 41:159–164, 1986

Hoyt MF: Therapist resistances to short-term dynamic psychotherapy. J Am Acad Psychoanal 13:93–112, 1985

Hoyt MF: Teaching and learning short-term psychotherapy, in Psychotherapy in Managed Health Care: The Optimal Use of Time and Resources. Edited by Austad CS, Berman WH. Washington, DC, American Psychological Association, 1991, pp 98–107

Hoyt MF, Austad CS: Psychotherapy in a staff model health maintenance organization: providing and assuring quality care in the future. Psychotherapy: Theory, Research and Practice 29:119–129, 1992

Hoyt MF, Rosenbaum R, Talmon M: Planned single-session psychotherapy, in The First Session in Brief Therapy. Edited by Budman S, Hoyt MF, Friedman S. New York, Guilford, 1992, pp 59–86

Hymowitz C, Pollock EJ: Psychobattle: cost-cutting firms monitor couch time as therapists fret. Wall Street Journal, July 13, 1995, p 1

Iglehart JK: Managed care and mental health. N Engl J Med 334:131–135, 1996

Johnson DH, Gelso CJ: The effectiveness in counseling and psychotherapy: a critical review. Counseling Psychology 9:70–83, 1980

Joyce AS, Duncan SC, Piper WE: Task analysis of "working" responses to dynamic interpretation in short-term individual psychotherapy. Psychotherapy Research 5:49–62, 1995

Karon BP: Provision of psychotherapy under managed health care: a growing crisis and national nightmare. Professional Psychology: Research and Practice 26:5–9, 1995

Kopta SM, Howard KI, Lowry JL, et al: Patterns of symptomatic recovery in psychotherapy. J Consult Clin Psychol 62:1009–1016, 1994

Koss MP, Shiang J: Research on brief psychotherapy, in Handbook of Psychotherapy and Behavior Change, 4th Edition. Edited by Bergin AE, Garfield SL. New York, Wiley, 1994

Koss MP, Butcher JN, Strupp HH: Brief psychotherapy methods in clinical research. J Consult Clin Psychol 54:60–67, 1986

Laiken M, Winston A, McCullough L: Intensive short-term dynamic psychotherapy, in Handbook of Short-Term Dynamic Psychotherapy. Edited by Crits-Christoph P, Barber JP. New York, Basic Books, 1991, pp 80–109

Levenson H: Time Limited Dynamic Psychotherapy: A Guide to Clinical Practice. New York, Basic Books, 1995

Levenson H, Bolter K: Short-term psychotherapy values and attitudes: changes with training. Paper presented at the American Psychological Association Convention, Atlanta, GA, August 1988

Levenson H, Butler S: Concise guide to brief dynamic psychotherapy. Washington, DC, American Psychiatric Press, 1997

Levenson H, Hales RE: Brief psychodynamically informed therapy for medically ill patients, in Medical-Psychiatric Practice, Vol 2. Edited by Stoudemire A, Fogel BS. Washington DC, American Psychiatric Press, 1993, pp 3–37

Levenson H, Overstreet D: Long-term outcome with brief psychotherapy. Paper presented at the annual meeting of Society for Psychotherapy Research Meeting, Pittsburgh, PA, June 1993

Levenson H, Speed J, Budman S: Therapists' experience, training, and skill in brief therapy: a bicoastal survey. Am J Psychother 49:95–117, 1995

Luborsky L, Crits-Christoph P: Understanding transference: the CCRT method. New York, Basic Books, 1990

Luborsky L, McLellan AT, Woody GE, et al: Therapist success and its determinants. Arch Gen Psychiatry 42:602–611, 1985

MacKenzie KR: Principles of brief intensive psychotherapy. Psychiatric Annals 21:398–404, 1991

Magnavita JJ: The evolution of short-term dynamic psychotherapy: treatment of the future? Professional Psychology: Research and Practice 24: 360–365, 1993

Malan DH: A Study of Brief Psychotherapy. London, Tavistock, 1963

Malan DH: The Frontier of Brief Psychotherapy. New York, Plenum, 1976

Malan DH: Individual Psychotherapy and the Science of Psychodynamics. London, Butterworth, 1979

Mann J: Time-Limited Psychotherapy. Cambridge, MA, Harvard University Press, 1973

Marmar CR, Gaston L, Gallagher D, et al: Alliance and outcome in late-life depression. J Nerv Ment Dis 177: 464–472, 1989

Marmor J: Short-term dynamic psychotherapy. Am J Psychiatry 136:149–155, 1979

Marziali E, Marmar C, Krupnick J: Therapeutic alliance scales: development and relationship to psychotherapy outcome. Am J Psychiatry 138:361–364, 1981

Mendelsohn R: Critical factors in short-term psychotherapy: a summary. Bull Menninger Clin 42:133–149, 1978

Mental Health: Does Therapy Help? Consumer Reports, November 1995, pp 734–739

Messer SB, Warren CS: Models of Brief Psychodynamic Therapy: A Comparative Approach. New York, Guilford, 1995

Miller IJ: Managed care is harmful to outpatient mental health services: a call for accountability. Profession Psychology: Research and Practice 27:349–363, 1996

Neff WL, Lambert MJ, Kirk ML, et al: Therapists' attitudes toward short-term therapy: changes with training. Employee Assistance Quarterly 11:67–77, 1996

Olfson M, Pincus HA: Outpatient psychotherapy in the United States, I: volume, costs, and other user characteristics. Am J Psychiatry 151:1281–1288, 1994

Orlinsky DE, Grawe K, Parks BK: Process and outcome in psychotherapy, in Handbook of Psychotherapy and Behavior Change, 4th Edition. Edited by Garfield SL, Bergin AE. New York, Wiley, 1994, pp 270–376

Peake TH, Bordin CM, Archer RP: Brief Psychotherapies: Changing Frames of Mind. Beverly Hills, CA, Sage, 1988

Perry S, Frances A, Klar H, et al: Selection criteria for individual dynamic psychotherapies. Psychiatr Q 55:3–16, 1983

Phillips LE: The ubiquitous decay curve: delivery similarities in psychotherapy, medicine and addiction. Professional Psychology: Research and Practice 18:650–652, 1987

Piper WE, Debbane EG, Bienvenu JP, et al: A comparative study of four forms of psychotherapy. J Consult Clin Psychol 52:268–279, 1984

Pumpian-Mindlin E: Consideration in the selection of patients for short-term therapy. Am J Psychother 7:641–652, 1953

Rachman AW: Rule of empathy: Sandor Ferenczi's pioneering contribution to the empathic method in psychoanalysis. J Am Acad Psychoanal 16:1–27, 1988

Rank O: Will Therapy (1929). Translated by Taft J. New York, Knopf, 1936

Reid WJ, Shyne AW: Brief and Extended Casework. New York, Columbia University Press, 1969

Rounsaville BJ, O'Malley S, Foley S, et al: Role of manual-guided training in the conduct and efficacy of interpersonal psychotherapy for depression. J Consult Clin Psychol 56:681–688, 1988

Safran JD, Muran JC, Samstag LW: Resolving therapeutic alliance ruptures: A task-analytic investigation, in The Working Alliance: Theory, Research and Practice. Edited by Hovath AO, Greenberg LS. New York, Wiley 1994, pp 225–255

Schacht TE, Binder JL, Strupp HH: The dynamic focus, in Psychotherapy in a New Key: A Guide to Time-Limited Dynamic Psychotherapy. Edited by Strupp HH, Binder JL. New York, Basic Books, 1984, pp 65–109

Seligman MEP: The effectiveness of psychotherapy: the Consumer Reports study. Am Psychol 50:965–974, 1995

Shapiro D, Rees A, Barkham M, et al: Effects of treatment duration and severity of depression on the maintenance of gains after cognitive-behavioral and psychodynamic-interpersonal psychotherapy. J Consult Clin Psychology 63:378–387, 1995

Shea MT, Pilkonis PA, Beckham E, et al: Personality disorders and treatment outcome in the NIMH Treatment of Depression Collaborative Research Program. Am J Psychiatry 147:711–718, 1990

Sifneos PE: Short-Term Psychotherapy and Emotional Crisis. Cambridge, MA, Harvard University Press, 1972

Sifneos PE: The teaching and supervision of STAPP, in Basic Principles and Techniques of Short-Term Dynamic Psychotherapy. Edited by Davanloo H. New York, Jason Aronson, 1978, pp 491–499

Sifneos PE: Short-Term Dynamic Psychotherapy: Evaluation and Technique. New York, Plenum, 1979

Sifneos PE: Short-Term Dynamic Psychotherapy: Evaluation and Technique, 2nd Edition. New York, Plenum, 1987

Silberschatz G, Fretter PB, Curtis JT: How do interpretations influence the process of psychotherapy? J Consult Clin Psychol 54:646–652, 1986

Small L: The Briefer Psychotherapies. New York, Brunner/Mazel, 1979

Speed JL: Therapists' practice, training, and skill in brief therapy: a survey of California and Massachusetts psychologists. Unpublished doctoral dissertation, Wright Institute Graduate School of Psychology, Berkeley, CA, 1992

Stern S: Managed care, brief therapy, and therapeutic integrity. Psychotherapy 30:162–175, 1993

Strupp HH: Problems of research, in Short-Term Dynamic Psychotherapy. Edited by Davanloo H. New York, Jason Aronson, 1980a, pp 379–392

Strupp HH: Success and failure in time-limited psychotherapy: a systematic comparison of two cases: comparison 1. Arch Gen Psychiatry 37:595–603, 1980b

Strupp HH: Success and failure in time-limited psychotherapy: a systematic comparison of two cases: comparison 2. Arch Gen Psychiatry 37:708–716, 1980c

Strupp HH: Success and failure in time-limited psychotherapy: further evidence (comparison 4). Arch Gen Psychiatry 37:947–954, 1980d

Strupp HH: Success and failure in time-limited psychotherapy: with special reference to the performance of a lay counselor. Arch Gen Psychiatry 37:831–841, 1980e

Strupp HH: The outcome problem in psychotherapy: contemporary perspectives, in Psychotherapy Research and Behavior Change. Edited by Harvey TH, Parks MM. Washington, DC, American Psychological Association, 1982, pp 39–71

Strupp HH: Time-limited dynamic psychotherapy: development and implementation of a training program, in Brief Therapy: Myths, Methods, and Metaphors. Edited by Zeig JK, Gillian SG. New York, Brunner/Mazel, 1990, pp 327–341

Strupp HH, Binder JL (eds): Psychotherapy in a New Key: A Guide to Time-Limited Dynamic Psychotherapy. New York, Basic Books, 1984

Strupp HH, Hadley SW: Specific vs nonspecific factors in psychotherapy: a controlled study of outcome. Arch Gen Psychiatry 36:1125–1136, 1979

Strupp HH, Butler SF, Rosser CL: Training in psychodynamic therapy. J Consult Clin Psychol 56:689–695, 1988

Thackrey M, Butler SF, Strupp HH: The Capacity for Dynamic Process Scale (CDPS), in A Collection of Psychological Scales. Edited by Canfield ML, Canfield JE. New York, Basic Books, 1993, pp 191–210

Therapy for the '90s. U.S. News and World Report, January 13, 1992, pp 55–56

Ursano RJ, Dressler DM: Brief vs long-term psychotherapy: a treatment decision. J Nerv Ment Dis 159:164–171, 1974

Ursano RJ, Dressler DM: Brief versus long-term psychotherapy: clinician attitudes and organizational design. Compr Psychiatry 18:55–60, 1977

Ursano RJ, Hales RE: A review of brief individual psychotherapies. Am J Psychiatry 143:1507–1517, 1986

Weiss J, Sampson H, Mount Zion Psychotherapy Research Group: The Psychoanalytic Process: Theory, Clinical Observations, and Empirical Research. New York, Guilford, 1986

Winokur M, Dasberg H: Teaching and learning short-term dynamic psychotherapy: techniques and resistances. Bull Menninger Clin 47:36–52, 1983

Wolberg LR: Handbook of Short-Term Psychotherapy. New York, Thieme-Stratton, 1980

CHAPTER 29

PSYCHOANALYSIS, PSYCHOANALYTIC PSYCHOTHERAPY, AND SUPPORTIVE PSYCHOTHERAPY

ROBERT J. URSANO, M.D.
EDWARD K. SILBERMAN, M.D.

Our health is directly and indirectly affected by our behavior: our thoughts, feelings, fantasies, and actions. Because of this effect, both increased morbidity and mortality can result from psychiatric illness. Frequently, psychopathology limits our ability to see options and exercise choices, leading to feelings, thoughts, fantasies, and actions that may be painful, restricted, and repetitive. Psychotherapy is directed toward changing these learned forms of behavior that affect health and performance. Personality is, in fact, a series of probable behaviors that each individual characteristically has in a given context (Ursano et al. 1996). Changing these response patterns can change the risk of disease, illness, and negative health behaviors, as well as interpersonal strategies that may decrease productivity and success.

Originally called the *talking cure*, psychotherapy is the generic term for a large number of treatment techniques that are directed toward changing behavior through verbal interchange. In the context of talking, psychotherapy provides understanding, support, new experiences, and new knowledge that can 1) result in learning, 2) increase the range of behaviors available to the patient, 3) relieve symptoms, and 4) alter maladaptive and unhealthy patterns of behavior. In the process of this reorganization, both perception and behavior change.

The target organ of psychotherapy is the brain. Feelings, thoughts, fantasies, and actions are brain functions. If behavior is to change, brain function and activity must alter at some basic level (Kandell 1979, 1989). If neuron A used to fire to neuron B, it must now fire to neuron C. Just as past life experience affects the development and maturation of the brain, and therefore brain activity, so too does present life experience, including the experience of psychotherapy.

Our social connectedness, a major focus of psychotherapeutic work, mediates both morbidity and mortality (House et al. 1988) and serves to regulate bodily function (Hofer 1984). The common observation that a phobic individual will approach the phobic object when accompanied by a supportive other illustrates the profound biological activities that accompany interpersonal relations and of which we know very little. How the "outside" (i.e., life experience) changes what is inside (i.e., our biology) is fundamental to an understanding of brain function and to the effectiveness of all psychotherapies. Our understanding of these processes, the science of behavior change, is only now emerging (Ursano and Fullerton 1991). Baxter et. al. (1992) showed that after psychotherapy, changes in the brain evident through positron-emission tomography are similar to those following treatment with fluoxetine.

Psychotherapy was defined by Harry Stack Sullivan (1954) as primarily a verbal interchange between two individuals in which one of these individuals is designated an expert and the other a help-seeker. These two persons work together to identify the patient's characteristic problems in living, with the hope of achieving behavioral change (Table 29–1). This definition of psychotherapy excludes a substantial number of activities that are inaccurately considered psychotherapy. First, psychotherapy by this definition is verbal. Certainly more than 90% of the interchange in psychotherapy is verbal. Although nonverbal communication can be important, it is never the primary activity of psychotherapy. Second, the requirement that one person be the help-seeker and the other an expert sets the roles, activities, and boundaries of this interchange. Two friends sharing a drink at a bar or restaurant do not fit this picture. In fact, in the bar or restaurant the social setting and rules are very different. In these settings, the rules of interaction dictate an equal sharing of one's problems. If one person is always the listener, the other begins to feel uncomfortable, because this is not the expected interchange. Rather, at the bar or restaurant, one person talks and then the other often says, "Oh yes, me too," or something similar. Not so in psychotherapy. Here the patient reveals his or her problems, but the physician-therapist provides help, not a reciprocal revelation of problems. The two settings have different rules governing the relationship (Epstein 1995).

All medical treatments, including psychotherapy, also show the effects of nonspecific curative factors in their outcomes (Table 29–2). These factors, also called *placebo effects*, include the presence of a confiding relationship, abreaction (i.e., the expression of intense feelings), the provision of new information, and the provision of a rationale or

meaning (i.e., diagnosis) that organizes seemingly unrelated symptoms and events and maximizes the patient's probability of success experiences (J. D. Frank 1971). Clinicians use these principles as part of the art and science of medical treatment to increase their patients' relief of pain and suffering.

In addition to these nonspecific factors, most medical treatments also have specific curative factors. Similarly, the psychotherapies identify specific technical interventions and procedures directed toward behavioral change.

As in other medical treatments, there are contraindications to and dangers in the use of psychotherapy (Crown 1983; Hadley and Strupp 1976). It is not sufficient in the present-day climate to take the position that "the operation was a success but the patient died"—to state that psychotherapy was a success but no change occurred. Although the therapist in individual psychotherapy does not "require" behavioral change and, depending on the type of psychotherapy, may or may not directly use technical procedures for behavioral change, the final result of the therapist's technical expertise is behavioral change, including alterations in the patient's well-being, physical health, social supports, and societal productivity, as well as symptomatic relief. What is dealt with in treatment is what the patient is able to bring into focus, what the patient can tolerate talking about, and what he or she can tolerate the therapist's talking about (Coleman 1968).

Psychotherapy is both efficacious and cost effective (Crits-Christoph 1992; Lazar 1997). The effectiveness of psychotherapy is not argued now as it had been in the past (Luborsky et al. 1975; Parloff 1982; Parloff et al. 1986; Shapiro and Shapiro 1982; Smith et al. 1980; Spiegel and Lazar 1997). However, the answer to the question of which psychotherapy for which patient and by which therapist is still unclear (Parloff 1982).

The cost-effectiveness of psychotherapeutic treatment is a focus of substantial research (Krupnick and Pincus 1992; Lazar 1997). Individual psychotherapy has been shown to result in fewer days of hospitalization for

TABLE 29-1. Individual psychotherapy

Consists of an interaction between two persons.

Interaction is primarily verbal.

One person is the help-seeker and the other an expert.

Goal of the interaction is to identify the characteristic patterns of behavior of the patient that are causing symptoms and problems in living.

Patient has the expectation of help and change.

TABLE 29-2. The nonspecific curative factors of medical intervention

Development of a confiding relationship

Maintaining the expectation of help and benefit

Providing opportunities for abreaction

Providing new information

Providing a rationale/organization/meaning (diagnosis) to seemingly unrelated symptoms and events

Maximizing the probability that the patient will experience a success

patients on medical and surgical services of a general hospital. In health clinics or health maintenance organizations, brief psychotherapy decreases the number of visits to primary health care providers, reduces the number of laboratory and X-ray studies, decreases the number of prescriptions given, and, overall, reduces direct health care costs (Longobardi 1981; Sharfstein et al. 1984). Mumford et al. (1984) summarized their meta-analysis of the cost-offset effects of outpatient mental health treatments, the majority of which were short-term. They found that outpatient psychotherapy resulted in an average reduction of 33% in use of medical care. Furthermore, these reductions occurred predominantly in the more expensive inpatient medical services.

In another study (Meyer et al. 1981), 72 patients with major emotional problems who had been treated only by internists in a general medical clinic were compared with 62 patients who, in addition to being treated by internists for medical problems, received 10 weekly psychotherapy visits. Both groups had approximately an equal degree of emotional disturbance. At 4-month and 1-year follow-ups, the brief psychotherapy group reported many more global improvements than did the nonpsychotherapy group. Also, more patients in the brief psychotherapy group than in the nonpsychotherapy group were employed at 1-year follow-up. This study suggests that there are specific beneficial effects of brief psychotherapy when it is used in a medical setting by skilled psychotherapists.

Combining psychotherapy with antidepressant medication has also been shown to produce the best outcome at 1-year follow-up when compared with either treatment alone (DiMascio et al. 1979; Weissman et al. 1981).

Smith and colleagues (Smith and Glass 1977; Smith et al. 1980) showed an effect size of psychotherapy of 0.68, a level equivalent to that of several clinical trials that were stopped early because it would have been unethical to withhold such a clearly effective treatment from patients. Crits-Christoph (1992) demonstrated somewhat larger effect sizes in a review of well-designed studies of brief psychodynamic psychotherapy. This review also found that after brief psychodynamic psychotherapy, patients were better off than 79% of those on a waiting list in terms of psychiatric symptom levels and social adjustment. Howard et al. (1986) found that 74% of patients in psychotherapy were improved after 26 sessions. For a comparison group with only general medical support, this degree of recovery required 2 years (McNeilly and Howard 1991).

Although at times we speak of psychotherapy as beginning as soon as the physician sees the patient, this hyperbole is used primarily to underscore the importance of interpersonal and transferential elements in the initial meeting with the patient. In fact, it is extremely important to distinguish the diagnostic interviews from the ongoing treatment. The evaluation process is distinct from, although related to, the psychotherapy itself. The interventions and technical procedures performed during the evaluation phase are substantially different from the technical procedures of psychotherapy itself. During the evaluation phase, the physician must assess the diagnosis and the patient's ego strength and physical health. In addition, the clinician must closely consider the selection criteria and the different treatment options, including "no treatment indicated" (Frances and Clarkin 1981). This phase constitutes, in Levinson's terminology, the *candidacy stage* (Levinson et al. 1967). Through negotiation with the patient, a treatment decision is reached and the psychotherapy begins.

Many patients do not make it through the evaluation phase of seeking help. Repeatedly, it has been shown that more than 50% of patients drop out by five sessions. It is inappropriate to consider those who drop out as having been in psychotherapy. Clearly, some of these patients experience benefit during their short contact with mental health professionals (Malan et al. 1975)—some through the nonspecific curative factors of help seeking and others through guidance and crisis intervention. In addition, many may drop out because they did not receive what they were looking for.

Psychotherapies can be distinguished by their overall goals, the techniques used, and the diagnostic categories to which the techniques can be applied. In this chapter we review psychoanalytically oriented treatments—psychoanalysis and psychoanalytically oriented (psychodynamic) psychotherapy—interpersonal psychotherapy, which has many psychodynamic elements, and, finally, supportive psychotherapy. The psychoanalytically oriented and supportive psychotherapies remain the most commonly used psychotherapies. Many of the principles of the psychodynamic/psychoanalytic treatments have been incorporated into other treatment modalities and into the clinical assessment process, medication management, and ward milieu work. Understanding the principles and phenomena observed in psychodynamic treatment, therefore, is often critical to success with other treatments and evaluation techniques (Gabbard 1990). In addition, skill in the briefer forms of psychotherapy is related to skill in the longer-term treatments, although these treatment approaches are not the same.

The psychoanalytically oriented treatments and supportive psychotherapy are applied to a wide array of diagnostic problems. Understanding the techniques and the phases of these therapies can also provide important knowledge and skills for assessment and management of medication, compliance, interpersonal stressors, and past and present family problems, all of which can greatly affect outcome, relapse, rehabilitation, and social function.

PSYCHOANALYTICALLY ORIENTED PSYCHOTHERAPIES

Primary to the psychodynamic (psychoanalytically oriented) treatments is the importance of the patient feeling engaged and involved in the work. Through the exploration of the patient's conflicts evidenced in symptoms, metaphors, and symbols, both defensive patterns and disturbances in present interpersonal relationships can be identified in the treatment setting as well as in the patient's life. The therapist's ability to hear what the patient has to say and to understand its meaning is central to all psychoanalytically oriented treatments. This facet of treatment demands skill in neutral listening and the ability to identify with the patient's perspective and worldview while not losing one's own.

The therapist is always listening for the continuity present, but hidden, between each session (Coleman 1968). The therapist operates on the hypothesis that each session is related to the previous one. The psychoanalyst and the psychodynamic psychotherapist listen to the patient's experience of the world and the resulting conflicts and defenses that result in the day-to-day changes in moods, thoughts, and behaviors (Mohl and McLaughlin 1996; Silberman and Certa 1996).

In the initial phase of treatment, the therapeutic alliance (i.e., the working alliance) is developed (Greenson 1965; Zetzel 1956). The therapeutic alliance is the reality-based relationship between the analyst (or the therapist) and the patient that forms the basis of working together in a cooperative manner. The therapeutic alliance is nurtured through the identification of the patient's initial anxieties about beginning treatment. Fostering the therapeutic alliance is a part of the therapist's establishment of the conditions under which the patient can favorably hear and deal with the interpretations that the therapist will give later in the treatment.

Few empirical studies of psychoanalytic treatment have been done (Bachrach et al. 1985; Kantrowitz et al. 1986, 1987, 1990; Kernberg et al. 1972; Wallerstein 1992). The brief psychodynamic treatments have a somewhat greater empirical database, but much further research is needed here as well (Crits-Christoph 1992; Gomes-Schwartz et al. 1978; Horowitz et al. 1986; Luborsky et al.

1975, 1988; Malan 1980; Strupp 1980a, 1980b, 1980c). In general, the studies that have been conducted support the efficacy of psychoanalytically oriented treatment approaches. However, methodological issues are prominent in most of the research in this area. Moreover, the difficulties of long-term studies are substantial. Handbooks for treatment will go far in improving research in the psychoanalytically oriented treatments (Luborsky 1984; Strupp and Binder 1984).

PSYCHOANALYSIS

Psychoanalysis was developed by Sigmund Freud beginning in the late nineteenth century. Originally, Freud used hypnosis to recover forgotten memories related to traumas of early childhood. Historically, he progressed from hypnosis to the "pressure technique" and finally to the modern approach of using free association. Perhaps Freud's most important and lasting discovery was the contribution of psychic reality to development and conflict formation. Freud found that it was the subjective experience of events in childhood—that is, the psychic reality of the events—rather than the presence or absence of the actual events, that affected development and conflict formation. This discovery led Freud to identify the role of the unconscious and unremembered experiences of childhood and to develop a mechanism, psychoanalysis, to discover and bring these memories into awareness.

The dangers of neglecting the actuality of traumatic events have been highlighted in recent years and must always be considered by the therapist. In the treatment of children this is particularly important because of the need to intervene to protect the child. Often a neglect of the reality of trauma results if the therapist does not understand that the patient's recall is a mixture of both subjective factors and objective fact, neither of which can be ignored.

Freud identified dreams, slips of the tongue, and free association as important windows on the influence of childhood and the present conflicts of the patient. From the psychoanalytic view, an understanding of the conflicts experienced in childhood is important to gaining knowledge of and changing present behavior (Brenner 1976). The conflicts of childhood are called the *childhood neurosis*.

Conflicts are patterns of feelings, thoughts, and behavior that were "learned" (i.e., incorporated into brain function and patterning) during childhood. "Neurotic" conflicts result in the patient's feelings of anxiety and depression; somatic symptoms; work, social, or sexual inhibition; and maladaptive interpersonal relations. Typically such conflicts are between libidinal (i.e., sexual/bodily) and aggressive wishes. Libidinal wishes can be thought of as longings for sexual and emotional gratification. Aggressive wishes are destructive desires that either are primary or result from frustration and deprivation.

The concept of sexual wishes is quite broad in psychoanalysis and is not limited to only genital feelings. Sexual wishes include wishes to be held and touched, to control, to eat, and many others. This concept of sexuality was another of Freud's major contributions: his discovery, and the subsequent confirmation through child observation, of the intimate relationship between children and their bodies. It is through their bodies that children come to know mother, father, and the world. It is hard to overemphasize the radical change in thinking that resulted from beginning to think of the child as having thoughts, feelings, and fantasies and as not being a "tabula rasa" or a "small adult."

The goal of psychoanalysis is the elucidation of the childhood neurosis (i.e., conflicts) as it presents in the transference neurosis (Table 29–3). This is a major undertaking that requires a reasonably psychiatrically healthy individual who can sustain the treatment. Psychoanalysis is frequently criticized for being used to treat reasonably psychiatrically healthy people. In fact, however, this is the tradition of medicine. For example, one may ask who receives triple bypass surgery: the individual with a single left main descending artery occlusion or the individual who is having a myocardial infarction and in the end stage of congestive heart failure? Clearly, the answer is the former. This under-

TABLE 29-3. Psychoanalysis

Goal	Resolution of the childhood neurosis as it presents itself in the transference neurosis
Selection criteria	Experiences conflict that is primarily oedipal
	Experiences conflict as internal
	Is psychologically minded
	Is able to obtain symptom relief through understanding
	Is able to experience and observe strong affects without acting out
	Has supportive relationships available in both the present and the past
Duration	Four to five sessions per week; 3–6 years, average duration
Techniques	Free association
	Therapeutic alliance
	Neutrality
	Abstinence
	Defense analysis
	Interpretation of transference

scores the frequently forgotten point that medical treatments are given to patients rather than to diseases. All medical treatments, including psychoanalysis, make certain requirements of the patient. These requirements must be considered when the treatment is prescribed. Psychoanalysis is very demanding of patients. It requires an individual who is able to access his or her fantasy life in an active, experiencing manner and is able to leave it behind at the end of a session.

Psychoanalysis focuses on the recovery of childhood experiences as they appear in the relationship with the analyst (Coltrera 1980; Freud 1912a/1958; Gill 1982; Greenson 1967). This re-creation in the doctor-patient relationship of a conflicted relationship with a childhood figure is the *transference neurosis*. Frequently, the transference is paternal or maternal, but it need not be. Sibling, aunt, uncle, and grandparent transferences are all important parts of psychoanalytic work. The transference neurosis (in contrast to transference phenomena) is the sustained appearance of the transference over time. When the transference neurosis is present, the patient experiences the analyst in a similar manner as he or she once did the significant figure from the past. Frequently, this experience is accompanied by other elements of the past being experienced in the patient's life.

Transference is a ubiquitous phenomenon that is increasingly able to be studied empirically (Fried et al. 1992; Luborsky and Crits-Christoph 1990). Several empirical studies support the importance of addressing the transference for a successful outcome of psychodynamic treatment (Brodaty 1983; Donovan 1984; Frances and Perry 1983; Luborsky and Crits-Christoph 1990; Malan 1975, 1976, 1980; Marziali 1984; Marziali and Sullivan 1980). Transference is the result of our tendency to see the past in the present, to exclude new information, and to see what is familiar to us (Table 29–4). This "looking for the familiar" results in our reacting and responding in ways that are characteristic of our relationships with significant figures from our past. The analyst's relative abstinence (i.e., avoiding gratifying wishes) and neutrality (i.e., not encouraging one side or another of the patient's conflict—either the wishes or the defenses and prohibitions) help create a setting in which the transference can emerge and, more important, in which it can be observed and understood by the analyst and the patient. It is the contrast between the patient's experience of the analyst in the transference and his or her experience in the therapeutic alliance that facilitates the recognition that the transference thoughts and feelings are self-generated.

The transference is not a total distortion of the doctor-patient relationship. Rather, it is often an elaboration

TABLE 29–4. Transference and countertransference

Transference	Seeing the past in the present
	Seeing the familiar
	Excluding new information
Countertransference	
Concordant	Identifying with the patient's feelings
	The therapist feels as though he or she were the patient
Complementary	Reacting to the patient's feelings
	The therapist feels as though he or she were the transference figure

(without confirming information) of an observation the patient has made about the analyst or his or her office. Reality serves as the seed on which the transference is constructed. The patient's understanding of the transference aids in the recall of the past and the recovery of lost feelings.

Countertransference is the analyst's transference response to the patient. At times, *countertransference* is also used to describe the analyst's specific neurotic responses to the patient's transference (Table 29–4). However, this is not clearly different from the first, more general, definition (Blum 1986; Sandler et al. 1973). Countertransference is also ubiquitous and it is not limited to the psychoanalytic setting. In fact, it can be an important part of any relationship, particularly the doctor-patient relationship; when present, it may be intense and enduring. Countertransference is increased by life stress and unresolved conflicts in the analyst. It can appear as either an identification with or a reaction to the patient's conscious and unconscious fantasies, feelings, and behaviors (Racker 1957). Through analysis of his or her own countertransference reactions, the analyst recognizes subtle aspects of the transference relationship and is better able to understand the patient's experience (Searles 1965). Skill in recognizing countertransference and transference is an important part of the psychiatrist's armamentarium in all treatment settings, particularly those involving consultation-liaison psychiatry, in which the doctor-patient or nurse-patient relationships can be the major reason a consultation was requested.

The design of the psychoanalytic treatment situation fosters the patient's observing capacity so that the transference neurosis can be analyzed (Stone 1961). Transference is not unique to the psychoanalytic situation. It occurs throughout life in all areas and is a frequent accompaniment to hospitalization of any kind. Entering a hospital, having one's clothes removed, having one's name forgotten, being required to eat when told, and having to submit to medical procedures constitute a highly regressive experience that facilitates the appearance of transferences. The ability to recognize transference phenomena as they appear in all doctor-patient relationships is very important. Psychoanalysis is unique in its efforts to establish a setting in which the transference, when it appears, can be used as a vehicle for understanding.

Modern psychoanalysis continues to require frequent meetings of the analyst and analysand—usually, four to five sessions per week. (Freud originally met with his patients six times per week.) This frequency of sessions is continued, on the average, for 3–6 years. This intensity of meetings is necessary for the patient to develop sufficient trust to explore his or her inner fantasy life. In addition, given the number of events that occur daily in a life, the frequent meetings enable the patient to explore fantasies rather than only the reality-based perceptions of life events (Freud 1912b/1958). Individuals who are in crisis and who therefore are very concerned and focused on the real events in their life are not good candidates to enter psychoanalysis. Psychoanalysis focuses on the patient's experience and fantasies of his or her life rather than on the real events. A crisis does not allow the patient the opportunity to explore fantasies. In general, the patient in psychoanalysis is encouraged to use the couch so that the patient's focus on fantasies rather than on reality will be further facilitated. In addition, the analyst usually sits out of view, allowing the patient better to elaborate his or her fantasies about the analyst.

Free association is a major element in the technique of psychoanalysis. Freud described free association through an analogy of a train ride (Freud 1913/1958). He suggested that if the analyst and analysand were riding together on a train and the analyst were blind, the analysand would not forget to describe the beautiful mountains or the ugly coal slags. This analogy is meant to convey the sense of the patient's reporting of all thoughts that come to mind without censorship and without dismissing them as too trivial. In point of fact, free association is difficult to attain, and much of the work of psychoanalysis is based on identifying those places where free association breaks down (i.e., the occurrence of a defense, clinically experienced by the analyst as resistance). When the patient is able to achieve the highest level of free association, the neurotic conflicts have been removed and termination is near.

Early in treatment, the analyst establishes a therapeutic alliance with the patient that allows for a reality-based consideration of the demands of the treatment and for a working collaboration between analyst and analysand toward the patient's understanding himself or herself

(Greenson 1965; Zetzel 1956). The analyst focuses on analyzing the defenses the patient uses to minimize conflict and disturbing affects (Freud 1912b/1958, 1913/1958, 1914/1958) (Table 29–5). Defenses such as intellectualization, reaction formation, denial, repression, and other neurotic cognitive mechanisms are identified and repeatedly interpreted to the patient. Through the analysis of defense, the working alliance strengthens and the patient's ability to observe internal fantasies increases. In addition, the patient's comfort with talking about his or her feelings with the analyst increases. In this way, the transference grows more available and can be analyzed.

The analysis of the patient's dreams is an important element of psychoanalytic treatment (Freud 1911/1958; Sharpe 1961; Ursano et al. 1997). Dreams, as well as slips of the tongue and symptoms, express the conflicts of the patient in "metaphor," evidencing the out-of-awareness (i.e., unconscious) elements of the conflict. The building blocks of dreams are recent life events. Dreams express both a present and a childhood conflict in much the same way that a rebus expresses a story. The grammar of the dream process is different from that of conscious thought. Rather than following logic and time sequence, dreams are constructed by condensation of multiple meanings and the use of symbols. There are no universal symbols. The symbols, perhaps better thought of as symbolic vehicles available to any given person, are from the "dictionary" of meanings developed as part of the individual's life experience, both in childhood and in adulthood. Thus, dreams (and slips of the tongue and symptoms) are a means for the patient to understand the feelings and thoughts that influence his or her life, that are out of awareness, and that often are derived from childhood experiences, beliefs, and views of the interpersonal world and familial behavior (Weiss and Sampson 1986).

The primary goal of psychoanalysis is the establishment of the transference relationship and the subsequent

analysis of this relationship. It is this primary focus that distinguishes psychoanalysis from psychodynamic psychotherapy. The specific treatment effects of psychoanalysis grow from the experience and analysis of the transference, reawakened affects, cognitions, and behaviors linked with significant individuals in the patient's past. In the context of the arousal associated with these figures and the simultaneous understanding of the experience, behavioral change occurs (Loewald 1980).

The analyst uses a number of techniques in his or her interventions, including interpretation and clarification (Bibring 1954; Glover 1968; Sandler et al. 1973). Classically, an interpretation is the linking together of the patient's experience of an event in the present with the transference experience of the analyst and the childhood-significant figure. Rarely are interpretations actually given in one sentence in one session. More frequently, interpretations occur over a period during which the past, the present, and the transference experiences are linked together.

Medications are infrequently used in psychoanalysis, although some analysts are attempting to use psychoanalysis with medication in the treatment of persons with affective disorders. Psychoanalysis is actually a highly supportive treatment for the individual who experiences frequent contact, quiet inquiry, and intellectual understanding as a supportive environment (de Jonghe et al. 1992; Wallerstein 1986, 1989). The supportive elements and their contribution to the treatment process have been less discussed in psychoanalysis than in other treatments. The need for medication may indicate the patient's need for greater support than can be provided in the psychoanalytic treatment.

The analyst operates under several guiding principles that facilitate the analysis of the transference. These principles include 1) neutrality, by which the analyst favors neither the patient's wishes (i.e., id) nor the condemnations of these wishes (i.e., superego); and 2) abstinence, whereby the analyst does not provide gratification to the patient similar to that of the wished-for object (Freud 1915 [1914]/1958) (Table 29–6). It is helpful in understanding the rule of abstinence to recognize a definition of transference used by Joseph Sandler. Sandler (1973) described transference as the role pressure placed on the analyst to conform to the behaviors of the significant individual from the past. Therefore, transference is experienced by the analyst as an expectation from the patient that the analyst will behave in a certain manner. Abstinence is the avoidance of becoming this figure *in reality* and gratifying these wishes or beliefs. The therapist's abstinence leads to his or her being somewhat silent but not withholding, in order better to observe how the patient organizes his or her psychic world. This stance must be explained and the patient educated

TABLE 29–5. Defense mechanisms

Repression	Intellectualization
Reaction formation	Regression
Displacement	Sublimation
Reversal	Splitting
Denial	Projection
Inhibition	Projected identification
Asceticism	Omnipotence
Isolation of affect	Devaluing
Identification with the aggressor	Primitive idealization

TABLE 29-6.   Principles of psychoanalytic technique

Neutrality	The analyst maintains a neutral stance favoring neither the patient's wishes (i.e., id) nor the patient's condemnations of these wishes (i.e., superego).
Abstinence	The analyst does not gratify the patient's desire or expectation that the analyst act like the person from the past. Rather, the analyst helps the patient see and understand this process.

about the reason for this stance.

The assessment of a patient for psychoanalysis must include diagnostic considerations as well as an assessment of the patient's ability to make use of the psychoanalytic situation for behavioral change. These considerations include the patient's psychological-mindedness; the availability of supports in his or her real environment to sustain the psychoanalysis, which can be felt as quite depriving; and the patient's ability to experience and simultaneously to observe highly charged affective states.

Because of the frequency of the sessions and the duration of the treatment, the cost of psychoanalysis can be prohibitive. Low-fee clinics frequently make available a substantial amount of treatment to some patients who could not otherwise afford it.

Psychoanalysis has been useful in the treatment of obsessional disorders, anxiety disorders, dysthymic disorders, and moderately severe personality disorders. Individuals with substantial preoedipal pathology, usually indicated by chaotic life settings and an inability to establish a supportive dyadic relationship, as is often seen in patients with narcissistic, borderline, schizoid, paranoid, and schizotypal personality disorders, are usually not thought to be candidates for traditional psychoanalysis. In the present climate of emphasis on cost-effectiveness, psychoanalysis is more frequently recommended after a course of brief psychotherapy has proved to be either ineffective or insufficient.

PSYCHOANALYTIC PSYCHOTHERAPY

Psychoanalytically oriented psychotherapy—also known as *psychoanalytic psychotherapy*, *psychodynamic psychotherapy*, and *explorative psychotherapy*—is a psychotherapeutic procedure that recognizes the development of transference and resistance in the psychotherapy setting (Bruch 1974; Fromm-Reichmann 1950). Both long-term and brief psychodynamic psychotherapy are possible. In the past, the terms *brief psychotherapy* and *long-term psychotherapy*

were frequently used synonymously with *supportive psychotherapy* and *explorative psychotherapy*, respectively. However, brief and long-term more accurately describe the duration rather than the technique, focus, or goal of psychoanalytically oriented psychotherapy (Budman and Gurman 1983; Errera et al. 1967; Ursano and Dressler 1977). Brief psychotherapy, in particular, requires the therapist to confront his or her own ambitiousness and perfectionism as well as any exaggerated ideal of personality structure and function. The time limits of brief psychotherapy give the therapy its unique characteristics and distinguish it from long-term psychotherapy and psychoanalysis (Ursano and Dressler 1974). Stierlin (1968) identified two treatment factors that are important to understanding the effectiveness of psychotherapy: the "propitious moment" and the "shared past." Brief psychotherapy uses the propitious moment to create personality change, whereas long-term treatment uses the shared past that develops between therapist and patient. Both the propitious moment and the shared past carry psychotherapeutic advantages and disadvantages, emphasizing certain technical possibilities and limiting others.

Following World War II, the interest in psychoanalysis resulted in a rapid growth in the demand for psychotherapy. This growing demand considerably increased the resultant pressure on psychiatrists to develop briefer and less intense forms of psychotherapy than psychoanalysis. In addition, the community mental health movement, and, more recently, the increasing cost of mental health care, have stimulated efforts to find briefer forms of psychotherapy. At present, brief psychotherapy is an important part of the psychiatrist's armamentarium. (See Chapter 28 for a detailed discussion of brief psychodynamic psychotherapy.)

Psychoanalytic psychotherapy is usually more focused than the extensive reworking of personality undertaken in psychoanalysis (Dewald 1978). In addition, psychoanalytic psychotherapy is oriented somewhat more to the here and now and there is less of an attempt to reconstruct the developmental origins of conflicts. Psychoanalytically oriented psychotherapy may take as its entire goal the analysis of a set of defenses that are interfering with the patient's development. The accomplishment of this task may substantially open up the patient's life and development.

Psychoanalytic psychotherapy recognizes and interprets transference when it occurs (Table 29–7). However, the entire treatment is not directed toward the establishment and analysis of the transference in the thorough manner of a psychoanalysis. Long-term psychodynamic psychotherapy includes more transference work than do the brief psychodynamic psychotherapies. Psychoanalytic psychotherapy also makes use of techniques that are not

TABLE 29–7.   **Psychoanalytic psychotherapy**

Goal	Defense and transference analysis with limited reconstruction of the past
Selection criteria	When a narrower focus and less comprehensive outcome is acceptable
	The same selection criteria as in psychoanalysis are used, but they can include more seriously disturbed patients who can use understanding to resolve symptoms when supportive elements are available in the treatment
Duration	One to three sessions per week for 1–6 years on average
Techniques	Therapeutic alliance
	Face to face
	Free association
	Defense and transference interpretation
	More use of clarification, suggestion, and learning through experience than in psychoanalysis
	Medication

available in psychoanalysis. This allows for its application to a broader range of patients, including those with psychotic regressive potentials such as borderline personality disorder.

Usually, patients in long-term psychoanalytic psychotherapy are seen one, two, or three times per week; twice per week is desirable in that this frequency allows for sufficient intensity for the transference to unfold and to be interpreted. Patient and therapist meet in face-to-face encounters and free association is encouraged. Psychoanalytic psychotherapy may extend from several months to several years, at times taking as long as a psychoanalysis. The length of treatment is determined by the number of focal problem areas undertaken in the treatment. Medications can be used in psychoanalytic psychotherapy and provide another means of titrating the level of regression a patient may experience. The therapist uses interpretations and clarifications as in psychoanalysis. In addition, however, the therapist may use other interpretative techniques such as suggestion, manipulation, and confrontation (Bibring 1954). Manipulation in this context refers to learning from experience, such as pointing out that the therapist does not respond in the expected transferential manner. Confrontation is not "fighting" but rather pointing out to the patient when something is being denied or avoided.

The same patients who are treated in psychoanalysis can be treated in psychoanalytic psychotherapy. However, the focus of the treatment is much narrower and the expected outcome less comprehensive. At times, the supportive elements of a psychoanalytic psychotherapy can interfere with the patient's full experience of his or her conflicts, which can be more evident to the patient in a psychoanalysis. The psychosocial problems and internal conflicts of patients who could not be treated in psychoanalysis, such as those with major depression, schizophrenia, and borderline personality disorder, can be addressed in a long-term psychoanalytic psychotherapy. The long-term contributions of psychoanalytic psychotherapy to the treatment of major depression and schizophrenia, for which biological treatments have proved efficacious for some of the major symptoms, require further study. Patients with these diagnoses use psychotherapy to modify illness-onset conditions and facilitate readjustment, recovery, and integration into family and community. In long-term psychoanalytic psychotherapy, the regressive tendencies of such patients can be titrated with greater elements of support, the use of medication as needed, and greater reality feedback through the face-to-face encounter with the therapist.

Strupp's studies of college students and Luborsky's work on the helping alliance confirm the importance of interactional variables and support to the outcome in psychotherapy (Butler and Strupp 1993; Horvath et al. 1993; Luborsky et al. 1988; Strupp 1980a, 1980b; Strupp and Binder 1984). Both investigators also found that the quality of the therapeutic interaction and the handling of the transference and countertransference are critical to success or failure in treatment. Strupp's studies indicate that patients treated by nonprofessionally trained therapists are as much improved, on average, as patients treated by professional therapists. However, they also show that such nonexperienced therapists run out of relevant material and soon become unwilling to continue to treat patients over an extended period (Strupp 1980c; Strupp and Hadley 1979). One of the important tasks of training in psychotherapy may be the development of the ability to "endure" with the patient and, over time, with numbers of patients. Technical training and a theoretical framework may allow the therapist to maintain a sense of competence, direction, and interest in the work that the nonprofessional therapist cannot.

The opening phase of psychodynamic psychotherapy is often marked by the activation of the magical expectations of the patient and the belief that past pains will now be resolved. During the initial phase, the therapist may make few comments and usually accepts the positive transference of the patient. Important aspects of the current problems, the patient's characteristic defense mechanisms and coping styles, and the developmental roots of the central issue become clearer during this phase. In the middle phase of treatment, resistance is likely to appear, as well as the negative transference. The patient experiences the frustration that all of the wished-for changes are not occurring. Defenses are identified and analyzed, and usually the transference is sufficiently evident to be worked with.

The patient must be educated about transference phenomena and develop sufficient observing ego to participate with the therapist in wondering about this aspect of his or her internal life. The transference is not suddenly interpreted to the patient, nor should one assume that the patient knows that it is expected or desirable to talk about feelings toward the therapist. It is the skill of the therapist that allows him or her to know when to introduce this topic to the patient and how to help the patient increasingly to explore this area of feelings and thoughts. In the end phase of treatment, termination and the patient's resistances to termination are prominent. Termination is based on having reached a series of life goals that allows the patient to continue on a normal developmental path. Ideal treatment goals are not the end point. Rather, the reestablishment of normal development and the removal of obstacles to the normal recovery processes are the goals of treatment. The patient's increased capacity to understand his or her conflicts and to analyze conflicts independently indicates that the end of treatment will occur shortly.

INTERPERSONAL PSYCHOTHERAPY

Interpersonal psychotherapy (IPT) is a psychotherapy developed by Klerman and colleagues (Klerman et al. 1984a, 1984b; Rounsaville et al. 1985b). Either brief or longer term, IPT focuses on current interpersonal problems in outpatient nonbipolar, nonpsychotic depressed individuals. IPT has been the major psychotherapeutic modality used in combined psychotherapy and pharmacological treatment studies. This psychotherapy has also been used in treating drug abuse. It did not, however, have a notable impact on outcome when patients were already participating in a well-run treatment program that included weekly group psychotherapy (Rounsaville et al. 1983, 1985a). IPT derives from the interpersonal school of psychiatry that originated with Adolf Meyer and Harry Stack Sullivan. The understanding of social supports and of attachment provides further theoretical underpinning for this form of psychotherapy. IPT focuses on reassurance, clarification of feeling states, improvement in interpersonal communication, testing of perception, and interpersonal skills rather than on personality reconstruction.

In IPT the therapist focuses on the patient's current social functioning (Table 29–8). A complete inventory of current and past significant interpersonal relationships, including the family of origin, friendships, and relations in the community, is a part of the evaluation phase. Patterns of authority, dominance and submission, dependency and autonomy, intimacy, affection, and activities are observed. Cognitions are generally seen as beliefs and attitudes about norms, expectations and roles, and role performance. Defense mechanisms may be recognized, but they are explored in terms of interpersonal relations. Similarly, dreams may be examined as a reflection of current interpersonal problems. In IPT, the therapist may explore distorted thinking by comparing what the patient says with what he or she does or by identifying the patient's view of an interpersonal relationship (Klerman et al. 1984b).

IPT has been primarily used in the treatment of depressed patients (A. F. Frank et al. 1991). In the opening phase of IPT, a detailed symptom history is taken, usually using a structured interview. The symptoms are reviewed with the patient, and the patient receives explicit information about the natural course of depression as a clinical condition. There is an emphasis on legitimizing the patient in the sick role. A second major task of this phase is the assessment of the patient's interpersonal problem areas. There is an attempt to identify one or more of four problem areas: grief reaction, interpersonal disputes, role transition, and interpersonal deficits. Each of these areas is thought to be related to depression.

The middle phase of treatment is directed toward resolving the problem area or areas. Clarifying positive and negative feeling states, identifying past models for relationships, and guiding and encouraging the patient in examining and choosing alternative courses of action constitute the basic techniques for handling each problem area (Weissman and Markowitz 1994). The focus is kept on current dilemmas and not past interpersonal relationships.

TABLE 29–8. Interpersonal psychotherapy

Goal	Improvement in current interpersonal skills
Selection criteria	Outpatient, nonbipolar, nonpsychotic depression
Duration	Short- and long-term Usually once-weekly meetings
Techniques	Reassurance Clarification of feeling states Improvement of interpersonal communication Testing perceptions Development of interpersonal skills Medication

Interpersonal events, rather than intrapsychic or cognitive events, are the focus of IPT.

Much of IPT is based on psychodynamic theory. The therapist's attitude is one of exploration, similar to the attitude in other insight-oriented psychotherapies when applied in a medical model. Applying the dictum of working "from the surface to the depths" results in much of the resemblance of IPT to psychodynamic psychotherapy. However, Klerman and colleagues found it useful to highlight the differences between these approaches to standardize a psychotherapeutic technique. Collaborative clinical trials have demonstrated the advantage of maintenance IPT in enhancing social functioning during recovery from depression and in reducing symptoms and improving functioning during the acute phase of a depressive episode. These effects require 6–8 months to become apparent. Depressed patients undergoing combined pharmacotherapy and IPT have the best outcomes (DiMascio et al. 1979; Weissman et al. 1981).

COMPARISON OF PSYCHODYNAMIC, INTERPERSONAL, AND COGNITIVE PSYCHOTHERAPIES

Because interpersonal and cognitive (see Chapter 30) psychotherapies are related to the psychodynamic model, there is a high degree of overlap in the problem areas identified in any given patient in these treatments. The conceptualization of the problem, however, is different. In many ways it is complementary rather than mutually exclusive. The psychoanalytic, interpersonal, and cognitive psychotherapies share explorative and change-oriented goals. Cognitive psychotherapy focuses on the patient's thinking; IPT on the patient's interpersonal relations and social supports; and psychoanalytically oriented treatments on the internal experience of the patient and its relationship to past experience. Cognitive and interpersonal psychotherapies are most frequently used to treat depression rather than to treat an entire range of psychopathology. No studies using well-defined psychodynamic psychotherapies and medication have been performed. In this area, IPT and cognitive psychotherapy have been more closely studied.

IPT, cognitive psychotherapy, and the more traditional psychodynamic psychotherapies can be compared (Table 29–9). All three modalities are complex methods of treatment that must be tailored to the individual patient. All demand a high degree of clinical judgment, and the therapist requires a considerable amount of time to acquire competency in administering these treatments (Beck et al. 1979).

The relationship between therapist and patient and the establishment of a therapeutic alliance are essential in IPT, cognitive psychotherapy, and the psychoanalytically oriented treatments. Extensive exploration of the patient's thoughts and feelings, including those involving the therapist, is a major portion of the work. In addition, in all three, the therapist attempts to maintain an investigative, collaborative, and nonjudgmental stance.

In practice, cognitive psychotherapy is similar to the analysis of defense in the psychodynamic approaches. Understanding defenses focuses the patient and therapist on the hidden cognitive distortions that result in the patient's faulty perception of both the internal and the external world. In the dynamic model, defense mechanisms are directed toward the control of anxiety resulting from conflict. The defenses, however, distort perception and cognition—resulting in distortions that are similar to those that are the focus of cognitive psychotherapy. In cognitive psychotherapy, cognitions are seen as the causative agent of the patient's distress. Much of the work in identifying these cognitions and alerting the patient to them is similar to the understanding and interpretation of defenses in the psychodynamic psychotherapies. The schemata underlying the faulty cognitions of cognitive psychotherapy are unconscious assumptions, which in the psychodynamic model are viewed as being derived from earlier experience. Both treatments share the importance of identifying these unconscious patterns of behavior and of making them known to the patient. To the extent that a psychodynamic psychotherapy focuses on the here-and-now experience of the patient rather than on the reconstruction of past experience, its similarity to cognitive psychotherapy increases. Frequently, the understanding of a defensive pattern used by a patient to handle an ongoing conflict can be the end point of a well-conducted psychodynamic psychotherapy. In such a case, the outcomes for cognitive and psychodynamic individual psychotherapy might be quite similar.

With regard to the degree of structure and directiveness, however, the two types of psychotherapy are different. In psychodynamic psychotherapy, the structure of the session is largely determined by the flow of the patient's thoughts and the interaction of these thoughts with the therapist's interpretive comments. In contrast, cognitive psychotherapy sessions are structured by an agenda that serves to focus the patient's thoughts and activities. In psychodynamic psychotherapy the role of the therapist is limited to that of an empathic interpreter and sharer of the patient's experiences, whereas in cognitive psychotherapy the therapist may direct, prescribe, enjoin, educate, train,

TABLE 29–9.   Comparison of psychoanalytic, interpersonal, and cognitive psychotherapies

	Psychoanalytic/ psychodynamic psychotherapy	Interpersonal psychotherapy	Cognitive psychotherapy
Treatment focus	Internal experience	Interpersonal relationships and social supports	Thoughts/cognitions
Primary diagnoses treated	Anxiety Depression Personality disorders	Depression Anxiety	Depression Anxiety
Skill needed by therapist	++++	++++	++++
Therapeutic alliance	++++	++++	++++
Nonjudgmental stance	++++	++++	++++
Focus			
Cognitive	+++ (defense mechanisms)	+	++++ (cognitive distortions)
Interpersonal	++++ (transference and past relationships)	++++ (interpersonal withdrawal, attachment and models)	+
Technique			
Nondirective	++++	+	+
Directive/behavioral interventions	+	++++	++++

Note.   Plus signs indicate degree, from small (+) to great (++++).

or role-play as well. Furthermore, in cognitive psychotherapy more emphasis is placed on directly altering psychopathology rather than on facilitating its alleviation through insight and resolution of inferred underlying conflicts.

IPT is most closely related to the psychodynamic object-relations perspective. Understanding internal objects rests on understanding the actual interpersonal relationships of the patient, including his or her relationship with the physician. Both interpersonal and psychodynamic psychotherapy share a focus on identifications and transference, which in IPT is defined as "past models for relationships." In addition, in IPT particular attention is paid to withdrawal and detachment, areas related to defenses in the psychodynamic model and to faulty cognitions in the cognitive model. Interpersonal rather than intrapsychic or cognitive events are identified in IPT. This frequently means that the interpersonal psychotherapist's attention is directed toward the same area of disturbance as is the cognitive or psychodynamic psychotherapist's. However, the identified "problem"—interpersonal deficits, faulty cognitions, or intrapsychic conflict—is different.

The differences in the interventions used by these psychotherapies are more striking than the differences in their goals or in the problems they target for treatment (DeRubeis et al. 1982). To what extent it is the differences in psychotherapeutic treatments, not the similarities, that produce behavioral change is not clear. Both cognitive and interpersonal psychotherapy use more directive and behavioral interventions than do psychodynamic approaches. IPT and cognitive psychotherapy make more use of teaching new behavioral skills. More than the cognitive and interpersonal treatments, the psychodynamic psychotherapies rely on the patient to activate and practice new behaviors without direction. The briefer psychotherapies (i.e., IPT, cognitive psychotherapy, and brief psychodynamic psychotherapy) lack the extended working-through and application period of psychoanalysis and of intensive (i.e., long-term) psychodynamic psychotherapy.

Empirical studies comparing well-defined psychodynamic psychotherapy with cognitive and interpersonal psychotherapies have not been undertaken. Future research must address which form of psychotherapy may be most helpful for which patient. To develop research strategies, it would be helpful to conceptualize this question as related to the mode or modes through which any particular patient can most effectively learn new behaviors. An individual's available learning path (e.g., through the study of cognitions, interpersonal relations, and/or subjective experience) is influenced by state, trait, and contextual variables. The process of learning in the psychotherapies and psychoanalysis, a process of altering neuronal organization through behavioral (primarily verbal) means, may be influenced by the patient's diagnosis, medications, history, cognitive style, developmental stage, and affective availability, as well as the doctor-patient match and other variables. The effectiveness of the therapist in any given modality is certainly a critical variable. The differences and similarities in the outcomes of cognitive, interpersonal, and psychodynamic treatments also require study.

SUPPORTIVE PSYCHOTHERAPY

Despite its ubiquitous use by psychiatrists, *supportive psychotherapy* has traditionally been viewed as a residual category to be prescribed to those patients not amenable to other forms of treatment. Until recently, supportive psychotherapy has been the subject of little conceptual scrutiny or empirical study. Several books and review articles devoted to the subject have now appeared (Pinsker et al. 1991; Rockland 1989a, 1989b; Werman 1984, 1988; Winston et al. 1986). Its techniques have often been defined negatively, that is, in terms of what to avoid rather than what to do (Wallace 1983; Winston et al. 1986).

Supportive psychotherapy can better be defined by its specific goal than by technical procedures. Supportive psychotherapy aims to help the patient maintain or reestablish his or her best possible level of functioning given the limitations of his or her illness, personality, native ability, and life circumstances (Table 29–10). In general, this goal distinguishes supportive psychotherapy from the change-oriented psychotherapies, which aim to reverse primary disease processes and symptoms or restructure personality. However, theorists in self psychology have pointed out that providing a "holding environment," listening empathically, and being a safe and reliable object of identification, which constitute the foundation of supportive therapy, may themselves lead to strengthening of the ego and increased independence of the patient (Ornstein 1986).

Thus, with regard to both techniques and outcome, the line between supportive and change-oriented psychotherapies may not always be clear. The situation is somewhat analogous to the medical treatment of viral versus bacterial infections. Treatment of the former is basically supportive in that it aims to maintain normal bodily functions (for example, treatment goals may include fever reduction, control of cerebral edema, or dietary compensation for liver failure) in the face of infection, whereas treatment of the latter aims to eliminate the infection. However, antibiotic treatment of bacterial infections itself is support-

TABLE 29–10.   Supportive psychotherapy

Goal	Support of reality testing
	Provision of ego support
	Maintenance or reestablishment of usual level of functioning
Selection criteria	Very healthy individual faced with overwhelming crises
	Patient with ego deficits
Duration	Days, months, or years—as needed
Techniques	Predictable availability of therapist
	Use of interpretation to strengthen defenses
	Maintenance of reality-based working relationship grounded in support, concern, and problem solving
	Suggestion, reinforcement, advice, reality testing, cognitive restructuring, reassurance, limit setting, and environmental interventions
	Medication
	Psychodynamic life narrative

ive in that it works as an adjunct to the body's natural immune system, without which the antibiotic treatment is relatively ineffective. Similarly, there are supportive elements in all effective forms of psychotherapy, and the terms *supportive* and *change-oriented* merely describe the balance of efforts in a particular case.

INDICATIONS

Because there are relatively few data to support the assignment of patients to one or another therapy type, personal predilection of the therapist often plays a prominent role in the prescription of supportive versus change-oriented psychotherapy. Most often, change- or insight-oriented therapy is automatically considered the treatment of first choice and supportive therapy is assigned to those patients who are not considered to be able to change. Some authors, however, have suggested that the two types of treatment should be considered on a more equal basis, because a briefer or less intense treatment may be in many patients' best interest as a treatment of first choice (Pinsker et al. 1991; Rockland 1989b). Such considerations become especially relevant as economic pressures force clinicians to prescribe the most efficient among potentially effective treatments.

In common clinical practice, patients at both ends of the health-sickness continuum receive supportive psychotherapy: those who are generally very psychiatrically healthy and well adapted but who have become impaired in response to stressful life circumstances and those who have serious illnesses that cannot be cured (Table 29–11). Supportive psychotherapy may be brief or long-term. The psychiatrically healthy individual, when faced with overwhelming stress or crises—particularly in the face of traumas or disasters—may seek help and be a candidate for supportive psychotherapy. The relatively psychiatrically healthy candidate for supportive psychotherapy is a well-adapted individual with good social support and interpersonal relations, flexible defenses, and good reality testing who is in acute crisis, making use of social supports, not withdrawing, and anticipating resolution of crisis. Although functioning below his or her usual level, this patient remains hopeful about the future and makes use of resources available for problem solving, respite, and growth. This patient uses supportive psychotherapy to reconstitute more rapidly, to avoid errors in judgment by "talking out loud," to relieve minor symptomatology, and to grow as an individual by learning about the world.

The more typical candidate for supportive psychotherapy has significant deficits in ego functioning, including the following:

1. *Poor reality testing.* The patient shows an inability to separate fact from fantasy and to recognize bound-

TABLE 29–11. Characteristics of candidates for supportive psychotherapy

Type I: *Patient impaired by overwhelming crisis, trauma, or disaster and functioning below usual level in response to a crisis.*

Generally very psychiatrically healthy

Well adapted

Good social supports

Good interpersonal relations

Flexible defenses

Good reality testing

Hopeful about future

Uses resources

Type II: *Patient has chronic ego deficits and impaired functioning.*

Impaired reality testing

Difficulty with impulse control

Limited ability to sublimate

Limited interpersonal relations

Frequently high levels of aggression

Limited ability to self-soothe/refuel

Low verbal ability and capacity for introspection

aries between self and others. Such patients may become psychotic under the stress of psychodynamic psychotherapy and develop psychotic transferences.

2. *Poor impulse control.* Typically, such patients need promptly to discharge affects through actions that are often destructive to themselves or others. Such discharge may be because of overwhelmingly intense affects or because the patient has a low ability to tolerate unpleasant affects. These patients are not able to contain and examine feelings as is required by more explorative, change-oriented psychotherapies—psychodynamic, interpersonal, or cognitive. At the least, such patients often bolt from psychotherapy when strong negative affects are aroused.

3. *Poor interpersonal relations.* This patient is unable to form and maintain stable relationships that include reasonable levels of trust and intimacy. Such patients are limited in their capacity to maintain therapeutic relationships as well, especially those that arouse powerful feelings.

4. *Poor balance of affects.* This category includes patients who are overwhelmed by anger or anxiety and those who experience little or no affect of any sort. Such patients generally form tenuous and unstable relationships.

5. *Lack of ability to sublimate.* These patients are unable to channel energy into creative and socially useful activities, reflecting their low ability to master affects and impulses pleasurably.

6. *Low capacity for introspection.* Because self-observation is a necessary step toward the attainment of insight, these patients do poorly in psychotherapies that require self-reflection and curiosity about one's self and one's interpersonal relations.

7. *Low verbal ability.* Most clinicians do not include high intelligence as a prerequisite for insight-oriented psychotherapy. However, patients for the psychodynamic, interpersonal, and cognitive psychotherapies do need to be able to identify and communicate their thoughts and feelings intelligibly to the therapist and, more important, to experience this verbal exchange as at least somewhat relieving and as a valued method of problem solving.

A variety of other factors have been proposed as exclusion criteria for insight-oriented psychotherapy and as possible indications for supportive psychotherapy. Motivation has been stressed by many authors as being of importance. However, it has yet to be determined whether motivation for symptom change, for behavioral change, for a relationship with the therapist, or for insight (among others) is crucial in assigning patients to explorative/ change-oriented (psychodynamic, interpersonal, and cognitive) versus supportive psychotherapy (Bloch 1979). Alexithymic patients are generally referred for supportive rather than insight psychotherapy. Such patients are characterized by an inability to find words to describe their emotions; they tend to describe situational details and symptoms rather than feelings (Sifneos 1975). These patients are thought to be prone to psychosomatic illnesses and likely to be unsuited for insight-oriented psychotherapy (Sifneos 1972, 1972–1973, 1974). However, studies of patients with the traditional psychosomatic illnesses have found these patients to be quite variable in their responses to psychotherapy (Kellner 1975). It remains to be determined to what extent other personality factors may account for the differences. Patients who are very passive and who lack the conviction that their own efforts are effective may be candidates for supportive rather than insight-oriented psychotherapy (Werman 1981). Patients who derive substantial practical benefit from their illness, such as financial or emotional support (i.e., secondary gain), may also be appropriate candidates for supportive psychotherapy rather than an insight-oriented approach (Persson and Alström 1983).

Ego strength and the ability to form relationships may be more important than diagnosis in the selection of patients for supportive psychotherapy (Werman 1984). The patient's ability to relate to the therapist and the patient's history of personal relationships, work and educational performance, and use of leisure time have important effects on the treatment recommendation. Almost no attention has been paid to which characteristics of the patient may predict a good result from supportive psychotherapy rather than merely a poor response to the change-oriented psychotherapies. Delineation of the minimum level of personal strengths needed to benefit from supportive individual psychotherapy is an important task for future research.

TECHNIQUES

Psychoanalytic psychology has provided the major contributions to the theory of the supportive aspects of psychotherapy (de Jonghe et al. 1994). In-depth psychological understanding of patients is as necessary in supportive psychotherapy as it is in the change-oriented, explorative psychotherapies (Pine 1976; Werman 1984). Indeed, although supportive therapy is often dismissed as mere "hand-holding" or "paid friendship," skillful practice of supportive psychotherapy may actually be more difficult than that of change-oriented psychotherapy because the patient may have less capac-

ity to engage beneficially with a therapist (Wallace 1983). Understanding unconscious motivation, psychic conflict, the patient-therapist relationship, and the patient's use of defense mechanisms is essential to comprehending the patient's strengths and vulnerabilities. This knowledge is critical to providing support as well as insight (Bellak and Siegel 1983; Karen Horney Clinic Medical Board 1981; Rockland 1989a).

The technique of supportive psychotherapy can be divided into aspects of the therapist-patient relationship and active interventions by the therapist (Pine 1976). The early mother-child relationship has special implications for supportive psychotherapy (Adler 1982; Pine 1976). The therapist who is predictably available and safe (i.e., who accepts the patient and puts aside his or her own needs in the service of the treatment) assumes some of the holding functions of the good parent. In such a therapeutic situation, the patient is able to identify with and incorporate the well-functioning aspects of the therapist—such as the capacity for self-observation and the ability to tolerate ambivalence (Pine 1976). The patient's use of the therapeutic relationship to achieve greater autonomy may in some ways parallel the child's growing independence as the child's image of the mothering figure is increasingly internalized (Adler 1982; Pine 1976). The use of the mothering figure as a mirror of internal reality or an object of idealization by the child may be necessary to the child's achievement of a cohesive, stable sense of self. Similarly, permitting the patient to see himself or herself "mirrored" in the therapist and as part of an idealized parental figure over long periods may stabilize new internal structures and behaviors. Such an approach is in contrast to psychoanalytically oriented psychotherapy, in which such attitudes are generally interpreted as a defense.

Patients in supportive psychotherapy frequently develop intensely dependent and ambivalent relationships with the therapist. This relationship often parallels the separation-individuation process of normal child development (Adler 1982). Patients may recapitulate with the therapist the alternating autonomy and rapprochement experienced with the parent. The therapist's respect for the patient's autonomy and need for "refueling" may be important in strengthening the patient's independence and return to health. The containment of affect is also an important supportive function (Adler 1982; Kernberg 1975, 1984). Patients in need of supportive psychotherapy typically fear the destructive power of their rage and envy. They may be helped to modulate their emotional reactions by the reliable presence of the therapist and a therapeutic relationship that remains unchanged in the face of emotional onslaughts.

The therapist uses interpretation to strengthen

defenses and fosters the supportive relationship by refraining from interpreting positive transference feelings and waiting until the intensity of feelings has abated before commenting about negative transference feelings (Buckley 1986). Interpretations of the negative transference are limited to those needed to ensure that the treatment is not disrupted. While maintaining a friendly stance toward the patient, the therapist must respect the patient's need to establish a comfortable degree of distance. The therapist must not push for a more intimate or emotion-laden relationship than the patient can tolerate (Robinson and Flaherty 1982). The rapport with the patient, which the supportive psychotherapist tries to establish, differs from the therapeutic alliance of insight-oriented therapy. The doctor-patient relationship in supportive psychotherapy does not require the patient to observe and report on his or her own feelings and behavior to the same extent as in the change-oriented, explorative psychotherapies. In addition, the therapist acts more as a guide and a mentor. There is virtually unanimous agreement among writers on supportive psychotherapy that fostering a good working relationship with the patient is the first priority. Studies indicate that in the case of more severely ill patients, this may take many months, in contrast to work with psychiatrically healthier patients, in which the therapeutic alliance tends to develop early or not at all (Docherty 1989; A. F. Frank and Gunderson 1990).

The therapist must be available to the patient in a way that is regular and predictable. Rather than approaching the patient as a "blank screen," the therapist must actively demonstrate concern, involvement, sympathy, and a supportive attitude (Stafford-Clark 1970; Werman 1984). In taking such an active stance, the therapist must especially guard against grandiosity and personal biases so that he or she does not "become an omnipotent decision maker" but rather acts as a "strong, benign individual who is reasonably available when needed" (Nurnberg 1984, p. 219). To the extent that the patient develops the capacity to observe himself or herself, the psychotherapy may proceed beyond support and take on features of the explorative and change-oriented psychotherapies.

Many of the active interventions of supportive psychotherapy are based on the principle of "substitutive psychotherapy" (Werman 1984), in which the psychotherapy substitutes for capacities that the patient lacks. This is sometimes stated as the therapist acting as an "auxiliary ego" for the patient. The deficient ego capacities for which substitution is needed may include basic elements of self-perception such as a stable sense of self over time and a clear recognition of boundaries between one's self and others. Techniques that may support the patients' deficient ego functions include suggestion, reinforcement, advice, reality testing, cognitive restructuring, reassurance, clarification, limit setting, environmental interventions, and concurrent use of medication (Dewald 1994; Rockland 1989b; Werman 1984).

The defenses of denial and avoidance may be handled by encouraging the patient to discuss alternative behaviors, goals, and interpretations of events (Castelnuovo-Tedesco 1986). In general, the therapist tries to reinforce the most adaptive defenses of which the patient is capable while discouraging use of the more primitive defenses. To do so effectively, the therapist must judge the capacities of the patient and the degree to which a primitive defense might be necessary for the patient's equilibrium. Thus, McGlashan (1982) advocated reinforcing the primitive defenses of patients with schizophrenia, whereas Kernberg (1984) emphasized modifying such defenses in those patients with severe personality disorders.

Reassurance takes a variety of forms in supportive psychotherapy, including supporting an adaptive level of denial (such as that which may be employed by a patient in coping with a terminal illness); the patient's experience of the therapist's empathic attitude; or the therapist's reality testing of the patient's negatively biased self-evaluations or evaluations of his or her situation (Werman 1984). Reassuring a patient is not easy (Peteet 1982). Reassurance requires a clear understanding of what the patient fears. Overt expressions of interest and concern may be reassuring to a patient who fears rejection but threatening to one who fears intrusion. In a similar vein, Rockland (1989a, 1989b) stressed the need to tailor interventions to fit the character traits and unconscious transferences of the patient. Thus, the therapist may stress independence in the case of a patient who fears passivity or loss of control and may give advice and direction to a clinging, dependent patient. Similarly, intellectualized language may be more effective with obsessional patients, and emotionally toned language with histrionic patients.

Communication of the therapist's knowledge of the patient and his or her circumstances is a pedagogical aspect of supportive psychotherapy (Werman 1981). The therapist uses simple, concrete language that has personal meaning for the patient. The therapist may discuss with the highly inhibited patient the advantages of being more assertive or spontaneous, or he or she may point out to the patient with poorly developed social controls the dangers of impulsive behavior. In this manner the therapist functions as an "auxiliary superego." In both the very constricted patient and the very impulsive patient, the therapist's recognition and accurate warning of the patient's affects may aid the patient in recognizing and differentiating emotional states, a necessary step in tolerating and modulating affect (Pine 1976).

Interpretive comments may be used by the supportive therapist, although the form and content of interpretations usually differ from those in psychoanalytically oriented psychotherapy. Interpretations in supportive psychotherapy are given in a manner consistent with the principle of decreasing (rather than increasing) anxiety and strengthening (rather than loosening) defenses. Thus, they deal with material close to the patient's awareness rather than with unconscious material that might be distressing or frightening, and they can often serve to strengthen the defenses of intellectualization and rationalization (Werman 1984). Interpretations are used not to open up new material to consciousness but to diminish anxiety and provide plausible explanations based on what is already conscious. Interpretations are framed in terms of current issues and situations using formulations that the patient can readily accept. Such interventions are sometimes referred to as *interpreting upward*. The therapeutic efficacy of this technique was first described by Glover (1931), who pointed out that incomplete or inexact interpretations often result in alleviation of symptoms.

The psychodynamic life narrative can be used as a supportive interpretation (Viederman 1983). The narrative is the formulation of the patient's current difficulties (often a life crisis) as the inevitable product of previous life experiences. The narrative uses only facts of which the patient is already aware and explanations that do not threaten self-esteem. It serves to give the patient a sense of control through understanding, to help him or her accept emotional responses as justifiable and inevitable, and to strengthen the alliance with the therapist, who is seen as giving something valuable. Such a narrative may be contraindicated in patients who can benefit from psychoanalytically oriented psychotherapy, because it will strengthen defensive intellectualization, close off avenues to greater understanding, and possibly stir powerful expectations of gratification from the therapist.

Intellectualized interpretations may be useful in discussing dreams in supportive psychotherapy (Werman 1978). In addition, these interpretations may foster an increased capacity for self-observation (Ermutlu 1977). A technique that has been used for the latter purpose consists of suggesting that pathological behavior is the product of a "sick part" of the patient that is distinct from the patient as a whole. This induced dichotomy of personality helps the patient recognize both the pathological behaviors and the better functioning aspects of himself or herself and fosters his or her identification with more mature, adaptive traits.

The suitability of an interpretation may depend more on the manner in which it is given than on the content (Pine 1986). In supportive psychotherapy, interpretations are phrased to relieve the patient of the pressure to make an immediate response. The therapist tries to communicate that although the interpretation may be painful, he or she will stick by the patient through the patient's discomfort. Interpretations can best be made at times of low emotional intensity. The patient can also be given advance warning that a potentially painful comment is going to be made. Such techniques are directed toward sufficiently modulating the patient's emotional response so that the interpretation can be tolerated and processed.

The therapist's expression of interest, advice giving, and facilitation of ventilation reinforce desired behaviors (P. R. Sullivan 1971). Expressions of interest and solicitude are positively reinforcing. Advice can lead to behavioral change if it is specific and applies to frequently occurring behaviors of the patient. Desired behaviors can be rewarded by the therapist's approval and by social reinforcement. Ventilation of emotions is useful only if the therapist can help the patient safely contain and limit these emotions, thus extinguishing the anxiety response to emotional expression. Cognitive and behavioral psychotherapeutic interventions that strengthen the adaptive and defensive functioning of the ego (e.g., realistic and logical thinking, social skills, containment of affects such as anxiety) can contribute to the supportive aspects of psychotherapy (Novalis et al. 1993).

Except in the case of brief treatment aimed at supporting the patient through a life crisis or traumatic event, termination in supportive psychotherapy is not a goal in the same sense as it is in change-oriented therapies. In the most usual situation, the patient's functional deficits necessitate ongoing, long-term support. In such a case, keeping the patient in treatment might be a more appropriate goal than terminating treatment. A second possibility is that the treatment may gradually evolve into a more change-oriented treatment, including modification of ego structure and improvement in function. When this happens, it may be appropriate to reevaluate goals with the patient and consider criteria for termination.

EFFICACY

Very little information is available on the effectiveness of supportive psychotherapy. Most data come from studies in which supportive psychotherapy has been used as a control in testing the efficacy of other treatments (Conte and Plutchik 1986). In such studies, the procedures used in supportive psychotherapy tend to be poorly specified, and no attempts are made to correlate individual supportive techniques with outcome. There are no studies in which supportive psychotherapy is compared with no treatment or minimal treatment.

Despite its limitations, the research literature offers some evidence that supportive psychotherapy is an effective treatment. The Menninger Psychotherapy Project assessed long-term (i.e., of up to 10 years) explorative and supportive psychotherapy in a group of patients with mixed symptomatic and personality pathology (Wallerstein 1986). A surprising result of the study was that the techniques of supportive therapy produced improvement in functioning and ego strength comparable to that with expressive and insight-oriented techniques. This result backs the suggestion that sophisticated support itself promotes change in some patients.

Studies of patients with anxiety disorders have also demonstrated the efficacy of supportive therapy. The effects of imipramine therapy plus behavior therapy have been compared with those of imipramine therapy plus supportive psychotherapy in a group of patients with agoraphobia, mixed phobia, or simple phobia (Klein et al. 1983; Zitrin et al. 1978). The supportive psychotherapy was nondirective and based on psychodynamic principles; the behavior therapy consisted of desensitization procedures and assertiveness training in addition to nondirective supportive techniques. The expected benefit of adding behavioral techniques to supportive psychotherapy was not found; patients in both groups fared equally well. Similar results were reported by Alström et al. (1984a), who found that psychodynamically oriented supportive psychotherapy was as effective as behavior therapy and more effective than infrequent educative sessions in the treatment of women with agoraphobia. Nine months after treatment, patients in the supportive psychotherapy group were doing better than those who had had other treatments. Supportive psychotherapy and prolonged exposure (behavior) therapies were equally effective in treating men and women with social phobia (Alström et al. 1984b). These results may indicate that the active ingredient in both supportive psychotherapy and behavioral treatments is the encouragement of the patient to expose himself or herself to the feared situation (Klein et al. 1983).

Research in the psychotherapy of schizophrenia has failed to demonstrate the benefit of explorative, expressive techniques (Gomes-Schwartz 1984). By contrast, the use of supportive techniques appears more promising. May (1968) found that inpatients with nonchronic schizophrenia had somewhat better outcomes when treated with supportive psychotherapy and antipsychotic medication than when treated with medication alone. When these approaches were used singly, however, medication was more

effective than psychotherapy. A more recent study compared explorative, insight-oriented psychotherapy with reality-adaptive supportive psychotherapy in patients with schizophrenia (Gunderson et al. 1984; Stanton et al. 1984). The patients, who were maintained on their usual medications, were followed during both inpatient and outpatient phases of their treatment. Although minor differences favored both of the groups, the two treatments proved equally effective on most outcome measures, and the cost-effectiveness of supportive psychotherapy was much higher. The study design did not permit estimation of the added benefit of either type of psychotherapy over medication management alone. Supportive therapy may not be equally useful at all phases of schizophrenic illness. For example, Hogarty et al. (1974) found that such treatment increased the rate of relapse in the first 6 months after discharge from the hospital but decreased it thereafter.

A larger body of research exists indicating that supportive psychotherapy is an effective component of the treatment of patients with a variety of medical illnesses. Karush and colleagues (1969) reported that ulcerative colitis patients with high dependency and low ego strength improved both somatically and emotionally after supportive psychotherapy but not after insight-oriented treatment. The best results were found in cases in which the therapist was viewed as warm, understanding, and optimistic and a positive working relationship had been formed. Forester et al. (1985) assessed the effects of supportive psychotherapy on patients undergoing radiation treatment. The psychotherapy, which consisted of educational clarification of emotional issues and ventilation of feelings, resulted in less emotional distress and fewer complaints of side effects than were evident in the control group, which received no psychotherapy. Mumford et al. (1982) reviewed controlled studies of psychotherapy treatment of patients recovering from myocardial infarction and surgery and found positive effects of the treatment on the experience of pain, cooperation with treatment, incidence of complications, speed of recovery, and number of days in the hospital. The psychotherapies centered around education of the patients about their illnesses and treatments but also included varying amounts of cognitive and behavioral techniques, ventilation, and reassurance in the context of a supportive relationship.

The evidence to date, though preliminary, suggests that supportive psychotherapy can be effective in both psychiatric and medical illnesses and is frequently more cost-effective than more intensive psychotherapies for some disorders. More research is needed regarding the indications, contraindications, and techniques of supportive psychotherapy.

EDUCATION

The importance of individual psychotherapy to the practicing clinician makes mandatory the inclusion of instruction on psychotherapy in psychiatric residency training. The skills learned in psychotherapy—both the ability to intervene and the ability to recognize transference, countertransference, and defense—are important in many other treatment modalities. The clinician skilled in recognizing these phenomena is better able to perform a wide array of treatments, including medication management, family therapy, inpatient psychiatric treatment, and consultation-liaison.

The fundamental skills of establishing the therapeutic alliance, understanding the relationship of transference to anxiety and regression, and providing support are central to psychiatric care. Learning psychodynamic psychotherapy provides the opportunity to work with a specific treatment modality as well as to become skilled in a wide array of areas central to clinical care. Learning long-term psychodynamic psychotherapy is not the equivalent of learning the brief psychotherapies or supportive psychotherapy; however, it may be true that the long-term psychotherapist is best prepared for using the briefer psychotherapy, in which there are fewer opportunities to make mistakes and to correct them. In this era of managed care, it is even more likely that the psychiatrist will be called on to supervise others conducting psychotherapy. For this reason also, skills in psychotherapy are necessary.

Psychiatric residents must develop skills to apply all psychotherapeutic treatment modalities and to understand their indications and contraindications. Psychoanalysis, with its extended intensive training requirements, is essentially a subspecialty area and is now generally pursued postresidency. It offers the opportunity for specific patients to gain broad-based understanding in a generally supportive environment. Supportive psychotherapy, the mainstay of psychiatric treatment, is much more complicated than is often recognized. The understanding of which patient for which treatment at which time is as critical for the prescription of psychotherapy as it is for the prescription of psychopharmacological agents (Frances et al. 1984). Given the decrease in the number of psychoanalysts in medical school education, learning the indications for referral for psychoanalysis may be increasingly difficult for future psychiatrists.

The brief psychotherapies (see Chapter 28) are best taught in conjunction with the discussion of the principles of long-term psychotherapy and in the context of learning psychodynamic formulations of pathology and the ways in which defenses, transferences, and countertransferences appear in the psychotherapeutic dyad. The resident can then begin to learn the unique constraints and advantages that accrue within a brief period as well as the unique advantages of long-term psychotherapeutic work. Through contrasting the psychotherapies, the trainee learns appropriate patient selection and technical procedures to accomplish psychotherapy. Such training requires both familiarity with the psychotherapy literature and supervised clinical experiences in the various psychotherapies. All physicians should be versed in brief supportive psychotherapy as a technique distinct from pure "counseling" and education.

The evaluation of the patient is an important part of initiating any psychotherapy. Seeing psychotherapy as a modality that must be prescribed in duration, focus, and intensity and with a plan similar to pharmacological treatment of a patient enhances the resident's sense of mastery, accomplishment, and competence in dealing psychotherapeutically with a broad range of patients (Luborsky and Auerbach 1985).

The teaching of supportive psychotherapy requires further development of the knowledge base in supportive psychotherapy and the description of the technical procedures. At present, supportive psychotherapy remains a neglected area of teaching despite its complexity. A clearer delineation of the technical procedures used in psychotherapy and their assessment on a supportive versus change-oriented/explorative continuum should be part of psychotherapy supervision. In addition, such clarification will facilitate comparison among the psychotherapies and foster appropriate research questions, including those concerning the use of supportive psychotherapy as part of medication management.

CONCLUSIONS

Individual psychoanalytically oriented and supportive psychotherapies are an effective treatment for a wide range of symptoms and disorders. These treatment modalities require accurate diagnosis, treatment planning, and consistent application of principles and technique. Various types of psychotherapy are now well described. Further research is needed to identify which psychotherapy is most effective for which patient. The identification of specific types of change associated with different psychotherapies may aid this process.

The psychoanalytic treatments—psychoanalysis and psychoanalytic psychotherapy—now span the range of approaches—from brief to long-term and focal to broad-based. Interpersonal psychotherapy has primarily been used in research, but highlighted in this form of therapy is the importance of focusing on the social relationships as an aspect of understanding the psychoanalytic components of personality and mind-brain interaction. Interpersonal psychotherapy, cognitive psychotherapy, and supportive psychotherapy have more of an empirical research base than do the more specific psychoanalytic treatments. Research studies with more rigorous designs and conducted over longer periods are needed. Supportive psychotherapy, probably the most widely practiced of the psychotherapies, continues to be lacking in specific research. Better delineation of the specific technique in supportive psychotherapy will aid this development.

Clinicians require training in each of the psychotherapy modalities better to recognize the relationship of the psychotherapies to each other and the potential therapeutic benefits and costs associated with each.

REFERENCES

Adler E: Supportive psychotherapy revisited. Hillside Journal of Clinical Psychiatry 4:3–13, 1982

Alström JE, Nordlund CL, Persson G, et al: Effects of four treatment methods on agoraphobic women not suitable for insight-oriented psychotherapy. Acta Psychiatr Scand 70:1–17, 1984a

Alström JE, Nordlund CL, Persson G, et al: Effects of four treatment methods on social phobic patients not suitable for insight-oriented psychotherapy. Acta Psychiatr Scand 70:97–110, 1984b

Bachrach HM, Weber JJ, Solomon M: Factors associated with the outcome of psychoanalysis (IV). International Review of Psycho-Analysis 12:379–389, 1985

Baxter C, Schwartz S, Berman K, et al: Caudate glucose metabolic rate changes with both drug and behavior therapy for obsessive-compulsive disorder. Arch Gen Psychiatry 49:681–689, 1992

Beck AT, Rush AJ, Shaw BF, et al: Cognitive Therapy of Depression. New York, Guilford, 1979

Bellak L, Siegel H: Handbook of Intensive, Brief, and Emergency Psychotherapy. Larchmont, NY, CPS, 1983

Bibring E: Psychoanalysis and the dynamic psychotherapies. J Am Psychoanal Assoc 2:745–770, 1954

Bloch S: Assessment of patients for psychotherapy. Br J Psychiatry 135:193–208, 1979

Blum HP: Countertransference and the theory of technique: discussion. J Am Psychoanal Assoc 34:309–328, 1986

Brenner C: Psychoanalytic Technique and Psychic Conflict. New York, International Universities Press, 1976

Brodaty JH: Techniques in brief psychotherapy. Aust N Z J Psychiatry 17:109–115, 1983

Bruch H: Learning Psychotherapy: Rationale and Ground Rules. Cambridge, MA, Harvard University Press, 1974

Buckley P: [Supportive psychotherapy] A neglected treatment. Psychiatric Annals 16:515–517, 521, 1986

Budman SH, Gurman AS: The practice of brief therapy. Professional Psychology 14:277–292, 1983

Butler SF, Strupp HH: Effects of training experienced dynamic therapists to use a psychotherapy manual, in Psychodynamic Treatment Research. Edited by Miller NE, Luborsky L, Barber JP, et al. New York, Basic Books, 1993, pp 191–210

Castelnuovo-Tedesco P: The Twenty-Minute Hour: A Guide to Brief Psychotherapy for the Physician. Washington, DC, American Psychiatric Press, 1986

Coleman JV: Aims and conduct of psychotherapy. Arch Gen Psychiatry 18:1–6, 1968

Coltrera JT: Truth from genetic illusion: the transference and the fate of the infantile neurosis, in Psychoanalytic Explorations of Technique: Discourse on the Theory of Therapy. Edited by Blum HP. New York, International Universities Press, 1980, pp 284–313

Conte HR, Plutchik R: Controlled research in supportive psychotherapy. Psychiatric Annals 16:530–533, 1986

Crits-Christoph P: The efficacy of brief dynamic psychotherapy: a meta-analysis. Am J Psychiatry 149:151–158, 1992

Crown S: Contraindications and dangers of psychotherapy. Br J Psychiatry 143:436–441, 1983

de Jonghe F, Rijnierse P, Janssen R: The role of support in psychoanalysis. J Am Psychoanal Assoc 40:475–499, 1992

de Jonghe F, Rijnierse P, Janssen R: Psychoanalytic supportive psychotherapy. J Am Psychoanal Assoc 42: 421–446, 1994

DeRubeis RJ, Hollon SD, Evans MD, et al: Can psychotherapies for depression be discriminated? A systematic investigation of cognitive therapy and interpersonal therapy. J Consult Clin Psychol 50:744–756, 1982

Dewald P: The process of change in psychoanalytic psychotherapy. Arch Gen Psychiatry 35:535–542, 1978

Dewald PA: Principles of supportive psychotherapy. Am J Psychiatry 48:505–518, 1994

DiMascio A, Weissman MM, Prusoff BA, et al: Differential symptom reduction by drugs and psychotherapy in acute depression. Arch Gen Psychiatry 36:1450–1456, 1979

Docherty JP: The individual psychotherapies: efficacy, syndrome-based treatments, and the therapeutic alliance, in Outpatient Psychiatry: Diagnosis and Treatment, 2nd Edition. Edited by Lazare A. Baltimore, MD, Williams & Wilkins, 1989, pp 624–644

Donovan JM: More on transference interpretations (letter). Am J Psychiatry 141:142, 1984

Epstein R: Boundaries. Washington, DC, American Psychiatric Press, 1995

Ermutlu I: Induced dichotomy of personality as a technique in supportive psychotherapy. Psychiatric Forum 7:19–22, 1977

Errera P, McKee B, Smith DC, et al: Length of psychotherapy: studies done in a university community psychiatric clinic. Arch Gen Psychiatry 17:454–458, 1967

Forester B, Kornfeld DS, Fleiss JL: Psychotherapy during radiotherapy: effects on emotional and physical distress. Am J Psychiatry 142:22–27, 1985

Frances A[J], Clarkin JF: No treatment as the prescription of choice. Arch Gen Psychiatry 38:542–545, 1981

Frances A[J], Perry S: Transference interpretations in focal therapy. Am J Psychiatry 140:405–409, 1983

Frances AJ, Clarkin J, Perry S: Differential Therapeutics in Psychiatry: The Art and Science of Treatment Selection. New York, Brunner/Mazel, 1984

Frank AF, Gunderson JG: The role of the therapeutic alliance in the treatment of schizophrenia: relationship to course and outcome. Arch Gen Psychiatry 47:228–236, 1990

Frank AF, Kupfer DJ, Wagner EF, et al: Efficacy of interpersonal psychotherapy as a maintenance treatment of recurrent depression. Arch Gen Psychiatry 48:1053–1059, 1991

Frank JD: Therapeutic factors in psychotherapy. Am J Psychother 25:350–361, 1971

Freud S: The handling of dream-interpretation in psycho-analysis (1911), in Standard Edition of the Complete Psychological Works of Sigmund Freud, Vol 12. Translated and edited by Strachey J. London, Hogarth Press, 1958, pp 89–96

Freud S: The dynamics of transference (1912a), in Standard Edition of the Complete Psychological Works of Sigmund Freud, Vol 12. Translated and edited by Strachey J. London, Hogarth Press, 1958, pp 97–108

Freud S: Recommendations to physicians practising psycho-analysis (1912b), in Standard Edition of the Complete Psychological Works of Sigmund Freud, Vol 12. Translated and edited by Strachey J. London, Hogarth Press, 1958, pp 109–120

Freud S: On beginning the treatment (further recommendations on the technique of psycho-analysis I) (1913), in Standard Edition of the Complete Psychological Works of Sigmund Freud, Vol 12. Translated and edited by Strachey J. London, Hogarth Press, 1958, pp 121–144

Freud S: Remembering, repeating and working-through (further recommendations on the technique of psycho-analysis II) (1914), in Standard Edition of the Complete Psychological Works of Sigmund Freud, Vol 12. Translated and edited by Strachey J. London, Hogarth Press, 1958, pp 145–156

Freud S: Observations on transference-love (further recommendations on the technique of psycho-analysis III) (1915[1914]), in Standard Edition of the Complete Psychological Works of Sigmund Freud, Vol 12. Translated and edited by Strachey J. London, Hogarth Press, 1958, pp 157–173

Fried D, Crits-Christoph P, Luborsky L: The first empirical demonstration of transference in psychotherapy, J Nerv Ment Dis 180:326–331, 1992

Fromm-Reichmann F: Principles of Intensive Psychotherapy. Chicago, IL, University of Chicago Press, 1950

Gabbard GO: Psychodynamic Psychiatry in Clinical Practice. Washington, DC, American Psychiatric Press, 1990

Gill M: The Analysis of Transference, I: Theory and Technique. New York, International Universities Press, 1982

Glover E: The therapeutic effect of inexact interpretation: a contribution to the theory of suggestion. Int J Psychoanal 12:397–411, 1931

Glover E: The Technique of Psychoanalysis. New York, International Universities Press, 1968

Gomes-Schwartz B: Individual psychotherapy of schizophrenia, in Schizophrenia: Treatment, Management, and Rehabilitation. Edited by Bellack AS. Orlando, FL, Grune & Stratton, 1984, pp 307–345

Gomes-Schwartz B, Hadley S, Strupp H: Individual psychotherapy and behavior therapy. Annu Rev Psychol 29:435–447, 1978

Greenson RR: The working alliance and the transference neurosis. Psychoanal Q 34:155–181, 1965

Greenson RR: The Technique and Practice of Psychoanalysis. New York, International Universities Press, 1967

Gunderson JE, Frank AF, Katz HM, et al: Effects of psychotherapy in schizophrenia, II: comparative outcome of two forms of treatment. Schizophr Bull 10:564–598, 1984

Hadley SW, Strupp HH: Contemporary views of negative effects in psychotherapy: an integrated account. Arch Gen Psychiatry 33:1291–1302, 1976

Hofer MA: Relationships as regulators: a psychobiologic perspective on bereavement. Psychosom Med 46:183–197, 1984

Hogarty GE, Goldberg SC, Schooler NR, et al: Drug and sociotherapy in the aftercare of schizophrenic patients, III: adjustment of nonrelapsed patients. Arch Gen Psychiatry 31:609–618, 1974

Horowitz MJ, Marmar CR, Weiss DS, et al: Comprehensive analysis of change after brief dynamic psychotherapy. Am J Psychiatry 143:582–589, 1986

Horvath A, Gaston L, Luborsky L: The therapeutic alliance and its measures, in Psychodynamic Treatment Research. Edited by Miller NE, Luborsky L, Barber JP, et al. New York, Basic Books, 1993, pp 247–273

House JS, Landis KR, Umberson D: Social relationships and health. Science 241:540–545, 1988

Howard KI, Kopta SM, Krause MS, et al: The dose-effect relationship in psychotherapy. Am Psychol 41:159–164, 1986

Kandell ER: Psychotherapy and the single synapse: the impact of psychiatric thought on neurobiologic research. N Engl J Med 301:1028–1037, 1979

Kandell ER: Genes, nerve cells, and the remembrance of things past. J Neuropsychiatry Clin Neurosci 1:103–125, 1989

Kantrowitz JL, Paolitto F, Sashin J, et al: Affect availability, tolerance, complexity, and modulation in psychoanalysis: follow up of a longitudinal, prospective study. J Am Psychoanal Assoc 34:529–559, 1986

Kantrowitz JL, Katz AL, Paolitto F, et al: Changes in the level and quantity of object relations in psychoanalysis: follow up of a longitudinal, prospective study. J Am Psychoanal Assoc 35:23–46, 1987

Kantrowitz JL, Katz AL, Paolitto F: Followup of psychoanalysis five to ten years after termination, I: stability of change. J Am Psychoanal Assoc 38:471–496, 1990

Karen Horney Clinic Medical Board: Guidelines for identifying therapeutic modalities. Am J Psychoanal 41:195–202, 1981

Karush A, Daniels GE, O'Connor JF, et al: The response to psychotherapy in chronic ulcerative colitis, II: factors arising from the therapeutic situation. Psychosom Med 31:201–226, 1969

Kellner R: Psychotherapy in psychosomatic disorders: a survey of controlled studies. Arch Gen Psychiatry 32:1021–1028, 1975

Kernberg OF: Borderline Conditions and Pathological Narcissism. New York, Jason Aronson, 1975

Kernberg OF: Severe Personality Disorders: Psychotherapeutic Strategies. New Haven, CT, Yale University Press, 1984

Kernberg OF, Burstein ED, Coyne L, et al: Psychotherapy and psychoanalysis: final report of the Menninger Foundation's Psychotherapy Research Project. Bull Menninger Clin 36:1–275, 1972

Klein DF, Zitrin CM, Woerner MG, et al: Treatment of phobias, II: behavior therapy and supportive psychotherapy: are there any specific ingredients? Arch Gen Psychiatry 40:139–145, 1983

Klerman GL, Weissman MM, Rounsaville BJ, et al: Interpersonal psychotherapy for depression, in Psychiatry Update: The American Psychiatric Association Annual Review, Vol 3. Edited by Grinspoon L. Washington, DC, American Psychiatric Press, 1984a, pp 56–67

Klerman GL, Weissman MM, Rounsaville BJ, et al: Interpersonal Psychotherapy of Depression. New York, Basic Books, 1984b

Krupnick JL, Pincus HA: The cost-effectiveness of psychotherapy: a plan for research. Am J Psychiatry 149:1295–1305, 1992

Lazar SG (ed): Extended dynamic psychotherapy: making the case in an era of managed care. Psychoanalytic Inquiry (suppl) 1997

Levinson DJ, Merrifield J, Berg K: Becoming a patient. Arch Gen Psychiatry 17:385–406, 1967

Loewald HW: On the therapeutic action of psychoanalysis, in Papers on Psychoanalysis. New Haven, CT, Yale University Press, 1980, pp 221–256

Longobardi PG: The impact of a brief psychological intervention on medical care utilization in an army health care setting. Med Care 19:655–671, 1981

Luborsky L: Principles of Psychoanalytic Psychotherapy: A Manual for Supportive Expressive Treatment. New York, Basic Books, 1984

Luborsky L, Auerbach AH: The therapeutic relationship in psychodynamic psychotherapy: the research evidence and its meaning for practice, in Psychiatry Update: The American Psychiatric Association Annual Review, Vol 4. Edited by Hales RE, Frances AJ. Washington, DC, American Psychiatric Press, 1985, pp 550–561

Luborsky L, Crits-Christoph P: Understanding Transference. New York, Basic Books, 1990

Luborsky L, Singer B, Luborsky L: Comparative studies of psychotherapies: is it true that "everyone has won and all must have prizes"? Arch Gen Psychiatry 32:995–1008, 1975

Luborsky L, Crits-Christoph P, Mintz J, et al: Who Will Benefit From Psychotherapy? New York, Basic Books, 1988

Malan DH: A Study of Brief Psychotherapy. New York, Plenum, 1975

Malan DH: The Frontier of Brief Psychotherapy. New York, Plenum, 1976

Malan DH: Toward the Validation of Dynamic Psychotherapy. New York, Plenum, 1980

Malan DH, Heath ES, Bacal HA, et al: Psychodynamic changes in untreated neurotic patients, II: apparently genuine improvements. Arch Gen Psychiatry 32:110–126, 1975

Marziali EA: Prediction of outcome of brief psychotherapy from therapist interpretive interventions. Arch Gen Psychiatry 41:301–304, 1984

Marziali EA, Sullivan JM: Methodological issues in the content analysis of brief psychotherapy. Br J Med Psychol 53:19–27, 1980

May PRA: Treatment of Schizophrenia: A Comparative Study of Five Treatment Methods. New York, Science House, 1968

McGlashan TH: DSM-III schizophrenia and individual psychotherapy. J Nerv Ment Dis 170:752–757, 1982

McNeilly CL, Howard KJ: The effects of psychotherapy: a re-evaluation based on dosage. Psychotherapy Research 1:74–78, 1991

Meyer E, Derogatis LR, Miller MJ, et al: Addition of time-limited psychotherapy to medical treatment in a general medical clinic: results at one-year follow-up. J Nerv Ment Dis 169:780–790, 1981

Mohl PC, McLaughlin GDW: Listening to the patient, in Psychiatry. Edited by Tasman A, Kaye J, Lieberman J. Philadelphia, WB Saunders, 1996, pp 3–18

Mumford E, Schlesinger H[J], Glass CV: The effects of psychological intervention on recovery from surgery and heart attacks: an analysis of the literature. Am J Public Health 72:141–151, 1982

Mumford E, Schlesinger HJ, Glass GV, et al: A new look at evidence about reduced cost of medical utilization following mental health treatment. Am J Psychiatry 141:1145–1158, 1984

Novalis PN, Rojceicz SJ Jr, Peele R: Clinical manual of supportive psychotherapy. Washington, DC American Psychiatric Press, 1993

Nurnberg HG: Survey of psychotherapeutic approaches to narcissistic personality disorder. Hillside Journal of Clinical Psychiatry 6:204–220, 1984

Ornstein A: Supportive psychotherapy: a contemporary view. Clinical Social Work Journal 14:14–30, 1986

Parloff MB: Psychotherapy research evidence and reimbursement decisions: Bambi meets Godzilla. Am J Psychiatry 139:718–727, 1982

Parloff MB, Lond P, Wolfe B: Individual psychotherapy and behavior change. Annu Rev Psychol 37:321–349, 1986

Persson G, Alström JE: A scale for rating suitability for insight-oriented psychotherapy. Acta Psychiatr Scand 68:117–125, 1983

Peteet JR: A closer look at the concept of support: some applications to the care of patients with cancer. Gen Hosp Psychiatry 4:19–23, 1982

Pine F: On therapeutic change: perspective from a parent-child model. Psychoanalysis and Contemporary Science 5:537–569, 1976

Pine F: [Supportive psychotherapy] A psychoanalytic perspective. Psychiatric Annals 16:526–529, 1986

Pinsker H, Rosenthal R, McCullough L: Dynamic supportive psychotherapy, in Handbook of Short-Term Dynamic Psychotherapy. Edited by Crits-Christoph P, Barben JP. New York, Basic Books, 1991, pp 220–247

Racker H: Meanings and uses of countertransference. Psychoanal Q 26:303–357, 1957

Robinson MV, Flaherty JA: Self-regulation of distance in supportive psychotherapy. Clinical Social Work Journal 10:209–217, 1982

Rockland LH: Psychoanalytically oriented supportive therapy: literature review and techniques. J Am Acad Psychoanal 17:451–462, 1989a

Rockland LH: Supportive Therapy: A Psychodynamic Approach. New York, Basic Books, 1989b

Rounsaville BJ, Glazer W, Wilber CH, et al: Short-term interpersonal psychotherapy in methadone-maintained opiate addicts. Arch Gen Psychiatry 40:629–636, 1983

Rounsaville BJ, Gawin F, Kleber H: Interpersonal psychotherapy adapted for ambulatory cocaine abusers. Am J Drug Alcohol Abuse 11:171–191, 1985a

Rounsaville BJ, Klerman GL, Weissman MM, et al: Short-term interpersonal psychotherapy (IPT) for depression, in Handbook of Depression: Treatment, Assessment and Research. Edited by Beckham EE, Leber WB. Homewood, IL, Dorsey Press, 1985b

Sandler J, Dare C, Holder A: The Patient and the Analyst: The Basis of the Psychoanalytic Process. New York, International Universities Press, 1973

Searles HF: Collected Papers on Schizophrenia and Related Subjects. New York, International Universities Press, 1965

Shapiro DA, Shapiro D: Meta-analysis of comparative therapy outcome studies: a replication and refinement. Psychol Bull 92:581–604, 1982

Sharfstein SS, Muszynski S, Myers E: Health Insurance and Psychiatric Care: Update and Appraisal. Washington, DC, American Psychiatric Press, 1984

Sharpe EF: Dream Analysis. London, Hogarth Press, 1961

Sifneos PE: Short-Term Psychotherapy and Emotional Crisis. Cambridge, MA, Harvard University Press, 1972

Sifneos PE: Is dynamic psychotherapy contraindicated for a large number of patients with psychosomatic diseases? Psychother Psychosom 21:133–156, 1972–1973

Sifneos PE: A reconsideration of psychosomatic symptom formations in view of recent clinical observations. Psychother Psychosom 24:151–155, 1974

Sifneos PE: Problems of psychotherapy of patients with alexithymic characteristics and physical disease. Psychother Psychosom 26:65–70, 1975

Silberman EK, Certa K: Psychiatric interview: settings and techniques, in Psychiatry. Edited by Tasman A, Kaye J, Lieberman J. Philadelphia, WB Saunders, 1996, pp 19–39

Smith ML, Glass GV: Meta-analysis of psychotherapy outcome studies. Am Psychol 32:752–760, 1977

Smith ML, Glass GV, Miller TI: The Benefits of Psychotherapy. Baltimore, MD, Johns Hopkins University Press, 1980

Spiegel D, Lazar SG: The need for psychotherapy in the medically ill. Psychoanalytic Inquiry (suppl) 45–50, 1997

Stafford-Clark D: Supportive psychotherapy, in Modern Trends in Psychological Medicine II. Edited by Price JH. New York, Appleton-Century-Crofts, 1970, pp 277–295

Stanton AH, Gunderson JG, Knapp P, et al: Effects of psychotherapy in schizophrenia, I: design and implementation of a controlled study. Schizophr Bull 10:520–563, 1984

Stierlin H: Short-term versus long-term psychotherapy in the light of a general theory of human relationships. Br J Med Psychol 41:357–367, 1968

Stone L: The Psychoanalytic Situation: An Examination of Its Development and Essential Nature. New York, International Universities Press, 1961

Strupp HH: Success and failure in time-limited psychotherapy: a systematic comparison of two cases: comparison 1. Arch Gen Psychiatry 37:595–604, 1980a

Strupp HH: Success and failure in time-limited psychotherapy: further evidence (comparison 4). Arch Gen Psychiatry 37:947–954, 1980b

Strupp HH: Success and failure in time-limited psychotherapy: with special reference to the performance of a lay counselor. Arch Gen Psychiatry 37:831–841, 1980c

Strupp HH, Binder J: Psychotherapy in a New Key: Time-Limited Dynamic Psychotherapy. New York, Basic Books, 1984

Strupp HH, Hadley SW: Specific vs nonspecific factors in psychotherapy: a controlled study of outcome. Arch Gen Psychiatry 36:1125–1136, 1979

Sullivan HS: The Psychiatric Interview. Edited by Perry HS, Gawel ML. New York, WW Norton, 1954

Sullivan PR: Learning theories and supportive psychotherapy. Am J Psychiatry 128:763–766, 1971

Ursano RJ, Dressler DM: Brief vs long term psychotherapy: a treatment decision. J Nerv Ment Dis 159:164–171, 1974

Ursano RJ, Dressler DM: Brief versus long-term psychotherapy: clinician attitudes and organizational design. Compr Psychiatry 18:55–60, 1977

Ursano RJ, Fullerton CS: Psychotherapy: medical intervention and the concept of normality, in The Diversity of Normal Behavior: Further Contributions to Normatology. Edited by Offer D, Sabshin M. New York, Basic Books, 1991, pp 39–59

Ursano, RJ, Epstein RS, Lazar SG: Behavioral responses to illness: personality and personality disorders, in Textbook of Consultation Liaison Psychiatry. Edited by Rundell JR, Wise MG. Washington, DC, American Psychiatric Press, 1996, pp 116–137

Ursano RJ, Sonnenberg SM, Lazar SG: Concise Guide to Psychodynamic Psychotherapy: Principles and Techniques in the Era of Managed Care. Washington, DC, American Psychiatric Press, 1997

Viederman M: The psychodynamic life narrative: a psychotherapeutic intervention useful in crisis situations. Psychiatry 46:236–246, 1983

Wallace ER: Dynamic Psychiatry in Theory and Practice. Philadelphia, Lea & Febiger, 1983

Wallerstein RS: Forty-Two Lives in Treatment: A Study of Psychoanalysis and Psychotherapy. New York, Guilford, 1986

Wallerstein RS: Psychoanalysis and psychotherapy: an historical perspective. Int J Psychoanal 70:563–591, 1989

Wallerstein RS: Follow up in psychoanalysis: what happens to treatment gains. J Am Psychoanal Assoc 40:665–690, 1992

Weiss J, Sampson H: The Psychoanalytic Process: Theory, Clinical Observation and Empirical Research. New York, Guilford, 1986

Weissman MM, Markowitz JC: Interpersonal psychotherapy. Arch Gen Psychiatry 51:599–606, 1994

Weissman MM, Klerman GL, Prusoff BA, et al: Depressed outpatients: results one year after treatment with drugs and/or interpersonal psychotherapy. Arch Gen Psychiatry 38:51–55, 1981

Werman DS: The use of dreams in psychotherapy: practical guidelines. Canadian Psychiatric Association Journal 23:153–158, 1978

Werman DS: Technical aspects of supportive psychotherapy. Psychiatric Journal of the University of Ottawa 6:153–160, 1981

Werman DS: The Practice of Supportive Psychotherapy. New York, Brunner/Mazel, 1984

Werman DS: On the mode of therapeutic action of psychoanalytic supportive psychotherapy, in How Does Treatment Help? On the Modes of Action of Psychoanalytic Psychotherapy. Edited by Rothstein A. Madison, CT, International Universities Press, 1988, pp 157–167

Winston A, Pinsker H, McCullough L: A review of supportive psychotherapy. Hospital and Community Psychiatry 37:1105–1114, 1986

Zetzel ER: Current concepts of transference. Int J Psychoanal 37:369–376, 1956

Zitrin CM, Klein DF, Woerner MG: Behavior therapy, supportive psychotherapy, imipramine, and phobias. Arch Gen Psychiatry 35:307–316, 1978

APPENDIX: GLOSSARY

Abstinence: Therapist's technical stance of being somewhat silent, although not withholding, in order better to observe how the patient organizes his or her psychic world. Requires explanation for and education of the patient.

Acting out: Expressing unconscious conflict in action rather than in words.

Asceticism: Denial of pleasure, including food, sleep, exercise, and sexual gratification, usually with an air of superiority or of doing good for someone else. Typical of adolescence.

Behavior: Thoughts (i.e., cognitions), feelings (i.e., affects), fantasies, and actions.

Brief psychodynamic psychotherapy: Psychodynamic psychotherapy that is focal and of limited duration, usually 12–20 sessions.

Cognitive psychotherapy: Psychotherapy that focuses on inappropriate and inaccurate cognitions and beliefs. Includes homework and behavioral interventions.

Complementary countertransference: Therapist's identification with a significant figure from the patient's past whom the patient is experiencing in the transference.

Concordant countertransference: Therapist's identification with the patient's emotional experience.

Countertransference (*see also* Complementary countertransference; Concordant countertransference): Psychotherapist's emotional experience of the patient. May be a help or an impediment to treatment. May be experienced by the therapist as pressure to act in a certain way with the patient.

Defense (*see* Mechanisms of defense)

Denial: Act of ignoring painful realities as though they were not present—for example, a man in an intensive care unit after a myocardial infarction refuses to believe he has had a heart attack and continues to run his business from his bed as though nothing had happened.

Devaluing: Minimizing and dismissing with an air of contempt.

Displacement: Act of focusing one's anxiety or feelings on a different object or person from the one to which or to whom these feelings are truly related—for example, kicking the dog when being angry with one's spouse.

Ego (*see also* Superego): Portion of the personality that mediates between the real world and the internal world. Includes autonomous functions such as thinking.

End phase of treatment (*see also* Termination): Last phase of a psychotherapy, which includes consolidation, recapitulation of symptoms and defenses, practice, and end setting.

Evaluation phase: Initial two to four sessions that are used to assess the patient and reach a treatment decision.

Explorative psychotherapy (*see* Psychodynamic psychotherapy)

Free association: Technical procedure of encouraging the patient to speak as freely as possible, to suspend judgment, and to say whatever comes to mind. Always only a relative term. Requires education of the patient.

Id: Wishful portion of the tripartite psychoanalytic personality model.

Identification with the aggressor: Act of behaving like a significant person in one's life who has been aggressive or violent toward oneself.

Inhibition: Constriction of thoughts, feelings, and/or behaviors to avoid internal conflict.

Insight-oriented psychotherapy (*see* Psychodynamic psychotherapy)

Intellectualization: Use of excessively intellectual, factual, and cognitive mechanisms to decrease anxiety.

Interpersonal psychotherapy: Psychotherapy focused on interpersonal relations and social functioning.

Interpretation: Technical procedure of making what is unconscious (i.e., out of the patient's awareness) conscious. May include linking the transference with a present experience and also with a past significant figure.

Isolation of affect: Separation of feelings from awareness. Related to intellectualization.

Long-term psychotherapy (*see* **Psychodynamic psychotherapy**)

Mechanisms of defense: Ways of thinking (i.e., cognitions) directed toward decreasing unpleasant affective states (anxiety) and maintaining unconscious conflicts out of awareness. Examples include intellectualization, repression, externalization, somatization, splitting, denial, and acting out.

Neurosis: Older term used in psychoanalytic writings to mean internal conflict.

Object relationships: Internal representational world of "people" as distinguished from the "real" persons; the experiential world of the patient, populated with meanings and perceptions rather than real events.

Objects (*see* **Object relationships**)

Omnipotence: Primitive defense in which one exaggerates one's own sense of power and ability.

Primitive idealization: Act of exaggerating the power, ability, and prestige of another person to relieve one's own anxiety.

Projection: Primitive defense in which one attributes one's own conflicted feelings and wishes to another person.

Projective identification: Primitive defense in which one projects one's own feelings onto another and then attempts to control those feelings in that person.

Psychic reality: The "internal world," that is, unconscious perceptions based on the meanings of events rather than on the actual events. Derives from biological givens and developmental experience.

Psychoanalysis: Psychotherapeutic treatment of great intensity, usually several years in length, directed at the elaboration of the patient's psychic reality and world of meaning through examination of the transference. Focuses on how these areas affect behavior. Term also used to describe the theory of mental functioning derived from this technique.

Psychoanalytic psychotherapy (*see* **Psychodynamic psychotherapy**)

Psychodynamic psychotherapy (*also called* **Explorative psychotherapy; Insight-oriented psychotherapy; Long-term psychotherapy; Psychoanalytic psychotherapy**):   The "talking cure" based on the principles of a psychoanalytic understanding of mental functioning (e.g., presence of defenses, transference, and psychic reality) as aspects of mental life. Primary goal is to make what is out of awareness available for conscious processing through identifying patterns of behavior derived from childhood.

Psychotherapy: The generic term for all "talking cures." Verbal interchange between an expert and a help-seeker, the goal of which is to alter characteristic patterns of behavior that are causing the help-seeker difficulties. Includes cognitive psychotherapy, interpersonal psychotherapy, and psychoanalysis, among others.

Reaction formation: Act of doing the opposite of what one feels (e.g., being overly ingratiating to people with whom one is angry).

Reality testing: An ego function. The capacity to distinguish reality from fantasy, and internal wishes and thoughts from external events.

Regression: Return to an earlier mode of functioning to avoid experiences of conflict in the present.

Repression: Act of removing conflicted thoughts and feelings from awareness; act of forgetting.

Resistance: Clinical term used to describe the therapist's experience of the patient's unconscious reluctance to experience disturbing affects related to childhood conflicts. Includes defense mechanisms, secondary gain, reinforcing nature of acting out, need to punish oneself, and need to thwart progress.

Reversal: Act of changing an impulse or wish from active to passive.

Splitting: Primitive defense that separates positive and negative self and object images so that individuals tend to be seen as all good or all bad.

Sublimation: Mature defense mechanism resulting in the application of the energy from previous conflicts in appropriate feelings, thought, and behaviors in the present.

Superego (*see also* **Ego**):   That part of the personality that includes one's conscience and one's goals.

Supportive psychotherapy: Psychotherapy directed toward helping the patient reestablish his or her previous best level of functioning. The most common form of psychotherapy, requiring thoughtful and skilled application of psychodynamic principles and techniques.

Termination (*see also* End phase of treatment): Act of ending psychotherapy. This phase of treatment is demanding for the therapist as well as for the patient.

Therapeutic alliance: Reality-based relationship of the therapist and the patient who are working together.

Transference: Experience of acting toward, feeling, and/or perceiving another person to be like a significant figure from one's past. Important area of learning in the psychoanalytic psychotherapies but not limited to therapy settings.

Transference neurosis: Prominent, substantial transference typical of psychoanalysis.

Working alliance (*see* Therapeutic alliance)

CHAPTER 30

BEHAVIOR THERAPIES

W. STEWART AGRAS, M.D.
ROBERT I. BERKOWITZ, M.D.

Behavior therapy developed as a scientific approach to human behavior change. The search for an understanding of the process of learning moved from the field of philosophy to the newly developing field of psychology late in the nineteenth century. Association theory had already been developed by the British school of philosophical empiricism, but it was Pavlov and his co-workers who demonstrated the basic principles of learning by contiguity and the way in which new connections could be acquired, generalized, and extinguished. In the United States, first Thorndike and then Skinner and his colleagues demonstrated how the environment alters behavior and introduced principles such as reinforcement, punishment, and stimulus control. In broad terms, Skinner postulated that the environmental consequences of behavior determined which actions would be strengthened and which would be weakened, over time.

These developments were contemporary with the development of psychoanalytic theory and practice, and beginning in the 1950s numerous attempts were made to integrate the more recently developed learning theories and psychoanalytic theory. These attempts failed to gain acceptance from either psychoanalytic theorists or learning theorists, perhaps because they did not lead to new testable propositions. Thus, behavior therapy developed as an alternative way of understanding and treating disordered behavior, being sparked by the failure to demonstrate the efficacy of psychoanalysis. Among the basic principles underlying the conceptual basis for behavior therapy are the following:

1. Both normal and abnormal behaviors are assumed to be learned and maintained in the same way; thus, procedures that alter normal behaviors will also be useful in altering deviant behaviors. An example of this is positive reinforcement, which affects a wide range of behaviors across a variety of different species and which has proven useful in modifying many problem behaviors.

2. The social environment plays a key role in the development and maintenance of both normal and abnormal behaviors. A consequence of this view is that the patients' environment may need to be altered to maintain newly acquired behaviors and prevent relapse.

3. The major focus of treatment is on the behavior problem itself, and, thus, specification of both the behaviors to be changed and the circumstances presently maintaining those behaviors is an important

facet of assessment and treatment. Behaviors requiring treatment will usually be broken up into discrete components, each of which will be treated using individually tailored procedures depending on the behavior and its antecedents and consequences.

4. Behavior therapy is based on a scientific approach to treatment. Treatment procedures must be well specified so that they can be replicated by others; this involves the development of detailed treatment manuals. Treatment procedures must be evaluated in controlled experiments and the active components of treatment separated from inactive components by additive clinical experimental designs.

Social-cognitive learning theory (Bandura 1986) has now become the most widely accepted theoretical underpinning of behavior therapy. This theory incorporates elements of both Pavlovian and Skinnerian theories but goes beyond these in postulating an interaction between environment, behavior, and cognitive processes. Not only does the environment affect the person, but the person can alter his or her personal environment, thus affecting future behavior. Reinforcement is viewed not as the automatic effect of reward but rather as a source of information about the potential effects of future behavior. Similarly, classical conditioning is no longer viewed as an automatic result of the occurrence of two stimuli occurring closely in time. Experimental work has demonstrated that prior experience and recognition of the relatedness of events are often crucial to this type of learning. Hence, cognitive processes are recognized as important modulators of behavior.

Basic research is beginning to unravel the biology of learning. It is now clear that learning leads to neurochemical changes in the central nervous system. Work with the simple organism Aplysia, a sea mollusk, has revealed that when this animal learns avoidance behavior, the chemical structure of cells in the nervous system is altered. When the avoidance behavior disappears—for example, through repeated exposure—the chemical changes are reversed (Kandel 1989). Hence, there is a reciprocal interaction between biological processes in the central nervous system and behavior changes resulting from environmental influences. Because psychotherapy involves learning new ways of behaving, and learning produces neurochemical changes, the behavior changes associated with therapy should be detectable by imaging methods. In a study of patients with obsessive-compulsive disorder (OCD), positron-emission tomography was used to investigate changes in rates of glucose metabolism in the cerebrum before and after treatment with behavior therapy (Baxter et al. 1992). Rates of glucose metabolism in the

right head of the caudate nucleus changed when the OCD was successfully treated but did not change in patients who did not respond to treatment. Moreover, these changes were similar to those produced by antidepressant treatment.

In addition to developments in theory and practice, behavior therapy has reached into new areas of endeavor. These include the development of behavioral pediatrics and behavioral medicine, which have in turn taken behavior therapy into preventive medicine. Another active area of research involves investigations of the interaction between behavior therapy and pharmacological treatments. Finally, the development of effective manualized therapies derived from perspectives other than behavior therapy not only allows comparisons of behavior therapy with these procedures, but also allows the testing of differing hypotheses regarding the processes by which therapeutic behavior change occurs.

It should be recognized that behavior therapy is not a monolithic procedure; rather, it involves the application of a variety of well-specified therapeutic procedures that have been packaged to treat or prevent a variety of disorders. The large number of applications of behavior therapy to the wide variety of psychiatric problems, and the extensive research literature, preclude a comprehensive account in this chapter. Thus, the focus will be on applications in a few common disorders.

THERAPEUTIC PROCEDURES

In the following paragraphs, some therapeutic procedures commonly used in behavior therapy are detailed. Many of these procedures form one component of a more complex therapeutic package that has been designed for a particular psychiatric disorder and tested in controlled outcome studies. It should be recognized that certain procedures common to all therapies are employed in such therapeutic packages—including a therapeutic rationale and therapeutic instructions—and that a satisfactory therapeutic relationship is as essential to behavior therapy as it is to other psychotherapies.

SYSTEMATIC DESENSITIZATION

Systematic desensitization, a procedure introduced by Wolpe (1958), is most often used in the treatment of phobias (see section on anxiety disorders). After a thorough exploration of the patient's phobia, a hierarchy of feared situations along one dimension is created—for example, for a patient with height phobia, looking down from the second floor of a building to looking down from a skyscraper, with many gradual steps in between. The patient is then taught deep muscle relaxation (see subsection on relaxation training) and next visualizes the first item in the hierarchy for some 20–30 seconds, signaling if any anxiety has been aroused. When the visualization of the first scene has produced no anxiety on two repetitions, the therapist moves on to the next item in the hierarchy. Because there may be some recrudescence of anxiety between sessions, it is usually wise to drop back a couple of items and to proceed forward from there.

Some patients have difficulty visualizing feared scenes and may need coaching (e.g., to imagine colors and specific details of a particular scene). Systematic desensitization is little used today, having been largely superseded by the use of direct exposure to the feared situation, as will be described in the next subsection. The procedure is useful, however, in extremely fearful patients who will not venture into the feared situation, when it is used before exposure to the feared situation.

EXPOSURE THERAPY (PROGRAMMED PRACTICE)

Exposure therapy, sometimes known as *programmed practice*, is one of the most investigated and frequently used therapies in the treatment of phobias, including agoraphobia. There are several variants of this therapeutic procedure, although all begin with the construction of a hierarchy of feared situations along a particular dimension. The simplest variant of exposure therapy is known as *exposure instructions*. The therapist helps the patient construct the first few steps in a hierarchy of the feared situation. For example, for the patient with agoraphobia who is housebound, this involves walking a few yards from the front door, then walking half a block, then walking a block, and so on. With the use of the hierarchy, a course is laid out along which the patient is instructed to walk alone. The instructions are to walk as far as possible until mild anxiety is evident. At least one session, lasting approximately 30 minutes, should be held each day. The patient repeats each walk until the anxiety has dissipated and then he or she begins to walk farther. A diary is kept for each trial. At the next session the diary is reviewed, progress is attended to and praised, and any stumbling blocks are discussed and a solution for them is found. Progress is usually slow at first, with occasional setbacks, but as the patient gains experience with the method, he or she is able to make faster progress and eventually can proceed on his or her own.

In *therapist-assisted exposure*, the therapist accompanies the patient to the feared situation and provides direct coaching on facing it. In such cases the therapist may chal-

lenge the patient to experience maximal anxiety levels. In addition, the therapist may explore the thoughts of the patient during the exposure experience so that distorted cognitions can be directly challenged.

Group exposure therapy combines individualized exposure instructions and practice with group education concerning the phobia (usually panic disorder with agoraphobia) and with a discussion of the participants' experiences during exposure to the feared situation. Such group sessions are usually 3 hours in duration, comprising a 30-minute educational session, an exposure session with individual practice, and a 45-minute debriefing session. Group sessions are often held daily for 10–14 days.

Flooding is a form of exposure therapy in which patients are exposed to the maximal phobic situation and kept in that situation until their fear dissipates. Although this form of treatment produces positive results more rapidly than does graduated exposure, it may be associated with much discomfort and therefore is rarely used today.

COGNITIVE THERAPY

Although behavior therapy, as its name implies, tends to focus on the current behavior of the patient, from the earliest days of behavior therapy there was at least some focus on the specific cognitions accompanying a particular disorder. The importance of distorted cognitions has been particularly recognized in the treatment of the anxiety disorders, depression, and the eating disorders. The typical approach to cognitive therapy involves a thorough exploration of the thoughts and feelings preceding, during, and following a particular behavior (e.g., binge eating or purging). For patients who have difficulty recalling such thoughts, self-monitoring is often useful. Once the cognitions have been clearly identified, the reality of such thoughts is considered in detail. When the patient recognizes the unrealistic nature of the thoughts, such thinking can be challenged in vivo by the patient or behavioral experiments designed further to test the reality of such thinking can be devised.

The following case history is an example of the use of cognitive therapy:

A philosophy student in her late 20s had a sudden panic attack while presenting a paper in her class. She then had several further attacks (apparently precipitated by thoughts of failure), lost her appetite, and began to lose weight. In addition, she began to avoid leaving home unless accompanied by her husband. She was evaluated within a month of the start of her symptoms. During the initial interview, it became clear that this ambitious young woman thought that her life was out of control, that she was a failure, that she could not continue with her projected career as a philosopher, and that her life was essentially over. She was particularly afraid that her wealthy and successful husband would divorce her and find a more suitable companion. Because she was a philosopher and supposedly a logical individual, the therapist asked her to examine the reality of her beliefs. Within the first session she was able to see that her beliefs were unrealistic. She immediately began practicing leaving home alone, challenging her unrealistic thinking when it recurred. Within a few sessions she no longer felt anxious, was able to resume her studies, had no phobic limitation, and once more felt secure in her marriage. At 1-year follow-up she remained, by her assessment, symptom free.

It should be noted that cognitive procedures are usually combined with behavior change procedures, and that many behavior therapies are now referred to as *cognitive-behavior* therapies.

REINFORCEMENT

Reinforcement consists of making an event contingent on the performance of a behavior that one wishes to change. *Positive reinforcement* is said to occur when the contingent application of the event strengthens the behavior. Positive reinforcers are usually viewed as pleasant (e.g., food, attention, praise, money). All therapists use verbal attention to reinforce particular themes during therapy sessions. Behavior therapists tend to use such reinforcement in a more precise manner, making attention or praise contingent on the occurrence of the behavior that is being strengthened. Although positive reinforcement is an aspect of all therapeutic encounters, it is most often used to strengthen prosocial behaviors in children with conduct disorder or in persons with schizophrenia (discussed later in this chapter). *Negative reinforcement* refers to a process by which a particular behavior removes the reinforcing event, thus strengthening the behavior. The events used in a negative reinforcement paradigm are usually regarded as unpleasant. For example, in the treatment of anorexia nervosa the often-used threat of tube-feeding serves as a negative reinforcer, because the patient can avoid the negative occurrence (i.e., tube-feeding) by eating and gaining weight.

In addition to using reinforcement within a therapeutic package of some kind, the psychiatrist must review patients' current behavior to identify reinforcers that might be maintaining the pathological behavior. It is also clear that staff attention to problem behaviors increases the frequency of such behaviors. Therefore, nursing and medical staff at all levels should be trained in the application of social reinforcement and extinction procedures. Research has shown that untrained nursing staff attend to problem behaviors more frequently than they attend to prosocial behaviors of patients. Such an approach causes an increase in the frequency of problem behaviors.

EXTINCTION

Removal of positive reinforcement weakens behavior and may lead to its total disappearance. This procedure is known as *extinction*. From a clinical viewpoint, extinction can be used only in environments such as an inpatient unit or a classroom in which reinforcement can be controlled, although relatives of patients can be taught to use extinction in the home. The withdrawal of positive reinforcement may lead to an *extinction burst*, in which the unwanted behavior briefly increases in frequency or strength. If the procedure is being applied by relatives in the home setting, it is important to warn them that an increase in the problem behavior may occur at first, so that they do not abandon the attempt to control the behavior through extinction.

PUNISHMENT

The punishment paradigm consists of the application of an aversive stimulus contingent on the unwanted behavior, with the aim of rapidly bringing the behavior under control. Punishment is used infrequently in behavior therapy and only in situations in which the behavior in question threatens physical harm and in which more benign procedures such as positive reinforcement or extinction have failed. An example of the application of punishment is given in the subsection on ruminative vomiting, a life-threatening condition in infancy. The use of punishment, because it raises difficult ethical issues, is usually supervised by a committee that should include an informed layperson. In addition, if the use of punishment does not bring the unwanted behavior rapidly under control, the punishment paradigm should be reviewed for the accuracy of its use and/or stopped.

AVERSION THERAPY

Aversion therapy, which should not be confused with punishment, is based on the principle of classical conditioning and involves pairing an aversive stimulus with the unwanted behavior. An example of such a paradigm is the pairing of nausea (induced with emetine) with the drinking of alcohol in the treatment of alcoholism. It has been shown that such classical conditioning is more powerful if it involves the same physiological system as the one involved in the unwanted behavior. Thus, drinking is paired with nausea in the case of alcoholism because both involve the gastrointestinal system. One of the problems with aversive therapy is that exposure to the original stimulus (in this case, drinking alcohol) tends to weaken the classically conditioned response and lead to relapse. Therefore, in the original application of such conditioning, booster sessions were found to delay relapse. Nonetheless, the tendency toward relapse after aversion therapy has led to a decrease in enthusiasm for the use of aversion therapy in general.

BIOFEEDBACK

The principal aim of biofeedback procedures is to magnify a response that is not accessible to a patient and to provide feedback regarding changes in that response over time. For example, small muscle contractions are not usually discriminable by patients. Such responses can be amplified through the use of electronic monitoring, and a signal can be displayed, either visually or in the form of a continuous tone, that is proportional to the muscle contraction being measured. In this way, the patient can be informed about the degree of contraction and can potentially learn either to increase or to decrease the contractions, depending on the aim of therapy. Thus, in the case of nerve or muscle damage the aim would be to increase contractions in selected muscles, whereas in the case of tension headache the aim would be to reduce tension in the affected muscles. Biofeedback has many potential applications—for example, in fecal incontinence, through training of the anal sphincter; in hypertension, through displaying blood pressure values and allowing patients to discover methods to control their blood pressure; and in Raynaud's disease, through enhancing temperature control. Using small portable biofeedback units, patients can practice in their own homes, and thus learning can be transferred from the office to the patients' own environment.

RELAXATION TRAINING

Relaxation training is a relatively simple therapeutic technique that is useful in a variety of conditions (discussed later in this chapter) and often forms a component of a behavior therapy treatment package. Patients are first presented with a rationale. For example, a patient who has tension headaches would be told that muscles tense up as a result of anxiety and this can lead to pain; if the patient were to learn to relax his or her muscles, such pain could be lessened. Patients are then seated comfortably in a chair and are taught to tense and then relax each muscle group

systematically. Soon they are able to induce relaxation fairly quickly simply by relaxing all their muscles. Patients are encouraged at the same time to visualize a pleasant relaxing scene or to use a simple mantra to control distracting thoughts. Patients are given a tape recording of relaxation instructions and are encouraged to use the tape for some 20 minutes each day at home. After several treatment sessions with intervening home practice, patients are taught rapid relaxation techniques. In this procedure, patients are taught to scan their bodies intermittently for tense muscles and to bring on the relaxation response rapidly using the word *relax*, which they have previously paired with a deeply relaxed state. This procedure can then be used during the course of their everyday lives.

MODELING

Modeling refers to a procedure in which a desired behavior is performed by a therapist with the aim of having a patient copy the performance. It may be necessary to break a complex behavior pattern into its component parts and model each piece of the behavior sequentially until the entire sequence can be performed by the patient. Reinforcement such as praise is used as the patient gradually masters the desired behavior. The patient is then encouraged to try out the behavior at home. Modeling has been used to treat children's phobias through encouragement to expose themselves to the feared situation; in social skills training in disorders such as schizophrenia; in marital counseling; and in training in better parenting skills.

SOCIAL SKILLS TRAINING

Social skills training is used in the rehabilitation of patients with schizophrenia (discussed later in this chapter); in the treatment of social phobia, particularly when the phobia is combined with avoidant personality disorder; and in any patient in whom a particular social skills deficit is apparent. The first step is to analyze the social skills deficit in concrete behavioral terms—for example, avoiding eye contact, a slumped body posture that is not conducive to interpersonal communication, or speaking too softly. More appropriate behavior is then gradually developed by means of modeling and social reinforcement, together with opportunities for the patient to practice the new behaviors (e.g., in a group setting). The patient is next encouraged to practice the new behaviors in his or her own environment. Videotapes of the patient performing the desired behavior may also be employed so that the therapist can give detailed feedback on progress.

ANXIETY DISORDERS

PANIC DISORDER WITH OR WITHOUT AGORAPHOBIA

Agoraphobia (and the simple phobias) have been a central focus of behavior therapy since Wolpe's description of systematic desensitization first appeared (Wolpe 1958). The work in this area is an excellent example of the continual refinement of therapeutic hypotheses and procedures based on the results of clinical trials. On the basis of his findings from animal experiments in which fear responses were induced and then treated, Wolpe formulated the hypothesis that if a response that inhibits anxiety occurs in an anxiety-provoking situation, then the anxiety response will be weakened—an example of the principle of *reciprocal inhibition*. In his animal experiments, Wolpe used food to inhibit fear while the animal was exposed to gradually intensifying fear-arousing situations. In humans, relaxation was used to inhibit anxiety; hence, in the clinical application of systematic desensitization, deep muscle relaxation is paired with the imagination of feared scenes presented in a graded hierarchy, beginning with those provoking the least fear and gradually progressing to more fear-arousing scenes. Research in the field was catalyzed by the development of an analog model of phobia, namely, snake fears (Lazovik and Lang 1960). This model allowed for a more rapid delineation of the active and inactive components of systematic desensitization than would have been possible if research had been limited to clinical populations.

Findings from analog research challenged the theory on which systematic desensitization was based. Therapeutic instructions were found to be an essential component of desensitization, and removal of such instructions from the therapeutic package weakened the efficacy of treatment. This finding was not entirely surprising, given that therapeutic instructions have been found to be a major component of all psychotherapies. Such instructions comprise information concerning the therapeutic rationale, a description of the therapeutic procedures to be used, and, perhaps most important, an assessment of the outcome that might be expected from treatment. More surprising was the finding that pairing relaxation with feared scenes was not essential for successful outcome, nor was a gradual approach to the feared situation in imagination. This finding challenged the central notion of reciprocal inhibition. Ultimately, exposure to the feared situation itself was found to be the critical ingredient for successful treatment.

Many controlled clinical trials have demonstrated the effectiveness of graded exposure therapy in the treatment of agoraphobia (Taylor and Arnow 1988). Long-term studies have shown that improvement is well maintained for periods of up to 7 years (Fava et al. 1995). Involving a spouse (or friend) in the treatment process adds to the effectiveness of exposure therapy, probably because the patient's practice in the feared situation is better supported. The addition of couples training in communication skills enhances maintenance of the effects of exposure therapy. Such enhanced communication may allow the couple to adjust better to the agoraphobic individual's newfound freedom of movement, a change that may be stressful for some couples. Overall, exposure therapy is associated with dropout rates of approximately 10%, and more than 80% of patients demonstrate marked improvement. However, exposure therapy may be less effective in reducing panic attacks than in reducing or eliminating phobic behavior.

Behavior Therapy for Panic Disorder

Several studies suggest that the catastrophic interpretation of panic symptoms rather than the frequency of panic attacks is the critical element associated with the severity of agoraphobia. Catastrophic cognitions fall into three categories: 1) fear of illness, 2) fear of loss of control, and 3) fear of embarrassment while having a panic attack. It is hypothesized that persons susceptible to such cognitions misinterpret either mild symptoms of anxiety or other body changes (e.g., dizziness on standing up suddenly) in a catastrophic manner, leading to spiraling anxiety that culminates in a panic attack. It follows that therapy aimed at correcting such misinterpretations should lead to a reduction in panic. Such therapy consists, first, in identifying the type of cognitions experienced by the patient and, second, having the patient expose himself or herself to situations in which the catastrophic cognitions occur, essentially demonstrating to himself or herself that the feared consequences do not occur in reality (e.g., despite a fear of having a heart attack because of an accelerating heart rate, no heart attack occurs). In addition, some physical symptoms leading to the catastrophic thinking patterns can be induced in the therapy situation (e.g., in the case of dizziness, spinning the patient in a chair) and the reality of the frightening thoughts can thus be directly disconfirmed.

Controlled studies have demonstrated the effectiveness of this treatment in reducing panic attacks; between 50% and 90% of patients achieved remission of their symptoms in the various studies (e.g., Barlow et al. 1989; Clark et al. 1994; Craske et al. 1995). Follow-up studies reveal some relapse in symptoms of panic, although, for the most part, maintenance of treatment effects is good.

Combination Therapy

In general, it appears that the most effective treatment for agoraphobia with panic is a combination of pharmacological treatment and exposure therapy. For example, in a recent study comparing exposure therapy with and without treatment with fluvoxamine, the addition of medication was found to enhance the outcome of exposure therapy (de Beurs et al. 1995). For patients with agoraphobia who have not experienced panic attacks, exposure therapy alone should suffice. Behavior therapy may also be useful in the discontinuation of treatment with alprazolam, as demonstrated in a study comparing a slow tapering of medication with and without behavior therapy. Patients receiving the combined treatment were more successful in discontinuing alprazolam therapy and were significantly less anxious and depressed after medication discontinuation than those not receiving behavior therapy (Bruce et al. 1995).

SIMPLE PHOBIA

Because medication appears to have little place in the treatment of simple phobia, the approach to this problem that is most often used is graded exposure therapy. Such treatment is usually fairly easy to arrange and involves the patient's gradually approaching the feared object or situation. Therapist-aided exposure may be used in which the therapist accompanies the patient into the phobic situation and directly arranges exposure trials, or the therapist may simply use instructions regarding the practice of exposure and request that the patient keep a record of such practice. This record is examined at subsequent treatment sessions and solutions to problems encountered by the patient are worked out. Most patients with simple phobia respond rapidly to such treatment, and follow-up studies suggest that gains are well maintained.

SOCIAL PHOBIA

The number of studies of the treatment of social phobia, once a rather neglected area of research, is now increasing (Heimberg and Barlow 1991; Heimberg et al. 1993). Findings of controlled studies suggest that the behavioral treatment of choice is a combination of exposure therapy and cognitive restructuring. One study found that the addition of cognitive restructuring to exposure therapy prevented relapse. The principal area of focus for cognitive change is in eliciting the details of the social phobic patient's fears of negative evaluation by others and challenging the reality of these ideas. Exposure therapy in social phobia is more difficult to arrange than in the case of simple phobia or agoraphobia because social situations are less controllable by the patient than other phobic situations and may become more intense than expected. Moreover, many social interchanges are of short duration and therefore do not provide the more prolonged exposure characteristic of the therapy for other phobias. Hence, careful planning of exposure situations, ensuring a sufficient number of opportunities for exposure, and providing support for failure experiences when the social situation is more intense than was planned are all important aspects of the treatment of social phobia.

OBSESSIVE-COMPULSIVE DISORDER

There have been remarkable advances in the treatment of obsessive-compulsive disorder (OCD) with behavior therapy, although the results of treatment are not completely satisfactory. Deriving from basic work concerning the relationship between anxiety and avoidance behaviors such as compulsions, *response prevention* of compulsive rituals has become one of the cornerstones of behavior therapy in this condition (Stanley and Turner 1995). The thesis is that the compulsive behavior does not allow for reality testing of the fear. Thus, patients' fear of contamination leading to illness and death is reinforced by the fact that they do not become sick or die as long as they engage in hand washing.

The main therapeutic procedure is to prevent the patient from engaging in compulsive acts such as hand washing after exposure to "contaminating" situations. This may be accomplished by means of a gradual approach on an outpatient basis in which the patient, perhaps aided by a relative, abstains from engaging in compulsive behavior after exposure to the feared situation. A hierarchical approach is taken, in which the patient begins with the easiest situation and gradually moves toward more difficult tasks. On an inpatient basis, a more intensive approach can be taken—for example, preventing the patient from engaging in hand washing for a period of several days while providing a supportive relationship. The efficacy of this approach was first demonstrated in controlled single-case studies and since then has been examined in a number of controlled clinical trials.

Although response prevention results in marked diminution in compulsive behavior, it does not usually eliminate the fear of contamination. Controlled studies have demonstrated that exposure to contaminating situations results in marked diminution in contamination fears but relatively little change in rituals (Steketee et al. 1982). The combination of the two treatments (exposure plus response prevention) is clearly superior to either one alone. Finally, it has been shown that the addition of desensitization in imagination—focusing on the imagined catastrophic consequences of contamination—results in superior maintenance of recovery. Thus, a three-part behavior therapy dealing with separate components of the disorder appears to be most effective: response prevention for rituals, exposure therapy for phobic anxiety, and imaginal desensitization for obsessive worry.

Relatively little is known about the efficacy of combinations of behavior therapy and pharmacological treatment. A review of the literature suggests that patients in medication studies drop out at higher rates and experience somewhat less positive results than do patients in studies involving behavior therapies. To date, however, there has been no direct comparison of exposure plus response prevention and medication, nor have studies adequately compared the effectiveness of combining the two treatments with the efficacy of either treatment alone, although there is some evidence that such a combination may be the preferred treatment for OCD.

MOOD DISORDERS

MAJOR DEPRESSION

The effectiveness of a cognitive-behavioral approach to the treatment of unipolar nonpsychotic depression has been studied extensively in controlled clinical trials. In this treatment, the contingencies maintaining the depressed mood, often conceptualized as a relative lack of environmental reinforcement, are examined. Among the therapeutic procedures used are 1) problem solving combined with the teaching of coping skills to enhance the reinforcement deficit and 2) an examination of self-defeating cognitions, followed by the psychiatrist's teaching the patient to recognize such thoughts, to challenge them, and to substitute more adaptive thinking. Because antidepressant therapy can be viewed as the standard treatment for major depression, much recent research has been aimed at clarifying the relative effectiveness of pharmacological therapy and cognitive-behavior therapy (CBT) and the effectiveness of the combined treatments (Clarkin et al. 1996).

In one of the first studies to examine this issue systematically, Kovacs et al. (1981) found that both imipramine therapy and CBT produced improvement in depressive symptomatology in a 12-week treatment period and that CBT was marginally superior. At 1-year follow-up, both groups of patients maintained their improvement; however, there was a suggestion that those receiving CBT showed less relapse than those receiving imipramine. In the recent large-scale National Institute of Mental Health Treatment of Depression Collaborative Research Program (Elkin et al. 1989) CBT, interpersonal therapy, and

antidepressant medication were compared in a multicenter trial. The results suggested that all three therapies were effective but that medication was more effective in cases of severe depression.

Other studies have found that of patients who respond to therapy, those receiving CBT in combination with a tricyclic antidepressant show less tendency to relapse than those receiving antidepressants alone (Simons et al. 1986). Given that patients receiving antidepressants tend to improve more quickly than those receiving CBT, the preferred treatment for major depression would seem to be a combination of CBT and an antidepressant.

Social skills training has also been used to treat major depression. Such training involves the teaching of more assertive behavior that would be expected to increase social interaction and strengthen environmental reinforcement. Controlled studies have shown that this approach is as effective as CBT. Indeed, one must conclude from a survey of the literature that behavior therapy, interpersonal therapy (IPT), and time-limited focused psychotherapy are all equally effective in the treatment of major depression, although superior maintenance has been demonstrated only in the case of CBT and IPT at this time. This raises the theoretical issue regarding what procedures might be shared by these different approaches to treatment and whether they affect depressed mood through the same or different psychological processes.

OTHER DEPRESSIVE DISORDERS

The place of behavior therapy in more severe depression (e.g., cases meeting research criteria for endogenous depression) is less certain, due to a relative lack of controlled treatment studies in this area. Early work suggests, however, that CBT may be quite effective in both outpatient and inpatient populations and may be a useful alternative to treatment with medication. This modality may perhaps be helpful in patients who are not able to tolerate adequate dosage of antidepressant medication or as an adjunctive treatment combined with medication. CBT has also appeared to be useful in the treatment of dysthymia in initial uncontrolled studies.

DISORDERS OF EATING

The three major disorders of eating are *anorexia nervosa*, *bulimia nervosa*, and *binge eating disorder* (BED), the latter often associated with obesity. The development of behavior therapy differs significantly between these three disorders for different reasons. In the case of anorexia nervosa, the relative rarity of the disorder has militated against the conduct of controlled clinical trials, and very little is known about the comparative effectiveness of different approaches to treatment over the long term. Bulimia nervosa, although common, markedly increased in prevalence toward the end of the 1970s, and clinical research is now in a state of relative maturity. BED has only recently attracted research attention, and therefore much less is known about the treatment of this disorder, although it would appear that treatments effective in bulimia nervosa are also effective in BED.

ANOREXIA NERVOSA

The behavioral approach to the treatment of anorexia nervosa is aimed at the restoration of normal body weight, usually within an inpatient setting. It is widely agreed that weight restoration in the severely emaciated patient is the first objective of treatment. Next, there should be an attempt to deal with whatever problems appear to have precipitated and are maintaining the eating disorder. Crisp et al. (1991) viewed anorexia nervosa as an avoidance of maturation (a weight and shape phobia); thus, weight restoration is viewed as exposing the patient to problems that are being avoided through starvation (i.e., an exposure therapy).

Single-case controlled research, a useful approach when dealing with a relatively rare disorder, has revealed three procedures that promote increased caloric intake: reinforcement of weight gain in small increments, feedback of information regarding progress (usually accomplished by daily weight and caloric consumption feedback), and the serving of large meals even though the patient will at first leave most of the food untouched. These procedures are used in the context of a carefully negotiated therapeutic contract and a well-designed ward milieu (Agras 1987). Such programs lead to steady weight gain, and studies suggest that behavior therapy is more efficient than other treatment approaches, resulting in shorter hospital stays for equal amounts of weight gain. The only large-scale controlled study of an inpatient behavioral approach to weight restoration suggested that behavior therapy may be relatively more effective in the less severe case of anorexia nervosa.

More recently, research has been directed toward evaluating outpatient treatments for anorexia nervosa. One study compared inpatient and outpatient care for anorexia nervosa in a randomized controlled trial (Crisp et al. 1991). Surprisingly, the results of outpatient care equaled those of inpatient care, in that weight gains in the patients receiving outpatient care were equivalent to those in the patients

receiving inpatient care, and weight gains in the patients in these groups were superior to those in patients who received no treatment. This study requires replication by other investigators because of methodological problems, including a high rate of dropout from the study. Nonetheless, in an era in which the duration of hospitalization for the anorexic patient is becoming ever shorter, this study may point the way to the future of treatment of anorexia.

BULIMIA NERVOSA

The upsurge in the number of young women seeking treatment for bulimic symptoms in the late 1970s presented clinicians with a difficult problem because no effective treatment methods had been described for this condition. The work of Fairburn (1981), who first described a CBT for bulimia, has led to the appearance of a large number of controlled trials in the last decade. It is generally agreed that the social pressure for women to remain thin has increased during the past 15 years. This pressure leads a subgroup of young women to restrict their caloric intake markedly and to form rigid rules relating to food, leading to an increased probability of binge eating and eventually, because of threatened weight increase, to purging. It is also probable that the most susceptible young women are those who markedly restrict their food intake despite being genetically programmed for having a fuller figure. Research has shown that some bulimic individuals have a markedly increased energy efficiency, maintaining normal body weight in the absence of purging on a mean daily caloric intake of approximately 1,400 calories. They also tend to eat very little early in the day, which sets the scene for binge eating later in the day.

CBT is aimed at overcoming the dietary restriction and distorted thinking patterns that are believed to maintain bulimia nervosa. The basic components of CBT include self-disclosure to significant others, thus increasing social control over the secretive bulimic behaviors; gradual reintroduction of the consumption of three adequate meals each day; slow introduction of "feared" binge foods to the diet; challenge of distorted cognitions regarding food intake; and a relapse prevention program (Agras 1987; Fairburn 1981). Controlled studies have demonstrated that CBT is more effective in reducing binge eating and purging than are a waiting-list control condition; a pill placebo; psychoeducational treatment; nondirective psychotherapy combined with self-monitoring of eating behavior; stress management; and, in some studies, behavior therapy (i.e., a treatment omitting the procedures aimed at correcting distorted thinking patterns). In other studies, CBT and behavior therapy have been found to be equivalent in effectiveness in reducing binge eating and purging, although patients receiving CBT almost always have psychiatrically healthier attitudes toward weight and shape, attitudes that are specifically targeted by CBT. Overall, some 55% of patients with bulimia recover with the use of CBT, and the majority maintain their gains over follow-up periods of up to 5 years (Fairburn et al. 1993). A substantial proportion of those not fully recovering have a subclinical eating disorder at follow-up.

Combination Therapy

Because both CBT and antidepressant medication have been used in the treatment of bulimia nervosa, the relative effectiveness of these different approaches to treatment and their combination has been investigated. Studies have shown that CBT is superior to antidepressant medication in reducing binge eating and purging and that the combined treatment is no more effective than CBT alone. It appears, however, that the combined treatment more effectively reduces depression and emotionally induced eating, and there is tentative evidence that, as in depression, the combined treatment leads to better maintenance of improvement (Agras et al. 1992; Mitchell et al. 1990). More recently, Walsh et al. (1997) conducted a study in which two antidepressants, desipramine and fluoxetine, were used. These investigators substituted fluoxetine when desipramine was ineffective; such a model is more similar to that used by practitioners. Walsh and colleagues found that the sequential use of these medications was as effective as CBT and that there was a marginally improved effectiveness when medication was combined with CBT.

Other Approaches to Treatment

It has been shown that an adaptation of interpersonal therapy (IPT)—an approach that was first demonstrated to be effective in the treatment of depression—to eating disorders is as effective as CBT (Fairburn et al. 1991). This is an interesting finding, given that no attention was paid to eating disturbances in the interpersonal treatment. This suggests that IPT and CBT may work by different processes. There is much evidence that negative affect, frequently arising from interpersonal conflicts, triggers binge eating. It may be that IPT works by reducing negative affect, whereas CBT works by reducing dietary restraint.

BINGE EATING DISORDER

The research in bulimia nervosa has resulted in the rediscovery of a subset of obese individuals who binge eat but do not purge. The proportion of overweight individuals who binge eat increases with increasing levels of adiposity, from 10% in mildly obese persons to more than 40% in severely obese persons. Moreover, it appears that these individuals are less successful in their weight loss attempts than are their non–binge-eating counterparts. The similarity of this disorder to bulimia nervosa suggests that treatments effective in that condition should be effective in BED. Initial research has shown this hypothesis to be true: both CBT and IPT have been demonstrated to be equally effective in reducing binge eating in controlled studies (Agras et al. 1994; Wilfley et al. 1993). As is the case with bulimia nervosa, although antidepressant medication appears effective, adding therapy with such medication to CBT does not result in a significant additional reduction in binge eating. However, those receiving antidepressant treatment lose more weight than those not receiving medication.

The optimal approach for treating the obese binge-eating patient is to begin treatment with CBT and follow this with weight loss treatment that does not demand overly restrictive dieting. Patients with BED who stop binge eating and who maintain abstinence also maintain their weight losses.

PSYCHOTIC DISORDERS

The behavioral approach to the treatment of psychotic disorders may be viewed as being adjunctive to pharmacological treatment and directed toward amelioration of specific problem behaviors or, more broadly, toward the social rehabilitation of the disturbed individual. These aims are accomplished using methods deriving from operant conditioning. Thus, precise definition of the problem behavior, combined with the use of reinforcement in various forms, is the core of the approach for patients with either disturbed behavior that does not improve with the use of medication or limitations in social and vocational skills secondary to the psychotic process.

Some of the first applications of behavior therapy were to severely disturbed individuals with chronic psychoses. The early successes of reinforcement therapy, demonstrated largely in single-case experiments, led to many applications in the mental hospital, in which a large number of problems, including aggressive and disruptive behavior, delusional behavior, depression, and apathy, were found susceptible to change (Kazdin 1977). Ayllon and Azrin (1965) demonstrated the effectiveness of using tokens with chronic psychotic patients, thus broadening the range of backup reinforcers that could be used to motivate individuals. One of the most sophisticated applications and testings of a token economy system was the experiment conducted by Paul and Lentz (1977) comparing a social-learning program with a more traditional milieu therapy program. This experiment had many noteworthy features, including the use of multiple outcome measures, continuous monitoring of staff behavior to ensure proper operation of programs, collection of long-term follow-up data, and computation of the cost-effectiveness of the two programs. Patients in both treatment programs showed progress, but those in the social-learning program showed significantly greater improvement across a range of prosocial behaviors, required less medication, and maintained their gains more successfully during the 18-month follow-up. Moreover, the social-learning program was the most cost-efficient of the two programs.

Whereas the token economy focused on generating skills useful to most patients, social skills training, delivered within complex and sophisticated rehabilitation programs and based on a detailed analysis of each patient's interpersonal deficits, now forms a more individualized approach to the patient with schizophrenia. Among the skills taught are maintaining eye contact, reacting more quickly to interpersonal communication, varying intonation, and reinforcing prosocial responses from others. Techniques such as modeling prosocial behaviors are often used. In addition, the patient and family members may be taught more effective conflict resolution through the use of role playing, video feedback, and practice. A number of controlled studies have demonstrated that clinically meaningful changes in behavior occur as a result of social skills training, improvements of up to 70% in social functioning are made, and hospital stays are shortened.

In recognition of the fact that environmental stress is a factor affecting the outcome of treatment in schizophrenic patients, the effectiveness of a behavioral family-based treatment has been studied intensively (Falloon et al. 1985). The main focus of such treatment has been problem solving at the family level. When families are unable to use the problem-solving approach successfully, training in communication skills is added to the program. Specific behavior problems impeding the process of therapy are dealt with using appropriate behavior change techniques. Compared with patients undergoing individual treatment, those receiving behavioral family therapy showed a 10-fold decrease in the number of days spent in the hospital or in jail during follow-up. In addition, the number of days spent in residential facilities decreased 30-fold. Thus, we may conclude that behavioral family treatment is an effective addition to the treatment of chronic schizophrenia.

BEHAVIORAL MEDICINE

Behavior therapy has been applied to a number of medical disorders, including essential hypertension, hypercholesterolemia, and obesity; headache; sleep disturbance; gastrointestinal problems; and asthma. In addition, therapeutic procedures have been developed for problems common to many medical disorders such as compliance with medication taking and the response to stress.

OBESITY

Behavioral treatment for mild to moderate obesity contains the following elements: 1) self-monitoring; 2) reinforcement of an increase in activity levels; 3) slowing of the eating rate; 4) narrowing of the stimuli associated with eating; 5) adherence to a low-fat, high-fiber, heart-healthy diet; and 6) the use of reinforcement and self-reinforcement to attain short-term goals. This treatment package has been shown to be more effective than more traditional dietary approaches to weight control, psychotherapy, and even pharmacological treatment in a large number of controlled studies. The degree of weight loss achieved by the average patient is modest, usually averaging approximately 0.5 kg per week of treatment. Treatment programs of 16 weeks' duration result in a mean weight reduction of 8–10 kg. Weight loss is enhanced when reinforcement procedures, such as refund of a monetary deposit depending on weekly weight loss, are used. There is, however, marked variability in weight loss between individuals: some patients do not lose weight, whereas others lose more than 15 kg over the same period. The reasons for such variability are unclear, although there is evidence that poor adherence to the treatment regimen and particularly to self-monitoring is associated with a poorer outcome. In addition, biological factors—for example, adaptation of basal metabolic rate to dietary restriction—may vary between individuals. Finally, as discussed earlier in this chapter, the obese binge-eating patient appears to have more difficulty in losing weight than does the obese non–binge-eating patient.

Group therapy is the most usual behavioral approach to the treatment of obesity and may have advantages over individual treatment in that a wide variety of problem situations and their solutions are presented in a group context. Maintenance of weight loss appears to depend on the continued practice of behaviors learned during treatment. The most crucial of these are adherence to a healthy diet and eating style and continued exercise. Patients who continue to practice these behaviors have been shown to maintain or even increase their initial weight losses up to 5 years after treatment. Those who do not continue such behaviors tend to regain all weight that they lost, and some regain even more weight.

Behavior therapy has also been used to enhance the maintenance of weight loss with a very-low-calorie diet (VLCD), a treatment regimen used in moderately to severely obese patients. VLCDs were initially associated with a series of deaths in obese patients undergoing such treatment. These deaths were caused by inadequate protein in the diet accompanied by potassium deficiency, which in susceptible individuals led to ventricular fibrillation. Modern variants of the diet with adequate protein, minerals, and vitamins have proved safe when used with careful medical supervision. One controlled study demonstrated that weight regain after completion of a 12-week VLCD was less in a group of patients who were also receiving behavior therapy than in a group of patients who were not receiving this adjunctive treatment. Clinical studies suggest that mean weight losses of 20 kg or more might be expected with this combination of treatments, as well as marked improvement in cardiovascular risk factors including blood pressure, serum cholesterol levels, and even sleep apnea.

Relapse Prevention and Longer-Term Treatment

Longer-term follow-up studies have demonstrated difficulty with weight regain after acute weight loss (Brownell and Wadden 1986; Stunkard and Penick 1979). The theory of relapse proposed for the addictions but applicable to the treatment of obesity suggests that relapse (i.e., a return to previous behaviors) occurs when a patient who has insufficient ways to cope is confronted by a high-risk situation, problem, or emotional state. Precipitants to overeating often include negative affective states while alone or positive affective states in social situations. Cognitive-behavioral approaches have begun to address the relapse issue.

In a study addressing long-term treatment, Perri et al. (1988) treated a group of obese patients using behavioral techniques. Participants were then randomized to a no-treatment control group and to four other groups, each of which used a variety of behavioral approaches. All of the behavioral groups had continued therapist contact biweekly for an additional year. Problem situations were discussed and new strategies developed to help patients cope without resorting to eating at high-risk times. The participants in the no-treatment control group regained approximately one-half the weight they had lost during the year, whereas the participants in all of the behavioral groups maintained weight losses. In sum, continued therapist contact, longer treatment, and cognitive-behavioral approaches appear necessary for greater weight loss maintenance.

Combined Treatments

As is the case with other disorders, the question arises with regard to whether the effects of behavior therapy and medication might be synergistic. Several studies involving the combination of appetite-suppressant drugs, such as fenfluramine, and behavior therapy have been reported. The most impressive of these found an advantage in terms of weight loss for the group receiving fenfluramine at the end of treatment (Craighead et al. 1981). However, at 1-year follow-up this result was reversed, with those receiving medication regaining more weight than those receiving behavior therapy. The combined-treatment group lost less weight at this time did than those who were treated with behavior therapy alone. It may have been the case that patients receiving medication attributed their weight losses to the medication and thus did not practice the behavior changes needed to maintain the weight losses. The withdrawal of fenfluramine and dexfenfluramine from the market because of their linkage with cardiac valvular damage in a substantial number of cases has reduced the number of available appetite suppressant agents. Sibutramine has recently been approved for use in the treatment of obesity, and phentermine remains on the market because there is no evidenc of a relationship between cardiac damage and the latter medication.

HEADACHE

The research literature on the treatment of both tension and migraine headache suggests that relaxation and biofeedback procedures are equally effective. Relaxation training is simpler to apply and should thus be the preferred treatment. Both relaxation training and biofeedback are more effective in reducing the number and intensity of tension or migraine headaches than either no treatment or treatment with various types of placebos. One study, however, suggests that patients who do not respond to relaxation training may benefit from biofeedback. Follow-up studies show good maintenance for patients who improved with treatment; however, a fairly large percentage of individuals, perhaps 40%, are nonresponders. For the responder, studies have suggested that booster sessions may lead to lowered relapse rates. The mechanism of action of relaxation training and related procedures in the treatment of headache is uncertain, although it seems likely that lowering of sympathetic nervous system activity is the basis for the effect.

PRIMARY INSOMNIA

Sleep disturbance uncomplicated by other psychiatric or physical disorders is a common problem in medical practice. Given the potential deleterious effects of long-term use of hypnotic agents, it should not be treated for longer than a few days with medication. Thus, the discovery and testing of nonpharmacological approaches to the treatment of sleep-onset insomnia are important.

Two behavior therapy approaches to sleep disturbance have been shown to be effective in controlled studies. Both of these approaches decrease the amount of time before sleep onset as measured by self-report and polysomnography. The first of these treatments, relaxation training, is based on the rationale that anxiety and other distractions preventing sleep onset can be controlled with such training. The second treatment, stimulus control, is based on the theory that sleep onset should be signaled by a narrow range of stimuli—that is, being in bed in a dark room and feeling drowsy—and that for many patients with sleep-onset disturbance the connection between these stimuli and sleep has broken down. Thus, stimulus control treatment consists of removing distractions such as books, television, and radio from the bedroom. In addition, patients are instructed to get up if they do not fall asleep within 10 minutes and are further instructed not to go back to bed until they are drowsy. It has been shown that this treatment is more effective than relaxation training (Lacks et al. 1983). The preferred treatment approach to uncomplicated sleep-onset disturbance should now be stimulus control training combined with discontinuance of hypnotic medication.

STRESS MANAGEMENT

Relaxation training is useful in ameliorating many symptoms of stress, including anxiety, tension headache, and sleep disturbance. In addition, relaxation training appears to modify the Type A behavior pattern, an independent risk factor for cardiovascular disease. Type A behavior, which may represent a maladaptive response to life stress, consists of aggressive striving, time urgency, irritability, and impatience. A long-term controlled study involving patients who had had myocardial infarction demonstrated that it was possible to modify this pattern of behavior with an educational treatment regimen based on relaxation training and that reduction in Type A behavior was associated with fewer recurrent myocardial infarctions (Friedman et al. 1984).

ADHERENCE TO A MEDICAL REGIMEN

A number of controlled studies have demonstrated that behavior change approaches can improve adherence to the medical regimen, particularly medication taking. Ap-

pointment keeping, one of the first steps in adherence, has been shown to improve with the use of simple reminder strategies (e.g., a telephone call or a reminder card). Controlled studies suggest that appointment keeping can be improved from levels of approximately 70% to levels of more than 90% with the use of these simple strategies, thereby improving the cost-effectiveness of medical care (Gates and Colborn 1976).

Compliance with medication taking has also been shown to be poor: approximately half of all patients take medication as prescribed, a further 20% take medication approximately 80% of the time, and the remainder take either no medication or very little medication. Behavior change strategies are aimed at several aspects of the problem (Agras 1989). First, the patient's expectancies regarding the effectiveness of the proposed treatment are explored. If the patient does not expect the treatment to work, he or she will be unlikely to adhere to the prescribed regimen. For example, a negative experience of a relative or friend with the prescribed treatment may affect the expectations of a patient regarding outcome. Education regarding the short- and long-term benefits of the medical regimen is important in helping to promote a positive expectation regarding treatment. Second, the complexity of the regimen should be examined, because it has been shown that the more complex the regimen, the poorer the compliance. This includes an examination of all the medications that the patient is currently taking and an attempt to fit the new medication into the current regimen. Third, it has been demonstrated that patients quickly forget instructions given by their physicians; this underlines the need for written instructions. Fourth, it appears important to tie medication taking to other regularly scheduled behaviors (e.g., mealtimes, bedtime) and to have the pills stored in such a way that they are easily accessible at such times. Finally, the early handling of side effects to medication appears critical in maintaining adequate adherence. Patients with preexisting symptoms similar to the side effects of a medication appear particularly likely to prematurely discontinue taking medication. Identification of such symptoms before beginning medication is therefore important.

CANCER

One important role of behavior therapy in the treatment of patients with cancer is the reduction of anxiety and nausea associated with cancer chemotherapy, an example of classical conditioning. Relaxation training can be used for patients who do not respond to modern antiemetic agents. Controlled studies demonstrate that such treatment is effective in reducing anxiety, nausea, and vomiting. Unfortunately, little is known about the comparative effects of medication and relaxation training in reducing nausea and vomiting or whether these two treatment modalities augment each other. A second role of behavior therapy is to enhance coping with cancer. In a randomized controlled study involving patients in whom malignant melanoma had been newly diagnosed, Fawzy et al. (1994) used a structured 6-week group-intervention having components including health education, stress management, coping skills, and supportive group psychotherapy. There were several interesting findings. First, the group receiving the intervention used significantly more active-coping methods than did the control (usual care) group. Second, the active-treatment group experienced notable immunological changes. Third, at 6-year follow-up there was a strong trend for recurrence to be lower, and survival to be longer, in the active-treatment group. These results are similar to those of Spiegel et al. (1989), who employed a 1-year program of supportive-expressive group psychotherapy in women with breast cancer. After 1 year of treatment, the group receiving active treatment showed markedly less anxiety and pain than did the control group. In addition, at 10-year follow-up, length of survival time was superior for the group receiving the active treatment. Because the two treatments differed from one another, it is possible that some common mechanism was responsible for the observed results.

DISORDERS OF CHILDHOOD

Behavior therapy for children's disorders has been based on the use of operant conditioning, particularly the application of reinforcement procedures. This model emphasizes that behavior is a function of its consequences. Maladaptive behaviors are hypothesized to be learned as a result of complex reinforcement and punishment schedules in specific social environments. By analyzing the contingencies surrounding a behavior, one may change it by altering those contingencies. More recently, therapeutic procedures found to be useful in adults (e.g., in the treatment of anxiety disorder, depression, and OCD) have been successfully applied to children. Selected areas in the treatment of children's disorders are reviewed in the following subsections.

AUTISM

Autism, a pervasive developmental disorder, is no longer considered to be psychogenic in origin and is now seen as a central nervous system disorder (Cohen and Shaywitz 1982). Lovaas et al. (1971, 1979) made an important contribution to our understanding of autism by identifying the perceptual problem of *stimulus overselectivity*. When a variety of stimuli are presented to autistic children, as is the case in almost every social contact, only one portion is attended to, and there is a lack of response to the complex stimulus and its meaning. In one study, normal children were able to respond to each component (auditory, visual, and tactile) of a complex cue, while the autistic child responded selectively to only one cue and not the others. Thus, the autistic child's response to situations often appears bizarre. No evidence of sensory deficits is found. When simple cues are presented to autistic children, behavioral responding is more consistent. When well-defined cues are used, along with immediate and tangible reinforcers, desired behaviors can gradually be shaped. Behavioral excesses (e.g., tantrums, aggression, self-stimulatory behaviors) may be either punished (using, for example, time-out from reinforcement, in which a child might be put in a room alone for a few minutes contingent on disruptive behavior) or, if mild, ignored with the aim of weakening them (an example of the removal of reinforcement, i.e., extinction). Therapists and parents can be trained to teach autistic children in this way, and environments can be designed to reinforce desired behaviors systematically. Lovaas (1977) also developed methods to teach language skills to autistic children. Such children are able to learn but require very specific programming. Verbal skills are taught progressively, first with the use of reinforcement for attending to the teacher, then by the use of imitation, then by labeling objects, followed by stating simple sentences. Autistic children are able to improve their language skills substantially with this method, although this improvement is also correlated with IQ and maintenance depends on continued reinforcement. Increasing language skills can also facilitate socialization in children with severe language deficiencies.

In a controlled study, Lovaas (1977) provided intensive treatment to young autistic children and their parents. Parents, along with children, applied a home-based program using operant procedures over a 2-year period. The children received reinforcement for learning, communication, and social behaviors. After the trial, 47% of the children in the intervention group had been placed in a regular first-grade classroom (and IQ levels had markedly increased compared with pretreatment levels), whereas none from the no-treatment control group were able to be placed in such a classroom setting. These results suggest that such early, intensive, and comprehensive treatment may be very useful in autism.

Combination Treatment

In a controlled study, Campbell et al. (1978) investigated the use of haloperidol or placebo versus contingent or noncontingent reinforcement in a language training program for hospitalized autistic children. Medication reduced stereotypical and withdrawn behavior in older, but not younger, children, whereas contingency management improved ward behaviors and compliance and imitation in the language training program. The group receiving haloperidol and contingent reinforcement showed the greatest improvement.

CONDUCT DISORDER

Parents often seek help for their children's behavior problems, including aggressiveness, destructiveness, oppositional behavior, temper tantrums, and other negative behaviors (e.g., whining, screaming, threatening). Numerous studies have described a high rate of what Patterson (1976) described as *coercive interactions* in families of these children. Parents of these children respond with coercive behaviors when attempting to control their children's misbehavior. Patterson described a negative reinforcement model in which the coercive behavior of the parent may be reinforced by the reduction of the aversive behavior of the child. Unfortunately, the parent also models punitive behaviors to the child, who is then trained to behave similarly. In addition, parents may, without intending to, positively reinforce the deviant behaviors, either by attending to them or by fulfilling a demand accompanied by the deviant behavior (Wahler 1976). Often a parent will spend considerable effort and time with a child in attempting to abort a temper tantrum, and this approach may in fact reinforce the behavior.

To address such problems, the primary research effort has been in training parents to use social learning techniques to shape more adaptive and prosocial behaviors in their children. Such programs (Patterson 1976) have taught parents to monitor both prosocial and deviant behaviors, develop positive reinforcement systems (e.g., contingent point systems for obtaining rewards), use extinction (i.e., "ignoring") for minor misbehaviors, and use punishment (e.g., time-out) for serious infractions. Christophersen et al. (1972) examined the use of a home reinforcement system (i.e., token economy) with observations by parents and reliability checks by the experimenters. The token economy is a systematic use of contingent reinforcement using tokens (often points or stars) earned by the child for prosocial behaviors and later used to purchase privileges or desired items. This approach led to a marked reduction in deviant behaviors and increase in prosocial behaviors.

Christophersen et al. (1976) also compared the parent training and home token economy system with conventional outpatient treatment for children with conduct disorder. Parents using the token economy reported a 67% reduction in deviant behavior, whereas those using traditional treatment reported only a 34% reduction. Similar systems have been designed and have been found useful in the classroom, psychiatric inpatient programs, and residential treatment programs for children with behavioral disturbances.

There are, however, limits to the efficacy of such programs. It has been shown, for example, that marital discord is associated with conduct disorder in children. In such cases, improvement is unlikely until the marital discord has been addressed. Other complicating parental factors may include depression, substance abuse, or other psychopathology that will require therapeutic attention for the child to improve using behavioral techniques.

Kazdin and colleagues (Kazdin 1987; Kazdin et al. 1987) reviewed in greater detail the behavioral treatments for conduct and oppositional disorders and suggested that the more severe the conduct disorder, the more guarded the outcome. He and his colleagues studied the combined effects of parent management training (using behavioral techniques described earlier in this chapter) and a cognitive-behavioral problem-solving skills training approach for the children, the latter approach aimed at improving maladaptive thinking patterns. Such patterns seen in aggressive children, Kazdin et al. noted, include the lack of problem-solving skills and the tendency to believe others are antagonistic toward them. Those children receiving the combined treatment exhibited less aggressive behavior at home and in school, along with greater overall prosocial behaviors, than did the contact-control group, both following treatment and at 1-year follow-up. Further controlled work is much needed so that more powerful therapies for this important disorder can be developed.

Kazdin (1987) and others advocated earlier treatment for children and their families, that is, treatment before the children became heavily involved in antisocial behaviors and involved in the juvenile justice system. Such research should focus on early intervention to minimize the severity of the conduct disorder and the frequency of antisocial behaviors.

One study (Dumas and Wahler 1985) evaluated mother-child dyads participating in a parent-training program for children with conduct disorder. Mothers who had a low level of community contact (i.e., insular mothers) used more aversive control toward their children than did mothers with a higher level of community contacts. Children of the insular mothers were more aggressive than those of noninsular mothers in general, and in particular when responding to negative maternal behavior. Increasing contacts with friends and social supports in the community may help reduce negative interpersonal interactions.

ATTENTION-DEFICIT/HYPERACTIVITY DISORDER

Attention-deficit/hyperactivity disorder (ADHD) and associated learning disabilities may occur in more than 5% of children in the United States. Hyperactive children demonstrate excessive motor activity, distractibility, and impulsivity, which causes adjustment difficulties both at home and in school. These children often have difficulty when concentration is required for task completion. Behavioral studies using contingent reinforcement of desired behaviors in this population demonstrated that when teachers differentially attended to and reinforced appropriate classroom behavior, deviant behavior was reduced (Becker et al. 1967). Children who were rewarded for increasing academic work through use of free time or through participation in preferred classroom activities made considerable academic gains that were well maintained. Maintenance in school-related gains has been enhanced by the addition of parental reinforcement (Ayllon et al. 1975). When children brought home a good-behavior letter, one indicating cooperation and a reduced level of deviant behavior, they could select home-based rewards (e.g., praise, more allowance money); failure to bring home the letter resulted in an earlier bedtime or withholding of allowances.

Ayllon et al. (1975) evaluated academic performance in children who had been taking methylphenidate and who continued to do poorly academically. When methylphenidate therapy was discontinued, their hyperactivity increased. A token program was instituted whereby first work in math and then work in both math and reading were reinforced. Not only did academic performance improve, but the hyperactivity decreased. The behaviors incompatible with learning were reduced if the child was successful academically. A number of studies have begun to evaluate whether interactive effects exist when both behavioral and pharmacological interventions are used. Controlled studies suggest that medication reduces hyperactive behaviors but does little for either the learning deficits or the impulsive and aggressive behaviors associated with this disorder (Gadow 1985). Thus, a combination of behavior therapy and medication is most commonly used in the treatment of ADHD.

RUMINATIVE VOMITING

Ruminative vomiting is seen in infants and in mentally retarded individuals of all ages. Milk, or food in the case of the older child, is regurgitated and spat out. Because in infancy this condition is often life-threatening, the principal approach to treatment has been within a punishment paradigm. Punishment is much less useful as a therapeutic procedure than the use of positive reinforcement, because there are unwanted side effects such as aggressive behavior and there is always the possibility of inflicting physical harm. For the most part, punishment is used only in situations in which the behavior to be changed threatens injury to the patient and only when procedures using positive reinforcement have been found not to lead to improvement. In institutions where punishment procedures are frequently used, it is essential that an oversight committee be appointed to monitor the use of punishment.

Infants with ruminative vomiting regurgitate their food mouthful by mouthful, which leads to malnutrition and dehydration and thus poses a threat to life. One approach to treatment is to use the principle of punishment, whereby an unpleasant event is made contingent on each episode of regurgitation. In one controlled study, a drop of lemon juice on the tongue was used as the unpleasant event. During baseline measurement, before treatment was begun, the infant ruminated between 40% and 70% of the time the infant was awake (Sajwaj et al. 1974). Once lemon juice was presented contingent on spitting up food, the rate of ruminative vomiting decreased steadily. Punishment was then briefly removed, and rumination quickly returned to original baseline levels, confirming the effectiveness of lemon juice as a punishing event. Reintroduction of punishment led to disappearance of the behavior and a return to normal weight, with no relapse at 1-year follow-up. Similar procedures have been used successfully in mentally retarded ruminating individuals.

CHILDHOOD DEPRESSION

The behavioral treatment of childhood depression has been modeled on the demonstratedly successful treatment of adult depression using either social skills training or a more comprehensive CBT package. The treatment package used with depressed children is similar to that used with adults and is aimed at decreasing depressive thinking, enhancing social skills, and increasing pleasant activities. Several controlled single-case studies have demonstrated the effectiveness of either the whole cognitive-behavioral package or an element of the package (e.g., social skills training). However, many of these studies focused their assessment of improvement on the specific skills taught, rather than on depression. In one controlled study, it was found that some 50% of adolescents no longer met criteria for depression after treatment, whereas little change was observed in the waiting-list control group. There was continued improvement over a 2-year follow-up: less than 10% met criteria for depression at 1 year, and less than 20% met criteria at 2 years. This finding suggests that although not everyone improves, the effects of treatment are long-lasting. Interestingly, adding therapy for the parents of these children produced no added benefits. Other studies suggest that younger children respond equally well to treatment, but, as with adults, there tends to be no difference between different types of active treatment.

BEHAVIORAL PEDIATRICS

As in the case of adults, behavioral approaches have been used increasingly in pediatric populations with medical problems. Chronic diseases in childhood often require complex behavior changes for optimal treatment. Such is the case, for example, for the child with insulin-dependent diabetes mellitus who must comply with medications, diet, and exercise. Epstein et al. (1981) developed an educational intervention aimed at increasing knowledge and skills, using instruction, feedback concerning performance, and reinforcement. The content included insulin dosage, diet, exercise, self-administration of insulin, and the signs and symptoms of hypoglycemia. Parents participated, encouraging child adherence. Substantial improvements were made: urine samples were negative for glucose in 27% of cases during treatment, 39% after treatment, and 45% at 2-month follow-up.

Reinforcement systems have also been used to help children adhere to the demands of hemodialysis (Magrab and Papadopoulou 1977). Children were encouraged to adhere to diet and were rewarded with prizes for improvements in weight and in potassium and blood urea nitrogen levels. Similar reinforcement approaches have been helpful in larger populations, such as for the encouragement of attendance at dental facilities by low-income families (Reiss et al. 1976).

Modeling has proved useful in reducing children's fears before medical procedures. Melamed and Siegel (1975), in a randomized, controlled study, studied children who were about to have surgery. One group of children in the study viewed a film about a child coping with hospitalization and medical procedures, whereas the control group saw a film on another topic. Directly after this film, the experimental group demonstrated more physiological arousal. However, before surgery and a month later, both self-report of fear and physiological arousal were notably less in the experimental group. Fewer children in the experimental group required pain medication after surgery or complained of side effects, and more returned to eating solid foods sooner. This procedure is an excellent example of the use of modeling to aid in adaptive coping with a stressful life event.

REFERENCES

Agras WS: Eating Disorders: Management of Obesity, Bulimia, and Anorexia Nervosa. New York, Pergamon Press, 1987

Agras WS: Understanding compliance with the medical regimen: the scope of the problem and a theoretical perspective. Arthritis Care & Research 2 (suppl):8–16, 1989

Agras WS, Rossiter EM, Arnow B, et al: Pharmacologic and cognitive-behavioral treatment for bulimia nervosa: a controlled comparison. Am J Psychiatry 149:82–87, 1992

Agras WS, Telch CF, Arnow B, et al: Weight loss, cognitive-behavioral, and desipramine treatments in binge eating disorder. An additive design. Behavior Therapy 25:209–238, 1994

Ayllon T, Azrin NH: The measurement and reinforcement of behavior of psychotics. J Exp Anal Behavior 8:357–383, 1965

Ayllon T, Layman D, Kandel HJ: A behavioral-educational alternative to drug control of hyperactive children. J Appl Behav Anal 8:137–146, 1975

Bandura A: Social Foundations of Thought and Action. Englewood Cliffs, NJ, Prentice-Hall, 1986

Barlow DH, Craske MG, Cerny JA, et al: Behavioral treatment of panic disorder. Behavior Therapy 20:261–282, 1989

Baxter LB, Schwartz JM, Bergman K, et al: Caudate glucose metabolic rate changes with both drug and behavior therapy for obsessive-compulsive disorder. Arch Gen Psychiatry 49:681–689, 1992

Becker WC, Madsen CH, Arnold CR, et al: The contingent use of teacher attention and praising in reducing classroom behavior problems. Journal of Special Education 1:287–307, 1967

Brownell KD, Wadden TA: Behavior therapy for obesity: modern approaches and better results, in Handbook of Eating Disorders: Physiology, Psychology and Treatment of Obesity, Anorexia, and Bulimia. Edited by Brownell KD, Foreyt JP. New York, Basic Books, 1986, pp 180–197

Bruce TJ, Spiegel DA, Gregg SF, et al: Predictors of alprazolam discontinuation with and without cognitive behavior therapy in panic disorder. Am J Psychiatry 152:1156–1160, 1995

Campbell M, Anderson L, Meier M, et al: A comparison of haloperidol and behavior therapy and their interaction in autistic children. J Am Acad Child Psychiatry 17:640–655, 1978

Christophersen ER, Arnold CM, Hill DW, et al: The home point system: token reinforcement procedures for application by parents of children with behavior problems. J Appl Behav Anal 5:485–497, 1972

Christophersen ER, Barnard JD, Ford D, et al: The family training program: improving parent-child interaction patterns, in Behavior Modification Approaches to Parenting. Edited by Mash EJ, Handy LC, Hamerlynck LA. New York, Brunner/Mazel, 1976, pp 137–155

Clark DM, Salkovskis PM, Hackmann A, et al: A comparison of cognitive therapy, applied relaxation and imipramine in the treatment of panic disorder. Br J Psychiatry 164:759–769, 1994

Clarkin JF, Pilkonis PA, Magruder K: Psychotherapy of depression: implications for reform of the health care system. Arch Gen Psychiatry 53:717–723, 1996

Cohen DJ, Shaywitz BA: Preface to special issue on neurobiological research in autism. J Autism Dev Disord 12:103–109, 1982

Craighead LW, Stunkard AJ, O'Brien R: Behavior therapy and pharmacotherapy of obesity. Arch Gen Psychiatry 38:763–768, 1981

Craske MG, Maidenberg E, Bystritsky A: Brief cognitive-behavioral versus non-directive therapy for panic disorder. J Behav Ther Exp Psychiatry 26:113–120, 1995

Crisp AH, Norton K, Gowers S, et al: A controlled study of the effects of therapies aimed at adolescent and family psychopathology in anorexia nervosa. Br J Psychiatry 159:325–333, 1991

de Beurs E, van Balkom AJ, Lange A, et al: Treatment of panic disorder with agoraphobia: comparison of fluvoxamine, placebo, and psychological panic management combined with exposure and of exposure in vivo alone. Am J Psychiatry 152:683–691, 1995

Dumas JE, Wahler RG: Indiscriminate mothering as a contextual factor in aggressive-oppositional child behavior: "Damned if you do and damned if you don't." J Abnorm Child Psychol 13:1–17, 1985

Elkin E, Shea T, Watkins J, et al: National Institute of Mental Health Treatment of Depression Collaborative Research Program: general effectiveness of treatment. Arch Gen Psychiatry 46:971–982, 1989

Epstein LH, Beck S, Figuera J, et al: The effects of targeting improvements in urine glucose on metabolic control in children with insulin dependent diabetes. J Appl Behav Anal 14:365–376, 1981

Fairburn CG: A cognitive-behavioral approach to the treatment of bulimia. Psychol Med 11:707–711, 1981

Fairburn CG, Jones R, Peveler RC, et al: Three psychological treatments for bulimia nervosa: a comparative trial. Arch Gen Psychiatry 48:463–469, 1991

Fairburn CG, Jones R, Peveler RC, et al: Psychotherapy and bulimia nervosa: longer-term effects of interpersonal psychotherapy, behavior therapy, and cognitive-behavior therapy. Arch Gen Psychiatry 50:419–428, 1993

Falloon IRH, Boyd JL, McGill CW, et al: Family management in the prevention of morbidity of schizophrenia. Arch Gen Psychiatry 42:887–896, 1985

Fava GA, Zielezny M, Savron G, et al: Long term effects of behavioral treatment for panic disorder with agoraphobia. Br J Psychiatry 166:87–92, 1995

Fawzy FI, Fawzy NW, Hyun CS, et al: Malignant melanoma: effects of an early structured psychiatric intervention, coping, and affective state on recurrence and survival 6 years later. Arch Gen Psychiatry 50:681–689, 1993

Friedman M, Thoresen CE, Gill JJ, et al: Alteration of Type A behavior and reduction in cardiac recurrences in postmyocardial infarction patients. Am Heart J 108:237–248, 1984

Gadow KD: Relative efficacy of pharmacological, behavioral, and combination treatments for enhancing academic performance. Clinical Psychology Review 5:513–533, 1985

Gates SJ, Colborn DK: Lowering appointment failures in a neighborhood health center. Med Care 14:263–267, 1976

Heimberg RG, Barlow DH: New developments in cognitive-behavioral therapy for social phobia. J Clin Psychiatry 52:21–30, 1991

Heimberg RG, Salzman DG, Holt CS, et al: Cognitive-behavioral group treatment for social phobia. Cognitive Therapy Research 14:1–23, 1993

Kandel ER: Genes, nerve cells, and the remembrance of things past. J Neuropsychiatry Clin Neurosci 1:103–107, 1989

Kazdin AE: The Token Economy: A Review and Evaluation. New York, Plenum, 1977

Kazdin AE: Conduct Disorder in Childhood and Adolescence. Newberry Park, CA, Sage, 1987

Kazdin AE, Esveldt-Dawson K, French NH, et al: Effects of parent management and problem solving skills training combined in a treatment of antisocial child behavior. J Am Acad Child Adolesc Psychiatry 26:416–424, 1987

Kovacs M, Rush AJ, Beck AT, et al: Depressed outpatients treated with cognitive therapy or pharmacotherapy: a one-year follow-up. Arch Gen Psychiatry 38:33–39, 1981

Lacks P, Bertelson AD, Gans L, et al: The effectiveness of three behavioral treatments for different degrees of sleep onset insomnia. Behavior Therapy 14:593–605, 1983

Lazovik AD, Lang PJ: A laboratory demonstration of systematic desensitization psychotherapy. Journal of Psychological Studies 11:238–247, 1960

Lovaas OI: Language Development Through Behavior Modification. New York, Wiley, 1977

Lovaas OI, Schreibman L, Koegel RI, et al: Selective responding by autistic children to multiple sensory input. J Abnorm Psychol 77:211–222, 1971

Lovaas OI, Koegel RL, Schreibman L: Stimulus overselectivity in autism: a review of research. Psychol Bull 86:1236–1254, 1979

Magrab PR, Papadopoulou ZL: The effect of a token economy on dietary compliance for children on hemodialysis. J Appl Behav Anal 10:573–578, 1977

Melamed BG, Siegel LJ: Reduction of anxiety in children facing hospitalization and surgery by use of filmed modeling. J Consult Clin Psychol 43:511–521, 1975

Mitchell JE, Pyle RL, Eckert ED, et al: A comparison study of antidepressants and structured intensive group psychotherapy in the treatment of bulimia nervosa. Arch Gen Psychiatry 47:149–157, 1990

Patterson GR: The aggressive child: victim and architect of a coercive system, in Behavior Modification and Families. Edited by Mash EJ, Hamerlynck LA, Handy LC. New York, Brunner/Mazel, 1976, pp 93–127

Paul GL, Lentz RG: Psychosocial Treatment of Chronic Mental Patients: Milieu Versus Social Learning Programs. Cambridge, MA, Harvard University Press, 1977

Perri MG, McAllister DA, Gange JJ, et al: Effects of four maintenance programs on the long-term management of obesity. J Consult Clin Psychol 56:529–534, 1988

Reiss M, Plotrowski WD, Bailey JS: Behavioral community psychology: encouraging low-income parents to seek dental care for their children. J Appl Behav Anal 9:387–398, 1976

Sajwaj T, Libet J, Agras WS: Lemon juice therapy: the control of life-threatening rumination in a six-month-old infant. J Appl Behav Anal 7:557–563, 1974

Simons AD, Murphy GE, Levine RD, et al: Cognitive therapy and pharmacotherapy for depression. Arch Gen Psychiatry 43:43–50, 1986

Spiegel D, Bloom JR, Kraemer HC, et al: Effect of psychosocial treatment on survival of patients with metastatic breast cancer. Lancet 2:888–891, 1989

Stanley MA, Turner SM: Current status of pharmacological and behavioral treatment of obsessive-compulsive disorder. Behavior Therapy 26:163–186, 1995

Steketee G, Foa EB, Grayson FB: Recent advances in the behavioral treatment of obsessive-compulsives. Arch Gen Psychiatry 39:1365–1371, 1982

Stunkard AF, Penick SB: Behavior modification in the treatment of obesity: the problem of maintaining weight loss. Arch Gen Psychiatry 36:801–806, 1979

Taylor CB, Arnow B: The Nature and Treatment of Anxiety Disorders. New York, Free Press, 1988

Wahler RG: Deviant child behavior within the family: developmental speculations and behavior change strategies, in Handbook of Behavior Modifications and Behavior Therapy. Edited by Leitenberg H. Englewood Cliffs, NJ, Prentice-Hall, 1976, pp 516–543

Walsh BT, Wilson GT, Loeb KL, et al: Medication and psychotherapy in the treatment of bulimia nervosa: preliminary findings. Am J Psychiatry 154:523–531, 1997

Weintraub M: Long-term weight control: the National Heart, Lung and Blood Institute funded multimodal intervention study. Clin Pharmacol Ther 51:586–594, 1992

Wilfley DE, Agras WS, Telch CF, et al: Group cognitive-behavioral therapy and group interpersonal therapy for the nonpurging bulimic: a controlled comparison. J Consult Clin Psychol 61:296–305, 1993

Wolpe J: Psychotherapy by Reciprocal Inhibition. Stanford, CA, Stanford University Press, 1958

CHAPTER 31

COGNITIVE THERAPY

JESSE H. WRIGHT, M.D., PH.D.
AARON T. BECK, M.D.

Cognitive therapy (CT) is a system of psychotherapy based on theories of pathological information processing in mental disorders. Treatment is directed primarily at modifying distorted or maladaptive cognitions and related behavioral dysfunction. Therapeutic interventions are usually focused and problem oriented. Although the use of specific techniques is a major feature of this approach, there can be considerable flexibility and creativity in the clinical application of cognitive therapy.

In this chapter we trace the historical origins of CT, explain basic cognitive theories, discuss experimental findings on cognitive pathology, and detail commonly used cognitive therapy techniques. The main focus is on the treatment of depression and anxiety disorders. Cognitive therapy procedures for eating disorders, characterological problems, and other psychiatric conditions also are described. Finally, the extensive research on the effectiveness of cognitive therapy is reviewed and summarized.

HISTORICAL BACKGROUND

The cognitive therapy approach to depression was first proposed by Beck in the early 1960s (A. T. Beck 1963,

1964). He had begun to study depression from a psychoanalytical perspective several years earlier, but had been struck by incongruities between the "retroflexed hostility" concept of psychoanalysis and his observations that depressed individuals usually hold negatively biased constructions of themselves and their environment (A. T. Beck 1963, 1964). Subsequently, a comprehensive cognitive therapy for depression was articulated, and the treatment model was extended to a variety of other conditions, including anxiety disorders (A. T. Beck 1967, 1976). Cognitive therapy was described in a fully developed form in *Cognitive Therapy of Depression* (A. T. Beck et al. 1979). This volume was the culmination of a series of treatment manuals developed at the Center for Cognitive Therapy at the University of Pennsylvania. The therapy interventions were designed to be compatible with the cognitive model of depression and were drawn from several sources including the clinical experiences of Beck and colleagues and the writings of behaviorists and post-Freudian analysts (A. T. Beck et al. 1979; Thase and Beck 1992).

Cognitive therapy is linked philosophically to the concepts of the Greek Stoic philosophers and eastern schools of thought such as Taoism and Buddhism (A. T. Beck et al. 1979). The writing of Epictetus in the *Enchiridion* ("Men are disturbed not by things, but by the views which they take of them.") captures the essence of the perspective that our ideas or thoughts are a controlling factor in our emotional lives. Modern philosophers also have endorsed the concept that conscious ideas are at the center of human experience and that the meanings attached to events are a primary source of our actions. The phenomenological approach to philosophy, as exemplified in the writings of Kant, Jaspers, Binswanger, and others has significantly influenced the development of cognitive therapy (A. T. Beck et al. 1979). Frankl's (1985) logotherapy and Mahoney's (1985) and Guidano and Liotti's (1983) theories on constructivism also have played a role in formulating cognitively oriented treatment models. These authors have emphasized the importance of cognitive factors in finding meaning in life and in promoting personal growth.

There have been a number of developments in the field of psychotherapy during the 20th century that have contributed to the formulation of the cognitive therapy approach. The neo-Freudians, such as Adler (1936), Horney (1950), Alexander (1950), and Sullivan (1953) focused on the importance of perceptions of the self and on the salience of conscious experience (Raimy 1975). Other contributions came from the field of developmental psychology (Bowlby 1985; Piaget 1954) and from Kelly's (1955) theory of personal constructs. These writers stressed the significance of schemas (cognitive templates) in perceiving, assimilating, and acting upon information from the environment.

Cognitive therapy also incorporates theories and treatment methods of behavior therapy. Procedures such as activity scheduling, graded task assignments, exposure, and social skills training play a fundamental role in cognitive therapy (A. T. Beck et al. 1979; Lewinsohn et al. 1982; Meichenbaum 1977). In addition, Ellis' rational emotive therapy (Ellis 1962, 1973) has helped promulgate CT and related treatments.

Investigations in the field of cognitive psychology have solidified the concepts originally proposed by Beck and have led to a refinement of the cognitive therapy approach (e.g., Dobson and Shaw 1986; Hollon and Kendall 1980; LeFebvre 1981; Nelson and Craighead 1977; Rizley 1978). Also, the utility of the cognitive model has been demonstrated in a number of outcome trials reviewed later in this chapter. Recent developments have included the description of cognitive and behavioral techniques for personality disorders (A. T. Beck et al. 1990a; J. Beck 1997; Perris 1994; Shearin and Linehan 1994), substance abuse (Barrett and Meyer 1993; A. T. Beck et al. 1992a; Caroll et al. 1994a 1994b; Fisher and Bentley 1996), geriatric patients (Beutler et al. 1987; Steuer et al. 1984; Wilson et al. 1995), and eating disorders (Agras et al. 1992; P. J. Cooper and

Steere 1995; Fairburn et al. 1991). Also, theories and procedures have been developed for combining cognitive therapy and pharmacotherapy (Rush 1988; J. H. Wright and Schrodt 1989; J. H. Wright and Thase 1992), applying CT principles in the treatment of psychotic patients (Alford and Correia 1994; Garety et al. 1994; Kingdon and Turkington 1991; Perris and Skagerlind 1994), implementing cognitively oriented inpatient treatment (Bowers 1989; Stuart et al. 1997; J. H. Wright et al. 1992a), and using CT in behavioral medicine (Bergdahl et al. 1995; Dworkin et al. 1994; Speckens et al. 1995; Payne and Blanchard 1995; Sensky and Wright 1992; White and Neilson 1995).

In a review of the evolution of cognitive therapy over the past 30 years, Beck (A. T. Beck 1993) observed that intensive efforts have been made to have CT fulfill the criteria for a system of psychotherapy (Table 31–1). These criteria include: 1) a comprehensive theory, 2) empirical data to support this theory, 3) an operationalized therapy that interlocks with theoretical concepts, and 4) demonstrated efficacy of the treatment (A. T. Beck 1993). The remainder of this chapter is devoted to describing basic cognitive theories and their experimental basis, the translation of theoretical constructs into clinical practice, and the validation of cognitive therapy in controlled research.

BASIC CONCEPTS

THE COGNITIVE MODEL

The cognitive model for psychotherapy is grounded on the theory that there are characteristic errors in information processing in depression, anxiety disorders, personality disturbances, and other psychiatric conditions (A. T. Beck 1976; A. T. Beck and Rush 1992). For example, Beck (A. T. Beck 1976; A. T. Beck and Rush 1992) has proposed that there are three major areas of cognitive distortion in depression (the negative cognitive triad of self, world, and future) and that patients with anxiety disorders habitually overestimate the danger or risk in situations. Cognitive distortions such as misperceptions, errors in logic, or misattributions are thought to lead to dysphoric

TABLE 31–1. **Criteria for a system of psychotherapy**

- A comprehensive theory
- Empirical support for the theory
- An operationalized therapy based on theoretical principles
- Empirical evidence for effectiveness of the psychotherapy

Source. Adapted from Beck (in press).

affect and maladaptive behavior. Furthermore, a "vicious cycle" is perpetuated when the behavioral response confirms and amplifies negatively distorted cognitions (J. H. Wright 1988). This point is illustrated by the case of Mr. S, a 45-year-old recently divorced, depressed man. After being rebuffed on his first attempt to ask a woman for a date, Mr. S had a series of dysfunctional cognitions such as, "You should have known better . . . . You're a loser . . . . There's no use trying." His subsequent behavioral pattern was consistent with these cognitions—he made no further social contacts and became more lonely and isolated. The negative behavior led to additional maladaptive cognitions (e.g., "No one will want me . . . . I'll be alone the rest of my life . . . . What's the use of going on?").

The cognitive therapy perspective can be summarized in a working model (Figure 31–1) that expands on the well known stimulus-response paradigm (J. H. Wright 1988). Cognitive mediation is given the central role in this model. However, an interactive relationship between environmental influences, cognition, emotion, and behavior is also recognized. It should be emphasized that this working model does not presume that cognitive pathology is the only cause of specific syndromes or that other factors such as genetic predisposition, biochemical alterations, or interpersonal conflicts are not involved in the etiology of psychiatric illnesses. Instead, the model is used simply as a guide for the actions of the cognitive therapist in clinical practice. It is assumed that most forms of psychopathology have complex etiologies involving cognitive, biological, social, and interpersonal influences, and that there are multiple, potentially useful, approaches to treatment (see, for example, Akiskal and McKinney 1975; Engel 1977; J. H. Wright and Thase 1992; J. H. Wright et al. 1992b). In addition, it is assumed that cognitive changes are accomplished through biological processes and that psychopharmacologic treatments can alter cognitions (J. H. Wright and Thase 1992). This position is consistent with outcome research on cognitive therapy and pharmacotherapy (Blackburn et al. 1981; Imber et al. 1990; Peselow et al. 1990; Simons et al. 1984) and with other studies that have documented neurobiological changes associated with conditioning in animals or psychotherapy in humans (Baxter et al. 1992; Kandel 1979; Kandel and Schwarz 1983; Mohl 1987; J. M. Schwartz et al. 1996).

The working model in Figure 31–1 posits a close relationship between cognition and emotion. The general thrust of cognitive therapy is that emotional responses are largely dependent upon cognitive appraisals of the significance of environmental cues. For example, sadness is likely when an event (or memory of an event) is perceived in a negative way (such as a loss, a defeat, or a rejection), and anger is common when it is judged that there are threats to one's self or loved ones (A. T. Beck and Rush 1992). The cognitive model also incorporates the effects of emotion on cognitive processing. Heightened emotion can stimulate and intensify cognitive distortion (Bower 1981; Greenburg and Safran 1984). Therapeutic procedures in cognitive therapy involve interventions at all points in the working model diagrammed in Figure 31–1. However, most of the effort is directed at stimulating either cognitive or behavioral change.

LEVELS OF DYSFUNCTIONAL COGNITIONS

Beck and colleagues (A. T. Beck 1976; A. T. Beck et al. 1979; Dobson and Shaw 1986) have suggested that there are two major levels of dysfunctional information processing: 1) automatic thoughts, and 2) basic beliefs incorporated in schemas. Automatic thoughts are the cognitions that occur rapidly while a person is in a situation (or is recalling an event). These automatic thoughts usually are not subjected to rational analysis and often are based on erroneous logic. Although the individual may be only subliminally aware of these cognitions, automatic thoughts are accessible through questioning techniques used in cognitive therapy (A. T. Beck et al. 1979; J. H. Wright and Beck 1983). The different types of faulty logic in automatic thinking have been termed *cognitive errors* (A. T. Beck et al. 1979). Descriptions of typical cognitive errors such as selective abstraction, arbitrary inference, and absolutistic thinking are found in Table 31–2.

Schemas are deeper cognitive structures that contain the basic rules for screening, filtering, and coding information from the environment (A. T. Beck et al. 1979; J. H. Wright and Beck 1983). These organizing constructs

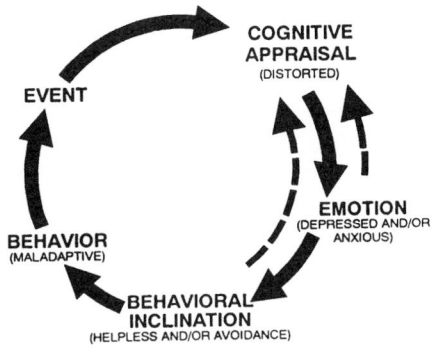

FIGURE 31–1. A working model for cognitive therapy. *Source.* Adapted from Wright 1988.

TABLE 31–2.　Cognitive errors

Selective abstraction (Sometimes termed "mental filter"): drawing a conclusion based on only a small portion of the available data.

Arbitrary inference: coming to a conclusion without adequate supporting evidence or despite contradictory evidence.

Absolutistic thinking ("All or none" thinking): categorizing oneself or personal experiences into rigid dichotomies (e.g., all good or all bad, perfect or completely flawed, success or total failure).

Magnification and minimization: over or undervaluing the significance of a personal attribute, a life event, or a future possibility.

Personalization: linking external occurrences to oneself (e.g., taking blame, assuming responsibility, criticizing oneself) when there is little or no basis for making these associations.

Catastrophic thinking: predicting the worst possible outcome while ignoring more likely eventualities.

Source.　Adapted from Beck et al. 1979; Wright and Beck 1983.

are developed through early childhood experiences and subsequent formative influences. Schemas can play a highly adaptive role in allowing rapid assimilation of data and appropriate decision making (Bowlby 1985). However, in psychiatric disorders there are clusters of maladaptive schemas that perpetuate dysphoric mood and ineffective or self-defeating behavior (A. T. Beck 1976; A. T. Beck et al. 1990a). Examples of adaptive and maladaptive schemas are included in Table 31–3.

One of the basic tenets of cognitive therapy is that maladaptive schemas often lie dormant until they are triggered by stressful life events (A. T. Beck et al. 1979; Miranda 1992). The newly emerged schema(s) then influences the more superficial level of cognitive processing so that automatic thoughts are consistent with the rules of the schema. This theory applies primarily to episodic disorders such as depression. In chronic conditions (for example, personality disturbances and eating disorders), schemas that pertain to the self may be present consistently and may be more resistant to change than in depression or anxiety disorders (A. T. Beck et al. 1990a; A. T. Beck and Rush 1992).

An example of the relationship between schemas and automatic thoughts can be found in the case of Mrs. C, a 39-year-old schoolteacher, married for the second time, who was functioning well until her husband made an unwise financial investment. When the family's economic situation changed, Mrs. C became depressed and started to have crying spells in her classroom. During the course of cognitive therapy, several important schemas were uncovered. One of these was the maladaptive belief: "You'll fail,

no matter how hard you try." This schema was associated with a host of negative automatic thoughts (e.g., "I messed up again. . . . We'll lose everything. . . . It's not worth the effort"). Although there had been a significant financial loss, and the marriage was stressed because of the situation, the emergence of Mrs. C's underlying schema led to an overgeneralization of the significance of the problem and a perpetuation of dysfunctional automatic thoughts.

COGNITIVE PATHOLOGY IN DEPRESSION AND ANXIETY DISORDERS

The role of cognitive functioning in depression and anxiety disorders has been studied extensively. Information processing also has been examined in eating disorders, characterological problems, and other psychiatric conditions. In general, the results of this investigative effort have confirmed Beck's hypotheses (A. T. Beck 1963, 1964, 1976; A. T. Beck and Rush 1992; A. T. Beck et al. 1979; J. H. Wright 1988; J. H. Wright and Beck 1983; Rush 1983). A full review of this research is not attempted here. However, a synthesis of results of significant studies on depression and anxiety is provided. These findings have played an important role in both confirming and shaping the treatment procedures used in cognitive therapy. Cognitive pathology in eating disturbances, personality disorders, and psychoses is described in the section on cognitive therapy applications.

TABLE 31–3.　Adaptive and maladaptive schemas

Adaptive	Maladaptive
No matter what happens, I can manage somehow.	I must be perfect to be accepted.
If I work at something, I can master it.	If I choose to do something, I must succeed.
I'm a survivor.	I'm a fake.
Others can trust me.	Without a woman, I'm nothing.
I'm lovable.	I'm stupid.
People respect me.	No matter what I do, I won't succeed.
I can figure things out.	Others can't be trusted.
If I prepare in advance, I usually do better.	I can never be comfortable around others.
I like to be challenged.	If I make one mistake, I'll lose everything.
There's not much that can scare me.	The world is too frightening for me.

Numerous studies have documented a negative cognitive bias in depression. For example, distorted automatic thoughts and cognitive errors have been found to be much more frequent in depressed persons than control subjects (Blackburn et al. 1986a; Dobson and Shaw 1986; Hollon et al. 1986; LeFebvre 1981; Watkins and Rush 1983). A selective recall bias also has been described. Depressed individuals are more likely to remember negative than positive self-referent information (D. M. Clark and Teasdale 1982; Gotlib 1981; Lloyd and Lishman 1975; Nelson and Craighead 1977; Teasdale and Fogarty 1979).

Substantial evidence has been collected to support the concept of the negative cognitive triad (J. H. Wright and Beck 1983; Haaga et al. 1991). A particularly well designed study in this area of research was performed by Blackburn and colleagues (1986a) who used the Cognitive Bias Questionnaire to test distortions in the three areas of the negative cognitive triad (self, world, and future). Depressed individuals scored more than twice as high on this scale as nondepressed control subjects. A large group of investigations has established that one of the elements of the negative cognitive triad, hopelessness, is highly associated with suicide risk (A. T. Beck et al. 1975, 1985b; Fawcett et al. 1987; Minkoff et al. 1973; Nekanda-Trepka et al. 1983; Prezant and Neimeyer 1988). Beck and colleagues (A. T. Beck et al. 1985b) found that hopelessness was the strongest predictor of ultimate suicide in a sample of depressed inpatients followed 10 years after discharge. Also, in a related study with outpatients, hopelessness was shown to predict ultimate suicides with a high degree of sensitivity (A. T. Beck et al. 1990b).

Research on schemas has been limited by problems in measuring these underlying cognitive structures (see for example, Bradley and Mathews 1982; Davis and Unruh 1981; Derry and Kuiper 1981). The most commonly used instrument, the Dysfunctional Attitude Scale (DAS; Weissman 1979) has been criticized because it appears to tap a general tendency for negatively biased thinking and may not directly assess schemas (Hollon et al. 1986). Further, Beck's theories indicate that schemas become dormant during remissions: therefore, these core beliefs would not be expected to be readily accessible with a self-rating instrument such as the DAS. Nevertheless, several investigations have found high DAS scores during periods of depression and marked reductions with symptomatic improvement (e.g., Blackburn et al. 1986a; DeRubeis et al. 1990; Simons et al. 1984). It has been suggested that small residual elevations in DAS scores after recovery from depression may indicate that this scale detects underlying schemas that are a marker for vulnerability to relapse (Blackburn et al. 1986a; D. E. Giles et al. 1989; Riskind and Steer 1984).

Abramson and colleagues (1978) have proposed that attributions to life events are negatively distorted in depression and that misattributions can play a role in the development of this disorder. The relevance of early research on attributions has been questioned because most investigations were performed with nonclinical experimental subjects (Peterson et al. 1985). Also, some studies of carefully diagnosed depressed patients found little or no evidence for attributional distortions (Hargreaves 1985; Miller et al. 1982). Nevertheless, the overall results of research on attributions indicate that clinically depressed individuals are prone to blame themselves for adverse life events, give global meaning to circumscribed occurrences, and believe that negative situations will last indefinitely. In contrast, individuals that do not suffer from depression commonly view noxious events as being due to external forces (e.g., fate, bad luck), as having isolated significance (limited only to the specific events), and being transient situations (Deutscher and Cimbolic 1990; Hammon et al. 1981; Raps et al. 1982; Zautra et al. 1985; Zimmerman et al. 1986).

Studies of responses to feedback have provided another perspective on dysfunctional information processing. Depressed individuals usually overestimate the amount of negative feedback and underestimate the amount of positive feedback that they receive (DeMonbreun and Craighead 1977; Gotlib 1983; Loeb et al. 1964; Nelson and Craighead 1977; Rizley 1978; Wenzloff and Grozier 1988). In analogue experiments, depressed subjects have expended decreased effort on subsequent trials after concluding that they have performed poorly on a task (Klein et al. 1976; Loeb et al. 1971). Interestingly, several studies have found a "positive self-serving bias" in nondepressed control subjects (Alloy and Ahrens 1987; Gotlib and Olson 1983; Rizley 1978). The tendency for nondepressed individuals to hear more positive and/or less negative feedback than they actually receive and to expend extra effort after being told they have not done well, may be an adaptive trait (Rizley 1978).

Although the research base for CT techniques has been primarily in the area of cognitive bias, findings from an additional field of investigation, learning and memory functioning, also have relevance for clinical practice (J. H. Wright 1988; J. H. Wright and Salmon 1990). Depressed individuals have been shown to have significant deficits in performing tasks that require abstract thinking, deep levels of memory, or sustained effort (Braff and Beck 1974; Danion et al. 1991; R. M. Glass et al. 1981; Golinkoff and Sweeney 1989; Weingartner et al. 1981). Most psychotherapies, including cognitive therapy, have a goal of helping the patient to gain insight. However, the results of research on learning and memory functioning indicate that overly ambitious therapeutic interventions, especially early in treatment, may overload the patient. It has been suggested that treatment interactions should be geared to the patient's cognitive capacity and that CT procedures such as structuring, pacing, agenda-setting, psychoeducation, and providing feedback should be used to counter deficits in learning and memory functioning (J. H. Wright 1988; J. H. Wright and Salmon 1990).

Studies of information processing in anxiety disorders have provided additional confirmation for the cognitive model of psychopathology. Anxious patients have been found to have an attentional bias in responding to potentially threatening stimuli (Matthews and MacLeod 1987). Individuals with significant levels of anxiety are more likely than nonanxious persons to have a facilitated intake of information about potential threat; and further, those with anxiety disorders are prone to interpret environmental situations as being unrealistically dangerous or risky (Fitzgerald and Phillips 1991; Mathews and MacLeod 1987). Anxious patients also have been shown to have an enhanced recall for memories associated with threatening situations or past anxiety states (Cloitre and Liebowitz 1991; Ingram and Kendall 1987). Thus, dysfunctional thinking in anxiety disorders spans over several phases of information processing, including attention, elaboration and inference, and retrieval from memory.

Automatic thoughts associated with themes of danger, threat, uncontrollability, or anticipated incompetence have been observed at much higher rates in patients with elevated levels of anxiety than those with low anxiety (Ingram and Kendall 1987; Kendall and Hollon 1989). In other studies of cognitive biasing in anxiety disorders, investiga-tors have noted high frequencies of negative self-statements (C. R. Glass and Furlong 1990), beliefs that social behavior is inadequate or standards of others cannot be met (Wallace and Alden 1991), misinterpretations of bodily stimuli (McNally and Foa 1987), and overestimates of future misfortune (Mizes et al. 1987).

Comparisons of depressed and anxious patients have revealed differences between the two groups and common features of the disorders (D. A. Clark et al. 1990; Ingram et al. 1987). In depression, cognitions about hopelessness, low self-worth, and failure are more frequent, whereas in anxiety, cognitive themes are usually related to anticipated harm or danger (D. A. Clark et al. 1990). Also, depressed patients are more likely to have absolute thoughts about negative themes, whereas those with anxiety disorders tend to have questioning thoughts concerning the uncertainty of future events (D. A. Clark et al. 1990; Ingram and Kendall 1987; Kendall and Hollon 1989). Although the content of thoughts may be different, depressed and anxious patients both have demoralization, self-absorption, a predominance of automatic information processing, and a reduction in the cognitive capacity needed for problem solving and task performance (D. A. Clark et al. 1990; Ingram and Kendall 1987; Ingram et al. 1987). Findings of studies on cognitive pathology in depression and anxiety disorders are summarized in Table 31–4.

THERAPEUTIC PRINCIPLES

GENERAL PROCEDURES

Cognitive therapy is usually a short-term treatment, lasting from 4 to 20 sessions (J. Beck 1995). In some instances,

TABLE 31–4. **Pathological information processing in depression and anxiety disorders**

Predominant in depression	Predominant in anxiety disorders	Common to both depression and anxiety disorders
Hopelessness	Fears of harm or danger	Demoralization
Low self-esteem	High sensitivity to information about potential threat	Self-absorption
Negative view of environment	Automatic thoughts associated with danger, risk, uncontrollability, incapacity	Heightened automatic information processing
Automatic thoughts with negative themes	Overestimates of risk in situations	Maladaptive schemas
Misattributions	Enhanced recall of memories for threatening situations	Reduced cognitive capacity for problem solving
Overestimates of negative feedback		
Enhanced recall of negative memories		
Impaired performance on cognitive tasks requiring effort, abstract thinking		

very brief treatment courses are used for patients with mild or circumscribed problems, or longer series of CT sessions are used for those with chronic or especially severe conditions. However, the typical patient with major depression or an anxiety disorder can be treated successfully within the short-term format. After completion of the initial course of treatment, intermittent booster sessions may be useful in some cases, particularly for individuals with a history of recurrent illness. Booster sessions can help maintain gains, solidify what has been learned in cognitive therapy, and decrease the chances of relapse (Thase 1992).

Although cognitive therapy is primarily directed at the "here and now," knowledge of the patient's family background, developmental experiences, social network, and medical history helps guide the course of therapy. Collecting a thorough history is an essential component of the early phase of treatment. History taking is often augmented in CT by asking the patient to write a brief "autobiography" as one of the early homework assignments. This material is then reviewed during a subsequent therapy session.

The bulk of the therapeutic effort in CT is devoted to working on specific problems or issues in the patient's present life. The problem-oriented approach is emphasized for several reasons. First, directing the patient's attention to current problems stimulates the development of action plans that can help reverse helplessness, hopelessness, avoidance, or other dysfunctional symptoms. Second, data on cognitive responses to recent life events are more readily accessible and verifiable than for events that happened years in the past. Third, practical work on present problems helps to prevent the development of excessive dependency or regression in the therapeutic relationship. Finally, current problems usually provide ample opportunity to understand and explore the impact of past experiences (J. H. Wright 1988).

THE THERAPEUTIC RELATIONSHIP

The therapeutic relationship in cognitive therapy is characterized by a high degree of collaboration between patient and therapist and an empirical tone to the work of therapy. The therapist and patient function much like an investigative team. They develop hypotheses about the validity of automatic thoughts and schemas or alternately about the effectiveness of patterns of behavior. A series of exercises or experiments is then designed to test the validity of the hypotheses and, subsequently, to modify cognitions or behavior. Beck and colleagues (A. T. Beck et al. 1979) have termed this form of therapeutic relationship *collaborative empiricism*. Methods of building a collaborative and empirical relationship are listed in Table 31–5.

The therapist usually is more active in CT than in most other psychotherapies. The degree of therapist activity varies with the stage of treatment and the severity of the illness. Generally, a more directive and structured approach is emphasized early in treatment, when symptoms are severe. For example, a markedly depressed patient who is beginning treatment may benefit from considerable direction and structure because of symptoms such as helplessness, hopelessness, low energy, and impaired concentration (J. H. Wright and Salmon 1990). As the patient improves and understands more about the methods of cognitive therapy, the therapist can become somewhat less active. By the end of treatment, the patient should be able to use self-monitoring and self-help techniques with little reinforcement from the therapist.

Collaborative empiricism is fostered throughout the therapy, even when directive work is required. Although the therapist may suggest specific strategies or give homework assignments designed to combat severe depression or anxiety, the patient's input is always solicited and the self-help component of CT is emphasized from the outset of treatment. Also, it is made clear that cognitive therapy is not an attempt to convert all negative thoughts to positive ones. In fact, bad things do occur to people, and some individuals have behaviors that are ineffective or self-defeating (Krantz 1985). It is emphasized that in CT one seeks to obtain an accurate assessment of 1) the validity of cognitions, and 2) the adaptive versus maladaptive nature of behavior. If cognitive distortions have occurred, then the patient and therapist will work together to develop a more rational perspective. On the other hand, if actual negative experiences or characteristics are identified, they will attempt to find ways to cope or to change.

The development of a collaborative working relationship is dependent on a number of therapist and patient

TABLE 31–5. **Methods of enhancing collaborative empiricism**

- Work together as an investigative team
- Adjust therapist activity level to match the severity of illness and phase of treatment
- Encourage self-monitoring and self-help
- Obtain accurate assessment of validity of cognitions and efficacy of behavior
- Develop coping strategies for real losses and actual deficits
- Promote essential "nonspecific," therapist variables (e.g., kindness, empathy, equanimity, positive general attitude)
- Provide and request feedback on regular basis
- Recognize and manage transference
- Customize therapy interventions
- Use gentle humor

characteristics. The "nonspecific" therapist variables that are important components of all effective psychotherapies (Barrett and Wright 1984; Davis and Wright 1994; Truax and Mitchell 1971) are equally significant in cognitive therapy (see Table 31–6). Professionals who are kind, understanding, and can convey appropriate empathy make good cognitive therapists. Other factors of significance are the ability of the therapist to generate trust, to demonstrate a high level of competence, and to exhibit equanimity under pressure (A. T. Beck et al. 1979; Thase and Beck 1992; J. H. Wright and Davis 1992). Cognitive therapists also must be able to maintain an energetic pace and to sustain their concentration throughout the treatment sessions.

Another characteristic that can influence the therapeutic relationship is the therapist's general attitude. Clinicians with a reasonably positive outlook on life and a belief that individual efforts can lead to significant change are likely to form more adaptive therapeutic relationships than those who may be overly discouraged or pessimistic. If the latter features are present, the therapist may require personal therapy to be able to forge the collaborative and empirical relationships that are necessary for effective CT.

Additional procedures that cognitive therapists use to encourage collaborative empiricism are 1) providing feedback throughout sessions, 2) recognizing and managing transference, 3) customizing therapy interventions, and 4) using gentle humor. The therapist gives feedback to keep the therapeutic relationship anchored in the "here and now," and to reinforce the working aspect of the therapy process. Comments are made frequently throughout the session to summarize major points, to give direction, and to keep the session on target. Also, questions are asked at several intervals in each session to determine how well the patient has understood a concept or has grasped the essence of a therapeutic intervention. Because cognitive therapy is highly psychoeducational, the therapist functions to some degree as a teacher. Thus, discreet positive feedback is given to help stimulate and reward the patient's efforts to learn. On a cautionary note, however, the cognitive therapist needs to avoid overzealous coaching or providing inaccurate or overdone positive feedback. Such actions will usually undermine the development of a good collaborative relationship.

Patients also are encouraged to give feedback throughout the sessions. In the beginning of treatment, patients are told that the therapist will want to hear from them regularly about how the sessions are going. What are the patient's reactions to the therapist? What things are going well? What would the patient like to change? What points are clear and make sense? What seems confusing?

A collaborative therapeutic relationship with frequent opportunities for two-way feedback generally discourages the formation of a transference neurosis. Cognitive therapy methodology and the short-term nature of treatment promote pragmatic working relationships as opposed to recapitulations of dysfunctional, early relationships. Nevertheless, significant transference reactions can occur. These are more likely with patients who have personality disorders or other chronic illnesses that require longer term treatment. The formation of negative or problematic transference reactions is rare in conventional, short-term CT of persons with uncomplicated depression or anxiety disorders. When transference reactions occur, the cognitive therapist applies CT procedures to understand the phenomenon and to intervene. Typically, automatic thoughts and schemas that pertain to the therapeutic relationship are identified, explored, and modified if possible.

Another feature of cognitive therapy that increases the collaborative nature of the therapeutic relationship is the customization of therapy interventions to meet the level of the patient's cognitive and social functioning. A profoundly depressed or anxious individual of low average intelligence may require a primarily behavioral approach, with limited efforts at understanding concepts such as automatic thoughts and schemas, especially in the beginning of treatment. Conversely, a less symptomatic patient with higher intelligence and ability to grasp abstract concepts may be able to profit from schema assessment early in therapy. If treatment procedures are pitched at a proper level, the patient is more likely to understand the material of therapy and to form a collaborative relationship with the therapist who is directing the treatment.

The therapeutic relationship also can be enhanced by using gentle humor during CT sessions. For example, the therapist may encourage the patient's sense of humor by providing opportunities to laugh together at some improbable situation or humorously distorted cognition. On occasion, the therapist may use hyperbole in a discreet manner to point out an inconsistency or an illogical conclusion. Humor needs to be injected carefully into the therapeutic relationship. Some patients respond quite well to humor. Others may be limited in their ability to use this feature of therapy. However, appropriate use of humor can

---

TABLE 31–6. Structuring procedures for cognitive therapy

- Set agenda for therapy sessions
- Give constructive feedback to direct the course of therapy
- Employ common CT techniques on regular basis
- Assign homework to link sessions together

strengthen the therapeutic relationship in cognitive therapy if patient and therapist are able to laugh with one another and to use humor to deflate exaggerated or distorted cognitions.

STRUCTURING THERAPY

Several of the structuring procedures commonly employed in cognitive therapy are listed in Table 31–6. One of the most important techniques for CT is the use of a therapy agenda. At the beginning of each session, the therapist and patient work together to derive a short list of topics, usually consisting of 2–4 items. Generally, it is advisable to shape an agenda that 1) can be managed within the time frame of an individual session, 2) follows up on material from earlier sessions, 3) reviews any homework from the previous session and provides an opportunity for new homework assignments, and 4) contains specific items that are highly relevant to the patient but are not too global or abstract.

Agenda setting helps to counteract hopelessness and helplessness by reducing seemingly overwhelming problems down into workable segments. The agenda setting process also encourages patients to take a problem-oriented approach to their difficulties. Simply articulating a problem in a specific manner often can initiate the process of change. In addition, the agenda keeps the patient focused on salient issues and encourages efficient use of the therapy time.

The agenda is set in a collaborative manner, and decisions to depart from the agenda are made jointly between therapist and patient. When work on an agenda item generates important information on a topic that was not foreseen at the beginning of the session, the therapist and patient discuss the merits of diverting or modifying the agenda. An excessively rigid approach to using a therapy agenda is not advocated. There must be sufficient flexibility to investigate promising new leads or to allow the patient to express significant thoughts or feelings that were unexpected at the beginning of the session. However, an overall commitment to setting and following the therapy agenda gives needed structure to patients who are unable to define problems clearly or think of ways to cope with them.

Feedback procedures described earlier are also used in structuring CT sessions. For example, the therapist may observe that the patient is drifting from the established agenda or is spending time discussing a topic of questionable relevance. In situations such as these, constructive feedback is given to direct the patient back to a more profitable area of inquiry. Heavy-handed, negatively oriented feedback is avoided. Instead, the therapist tends to give encouraging remarks that point the patient to issues that provide significant opportunities for change.

Commonly used CT techniques add an additional structural element to the therapy. Examples include activity scheduling, thought recording, and graded task assignments. These interventions, and others of similar nature, provide a clear and understandable method for reducing symptoms. Repeated use of procedures such as recording, labeling, and modifying automatic thoughts helps to link sessions together, especially if they are introduced in therapy and then assigned as homework.

PSYCHOEDUCATION

Psychoeducational procedures are a routine component of cognitive therapy. One of the major goals of the treatment approach is to teach patients a new way of thinking that can be applied in resolving current symptoms and in managing problems that will be encountered in the future. The psychoeducational effort usually begins with the process of socializing the patient to therapy. In the opening phase of treatment, the therapist explains the basic concepts of cognitive therapy and introduces the patient to the format of CT sessions. The therapist also devotes time early in treatment to discussing the therapeutic relationship in CT and the expectations for both patient and therapist. Often, reading assignments are given to reinforce learning and to deepen the patient's understanding of cognitive therapy principles. Examples of common reading assignments include *Coping With Depression* (A. T. Beck and Greenberg 1974), selections from *Feeling Good* (Burns 1980) or *The Feeling Good Handbook* (Burns 1990), or *Coping With Anxiety* (included in A. T. Beck et al. 1985a).

The major portion of the psychoeducational work in CT involves brief explanations or illustrations coupled with homework assignments. These activities are woven into treatment sessions in a manner that emphasizes a collaborative, active learning approach. Some cognitive therapists have described the use of "mini-lectures," (Epstein et al. 1988) but a heavily didactic approach is generally avoided. In some instances audio and videotape educational material is used in cognitive therapy. Also, group sessions have been used to educate patients about CT (Covi and Lipman 1987; Covi et al. 1982; Freeman et al. 1992). Computerized CT is one of the more interesting and potentially useful methods of psychoeducation (see section on computer-assisted cognitive therapy in this chapter).

COGNITIVE TECHNIQUES

Identifying Automatic Thoughts

Much of the work of cognitive therapy is devoted to recognizing and then modifying negatively distorted or illogical automatic thoughts (see Table 31–7). The most powerful way of introducing the patient to the effects of automatic thoughts is to find an in vivo example of how automatic thoughts can influence emotional responses. Mood shifts during the therapy session are almost always good places to pause to identify automatic thoughts. The therapist observes that a strong emotion such as sadness, anxiety, or anger has appeared and then asks the patient to describe the thoughts that "went through your head" just prior to the mood shift. This technique is illustrated in the example of Mr. B, a 50-year-old depressed man who had suffered several recent losses and had developed extremely low self-esteem.

Therapist: "How did you react to your wife's criticism?"

Mr. B: (Suddenly appears much more sad and anxious) "It was just too much to take."

Therapist: "I can see this really upsets you. Can you think back to what went through your mind right after I asked you the last question? Just try to tell me all the thoughts that popped into your head."

Mr. B: (Pause, then recounts) "I'm always making mistakes. I can't do anything right. There's no way to please her. I might as well give up."

Therapist: "I can see why you felt so sad. When these kinds of thoughts just automatically pop into your mind, you don't stop to think if they are accurate or not. That's why we call them automatic thoughts."

Mr. B: "I guess you're right. I hardly realized I was having those thoughts until you asked me to say them out loud."

Therapist: "Recognizing that you're having automatic thoughts is one of the first steps in therapy. Now let's see what we can do to help you with your thinking and with the situation with your wife."

TABLE 31–7. Methods for identifying and modifying automatic thoughts

- Socratic questioning (guided discovery)
- Use of mood shifts to demonstrate automatic thoughts in vivo
- Imagery exercises
- Role play
- Thought recording
- Generating alternatives
- Examining the evidence
- Decatastrophizing
- Reattribution
- Cognitive rehearsal

Beck has described emotion as the "royal road to cognition" (A. T. Beck 1989). The patient usually is most accessible during periods of affective arousal, and cognitions such as automatic thoughts and schemas generally are more potent when they are associated with strong emotional responses. Hence, the cognitive therapist capitalizes on spontaneously occurring affective states during the interview and also pursues lines of questioning that are likely to produce intense affect. One of the myths about CT is that it is an overly intellectualized form of therapy. In fact, cognitive therapy, as formulated by Beck and colleagues (A. T. Beck et al. 1979) involves efforts to increase affect and to use emotional responses as a core ingredient of therapy (J. H. Wright 1988).

One of the most frequently used procedures in CT is Socratic questioning (also termed *guided discovery*). There is no set format or protocol for this technique. Instead, the therapist must rely on his or her experience and ingenuity to formulate questions that will help patients move from having a "closed mind" to a state of inquisitiveness and curiosity. Socratic questioning stimulates recognition of dysfunctional cognitions and development of a sense of dissonance about the validity of strongly held assumptions.

Socratic questioning usually involves a series of inductive questions that are likely to reveal dysfunctional thought patterns. The use of this technique to identify automatic thoughts is illustrated in the case of Ms. W, a 42-year-old woman with an anxiety disorder.

Therapist: "What things seem to trigger your anxiety?"

Ms. W: "Everything. It seems like no matter what I do I'm nervous all the time."

Therapist: "I suppose that 'everything' could trigger your anxiety and that you have no control over it. But, let's stop for a moment and see if there are any other possibilities. Is that okay?"

Ms. W: "Sure."

Therapist: "Then try to think of a situation where your anxiety is very high and one where it's much lower."

Ms. W: "Well, a high anxiety time would be whenever I try to go out in public, like to go shopping or to a party. And a low anxiety time would be sitting at home watching TV."

Therapist: "So there's some variation depending on what you are doing at the time."

Ms. W: "I guess that's right."

Therapist: "Would you like to find out what's behind the variation?"

Ms. W: "I guess. But I suppose it's just because being out with people makes me nervous and being at home feels safe."

Therapist: "That's one explanation. I wonder if there might be any others—ones that would give you some clues on how to get over the problem?"

Ms. W: "I'm willing to look."

Therapist: "Well then, let's try to find out something about the different thoughts that you have about these two situations. When you think of going out to a party, what comes to mind?"

Ms. W: "I'll be embarrassed. I won't have any idea what to say or do. I'll probably panic and run out the door."

This example depicts the typical use of Socratic questions early in the therapy process. Further questioning would be required to help the patient fully understand how dysfunctional cognitions are involved in her anxiety responses and how changing these cognitions could dampen her anxiety and promote a higher level of functioning.

Imagery and role play are used as alternate methods of uncovering cognitions when direct questions are unsuccessful in generating suspected automatic thinking (A. T. Beck et al. 1979). These techniques also are selected when only a limited amount of automatic thoughts can be brought out through Socratic questioning, and the therapist expects that more important automatic thoughts are present. Some patients may be able to use imagery procedures with few prompts or directions. In this case, the clinician only may need to ask the patient to imagine himself or herself back in a particularly troubling or emotion-provoking situation and then to describe the thoughts that occurred. However, most patients, particularly in the early phases of therapy, can benefit from "setting the scene" for the use of imagery (J. H. Wright 1988). The patient is asked to describe the details of the setting. When and where did it take place? What happened immediately before the incident? How did the characters in the scene appear? What were the main physical features of the setting? Questions such as these help bring the scene alive in the patient's mind and facilitate recall of cognitive responses to the situation.

Role play is a related technique for evoking automatic thoughts. When this procedure is used, the therapist first asks a series of questions to try to understand a vignette involving an interpersonal relationship or other social interchange that is likely to stimulate dysfunctional automatic thinking. Then, with the permission of the patient, the therapist briefly steps into the role of the individual in the scene and facilitates the playing out of a typical response set. Role play is used less frequently than Socratic questioning or imagery and is best suited to therapeutic situations in which there is an excellent collaborative relationship and the patient is unlikely to respond to the role play exercise with a negative or distorted transference reaction.

Thought recording is one of the most frequently used CT procedures for identifying automatic thoughts (J. Beck 1995). Patients can be asked to log their thoughts in a number of different ways. The simplest method is the two column technique—a procedure that often is used when the patient is just beginning to learn how to recognize automatic thoughts. The two column technique is illustrated in Table 31–8. In this case, the patient was asked to write down automatic thoughts that occurred in stressful or upsetting situations. Alternately, the patient could try to identify emotional reactions in one column and automatic thoughts in the other. A three column exercise could include a description of the situation, a list of automatic thoughts, and a notation of the emotional response. Thought recording helps the patient to recognize the effects of underlying automatic thoughts and to understand how the basic cognitive model (i.e., relationship between situations, thoughts, feelings, and behaviors) applies to his or her own experiences. This procedure also initiates the process of modifying dysfunctional cognitions.

Thought recording is usually explained and illustrated in a therapy session and then additional exercises are assigned for homework. Depending on the case conceptualization, the therapist may suggest that the patient pay special attention to certain situations or issues (e.g., panic-inducing environmental cues, recurrent interpersonal problems, or dysfunctional behavioral responses). Also, specific assignments may be made to set up an in vivo experience that is likely to generate automatic thoughts. Examples might include discussing a troubling situation with a family member or attempting to engage in an anxiety provoking situation or behavior that is usually avoided. Automatic thoughts that are recorded during these homework assignments are brought to the next session for review and discussion.

TABLE 31–8. Two-column thought recording

Situation	Automatic thoughts
Call from boss to submit a report	I can't do this. I don't know what to do. It won't be acceptable.
My wife asks me to help more around the house	Nothing I do is ever enough. She thinks I don't try.
Car won't start	I was stupid to buy this car. Nothing works right anymore. This is the last straw.

MODIFYING AUTOMATIC THOUGHTS

There usually is no sharp division in cognitive therapy between the phases of eliciting and modifying automatic thoughts. In fact, the processes involved in identifying automatic thoughts often are enough to initiate substantive change. As the patient begins to recognize the nature of his or her dysfunctional thinking, there typically is an increased degree of skepticism regarding the validity of automatic thoughts. Although patients can start to revise their cognitive distortions without specific additional therapeutic interventions, modification of automatic thoughts can be accelerated if the therapist applies Socratic questioning and other basic CT procedures to the change process (Table 31–7).

Techniques used for revising automatic thoughts include 1) generating alternatives, 2) examining the evidence, 3) decatastrophizing, 4) reattribution, 5) thought recording, and 6) cognitive rehearsal (A. T. Beck et al. 1979; J. H. Wright 1988; J. Beck 1995). Socratic questioning is used in all of these procedures. *Generating alternatives* is illustrated in the case of Ms. D, a 32-year-old woman with major depression. The therapist's questions were pointed toward helping Ms. D to see a broader range of possibilities than she had originally considered.

Ms. D: "Every time I think of going back to school, I panic."

Therapist: "And when you start to think of going to school, what thoughts come to mind?"

Ms. D: "I'll botch it up. I won't be able to make it. I'll feel so ashamed when I have to drop out."

Therapist: "What else could happen? Anything even worse, or are there any better possibilities?"

Ms. D: "Well it couldn't get much worse unless I never even tried at all."

Therapist: "How would that be so bad?"

Ms. D: "Then I'd just be the same—stuck in a rut, not going anywhere."

Therapist: "We can take a look at that conclusion later—that not going to school would mean that you would stay in a rut; but for now let's look at the other possibilities if you do try to go to school again."

Ms. D: "Okay. I guess there's some chance that it would go pretty well, but it'll be hard for me to manage school, the house, and all my family responsibilities."

Therapist: "When you try to step back from the situation and not listen to your automatic thoughts, what's the most likely outcome of your going back to school?"

Ms. D: "It will be a difficult adjustment, but it's something I want to do. I have the intelligence to do it if I apply myself."

Examining the evidence is a major component of the collaborative empirical experience in CT. Specific automatic thoughts or clusters of related automatic thoughts are set forth as hypotheses, and the patient and therapist then search for evidence both for and against the hypothesis. In the case of Ms. D, the thought "If I don't go to school, I'd just be the same—stuck in a rut, not going anywhere" was selected for an examining the evidence exercise. The therapist believed that returning to school was probably an adaptive action for the patient to take. However, it also was thought that seeing further education as the only route to change would excessively load this activity with a "make or break" mentality and would promote a disregard for other modifications that might increase self-esteem and self-efficacy.

Decatastrophizing involves efforts to reconceptualize feared outcomes in a manner that encourages coping and problem solving. This technique can be effective even if there is a reasonably high likelihood that a negative prediction will actually occur. For example, a man might correctly judge his marriage to be so troubled that his wife may ask for a divorce. In this instance, the therapist would help the patient to recognize distorted cognitions about his ability to manage a possible breakup of the marriage. The patient might think, "I couldn't make it without her" or "I'd lose everything." The decatastrophizing procedure would involve examining negative automatic thoughts for their validity; looking for previously unrecognized attributes, interests, or coping mechanisms; reviewing the ways that the patient had managed losses in the past; and stimulating the patient to think beyond the immediate situation. The use of *reattribution techniques* is based on findings of studies on the attributional process in depression explained earlier in this chapter. Depressed individuals have been found to have negatively biased attributions in three dimensions: global versus specific, internal versus external, and fixed versus variable (Abramson et al. 1978). Several different types of reattribution procedures are employed, including psychoeducation about the attributional process, Socratic questioning to stimulate reattribution, written exercises to recognize and reinforce alternate attributions, and homework assignments to test out the accuracy of attributions.

The Daily Record of Dysfunctional Thoughts (DRDT) (A. T. Beck et al. 1979) or other similar thought records are standard tools used in modification of automatic thoughts. The DRDT is a five-column thought-recording device used to encourage both identification and change of dysfunctional cognitions. A fourth (rational thoughts) and fifth (outcome) column are added to the three-column thought record described earlier. The patient is instructed to use this form to capture and change automatic thoughts. Either a stressful event or a memory of an event or situation is noted in the first column. Automatic thoughts are recorded in the second column and are rated for degree of belief (how much the patient believes them to be true at the moment they occur) on a 0–100 scale. The third column is used to observe the emotional response to the automatic thoughts. The intensity of emotion is rated on a 1–100 scale. The fourth column, rational thoughts, is the most critical part of the DRDT. The patient is asked to stand back from the automatic thoughts, assess their validity, and then write out a more rational or realistic set of cognitions. There are a wide variety of procedures that can be used to facilitate the development of rational thoughts for the DRDT.

Most patients can learn about cognitive errors and can start to label specific instances of erroneous logic in their automatic thoughts. This is often the first step in generating a more rational pattern of cognitive responses to life events. This process is illustrated in the case of Mr. E, a 58-year-old man with major depression, who completed a DRDT during the middle phase of cognitive therapy (Table 31–9). He had learned how to use the DRDT during prior therapy sessions and had been acquainted with the concept of cognitive errors through therapy experiences and from reading *Feeling Good* (Burns 1980). Mr. E noted the particular cognitive errors involved with each of his automatic thoughts and wrote out a more rational set of cognitions.

Previously described techniques such as generating alternatives, examining the evidence, and reattribution also are used by the patient in a self-help format when the DRDT is assigned for homework. In addition, the therapist often is able to help the patient refine or add to the list of rational thoughts when the DRDT is reviewed at a subsequent therapy session. Repeated attention to generating rational thoughts on the DRDT is very helpful in breaking maladaptive patterns of automatic and negatively distorted thinking.

The fifth column of the DRDT, outcome, is used to record any changes that have occurred as a result of revising and modifying automatic thoughts. In the case of Mr. E, there was a significant decrease in dysphoric affect. Although the use of the DRDT will usually lead to the development of a more adaptive set of cognitions and a reduction in painful affect, on some occasions the initial automatic thoughts will prove to be accurate. In such situations, the therapist helps the patient take a problem solving approach, including the development of an action plan, to manage the stressful or upsetting event.

Cognitive rehearsal is used to help uncover potential negative automatic thoughts in advance and to coach the patient in ways of developing more adaptive cognitions. First, the patient is asked to use imagery or role play to identify possible distorted cognitions that could occur in a stressful situation. Second, the patient and therapist work together to modify the dysfunctional cognitions. Third, imagery or role play is used again, this time to practice the more adaptive pattern of thinking. Finally, for a homework assignment, the patient is asked to try out the newly acquired cognitive patterns in vivo.

IDENTIFYING AND MODIFYING SCHEMAS

The process of identifying and modifying schemas is somewhat more difficult than changing negative automatic thoughts because these core beliefs are more deeply embedded, may be largely out of the patient's awareness, and usually have been reinforced through years of life experience. However, many of the same techniques described for automatic thoughts are employed successfully in therapeutic work at the schema level (A. T. Beck et al. 1979; Thase and Beck 1992; J. H. Wright 1988). Procedures such as Socratic questioning, imagery, role play, and thought recording are used to uncover maladaptive schemas (Table 31–10).

As the patient gains experience in recognizing automatic thoughts, repetitive patterns begin to emerge that may suggest the presence of underlying schemas. Therapists have several options at this point. A psychoeducational approach can be used to explain the concept of schemas (may be alternately termed core beliefs or basic assumptions) and their linkage to more superficial, automatic thoughts (Dobson and Shaw 1986). Patients may then start to recognize schemas on their own. However, when the patient first starts to learn about basic assumptions, the therapist may need to suggest that certain schemas might be operative and then engage the patient in collaborative exercises that test these hypotheses.

Modification of schemas may require repeated attention, both in and out of therapy sessions. One commonly used procedure is to ask the patient to keep a list in a therapy notebook of all the schemas that have been identified to date. The schema list can be reviewed before each session. This technique promotes a high level of awareness of schemas and usually encourages the patient to place issues pertaining to schemas on the agenda for therapy.

Cognitive therapy interventions that are particularly helpful in modifying schemas include examining the evidence, listing advantages and disadvantages, generating alternatives, and cognitive rehearsal. After a schema has been identified, the therapist may ask the patient to do a pro-con analysis (examining the evidence) using a double-column

TABLE 31–9.   Daily record of dysfunctional thoughts—an example

Situation	Automatic thought(s)	Emotion(s)	Rational response	Outcome
Describe: a. Actual event leading to unpleasant emotion; *or* b. Stream of thoughts, daydream, or recollection leading to unpleasant emotion; *or* c. Unpleasant physiological sensations	a. Write automatic thought(s) that preceded emotion(s); rate belief in automatic thought(s), 0–100%	a. Specify sad, anxious, angry, etc. b. Rate degree of emotion, 1–100%	a. Identify cognitive errors b. Write rational response to automatic thought(s) c. Rate belief in rational response, 0–100%	a. Once again, rate belief in automatic thought(s), 0–100% b. Specify and rate subsequent emotion(s) 0–100%
Date: 4/15/98				
I wake up and I'm immediately troubled. I start to worry about work.	1. I can't face another day. (90%)	Sad: 90% Anxious: 80%	1. *Magnification.* Even though it has been rough, I have been able to get to work every day. Get a shower and make breakfast—that will get things started. (80%)	Sad: 30% Anxious: 40%
	2. The big project is due in 2 weeks; I'll never get it done. (100%)		2. *Catastrophizing, all-or-none thinking.* About half of the work is done. Don't panic. Break it down into pieces. Taking one step at a time helps. (95%)	
	3. Everybody knows I'm ready to fall apart. (90%)		3. *Overgeneralization, magnification.* Some people know I've been in trouble, but they haven't gotten down on me. I'm the one who puts me down. (95%)	
	4. It's hopeless. (85%)		4. *Magnification.* I know my job well and have a good track record. If I stick with this, I can probably make it. (90%)	

Source.   Adapted from Beck et al. 1979.

TABLE 31–10. Methods for identifying and modifying schemas

- Socratic questioning
- Imagery and role play
- Thought recording
- Identifying repetitive patterns of automatic thoughts
- Psychoeducation
- Listing schemas in therapy notebook
- Examining the evidence
- Listing advantages and disadvantages
- Generating alternatives
- Cognitive rehearsal

procedure. This technique usually induces the patient to doubt the validity of the schema and to start to think of alternate explanations. An examining-the-evidence intervention is illustrated in the case of Ms. R, a 24-year-old woman with depression and bulimia (Table 31–11). During the course of her cognitive therapy, Ms. R identified an important schema that was affecting both the depression and the eating disorder ("I must be perfect to be accepted."). By examining the evidence, Ms. R was able to see that her schema was based at least in part on faulty logic.

Ms. R also used the listing advantages and disadvantages technique as part of the strategy to modify this maladaptive schema (Table 31–12). Some schemas appear to have few, if any, advantages (e.g., "I'm stupid"; "I'll always lose in the end") but many schemas have both positive and negative features (e.g., "If I decide to do something, I must succeed"; "I always have to work harder than others or I'll fail"). The latter group of schemas may be maintained even in the face of their dysfunctional aspects because they encourage hard work, perseverance, or other behaviors that are adaptive. Yet, the absolute and demanding nature of the schemas ultimately leads to excessive stress, failed expectations, low self-esteem, or other deleterious results. Listing advantages and disadvantages helps the patient to examine the full range of effects of the schema and often encourages modifications that can make the schema both more adaptive and less damaging. In Ms. R's case, this exercise set the stage for another step of schema modification, generating alternatives (Table 31–13).

The list of alternative schemas will usually include several different options, ranging from rather minor adjustments to extensive revisions in the schema. The therapist uses Socratic questioning and other cognitive therapy techniques such as imagery and role play to help the patient recognize potential alternative schemas. A "brainstorming" attitude is encouraged. Instead of trying to be sure that a revised schema is entirely accurate at first glance, the

TABLE 31–11. Schema modification through examining the evidence

Schema: "I must be perfect to be accepted."	
Evidence for	**Evidence against**
The better I do, the more people seem to like me.	Others who aren't "perfect" seem to be to be loved and accepted. Why should I be different?
Women who have a perfect figure are most attractive to men.	You don't have to have a perfect figure. Hardly anybody has one—just the models on television.
My parents have the highest standards, they are always pushing me to do better.	My parents want me to do well. But they'll probably accept me as long as I try to do my best, even if I don't meet all of their expectations. This statement is absolute and sets me up for failure because no one can be perfect all the time.

TABLE 31–12. Schema modification through listing advantages and disadvantages

Schema: "I must be perfect to be accepted."	
Advantages	**Disadvantages**
I've tried very hard to be the best.	I never really feel accepted because I've never reached perfection.
I've received top marks in school.	I'm always down on myself. I've developed bulimia. I'm obsessed with my body size.
I'm in lots of activities, and I've won dancing competitions.	I have trouble accepting my successes. I drive myself too hard and can't enjoy ordinary things.

therapist usually suggests that they try to generate a variety of modified schemas without initially considering their validity or practicality. This stimulates creativity and gives the patient further encouragement to step aside from rigid long-standing schemas.

After alternatives are generated and discussed, the therapy turns toward examining the potential consequences of changing basic attitudes. Cognitive rehearsal can be used in the therapy session to test a schema modification. This may be followed by a homework assignment to try out the revised schema in vivo. Therapist and patient

TABLE 31–13.　Schema modification though generating alternatives

Schema: "I must be perfect to be accepted."
Possible alternatives
People that are successful are more likely to be accepted.
If I try to do my best (even if it's not perfect), others are likely to accept me.
I would like to be perfect, but that's an impossible goal. I'll choose certain areas to try to excel (school, work, career) and not demand perfection everywhere.
You don't need to be perfect to be accepted.
I'm worthy of love and acceptance without trying to be perfect.

work together to choose the most reasonable modifications for underlying schemas and to reinforce learning these new constructs through multiple practice sessions in therapy sessions and in real-life experiences.

BEHAVIORAL PROCEDURES

Behavioral interventions are used in CT to 1) change dysfunctional patterns of behavior (e.g., helplessness, isolation, phobic avoidance, inertia, bingeing and purging); 2) reduce troubling symptoms (e.g., tension, somatic and psychic anxiety, intrusive thoughts); and 3) assist in identifying and modifying maladaptive cognitions (see Table 31–14 for listing of behavioral techniques). As discussed earlier in this chapter, the cognitive model for therapy (Figure 31–1) suggests that there is an interactive relationship between cognition and behavior. Thus, behavioral initiatives should influence cognition, and cognitive interventions should have an impact on behavior.

The Socratic questions used in cognitively oriented procedures have a direct parallel when the emphasis is on behavioral change. The therapist asks a series of questions that help differentiate actual behavioral deficits from negatively distorted accounts of behavior (J. H. Wright 1988). Depressed and anxious patients usually overreport their symptomatic distress or the difficulties they have in managing situations. Often, well framed questions can reveal cognitive distortions and also stimulate change as the patient considers the negative impact of dysfunctional behavior. Two specific behavioral techniques, activity scheduling and graded task assignments, are explained below.

Activity scheduling is a structured method of learning about the patient's behavioral patterns, encouraging self-monitoring, increasing positive mood, and designing strategies for change (A. T. Beck et al. 1979; J. H. Wright

and Beck 1983; Thase and Beck 1992). A daily or weekly activity log is employed in which the patient is asked to record what he or she does during each hour of the day and then to rate each activity for mastery and pleasure on a 0–10 scale. When the activity record is first introduced, the patient usually is asked to make a record of baseline activities without attempting to make any changes. The data are then reviewed in the next therapy session.

Almost invariably, the patient rates some activities higher than others on mastery and/or pleasure. For example, Mr. G, a 48-year-old depressed man, who had told his therapist that "I don't enjoy anything anymore" described several activities on his Daily Activity Schedule that contradicted this statement. Reading while sitting alone was rated as a 6 on mastery and 8 on pleasure, and attending his son's choir concert was rated as 7 on mastery and 10 on pleasure. Conversely, attempting to work in his home office was rated as a 1 on mastery and a 0 on pleasure. Discussion of the activity scheduling assignment with Mr. G helped him to see that he was still capable of performing reasonably well in certain activities and also that he was able to derive considerable enjoyment from some of his actions. In addition, the schedule was used to target problem areas (e.g., working in his home office) that would require further work in therapy. Finally, the activity schedule provided data that could be used in adjusting Mr. G's daily routine to promote a heightened sense of mastery and greater enjoyment.

Another behavioral procedure, the graded task assignment, can be used when the patient is facing a situation that seems excessively difficult or overwhelming. A challenging behavioral goal is broken down into small steps that can be taken one at a time. When used to promote exposure to a feared object or situation, the graded task assignment is quite similar to the systematic desensitization protocols that are used in traditional behavior therapy (Wolpe 1969).

TABLE 31–14.　Behavioral procedures used in cognitive therapy

- Questioning to identify behavioral patterns
- Activity scheduling with mastery and pleasure recording
- Self-monitoring
- Graded task assignments
- Behavioral rehearsal
- Response prevention
- Distraction
- Relaxation exercises
- Respiratory control
- Assertiveness training
- Modeling
- Social skills training

However, a cognitive component is added to the methodology. There is an added emphasis placed on improving self-esteem and self-efficacy, countering hopelessness and helplessness, and using the graded task assignment to disprove maladaptive thoughts and schemas. With depressed individuals, the graded task assignment typically is used as a problem-solving technique. This step-wise approach, coupled with cognitive techniques such as Socratic questioning and thought recording, can reactivate the patient and focus his or her energy in a productive manner.

An example of the use of a graded task assignment can be found in the case of Mr. G, the 48-year-old man described in the section on activity scheduling. One of the particularly troublesome items uncovered with activity scheduling was the patient's difficulty in getting to work at his home office. Socratic questioning revealed that Mr. G had been unable to work in his home office for over 6 weeks. Mail, bills, and correspondence with friends were piled up to the point that he saw the situation as impossible. Cognitions related to this problem included automatic thoughts such as "It's too much . . . . I've procrastinated too long this time . . . . I'm totally swamped . . . . I can't handle it."

The therapist and patient constructed a series of steps that encouraged Mr. G to approach the task and eventually master the problem. The graded task assignment included the following steps: 1) walk into the office and sit down at the desk for at least 15 minutes; 2) spend at least 20 minutes sorting mail into categories; 3) open and discard any junk mail; 4) open and read any personal letters, and write list of responses required; 5) open and stack all bills; 6) clean office; 7) respond in writing to at least one letter; 8) balance checkbook; 9) pay all current or overdue bills; 10) respond to additional letters if necessary. Reasonable goals for specific time intervals were discussed, and the therapist used coaching, Socratic questioning, and other cognitive techniques to help Mr. G accomplish the task.

Other behavioral techniques used in CT include behavioral rehearsal (a procedure that is usually combined with cognitive rehearsal described earlier), graded exposure to feared stimuli, response prevention (a collaborative exercise in which the patient agrees to stop a dysfunctional behavior, such as prolonged crying spells, and to monitor cognitive responses), distraction (alternate activities that can temporarily divert a patient from intrusive thoughts, depressive ruminations, or other dysfunctional cognitions), relaxation exercises, respiratory control, assertiveness training, modeling, and social skills training (D. M. Clark et al. 1985; Meichenbaum 1977; J. H. Wright 1988; J. H. Wright and Beck 1983; Thase and Wright 1991; Young and Beck 1982).

COMPUTER-ASSISTED COGNITIVE THERAPY

Several forms of computer-assisted cognitive therapy are now available for clinical use. Selmi and colleagues (1990, 1991) developed a text-based program that teaches patients how to use cognitive therapy to cope with depression. An outcome study demonstrated that patients with mild to moderate depression responded well to the computer program (Selmi et al. 1991). Subjects who received the computerized therapy improved as much as those who were treated with standard CT, and both active treatments were superior to a wait list control. Colby and Colby (1990) have produced a computer program that incorporates some of the principles of cognitive therapy but does not cover the major CT interventions in depth. One of the interesting features of the Colby and Colby program is a dialogue mode in which the computer attempts to carry on a therapeutic conversation with the patient using "natural language." Although this dialogue is highly inventive, it does not simulate the typical therapeutic interview in cognitive therapy. Also, problems in understanding the patient's typed responses and in giving accurate feedback were observed in an empirical study of this software (Stuart and Larue 1996). One research group (Bowers et al. 1993) found that the Colby and Colby program was ineffective in treating severely ill inpatients, but Colby (1995) has reported very high patient satisfaction among a large number of users of this program.

Both the Selmi et al. and Colby and Colby forms of computer-assisted therapy have the disadvantage of being text based. These programs require the patient to type responses and to read large amounts of written material. J. H. Wright, Salmon, Wright, and Beck (1995a, 1995b, 1996) have recently introduced a multimedia form of computer-assisted cognitive therapy that is designed to be "user friendly" and to be suitable for a wide range of patients, including those with no previous computer or keyboard experience. J. H. Wright and colleagues (1995b, 1996) have suggested that computer-assisted learning can be used as a tool to help patients acquire cognitive therapy skills, practice self-help, and build self-esteem. Possible contributions of computer-assisted CT may include decreased cost of treatment, increased access to therapy, more rapid socialization to treatment procedures and techniques, and a reduced burden on therapists to teach basic CT concepts (Colby 1995; J. H. Wright et al. 1996). Pressures from managed care for improved efficiency and cost of treatment, together with advances in design of computer programs, may promote a growth in the use of computer-assisted cognitive therapy in clinical practice.

SELECTING PATIENTS FOR COGNITIVE THERAPY

Cognitive therapy procedures have been described for a large number of diagnostic categories (A. T. Beck 1993; Freeman and Dattilio 1992; Freeman et al. 1989; F. D. Wright et al. 1993). Although there are no contraindications to using this treatment approach, cognitive therapy is usually not attempted with patients who have a substantial degree of organic brain disease (e.g., mental retardation, dementia, or delirium). Ludgate and colleagues (1992) have suggested that CT should be considered a primary treatment for 1) disorders where it has been proven to be effective in controlled research (e.g., unipolar depression [nonpsychotic], anxiety disorders, eating disorders, and psychophysiological disorders), and 2) other conditions for which a clearly detailed treatment method has been developed (e.g., personality disorders, substance abuse), there is some evidence for effectiveness, and there is no substantive research data to support the superiority of other treatment approaches. Cognitive therapy should be considered an adjunctive therapy for disorders such as major depression with psychotic features, bipolar illness, and schizophrenia where there is clear evidence for the effectiveness of biological treatments, and the effects of CT alone compared with pharmacotherapy have not been studied.

Several studies have examined possible predictors for outcome in CT. Simons and colleagues (1985) observed that high scores on a test of self-control predicted an enhanced response to CT compared with a tricyclic antidepressant. However, this finding was not replicated in later studies (Jarrett et al. 1991; Wetzel et al. 1992). Miller and colleagues (1989) found that high levels of cognitive dysfunction in depressed inpatients were associated with a superior response to CT. Another group of investigators has reported that patients with chronic or especially severe depression may respond somewhat less well to CT than individuals with lower levels of symptoms. (Thase et al. 1993; Thase et al. 1994b). The research of Thase and colleagues (1993, 1994b) did not include control groups. When CT has been compared directly with pharmacotherapy, most studies have found no relationship between severity or endogenous subtype and treatment outcome (see "Effectiveness of Cognitive Therapy," in this chapter).

Investigations of biological predictors have yielded conflicting results. Dexamethasone nonsuppression has been associated with a reduced response to both CT and pharmacotherapy (Corbishley et al. 1990; McKnight et al. 1992). In a recent study, Thase and colleagues (1996b) found that the DST did not reliably discriminate between responders and nonresponders to CT in group of severely ill inpatients, but high urinary free cortisol levels were associated with a diminished response to CT. EEG sleep studies usually have not differentiated CT responders and nonresponders (Corbishley et al. 1990; Jarrett et al. 1990; Simons and Thase 1992; Thase et al. 1994a). One large study of 90 outpatients treated with CT found that EEG sleep abnormalities were associated with a lower recovery rate and higher risk for relapse (Thase et al. 1996a). Although studies of biological markers suggest that cortisol levels or EEG findings may help predict treatment response in some cases, the overall findings of research in this area do not support the use of laboratory tests to select patients for cognitive therapy.

Clinical experience has suggested that patients who are free of severe character pathology (especially borderline or antisocial features) have previously formed strong, trusting relationships with significant others, have a belief in the importance of self-reliance, and have a curious or inquisitive nature are especially suitable for cognitive therapy (Thase and Beck 1992). Average or above-average intelligence also can be helpful, but cognitive therapy procedures can be simplified for those with subnormal intellectual skills or impaired learning and memory functioning (Casey and Grant 1992; Thompson 1996; J. H. Wright and Salmon 1990). Of course, most patients do not have a full combination of the ideal features noted above. A flexible approach can be employed in which cognitive therapy procedures are customized to match the special characteristics of the patient's social background, intellectual level, personality structure, and clinical disorder (Freeman and Dattilio 1992).

COGNITIVE THERAPY APPLICATIONS

The basic procedures described in this chapter are used in all cognitive therapy applications. However, the targets for change, selection of techniques, and timing of interventions may vary depending upon the condition being treated and the format for therapy. A full discussion of the multiple applications and formats for CT is beyond the scope of this chapter. The reader is referred to comprehensive books on cognitive therapy for a more detailed accounting of the modifications of this treatment approach for different clinical disorders (Freeman and Dattilio 1992; Freeman et al. 1989; Salkovskis 1996; F. D. Wright et al. 1993). Cognitive therapy methods have been outlined for a number of clinical problems not covered here, including conditions such as substance abuse (Barrett and Meyer 1992; Caroll et al. 1994a, 1994b; Fisher and Bentley

1996; Oei et al. 1991; Thase 1997), chronic depression (Scott 1992; Scott et al. 1992), hypochondriasis (Warwick and Salkovskis 1990), body dysmorphic disorder (N. B. Schmidt and Harrington 1995), gambling addiction (Bujold et al. 1994; Sharpe and Tarrrier 1993), and psychophysiological disorders (Bergdahl et al. 1995; Dworkin et al. 1994; Payne and Blanchard 1995; Speckens et al. 1994; White and Neilson 1995). Group cognitive therapy techniques have been described by Covi and Primakoff (1988) and Freeman and colleagues (1992); and procedures for marital and family cognitive therapy have been set forth by Beck (A. T. Beck 1988), Epstein and colleagues (1988), and Wright and Beck (J. H. Wright and Beck 1993). Also, strategies have been developed for using cognitive therapy as a comprehensive model for inpatient treatment (F. D. Wright et al. 1993). In this portion of the chapter, we briefly examine the distinctive features of cognitive therapy for five common psychiatric illnesses—depression, anxiety disorders, eating disturbances, personality disorders, and psychosis.

DEPRESSION

In the opening phase of treatment of depression, the cognitive therapist focuses on establishing a collaborative relationship and introduces the patient to the cognitive model. Agendas, feedback, and psychoeducational procedures are used to structure sessions. The emphasis is placed on two major forms of cognitive dysfunction: negatively distorted thinking and deficits in learning and memory functioning (Thase and Beck 1992). Early in therapy, a special effort may be placed on relieving hopelessness because of the close link between this element of the negative cognitive triad and suicide risk. Also, reduction in hopelessness can be an important step in reactivating and reenergizing the depressed patient.

Problems with learning and memory functioning are countered with the aforementioned structuring procedures and with learning reinforcement techniques such as written therapy notes, diagrams, and homework assignments (Thase and Wright 1991; J. H. Wright 1988). The clinician carefully matches the therapeutic work to the patient's level of cognitive functioning so that learning is encouraged and the patient is not overwhelmed with the material of therapy. Behavioral techniques, such as activity scheduling and graded task assignments, often are a major component of the opening phase of cognitive therapy of depression (Thase and Wright 1991).

The middle portion of treatment is usually devoted to eliciting and modifying negatively distorted automatic thoughts. Behavioral techniques continue to be used in most cases. By this point in the therapy, patients should understand the cognitive model and be able to employ thought monitoring techniques to reverse all three elements of the negative cognitive triad (self, world, and future). Typically, the patient is taught to identify cognitive errors (e.g., selective abstraction, arbitrary inference, absolutistic thinking) and to use procedures such as generating alternatives and examining the evidence to alter negatively distorted thinking.

Work on eliciting and testing automatic thoughts continues during the latter portion of treatment. However, if there have been gains in functioning and the patient has grasped the basic principles of CT, therapy can turn primarily to identifying and altering maladaptive schemas. The concept of schemas usually has been introduced earlier in therapy, but the principal efforts at changing these underlying structures are reserved for the late phase of treatment when the patient is more likely to grasp and retain complex therapeutic initiatives. Before therapy concludes, the therapist helps the patient review what has been learned during the course of treatment and also suggests thinking ahead to possible circumstances that could trigger a return of depression. The potential for relapse is recognized, and problem-solving strategies are developed that can be employed in future stressful situations (Thase 1992).

ANXIETY DISORDERS

Although the techniques used in CT for anxiety disorders are similar to those employed in the treatment of depression, treatment efforts are directed toward altering four major types of dysfunctional anxiety-producing cognitions: 1) overestimates of the likelihood of a feared event, 2) exaggerated estimates of the severity of a feared event, 3) underestimation of personal coping abilities, and 4) unrealistically low estimates of the help that others can offer (D. M. Clark and Beck 1988). Most authors have recommended that a mixture of cognitive and behavioral measures be used in patients who suffer from anxiety disorders (Alford et al. 1990; Barlow and Cerney 1988; A. T. Beck et al. 1985a; D. M. Clark and Beck 1988).

In panic disorder, the emphasis is placed on helping the patient to recognize and change grossly exaggerated estimates of the significance of physiological responses or fears of imminent psychological disaster (A. T. Beck et al. 1985a, 1992b; D. M. Clark 1986). For example, an individual with panic disorder may begin to perspire or breathe more rapidly, after which cognitions such as "I can't catch my breath . . . . I'll pass out . . . . I'll have a stroke," increase the intensity of the autonomic nervous system activity. The vicious cycle interaction between catastrophic cognitions and physiological arousal can be broken in two complimentary ways: 1) altering the dysfunctional cognitions and 2) interrupting the cascading autonomic hyperactivity. Commonly used cognitive interventions include Socratic questioning, imagery, thought recording, generating alternatives, and examining the evidence. Behavioral measures such as relaxation training and respiratory control are used to dampen the physiological arousal associated with panic (D. M. Clark et al. 1985). Also, when panic attacks are stimulated by specific situations (e.g., driving, public speaking, crowds), graded exposure may be particularly useful in helping patients to both master a feared task and overcome their panic symptoms.

Cognitive therapy of phobic disorders centers on modifying unrealistic estimates of risk or danger in situations and engaging the patient in a series of graded exposure assignments. Generally, cognitive and behavioral procedures are used simultaneously. For example, a graded task assignment for an individual with agoraphobia might include a step-wise increase in experiences in a social setting accompanied by use of the Daily Record of Dysfunctional Thoughts to record and revise maladaptive automatic thinking. Patients with generalized anxiety disorder usually have diffuse cognitive distortions about many circumstances in their lives (e.g., physical health, finances, loss of control, family issues) coupled with persistent autonomic overarousal (A. T. Beck et al. 1985a; J. H. Wright and Borden 1992). The cognitive therapy approach to generalized anxiety disorder is closely related to methods used for panic disorder and phobias. However, special attention is paid to defining the stimuli that are associated with increased anxiety. Breaking down the generalized state of anxiety into workable segments can help the patient gain mastery over what initially appears to be an uncontrollable situation.

Behavioral techniques such as exposure and response prevention are used together with cognitive restructuring for patients with obsessive-compulsive disorder (OCD) (Emmelkamp and Beens 1991; James and Blackburn 1995; Salkovskis 1985). Cognitive interventions include thought stopping, challenging the validity of obsessional thoughts, attempting to replace dysfunctional cognitions with positive self-statements, and modifying negative automatic thoughts (James and Blackburn 1995). Salkovskis and Warwick (1985) have noted that cognitive procedures may be needed in some cases to help the patient engage in exposure and response prevention.

EATING DISORDERS

Individuals with eating disorders may have many of the cognitive distortions that are seen in depression. However, they have an additional cluster of cognitive biases about body image, eating behavior, and weight (D. A. Clark et al. 1989; Schlesier-Carter et al. 1989; Zotter and Crowther 1991). Patients with eating disorders usually place inordinate value on body shape as a measure of self-worth and as a condition for acceptance (e.g., "I must be thin to be accepted" . . . "If I'm overweight, nobody will want me" . . . "Fat people are weak"). They also may believe that any variance from their excessive standards means a total loss of control.

Cognitive therapy interventions are used to subject these maladaptive cognitions to empirical testing (Agras et al. 1992; P. J. Cooper and Steere 1995; Fairburn 1985; Garner 1992; Garner and Bemis 1985). Commonly used procedures include eliciting and testing automatic thoughts, examining the evidence, reattribution, and in vivo homework assignments (Bowers 1992). In addition, behavioral techniques are used to stimulate more adaptive eating behavior and to uncover significant cognitions related to eating (Bowers 1992; Garner 1992). As in treatment of other disorders, the relative emphasis on cognitive procedures compared with behavioral measures is dictated by the severity of the illness and the phase of treatment. An individual with anorexia nervosa who is malnourished and has an electrolyte imbalance may require hospitalization during the initial part of treatment for a contingency management program (Bowers 1992). Patients with this level of illness may have a significant impairment in learning and memory functioning and therefore have limited capacity to understand thought recording or other cognitive interventions. In contrast, a patient with uncomplicated bulimia nervosa may be able to benefit from relatively demanding cognitively oriented procedures early in treatment.

One of the critical factors in treating patients with eating disorders is the development of an effective working relationship. Compared with individuals with depression or anxiety disorders, those with eating disturbances often are reluctant to fully engage in therapy. Frequently, they have long-standing patterns of hiding their behavior from others and have developed elaborate methods of maintaining their dysfunctional approach to meals, body weight, and exercise. Thus, the patient with an eating disorder poses a special problem for the cognitive therapist. A thorough psychoeducational effort and considerable patience are usually required for the formation of a collaborative empirical relationship. Also, if the therapist focuses in the beginning on problem areas that the patient clearly wants to change (e.g., low self-esteem, hopelessness, loss of interest), struggles over control of eating disorders can be avoided until there have been successful experiences in working together in therapy.

PERSONALITY DISORDERS

Beck and colleagues (A. T. Beck et al. 1990a) have articulated a cognitive therapy approach to personality disorders that is based on a cognitive conceptualization of characterological disturbances. They suggest that the different personality types have idiosyncratic cognitions in four main areas: basic beliefs, view of self, view of others, and strategies for social interaction. For example, an individual with a narcissistic personality might believe, "I'm special . . . . I'm better than the rest . . . . Ordinary rules don't apply to me." This cognitive set leads to behavioral strategies such as manipulativeness, breaking rules, and exploiting others (A. T. Beck et al. 1990a). In contrast, a person with a dependent personality disorder might have core beliefs such as, "I need others to survive . . . . I can't manage on my own . . . . I can't be happy if I'm alone." The interpersonal strategies associated with these beliefs would include efforts to cling to or entrap others (A. T. Beck et al. 1990a).

Cognitive therapy methods typically employed in treatment of affective disorders may not be successful with characterological problems (A. T. Beck et al. 1990a; Persons et al. 1988; Pretzer and Beck 1992). Recommendations that have been made for modifying CT for treatment of personality disorders are summarized in Table 31–15 (A. T. Beck et al. 1990a; J. Beck 1997; Linehan 1987, 1993; Shearin and Linehan 1994). The problem-oriented, structured, and collaborative empirical characteristics of CT are retained in therapeutic work with patients who have personality disturbances, but there is an added emphasis on the therapeutic relationship. Persons with characterological disorders often recapitulate in the therapy encounter the impaired relationships that they have had with significant others in the past.

TABLE 31–15.   Modifications of cognitive therapy for personality disorders

- Pay special attention to the therapeutic relationship
- Attend to one's own (the therapist's) cognitive responses and emotional reactions
- Develop an individualized case conceptualization (including an assessment of the impact of developmental experiences, significant traumas, and environmental stresses)
- Place an initial focus on increasing self-efficacy
- Use behavioral techniques, such as rehearsal and social skills training, to reverse actual deficits in interpersonal functioning
- Set firm, reasonable limits
- Set realistic goals
- Anticipate compliance problems
- Review and repeat treatment interventions

Treatment of personality disorders with CT may take considerably longer than therapy of more circumscribed problems such as depression or anxiety. Patients with personality disturbances have deeply ingrained schemas that are unlikely to change within the short-term format used for other disorders (J. Beck 1997; Perris 1994; Young and Lindemann 1992). When the course of therapy lengthens, there is a greater chance for development of transference and countertransference reactions. In cognitive therapy, transference is viewed as a manifestation of underlying schemas. Therefore, transferential phenomena are recognized as opportunities for examining and modifying core beliefs.

An individualized case conceptualization is used. This formulation includes hypotheses on the role of maladaptive schemas in symptom production. Consideration also is given to the influences of parent-child conflicts, traumatic experiences, and the current social network on cognitive and behavioral pathology. Patients with personality disorders often have significant real-life problems, including severely disturbed interpersonal relationships and pronounced social skills deficits.

Although an ultimate goal of treatment is to modulate ineffective or maladaptive schemas, initial efforts (using procedures such as behavioral techniques or thought recording) may be directed at more readily accessible targets such as increasing self-efficacy or decreasing dysphoric mood. Self-monitoring, self-help exercises, and the structuring procedures used in cognitive therapy help prevent excessive dependency. However, patients with character disorders (especially those with borderline, narcissistic, or dependent personalities) are prone to have excessive expectations, to be overly demanding, or to exhibit manipulative behavior. Thus, the cognitive therapist needs to set firm but reasonable limits and to help the patient articulate realistic treatment goals (A. T. Beck et al. 1990a).

Adherence to treatment recommendations can be another problem in CT of personality disorders. The therapist can use procedures such as Socratic questioning or schema identification to uncover the reasons for noncompliance and help the patient follow through with homework assignments or other therapeutic work. Reviewing and repeating treatment interventions is another important component of CT for personality disorders. Considerable patience and persistence is required from the therapist as efforts are made to help the patient reverse chronic, deeply imbedded psychopathology.

PSYCHOSIS

Psychotic illnesses are one of the indications for adjunctive cognitive therapy (Ludgate et al. 1992). Although biological treatments are the accepted form of therapy for psychotic patients, cognitive psychotherapy can help these individuals understand their disorders, adhere to treatment recommendations, and develop more effective psychosocial functioning (Cochran 1986; Eckman et al. 1992; Fowler and Morley 1989; Kingdon and Turkington 1991; Lecompte 1995; Perris 1989; Perris and Skagerlind 1994; J. H. Wright and Schrodt 1989). Also, there have been reports that CT can be used to decrease delusions and hallucinations (Chadwick and Birchwood 1994; Chadwick and Lowe 1994; Fowler and Morley 1989; Garety et al. 1994; Kingdon and Turkington 1991; Tarrier et al. 1993).

In cognitive therapy of patients who have psychotic symptoms, the therapist conveys that maladaptive cognitions and reactions to life stress may interact with biological factors in the expression of the illness (Scott et al. 1992). Therefore, attempts to develop more adaptive cognitions or to learn how to cope better with environmental pressures can assist with efforts toward managing the disorder. During the early part of therapy with a psychotic patient, there is a strong emphasis on building a therapeutic alliance (Alford and Beck 1994; Scott et al. 1992). The rationale for neuroleptic medication is explained, and the therapist tries to stimulate hope by modifying intensely negative cognitions about the illness or its treatment (e.g., "I'm to blame . . . . Nothing will help . . . . Drugs don't work.") Usually, attempts to challenge hallucinations or delusions directly are delayed until a solid therapeutic relationship has been established. However, efforts are made to reverse delusional self-destructive cognitions as early as possible in the treatment process (Ludgate et al. 1992).

Reality testing is performed in a gentle, nonconfrontational manner (Kingdon and Turkington 1991; Ludgate et al. 1992). Usually delusions with lowest level of conviction are targeted first (Alford and Beck 1994). The therapist uses guided discovery as the major intervention, but also may help the patient to record and change distorted automatic thoughts (Scott et al. 1992). Eliciting and testing maladaptive automatic thoughts and schemas may be particularly useful for chronic patients who have dysfunctional information processing associated with low self-esteem or ineffective social functioning (J. H. Wright and Schrodt 1989). Behavioral techniques such as activity scheduling, graded task assignments, and social skills training also are used with psychotic patients. These procedures can be used to provide needed structure or to teach adaptive behaviors. Initiatives that can reduce the risk of relapse are another component of the CT approach to psychotic disorders. Recommended interventions include 1) use of CT techniques that enhance medication compliance (see for example Lecompte 1995; J. H. Wright and Thase 1992),

2) identification of potential triggers for symptom exacerbation, 3) development of cognitive and behavioral strategies to manage stressful life events, and 4) extension of cognitive therapy to the entire family unit (Scott et al. 1992).

EFFECTIVENESS OF COGNITIVE THERAPY

DEPRESSION—ACUTE TREATMENT PHASE STUDIES

Cognitive therapy has been investigated in many carefully designed outcome trials that have documented the effectiveness of this treatment approach. The most intensive research has been directed at cognitive therapy of depression and anxiety disorders. Meta-analyses of the numerous outcome studies of CT for depression have found that this form of therapy compares well with other treatments for depression (Dobson 1989; Gaffan et al. 1995; Robinson et al. 1990). For example, Dobson (1989) concluded that CT was at least as effective as pharmacotherapy for depression and that there was some evidence for superiority of CT when all studies were considered together. In a subsequent review, Hollon and colleagues (1991) argued that some studies have been biased either toward cognitive therapy or pharmacotherapy and thus suggested that firm conclusions on the relative efficacy of these treatments were still premature. A recent meta-analysis of 65 studies of CT for depression attempted to control for potential bias of the investigator by rating all studies on a researcher allegiance scale (Gaffan et al. 1995). Even when researcher allegiance was taken into account, the results of Dobson's (1989) original meta-analysis were upheld.

Studies of cognitive therapy for depression have been the subject of a detailed review by Thase (1995). Several of the more important investigations are noted here. The first major comparison of CT and pharmacotherapy was performed at the Center for Cognitive Therapy at the University of Pennsylvania (Rush et al. 1977). In this study, cognitive therapy was found to be superior to imipramine in the treatment of depressed outpatients. However, results of this study have been questioned because of the "Lourdes effect" and because imipramine was tapered and stopped before the end of the trial (Rush et al. 1977). Two later studies, both performed in the United Kingdom, also found CT to be an effective treatment for depression (Blackburn et al. 1981; Teasdale et al. 1984). Blackburn et al. (1981) performed the first outcome trial at a facility other than the center where cognitive therapy was developed. Patients from one of two settings, hospital outpatient or general practice clinics, were randomly assigned to CT, pharmacotherapy with amitriptyline or clomipramine, or a combination of CT and pharmacotherapy. Cognitive therapy was more effective than pharmacotherapy in the general practice patients, but doubts have been raised about the adequacy of the drug treatment in this sample (Hollon et al. 1991). Patients treated in the hospital outpatient setting responded equally well to all three treatments. There was a trend for the combined treatment to provide greater symptom reduction. Teasdale et al. (1984) compared "treatment as usual" (some, but not all patients treated with antidepressants) in a family practice setting to the same form of treatment plus cognitive therapy. Patients who received the added CT component were significantly less depressed at the end of the trial.

Two major investigations in the United States attempted to replicate and extend the original Rush et al. (1977) study. Murphy et al. (1984) at Washington University in St. Louis randomly assigned depressed outpatients to treatment with CT alone, nortriptyline alone, CT plus placebo, or combined CT and nortriptyline. The results of this study indicated that all treatments were effective for short-term symptom reduction. Similar findings were obtained in an outcome trial completed at the University of Minnesota. Hollon et al. (1992a) assessed the relative efficacy of cognitive therapy alone, imipramine, and combined treatment with CT and imipramine. As in the Murphy et al. (1984) study, there were no significant differences found between the treatments in the acute phase of the research. Nonsignificant trends were observed for the combined treatment to be superior to either condition alone.

The National Institute of Mental Health (NIMH) Treatment of Depression Collaborative Research Project (Elkin et al. 1989) also examined the relative efficacy of CT and pharmacotherapy. Additional comparisons were made with another focused psychotherapy for depression, interpersonal therapy, and with placebo plus clinical management. All four treatments, including placebo plus clinical management, were associated with significant improvement in this trial. In the primary statistical analysis, there were no differences found between either of the psychotherapies and imipramine (plus clinical management). However, when patients were stratified by level of initial severity, CT was somewhat less effective (in the more severely affected patients) than the other active treatments. This finding is inconsistent with results of other trials that compared CT with pharmacotherapy. No association between severity of depression (or endogenous subtype) and treatment outcome was found in these studies (Blackburn et al. 1981; Hollon et al. 1992a; Kovacs et al. 1981; Teasdale et al. 1984).

The most recent outcome study that compared CT with medication for depression found that two forms of psychotherapy, CT and applied relaxation (AR), were both superior to desipramine (Murphy et al. 1995). The psychotherapies were conducted over 16 weeks and consisted of up to 20 sessions. Desipramine was given at therapeutic doses, and plasma levels were monitored. The percentages of patients in each treatment group who experienced a remission of depression were 82% for CT, 73% for AR, and 29% for desipramine. The authors suggested that a possible explanation for the low rate of treatment response in patients who received desipramine was the lack of psychotherapy in the medication group. Although patients on desipramine saw a pharmacotherapist for 20-minute sessions on a weekly or biweekly basis, the physician was specifically instructed not to engage in psychotherapy (Murphy et al. 1995). Results of the Murphy et al. (1995) study suggest that some element of psychotherapy may be required for optimal response to antidepressant medication and that pharmacotherapy may be disadvantaged in comparison to CT if psychotherapy is not provided. Blackburn et al. (1981) reported a similar poor outcome for pharmacotherapy alone in subjects treated in a primary care setting.

Further evidence for the effectiveness of cognitive therapy for depression has come in studies of group cognitive therapy (Covi and Lippman 1987; Free et al. 1991; Zettle and Rains 1989), geriatric depressed patients (Beutler et al. 1987; Riskind et al. 1985; Steuer et al. 1984; Wilson et al. 1995), and hospitalized depressive patients (Bowers 1990; Miller et al. 1989; Stuart and Bowers 1995; Thase et al. 1991; Whisman et al. 1991). The overall results of CT outcome studies indicate that cognitive therapy is an effective treatment for depression and is comparable to antidepressants in producing acute symptomatic relief. Studies in which CT was found to be more effective than antidepressants have been questioned because of possible inadequacies in the pharmacotherapy regimens. Conversely, the single controlled study that suggested the possibility that CT might be less effective than medication for severe depression (Elkin et al. 1989) has been criticized because of questions about supervision of cognitive therapists and varied responses at different treatment sites (Hollon et al. 1991; Thase and Beck 1992).

DEPRESSION—LONG-TERM OUTCOME STUDIES

Several of the investigations reviewed above measured the effects of the short-term therapies one and two years after treatment was completed. Results of these studies have generally favored cognitive therapy in preventing relapse. Kovacs et al. (1981) found that patients treated with CT in the Rush et al. (1977) study had a 31% relapse rate at 1 year compared with a 65% relapse rate for those treated with imipramine. An even higher differential relapse rate was described by Blackburn and colleagues (1986b). A 2-year naturalistic follow-up investigation of patients treated in the Blackburn et al. (1981) study found a substantially lower relapse rate in patients treated with CT alone (23%) or combined therapy (21%) as compared with pharmacotherapy alone (78%). Although the adequacy of the pharmacotherapy has been questioned because some patients were treated in a general practice setting, the Blackburn and colleagues (1986b) study provides information on outcome in patients who receive a refined form of psychotherapy as compared with practice as usual.

Simons et al. (1986), who followed patients 1 year after their study, found the lowest relapse rates in patients who received CT alone (20%) or CT plus placebo (18%). Combined treatment was associated with a 43% rate of relapse, and pharmacotherapy alone led to the highest rate of relapse (67%). Patients in the Hollon et al. (1992) study showed the same pattern of long-term response to treatment (Evans et al. 1992). The relapse rate for those treated with pharmacotherapy (without medication maintenance) was over twice the rate for patients who received CT or combined treatment.

The only investigation that did not find a superiority for cognitive therapy in preventing relapse was the NIMH Collaborative Study (Elkin et al. 1989; Shea et al. 1992). However, patients treated with CT were less likely to require treatment in the follow-up period than any of the other therapies, and relapse rates were lower for CT (36%) than imipramine plus clinical management (50%) 18 months after the study was completed. During the acute treatment phase of the NIMH Collaborative Study, CT was found to be less effective than imipramine for severe depression (Elkin et al. 1989). In contrast, no differences were detected in the effectiveness of treatments for more severely ill patients at follow-up (Shea et al. 1992). A recently completed study examined the usefulness of CT in treating residual symptoms of depression in patients who did not respond fully to antidepressants (Fava et al. 1996). During a 4-year follow-up period, the relapse rate was 35% for CT and 70% for routine clinical management. Taken together, results of investigations of the long-term effects of cognitive therapy support the use of this treatment to help reduce relapse and recurrence.

ANXIETY DISORDERS

Cognitive therapy also has been found to be an effective therapy for anxiety disorders. Especially strong evidence has been collected to support the utility of CT and related therapies in treatment of panic disorder. Two major forms of therapy have been developed: *panic control treatment* (PCT)—a combination of relaxation training, cognitive restructuring, and exposure (Barlow and Cerney 1988), and *focused cognitive therapy*—a more cognitively oriented treatment that uses exposure but places less emphasis on behavioral interventions than PCT (A. T. Beck et al. 1985a).

Barlow and colleagues (1989) reported that 87% of patients who completed a course of PCT were panic free after treatment and that PCT was significantly more effective than either relaxation training alone or a waiting list control condition. In a related investigation that compared PCT and alprazolam for panic disorder, this research group observed that PCT was superior to a waiting list control or placebo (Klosko et al. 1990). Of those completing the study, 87% who received PCT were free of panic attacks compared with 50% for alprazolam, 33% for the waiting list control, and 36% for placebo. The treatment protocol designed by Barlow and Cerney (1988) also was efficacious in an open trial of therapy administered by pharmacologically oriented clinicians who received training in this approach (Welkowitz et al. 1991). Shear et al. (1991a) noted that a cognitive and behavioral treatment package closely related to PCT was highly effective in clinical practice and, in addition, was capable of reversing vulnerability to sodium lactate–induced panic (Shear et al. 1991b).

Focused cognitive therapy, as described by Beck and colleagues (A. T. Beck et al. 1985a), also has fared well in outcome studies. Sokol et al. (1989) reported dramatic reductions in panic frequency (mean of 4.5 panic attacks a week before treatment to zero attacks per week after treatment) in an uncontrolled study of patients treated at the Center for Cognitive Therapy, University of Pennsylvania. Subsequently, Beck and colleagues (A. T. Beck et al. 1992b) studied panic disorder patients who were randomly assigned to CT or supportive psychotherapy. Results strongly favored cognitive therapy. After 8 weeks, almost three times as many patients who received CT than supportive therapy were panic free. An additional study compared focused CT, relaxation training, imipramine, and a waiting list control in the treatment of panic disorder (D. M. Clark et al. 1994). All three active treatments were superior to the control condition, but CT led to greater reductions in anxiety levels, catastrophic cognitions, and frequency of panic attacks.

Other investigators also have documented the effectiveness of cognitive and behavioral treatment programs for panic disorder with or without agoraphobia (Arntz and Van Den Hout 1996; J. G. Beck et al. 1994; Bouchard et al.

1996; Craske et al. 1995; Laberge et al. 1993; Ost et al. 1993; Otto et al. 1993; Pollack et al. 1994; Westling and Ost 1995). Otto and colleagues (1993) have demonstrated that CT is more effective than standard clinical management in helping panic disorder patients discontinue benzodiazepines. Also, studies that have examined the long-term effects of treatment for panic disorder have found significant relapse prevention effects for cognitive therapy (Otto and Whittal 1995).

Only one investigation found any evidence that CT may be less effective than other treatments. Black et al. (1993) compared a shortened form of CT (8 sessions) to fluvoxamine and placebo in patients with panic disorder. CT subjects were significantly improved compared with placebo on some (e.g., Clinical Global Impression [CGI] scores, panic attack severity scores) but not all ratings. Evidence was found for superiority of fluvoxamine on several clinical measures; however, the panic attack severity score was lowest for CT subjects at the end point analysis (CT = 6.8, fluvoxamine = 8.1, placebo = 15.3).

Although early trials of CT for generalized anxiety disorder (GAD) reported evidence for treatment effectiveness (e.g., Blowers et al. 1987; Durham and Turvey 1987), differences were not always found between cognitive therapy and supportive or more traditional behavioral approaches (Hollon and Beck 1994). Initial studies of CT for generalized anxiety were marred by design problems such as lack of specificity in the treatment approaches, use of unsophisticated or truncated forms of cognitive therapy, and selection of cognitive therapists with limited training or experience. Nevertheless, most studies of CT (or combined CT and behavioral therapy) for GADs have found cognitive therapy to be efficacious (Hollon and Beck 1994).

Later trials of CT for generalized anxiety used more precise research designs. Power and colleagues (1990) randomly assigned patients with GAD to diazepam, placebo, CT, diazepam plus CT, or placebo plus CT. Individuals treated in any of the three cognitive therapy conditions were substantially improved by the end of the study. Diazepam alone also showed significant treatment effects as compared with placebo, but this was less marked than for cognitive therapy.

Butler and colleagues (1991) performed a carefully designed study of CT for generalized anxiety. This research group had extensive previous experience in behavior therapy practice and research. In addition, they received intensive training in CT (including supervision at the Center for Cognitive Therapy, University of Pennsylvania). Adherence to the treatment models (both CT and behavior therapy) was monitored by independent raters. Results of this study indicated that CT was clearly superior to behavior therapy or a waiting list control. Furthermore, patients treated with cognitive therapy had significantly more change in measures of dysfunctional cognition, including anxious thoughts and maladaptive beliefs. Another well designed study compared CT with analytic psychotherapy (AP) and anxiety management training (AMT, a psychoeducation-based therapy that teaches anxiety coping strategies) for treatment of 110 patients with GAD (Durham et al. 1994). CT was clearly superior to the other treatments. The differential response between CT and AP was so dramatic that the authors questioned whether analytic therapy was suitable for persons with GAD.

Several well executed studies have found evidence for the effectiveness of CT for social phobia (Gelernter et al. 1991; Heimberg et al. 1990; Hope et al. 1995). Heimberg's group cognitive and behavioral method has been the most widely studied (Juster and Heimberg 1995). Overall results of multiple studies indicate that treatment response is best when cognitive and exposure procedures are combined in therapy of social phobia (Juster and Heimberg 1995; Taylor 1996).

Although behavioral treatments have been shown to be effective for OCD (James and Blackburn 1995; Salkovskis and Westbrook 1989), only one outcome trial has been completed in which CT was compared directly with behavioral therapy (Van Oppen et al. 1995). Seventy-one patients with OCD who were not taking antidepressants were randomly assigned to Beck's form of CT or exposure plus response prevention (ERP). Both treatments led to statistically significant improvement, but CT was superior to ERP in reducing symptoms of OCD. Cognitive restructuring and behavioral methods are often combined in treating obsessive-compulsive patients (James and Blackburn 1995; J. M. Schwartz et al. 1996). It is still unclear whether a full package of cognitive and behavioral techniques offers significant advantages over either treatment alone.

EATING DISORDERS

A large number of experimental trials have found that CT significantly improves the symptoms of bulimia (Agras et al. 1992, 1994; P. J. Cooper and Steere 1995; P. J. Cooper et al. 1996; Fairburn et al. 1991, 1993, 1995; Garner 1992; Leitenberg et al. 1994; Thackwray et al. 1993). Authors of a recent review of 21 studies of psychotherapy for bulimia nervosa concluded that there was convincing evidence for the efficacy of cognitive-behavioral treatment (Mitchell et al. 1996). Agras and colleagues (1992) found that cognitive-behavioral therapy and CT combined with desipramine were superior to desipramine alone in treatment of bulimia nervosa. In another study, Fairburn and colleagues (1991, 1993) compared CT with behavioral treatment and interpersonal therapy. Although all three psychological treatments used by Fairburn and colleagues led to improvement in bulimic symptoms, CT and interpersonal therapy were superior to behavior therapy, and CT was the most effective in modifying extreme dieting, emesis, and dysfunctional attitudes (Fairburn et al. 1991, 1993). Thackwray and colleagues (1993) observed that bulimic patients treated with a full package of cognitive and behavioral therapy fared much better over time than those who received behavior therapy alone. Six months after treatment, 69% of the subjects treated with cognitive-behavioral therapy were abstinent from binge eating and purging. The abstinence rate for behavior therapy and an attention placebo group were 38% and 15%, respectively. Thus, combined cognitive and behavioral therapy appears to offer advantages over a purely behavioral approach to bulimia.

Two studies have investigated the utility of CT self-help manuals in the treatment of bulimia. Schmidt and colleagues (U. Schmidt et al. 1993) gave 28 bulimic patients a CT handbook and no other treatment. Twenty of the subjects were judged to be much improved (*n* = 12) or somewhat improved (*n* = 8) after using the workbook for 4–6 weeks. Another research group reported that a CT program of 8 sessions of 20–30 minutes with a social worker plus use of a self-help manual led to an 80% reduction in the frequency of bulimic episodes (P. J. Cooper et al. 1996). Although these studies were uncontrolled, the results suggest that it may be possible to lower the cost of CT and increase access to treatment for bulimia by using self-help methods.

OUTCOME RESEARCH FOR OTHER DISORDERS

The majority of CT outcome research has been concerned with depression, anxiety disorders, and eating disorders. However, a substantial amount of investigative work has been completed on the efficacy of cognitive therapy for other conditions such as psychophysiological disorders, substance abuse, psychoses, and personality disorders. A broad range of studies have examined the utility of CT in behavioral medicine (Sensky et al. 1993). In one investigation, depressed multiple sclerosis patients treated with cognitive therapy had significantly improved psychological functioning as compared with a no-treatment control condition (Larcombe and Wilson 1984). In another study, cancer patients who received mastectomies experienced

reduced psychological distress after a course of cognitively oriented therapy (Tarrier and Maguire 1984). Several groups have reported that cognitive therapy can be a helpful approach in the management of chronic pain (Phillips 1987; Skinner et al. 1990; Turner and Clancy 1986). The cognitive treatment model for chronic pain has been described in detail by Turk and colleagues (1983).

Other investigators have observed that CT can be useful in the treatment of skin disorders (Horne et al. 1989), epilepsy (Goldstein 1990), asthma (Maes and Schlosser 1988), inflammatory and irritable bowel syndromes (Payne and Blanchard 1995; S. P. Schwartz and Blanchard 1991), myocardial infarction (Friedman et al. 1986), temporomandibular disorders (Dworkin et al. 1994), fibromyalgia (White and Nielson 1995), and medically unexplained physical symptoms (Speckens et al. 1995). Attempts at using CT to help patients with rheumatoid arthritis have met with mixed results (Keefe and Van Horn 1993; Kraaimaat et al. 1995). Although there is some evidence that CT has short-term positive effects in this group of patients, the progressive course of the illness tends to reduce gains over time. Generally, results of studies in behavioral medicine indicate that CT can improve psychophysiological functioning, subjective well being, and/or coping with illness.

Applications of CT for substance abuse, psychotic disorders, and characterological disturbances have not yet been studied extensively under controlled conditions. However, several important findings have been reported, and a significant amount of research is currently underway. An early investigation for substance abuse suggested that CT (plus paraprofessional drug counseling) may be superior to drug counseling alone in treatment of heroin addicts (Woody et al. 1983). In a large study of treatment for cocaine abuse, Wells et al. (1994) found that a relapse prevention program, based in part on cognitive-behavioral methods and a 12-step approach were equally effective in decreasing both cocaine and alcohol use. The patients who received relapse prevention had a lower use of alcohol than those treated with the 12-step approach at the follow-up assessment.

Another study of CT-based relapse prevention program found that cognitive-behavioral therapy was more effective than desipramine or clinical management in reducing cocaine behaviors and fostering abstinence (Carroll et al. 1995). Carroll et al. (1994a, 1994b) observed no differences immediately after treatment in subjects with cocaine dependence who received CT (relapse prevention), desipramine, or placebo. However, the CT subjects had a significantly improved response at the 1-year follow-up. The authors concluded that this effect was likely due to "implementation of the generalizable coping skills conveyed through that treatment." Limited research has been completed on CT for alcohol abuse, but preliminary studies have shown that alcoholic individuals, even those with significant Axis II pathology, can respond well to a cognitive therapy approach (Fisher and Bentley 1996; Longabaugh et al. 1994; Schonfeld and Dupree 1995; Sitharthan et al. 1996).

There has been a growing interest in studying the use of CT and related therapies for psychotic disorders. In several uncontrolled studies, cognitive therapy has been reported to reduce schizophrenic symptoms (Chadwick and Birchwood 1994; Chadwick and Lowe 1994; Fowler and Morley 1989; Kingdon and Turkington 1991; Perris and Skagerlind 1994). Two groups of investigators have compared CT with a waiting list control; however randomized assignment was not used (Garety et al. 1994; Tarrier et al. 1993). Tarrier and colleagues (1993) studied treatment with CT in a group of 27 schizophrenic subjects. The subjects served as their own control by being placed on a waiting list prior to beginning treatment. After treatment with CT, significant improvement was observed in psychotic symptoms measured by the Brief Psychiatric Rating Scale (BPRS). Garety et al. (1994) described a preliminary investigation of schizophrenic patients treated with an average of 16 sessions of CT as compared with subjects who were placed on a waiting list. Results of this study were mixed. Delusions, general symptom scores, and depression were significantly improved with treatment, but no changes were noted in measures of social functioning. Contrasting results were observed in a study of a skills training approach that uses some features of cognitive therapy but does not focus on challenging positive symptoms or modifying negative automatic thoughts (Eckman et al. 1992). The "modular skills training" approach developed by Liberman was found to be superior to supportive group therapy for schizophrenia in a randomized trial (Eckman et al. 1992). However, significant effects were observed only for improved skill level. There were no significant differences between groups in BPRS scores.

The most recent investigation of CT for psychosis found substantial improvement in positive symptoms and reduced time required for recovery (Drury et al. 1996a, 1996b). Forty patients with nonaffective psychosis were randomly assigned to CT plus standard clinical management or treatment as usual. The percentages of patients who had moderate to severe residual symptoms after treatment were 5% for those who received the added CT compared with 56% for subjects who were treated with standard therapy. Taken together, results of studies of CT for psychosis suggest that a comprehensive treatment program that incorporates cognitive, behavioral, and social

skills training might be best suited for reducing the pervasive symptoms of these disorders.

One of the important potential targets for CT of severe and chronic mental disorders is treatment adherence (Scott and Wright 1997). Cognitive therapy has been shown to improve adherence to lithium carbonate regimens in patients with bipolar disorder (Cochran 1986), and CT appeared to enhance medication compliance in an uncontrolled study of schizophrenic patients treated in small group homes (Perris and Skagerlind 1994). Additional research is clearly needed on the use of CT for treatment adherence. CT methods have been described as especially well suited for helping clinicians and patients to collaborate effectively in promoting adherence to treatment recommendations (Lecompte 1995; Rush 1988; Scott and Wright 1997).

Outcome research on cognitive therapy for personality disorders is the beginning stage of development. Results of preliminary studies indicate that the presence of an Axis II disorder may complicate the treatment of depression, anxiety disorders, or eating disorders with CT (T. R. Giles et al. 1985; Mavissakalian and Hammon 1987; Persons et al. 1988; Rush and Shaw 1983). However, a large randomized trial of CT for alcohol abuse found that patients who had antisocial personality disorder responded well to treatment, and in some cases actually did better than subjects without personality disorder (Longabaugh et al. 1994). Also, patients with body dysmorphic disorder and comorbid Axis II disorders were observed to have highly significant and substantial improvement after treatment with cognitive therapy (Neziroglu et al. 1996).

The most notable research on a cognitive-behavioral approach to personality disorders has been conducted by Linehan and colleagues (Linehan 1993; Linehan et al. 1991, 1993, 1994; Shearin and Linehan 1994). This group has developed an innovative approach to borderline personality disorder that incorporates cognitive and behavioral procedures. Linehan's dialectical behavior therapy (DBT) uses modeling, directive and supportive techniques, coaching, skills training, and behavioral rehearsal in an intensive program of weekly individual therapy and telephone consultation (Shearin and Linehan 1994). In a randomized trial of 44 borderline patients treated with DBT or treatment as usual, significant reductions in suicidal acts and the medical risk for suicide were observed in those who received DBT (Linehan et al. 1991). At the 6-month posttreatment assessment, DBT was still superior to treatment as usual, but these differences had disappeared by the time of the 12-month assessment (Linehan et al. 1993). Subjects treated with DBT had fewer days of inpatient hospitalization than control subjects during the year after completion of therapy.

Another analysis of data from Linehan's studies indicated that DBT had mixed effects on social and interpersonal functioning (Linehan et al. 1994). In a group of 26 patients with borderline personality and chronic suicidal activities treated with DBT or treatment as usual, DBT was found to significantly improve measures of anger and interviewer rated social adjustment. Global life satisfaction was not different in the two experimental groups. In a review of Linehan's work, Perris (1994) observed that DBT emphasizes behavioral change more than revision of dysfunctional schemas. He suggested that improvements in interpersonal skills are more likely to be long-lasting if patients learn functional "personal rules of living."

A limited number of other studies of CT for personality disorders have been conducted. Two groups investigated the usefulness of group therapy based on DBT (Shearin and Linehan 1994; Springer et al. 1996). In a study of inpatients with a variety of Axis II diagnoses, DBT was no more effective than supportive group therapy (Springer et al. 1996). The treatment program was quite short compared with the DBT described by Linehan, and a variety of other treatments were used for this inpatient sample. Thus, the study by Springer and colleagues (1996) does not appear to be an adequate test of DBT. Shearin and Linehan (1994) have described a small study in which they attempted to teach the skills training component of DBT in a group format. They concluded that DBT cannot be effectively delivered in an abbreviated package of skills training only.

Beck's model for CT of personality disorders has not been tested in controlled trials. Two recent case series have been reported in which CT appeared to be useful in treatment of personality disorders (Davidson and Tyer 1996; Nelson-Gray et al. 1996). Outcome research has been extremely limited for any type of psychotherapy of personality disorders. These conditions are notoriously difficult to treat under controlled conditions because of pervasive interpersonal and skills deficits and a frequent need for long-term therapy. Linehan's groundbreaking research has stimulated hope that additional studies will help elucidate the most effective methods of treating this challenging group of patients.

CONCLUSIONS

Cognitive therapy is a recently developed system of psychotherapy that is linked philosophically with a long tradition of viewing cognition as a primary determinant of emotion and behavior. The theoretical constructs of CT are supported by a large body of experimental findings regarding dysfunctional information processing in psychiatric disorders. In clinical practice, cognitive therapy is usually short-term, problem oriented, and highly collaborative. Therapists and patients work together in an empirical style, seeking to identify and modify maladaptive patterns of thinking. Behavioral techniques are used to uncover distorted cognitions and to promote more effective functioning. Also, psychoeducational procedures and homework assignments help reinforce concepts learned in therapy sessions. The goals of cognitive therapy include both immediate symptom relief and the acquisition of cognitive and behavioral skills that will decrease the risk for relapse.

The efficacy of cognitive therapy for depression, generalized anxiety, panic disorder, eating disorders, and other conditions has been established in a wide range of outcome studies. Newer applications for cognitive therapy, such as personality disorders, substance abuse, and psychosis are beginning to receive attention from investigators. Detailed treatment manuals or other guidelines for therapy have been described for most psychiatric illnesses.

Cognitive therapy has rapidly evolved into one of the major psychotherapeutic orientations in modern psychiatric treatment. Future challenges for this therapy model include study of the relative importance of treatment components, detailed examination of predictors for outcome, elucidation of the interface between biological and cognitive processes, and incorporation of new developments in computer-assisted learning. The empirical nature of cognitive therapy should promote further exploration of the potential uses for this treatment approach.

REFERENCES

Abramson LY, Seligman MEP, Teasdale J: Learned helplessness in humans: critique and reformulation. J Abnorm Psychol 87:49–74, 1978

Adler A: The neurotic's picture of the world. International Journal of Individual Psychology 2:3–10, 1936

Agras WS, Rossiter EM, Arnow B, et al: Pharmacologic and cognitive-behavioral treatment for bulimia nervosa: a controlled comparison. Am J Psychiatry 149:82–87, 1992

Agras WS, Rossiter EM, Arnow B, et al: One-year follow-up of psychosocial and pharmacologic treatments for bulimia nervosa. J Clin Psychiatry 55:179–183, 1994

Akiskal HS, McKinney WT: Overview of recent research in depression: integration of ten conceptual models into a comprehensive clinical frame. Arch Gen Psychiatry 32:285–305, 1975

Alexander F: Psychosomatic Medicine: Its Principles and Applications. New York, WW Norton, 1950

Alford BA, Beck AT: Cognitive therapy of delusional beliefs. Behav Res Ther 32:369–380, 1994

Alford BA, Correia CJ: Cognitive therapy of schizophrenia: theory and empirical status. Behavior Therapy 25:17–33, 1994

Alford BA, Freeman A, Beck AT, et al: Brief focused cognitive therapy of panic disorder. Psychotherapy 27:230–234, 1990

Alloy LB, Ahrens AH: Depression and pessimism for the future: biased use of statistically relevant information in predictions for self versus others. J Pers Soc Psychol 52:366–378, 1987

Arntz A, Van Den Hout M: Psychological treatments of panic disorder without agoraphobia: cognitive therapy versus applied relaxation. Behav Res Ther 34:113–121, 1996

Barlow DH, Cerney JA: Psychological Treatment of Panic. New York, Guilford, 1988

Barlow DH, Craske MG, Cerney JA, et al: Behavioral treatment of panic disorder. Behavior Therapy 20:261–268, 1989

Barrett CL, Meyer RG: Cognitive therapy with alcoholism, in Cognitive Therapy with Inpatients: Developing a Cognitive Milieu. Edited by Wright JH, Thase ME, Beck AT, et al. New York, Guilford, 1993, pp 315–336

Barrett CL, Wright JH: Therapist variables, in Issues in Psychotherapy Research. Edited by Hersen M, Nichelson L, Bellack AS. New York, Plenum, 1984, pp 361–391

Baxter LR Jr, Schwartz JM, Bergman KS, et al: Caudate glucose metabolic rate changes with both drug and behavior therapy for obsessive-compulsive disorder. Arch Gen Psychiatry 49:681–689, 1992

Beck AT: Thinking and depression. Arch Gen Psychiatry 9:324–333, 1963

Beck AT: Thinking and depression, II: theory and therapy. Arch Gen Psychiatry 10:561–571, 1964

Beck AT: Depression: Clinical, Experimental, and Theoretical Aspects. New York, Harper & Row, 1967

Beck AT: Cognitive Therapy and the Emotional Disorders. New York, International Universities Press, 1976

Beck AT: Love is Never Enough. New York, Harper & Row, 1988

Beck AT: Cognitive therapy and research: a 25-year retrospective. Presented at World Congress of Cognitive Therapy. Oxford, England, 1989

Beck AT: Cognitive therapy: past, present, and future. J Consult Clin Psychol 61:194–198, 1993

Beck AT: Cognitive therapy: a status report. J Clin Psychol Psychopathology (in press)

Beck AT, Greenberg RL: Coping with depression (a booklet). New York, Institute for Rational Living, 1974

Beck AT, Rush AJ: Cognitive therapy, in Comprehensive Textbook of Psychiatry, 6th Edition. Edited by Kaplan HI, Sadock BJ. Baltimore, MD, Williams & Wilkins, 1992, pp 1847–1857

Beck AT, Kovacs M, Weissman A: Hopelessness and suicidal behavior—an overview. JAMA 234:1146–1149, 1975

Beck AT, Rush AJ, Shaw BF, et al: Cognitive Therapy of Depression. New York, Guilford, 1979

Beck AT, Emery GD, Greenberg RL: Anxiety Disorders and Phobias: A Cognitive Perspective. New York, Basic Books, 1985a

Beck AT, Steer RA, Kovacs M, et al: Hopelessness and eventual suicide: a 10-year prospective study of patients hospitalized with suicidal ideation. Am J Psychiatry 142:559–562, 1985b

Beck AT, Freeman A, et al: Cognitive Therapy of Personality Disorders. New York, Guilford, 1990a

Beck AT, Brown G, Berchick RJ, et al: Relationship between hopelessness and ultimate suicide: a replication with psychiatric outpatients. Am J Psychiatry 147:190–195, 1990b

Beck AT, Wright JH, Neuman C: Cocaine abuse, in Comprehensive Casebook of Cognitive Therapy. Edited by Freeman A, Dattilio FM. New York, Plenum, 1992a, pp 185–192

Beck AT, Sokol L, Clark DA, et al: A cross-over study of focused cognitive therapy for panic disorder. Am J Psychiatry 149:778–783, 1992b

Beck J: Cognitive Therapy: Basics and Beyond. New York, Guilford, 1995

Beck JG, Stanley MA, Baldwin LE, et al: Comparison of cognitive therapy and relaxation training for panic disorder. J Consult Clin Psychol 62:818–826, 1994

Bergdahl J, Anneroth G, Perris H: Cognitive therapy in the treatment of patients with resistant burning mouth syndrome: a controlled study. J Oral Pathol Med 24:213–215, 1995

Beutler LE, Scogin F, Kinkish P, et al: Group cognitive therapy and alprazolam in the treatment of depression in older adults. J Consult Clin Psychol 55:550–556, 1987

Black DW, Wesner R, Bowers W, et al: A comparison of fluvoxamine, cognitive therapy, and placebo in the treatment of panic disorder. Arch Gen Psychiatry 50:44–50, 1993

Blackburn IM, Bishop S, Glen AIM, et al: The efficacy of cognitive therapy in depression: a treatment trial using cognitive therapy and pharmacotherapy, each alone and in combination. Br J Psychiatry 139:181–189, 1981

Blackburn IM, Jones S, Lewin RJP: Cognitive style in depression. Br J Clin Psychol 25:241–251, 1986a

Blackburn IM, Eunson KM, Bishop S: A two-year naturalistic follow-up of depressed patients treated with cognitive therapy, pharmacotherapy, and a combination of both. J Affect Disord 10:67–75, 1986b

Blowers C, Cobb J, Mathews A: Generalized anxiety: a controlled treatment study. Behav Res Ther 25:493–502, 1987

Bouchard S, Gauthier J, Laberge B, et al: Exposure versus cognitive restructuring in the treatment of panic disorder with agoraphobia. Behav Res Ther 34:213–224, 1996

Bower GH: Mood and memory. Am Psychol 36:129–148, 1981

Bowers WA: Cognitive therapy with inpatients, in Handbook of Cognitive Therapy. Edited by Freeman A, Simon KM, Arkowitz H, et al. New York, Plenum, 1989, pp 583–596

Bowers WA: Treatment of depressed inpatients: cognitive therapy plus medication, relaxation plus medication, and medication alone. Br J Psychiatry 156:73–78, 1990

Bowers WA: Inpatient cognitive therapy for eating disorders, in Cognitive Therapy with Inpatients: Developing a Cognitive Milieu. Edited by Wright JH, Thase ME, Beck AT, et al. New York, Guilford, 1992, pp 337–356

Bowers W, Stuart S, MacFarlane R, et al: Use of computer-administered cognitive-behavior therapy with depressed inpatients. Depression 1:294–299, 1993

Bowlby J: The role of childhood experience in cognitive disturbance, in Cognition and Psychotherapy. Edited by Mahoney MJ, Freeman A. New York, Plenum, 1985, pp 181–200

Bradley B, Mathews A: Negative self-schemata in clinical depression. Br J Clin Psychol 22:173–181, 1982

Braff DL, Beck AT: Thinking disorder in depression. Arch Gen Psychiatry 31:456–459, 1974

Bujold A, Ladouceur R, Sylvain C, et al: Treatment of pathological gamblers: an experimental study. J Behav Ther Exp Psychiatry 25:275–282, 1994

Burns DD: Feeling Good. New York, William Morrow, 1980

Burns DD: The Feeling Good Handbook. New York, Penguin, 1990

Butler G, Fennell M, Robson P, et al: Comparison of behavior therapy and cognitive behavior therapy in the treatment of generalized anxiety disorder. J Consult Clin Psychol 59:167–175, 1991

Carroll KM, Rounsaville BJ, Nich C, et al: One-year follow-up of psychotherapy and pharmacotherapy for cocaine dependence. Arch Gen Psychiatry 51:989–997, 1994a

Carroll KM, Rousaville BJ, Gordon LT, et al: Psychotherapy and pharmacotherapy for ambulatory cocaine abusers. Arch Gen Psychiatry 51:177–187, 1994b

Carroll KM, Nich C, Rounsaville BJ: Differential symptom reduction in depressed cocaine abusers treated with psychotherapy and pharmacotherapy. J Nerv Ment Dis 183:251–259, 1995

Casey DA, Grant RW: Cognitive therapy with depressed elderly inpatients, in Cognitive Therapy with Inpatients: Developing a Cognitive Milieu. Edited by Wright JH, Thase ME, Beck AT, et al. New York, Guilford, 1992, pp 295–314

Chadwick P, Birchwood M: The omnipotence of voices: a cognitive approach to auditory hallucinations. Br J Psychiatry 164:190–201, 1994

Chadwick PDJ, Lowe CF: A cognitive approach to measuring and modifying delusions. Behav Res Ther 32:355–367, 1994

Clark DA, Feldman J, Channon S: Dysfunctional thinking in anorexia and bulimia nervosa. Cognitive Therapy and Research 13:377–387, 1989

Clark DA, Beck AT, Stewart B: Cognitive specificity and positive-negative affectivity: complementary or contradictory views on anxiety and depression? J Abnorm Psychol 99:148–155, 1990

Clark DM: A cognitive approach to panic. Behav Res Ther 24:461–470, 1986

Clark DM, Beck AT: Cognitive approaches, in Handbook of Anxiety Disorders. Edited by Last CG, Hersen M. New York, Pergamon, 1988, pp 362–385

Clark DM, Teasdale JD: Diurnal variation in clinical depression and the accessibility of memories of positive and negative experiences. J Abnorm Psychol 91:87–95, 1982

Clark DM, Salkovskis PM, Chalkley AJ: Respiratory control as a treatment for panic attacks. J Behav Ther Exp Psychiatry 16:23–30, 1985

Clark DM, Salkovskis PM, Hackmann A, et al: A comparison of cognitive therapy, applied relaxation and imipramine in the treatment of panic disorder. Br J Psychiatry 164:759–769, 1994

Cloitre M, Liebowitz MR: Memory bias in panic disorder: an investigation of the cognitive avoidance hypothesis. Cognitive Therapy and Research 15:371–386, 1991

Cochran SD: Compliance with lithium regimens in the outpatient treatment of bipolar affective disorders. Journal of Compliance in Health Care 1:151–169, 1986

Colby KM: A computer program using cognitive therapy to treat depressed patients. Psychiatr Serv 46:1223–1225, 1995

Colby KM, Colby PM: Overcoming Depression. Malibu, CA, Artifactual Intelligence Works, 1990

Cooper PJ, Steere J: A comparison of two psychological treatments for bulimia nervosa: implications for models of maintenance. Behav Res Ther 33:875–885, 1995

Cooper PJ, Coker S, Fleming C: An evaluation of the efficacy of supervised cognitive behavioral self-help for bulimia nervosa. J Psychosom Res 40:281–287, 1996

Corbishley M, Beutler L, Quan S, et al: Rapid eye movement density and latency and dexamethasone suppression as predictors of treatment response in depressed older adults. Current Therapeutic Research 47:846–859, 1990

Covi L, Lipman RS: Cognitive behavioral group psychotherapy combined with inipramine in major depression. Psychopharmacol Bull 23:173–176, 1987

Covi L, Primakoff L: Cognitive group therapy, in The American Psychiatric Press Review of Psychiatry. Edited by Frances AJ, Hales RE. Washington, DC, American Psychiatric Press, 1988, pp 608–616

Covi L, Roth D, Lipman RS: Cognitive group psychotherapy of depression: the close-ended group. Am J Psychother 36:459–469, 1982

Craske MG, Maidenberg E, Bystritsky A: Brief cognitive-behavioral versus nondirective therapy for panic disorder. J Behav Ther Exp Psychiatry 26:113–120, 1995

Danion JM, Schroeder DW, Zimmerman MA, et al: Explicit memory and repetition priming in depression. Arch Gen Psychiatry 48:707–711, 1991

Davidson KM, Tyrer P: Cognitive therapy for antisocial and borderline personality disorders: single case study series. Br J Clin Psychol 35:413–429, 1996

Davis H, Unruh WR: The development of the self-schema in adult depression. J Abnorm Psychol 90:125–133, 1981

Davis D, Wright JH: The therapeutic relationship in cognitive-behavioral therapy: patient perceptions and therapist responses. Cognitive and Behavioral Practice 1:25–45, 1994

DeMonbreun BG, Craighead WE: Distortion of perception and recall of positive and neutral feedback in depression. Cognitive Therapy and Research 1:311–329, 1977

Derry PA, Kuiper NA: Schematic processing and self-reference in clinical depression. J Abnorm Psychol 90:286–297, 1981

DeRubeis RJ, Evans MD, Hollon SD, et al: How does cognitive therapy work? Cognitive change and symptom change in cognitive therapy and pharmacotherapy for depression. J Consult Clin Psychol 58:862–869, 1990

Deutscher S, Cimbolic P: Cognitive process and their relationship to endogenous and reactive components of depression. J Nerv Ment Dis 178:351–359, 1990

Dobson KS: A meta-analysis of the efficacy of cognitive therapy for depression. J Consult Clin Psychol 57:414–419, 1989

Dobson KS, Shaw BF: Cognitive assessment with major depressive disorders. Cognitive Therapy and Research 10:13–29, 1986

Drury V, Birchwood M, Cochrane R, et al: Cognitive therapy and recovery from acute psychosis: a controlled trial I; impact on psychotic symptoms. Br J Psychiatry 169:593–601, 1996a

Drury V, Birchwood M, Cochrane R, et al: Cognitive therapy and recovery from acute psychosis: a controlled trial II; impact on recovery time. Br J Psychiatry 169:602–607, 1996b

Durham RC, Turvey AA: Cognitive therapy vs. behavior therapy in the treatment of chronic general anxiety. Behav Res Ther 25:229–234, 1987

Durham RC, Murphy T, Allan T, et al: Cognitive therapy, analytic psychotherapy and anxiety management training for generalised anxiety disorder. Br J Psychiatry 165:315–323, 1994

Dworkin SF, Turner JA, Wilson L, et al: Brief group cognitive-behavioral intervention for temporomandibular disorders. Pain 59:175–187, 1994

Eckman TA, Wirshing WC, Marder SR, et al: Technique for training schizophrenic patients in illness self-management: a controlled trial. Am J Psychiatry 149:1549–1555, 1992

Elkin I, Shea MT, Watkins JT, et al: NIMH Treatment of Depression Collaborative Research Program: 1; general effectiveness of treatments. Arch Gen Psychiatry 46:971–982, 1989

Ellis A: Reason and Emotion in Psychotherapy. New York, Lyle Stuart, 1962

Ellis A: Humanistic Psychotherapy: The Rational-Emotive Psychotherapy. New York, McGraw-Hill, 1973

Emmelkamp PMG, Beens H: Cognitive therapy with obsessive-compulsive disorder: a comparative evaluation. Behav Res Ther 29:293–300, 1991

Engel GL: The need for a new medical model: a challenge for biomedicine. Science 196:129–136, 1977

Epstein N, Schlesinger SE, Dryden W: Cognitive-Behavioral Therapy With Families. New York, Bruner-Mazel, 1988

Evans MD, Hollon SD, DeRubeis RJ, et al: Differential relapse following cognitive therapy and pharmacotherapy for depression. Arch Gen Psychiatry 49:802–808, 1992

Fairburn CG: Cognitive-behavioral treatment for bulimia, in Handbook of Psychotherapy for Anorexia Nervosa and Bulimia. Edited by Garner DM, Garfinkel PE. New York, Guilford, 1985, pp 160–169

Fairburn CG, Jones R, Peveler RC, et al: Three psychological treatments for bulimia nervosa. Arch Gen Psychiatry 48:463–469, 1991

Fairburn CG, Jones R, Peveler RC, et al: Psychotherapy and bulimia nervosa. Arch Gen Psychiatry 50:419–428, 1993

Fairburn CG, Norman PA, Welch SL, et al: A prospective study of outcome in bulimia nervosa and the long-term effects of three psychological treatments. Arch Gen Psychiatry 52:304–312, 1995

Fava GA, Grandi S, Zielezny M, et al: Four-year outcome for cognitive behavioral treatment of residual symptoms in major depression. Am J Psychiatry 153:945–947, 1996

Fawcett J, Scheftner W, Clark D, et al: Clinical predictors of suicide in patients with major affective disorders: a controlled prospective study. Am J Psychiatry 144:35–40, 1987

Fisher MS, Bentley KJ: Two group therapy models for clients with a dual diagnosis of substance abuse and personality disorder. Psych Serv 47:1244–1250, 1996

Fitzgerald TE, Phillips W: Attentional bias and agoraphobic avoidance: the role of cognitive style. J Anxiety Disord 5:333–341, 1991

Fowler D, Morley S: The cognitive-behavioral treatment of hallucinations and delusions: a preliminary study. Behavioral Psychotherapy 17:262–282, 1989

Frankl VE: Logos, paradox, and the search for meaning, in Cognition and Psychotherapy. Edited by Mahoney MJ, Freeman A. New York, Plenum, 1985, pp 3–49

Free ML, Oei TPS, Sanders MR: Treatment outcome of a group cognitive therapy program for depression. International Journal of Group Psychotherapy 41:533–547, 1991

Freeman A, Dattilio FM: Comprehensive Casebook of Cognitive Therapy. New York, Plenum, 1992

Freeman A, Simon KM, Beutler LE, et al (eds): Comprehensive Handbook of Cognitive Therapy. New York, Plenum, 1989

Freeman A, Schrodt GR, Gilson M, et al: Cognitive group therapy with inpatients, in Cognitive Therapy With Inpatients: Developing a Cognitive Milieu. Edited by Wright JH, Thase ME, Beck AT, et al. New York, Guilford, 1992, pp 121–153

Friedman M, Thorensen CD, Gill JJ, et al: Alteration of type A behavior and its effect on cardiac recurrences in post myocardial infarct patients: summary results of the recurrent coronary prevention project. Am Heart J 112:653–665, 1986

Gaffan EA, Tsaousis I, Kemp-Wheeler SM: Researcher allegiance and meta-analysis: the case of cognitive therapy for depression. J Consult Clin Psychol 63:966–980, 1995

Garety PA, Kuipers L, Fowler D, et al: Cognitive behavioral therapy for drug-resistant psychosis. Br J Med Psychol 67:259–271, 1994

Garner DM: Psychotherapy for eating disorders. Current Opinion in Psychiatry 5:391–395, 1992

Garner DM, Bemis KM: A cognitive-behavioral approach to anorexia nervosa. Cognitive Therapy Research 6:123–150, 1985

Gelernter CS, Uhde TW, Cimbolic P, et al: Cognitive-behavioral and pharmacological treatments of social phobia: a controlled study. Arch Gen Psychiatry 48: 938–945, 1991

Giles DE, Etzel BA, Biggs MM: Long-term effects of unipolar depression on cognitions. Compr Psychiatry 30:225–230, 1989

Giles TR, Young RR, Young DE: Behavioral treatment of severe bulimia. Behavior Therapy 16:393–405, 1985

Glass CR, Furlong M: Cognitive assessment of social anxiety: affective and behavioral correlates. Cognitive Therapy and Research 14:365–384, 1990

Glass RM, Uhlenhuth EH, Hartel FW, et al: Cognitive dysfuntion and imipramine in outpatient depressives. Arch Gen Psychiatry 38:1048–1051, 1981

Goldstein LH: Behavioral and cognitive-behavioral treatments for epilepsy: a progress review. Br J Clin Psychol 29:257–269, 1990

Golinkoff M, Sweeney JA: Cognitive impairments in depression. J Affect Disord 17:105–112, 1989

Gotlib IH: Self-reinforcement and recall: differential deficits in depressed and nondepressed psychiatric inpatients. J Abnorm Psychol 90:521–530, 1981

Gotlib IH: Perception and recall of interpersonal feedback: negative bias in depression. Cognitive Therapy and Research 7:399–412, 1983

Gotlib IH, Olson JM: Depression, psychopathology, and self-serving attributions. Br J Clin Psychol 22:309–310, 1983

Greenberg LS, Safran JD: Integrating affect and cognition: a perspective on the process of therapeutic change. Cognitive Therapy and Research 8:559–578, 1984

Guidano VF, Liotti G: Cognitive Processes and Emotional Disorders: A Structural Approach to Psychotherapy. New York, Guilford, 1983

Haaga DA, Dyck MJ, Ernst D: Empirical status of cognitive theory of depression. Psychol Bull 110:215–236, 1991

Hammon C, Krantz SE, Cochran SD: Relationships between depression and causal attributions about stressful life events. Cognitive Therapy and Research 5:351–358, 1981

Hargreaves IR: Attributional style and depression. Br J Clin Psychol 24:65–66, 1985

Heimberg RG, Dodge CS, Hope DA, et al: Cognitive behavioral group treatment for social phobia: comparison with a credible placebo control. Cognitive Therapy and Research 14:1–23, 1990

Hollon SD, Beck AT: Cognitive and cognitive-behavioral therapies, in Handbook of Psychotherapy and Behavior Change: An Empirical Analysis, 4th Edition. Edited by Garfield SL, Bergin AE. New York, John Wiley, 1994, pp 428–466

Hollon SD, Kendall PC: Cognitive self-statements in depression: development of an automatic thought questionnaire. Cognitive Therapy and Research 4:383–395, 1980

Hollon SD, Kendall PC, Lumry A: Specificity of depressotypic cognitions in clinical depression. J Abnorm Psychol 95:52–59, 1986

Hollon SD, Shelton RC, Loosen PT: Cognitive therapy and pharmacotherapy for depression. J Consult Clin Psychol 59:88–99, 1991

Hollon SD, DeRubeis RJ, Evans MD, et al: Cognitive therapy and pharmacotherapy for depression: singly and in combination. Arch Gen Psychiatry 49:774–782, 1992a

Hollon SD, DeRubeis RJ, Seligman MEP: Cognitive therapy and the prevention of depression. Applied and Preventive Psychology 1:89–95, 1992b

Hope DA, Heimberg RG, Bruch MA: Dismantling cognitive-behavioral group therapy for social phobia. Behav Res Ther 33:637–650, 1995

Horne DJ, White AW, Varigos GA: A preliminary study of psychological therapy in the management of atopic eczema. Br J Med Psychol 62:241–248, 1989

Horney K: Neurosis and Human Growth: The Struggle Toward Self-Realization. New York, WW Norton, 1950

Imber SD, Pilkonis PA, Sotsky SM, et al: Mode-specific effects among three treatments for depression. J Consult Clin Psychol 58:353–359, 1990

Ingram RE, Kendall PC: The cognitive side of anxiety. Cognitive Therapy and Research 11:523–536, 1987

Ingram RE, Kendall PC, Smith TW, et al: Cognitive specificity in emotional distress. J Pers Soc Psychol 53:734–742, 1987

James IA, Blackburn IM: Cognitive therapy with obsessive-compulsive disorder. Br J Psychiatry 166:444–450, 1995

Jarrett R, Rush AJ, Khatami M, et al: Does the pretreatment of polysomnogram predict response to cognitive therapy in depression outpatients? A preliminary report. Psychiatry Res 33:285–299, 1990

Jarrett R, Giles D, Gullion C, et al: Does learned resourcefulness predict repsonse to cognitive therapy in depressed outpatient? J Affect Disord 23:223–229, 1991

Juster HR, Heimberg RG: Social phobia: longitudinal course and long-term outcome of cognitive-behavioral treatment. Psychiatr Clin North Am 18:821–842, 1995

Kandel ER: Psychotherapy and the single synapse: the impact of psychiatric thought on neurobiologic research. N Engl J Med 301:1028–1037, 1979

Kandel ER, Schwartz JH: Molecular biology of learning: modulation of transmitter release. Science 218:433–443, 1983

Keefe FJ, Van Horn Y: Cognitive-behavioral treatment of rheumatoid arthritis pain. Arthritis Care and Research 6:213–222, 1993

Kelly G: The Psychology of Personal Constructs. New York, WW Norton, 1955

Kendall PC, Hollon SD: Anxious self-talk: development of the Anxious Self-Statements Questionnaire (ASSQ). Cognitive Therapy and Research 13:81–93, 1989

Kingdon D, Turkington D: The use of cognitive behavior therapy with a normalizing rationale in schizophrenia. J Nerv Ment Dis 179:207–211, 1991

Klein DC, Fencil-Morse E, Seligman MEP: Learned helplessness, depression, and the attribution of failure. J Pers Soc Psychol 33:508–516, 1976

Klosko JS, Barlow DH, Tassinari R, et al: A comparison of alprazolam and behavior therapy in treatment of panic disorder. J Consult Clin Psychol 58:77–84, 1990

Kovacs M, Rush AJ, Beck AT, et al: Depressed outpatients treated with cognitive therapy or pharmacotherapy. Arch Gen Psychiatry 38:33–39, 1981

Kraaimaat FW, Brons MR, Geenen R, et al: The effect of cognitive behavior therapy in patients with rheumatoid arthritis. Behav Res Ther 33:487–495, 1995

Krantz SE: When depressive cognitions reflect negative realities. Cognitive Therapy and Research 9:595–610, 1985

Laberge B, Gauthier JG, Cote G, et al: Cognitive-behavioral therapy of panic disorder with secondary major depression: a preliminary investigation. J Consult Clin Psychol 61:1028–1037, 1993

Larcombe NA, Wilson PH: An evaluation of cognitive-behavior therapy for depression in patients with multiple sclerosis. Br J Psychiatry 145:366–371, 1984

Lecompte D: Drug compliance and cognitive-behavioral therapy in schizophrenia. Acta Psychiatrica Belgica 95:91–100, 1995

LeFebvre MF: Cognitive distortion and cognitive errors in depressed psychiatric and low back pain patients. J Consult Clin Psychol 49:517–525, 1981

Leitenberg H, Rosen J, Wolf R, et al: Comparison of cognitive-behavioral therapy and desipramine in the treatment of bulimia nervosa. Behav Res Ther 32:37–45, 1994

Lewinsohn PM, Sullivan JM, Grosscup SJ: Behavioral therapy: clinical applications, in Short-Term Psychotherapies for Depression. Edited by Rush AJ. New York, Guilford, 1982, pp 50–87

Linehan MM: Dialectical behavior therapy for borderline personality disorder: theory and method. Bull Menninger Clin 51:261–276, 1987

Linehan MM: Cognitive-Behavioral Treatment of Borderline Personality Disorder. New York, Guilford, 1993

Linehan MM, Armstrong HE, Suarez A, et al: Cognitive-behavioral treatment of chronically parasuicidal borderline patients. Arch Gen Psychiatry 48:1060–1064, 1991

Linehan MM, Heard HL, Armstrong HE: Naturalistic follow-up of a behavioral treatment for chronically parasuicidal borderline patients. Arch Gen Psychiatry 50:971–974, 1993

Linehan MM, Tutek DA, Heard HL, et al: Interpersonal outcome of cognitive behavioral treatment for chronically suicidal borderline patients. Am J Psychiatry 151:1771–1776, 1994

Lloyd GG, Lishman WA: Effect of depression on the speed of recall of pleasant and unpleasant experiences. Psychol Med 5:173–180, 1975

Loeb A, Beck AT, Feshbach S, et al: Some effects of reward on the social perception and motivation of psychiatric patients varying in depression. Journal of Abnormal Social Psychology 68:609–616, 1964

Loeb A, Beck AT, Diggory J: Differential effects of success and failure on depressed and nondepressed patients. J Nerv Ment Dis 152:106–114, 1971

Longabaugh R, Rubin A, Malloy P, et al: Drinking outcomes of alcohol abusers diagnosed as antisocial personality disorder. Alcoholism: Clinical and Experimental Research 18:778–785, 1994

Ludgate JW, Wright JH, Bowers W, et al: Individual cognitive therapy with inpatients, in Cognitive Therapy with Inpatients: Developing a Cognitive Milieu. Edited by Wright JH, Thase ME, Beck AT, et al. New York, Guilford, 1992, pp 91–120

Maes S, Schlosser M: Changing health behavior outcomes in asthmatic patients: a pilot study. Soc Sci Med 26:359–364, 1988

Mahoney MJ: Psychotherapy and human change processes, in Cognition and Psychotherapy. Edited by Mahoney MJ, Freeman A. New York, Plenum, 1985

Mathews A, MacLeod C: An information-processing approach to anxiety. Journal of Cognitive Psychotherapy: An International Quarterly 1:105–115, 1987

Mavissakalian M, Hamman MS: DSM-III personality disorder in agoraphobia, II; changes with treatment. Compr Psychiatry 28:356–361, 1987

McKnight DL, Nelson-Gray RO, Barnhill J: Dexamethasone suppression test and response to cognitive therapy and antidepressant medication. Behavior Therapy 1:99–111, 1992

McNally RJ, Foa EB: Cognition and agoraphobia: bias in the interpretation of threat. Cognitive Therapy and Research 11:567–581, 1987

Meichenbaum DB: Cognitive-Behavior Modification: An Integrative Approach. New York, Plenum, 1977

Miller IW, Norman WH, Keitner GI, et al: Cognitive-behavioral treatment of depressed inpatients. Behavior Therapy 20:25–47, 1989

Miller IW, Klee SH, Norman WH: Depressed and nondepressed inpatients' cognitions of hypothetical events, experimental tasks, and stressful life events. J Abnorm Psychol 91:78–81, 1982

Minkoff K, Bergman E, Beck AT, et al: Hopelessness, depression, and attempted suicide. Am J Psychiatry 130:455–459, 1973

Miranda J: Dysfunctional thinking is activated by stressful life events. Cognitive Therapy and Research 16:473–483, 1992

Mitchell JE, Hoberman HN, Peterson CB, et al: Research on the Psychotherapy of Bulimia Nervosa: Half Empty or Half Full. Int J Eat Disord 20:219–229, 1996

Mizes JS, Landolf-Fritsche B, Grossman-McKee D: Patterns of distorted cognitions in phobic disorders: an investigation of clinically severe simple phobics, social phobics, and agoraphobics. Cognitive Therapy and Research 11:583–592, 1987

Mohl PC: Should psychotherapy be considered a biological treatment? Psychosomatics 28:320–326, 1987

Murphy GE, Simons AD, Wetzel RD, et al: Cognitive therapy and pharmacotherapy, singly and together in the treatment of depression. Arch Gen Psychiatry 41:33–41, 1984

Murphy GE, Carney RM, Knesevich MA, et al: Cognitive behavior therapy, relaxation training, and tricyclic antidepressant medication in the treatment of depression. Psychol Rep 77:403–420, 1995

Nekanda-Trepka CJS, Bishop S, Blackburn IM: Hopelessness and depression. Br J Clin Psychol 22:49–60, 1983

Nelson RE, Craighead WE: Selective recall of positive and negative feedback, self—control behaviors and depression. J Abnorm Psychol 86:379–388, 1977

Nelson-Gray RO, Johnson D, Foyle LW, et al: The effectiveness of cognitive therapy tailored to depressives with personality disorders. J Pers Disord 10:132–152, 1996

Neziroglu F, McKay D, Todaro J, et al: Effect of cognitive behavior therapy on persons with body dysmorphic disorder and comorbid Axis II diagnoses. Behavior Therapy 27:67–77, 1996

Oei TPS, Lim B, Young RM: Cognitive processes and cognitive behavior therapy in the treatment of problem drinking. J Addict Dis 10:63–80, 1991

Ost LG, Westling BE, Hellstrom K: Applied relaxation, exposure in vivo and cognitive methods in the treatment of panic disorder with agoraphobia. Behav Res Ther 31: 383–394, 1993

Otto MW, Pollack MH, Sachs GS, et al: Discontinuation of benzodiazepine treatment: efficacy of cognitive-behavioral therapy for patients with panic disorder. Am J Psychiatry 150:1485–1490, 1993

Otto MW, Whittal ML: Cognitive-behavior therapy and the longitudinal course of panic disorder. Psychiatr Clin North Am 18:803–820, 1995

Payne A, Blanchard EB: A controlled comparison of cognitive therapy and self-help support groups in the treatment of irritable bowel syndrome. J Consult Clin Psychol 63:779–786, 1995

Perris C: Cognitive Therapy With Schizophrenic Patients. New York, Guilford, 1989

Perris C, Skagerlind L: Cognitive therapy with schizophrenic patients. Acta Psychiatr Scand 89 (suppl 382):65–70, 1994

Perris C: Cognitive therapy in the treatment of patients with borderline personality disorders. Acta Psychiatr Scand 89 (suppl 379):69–72, 1994

Persons JB, Burns BD, Perhoff JM: Predictors of drop-out and outcome in cognitive therapy for depression in a private practice setting. Cognitive Therapy and Research 12:557–575, 1988

Peselow ED, Robins C, Block P, et al: Dysfunctional attitudes in depressed patients before and after clinical treatment and in normal control subjects. Am J Psychiatry 147:439–444, 1990

Peterson C, Villanova P, Raps CS: Depression and attributions: factors responsible for inconsistent results in the published literature. J Abnorm Psychol 94:165–168, 1985

Phillips HC: The effects of behavioral treatment on chronic pain. Behav Res Ther 25:365–377, 1987

Piaget J: The Construction of Reality in the Child. New York, Basic Books, 1954

Pollack MH, Otto MW, Kaspi SP, et al: Cognitive behavior therapy for treatment-refractory panic disorder. J Clin Psychiatry 55:200–205, 1994

Power KG, Simpson RJ, Swanson V, et al: Controlled comparison of pharmacological and psychological treatment of generalized anxiety disorder in primary care. British Journal of General Practice 40:289–294, 1990

Pretzer J, Beck AT: A cognitive theory of personality disorders, in Major Theories of Personality Disorder. Edited by Clarkin J, New York, Guilford, 1996, pp 36–105

Prezant DW, Neimeyer RA: Cognitive predictors of depression and suicide ideation. Suicide Life Threat Behav 18:259–264, 1988

Raimy V: Misunderstandings of the Self. San Francisco, CA, Jossey Bass, 1975

Raps CS, Peterson C, Reinhard KE, et al: Attributional style among depressed patients. J Abnorm Psychol 91:102–108, 1982

Riskind JH, Steer R: Do maladaptive attitudes "cause" depression? Misconception of cognitive theory. Arch Gen Psychiatry 41:1111, 1984

Riskind JH, Beck AT, Steer RA: Cognitive-behavioral therapy in geriatric depression: comment on Steuer et al. J Consult Clin Psychol 53:944–947, 1985

Rizley R: Depression and distortion in the attribution of causality. J Abnorm Psychol 87:32–48, 1978

Robinson LA, Berman JS, Neimeyer RA: Psychotherapy for the treatment of depression: a comprehensive review of controlled outcome research. Psychol Bull 108:30–49, 1990

Rush AJ: Cognitive therapy of depression: rationale, techniques, and efficacy. Psychiatr Clin North Am 6:105–127, 1983

Rush AJ: Cognitive approaches to adherence, in The American Psychiatric Press Review of Psychiatry. Edited by Francis AJ, Hales RE. Washington, DC, American Psychiatric Press, 1988, pp 627–642

Rush AJ, Shaw BF: Failure in treating depression by cognitive therapy, in Failures in Behavior Therapy. Edited by Foa EB, Emmelkamp PGM. New York, Wiley, 1983, pp 213–224

Rush AJ, Beck AT, Kovacs M, et al: Comparative efficacy of cognitive therapy and pharmacotherapy in the treatment of depressed outpatients. Cognitive Therapy and Research 1:17–37, 1977

Salkovskis PM: Obsessional-compulsive problems: a cognitive-behavioral analysis. Behav Res Ther 25:571–583, 1985

Salkovskis PM (ed): Frontiers of Cognitive Therapy. New York, Guilford, 1996

Salkovskis PM, Warwick HM: Cognitive therapy of obsessive-compulsive disorder: treating treatment failures. Behavioural Psychotherapy 13:243–255, 1985

Salkovskis PM, Westbrook D: Behavior therapy and obsessional ruminations: can failure be turned into success? Behav Res Ther 27:149–160, 1989

Schlesier-Carter B, Hamilton SA, O'Neil PM, et al: Depression and bulimia: the link between depression and bulimic cognitions. J Abnorm Psychol 98:322–325, 1989

Schmidt NB, Harrington P: Cognitive-behavioral treatment of body dysmorphic disorder: a case report. J Behav Ther Exp Psychiatry 26:161–167, 1995

Schmidt U, Tiller J, Treasure J: Self-treatment of bulimia nervosa: a pilot study. Int J Eat Disord 13:273–277, 1993

Schonfeld L, Dupree LW: Treatment approaches for older problem drinkers. The International Journal of the Addictions 30:1819–1842, 1995

Schwartz JM, Stoessel PW, Baxter LR Jr, et al: Systematic changes in cerebral glucose metabolic rate after successful behavior modification treatment of obsessive-compulsive disorder. Arch Gen Psychiatry 53:109–113, 1996

Schwartz SP, Blanchard EB: Evaluation of psychological treatment for inflammatory bowel disease. Behav Res Ther 29:167–177, 1991

Scott J: Chronic depression: can cognitive therapy succeed when other treatments fail? Behavioural Psychotherapy 20:25–36, 1992

Scott J, Wright JH: Cognitive therapy for chronic and severe mental disorders, in American Psychiatric Press Review of Psychiatry, Vol 16. Edited by Dickstein LJ, Riba MB, Oldham JM. Washington, DC, American Psychiatric Press, 1997, pp 1135–1170

Scott J, Byers S, Turkington D: The chronic patient, in Cognitive Therapy with Inpatients: Developing a Cognitive Milieu. Edited by Wright JH, Thase ME, Beck AT, et al. New York, Guilford, 1992, pp 357–390

Selmi PM, Klein MH, Greist JH, et al: Computer-administered therapy for depression. Am J Psychiatry 147:51–56, 1990

Selmi PM, Klein MH, Greist JH, et al: Computer-administered therapy for depression. M.D. Computing 8:98–102, 1991

Sharpe L, Tarrier N: Towards a cognitive-behavioural theory or problem gambling. Br J Psychiatry 162:407–412, 1993

Shea MT, Elkin I, Imber SD, et al: Course of depressive symptoms over follow-up: findings from the NIMH treatment of depression collaborative research program. Arch Gen Psychiatry 49:782–787, 1992

Shear MK, Ball G, Fitzpatrick M, et al: Cognitive-behavioral therapy for panic: an open study. J Nerv Ment Dis 179:468–472, 1991a

Shear MK, Fyer AJ, Ball G, et al: Vulnerability to sodium lactate in panic disorder patients given cognitive-behavioral therapy. Am J Psychiatry 148:195–197, 1991b

Shearin EN, Linehan MM: Dialectical behavior therapy for borderline personality disorder: theoretical and empirical foundations. Acta Psychiatr Scand 89 (suppl 379):61–68, 1994

Simons AD, Thase ME: Biological markers, treatment outcome, and 1 year follow-up in endogenous depression: electroencephalographic sleep studies and cognitive therapy. J Consult Clin Psychol 60:392–401, 1992

Simons AD, Garfield SL, Murphy CE: The process of change in cognitive therapy and pharmacotherapy for depression. Arch Gen Psychiatry 41:45–51, 1984

Simons AD, Lustman PJ, Wetzel RD, et al: Predicting response to congitive therapy of depression: the role of learned resourcefulness. Cognitive Therapy and Research 9:79–89, 1985

Simons AD, Murphy GE, Levine JE, et al: Cognitive therapy and pharmacotherapy for depression: sustained improvement over one year. Arch Gen Psychiatry 43:43–49, 1986

Sitharthan T, Kavanagh DJ, Sayer G: Moderating drinking by correspondence: an evaluation of a new method of intervention. Addiction 91:345–355, 1996

Skinner JB, Erskine A, Pearce S, et al: The evaluation of a cognitive-behavioral treatment program in outpatients with chronic pain. J Psychosom Res 34:13–19, 1990

Sokol L, Beck AT, Greenberg RL, et al: Cognitive therapy of panic disorder: a nonpharmacological alternative. J Nerv Ment Dis 177:711–716, 1989

Speckens AEM, van Hemert AM, Spinhoven P, et al: Cognitive behavioural therapy for medically unexplained physical symptoms: a randomised controlled trial. BMJ 311:1328–1332, 1995

Springer T, Lohr NE, Buchtel HA, et al: A preliminary report of short-term cognitive-behavioral group therapy for inpatients with personality disorders. The Journal of Psychotherapy Practice and Research 5:57–71, 1996

Steuer JL, Mintz J, Hammen CL, et al: Cognitive-behavioral and psychodynamic group psychotherapy in treatment of geriatric depression. J Consult Clin Psychol 52:180–189, 1984

Stuart S, Bowers WA: Cognitive therapy with inpatients: review and meta-analysis. Journal of Cognitive Psychotherapy: An International Quarterly 9:85–92, 1995

Stuart S, LaRue S: Computerized cognitive therapy: the interface between man and machine. Journal of Cognitive Psychotherapy: An International Quarterly 10:181–191, 1996

Stuart S, Wright JH, Thase ME, et al: Cognitive therapy with inpatients. General Hospital Psychiatry 19:42–50, 1997

Sullivan HS: Interpersonal Theory of Psychiatry. New York, WW Norton, 1953

Tarrier N, Maguire P: Treatment of psychological distress following mastectomy: an initial report. Behav Res Ther 22:81–84, 1984

Tarrier N, Beckett R, Harwoods S, et al: A trial of two cognitive-behavioral methods of treating drug-resistant residual psychotic symptoms in schizophrenic patients; I: outcome. Br J Psychiatry 162:524–532, 1993

Taylor S: Meta-analysis of cognitive-behavioral treatments for social phobia. J Behav Ther Exp Psychiatry 27:1–9, 1996

Teasdale JD, Fogarty SJ: Differential effects of induced mood on retrieval of pleasant and unpleasant events from episodic memory. J Abnorm Psychol 88:248–257, 1979

Teasdale JD, Fennell MJV, Hibbert GA, et al: Cognitive therapy for major depressive disorder in primary care. Br J Psychiatry 144:400–406, 1984

Thackwray DE, Smith MC, Bodfish JW, et al: A comparison of behavioral and cognitive-behavioral interventions for bulimia nervosa. J Consult Clin Psychol 61:639–645, 1993

Thase ME: Transition and aftercare, in Cognitive Therapy With Inpatients: Developing a Cognitive Milieu. Edited by Wright JH, Thase ME, Beck AT, et al. New York, Guilford, 1992, pp 414–435

Thase ME: Reeducative psychotherapies, in Treatments of Psychiatric Disorder. Edited Gabbard GO. Washington, DC, American Psychiatric Press, 1995, pp 1199–1204

Thase ME: Cognitive-behavioral therapy for substance abuse disorders, in Review of Psychiatry, Vol 16. Edited by Dickstein LJ, Riba MB, Oldham JM. Washington, DC, American Psychiatric Press, 1997, pp I45–I71

Thase ME, Beck AT: An overview of cognitive therapy, in Cognitive Therapy With Inpatients: Developing a Cognitive Milieu. Edited by Wright JH, Thase ME, Beck AT, et al. New York, Guilford, 1992, pp 3–35

Thase ME, Wright JH: Cognitive behavioral therapy with depressed inpatients: an abridged treatment manual. Behavior Therapy 22:579–595, 1991

Thase ME, Bowler K, Harden T: Cognitive behavior therapy of endogenous depression, part 2; preliminary findings in 16 unmedicated patients. Behavior Therapy 22:469–477, 1991

Thase ME, Simons AD, Reynolds III CF: Psychobiological correlates of poor response to cognitive behavior therapy: potential indications for antidepressant pharmacotherapy. Psychopharmacol Bull 29:293–301, 1993

Thase ME, Reynolds III CF, Frank E, et al: Polysomnographic studies of unmedicated depressed men before and after cognitive behavioral therapy. Am J Psychiatry 151:1615–1622, 1994a

Thase ME, Reynolds III CF, Frank E, et al: Response to cognitive-behavioral therapy in chronic depression. Journal of Psychotherapy Practice and Research 3:204–214, 1994b

Thase ME, Simons AD, Reynolds III CF: Abnormal electroencephalographic sleep profiles in major depression. Arch Gen Psychiatry 53:99–108, 1996a

Thase ME, Dube S, Bowler K, et al: Hypothalamic-pituitary-adrenocortical activity and response to cognitive behavior therapy in unmedicated, hospitalized depressed patients. Am J Psychiatry 153:886–891, 1996b

Thompson LW: Cognitive-behavioral therapy and treatment for late-life depression. J Clin Psychiatry 57 (suppl 5):29–37, 1996

Traux CB, Mitchell KM: Research on certain therapist interpersonal skills in relation to process and outcome, in Handbook of Psychotherapy and Behavior Change: An Empirical Analysis. Edited by Bergin AE, Garfield SL. New York, Wiley, 1971, pp 299–344

Turk DC, Meichenbaum D, Genest M: Pain and behavioral medicine: a cognitive-behavioral perspective. New York, Guilford, 1983

Turner JA, Clancy S: Strategies for coping with chronic low back pain: relationship to pain and disability. Pain 24:355–364, 1986

Van Oppen P, De Haan E, Van Balkom AJLM, et al: Cognitive therapy and exposure in vivo in the treatment of obsessive compulsive disorder. Behav Res Ther 33:379–390, 1995

Wallace ST, Alden LE: A comparison of social standards and perceived ability in anxious and nonanxious men. Cognitive Therapy and Research 15:237–254, 1991

Warwick HM, Salkovskis PM: Hypochondriasis. Behav Res Ther 28:105–117, 1990

Watkins JT, Rush AJ: Cognitive response test. Cognitive Therapy and Research 7:125–126, 1983

Weingartner H, Cohen RM, Murphy DL, et al: Cognitive processes in depression. Arch Gen Psychiatry 38:42–47, 1981

Weissman AN: The dysfunctional attitude scale: a validation study. Dissertation Abstracts International 40:1389B–1390B, 1979

Welkowitz LA, Papp LA, Cloitre M, et al: Cognitive-behavior therapy for panic disorder delivered by psychopharmacologically oriented clinicians. J Nerv Ment Dis 179:473–477, 1991

Wells EA, Peterson PL, Gainey RR, et al: Outpatient treatment for cocaine abuse: a controlled comparison of relapse prevention and twelve-step approaches. Am J Drug Alcohol Abuse 20:1–17, 1994

Wenzloff RM, Grozier SA: Depression and the magnification of failure. J Abnorm Psychol 97:90–93, 1988

Westling BE, Ost L: Cognitive bias in panic disorder patients and changes after cognitive-behavioral treatments. Behav Res Ther 33:585–588, 1995

Wetzel R, Murphy G, Carney R, et al: Prescribing therapy for depression: the role of learned resourcefulness, a failure to replicate. Psychol Rep 70:803–807, 1992

Whisman MA, Miller IW, Norman WH, et al: Cognitive therapy with depressed inpatients: specific effects on dysfunctional cognitions. J Consult Clin Psychol 59:282–288, 1991

White KP, Nielson WR: Cognitive behavioral treatment of fibromyalgia syndrome: a follow-up assessment. J Rheumatology 22:717–721, 1995

Wilson KCM, Scott M, Abou-Saleh M, et al: Long-term effects of cognitive-behavioural therapy and lithium therapy on depression in the elderly. Br J Psychiatry 167:653–658, 1995

Wolpe J: The Practice of Behavior Therapy. New York, Pergamon, 1969

Woody GE, Luborsky L, McLellan AT, et al: Psychotherapy for opiate addicts: does it help? Arch Gen Psychiatry 40:639–645, 1983

Wright FD, Beck AT, Newman CF, et al: Cognitive therapy of substance abuse: theoretical rationale. NIDA Res Monogr 137:123–146, 1993

Wright JH: Cognitive therapy of depression, in The American Psychiatric Press Review of Psychiatry, Vol 7. Edited by Frances AJ, Hales RE. Washington, DC, American Psychiatric Press, 1988, pp 554–590

Wright JH, Beck AT: Cognitive therapy of depression: theory and practice. Hospital and Community Psychiatry 34:1119–1127, 1983

Wright JH, Beck AT: Family cognitive therapy with inpatients, in Cognitive Therapy With Inpatients: Developing a Cognitive Milieu. Edited by Wright JH, Thase ME, Beck AT, et al. New York, Guilford, 176–191, 1992

Wright JH, Borden J: Cognitive therapy of depression and anxiety. Psychiatric Annals 21:424–428, 1992

Wright JH, Davis MH: Hospital psychiatry in transition, in Cognitive Therapy With Inpatients: Developing a Cognitive Milieu. Edited by Wright JH, Thase ME, Beck AT, et al. New York, Guilford, 1992, pp 193–218

Wright JH, Salmon PG: Learning and memory in depression, in Depression: New Directions in Theory, Research, and Practice. Edited by McCann CD, Endler NS. Toronto, Canada, Wall & Thompson, 1990, pp 211–236

Wright JH, Schrodt GR Jr: Combined cognitive therapy and pharmacotherapy, in Handbook of Cognitive Therapy. Edited by Freeman A, Simon MK, Arkowitz H, et al. New York, Plenum, 1989, pp 267–283

Wright JH, Thase ME: Cognitive and biological therapies: a synthesis. Psychiatric Annals 22:451–458, 1992

Wright JH, Wright AS: Performance tracking in computer-assisted cognitive therapy. Presented at the Annual Meeting of the American Psychiatric Association, New York, NY, May 1996

Wright JH, Wright AS: Computer-assisted psychotherapy. J Psychother Pract Res 6:315–329, 1997

Wright JH, Thase ME, Beck AT, et al (eds): Cognitive Therapy With Inpatients: Developing a Cognitive Milieu. New York, Guilford, 1992a

Wright JH, Thase ME, Sensky T: Cognitive and biological therapies: a combined approach, in Cogntive Therapy With Inpatients: Developing a Cognitive Milieu. Edited by Wright JH, Thase ME, Beck AT, et al. New York, Guilford, 1992b, pp 193–218

Wright JH, Salmon P, Wright AS, et al: Cognitive Therapy: A Multimedia Learning Program. Louisville, KY, MindStreet, 1995a

Wright JH, Salmon P, Wright AS, et al: Cognitive Therapy: A Multimedia Learning Program. Presented at the Annual Meeting of the American Psychiatric Association, Miami Beach, FL, May 1995b

Young JE, Beck AT: Cognitive therapy: clinical applications, in Short-Term Psychotherpies for Depression. Edited by Rush, AJ. New York, Guilford, 1982, pp 182–214

Young JE, Lindemann MD: An integrative schema-focused model for personality disorders. Journal of Cognitive Psychotherapy: An International Quarterly 6:11–23, 1992

Zautra JH, Guenther RT, Chartier GM: Attributions for real and hypothetical events: their relation to self-esteem and depression. J Abnorm Psychol 94:530–540, 1985

Zettle RD, Rains JC: Group cognitive and contextual therapies in treatment of depression. J Clin Psychol 45:436–445, 1989

Zimmerman M, Coryell W, Corenthal C, et al: Dysfuntional attitudes and attribution style in healthy controls and patients with schizophrenia, psychotic depression, and nonpsychotic depression. J Abnorm Psychol 95:403–405, 1986

Zotter DL, Crowther JH: The role of cognitions in bulimia nervosa. Cognitive Therapy and Research 15:413–426, 1991

CHAPTER 32

HYPNOSIS

DAVID SPIEGEL, M.D.
JOSE R. MALDONADO, M.D.

Hypnosis is a natural state of aroused, attentive focal concentration with a relative suspension of peripheral awareness. It involves an intensity of focus that allows the hypnotized person to make maximal use of innate abilities to control perception, memory, and somatic function. Hypnotic capacity represents both a potential vulnerability to certain kinds of psychiatric illness, such as posttraumatic stress and dissociative disorders, and an asset, in that it facilitates various psychotherapeutic strategies. Because it is a normal and widely distributed trait, and because entry into hypnotic states occurs spontaneously, hypnotic phenomena occur frequently. Even psychiatrists who make no formal use of hypnosis can enhance their effectiveness by learning to recognize and take advantage of hypnotic mental states.

HISTORY

Trance experiences have been described at least as far back as the time of the ancient Greeks, often as vehicles for treatment of mental or physical illness. In non-Western cultures, such experiences tended to be the domain of the healer, who entered a dissociative state as part of the healing ceremony. Frequently, however, these ceremonies were public and invited both patient and observers to enter the trance state as well.

Hypnosis was identified as a formal phenomenon of psychotherapeutic interest in the 18th century. Franz Anton Mesmer employed it as an alternative treatment for many ills that we would now label as stress-related or psychosomatic (Lopez 1993). His work is credited with being the first Western conceptualization of a psychotherapy (Ellenberger 1970), a therapeutic talking interaction between doctor and patient. Shortly thereafter, Louis XVI (1784) appointed two commissions to investigate the phenomenon (known as "animal magnetism") and Mesmer's claims of medical efficacy. The infamous Dr. Guillotin headed one commission; the other, made up of five members of the Academy of Sciences, was headed by Benjamin Franklin, American ambassador to France. Both commissions concluded that the success of mesmerism was due to the manipulation of the imagination. Nevertheless, the panel acknowledged that the phenomenon of suggestion, the influence of one individual on another, was at the root of social order as well as personal change. Despite this official rejection, hypnosis persisted in one form or another for two centuries as a treatment tool involving the therapeutic use of this special alteration in consciousness.

In the 19th century, interest in hypnosis persisted in this country as evidenced by the writings of William James (1890), Boris Sidis (1898), and Morton Prince (founder of the *Journal of Abnormal Psychology*), all of whom were fascinated by the extreme symptoms observed in patients with such dissociative symptoms as multiple personality disorder (renamed *dissociative identity disorder* in DSM-IV [American Psychiatric Association 1994]). On the Continent, serious practitioners such as Braid (1843) and Esdaile (Ernst 1995; Esdaile 1846/1957) used hypnosis to treat symptoms, which included pain and anxiety. Janet (1907) built a theory of the unconscious involving compartmentalization of memory that differed from Freud's model in that it was horizontal rather than vertical and archaeological (E. R. Hilgard 1977). Information kept out of awareness was relatively untransformed and could be accessed directly, using techniques such as hypnosis, which Janet also utilized as evidence of experimentally induced pathology. Breuer and Freud (1893–1895/1955) used hypnotic age regression to treat hysterical symptoms and began to develop their theory linking unconscious determinants to conscious symptoms. They considered "hypnoid" states the building blocks of hysterical symptomatology and accurately observed that hypnotic processes could be normal and yet were often mobilized in the service of resolving an unconscious conflict. Hypnoid states were seen as the vehicle for expressing conflicts rather than the cause of them or pathological in themselves. Later, attributing the phenomenon to transference, Freud (1925[1924]/1959) abandoned hypnosis as a technique in favor of free association after a patient emerging from a hypnotic session threw her arms around him.

In the early part of the 20th century, there was relatively little clinical use of hypnosis, although new treatment techniques were developed and promulgated (cf. Erickson 1967). Interest revived during World War II, when army psychiatrists found the technique helpful in treating what was then called "traumatic neurosis" (Kardiner and Spiegel 1947). An era of serious laboratory investigation of the phenomenon began in the 1950s with the development of several hypnotizability scales (Stanford Hypnotic Susceptibility Scales [E. R. Hilgard 1965; Weitzenhoffer and Hilgard 1959, 1962]). By the 1970s, several shorter hypnotizability scales were in use in clinical settings (Stanford Hypnotic Clinical Scale [E. R. Hilgard and Hilgard 1975], Hypnotic Induction Profile [H. Spiegel and Spiegel 1987]). Investigations ranged from studies of the relationships among hypnotizability, placebo response, and acupuncture, to studies of the differential hypnotizability of patients with psychosis and other psychiatric disorders, to investigations to determine neurophysiological correlates of the hypnotic state and hypnotic capacity, all with varying success.

In the mid-1950s, the American Medical Association and the American Psychiatric Association officially recognized hypnosis as a legitimate therapeutic tool. Two professional hypnosis societies have emerged—the Society for Clinical and Experimental Hypnosis, which emphasizes research in the field, and the American Society for Clinical Hypnosis—and each publishes a journal. Hypnosis is now taught in many major medical schools. A division of the American Psychological Association (Division 30) is devoted to the study of hypnosis, and the use of hypnosis in clinical and investigational areas is increasing.

DEFINITION

Alterations in consciousness occur frequently in the course of ordinary life: at moments of physical or psychological stress, as a result of formal instruction or direction, in the diurnal sleep-wake cycle, and with the use of a variety of psychoactive substances (H. Spiegel 1963). Indeed, such cyclic variation is the norm, not the exception. Sleep is requisite for normal attention, and it may also be that alterations within wakefulness optimize attentional processes. Certain variations in consciousness may change the relationship between mental and physical states and alter the degree to which concentration is focused. One of these alterations in consciousness is *hypnosis*, a naturally occurring phenomenon in which focal concentration is intensified at the expense of peripheral awareness.

Hypnosis is a state of attentive, receptive concentration with a relative suspension of peripheral awareness. Hypnotic phenomena occur spontaneously, and the alteration of consciousness that hypnotized individuals experience has a variety of therapeutic applications. Hypnotic experience involves three main factors: absorption, dissociation, and suggestibility. Each of these factors is discussed here (see Figure 32–1).

ABSORPTION

Absorption is immersion in a central experience at the expense of contextual orientation (J. R. Hilgard 1970; Tellegen 1981; Tellegen and Atkinson 1974). When one is intensely involved in a central object of consciousness, one tends to ignore perceptions, thoughts, memories, or motor activities at the periphery. Hypnotized individuals are intensely absorbed in their trance experience. In a hypnotic age regression, subjects act as though they were younger, suspending awareness that they really are

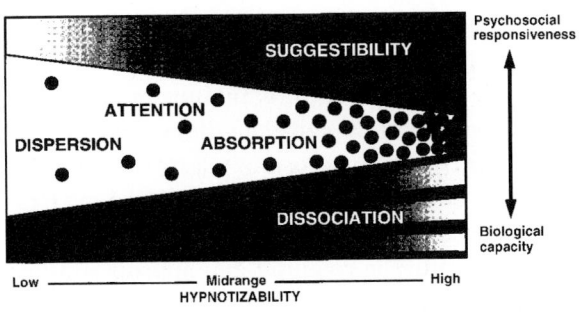

FIGURE 32-1. Continuum of attention and dissociation. This diagram depicts the spectrum of normal attentional focus. Hypnotic phenomena are characterized by intense absorption, with accompanying enhanced dissociation and suggestibility.

decades older than the assumed age. The subjects are aware of the incongruity of the situation or suggestion, yet they easily ignore it. This makes the experience of acting like a 3-year-old more vivid, because it is not plagued by disbelief and critical evaluation.

Research has shown a correlation between hypnotizability and a spontaneous tendency for people to undergo absorbing experiences (Tellegen and Atkinson 1974). Thus, those who tend to get so caught up in a movie that they lose awareness of being in a theater are in a trancelike state and are relatively more hypnotizable. What a person in a hypnotic trance concentrates on is attended to relatively completely.

DISSOCIATION

This intense absorption means that many routine experiences that would ordinarily be conscious occur out of ordinary conscious awareness. Even complex emotional states or sensory experiences may be dissociated. These experiences may range from the simple, such as a feeling that the hand is not as much a part of the body as usual, to the complex. Some involve memory alterations, such as dissociative amnesia for a traumatic event, whereas others pertain to identity and motor function, as in a fugue episode in which for a period of hours to months an individual functions as though he or she had a different name and residence. Such experiences can be both induced and reversed with the structured use of hypnosis.

Dissociated information is temporarily and reversibly unavailable to consciousness but may nonetheless influence conscious (or other unconscious) experience. A rape victim may have no conscious memory of the crime but may become anxious when exposed to stimuli reminiscent of the event. Absorption and dissociation are complemen-

tary constructs. Intense focal attention facilitates putting other information outside conscious awareness.

SUGGESTIBILITY

Suggestibility is enhanced in hypnosis. Because of their intense absorption in the trance experience, hypnotized individuals usually accept instructions relatively uncritically (hence the term *suggestibility*). Although hypnotized individuals are not deprived of their will, they do have a tendency to accept instructions in a trance uncritically, suspending the usual conscious editing function that raises the question "Why?" when an instruction is given. Thus, hypnotized individuals are more prone to accept directions, no matter how irrational. They are also less prone to distinguish an instruction as coming from another rather than from themselves (i.e., hypnotic source amnesia) and so will tend to act on another person's ideas as though they were their own. Thus, a hypnotized individual is especially vulnerable to the nature of the therapeutic intervention; the trance state can enhance responsiveness, either for good or for ill.

MYTHS DISPELLED

There are a variety of common "mythunderstandings" about hypnosis (Table 32–1).

1. **Hypnosis is not sleep.** The most prevalent misunderstanding derives from the name itself: the Greek root *hypnos* means "sleep." The hypnotized individual is not asleep but rather is awake and alert. Like a sleeping person, a hypnotized individual has suspended peripheral awareness but, in contrast to what occurs in sleep, his or her focal attention is intense and carefully controlled. The power spectral electroencephalogram (EEG) of hypnotized individuals shows a pattern consistent with resting alertness rather than sleep.

TABLE 32-1. Corrections of common myths about hypnosis

Hypnosis is not sleep.

Hypnotizability is a trait: not everyone is hypnotizable.

Hypnosis is not something *done to* a subject or patient.

Hypnotizability is *not* a susceptibility or a sign of weak-mindedness.

There is nothing intrinsically dangerous about hypnosis.

There is nothing intrinsically therapeutic about hypnosis.

2. **Hypnotizability is a trait: not everyone is hypnotizable.** Hypnotizability is a capacity that varies considerably from one individual to another. Indeed, hypnotizability is a stable and measurable trait, as consistent over a 25-year interval in adulthood as is intelligence (Piccione et al. 1989). Hypnotizability is greatest in late childhood and decreases gradually throughout adulthood. About 1 of 4 adults is not hypnotizable, and 1 of 10 is highly hypnotizable (H. Spiegel and Spiegel 1987).

3. **Hypnosis is not something *done to* a subject or patient.** Recognition of this fact is helpful for demystifying hypnosis and reducing anxiety on the part of both the doctor inducing hypnosis and the patient. The doctor is not doing something *to* the patient. Rather, a doctor inducing hypnosis is in the position of the Socratic teacher, one who helps students discover what they already know. A correctly performed hypnotic induction allows the patient and doctor to assess and explore the patient's hypnotic capacity or lack of it. This approach tends to minimize power struggles between doctor and patient. For example, there is less chance of misinterpreting a patient's inability to experience a hypnotic trance as resistance. On the other hand, some therapists become frightened when working with an extremely hypnotizable patient, because they think that they have imposed an extreme transformation of consciousness on the patient, when in fact they have merely identified and mobilized it. There are no apparent gender differences in hypnotizability—men and women are equally hypnotizable (Stern et al. 1979).

4. **Hypnotizability is *not* a susceptibility or a sign of weak-mindedness.** Rather, it is an intact capacity for focused concentration that is often associated with, if anything, the absence of serious psychotic and neurological disorders.

5. **There is nothing intrinsically dangerous about hypnosis.** Hypnosis is a benign procedure that is tolerated well by patients. The same cognitive flexibility that allows patients to enter the trance facilitates their exit from it with clear structure and support from the therapist. There are few serious contraindications for the use of hypnosis. It is not in itself a dangerous procedure. Indeed, most patients find it relaxing. An occasional patient is slow in exiting from the hypnotic state. Calm reassurance never fails to complete the termination of the trance procedure. Rarely, a paranoid patient may incorporate the attempted hypnotic induction into a delusional system, although careful explanation of the procedures in advance and the use of a hypnotizability test as an initial encounter tend to minimize the likelihood of this occurring. A suicidally depressed patient may view the use of hypnosis as a last resort and become dangerously disappointed if he or she perceives it as a failure. As with any intervention, careful basic clinical screening is required and appropriate management is necessary, but the procedure itself is, in general, benign and well accepted by patients.

6. **There is nothing intrinsically therapeutic about hypnosis.** Hypnosis is not in and of itself a therapy. Many patients find it a relaxing and comfortable state and may be reassured by the fact that they can produce in a formal state of hypnosis some or all of the symptoms they have experienced spontaneously, such as conversion symptoms, hysterical seizures, or fugue episodes. The use to which the trance state is put, however, is the crucial issue in determining treatment outcome.

MEASURING HYPNOTIZABILITY

RATIONALE

Because hypnotizability is a stable and measurable trait, a clinical assessment of hypnotizability can be a helpful starting point for the use of hypnosis in treatment (H. Spiegel and Spiegel 1987). This approach combines a hypnotic induction with a procedure that provides the psychiatrist with a deduction of the patient's hypnotic ability. It has several advantages:

1. Hypnotizability testing helps to clarify the hypnotic interaction. It is the therapist's role to assess systematically patients' ability to respond rather than to push them to respond in a certain manner. Such a dispassionate hypnotic induction reduces pressure on therapists to prove their ability to put a patient into a hypnotic state. Likewise, it reduces the sense of pressure on the patient to either comply or resist. Rather, the testing setting creates an atmosphere of scientific exploration that encourages rather than coerces involvement.

2. The use of such a standardized interaction with a large number of patients allows the psychiatrist to make informed inferences about variations in patient response. Patients' relative ability (or inability) to allow the therapist to restructure their inner experience via hypnosis also provides helpful information about their general interpersonal style. For example,

highly hypnotizable individuals generally rate themselves as more trusting than do those who are not hypnotizable (Roberts and Tellegen 1973). In addition, hypnotizability testing provides information of relevance to differential diagnosis, as will be discussed later in this chapter.

3. Hypnotizability testing provides data about the patient's ability to respond to a treatment that employs hypnosis. Highly hypnotizable individuals can be rationally encouraged. Nonhypnotizable individuals can be offered an alternative approach that is likely to be more efficacious, such as one of the behavioral therapies, biofeedback, or relevant psychoactive medication.

HYPNOTIZABILITY SCALES

Hypnotizability scales have existed since the early part of the century and have been widely used in research—for example, the Stanford Hypnotic Susceptibility Scales, Forms A and B (SHSS:A) and Form C (SHSS:C) (E. R. Hilgard 1965; Weitzenhoffer and Hilgard 1959, 1962). These scales involve a structured hypnotic induction and an assessment of the subject's response to a variety of instructions, including alterations in control over movement, sensation, temporal orientation, and perception, such as hallucinatory experiences. More recently, hypnotizability scales have been developed for clinical use (Hypnotic Induction Profile [HIP; H. Spiegel and Spiegel 1987], Stanford Hypnotic Clinical Scale [SHCS; E. R. Hilgard and Hilgard 1975]). These scales are briefer (5–10 minutes for the HIP and 20 minutes for the SHCS, compared with 1 hour for the Stanford research scales) and are designed for use even with patients who have severe psychiatric disturbances.

The HIP calls for rapid induction commencing with upward gaze and lowering of the eyelids, followed by a series of instructions to the subject to elevate the left hand and keep it in the air, even if the examiner pulls the hand down. Subjects are rated on five items assessing cognitive and behavioral aspects of the hypnotic experience (Table 32–2): 1) their ability to experience a sense of *dissociation* of

TABLE 32–2. Responses measured in the Hypnotic Induction Profile

Dissociation

Movement

Involuntariness

Cut-off signal ending hypnotic instruction

Sensory alteration

the left hand from the body; 2) *movement* of the hand, its floating back up in the air after being pulled down, accompanied by 3) a sense of *involuntariness* during elevation of the hand; 4) response to the *cut-off signal* ending the hypnotic experience; and 5) a *sensory alteration* in the hand or elsewhere in the body. The entire procedure can be administered and the scoring done in less than 10 minutes. It predicts responsiveness to a variety of treatments and facilitates differential diagnosis (see Figure 32–2) (H. Spiegel and Spiegel 1987; D. Spiegel et al. 1982, 1988).

PREDICTION OF TREATMENT RESPONSIVENESS

Because hypnotic trance involves an intensification of concentration and an increase in receptiveness, it would make sense that the capacity to experience hypnosis should be correlated with responsiveness to treatment. Indeed, this has been found to be the case in treatment with hypnosis of problems such as pain (E. R. Hilgard and Hilgard 1975), smoking cessation (H. Spiegel and Spiegel 1987; D. Spiegel et al. 1993a), and asthma (Collison 1975). Hypnotizability is also correlated with the increased likelihood of responding even to treatments that do not explicitly employ hypnosis, such as acupuncture (Katz et al. 1974).

HYPNOTIZABILITY AND PSYCHIATRIC DISORDERS

One of the most interesting theoretical areas of research in hypnosis is the relationship between hypnotizability and

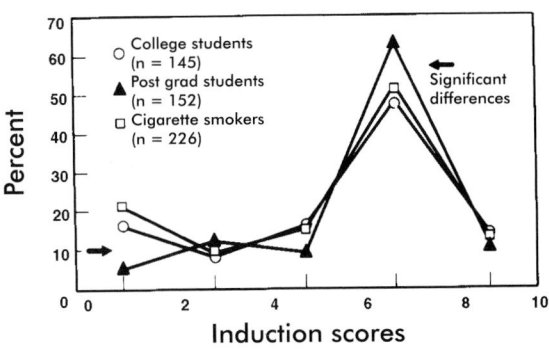

FIGURE 32–2. Hypnotizability as measured by the Hypnotic Induction Profile in three populations. The variance accounted for by motivational differences may be reflected in the slightly higher scores of postdoctoral students enrolled in a hypnosis course.

Source. D. Spiegel, E. Frischholz, unpublished data, 1980.

psychopathology (Figure 32–3). There is accumulating evidence that high hypnotizability is associated with some serious psychiatric disorders.

HYPNOTIZABILITY IN DISSOCIATIVE IDENTITY DISORDER

Clinicians have long observed that it is unusual to find a patient with a severe dissociative disorder such as fugue, amnesia, or dissociative identity disorder (i.e., multiple personality disorder) who is not highly hypnotizable (see also Chapter 18 in this textbook; Frischholz 1985; Maldonado and Spiegel 1997). The recent literature on dissociative identity disorder indicates that most patients with this disorder are highly hypnotizable and report a history of severe physical and sexual abuse in childhood (Braun and Sachs 1985; Kluft 1985; Maldonado and Spiegel 1997; Maldonado et al. 1997; D. Spiegel 1984). This observation has led to the recognition that the capacity to dissociate—to separate, for example, psychological from physical experience—is mobilized both during and after periods of extreme physical duress such as assault (Bremner and Brett 1997; Butler et al. 1996; Eriksson and Lundin 1996; Kluft 1984a, 1984b; Koopman et al. 1995; Putnam 1985; D. Spiegel 1984, 1986, 1988, 1990; D. Spiegel et al. 1988; van der Kolk and van der Hart 1989; Wood and Sexton 1997). In some cases, especially cases of repeated, severe assault in childhood, a temporary dissociation that allows

the child to tolerate overwhelming fear and pain becomes an ongoing part of the personality structure, and thus the posttraumatic stress disorder (PTSD) takes the form of dissociated selves, one of whom suffered and, indeed, in the unconscious, "deserved" the pain and humiliation, others of whom take the stance of protecting the patient from further injury. Because the hypnotic state can be induced in a matter of seconds, and hypnotizability is associated with a higher frequency of spontaneously occurring hypnotic-like experiences, it makes sense that individuals who are highly hypnotizable will have spontaneously mobilized this capacity, especially in the face of serious environmental stress, as in the following example:

> A 16-year-old girl had been beaten by her father during a dispute with her mother when the patient was 4 years old. The girl began developing dissociative episodes in which she would suddenly act and talk like a 4-year-old child. She had no memories of these episodes after they occurred, and they could last for several hours.

[The dissociation between her normal and dissociated mental state is illustrated in Figure 32–4. Both drawings of the same theme, the patient standing next to a tree with her mother, were drawn within a 10-minute period—the former during hypnotically induced dissociation, the latter afterward. The difference in drawing style is clear, as is the disturbed nature of the "4-year-old's" drawing. *Faceless people are floating in air, and the sky merges with the tree.* The other drawing is more age appropriate, and the figures have a kind of stiff placidity (D. Spiegel and Rosenfeld 1984).]

> The patient had dissociated memories and affects associated with this assault by her father. They reemerged much later when she was sexually exploited by an employer. After months of hospitalization, she learned to use self-hypnosis not only to face past traumatic experiences but also in an effort to protect herself. She came to experience the dissociated state as a "protective light" that surrounded her.

Hypnosis is useful early in the treatment of such patients, first, in determining whether they have a dissociative disorder, and, second, in providing rapid access to these dissociated states. This process can be used to demonstrate for these patients how to control dissociation and to begin a process of communication that in the context of well-structured psychotherapy can eventually lead to a reduction in such spontaneous dissociative symptoms. It is important that the impact of whatever physical trauma occurred be recognized and taken into account in the therapy and that the therapy help such patients work through their reactions to that impact. Recognizing and teaching

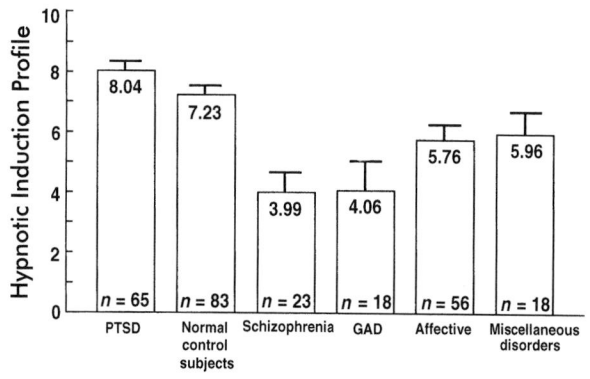

FIGURE 32–3. Psychopathology and hypnotizability. Hypnotic Induction Profile scores indicate higher than normal responsiveness among patients with posttraumatic stress disorder but lower responsiveness among other psychiatric patient groups. PTSD = posttraumatic stress disorder; GAD = generalized anxiety disorder.
Source. Reprinted with permission from Spiegel D, Hunt T, Dondershine HE: "Dissociation and Hypnotizability in Posttraumatic Stress Disorder." *American Journal of Psychiatry* 145:301–305, 1988.

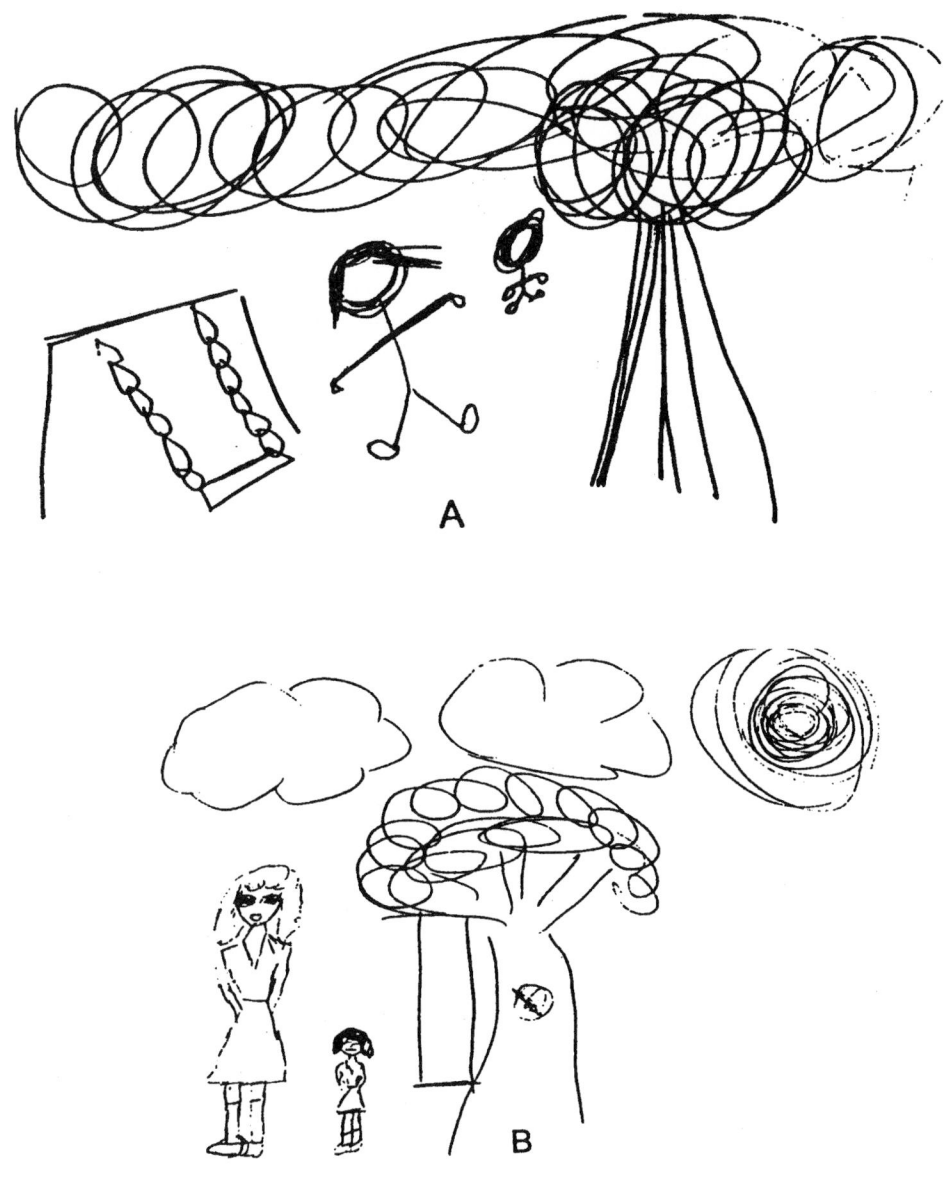

FIGURE 32–4. Hypnotic age regression. Drawings made during *(A)* and after *(B)* hypnotically induced dissociation during which this 16-year-old patient experienced herself as 4 years old.

patients with dissociative disorders how to master this capacity is an important psychotherapeutic task (see Chapter 18).

The capacity for hypnotic dissociation has been found to be relevant to a milder but pronounced cluster of symptoms labeled the "Grade 5 syndrome" (H. Spiegel 1974). This cluster has many similarities to the DSM Axis II histrionic personality disorder diagnosis. Patients with these symptoms, who are highly hypnotizable, repeatedly establish naive and dependent relationships, often express symptoms in dramatic ways, are sluggish in reorienting to internal rather than external cues, and form intense affiliations with new ideas and persons, affiliations that tend not to last over time. These patients require a tightly structured, supportive psychotherapy that recognizes their tendency unwittingly to build relationships in which they are vulnerable to control by others. One such patient described herself as a "disciple in search of a teacher." Individuals who in the setting of hypnotizability testing are less able to allow the therapist to restructure their internal world may, in general, be more defended against the influence of other people, whereas those who are highly hypnotizable on formal testing may in less formal circumstances likewise allow other people to reorient them in a hypnotic-like way. In this sense, the hypnotic encounter can be seen as a kind of crystallized transference, a sample of the patient's general style of relating to others.

HYPNOTIZABILITY IN PHOBIC AND ANXIETY DISORDERS

Several studies have proffered evidence that phobic individuals are more highly hypnotizable than are control populations (Frankel and Orne 1976; Gerschman et al. 1979), although other studies have failed to replicate this finding (Frischholz et al. 1982). It is possible that some kinds of phobic symptoms mobilize dissociative capacity, with the symptom representing absorption in the fear of the situation and suspension of critical judgment about it. However, patients with generalized anxiety disorder (GAD) have markedly lower scores than do subjects without the disorder (D. Spiegel et al. 1982). Those patients with GAD who take benzodiazepines tend to have higher hypnotizability scores than do those who are untreated (D. Spiegel 1980).

HYPNOTIZABILITY IN EATING DISORDERS

Pettinati and colleagues (1990) administered both the SHSS:C and the HIP to patients with bulimia and anorexia nervosa. The authors observed higher hypnotizability in the bulimic patients than in the restricting patients. These researchers noted that many of the bulimic patients reported that they were in a trancelike state when they engaged in their compulsive bingeing and purging behavior. Vanderlinden et al. (1995) found that compared with control subjects, eating disorder patients scored significantly higher on the Dissociation-Questionnaire (DIS-Q) and the Stanford Hypnotic Clinical Scale (SHCS). Covino et al. (1994) examined the levels of hypnotizability and dissociation in an outpatient sample of bulimic women of normal weight and compared these levels with those of healthy controls. They found that bulimic patients were significantly more hypnotizable than were controls and that they scored higher on self-report scales of dissociative experiences. These findings suggest a possible opportunity for intervention employing hypnosis in controlling this form of eating disorder (Gross 1984).

HYPNOTIZABILITY IN SCHIZOPHRENIA AND AFFECTIVE DISORDERS

As far back as 1937, Copeland and Kitching observed that presumedly psychotic patients who were hypnotizable were not genuinely psychotic. Given the complex cognitive tasks involved in tests of hypnotic responsiveness, it makes sense theoretically that patients experiencing delusions, loose associations, and hallucinations might score more poorly on tests of hypnotizability, as they do on most other psychological tests. On the other hand, because hallucinations can be produced artificially in hypnotic states, some investigators have predicted that schizophrenic individuals should be equally or even more hypnotizable than subjects without schizophrenia. More than 20 studies have been conducted on the issue, and the findings have generally shown somewhat lower, and the absence of very high, hypnotizability among schizophrenic patients (Lavoie and Sabourin 1980; Pettinati 1982). Schizophrenic patients show a more restricted range of scores, and those who do better on psychological tests such as the Rorschach are more hypnotizable than those who display more thought disorganization.

Psychotic patients, especially those with schizophrenia, score differently on hypnotizability scales than do nonpsychotic individuals. Their scores on the HIP are substantially lower than those of control samples (Pettinati 1982; Pettinati et al. 1990; D. Spiegel et al. 1982). Mean scores of schizophrenic patients have not been found to be lower than those of psychiatrically healthy individuals in studies employing the SHSS (Lavoie and Elie 1985; Lavoie and Sabourin 1980; Pettinati 1982; Pettinati et al. 1990). However, these studies show lower variance in scores, which means there is a relative absence of very high hypnotizability among schizophrenic patients. Furthermore, Lavoie and Elie (1985) found significantly fewer autistic forms of primary process on the Rorschach tests of the more hypnotizable schizophrenic patients. Thus, schizophrenic patients show impairment that interferes with hypnotic concentration: scores on some scales indicate that these individuals are substantially less hypnotizable, and scores on all measures show very few of them to be highly hypnotizable.

Studies using the HIP have in particular shown substantially lower hypnotizability scores for schizophrenic individuals compared with psychiatrically healthy subjects (Pettinati 1982; D. Spiegel et al. 1982), whereas those employing the Stanford scales (SHSS:A and SHSS:C; Weitzenhoffer and Hilgard 1959, 1962) have tended to show a restricted range of scores among schizophrenic patients but mean scores that are not significantly lower than those of comparison groups (Lavoie and Sabourin 1980; Pettinati 1982). In addition, patients with major affective disorders have been found to score higher than schizophrenic patients but lower than subjects without schizophrenia (D. Spiegel et al. 1982) (Figure 32–3). These findings were independent of psychoactive medication use (D. Spiegel 1980). Thus, several psychiatric syndromes—schizophrenia, generalized anxiety disorder, and, to a lesser extent, major affective disorder—have been found to be associated with generally lower hypnotic responsiveness. The symptoms of the illness apparently impair expression of a patient's native capacity for hypnotic concentration.

Given these findings, the possibility exists that hypnotizability testing can in certain cases be used to clarify differential diagnosis. For example, it has been increasingly recognized, in part on the basis of genetic data, that an acute psychotic episode is a manifestation of an illness other than chronic and borderline schizophrenia. There is considerable phenomenological overlap among acute psychoses. However, patients with hysterical psychosis or a dissociative disorder should be extremely hypnotizable (D. Spiegel and Fink 1979; Steingard and Frankel 1985; van der Hart and Spiegel 1993). On the other hand, patients with chronic or borderline schizophrenia score at the other end of the hypnotizability spectrum (Lavoie and Sabourin 1980; Pettinati 1982; Pettinati et al. 1990; D. Spiegel and Fink 1979; D. Spiegel et al. 1982; van der Hart and Spiegel 1993).

HYPNOSIS IN TREATMENT

INDICATIONS AND CONTRAINDICATIONS

Hypnosis has been shown to be an effective adjunct to the treatment of a variety of symptoms and problems (Table 32–3). As noted earlier, hypnosis has an important place in the treatment of dissociative disorders—for example, in identifying and controlling dissociative fugue, amnesia, and identity disorder—and in treating PTSD and conversion disorder. Hypnosis also has been widely used in the treatment of anxiety disorders and phobias. A number of studies have demonstrated the efficacy of hypnosis in the treatment of pain. Hypnosis has been useful in the control of such psychosomatic problems as asthma and psoriasis. It has been extensively used in habit control, especially for smoking, and to a lesser extent for weight control.

Use of hypnosis should be considered if the patient has the requisite hypnotizability, indicates he or she will be cooperative during the procedure, and has a problem for which hypnosis has been shown to be of adjunctive utility. The first criterion is measured by hypnotizability testing as discussed above. The second criterion can be met by a brief but frank discussion with the patient about the nature of hypnosis, with clarification of the fact that in hypnosis the doctor does not control the patient but rather explores the patient's capacity to focus and intensify concentration. The therapist should be no more interested in using hypnosis than the patient is, and the extremely rare problems arising from the use of hypnosis can generally be avoided if the procedure is never forced on an unwilling or ambivalent patient.

Although transference and other relationship factors must be taken into account when hypnosis is used in psychotherapy, artificial enhancement of transference distortions can be avoided by this dispassionate approach to hypnotic induction and assessment.

TABLE 32–3. **Uses of hypnosis in psychiatric disorders**

Psychiatric disorder	Hypnotic technique(s)	Goal(s)
Bulimia nervosa	Restructuring relationship to body and eating	To control spontaneous dissociative aspects of impulsive behavior
Conversion disorder	Hypnotizability testing, symptom enhancement, symptom alteration	To help make differential diagnosis and to identify, control, and reduce symptoms
Dissociative disorder	Hypnotizability testing, symptom elicitation, regression, restructuring	To clarify diagnosis, enhance symptom control, facilitate access to dissociative states, and facilitate working through
Phobic and anxiety disorders	Dissociating psychological from somatic distress, screen technique, desensitization	To reduce somatic amplification of anxiety, restructure anxiety-inducing stimuli, and separate stimuli from conditioned response
Posttraumatic stress disorder	Regression, abreaction, restructuring	To enhance control over access to traumatic memories, reduce spontaneous "flashbacks," and facilitate working through
Schizophrenia	Hypnotizability testing	To help make differential diagnosis

APPLICATIONS OF HYPNOSIS IN PSYCHOTHERAPY

Although some psychoanalysts view hypnosis as a contaminant of therapy, Freud himself speculated toward the end of his career that the pure gold of analysis might well have to be alloyed with the baser metal of suggestion. Indeed, the early influence of Charcot as Freud's hypnosis teacher (von Plessen 1996) had a lasting effect; over the psychoanalytic couch in his last office in London, Freud placed a drawing of Charcot inducing hypnosis. Psychotherapies employing hypnosis can use, rather than merely analyze, transference. Hypnosis has been used in intensive psychotherapy as a means of gaining access to repressed memories that have not emerged through use of other techniques—for example, when both the patient and the psychotherapist have worked on resistance issues and believe that some additional leverage is necessary. Such a use of hypnosis comes up particularly in regard to traumatic events that may have occurred during childhood and have been dissociated.

Dissociative Disorders

Hypnosis can be a helpful tool in the psychotherapy of dissociative disorders. Patients with these disorders experience their fugue states, dissociated identities, and conversion symptoms as occurring suddenly and beyond their control. Hypnosis used formally can serve therapeutic as well as diagnostic purposes (Kluft 1993; see also Chapter 18). The controlled access to the hypnotic state often spontaneously triggers the dissociative symptom (e.g., hysterical pseudoseizures). It is possible to induce the symptom—for example, by using age regression and having the patient reexperience the last time the dissociative symptom was present. In this structured manner, the patient can be taught to practice bringing on the symptom and thereby learn to control it, as in the following example:

> A 16-year-old boy was brought to the emergency room writhing and screaming that he was possessed by "demons of Satan." He was initially diagnosed as having schizophrenia and was given antipsychotic medication, to which he did not respond. His history indicated that he had been well until several months earlier, when his girlfriend had left him and he had made a suicide gesture in front of her home. She took him to the local pastor, who referred to the suicide attempt as "Satan's work." The boy then began having possession episodes in which he growled in a strange voice that threatened to put a curse on the patient and to transfer the curse to anyone who tried to interfere. The patient was amnesic for each episode afterward.
>
> The patient was examined with the HIP and scored 10 of 10 points, indicating high hypnotizability. He was then age-regressed to the last possession episode, and he changed abruptly from being polite and subdued, and harboring the delusional belief that he was possessed by a demon, to laughing in a bizarre manner, sniffling, and growling. The regression was ended and he reassumed his more restrained demeanor. He was congratulated for having been able to bring on the possession episode. His parents were encouraged not to panic as they had previously when these episodes occurred and also to change the bedroom arrangement in the home. He had been sharing a room with an older sister, who it turned out had been sexually active with her boyfriend. Within a few weeks the possession episodes stopped, and the patient maintained his improvement for years afterward without the use of antipsychotic medications.

This patient would have met DSM-IV criteria for dissociative identity disorder, although the presentation was atypical in that the symptoms did not begin in early childhood and were circumscribed and resolved fairly rapidly. This assessment and intervention prevented an incorrect diagnosis from being made and the patient's being treated for schizophrenia (D. Spiegel and Fink 1979).

Posttraumatic Stress Disorder

The use of hypnosis in the psychotherapy of trauma was initially thought to be limited to abreaction, based on Freud's cathartic method. The idea was that some intense affect associated with the traumatic event needed to be released and that simply repeating the event with its associated emotion in the trance state would suffice to resolve the symptoms. However, it became clear to Freud (1914/1958) that conscious, cognitive work must be done on the material for it to be successfully worked through.

For therapy to be effective, the patient must reexperience the traumatic events with an enhanced sense of control over the memories of the experience. This may take the form of a symbolic restructuring of the traumatic experiences in hypnosis (H. Spiegel and Spiegel 1987), with the use of a grief work model (D. Spiegel 1981). Hypnosis can be used to provide controlled access to the dissociated or repressed memories of the traumatic experience and then to help patients restructure their memories of the events.

Given the growing evidence that many people enter a dissociated state during physical trauma (Butler et al. 1996; Cardeña and Spiegel 1993; D. Spiegel and Cardeña 1991; van der Kolk and Fisler 1995; van der Kolk et al. 1994), it makes sense that enabling them to enter a structured dissociative state in therapy would facilitate their access to memories of the traumatic experience, memories that must be worked through to resolve the posttraumatic symptomatology. Hypnosis can be helpful in allowing the victim to review aspects of the trauma in a controlled manner. The memories can be experienced for a time with the assurance that they can be put aside afterward. In a trance, patients can be quickly taught how to produce a state of physical relaxation despite whatever psychological stress they experience. They can then find a condensation image that symbolizes some aspect of the trauma.

It is often helpful to have them do this on an imaginary screen, which gives them some sense of distance from the event. It is also useful to divide the screen in half, having the patient picture on one side some aspect of the event (e.g., a rape victim's image of the assailant) and on the other side of the screen something he or she did to protect himself or herself (e.g., struggling with the assailant, talking with him, running away). This enables the patient to restructure his or her view of the assault, facing it, but not simply in the familiar terms of the humiliation, pain, and fear with which it was initially associated. Victims can better acknowledge their helplessness when they also recognize their efforts to protect themselves. Bereaved individuals can picture themselves at the graveside on one side of the screen and at an earlier moment of joy with the deceased on the other side of the screen. They can then be taught a self-hypnosis exercise in which they grieve and work through traumatic memories while enhancing their sense of control over the process (D. Spiegel 1981).

The most distressing thing about a traumatic event is the sense of absolute helplessness that it engenders. This helplessness is reenacted in a PTSD through loss of control over state of mind, with spontaneous dissociative states, startle reactions, or intrusive recollections of the event. Furthermore, such patients may tend to identify the therapist with the assailant and feel that the therapy amounts to a reinflicting of the trauma. It is crucial that the therapy, especially when a technique such as hypnosis is used, be structured so that the process enhances patients' sense of control. This approach can allow patients to integrate the image of themselves as victims with the ongoing, more global image of themselves as persons coping effectively with severe stress, making the repressed material conscious and therefore less powerful and enabling them to establish a new, more congruent self-image and absorb the loss into the ongoing flow of their lives.

The principles of this kind of psychotherapy (Table 32–4) can be summarized with the following eight *C*s:

1. **Confrontation.** It is important to confront the traumatic events directly rather than attribute the symptoms to some long-standing personality problem.

2. **Confession.** It is often necessary to allow such patients to confess deeds or emotions that are embarrassing to them and at times repugnant to the therapist. It is important to help these patients distinguish between misplaced guilt and real remorse. There is always a retrospective wish to change traumatic circumstances through a fantasy that such circumstances could have been controlled. The price is irrational guilt: "I should have known."

3. **Consolation.** The intensity of these experiences requires an actively consoling approach from the therapist, lest he or she be perceived as being judgmental or as collaborating in the pain inflicted on the patient. A kind of traumatic transference can develop in which, for example, rape victims may believe that their therapists are reinflicting the trauma during the "working through" phase. Appropriate expressions of sympathy and concern can be helpful in acknowledging and diffusing this common reaction.

4. **Condensation.** It is important to find an image that condenses a crucial aspect of the traumatic experience. This representation can make the overwhelming aspects of the trauma more manageable by giving them concrete, symbolic form. Furthermore, this approach can be used to facilitate a restructuring of the experience by joining previously disparate images—for example, linking the pain associated with the death of a buddy in combat with the happiness experienced during some earlier shared time. This allows patients to alter the pain of the loss by attending to positive aspects of the lost relationship that remain in memory.

5. **Consciousness.** In a gradual manner, so that the patient is not overwhelmed, the therapist must make conscious previously dissociated traumatic memories.

6. **Concentration.** Use of the intense concentration characteristic of the hypnotic state is helpful in reinforcing the boundaries of the traumatic experience and of the painful affect associated with it. Through sharply focusing attention on the loss, the inference is made that when the hypnotic state is ended, attention can be shifted away from the traumatic experience.

TABLE 32–4. Principles of psychotherapy for trauma victims: the eight *C*s

Confrontation	Consciousness
Confession	Concentration
Consolation	Control
Condensation	Congruence

7. **Control.** Because the most painful aspect of severe trauma is the sense of absolute helplessness, the loss of control over one's body and the course of events, it is especially important that the process of the therapeutic intervention enhance the patient's sense of control over the memories. The experience should be structured so that patients are given the opportunity to terminate the working through when they feel they have had enough, can remember as much from the hypnosis as they care to, and feel they are in charge of the self-hypnosis experience. They should learn to use it on their own as a self-hypnosis exercise as well as with the therapist. Such procedures help patients to deal with traumatic memories with a greater sense of control and mastery.

8. **Congruence.** The goal of the therapy is to help patients integrate dissociated or repressed traumatic material into conscious awareness in such a way that they can tolerate experiencing the memories as part of themselves, so that the traumatic past is not disjunctive and incompatible with the present. Patients should emerge from therapy having reviewed not only what was done to them but what they did to protect themselves, not only what they lost but what they had had that made the loss so painful.

FORENSIC USES

A major application of hypnosis in the legal setting has been for the purpose of refreshing recollection of witnesses and victims of crimes (Gravitz 1995). There have been some positive results with this technique—for example, the case involving the driver of a hijacked school bus in Chowchilla, CA (*People v. Schoenfeld* 1980). Under hypnosis, and not previously, the driver was able to recall the numbers and letters on the license plate of the car that overtook the bus. This led to the arrest and conviction of the kidnappers.

Nonetheless, there has been serious criticism of the use of hypnosis with witnesses and victims. Two charges are leveled at the technique. One is *confabulation*—that a hypnotized witness will make up material (Laurence and Perry 1983) and become what has been called an "honest liar" (H. Spiegel 1980), someone who believes his or her misstatement out of a desire to please the hypnotist or simply as a result of being in the nonrational hypnotic state itself. The other is *concreting*—that having gone through the process of hypnosis, even if new information is not made up, the subject will emerge with an enhanced conviction that his or her memories are correct and that the subject will therefore be more convincing to a jury than he or she should be (Diamond 1980; Dywan 1995; McConkey 1992; Orne 1979; D. Spiegel and Scheflin 1994; D. Spiegel and Spiegel 1986). There is evidence that under hypnosis people are more likely to make confident errors—the accuracy of the memories they produce is no better than usual but their confidence in the accuracy of their memories increases (McConkey 1992).

Courts have been uniformly unwilling to admit the testimony of a person hypnotized while testifying. More recently, however, courts have also begun to exclude testimony of witnesses who have previously been hypnotized about the event in question. The case law has provided some examples of egregious misuses of hypnosis. For example, in *People v. Shirley* (1982), a woman whose memory of the details of a questionable sexual assault was obscured because of her having ingested a substantial amount of alcohol was hypnotized by a member of the prosecution team the night before she was to testify. Her testimony improved dramatically. The conviction was overturned by the California Supreme Court, which ruled that any witness or victim who had been hypnotized about the facts of a crime could not subsequently testify. In other words, the use of hypnosis created an issue of admissibility rather than weight given to testimony. The court excluded defendants from this prohibition. In a subsequent case, *People v. Guerra* (1984), the conviction of a rapist was likewise overturned, because critical details regarding the nature of the attack were provided by the witness only during a hypnosis session in which considerable pressure was applied for her to remember penetration by the assailant. However, in this case the California Supreme Court left open the possibility that the testimony of a witness whose story had not changed despite a hypnotic interrogation might be salvaged. The Arizona Supreme Court (State ex rel. *Collins v. Superior Court* 1982) retreated from its extreme position and adopted a standard that holds in New York (*People v. Hughes* 1983) and New Jersey (*People v. Hurd* 1980), among other states, which is that such witnesses may testify about their prehypnotic recollection of events. The United States Supreme Court, in *Rock v. Arkansas* (1987), ruled that a defendant could testify about his or her prehypnotic recollection of events, thereby rejecting a per se exclusion of testimony that could have been influenced by hypnosis.

From a practical point of view, it is wise to caution attorneys and witnesses that the use of hypnosis might leave open the possibility of challenge to witnesses' credibility or even to their admissibility as witnesses (Scheflin and Shapiro 1989; D. Spiegel and Scheflin 1994). Taking note of this problem, the California Legislature (1985) passed a law stating that witnesses would be allowed to testify after hypnotic interrogation if certain guidelines were followed. These guidelines include the use of an independent expert psychiatrist or psychologist as a hypnosis consultant, careful documentation of the witness's memory before hypnosis, and electronic recording of all interaction preceding, during, and after hypnosis sessions (Maldonado and Spiegel 1997; D. Spiegel and Spiegel 1986). The kind of situation in which hypnosis is most likely to be worth the risk is one in which there is a traumatic amnesia for the events of a crime or in which all other avenues of exploration have been exhausted. Hypnosis should not be used as a replacement for routine police work.

The Council on Scientific Affairs of the American Medical Association convened a panel of experts to examine the research evidence relevant to this problem. The report issued by the panel (Orne et al. 1985) concluded that what evidence exists indicates that the use of hypnosis tends to increase the productivity of witnesses, resulting in new memories, some of which are true and some of which are incorrect. Furthermore, some studies showed an increase in the confidence assigned by hypnotized subjects to their memories despite the fact that the percentage of correct responses had not improved. The panel noted that the analogy between the laboratory setting in which most of the studies were done and the real-life situation in the courtroom must be drawn with great caution and that situations in which extreme emotional and physical trauma had occurred differ markedly. The panel recommended that careful guidelines similar to the ones outlined in the California law be followed when hypnosis is used in the forensic setting (Bloom 1994; Maldonado and Spiegel 1997; D. Spiegel and Spiegel 1986).

Certainly, it is clear that hypnosis is no truth serum and that the courts must weigh the effects of any hypnotic induction on a witness. At the same time, hypnosis may in certain cases help a traumatized and amnesic witness to recall details not brought forward through conventional interrogation methods (Brown et al. 1998).

BRIEF TREATMENT: SYMPTOM RESTRUCTURING WITH HYPNOSIS

Hypnosis has been used as an adjunctive tool in the treatment of a variety of common psychiatric and medical problems, including habit disorders, anxiety and phobic states, psychosomatic problems, and pain. Because the hypnotic state involves an enhanced and altered state of concentration with an ability to produce changes in perception and certain body functions, it makes sense that it would be an effective tool in managing these psychosomatic problems. A variety of techniques have been employed in symptom-oriented treatment using hypnosis. One is the so-called ego-strengthening approach, in which hypnosis is used to provide positive reinforcement for behavior change (Crasilneck and Hall 1985). Erickson (1967) made use of a "therapeutic bind," mobilizing the patient's resistance to treatment by intensifying, or "prescribing," symptoms. The patient would then construe eliminating the symptom as a victory over the therapist. This approach, although not necessary among patients who are well motivated and who have resolved their ambivalence about symptom reduction, has the virtue of demonstrating to patients their ability to modulate symptoms, bypassing defensiveness by worsening rather than lessening them (Erickson 1967). Other therapists employ simple instructions that a symptom will disappear. This authoritarian approach often puts both therapist and patient in an awkward situation—it is unwise to tell a patient something one is not certain is true, whether or not the patient is in a trance. No one can be certain that a symptom will disappear, even in the case of a highly hypnotizable patient.

More recent approaches to the use of hypnosis have emphasized the educational aspects of the experience. In particular, it is most efficient to structure the intervention as a lesson in self-hypnosis that the patient can learn to employ in the service of symptom reduction. Also, it is useful to teach patients a cognitive strategy that alters their perspective on the problem, reinforced by the self-hypnosis. One such approach is *restructuring* (H. Spiegel and Spiegel 1987). Restructuring in hypnosis involves using the intense concentration characteristic of the trance state to help patients develop a strategy for change that amounts to an affirmation experience rather than a struggle, focusing on what they are for rather than what they are against. For example, instead of telling themselves not to smoke or that cigarettes taste bad, patients use the self-hypnosis exercise to focus on a broader commitment to protect their body in the same way that they would protect a child from poison, viewing their bodies as trusting, innocent creatures that depend on them for their protection. In this approach, mind and body are viewed as distinct but interdependent, and the goal is to change the relationship to the body rather than to prevent smoking (Figure 32–5). Thus, these patients' perspective on the problem is enlarged, which makes the resolution of the problem itself an example of a broader pattern of relating to one's body. This therapeutic focus avoids the trap of increasing attention to the problem, in this case smoking, that can actually increase the desire to engage in the activity (e.g., to smoke) (similar to telling oneself,

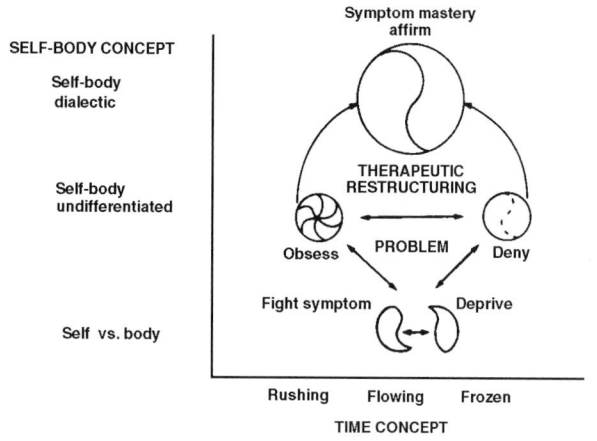

FIGURE 32–5.   Model for constructing a restructuring treatment strategy using hypnosis. This model emphasizes a commitment to affirm a restructured relationship of respect for one's body rather than fight against the symptom, which only amplifies it.

"Don't think about purple elephants").

This kind of restructuring strategy can be applied to other problems as well, such as mild to moderate overeating (Barabasz and Spiegel 1989), and to the treatment of pain (Brose et al. 1997; E. R. Hilgard and Hilgard 1975; D. Spiegel 1985). In the latter case, patients are taught to transform the pain signal by making the affected body area colder or warmer, or numb, or to focus on a sensation in some other part of the body. The management of anxiety or panic attacks is not taught by an instruction to relax or not be anxious; rather, patients learn to affiliate with a physical metaphor that connotes relaxation, such as floating in water. In this way, patients can overcome urges or symptoms not by struggling against them but by subsuming them under a commitment to a new way of relating to the body, or through a hypnotically developed capacity to transform sensation (H. Spiegel and Spiegel 1987).

ANXIETY DISORDERS AND PHOBIAS

The Epidemiologic Catchment Area study sponsored by the National Institute of Mental Health demonstrated that anxiety disorders are among the most widely prevalent psychiatric disturbances, affecting as much as 15% of the population (Myers et al. 1984). Anxiety is a state of psychosomatic discomfort experienced by patients largely in physical terms, with increases in heart rate, gastrointestinal and thoracic discomfort, diaphoresis, and motor restlessness. Panic attacks (i.e., sudden and intense states of this kind of discomfort) may be associated with irrational

avoidance behavior (i.e., phobias). On the other hand, a more chronic state may inhibit psychological comfort and social functioning, as in generalized anxiety disorder (GAD).

A number of articles have been published concerning the use of hypnosis as adjunct to dental procedures and in the treatment of dental phobia (Hammarstrand et al. 1995; Lu 1994; Moore et al. 1996; Peretz 1996; Robb 1996; Rustvold 1994; Shaw and Niven 1996; Shaw and Welbury 1996; Wilks 1994). The success of use of hypnotic techniques in dental work has created a new interest in teaching these techniques in American dental schools (J. H. Clarke 1996; Herod 1995).

Similarly, hypnotic techniques have been successfully used to assist phobic patients undergoing a number of medical/surgical and diagnostic procedures, thus diminishing the need for excessive anesthesia or antianxiety medication, improving compliance, and eliminating trauma to patients (Cadranel et al. 1994; Chandler 1996; Ellis and Spanos 1994; J. R. Hilgard and LeBaron 1982; Kessler and Dane 1996; Lambert 1996; Lang et al. 1996; Mize 1996; Rape and Bush 1994).

Hypnosis has also been reported to be useful in the treatment of anxiety and phobias (J. C. Clarke and Jackson 1983; Erickson 1967; J. R. Hilgard and LeBaron 1982; Maldonado and Spiegel 1996; McGuinness 1984; Somer 1995; D. Spiegel et al. 1981b; Stanton 1993). Hypnosis may be especially helpful as an adjunctive tool for treating these anxiety states because of the ability of the hypnotized person to control somatic response. For example, in a recent randomized trial of self-hypnotic analgesia and patient-controlled (pharmacological) analgesia (PCA) versus PCA alone among patients undergoing invasive radiological procedures, those in the hypnosis condition used one-ninth the amount of medication, experienced less pain and anxiety, and had fewer medical complications compared with patients in the second group (Lang et al. 1996). Whereas, as noted earlier, the hypnotizability of patients with GAD is low, studies show that phobic patients are at least normally and perhaps highly hypnotizable (Frankel and Orne 1976).

A variety of treatment strategies employing hypnosis have in common a restructuring of cognition by combining imagery with physical relaxation. Anxious patients are instructed to maintain such a sense of floating relaxation while picturing feared situations on an imaginary screen in the trance state. This approach clearly has elements in common with systematic desensitization (Marks et al. 1968), the difference being that in the former the induction of physical relaxation coupled to a noxious stimulus can be included very quickly without the development and working through of a hierarchy.

The hypnotic session may be used initially to demonstrate to patients that they have a greater degree of control over somatic responsiveness than they imagine. It may also be useful to teach these patients to picture on the screen a place that they find intrinsically relaxing so that they can use their memory of, for example, a mountain lake or the beach as a means of providing a respite from anxious preoccupation. They may use the same trance state as a means of facing their concerns, placing an image of an upcoming performance, for example, on one side of the screen while on the other side testing out various strategies for mastering the situation. The pleasant image may be especially useful for medical patients having to undergo procedures. Both in preparation and while in the clinic or hospital they can enter a state of self-hypnosis and imagine being somewhere they enjoy, thereby dissociating their psychological experience from the physical aspects of the procedure, as in the following case:

A 39-year-old woman with a brain tumor found herself unable to tolerate the magnetic resonance imaging (MRI) scanner. She felt a sense of panic when she was enclosed in the scanner, and the noise added to her discomfort. She admitted that she was anxious about the result, a possible recurrence of the tumor, but said she was prepared for that and knew she needed to have the scan. She proved to be moderately hypnotizable (6/10 on the HIP) and was taught to enter a state of self-hypnosis in which she imagined that she was water-skiing, her favorite sport. She practiced this several times a day and went into that state in the scanner. Imagining that the clanking sound of the scanner was the boat engine, she tolerated the procedure well.

Specific phobias call for variation in cognitive strategy. Patients with flying phobia, for example, can be taught to combine the hypnotically induced physical sense of floating with the concept of floating with the airplane. They can then focus on the idea of the plane as an extension of the body, instead of feeling trapped inside the plane, and also concentrate on the difference between a possibility and a probability. The mere fact that a crash is possible does not make it likely. This is a technique that can be employed by patients before and during the airplane flight.

Individuals with acrophobia can be taught in the trance state to view gravity not as something likely to pull them off a cliff or building but rather as something that roots them to the ground. Agoraphobic patients may find it useful to imagine a plastic bubble surrounding them that they can take with them even when they leave their protective environment. Thus, whatever sense of safety they feel at home can sometimes be carried with them. Patients with animal phobias can be taught to feel more in control of a situation with an animal by first learning to control their own somatic response to it. Cognitively, they can concentrate on the difference between dangerous and tame animals (D. Spiegel and Spiegel 1988; H. Spiegel and Spiegel 1987). Other approaches using hypnosis have included instructing patients in a trance to imagine that they are literally somewhere else, away from the fearful stimulus (Erickson 1967) or that their capacity to master the situation and their response to it will improve (Crasilneck and Hall 1985). There is generally less attention paid to uncovering techniques that seek to link the complaint of anxiety to some early traumatic experience, although this is most applicable, as noted earlier, to clear cases of PTSD, as opposed to phobic and anxiety disorders.

INSOMNIA

The use of hypnosis to treat insomnia overlaps considerably with the treatment of anxiety disorders. Because hypnosis is not sleep but a form of concentration, it might seem paradoxical to use hypnosis to help people fall asleep. However, it can be helpful for inducing a state of physical relaxation that is at least compatible with sleep, diminishing the sympathetic arousal usually associated with anxious preoccupation. Thus, patients can be instructed to go into a state of self-hypnosis and induce a sense of floating relaxation physically; then, if preoccupied with arousing or uncomfortable thoughts, they can project these thoughts onto an imaginary screen in the trance state. Patients are instructed to become "traffic directors" for their own thoughts, to deal with them on the screen, thereby dissociating them from the evoked physical response (H. Spiegel and Spiegel 1987). Such approaches can be helpful in conjunction with standard sleep laboratory approaches, which include keeping the bedroom as a place where work and other anxiety-arousing activities do not occur and avoiding constantly looking at the clock when awakened. It is also important to distinguish routine insomnia due to situational reactions and anxiety from the more severe early morning awakening associated with depression or from the repeated arousals from sleep that are associated with sleep apnea syndrome. Few results of formal studies have been reported, but most case reports suggest that hypnosis is useful in the treatment of not only primary insomnia but other sleep disturbances as well (Bauer and McCanne 1980; Becker 1993; Schenck and Mahowald 1995).

GASTROINTESTINAL DISORDERS

Relaxation instructions have been helpful for some patients with stress-related bowel disease, such as ulcerative colitis and regional enteritis. Patients have found it helpful to imagine in trance something soothing in the gut; such imagining giving them a sense of control over a symptom that makes them feel especially helpless, thereby diminishing the cycle of reactive anxiety. A well-conducted randomized trial (Whorwell et al. 1984, 1987) showed that 15 patients with irritable bowel syndrome who were treated with hypnosis reported significant improvement in pain, abdominal distension, and diarrhea, as well as emotional well-being, compared with a control group of 15 patients. An 18-month follow-up of 15 of these patients showed continued remission, and the authors reported similar improvement in 35 additional patients (Houghton et al. 1996).

Hypnosis has been repeatedly used with great success in the treatment of emesis, of all causes and in both children (Keller 1995) and adults (Covino and Frankel 1993; Faymonville et al. 1995). Zeltzer et al. (1984) reported significant reduction in chemotherapy-induced nausea and vomiting among 19 patients who had been taught hypnosis. Hypnosis has been reported not only to help in the treatment of acute emesis associated with chemotherapy treatment (Genuis 1995; J. R. Hilgard and LeBaron 1982; Jacknow et al. 1994) but also to prevent anticipatory anxiety and emesis associated with cancer therapy (Redd et al. 1982). Even hyperemesis gravidarum has been reported to respond well to hypnotic intervention (Baram 1995; Fuchs et al. 1980; Iancu et al. 1994; Torem 1994).

Klein and Spiegel (1989) observed significant hypnotic control of gastric acid secretion among 28 highly hypnotizable subjects. When these patients were hypnotized and instructed to eat an imaginary meal, basal acid output increased 89%. In another trial designed to test reduction in acid output, subjects were instructed to use hypnosis to experience deep relaxation. There was a notable 39% decrease in basal acid output. In a third trial, subjects were given an injection of pentagastrin, which stimulates maximal parietal cell output. There was still a marked 11% reduction in pentagastrin-stimulated peak acid output during hypnosis. This study further emphasizes the fact that high hypnotizability is a two-edged sword, in that it may increase or decrease a given physiological parameter, depending on the mental content during the hypnotic state. That these observations may have clinical relevance is illustrated by the findings of a controlled trial of hypnosis in relapse prevention of duodenal ulcers (Colgan et al. 1988). Thirty patients with rapidly relapsing ulcer disease were randomly assigned, after administration of ranitidine, to hypnosis treatment or no treatment. All of the control subjects but only 53% of the hypnosis patients relapsed. More recently, several articles reported the benefits of hypnosis

in the treatment of ulcer disease (Francis and Houghton 1996). Thus, hypnosis seems to be an effective adjunct to the management of some gastrointestinal disorders.

TREATMENT OUTCOME STUDIES

Outcome studies have generally shown hypnosis to be efficacious and hypnotizability to be predictive of treatment response. A 7-year follow-up of 178 patients treated with a single session of self-hypnosis for flying phobia indicated that 52% were either improved or cured. Employing hypnosis in the treatment of warts has resulted in a success rate ranging from 27% (Johnson and Barber 1978) to 80% (Ewin's 1992). In most cases, hypnotizability predicts responsiveness to treatment (D. Spiegel et al. 1981b). There have been comparatively few well-controlled studies comparing hypnosis as an adjunct with other techniques. Those studies conducted among patient populations tend to show use of hypnosis to be an advantage, especially when patients request it (Glick 1970; Lazarus 1973). Studies among student volunteers who are symptomatic tend to show no clear advantage for hypnosis versus desensitization, whereas those studies in which stress is induced in nonsymptomatic volunteers show some advantage for relaxation training over hypnosis (Marks et al. 1968).

In general, outcome studies show some overlap between behavioral techniques and hypnosis in both structure and outcome. For example, Kirsch and colleagues (Kirsch 1996; Kirsch et al. 1995) conducted a meta-analysis of 18 studies in which a cognitive-behavior therapy was compared with the same therapy supplemented by hypnosis. The results indicated that the addition of hypnosis substantially enhanced treatment outcome. The average patient receiving cognitive-behavior therapy with hypnosis showed greater improvement, about twice the weight loss, than at least 70% of patients receiving nonhypnotic treatment (mean weight loss was 11.83 lb [5.37 kg] for the hypnosis group and 6.00 lb [2.72 kg] for the group receiving cognitive treatment without hypnosis). The effects of hypnotic intervention seemed especially pronounced at long-term follow-up, which indicates that unlike those in nonhypnotic treatment, patients in whom the hypnotic state had been induced continued to lose weight after the treatment ended ($r = .74$). Both approaches—behavioral techniques and hypnosis—involve the use of imagery and restructuring of cognition about the feared stimulus coupled with a means of producing physical relaxation. Hypnosis can be most effective when it is used to enhance patients' sense of mastery and control over psychological experience as well as their somatic response to such experience.

PAIN SYNDROMES

Pain is the ultimate psychosomatic phenomenon, always representing both tissue injury and the psychological reaction to such injury. The first formal study of the use of hypnosis in pain was performed more than a century ago in India, when a Scottish surgeon named Esdaile (1846/1957) reported 80% surgical anesthesia for amputations using hypnosis. He was immediately censured by his colleagues and 10 years later withdrew the findings when a report came out from Massachusetts General Hospital that ether anesthesia had been 90% effective. Indeed, one of the surgeons strode to the front of the amphitheater and announced, "Gentlemen, this is no humbug!" to distinguish the use of ether from hypnosis.

Nonetheless, it is clear that psychological factors are major variables in the intensity of the pain experience. A century later, at the same hospital, Beecher (1956) demonstrated that the intensity of pain was directly associated with its meaning. To the extent that pain represented threat and the possibility of future disability, it was more intense among civilian surgical patients than it was among a group of combat soldiers to whom the pain of injury meant that they were likely to get out of combat alive.

Behavioral approaches to pain control emphasize changing patterns of social reinforcement that are contingent on pain-related behavior (Fordyce et al. 1973). Pain is classified as primarily operant (i.e., influenced by secondary gain) or respondent (i.e., driven by a noxious physical stimulus). Respondent pain may gradually be transformed into operant pain as attention and sympathy reinforce pain behavior. This process can be reversed through use of positive reinforcement for nonpain behavior. For example, nurses and family members can be trained to pay a great deal of attention to such patients when they increase their activity level or converse about subjects other than their pain. Social contacts involving the pain itself, such as demands for medication, are best kept brief and formal. This approach can be helpful, especially in chronic pain syndromes, in increasing levels of physical activity and diminishing excessive analgesic medication use.

Hypnosis facilitates alteration of the subjective experience of pain (Brose et al. 1997). The techniques most often employed involve physical relaxation coupled with imagery that provides a substitute focus of attention for the painful sensation (Table 32–5). Patients can be taught to develop a comfortable, floating sensation, and highly hypnotizable individuals may simply imagine receiving an injection of novocaine in the affected area, producing a sense of tingling numbness. Some patients prefer to imagine moving the pain to another part of their body or to develop a sensation of floating above their own bodies, creating distance between themselves and the painful sensation. More moderately hypnotizable patients often prefer to focus on a change in temperature, either warmth or coolness, imagining that they are floating in a warm bath or a mountain stream or immersing a painful hand in a bucket of ice chips. That temperature metaphors are usually effective may be related to the fact that pain and temperature fibers run together in the lateral spinothalamic tract, separate from other sensory fibers. Less hypnotizable patients may benefit from distraction techniques in which they concentrate hard on sensations in other parts of their bodies.

Regardless of the metaphor selected, certain general principles can be employed with all uses of hypnosis for pain control. The first principle is to teach patients to filter the hurt out of the pain. Patients learn to transform the pain experience by acknowledging that even though it may exist, there is a distinction between the signal itself and the discomfort the signal causes. The hypnotic metaphor helps them transform the signal into one that is less uncomfortable. The second principle is to expand the perceptual options available to patients by having them change from an experience in which either the pain is there or it is not, to one in which they see a third option, which is that the pain is there but it is transformed by the presence of such competing sensations as tingling, numbness, warmth, or coolness. The third principle is to teach patients not to fight the pain. Fighting pain only enhances the pain by focusing attention

TABLE 32–5. Steps used in hypnotic analgesia

1. Induce physical relaxation through use of a metaphor such as floating.

2. Alter perception of the pain by:
   Inducing dissociation from current sensory experience
   Imagining a sense of warmth, coolness, tingling, or numbness
   Focusing attention on sensation in a nonpainful part of the body

3. Transform the pain.

4. Provide positive reinforcement for symptom improvement.

5. Use a rehabilitation model for treatment.

6. Reduce secondary gain for symptom maintenance.

7. Treat amplifying comorbid conditions:
   Anxiety related to disease progression
   Depression

on it, by enhancing related anxiety and depression, and by increasing physical tension that can literally put traction on painful parts of the body and increase the pain signals generated peripherally:

A world-class competition swimmer had collapsed in an alley as a result of hemorrhaging of an undiagnosed lymphoma in his abdomen. During his chemotherapy he lay writhing in his bed, screaming with pain and demanding increasing amounts of analgesic medication, even while he was receiving high doses of opiates. The nursing staff refused to care for him on regular rotation because he was so difficult to be with. Found to be moderately hypnotizable, he was taught a self-hypnosis exercise that involved his imagining that he was somewhere he preferred to be.

"I'm a great swimmer, but I've never surfed," he said.

"Good, let's go to Hawaii," the physician suggested.

He continued to wince, but there was a different tone in his voice.

"What happened?" the physician asked.

"I fell off the surfboard," he responded.

"This time, do it right," the physician replied.

He did this self-hypnosis exercise regularly, and 48 hours later he was no longer taking any pain medications and was joking with the nurses in the hallway. The nurses resumed caring for him on regular shift rotations. A subsequent notation in the medical record stated: "Patient off of pain medication: tumor must be regressing."

For children undergoing painful procedures, the main focus is on imagery rather than relaxation, because they are highly hypnotizable and are easily absorbed in images. Some find it helpful to play in an imaginary baseball game, to picture themselves going to another room in the house, or to imagine themselves watching a favorite television show. This enables them to restructure their experience of what is going on and dissociate themselves psychologically from pain and fear of the procedure. It is helpful to have parents assisting and to go through several rehearsals of the procedure so that the children do not encounter anything unfamiliar. Hypnosis has successfully been used in children to reduce significantly the pain associated with invasive procedures (J. R. Hilgard and LeBaron 1982; Zeltzer and LeBaron 1982). The use of imagery techniques with suggestions for a favorable postoperative course has been associated with markedly lower postoperative pain ratings and shorter hospital stays (Lambert 1996).

Hypnotic analgesia seems to work through two mechanisms: *physical relaxation* and *attention control*. Patients in pain tend to splint the painful area instinctively, and yet this enhanced muscle tension around a painful area often increases pain. Most patients find that they can enhance their physical response by focusing on a variety of images that connote physical relaxation, such as a sense of floating. Second, because hypnosis involves an intensification and narrowing of the focus of attention, it allows individuals to place pain at the periphery of their awareness by putting some competing metaphor or sensation at the center of their attention. Thus, by focusing on a memory of dental anesthesia and spreading that numbness to the affected area, making the area warmer or cooler, substituting a sense of tingling or lightness, or focusing on sensation in some nonpainful part of the body, hypnotized individuals can diminish the amount of attention they pay to painful stimuli.

Miller and Bowers (1993) challenged the notion of pure social compliance as the mechanism of action of hypnotic analgesia. They compared the extent of pain reduction produced by hypnotic analgesia with that produced by a stress-inoculation procedure, in a group of highly and poorly hypnotizable subjects. They found that stress inoculation but not hypnotic analgesia impaired performance of a cognitively demanding task that competed with pain reduction for cognitive resources. This finding suggests that hypnotic analgesia occurs with little or no cognitive effort to reduce pain. The results do support the notion of dissociated control, which proposes that suggestions for analgesic relief during hypnosis directly activate pain reduction and thereby avert the need for cognitive strategies to reduce pain. That this hypnotic analgesia is not merely social compliance but involves neurophysiological changes in information processing is suggested by the cortical event–related potential studies. In these studies, highly hypnotizable individuals could diminish the P100 and P300 components of their event-related response to a somatosensory stimulus by focusing on a hallucinated image that would block their perception of the stimulus (D. Spiegel et al. 1989; Figure 32–6). This cortical attention deployment mechanism is at the moment the most plausible explanation, although a number of studies have tested the idea that endogenous opiates are involved in hypnotic analgesia. With one partial exception (Frid and Singer 1979), studies with both volunteers (Goldstein and Hilgard 1975) and patients in chronic pain (D. Spiegel and Albert 1983) have shown that hypnotic analgesia is not blocked and reversed by a substantial dose of naloxone given in double-blind, crossover fashion (Figure 32–7).

More recently, Kiernan and colleagues (1995) reported that hypnotic analgesia may act through one of two neurological mechanisms: a reduction of R-III nociceptive reflex, which is related to spinal cord antinociceptive mechanisms; or reductions in pain sensation over and beyond reductions in R-III, which may be related to brain

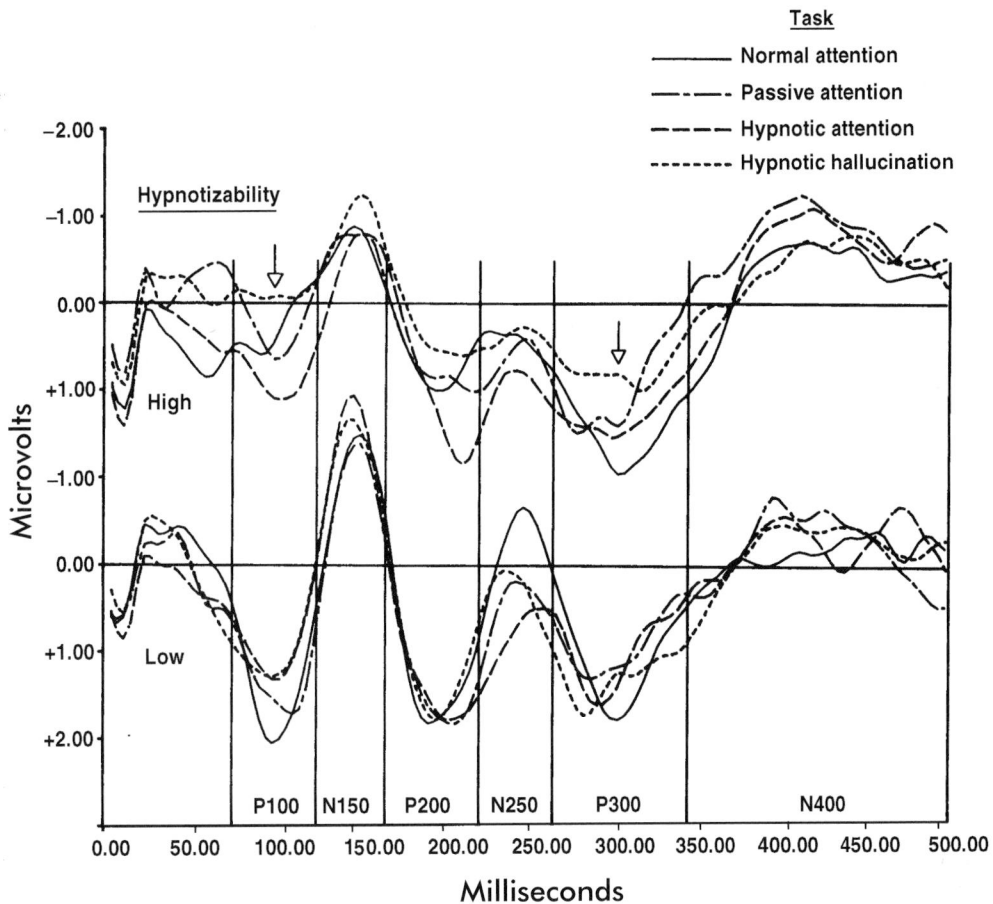

FIGURE 32-6. Somatosensory event–related potentials among 10 highly hypnotizable and 10 poorly hypnotizable individuals. Hypnotic obstructive hallucination results in reduction of P100 and P300 amplitudes, whereas hypnotic attention is associated with an increase in P100 amplitude.

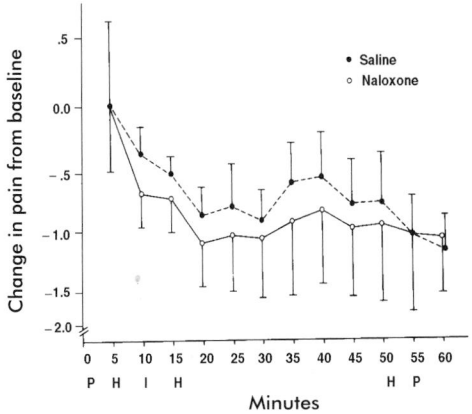

FIGURE 32-7. Effect of naloxone on the hypnotic reduction in clinical pain. Hypnotic reduction in physical pain is not blocked by naloxone: 10 mg of naloxone, given in a double-blind, crossover design, does not block and reverse hypnotic analgesia. P = mood assessment; H = hypnotic analgesia exercise; I = injection of naloxone or saline.

mechanisms that serve to prevent awareness of pain signals once nociception has reached higher centers. Whatever the mechanism, hypnotic analgesia is efficacious (Dahlgren et al. 1995; Faymonville et al. 1995; Genuis 1995; Hargadon et al. 1995). Systematic studies have demonstrated that hypnosis is superior to an attentional control condition for analgesia among children undergoing painful procedures (Zeltzer and LeBaron 1982). Furthermore, in a randomized prospective study, a combination of hypnosis and group psychotherapy was shown to result in a 50% reduction in pain among metastatic breast cancer patients (D. Spiegel and Bloom 1983; Figure 32–8), and there was a corresponding reduction in mood disturbance (D. Spiegel et al. 1981a). Hypnotic analgesia has also been shown to be more potent than either placebo analgesia (McGlashan et al. 1969) or acupuncture analgesia (Knox and Shum 1977), although there is a correlation between hypnotizability and responsiveness to acupuncture (Katz et

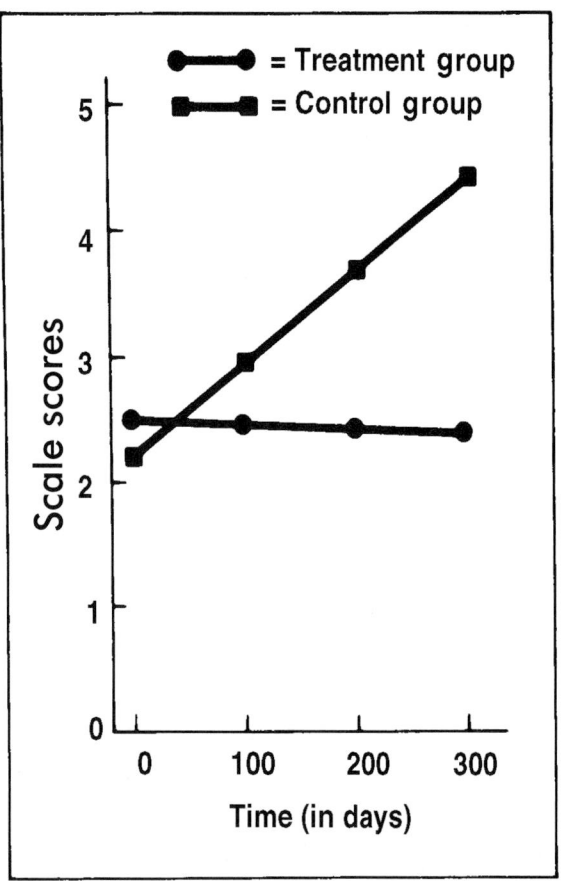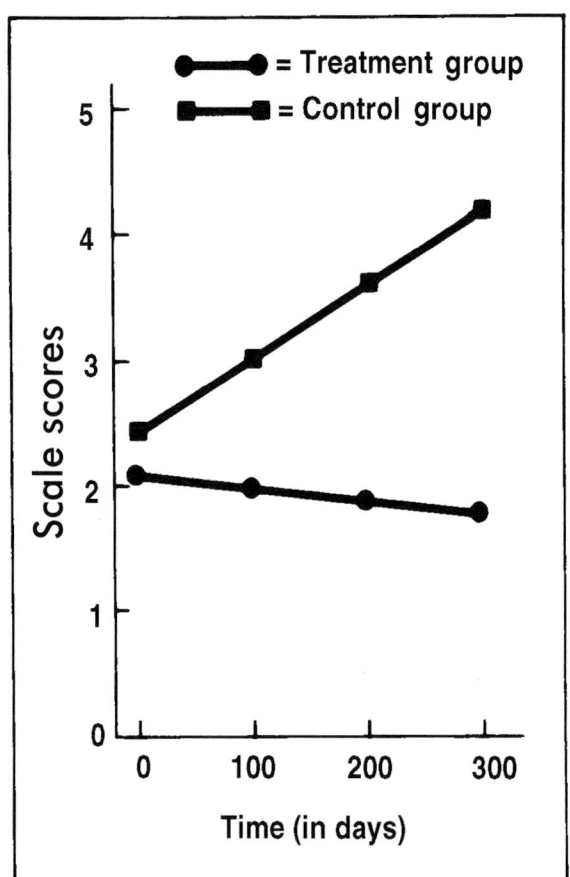

FIGURE 32–8. Reduction of cancer pain with hypnosis. Changes in pain sensation (left) and suffering (right) among 54 women with metastatic breast cancer randomized to weekly treatment with group support and training in self-hypnosis or to a control condition. Note doubling of pain during the year in the control group but reduction of pain in the treatment group.
Source. Reprinted with permission from Spiegel D: "The Use of Hypnosis in Controlling Cancer Pain." *CA: A Cancer Journal for Clinicians* 35:221–231, 1985.

al. 1974). Thus, hypnotic mechanisms of pain control may be mobilized by other treatment techniques, but the explicit use of hypnosis with hypnotizable patients has proved to be a more powerful means of controlling pain.

In a review of studies, E. R. Hilgard and Hilgard (1975) estimated a .5 correlation between hypnotizability and treatment responsiveness for pain control. The ability of hypnotizable individuals to focus their attention and alter their response to perception while at the same time produce a physical state of relaxation allows them to restructure their experience of pain and thereby develop a sense of mastery over it. Because the pain experience is both psychological and physical, this technique mobilizes and focuses cognitive experience while producing a sense of physical relaxation.

PSYCHOSOMATIC DISORDERS

Because highly hypnotizable individuals show an unusual capacity for psychological control over somatic function, it makes sense that hypnotic phenomena may be involved both in the etiology of some psychosomatic symptoms and in their control (D. Spiegel 1994; D. Spiegel and Vermutten 1994). For example, Andreychuk and Skriver (1975) found that hypnotizability not only was a predictor of treatment response for migraine headaches, but also was a correlate of pretreatment symptom severity. That is, more highly hypnotizable individuals complained of more severe migraine symptoms before treatment but responded better to intervention. Highly hypnotizable individuals have been shown to have the capacity to control peripheral skin temperature and blood flow (Grabowska

1971; Zimbardo et al. 1970) and to be able to suppress cortical evoked response to a perceptual stimulus while hallucinating an obstruction to that stimulus (D. Spiegel et al. 1985, 1989). Certain classic conversion disorders such as hysterical paralysis may well represent dissociative phenomena, because profound alterations in sensation and experience of control over motor function are standard hypnotic phenomena (D. Spiegel 1994; D. Spiegel and Vermutten 1994). Nonetheless, these disorders have been documented rarely.

In general, hypnosis is useful in two senses, one diagnostic, the other therapeutic. Patients who are highly hypnotizable are more likely to have conversion symptoms, such as hysterical pseudoseizures, than those who are not, especially if hypnotic induction tends to bring on the symptom, worsen it, or ameliorate it. Such changes in the symptom during or after a trial of hypnosis can be used constructively to teach the patient to utilize self-hypnosis as a means of enhancing control over the severity of the symptom. This makes the symptom seem less alien and threatening. However, even among highly hypnotizable patients it is rare for a conversion symptom simply to disappear, and, indeed, pushing patients to relinquish it too quickly may humiliate them, because this conveys the message that the problem was "all in their head." Hypnosis can be appropriately used as part of a rehabilitation strategy, particularly insofar as it can help patients master the reactive anxiety that is associated with real physical dysfunction as well as conversion symptoms. A patient can be taught to use a state of self-hypnosis to develop the sense of floating relaxation while picturing bothersome problems on an imaginary screen. The patient can then work on, for example, improving use of a dysfunctional hand by developing tremors that gradually build up strength and circulation. One patient with persistent contractures of the entire hand secondary to a compound fracture of the index finger had been treated with a variety of techniques for 3 years with no improvement. He then used this kind of self-hypnosis exercise to focus on rehabilitation rather than seek further information about causation. At the end of another year of daily exercise, he regained full function of the hand and returned to work (D. Spiegel and Chase 1980; Figure 32–9).

Hypnosis has been effective in helping asthmatic patients (Aronoff et al. 1975; Ewer and Stewart 1986; Inoue et al. 1995; Kohen 1986; Kohen and Wynne 1997; Maher-Loughan 1970; Morrison 1988). They can learn to use it as a first resort rather than medication when they begin to feel an attack coming on, thereby interrupting the vicious cycle of anxiety and bronchoconstriction. It is often helpful to have asthmatic patients enter a state of self-hypnosis and imagine that they are in a place where

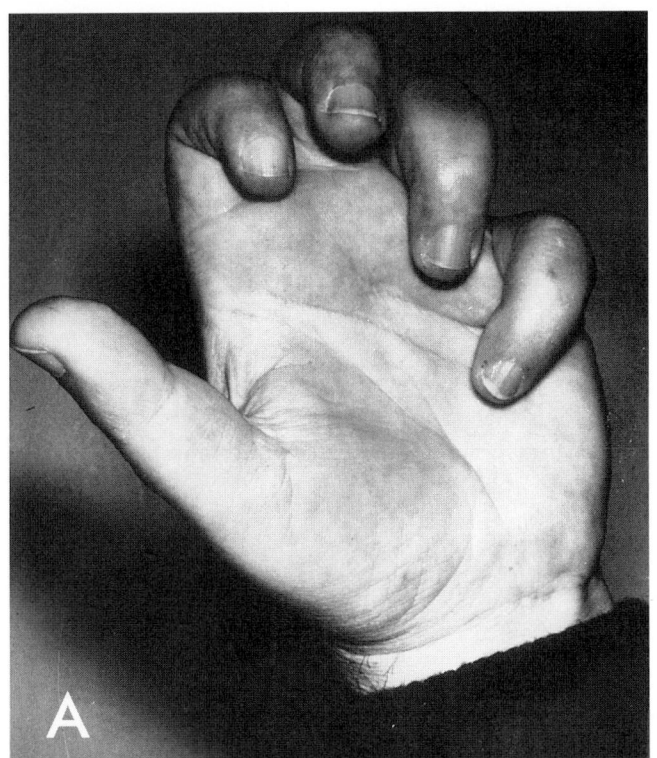

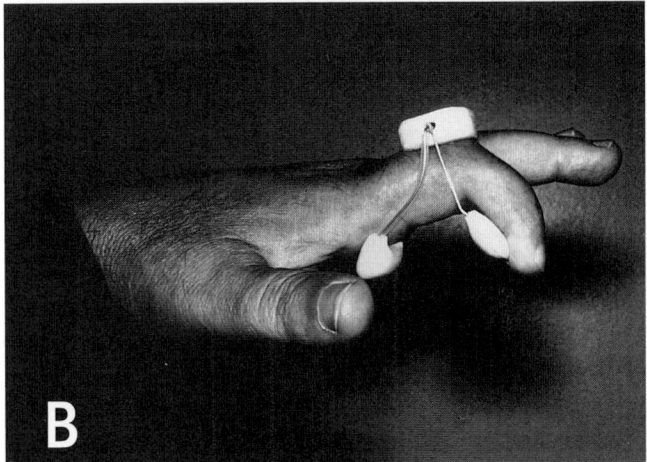

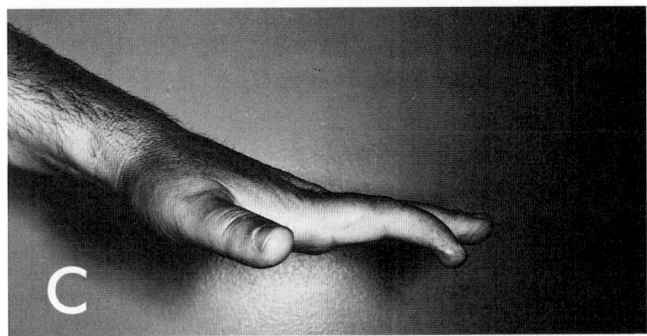

FIGURE 32-9.   Treatment of contractures of the hand using self-hypnosis. Hand in maximal extension before (A), during (B), and after (C) treatment using self-hypnosis exercises and dynamic splinting.

they naturally breathe easily—for example, in the mountains or near the ocean (H. Spiegel and Spiegel 1987). Hypnotizability is correlated with treatment response (Collison 1975).

Similarly, warts have been treated using hypnosis (Ewin 1992) and one carefully controlled study demonstrated that simple hypnotic instructions to the effect that the warts would tingle and disappear resulted in a rate of improvement that was substantially better than the spontaneous rate of remission of warts (Surman et al. 1973). Thus, hypnosis can be helpful in controlling the psychosomatic interaction that can lead to either deterioration or improvement of somatically related symptoms. Other studies have shown specific benefits of hypnosis over simple task-motivating instructions in the elimination of warts (Spanos et al. 1988, 1990).

SMOKING CESSATION

Hypnosis has been employed as an adjunctive tool with a variety of habit control strategies, primarily for smoking cessation (Table 32–6). It has been used to 1) provide a kind of substitute physical relaxation for the momentary respite that accompanies inhaling a cigarette, 2) enhance self-observation and self-monitoring, 3) provide positive reinforcement for behavior change, 4) diminish the positive reinforcement provided by smoking itself, and 5) facilitate cognitive restructuring of the smoking habit. Hypnosis has been employed in group and individual settings. More recently, the emphasis has been on teaching patients self-hypnosis rather than having multiple sessions with a therapist. Although some dramatic, immediate results can occur when the patient is being instructed that he or she will find the cigarette distasteful or feel physically uncomfortable while inhaling, such approaches can create unnecessary dependency on the therapist. It is helpful to find a strategy that is intrinsically self-reinforcing and meaningful to the patient and that can be practiced whenever the urge to smoke comes on the patient. One cognitive restructuring model involves emphasizing that smoking is

destructive specifically to the patient's body and thereby limits what the patient can do with his or her life. The focus in hypnosis is then on protecting the patient's body from poison in the same way that the patient would protect an infant or a pet from ingesting noxious food. This approach enables the patient to balance the urge to smoke against the urge to protect his or her body from damage—in other words, the focus is on what the patient is *for* rather than what he or she is *against* (H. Spiegel 1970).

Factors that account for the utility of hypnosis as an adjunct to smoking cessation treatment include 1) enhanced responsiveness to suggestion (Rabkin et al. 1984; H. Spiegel and Spiegel 1987); 2) alteration of unconscious motivation to smoke (Rabkin et al. 1984); 3) immediate symptom relief (Orne 1977); 4) nonspecific ceremonial, expectational, and placebo factors (Orne 1977); 5) enhanced ability to focus attention on the treatment strategy (Frischholz and Spiegel 1986); and 6) facilitation of ongoing self-administration through self-hypnosis (H. Spiegel and Spiegel 1987).

The generally accepted criterion for evaluating treatment interventions for smoking is complete abstinence at 6 months rather than reduction in smoking. Results of various trials of hypnosis in treatment indicate quit rates ranging from 13% to 64% with individual interventions and a follow-up time of at least 6 months (Holroyd 1980, 1991; Schwartz 1987). The single-session approach developed by H. Spiegel (1970) is widely used (Schwartz 1987) and produces long-term complete abstinence rates of 20%–35% when undertaken by him (H. Spiegel 1970; H. Spiegel and Spiegel 1987) and others (Barabasz et al. 1986; Berkowitz et al. 1979; Frank et al. 1986; see Figure 32–10). Abstinence rates as high as 40% at 6 months have been

---

TABLE 32–6. Objectives of the use of hypnosis in smoking cessation treatment

1. To provide an alternative means of inducing physical relaxation
2. To enhance self-observation and self-monitoring
3. To provide positive reinforcement for behavior change
4. To diminish the positive reinforcement provided by smoking itself
5. To facilitate cognitive restructuring of the smoking habit

---

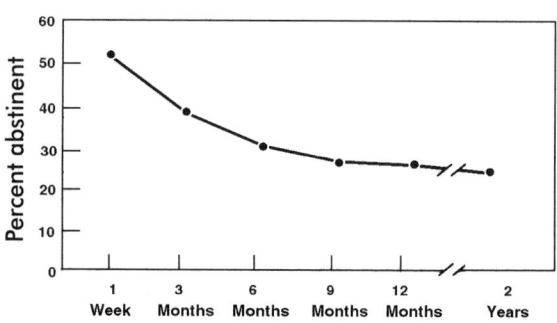

FIGURE 32–10. Percentage of patients taught a single-session, self-hypnosis restructuring strategy to stop smoking who remained continuously abstinent up to follow-up at 2 years.

reported (Hyman et al. 1986; Williams and Hall 1988).

These abstinence rates are superior to the rates of unassisted quitting (Gritz and Bloom 1987). In addition, hypnotizability has been shown to predict better outcome (Barabasz et al. 1986; D. Spiegel et al. 1993a; H. Spiegel and Spiegel 1987). Thus, although in general there is no evidence that treatments employing hypnosis are more effective than other interventions for smoking, they may well be more efficient, in that they enable patients to employ self-hypnosis to reinforce a cognitive restructuring strategy while at the same time they provide an episode of physical relaxation.

WEIGHT CONTROL

Hypnosis has been employed as an adjunct to a comprehensive dietary and exercise control program for weight reduction and management. The same restructuring principles discussed previously can be applied to overeating: experiencing an excess of food as damaging to the body, and learning to eat with respect for one's body. This again involves focusing on what the patient is *for*—rather than being against food. Indeed, an important component of such an approach can be to teach the patient to use self-hypnosis training to control the urge to overeat by preparing a list of foods that constitute eating with respect and then comparing an urge with the foods on the list. If the desired food is on the list, the patient is encouraged to eat it like a gourmet, focusing intently on all aspects of the eating experience. If the food is not on the list, rather than fight the urge the patient is encouraged to use self-hypnosis to compare it with his or her overall commitment to treat the body with respect and therefore to eat with respect. Patients can thus deal with the desire to eat not as an occasion to feel deprivation but rather as one in which they are enhancing their mastery of the urge by focusing on protecting their body. In addition, hypnosis can be used to help patients provide positive self-reinforcement for compliance with a revised eating regimen (Crasilneck and Hall 1985).

Clinical experience suggests that persons within 20% of their ideal body weight may obtain some benefit from such restructuring techniques with self-hypnosis in addition to careful attention to diet and exercise. There is evidence that treatment employing hypnosis is effective (Barabasz and Spiegel 1989). In a meta-analysis of studies on the effect of adding hypnosis to cognitive-behavioral treatments for weight reduction, Kirsch (1995, 1996) found that the mean weight loss in the hypnosis group was twice that of the group treated without hypnosis. His findings further indicated that the benefits of hypnosis increase

substantially over time. Furthermore, hypnotizability has been shown to be correlated with weight reduction in some studies (Anderson 1985).

NEUROPHYSIOLOGICAL ASPECTS OF HYPNOSIS

Efforts to identify neurobiological correlates of the hypnotic state and trait have been frustrating but not unrewarding. The belief that hypnotizability is biologically based dates at least as far back as Rudolf Heidenhain (1880), who explained hypnosis physiologically in terms of cortical inhibition. Between 1877 and 1884 Pavlov studied, under Heidenhain, hypnotic phenomena during conditional reflex experiments. Later, Pavlov (1910) described hypnotic states and explained them in terms of partial inhibition of the cortex (Windholz 1996). Subsequently, the debate regarding the mechanisms mediating the hypnotic phenomenon continued between Charcot (1890; Wildocher and Dantchev 1994) and Bernheim (1889/1964).

Power spectral analysis, the study of resting patterns of electrical activity in the brain, has been relatively unenlightening with regard to hypnosis. There has been some indication of more alpha activity among highly hypnotizable persons, whether or not they are in a trance, and of an alpha laterality difference favoring the left hemisphere among this population (Morgan et al. 1974). This difference suggests that hypnosis may differentially involve the right cerebral hemisphere; alpha is the noise the brain makes when resting but alert, so relatively less alpha on the right suggests more activity. This hypothesis is supported by observations that highly hypnotizable persons tend to be "left-lookers," preferring to activate their right hemispheres (Bakan 1969; Gur and Reyher 1973). More recent studies of power spectral analysis suggest that theta power, especially in the frontal region, best differentiates highly hypnotizable from poorly hypnotizable individuals (Sabourin et al. 1990). Graffin and colleagues (1995) obtained electroencephalographic measures in both highly and poorly hypnotizable subjects under three separate conditions: an initial baseline period; just preceding and following a standard hypnotic induction; and during the induction. They found that there was a differential pattern of electroencephalographic activity between highly hypnotizable subjects and poorly hypnotizable subjects during the baseline period, characterized by greater theta power in the more frontal areas of the cortex for the former group. They also observed that in the period just preceding and following the hypnotic induction, poorly hypnotizable subjects displayed an increase in theta activity, whereas highly hypnotizable subjects displayed a decrease. Furthermore, during the actual hypnotic induction itself, theta power increased markedly for both groups in the more posterior areas of the cortex, whereas alpha activity increased across all sites. These findings suggest that anterior/posterior cortical differences may be more important than hemispheric laterality for understanding the hypnotic processes.

Although early results were mixed, studies of the effects of hypnotic hallucination on event-related potentials (ERPs) have since yielded more promising results. The basic premise of these experiments is that because hypnotized individuals can experience perceptual alterations, including hallucinations, these changes might be reflected in corresponding alterations in the amplitude of the cortical evoked response to stimuli. Whereas some early studies showed no such effects (e.g., Amadeo and Yanovski 1975; Halliday and Mason 1964), others did (e.g., Clynes et al. 1964; Wilson 1968) but were hampered by small sample sizes, nonquantitative analysis of electroencephalograms (EEGs), limited use of hypnotizability testing, and use of subjects with neurological or psychiatric impairments. However, there is accumulating evidence that highly hypnotizable individuals experiencing a hypnotic hallucination that alters their perception of a stimulus have corresponding amplitude changes in the response evoked by that stimulus. For example, D. Spiegel et al. (1985) found that six highly hypnotizable subjects who experienced a hallucination of a cardboard box obstructing their view of a stimulus generator had significant reductions in P300 amplitude throughout the scalp and in N200 amplitude in the occipital region as well. These alterations occurred in no other hypnotic condition and did not occur among a group of individuals with low hypnotizability who were attempting to experience the same perceptual alteration. Furthermore, the reduction in P300 amplitude was significantly greater in the right than in the left occipital region, a finding that again implicates the right cerebral hemisphere in hypnotic experience. However, more recent visual ERP research has in fact implicated the left cerebral hemisphere in hypnotic perceptual alteration. These studies indicated greater reduction of occipital P200 amplitude during hypnotic obstructive hallucination when visual stimuli were presented to the right visual field than when they were presented to the left visual field, which demonstrates a stronger hypnotic effect of imagery in the left than the right occipital cortex. The automaticity noted in hypnotic response to instructions may selectively involve left hemisphere language areas or the specialization of the left hemisphere for image generation (Farah 1986).

Allen and colleagues (1995) studied the effect of posthypnotic amnesia using ERPs between simulators and hypnotized subjects. All participants demonstrated larger late positive component (LPC) amplitudes (compared with baseline) when confronted with learned words than when confronted with unlearned words, regardless of whether amnesia was reported. Nevertheless, the highly hypnotizable participants who reported recognition amnesia had significant changes in attention-related (P1 and N1) and recognition-related (N400 and LPC) ERP component amplitudes as a function of whether amnesia was reported, which suggests that posthypnotic amnesia may involve alterations in the processes of attention, selection, and accessibility.

Similar alteration in ERP amplitude congruent with hypnotic perceptual alteration has also been found when somatosensory stimuli are used (D. Spiegel et al. 1989; Figure 32–8). The hypnotic instruction is analogous to that used clinically for pain control. Each subject was told that his or her hand would be cool and numb and that this numbness would filter out any other sensations in the affected area. There was a significant reduction in P300 amplitude and also in P100 amplitude, suggesting earlier filtering of this somatosensory signal in the hypnotic hallucination condition. Thus, these subjects responded cortically as though the stimulus were less intense as well as less relevant. In another condition, subjects were told that the stimuli were pleasant and interesting and they should pay full attention to them. This yielded a significant increase in P100 amplitude but not P300 amplitude in hypnosis. Thus, highly hypnotizable subjects were capable of producing bidirectional changes in ERP amplitude to sensory stimuli, depending on the cognitive task employed during hypnosis. Poorly hypnotizable subjects showed no such changes, even though they were given an identical set of instructions by an experimenter blind to their hypnotizability.

Similar results have been obtained in the auditory system. Sigalowitz and colleagues (1991) found P300 amplitude differences among highly hypnotizable individuals hallucinating a reduction or increase in tones, whereas poorly hypnotizable persons did not show such a change. The amplitude reduction did not reach statistical significance, but the increase during positive hallucination did.

BRAIN IMAGING

There has been little study of hypnosis using newer brain imaging techniques such as positron-emission tomography (PET), single photon emission computed tomography (SPECT), and magnetic resonance imaging (MRI). However, a recent positron emission tomography (PET) study indicates that hypnotic reduction of the perceived unpleasantness of a stimulus was associated with significant changes in pain-evoked activity within anterior cingulate but not somatosensory cortex (Rainville et al. 1997). In addition, Szechtman and colleagues (1998) measured regional cerebral blood flow (rCBF) using PET, whereas highly hypnotizable subjects were hypnotized and asked to produce vivid auditory hallucinations. Subjects who could produce the hallucinations (8 of the 14 tested) had increased rCBF in the right anterior cingulate gyrus, and the "externality" and "clarity" of the hallucinations were highly correlated with blood flow in this region (Szechtman et al. 1998). Thus there is evidence of effects of hypnotic perceptual alteration on cerebral blood flow, which may involve activity of frontal attentional regions. Evidence of involvement of primary sensory (temporal) cortex was found in the Szechtman et al. study as well.

These techniques have proven useful in identifying subsystems within the brain devoted to specific types of perceptual and cognitive processing—for example, activation of the left inferior frontal cortex and anterior cingulate gyrus in response to visual and auditory presentation of words (Volkow and Tancredi 1991). This brain imaging work has led to the parsing of attentional processes into a series of components with different neuroanatomic localizations, using PET imaging of brain responses to various attentional tasks (Posner and Peterson 1990). The posterior attentional system involves orienting, with activation of the posterior or prestriate cortex. Focusing of attention—for example, detecting a faint blip on a radar screen—is associated with activity in the anterior cingulate gyrus. Arousal involves activity in the right frontal cortex. These new theories and the data that support them offer the possibility of greater specificity in identifying the neurophysiological basis of hypnotic processes. For example, the majority of observations of a connection between hypnosis and alteration in ERP amplitude have involved changes in the P300 amplitude, which is maximal over the frontal and central cortex. This would suggest some specific involvement of the anterior attentional systems in hypnotic concentration. These systems include focusing (anterior cingulate) and arousal (frontal, especially on the right), phenomena that are consistent with the fact that hypnosis involves intense absorption, or focal attention, and a state of resting alertness or arousal.

NEUROTRANSMITTERS

Further indirect evidence for the involvement of the frontal cortex in hypnotic phenomena derives from a finding that hypnotizability is significantly correlated with cerebrospinal fluid (CSF) levels of homovanillic acid (HVA), a metabolite of dopamine (D. Spiegel and King 1992; Figure 32–11). High levels of HVA in the CSF primarily reflect activity in the frontal cortex and basal ganglia, regions rich in dopaminergic synapses. Administration of amphetamine, which stimulates the release of dopamine, has been shown to enhance hypnotizability (Sjoberg and Hollister 1965). Although at first the basal ganglia might seem irrelevant to such attention-deployment mechanisms, the automaticity observed in hypnotic motor behavior could represent an activation of this region (D. Spiegel et al. 1993b), which is involved in both implicit memory (Mishkin 1991; Schacter 1987) and routine motor activity, especially of large muscle groups.

CONCLUSIONS

Hypnotizability is a stable and measurable trait, one that connotes the presence of an intact ability to concentrate intensely, a receptivity to new information, and a flexibility in changing behavior. Thus, the capacity to experience hypnosis constitutes a therapeutic resource in the patient that can be mobilized by formal hypnosis during the therapy session and by self-hypnosis exercises afterward. It is this cognitive flexibility that makes hypnotizable individu-

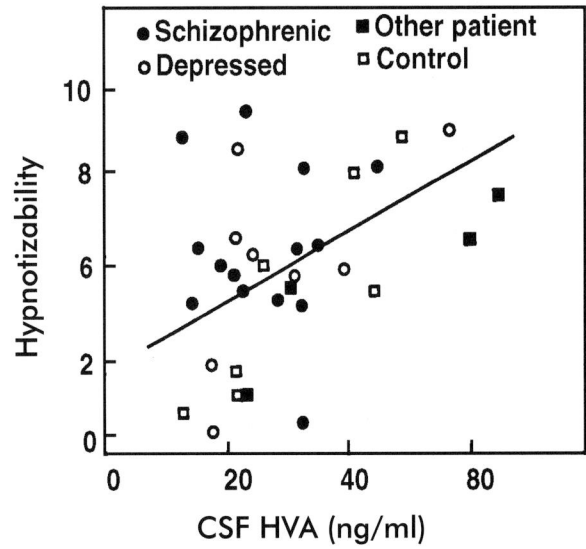

FIGURE 32–11. Hypnotizability as a function of homovanillic acid (HVA) in the cerebrospinal fluid (CSF), with regression line.

als adept at employing strategies such as restructuring that can help them alter their perspective on their symptoms by experiencing symptom resolution as an occasion to enhance their sense of mastery, rather than as submission to the will of the therapist.

Many therapeutic approaches using hypnosis involve patients' changing their perspective on the relationship between their psychological and physical state, dissociating mental from physical stress, adopting a stance of protectiveness toward their body rather than fighting destructive urges, or learning to see sudden discontinuities in consciousness as understandable and controllable hypnotic phenomena. This alteration in consciousness that has long been associated with a myth about losing control can actually be mobilized as a powerful therapeutic tool in enhancing patients' control over their behavior, perceptions, somatic functions, and cognition.

REFERENCES

Allen JJ, Iacono WG, Laravuso JJ, et al: An event-related potential investigation of posthypnotic recognition amnesia. J Abnorm Psychol 104:421–430, 1995

Amadeo M, Yanovski A: Evoked potentials and selective attention in subjects capable of hypnotic analgesia. Int J Clin Exp Hypn 23:200–210, 1975

American Psychiatric Association: Diagnostic and Statistical Manual of Mental Disorders, 4th Edition. Washington, DC, American Psychiatric Association, 1994

Anderson MS: Hypnotizability as a factor in the treatment of obesity. Int J Clin Exp Hypn 33:150–159, 1985

Andreychuk T, Skriver C: Hypnosis and biofeedback in the treatment of migraine headache. Int J Clin Exp Hypn 23:172–183, 1975

Aronoff GM, Aronoff S, Peck LW: Hypnotherapy in the treatment of bronchial asthma. Ann Allergy 42:356–362, 1975

Bakan P: Hypnotizability, laterality of eye movements, and functional brain asymmetry. Percept Mot Skills 28:927–932, 1969

Barabasz AF, Baer L, Sheehan DV, et al: A three-year follow-up of hypnosis and restricted environmental stimulation therapy for smoking. Int J Clin Exp Hypn 34:169–181, 1986

Barabasz M, Spiegel D: Hypnotizability and weight loss in obese subjects. Int J Eat Disord 8:335–341, 1989

Baram DA: Hypnosis in reproductive health care: a review and case reports. Birth 22:37–42, 1995

Bauer KE, McCanne TR: An hypnotic technique for treating insomnia. Int J Clin Exp Hypn 28:1–5, 1980

Becker PM: Chronic insomnia: outcome of hypnotherapeutic intervention in six cases. Am J Clin Hypn 36:98–105, 1993

Beecher HK: Relationship of significance of wound to pain experienced. JAMA 161:1609–1616, 1956

Berkowitz B, Ross-Townsend A, Kohberger R: Hypnotic treatment of smoking: the single-treatment method revisited. Am J Psychiatry 136:83–85, 1979

Bernheim H: Hypnosis and Suggestion in Psychotherapy: A Treatise on the Nature of Hypnotism (1889). Translated by Herter CA. New Hyde Park, NY, University Books, 1964

Bloom PB: Clinical guidelines in using hypnosis in uncovering memories of sexual abuse: a master class commentary. Int J Clin Exp Hypn 42:173–178, 1994

Braid J: Neurohypnology, or the Rationale of Nervous Sleep Considered in Relation With Animal Magnetism, Illustrated by Numerous Cases of Its Successful Application in the Relief and Cure of Disease. London, John Churchill, 1843

Braun BG, Sachs RG: The development of multiple personality disorder: predisposing, precipitating, and perpetuating factors, in Childhood Antecedents of Multiple Personality Disorder. Edited by Kluft RP. Washington, DC, American Psychiatric Press, 1985, pp 37–64

Bremner JD, Brett E: Trauma-related dissociative states and long-term psychopathology in posttraumatic stress disorder. J Trauma Stress 10:37–49, 1997

Breuer J, Freud S: Studies on hysteria (1893–1895), in The Standard Edition of the Complete Psychological Works of Sigmund Freud, Vol 2. Translated and edited by Strachey J. London, Hogarth Press, 1955, pp 1–319

Brose WG, Gaeta R, Spiegel D: Neuropsychiatric aspects of pain management, in American Psychiatric Press Textbook of Neuropsychiatry, 3rd Edition. Edited by Yudofsky SC, Hales RE. Washington, DC, American Psychiatric Press, 1997, pp 245–275

Brown DP, Scheflin AW, Hammond DC: Memory, trauma treatment, and the law. New York, WW Norton, 1998

Butler LD, Duran RE, Jasiukaitis P, et al: Hypnotizability and traumatic experience: a diathesis-stress model of dissociative symptomatology. Am J Psychiatry 153 (suppl 7):42–63, 1996

Cadranel JF, Benhamou Y, Zylberberg P, et al: Hypnotic relaxation: a new sedative tool for colonoscopy? J Clin Gastroenterol 18:127–129, 1994

California Legislature: AB 2669 Chapter 7, Hypnosis of Witnesses, added to Chapter 7, Division 6, of the Evidence Code, Enacted January 1, 1985

Cardeña E, Spiegel D: Dissociative reactions to the San Francisco Bay Area earthquake of 1989. Am J Psychiatry 150:474–478, 1993

Chandler T: Techniques for optimizing MRI relaxation and visualization. Administrative Radiology Journal 15:16–18, 1996

Charcot JM: Oeuvres complètes de JM Charcot, Tome IX. Paris, Lecrosnier et Babe, 1890

Clarke JC, Jackson JA: Hypnosis and Behavior Therapy: The Treatment of Anxiety and Phobias. New York, Springer, 1983

Clarke JH: Teaching clinical hypnosis in U.S. and Canadian dental schools. Am J Clin Hypn 39:89–92, 1996

Clynes M, Kohn M, Lifshitz K: Dynamics and spatial behavior of light-evoked potentials, their modification under hypnosis, and on-line correlation in relation to rhythmic components. Ann N Y Acad Sci 112:468–509, 1964

Colgan SM, Faragher EB, Whorwell PJ: Controlled trial of hypnotherapy in relapse prevention of duodenal ulceration. Lancet 1:1299–1300, 1988

Collison DR: Which asthmatic patients should be treated by hypnotherapy? Med J Aust 1:776–781, 1975

Copeland MD, Kitching EH: Hypnosis in mental hospital practice. Journal of Mental Science 83:316–329, 1937

Covino NA, Frankel FH: Hypnosis and relaxation in the medically ill. Psychother Psychosom 60:75–90, 1993

Covino NA, Jimerson DC, Wolfe BE, et al: Hypnotizability, dissociation, and bulimia nervosa. J Abnorm Psychol 103:455–459, 1994

Crasilneck HD, Hall JA: Clinical Hypnosis: Principles and Applications, 2nd Edition. New York, Grune & Stratton, 1985

Dahlgren LA, Kurtz RM, Strube MJ, et al: Differential effects of hypnotic suggestion on multiple dimensions of pain. J Pain Symptom Manage 10:464–470, 1995

Diamond BL: Inherent problems in the use of pretrial hypnosis on a prospective witness. California Law Review 68:313–349, 1980

Dywan J: The illusion of familiarity: an alternative to the report-criterion account of hypnotic recall. Int J Clin Exp Hypn 43:194–211, 1995

Ellenberger H: The Discovery of the Unconscious: The History and Evolution of Dynamic Psychiatry. New York, Basic Books, 1970

Ellis JA, Spanos NP: Cognitive-behavioral interventions for children's distress during bone marrow aspirations and lumbar punctures: a critical review. J Pain Symptom Manage 9:96–108, 1994

Erickson MH: Advanced Techniques of Hypnosis and Therapy: Selected Papers of Milton H. Erickson, M.D. Edited by Haley J. New York, Grune & Stratton, 1967

Eriksson NG, Lundin T: Early traumatic stress reactions among Swedish survivors of the Estonia disaster. Br J Psychiatry 169:713–716, 1996

Ernst W: 'Under the influence' in British India: James Esdaile's Mesmeric Hospital in Calcutta, and its critics. Psychol Med 25:1113–1123, 1995

Esdaile J: Hypnosis in Medicine and Surgery (1846). New York, Julian Press, 1957

Ewer TC, Stewart DE: Improvement in bronchial hyper-responsiveness in patients with moderate asthma after treatment with a hypnotic technique: a randomized controlled trial. British Medical Journal of Clinical Research and Education 293:1129–1132, 1986

Ewin DM: Hypnotherapy for warts (verruca vulgaris): 41 consecutive cases with 33 cures. Am J Clin Hypn 35:1–10, 1992

Farah M: The laterality of mental image generation: a test with normal subjects. Neuropsychologia 24:541–551, 1986

Faymonville ME, Fissette J, Mambourg PH, et al: Hypnosis as adjunct therapy in conscious sedation for plastic surgery. Reg Anesth 20:145–151, 1995

Fordyce WE, Fowler RS, Lehmann JR: Operant conditioning in the treatment of chronic pain. Arch Phys Med Rehabil 54:399–408, 1973

Francis CY, Houghton LA: Use of hypnotherapy in gastrointestinal disorders. Eur J Gastroenterol Hepatol 8:525–529, 1996

Frank RG, Umlauf RL, Wonderlich SA, et al: Hypnosis and behavioral treatment in a worksite smoking cessation program. Addict Behav 11:59–62, 1986

Frankel FH, Orne MT: Hypnotizability and phobic behavior. Arch Gen Psychiatry 33:1259–1261, 1976

Freud S: Remembering, repeating and working-through (further recommendations on the technique of psycho-analysis II) (1914), in The Standard Edition of the Complete Psychological Works of Sigmund Freud, Vol 12. Translated and edited by Strachey J. London, Hogarth Press, 1958, pp 145–156

Freud S: An autobiographical study (1925[1924]), in The Standard Edition of the Complete Psychological Works of Sigmund Freud, Vol 20. Translated and edited by Strachey J. London, Hogarth Press, 1959, pp 1–74

Frid M, Singer G: Hypnotic analgesia in conditions of stress is partially reversed by naloxone. Psychopharmacology (Berl) 63:211–215, 1979

Frischholz EJ: The relationship among dissociation, hypnosis, and child abuse in the development of multiple personality disorder, in Childhood Antecedents of Multiple Personality Disorder. Edited by Kluft RP. Washington, DC, American Psychiatric Press, 1985, pp 99–126

Frischholz EJ, Spiegel D: Adjunctive uses of hypnosis in the treatment of smoking. Psychiatric Annals 16:87–90, 1986

Frischholz EJ, Spiegel D, Spiegel H, et al: Differential hypnotic responsivity of smokers, phobics, and chronic-pain control patients: a failure to confirm. J Abnorm Psychol 91:269–272, 1982

Fuchs K, Paldi E, Abramovici H, et al: Treatment of hyperemesis gravidarum by hypnosis. Int J Clin Exp Hypn 28:313–323, 1980

Genuis ML: The use of hypnosis in helping cancer patients control anxiety, pain, and emesis: a review of recent empirical studies. Am J Clin Hypn 37:316–325, 1995

Gerschman J, Burrows GD, Reade P, et al: Hypnotizability and the treatment of dental phobic illness, in Hypnosis. Edited by Burrows GD, Collison DR, Dennerstein L. Amsterdam, Elsevier North-Holland Biomedical, 1979, pp 33–39

Glick BS: Conditioning therapy with phobic patients: success and failure. Am J Psychother 24:92–101, 1970

Goldstein E, Hilgard E: Failure of opiate antagonist naloxone to modify hypnotic analgesia. Proc Natl Acad Sci U S A 71:1041–1043, 1975

Grabowska MJ: The effect of hypnosis and hypnotic suggestions on the blood flow in the extremities. Pol Med J 10:1044–1051, 1971

Graffin NF, Ray WJ, Lundy R: EEG concomitants of hypnosis and hypnotic susceptibility. J Abnorm Psychol 104:123–131, 1995

Gravitz MA: First admission (1846) of hypnotic testimony in court. Am J Clin Hypn 37:326–330, 1995

Gritz E, Bloom J: Psychosocial sequelae of cancer in long-term survivors and their families. Paper presented at the Western Regional Conference of the American Cancer Society, Los Angeles, CA, January 1987

Grond M, Pawlik G, Walter H, et al: Hypnotic catalepsy-induced changes of regional cerebral glucose metabolism. Psychiatry Res 61:173–179, 1995

Gross M: Hypnosis in the therapy of anorexia nervosa. Am J Clin Hypn 26:175–181, 1984

Gur R, Reyher J: Relationship between style of hypnotic induction and direction of lateral eye movements. J Abnorm Psychol 82:499–505, 1973

Halliday AM, Mason AA: Cortical evoked potentials during hypnotic anaesthesia. Electroencephalogr Clin Neurophysiol 16:312–314, 1964

Hammarstrand G, Berggren U, Hakeberg M: Psychophysiological therapy vs. hypnotherapy in the treatment of patients with dental phobia. Eur J Oral Sci 103:399–404, 1995

Hargadon R, Bowers KS, Woody EZ: Does counterpain imagery mediate hypnotic analgesia? J Abnorm Psychol 104:508–516, 1995

Herod EL: Psychophysical pain control during tooth extraction. General Dentistry 43:267–269, 1995

Hilgard ER: Hypnotic Susceptibility. New York, Harcourt, Brace & World, 1965

Hilgard ER: Divided Consciousness: Multiple Controls in Human Thought and Action. New York, Wiley, 1977

Hilgard ER, Hilgard JR: Hypnosis in the Relief of Pain. Los Altos, CA, William Kaufmann, 1975

Hilgard JR: Personality and Hypnosis: A Study of Imaginative Involvement. Chicago, IL, University of Chicago Press, 1970

Hilgard JR, LeBaron S: Relief of anxiety and pain in children and adolescents with cancer: quantitative measures and clinical observations. Int J Clin Exp Hypn 30:417–442, 1982

Holroyd J: Hypnosis treatment for smoking: an evaluative review. Int J Clin Exp Hypn 28:341–357, 1980

Holroyd J: The uncertain relationship between hypnotizability and smoking treatment outcome. Int J Clin Exp Hypn 39:93–102, 1991

Houghton LA, Heyman DJ, Whorwell PJ: Symptomatology, quality of life and economic features of irritable bowel syndrome—the effect of hypnotherapy. Aliment Pharmacol Ther 10:91–95, 1996

Hyman GJ, Stanley RO, Burrows GD, et al: Treatment effectiveness of hypnosis and behaviour therapy in smoking cessation: a methodological refinement. Addict Behav 11:355–365, 1986

Iancu I, Kotler M, Spivak B, et al: Psychiatric aspects of hyperemesis gravidarum. Psychother Psychosom 61:143–149, 1994

Inoue H, Kobayashi H, Chiba T: Classification for bronchial asthma from the viewpoint of autonomic nerve function and airway hyperreactivity [in Japanese]. Nippon Kyobu Shikkan Gakkai Zasshi 33 (suppl):104–105, 1995

Jacknow DS, Tschann JM, Link MP, et al: Hypnosis in the prevention of chemotherapy-related nausea and vomiting in children: a prospective study. J Dev Behav Pediatr 15:258–264, 1994

Janet P: The Major Symptoms of Hysteria: Fifteen Lectures Given in the Medical School of Harvard University. New York, Macmillan, 1907

Johnson RF, Barber TX: Hypnosis, suggestions, and warts: an experimental investigation implicating the importance of "believed-in efficacy." Am J Clin Hypn 20:165–174, 1978

Kardiner A, Spiegel H: War Stress and Neurotic Illness. New York, Paul Hoeber, 1947

Katz RL, Kao CY, Spiegel H, et al: Pain, acupuncture, and hypnosis. Adv Neurol 4:819–825, 1974

Keller VE: Management of nausea and vomiting in children. J Pediatr Nurs 10:280–286, 1995

Kessler R, Dane JR: Psychological and hypnotic preparation for anesthesia and surgery: an individual differences perspective. Int J Clin Exp Hypn 44:189–207, 1996

Kiernan BD, Dane JR, Phillips LH, et al: Hypnotic analgesia reduces R-III nociceptive reflex: further evidence concerning the multifactorial nature of hypnotic analgesia. Pain 60:39–47, 1995

Kirsch I: Hypnotic enhancement of cognitive-behavioral weight loss treatments—another meta-reanalysis. J Consult Clin Psychol 64:517–519, 1996

Kirsch I, Montgomery G, Sapirstein G: Hypnosis as an adjunct to cognitive-behavioral psychotherapy: a meta-analysis. J Consult Clin Psychol 63:214–220, 1995

Klein KB, Spiegel D: Modulation of gastric acid secretion by hypnosis. Gastroenterology 96:1383–1387, 1989

Kluft RP: An introduction to multiple personality disorder. Psychiatric Annals 14:19–24, 1984a

Kluft RP: Treatment of multiple personality disorder: a study of 33 cases. Psychiatr Clin North Am 7:9–29, 1984b

Kluft RP: Childhood multiple personality disorder: predictors, clinical findings, and treatment results, in Childhood Antecedents of Multiple Personality Disorder. Edited by Kluft RP. Washington, DC, American Psychiatric Press, 1985, pp 167–196

Kluft RP: The treatment of dissociative disorder patients: an overview of discoveries, successes and failures. Dissociation 7:135–137, 1993

Knox VJ, Shum K: Reduction of cold-pressor pain with acupuncture analgesia in high- and low-hypnotic subjects. J Abnorm Psychol 86:639–643, 1977

Kohen DP: Application of relaxation/mental imagery (self-hypnosis) to the management of asthma: report of behavioral outcomes of a two-year, prospective controlled study. Am J Clin Hypn 34:283–294, 1986

Kohen DP, Wynne E: Applying hypnosis in a preschool family asthma education program: uses of storytelling, imagery, and relaxation. Am J Clin Hypn 39:169–181, 1997

Koopman C, Classen C, Cardeña E, et al: When disaster strikes, acute stress disorder may follow. J Trauma Stress 8:29–46, 1995

Lambert SA: The effects of hypnosis/guided imagery on the postoperative course of children. J Dev Behav Pediatr 17:307–310, 1996

Lang EV, Joyce JS, Spiegel D, et al: Self-hypnotic relaxation during interventional radiological procedures: effects on pain perception and intravenous drug use. Int J Clin Exp Hypn 44:106–119, 1996

Laurence JR, Perry C: Hypnotically created memory among highly hypnotizable subjects. Science 222:523–524, 1983

Lavoie G, Elie R: The clinical relevance of hypnotizability in psychosis, with reference to thinking processes and sample variances, in Modern Trends in Hypnosis. Edited by Waxman D, Misra P, Gibson M, et al. New York, Plenum, 1985, pp 41–66

Lavoie G, Sabourin M: Hypnosis and schizophrenia: a review of experimental and clinical studies, in Handbook of Hypnosis and Psychosomatic Medicine. Edited by Burrows GD, Dennerstein L. Amsterdam, Elsevier North-Holland Biomedical, 1980, pp 377–420

Lazarus AA: "Hypnosis" as a facilitator in behavior therapy. Int J Clin Exp Hypn 21:25–31, 1973

Lopez CA: Franklin and Mesmer: an encounter. Yale J Biol Med 66:325–331, 1993

Lu DP: The use of hypnosis for smooth sedation induction and reduction of postoperative violent emergencies from anesthesia in pediatric dental patients. ASDC J Dent Child 61:182–185, 1994

Maher-Loughan GP: Hypnosis and autohypnosis for the treatment of asthma. Int J Clin Exp Hypn 18:1–14, 1970

Maldonado JR, Spiegel D: Hypnosis, in Psychiatry. Edited by Tashman A, Kay J, Lieberman J. Philadelphia, PA, WB Saunders, 1996, pp 1475–1499

Maldonado JR, Spiegel D: Trauma, dissociation and hypnotizability, in Trauma: Memory and Dissociation. Edited by Marmar R, Bremmer D. Washington, DC, American Psychiatric Press, 1998, pp 57–106

Maldonado JR, Butler L, Spiegel D: Treatment of dissociative disorders, in A Guide to Treatments That Work. Edited by Nathan PE, Gorman JM. New York, Oxford Press, 1997, pp 423–446

Marks IM, Gelder MG, Edwards G: Hypnosis and desensitization for phobias: a controlled prospective trial. Br J Psychiatry 114:1263–1274, 1968

McConkey KM: The effects of hypnotic procedures on remembering, in Contemporary Hypnosis Research. Edited by Fromm E, Nash MR. New York, Guilford, 1992, pp 405–426

McGlashan TH, Evans FJ, Orne MT: The nature of hypnotic analgesia and the placebo response to experimental pain. Psychosom Med 31:227–246, 1969

McGuinness TP: Hypnosis in the treatment of phobias: a review of the literature. Am J Clin Hypn 26:261–272, 1984

Miller ME, Bowers KS: Hypnotic analgesia: dissociated experience or dissociated control? J Abnorm Psychol 102:29–38, 1993

Mishkin M: Cerebral memory circuits, in 1990 Yakult International Symposium: Perception, Cognition and Brain. Yakult Honsha Co, Tokyo, August 1991

Mize WL: Clinical training in self-regulation and practical pediatric hypnosis: what pediatricians want pediatricians to know. J Dev Behav Pediatr 17:317–322, 1996

Moore R, Abrahamsen R, Brodsgaard I: Hypnosis compared with group therapy and individual desensitization for dental anxiety. Eur J Oral Sci 104:612–618, 1996

Morgan AH, MacDonald H, Hilgard ER: EEG alpha: lateral asymmetry related to task and hypnotizability. Psychophysiology 11:275–282, 1974

Morrison JB: Chronic asthma and improvement with relaxation induced by hypnotherapy. J R Soc Med 81:701–704, 1988

Myers JK, Weissman MM, Tischler GL, et al: Six-month prevalence of psychiatric disorders in three communities: 1980 to 1982. Arch Gen Psychiatry 41:959–967, 1984

Orne MT: Hypnosis in the treatment of smoking, in Proceedings of the 3rd World Conference on Smoking and Health, Vol 2 (DHEW NIH 77-1413). Washington, DC, Department of Health, Education and Welfare, 1977, pp 489–507

Orne MT: The use and misuse of hypnosis in court. Int J Clin Exp Hypn 27:311–341, 1979

Orne MT, Axelrad AD, Diamond BL, et al: Scientific status of refreshing recollection by the use of hypnosis. JAMA 253:1918–1923, 1985

People v Guerra, C-41916 Supreme Court, CA, Orange Co (1984)

People v Hughes, 59 NY2d 523, 466 NYS2d 255, 543 NE2d, 484 (1983)

People v Hurd, Supreme Court, NJ, Somerset Co, April 2, 1980

People v Schoenfeld, 168 Cal Rptr 762, 111 CA3d 671 (1980)

People v Shirley, 31 Cal 3d 18, 641 P2d 775 (1982), modified 918a (1982)

Peretz B: Relaxation and hypnosis in pediatric dental patients. Journal of Clinical Pediatric Dentistry 20:205–207, 1996

Pettinati HM: Measuring hypnotizability in psychotic patients. Int J Clin Exp Hypn 30:404–416, 1982

Pettinati HM, Kogan LG, Evans FJ, et al: Hypnotizability of psychiatric inpatients according to two different scales. Am J Psychiatry 147:69–75, 1990

Piccione C, Hilgard ER, Zimbardo PG: On the degree of stability of measured hypnotizability over a 25-year period. J Pers Soc Psychol 56:289–295, 1989

Posner MI, Peterson SE: The attention system of the human brain. Annu Rev Neurosci 13:25–42, 1990

Putnam FW Jr: Dissociation as a response to extreme trauma, in Childhood Antecedents of Multiple Personality Disorder. Edited by Kluft RP. Washington, DC, American Psychiatric Press, 1985, pp 65–97

Rabkin SW, Boyko E, Shane F, et al: A randomized trial comparing smoking cessation programs utilizing behaviour modification, health education or hypnosis. Addict Behav 9:157–173, 1984

Rainville P, Duncan GH, Price DD, et al: Pain affect encoded in human anterior cingulate but not somatosensory cortex. Science 277:968–971, 1997

Rape RN, Bush JP: Psychological preparation for pediatric oncology patients undergoing painful procedures: a methodological critique of the research. Childrens Health Care 23:51–67, 1994

Redd WH, Andresen GV, Minagawa RY: Hypnotic control of anticipatory emesis in patients receiving cancer chemotherapy. J Consult Clin Psychol 50:14–19, 1982

Robb ND, Crothers AJ: Sedation in dentistry, part 2: management of the gagging patient. Dental Update 23:182–186, 1996

Roberts AH, Tellegen A: Ratings of "trust" and hypnotic susceptibility. Int J Clin Exp Hypn 21:289–297, 1973

Rock v Arkansas, 107 S Ct 2704, 97 LEd 2d 37 (1987)

Rustvold SR: Hypnotherapy for treatment of dental phobia in children. General Dentistry 42:346–348, 1994

Sabourin ME, Cutcomb SD, Crawford HJ, et al: EEG correlates of hypnotic susceptibility and hypnotic trance: spectral analysis and coherence. Int J Psychophysiol 10:125–142, 1990

Schacter DL: Implicit memory: history and current status. J Exp Psychol Learn Mem Cogn 13:501–518, 1987

Scheflin AW, Shapiro JL: Trance on Trial. New York, Guilford, 1989

Schenck CH, Mahowald MW: Two cases of premenstrual sleep terrors and injurious sleep-walking. J Psychosom Obstet Gynaecol 16:79–84, 1995

Schwartz JL: Smoking Cessation Methods: United States and Canada, 1978–85 (USPHS NIH 87–2940). Washington, DC, Division of Cancer Prevention and Control, National Cancer Institute, 1987

Schwartz JL: Methods for smoking cessation. Clin Chest Med 12:737–753, 1991

Shaw AJ, Niven N: Theoretical concepts and practical applications of hypnosis in the treatment of children and adolescents with dental fear and anxiety. Br Dent J 180:11–16, 1996

Shaw AJ, Welbury RR: The use of hypnosis in a sedation clinic for dental extractions in children: report of 20 cases. ASDC J Dent Child 63:418–420, 1996

Sigalowitz SJ, Dywan J, Ismailos L: Electrocortical evidence that hypnotically induced hallucinations are experienced. Paper presented at the Society for Clinical and Experimental Hypnosis Meeting, New Orleans, LA, October 1991

Sjoberg BM, Hollister LE: The effects of psychotomimetic drugs on primary suggestibility. Psychopharmacologia 8:251–262, 1965

Somer E: Biofeedback-aided hypnotherapy for intractable phobic anxiety. Am J Clin Hypn 37:54–64, 1995

Spanos NP, Stenstrom RJ, Johnston JC: Hypnosis, placebo and suggestion in the treatment of warts. Psychosom Med 50:245–260, 1988

Spanos NP, Williams V, Gwynn MI: Effects of hypnotic, placebo, and salicylic acid treatments on wart regression. Psychosom Med 52:109–114, 1990

Spiegel D: Hypnotizability and psychoactive medication. Am J Clin Hypn 22:217–222, 1980

Spiegel D: Vietnam grief work using hypnosis. Am J Clin Hypn 24:33–40, 1981

Spiegel D: Multiple personality as a post-traumatic stress disorder. Psychiatr Clin North Am 7:101–110, 1984

Spiegel D: The use of hypnosis in controlling cancer pain. CA Cancer J Clin 35:221–231, 1985

Spiegel D: Dissociating damage. Am J Clin Hypn 29:123–131, 1986a

Spiegel D: Dissociation, double binds, and posttraumatic stress in multiple personality disorder, in Treatment of Multiple Personality Disorder. Edited by Braun BG. Washington, DC, American Psychiatric Press, 1986b, pp 61–77

Spiegel D: Dissociation and hypnosis in posttraumatic stress disorders. Journal of Traumatic Stress 1:17–33, 1988

Spiegel D: Hypnosis, dissociation, and trauma: hidden and overt observers, in Repression and Dissociation: Implications for Personality Theory, Psychopathology, and Health. Edited by Singer JL. Chicago, IL, University of Chicago Press, 1990a, pp 121–142

Spiegel D: Trauma, dissociation, and hypnosis, in Incest-Related Syndromes of Adult Psychopathology. Edited by Kluft RL. Washington, DC, American Psychiatric Press, 1990b, pp 247–261

Spiegel D, Albert L: Naloxone fails to reverse hypnotic alleviation of chronic pain. Psychopharmacology (Berl) 81:140–143, 1983

Spiegel D, Bloom JR: Group therapy and hypnosis reduce metastatic breast carcinoma pain. Psychosom Med 45:333–339, 1983

Spiegel D, Cardeña E: Disintegrated experience: the dissociative disorders revisited. J Abnorm Psychol 100:366–378, 1991

Spiegel D, Chase RA: The treatment of contractures of the hand using self-hypnosis. J Hand Surg [Am] 5:428–432, 1980

Spiegel D, Fink R: Hysterical psychosis and hypnotizability. Am J Psychiatry 136:777–781, 1979

Spiegel D, King R: Hypnotizability and CSF HVA levels among psychiatric patients. Biol Psychiatry 31:95–98, 1992

Spiegel D, Rosenfeld A: Spontaneous hypnotic age regression: case report. J Clin Psychiatry 45:522–524, 1984

Spiegel D, Scheflin AW: Dissociated or fabricated? Psychiatric aspects of repressed memory in criminal and civil cases. Int J Clin Exp Hyp 42:411–432, 1994

Spiegel D, Spiegel H: Forensic uses of hypnosis, in Handbook of Forensic Psychology. Edited by Weiner IB, Hess AK. New York, Wiley, 1987, pp 490–507

Spiegel D, Spiegel H: Assessment and treatment using hypnosis, in Handbook of Anxiety Disorders. Edited by Last CG, Hersen M. New York, Pergamon, 1988, pp 401–412

Spiegel D, Vermutten E: Effects of hypnosis on somatic functions, in Dissociation: Culture, Mind, and Body. Edited by Spiegel D. Washington, DC, American Psychiatric Press, 1994, pp 185–209

Spiegel D, Bloom JR, Yalom I[D]: Group support for patients with metastatic cancer: a randomized prospective outcome study. Arch Gen Psychiatry 38:527–533, 1981a

Spiegel D, Frischholz EJ, Maruffi B, et al: Hypnotic responsivity and the treatment of flying phobia. Am J Clin Hypn 23:239–247, 1981b

Spiegel D, Detrick D, Frischholz E[J]: Hypnotizability and psychopathology. Am J Psychiatry 139:431–437, 1982

Spiegel D, Cutcomb S, Ren C, et al: Hypnotic hallucination alters evoked potentials. J Abnorm Psychol 94:249–255, 1985

Spiegel D, Hunt T, Dondershine HE: Dissociation and hypnotizability in posttraumatic stress disorder. Am J Psychiatry 145:301–305, 1988

Spiegel D, Bierre P, Rootenberg J: Hypnotic alteration of somatosensory perception. Am J Psychiatry 146:749–754, 1989

Spiegel D, Frischholz EJ, Fleiss JL, et al: Predictors of smoking abstinence following a single-session restructuring intervention with self-hypnosis. Am J Psychiatry 150:1090–1097, 1993a

Spiegel D, Frischholz EJ, Spira J: Functional disorders of memory, in American Psychiatric Press Review of Psychiatry, Vol 12. Edited by Oldham JM, Riba MB, Tasman A. Washington, DC, American Psychiatric Press, 1993b, pp 747–782

Spiegel H: The dissociation-association continuum. J Nerv Ment Dis 136:374–378, 1963

Spiegel H: Termination of smoking by a single treatment. Arch Environ Health 20:736–742, 1970

Spiegel H: The Grade 5 syndrome: the highly hypnotizable person. Int J Clin Exp Hypn 22:303–319, 1974

Spiegel H: Hypnosis and evidence: help or hindrance? Ann N Y Acad Sci 347:73–85, 1980

Spiegel H, Spiegel D: Trance and Treatment: Clinical Uses of Hypnosis. Washington, DC, American Psychiatric Press, 1987

Stanton HE: Using hypnotherapy to overcome examination anxiety. Am J Clin Hypn 35:198–204, 1993

State ex rel Collins v Superior Court, 132 Ariz 180, 644 P2d 1266 (1982), supplemental opinion filed May 4, 1982

Steingard S, Frankel FH: Dissociation and psychotic symptoms. Am J Psychiatry 142:953–955, 1985

Stern DL, Spiegel H, Nee JCM: The Hypnotic Induction Profile: normative observations, reliability, and validity. Am J Clin Hypn 21:109–132, 1979

Surman OS, Gottlieb SK, Hackett TP, et al: Hypnosis in the treatment of warts. Arch Gen Psychiatry 28:439–441, 1973

Szechtman H, Woody E, Bowers KS, et al: Where the imaginal appears real: a positron emission tomography study of auditory hallucinations. Proceedings of the National Academy of Sciences 95:1956–1960, 1998

Tellegen A: Practicing the two disciplines for relaxation and enlightenment: comment on "Role of the Feedback Signal in Electromyograph Biofeedback: The Relevance of Attention," by Qualls and Sheegan. J Exp Psychol Gen 110:217–226, 1981

Tellegen A, Atkinson G: Openness to absorbing and self-altering experiences ("absorption"), a trait related to hypnotic susceptibility. J Abnorm Psychol 83:268–277, 1974

Torem MS: Hypnotherapeutic techniques in the treatment of hyperemesis gravidarum. Am J Clin Hypn 37:1–11, 1994

Ulich P, Meyer HJ, Biehl B, et al: Cerebral blood flow in autogenic training and hypnosis. Neurosurg Rev 10:P305–P307, 1987

van der Hart O, Spiegel D: Hypnotic assessment and treatment of trauma-induced psychoses: the early psychotherapy of H. Breukink and modern views. Int J Clin Exp Hypn 41:191–209, 1993

van der Kolk BA, Fisler R: Dissociation and the fragmentary nature of traumatic memories: overview and exploratory study. J Trauma Stress 8:505–525, 1995

van der Kolk BA, van der Hart O: Pierre Janet and the breakdown of adaptation in psychological trauma. Am J Psychiatry 146:1530–1540, 1989

van der Kolk BA, Hostetler A, Herron N, et al: Trauma and the development of borderline personality disorder. Psychiatr Clin North Am 17:715–730, 1994

Vanderlinden J, Spinhoven P, Vandereycken W, et al: Dissociative and hypnotic experiences in eating disorder patients: an exploratory study. Am J Clin Hypn 38:97–108, 1995

Volkow ND, Tancredi LR: Biological correlates of mental activity studied with PET. Am J Psychiatry 148:439–443, 1991

von Plessen K: Jean Martin Charcot and his controversial research on hysteria. Tidsskr Nor Laegeforen 116:3633–3635, 1996

Weitzenhoffer AM, Hilgard ER: Stanford Hypnotic Susceptibility Scale, Forms A and B. Palo Alto, CA, Consulting Psychologists Press, 1959

Weitzenhoffer AM, Hilgard ER: Stanford Hypnotic Susceptibility Scale, Form C. Palo Alto, CA, Consulting Psychologists Press, 1962

Whorwell PJ, Prior A, Faragher EB: Controlled trial of
hypnotherapy in the treatment of severe refractory irrita-
ble-bowel syndrome. Lancet 1:1232–1234, 1984

Whorwell PJ, Prior A, Colgan SM: Hypnotherapy in severe irritable bowel syndrome: further experience. Gut 28:
423–425, 1987

Widlocher D, Dantchev N: Charcot and hysteria. Rev Neurol
(Paris) 150:490–497, 1994

Wilks CG: The use of hypnosis in the management of gagging
and intolerance to dentures (letter). Br Dent J 176:332,
1994

Williams JM, Hall DW: Use of single session hypnosis for
smoking cessation. Addict Behav 13:205–208, 1988

Wilson NJ: Neurophysiologic alterations with hypnosis. Diseases of the Nervous System 29:618–620, 1968

Windholz G: Hypnosis and inhibition as viewed by Heidenhain
and Pavlov. Integr Physiol Behav Sci 31:155–162, 1996

Wood DP, Sexton JL: Self-hypnosis training and captivity survival. Am J Clin Hypn 39:201–211, 1997

Zeltzer L, LeBaron S: Hypnosis and nonhypnotic techniques
for reduction of pain and anxiety during painful procedures
in children and adolescents with cancer. J Pediatr 101:
1032–1035, 1982

Zeltzer L, LeBaron S, Zeltzer PM: The effectiveness of behavioral intervention for reduction of nausea and vomiting in
children and adolescents receiving chemotherapy. J Clin
Oncol 2:683–690, 1984

Zimbardo PG, Maslach C, Marshall G: Hypnosis and the Psychology of Cognitive and Behavioral Control. Stanford,
CA, Department of Psychology, Stanford University, 1970

CHAPTER 33

GROUP THERAPY

SOPHIA VINOGRADOV, M.D.
PAUL D. COX, M.D.
IRVIN D. YALOM, M.D.

Interpersonal relationships are of crucial importance to human psychological development. There are many psychiatric and therapeutic implications to this simple premise. Personality and patterns of behavior can be seen as the result of early interactions with other significant human beings. Modern schools of dynamic psychotherapy underscore the link between psychopathology and distorted interpersonal relationships and emphasize that psychiatric treatment must be directed toward understanding and correcting these distortions. Although this can of course take place in the context of the therapist-patient dyad, it is self-evident that a group of people can serve as an immensely specific therapeutic tool. In such a group setting, patients are provided with a varied array of interpersonal relationships that, with proper guidance, will permit them to identify, explore, and alter maladaptive interpersonal behavior.

Furthermore, the group setting is at once a ubiquitous and elusive phenomenon in our society. After all, groups are everywhere around us throughout our lives, from our early family units, to the classroom and our classmates, to the persons we surround ourselves with at work, at play, and at home. At the same time, we hear complaints about increasing interpersonal alienation in modern life—a sense of isolation, anonymity, and even social fragmentation. Perhaps because of this, and because it can provide such a powerful and unique therapeutic experience, the group setting is being used more and more not only by mental health professionals but by laypersons. Alcoholics Anonymous, Parents Without Partners, Recovery, Inc., Overeaters Anonymous, Mended Hearts, and Compassionate Friends are but a few of the current specialized and self-help groups available in the lay setting.

A number of specialized groups have been developed to function in a supportive and occasionally highly therapeutic mode in nonpsychiatric medical settings as well. The groundbreaking work of Spiegel et al. (1989) demonstrated a twofold increase in survival rate for patients with metastatic breast carcinoma who participated in a long-term psychodynamically oriented support group. Fawzy and colleagues (1993) found an improvement both in use of coping strategies and in immune function in patients with malignant melanoma who participated in a short-term group intervention.

CLINICAL RELEVANCE OF GROUP THERAPY

Although the general principles of group therapy are increasingly being employed by the self-help group movement and by other mental health professions, mainstream psychiatric education has de-emphasized the teaching and practice of group therapy. Perhaps the remedicalization of psychiatry, with its emphasis on biological modes of treatment for mental illness, accounts for this trend. Also, some psychiatrists may be alienated by the fact that the group treatment modality is being used so often by laypersons in settings that are, strictly speaking, nonpsychiatric. The estrangement of psychiatrists from group work is of some concern; after all, group therapy is a widely practiced mode of psychotherapy that is employed in a vast number of clinical settings with a proven degree of clinical effectiveness. The advent of widespread managed care and population-based care systems will probably necessitate increased use of groups and therefore the teaching of groups.

EFFICACY

First and foremost, group therapy is effective treatment. Multiple outcome studies of varying sophistication and methodological design have been performed since the early 1960s. Considerable clinical consensus and research evidence have accumulated indicating that various forms of group therapy are beneficial to their participants (Dies 1979, 1993; Kaul and Bednar 1986; MacKenzie 1997; Orlinsky and Howard 1986; Smith et al. 1980; Yalom 1983, 1985). Investigators over the years have concluded that group treatment is as effective as individual therapy in treating psychological disorders (D. A. Shapiro and Shapiro 1982; Smith et al. 1980). Recently, 32 studies that directly contrasted individual and group treatments were analyzed (Tillitski 1990; Toseland and Siporin 1986); in 24 of the studies, no major differences were found between the two modalities. In the remaining 8 studies, group therapy was found to be more effective than individual therapy.

NUMBERS OF GROUP THERAPY PATIENTS

Enormous numbers of psychiatric patients receive their sole or primary treatment in groups. This is particularly true in institutional settings and for chronically mentally ill persons. At least one-half of all psychiatric hospitals and one-quarter of all correctional institutions, not to mention the vast majority of community mental health centers, use group treatments (J. L. Shapiro 1978). Many health maintenance organizations make substantial use of group therapy as well (Cheifetz and Salloway 1984; MacKenzie 1997; Spitz 1997). Altogether, hundreds of thousands of patients undergo group therapy. Furthermore, patients most often found in institutional settings—the chronically ill—represent one of the greatest current challenges to the psychiatric profession and to social policy regarding the mentally ill. When compared with these populations, patients receiving routine individual therapy are a relatively insignificant subset, in terms of both large-scale mental health policy and sheer numbers.

NONPSYCHIATRIC GROUPS

New orders of magnitude occur when we consider the staggering number of nonpsychiatric clients who receive treatment in specialized therapy groups or in one of the vast number of self-help groups. For example, the use of groups for patients with particular medical conditions—such as cancer support groups, post–myocardial infarction groups, and diabetes education groups—is burgeoning in the health care setting (Stern 1993). In 1983, perhaps 12 million to 14 million individuals attended some form of self-help group (e.g., Alcoholics Anonymous, Compassionate Friends, Recovery, Inc.) (Lieberman 1990). And hundreds of thousands of Americans continue to seek involvement in large group awareness training such as Lifespring. Inevitably, the practicing therapist of nearly every persuasion will encounter clients who have had contact with some form of group experience.

PRACTICAL ASPECTS OF GROUP THERAPY: COST-EFFECTIVENESS AND EFFICIENCY

At its inception, group therapy was grounded in practical aspects. To facilitate the treatment of large numbers of tuberculosis patients at the turn of the century, a Boston internist named Joseph Pratt developed a workable, efficient treatment format: group meetings. Many of Dr. Pratt's patients were indigent and could not afford private care; many were debilitated, despondent, and ostracized in the healthy community. Needing to work with many different individuals in a highly efficient manner, Dr. Pratt began organizing groups of 20 or 30 patients and lecturing them once or twice a week (Pratt 1922). Even today, of course, group therapy retains this advantageous feature of expediency. Large numbers of patients can be treated and efficient use can be made of time and other resources.

Cost-effectiveness played an important role in the early development of group therapy as well. As noted in the previous paragraph, Pratt himself worked with indigent patients, and several other early pioneers in the group-lecture approach treated psychotic individuals who could afford only institutional care. Alfred Adler, an Austrian psychiatrist who became interested in theories of group behavior and of social interest, also spoke of "bringing psychology to the people" (Ansbacher 1980, p. 733). In England during and after World War II, the overwhelming number of psychiatric casualties and the limited hospital staff available made group treatment the most practical modality and led to an explosion in group therapy practice and research, which included the work of Wilfred Bion and the Tavistock model of group behavior and of S. H. Foulkes and group analysis (Pines and Hutchinson 1993). The same situation holds true today in many understaffed community agencies or institutional settings: treatment groups permit more efficient use of limited staff. Leadership in managed care supports the use of groups in large part for reasons of expediency.

Fortunately, the rationale for group therapy goes well beyond economics and savings in staff time. In examining nine studies comparing the differential efficiency of individual and group therapy, Toseland and Siporin (1986) concluded that group treatment is more consistently efficient and/or cost-effective. As efforts to maintain or improve outcomes while containing costs continue, these practical considerations of expediency and cost and staff efficiency will undoubtedly take on more weight. In fact, more than one group therapist has suggested that clinicians soon may need to justify individual therapy and defend their decision not to use the more cost-effective group therapy (Dies 1986; MacKenzie 1997). However, although group therapy is more cost-efficient, its advantages transcend simple economic considerations: it is a form of treatment that makes use of unique therapeutic properties not shared by other psychotherapies.

SCOPE OF CURRENT GROUP THERAPY PRACTICE

Current group therapy practice encompasses a wide spectrum, ranging from the long-term interactional outpatient group and the medication-support group to the time-limited psychoeducational group to the acute crisis drop-in group (MacKenzie 1997; Vinogradov and Yalom 1989). Therapy groups can be categorized by means of four interrelated characteristics (Table 33–1): the setting of the group, its duration, its goals, and its techniques.

SETTING

One distinguishing feature among groups is their clinical setting. A particularly clear distinction can be made between psychiatric inpatient and outpatient groups. Inpatient groups on a psychiatric ward tend to meet daily, are usually composed of individuals with acute psychiatric problems, and often involve mandatory participation; turnover is great, with membership fluctuating widely because of the short duration of hospitalization. Psychiatric outpatient groups, in contrast, meet once weekly, consist of individuals who show more similar and more stable levels of functioning, and involve voluntary participation; membership tends to be more stable. There can be exceptions, of course. Some inpatient wards attempt to form more homogeneous groups that are based on level of functioning, although their membership will still vary widely. And psychiatric outpatient groups encompass many variations, ranging from the monthly drop-in group for chronically ill patients in a medication clinic to the twice-weekly interactional group run in a private practitioner's office.

Inpatient versus outpatient is but one distinction. Group therapy is also practiced in a myriad of other clinical settings, extending from the daily small groups in a psychiatric day hospital, to weekly probation groups, to staff retreats or support groups. Specialized groups for medical syndromes, such as diabetes education groups or lupus support groups, often meet in a hospital or clinic setting, whereas other types of specialized groups (e.g., rape crisis groups, Vietnam veterans' groups), may be associated with a center that offers counseling services (e.g., rape trauma center, veterans' outreach center).

DURATION

A second consideration for any therapy group is its duration. Most inpatient groups are an integral part of the treatment program and are thus indefinitely self-sustaining; the ward census may change, different kinds of patients may be hospitalized, but the group meets every day. Outpatient groups have more latitude with regard to duration. They can exist for one session only (e.g., a drop-in crisis group that meets as needed at a student health center), or they can be open-ended and long-term in nature and periodically renew their membership over the years. In an interactionally oriented outpatient group, members will usually stay in therapy for 1–3 years, and "graduating" members are replaced as they leave so that

TABLE 33–1. Scope of current group therapy practice

Type of group	Life of group	Attendance	Average length of stay in group	Goals	Major therapeutic factors/techniques	Membership criteria
Prototypic interactionally oriented groups	Indefinite; as permitted by professional schedule of group leaders	Voluntary, but regular attendance essential	1–2 years	Character change; symptom relief	Interpersonal learning; corrective recapitulation of primary family group	Higher-functioning patients; interpersonal pathology; desire to change, able to tolerate interpersonal focus; able to attend all sessions
Acute inpatient groups	Indefinite; usually integral part of ward program	Generally mandatory during hospitalization; will show higher turnover	1–2 days to several weeks, depending on length of hospitalization	Restoration of function	Instillation of hope; socialization techniques; altruism; existential factors	Patients may be placed in different groups by level of functioning; membership will fluctuate widely
Follow-up or after-care groups; discharge planning groups; day hospital groups; probation groups	Indefinite; usually associated with a specific program	Often mandatory	Usually fixed number of sessions	Deinstitution-alization	Instillation of hope; imparting of information; imitative behavior; socializing techniques	Patients require follow-up care or aftercare; able to tolerate group setting and attend required sessions
Medication or clinic groups	Indefinite; usually part of clinic program	Voluntary; often occurring on a drop-in basis	Indefinite; depends on patient's enrollment in clinic	Support; education; maintenance of functions	Imparting of information; socializing techniques	Patients on long-term psychiatric medication; able to tolerate group setting
Behaviorally oriented groups (e.g., eating disorders group)	Time-limited, often 6–12 sessions; some groups are ongoing	Voluntary, but regular attendance generally prerequisite for group participation	Life of group	Discrete behavior change	Techniques of behavior modification; universality; imitative behavior	Patients with specific behavioral problem; desire to change
Specialized groups for medical disorders (e.g., diabetes, heart disease)	Time-limited, often 6–12 sessions; some groups are ongoing	Voluntary; often drop-in basis	Life of group or fixed number of sessions	Education; support; socialization	Universality; cohesiveness; imparting of information; imitative behavior; altruism; existential factors	Patients with specific medical problems; desire for further education and support
Specialized groups for life events: bereavement groups, divorce groups	Tend to be time-limited, 8–12 sessions	Voluntary; often flexible	Life of group	Support; catharsis; socialization	Cohesiveness; altruism; existential factors	Patients or clients who have undergone life event; desire for group experience
Specialized support groups: Vietnam veterans' outreach groups, rape crisis groups, student center drop-in groups, professional support groups, professional retreats	Indefinite; ongoing for professional retreats, which usually last 1–3 days	Usually drop-in basis; for staff support groups, especially during retreats, all members of staff should attend	Variable	Support; catharsis	Cohesiveness; altruism; occasional interpersonal learning	Patients or clients who belong to specialized situation; desire for support

the size of the group remains approximately constant. A sizable number of groups in the outpatient setting, however, choose a time-limited format, especially if they are focusing on a specific problem. For example, an educational-behavioral group for patients with eating disorders may be designed to meet for six sessions.

GOALS

A third factor that can be used to characterize the different kinds of group therapy pertains to the goals of the group, which may be conceptualized as existing along a spectrum. At one end of this spectrum are the ambitious goals of long-term interactional groups: symptom relief and character change. At the other end, there is the more limited but crucial goal of restoration of function: the deinstitutionalizing role of acute inpatient therapy groups. Between these two extremes lie the goals of the large majority of therapy groups. For some, such as medication clinic groups or inpatient and outpatient groups for chronically mentally ill persons, the most important goal will be maintenance of appropriate psychosocial functioning. Numerous others, including social skills training groups and specialized and self-help groups, attempt to provide education, socialization, and support. Many symptom-oriented short-term groups that are behaviorally focused (e.g., groups centered on bulimia, agoraphobia, or smoking cessation) have the goal of discrete behavior change.

THEORETICAL ORIENTATION AND TECHNIQUES

A fourth aspect of any therapy group is its theoretical orientation and the techniques employed by the therapist. This aspect is closely entwined with the goals of the group. An eating disorders group with the goal of discrete behavior change, for example, may have a cognitive-behavioral orientation and may focus on identifying cognitive distortions and triggers to behavioral responses. An analytic therapy group that has the goal of improving patients' ego functioning, on the other hand, may focus on the analysis of transference and resistance.

A wide range of theories and techniques inform the current practice of group therapy (Alonso and Swiller 1993). In this chapter, we will for the most part describe an understanding and an application of group therapy that are based on an interpersonal model of psychological functioning. This interpersonal orientation has a sound clinical and empirical foundation and translates into a set of clear and coherent tasks and techniques for the group therapist.

MEMBERSHIP CRITERIA

As can be seen from Table 33–1, the specific membership criteria for a given therapy group can vary widely from one type of group to another and are intimately linked to the goals of the group. In a behaviorally oriented group for patients with obsessive-compulsive disorder, for example, inclusion criteria are obsessive-compulsive symptomatology and a desire to change. The exclusion criterion is simply an inability to partake in a group experience (an extremely paranoid and obsessive individual would be excluded, for example). In contrast, a prototypic interactionally oriented group has much more stringent inclusion criteria: a member must admit to some interpersonal pathology, must have the ego strength and functioning necessary to tolerate an interpersonal focus, and must commit to regular attendance.

From these examples, the underlying principle for membership is made clear: whatever the specific nature of the group, a member must be able to perform the group task as the group works toward its goals. A member must therefore have problem areas that are compatible with the goals of the group and must have some motivation to change. Exclusion criteria include any factors that may interfere with the group task, such as marked incompatibility with group norms or with one or more group members, inability to tolerate the group setting, or a tendency to assume a deviant role in the group. These general criteria are outlined in Table 33–2 and are discussed further in the section on selecting patients and composing a therapy group.

In sum, the scope of current group therapy practice is wide indeed; those persons receiving treatment range from severely ill hospitalized psychiatric patients, to high-functioning outpatients, to persons with specific nonpsychiatric problems. Group therapy is a highly flexible psychotherapeutic modality, one that can be adapted to a variety of settings, time constraints, goals, and techniques.

TABLE 33–2. General membership criteria for group therapy

Inclusion criteria

Ability to perform group task

Problem areas compatible with group goals

Motivation to change

Exclusion criteria

Marked incompatibility with group norms for acceptable behavior

Inability to tolerate group setting

Severe incompatibility with one or more members

Tendency to assume deviant role

THERAPEUTIC FACTORS IN GROUP THERAPY: THE INTERPERSONAL FOCUS

Consider for a moment a hypothetical therapy group—let us say an outpatient group with eight members. Psychotherapy with one individual patient is a complex enough undertaking, but a group of patients is a potential Tower of Babel! Eight individuals intensively interact together, each with a different presenting complaint, varying psychological needs, unique problems in living, and, of course, a distinct character structure. Certain theorists would even argue that a new entity, with its own personality and characteristics, has been formed: the group itself.

The complexity of understanding and making sense of this enterprise often seems overwhelming to the neophyte therapist. What is needed is some simplifying principle, some mode of distinguishing between the truly essential, mutative aspects of the therapy group experience and those elements that represent the accessory characteristics of conscious and unconscious interaction in the group. We need to ask this question: Of all the dizzying, complex events in a group's transactions, which truly help the patient to change? We must identify the actual mechanisms of change in group therapy.

IDENTIFYING THE THERAPEUTIC FACTORS IN GROUP THERAPY

Group therapy was practiced for nearly half a century before researchers took steps to determine which factors actually help patients to change. Since the 1950s, a variety of research approaches have been used, including the interview and testing of group therapy patients with successful outcomes, as well as questionnaires directed at experienced group therapists and trained observers. Using these methods, researchers have identified a number of mechanisms of change in group therapy, that is, the curative or therapeutic factors.

There is usually a high degree of overlap among the various classification systems proposed by different investigators (Bloch 1986; Bloch and Crouch 1985; Butler and Fuhriman 1983; Corsini and Rosenberg 1955; Dies 1993; Fuhriman and Burlingame 1990; Yalom 1970). Yalom (1995) derived an atheoretical, 11-factor inventory of the therapeutic mechanisms operating in group therapy (Table 33–3): 1) instillation of hope, 2) universality, 3) imparting of information, 4) altruism, 5) development of socializing techniques, 6) imitative behavior, 7) catharsis, 8) corrective recapitulation of the primary family group, 9) existential factors, 10) group cohesiveness, and 11) interpersonal

learning. Yalom suggested that these primary factors, derived from extensive clinical and research evidence, serve as provisional guidelines for determining how group therapy helps patients to change. Furthermore, these factors can constitute the basis for an effective technical approach to therapy. In his comprehensive text on group therapy, *The Theory and Practice of Group Psychotherapy*, Yalom (1995) utilized these therapeutic factors as a central organizing principle.

Let us define and briefly discuss each of these factors. The last factor—the powerful but often misunderstood mechanism of interpersonal learning—will be discussed in greater detail.

Instillation of Hope

Instilling and maintaining hope is crucial in all psychotherapies and plays a unique role in group therapy. Clinical sentiment and research evidence alike indicate that faith in the treatment mode can in itself be therapeutically effective, both when the patient has a high expectation of help and when the therapist believes in the efficacy of the treatment (Bloch and Crouch 1985). In therapy groups of every ilk, there will be patients who have improved as well as members who are at a low ebb; patients will often remark at the end of therapy how important it was for them to observe the improvement of others and thus to hope for their own improvement. Many of the self-help groups that emerged in the 1970s and 1980s, such as Compassionate Friends for bereaved parents or Mended Hearts for cardiac surgery patients, also place a heavy emphasis on the instillation of hope. Groups such as Alcoholics Anonymous that are aimed at substance abuse often use the testimonials of former alcoholic or recovered addicted persons to inspire hope in new members.

TABLE 33–3. **Yalom's inventory of the therapeutic factors in group therapy**

Instillation of hope

Universality

Imparting of information

Altruism

Development of socializing techniques

Imitative behavior

Catharsis

Corrective recapitulation of the primary family group

Existential factors

Group cohesiveness

Interpersonal learning

Universality

Many patients go through life with a sense of isolation. Secretly convinced that they are unique in their loneliness or their wretchedness, that they alone have certain unacceptable problems or impulses, these persons remain socially isolated and have few opportunities for frank and candid consensual validation. In a therapy group, especially in its early stages, the disconfirmation of a patient's sense of uniqueness comes as a powerful sense of relief. Some specialized groups, in fact, are focused on helping individuals for whom secrecy has been an especially important and isolating part of life. For example, short-term structured groups for bulimic patients require open disclosure about attitudes toward body image and detailed accounts about bingeing and purging behavior. As a rule, patients experience a great sense of relief when they discover that they are not alone, that some of their problems are "universal," and that other group members share the same dilemmas. Often, the degree of relief is directly related to the degree of reluctance to disclose.

Imparting of Information

The imparting of information occurs in a group whenever a therapist gives didactic instruction to patients about mental functioning or whenever advice or direct guidance about life problems is offered either by the leader or by other group members. Although long-term interactional groups generally do not value the use of didactic education or advice, other types of groups rely more or less heavily on these two manners of imparting information. Let us briefly examine each of them in turn.

Many self-help groups such as Recovery, Inc. (for psychological problems), Make Today Count (for cancer patients), and Gamblers Anonymous emphasize *didactic instruction*. Experts are often invited to address the group, and members are strongly encouraged to exchange information among themselves. Most, if not all, specialized groups led by professionals rely heavily on this procedure as well; groups aimed at patients with a specific disorder or facing a specific life crisis (e.g., obesity, trauma such as rape, epilepsy, chronic pain) build in a teaching component and offer explicit instruction about the nature of the patient's illness or life situation. Many day-treatment groups or social skills training groups for chronically mentally ill persons also use teaching and instruction.

Unlike explicit didactic instruction from the therapist, *direct advice* from other members occurs without exception in every kind of therapy group. In dynamic interactional therapy groups, it is invariably part of the early life of the group but is generally of limited value to members. Later, when the group has moved beyond an initial "problem-solving" stage and has begun to engage in true interactional work, the reappearance of advice seeking or advice giving around a given issue is an important clue to resistance in the group. In contrast, noninteractionally focused groups often make explicit and effective use of direct suggestions and guidance. For example, members of behavior-shaping groups, discharge groups (those that prepare patients for discharge from the hospital), Recovery, Inc., and Alcoholics Anonymous offer one another considerable direct advice. Discharge groups may discuss the events of a patient's trial home visit and offer suggestions for alternative behavior, whereas Alcoholics Anonymous and Recovery, Inc., use guidance and directive slogans. Research on a behavior-shaping group of male sex offenders found that the most effective form of guidance was either systematic operationalized instructions or alternative suggestions from peers about how to reach a desired goal (Flowers 1979).

Altruism

In a therapy group, patients become enormously helpful to one another: they share similar problems and offer one another support, reassurance, suggestions, and insight. To the patient starting therapy who is demoralized and who feels that he or she has nothing of value to offer anyone, the experience of being helpful to other members of the group can be surprisingly rewarding. Not only does the altruistic act boost self-esteem, it also distracts patients who spend much of their psychic energy immersed in morbid self-absorption. By its very structure, the therapy group fosters the act of being helpful to others and counters overly solipsistic preoccupation.

Development of Socializing Techniques

Social learning—the development of basic social skills—is a therapeutic factor that operates in all therapy groups, although the nature of the skills taught and the explicitness of the process vary greatly according to the type of group therapy. In some groups, such as those preparing long-term hospitalized patients for discharge or those for adolescents with behavioral problems, there may be explicit emphasis on the development of social skills. Role-playing is often employed, in which patients learn to approach prospective employers for a job or adolescent boys learn to invite a girl to a dance. In groups that are more interactionally oriented, patients often learn about maladaptive social behavior from the open feedback they offer one another. A patient may, for example, learn about a disconcerting tendency to avoid eye contact during conversation, or about the effect that his or her whispery voice and constantly folded arms have on others, or about a host of other social habits that, unbeknownst to the patient, have been undermining his or her social relationships.

Imitative Behavior

The importance of imitative behavior as a therapeutic factor in groups is difficult to gauge, but there is some evidence from social psychological research that therapists may underestimate its importance. Bandura et al. (1969), for example, experimentally demonstrated nearly 30 years ago that imitation of healthy behavior is an effective therapeutic force in the treatment of certain phobias. In group therapy we often observe patients who benefit by observing the therapy of another patient with a similar problem constellation, a phenomenon of "vicarious learning." A timid, somewhat repressed female member might observe another woman in the group begin to improve as the woman experiments with more engaging behavior and perhaps a more attractive appearance; the timid patient may then try new ways of presenting herself as well.

Catharsis

Catharsis, or the ventilation of emotions, is a complex therapeutic factor that is linked to other processes in the group, particularly universality and cohesiveness. The sheer act of ventilation, by itself, although often accompanied by a sense of emotional arousal and relief, rarely promotes lasting change for a patient. It is the affective sharing of one's inner world, and then the acceptance by others, that is of paramount importance. Being accepted by others after expressing strong emotions brings into question one's belief that one is basically repugnant, unacceptable, or unlovable. Therapy is both an emotional and a corrective experience; for change to take place, a patient must experience something strongly in the group setting and then understand the implications of that emotional experience. We will return to this fundamental premise later when we discuss the here-and-now focus of group therapy.

Corrective Recapitulation of the Primary Family Group

Patients often enter group therapy with a history of unsatisfactory experiences in their first and most important group experience, the primary family. Because group therapy offers such a vast array of recapitulative possibilities, patients may begin to interact with leaders or other members as they once interacted with parents and siblings (Baker and Baker 1993). A helplessly dependent patient

may ascribe unrealistic knowledge and power to the leader. A rebellious and defiant individual may see the therapist as someone who blocks autonomy in the group or who strips members of their individuality. The "primitive" or chaotic patient might attempt to split the cotherapists or even the entire group, igniting fires of bitter disagreement and rivalry. The competitive patient will compete with other members for the therapist's attention or perhaps seek allies in an effort to topple the therapist(s). And a self-effacing individual or one with poor self-esteem may neglect his or her own interests in a seemingly selfless effort to placate or provide for other members. All of these patterns of behavior can represent a recapitulation of early family experiences.

What is of capital importance in interactional group therapy (and to a lesser degree in other group settings that make use of psychological insight) is not only that these kinds of early familial conflicts are reenacted but that they are understood and corrected. The group leader must not permit these growth-inhibiting relationships to freeze into the rigid, impenetrable system that characterizes many family structures. Instead, the leader must constantly explore and challenge fixed roles in the group and must constantly encourage members to test new behaviors. By exploring and altering ingrained patterns of behavior with leaders and other group members, the patient is liberated from the yoke of unfinished business from the past.

Existential Factors

An existential approach to the understanding of patients' concerns posits that the human being's paramount struggle is with the givens of existence: death, isolation, freedom, and meaninglessness (Yalom 1980). In certain kinds of therapy groups, particularly those centered around patients with cancer or chronic and life-threatening medical illnesses, or in bereavement groups, members will often begin to confront some of these existential issues. They will realize that there is a limit to the guidance and support they can receive from others. They may find that the ultimate responsibility for the conduct of their lives is their own. They will often learn that although one can be close to others, there is nonetheless a basic aloneness to existence that cannot be avoided. As they accept some of these issues, many patients who are confronting death learn to face their limitations and their mortality with greater candor and courage. In group therapy, the sound and trusting relationship among members—the basic, intimate encounter—has an intrinsic value in that it provides presence and a "being with" in the face of these harsh existential realities (Benioff and Vinogradov 1993; Yalom and Vinogradov 1988).

Group Cohesiveness

Although it is discussed near the end of this brief description of therapeutic factors, group cohesiveness is one of the more complex and absolutely integral features of a successful therapy group (Dies 1993). Cohesiveness in a group context refers to the affinity that members have for their group and for the other members. The members of a cohesive group are accepting of one another, supportive, and inclined to form meaningful relationships in the group; they are ready to perform the group task. As such, cohesiveness can be conceptualized as a necessary precondition for change rather than a true mechanism of change. And yet, many if not most psychiatric patients have had an impoverished history of belonging; never before have they been a valuable, integral, participating member of any kind of group, and the successful negotiation of a group therapy experience may in itself be curative. For these patients, group cohesiveness appears to be a true therapeutic factor. Furthermore, the social behavior required for members to be esteemed by a cohesive group tends also to be adaptive for the individual in his or her social life outside the group.

How else does group cohesiveness set the stage for change? Quite simply, by providing conditions of acceptance and understanding. Under cohesive conditions, patients are more inclined to express and explore themselves, to become aware of and integrate hitherto unacceptable aspects of themselves, and to relate more deeply to others. Cohesiveness in a group thus favors self-disclosure, risk taking, and the constructive expression of confrontation and conflict—all phenomena that facilitate successful therapy.

Highly cohesive groups are stable groups with better attendance, more active patient commitment and participation, and less membership turnover than groups that have not cohered. Some groups in certain settings, such as those specializing in a particular problem or disorder (e.g., a cancer support group or a group for women law students that is run by a university health center), will by their very nature develop a great deal of cohesiveness. In other kinds of groups, especially those in which membership changes frequently, the leader may need actively to facilitate the development of this important therapeutic factor. We will discuss means of fostering cohesiveness in the sections exploring the group therapist's tasks and techniques.

Interpersonal Learning

Group therapy may make use of any number of the therapeutic factors described here, but its cardinal feature is that it draws together a number of different individuals who wish to change something about themselves or their situations. This provides each member in the group with a unique ensemble of interpersonal interactions to explore. R. D. Laing (1967) suggested, "My experience and my action occur in a social field of reciprocal influence and interaction. I experience myself . . . as experienced by and acted upon by others . . ." (p. 9). Surprisingly, this potent mechanism for change in group therapy—interpersonal learning—is often overlooked, misapplied, or misunderstood by leaders, perhaps because the encouragement of interpersonal exploration requires considerable therapist skill and experience. To place the use of interpersonal learning into its full context, we will examine three underlying concepts: the importance of interpersonal relationships, the group as a social microcosm, and learning from behavioral patterns in the social microcosm.

Importance of interpersonal relationships. Humans are gregarious creatures committed for life to a social existence based on interpersonal communication through language. Harry Stack Sullivan (1953) contended that the need for interpersonal acceptance and security is basic and, given the prolonged period of helplessness during infancy, may be as crucial to survival as any biological need. To ensure and promote this interpersonal acceptance, a developing child will accentuate those aspects of behavior that meet with approval or obtain desired ends and will suppress those aspects that engender punishment or disapproval. The human personality can thus be seen as shaped almost entirely by interaction with other significant beings. Goffman (1961) noted: "There seems to be no agent more effective than another person in bringing a world for oneself alive, or, by a glance, a gesture, or a remark, shriveling up the reality in which one is lodged" (p. 41). Psychopathology arises when these interactions have resulted in distortions in how one perceives others and in how one reacts to them.

Psychotherapists who use an interpersonal frame of reference—and what psychotherapist does not do so at one time or another?—concentrate on the interpersonal pathology that underlies or arises from a particular symptom complex. The therapist translates symptoms into interpersonal language. For example, the psychotherapist rarely addresses "depression" per se. The typical symptom cluster of dysphoric mood and neurovegetative signs does not in and of itself offer a handhold for beginning the process of psychotherapeutic change. Instead, the clinician forms a relationship with the person who is depressed and ascertains the underlying interpersonal problems that arise from the depression and that most certainly also exacerbate it (problems such as dependency, obsequiousness, inability to express rage, and hypersensitivity to rejection). Once these maladaptive interpersonal themes have been identified, the therapist and the patient can undertake the work of understanding and altering them.

The group as a social microcosm. Sooner or later, given enough time and freedom, each person in the group will begin to interact with other group members in the same way that he or she interacts with persons outside the group. In other words, participants create in the group the same type of interpersonal world they inhabit on the outside. The group becomes a laboratory experiment in which interpersonal strengths and weaknesses unfold "in miniature." Slowly but predictably, each individual's interpersonal pathology comes to be displayed in the group. Arrogance, impatience, narcissism, grandiosity, sexualization—all such traits eventually surface. There is hardly any need for members to describe their past or to report present difficulties with relationships in their outside life. Group behavior provides far more accurate and immediate data. Members act out their interpersonal problems before the eyes of everyone in the group, and a freely interacting group will, in time, develop into a social microcosm of each of the members of that group. The following vignettes illustrate this principle:

> John, a busy and successful dentist, had serious marital problems and was "coerced" into group therapy by his wife and marriage counselor. His wife complained that he was detached and uninvolved and that she had to throw a "tantrum" to get him to respond. John believed that his wife was always angry and critical toward him for no reason. Although John was polite and ingratiating, his participation in the group remained at a superficial level even after several months. He felt distant and a bit disdainful of the group that he was "forced" to attend. Soon the female members were prodding him, complaining that he wasn't engaged in the group work, asking, "Where is John really at?" They grew angry and more shrill in their interactions with John (just like his wife) in order to elicit a response, any response, from him—a reflection in miniature of the problems in his marriage.

> Elizabeth was a very attractive woman who, after her husband's job promotion and transfer, had left a high-powered career and had a baby; she soon entered a severe depression and felt overwhelmed by pain she could not express. She found her life lacking in intimacy, and her outside relationships, as well as her marriage, felt superficial and inauthentic to her. In the group, Elizabeth was very popular. She was charming, sensitive, and concerned about everyone. However, she rarely let the group glimpse behind her composed facade and into the depths of her pain and despair. Her great shame about her depression (after all,

she "had it so good") and even deeper shame about the childhood of poverty and abuse from which she had risen resulted in her recreating in the group the same type of cordial but distant and unnourishing relationships she had established in her social life and marriage.

> Mark joined the group after his divorce and a string of unsuccessful romantic encounters. He had no close friends, male or female. He was sexually compulsive and competitive, and although he dated frequently, the thrill of the initial sexual conquest would inevitably pall, leaving him with a feeling of emptiness. Mark soon recreated this behavior in the therapy group. Although an active and involved member, he devoted himself almost exclusively to courting the attractive women in the group, including the female cotherapist. The female members began to feel sexualized and withdrew from him. Because he had also adopted an exceedingly competitive stance with the men in the group (especially powerful men, such as the male cotherapist), Mark quickly succeeded in isolating himself from all fulfilling relationships in the social microcosm of the group.

Learning from behavioral patterns in the social microcosm. These preceding concepts interrelate in the process of group therapy to provide the therapist with an extremely powerful tool for change: interpersonal learning. In this process, psychopathology emerges from and is embodied in distorted interpersonal interactions, in which the group becomes a social microcosm as each member displays his or her interpersonal pathology, and in which feedback allows members to identify and change their interpersonal behavior. This process is described here and is schematically outlined in Figure 33–1 (Yalom 1985, 1986, 1995).

1. *Displaying interpersonal pathology:* Members display their characteristic interpersonally distorted behavior.
2. *Providing feedback and self-observation:* Members share observations of each other and discover some of their own blind spots.
3. *Sharing reactions:* Members point out one another's blind spots and point out how each member's behavior makes them feel.
4. *Examining results of sharing reactions:* Each member begins to have a more objective picture of his or her own behavior and of the impact it has on others.
5. *Understanding one's opinion of oneself:* Each member becomes aware of how one's own behavior influences the opinions of others and, hence, one's opinions of oneself.

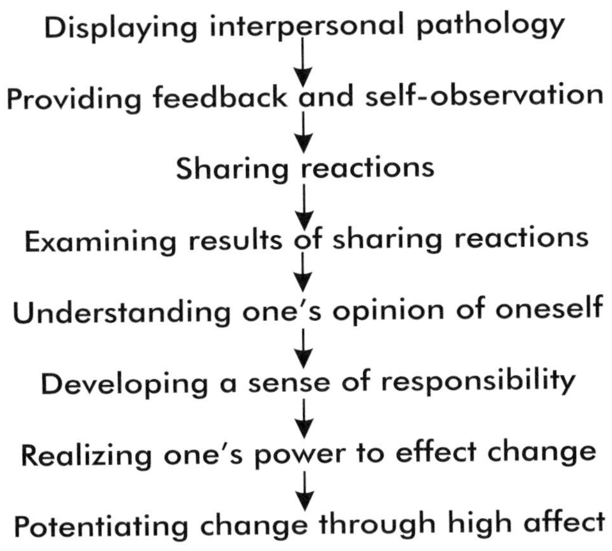

Displaying interpersonal pathology

↓

Providing feedback and self-observation

↓

Sharing reactions

↓

Examining results of sharing reactions

↓

Understanding one's opinion of oneself

↓

Developing a sense of responsibility

↓

Realizing one's power to effect change

↓

Potentiating change through high affect

FIGURE 33–1. Learning from behavioral patterns in the social microcosm of the therapy.

6. *Developing a sense of responsibility:* As a result of understanding how one's behavior influences one's sense of self-worth, one becomes more fully aware of responsibility for one's interpersonal life.

7. *Realizing one's power to effect change:* With the acceptance of responsibility for life's interpersonal dilemmas, each member begins to realize that one can change what one has created.

8. *Potentiating change through high affect:* The more emotionally laden are the events of this sequence, the greater is the potential for change.

Interpersonal learning is the primary mechanism for change in unstructured, longer-term, high-functioning interaction groups; in these settings, in fact, the elements of interpersonal learning are typically ranked by members as being the most helpful aspect of the group therapy experience (Butler and Fuhriman 1980; Freedman and Hurley 1980; Lieberman et al. 1973; Yalom 1995). Of course, not all therapy groups concentrate in an explicit manner on interpersonal learning. However, interpersonal interaction, with its rich potential for learning and change, does occur any time a group assembles.

FORCES THAT MODIFY THE THERAPEUTIC FACTORS IN GROUP THERAPY

We have applied a simplifying principle to the group therapeutic process and have identified a comprehensive set of

therapeutic factors that operate in group therapy. And yet, group therapy is obviously a forum for change whose form, content, and process vary considerably both across groups and within the same group at any given time. In other words, different types of groups will make use of different clusters of therapeutic factors (see Table 33–1), and, furthermore, as a group evolves, different sets of factors come into play (Dies 1993). Thus, we need to be aware that three modifying forces can influence the therapeutic mechanisms at work in any given group: the type of group, the stage of therapy, and individual differences among patients.

Type of Group

Research on long-term interactional outpatient group therapy indicates that group members consistently select a constellation of three factors—interpersonal learning, catharsis, and self-understanding—as those elements of group therapy most helpful to them (Yalom 1995). Inpatients, in contrast, tend to identify other mechanisms: the instillation of hope and the existential factor of assumption of responsibility (Leszcz et al. 1985; Yalom 1983). This difference in emphasis is due to the fact that inpatient groups have high member turnover and are heterogeneous in clinical composition (i.e., patients with greatly differing ego strength, motivation, goals, and psychopathology meet in the same group for varying lengths of time). Furthermore, psychiatric patients usually enter the hospital in a state of despair, after they have exhausted other available resources. Groups that are centered around self-help concepts, such as Alcoholics Anonymous, Recovery, Inc., or support groups for bereaved parents, rely on the mechanisms of universality, guidance, altruism, and cohesiveness (Lieberman and Borman 1979).

Stage of Therapy

Patients' needs and goals change during the course of therapy and so, too, do the therapeutic factors that are most helpful to them. In its early stages, an outpatient group is most concerned with establishing boundaries and maintaining membership, and factors such as instillation of hope, guidance, and universality loom most important. Other factors, such as altruism and group cohesiveness, will operate throughout the duration of therapy, but their nature changes with the stage of the group. In the case of altruism, for example, early in the group, patients will offer suggestions to each other, ask appropriate questions, and show concern and attention. Later, they will be able to express a deeper caring and greater support for each other and exhibit a true sharing of emotion.

Initially, group cohesiveness occurs through group support and acceptance, whereas later in the life of the group it facilitates self-disclosure. Ultimately, group cohesiveness makes it possible for members to explore issues of confrontation and conflict, issues so essential to interpersonal learning. The longer patients participate in a group, the more they value the therapeutic factors of cohesiveness, self-understanding, and interpersonal interaction (Butler and Fuhriman 1983).

Differences Among Patients

As mentioned at the beginning of this section, each patient in group therapy is different, and patients with different levels of functioning will find different therapeutic factors beneficial. Higher-functioning patients tend to value interpersonal learning more than do lower-functioning patients in the same group. In one study of inpatient groups, both types of patients chose awareness of responsibility and catharsis as helpful elements of group therapy; however, the lower-functioning patients also valued the instillation of hope, and higher-functioning patients selected universality, vicarious learning, and interpersonal learning as additional useful experiences (Leszcz et al. 1985). A group experience is something of a therapeutic cafeteria: many different mechanisms of change are available, but each individual patient will make the most use out of those particular factors that are most suited to his or her needs and problems. A passive, repressed individual may benefit from experiencing and expressing strong affect, through catharsis, for example; whereas someone with impulse dyscontrol may profit from self-restraint and an intellectual structuring of the affective experience through imitative behavior. Some patients need to develop very basic social skills through the development of socializing techniques, whereas others benefit from the identification and exploration of much subtler interpersonal issues—for example, the patient who exaggerates helplessness and irrationality as a means of controlling other persons.

THERAPEUTIC FACTORS: SUMMARY

In sum, the comparative usefulness and potency of these simplified therapeutic factors are complex and change across groups, across members of the same group, and across time. Research indicates that different types of groups make use of different therapeutic factors, and therapists who are leading groups must have a firm grasp of those factors that are most compatible with the needs and capacities of their group members. An emphasis on interpersonal learning is not appropriate for a behaviorally oriented group for persons with bulimia nervosa, just as time taken for didactic education would frustrate the members of a long-term, intensive interactional group. The therapist thus has the basic task not only of understanding the appropriate mechanisms and goals for change in any given group, but also—as we shall explore in the next section—of establishing and maintaining the group within the setting of those goals.

THE THERAPIST'S BASIC TASKS IN GROUP THERAPY

When a therapist begins individual psychotherapy with a new client, the therapist-patient dyad exists ipso facto, and the initial work of therapy unfolds from this point. But when a therapist starts a therapy group, the process is quite different. Long before the first meeting, the leader will have been hard at work, for the group therapist's initial task is to create a physical entity where none existed. The leader assembles a group and offers the professional help that is the initial raison d'être for the group. The leader selects the members and sets the time, place, and tone for the meetings. In sum, the therapist has the basic tasks of establishing and maintaining the group and resolving the problems typically encountered in the group setting (Table 33–4).

Let us explore some of these general principles of group format, composition, and maintenance, keeping in

---

TABLE 33–4.   Therapist's basic tasks in group therapy

1. The decision to establish a therapy group:
   a. Determine setting and size of the group.
   b. Choose frequency and length of group sessions.
   c. Decide on open versus closed group.
   d. Select a co-therapist for the group.
2. The act of creating a therapy group:
   a. Formulate appropriate goals.
   b. Select patients who can perform the group task.
   c. Prepare patients for group therapy.
3. The construction and maintenance of a therapeutic environment:
   a. Build the culture of the group explicitly and implicitly.
   b. Identify and resolve common problems (membership turnover, subgrouping, conflict).
   c. Use procedural aids as appropriate.

mind that these basic tasks can be modified to suit the needs of particular kinds of therapy groups.

ESTABLISHING A THERAPY GROUP

Setting and Size

Before the first group meeting takes place, the therapist makes certain decisions about its circumstances. The most pragmatic of these involves choosing an appropriate meeting place. A setting that provides privacy and freedom from distraction is essential, of course, but a group meeting room should also be consistently available and of adequate size and have comfortable seating. A circular seating arrangement is necessary: all of the members must be able to see one another. The use of inpatient wards with long sofas does not permit good interaction. If three or four members sit in a row, they cannot see one another, and consequently most remarks in such groups are directed to the therapist, the one person visible to all. Furniture in the center of the room may hide nuances of body behavior; a table, for example, might mask the clenched fists of a member with a stoic facial expression. Some therapists provide coffee and tea at the meeting place; one effect of this is to increase the sociability of the setting, at least before the actual session.

The optimal size of a group is a function of its therapeutic goals. Organizations such as Alcoholics Anonymous and Recovery, Inc., that operate with group settings of up to 80 members rely heavily on inspiration, guidance, and suppression to change members' behavior. But leaders working in a large therapeutic community (e.g., in a residential halfway house) might wish to make use of a different set of factors, such as group pressure and interdependence to foster reality testing or to instill a sense of individual responsibility to the social community. In this setting, groups of 15 or so members may be more appropriate.

The ideal size for a prototypic interactional group is 7 or 8 members, and certainly no more than 10. Too few members will not provide the critical mass necessary for interpersonal interactions. In a group that is too small, there will not be enough opportunities for broad consensual validation of different viewpoints, and patients will tend to interact one at a time with the therapist rather than with one another. Anyone who has ever tried to conduct a group with only two or three patients knows the frustration of this enterprise. In a group with more than 10 members, however, there may be ample fruitful interaction, but some members will be left out. There will simply be insufficient time to examine and understand all of the interactions.

When the therapist is working with inpatients or leading specialized outpatient groups, his or her focus may not be as explicitly interpersonally oriented as in the prototypic interaction group, but the therapist will still want to aim for a lively and engaging group, one that encourages active participation by as many members as possible. In our clinical experience, the optimal group size that allows members to share experiences with one another ranges from a minimum of 4 or 5 to a maximum of 12; groups of 6–8 members seem to offer the greatest opportunity for verbal exchange among all patients.

Time Constraints and Use of Open Versus Closed Groups

The late 1960s and early 1970s saw a great deal of experimentation with the time variable in group therapy. Weekly 4- to 8-hour groups were not unheard of, and marathon weekend sessions were common. Research has failed to demonstrate any superiority of the time-extended meeting, and today there is a clinical consensus that the optimal duration for a session in ongoing group therapy is between 60 and 120 minutes (Yalom 1995). Usually 20–30 minutes are required for the group to warm up, and at least 60 minutes are needed to work through the major themes of the session. After about 2 hours, most therapists find they begin to fatigue and the group becomes weary and repetitious. Groups that meet frequently, such as daily inpatient groups, or groups that consist of lower-functioning patients who can tolerate only limited social stimuli, do well with briefer sessions. Groups that meet less often or that are centered on higher-functioning interactional work require at least 90 minutes per session in order to be fruitful.

The frequency of meetings can vary from once a day—typically in the inpatient setting, where therapy groups meet from three to six times a week—to once a month, as in clinic medication-support groups. A once-weekly schedule is most common in outpatient group work and seems well suited to supportive or specialized groups. Long-term interactional groups also tend to meet once per week, although clinical experience suggests that twice-weekly sessions, when feasible, increase the intensity and productivity of this kind of group.

The decision to make a group open or closed is related to the goals of the group and its identified life span. A closed group meets for a predetermined number of sessions, begins with a fixed number of members, and, as of the first session, closes its doors and accepts no new members. For example, therapists working with a specialized group of bereaved spouses or of patients with eating disorders may take in a fixed number of patients for a preset number of sessions, usually 8–12 meetings. In such time-limited groups, each session may follow a predetermined protocol. External time constraints can also influence the format of a group. For example, in a university health center, a support group for graduate students having trouble with their dissertations may be set up to run the length of an academic semester.

In contrast, open groups either are more flexible about size—consider the ongoing inpatient group on a psychiatric ward, which reflects ward census—or may maintain a consistent size by replacing members as they leave the group. Open groups usually have a broader set of therapeutic goals and generally meet indefinitely; although members come and go, the group has a life of its own. Such ongoing outpatient groups at psychiatric teaching centers have been known to continue for more than 20 years and to have been the training ground for generations of residents!

Use of a Cotherapist

Most group therapists prefer to work with a cotherapist. Cotherapists complement and support each other. As the therapists share points of view and examine hunches together, each therapist's observational range is broadened. There is much agreement among clinicians that a male-female cotherapist team has unique advantages. It recreates the parental configuration of the primary family, which for many members increases the affective charge of the group. Many patients can benefit from observing a male therapist and a female therapist working together with mutual respect and without the derogation, exploitation, or sexualizing that the patients too often take for granted in male-female relationships. Moreover, the group is provided with a wider array of transferential possibilities, for patients will differ in their reactions to each of the cotherapists and to the cotherapists' relationship. In a group led by a male-female cotherapist team, for example, a somewhat histrionic female member may pander to the male leader and ignore his female counterpart, a pattern that would not emerge as clearly in a group led by one therapist. Other members may have fantasies about the relationship between the two cotherapists.

The cotherapy format seems particularly helpful for beginning therapists and for experienced therapists working with an especially difficult patient population. In addition to clarifying transference distortions of each other's presentation in the group, cotherapists can support each other in maintaining objectivity in the face of massive group pressure. We had occasion to work at one point with a lonely female member of a group, a hospital volunteer who became romantically involved with one of her psychiatric patients; she discussed this in a group session and then verbally flagellated herself. In an effort to be supportive, the other members unanimously and vociferously condoned her behavior and attempted to pressure the leaders into a noncritical stance as well. As cotherapists, we were better able to resist the powerful group pressure and maintain our professional objectivity about this woman's behavior.

Similarly, cotherapists are invaluable in helping each other constructively weather an attack from group members. A therapist under the gun may be too threatened either to clarify the attack or to encourage further exploration without appearing defensive or condescending. There is nothing more squelching than when a leader under fire says, "It's really great that you're expressing your feelings and attacking me. Keep it going!" It is usually the cotherapist who can best help members channel and express their anger in an appropriate manner and who can then lead members to examine the source and the meaning of that anger.

There is some question whether cotherapists should openly reveal their differences of opinion during the group session. Two factors to consider are the level of functioning of the group and the maturity of the group. Patients who are lower functioning and who are more fragile or unstable overall should generally not be exposed to conflict between the cotherapists, no matter how gently it is expressed. Likewise, cotherapist disagreement is not helpful early in the work with even higher-functioning patients, for a beginning group usually is not stable or cohesive enough to tolerate divisiveness in leadership. Later in such a group, however, the therapists' honesty about disagreement can contribute substantially to the potency and honesty of the group. Members observe the leaders they respect disagreeing openly and resolving their differences with honesty and tact. Members also experience the therapists not as infallible authority figures but as humans with imperfections, and they thus learn to differentiate others according to individual attributes rather than stereotyped roles.

The major disadvantages of the cotherapy format flow from problems in the cotherapy relationship itself. If coleaders are uncomfortable with each other, closed and competitive, or in wide disagreement about style and strategy, there is little chance that their group will be able to work effectively. Research has demonstrated that the major cause of failure is cotherapists' embracing vastly different ideological positions (Paulson et al. 1976). Therefore, when choosing a coleader it is important to select someone who is different enough in personal style to be complementary but who is similar in theoretical orientation.

Whenever two therapists of vastly different levels of experience lead a group together, it is important that they be open-minded and mature, comfortable with each other, and comfortable in their roles as co-workers or as teacher and apprentice. Splitting is a phenomenon that often occurs in groups led by cotherapists, and some patients are very perceptive about tensions in the cotherapists' relationship. For example, if a neophyte therapist feels jealous of a senior cotherapist's clinical experience and wisdom, a member might marvel at everything the older therapist says and denigrate the younger therapist's interventions. Occasionally the entire group can become split into two factions, with each cotherapist having a "team" of patients aligned with him or her; this may occur because the patients believe they have a special relationship with one or the other of the therapists or because they believe that one of the therapists is more intelligent, more senior, or more attractive or has a similar ethnic background. Splitting, like the problem of subgrouping that we will discuss later, should always be noted and openly interpreted in the group.

Combining Group Therapy With Other Therapeutic Modalities

The standard group therapy format, in which one therapist meets with six to eight patients, is often combined with other therapeutic modalities. For example, some or all of the patients in a given group may also be involved in concurrent individual psychotherapy with other therapists; this is often described as *conjoint therapy* and is one of the more preferable means for combining psychotherapies. Occasionally, all or some of the members in a group are in concurrent individual therapy with the group therapist in what is known as *combined therapy*. This latter therapy usually arises when a psychotherapist in solo private practice forms a group from the ranks of his or her individual patients. Both conjoint and combined therapies are frequently encountered by therapists who run groups in clinics or on inpatient wards. Amaranto is developing models to incorporate the advantages of both.

When is it useful to combine psychotherapeutic modalities? Some patients may go through a life crisis so severe that they require temporary individual support in addition to group therapy. Others may be so chronically disabled by fear, anxiety, or aggression that they require individual therapy to participate effectively in the group and avoid becoming locked into a stereotyped role. At times, active individual intervention is necessary simply to explore the patient's conflicts in group therapy and thus prevent him or her from having an unprofitable experience or from dropping out of the group. Individual or group therapy approaches complement each other most effectively when the individual and group therapists support each other and are in frequent contact and when the individual therapy is interpersonally oriented and explores feelings and incidents related to current group meetings.

Concurrent individual therapy can hinder group therapy in several ways. When there is a marked difference in approach between the individual therapist and the group therapist, patients may become confused and the two therapies may work at cross-purposes. The patient who is used to the support and narcissistic gratification of individual therapy—who is accustomed to exploring fantasies, dreams, associations, and memories and to being the exclusive center of attention of a therapist—may become frustrated by initial group meetings. Early sessions usually offer less personal support and may be dedicated more to building a cohesive unit and to examining here-and-now interactions than to deep exploration of each member's life. Individual therapy and group therapy can also interfere with each other if patients use their individual therapy to drain off affect from the group, reacting to emotionally laden events in the group only later in the sanctum of their individual therapy hour.

Another combination is the use of group therapy with medication clinics, a practical and humane combination of modalities most often, but not exclusively, used with chronic psychiatric patients (Brook 1993). In this approach, patients who attend biweekly or monthly medication clinics, usually to receive prescriptions for antipsychotic medication or for mood stabilizers, also participate in a group meeting associated with the clinic. Sessions are generally highly structured and focus on educating patients about their medications, on solving practical problems, and on sharing a difficult plight. A chronically psychotic patient who lives in relative social isolation can use these groups to practice some basic social skills and to receive support for his or her efforts. Group therapy is used to personalize, enhance, and reinforce the patient's experience in a medication clinic.

CREATING A THERAPY GROUP

Formulating Goals

As a first step to creating a therapy group, the therapist must carefully examine all of the clinical facts of life that will bear on the group. The *intrinsic* factors (e.g., mandatory attendance for patients on legal probation, duration of treatment in a ward group of hospitalized patients with cancer) are built into the clinical situation and cannot be changed; the group leader must adapt to them. The *extrinsic* factors are those that have become tradition or policy in a given setting—an example might be an inpatient ward's fixed program of daily community meetings. Extrinsic factors are arbitrary and within the power of the therapist to change.

Once a clear view of the clinical facts of life has been obtained, the leader's second step is to construct a reasonable set of clinical goals for the group. This is the most important step in creating a therapy group, for the selection of inappropriate or vaguely defined goals is sure to result in failure. The goals of a long-term outpatient group are ambitious: to offer symptomatic relief and to change character structure. An attempt to apply these same goals to an aftercare group of patients with chronic schizophrenia would result in therapeutic nihilism.

Goals must be shaped that are appropriate to the clinical situation and achievable in the amount of time available. In time-limited, specialized groups, the goals must be focused, achievable, and tailored to the capacity and potential of the group members. It is important that the therapy group be a success experience; patients enter therapy feeling defeated and demoralized, and the last thing they need is another failure.

Selecting Patients and Composing a Therapy Group

Once the therapist has a clear idea of the goals of the group—in other words, a clear idea of the group task—he or she must select members who can achieve these goals and perform the group task. The leader's expertise in the selection and preparation of members will greatly affect the group's fate. The therapist must create a group that coheres, and, because nothing threatens a group's cohesiveness more than the presence of a grossly deviant member, the selection of members must be guided by the notion of group integrity and the avoidance of deviancy. A group of board-and-care-home residents with chronic schizophrenia cannot cohere effectively in the presence of an exploitative and manipulative member with a personality disorder; nor can a high-functioning group of outpatients function well together in the presence of a patient who frequently goes into dissociative states.

The single most important criterion for member selection, no matter what the group, is an ability to perform the group task. Study of group failures reveals that deviancy (i.e., an inability or refusal to engage in the group task) is negatively related to outcome. An individual who considers himself or herself (or is considered by other members) to be "out of the group" or a deviant or mascot has little likelihood of profiting from the group and there is a fair chance of negative outcome for that person (Lieberman et

al. 1973). Therefore, selection for group therapy is, in practice, conducted by the process of elimination. Group therapists exclude certain patients from consideration (most often because the therapist predicts the patient will assume a deviant role or because the patient lacks motivation for change) and accept remaining patients.

Once a leader determines that a patient could benefit from group therapy, how does he or she go about actually composing a group? How is it decided which patients will work well together? Above all, the therapist must be concerned about the group's *integrity*. Members selected must be committed to the task of therapy and to regular attendance in the group. To attempt to refine the process of composition even more—to form a group ideally composed to interact therapeutically—is every group therapist's dream, yet we lack the knowledge and instruments necessary to permit us to realize this dream. Perhaps the key concept is group cohesiveness. An effective rule of thumb for longer-term outpatient groups is "homogeneity in ego strength, heterogeneity in problem areas" (Whitaker and Lieberman 1964). In other words, patients profit from a mixture of personality styles, ages, and problem areas—all factors that enrich the broth of the ensuing group interaction—but the group coheres best if all members possess the ego strength necessary to participate equally in the group task.

The situation is different in specialized or symptom-oriented groups; in these cases, members always share at least one major problem area (e.g., an eating disorder, bereavement, chronic pain), but they may be heterogeneous in terms of ego strength. Whenever possible, the therapist aims for similar levels of motivation and psychological-mindedness in the composition of the group. Having one or two members who are fragile, brittle, or work avoidant impedes the work of a fast-paced, highly motivated group. Likewise, a stolid group of more concrete chronically ill psychiatric patients can become destabilized if pushed too hard too fast by a confrontational, agitated, or manic individual (Kahn 1984; Kanas 1985, 1986). Beyond this, leaders may wish to try to balance the group composition along various parameters, such as by composing a group with an equal number of men and women, a wide age range, or varied interpersonal activity levels.

Often (as in, for example, mandatory inpatient groups or a group in a correctional institution) the therapist has minimal influence over group membership. At the very least, he or she must exercise the group therapist's prerogative and exclude those patients who are markedly incompatible with the prevailing group norms for acceptable behavior. Examples might include the physically agitated patient or the manic patient. Patients who cannot tolerate the stress of a group setting, such as extremely paranoid individuals, and patients who are absolutely incompatible with at least one other member also should not be included in the group. Group member screening is even more complicated in managed care settings. On the one hand, therapists often feel pressure from administration to fit patients into a group, and a higher risk of poor fit is tolerated. On the other hand, large institutional settings with large group programs are more likely to have a group that is suitable for any given patient. Unfortunately, the former situation is more common early in group program development.

One reason it is so difficult to compose an ideal group is that it is extremely difficult to predict subsequent group behavior from information available at the time of the screening procedure. An important source of information is the candidate's previous experience in groups. Another important source is the screening procedure itself. In the one or two intake interviews, the therapist should focus on the candidate's interpersonal functioning: past, present, and in the interview itself. The therapist must assess the individual's ability to tolerate interpersonal interactions and to reflect on them. Suitable questions might include the following: "How has the interview been for you so far today?" "Were there any parts that made you uncomfortable?" "What is it like for you to reveal things about yourself to a relative stranger?"

Preparing Patients for Group Therapy

Preparation of the patient for group therapy is another one of the therapist's essential tasks. A great deal of powerful research evidence has demonstrated that pregroup preparation decreases the number of dropouts, increases cohesiveness, and accelerates the work of therapy (Piper and Perrault 1989; Piper et al. 1982; Yalom 1966, 1995). In some settings, such as an inpatient ward or a medication-support group, this preparation will of necessity be minimal and will consist mainly of orienting the patient to the time, location, composition, procedure, and goals of the group. But even this brief preparation helps to orient patients to the group experience and provides guidelines about how to benefit from the group.

For most outpatient groups, preparation is best accomplished during one or two individual sessions with each patient before he or she begins group therapy. After deciding during an intake interview that the patient is a suitable candidate for group therapy, the therapist may then proceed to prepare the patient for the group. Patients have ample amounts of primary anxiety, and therapists must avoid adding yet more—the secondary anxiety that arises from being thrown into an ambiguous, intrinsically threatening situation. Therefore, providing clarity is the chief aim of the pregroup preparatory procedure. The therapist provides patients with a cognitive structure that enables them to participate more effectively in the group from the start.

Many patients hold misconceptions about group therapy's worth and efficacy; they believe that it is cheaper or diluted therapy and therefore not as worthwhile as individual therapy. These negative expectations must be addressed openly and corrected so that the patient will engage fully in treatment. Other patients express concerns about procedure and process: the size of the group, the type of members, the amount of negative confrontation, confidentiality. One of the most pervasive fears is the fear of having to reveal oneself and confess shameful transgressions to an audience of hostile strangers. Another common worry is a fear of mental contagion, of being made sicker through association with other psychiatric patients. Often this fear is a preoccupation of schizophrenic or borderline patients, although the fear may also be observed in patients who project their own feelings of self-contempt or hostility onto others.

A cognitive approach to group therapy preparation has several goals (Table 33–5):

- To provide a rational explanation to the patient about the group therapy process
- To describe what types of behavior are expected of patients in the group
- To establish a treatment contract
- To raise expectations about the effects of the group
- To predict some of the problems, discouragement, and frustration that may be encountered in early meetings

Underlying everything the therapist says is a process of demystification and the establishment of a therapeutic alliance. This comprehensive preparation enables the patient to make an informed decision to enter the therapy group and enhances commitment to the group from the beginning.

TABLE 33–5. Rationale behind group therapy preparation

To provide a rational explanation to the patient about the group therapy process.

To describe the behavior expected of patients in the group.

To establish an attendance contract.

To raise expectations about the effects of the group.

To predict some of the common problems and discouragement that may be encountered in early meetings.

CONSTRUCTING AND MAINTAINING A THERAPEUTIC ENVIRONMENT

Building the Culture of the Group

Once the group is a physical reality and the first meeting is under way, the leader must establish behavioral norms that will guide the interactions of the newly formed group. In individual therapy the therapist is the sole designated agent of direct change, but in group therapy the situation is more complex. Ideally, *all* of the members of the group will provide support, a sense of universality, and interpersonal feedback—in other words, the members themselves will be important agents of change. Any time a group of people assembles, be it in a professional, social, or even family setting, it will develop a "culture," a set of unwritten rules or norms that determine the acceptable behavioral procedure of the group. In group therapy, it is the leader's task to create a group culture maximally conducive to effective group interaction and to the development of the various therapeutic factors.

Norms constructed early in the group are important. They are shaped both by the expectations of the members as they start the group and by the behavior of the therapist during the early sessions. The therapist influences this process of norm setting in two different ways. First, the leader, in the role of technical expert, can *explicitly* shape the group norms. During early preparation of patients for group therapy, for example, patients can be given explicit instructions about the rules for appropriate behavior in the group, such as sharing concerns about body image in an eating disorders group. Once a group gets under way, the leader may reward desirable behavior through social reinforcement. If a usually shy member begins to participate, or if members start to offer one another spontaneous and honest feedback, this new behavior may be shaped and rewarded verbally or nonverbally through changes in the therapist's body language, eye contact, and facial expression.

The second way the therapist shapes therapeutic norms in the group is through model setting. In an acute inpatient therapy group, for example, leaders offer a model of nonjudgmental acceptance and appreciation of members' strengths as well as problem areas, helping to shape a group that is health oriented. In a social skills training group for schizophrenic patients, the leader might choose to model simple, direct, socially rewarding conversation. No matter what the level and functioning of the group, the effective leader sets a model of interpersonal honesty and spontaneity for his or her group members. But the therapist's honesty must take place in the service of his or her background responsibility; nothing takes precedence over the goal of being helpful to the patient.

There are several basic therapeutic group norms that should be encouraged in any group setting, regardless of its orientation. The first of these is the norm of the *self-monitoring group*, in which the group itself learns to assume responsibility for its own functioning. Any therapist who has ever worked in a group in which the members are completely dependent on the leader for direction knows firsthand the signs of the passive group. The patients seem to be an audience at a play; they appear to be waiting for the leader to make the curtain rise and the action begin. The group begins to feel stilted, heavy, and forced. After every meeting, the leader feels fatigued, powerless, and irritated by the burden of making it all work.

How can the therapist build a culture that encourages the development of a self-monitoring group? This can be accomplished by keeping in mind that initially, only the leader knows when a group has been productive. The therapist must start to share this knowledge with the patients at the very inception of a group and slowly educate them to recognize a good session. The therapist might say, "This was an exciting meeting today and everyone shared a lot. I hate to see it end." The evaluative function can then be shifted to the patients by the therapist's saying, "How is the group going so far today? What's been the most satisfying part?" And, finally, members can be taught that they have the ability to influence the course of a session; the therapist could say, "Things have been slow today. What could we do to make it different?"

There are several other basic norms that influence the therapy. *General procedural norms* must always be actively shaped by the leader. Ideally, the most therapeutic procedural format of a group is one that is unstructured, unrehearsed, and freely flowing. The therapist must intervene actively to preclude the development of a nontherapeutic procedure, for example, a "taking turns" format in which members figuratively line up to discuss specific problems or life crises one after another by rote. In such an instance, the therapist might interrupt and ask how the practice got started or what effect it has on the group. The leader could also indicate that the group has many other procedural options from which to choose.

When *members consider the group important*, group therapy becomes more effective, and the leader who reinforces this norm increases the therapeutic potency of his or her group. Likewise, the therapist augments the power of the group by increasing *the continuity between meetings*. It is the task of the therapist, as the group "time-binder, to call attention to behavioral patterns developing over several meetings. Finally, a group functions best when it sees its *members as agents of help and support*; a truly therapeutic culture implies, both explicitly and implicitly, that members will learn the most and receive the most help from one another.

Identifying and Resolving Common Problems in Group Therapy

Membership problems.   The early developmental sequence and potency of a therapy group are strongly affected by *membership problems.* Turnover in membership, tardiness, and absence are facts of life in all groups, yet these events will threaten a group's stability and integrity. Considerable absenteeism will redirect an outpatient group's attention and energy from its developmental tasks to the problem of maintaining membership, whereas continual turnover in inpatient groups powerfully affects group cohesiveness. Tardiness and irregular attendance must be discouraged in all group settings and should be regarded in the same way in which one regards these phenomena in individual therapy.

Leaders of long-term outpatient therapy groups should keep in mind that in the normal course of such groups, 10%–35% of the members will drop out in the first 12–20 meetings (Yalom 1966, 1995). In an open group it is the therapist's task to replace dropouts by adding new members. Dropouts are threatening to the group's stability for two reasons: they impede the development of cohesiveness, and they implicitly (and sometimes explicitly) devalue the group. Dropouts are also threatening to the leader, especially to the neophyte, and the therapist may unwittingly adopt a seductive posture in an effort to keep a patient in the group. The drop-out rate can be reduced through vigorous pretherapy selection and preparation (Connelly et al. 1986; McCallum et al. 1992; Orlinsky and Howard 1986; Piper and Perrault 1989). If predictions of the general problems and frustrations that can arise early in a group are made to new members ahead of time, there is less likelihood that dropping out will occur.

Subgrouping.   A second problem commonly encountered in group therapy is *subgrouping*—the splitting off of smaller units. A subgroup usually arises from the belief by two or more members that these members can derive more gratification from a relationship with one another than from one with the entire group. Extragroup socializing, which often occurs in outpatient groups (and almost invariably in inpatient groups), is often the first stage of subgrouping. A clique of three or four members will begin to have telephone conversations, to have coffee or dinner, and to share separate observations and interactions with one another. Occasionally, two members will become sex-

ually involved. A subgroup may also coalesce completely within the confines of the group therapy room, as members who perceive themselves to be similar form coalitions based on age, similar values, comparable education, and the like. Remaining group members, excluded from the clique, generally do not possess effective social skills and do not usually coalesce into a second subgroup. This phenomenon of "ingroup" versus "outgroup" can often be strikingly observed in inpatient settings.

The members of a subgroup can be recognized by a code of behavior: they agree with one another regardless of the issue and they avoid confrontations among their own membership; they exchange knowing glances when a member who is not in the clique speaks; they arrive and depart from the meeting together. Complications arise for all members of the therapy group, whether they belong to the subgroup or not. If a member belongs, loyalty to the subgroup is a major issue, secrets begin to be kept, and the free and honest discussion of feelings becomes inhibited. If a member has been excluded from the subgroup, complex feelings of envy, competition, and inferiority are aroused. Unfortunately, as these emotions and the anxiety associated with earlier exclusion experiences are evoked, it becomes exceptionally difficult for members to comment on their feelings of exclusion.

It is not the extragroup socializing that is crippling to a group per se; rather, it is the conspiracy of silence around it that becomes dangerous. The primary task in the group is to examine in depth the interpersonal relationships among all of the members, and extragroup socializing inhibits this examination. Important material—the relationship between members who are interacting outside the group, feelings of exclusion in patients who are not part of this interaction—remains covert, and the task of the group is sabotaged. Patients who violate group norms through the pursuit of subgrouping or through secret extragroup liaisons are opting for immediate-need gratification rather than for involvement in interpersonal learning and change. Subgrouping or extragroup behavior that remains covert—that is not examined in the group session—becomes a potent form of resistance. It hobbles the therapist and makes a travesty of other members' efforts to be revealing, to give honest feedback, and to participate fully and authentically in the group process.

Subgrouping represents a situation that contains both high risk and high gain. In pregroup preparation, the therapist attempts to prevent its occurrence by actively encouraging the development of group norms whereby all extragroup behavior is subsequently brought back into the group for discussion. When it does take place, subgrouping must be explicitly identified—usually by the leader—and explored in the light of the group task, which is the in-depth examination of the interpersonal relationships among all members. When the powerful issues that give rise to subgrouping are confronted by the group, discussed openly, and worked through, they can prove to be of considerable therapeutic import in the very group they were hampering.

In fact, deliberate use of subgrouping is part of the conceptual heart of systems-centered therapy. Agazarian (1997) utilized systems theory and directed therapeutic efforts mostly toward subgroups. The group-as-a-whole is a supra-entity (it contains the subgroup) and the individual members are part of subgroups (subgroups of the subgroup). Changes occurring at the level of the subgroup influence the nature of the group-as-a-whole as well as the participating individuals. Such parsimony of effort is further enhanced by the deliberate addressing of details of subgrouping. Noting changes in the "boundaries" between subgroups (e.g., splits, containing and integrating differences) and the direction of the systems or subsystem's energy (vectors) can be the basis for interventions. These interventions placed in a framework that Agazarian (1997) called "defense modification" appear to move forward quickly the work of the group-as-a-whole as well as that of the individuals. Subgrouping, like any powerful phenomenon, can be destructive if unaddressed. However, it is also potentially instructive and productive. Agazarian enhanced group therapists' ability to use subgrouping effectively.

Conflict.   *Conflict*, a third common problem, is inevitable in the course of a group's development. The task of the therapist is to identify conflict as it arises and to harness it in the service of the group task. Conflict resolution is virtually impossible in the presence of off-target or oblique hostility, and, once again, it is the therapist's task to identify and render overt that which has been covert. For example, he or she might say, "Bob, I've noticed that you've cut off Mary a couple of times today. I wonder if you're feeling a little angry because of the feedback the women in the group gave you last week."

How can the therapist harness conflict in the group and use it in the service of interpersonal growth? One important step is to find the right level for the group at hand. Too much conflict is threatening and counterproductive for just about any group of individuals, but too little conflict—especially with higher-functioning patients—leaves the group stagnant, excessively cautious, and superficial. Here, a judicious amount of confrontation, anger, and conflict resolution can provide an affectively charged learning experience for the group members.

Group cohesiveness is the prime prerequisite for the successful management of conflict. Members must have developed a feeling of mutual respect and trust and must value the group sufficiently to be able to tolerate confrontational or uncomfortable interactions. The leader will need to emphasize that open communication must be maintained if the group is to survive; all members must continue to deal directly with one another, no matter how angry they become. Norms must be established in which it is made clear that group members are there to understand themselves, not to outdo, defeat, or ridicule one another. Furthermore, every member is to be taken seriously. When a group begins to treat one person as someone whose opinions and anger are to be lightly regarded, the hope of effective treatment for that patient has all but officially been abandoned.

Not all groups tolerate the same level of conflict. The open, conflictual confrontation that might take place between two members of a long-term outpatient group would be devastating in a group for schizophrenic patients (Kanas 1985, 1996). Gentle, cautious disagreement would be appropriate in a time-limited group for patients with panic disorder, whereas such disagreement would be seen as an avoidance of the real issues in a long-term outpatient group. Furthermore, even the same group may not tolerate the same level of conflict at different points in its development. Early on, a prototypic group needs to invest its energy in the development of cohesiveness, trust, and support. In its middle phases, such a group will begin the constructive exploration of disagreement and confrontation. Much later, as members are terminating therapy, they may wish to focus again on the positive, more intimate aspects of the group experience rather than the divisive ones.

Finally, therapists should remember that conflict easily gets out of hand, no matter what the group setting. Leaders will often have to intervene vigorously to keep conflict within constructive bounds. Most often, this will include helping patients to express anger more directly and more fairly and ensuring that everyone gets a turn to respond to the anger. As with any affectively charged experience in the group, the therapist will need to encourage active feedback and consensual validation from all of the group members and, more than ever, will need to help patients process the meaning of that experience within the context of the group.

TECHNIQUES OF THE GROUP THERAPIST

Although individual and group therapists often use similar psychotherapeutic techniques, a number of interventions are unique to group therapy. These interventions include working in the here and now, using therapist transparency, and employing various procedural aids that can enhance the group work. We shall briefly examine each of these group therapy techniques and then describe how fundamental group therapy technology can be modified to suit a specialized group setting.

WORKING IN THE HERE AND NOW

Even in the absence of direct leadership—for example, in a self-help group with no designated leader—an environment can develop in which nearly all of the therapeutic factors, from universality to altruism, will operate. The one important exception is the factor of interpersonal learning. In group therapy, interpersonal learning requires the presence of a leader, one who is well versed in the specific therapeutic techniques of working in the here and now. The principles of working in the here and now and the use of interpersonal learning are of most consequence in prototypic interactional groups, but these fundamental concepts can be modified to suit the needs of other kinds of groups and form an essential part of any group therapist's armamentarium (Dies 1993; Kahn 1984; Rothke 1986).

Goals

The primary goal of the long-term outpatient therapy group, and, to a lesser extent, of many other kinds of groups, is to help each individual understand as much as possible about his or her interactions with the other members of the group, therapists included. To accomplish this, members must learn to focus on the immediate interpersonal transactions occurring in the group. For the therapist, this means that the most fundamental principle of technique is to focus on the present, on what takes place in the therapy room in the here and now of the group interaction. By directly focusing on the here and now, the leader solicits and engages the active participation of all the members and maximizes the power and efficiency of the group. In other words, the therapy group focus is most powerful if it is basically ahistoric—that is, if it de-emphasizes the historical past and even the current outside life of the individual members in favor of the here-and-now events in the group. De-emphasis does not imply that history is unimportant; rather, it implies that groups work most efficiently on the interactions occurring in the immediate present.

If it is to be therapeutically effective, a group experience must contain both an affective and a cognitive component. That is, the group members must be involved with one another in an affective matrix: they must interact freely, they must reveal a great deal of themselves, and they must experience and express important emotions. But they must also step outside that experience and examine, understand, and integrate the meaning of the emotional experience they have just undergone (Yalom and Vinogradov 1993). Thus, a here-and-now focus consists of a rotating sequence of affect evocation and affect examination (Figure 33–2).

The absence of either the affective or the cognitive components of the here-and-now experience jeopardizes therapy. Encounter groups were often powerful and exciting events in the 1960s and 1970s, but many participants found that a strong emotional occurrence without subsequent examination promoted little real learning. No real therapeutic change occurs unless group members can integrate what they have learned in the here and now and then transfer that learning to their real-life situation. Likewise, leaders who focus exclusively on explanations and intellectual integration can end up squelching all expression of spontaneous affect and create a lifeless, sterile group.

Techniques

These two stages of the here-and-now focus—affect evocation followed by affect examination—are different in character and demand two very distinct sets of techniques. For the first stage, the stage of emotional experience, the therapist needs a set of techniques that will plunge the group into the immediate interpersonal interactions. For the second stage, clarification and understanding of the emotional experience, the therapist needs a set of techniques that will help the group transcend itself to examine and interpret its own experience. Let us consider each of these stages in turn.

Plunging the group into the here and now.   The starting place for shaping a group focused on the here and now is the pregroup preparation. The leader can offer the patient a rationale of the here-and-now approach through a

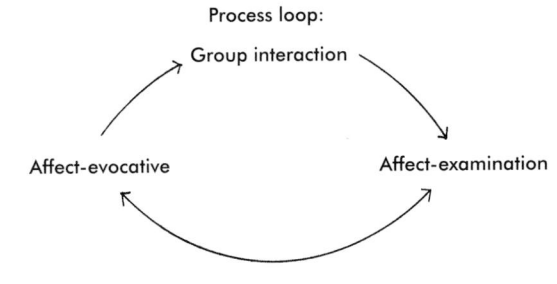

FIGURE 33–2.   Schematic representation of the here-and-now technique in group therapy.

brief, simplified discussion of the interpersonal approach to therapy. Patients benefit from an explicit description of how various kinds of psychological problems arise from (and are manifested in) patients' relationships with others and how group therapy is an ideal setting to take a close look at interpersonal relationships. Without this preparation, patients may be confused by the here-and-now focus of the group. After all, they sought therapy to deal with painful feelings such as anxiety, anger, or depression; how can they not be puzzled to find themselves in a group in which the therapist is asking them to reveal their feelings toward seven strangers? To alleviate this kind of confusion and to ensure that patients participate fully, the therapist must provide a cognitive bridge for incoming members.

After laying these foundations for the here-and-now focus in the pregroup preparation, the leader continues to reinforce this focus throughout therapy. Experienced group therapists think "here and now" at all times and consider themselves as shepherds keeping the group at work grazing on current interactions. All strays into the past, into outside life, or into intellectualization must be headed off or gently nudged back into the present. Whenever the group engages in some "there-and-then" discussion, for example, the group leader must think, "How can I bring this back into the here and now?"

The therapist must begin to steer the group into the here and now in its very first session. Consider for a moment the beginning of any therapy group. Typically, some member will get things started by sharing with the group a major life problem or concern and the reasons why he or she is now in this therapy group. Usually this disclosure begets both some support and some similar disclosure from others, and in a short period the group members have begun to share a great deal.

To plunge the group into the here and now, the interactionally oriented therapist may intervene with a comment such as "This group has made a good start, and many of you have shared some important things about yourselves. However, I have a hunch that something else has been happening here today as well. [It is of course more than a hunch. The therapist knows perfectly well that what he or she is about to say has occurred.] Each of you has found himself or herself thrown together with a group of strangers. No doubt you've been observing and sizing up one another and making first impressions." By this time, some persons in the group will be nodding in agreement, and the therapist may then set the task of the group: "Perhaps we could spend the rest of the meeting today discussing what each of you has come up with so far." Or, in a more fragile, lower-functioning group in which members might find this open-ended task threatening, an alternative sug-

gestion could be, "Perhaps we could share what we liked the most about each other's participation so far." Now, this is no subtle intervention. It is a heavy-handed, explicit instruction to begin the process of here-and-now interaction. And yet the vast majority of groups, no matter what their composition or orientation, respond favorably to this intervention. Even groups of hospitalized patients, if proper boundaries are placed, accomplish this task with considerable ease and reward.

Group therapists must be active and continue diligently from session to session to bring the group discussion into the here and now. They must shift the content of the material from outside the group to inside the group, from abstract reflections on problems to specific revelations, from generic statements to personal disclosure. When a patient states that he or she is embarrassed to talk about certain things in the group, the therapist might ask what the patient anticipates happening if he or she were to take the risk and talk about something "embarrassing." If the patient supposes that people might laugh or be judgmental, the leader could then ask, "Who here in the group do you feel would laugh at you?" Once the group member reveals his or her guesses about others' reactions, the door is open to good interactional work. Other group members can confirm or, as is more often the case, disconfirm those guesses.

A useful technique for activating the here and now is to identify an ingroup analogue for some outgroup problem and then to work on the ingroup analogue rather than the outgroup situation. If, for example, a male patient brings in an account of an argument he had with his wife in which she accused him of being unfeeling, it is incumbent on the group leader to search for some type of here-and-now manifestation of that conflict. The therapist might reflect on recent interactions in the group in which members wondered whether this patient was really empathic to their problems. Or the therapist might ask some of the female members of the group to picture being married to this patient. To what degree of close emotional contact could they imagine being in with him? Without an intervention of this sort, the group will spend its energies on helping the patient solve the problems that led to the argument with his wife—an inefficient use of a group's time. Generally presented with incomplete or biased data, groups are almost always destined to fail to solve outside problems, and members end up feeling frustrated or discouraged.

The therapist who is experienced in working in the here and now is able to use almost every incident as a springboard for interactional exploration. If a patient monopolizes the group with a long 20-minute convoluted account of some painful period in his past life, the leader should start to reflect, "What are the interactional aspects of this behavior?" The leader may recall that in the first session, this patient said he often feels others don't listen to him. "Is it possible," the therapist could ask aloud, "that this is one of those times?" Another tack might be to ask why the patient chose to deliver this monologue today in the group. "What do the rest of you think? Could it be related to a feeling of being misunderstood in last week's meeting?" Or the patient could be encouraged to guess how the rest of the group is reacting to what he has been saying. Any one of these approaches has the same effect: it moves the group members away from a content-oriented monologue in which they cannot participate to a discussion of the relationships among members.

Individuals do not engage naturally and easily in the here and now. The experience is new and frightening, especially for the many patients who have not previously had close and honest relationships or who have spent their lives keeping certain thoughts and feelings—anger, pain, intimacy—covert. The therapist must offer much support, reinforcement, and explicit training. A first step is to help patients understand that the here-and-now focus is not synonymous with confrontation and conflict. In fact, many patients have problems not with anger or rage but with closeness and the honest and nondemanding or nonmanipulative expression of positive sentiments. Accordingly, it is important early in the group to encourage the expression of positive feelings as well as critical ones (Yalom and Vinogradov 1993).

The leader must teach group members how to request and how to offer feedback that is centered within the group's interactions and that is specific and personal. Observations or requests that have to do with there-and-then problems or that are global and abstract—such as "What should I do about my fights with my boyfriend?" or "You're really nice" or "Am I a boring person?"—are always unhelpful. The more specific the question or feedback, the more useful and potent it is. Much more fruitful are requests such as "I'd like to explore why I keep locking horns with the men in this group," and feedback such as "I feel closest to you when you share your pain with me, but I get turned off when you present yourself as having it all together and needing very little from the group."

Understanding the here and now.   The second stage of the here-and-now focus requires an entirely different set of functions and techniques from the therapist. If the first stage demands activation and plunging of the group into the present affective experience, the second stage demands reflection, explanation, and interpretation. Often this latter phase of the group work is referred to as *group*

process. If several individuals engage in a discussion, the content of their discussion is obvious; the discussion consists of the actual words spoken and the substantive issues addressed. But the process of the discussion is entirely different. The process refers to how this content was expressed and what it reveals about the nature of the relationship of the individuals holding the discussion.

The group therapist must always attend to the process of the communication in the group—that is, he or she must examine how the words exchanged shed light on the relationships among the participants. Consider, for example, the patient who suddenly reveals in a meeting that as a child she was sexually molested by her stepfather. The group members will probably probe for more "vertical disclosure," for more details such as how long the abuse lasted, what role her mother played, and whether the abuse affected the patient's relationship with men. A process-oriented therapist is more concerned about "horizontal disclosure" (i.e., disclosure about the disclosure) and, accordingly, will attend to the relational aspects of the patient's disclosure (Vinogradov and Yalom 1989). The leader may then pose questions such as "Why is Betty revealing this to us today rather than some other day?" or "What has permitted her to take this risk today?" or "What prevented her from telling us this earlier?" or "How does she anticipate the group will respond?"

The recognition of process is part of the art of psychotherapy and often requires a long apprenticeship. To understand process, one needs to register continually all of the available data. Who chooses which seat? Who is always late? At whom do members look when talking with each other? Who meets with whom at the end of the group? How does the group change when a particular member is absent? Some of the most valuable data are the therapist's own reactions. Feelings of impatience, frustration, or boredom in a group session represent valuable information and should be put to use. Likewise, when the leader feels engaged or excited by the group interactions, this is often the sign of a potent, hard-working meeting.

To recognize and understand the process in the here and now, it is helpful to keep in mind that certain tensions and processes will be present to some degree in every therapy group. One of the most fundamental of these is the struggle for dominance. Others include basic group conflicts faced by each member: the conflicts between sibling rivalry and the need for mutual support, between self-interest and the desire to help another person, and between the wish to immerse oneself in the comforting body of the group on the one hand and the fear of losing one's precious autonomy on the other. Certain theoretical models of group behavior have been developed, by Bion (1959) and others, to describe and explain these basic conflicts.

The therapist who recognizes and identifies these fundamental tensions when they manifest themselves in the group will have illuminated an important part of the here-and-now process. As an example, we once had occasion to work with an articulate and provocative young man who had long enjoyed the role of dominant member of a group. When an older, very successful and aggressive man joined as a new member, the younger man gradually became withdrawn and depressed and soon announced his intention of leaving the group. It was not until the therapist called attention to the struggle for dominance that the patient began to explore some of his feelings about competition and envy.

USE OF TRANSFERENCE AND THERAPIST TRANSPARENCY

Transference

Group members regard group therapists in an unrealistic light for many reasons. True transference or displacement of affect from some prior object, such as an early parental figure, is one reason. Conflicted attitudes toward authority as represented by the leader (e.g., dependency, autonomy, rebellion) are another. And still another reason is the patient's tendency to ascribe superhuman features to therapists so that the patient can use the therapists as a shield against existential anxiety. One realistic source of strong feelings lies in the members' explicit or intuitive appreciation of the great power that group therapists wield. The therapists' consistent presence and impartiality are essential for group survival and stability. Group therapists cannot be exposed; they can add new members, expel old members, and mobilize enormous group pressure around any issue they wish.

True transference does, of course, occur in therapy groups; indeed, it is powerful and radically influences the nature of the group discourse. But just as there will be, in any group, patients whose therapy hinges on the resolution of transference distortion, so there will also be many others whose improvement depends on interpersonal learning stemming not from transferential work with the therapist but from peer-oriented work with another member around such issues as competition, exploitation, or sexual and intimacy conflicts. Thus, if leaders ignore transference considerations, they may seriously misunderstand some important transactions; if, on the other hand, they see only the transference aspects of the group, they will fail to encourage the exploration of many other important interactions and may also fail to relate authentically to many of the

group members. The cardinal rule is to maintain flexibility. Group therapists have a variety of tasks: they must make good use of any irrational attitudes toward them without at the same time neglecting a leader's many other functions in the group.

To work effectively with transference in the therapy group, leaders must help patients recognize, understand, and change their distorted attitudes. Two major approaches or techniques facilitate transference resolution in the therapy group. The first of these involves consensual validation (or, as is more often the case, consensual invalidation) by other group members of the patient's distorted views. The second, which shall be discussed separately, makes use of increased therapist transparency.

In consensual validation, a group leader encourages a patient to validate his or her impressions against those of other members. If many or all of the group members concur in the patient's view of and feelings toward the leader (say, that the leader is "too autocratic"), it can be concluded either that the patient's reaction to the therapist stems from global group forces related to the leader's role or that the reaction is not an unrealistic one at all and the patient is perceiving the leader accurately. Therapists, too, have blind spots. If, on the other hand, one member alone possesses a particular view of the therapist, then this member may be helped to examine the possibility that he or she sees the group leader, and perhaps other persons too, through an internal distorting prism.

Therapist Transparency

Group therapists can also allow a patient to confirm or disconfirm irrational impressions by gradually revealing more of themselves, reacting to the patient as a real person in the here and now. Leaders can thus respond to their patients authentically, share their feelings in a judicious and responsible manner, and acknowledge or refute motives and feelings attributed to them. In this approach, they look at their own blind spots and demonstrate respect for the feedback members offer them. In the face of mounting reality-based data about the therapist, it becomes increasingly difficult for members to maintain their fictitious beliefs about the group leader (Vinogradov and Yalom 1990).

One fear that therapists sometimes have concerning personal self-disclosure is the fear of escalation—the fear that once they reveal themselves, the insatiable group will demand even more. But strong forces in the group oppose this trend. Although members are enormously curious about their group leader, they also wish the therapist to remain unknown and all-powerful. Although they appreciate the responsible and growth-promoting use of interpersonal feedback from their leader, few want the therapist to discuss his or her personal problems.

There are many different approaches to therapist transparency, depending on the therapist's personal style and the goals in the group at a particular time. It is helpful to ask oneself what the purpose of self-disclosure is at any given point in the group: "Am I trying to facilitate transference resolution? Am I providing a model in an effort to create therapeutic norms? Am I attempting to assist the interpersonal learning of members by working on their relationship with me? Am I attempting to support and demonstrate my acceptance of members by saying, in effect, 'I value and respect you and demonstrate this by giving of myself'?" At all times, the therapist must consider whether transparency is consonant with other group therapy tasks (Vinogradov and Yalom 1990).

Although therapist self-disclosure generally facilitates group interaction, it is important to keep in mind that the group therapist's primary raison d'être is not to be fully self-disclosing. Furthermore, leader self-revelation must be guided by the different needs of each group member. Not all patients need the same thing, either from the therapist or from the group. Some patients need to relax controls and to learn how to express their emotions in an honest and responsible manner, whether they be anger, love, tenderness, envy, or other emotions. Other patients need the opposite, in that they need to gain impulse control and to accept limits to the expression of their emotions; their lifestyles may already be characterized by labile and immediately acted-on affect. Even the transparent and authentically self-disclosing therapist must provide some cognitive structuring—some intellectual integration to the group experience. Only in this manner can patients learn to generalize their experiences to outside life.

The leader's role undergoes a gradual metamorphosis during the life of any relatively stable interactional group. In the beginning, therapists busy themselves with the many functions necessary for the creation of the group, the development of a social system in which the many therapeutic factors may operate, and the activation and illumination of the here and now. Gradually, the leader begins to interact with each of the members, and the members' early stereotypes of the therapist become more difficult to maintain. This process between the therapist and each of the members is not qualitatively different from the interpersonal learning that ensues as a result of each member's relationship with other members. After all, therapists have no monopoly on authority, dominance, sagacity, or aloofness, and many members work out their conflicts in these areas not only with the leader but with other members who have these attributes.

PROCEDURAL AIDS

A group leader's therapeutic armamentarium can be expanded through the use of procedural aids—specialized techniques that are not essential but may facilitate the course of therapy. We will discuss three such approaches: written summaries, videotaping, and structured exercises.

Written Summaries

The course of most outpatient therapy groups, especially interactionally oriented groups, is facilitated by the use of written summaries (Yalom 1995; Yalom et al. 1975). The most useful procedure is for the group leader to dictate a candid, concise description of the group session after each meeting and to have a transcription (of approximately two to three single-spaced pages) sent out to the group members the following day. These summaries serve to extend the effect of the group's here-and-now interactions during the week between meetings. Patients have been unanimous in their positive evaluation of this technique. Most await the arrival of the weekly summary with anticipation and read and consider it seriously. Many members reread the summaries several times, and almost all file them for future review. The patients' therapeutic perspectives and commitment are deepened, and the patient-therapist relationship is strengthened. No serious transference complications, breaks in confidentiality, or other adverse consequences have been noted to occur by practitioners of this method.

Weekly summaries are most valuable if they are honest and straightforward about the process of therapy in the group. They are virtually identical to the summaries therapists make for their own files and are based on the assumption that each patient is a full collaborator in the therapeutic process—that psychotherapy is strengthened and not weakened by demystification. The orientation of the material in the summary reflects the therapeutic orientation of the group. In a long-term interaction group, the summary focuses on the interpersonal transactions that occurred in the meeting and the therapist's reflections on some of the dynamics and implications of those transactions. In a time-limited outpatient group for bereaved spouses, the summaries are more descriptive in nature and underline some of the members' modes of coping with bereavement: loneliness, change in social role, disposition of the effects of the dead spouse, and confrontation with existential issues such as death, aloneness, meaning in life, and regret (Yalom and Vinogradov 1988).

The summary serves several functions (Table 33–6). It provides an understanding of the here-and-now events of the session and facilitates the integration of powerful affec-

TABLE 33-6. Benefits of weekly written summary of group therapy session

1. Provides a further understanding of the here-and-now events of the session.
2. Helps integrate powerful affective experiences.
3. Labels the session as good or resistive.
4. Notes and rewards patient gains.
5. Predicts undesirable developments.
6. Increases group cohesiveness by emphasizing similarities among members.
7. Underscores caring or positive emotions.
8. Provides continuity from meeting to meeting.
9. Allows interpretations.
10. Provides a view of the group's long-term development.

Note. Weekly written summaries are sent to all members between sessions.

tive experiences. It labels sessions as good or resistive, notes and rewards patient gains in the group, and predicts undesirable developments in the group, thus minimizing their impact. It increases group cohesiveness by emphasizing similarities among members, by underscoring the expressing of caring or other positive emotions, and by providing continuity from one meeting to another. The summary is also an ideal forum for interpretations, either for interpretations made during the session (which may have fallen on deaf ears if delivered in the midst of a heated discussion) or for new interpretations that have occurred to the therapist after the meeting. Finally, the summary provides hope to the patients by helping them realize that the group is an orderly process and that the therapist has some coherent sense of the group's long-term development.

Videotaping

Modern scientific technology has no doubt contributed to the dehumanization of present-day society; to the deconstitution of stable, support-giving social, work, and kinship groups; and, consequently, to the necessity for group therapy. However, it has also created an instrument, the videotape recorder, that has considerable potential benefit for the teaching, practice, and understanding of group therapy. Some therapists make the videotape recording a central feature of therapy; they may arrange for immediate playback of certain segments during a meeting or set up regularly scheduled playback sessions. Other therapists, ourselves included, find the technique of value but prefer to use it as a teaching device or occasionally as an auxiliary aid in the therapeutic process.

Although feedback from others about one's behavior is important, it is never as convincing as information one discovers for oneself, and videotape provides feedback that is not mediated through a second person. Often a patient's cherished self-image is radically challenged by a videotape playback. It is not unusual for a patient suddenly to recall and to accept previous feedback he or she has received from other members. The patient realizes that the group has been honest and, if anything, overprotective in previous confrontations.

Often profound realizations occur: for the first time, patients observe with their own eyes their full behavior and its impact on others. Many initial playback reactions are concerned with physical attractiveness and mannerisms, whereas in subsequent playback sessions patients begin to make more careful note of their interactions with others, their withdrawal or timidity, and their self-preoccupation or aloofness or their hostility.

Patients who will be able to view the playback are usually receptive to the suggestion of videotaping. Often, however, they are concerned about confidentiality and need reassurance on this issue. If the videotape is to be viewed by anyone other than group members (e.g., students, researchers, supervisors), the therapist must be explicit about the purpose of the viewing and the identity of the viewers and must obtain written permission from all of the members.

Structured Exercises

The term *structured exercises* refers to the many group activities in which members follow some specific set of orders, generally prescribed by the leader. These kinds of exercises play a more important role in brief, specialized therapy groups than in long-term general outpatient groups (Lieberman et al. 1973; McKay and Paleg 1992; Yalom 1985; Yalom et al. 1975). The precise rationale of the procedures varies, but in general, structured exercises are meant to be accelerating devices. Some structured exercises (warm-up procedures) permit a bypassing of hesitant, uneasy first steps of the group; others speed up interaction through assignment to individuals of interactional tasks that circumvent cautious, ritualized social behavior; still others speed up individual work by helping members get in touch with suppressed emotions, with unknown or hidden parts of themselves, and with their physical bodies.

A structured exercise may require only a few minutes, or it may consume an entire meeting. Although the exercise may be predominantly nonverbal in nature, there is always a verbal component in that the exercise generates data that subsequently can be discussed by the group. The exercise can involve the group as a whole; for example, a group of chronically mentally ill day-treatment patients may be asked to plan an outing. Or it can involve one member vis-à-vis the group: in a trust exercise, used in an encounter-type group, one member stands, with eyes closed, in the center of the group circle and then falls, allowing the group to support him or her. Exercises can include each individual within the group, such as a "go around," in which each member is asked to give initial impressions of everyone else. In another type of go around that is useful in the early life of a group, each member shares some background history. In working with bereaved spouses, we ask members during an early session to bring in a wedding photograph to share with the rest of the group.

Many of the therapist tasks and techniques that we have already described—norm setting, here-and-now activation, understanding the here and now—involve approaches that have a prescriptive quality (approaches in the form of such questions as "Whose opinion in the group especially matters to you?" or "Can you look at Mary as you talk to her?" or "What has it been like for you to share that with us?" or "On a risk-taking scale of 1 to 10, how much have you risked with us today?"). Every experienced group leader uses some structured exercises, at times in a subtle and spontaneous manner. For example, if a group is tense and blocked and experiences a silence of a minute or two (a minute's silence feels very long in a group!), the leader might ask for a quick go around in which each member says briefly what he or she had been feeling or had thought of saying, but did not, in that silence. Such an exercise usually generates much valuable data.

Although the judicious use of structured exercises can facilitate the course of group therapy, excessive use of such exercises is counterproductive. In long-term group therapy, members make more therapeutic headway if the leaders encourage them to experience their timidity or suspiciousness and to understand the underlying dynamics rather than if the leaders prescribe an exercise that plunges members willy-nilly into deep disclosure or expression (Flowers 1990). In acute or short-term settings such as inpatient groups and certain specialized outpatient groups, the situation is more complex. Faced with a limited amount of time in which to be helpful to many different patients, therapists may find that structured exercises are extremely useful: the exercises increase patient participation, provide a discrete, appropriate group task, and increase group efficiency. But there is a pitfall to be avoided. Whenever therapists prescribe structured tasks for a group, even during a single meeting, they run the risk of infantilizing members and establishing norms that block the group from developing into a potent therapeutic force. Members of a highly structured, leader-centered group begin to feel that all help emanates from the leader. They passively await their turn to work with the therapist. They de-skill themselves from an interpersonal point of view and cease to avail themselves of the help and resources that other group members can provide. Although it is useful to impose structure judiciously when working with brief, specialized groups, it is essential to use that structure in a way that encourages each member's autonomous functioning.

MODIFICATION OF BASIC TECHNIQUES FOR A SPECIALIZED CLINICAL SETTING: THE ACUTE INPATIENT THERAPY GROUP

The therapist faced with the task of organizing a therapy group in a specialized clinical situation must learn to modify fundamental group principles and techniques. We suggest these three basic steps:

1. *Assessment of the clinical setting:* Determine the immutable clinical restraints surrounding the group.
2. *Formulation of goals:* Develop goals that are appropriate and achievable within the existing clinical restraints.
3. *Modification of traditional technique:* Retain the basic principles of group therapy but alter techniques to adapt them to the clinical setting and to achieve the specified goals.

We shall illustrate these steps by discussing a highly specialized group setting: the acute inpatient therapy group. We have chosen this setting for two reasons. First, the clinical challenge of inpatient group therapy is severe, and radical modifications of technique and strategy are required in order to lead effective groups in this setting (Kibel 1993). Second, the inpatient group is the most commonly encountered specialized group and is found on virtually every acute psychiatric ward in the country.

Assessment of the Clinical Setting

The clinical setting facing the inpatient therapist appears highly inhospitable to the practice of traditional group therapy. Intrinsic limitations over which the therapist has no control include the rapid turnover of patients (patients will often be present for only a single group meeting) and the severity and heterogeneity of psychopathology among hospitalized patients. Extrinsic constraints that affect the formation of an inpatient group are represented by such matters as ward policy, staffing, and administrative support (or lack thereof) for group therapy.

The therapist must carefully delineate both the intrinsic and extrinsic limitations of the clinical setting and then take steps to change those extrinsic factors that might hinder the group. On an inpatient ward, for example, the therapist can enlist the support of administrative and clinical staff to ensure that group therapy is a part of the ward program, that group time is set aside and protected for all patients, and that there are adequate group meeting facilities.

Formulation of Goals

Taking into account the clinical facts of life or constraints of the inpatient setting, the therapist must proceed to formulate appropriate goals for an inpatient therapy group (Table 33–7). Six achievable goals for the inpatient setting have been highlighted (Yalom 1983):

1. *To engage patients in the therapeutic process:* Patients are helped to become involved in a process that they find constructive and supportive and will wish to continue after discharge from the hospital.
2. *To teach patients that talking helps:* Patients are exposed to the benefits of psychotherapy and of improved communication skills.
3. *To spot problems:* Patients are helped to learn to identify their maladaptive interpersonal behavior.
4. *To decrease patients' sense of isolation:* Patients are encouraged to develop satisfying social contacts.
5. *To allow patients to be helpful to others:* Patients are allowed to see that they can contribute to the lives of people around them.
6. *To alleviate hospital-related anxiety:* Patients are encouraged to share concerns about the stigma of psychiatric hospitalization, to discuss distressing events on the ward (e.g., bizarre behavior of other patients, staff tensions, acutely disturbed patients), and to achieve reassurance from other group members.

Modification of Traditional Technique

Once appropriate goals have been established, therapists must modify their standard group therapy techniques in

TABLE 33–7. Goals for acute inpatient therapy groups

To engage patients in the therapeutic process.
To teach patients that talking helps.
To spot problems.
To decrease isolation.
To allow patients to be helpful.
To alleviate hospital-related anxiety.

order to lead effective groups on the acute psychiatric inpatient ward (Table 33–8). Four essential modifications that we will discuss are 1) the shortening of the time frame, 2) the use of direct support, 3) emphasis on the here and now, and 4) the provision of structure.

Shortening of time frame.   The first and most fundamental modification the inpatient group leader makes is to shorten the time frame radically. The therapist in an acute inpatient group must consider the life of the group to be only a single session and must strive to offer something useful for as many patients as possible during that session. Naturally, a single-session time frame demands efficiency. There is no time to waste: the leader has only a single opportunity to engage each patient and must not squander that opportunity. This need for efficiency demands heightened therapist activity. The therapist must be prepared to activate the group, to call on members, to support them, and to interact personally with them.

Use of direct support.   Inpatient group therapists must also learn to offer support quickly and directly. The most direct manner of offering support is simply to acknowledge openly each patient's efforts, intentions, strengths, positive contributions, and risks. If, for example, a member states that he finds a woman in the group very attractive, the leader must judiciously support this patient for the risk he has taken. The leader may wonder whether the group member has previously been able to express his admiration of another person so openly or may note that his openness encourages other members to take risks and reveal important feelings. Inpatient group therapists must try to emphasize the positive rather than the negative aspects of a person's behavior or defense. For example, rather than confront the patient who insists on playing "assistant therapist," the therapist may instead make positive comments on how helpful this patient has been to others. The stage is then set for a gentle remark on the patient's selflessness and reluctance to ask for something personal from the group.

The supportive therapist also makes it a point to help patients—especially objectionable or irritating pa-

TABLE 33–8. Modifications of basic techniques for acute inpatient therapy groups

Shortening of the time frame.
Use of direct support.
Emphasis on the here and now.
Provision of structure.

tients—obtain support from the group. A self-centered patient who incessantly complains about a health condition or an insoluble situational problem will quickly alienate any group. When the therapist identifies such behavior, he or she must intervene quickly to circumvent the development of group animosity and rejection. The therapist may, for example, assign the patient the task of introducing new members into the group, giving positive feedback to other members, or attempting to guess and express what each member's evaluation of the group is that day. Or the leader may reframe the patient's irritating behavior: "Perhaps you have needs, too, but have trouble expressing them. I wonder if your preoccupation with your health [finances, spouse] isn't a way of asking for something from the group." Helping the patient to formulate a specific request for attention from the group often generates a positive response from the other members.

Another approach is to focus on making the group safe. Whereas some conflict and tension are necessary to the therapeutic work in a long-term outpatient group, inpatients are much too vulnerable to tolerate the additional anxiety of group conflict. The group therapist must anticipate and avoid confrontation and conflict whenever possible. If patients are irritable or critical, the leader can channel that work onto himself or herself. If two patients are locked into an adversarial position, the leader can remind them that sparks often fly between two persons who have similarities or who have envious feelings toward each other. Then each of the patients can be invited to talk about those aspects of the other that he or she admires or envies or to discuss the ways that he or she resembles the other.

When the therapist leads a group of severely regressed patients, he or she must provide even more support, in an even more direct fashion. The patients' behavior must be examined and then reframed in some positive way. The therapist can, for example, support the mute patient for staying the whole session, compliment the patient who leaves early for having stayed 20 minutes, or support inactive patients for having paid attention throughout the meeting. At times the therapist must even label inappropriate or bizarre statements as attempts to communicate with the group.

Emphasis on the here and now.   These foregoing considerations of therapist efficiency, activity, and support in the inpatient setting do not make the here-and-now focus any less important than in outpatient therapy. Such a focus helps inpatients learn many important interpersonal skills: those of communicating more clearly, getting closer to others, expressing positive feelings, noticing personal mannerisms that push people away, listening, offering support, revealing oneself, and forming friendships. However, the clinical conditions of extremely brief treatment duration and more severe pathology demand modifications in basic technique. There is insufficient time to work through interpersonal issues. Instead, the therapist simply helps patients to spot major interpersonal problems and to reinforce interpersonal strengths. Explicit instruction must be provided about the relevance of the here and now by, for example, explaining that group therapy focuses on the way people relate to one another because that is what group therapy does best; and that, furthermore, groups do this most effectively by examining the relationships between members of the group. The group leader must emphasize that even though patients may enter the hospital for many different reasons, everyone can benefit from learning how to get more out of their relationships with others.

Provision of structure.   Finally, work with the acute inpatient group requires structure, and just as there is no place in acute inpatient group work for the inactive therapist, there is also no place for the nondirective therapist. Group leaders provide structure for the inpatient group in several ways: by instructing patients about and orienting them to the nature and purpose of the meeting, by establishing clear spatial and temporal boundaries for the group, and by using a lucid and confident personal style that reassures confused or anxious patients and contributes to a sense of structure. One of the most potent ways of providing structure is to build into each session a consistent, explicit sequence. Although different group sessions will have different sequences depending on the composition and task of the group, the following are natural lines of division:

1. *The first few minutes:* The therapist provides explicit structure for the group. If there are new members (and there usually are in the acute inpatient group), this is the time to orient them to therapy.
2. *Definition of the task:* The therapist determines the most profitable direction for the group to take in a particular session. The leader may, for example, listen to get a sense of the urgent issues on the ward that day. Or the leader may provide a structured exercise, such as having each patient formulate (with the leader's help) an agenda to follow during that session (Yalom 1983). For example, an agenda of a shy and inhibited young depressed woman might be to try to express some positive feelings in the group.
3. *Accomplishing the task:* The therapist helps the group to address the broad issues raised at the start of the

session and, in the process, attempts to have as many patients participate as possible. If the group uses an agenda format, this is the "agenda-filling" stage: the shy patient is helped to identify the members toward whom she feels positively and to express those feelings.

4. *The final few minutes:* The leader indicates that the work phase is over and the remaining time is devoted to review and analysis of the meeting. This is the summing-up period and the self-reflective loop of the here-and-now process, in which the therapist attempts to clarify the group interaction that occurred in the session. How, for example, did the group respond when a usually shy and inhibited member openly expressed some positive sentiments?

GROUP THERAPY PROGRAMS AND MANAGED CARE SYSTEMS

It is the larger work that defines practice and establishes the parameters within which change and adaptation occur. That being the case, we find it puzzling that physicians pay so little attention to how changes in the larger work world affect their lives. (Tischleer and Astrachan 1996, p. 959)

The importance of group therapy is growing in today's managed care environment. Community mental health programs, the military, and the Veterans Administration use systematic approaches to the delivery of mental health care. However, group therapy is moving beyond the public sector and the private office to the private sector, which is sensitive to resource allocation, vigilant about empirical results, and concerned with user satisfaction (both patient and referring source). As mental health care delivery systems replace the individual practitioner or the small group practice, group therapy programs must become more sophisticated. As systems and subsystems (i.e., group programs in mental health divisions in health care systems) enlarge, the number of permutations of pairings increases geometrically with more pieces. Therapists and administrators must accept the associated increased administrative needs. The extra cost will be more than adequately recouped in terms of dollars and better patient care. Group treatment modalities and preventive strategies will become ever more important both in mental health care settings and in health programs in general. Group therapy is becoming central to employees and leaders of clinical enterprises competing in today's marketplace. To best serve patients, employees, and systems, everyone must cooperate in group program development.

The most obvious economic reason for increased utilization of group therapy is efficiency of use of staff time (number of patients per staff hour). However, group therapy as a labor-saving strategy is prone to being overused and exploited. Incorporation of managed care is expanding the use of group therapy to serve large populations effectively and efficiently. Therapists as well as administrators and staff must change the institutional culture and protocols to implement a group therapy program and other explicit cost-cutting strategies (i.e., pre-authorization and concurrent utilization review). When something new is being started, extensive changes often feel like "blunt blows." Eventually, the technique for changing old patterns is refined (Bennett 1993). In many sectors of health care delivery, both the process of starting a group therapy program and the process of shifting utilization patterns are just beginning. Despite the current changes being logical responses to economic realities, institutions are adapting slowly and facing substantial internal resistance.

As the norms regarding delivery of mental health care broaden to accommodate economic realities, the emphasis shifts from methods involving forcing behavior change from the outside (by pre-authorization and concurrent review) to methods by which the treatment clinic and providers take on increasing responsibility and risk for providing both efficient and effective care (as measured by capitation and case rates) (Bennett 1993). The responsibility of structuring care systems is shifted from the payers back to the providers. Deciding which patients require more care is made by a team in the clinic closest to the situation. To absorb costs associated with exceptional circumstances, one must cover large populations—thus spreading the cost of one expensive patient over many inexpensive patients. Performing actuarial assessments based on populations of more than 5,000 greatly improves the chances of reliably predicting infrequent but expensive episodes of acute mental illness. Today, business managers as well as clinician-employees rely on accurate assessment of actuarial risk. Managed care works best among large populations of potential patients who stay well. Developing a group program facilitates preventive care for large populations, by preventing full-blown illness and decreasing morbidity through secondary prevention.

STARTING A GROUP PROGRAM

Institutional edicts concerning group therapy must be accompanied by facilitation and reinforcement of behavior change. Initial attempts may even be awkward. Some clinicians may find the shift from "Why group therapy?" to "Why not group therapy?" a shock. New programs usually start small, and as the system encourages referral to groups, individual patients for whom there is no obvious group may end up in the proverbial procrustean bed. Not everyone can be effectively treated in the same type of group therapy, and the process of deciding which patient belongs in which group is still being refined (Harwood 1996).

Therefore, at the start, everyone may find starting a group program challenging. With each early referral there are risks of refusal by the patient, the receiving clinician or group therapist, or the group, and a delicate balancing of priorities is required. Referral failures discourage the referring clinician and dropouts as well as the overwhelmed neophyte group therapist. Initially, the effort put into making decisions such as those concerning which groups to start, when to start them, and how to match patients and groups will be out of proportion to the savings that a small group program produces. As a group program enlarges, fit-and-matching issues become less problematic but still require a coherent, thoughtful approach. Group program coordinators perform many of the essential executive, practical, and educational tasks necessary to develop, enlarge, and maintain a group program.

Which patients can best be treated in a group remains to be definitively delineated. Evaluations and crisis stabilization are almost always performed individually. After that, group or individual approaches may be used for secondary prevention—either time-limited treatments or maintenance treatments. Preventive efforts, although historically underemphasized, are gaining in esteem as their value in capitation systems becomes apparent. Given the absence of a litmus test for likelihood to fail in group therapy, one could argue that referral to a group should always be a part of the initial treatment plan. Rather than "Who will fail in group treatment?" the question may be, "How can we prepare everyone to benefit from some form of group treatment, even when individual sessions are being utilized as well?"

Long-term groups with highly impaired populations appear economical (Gabbard et al. 1997; MacKenzie 1997). Time-limited groups focus on a different patient population and offer increased flexibility. In settings where the shift to using group therapy is well under way, clinicians and administrators must continue to refine their efforts. Wherever group therapy is not being used, it is essential that staff members encourage each other to ask the question "Why not group therapy?" rather than "Why group therapy?" This is a first step toward shifting the institutional culture.

The next sections briefly touch on the history of changes in delivery systems influencing the practice of group therapy, the nature of the current stimuli, the current status of response by the mental health care delivery system, and the implications for systems of training as well as for systems seeking to deliver the best care possible on a per-dollar basis.

DELIVERY SYSTEMS AND GROUP THERAPY

The penetration of group psychotherapy into clinical services has always been dependent on social and political trends related to access. (MacKenzie 1996, p. 102)

As noted earlier, the first therapy group is credited to the internist Joseph Pratt. At a time when tuberculosis was common, Pratt brought his sanitarium patients together for classes. Soon other practitioners, including early psychoanalysts, began seeing patients in group settings. Over the course of the next several decades, changes in the need for mental health care led to creative work and change in group therapy practice. During World War II, Wilfred Bion, a British psychoanalyst, used group process to care for patients with psychiatric problems brought about by the war. His ideas as described earlier in this chapter continue to influence courses in institutional dynamics, basic group therapy, and organizational change.

During the 1970s, there was a shift from care in locked institutions to community mental health care, and T-groups and encounter groups were created. Although this was a productive period in many ways, many programs were inadequately funded. Poorly formulated systems often used group gatherings as a panacea. Theories regarding the appropriate leadership style or group therapy for a population had not evolved sufficiently to allow consistently appropriate referrals. Thus, the schizophrenia of some patients became worse with the use of overly stimulating and anxiety-producing forms of group therapy. Poorly trained group leaders led risky endeavors that resulted in boundary violations and other negative outcomes. During this period, Yalom's empirical research (described earlier in this chapter) led to the creation of a list of therapeutic factors as well as interpersonal group psychotherapy. Group therapy, popularized and overextended during the free-love 1960s, reentered the health care arena.

Current Health Care Delivery as a Stimulus

Application is quite uneven because of lack of expertise in designing and implementing group programs and because of a lack of adequately trained providers. (MacKenzie 1996, p. 104)

Now in the 1990s, there again exists an incentive for developing groups. As in the past, we face the risk of poorly thought out expansions of the use of group therapy. What is different now? Why would we try to improve on what people as brilliant as Bion and Yalom developed? What will make such improvement possible?

Changes inside and outside the field of group therapy will stimulate further development. Bion and Yalom were able to outline truths of group behavior in institutional and small group settings. Their theories are valid for patient treatment groups but are not enough in the case of group program development for primary and secondary prevention. Furthermore, treating brain disease requires integration of group behavior theory and the latest treatments (e.g., therapy with new medication, cognitive therapy for drug abuse, interpersonal therapy for eating disorders) (Verhulst 1996). Changes in the health care delivery system will likely stimulate new inquiries into overlooked or underdeveloped applications of group behavior (e.g., psychoeducational groups, medication-support groups). Unlike 20 years ago, today's improved information systems permit increased vigilance about using treatments that work. Even the modest systems currently in place will mitigate against the most egregious misuses and overuses of group therapy.

There are many different ways to use group process to enhance patients' treatment. Group analysis focuses on treatment through the group. This approach continues to influence other forms of group therapy. Yalom's therapeutic factors provide a framework for therapists to enhance the efficacy of cognitive, behavioral, and psychoeducational approaches. In group therapy, universality, altruism, increased opportunity for positive modeling, and lending of hope all can amplify the impact that other approaches rely on to help patients. Increasing pressure to provide efficient care changes the direction of development and innovation. For example, homogenous groups cohere more rapidly. This contributed to the development of symptom-specific, illness-specific, and developmental stage–specific groups. The need for resource-sensitive methods has led to the development of different types of time-limited groups. The need for a new way to incorporate group therapy will undoubtedly influence what aspects of group therapy receive the most attention in research and development circles.

Although group therapists in private practice have always believed in the efficacy of their treatment, they still struggle to gather enough patients—particularly in the case of less common disorders—to form a viable group. In larger populations, infrequently occurring illnesses turn up at predictable rates, which facilitate planning care for systems and forming of groups.

Group Programs

Despite the advantage of having multiple groups from which to choose, rarely do group therapists combine forces. However, a few systems such as the Tavistock clinic and New York Group Psychoanalytic Society have increased the number of options available for referral by the evaluating clinician. With adequate communication, a better match between patient and group is possible in this type of system. The group therapy systems mentioned offer a narrow array of group therapies, and the potential members probably self-select and represent a narrow array of illnesses. Group programs at health maintenance organizations (HMOs) such as Harvard Community Health Plan and Kaiser Permanente offer a broader spectrum but rarely include all of the possible types of group therapies that have been shown to be efficacious. A triage system for different types of group therapies remains to be effectively developed. Communication systems often fail to convey sufficient information about the patients to match groups and patients carefully. Nonetheless, every effort should be made to convey to all clinicians, especially those providing initial assessment, the type and nature of the groups available (Crosby 1995). Predicting better outcomes in particular groups will require more research. Although integration of an assessment and triage process, and developing a communication system, an information system, and an outcome data system are challenging, few investments in human resources and systems development will provide higher dividends for the corporate board and be more advantageous to the patient.

New information systems are allowing and patterns of reimbursement are encouraging more thoughtful utilization of group therapists. Administrative staff use larger, more sophisticated information systems to track the clinical needs of larger and larger populations. Managed care payers reward clinicians for keeping people healthy and intervening more quickly in chronic illnesses by maintaining a framework of regular contact. Although developments in group theory have been substantial and influential, the recent changes outside the field are currently more important.

THE CURRENT RESPONSE

Under the leadership of the American Group Psychotherapy Association, a National Registry of Certified Group Psychotherapists attempts to ensure that group therapists have appropriate levels of training and experience, so that the likelihood of excesses such as application of the wrong type of group treatment to a patient (i.e., psychoanalytic for schizophrenia) is reduced. But we must still improve treatment-patient matching, pregroup preparation, and methods of structuring a group program. Most clinicians and academicians focus on developing new treatment frameworks for specific types of illness rather than on developing systems to use what is available more effectively.

Staff model HMOs lead the effort to identify which types of groups are most useful in treating large populations. Group coordinators focus on time-limited groups, especially psychoeducational groups, that help people avoid developing full-blown illness. For example, Kaiser Permanente in Portland, OR, has more than 100 different types of groups each year.

In the past, groups for chronically, persistently, and severely mentally ill patients were almost exclusively the province of public mental health programs. With the advent of new forms of reimbursement by Medicaid and Medicare, books have been written on treating such patients in groups. Bauer and McBride (1996), Kanas (1996), and Stone (1996) wrote on group therapy for severely mentally ill patients (bipolar affective disorder, schizophrenia, and chronic mental illness, respectively). Linehan (1993), MacKenzie (1997), and Budman et al. (1996), among others, developed models for treating severe personality disorders in groups and empirically tested the models for efficacy.

Several approaches to time-limited group treatment for common disorders are well developed and are published in both book and workbook form. Many utilize tenets of cognitive or behavioral group therapy (e.g., Padesky on depression, Zueker-White on panic disorder). The theoretical basis and layout of the books lend the books to a structured, focused group approach. The reader can often use the pretreatment and posttreatment assessments in these books. Adding tests to assess parameters such as locus of control, motivation, social competence, learned resourcefulness, ego strength, coping style (Piper and Joyce 1996), psychological-mindedness (McCallum and Piper 1996), and psychological defenses (Tasca et al. 1994) to the pretest may facilitate the matching of patients and groups.

Medication-support group therapy and time-limited interpersonal group therapy are two types of group therapy that are relatively underdeveloped. Psychiatrists can provide secondary prevention with medication-support groups. Such groups offer members regular contact with highly trained mental health professionals. Because they are more efficient in terms of numbers of patients seen, visits can be more frequent than individual medication checks. Yet the task is different than in a therapy group; therefore, these groups need not meet weekly. In a medication-support group, the clinician can observe the patient's level of function in an environment that is probably more like the outside world than the environment of dyadic interactions and is not limited by the patient's descriptions of outside events. Additionally, group therapy offers the patient the opportunity to benefit from Yalom's therapeutic factors: universality, altruism, and sharing of information. Psychiatrists such as Dr. Ana-Marie Indio are working on new models of medication groups at staff model HMOs.

Another relatively overlooked area of group therapy is time-limited interpersonal group therapy that would lend itself to ease of referral by virtue of being generic, of having frequent points of entry, and of taking place as well with eight members as with five. Thus referral to a group does not need to be as rigorously assessed for its resource utilization (no additional clinician time is taken up by having an eighth member versus another individual patient requires scheduling and additional time slot.) So there is less pressure to limit future visits and only provide crisis stabilization (as per many managed care contracts). Time-limited groups can enhance acute crisis benefits. The current trend of awarding a contract to the lowest bidder will eventually be replaced when it is recognized that inexpensive ways to enhance benefit pay off in increased customer satisfaction. Time-limited interpersonal group therapy may be one way to provide benefit to the patient as well as secondary prevention, all at little additional cost.

A well-run time-limited interpersonal group can be very effective in helping people resolve interpersonal difficulties. Relationship problems both lead to and arise from acute psychiatric decompensations. Addressing relationship problems can be viewed as both part of the healing from the last episode and preventive work for the next potential episode. A therapist can run such a group as well with nine patients as with only five. Little extra cost is incurred in entering a few more patients in the group, with the exception of the costs involved in writing notes, fielding phone calls, and turning up problems earlier that may otherwise have gone unnoticed until later.

Resistance

Clinicians are responsible for overcoming not only their patients' reservations but also their own. Although this additional work required is not equivalent to that involved in treating a full-time weekly patient, it does add up, and rewarding group therapists for their effort is essential. Administrators must credit group therapists for a higher overhead per clinical hour. The institution will still benefit, through increased number of patients seen in a day and secondary prevention (Dick and Wooff 1986).

Clinicians must educate their patients about mental illness, treatment, and group therapy. The fact that group therapy is as effective as individual therapy is not widely known even among therapists, and a sense of certainty about the effectiveness of group therapy must be conveyed to patients. In addition, patients may fear that the group will reject them. Such fear must be addressed. Inexperienced group therapists—even if they are experienced clinicians—are like their patients in that they too fear public exposure of and shame about their mistakes. Neophyte group therapists face learning (or at least adapting to) a whole new set of treatment parameters. For both patients and therapists, adequate appreciation of the issues leads to the understanding that although group work initially seems threatening, it is ultimately therapeutic.

The extent to which patients expect humiliation often predicts the degree of relief they will feel when they find out that other people have similar problems and struggles. Similarly, group therapists who are aware of the potential levels and types of complexity in a group are more likely to recognize opportunities that can influence the group process. Just as a new patient entering a group is anxious, a reality-based neophyte group therapist should be both excited and daunted by the task ahead. A greater awareness of the underlying complexity, when it is thoughtfully reflected on and when the therapist receives appropriate supervision, will enhance the group therapist's efforts.

An increasingly common strategy in group therapy is the use of treatment manuals written by experts based on research. Often these focus on specific illnesses or issues and employ a wide variety of theoretical frameworks. Developing a manual to guide neophyte group therapists not only permits the outlining of what works well in group therapy, but also reduces the anxiety of the inexperienced group therapists. Perhaps such eclectic statements as the following will become common.

> Therefore, specific portions of those interventions that were found to be effective and appropriate were combined in a 6 week, structured group intervention that was tailored to encompass health education, stress management, coping skills, and supportive group psychotherapy. (Fawzy et al. 1995, p. 111)

THE FUTURE

The number of health services studies looking at the economic efficiency of different treatment systems is growing. University researchers and managed care companies are seeking to clarify which treatments work under which circumstances. Universities have an interest in and a devotion to acquiring knowledge but lack the effective administrative infrastructure to care for a large population effectively. Large managed care organizations (MCOs) have an interest in and a devotion to saving money and a growing interest in clarifying how to deliver the most efficacious and efficient care. Most important, managed care companies are ahead of universities in the development of information systems and administrative infrastructure for large systems of care that thoroughly test economic and clinical efficiency and efficacy of treatment. Leadership, employee-clinicians, and patient-consumers will all benefit from such infrastructure. Clinic directors, group coordinators, and outpatient clinicians working together will better delineate the benefits of different types of group therapy and patterns of implementation for patients with various disorders. To answer the many remaining questions about helping patients by using group therapy, researchers, clinic administrators, and clinicians will need to collaborate.

Academic medical centers seeking to replace old revenue sources (grants and indirect Medicare funds) are developing new types of relationships with the health care industry. Private sector MCOs can work with medical centers or with research consulting companies. Additionally, academic medical centers can develop their own MCOs. These three different models and mixes of academia and industry offer multiple possibilities for how the current challenges can be met. Large group therapy programs should be integrated into mental health care delivery systems and will offer opportunities to test hypotheses. Addressing questions of program structure will require the combination of academic skills and knowledge with private industry's administrative infrastructure and capital.

Even before the ascent of managed care, several prominent authors had written books and articles on developing and maintaining group therapy training programs. Administrative sanction, effective leadership of the group program, and effective coordination of multiple practitioners are some of the essential factors of a successful group therapy training program (Lonergan 1991, 1995). With the advent of managed care, obtaining administrative support for group programs and even hiring group program coordinators to lead and coordinate such efforts have become easier. Training programs (e.g., in academic medical centers) that are developing the capacity to meet managed care contracts are relying on the efficiency of group therapy to compensate for the inherent inefficiency of some necessary training experiences such as those involving long-term individual treatment of mild to moderately ill patients.

CONCLUSIONS

Group therapy is a widely practiced mode of treatment that is used effectively in a vast number of clinical settings.

It involves a host of therapeutic factors or mechanisms of change, many of which are unique to group therapy. These mechanisms range from the therapeutic factors widely encountered in many different kinds of groups (such as universality, altruism, catharsis, and the imparting of information) to the potent but often misunderstood factor of interpersonal learning, which requires a skilled and experienced therapist working in a specialized interactional setting. Various constellations of these therapeutic factors operate in different types of groups at any given time. Therapists must understand the particular mechanisms of change at work in different kinds of groups and employ appropriate techniques to facilitate such mechanisms and complete the group task.

Group leaders make use of specific techniques and interventions, and all clinicians should be familiar with the technology used in group therapy. Some of these unique interventions include working in the here and now, therapist transparency, and the use of various procedural aids. These fundamental techniques can be modified to suit any specialized group setting, from the acute inpatient group to the symptom-oriented outpatient group. Indeed, the power of group therapy lies in its adaptability. Highly flexible and efficient, it may be the only mode of psychotherapy that can accommodate an almost infinite variety of setting, goals, and patients.

REFERENCES

Agazarian YM: Systems-Centered Therapy for Groups. New York, Guilford, 1997

Alonso A, Swiller HI: Introduction: the case for group therapy, in Group Therapy in Clinical Practice. Edited by Alonso A, Swiller HI. Washington, DC, American Psychiatric Press, 1993, pp xxi–xxv

Amaranto EA, Benden S: Individual psychotherapy as an adjunct to group psychotherapy. Int J Group Psychother 40:91–101, 1990

Ansbacher HL: Alfred Adler, in Comprehensive Textbook of Psychiatry/III, 3rd Edition, Vol 1. Edited by Kaplan HI, Freedman AM, Sadock BJ. Baltimore, MD, Williams & Wilkins, 1980, pp 729–740

Baker MN, Baker HS: Self psychological contributions to the theory and practice of group psychotherapy, in Group Therapy in Clinical Practice. Edited by Alonso A, Swiller HI. Washington, DC, American Psychiatric Press, 1993, pp 49–68

Bandura A, Blanchard EB, Ritter B: Relative efficacy of desensitization and modeling approaches for inducing behavioral, affective, and attitudinal changes. J Pers Soc Psychol 13:173–199, 1969

Bauer MS, McBride L: Structured Group Psychotherapy for Bipolar Disorder: The Life Goals Program. New York, Springer, 1996

Benioff L, Vinogradov S: Group psychotherapy with cancer patients and the terminally ill, in Comprehensive Textbook of Group Psychotherapy, 3rd Edition. Edited by Kaplan HI, Sadock BJ. Baltimore, MD, Williams & Wilkins, 1993, pp 477–489

Bennett MJ: View from the bridge: reflections of a recovering staff model HMO psychiatrist. Psychiatr Q 64:45–75, 1993

Bion WR: Experience in Groups. New York, Basic Books, 1959

Bloch S: Therapeutic factors in group psychotherapy, in Psychiatry Update: American Psychiatric Association Annual Review, Vol 5. Edited by Frances AJ, Hales RE. Washington, DC, American Psychiatric Press, 1986, pp 678–698

Bloch S, Crouch E: Therapeutic Factors in Group Psychotherapy. Oxford, UK, Oxford University Press, 1985

Brook DW: Medication groups, in Group Therapy in Clinical Practice. Edited by Alonso A, Swiller HI. Washington, DC, American Psychiatric Press, 1993, pp 155–170

Budman SH, Cooley S, Demby A, et al: A model of time-effective group psychotherapy for patients with personality disorders: the clinical model. Int J Group Psychother 46:329–355, 1996

Butler T, Fuhriman A: Patient perspective on the curative process: a comparison of day treatment and outpatient psychotherapy groups. Small Group Behavior 11:371–388, 1980

Butler T, Fuhriman A: Curative factors in group therapy: a review of the recent literature. Small Group Behavior 14:131–142, 1983

Cheifetz DI, Salloway JC: Patterns of mental health services provided by HMOs. Am Psychol 39:495–502, 1984

Connelly JL, Piper WE, De Carufel FL, et al: Premature termination in group psychotherapy: pretherapy and early therapy predictors. Int J Group Psychother 36:145–152, 1986

Corsini R, Rosenberg B: Mechanisms of group psychotherapy: processes and dynamics. J Abnorm Soc Psychol 51:406–411, 1955

Crosby G, Sabin J: Developing and marketing time-limited therapy groups. Psychiatr Serv 46:7–8, 1995

Dick BM, Wooff K: An evaluation of a time-limited programme of dynamic group psychotherapy. Br J Psychiatry 148:159–164, 1986

Dies RR: Group psychotherapy: reflections on three decades of research. Journal of Applied Behavioral Sciences 15:361–373, 1979

Dies RR: Practical, theoretical, and empirical foundations for group psychotherapy, in Psychiatry Update: American Psychiatric Association Annual Review, Vol 5. Edited by Frances AJ, Hales RE. Washington, DC, American Psychiatric Press, 1986, pp 659–667

Dies RR: Research on group psychotherapy: overview and clinical applications, in Group Therapy in Clinical Practice. Edited by Alonso A, Swiller HI. Washington, DC, American Psychiatric Press, 1993, pp 473–518

Fawzy FI, Fawzy NW, Hyun CS, et al: Malignant melanoma: effects of an early structured psychiatric intervention, coping, and affective state on recurrence and survival 6 years later. Arch Gen Psychiatry 50:681–689, 1993

Fawzy FI, Fawzy NW, Arndt LA, et al: Critical review of psychosocial interventions in cancer care. Arch Gen Psychiatry 52:100–113, 1995

Flowers JV: The differential outcome effects of simple advice, alternatives and instructions in group psychotherapy. Int J Group Psychother 29:305–316, 1979

Flowers JV, Booraem CD: The frequency and effect on outcome of different types of interpretation in psychodynamic and cognitive-behavioral group psychotherapy. Int J Group Psychother 40:203–214, 1990

Freedman S, Hurley J: Perceptions of helpfulness and behavior in groups. Group 4:51–58, 1980

Fuhriman A, Burlingame GM: Consistency of matter: a comparative analysis of individual and group process variables. The Counseling Psychologist 18:60–63, 1990

Gabbard GO, Lazar SG, Hornberger J, et al: The economic impact of psychotherapy: a review. Am J Psychiatry 154:147–155, 1997

Goffman E: Encounters: Two Studies in the Sociology of Interaction. Indianapolis, IN, Bobbs-Merrill, 1961

Harwood I: Towards optimum group placement from the perspective of self and group experience. Group Analysis 29:199–218, 1996

Kahn EM: Group treatment interventions for schizophrenics. Int J Group Psychother 34:149–153, 1984

Kanas N: Inpatient and outpatient group therapy for schizophrenic patients. Am J Psychother 39:431–439, 1985

Kanas N: Group therapy with schizophrenics: a review of controlled studies. Int J Group Psychother 36:339–351, 1986

Kanas N: Group Therapy for Schizophrenic Patients. Washington, DC, American Psychiatric Press, 1996

Kaul TJ, Bednar RL: Experiential group research: results, questions, and suggestions, in Handbook of Psychotherapy and Behavior Change, 3rd Edition. Edited by Garfield SL, Bergin AE. New York, Wiley, 1986, pp 671–714

Kibel HD: Inpatient group psychotherapy, in Group Therapy in Clinical Practice. Edited by Alonso A, Swiller HI. Washington, DC, American Psychiatric Press, 1993, pp 93–111

Laing RD: The Politics of Experience. New York, Pantheon, 1967

Leszcz M, Yalom ID, Norden M: The value of inpatient group psychotherapy: patients' perceptions. Int J Group Psychother 35:411–433, 1985

Lieberman MA: A group therapist perspective on self-help groups. Int J Group Psychother 40:251–278, 1990

Lieberman MA, Borman L: Self-help groups for coping with crisis. San Francisco, CA, Jossey-Bass, 1979

Lieberman MA, Yalom ID, Miles MB: Encounter Groups: First Facts. New York, Basic Books, 1973

Linehan MM: Cognitive-Behavioral Treatment of Borderline Personality Disorder. New York, Guilford, 1993

Lonergan E[C]: Keeping a group psychotherapy program alive and well within a psychiatry residency. Group 15:168–180, 1991

Lonergan EC: Discussion. Group 19:100–107, 1995

MacKenzie KR: Time-limited group psychotherapy: has Cinderella found her prince? Group 20:95–111, 1997

MacKenzie KR: Time-Managed Group Psychotherapy: Effective Clinical Applications. Washington, DC, American Psychiatric Press, 1997

McCallum M, Piper WE: Psychological mindedness. Psychiatry: Interpersonal and Biological Processes 59:48–64, 1996

McCallum M, Piper WE, Joyce AS: Dropping out from short-term group therapy. Psychotherapy 29:206–252, 1992

McKay M, Paleg K: Focal Group Psychotherapy. Oakland, CA, New Harbinger, 1992

Orlinsky DE, Howard KI: Process and outcome in psychotherapy, in Handbook of Psychotherapy and Behavior Change, 3rd Edition. Edited by Garfield SL, Bergin AE. New York, Wiley, 1986, pp 311–381

Paulson I, Burroughs JC, Gelb CB: Cotherapy: what is the crux of the relationship? Int J Group Psychother 26:213–224, 1976

Pines M, Hutchinson S: Group analysis, in Group Therapy in Clinical Practice. Edited by Alonso A, Swiller HI. Washington, DC, American Psychiatric Press, 1993, pp 29–47

Piper W[E], Joyce A: A consideration of factors influencing the utilization of time-limited, short-term group therapy. Int J Group Psychother 46:311–328, 1996

Piper WE, Perrault EL: Pretherapy preparation for group members. Int J Group Psychother 39:17–34, 1989

Piper WE, Debbane EG, Bienvenu J-P, et al: A study of group pretraining for group psychotherapy. Int J Group Psychother 32:309–325, 1982

Piper WE, McCallum M, Azim HFA: Adaptation to Loss Through Short-Term Group Psychotherapy. New York, Guilford, 1992

Pratt JH: The principles of class treatment and their application to various chronic diseases. Hospital Social Service 6:404, 1922

Rothke S: The role of interpersonal feedback in group psychotherapy. Int J Group Psychother 36:225–240, 1986

Shapiro DA, Shapiro D: Meta-analysis of comparative therapy outcome studies: a replication and refinement. Psychol Bull 92:581–604, 1983

Shapiro JL: Methods of Group Psychotherapy and Encounter. Itasca, IL, Peacock, 1978

Smith ML, Glass GV, Miller TI: The Benefits of Psychotherapy. Baltimore, MD, Johns Hopkins University Press, 1980

Spiegel D, Bloom JR, Kraemer HL, et al: Effect of psychosocial treatment on survival of patients with metastatic breast cancer. Lancet 2:888–891, 1989

Spitz HI: Group Psychotherapy and Managed Mental Health Care: A Clinical Guide for Providers. New York, Brunner/Mazel, 1996

Spitz HI: The effect of managed mental health care and group psychotherapy: treatment, training, and therapist-morale issues. Int J Group Psychother 47:23–30, 1997

Stern MJ: Group therapy with medically ill patients, in Group Therapy in Clinical Practice. Edited by Alonso A, Swiller HI. Washington, DC, American Psychiatric Press, 1993, pp 185–199

Stone W: Group Psychotherapy for People With Chronic Mental Illness. New York, Guilford, 1996

Sullivan HS: The Interpersonal Theory of Psychiatry. New York, WW Norton, 1953

Tasca GA, Russell V, Busby K: Characteristics of patients who choose between two types of group psychotherapy. Int J Group Psychother 44:499–508, 1994

Tillitski CJ: A meta-analysis of estimated effect sizes for group versus individual control treatments. Int J Group Psychother 40:215–224, 1990

Tischler G, Astrachan B: A funny thing happened on the way to reform. Arch Gen Psychiatry 52:959–963, 1996

Toseland RW, Siporin M: When to recommend group treatment: a review of the clinical and the research literature. Int J Group Psychother 36:171–201, 1986

Verhulst J: The role of the psychiatrist: defining methods, theories, and practice in the time of managed care. Academic Psychiatry 20:195–204, 1996

Vinogradov S, Yalom ID: Concise Guide to Group Psychotherapy. Washington, DC, American Psychiatric Press, 1989

Vinogradov S, Yalom ID: Self-disclosure in group psychotherapy, in Self-Disclosure in the Therapeutic Relationship. Edited by Stricker G, Fisher N. New York, Plenum, 1990, pp 191–203

Whitaker DS, Lieberman MAL: Psychotherapy Through the Group Process. New York, Atherton Press, 1964

Yalom ID: A study of group therapy dropouts. Arch Gen Psychiatry 14:393–414, 1966

Yalom ID: The Theory and Practice of Group Psychotherapy. New York, Basic Books, 1970

Yalom ID: Existential Psychotherapy. New York, Basic Books, 1980

Yalom ID: Inpatient Group Psychotherapy. New York, Basic Books, 1983

Yalom ID: The Theory and Practice of Group Psychotherapy, 3rd Edition. New York, Basic Books, 1985

Yalom ID: Interpersonal learning, in Psychiatry Update: American Psychiatric Association Annual Review, Vol 5. Edited by Frances AJ, Hales RE. Washington, DC, American Psychiatric Press, 1986, pp 699–713

Yalom ID: The Theory and Practice of Group Psychotherapy, 4th Edition. New York, Basic Books, 1995

Yalom ID, Vinogradov S: Bereavement groups: techniques and themes. Int J Group Psychother 38:419–457, 1988

Yalom ID, Vinogradov S: Interpersonal group psychotherapy, in Comprehensive Textbook of Group Psychotherapy, 3rd Edition. Edited by Kaplan HI, Sadock BJ. Baltimore, MD, Williams & Wilkins, 1993, pp 185–195

Yalom I[D], Brown S, Bloch S: The written summary as a group psychotherapy technique. Arch Gen Psychiatry 32:605–613, 1975

CHAPTER 34

MARITAL AND FAMILY THERAPY

LESLIE B. KADIS, M.D.
RUTH MCCLENDON, M.S.W.

Judging from our recent meta-analysis, it is clear that marital and family therapy works. The literature support-ing that conclusion is at least as strong as it is for other forms of psychotherapy.

—Shadish et al. 1995, p. 345

We live in a complex world, a world of numerous reciprocal relationships. Most of us interact daily with our partners, children, col-leagues, and neighbors, as well as with numerous people who provide the services for living life. All of these inter-actions have an impact on us, and we in turn have an im-pact on them. When they support a positive view of our-selves, we feel at peace; when they do not, we feel anxious.

The individual approach in therapy is one of helping people manage the anxiety derived from the difficult inter-actions of daily life by focusing on the internalized compo-nents of those interactions as revealed by each patient. An-other approach in therapy is to focus on the relationships between the people themselves. Each approach has its ad-vantages and disadvantages. Each has its place.

Although the focus here is on therapy with families and couples—nowadays encompassed by the field of marital and family therapy (MFT)—this chapter is really about changing relationships through changing the interactions among the people who make up the family or marital unit. However, it is important to note that the ideas we discuss are frequently applied outside the MFT setting. For in-stance, consultants use the principles and techniques in both corporate and family business environments. Attor-neys use the ideas and techniques of relationship therapy to facilitate arbitration, and social scientists draw on the theo-ries of family therapy to understand better the complex web of entire cultures. Despite the setting, these therapists, consultants, facilitators, and scholarly observers of society are *thinking family*, or, in other words, thinking about the family as a system—they have in mind the complex web of relationships, the pattern of transactions that repeat themselves, and the unspoken rules that drive these transactions, regardless of which aspect of the family they are addressing.

In this chapter we develop this idea of *thinking family*. We present an integrated view of the field of relationship therapy and describe some of the tools of the trade that help couples, families, and other relationships heal. We discuss the history of MFT, summarize the different relevant theories, and place the ideas of relationship therapy within the context of the various forms of psychotherapy. Finally, we describe a model for relationship therapy. Drawing on and integrating aspects of several theoretical approaches, this model offers a structure that can be helpful in most psychotherapeutic orientations.

Our goal is to present both the theoretical and the practical cornerstones of relationship therapy that help us move a family or couple toward healing. As M. Pipher (1996) said,

> Therapists have enormous power to do good or ill in families. We are called upon to explain behavior and to say something is happening. When a delinquent adolescent boy comes in, we can ask about his parents' relationship, his friends, the music he listens to or the school he attends. When a woman comes in depressed, we can ask questions about her exercise, diet and use of chemicals, her health, her marriage, her work or her childhood. Our questions suggest causes and lead clients toward solutions. We can ask questions that pull for pathology or questions that bring out strengths. We can ask questions that increase distancing and scapegoating of family members. Or we can ask questions that begin the healing. (Pipher 1996, p. 27)

What we as marital and family therapists do with our power is up to each one of us.

DEFINITIONS

Definitions are important. Too often, particularly in the context of relationships, we think we agree about the meaning of our words, only to find later that we were wrong. Let us look now at what is meant today by the terms *family*, *marital and family therapy* or *relationship therapy*, and *family systems*, and explore the relatively new concept of *thinking family*.

FAMILY

Defining *family* presents some difficulty because in the modern-day world each of us has a different concept of family. Our unique understanding of family is born out of current experiences with our nuclear families as well as our history with our family of origin. Both are tempered by contemporary sociocultural realities. Fewer than 51% of American children living today will grow up in traditional two-parent, nuclear families. For the other 49% of children, other types of families or situations have become the norm: single-parent families, stepfamilies or blended families, adoptive families, families in which grandparents serve as guardians, foster families, families in which both parents are the same gender, and even group homes.

The ever-increasing prevalence of working mothers has made another major change in American families. In fact, sociologists point out that the traditional family with a stay-at-home wife and mother is becoming an unattainable ideal. The evidence for this seemingly radical position is the observation that "more than three-fifths of married women with dependent children are in the labor force, as well as a majority of mothers of infants, while there are more than twice as many single-mother families as married, homemaker-mom families" (Stacey 1996, p. 6). The trends in most of the Western world are comparable.

Given this diversity of both form and function, it is difficult to derive a definition of family. Many who write about family therapy consider the family to be a group of people who have a kinship bond and who share a common current experience. This definition is, on the one hand, still too narrow to take in the full range of family configurations; yet, on the other hand, this definition is useful because it distinguishes the family from other affinity groups. A work group, for example, shares a current experience and may have a long history as a group but rarely shares a kinship bond. Similarly, friendship groups, as well as groups that come together because of a common religious or other affiliation, meet some but not all of the requirements.

We have chosen to permit our own intuition about what a family is to guide us. If a group of people think of themselves as a family, then as family therapists interested in the nature of the relationship, we consider this an appropriate unit to investigate.

FAMILY THERAPY

It is equally difficult to define family therapy. The generally accepted definition is "any psychotherapeutic endeavor that explicitly focuses on altering the interaction between or among family members and seeks to improve the functioning of the family as a unit, or its subsystems and/or the functioning of individual members of the family" (Gurman 1986, p. 565). We accept and follow this definition with one caveat: it is not necessary to meet with the entire family to alter or improve the functioning of the family unit. The reason for this dictum will become apparent when we discuss the concept of *thinking family*.

FAMILY SYSTEMS

The idea that the family—any and every family—operates as a system is the defining concept for MFT. This systems approach, not the number of people in the room, is what differentiates MFT from individual therapy. Similarly, the idea of systems, not the format of the therapy, also differentiates MFT from group therapy. But it is difficult for many of us to obtain a working understanding of systems because the Western world thinks in a linear fashion. We think in terms of beginnings and endings, cause and effect. Systems, however, are anything but linear.

Conceptually, a system is something that is made up of interacting parts. Thus, we can talk about a machine as a system, a government as a system, a single-cell organism as a system, or a group of people as a system (von Bertalanffy 1969). When any particular system is discussed, it is described from the perspective of the way the various parts interact rather than of the individual parts themselves. Although a car engine contains cylinders and pistons and many other parts, we think of it as a car engine and describe it from the perspective of how all the parts interact to enable the engine to work.

Systems theorists recognize that a car engine is very different from what one might expect on seeing the components laid out on a table. A therapist recognizes that any family is different from what might be envisaged from knowing the individual persons who make up the family. The family has its own structure, its own rules, and a unique memory of the history of how it has managed through the ups and downs of life. A unique system unto itself, any family inevitably differs from all other families in what it is and how it works. Yet, a family also operates according to basic generic functions required of any family unit; therefore, *thinking family* means thinking about how structure, rules, methods of problem solving, and patterns of interaction might operate within the family in treatment. These insights then can be applied regardless of which members may be in the room.

One way of describing a system is through describing the style or pattern of interactions. Focusing on the pattern of interactions is one of the most important contributions that MFT has made to psychotherapy. It has changed the nature of the dialogue between patient and therapist from a focus on the intrapsychic content—that is, what the patient is telling the therapist—to a focus on the interpersonal process. This emphasis is similar to attending primarily to group process rather than to the individuals in the group.

Unfortunately, however, it is extremely difficult to describe this shift in emphasis, because we do not have an adequate language. Let us go back to the story of the expulsion of Adam and Eve from the Garden of Eden; a key parable in Western civilization, it exemplifies our customary thinking in terms of cause and effect. In contrast, the systems approach requires us to shift from cause and effect to circular thinking (Selvini-Palazzoli 1980). If this story is viewed from a linear perspective, as it usually is, it indicates that Eve gave Adam the apple and this act resulted in their expulsion. But when the story is viewed from a circular perspective, there is the possibility that Eve may have been responding to Adam's want and that Adam in turn may have been helping her manifest her love of giving.

In systems terms, A does not cause B; instead, A and B reciprocally interact and have an impact on each other. We have all heard the typical couple dialogue: (A) "I wouldn't yell if he listened to me." (B) "I can't listen when she yells."

Individual therapists for each of these people would be drawn to one or the other side of the argument, depending on how the problem was presented to them. Systems therapists, on the other hand, think of this sequence as a circular process in which A and B are each reacting to the other (Jackson 1965; Miller 1955). There is no beginning and no end. One important corollary of the idea of circular causality is that the therapist's description of the problem—how the therapist talks about it and how he or she intervenes—depends on how the therapist punctuates the A-causes-B-causes-A sequence. Systems therapists are ever aware that their personal viewpoints introduce important variables into the understanding of the relationship (Watzlawick 1974).

Within this oversimplified version of a typical interpersonal dilemma, the task of the systems therapist is to describe the sequence of interactions in such a way that an appropriate intervention can result in positive change. There are several ways to do this—and, as we discuss later in the chapter, the differences have more to do with style, or therapist/theorist preference, than with substance. Faced with the A and B example above, the systems theorist could describe the recursive nature of those specific transactions (and others like it that would invariably be discovered) and use a term such as *symmetrical relationship*, which indicates that each statement is matched by a subsequent statement, so that there is continuous escalation (Watzlawick et al. 1974). The expanding, intensifying, or ongoing fight between a couple or between siblings is typical of a symmetrical relationship.

One characteristic of the systems approach is that descriptions do not suggest cause. They do, however, allow different possibilities to intervene. A classic systems intervention is to prescribe fighting, but fighting that is carried on in a ritualized way. This brings an uncontrolled experience under control without the therapist's ever entering the argument. A different systems therapist/theorist, working with the same couple, might attend to the structure of the relationship (Minuchin et al. 1967; Minuchin 1974).

In looking at relationship structure, a possible observation might be that the partners finish each other's statements. This would indicate unclear interpersonal boundaries. In this case the therapist could introduce exercises during sessions and suggest homework that will promote differentiation. Alternatively, a therapist interested in structure might notice that each of the partners does not hear the other person at all. This would indicate boundaries that are too rigid, which might soften under the protection of traditional communication training.

Finally, it is possible to decipher the hidden rules that govern the operations of all recursive patterns and then to conclude that this couple acts as though they believe "You have to yell to be heard" or "No one listens" or, perhaps, "It's not okay to talk about hurts" (Aponte and Hoffman 1973). Belief systems might be addressed directly through use of a historical approach or indirectly with a behavioral approach that reinforces and rewards listening. Whichever approach the relationship therapist chooses, he or she will be adopting a broader perspective than that provided by merely listening to the content, heeding the intrapsychic conflicts, or attending to the defenses.

THINKING FAMILY

Lastly, we want to define how the important concept of *thinking family* applies to treatment. Earlier, the prevailing belief in the field of family counseling required a family and marital therapist to have the entire relationship unit in the office model to evaluate the system and design the appropriate intervention. This requirement is no longer operative because we have learned to respect the power of one individual to affect the entire family unit. Making the most of this power requires *thinking family*: keeping the entire current family system in mind regardless of who is in the office.

Understanding the reciprocal interactions between the family as a system and the individual has led to a broadening of the focus for interventions in relationship therapy to include the individual. If we keep the systems perspective in mind, even when we are working with just one patient, we will be thinking family and doing relationship therapy.

The shift in the focus of MFT to include the individual, while *thinking family*, is both historically and conceptually important. Early in the history of the field, interventions were designed mainly to change the interactional pattern, because it was believed that the pattern itself was the source of the problem. Although this belief continues to be true to some extent today, modern-day practitioners, as mentioned, have included interventions targeted toward specific individuals in the family unit as well.

Some theorists, wanting to separate the individual from what has been called the *undifferentiated ego mass* (Bowen 1978), focus on the individual with their eye to the family system. Others in the field do this from a strategic standpoint, holding to the view that if one individual changes, the interactional pattern of the family will change. These two viewpoints have led to the development of schools of thinking that believe it is possible to conduct marital therapy when only one partner is present (Bowen 1978; Wiener-Davis 1992).

The essential point is that *marital and family therapy* refers as much to a way of conceptualizing a therapeutic framework as to a specific therapeutic modality or school of therapy. In other words, even though many family therapists do not meet with the family as a whole, the ideas and approaches of family therapy are paramount in their approaches because they *think family*.

This idea of *thinking family* is particularly useful for individually oriented psychotherapists because it opens the door to different ways of conceptualizing the mental models of their patients. *Thinking family* is a matter of adopting a broader perspective with whoever is in the office and thereby using a systems approach to affect the entire social unit.

INDICATIONS AND CONTRAINDICATIONS

Relationship therapy was first thought of as a panacea for the patient's ills. This therapy took hold partly in reaction to the long-term psychoanalytic approach that had been the dominant paradigm for psychotherapy in the preceding years and partly because the emerging data describing seriously disturbed communications in the families of schizophrenic patients (Wynne and Singer 1963) pointed away from intrapsychic causality.

These data led to one popular early formulation: the idea of the "schizophrenogenic mother." Hence, it is not surprising that at that time the family was often considered the root of individual problems; therefore, family therapy was indicated. However, over time, with more thorough research and a better understanding of biologic factors, including their interaction with psychosocial factors, it became clearer when and when not to prescribe some form of relationship therapy.

Today, outcome research provides some criteria for prescribing relationship therapy. Based on meta-analysis either marital or family therapy is specifically indicated to facilitate the treatment of a severely mentally ill family member, whether to foster compliance with medication, mobilize resources, minimize the likelihood of rehospitalization, or ameliorate stress in the caregivers (Pinsoff and Wynne 1995). In other similar studies, therapy aimed at improving the couple relationship is also specifically indicated when one of the members is depressed; and with the family when a conduct disorder is evident or there is substance abuse (Prince and Jacobson 1995).

An important indication for initiating one or more relationship interviews—a relative indication—is the presence of a psychophysiologic disorder. Some of the earliest research work in the field of family therapy demonstrated that juvenile diabetics were more stable following family therapy and that anorexic patients gained and maintained their weight when family therapy was part of the therapeutic strategy (Minuchin et al. 1978).

Overall, there is usually good cause for a therapist to test the waters for relationship therapy by meeting for at least one conjoint session with the partner or the entire family of any primary patient. The general indications and contraindications are summarized in Table 34–1.

The specific indications for family therapy are similar. Family therapy is specifically indicated when it is requested by the family, when an individual family member in treatment is not making progress, when the onset of symptoms

TABLE 34–1. Indications and contraindications

Relationship therapy is indicated

When there is a crisis or major life transition in the relationship

When the onset of symptoms is connected to relationship disharmony

When the patient is a child or adolescent, and there are health, educational or legal problems

As an adjunct to medical treatment or psychotherapy— to gather or impart information

Relationship therapy is contraindicated

When the therapeutic environment is not safe and someone will be harmed by information, uncontrolled anxiety, or hostility

When there is a lack of willingness to be honest

When there is an unwillingness to maintain confidentiality

in one or more family members relates to obvious family disharmony, when one or more family members are distressed during a current major family life transition, or when a minor child is in serious difficulty.

On the basis of meta-analysis of the outcome research, family therapy is also specifically indicated to facilitate the treatment of a severely mentally ill family member, whether to foster compliance with medication, to mobilize resources, to minimize the likelihood of rehospitalization, or to ameliorate stress in the caregivers (Pinsoff 1995). And on the basis of similar studies, therapy aimed at improving the couple relationship is also specifically indicated when one of the members is depressed; and family therapy is also specifically indicated when a conduct disorder is evident or substance abuse exists (Prince 1995).

An important indication for one or more relationship interviews is the presence of a psychophysiological disorder. Some of the earliest research work in the field of family therapy demonstrated that juvenile diabetic patients were more stable after undergoing family therapy and that anorexic patients gained and maintained their weight when family therapy was part of the therapeutic strategy (Minuchin 1978). This early work has been validated more recently (Ryden 1994).

Overall, there is usually good cause for a therapist to test the waters for relationship therapy by meeting for at least one conjoint session with the partner or the entire family of the primary patient. However, it may quickly become clear, perhaps as early as the first or second interview, that relationship therapy will not work.

CONTRAINDICATIONS

Relationship therapy is relatively contraindicated, in the case of the couple relationship, when there is an obvious lack of commitment to the relationship, when one partner is secretly involved with another person and is unwilling either to stop the affair or to discuss the affair openly, and when the therapeutic environment itself becomes unsafe because of an inability to control the hostility or anxiety generated there.

Family therapy is contraindicated when one of the parents is not committed to the family or the process, when the hostility present would be hurtful to one of the family members, and when the issues discussed might be injurious to the children in some way.

About this last point, however, there is disagreement in the field. The literature is filled with a lively debate on the question of what subjects should and should not be discussed when children are present. Actually, discussing whether to include the children is sometimes productive for the parents and the therapist, even when the final decision is not to include them. For instance, although it may be painful for the family to realize the extent of the disaffection or hostility of one of its members, an open discussion of the problem may serve to clarify the situation. Similarly, it is often useful for the therapist to validate either the high level of hostility or the lack of commitment to the relationship. Putting the cards on the table can pave the way for change.

Another important contraindication for relationship therapy is lack of skill on the part of the MFT therapist. Even this, however, is only a relative contraindication, because a therapist who is unskilled in MFT but familiar with the ideas and experience of his or her own personal reactions to the family and its style (e.g., countertransference) can still be successful in treating patients with relationship problems.

HISTORY AND DEVELOPMENT OF RELATIONSHIP THERAPY

The history of MFT is itself a metaphor for the complexity and ambiguity of the field. Although the actual time line of the development of the field is short—from the early 1950s to the present—the number of different ideas is large and the creativity within the field is exciting.

Although family therapy and marital therapy today have enough in common to be considered one topic, they developed along completely separate lines and within wholly different time frames. The origins of marital therapy are much older than are the origins of family therapy; they can be traced back to biblical times, when marital therapy took the form of guidelines for conducting oneself with a partner. Marital therapy began as marriage counseling, originally in the form of advice giving and counseling—most often, pastoral counseling. Later, peer counseling, marriage enhancement, sex therapy, coaching, family life education, and psychoeducation became part of marital counseling. It was not until 1970 that marital therapy was considered a separate entity and the name was changed from *marriage counseling.*

Family therapy, by comparison, is a relative newcomer, having entered the scene in the 1950s (Broderick and Schrader 1991). The impetus for the development of the field of family therapy, as distinct from that of marital therapy, was its founders' clinical experiences. In the mid-1950s two separate areas of investigation sprang up. One area grew out of findings by a few dynamically trained therapists who were meeting with the families of their individual pa-

tients. In these meetings the therapists frequently found discrepancies between what their patients were telling them and their own observations. In addition, events, perceptions, and recollections were often not what they appeared to be, and the therapists' explanatory models did not account for these discrepancies.

Concurrently, another area of investigation was created when other clinicians who were gathering experience with hospitalized patients, particularly those with schizophrenia, noted that patients frequently relapsed shortly after their return home—which pointed to some important negative influence exerted within the family (Wynne 1963). Many years later, the first research-based explanations of this phenomenon were proposed, and in 1985 it was discovered that the highest relapse rates for patients with schizophrenia occurred in families that were close yet covertly hostile and critical (Leff 1985). This variable, labeled *expressed emotion,* is an important tool used in evaluating how the family's process can trigger the onset of mental illness.

In the fable about the blind men and the elephant, each of the four men touched only one part of the elephant; as a result, they created four different impressions of the whole creature. In the case of relationships, the phenomenon is different. Each person present might experience an identical event, but each individual would experience it through his or her own personal lens. In the instance of a marriage or a family, even when the experience is similarly described by the participants, the meaning attributed to the events can be decidedly different. To add to the complexity, an outside observer such as a therapist will likely attribute a still different meaning to the events.

The early family therapists sought to understand and explain this uniqueness of perception. Many different schools of MFT proliferated in the early days and have continued into the present. Exploring the interpersonal world of the patient was not such a new idea, of course; the important point was that MFT therapists began to realize that what their patients told them was only one possible view.

In the early days of MFT, it was thought that the source of all pathology resided in the malfunctioning system (Hoffman 1981). Some early research correlated specific family patterns with individual perceptions (Reiss 1971). Since then, that thinking has been modified, leading to a more balanced view in which both individual and relationship factors are considered important and are believed to affect each other.

Part of this change occurred because research made it abundantly clear that individual pathology can develop in healthy as well as malfunctioning relationships. Another part of the change evolved because of the inability to carry out clinically some of the basic tenets of the pure systems theorists.

Finally, an important contributor to the change in direction was the new feminist-informed theory. This theory pointed out the importance of power, and the potential for the abuse of that power, within the family. It also served as a reminder that people sometimes do bad things, an therapists began realizing that it is not always possible, safe, or even useful to maintain the strict therapeutic neutrality espoused by the pure systems therapists (Gilligan 1982; Goldner 1988; Philpot and Brooks 1995; Walker 1985).

Throughout the development of the field of relationship therapy, the idea has remained constant that each person exists in the context of a larger system and that one's behavior affects the system and the system reciprocally affects oneself (Miller 1955). Typically, the most important system is one's current family—be it the marital dyad, the immediate or extended family, the family of origin, or one's mental model of a family.

It follows, then, that any mental health professional who seeks to help the individual patient is best served if he or she understands the family system of the patient and uses the tool of *thinking family*.

CURRENT STATE OF THE FIELD

A tennis instructor once pointed out that there are countless ways of holding the racket, different styles for the backhand and the follow-through, and multiple ways for the player to stand. The pros demonstrate and win with many of them. The instructor then went on to say that when it comes time to hit the ball, the laws of physics take over and the ball goes where the racket sends it.

The many different approaches to MFT are something like the many different approaches in tennis. Treatment possibilities have become too numerous to count—even though there are fewer than the reputed 400 different approaches to psychotherapy in general. All the while, relationship therapists are always working to further understand and organize the "laws of physics" as they apply to helping marital and family relationships change in positive ways.

Fortunately, outcome research points the way to a system that organizes the different approaches of MFT through a combination of theory and commonality of approach. According to the research, there are two basic forms of MFT: insight-oriented marital and family therapy and behavioral marital and family therapy (Snyder 1991). Surprisingly, virtually all of the theoretical approaches or

schools fall into these two categories. A few integrative approaches successfully combine elements of both insight-oriented and behavioral approaches; because these approaches tend to be more practical than theoretical, they will be addressed separately.

INSIGHT-ORIENTED MARITAL AND FAMILY THERAPY

The approaches classified under the heading of insight-oriented marital and family therapy (IOMFT) (also known as the *growth-oriented* or *developmentally oriented approaches*) have their roots firmly planted in psychoanalytic theory. Although they do not necessarily use the psychoanalytic method, understanding is their target. Typically, the insight-oriented approaches first locate the important affect and then trace the roots of the affect to the early experience and finally to understand the current conflict in the context of that early experience.

The methods for uncovering affect and developing insight are specific for each approach, but when it comes to *hitting the ball*, the *laws of physics take over*. Through an insight-oriented approach to relationship therapy, family members or marital partners gain a new understanding of the person who is the current focus. In addition, in accordance with the ideas of MFT, the person who is the focus is affected by the attitudinal and possibly behavioral changes of other family members.

Here are brief sketches of the six major insight-oriented approaches to relationship therapy:

Psychodynamic Therapy

The *psychodynamic* model is probably the most familiar of the insight-oriented approaches (Ackerman 1958; Byng-Hall 1988; Gadlin 1985; Slipp 1988). Affect leads to insight, and insight leads to transformation. The main foci include understanding the defensive patterns of the family and each of its individual members and understanding the transferential nature of relationships between the family members as well as with the therapist. The primary techniques used draw on the techniques of psychodynamic individual therapy: building the therapeutic alliance over time, encouraging free association, and working toward insight through interpretation.

Psychodynamically oriented relationship therapy includes some of the same principles that inform the similarly oriented group therapies as well. It is not too much of a stretch to recognize transference as a here-and-now phenomenon and, by extension, to recognize that families will go to great lengths to stabilize those relationships by avoiding change. Psychodynamically oriented relationship therapists encourage free association by structuring the environment so that it is safe to say anything and everything. They then confront the resistance to open communication.

Transference to the group is a generally accepted prerequisite for successful group therapy. It manifests in family life as cohesiveness. Because cohesiveness is perhaps the single most consistent factor that defines the healthy family, the development of cohesiveness is an important therapeutic goal. In psychodynamically oriented family therapy, this development occurs when people reveal their innermost thoughts, dreams, and fantasies and allow the exploration of unconscious material.

In the earliest forms of psychodynamic family therapy, therapists interviewed a family member while other members of the family were present and then explored the family members' reactions, again from a psychodynamic perspective. This technique acquired new life in the 1960s and 1970s with the "fishbowl" technique promoted by the National Training Laboratory, itself a forerunner of the human potential movement.

The fishbowl is characterized by an inner and outer circle. The inner circle is the working group; the outer circle is the observers. After a designated amount of time, the working group changes places with the observers, and the observers then process what they saw and heard while the previous working group looks on. This technique is used by some relationship therapists who work with multiple family groups (Kadis and McClendon 1981) or other affinity groups in different settings. It has also become part of the reflecting team approach, in which members of the team of therapists sit behind a one-way mirror until some crucial point in the proceedings, at which time they enter the consultation room and report their observations to the family and to the therapists who remained in the room.

Relationship therapists differ in both style and focus in their use of the psychodynamic approach. Paul and Paul (1975) focused on the unresolved grieving process, Stierlin (1974) addressed the adolescent struggle for independence, and Framo (1965, 1980) focused on the spousal or familial reenactment of conflicts that occurred in the family of origin. The same is true for marital therapy. Using a model rooted in developmental theory, Bader and Pearson (1988) aimed to facilitate individuation in the couple. Irrespective of the styles of different therapists or whether their focus is the couple or the family, the goal of psychodynamically oriented relationship therapy is to uncover the affect, track it to the early belief, expose the belief, and create a new understanding.

Object Relations Therapy

The *object relations approach* is probably the most prevalent of the psychodynamically oriented forms of relationship therapy, possibly because of the thoughtful writings of its main proponents, D. Scharff and J. Scharff (1986). Object relations family therapists emphasize the importance of projection and projective identification in maintaining the distortions that confound marital and family interactions (Givelber 1990; Scharff 1986). They theorize that because the objects, as defined by the theory, are simultaneously real and unconscious, projection and projective identification occur in real time in the relationship therapist's office. In this approach, projective identification is addressed directly through interpretation, maintaining the basic tenet of the insight-oriented therapies, that insight and understanding lead to transformation.

Family-of-Origin Therapy

Using a developmental or intergenerational paradigm, Murray Bowen (1978) focused on the issues of separation and individuation. In this formulation, *family-of-origin therapy*, the primary task of the individual is to separate and individuate from the undifferentiated ego mass of his or her family of origin. Failure to do so results in failure to acquire clear self boundaries; it is associated with anxiety and affects the entire family unit.

Understanding Bowen's approach depends on understanding the nature and impact of transgenerational patterns and bonds. Bowen's ideas of a family emotional system, of multigenerational transmission of symptoms, beliefs, and attitudes, and of triangulation have become part of the thinking of most contemporary family therapists (Friedman 1991).

The term *triangulation* refers to a process in which two people in conflict reduce the tension by incorporating a third person in the relationship. For example, when a couple is in open conflict, one partner may develop a special relationship with one of the children to defuse the conflict. Triangulation can also be brought into play when one or both partners have difficulties with closeness or distance. This dynamic is commonly present when there is an extramarital affair. The third person can meet the need for closeness in one person and/or divert the anxiety over closeness in the other. Triangles can be used in this way to help manage both internal and interpersonal stress. Partners ideally provide structure for each other, and in doing so help to reduce anxiety. When one partner is unavailable for whatever reason, the third person in the triangle can fill the need for structure and reduce the intrapsychic tension.

A tool for managing triangulation is the *genogram*, the

use of which is one of the most important techniques of relationship therapy (McGoldrick and Gerson 1985). This instrument was developed because of Bowen's belief in the need for individuals to separate from their family of origin. The genogram puts the entire family of origin in both historical and emotional perspective. It is a graphic representation of three generations of the family of origin of one of the family members that is constructed in the presence of the couple or entire family. Constructing the genogram serves many purposes. It shifts and defuses the interpersonal conflict by moving the focus from the interpersonal to the intrapsychic; it enables the central person to see his or her family of origin in a new light; and it allows alternate explanations to be given for current behavior. Moreover, as a result of these alternate explanations, the genogram process helps other family members view the focal person differently.

Bowen, one of the founders of the field of MFT, was among the first to promote the idea that a therapist could conduct a course of family therapy without working with the entire family unit. This is done by turning attention to the family of origin. Bowen also taught us as therapists that whenever we think about the different triangles, we are in effect thinking about the family as a system—we are *thinking family*.

Contextual Therapy

Recognizing the interrelatedness of the individual and his or her relationship, Boszormenyi-Nagy and colleagues (Boszormenyi-Nagy and Spark 1973) explored a new paradigm in which the therapeutic contract was thought of as multilateral. *Contextual therapy* recognizes that family members interact as individuals with the entire family as a system, as well as with each other individually, and that the family also functions as a unit. Multilateral contracts are formed that honor the multiplicity of obligations and responsibilities that follow from this arrangement. This situation is known as *multidirected partiality* and is an alternative to therapeutic neutrality.

Contextual therapy is a variation on the developmental theme and focuses on similar family systems issues, as do the other insight-oriented therapies, but it does so from the ethical perspective of the obligations and responsibilities that various members of the family have to or for one another. In contextual therapy, attention is directed to the bargains people make to get their needs met; the implicit quid pro quo becomes the focus. This form of relationship therapy is unique among the insight-oriented approaches in that it incorporates a large component of education along with insight.

Postmodern Therapies

Another way of thinking about insight is from the perspective of the stories we tell ourselves about ourselves, about our history, and about our world. As children we all made up stories, often out of awareness. We made up stories about who we were, where we came from, how we fit first into our families and later into the world; stories about loss and death; stories about order and chaos. These stories serve to orient us, guide us, and sustain us because they help us explain the events in our world. They help us make sense of the unexpected and they bring order to chaos.

The *postmodern therapies*, which include constructivist therapy and *narrative therapy*, were developed to account for individual stories as well as the observation that because each individual's perceptions are unique, in essence each person constructs his or her own reality (Anderson and Goolishian 1988; Hoffman 1990; White and Epston 1993). In this formulation, interpersonal conflict is a consequence of differing realities' bumping against each other. In the postmodern approach the common factor is, again, insight, although the understanding required is understanding about the stories rather than about the defenses or projections.

The postmodern therapist thinks of himself or herself as a cocreator and believes that the therapeutic element is the active structuring of questions. The questions themselves are thought to be the main therapeutic intervention (Silverstein 1996). In an effort to elucidate the underlying story, a postmodern therapist might say to a man who has abused his wife, "So you think it is all right to yell at your wife when you are upset. . . . Where in your family did you learn that?" The postmodern therapies return the focus to one of the original concepts of family therapy: everybody in a family sees things differently, and these differences create communication deviances that ultimately lead to the development of symptoms. Because each person constructs his or her own reality, the goal of postmodern relationship therapy becomes the creation of a new story (or narrative) for the family.

It has been suggested that because the approaches that rely on systems theory, with their orientation in the here-and-now, focus on circular causality and therapeutic neutrality, such approaches lack the ability to predict future behavior. As a result, they are less subject to experimental verification and less able to deal with situations that require a judgment. The postmodern therapies, however, may be better able to deal with the turbulence and violence that plague the contemporary family, because they consider how each person views the world and address those views individually (Fraenkel 1995).

Experiential Therapy

At first glance, the *experiential approaches* appear different from the other forms of IOMFT because the insight component is not as obvious. They are, however, similar to these other forms. Experiential approaches use affect as the guide to the early experiences to develop insights into the current conflict and into the self. But these insights are gained on the experiential rather than cognitive level. The work of Virginia Satir and that of Carl Whitaker are the most prominent examples of work in this subgroup of IOMFT.

Satir (1964) strongly believed that the way each family member originally experienced the family environment created defensive attitudes and feelings of shame. These entrenched experiences and feelings ultimately lead to the presenting problem or problems. Her goal was to help the couple or family create and maintain new experiences that would be markedly different from the ones they had when they were left to their own devices. To this end, she developed a multiplicity of techniques that touched all the senses and evoked emotions, which she then helped the family to handle in a productive way.

Many of the techniques Satir devised depend to a large extent on the effective communication of feelings and thoughts. These communication techniques are a major part of the armamentarium of most modern-day relationship therapists. Her work also stands out because it is accessible; patients intuitively understand and can easily translate her ideas into their own frame of reference.

Carl Whitaker's work is different from that of Virginia Satir in that his style was extremely personal (Napier and Whitaker 1978). He depended on the force of his personality, the uniqueness of his vision, and the courage to do and say the unthinkable in the family setting. He had the ability to shake up the family in such a way that it became difficult for them to ever operate as they had before. The new experiences he created for the family led, as they did with Satir, to intuitive understandings and to lasting change.

BEHAVIORAL MARITAL AND FAMILY THERAPY

Whereas the insight-oriented family therapist holds to the view that change occurs through understanding—or, in other words, emotional change precedes behavioral change—the behaviorally oriented marital and family therapist takes the opposite view. Behavioral therapists believe that change in behavior promotes change in attitudes and that emotional change follows behavioral change.

A large group of therapists and a sizable number of research-based outcome studies suggest that behavioral marital and family therapy (BMFT) is successful in promoting and maintaining change (Baucom et al. 1990; Beck 1988; Jacobson 1981; Jacobson and Addis 1993; Jacobson and Margolin 1979). As in the case of IOMFT, there are many different approaches to promoting behavioral change in relationships.

Some of the approaches briefly described here are behavioral in that they depend on various aspects of the behavior-exchange model. Others are behavioral in that they focus on changing the way people interact. And still others are behavioral in that they provide information about the problem, about various options for solving the problem, or about communication and other skills. All of these approaches depend on the principle that behavior change precedes affective change.

Structural Family Therapy

Salvador Minuchin (Minuchin 1974; Minuchin 1967) at the Philadelphia Child Guidance Clinic developed a model of family therapy based on his understanding of the structure of the family. This structural approach focuses on both the hierarchy of relationships in the family and the rules of relating that define the boundaries between the subsystems of the family. In *structural family therapy* the recursive nature of the transactions is used to intuit the rules of the system; this information in turn helps clarify the structure of the system.

By attending to the structure of the family and designing interventions to modify the structure, Minuchin and his followers (Minuchin et al. 1978) have been able to treat some of the most entrenched multiproblem families. Such families often have little psychological insight and present with difficult psychosomatic problems, such as anorexia nervosa.

Working from a behavioral standpoint, structural family therapy maps the interpersonal dynamics of a family by focusing on the psychological boundaries, or the interpersonal transactions that create the psychological boundaries between people. Structural family therapists are most interested in boundaries: those that separate and distinguish the generations, those that separate and distinguish sibling and individual subsystems, and those that define the alliances and coalitions within the family.

Structural family therapy introduces form and order into some of the most chaotic and difficult relationships, possibly because focusing on the structure of the family prevents both family members and the therapist from getting lost in the details of the very serious problems. Once form and order are established, a wide range of clinical symptoms may abate; even some biochemical parameters, such as blood sugar in brittle diabetic patients, can revert toward normal.

Strategic Family Therapy

Working from a systems-based model, Jay Haley (1971) and other strategic therapists (Madanes 1981) suggested that understanding, emotions, and transference have no place in family therapy but that the repetitive and maladaptive interactional patterns need to be changed instead, through *strategic family therapy*. They paid no particular attention to the cause. Although the therapist must understand these patterns from the perspective of being able to define them, merely understanding the cause of the patterns may be considered worse than not useful; it can even be thought of as counterproductive. Strategic therapists often keep the details of the perceived patterns or intervention tactics from the family or couple (Haley 1976).

Haley and his followers developed a host of ingenious techniques for modifying maladaptive interactional patterns. These strategic interventions, often combined with structural interventions, are particularly useful when families are entrenched in a particular point of view or are negatively disposed toward therapy. A family in a constant state of uproar may be instructed, for example, to continue fighting but to fight only at prescribed times or on prescribed days. Following this prescription changes nothing, yet changes everything, because the very act of deciding when to fight introduces order and forethought into the chaotic picture.

Like the structural therapist, the strategic therapist strives to change only the behavior—he or she is confident that affective change, feelings of closeness, and the ability to solve problems will change along the way. Some of Haley's ideas were drawn from the work of Milton Erickson (Haley 1973). Erickson's genius as a therapist lay in his ability to invent interventions that bypassed rather than confronted a person's defenses. Strategic therapists make use of creative, often paradoxical prescriptions. Ericksonian therapists, generally considered to be strategic therapists, find ways to deliver these prescriptions to the entire family through the use of metaphor and trance (Lankton and Lankton 1986).

Brief Family Therapy

Brief family therapy has been a work in progress since the earliest days of family therapy. Long before this therapy was either fashionable or mandated by health insurance and health maintenance organization cost-containment strategies, the brief family therapists at the Mental Research Institute in Palo Alto, CA (also known as the Palo Alto Group), experimented with and refined techniques for completing therapy within 10 sessions (Hudson and O'Hanlon 1994; Watzlawick et al. 1974; Weakland et al. 1974). Using an orthodox systems approach, they attended to the way a family solves its problems rather than to the reasons for the problem or the individual pathology that might be present. Their model expanded a communications-based approach founded in cybernetics. Practical and solution-oriented, its approach and techniques are a cornerstone of what is now thought of as brief therapy. This model, with its focus on the regulation of family patterns by the family rules, represents one of the purist systems-based approaches.

The Milan school, an outgrowth of the Mental Research Institute model, presents another example of a pure systems approach. Developed by M. Selvini-Palazzoli, this group examines every aspect of the present relationship, focusing on the way each person tries to help the family (Selvini-Palazzoli et al. 1978). Even the most outrageous behavior is brought under the umbrella of helping the family. It makes the unconscious conscious and creates a situation in which it is very difficult for family members to maintain unwanted patterns (Selvini-Palazzoli et al. 1980).

Both of these approaches also promote the idea of cotherapy and the use of therapist teams with teams in the room and teams behind the one-way screen working together. The influence of this group of family therapists can be felt in every MFT setting.

Solution-Focused Therapy

The brief family therapy approach led naturally to the development of the *solution-focused family therapy* approach. Again, the format is brief therapy, and the attitude is entirely present-centered. The interventions are typically strategic; most important, the philosophy and techniques are usually practical. Not surprisingly, solution-focused approaches (de Shazer 1988; Hudson and O'Hanlon 1994; Wiener-Davis 1992) have found a home in the current managed-care environment.

The brief therapy approach, along with solution-focused approaches, works best in high-functioning families that are relatively flexible, as compared with families with firmly entrenched styles. These two therapies also work best when the family members or partners in a couple already have some skills to manage their own lives. Both brief and solution-focused therapies may be usefully combined with psychoeducational therapy, behavioral therapy, and other forms of therapy that lead to the acquisition of needed skills.

Behavioral Marital and Family Therapy

Within the entire category of BMFT is a specific approach also called *behavioral marital and family therapy*. This subset of BMFT uses a behavioral-exchange model, postulating the existence of a storehouse of items each of us wants: love, sex, status, and support. We trade with each other for these commodities, and the nature of the trade defines the relationship. For most families and couples, all the commodities are in the same location and each exchange affects the other (Jacobson 1979; Patterson 1975).

Behavioral-exchange theory helps us to understand both the properties and the context of interpersonal relationships by placing them into a framework of the rational bargains that partners make. Understanding this leads directly to a social-learning approach to facilitating improved relations. Behaviorally oriented relationship therapists help families in such ways as identifying antecedent events; structuring agreements; teaching the principles of reinforcement and, in certain circumstances, the use of punishment (aversive conditioning); and anticipating and planning for future possible sources of stress. These approaches are particularly useful when school-age children are involved and conduct problems predominate. They are also useful in certain marital situations, such as situations of sexual dysfunction and marriage enrichment.

Psychoeducational approaches. One of the most important recent developments in the field has been the recognition of the role of educational approaches in treating and managing serious mental illness and in helping families when a family member has a chronic illness. Although it is common for relationship therapists to incorporate educational components into their approach, current data suggest the existence of definite benefits for many families from a comprehensive educational program instituted early in the course of treatment.

There are three main *psychoeducational approaches*: parent management training (Estrada and Pinsoff 1995; Kazdin 1993), family group education (Stanton and Todd 1982; Steinglass et al. 1987), and relapse prevention training (Falloon et al. 1984; Goldstein et al. 1978; Goldstein and Miklowitz 1995; Gonzalez et al. 1989). Detailed protocols are available for use with parents who have a child with conduct disorder and with families in which there is a chronic disability, a hospitalized schizophrenic patient, or a problematic substance abuser. These protocols, subjected to rigorous testing, have proven to be valuable.

In *parent management training*, parents are trained to be therapists for their child with conduct disorder; in the process, they develop a new set of parenting skills. Parents learn to recognize and assess problem behaviors and learn how to apply various social-learning procedures such as positive reinforcements, contingency contracting, and aversive conditioning. The teaching methods included are ones the parents will themselves use with the child. The latter include modeling, role-playing, contracting, feedback, and practice. Parent management training has proven helpful for families in which a child either has conduct disorder or is autistic. It has also proven to be of some help for children with attention-deficit/hyperactivity disorder. It has been less effective when the child has an anxiety disorder (Estrada and Pinsoff 1995).

Family group education—specifically devised as family centered interventions for people with chronic disabilities—uses an eight-session multiple-family discussion group format. Included in this program are instructional presentations, which are followed by group discussion. The group-interaction component is developed through the use of instructional material or other disability-related information (Gonzalez et al. 1989).

Relapse prevention training programs for patients with psychotic disorders have recently been reviewed by Goldstein and Miklowitz (1995). The review concluded that such programs can reduce relapse rate. Although this review was specific, it seems likely that the family education protocol approach—the guidelines for which are outlined here—can be applied to substance-abuse problems and other severe but nonpsychotic disorders. This is particularly relevant when psychosocial stressors are known to play an important role in the course of the illness.

One set of guidelines for psychoeducational interventions when a family member has a serious mental illness requires that the therapist understand the impact of the disorder on the family and the way the family's response supports the maintenance of the symptom. Some families expect more of the individual than is realistic, whereas others expect too little and therefore hinder progress. Often families also fear change. Fortunately, families can be taught to respond differently (Perlmutter 1996).

Goldstein and Miklowitz (1995) believed that some goals are especially critical in a psychotherapeutic program. These goals are integration of the psychotic experience, acceptance of vulnerability to future episodes, acceptance of dependence on psychotropic medications for symptom control, anticipation of stressful life events that act as triggers for recurrence of the disorders, and distinguishing of personality traits from symptoms of the disorder. They also concluded that it is important to engage the family of the psychotic patient early in the process, to educate them about the illness, make specific recommendations for coping, communication, and problem solving, and prepare them for early crisis intervention.

MARITAL THERAPY

Although marital therapy is rightly included as a subset of family therapy, the dyadic bond has enough unique features to merit special attention (Johnson 1986). Forming a partnership with another person is one of life's most important transitions. It is a marker of entrance into adulthood and brings to mind the parental models of both partners. Committed partnering also presents the special challenge of walking the fine line between autonomy and dependence; it is the adult-stage variation of the earlier separation-individuation developmental landmark.

The issue of independence versus dependence is addressed in every form of marital theory and therapy. Bowen-derived theory addresses this conflict with the focus on differentiating from the undifferentiated ego mass; structural therapy addresses it in the context of boundaries between subsystems; the experiential therapies and the insight-oriented therapies address the conflict through the various forms of projection and transference. Even the psychoeducational therapies strive to facilitate independence as they teach parents how to manage children and, in the process, how to be separate from the children and from each other.

As previously mentioned, there are several ways of managing the tension related to the separation-individuation conflict. Distancing in the form of withdrawing by some form of pushing or pulling away and distancing by some form of triangulating are the most common. When partners use these mechanisms in an agreed-on way, the relationship is stable. Problems develop when their needs for distance and closeness are out of balance. If one person has a greater need for distance at any given time, pulling away is usually experienced as loss by the other person, and the ensuing attempts to close the distance will often raise the conflict level.

Again, virtually all of the specific marital therapies are designed to address this dynamic. Jacobson (1981) negotiated reciprocal agreements with the partners in addition to teaching skills to manage affect. Gottman (Gottman 1993, 1994; Gottman and Levinson 1985) used psychoeducational behavioral methods to manage affect. On the other hand, Hendrix (1988) tracked self-image as a way of facilitating individuation, whereas Bader and Pearson (1988) used an integrative systems/insight-oriented approach that directly addresses the discrepancy between the partners' level of attained separation-individuation.

These are but a few of the many ways marital therapists help clients manage difficulties in sustaining a partnership. Marital therapists also help divorcing couples (Kaslow 1995), provide sex therapy (LoPiccolo and Miller 1975; Schnarch 1995), and help couples deal with serious illness. These are situations in which the dependency needs of one or both of the partners is seriously threatened. The approach is geared toward separating the individuals from the emotional tangle while at the same time building individual strengths (Gonzalez 1989).

Probably the most important aspect of marital therapy is, again, the idea of *thinking family*. In the current context, *thinking family* not only applies to the concept of circular causality but also helps the therapist remember that what he or she sees when meeting with the couple may be very different from what the couple experiences at home when children (if there are children) or other family members are present.

NEW DIRECTIONS

Relationship therapy works: people change, and difficult problems get resolved. We know that for certain and, in fact, have known that for a long time. However, we are only now understanding how the therapy works and what therapeutic techniques specifically promote positive change.

Current research outlines two elements that need to be present in psychotherapy for change to occur, for change to occur in a reasonable length of time, and for change to endure. These elements are 1) a definite focus for the therapy and 2) a clear connection between presenting problems and the associated feelings, childhood experiences, and cognitive processing (Greenberg et al. 1988; Jacobson and Addis 1993; Johnson and Greenberg 1985; McClendon and Kadis 1990; Snyder et al. 1991).

This research suggests that insight or understanding alone is not sufficient to promote lasting change and that the expression of affect or emotion is essential. However, emotions alone, in and of themselves, are not sufficient either. What seems necessary for success is 1) mobilizing present affect, 2) linking that affect to the dynamics of the past, and 3) making the whole package relevant to the present.

Placing this prescription for success in MFT in the context of the climate for mental health in the late 1990s raises questions about what direction relationship therapy will take in future years. It seems likely that new approaches will blend different components into coherent and flexible models and that these integrated approaches will include elements of different therapeutic strategies. For example, the therapeutic modalities can combine systems and individual models or integrate behavioral and insight-oriented approaches.

Alternatively, we can integrate along the dimension of readiness to change. Exploring a "transtheoretical approach," Prochaska and DiClemente (1992) focused on how ready the individual or system is to change; interventions are then tailored to the stage of readiness. It is also possible to look at the type of pathology—or, as it is currently called, dysfunctionality—and develop an integrated approach that addresses the relationship in this way.

Each integrative view has its advantages and disadvantages, as well as its proponents and detractors. As yet, there is no agreed-on method of integrating. However, there is a growing sense that the integration of various suitable therapeutic modalities is most likely to address the individual patient's needs.

REDECISION RELATIONSHIP THERAPY

It may be helpful to present an outline of a working model for relationship therapy. This model has been chosen not only because of its familiarity to the two authors, but, more important, because the structure of the model allows for integration along many different lines as well as for flexibility in its application.

Redecision therapy with individuals originated with the Gouldings (Goulding and Goulding 1978) more than 25 years ago. Early decisions are the representations of the child's attempt to make sense of his or her world in the face of genetic endowment, specific skills, and experiences in his or her family of origin. These early decisions usually take the form of beliefs about the self. Redecisions are cognitive and affective reinterpretations of these beliefs about the self. Redecisions begin when individuals recognize the intrusion of childhood thinking and feeling into present circumstances. Drawing on the abilities acquired by the evolution of adult perceptions and resources, individuals are helped to recognize the value and importance of the early decisions made in childhood and then to develop new perceptions and conclusions about themselves. The redecision occurs with the incorporation of updated and current information about one's self and circumstances.

Within a unified structure, redecision relationship therapy (RRT) delineates a focus, utilizes contracts, and combines systems and individual redecision work. The model can be used in many different therapeutic structures, from long-term treatment or intensive multiple-family group therapy to brief and even single-session interventions. It gives direction and structure to the treatment process, encourages many forms of psychotherapeutic intervention, and enables interventions to be determined by the situation or the relationship. RRT addresses the ongoing, continuous, and dynamic interaction of the system and the individuals who make up the system. McClendon (1977) first described this three-stage model as *redecision family therapy*.

This approach was further developed by both of us (McClendon and Kadis 1983). We observed that current behavior (in the form of interactional patterns) and personal history (in the form of early decisions) operate in a reciprocal relationship. As a result, we work first on one aspect and then on the other, in the belief that dealing with both is essential to relationship therapy.

Although the three-stage model is presented as a linear progression, in real life it is more of a flexible entity that accommodates relationships and circumstances as they are. As with any form of therapy, the presenting circumstances and the depth of the pathology drive the model. In other words, although the three stages are described as distinct entities, they are rarely clearly demarcated. For example, while a family is involved directly in the work of one stage, the work on the other stages may be going on as well. Back-and-forth movement among the three stages is continual. A progression through the stages can occur within one interview, just as it occurs over the entire treatment process.

In addition, research on the model (Bader 1976) has demonstrated that it is not necessary for each individual in the relationship to do the intrapsychic work of stage 2 (described later in this section). Systems and relationships can change with the change of only one person.

With any form of therapy or any move in life, destinations define the journey. In relationship therapy, the patients' vision of what is healthy for them is used to define the overall direction of the work. In the RRT, this vision is combined with research work on healthy relationships that has clearly delineated many of the elements of healthy systems (Lewis 1976; Olson 1989). RRT incorporates what constitutes a healthy family into its framework in that it focuses on the family's ability to address and manage whatever life brings.

But there is more to life than the executive functions. Because there is also the need for intimacy, this too is incorporated into RRT. Sidney Jourard (1971) described the healthy relationship as one in which members know about each other, care about each other, respond to each other, and respect each other. These are the essential elements in emotional intimacy. RRT targets the development of solid executive functions along with a healthy emotional tone.

Finally, an important challenge of relationship therapy is to create the environment in which system members will reveal themselves. This is sometimes quite a task, because people usually restrict or distort their behaviors, thoughts, and feelings when outsiders, even other family members, are present. Much of RRT is devoted to creating this safe environment in which family members can be themselves and show themselves, not only to the therapist but, even more important, to one another. Here are some guidelines to facilitate this process:

- Know where you are going and keep the direction positive.
- Focus on current interactions and how they impede relationship health.
- Help each person learn how his or her behavior affects others.
- Motivate people to take responsibility for their own decisions and change.
- Create new relationship dynamics by teaching new skills, behaviors, and guidelines for relationships.

Stage 1 of RRT is a systems stage, in which the focus is on symptom or problem resolution through changes in both the structure and function of the system. The purpose of stage 1 is the emancipation of the individual from the emotional tangle and problems that dominate the relationship. In stage 1, the ongoing and continuous interactional patterns that negatively affect problem-solving behavior, positive coping skills, task mastery, social competence, and intimacy are examined and then interrupted. The interface of defenses, mental models, or early decisions and how they manifest themselves in the present are delineated. The strategies and techniques of behavioral marital and family therapy are typically incorporated into this stage.

Stage 2 is the intrapersonal or intrapsychic stage. In stage 2, the main focus shifts to the transformation of internal models. This process involves helping the individual confront his or her past to gain the confidence to master the present and decide on the future. The focal point for changing internal models or making redecisions (Goulding and Goulding 1978) is derived from the individual's process and participation with other system members. The depth-oriented strategies and techniques drawn from insight-oriented marital and family therapy are applicable during this stage.

Stage 3, reintegration, is focused on the prevention of future disablement, both individual and systemic, through teaching new, effective, and healthy ways to function within the interpersonal system. Psychoeducational and specific behavioral interventions that provide information

and teach new skills are particularly valuable in the third stage, when the emotional temperature has been lowered.

RRT integrates interpersonal and intrapersonal perspectives. It stresses the dignity of each person and his or her ability to change. As a treatment approach, redecision relationship therapy brings action, vitality, and humor to the process, emphasizes the positive, and uses the strengths of the relationship.

CONCLUSIONS

Recently, the *Journal of Marital and Family Therapy* devoted an entire issue to a review of the outcome research in the field. According to this outcome research, MFT tends to work best in the following situations: 1) the child is the patient and the disorder is one of conduct, 2) the wife in the couple is depressed, 3) a substance-abusing person enters treatment and is then maintained after treatment, and 4) a schizophrenic individual is the patient and MFT is used to reduce relapse rates.

This summary of outcomes in therapy is a good beginning, yet many important questions remain unanswered. As is true for psychotherapy research in general, much of the MFT research was completed in the laboratory setting rather than in the clinical setting. In the laboratory, the population is carefully selected and the various parameters are subjected to rigorous control. Because this approach is rarely possible outside the laboratory, clinical experience inevitably and frequently is at odds with research findings.

This dilemma leads to a few crucial questions. First, which form of relationship therapy is the most effective in the clinical setting? At the moment, it is not clear that any one form of therapy works better than any other.

Second, what is the best recipe for successful relationship therapy? Insight alone does not result in major changes, and behavioral change by itself may not be long-lasting either. So far, what appears to be the right mix of ingredients is a focused approach that 1) attends to the relationship's current reality, 2) uses emotions relevant to the current process (not necessarily the current situation) as a way of gaining access to the intrapsychic past of the individuals in the relationship, and 3) builds a new working relationship in the present.

It has been observed that skilled clinicians employ these therapeutic strategies, regardless of their own theoretical orientation. In addition, it is known that MFT works best when the procedures are standardized. This observation may also explain some of the discrepancies between research findings and clinical experience. Therapy in research settings often follows a set protocol; in a clinical setting, it rarely does.

This discussion leads us finally to a third unanswered question: What are the therapist variables that affect the outcome of relationship therapy? As yet, we have no good answers to this question.

Because every relationship is unique, no single set of skills or any total theory can apply to all of them. The different theories and different modes of approaching relationships simply serve to guide us in our attempts to respond to particular situations in ways that will be both efficient and effective.

We therapists have the power to help patients heal. How we choose to use that power in the situations that confront us is both a professional and a personal decision—influenced by theoretical training and tempered by practical experience.

REFERENCES

Ackerman N: The Psychodynamics of Family Life. New York, Basic Books, 1958

Anderson H, Goolishian H: Human systems as linguistic systems: preliminary and evolving ideas about the implications for clinical theory. Fam Process 27:371–393, 1988

Aponte H, Hoffman L: The open door: a structural approach to a family with an anorectic child. Fam Process 12:1–44, 1973

Bader E: Redecisions in family therapy: a study of change in an intensive family workshop. Dissertation Abstracts: Ann Arbor, MI, University No. 7625064, 1976

Bader E, Pearson P: In Quest of the Mythical Mate. New York, Brunner/Mazel, 1988

Baucom D, Sayers S, Sher T: Supplementing behavioral marital therapy with cognitive restructuring and emotional expressiveness training: an outcome investigation. J Consult Clin Psychol 58:636–645, 1990

Beck A: Love Is Never Enough. New York, Harper & Row, 1988

Boszormenyi-Nagy I, Spark G: Invisible Loyalties: Reciprocity in Intergenerational Family Therapy. New York, Harper & Row, 1973

Bowen M: Family Therapy in Clinical Practice. New York, Jason Aronson, 1978

Broderick C, Schrader S: The history of professional marriage and family therapy, in Handbook of Family Therapy II. Edited by Gurman A, Kniskern D. New York, Brunner/Mazel, 1991, pp 3–40

Byng-Hall J: Scripts and legends in families and family therapy. Fam Process 27:167–180, 1988

de Shazer S: Clues: Investigating Solutions in Brief Therapy. New York, WW Norton, 1988

Estrada A, Pinsoff W: The effectiveness of family therapies for selected behavioral disorders of childhood. Journal of Marital and Family Therapy 21:403–440, 1995

Falloon I, Boyd J, McGill C: Family Care of Schizophrenia: A Problem-Solving Approach to the Treatment of Mental Illness. New York, Guilford, 1984

Fraenkel P: The nomothetic-ideographic debate in family therapy. Fam Process 34:113–121, 1995

Framo J: Rationale and techniques of intensive family therapy, in Intensive Family Therapy: Theoretical and Practical Aspects. Edited by Boszormenyi-Nagy I, Framo J. New York, Harper & Row, 1965, pp 201–243

Framo J: Family of origin as a therapeutic resource for adults in marital and family therapy: you can and should go home again. Fam Process 15:193–210, 1980

Friedman D: Bowen theory and therapy, in Handbook of Family Therapy II. Edited by Gurman A, Kniskern D. New York, Brunner/Mazel, 1991, pp 134–170

Gadlin W: Psychiatric consultation to the medical ward: a group analytic and general systems theory point of view. Int J Group Psychother 35:263–278, 1985

Gilligan C: In a Different Voice. Cambridge, MA, Harvard University Press, 1982

Givelber F: Object relations and the couple: separation-individuation, intimacy and marriage, in One Couple, Four Realities: Multiple Perspectives on Couples Therapy. Edited by Chasin R, Grunebaum H, Herzig M. New York, Guilford, 1990, pp 171–190

Goldner V: Generation and gender: normative and covert hierarchies. Fam Process 27:17–31, 1988

Goldstein M, Miklowitz D: The effectiveness of psychoeducational family therapy in the treatment of schizophrenic disorders. Journal of Marital and Family Therapy 21:361–376, 1995

Goldstein M, Rodnick E, Evans J, et al: Drug and family therapy in the aftercare treatment of acute schizophrenics. Arch Gen Psychiatry 35:1169–1177, 1978

Gonzalez S, Steinglass P, Reiss D: Putting the illness in its place: discussion groups for families with chronic medical illnesses. Fam Process 28:69–87, 1989

Gottman J: Theory of marital dissolution and stability. Journal of Family Psychology 7:57–75, 1993

Gottman J: Why Marriages Succeed or Fail. New York, Simon & Schuster, 1994

Gottman J, Levinson R: A valid procedure for obtaining self affect and marital interaction. J Consult Clin Psychol 53:151–160, 1985

Goulding R, Goulding M: Changing Lives Through Redecision Therapy, 2nd Edition. New York, Brunner/Mazel, 1978

Greenberg L, James P, Conry R: Perceived change processes in emotionally focused couples therapy. Journal of Family Psychology 2:5–23, 1988

Gurman A, Kniskern D, Pinsof W: Research on the process and outcome of family therapy, in Handbook of Psychotherapy and Behavior Change, 3rd Edition. Edited by Garfield S, Bergin A. New York, Wiley, 1986, pp 565–624

Haley J: Changing Families. New York, Grune & Stratton, 1971

Haley J: Uncommon Therapy: The Psychiatric Techniques of Milton H. Erickson, M.D. New York, WW Norton, 1973

Haley J: Problem-Solving Therapy: New Strategies for Effective Family Therapy. San Francisco, CA, Jossey-Bass, 1976

Hendrix H: Getting the Love You Want. New York, Henry Holt, 1988

Hoffman L: Foundations of Family Therapy: A Conceptual Framework for Systems Change. New York, Basic Books, 1981, pp 105–125

Hoffman L: Constructing realities: an art of lenses. Fam Process 29:1–12, 1990

Hudson P, O'Hanlon W: Rewriting Love Stories: Brief Marital Therapy. Philadelphia, WW Norton, 1994

Jackson D: Family rules: marital quid pro quo. Arch Gen Psychiatry 12:589–594, 1965

Jacobson N: Behavioral marital therapy, in Handbook of Family Therapy. Edited by Gurman A, Kniskern D. New York, Brunner/Mazel, 1981, pp 556–591

Jacobson N, Addis M: Research on couples and couple therapy: what do we know? Where are we going? J Consult Clin Psychol 61:85–93, 1993

Jacobson N, Margolin G: Marital Therapy: Strategies Based on Social Learning and Behavior Exchange Principles. New York, Brunner/Mazel, 1979

Johnson S: Bonds or bargains: relationship paradigms and their significance for marital therapy. Journal of Marital and Family Therapy 12:259–268, 1986

Johnson S, Greenberg L: Emotionally focused couples therapy. Journal of Marital and Family Therapy 11:313–317, 1985

Jourard S: The Transparent Self. New York, Van Nostrand Reinhold, 1971

Kadis L, McClendon R: Redecision family therapy: its use with intensive multiple family groups. American Journal of Family Therapy 9:75–83, 1981

Kaslow F: The dynamics of divorce therapy, in Integrating Family Therapy: Handbook of Family Psychology and Systems Theory. Edited by Mikesell R, Lusterman D, McDaniel C. Washington, DC, American Psychological Association, 1995, pp 271–285

Kazdin A: Treatment of conduct disorder: progress and directions in psychotherapy research. Development and Psychopathology 5:277–310, 1993

Lankton S, Lankton C: Enchantment and Intervention in Family Therapy: Training in Ericksonian Approaches. New York, Brunner/Mazel, 1986

Leff J, Vaughn C: Expressed Emotion in Families. New York, Guilford, 1985

Lewis J, Beavers R, Gosett J, et al: No Single Thread: Psychological Health in Family Systems. New York, Brunner/Mazel, 1976

LoPiccolo J, Miller V: Procedural outline for sexual enrichment groups. Consulting Psychology 5:46–49, 1975

Madanes C: Strategic Family Therapy. San Francisco, CA, Jossey-Bass, 1981

McClendon R: My mother drives a pickup truck, in TA After Eric Berne: Recent Advances in Transactional Analysis. Edited by Barnes G. New York, Harpers College Press, 1977, pp 99–113

McClendon R, Kadis L: Chocolate Pudding and Other Approaches to Intensive Multiple Family Therapy. Palo Alto, CA, Science and Behavior Books, 1983

McClendon R, Kadis L: A model of integrating individual and family therapy: the contract is the key, in Brief Therapy: Myths, Methods and Metaphors. Edited by Zeig J, Munion W. New York, Brunner/Mazel, 1990, pp 135–150

McGoldrick M, Gerson R: Genograms in Family Assessment. New York, WW Norton, 1985

Miller J: Toward a general theory for the behavioral sciences. Am Psychol 10:695–704, 1955

Minuchin S: Families and Family Therapy. Cambridge, MA, Harvard University Press, 1974

Minuchin S, Montalvo B, Guerney B, et al: Families of the Slums: An Exploration of Their Structure and Treatment. New York, Basic Books, 1967

Minuchin S, Rosman B, Baker L: Psychosomatic Families: Anorexia Nervosa in Context. Cambridge, MA, Harvard University Press, 1978

Napier A, Whitaker C: The Family Crucible. New York, Harper & Row, 1978

O'Hanlon W, Weiner-Davis M: In Search of Solutions in Brief Therapy. New York, WW Norton, 1989

Olson D, Russell C, Speckle D: Circumplex Model: Systemic Assessment of Families, 2nd Edition. New York, Haworth, 1989

Patterson G, Reid J, Jones R, et al: A Social Learning Approach to Family Intervention. Eugene, OR, Castalia, 1975

Paul N, Paul B: A Marital Puzzle: Transgenerational Analysis in Marriage. New York, WW Norton, 1975

Perlmutter R: A Family Approach to Psychiatric Disorders. Washington, DC, American Psychiatric Press, 1996

Philpot C, Brooks G: Intergender communication and gender-sensitive family therapy, in Integrating Family Therapy: Handbook of Family Psychology and Systems Theory. Edited by Mikesell R, Lusterman D, McDaniel C. Washington, DC, American Psychological Association, 1995, pp 303–326

Pinsoff W, Wynne L: The efficacy of marital and family therapy: overview and conclusions. Journal of Marital and Family Therapy 21:585–616, 1995

Pipher M: The Shelter of Each Other: Rebuilding Our Families. New York, GB Putnam's Sons, 1996

Prince S, Jacobson N: A review and evaluation of marital and family therapy for affective disorders. Journal of Marital and Family Therapy 21:377–402, 1995

Prochaska J, DiClemente C: Stages of change in the modification of problem behaviors. Prog Behav Modif 28:183–218, 1992

Reiss D: Varieties of consensual experience. Fam Process 10:1–35, 1971

Ryden O, Nevander L, Johnsson H, et al: Family therapy in poorly controlled juvenile IDDM: effects on diabetic control, self-evaluation, and behavioral symptoms. Acta Peadiatr 83:285–291, 1994

Satir V: Conjoint Family Therapy. Palo Alto, CA, Science and Behavior Books, 1964

Scharff D, Scharff J: Object Relations Family Therapy. New York, Jason Aronson, 1986

Schnarch D: A family systems approach to sex therapy and intimacy, in Integrating Family Therapy: Handbook of Family Psychology and Systems Theory. Edited by Mikesell R, Lusterman D, McDaniel C. Washington, DC, American Psychological Association, 1995, pp 239–258

Selvini-Palazzoli M, Boscolo L, Cecchin G, et al: Paradox and Counterparadox. New York, Jason Aronson, 1978

Selvini-Palazzoli M, Boscolo L, Ceechi G, et al: Hypothesizing-circularity-neutrality. Fam Process 19:3–12, 1980

Shadish W, Ragsdale K, Glasser R, et al: The efficacy and effectiveness of marital and family therapy: a perspective from meta-analysis. Journal of Marital and Family Therapy 21:345–360, 1995

Silverstein O: Genograms and couples therapy. Paper presented at the Brief Therapy Conference, San Francisco, CA, December 1996

Slipp S: The technique and practice of object relations family therapy. Northvale, NJ, Jason Aronson, 1988

Snyder D, Wills R, Grady-Fletcher A: Long-term effectiveness of behavioral versus insight-oriented marital therapy: a 4 year follow-up study. J Consult Clin Psychol 59:138–141, 1991

Stacey J: In the Name of the Family: Rethinking Family Values in the Postmodern Age. Boston, Beacon, 1996

Stanton M, Todd T: The Family Therapy of Drug Abuse and Addiction. New York, Guilford, 1982

Steinglass P, Bennett L, Wolin S, et al: The Alcoholic Family. New York, Basic Books, 1987

Stierlin H: Separating Parents and Adolescents: A Perspective on Running Away, Schizophrenia, and Waywardness. New York, Quadrangle/New York Times Book Co, 1974

von Bertalanffy L: General System Theory: Essays on Its Foundation and Development, Revised Edition. New York, Braziller, 1969

Walker L: The Battered Woman. New York, Harper & Row, 1985

Watzlawick P, Weakland J, Fisch R: Change: Principles of Problem Formation and Problem Resolution. New York, WW Norton, 1974

Weakland J, Fisch R, Watzlawick P, et al: A brief therapy: focused problem resolution. Fam Process 13:141–168, 1974

White M, Epston D: Narrative Means to Therapeutic Ends. New York, WW Norton, 1993

Wiener-Davis M: Divorce Busting. New York, Fireside, 1992

Wynne L, Singer M: Pseudo-mutuality in the family relations of schizophrenics. Arch Gen Psychiatry 9:161–206, 1963

CHAPTER 35

TREATMENT OF CHILDREN AND ADOLESCENTS

STEPHEN J. COZZA, M.D.
MINA K. DULCAN, M.D.

This chapter provides an overview of and an orientation to the psychiatric treatment of children and adolescents. Treatment modalities as they apply to adults are covered in the other chapters in Section IV of this textbook. This chapter focuses on what is different or unique in the treatment of children and adolescents. Popper and Steingard, in Chapter 23 ("Disorders Usually First Diagnosed in Infancy, Childhood, or Adolescence"), address childhood psychopathology and outline the treatment methods used for each disorder. Throughout this chapter, the terms *child* and *children* refer to children of all ages, to include adolescents, unless otherwise stated.

Techniques used in the treatment of child psychiatric conditions have developed from two different sources: the traditions of understanding and treating children based upon developmental uniqueness, and treatments that were originally designed for adults and were then applied to children and adolescents. Increasingly, more rigorous evaluation and diagnostic procedures have allowed greater specificity in the application of treatments to our younger patients. In addition, expanding research on the efficacy of specific therapeutic approaches continues to enlarge our armamentarium of empirically tested interventions.

The goals of all treatments are to reduce symptoms, to improve emotional and behavioral functioning, to remedy skill deficits, and to remove obstacles to normal development. In contrast to the treatment of adults, a child is usually brought by someone else, and in each case there are at least two clients: the parent and the child, whose needs and desires may conflict. In comparison with adults, children are more dependent on others for meeting their basic needs, they have fewer choices of residence or activities, and they are required to attend school.

EVALUATION

Psychiatric treatment should be preceded by a comprehensive clinical evaluation. In an emergency situation, treatment may have to be initiated following a brief expedient assessment of the child's medical and psychological status. A more thorough evaluation should be accomplished as soon as possible. True emergencies are, fortunately, uncommon, and in most cases the evaluation will be completed before treatment is begun. Of course, the process of assessment does not end with the initiation of treatment but continues throughout.

The American Academy of Child and Adolescent Psychiatry (AACAP) is producing an increasing number of practice parameters as guides to evaluation and treatment of specific disorders. Guidelines for attention-deficit/hyperactivity disorder (ADHD), conduct disorders, anxiety disorders, schizophrenia, bipolar disorder, and forensic evaluation of physical or sexual abuse have been completed (American Academy of Child and Adolescent Psychiatry Work Group on Quality Issues 1992, 1993, 1997a, 1997b, 1997c; McClellan and Werry 1994). Other documents are in various stages of preparation. In addition, AACAP published "Practice Parameters for the Psychiatric Assessment of Children and Adolescents" (American Academy of Child and Adolescent Psychiatry Work Group on Quality Issues 1995). The component guidelines discussed in that document are outlined in Table 35–1.

The purpose of the comprehensive psychiatric assessment of children is similar to the assessment of adults: to determine the presence of one or more psychiatric disorders and to recommend a well-formulated treatment plan that addresses the disorder. Special considerations for children make evaluation different from that for adult patients. Practitioners must have a clear understanding of normal development and the differences that may exist among children at the same or different ages in order to distinguish normal from pathological behaviors. Also, practitioners must be able to apply developmental understanding in the diagnostic interview of the child, using approaches like imaginative play and projective techniques with younger children or with those who are less skilled in verbal communication.

Information from the school is always useful and is essential when there is concern about learning or behavior in school or peer functioning. With parental consent, the clinician talks with the teacher; obtains records of testing, grades, and attendance; and requests completion of a standardized checklist, such as the Teacher Report Form of the Child Behavior Checklist (Achenbach 1991). Even better, though less convenient, is a visit to the school to observe the youngster with peers in the classroom and on the playground and to talk with teachers and counselors.

A referral to another provider such as a pediatrician, pediatric neurologist, child psychologist, or speech and language specialist may be necessary to complete the assessment. Psychological evaluation, including an intelligence test and achievement tests, should be obtained when there is any question about learning or IQ, with additional testing as indicated.

TABLE 35–1. Psychiatric assessment of children and adolescents

Purpose of assessment
- Address the presenting complaint
- Understand the nature of the problem
- Recommend an appropriate treatment plan

Sources of information
- Use a variety of informants to include parents, child, and school
- Contact other agencies (i.e., child protective services, juvenile justice system) when appropriate
- Review appropriate records (i.e., prior treatment, hospitalization, psychological testing, school records)

Parent interview
- Include both parents when possible
- Discuss parameters of evaluation (i.e., number of sessions required, release of information, confidentiality, cost)
- Review history of presenting problem
- Obtain developmental and medical histories
- Review areas of function (i.e., school, family, peers)
- Obtain family and parental histories

Child interview
- Preparation of the child by the parent
- Interview using developmentally appropriate techniques
- Developmental mental status examination

Further consultation or procedures
- Psychological and psychoeducational testing
- Pediatric or pediatric subspecialty consultation
- Speech and language services
- Other laboratory or imaging studies

Formulation and communication of findings

Source. Adapted from American Academy of Child and Adolescent Psychiatry Work Group on Quality Issues 1995.

TREATMENT PLANNING

The planning of a treatment regimen takes into consideration psychiatric diagnosis, target emotional and behavioral symptoms, and the strengths and weaknesses of the patient and family. Resources and risks in the school, neighborhood, and social support network, and any religious group affiliation, also influence the selection of treatment strategies.

In making a plan, the clinician should consider any modality or a combination of the modalities presented in this chapter. The practice of offering a single treatment to all patients, chosen because of the clinician's own training and theoretical beliefs or because that is what the facility offers, is to be avoided, whether that modality is individual therapy, family therapy, pharmacotherapy, hospitalization, or any other form of treatment. Treatments not in the repertoire of the clinician or those requiring additional staff and/or structure should be arranged by referral. Unfortunately, the practical realities of the quality and availability of community resources and the family's ability to pay for treatment often force the clinician to make compromises to an ideal plan.

The clinician must decide which treatment is likely to be the most efficient or to have the highest benefit-risk ratio and whether treatments should be administered simultaneously or in sequence. Unfortunately, very few systematic prospective studies have been conducted comparing well-defined treatments for carefully described groups of child patients.

Parents are best included in the choice of treatment strategies, with the strength of the clinician's recommendation depending on the clarity of the indications. The skilled clinician presents the probable course of the disorder if untreated, as well as the best estimate of benefits and risks of all available treatments for a particular child. The child patient is included in decision making as appropriate. The motivation and ability of the responsible adults to carry out the treatment should be considered because the best treatment has little chance of success without the cooperation of the family.

Treatment planning is an ongoing process, with reevaluations done as interventions are attempted and their results observed and as additional information about the child and family comes to light.

INFORMED CONSENT

The implementation of any treatment plan requires a carefully obtained informed consent from parents before the plan is initiated. The concept of informed consent is more complicated with children because of legal lack of competency. Although parents provide informed consent for children, clinicians should strive to obtain assent from child patients before initiating any treatment. The challenge may be even greater when pharmacotherapy is considered (Krener and Mancina 1994). Such a consent should include a general discussion of the selected therapeutic modality, its intended purpose, the availability of any alternative treatments (to include a choice of no treatment), and the nature of any adverse reactions that could result. An open discussion of any questions or concerns not only meets the legal obligations of practice, but also can

safeguard the therapeutic alliance should undesirable side effects occur. Although not always necessary, parents' written consent may be useful in some situations. Printed materials to supplement discussion with the physician in educating parents and children regarding a variety of treatments are now available (Bastiaens and Bastiaens 1993; Dulcan 1998).

CONFIDENTIALITY

It is essential that the guidelines for confidentiality and for sharing information between parent and child be clear. Adolescents are usually more sensitive to this issue than younger children. In general, either party should be told when information from one party's session will be relayed to the other. In some situations, parents and children may participate in the decision. When children are engaged in potentially dangerous activities or have serious thoughts of harming themselves or others, parents must be informed. Carefully planned family sessions in which the therapist coaches and supports a parent or child in sharing information may be more useful than secondhand reports.

An area of increasing concern for clinicians is the impingement of managed care practices on the ability to maintain confidentiality. Clinicians should ensure that they inform children and parents of the possible need to share some information with third-party entities and make prudent choices as to the nature and quantity of information that are appropriate to pass on.

PSYCHOPHARMACOLOGY

This necessarily brief and relatively superficial section focuses on how drug treatment of children is different from that of adults (see Chapter 27 for psychopharmacological treatment of adults and shared mechanisms of action and side effects). The reader is referred to other brief (M. Campbell and Cueva 1995a, 1995b) and comprehensive (Riddle 1995a, 1995b) reviews of pediatric psychopharmacology.

Important general principles of pediatric psychopharmacology include minimizing polypharmacy and virtually never using medication as the only treatment. Most disorders of children and adolescents that require medication are either chronic (e.g., ADHD, autistic disorder, or Tourette's disorder) or likely to have recurrent episodes (e.g., mood disorders), and a long-term relationship with the physician is crucial. It is important to educate the family regarding the disorder, its treatment, and the different needs at each developmental stage. The physician must consider the meaning of the prescription and administration of a medication to the child, the family, the school, and the child's peer group.

Medication types are classified rather roughly by functional effect (e.g., antidepressant). This classification ignores the fact that no agent has only one effect. In pediatric psychopharmacology, the category name may even be inaccurate for the actual use and clinical effect, as in the treatment of ADHD with "stimulant" medications.

SPECIAL ISSUES FOR CHILDREN AND ADOLESCENTS

Pharmacokinetics and Pharmacodynamics

Pharmacokinetics is the study of the movement of drugs into, around, and out of the body by the processes of absorption, distribution, metabolism, and elimination. Although children share some similarities in the physiological processing of medications with adults, developmental differences are clinically relevant, particularly in regard to drug distribution and metabolism.

Factors that most greatly impact on the developmental differences of distribution of drugs in children are differences in proportion of extracellular water volume and body fat. Extracellular water volume decreases substantially from birth through early adolescence. This decrease results in a larger distribution volume for water-soluble drugs in younger children requiring a relatively higher dose to achieve a comparable plasma concentration (Clein and Riddle 1995).

In general, children have lower proportional body fat than adults, thus reducing the distribution volume for lipid-soluble medications. Although this would result in an expected increase in plasma concentrations of such medications in children compared with adults using weight-adjusted dosages, lower plasma levels in children have been reported. This finding indicates that other pharmacokinetic differences, presumably increased metabolism in children, offset this effect (Clein and Riddle 1995).

By late infancy to early childhood, hepatic metabolic activity is at its peak. This substantially greater metabolic rate is related to the proportionally larger liver size of children compared with adults. Relative to body weight, the liver of a toddler is 40%–50% greater and that of a 6-year-old is 30% greater than the liver of an adult. This greater metabolic rate has been postulated as the principal factor contributing to decreased drug plasma concentration levels and decreased drug half-lives in children com-

pared with adults (Clein and Riddle 1995).

Medication dosage also is determined by pharmacodynamics, or how the biological system responds to the drug. For example, interaction with receptors is determined by receptor number, distribution, structure, function, sensitivity, and mechanism of action. Little is known about the influence of growth and development on these variables.

Ideally, medication doses in children should be derived from studies of children rather than adults, but studies of children often are not possible. Protocols using healthy children are not permitted, and few dosage studies have been done in symptomatic children. Dosage may be determined empirically or by weight or surface area. Generally, children are anticipated to require a higher weight-adjusted dose to achieve the same blood levels and therapeutic effects as adults. However, clinicians should remain alert to the possibility that such practice occasionally results in toxicity.

Side Effects

Side effects are common in children being treated with psychiatric medications. Clinicians must actively look for adverse reactions, as children often will not report them and parents may not notice. Occasionally, children will develop an uncharacteristic or paradoxical response to a particular medication. Such a response may be extremely individual in its manifestation, affecting one child but not another. *Behavioral toxicity* is a term that is used to describe a response to medication in which a child demonstrates behavioral or symptomatic aggravation caused by a particular medication (Van Putten and Marder 1987).

Measurement of Outcome

Effective medication management in children requires the identification of clear target symptoms that are monitored during the course of a medication trial. The physician must obtain emotional, behavioral, and physical baseline and posttreatment data. Therapeutic effects can be assessed by interviews and rating scales, direct observation, collection of data from outside sources (e.g., teachers), or specific tests evaluating attention or learning (Conners 1985).

In reading the psychopharmacology literature, it is important to distinguish between *statistically* significant effects and *clinically* significant ones and to know whether the target symptoms are reduced to near normal levels, or merely changed, and the clinical meaning of the change. The percentage of patients who improve may be more important than changes in group means. Some patients may improve and others worsen, resulting in nonsignificant group data. On the other hand, statistically significant group changes may translate into only modest changes in individual patient functioning that may not be worth the risk of medication.

Developmentally Disabled Patients

Medication effects are even more difficult to assess in children and adolescents with mental retardation or pervasive developmental disorders (PDDs). Their impaired ability to verbalize symptoms is relevant to diagnosis, measurement of efficacy, and detection of side effects. These individuals are prone to physical side effects and are at risk for idiosyncratic behavioral effects or simply less prominent therapeutic effects.

Heterogeneity of samples of autistic children in language development, motor activity, severity of stereotypies, affective range and lability, chronological age, and IQ may lead to variable drug effects. Autistic youngsters are even more likely to react differently to specific drugs than do children with other psychiatric disorders, even when the target symptoms seem similar.

Compliance

Taking medication as directed can be particularly problematic for children because the cooperation of two people, parent and child, and often school personnel as well, is required. In general pediatric practice, high compliance to medication regimens is associated with the degree of parental concern about the seriousness of their child's illness, the severity of the child's symptoms, and prior high compliance to treatment (Lewis 1995). Compliance appears inversely related to the complexity of the medication regimen (including the number of medicines used and the frequency of dosing). Although experiences in general pediatrics and adult psychiatry indicate that educational efforts may improve compliance, administration of psychotropic medications in children is more complex. Bastiaens (1992) found no correlation between knowledge of medications and compliance in a group of inpatient children and adolescents. In a later study, he found that compliance in a group of inpatient adolescents correlated better with attitudes than with knowledge of pharmacotherapy, indicating a need to examine and explore a child's feelings about taking medication (Bastiaens 1995).

Ethical Issues

Those physicians who treat children with pharmacotherapy face significant ethical challenges (Coffey 1995). The practice of pharmacotherapy of children is often modeled on adult treatments because rigorous, controlled double-blind studies in children are few. Pharmaceutical companies often do not go to the expense and trouble of testing drugs in children and adolescents. Although it is important to note that U.S. Food and Drug Administration (FDA) guidelines as published in the *Physicians' Desk Reference* (PDR) are not meant to regulate the clinical practice of physicians (Popper 1987), the clinician must be responsible for the careful use of medications in the child population, basing decisions upon a thorough understanding of the scientific literature. The lack of knowledge of the potential impact of medications on the neural development of children further complicates the issue. A clinician must balance multiple factors: the risks of the untreated disorder, the relative efficacy of medications, and the potential adverse outcomes or unknowns of medication use.

The interaction between pharmacotherapy and the environment is an issue for adult patients but even more so for children and adolescents because their immature developmental status places them in the care of adults, whether parents, teachers, or staff in an inpatient unit or residential treatment setting. There is a danger of misinterpreting the youngster's response to the family, school, or institutional milieu as an exacerbation requiring medication or as improvement due to a medication. Many adults seek to use drugs to control or eliminate troublesome behavior rather than instituting more time-consuming and difficult therapeutic or behavioral management strategies. The physician must therefore evaluate and monitor the environment as well as the patient.

STIMULANTS

This category of medications, which includes methylphenidate, dextroamphetamine, and magnesium pemoline, is the most studied and most used in pediatric psychopharmacology and is most often prescribed by non-child psychiatrists such as pediatricians and general practitioners.

Contrary to prevailing mythology, hyperactive boys, healthy boys, and healthy adults have similar cognitive and behavioral responses to comparable doses of stimulants. Although it is clear that stimulants do *not* have a "paradoxical" effect in ADHD, the actual mechanism of action remains unclear. It is likely that stimulant therapeutic effect is related to augmentation of dopaminergic and adrenergic activity in the central nervous system (CNS). One theory suggests that stimulants act by reducing the excessive, poorly synchronized variability in the various dimensions of arousal and reactivity seen in ADHD (Evans et al. 1986).

Stimulants reduce the performance decrement seen as patients with ADHD perform tasks, perhaps by improving motivation and focusing effort.

Indications and Efficacy

The most established indication for stimulant use is in the treatment of ADHD. The vast majority of the literature on this topic has focused on the efficacy of stimulants in school-age white males. Although data have been extrapolated to the treatment of other populations, a relatively limited body of literature is available on preschoolers and adolescents (T. Spencer et al. 1996b). In preschool-age children, stimulant efficacy is more variable, and the rate of side effects, especially sadness, irritability, clinginess, insomnia, and anorexia, is higher (S. B. Campbell 1985). Previous practices calling for discontinuation of stimulant treatment in adolescents have been abandoned. Most recently, T. Spencer et al. (1996b) reviewed studies of stimulant treatment in adolescents and concluded that, although limited, results indicate that stimulants are equally effective in adolescents as in school-age children.

Stimulants have been found to be effective in treating ADHD symptoms in the mentally retarded population (Aman et al. 1991). Of concern, however, is the fact that this population may be prone to more serious side effects, particularly those children who are more severely impaired (Handen et al. 1991). Children with fragile X syndrome also have been shown to benefit significantly from stimulant treatment of ADHD symptoms (Hagerman et al. 1988). Despite previous concern about treating children with PDDs with stimulants, Birmaher et al. (1988) described the effective use of this medication in a group of nine autistic children who did not develop significant side effects or show worsening of stereotypies.

The use of stimulants in patients with tics or Tourette's disorder remains controversial. The greatest concern is precipitating new tics. Often, however, patients with Tourette's disorder are far more disabled by their inattention, impulsivity, low frustration tolerance, and oppositional behavior than by the tics. Data suggest that in children who already have Tourette's disorder, methylphenidate improves behavior without significantly worsening tics (Gadow et al. 1992). Stimulants should be used with caution in patients with a history of tics or Tourette's disorder, either in themselves or their families, and should be discontinued if persistent new tics develop.

The short-term efficacy of stimulants in ADHD is well documented. Global judgments by parents, teachers, and clinicians rate 65%–75% of hyperactive children improved on stimulants, with placebo response reported between 2%

and 39% (Wilens and Biederman 1992). Those 25%–35% of nonresponders demonstrate no change or worsening of symptoms, or they have intolerable side effects to the medications. A study using a wide range of doses of methylphenidate and dextroamphetamine found that 96% of the sample improved behaviorally in response to one or both drugs, although some children did not continue on medication because of adverse effects (Elia et al. 1991). Stimulant effects on various domains (cognitive, behavioral, social) are highly variable within and among individuals. A dose that produces improvement in one domain may have no effect or may even lead to worsening in another. Higher doses of stimulants, in some studies, have been shown to improve behavior but impair cognitive functioning (Sprague and Sleator 1977). Even more puzzling, the response may differ between measures (e.g., math and read-

TABLE 35–2. Therapeutic effects of stimulant medications in attention-deficit/hyperactivity disorder responders

Cognitive effects[a]
- Improve sustained attention
- Improve reaction time
- Reduce impulsivity
- Enhance sensitivity and style of cognitive response
- Improve short-term memory

Motor effects
- Reduce excessive motor behavior

Classroom effects
- Decrease off-task behavior
- Decrease inappropriate verbalizations
- Improve on-task seat work
- Improve academic performance
- Improve compliance

Effects on aggressivity
- Reduce physical aggression
- Reduce verbal aggression
- May reduce covert aggression (i.e., vandalism, stealing)

Effects on mother/family-child interaction
- Increase maternal warmth
- Decrease maternal criticism
- Increase verbal interactions
- Enhance positive family interactions

Effects on peer relationships
- Improve peer cooperation
- Partially "normalize" peer interaction

[a]Higher doses of stimulant medications may rarely cause cognitive deterioration.
Source. Adapted from Greenhill 1995.

ing), even in the same domain. Specific effects documented in groups of ADHD stimulant responders are listed in Table 35–2.

Stimulants have been demonstrated to have no effect on learning disabilities in the absence of an attention deficit (Gittelman et al. 1983). The use of stimulants in populations with comorbid ADHD and learning disorders appears to have a role in treating the underlying ADHD- related attentional and behavioral symptoms (Gadow 1983).

Stimulants have not yet been demonstrated to have long-term therapeutic effects, but all existing studies have serious methodological problems, including inappropriate control groups; short duration; premature drug discontinuation; excessive, inadequate, or poorly timed doses; questionable compliance with medication; lack of attention to individual variation in response; insensitive outcome measures; and no treatment of associated academic, social, or family problems (Pelham 1983). The ongoing National Institute of Mental Health Collaborative Multisite Multimodal Treatment Study of ADHD children has been designed to address these areas of weakness (Richters et al. 1995). It is clear that medication alone is rarely sufficient treatment. Even children who respond positively continue to show deficits in some areas. Specific learning disabilities and gaps in knowledge and skills due to inattention require educational remediation. Social skills deficits and family pathology may need specific treatment. Parent education and training in techniques of behavior management are virtually always indicated.

Initiation and Maintenance

The decision to medicate a child or adolescent with a stimulant is based on the presence of persistent target symptoms that are sufficiently severe to cause functional impairment at school and usually also at home and with peers. Parents must be willing to monitor medication and to attend appointments. Other interventions are generally implemented first, unless severe impulsivity and noncompliance create an emergency situation. Efforts to predict drug responsiveness among a group of hyperactive children have been largely unsuccessful. Comorbid anxiety disorder may suggest lesser likelihood of improvement (Pliszka 1989), whereas children with more severe inattention may have a greater positive response to medication (Rapoport and DuPaul 1986).

Multiple outcome measures, determined by using more than one source, setting, and method of gathering data and including premedication baseline school data on behavior and academic performance, are essential. Education for the child, family, and teacher is helpful before the start of medication (see Bastiaens and Bastiaens 1993; Dulcan 1998). The physician should explicitly debunk common myths about stimulant treatment—for example, that stimulants have a paradoxical sedative action, that they lead to drug abuse, and that they are not needed or ineffective after puberty. The physician should work closely with parents on dose adjustments and obtain annual academic testing and more frequent reports from teachers.

No patient characteristics are helpful in suggesting which stimulant drug is best for a particular child. Twenty-five percent of a sample of boys with ADHD taking both methylphenidate and dextroamphetamine were behaviorally positive responders to one of the drugs but not the other. Of the nonresponders to each drug, the majority responded to the other drug (Elia et al. 1991). Methylphenidate is the most commonly used and best studied. Dextroamphetamine is less expensive but is not included in many third-party formularies. Disadvantages of dextroamphetamine include negative attitudes of pharmacists, including some who are unwilling to stock it; greater risk of growth retardation; and higher potential for abuse.

Longer-acting preparations of methylphenidate (Ritalin Sustained Release [Ritalin-SR]) and dextroamphetamine (Dexedrine Spansule) are available. These particular medications are appealing for children who experience a brief duration of action of the standard formulations (2½–3 hours) or severe rebound or when administering medication every 4 hours is inconvenient, stigmatizing, or impossible. Parents and children should be warned by clinicians that breaking or chewing either long-acting preparation will destroy the sustained release packaging and could result in excessively high doses of medication.

There have been concerns about the efficacy of the long-acting preparations of both Dexedrine Spansule (G. L. Brown et al. 1980) and Ritalin-SR (Pelham et al. 1987, 1990). Of the two preparations, Ritalin-SR more often has been identified as less reliable and less effective, although in a more recent review, Greenhill (1995) inferred equal clinical efficacy of these long-acting compounds based upon available controlled studies. An innovative strategy for difficult-to-manage cases is the combination of short-acting and longer-acting medication forms (Fitzpatrick et al. 1992).

Magnesium pemoline is a longer-acting CNS stimulant that is structurally dissimilar to methylphenidate and dextroamphetamine. Pemoline may be able to be given once a day and has the least abuse potential. Sallee et al. (1992) report that although bioavailability of pemoline may vary by 200% among subjects, therapeutic plasma concentrations result in effective clinical outcome when children are dosed appropriately. Similarly, in a double-blind crossover study, Pelham et al. (1995) identified the effectiveness of pemoline as a long-acting stimulant medication with rapid onset when appropriately dosed and titrated. In their report, Pelham et al. (1995) described no increased incidence of side effects when doses were increased every 2–3 days rather than the traditional weekly titration, allowing for a much more rapid onset of action. The possibility of pemoline-induced chemical hepatitis requires baseline measurement of liver function and regular clinical monitoring. Recent information released by Abbott Laboratories (1996) (manufacturer of Cylert) identified 13 cases of acute hepatic failure reported to the FDA since 1975 as a result of treatment with this compound. For this reason, pemoline should not be considered as a first-line therapy for ADHD.

Stimulant medication should be initiated with a low dose and titrated within the recommended range every week or two according to response and side effects, with body weight as a rough guide (Table 35–3). When children reach age 3 years, their absorption, distribution, protein binding, and metabolism of stimulants are similar to those of an adult (Coffey et al. 1983), although adults have more side effects than do children at the same mg/kg dose. Giving medication after meals minimizes anorexia. Preschool-age children or patients with ADHD, predominantly inattentive type; mental retardation; or PDDs may benefit from (and have fewer side effects with) lower doses

than those patients with ADHD with prominent symptoms of hyperactivity or impulsivity. Starting with only a morning dose may be useful in assessing drug effect by comparing morning and afternoon school performance. The need for an after-school dose or medication on weekends should be individually determined. Behavioral checklists such as the Child Attention Profile (CAP) (Edelbrock 1991) (Tables 35–4 and 35–5), the Conners Teacher Rating Scale (CTRS), and the Conners Parent Rating Scale (CPRS) (Conners and Barkley 1985) are useful in monitoring the efficacy of medications in a variety of settings.

If symptoms are not severe outside of the school setting, children should have an annual drug-free trial in the summer, at least 2 weeks' duration but longer if possible. If school behavior and academic performance are stable, a carefully monitored trial off medication during the school year (but *not* at the beginning) will provide data on whether medication is still needed.

Tolerance is reported anecdotally, but compliance is often irregular and should be the first possibility considered when medication appears ineffective. Children should not be responsible for their medication because youngsters are impulsive and forgetful at best, and most dislike the idea of taking medication, even when they can verbalize its positive effects and cannot identify any side effects. They will often avoid, "forget," or simply refuse medication. Lower efficacy of a generic preparation may be

TABLE 35–3.   Clinical use of stimulant medications

	Methylphenidate (Ritalin)	Dextroamphetamine (Dexedrine)	Pemoline (Cylert)
How supplied (mg)	5, 10, 20 Sustained release 20	5, 10 Elixir (5 mg/5 mL) Spansules 5, 10, 15	18.75, 37.5, 75.0
Usual single dose range (mg/kg/dose)	0.3–0.7	0.15–0.5	0.5–2.5
Usual daily dose range (mg/day)	10–60	5–40	37.5–112.5
Usual starting dose (mg)	5–10 qd or bid	2.5 or 5 qd or bid	37.5–56.25 qd[a]
Maintenance number of doses per day	2–3	2–3	1–2
Monitor	Pulse Blood pressure Weight Height Dysphoria Tics	Pulse Blood pressure Weight Height Dysphoria Tics	Pulse Blood pressure Weight Height Dysphoria Tics Liver function

Source.   Adapted from Dulcan and Martini 1998 and [a]Pelham et al. 1995.

TABLE 35–4. Child Attention Profile (CAP)

Child's name:_____   Child's age:_____

Today's date:_____   Child's sex: M [ ]   F [ ]

Filled out by:_____

Below is a list of items that describes pupils. For each item that describes the pupil **now or within the past week,** check whether the item is **Not True, Somewhat or Sometimes True, or Very or Often True.** Please check all items as well as you can, even if some do not seem to apply to this pupil.

	Not true	Somewhat or sometimes true	Very or often true
	[ ]	[ ]	[ ]
1. Fails to finish things he/she starts	[ ]	[ ]	[ ]
2. Can't concentrate, can't pay attention for long	[ ]	[ ]	[ ]
3. Can't sit still, restless, or hyperactive	[ ]	[ ]	[ ]
4. Fidgets	[ ]	[ ]	[ ]
5. Daydreams or gets lost in his/her thoughts	[ ]	[ ]	[ ]
6. Impulsive or acts without thinking	[ ]	[ ]	[ ]
7. Difficulty following directions	[ ]	[ ]	[ ]
8. Talks out of turn	[ ]	[ ]	[ ]
9. Messy work	[ ]	[ ]	[ ]
10. Inattentive, easily distracted	[ ]	[ ]	[ ]
11. Talks too much	[ ]	[ ]	[ ]
12. Fails to carry out assigned tasks	[ ]	[ ]	[ ]

Please feel free to write any comments about the pupil's work or behavior in the last week.

Source. Reprinted with the permission of Craig Edelbrock, Ph.D., University of Massachusetts Medical Center, Worcester, Massachusetts.

another possibility. Decreased drug effect also may be due to a reaction to a change at home or school. Greenhill (1995) uses the term *pseudotolerance* to define circumstances in which increased symptomatology is inaccurately ascribed to decreased medication efficacy (e.g., when symptoms are exacerbated due to changes in a child's life rather than changes in response to medication). True tolerance may be more likely with the long-acting formulations (Birmaher et al. 1989); if it occurs, another of the stimulants may be substituted.

Risks and Side Effects

Most side effects are similar for all stimulants (Table 35–6). Insomnia may be due to drug effect, to rebound, or to a preexisting sleep problem. Stimulants may worsen or improve irritable mood (Gadow 1992). Black male adoles-

TABLE 35–5. Child Attention Profile (CAP) scoring

Each of the 12 items is scored 0, 1, or 2.

Total score = sum of the scores on all items

Subscores:

Inattention: Sum of scores on items 1, 2, 5, 7, 9, 10, and 12

Overactivity: Sum of scores on items 3, 4, 6, 8, and 11

Scores recommended as the upper limit of the normal range (93rd percentile):

	Boys	Girls
Inattention	9	7
Overactivity	6	5
Total score	15	11

Source. Reprinted with the permission of Craig Edelbrock, Ph.D., University of Massachusetts Medical Center, Worcester, Massachusetts.

TABLE 35–6. Side effects of stimulant medications

Common initial side effects (try dose reduction)

Anorexia

Weight loss

Irritability

Abdominal pain

Headaches

Emotional oversensitivity, easy crying

Less common side effects

Insomnia

Dysphoria (especially at higher doses)

Decreased social interest

Impaired cognitive test performance (especially at
    very high doses)

Less than expected weight gain

Rebound overactivity and irritability (as dose wears off)

Anxiety

Nervous habits (e.g., picking at skin, pulling hair)

Hypersensitivity rash, conjunctivitis, or hives

Withdrawal effects

Insomnia

Rebound ADHD symptoms

Depression (rare)

Rare but potentially serious side effects

Motor or vocal tics

Tourette's disorder

Depression

Growth retardation

Tachycardia

Hypertension

Psychosis with hallucinations

Stereotyped activities or compulsions

Side effects reported with pemoline only

Choreiform movements

Dyskinesias

Night terrors

Lip licking or biting

Chemical hepatitis–elevated SGOT and SGPT,
    jaundice, epigastric pain (J. F. Patterson 1984)

Note. ADHD = attention-deficit/hyperactivity disorder;
SGOT = serum glutamic-oxaloacetic transaminasse;
SGPT = serum glutamic-pyruvic transaminase.
Source. Adapted from Dulcan and Martini 1998.

cents who take stimulants may be at higher risk for elevated blood pressure (R. T. Brown and Sexson 1989).

Although stimulant-induced growth retardation has been a significant concern, decrease in expected weight gain is small and may be clinically insignificant, despite statistical significance. The magnitude is dose related and appears to be greater with dextroamphetamine than with methylphenidate or pemoline. Effect on height can be minimized by using "drug holidays." The mechanism does not appear to be mediated via effects on growth hormone (Greenhill et al. 1981, 1984). Some authors have suggested that growth delays in ADHD children may be related to dysmaturity inherent to the disorder itself rather than medication effects (T. Spencer et al. 1996a).

Rebound effects, consisting of increased excitability, activity, talkativeness, irritability, and insomnia, beginning 4–15 hours after a dose, may be seen as the last dose of the day wears off or for up to several days after sudden withdrawal of high daily doses of stimulants. This effect may resemble a worsening of the original symptoms (Zahn et al. 1980).

Attention is required to avoid possible emanative effects of medication—that is, indirect and inadvertent cognitive and social consequences, such as lower self-esteem and self-efficacy; attribution by child, parents, and teachers of both success and failure to the medication rather than to the child's effort; stigmatization by peers; and dependence by parents and teachers on medication rather than making needed changes in the environment (Whalen and Henker 1991). Both patients and relevant adults can be instructed that medication enables the patients to accomplish what they wish to do; it does not *make* them do anything. Children and adolescents should be given full credit for improvement and helped to take an appropriate amount of responsibility for problems.

Although there is a commonly held notion that stimulants lower the seizure threshold, there is no evidence that stimulants produce an increase in seizure activity. Addiction has *not* been found to result from the prescription of stimulants for ADHD.

A cautionary note: Earlier literature recommended adding imipramine if children developed depression while taking methylphenidate. This combination has been associated with a syndrome of confusion, affective lability, marked aggression, and severe agitation (Grob and Coyle 1986). The mechanism may be via methylphenidate's interference with the hepatic metabolism of imipramine, resulting in a longer half-life and elevated blood levels. There are now better medication choices for the treatment of depressed children with ADHD.

CLONIDINE

Clonidine is an α-noradrenergic agonist approved for the treatment of hypertension.

Indications and Efficacy

Tourette's disorder. Clonidine modestly decreases complex motor and vocal tics (Leckman et al. 1991). Although the effect is less powerful than that of neuroleptics, the side-effect profile is far more benign, making it a good first-line medication choice for Tourette's disorder. Clonidine is most useful in reducing subjective distress and the behavioral symptoms of hyperactivity and impulsivity that often accompany Tourette's disorder. Clonidine may be combined with small doses of haloperidol or pimozide for patients who cannot be treated satisfactorily by either medication alone.

Attention-deficit/hyperactivity disorder. Clonidine is useful in modulating mood and activity level and in improving cooperation and frustration tolerance in a subgroup of children with ADHD, especially those who are highly aroused, hyperactive, impulsive, defiant, and labile (Hunt et al. 1990). Steingard et al. (1993) report that children with ADHD and comorbid tics may have a more positive response to clonidine than children who have ADHD without tics. Although not effective in treating inattention per se, clonidine may be used alone for children who have tics or for those who are nonresponders or negative responders to stimulants. It may be most useful in combination with a stimulant when stimulant response is only partial or when stimulant dose is limited by side effects; the combination may allow a decrease in dose of stimulant medication of up to 40% (Hunt et al. 1990). Clonidine often improves a child's ability to fall asleep, whether insomnia is due to ADHD overarousal, oppositional refusal to go to bed, or stimulant effect or rebound.

Other uses. Recently, clonidine has been described as beneficial in a small open study of preschool children with severe posttraumatic stress disorder (PTSD; Harmon and Riggs 1996). Fankhauser et al. (1992) reported a double-blind, placebo-controlled study in which transdermal clonidine was found to reduce hyperarousal and improve social relating in a group of seven children and two adults with autism. These findings are preliminary and require further investigation before clonidine is used routinely for these purposes in children.

Initiation and Maintenance

Blood pressure and pulse should be measured before a patient starts taking clonidine. An electrocardiogram (ECG) and baseline laboratory blood studies (especially fasting glucose) may be considered. Clonidine is initiated at a low dose of .05 mg (one-half of the smallest manufactured tablet) at bedtime. This low dose converts the side effect of initial sedation into a benefit. An alternate strategy is to begin with .025 mg qid. Either way, the dose is then titrated gradually over several weeks to .15–.30 mg/day (.003–.01 mg/kg/day) in three or four divided doses. Young children (ages 5–7 years) may require lower initial and maintenance doses. The transdermal form (skin patch) may be useful to improve compliance and reduce variability in blood levels. It lasts only 5 days in children (compared with 7 days in adults) (Hunt et al. 1990). Once the daily dose is determined using pills, an equivalent-size patch may be substituted (.1, .2, .3 mg/day). The patch may be cut to adjust the dose. Unfortunately, patches do not adhere well in hot, humid climates.

Clonidine has a slow onset of therapeutic action, in part because of the gradual dose increase needed to minimize side effects and perhaps because of the time required for receptor downregulation (Hunt et al. 1991). Significant clinical response is not seen for as long as a month, and maximal effect may be delayed for another several months.

When clonidine is discontinued, it should be tapered over several days to a week, rather than stopped suddenly, to avoid a withdrawal syndrome consisting of increased motor restlessness, headache, agitation, elevated blood pressure and pulse rate, and (in patients with Tourette's disorder) exacerbation of tics (Leckman et al. 1986).

Risks and Side Effects

Sedation is a troublesome side effect, although it tends to decrease after several weeks. Dry mouth, nausea, and photophobia have been reported, with hypotension and dizziness possible at high doses. The skin patch often causes local pruritic dermatitis. Depression may occur, often in patients with a history of depressive symptoms in themselves or their families (Hunt et al. 1991). Glucose tolerance may decrease, especially in those patients at risk for diabetes.

Recent reports of serious adverse drug reactions (including sudden death) in children treated with clonidine, alone or in combination with methylphenidate, have raised concerns about the safety of this medication in the pediatric population (Cantwell et al. 1997; Popper 1995). Popper (1995) identified no clear evidence that the combination of clonidine and methylphenidate is unsafe. However, he also warned that there was little scientific evidence available to comment on either the potential benefits or risks of methylphenidate-clonidine treatment and that clinicians should proceed with caution. These authors recommended thorough cardiovascular screening and monitoring of children treated with clonidine, as well as gradual titration and tapering of dose to reduce cardiovascular side effects. Clonidine should only be used when good compliance with the medication regimen is demonstrated.

GUANFACINE

Guanfacine, another centrally acting antihypertensive medication, is a more selective α_2-agonist than clonidine and appears to be longer acting and less sedating. It has been demonstrated effective in two open trials of children with ADHD (Hunt et al. 1995) and comorbid ADHD and Tourette's disorder (Chappell et al. 1995). Controlled investigation is needed to determine the efficacy and safety (given its similarity to clonidine) of guanfacine in children.

TRICYCLIC ANTIDEPRESSANTS

Indications and Efficacy

Depression. Despite promising anecdotal data and open trials, only one study has documented superiority of a tricyclic antidepressant (TCA) over placebo. Even with statistical significance, however, clinical significance appeared small. The strongest evidence of efficacy is in hospitalized prepubertal children with major depression who are dexamethasone nonsuppressors (Preskorn et al. 1987).

Attention-deficit/hyperactivity disorder. TCAs are indicated for those patients who do not respond to stimulants or who develop significant depression while taking stimulants, or for the treatment of ADHD symptoms in patients with tics or Tourette's disorder. Patients with ADHD and comorbid anxiety disorder may respond better to a TCA than to a stimulant (Kutcher et al. 1992). The longer duration of action of TCAs prevents a dose having to be taken at school, and rebound is not a problem. Efficacy in improving cognitive symptoms does not appear to be as great as for stimulants. Initial studies used imipramine; however, desipramine has less anticholinergic effect and well-documented sustained efficacy (Biederman et al. 1989). Nortriptyline produced improved attitude followed by an increase in attention span and a decrease in impulsivity in an open trial of 60 children who had a poor response to stimulants or an initial score on the Children's Depression, Inventory (Kovacs 1985) of greater than 9 (Saul 1985). Drawbacks include possible difficulty maintaining the effect over time; serious potential cardiac side effects, especially in prepubertal children; and danger of accidental or intentional overdose. Availability of other useful and safe medications in the treatment of ADHD should make TCAs a second- or third-line medication in treating this disorder in children.

Obsessive-compulsive disorder. Clomipramine (but not other TCAs), a serotonin reuptake inhibitor, is useful in the treatment of obsessive-compulsive disorder (OCD) in children, independent of antidepressant activity (DeVeaugh-Geiss et al. 1992; Leonard et al. 1989). Symptoms are rarely eliminated entirely, but when the medication is effective, the force of obsessions and compulsions is reduced sufficiently to improve quality of life. Combined medication treatment with cognitive-behavior therapy may be optimal (March et al. 1994).

Autistic disorder. Gordon et al. (1993) reported a double-blind study in which clomipramine was significantly more effective than either placebo or desipramine in improving several autistic symptoms (obsessive-compulsive symptoms, reciprocal social interactions, stereotypies, and self-injury). There was no difference between desipramine and placebo noted. In a recent open study examining the use of clomipramine in treating young children (ages 3.5–8.7 years), Sanchez et al. (1996) reported no therapeutic effect. Significant adverse reactions were noted (urinary retention), but further research is required.

Enuresis. All of the TCAs have been found to be equally effective in the treatment of nocturnal enuresis. The mechanism remains unclear, but it does not seem to be by altering sleep architecture, or by treating depression, or via peripheral anticholinergic activity. In 80% of patients, within the first week, TCAs reduce the frequency of bed-wetting. Total remission, however, occurs in relatively few cases. Wetting returns when the drug is discontinued. Behavioral treatments that avoid drug side effects and have higher remission rates are the best first choice. Imipramine may be useful on a short-term basis or for special occasions (e.g., overnight camp).

Anxiety disorders. The majority of the work has examined the use of TCAs for separation anxiety disorder and school absenteeism. The original open study demonstrating efficacy of imipramine in treating children with separation anxiety disorder and school absenteeism has not been replicated (Gittelman-Klein and Klein 1971). The efficacy of imipramine in patients with anxiety disorders is controversial (Bernstein et al. 1990; Klein et al. 1992). Medication may be useful as an adjunct if psychosocial treatment is ineffective. Several case studies of the effectiveness of TCAs in treating childhood panic disorder have been reported (Black and Robbins 1989; Garland and Smith 1990).

Initiation and Maintenance

Pharmacokinetics for TCAs is different in children than in adolescents or adults. The smaller fat-to-muscle ratio in children leads to a decreased volume of distribution, and children are not protected from excessive dosage by a large volume of fat in which the drug can be stored. Children have larger livers relative to body size, leading to faster metabolism (Sallee et al. 1986), more rapid absorption, and lower protein binding than in adults (Winsberg et al. 1974). As a result, children are likely to need a higher weight-corrected dose of imipramine than adults. Prepubertal children are prone to rapid dramatic swings in blood levels from toxic to ineffective and should have divided doses to produce more stable levels (Ryan 1992). Parents must be reminded to supervise closely the administration of medication and to keep pills in a safe place. Guidelines for monitoring the cardiovascular effects of TCAs are given in Table 35–7.

The usefulness of plasma levels is limited by the relative rarity of laboratories able to perform them satisfactorily. Medication cannot be safely titrated by plasma level, as there is no known level below which toxicity can be ensured not to occur. Plasma levels (drawn 9–11 hours after the last dose) can identify rapid and slow metabolizers. Determination of levels is recommended for patients who fail to respond to usual doses (possibly low levels) or those who have severe side effects at usual doses (possibly very high levels). Chlorpromazine, even in low doses, increases plasma levels of nortriptyline (Geller et al. 1985). TCA levels often increase during febrile illnesses because of an increased amount of plasma protein that binds to the drug. The amount of free drug is not increased, however, and these higher levels do not lead to toxicity (Fetner and Geller 1992).

If the patient's history suggests head trauma or seizures, an electroencephalogram (EEG) is indicated before starting treatment.

Depression. For imipramine, the starting dose is 25 mg/day, which may be increased every 4 days by 1 mg/kg/day to a maximum dose of 5 mg/kg/day. Optimum plasma level of imipramine plus desipramine appears to be 150–250 ng/mL (Preskorn et al. 1987; Ryan 1990).

Nortriptyline may have fewer side effects and a more precise therapeutic window of 75–150 ng/mL, usually attained at .5 to 2.0 mg/kg/day (Ryan 1990). It has a longer half-life than imipramine and may be given twice a day in children. Variability in metabolism is greater for nortriptyline than for imipramine (Geller et al. 1986).

Attention-deficit/hyperactivity disorder. Imipramine is begun with 10 or 25 mg/day and increased weekly. The maximum dose is 5 mg/kg/day (divided tid in children). Plasma levels do not predict efficacy. Some patients respond to a daily dose as low as 2 mg/kg. Nortriptyline is given at 25–75 mg/day in two divided doses (Saul 1985).

Obsessive-compulsive disorder. Doses of clomipramine used to treat OCD are generally lower than TCA doses used for depression. Response is delayed for 10–14 days, as in the treatment of depression, and is unlike the immediate response seen in the treatment of ADHD or enuresis (Rapoport 1986). Clomipramine is started at 25 mg/day (or every other day) and gradually increased over 2 weeks to a maximum of 100 mg/day or 3 mg/kg/day, whichever is less. If necessary, the dose may be gradually increased up to a maximum of 200 mg/day in children or 250 mg/day in adolescents, or 3.5 mg/kg/day, whichever is less (Green 1991). Divided doses are preferable during titration. Chronic treatment (years) is required.

Enuresis. Daily charting of wet and dry nights is used before starting medication to obtain a baseline and subsequently to monitor progress. Much lower doses are needed than for the treatment of depression. Imipramine is started at 10–25 mg at bedtime and increased by 10- to 25-mg increments weekly to 50 mg (75 mg in preadolescents), if

TABLE 35–7. Suggested guidelines for monitoring electrocardiograms and vital signs of children and adolescents receiving tricyclic antidepressants

Parameter	Children	Adolescents
Vital signs		
Heart rate	< = 110–130 beats/min[a]	< = 110–120 beats/min[a]
Blood pressure	< 120/80 mm Hg	< 140/90 mm Hg
Electrocardiogram		
P-R interval	< 200 msec	< 200 msec
QRS interval	< = 120 msec ± > 30% over baseline	± 120 msec
QTc interval	< = 460–480 msec	< = 460–480 msec

[a]For 2 consecutive weeks.
Source. Reprinted with permission from Wilens TE, Biederman J, Baldessarini RJ, et al.: "Cardiovascular Effects of Therapeutic Doses of Tricyclic Antidepressants in Children and Adolescents." *Journal of the American Academy of Child and Adolescent Psychiatry* 35:1491–1501, 1996. Copyright 1996, American Academy of Child and Adolescent Psychiatry.

necessary. Maximum dose is 2.5 mg/kg/day (Ryan 1990). Tolerance may develop, requiring a dose increase. For some children, TCAs lose their effect entirely. If medication is used chronically, the child or adolescent should have a drug-free trial at least every 6 months because enuresis has a high spontaneous remission rate.

Anxiety disorders.   In separation anxiety disorder and school nonattendance, psychological interventions such as family therapy, work with school personnel, and desensitization should be used before and along with medication. For children with school phobia, McDaniel (1986) recommends 125 mg as the maximum dose of imipramine. The starting dose for children ages 6–8 years is 10 mg at bedtime and for older children, 25 mg at bedtime. The dose may be increased by 10–50 mg/day, but those with school avoidance require at least 75 mg/day. Some patients require a higher dose for complete response, but if there is no detectable positive response at 125 mg/day, improvement at higher doses is unlikely. After clinical response (6–8 weeks), medication is continued at least another 8 weeks and then gradually withdrawn.

Risks and Side Effects

The quinidine-like effect of TCAs slows cardiac conduction time and repolarization. At doses of more than 3 mg/kg/day of imipramine or desipramine, children and adolescents may develop an increased pulse and small but statistically significant ECG changes (intraventricular conduction defects, such as lengthened P-R interval, that may progress to a first-degree atrioventricular heart block and occasional widening of the QRS complex) (Wilens et al. 1996). In one carefully monitored group of nearly 200 children and adolescents, desipramine in doses of up to 5 mg/kg/day produced increases in diastolic blood pressure, heart rate, and ECG conduction parameters that were statistically significant but not symptomatic or clinically meaningful (Biederman 1991). Prolongation of the QTc interval may be a sensitive indicator of cardiac effect (Wiles et al. 1991). The tendency of prepubertal children to have wider swings in blood levels may place them at higher risk for serious cardiac conduction changes. A minority of the population has a genetic defect in TCA metabolism, increasing risk for toxicity.

Five cases of sudden death have been reported in children being treated with desipramine, three of whom died immediately after physical exertion (Popper and Zimnitzky 1995). A causal relationship between the medication and the deaths has not been established. Cardiac etiology is often concluded; however, a recent review of cardiovascu-

lar changes in children treated with TCAs (Wilens et al. 1996) concluded that although changes in blood pressure, heart rate, and ECG parameters are identifiable, they are probably of minor significance. Nevertheless, since other safe and effective medications are available (to include other TCAs), the routine use of desipramine in children is discouraged.

Anticholinergic side effects may occur in children, although less commonly than in adults. Most of these side effects are transient and/or respond to a decrease in dose. Of particular importance for children are dry mouth (which may lead to an increase in dental caries in long-term use [Herskowitz 1987]), drying of bronchial secretions (especially problematic for asthmatic children), sedation, anorexia, constipation, nausea, tachycardia, palpitations, and increased diastolic blood pressure.

Other reported side effects include abdominal pain, chest pain, headache, orthostatic hypotension (rare in young patients), syncope, mild tremors of hands and fingers, weight loss, and tics. The seizure threshold may be lowered, with worsening of preexisting EEG abnormalities and rarely a seizure. Seizures appear to be more common with clomipramine. Side effects with a probable allergic mechanism include rash, worsening of eczema, and rarely thrombocytopenia (M. Campbell et al. 1985).

Behavioral toxicity may be manifested by irritability, worsening of psychosis, mania, agitation, anger, aggression, forgetfulness, or confusion. CNS toxicity may be mistaken for exacerbation of the primary condition. A drug blood level is often required to differentiate the two. As depressed children, especially those who are anergic and withdrawn, improve with TCA treatment, crying and verbalizations of sadness and anger may transiently increase.

Sudden cessation of moderate or higher doses results in flulike anticholinergic withdrawal syndrome, with nausea, cramps, vomiting, headaches, and muscle pains. Other manifestations may include social withdrawal, hyperactivity, depression, agitation, and insomnia (Ryan 1990). TCAs should therefore be tapered over a 2- to 3-week period. The short half-life of TCAs in prepubertal children often produces daily withdrawal symptoms if medication is given only once a day. These symptoms also may indicate that poor compliance is resulting in missed doses. Because of the predictability of TCA-induced electrocardiographic changes, a rhythm strip is useful in monitoring compliance.

The physician should be alert to the risk of intentional overdose or accidental poisoning, not only by the patient but by other family members, especially young children.

OTHER ANTIDEPRESSANTS

Selective Serotonin Reuptake Inhibitors

Fluoxetine. The most well-supported indication for the use of fluoxetine in children is in the treatment of obsessive-compulsive disorder as evidenced by the controlled study completed by Riddle et al. (1992). In this study, 14 children (ages 8–15 years) diagnosed with obsessive-compulsive disorder demonstrated significant improvement on the Clinical Global Impressions—Obsessive-Compulsive Scale (CGI-OCD) but not the Children's Yale-Brown Obsessive Compulsive Scale (CY-BOCS) with fluoxetine compared with placebo.

Use of fluoxetine in childhood depression is less clear. Although fluoxetine was found to benefit depressed adolescents in an open trial by Boulos et al. (1992), no significant difference was reported in a double-blind, placebo-controlled study of depressed adolescents (Simeon et al. 1990). A complication of the latter study is that high fixed doses of medication (60 mg/day) may have led to medication nonresponse. In a more recent study, Colle et al. (1994) reported reduction of depressed symptoms in an extended open trial of fluoxetine treatment in depressed teenagers, indicating that clinical response may improve in trials lasting longer than 8 weeks. One rigorous double-blind, placebo-controlled trial in children and adolescents with depression found that fluoxetine yielded improvement in depressive symptoms significantly greater than did placebo (Emslie et al. 1995). Further controlled investigation is required.

Fluoxetine has been used in the treatment of a variety of other disorders. Anecdotal reports suggest that fluoxetine may be useful in the treatment of ADHD (Barrickman et al. 1991). Gammon and Brown (1993) reported both safety and benefit in the combined use of fluoxetine and methylphenidate in the treatment of children with ADHD who had demonstrated inadequate response to methylphenidate alone. Cook et al. (1992) reported improvement of perseverative behaviors in an open study of fluoxetine treatment in children and adults with autism and mental retardation. Birmaher et al. (1994) reported marked to moderate improvement in children and adolescents with mixed anxiety disorders treated with fluoxetine in an open study. Although fluoxetine was initially reported effective in the treatment of obsessions and compulsions in Tourette's disorder (Como and Kurlan 1991; Riddle et al. 1990), a double-blind study failed to confirm these earlier findings (Kurlan et al. 1993). A double-blind, placebo-controlled study examining the effectiveness of fluoxetine in the treatment of elective mutism in a small group of children showed mixed results (Black and Uhde 1994). Further research is required in these areas.

Fluoxetine is begun at a dose of 5–10 mg/day, usually in the morning. Relatively few patients require a dose greater than 20 mg/day and are often well managed at lower doses. Dose adjustments may require the use of alternate-day regimens, the use of the new liquid formulations, or dissolving medication in juice and dispensing aliquots.

Although fluoxetine has relatively few somatic side effects (anorexia, weight loss, headaches, nausea, vomiting, tremor), behavioral toxicity is common. Symptoms include restlessness, insomnia, social disinhibition, agitation (Riddle et al. 1990–1991), mania (Venkataraman et al. 1992), and suicidal ideation or behavior (King et al. 1991). Akathisia may contribute to the etiology of these effects.

Sertraline. No controlled studies have yet been published that examine the efficacy of sertraline treatment in children. Two uncontrolled studies have demonstrated improvement in children with major depressive disorder treated with sertraline (McConville et al. 1996; Tierney et al. 1995). Of concern is "behavioral activation," including the development of mania observed in 21% of the Tierney et al. (1995) study group. Reports of behavioral activation and mania associated with sertraline treatment in children have become common in the literature (Ghaziuddin 1994; Guile 1996; Minnery et al. 1995), requiring a cautious approach to its use in this population. Sertraline is begun at 25 mg/day, with usual therapeutic doses in the range of 50–200 mg/day.

Fluvoxamine. A preliminary report of the use of fluvoxamine, a selective serotonin reuptake inhibitor (SSRI) relatively new to the United States, indicates that it may be effective and safe in the treatment of OCD and depression in adolescents (Apter et al. 1994). This finding was corroborated by a much larger multicenter, double-blind, placebo-controlled investigation examining the use of fluvoxamine in the treatment of children and adolescents with OCD (Walkup 1996). The results of the study suggested the relative safety of this medication in the pediatric population during short-term use.

Bupropion

Bupropion is a compound of the aminoketone class and is structurally unrelated to other antidepressants. Small controlled studies have demonstrated the superiority of bupropion to placebo in the treatment of ADHD in children (Casat et al. 1987; Clay et al. 1988; Simeon et al. 1986). More recently, Conners et al. (1996) reported the findings of a multisite, double-blind, placebo-controlled study corroborating these previous results, confirming that bupropion can be beneficial in the treatment of ADHD and possibly conduct disorder. Another study found the efficacy of bupropion in treating ADHD to be not statistically significantly different from methylphenidate (Barrickman et al. 1995). Bupropion may prove to be a safe and effective treatment of depression in children with ADHD, as it appears to have less cardiac side effects than do TCAs. In addition, substance-abusing adolescent patients with ADHD may benefit from treatment with bupropion because of its lack of abuse potential. Bupropion has been reported to exacerbate tics in children with comorbid ADHD and Tourette's disorder and may not be suitable for use in this population (T. Spencer et al. 1993).

Bupropion is administered in two or three daily doses, beginning with a low dose (37.5 or 50 mg bid), with titration over 2 weeks to a usual maximum of 250 mg/day (300–400 mg/day in adolescents). A long-acting preparation of this medication is now available allowing once or twice daily dosing. The most serious side effect is a decrease in the seizure threshold, seen most frequently in patients with an eating disorder. Bupropion is contraindicated in this population. Other side effects in children include skin rash, perioral edema, nausea, increased appetite, agitation, and exacerbation of tics.

Monoamine Oxidase Inhibitors

Clinical experience suggests that monoamine oxidase inhibitors (MAOIs) may be useful in the treatment of depressed adolescents who do not respond to TCAs (Ryan et al. 1988b), as well as in children with ADHD (Zametkin et al. 1985). The availability of other safe and effective treatments for these disorders makes MAOIs a more distant therapeutic choice. In using MAOIs, suicidal and impulsive outpatients should be excluded because of the risk of severe reactions with dietary indiscretions or drug interaction. In any case, careful dietary instruction and review are necessary. Caution is indicated because of the multiple interactions between MAOIs and other medications.

LITHIUM CARBONATE

Indications and Efficacy

Lithium may be considered in the treatment of children and adolescents with bipolar affective disorder, mixed or manic (Strober et al. 1990; Varanka et al. 1988). It is not indicated for prophylaxis in bipolar disorder in children and

adolescents unless there is well-documented history of recurrent episodes. Lithium augmentation has been effective in some open trials with adolescents who have tricyclic-refractory depression (Ryan et al. 1988a; Strober et al. 1992). However, fewer adolescents than adults respond to this strategy. It is not yet clear whether lithium is efficacious for the treatment of behavior disorders without an apparent mood disorder in children of bipolar parents or for children and adolescents who have behavior disorders accompanied by mood swings. The combination of lithium and methylphenidate may be more effective in the treatment of combined disruptive behavior disorders (ADHD/conduct disorder) and mood disorders than either medication used alone (Carlson et al. 1992).

In children with severe impulsive aggression, especially when it is accompanied by explosive affect, lithium is equal or superior to haloperidol in reducing aggression, hostility, and tantrums, with fewer side effects (M. Campbell et al. 1984). These positive findings were more recently replicated, although with more modest lithium effect (M. Campbell et al. 1995). Lithium also may be useful in mentally retarded or autistic youths with severe aggression directed toward themselves or others or with symptoms suggestive of bipolar disorder (M. Campbell et al. 1985; Kerbeshian et al. 1987; Steingard and Biederman 1987).

Initiation and Maintenance

Lithium should not be prescribed unless the family is willing and able to comply with regular multiple daily doses and with blood monitoring of lithium levels. In addition to the usual detailed medical history and physical examination, complete blood count (CBC) with differential, liver function tests, electrolytes, serum thyroxine and thyroid-stimulating hormone (TSH), blood urea nitrogen (BUN), creatinine, and ECG should be determined before starting lithium. Some clinicians recommend determining renal concentrating ability (urine specific gravity or osmolality after overnight fluid deprivation) (C. Popper, personal communication, 1992). A patient with a history suggesting increased risk of seizures warrants an EEG. Height, weight, TSH, creatinine, and morning urine specific gravity (or osmolality) should be obtained every 3–6 months.

Lithium levels, drawn 10–12 hours after the last dose, should be obtained twice weekly during initial dose adjustment and monthly thereafter. Three to four days are required to reach steady-state levels after a dose change. Therapeutic levels are the same as for adults, .6–1.2 mEq/L, which can usually be attained with 900–1,200 mg/day, in divided doses, although daily doses of up to 2,000 mg may be required (M. Campbell et al. 1985). The starting dose is 150–300 mg/day, gradually titrated upward in divided doses according to serum levels and clinical effects. Because lithium excretion occurs primarily through the kidney, and most children have more efficient renal function than adults, they may require higher doses for body weight than do adults (Weller et al. 1986). In prepubertal children, dose may be titrated more rapidly using a regimen based on body weight (Weller et al. 1986) or on a serum level drawn 24 hours after a single 600-mg dose (Fetner and Geller 1992). More steady blood levels may be obtained by using a slow-release formulation. Lithium should be taken with food to minimize gastrointestinal distress. Some difference may be present in pharmacokinetics between lithium carbonate and lithium citrate, and clinicians should not assume equal dosing when shifting between the two forms (Reischer and Pfeffer 1996).

Following lithium treatment of an acute manic episode, medication may be gradually discontinued after 6–12 months and the patient observed closely for possible relapse.

Risks and Side Effects

The younger the child, the more likely the occurrence of side effects (M. Campbell et al. 1991). Autistic children have more frequent and severe side effects from lithium than do children with conduct disorder, even at lower doses (M. Campbell et al. 1991). Children may experience side effects at serum levels that are lower than those in adults: most commonly, weight gain, vomiting, headache, nausea, tremor, enuresis, stomachache, weight loss, sedation, and anorexia (M. Campbell et al. 1991). Common, early-onset side effects, which seem to be related to rapid increase in serum level, include nausea, diarrhea, muscle weakness, thirst, urinary frequency, a dazed feeling, and hand tremor. Polydipsia and polyuria secondary to vasopressin-resistant diabetes insipidus may result in enuresis, especially in institutionalized retarded patients (M. Campbell et al. 1985). In growing children, the consequences of hypothyroidism (which could resemble retarded depression) are potentially more severe than in adults. Because of its teratogenic potential, lithium is relatively contraindicated in sexually active girls. The calcium mobilization from bones that has been noted in adults might cause a significant problem in growing children (Herskowitz 1987). Lithium's tendency to aggravate acne may be especially significant for adolescents. Isotretinoin, used in adults to treat severe acne, should not be used in sexually active girls due to teratogenicity (Herskowitz

1987). Lithium effects on glucose are controversial, but both hyperglycemia and exercise-induced hypoglycemia are possible. Rarely, lithium may cause extrapyramidal symptoms (EPS) in children (Samuel 1993).

Toxicity is closely related to serum levels, and the therapeutic margin is narrow. Symptoms of lithium toxicity include vomiting, drowsiness, hyperreflexia, sluggishness, slurred speech, ataxia, anorexia, convulsions, stupor, coma, and death. Adequate salt and fluid intake is necessary to prevent levels rising into the toxic range. The family should be instructed in the importance of preventing dehydration from heat or exercise and in the need to stop the lithium and contact the physician if the child or adolescent develops an illness with fever, vomiting, diarrhea, and/or decreased fluid intake. The erratic consumption of large amounts of salty snack foods may cause fluctuations in lithium levels (Herskowitz 1987). Lithium levels may be increased to toxic levels by nonsteroidal anti-inflammatory agents (often taken by adolescent girls to treat menstrual symptoms) (Fetner and Geller 1992).

NEUROLEPTIC DRUGS

Indications and Efficacy

Neuroleptic medications, also termed antipsychotic medications or major tranquilizers, are more fully discussed in Chapter 27. Their use in children and adolescents has been reviewed by Teicher and Glod (1990) and more recently by Findling et al. (1996). The recent introduction of "atypical" antipsychotic medications (clozapine and risperidone) has added significantly to the child and adolescent psychiatrist's pharmaceutical armamentarium.

Schizophrenia.   Few studies examining the efficacy of typical antipsychotic medications in schizophrenic children exist (Findling et al. 1996). Of the two investigations with more stringent diagnostic admission criteria, both controlled studies (Pool et al. 1976; Realmuto et al. 1984) demonstrated moderate effectiveness of antipsychotic medication in adolescent schizophrenic patients. Medication-induced side effects in both studies were substantial, particularly sedation (in low-potency agents) and EPS (in high-potency agents), supporting the belief that children may be at higher risk than adults for developing side effects. E. K. Spencer et al. (1992) reported preliminary results of the first double-blind, placebo-controlled trial of haloperidol in schizophrenic prepubertal children. Findings similarly support moderate improvement of symptoms in those taking haloperidol rather than placebo.

The more limited effect of typical antipsychotic medications, coupled with higher side-effect profiles (to include tardive dyskinesia), in children has led clinicians to consider the use of atypical antipsychotics in the treatment of the pediatric population. Open trial and double-blind controlled studies examining the efficacy of clozapine in treatment-resistant, childhood-onset adolescent schizophrenic patients (Frazier et al. 1994; Kumra et al. 1996; Remschmidt et al. 1994) have consistently demonstrated the superiority of clozapine to standard treatments, specifically haloperidol. As treatment with clozapine is compounded by possible serious side effects (agranulocytosis, seizures, and significant weight gain), its use is reserved for treatment of those select pediatric patients who have failed to respond to trials of standard antipsychotics.

Information regarding the use of risperidone in the treatment of schizophrenia in the pediatric population is limited to several case reports and open-label studies (Armenteros et al. 1997; Grcevich et al. 1996; Quintana and Keshavan 1995) in which positive and negative symptoms of the disorder appeared to have improved. As an atypical agent, risperidone may eventually prove to have greater efficacy than current standard treatments; however, controlled investigation is required.

Autistic disorder and pervasive developmental disorder. In some hyper- or normoactive autistic children, haloperidol (in doses of 0.5–4.0 mg/day) has been found to decrease behavioral target symptoms such as hyperactivity, aggressiveness, temper tantrums, withdrawal, and stereotypies (L. T. Anderson et al. 1989). Efficacy in enhancing learning is controversial but clearly will not occur in the absence of a highly structured behavioral/educational program. The majority of hypoactive autistic children do not respond well to haloperidol (M. Campbell et al. 1985) but may do better with pimozide (Ernst et al. 1992). Two open trials (totaling 34 patients) have described the effectiveness of risperidone in the treatment of disruptive behaviors in children with severe developmental disorders (Fisman and Steele 1996; Hardan et al. 1996).

Tourette's disorder. Efficacy of neuroleptic medications is often difficult to evaluate in patients with Tourette's disorder because of the natural waxing and waning of symptoms. Haloperidol in low doses is initially effective for up to 70% of patients (Cohen et al. 1992). Unfortunately, side effects often limit haloperidol's usefulness, and withdrawal of the drug may lead to severe exacerbation of symptoms for up to several months. Pimozide, a high-potency neuroleptic that also blocks calcium channels, has been demonstrated to be effective in the treatment of Tourette's disorder. Although considered an alternative medication to haloperidol and clonidine,

one study suggests that pimozide may result in less cognitive impairment than haloperidol when prescribed at effective lower doses (Sallee and Rock 1994). Risperidone recently has been reported as effective in reducing symptoms in two open-label studies of chronic tic/Tourette's disorder (Bruun and Budman 1996; Lombroso et al. 1995).

Conduct disorder. Studies of hospitalized, severely aggressive children, ages 6–12 years, have demonstrated short-term efficacy of haloperidol (1–6 mg/day or .04–.21 mg/kg/day), thioridazine (mean = 170 mg/day), and molindone (mean = 26.8 mg/day) compared with placebo in reducing, although not eliminating, aggression, hostility, negativism, and explosiveness. Chlorpromazine leads to unacceptable sedation at relatively low doses (M. Campbell et al. 1985; Greenhill et al. 1985).

Initiation and Maintenance

Medication should not be used as the sole treatment in the aforementioned complex disorders. Before medication is initiated, a complete physical examination and baseline laboratory workup, including CBC, differential, liver profile, and urinalysis, should be done. A baseline EEG is recommended in children being treated with clozapine, and a weekly WBC with differential is mandatory. Doses must be titrated individually, with careful attention to positive and negative effects. Age, weight, and severity of symptoms do not provide clear guidelines. The initial dose should be very low, with gradual increments no more than once or twice a week. Although divided doses are often used during titration, in most cases, once a therapeutic dosage has been reached, a single daily dose (usually at bedtime) can be used. Children metabolize these drugs more rapidly than do adults but also require lower plasma levels for efficacy (Teicher and Glod 1990). Neuroleptics interact with a wide variety of other drugs (Teicher and Glod 1990).

Schizophrenia. Older adolescents with schizophrenia may require doses of neuroleptics in the adult range. Young adolescents fall in between, and doses must be empirically determined because there are few data. To avoid sedation or cognitive blunting that interferes with learning, one of the higher-potency drugs, such as haloperidol, fluphenazine, trifluoperazine, or perphenazine, may be best. It may require several weeks for full efficacy to be achieved. Clozapine should be started at very low doses—12.5 mg/day or 25 mg/day—and titrated slowly to minimize side effects to an expected dosage range of 25–500 mg/day. Risperidone should be initiated at low doses (.5–1.0 mg) and titrated slowly, to prevent development of EPS, to an expected dosage range of 2.0–4.0 mg/day.

Autistic disorder. It is important to give a trial of sufficient length to determine if the drug is efficacious, barring serious side effects requiring immediate discontinuation. Typical daily doses are 0.5–4 mg haloperidol. If the drug appears to be helpful, it should be continued for at least several months. At 3- to 6-month intervals, the drug should be discontinued to observe for withdrawal dyskinesias and to determine if the drug continues to be necessary. Some children may have physical withdrawal symptoms or a rebound phenomenon consisting of worsening of behavior for up to 8 weeks after the medication is stopped (M. Campbell et al. 1985). Developmentally disturbed children treated with risperidone may benefit from doses as low as 0.5–1.0 mg/day (Fisman and Steele 1996).

Tourette's disorder. Careful monitoring of patients with Tourette's disorder for several months before starting medication is possible, since this is a chronic disorder and not usually an emergency. This monitoring permits the clinician to establish a baseline of symptoms and to assess the need for psychological and educational interventions. An initial dose of haloperidol is .5 mg/day. It may be slowly increased up to 1–3 mg/day, divided in twice-daily doses (Cohen et al. 1992). Pimozide, which may be given in a single daily dose, is started at 1 mg/day and may be gradually increased to a maximum of 6–10 mg/day (.2 mg/kg). The usual dose range is 2–6 mg/day (Cohen et al. 1992). Risperidone doses in the range of 1.0–2.5 mg/day appear to be useful (Lombroso et al. 1995).

Risks and Side Effects

Acute EPS, including dystonic reactions, parkinsonian tremor, rigidity and drooling, and akathisia, occur as in adults. Laryngeal dystonia is potentially fatal. Acute dystonia may be treated with oral or intramuscular diphenhydramine, 25 mg or 50 mg, or benztropine mesylate, .5–2.0 mg. Adolescent boys seem to be more vulnerable to acute dystonic reactions than are adult patients, so the physician may be more inclined to use prophylactic antiparkinsonian medication. In children, however, reduction of neuroleptic dose is preferable to the use of antiparkinsonian agents (M. Campbell et al. 1985).

For treatment or prevention of parkinsonian symptoms, adolescents may be given the anticholinergic drug benztropine mesylate, 1–2 mg/day, in divided doses. Chronic parkinsonian symptoms are often drastically

underrecognized by clinicians (Richardson et al. 1991). The neuromuscular consequences may impair the performance of age-appropriate activities, and the subjective effects may lead to noncompliance with medication. Akathisia may be especially difficult to identify in young patients or those with limited verbal abilities.

Tardive or withdrawal dyskinesias, some transient but others irreversible, seen in 8%–51% of neuroleptic-treated children and adolescents (M. Campbell et al. 1985), mandate caution regarding casual use of these drugs. Tardive dyskinesia has been documented in children and adolescents after as brief a period of treatment as 5 months (Herskowitz 1987) and may appear even during periods of constant medication dose. One case of tardive dyskinesia was recently reported in an adolescent treated with risperidone (Feeney and Klykylo 1996), indicating that those patients treated with atypical neuroleptics may not be immune to this serious adverse reaction. In children with autism or Tourette's disorder, it may be especially difficult to distinguish medication-induced movements from those characteristic of the disorder. Before patients begin taking a neuroleptic, they should be examined carefully for abnormal movements by using a scale such as the Abnormal Involuntary Movement Scale (AIMS 1988) and should be periodically reexamined. Parents and patients (if they are able) should receive regular explanations of the risk of movement disorders.

Potentially fatal neuroleptic malignant syndrome has been reported in children and adolescents (Latz and McCracken 1992), with a presentation similar to that seen in adults.

Weight gain may be problematic with the long-term use of the low-potency neuroleptics. Abnormal laboratory findings seem to be reported less often for children than for adults, but the clinician should be alert to the possibility, especially of agranulocytosis or hepatic dysfunction. If an acute febrile illness or easy bruising occurs, medication should be withheld and CBC with differential and liver enzymes should be determined (M. Campbell et al. 1985).

Another concern is behavioral toxicity, manifested as worsening of preexisting symptoms or development of new symptoms such as hyperactivity or hypoactivity, irritability, apathy, withdrawal, stereotypies, tics, or hallucinations (M. Campbell et al. 1985). Low-potency antipsychotic drugs such as chlorpromazine and thioridazine can produce cognitive dulling and sedation that interfere with the patient's ability to benefit from school (M. Campbell et al. 1985) and are probably best avoided. Children and adolescents are more sensitive than adults to this sedation (Realmuto et al. 1984). Children may be at greater risk of neuroleptic-induced seizures than adults because of their immature nervous systems and the high prevalence of abnormal EEGs in seriously disturbed children (Teicher and Glod 1990).

Anticholinergic side effects such as hypotension, dry mouth, constipation, nasal congestion, blurred vision, and urinary retention are unusual. Miscellaneous side effects include abdominal pain, enuresis (Realmuto et al. 1984), photosensitivity, and various neuroendocrine effects that may be especially distressing to adolescents.

Kumra et al. (1996) reported a high incidence of serious adverse effects (neutropenia and seizure activity) in children who were treated with clozapine, indicating a need for extremely close monitoring of children treated with this medication.

Side effects are a significant problem of long-term use of haloperidol for Tourette's disorder. Frequent complaints include lethargy, feeling like a "zombie," dysphoria, personality changes, weight gain, parkinsonian symptoms, akathisia, and intellectual dulling (Cohen et al. 1992). Dysphoria and school avoidance also have been reported (Mikkelsen et al. 1981). Pimozide appears to have a similar but less severe side-effect profile.

Pimozide causes ECG changes in up to 25% of patients (T-wave inversion, U waves, QTc prolongation, and bradycardia), although these appear to be less clinically significant than originally thought. The ECG should be evaluated at baseline and monitored monthly during dosage increases and at 3-month intervals thereafter (Cohen et al. 1992).

For a more detailed discussion of neuroleptic side effects and their management, see Chapter 27 of this textbook and Whitaker and Rao (1992).

ANXIOLYTICS, SEDATIVES, AND HYPNOTICS

There are few data on the safety and efficacy of anxiolytics and sedative-hypnotics in children and adolescents, although this population appears to respond similarly compared with adult patients' responses (T. Spencer et al. 1995). In most cases, psychosocial interventions should precede and accompany pharmacotherapy.

Benzodiazepines

Indications and efficacy. Benzodiazepines may be used in the short-term treatment of children with severe anticipatory anxiety. Although an open trial of alprazolam for children with avoidant and overanxious disorders was promising, a double-blind study did not find superiority of this drug over placebo in the context of an intensive treatment program (Simeon et al. 1992). Efficacy may have been limited by low

doses and the short duration of treatment.

Preliminary evidence suggests that clonazepam may be useful in the treatment of panic disorder and neuroleptic-induced akathisia in adolescents (Biederman 1987; Kutcher et al. 1987, 1992). In a small open trial, clonazepam was found effective in diminishing tics in children with ADHD and comorbid tic disorders when used adjunctively with clonidine (Steingard et al. 1994). In a double-blind, placebo-controlled study, Graae et al. (1994) reported the clinical effectiveness of clonazepam in the treatment of anxiety disorders (predominantly separation anxiety disorder) in children. However, statistical superiority over placebo was not found, and most children evidenced side effects, notably sedation and disinhibition.

Initiation and maintenance. Infants and children absorb diazepam faster and metabolize it more quickly than do adults (Simeon and Ferguson 1985). Usual daily dose ranges for children and adolescents are as follows: lorazepam, .25–6 mg; diazepam, 1–20 mg; and alprazolam, 0.25–4 mg. Clonazepam has been used at .5–3 mg/day. Dosage schedule depends on age (more frequent in children) and the specific drug (Coffey 1990; Kutcher et al. 1992). When the medication is being discontinued, the dose needs to be tapered gradually to avoid withdrawal seizures or rebound anxiety.

Risks and side effects. In addition to the risks of substance abuse and physical or psychological dependence, side effects include sedation, cognitive dulling, ataxia, confusion, emotional lability, and worsening of psychosis. Paradoxical or disinhibition reactions may occur, manifested by acute excitation, irritability, increased anxiety, hallucinations, increased aggression and hostility, rage reactions, insomnia, euphoria, and/or incoordination (Coffey 1990; Graae et al. 1994; Reiter and Kutcher 1991; Simeon and Ferguson 1985).

Antihistamines

Indications and efficacy. Diphenhydramine or hydroxyzine may be used for severe difficulty falling asleep that has not responded to psychological interventions. Medication should be used only for a short time, to break the cycle and to give parents a rest and energy to pursue other solutions. Diphenhydramine is used in the treatment of acute dystonic reactions. Antihistamines are probably not effective when used as a prn medication for behavioral control (Vitiello et al. 1991).

Initiation and maintenance. An initial dose of diphenhydramine or hydroxyzine in children and adolescents is

10 or 25 mg/day. Either drug is titrated gradually up to a maximum of 200–300 mg/day (5 mg/kg/day) (Coffey 1990).

Side effects. The most common side effects of antihistamines are dizziness and oversedation. Some children become paradoxically agitated. Occasionally, incoordination, blurred vision, dry mouth, nausea, abdominal pain, or agitation is seen. With high doses of antihistamines, the seizure threshold is lowered. Leukopenia and agranulocytosis are extremely rare. Antihistamines have been reported to cause acute dystonic reactions, tics, and possibly (with chronic administration) tardive dyskinesia. They should not be used for asthmatic patients because of drying of mucous membranes, or in the presence of glaucoma or bladder neck obstruction because of anticholinergic effects.

Buspirone

Buspirone is a relatively new nonbenzodiazepine anxiolytic that is reported to be less sedating and have less risk of abuse or dependence than do the benzodiazepines. It also has been reported possibly to have weak antidepressant efficacy.

Indications and efficacy. All data on buspirone treatment in children are anecdotal. Suggested uses are for generalized anxiety disorder (Kutcher et al. 1992), for mixed anxiety disorders (Simeon et al. 1994), as a supplementary drug in the treatment of OCD, and for reducing aggression and anxiety in patients with mental retardation (Ratey et al. 1991), autistic disorder (Realmuto et al. 1989), or conduct disorder.

Initiation and maintenance. Tentative guidelines for children and adolescents suggest a starting dose of 2.5–5 mg/day, increasing to three times a day over 2–3 days (Kutcher et al. 1992). The dose may be increased gradually to a maximum of 20 mg/day in children and 60 mg/day in adolescents, in three divided doses. The therapeutic effects may be delayed for 1–2 weeks after reaching the proper dose, with maximal effects not seen for an additional 2 weeks (Coffey 1990).

Risks and side effects. Reported adverse effects include insomnia, dizziness, anxiety, nausea, headache, restlessness, agitation, depression, and confusion (Coffey 1990). Possible psychotic symptoms were reported in two children treated with buspirone (Soni and Weintraub 1992), indicating that clinicians should closely monitor children who are prescribed this medication.

ANTICONVULSANTS

The antiepileptic drugs carbamazepine, valproic acid, and clonazepam are used for a variety of (non-FDA approved) psychiatric indications. Efficacy may be unrelated to anticonvulsant effect. Wide variations in bioavailability and rate of absorption of generic products have led to recommendations that the brand name (or at least a single generic) product be prescribed. Data on children and adolescents generally are far more limited than those from studies of adults, but side-effect patterns appear to be similar. Clonazepam has been discussed previously in the section on benzodiazepines and therefore is not discussed in this section.

All of the anticonvulsants have complex interactions with multiple other drugs.

Carbamazepine

Indications and efficacy. Patients with severe impulsive aggression with emotional lability and irritability who have an abnormal EEG or a strong clinical suggestion of episodic phenomena may deserve a trial of carbamazepine (Evans et al. 1987). Preliminary data suggest this drug's efficacy in children with severe explosive aggression, even in the absence of neurological findings (Kafantaris et al. 1992). Carbamazepine also may be useful in the treatment of psychiatric symptoms associated with temporal lobe epilepsy (Trimble 1990). Satisfactory data on the use of carbamazepine in young bipolar patients are lacking, although some clinicians consider its use in manic adolescents who are not responding to lithium or who are rapid cyclers. An anecdotal report of the effective response to carbamazepine in 28 children and adolescents with the diagnosis of PTSD is encouraging (Loof et al. 1995) but requires further investigation.

Initiation and maintenance. Hemoglobin, hematocrit, WBC, platelets, liver function, BUN, and creatinine should be measured before the patient begins taking carbamazepine. The degree of laboratory monitoring necessary is controversial. A conservative recommendation includes CBC and liver function studies weekly for the first 4 weeks, monthly for 4 months, and every 3 months thereafter (Silverstein et al. 1983). A more modest regimen is CBC (with differential and platelet count), serum iron, BUN, and creatinine after the first month and then every 3–6 months (Trimble 1990). Tests always should be done if a rash, sore throat, fever, malaise, lethargy, weakness, vomiting, increased urinary frequency, anorexia, jaundice, easy bruising, bleeding, or mouth ulcers develop. If the neutrophil count drops below 1,000, or if hepatitis occurs, the drug should be stopped (Silverstein et al. 1983).

The initial dose of carbamazepine is 100 mg/day with food. Children eliminate carbamazepine more rapidly than do adults (Jatlow 1987), and plasma levels (drawn approximately 12 hours after the last dose) are crucial because dosage calculated by weight correlates poorly with plasma concentration. Titration is gradual (weekly increase of 100 mg/day), guided by plasma levels, to a usual plateau of 8–12 µg/mL. The usual daily dose range is 10–50 mg/kg, divided into three doses for children and two for older adolescents. Autoinduction of hepatic enzymes may lead to declining plasma concentration, especially in the first 6 weeks, requiring an increase in dose. Carbamazepine deteriorates if stored under humid conditions.

Risks and side effects. The most common adverse effects of carbamazepine are drowsiness, nausea, rash, diplopia, nystagmus, and reversible dose-related leukopenia. Other side effects include vomiting, vertigo, ataxia, tics, muscle cramps, exacerbation of seizures, rare blood dyscrasias, hepatotoxicity, severe skin reactions (e.g., Stevens-Johnson or systemic lupuslike syndromes), and inappropriate secretion of antidiuretic hormone (in rare cases leading to acute renal failure) (Evans et al. 1987; Trimble 1990). Teratogenic effects have been demonstrated. Adverse behavioral reactions, such as extreme irritability, agitation, insomnia, obsessive thinking, hallucinations, delirium, psychosis, paranoia, hyperactivity, aggression, and mania, may be seen during the first 1–4 weeks of treatment (Evans et al. 1987; Herskowitz 1987; Pleak et al. 1988).

Valproic Acid

Two open-label, uncontrolled trials of valproic acid in the treatment of adolescents with mania have been reported (Papatheodorou et al. 1995; West et al. 1994). Both studies found that valproic acid was generally well tolerated and beneficial in this population. Although valproic acid may be beneficial in the treatment of mania, larger controlled studies are required to establish efficacy in comparison with established treatments.

Monitoring serum valproate levels is less useful than for other anticonvulsants (Trimble 1990). The initial laboratory workup is the same as for carbamazepine. Liver function tests and CBC may be repeated weekly for the first month, then every 4–6 months. For children younger than age 10 years, monthly liver function tests are advisable (Trimble 1990).

The most frequent adverse effects are nausea, vomiting, and gastrointestinal distress (which may be diminished by using enteric-coated divalproex sodium), sedation, weight gain, and tremor (Trimble 1990). Acute hepatic failure is almost always restricted to children younger than age 3 years, especially those with mental retardation or who are following a regimen of anticonvulsant polytherapy. Other side effects are similar to those seen in adults. Of uncertain significance is the report of menstrual disturbances, polycystic ovaries, and hyperandrogenism in a series of women treated with valproic acid for epilepsy (Isojarvi et al. 1993). Although these problems may be attributable to epilepsy in this population, the impact of long-term valproic acid use on female reproduction in adolescent manic patients requires further investigation.

BETA-BLOCKING AGENTS

Indications and Efficacy

β-adrenergic blockers may be useful in patients with otherwise uncontrollable rage reactions and impulsive aggression or self-injurious behavior, especially those with evidence of organicity. In a recent comprehensive review of the literature on this topic, Connor (1993) commented on the lack of methodologically controlled studies of these medications in the pediatric population. Propranolol has been found to be effective in daily doses of 50–960 mg, with a median of 160 mg (Williams et al. 1982). Anecdotal reports suggest that propranolol may be effective in the treatment of agitated, hyperaroused children and adolescents with PTSD (Famularo et al. 1988) and children and adolescents with "hyperventilation attacks" (Joorabchi 1977). In an open trial, a single dose of 40 mg propranolol appeared to be helpful in reducing test anxiety and improving performance in high school students (Faigel 1991). Pindolol and nadolol, with fewer side effects and longer half-lives, have been suggested as alternatives. Other than a single case report of the benefit of nadolol in a child with PDD (Connor 1994), these medications have not been tested in children.

Initiation and Maintenance

Initial workup should include a recent history and physical examination, with particular attention to medical contraindications: asthma, diabetes, bradycardia, heart block, cardiac failure, or hypothyroidism. Fasting blood sugar and glucose tolerance test may be indicated if there is risk of diabetes. An ECG may be considered.

In children and adolescents, the initial dose of propranolol is 10 mg tid, increasing by 10–20 mg every 3–4 days, and pulse and blood pressure should be monitored (minimum pulse 50, blood pressure 80/50). The standard daily dose range is 10–120 mg for children and 20–300 mg for adolescents, divided into three doses (2–8 mg/kg/day) (Coffey 1990). The short elimination half-life in children (2–3 hours) may necessitate four doses daily. Dose is titrated to clinical effect or side effects. Maximum improvement at a given dose may not be seen for up to 8 weeks. If a β-blocker is to be discontinued, it should be tapered gradually to avoid rebound hypertension and tachycardia. When β-blockers are used together with chlorpromazine or thioridazine (but not haloperidol), blood levels of patients taking these drugs are elevated.

Risks and Side Effects

Side effects of β-blockers are generally the same as in adults. Tiredness, mild hypotension, and bradycardia are the most common. Decreased sexual interest and performance, dysphoria, insomnia, nightmares, or hypoglycemia (in patients with diabetes) may occur.

NALTREXONE

Abnormalities of endogenous opioids have been suggested to occur in persons who have autism and in mentally retarded persons who engage in self-injurious behavior. Naltrexone, a potent opiate antagonist, has been found to be effective in the treatment of hyperactivity in autistic children in several double-blind and placebo-controlled studies (M. Campbell et al. 1993; Kolmen et al. 1995; Willemsen-Swinkels et al. 1996). Although earlier reports suggested that naltrexone treatment increased social interaction and decreased self-injury in autistic patients, these later controlled studies failed to demonstrate statistical difference from response to placebo in regard to these behaviors. In doses of .5–2.0 mg/kg/day, naltrexone appears to be safe, with only mild side effects noted. No changes in any laboratory measures, ECG, or vital signs have been demonstrated in children or adolescents. Clearly, further controlled trials are needed, but cautious clinical use of naltrexone in patients with severe behavioral symptoms may be indicated, particularly given its benign side-effect profile.

DESMOPRESSIN

Desmopressin (DDAVP) is an analog of antidiuretic hormone administered as a nasal spray to treat nocturnal enuresis. Onset of action is rapid, and side effects are mild (nasal mucosal dryness or irritation, headache, epistaxis, and nausea) in patients with normal electrolyte regulation.

DDAVP acts by increasing water absorption in the kidneys, thereby reducing the volume of urine. Water intoxication is rare, but children should be encouraged to limit fluid intake in the evenings when taking desmopressin. In a review of the recent literature, Thompson and Rey (1995) concluded that desmopressin is not as effective as alarm methods, is more effective than placebo (approximately the same as imipramine), and may be best used occasionally (e.g., sleep-overs) for children who are known to respond. In children who wet the bed four nights during the week, a one-third reduction in enuresis can be expected (Thompson and Rey 1995). No predictors of response have been identified. The usual dose is 10–40 µg intranasally at bedtime. Relapse is likely upon discontinuation of treatment.

ELECTROCONVULSIVE THERAPY

Experience in the use of electroconvulsive therapy (ECT) in adolescents is limited and is extremely rare in prepubertal children. Understandably, many clinicians are reluctant to use a procedure that induces seizures in a developing brain, particularly when long-term effects are not clear. The American Psychiatric Association Task Force on ECT (1990) does not reject the use of ECT in the pediatric population but recommends it be reserved for clinical situations when other treatment choices have been exhausted or are unacceptable. Bertagnoli and Borchardt's (1990) comprehensive review of the literature discussing ECT in children concluded that ECT benefits children and adolescents with bipolar disorder and depression. Similarly, in an institutional record review of 13 adolescents treated with ECT, Moise and Petrides (1996) concluded that ECT is a useful, effective treatment for adolescents with severe psychiatric disorders when first- and second-line treatments are ineffective. Complications of ECT in the pediatric population include brief cognitive impairment, increase in seizure threshold, behavioral disinhibition, and post-ECT anxiety (Bertagnoli and Borchardt 1990). More information regarding the effectiveness and side effects of ECT in children and adolescents is needed.

CATEGORIES OF PSYCHOTHERAPY

Psychotherapies can be classified in different ways (Table 35–8). There are few data to guide the selection of type of therapy for a particular disorder or patient.

TABLE 35-8.   Varieties of psychotherapy

Theoretical foundations

  Psychoanalytic

  Behavioral or social learning

  Developmental

  Ecological

  Family systems

  Cognitive

Target of intervention

  Individual

  Parent

  Family

  Group

Duration

  Short (4–6 sessions)

  Intermediate (up to 6 months)

  Long (6 months to years)

Goals of therapy

  Crisis intervention

  Support

  Symptom removal

  Personality reconstruction

INDIVIDUAL PSYCHOTHERAPY

All individual therapies have certain common themes (Strupp 1973):

■ Relationship with a therapist who is identified as a helping person and who has some degree of control and influence over the patient

■ Instillation of hope and improved morale

■ Use of attention, encouragement, and suggestion

■ Goals of helping the patient to achieve greater control, competence, mastery, and/or autonomy; to improve coping skills; and to abandon or modify unrealistic expectations of himself or herself, others, and the environment

In the treatment of children, it is essential to consider the patients' environment and family dynamics. In most cases, work with parents and school, and often pediatricians, welfare agencies, courts, or recreation leaders, must accompany individual therapy. The cooperation of parents, and often teachers, is required to maintain the child in treatment and to remove any secondary gain resulting from the symptoms. The therapist must be aware of a patient's level of physical, cognitive, and emotional development in order to understand the symptoms, set appropriate goals, and tailor effective interventions.

Behavior modification, cognitive-behavior therapy, and even indirect family therapy can be conducted in individual sessions and are covered in subsequent subsections of this chapter.

Communication With Children and Adolescents

Children are less able to use abstract language than are adults. They use play to express feelings, to narrate past events, to work through trauma, and to regress. It is less threatening and anxiety provoking if the therapist works in the displacement, uses the metaphor of the play, and bases questions and comments on characters in the play rather than on the child (even if the connection is clear to the therapist). Effective communications are tailored to the child's stage of language, cognitive, and affective development. The therapist must be aware that the vocabulary of some bright and precocious children exceeds their emotional understanding of events and concepts.

Dramatic play with dolls or puppets, drawing, painting, or modeling with clay, as well as questions about dreams, wishes, or favorite stories or television shows, can provide access to children's fantasies, emotions, and concerns. Adolescents may prefer creative writing or more complex expressive art techniques.

Resistant Child or Adolescent

It is not surprising that many children or adolescents do not cooperate in therapy because most are brought to treatment by adults. These young patients often do not wish to change themselves or their behaviors and view their parents' and teachers' complaints as unreasonable or unfair. In addition, a child or adolescent may refuse to participate in or may attempt to sabotage therapy for a variety of dynamic reasons (Gardner 1979). Effective interventions are tailored to the cause of the resistance.

A child who is anxious or having difficulty separating from a parent may be helped by initially permitting the parent to remain in the therapy room. When a child or adolescent does not talk, whether from anxiety or opposition, the therapist often addresses this reluctance, either directly or through play. Long silences are not generally helpful and tend to increase anxiety or battles for control. Attractive play materials help to make therapy less threatening and to encourage participation while the therapist builds an alliance. However, the therapist must guard against the danger of sessions becoming mere play or recreation instead of therapy. Gardner (1979) has developed a variety of techniques that incorporate therapeutic activities with story-telling, drama, and game boards. Using behavioral contingencies in therapy also may improve motivation, especially of materially deprived children.

Schizophrenic Child

Individual psychotherapy may be useful as part of a comprehensive treatment plan for children who are schizophrenic or very fragile (Cantor and Kestenbaum 1986). The therapist must be prepared to provide structure, to limit regression and fantasy, and to focus on reality testing and development of stronger defense mechanisms and healthier coping skills. The relationship with the therapist may be especially crucial for these youngsters.

Types of Individual Psychotherapy

Psychoanalysis. In this relatively infrequently used modality for children and adolescents, neurotic symptoms are viewed as arising from internalized intrapsychic conflict, nonorganic developmental arrest, or regression. The goals are to remove these symptoms that have become independent of their original context, through structural changes in defensive organization and personality. The analyst functions as a transference object. The principal technique for producing change is interpretation of unconscious content, resulting in greater conscious awareness and adaptive control of emotions and behavior.

The family must be able to sustain a process that is expensive, lasts for years, and requires sessions four to five times a week. The patient must have sufficient intelligence, capacity for verbalization and insight, and frustration tolerance. Psychoanalysis is contraindicated for psychotic youth or those with serious cognitive or ego deficiencies (Sours 1978).

Psychodynamically oriented psychotherapy. This treatment is grounded in psychoanalytic theory but is more flexible and emphasizes the real relationship with the therapist and the provision of a corrective emotional experience as well as the transference. Frequency is typically once or twice a week, most commonly over a period of 1–2 years. Interaction between the parents and the therapist is more active. Goals of therapy include symptom resolution, change in behavior, and return to normal developmental process. Change occurs via transference interpretation and maturation of defenses, catharsis, development of insight, ego strengthening, improved reality testing, and sublimation (Adams 1982). The therapist forms an alliance with the child or adolescent, reassures, promotes

controlled regression, identifies feelings, clarifies thoughts and events, makes interpretations, judiciously educates and advises, and acts as an advocate for the patient (Adams 1982).

Dynamically oriented individual therapy alone is much more likely to be effective for children and adolescents who are in emotional distress or who are struggling to deal with a stressor than for those children with behavior problems. Children and adolescents with attention-deficit, oppositional, or conduct disorders rarely acknowledge their problem behaviors and are usually better treated in family or group therapy, by parent training in behavior management, or in a structured milieu. Youngsters with ADHD have little insight into their behavior and its effect on others, and they may be genuinely unable to report their problems or to reflect on them. However, insight-oriented therapy may be useful for some of these youngsters to address comorbid anxiety or depression or symptoms resulting from psychological trauma.

Recently, Bleiberg et al. (1997) have argued the applicability of psychoanalytically oriented psychotherapy for more disturbed children. Such treatment is designed to help the child reflect on his or her inner affective states, establish accurate representations of self and others, appreciate realistic causal relationships, and build flexibility of response to environmental situations.

Supportive therapy. This type of therapy has less ambitious goals and may be especially useful for children and adolescents who do not have satisfying relationships with adults because parents are unavailable or mismatched or the youngsters' symptoms make it difficult to establish a positive relationship. For the patient in crisis, the therapist provides support until a stressor resolves, a developmental crisis has passed, or the patient or environment changes sufficiently so that other adults can take on the supportive role. There is a real relationship with the therapist, who facilitates catharsis and provides understanding and judicious advice.

Time-limited therapy. All of the various models of time-limited therapy have in common a planned, relatively brief duration; a predominant focus on the presenting problem; a high degree of structure and attention to specific, limited goals; and active roles for both therapist and patient. Length of treatment varies among models from several sessions to 6 months. The short duration is used to increase patient motivation, participation, and reliance on resources within the patient's world rather than on the therapist (Kisch 1997). Theoretical foundations include psychodynamic, crisis, family systems, cognitive, behavioral or social learning and guidance, or educational theories (Dulcan 1984; Dulcan and Piercy 1985).

The limited outcome data available indicate that time-limited treatment is at least as effective for some patients as longer-term therapy. These methods have been recommended for both multiproblem families in crisis who are unlikely to persist in longer-term treatment and well-functioning children and families with circumscribed problems of relatively recent onset.

Although time-limited treatment is designed to be brief, children or families may return to a therapist should other problems or symptoms develop for an additional "round" of treatment. Such intermittent interaction can remain problem-focused and reduce dependency on the therapist (Kisch 1997).

A model of interpersonal psychotherapy has been modified for depressed adolescents (IPT-A; Mufson et al. 1994). This 12-week treatment focuses on improving interpersonal relationships in the lives of depressed adolescents through role clarification and enhanced communication. This modality has been elaborated in a treatment manual and has demonstrated efficacy in preliminary study.

Cognitive therapy.   The cognitive therapy techniques developed for the treatment of depression in adults have been adapted for adolescents (Wilkes and Rush 1988). Caution is needed to ensure that homework assignments that are an integral part of this therapy are not perceived as aversive when added to homework assigned in school. Prepubertal children's more concrete cognitive processes may make this rather intellectual model impractical, although creative adaptations and the incorporation of behavioral techniques can render this approach accessible (Emery et al. 1983). Cognitive self-control training may be effective in reducing aggressive behavior in adolescents, although compliance with self-monitoring procedures is often poor (Dangel et al. 1989).

PARENT COUNSELING

Parent counseling or guidance is primarily a psychoeducational intervention, conducted in a mental health setting. It may be conducted with a single parent or couple or in groups. Parents learn about normal child and adolescent development. Efforts are made to help parents understand their child and his or her problems and to modify practices that seem to be contributing to the current difficulties (whatever their original cause). The therapist's understanding of the parents' point of view and of the hardships of living with a disturbed child is crucial. For some

parents who have serious difficulties of their own, parent counseling may merge into or pave the way for individual treatment of the adult or couple.

Virtually all parents of children with psychiatric or learning problems need and deserve education in the nature of their children's disorders and in selecting treatments and managing difficult behaviors. Parents spend far more time with their children than the therapist and can powerfully assist or impede treatment. Parents of children with chronic problems must become skilled advocates to ensure that their children receive the treatment and schooling they need. Carefully selected reading material may be extremely useful to parents (see the appendix to this chapter).

BEHAVIOR THERAPY

In behavior therapy, symptoms are viewed as resulting from bad habits, faulty learning, or inappropriate environmental responses to behavior rather than as stemming from unconscious or intrapsychic motivation. Attention is focused on observable behaviors, psychophysiological responses, and self-report statements. Behavioral approaches are characterized by detailed assessment of problematic responses and the environmental conditions that elicit and maintain them, the development of strategies to produce change in the environment and therefore in the patient's behavior, and repeated assessment to evaluate the success of the intervention.

In an operant approach, positive and negative environmental contingencies that increase and decrease the frequency of behaviors are identified and then modified in an attempt to decrease problem behaviors and increase adaptive ones. The token economy uses points, stars, or tokens that can be earned for desirable behaviors (and lost for problem behaviors) and exchanged for backup reinforcers. These reinforcers may be money, food, toys, privileges, or time with an adult in a pleasant activity. Token economies can be successfully used by parents, teachers, and therapists (with groups or individuals) and by staff on inpatient units.

Social learning theory integrates conditioning theory with cognitive processes and emphasizes the importance of learning by observing or imitating the behavior of others. Modeling of behaviors is used in treating children's anxiety and fears, in decreasing social withdrawal (Kendall and Morison 1984), and in teaching positive skills.

Indications and Efficacy

Behavior therapy is by far the most thoroughly evaluated psychological treatment for children. Maximally effective programs require home and school cooperation, focus on specific target behaviors, and ensure that contingencies follow behavior quickly and consistently.

Behavior therapy is the most effective treatment for simple phobias, for enuresis and encopresis, and for the noncompliant behaviors seen in oppositional defiant disorder and conduct disorder. For youngsters with ADHD, behavior modification can improve both academic achievement and behavior, if specifically targeted. Both punishment (time-out and response cost) and reward components are required. Behavior modification is more effective than medication in improving peer interactions, but skills may need to be taught first. Many youngsters require programs that are consistent, intensive, and prolonged (months to years). A wide variety of other childhood problems, such as motor and vocal tics, trichotillomania, and sleep problems, are treated by behavior modification, either alone or in combination with pharmacotherapy.

The greatest weaknesses of behavior therapy are lack of maintenance of improvement over time and failure of changes to generalize to situations other than the ones in which training occurred. Generalization and maintenance can be maximized by conducting training in the settings in which behavior change is desired, at multiple times and places, facilitating transfer to naturally occurring reinforcers and gradually fading reinforcement on an intermittent schedule (Stokes and Baer 1977).

Parent Management Training

Effective training packages, based on social learning theory, have been developed for parents of noncompliant, oppositional, and aggressive children (Forehand and McMahon 1981; G. R. Patterson 1975) and delinquent adolescents (G. R. Patterson and Forgatch 1987). Such behaviors in children have been found to lead to inappropriately harsh or ineffective parental responses. Through training, parents are taught to give clear instructions, to positively reinforce good behavior, and to use punishment effectively. One frequently used negative contingency is the time-out, so called because it puts the child in a quiet, boring area where there is a time-out from accidental or naturally occurring positive reinforcement. The most powerful parent training programs use a combination of written materials and verbal instruction in social learning principles and contingency management, modeling by the therapist, and behavioral rehearsal of skills to be used. Families with low socioeconomic status, parental psychopathology (such as depression), marital conflict, and lack of a social support network require maximally potent interventions, with attention to parental problems as

necessary. Other families may be able to succeed with written materials only or with manuals supplemented by group lectures.

Behavioral intervention can be done in the context of family therapy in which the family learns how to negotiate and to solve problems together. A key technique is parent-child contingency contracting, which entails a written social contract between parent and child to change behaviors in both parties, with specified contingencies (Blechman 1981).

Classroom Behavior Modification

Techniques for behavior modification in schools include token economies, class rules, and attention to positive behavior, as well as response cost programs in which reinforcers are withdrawn in response to undesirable behavior. Although teachers often resist what they perceive as extra work, an effective program for children with attention and conduct problems required only that teachers observe every 30 minutes whether children were on-task and provide verbal feedback (Pelham and Murphy 1986). Reinforcers such as positive recognition or stars on a chart may be dispensed by teachers or more tangible rewards or privileges by parents through the use of daily report cards. Even special education teachers rarely have sophisticated skills in behavior modification, and therapists may need to work closely with teachers and other school staff to develop appropriate programs.

Behavioral Treatment of Specific Symptoms

Following an evaluation for psychiatric disorders or sexual abuse and a complete medical history, physical examination, and any necessary laboratory tests to rule out a medical disorder, the treatment of choice for enuresis or encopresis is behavioral.

Enuresis. In younger children, especially those who wet only at night, enuresis is largely a consequence of delayed maturation. While waiting for the child to outgrow it, the most useful strategy is to minimize secondary symptoms by discouraging the parents from punishing or ridiculing the child. Older children can be taught to change their own beds, thus reducing expectable negative reactions from parents. A simple monitoring and reward procedure that includes a chart with stars to be exchanged for rewards may be effective for some children who are motivated to stop wetting the bed.

Two additional programs found to be effective in treating nocturnal enuresis are the urine alarm device and dry bed training (DBT). The urine alarm is a conditioning treatment that results in dryness in up to two-thirds of children (Schmitt 1982). The success rate can be increased and relapses minimized by the addition of contingencies for wet and dry nights, diminished gradually once urinary control is achieved (Kaplan et al. 1989). DBT (Azrin et al. 1974) is an equally effective, but somewhat more cumbersome, behavioral program that includes positive practice, contingent response, and the urine alarm in combination. A DBT parent training manual is available (see Azrin and Foxx 1974 under "Enuresis" in the appendix).

Children who are secondarily enuretic (having previously been dry) and those who have accompanying psychiatric problems are more difficult to treat. Other interventions may be necessary before they are motivated to participate in or be responsive to behavioral techniques.

Encopresis.   The treatment of encopresis is somewhat more complex because encopresis frequently results from chronic constipation and stool withholding, which creates physiological consequences requiring medical treatment. In addition, children with encopresis more commonly have associated psychiatric disorders than do those with enuresis.

Behavioral treatment of encopresis must be integrated into a plan that also includes educational and psychological approaches (Levine 1982). Because encopresis often results in stool retention and impaction, an initial bowel cleanout is sometimes required. This regimen is followed by a bowel "retraining" program using oral mineral oil, a high-roughage diet, ample fluid intake, and a mild suppository. The behavioral program focuses on the development of a regular toileting routine with scheduled positive toilet practicing. Behaviors that progressively approximate the appropriate passing of feces in the toilet are rewarded. Routine pants checks followed by contingent positive or negative response are often included. Administration of enemas by parents is contraindicated, as that alone does not improve bowel function and is toxic to the parent-child relationship.

Anxiety disorders.   Desensitization, in vivo or in fantasy, is the treatment of choice for simple phobias, often supplemented by modeling. The principles and techniques are essentially the same as those used with adults, with modification for developmental level. In vivo desensitization, often combined with contingency management and parent guidance, may be effective in the treatment of school avoidance (school phobia) resulting from separation anxiety disorder.

Behavioral approaches using exposure and response prevention (E/RP) appear to be effective in the treatment of obsessive-compulsive disorder in children and adolescents.

March et al. (1994) have developed a protocoled, time-limited E/RP treatment that has demonstrated therapeutic effect in an open trial with children and adolescents with OCD. Further research examining this method is under way.

Cognitive-Behavior Modification or Problem-Solving Therapy

Cognitive-behavior modification (CBM) or problem-solving therapy may be administered individually or in a group. The teaching of cognitive strategies such as stepwise problem solving and self-monitoring is combined with the behavior modification techniques of contingent reinforcement and modeling. CBM was developed in an attempt to improve the generalization and durability of behavior modification techniques. CBM is theoretically appealing because it directly addresses presumed deficits in control of impulsivity and problem solving and provides a structure for work with children who would otherwise gain little benefit from therapy.

Although early studies of CBM with aggressive, impulsive, and hyperactive children found improvement on measures of cognitive impulsivity and social behavior, subsequent results in hyperactive children have been disappointing and have not demonstrated that CBM improves outcome when added to stimulant medication (Abikoff 1985). Possible reasons for this lack of improvement are inappropriate patient selection, lack of attention to generalization, omission of behavioral contingencies from the training, and insufficiently intensive and extensive training. Problem-solving skills training has been shown to be additive to milieu treatment and superior to conventional individual therapy in improving the behavior of hospitalized children with conduct problems (Kazdin et al. 1987). Cognitive-behavioral techniques also are used for the treatment of socially isolated and anxious children (Kane and Kendall 1989; Kendall and Morison 1984).

Behavioral Medicine Techniques

Behavioral methods can be used to treat somatic symptoms. These interventions should be carried out in collaboration with the primary physician and any necessary medical specialists. Children are just as sensitive as adults are to implications that their symptoms are not "real," so care must be taken to explain the interaction of psychological processes and physical symptoms and to develop a working alliance.

A variety of techniques have been used for children, in much the same way as for adults, but with adaptations for the children's level of cognitive or emotional development.

Especially important is an understanding of any misconceptions youngsters may have about the disease state and its treatment. These notions vary according to a patient's stage of cognitive development and his or her unique experience.

Hypnotherapy. Children are more hypnotizable than are adults (Williams 1979). Although hypnosis is occasionally used to facilitate insight in dynamic psychotherapy or to remove a behavioral symptom or habit, for children the most common uses of hypnosis are in the treatment of physical symptoms with a psychological component or to help a child manage pain or nausea associated with a physical disorder or its treatment. Successful use of hypnosis to reduce pain and anxiety has not been reported in children younger than age 6 years (Varni et al. 1986).

Relaxation training. Four types of relaxation procedures are applicable to children and adolescents: progressive muscle relaxation, meditative breathing, autogenics (i.e., silently repeating commands or statements), and imagery-based techniques (Masek et al. 1984). The choice is determined by the characteristics of the child or adolescent and of the disorder being treated. For example, asthmatic children or adolescents may have difficulty using breathing techniques. Imagery may fit particularly well with most children's interest in fantasy. Relaxation training has been used in the treatment of pediatric migraine, juvenile rheumatoid arthritis, and hemophilia. These techniques, also called cognitive-behavioral self-regulation of pain perception, can result not only in decreased subjective experience of pain and reduced need for analgesics, but also in improved mood, self-esteem, and physical and social functioning (Varni et al. 1986). Similar techniques also have been used in the treatment of children and adolescents with asthma or cystic fibrosis.

Pain behavior management. The strategy of pain behavior management is to use operant techniques in the treatment of chronic pain. For example, the antecedents and consequences of headaches are determined by observation and by keeping a pain diary (if the child is old enough), and then attempts are made to modify those situations and events that seem to precipitate or positively reinforce pain as the therapist works with the patient, parents, teachers, pediatrician, and significant others. Emphasis is placed on stress management techniques (Masek et al. 1984) and on functioning normally despite pain. With reduced pain and pain-related behaviors, patients experience an increased sense of control and mastery and an increase in age-appropriate positive activities

(Varni et al. 1986). These techniques have been adapted to the treatment of respiratory symptoms in children and adolescents with asthma or cystic fibrosis.

Stress inoculation. Stress inoculation is a multicomponent cognitive-behavioral approach that combines education, modeling procedures, systematic desensitization, hypnosis, contingency management, and training and practice in coping skills such as imagery and breathing exercises. It is useful in preventing stress and anxiety in children before medical and dental procedures and in chronically ill children for reducing anxiety, pain, or other discomfort related to repeated procedures such as spinal taps, bone marrow aspirations, and chemotherapy injections. Before a therapist implements such a program, the medical procedure is analyzed in detail, including the rationale, details of the procedure and its sensations and side effects, and portions likely to be perceived as uncomfortable or frightening. Also important are the characteristics and previous direct or vicarious experience of the patient (Melamed et al. 1984; Varni et al. 1986).

FAMILY TREATMENT

Attempts to treat children and adolescents without considering the persons with whom they live and the patients' relationships with other significant persons are doomed to failure. Any change in one family member, whether resulting from a psychiatric disorder, psychiatric treatment, a normal developmental process, or an outside event, is likely to produce change in other family members and in their relationships. Family constellations vary widely from the traditional nuclear family, to single-parent family, a blended or step-family, an adoptive or foster family, or a group home. The term *parents* in this chapter applies to adults filling the parenting role, whatever their actual relationship to the patient.

Evaluation of Families

Data should be gathered on each person living with the patient, as well as on others who may be important or have been so in the past (e.g., noncustodial parents, grandparents, or siblings who are no longer living at home). It is often useful to have at least one session that includes all significant family members. For families with young children, techniques such as the use of family drawings or puppet play or the assignment of family tasks to be carried out in the session are often useful. A variety of schemas exist by which to assess a family's structure and dynamic functioning.

TABLE 35–9.   Family tasks

- Forming a "marital coalition" to meet the needs of the adults for intimacy, sexuality, and emotional support
- Establishing a parental coalition capable of flexible relationships with the children and presenting a consistent disciplinary front
- Nurturance, enculturation, and emancipation of children
- Coping with crisis

Source.   Adapted from Fleck 1976.

The family's developmental stage offers a clue to predictable transitional crises as children are born, become adolescents, and are launched from the nuclear family (Carter and McGoldrick 1980). Important tasks for all families are listed in Table 35–9.

The McMaster Model (developed by Epstein and his colleagues at McMaster University in Hamilton, Ontario) focuses on the family's current functioning in regard to problem solving, communication, suitability of family roles, ability of family members to respond appropriately to emotional stimuli, extent to which family members are involved in and value each other's interests and activities, and style and success of controlling behavior of family members (Barker 1981).

Tasks of the initial session of a family assessment include establishing an alliance with family members; gathering data by direct questions, by observing, and by assessing the impact of trial interventions; and proposing a provisional plan for treatment.

Family Therapy

In the most general sense, family therapy is psychological treatment conducted with an identified patient and at least one biological or functional (i.e., by marriage, adoption, and so forth) family member. Related techniques include therapy with an individual patient that takes a family systems perspective or therapy sessions with family members other than the identified patient, based on noncompliance with treatment, severity of illness, or other factors. Some family therapists insist that all family members attend sessions, but this requirement can be unnecessarily rigid in some cases. Family therapy addresses primarily the interaction *among* family members rather than the processes *within* an individual.

Although some advocate family therapy as the best and only treatment for all disorders, most clinicians would agree that there are some situations in which family therapy is preferred over other treatments, others in which it should be combined with other treatments, and still others

in which it is not possible or is relatively contraindicated. Research on this topic is limited, so accumulated clinical judgment and experience must prevail.

Family therapy may be particularly useful when there are dysfunctional interactions or impaired communication within the family, especially when these appear to be related to the presenting problem. It also may be useful when symptoms seem to have been precipitated by difficulty with a developmental stage for an individual or the family or by a change in the family such as divorce or remarriage. If more than one family member is symptomatic, family therapy may be both more efficient and more effective than multiple individual treatments. Family therapy should be considered when one family member improves with treatment but another, not in treatment, worsens. In any case, the family must have, or be induced to have, sufficient motivation to participate. When the identified patient is relatively unmotivated to participate or to change, family therapy is likely to be more effective than individual therapy. Attention to family systems issues also may be useful when progress is blocked in individual therapy or in behavior therapy.

Family therapy is contraindicated as a sole treatment method in cases of clearly organic physical or mental illness or if the family equilibrium is precarious and one or more family members are at serious risk of decompensation. In these situations, family therapy may be useful in combination with other treatments, such as medication or hospitalization. It is counterproductive to include in family therapy sessions a patient who is acutely psychotic, violent, or delusional regarding the family. Family sessions may not be helpful when a parent has severe, intractable, or minimally relevant psychopathology or when the child strongly prefers individual treatment. Children should not be included in sessions in which parents persist (despite redirection) in criticizing the children or in sharing inappropriate information, when the most critical need is marital therapy, or when parents primarily need specific, concrete help with practical affairs.

A variety of family therapies are considered when treating children and adolescents (Table 35–10).

Structural therapy.   Structural therapy has been the model most used and studied when a child or adolescent is the identified patient. Developed by Salvador Minuchin

TABLE 35–10.   Models of family therapy

- Structural	- Behavioral
- Multigenerational	- Psychoeducational
- Strategic	- Multiple family group

and his colleagues at the Philadelphia Child Guidance Clinic, it has been used extensively with families of children and adolescents with eating disorders and psychophysiological disorders such as asthma. Focus is on the present, in which the identified patient's symptoms are presumed to serve a function for the family. The process of assessment includes mapping patterns of communication and the structure of the family, including the location and permeability of boundaries between family members and around the family and its subsystems. Other important variables are the character and flexibility of alignments of family members, including alliances (joining together of two or more members in a common interest or task) and coalitions (joint actions directed against one or more family members). Data are gathered on the distribution of power within the family and on the family's sources of stress and support in the environment.

The therapist uses assigned tasks and his or her interactions with family members to provoke change in the family structure and thereby its functioning. When the symptom is no longer needed, it disappears. Relabeling (i.e., redefining a behavior or symptom to have a different, less negative meaning) opens alternative pathways for family interactions.

Multigenerational family therapy. Pioneered by Murray Bowen, multigenerational family therapy emphasizes how current patterns in families are repetitions of the past. Change results from insights gained in the exploration of parents' families of origin and the relationships over several generations of the nuclear family to the extended family. Grandparents are often involved indirectly or even included in sessions.

Strategic family therapy. Strategic family therapy, developed by Haley and by Palazolli and her colleagues, produces change through a complex and indirect plan of action that is not fully shared with the family. In practice, paradoxical instructions are devised to upset the family equilibrium and permit change, especially in families resistant to more straightforward techniques. This potentially powerful model should be used only by experienced therapists.

Behavioral family therapy. Models of behavioral family therapy include G. R. Patterson's (1975), based on social learning theory, and Alexander's functional family therapy, both of which are used in the treatment of children and adolescents with conduct disorder. Henggeler and Borduin (1990) extended this model to a multisystemic approach that uses energetic outreach into the home, neighborhood, and school and adds peer group and school-based interventions to family treatment of adolescent delinquents.

Psychoeducational family therapy. A psychoeducational approach to family therapy has been most extensively developed in the treatment of families of adult schizophrenic patients (C. M. Anderson et al. 1980), but it has been extended to a number of childhood disorders, such as eating disorders, ADHD, and depression. Detailed didactic presentations about the disorder, in the setting of a multiple family group, are designed to improve the family's coping skills through increased understanding of the illness and its treatment, to teach home behavior management techniques, and to enhance family support networks. Ongoing treatment of individual families includes family systems interventions when educational and behavioral techniques are blocked by dysfunctional family structures or processes. The identified patient is included in family sessions when his or her clinical status permits.

Multiple family therapy. The multifamily approach combines features of group and family therapy. Sessions include three to five families with similar problems who may be isolated from other supports and who can benefit from the interaction with other families.

GROUP THERAPY

Indications

Group therapy is particularly appropriate for children, who are often more willing to reveal their thoughts and feelings to peers than to adults. Establishing rewarding social relationships, a crucial developmental task for children of all ages, is especially difficult for those youths with a psychiatric disorder. Group therapy offers unparalleled opportunities for the clinician to evaluate youths' behavior with peers, to model and facilitate practice of important skills, and to provide youngsters with companionship and mutual support. Interventions by peers may be far more acute and powerful in their effect than those by an adult therapist. An additional benefit is the larger number of patients who can benefit from limited therapist time.

Target symptoms include absent or conflictual peer relationships, aggression, withdrawal, timidity, difficulty with separation, and deficient social interactive or problem-solving skills. These problems often are not apparent or accessible to intervention in individual therapy sessions. Group therapy can be a powerful modality in the treatment of adolescents with eating disorders or substance abuse.

On the negative side, forming an outpatient group is often tedious and time consuming. Diverse schedules and lack of transportation make gathering a sufficient number of patients difficult. More space and preparation are required than for individual or family therapy.

Group psychotherapy is contraindicated for those who are acutely psychotic, paranoid, or actively suicidal. Adolescents with sociopathic traits or behaviors should not be included in groups with teenagers who might be victimized or intimidated. Severely aggressive or hyperactive children probably should not be included in outpatient groups because of the difficulty in controlling their behavior, the contagion of problem behaviors, and the intimidation of less assertive children. Groups should *not* be used as a repository for unmotivated, nonverbal, difficult patients.

Although group therapy may be used as the sole treatment modality, it is often used in combination with another intervention. Groups also may serve an evaluation function, particularly for preschool- and school-age children (Scheidlinger 1984).

Technical Considerations

Theoretical models. All of the theoretical models used in individual therapy may be used with groups. Therapy may be exclusively verbal, or it may include expressive arts techniques, psychodrama, arts and crafts, and sports activities; behavioral techniques such as modeling or overt practice; or cognitive-behavioral strategies for depression (Lewinsohn et al. 1990). The skilled group therapist has an understanding of systems theory and group process, whatever the model of intervention. Contingency management (i.e., rewards and consequences) may be an essential adjunct for groups that include children with behavior disorders.

Group size. Groups range from 4 to 10 patients, with the number varying according to the number of leaders, the age and type of pathology of the group members, and the number of suitable candidates available.

Group composition. The composition of the group depends on its purpose. Patients in support groups are chosen because they share a single stressor—for example, sexual abuse, parental divorce, or chronic physical illness. Other groups are specifically targeted to a single disorder. Groups that focus on social skills work best with a mixture of patients.

Groups that are conducted with patients in special schools, inpatient units, or day hospitals typically include all children or adolescents enrolled in the program, although the patients may be divided by age or level of functioning. Special topic groups, such as treatment of substance abuse, or predischarge groups also may be offered in these settings.

It is useful for the group therapist to interview prospective group members individually, to assess suitability for the group, to orient patients to the goals and methods of the group, to learn more about the children or adolescents, and to begin to develop a therapeutic alliance between the patients and the leader. It also is helpful to interview the parent(s) for similar reasons. The younger the child, the more important is parental cooperation.

Group members should be in the same or adjacent developmental stage. Children change so dramatically as they develop that an age span broader than 2–3 years is unlikely to result in a therapeutic group process. In forming groups for pre- and early adolescents, developmental stage is often more important than chronological age because girls are approximately 2 years ahead of boys in physical and social development, and there is great variability among youngsters of the same sex. The dynamic issues differ at various developmental stages.

Opinions on the mixing of boys and girls differ. Although some issues are easier to handle in single-sex groups, children and adolescents need to learn to get along with the opposite sex in school and in the neighborhood and often with siblings. Therefore, mixing boys and girls, although initially more difficult, may be productive.

Frequency, duration, and goals. For convenience, outpatient groups typically meet once a week. Frequency of group meetings on inpatient units varies from one to seven times per week. Groups may have a defined, limited duration from several months to an academic year or may be open-ended. Short-term groups focus on "current and explicit behavior, adaptation, coping, competency, strengths and growth . . . [with] emphasis on the dynamics of the 'here-and-now' corrective emotional experience, [and] on the patients' active participation in the change effort. . . . " (Scheidlinger 1984, p. 581). Long-term groups are more likely to aim for the promotion of insight, the resolution of unconscious conflicts, and the removal of developmental arrests. Although there are exceptions, short-term groups generally have a defined membership, with no new members added once the group begins. Long-term groups more often have changing membership, with patients entering and leaving as their clinical status dictates.

Group leadership. Of all modalities of therapy, the need for cotherapists is most clear in group treatment.

Groups are complex, with many events occurring simultaneously, and a second observer is valuable. This arrangement also allows continuity of treatment when one leader needs to be absent. In groups of younger children, an extra pair of hands is needed. Coleaders who differ in age, sex, race, and ethnicity expand the opportunity for different types of patient-therapist relationships.

Group rules. The nature of the group and the patients determines the optimal degree of structure. A psychodynamically oriented group composed of depressed or anxious adolescents will need far fewer rules than a group whose goal is to teach social skills to school-age boys with conduct problems. The leaders are responsible for maintaining control of behavior within the group. At times, this control may even require strategies such as the time-out.

The leader(s) must make explicit the rules of confidentiality for the group, as the group setting expands the risk of breach of confidentiality to include the patients' peers. This breach is of most concern to adolescents and preadolescents.

Family contact. Involving parents is especially important for preschool- and school-age children to discover important events in the children's lives and to assess progress. Adolescents are more willing and able to report and are also more sensitive to confidentiality issues. All parents should be kept apprised of the goals of the group, both in general and specifically for their child. Parent education in development and behavior management can be provided efficiently by grouping parents together. Parents also may appreciate the opportunity to meet with others whose children have similar problems.

Developmental Issues

Preschool-age groups. Young children are less able to verbalize and thus require more structure and planned activities. A group can provide a powerful context for the teaching of social skills and language, especially for children who are autistic or severely delayed.

School-age groups. Because school-age children have great difficulty bringing in outside material for discussion or engaging in introspection, verbal portions of the group are best focused on events that occur in the group itself. Games and craft activities can provide a useful framework, but the leaders must ensure that recreation does not become the only function of the group. Behavior modification and cognitive problem-solving techniques are especially useful for children this age.

Many child patients will not spontaneously attempt to relate to other children. Others have been rejected or scapegoated by peers. If the group is successful, the children will use the skills they have learned to form relationships with peers at school and in their neighborhoods.

Children with ADHD are often referred to group therapy because of their difficulty with peer relations and their lack of insight into their difficulties. Those children who are being treated with stimulant medication should receive a dose before the group meets to help them benefit from the therapy and not disrupt it for others.

Adolescent groups. Scheidlinger (1985) identifies four major categories of group work with adolescents:

1. *Group psychotherapy:* treatment of a balanced selection of patients, using the group as the primary modality, with goals of relief of psychological distress, modification of pathological modes of functioning, and amelioration of personality dysfunction
2. *Therapeutic groups for patients in mental health, medical, or residential settings:* used as ancillary treatment or as an aid in rehabilitation
3. *Human development and training groups:* offered to youths who are not psychiatric patients and focus on prevention and enrichment
4. *Self-help and mutual help groups:* may or may not have professional leaders and consist of peers working together to satisfy a shared need or overcome a common handicap; extensively used in the treatment of substance abuse

Although activities may be useful, many adolescent groups can be conducted in an exclusively verbal format. If both boys and girls are included in the same group, the leader must be alert to sexual undercurrents and acting out while facilitating the discussion of sexual concerns and practicing of heterosexual social skills (Scheidlinger 1985). To avoid scapegoating, it is important that the proportion of boys to girls not be too unequal.

HOSPITAL AND RESIDENTIAL TREATMENT

Indications

Because children should be treated in the setting that is least restrictive and disruptive to their lives, hospital or residential treatment is indicated only in emergencies or for youngsters who have not responded to efforts at outpatient treatment because of severity of the disorder, lack of motivation, resistance, or disorganization of patients and/or family. Programs vary widely in their criteria for admission.

Placement in a residential treatment center may be indicated for children and adolescents with chronic behavior problems such as aggression, running away, truancy, substance abuse, school phobia, or self-destructive acts that the family, foster home, and/or community cannot manage or tolerate. Some parents harbor negative attitudes toward their children or adolescents or have severe psychopathology of their own. Children for whom it is not advisable to return home—because of factors in the youngsters, their families, or both—may be referred to a residential treatment center following a hospital stay. Because of the increase in managed care environments, admission criteria have become increasingly restricted and lengths of stay have been substantially reduced.

Short-term hospitalization is more often an acute event, stemming from immediate physical danger to self or others, acute psychosis, a crisis in the environment that reduces the ability of the caregiving adults to cope with the child or adolescent, or the need for more intensive, systematic, and detailed evaluation and observation of the patient and family than is possible on an outpatient basis or in a day program. Managed care pressures have forced hospital lengths of stay to decrease significantly, often allowing only clinical stabilization of the patient before his or her discharge from the hospital. Briefer hospitalizations of severely ill child psychiatric patients require well-coordinated transfer to lesser levels of care in the clinical continuum (residential, day, and intensive outpatient treatments) to ensure maintenance of clinical stability.

Longer-term hospitalization may be indicated for those patients who do not improve sufficiently in a brief period and who continue to require a secure setting and intensive treatment.

Efficacy

Systematic outcome evaluation is extremely difficult because of the complexity of the cases and the need for crisis intervention. Controlled studies that would be considered methodologically adequate comparing 24-hour treatment with no treatment or other types of treatment may not even be ethical or feasible. In general, more severely ill patients with fewer individual and family resources have a poorer outcome.

Differences in Settings

Residential treatment centers, compared with hospital units, tend to be longer term, tend to be more open to and integrated with the community, and tend not to use the medical model. Usually, residential centers have a lower staff-to-patient ratio and less highly trained personnel. These centers are more likely to be organized based on a family group model and organized by sections or cottages.

Facilities may be under the auspices of a state, county, or city; part of a medical school; or in a private, a nonprofit, or an investor-owned hospital. Inpatient units may be located in a general hospital, pediatric specialty hospital, or psychiatric hospital. Most settings separate children and adolescents, but others mix age groups. A relatively recent development is the psychosomatic or pediatric medical-psychiatric unit for children and adolescents with coexisting physical and psychiatric problems.

Some units are locked and can accommodate involuntary patients, as well as runaways, and highly impulsive, psychotic, or actively suicidal youths who require more security. Other units are open and admit only voluntary patients. Intensity of staffing varies widely. Units that are part of a medical school are the most intensively staffed because of the presence of a variety of trainees. Programs operated by state or county governments often have fewer professional staff because of budget restraints and problems in recruiting.

Inpatient units for children can be classified according to the usual length of stay on such units. The lengths of stay on brief-stay or crisis intervention units average 1–2 weeks. These units emphasize rapid evaluation, triage, stabilization, and development of a treatment plan that will be implemented on an outpatient basis or in another facility. Stays on intermediate units last several weeks to months, and more definitive treatment can be conducted. Children may stay on long-term units from several months to longer than 1 year. On these units, care for the most severely impaired youth is provided. Increasing financial pressures have resulted in reduced overall lengths of stay in all types of units.

Treatment Planning

Ideally, hospitalization forms part of a comprehensive continuum of care for children. With ever-shorter lengths of stay, rapid and efficient planning and execution of evaluation and treatment strategies are essential. The goal is not to eliminate all psychopathology but to address the "focal problem" that precipitated hospitalization and then to discharge the patient to home, residential treatment, or foster placement, where he or she can receive outpatient or day treatment (Harper 1989).

Components of Treatment

The relative emphasis placed on each treatment modality differs according to the philosophy of treatment, the nature of the patient population, the usual length of stay, and the availability of highly specialized staff. All of the following should be present in some form.

Psychopharmacology. Hospitalization offers an ideal opportunity for systematic trials of medication in children or adolescents who have not responded to conventional treatment, who are diagnostically puzzling, who have medical problems complicating pharmacotherapy, or whose parents are noncompliant, disorganized, or unreliable reporters of efficacy or side effects. Systematic drug trials for individual patients can be designed using single- or double-blind methods evaluated by observations on the ward and in the classroom. As-needed (i.e., prn) medications, used to control aggression or other behavior problems, should be used only for brief periods until more effective, ongoing treatments are begun.

Individual psychotherapy. As newer treatment methods evolve and hospital stays become ever shorter, individual psychotherapy is less often a primary treatment modality than in the past. However, regularly scheduled individual sessions with a therapist with whom the child or adolescent can develop a special relationship continue to be essential in developing a more complete understanding of the patient's intrapsychic, familial, and social dynamics and in assisting him or her to develop more adaptive methods of coping with strong emotions. The therapist may be able to help the patient to deal with past traumas and losses, to better understand his or her current difficulties, and to make use of the other treatments offered. The confidentiality that is usual in outpatient therapy is not present in a hospital or residential setting, since all staff participate as a treatment team.

Milieu therapy. Milieu therapy includes the total environment of a structured schedule for meals, sleep, and so forth and a program of activities. The patient can be observed over an extended period of time in school, free play with peers, meals, sleep, and self-care. In the most effective milieus, all activities and interactions with staff are consistent with the treatment plan. Goals of the milieu include promoting a feeling of security, by clarity of rules and regularity of schedule, and increased self-esteem and competence through learning of skills. Most settings include a token economy or levels program, which also may be used for specific treatment, for management of behavior (e.g., encouraging a patient with anorexia nervosa to eat).

Group therapy. In addition to general or special topic groups (e.g., 12-step models, survivors of abuse), group therapy may include community meetings in which privileges and rules are decided, social skills are practiced, and patients learn to observe their own and others' behavior and to recognize the impact of their behavior on others.

Education. Virtually all children who require psychiatric hospitalization have had problems in school. The small classes and highly trained teachers of a hospital unit can provide a detailed evaluation of a youngster's academic strengths and weaknesses, incorporating data from intelligence and achievement tests and special tests for learning disabilities into direct observation of classroom behavior and learning. Educational strategies can be developed and tested. One of the most important parts of discharge planning is arranging for an appropriate educational placement and working with the new teacher to continue progress made in the hospital. The hospitalization often allows child or adolescent patients their first opportunity to experience academic success.

Many residential treatment centers have their own schools on the centers' grounds. As youngsters improve, they are gradually integrated into special education or mainstream programs in local public or private schools.

Family treatment. Work with families is an essential part of hospital treatment, including intensive evaluation of family functioning and deciding where the child should reside. Interventions may include family therapy, parent counseling in behavior management, and education about the nature of their child's disorder. Parents may require marital therapy, individual medical or psychiatric assessment and treatment, or help with housing or income.

Additional services. Medical evaluation and treatment must be provided. The following more specialized resources should be available through consultation as necessary: neurological evaluation and treatment, speech and language assessment and therapy, physical therapy, and occupational therapy.

Disposition planning and aftercare. Disposition planning and follow-up may be the most important parts of the treatment if gains made are to be maintained and continued. A complete disposition plan includes consideration of where the child should live, school placement, and continuation of individual therapy, family therapy, and/or pharmacotherapy.

DAY TREATMENT

Indications

A day program may be best for the child who requires more intensive intervention than can be provided in outpatient visits but who is able to live at home. Day treatment is less disruptive to the patient and family than hospitalization or residential placement and can offer an opportunity for more intensive work with parents, who may even attend the program on a regular basis. A day program may be used as a transition for a child who has been hospitalized or to avert a hospitalization. It may be implemented in combination with placement in a foster or group home.

Programs

Some programs involve a full day, 5 days a week, and include a school or therapeutic nursery school program. There are decided advantages in being able to integrate the treatment plan and therapeutic focus into the entire day. Other programs may meet in the late afternoon and evening hours, after patients attend community schools. It is desirable to offer all of the treatment modalities that are available on an inpatient unit.

Innovative, intensive summer treatment programs have been developed for children with ADHD and associated behavior and learning problems (Pelham and Hoza 1987). These programs provide positive social and recreational experiences for children who otherwise would not be able to participate in camp, while teaching parents behavior modification techniques, supplementing classroom work, and rigorously assessing medication efficacy and side effects.

ADJUNCTIVE TREATMENTS

At times, an intervention that is not a psychiatric treatment may be recommended as part of a treatment plan. These programs may be crucial for the child's well-being and/or the treatment of the psychiatric disorder, or they may be facilitative, speeding progress or improving level of function.

PARENT SUPPORT GROUPS

Parents of children with psychiatric disorders, together with mental health professionals and teachers, have established groups that provide education and support for parents, as well as advocacy for services and fund-raising for research. National organizations with local chapters include Parents Anonymous, for abusive or potentially abusive parents; the Association for Retarded Citizens; the Autism Society of America; Children with Attention Deficit Disorders (CHADD); and the Learning Disabilities Association of America. Recently, the National Alliance for the Mentally Ill (NAMI) established a Child and Adolescent Network (NAMI-CAN) as its concerns broadened to include children and adolescents. Local groups focused on a particular disorder or on more generic issues can provide a powerful adjunct to direct clinical services.

SPECIAL EDUCATION

Modified school programs are indicated for those children who cannot perform satisfactorily in regular classrooms or who need special structure or teaching techniques to reach their academic potential. These programs range in intensity from tutoring or resource classrooms several hours a week, to special classrooms in mainstream schools, to public or private schools that serve only children with special educational needs. Resources differ from community to community, but most communities have programs for mentally retarded youth, for those with learning disabilities (specific developmental disorders), and for those whose emotional and/or behavioral problems require a special setting for learning or for the control of their behavior. Classes are small, with a high teacher-to-student ratio and teachers who are specially trained.

Before being placed in a special class, youngsters must have an individually administered battery of psychological tests, including an intelligence test, achievement tests, and an evaluation for learning disabilities. Federal law requires that all children who need them receive special services and that services be provided in the least-restrictive environment (i.e., as much in the mainstream with other children and adolescents as possible).

Boarding schools may be useful when there is a problem between parent and child that is unresponsive to treatment. Some of these schools have special programs for children with learning disabilities or psychiatric disorders.

RECREATION

Learning a sport or skill at which one can do well is an important adjunct in the treatment of a child who lacks positive relationships with peers or adults because of social isolation or withdrawal or who is ignored or actively rejected. A relationship with an adult such as a Big Brother or a Young Men's Christian Association (YMCA) counselor, and an opportunity to interact with a normal peer group under supervision, may provide support and build self-esteem until the child is sufficiently improved to establish relationships independently. Some families have employed a high school or college student one or more afternoons a week to teach social and play skills, develop a relationship, and provide structured time. This approach also gives parents a respite and an opportunity to spend time with their other children.

Day or overnight summer camps may present opportunities for psychological growth in multiple domains. Some youngsters can attend regular camp, whereas others need a special program for children and adolescents with psychiatric or medical problems.

FOSTER CARE

Placement in a foster home may be needed when parents are unwilling or unable to care for a child. Indications are clearest in cases of physical neglect or physical or sexual abuse. Other families may be unable to provide the appropriate emotional or physical environment. Court intervention is required for placement. Although foster placement can be a suitable and effective intervention, children in foster care may have a variety of unmet physical, developmental, and mental health needs, often making foster care less than optimal and clearly unsatisfactory as a long-term solution (Rosenfeld et al. 1997). Unfortunately, child welfare agencies in many communities are overwhelmed, and children and adolescents may require advocacy either to accomplish removal from home to a foster placement or for termination of foster placement and return to parents, group home placement, or release for adoption.

Children with severe behavioral or physical problems, or older adolescents who are difficult to place or maintain in foster or adoptive homes, may be admitted to group homes. These homes vary in staffing and intensity of their programs. Some approach residential treatment, whereas others simply provide a supervised residence.

DIETARY TREATMENTS

Since the mid-1970s, advocates of dietary treatment of behavioral problems have been remarkably persistent, despite the lack of scientific evidence. A variety of food additives and food allergens have been proposed as contributory or even causal in childhood behavior disorders, especially hyperactivity and autism. Reviews of the methodologically adequate studies show that, at most, 5% of hyperactive children may show behavioral or cognitive improvement on the Kaiser-Permanente Diet, but these changes are not as dramatic as those induced by stimulants (Wender 1986). The only characteristic associated with greater likelihood of response is age less than 6 years. There are no data to support dietary treatments for autism.

Parents and primary care practitioners find dietary treatment appealing because it is more "natural" than medication. However, special diets demand extra work and often additional expense from a family already disrupted by a child's behavior problems. Given the minimal evidence of efficacy and the extreme difficulty inducing children to comply with restricted diets, such diets should not be recommended. Families who insist on trying a diet should be permitted to do so, provided the diet is nutritionally sound, because initial attempts to dissuade them may disrupt the therapeutic alliance.

Controlled studies have been unable to demonstrate that ingesting sugar has an effect on activity or aggression in healthy or hyperactive children, even those identified by their parents as sugar responsive (Milich et al. 1986; Wender and Solanto 1991). Clinically insignificant effects on attention have been demonstrated only in young children and only after a high-carbohydrate breakfast (Wender and Solanto 1991).

Caffeine, in the form of coffee or cola, has been popularly recommended by nonprofessionals for the treatment of hyperactivity, despite significant side effects and no demonstration of efficacy.

Megavitamin therapy, the prescription of vitamins in quantities greatly in excess of the recommended daily allowance (RDA) guidelines, has been suggested as a treatment for schizophrenia, autism, hyperactivity, and learning disabilities. Extreme claims have been made from uncontrolled studies. Not only is scientific evidence of effectiveness lacking, but toxic effects also are possible (Harley 1980). Parents, particularly those of autistic children, may pursue this treatment out of desperation.

INTEGRATION OF MULTIPLE MODALITIES

Sophisticated simultaneous or sequential use of different techniques offers substantial promise of improved treatment outcome. There is a clear need for more power and wider coverage of symptoms than any single treatment alone provides. The following are some examples.

COLLABORATIVE THERAPY

In general, treatment by a single therapist is most efficient and effective. Indications for collaborative treatment (two or more therapists working as a team) in the outpatient setting include a child who is unusually concerned about confidentiality; the need for several different types of skills (e.g., individual psychotherapy, family therapy and pharmacotherapy), which a single therapist does not have; or clear indications for different qualities in a patient's and parent's therapists (e.g., a boy who would benefit from a male role model but whose mother has great difficulty relating to men).

In collaborative treatment, in order to maintain free and open communication and to discuss and agree on treatment plans, it is essential for the therapists to avoid aligning into competitive teams. Conflicts over relative power and authority of the therapists can sabotage treatment. It is fundamentally important that the child and adolescent psychiatrist not allow himself or herself to be relegated solely to the role of pharmacotherapist.

COMBINED TREATMENTS

It is increasingly clear that child psychiatric patients do not benefit from a "purist" approach to treatment that makes use of a single modality. A clinician must be able to weave together flexibly a treatment that draws from psychodynamic, behavioral, family systems, and pharmacotherapeutic approaches in order to address a child's specific disorder at his or her specific developmental level (Lewis 1997).

Combined Psychotherapies

A highly structured and effective model has been developed from a theoretical framework of ego psychoanalytic object-relations theory for children with oppositional or conduct disorders who have some social bonds and a capacity for guilt. Interventions include individual supportive-expressive play psychotherapy, parent training, and play group psychotherapy, according to the child's presenting problems (Kernberg and Chazan 1991).

An ingenious model of child psychotherapy developed by Strayhorn (1988) makes explicit the identification of "psychological skills" or competencies expected for the child's age that are lacking. In this model, specific interventions are designed to address the missing skills, including verbal and play therapy, education of child and parent, and behavioral techniques such as modeling and contingency management.

Medication Plus Psychotherapeutic Intervention

Traditionally, the use of medications and psychotherapy was seen as an either-or phenomenon in which proponents of either modality saw their own as more valuable and the other as unnecessary or even harmful. Increasingly, we are aware of the potential synergistic effect from combining medication with psychotherapeutic interventions, as these treatments may address different aspects of a single disorder (O'Brien and Perlmutter 1997).

Attention-deficit/hyperactivity disorder. The implementation of a multimodal treatment for ADHD has traditionally been clinically encouraged. Such treatment combines medication management (most often stimulants), behavioral interventions, parent management training, appropriate school placement and school-based interventions, as well as child-focused treatments (psychotherapy, cognitive-behavioral treatment, and social skills training). More recent reports have questioned the benefit of multimodal treatment over medication alone (American Academy of Child and Adolescent Psychiatry Work Group on Quality Issues 1997a). An ongoing, multicenter study examining the long-term benefit of multimodal treatments for ADHD should assist in clarifying this issue (Richters et al. 1995).

Autistic disorder. Children with autism require a comprehensive therapeutic plan that may include psychoeducation of the parents and family, special education placement, speech and language therapies, behavioral management approaches, social skills training, and pharmacotherapy. An individualized treatment should take into account the particular deficits of the child, as well as individual and family strengths (M. Campbell et al. 1996).

Depression. Current recommendations for treatment of depression include cognitive-behavior therapy, psychodynamic psychotherapy, parental and family therapies, as well as pharmacotherapy, either alone or in combination (Birmaher et al. 1996). Treatments should be individualized, based upon presumed etiology, severity of illness, and individual/family strengths.

Anxiety disorders. Recently suggested approaches to treatment of older children and adolescents with anxiety disorders include the combined use of cognitive-behavior, psychodynamic, and supportive psychotherapies; family therapy; and pharmacotherapy tailored to the child's clinical needs (Bernstein et al. 1996).

Obsessive-compulsive disorder. The combination of cognitive-behavior therapy and pharmacotherapy appears optimal in the treatment of OCD. One preliminary study suggests that both cognitive-behavior therapy and pharmacotherapy in the treatment of children and adolescents with OCD may be superior to medication alone (March et al. 1994); however, controlled studies are required.

CONCLUSIONS

The treatment of psychiatric disorders in children and adolescents is both an art and a science. Research on assessment and diagnosis, biological correlates of disorders, and outcome of traditional and newly developed techniques will continue to improve the specificity and outcome of treatment. However, a need always will exist for clinical skills in tailoring and applying psychosomatic techniques to individual patients and their families.

REFERENCES

Abbott Laboratories: Press Release: Focus on Cylert, 1996

Abikoff H: Efficacy of cognitive training interventions in hyperactive children: a critical review. Clin Psychol Rev 5: 479–512, 1985

Abnormal Involuntary Movement Scale (AIMS). Psychopharmacol Bull 24:781–783, 1988

Achenbach TM: Manual for the Teacher's Report Form and 1991 Profile. Burlington, VT, University of Vermont, Department of Psychiatry, 1991

Adams PL: A Primer of Child Psychotherapy, Second Edition. Boston, MA, Little, Brown, 1982

Aman MG, Marks RE, Turbott SH, et al: Clinical effects of methylphenidate and thioridazine in intellectually subaverage children. J Am Acad Child Adolesc Psychiatry 30:246–256, 1991

American Academy of Child and Adolescent Psychiatry Work Group on Quality Issues: Practice parameters for the assessment and treatment of conduct disorders. J Am Acad Child Adolesc Psychiatry 31:iv–vii, 1992

American Academy of Child and Adolescent Psychiatry Work Group on Quality Issues: Practice parameters for the assessment and treatment of anxiety disorders. J Am Acad Child Adolesc Psychiatry 32:1089–1098, 1993

American Academy of Child and Adolescent Psychiatry Work Group on Quality Issues: Practice parameters for the psychiatric assessment of children and adolescents. J Am Acad Child Adolesc Psychiatry 34:1386–1402, 1995

American Academy of Child and Adolescent Psychiatry Work Group on Quality Issues: Practice parameters for the assessment and treatment of children, adolescents, and adults with attention-deficit/hyperactivity disorder. J Am Acad Child Adolesc Psychiatry 36:1S–37S, 1997a

American Academy of Child and Adolescent Psychiatry Work Group on Quality Issues: Practice parameters for the forensic evaluation of children and adolescents who may have been physically or sexually abused. J Am Acad Child Adolesc Psychiatry 36:423–442, 1997b

American Academy of Child and Adolescent Psychiatry Work Group on Quality Issues: Practice parameters for the assessment and treatment of children and adolescents with bipolar disorder. J Am Acad Child Adolesc Psychiatry 36:138–157, 1997c

American Psychiatric Association Task Force on ECT: The practice of ECT: recommendations for treatment, training and privileging. Convulsive Therapy 6:85–120, 1990

Anderson CM, Hogarty GE, Reiss DJ: Family treatment of adult schizophrenic patients: a psycho-educational approach. Schizophr Bull 6:490–505, 1980

Anderson LT, Campbell M, Adams P, et al: The effects of haloperidol on discrimination learning and behavioral symptoms in autistic children. J Autism Dev Disord 19:227–239, 1989

Apter A, Ratzoni G, King RA, et al: Fluvoxamine open-label treatment of adolescent inpatients with obsessive-compulsive disorder or depression. J Am Acad Child Adolesc Psychiatry 33:342–348, 1994

Armenteros JL, Whitaker AH, Welikson M, et al: Risperidone in adolescents with schizophrenia: an open pilot study. J Am Acad Child Adolesc Psychiatry 36:694–700, 1997

Azrin NH, Sneed TJ, Foxx RM: Dry-bed training: rapid elimination of childhood enuresis. Behav Res Ther 12:147–156, 1974

Barker P: Basic Family Therapy. Baltimore, MD, University Park Press, 1981

Barrickman LL, Noyes R, Kuperman S, et al: Treatment of ADHD with fluoxetine: a preliminary trial. J Am Acad Child Adolesc Psychiatry 30:762–767, 1991

Barrickman LL, Perry PJ, Allen AJ, et al: Bupropion versus methylphenidate in the treatment of attention-deficit hyperactivity disorder. J Am Acad Child Adolesc Psychiatry 34:649–657, 1995

Bastiaens L: Knowledge, expectations and attitudes of hospitalized children and adolescents in psychopharmacological treatment. J Child Adolesc Psychopharmacol 3:157–171, 1992

Bastiaens L: Compliance with pharmacotherapy in adolescents: effects of patients' and parents' knowledge and attitudes toward treatment. J Child Adolesc Psychopharmacol 5:39–48, 1995

Bastiaens L, Bastiaens DK: A manual of psychiatric medications for teenagers. J Child Adolesc Psychopharmacol 3:M1–M59, 1993

Bernstein GA, Garfinkel BD, Borchardt CM: Comparative studies of pharmacotherapy for school refusal. J Am Acad Child Adolesc Psychiatry 29:773–781, 1990

Bernstein GA, Borchardt CM, Perwien AR: Anxiety disorders in children and adolescents: a review of the past 10 years. J Am Acad Child Adolesc Psychiatry 35:1110–1119, 1996

Bertagnoli MW, Borchardt CM: A review of ECT for children and adolescents. J Am Acad Child Adolesc Psychiatry 29:302–307, 1990

Biederman J: Clonazepam in the treatment of prepubertal children with panic-like symptoms. J Clin Psychiatry 48 (suppl):38–41, 1987

Biederman J: Sudden death in children treated with a tricyclic antidepressant. J Am Acad Child Adolesc Psychiatry 30:495–498, 1991

Biederman J, Baldessarini RJ, Wright V, et al: A double-blind placebo controlled study of desipramine in the treatment of ADD, I: efficacy. J Am Acad Child Adolesc Psychiatry 28:777–784, 1989

Birmaher B, Quintana H, Greenhill LL: Methylphenidate treatment of hyperactive autistic children. J Am Acad Child Adolesc Psychiatry 27:248–251, 1988

Birmaher B, Greenhill LL, Cooper TB, et al: Sustained release methylphenidate: pharmacokinetic studies in ADHD males. J Am Acad Child Adolesc Psychiatry 28:768–772, 1989

Birmaher B, Waterman GS, Ryan N, et al: Fluoxetine for childhood anxiety disorders. J Am Acad Child Adolesc Psychiatry 33:993–999, 1994

Birmaher B, Ryan ND, Williamson DE, et al: Childhood and adolescent depression: a review of the past 10 years, II. J Am Acad Child Adolesc Psychiatry 35:1575–1583, 1996

Black B, Robbins DR: Case study: panic disorder in children and adolescents. J Am Acad Child Adolesc Psychiatry 29:36–44, 1989

Black B, Uhde TW: Treatment of elective mutism with fluoxetine: a double-blind, placebo-controlled study. J Am Acad Child Adolesc Psychiatry 33:1000–1006, 1994

Blechman EA: Toward comprehensive behavioral family intervention: an algorithm for matching families and interventions. Behav Modif 5:221–236, 1981

Bleiberg E, Fonagy P, Target M: Child psychoanalysis: critical overview and a proposed reconsideration. Child Adolesc Psychiatr Clin N Am 6:1–38, 1997

Boulos C, Kutcher S, Gardner D, et al: An open naturalistic trial of fluoxetine in adolescents and young adults with treatment-resistant major depression. J Child Adolesc Psychopharmacol 2:103–111, 1992

Brown GL, Ebert MH, Mikkelsen EJ, et al: Behavior and motor activity response in hyperactive children and plasma amphetamine levels following a sustained release preparation. J Am Acad Child Psychiatry 19:225–239, 1980

Brown RT, Sexson SB: Effects of methylphenidate on cardiovascular responses in attention deficit hyperactivity disordered adolescents. Journal of Adolescent Health Care 10:179–183, 1989

Bruun RD, Budman CL: Risperidone as a treatment for Tourette's disorder. J Clin Psychiatry 57:29–31, 1996

Campbell M, Cueva JE: Psychopharmacology in child and adolescent psychiatry: a review of the past seven years, I. J Am Acad Child Adolesc Psychiatry 34:1124–1132, 1995a

Campbell M, Cueva JE: Psychopharmacology in child and adolescent psychiatry: a review of the past seven years, II. J Am Acad Child Adolesc Psychiatry 34:1262–1272, 1995b

Campbell M, Small AM, Green WH, et al: Behavioral efficacy of haloperidol and lithium carbonate. Arch Gen Psychiatry 41:650–656, 1984

Campbell M, Green WH, Deutsch SI: Child and Adolescent Psychopharmacology. Beverly Hills, CA, Sage, 1985

Campbell M, Silva RR, Kafantaris V, et al: Predictors of side effects associated with lithium administration in children. Psychopharmacol Bull 27:373–380, 1991

Campbell M, Anderson LT, Small AM, et al: Naltrexone in autistic children: behavioral symptoms and attentional learning. J Am Acad Child Adolesc Psychiatry 32:1283–1291, 1993

Campbell M, Adams PB, Small AM, et al: Lithium in hospitalized aggressive children with conduct disorder: a double-blind and placebo-controlled study. J Am Acad Child Adolesc Psychiatry 34:445–453, 1995

Campbell M, Schopler E, Cueva JE, et al: Treatment of autistic disorder. J Am Acad Child Adolesc Psychiatry 35:134–143, 1996

Campbell SB: Hyperactivity in preschoolers: correlates and prognostic implications. Clin Psychol Rev 5:405–428, 1985

Cantor S, Kestenbaum C: Psychotherapy with schizophrenic children. Journal of the American Academy of Child Psychiatry 25:623–630, 1986

Cantwell DP, Swanson J, Connor DF: Case study: adverse response to clonidine. J Am Acad Child Adolesc Psychiatry 36:539–544, 1997

Carlson GA, Rapport MD, Kelly KL, et al: The effects of methylphenidate and lithium on attention and activity level. J Am Acad Child Adolesc Psychiatry 31:262–270, 1992

Carter E, McGoldrick M (eds): The Family Life Cycle: A Framework for Family Therapy. New York, Gardner Press, 1980

Casat CD, Pleasants DZ, Van Wyck Fleet J: A double-blind trial of bupropion in children with attention deficit disorder. Psychopharmacol Bull 23:120–122, 1987

Chappell PB, Riddle MA, Scahill L, et al: Guanfacine treatment of comorbid attention-deficit hyperactivity disorder and Tourette's syndrome: preliminary clinical experience. J Am Acad Child Adolesc Psychiatry 34:1140–1146, 1995

Clay TH, Gualtieri CT, Evans RW, et al: Clinical and neuropsychological effects of the novel antidepressant bupropion. Psychopharmacol Bull 24:143–148, 1988

Clein PD, Riddle MA: Pharmacokinetics in children and adolescents. Child Adolesc Psychiatr Clin N Am 4:59–75, 1995

Coffey BJ: Anxiolytics for children and adolescents: traditional and new drugs. J Child Adolesc Psychopharmacol 1:57–83, 1990

Coffey BJ: Ethical issues in child and adolescent psychopharmacology. Child Adolesc Psychiatr Clin N Am 4:793–807, 1995

Coffey BJ, Shader RI, Greenblatt DJ: Pharmacokinetics of benzodiazepines and psychostimulants in children. J Clin Psychopharmacol 3:217–225, 1983

Cohen DJ, Riddle MA, Leckman JF: Pharmacotherapy of Tourette's syndrome and associated disorders. Psychiatr Clin North Am 15:109–129, 1992

Colle LM, Belair JF, DiFeo M, et al: Extended open-label fluoxetine treatment of adolescents with major depression. J Child Adolesc Psychopharmacol 4:225–232, 1994

Como PG, Kurlan R: An open-label trial of fluoxetine for obsessive-compulsive disorder in Gilles de la Tourette's syndrome. Neurology 41:872–874, 1991

Conners CK: Methodological and assessment issues in pediatric psychopharmacology, in Diagnosis and Psychopharmacology of Childhood and Adolescent Disorders. Edited by Wiener JM. New York, Wiley, 1985, pp 69–110

Conners CK, Barkley RA: Rating scales and checklists for child psychopharmacology. Psychopharmacol Bull 21:816–832, 1985

Conners CK, Casat CD, Gualtieri CT, et al: Bupropion hydrochloride in attention deficit disorder with hyperactivity. J Am Acad Child Adolesc Psychiatry 35:1314–1321, 1996

Connor DF: Beta blockers for aggression: a review of the pediatric experience. J Child Adolesc Psychopharmacol 3:99–114, 1993

Connor DF: Nadolol for self-injury, overactivity, inattention, and aggression in a child with pervasive developmental disorder. J Child Adolesc Psychopharmacol 4:101–111, 1994

Cook EH Jr, Rowlett R, Jaselskis C, et al: Fluoxetine treatment of children and adults with autistic disorder and mental retardation. J Am Acad Child Adolesc Psychiatry 31:739–745, 1992

Dangel RF, Deschner JP, Rasp RR: Anger control training for adolescents in residential treatment. Behav Modif 13:447–458, 1989

DeVeaugh-Geiss J, Moroz G, Biederman J, et al: Clomipramine hydrochloride in childhood and adolescent obsessive-compulsive disorder: a multicenter trial. J Am Acad Child Adolesc Psychiatry 31:45–49, 1992

Dulcan MK: Brief psychotherapy with children and their families: the state of the art. Journal of the American Academy of Child Psychiatry 23:544–551, 1984

Dulcan MK (ed): Understanding Drug Medications for Behavioral and Emotional Problems: Guidance for Parents, Youths and Teachers. Washington, DC, American Psychiatric Press, 1998

Dulcan MK, Martini DR: Concise Guide to Child and Adolescent Psychiatry, Second Edition. Washington, DC, American Psychiatric Press, 1998

Dulcan MK, Piercy PA: A model for teaching and evaluating brief psychotherapy with children and their families. Professional Psychology: Research and Practice 16:689–700, 1985

Edelbrock CS: Child Attention Profile, in Attention-Deficit Hyperactivity Disorder: A Clinical Workbook. Edited by Barkley RA. New York, Guilford, 1991

Elia J, Borcherding BG, Rapoport JL, et al: Methylphenidate and dextroamphetamine treatments of hyperactivity: are there true nonresponders? Psychiatry Res 36:141–155, 1991

Emery G, Bedrosian R, Garber J: Cognitive therapy with depressed children and adolescents, in Affective Disorders in Childhood and Adolescence: An Update. Edited by Cantwell DP, Carlson GA. New York, Spectrum, 1983, pp 445–471

Emslie G, Weinberg W, Kowatch R, et al: A double-blind, placebo-controlled study of fluoxetine in depressed children and adolescents. Paper presented at the Symposium on Selective Serotonin Reuptake Inhibitors in Children and Adolescents at the annual meeting of the New Clinical Drug Evaluation Unit (NCDEU), Orlando, FL, May 31–June 3, 1995

Ernst M, Magee HJ, Gonzalez NM, et al: Pimozide in autistic children. Psychopharmacol Bull 28:187–191, 1992

Evans RW, Gualtieri CT, Hicks RE: A neuropathic substrate for stimulant drug effects in hyperactive children. Clin Neuropharmacol 9:264–281, 1986

Evans RW, Clay TH, Gualtieri CT: Carbamazepine in pediatric psychiatry. Journal of the American Academy of Child Psychiatry 26:2–8, 1987

Faigel HC: The effect of beta blockade on stress-induced cognitive dysfunction in adolescents. Clin Pediatr (Phila) 30:441–445, 1991

Famularo R, Kinscherff R, Fenton T: Propranolol treatment for childhood posttraumatic stress disorder, acute type. Am J Dis Child 142:1244–1247, 1988

Fankhauser MP, Karumanchi VC, German ML, et al: A double-blind, placebo-controlled study of the efficacy of transdermal clonidine in autism. J Clin Psychiatry 53:77–82, 1992

Feeney DJ, Klykylo W: Risperidone and tardive dyskinesia. J Am Acad Child Adolesc Psychiatry 35:1421–1422, 1996

Fetner HH, Geller B: Lithium and tricyclic antidepressants. Psychiatr Clin North Am 15:223–241, 1992

Findling RL, Grcevich SJ, Lopez I, et al: Antipsychotic medications in children and adolescents. J Clin Psychiatry 57 (suppl 9):19–23, 1996

Fisman S, Steele M: Use of risperidone in pervasive developmental disorders: a case series. J Child Adolesc Psychopharmacol 6:177–190, 1996

Fitzpatrick PA, Klorman F, Brumaghim JT, et al: Effects of sustained-release and standard preparations of methylphenidate on attention deficit disorder. J Am Acad Child Adolesc Psychiatry 31:226–234, 1992

Fleck S: A general systems approach to severe family pathology. Am J Psychiatry 133:669–673, 1976

Forehand RL, McMahon RJ: Helping the Noncompliant Child: A Clinician's Guide to Parent Training. New York, Guilford, 1981

Frazier JA, Gordon CT, McKenna M, et al: An open trial of clozapine in 11 adolescents with childhood-onset schizophrenia. J Am Acad child Adolesc Psychiatry 33:658–663, 1994

Gadow KD: Effects of stimulant drugs on academic performance in hyperactive and learning disabled children. Journal of Learning Disabilities 16:290–299, 1983

Gadow KD: Pediatric psychopharmacology: a review of recent research. J Child Psychol Psychiatry 33:153–195, 1992

Gadow KD, Nolan EE, Sverd J: Methylphenidate in hyperactive boys with comorbid tic disorder, II: short-term behavioral effects in school settings. J Am Acad Child Adolesc Psychiatry 31:462–471, 1992

Gammon GD, Brown TE: Fluoxetine and methylphenidate in combination for treatment of attention deficit disorder and comorbid depressive disorder. J Child Adolesc Psychopharmacol 3:1–10, 1993

Gardner RA: Helping children cooperate in therapy, in Basic Handbook of Child Psychiatry, Vol 3: Therapeutic Interventions. Edited by Harrison SI. New York, Basic Books, 1979, pp 414–433

Garland EJ, Smith DH: Case study: panic disorder on a child psychiatric consultation service. J Am Acad Child Adolesc Psychiatry 29:785–788, 1990

Geller B, Cooper TB, Farooki ZQ, et al: Dose and plasma levels of nortriptyline and chlorpromazine in delusionally depressed adolescents and of nortriptyline in nondelusionally depressed adolescents. Am J Psychiatry 142:336–338, 1985

Geller B, Cooper TB, Chestnut EC, et al: Preliminary data on the relationship between nortriptyline plasma level and response in depressed children. Am J Psychiatry 143:1283–1286, 1986

Ghaziuddin M: Mania induced by sertraline in a prepubertal child (letter). Am J Psychiatry 151:944, 1994

Gittelman R, Klein DF, Feingold I: Children with reading disorders, II: effects of methylphenidate in combination with reading remediation. J Child Psychol Psychiatry 24:193–212, 1983

Gittelman-Klein R, Klein DF: Controlled imipramine treatment of school phobia. Arch Gen Psychiatry 25:204–207, 1971

Gordon CT, State RC, Nelson JE, et al: A double-blind comparison of clomipramine, desipramine, and placebo in the treatment of autistic disorder. Arch Gen Psychiatry 50:441–447, 1993

Graae F, Milner J, Rizzotto L, et al: Clonazepam in childhood anxiety disorders. J Am Acad Child Adolesc Psychiatry 333:372–376, 1994

Grcevich SJ, Findling RL, Rowane WA, et al: Risperidone in the treatment of children and adolescents with schizophrenia: a retrospective study. J Child Adolesc Psychopharmacol 6:251–257, 1996

Green WH: Child and Adolescent Clinical Psychopharmacology. Baltimore, MD, Williams & Wilkins, 1991

Greenhill LL: Attention-deficit hyperactivity disorder. Child Adolesc Psychiatr Clin N Am 4:123–168, 1995

Greenhill LL, Puig-Antich J, Chambers W, et al: Growth hormone, prolactin, and growth responses in hyperkinetic males treated with d-amphetamine. J Am Acad Child Adolesc Psychiatry 20:84–103, 1981

Greenhill LL, Puig-Antich J, Novacenko H, et al: Prolactin, growth hormone and growth responses in boys with attention deficit disorder and hyperactivity treated with methylphenidate. J Am Acad Child Adolesc Psychiatry 23:58–67, 1984

Greenhill LL, Solomon M, Pleak R, et al: Molindone hydrochloride treatment of hospitalized children with conduct disorder. J Clin Psychiatry 46:20–25, 1985

Grob CS, Coyle JT: Suspected adverse methylphenidate-imipramine interactions in children. J Dev Behav Pediatr 7:265–267, 1986

Guile JM: Sertraline-induced behavioral activation during the treatment of an adolescent with major depression. J Child Adolesc Psychopharmacol 6:281–285, 1996

Hagerman RJ, Murphy MA, Wittenberg MD: A controlled trial of stimulant medication in children with the fragile X syndrome. Am J Med Genet 30:377–392, 1988

Handen BL, Feldman H, Gosling A, et al: Adverse side effects of methylphenidate among mentally retarded children with ADHD. J Am Acad Child Adolesc Psychiatry 30:241–245, 1991

Hardan A, Johnson K, Johnson C, et al: Case study: risperidone treatment of children and adolescents with developmental disorders. J Am Acad Child Adolesc Psychiatry 35:1551–1556, 1996

Harley JP: Dietary treatment of behavioral disorders. Advances in Behavioral Pediatrics 1:129–151, 1980

Harmon RJ, Riggs PD: Clonidine for posttraumatic stress disorder in preschool children. J Am Acad Child Adolesc Psychiatry 35:1247–1249, 1996

Harper G: Focal inpatient treatment planning. J Am Acad Child Adolesc Psychiatry 28:31–37, 1989

Henggeler SW, Borduin CM: Family Therapy and Beyond: A Multisystemic Approach to Treating the Behavior Problems of Children and Adolescents. Belmont, CA, Brooks/Cole, 1990

Herskowitz J: Developmental neurotoxicology, in Psychiatric Pharmacosciences of Children and Adolescents. Edited by Popper C. Washington, DC, American Psychiatric Press, 1987, pp 81–123

Hunt RD, Capper S, O'Connell P: Clonidine in child and adolescent psychiatry. J Child Adolesc Psychopharmacol 1:87–102, 1990

Hunt RD, Lau S, Ryu J: Alternative therapies for ADHD, in Ritalin: Theory and Patient Management. Edited by Greenhill LL, Osman BB. New York, Mary Ann Liebert, 1991, pp 75–95

Hunt RD, Arnsten AF, Asbell MD: An open trial of guanfacine in the treatment of attention-deficit hyperactivity disorder. J Am Acad Child Adolesc Psychiatry 34:50–54, 1995

Isojarvi JI, Laatikainen TJ, Pakarinen AJ, et al: Polycystic ovaries and hyperandrogenism in women taking valproate for epilepsy. N Engl J Med 329:1383–1388, 1993

Jatlow PI: Psychotropic drug disposition during development, in Psychiatric Pharmacosciences of Children and Adolescents. Edited by Popper C. Washington, DC, American Psychiatric Press, 1987, pp 27–44

Joorabchi B: Expressions of the hyperventilation syndrome in childhood. Clin Pediatr (Phila) 16:1110–1115, 1977

Kafantaris V, Campbell M, Padron-Gayol MV, et al: Carbamazepine in hospitalized aggressive conduct disorder children: an open pilot study. Psychopharmacol Bull 28: 193–199, 1992

Kane MT, Kendall PC: Anxiety disorders in children: a multiple-baseline evaluation of a cognitive-behavioral treatment. Behavior Therapy 20:499–508, 1989

Kaplan SL, Breit M, Gauthier B, et al: A comparison of three nocturnal enuresis treatment methods. J Am Acad Child Adolesc Psychiatry 28:282–286, 1989

Kazdin AE, Esveldt-Dawson K, French NH, et al: Problem-solving skills training and relationship therapy in the treatment of antisocial child behavior. J Consult Clin Psychol 55:76–85, 1987

Kendall PC, Morison P: Integrating cognitive and behavioral procedures for the treatment of socially isolated children, in Cognitive Behavior Therapy With Children. Edited by Meyers AW, Craighead WE. New York, Plenum, 1984, pp 261–288

Kerbeshian J, Burd L, Fisher W: Lithium carbonate in the treatment of two patients with infantile autism and atypical bipolar symptomatology. J Clin Psychopharmacol 7: 401–405, 1987

Kernberg PF, Chazan SE: Children With Conduct Disorders: A Psychotherapy Manual. New York, Basic Books, 1991

King RA, Riddle MA, Chappell PB, et al: Emergence of self-destructive phenomena in children and adolescents during fluoxetine treatment. J Am Acad Child Adolesc Psychiatry 30:179–186, 1991

Kisch EH: Brief psychotherapy with children, adolescents, and their families. Child Adolesc Psychiatr Clin N Am 6:137–150, 1997

Klein RG, Koplewicz HS, Kanner A: Imipramine treatment of children with separation anxiety disorder. J Am Acad Child Adolesc Psychiatry 31:21–28, 1992

Kolmen BK, Feldman HM, Handen BL, et al: Naltrexone in young autistic children: a double-blind, placebo-controlled crossover study. J Am Acad Child Adolesc Psychiatry 34:223–231, 1995

Kovacs M: The Children's Depression, Inventory (CDI). Psychopharmacol Bull 21:995–998, 1985

Krener PK, Mancina RA: Informed consent or informed coercion? Decision-making in pediatric psychopharmacology. J Child Adolesc Psychopharmacol 4:183–200, 1994

Kumra S, Frazier JA, Jacobsen LK, et al: Child-onset schizophrenia: a double-blind clozapine-haloperidol comparison. Arch Gen Psychiatry 53:1090–1097, 1996

Kurlan R, Como PG, Deeley C, et al: A pilot controlled study of fluoxetine for obsessive-compulsive symptoms in children with Tourette's syndrome. Clin Neuropharmacol 16:167–172, 1993

Kutcher SP, MacKenzie S, Galarraga W, et al: Clonazepam treatment of adolescents with neuroleptic-induced akathisia. Am J Psychiatry 144:823–824, 1987

Kutcher SP, Reiter S, Gardner DM, et al: The pharmacotherapy of anxiety disorders in children and adolescents. Psychiatr Clin North Am 15:41–67, 1992

Latz SR, McCracken JT: Neuroleptic malignant syndrome in children and adolescents: two case reports and a warning. J Child Adolesc Psychopharmacol 2:123–129, 1992

Leckman JF, Ort S, Caruso KA, et al: Rebound phenomena in Tourette's syndrome after abrupt withdrawal of clonidine: behavioral, cardiovascular, and neurochemical effects. Arch Gen Psychiatry 43:1168–1176, 1986

Leckman JF, Hardin MT, Riddle MA, et al: Clonidine treatment of Gilles de la Tourette's syndrome. Arch Gen Psychiatry 48:324–328, 1991

Leonard HL, Swedo SE, Rapoport JL, et al: Treatment of obsessive-compulsive disorder with clomipramine and desipramine in children and adolescents: a double-blind crossover comparison. Arch Gen Psychiatry 46: 1088–1092, 1989

Levine MD: Encopresis: its potentiation, evaluation and alleviation. Pediatr Clin North Am 29:315–330, 1982

Lewinsohn PM, Clarke GN, Hops H, et al: Cognitive-behavioral treatment for depressed adolescents. Behavior Therapy 21:385–401, 1990

Lewis O: Psychological factors affecting pharmacologic compliance. Child Adolesc Psychiatr Clin N Am 4:15–22, 1995

Lewis O: Integrated psychodynamic psychotherapy with children. Child Adolesc Psychiatr Clin N Am 6:53–68, 1997

Lombroso PJ, Scahill L, King RA, et al: Risperidone treatment of children and adolescents with chronic tic disorders: a preliminary report. J Am Acad Child Adolesc Psychiatry 34:1147–1152, 1995

Loof D, Grimley P, Kuller F, et al: Carbamazepine for PTSD. J Am Acad Child Adolesc Psychiatry 34:703–704, 1995

March JS, Mulle K, Herbel B: Behavioral psychotherapy for children and adolescents with obsessive-compulsive disorder: an open trial of a new protocol-driven treatment package. J Am Acad Child Adolesc Psychiatry 33:333–341, 1994

Masek BJ, Spirito A, Fentress DW: Behavioral treatment of symptoms of childhood illness. Clin Psychol Rev 4:561–570, 1984

McClellan J, Werry J: Practice parameters for the assessment and treatment of children and adolescents with schizophrenia. J Am Acad Child Adolesc Psychiatry 33:616–635, 1994

McConville BJ, Minnery KL, Sorter, MT, et al: An open study of the effects of sertraline on adolescent major depression. J Child Adolesc Psychopharmacol 6:41–51, 1996

McDaniel KD: Pharmacologic treatment of psychiatric and neurodevelopmental disorders in children and adolescents, I. Clin Pediatr (Phila) 25:65–71, 1986

Melamed BG, Klingman A, Siegel LJ: Individualizing cognitive behavioral strategies in the reduction of medical and dental stress, in Cognitive Behavior Therapy With Children. Edited by Meyers AW, Craighead WE. New York, Plenum, 1984, pp 289–313

Mikkelsen EJ, Detlor J, Cohen DJ: School avoidance and social phobia triggered by haloperidol in patients with Tourette's disorder. Am J Psychiatry 138:1572–1576, 1981

Milich R, Wolraich M, Lindgren S: Sugar and hyperactivity: a critical review of empirical findings. Clin Psychol Rev 6:493–513, 1986

Minnery KL, West SA, McConville BJ, et al: Sertraline-induced mania in an adolescent. J Child Adolesc Psychopharmacol 5:151–153, 1995

Moise FN, Petrides G: Case study: electroconvulsive therapy in adolescents. J Am Acad Child Adolesc Psychiatry 35:312–318, 1996

Mufson L, Moreau D, Weissman MM, et al: Modification of interpersonal psychotherapy with depressed adolescents (IPT-A): phase I and II studies. J Am Acad Child Adolesc Psychiatry 33:695–705, 1994

O'Brien JD, Perlmutter I: The effect of medication on the process of psychotherapy. Child Adolesc Psychiatr Clin N Am 6:185–196, 1997

Papatheodorou G, Kutcher SP, Katic M: The efficacy and safety of divalproex sodium in the treatment of acute mania in adolescents and young adults: an open clinical trial. J Clin Psychopharmacol 15:110–116, 1995

Patterson GR: Families: Applications of Social Learning to Family Life. Champaign, IL, Research Press, 1975

Patterson GR, Forgatch M: Parents and Adolescents Living Together. Eugene, OR, Castalia, 1987

Patterson JF: Hepatitis associated with pemoline (letter). South Med J 77:938, 1984

Pelham WE Jr: The effects of psychostimulants on academic achievement in hyperactive and learning-disabled children. Thalamus 3:1–47, 1983

Pelham WE Jr, Hoza J: Behavioral assessment of psychostimulant effects on ADD children in a summer day treatment program, in Advances in Behavioral Assessment of Children and Families, Vol 3. Edited by Prinz R. Greenwich, CT, JAI Press, 1987, pp 3–33

Pelham WE Jr, Murphy HA: Attention deficit and conduct disorders, in Pharmacological and Behavioral Treatment: An Integrative Approach. Edited by Hersen M. New York, Wiley, 1986, pp 108–148

Pelham WE Jr, Sturges J, Hoza J, et al: Sustained release and standard methylphenidate effects on cognitive and social behavior in children with attention deficit disorder. Pediatrics 80:491–501, 1987

Pelham WE Jr, Greenslade KE, Vodde-Hamilton M, et al: Relative efficacy of long-acting stimulants on children with attention deficit-hyperactivity disorder: a comparison of standard methylphenidate, sustained-release methylphenidate, sustained-release dextroamphetamine, and pemoline. Pediatrics 86:226–237, 1990

Pelham WE Jr, Swanson JM, Furman MB, et al: Pemoline effects on children with ADHD: a time-response by dose-response analysis on classroom measures. J Am Acad Child Adolesc Psychiatry 34:1504–1513, 1995

Pleak RR, Birmaher B, Gavrilescu A, et al: Mania and neuropsychiatric excitation following carbamazepine. J Am Acad Child Adolesc Psychiatry 27:500–503, 1988

Pliszka SR: Effect of anxiety on cognition, behavior, and stimulant response in ADHD. J Am Acad Child Adolesc Psychiatry 28:882–887, 1989

Pool D, Bloom W, Mielke DH, et al: A controlled evaluation of Loxitane in seventy-five adolescent schizophrenic patients. Curr Ther Res Clin Exp 19:99–104, 1976

Popper C: Medical unknowns and ethical consent: prescribing psychotropic medications for children in the face of uncertainty, in Psychiatric Pharmacosciences of Children and Adolescents. Edited by Popper C. Washington, DC, American Psychiatric Press, 1987, pp 125–161

Popper CW: Combining methylphenidate and clonidine: pharmacologic questions and news reports about sudden death. J Child Adolesc Psychopharmacol 5:157–166, 1995

Popper CW, Zimnitzky B: Sudden death putatively related to desipramine treatment in youth: a fifth case and a review of speculative mechanisms. J Child Adolesc Psychopharmacol 5:283–300, 1995

Preskorn SH, Weller EB, Hughes CW, et al: Depression in prepubertal children: dexamethasone nonsuppression predicts differential response to imipramine versus placebo. Psychopharmacol Bull 23:128–133, 1987

Quintana H, Keshavan M: Case study: risperidone in children and adolescents with schizophrenia. J Am Acad Child Adolesc Psychiatry 34:1292–1296, 1995

Rapoport JL: Antidepressants in childhood attention deficit disorder and obsessive-compulsive disorder. Psychosomatics 27 (suppl):30–36, 1986

Rapoport JL, DuPaul GJ: Hyperactivity and methylphenidate: rate-dependent effects on attention. Int Clin Psychopharmacol 1:45–52, 1986

Ratey J, Sovner R, Parks A, et al: Buspirone treatment of aggression and anxiety in mentally retarded patients: a multiple-baseline, placebo lead-in study. J Clin Psychiatry 52:159–162, 1991

Realmuto GM, Erickson WD, Yellin AM, et al: Clinical comparison of thiothixene and thioridazine in schizophrenic adolescents. Am J Psychiatry 141:440–442, 1984

Realmuto GM, August GJ, Garfinkel BD: Clinical effect of buspirone in autistic children. J Clin Psychopharmacol 9:122–125, 1989

Reischer H, Pfeffer CR: Lithium pharmacokinetics. J Am Acad Child Adolesc Psychiatry 35:130–131, 1996

Reiter S, Kutcher SP: Disinhibition and anger outbursts in adolescents treated with clonazepam (letter). J Clin Psychopharmacol 11:268, 1991

Remschmidt H, Schultz E, Martin M: An open trial of clozapine in thirty-six adolescents with schizophrenia. J Child Adolesc Psychopharmacol 4:31–41, 1994

Richardson MA, Haugland G, Craig TJ: Neuroleptic use, parkinsonian symptoms, tardive dyskinesia, and associated factors in child and adolescent psychiatric patients. Am J Psychiatry 148:1322–1328, 1991

Richters JE, Arnold E, Jensen PS, et al: NIMH collaborative multisite multimodal treatment study of children with ADHD, I: background and rationale. J Am Acad Child Adolesc Psychiatry 34:987–1000, 1995

Riddle M (ed): Pediatric Psychopharmacology, I (Child and Adolescent Psychiatric Clinics of North America). Philadelphia, WB Saunders, 1995a

Riddle M (ed): Pediatric Psychopharmacology, II (Child and Adolescent Psychiatric Clinics of North America). Philadelphia, WB Saunders, 1995b

Riddle M, Hardin MT, King R, et al: Fluoxetine treatment of children and adolescents with Tourette's and obsessive-compulsive disorders: preliminary clinical experience. J Am Acad Child Adolesc Psychiatry 29:45–48, 1990

Riddle M, King RA, Hardin MT, et al: Behavioral side effects of fluoxetine in children and adolescents. J Child Adolesc Psychopharmacol 1:193–198, 1990–1991

Riddle M, Scahill L, King RA, et al: Double-blind, crossover trial of fluoxetine and placebo in children and adolescents with obsessive-compulsive disorder. J Am Acad Child Adolesc Psychiatry 31:1062–1069, 1992

Rosenfeld AA, Pilowsky DJ, Fine P, et al: Foster care: an update. J Am Acad Child Adolesc Psychiatry 36:448–457, 1997

Ryan ND: Heterocyclic antidepressants in children and adolescents. J Child Adolesc Psychopharmacol 1:21–31, 1990

Ryan ND: The pharmacologic treatment of child and adolescent depression. Psychiatr Clin North Am 15:29–40, 1992

Ryan ND, Meyer V, Dachille S, et al: Lithium antidepressant augmentation in TCA-refractory depression in adolescents. J Am Acad Child Adolesc Psychiatry 27:371–376, 1988a

Ryan ND, Puig-Antich J, Rabinovich H, et al: MAOIs in adolescent major depression unresponsive to tricyclic antidepressants. J Am Acad Child Adolesc Psychiatry 27:755–758, 1988b

Sallee F, Rock CM: Effects of pimozide on cognition in children with Tourette syndrome: interaction with comorbid attention-deficit hyperactivity disorder. Acta Psychiatr Scand 90:4–9, 1994

Sallee F, Stiller R, Perel J, et al: Targeting imipramine dose in children with depression. Clin Pharmacol Ther 40:8–13, 1986

Sallee F, Stiller RL, Perel JM: Pharacodynamics of pemoline in attention deficit disorder with hyperactivity. J Am Acad Child Adolesc Psychiatry 31:244–251, 1992

Samuel RZ: EPS with lithium (letter). J Am Acad Child Adolesc Psychiatry 32:1078, 1993

Sanchez LE, Campbell M, Small AM: A pilot study of clomipramine in young autistic children. J Am Acad Child Adolesc Psychiatry 35:537–544, 1996

Saul RC: Nortriptyline in attention deficit disorder. Clin Neuropharmacol 8:382–384, 1985

Scheidlinger S: Short-term group psychotherapy for children: an overview. Int J Group Psychother 34:573–585, 1984

Scheidlinger S: Group treatment of adolescents: an overview. Am J Orthopsychiatry 55:102–111, 1985

Schmitt BD: Nocturnal enuresis: an update on treatment. Pediatr Clin North Am 29:21–36, 1982

Silverstein FS, Boxer L, Johnson MV: Hematological monitoring during therapy with carbamazepine in children. Ann Neurol 13:685–686, 1983

Simeon JG, Ferguson HB: Recent developments in the use of antidepressant and anxiolytic medications. Psychiatr Clin North Am 8:893–907, 1985

Simeon JG, Ferguson HB, Van Wyck Fleet J: Bupropion effects in attention deficit and conduct disorders. Can J Psychiatry 31:581–585, 1986

Simeon JG, Dinicola V, Phil M, et al: Adolescent depression: a placebo-controlled fluoxetine treatment study and follow-up. Prog Neuropsychopharmacol Biol Psychiatry 14:791–795, 1990

Simeon JG, Ferguson HB, Knott V, et al: Clinical, cognitive, and neurophysiological effects of alprazolam in children and adolescents with overanxious and avoidant disorders. J Am Acad Child Adolesc Psychiatry 31:29–33, 1992

Simeon JG, Knott VJ, Dubois C, et al: Buspirone therapy of mixed anxiety disorders in childhood and adolescence: a pilot study. J Child Adolesc Psychopharmacol 4:159–170, 1994

Soni P, Weintraub AL: Case study: buspirone-associated mental status changes. J Am Acad Child Adolesc Psychiatry 31:1098–1099, 1992

Sours JA: The application of child analytic principles to forms of child psychotherapy, in Child Analysis and Therapy. Edited by Glenn J. New York, Jason Aronson, 1978, pp 615–646

Spencer EK, Kafantaris V, Padron-Gayol MV, et al: Haloperidol in schizophrenic children: early findings from a study in progress. Psychopharmacol Bull 28:183–186, 1992

Spencer T, Biederman J, Steingard R, et al: Bupropion exacerbates tics in children with attention-deficit hyperactivity disorder and Tourette's syndrome. J Am Acad Child Adolesc Psychiatry 32:211–214, 1993

Spencer T, Wilens T, Biederman J: Psychotropic medication for children and adolescents. Child Adolesc Psychiatr Clin N Am 4:97–121, 1995

Spencer T, Biederman J, Harding M, et al: Growth deficits in ADHD children revisited: evidence for disorder-associated growth delays? J Am Acad Child Adolesc Psychiatry 35:1460–1469, 1996a

Spencer T, Biederman J, Wilens T et al: Pharmacotherapy of attention-deficit hyperactivity disorder across the life cycle. J Am Acad Child Adoles Psychiatry 35:409–432, 1996b

Sprague RL, Sleator EK: Methylphenidate in hyperkinetic children: differences in dose effects on learning and social behavior. Science 198:1274–1276, 1977

Steingard R, Biederman J: Lithium responsive manic-like symptoms in two individuals with autism and mental retardation. Journal of the American Academy of Child Psychiatry 26:932–935, 1987

Steingard R, Biederman J, Spencer TJ, et al: Comparison of clonidine response in the treatment of attention-deficit hyperactivity disorder with and without comorbid tic disorders. J Am Acad Child Adolesc Psychiatry 32:350–353, 1993

Steingard R, Goldberg M, Lee D, et al: Adjunctive clonazepam treatment of tic symptoms in children with comorbid tic disorders and ADHD. J Am Acad Child Adolesc Psychiatry 33:394–399, 1994

Stokes TF, Baer DM: An implicit technology of generalization. J Appl Behav Anal 10:349–367, 1977

Strayhorn JM Jr: The Competent Child: An Approach to Psychotherapy and Preventive Mental Health. New York, Guilford, 1988

Strober M, Morrell W, Lampert C, et al: Relapse following discontinuation of lithium maintenance therapy in adolescents with bipolar I illness: a naturalistic study. Am J Psychiatry 147:457–461, 1990

Strober M, Freeman R, Rigali J, et al: The pharmacotherapy of depressive illness in adolescence, II: effects of lithium augmentation in nonresponders to imipramine. J Am Acad Child Adolesc Psychiatry 31:16–20, 1992

Strupp HH: Psychotherapy: Clinical, Research, and Theoretical Issues. New York, Jason Aronson, 1973

Teicher MH, Glod CA: Neuroleptic drugs: indications and guidelines for their rational use in children and adolescents. J Child Adolesc Psychopharmacol 1:33–56, 1990

Thompson S, Rey JM: Functional enuresis: is desmopressin the answer? J Am Acad Child Adolesc Psychiatry 34:266–271, 1995

Tierney E, Joshi PT, Llinas JF, et al: Sertraline for major depression in children and adolescents: preliminary clinical experience. J Child Adolesc Psychopharmacol 5:13–27, 1995

Trimble MR: Anticonvulsants in children and adolescents. J Child Adolesc Psychopharmacol 1:33–56, 1990

Van Putten T, Marder SR: Behavioral toxicity of antipsychotic drugs. J Clin Psychiatry 48 (suppl):13–19, 1987

Varanka TM, Weller RA, Weller EB, et al: Lithium treatment of manic episodes with psychotic features in prepubertal children. Am J Psychiatry 145:1557–1559, 1988

Varni JW, Jay SM, Masek BJ, et al: Cognitive-behavioral assessment and management of pediatric pain, in Handbook of Psychological Treatment Approaches. Edited by Holvman AD, Turk ED. New York, Pergamon, 1986, pp 168–192

Venkataraman S, Naylor MW, King CA: Mania associated with fluoxetine treatment in adolescents. J Am Acad Child Adolesc Psychiatry 31:276–281, 1992

Vitiello B, Hill JL, Elia J, et al: PRN medications in child psychiatric patients: a pilot placebo-controlled study. J Clin Psychiatry 52:499–501, 1991

Walkup JT: Fluvoxamine for children and adolescents with obsessive compulsive disorder. American Academy of Child and Adolescent Psychiatry News, July/August 1996, pp 12–13

Weller EB, Weller RA, Fristad MA: Lithium dosage guide for prepubertal children: a preliminary report. Journal of the American Academy of Child Psychiatry 25:92–95, 1986

Wender EH: The food additive-free diet in the treatment of behavior disorders: a review. J Dev Behav Pediatr 7:35–42, 1986

Wender EH, Solanto MV: Effects of sugar on aggressive and inattentive behavior in children with attention deficit disorder with hyperactivity and normal children. Pediatrics 88:960–966, 1991

West SA, Keck PE, McElroy SL: Open trial of valproate in the treatment of adolescent mania. J Child Adolesc Psychopharmacol 4:263–267, 1994

Whalen EH, Henker B: Social impact of stimulant treatment for hyperactive children. Journal of Learning Disabilities 24:231–241, 1991

Whitaker A, Rao U: Neuroleptics in pediatric psychiatry. Psychiatr Clin North Am 15:243–276, 1992

Wilens TE, Biederman J: The stimulants. Psychiatr Clin North Am 15:191–222, 1992

Wilens TE, Biederman J, Baldessarini RJ, et al: Cardiovascular effects of therapeutic doses of tricyclic antidepressants in children and adolescents. J Am Acad Child Adolesc Psychiatry 35:1491–1501, 1996

Wiles CP, Hardin MT, King RA, et al: Antidepressant-induced prolongation of QTc interval on EKG in two children, in Abstracts of the Annual Meeting of the American Academy of Child and Adolescent Psychiatry. Washington, DC, 1991, p 70

Wilkes TCR, Rush AJ: Adaptations of cognitive therapy for depressed adolescents. J Am Acad Child Adolesc Psychiatry 27:381–386, 1988

Willemsen-Swinkels SH, Buitelaar JK, van Engeland H: The effects of chronic naltrexone treatment in young autistic children: a double-blind placebo-controlled crossover study. Biol Psychiatry 39:1023–1031, 1996

Williams DT: Hypnosis as a psychotherapeutic adjunct, in Basic Handbook of Child Psychiatry, Vol 3: Therapeutic Interventions. Edited by Harrison SI. New York, Basic Books, 1979, pp 108–116

Williams DT, Mehl R, Yudofsky S, et al: The effect of propranolol on uncontrolled rage outbursts in children and adolescents with organic brain dysfunction. Journal of the American Academy of Child Psychiatry 21:129–135, 1982

Winsberg BG, Perel JM, Hurwic MJ, et al: Imipramine protein binding and pharmacokinetics in children, in The Phenothiazines and Structurally Related Drugs. Edited by Forrest IS, Carr CJ, Usdin E. New York, Raven, 1974, pp 425–431

Zahn TP, Rapoport JL, Thompson CL: Autonomic and behavioral effects of dextroamphetamine and placebo in normal and hyperactive prepubertal boys. J Abnorm Child Psychol 8:145–160, 1980

Zametkin A, Rapoport JL, Murphy DL, et al: Treatment of hyperactive children with monoamine oxidase inhibitors, I: clinical efficacy. Arch Gen Psychiatry 42:962–966, 1985

SUGGESTED READINGS

Abramowitz AJ, O'Leary SG: Behavioral interventions for the classroom: implications for students with ADHD. School Psychology Review 20:220–234, 1991

Barker P: Basic Family Therapy, Second Edition. Baltimore, MD, University Park Press, 1986

Barkley RA: Defiant Children: A Clinician's Manual for Parent Training. New York, Guilford, 1987

Barkley RA: Attention Deficit Hyperactivity Disorder: A Handbook for Diagnosis and Treatment. New York, Guilford, 1990

Cohen DJ, Bruun RD, Leckman JF: Tourette's Syndrome and Tic Disorders: Clinical Understanding and Treatment. New York, Wiley, 1988

Coppolillo HP: Psychodynamic Psychotherapy of Children: An Introduction to the Art and the Technique. Madison, CT, International Universities Press, 1987

Dulcan MK, Martini DR: Concise Guide to Child and Adolescent Psychiatry, Second Edition. Washington, DC, American Psychiatric Press, 1998

Ghuman HS, Sarles RM: Handbook of Adolescent Inpatient Psychiatric Treatment. New York, Brunner/Mazel, 1994

Greenhill LL, Osman BB: Ritalin: Theory and Patient Management. New York, Mary Ann Liebert, 1991

Harris JC: Developmental Neuropsychiatry: The Fundamentals Vol 1. New York, Oxford University Press, 1995

Harris JC: Developmental Neuropsychiatry: Assessment, Diagnosis, and Treatment of Developmental Disorders, Vol 2. New York, Oxford University Press, 1995

Kratochwill TR, Morris RJ (ed): Handbook of Psychotherapy With Children and Adolescents. Needham Heights, MA, Allyn & Bacon, 1993

Kutcher SP: Child and Adolescent Psychopharmacology. Philadelphia, WB Saunders, 1997

Lewis M (ed): Child and Adolescent Psychiatry: A Comprehensive Textbook, Second Edition. Baltimore, MD, Williams & Wilkins, 1996

Wiener JM (ed): Textbook of Child and Adolescent Psychiatry. Washington, DC, American Psychiatric Press, 1991

APPENDIX: BOOKS FOR PARENTS

ATTENTION-DEFICIT/HYPERACTIVITY DISORDER

Alexander-Roberts C: ADHD and Teens: A Parent's Guide to Making It Through the Tough Years. Dallas, TX, Taylor Publishing Company, 1995

Hallowell EM, Ratey JJ: Driven to Distraction: Recognizing and Coping With Attention Deficit Disorder From Childhood Through Adulthood. New York, Simon & Schuster, 1995

Silver LM, Silver LB: Dr. Larry Silver's Advice to Parents on Attention-Deficit Hyperactivity Disorder. Washington, DC, American Psychiatric Press, 1992

Wender P: The Hyperactive Child, Adolescent and Adult: Attention Deficit Disorder Through the Lifespan. New York, Oxford University Press, 1987

AUTISM

Siegel B: The World of the Autistic Child. New York, Oxford University Press, 1996

DEPRESSION

Cytryn L, McKnew DH Jr, Cytryn LW: Growing Up Sad: Childhood Depression and Its Treatment. New York, WW Norton, 1996

ENURESIS

Azrin N, Foxx R: Toilet Training in Less Than a Day. New York, Simon & Schuster, 1974

LEARNING DISABILITIES

Silver LB: The Misunderstood Child: A Guide for Parents of Learning Disabled Children. New York, McGraw-Hill, 1984

MANAGING CHILD BEHAVIOR

Greenspan SI, Salmon J: The Challenging Child: Understanding, Raising, and Enjoying the Five "Difficult" Types of Children. Reading, MA, Addison-Wesley, 1996

Sears W, Sears M: The Discipline Book: Everything You Need to Know to Have a Better-Behaved Child: For Birth to Age Ten. Boston, Little, Brown, 1995

Turecki S, Tonner L: The Difficult Child. New York, Doubleday Dell, 1989

MENTAL ILLNESS

McElroy E (ed): Children and Adolescents With Mental Illness: A Parent's Guide. Washington, DC, Woodbine, 1988

OBSESSIVE-COMPULSIVE DISORDER

Rapoport JL: The Boy Who Couldn't Stop Washing: The Experience and Treatment of Obsessive-Compulsive Disorder. New York, Penguin Books, 1990

POSTTRAUMATIC STRESS DISORDER

Terr L: Too Scared to Cry: Psychic Trauma in Childhood. New York, Harper & Row, 1990

SCHIZOPHRENIA

Cantor S: The Schizophrenic Child: A Primer for Parents and Professionals. Montreal, Quebec, Eden Press, 1982

SPECIAL TOPICS

CHAPTER 36

SUICIDE

T. B. GHOSH, M.D.
BRUCE S. VICTOR, M.D.

Suicide can be understood from many different perspectives, from religious, philosophical, and sociological, to psychological and biological.

Historically, the meaning of suicide has reflected the religious tradition of a given culture (Stevenson 1988). The Judeo-Christian tradition has held that life is a gift from God and that the taking of it is strictly forbidden. These influences still exist and may contribute to the lower suicide rates in more traditionally Catholic countries such as Italy, Spain, and Ireland.

More recently, secular philosophy has influenced how suicide is received in our society. Respect for the individual's will and personal rights has led some to view suicide as a rational act, a choice of death over pain. This view has led to movements that support suicide as a right of terminally ill patients and has been taken one step further with physician-assisted suicides in the terminally ill. Referenda on this issue in several states have been defeated, yet the decreasing margins of defeat reflect growing support by many in our society.

The critical issue facing the psychiatric clinician is suicide as a "rational" act. Can it be a rational act in someone who has a psychiatric illness? The overwhelming majority of suicides, more than 90%, are in individuals who are psychiatrically ill at the time of suicide (Black and Winokur 1990; E. Robins et al. 1959).

Hence, our focus in this chapter will be to review suicide from a clinical psychiatric viewpoint rather than from a religious, philosophical, or sociological perspective. We review the epidemiology and demographics of suicide and then discuss the psychiatric syndromes and psychological factors most correlated with suicide. We then discuss the emerging neurobiological factors in suicide and, at the end of the chapter, review the assessment and management of the suicidal patient.

EPIDEMIOLOGY AND DEMOGRAPHICS

A knowledge of the epidemiology and demographics of suicide is essential to the clinician for assessing the suicidal patient. Suicide is the ninth leading cause of death in the United States, resulting in 30,000 deaths annually. The rate is almost 11.6 per 100,000 people. Despite suicide prevention programs, more recognition of depression, hospitalization, and advances in biological treatments for depression, the *overall* rate of suicide has not changed over the last several decades; it has remained in the range of 11–12 per 100,000 (Sainsbury 1986b; Stevenson 1988).

One of the few identified factors that correlate with the overall rate of suicide is the availability of the means to suicide. This correlation was first demonstrated in England earlier in the century: when the toxicity of gas supplied in the homes was reduced, the suicide rate diminished concomitantly. The availability of firearms also appears to correlate with suicide risk. In a recent study involving five New York counties, Marzuk et al. (1992a) demonstrated that the differences in overall suicide risk among counties were explained by differentially available lethal means of injury.

Although the overall rate of suicide has remained constant over the last several decades, rates among different subgroups of age, sex, and race have changed. The highly publicized increase in adolescent and youth suicide appears to have been offset by a declining rate of suicide among older adults (L. N. Robins and Kulbok 1988); however, the rates of suicide among elderly persons still remain high.

Figure 36–1 provides a breakdown of suicide rates per 100,000 people on the basis of race, sex, and age group. The rates for both white and black females are relatively constant and low compared with that for males. The rate for black males peaks between ages 20 and 40, declines, and then increases again after age 75. Finally, and most strikingly, the high rate of completed suicides in white males, initially peaking between ages 20 and 40, levels off between ages 40 and 65 and then rapidly increases after age 65. The suicide rate is extraordinary for white males at ages 85 and older (i.e., 50 suicides per 100,000).

The general demographics for persons at low or high risk for completed suicide are presented in Table 36–1. Patients younger than age 45 are at low risk compared with patients older than age 45; female patients are at low risk compared with male patients. With regard to ethnicity, most studies demonstrate that Caucasians are at highest risk for suicide, followed by Native Americans, African Americans, Hispanic Americans, and Asian Americans. Patients who live with others or who are married are at lower risk than patients who live alone or who are divorced or widowed. Good health correlates with low risk and poor health with high risk. The incidence of suicide differs by geographic location in the United States, with middle-Atlantic regions having lower rates compared with the western mountain states. Although this difference may be artifactual and may reflect differential reporting and autopsy examinations, the different rates are striking: 18.4 per 100,000 in middle-Atlantic states versus 32.2 per 100,000 in western mountain states. From an international perspective, the United States suicide rate is average and analogous to the rates in Great Britain and Canada. The highest rates are in Germany, Scandinavia, Eastern Europe, and Japan, whereas the lowest rates, as mentioned previously, are in the traditionally Catholic countries (i.e., Italy, Spain, and Ireland) (Sainsbury 1986b).

PARASUICIDE

Self-destructive behavior and nonfatal suicide attempts, although difficult to categorize, have been conceptualized as *parasuicide*. The distinction between parasuicide and complete suicide is important: parasuicidal patients usually recognize that the means are nonlethal, and these patients have different characteristics than patients who display lethal suicidal behavior. Moscicki (1989) reported on the annual rate of suicide attempts found in the National Institute of Mental Health (NIMH) Epidemiologic Catchment Area (ECA) study of more than 18,000 United States residents. Although the rates varied between the sample communities, the overall rate was .3%. Extrapolating from the rate of completed suicides (i.e., 12 per 100,000), one would estimate that about 23 persons

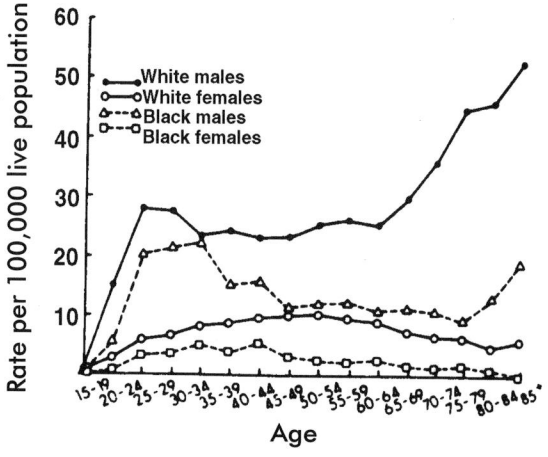

FIGURE 36–1. Suicide rates in the United States by age, sex, and color, 1980.
Source. Mortality Statistics Branch, National Center for Health Statistics (based on published and unpublished data). Used with permission of George E. Murphy, M.D.

TABLE 36–1. **Suicide risk: general demographics**

Low risk	High risk
Under age 45	Over age 45
Female	Male
Nonwhite	White
Lives with others	Lives alone
Good health	Poor health

attempted suicide for every 1 who completed it.

The general distinctions between those persons who attempt suicide and those who complete suicide are shown in Table 36–2. Suicide attempts are more likely in females, whereas completions are more likely in males. Suicide attempters are more likely to be young (younger than age 35), whereas completers are more likely to be older (older than age 60). The attempters' methods tend to be of low lethality—for example, so-called pill underdosages or wrist lacerations—compared with highly lethal methods such as firearms or hanging. The setting also distinguishes attempts from completions. The patient who makes the suicide attempt at home or where he or she can be discovered contrasts with the patient who chooses an isolated setting where there is a very low chance for rescue. The method and the setting are important in the determination of the risk-to-rescue fantasy ratio: the higher the ratio, the more serious and potentially lethal the attempt. Finally, certain psychiatric diagnoses in suicidal patients have been found to be associated with either suicide attempt or suicide completion. Suicidal patients with adjustment disorders and personality disorders (especially cluster B personality disorders) are more likely to make nonlethal suicide attempts, whereas suicidal patients with mood disorders, psychoses, and substance abuse problems tend to be completers.

One cannot discount the importance of parasuicide because 10% of attempters ultimately will complete suicide.

SUICIDE AND PSYCHIATRIC ILLNESS

In addition to outlining the social factors in suicide, epidemiological surveys have demonstrated that the vast majority of completed suicides are in patients with diagnosable psychiatric conditions. In their classic study, E. Robins et al. (1959) demonstrated that 94% of individuals who completed suicide were psychiatrically ill, mainly from affec-

TABLE 36–2. **Suicide attempts versus completions: demographics**

	Attempts	Completions
Sex	Female	Male
Age	Under 35	Over 60
Means	Low lethality (e.g., wrist laceration)	High lethality (e.g., firearms, hanging)
Setting	High chance of rescue	Low chance of rescue
Diagnosis	Adjustment disorder, personality disorder	Mood disorder, substance abuse

tive disorders or alcoholism. More recently, Black and Winokur (1990) found a similar result based on a review of studies of completed suicides: 90% of the persons who completed suicide were psychiatrically ill at the time of death. A small percentage of suicides are by people who have suffered a particular interpersonal loss, a financial loss, or a loss in social status. There also is an incidence of suicides in nonpsychiatric patients with terminal medical illness (e.g., cancer), but even suicide in those with terminal illness accounts for only about 5% of the total number of suicides. The vast majority of suicides occur in patients with psychiatric disturbances that probably, in most cases, are treatable.

Suicide and Mood Disorders

Mood disorder is the diagnostic category most often represented among persons who suicide. Studies show that the presence of a mood disorder in persons who suicide ranges from 45% to as high as 77% (Barraclough et al. 1974; E. Robins et al. 1959). It has been estimated that about 15% of patients with mood disorders will go on to commit suicide (Sainsbury 1986a). However, many studies that support the 15% figure combined both unipolar depression and bipolar depression. In a review of 30 studies of patients with depressive illness, including "neurotic depression" (now subsumed under the category dysthymic disorder), Miles (1977) concluded that 15% ultimately suicided. The suicide rate among persons with dysthymic disorder would be difficult to estimate, given the heterogeneity of the diagnosis and the difficulty in applying this new classification to previous studies of affective illness. However, another depressive subtype—psychotic depression—has been studied with regard to suicide risk. Patients with delusional depressive features are at five times greater risk for suicide than are patients with other mood disorders (Roose et al. 1983).

The first 3 months after the onset of a major depressive episode and the first 5 years after the lifetime onset of major depressive disorder represented the highest-risk period for attempted suicide, independent of the severity or duration of depression. Familial and genetic factors, early-life loss experiences, and comorbid alcoholism may be causal factors (Malone et al. 1995).

The rate of suicide completion associated with untreated bipolar disorder has been noted to be as high as 20% (Goodwin and Jamison 1990). Another study (Winokur and Tsuang 1975) examined the risk differential between bipolar and unipolar patients. In a 30- to 40-year follow-up of 76 bipolar patients and 182 unipolar patients, the suicide rates were 8.5% and 10.6%, respectively. Most authors agree that the predisposing factor is not the manic state itself but rather the presence of depression that accompanies a mixed bipolar state. Clinical experience suggests that the mixed bipolar state is associated with a particularly high risk of suicide because of the dangerous combination of highly dysphoric mood and a high level of energy and perturbation. Also, the bipolar II patient group is frequently associated with suicide (Goldring and Fieve 1984). In the absence of frank mania, the bipolar II patient's condition may be underdiagnosed, and the patient may inadvertently be denied a trial of mood stabilizers; consequently, persistent cycling and affective lability may predispose the patient to suicide.

In summary, about 15%–20% of patients with mood disorders will commit suicide, making these disorders among the most lethal of medical conditions. Many studies that support these conclusions are based on epidemiological data that are drawn from a mixture of treated and untreated populations. Although sparse data are available on the rate of suicide in a treated population, clinical experience suggests that it is significantly less than 15%. For example, in the NIMH Collaborative Program on the Psychobiology of Depression (Fawcett et al. 1990), the rate of completed suicide was only 3% over 10 years.

Suicide and Anxiety

One of the most important findings of recent years is that anxiety, particularly panic attacks, is a major short-term risk factor in suicide. Fawcett et al. (1990) reported results of a 10-year follow-up from the NIMH Collaborative Program on the Psychobiology of Depression. The sample consisted of 954 patients with major affective disorders. The authors outlined nine factors that were correlated with suicide. Six of the factors were correlated with suicide within the first year of the follow-up: panic attacks, severe psychic anxiety, diminished concentration, global insomnia, alcohol abuse, and anhedonia. These factors, including the possibility of alcohol as a self-medication for anxiety, demonstrated the importance of anxiety symptoms as markers of short-term suicide risk. The three factors that were found to correlate with suicide *after* the first year, in the subsequent 9 years of the study, were the risk factors that had been identified in prior studies: history of previous suicide attempts, suicidal ideation, and hopelessness. These findings have a major importance clinically because they are factors that can be modified, which highlights the importance of aggressively treating anxiety, panic, and insomnia in patients with mood disorders.

Weissman et al. (1989), in their analysis of the re-

nowned ECA study of 18,011 adults across the United States, found that 20% of subjects with panic disorder and 12% of subjects with panic attacks had made suicide attempts. These results could not be explained by any coexistence of depression or of substance abuse. Other investigators have challenged the significance of these findings. In a retrospective study of outpatients, Beck et al. (1991) found only one suicide attempt among 151 panic disorder patients. Friedman et al. (1992) and Henriksson et al. (1996) found noncomorbid panic disorder, in particular, appeared to be rare among completed suicides. Suicide in persons with panic disorder is associated with superimposed major depression and substance abuse and with personality disorders. The differences between these studies and Weissman et al.'s study may have to do with clinical versus community sampling. Further research is needed to determine which specific subgroups of panic patients are at higher risk for suicide. At present, when the above findings are considered in conjunction with Fawcett et al.'s findings, it should be noted that patients with severe anxiety and panic attacks may be at higher risk for suicide, and clinicians should be alert to this possibility.

Suicide and Chemical Dependence

Chemical dependence, on either alcohol or drugs, increases the suicide risk in a patient fivefold. It is important to note in this diagnostic group that although alcohol is the single most prevalent substance, the majority of suicides occur in those persons with multiple substance abuse. After mood disorders, chemical dependence represents the most frequently encountered diagnosis among those who suicide (Marzuk and Mann 1988). About 25% of persons who suicide in the United States have been found to have alcoholism (Murphy and Wetzel 1990). However, mixed substance abuse is even more closely associated with suicide. In the San Diego Suicide Study (Rich et al. 1986), mixed substance abuse was identified in 67% of completed suicides in youths and young adults and in 46% of suicides in adults ages 30 and older. In recent years, the prevalence of crack cocaine use has increased dramatically, with a subsequent increase in cocaine-related suicide. In a recent study of completed suicides in New York City, one in five individuals had used cocaine within days of the suicide (Marzuk et al. 1992b).

There are some general characteristics of chemically dependent persons who complete suicide (Table 36–3). These persons tend to be young males who use alcohol and other drugs *concurrently*, who have a history of overdoses, and who have comorbid psychiatric disorders, especially depressive disorders. Although suicide in persons who

TABLE 36–3. Characteristics of substance abusers who commit suicide

Age: 20s–30s
Sex: Male
Concurrent alcohol abuse and use of multiple substances especially

> Opiates
>
> Sedatives
>
> Amphetamines
>
> Cocaine

Mean age at onset of disorder: 15 years
Mean duration of disorder: 9 years
Chronic use
History of drug overdoses
Comorbid psychiatric syndromes especially

> Depression
>
> Borderline personality disorder
>
> Psychoses

Recent (< 6 weeks) interpersonal loss
Childhood history of hyperactivity
Incorrigibility
Family financial difficulties
Family suicidal behaviors
Parental abuse
Living in foster homes
Family history of

> Depression
>
> Suicide
>
> Alcoholism

Source. Adapted with permission from Marzuk and Mann 1988.

abuse substances occurs after many years into the illness, it tends to occur abruptly, often within 6 weeks of interpersonal loss.

Roy et al. (1990) studied 298 alcoholic subjects who had attempted, but not completed, suicide and compared these findings with data on suicide completers obtained in other studies. Several similarities were found between substance-abusing suicide completers and attempters—namely, the presence of psychiatric diagnosis, especially major depression, antisocial personality disorder, mixed substance abuse, panic disorder, phobic disorder, or generalized anxiety disorder. Like suicide completers, attempters had a family history of alcoholism and had experienced the onset of alcohol-related problems at an earlier age, usually in their early 20s. The main difference between the attempter group in this study and the completer groups reported in other studies was that attempters were more likely to be female. In Roy et al.'s (1990) study of alcoholic subjects, 30.6% of females attempted suicide compared with 14.6% of males.

Depressive disorder and substance abuse constitute a particularly lethal combination (Jaffe and Ciraulo 1986), one that highlights the importance of recognizing depression in the alcoholic patient. These depressive symptoms can be the result of underlying affective illness but also can result from the direct toxic effects of alcohol, impaired hepatic function, and poor nutrition, as well as organic brain syndromes from head trauma. Another problem is that patients with comorbid psychiatric and substance use disorders exhibit poor compliance with their medication regimen (Drake et al. 1989). Moreover, comorbid psychiatric conditions, especially affective illness, are often undertreated, consequently increasing the likelihood of suicidal behavior.

In addition to the underlying risk for suicidal behavior due to alcohol dependence itself, acute intoxication also increases suicide risk. Alcohol and drugs may produce disinhibition and remove the remaining constraints to suicide in a given chemically dependent individual and thus serve as an acute precipitant to suicide. Furthermore, the disinhibition and poor judgment associated with the intoxicated state can result in high-risk behaviors such as auto accidents and drug overdoses. Such events are sometimes considered "accidental" suicidal behavior in this fatalistic population. These accidental suicides occur not only among persons driving while intoxicated, and particularly in accidents involving a single vehicle, but also among pedestrians who are intoxicated; a high percentage of pedestrians killed in traffic accidents were noted to have been intoxicated at the time of the accident (Weiss and Stephens 1992).

Another mechanism for the enhanced suicide risk in the substance-abusing population may be related to serotonergic functioning, as is discussed in more detail later in this chapter. Recent studies have demonstrated the link between hypoactive serotonin function and violent suicide attempts (Brown et al. 1982). There may be a connection, as well, between serotonin dysfunction and alcoholism. Linnoila et al. (1989) noted a high prevalence of alcoholism in impulsive patients and found that those subjects with alcoholic fathers had low cerebrospinal fluid (CSF) levels of 5-hydroxyindoleacetic acid (5-HIAA).

Suicide and Schizophrenia

Approximately 10% of patients with schizophrenia complete suicide (Miles 1977). The majority of the suicides in schizophrenic patients are in young males (Table 36–4): in

TABLE 36–4. **Age and sex ratio in patients with chronic schizophrenia who commit suicide: studies since 1980**

Study	Suicides (N)	Mean age (years)	Male (%)
Cheung 1981	12	31.0	83.3
Roy 1982	30	27.9	80.0
Hogan and Awad 1983	67	35.5	80.6
Breier and Astrachan 1984	20	30.3	90.0
Wilkinson and Bacon 1984	17	42.0	47.0
Allebeck and Wistedt 1986	33	35.9	54.0
Drake and Cotton 1986	15	31.7	60.0
Nyman and Jonsson 1986	10	30.4	90.0
Meta-analysis	204	33.0	73.1

Source. Adapted with permission from Weiden and Roy 1992.

a review of studies from the 1980s, 73% of those who completed suicide were male, and the mean age at death was 33 (Weiden and Roy 1992). Also of interest is that in schizophrenia, suicide risk is *not* greatest during the active hallucinatory phase; schizophrenic patients are more likely to complete suicide when the psychosis is under control and they are in a depressive recovery phase of the illness. (In this regard, schizophrenia can be contrasted to depression, in which suicide risk is increased during the psychotic delusional phase.) Schizophrenic patients at greatest risk are young men, usually in the first few years of the illness, who are in remission and nonpsychotic but who remain depressed and perhaps have come to the recognition that their life is fundamentally different than it used to be.

The recognition of loss of functioning, especially in individuals with high premorbid achievement and high self-expectations, appears to correlate with suicide completion. For example, one study found that a higher percentage of schizophrenic patients who suicided had college educations, awareness of the extent of their pathology, and fears of further deterioration compared with schizophrenic patients who had not suicided (Drake and Cotton 1986). These authors also noted that the secondary depression in schizophrenic patients that predisposed them to suicide was better characterized as psychological distress and hopelessness rather than major depressive disorder with vegetative signs. Once again, hopelessness was found to be a key factor in the schizophrenic population and, further-

more, appears to cut across all psychiatric diagnoses as a suicide predictor.

Data on the suicide risk in the actively psychotic schizophrenic patient have been compiled. All clinicians ask the schizophrenic patient about command hallucinations for self-harm and view this state as one of high suicide risk. A meta-analysis of studies (Breier and Astrachan 1984; Drake et al. 1984; Roy 1982) revealed that of 65 completed suicides among schizophrenic patients, only 2 could be attributed to command hallucinations; however, Weiden and Roy (1992) suggest that these meta-analyses may be biased by secondary treatment effects. These authors note that clinicians are more likely to hospitalize schizophrenic persons for psychotic symptoms than for depressive symptoms. The net effect of these practices is that the schizophrenic person who is actively experiencing command hallucinations is hospitalized and the suicide is prevented; in contrast, the demoralized psychologically distressed patient tends not to be hospitalized and thus may not be protected from suicidal behavior. The clinical implication of this finding is not to reverse the convention of hospitalizing the command-hallucinating schizophrenic patient but rather to be equally vigilant about the nonpsychotic demoralized schizophrenic patient.

Also, of note is that in a recent study of schizophrenic outpatients, although command hallucinations had minimal influence on the outcome of schizophrenia, those in the study that committed suicide had command hallucinations. Therefore, in outpatients with schizophrenia who have a history of suicide attempts, suicidal command hallucinations should be taken seriously (Zisook et al. 1995). In the psychiatric hospital setting, the inpatients most at risk for suicide had previously exhibited suicidal behavior, had schizophrenia, had been admitted involuntarily, and had lived alone. It was noted that the risk of suicide persists among long-stay schizophrenic patients (Roy et al. 1995)

Suicide risk in schizophrenia, as with other disorders, appears to be greatest during the post–inpatient hospitalization period. This finding is consistent with the observation that the greatest risk occurs not during the psychotic period but more often after the psychosis has resolved. At that time, patients actually have more insight into their condition and more clearly may recognize the reality of their situation. Later, in their outpatient course, patients may have developed better coping strategies and adapted to their new life circumstance. The clinical implication is that in the postdischarge phase, in the first few weeks up to the first 3 months after discharge, a clinician must be very alert to patients' self-perceptions, recognition of reality, coping strategies, and support systems.

Suicide and Borderline Personality Disorder

Suicidal behavior in a patient with borderline personality disorder represents a particular challenge for the clinician, especially when making the distinction between, on the one hand, a potentially lethal attempt and, on the other, chronic self-mutilation or suicide attempts as a way of life. The incidence of completed suicide in borderline patients ranges from 3% to 8% (McGlashan and Heinssen 1988; Stone et al. 1987). Thus, the overall rate of completed suicide in this group is less than that in patients with primary affective disorders, substance abuse, or schizophrenia; however, the borderline personality disorder diagnosis comprises a heterogeneous group of individuals who may have coexisting Axis I disorders, and the literature is inconclusive about whether coexisting Axis I disorders place the borderline patient at higher risk for suicide completion. Moreover, although suicide attempts in personality disorder patients are often viewed as manipulative, they can be quite serious.

Corbitt et al. (1996) found that subjects with comorbid major depressive disorder and borderline personality disorder were more likely than other patients to have a history of multiple suicide attempts and were equally likely to have made a highly lethal attempt. Number of borderline personality disorder and other cluster B (dramatic/erratic) criteria were better predictors of past suicidal behavior than were depressive symptoms. The authors concluded that patients with borderline personality disorder symptomatology are at risk for serious suicide attempts. Hence, severity of comorbid cluster B personality disorder psychopathology should be considered in assessing suicide risk in patients with major depression.

Jacobs (1992) has proposed a model of assessment of suicide in the borderline patient that focuses on three areas (Figure 36–2):

1. The specific dynamics of the borderline individual that would place the person at higher risk
2. The coexistence of other psychiatric disorders that would place the individual at high risk
3. The suicide perspective, which includes identification of psychological commonalities of suicide and objectification of suicidal intent and behavior

With regard to specific borderline psychopathology, Kernberg (1984) outlines particular characteristics that are associated with high risk for suicide: impulsivity, hopelessness, despair, antisocial features, and interpersonal aloofness. He also describes characteristics of patients for whom chronic self-mutilation and suicide attempts are a "way of life" and that thus may predispose patients more to parasuicide than to completed suicide. "Infantile masochistic" patients use suicidal behavior to maintain connection. These behaviors tend to arise at times of intense rage attacks or rage mixed with temporary depressive flare-ups. The behaviors are designed to establish control over the environment by evoking guilt feelings in others, for example, after the breakup of an interpersonal relationship. At times, the behavior may be an expression of unconscious guilt over success or over the deepening of a psychotherapeutic relationship. Infantile masochistic patients exhibiting this form of negative therapeutic reaction are at particularly high risk for suicide attempts.

Another group of patients exhibit suicidal behavior that reflects malignant narcissism. These patients experience increased self-esteem and confirmation of their pathological grandiosity in suicidal behavior. They may convey a sense of calm and "triumph" over the fear of destruction, in contrast to the fearful, pleading efforts of staff and relatives to keep the patients from harming themselves (Kernberg 1984).

The second component of the model is the evaluation of coexisting psychiatric disorders. Although it is unclear whether comorbid disorders in fact increase the suicide risk, it is clinically important to recognize and vigorously treat these conditions in borderline patients. Particular attention should be paid to comorbid affective illness, substance abuse, eating disorders, and posttraumatic stress disorder (PTSD).

The third component of the tripartite assessment

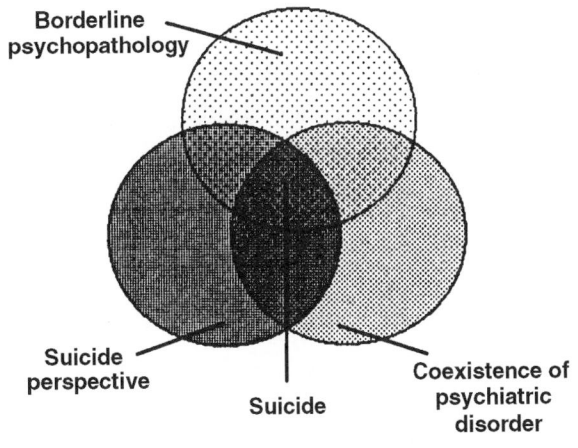

FIGURE 36–2. Tripartite model of suicide assessment in the patient with borderline personality disorder.
Source. Reprinted with permission from Jacobs D: "Evaluating and Treating Suicidal Behavior in the Borderline Patient," in *Suicide and Clinical Practice.* Edited by Jacobs D. Washington, DC, American Psychiatric Press, 1992, pp. 115–130.

model, the suicide perspective, consists of objectification of suicidal intent and identification of specific psychological commonalities and psychodynamic formulations. After identifying suicidal ideation, it is important that the clinician measure actual suicide intent. The clinician needs to determine the patient's ability to control suicidal thoughts, distinguish between active suicidal thoughts and passive suicidal thoughts, determine the patient's reasons for living and dying, determine the degree to which a suicidal plan has been developed, and evaluate the deterrents to carrying out such a plan (e.g., impact on family, loved ones). Common psychological factors are reviewed later in this chapter.

Along with the tripartite assessment, treatment for the borderline suicidal patient requires a high degree of creativity and individualization for the patient's specific circumstances. First, if there is any doubt about the strength of the therapeutic relationship or of the possibility of a negative therapeutic reaction, the patient should be hospitalized. Hospitalization can be focused on reestablishing the therapeutic alliance. Many clinicians advocate the use of brief hospitalizations to minimize the possibility of institutional dependence in this patient group. Pharmacotherapy is recommended for any overlaying Axis I condition. However, even in the absence of a definable Axis I condition, a variety of psychotropics have been useful to help with specific symptoms in borderline patients. Although the psychotropics that have been useful run the gamut of the entire spectrum of agents, one study offers guidelines for the differential use of carbamazepine, tranylcypromine, and alprazolam in borderline patients (Cowdry and Gardner 1988). Psychological tools in working with the suicidal borderline patient that are particularly important include empathy and the development of an antisuicide contract. The so-called no self-harm contract should not be taken literally as a contract to eliminate suicidal feelings. Rather, it serves to communicate the patient's *loss of control over suicidal feelings* and the importance of maintaining communication between the patient and the psychiatrist.

PSYCHOLOGICAL FACTORS IN SUICIDAL BEHAVIOR

Given that suicide is not a diagnosis of a specific problem, what are the underlying psychological factors? A central factor is the issue of hopelessness. There is a high association with hopelessness in long-term suicide risk. Not specific to depression, hopelessness can accompany demoralization with a number of other syndromes: schizophrenia, anxiety disorders, and chronic conditions, including medical conditions. This factor can be measured with the Beck

Hopelessness Scale, which is a 20-item self-report instrument that assesses the degree to which a person holds negative expectations about the future (Beck and Steer 1988). In a prospective study of 1,958 outpatients, Beck et al. (1990) found that hopelessness was highly correlated with eventual suicide. A scale cutoff score of 9 or above identified 16 (94.2%) of the 17 patients who completed suicide. Assessment of hopelessness is one of the key aspects in the management of the suicidal patient.

In addition to hopelessness, Hendin (1991) has identified desperation as another important factor in suicide. Desperation implies not only a sense of hopelessness about change but a sense that life is impossible without such change. Guilt also was found to be another affective component of desperation. In a study of Vietnam veterans with PTSD, guilt was found to be prominent in those veterans exhibiting suicidal behavior. This guilt stemmed from self-hatred and a need for punishment, attributable in part to perceived guilt from actions committed during combat and in part to survivor guilt. These findings can be extended to certain disorders other than PTSD, especially depression, a component of which is the guilt that derives from the self-recriminatory state of the depressed person.

Aggression and violence are important in understanding suicide. Classical psychoanalytic theory postulated the importance of aggression toward the self in suicidal behavior. Freud (1917 [1915]/1957) described suicide as a murderous attack on an internalized object that had become a source of ambivalence. Thus, from a psychological sense, the introjected love object is the focus of the attack. Recent studies, however, demonstrate that aggression toward others—that is, violent behavior—often goes hand in hand with suicidal behavior. Suicide usually was associated with conscious rage in the violent individuals studied, and rage should therefore be viewed as an important psychological factor underlying suicidal behavior (Hendin 1991). Apter et al. (1991) studied suicide risk in patients with a history of violent behavior and in those without a history of violence. Their findings demonstrated that the two groups had similar correlates of suicide risk with regard to several psychological factors: anger, fear, anxiety, impulse dyscontrol, suspiciousness, and rebelliousness. However, of particular note, there was a correlation between sadness and suicide risk in the nonviolent patients; no such correlation was found in the violent patients.

Hendin (1991) has reviewed some of the common meanings of death ascribed to patients who commit suicide: death as reunion, rebirth, retaliatory abandonment, revenge, and self-punishment or atonement. The fantasy of reunion with a lost object through death may account for the phenomenon of anniversary suicides, as well as suicides that occur during bereavement. The fantasy of rebirth is related to the fantasy of identification with the lost object: patients view themselves as incomplete in the absence of the missing object and view the reunion through suicide as a form of rebirth. Suicide and suicide attempts as retaliatory abandonment are seen in patients who feel that the only way they can have mastery over a situation is through control of living or dying. This illusion of mastery and maintenance of control may account for individuals who keep the means for suicide readily available even if they never attempt suicide. Suicide as revenge correlates with the classical Freudian observation of the unconscious wish to kill the ambivalently regarded lost object. As an extension of this unconscious wish, unconscious rage and murderous impulse are seen as the need for self-punishment or atonement. The patient feels guilty about his or her hatred of the object, and suicide not only serves as revenge but also accomplishes atonement.

Shame and humiliation are two other factors that sometimes underlie suicide. Certain individuals may view suicide as a face-saving mechanism after suffering a social humiliation (e.g., a sudden loss of status or income). This form of suicide is rare in individuals not suffering from psychiatric illness. However, psychiatrically ill patients may feel shame related to suicidal ideation and may be reluctant to seek treatment or rely on support systems. The existence of a support system is not sufficient; the patient must be willing to rely on it. Often, shameful feelings inhibit this process. Therefore, it is important to be alert to these feelings in patients.

Finally, stressors predisposing to suicide coincide with developmental phases over the life cycle (Rich et al. 1991). Three common stressors are 1) conflict, separation, and rejection; 2) economic problems; and 3) medical illness. In the San Diego Suicide Study, interpersonal conflicts, separations, and rejections were the predominant stressors for adolescents and individuals in early adulthood. Although these issues remained as significant stressors for those who completed suicide in middle adulthood, for the 40- to 60-year-old group, economic problems were deemed the principal stressor. In patients older than age 60 years, medical illness played an increasingly important role and was considered the most significant predisposing factor in patients older than age 80.

SUICIDE IN SPECIAL POPULATIONS

SUICIDE AND THE ELDERLY

As was shown in Figure 36–1, the suicide rate doubles to quadruples in patients older than age 65 years, especially in white males. Factors predisposing older individuals to suicide are social isolation, loss of spouse, anxiety due to financial instability, and finally, undertreated mood disorders. The prevalence of mood disorders is probably not higher in this age group, but the disorders probably are underrecognized and undertreated. In a cross-section of older patients, primary depression was present in about 3.7%, with a total of 14% complaining of a dysphoric state (Blazer and Williams 1980); however, in a cohort of suicidal older individuals, the presence of depression was reported to be as high as 80% (Morgan 1989). Depression may go underrecognized in older persons because of the atypical features in this population, including masked depression (primarily multiple somatic complaints or continued unfounded fearfulness of somatic illness) and pseudodementia (i.e., the artificially reduced cognitive capacities resulting from a primary depressive condition).

Skoog et al. (1996) studied the frequency of suicidal feelings among a population sample of 85-year-olds who did not have dementia. They found that figures for suicidal feelings were significantly higher among subjects with mental disorders. Women who felt that life was not worth living had a higher 3-year mortality rate than did women without these feelings (43.2% versus 14.2%, respectively). This finding was independent of concomitant physical and mental disorders. The substantially higher mortality rate in women who felt that life was not worth living compared with women who did not feel the same suggested these feelings must be taken seriously.

Finally, indirect self-destructive behavior is often seen in institutional settings for older individuals when they refuse to accept medications or medical care, refuse to take part in activities, and struggle for control with caregivers. These behaviors should alert the clinician and caregivers to the presence of an underlying depression (Morgan 1989). Because the percentage of older persons in the United States population is growing, the issues of recognizing underlying conditions, implementing vigorous treatment, and managing suicidality in older persons will be increasingly important in the future.

SUICIDE AND YOUTH

The rate of adolescent suicide has increased dramatically since 1960 (Figure 36–3). The rate of suicide in adolescent males (white and nonwhite) from 1960 to 1980 almost tripled. Adolescent female suicides have increased two- to threefold.

Factors that may have contributed to this increase are the rise in depressive disorders among youths (severe

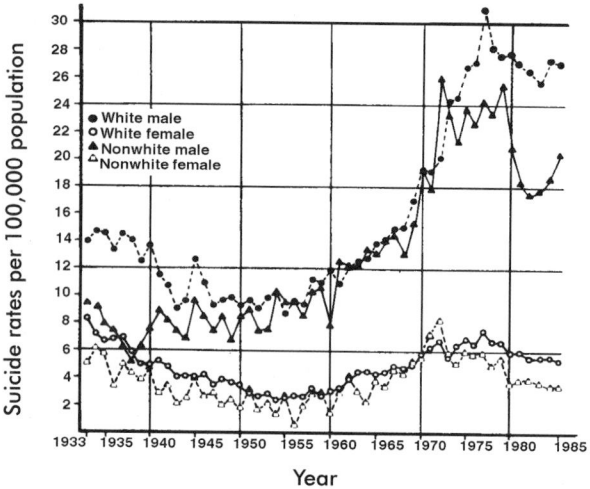

FIGURE 36–3.   Suicide rates among 15- to 19-year-olds in the United States, 1933–1985.

depression is the most prevalent characteristic of the suicidal adolescent), the rise in the divorce rate, the dissolution of the nuclear family, and the availability of firearms (Pfeffer 1988). Males are at greater risk than females and whites are at greater risk than nonwhites for *completed* suicide. In a recent large controlled study using the psychological autopsy methodology, several other notable risks were identified; these derived from school problems, a family history of suicidal behavior, poor parent-child communication, and stressful life events (Gould et al. 1996).

Exposure to suicide also may be a factor: for certain individuals, experiencing suicide in a family member or friend appears to make suicide more "permissible." This phenomenon may be at play in the "cluster" suicides observed in youth, although this point is still controversial. Brent et al. (1996), in a 3-year controlled follow-up reported that exposure to suicide does not result in an increased risk of suicidal behavior among friends and acquaintances, but it has a relatively long impact in terms of increased incidence of depression, anxiety, and PTSD.

Although there are environmental and sociocultural factors, the importance of psychopathology in youth suicide cannot be overestimated. In the adolescent, the main diagnoses are depression and conduct disorder, especially with antisocial behaviors. Hostility, aggression, and assaultiveness also are correlated with suicide. Suicide in youth, as in other populations, often goes hand in hand with hostility, not only toward the self but toward others. A correlation between suicidality and aggressive behavior has been found in adolescents in many instances when there is parental substance abuse.

SUICIDE IN PATIENTS WITH HUMAN IMMUNODEFICIENCY VIRUS/ACQUIRED IMMUNODEFICIENCY SYNDROME

Among the most unique medical phenomena identified in the last decade has been the epidemic of infection with human immunodeficiency virus (HIV) and subsequent progression to acquired immunodeficiency syndrome (AIDS). This epidemic also has implications in the field of suicidology because of the unique impact on primarily young people with chronic and life-threatening illness. In clinical practice, there is a high prevalence of suicidal ideation among patients afflicted with HIV. Oftentimes, suicidal ideation comes in the form of a need to maintain control, especially in a syndrome such as AIDS in which a patient can rapidly develop encephalopathy and dementia. These patients often have seen others in their peer group become, over a short period of time, demented and unable to care for themselves. Patients may develop a view of suicide as a legitimate way out before the demise into debilitation or dementia. Clinical experience suggests that suicide appears to have acceptance in the AIDS population. Breitbart et al. (1996) found HIV-infected patients supported policies favoring physician-assisted suicide at rates comparable to those in the general public. Patients' interest in physician-assisted suicide appeared to be more a function of psychological distress and social factors than physical factors. These findings highlight the importance of psychiatric and psychosocial assessment and intervention in the care of patients who express interest in or request physician-assisted suicide.

However, whether or not the patient actually completes suicide, maintaining suicidal ideation as a source of control over his or her illness appears to be fairly prevalent.

The actual risk of suicide in persons with AIDS is greater than that in the general population (Zeck et al. 1988). In an epidemiological study of New York City residents, the suicide rate for men with AIDS was 680 per 100,000 persons per year, whereas for a comparison group of men ages 20–59 without a diagnosis of AIDS the suicide rate was 18 per 100,000 persons per year. The suicide rate in the AIDS patients was 36 times that in age-matched men without AIDS (Marzuk et al. 1988). Interestingly, a later study (McKegney and O'Dowd 1992) found that a group of psychiatric consultation patients with diagnosed AIDS were significantly *less* suicidal than a group of patients who were HIV-positive but had not yet developed AIDS. The authors postulated that the prevalence of delirium and dementia in the AIDS patients may have led to organicity, which might have actually reduced the suicide risk in the diagnosed AIDS patients compared with the HIV patients.

Nevertheless, in clinical work it is important to keep in mind the suicide potential in the AIDS patient group. One should carefully evaluate depression and organicity, as well as the value system the patient may have about suicide, while keeping in mind that there appears to be acceptance of suicide in this population.

BIOLOGICAL ASPECTS OF SUICIDAL BEHAVIOR

Psychiatry is a medical discipline that often deals in fatal illness. Studies detailing various nonbiological methods of predicting suicide have been almost universally negative. Indeed, even the demographic risk factors covered earlier in this chapter have not led to accurate predictions of who might commit suicide. Furthermore, organized programs of suicide prevention utilizing only psychotherapeutic and psychosocial intervention have been disappointing (Chowdhury et al. 1973; Ettinger 1980). These failures regarding the assessment and prediction of suicidal behavior have made the identification of biological factors in the genesis of this behavior especially clinically compelling.

The importance of biological factors in suicidal behavior was suggested by studies of completed suicide demonstrating a much higher concordance rate for monozygotic twins than dizygotic twins. Interestingly, significantly more living monozygotic than dizygotic co-twins of twins who complete suicide attempt suicide (Roy et al. 1995). Later studies examining biological relatives of adoptees who committed suicide found a significantly higher incidence of suicide than in the biological relatives of control subjects (Schulsinger et al. 1979). As such, these results support the argument for the possible existence of a genetic predisposition toward suicidal behavior.

But what is the nature of this predisposition? In the last decade, there has been a proliferation of studies detailing more direct examination of the neurochemical functioning of suicidal patients that further distinguishes them from nonsuicidal patients. Although several neurochemical factors have been implicated, the main focus has been on alterations in serotonergic transmission in the central nervous system (CNS). We review these studies below for the clinician to gain an appreciation of the neurobiological underpinnings of suicidal behavior.

POSTMORTEM STUDIES OF SUICIDE VICTIMS

The initial postmortem studies of brains of suicide victims began as a quest to determine underlying biochemical de-

rangements in depressed patients because, at that time, it was assumed that all suicide victims were depressed. As can be seen in Table 36–5, serotonin and its major metabolite, 5-HIAA, are decreased in the brain stem and in other subcortical nuclei. Yet, interestingly, alterations in these levels were not found in cortical regions. Part of the reason for this phenomenon may well have to do with some of the variables involved in the actual performance of these studies. Specifically, actual amounts of serotonin and 5-HIAA are influenced by factors such as diet and the digestion of drugs or alcohol. Other factors include the amount of postmortem delay and the toxicity of the mode of suicide (such as carbon monoxide poisoning).

The influences of the above-listed factors are minimized by the utilization of *receptor binding assay*. Stemming from research involving platelets, it was found that imipramine binding might well serve as a measure of presynaptic serotonergic functioning. Four of five studies demonstrated decreased imipramine binding not only in the cortex but also in the hypothalamus (Table 36–6), suggesting decreased presynergetic serotonergic transmission in persons who suicide. A recent study demonstrated lowered cortical serotonin transporter binding—also a

TABLE 36–5. Postmortem neurotransmitter and metabolite studies of completed suicides

Study	Findings
Shaw et al. 1967	⇓ Brain-stem 5-HT
Beskow et al. 1976	⇓ Brain-stem 5-HIAA
Bourne et al. 1968	⇓ Brain-stem 5-HIAA
Pare et al. 1969	⇓ Brain-stem 5-HT
Lloyd et al. 1974	⇓ Brain-stem 5-HT
Korpi et al. 1986	⇓ Hypothalamus 5-HT
	⇓ Nucleus accumbens 5-HIAA
Cochran et al. 1976	No change in brain 5-HT
Stanley et al. 1983	No change in 5-HIAA or 5-HT levels in frontal cortex
Crow et al. 1984	No change in 5-HIAA or 5-HT levels in frontal cortex
Owen et al. 1983	No change in 5-HIAA levels in frontal cortex

Note. 5-HT = 5-hydroxytryptamine (serotonin); 5-HIAA = 5-hydroxyindoleacetic acid.
Source. Adapted with permission from Winchel RM, Stanley B, Stanley M: "Biochemical Aspects of Behavior," in *Suicide Over the Life Cycle: Risk Factors, Assessment, and Treatment of Suicidal Patients.* Edited by Blumenthal SJ, Kupfer DJ. Washington, DC, American Psychiatric Press, 1990, pp. 97–126.

TABLE 36–6. Postmortem receptor studies of completed suicides: serotonergic receptor findings

Study	Findings
Imipramine binding	
Stanley et al. 1982	⇓ [^{3}H]imipramine binding in cortex
Paul et al. 1984	⇓ [^{3}H]imipramine binding in hypothalamus
Perry et al. 1983[a]	⇓ [^{3}H]imipramine binding in cortex
Crow et al. 1984	⇓ [^{3}H]imipramine binding in cortex
Myerson et al. 1982	⇑ [^{3}H]imipramine binding in cortex
5-HT$_2$ binding	
Stanley and Mann 1983	⇑ 5-HT binding in cortex
Mann et al. 1986	⇑ 5-HT binding in cortex
Meltzer et al. 1987	⇑ 5-HT binding in cortex
Owen et al. 1983	[Nonsignificant increase in 5-HT binding in cortex]
Cheetam et al. 1987	⇓ 5-HT binding in cortex

Note. 5-HT = 5-hydroxytryptamine (serotonin).
[a]Depressed patients dying of natural causes.

presynaptic measure—in the ventrolateral prefrontal cortex in the brains of suicide victims (Arango et al. 1995).

By using ligands such as ^{3}H-labeled spiroperidol, ^{3}H-labeled ketanserin, or ^{125}I-labeled LSD, it is possible to measure postsynaptic serotonin binding sites. Several studies (Table 36–6) have noted an increase in serotonin$_2$ (5-HT$_2$) receptor binding in the frontal and prefrontal cortices of suicide victims. These findings suggest that there is a postsynaptic compensation for the overall decrease in serotonergic transmission in suicidal patients.

However, postmortem studies of suicide victims have focused on other neurotransmitter systems. One study cited an increase in muscarinic cholinergic receptor bindings (Myerson et al. 1982). More interestingly, other studies of suicide victims found increases in β-adrenergic receptor binding not only in the prefrontal cortex but also in the temporal cortex (Mann et al. 1986; Zanko and Bigeon 1983). In the one study in which *both* 5-HT$_2$ and β-adrenergic binding were compared, there were no victims who were found to have low levels of both receptors. Therefore, the consideration of abnormalities in multiple neurotransmitter systems will greatly aid in our ability to identify those patients at greatest risk for suicide.

One study found that binding sites for corticotropin-releasing factor (CRF) were reduced in the frontal cortex of persons who committed suicide (Nemeroff et al. 1988). This finding is consistent with previous research which found that patients with clinically significant depression have increased CRF in the CSF, suggesting that the reduction of CRF binding sites in the postmortem study represents a downregulation in response to the increase in CRF (Nemeroff et al. 1984). This finding also dovetails with some studies that suggest an increased capacity for the dysregulation of the hypothalamic-pituitary-adrenal axis as measured by the dexamethasone suppression test (Targum et al. 1983).

CEREBROSPINAL FLUID STUDIES OF SUICIDE ATTEMPTERS

Although it can be argued that the study of biogenic amines and their breakdown products in the CSF reflects a somewhat derivative measure of actual neuronal transmission, a very high positive correlation between 5-HIAA found in the brain at autopsy and in the CSF has been demonstrated. Therefore, the spate of studies of CSF 5-HIAA can be considered reflective of CNS functioning, further corroborating the postmortem literature cited previously regarding underlying neurobiological dysfunction in suicidal patients.

The initial studies of CSF in depressed patients also attempted to distinguish between biochemically distinct forms of depression. That patients who had made suicide attempts had low levels of 5-HIAA was significant not only from the standpoint of biochemically distinguishing those patients who had attempted suicide, but also from the perspective of predicting future suicidal behavior. One of the initial studies demonstrated that 21% of patients who had been hospitalized after a suicide attempt and had been found to have low levels of CSF 5-HIAA actually committed suicide within 1 year after the original evaluation (Åsberg et al. 1976). Several other studies corroborated the initial finding that depressed patients whose CSF levels of 5-HIAA were subnormal were more likely to have attempted suicide (Agren 1980; Banki 1981; Träskman et al. 1981).

Interestingly, however, suicidal and nonsuicidal patients with *bipolar* disorder could not be distinguished on the basis of their CSF 5-HIAA (Berrettini et al. 1986). This finding, which contrasts with results from the studies previously discussed regarding patients with unipolar depression, is somewhat perplexing, given the high rate of suicide in patients with bipolar disorder. Goodwin (1986) has posited that because serotonergic dysregulation is probably central to the genesis of bipolar disorder, this may overshadow any singular relationship between serotonergic hypofunction and suicide in these patients.

Decreases in CSF 5-HIAA also have been shown to distinguish between schizophrenic patients who had attempted suicide and those who had not (Banki et al. 1983; Ninan et al. 1984; Roy et al. 1985). This measure also distinguished suicidal patients with personality disorders as well as alcoholic patients with a history of suicide attempts (Banki et al. 1984; Brown et al. 1979). These findings further support not only the idea that suicidal behavior is not merely an end result of clinical depression, but also that serotonergic dysfunction may well underlie suicidal behavior in patients across diagnoses. That low levels of 5-HIAA actually may represent a trait disorder is further suggested by the lack of a temporal relationship between the suicide attempt and the CSF 5-HIAA level.

Both human and animal studies correlate aggressive behavior with serotonergic hypofunction. This hypofunction may not signify a specific diathesis for suicide but rather reflects a decreased threshold for aggressive behavior whether directed against others or oneself. Yet it is clear that successful suicide attempts are often predicated on systematic planning rather than a momentary loss of impulse control; indeed, violent methods of suicide often involve *more* planning. Thus, it is difficult to determine which aspects of suicidal behavior specifically correlate with decreased levels of CSF 5-HIAA.

Most recently, a study of violent suicide attempters demonstrated not only lower levels of CSF 5-HIAA but also significantly increased CSF levels of 3-methoxy-4-hydroxyphenylglycol (MHPG), the chief metabolic breakdown product of norepinephrine (Träskman-Bendz et al. 1992). This finding appears to corroborate previous research suggesting that serotonin is an inhibitory neurotransmitter of the noradrenergic system and that heightened noradrenergic turnover in the face of diminished serotonergic input may well represent a significant part of the biochemical underpinnings of violent suicide.

In addition, some patients with depression who had attempted suicide also were found to have decreased CSF levels of homovanillic acid (HVA), the metabolite of dopamine. In a 5-year follow-up study, those patients who went on to attempt suicide again after the initial evaluation were found to have significantly lower CSF levels of 5-HIAA and HVA (Roy et al. 1986). It is interesting to note that a recent study also demonstrated that both decreased 5-HIAA and HVA correlated with a history of suicide attempts resulted in greater medical damage (Mann et al. 1996).

Taken together, these findings suggest, first, that it is important to consider more than just serotonergic abnor-

malities and, second, that increasing the sensitivity and specificity of possible biological predictors of suicidal behavior will involve an analysis of a cluster of biochemical variables.

FINDINGS IN THE PERIPHERY: PHARMACOLOGICAL CHALLENGE TESTS; PLATELET, URINE, AND SERUM STUDIES

Because lumbar puncture is generally not performed in the office, investigators have recently searched for alternative methods of assessing the neurochemical functioning. One method of testing the integrity of the serotonergic system is to measure prolactin or cortisol release in response to pharmacological agents such as fenfluramine, precursors such as L-tryptophan or 5-hydroxytryptophan, or serotonin receptor antagonists such as metachlorophenyl-piperazine (mCPP) or MK-212. Recent studies have demonstrated that prolactin response to fenfluramine is blunted in patients who have attempted suicide (Coccaro et al. 1989; De Meo et al. 1988). One study has demonstrated a heightened cortisol response to 5-hydroxy-tryptophan, which may reflect receptor supersensitivity (Mann and Arango 1992).

Studies have demonstrated that the number of platelet 5-HT$_2$ receptors is increased in suicidal patients (Pandey et al. 1990, 1995). There also have been recent studies suggesting platelet manifestations of presynaptic serotonergic hypofunction: specifically, decreased platelet serotonin uptake and ^{3}H imipramine binding (Marazitti et al. 1995). One study demonstrated that platelet imipramine binding showed significant seasonal variation in adolescents who attempted suicide, with the nadir occurring in late winter/early spring (Pine et al. 1995). These findings are interesting not only because of the consistency with similar changes in the CNS, but also because the relative ease of a venipuncture may provide a more accessible avenue for assessment of serotonergic functioning.

Measuring urine metabolites of neurochemicals might provide another peripheral measure of underlying biological differences among suicidal and nonsuicidal patients. Indeed, one of the first studies of possible biological markers for suicidal behavior found increased amounts of 17-hydroxycorticosteroids in the urine of depressed patients who had attempted suicide (Bunney and Fawcett 1965). Subsequent studies demonstrated increased urinary cortisol, particularly among patients who attempted suicide by violent means (i.e., hanging, firearms). Most recently, one group found that patients with depression who attempted suicide had significantly lowered levels of dopamine, HVA, and dihydrophenylacetic acid (DOPAC) compared with nonsuicidal depressed patients (Roy et al. 1992).

There recently has been the intriguing suggestion that lowered serum cortisol is associated with suicide attempts: in one large study, male psychiatric patients with low serum cholesterol levels were twice as likely to have made a serious suicide attempt as men with cholesterol levels above the 25th percentile (Golier et al. 1995). In an emergency room setting, patients who were admitted following a suicide attempt were found to have significantly lower serum cholesterol than were nonsuicidal psychiatric inpatients (Kunugi et al. 1997). Explanations for this finding have included both possible modifications of serotonin metabolism and interleukin-2 (Penttinen 1995). However, there is conflicting evidence regarding the interrelationship between cholesterol levels and decreased serotonin activity in the brain, perhaps pointing again to the necessity for examining other neurochemical or neuroendocrine processes that might also underlie suicidal behavior.

Taken together, these findings may one day yield a biological suicide-potential workup for patients who might have other demographic or clinical risk factors. Future research will focus on the identification and prediction of suicidal behavior that may come with consideration of a clustering of these biological variables.

ASSESSMENT OF THE SUICIDAL PATIENT

It has been written that "during a cardiac arrest, the first procedure is to take your own pulse" (Shem 1978). Facetious as this statement sounds, it exhorts the clinician to monitor his or her own reactions to a potentially life-threatening situation, particularly as they might interfere with his or her ability to assess such a situation accurately. Indeed, the suicidal patient may provoke a panoply of unpleasant emotions, such as hate, fear, and restlessness, in the evaluating clinician that might interfere with the ability to establish adequate rapport. As a result, inquiries regarding suicidal ideation or intent may be rushed, put off until the end of the interview, or not ventured at all. It is of paramount importance, then, that the evaluating clinician acknowledge in a nonjudgmental way his or her own countertransferential reaction to a suicidal patient. In this way, the evaluator can maximize his or her ability to interact with the suicidal patient so as to "blend enough compassion so that the suicidal person experiences the clinician as an ally and enough detachment so that the clinician is not overwhelmed by his or her own responses to the patient's pain" (Doyle 1990, p. 381).

The evaluation of suicidal ideation or behavior is done in a manner similar to the investigation of any symptom cluster that might have adverse medical consequences. First, the clinician maintains an index of suspicion stemming from the demographic characteristics reviewed earlier in this chapter. Then, the clinician must individualize the assessment to the patient—specifically by considering personal and family history, assessing current medical and psychiatric status, determining psychosocial assets and liabilities, and taking into consideration prior response to treatment.

In taking a personal history of a patient to assess suicidal ideation, it is quintessential to evaluate the patient's level of intention of acting upon such ideation. Furthermore, one must always inquire as to the presence of a plan of suicide action, paying particular attention to the steps already taken to implement such a plan and assessing its potential lethality. The availability of means must be assessed, ranging from stockpile medications to firearms. One should also inquire as to whether the patient has taken any specific actions in preparation for death such as purchasing a gun, writing a will, or giving away prized objects. It is also important to inquire about the presence of other symptoms that have been associated with a higher suicide risk. These include delusional symptoms (particularly command hallucinations), anhedonia, hopelessness, and severe anxiety.

It is essential to obtain a history of prior suicide attempts as well as a history of violence and impulsivity. In addition, the presence of substance abuse should be assessed because, as noted earlier in this chapter, it also has been associated with an increased risk of suicide. Patients with a family history of suicide as well as violence might also alert the clinician to the presence of a liability to more dangerous suicidal behavior. The clinician also must inquire about the circumstances of previous violence as well as whether the patient thinks this behavior is abnormal or unusual. The clinician also should attempt to determine whether the violence is tied to a specific mood state.

A complete evaluation for suicide potential also will include the assessment of an individual's strengths. Despite the presence of suicidal behavior, it may well be that an individual has a proven ability not only to control his or her behavior but also to bring familial or financial resources to bear upon his or her situation. A *motivation to seek help in general*, and meaningful psychiatric treatment in particular, should be determined. As part of this assessment, the clinician should become familiar with the patient's prior responses to treatment, including responses to pharmacotherapeutic intervention as well as psychotherapy and psychosocial support.

Several more formal methods of suicide risk assessment have been used in research settings with varying degrees of success. One of the best developed scales is the Risk Estimator Scale for Suicide (Motto et al. 1985). This scale was the result of a 2-year prospective study of 2,753 patients with depression or suicidality in which completed suicides were noted. Fifteen variables were incorporated into a scale that gives an estimated risk of suicide in 2 years (Table 36–7). These variables included demographics, psychiatric history, and stressors, as well as interpreted factors such as the interviewer's reaction to the subject. Other scales for the measurement of suicidal ideation include the Scale for Suicidal Ideation and the Suicide Intent Scale, both developed by Beck et al. (1975). Also, because hopelessness has been identified by Beck and his group as being central to suicidal intent, the Beck Hopelessness Scale (Beck and Steer 1988) also might be considered to have clinical utility. These scales also underscore the need to consider a large number of factors that might increase suicide risk; this is particularly true in light of the recent sobering study that suggested that more than three-fourths of patients who ultimately commit suicide do not communicate their intent to do so in appointments with health care professionals that took place within 28 days of the actual suicide.

TREATMENT OF THE SUICIDAL PATIENT

As mentioned earlier, suicidal behavior is a syndrome that cuts across rigid diagnostic lines. As such, it is important that this behavior be addressed apart from, and in addition to, the ostensible underlying psychiatric condition.

The clinician must first confront his or her own feelings, however unpleasant or embarrassing, regarding the patient. As Doyle (1990) points out, "The clinician's experience of anxiety, anger, sadness, or confusion may reflect

TABLE 36–7. Final set of variables from Risk Estimator Scale for Suicide (Motto et al. 1985)

Variable	High-risk category	Coefficient (weight)	Standard error	P
1. Age	Risk increases with age	0.273[a]	.092	.001
2. Occupation	Executive, administrator, owner of business, professional, semiskilled worker	0.515	.206	.013
3. Financial resources	Risk increases with resources	0.373	.120	.002
4. Emotional disorder in family	Depression, alcoholism	0.486	.195	.013
5. Sexual orientation	Bisexual, active; homosexual, inactive	0.692	.252	.006
6. Previous psychiatric hospital admissions	Risk increases with number of admissions	0.228	.079	.004
7. Result of previous efforts to obtain help	Negative or variable	0.593	.199	.003
8. Threatened financial loss	Yes	0.674	.271	.013
9. Special stress	Severe	0.676	.191	.000
10. Sleep (hours per night)	Risk increases with number of hours per night	0.395	.161	.014
11. Weight change, present episode	Gain or 1%–9% loss	0.646	.241	.013
12. Ideas of persecution or reference	Yes	0.636	.198	.014
13. Suicidal impulses	Yes	1.071	.227	.000
14. Seriousness of present suicide attempt—intent	Unambivalent or ambivalent but weighted toward suicide	0.943	.201	.000
15. Interviewer's reaction to subject	Risk increases with negativity of reaction	0.454	.163	.006

[a]Applied to square root of age.

the patient's internal milieu and suggest areas for exploration and intervention. . . . Rather than avoiding or denying feelings, the clinician uses them to form hypotheses about the patient that deserve further investigation" (p. 383).

Initially, it may seem to the patient that his or her alliance with the clinician is his or her only tie to life. Ultimately, the patient and clinician must arrive at a mutually agreeable contract regarding further courses of action to be taken based on their alliance.

Principles of acute intervention, as delineated by Blumenthal (1990), begin with adequate supervision of the suicidal patient. If this supervision cannot be sufficiently accomplished in an outpatient setting, hospitalization, whether on a voluntary or involuntary basis, should be considered. It is also necessary to limit the patient's access to potentially self-destructive methods, principal among which is antidepressant medication. It is a poignant irony that medicinal compounds specifically designed to combat conditions leading to suicide are extremely lethal when taken in overdosage. The clinician should be keenly aware of lethal indexes of medications and prescribe only small amounts at a time. For example, with tricyclic antidepressants, less than 1 g total should be dispensed at any given time. Although the clinician cannot eliminate all other potential means to suicide, he or she must make an effort to reduce the risk. This effort may involve, for example, contracting with the patient for him or her to give up access to firearms that may be in his or her possession and, at times, even convincing the patient to agree to have knives and other sharp instruments under another person's lock and key.

SOMATIC TREATMENT

In general, the aim of biological therapy in the treatment of suicidal patients has been to treat the diagnosed psychiatric condition. As a result, there have been few studies describing the response of suicidal behavior per se to specific pharmacotherapeutic interventions.

The role of dopamine in suicidal behavior seemed to be given more weight by two studies that indicated that postsynaptic dopaminergic blocking agents appeared to decrease suicidal behavior in patients with severe character disorders (Cowdry and Gardner 1988; Soloff et al. 1986).

As might be expected, however, much focus has been placed on interventions affecting the serotonergic system. With the advent of medications that selectively affect the serotonergic system, one might expect these medications to be associated with more significant amelioration of suicidal behavior than either tricyclic antidepressants or antidepressants that promote noradrenergic transmission. Some, although not all, of the early comparison studies

suggested an earlier improvement in suicidality in the group treated with serotonergic agents (de Wilde et al. 1985; Montgomery et al. 1981; Mullin et al. 1988).

However, Teicher et al. (1990) reported six cases of the emergence of severe suicidal preoccupation in patients undergoing treatment with fluoxetine, a selective serotonin reuptake inhibitor (SSRI). Another study noted the emergence of self-destructive behavior in six children and adolescents receiving fluoxetine (King et al. 1991). The dramatic impact of these studies was to draw attention to the possibility of "paradoxical reactions" of antidepressants: the agents appeared to produce or intensify the symptoms that they were ostensibly introduced to treat. Although the aforementioned studies seemed to popularize the notion of such paradoxical reactions, the emergence of new-onset suicidality, intensification of previously existing suicidality, and increased assaultiveness had already been reported with tricyclic antidepressants (Damluji and Ferguson 1988; Rampling 1978; Soloff et al. 1987), maprotiline (Rouillon et al. 1989), and alprazolam (Gardner and Cowdry 1985).

Larger studies have since assessed the worsening of suicidal ideation upon initiation of antidepressant therapy. One study, a retrospective chart review of more than 1,000 patients who were treated with antidepressants, demonstrated no difference in any single antidepressant medication in the seeming production of suicidal ideation (Fava and Rosenbaum 1991), whereas another analysis revealed a worsening of suicidal ideation in fluoxetine-treated patients (Mann and Kapur 1991). Another large study revealed that the emergence of suicidality was less frequent in patients receiving fluoxetine than in patients receiving other antidepressant treatments or placebo (Beasley et al. 1991). In a recent study of more than 600 patients being treated for anxiety disorders, there was no evidence that fluoxetine was associated with increased risk of suicide attempts or gestures; in fact, of those patients who were also diagnosed as having a major depressive disorder at intake, there was a statistically lower probability of suicide attempts or gestures for those taking fluoxetine than for those not taking fluoxetine (Warshaw and Keller 1996).

It should be evident that the appearance or worsening of suicidal behavior exists with a wide variety of antidepressants, although this phenomenon probably affects fewer than 6% of the patients treated (Mann and Kapur 1991). What mechanisms might explain the production of this paradoxical effect? One explanation is that this phenomenon occurs as a result of drug-induced akathisia. In fact, neuroleptic-induced akathisia, which is initially indistinguishable from that induced by some antidepressants, has been associated with increased acting-out behaviors and increased suicide attempts (Drake and Ehrlich 1985; Siris 1985). Another possible mechanism might be a paradoxical lowering of serotonin. Electrophysiological studies have demonstrated that medications that block the reuptake of serotonin in the synaptic cleft actually cause an initial decrease in the firing of serotonergic neurons (Blier et al. 1990; de Montigny et al. 1990). It is conceivable that in an unfortunate minority of individuals, this initial phase may be prolonged to a clinically deleterious degree.

Interestingly, other studies suggest that serotonergic agents may selectively decrease suicidality and impulsiveness not only in patients with major depressive disorder (Muijen et al. 1988), but also in patients with borderline personality disorder (Cornelius et al. 1991; Norden 1989). One study compared the relative effectiveness of serotonergic antidepressants with that of noradrenergic antidepressants in the treatment of patients with major depressive disorders who had already made suicide attempts; the serotonergic antidepressants were found to be significantly more effective in the treatment of these patients (Sacchetti et al. 1991). This is an intriguing finding in light of the posited serotonergic hypofunction in suicidal patients. However, literature to date is too preliminary to support the hypothesis that SSRIs are the antidepressants of choice in the suicidal patient because of their neurotransmitter action. Rather, SSRIs and other new-generation antidepressants may be viewed as more prudent choices over tricyclic antidepressants because of their low lethality index.

Finally, the role of electroconvulsive therapy cannot be overemphasized as a safe and relatively rapid somatic treatment for the acutely suicidal depressed patient.

PSYCHOTHERAPY WITH THE SUICIDAL PATIENT

In his classic treatise on suicide, Durkheim (1897/1951) noted that the risk of suicide varied inversely to the degree of connectedness with family and society as a whole. Indeed, as discussed earlier in this chapter, the risk of suicide seems to correlate inversely with the maintenance of ongoing personal and professional relationships. Thus, one of the daunting tasks in the psychotherapy of the suicidal patient is the realization that the psychotherapist may be perceived as the last ballast of hope that human connectedness may be yet something worth striving for. The establishment of the therapeutic alliance, then, is the singularly most important task in the treatment of the suicidal patient.

The establishment of the therapeutic alliance is common to all of the psychotherapeutic traditions. Also common to all psychotherapeutic traditions is the role of the empathic method (Jacobs 1989) in the treatment of suicidal patients. There is no "suicide-specific" psychotherapy, and clinicians are increasingly aware of the value of integrating principles from psychodynamic and cognitive-behavior therapy. An important contribution of cognitive psychology has been the identification of hopelessness as the psychological factor most consistent with suicidal intent—even more so than the subjective experience of depression (Beck et al. 1975; Weisman et al. 1979; Wetzel 1976). The emphasis in cognitive therapy of suicidal behavior is the correction of cognitive distortions that may have resulted in the perception of hopelessness, and the therapist strives to instill hope in this process. Also, to the degree that depression or hopelessness has led to deterioration of problem-solving abilities, therapy is geared to the enhancement of those skills, including increasing the patient's capacity to view options and alternatives to suicide.

Psychodynamic psychotherapies have stemmed from an understanding of the dynamics of the individual's suicidal motivation, as well as of the act of suicide itself (Dulit and Michels 1992; Hendin 1991). In addition, the psychodynamic literature offers useful insights regarding countertransference pitfalls in the treatment of suicidal patients. It is necessary for therapists to address countertransferential feelings in themselves. Addressing countertransferential feelings is necessary less to expunge oneself of "incorrect" feelings than to realize how one's refusal to acknowledge them might lead to the subversion of the therapeutic alliance (Maltsberger and Buie 1974).

As mentioned previously, psychosocial interventions have had little impact on the rate of suicide. In fact, some of the proposed treatments have been thought to exacerbate suicidal intent (Chowdhury et al. 1973; Liberman and Eckman 1981). As such, psychotherapy per se must be seen as yet another procedure administered to a patient who has a potentially terminal outcome—something that has the capacity to render either better clinical improvement or deterioration. What is necessary, however, is to determine the actual efficacy of specialized psychotherapeutic techniques both alone and in combination with pharmacotherapeutic interventions. Only by determining this efficacy can we expect to have an impact on the suicide rate, a rate that has not changed in 45 years.

CONCLUSIONS

Suicide is a complex, multidimensional phenomenon that has been studied from philosophical, sociological, and clinical perspectives. In this chapter we have focused on suicide from a clinical perspective, emphasizing psychiatric illness, psychological factors, and neurobiological correlates of suicidality. We have given an overview of management of suicidal patients, including risk assessment, pharmacotherapy, and psychotherapy.

As reiterated throughout this chapter, the overall rate of suicide has not changed in 45 years. However, it is clear that in treated populations the risk of suicide can be reduced. Our role as clinicians is to hone our skills at recognition and treatment to prevent suicide in any patient. However, ultimately, to have an impact on the overall rate, we need to advance our efforts in *primary* prevention through education—in schools, in the workplace, and through the media. Because, as noted suicidologist Edwin Shneidman (1986) writes, "In the end, effective prevention of suicide is everybody's business" (p. 16).

REFERENCES

Agren H: Symptom patterns in unipolar and bipolar depression correlating with monoamine metabolites in the cerebrospinal fluid, II: suicide. Psychiatry Res 3:225–236, 1980

Allebeck P, Wistedt B: Mortality in schizophrenia. Arch Gen Psychiatry 43:650–653, 1986

Apter A, Kotler M, Sevy S, et al: Correlates of risk of suicide in violent and nonviolent psychiatric patients. Am J Psychiatry 148:883–887, 1991

Arango V, Underwood M, Gubbi A, et al: Localized alterations in pre- and postsynaptic serotonin binding sites in the ventrolateral prefrontal cortex of suicide victims. Brain Res 688:121–133, 1995

Åsberg M, Thorän P, Träskman L, et al: Serotonin depression: a biochemical subgroup within affective disorders? Science 191:478–480, 1976

Banki CM: Factors influencing monoamine metabolites and tryptophan in patients with alcohol dependence. J Neural Transm 50:89–101, 1981

Banki CM, Arat M, Papp Z, et al: The effect of dexamethasone on cerebrospinal fluid metabolites in psychiatric patients. Pharmacopsychiatrics 16:77–81, 1983

Banki CM, Arat M, Papp Z, et al: Biochemical markers in suicidal patients: investigations with cerebrospinal fluid amine metabolites and neuroendocrine tests. J Affect Disord 6:341–350, 1984

Barraclough B, Bunch J, Nelson B, et al: A hundred cases of suicide: clinical aspects. Br J Psychiatry 125:355–373, 1974

Beasley CM Jr, Dornseif BE, Bosomworth JC, et al: Fluoxetine and suicide: a meta-analysis of controlled trials of treatment for depression. BMJ 303:685–692, 1991

Beck AT, Steer RA: Manual for the Beck Hopelessness Scale. San Antonio, TX, Psychological Corporation, 1988

Beck AT, Beck R, Kovacs M: Classification of suicidal behaviors, I: quantifying intent and medical lethality. Am J Psychiatry 132:285–287, 1975

Beck AT, Brown G, Berchick RJ, et al: Relationship between hopelessness and ultimate suicide: a replication with psychiatric outpatients. Am J Psychiatry 147:190–195, 1990

Beck AT, Steer RA, Sanderson WC, et al: Panic disorder and suicidal ideation and behavior: discrepant findings in psychiatric outpatients. Am J Psychiatry 148:1195–1199, 1991

Berrettini WH, Nurnberger JI Jr, Narrow W, et al: Cerebrospinal fluid studies of bipolar patients with and without a history of suicide attempts. Ann N Y Acad Sci 487:197–201, 1986

Beskow J, Gottfires CG, Roos BE, et al: Determination of monoamine and monoamine metabolites in the human brain: post-mortem studies in a group of suicides and a control group. Acta Psychiatr Scand 53:7–20, 1976

Black DW, Winokur G: Suicide and psychiatric diagnosis, in Suicide Over the Life Cycle: Risk Factors, Assessment, and Treatment of Suicidal Patients. Edited by Blumenthal SJ, Kupfer DJ. Washington, DC, American Psychiatric Press, 1990, pp 135–153

Blazer D, Williams CP: Epidemiology of dysphoria and depression in an elderly population. Am J Psychiatry 137:439–444, 1980

Blier P, de Montigny C, Chaput Y: A role for the serotonin system in the mechanism of action of antidepressant treatments: preclinical evidence. J Clin Psychiatry 51 (suppl):14–21, 1990

Blumenthal SJ: An overview and synopsis of risk factors, assessment, and treatment of suicidal patients over the life cycle, in Suicide Over the Life Cycle: Risk Factors, Assessment, and Treatment of Suicidal Patients. Edited by Blumenthal SJ, Kupfer DJ. Washington, DC, American Psychiatric Press, 1990, pp 685–733

Bourne HR, Bunney WE, Colburn RW, et al: Noradrenaline, 5-hydroxytryptamine, and 5-hydroxyindoleacetic acid in the hindbrains of suicidal patients. Lancet 2:805–808, 1968

Breier A, Astrachan BM: Characterization of schizophrenic patients who commit suicide. Am J Psychiatry 141:206–209, 1984

Breitbart W, Rosenfeld BD, Passik SD: Interest in physician-assisted suicide among ambulatory HIV-infected patients. Am J Psychiatry 153:238–242, 1996

Brent DA, Moritz G, Bridge J, et al: Long-term impact of exposure to suicide: a three-year controlled follow-up. J Am Acad Child Adolesc Psychiatry 35:646–653, 1996

Brown GL, Goodwin FK, Ballenger JC, et al: Aggression in humans correlates with cerebrospinal fluid amine metabolites. Psychiatry Res 1:131–139, 1979

Brown GL, Ebert MH, Goyer PF, et al: Aggression, suicide, and serotonin: relationship to CSF amine metabolites. Am J Psychiatry 139:741–746, 1982

Bunney WE Jr, Fawcett JA: Possibility of a biochemical test for suicidal potential: an analysis of endocrine findings prior to three suicides. Arch Gen Psychiatry 13:232–239, 1965

Cheetam SC, Cross AJ, Crompton MR, et al: Serotonin and GABA function in depressed suicide victims. Paper presented at the International Conference on New Directions in Affective Disorders, Jerusalem, 1987

Cheung HK: Schizophrenics fully remitted on neuroleptics for 3–5 years: to stop or continue drugs? Br J Psychiatry 138:490–494, 1981

Chowdhury N, Hicks RC, Keitman N: Evaluation of an aftercare service for parasuicide (attempted suicide) patients. Social Psychiatry 8:67–81, 1973

Coccaro EF, Siever LJ, Klar HM, et al: Serotonergic studies in patients with affective and personality disorders: correlates with suicidal and impulsive aggressive behavior. Arch Gen Psychiatry 46:587–599, 1989

Cochran E, Robins E, Grote S: Regional serotonin levels in brain: a comparison of depressive suicides and alcoholic suicides with controls. Biol Psychiatry 11:283–294, 1976

Corbitt EM, Malone KM, Haas GL, et al: Suicidal behavior in patients with major depression and comorbid personality disorders. J Affect Disord 39:61–72, 1996

Cornelius JR, Soloff PH, Perel JM, et al: A preliminary trial of fluoxetine in refractory borderline patients. J Clin Psychopharmacol 11:116–120, 1991

Cowdry RW, Gardner DL: Pharmacotherapy of borderline personality disorder: alprazolam, carbamazepine, trifluoperazine, and tranylcypromine. Arch Gen Psychiatry 45:111–119, 1988

Crow TJ, Cross A, Cooper SJ, et al: Neurotransmitter receptors and monoamine metabolites in the brains of patients with Alzheimer-type dementia and depression, and suicides. Neuropharmacology 23:1561–1569, 1984

Damluji NF, Ferguson JM: Paradoxical worsening of depressive symptomatology caused by antidepressants. J Clin Psychopharmacol 8:347–349, 1988

De Meo MD, McBride PA, Mann JJ, et al: Fenfluramine challenge in major depression, in New Research and Abstracts, 141st annual meeting of the American Psychiatric Association, Montreal, Quebec, May 1988, NR169, p. 91

de Montigny C, Chaput Y, Blier P: Modification of serotonergic neuron properties by long-term treatment with serotonin reuptake blockers. J Clin Psychiatry 51 (suppl B):4–8, 1990

de Wilde J, Mertens C, Fredricson Overø K, et al: Citalopram versus mianserin: a controlled, double-blind trial in depressed patients. Acta Psychiatr Scand 72:89–96, 1985

Doyle BB: Crisis management of the suicidal patient, in Suicide Over the Life Cycle: Risk Factors, Assessment, and Treatment of Suicidal Patients. Edited by Blumenthal SJ, Kupfer DJ. Washington, DC, American Psychiatric Press, 1990, pp 381–423

Drake RE, Cotton PG: Depression, hopelessness and suicide in chronic schizophrenia. Br J Psychiatry 148:554–559, 1986

Drake RE, Ehrlich J: Suicide attempts associated with akathisia. Am J Psychiatry 142:499–501, 1985

Drake RE, Gates C, Cotton PG, et al: Suicide among schizophrenics: who is at risk? J Nerv Ment Dis 172:613–617, 1984

Drake RE, Osher FC, Wallach MA: Alcohol use and abuse in schizophrenia: a prospective community study. J Nerv Ment Dis 177:408–414, 1989

Dulit RA, Michels R: Psychodynamics and suicide, in Suicide and Clinical Practice. Edited by Jacobs D. Washington, DC, American Psychiatric Press, 1992, pp 43–53

Durkheim E: Suicide: A Study in Sociology (1897). Translated by Spaulding JA, Simpson G. New York, Free Press, 1951

Ettinger R: A follow-up investigation of patients after attempted suicide, in The Suicide Syndrome. Edited by Farmer R, Hirsh S. London, Croon Helm, 1980, pp 167–172

Fava M, Rosenbaum JP: Suicidality and fluoxetine: is there a relationship? J Clin Psychiatry 52:108–111, 1991

Fawcett J, Scheftner WA, Fogg L, et al: Time-related predictors of suicide in major affective disorder. Am J Psychiatry 147:1189–1194, 1990

Freud S: Mourning and melancholia (1917[1915]), in Standard Edition of the Complete Psychological Works of Sigmund Freud, Vol 14. Translated and edited by Strachey J. London, Hogarth, 1957, pp 237–260

Friedman S, Jones JC, Chernen L, et al: Suicidal ideation and suicide attempts among patients with panic disorder: a survey of two outpatient clinics. Am J Psychiatry 149:680–685, 1992

Gardner DL, Cowdry RW: Alprazolam-induced dyscontrol in borderline personality disorder. Am J Psychiatry 142:98–100, 1985

Goldring N, Fieve RR: Attempted suicide in manic-depressive disorder. Am J Psychother 38:373–383, 1984

Golier J, Marzuk P, Leon A, et al: Low serum cholesterol and attempted suicide. Am J Psychiatry 152:419–423,1995

Goodwin FK: Suicide, aggression, and depression: a theoretical framework for future research. Ann N Y Acad Sci 487:351–355, 1986

Goodwin FK, Jamison KR: Manic-Depressive Illness. New York, Oxford University Press, 1990

Gould MS, Fisher P, Parides M, et al: Psychosocial risk factors of child and adolescent completed suicide. Arch Gen Psychiatry 53:1155–1162, 1996

Hendin H: Psychodynamics of suicide, with particular reference to the young. Am J Psychiatry 148:1150–1158, 1991

Henriksson MM, Isometsa ET, Kuoppasalmi KI, et al: Panic disorder in completed suicide. J Clin Psychiatry 57:275–81, 1996

Hogan TP, Awad AG: Pharmacotherapy and suicide risk in schizophrenia. Can J Psychiatry 28:277–281, 1983

Jacobs D: Psychotherapy with suicidal patients, in Suicide: Understanding and Response. Edited by Jacobs D, Brown HN. Madison, CT, International Universities Press, 1989, pp 329–342

Jacobs D: Evaluating and treating suicidal behavior in the borderline patient, in Suicide and Clinical Practice. Edited by Jacobs D. Washington, DC, American Psychiatric Press, 1992, pp 115–130

Jaffe JH, Ciraulo DA: Alcoholism and depression, in Psychopathology and Addictive Disorders. Edited by Meyer RE. New York, Guilford, 1986, pp 293–320

Kernberg OF: Severe Personality Disorders: Psychotherapeutic Strategies. New Haven, CT, Yale University Press, 1984

King RA, Riddle MA, Chappell PB, et al: Emergence of self-destructive phenomena in children and adolescents during fluoxetine treatment. J Am Acad Child Adolesc Psychiatry 30:179–186, 1991

Korpi ER, Kleinman JE, Goodman SI, et al: Serotonin and 5-hydroxyindoleacetic acid in brains of suicide victims: comparison in chronic schizophrenic patients with suicide as cause of death. Arch Gen Psychiatry 43:594–600, 1986

Kunugi H, Takei, Aoki H, et al: Low serum cholesterol in suicide attempters. Biol Psychiatry 41:196–200, 1997

Liberman RP, Eckman T: Behavior therapy versus insight-oriented therapy for repeated suicide attempters. Arch Gen Psychiatry 38:1126–1130, 1981

Linnoila M, De Jong J, Virkkunen M: Family history of alcoholism in violent offenders and impulsive fire setters. Arch Gen Psychiatry 46:613–616, 1989

Lloyd KG, Farley IJ, Deck H, et al: Serotonin and 5-hydroxyindoleacetic acid in discrete areas of the brainstem of suicide victims and control patients. Adv Biochem Psychopharmacol 11:387–397, 1974

Malone KM, Haas GL, Sweeney JA, et al: Major depression and the risk of attempted suicide. J Affect Disord 34:173–185, 1995

Maltsberger JT, Buie DH: Countertransference hate in the treatment of suicidal patients. Arch Gen Psychiatry 30:625–633, 1974

Mann JJ, Arango V: Integration of neurobiology and psychopathology in a unified model of suicidal behavior. J Clin Psychopharmacol 12(suppl):2S–7S, 1992

Mann JJ, Kapur S: The emergence of suicidal ideation and behavior during antidepressant pharmacotherapy. Arch Gen Psychiatry 48:1027–1033, 1991

Mann JJ, Stanley M, McBride PA, et al: Increased serotonin₂ and β-adrenergic receptor binding in the frontal cortices of suicide victims. Arch Gen Psychiatry 43:954–959, 1986

Mann JJ, Malone K, Psych M, et al: Attempted suicide characteristics and cerebrospinal fluid amine metabolites in depressed inpatients. Neuropsychopharmacology 15:576–586, 1996

Marazitti D, Presta S, Silvestri S, et al: Platelet markers in suicide attempters. Prog Neuropsychopharmacol Biol Psychiatry 19:375–383, 1995

Marzuk PM, Mann JJ: Suicide and substance abuse. Psychiatric Annals 18:639–645, 1988

Marzuk PM, Tierney H, Tardiff K, et al: Increased risk of suicide in persons with AIDS. JAMA 259:1333–1337, 1988

Marzuk PM, Leon AC, Tardiff K, et al: The effect of access to lethal methods of injury on suicide rates. Arch Gen Psychiatry 49:451–458, 1992a

Marzuk PM, Tardiff K, Leon AC, et al: Prevalence of cocaine use among residents of New York City who committed suicide during a one-year period. Am J Psychiatry 149:371–375, 1992b

McGlashan TH, Heinssen RK: Hospital discharge status and long-term outcome for patients with schizophrenia, schizoaffective disorders, borderline personality disorder, and unipolar affective disorder. Arch Gen Psychiatry 45:363–368, 1988

McKegney FP, O'Dowd MA: Suicidality and HIV status. Am J Psychiatry 149:396–398, 1992

Meltzer HY, Nash JF, Ohmori T, et al: Neuroendocrine and biochemical studies in serotonin and dopamine in depression and suicide. Paper presented at the International Conference on New Directions in Affective Disorders, Jerusalem, 1987

Miles CP: Conditions predisposing to suicide: a review. J Nerv Ment Dis 164:231–246, 1977

Montgomery SA, McAuley R, Rani SJ, et al: A double blind comparison of zimelidine and amitriptyline in endogenous depression. Acta Psychiatr Scand Suppl 63 (suppl 290):314–329, 1981

Morgan AC: Special issues of assessment and treatment of suicide risk in the elderly, in Suicide: Understanding and Response. Edited by Jacobs D, Brown HN. Madison, CT, International Universities Press, 1989, pp 239–256

Moscicki EK: Epidemiology surveys as tools for studying suicidal behavior: a review. Suicide Life Threat Behav 19:131–146, 1989

Motto JA, Heilbron DC, Juster RP: Development of a clinical instrument to estimate suicide risk. Am J Psychiatry 142:680–686, 1985

Muijen M, Roy D, Silverstone T, et al: A comparative clinical trial of fluoxetine, mianserin and placebo in depressed outpatients. Acta Psychiatr Scand 78:384–390, 1988

Mullin JM, Pandita-Gunawerdina UR, Whitehead AM: A double-blind comparison of fluvoxamine and dothiepin in the treatment of major affective disorders. Br J Clin Pract 42:51–55, 1988

Murphy GE, Wetzel RD: The lifetime risk of suicide in alcoholism. Arch Gen Psychiatry 47:383–392, 1990

Myerson LR, Wennogle LP, Abel MS, et al: Human brain receptor alterations in suicide victims. Pharmacol Biochem Behav 17:159–163, 1982

Nemeroff CB, Widerlov E, Bissette G, et al: Elevated concentrations of CSF corticotropin releasing factor–like immunoreactivity in depressed patients. Science 226:1342–1344, 1984

Nemeroff CB, Owens MJ, Bissette G, et al: Reduced corticotropin releasing factor binding sites in the frontal cortex of suicide victims. Arch Gen Psychiatry 45:577–579, 1988

Ninan PT, van Kammen DP, Scheinin M, et al: CSF 5-hydroxyindoleacetic acid levels in suicidal schizophrenic patients. Am J Psychiatry 141:566–569, 1984

Norden MJ: Fluoxetine in borderline personality disorder. Prog Neuropsychopharmacol Biol Psychiatry 13:885–893, 1989

Nyman A, Jonsson H: Patterns of self-destructive behavior in schizophrenia. Acta Psychiatr Scand 73:252–262, 1986

Owen F, Cross A, Crow TJ, et al: Brain 5-HT₂ receptors and suicide. Lancet 2:1256, 1983

Pandey GN, Pandey SC, Janicak PG, et al: Platelet serotonin-2 receptor binding sites in depression and suicide. Biol Psychiatry 28:215–222, 1990

Pandey G, Pandey S, Duvivedi Y, et al: Platelet serotonin$_{2A}$ receptors: a potential biological marker for suicidal behavior. Am J Psychiatry 152:850–855, 1995

Pare CMB, Yeung DP, Brice K, et al: 5-Hydroxytryptamine, noradrenaline and dopamine in brainstem, hypothalamus and caudate nucleus of controls and of patients committing suicide by coal gas poisoning. Lancet 2:133–135, 1969

Paul SM, Rehavi M, Skolnick P, et al: High affinity binding of antidepressants to a biogenic amine transport site in human brain and platelet: studies in depression, in Neurobiology of Mood Disorders. Edited by Post RM, Ballenger JC. Baltimore, MD, Williams & Wilkins, 1984, pp 845–853

Perry EK, Marshall EF, Blessed G, et al: Decreased imipramine binding in the brains of patients with depressive illness. Br J Psychiatry 142:188–192, 1983

Penttinen J: Hypothesis: low serum cholesterol, suicide, and interleukin-2 Am J Epidemiol 141:716–718, 1995

Pfeffer CR: Risk factors associated with youth suicide: a clinical perspective. Psychiatric Annals 18:652–656, 1988

Pine D, Trautman P, Shaffer D, et al: Seasonal rhythm of platelet [³H] imipramine binding in adolescents who attempted suicide. Am J Psychiatry 152:923–925, 1995

Rampling D: Aggression: a paradoxical response to tricyclic antidepressants. Am J Psychiatry 135:117–118, 1978

Rich CL, Young D, Fowler RC: San Diego Suicide Study, I: young versus old subjects. Arch Gen Psychiatry 43:577–582, 1986

Rich CL, Warsradt GM, Nemiroff RA, et al: Suicide, stressors, and the life cycle. Am J Psychiatry 148:524–527, 1991

Robins E, Murphy GE, Wilkinson RH, et al: Some clinical considerations in the prevention of suicide based on a study of 134 successful suicides. Am J Public Health 49:888–899, 1959

Robins LN, Kulbok PA: Epidemiological studies in suicide. Psychiatric Annals 18:619, 623–627, 1988

Roose SP, Glassman AH, Walsh BT, et al: Depression, delusions, and suicide. Am J Psychiatry 140:1159–1162, 1983

Rouillon F, Phillips R, Seurvier D, et al: Rechutes de depression unipolaire et ellicacite de la maprotiline. Encephale 15:527–534, 1989

Roy A: Suicide in chronic schizophrenia. Br J Psychiatry 141:171–177, 1982

Roy A, Ninan P, Mazonson A, et al: CSF monoamine metabolites in chronic schizophrenic patients who attempt suicide. Psychol Med 15:335–340, 1985

Roy A, Agren H, Pickar D, et al: Reduced CSF concentrations of homovanillic acid and homovanillic acid to 5-hydroxyindoleacetic acid ratios in depressed patients: relationship to suicidal behavior and dexamethasone nonsuppression. Am J Psychiatry 143:1539–1545, 1986

Roy A, Lamparski D, DeJong J, et al: Characteristics of alcoholics who attempt suicide. Am J Psychiatry 147:761–765, 1990

Roy A, Karoum F, Pollack S: Marked reduction in indexes of dopamine metabolism among patients with depression who attempt suicide. Arch Gen Psychiatry 49:447–450, 1992

Roy A, Segal N, Sarchiapone M: Attempted suicide among living co-twins of twin suicide victims. Am J Psychiatry 152:1075–1076, 1995

Sacchetti E, Vita A, Guarneri L, et al: The effectiveness of fluoxetine, clomipramine, nortriptyline, and desipramine in major depressives with suicidal behavior: preliminary findings, in Serotonin Related Psychiatric Syndromes. Edited by Cassano GB, Akiskal HS. London, Royal Society of Medicine Services, 1991, pp 47–53

Sainsbury P: Depression, suicide, and suicide prevention, in Suicide. Edited by Roy A. Baltimore, MD, Williams & Wilkins, 1986a, pp 73–88

Sainsbury P: The epidemiology of suicide, in Suicide. Edited by Roy A. Baltimore, MD, Williams & Wilkins, 1986b, pp 17–40

Schulsinger F, Kety SS, Rosenthal D, et al: A family study of suicide, in Origin, Prevention and Treatment of Affective Disorders. Edited by Schon M, Stromgren E. New York, Academic Press, 1979, pp 277–287

Shaw DM, Camps FE, Eccleston EG: 5-Hydroxytryptamine in the hind-brain of depressive suicides. Br J Psychiatry 113:1407–1411, 1967

Shem S: The House of God. New York, Richard Marek Publishers, 1978

Shneidman ES: Some essentials of suicide and implications for response, in Suicide. Edited by Roy A. Baltimore, MD, Williams & Wilkins, 1986, pp 1–16

Siris SG: Three cases of akathisia and "acting out." J Clin Psychiatry 46:395–397, 1985

Skoog I, Aevarsson O, Beskow J, et al: Suicide in the elderly. Am J Psychiatry 153:1015–1020, 1996

Soloff PH, George A, Nathan RS, et al: Progress in pharmacotherapy of borderline disorders: a double-blind study of amitriptyline, haloperidol, and placebo. Arch Gen Psychiatry 43:691–697, 1986

Soloff PH, George A, Nathan RS, et al: Behavioral dyscontrol in borderline patients treated with amitriptyline. Psychopharmacol Bull 23:177–181, 1987

Stanley M, Mann JJ: Increased serotonin-2 binding sites in frontal cortex of suicide victims. Lancet 1:214–216, 1983

Stanley M, Virgilio JJ, Gerson S: Tritiated imipramine binding sites are decreased in the frontal cortex of suicides. Science 216:1337–1339, 1982

Stanley M, McIntyre I, Gershon S: Post-mortem serotonin metabolism in suicide victims. Paper presented at the American College of Neuropsychopharmacology, San Juan, Puerto Rico, December 1983

Stevenson JM: Suicide, in The American Psychiatric Press Textbook of Psychiatry. Edited by Talbot JA, Hales RE, Yudofsky SC. Washington, DC, American Psychiatric Press, 1988, pp 1021–1035

Stone MH, Stone DK, Hurt SW: Natural history of borderline patients treated by intensive hospitalization. Psychiatr Clin North Am 10:185–206, 1987

Targum SD, Rosen L, Capodanno AE: The dexamethasone suppression test in suicidal patients with unipolar depression. Am J Psychiatry 140:877–879, 1983

Teicher MH, Glod C, Cole JO: Emergence of intense suicidal preoccupation during fluoxetine treatment. Am J Psychiatry 147:207–210, 1990

Träskman L, Åsberg M, Bertilsson L, et al: Monoamine metabolites in CSF and suicidal behavior. Arch Gen Psychiatry 38:631–636, 1981

Träskman-Bendz L, Alling C, Oreland L, et al: Prediction of suicidal behavior from prologic tests. J Clin Psychopharmacol 12 (suppl):21S–26S, 1992

Warshaw M, Keller M: The relationship between fluoxetine use and suicidal behavior in 654 subjects with anxiety disorders. J Clin Psychiatry 57:158–166, 1996

Weiden P, Roy A: General versus specific risk factors for suicide in schizophrenia, in Suicide and Clinical Practice. Edited by Jacobs D. Washington, DC, American Psychiatric Press, 1992, pp 75–100

Weisman A, Beck AT, Kovacs M: Drug abuse, hopelessness and suicidal behavior. International Journal of Addiction 14:451–464, 1979

Weiss RD, Stephens PS: Substance abuse and suicide, in Suicide and Clinical Practice. Edited by Jacobs D. Washington, DC, American Psychiatric Press, 1992, pp 101–114

Weissman MM, Klerman GL, Markowitz JS, et al: Suicidal ideation and suicide attempts in panic disorder and attacks. N Engl J Med 321:1209–1214, 1989

Wetzel RD: Hopelessness, depression, and suicide intent. Arch Gen Psychiatry 33:1069–1073, 1976

Wilkinson G, Bacon N: A clinical and epidemiological survey of parasuicide and suicide in Edinburgh schizophrenics. Psychol Med 14:899–912, 1984

Winchel RM, Stanley B, Stanley M: Biochemical aspects of behavior, in Suicide Over the Life Cycle: Risk Factors, Assessment, and Treatment of Suicidal Patients. Edited by Blumenthal SJ, Kupfer DJ. Washington, DC, American Psychiatric Press, 1990, pp 97–126

Winokur G, Tsuang M: The Iowa 500: suicide in mania, depression, and schizophrenia. Am J Psychiatry 132:650–651, 1975

Zanko MT, Bigeon A: Increased β-adrenergic receptor binding in human frontal cortex of suicide victims. Paper presented at the annual meeting of the Society for Neuroscience, Boston, 1983

Zeck PM, Tierney H, Tardiff K, et al: Increased risk of suicide in persons with AIDS. JAMA 259:1333–1337, 1988

Zisook S, Byrd D, Kuck J, et al: Command hallucinations in outpatients with schizophrenia. J Clin Psychiatry 56:462–465, 1995

CHAPTER 37

VIOLENCE

KENNETH TARDIFF, M.D., M.P.H.

Violence by psychiatric patients has become a public concern because of publicity around murders committed by psychiatric patients. We are all familiar with newspaper and television reports about a former patient who has been discharged from a hospital and kills his wife, or a man with a history of psychiatric problems who kills a number of people in a public place, or a depressed woman who kills her children and then herself. In reality, severely disturbed psychiatric patients are responsible for a small percentage of homicides and other violence occurring in society. Although psychiatric patients are not responsible for many homicides or violence in society, there is evidence that a relationship exists between having some mental disorders and increased risk of violence (Monahan 1992).

Psychiatrists should be able to evaluate and treat violent patients. A number of studies indicate that approximately 10% of the patients seen in psychiatric hospitals have manifested violent behavior toward others just before being admitted to these hospitals (Davis 1991; Tardiff 1983), a finding that is true for private as well as public hospitals. A more recent study found that the percentage of patients who are violent before admission approaches 15% (Tardiff et al. 1997). Furthermore, the occurrence of violent behavior even among chronic inpatients is still appreciable. Learning how to evaluate and manage violent pa-

tients is important not only for the safety of society and of patients in treatment settings, but also for the safety of mental health professionals who themselves are at high risk of being assaulted (American Psychiatric Association 1993; Thackrey 1987).

In this chapter, I discuss the topic of violence from the perspective of the clinician. (For more detailed and extensive coverage of this topic, see Tardiff 1988, 1996.)

CAUSES OF VIOLENCE

Before the clinical aspects of evaluation and management of the violent patient can be discussed, it is important to appreciate that a broad spectrum of factors interact to produce violent behavior in humans. One can conceptualize, although somewhat artificially, a group of internal or innate factors within the individual and external factors present during child development or in the environment that interact to either increase or decrease an individual's propensity for violent behavior. Appreciation of these innate and environmental factors is essential to prepare the clinician to see the evaluation and treatment of the violent patient in the context of society. Conversely, the clinician should realize that much violence in society is related to factors such as economics, drug dealing, and other criminal activities not within the usual realm of psychiatric expertise, thus posing the question of psychiatry's involvement in such matters (Tardiff 1992).

NEUROPHYSIOLOGICAL FACTORS

Since 1970, researchers have focused on the temporal lobe as the area of the brain responsible for aggressive behavior, based on cases of patients with partial complex seizures who manifested violent behavior (Mark and Ervin 1970; Monroe 1970). Yet, the role of the temporal lobe and of epilepsy in violence has remained controversial. Delgado-Escueta et al. (1981) conducted a large international collaborative study and found that violence was rare among epileptic patients. Hermann and Whitman (1984) have reviewed the literature and found no overall difference in levels of violence between persons with or without epilepsy. Despite this, some investigators (Monroe 1985; Weiger and Bear 1988) continue to emphasize the importance of epilepsy and limbic ictus in episodic dyscontrol and violence by maintaining that the surface electroencephalogram (EEG) is a crude and ineffective measurement of subcortical activity and that patients with episodic dyscontrol often respond to anticonvulsant medication. With recent advances in imaging using magnetic resonance, there is evidence that subtle damage to the amygdaloid nucleus is associated with violence (Tonkonogy 1991). Elliot (1992) has presented an excellent summary of studies pointing to neurological dysfunction as a factor in violence. Also, Eichelman (1992) has summarized the basic science literature on animal and human aggression.

GENETIC DETERMINANTS

In the past two decades there has been a great deal of interest in and research on sex chromosome abnormalities and violent behavior, particularly the XYY abnormality. Schiavi et al. (1984), having reviewed the literature, conducted a double-blind controlled study and found no association between XYY or XXY chromosome abnormalities and violence. The role of these chromosomal abnormalities is doubtful, and any association with arrest for crimes is probably linked to other factors such as low intelligence. Twin studies showing increased criminal behavior in monozygotic twins were subject to a number of methodological problems, and a study by Bohman et al. (1982) of adopted men in Sweden failed to show that the violent crimes committed by these men were related to violence in their biological or adoptive parents. Other studies of twins

reared apart have found that inheritance is an important factor in the expression of aggression (Tellegen et al. 1988). Thus, genetic determinants deserve further study.

HORMONES

Violence may be associated with gross endocrine disease such as Cushing's disease or hyperthyroidism, but the role of androgens, hypoglycemia, and premenstrual syndrome is more controversial. Studies have not found a relationship between androgens and violent behavior (Rada et al. 1983). This finding leaves us with the probable conclusion that increased rates of violence by men in society are accounted for by other factors such as role expectations in society. Studies of hypoglycemic patients as well as habitually violent defenders have indicated that hypoglycemia may play a role in extreme cases of violence and fire setting (Virkkunen 1982; Virkkunen et al. 1989). Low glucose levels were not found in a later, larger study of violent criminals (De Jong et al. 1992). Perhaps in some individuals with certain personality and environmental precipitants, the hypoglycemic state may tip the balance toward aggressive behavior. Premenstrual syndrome has been used as a defense in crimes of manslaughter, arson, and assault in Europe (Dalton 1980). R. L. Reid and Yen (1981) did an extensive search of the literature and found little or no research evidence that premenstrual syndrome is a direct contributing factor to criminal activity or even that it is a nonspecific factor perhaps producing irritability that tips the balance in the case of an individual predisposed to violence.

NEUROTRANSMITTERS

Brown et al. (1982) found that a history of aggressive behavior and a history of suicidal behavior were both related to decreased cerebrospinal fluid (CSF) 5-hydroxyindoleacetic acid (5-HIAA) levels. Lidberg et al. (1985) found that men who were convicted of criminal homicide and a group of men who committed suicide both had lower levels of 5-HIAA in their spinal fluid than did male control subjects. Linnoila et al. (1983) found that among offenders who killed with unusual cruelty, those who were impulsive had significantly lower CSF 5-HIAA concentrations than did nonimpulsive offenders, the latter group being defined as those who premeditated their crimes. The central serotonergic system has continued to be the focus of attention in research on violent individuals (Coccaro 1992). This finding is in agreement with other studies of suicide and serotonin metabolism (Apter et al. 1991; Belfrage et al. 1992; Braverman and Pfeiffer 1985; Coccaro et al. 1989;

Fishbein et al. 1989). Thus, low CSF 5-HIAA may be a marker of impulsivity rather than of a specific type of violence (i.e., suicide or externally directed aggression).

PSYCHIATRIC DISORDERS

Rabkin (1979) reviewed a number of studies and concluded that arrests and conviction rates for violent crimes among psychiatric patients are greater than those for the general population. Yet, psychiatric patients should not be regarded as a homogeneous group. Diagnosis per se should not be used as an indicator of potential for violence. There are, however, certain categories that are overrepresented in groups of patients who are violent. Paranoid schizophrenia is one of these diagnostic categories (Calcedo-Barba and Calcedo-Ordonez 1994; Lindqvist and Allebeck 1990; Tardiff 1983). The fact that patients with psychotic disorders pose a higher risk of violent behavior has been confirmed by a number of other studies (Humphreys et al. 1992; Krakowski et al. 1986). When one looks at violent patients in a different setting—that is, the outpatient clinic—nonpsychotic disorders are often associated with violent behavior (Binder and McNeil 1990; Kay et al. 1988; Tardiff and Koenigsberg 1985). Personality disorders, particularly the borderline and antisocial types, are associated with increased rates of violence (Bland and Orn 1986; Hare and McPherson 1984; Hart and Hare 1991). A number of cognitive impairment disorders with delirium, dementia, or other pathology can be associated with violent behavior (Deutsch et al. 1991; W. H. Reid and Balis 1987). The role of psychopathology and psychiatric disorders is elaborated on later in this chapter in the section on evaluation of the violent patient.

ALCOHOL AND DRUGS

Alcohol is well known for its association with violence through its ability to lessen inhibition against antisocial and violent behavior and to decrease perceptual and cognitive alertness, with resulting impairment of judgment. A number of epidemiological studies have found a strong link between alcohol use and certain types of homicide involving disputes (Goodman et al. 1986; Tardiff et al. 1986). Clinical studies have found that alcohol produces violence through its pharmacological effects (Bushman and Cooper 1990). Many street drugs of abuse have been found to be associated with violent behavior, including amphetamines, cocaine, hallucinogens, and minor tranquilizer-sedatives (Holcomb and Ahr 1988; Honer et al. 1987; Nurco et al. 1985; Swanson et al. 1990). In a study of homicides in Manhattan, it was found that opiate drug abuse was

related to violence indirectly and not in terms of a primary psychopharmacological effect. Narcotics played a key role because of the activities aimed at obtaining these drugs (Tardiff et al. 1986). In a latter study of homicides, one-third of homicide victims were found to be positive for cocaine or its metabolite on toxicological tests (Tardiff et al. 1994). Crack cocaine has become an important factor, especially in urban settings, in increased rates of homicides. A large proportion of this violence is related to the business of buying and selling cocaine (Goldstein et al. 1989).

DEVELOPMENTAL FACTORS

Kempe and Helfer (1980) have found that being abused as a child is related to becoming physically abusive as an adult. In fact, even witnessing intrafamily violence, as in spouse abuse, is related to increased problems with violence among children (Jaffe et al. 1986). There has been criticism of studies on the effect of past child abuse and other familial violence because of their retrospective designs (Widom 1989b). A prospective cohort study has confirmed that being abused and neglected as a child does increase one's risk for adult violence (Widom 1989a). Others have pointed out that the link could be a genetic one, with abusing parents being criminals and the risk for violence being inherited (Di Lalla and Gottesman 1991). Violence need not take place in the home to have a possible influence on the child and adolescent because there is evidence that television violence could be related to later aggressive behavior (National Institute of Mental Health 1982). However, Freedman (1984) has criticized this research. Research should be done in naturalistic settings, and the long-term effects of television violence should be studied further. In light of the high rate of child abuse, intrafamily violence, and violence depicted in the mass media, there should be great concern that we are raising the next generation of violent adults. Monitoring and regulating violence in the media are essential to prevent this outcome (Centerwall 1992).

SOCIOECONOMIC FACTORS

The nonwhite population in the United States has high rates of violence as perpetrators as well as victims. This has been explained in terms of the necessity to fight rather than being able to achieve through verbal or economic means, given the widespread poverty in black ghettos. Added to this is the breakup of families, alienation, discrimination, and frustration (Wilson 1987). Some researchers have courted the hypothesis that blacks and Hispanics live in a violent subculture (Wolfgang 1981). Others have found that in violence there is no difference between blacks and whites when socioeconomic status is taken into consideration (Centerwall 1984).

There have been ongoing debates and conflicting findings as to whether economic inequality as opposed to absolute poverty is responsible for high rates of homicide and other crimes among blacks (Blau and Blau 1982; Williams 1984). The former theory states that violence occurs because of hostility in one person who perceives he or she is disadvantaged relative to other persons, whereas the latter theory holds that deprivation itself causes violence. These contradictory findings are probably due to the use of large metropolitan areas as units of analysis. A study by Messner and Tardiff (1986) used neighborhoods as small units of analysis, which were more naturalistic, to test the hypothesis that economic inequality was related to homicide. The authors found that economic inequality and race were not related to homicide, but rather the prime determinants were absolute poverty and marital disruption. There appears to be a cycle of poverty, deprivation, disruption of families, unemployment, and further difficulty maintaining personal ties, family structures, and social control.

FIREARMS

There is evidence that the number of homicides associated with firearms has increased significantly in this century, particularly since 1960 (Tardiff et al. 1994). Firearms are important because they turn what would have been an assault into a homicide. It is difficult to determine whether this increase in homicides is due to increased availability of firearms because the import and export of firearms are not accurately measured. There is evidence, however, that gun control legislation is effective in decreasing the rate of homicides involving firearms (Cook 1982). Knowing whether there is a gun in the home is important in the evaluation of violence potential because it increases the probability of serious violence and death (Saltzman et al. 1992; U.S. General Accounting Office 1991).

PHYSICAL ENVIRONMENT

Physical crowding may be related to violence through increased contact and decreased defensible space, whereas an increased number of persons without crowding may result in increased social control and decreased violence (Anderson 1982; Sampson 1983). These principles in society are similar to what is found on psychiatric inpatient units, namely, that increased numbers of patients are associated with increased violence (Palmstierna at al. 1991). The

number of bystanders available for surveillance and intervention may prevent the commission of crimes, including homicide (Messner and Tardiff 1985). Thus, the effect of bystanders on the level of violence in the community may be positive through such programs as Crime Watch and other efforts at community organization.

Bell and Baron (1981), in reviewing a number of ecological and ethological studies, as well as laboratory studies, concluded that there is a relationship between heat and aggression that is curvilinear: moderately uncomfortable ambient temperatures produce an increase in aggression, whereas extremely hot temperatures decrease aggression. The implications of these environmental findings for the community of the inpatient unit are obvious. With overcrowding, inadequate numbers of staff, heat, and disruptive rather than supportive patients, one would anticipate that violence would increase on such inpatient units.

SUMMARY

Violence is the result of an interaction between characteristics of the individual and factors in the environment. Biological or innate factors such as neurophysiological dysfunction, hormones, inheritance, and neurotransmitter abnormalities are nonspecific in the way they cause violence. Rather than a specific mechanism, they tip the balance by impairing the person's ability to achieve goals by a nonviolent means or by increasing impulsivity, irritability, irrationality, or disorganization of behavior. The environment may influence the individual during development, for example, by the child's being subjected to abuse or having to witness violence either within one's family or subculture or on television and other mass media. Poverty and other adverse social conditions have a damaging impact on the family and the social network as well as on the individual. Use of alcohol and drugs and the availability of weapons kindle an explosion of violence in the individual. For the individual patient, some biological and environmental factors may be more important than others, but the clinician should weigh all of these factors in the evaluation of the patient and for the purpose of planning and implementing treatment.

ACUTE MANAGEMENT

SAFETY

At one time or another, all of us are faced with the situation, whether in the emergency room, the inpatient unit, or even the outpatient clinic, in which we will be summoned to deal with a patient who has just struck someone or thrown something or who is threatening violence. Often, a group of people—either staff, police, patients, or other observers—have gathered around the patient. The psychiatrist or other professional presiding in that setting is expected to take charge and "do something." In defusing the situation and evaluating future potential for violence, the ideal situation is to be alone with the patient in a closed room. Obviously, this situation may not always be advisable for safety reasons. The foremost thought in the psychiatrist's mind at that point should be, Do I feel safe (Eichelman and Hartwig 1995)? The psychiatrist must feel safe with the patient or else this insecurity will interfere with the evaluation and may result in physical injury or death. In talking to the patient, a wide range of options should be considered, from being alone with the patient with the door closed, to being alone with the door open, to being alone with aides outside of the room, to being alone with aides inside of the room, to the most extreme option, that is, interviewing the patient while the patient is in physical restraints. The psychiatrist should not feel omnipotent despite the thought that others expect him or her to have magical powers in calming violent patients as is sometimes portrayed in the movies. In addition to relying on one's feelings concerning safety, one should take into consideration the possibility of countertransference reactions or other inappropriate reactions such as denial that will interfere with the effective management of a particular patient. These reactions are discussed at length later in this chapter.

INSTANT DIFFERENTIAL DIAGNOSIS

In deciding how to proceed in terms of talking to the patient or using physical means of control, the clinician should make an instant differential diagnosis and categorize the patient's condition into one of three groups:

1. *Organic mental disorders:* For patients with cognitive impairment disorders and substance-related disorders who are having a violent episode, it is frequently impossible to intervene effectively and influence them through verbal means. One should treat the underlying medical or other physical disorder rather than only relying on neuroleptics to control violence. If the etiology of the disorder is unknown and if there is actual violence or imminent violence, the patient probably should be restrained as the laboratory tests and evaluation proceed.
2. *Psychotic disorders:* The violent patients in this group are usually schizophrenic or manic and are again difficult to influence through verbal means. Neuroleptic medication rapidly administered is usually the

treatment of choice for these patients, although they may have to be restrained or secluded until it takes effect.
3. *Nonpsychotic, nonorganic disorders:* The patients in this group are primarily those with personality disorders or intermittent explosive disorder who are often amenable to verbal intervention without seclusion or restraint. One may want to offer medication to a patient in this group and give him or her the option of either accepting or rejecting the medication, thus giving the patient a sense of control in the situation. In deciding to use physical means of control, the psychiatrist can assess the patient's degree of impulse control by the patient's compliance with routine requests and procedures in the clinic or emergency room (Table 37–1).

VERBAL INTERVENTION

Verbal means of intervention and even prevention should receive serious consideration (Table 37–2). In terms of prevention, it is essential that an inpatient unit have adequate, well-trained staff to ensure implementation of ongoing treatment programs and also for the prevention of violence. In the emergency situation, the staff should be adequate in number and trained to implement seclusion and restraint techniques effectively, appropriately, and safely. Most important, the staff should be caring and nonauthoritarian yet at the same time should act as part of the ward milieu, demonstrating social norms and limits. This balance is difficult to achieve, but nevertheless, it is essential in the prevention of violent behavior on inpatient units. The staff should talk to patients in a calm, nonprovocative manner and listen to patients. As tension increases before violence occurs, even the most psychotic

TABLE 37-1. Types of violent patients and emergency responses

Type	Response
Organic mental disorders	Patient generally requires restraint until etiology known.
	Not usually amenable to talk.
Psychotic disorders	Patient generally requires restraint and neuroleptic.
	Not usually amenable to talk.
Nonpsychotic, nonorganic disorders	Patient generally responds to talk with de-escalation.
	Staff for restraint and/or medication should be available nearby.

TABLE 37–2. Verbal management of violent patients

- Be concerned for your safety.
- Appear calm and in control.
- Speak softly in a nonprovocative, nonjudgmental manner.
- Both patient and clinician sit, if possible.
- Do not tower over patient or stare at the patient.
- When the patient begins to talk, listen.

schizophrenic patient may respond to nonprovocative interpersonal contact and expression of concern and caring. It is important that staff recognize for a particular patient the warning signs of violence that have preceded violent acts in the past. A patient may have manifested a specific pattern of behavior or speech before an explosive episode. It may be in the form of pacing in front of the nursing station, repeating the same word or phrase, or some other warning sign.

SECLUSION AND RESTRAINT

In 1982, the Supreme Court ruled in the case of *Youngberg v. Romeo* that Mr. Romeo, a violent, profoundly mentally retarded man who was institutionalized, could be deprived of his liberty in terms of being restrained if it could be justified to protect others or himself and, most important, if the decision was based on a professional's clinical judgment that is not a substantial departure from professional standards. The importance of this case is that the Court deferred to professional judgment rather than to a rigid hierarchy of restrictiveness in the management of violence by patients. At the time the court decision was rendered, I was chairing a task force of the American Psychiatric Association (APA) to develop guidelines for the psychiatric uses of seclusion and restraint. The guidelines have been approved by the APA and have set reasonable, minimal clinical standards for management of violence using seclusion and restraint in the context of verbal intervention, involuntary medication, and other factors in the treatment environment. The guidelines are expanded on in a book by members of the task force (Tardiff 1984; see Table 37–3).

TABLE 37–3. Indications for seclusion or restraint

- To prevent harm to others
- To prevent harm to the patient
- To prevent serious disruption of treatment environment
- As ongoing behavioral treatment
- At the patient's request if appropriate clinically
- To decrease stimulation (for seclusion only)

Indications for emergency use of seclusion and restraint are as follows:

1. To prevent imminent harm to others—namely, staff and other patients—if other means are not effective and appropriate
2. To prevent imminent harm to the patient if other means of control are not effective or appropriate
3. To prevent serious disruption of the treatment program or significant damage to the environment
4. As part of an ongoing behavior treatment program
5. To decrease the amount of stimulation that the patient receives (for seclusion)
6. At the patient's request (for seclusion)

These indications for the emergency use of seclusion and restraint state that violence need not actually occur but that the staff may use these measures for imminent violence, as in the case discussed earlier in which a patient's past pattern of escalation to violence is known or if it is apparent that a patient is on the verge of exploding.

The decision as to whether seclusion, restraint, or involuntary medication is used is a clinical one and should be based on the individual needs and status of the patient. For example, restraint probably would be preferable if the patient is delirious and the etiology of the delirium is unknown. In this case, one would prefer to keep the patient free of drugs, certainly neuroleptics, until the underlying etiology is determined, and seclusion would not be appropriate because the sensory deprivation may worsen the patient's delirium. Restraint also might be preferred if close medical monitoring is necessary, as is for patients with heart disease, infections, metabolic illness, drug overdoses, or other medical problems. On the other hand, seclusion may be the method of choice in the case of a manic person who needs a decrease of stimulation. Involuntary medication may be the preferred method of control, perhaps with seclusion or restraint, for the paranoid schizophrenic patient who has stopped taking medications and has become violent or is imminently so. Rapid tranquilization is discussed later in this chapter. A combination of the control measures may be used, for example, in the case of the violent manic patient with a history of epilepsy who may be secluded and given lower doses of involuntary medication, such as haloperidol, than are usually prescribed because of a concern about decreased seizure threshold resulting from the neuroleptic medication. The reasons for using seclusion, restraint, or other physical means of control and subsequent monitoring must be documented in the patient's record.

As with any medical procedure, there are contraindications as well as indications (Table 37–4). Seclusion and restraint should never be used to punish a patient as retribution for a particular act. Although this type of retribution may be the philosophy of a penal institution, it has no place in a treatment setting. Seclusion and restraint should never be used solely for the convenience of the staff or of other patients on the inpatient unit, or solely for the sake of the treatment programs on the ward. If seclusion and restraint are used for these reasons, then the treatment plan for the patient should be reviewed and a change of treatment program or setting should be considered. Seclusion and re-

TABLE 37–4. Guidelines for seclusion and restraint

- Not used to punish a patient or solely for the convenience of staff or other patients.
- Psychiatrist/staff must take into consideration the medical and psychiatric status of the patient (e.g., drug overdose, medical disease, self-mutilation).
- Psychiatrist/staff must follow written guidelines of institution.
- Adequate staff must be present (at least four) for implementation.
- Once decision is made to use seclusion or restraint, patient should be given seconds to comply by walking to seclusion room.
- If patient does not comply, each staff member should grab a limb and bring patient backward to the ground.
- Restraint devices are applied, or patient is carried to seclusion by four staff members.
- Patient is searched for belts, pins, watches, and other dangerous objects and is placed in gown.
- Physician sees patient for first episode, preferably within 1 hour and definitely within 3 hours.
- Physician is contacted for subsequent episodes and may elect not to see patient.
- Physician sees a patient in seclusion or restraint at least every 12 hours.
- A review by persons outside the unit should be done if patient is secluded or restrained continuously over 72 hours.
- Nursing staff should observe patient at least every 15 minutes.
- Nursing staff should visit patient at least every 2 hours.
- Meals (without utensils), fluids, and toileting should be provided at appropriate times and with caution.
- With four-point restraints, each limb should be released or restraint loosened every 15 minutes.
- Patient should be gradually released from seclusion or restraint.
- Each decision, observation, and measurement, as well as care, must be documented in detail in the patient's record or in a log.
- Patients and staff should discuss the seclusion or restraint after each episode.

straint should never be used inappropriately as the result of the dynamics of the ward. Seclusion should not be used if the patient needs close medical monitoring, is self-mutilative, or wants to be secluded so as to avoid participating in the treatment program. A patient should not be secluded if seclusion rooms are unable to be cooled, particularly when the patient is taking neuroleptic medication, because a hot room interferes with regulation of body temperature, resulting in death in some instances on hot days.

The APA Task Force on Psychiatric Uses of Seclusion and Restraint did not recommend specific techniques for approaching patients or for using restraint devices but indicated that seclusion and restraint should be considered analogous to cardiopulmonary resuscitation in an institution in that there should be

- Written, specific guidelines and a manual for the use of these procedures
- Approval of the guidelines by the administrators of the hospital, their lawyers, and the state
- Education of the staff in terms of the guidelines and actual rehearsal of the techniques
- Feedback from staff regarding problems with the guidelines, with revisions following accordingly

Once the decision to seclude or restrain a patient has been made, a clinical staff member should be chosen to be the leader for the procedure. This leader need not be the most senior staff member but should be the most appropriate person for that patient. In addition, sufficient force in the form of four staff members should be assembled behind the leader as the patient is approached. The staff should appear ready, confident, and emotionally detached but not provocative. If possible, another staff person should be available to clear the area of patients as well as to observe and monitor how the procedure is carried out. Further verbal interchange with the patient is inappropriate, except for a clear statement by the leader that the patient will be secluded or restrained because the patient is out of control. The patient may be asked to walk quietly with or without underarm support to the seclusion room and given a few seconds to respond (Figure 37–1).

Verbal interchange with the patient at this point often leads to debate, violence by the patient, and a generally chaotic situation, and it increases the possibility that someone will be injured. If the patient does not immediately respond, each staff member should seize one of the patient's limbs in a plan agreed to beforehand. The patient should be brought backward to the ground, and the patient's head should be controlled to avoid biting (see Figure 37–2). Staff should avoid hurting the patient, twisting extremities out

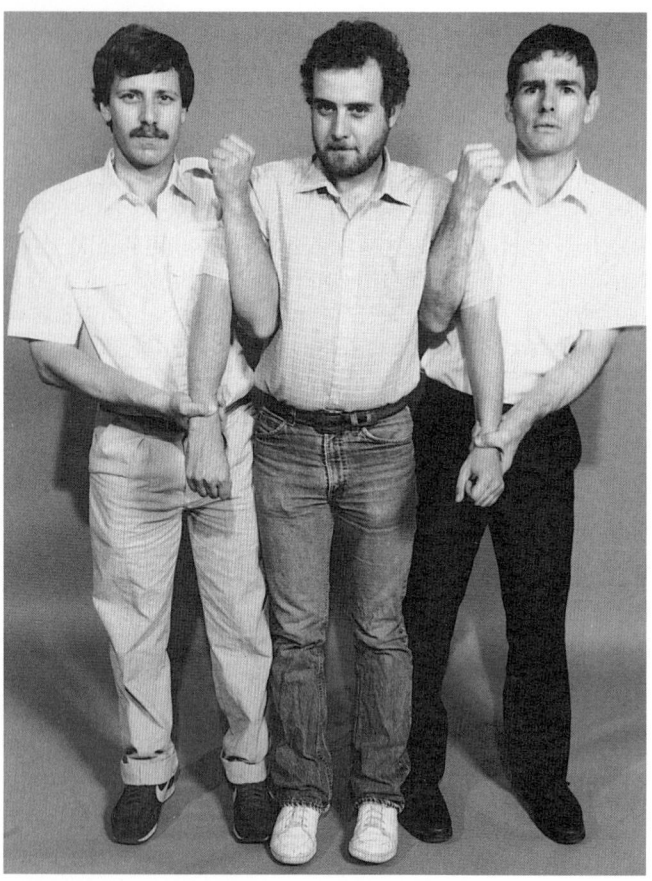

FIGURE 37–1. Walking the patient to the seclusion room with underarm support.
Source. Reprinted with permission from Thackrey M: *Therapeutics for Aggression: Psychological/Physical Crisis Intervention.* New York, Human Sciences Press, 1987. Copyright 1987, Human Sciences Press.

of the range of normal motion, sitting on the patient, cursing, or other disrespectful behavior. At this point, restraint devices should be applied, or if the patient is to be taken into seclusion, the staff should grab the patient's legs at the knees and grab the arms around the elbow with underarm support (see Figure 37–3). Variations on this basic approach have been recommended and illustrated with photographs by Thackrey (1987). These variations may be of interest to clinicians, but again the specific techniques to be used are the prerogative of each institution and must be clearly stated and rehearsed.

If the patient is to be placed in seclusion, he or she should be searched thoroughly. Belts, pins, rings, matches, and other objects should be removed. It is often advisable to remove the patient's street clothes and place an appropriate gown on the patient. If medication is to be used, it can be injected at this time. The patient should be placed in the seclusion room on his or her back with the head to the

door or face down with the head away from the door. Gradually, staff should leave the patient, with the last person controlling the patient's arms and legs.

In most cases, the seclusion and restraint will take place without the physician being present. Each state (and institution) has varying time parameters as to when a physician must see a patient in seclusion or restraint. The parameters that follow are the recommendations of the APA Task Force on Psychiatric Uses of Seclusion and Restraint that were made as representing minimal standards (Tardiff 1984).

The physician should see the patient preferably within 1 hour. This 1-hour time frame is essential because the patient's medical and psychiatric status must be assessed by a physician, and the appropriateness of seclusion and restraint must be approved, as well as any special monitoring of the patient. These recommendations have provoked some hospitals to complain that an undue burden is placed on their psychiatrists; however, the task force maintained that it is good medical practice for a physician to see a patient for the first episode of seclusion or restraint within a short period of time. A physician should visit a patient at least every 4 hours. If a patient is in seclusion or restraint

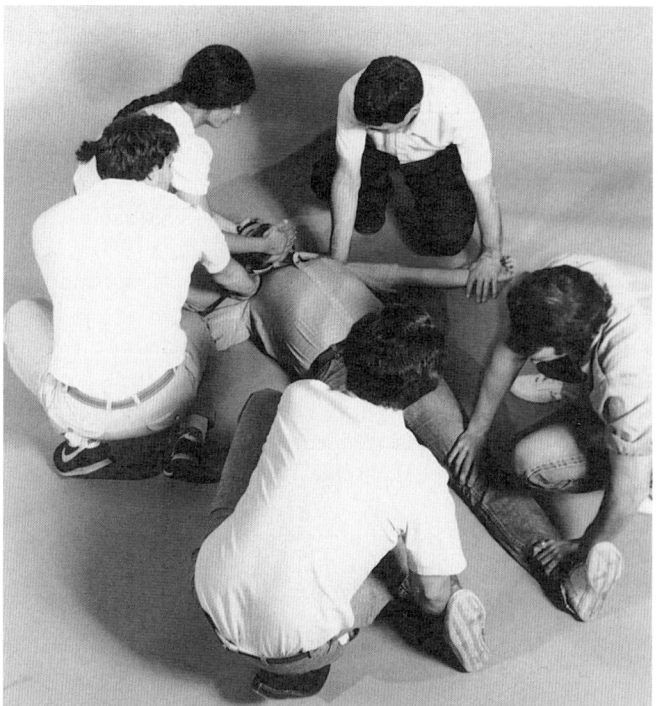

FIGURE 37–2. Patient restrained supine with staff holding each limb and controlling head to prevent biting.
Source. Reprinted with permission from Thackrey M: *Therapeutics for Aggression: Psychological/Physical Crisis Intervention.* New York, Human Sciences Press, 1987. Copyright 1987, Human Sciences Press.

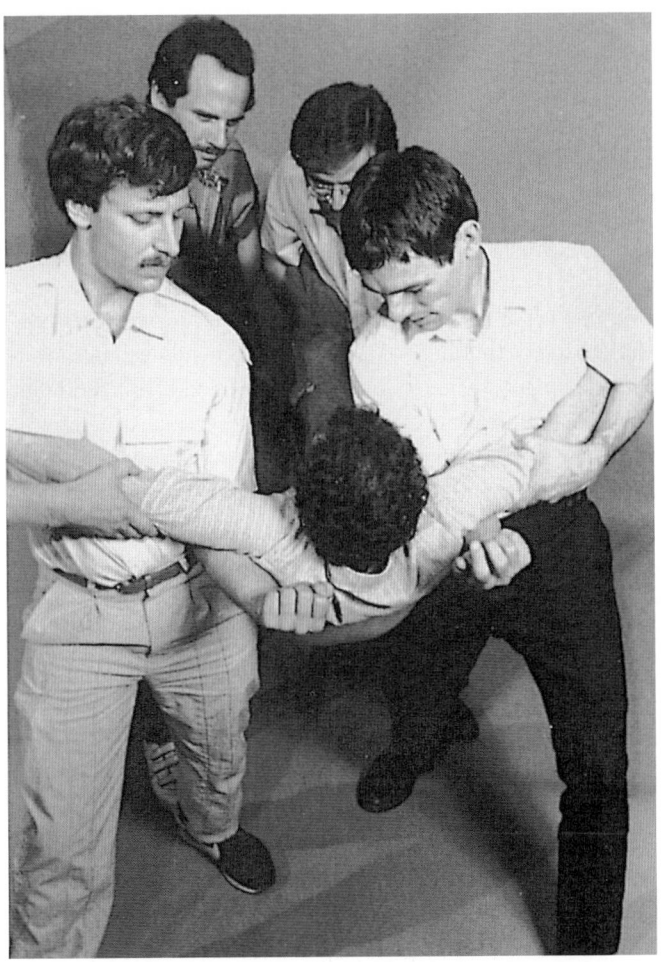

FIGURE 37–3. Transporting the patient to the seclusion room with each limb restrained and support under arms. *Source.* Reprinted with permission from Thackrey M: *Therapeutics for Aggression: Psychological/Physical Crisis Intervention.* New York, Human Sciences Press, 1987. Copyright 1987, Human Sciences Press.

continuously for more than 72 hours, there should be a review of the case by persons outside of the treatment unit.

The patient should be observed by the nursing staff at least every 15 minutes, and his or her behavior and status should be documented in writing at each observation. In fact, in many units, once a patient is in seclusion or restraint, constant observation or one-to-one observation by staff is automatically triggered. The placement of a patient in seclusion should not be a reason for abandoning the patient but should increase the amount of attention from staff. There should be a visit in the room by the nursing staff at least every 2 hours, especially if there is the question of drug overdose or if medication has been given for very agitated persons. Toileting for the patient should be done every 4 hours. As with a direct visit with a patient, toileting may be dangerous and may require more force and staff

equal to the number present when the patient was originally placed in seclusion or restraint. Meals should be served when the ward meals are served. There should be no forks or knives, even plastic ones, because these can be used as weapons. It is preferable to have a staff member sit with the patient during mealtime, not only for purposes of social interaction but also for evaluation of the degree of control manifested by the patient. The latter point is important in determining when the patient will be removed from seclusion. For four-point restraints of the extremities, each extremity should be released or loosened every 15 minutes, and if the patient is on his or her back, he or she should be constantly observed to prevent aspiration.

The patient is not abruptly removed from seclusion or restraint. Rather, from the very beginning of the episode, staff should be testing the patient's degree of control—for example, the patient's complying with simple requests such as to sit in the corner when staff visit or bring meals. As the patient manifests an increased level of control, the seclusion room door may be left open with staff outside of the door, and gradually the patient is reintroduced to his or her room and then the general ward setting.

STAFF FEELINGS ABOUT VIOLENCE

The staff should know their own feelings about violence in general and about specific violent patients based on countertransference reactions or other emotional reactions to patients (Eichelman and Hartwig 1995; Lion and Pasternak 1973). Negative or inappropriate feelings about patients must be recognized so as not to act on them. In addition, the staff should be constantly monitoring the ward dynamics, particularly in terms of staff conflict that may translate into inappropriate patient care in the management of violence. The staff know their own past experiences with violence and how this may affect their treatment of patients. Anger toward a patient for a particular act may be justified, or it may be the result of countertransference in which the patient resembles an abusive parent or spouse.

A number of defense mechanisms may interfere with the treatment of violent patients and in fact may pose a danger to the therapist and others. Denial of a patient's dangerousness may occur because of the therapist's past experiences with violence or because the patient may be particularly attractive or interesting. To the contrary, a patient may be viewed as more dangerous than he or she actually is because of staff anxiety that is projected onto the patient. Displacement can occur from one patient who is really dangerous to another who is not dangerous but who serves as an acceptable scapegoat for a staff member.

Negative emotional reactions about patients may exist because of bias and prejudice, which obviously are not acceptable. In addition, ward dynamics may result in the inappropriate treatment of violent patients. For example, nursing staff feeling abandoned by the administration or medical staff inappropriately may seclude or restrain a particular patient so as to activate procedures for which the psychiatrist is required to be on the ward and to examine the patient.

To address some of these concerns about the psychodynamics of the staff as well as patients, it is important to discuss a violent episode once it has occurred. Contrary to what staff usually wish to do, this discussion should be done among the staff as well as with the patient who was violent and among other patients on the ward. Often, once the episode is finished, staff members are content to forget about it or deny it. Instead, the violent episode should be discussed in terms of what happened, what would have prevented it, why seclusion or restraint was used (if it was), and how the patient or the staff felt in terms of using seclusion and restraint. It is important to recognize that most patients will have negative reactions to being secluded and restrained; the most positive reaction from a patient is usually, "I must have really been out of control or crazy to deserve something like that." Among other patients on the ward, it is important to talk about the violent episode and discuss why seclusion and restraint were used for that particular patient so as to allay other patients' fears that they could be secluded or restrained for no apparent reason in the future.

MEDICATION IN EMERGENCIES

There are useful reviews of the literature on the use of medication in the emergency situation (Brizer 1988; Dubin et al. 1986; Eichelman 1986; Soloff 1987; Tardiff 1996). The most common types of medication used are the neuroleptics (Table 37–5). These are most often used for patients with schizophrenia or mania, but they may be used, with some reservations, on an emergency basis for patients with cognitive impairment, organic mental disorders, personality disorders, and mental retardation. The following concerns should be borne in mind. In terms of cognitive impairment disorders, the sedative or anticholinergic effects of neuroleptics may aggravate delirious or toxic metabolic confusional states. Intoxication with alcohol or sedative drugs is a relative contraindication to the use of neuroleptic medications, particularly rapid tranquilization neuroleptics, until one can make certain that the patient's level of consciousness is worsening. Overdose with anticholinergic drugs can produce delir-

ium that would be increased by neuroleptics. In such situations and if the etiology of the cognitive impairment disorder is unknown, one should consider using physical restraint until, in the latter case, one can determine the etiology of the disorder. If the patient is restrained, one can draw blood for a toxic screen for alcohol and other drugs.

There is less concern about the short-term use of neuroleptics to control violence among patients with personality disorders or mental retardation; however, prolonged use of this class of medication is ill advised in the absence of psychotic psychopathology because of side effects. Also, in mentally retarded persons there is interference with learning, which is the main problem with this group of patients. Alternate means of management should be seriously considered, including verbal intervention and behavior therapy, described later in this chapter.

For the schizophrenic or manic patient who is out of control and violent, rapid tranquilization has been found to be safe and effective, despite possible side effects, which include sedation, orthostatic hypotension, anticholinergic effects, seizures, and severe extrapyramidal symptoms. Soloff (1987) describes this technique as an intensive care procedure to be used only with adequate staff and monitoring of vital signs and behavior. Decrease of violent behavior occurs usually within 20 minutes, and improvement of psychotic symptomatology occurs within 6 hours.

Rapid tranquilization can be carried out in many different ways. High-potency neuroleptics, usually haloperidol, can be given in a low-dose strategy (5 mg intramuscularly every 4–8 hours for a maximum of 15–30 mg/day). On

TABLE 37–5. **Medications in emergencies for violence**

Drug	Dosage	Special considerations
Haloperidol	15 mg im every 4 hours to 10 mg im every 30 minutes	Maximum of 100 mg/day; caution in delirious patients and alcohol/drug toxic or withdrawal states
Chlorpromazine	25 mg im every 4 hours to 75 mg im every 4 hours	Maximum of 400 mg/day; caution in delirium and alcohol/drug states; observe for postural hypotension
Lorazepam	2–4 mg im or by mouth and repeat every hour if im or 4–6 hours if by mouth	Maximum of 10 mg/day

the other hand, haloperidol may be administered in a high-dose strategy (10 mg intramuscularly every 30 minutes, with a maximum 24-hour total daily dose of 45–100 mg). If a low-potency neuroleptic such as chlorpromazine is used, a test dose of 10–25 mg intramuscularly is recommended to rule out excessive sensitivity to orthostatic hypotension. If orthostatic hypotension is not a problem after an hour, chlorpromazine is given 25 mg intramuscularly every 4 hours in a low-dose strategy, or up to 75 mg intramuscularly every 4 hours in a high-dose strategy, for a maximum dose of 400 mg in 24 hours. If severe orthostatic hypotension occurs with a low-potency neuroleptic, that medication should be discontinued. If a severe hypotensive crisis occurs, treatment includes intravenous fluids and the use of vasopressors such as metaraminol bitartrate or levarterenol bitartrate. Epinephrine is contraindicated because it may lower blood pressure further in neuroleptic-induced orthostatic hypotension. Another untoward effect of rapid neuroleptics is a paradoxical increase in agitation as the result of akathisia or the feeling that there has been a loss of control as the patient becomes more sedated.

Some authors have not recommended benzodiazepines for management of the acutely violent patient for fear of further decreasing inhibition, particularly in those patients with personality disorders. However, benzodiazepines are the treatment of choice in withdrawal from alcohol, even with associated psychotic psychopathology, because the use of neuroleptic medications in such patients would decrease seizure threshold and increase the risk of seizures. Obviously, restraint or closely monitored seclusion probably would be indicated also in the management of such patients.

For the emergency use of benzodiazepines, lorazepam also is useful because it produces sedation for a longer period of time than diazepam (the former remaining in the circulation rather than being absorbed into tissues). On the other hand, the half-life of lorazepam is 12 hours—much shorter than that of diazepam—so accumulation is not as problematic as it is with diazepam. Lorazepam given by intramuscular injection rapidly begins to enter the circulation and produces sedation within an hour. The oral administration of lorazepam produces more gradual effects, with sedation occurring usually in more than 1 hour and in less than 4 hours after administration. The dose is 2–4 mg by mouth or intramuscularly. A subsequent 2- to 4-mg dose can be repeated if there is continued agitation and aggression, with the timing dependent on the route of administration (i.e., in an hour or so if administered intramuscularly or 4–6 hours if administered orally). Often, this approach is sufficient to manage violence in the emergency situation.

After the emergency has subsided, lower maintenance levels of lorazepam with or without neuroleptics to a maximum of 10 mg/day in three divided doses can be given.

POTENTIAL FOR VIOLENCE IN THE NEAR FUTURE

In interviewing the patient who has been violent or who is threatening violence, one should appear calm and in control and speak softly in a nonprovocative, nonjudgmental manner. One should begin commenting in a neutral, concrete manner about the obvious (e.g., "You look angry" or "Could you tell me what you are concerned about?"). Comments such as "Why did you do that?" or "Act like a man!" should not be used because they are provocative and most certainly will result in further violence. This is not the time for giving the patient insight or dynamic interpretations. Both the evaluator and the violent patient should be sitting or both should be standing. It is important that the evaluator not tower over the patient and that he or she allow enough space between the patient and himself or herself. The evaluator should attempt to project passivity and yet a sense of control in the situation. When the patient starts to talk, the evaluator should listen in an empathic and concerned manner. Again, the evaluator may want to offer medication because it gives the patient a sense of control in terms of choosing whether to accept or reject it.

The evaluation of a patient's violence or homicide potential is done to determine whether to admit the patient to a hospital, is done at the time of the patient's discharge, or is done in outpatient therapy in *Tarasoff*-like situations, with the duty to protect potential victims of the patient (Beck 1985). In making a decision about violence potential, one should interview the patient as well as family members, police, and other persons with information about the patient because patients may minimize threats or violent acts that have preceded the interview. The evaluation of violence potential is analogous to that of suicide potential. If the patient does not express thoughts of violence, one should begin the evaluation by asking a subtle question such as "Have you ever lost your temper?" If the answer is yes, then the evaluation should proceed in terms of how, when, and so on. In the same manner, one would begin the evaluation of suicide potential by asking, "Have you ever felt that life was not worth living?" If the answer is yes, one would proceed with the evaluation of suicide.

Similar to evaluating suicide potential, evaluating violence potential includes assessing how well planned the threat is (Tardiff 1989, 1996). Vague threats of killing someone are not as serious as saying "I'm going to kill my boss because he doesn't appreciate my work and plans to fire me." As is done in the evaluation of suicide potential, determining availability of a means to inflict injury is important in the evaluation of violence potential. For example, if the patient has recently purchased or owns a gun, one should obviously take the threat more seriously. A history of violence or other impulsive behavior is often predictive of future violence. One should ask about injuries to other persons, destruction of property, reckless driving, reckless spending, sexual acting out, and other impulsive behaviors. One should assess the degree of a patient's past injuries (e.g., broken bones and lacerations), as well as injuries of those toward whom the violence had been directed and the circumstances of the injuries. Often there is a pattern of past violent behavior in specific circumstances (e.g., escalation of a dispute between a husband and wife about issues of money, esteem, or sexuality). On an inpatient unit, if a patient has been violent, staff should look for characteristic patterns of behavior before violent episodes or specific situations that have triggered violence. As is done in the evaluation of suicidal patients, in violent patients the presence of alcohol or drug abuse should be determined and should alert the evaluator to an increased risk of violent behavior.

Alcohol, sedatives, and minor tranquilizers decrease inhibition and make it more probable that someone will act on his or her thoughts rather than control his or her behavior. (Drugs are discussed later in this chapter.) The importance of immediately getting blood and urine samples for assay in the emergency situation, or unannounced in the more prolonged evaluation of a patient, cannot be overemphasized. The presence of psychosis (in the case of a violent patient, usually paranoid delusional thinking or more disorganized psychosis) should warn the evaluator that threats of violence must be taken seriously and handled accordingly (Table 37–6).

TABLE 37–6. Assessment of violence potential (following increased risk)

- How well planned is a threat?
- Are means for harming others available?
- Is there a history of previous violence or other impulsive behaviors?
- If so, what were the precipitants, who were the victims, and how serious were the injuries?
- Is there a history of being abused as a child?
- Is there alcohol or drug abuse?
- Is there psychosis?

MORE EXTENDED EVALUATION OF THE VIOLENT PATIENT

Once the acute violent episode has been managed and the patient is safely in the hospital, one may collect more data in terms of the history, physical examination, laboratory tests, and psychological testing.

ORGANIC MENTAL DISORDERS

A number of organic disorders are associated with violent behavior, including substance abuse, central nervous system (CNS) disorders, systemic disorders, and seizure disorders (Eichelman 1992; Elliot 1992; W. H. Reid and Balis 1987; Tardiff 1996). In addition to the usual sensorium disturbances, one should look for dysarthria, nystagmus, unsteady gait, dilated pupils, tachycardia, and tremors, all of which may indicate that a substance use disorder is present. Substances that can produce violent behavior as a result of the intoxicated state as well as during withdrawal include alcohol, barbiturates, other sedatives, and anxiolytics. Other substances that can produce violence when the patient is intoxicated include amphetamines and other sympathomimetics, cocaine, phencyclidine (PCP) and other hallucinogens, anticholinergics, glue (sniffing), and other drugs such as steroids.

CNS disorders that have been associated with violent behavior include traumatic brain injuries, including birth injury as well as adult trauma acutely and in the postconcussion syndrome; intracranial infections, including encephalitis and postencephalitic syndrome; brain tumors; cerebrovascular disorders; Alzheimer's disease; Wilson's disease; multiple sclerosis; and normal-pressure hydrocephalus. Systemic disorders affecting the CNS include metabolic disorders, such as hypoglycemia; electrolyte imbalances; hypoxia; uremia; Cushing's disease; vitamin deficiencies, such as pernicious anemia; systemic infections; systemic lupus erythematosus; porphyria; and industrial poisoning, such as with lead.

As previously mentioned, violence during a partial complex seizure is rare and clinically is often nonpurposeful and not serious (Delgado-Escueta et al. 1981). Interictal violence has not been found to be significant and when it occurs, it is usually the result of underlying psychopathology. Violence during postseizure encephalopathy is more subtle but does occur. Nevertheless, a violent individual with a history of episodic violence should receive an EEG while awake and asleep using nasopharyngeal leads, as well as a brain scan and magnetic resonance imaging to look for tumors, atrophy, or hydrocephalus. In addition to the routine complete blood count, blood chemistries, and urinalysis, there should be a toxic screen of blood and urine as soon as possible to assay for alcohol, barbiturates, minor tranquilizers, amphetamines, marijuana, hallucinogens, and over-the-counter antihistamines and anticholinergics. Two types of assays should be done on each sample (e.g., radioimmunoassay and liquid or gas chromatography) for purposes of confirmation. Other laboratory studies to be considered include serum B_{12} and folate, thyroid function tests, tests for syphilis and human immunodeficiency virus (HIV) infection, glucose tolerance tests, ceruloplasmin, urine porphobilinogen, and other chemistries as indicated by the history and physical examination.

Psychological tests are useful to evaluate organicity and intelligence. The Bender Gestalt (Lacks 1984) is used as an initial screening measure, to be followed later by more sophisticated tests, such as the Halstead-Reitan battery (Reitan 1955).

PSYCHOTIC DISORDER

The paranoid schizophrenic patient poses a number of problems. First, paranoid delusions may be very subtle, and the patient may attempt to hide these. Therefore, the evaluator must listen for subtle clues and follow up regarding the assessment of violence toward others. Another problem with the violent paranoid schizophrenic patient is aftercare once the patient has been stabilized with medication and is no longer threatening violence or no longer appears to be violent toward others. Among violent patients who are admitted to hospitals, paranoid schizophrenic patients often are seen as the most appropriate for community placement once treatment has occurred in the hospital. However, noncompliance with medication is often a problem after the patients are discharged. In some states, programs of aftercare have been mandated that involve formerly violent patients being involuntarily returned to the hospital if they do not comply with outpatient treatment (e.g., weekly depot fluphenazine or haloperidol injections). There are problems in implementing these programs. First, the staff may not view themselves as police or agents of the police in terms of reporting patients. Second, there is a legitimate fear of approaching a patient who has not appeared for treatment knowing that the patient has been violent in the past and may be armed.

Other patients with schizophrenia have more disorganized symptomatology, and violence may be the result of that or delusional or hallucinatory symptoms, particularly command hallucinations. It is important to realize that schizophrenic patients can be violent for reasons that have nothing to do with schizophrenia (e.g., to manipulate others or for sadistic motives). Manic patients also are disorganized and less intentional in terms of their violent behavior. Depressed patients are rarely violent; however, when they are, they usually have psychotic depressions and murder their spouse and/or children and then commit suicide.

NONORGANIC, NONPSYCHOTIC DISORDERS

Among patients with nonorganic, nonpsychotic disorders, a number with personality disorders are violent, and psychodynamic considerations are important. These patients tend to act rather than talk about conflicts. Patients with the best prognoses are those who have the diagnosis of intermittent explosive disorder. These patients should be distinguished from persons with other types of personality disorders associated with violent behavior. Intermittent explosive disorder consists of several discrete episodes of loss of control involving violence toward others or destruction of property. A violent episode may have little apparent precipitating cause or may be linked to predictable patterns of escalation of conflict between the patient and others, usually family members. In any case, violence is out of proportion to any precipitating factors. The violence may occur for a few minutes or an hour and is often associated with alcohol use. It is followed by remorse and feelings of guilt concerning the beating of a spouse, child, or other family member. Remorse and the threat of marital dissolution often motivate the patient into psychotherapy. Between episodes there are few problems with impulse control or violence.

In distinction to intermittent explosive disorder is antisocial personality disorder, in which there are intermittent episodes of violent behavior. Between these violent outbursts there is pervasive antisocial behavior and violence on an ongoing basis (e.g., theft, drug dealing, job problems, lying, reckless driving, and other impulsive behaviors).

Differing from patients with intermittent explosive disorder are those who have borderline personality disorder, which manifests, in addition to episodic violence, a broad instability of interpersonal relationships as well as profound mood and identity problems. Violence is just one of many impulsive behaviors, including sexual acting out, overspending, overeating, suicide attempts, drug and alcohol abuse, and stealing.

There are two types of murderers who may not appear psychotic but who kill large numbers of people. Fortunately, mass murders are not frequent occurrences. The murderer with isolated explosive disorder typically commits a single unexpected episode of profound vio-

ble, mass murder with a gun in a restaurant —and usually there is no history of prior vi-perpetrator appears to be a respected, or , member of society or else an isolated person. As Dietz (1987) points out, there also is often a preoccupation with guns and militaristic themes. The second type of mass murderer is the serial murderer. Again, the perpetrator may seem to be a solid member of society, and often the victims are women or, in the case of the "Atlanta murderer" in the mid-1980s, children. Preoccupations in the serial murderer follow sexual rather than militaristic themes.

LONG-TERM TREATMENT

As with many problems in psychiatry, treatment of violent patients must adhere to the biopsychosocial model. Not all violent patients need medication, but it should be considered in the formulation of the treatment plan. Psychological intervention may be in the form of behavior therapy or psychotherapy. The impact of the patient's violence on various levels of the social order, from the family to society, must be addressed in treatment, as should the role of social factors in causation of the patient's violence.

LONG-TERM MEDICATION

There is no one drug for treatment of violence because the underlying etiology for violence differs among patients. In the following discussions, I describe drugs that have some proven efficacy in the management of violent behavior, the types of patients in whom these medications have been most effective, dose and route of administration, and side effects.

Before one considers using a drug for a violent patient, there must be an established baseline for the violence manifested by the patient. A good measure of the frequency, severity, and target of the violent behavior is the Overt Aggression Scale (Yudofsky et al. 1986). Since the buildup, maintenance, and withdrawal phases in the use of medications (particularly propranolol, lithium, and the anticonvulsants) will be long, there must be a quantitative measurement of response (see Table 37–7).

Antipsychotics or neuroleptics. The antipsychotic medications are used for schizophrenia and mania and in some organic disorders for delusional thinking or control of violence. Antipsychotics are used as long-term medication primarily for schizophrenic patients. Especially for paranoid schizophrenic patients who have manifested violent behavior or made threats of violence, compliance with

medication is notoriously bad (Young et al. 1986). Thus, clinicians should consider using long-acting depot forms of antipsychotic medication. Antipsychotic medication should not be used for violent mentally retarded patients unless there is psychotic symptomatology. Using long-term antipsychotics for these patients raises the risk of side effects (e.g., tardive dyskinesia) and the concern that learning may be impaired in this group of patients for whom learning is already a major problem.

On inpatient units, haloperidol and fluphenazine are popular because of their ability to be administered rapidly in high doses with minimal side effects and with safety in terms of not decreasing the seizure threshold in epileptic patients. This latter point is important for patients with schizophrenia and coexisting subictal activity. Equally important to their use in combating noncompliance with medication, there is a smooth transition from using haloperidol and fluphenazine in an emergency situation, to oral maintenance doses, to long-term depot use (Kane 1985).

If the clinician wishes to choose an antipsychotic with more sedative side effects or if extrapyramidal side effects are problematic, chlorpromazine or other low-potency antipsychotics are recommended. I do not recommend thioridazine for violent psychotic patients because clinicians may want to use propranolol for these patients, and as is discussed later, propranolol increases blood levels of thioridazine and the risk of pigmentary retinopathy. Clozapine and risperidone have been found to be effective in the treatment of violent psychotic patients who do not respond to other antipsychotic medication (Ratey et al. 1993; Volavka and Meibach 1995; Volavka et al. 1993). Clozapine and risperidone may have an antiaggressive effect separate from their antipsychotic effect.

Anxiolytic drugs. The use of standard anxiolytic drugs such as diazepam or lorazepam for the control of violence over a long period of time is generally not recommended. This guideline stems from a concern that long-term use of these medications will result in drug abuse, dependency, and tolerance. In addition, these drugs can produce disinhibition and confusion. Buspirone has been shown to be as effective as diazepam and other benzodiazepines in managing anxiety. Buspirone appears to lack the hypnotic and abuse potential of other antianxiety agents. It does not appear to interact with other sedating drugs, including alcohol. There should be clear-cut indications (e.g., anxiety) for the long-term use of anxiolytic agents (Shader and Greenblatt 1993). Indications for long-term use of anxiolytics are distinct from indications for their short-term emergency use, when sedative side effects are sought in the

TABLE 37-7. **Medications for long-term management of violence**

Drug	Dosage	Special considerations
Neuroleptics	Doses used for schizophrenicpatients.	Indicated for schizophrenic and other psychotic states.
		Not for personality disorders or mental retardation.
		Akathisia may be associated with violence.
		Depot forms recommended.
Lithium	Doses and blood levels used.	Indicated for violence, especially that accompanying bipolar disorder and mental retardation.
		Testing for thyroid, renal, and cardiac function.
Anticonvulsants (e.g., carbamazepine, valproate, and clonazepam)	Doses for epilepsy and blood level used.	Indicated for epilepsy and serious episodic violence without electroencephalogram abnormalities.
		Regular hematological and liver testing.
Propranolol	20 mg three times daily and increase by 60 mg every 4 days.	Contraindications are bronchialasthma, chronic obstructivepulmonary disease, insulin-dependent diabetes, cardiacdisease, peripheral vasculardisease, renal disease, and hyperthyroidism.
	Doses held or cut back if blood pressure below 90/60 mmHg, pulse below 50, or wheezing occurs.	Caution with concurrent neuroleptics because propranolol increases blood levels three to four times.
	Decrease dose gradually.	

management of violence. I have found clonazepam to be effective in managing episodic violence in patients with intermittent explosive disorder and some personality disorders when there is no serious history of drug abuse. Clonazepam is used to enhance self-control rather than to alleviate anxiety. This drug is used in conjunction with psychotherapy. Low doses in the range of .5 mg two or three times daily on a regular basis are often effective. Higher doses may produce disinhibition.

The problems associated with anxiolytic agents and sedatives, particularly in patients with a history of violence and personality disorders, are abuse and dependence. Physical dependence results in a withdrawal reaction if these medications are discontinued rapidly. This withdrawal reaction may involve aggression and violent behavior, as well as other symptoms such as anxiety, irritability, insomnia, tremors, headache, dizziness, anorexia, nausea, vomiting, diarrhea, incoordination, seizures, and depression. The onset of the withdrawal reaction depends on the particular medication and may be anywhere from a day for a short-acting drug such as lorazepam up to 1 week following cessation of other longer-acting drugs. A gradual reduction of dosage is recommended, namely 5%–10% a day for 10–14 days. A long-acting benzodiazepine may be substituted for shorter-acting benzodiazepines. Patients with a history of seizures, alcohol abuse, or abuse of other drugs should be hospitalized for detoxification.

Carbamazepine and other anticonvulsants. There have been a number of case studies and open drug trials that have indicated that carbamazepine is probably effective for the management of aggression in a number of different types of psychiatric patients (Evans and Gualtieri 1985). In a double-blind, crossover study of 13 chronic psychiatric patients, 10 of whom were schizophrenic patients, there were beneficial effects in terms of decreasing aggressive episodes (Neppe 1983). Although the patients were not epileptic, they did have temporal lobe EEG abnormalities. The patients were treated with antipsychotics, anticholinergics, antidepressants, and benzodiazepines. Luchins (1983) reported on an open carbamazepine trial in seven chronic psychiatric inpatients, six of whom were schizophrenic patients. None of the patients had EEG abnormalities. He reported that six of the seven patients had fewer aggressive episodes while taking carbamazepine than they did either before or after taking the drug. All the patients were concurrently treated with antipsychotic drugs. Mattes et al. (1984) found that carbamazepine is effective in decreasing aggression in patients with psychiatric diagnoses other than schizophrenia. These diagnoses include personality disorders, conduct disorders, and some organic disorders. Later noncontrolled studies have confirmed that carbamazepine is effective for violent patients without epilepsy (Mattes 1984; Mattes 1990; Neppe 1991). There is evidence that carbamazepine may be effective in terms of managing aggression and irritability in patients with overt seizures, both complex partial seizures and generalized seizures; in schizophrenic patients with and without EEG abnormalities; and with other types of patients who have episodic violence but do not have gross brain damage or mental retardation.

Patients without seizure disorders have benefited from carbamazepine at doses of approximately 600 mg/day. Once the therapeutic level (8–12 ng/mL) is reached and a response is obtained, blood levels of carbamazepine should be monitored every month for the first 3 months and then every 3 months thereafter.

Other anticonvulsants have been tried in the control of aggression with inconsistent results (Brizer 1988). Positive findings have included the use of diphenylhydantoin in the treatment of aggressive mentally retarded children, violent nonepileptic male adults (half of whom had EEG abnormalities), and adults with episodic dyscontrol syndrome (Barratt 1993; Barratt et al. 1991). Valproate has been found to be effective for violent patients who cannot be treated with carbamazepine (Brizer 1988).

Propranolol and other β-blockers. Silver and Yudofsky (1985) reviewed a number of control studies, open trials, and case reports on the effectiveness of propranolol in the management of aggressive behavior. Most of the patients studied and responding to propranolol were those with organic brain disease, often with gross impairment secondary to trauma, tumor, alcoholism, encephalitis, Huntington's disease, dementia, Wilson's disease, Korsakoff's psychosis, and mental retardation. In addition, some patients with minimal brain dysfunction or attention deficit also have been reported to respond to propranolol. Nearly all of the patients in these studies were refractory to other medications, including antipsychotics, anxiolytics, anticonvulsants, and lithium. In a number of cases, concurrent antipsychotic medication was used. β-blockers are effective for violence associated with traumatic brain injury when psychosis is present, since a number of neurological side effects of antipsychotic drugs may be avoided. On the other hand, propranolol can be used in conjunction with antipsychotic drugs for the management of violence in other types of psychotic disorders.

Before using propranolol, there should be a thorough medical evaluation of the patient. Patients with the following diseases should be excluded from treatment with propranolol: bronchial asthma; chronic obstructive pulmonary disease; insulin-dependent diabetes; cardiac diseases, including angina or congestive heart failure; diabetes mellitus; significant peripheral vascular disease; severe renal disease; and hyperthyroidism. Hypertensive patients should be given propranolol with caution because sudden discontinuation of propranolol may result in rebound hypertension.

In other case studies, β-blockers other than propranolol have been used (Ratey et al. 1992; Silver and Yudofsky 1988). These other drugs include nadolol, used in the treatment of aggressive patients with chronic paranoid schizophrenia. Pindolol has been reported to be effective in the treatment of aggression in patients with organic brain syndrome. Metoprolol has been reported effective with two patients: one with intermittent explosive disorder related to meningitis and alcohol abuse, and the other with a penetrating brain trauma with temporal lobe epilepsy.

Lithium. Long-term use of lithium helps to prevent manic episodes and associated hyperactive aggressive behavior. In a double-blind trial testing the effectiveness of lithium in the treatment of aggression in adult mentally retarded patients, Craft et al. (1987) found that 73% of patients showed a reduction in aggression during treatment. The use of lithium was the same as that for the management of bipolar patients. Although there have been other reports of the use of lithium in patients with other disorders, there is a sparsity of double-blind controlled studies (Glenn et al. 1989; Luchins and Dojka 1989; Sheard 1975; Sheard et al. 1976; Tupin et al. 1973). These patients with other disorders include those who have organic brain syndrome or head injury; aggressive schizophrenic patients; nonpsychotic, aggressive prisoners; and delinquents and children with conduct or attention-deficit/hyperactivity disorders. Because lithium affects many organ systems in the body, an extensive medical examination is recommended before beginning lithium and during the course of treatment (Silver and Yudofsky 1988).

Psychostimulants. Brizer (1988) reviewed the literature on the use of psychostimulants for the treatment of violent behavior. The use of amphetamines is accepted in controlling aggressive behavior associated with attention-deficit/hyperactivity disorder. There have been some reports of the successful use of amphetamines to control aggression in adults with a history of this disorder as well. In addition, there were two studies reporting the successful use of amphetamines in delinquent youths: one to control aggression in a group of hospitalized black aggressive delinquents, and the other to decrease violence in the classroom for a group of aggressive outpatient boys with antisocial behavior. Further studies are indicated, and the clinician should proceed with caution in prescribing amphetamines because there is great potential for addiction, abuse, and the production of violent behavior through hyperactivity, emotional lability, or delusional thinking as a result of abuse of psychostimulants.

Serotonergic drugs. The development of selective serotonin reuptake inhibitors has opened the door for a clinical test of the theory that serotonin is responsible for impulsive violent behaviors. Earlier, the antidepressant trazodone was found to reduce violence in patients without symptoms of depression (Wilcock 1987). Fluoxetine has been used successfully to treat impulsive violent patients with personality disorders and patients with chronic schizophrenia (Coccaro et al. 1990; Goldman and Janecek 1990) without depression. With the introduction of sertraline, paroxetine, and other drugs, more research on the use of serotonergic drugs for the treatment of violent patients is anticipated.

BEHAVIOR THERAPY

Liberman and Wong (1984) have succinctly described the use of behavioral analysis and therapy in the management of violent behavior. They caution that such a program of treatment should be planned and conducted only by clinicians skilled in behavioral analysis and therapy and that there should be standardized policies and review processes to prevent abuse of patients. Programs of behavioral management for patients with violent behavior should definitely not be ad hoc attempts on inadequately staffed and trained general inpatient units.

The target behaviors of the behavioral treatment program must be clearly specified. General terms such as assault or violence are not sufficient; instead, behaviors such as pushing, shoving, hitting, pulling hair, and so forth must be clearly defined. Consequences of such behavior also must be clearly specified.

The consequences include a broad spectrum of procedures ranging from a token economy and other means of positive reinforcement and social training skills, to more restrictive procedures such as social extinction, sensory extinction, contingent observation, required relaxation, seclusionary time-out, and contingent restraint. Usually, one begins with a positive reinforcement and later turns to more restrictive procedures, such as time-out and restraint.

However, severe violent behavioral problems usually necessitate use of the more restrictive procedures earlier in the treatment plan.

Positive reinforcement may occur as frequently as every 10–20 seconds in seriously aggressive patients in the manner of giving food and attention to reward and reinforce nonassaultive and nondestructive behavior. This approach is termed *differential reinforcement of other behavior*, and the frequency of reinforcement is gradually spaced out over longer intervals as the patient becomes more cooperative. For less severe violent behavior and more cooperative patients, a token economy program is used to motivate patients toward prosocial behavior. Tokens serving as currency are given for nonviolent and prosocial behavior. These tokens are exchanged for cigarettes, snacks, privileges, and other luxuries.

As noted earlier in this chapter, violent behavior could be the result of an inability to communicate and a lack of other social skills. In social skills training, patients are taught how to satisfy their needs through appropriate behavior rather than violent behavior. Training involves instruction describing a rationale for the behavior desired, demonstration of the desired behavior, rehearsal of the behavior, and reinforcement for performing the behavior. Social extinction is the withdrawal of attention from the patient when the patient manifests some undesirable behavior, such as violence. Obviously, the violent behavior cannot be dangerous, and all members of the treatment team must be consistent in ignoring it. Sensory extinction is used for predominantly self-mutilative or injurious behavior, for example, in patients who bang their heads or scratch their faces. In such patients, helmets and foam-padded gloves would be used to protect the patient as well as decrease the sensory consequences of such behavior. Contingent observation is the removal of a patient from an activity for a short period of time following an episode of violence or other inappropriate behavior. This approach is usually taken for minor disruptive behavior such as verbal aggression. It involves placing the patient near the ongoing activity, for example, in a chair for a few minutes while watching the appropriate behavior of other patients.

A more restrictive procedure, required relaxation involves physically placing a patient in a supine position and restraining the patient's arms, legs, and body, if necessary, while the patient is assisted in relaxation. This process lasts for about 10 minutes. Seclusionary time-out or time-out–form reinforcement involves placing the patient in an area isolated from other patients. In distinction to seclusion used in the emergency situation, seclusionary time- out is often brief, usually 5 minutes and rarely longer than 1 hour. Contingent restraint is also more restrictive in that it involves immobilizing part or all of the patient's body by restraints, such as cuffs and belts, a Posey jacket, or other ties, or by a therapist physically holding a patient for a brief period of time following violent behavior. These seclusionary and restraintlike procedures, in addition to being shorter in duration than are seclusion and restraint in the emergency situation, need not involve a physician each time procedures are used because they are part of an ongoing planned treatment program.

LONG-TERM OUTPATIENT PSYCHOTHERAPY

The frequency of violence among patients in outpatient treatment settings is less than that for patients admitted to inpatient units. For example, approximately 3% of patients seen in clinics in the New York City area had a history of recent violence toward others. Patients who are violent in outpatient settings are more likely to be those with personality disorders, child or adolescent disorders, or mental retardation. Again, male patients are more likely to be violent than are female patients, and violence is greater among the younger patients. The spouse, mate, or other family members are the targets of violence in more than half of the cases (Tardiff and Koenigsberg 1985).

Although psychotherapy of the violent patient may be on an individual basis, often therapists involve the spouse or family in treatment. This approach is advisable because of the role of the family in the dynamics of violence. Such an approach is intended not to blame the victim(s) but to analyze interactions that lead to violence. In addition, it is important to get information from persons other than the patient to make certain that problems with violence are not minimized by the patient. Finally, even if violence does not appear to be related to the spouse or family, underlying dynamics may be. For example, a young man assaulted an unknown woman. With further analysis of the man's marriage and conflict with his wife, it was apparent that this was a displacement of violence from his wife to the unknown woman. Some therapists prefer group therapy for violent patients because it is less threatening to the patient than a one-to-one relationship and allows the patient to appreciate that other people have problems with violence. The group is often supportive, yet at the same time the group can confront a patient rather than have the therapist do so. Usually, groups are led by two therapists, which makes it less stressful for each leader.

Lion and Tardiff (1987) have reviewed the principles of using psychotherapy for problems with aggression:

1. The motivation of the patient and the patient's reason for psychotherapy must be evaluated. An inappropriate reason to enter psychotherapy is an attempt to impress the court before a trial for some violent crime. A more appropriate reason is because the patient's marriage, job, or another aspect of his or her life is being jeopardized by the violent behavior and/or because the patient feels guilty about his or her behavior.

2. The patient must develop a sense of self-control of emotions and behavior. At first, the patient relies on the strength and self-control of the therapist. The therapist may give the patient his or her telephone number or the telephone number of the emergency room to call if the patient fears impending violence. The therapist and the patient must be aware that following this honeymoon period in psychotherapy, subsequent violent episodes will occur, and they must be prepared to analyze such episodes without feelings of disappointment. The nature of the transference must be constantly analyzed. Particularly for borderline and psychotic patients, the therapist must look for signs of negative transference that may pose a danger to the therapist. As has been discussed earlier in this chapter, countertransference and negative feelings toward patients are particularly common problems in the treatment of violent patients because violence provokes strong emotions in the therapist that may activate past experience as well as a number of mechanisms of defense. Thus, it is important that the therapist know his or her feelings and not allow them to interfere with treatment.

3. Verbal communication should be facilitated. The patient should be encouraged to talk rather than act to express concerns and weaknesses without fear of retaliation or humiliation, which often occurred when such concerns were shared in the past with spouse, family, or friends.

4. The patient should develop an understanding of the consequences of violent behavior. For example, the patient should be encouraged to fantasize about what it would be like to be in jail or what it would be like to be divorced if spouse abuse continues.

5. The patient should gain insight about the dynamics of violence and early warning signs—for example, flushing of the face, rapid heartbeat, sweating, and a feeling of tension. The patient should be encouraged to avoid a violent situation at first by taking a walk or calling the therapist and eventually to develop insight in dealing with a potentially violent situation psychologically.

SPECIAL CONCERNS IN THE TREATMENT OF VIOLENT PATIENTS

DANGER TO THE THERAPIST

The first concern in treating violent patients is danger to the therapist. Any threat, even if made in a joking manner, must be taken seriously and evaluated. The therapist should acknowledge to the patient that these threats are frightening, and together they must identify and address the problem if treatment is to continue.

There should be some way for the therapist to communicate that he or she is in trouble inside an office or, conversely, for a receptionist to warn the therapist that there is a potential problem with violence before a patient enters the therapist's office (e.g., if a patient is agitated or appears to have been drinking). This warning can be done through an electrical device such as a buzzer or in other ways such as using code words or prearranged signals to communicate trouble either by the therapist or by the receptionist. Even in outpatient settings where few violent patients are seen, there should be a plan of response to a violent situation, including hostage-taking situations. This plan should be written and rehearsed by all involved in the response to such situations. In addition, in emergency rooms, patients should be searched for weapons. Offices should not contain heavy objects such as ashtrays and should contain pillows or a light chair that may be used as shields in case of violence, particularly if the patient has a knife or weapon other than a gun. If a patient appears with a gun in the waiting room and it is possible for the psychiatrist to escape, he or she should do so. If a patient produces a gun in the office and escape is impossible, the therapist should remain outwardly calm and comply with any requests in the early phase of this emergency. Eventually, the therapist should ask the patient to put the gun on the desk or table rather than reach for the gun or ask the patient to drop the gun, both of which may result in the gun discharging.

Concern for the safety of staff includes injuries caused by patients, particularly on inpatient units or in the emergency room. Thackrey (1987) has described and illustrated through photographs a number of physical techniques for self-protection. He has included techniques that are effective and safe for the therapist as well as the patient. He maintains that they require a minimum amount of training and practice for proficiency. It should be emphasized that reading about these techniques should not replace specific guidelines for, and rehearsal of, physical techniques within each institution.

Thackrey (1987) describes a nonthreatening, protective posture that, in essence, is a sideward stance that mini-mizes the amount of body area that would be the target of violent attack and is less threatening to a potentially violent patient than facing the patient. Furthermore, one must anticipate a punch, kick, or other form of attack and either escape out of reach of the patient or, conversely, approach the patient so closely that an effective punch or kick is not possible. The author illustrates various ways of deflecting a punch or kick with the arms or legs and describes various means of escaping from holds of patients. For example, if a patient grabs at the wrist, the clinician bends the arms at the elbow for added strength and swiftly turns the arm against the patient's thumb to release the clinician's arm. Thackrey describes movements to escape if the patient grabs one's hair by establishing control on the grabbing hand of the patient to minimize further damage and then moving the patient's hand into a mechanically inferior position. Escape from choking has as a key aspect of survival tucking of the chin downward, thus protecting critical air and blood circulation structures and making it more difficult for the patient to get a solid grip around the neck. Protection of these structures is essential to avoid losing consciousness and to gain time in terms of release from a choking hold. Escape from biting of an extremity, for example, is effected by pushing the bitten part deeper into the patient's mouth and closing the patient's nostrils, thus forcing the patient to take a gasp of air and giving the clinician a chance to escape.

DUTY TO PROTECT POTENTIAL VICTIMS

Another concern is danger to others and the responsibility of the clinician to protect intended victims of violent patients. Mills et al. (1987) have reviewed court decisions and legislation in the decade following the *Tarasoff* decision in California. The details and ramifications of this case are discussed in Chapter 41 of this textbook, but a few words about the clinical aspects of the duty to protect are relevant here. A central issue is a balance between the confidentiality and privileged information given to the physician and the duty to protect the community. This balance of responsibility has long been rooted in medical practice. Mills et al. (1987) point out that the duty to protect need not involve warning the intended victim or the police but instead should involve change of treatment standards, including civil commitments. A shift of burden of decision making to the courts may be sufficient. Mills and his colleagues argue that a standard of liability for a professional requires that there not be a substantial departure from clinical standards of decision making.

Appelbaum (1985) has a model for meeting the requirements imposed by the *Tarasoff* doctrine. He recommends viewing the fulfillment of the duty to protect in three stages. First, there must be an assessment of the potential for harm in that the therapist must gather data relevant to the evaluation of dangerousness, and the determination of this dangerousness must be made based on these data. Appelbaum (1985) reassures us that in many Tarasoff-like cases, therapists have not been faulted for inaccurate predictions but rather for failing to gather data and to document how the decision concerning homicide or danger potential was made.

The basic model recommended earlier in this chapter in the discussion of short-term evaluation of violence potential could serve in Appelbaum's model. Analogous to assessment of suicide risk, the determination of dangerousness in the immediate future would be made for the next few days or week at most. Reasons for risk of immediate dangerousness should be documented on the patient's record for the specified period of time and then a reevaluation should be done when the patient is next seen.

The second stage in Appelbaum's model for meeting the requirements imposed by the *Tarasoff* decision is a formulation of a course of action to protect the intended victim. This course of action may involve changing or increasing the patient's medication, hospitalizing the patient, increasing security on the inpatient unit, or warning the intended victim or the police.

The third stage of this model is directly warning the intended victim. Mills (1984) points out the problems in determining which steps to warn an intended victim are reasonable and under what circumstances. Beyond issues of confidentiality and the effect on the therapy of the patient if the victim is warned, there are questions about how to warn a victim (i.e., should the therapist take time to visit the intended victim, merely telephone, or send a letter?). Issues about possibly causing needless distress for the intended victim and what actions the victim or police really can take to prevent violence must be considered.

Beck (1985) has noted, based on a review of cases, especially those outside of California, that the duty to protect or warn exists only if there is evidence that the patient is posing a serious threat to do bodily harm to a specific person. If careful assessment, documented in writing, fails to reveal such evidence, there is no liability for the therapist. In fact, even if *Tarasoff*-like laws do not exist, such documentation should be done as part of professional clinical care.

CONCLUSIONS

Violence is a frequent and serious problem in institutions. The causes of violence involve a balance of factors within the patient, usually nonspecific, and factors surrounding the patient. There is never one cause and never one treatment; instead, a balance of biological, social, and psychological factors is responsible for a violent act. Treatment of the violent patient on inpatient units should first address prevention in terms of adequately trained staff who are aware of their feelings and the psychodynamics operating in themselves as well as in patients. The environment should be therapeutic and uncrowded, with a balance of humanistic caring and a sense of social order. The opportunity for patients to talk to, or at least be with, staff is important. Verbal contact with potentially violent patients should be done in a nonprovocative, calm manner. If a violent episode occurs, there should be an instant differential diagnosis and classification of the patient's condition into one of three categories: organic mental disorders, functional psychotic disorders, or nonpsychotic, nonorganic disorders. The last category is the most amenable to verbal intervention.

If physical controls are used, the decision to use involuntary medication, seclusion, or restraint should be based on the needs of the individual patient and situation and not on a legal hierarchy of restrictiveness. Seclusion and restraint should be used in keeping with accepted professional guidelines, most notably those of the APA (Tardiff 1984). If common sense and good professional judgment are used, the therapist is protected under the law for injury to the patient while seclusion or restraint is being used, and the number of injuries would be expected to diminish.

In terms of managing violent patients with medication, rapid neuroleptization is effective for a large proportion of patients in the emergency situation, with certain caveats for patients with organic mental disorders with unknown etiology and those with intoxication or withdrawal from alcohol or sedative drugs. In terms of the long-term treatment of the violent patient, no one medication is specified, but medication is targeted to the underlying disorder.

Behavioral treatment is effective for the management of violent behaviors in certain types of patients; however, such treatment should be planned by clinicians experienced with behavioral analysis and therapies and implemented by a large number of experienced staff.

There are definite principles and goals of outpatient psychotherapy for the violent patient and his or her family. Issues of transference and countertransference must be monitored and attended to actively.

Two overriding concerns in the treatment of violent patients are fear for one's safety and a concern for the safety of others. The treatment of violent patients need not be perilous as long as certain safeguards are kept in mind. The responsibility to protect intended victims of violence should include assessment of a patient's violence potential, which is analogous to the assessment of suicide potential. This assessment should be documented clearly in the patient's records and reevaluated at the next visit. If the patient is found to pose a substantial threat to others, then in most states the clinician has the duty to protect, although not necessarily warn, intended victims.

FUTURE DIRECTIONS IN RESEARCH

Future research should use clear phenomenological definitions of violence, that is, specific behaviors rather than subjective definitions of violence such as "verbal aggression." Research on the biology of violence should include finding more sensitive measures of neurophysiological and biochemical dysfunction of the brain and using technology such as nuclear magnetic resonance imaging, positron-emission tomography, single photon emission computed tomography, regional cerebral blood flow, and brain electrical mapping. In addition, studies should be using new techniques for the study of neurotransmitters such as digital subtraction autoradiography for brain dopamine and serotonin receptors (Altar et al. 1985). Drugs that increase serotonin levels should be studied in terms of their effects on violent, and particularly impulsive, behavior. Epidemiological studies should use more sophisticated techniques and data systems concerning crime and violence with a goal of accurate reporting of domestic violence, child abuse, and linkage of homicides to detect serial murderers. There should be prospective studies so as to develop a better ability to predict violence in the near and distant future.

Although beyond the scope of psychiatry alone, intervention programs aimed at decreasing child and spouse abuse, relieving poverty and unemployment, and decreasing drug and alcohol use will decrease the incidence of violence in our society. Such efforts must be supported by all citizens of our society.

REFERENCES

Altar CA, O'Neil SO, Walter RJ, et al: Brain dopamine and serotonin receptor sites revealed by digital subtraction autoradiography. Science 228:597–600, 1985

American Psychiatric Association: Clinician Safety: Report of the American Psychiatric Association Task Force on Clinician Safety. Washington, DC, American Psychiatric Association, 1993

Anderson AC: Environmental factors and aggressive behavior. J Clin Psychiatry 43:280–283, 1982

Appelbaum PS: Tarasoff and the clinician: problems in fulfilling the duty to protect. Am J Psychiatry 142:425–429, 1985

Apter A, Kotler M, Sevy S, et al: Correlates of risk of suicide in violent and nonviolent psychiatric patients. Am J Psychiatry 148:883–887, 1991

Barratt ES: The use of anticonvulsants in aggression and violence. Psychopharmacol Bull 29:75–81, 1993

Barratt ES, Kent TA, Bryant SG, et al: A controlled trial of phenytoin in impulsive aggression. J Clin Psychopharmacol 11:388–389, 1991

Beck JC (ed): The Potentially Violent Patient and the Tarasoff Decision in Psychiatric Practice. Washington, DC, American Psychiatric Press, 1985

Belfrage H, Lidberg L, Oreland L: Platelet monoamine oxidase activity in mentally disordered violent offenders. Acta Psychiatr Scand 85:218–221, 1992

Bell PA, Baron RA: Ambient temperature and human violence, in Multidisciplinary Approaches to Aggression Research. Edited by Brain PF, Benton D. Amsterdam, Elsevier/North Holland Biomedical, 1981, pp 76–88

Binder RL, McNeil DE: The relationship of gender to violent behavior in acutely disturbed psychiatric patients. J Clin Psychiatry 51:110–114, 1990

Bland R, Orn H: Family violence and psychiatry. Can J Psychiatry 31:129–137, 1986

Blau JR, Blau PM: The cost of inequality: metropolitan structure and violent crime. American Sociological Review 47:114–129, 1982

Bohman M, Cloninger CR, Sigvardsson S, et al: Predisposition to petty criminality in Swedish adoptees, I: genetic and environmental heterogeneity. Arch Gen Psychiatry 39:1233–1241, 1982

Braverman ER, Pfeiffer CC: Suicide and biochemistry. Biol Psychiatry 20:123–124, 1985

Brizer DA: Psychopharmacology and the management of violent patients. Psychiatr Clin North Am 11:551–568, 1988

Brown GL, Ebert MH, Goyer PF, et al: Aggression, suicide, and serotonin: relationships to CSF amine metabolites. Am J Psychiatry 139:741–746, 1982

Bushman BJ, Cooper HM: Effects of alcohol on human aggression: an integrative research review. Psychol Bull 107:341–354, 1990

Calcedo-Barba AL, Calcedo-Ordonez A: Violence and paranoid schizophrenia. Int J Law Psychiatry 17:253–263, 1994

Centerwall BS: Race, socioeconomic status and domestic homicide: Atlanta, 1971–1972. Am J Public Health 74:813–815, 1984

Centerwall BS: Television and violence: the scale of the problem and where to go from here. JAMA 267:3059–3063, 1992

Coccaro EF: Impulsive aggression and central serotonergic system function in humans: an example of a dimensional brain-behavior relationship. Int Clin Psychopharmacol 7:3–12, 1992

Coccaro EF, Siever LJ, Klar HM, et al: Serotonergic studies in patients with affective and personality disorders: correlates with suicidal and impulsive aggressive behavior. Arch Gen Psychiatry 46:587–599, 1989

Coccaro EF, Astill JL, Herbert JL, et al: Fluoxetine treatment of impulsive aggression in DSM-III-R personality disorder patients. J Clin Psychopharmacol 10:373–375, 1990

Cook PJ: The role of firearms in violent crime: an interpretive review of the literature, in Criminal Violence. Edited by Wolfgang ME, Weiner NA. Beverly Hills, CA, Sage, 1982, pp 236–291

Craft M, Ismail IA, Krishnamurti D, et al: Lithium in the treatment of aggression in mentally handicapped patients: a double-blind trial. Br J Psychiatry 150:685–689, 1987

Dalton K: Cyclical criminal acts in premenstrual syndrome. Lancet 2:1070–1071, 1980

Davis S: Violence by psychiatric inpatients: a review. Hospital and Community Psychiatry 42:585–590, 1991

De Jong J, Virkkunen M, Linnoila M: Factors associated with recidivism in a criminal population. J Nerv Ment Dis 180:543–550, 1992

Delgado-Escueta AV, Mattson RH, King L, et al: The nature of aggression during epileptic seizures. N Engl J Med 305:711–716, 1981

Deutsch LH, Bylsma FW, Rovner BW, et al: Psychosis and physical aggression in probable Alzheimer's disease. Am J Psychiatry 148:1159–1163, 1991

Dietz PE: Patterns in human violence, in Psychiatry Update: American Psychiatric Association Annual Review, Vol 6. Edited by Hales RE, Frances AJ. Washington, DC, American Psychiatric Press, 1987, pp 465–490

Di Lalla LF, Gottesman I: Biological and genetic contributors to violence: Widom's untold tale. Psychol Bull 109:125–129, 1991

Dubin WR, Weiss KJ, Dorn JM: Pharmacotherapy of psychiatric emergencies. J Clin Psychopharmacol 6:210–222, 1986

Eichelman BS: Toward a rational pharmacotherapy for aggressive and violent behavior. Hospital and Community Psychiatry 39:31–39, 1986

Eichelman BS: Aggressive behavior: from laboratory to clinic: quo vadit? Arch Gen Psychiatry 49:488–492, 1992

Eichelman BS, Hartwig AC (eds): Patient Violence and the Clinician. Washington, DC, American Psychiatric Press, 1995

Elliot FA: Violence: the neurologic contribution. Arch Neurol 49:595–603, 1992

Evans RW, Gualtieri CT: Carbamazepine: a neuropsychological and psychiatric profile. Clin Neuropharmacol 8:221–241, 1985

Fishbein DH, Lozovsky D, Jaffe JH: Impulsivity, aggression, and neuroendocrine responses to serotonergic stimulation in substance abusers. Biol Psychiatry 25:1049–1066, 1989

Freedman JL: Effects of television violence on aggressiveness. Psychol Bull 96:227–246, 1984

Glenn MB, Wroblewski B, Parziale J, et al: Lithium carbonate for aggressive behavior or affective instability in ten brain-injured patients. Am J Phys Med Rehabil 68:221–226, 1989

Goldman MB, Janecek HM: Adjunctive fluoxetine improves global function in chronic schizophrenia. J Neuropsychiatry Clin Neurosci 2:429–431, 1990

Goldstein PJ, Brounstein HH, Ryan PJ, et al: Crack and homicide in New York City, 1988: a conceptually based event analysis. Contemporary Drug Problems 5:651–687, 1989

Goodman RA, Mercy JA, Loya F, et al: Alcohol use and interpersonal violence: alcohol detected in homicide victims. Am J Public Health 76:144–149, 1986

Hare RD, McPherson LM: Violent and aggressive behavior by criminal psychopaths. Int J Law Psychiatry 7:35–50, 1984

Hart SD, Hare RD: Psychopathology and the DSM-IV criteria for antisocial personality. J Abnorm Psychol 100:391–398, 1991

Hermann BP, Whitman S: Behavioral and personality correlates of epilepsy: a review, methodological critique and conceptual model. Psychol Bull 95:451–497, 1984

Holcomb WR, Ahr PR: Arrest rates among young adult psychiatric patients treated in inpatient and outpatient settings. Hospital and Community Psychiatry 39:52–57, 1988

Honer WE, Gewirtz E, Turey M: Psychosis and violence in cocaine smokers (letter). Lancet 1:451, 1987

Humphreys MS, Johnstone EC, MacMillan JF, et al. Dangerous behavior preceding first admission for schizophrenia. Br J Psychiatry 161:501–505, 1992

Jaffe P, Wolfe D, Wilson SK, et al: Family violence and child adjustment: a comparative analysis of girls' and boys' behavioral symptoms. Am J Psychiatry 143:74–77, 1986

Kane JM: Compliance issues in outpatient treatment. J Clin Psychopharmacol 5 (suppl):22S–27S, 1985

Kay SR, Wolkenfeld F, Murrill LM: Profiles of aggression among psychiatric patients, II: covariates and predictors. J Nerv Ment Dis 176:547–557, 1988

Kempe CH, Helfer RE (eds): The Battered Child, 3rd Edition, Revised and Expanded. Chicago, IL, University of Chicago Press, 1980

Krakowski M, Volavka J, Brizer D: Psychopathology and violence: a review of literature. Compr Psychiatry 27:131–148, 1986

Lacks P: Bender Gestalt Screening for Brain Dysfunction. New York, Wiley, 1984

Liberman RP, Wong SE: Behavior analysis and therapy procedures related to seclusion and restraint, in The Psychiatric Uses of Seclusion and Restraint. Edited by Tardiff K. Washington, DC, American Psychiatric Press, 1984, pp 35–67

Lidberg L, Tuck JR, Åsberg M, et al: Homicide, suicide and CSF 5-HIAA. Acta Psychiatr Scand 71:230–236, 1985

Lindqvist P, Allebeck P: Schizophrenia and crime: a longitudinal follow-up of 644 schizophrenics in Stockholm. Br J Psychiatry 157:345–350, 1990

Linnoila M, Virkkunen M, Scheinin M, et al: Low cerebrospinal fluid 5-hydroxyindoleacetic acid concentration differentiates impulsive from nonimpulsive violent behavior. Life Sci 33:2609–2614, 1983

Lion JR, Pasternak SA: Countertransference reactions to violent patients. Am J Psychiatry 130:207–210, 1973

Lion JR, Tardiff K: The long-term treatment of the violent patient, in Psychiatry Update: American Psychiatric Association Annual Review, Vol 6. Edited by Hales RE, Frances AJ. Washington, DC, American Psychiatric Press, 1987, pp 537–548

Luchins DJ: Carbamazepine in violent nonepileptic schizophrenics. Psychopharmacol Bull 20:569–571, 1983

Luchins DJ, Dojka D: Lithium and propranolol in aggression and self-injurious behavior in the mentally retarded. Psychopharmacol Bull 25:372–375, 1989

Mark VH, Ervin FR: Violence and the Brain. New York, Harper & Row, 1970

Mattes JA: Comparative effectiveness of carbamazepine and propranolol for rage outbursts. J Neuropsychiatry Clin Neurosci 2:159–164, 1990

Mattes JA, Rosenberg J, Mays D: Carbamazepine versus propranolol in patients with rage outbursts: a random assignment study. Psychopharmacol Bull 20:98–100, 1984

Messner S, Tardiff K: The social ecology of urban homicide: an application of the routine activities approach. Criminology 23:241–267, 1985

Messner S, Tardiff K: Economic inequality and levels of homicide: an analysis of urban neighborhoods. Criminology 24:297–317, 1986

Mills MJ: The so-called duty to warn: the psychotherapeutic duty to protect third parties from patients' violent acts. Behav Sci Law 2:237–257, 1984

Mills MJ, Sullivan G, Eth S: Protecting third parties: a decade after Tarasoff. Am J Psychiatry 144:68–74, 1987

Monahan J: Mental disorder and violent behavior: perceptions and evidence. Am Psychol 47:511–521, 1992

Monroe RR: Episodic Behavioral Disorders. Cambridge, MA, Harvard University Press, 1970

Monroe RR: Episodic behavioral disorders and limbic ictus. Compr Psychiatry 26:466–479, 1985

National Institute of Mental Health: Television and behavior: ten years of scientific progress and implications for the eighties, Vol 1: summary report (DHHS Publ No ADM-82-1195). Rockville, MD, National Institute of Mental Health, 1982

Neppe VM: Carbamazepine as adjunctive treatment in nonepileptic chronic inpatients with EEG temporal lobe abnormalities. J Clin Psychiatry 44:326–331, 1983

Neppe VM, Bourman BR, Lawchuck KS: Carbamazepine for atypical psychosis with episodic hostility. J Nerv Ment Dis 179:439–441, 1991

Nurco DN, Ball JC, Shaffer JW, et al: The criminality of narcotic addicts. J Nerv Ment Dis 173:94–102, 1985

Palmstierna T, Huitfeldt B, Wistedt B: The relationship of crowding and aggressive behavior on a psychiatric intensive care unit. Hospital and Community Psychiatry 42:1237–1240, 1991

Rabkin JG: Criminal behavior of discharged mental patients: a critical review of the research. Psychol Bull 86:1–27, 1979

Rada RT, Kellner R, Stivastava C, et al: Plasma androgens in violent and nonviolent sex offenders. Bulletin of the American Academy of Psychiatry and the Law 11:149–158, 1983

Ratey JJ, Sorgi P, O'Driscoll GA, et al: Nadolol to treat aggression and psychiatric symptomatology in chronic psychiatric inpatients: a double-blind, placebo-controlled study. J Clin Psychiatry 53:41–46, 1992

Ratey JJ, Leveroni C, Kilmer D, et al: The effects of clozapine on severely aggressive psychiatric inpatients in a state hospital. J Clin Psychiatry 54:219–223, 1993

Reid RL, Yen SC: Premenstrual syndrome. Am J Obstet Gynecol 139:85–104, 1981

Reid WH, Balis GU: Evaluation of the violent patient, in Psychiatry Update: American Psychiatric Association Annual Review, Vol 6. Edited by Hales RE, Frances AJ. Washington, DC, American Psychiatric Press, 1987, pp 491–509

Reitan RM: Investigation of the validity of Halstead's measures of biological intelligence. Archives of Neurology and Psychiatry 48:474–477, 1955

Saltzman LE, Mercy JA, O'Carroll PW, et al: Weapon involvement and injury outcomes in family and intimates assaults. JAMA 267:3043–3047, 1992

Sampson RJ: Structural density and criminal victimization. Criminology 21:276–293, 1983

Schiavi RC, Theilgaard A, Owen DR, et al: Sex chromosome anomalies, hormones, and aggressivity. Arch Gen Psychiatry 41:93–99, 1984

Shader RI, Greenblatt DJ: Drug therapy: use of benzodiazepines in anxiety disorders. N Engl J Med 328:1398–1405, 1993

Sheard MH: Lithium in the treatment of aggression. J Nerv Ment Dis 160:108–118, 1975

Sheard MH, Marini JL, Bridges CI, et al: The effect of lithium in impulsive aggressive behavior in man. Am J Psychiatry 133:1409–1413, 1976

Silver JM, Yudofsky S: Propranolol for aggression: literature review and clinical guidelines. International Drug Therapy Newsletter 20:9–12, 1985

Silver JM, Yudofsky SC: Psychopharmacology and electroconvulsive therapy, in The American Psychiatric Press Textbook of Psychiatry. Edited by Talbott JA, Hales RE, Yudofsky SC. Washington, DC, American Psychiatric Press, 1988

Soloff PH: Emergency management of violent patients, in Psychiatry Update: American Psychiatric Association Annual Review, Vol 6. Edited by Hales RE, Frances AJ. Washington, DC, American Psychiatric Press, 1987, pp 510–536

Swanson JW, Holzer CE, Ganju VK, et al: Violence and psychiatric disorder in the community: evidence from the Epidemiologic Catchment Area surveys. Hospital and Community Psychiatry 41:761–770, 1990

Tardiff K: A survey of assault by chronic patients in a state hospital system, in Assaults Within Psychiatric Facilities. Edited by Lion JR, Reid WH. New York, Grune & Stratton, 1983, pp 3–19

Tardiff K (ed): The Psychiatric Uses of Seclusion and Restraint. Washington, DC, American Psychiatric Press, 1984

Tardiff K (ed): The violent patient. Psychiatr Clin North Am Vol 11, No 4, 1988

Tardiff K: A model for the short-term prediction of violence potential, in Current Approaches to the Prediction of Violence. Edited by Brizer DA, Crowner ML. Washington, DC, American Psychiatric Press, 1989, pp 1–12

Tardiff K: The current state of psychiatry in the treatment of violent patients. Arch Gen Psychiatry 49:493–499, 1992

Tardiff K: Concise Guide to Assessment and Management of Violent Patients, 2nd Edition. Washington, DC, American Psychiatric Press, 1996

Tardiff K, Koenigsberg HW: Assaultive behavior among psychiatric outpatients. Am J Psychiatry 142:960–963, 1985

Tardiff K, Gross EM, Messner SF: A study of homicides in Manhattan, 1981. Am J Public Health 76:139–143, 1986

Tardiff K, Marzuk PM, Leon AJ, et al: Homicide in New York City: cocaine use and firearms. JAMA 272:43–46, 1994

Tardiff K, Marzuk PM, Leon AJ, et al: Violence by patients admitted to a private psychiatric hospital. Am J Psychiatry 154:88–93, 1997

Tellegen A, Lykken DT, Bouchard TJ, et al: Personality similarity in twins reared apart and together. J Pers Soc Psychol 54:1031–1039, 1988

Thackrey M: Therapeutics for Aggression: Psychological/Physical Crisis Intervention. New York, Human Sciences Press, 1987

Tonkonogy JM: Violence and temporal lobe lesion: head CT and MRI data. J Neuropsychiatry Clin Neurosci 3:189–196, 1991

Tupin JP, Smith DB, Clanon TL, et al: The long-term use of lithium in aggressive prisoners. Compr Psychiatry 14:311–317, 1973

U.S. General Accounting Office: Many deaths and injuries caused by firearms could be prevented (Publ No GAO/PEMD-91-9). Washington, DC, U.S. Government Printing Office, 1991

Virkkunen M: Reactive hypoglycemia tendency among habitually violent offenders: a further study by means of the glucose tolerance test. Neuropsychobiology 8:35–40, 1982

Virkkunen M, De Jong J, Bartko J, et al: Psychobiological concomitants of history of suicide attempts among violent offenders and impulsive fire setters. Arch Gen Psychiatry 46:604–606, 1989

Volavka J, Meibach RC: Effect of risperidone on hostility in schizophrenia. J Clin Psychopharmacol 15:243–249, 1995

Volavka J, Zito JM, Vitrai J, et al: Clozapine effects on hostility and aggression in schizophrenia. J Clin Psychopharmacol 13:287–288, 1993

Weiger B, Bear D: An approach to the neurology of aggression. J Psychiatr Res 22:85–89, 1988

Widom CS: The cycle of violence. Science 244:160–171, 1989a

Widom CS: Does violence beget violence? A critical examination of the literature. Psychol Bull 106:3–25, 1989b

Wilcock G: Trazodone for aggressive behavior. Lancet 1:929–930, 1987

Williams K: Economic sources of homicide: reestimating the effects of poverty and inequality. American Sociological Review 49:283–289, 1984

Wilson WJ: The Truly Disadvantaged: The Inner City, The Underclass and Public Policy. Chicago, University of Chicago Press, 1987

Wolfgang ME: Sociocultural overview of criminal violence, in Violence and the Violent Individual. Edited by Hoys JR, Robert TK, Solway KS. New York, SP Medical and Scientific Books, 1981, pp 153–170

Young JL, Zonana HV, Shepler L: Medication noncompliance in schizophrenia: codification and update. Bulletin of the American Academy of Psychiatry and the Law 14:105–122, 1986

Yudofsky SC, Silver JM, Jackson W: The Overt Aggression Scale: an operationalized rating scale for verbal and physical aggression. Am J Psychiatry 143 (suppl):35–39, 1986

CHAPTER 38

PSYCHIATRIC ASSESSMENT OF FEMALE PATIENTS

VIVIEN K. BURT, M.D., PH.D.
VICTORIA HENDRICK, M.D.

Recently there has been a growing awareness that there is diagnostic and therapeutic value to addressing female-specific differences in psychiatric disorders. For example, the prevalence of depressive and anxiety disorders is twice as high in women as in men (Kessler et al. 1994; Weissman et al. 1991). Psychosocial reasons for women's greater vulnerability to these disorders include their relatively lower income, caregiving responsibilities, greater likelihood of experiencing sexual and domestic violence, and disadvantaged social status. Biologically, gonadal steroids are known to have psychoactive effects and may contribute to gender differences (McGlone 1980; Vogel et al. 1978). For example, estrogen produces antidopaminergic and serotonin-enhancing effects, and progesterone metabolites modulate γ-aminobutyric acid (GABA) receptors (Freeman et al. 1993; Seeman and Lang 1990; Sherwin 1990).

Female-specific elements of a psychiatric evaluation include an assessment of the temporal relationship of symptoms with the patient's menstrual cycle. Thus, for some women treated with psychotropic medications who experience premenstrual exacerbation or recurrence of symptoms, it may be worthwhile to check plasma levels of medication, as they may fluctuate across the menstrual cycle (Kimmel et al. 1992). It is important to consider the possibility that a woman of childbearing age may be pregnant and to assess her use of contraception and her plans for pregnancy, as these factors influence treatment recommendations. A history of reproductive-related mood changes (e.g., oral contraceptive dysphoria, premenstrual mood symptoms, postpartum and perimenopausal depression) predicts future reproductive-related mood changes and may guide treatment decisions (Stewart and Boydell 1993). A patient's use of exogenous hormones (e.g., oral contraceptive or hormone replacement therapy) should be assessed, as these may influence plasma levels of medications. Estrogen has an inhibitory effect on oxidative hepatic metabolism, thus potentially increasing blood levels of drugs that are oxidatively metabolized (e.g., many tricyclic antidepressants [TCAs], diazepam, clonazepam, chlordiazepoxide). On the other hand, drugs that undergo conjugative metabolism (e.g., lorazepam, oxazepam, temazepam) may be cleared more rapidly, as estrogen appears to induce hepatic conjugative enzymes. For a middle-aged woman reporting sleep impairment, the clinician should inquire about the occurrence of perimenopausal night sweats that may cause sleep disruption. The presence of seasonal affective disorder, which predominates in women, should be explored.

The psychiatric evaluation of female patients should include certain laboratory examinations, particularly a thyroid panel for women reporting changes in energy level, weight, or temperature tolerance. Autoimmune thyroid disorders occur primarily in women and have an estimated prevalence of 16% in women older than age 65 years. A follicle-stimulating hormone (FSH) level may identify perimenopausal/menopausal status in middle-aged women. It is prudent to measure a serum β-human chorionic gonadotropin (HCG) to rule out pregnancy for women of reproductive age who are considering a trial of pharmacotherapy. If menstrual cycling is irregular, a serum prolactin level and thyroid-stimulating hormone (TSH) should be obtained, as both hyperprolactinemia and hypothyroidism may produce amenorrhea or irregular bleeding. Although hyperprolactinemia is a common sequela of neuroleptic medication in female patients, this condition may require an endocrinological evaluation and a brain imaging study to assess for the presence of a prolactin-producing pituitary tumor.

For women with symptoms of an eating disorder, additional laboratory evaluations include serum albumin, total protein, and glucose to assess nutritional status; serum amylase levels to assess the extent of self-induced vomiting; serum electrolytes, blood urea nitrogen, and creatinine to determine fluid/electrolyte abnormalities; and a complete blood count to assess for anemia from nutritional deficiency and from internal bleeding (e.g., due to esophageal tears resulting from self-induced vomiting). An electrocardiogram may reveal cardiac conduction abnormalities from electrolyte imbalance, malnutrition, or ipecac-induced cardiomyopathy.

PREMENSTRUAL DYSPHORIC DISORDER

In DSM-IV (American Psychiatric Association 1994), premenstrual dysphoric disorder (PMDD) is listed as a mood disorder not otherwise classified and describes the recurrent physical and emotional symptoms restricted to the late luteal phase of the menstrual cycle and remitting within the first day or two following the onset of menstruation. Although PMDD is best determined by prospective daily symptom ratings over a 2-month interval, in clinical practice, PMDD often is provisionally diagnosed and treatment is begun even as prospective daily ratings are in progress. Although most women of childbearing age experience some symptoms of PMDD over the course of some of their menstrual cycles, only about 5%–9% of childbearing-age women meet the criteria needed to establish the diagnosis of PMDD. It is important to identify other psychiatric disorders, including unipolar depression, dysthymia, or an anxiety disorder, which may exacerbate premenstrually, because treatment approaches may necessitate medication or behavioral modification to address premenstrual worsening of symptoms that occur throughout the month (Hendrick et al. 1996).

EVALUATION AND TREATMENT OF PREMENSTRUAL DYSPHORIC DISORDER

The evaluation for PMDD includes a full psychiatric evaluation, especially documentation of course of presenting symptoms, possible precipitants, and previous treatment approaches and responses. Medical evaluation should rule out those physical conditions that may cause symptoms in association with times in the menstrual cycle (e.g., thyroid abnormalities, endometriosis, fibrocystic breast disease). Family psychiatric history, particularly any history of premenstrual symptoms and effective treatments in female relatives, is useful to guide treatment in the patient with PMDD. Medication use, including both prescribed and over-the-counter medications, should be recorded, and substances that may produce psychiatric side effects should be noted. The use of caffeine, salt, alcohol, and nicotine should be assessed because these may cause symptoms that mimic those of PMDD.

Treatment should be based on the severity and nature of symptoms, the patient's desire to be treated continuously throughout the cycle or only on symptomatic days, and the patient's views regarding the use of psychotropic versus other palliative agents. Mild premenstrual symptoms often can be treated with nonpharmacological interventions (e.g., sleep hygiene education, with emphasis on adequate sleep during the symptomatic premenstrual days). Completion of prospective ratings on a daily basis often alerts the patient to high-risk days during which it is best to avoid difficult decisions and to minimize caffeine, salt, alcohol, and nicotine. Such nonpharmacological interventions are also useful to address symptoms while awaiting the results of prospective symptom rating.

Of the pharmacological treatments, the most promising include serotonergic medications such as fluoxetine to treat premenstrual dysphoria, irritability, and tension (Altshuler et al. 1995c; Steiner et al. 1995). To be effective, serotonergic medications are given throughout the month, although administration of fluoxetine only during the two premenstrual weeks has met with some success. Other psychotropic medications that have been effective at standard doses include nortriptyline, nefazodone, and clomipramine (Altshuler et al. 1995c). Premenstrual anxiety and irritability may be treated with anxiolytics such as buspirone and alprazolam (Xanax).

Although progesterone supplementation is a popular treatment, controlled studies have failed to prove its effectiveness in alleviating symptoms of PMDD. Subcutaneous or transdermal estrogen has been somewhat successful, although side effects include nausea, weight gain, and mastalgia. The synthetic androgen danazol and gonadotropin-releasing hormone (GnRH) agonists such as leuprolide produce an anovulatory state by suppressing the hypothalamic-pituitary-ovarian axis and successfully treat the symptoms of PMDD. However, these drugs, in addition to causing significant side effects, produce a hypoestrogenemic state and thus increase the risk of osteoporosis and possibly heart disease. Therefore, these treatments are rarely used for PMDD.

Other pharmacological modalities include vitamin B_6 (pyridoxine) at doses of 50 mg/day. Doses greater than 100 mg/day should be avoided because higher doses may cause peripheral neuropathy.

Less clearly useful, but benign and worth a try, are primrose oil, calcium, magnesium, and vitamin E. Diuretics (e.g., spironolactone, hydrochlorothiazide) are useful for the treatment of women with premenstrual edema and bloating. The use of the anti-inflammatory prostaglandin inhibitors (e.g., mefenamic acid, naproxen) is effective for the treatment of premenstrual pelvic pain, cramping, and headache. Other medications that have been reported to be helpful include atenolol, clonidine, and naltrexone.

HORMONAL CONTRACEPTION AND EFFECTS ON MOOD

Hormonal contraceptive agents include oral contraceptives, or birth control pills, and long-acting agents (implants and injections). Oral contraceptives are more than 99% effective when properly used, ensure regular menses, and reduce the risks for endometrial and ovarian cancer, ovarian cysts, ectopic pregnancy, and iron deficiency anemia.

Birth control pills are composed of either a combination of an estrogen and progestin or progestin only. Monophasic combination birth control pills contain fixed doses of estrogen and progestin throughout the cycle, whereas biphasic or triphasic agents contain doses of hor-

mones that vary according to different times in the cycle. Although progestin-only pills are somewhat less effective than combination agents and may cause menstrual irregularities, they are nevertheless indicated for breast-feeding women or women for whom estrogen is contraindicated (e.g., hypertension or breast cancer).

Oral contraceptive agents also can be categorized according to their levels of estrogenic, progestational, and androgenic activities. Estrogenic side effects include nausea, mastalgia, headaches, elevated blood pressure, and uterine fibroid enlargement. Side effects of progestational agents are weight gain, diminished libido, headaches, and irregular bleeding. Androgen-associated side effects include hirsutism, acne, and weight gain.

Recently, the long-acting progestational contraceptive agents Norplant (levonorgestrel implants) and Depo-Provera (medroxyprogesterone acetate injections) have gained acceptance because of their ease of use and long-lasting effectiveness. Norplant, a subdermal implant, provides up to 5 years of contraception, and Depo-Provera, an injectable agent, is injected every 3 months. Like the oral progestational agents, the side effects of these long-lasting progestational contraceptives include irregular bleeding and weight gain.

EFFECTS OF HORMONAL CONTRACEPTIVES ON MOOD

New-onset depression occurring in women without an affective history does not appear to be associated with the use of oral contraceptives. However, the use of oral contraceptives may precipitate a recurrence in women with a history of depression or premenstrual dysphoria (Bancroft and Sartorius 1990; Kendler et al. 1988). It is also possible that oral contraceptive use may be associated with subclinical depressive syndromes (Bancroft and Sartorius 1990; Parry and Rush 1979). Especially for women with histories of premenstrual depression, the triphasic oral contraceptive agents may cause negative moods (Bancroft and Rennie 1993; Bancroft et al. 1987). Because oral contraceptives may produce a functional vitamin B_6 deficiency, supplementation with vitamin B_6 (25–50 mg/day) may counteract oral contraceptive–induced dysphoria (Winston 1973). Unrelated to depression, diminished libido has been reported in relation to the use of oral contraceptives (Graham and Sherwin 1992).

Despite reports that mood enhancement may occur in some women who take birth control pills, there are no prospective studies that have shown consistently elevated mood in women with PMDD who are taking oral contraceptives (Graham and Sherwin 1992).

Norplant (levonorgestrel implants) has been reported to cause new-onset depression and panic attacks (Wagner and Berenson 1994), and although Depo-Provera (medroxyprogesterone acetate injections) has been anecdotally associated with depression, this finding has not been supported by the results of a single study (Westhoff et al. 1995).

For women with new-onset mood changes who have recently begun to use hormonal contraception, consideration should be given to switching agents or using another form of birth control.

PSYCHIATRIC DISORDERS IN PREGNANCY

Although pregnancy has in the past been believed to protect against psychiatric illness, a growing body of literature shows that this is not the case. When women with psychiatric disorders plan their pregnancies, there is time to discuss treatment options and to switch, if necessary, to medications that appear safer in pregnancy. For patients who become pregnant while taking psychotropic agents, if clinically feasible, an attempt should be made to discontinue the medication. Because the uteroplacental circulation does not fully form until approximately 2 weeks following conception, the developing embryo most likely will not be exposed to a medication taken during the time between conception and the first missed menstrual period.

For the pregnant patient with psychiatric symptoms, nonpharmacological interventions should be attempted whenever possible. Caffeine, nicotine, and alcohol should be discouraged; environmental stressors should be minimized as much as possible; and the need for adequate nutrition and sleep, and strategies to achieve these, should be emphasized and discussed. Psychotherapy, group support, and family and marital counseling should be initiated when appropriate. However, for women with brittle psychiatric conditions, discontinuation of medication may precipitate a risk of relapse. Although the consequences of relapse vary for different disorders, for many women a relapse may result in alcohol or substance use, impulsive behavior, and inattention to a regimen of good prenatal care.

Before a psychotropic agent is administered to a pregnant patient, risks and benefits to both the mother and the fetus should be evaluated and shared with the patient; her partner, whenever possible; and her obstetrician. Discussions should be documented, and the clinician should assess and note the patient's understanding and capacity to consent to the treatment plan.

TREATMENT OF DEPRESSION DURING PREGNANCY

Approximately 10% of pregnant women experience major or minor depression, a rate similar to that of nonpregnant women. Depression during pregnancy is associated with poor prenatal care, inadequate nutrition, a significantly elevated risk of postpartum depression (O'Hara 1993), suicide, greater incidence of preterm deliveries, and small-for-gestational-age babies (Steer et al. 1992). If the patient has severe symptoms that do not improve with nonpharmacological means and that pose a threat to herself or the pregnancy (i.e., she is suicidal, psychotic, or not gaining weight), it may be necessary to initiate a trial of pharmacotherapy.

For some patients who are likely to relapse if they do not take their medication during the entire pregnancy, it may be possible to avoid medication during the first trimester, which is the time of greatest vulnerability for major congenital malformations of the fetus. When a medication is used during pregnancy, the dosage should be kept at the minimum necessary for symptom control.

To date, a greater body of literature exists on the use of TCAs in pregnancy than any other antidepressants. Available data show no TCA-associated congenital anomalies, although transient perinatal toxicity or withdrawal symptoms have been reported when these agents are used near the time of birth (Altshuler et al. 1996). Symptoms include jitteriness, irritability, lethargy, decreased muscle tone, and anticholinergic effects such as constipation, tachycardia, and urinary retention.

If the decision is made to treat with a TCA, nortriptyline or desipramine is preferable because there is less likelihood of anticholinergic and hypotensive side effects. Antidepressant dosages may need to be adjusted over the course of pregnancy, as blood levels may fall, particularly after the patient begins the third trimester (Altshuler and Hendrick 1996).

There does not appear to be a greater risk of major congenital anomalies associated with the use of fluoxetine in pregnancy (Chambers et al. 1996; Pastuszak et al. 1993). Although a recent report has suggested that fluoxetine use may be associated with a greater likelihood of premature delivery and lower infant birth weight (Chambers et al. 1996), this finding actually may be the result of primary depression rather than fluoxetine use.

To date, no studies exist on the use of sertraline, paroxetine, fluvoxamine, bupropion, trazodone, venlafaxine, or nefazodone in pregnancy. The monoamine oxidase inhibitors (MAOIs) should not be used in pregnant women because of the risk of hypertensive crisis. Additionally, MAOIs interact adversely with tocolytic agents (e.g., terbutaline), which may be necessary to forestall premature labor.

With regard to neurobehavioral sequelae, a recent study suggests that exposure to either TCAs or fluoxetine in utero does not appear to result in significant differences in IQ, temperament, mood, activity, or distractibility in children up to age 86 months (Nulman et al. 1997).

TREATMENT OF BIPOLAR DISORDER DURING PREGNANCY

No studies have prospectively assessed the course of bipolar disorder across pregnancy. The incidence of Ebstein's anomaly, a serious defect in the formation of the tricuspid valve of the heart, is raised from the estimated rate of 1 per 20,000 in the general population to a rate of approximately 1 per 1,000 by first-trimester use of lithium (Altshuler et al. 1996; Cohen et al. 1994). Other potential adverse consequences of lithium use in pregnancy include hypotonia, poor suck reflex, hypoglycemia, cyanosis, neonatal goiter, and diabetes insipidus (Miller 1994a; Woody et al. 1971).

Use of valproic acid and carbamazepine in the first trimester is associated with an increased risk of neural tube defects, including spina bifida (up to 5% for valproic acid and 1% for carbamazepine), and with developmental delay, craniofacial defects, and fingernail hypoplasia.

Thus, for patients with relatively stable bipolar disorder, an attempt should be made to discontinue mood stabilizing medications before conception. Gradual medication taper appears less likely to produce relapse than does abrupt discontinuation (Faedda et al. 1993). However, for women with more brittle illnesses, mood stabilizers may need to be continued during pregnancy. Lithium is preferable to carbamazepine and valproic acid because it is associated with a lower risk of teratogenicity. It should be administered in multiple daily dosing to avoid peak blood levels, and levels should be monitored closely. The lithium dose may require adjustment because blood levels often drop as pregnancy progresses. At week 18, a level II ultrasound may be obtained to assess for potential cardiovascular anomalies. To reduce the risk of lithium toxicity in the mother due to the rapid drop in plasma volume after childbirth, lithium should be tapered by approximately 50% in the 1–2 weeks before the estimated date of delivery.

If carbamazepine or valproic acid must be continued in pregnancy, an amniotic α-fetoprotein analysis at week 16 and an ultrasound at week 18–22 should be obtained to assess for neural tube defects. The risk of neural tube defects may be reduced by dietary folate supplementation. For women who experience an exacerbation or escalation of symptoms, electroconvulsive therapy (ECT) is another option.

TREATMENT OF SCHIZOPHRENIA DURING PREGNANCY

The course of schizophrenia throughout pregnancy is variable and unpredictable. Pregnant schizophrenic women require close management, as psychotic symptoms have been associated with fetal abuse or neonaticide, failure to obtain prenatal care, paranoid delusions regarding necessary medical procedures that therefore prevent cooperation, impaired self-care, inability to recognize labor, and greater risk of adverse pregnancy outcomes (prematurity, low birth weight, low Apgar scores). Patients should be screened for substance abuse, psychosocial stressors, housing and financial resources, and other factors that negatively impact parenting ability.

As with all psychotropic medications, neuroleptic medications should be used in pregnancy only when necessary (e.g., for patients with psychotic symptoms that pose a risk to the patient or fetus). Neuroleptic use on an as-needed basis may help reduce the overall dose exposure of the fetus. However, daily dosing is often necessary for severely ill patients.

The limited data on antipsychotic agents in pregnancy show no increased risk of congenital malformations with the use of high-potency neuroleptics (e.g., haloperidol and trifluoperazine). Low-potency phenothiazines, on the other hand, have been implicated in a higher incidence of nonspecific congenital anomalies and neonatal jaundice. A single case report of clozapine used in pregnancy showed no adverse sequelae (Waldman and Safferman 1993). No information exists to date on risperidone or olanzapine used during pregnancy. For infants exposed to neuroleptics in utero near the time of delivery, a transient syndrome of motor restlessness, tremor, hypertonia, hyperreflexia, irritability, dyskinesia, and poor feeding has been noted (Altshuler et al. 1996).

Agents to treat extrapyramidal side effects should be avoided in pregnancy because they are associated with major and minor congenital anomalies. The anticholinergic agents trihexyphenidyl and benztropine have been associated with minor congenital malformations and anticholinergic symptoms in the newborn, including functional bowel obstruction and urinary retention. Diphenhydramine has been linked with a greater risk of orofacial clefts and with perinatal withdrawal symptoms. Animal studies have reported cardiovascular malformations following in utero exposure to amantadine (Altshuler et al. 1996). Alternative strategies for patients who experience extrapyramidal symptoms include reduction of the neuroleptic dose or switching to a lower-potency agent.

TREATMENT OF ANXIETY DISORDERS DURING PREGNANCY

For women with preexisting panic disorder, symptoms may improve during pregnancy, may continue unchanged, or may worsen. Obsessive-compulsive disorder (OCD) has been reported to worsen during pregnancy (Buttolph and Holland 1990). Nonpharmacological interventions for anxiety disorders include cognitive-behavior therapy, elimination of caffeine and nicotine, reduction of psychosocial stressors, and couples therapy. TCAs and fluoxetine are reasonable treatment options for severe intractable symptoms that do not respond to these measures. Until these medications take effect, small, occasional doses of benzodiazepines may be necessary. Intermittent use of low doses of benzodiazepines during pregnancy, particularly after the first trimester, does not appear to increase the risk of adverse neonatal sequelae. Nevertheless, the use of benzodiazepines in pregnancy is controversial, with some researchers noting a significant risk of oral clefts, particularly with diazepam and alprazolam (Altshuler et al. 1996). Other studies, however, have not found this association. Thus, an attempt should be made to avoid benzodiazepines during gestational weeks 5–9, as this is the period when fetal formation of the palate occurs. Transient perinatal syndromes, including hypotonia, failure to feed, temperature dysregulation, apnea, and low Apgar scores, have been noted with last-trimester use of benzodiazepines. Near term, the use of benzodiazepines should generally be kept at a minimum. Whenever possible, benzodiazepine dose changes should be gradual to avoid precipitating in utero withdrawal.

ELECTROCONVULSIVE THERAPY DURING PREGNANCY

ECT is a reasonable treatment option for pregnant patients with severe mood disorders, as it appears safe and effective and exposes the developing fetus to a minimum of psychoactive medication (Miller 1994b). Special considerations in the administration of ECT to pregnant women include the need for a pelvic examination and uterine tocodynamometry to exclude uterine contractions and elevation of the right hip to ensure adequate placental perfusion. The muscle relaxant succinylcholine and the anticholinergic agent glycopyrrolate appear relatively safe to use in pregnancy (Miller 1994b). Following the procedure, external fetal monitoring should continue for several hours.

SUBSTANCE ABUSE DURING PREGNANCY

In addition to premature labor, abruptio placentae, stillbirth, and other obstetrical complications, teratogenic effects are associated with alcohol and its metabolite acetaldehyde. Infants exposed in utero to alcohol are at risk for fetal alcohol syndrome, a disorder characterized by mental retardation, microcephaly, hypoplastic philtrum and maxilla, thinned upper vermilion, shortened palpebral fissures, and attention deficit with hyperactivity in childhood.

Cocaine use during pregnancy is associated with reduced placental blood flow, intrauterine growth retardation, and genitourinary tract malformations. Preterm labor, abruptio placentae, and other obstetrical complications may occur as a result of cocaine's vasoconstrictive effect. Neonates may experience a withdrawal syndrome lasting several months.

Like cocaine, heroin use during pregnancy is frequently associated with obstetrical complications and a perinatal withdrawal syndrome characterized by irritability, poor feeding, respiratory difficulties, and tremulousness. In utero exposure to opiates also has been linked with a greater risk of sudden infant death syndrome (SIDS).

POSTPARTUM PSYCHIATRIC DISORDERS

For some women, the first six postpartum months represent a time of increased vulnerability for postpartum disorders (Kendell et al. 1987). The burden of postpartum illness is significant because postnatal psychiatric illnesses have a negative impact on family life and infant development and increase the likelihood that the mother will experience further psychiatric illness in the future. Classically, emotional conditions occurring during the postpartum period include postpartum blues, postpartum depression, and postpartum psychosis. More recently, postpartum anxiety disorders have been recognized. Postpartum panic disorder with or without agoraphobia appears to be the most frequently reported anxiety condition (Wisner et al. 1993). Postpartum OCD also recently has been described (Sichel et al. 1993). Although no specific etiology has been found to explain the onset of psychiatric illness during the postpartum period, the causes probably reside in a combination of biological/endocrine and psychosocial factors. Because the literature to date on postpartum anxiety disorders is sparse, the following discussions on postpartum mood disorders include only postpartum mood conditions.

POSTPARTUM BLUES

Up to 85% of mothers experience postpartum blues (O'Hara 1987), a temporary condition beginning in the first 2–4 days following birth, peaking between postpartum days 5–7, and dissipating by the end of the second postpartum week. Symptoms include tearfulness, mood lability, irritability, and anxiety. That this condition is part of the affective spectrum of psychiatric disorders is supported by the findings that risk factors include a history of PMDD and depression (especially during pregnancy), as well as a family history of depression (O'Hara et al. 1991). Because postpartum blues resolve spontaneously, this condition does not require active aggressive treatment. However, because new mothers are generally discharged from the hospital before the onset of postpartum blues, all prospective and new parents should be counseled regarding information about its existence. Therefore, partners, other family members, and health care providers will be prepared to provide needed support and reassurance.

POSTPARTUM DEPRESSION

Although major depression occurring during the postpartum period has a prevalence of approximately 10%, similar to that of the general population, it appears that postpartum women have increased rates of depressive symptomatology. Full-blown postpartum depression and postpartum depressive symptoms that do not meet major depressive criteria often cause great distress within the family and have a negative impact on the emotional and cognitive development of the baby (O'Hara 1987; Stein et al. 1991). Both behavioral and cognitive deficits have been seen in 3- and 4-year-old children of postnatally depressed mothers (Holden 1991). Having a history of major depression increases the risk for postpartum depression to 24% (O'Hara 1993), whereas depression during pregnancy increases the likelihood of postpartum depression to 35% (O'Hara 1993). Women who have had a previous postpartum depression are at 50% risk of postpartum depression (Garvey et al. 1983). Other risk factors for postpartum depression include stressful life events and lack of support from partner, spouse, or others.

Treatment of postpartum depression is multimodal and includes individual and group psychotherapy, psychopharmacology, psychoeducation, and support. A combination of individual psychotherapy, particularly in the form of cognitive therapy, and standard pharmacotherapy to treat depression and secondary anxiety is an effective treatment strategy. Lay advocacy groups (e.g., Postpartum Support International, Depression After De-

livery) offer assistance in the form of group therapy and mutual support. If there are interpersonal difficulties between the patient and her partner, conjoint therapy provides an important adjunct. Assistance with household duties and child care is essential, as this provides the patient with opportunities to reduce sleep deprivation. Educating the patient and the members of her family that postpartum disorders are fairly common and treatable is reassuring and offers everyone the opportunity to talk together about practical strategies to reduce stress in the home and provide assistance with day-to-day household duties. For those patients who have a history of depression, particularly postpartum depression, prophylaxis with antidepressant medication may forestall a recurrence (Wisner and Wheeler 1994).

The issue of whether or not to breast-feed should be discussed thoroughly because nursing may alter the treatment modality or may influence the choice of medication should pharmacotherapy be indicated. For those patients whose depression is characterized by psychosis or suicidality, when maternal or infant health is compromised or when the illness is refractory to psychopharmacological intervention, ECT is often the treatment of choice to hasten rapid improvement. Such cases generally require hospitalization until stabilization is achieved.

POSTPARTUM PSYCHOSIS

The most serious postpartum illness, postpartum psychosis, occurs in 1–2 of every 1,000 births (O'Hara 1987). The condition is characterized by mood lability, agitation, confusion, thought disorganization, hallucinations, and disturbed sleep. Women who have had an episode of postpartum psychosis are at risk for subsequent bipolar disorder, suggesting that postpartum psychosis may be a subcategory of bipolar disorder. Having a history of bipolar disorder confers a 35% risk of developing postpartum psychosis (Rohde and Marneros 1992). A history of postpartum psychosis confers a relapse risk of 20%–33% (Davidson and Robertson 1985; Kendell et al. 1987; Sichel 1992). Having both bipolar disorder and a prior postpartum psychotic episode increases the risk of a subsequent postpartum psychosis to 50% (Kendell et al. 1987). Primiparity and a family history of bipolar disorder also appears to heighten the risk for postpartum psychosis (O'Hara 1987).

Because postpartum psychosis carries with it the risk of suicide, infant neglect, or infanticide (1 in 50,000) (Rohde and Marneros 1993), patients are generally hospitalized. The initial workup includes a medical assessment to rule out organic etiologies such as postpartum thyroiditis,

Sheehan's syndrome, pregnancy-related autoimmune disorders, human immunodeficiency virus (HIV)–related infection, intoxication/withdrawal states, or an intracranial mass. Acute pharmacological treatment includes the use of a mood stabilizer, a neuroleptic for psychosis, and a benzodiazepine for agitation. Antidepressants should be administered with great caution because these may provoke rapid cycling (Altshuler et al. 1995a; Sichel 1992). Maintenance treatment for the patient whose postpartum psychosis was preceded by chronic recurrent affective illness generally involves long-term treatment with a mood stabilizer. For those patients without a psychiatric history other than a single episode of postpartum psychosis, medications are often tapered and discontinued by 1 year of treatment. It is prudent for patients with a history of postpartum psychosis who subsequently become pregnant to be placed on a prophylactic mood stabilizer either during the third trimester or at delivery. Because women with bipolar disorder are at significant risk for postpartum psychosis, a mood stabilizer is best administered during the last trimester or immediately upon delivery (Stewart et al. 1991). Women whose first psychotic episode occurs in the postpartum period have a 60% risk of recurrent affective illness (Davidson and Robertson 1985; Videbech and Gouliaev 1995) and therefore should be followed over the course of several years.

BREAST-FEEDING AND PSYCHOTROPIC MEDICATIONS

Approximately one-half of new mothers breast-feed, and of these, roughly 28,000 are estimated to have postpartum depression (Stowe 1996). Although it is accepted that breast-feeding enhances maternal-infant bonding and is also an excellent source of nutrition for infants during the first 6 months of life, for women who require psychotropic treatment for postpartum disorders, the decision of whether to forgo breast-feeding or to proceed despite nursing is a difficult one.

The data regarding the safety of the use of psychotropic medications by breast-feeding mothers are limited to case reports and small naturalistic studies. Some women are reluctant to risk any possible exposure of their babies to medications in breast milk and therefore elect to bottle-feed. Nevertheless, for other nursing mothers, the desire to breast-feed is so strong that they would prefer to forgo treatment rather than bottle-feed. For these women, treatment of a postpartum disorder while continuing to breast-feed may be carried out after discussing the available data on breast-feeding and psychotropic medication use and thoroughly reviewing risks and benefits.

Guidelines for using psychotropic medication in breast-feeding mothers include apprising the infant's pediatrician of the need to monitor the infant carefully for potential adverse effects. The infant's baseline of behavior and sleep and feeding patterns should be assessed before the nursing mother uses the medication. Medication exposure should be minimized by prescribing the lowest dosage of medication that achieves remission of psychiatric symptoms. Short-acting rather than long-acting medications are preferable, and supplementation of breast milk with formula reduces the infant's exposure to the drug. Noting the time of dose administration and measuring breast milk concentrations of medication over a 24-hour period may reveal those times in the day when milk drug concentrations peak and breast-feeding is best avoided.

Once steady state has been reached in the maternal serum, infant serum should be assayed to the lowest limits of sensitivity to determine the concentration of drug in the mother as well as active metabolites. In cases where infant drug levels are nondetectable and the infant is free of adverse effects, breast-feeding may be continued. Nevertheless, since the clinical significance of any exposure to the baby of even small (and nondetectable) doses of psychotropic agents is unknown, the baby's clinical status should be continually monitored.

Most medications, including TCAs, benzodiazepines, and neuroleptics, have been classified by the American Academy of Pediatrics as "drugs whose effect on nursing infants is unknown but may be of concern" (American Academy of Pediatrics, Committee on Drugs 1994). Data on the use of selective serotonin reuptake inhibitors (SSRIs) while nursing is conflicting. Although some reports suggest that fluoxetine is safe during breast-feeding, a single case report of fluoxetine and norfluoxetine accumulation in an infant's serum and associated colic has resulted in revision of U.S. Food and Drug Administration (FDA) labeling to recommend against the use of this drug in breast-feeding women (Lester et al. 1993). A single study of the use of sertraline while breast-feeding is reassuring, as sertraline levels were nondetectable (Altshuler et al. 1995b). MAOIs are best avoided because they may cause hypertension in the infant.

Lithium is contraindicated by the Academy's Committee on Drugs because adverse effects have been noted in breast-fed infants. Although valproic acid and carbamazepine are considered by the committee to be compatible with breast-feeding, there are two reported cases of hepatic dysfunction in infants exposed to carbamazepine via breast milk (Frey et al. 1990; Merlob et al. 1992), and although valproic acid accumulates in breast milk to a lesser extent than carbamazepine (von Unruh et al. 1984), it should be used with caution in breast-feeding mothers because this medication has been associated with infant hepatotoxicity.

ELECTIVE ABORTION

Since the Supreme Court decision of *Roe v. Wade* in 1973, first-trimester abortions have been a woman's legal right. In the United States, most women who elect to terminate a pregnancy by abortion are younger than age 25, single, and have no children. Approximately 1.5 million abortions are performed in the United States each year (Frye et al. 1994).

Most abortions are performed by dilation and evacuation of uterine contents by means of vacuum aspiration or curettage and are associated with a mortality rate of approximately .4 per 100,000 procedures. This rate is 25 times lower than the rate associated with carrying a pregnancy to term.

Reasons for termination of pregnancy include poor partner support, inability to provide financial support for a child, and inability or lack of desire to bear responsibility for a child. A woman may be reluctant to carry the pregnancy to term if a fetal congenital anomaly has been diagnosed or if the pregnancy resulted from rape or incest.

For most women, abortion is followed by feelings of relief. However, adverse psychological sequelae may result if there was ambivalence about the decision, if the abortion was performed beyond the first trimester, or if there is a psychiatric history (Dagg 1991; Zolese and Blacker 1992). Thus, abortion counseling should be offered before the procedure. Counseling provides an opportunity for a woman and her partner to obtain information regarding the likelihood of pain, discomfort, or other adverse sequelae following the abortion and to learn effective contraceptive methods to prevent future unwanted pregnancies. For women whose pregnancy is the result of a rape, counseling is an important part of the recovery from the trauma of the assault.

For a woman undergoing an abortion because of a fetal diagnosis of congenital deformity or impending fetal demise, feelings may include mourning for the loss of a wished-for baby and self-blame about having produced a deformed fetus. She may experience anxiety and ambivalence about becoming pregnant in the future and will benefit from sensitive education and support. Whenever possible, the woman's partner should be included in therapy, particularly because he also may be grieving.

When a chronically mentally ill woman seeks an abortion, a careful psychiatric evaluation should be undertaken to assess delusions and paranoid feelings that may be influencing her decision. Her ability to understand her condition and the options available to her should be assessed. Before the pregnancy is terminated, the patient's psychiatric condition should be stabilized.

PSYCHOLOGICAL ASPECTS OF INFERTILITY

Ten to 15% of all couples in the United States have difficulties in achieving pregnancy; when pregnancy does not occur following 1 year of unprotected intercourse, the couple is said to be infertile (LaPane et al. 1995). Infertility may be caused by ovulatory dysfunction, uterine or tubal disease, cervical problems, infectious disease, and immunological factors. Male factors are believed to underlie infertility in 40%–60% of cases (Jones and Toner 1993; McCartney and Downey 1993). With the exception of anorexia nervosa, psychiatric syndromes are not believed to contribute significantly to infertility. However, infertility may produce significant psychiatric and psychological symptoms, including a loss of self-esteem (Facchinetti et al. 1992).

Some women may feel a loss of femininity. They tend to be more emotionally affected than their male partners. However, some men may feel inhibited by the demands to perform sexually at scheduled times. Both members of the couple may suffer from diminished libido and may experience a loss of sexuality. Often there is a sense of isolation from friends whose social activities involve children. The financial burden of both evaluation and treatment for infertility is an additional significant source of stress and may mean alterations in major decisions such as the purchase of a home or car or vacations.

The evaluation of infertility involves assessment of both members of the couple and includes screening for sexually transmitted diseases and normal endocrine functioning. The infertility workup includes assessment of ovulation, quantity and quality of sperm, visualization of the woman's anatomy, and determination of patency of ductile systems in the woman and/or man. Tests are often repeated at different intervals over a single menstrual cycle and at subsequent menstrual cycles. The assessment invariably requires substantial reorganization of the day-to-day lives of both partners, with office visits dictated by responses to treatment, dates of ovulation, and physicians' schedules.

TREATMENT OF INFERTILITY AND PSYCHOLOGICAL IMPLICATIONS

The choice of treatment depends on the etiology of infertility. If mechanical blockage in the female reproductive tract is identified, it can be corrected with surgery or at the time of the laparoscopy. For endometriosis, GnRH agonists such as leuprolide (Lupron) are helpful. If ovulatory dysfunction is identified as etiological, clomiphene citrate can be used to induce ovulation. If clomiphene citrate is unsuccessful, human menopausal gonadotropins (Pergonal [FSH and luteinizing hormone (LH)] or Metrodin [FSH]) are the next step. Unlike clomiphene citrate, which is orally administered, the human menopausal gonadotropins are administered by daily injections. These require daily visits to the physician unless the woman or her partner feel comfortable administering the injections. Side effects may include fatigue, nausea, headache, diarrhea, and weight gain. Clomiphene citrate is associated with a 5% incidence of multiple gestation. This incidence rises to 20% with human menopausal gonadotropins.

If these treatments do not enable the couple to achieve pregnancy, they may opt for assisted reproductive technology, such as gamete intrafallopian transfer (GIFT) or zygote intrafallopian transfer (ZIFT). In the former method, oocytes and sperm are combined in vitro and immediately deposited in the woman's fallopian tubes; in the latter, eggs are fertilized in vitro and the resultant zygotes are placed in the fallopian tubes. In the case of in vitro fertilization (IVF), fertilized embryos are placed directly into the uterus. Serial ultrasounds are necessary to monitor ovulation and posttransfer embryological development and to assess for the development of ovarian hyperstimulation. These procedures are expensive and have limited success rates: IVF has a 14% success rate, GIFT a 23% rate, and ZIFT a 15% rate (McCartney and Downey 1993). The risk of multiple gestation is approximately 25%, and there is a 6% chance of severe ovarian hyperstimulation syndrome, a potentially life-threatening complication.

When infertility results from an untreatable male factor, artificial insemination by a donor (AID), also called therapeutic donor insemination (TDI), may be attempted. Intracytoplasmic sperm injection (ICSI) followed by artificial insemination is an alternative in cases of male-factor infertility. For a woman who is unable to ovulate, egg donation is an option. Medications are administered to both the donor and the infertile woman in order to synchronize cycles. The donor eggs are then fertilized with sperm through the procedures of IVF or GIFT and transferred to the infertile woman, who then carries the pregnancy. In the case of a woman who is able to ovulate but cannot carry the pregnancy, a fertilized egg may be inseminated in a surrogate mother, who then will carry the pregnancy.

Thus, infertility treatment is an arduous and demanding process. The medical interventions in the couple's sexual activities often have a negative impact on intimacy and spontaneity, and the daily monitoring of reproductive-related bodily functions can distract from other aspects of their lives. The relatively modest success rates and the high cost of the procedures add to the stress of treatment. A woman who postponed pregnancy for career concerns may experience significant guilt and self-blame. Complicating the situation, the medications used (clomiphene citrate, human menopausal gonadotropins, GnRH agonists) may produce negative mood changes, anxiety, and insomnia, in addition to myriad physical side effects. Infertility is not associated with the development of major depressive disorder (Downey and McKinney 1992), but it does produce negative mood changes and may exacerbate preexisting psychiatric disorders. Thus, psychiatric evaluation and treatment may be indicated. A psychiatrist additionally can play a role in exploring alternative options, including adoption. The psychiatrist should encourage both members of the couple to participate in therapy, either jointly or individually. A referral to RESOLVE, the national self-help organization for infertile couples that sponsors groups and workshops, can help the couple feel less isolated and overwhelmed.

PERIMENOPAUSE AND MENOPAUSE

Menopause refers to the cessation of ovulation and menstrual cycling and usually occurs between ages 44 and 55 (average age, 51.4 years). *Perimenopause* and *climacteric* are interchangeable terms that describe the years before menopause when ovarian function begins to decline.

As ovarian production of estrogen declines, the pituitary hormones LH and FSH rise. An elevated serum FSH level, especially if obtained shortly after the onset of menses (when FSH levels should be at their nadir), suggests a woman is perimenopausal. Elevated FSH levels (i.e., 40 mU/mL or above, obtained later in the cycle) can be misleading because this hormone may rise into the menopausal range in premenopausal women, particularly at midcycle. Levels of estradiol, the biologically active form of estrogen, remain under 25 pg/mL following menopause.

Physiological changes resulting from low estrogen levels begin to manifest during the perimenopausal years and include hot flushes and cold sweats. These symptoms occur in 80% of perimenopausal women and may persist for years after the last menstrual period. Hot flushes are sensations of heat that develop in the face and body and last up to several minutes; they often are associated with perspiration, breathlessness, dizziness, and tachycardia. These symptoms may be confused with a panic attack, particularly because they occur unexpectedly and may be associated with some anxiety. Night sweats may produce sleep deprivation, which subsequently may lead to decreased concentration, fatigue, and irritability. Other signs of declining ovarian estrogen production include atrophy of the urogenital tract lining, sometimes leading to infection, urinary frequency and urgency, and occasional stress incontinence. Women may experience painful intercourse and reduced libido. Particularly serious long-term consequences of low estrogen levels are osteoporosis and cardiovascular disease.

Large epidemiological studies have found that most women are not at greater risk for depression during their perimenopausal years compared with other times in their lives (Kaufert et al. 1992; Matthews et al. 1990), thus discrediting the term *involutional melancholia* coined by Kraepelin in 1890 to describe a depressive syndrome occurring in association with menopause.

It appears that there are subgroups of women whose risk for depressive mood changes rises at perimenopause. These include women with histories of previous reproductive-related mood syndromes (e.g., oral contraceptive–related mood changes, premenstrual dysphoria, and postpartum depression) (Stewart and Boydell 1993) and women who experience severe vasomotor symptoms (hot flushes, night sweats). With the lessening of physical symptoms, mood symptoms tend to resolve. Other risk factors for depressive symptoms at menopause include being divorced, widowed, or separated; having significant caregiving responsibilities; and experiencing a chronic illness (Avis and McKinlay 1991, 1995).

EVALUATION AND TREATMENT OF DEPRESSION IN PERIMENOPAUSAL AND MENOPAUSAL WOMEN

The evaluation of depression in a middle-aged woman should include a descriptive assessment of menstrual status. Thus, the evaluation should document menstrual cycle patterns, vasomotor symptoms, and sexual function. The laboratory workup should include serum FSH and a thyroid panel. A full physical examination will exclude other medical disorders (e.g., autoimmune disorders, endocrine disorders, heart disease, cancer) that may produce depressive symptoms.

For perimenopausal women with major depression, standard antidepressant treatment, including psychotherapy and/or antidepressants is essential. If vasomotor symptoms also are present, estrogen replacement effectively will treat this syndrome and reduce sleep disturbance due to middle-of-the-night awakening secondary to the physical symptoms of endogenous estrogen decline. For perimenopausal women with severe hot flushes or night sweats

who report subclinical depression and lethargy, institution of hormone replacement therapy may relieve the psychological symptoms as the vasomotor symptoms become less distressing. As women experience relief from vasomotor symptoms (usually within 2 weeks of beginning hormone replacement), depressive symptoms also should improve.

For most women, hormone replacement involves the administration of both estrogen and progestin. The purpose of the progestin is to counteract the endometrial proliferation that occurs with estrogen and which increases the risk of endometrial cancer. Women who have had a hysterectomy do not require progestin supplementation. The progestin is taken either on a daily basis with the estrogen (continuous regimen) or at a higher dose only during 12–14 days of each month (cyclic regimen). The cyclic regimen produces vaginal bleeding following withdrawal of the progestin. No monthly bleeding occurs with the continuous regimen, but irregular spotting may occur that requires endometrial biopsy to rule out hyperplasia or malignancy.

Estrogen and progesterone supplementation is available in a variety of preparations, including conjugated equine estrogen (Premarin) .625–1.25 mg and medroxyprogesterone acetate (Provera) 2.5–10 mg. Alternative preparations include formulations in which a small amount of testosterone supplementation is added to the estrogen (e.g., Estratest) and may be helpful for women who have experienced diminished libido.

In addition to providing relief of vasomotor symptoms, estrogen replacement helps protect against osteoporotic bony changes and cardiovascular disease. Estrogen has been reported to produce a mood-elevating effect, particularly in surgically menopausal women (Sherwin 1988). However, estrogen alone is not currently accepted as effective monotherapy for clinical depression. Thus, if a patient continues to feel depressed after resolution of the vasomotor symptoms, standard psychiatric treatment should be initiated. Psychosocial factors that may contribute to depressed mood also should be addressed, including caring for aging parents, new-onset health problems in herself or her spouse, financial difficulties, and changes in sexuality of the patient or her partner.

GENDER ISSUES IN THE TREATMENT OF MAJOR MENTAL ILLNESS

SCHIZOPHRENIA IN WOMEN

Although the incidence of schizophrenia does not differ between the sexes, the onset of the disorder tends to occur approximately 5 years later in women (ages 20–29 years in women versus 15–24 years in men). Furthermore, approximately 15% of schizophrenic women develop new-onset symptoms of schizophrenia in their mid- to late 40s (Goldstein and Link 1988).

Women are less likely to have a poor premorbid history and tend to display more affective and positive symptoms and fewer negative symptoms than do men. Neuroanatomical studies suggest that structural brain abnormalities are more likely to be found in men than in women. More relatives of schizophrenic women than relatives of schizophrenic men are likely to develop the disorder. This suggests that heredity may be more important for schizophrenic women but that environment may play a relatively greater role for schizophrenic men.

Among gender-specific differences in the treatment of schizophrenia, women appear to be more responsive to treatment and to require lower doses of medication than do men. Thus, it has been suggested that estrogen, which in animals has antidopaminergic effects (Bedard et al. 1983), may have a protective effect against schizophrenia (Szymanski et al. 1995). This finding is also supported by observations that schizophrenia is exacerbated during low-estrogen phases of the menstrual cycle (Seeman and Lang 1990; Szymanski et al. 1995) and in perimenopausal years (Seeman 1986).

Hyperprolactinemia induced by neuroleptics frequently causes menstrual irregularities and amenorrhea. For nonpregnant amenorrheic women of childbearing age, nonneuroleptic-induced causes of menstrual cycle disturbances include hypothyroidism, stress, weight loss, opiate use, oral contraceptives, and primary hyperprolactinemia. However, the most frequent cause of menstrual irregularity (and galactorrhea) in schizophrenic women is neuroleptic-induced hyperprolactinemia with secondary hypoestroginemia. Amenorrhea tends to occur with prolactin levels greater than 60 ng/mL (normal prolactin levels = 5–25 ng/mL). If prolactin levels exceed 100 ng/mL, an endocrine consultation should be requested to assess the possibility of a pituitary adenoma.

For neuroleptic-induced hyperprolactinemia, consideration should be given to reducing the dose of medication. If the administered dose is necessary to control psychotic symptoms, the dopamine agonist bromocriptine, 2.5–7.5 mg bid, may be given. Although bromocriptine is a dopamine agonist, the low doses needed to treat hyperprolactinemia do not generally cause psychotic effects. The troublesome side effect of severe nausea with oral bromocriptine may be counteracted by taking the drug with food. A third approach is the use of an oral contraceptive, which has the triple effects of restoring menstrual cycle regularity, providing contraception, and protecting against the long-term hypoestrogenemic effects of osteoporosis and heart disease. Of note, despite the frequency of anovulatory cycles in neuroleptic-treated schizophrenic women, schizophrenic women nevertheless may become pregnant. Schizophrenic women should therefore be counseled about birth control and provided with behavioral approaches to avoid unwanted sexual advances.

DEPRESSION IN WOMEN

Depression is more prevalent in women than in men by a factor of 1.7 to 2, respectively (Kessler et al. 1993, 1994; Weissman et al. 1991). Dysthymia is twice as prevalent in women than in men (Weissman et al. 1984). Seasonal affective disorder is also more frequent in women than men (Rosenthal et al. 1992). It appears that women with a history of one or more reproductive-related depressive conditions (e.g., oral contraceptive–induced depression, postpartum depression, PMDD, perimenopausal depression) are at increased risk for other reproductive-related depressive episodes.

Women of childbearing age who are planning to become pregnant and are likely to need continued psychotropic treatment during pregnancy and the postpartum period are best placed on a medication whose safety is such that it will not be necessary to alter medications should pregnancy occur. For those women whose depressive condition occurs throughout the month but with premenstrual exacerbation, charting of symptoms is often a useful way to document those days when an increase in antidepressant dose or addition of another agent may protect against decompensation during the premenstrual days. Since women with histories of depression are at increased risk for postpartum depression, consideration should be given to preventing an episode of depression in the postpartum period. Even for women who are asymptomatic during pregnancy, a history of recurrent major depression (particularly occurring in prior postpartum intervals) often calls for initiation of prophylactic antidepressant treatment in late pregnancy or immediately upon delivery.

BIPOLAR DISORDER IN WOMEN

Bipolar disorder is equally prevalent in men and women. However, bipolar women experience more depressions and fewer manic episodes than bipolar men do, and mixed states are more common in women than men. Rapid cycling is three times as common in women than men. It has been suggested that since bipolar women tend to experience recurrent depressions, they are often treated with antidepressants, and this treatment may precipitate rapid cycling. Additionally, thyroid dysfunction is more common in women and may precipitate rapid cycling.

For some bipolar women, premenstrual relapse or exacerbation of symptoms occurs. Some reports have indicated that lithium levels fluctuate across the menstrual cycle (Hendrick et al. 1996). If symptoms change over the course of the menstrual cycle, serum lithium levels may be taken during symptomatic days, and adjustments in lithium dosage may be made accordingly.

Because the risk for hypothyroidism is greater for women than for men, particularly in the over-40 age group, women taking lithium should be monitored for thyroid dysfunction at least every 6 months. Carbamazepine induces hormone clearance and metabolism, thereby diminishing oral contraceptive efficacy. In addition, women who take carbamazepine and who receive hormone replacement therapy following menopause may require higher doses of estrogen to treat menopause-related vasomotor symptoms effectively.

ANXIETY DISORDERS IN WOMEN

Women are particularly prone to anxiety disorders, and for those women who suffer from anxiety disorders, comorbid depression is common. Women are twice as likely as men to use anxiolytic medication, and in large part, women do so because of the predominance of anxiety disorders in women (Baum et al. 1984). For example, women are twice as likely as men to have posttraumatic stress disorder and are two to three times as likely to experience panic disorder with agoraphobia (Bourdon et al. 1988; Robins et al. 1984; Schneier et al. 1992). Panic disorder with agoraphobia is more common in alcoholic women than alcoholic men (Task Force on Panic Anxiety and Its Treatments 1993). Although OCD prevalence rates are roughly equal between the sexes, the onset of the illness tends to be earlier in women than men (age 25 years in women versus age 20 years in men) (Flament and Rapoport 1984). The evaluation for anxiety should rule out medical conditions that mimic anxiety symptoms (e.g., cardiovascular disease, thyroid disorders, lupus, and iron deficiency anemia). Caffeine and nicotine use also causes anxiety symptoms in some patients. Medications such as nonsteroidal anti-inflammatory agents, decongestants, steroids, and appetite suppressants may precipitate anxiety attacks. In some perimenopausal women, vasomotor symptoms may be mistaken for panic attacks.

ALCOHOL ABUSE AND SUBSTANCE ABUSE IN WOMEN

Although alcohol abuse is at least twice as common in men than in women (Blume 1994), for an equal amount of alcohol per unit of body weight, women tend to become more intoxicated than men. The increased susceptibility to alcohol abuse in women versus men may be explained because in women, alcohol dehydrogenase is less active and also because women have less body water (and more body fat) than men have. Complications from alcohol abuse, such as peptic ulcer, liver disease, anemia, and cerebral atrophy, develop more quickly in women, and women are more likely to die from alcoholism than are men. Risk factors for alcoholism in women include a history of sexual abuse, substance abuse, adult antisocial personality disorder, and depression.

Although hallucinogen and opiate abuse predominates in men, prevalence rates for cocaine and amphetamine abuse are equal. Women often use stimulants for weight control. Women substance abusers are more likely to experience comorbid psychiatric disorders. Because many women drink to self-medicate premenstrual tension, it is important to assess for premenstrual symptoms in alcohol and drug use (Hendrick et al. 1996). Risk factors for drug abuse in women include a family history of substance abuse, antisocial personality disorder, depression, and being in a relationship with a drug-abusing or dependent partner.

Treatment includes referral to self-help groups such as Alcoholics Anonymous, Cocaine Anonymous, and the all-women support group Women for Sobriety. Family and marital conflicts should be evaluated and addressed carefully, since the likelihood of a woman remaining sober is often dependent on the sobriety of significant others.

FEMALE-SPECIFIC CANCERS

Both breast cancer and gynecological cancers tend to be particularly stressful to women because they affect the organs of reproduction, sexuality, and femininity. Treatment strategies include surgery, radiation therapy, and chemotherapy. Sexual problems may emerge following treatment because of the direct physical effects of these modalities, fears of recurring cancer, or a decreased sense of femininity. Partners' attitudes are particularly important because women with these types of cancer need support and encouragement.

A psychiatric consultation may be requested for women undergoing treatment for breast or gynecological cancer. For women in whom organic etiologies for mood disorders have been excluded, psychotherapy is a useful modality, particularly supportive or cognitive approaches to improve a sense of control. Standard antidepressant medications may be useful to increase appetite and sleep. Additionally, TCAs and SSRIs may be useful to reduce pain. Since tamoxifen may reduce serum TCAs (Jefferson 1995), for antidepressant-treated cancer patients who do not appear to be responding as well as expected, it is prudent to assess serum levels of parent and metabolite compounds and to compare these levels with pre-tamoxifen-treated levels. If antidepressant medication is necessary for a tamoxifen-treated cancer patient, consideration should be given to increasing the dose of antidepressant to achieve clinical efficacy.

Many women with breast or gynecological cancer experience anxiety in response to the stress of difficult or uncomfortable treatment regimens and in response to a sense of loss of control with regard to exogenous stressors and toll of the illness. Guided imagery and progressive relaxation techniques, in conjunction with the use of low doses of anxiolytic medication, may be helpful in the acute phase of treatment. For sleep difficulties, reviewing the basic techniques of sleep hygiene are helpful; if insomnia persists, short-acting benzodiazepines or low-dose trazodone also may be useful. Women with cancer who have a history of alcohol or substance abuse or dependence are at risk for a recurrence. Encouraging these women to participate in lay advocacy groups (e.g., Alcoholics Anonymous or Narcotics Anonymous) and providing them with the opportunity to discuss their fear, anger, and sadness in individual therapy are particularly important. Women with breast or gynecological cancer sometimes experience a change in the quality of their sexual or marital relationships. For women whose surgery was extensive, their sense of sexuality and femininity may be called into question. Induced menopause secondary to radical hysterectomy or vasomotor symptoms due to tamoxifen may cause additional discomfort and may cause further sleep disruptions, with depression, irritability, and anxiety. Frequently, the partner also experiences a sense of loss and fear and may have difficulty viewing surgical or radiation scars. Conjoint education and counseling are often helpful.

Group support, in the form of advocacy groups such as Reach to Recovery or groups sponsored by the American Cancer Society, is helpful because it offers group members the opportunity to share common concerns, practical advice, and appreciation of the implications of having a diagnosis of cancer. Participation in support groups has been reported to improve 10-year survival rates for women with metastatic breast cancer (Spiegel et al. 1989).

CONCLUSIONS

The comprehensive assessment and management of psychiatric disorders in women should include an evaluation of those aspects of the patients' conditions that are female specific. These gender-specific etiological aspects are undoubtedly the result of genetic differences, endocrinological differences, and psychosocial stressors that tend to affect women more than men. By maintaining an awareness of the vulnerable times in a woman's life when she is likely to experience a psychiatric illness, the mental health clinician can proactively provide treatment and therefore may prevent a recurrence or relapse.

REFERENCES

Altshuler LL, Hendrick V: Pregnancy and psychotropic medication: changes in blood levels. J Clin Psychopharmacol 16:78–80, 1996

Altshuler LL, Post RM, Leverich GS, et al: Antidepressant-induced mania and cycle acceleration: a controversy revisited. Am J Psychiatry 152:1124–1129, 1995a

Altshuler LL, Burt VK, McMullen M, et al: Breastfeeding and sertraline: a 24-hour analysis. J Clin Psychiatry 56: 243–245, 1995b

Altshuler LL, Hendrick V, Parry B: Pharmacologic management of premenstrual disorder. Harv Rev Psychiatry 2:223–245, 1995c

Altshuler LL, Cohen L, Szuba MP, et al: Pharmacologic management of psychiatric illness in pregnancy: dilemmas and guidelines. Am J Psychiatry 153:592–606, 1996

American Academy of Pediatrics, Committee on Drugs: Transfer of drugs and other chemicals into human milk. Pediatrics 93:137–251, 1994

American Psychiatric Association: Diagnostic and Statistical Manual of Mental Disorders, 4th Edition. Washington, DC, American Psychiatric Association, 1994

Avis NE, McKinlay SM: A longitudinal analysis of women's attitudes towards menopause: results from the Massachusetts Women's Health Study. Maturitas 13:65–79, 1991

Avis NE, McKinlay SM: The Massachusetts Women's Health Study: an epidemiologic investigation of the menopause. J Am Med Womens Assoc 50:45–49, 1995

Bancroft J, Rennie D: The impact of oral contraceptives on the experience of perimenstrual mood, clumsiness, food craving and other symptoms. J Psychosom Res 37:195–202, 1993

Bancroft J, Sartorius N: The effects of oral contraceptives on well-being and sexuality. Oxford Review of Reproductive Biology 12:57–92, 1990

Bancroft J, Sanders D, Warner P, et al: The effects of oral contraceptives on mood and sexuality: a comparison of triphasic and combined preparations. J Psychosom Obstet Gynaecol 7:1–8, 1987

Baum C, Kennedy DL, Forbes MB, et al: Drug use in the United States in 1981. JAMA 251:1293–1297, 1984

Bedard P, Boucher R, DiPolo T, et al: Biphasic effect of estradiol and domperidone on lingual dyskinesia in monkeys. Exp Neurol 82:172–182, 1983

Blume SB: Gender differences in alcohol-related disorders. Harv Rev Psychiatry 2:7–14, 1994

Bourdon KH, Boyd JH, Rase DS, et al: Gender differences phobias: results of the ECA community survey. J Anxiety Disord 2:227–241, 1988

Buttolph ML, Holland DA: Obsessive-compulsive disorders in pregnancy and childbirth, in Obsessive Compulsive Disorders: Theory and Management. Edited by Jenike MA, Baier L, Minichiello WE. Chicago, Year Book Medical, 1990, pp 89–95

Chambers CD, Johnson KA, Dick LM, et al: Birth outcomes in pregnant women taking fluoxetine. N Engl J Med 155:1010–1015, 1996

Cohen LS, Friedman JM, Jefferson JW, et al: A re-evaluation of risk of in utero exposure to lithium. JAMA 271:146–150, 1994

Dagg PKB: The psychological sequelae of therapeutic abortion—denied and completed. Am J Psychiatry 148:578–585, 1991

Davidson J, Robertson E: A follow-up study of postpartum illness, 1946–1978. Acta Psychiatr Scand 71:451–457, 1985

Downey J, McKinney M: The psychiatric status of women presenting for infertility evaluation. Am J Orthopsychiatry 62:196–205, 1992

Facchinetti F, Demyttenaere K, Fioroni L, et al: Psychosomatic disorders related to gynecology. Psychother Psychosom 58:137–154, 1992

Faedda GL, Tondo L, Baldessarini RJ, et al: Outcome after rapid versus gradual discontinuation of lithium treatment in bipolar disorders. Arch Gen Psychiatry 50:448–455, 1993

Flament MF, Rapoport JL: Childhood obsessive-compulsive disorder, in New Findings in Obsessive-Compulsive Disorder. Edited by Insel TR. Washington, DC, American Psychiatric Press, 1984, pp 23–43

Freeman W, Purdy RH, Coutifaris C, et al: Anxiolytic metabolites of progesterone: correlation with mood and performance measures following oral progesterone administration to healthy female volunteers. Clinical Neuroendocrinology 58:478–484, 1993

Frey B, Schubiger G, Musy JP: Transient cholestatic hepatitis in a neonate associated with carbamazepine exposure during pregnancy and breastfeeding. Eur J Pediatr 150:136–138, 1990

Frye AA, Atrash HK, Lawson HW, et al: Induced abortion in the United States: a 1994 update. J Am Med Womens Assoc 49:131–136, 1994

Garvey MJ, Tuason VB, Lumry AE, et al: Occurrence of depression in the postpartum state. J Affect Disord 5:97–101, 1983

Goldstein JM, Link BG: Gender and the expression of schizophrenia. J Psychiatr Res 22:141–155, 1988

Graham CA, Sherwin BB: A prospective treatment study of premenstrual symptoms using a triphasic oral contraceptive. J Psychosom Res 36:257–266, 1992

Hendrick V, Altshuler LL, Burt VK: Course of psychiatric disorders across the menstrual cycle. Harv Rev Psychiatry 4:200–207, 1996

Holden JM: Postnatal depression: its nature, effects, and identification using the Edinburgh Postnatal Depression Scale. Birth 18:211–221, 1991

Jefferson JW: Tamoxifen-associated reduction in tricyclic antidepressant levels in blood. J Clin Psychopharmacol 15:223–224, 1995

Jones HW, Toner JP: The infertile couple. N Engl J Med 23:1710–1715, 1993

Kaufert PA, Gilbert P, Tate R: The Manitoba Project: a reexamination of the link between menopause and depression. Maturitas 14:143–155, 1992

Kendell RE, Chalmers JC, Platz C: Epidemiology of puerperal psychoses. Br J Psychiatry 150:662–673, 1987

Kendler KS, Martin NS, Heath AC, et al: A twin study of the psychiatric side effects of oral contraceptives. J Nerv Ment Dis 176:153–160, 1988

Kessler RC, McGonagle KA, Swartz M, et al: Sex and depression in the National Comorbidity Survey, I: lifetime prevalence, chronicity, and recurrence. J Affect Disord 19:85–96, 1993

Kessler RC, McGonagle KA, Zhao S, et al: Lifetime and 12-month prevalence of DSM-III-R psychiatric disorders in the United States: results from the National Comorbidity Survey. Arch Gen Psychiatry 51:8–19, 1994

Kimmel S, Gonsalves L, Youngs D, et al: Fluctuating levels of antidepressants. J Psychosom Obstet Gynaecol 2:109–115, 1992

LaPane KL, Zierler S, Lasater TM, et al: Is a history of depressive symptoms associated with an increased risk of infertility in women? Psychosom Med 57:509–513, 1995

Lester BM, Cucca J, Andreozzi BA, et al: Possible association between fluoxetine hydrochloride and colic in an infant. J Am Acad Child Adolesc Psychiatry 32:1253–1255, 1993

Matthews KA, Wing RA, Kuller LH: Influences of natural menopause on psychological characteristics and symptoms of middle-aged healthy women. J Consult Clin Psychol 58:345–351, 1990

McCartney CF, Downey J: New reproductive technologies, in Medical Psychiatric Practice. Edited by Stoudemire A, Fogel PS. Washington, DC, American Psychiatric Press, 1993, p 302

McGlone J: Sex differences in human brain asymmetry: a critical survey. Behav Brain Sci 3:215–263, 1980

Merlob P, Mor N, Litwin A: Transient hepatic dysfunction in an infant of an epileptic mother treated with carbamazepine during pregnancy and breastfeeding. Ann Pharmacother 26:1563–1565, 1992

Miller LJ: Psychiatric medication during pregnancy: understanding and minimizing risks. Psychiatric Annals 24:69–75, 1994a

Miller LJ: Use of electroconvulsive therapy during pregnancy. Hospital and Community Psychiatry 45:444–450, 1994b

Nulman I, Rovet J, Stewart DE, et al: Neurodevelopment of children exposed in utero to antidepressant drugs. N Engl J Med 336:258–262, 1997

O'Hara MW: Post-partum "blues," depression, and psychosis: a review. J Psychosom Obstet Gynaecol 7:203–227, 1987

O'Hara MW: Summary and implications, in Postpartum Depression: Causes and Consequences. Edited by O'Hara MW. New York, Springer-Verlag, 1993, pp 168–194

O'Hara MW, Schlechte JA, Lewis DA, et al: Prospective study of postpartum blues. Arch Gen Psychiatry 48:801–806, 1991

Parry BL, Rush AJ: Oral contraceptives and depressive symptomatology: biologic mechanisms. Compr Psychiatry 20:347–358, 1979

Pastuszak A, Schick-Boschetto B, Zuber C, et al: Pregnancy outcome following first-trimester exposure to fluoxetine (Prozac). JAMA 269:2246–2248, 1993

Robins LN, Helzer JE, Weissman MM, et al: Lifetime prevalence of specific disorders in three sites. Arch Gen Psychiatry 41:949–958, 1984

Rohde A, Marneros A: Schizoaffective disorders with and without onset in the puerperium. Eur Arch Psychiatry Clin Neurosci 242:27–33, 1992

Rohde A, Marneros A: Postpartum psychoses: onset and long-term course. Psychopathology 26:203–209, 1993

Rosenthal NE, Sack DA, Gillin JC, et al: Seasonal affective disorder: a description of the syndrome and preliminary findings with light therapy. Arch Gen Psychiatry 53:289–292, 1992

Schneier FR, Johnson J, Hornig CD, et al: Social phobia: comorbidity and morbidity in an epidemiologic sample. Arch Gen Psychiatry 49:282–288, 1992

Seeman MV: Current outcome in schizophrenia: women versus men. Acta Psychiatr Scand 73:609–617, 1986

Seeman MV, Lang ML: The role of estrogens in schizophrenia gender differences. Schizophr Bull 16:185–194, 1990

Sherwin BB: Affective changes with estrogen and androgen replacement therapy in surgically menopausal women. J Affect Disord 14:177–187, 1988

Sherwin BB: Up-regulatory effect of estrogen on platelet ^{3}H-imipramine binding sites in surgically menopausal women. Biol Psychiatry 28:339–348, 1990

Sichel DA: Psychiatric issues in the postpartum period. Currents in Affective Illness 11:5–12, 1992

Sichel DA, Cohen LS, Dimmock JA, et al: Postpartum obsessive-compulsive disorder: a case series. J Clin Psychiatry 54:156–159, 1993

Spiegel D, Bloom JR, Kraemer HC, et al: Effect of psychosocial treatment on survival of patients with metastatic breast cancer. Lancet 2:888–891, 1989

Steer RA, Scholl TO, Hediger ML, et al: Self-reported depression and negative pregnancy outcomes. J Clin Epidemiol 45:1093–1099, 1992

Stein A, Gath D, Bucher J, et al: The relationship between post-natal depression and mother-child interaction. Br J Psychiatry 158:46–52, 1991

Steiner M, Steinberg S, Stewart D, et al: Fluoxetine in the treatment of premenstrual dysphoria. N Engl J Med 332:1529–1534, 1995

Stewart DE, Boydell KM: Psychologic distress during menopause: associations across the reproductive life cycle. Int J Psychiatry Med 23:157–162, 1993

Stewart DE, Klompenhouwer JL, Kendell BF, et al: Prophylactic lithium in puerperal psychosis. Br J Psychiatry 158:393–397, 1991

Szymanski S, Lieberman JA, Alvir JM, et al: Gender differences in onset of illness, treatment response, course, and biologic indexes in first-episode schizophrenic patients. Am J Psychiatry 152:698–703, 1995

Task Force on Panic Anxiety and Its Treatments: Panic anxiety and panic disorder, in Panic Anxiety and Its Treatments. Edited by Klerman GL, Hirschfield RMA, Weissman MM, et al. Washington, DC, American Psychiatric Press, 1993, pp 3–38

Videbech P, Gouliaev G: First admission with puerperal psychosis: 7–14 years of follow up. Acta Psychiatr Scand 91:167–173, 1995

Vogel W, Klaiber EL, Broverman DM: The role of gonadal steroid hormones in psychiatric depression in men and women. Progress in Neuropsychopharmacology 2:487–503, 1978

von Unruh GE, Froescher W, Hoffman F, et al: Valproic acid in breast milk: how much is really there? Ther Drug Monit 6:272–276, 1984

Wagner KD, Berenson AB: Norplant-associated major depression and panic disorder. J Clin Psychiatry 55:478–480, 1994

Waldman M, Safferman A: Pregnancy and clozapine. Am J Psychiatry 150:168–169, 1993

Weissman MM, Leaf PJ, Holzer CE III, et al: The epidemiology of depression: an update on sex differences in rates. J Affect Disord 7:179–188, 1984

Weissman MM, Bruce MI, Leaf PJ, et al: Affective disorders, in Psychiatric Disorders in America. Edited by Robins LN, Regier DA. New York, Free Press, 1991, pp 53–80

Westhoff C, Wieland D, Tiezzi L: Depression in users of depo-medroxyprogesterone acetate. Contraception 51:351–354, 1995

Winston F: Oral contraceptives, pyridoxine, and depression. Am J Psychiatry 130:1217–1221, 1973

Wisner KL, Wheeler SB: Prevention of recurrent postpartum major depression. Hospital and Community Psychiatry 45:1191–1196, 1994

Wisner KL, Peindl K, Hanusa BH: Relationship of psychiatric illness to childbearing status: a hospital-based epidemiologic study. J Affect Disord 28:39–50, 1993

Woody JN, London WL, Wilbanks GD: Lithium toxicity in a newborn. Pediatrics 47:94–96, 1971

Zolese G, Blacker CVR: The psychological complications of therapeutic abortion. Br J Psychiatry 160:742–749, 1992

CHAPTER 39

GERIATRIC PSYCHIATRY

DAN BLAZER, M.D., PH.D.

Psychiatrists who work with older adults encounter diagnostic and therapeutic problems that are more complex than those encountered in young adult and middle-aged patients. Most older patients with psychiatric disorders do not fit easily into the diagnostic categories of DSM-IV (American Psychiatric Association 1994) because they experience multiple symptoms that affect both physical and psychiatric functioning. Once the problem is formulated by the clinician, usual treatment approaches must be modified to manage the functional disability that results from the psychiatric problem as well as to reverse the underlying disorder.

Multiple system involvement and functional impairment are not unique to geriatric psychiatry. Geriatricians must manage equally complex disease presentations that involve a range of dysfunctions, from the molecular to the psychosocial. For example, the onset of Type II diabetes mellitus in an older adult disrupts not only glucose metabolism but also lifelong patterns of food intake and exercise. Educational and psychotherapeutic interventions, as well as diet and medication prescription, are necessary to treat the patient successfully. Type II diabetes cannot be cured, so the goal for the clinician is to maintain overall function of the older adult in the presence of the chronic illness.

In an era when there is emphasis upon specific disorders in modern psychiatry, psychiatrists working with older adults can benefit from the syndromal approach to impairment, a paradigm shift developed by geriatricians to structure diagnostic and therapeutic strategies for older patients. Geriatricians de-emphasize specific *diagnoses* and concentrate instead on *geriatric syndromes,* which include incontinence, dizziness, falling, failure to thrive, and constipation. In this chapter, I follow this syndromal approach, identifying seven psychiatric syndromes that are most prevalent among older individuals and describing them within the context of the management of the resultant impairment: acute confusion, memory loss, insomnia, anxiety, suspiciousness, depression, and hypochondriasis (Table 39–1). Because the psychiatric disorders that contribute to these syndromes are described elsewhere in this text, emphasis will be placed on those aspects of the syndromes that are unique to late life and on the management of the older adult experiencing these syndromes.

ACUTE CONFUSION

Acute confusion, or delirium, is a transient organic brain syndrome characterized by acute onset and global impairment of cognitive function. The older person experiencing acute confusion exhibits a decreased ability to maintain attention to environmental stimuli and has difficulty shift-

TABLE 39–1. **Geriatric psychiatric syndromes**

Acute confusion	Memory loss
Insomnia	Anxiety
Suspiciousness	Depression
Hypochondriasis	

ing attention from one set of stimuli to another. Thinking is disorganized, speech becomes rambling, and he or she exhibits a decreased level of consciousness. Emotional disturbances often, but not always, accompany acute confusion and may be the presenting problem in late life. These emotional disturbances include anxiety, fear, irritability, and anger. Some older persons, in contrast, are apathetic and withdrawn during an episode of delirium, and therefore these individuals are much more difficult to diagnose. Acute confusion, by definition, is brief, usually lasting a few hours but possibly lasting weeks, such as in the case of confusion secondary to medications.

The frequency of delirium among the older population is difficult to estimate, as many episodes are undetected because of their brevity. Most estimates of prevalence range from 15% to 25% on medical and surgical wards (Beresin 1988). The prevalence is higher on intensive care units and higher among persons who are recovering from cardiovascular surgery. When delirium is diagnosed in an older patient who has been hospitalized, the hospitalization is usually prolonged, and both inhospital and posthospital mortality rates are increased. Mortality at 2-year follow-up nears 50%.

Acute confusion in late life is the common outcome of a cascade of biological, cognitive, and environmental contributors. Biological brain function declines with age, although functional capacity varies greatly within age groups. Degenerative changes, such as those characteristic of Alzheimer's disease, render the older person more susceptible to physiological changes secondary to aging and disease. These physiological changes include drug intoxication, electrolyte disturbance, infection, hypoalbuminemia, and hypoxia. For example, an older adult with early primary degenerative dementia may experience congestive heart failure. The vulnerable brain cannot adapt to the decreased delivery of oxygen and glucose during failure because of a decreased reserve capacity, and acute confusion emerges. Common external biological stressors that precipitate acute confusion in older adults at risk are listed in Table 39–2.

Cognitive contributors to delirium include a predisposition to hallucinations and delusions, such as that in an aging patient who has a history of schizophrenia. Environmental contributors include the unfamiliar surroundings of a hospital or long-term care facility and social isolation. Therefore, the hospital, where the convergence of these contributors is likely, is a high-risk environment for delirium.

General therapy for the confused older individual, to be administered in parallel with specific therapy for the underlying cause of the acute confusion, begins with medical support. Vital signs and level of consciousness should be closely monitored. Vasopressor agents may be needed to increase blood pressure, and excessive fever should be treated with ice baths and alcohol sponges. Once the syndrome of acute confusion is recognized and the precipitant of the confusion is established through history, physical

TABLE 39–2. **Common external biological stressors that precipitate acute confusion in the at-risk older adult**

Intoxication
  Drugs (anticholinergic agents, sedative-hypnotics, anxiolytics, hypertensive agents)
  Alcohol
Withdrawal symptoms
  Medications (sedative, hypnotic, anxiolytic)
  Alcohol
Metabolic disorders
  Hypoxia
  Hypoglycemia
  Failure of vital organs, such as the liver and kidney
Nutritional disorders
  Vitamin deficiency (thiamine, vitamin B_{12}, folate)
Fluid and electrolyte imbalance
  Dehydration
  Alkalosis or acidosis
  Hypernatremia or hyponatremia
Endocrine disorders
  Hyperthyroidism or hypothyroidism
  Addison's disease or Cushing's syndrome
  Pituitary hypofunction
Cardiovascular disorders
  Congestive heart failure
  Cardiac arrhythmia
  Myocardial infarction
Infections
  Pneumonia
  Influenza
  Acquired immunodeficiency syndrome
Physical injury
  Hyperthermia or hypothermia

examination, and laboratory studies, the clinician can begin therapy. Acute confusion may present as a psychiatric emergency that threatens permanent brain damage. Severe hypoglycemia, hypoxia, and hyperthermia are examples of critical conditions that may present as acute confusion. Therefore, the initial treatment should include the establishment of an adequate airway to ensure that the patient is breathing and the administration of 100 mL 50% dextrose plus 100 mg thiamine intravenously if hypoglycemia and Wernicke's encephalopathy cannot be ruled out.

The clinician also must pay special attention to reducing the demands that excess and conflicting environmental stimuli make on the patient's cerebral function. Order and simplicity in the environment are critical to the management of the confused older patient, who should be maintained in a quiet, simply furnished, and well-lighted room. Lights should be left on at night. Care can best be facilitated by constant attention from familiar persons such as family members, who frequently should orient the patient to time, place, and person. Physicians, nurses, and other hospital personnel should explain all procedures. Restraints should be kept to a minimum. Behavioral agitation generally can be managed by judicious use of antipsychotic medications, such as haloperidol, in low doses (administered either intramuscularly or orally).

MEMORY LOSS

The syndrome of memory loss (the dementia syndrome) is one of the more frequent and disabling syndromes experienced by older adults. Late-life memory loss is usually accompanied by a more or less sustained decline in cognitive function from a previously obtained intellectual level, usually with an insidious onset. Other cognitive capacities that decline with memory include language, spatial or temporal orientation, judgment, and abstract thought. There is usually no alteration of state of consciousness until very late in the memory loss syndrome, which is in contrast with acute confusion.

Disabling memory loss may begin in mid-life, but it is much more frequent in persons older than age 75 years than it is in persons between ages 65 and 74. Prevalence estimates from community samples of memory impairment are generally 5%–15%, with most investigators estimating memory impairment in at least 5% of persons older than age 65 years in the community and in 30%–50% of institutional residents (Katzman and Jackson 1991). *Alzheimer's disease*, the most common disorder contributing to the dementia syndrome, has been estimated to be prevalent in

11% of community-based persons older than age 65 years, with more than 40% of persons age 85 years or older experiencing Alzheimer's disease (Evans et al. 1989). Prevalence estimates of Alzheimer's disease include both mild and severe cases, so significant memory impairment may be found in only a proportion of persons identified as having Alzheimer's disease in community samples.

Memory loss is usually progressive. Until age 75, the life expectancy of persons experiencing Alzheimer's disease or multi-infarct dementia is reduced by about one-half. After age 75, life expectancy is less affected by memory loss. Some dementing disorders, however, do not lead to inevitable decline in function. For example, alcohol-induced amnestic disorder can be arrested if the older person stops drinking and returns to a nutritional diet. Even those persons who have Alzheimer's disease and vascular dementias, such as multi-infarct dementia, may experience significant decline over an interval, only to enter a "plateau" in functioning for a subsequent interval that may last for many months.

More than 50% of persons experiencing chronic memory loss will, at autopsy, exhibit the changes of Alzheimer's disease only. The next most common contributors to the syndrome are the vascular dementias, especially multi-infarct dementia. Clinically and pathophysiologically, it is difficult to disaggregate the vascular dementias. (For example, it is difficult to distinguish multi-infarct dementia from Binswanger's disease.) Multi-infarct dementia also frequently is comorbid with Alzheimer's disease (Tomlinson et al. 1970). In contrast to Alzheimer's disease, however, multi-infarct dementia is more common in males than in females. Many patients with Parkinson's disease develop brain changes late in the course of their disease similar to those changes found in Alzheimer's disease. Clinically, except for their parkinsonian symptoms, these patients cannot be distinguished from patients experiencing Alzheimer's disease. In addition, many patients with Alzheimer's disease exhibit changes in the substantia nigra at autopsy. Approximately 5% of older persons experience memory loss as a result of alcohol-induced amnestic disorder (Cutting 1978; Lishman 1981).

The primary risk factor for Alzheimer's disease is age, with the prevalence of Alzheimer's, as mentioned previously, being an exponential function of age. Other risk factors for Alzheimer's disease include Down's syndrome, family history of Alzheimer's disease, head trauma, and possibly lack of education. Genetic risk factors have received much attention in recent years, especially the relationship between the disease and apolipoprotein E (APOE) genotype (Roses 1994) The APOE genotype expresses itself in three alleles (2, 3, and 4). Persons with an APOE genotype of 4/4 are at much greater risk for developing Alzheimer's disease than are persons with a 2/2 genotype, with a range of risk between the most vulnerable (4/4) and the most protective (2/2). Most cases of Alzheimer's disease, however, cannot be attributed to one etiological agent. Male sex, hypertension, and possibly black race are risk factors for multi-infarct dementia. Alcohol use regularly over many years is the primary cause of alcohol-induced amnestic disorder.

The diagnostic workup of the older adult who has memory loss begins with a history, the most important component of the evaluation. A history should be obtained from both family members and the patient. The nature and severity of memory loss should be assessed in conjunction with a chronological account of the onset of the older adult's problems and specific behavioral changes. Patient and family should be asked about common problems resulting from memory loss, such as becoming lost in a familiar place, having difficulties with driving, becoming repetitious, and losing objects. Medical history should include inquiries about relevant systemic diseases, trauma, surgery, psychiatric problems, diet, and alcohol and drug use. (A thorough documentation of prescription and over-the-counter drugs is essential.) Family history should include questions about relatives who have memory loss, Down's syndrome, alcohol problems, and psychiatric disorders. The physical examination should include not only a thorough neurological examination, but also a general physical workup to determine the health of the patient.

The nature and degree of the cognitive dysfunction should be assessed by both a thorough mental status examination and objective cognitive testing. Standardized mental status examinations such as the Mini-Mental State Examination (MMSE; Folstein et al. 1975) and the Blessed Information-Memory-Concentration Test (Blessed et al. 1968) are available and are useful quantitative means of documenting memory loss at the initial evaluation.

The in-office or hospital-based initial assessment of memory and cognitive functioning is followed by a more in-depth evaluation of cognition with instruments such as the Reitan Battery, the Trail-Making Test, and tests of functions such as delayed recall and spatial ability (Reitan 1955). Performance on the short screening and on the more in-depth neuropsychological testing provides a baseline from which decline in function and/or response to therapeutic intervention can be determined. Laboratory tests to assess memory loss, such as that seen in Alzheimer's disease, are listed in Table 39–3. There is no justification for genotyping either a patient with Alzheimer's disease or family members at this time, despite the emerging evidence of a hereditary predisposition for certain genotypes such as APOE 4/4.

The purpose of the comprehensive diagnostic workup of the older adult who has memory loss is to establish the baseline functional impairment as well as to rule out reversible causes of the dementia syndrome. Although screening for reversible causes is essential, the yield from many of these tests is sparse. Reports suggesting that a large percentage of patients who initially see clinicians because of memory loss and who experience a return to previous function with treatment are misleading.

Although no definitive treatment for cognitive decline in Alzheimer's disease has been discovered, many clinical trials are currently under way to establish the efficacy of agents that might retard the progression of memory problems in older persons. Most of these therapies are based on the cholinergic hypothesis of memory and include the use of cholinergic precursors such as 1) lecithin, a dietary supplement rich in choline; and 2) cholinergic agonists, such as tetrahydroaminoacridine (THA) and physostigmine. THA and donepezil are available to physicians in office-based practice. Patients in late life who have memory loss may be referred to specialized centers (memory disorder clinics) where they can be evaluated and, if they meet criteria, enrolled in a clinical trial where they may receive a number of experimental agents, including estrogens.

Psychotropic medications are used extensively in patients suffering from memory loss, primarily because of secondary symptoms such as verbal or physical aggression, anxiety, depression, psychoses, and severe agitation or

TABLE 39–3.   Laboratory tests to assess memory loss

Standard diagnostic tests

Complete blood count, electrolyte panel, screening metabolic panel, thyroid function test (T3, T4, free thyroxine index, thyroid-stimulating hormone)

Vitamin B_{12} and folate levels

Tests for syphilis

Urinalysis

Electrocardiogram

Chest X ray

Elective tests

Magnetic resonance imaging or computed tomography

Electroencephalogram

Formal neuropsychological assessment

Cerebral blood flow studies

Lumbar puncture

Event-related potentials

regressive behavior. Other secondary behaviors, however, such as wandering, inappropriate verbalization, repetitive activities (touching), obstinacy in following suggestions or commands, hoarding materials, stealing, and inappropriate voiding, are not as amenable to medication. Therefore the first step for the clinician treating the patient with memory loss is to assess what symptoms might be responsive to a medication.

After determining that the behavioral problem that has emerged cannot be handled by nonpharmacological means and is an ongoing behavioral problem, medication should be prescribed. The specifics of medication use can be found in other portions of this textbook. Agitation and anxiety can be treated with antianxiety agents (such as short-acting benzodiazepines), neuroleptics (generally the high-potency neuroleptics are preferred in low doses), anticonvulsants (such as carbamazepine), β-blockers, lithium, buspirone, and occasionally low doses of antidepressant agents (such as trazodone) at night. Clonazepam has been reported to be of benefit in agitated patients with multi-infarct dementia; however, the episodic mood swings and acute confusion that often accompany such dementia are not as responsive to medications.

The neuroleptics are the most effective psychotropics for controlling severe agitation, aggressive behavior, and psychoses. Most neuroleptics are effective but produce side effects, and, therefore, the selection of a drug is usually determined by the side-effect profile least adverse for a given patient. For example, thioridazine is a more sedating drug and less likely to cause parkinsonian effects, whereas haloperidol is a drug much less likely to produce anticholinergic effects and postural hypotension. The new generation antipsychotic agents olanzapine and risperidone are probably less prone to side effects, yet empirical studies in the elderly are scarce to date. The most troublesome side effects that ensue from using neuroleptic agents are postural hypotension (and the risk of falling) and tardive dyskinesia. These side effects may be avoided by using agents such as buspirone and carbamazepine, although the potency of these agents is lower than that of the neuroleptics.

Because depression (even the syndrome of major depression) is frequent among patients with chronic memory loss, the use of an antidepressant agent is often indicated. In general, the antidepressant agent will not lead to an improvement in memory. Postural hypotension is a major concern when using the antidepressant medications. Despite theoretical concerns regarding anticholinergic effects, most tricyclic antidepressants with low to moderate anticholinergic effects (such as desipramine and nortriptyline) can be prescribed to demented elderly patients without the risk of increasing their memory dysfunction. Selective serotonin reuptake inhibitors (SSRIs), however, are usually preferred.

Whatever medication is prescribed to the older adult with memory loss, it should be tapered slowly on a periodic basis to determine if the medication continues to be required. If the drug is not required, then an unnecessary and potentially dangerous drug can be eliminated from the medication regime. Careful documentation of the target symptoms for the medication and monitoring of the effectiveness of the medication in reversing these symptoms assists physicians and nursing staff to identify drugs that can be discontinued.

The behavioral management of the patient with memory loss not only is useful to the patient but provides the family with the sense of accomplishment in the presence of an illness that tends to leave the family helpless and bewildered. The family and the physician should develop behaviors that promote both patient and family security. Familiar routines and consistent repetition of instructions usually enhance security. The family, as much as possible, should provide moments of fun with the patient suffering from memory loss, even when these brief moments of relief are quickly forgotten by the patient. Families can substitute for the patient's lost ability by performing tasks for the patient such as putting out clothes in the morning. Families should not hesitate to "do for" these patients, for patients with memory loss are truly more dependent than other elderly persons. Families must also compensate for the loss of impulse control that accompanies memory loss. One means is distraction; the patient who is about to remove his or her clothes or masturbate in public can be distracted by getting the patient's attention through conversation or asking the patient to walk with a family member. Patients with memory loss can usually assist in household tasks, even when the disorder is moderately severe. Even though the older adult with memory loss cannot prepare a meal by himself or herself, nevertheless, the elderly person can work with the spouse or other family members in routine tasks.

Management of memory loss must include a review of the patient's environment for problems in safety. Typical safety problems include becoming lost, wandering into busy traffic, erratic or accidental use of medicines, falls (secondary to poor lighting or slippery surfaces), accidents while driving, and leaving things unattended (such as leaving appliances turned on). Home visits by geriatric nurse specialists are most hopeful in reviewing the household for potential problems.

Perhaps the most important long-term component for managing the older adult with memory loss is support of the family. Families are the primary caregivers of elderly persons with memory loss until the memory loss becomes severe enough to lead to institutionalization. With proper support, the older person can remain at home for a longer period of time and the family can function more effectively in the midst of the devastation of the severe memory loss. Education of the family regarding the expected progression of memory loss and the many behaviors that accompany such loss, but which may not be intuitively recognized as resulting from the illness, is key to family support. Excellent educational materials are available and support groups are located throughout the world to assist the family of the patient with memory loss. In addition, families must be monitored for caregiver stress. If the clinician is not sensitive to the potential for the stress in caregivers, then family members may exceed their limits and experience "burnout," which could lead to neglect and/or abuse of the older adult. Respite for the caregiver, education, and therapy are essential in keeping the care system operative.

INSOMNIA

Insomnia is more frequent in the elderly population than in any other age group. Older persons tend to experience more nighttime sleep disturbances and use larger quantities of sedative-hypnotics than do persons in midlife. Both the lack of sleep and the subsequent medication use frequently lead to deterioration in daytime alertness and functioning. The most common sleep disturbances leading to insomnia in the elderly are

1. *Primary insomnia:* a persistent difficulty in initiating and maintaining sleep that is not related to another mental disorder or known organic factor
2. *Sleep-disordered breathing* (i.e., sleep apnea)
3. *Nocturnal myoclonus:* periodic leg movements that disturb sleep
4. *Sleep-wake schedule disorder:* a mismatch between the normal sleep-wake schedule for the elderly person's environment and his or her sleep-wake pattern

Secondary causes of insomnia are frequent in late life and include anxiety disorders, depressive disorders, dementing disorders, and physical illnesses such as chronic or obstructive pulmonary disease and, most frequently, nocturia.

Sleep changes characteristic in late life include decreased total sleep time, frequent arousals, increased percentages of Stage 1 and Stage 2 sleep, decreased percentages of Stage 3 and Stage 4 sleep, decreased rapid eye movement (REM) latency, decreased absolute amounts of

REM sleep, and a tendency to exhibit a redistribution of sleep across the 24-hour day (e.g., napping during the day). Many of these sleep changes are similar to those that occur in depression and in dementing disorders, although not as severe. Older persons are also more likely to phase-advance in the sleep cycle, with a tendency toward "morningness."

Nearly 35% of older persons report sleep-related problems in community surveys. Even though older persons comprise only 11% of the United States population, they are estimated to take between 25% and 40% of the sedative-hypnotics prescribed (National Institutes of Health Consensus Development 1990). The proportion of older persons living in long-term care facilities experiencing sleep problems and taking sedative-hypnotic agents is much higher. Sleep apnea is more prevalent in elderly men than women, with the apnea index (i.e., the number of apneas per hours of sleep) being 5 or greater in 25%–35% of elderly persons in the community (Berry and Phillips 1988). The prevalence of myoclonus probably ranges from 25% to 50% among healthy elderly persons in the community (Dickel et al. 1986). There is no adequate study of the prevalence of sleep-wake schedule disorder, but the experience of this disorder is frequently reported by elderly persons, especially in long-term care facilities.

The diagnostic workup of an older person experiencing insomnia begins with a recognition of the severity of the sleep disturbance. Screening questions during the interview should include an assessment of the patient's satisfaction with his or her sleep, daytime napping, fatigue during usual daily activities, and complaint by a bed partner or other observer of unusual behavior during sleep (such as snoring, pauses in breathing, or periodic myoclonic movements). A careful medical and psychiatric history is necessary to identify or rule out serious diseases that contribute to the sleep problem.

Medication history is essential in determining the etiology of insomnia. Prescribed medications, especially sedative-hypnotics and anxiolytics, as well as alcohol, have significant effects on sleep and also may impair cardiopulmonary function. Symptoms of the major psychiatric disorders affecting older persons, such as dementia, depression, or severe anxiety, may also lead to insomnia. If a sleep-wake cycle dysfunction is suspected, then patients may be asked to keep a log of napping, going to sleep, and awakening. Physical and neurological examinations are necessary, especially when sleep apnea is suspected. Heavy snoring requires a thorough examination of the nose and throat, usually by an otolaryngologist.

Although primary care physicians can usually recognize most sleep disorders and manage them effectively, specialized evaluation of sleep disorders is sometimes required. Referral to a psychiatrist or neurologist with special interest in sleep disorders is indicated. Upon referral, most patients, after a thorough history/physical examination and withdrawal from medication, are evaluated by polysomnography. Polysomnographic techniques have been improved in recent years; the older person can now be fitted with a portable recording instrument and returned home to sleep for two evenings. Polysomnography, followed by a multiple sleep latency test, can be used to establish the diagnosis of narcolepsy and to quantify daytime sleepiness as well as to document sleep apnea.

Following a thorough diagnostic workup, the clinician must distinguish between the causes of insomnia in the elderly patient, many occurring simultaneously in the same patient. These include

- Normal age-dependent changes in sleep
- Sleep-disordered breathing and nocturnal myoclonus
- Sleep-phase alterations
- Psychiatric disorders such as Alzheimer's disease or major depression
- Medical problems contributing to sleep difficulties such as chronic pain
- Effects of medications such as the prolonged use of a sedative-hypnotic agent
- Poor sleep hygiene such as excessive stimulation prior to bedtime
- Environmental factors that prevent sleep such as excessive heat or noise
- Psychological factors such as loneliness or boredom

In addition, many elderly persons experience primary insomnia with no organic or psychological explanation.

The cornerstones of effective treatment of insomnia in late life are the management of the underlying causes of the sleep disturbance and improved sleep hygiene. For example, a significant portion of older adults experiencing chronic insomnia also experience psychiatric disorders, especially depression and alcohol problems. Both of these conditions are responsive to therapy. Physical problems such as hypothyroidism or arthritis may not be reversed, but the symptoms can be relieved with medications or other therapeutic interventions. Nocturnal myoclonus or restless leg syndrome may respond to medication such as tryptophan or clonazepam. Sleep-apnea syndrome that does not respond to conservative management may require surgery to improve flow in the nasopharyngeal region.

Institution of good sleep hygiene is the next step in managing insomnia among elderly patients. First, the patient should be encouraged to initiate sleep at the same time every night, preferably at a later rather than an earlier time (to prevent early-morning wakefulness). The bedroom should be used primarily for sleeping and not for napping. Therefore, if the elderly patient has difficulty sleeping at night, the bed should be made up in the morning and the patient should be encouraged not to nap in the bed and to spend as little time as possible in the bedroom during the day. Exercising can facilitate sleep, but exercise should not be initiated after later afternoon. Alcohol and caffeine should be avoided in the evenings, and the evening meal should be moderate and at least 2–3 hours before bedtime. Food intake should also be limited during the 2–3 hours prior to bedtime (to prevent nocturia).

Bedrooms should generally be maintained at a temperature between 65° and 72°F. To maintain a cool bedroom, many elderly persons who cannot afford air conditioning are forced to leave their windows open at night, possibly exposing them to noises that are likely to disturb sleep. One means for decreasing the potential of noise to disrupt the night's sleep is to institute "white noise" with specially built devices to emit white noise (such as waterfall or rain sounds) or by running a fan during the night. If the elderly person still cannot sleep at night, he or she is encouraged to get up, go to another room, and engage in some non-stimulating activity (such as reading or listening to music). When the elderly person again becomes drowsy, he or she should return to the bedroom and attempt to initiate sleep once again. If the individual experiences a difficult night of sleep, he or she should make extra efforts the next day to avoid napping.

Methods of relaxation training can be used successfully in enabling the insomniac elderly patient to initiate sleep. Progressive relaxation involves the alternate tensing and relaxing of muscle groups coupled with visualizing a relaxing scene. Elderly patients can be trained in such relaxation techniques by means of training tapes (instructing in progressive relaxation) or directly by a health care professional. However, an elderly patient should not habitually use training tapes to initiate sleep but rather be encouraged to shift to autoregulation of sleep.

A number of medications can be used to facilitate sleep in the elderly population, yet these medications should be used with care. If the elderly patient is taking medications that adversely affect sleep (such as long-term use of a sedative-hypnotic agent), then the pharmacological approach to treatment is to discontinue that medication (usually over about 10 days for a sedative-hypnotic). If the sleep problem is secondary to a medical problem, then optimal management of the medical problem with medications can assist the patient with sleep. For example, adequate treatment of arthritis with analgesics can improve sleep.

The antidepressant agents not only are useful in managing the older adult with insomnia secondary to depression but can but can be used as sedative agents as well, especially if prescribed in low dose. For example, 25–50 mg trazodone or 25 mg amitriptyline may be preferable to using a benzodiazepine on a long-term basis if chronic use of a sedative is indicated. In general, the benzodiazepines that are short to medium acting are preferred over those that are more extended in length of action. Therefore, temazepam (15 mg) is preferred to flurazepam (15 mg) as a sedative-hypnotic. The benzodiazepines also can be used in individuals with nocturnal myoclonus. This therapy does not suppress the myoclonus but rather overrides the arousal effect of the muscle jerks.

ANXIETY

Anxiety is a frequent symptom among older persons, either secondary to other problems, such as hyperthyroidism, or as the primary symptom of a disorder such as generalized anxiety disorder. Many of the anxiety disorders, however, are relatively less frequent in late life. Although phobia disorders can affect persons at all stages of the life cycle, the more severe phobias, such as agoraphobia and social phobia, begin early in life and are more common in children and young adults than in older persons. Generalized anxiety disorder is a frequent diagnosis regardless of age, yet generalized anxiety is often comorbid with other psychiatric disorders such as major depression. Panic disorder is relatively frequent and severe among younger persons but much less so among older persons (although data documenting a lower prevalence among older persons are sparse). Posttraumatic stress disorder can occur at any age but is found more frequently in younger persons than older persons. Obsessive-compulsive traits are common throughout the life cycle, although the severe manifestations of this disorder are less likely to be observed in older persons. Therefore, the management of anxiety symptoms in older persons usually consists of managing the symptoms of generalized anxiety that are the primary problem or comorbid with other disorders.

Community surveys of individuals experiencing anxiety symptoms estimate that approximately 5% of older persons meet DSM-III (American Psychiatric Association 1980) criteria for the diagnosis of generalized anxiety disorder. (There have been no large community studies of the anxiety disorders using DSM-IV criteria, but a comparison of criteria suggests that the prevalence of generalized anxiety would be somewhat lower using the newer criteria.) Approximately 20% of older persons report some cognitive or somatic symptoms of anxiety in community surveys, with somatic symptoms being more prevalent than cognitive symptoms. DSM-III simple phobia, in a survey in North Carolina, was found in 10% of persons age 65 years or older compared with 13% of persons in middle age. Agoraphobia was found in 5% of the 65-or-older age group compared with 7% of the middle-age group (Blazer et al. 1991).

Anxiety results from a number of medical and psychiatric conditions. Hyperthyroidism, with an atypical presentation, may be mistaken for a psychogenic anxiety disorder. Cardiac arrhythmias may produce palpitations and shortness of breath in older persons in a syndrome resembling generalized anxiety disorder, with episodic exacerbations and remissions depending on the status of the heart. Pulmonary emboli, if not severe, may present as shortness of breath and subjective anxiety.

Many medications lead to symptoms of anxiety. Caffeine is a frequent cause of anxiety, and older persons are frequently not aware of the multiple sources of caffeine in their diet. Over-the-counter sympathomimetic medications (such as ephedrine) may lead to palpitations and subsequent subjective symptoms of anxiety. Anticholinergic agents, when they impair memory, lead to anxiety that is secondary to the memory loss and confusion. Older persons also may experience significant anxiety upon withdrawal from certain medications, especially alcohol and anxiolytic agents. Postural hypotension may lead to dizziness and shortness of breath, which may be interpreted by the older person as episodic anxiety. Hypoglycemia 4–5 hours after a large meal is another contributor to anxiety.

Many psychiatric disorders are manifested, in part, by symptoms of anxiety. Moderate to severe acute confusion is usually associated with anxiety and agitation, especially when the older person is in an unfamiliar place. Anxiety is a common accompaniment of major depression; older patients who experience major depression also meet the criteria for generalized anxiety disorder in more than 50% of the cases. Hypochondriasis is associated with anxiety, especially when dependency needs are not met by family and health care professionals. Dementing disorders, especially in the early and middle stages, are associated with anxiety and agitation. Later in the dementing disorder, the agitation is episodic, and the cognitive, subjective anxiety is less well documented. Late-life schizophrenia with acute paranoid ideation is usually accompanied by agitation and anxiety, especially in the evenings when the older person is home alone. In addition, some older persons experience acute panic attacks and meet the criteria for panic disorder, and some exhibit symptoms of generalized anxiety, without apparent biological or psychosocial causation.

The perceptive clinician must not overlook the possibility that the anxiety symptoms may be secondary to appropriate fear. Many older persons must expose themselves daily to situations that threaten their security. Older adults living in inner cities often fear being attacked as they walk the streets. Older individuals with memory loss who live alone may fear that they will get lost driving to the doctor's office. Those who have lost the acuteness of their reflexes fear driving on busy, crowded highways.

The use of nonpharmacological therapies such as relaxation training, cognitive restructuring, and activity structuring for the treatment of anxiety in older adults has not been studied extensively. Nevertheless, the danger of medication, as well as the successful application of cognitive-behavior therapies to other psychiatric disorders in late life, especially depression, suggests that nonpharmacological therapies also may be applicable to anxiety disorders. Older persons who do not have cognitive dysfunction are good candidates for relaxation training and biofeedback. No evidence has been forthcoming to suggest that older persons are less capable of taking advantage of these therapies than are middle-aged persons. Cognitive restructuring, based on the cognitive therapy described originally for depression, has not been adapted for anxiety in older adults to date. However, there is little evidence that nonstructured psychotherapy is of benefit in treating generalized anxiety or panic episodes in late life.

The cornerstone of pharmacological therapy for the anxiety disorders is benzodiazepines. These drugs repeatedly have been demonstrated to be effective for the control of anxiety when compared with a placebo and are relatively free of side effects. They are generally well tolerated by persons of all ages but present unique problems when prescribed to older persons. For example, the half-life of the benzodiazepines may be increased dramatically in late life, with diazepam (2.5–5 mg) having a half-life nearing 4 days in persons in their 80s. Older persons are also more susceptible to potential side effects of benzodiazepines such as fatigue, drowsiness, motor dysfunction, and memory impairment. Clinicians must be especially careful when prescribing benzodiazepines to older individuals who drive. Therefore, the shorter-acting benzodiazepines, such as alprazolam (.125 mg), oxazepam (15 mg), and lorazepam (2 mg), given two to three times a day, have been preferred agents in late life. Nevertheless, short-acting drugs in some older patients may lead to brief withdrawal episodes during the day and a rebound of anxiety.

Other agents are generally less effective in controlling late-life anxiety. Buspirone (10 mg tid) is relatively safe, with few side effects, and does not appear to lead to abuse or dependency. Nevertheless, it takes 3–4 weeks for the therapeutic effect to become manifest. Older adults who perceive that they have benefited from benzodiazepines generally do not accept buspirone as an alternative. The antidepressant agents are useful in treating anxiety mixed with depression. Nevertheless, in many older persons with a mixed anxiety-depression syndrome, the depressive symptoms improve while the antidepressant is being used, yet the anxiety symptoms persist. Therefore, a combination of a benzodiazepine and an antidepressant is sometimes used. Some have suggested that β-blockers such as propranolol (10 mg bid) are valuable in treating anxiety disorders. These drugs must be monitored carefully, given their propensity to slow the heart rate. Buspirone and the β-blockers may be more effective in controlling agitation and behavioral problems in dementia patients than in controlling generalized anxiety.

SUSPICIOUSNESS

A frequent symptom in older adults, especially older adults experiencing cognitive impairment, is suspiciousness, which may range from increased cautiousness and distrust of family and friends to overt paranoid delusions. Of the suspicious or paranoid older persons, a unique group has been described, especially in the European literature, for many years. *Late-life paraphrenia* has been distinguished from both chronic schizophrenia and dementia and is characterized by marked paranoid delusions in older adults who nevertheless maintain function in the community for months or even years (Almeida et al. 1995). Persons experiencing paraphrenia are predominantly women and often live alone. However, marked suspiciousness in conjunction with cognitive impairment is a more common manifestation of the syndrome. These persons would usually be diagnosed as having late-onset delusional disorder according to DSM-IV criteria.

The predominant delusions that are encountered in older persons are persecutory delusions and somatic delusions. Persecutory delusions often revolve around a single theme or a series of connected themes, such as family and neighbors conspiring against the delusional older person. Somatic delusions often involve the gastrointestinal tract and frequently reflect the older person's fear that he or she is experiencing cancer. Regardless of the etiology of suspiciousness and paranoid delusions, when older persons believe they are threatened from the social environment, often because they do not understand what is happening in that environment, agitation becomes paramount. Agitation in the suspicious older person is an acute symptom that may require emergency management as described later in this discussion.

Suspiciousness and paranoid behavior were found in 17% of persons in one community survey (Lowenthal 1964), and a sense of persecution was reported in 4% in another survey (Christenson and Blazer 1984). Therefore, the perception by older persons that they live in a hostile social environment is common and represents a much larger proportion of older individuals than those who would be diagnosed as having schizophrenia or a late-life paranoid disorder such as late-life paraphrenia. Some of these suspicions may be justified if the older person lives in an unsafe community or has been the victim of fraud. Among persons in the community, fewer than 1% have schizophrenia or a paranoid disorder.

Many different disorders may lead to suspiciousness, delusions, and agitation. Chronic schizophrenic disorder, which has its onset earlier in life and persists into late life, is perhaps the most easily identified cause of late-life suspiciousness. As schizophrenia tends to be characterized by a decline in social function over the life cycle and a shorter life expectancy (although the prognosis of schizophrenia varies greatly from individual to individual), chronic schizophrenia that persists into late life and yet leaves the older person relatively free of other symptoms is uncommon. Nevertheless, persons may experience severe symptoms of schizophrenia in early or mid-life and then enter a period of remission from which they do not relapse with further schizophrenic behavior until late life. Schizophrenic-like illness also may have its first onset in late life, and the pattern is similar to that described previously for late-life paraphrenia. Usually, depression and organic mental disorders do not contribute to these late-onset schizophrenic-like states. In contrast, organic mental disorders and late-onset depression are frequently associated with some psychotic symptoms.

Late-onset delusional disorder, with mild to moderate symptomatology, is a more frequent cause of suspiciousness in late life. Delusions, often of being persecuted by family and friends, usually center on a single theme or a connection of themes. For example, an older woman may become convinced that her daughter was instrumental in the death of her husband (or that the daughter neglected her father during a chronic illness). That woman, in turn, may not listen to reason regarding the daughter's behavior and may never forgive the daughter for the perceived abuse or neglect. These delusions may lead to a withdrawal of affection, financial support, and social contact with the daughter.

Another common cause of suspiciousness in late life is organic delusional syndrome. These delusions, in contrast

to late-onset delusional disorder, wax and wane through time in severity and in content. Persecutory delusions are most common and often emerge when the older person's environment is changed. Organic delusional syndrome often emerges from medications or from localized brain damage (such as in Huntington's chorea and alcohol abuse). Suspiciousness also may result from the dementing disorders. For some persons experiencing Alzheimer's disease, paranoid thoughts may dominate other symptoms of the dementing illness, especially in the early stages. Perhaps the most common encounter psychiatrists have with suspicious older persons is with demented patients who have become a management problem because of suspiciousness and agitation.

Despite the range of disorders that may lead to suspiciousness in older persons, some investigators have suggested common psychobiological contributors to the syndrome in late life. A family history of suspiciousness and delusional thought is uncommon among suspicious older persons, and therefore, hereditary contributions are probably less important than at earlier stages of the life cycle. Degeneration of subcortical tissues with aging may disrupt neurotransmission and higher brain functions, which in turn contributes to a deficiency in maintaining attention and filtering information, symptoms that have been associated with psychotic thinking. That women are more likely to experience more severe syndromes of suspiciousness than men in late life (in contrast to the equal sex distribution of psychoses earlier in life) has led some investigators to suggest that menopause and the resultant decrease in estrogen binding to dopamine receptors may place women at risk who were previously protected from developing suspicious thinking. Sensory deprivation also has been identified as a potential risk factor for suspiciousness, regardless of the underlying disorder. Social isolation also may contribute to suspiciousness.

The key to the diagnostic workup of the suspicious older person is the psychiatric evaluation. Delusional thinking and agitation usually render the patient's history inaccurate, and therefore family members should be interviewed to review the patient's behavior, especially any change in behavior. Previous psychotic or delusional episodes should be documented, as well as previous treatment. Clinicians evaluating the suspicious older person should remember that older adults are occasionally abused by family members, and the seemingly delusional description of family behavior by the older individual may contain some truth.

The management of suspiciousness and agitation in older adults requires 1) ensuring a safe environment; 2) initiating a therapeutic alliance; 3) considering and, if appropriate, instituting pharmacological therapy; and 4) managing acute behavioral crises. When the older patient is determined to be suspicious and agitated, the clinician must first decide whether hospitalization is necessary. In general, paranoid older persons do not adapt well to the hospital. Change from familiar surroundings and interaction with strange persons tend to exacerbate the suspiciousness. Nevertheless, older patients often are so disabled in their behavior secondary to schizophrenic or delusional disorder that hospitalization is necessary.

Once the older patient is hospitalized, the clinician must initiate a therapeutic alliance. With the older patient, this alliance is best accomplished by taking a medical approach to the patient and expressing concern about all of the patient's physical and emotional concerns. Most suspicious older patients are quite accepting of medical care and are trusting of physicians. It is rarely necessary for clinicians to confront patients regarding suspicions or delusional thinking; therefore, older patients' responses to questions can be supportive, and clinicians do not need to agree with statements made by the patients that are known to be untrue.

The cornerstone of managing the moderately to severely suspicious older patient is medication, especially antipsychotic agents. Medications most frequently used to treat older persons are thioridazine (10–25 mg po tid), haloperidol (.5–2 mg po tid), thiothixene (5 mg po tid), and loxapine (10 mg po tid). Newer agents such as risperidone (2 mg po bid) and olanzapine 10 mg/day) also are used. Dosage of these agents is relatively small initially, and one-half of the dose should be given during the evening. If thioridazine is used, then 10 mg tid and 25 mg at night may be adequate to control moderately suspicious thoughts and agitated behavior. Haloperidol may be given .5 mg po bid and 2 mg po qhs. Doses can be increased significantly if necessary. Physicians who prescribe antipsychotic medications for the treatment of suspiciousness in an older adult should monitor carefully the success of these agents. If the drug is deemed not successful—for example, if the target symptoms do not change with the medication—then it should be discontinued, given the significant side effects that may result.

Finally, the physician must be prepared to deal with severe agitation and violent behavior. Medications alone will not control these behaviors. Physicians must work with the nursing staff to prevent such behavior in patients at risk while they are in the hospital and to instruct families regarding methods of prevention when these patients are at home. Suggestions for preventing violent behavior are listed in Table 39–4.

Periods of severe agitation are usually brief and, if

TABLE 39–4. Suggestions for preventing aggressive and violent behavior in the suspicious older adult

- Psychologically disarm the older patient by assisting him or her to express his or her fears.
- Distract the attention of the older patient. One person should calmly speak to the agitated older patient to distract attention from perceived threats in the patient's surroundings.
- Provide directions to the older patient in simple terms for even the most simple behaviors. Suspicious older patients have difficulty interpreting complex procedures.
- Communicate clearly and concisely. The suspicious older patient has a decreased ability to receive and organize complex information.
- Communicate expectations. A firm command to the suspicious older patient in simple terms is essential for controlling aggressive behavior.
- Avoid arguing and defending. Arguments between staff and an agitated older patient only increase fear and agitation in the patient.
- Avoid threatening body language. Staff should move slowly, predictably, and respectfully in the personal space of the suspicious older patient. Threatening gestures (such as clenched fists) must be avoided.
- Remain at a safe distance from the agitated older patient until help is available. A staff member should not attempt to single-handedly control even a small agitated older person.

managed properly, are soon forgotten by the older patient. Then the physician once more can work toward establishing a sustained therapeutic relationship with the patient.

DEPRESSION

Depression is one of the more frequent and the second most disabling geriatric psychiatry syndrome (after memory loss) experienced by older adults. Late-life depression is characterized by symptoms similar to those experienced at earlier stages of the life cycle, with some significant differences. The depressed mood is usually apparent in the older adult but may not be a spontaneous complaint. Older persons are more likely to experience weight loss (as opposed to weight gain or no change in weight) during a major depressive episode and are less likely to report feelings of worthlessness or guilt. Although older persons experience more difficulty with cognitive performance tests during a depressive episode, they are no more likely than persons in mid-life to report cognitive problems subjectively.

Complaints of cognitive dysfunction are common to more severe depressive episodes regardless of the person's age. Persistent anhedonia associated with a lack of response to pleasurable stimuli is a common and central symptom of late-life depression. Older persons are also more likely to exhibit psychotic symptoms during a depressive episode than are younger persons.

In community surveys, older adults are less likely to be diagnosed as having major depression than are persons in young adulthood or middle age. Depressive symptoms, however, are about equally prevalent across the life cycle. Standardized interviews reveal that 1%–2% of persons in the community are diagnosed as experiencing major depression, whereas an additional 2% are diagnosed as having dysthymia (Blazer et al. 1987). Major depression is much more prevalent among older persons in the hospital and in long-term–care facilities, ranging from 10% to 20% (Koenig et al. 1988).

Late-life depression fits well in the biopsychosocial model of psychiatric disorders. Although a hereditary predisposition to depression is less likely among persons in late life experiencing a first onset of depression, a number of biological factors are associated with late-life depression. Poor regulation of the hypothalamic-pituitary-adrenal axis, as well as disruption of the sleep cycle and other circadian rhythms, is more likely to be present among older persons than among younger persons. These problems also have been associated with major depression. Most older persons are satisfied with their lives and are not psychologically predisposed to depression. Nevertheless, some experience a demoralization and a despair resulting not only from incapacities due to aging, but also from a sense of not having fulfilled their life expectations. Older persons must adapt to many adverse life experiences, especially losses of relatives and friends, yet they are often more likely to respond to these losses without difficulty than are persons who are younger. Older persons, for example, expect that they will lose family and friends through death. And those family and friends that they do lose often have suffered chronic illnesses for some time, thus permitting older persons to grieve the loss, in part, before the actual loss.

Major depression is relatively infrequent among older persons yet is the most challenging of the late-life mental disorders to manage. Older persons also may experience bipolar disorder, with a first-onset manic episode after age 65. Psychotic depressions are more common in late life than at other stages of the life cycle. Other common causes of late-life depression include organic mood disorder, such as a depressed mood secondary to antihypertensive medications, and the depression associated with the common dementing disorders, such as primary degenerative dementia and multi-infarct dementia. Medical illness, such as hypothyroidism, frequently leads to an organic mood disorder. An adjustment disorder with depressed mood secondary to physical disability and/or chronic illness is among the most frequent causes of depressed mood among older individuals.

As with the diagnosis of other geriatric psychiatry syndromes, the patient's history and a collateral history from a family member are the keys to making the diagnosis of depression in late life. Although older persons may exhibit some tendency to "mask" their depressive symptoms, a careful interview almost invariably reveals significant depression if it is present. The history should be complemented by a thorough mental status examination with attention directed to disturbances of motor behavior, perception, presence or absence of hallucinations, disturbances of thinking, and thorough cognitive testing. Psychological testing may be implemented to distinguish depression from dementia but should not be performed in the midst of a severe depressive episode. The laboratory workup of the depressed older adult is presented in Table 39–5.

Some tests, such as the blood count and measurement of B_{12} and folate levels, are useful in screening for medical illness that may present with depressive symptoms. The thyroid panel is essential in the diagnosis of the depressed older patient, given that subclinical hypothyroid disorders are frequently uncovered in the workup. The dexamethasone suppression test is not especially valuable in making the diagnosis of late-life depression but may provide information regarding response to therapy, such as pharma-

TABLE 39–5.   Laboratory workup of the depressed older adult

Routine

Complete blood cell count

Urinalysis

T3, T4, free thyroxine index, thyroid-stimulating hormone

Venereal Disease Research Laboratory test

Vitamin B_{12} and folate assays

Chemistry screen (sodium, chlorine, potassium, blood urea nitrogen, calcium, glucose, creatinine)

Electrocardiogram

Elective

Dexamethasone suppression test

Polysomnography

Magnetic resonance imaging (or computed tomography)

Cerebrospinal fluid assays

Thyroid-releasing hormone stimulation test

cotherapy or electroconvulsive therapy (ECT), if repeated after the therapy has been initiated for a few days. Although the abnormalities in sleep associated with depression frequently parallel those associated with normal aging, experienced polysomnographers can distinguish them. Cerebral atrophy and subcortical leukoencephalopathies are often found on magnetic resonance imaging (MRI) scanning in older persons who experience major depression without demonstrative cognitive dysfunction. The diagnostic significance of these findings, however, has yet to be determined. The physician ordering laboratory tests for a depressed older patient also must consider the potential adverse health consequences for an older adult experiencing a severe or chronic mood disorder. For example, major depression is associated with decreased bone mineral density, placing older women with depression at greater risk for osteoporosis (Michelson et al. 1996).

Clinical management involves pharmacotherapy, ECT, psychotherapy, and work with the family. Despite the advent of a new generation of antidepressants, many geriatric psychiatrists still prefer to first administer one of the secondary amines, such as nortriptyline or desipramine, to healthy older adults. Each has relatively low anticholinergic effects and is known to be an effective antidepressant. Postural hypotension and the potential for serious health consequences are the most troublesome side effects that older adults usually encounter when treated with the tricyclic antidepressants. Given that Medicare does not reimburse the older adult for medications, the lower cost of the tricyclic antidepressants compared with the cost of newer agents is a major factor in prescribing them. The SSRIs fluoxetine, sertraline, paroxetine, and nefazodone can be used at a somewhat lower dose than is prescribed at earlier stages of the life cycle (e.g., 10 mg/day fluoxetine or 200 mg bid nefazodone). The most common adverse effects that limit the use of SSRIs are agitation and persistent weight loss. The older person who does not respond to the antidepressant medications or who experiences significant side effects from the medications may be a candidate for ECT. Depressed older persons who are candidates for ECT should be experiencing a severe depressive episode and are especially likely to respond if they are experiencing psychotic symptoms. With proper medical support, ECT is a safe and effective treatment for older adults.

A number of studies have demonstrated the effectiveness of cognitive and behavioral therapies in outpatient treatment of older persons who have major depression without melancholia (Koder et al. 1996). Cognitive therapy also may be an adjunct for severe melancholic depressions that are treated concomitantly with medications.

Cognitive-behavior therapy is well tolerated by older people because of its limited duration and educational orientation, as well as the active interchange between the therapist and the patient.

Any effective therapy for depression with older persons must include work with the family. Families are often the most important allies of the clinician working with depressed older patients. Families should be informed as to the danger signs, such as potential for suicide, in a severely depressed older family member. In addition, the family can provide structure for reengaging a withdrawn and depressed older person into social activities.

HYPOCHONDRIASIS

Hypochondriasis among older persons is one of the more common and frustrating of the somatoform disorders encountered by health care professionals. An essential feature of hypochondriasis in older persons is their belief that they have one or a number of serious illnesses. This belief derives from an exaggerated interpretation of physical signs and sensations. The medical workup often will reveal some physical abnormality but does not support a medical diagnosis that can account for the severity and breadth of symptoms experienced. However, hypochondriacal symptoms do not reach the level of somatic delusions. The distinction between a psychotic disorder manifested by somatic delusions and hypochondriasis is usually easy to make because the delusion is either unrelated to any physical sensation or in no way relates to the symptoms reported. To meet criteria for a diagnosis of hypochondriasis, older persons must experience the disorder for at least 6 months; when most physicians encounter hypochondriacal older patients, their symptoms have lasted far longer than 6 months. Hypochondriacal symptoms in older persons usually are described as being in the gastrointestinal or genitourinary area. Exaggerated concerns regarding constipation, difficulty with eating because of gastric problems, abdominal pain, and genitourinary pain are among the most frequent. As with individuals who have hypochondriasis at other stages of life, older persons with this disorder do not experience relief when assured by a physician that the medical problem is not severe.

In community surveys, exaggerated concern about health is found among 10% of older persons (Blazer and Houpt 1979). In contrast, another 10% usually perceive their health as being significantly better than it actually is. The majority of older persons assessed their health accurately, with no "trend" for older individuals inaccurately to perceive their health as being worse than it actually is. There are no community surveys that accurately estimate the prevalence of hypochondriasis. That hypochondriacal older persons are frequently encountered by primary care physicians should not lead to the assumption that hypochondriasis is a common problem among this population. Hypochondriacal older persons overuse health care services, and therefore, one or two hypochondriacal older patients in a primary care physician's practice may occupy an appreciable amount of time, leading the physician to believe that hypochondriasis is one of the most common conditions that he or she encounters.

The etiology of hypochondriasis is, by definition, not biological. This does not mean, however, that hypochondriacal older persons do not experience physical illness or that the symptoms reported by some older individuals are not, to some degree, the expression of actual physical problems. Exaggeration of symptoms (as opposed to the invention of symptoms) is the manifestation of hypochondriasis.

A number of mechanisms may contribute to hypochondriasis in older persons. First, the symptoms may be used to shift anxiety from specific psychological conflicts to more concrete problems with body functioning. An older person may fear the loss of his or her mind, the loss of a spouse, the loss of personal capabilities, or the loss of a social role. Fear of these losses is then replaced by a preoccupation with physical health in hypochondriasis. Some older persons may use hypochondriacal symptoms as a means of punishing themselves for unacceptable, hostile feelings or behaviors in the past for which they now feel guilty. If an older person has engaged in some type of indiscretion, such as a sexual indiscretion, genitourinary pains or concerns may predominate as hypochondriacal symptoms later in life. Unfortunately, interpreting the connection between past guilt and present concern usually does not alleviate the problem of hypochondriasis.

Social factors are probably the major reason that aging persons are at risk for developing hypochondriasis. Older persons often have difficulty meeting personal and/or social expectations. Family members may wish the older family member to participate in activities that are beyond his or her capability, such as a long walk, lifting luggage, or preparing a meal. Failure to meet these family expectations, or perhaps anger at the family for insisting that these expectations be met, can lead the older person to focus on his or her physical problems to the exclusion of facing the issue directly. Older persons also use hypochondriasis as a means of adapting to the real problem of isolation. Preoccupation with physical problems and obtaining help for those physical problems in some cases become the center of the older person's life. Frequent visits to the physician require assis-

tance with transportation from family or friends and provide social contact with persons in the health care professional's office. The older patient also learns that physical complaints facilitate communicating with others because they provide the individual with a topic of conversation. Isolated older persons may feel they have little else to contribute to conversations and, therefore, focus upon their physical problems.

The clinician working with a hypochondriacal older patient must be vigilant for the presence of more severe psychopathology. Depression is frequently accompanied by exaggerated physical concerns, regardless of age. If an older person exhibits both significant depressive symptoms and symptoms of hypochondriasis, then the clinician must be alert to the possibility of suicide. Suicide has been demonstrated to be more common in persons exhibiting both depression and exaggerated physical concerns compared with depressive symptoms alone. Hypochondriasis also may mask emerging difficulties with memory. Older persons may avoid direct challenges to their cognitive status by focusing on their physical concerns.

The diagnostic workup of the hypochondriacal older patient consists of a thorough history and a routine physical examination. Routine laboratory studies should be performed, but once the clinician is assured that the patient does not have a severe or undetected physical problem that contributes to the symptoms, then he or she should limit further laboratory studies. The differential diagnosis includes major depression and dysthymia, anxiety disorders (both generalized anxiety and panic), schizophrenic disorder (if the exaggerated physical concern expressed by the patient borders on delusional thinking), and dementing disorders. The diagnosis of hypochondriasis does not exclude the diagnosis of other psychiatric disorders. Many older persons with hypochondriasis meet criteria for a somatoform disorder and, for example, a dementing disorder.

Working with the hypochondriacal older patient requires both tact and patience. The development of a management strategy should be based on management goals (see Table 39–6). Older patients with hypochondriasis are best managed by a primary care physician as opposed to a psychiatrist. After the initial evaluation, the hypochondriacal older patient should be seen for relatively brief but regularly scheduled visits, in general lasting no more than 10–20 minutes each. Emphasis during the follow-up visits initially should be on a brief review of interval historical information coupled with a brief physical examination (including checking pulse and blood pressure). The remainder of the visit should be relatively unstructured and should focus on events in the patient's life. The clinician should refrain from interpretations connecting the physical problems with specific life events, instead encouraging the patient to discuss concerns about family, friends, perceived isolation, and so forth. The clinician may prescribe medications but must recognize that older patients with hypochondriasis are at increased risk for becoming dependent on psychotropic medications. Placebos are generally not appropriate because discovery that a placebo has been prescribed undoubtedly will destroy the relationship between patient and doctor.

Medications that can be used for treating the hypochondriacal older patient include those with relatively few side effects and those that have been demonstrated to be at least minimally effective for alleviating the symptoms expressed by the patient. For example, L-tryptophan can be prescribed for problems with sleeping (2 g of this drug at night would be an appropriate dose). Another mildly sedating drug is diphenhydramine, given at 25–50 mg at night. Neither of these drugs will lead to habituation.

The concept of "treatment" for hypochondriasis is actually misleading. Whatever treatment plan is instituted, it, in fact, is a management plan with the goals of 1) controlling and decreasing the use of health services, 2) decreasing the concern and anxiety expressed by the hypochondriacal older person about the availability and commitment of health care professionals, 3) decreasing strain on the family, 4) increasing the capabilities of the family to provide a supportive environment to the hypochondriacal older person, 5) decreasing conflicts within the family, and 6) decreasing anxiety expressed by the hypochondriacal older person. Given these goals, it is essential that the hypochondriacal older person be treated within the context of the family when family members are available. Hypochondriacal symptoms often disappear during the process of aging. As older persons resolve conflicts with family, and as they accept their one and only life for what it is, anxiety decreases and appropriate social interactions increase.

TABLE 39-6. Goals for managing hypochondriasis in the older adult

- Control excessive use of health care services.
- Decrease concern and anxiety of the hypochondriacal older person.
- Assure hypochondriacal older person of professional commitment to managing his or her condition.
- Decrease family stress and facilitate the family as social support.
- Decrease anxiety, anger, and frustration of the health care professional treating the hypochondriacal patient.

CONCLUSIONS

The seven geriatric syndromes discussed in this chapter account for the majority of the psychopathology that both psychiatrists and geriatricians encounter while working with older adults. The syndromal approach permits the clinician to focus on the functional impairment that results from psychopathology and on the day-to-day management of the older person in both the hospital and the outpatient clinic. A syndromal approach also provides a more realistic conceptualization of late-life psychopathology, which often is comorbid across psychiatric diagnoses and comorbid with physical illnesses.

REFERENCES

Almeida OP, Howard RJ, Levy R, et al: Psychotic states arising in late life (late paraphrenia): psychopathology and nosology. Br J Psychiatry 166:205–214, 1995

American Psychiatric Association: Diagnostic and Statistical Manual of Mental Disorders, 3rd Edition. Washington, DC, American Psychiatric Association, 1980

American Psychiatric Association: Diagnostic and Statistical Manual of Mental Disorders, 4th Edition. Washington, DC, American Psychiatric Association, 1994

Beresin EV: Delirium in the elderly. J Geriatr Psychiatry Neurol 1:127–143, 1988

Berry DTR, Phillips BA: Sleep-disordered breathing in the elderly: review and methodological comment. Clin Psychol Rev 8:101–120, 1988

Blazer DG, Houpt JL: Perception of poor health in the healthy older adult. J Am Geriatr Soc 27:330–336, 1979

Blazer DG, Hughes DC, George LK: The epidemiology of depression in an elderly community population. Gerontologist 27:281–287, 1987

Blazer DG, George LK, Hughes DC: The epidemiology of anxiety disorders: an age comparison, in Anxiety Disorders in the Elderly. Edited by Salzman C, Lebowitz B. New York, Springer, 1991, pp 17–30

Blessed G, Tomlinson BE, Roth M: The association between quantitative measures of dementia and of senile change in the cerebral grey matter of elderly subjects. Br J Psychiatry 114:797–811, 1968

Christenson R, Blazer D: Epidemiology of persecutory ideation in an elderly population in the community. Am J Psychiatry 141:1088–1091, 1984

Cutting J: The relationship between Korsikov's syndrome and "alcoholic dementia." Br J Psychiatry 132:240–251, 1978

Dickel MJ, Sassin J, Mosko S: Sleep disorders in an aged population: preliminary findings of a longitudinal study. Sleep Research 15:116–123, 1986

Evans IA, Funkenstein H, Albert MS, et al: Prevalence of Alzheimer's disease in a community population of older persons higher than previously reported. JAMA 262:2551–2556, 1989

Folstein MF, Folstein SE, McHugh PR: Mini-Mental State: a practical method for grading the cognitive state of patients for the clinician. J Psychiatr Res 12:189–198, 1975

Katzman R, Jackson JE: Alzheimer's disease: basic and clinical advances. Journal of Geriatric Psychiatry 39:516–525, 1991

Koder D, Brodaty H, Anstey K: Cognitive therapy for depression in the elderly. Int J Geriatr Psychiatry 11:97–107, 1996

Koenig HG, Meador KG, Cohen HJ, et al: Self-rated depression scales and screening for major depression in the older hospitalized patient with medical illness. J Am Geriatr Soc 36:699–706, 1988

Lishman WA: Cerebral disorder in alcoholism: syndromes of impairment. Brain 104:1–20, 1981

Lowenthal MF: Lives in Distress. New York, Basic Books, 1964

Michelson D, Stratakis C, Hill L, et al: Bone mineral density in women with depression. N Engl J Med 335:1176–1181, 1996

National Institutes of Health Consensus Development: The Treatment of Sleep Disorders in Older Persons. Washington, DC, U.S. Government Printing Office, 1990

Reitan RM: The distribution according to age of a psychologic measure dependent upon organic brain functions. Journal of Gerontology 10:338–340, 1955

Roses AD: Apolipoprotein E affects the rate of Alzheimer disease expression: β-amyloid burden is a secondary consequence dependent on APOE genotype and duration of disease. J Neuropathol Exp Neurol 53:429–437, 1994

Tomlinson E, Blessed G, Roth M: Observations on the brains of demented old people. J Neurol Sci 11:205–242, 1970

SUGGESTED READINGS

Birren JE, Sloane RB, Cohen GD: Handbook of Mental Health and Aging, 2nd Edition. New York, Academic, 1992

Blazer DG: Depression in Late Life. St Louis, MO, CV Mosby, 1982

Blazer DG: Hypochondriasis, in A Family Approach to Health Care in the Elderly. Edited by Blazer DG, Siegler IC. Menlo Park, CA, Addison-Wesley, 1984, pp 140–156

Blazer DG: Depression in the elderly. N Engl J Med 320:164–166, 1989

Blazer DG: Anxiety disorders, in The Merck Manual of Geriatrics. Edited by Abrams WB, Berkow R. Rathway, NJ, Merck, Sharp & Dohme, 1990, pp 1007–1111

Blazer DG: Emotional Problems in Later Life: Intervention Strategies for Professional Caregivers. New York, Springer, 1990

Busse EW: Somatoform and psychosexual disorders, in Geriatric Psychiatry, 2nd Edition. Edited by Busse EW, Blazer DG. Washington, DC, American Psychiatric Press, 1996, pp 291–312

Busse EW, Blazer DG (eds): Geriatric Psychiatry, 2nd Edition. Washington, DC, American Psychiatric Press, 1996

Coffey CE, Figiel GS, Djang WT, et al: Effects of ECT on brain structure: a pilot prospective magnetic resonance imaging study. Am J Psychiatry 145:701–706, 1988

Gallagher D, Thompson LW: Differential effectiveness of psychotherapies for the treatment of major depressive disorder in older adult patients. Psychotherapy 19:482–490, 1982

Gublin MJ: Managing sleep disturbance of the elderly without drug therapy. Geriatric Medicine Today 4:72–85, 1985

Gwyther LP: Care of Alzheimer's Patients. New York, Alzheimer's Disease and Related Disease Association/American Health Care Association, 1985

Hoch CC, Busse DG, Monk TH, et al: Sleep disorders and aging, in Handbook of Mental Health and Aging, 2nd Edition. Edited by Birren JE, Sloane RB, Cohen GD. New York, Academic, 1992, pp 557–582

Koder D, Brodaty H, Anstey K: Cognitive therapy for depression in the elderly. Int J Geriatr Psychiatry 11:97–107, 1996

Larson EB, Lo B, Williams ME: Evaluation and care of elderly patients with dementia. J Gen Intern Med 1:116–125, 1986

Lipowski ZJ: Delirium in the elderly patient. N Engl J Med 320:578–582, 1989

Maletta GJ: Pharmacologic treatment and management of the aggressive demented patient. Psychiatric Annals 20:446–455, 1990

Massey EW, Coffey CE: Delirium: diagnosis and treatment. South Med J 76:1147–1150, 1983

National Institutes of Health Consensus Development: Differential diagnosis of dementing diseases. National Institutes of Health Consensus Development Conference Statement 6(11):1–9, 1987

Reynolds CF III, Kupfer DJ, Hoch CC, et al: Sleeping pills for the elderly: are they ever justified? J Clin Psychiatry 46 (No 2, Sec 2):9–12, 1985

Roses AD: Apolipoprotein E affects the rate of Alzheimer Disease Expression: β-amyloid burden is a secondary consequence dependent on APOE genotype and duration of disease. J Neuropathol Exp Neurol 53:429–437, 1994

Sheikh JI: Anxiety and its disorders in old age, in Handbook of Mental Health in Aging, 2nd Edition. Edited by Birren JE, Sloane RB, Cohen GD. New York, Academic, 1992, pp 410–432

Wells CE: Delirium in dementia, in Basic Psychiatry for the Primary Care Physician. Edited by Abrams H. New York, Basic Books, 1976, pp 37–61

CHAPTER 40

THE BASICS OF CULTURAL PSYCHIATRY

EZRA E. H. GRIFFITH, M.D.
CARLOS A. GONZÁLEZ, M.D.
HOWARD C. BLUE, M.D.

Culture as it informs contemporary psychiatric diagnosis and practice is not a "visible" or "exotic" difference in symbolic orientation, but rather a subtle all pervasive frame of reference that the psychiatrist may or may not share with his/her patient, and that involves the construction of persons, the assessment of behavior, the choice of a therapeutic rationale and a suitable 'end stage' of adaptive function that is targeted as and/or signals a cure.

—Fabrega 1992, p. 100

Cultural psychiatry has gained considerable visibility and prestige as a discipline in the last few decades because of an increased recognition that culture plays a significant role in individuals' lives and has considerable impact on the development of their self-concept. Such understanding has directly resulted from the collaborative efforts of psychiatrists, anthropologists, sociologists, and individuals from other professional groups. The pressure for such interdisciplinary thinking and problem solving has come, too, from society's wish to understand the nature of certain problems that are vexing, peculiarly difficult to resolve, and evidently linked to culture. How and to what extent, for example, do the differences in lifestyle and values of ethnic groups in the United States account for the contrasting health and mental health status of these groups? Are there specific cultural elements that determine why certain national groups form suicide squads to perform terrorist actions? Are there cultural determinants of the recently perceived rise in intragroup violence in the United States and intergroup violence abroad? Why is it that certain emotional disorders found in Asia baffle psychiatrists trained in North America? How is it that differences in religious beliefs can seem to fuel protracted strife among groups of people? Such questions reflect the key assumption that their solution does not lie simply in some biological framework but at least partly in understanding the role of culture as an integral component of human existence and behavior.

DEFINITIONS OF CULTURAL PSYCHIATRY

Certain key concepts have been consistently critical to the understanding of cultural psychiatry. First is *society*, which Leighton and Murphy (1965) defined as a group of human beings who live together in a system of social relationships. Obviously, the structural organization of every group is an important characteristic and influences the values and activities of the group. For example, the organization of the family is often linked to the child-rearing practices of the group.

A second crucial concept is *culture*, which Leighton and Murphy (1965) considered to be an abstract concept that describes a particular society's entire way of living. The notion encompasses shared patterns of belief, feeling, and knowledge that ultimately guide everyone's conduct and definition of reality. Culture refers to a multiplicity of elements that define human life, such as social relationships, religion, technology, and economics. Furthermore, it is an ever-changing concept, one that is learned, taught by one generation to the next, and obviously an integral part of all societies. *Ethnicity* is a somewhat narrower term, in that it encompasses the notion that people identify with each other because of a shared heritage. In a technical sense, distinctions exist between social structure and cultural processes. However, it is often the case in the psychiatric arena that social and cultural components are combined to facilitate conceptualizations.

Another important definition centers on *environment*, which refers to physical circumstances of climate, altitude, natural resources, and the presence or absence of noxious agents. In this context, it is to be understood that, for example, a tropical climate has considerable influence on the games played by adolescents and favors the use of the outdoors. Similarly, a severely cold climate influences the dating practices of young lovers, because activities outdoors would be circumscribed. In the Caribbean, West Indian males like the year-round habit of standing for hours in groups talking about politics, sports, women, and other pressing topics of the day. They call it "liming." West Indians who have lived in cold climates speak disparagingly of the inability to lime where it is cold and snowing. Regarding the effect of noxious agents on those living in a particular area, it is well recognized that persons living in areas plagued by snakes, for example, are preoccupied with protecting themselves from intrusions by reptiles. In addition, special myths and fantasies that carry a central snake theme may then develop in that particular population. Closer to home, various workers have commented about the effect on children of their growing up while being chronically exposed to an environment that is characterized by such noxious agents as violence, crime, poverty, and drug abuse.

These definitions lead to a clearer appreciation of the notion that cultural psychiatry concerns itself with the relationship between psychiatric disorders and the matrix created by the interplay of society, culture, and environment. The more restrictive term *cross-cultural* (or *transcultural*) implies that a psychiatric problem in two different cultures is being compared in some way or that a psychiatric question in a particular culture is being studied or approached by someone who is from another culture.

Another important consideration in cultural psychiatry is the difference between the *emic* and the *etic* perspective. Simply stated, the term *emic* refers to the ways people in a given culture view a phenomenon occurring within that culture. The term *etic* refers to a culture-general or universal approach to the viewing of psychiatric problems. Westermeyer (1985) has warned against thinking that a diagnosable phenomenon is either emic or etic in nature, but rather states the issue as the extent to which a given diagnostic entity is emic versus the extent to which it is etic. Consequently, observers from culture A may impose their cultural perspectives on their observations about culture B. The result is a "pseudoetic" or "imposed etic" view that may very well include a number of distortions about culture B. Berry (1975) has argued that an observer from culture A should temper this imposed etic view with emic considerations acquired through observation of culture B in order to eventually achieve a "derived etic" view of the specific psychiatric issue that is being considered within culture B.

SCOPE OF THE DISCIPLINE

Interest in cultural psychiatry has spread around the globe and has led to significant widening of its scope (Table 40–1). Broadly speaking, the discipline now includes such

---

TABLE 40–1. The scope of cultural psychiatry

- The study of people in their natural habitats
- The relationship of cultural factors to specific psychiatric disorders
- The relationship of psychiatric disorders and processes to human universals such as gender and age
- The impact of culture on personality development
- The investigation of culture-bound syndromes
- Comparative studies of diagnostic entities
- The influence of culture on healing systems
- The impact of culture on social roles
- The interplay of culture and psychotherapy
- The impact of race and ethnicity on response to psychotropic medications

themes as the study of people in their natural habitats, the relationship of cultural factors to specific psychiatric disorders, the relationship of psychiatric disorders and processes to human universals such as gender and age, culture and personality development, culture-bound syndromes, comparative studies of diagnostic entities, culture and healing systems, culture and social roles, culture and psychotherapy, and the impact of race and ethnicity on response to psychotropic medications (Draguns 1981; Kiev 1964; Leighton and Murphy 1965).

BRIEF HISTORICAL REVIEW

EARLY OBSERVATIONS

Although cultural psychiatry's recognition as a discipline may be fairly recent, there are many examples to demonstrate that observers have long been concerned with the relationship of culture and medicine and with the influence of culture on behavior. Williams (1986) pointed out how data were published in the mid-19th century purportedly showing that free African Americans living in Northern states had high rates of admission to state insane asylums. The figures were ultimately intended to show that African Americans lacked the ability to exist in a free society and consequently needed slavery to protect them from psychosocial stresses. Such an argument, though deeply flawed, was already clearly linking individuals' experiences with psychosocial institutions and the emergence of mental disorders.

FREUD AND OTHER CONTRIBUTORS

In a more formal sense, cultural psychiatry could be properly envisaged as not predating the contributions of Freud. In this regard, Foulks (1977) has provided an incisive review of the early linkage of culture and psychiatry by focusing on the development of relationships between anthropology and psychiatry. Only a few themes in this collaboration can be mentioned here. Sigmund Freud and Carl Jung, among others, were interested in proving that certain psychological phenomena existed across all cultures. Foulks considered that Freud's most serious use of anthropology was evident in Freud's claim that the Oedipus complex was to be found universally. Freud pointed out that the totem was the symbolic representative of an ancestor to whom individuals have special obligations, among which was interdiction of the killing of living representatives of the totem. Foulks interpreted Freud as having argued that the origin of this basic social system existed in actual events in prehistory; the patriarch dominated the females, and sons ultimately overthrew the father and killed him. Consequently, Freud utilized anthropological observations to conclude that in the primitive period of human evolution an actual situation became a part of all of our inheritance. Although Jung agreed with Freud on the universality of the Oedipus complex and considered it part of the collective unconscious, Horney (1937) challenged this hypothesis and argued that Oedipus was influenced by sociocultural forces. Still others (Chodoff 1966; Friedman and Downey 1995; Schrut 1994) have raised questions about the theoretical basis for Oedipus and have further questioned its universality and its significance for psychological development. Recently, Erickson (1993), using anthropological and sociobiological data, has challenged the notion of children's innate incestuous wishes, one of the major tenets of the Oedipus constellation. His data suggest that incestuous wishes might not be intense or even present among children who experienced consistently secure early bonding.

Other important themes and ideas in psychiatry have evolved from anthropologists' observations of societies and cultures. For example, Ruth Benedict's (1959) research in the field led to her formulation of the notion of *ethos*, which seemed to characterize the temperament of groups. On a comparative basis, Benedict appreciated that whereas an individual belonging to a particular group was likely to be stoic and unemotive, a member of a different group might be more inclined to be excitable, emotive, and impulsive. Such observations clearly had implications for the psychiatrist's definition of psychopathology.

Foulks (1977) included in his review the important contributions of Margaret Mead, only one of which was her rejection of the ideas that adolescence is inexorably characterized by rebellion. Mead used her Samoan observations to conclude that in a particular culture adolescence was not a conflictual period, as seen at that time in the West. She attributed the lack of conflict to the cultural continuity between child and adult roles in Samoa. Interestingly, this preceded the work of Offer (1969) in the United States, which put to rest the theory of adolescence as a period of inevitable tempestuousness. Offer's observations suggest that there is value in using a culture-free approach even when evaluating phenomena within one's culture of origin.

Foulks also mentioned the important contributions of workers such as Malinowski, Kardiner, Linton, Bettelheim, and Cawte to this particular interplay of anthropology and psychiatry, especially in regard to the formulation of psychoanalytic concepts.

RECENT CONTRIBUTORS

In the last two decades, cultural and transcultural psychiatry has seen a veritable explosion of knowledge in areas only peripherally related to psychoanalysis. Workers such as Manson et al. (1987) and Shore (1975) have provided substantial observations of Native Americans and their adjustment to contact with the dominant American culture. Separate analyses of religious rituals and their psychotherapeutic effects have been provided by Griffith et al. (1984), Ruiz and Langrod (1976), and Ness and Wintrob (1980). J. P. Spiegel (1983) and others (McGoldrick et al. 1982) have concentrated on elucidating the family structures and interactions of different ethnic groups.

Several workers (Blue and González 1992; Comas-Díaz and Jacobsen 1991; Gorkin 1986) have examined the impact of culture on the traditional clinical arena. Yamamoto (1977), Tseng (1973), Westermeyer (1979), and Kleinman (1982) have opened the window on Asian and Asian-American cultures. Guarnaccia et al. (1989b, 1990) have described the limitations of using standardized diagnostic instruments cross-culturally.

Kleinman (1980, 1988) has articulated more elaborate concepts for understanding the relationship of culture to sickness and care, and he has encouraged clinicians to think further about such notions as the sick role, illness behavior, doctor-patient communication, and patient and practitioner explanatory models of sickness. In addition, the McGill University group, through the *Transcultural Psychiatric Research Review* (recently renamed *Transcultural Psychiatry*) has done much to keep before us notions of transcultural psychiatry, including the development of recommendations and guidelines for the teaching of cultural psychiatry to psychiatric residents (Moffic et al. 1987).

Indeed, cultural psychiatry has seemed to flourish in recent years, as evidenced by the attention given it in different contexts by a number of scholars. For example, an entire issue of *Psychiatric Clinics of North America* (September 1995) was recently devoted exclusively to cultural psychiatry. The journal, *Culture, Medicine, and Psychiatry*, now features a cultural case studies section and a new journal, *Cultural Diversity and Mental Health*, has begun publication. Pedro Ruiz (1995) edited a section comprised of six chapters addressing different issues in cross-cultural psychiatry in Volume 14 of the *American Psychiatric Press Review of Psychiatry*. Other workers have also specifically highlighted the interaction of culture and clinical care, particularly with regard to the treatment of ethnic minorities found in the United States (Gaw 1993; González et al. 1995). An arena recently gaining prominence has been the study of racial and gender differences in response to psychotropic medications (Dawkins and Potter 1991; Lin et al. 1991; Mendoza et al. 1991; Strickland et al. 1991, 1995) to the point where an entire issue of the journal *Psychopharmacology Bulletin* has been devoted to the topic (Rudorfer 1996).

In 1991, the National Institute of Mental Health (NIMH) convened a group of experts on cultural psychiatry and asked them to develop recommendations that would be used by the American Psychiatric Association's (APA) Task Force preparing the *Diagnostic and Statistical Manual of Mental Disorders*, 4th Edition (DSM-IV; American Psychiatric Association 1994). The results of this collaborative effort by an international group of mental health professionals were detailed in *Culture and Diagnosis: A DSM-IV Perspective* (Mezzich et al. 1996), as well as in *DSM-IV Sourcebook* (Widiger et al. 1997). The group's contributions included a culturally informed addition to the introduction of the manual, inclusion of "specific cultural features" as a section in the description of most disorders, a set of guidelines to be used in the creation of a cultural formulation that takes into account the individual's cultural identity and worldview, and a glossary of "culture-bound" syndromes from around the world. Although dissatisfaction with the extent of changes has been voiced by some group members (Lewis-Fernández and Kleinman 1995), the impact of the work of this group on DSM-IV reaffirms the growing view of culture as a crucial consideration in the practice of psychiatry and other mental health disciplines.

CULTURE AND PERSONALITY

DEVELOPMENTAL ISSUES

Culture plays a paramount role in the development of long-standing personality traits and should not be neglected when one is considering children's maturation and character formation. Stoller and Herdt (1982) described at length the socially prescribed way that male children are raised by the Sambia, a tribal people of New Guinea who hold in the highest esteem the maleness and warriorhood of its men. The authors outlined the ways in which the Sambia established first a strong and prolonged bond between mother and son, then went through unique and elaborate rituals to break that bond and ultimately develop strong heterosexual males. The clarity of the cultural expectation and reinforcing value of the rituals ensured the social outcome of heterosexual maleness.

Other workers have addressed issues such as the influence of culture on the development of dependency traits among West Indians (Allen 1985) and the culturally determined socialization toward trance and dissociative states among particular groups (Bateson 1975; Koss 1975).

In the inner cities, the cultural milieu often includes poverty, chronic exposure to crime, street and domestic violence, and substance abuse, as well as a predominance of young, undersupported single mothers who are heads of households. The impact of this upbringing cannot be overlooked when viewing a child from these origins. It has been stated that traits that are routinely characterized as antisocial may be culturally appropriate and defensive in nature within this culture (Reid 1985). However, other workers (Cohen and Brook 1987) have found such phenomena as family instability and parental inconsistency to be risk factors for later psychopathology in children, such as immature behavior and conduct disorder, the latter a known precursor to antisocial personality disorder. It is unclear what the long-term effects will be of protracted exposure to the chronic stress of such an environment. Nevertheless, Westermeyer (1995) suggested one possibility when he described enculturation as the process by which a well-functioning family passes on its culture to its offspring. He hypothesized that circumstances impairing the family's ability to enculturate their children adequately may result in individuals who are less able to resist substance abuse.

The positive impact of the extended family on the development of otherwise disadvantaged youth has been cited as an important compensatory factor, although its precise long-term effect has yet to be ascertained (Wilson 1989). Comer, in his well-known work toward enhancing the school's role in the development of children, has shown significant enhancement of the self-concept of students participating in his School Development Program (Haynes and Comer 1990).

Despite all we know about the relationship between culture and individual development, longstanding assumptions still deserve constant scrutiny and even occasional revision. This has been particularly evident in recent work on the theories of homosexual development and on the relationship between culture and gender identity. Litzenberger and Buttenheim (1998) have recently pointed out that current dominant cultural assumptions about gender, sexual orientation, and mental health must be reconsidered. This is especially necessary because of the degree to which societal assumptions about heterosexuality have so permeated psychological theories about gender and sexual orientation.

EFFECT ON INTRAPSYCHIC DEVELOPMENT

The influence of culture on intrapsychic development has been an important theme, and nowhere has this been more evident than in the work generated about the development of self-concept. As would be expected, this has been of special interest to minority groups in this country. It is an old hypothesis that, for example, American blacks possess significant self-hatred. This negative self-concept has been thought to be reinforced by the white dominant American culture that defines blackness as bad and inferior. Spurlock (1986) reviewed the research that focused on the development of self-concept in African American children, pointing out how the early conclusions have been subsequently challenged. Baldwin (1979) also reviewed the theoretical models and research that relate to this important question of black self-hatred and questioned the methodology and subsequent conclusions of the research. Margaret Beale Spencer's (1982, 1988) work has been instrumental in our reconceptualization of the influence of the cultural context on the development of self-concept in African American children. Much of her research has focused on the nature of the interrelationship among race awareness, race dissonance (white-biased preferences [e.g., Black children's preferential selection of white dolls over black dolls]), and self-concept. Prior to Spencer's research, findings of race dissonance in African American children had been interpreted as evidence of a negative self-concept for blacks, thus supporting the black self-hatred hypothesis. Her data have demonstrated that race dissonance and negative self-concept are not necessarily correlated. Instead, race dissonance among African American children may be a product of social learning that attributes negative characteristics to black people and things, rather than an expression of low self-esteem. Close scrutiny has therefore led to a view of the black self-hatred hypothesis as based on incomplete evidence and faulty interpretations of the data.

Other investigators have written eloquently about the process of developing and refining a positive racial identity (Cross 1991, 1995; Parham 1989; Phinney 1989). Cross has used the term *nigrescence* to refer to a process of resocialization or identity change that ideally leads a person to overcome a negative internalized racial self-concept. He concedes that such a process is not necessary if an African American already possesses a positive racial self-concept or relies on some aspect of personal identity other than race/ethnicity to derive positive self-esteem. However, an African American with a racial attitude ranging from race neutral to antiblack may begin the process of nigrescence following an encounter that challenges his or her racial belief system and values. Whether the encounter is positive in quality (e.g., a trip to an African country) or negative (e.g., the direct experience of racial discrimination), such an event would catalyze initiation of the process and eventually lead to a reconfiguration of the person's racial identity. Cross believed that nigrescence is not necessarily a one-time occurrence; subsequent encounters may initiate new cycles of nigrescence, leading to further progression towards a positive self-image. The theory of racial identity development has been validated through empirical testing and has indeed served as a model for understanding self-concept development of other socioracial and sociocultural groups (Downing and Roush 1985; Finnegan and McNally 1987).

Other equally important issues have been studied in regard to the effect of culture on intrapsychic development. Considerable work has been done on the cultural stimuli in American society that lead women to conceptualize their status as secondary to the male's position (Carmen et al. 1981). The assumption has been that cultural values and stereotypes have been at the core of the notions that women are, for example, unable to be first-rate airplane pilots or surgeons. In general, many workers have taken the position that restructuring such distorted values could lead to significant change in the way future generations of women will think about themselves. Authors such as Gilligan (1982) have shown how previously accepted hypotheses relating to intrapsychic development, identity formation, and even morality have been developed largely from the male perspective, resulting in a view of the female as lacking idealized male qualities, rather than as possessing desirable abilities and attributes.

In cultures where the inequities between the sexes are more explicit, more salient, and more rigid, women may resort to alternative ways of developing and wielding power. Constantinides (1985) has described the *zar* spirit possession cult in Ethiopia and Sudan as offering such an alternative. A woman possessed by a zar is able to act in a manner that is not routinely acceptable in a nonafflicted woman, and she may make demands upon her husband that would not be allowed under any other circumstances.

There are, of course, many values and taboos that a specific culture holds dear. The aggressiveness with which the culture makes clear that the values are important ultimately affects the basic mode of thinking and behavior of the individual. Many Caribbean cultures emphasize that sickness is a manifestation of one's standing with God or other spirits. Such belief enhances the individual's use of projection as an explanatory coping mechanism, but it also finally conditions the help-seeking behavior of the person and influences his or her degree of hope for recovery.

EFFECT ON INTERPERSONAL RELATIONSHIPS

It should follow that the work on culture and its effect on developmental and intrapsychic tasks might be extrapo-

lated to conclusions or hypotheses about interpersonal relationships. Consequently, observations that led to assertions about the development of masculinity in particular societies were also ultimately used to clarify theories about homosexual and transsexual behavior. In the Sambia observations, the powerful and intense initiation rituals, coupled with the values and behavioral interventions of the males, led to the exclusion of transsexual behavior in that culture.

Similarly, females in American culture, who have thought of themselves as unable to perform certain jobs that have traditionally been held by males, have then in turn related hesitantly to the males, who have naturally been viewed as having all the power. Delgado et al. (1985) have pointed out that in the business world it has long been assumed that females are submissive, dependent, not adventurous, suggestible, noncompetitive, excitable when facing crises, likely to have their feelings hurt, emotional, and conceited about their appearance. The expectation has also been that such traits render a woman unable to make managerial decisions with confidence and dispatch. Alternatively, it has been argued that the female business manager who, in effect, behaves like a man in this type of job would be considered a "castrating woman."

It is in fact fairly easy to demonstrate that society, through its enunciation of values and beliefs, can affect and order the nature of interpersonal relationships. For example, a group's view of the aging members of their population can influence whether old people are revered or put away to die. The ancient problem of war has also been frequently thought to be a function of how some cultures revere belligerence and the domination of other groups, not to mention how the perception of intergroup differences can lead to hatred and ethnic strife. Similarly, the process whereby specific subgroups such as the deaf population are stigmatized is a culture-mediated process. It is the values and stereotypes held by the hearing majority group that leads to the interpersonal difficulties between stigmatizer and stigmatized.

Nevertheless, it cannot be assumed that one can draw a straight line of linkage from a baby's early experiences with his or her mother, who is the very embodiment of that culture's values, to the specific type of personality that characterizes the adult the baby has become. Schweder (1979) has pointed out that it is indeed difficult to be sure how specific child-rearing practices can lead to adult behavior that is predictable in a multiplicity of contexts. Such caution is a useful reminder that culture, as a single element, should never be taken as the only determinant of thinking or behavior.

FREQUENCY OF PSYCHIATRIC DISORDERS

Attempts to establish the frequency of psychiatric disorders across cultures have been fraught with difficulties. Some of the problems discussed in the section on symptom expression account for the complexities encountered here. Another significant issue arises from the fact that researchers and clinicians have been unable to agree about diagnostic categories. On the one hand, there are country-specific diagnoses, such as the classic *bouffées délirantes* of the French. This is an acute psychotic state that Americans would view as schizophrenia or bipolar illness. On the other hand, it has been well established that schizophrenia tends to be a broader category in the United States than it is in many other countries. There are diagnoses such as involutional paraphrenia that are used in other countries but that do not find currency in the United States. Establishing the frequency of disorders has now become a complex undertaking, because in one culture, for example, the abuse of alcohol may not be viewed in quite the same way as in another culture. Consequently, groups may tend to report it with differing frequency. As Westermeyer (1985) has pointed out, diagnosis in many countries may be a function of attitudes, political beliefs, historical influences, and even economic factors. Recently, Weissman et al. (1996) published the results of a cross-national epidemiologic study. Their population-based study involved 10 national sites and 38,000 community subjects. The study demonstrated great variability of the lifetime rates of depression across countries ranging from 1.5% in Taiwan to 19% in Lebanon; rates of bipolar disorder were more uniform. The variability of depression rates raised questions about whether cultural differences or different risk factors affected the expression of this disorder.

In the United States, significant problems have been associated with health care surveys of all the minority populations, specifically those of Native American, Hispanic, African, and Asian heritage. Much has been said about the task of identifying and sampling such groups, the complexity of achieving their cooperation, the tendency among many of the subgroups simply to answer yes to any interviewer's questions, the difficulty in designing valid interview protocols, and the complexity of controlling the bias of interviewers. In addition, there have often been technical difficulties associated with the preparation of interviewers who may not use the language of their respondents. The survey instruments may have been developed and validated using populations other than the minority groups. Even in this country, much of the work done has reflected contradictory results, some of which seem related to either the sampling or the methodologies used.

Williams (1986), reviewing the epidemiology of mental illness in African Americans, noted emerging difficulties in the NIMH-sponsored Epidemiologic Catchment Area (ECA) program. For example, the ECA surveys attempted to obtain good samples of African Americans by including inner-city communities. However, Williams suggested this was biased in favor of low-income African American males. Consequently, he questioned whether middle-class and other African Americans would be surveyed.

There were early claims that depression was rare among American blacks (Schwab 1978), and, indeed, conclusions have been drawn from these original data that few African Americans commit suicide (Prudhomme 1938). More recent work consistently contradicted such earlier findings (King 1982) and suggested that those earlier conclusions were a function of the bias of the observers who were conducting such work. Serious consideration of all this cross-cultural scholarship leads inevitably to the conclusion that relatively little is understood about the incidence and prevalence of psychiatric disorders across different nations and cultures. It is also equally difficult to sort out in a specific group what influence culture may have on the finding that a particular psychiatric disorder occurs commonly whereas another disorder is rarely encountered. Part of the complexity may stem from the fact that it is not clear whether the high rates of one disorder exert a protective effect that results in the low rates of the other disorder, or whether the disorder with high rates masks the expression of the other disorder. This is seen, for example, in some cultures where extensive alcohol abuse appears to mask the expression of depression or schizophrenia.

Hatch and Friedman (1996) recently argued that at the clinical practice level it may be quite difficult to appreciate the true frequency of a psychiatric disorder because of interference from cultural elements. They gave obsessive-compulsive disorder (OCD) as an example and pointed out that OCD was thought to be evenly distributed across racial groups. Yet, African Americans with OCD were difficult to find in clinical settings. The authors suggested that cultural differences influenced both the relatively low help-seeking behavior by blacks and the tendency for underdiagnosis of OCD in the same population.

It is hoped that the recent efforts to make DSM-IV a more culturally informed work has led to diagnostic categories that will retain more of their meaning in cross-cultural diagnostic endeavors.

CULTURE, SYMPTOMS, AND DIAGNOSIS

SYMPTOM EXPRESSION

The International Pilot Study of Schizophrenia (IPSS) was a transcultural psychiatric investigation of 1,202 patients in nine countries: Colombia, the former Czechoslovakia, Denmark, India, Nigeria, Taiwan, the former Soviet Union, Great Britain, and the United States. Although it was not an epidemiological survey, a major task of the project was to engender methods that might be used in different cultures to evaluate patients (Strauss et al. 1976). Specific interview schedules were used to collect data on patients who had already been admitted to treatment facilities.

Some conclusions from the IPSS merit consideration (Table 40–2). Certain symptoms (e.g., phenomena reported by patients, such as hallucinations and delusions) were the object of greatest interrater reliability, although the reliability was better for raters from the same center than for raters from different centers. In contrast to this finding, the data showed that the rating of signs gathered by observation rather than by self-report, such as flatness of affect or incongruity of affect, was below acceptable reliability ranges. Historical information, such as that having to do with patients' prior level of functioning, personality traits, work history, and social relationships, showed even more cross-cultural variability. This work suggested that some cross-cultural psychiatric information might be reliable, although it depended on what type of information one was collecting. Symptoms reported by patients would be a more useful reference point for comparison than signs rated by observers, and premorbid history may be misleading when viewed by a clinician from a culture different from the patient's. Consequently, the cross-cultural diagnosis of paranoid schizophrenia (for which there is substantial reliance on symptomatology) might be more reliable than the cross-cultural diagnosis of catatonic schizophrenia (for which the physician relies on observation of signs).

The IPSS project also found that across the nine centers, depressed patients with psychotic symptoms were among the most similar of any diagnostic category. Symptoms that characterized these patients in different centers were depressed mood, gloomy thoughts, hopelessness, early morning waking, delusions of self-depreciation, and sleep problems. These findings demonstrated that through the use of specific interview techniques, it was possible to rely on symptom expression to delineate certain disorders such as paranoid schizophrenia and psychotic depression. However, the researchers did point out that better instruments were needed to collect data that could be used in establishing relationships between symptomatology and social functioning.

Adebimpe et al. (1982) participated in a 5-year international study of schizophrenic patients. Analyzing a subset of the U.S. data, these authors looked at differences in severity of symptoms between black and white patients and between urban and rural patients. Their schizophrenic patients included several subtypes, and the raters used the Brief Psychiatric Rating Scale, the Itil-Keskiner Psychopathological Rating Scale, and structured in-person interviews. African American patients were found to exhibit the following severe symptoms when compared with white patients: auditory hallucinations, memory disturbances, disorientation, angry outbursts, and impulsiveness. The urban schizophrenic patients were less angry, aggressive, silly, negativistic, and uncooperative than the rural patients, while exhibiting more anxiety, rigidity, ambivalence, posturing, and asocial behavior. Although the authors appropriately expressed caution regarding some of the differential manner in which clinicians perceived black as opposed to white patients or rural as opposed to urban patients, they felt their findings could be seen as reflecting a differentiation of emotional states that was linked to contrasts in the culture of the patients. Studies such as this one have suggested quite strongly that the symptomatic expressions of specific psychiatric disorders may vary as a function of the culture of the patients. This possibility should not be seen as being at odds with the IPSS findings that clinicians from different cultures may be able to agree in their delineation of a subgroup of

TABLE 40–2. General trends in cross-cultural diagnosis (International Pilot Study on Schizophrenia)

Diagnostic information	How obtained	Reliability
Symptoms (e.g., hallucinations, delusions)	Patient report	Acceptable
Signs (e.g., flatness of affect, incongruity of affect)	Observation	Unacceptable
Historical data (e.g., work history, social relationships)	Synthesis of cross cultural exchange	Least acceptable

individuals who carry a similar diagnosis.

Marsella (1988) has elaborated a view of the interplay of biology, psychology, and culture that describes an inverse relationship between the extent that a disorder is biologically based (i.e., internal) and the impact of environmental (external) factors on a disorder's clinical presentation (Table 40–3). Marsella posited that a disorder primarily shaped by biological forces will have less variability between cultures than a disorder whose primary causation is social or environmental. Such a model predicts that the presentation of a cerebrovascular accident, for example, would have much less cross-cultural variability than would a dissociative disorder, the latter having a much larger presumed component from the social and environmental sphere. Psychotic and mood disorders, thought to have a sizable biological determinant but also to be strongly influenced by the sociocultural milieu, should fall between these two extremes with regard to their degree of cross-cultural variability.

In regard to the more basic notion of how culture may affect the expression of distress, studies and other observations of Puerto Ricans have been particularly interesting. Rates of reported symptoms among Puerto Ricans seem to have remained high in all socioeconomic classes and were noted to be higher when compared in the same studies with respondents from other cultural groups. Haberman (1976) specifically attempted to explain the finding that Puerto Ricans living and surveyed in Puerto Rico had higher symptom scores than did Puerto Ricans surveyed in New York City. Also, the severity of the psychiatric symptom scores of the Puerto Ricans in New York lessened as the length of time that the individuals had lived in the city increased. After considering other possible arguments, Haberman concluded that culture seemed to account for the Puerto Ricans' willingness to express their subjective distress; as they acculturated to New York City, their traditional response style was tempered.

The ECA study, conducted in the last decade, appeared to confirm that Puerto Ricans reported somatic symptoms out of proportion to the rest of the population, resulting in a higher mean number of somatization symptoms detected by the Diagnostic Interview Schedule (Escobar 1987). Guarnaccia et al. (1989b) subsequently reviewed these data after having created a measure to quantify the existence of *ataques de nervios*, a culturally accepted syndrome used to express personal distress. Their results implied that the "excessive" somatic symptoms picked up by the structured interview were related to the presence of *ataques de nervios* in this population, a syndrome that the interview schedule was not looking for and consequently did not find. In a similar way, Malgady et al. (1996) conducted focus groups of Puerto Rican adults aimed at developing meaningful idioms of expression. They then compared a group of clinic subjects to a group of nonpatients with regard to the presence of idioms of anger. An idiom of vindictive hostility, such as "It pays to remember who your enemies are," was found to correlate weakly with symptoms of anxiety and depression but was not predictive of a person's clinical status. An idiom of aggression, however, such as "At times, it is difficult to control my temper," was more strongly correlated with both anxiety and depression, and also predicted clinical status. It follows that when these idioms are not "seen" by diagnostic tools that do not anticipate their existence, it can influence the rate of diagnosis of anxiety and depressive disorders in this population. Caution therefore suggests that the use of etic diagnostic systems that are not tempered by knowledge of indigenous (i.e., emic) categories may lead to unexplainable or meaningless results. Not only does culture affect the expression of distress, but it can also act to hamper one's ability to identify and characterize distress in an individual from another culture.

CULTURE AND DIAGNOSTIC CLASSIFICATION

It has been a general assumption that culture has a significant effect on the determination of diagnostic categories. This axiom stems at least partly from the observation that different cultures are often in disagreement as to what behavior they label normal or abnormal. Wig (1983), in suggesting that culture has powerfully influenced diagnostic classification systems, noted that current American and European classification systems have elevated emotions such as anxiety and depression to the level of specific disor-

TABLE 40–3. Hypothesized impact of internal (biological) and external (psychosocial) factors on cross-cultural variability of clinical presentation

Clinical entity	Biological factors	Psychosocial factors	Cross-cultural variability
Cerebrovascular accident	***	*	Low
Psychotic disorders	**	**	Moderate
Dissociative disorders	*	***	High

ders. But he wondered why other emotions such as jealousy or hatred have not been treated in the same way. Wig was making the point that jealousy and hatred might be treated with much more emphasis in other cultures and therefore in a non–Euro-American system could be considered worthy of consideration as specific disorders.

The categorization or definition of normal behavior is, of course, a culture-bound phenomenon. Consequently, someone who suffers from hysterical drop attacks might be considered in one culture to be an individual who has received a special blessing, rather than someone in need of medical or psychiatric attention. Another such example has centered on the phenomenon of homosexuality. Even within the United States, the question of whether homosexuality is abnormal behavior has been the topic of significant discussion and disagreement among the lay public. Psychiatrists have not been exempt from this disagreement, eventually changing the "diagnosis" from homosexuality to "ego-dystonic" homosexuality (American Psychiatric Association 1980, p. 281), until arriving at the classification of "persistent and marked distress about one's sexual orientation" as a sexual disorder not otherwise specified (NOS) in DSM-III-R (American Psychiatric Association 1987, p. 296), which did not change in DSM-IV. An important criterion that has been reaffirmed by such changes is that any syndrome must be associated with subjective distress and/or help-seeking behavior in order to be classified as a disorder.

Fabrega (1992) has warned us quite eloquently of the inherent cultural character of biomedical psychiatry, and has introduced, as an alternative to the biomedical "disease" concept, the culturally neutral concept of the "Human Behavioral Breakdown (HBB)" as "sustained anomalies of behavior [that are] not willful and evaluated negatively [from within the culture]" (Fabrega 1992, p. 93). Using this model, he strongly advocated a view of illness that is guided by what he termed "symbolic, culturally relevant parameters of social behavior" (p. 100).

The way in which a particular culture defines hallucinations has also led to extended debate over the years. A Caribbean case example is particularly relevant here. A West Indian child voiced complaints about visual hallucinations that she was experiencing. This young girl was a member of a very fundamentalist religious group. She had been taken by her mother to the pastor of the group because the child had recounted stories of having seen strange figures that no one else could see. The pastor listened attentively to both child and mother and then spent considerable time in calming the mother's fears. Then he reinterpreted the hallucinations and restructured them in a context that was acceptable to the mother and consonant with the religious beliefs of the group to which they all belonged. In fact, the pastor attributed special religious characteristics to the objects that had been perceived in the visual hallucinations and convinced the mother that the child was especially chosen by Christ to have the experience. All of this clearly led to a redefinition of symptomatology that might have been perceived as abnormal. The child was not subsequently referred to a physician, and the whole affair was concluded in a manner that was at least temporarily satisfactory to everyone. The child's experience had been redefined as being normal.

Such differences over the definitions of normal and abnormal are not simply academic and do not relate only to settling what appears at first to be a straightforward disagreement. There are other important implications that flow from the resolution of this basic question. As mentioned above, general health behavior and help-seeking behavior are products of the process that defines normality. Waxler (1974) has reminded us that the views of the society not only influence the diagnosis of the disorder but, in fact, also condition the treatment and even the prognosis of what might be ultimately diagnosed as normal. In the case of the West Indian child above, both the mother's help-seeking behavior and her satisfaction with the diagnosis derived from a cultural world view that she accepted. In this case, even the short-term prognosis was a by-product of the cultural context, because the mother, as a result of the pastor's intervention, rejected a sick role for her daughter.

There are, of course, limitations to the power of redefining emotions and behavior in the context of the person's culture in order to "depathologize" them. The idea that all pathology stems from cultural incongruities is just as implausible as attributing all psychopathology to biological processes while ignoring social and environmental influences. Several workers (Levy et al. 1979; Neutra et al. 1977) followed the lives of Navajo persons with epilepsy who presented with "hand-trembling," a symptom viewed by the Navajo as a positive sign of power and ability to become a "shaman-like diagnostician" (Neutra et al. 1977, p. 256). These authors discovered no evidence that the culture provided any protection from physical suffering or that it allowed the sufferer continued privileged status or problem-free function within Navajo society.

Culture has possibly influenced diagnostic practices in ways that still await further clarification. For example, little attention has been given to how sociocultural factors such as poverty might influence the expression of psychiatric disorders. Poverty can produce malnutrition that in turn could potentially influence the expression of psychiatric illness. As mentioned earlier, poverty can lead to exposure to a multitude of stressors besides that of material need. Inner-city neighborhoods have more than their share of violence, chemical dependence, and crime, all of which can affect an individual's view of life, and all of which need to be taken into consideration by a culturally informed clinician.

The issue of diagnostic reliability across different cultures has already been dealt with earlier in the discussion of the World Health Organization's multicenter pilot study of schizophrenia that took place in several countries. It should be reemphasized here that clinicians across cultures can reach agreements in some areas, but, as has been previously noted, they find it difficult to agree in others.

Particular problems have been posed by the phenomenon of bereavement. American psychiatrists have tried to delineate carefully where uncomplicated bereavement ends and clinical depression starts. However, such attempts at categorization seem to fall short when the culture sanctions a recently bereaved individual's hearing the voice or the footsteps of the deceased relative. An appreciation of the specific culture's view of bereavement and a careful delineation of the patient's relationship to the dead relative in the context of the culture can help the psychiatrist avoid the error of diagnosing a psychotic depression when uncomplicated bereavement really exists. Eisenbruch (1984) has provided an extensive review of the ethnic and cultural variations in the development of bereavement practices that should be useful to clinicians interested in this complex phenomenon.

Significant cultural variability exists in the manner in which an individual is able or chooses to express inner turmoil. Many workers (Florsheim 1990; Katon et al. 1982; White 1982) have noted that the phenomenon of expressing distress verbally and emotionally, seen predominantly in North American and Western European societies, is not a cultural given for the rest of the world. The experience and expression of distress not only as a mental but also as a bodily dysfunction, dubbed "somatization" by Western cultures, seems to be the global rule, not the exception. "Psychologization," or the experience and expression of distress in primarily mental or psychological terms, seems to be a culture-bound phenomenon in the West, perhaps a vestige of outdated theories of mind-body duality (Goodman 1991). Problems have arisen when individuals subscribing to one of these views attempt to diagnose those individuals whose culture leads them to experience the world differently. Recently, Weiss et al. (1995) reported on a group of patients in India who were studied using both the Structured Clinical Interview for DSM-III-R (SCID; Spitzer et al. 1990) and the Explanatory Model Interview Catalogue (EMIC; Weiss et al. 1986), the latter being a semistructured interview designed to produce a view of illness from the patient's perspective. They commented that, although it was the style of most patients to complain of symptoms that were somatic in nature, the SCID, based on the Western diagnostic schema, had a strong tendency to interpret these complaints into a diagnosis of depression. Thus, recent Western diagnostic systems and classifications may yield results that reflect their ethnocentric bias at the expense of clinical accuracy.

Language, as a subset of culture, has a more concrete influence on diagnosis. For example, questions have been raised about the existence of depression as a concept in some languages. Some cultures facilitate the expression of complaints, whereas other cultures may inhibit the communication of inner feelings to health professionals. But in a transcultural context, language is also thought to have another special influence. This occurs when a health professional performs the assessment of a patient whose language is different from that of the clinician. Marcos (1975) found marked distortions when evaluations of patients were conducted through interpreters, even when such interpreters were proficient. Westermeyer (1985) noted that interpreters do fairly well in obtaining the pertinent factual information in a case but do considerably less well when asked to interpret affect. Both minimization and exaggeration of symptoms have been mentioned as results of such interviews. To lessen distortions, translators should be well versed in psychiatry, should not be family members, should be familiar with the patient's culture, and should attempt to translate all utterances of both participants verbatim. In addition, the interviewing clinician should meet with the translator both before and after the interview, as a way of processing some of the intangible, nonverbal components of the interview.

DSM-IV and the Cultural Context

As mentioned earlier, the Task Force on DSM-IV and, specifically the large group of cultural advisors to the Task Force, labored extensively over the 3 years prior to the work's publication to help produce a diagnostic classification that was more clinically accurate and contained a better integration of biomedical, social, psychological, and cultural concepts of illness and diagnosis.

An important result of these efforts has been the *cultural formulation*, devised as a way of integrating an individual's cultural and experiential context into the scope of diagnosis (Mezzich and Good 1997). An explanatory outline for deriving the cultural formulation can be found in Appendix I of DSM-IV (American Psychiatric Association 1994). It focuses the diagnostician's attention on five components of cultural data (Table 40–4), the synthesis of which then produces a more complete view of the individual within the cultural context. These five components include the following:

1. The cultural identity of the individual, including the contrast between culture of origin and host culture in immigrant or ethnic minority individuals
2. Cultural explanations of the individual's illness, such as idioms of distress, culturally based meaning of symptoms, and perceived causes or models for illness
3. Cultural factors related to psychosocial environment, including culturally informed interpretations of problems with social support and environmental stressors
4. Cultural aspects of the relationship between individual and clinician, including potential barriers to understanding and assessing the meaning of symptoms
5. An overall assessment of how the cultural context influences the diagnosis and the approaches to treatment

Mezzich (1996) has commented that the sparse presentation of the appendix and its somewhat recondite placement in the DSM as the ninth appendix (the "I" is a letter, not a roman numeral) has limited the accessibility to clinicians of concepts that are perhaps worthy of their own axis in the multiaxial schema (Guarnaccia 1996; Mezzich 1996; Weiss 1996).

Within the text of DSM-IV, reference to cultural variability was quite explicitly made in sections that describe possible culturally based presentations for each major category of illness. An attempt was therefore made to avoid an ethnocentric approach to diagnosis. For example, the section on mood disorders mentions the variable meaning of somatic complaints, a number of culturally derived attribu-

TABLE 40–4. Components of the cultural formulation

- Cultural identity of individual, including contrast between culture of origin and host culture
- Cultural explanations of individual's illness (e.g. idioms of distress, culturally based meaning of symptoms, perceived causes or models for illness)
- Cultural factors related to psychosocial environment, including culturally informed interpretations of problems with social support, environmental stressors
- Cultural aspects of relationship between individual and clinician, including potential barriers to understanding the meaning of symptoms
- Overall assessment of how cultural context influences diagnosis and approaches to treatment

tions of illness, and warns about the inappropriateness of interpreting idioms of distress as hallucinations or delusions.

Also important are the comments added to the section on personality disorders, the diagnosis of which is known to have some relative difficulty with interrater reliability. In particular, the DSM now warns that the cluster A disorders may be overdiagnosed in individuals whose culture, ethnicity, or status as immigrants or minorities may promote a paranoid or schizoid, but nevertheless adaptive, personality style. Antisocial personality disorder, in cluster B, may also be prone to overuse in oppressed subsets of the population in which such a stance is adaptive. The diagnosis of dependent personality disorder and avoidant personality disorder should also not be made without taking into account cultural norms for behavior and communication and the cultural stressors of migration, respectively.

RACE AND DIAGNOSIS

Race differs from culture in that, by definition, it is generally outwardly evident and therefore may be the first thing that a clinician usually knows about a patient (and that a patient knows about a clinician). If these two individuals happen to reside in a setting where the race of one is privileged in comparison with the race of the other, then differences take on further clinical significance.

Adebimpe (1981) described how African American patients in the United States were overdiagnosed in some categories and underdiagnosed in others. It is an important claim that was suggested earlier by Bell and Mehta (1980) and amplified and reviewed by Jones and Gray (1986). Adebimpe had reviewed several studies and concluded from the data that the apparent misdiagnosis of African Americans in comparison with whites resulted in African Americans' being found more often to be schizophrenic and less often to have mood disorders. However, Adebimpe realized that the data did not provide an answer to whether African American clinicians made the errors less often than white clinicians. There are also obvious implications here that erroneous diagnosing ultimately suggests the execution of inappropriate treatment plans and the communication of negative prognoses to the African American patients. In addition, the overdiagnosis of schizophrenic disorders in bipolar African American patients may result in their undue exposure to long-term treatment with antipsychotics, thereby increasing these patients' risk of developing tardive dyskinesia.

Several reasons have been given for these alleged errors in diagnosis (Adebimpe 1981; Jones and Gray 1986), all of which are related to the amount of social and cultural distance between patient and clinician, which in part is dependent on race. These differences are manifested in the areas of vocabulary, styles of interaction, values, and modes of communicating distress. Stereotypes of African-American psychopathology have also been evoked as partially responsible. For example, Jones and Gray (1986) reminded us of the long-held belief that African Americans are always cheerful and that having so little, they are unable to experience object loss. Also, differences in African Americans' expression of depression may lead to missing the diagnosis. It has been suggested that African Americans somatize a great deal more than white patients. Racial differences can also lead to misperceptions of the clinician by the patient. It is not unlikely that a patient from a nondominant race will react to a clinician from the majority race with feelings of suspicion and anger, which in turn may be interpreted by the clinician as paranoia, lability, or avoidance.

An interesting example is the recent case of a black American psychiatrist attempting to diagnose depression in a black African simply by looking at the African's face. The psychiatrist had not talked to the African but pointed out that because the African had to be an oppressed individual, the saddened face was ample proof of a depressive disorder. Such obviously problematic reasoning points out that no particular cultural group is above making arrogant assumptions about another group that eventually lead to erroneous diagnoses and problematic treatment.

Considerable emphasis has been placed on the bias inherent in the instruments that are used to aid clinicians in making diagnostic conclusions. African Americans have been noted to score higher than whites on several scales of the Minnesota Multiphasic Personality Inventory (MMPI), including the schizophrenia scale (Gynther 1972). This finding has been used to raise questions about the conclusions clinicians may reach from the use of scales that have not been originally validated on African American populations (Greene 1987). Dana and Whatley (1991) cited a number of reasons that the MMPI has limited utility in interracial diagnosis. These include the inventory's lack of social, economic, and political considerations; the intrinsic limitations of comparative norms; the use of stereotypes; and neglect of the impact of the assessor's role on interpretation.

Indeed, there have been extensive arguments on the topic of intelligence testing in the African American community, and a most incisive summary has been provided by Samuda (1973). Williams (1987) also has summarized the general issues relating to the psychological testing of minority patients. On the one hand, it has been pointed out that the definition of the intelligence quotient is precise

and that there is nothing wrong with the use of intelligence tests, even if the tests do nothing but measure the adaptation of a black individual to a white middle-class view of American life. Others have taken opposing views and emphasized that intelligence testing of blacks should be discontinued because the tests were standardized and normalized on white middle-class individuals. Furthermore, such opponents of the use of intelligence testing often have pointed out that the test results are misapplied and that the reference bases for the tests are obscure. Finally, they have frequently underlined the point that the test scores are inappropriately applied to predictions about African Americans that often spell a dim future for this already disadvantaged subgroup of the population.

Neighbors et al. (1989) reviewed research on race and diagnosis and highlighted two opposing viewpoints, neither of which has been unequivocally supported by recent studies. According to Neighbors and colleagues, workers have either 1) taken the position that diagnosticians assume racially based differences where there is none, or 2) assumed that racially based differences do exist but are unwittingly ignored by those making a diagnosis. Both hypotheses obviously would result in misdiagnosis, and the authors emphasized the need for further empirical research to resolve this dilemma.

Finally, it is important to remember that the concept of "race," based on overt physical differences between groups, cannot be taken to imply clinical uniformity. For example, it would be meaningless to group together people from Japan and China as "Asian" and expect that they feel, think, and behave in some racially determined pattern. In the same vein, Cohen et al. (1997) found remarkable differences in clinical presentation between African American and African Caribbean psychiatric outpatients, highlighting the importance of cultural, rather than racial factors in symptom expression and presentation.

GENDER AND DIAGNOSIS

Although a thorough discussion of the impact of gender differences on diagnosis is beyond the scope of this chapter, some mention must be made of recent developments and thinking regarding this topic.

An interesting trend within cultural psychiatry has been to examine gender differences in the presentation of some culture-bound syndromes. Some authors (Constantinides 1985; Littlewood and Lipsedge 1987) have commented that although sexism is a global issue, there are cultural differences in the way that women respond to gender discrimination or oppression. Various others (Bemporad et al. 1988; Gremillion 1992) have viewed anorexia nervosa as a culture-specific manifestation of conflict in women who are reacting to unrealistic expectations imposed by the present "Western" culture. As previously mentioned, Constantinides (1985) viewed some forms of spirit possession predominant in women in Somalia and Ethiopia as a culturally accepted manner of achieving a modicum of power within an otherwise sexually oppressive society. Littlewood and Lipsedge (1987) hypothesized that, just as the world of the Somali and Ethiopian women is dominated by the male-run Islam, the world of "Western" women is similarly dominated by male-run "biomedicine," in which response to gender differences may tend toward pathologizing women's behavior.

It has been argued that the whole gamut of personality disorders reflects an inherent bias of male psychiatrists against females. Consequently, males in this society would tend to approve the competitive style of male professionals while condemning and labeling the same behavior in females as narcissistic and destructive. Many workers have also felt that the definition of sexual dysfunctions has really been based on male conceptions of female sexuality. Once again, the increasing participation and outspokenness of females in the general society have led to a redefinition and reconsideration of the standards for defining normal sexual functioning in females.

It is commonplace to point out how male therapists, rooted in their culture-bound views of maleness, make errors in dealing with female patients. But it is also important to emphasize that female therapists can make similar mistakes. For example, American female therapists have difficulty understanding the dependency that women from other cultures show toward their men. Such female therapists may give clear prescriptive guidelines to foreign women to stop being subservient and to treat their men as equals. The clinician in these cases may be unconcerned about the impact that such advice would have on a woman coming from a family that was culturally different from that of the therapist.

CULTURE-SPECIFIC SYNDROMES

Considerable work has been done on the description of syndromes that psychiatrists consider either to be unique to certain cultures or to occur with special frequency among a defined group of people. As would be expected, questions remain as to whether there are special elements in a given culture that favor the development of endemic clinical entities. It also remains to be clarified whether syndromes seemingly particular to one culture or geographic distribution have clinical counterparts in other areas or cultures.

The DSM-IV defines *mental disorder* as a "clinically significant behavioral or psychological syndrome or pattern that . . . is associated with present distress (e.g., a painful symptom) or disability (impairment in . . . functioning) or with a significantly increased risk of suffering death, pain, disability, or an important loss of freedom" (American Psychiatric Association 1994, p. xxi). Recent questions have arisen about why clinically significant and distressing symptom patterns seen as "bound" to non-Western cultures retain the status of syndrome, whereas other symptom patterns, seen as clearly bound to Western culture, are reified as "disorders" (Hughes 1996). With this in mind, it is important to understand that the separate discussion of culture-bound syndromes is arbitrary, because at the present time there is no good reason for some of the entities discussed below to be excluded as disorders from the current diagnostic schema used in the United States.

It is also interesting that many of the syndromes classified as "culture-bound" have components of either somatization, dissociation, or both. Of all diagnostic categories in the DSM, those of somatoform and dissociative disorders are the ones most likely to be influenced by environmental and social forces. To make the diagnosis of a somatoform disorder, one must first exclude any biological component. History of social or environmental trauma or conflict predisposes an individual to dissociative disorders. It therefore makes sense that phenomena that demonstrate either dissociative or somatoform pathology would show the most cross-cultural variability, as theorized by Marsella (1988) and previously shown in Table 40–3.

Difficulty in the clarification and understanding of syndromes thought to be specific or bound to a given culture can be appreciated when one attempts to examine anxiety states or the mourning phenomenon across cultures. Most of us would agree that anxiety is a ubiquitous human experience. However, its clinical forms are well known to vary considerably from one country to another. It is unclear whether the anxious West Indian who somatizes is experiencing the same condition as the American who panics. Are these two conditions correspondingly equivalent states, and is culture the major differentiating element? Furthermore, there may be a specific cultural belief that strongly permeates the clinical entity. Consequently, a West Indian may see his or her somatic complaints as the result of having been hexed. It is often the existence of a framework of special meaning in which the symptoms have been couched that makes observers so commonly confident that the clinical syndrome is unique and lacking an equivalent state in another culture.

The following are some examples of culture-bound syndromes (see also Table 40–5):

TABLE 40–5. **Culture-specific syndromes**

Syndrome	Geographic or ethnic distribution	Clinical presentation
Ataques de nervios	The Americas, people of Hispanic heritage	Socially sanctioned display of grief or conflict, characterized by agitation, unfocused aggression, lability of mood, fluctuating levels of consciousness, difficulty moving limbs, hyperventilation.
"Falling out" "Blacking out" *Indisposition*	African Americans Bahamians Haitians	Occurs in response to great emotional excitement, characterized by collapse, inability to move, loss of volitional movement without loss of sensory consciousness or of bowel or bladder control.
Amok	Various locations and ethnicities, including Asia, Africa, New Guinea	Follows a personal humiliation, characterized by prodromal brooding, followed by sudden, uncontrollable homicidal rage, then full or partial amnesia for the episode.
Pibloktoq *Chakore* *Grisi siknis* "Frenzy witchcraft"	Arctic natives Ngawbere tribe, Panama Miskito tribe, Nicaragua Navajo, United States	Prodromal lethargic, depressed, anxious state, followed by agitated, seemingly purposeless running, ending in exhaustion, sleep, and amnesia for the episode.
Koro	Various countries in Asia	Feelings of panic brought about by the conviction that one's genitalia are retracting into the abdomen and that this phenomenon will result in death.
Anorexia, bulimia	North America	Bizarre eating patterns, apparently resulting from distorted body image, characterized either by severe caloric restriction, food bingeing and/or purging.
Spirit possession	Numerous cases reported in Asia, Africa	Brief, reversible episodes of dissociation, characterized by the victim's behaving as if possessed by a spirit or deity, and followed by amnesia for the episode.
Multiple personality disorder	Primarily North America, Western Europe	Chronic dissociative syndrome, usually associated with severe abuse in childhood, characterized by the sufferer's experience of two or more "personalities" coexisting and vying for control of the individual.
Hwa-byung	Korean nationals and Korean Americans	Ascribed to "excess anger," chronic frustration, adversity. Characterized by sensation of an epigastric mass, anorexia, anxiety, dyspnea, epigastric pain.
Generalized somatic syndromes ("brain-fag," *Ode Ori, shinkeishitsu*, neurasthenia, others)	Asia, Africa, the Americas	Characterized by low mental and physical energy, poor sleep, vague somatic complaints.

Ataques de Nervios

Described in Puerto Rican and other Hispanic groups (Guarnaccia et al. 1989a, 1989b), *ataques de nervios* refers to a socially sanctioned display of grief or great conflict characterized by "difficulty moving limbs, loss of consciousness or mind going blank, memory loss, [and symptoms of hyperventilation in which] . . . the person begins to shout, swear and strike out at others, [then] falls to the ground and either experiences convulsive body movements or lies 'as if dead'" (Guarnaccia et al. 1989b, p. 280). Generally, the episode is self-limited and may last only minutes. At other times, it is severe and extends to a few days, or the victim may suffer frequent attacks with few precipitating stressors, leading to distress and help-seeking behavior. Recent workers (González and Griffith 1996) have advocated the classification of this syndrome under the general category of dissociative disorders, whereas others have focused on the somatic and pseudoepileptiform aspects to favor its being classified as a somatoform disorder. The mere fact that a syndrome exists that straddles these two categories questions the wisdom of making hard distinctions between somatoform and dissociative disorders.

"Falling Out"

Seen among black Americans but also called "blacking out" by Bahamians and *indisposition* by Haitians in Miami (Kirmayer et al. 1995; Philippe and Romain 1979), "falling out" characteristically occurs in response to a high degree of emotional excitement, such as may occur in the setting of a religious ceremony, during an argument, in fear-producing situations, or in "profound sexual conflict" (Weidman 1979, p. 99). Those who manifest this syndrome often simply collapse but without biting the tongue or losing the contents of bowel or bladder. There is an accompanying lack of ability to speak or move, even though the individual hears and understands. Although some have favored the addition of trance and possession trance disorder to the section on dissociative disorders in DSM-IV (González et al. 1997), the present decision to include the syndrome's description under dissociative disorder NOS is still a substantial improvement in the manual's cross-cultural scope.

Amok

This phenomenon was traditionally associated with Malaya (Carr 1978), but has been described as occurring also in Africa and more rarely in Papua, New Guinea (Burton-Bradley 1968). Often, there is a prodromal period of brooding after an incident during which the victim (almost always male) has felt slighted or humiliated. What follows is a sudden, uncontrollable rage that leads to the individual's aimlessly running around with a weapon that is ultimately used to kill a number of people or animals. Sometimes the perpetrator then kills himself. Those captured alive have claimed no memory of the killing (Schmidt et al. 1977). Although some studies have shown the syndrome to be associated with psychotic disorders (Tan and Carr 1977), this does not appear to be a uniform finding. Although some workers (Gaw and Bernstein 1992; Spiegel and Cardeña 1991) have favored the inclusion of *amok* as an impulse control disorder, the final outcome of discussions is its mention under dissociative disorder NOS in DSM-IV; a cardinal feature of the syndrome is a temporary alteration in consciousness.

"Running" Syndromes

Simons (1985) has used the term *running taxon* to describe several similar syndromes characterized by prodromal lethargy, depression, or anxiety, followed by a high level of activity, a trancelike state, potentially dangerous behavior in the form of running or fleeing, and ensuing exhaustion, sleep, and amnesia for the episode. Among such syndromes are *pibloktoq* among native peoples of the Arctic (Gussow 1960), *chakore* in the Ngawbere of Panama (Bletzer 1985), *grisi siknis* among the Miskito of Nicaragua (Dennis 1985), and Navajo "frenzy" witchcraft (Neutra et al. 1977). Although present diagnostic schema are only able to place such syndromes in the sphere of dissociative disorder NOS, it is possible that future versions of the DSM will allow for the diagnosis of psychogenic fugue in some of these cases.

Koro

Various reports from Asia, including Hong Kong (Yap 1965), Singapore (Ngui 1969), India (Nandi et al. 1983), China (Tseng et al. 1988), and Malaysia (Adityanjee et al. 1991), have referred to the syndrome of *koro*, or *suo-yang*. This syndrome occurs either singly or in epidemics and is characterized by acute and prominent paniclike symptoms brought about by the sudden onset of fear that one's genitalia are retracting into the abdomen and that this will result in death. Although similar syndromes have also been described in Western settings, these have always been associated either with major (Axis I) diagnoses such as schizophrenia (Ede 1976; Edwards 1970) or with neurological/organic etiologies such as brain tumor (Lapierre 1972) or toxic states (Dow and Silver 1973). In contrast, reports from Asia suggest that *koro* presents as a generally benign, time-limited illness without association to additional psychopathology and with a good prognosis. Bernstein and Gaw (1990) have outlined a classification scheme for *koro* as a "genital retraction disorder" under the section of somatoform disorders. The proposed criteria would exclude organic factors and Axis I disorders other than somatoform disorders, and would ask for the determination of whether the case occurred within or outside of the cultural context.

Anorexia Nervosa and Bulimia Nervosa

Recently, bulimia nervosa has been argued to be most common among middle-class American white females, although it seems to be appearing also among black females from a similar socioeconomic background. This syndrome is characterized by excessive food intake that is then followed by self-induced vomiting. It is often associated with depression and anorexia. Although classified among the eating disorders by U.S. psychiatrists, these disorders are thought to represent American culture-bound syndromes, because they exist rarely, if at all, in other parts of the world. British psychiatrists have also been struck by the infrequent appearance of black subjects among their cases of anorexia nervosa or bulimia nervosa (Thomas and Szmukler 1985).

Spirit Possession and Dissociative Identity Disorder

Globally, there are a number of syndromes of "spirit possession," or possession trance (Akhtar 1988; Chandrashekar 1989; Gussler 1973; Kleinman 1980; Salisbury 1968; Sharp 1994; Stoller 1989; Suryani 1984; Suwanlert 1976; Yap 1960). These syndromes, which are characterized by the belief that the victim's body is taken over by a spirit, are manifested by identity confusion, an inability to control one's actions, a temporary change in the personality of the victim, and partial or total amnesia for the episode. In India, this disorder appears to be more prevalent among women (Chandrashekar 1989; Saxena and Prasad 1989) and among individuals having experienced chronic or acute interpersonal conflict or a recent loss. It is often reversible, with the longest episodes lasting days to weeks. In many cases, an episode of possession trance makes the person in such a trance more likely to be possessed again in the future.

The various accounts of possession trance reveal substantial differences from dissociative identity disorder as described in DSM-IV. The association with childhood abuse has hardly been mentioned with regard to pathological possession trance, but it has also not been systematically studied. Although both dissociative identity disorder and possession trance involve the coexistence within a person of different personalities, a key phenomenological difference between the two is the presumed origin of this other personality: in dissociative identity disorder the personality is understood by the victim as part of him or her, whereas in the possessed person the phenomenon is viewed as the effect of an external, supernatural entity. In addition, cases of pathological possession trance are often episodic and remitting, in contrast to the chronic nature of dissociative identity disorder. Furthermore, reports of simultaneous possession by several coconscious "spirits" are rare. The relationship between these two syndromes is presently uncertain, with authors (Adityanjee et al. 1989; Varma et al. 1981) suggesting that the syndromes may share common mechanisms, whereas "the pathoplastic influence of the prevailing culture may be important in causing [the] . . . differences" in presentation (Adityanjee et al. 1989, p. 1610). The inclusion of dissociative trance disorder in DSM-IV as a criteria set for further study (American Psychiatric Association 1994, p. 727) incorporates many of the findings cited previously, so as to allow collection of further data on pathological spirit possession and similar syndromes.

Hwa-Byung

This syndrome of somatic complaints, ascribed by Korean folklore to excess anger—the word *hwa* means "fire" or "anger," and the word *byung* means illness—is typically characterized by a sensation of an epigastric mass, anorexia, anxiety, dyspnea, and epigastric pain (Lin 1983). It is said to be primarily an illness of women and to be attributed by the affected persons themselves to adverse social circumstances such as "disappointments, sadness, miseries, hostility, grudges, and unfulfilled dreams and expectations" (Pang 1990, p. 496). Partial response of the syndrome to antidepressants has been reported (Lin 1983).

Generalized Somatic Syndromes

This term *generalized somatic syndromes* is meant to cover several illness behaviors that have in common the symptoms of low energy, poor ability to concentrate, poor sleep, headaches, and vague somatic complaints. The Nigerian syndromes of "brain fag" in students, described by Prince (1985), and *ode ori*, described by Makanjuola (1987) among the Yoruba, qualify as part of this group. Sufferers of *ode ori* who were examined with the Present State Examination (Wing et al. 1967) commonly exhibited depressed mood, "tension pains," complaints of ill health, delayed sleep, anxiety, and low energy.

Another generalized somatic syndrome with a strong component of mood dysregulation is that of *neurasthenia* in China (Kleinman 1982; Lin 1989; Ming-Yuan 1989), also known in Japan by the name of *shinkeisuijaku*, or "ordinary" *shinkeishitsu* (Russell 1989; Suzuki 1989). The term *neurasthenia* was used in the late 19th century by the American physician George M. Beard to describe a syndrome of headaches, insomnia, gastrointestinal symptoms, and vague somatic complaints, which Beard believed derived from an exhaustion of the victim's nervous system. Although the diagnosis eventually fell into disuse in its country of origin, it quickly caught on in the rest of the world throughout the 20th century, to the point that in 1968 it was reinstituted as a type of neurosis in DSM-II (American Psychiatric Association 1968), after having not been listed in DSM-I (American Psychiatric Association 1952; Lin 1989). Of note, Kleinman (1982) studied 100 patients diagnosed as neurasthenic in China with the use of a culturally adapted version of the Schedule for Affective Disorders and Schizophrenia (SADS), and determined that the vast majority of these persons, although complaining primarily of somatic ailments, were suffering from "clinical depression" and could benefit from antidepressant medication.

The generalized somatic syndromes described above are suspected of being culturally specific illness behaviors that occur as reactions to the biologically based disorder known in the West as depression, much as Kleinman's (1982) work with neurasthenia in China seemed to show.

There are many other culture-specific syndromes excluded here simply because of space limitations. Although they may appear "exotic" when viewed from outside the culture from which they originate, it is important to remember that understanding each of these syndromes necessitates having a good knowledge of its cultural context.

Significant research is still needed to allow for the eventual elimination of the term *culture-bound* from our diagnostic schema. Clinical and theoretical work must focus on the clear delineation of these syndromes, with the goals of improving our understanding of how patients afflicted with these entities should be treated, and enhancing our ability to determine their ultimate prognosis. It should be seen as a step forward that the APA Task Force on DSM-IV took an interest in improving the cross-cultural scope of the manual by adding material regarding cultural variation in clinical presentation as well as descriptions of many so-called culture-specific syndromes, both as an appendix and as potential presentations of "not otherwise specified" disorders. This will undoubtedly aid those involved in research on cross-cultural diagnosis.

MIGRATION AND PSYCHIATRIC DISORDERS

EFFECT ON FAMILIES AND INDIVIDUALS

It is no secret that migration has for many years been regarded as a cause of pathology. The movement of individuals from a cultural context in which they have been surrounded by family, friends, and familiar institutions to a different geographic area that distances these people from their usual support systems has generally been seen as seriously stressful. Such dislocation of human beings from their own cultural groups has frequently been a contributory element to the emergence of psychopathology in the individual who has moved. Clinicians have been so confident of this that they have often recommended that the patient then be sent back to his or her hometown or country, presumably with the idea that reentry into the home context would have a therapeutic effect on the patient. However, Hickling (1991) has recently suggested that this reentry into the home environment may also be stressful and problematic.

Littlewood and Lipsedge (1981) have described the situation of 16 Caribbean immigrants in London who were socially isolated, working-class women with children. These individuals all experienced a severely traumatic encounter with overt racism, problems with housing, or unemployment. Subsequently, they developed psychological difficulties that were characterized by rapid mental status changes and the elaboration of persecutory symptoms that involved neighbors. A 3-year follow-up showed that the women had continued to have significant psychiatric symptoms. These difficulties can be seen as the direct result of an unsuccessful adaptive response to the stress of confronting a new culture. This phenomenon whereby an individual from one culture comes in contact with another culture has been termed *psychological acculturation*.

The stress on families who are acculturating to a new sociocultural context can be expected to have serious problems for the families concerned. Canino and Canino (1980) have effectively described the complex process of acculturation for Puerto Rican families who migrated to the United States. Although they focused on the urban, low-income Puerto Rican family in the United States, their observations have wide applicability, because most migrants do suffer at least a temporary drop in their socioeconomic standing as a consequence of moving to a foreign land. Canino and Canino described the traditional pattern of the Puerto Rican family as characterized by the presence of an authoritarian father and a submissive, self-sacrificing mother; a great deal of involvement; dependence; and little emphasis on self-differentiation. The authors pointed out that independent behavior, especially in adolescent girls, was neither expected nor well tolerated. They emphasized that such a structure in the context of Puerto Rico remains normal and functional. However, the Puerto Rican family that has migrated to the United States then has to confront poverty, discrimination, and minimal political influence, as well as a host of cultural values that are significantly different from those they left behind. The American culture may be hostile to the authoritarian attitudes of the Puerto Rican father, encourage the mother to abandon her submissive style, and foster a sense of autonomy and independence in the adolescent daughter. If the family has to depend on the welfare system, this may further destabilize the prior structure by making the woman the recipient of financial assistance. In an effort to cope with his threatened traditional role, the father may attempt to reassert his authority, resulting in a family structure that is more rigid and less responsive to the stress of adaptation. This renders the family dysfunctional and pathological in this new cultural context.

The problem of migration is most easily conceptualized in terms of movement of families or individuals from one country to another. But clinicians need to remember that it is also an issue at home in the United States. On several occasions, the lead author has observed clinicians dealing with African American university students studying in predominantly white universities. The African American students previously only frequented predominantly African American institutions. In moving to the white university, they felt dislocated, rootless, and overwhelmed by a sensation of inferiority and of being an outsider. This in turn led to their becoming increasingly suspicious, defensive, and withdrawn. Obviously, their academic performance suffered. Once the therapist understands the role that is being played by cultural dissonance, he or she can then set about structuring ways of facilitating the adjustment of the student to the new culture.

PROCESS OF ACCULTURATION

Anthropologists worked in the early years on the concept of *acculturation* as a way of studying how two groups with different cultures come in contact and interact with each other. Often, one of the groups was numerically, politically, and economically stronger than the other. In recent years, it has been noted that groups, families, and individuals participate in this process of adaptation to a different culture.

The acculturation of groups can have effects that are physically obvious, such as one group's having access only to inferior housing or transportation. Biological changes may result from intermarriage of the two groups in contact; political, economic, linguistic, religious, and other changes are equally possible. It was commonly suggested in the past that the stress that resulted from the acculturation phenomenon would be borne principally by the nondominant group. However, we now know that the nature of the interaction between a dominant and a nondominant group depends on a series of elements; consequently, group tension and individual anxieties might be felt by members of both groups.

Berry and Kim (1988) have theorized that there is a systematic course to acculturation characterized by contact of the two groups, conflict between them, and adaptation to the interaction. Conflict occurs especially when there is resistance to the process by either of the two groups. Such stress ultimately influences the type of acculturative outcome.

The result of acculturation for the groups and the individuals concerned depends on a number of interacting factors, such as the phase of acculturation, the mode of acculturation, the type of acculturating group, the nature of the dominant cultural group, social and cultural characteristics of the less dominant group, and psychological characteristics of the individuals involved in the process.

Berry and Kim have constructed a theoretical model (Table 40–6) that is useful when one is attempting to understand how the various outcomes of the acculturation process differ in the level of stress that they generate for the individual and the group. These theorists have suggested that when a nondominant group comes in contact with a dominant group, members of the nondominant group must respond to two important questions. The first is whether the nondominant individual's cultural identity has such value that it should be retained. The second question is whether positive relations with the majority dominant group ought to be sought. Potentially, the varieties of answers to these two questions would influence the extent of stress present in the acculturative process, both for the individual and for the group.

In the application of this model to acculturation, Berry and Kim have carefully asserted that this theoretical framework is still subject to influence by elements such as the psychology of the individuals, economics, and politics. Thus, for example, the minority group may seek to pursue a strategy of *integration* by answering yes to both questions. In doing this, they may be purposefully looking for a style of acculturative adjustment that has minimal stress. Nevertheless, the majority group may simultaneously be following a political goal of blocking such integration because of a wish to deny the importance of the minority group's identity. In such a case, the integration approach would indeed produce significant stress for the nondominant group.

Another possible adaptive response is *marginality*. In this case, both of the questions would be answered in the negative. Marginality represents a hopeless and negative view of life, and individuals who subscribe to this position are most likely to be functioning on the very periphery of the society. By answering no to both questions, these indi-

TABLE 40–6. Potential outcome of acculturative interaction between dominant and nondominant groups

Nondominant individual's cultural identity valuable	Positive relations sought with dominant group	Outcome of acculturation
Yes	Yes	Integration
No	No	Marginality
Yes	No	Resistance
No	Yes	Assimilation

Source. Adapted from Berry and Kim 1988.

viduals reject any compromise with the dominant group and also see no value in their individual or group identity. It would seem evident that a consequence of this position would be intense identity conflict and confusion, both personally and politically.

In contrast to marginality, integration is characterized by affirmation of the value of the minority group's identity as well as the need to seek positive relations with the majority dominant group. Berry and Kim (1988) have hypothesized that this modality represents the least stressful adaptive response to acculturation because it is characterized by healthful ego adaptation and also places a positive premium on minority group institutions. At the same time, the seeking of positive relations with the majority group is a political approach that seeks compromise and consequently sets up a terrain for constructive interaction. This is not to suggest that the integrationist stance may not be full of problems when the dominant group is intent on frustrating the decisions and pursuits of the nondominant group. This is particularly evident in the political arena, as in the case of southern white supremacists who seek to block any political negotiations with African American leaders.

There are two other possibilities of adaptive response to the difficulties of acculturation: *resistance* and *assimilation*. In the context of the theory described above, both of these would be predictive of considerable acculturative stress. In the case of resistance, the individual answers affirmatively to the question of whether his or her nondominant group's identity is of value and answers in the negative to the question of whether positive relations should be sought with the majority group. In this situation, resistance implies a state of perpetual conflict with the dominant group. Although it is true that resistive acculturation could provide group support and enhancement of self-esteem, opposition to the seeking of positive relations with the dominant group would be expected to take its toll in the political and economic arena. One could argue that the Black Panther party was an example, par excellence, of the resistance pattern.

The posture of assimilation is an adaptive response in which the individual responds in the negative to the question of whether the nondominant group's identity is of value and answers affirmatively to the question of whether positive relations should be sought with the dominant group. Although resistive acculturation could potentially lead to caustic and difficult interactions with the dominant group, the assimilation stance still leads to a repudiation of the nondominant group's self-esteem and potentially results in what Bush (1976) has considered to be the "depreciated character." Clearly, Bush would argue that any refutation of a nondominant group's sense of self would

inevitably lead to a pervasive feeling of hopelessness. Consequently, one could argue that the assimilationist position is by definition self-destructive, particularly in the psychological sphere.

The importance of such a model lies in its potential applicability to the study of groups, families, and individuals. The model serves to highlight the complexity of the process of acculturation, its influence on the emergence of psychopathology at different unitary levels, and the various adaptive mechanisms available to a group to cope with the stress of migration. The Committee on Cultural Psychiatry of the Group for the Advancement of Psychiatry has used this model to generate hypotheses that explain the suicide rates of certain ethnic groups in the United States who are struggling with the task of adapting to the dominant culture (Group for the Advancement of Psychiatry 1989).

ETHNOCULTURE, RACE, AND PSYCHIATRIC TREATMENT

CULTURE AND PSYCHOTHERAPY

All societies have developed ways of confronting physical and psychological suffering. Psychotherapy in its broadest sense should be seen as a curing system for psychological ills. The technical ways in which psychotherapy is applied or practiced obviously vary from one culture to another. However, Frank (1963) has postulated that six elements lie at the core of all nonmedical healing and should exist independently of the cultural context in which the healing is practiced: 1) the emotional stirring of the individual, 2) the existence of a healer on whom the individual depends for help and who holds out hope of relief, 3) the arousal of the individual's expectations by the healer's personal attributes, 4) the evocation of hope in the individual, 5) the bolstering of the individual's self-esteem, and 6) the strengthening of the individual's ties with a supportive group (Table 40–7).

TABLE 40–7.   Core elements of nonmedical healing

- Emotional stirring of the individual
- Existence of healer on whom the individual depends
- Arousal of individual's expectations by healer's personal attributes
- Evocation of hope
- Bolstering of self-esteem
- Strengthening of the individual's ties with a supportive group

Source.   Adapted from Frank 1963.

Griffith and colleagues (Griffith and Mahy 1984; Griffith et al. 1980) have pursued the clarification of mechanisms that individuals employ in church for therapeutic purposes. Griffith and Mahy (1984) reported on the ceremony called "mourning" that is practiced in the Spiritual Baptist Church in the West Indies. The ritual involves praying, fasting, and the experiencing of dreams and visions while in isolation. In their analysis of the practice and their interviews of a group of individuals who had gone through the mourning ceremony, the authors concluded that mourning is a viable psychotherapeutic practice for the church members. Griffith and Mahy also were able to show how the mourning experience satisfies the requirements of nonmedical healing that had been established by Frank. Indeed, the authors pointed out that the use of the church as an institution in which one can engage in a psychotherapeutic experience requires a specific cultural world view that includes a view of life and of health as being positively influenced by a special commitment and relationship to God.

The importance of structuring a psychotherapeutic ritual around a belief system has been emphasized by Wittkower and Warnes (1974). These authors underlined the relevance of cultural factors in the application of psychotherapeutic practices. They showed how a belief in supernatural forces as the cause of psychological suffering would lead the patients away from Western medicine and toward increased reliance on other systems such as churches or other spiritual healing rituals. Numerous authors have emphasized the healing qualities of such native systems as the *Umbanda* cult in Brazil (Pressel 1973), *Espiritismo* in Puerto Rico (Comas-Díaz 1981; Koss 1975), and *Vodun* in Haiti (Métraux 1972) as being parallel in function and intent to the practice of psychodynamic psychotherapy in North America.

Within the United States, J. P. Spiegel (1976) described the problems created by cultural factors even when traditional psychoanalytically trained psychotherapists were at work. He outlined the problems that confronted middle-class American therapists who were seeking to establish a psychotherapeutic relationship with members of Irish-American families. Spiegel emphasized that the middle-class American therapists held values that were different from those of the Irish-American patients. These therapists approached their work with expectations that the patients would, for example, develop relative independence from their families and from other pressures for conformity to Irish-American values. The therapists also expected to maintain benevolent neutrality in the moral arena while hoping to have their patients be less under the domination of their own superego pressures. There

seemed to be a clear expectation that the patients would identify with and accept the goals and values of the therapists. However, this did not happen, and the result of the experimental work was that the therapists ultimately had to modify their own goals and procedures, this being the only alternative to abandoning the research and accepting failure. For example, the therapists had to accept the limitations on autonomy and independence within the general framework of the Irish family.

More recently, Blue and González (1992) have commented on the fallacy of seeing psychodynamic psychotherapy as being independent of culture, noting that psychodynamic thinking is rather a culture unto itself, and intimating that even psychodynamic psychotherapy that is intraracial and intraethnic is vulnerable to cross-cultural distortions. Others (Dien 1983; Florsheim 1990; Tung 1991) have mentioned that the view of the individual as an autonomous, independent being, as idealized by "Western" based psychological thought, is not consistent with the prevailing worldview elsewhere, in which considering the individual without looking at how this individual fits into his or her social context is meaningless.

Comas-Díaz and Jacobsen (1991) have carefully examined the notable impact of ethnic, racial, and cultural differences on the psychotherapeutic relationship, from the view of both transference and countertransference. Possible signs of interethnic transference include over-compliance, denial of ethnocultural differences, and the more understandable feelings of mistrust and hostility in a patient from an oppressed group. Intraethnic transference, in turn, can be characterized by idealization of the therapist, by viewing the therapist as a "traitor" to his or her race or culture, or by fear of merging with the therapist. Countertransferential reactions in an interethnic psychotherapeutic relationship can be characterized by denial of differences, excessive cultural curiosity, and guilt or pity when the patient is from a highly disadvantaged group. Intraethnic relationships are susceptible to countertransference reactions such as overidentification and collusion, as well as anger, especially when work with the patient touches on the therapist's unresolved feelings about oppression and prejudice.

The successful resolution of many of the difficulties resulting from cultural differences requires from therapists openness, flexibility, curiosity, and a willingness to acknowledge and explore the cross-cultural components of transference and countertransference.

Not all therapists may be capable of such stances. The traditional stance of having the therapist leave value choices ultimately and completely to the patient may only be theoretically possible in a vacuum. As the therapy unfolds, the therapist may indeed be sneaking into the exercise his or her own value representations. Ultimately, the emphasis on individualism and autonomy that is so much a part of American psychotherapy may have to be replaced by what J. P. Spiegel (1976) considered to be horizontal, collaborative decision making.

RACE AND PSYCHOTHERAPY

Whereas workers such as Jones (1982) have provided significant research impetus to the area of race and psychotherapy, Bradshaw (1982) emphasized effectively the clinical problems that have emerged as a function of the role that race plays in psychotherapy. He concentrated entirely on the problems of the black-white dichotomy. However, the issues that he outlined are applicable to other potential dichotomies in the patient-therapist context. Certain errors seem specific to the white therapist–black patient dyad. Bradshaw showed how the therapist could be influenced by common myths such as that of the African American family as a repository of severe pathology, the one-parent family as leading unavoidably to psychopathology, African Americans as having a poor self-image, African Americans as being sexually promiscuous, and African American patients as unable to be treated by traditional psychotherapy.

The maintenance of such myths seems partly related to the fact that white therapists are frequently ignorant of the reasons that African American patients present themselves as passive and inarticulate. In addition, the situation can be rendered more complex if the therapist's position is countenanced and reinforced by a white supervisor. Obviously, a white therapist's countertransference can be stimulated by antiwhite hostility coming from the patient.

Bradshaw also saw the black therapist–white patient dyad as having the potential for certain difficulty. In this context, both individuals may be unable to deal with the meaning of race in the therapeutic relationship. Blue and González (1992) have viewed the stress on African American therapists as the result, in part, of their sense of distance from both their culture of origin and the dominant culture, as represented by the patient. For the therapist, they have advocated careful self-examination and reliance on supervision, with the intent of focusing on racial transference as a way of addressing the patient's conflict, rather than as something to be avoided or ignored. Helms (1990), with influence from racial identity theory, proposed a racial identity interaction model for understanding the impact of race and ethnicity on the psychotherapeutic process. She theorized that the racial identity stage of each participant in a treatment dyad affects his or her reactions to the other

and that the nature of the therapeutic alliance is a function of the interplay of their expressed racial identities. Helms hypothesized that whites and people of color undergo racial identity change processes that influence how they handle racial material. There is a continuum of possible attitudes, perspectives, and outcomes of these processes. She suggested that the optimal outcome for whites involved abandoning entitlements associated with being white and relinquishing the myth of white superiority; for people of color it would involve overcoming internalized racism and negative self-concepts. In a treatment arrangement between a white person and a person of color, the position of each along this racial identity continuum would have a profound impact on the relationship. For example, a white therapist whose racial identity stage is manifested by denials that racism has significant impact on people's lives may have difficulty treating an African American client whose racial identity stage is characterized by firm beliefs that racism circumscribes his opportunities in life. This would continue to hold true for a dyad consisting of racially similar participants who may differ with regard to their own specific racial identity stage.

For example, the black therapist–black patient dyad is not exempt from having specific difficulties. African American therapists may also accept the myth that African American patients are "bad" patients. The patient may be seen as having so many social problems that he or she cannot benefit from psychotherapy. African American therapists who are not of the same social class as the African American patient may also react negatively to the patient's mannerisms and style that reflect a linkage to the lowest social and educational level. Black therapists and black patients may also establish a quick relationship that can lead to taking certain things for granted. For example, they may collude in attributing all the problems to the white society. Another possibility may be that the black therapist becomes angry at the black patient who expresses negative feelings about black people in general.

Although Bradshaw limited his comments to the therapeutic process that unfolds in the relationships established by specific types of patients and therapists, the situations are far more complex when the element of economics is introduced. African American patients, for example, may be rich or poor. Similarly, African American therapists may come from a variety of socioeconomic backgrounds. The same can be said of white therapists and white patients. Consequently, the element of race is likely to be complicated significantly by the element of class and indeed of education. Blumenthal and colleagues (1985) have pointed out that the research conducted on the problems created by these dichotomies remains unfortunately inconclusive.

The white clinician–black patient dyad has served as a useful model for reflecting on countertransference problems in cross-cultural psychotherapy. Indeed, this dyad has been a framework for others, such as the example of Jewish therapist and Arab patient. Gorkin (1986) outlined how to manage certain types of countertransference that emerge in this unique situation. In particular, he noted how a Jewish therapist might experience guilt and aggression while in the process of treating an Arab patient.

Hatch and Friedman (1996) reminded us that relatively little work has been done on the use of cognitive behavioral treatments with different ethnic and racial groups. In their own clinical work with African Americans and Afro-Caribbean residents in New York City, they recognized that there were certain distinctive elements in their treatment relationship with these patients that forced the authors to develop a unique approach to the care of these patients' obsessive-compulsive disorder. The elements were the patients' secretiveness about their disorder, their reluctance to take medication and to involve their families in the treatment enterprise, their pronounced misunderstanding of the disorder, and their discomfort with white clinicians.

GENDER AND PSYCHOTHERAPY

The problems created by the black-white dyad are analogous in many ways to those seen in the male-female therapy dyad. Although some analysts have defended vehemently the idea that social and cultural issues are but peripheral to psychoanalytic treatment, it seems likely that the differences in male and female development, their identity formation, and their worldview may have a differential impact on the context of therapy. Lester (1990) mentioned that male patients are more likely than female patients to resist transferential feelings to merge with and depend on the analyst. Speaking of countertransference, she stated that female analysts may be more tolerant of a client's "demands for maternal care" (p. 438), whereas a male therapist might become anxious and be more likely to attempt to distance himself from the patient when he faced such wishes from a patient. Cases in which the therapist is a man and the patient is a woman have also been thought to replicate and reinforce the inequitable power distribution that women have experienced throughout their lives in relationships such as with fathers, husbands, and work associates (Carmen et al. 1981).

Carmen and colleagues (1981) have described the culture-bound view that women's anger is inappropriate. Women themselves may have particular conflict about expressing their own anger, just as men have problems about having women express their anger. It is possible that a male therapist's countertransference will lead him to view an assertive or angry woman as "castrating," whereas this might be less likely to occur to him were he dealing with a male patient who behaved in a similar fashion. There is also the increasingly evident problem of the sexual abuse of female patients by male therapists. Such behavior from therapists has been condemned by the APA without regard to what role the female patient may have played. But not surprisingly, cases are beginning to appear in which male patients have accused female therapists of sexual abuse; similarly, there have been complaints in cases where patient and therapist are of the same gender.

Bradshaw (1982) raised squarely the problems that are possible in the dyad in which both patient and therapist are black. This makes it worthwhile to speculate that similar problems can occur in the dyadic context in which both patient and therapist are female. For example, a female therapist might encourage women to express inordinate anger against men or to participate in activities that may in fact be expressing the therapist's wishes and value system. One could also expect that the female patient and therapist could collude to project all of the problems onto males in the general society. Bernstein (1991) posited that a female therapist may overvalue a female patient's efforts in the workplace at the expense of unwittingly contributing to the patient's shame in obtaining pleasure from more traditional female roles, such as mothering. The author also added that therapy with a female patient may awaken within a female therapist the countertransferential reaction of competitiveness with her own mother, to the point where the therapist then injects these feelings into the patient's situation.

GENDER AND PHARMACOTHERAPY

Recent work has emphasized the influence of culture and culturally derived views of sex and gender on the focus of health research in general and mental health research specifically.

Krieger and Fee (1994) have argued that the use of sex and gender as variables has served to restrict the focus of medical research about women to reproductive health, largely ignoring nonreproductive issues such as hypertension, heart disease, cancer, and AIDS. They added that the primary focus on race and sex/gender as variables has impeded the investigation of the impact of social class on the health of both women and men.

Weissman and Olfson (1995) commented on current, significant knowledge gaps with regard to the development and treatment of major depression in women, despite the world-wide disproportionate incidence of this disorder in women. They mentioned that, despite well-documented physiological differences between men and women, studies remain to be done to explore differences in drug bioavailability and how they relate to sex-based differential responses to medication. In addition, they cited the potential influence of social and economic factors in promoting gender bias in medical treatment and research. For example, women were more likely than men to suffer disruptions in their medical insurance coverage, in part because a woman insured as a dependent is likely to lose this coverage in the event of divorce or death of her spouse. Moreover, women may be disproportionately underinsured or uninsured due to their higher representation in part-time work or in positions with companies too small to offer adequate insurance. It is quite possible that these gender-based social and financial inequities result not only in undertreatment but also in a certain amount of invisibility for women in clinical and research settings.

RACE AND PHARMACOTHERAPY

Lin et al. (1991) have reviewed the response of Asians to various psychotropics. They mentioned the well-known enzyme polymorphisms of alcohol dehydrogenase and aldehyde dehydrogenase, more prevalent in Asian populations, which are responsible, respectively, for some of the increased sensitivity to alcohol and the flushing response observed in many people of Asian descent or origin. A great majority of Asians are estimated to be "fast acetylators," in comparison with approximately 50% of Caucasians and African Americans. This may have an impact on Asians' metabolism of such drugs as clonazepam, caffeine, and phenelzine. In addition, differences in the activity of catechol-*O*-methyltransferase, have been linked to the higher incidence of dyskinesia in Asian parkinsonian patients treated with L-dopa. Racial differences in metabolism have also been confirmed as being responsible for the increased susceptibility of Asians to antipsychotics, antidepressants, and benzodiazepines.

Mendoza et al. (1991) recently reviewed studies on psychopharmacological treatment of Hispanic and Native Americans, finding that although some interesting differences have been found in various pathways of drug metabolism (debrisoquine and S-mephenytoin metabolism, acetylation, protein binding), little in the way of clinical correlation has occurred. In addition, clinical studies have suffered from the fact that diagnosis and outcome measures are hampered by wide cultural differences in symptom expression.

Strickland et al. (1991) reviewed psychopharmacological studies in African American populations and commented on the replicated finding that black Americans develop higher plasma levels and faster clinical responses to tricyclic antidepressants than do white populations. More specifically, the intracellular concentration of lithium in red blood cells was higher in African Americans than in Caucasians, apparently the result of a less efficient lithium-sodium counter transport system (Strickland et al. 1995). This may necessitate the use of lower doses of lithium in the treatment of bipolar disorder in this group and perhaps the use of alternative antimanic agents such as valproate and carbamazepine. Studies looking at differences in the metabolism of antipsychotics, however, have been inconclusive, in part because of what seems to be a bias toward blacks being diagnosed as schizophrenic more often than whites. Lawson (1996) argues that successful treatment outcomes for African Americans may be compromised by a combination of the aforementioned problem of misdiagnosis, the use of higher dosages of psychotropic medications with the attendant increased likelihood of side effects, the greater use of prn medications, poorer treatment compliance, and greater reluctance on the part of African Americans to seek psychiatric care. Hence, race and ethnicity must be considered seriously if one is to maximize pharmacotherapy and improve treatment outcomes.

Dawkins and Potter (1991) have commented on the dearth of information available on gender differences in the response to psychopharmacological treatment, given that animal studies have shown important differences, related in part to sex hormone levels. These authors attributed the lack of research on women to the delicate issue of the possible far-reaching effects of medication on women of childbearing age.

Medication obviously meets with varying levels of approval among different groups. In the Caribbean, many patients view psychiatrists as medical practitioners and therefore practically demand a prescription for some type of medication regardless of the nature of their complaint. Nevertheless, other Caribbean patients who belong to fundamentalist religious groups see God as the final healer. They refuse to take almost any medication and are convinced that prayer makes it unnecessary to swallow pills of any sort. Still others see the physician as the intermediary through whom God acts. These patients therefore pray and take pills. Such differing responses to pharmacotherapy from patients growing up in the same island show the complexity of the healing enterprise.

CONCLUSIONS

It should be clear from this chapter that culture plays an important role in psychiatry and all of medicine. The influence of culture extends from the etiological conception of sickness to the implementation of a treatment plan and even the prognosis. Culture, ethnicity, race, and gender require serious consideration by students of psychiatry who wish to become effective healers of mental disorders. Patients present complaints that stem from a matrix that is not purely biological. Culture influences this matrix as powerfully as does the biological heritage. Openness to considering the role of culture in the healing process is a hallmark of the thoughtful healer.

REFERENCES

Adebimpe VR: Overview: white norms and psychiatric diagnosis of black patients. Am J Psychiatry 138:279–285, 1981

Adebimpe VR, Chu C-C, Klein HE, et al: Racial and geographic differences in the psychopathology of schizophrenia. Am J Psychiatry 139:888–891, 1982

Adityanjee, Raju GSP, Khandelwal SK: Current status of multiple personality disorder in India. Am J Psychiatry 146:1607–1610, 1989

Adityanjee, Zain AM, Subramaniam M: Sporadic koro and marital disharmony. Psychopathology 24:49–52, 1991

Akhtar S: Four culture-bound psychiatric syndromes in India. Int J Soc Psychiatry 34:70–74, 1988

Allen EA: Psychological dependency among students in a "cross-roads" culture. West Indian Medical Journal 34:123–127, 1985

American Psychiatric Association: Diagnostic and Statistical Manual: Mental Disorders. Washington, DC, American Psychiatric Association, 1952

American Psychiatric Association: Diagnostic and Statistical Manual of Mental Disorders, 2nd Edition. Washington, DC, American Psychiatric Association, 1968

American Psychiatric Association: Diagnostic and Statistical Manual of Mental Disorders, 3rd Edition. Washington, DC, American Psychiatric Association, 1980

American Psychiatric Association: Diagnostic and Statistical Manual of Mental Disorders, 3rd Edition, Revised. Washington, DC, American Psychiatric Association, 1987

American Psychiatric Association: Diagnostic and Statistical Manual of Mental Disorders, 4th Edition. Washington, DC, American Psychiatric Association, 1994

Baldwin JA: Theory and research concerning the notion of black self-hatred: a review and reinterpretation. Journal of Black Psychology 5:51–77, 1979

Bateson G: Some components of socialization for trance. Ethos 3:143–155, 1975

Bell CC, Mehta H: The misdiagnosis of black patients with manic-depressive illness. J Natl Med Assoc 72:141–145, 1980

Bemporad JR, Ratey JJ, O'Driscoll G, et al: Hysteria, anorexia and the culture of self-denial. Psychiatry 51:96–103, 1988

Benedict R: Patterns of Culture. New York, Mentor Books, 1959

Bernstein DH: Gender-specific dangers in the female dyad in treatment. Psychoanal Rev 78:37–48, 1991

Bernstein RL, Gaw AC: Koro: proposed classification for DSM-IV. Am J Psychiatry 147:1670–1674, 1990

Berry JW: Ecology, cultural adaptation and psychological differentiation: traditional patterning and acculturative stress, in Cross-Cultural Perspectives on Learning. Edited by Brislin R, Bochner S, Lonner W. New York, Wiley, 1975, pp 207–231

Berry JW, Kim U: Acculturation and mental health, in Health and Cross-Cultural Psychology: Toward Applications. Edited by Dasen P, Berry JW, Sartorius N. Newberry Park, CA, Sage, 1988, pp 207–236

Bletzer KV: Fleeing hysteria (chakore) among Ngawbere of northwestern Panama: a preliminary analysis and comparison with similar illness phenomena in other settings. Med Anthropol 9:297–318, 1985

Blue HC, González CA: The meaning of ethnocultural difference: its impact on and use in the psychotherapeutic process, in Treating Diverse Disorders With Psychotherapy (New Dir Ment Health Serv No 55). Edited by Greenfeld D. San Francisco, CA, Jossey-Bass, 1992, pp 73–84

Blumenthal SJ, Jones EE, Krupnick JL: The influence of gender and race on the therapeutic alliance, in Psychiatry Update: American Psychiatric Association Annual Review, Vol 4. Edited by Hales RE, Frances AJ. Washington, DC, American Psychiatric Press, 1985, pp 586–606

Bradshaw WH Jr: Supervision in black and white: race as a factor in supervision, in Applied Supervision in Psychotherapy. Edited by Blumenfield M. New York, Grune and Stratton, 1982, pp 200–220

Burton-Bradley BG: The amok syndrome in Papua and New Guinea. Med J Aust 1:252–256, 1968

Bush JS: Suicide and blacks: a conceptual framework. Suicide Life Threat Behav 6:216–219, 1976

Canino IA, Canino G: Impact of stress on the Puerto Rican family: treatment considerations. Am J Orthopsychiatry 50:535–541, 1980

Carmen E[H], Russo NF, Miller JB: Inequality and women's mental health: an overview. Am J Psychiatry 138:1319–1330, 1981

Carr JE: Ethno-behaviorism and the culture-bound syndromes: the case of amok. Cult Med Psychiatry 2:269–293, 1978

Chandrashekar CR: Possession syndrome in India, in Altered States of Consciousness and Mental Health. Edited by Ward CA. Newbury Park, CA, Sage, 1989, pp 79–95

Chodoff P: A critique of Freud's theory of infantile sexuality. Am J Psychiatry 123:507–518, 1966

Cohen CI, Berment F, Magai C: A comparison of US-born African-American and African-Caribbean psychiatric outpatients. J Natl Med Assoc 89:117–123, 1997

Cohen P, Brook J: Family factors related to the persistence of psychopathology in childhood and adolescence. Psychiatry 50:332–345, 1987

Comas-Díaz L: Puerto Rican espiritismo and psychotherapy. Am J Orthopsychiatry 51:636–645, 1981

Comas-Díaz L, Jacobsen FM: Ethnocultural transference and countertransference in the therapeutic dyad. Am J Orthopsychiatry 61:392–402, 1991

Constantinides P: Women heal women: spirit possession and sexual segregation in a Muslim society. Soc Sci Med 21:685–692, 1985

Cross WE: Shades of Black: diversity in African American identity. Philadelphia, PA, Temple University Press, 1991

Cross WE: In search of Blackness and Afrocentricity: the psychology of black identity change, in Racial and Ethnic Identity: Psychological Development and Creative Expression. Edited by Harris HW, Blue HC, Griffith EEH. New York, Routledge Publications, 1995, pp 53–72

Dana RH, Whatley PR: When does a difference make a difference? MMPI scores and African Americans. J Clin Psychol 47:400–406, 1991

Dawkins K, Potter WZ: Gender differences in pharmacokinetics and pharmacodynamics of psychotropics: focus on women. Psychopharmacol Bull 27: 417–426, 1991

Delgado AK, Griffith EEH, Ruiz P: The black woman mental health executive: problems and perspectives. Administration in Mental Health 12:246–251, 1985

Dennis PA: Grisi Siknis in Miskito culture, in The Culture-Bound Syndromes: Folk Illnesses of Psychiatric and Anthropological Interest. Edited by Simons RC, Hughes CC. Dordrecht, The Netherlands, D Reidel, 1985, pp 289–306

Dien DS: Big Me and Little Me: a Chinese perspective on self. Psychiatry 46:281–286, 1983

Dow TW, Silver DA: Drug-induced koro syndrome. J Fla Med Assoc 60:32–33, 1973

Downing NE, Roush KL: From passive acceptance to active commitment: a model of feminist identity development for women. Journal of Counseling Psychology 13:695–709, 1985

Draguns JG: Cross-cultural counseling and psychotherapy: history, issues, current status, in Cross-Cultural Counseling and Psychiatry. Edited by Marsella J, Pedersen P. New York, Pergamon, 1981, pp 3–27

Ede A: Koro in an Anglo-Saxon Canadian. Canadian Psychiatric Association Journal 21:389–392, 1976

Edwards JG: The koro pattern of depersonalization in an American schizophrenic patient. Am J Psychiatry 126: 1171–1173, 1970

Eisenbruch M: Cross-cultural aspects of bereavement, II: ethnic and cultural variations in the development of bereavement practices. Cult Med Psychiatry 8:315–347, 1984

Erickson MT: Rethinking oedipus: an evolutionary perspective of incest avoidance. Am J Psychiatry 150:411–416, 1993

Escobar JI: Cross-cultural aspects of the somatization trait. Hospital and Community Psychiatry 38:174–180, 1987

Fabrega H: The role of culture in a theory of psychiatric illness. Soc Sci Med 35:91–103, 1992

Finnegan DG, McNally EB: Dual identities: counseling chemically dependent gay men and lesbians. Center City, MN, Hazelton, 1987

Florsheim P: Cross-cultural views of self in the treatment of mental illness: disentangling the curative aspects of myth from the mythic aspects of cure. Psychiatry 53:304–315, 1990

Foulks EF: Anthropology and psychiatry: a new blending of an old relationship, in Current Perspectives in Cultural Psychiatry. Edited by Foulks EF, Wintrob RM, Westermeyer J, et al. New York, Spectrum, 1977, pp 5–18

Frank JD: Persuasion and Healing: A Comparative Study of Psychotherapy. Baltimore, MD, Johns Hopkins Press, 1963

Friedman RC, Downey JI: Biology and the oedipus complex. Psychoanal Q 64(2):234–264, 1995

Gaw AC (ed): Culture, Ethnicity, and Mental Illness. Washington, DC, American Psychiatric Press, 1993

Gaw AC, Bernstein RL: Classification of amok in DSM-IV. Hospital and Community Psychiatry 43:789–793, 1992

Gilligan C: In a Different Voice: Psychological Theory and Women's Development. Cambridge, MA, Harvard University Press, 1982

González CA, Griffith EEH: Culture and the diagnosis of somatoform and dissociative disorders, in Culture and Psychiatric Diagnosis: A DSM-IV Perspective. Washington, DC, American Psychiatric Press, 1996, pp 137–149

González CA, Griffith EEH, Ruiz P: Cross-cultural issues in psychiatric treatment, in Treatments of Psychiatric Disorders. Edited by Gabbard GO. Washington, DC, American Psychiatric Press, 1995, pp 57–87

González CA, Lewis-Fernández R, Griffith EEH, et al: Impact of culture on dissociation: enhancing the cultural suitability of DSM-IV, in DSM-IV Sourcebook, Vol 3. Edited by Widiger TA, Frances AJ, Pincus HA et al. Washington, DC, American Psychiatric Press, 1997, pp 943–949

Goodman A: Organic unity theory: the mind-body problem revisited. Am J Psychiatry 148:553–563, 1991

Gorkin M: Countertransference in cross-cultural psychotherapy: the example of Jewish therapist and Arab patient. Psychiatry 49:69–79, 1986

Greene RL: Ethnicity and MMPI performance: a review. J Consult Clin Psychol 55:497–512, 1987

Gremillion H: Psychiatry as social ordering: anorexia nervosa, a paradigm. Soc Sci Med 35:57–71, 1992

Griffith EEH, Mahy GE: Psychological benefits of Spiritual Baptist "mourning." Am J Psychiatry 141:769–773, 1984

Griffith EEH, English T, Mayfield V: Possession, prayer, and testimony: therapeutic aspects of the Wednesday night meeting in a black church. Psychiatry 43:120–128, 1980

Griffith EEH, Young JL, Smith DL: An analysis of the therapeutic elements in a black church service. Hospital and Community Psychiatry 35:464–469, 1984

Group for the Advancement of Psychiatry, Committee on Cultural Psychiatry: Suicide and Ethnicity in the United States. New York, Brunner/Mazel, 1989

Guarnaccia PJ: Cultural comments on multiaxial issues, in Culture and Psychiatric Diagnosis: A DSM-IV Perspective. Edited by Mezzich JE, Kleinman A, Fabrega H, et al. Washington, DC, American Psychiatric Press, 1996, pp 335–338

Guarnaccia PJ, de la Cancela V, Carrillo E: The multiple meanings of ataques de nervios in the Latino community. Med Anthropol 11:47–62, 1989a

Guarnaccia PJ, Rubio-Stipec M, Canino G: Ataques de nervios in the Puerto Rican Diagnostic Interview Schedule: the impact of cultural categories on psychiatric epidemiology. Cult Med Psychiatry 13:275–295, 1989b

Guarnaccia PJ, Good BJ, Kleinman AM: A critical review of epidemiological studies of Puerto Rican mental health. Am J Psychiatry 147:1449–1456, 1990

Gussler J: Social change, ecology and spirit possession among the South African Nguni, in Religion, Altered States of Consciousness, and Social Change. Edited by Bourguignon E. Columbus, OH, Ohio State University Press, 1973, pp 88–126

Gussow Z: Pibloktoq (hysteria) among the polar Eskimo. The Psychoanalytic Study of Society 1:218–236, 1960

Gynther MD: White norms and black MMPIs: a prescription for discrimination? Psychol Bull 78:386–402, 1972

Haberman PW: Psychiatric symptoms among Puerto Ricans in Puerto Rico and New York City. Ethnicity 3:133–144, 1976

Hatch ML, Friedman S: Behavioral treatment of obsessive-compulsive disorder in African Americans. Cognitive and Behavioral Practice 3:303–315, 1996

Haynes NM, Comer JP: The effects of a school development program on self-concept. Yale J Biol Med 63:275–283, 1990

Helms JE: Black and White Racial Identity: Theory, Research, and Practice. Westport, CT, Greenwood, 1990

Hickling FW: Double jeopardy: psychopathology of black mentally ill returned migrants to Jamaica. Int J Soc Psychiatry 37:80–89, 1991

Horney K: The Neurotic Personality of Our Time. New York, Norton, 1937

Hughes CC: The culture-bound syndromes and psychiatric diagnosis, in Culture and Psychiatric Diagnosis: a DSM-IV perspective. Edited by Mezzich JE, Kleinman A, Fabrega H, et al. Washington, DC, American Psychiatric Press, pp 289–305, 1996

Jones BE, Gray BA: Problems in diagnosing schizophrenia and affective disorders among blacks. Hospital and Community Psychiatry 37:61–65, 1986

Jones EE: Psychotherapists' impressions of treatment outcome as a function of race. J Clin Psychol 38:722–731, 1982

Katon W, Kleinman A, Rosen G: Depression and somatization: a review. Am J Med 72:127–135, 1982

Kiev A: The study of folk psychiatry, in Magic, Faith and Healing. Edited by Kiev A. London, Free Press of Glencoe, 1964, pp 3–35

King LM: Suicide from a "black reality" perspective, in The Afro-American Family: Assessment, Treatment, and Research Issues. Edited by Bass BA, Wyatt GE, Powell GJ. New York, Grune & Stratton, 1982, pp 221–236

Kirmayer LJ, Young A, Hayton BC: The cultural context of anxiety disorders. Psychiatr Clin North Am 18:503–21, 1995

Kleinman A: Patients and Healers in the Context of Culture: An Exploration of the Borderland Between Anthropology, Medicine, and Psychiatry. Berkeley, CA, University of California Press, 1980

Kleinman A: Neurasthenia and depression: a study of somatization and culture in China. Cult Med Psychiatry 6:117–189, 1982

Kleinman A: Rethinking Psychiatry: From Cultural Category to Personal Experience. New York, Free Press, 1988

Koss JD: Therapeutic aspects of Puerto Rican cult practices. Psychiatry 38:160–171, 1975

Krieger N, Fee E: Man-made medicine and women's health: the biopolitics of sex/gender and race/ethnicity. Int J Health Serv 24(2):265–283, 1994

Lapierre YD: Koro in a French Canadian. Canadian Psychiatric Association Journal 17:333–334, 1972

Lawson WB: Clinical issues in the pharmacotherapy of African Americans. Psychopharmacol Bull 32(2):275–282, 1996

Leighton AH, Murphy JM: Cross-cultural psychiatry, in Approaches to Cross-Cultural Psychiatry. Edited by Murphy JM, Leighton AH. New York, Cornell University Press, 1965, pp 3–20

Lester EP: Gender and identity issues in the analytic process. Int J Psychoanal 71:435–444, 1990

Levy JE, Neutra R, Parker D: Life careers of Navajo epileptics and convulsive hysterics. Soc Sci Med 13B:53–66, 1979

Lewis-Fernández R, Kleinman A: Cultural psychiatry: theoretical, clinical, and research issues. Psychiatr Clin North Am 18:433–448, 1995

Lin K-M: Hwa-Byung: a Korean culture-bound syndrome? Am J Psychiatry 140:105–107, 1983

Lin K-M, Poland RE, Smith MW, et al: Pharmacokinetic and other related factors affecting psychotropic responses in Asians. Psychopharmacol Bull 27:427–439, 1991

Lin K-M, Anderson D, Poland RE: Ethnicity and psychopharmacology. Psychiatr Clin North Am 18:635–647, 1995

Lin T: Neurasthenia revisited: its place in modern psychiatry. Cult Med Psychiatry 13:105–129, 1989

Littlewood R, Lipsedge M: Acute psychotic reactions in Caribbean-born patients. Psychol Med 11:303–318, 1981

Littlewood R, Lipsedge M: The butterfly and the serpent: culture, psychopathology and biomedicine. Cult Med Psychiatry 11:289–335, 1987

Litzenberger BW, Buttenheim MC: Sexual orientation and family development: introduction. Am J Orthopsychiatry 68:344–351, 1998

Makanjuola ROA: "Ode Ori": a culture-bound disorder with prominent somatic features in Yoruba Nigerian patients. Acta Psychiatr Scand 75:231–236, 1987

Malgady RG, Rogler LH, Cortés DE: Cultural expressions of psychiatric symptoms: idioms of anger among Puerto Ricans. Psychological Assessment 8:265–268, 1996

Manson SM, Walker RD, Kivlahan DR: Psychiatric assessment and treatment of American Indians and Alaska Natives. Hospital and Community Psychiatry 38:165–173, 1987

Marcos LR: Effects of interpreters on the evaluation of psychopathology in non–English-speaking patients. Am J Psychiatry 136:171–174, 1975

Marsella AJ: Cross-cultural research on severe mental disorders: issues and findings. Acta Psychiatr Scand Suppl 78 (No 344):7–22, 1988

McGoldrick M, Pearce JK, Giordano J (eds): Ethnicity and Family Therapy. New York, Guilford, 1982

Mendoza R, Smith MW, Poland RE, et al: Ethnic psychopharmacology: the Hispanic and Native American perspective. Psychopharmacol Bull 27:449–461, 1991

Métraux A: Voodoo in Haiti. New York, Schocken Books, 1972

Mezzich JE: Culture and multiaxial diagnosis, in Culture and Psychiatric Diagnosis: A DSM-IV Perspective. Edited by Mezzich JE, Kleinman A, Fabrega H, et al. Washington, DC, American Psychiatric Press, 1996, pp 327–334

Mezzich JE, Good BJ (eds): On culturally enhancing the DSM-IV multiaxial formulation, in DSM-IV Sourcebook, Vol 3. Edited by Widiger TA, Frances AJ, Pincus HA, et al. Washington, DC, American Psychiatric Press, 1997, pp 983–989

Mezzich JE, Kleinman A, Fabrega H, et al: Culture and Psychiatric Diagnosis. Washington, DC, American Psychiatric Press, 1996

Ming-Yuan Z: The diagnosis and phenomenology of neurasthenia: a Shanghai study. Cult Med Psychiatry 13:147–161, 1989

Moffic HS, Kendrick EA, Lomax JW, et al: Education in cultural psychiatry in the United States. Transcultural Psychiatric Research Review 24:167–187, 1987

Nandi DN, Banerjee G, Saha H, et al: Epidemic koro in West Bengal, India. Int J Soc Psychiatry 29:265–268, 1983

Neighbors HW, Jackson JS, Campbell L, et al: The influence of racial factors on psychiatric diagnosis: a review and suggestions for research. Community Ment Health J 25:301–311, 1989

Ness RC, Wintrob RM: The emotional impact of fundamentalist religious participation: an empirical study of intragroup variation. Am J Orthopsychiatry 50:302–315, 1980

Neutra R, Levy JE, Parker D: Cultural expectations versus reality in Navajo seizure patterns and sick roles. Cult Med Psychiatry 1:255–275, 1977

Ngui PW: The koro epidemic in Singapore. Aust N Z J Psychiatry 3:263–266, 1969

Offer D: The Psychological World of the Teen-Ager: A Study of Normal Adolescent Boys. New York, Basic Books, 1969

Pang KYC: Hwa byung: the construction of a Korean popular illness among Korean elderly immigrant women in the United States. Cult Med Psychiatry 14:495–512, 1990

Parham TA: Cycles of psychological nigrescence. The Counseling Psychologist 17(2):187–226, 1989

Philippe J, Romain JB: Indisposition in Haiti. Soc Sci Med 13B:129–133, 1979

Phinney J: Stages of ethnic identity development in minority group adolescents. Journal of Early Adolescence 9:34–49, 1989

Pressel E: Umbanda in Sao Paulo: religious innovation in a developing society, in Religion, Altered States of Consciousness, and Social Change. Edited by Bourguignon E. Columbus, OH, Ohio State University Press, 1973, pp 264–318

Prince R: The concept of culture-bound syndromes: anorexia nervosa and brain-fag. Soc Sci Med 21:197–203, 1985

Prudhomme C: The problem of suicide in the American Negro. Psychoanal Rev 25:372–391, 1938

Reid WH: The antisocial personality: a review. Hospital and Community Psychiatry 36:831–837, 1985

Rudorfer MV (ed): Ethnicity in the pharmacologic treatment process. Psychopharmacol Bull 32(2):181–289, 1996

Ruiz P (ed): Cross-cultural psychiatry (Section IV), in American Psychiatric Press Review of Psychiatry, Volume 14. Edited by Oldham JM, Riba MB. Washington, DC, American Psychiatric Press, 1995, pp 461–630

Ruiz P, Langrod J: Psychiatry and folk healing: a dichotomy? Am J Psychiatry 133:95–97, 1976

Russell JG: Anxiety disorders in Japan: a review of the Japanese literature on Shinkeishitsu and taijinkyofusho. Cult Med Psychiatry 13:391–403, 1989

Salisbury RF: Possession in the New Guinea highlands. Int J Soc Psychiatry 14:85–94, 1968

Samuda RJ: Psychological Testing of American Minorities. New York, Harper & Row, 1973

Saxena S, Prasad KVSR: DSM-III subclassification of dissociative disorders applied to psychiatric outpatients in India. Am J Psychiatry 146:261–262, 1989

Schmidt K, Hill L, Guthrie G: Running amok. Int J Soc Psychiatry 23:264–274, 1977

Schrut AH: The oedipus complex: some observations and questions regarding its validity and universal existence. J Am Acad Psychoanal 22(4):727–751, 1994

Schwab JJ: Nineteenth-century studies of mental illness in Southern blacks. Interaction 1(4):21–25, 1978

Schweder RA: Rethinking culture and personality theory, Part 1. Ethos 7:255–278, 1979

Sharp LA: Exorcists, psychiatrists, and the problems of possession in northwest Madagascar. Soc Sci Med 38:525–542, 1994

Shore JH: American Indian suicide: fact and fantasy. Psychiatry 38:86–91, 1975

Simons RC: Sorting the culture-bound syndromes, in The Culture-Bound Syndromes: Folk Illnesses of Psychiatric and Anthropological Interest. Edited by Simons RC, Hughes CC. Dordrecht, The Netherlands, D Reidel, 1985, pp 25–38

Spencer MB: Preschool children's social cognition and cultural cognition: a cognitive developmental interpretation of race dissonance findings. J Psychol 112:275–296, 1982

Spencer MB: Self-concept development, in Perspectives in Black Child Development. Edited by Slaughter DT. San Francisco, CA, Jossey-Bass Press, 1988, pp 59–72

Spiegel D, Cardeña E: Cultural diversity of dissociative and somatoform disorders. Paper presented at the NIMH Conference on Culture and Diagnosis, Pittsburgh, PA, April 1991

Spiegel JP: Cultural aspects of transference and countertransference revisited. J Am Acad Psychoanal 4:447–467, 1976

Spiegel JP: Community therapy in a Fiji village. Journal of Operational Psychiatry 1:28–34, 1983

Spitzer RL, Williams JBW, Gibbon M, et al: Structured Clinical Interview for DSM-III-R. Washington, DC, American Psychiatric Press, 1990

Spurlock J: Development of self-concept in Afro-American children. Hospital and Community Psychiatry 37:66–70, 1986

Stoller P: Fusion of the Worlds. Chicago, IL, University of Chicago Press, 1989

Stoller RJ, Herdt GH: The development of masculinity: a cross-cultural contribution. J Am Psychoanal Assoc 30:29–59, 1982

Strauss JS, Carpenter Jr WT, Bartko JJ: A review of some findings from the international pilot study of schizophrenia, in Annual Review of Schizophrenic Syndrome, Vol 4. Edited by Cancro R. New York, Brunner/Mazel, 1976, pp 74–88

Strickland TL, Ranganath V, Lin K-M, et al: Psychopharmacologic considerations in the treatment of black American populations. Psychopharmacol Bull 27:441–448, 1991

Strickland TL, Lin K-M, Fu P, et al: Comparison of lithium ratio between African American and Caucasian bipolar patients. Biol Psychiatry 37(5):325–330, 1995

Suryani LK: Culture and mental disorder: the case of bebainan in Bali. Cult Med Psychiatry 8:95–113, 1984

Suwanlert S: Neurotic and psychotic states attributed to Thai "Phii Pob" spirit possession. Aust N Z J Psychiatry 10:119–123, 1976

Suzuki T: The concept of neurasthenia and its treatment in Japan. Cult Med Psychiatry 13:187–202, 1989

Tan EK, Carr JE: Psychiatric sequelae of amok. Cult Med Psychiatry 1:59–67, 1977

Thomas JP, Szmukler GI: Anorexia nervosa in patients of Afro-Caribbean extraction. Br J Psychiatry 146:653–656, 1985

Tseng W-S: The development of psychiatric concepts in traditional Chinese medicine. Arch Gen Psychiatry 29:569–575, 1973

Tseng W-S, Kan-Ming M, Hsu J, et al: A sociocultural study of koro epidemics in Guangdong, China. Am J Psychiatry 145:1538–1543, 1988

Tung M: Insight-oriented psychotherapy and the Chinese patient. Am J Orthopsychiatry 61:186–194, 1991

Varma VK, Bouri M, Wig NN: Multiple personality in India: comparison with hysterical possession state. Am J Psychother 35:113–120, 1981

Waxler NE: Culture and mental illness: a social labeling perspective. J Nerv Ment Dis 159:379–395, 1974

Weidman HH: Falling-out: a diagnostic and treatment problem viewed from a transcultural perspective. Soc Sci Med 13B:95–112, 1979

Weiss MG: Cultural comments on somatoform and dissociative disorders: II, in Culture and Psychiatric Diagnosis: A DSM-IV Perspective. Edited by Mezzich JE, Kleinman A, Fabrega H, et al. Washington, DC, American Psychiatric Press, 1996, pp 159–161

Weiss MG, Sharma SD, Guar RK, et al: Traditional concepts of mental disorders among Indian psychiatric patients. Soc Sci Med 23:379–386, 1986

Weiss MG, Raguram R, Channabasavanna SM: Cultural dimensions of psychiatric diagnosis: a comparison of DSM-III-R and illness explanatory models in south India. Br J Psychiatry 166:353–359, 1995

Weissman MM, Olfson M: Depression in women: implications for health care research. Science 269:799–801, 1995

Weissman MM, Bland RC, Canino GJ, et al: Cross-national epidemiology of major depression and bipolar disorder. JAMA 276:293–299, 1996

Westermeyer J: Folk concepts of mental disorder among the Lao: continuities with similar concepts in other cultures and in psychiatry. Cult Med Psychiatry 3:301–317, 1979

Westermeyer J: Psychiatric diagnosis across cultural boundaries. Am J Psychiatry 142:798–805, 1985

Westermeyer J: Cultural aspects of substance abuse and alcoholism. Psychiatr Clin North Am 18:589–605, 1995

White GM: The role of cultural explanations in "somatization" and "psychologization." Soc Sci Med 16:1519–1530, 1982

Widiger TA, Frances AJ, Pincus HA, et al (eds): The DSM-IV Sourcebook, Vol 3. Washington, DC, American Psychiatric Press, 1997

Wig NN: DSM-III: a perspective from the third world, in International Perspectives on DSM-III. Edited by Spitzer RL, Williams JBW, Skodol AE. Washington, DC, American Psychiatric Press, 1983, pp 79–89

Wing JK, Birley JLT, Cooper JE, et al: Reliability of a procedure for measuring and classifying "present psychiatric state." Br J Psychiatry 113:499–515, 1967

Williams CL: Issues surrounding psychological testing of minority patients. Hospital and Community Psychiatry 38:184–189, 1987

Williams DH: The epidemiology of mental illness in Afro-Americans. Hospital and Community Psychiatry 37:42–49, 1986

Wilson MN: Child development in the context of the Black extended family. Am Psychol 44:380–385, 1989

Wittkower ED, Warnes H: Cultural aspects of psychotherapy. Am J Psychother 28:566–573, 1974

Yamamoto J: An Asian view of the future of cultural psychiatry, in Current Perspectives in Cultural Psychiatry. Edited by Foulks EF, Wintrob RM, Westermeyer J, et al. New York, Spectrum, 1977, pp 209–215

Yap PM: The possession syndrome: a comparison of Hong Kong and French findings. Journal of Mental Science 106:114–137, 1960

Yap PM: Koro: a culture-bound depersonalization syndrome. Br J Psychiatry 111:43–50, 1965

CHAPTER 41

THE LAW AND PSYCHIATRY

ROBERT I. SIMON, M.D.

The body of law applied to the practice of psychiatry does not differ from that of medicine in general. Nevertheless, the diagnosis, treatment, and management of patients with psychiatric disorders present not only unique clinical and ethical concerns but unique legal considerations as well. For instance, determinations of a patient's competency, as well as the patient's ability to manage his or her personal affairs, may be required to determine the patient's mental capacity to make health care decisions. Currently, competency determinations are particularly relevant for patients suffering from Alzheimer's disease or dementia related to acquired immunodeficiency syndrome (AIDS). Accordingly, ethical and legal issues such as informed consent, the right to treatment, the right to refuse treatment, substitute decision making, and advance directives are commonly confronted in treating psychiatric patients.

Individuals who have been criminally charged must be legally competent to stand trial. Defendants with psychiatric impairments may not meet the competency standard. Therefore, such persons may require pretrial evaluations of their mental capacity to understand the charges against them and their ability to assist counsel in their own defense. Moreover, depending on the nature and duration of a psychiatric disorder, criminal defendants may seek acquittal or have the charges against them reduced on the basis of the argument that they were legally insane at the time the offense occurred.

Vulnerability to psychiatric malpractice suits has increased, more so in specific areas of psychiatric practice. Table 41–1 reveals the recent malpractice claims experience of the Psychiatrists Purchasing Group, the liability insurer of members of the American Psychiatric Association ("Benefacts" 1996). The increased use of somatic therapies, the assessment and management of violent patients, use of techniques to recover memories of sexual abuse, sexual misconduct, boundary violations, premature discharge of potentially violent patients, and managed care settings all represent areas of heightened liability for the psychiatric practitioner.

The chance of a psychiatrist being sued in the 1980s was 1 in 25 per year ("Benefacts" 1996). Through 1995, however, the odds have increased to about 1 out of every 12 psychiatrists. In some states, psychiatrists are sued at the rate of 1 in 6 every year. Psychiatrists in Massachusetts have moved from 20th to 12th among the most frequently sued specialists within a period of 3 years.

The American Psychiatric Association–sponsored Professional Liability Insurance Program identifies a number of factors to account for the increase in malpractice suits:

TABLE 41–1. Recent allegations of malpractice (approximate frequency of claims)

Allegation	Frequency (%)
Incorrect treatment	33
Attempted/completed suicide	20
Incorrect diagnosis	11
Improper supervision	7
Medication error/drug reaction	7
Improper commitment	5
Breach of confidentiality	4
Unnecessary hospitalization	4
Undue familiarity	3
Libel/slander	2
Other (e.g., abandonment, electroconvulsive therapy, third-party injury)	4

Source. Data from "Benefacts" 1996.

1. Psychiatrists are treating "sicker" patients in managed care settings.
2. Representatives of the media have scrutinized so-called recovered memories and ritual satanic abuse cases.
3. Tort reform legislation has failed.
4. Psychiatrists are specializing in new practice areas such as geriatric psychopharmacology, adolescent addiction medicine, multiple personality disorder, pain management, and adult children of alcoholics.
5. Psychiatrists are providing more primary care, such as in the management of patients with diabetes, hypertension, and a wide variety of acute general medical illnesses.

With the advent of managed care, psychiatrists treat a large volume of patients for brief visits and are more likely to be sued. When the psychiatrist spends less time with a patient, a working alliance is less likely to develop. Among primary care physicians it was reported that those with no malpractice claims used more statements of orientation, laughed and used more humor, and engaged patients more in a give-and-take dialogue than did colleagues who had been sued(Levinson et al. 1997). Primary care physicians with no claims also spent more time in routine visits than did sued primary care physicians (mean, 18.3 vs. 15.0 minutes). The length of the visit was an independent factor in predicting claims status.

In spite of the growth of malpractice claims, psychiatrists prevail in seven out of eight suits brought against them. A plaintiff has the heavy burden of proving his or her malpractice claim.

In addition, lawsuits involving psychological injuries and head trauma have increased annually and have become a major source of personal injury litigation. Because of the complexities often associated with establishing the extent and cause of a plaintiff's damages, forensic expertise in psychiatry is frequently needed by the courts.

PSYCHIATRIC MALPRACTICE: SOMATIC THERAPIES

Psychiatric malpractice is medical malpractice. *Malpractice* is the provision of substandard professional care that causes a compensable injury to a person with whom a professional relationship existed. Although this concept may seem relatively clear and simple, it has its share of conditions and caveats. For example, the essential issue is *not* the existence of substandard care per se, but whether there is compensable liability.

Medical malpractice is a tort (i.e., a wrong that is noncriminal and not related to a contract): it is a type of civil wrong committed as a result of negligence by a physician that causes injury to a patient in his or her care. *Negligence*, the fundamental concept underlying a malpractice lawsuit, is simply described as doing something that a physician with a duty of care (to the patient) should not have done or failing to do something that a physician with a duty of care should have done. The fact that a psychiatrist commits an act of negligence does not automatically make him or her liable to the patient bringing the lawsuit.

For a psychiatrist to be found *liable* to a patient for malpractice, four fundamental elements (Table 41–2) must be established by a preponderance of the evidence: 1) that there was a duty of care owed by the defendant, 2) that the duty of care was breached, 3) that the plaintiff (i.e., patient) suffered actual damages, and 4) that the deviation was the direct cause of the damages. Each of these four elements must be met or there can be no finding of liability, regardless of any finding of negligence. A psychiatrist may be neg-

TABLE 41–2. The four Ds of malpractice

Duty	There was a duty of care owed by the doctor.
Deviation	The duty of care was breached.
Damages	The patient suffered actual damages.
Direct causation	The deviation was the direct cause of the damages.

ligent but still not found to be liable. For example, if the patient suffered no real injuries because of the negligence, or if there was an injury but it was not directly due to the psychiatrist's negligence, a claim of malpractice will be defeated.

Critical to the establishment of a claim of professional negligence is the requirement that the defendant's conduct was substandard or was a deviation in the standard of care owed to the plaintiff. Except in the case of "specialists," the law presumes and holds all physicians to a standard of *ordinary care*, which is measured by its *reasonableness* according to the clinical circumstances in which it is provided.

The use of a somatic therapy, including electroconvulsive therapy (ECT), is evaluated no differently from use of any other medical treatment or procedure with respect to potential liability. The same general standard of *ordinary* and *reasonable care* governs the assessment of whether a psychiatrist's use of or failure to use a somatic intervention is legally actionable (Annotation 1979, 1985).

It is generally acknowledged within the psychiatric profession that there is no *absolute standard* protocol for the administration of psychotropic medication or ECT. Nevertheless, the existence of professional treatment guidelines and procedures that are generally accepted or used by a significant percentage of psychiatrists should alert clinicians to consider such guidelines as practice reference sources. For example, the American Psychiatric Association (APA) has published comprehensive findings and guidelines in the form of task force reports concerning ECT (American Psychiatric Association 1990) and tardive dyskinesia (American Psychiatric Association 1992b). Nevertheless, official guidelines must not preempt sound professional judgment in attending to the clinical needs of individual patients.

Official guidelines and procedures publications do not, per se, establish the standard of care by which a court might evaluate a psychiatrist's treatment. They do represent a credible source of information with which a reasonable psychiatrist at least should be familiar and should have considered (*Stone v. Proctor* 1963). In addition to expert testimony, courts generally consider official guidelines and the professional literature that establishes contemporary psychiatric practices in determining the standard of care.

There is some evidence that there is less professional autonomy and flexibility associated with the use of ECT. Normally, the "reasonable care" standard that is applied to psychiatric treatment is construed in a fairly broad manner because psychiatry is currently considered inexact. Some psychiatric treatments, however, such as ECT, appear to be more rigidly regulated than others. For instance, the Joint Commission on Accreditation of Healthcare Organiza-

tions (JCAHO) considers ECT a *special treatment* procedure, to be regulated by written policies. Whenever ECT is used, the procedure must be adequately justified and documented in the patient's medical chart (Joint Commission on Accreditation of Healthcare Organizations 1998, TX.7.2). These policies, coupled with any additional regulations that a facility might have promulgated regarding ECT, can serve as establishing the basis for liability if violated.

The "standard" for judging the use and administration of medication, on the other hand, appears to be consistent with the more flexible and general "reasonable care" requirement. Another reference source that bears highlighting is the *Physicians' Desk Reference* (PDR), which may be used to establish or dispute a psychiatrist's pharmacotherapy procedures. The PDR is a commercially distributed, privately published reference regarding medication products used in the United States. The Food and Drug Administration (FDA) requires that drug manufacturers have their official package inserts reported in the PDR (Simon 1992a). Accordingly, psychiatrists consult publications like the PDR as needed to keep abreast of current and accurate medication information. Although numerous courts have cited the PDR as a credible source of medication-related information in the medical profession, the PDR does not by itself establish *the* standard of care (*Gowan v. United States* 1985; *Witherell v. Weimer* 1986/1987). Instead, it may be used as one piece of evidence to establish the standard of care in a particular situation (*Callan v. Norland* 1983; *Doerr v. Hurley Medical Center* 1984). Courts generally follow the reasoning in *Ramon v. Farr* (1989), holding that drug inserts alone do not set the standard of care. They are only one element to be considered along with previous clinical experience, the scientific literature, approvals in other countries, expert testimony, and other pertinent factors. The presence of a substantial scientific literature that justifies the clinician's treatment is vastly more persuasive than FDA approval. The PDR or any other reference, however, cannot serve as a substitute for the psychiatrist's sound clinical judgment.

Fortunately, courts recognize the importance of professional judgment and give psychiatrists, like other medical specialists, some latitude in explaining special diagnostic or treatment considerations that guided their decision making. For instance, the clinical data regarding pharmacological treatment of rapid cycling bipolar disorder indicate that there is a variety of potentially useful drug therapies, some of which are considered experimental or on the cutting edge (Simon 1997). For instance, various drugs and hormones are clinically useful as mood stabilizers, such as carbamazepine, clozapine, thyroid and estrogen replacement, calcium channel blockers, antihypertensives, neuro-leptics, atypical antipsychotics, and other anticonvulsants (phenytoin, clonazepam, primidone). Yet none of these drugs are presently approved as mood stabilizers by the FDA.

The courts consider the fact that no one treatment of choice exists and that treatment applications are still being developed. Moreover, evidence that a treatment procedure is accepted by at least a respectable minority of profession-als in the field can establish that a particular treatment is a reasonable professional practice (Simon 1993). The stan-dard of care associated with the use of a somatic therapy to treat a psychiatric patient, *at a minimum*, should include some variation of the following considerations and mea-sures:

PRETREATMENT

- Complete clinical history (medical, psychiatric) (Tay-lor et al. 1987)
- Complete physical examination, as clinically indi-cated (preferably performed by another physician or, if necessary, by the psychiatrist)
- Administration of necessary laboratory tests and re-view of past test results (Daniel et al. 1992)
- Disclosure of sufficient information to obtain in-formed consent, including information regarding the risks and benefits both for receiving treatment and for *not* receiving treatment
- Thorough documentation of all decisions, informed consent information, pertinent patient responses, and other relevant treatment data

POSTTREATMENT

- Careful monitoring of the patient's response to treat-ment, including adequate follow-up evaluations and appropriate laboratory testing (Daniel et al. 1992)
- Prompt adjustments in treatment, as clinically indi-cated
- Arrangement for additional informed consent when treatment is altered appreciably or new treatment is initiated

The final word regarding treatment measures depends on the clinician, not the law. The preceding considerations should be viewed as general guidelines that are commonly associated with reasonable care when somatic therapies are implemented.

THEORIES OF LIABILITY

The term *psychiatric malpractice* is not a useful one, because the same basic legal principles are applied to any lawsuit al-leging malpractice by a physician, regardless of medical subspecialty. Use of descriptive terms such as *psychiatric* or *neuropsychiatric* reflects the general recognition that the theories of liability to be discussed represent the most common areas of malpractice associated with that subspecialty. The following is a limited review of the most common litigation areas in the somatic treatment of psy-chiatric patients.

The potential for negligence by a psychiatrist appears to be greatest in clinical situations involving the use of psychotropic medication. Although no reliable compila-tion of malpractice claims data has been published, anec-dotal information suggests that medication-related law-suits *do* constitute a significant share of the litigation filed against psychiatrists. As noted earlier, recent claims data from the APA Professional Liability Insurance Program showed that medication error and drug reaction consti-tuted 7% of malpractice allegations. However, allegations of drug mismanagement are likely a major contributor to the most common malpractice allegations of incorrect treatment (33%).

A review of the relevant case law indicates that a variety of mistakes, omissions, and poor medication treatment practices commonly result in malpractice actions brought against psy-chiatrists. The following discussion, although not intended to be exhaustive, provides a framework for identifying problem areas associated with medication treatment.

Failure to Evaluate Properly

Sound clinical practice requires that before any form of treatment is initiated, the patient should be properly eval-uated. The nature and extent of an evaluation is largely dic-tated by the type of treatment being contemplated and the medical condition of the patient. A physical examination should be conducted or obtained, if clinically indicated. A recently performed physical examination may suffice, or patients may be referred elsewhere by psychiatrists who do not perform physical examinations. Moreover, the duty to ensure that proper informed consent is obtained can also be fulfilled at this time.

A number of lawsuits have resulted from the failure to evaluate a patient properly before administering medica-tions (*Blanchard v. Levine* 1985; *Shaughnessy v. Spray* 1983). As a result of this omission, the patient's condition is mis-diagnosed and remains untreated. In addition, the patient is exposed to unnecessary side effects and risks of inappro-priate medications.

Failure to Monitor

Probably the most common act of negligence associated with pharmacotherapy is the failure to monitor the patient's progress while he or she is taking medication, including carefully following the patient for adverse side effects.

Once psychotropic medication has been prescribed, it is the psychiatrist's duty to monitor the patient. Consultation or referral may be necessary according to the clinical needs of the patient. Monitoring may require the use of laboratory testing. Serum drug levels are now obtainable for a number of psychotropic medications. The primary indications for these laboratory tests include assessment of therapeutic and toxic levels of medication and of patient compliance with treatment. The use of carbamazepine, valproic acid, and clozapine requires close monitoring of the hematopoietic system and the liver. A failure to supervise patients taking psychotropic medication properly can unnecessarily subject them to harmful side effects and can delay a change to more effective treatment. If a patient is harmed from these omissions, a malpractice action might result (*Chaires v. St. John's Episcopal Hospital* 1984; *Clifford v. United States* 1985; *Kilgore v. County of Santa Clara* 1982).

Split Treatment

In managed care or similar treatment settings, the mere prescribing of medication apart from a working doctor-patient relationship does not meet generally accepted standards of good clinical care. It is a prime example of fragmented care. Such a practice may diminish the efficacy of the drug treatment itself or even lead to the patient's failure to take the prescribed medication. Fragmented care, in which the psychiatrist functions only as a prescriber of medication while remaining uninformed about the patient's overall clinical status, constitutes substandard treatment that may lead to a malpractice action.

Split treatment situations require that the psychiatrist stay fully informed of the patient's clinical status as well as of the nature and quality of treatment the patient is receiving from the nonmedical therapist. In a collaborative relationship, responsibility for the patient's care is shared according to the qualifications and limitations of each discipline. The responsibilities of each discipline do not diminish those of the other disciplines. Patients should be informed of the separate responsibilities of each discipline. Periodic evaluation by the psychiatrist and the nonmedical therapist of the patient's clinical condition and needs is necessary to determine whether the collaboration should continue. On termination of the collaborative relationship, the patient should be informed by the clinicians either separately or jointly. In split treatments, if negligence is claimed on the part of the nonmedical therapist, it is likely that the collaborating psychiatrist will be sued, and vice versa (Woodward et al. 1993).

Psychiatrists who prescribe medications in split treatment arrangements should be able to hospitalize patients if necessary. If the psychiatrist does not have admitting privileges, prearrangements should exist with other psychiatrists who can hospitalize patients if emergencies arise.

Split treatment is increasingly used by managed care companies and is a potential malpractice minefield. Increasingly in managed care settings, psychiatrists are required to prescribe medications from a restrictive or closed formulary. For example, selective serotonin reuptake inhibitors (SSRIs) are currently considered first-line treatment for depression. However, a number of managed care companies allow the prescribing of tricyclic antidepressants (TCAs) only, which have a much greater lethality than SSRIs for patients who overdose. Psychiatrists, in their professional discretion, should determine which medications will be prescribed according to the special clinical needs of the patient.

Negligent Prescription Practices

The selection of a medication, the determination of initial dosage and form of administration, and other related procedures are all decisions left to the professional discretion of the treating psychiatrist. For example, in managed care settings, psychiatrists should vigorously resist attempts to restrict their choices of drugs by a restrictive or closed formulary or by therapeutic substitution (interchanging different chemical agents from the same therapeutic class, e.g., a TCA substituted for an SSRI). The prescribing of specific medications should be determined only by the psychiatrist and should be based on the clinical needs of the patient. An appeal should be filed if a drug that is not formulary approved is denied. The law recognizes that the physician is in the best position to "know the patient" and to determine what course of treatment is best under the circumstances. Accordingly, the standard by which a psychiatrist's prescription practices will be evaluated is reasonableness. In administering psychotropic medication, psychiatrists need only conform their procedures and decision making to those that are *ordinarily* practiced by other psychiatrists under similar circumstances.

A review of cases involving allegations of negligent prescription procedures reveals several common practices representing possible deviations from generally accepted treatment practice:

- Exceeding recommended dosages without clinical indications
- Negligently prescribing multiple drugs (i.e., "polypharmacy")
- Negligently prescribing medication for unapproved uses
- Negligently prescribing "unapproved" medications
- Negligently failing to disclose medication risks

As stated earlier, any physician who prescribes medication has a duty initially to obtain the informed consent of the patient (Table 41–3). Obtaining competent informed consent may be complicated by the fact that some psychiatric patients have a compromised mental capacity for health care decision making due to mental illness. Patients lacking such decision-making capacity require consent for treatment by substitute decision makers (Table 41–4).

Each time a medication is changed and a new drug is introduced, informed consent should be obtained. A failure to inform a patient properly of the risks and consequences of a prescribed medication can be grounds for a malpractice action if the patient is injured as a result (*Karasik v. Bird* 1984; *Moran v. Botsford General Hospital* 1984; *Wright v. State* 1986).

Other areas of negligence involving medication that have resulted in legal action include 1) failure to treat side effects once they have been recognized or should have been recognized, 2) failure to monitor a patient's compliance with prescription limits, 3) failure to prescribe medication

TABLE 41–3. Informed consent: reasonable information to be disclosed

Although there exists no consistently accepted set of information to be disclosed for any given medical or psychiatric situation, as a rule of thumb, five areas of information are generally provided:

1.	Diagnosis	Description of the condition or problem
2.	Treatment	Nature and purpose of proposed treatment
3.	Consequences	Risks and benefits of the proposed treatment
4.	Alternatives	Viable alternatives to the proposed treatment including risks and benefits
5.	Prognosis	Projected outcome with and without treatment

Source.   Reprinted with permission from Simon RI: *Clinical Psychiatry and the Law*, 2nd Edition. Washington, DC, American Psychiatric Press, 1992. Copyright 1992, American Psychiatric Press, Inc.

TABLE 41–4. Common consent options for patients lacking the mental capacity for health care decisions

Proxy consent of next of kin

Adjudication of incompetence, appointment of a guardian

Institutional administrators or committees

Treatment review panels

Substituted consent of the court

Advance directives (living will, durable power of attorney, health care proxy)

Statutory surrogates (spouse or court-appointed guardian)[a]

[a]Medical statutory surrogate laws (when treatment wishes of patient are unstated).
Source.   Reprinted with permission from Simon RI: *Clinical Psychiatry and the Law*, 2nd Edition. Washington, DC, American Psychiatric Press, 1992. Copyright 1992, American Psychiatric Press, Inc.

or appropriate levels of medication according to the treatment needs of the patient, 4) failure to refer a patient for consultation or treatment by a specialist, and 5) negligent withdrawal from medication.

TARDIVE DYSKINESIA

The development of neuroleptic medications in the mid-1950s dramatically improved the treatment and management of schizophrenic patients. Shortly after the introduction of neuroleptic medications as therapeutic agents, however, researchers and clinicians observed unusual muscle movements in some patients, referred to as *tardive dyskinesia* (TD).

The number of psychiatric patients treated with neuroleptics is quite high (H. J. Parry et al. 1973). The risk of developing TD is approximately 4%–7% per year of neuroleptic use (Lohr et al. 1986). These projections are even higher for elderly patients (Kane et al. 1982; Klawans and Barr 1982). As the newer antipsychotic drugs are used more frequently, the risk of developing TD is expected to be lower.

Given these data, the potential for *TD litigation* is clear. Despite the possibility of a large number of TD-related lawsuits, relatively few psychiatrists have been sued under this cause of action. One reason may be that patients who develop TD may not have the physical and psychological stamina required to pursue litigation.

Cases involving allegations of negligence after a patient develops TD are based on the same legal elements as any other malpractice action. Moreover, the bases for negligence mirror those that have been previously identified with general medication cases. These areas include, but are not limited to, the following:

- Failure to evaluate and monitor a patient properly.
- Failure to obtain informed consent.
- Negligent diagnosis of a patient's condition. For instance, in *Hyde v. University of Michigan Board of Regents* (1986/1986), a woman was awarded $1,000,000 from a medical center for misdiagnosis of her condition as Huntington's chorea instead of tardive dyskinesia. The verdict was later reversed on the basis of a subsequent case that expanded the state's sovereign immunity coverage.
- Wrongful prescription of neuroleptic medication. For example, in *Dovido v. Vasquez* (1986), a net award of $700,000 went to a 42-year-old plaintiff who suffered from tardive dyskinesia as a result of the defendant psychiatrist's negligent prescription of extremely high doses of fluphenazine.
- Failure to monitor medication side effects. For example, in *Clites v. State* (1982), the plaintiff was a mentally retarded man who had been institutionalized since age 11 and treated with major tranquilizers from age 18 to 23. Tardive dyskinesia was diagnosed at age 23, and the family subsequently sued. The family claimed that the defendants negligently prescribed medication, did not inform the patient of the possibility of developing TD, and failed to monitor and subsequently treat the patient's resulting side effects. The jury returned a verdict for the plaintiff and awarded damages in the amount of $760,165. This award was affirmed on appeal. The court ruled that the defendants were negligent because they deviated from the standards of the "industry." Specifically, the court cited a variety of omissions in ordinary psychiatric practice that, they concluded, reasonable psychiatrists would have provided. Among the "deviations" they noted were a failure to conduct regular physical examinations and laboratory tests, a failure to intervene at the first sign of TD, the inappropriate use of multiple medications at the same time, the use of drugs for convenience (e.g., "behavior management") rather than therapy, and the failure to obtain *informed* consent.

Patients receiving neuroleptic medication need to be frequently monitored. No stock answer can be given to the question of how frequently the psychiatrist should see a patient. Generally, psychiatrists should schedule return visits with a frequency that accords with the patient's clinical need. The longer the time between visits, however, the greater the risk of adverse drug reactions and untoward developments in the patient's condition. The interval between visits ordinarily should not be longer than 6 months.

Psychiatrists who do not follow patients according to their clinical needs may be subject to legal claims of failure to monitor patients properly.

The defenses and preventive measures applicable to TD-related malpractice claims are consistent with those used in any case alleging negligent drug treatment. Generally speaking, the application of sound clinical practice that is appropriately communicated to the patient and documented in the medical chart serves as an effective foil to any allegations of negligence should TD develop (*Frasier v. Department of Health and Human Resources* 1986; *Radank v. Heyl* 1986; *Rivera v. NYC Health and Hospitals* 1988). Moreover, for the psychiatrist who is treating *chronic aggression* with antipsychotic drugs, it is important to consider the warning by Yudofsky et al. (1987) that

> the use of antipsychotic medications in treating chronic aggression involves a substantial risk of the emergence of tardive dyskinesia, because the prevalence of tardive dyskinesia among patients on long-term neuroleptic treatment is about 25%....
>
> While antipsychotic agents are the treatment of choice for aggression due to psychosis and also may be helpful in the acute short-term management of violence through sedative action, we do *not* recommend their use in the long-term management of aggression, especially that which is secondary to organic brain syndrome. (p. 400)

ELECTROCONVULSIVE THERAPY

Although a significant proportion of psychiatrists believe that ECT is a viable treatment for certain mental disorders (O'Connell 1982), it has been estimated that *no more* than 3%–5% of all psychiatric inpatients in the United States receive this treatment (Weiner 1979). It can be expected from these figures that legal actions alleging negligence associated with ECT are likely to be infrequent. The low incidence of ECT-related malpractice suits has corroborated this suspicion (Krouner 1975; Perr 1980). Despite this low malpractice potential, lawsuits involving ECT are occasionally brought. Cases involving ECT-related injuries have represented a variety of circumstances in which negligence has occurred. These cases can be categorized into three groups: pretreatment, treatment, and posttreatment.

Pretreatment

Although there is some variation in pre-ECT evaluations, the following procedures recommended by the APA Task Force on Electroconvulsive Therapy (American Psychiatric Association 1990) generally should be performed:

1. A psychiatric history and examination to evaluate the indications for ECT
2. A medical examination to determine risk factors
3. Anesthesia evaluation
4. Informed consent (written)
5. An evaluation by a physician privileged to administer ECT

Although these recommendations by the APA Task Force on ECT do not define in absolute terms the standard of care for ECT, they may be proffered as evidence of the standard of care by attorneys in malpractice suits involving ECT. Official treatment guidelines, however, should never be a substitute for the psychiatrist's sound clinical judgment. Nevertheless, failure to conduct appropriate *pretreatment* procedures could endanger the welfare of the patient and ultimately result in a lawsuit for negligence.

Treatment

It is well established that psychiatrists are not held liable for a mere mistake in judgment, nor is a psychiatrist held to a standard of 100% accuracy or perfect performance (Smith 1986, p. 68; see also *Holton v. Pfingst* 1976). Therefore, a bad result does not automatically establish a claim for malpractice (*Howe v. Citizens Memorial Hospital* 1968). Instead, a patient must prove, by a preponderance of the evidence, that the psychiatrist deviated from the standard of care and that the deviation proximately caused the patient some injury or damage. The procedure for evaluating the care and treatment afforded a patient when ECT is used is no different. Cases involving ECT-related injuries in which the negligence has been related to the actual *treatment process* include the following errors:

■ Failure to use a muscle relaxant to reduce the chance of a bone fracture
■ Negligent administration of the procedure
■ Failure to conduct an evaluation of the patient, including the use of X rays, before continuing treatment

Posttreatment

It is common for patients treated with ECT to experience side effects such as temporary confusion, disorientation, and memory loss following its administration (O'Connell 1982). Because of these temporary debilitating effects, sound clinical practice requires that psychiatrists provide reasonable posttreatment care and safeguards. Courts have held that the failure to attend properly to a patient for a period of time following the administration of ECT can

result in malpractice liability. The following are examples of posttreatment circumstances that may constitute a negligence cause of action:

■ Failure to evaluate complaints of pain or discomfort following treatment
■ Failure to evaluate a patient's condition before resuming ECT treatments
■ Failure to monitor a patient properly to prevent falls
■ Failure to supervise properly a patient who was injured as a result of ECT

As a source of *civil liability*, ECT-related lawsuits today are quite rare and are not likely to represent a significant problem area for psychiatrists. However, as Perlin (1989) cautioned, "recent developments in right-to-refuse treatment law and statutory regulation of intrusive therapy are likely to insure that any future ECT litigation will still be considered carefully" (pp. 47–48).

RIGHT TO REFUSE TREATMENT

The developing concept that an institutionalized mentally disabled person has a right to refuse treatment is probably the most slippery issue in mental health law today. Buttressed by constitutionally derived rights to privacy and freedom from cruel and unusual punishment, the common law tort of battery, and the doctrine of informed consent, mentally disabled persons are increasingly being afforded protections traditionally reserved for the legally competent. This "new freedom" often runs directly counter to the dictates of clinical judgment (i.e., to treat and protect). As a result of this conflict, the courts vary considerably regarding the parameters of this right and the procedures to be followed.

Two landmark cases illustrate this point. In *Rennie v. Klein* (1978), the Third Circuit Court of Appeals recognized a right to refuse treatment in the state of New Jersey. The court, after extended litigation, found that this right could be overridden and antipsychotic drugs administered "whenever, in the exercise of professional judgment, such an action is deemed necessary to prevent the patient from endangering himself or others." In the second case, *Rogers v. Commissioner of Department of Mental Health* (1983), the court decided that in the absence of an emergency (e.g., serious threat of extreme violence or personal injury), any person who has not been adjudicated incompetent has a right to refuse antipsychotic medication. Incompetent persons have a similar right, but it must be exercised through a "substituted judgment treatment plan" that has been reviewed and approved by the court.

These two decisions are often viewed as legal bookends to the issue of the right to refuse treatment. The cases suggest parameters for other courts attempting to define such a right. The *Rennie* case became the model for subsequent legal decisions that adopted a treatment-driven rationale for the right to refuse treatment. *Rogers* became the basis for rights-driven approaches taken by some courts in litigating the right to refuse treatment.

Numerous state and federal decisions have tackled some aspect of this issue. Generally speaking, there is near-judicial recognition of an involuntarily hospitalized patient's right to refuse medication absent an emergency. Case law criteria for emergencies range from a risk of imminent harm to self or others to a deterioration in the patient's mental condition if treatment is halted. Until either more states enact legislation or the United States Supreme Court squarely rules on this issue, jurisdictions will continue to vary regarding the substance of the right to refuse treatment and the procedures by which such a right can be implemented.

THE SUICIDAL PATIENT

The most common legal action involving psychiatric care is the failure to provide reasonable protection to patients from harming themselves. Theories of negligence involving suicide can be grouped into three broad categories: failure to diagnose properly (i.e., assess the potential for suicide); failure to treat (i.e., use reasonable treatment interventions and precautions); and failure to implement (i.e., carry out treatment properly and not negligently).

These theories, each of which applies to inpatient and outpatient settings, are based on the practitioner's failure to act reasonably in exercising the appropriate duty of care owed to the patient. Wrongful death suits as a result of patient suicides are based on the legal concepts of foreseeability and causation. A typical lawsuit argues that a patient with the potential for suicide was not diagnosed and treated properly, resulting in the patient's death.

As a general rule, a psychiatrist who exercises reasonable care in compliance with accepted medical practice will not be held liable for any resulting injury. Normally, if a patient's suicide was not reasonably foreseeable, or when the suicide occurred as a result of intervening factors, this rule will apply.

FORESEEABLE SUICIDE

The evaluation of suicide risk is one of the most complex, difficult, and challenging clinical tasks in psychiatry. Suicide is a rare event with low specificity (high false-positive rates). A comprehensive assessment of a patient's suicide risk is critical to a sound clinical management plan. Using reasonable care in assessing suicide risk can preempt the problem of predicting the actual occurrence of suicide, for which professional standards do not yet exist. Standard approaches to the assessments of suicide risk are described in the psychiatric literature (Blumenthal 1990; Chiles and Strohsall 1995; Maris et al. 1992; Simon 1992a). Short-term (24–48 hours) suicide risk assessments are more reliable than long-term assessments.

As an accepted standard of care, an evaluation of suicide risk should be done with all patients, regardless of whether they present with overt suicidal complaints. A review of case law shows that reasonable care requires that a patient who is either suspected of being or confirmed to be suicidal must be the subject of certain affirmative precautions. A failure either to assess reasonably a patient's suicidality or to implement an appropriate precautionary plan, once the suicide potential becomes foreseeable, is likely to render a practitioner liable if the patient is harmed because of a suicide attempt. The law tends to assume that suicide is preventable if it is foreseeable. Foreseeability, however, should not be confused with preventability. In hindsight, many suicides seem preventable that were clearly not foreseeable.

When suicide risk assessments are competently performed and recorded, the psychiatrist demonstrates that he or she was careful and thorough in the management of the suicidal patient. Moreover, evidence of a reasonable suicide risk assessment also demonstrates that the psychiatrist adhered to the prevailing standard of care. Although psychiatrists cannot ensure favorable outcomes with suicidal patients, they can ensure that the process of suicide risk assessment was competently performed.

Inpatients

Intervention in an inpatient setting usually requires the following:

- Screening evaluations
- Case review by clinical staff
- Development of an appropriate treatment plan
- Implementation of that plan

Careful documentation of assessments and management interventions with changes responsive to the patient's clinical situation should be considered evidence of clinically and legally sufficient psychiatric care. Assessing suicide risk is only half the equation. Documenting the benefits of a psychiatric intervention (e.g., ward change, pass, discharge) against the risk of suicide permits an even-handed approach to the clinical management of the patient. Consideration only of a patient's suicide risk is a manifestation of defensive psychiatry that usually interferes with good clinical care, further exposing the psychiatrist to a potential malpractice suit.

Psychiatrists are more likely to be sued when a psychiatric inpatient commits suicide. The law presumes that the opportunities to foresee (i.e., anticipate) and control (i.e., treat and manage) suicidal patients are greater in the hospital.

Outpatients

Outpatient therapists face a somewhat different situation. Psychiatrists are expected to assess the severity and imminence of a foreseeable suicidal act. The result of the assessment dictates the nature of the duty-of-care options. Courts have reasoned that when an outpatient commits suicide, the therapist has not necessarily breached a duty to safeguard the patient from foreseeable self-harm because of the difficulty in controlling the patient (*Speer v. United States* 1981). Instead, the reasonableness of the psychiatrist's efforts is determinative.

SUICIDE PREVENTION PACTS

Suicide prevention "contracts" created between the clinician and the patient attempt to develop an expressed understanding that the patient will call for help rather than act out suicidal thoughts or impulses. These "contracts" have no legal authority; although they may be helpful in solidifying the therapeutic alliance, they may falsely reassure the psychiatrist. Suicide prevention agreements between psychiatrists and patients must not be used in place of adequate suicide assessment (Simon 1991b).

LEGAL DEFENSES

One legal defense that has created a split in the courts involves the use of the "open door" policy in which patients are allowed freedom of movement for therapeutic purposes. In these cases, the individual facts and reasonableness of the staff's application of the "open door" policy appear to be paramount. Nevertheless, courts have difficulty with abstract treatment notions such as personal growth when faced with a dead patient.

Another defense, the doctrine of sovereign or governmental immunity, may statutorily bar a finding of liability against a state or federal facility. An intervening cause of suicide over which the clinician has no control is another

valid legal defense. For example, a court may find a psychiatrist not liable for the suicidal act of a borderline patient who experienced a significant rejection between therapy sessions and then impulsively attempted suicide without trying to contact the psychiatrist. The court may rule that the suicide was caused by the superseding intervening variable of an unforeseen rejection and not by the psychiatrist's negligence.

Finally, the best-judgment defense has been used successfully when the patient was properly assessed and treated for suicide risk but he or she committed suicide anyway (Robertson 1991).

THE VIOLENT PATIENT

As a general rule, one person has no duty to control the conduct of a second person to prevent that person from physically harming a third person (Restatement [Second] of Torts 315(a) [1965]). Applying this rule to psychiatric care, psychiatrists traditionally have had only a limited duty to control hospitalized patients and to exercise due care on discharge. Within the last two decades, this rule has changed. After *Tarasoff* (*Tarasoff v. Regents of the University of California* 1976), the therapist's legal duty and potential liability significantly expanded. In *Tarasoff*, the California Supreme Court first recognized that a duty to protect third parties was imposed only when a special relationship existed between the victim, the individual whose conduct created the danger, and the defendant. The court stated that "the single relationship of a doctor to his patient is sufficient to support the duty to exercise reasonable care to protect others [from the violent acts of patients]."

Psychiatrists do not have the ability to predict violence with any accuracy. Violent behaviors are the result of the complex interplay among social, clinical, and personality factors that vary significantly across situations and time (Widiger and Trull 1994). Nonetheless, clinical methods for assessing the risk of violence exist that reflect the current standard of care (Baxter and Beck 1998; Monahan and Steadman 1994; Simon 1992a; Tardiff 1989).

The assessment of the risk of violence is essentially a clinical judgment. Because the validity of violence risk assessments is only modestly greater than chance, the MacArthur Violence Risk Assessment Study was established. The purpose of the study is to improve clinical risk assessment validity, to enhance effective clinical risk management, and to provide data on mental disorders and violence for informing mental health law and policy ("The MacArthur Violence Risk Assessment Study" 1996). Until more studies are available, sound clinical practice requires that thorough violence risk assessments be routinely performed on potentially violent patients on the basis of current knowledge of violence risk factors. Although violence risk assessments need to be made at such critical points as the initiation of ward status changes, passes, and discharge, violence risk assessment is more of a continuing process than a solitary event. All such assessments should be duly recorded.

The index of suspicion for potential violence should be high in patients with a past history of violence who are making current, serious threats of harm toward specific individuals. The potential for violence is further heightened if the patient is acutely psychotic, substance abusing, angry, fearful of being harmed, and experiencing delusions of being controlled or influenced (Link and Stueve 1994).

A majority of courts have found no duty to protect without an imminent threat of serious harm to a foreseeable victim. Only a small minority of courts have held that a duty to protect exists for the population at large. Despite the fact that the Tarasoff duty still is not law in some jurisdictions and is subject to different interpretations by individual courts, the duty to protect is, in effect, a national standard of practice.

In some jurisdictions, courts have held that the need to safeguard the public well-being overrides all other considerations, including confidentiality. Although a few courts have declined to find a *Tarasoff* duty in a specific case, a growing number of courts have recognized some variation of the original *Tarasoff* duty. No court has rejected the duty outright as legally invalid.

A number of states have enacted immunity statutes that protect the psychiatrist from legal liability caused by a patient's violent acts toward others (Appelbaum et al. 1989). The majority of these statutes define the therapist's duty in terms of warning the endangered third party and/or notifying the authorities. The duty-to-protect language stated in some statutes allows for a greater variety of clinical interventions.

RELEASE OF POTENTIALLY VIOLENT PATIENTS

Under managed care, discharging violent or potentially violent inpatients presents unique challenges for treating psychiatrists (Simon 1988). The treatment of psychiatric inpatients has changed dramatically in the managed care era (Lazarus and Sharfstein 1994). Most psychiatric units, particularly in general hospitals, have become short-stay,

acute care psychiatric facilities. Generally, only suicidal, homicidal, or gravely disabled patients with major psychiatric disorders pass strict precertification review for hospitalization (Tischler 1990). Close scrutiny by utilization reviewers permits only short hospitalization for these patients (Wickizer et al. 1996). The purpose of hospitalization is crisis intervention and management to stabilize patients and to ensure their safety. The treatment of these patients is being provided by a variety of mental health professionals. Nonetheless, the psychiatrist often must bear the ultimate burden of liability for treatments gone awry ("Why Are Liability Premiums Rising?" 1996). Limited opportunity usually exists during the hospital stay to develop a therapeutic alliance with patients. The ability to communicate with patients, the psychiatrist's stock-in-trade, is often severely curtailed. All these factors contribute to a greatly increased risk of malpractice suits against psychiatrists alleging premature or negligent discharge of patients due to cost-containment policies.

There is more control over the patient in the hospital than is available in an outpatient setting. Courts closely evaluate decisions made by psychiatrists who treat inpatients that adversely affect the patient or a third party. Liability imposed on psychiatric facilities that had custody of patients who injured others outside the institution following escape or release is clearly distinguishable from the factual situation of *Tarasoff*. Duty-to-warn cases generally involve patients in outpatient treatment, and liability arises from the inaction of the therapist who fails to take affirmative measures to warn or protect endangered third persons. In negligent-release cases, on the other hand, liability may arise from the allegation that the institution's affirmative act in releasing the patient caused injury to the third party. Nonetheless, allegations may be made that a psychiatrist or hospital personnel failed to warn individuals known to be at risk of harm from an inpatient prior to discharge. Lawsuits stemming from the release of foreseeably dangerous patients who subsequently injure or kill others are roughly five to six times more common than outpatient duty-to-warn litigation (Simon 1992b).

The psychiatrist's liability is determined by reference to professional standards. Consultation with other psychiatrists may provide additional protection when the discharge of a potentially violent patient appears problematic. Consulting with an attorney may help clarify legal obligations. Lawyers, however, tend to be highly risk averse and conservative when making recommendations. Clinicians must not abandon their professional judgment. Sound legal advice may not necessarily accord with the clinical realities surrounding the management of a specific patient.

The patient's willingness to cooperate with the psychiatrist is critical to maintaining follow-up treatment. The psychiatrist's obligation focuses on structuring the follow-up visits in such a manner to encourage compliance. A study of Veterans Administration (VA) inpatient referrals to a VA mental health outpatient clinic showed that of 24% of inpatients referred, approximately one-half failed to keep their first appointments (Zeldow and Taub 1981). Nevertheless, limitations do exist on the extent of the psychiatrist's ability to ensure follow-up care. Most patients retain the right to refuse treatment. These limitations must be acknowledged by both the psychiatric and legal communities (Simon 1992a). The American Medical Association Council on Scientific Affairs has developed evidence-based discharge criteria for safe discharge from the hospital (American Medical Association 1996).

In either the outpatient or inpatient situation, psychiatrists are in compliance with the responsibility to warn and protect others from potentially violent patients if they reasonably assess a patient's *risk* for violence and act in a clinically appropriate manner on the basis of their findings. Professional standards do exist for the assessment of the risk factors for violence (Simon 1992c). No standard of care exists, however, for the prediction of violent behavior. The clinician should assess the risk of violence frequently, updating the risk assessment at significant clinical junctures (e.g., room and ward changes, passes, discharge). A risk-benefit assessment should be conducted and recorded before a pass or discharge is issued. However, assessing the risk of violence is a "here and now" determination performed at the time of discharge. Once the patient is discharged, the potential for violence depend on the patient's mental state at any given time combined with concurrent situational factors.

INVOLUNTARY HOSPITALIZATION

A person may be involuntarily hospitalized only if certain statutorily mandated criteria are met. Three main substantive criteria serve as the foundation for all statutory commitment requirements: that the individual 1) be mentally ill, 2) be dangerous to self or others, and/or 3) be unable to provide for his or her basic needs. Generally, each state spells out which criteria are required and what each means. Terms such as *mentally ill* are often loosely described, thus placing the responsibility for proper definition onto the clinical judgment of the petitioner.

In addition to individuals with mental illness, certain states have enacted legislation that permits the involuntary hospitalization of three other distinct groups: developmentally disabled (mentally retarded) persons, individuals who are addicted to a substance or substances (alcohol, drugs), and mentally disabled minors. Special commitment provisions may exist governing requirements for the admission and discharge of mentally disabled minors as well as numerous due-process rights afforded these individuals (*Parham v. J. R.* 1979).

Involuntary hospitalization of psychiatric patients usually arises when violent behavior threatens to erupt toward self or others and when patients become unable to care for themselves. These patients frequently manifest mental disorders and conditions that readily meet the substantive criteria for involuntary hospitalization.

Clinicians must remember that they do not commit patients. This is done solely under the jurisdiction of the court. The psychiatrist merely initiates a medical certification that brings the patient before the court, usually after a brief period of hospitalization for evaluation. Clinicians should not attempt to second-guess the court's ultimate decision concerning involuntary hospitalization. The psychiatrist must be guided by the treatment needs of the patient in seeking medical certification.

Commitment statutes do not require involuntary hospitalization but are permissive (Appelbaum et al. 1989). The statutes enable mental health professionals and others to seek involuntary hospitalization for persons who meet certain substantive criteria. On the other hand, the duty to seek involuntary hospitalization is a standard-of-care issue. Patients who are mentally ill and pose an imminent, serious threat to themselves or others may require involuntary hospitalization as a primary psychiatric intervention.

LIABILITY

The most common cause of a malpractice action involving involuntary hospitalization is the failure of a psychiatrist to adhere in good faith to statutory requirements, leading to a wrongful commitment. Oftentimes, these lawsuits are brought under the theory of false imprisonment. Other areas of liability that may arise from wrongful commitment include assault and battery, malicious prosecution, abuse of authority, and intentional infliction of emotional distress (Simon 1992a, pp. 170–173).

In many states, psychiatrists are granted immunity from liability as long as they use reasonable professional judgment and act in good faith when petitioning for commitment (Mishkin 1989). Performing a careful examination of the patient, abiding by the requirements of the law, and ensuring that sound reasoning motivates the certification of the patient is primarily good clinical practice and, only secondarily, good risk management. However, evidence of willful, blatant, or gross failure to adhere to statutorily defined commitment procedures may expose a psychiatrist to a lawsuit.

RIGHTS OF INVOLUNTARILY HOSPITALIZED PATIENTS

A majority of states recognize the right of inpatients to refuse treatment. Even though the patient is involuntarily hospitalized, the hospitalization does not negate a presumption of competence. In most states, patients involuntarily hospitalized who refuse medication require a separate court hearing for an adjudication of incompetence and the provision of substituted consent by the court. Recently, persons hospitalized under criminal commitment have been accorded the right to refuse treatment. The courts have found that incarcerated patients' constitutional right to due process is adequately protected by the exercise of professional judgment within the medical peer review process of the institution.

Hospitalized patients possess other rights. Patients possess rights of visitation, although these rights can be temporarily suspended for proper cause relating to the patient's care and treatment. Free communications of hospitalized patients through mail, telephone, or visitors are considered a right, unless protection of the patient or others requires supervision of communications. The right to privacy includes allowing patients to have secure locker space, private toilet and shower facilities, and a minimum square footage of floor space. Protection of confidentiality is also included. Economic rights include the right to have and spend money and to handle one's own financial affairs responsibly. In most jurisdictions, involuntarily hospitalized patients do not lose their civil rights, such as the right to manage their own money. Hospitalized patients must be paid for their work in certain jurisdictions unless it is truly therapeutic labor (i.e., work not connected with maintenance of the hospital). "Patients' rights" are not absolute and often must be tempered by the clinical judgment of the mental health professional. Inevitably, disputes over perceived or real violations of patients' rights arise. In some jurisdictions, a civil rights officer or ombudsman is mandated by statute to mediate these disputes.

RECOVERED MEMORIES CASES

The clamorous controversy concerning recovered memories of sexual abuse threatens to undermine the credibility of the mental health professions. The debate continues to generate intense passions that drive an increasing number of recovered memory cases into the courts. Patients who allege recovered memories of abuse have sued parents and other alleged perpetrators. In a turnabout, the alleged victimizers have sued therapists whom they claim negligently induced false memories of sexual abuse. In some cases, patients have recanted and joined forces with others (usually their parents) to sue their therapists.

The memory debate has polarized many therapists into "believers" and "disbelievers." Most therapists hold personal beliefs about the validity of recovered memories of sexual abuse that are somewhere between the extremes. Strongly held personal biases about recovered memories represent a new occupational hazard for clinicians that can undermine the therapist's duty of neutrality to patients, creating deviant treatment boundaries and increasing the risk of incurring liability.

Litigation in recovered memory cases is expected to explode in the coming years. Multimillion dollar verdicts against mental health practitioners are anticipated. The basic allegation in these cases is that the therapist abandoned a position of neutrality to suggest, persuade, coerce, and implant false memories of childhood sexual abuse. The guiding principle of clinical risk management in recovered memory cases is to maintain therapist neutrality and establish sound treatment boundaries.

Complicating the situation is the empirical evidence about memory mechanisms, which, as is typical for any emerging science, reveals contradictory findings about how and what persons in various settings retain in memory and forget. Empirical studies frequently fail to distinguish whether allegedly repressed memories are not retrieved or simply not reported to researchers.

Sound risk management rests solidly on a clinical footing and is secondarily informed by awareness of the pertinent legal issues (Gutheil and Simon 1997). Risk management principles that should be considered when evaluating or treating a patient who recovers memories of abuse in psychotherapy include the following:

- Maintain therapist neutrality—do not suggest abuse.
- Stay clinically focused—provide adequate evaluation and treatment for patient's presenting problems and symptoms.
- Carefully document the memory recovery process.
- Manage personal biases and countertransference.
- Avoid mixing treater and expert witness roles.
- Closely monitor supervisory and collaborative therapy relationships.
- Clarify nontreatment roles with family members.
- Avoid use of special techniques (e.g., hypnosis or sodium amytal) unless clearly indicated; obtain consultation before proceeding.

- Stay within professional competence—do not take cases beyond your expertise.
- Distinguish between narrative truth and historical truth; in therapy, the therapist is largely attuned to the patient's perception of reality.
- Obtain consultation in problematic cases.
- Foster patient autonomy and self-determination. Do not suggest lawsuits; this should be the patient's decision after careful consideration.
- In managed care settings, inform patients with recovered memories that more than brief therapy may be required.
- When making public statements, distinguish personal opinions from scientifically established facts.
- If uncomfortable with a patient recovering memories of childhood abuse, stop and refer.
- Do not be reluctant to ask about abuse as part of a competent psychiatric evaluation.

SEXUAL MISCONDUCT

Therapist-patient sex is usually preceded by progressive boundary violations in treatment (Simon 1989). As a consequence, patients are frequently psychologically damaged by the precursor boundary violations as well as the eventual sexual misconduct of the therapist (Simon 1991a). An excellent account of the gradual erosion of treatment boundaries leading to near loss of control with a client is given by Rutter (1989).

General boundary guidelines exist for conducting psychiatric treatment (Simon 1992d). Awareness of these guidelines and of their transgression may help alert the therapist to progressive boundary violations (Simon 1994). Sexual misconduct does not occur in isolation but usually involves a variety of negligent acts of omission and commission.

CIVIL LIABILITY

Psychiatrists who sexually exploit their patients are subject to civil and criminal actions as well as ethical and professional licensure revocation proceedings. "The Principles of Medical Ethics With Annotations Especially Applicable to Psychiatry" states that sex with a current or former patient is unethical (section 2, annotation 1). Malpractice is the most common area of liability.

In a sexual exploitation case, the plaintiff has the difficult burden of proving, by a preponderance of the evidence (i.e., "more likely than not"), that the exploitation actually took place. This burden can be met when the plaintiff can provide corroborating evidence to support the claim, such as testimony from other abused (former) patients, letters, pictures, hotel or motel receipts, and identification of incriminating body marks. If the defendant practitioner admits to the exploitation, the plaintiff is left with the responsibility of showing that he or she sustained injuries as a result of the sexual activity. Typically, patient injury occurs in the form of emotional injury (i.e., worsened psychiatric condition). Expert psychiatric testimony usually is required to establish the type and extent of psychological damages, as well as to establish whether a breach of the standard of care occurred.

An increasing number of states have statutorily made sexual activity both civilly and criminally actionable. For instance, Minnesota enacted legislation that states the following:

> A cause of action against a psychotherapist for sexual exploitation exists for a patient or former patient for injury caused by sexual contact with the psychotherapist if the sexual contact occurred: 1) during the period the patient was receiving psychotherapy . . . or 2) after the period the patient received psychotherapy . . . if a) the former patient was emotionally dependent on the psychotherapist; or b) the sexual contact occurred by means of therapeutic deception. (Minn Stat Ann 148A.02 [West 1989])

A few states have enacted civil statutes proscribing sexual misconduct (Simon 1992a). A number of states make therapist sexual misconduct a crime (Bisbing et al. 1995, pp. 833–855). Some states prosecute sexual exploitation suits using their sexual assault statutes. Legislatures in a number of states have enacted statutes that provide civil or criminal remedies to patients who were sexually abused by their therapists (Appelbaum 1990; Strasburger et al. 1991).

Three types of remedies have been codified: reporting, civil liability, and criminal prosecution. *Reporting statutes* require a therapist who learns of any past or current therapist-patient sex to disclose this information. A few states have *civil statutes* proscribing sexual misconduct (Bisbing et al. 1995, pp. 155–180). Civil statutes incorporate a standard of care and make malpractice suits easier to pursue. For example, Minnesota's statute provides a specific cause of action against psychiatrists and other psychotherapists for injury caused by sexual contact with a patient (Minn Stat Ann 148A.02 [West 1989]). Some of these statutes also restrict unfettered discovery of the plaintiff's past sexual history. *Criminal sanctions* may be the only remedy for exploitative therapists without malpractice insurance, for therapists who are unlicensed, or for therapists who do not belong to professional organizations.

OTHER CIVIL THEORIES AND DEFENSES

A variety of causes of action may be asserted by a plaintiff who has been sexually exploited by a psychotherapist. In a minority of states, spouses of the injured patient also have legal standing to initiate their own cause of action against an exploitative practitioner on the grounds of loss of consortium (i.e., interference with the marital relationship).

A variety of defenses have been raised to diminish or protect against liability, but, to date, few have been legally successful (Table 41–5). For instance, the contention that the patient was aware that sex was not a part of treatment, that the sex occurred outside the treatment setting, that treatment ended before the sexual relationship began, or that the patient "consented" to the sexual contact have all been rejected by the courts. Patients cannot consent to malpractice. Moreover, in sexual misconduct cases, the issue is never patient consent but always breach of fiduciary trust by the therapist.

There is no "respected minority" in the profession that claims sexual relations with patients is therapeutic. This position had a few adherents at one time but is no longer publicly advocated by credible mental health professionals.

TABLE 41–5. Legal defenses asserted by defendants in sexual misconduct cases

1. Denial of plaintiff's allegations of sexual misconduct
2. Suit barred by statute of limitations
3. No doctor-patient relationship
4. Terminated patient—no legal fault under immunity statute
5. No causation of harm (psychological symptoms reflect inherent course of mental disorder)
6. No damages (no psychological harm caused by sex with patient)
7. Superseding intervening variable (not sex with patient) causing harm
8. Contributory and comparative negligence (plaintiff's "contribution" to sexual misconduct)
9. Liability in supervision of offending therapist: sexual misconduct of a supervisee is beyond the scope of employment ("detour and frolic")
10. Marriage to patient
11. Improper pleading by plaintiff
12. Consent in sexual assault claims

Source. Reprinted with permission from Simon RI: *Clinical Psychiatry and the Law,* 2nd Edition. Washington, DC, American Psychiatric Press, 1992. Copyright 1992, American Psychiatric Press, Inc.

CRIMINAL SANCTIONS

Sexual exploitation of a patient, under certain circumstances, may be considered rape or some analogous sexual offense and may therefore be criminally actionable (Hoge et al. 1995). Typically, the criminality of the exploitation is determined by one of three factors: the practitioner's means of inducement, the age of the victim, or the availability of a relevant state criminal code.

Sex with a current patient may be criminally actionable under sexual assault statutes if the state can prove beyond a reasonable doubt (i.e., with 90%–95% certainty) that the patient was coerced into engaging in the sexual act. Typically, this type of evidence is limited to the use of some form of substance (e.g., medication) either to induce compliance or to reduce resistance. Anesthesia, electroconvulsive treatment, hypnosis, drugs, force, and threat of harm have been used to coerce patients into sexual submission (Schoener et al. 1989, p. 331). To date, claims of "psychological coercion" through the manipulation of transference phenomena have not been successful in establishing the coercion necessary for a criminal case. In cases involving a minor patient, the issue of consent or coercion is irrelevant, because minors and adult incompetent persons are considered unable to provide valid consent. Therefore, sex with a child or an incompetent person is automatically considered a criminal act.

PROFESSIONAL DISCIPLINARY ACTION

For the purposes of adjudicating allegations of professional misconduct, licensing boards are typically granted certain regulatory and disciplinary authority by state statutes. As a result, state licensing organizations, unlike professional associations, may discipline an offending professional more effectively and punitively by suspending or revoking his or her license. Because licensing boards are not as restrained as the courts in civil and criminal actions by rigorous rules of evidence in trial procedures, it generally is easier for the patient to seek redress through this means. A review of published reports of sexual misconduct cases adjudicated before licensing boards revealed that in a vast majority of cases the evidence was reasonably sufficient to substantiate a claim of exploitation, leading to revocation of the professional's license or suspension from practice for varying lengths of time, including permanent suspension.

Patients can bring ethical charges against psychiatrists before the district branches of the American Psychiatric Association. Ethical violators may be reprimanded, suspended, or expelled from the APA. All national organizations of mental health professionals have ethically proscribed sexual relations between therapist and patient. Ethical charges can be filed only against members of a professional group; therefore, this option is not available to patients whose therapists do not belong to a professional organization.

CONFIDENTIALITY AND TESTIMONIAL PRIVILEGE

Confidentiality refers to the right of a patient to have communications spoken or written in confidence undisclosed to outside parties without implied or expressed authorization. *Privilege*, or more accurately *testimonial privilege*, can be viewed as a derivation of the right of confidentiality. Testimonial privilege is a statutorily created rule of evidence that permits the holder of the privilege (e.g., the patient) to exercise the right to prevent the person to whom confidential information was given (e.g., the psychiatrist) from disclosing it in a judicial proceeding.

CONFIDENTIALITY

Clinical-Legal Foundation

The basis for recognizing and safeguarding patient confidences is derived from four general sources. First, states have acknowledged this right of protection by including confidentiality provisions in either professional licensure laws or confidentiality and privilege statutes. The second source, and probably the most traditional, comprises the ethical codes of the various mental health professions. Third, the common law recognizes an attorney-client privilege, but developing case law also has carved out this source of protection for physicians and psychotherapists. In 1996, the Supreme Court ruled that communications between psychotherapist and patient are confidential and need not be disclosed in federal trials (*Jaffe v. Redmond* 1996). Fourth, the right of confidentiality may be subsumed under the right of privacy.

Breaching Confidentiality

Regardless of the basis of the right of confidentiality, once the doctor-patient relationship has been created, the professional assumes an automatic duty to safeguard a patient's disclosures. This duty is not absolute, and there are circumstances in which breaching confidentiality is both ethical and legal.

Patients also waive confidentiality in a variety of situations, especially in managed care settings. Medical records

are regularly sent to potential employers or to insurance companies when benefits are requested. A limited waiver of confidentiality ordinarily exists when a patient participates in group therapy. Whether one group member can be compelled in court to disclose information shared by another group member during group therapy is still unsettled legally. Many state confidentiality statutes provide statutory exceptions to confidentiality between the psychiatrist and the patient in one or more situations (Brakel et al. 1985, pp. 592–596; Table 41–6).

Patients' access to their own records is normally controlled by statutes. These statutory provisions are found under the heading of "medical records" or the much broader term "privilege."

If a patient gives the psychiatrist good reason to believe that a warning should be issued to an endangered third party, the confidentiality of the communication that gave rise to the warning may be lost. Because of the requirement to warn endangered third parties, psychiatrists who have issued warnings have been compelled to testify in criminal cases (Leong et al. 1992).

TESTIMONIAL PRIVILEGE

The patient—not the psychiatrist—is the holder of the privilege that controls the release of confidential information. Because privilege applies only to the judicial setting, it is called *testimonial privilege*. Privilege statutes represent the most common recognition by the state of the importance of protecting information provided by a patient to a psychotherapist. This recognition moves away from the essential purpose of the American system of justice (e.g., "truth finding") by insulating certain information from disclosure in court. This protection is justified on the basis that the special need for privacy in the doctor-patient relationship outweighs the unbridled quest for an accurate outcome in court.

TABLE 41–6.   Common statutory exceptions to confidentiality between psychiatrist and patient

Child abuse

Competency proceedings

Court-ordered examination

Dangerousness to self or others

Patient-litigant exception

Intent to commit a crime or harmful act

Civil commitment proceedings

Communication with other treatment providers

Privilege statutes usually are drafted with reference to one of the following four relationships, depending on the type of practitioner:

- Physician-patient (general)
- Psychiatrist-patient
- Psychologist-patient
- Psychotherapist-patient

Cases have been successfully litigated in which the broader physician-patient category has been applied to the psychotherapist when an applicable statute did not exist.

Exceptions to Testimonial Privilege

Privilege statutes also specify exceptions to testimonial privilege. Although exceptions vary, the most common include the following:

- Child abuse reporting
- Civil commitment proceedings
- Court-ordered evaluations
- Cases in which a patient's mental state is in question as a part of litigation

The last exception, known as the *patient-litigant exception*, commonly occurs in will contests, workers' compensation cases, child custody disputes, personal injury actions, and malpractice actions in which the therapist is sued by the patient.

LIABILITY

An unauthorized or unwarranted breach of confidentiality can cause a patient considerable emotional harm. As a result, a psychiatrist typically can be held liable for such a breach on the basis of at least four theories:

- Malpractice (breach of confidentiality)
- Breach of statutory duty
- Invasion of privacy
- Breach of (implied) contract

INFORMED CONSENT AND THE RIGHT TO REFUSE TREATMENT

Informed consent is a legal theory in medical malpractice. It provides a patient with a cause of action for not being adequately informed about the nature and consequences of a particular medical treatment or procedure undertaken.

This theory is founded on two distinct legal principles. The first is the right of every patient to determine what will or will not be done to his or her body, often referred to as the *right of self-determination* (*Schloendorff v. Society of New York Hospital* 1914). The second principle emanates from the fiduciary nature of the doctor-patient relationship. Inherent in a physician's duty of fiduciary care is the responsibility to disclose honestly and in good faith all requisite facts concerning a patient's condition. Included among factors to be disclosed are any treatment risks, alternatives, and consequences. The primary purpose of the doctrine of informed consent is to promote individual autonomy; secondarily, it is intended to promote rational decision making (Appelbaum et al. 1987).

There are three essential elements to the doctrine of informed consent:

- Competency
- Information
- Voluntariness

Usually, clinicians provide the first level of screening in identifying patient competency and in deciding whether to accept a patient's treatment decision. The patient or a bona fide representative must be given an adequate description of the treatment. If the patient who refuses treatment appears to lack health care decision-making capacity, it does not mean that the patient cannot be treated. An appropriate substitute decision maker can provide (or withhold) consent. To be able to provide informed consent, the patient or substitute decision maker should be told about the risks, benefits, and prognosis both with and without treatment, as well as alternative treatments and their risks and benefits. In addition, the competent patient must voluntarily consent to or refuse the proposed treatment or procedure.

COMPETENCY

It is clinically useful to distinguish the terms *incompetence* and *incapacity*. Incompetence refers to a court adjudication, whereas incapacity indicates a functional inability as determined by a clinician (Mishkin 1989). Legally, only competent persons may give informed consent. An adult patient is considered legally competent unless adjudicated incompetent or temporarily incapacitated because of a medical emergency. Incapacity does not prevent treatment; it merely requires the clinician to obtain substitute consent. Treating an incompetent patient without substituted consent is the same as treating a competent patient against his or her will.

Legal competence is narrowly defined in terms of cognitive capacity. The definition derives largely from the laws governing transactions. Important clinical concepts such as affective incompetence are not usually recognized by the law unless cognitive capacity is significantly diminished. For example, a severely depressed but cognitively intact patient may refuse antidepressant medication owing to profound feelings of hopelessness, helplessness, and worthlessness. Manic patients emphasize risks of medications while downplaying benefits. Schizophrenic patients tend to be fearful that medication will cause them serious harm. They are often unable to make a balanced assessment that considers both risks and benefits of a proposed drug. One study, in which three instruments were used to assess competency for treatment decisions, found that the schizophrenia and depression groups demonstrated poorer understanding of treatment disclosures, poorer reasoning in decision making regarding treatment, and a greater likelihood of failing to appreciate their illness or the potential treatment benefits (Grisso and Appelbaum 1995a). Denial of illness often interferes with insight and the ability to appreciate the significance of information provided to the patient. In *In The Guardianship of John Roe* (1992), the Massachusetts Supreme Judicial Court recognized that denial of illness can render a patient incompetent to make treatment decisions.

Competency is not a scientifically determinable state and is situation specific. The issue of competency arises in a number of civil, criminal, and family law contexts. Although there are no hard-and-fast definitions, the patient's ability to do the following is legally germane to determining competency:

- Understand the particular treatment choice being proposed
- Make a treatment choice
- Communicate that choice verbally or nonverbally

This standard obtains only a simple consent from the patient rather than an informed consent, however, because alternative treatment choices are not provided.

A review of case law and scholarly literature reveals four standards for determining incompetency in decision making (Appelbaum et al. 1987). In order of levels of mental capacity required, these standards include the following:

- Communication of choice
- Understanding of relevant information provided
- Appreciation of available options and consequences
- Rational decision making

Severely mentally disordered patients frequently deny their illnesses. Although they may communicate a choice and understand the information provided, these patients may lack the insight or ability to appreciate the information provided. Rational decision making is impaired as well. For example, schizophrenic patients tend to fear harm from the treatment while ignoring the risk of medication side effects. Grisso and Appelbaum (1995b), using three instruments for assessing competency to make treatment decisions, found that the schizophrenia and depression groups demonstrated poorer understanding of treatment disclosures, poorer reasoning in decision making regarding treatment, and a greater likelihood of failing to appreciate their illnesses or the potential treatment benefits.

Psychiatrists generally feel most comfortable with a rational decision-making standard in determining incompetency. Most courts prefer the first two standards above but often combine competency standards. A truly informed consent that considers the patient's autonomy, personal needs, and values occurs when rational decision making is applied by the patient to the risks and benefits of appropriate treatment options provided by the clinician.

Grisso and Appelbaum (1995a) found that the choice of standards determining competence affected the type and proportion of patients classified as impaired. When compound standards were used, the proportion of patients identified as impaired increased. These authors advised that clinicians be aware of the applicable standards in their jurisdictions.

A valid consent can be either *expressed* (oral or in writing) or *implied* from the patient's actions. The competency issue is particularly sensitive when dealing with minors or mentally disabled persons who lack the requisite cognitive capacity for health care decision making. In both cases, it is generally recognized in the law that an authorized representative or guardian may consent for the patient (see Table 41–4).

INFORMATION

The standard for exercising a legally sufficient disclosure varies from state to state. Traditionally, the duty to disclose was measured by a professional standard: either what a reasonable physician would disclose under the circumstances or the customary disclosure practices of physicians in a particular community. In the landmark case *Canterbury v. Spence* (1972), a patient-oriented standard was applied. This standard focused on the "material" information that a *reasonable* person in the patient's position would want to know to make a reasonably informed decision. An increasing number of courts have applied this standard, and some have expanded "material risks" to include information regarding the consequences of not consenting to the treatment or procedure (*Truman v. Thomas* 1980). Even in patient-oriented jurisdictions, there is no duty to disclose every possible risk. A material risk is defined as one in which a physician knows or should know what would be considered significant by a reasonable person in the patient's position. The issue of how much information a patient has to comprehend for consent to be valid is normally resolved by requiring a doctor to convey all appropriate information in terms that the average patient would understand.

VOLUNTARINESS

For a consent to be considered legally voluntary, it must be given freely by the patient and without the presence of any form of coercion, fraud, or duress that impinges on the patient's decision-making process. In evaluating whether a consent is truly voluntary, the courts typically examine all the relevant circumstances, including the psychiatrist's manner, the environmental conditions, and the patient's mental state.

EXCEPTIONS AND LIABILITY

There are four basic exceptions to the requirement of obtaining informed consent (Table 41–7). When immediate treatment is necessary to save a life or prevent imminent serious harm and it is impossible to obtain either the patient's consent or that of someone authorized to provide consent for the patient, the law typically "presumes" that the consent would have been granted. Two distinctions must be understood when applying this exception. First, the emergency must be serious and imminent; second, the patient's condition, not the surrounding circumstances (e.g., adverse environmental conditions), determines the existence of an emergency.

A second exception exists when a patient lacks sufficient mental capacity to give competent consent or is found

TABLE 41–7. Basic exceptions to obtaining informed consent

Emergencies

Incompetency

Therapeutic privilege

Waiver

Source. Reprinted with permission from Simon RI: *Concise Guide to Clinical Psychiatry and the Law.* Washington, DC, American Psychiatric Press, 1992. Copyright 1992, American Psychiatric Press, Inc.

to be legally incompetent. Someone who is incompetent is incapable of giving informed consent. Under these circumstances, consent must be obtained from a substitute decision maker.

The third exception, *therapeutic privilege*, is the most difficult to apply. Informed consent may not be required if a psychiatrist determines that a complete disclosure of possible risks and alternatives might have a deleterious impact on the patient's health and welfare. Jurisdictions vary in their application of this exception. Absent specific case law or statutes outlining the factors relevant to such a decision, a doctor must substantiate a patient's inability psychologically to withstand being informed of the proposed treatment. Some courts have held that therapeutic privilege may be invoked only if informing the patient will worsen his or her condition or so frighten the patient that rational decision making is precluded (*Canterbury v. Spence* 1972; *Natanson v. Kline* 1960). Therapeutic privilege cannot be used as a means of circumventing the legal requirement for obtaining informed consent from the patient before initiating treatment.

Finally, a physician need not disclose risks of treatment when the patient has competently, knowingly, and voluntarily waived his or her right to be informed (e.g., when the patient does not want to be informed of drug risks).

Absent a situation allowing one of the four exceptions, a psychiatrist who physically treats a patient without first obtaining informed consent is subject to legal liability. In some jurisdictions, a lack-of-informed-consent action may be defeated if case law or statute provides that a reasonable person under the given circumstances would have consented to treatment. As a rule of thumb, treatment without any consent or against a patient's wishes may constitute a battery (intentional tort), whereas treatment commenced with an inadequate consent will be treated as an act of medical negligence.

SECLUSION AND RESTRAINT

The psychiatric legal issues surrounding seclusion and restraint are complex. Seclusion and restraint have both indications and contraindications as clinical management tools (see Tables 41–8 and 41–9). The legal regulation of seclusion and restraint has become increasingly more stringent over the past decade.

Legal challenges to the use of restraints and seclusion have been made on behalf of the institutionalized mentally ill and the mentally retarded. Normally, these lawsuits do not stand alone but are part of a challenge to a wide range of alleged abuses within a hospital.

TABLE 41–8.   Indications for seclusion and restraint

1. Prevent clear, imminent harm to the patient or others.
2. Prevent significant disruption to treatment program or physical surroundings.
3. Assist in treatment as part of ongoing behavior therapy.
4. Decrease sensory overstimulation (seclusion only).
5. Respond to patient's voluntary reasonable request.

Source.   Reprinted with permission from Simon RI: *Concise Guide to Clinical Psychiatry and the Law.* Washington, DC, American Psychiatric Press, 1992. Copyright 1992, American Psychiatric Press, Inc.

TABLE 41–9.   Contraindications to seclusion and restraint

1. Extremely unstable medical and psychiatric conditions[a]
2. Delirious or demented patients unable to tolerate decreased stimulation[a]
3. Overtly suicidal patients[a]
4. Patients with severe drug reactions or overdoses or those patients requiring close monitoring of drug dosages[a]
5. For punishment or for convenience of staff

[a]Unless close supervision and direct observation are provided.
Source.   Reprinted with permission from Simon RI: *Concise Guide to Clinical Psychiatry and the Law.* Washington, DC, American Psychiatric Press, 1992. Copyright 1992, American Psychiatric Press, Inc.

Generally, courts hold, or consent decrees provide, that restraints and seclusion can be implemented only when a patient presents a risk of harm to self or others and no less restrictive alternative is available. Additional considerations include the following:

1. Restraint and seclusion can be implemented only by a written order from an appropriate medical official.
2. Orders are to be confined to specific, time-limited periods.
3. A patient's condition must be regularly reviewed and documented.
4. Any extension of an original order must be reviewed and reauthorized.

In addition to these guidelines, some courts and state statutes outline certain due process procedures that must be followed before a restraint or seclusion order can be implemented. Notably, patient due process protections are required only in cases in which restraint and seclusion are used for disciplinary purposes. Typical due process considerations include some form of notice, a hearing, and the involvement of an impartial decision maker. Absent language to the contrary, these procedures may be eased in cases of emergency.

The acceptability of restraint or seclusion for the purposes of training was recognized in the landmark case *Youngberg v. Romeo* (1982). *Youngberg* involved a challenge to the "treatment" practices at the Pennhurst State School and Hospital in Pennsylvania. The United States Supreme Court held that patients could not be restrained except to ensure their safety or, in certain undefined circumstances, "to provide needed training." Although it recognized that the defendant had a liberty interest in safety and freedom from bodily restraint, the Court added that these interests were not absolute and were in conflict with the need to provide training. The Court also held that decisions made by appropriate professionals regarding restraining the patient would presumptively be considered correct. *Youngberg* is viewed as the first step in the right direction by advocates for the developmentally disabled. In addition, psychiatrists and other mental health professionals have lauded the decision because the Court recognized that professionals, rather than the courts, are best able to determine the needs of patients, including when restraint is appropriate.

Most states have enacted statutes regulating the use of restraints, normally specifying the circumstances in which restraints can be used. Most often, those circumstances occur only when a risk of harm to self or danger to others is imminent. Statutory regulation of the use of seclusion is far less common. Only about one-half of the states have laws related to seclusion. The majority of states with laws regarding seclusion and restraint require some type of documentation of their use.

National guidelines for the proper use of seclusion and restraints have been established by the American Psychiatric Association Task Force on the Psychiatric Uses of Seclusion and Restraint (American Psychiatric Association 1984). The JCAHO has promulgated detailed guidelines for hospitals regarding seclusion and restraint requirements (Joint Commission on Accreditation of Healthcare Organizations 1997, Tx-47–Tx-57). Professional opinion concerning the clinical use of physical restraints and seclusion varies considerably. Unless precluded by state and federal freedom from restraint and seclusion statutes or JCAHO and hospital policies, a variety of uses for seclusion can be justified on both clinical and legal grounds (Simon 1992a).

NATIONAL PRACTITIONER DATA BANK

On September 1, 1990, the National Practitioner Data Bank established by the Health Care Quality Improvement Act of 1986 went into effect. The data bank tracks disciplinary actions, malpractice judgments, and settlements against physicians, dentists, and other health care professionals (Johnson 1991).

Hospitals, health maintenance organizations (HMOs), professional societies, state medical boards, and other health care organizations are required to report any disciplinary action taken against providers lasting more than 30 days. Disciplinary actions include limitation, suspension, or revocation of privileges or professional society membership. Under the Health Care Quality Improvement Act, immunity from liability is granted for health care entities and providers making peer review reports in good faith (Walzer 1990).

Hospitals are required to request information from the data bank concerning all physicians applying for staff privileges. Every 2 years, a query of the data bank is required concerning each physician or other practitioner on the hospital staff. Hospitals that do not comply face loss of immunity for professional peer review activities.

The public will not have access to the data bank. Plaintiffs' attorneys can have access to the data bank only if they can prove that the hospital failed to query the data bank regarding the physician in question. The information obtained can be used only to sue the hospital for negligent credentialing. Physicians can request information from the data bank about their own file.

COMPETENCY: THE BASIC CONCEPT

Nearly every area of human endeavor is affected by the law and, as a fundamental condition, requires one to be mentally competent. Essentially, competency is defined as "having sufficient capacity, ability . . . [or] possessing the requisite physical, mental, natural, or legal qualifications" (Black 1990, p. 284). This definition is deliberately vague and ambiguous because the term *competency* is a broad concept encompassing many different legal issues and contexts. As a result, its definition, requirements, and application can vary widely depending on the circumstances in which it is being measured (e.g., health care decisions, executing a will, or confessing to a crime).

In general, *competency* refers to some *minimal* mental, cognitive, or behavioral ability, trait, or capability required to perform a particular legally recognized act or to assume some legal role. Incompetency is a judicial determination. The term *incapacity*, which is often interchanged with the word *incompetency*, refers to an individual's functional inability to understand or to form an intention with regard to some act as determined by health care providers (Mishkin 1989).

The legal designation of "incompetent" is applied to an individual who fails one of the mental tests of capacity and is therefore considered *by law* not mentally capable of performing a particular act or assuming a particular role. The adjudication of incompetence by a court is subject or issue specific. In other words, the fact that a psychiatric patient is adjudicated incompetent to execute a will does not automatically render that patient incompetent to do other things, such as consent to treatment, testify as a witness, marry, drive, or make a legally binding contract.

Generally, the law recognizes only the decisions or choices that have been made by a competent individual. The law seeks to protect incompetent individuals from the harmful effects of their acts. Persons over the age of majority, which is now 18 (U.S. Dept. of Health and Human Services 1981), are presumed to be competent (*Meek v. City of Loveland* 1929). This presumption, however, is rebuttable by evidence of an individual's incapacity (*Scaria v. St. Paul Fire & Marine Insurance Company* 1975). For the psychiatric patient, perception, short- and long-term memory, judgment, language comprehension, verbal fluency, and reality orientation are mental functions that a court will scrutinize regarding "capacity" and "competency."

The issue of competency, whether in a civil or criminal context, is commonly raised in two situations: when the person is a minor and when he or she is mentally disabled. In many situations, minors are not considered legally competent and therefore require the consent of a parent or designated guardian. However, there are exceptions to this general rule, such as when minors are considered emancipated (Smith 1986, p. 178) or mature (*Gulf S I R Company v. Sullivan* 1928), or in some cases of medical need (abortion: *Planned Parenthood v. Danforth* 1976; mental health counseling: Ill Ann Stat 1990; *Jehovah's Witnesses v. King County Hospital* 1967, 1968).

The mentally disabled, including mentally impaired psychiatric patients, present a slightly different problem in evaluating competency. Lack of capacity or competency *cannot* be presumed from either treatment for mental illness (*Wilson v. Lehman* 1964) or institutionalization of such persons (*Rennie v. Klein* 1978). Mental disability or illness does *not* necessarily render a person incompetent in any or in all areas of functioning. Instead, scrutiny is given to determine whether there are specific functional incapacities that render a person incapable of making a particular kind of decision or performing a particular type of task.

Respect for individual autonomy (*Schloendorff v. Society of New York Hospital* 1914) demands that individuals be allowed to make decisions of which they are capable, even if they are seriously mentally ill, developmentally arrested, or organically impaired. As a rule, a patient with a psychiatric disorder that produces mental incapacity generally must be declared judicially incompetent before exercise of that patient's legal rights can be abridged. The person's current or past history of physical and mental illness is but one factor to be weighed in determining whether a particular test of competency is met.

HEALTH CARE DECISION MAKING

Because psychiatric patients frequently suffer from impaired mental capacity, the difficulty associated with obtaining a valid informed consent to proposed diagnostic procedures and treatments can be both challenging and frustrating. The need to obtain competent, informed consent is not negated simply because it "appears" that the patient is in need of medical intervention or would likely benefit from it. Instead, clinicians must assure themselves that the patient or an appropriate substitute decision maker has given a competent consent before proceeding with treatment. An increasing number of states require a judicial determination of incompetence and the court's substituted consent prior to the administration of neuroleptic treatment to a patient who is deemed by a health care provider to lack the functional mental capacity to consent (Simon 1992a).

Only a *competent* person is legally recognized as being able to give informed consent. Competent patients must not be treated against their objections. This is particularly important for health care providers working with patients who sometimes are of questionable competence because of mental illness, narcotic abuse, or alcoholism. When psychiatrists treat patients with neuropsychiatric deficits, the responsibility to obtain a valid informed consent can be clinically daunting because of the vacillating and unpredictable mental states associated with many central nervous system disorders.

Psychiatric patients who have been determined to lack the requisite functional mental capacity to make a treatment decision, except in cases of an emergency (*Frasier v. Department of Health and Human Resources* 1986), must have an authorized representative or guardian appointed to make health care decisions on their behalf (*Aponte v. United States* 1984). A number of consent options may be available for such patients, depending on the jurisdiction (see Table 41–4).

RIGHT TO DIE

Legal decisions addressing the issue of a patient's "right to die" fall into one of two categories: decisions dealing with

individuals who were incompetent at the time that removal of life-support systems is sought (*In re Conroy* 1985; *In re Quinlin* 1976) and decisions dealing with competent patients.

INCOMPETENT PATIENTS

In what was hoped to be the "final word" on this difficult and personal question of patient autonomy, the United States Supreme Court ruled, in *Cruzan v. Director, Missouri Department of Health* (1990), that the state of Missouri may refuse to remove a food and water tube surgically implanted in the stomach of Nancy Cruzan without clear and convincing evidence of her wishes. Ms. Cruzan was in a persistent vegetative state for 7 years. Without clear and convincing evidence of a patient's decision to have life-sustaining measures withheld in a particular circumstance, the state has the right to maintain that individual's life, even to the exclusion of the family's wishes.

Although it seemed to leave unanswered more questions than it answered, the Court's decision buttressed the position of "right-to-refuse" treatment advocates in three significant ways:

1. The Court seemed to give constitutional status to a competent person's right to refuse treatment:

   > . . . those competent to express their wishes do enjoy a constitutional right to refuse life-sustaining medical treatment . . . and . . . if people appoint relatives or friends to make decisions about medical treatment in the event they become incompetent, states "may well be constitutionally required" to defer to the wishes of such "surrogate decision-makers." (Marcus 1990)

2. The Court did not distinguish between artificially administered food and water and other life-sustaining measures, such as respirators. This distinction was a hotly contested sticking point in some previous lower court decisions.

3. An incompetent person who makes his or her wishes known in advance, such as through a living will, may have a constitutional right to halt life-sustaining intervention, depending on the proof of those wishes.

The importance of the *Cruzan* decision for physicians treating severely or terminally impaired patients is that physicians must seek clear and competent instructions regarding foreseeable treatment decisions. For example, a psychiatrist treating a patient with progressive degenerative diseases should attempt to ascertain the patient's wishes regarding the use of life-sustaining measures *while that patient can still competently articulate those wishes.* This information is best provided in the form of a living will, durable power-of-attorney agreement, or health care proxy. However, any written document that clearly and convincingly sets forth the patient's wishes can serve the same purpose.

Although physicians fear civil or criminal liability for stopping life-sustaining treatment, liability may now arise from overtreating critically or terminally ill patients (Weir and Gostin 1990). Legal liability may occur for providing unwanted treatment to an autonomous patient or treatment that is against the best interests of a nonautonomous patient.

COMPETENT PATIENTS

A small but growing body of cases has emerged involving *competent* patients—usually suffering from excruciating pain and terminal diseases—who seek the termination of further medical treatment. The single most significant influence in the development of this body of law is the doctrine of informed consent. Beginning with the fundamental tenet that "no right is held more sacred . . . than the right of every individual to the possession and control of his own person" (*Schloendorff v. Society of New York Hospital* 1914; *Union Pacific Realty Company v. Botsford* 1891), courts have fashioned the present-day "informed consent" doctrine and applied it to "right-to-die" cases.

Notwithstanding these principles, the right to decline life-sustaining medical intervention, even for a competent person, is not absolute. As noted in *In re Conroy* (1985), four countervailing state interests generally exist that may limit the exercise of that right: 1) preservation of life, 2) prevention of suicide, 3) safeguarding the integrity of the medical profession, and 4) protection of innocent third parties (*In re Conroy* 1985). In each of these situations, and depending on the surrounding circumstances, the trend has been to support a competent patient's right to have artificial life-support systems discontinued (*Bartling v. Superior Court* 1984; *Bouvia v. Superior Court* 1986; *In re Farrell* 1987; *In re Jobes* 1987; *In re Peter* 1987; *Tune v. Walter Reed Army Medical Hospital* 1985).

As a result of the *Cruzan* decision, courts now focus primarily on the reliability of the evidence proffered in establishing the patient's competence, specifically the clarity and certainty with which a decision to withhold medical treatment is made. Assuming that a terminally ill patient has chosen to forgo any further medical intervention *and* the patient is competent at the time this decision is made, courts are unlikely to overrule or subvert the patient's right to privacy and autonomy.

ADVANCE DIRECTIVES

The use of advance directives such as a living will, health care proxy, or durable medical power of attorney is recommended to avoid ethical and legal complications associated with requests to withhold life-sustaining treatment measures (Simon 1992a; Solnick 1985). The Patient Self-Determination Act, which took effect on December 1, 1991, requires hospitals, nursing homes, hospices, managed care organizations, and home health care agencies to advise patients or family members of their right to accept or refuse medical care and to execute an advance directive (LaPuma et al. 1991). These advance directives provide a method for individuals, while competent, to choose proxy health care decision makers in the event of future incompetency. A living will can be contained as a subsection of a durable power-of-attorney agreement. In the ordinary power of attorney created for the management of business and financial matters, the power of attorney generally becomes null and void if the person creating it becomes incompetent.

Because federal law does not specify the right to formulate advance directives, state law applies. Recently, state legislators have recognized that individuals may want to indicate who should make important health care decisions in case they become incapacitated and unable to act in their own behalf. All 50 states and the District of Columbia permit individuals to create a *durable* power of attorney (i.e., one that endures even if the competence of the creator does not) (*Cruzan v. Director, Missouri Department of Health* 1990, n. 3). A number of states, including the District of Columbia, do have durable power-of-attorney statutes that expressly authorize the appointment of proxies for making health care decisions (*Cruzan v. Director, Missouri Department of Health* 1990, n. 2).

Generally, durable power of attorney has been construed to empower an agent to make health care decisions. Such a document is much broader and more flexible than a living will, which covers only the period of a diagnosed terminal illness, specifying only that no "extraordinary treatments" be used that would prolong the act of dying (Mishkin 1985). To rectify the sometimes uncertain status of the durable power of attorney as applied to health care decisions, a number of states have passed or are considering passing health care proxy laws. The health care proxy is a legal instrument akin to the durable power of attorney but specifically created for health care decision making. Despite the growing use of advance directives, there is increasing evidence that physician values rather than patient values are more decisive in end-of-life decisions (Orentlicher 1992).

In a durable power of attorney or health care proxy, general or specific directions are set forth about how future decisions should be made in the event one becomes unable to make these decisions. The determination of a patient's competence, however, is not specified in most durable power-of-attorney and health care proxy statutes. Because this is a medical or psychiatric question, the examination by two physicians to determine the patient's ability to understand the nature and consequences of the proposed treatment or procedure, ability to make a choice, and ability to communicate that choice is usually minimally sufficient. This information, like all significant medical observations, should be clearly documented in the patient's file.

Because of the frequent absence of advance directives, a number of states have enacted statutory surrogate laws. These laws authorize certain persons, such as a spouse or a court-appointed guardian, to make health care decisions when the patient has not stated his or her wishes in writing.

The application of advance directives to psychiatric patients presents some difficulties. The classic example arises when a currently asymptomatic patient with an organic personality disorder and occasional bouts of severe affective instability draws up a durable power-of-attorney agreement or health care proxy directing the following: "If I become mentally unstable again, administer medications even if I strenuously object or resist." T. G. Gutheil (personal communication, September 1985) has described this as the "Ulysses Contract." In Greek mythology, Ulysses was bound to the mast of his ship so he could hear the beautiful, though lethal, sirens' song. All the other sailors covered their ears. When Ulysses heard the irresistible song of the sirens, he tried to struggle loose. When that failed, he demanded to be untied. Similarly, when mood instability recurs, the patient with an organic personality disorder may strenuously object to treatment.

Because durable power-of-attorney agreements or health care proxies can be easily revoked, the treating psychiatrist or institution has no choice but to honor the patient's refusal, even if there is reasonable evidence that the patient is incompetent. Legal consultation should be considered at this point. If the patient is grossly disordered and is an immediate danger to self and others, the physician or hospital is on firmer ground medically and legally to override the patient's treatment refusal temporarily. Otherwise, it is generally better to seek a court order for treatment than risk legal entanglement with the patient by attempting to enforce the original terms of the advance directive. Unless there are compelling medical reasons to do otherwise, courts generally honor the patient's original treatment directions that were given when he or she was competent.

GUARDIANSHIP

Guardianship is a method of substitute decision making for individuals who have been judicially determined to be unable to act for themselves (Brakel et al. 1985, p. 370). Historically, the state or sovereign possessed the power and authority to safeguard the estate of incompetent persons (Regan 1972).

This traditional role still reflects the purpose of guardianship today. In some states, there are separate provisions for the appointment of a "guardian of one's person" (e.g., health care decision making) and for a "guardian of one's estate" (e.g., authority to make contracts to sell one's property; Sale et al. 1982). The latter type of guardian is frequently referred to as a *conservator*, although this designation is not uniformly used throughout the United States. A further distinction, also found in some jurisdictions, is between *general (plenary)* and *specific* guardianship (Sale et al. 1982). As the name implies, the specific guardian is restricted to exercising decisions about a particular subject area. For instance, he or she may be authorized to make decisions about major or emergency medical procedures, with the disabled person retaining the freedom to make decisions about all other medical matters. General guardians, in contrast, have total control over the disabled individual's person, estate, or both (Sale et al. 1982).

Guardianship arrangements are increasingly used with patients suffering from dementia, particularly AIDS-related dementia and Alzheimer's disease (Overman and Stoudemire 1988). Under the Anglo-American system of law, an individual is presumed to be competent unless adjudicated incompetent. Thus, incompetence is a legal determination made by a court of law on the basis of evidence provided by health care providers and others that the individual's functional mental capacity is significantly impaired. The Uniform Guardianship and Protective Proceeding Act (UGPPA) or the Uniform Probate Code (UPC) is used as a basis for laws governing competency in many states (Mishkin 1989). Drafted by legal scholars and practicing attorneys, the uniform acts serve as models for the purpose of achieving uniformity among the state laws by enactment of model laws (UGPPA § 5-101).

General incompetency is defined by the UGPPA as meaning "impaired by reason of mental illness, mental deficiency, physical illness or disability, advanced age, chronic use of drugs, chronic intoxication, or other cause (except minority) to the extent of lacking sufficient understanding or capacity to make or communicate reasonable decisions."

Some patients suffering from psychiatric disorders

may meet the preceding definition. Generally, the appointment of a guardian is limited to situations in which the individual's decision-making capacity is so impaired that he or she is unable to care for personal safety or provide such necessities as food, shelter, clothing, and medical care, with the likely result of physical injury or illness (*In re Boyer* 1981). The standard of proof required for a judicial determination of incompetency is *clear and convincing evidence*. Although the law does not assign percentages to proof, clear and convincing evidence is in the range of 75% certainty (Simon 1992a, p. 160).

States vary concerning the extent of their reliance on psychiatric assessments. Nonmedical personnel such as social workers, psychologists, family members, friends, colleagues, and even the individual who is the subject of the proceeding may testify.

SUBSTITUTED JUDGMENT

Psychiatrists often find that the time required to obtain an adjudication of incompetence is unduly burdensome and that the process frequently interferes with the provision of quality treatment. Moreover, families are often reluctant to face the formal court proceedings necessary to declare their family member incompetent, particularly when sensitive family matters are disclosed. A common solution to both of these problems is to seek the legally authorized *proxy consent of a spouse or relative serving as guardian* when the refusing patient is believed to be incompetent. Proxy consent, however, is becoming less available as a consent option (Simon 1992a, pp. 108–114). Many states exclude surrogate authorizations for the treatment of mental disorders.

There are clear advantages associated with having the family serve as decision makers (Perr 1984). First, use of responsible family members as surrogate decision makers maintains the integrity of the family unit and relies on the sources who are most likely to know the patient's wishes. Second, it is more efficient and less costly than an attempt to prove incompetency. There are some disadvantages, however. Proxy decision making requires synthesizing the diverse values, beliefs, practices, and prior statements of the patient for a given specific circumstance (Emanuel and Emanuel 1992). As one judge characterized the problem, any proxy decision making in the absence of specific directions is "at best only an optimistic approximation" (*In re Jobes* 1987). Ambivalent feelings, conflicts within the family and with the patient, and conflicting economic interest may make certain family members suspect as guardians

(Gutheil and Appelbaum 1980). Also, relatives may not be available or want to get involved. Moreover, next of kin may possess dubious competence or even less competence than the patient.

The President's Commission for the Study of Ethical Problems in Medicine and Biomedical and Behavioral Research (1982) has recommended that the relatives of incompetent patients be selected as proxy decision makers for the following reasons:

1. The family is generally most concerned about the good of the patient.
2. The family is usually most knowledgeable about the patient's goals, preferences, and values.
3. The family deserves recognition as an important social unit, to be treated, within limits, as a single decision maker in matters that intimately affect its members.

A number of states permit proxy decision making by statute, mainly through informed-consent statutes (Solnick 1985). Some state statutes specify that another person may authorize consent on behalf of the incompetent patient, whereas others mention specific relatives.

Unless proxy consent by a relative is provided by statute or by case law authority in the state where the psychiatrist practices, it is not recommended that the good-faith consent by next of kin be relied on in treating a patient believed to lack health care decision-making capacity (Klein et al. 1983). The legally appropriate procedure to follow is to seek judicial recognition of the family member as the substitute decision maker.

Some patients treated in an emergency are expected to recover competency within a few days. As soon as the patient is able to competently consent to further treatment, such consent should be obtained directly from the patient. For the patient who continues to lack mental capacity for health care decisions, an increasing number of states provide administrative procedures authorized by statute that permit involuntary treatment of the incompetent and refusing mentally ill patients who do not meet current standards for involuntary civil commitment (Hassenfeld and Grumet 1984; Zito et al. 1984). In most jurisdictions, a durable power-of-attorney agreement permits the next of kin to consent through durable power-of-attorney statutes (Solnick 1985). However, in some instances, this procedure may not meet judicial challenge. To avoid this problem, a number of states have created health care proxies specifically for advance health care decision making.

PHYSICIAN-ASSISTED SUICIDE

With increasing legal recognition of physician-assisted suicide (PAS), psychiatrists are likely to be called on to become gatekeepers. Such a role would be a radical departure from the physician's code of ethics, in which doctors are prohibited from participating in any intervention that hastens death. Previously, the Supreme Court ruled in *Cruzan* that terminally ill persons could refuse life-sustaining medical treatment. Courts and legislatures will determine whether hastening death is an unwarranted extension of the right to refuse treatment. Every proposal for PAS requires a psychiatric screening or consultation to determine the terminally ill person's competence to commit suicide. The presence of psychiatric disorders associated with suicide, particularly depression, will have to be ruled out as the driving factor behind PAS. Much controversy rages over the ethics of this gatekeeping function (American Medical Association 1994).

CRIMINAL PROCEEDINGS

Individuals charged with committing crimes frequently display significant psychiatric and neurological impairment. A history of severe head injury may be present. The possibility of a neuropsychiatric disorder must be thoroughly investigated. For example, Lewis et al. (1986) examined 15 death-row inmates who were chosen for examination because of imminent execution rather than evidence of neuropathology. In each case, evidence of severe head injury and neurological impairment was found.

The causal connection between brain damage and violence remains frustratingly obscure. Violent behavior spans a wide spectrum from a normal response to a threatening situation to violence emanating directly from an organic brain disorder such as Klüver-Bucy syndrome, hypothalamic tumors, or temporal lobe epilepsy (Strub and Black 1988). Moreover, violent behavior is often the result of the interaction between an individual and a specific situation. Brain damage and mental illness may or may not play a significant role in this equation. Psychiatrists must acknowledge limitations in their expertise concerning the possible connection between brain damage and violence.

CRIMINAL INTENT (MENS REA)

Under the common law, the basic elements of a crime are 1) the mental state or level of intent to commit the act (known as the *mens rea*, or guilty mind), 2) the act itself or conduct associated with committing the crime (known as *actus reus*, or guilty act), and 3) a concurrence in time between the guilty act and the guilty mental state (*Bethea v. United States* 1977). To convict a person of a particular crime, the state must prove beyond a reasonable doubt that the defendant committed the criminal act with the requisite intent. All three elements are necessary to satisfy the threshold requirements for the imposition of criminal sanctions.

The question of intent is a particularly vexing problem for the courts. For example, everyone would agree that killing another person is deplorable conduct. But should the accidental death of child in a car accident, the heat-of-passion shooting by a husband of his wife's lover, and the "cold-blooded" murder of a bank teller by a robber all be punished in the same way? The determination of the defendant's intent, or *mens rea*, at the time of the offense is the law's "equalizer" and trigger mechanism for deciding criminal culpability and the appropriate assessment of retribution. For instance, a person who deliberately plans to commit a crime is more culpable than one who accidentally commits one.

There are two classes of intent used to categorize *mens rea*: specific and general. Specific intent refers to the *mens rea* in crimes in which a *further intention* exists beyond the presence of a general criminal intent. For instance, the courts frequently state that the intent necessary for first-degree murder includes a "specific intent to kill"; on the other hand, a person might commit an assault "with the intent to rape" (Melton et al. 1987). Unlike general criminal intent, specific criminal intent cannot be presumed from the unlawful criminal act but must be proved independently.

General criminal intent is more elusive. Such intent may be presumed from commission of the criminal act. The concept usually is used by the law to explain criminal liability in which a defendant was merely conscious or should have been conscious of his or her physical actions at the time of the offense (Melton et al. 1987). For example, general criminal intent would apply to a person who intended to violate the law by holding up a bank. General criminal intent is presumed by commission of the criminal act. To deal with the vagueness of these two standards, many states have enacted their own definitions of intent.

Persons with certain mental handicaps or impairments represent an interesting challenge for prosecutors, defense counsel, and judges in determining what, if any, retribution is justifiable. Mental impairment often raises serious questions about the intent to commit a crime and the appreciation of its consequences.

In addition to *mens rea*, a person's mental status can

play a deciding role in whether he or she is ordered to stand trial to face the criminal charges (*Dusky v. United States* 1960), acquitted of the alleged crime (*M'Naughten's Case* 1843; *United States v. Brawner* 1972), sent to prison, hospitalized (*Commonwealth v. Robinson* 1981; *Mental Aberration and Post Conviction Sanctions* 1981; *State v. Hehman* 1974), or, in some extreme cases, sentenced to death ("Eighth Amendment and the Execution of the Presently Incompetent" 1980; *Ford v. Wainwright* 1986). Before any defendant can be criminally prosecuted, the court must be satisfied that the accused is competent to stand trial, that is, he or she understands the charges brought against him or her and is capable of rationally assisting counsel with the defense.

COMPETENCY TO STAND TRIAL

In every situation in which competency is in question, the law seeks to reiterate a common theme: that only the acts of a rational individual are to be given recognition by society (*Neely v. United States* 1945). In doing so, the law attempts to reaffirm the integrity of the individual and of society in general.

The legal standard for assessing pretrial competency was established by the United States Supreme Court in *Dusky v. United States* (1960). Throughout involvement with the trial process, the defendant must have "sufficient present ability to consult with his lawyer with a reasonable degree of rational understanding and whether he has a rational as well as factual understanding of the proceedings against him" (*Dusky v. United States* 1960).

Typically, the impairment that raises the question of the defendant's competence is associated with a mental disease or defect. It is settled, however, that a person may be held to be incompetent to stand trial even if he or she does not suffer from a mental disease or defect as defined by the American Psychiatric Association (1994) in DSM-IV. For example, children under a certain age ordinarily are deemed incompetent to stand trial.

Although the majority of impairments implicated in competency examinations are functional rather than organic (Reich and Wells 1985), various forms of neuropsychiatric impairments typically raise questions about a defendant's competency to stand trial. In *Wilson v. United States* (1968), the defendant had no memory regarding the time of an alleged robbery because he had permanent retrograde amnesia. This impairment was caused by injuries he suffered in an automobile accident that occurred as he was being pursued by the police following the offense. Of the various criteria that the court established in determining the defendant's competency to stand trial, the following

are directly relevant to the issue of neuropsychiatric impairment:

1. The extent to which the amnesia affected the defendant's ability to consult with and assist his lawyer, and
2. The extent to which the amnesia affected the defendant's ability to testify in his own behalf. (*Wilson v. United States*)

Any disorder, whether functional or organic, that significantly impairs a defendant's cognitive and communicative abilities is likely to have impact on competency. Nevertheless, it is the actual *functional* mental capability to meet the minimal standard of trial competency, and not the severity of the deficits, that determines whether an individual is cognitively capable to be tried.

For example, Slovenko (1995) questioned whether psychiatric diagnosis is relevant to competency to stand trial. The presence or absence of a mental illness is irrelevant if the defendant is capable of meeting competency requirements. It is legal criteria, not medical or psychiatric diagnosis, that governs competency. Diagnosis is relevant only to the question of restoring the defendant's competency to stand trial with treatment.

Checklists and structured interviews have been developed to assess specific psychological factors applicable to the competency standards established in *Dusky*. The Interdisciplinary Fitness Interview, designed for use by lawyers and mental health professionals (Schreiber et al. 1987), provides for a detailed examination of psychopathology and legal knowledge, using explicit scales for rating each response to the competency evaluation. *Evaluating Competencies: Forensic Assessments and Instruments*, by Thomas Grisso (1986), is a standard reference in the field.

A defendant's impairment in one particular function, however, does not automatically render the accused incompetent. For example, the fact that the defendant is manifesting certain deficits because of damage to the parietal lobe does not necessarily mean that he or she lacks the requisite cognitive ability to aid in his or her own defense at trial (Tranel 1992). The ultimate determination of incompetency is solely for the court to decide (*United States v. David* 1975). Moreover, the impairment must be considered in the context of the particular case or proceeding. Mental impairment may render an individual incompetent to stand trial in a complicated tax fraud case but not incompetent for a misdemeanor trial.

Psychiatrists and psychologists who testify as expert witnesses regarding the effect of psychiatric problems on a defendant's competency to stand trial are most effective if their findings are framed according to the degree to which the defendant is cognitively capable of meeting the standards enunciated in *Dusky*.

INSANITY DEFENSE

One of the most controversial issues in American jurisprudence is the insanity defense. Defendants with functional or organic mental disabilities who are found competent to stand trial may seek acquittal on the basis that they were not criminally responsible for their actions because of insanity at the time the offense was committed.

Criminals commit crimes for many reasons, but the law presumes that all of them do so rationally and with their own free will. As a result, the law concludes that they are deserving of some form of punishment. Some offenders, however, are so mentally disturbed in their thinking and behavior that they are thought to be incapable of acting rationally. Under these circumstances, civilized societies have deemed it unjust to punish a "crazy" or insane person (Blackstone 1769; Coke 1680). This is in part due to fundamental principles of fairness and morality. In addition, the punishment of a person who cannot rationally appreciate the consequences of his or her actions thwarts the two major tenets of punishment: retribution and deterrence. The insanity defense is rarely used, and a successful insanity defense is even rarer. Approximately 1% of criminal defendants plead not guilty by reason of insanity; of these, only 10%–25% are successful. The chance of exculpation is greatest when the criminal defendant was found to be psychotic at the time of the crime by the pretrial assessment (Brakel et al. 1985, p. 720).

A generally accepted, precise definition of legal insanity does not exist. Over the years, tests of insanity have been subject to much controversy, modification, and refinement (Brakel et al. 1985, p. 707). The development of the insanity defense standard in the United States has had four basic elements (Table 41–10). The existence of a mental disorder has remained a consistent core of the insanity defense, whereas the three other elements have varied over time (Brakel et al. 1985, p. 709). Thus, there is variability in the

TABLE 41–10. Basic elements of insanity defense

Presence of a mental disorder

Presence of a defect of reason

A lack of knowledge of the nature or wrongfulness of the act

An incapacity to refrain from the act

Source. Reprinted with permission from Simon RI: "Legal and Ethical Issues in Traumatic Brain Injury," in *Traumatic Brain Injury.* Edited by Silver JM. Washington, DC, American Psychiatric Press, 1994.Copyright 1994, American Psychiatric Press, Inc.

insanity defense standard in the United States, depending on which state or jurisdiction has control over the defendant raising the defense.

Following the acquittal by reason of insanity of John Hinckley, Jr., on charges of attempting to assassinate President Reagan and murder others, an outraged public demanded changes in the insanity defense. Federal and state legislation to accomplish that result ensued. Between 1978 and 1985, approximately 75% of all states made some sort of substantive change in their insanity defense (Perlin 1989, p. 404). Nevertheless, a number of states continued to adhere to the American Law Institute (ALI) insanity defense standard or a version of it. The ALI test provides that

a person is not responsible for criminal conduct if at the time of such conduct as a result of mental disease or defect he lacks substantial capacity either to appreciate the criminality (wrongfulness) of his conduct or to conform his conduct to the requirements of law. As used in this Article, the terms "mental disease or defect" do not include an abnormality manifested only by repeated criminal or otherwise antisocial conduct. (Model Penal Code § 4.01 [1962]; 10 ULA 490-91 [1974])

This standard contains both a cognitive and a volitional prong. The *cognitive prong* derives from the 1843 M'Naughten rule exculpating the defendant who does not know the nature and quality of the alleged act or does not know the act was wrong. The *volitional prong* is a vestige of the irresistible impulse rule, which states that the defendant who is overcome by an irresistible impulse that leads to an alleged act is not responsible for that act. It is on the volitional prong that experts disagree the most in individual cases.

By contrast, defendants tried in a federal court are governed by the standard enunciated in the Comprehensive Crime Control Act (CCCA) of 1984 (P. L. No. 98-473, 98 Stat. 1837 [1984]). The CCCA provides that it is an affirmative defense to all federal crimes that, at the time of the offense, "the defendant, as a result of a severe mental disease or defect, was unable to appreciate the nature and quality or the wrongfulness of his acts. Mental disease or defect does not otherwise constitute a defense" (Model Penal Code § 402, 98 Stat., p. 2057). This codification eliminates the volitional or irresistible impulse portion of the insanity defense. That is, it does not allow an insanity defense based on a defendant's inability to conform his or her conduct to the requirements of the law. The defense is now limited to defendants who are unable to appreciate the wrongfulness of their acts (i.e., the *cognitive portion* of the defense). The burden of proof varies among the states. In a minority of states, the prosecution has the burden of proving beyond a reasonable doubt that the defendant was sane. In a majority of states and all federal courts, the defendant must bear the burden of proving by a preponderance of the evidence that she or he was insane (Melton et al. 1987). Nevada (Section 33, Nevada Revised Statutes 193.220) recently joined Montana, South Dakota, and Utah in abolishing the special plea of insanity. At the same time, it established the plea of guilty but mentally ill. In Montana, evidence of insanity is admissible to negate *mens rea*.

The threshold issue in making an insanity determination is not the existence of a mental disease or defect per se, but the lack of substantial mental capacity because of it. Therefore, the lack of capacity due to mental defects other than mental illness may be sufficient. For instance, mental retardation may represent an adequate basis for the insanity defense under certain circumstances.

The impulse disorders—intermittent explosive disorder, kleptomania, pathological gambling, and pyromania—generally have not fared well under an insanity defense. Persons with these conditions do not meet the criteria for the cognitive prong of an insanity defense. Presumably, the volitional prong would be applicable, but it is usually insufficient by itself. Moreover, courts and juries tend to view criminal acts arising from impulse disorders as impulses not resisted rather than irresistible impulses.

Pathological gambling no longer serves as a basis for an insanity defense (Rosenthal and Lorenz 1992). McGarry (1983) pointed out that the lack of volitional control over the isolated act of gambling does not assume a lack of control concerning criminal acts committed in the service of the impulse to gamble. Compulsive gambling, however, is being raised as a mitigating factor at sentencing (Rosenthal and Lorenz 1992). Less severe punishment is feasible through a court's willingness to consider treatment, community service, restitution, and the possibility of probation.

Depending on the severity of the functional or organic mental disorder and its impact on an offender's cognitive and affective processes, a defense of insanity might be warranted. At the least, the presence of a psychiatric disorder should be investigated as a *mitigating* factor that may have caused the offender to suffer from "diminished" capacity.

DIMINISHED CAPACITY

It is possible for a person to have the required *mens rea* yet be declared legally insane. For instance, a defendant's actions may be considered so "crazy" as to convince a jury that he or she was criminally insane and therefore not legally responsible. Yet his or her knowledge of the criminal act (e.g., committing a murder) was relatively intact. From this distinction, the law recognizes that there are "shades" of mental impairment that obviously can affect *mens rea*, but not necessarily to the extent of completely nullifying it. In recognition of this fact, the concept of *diminished capacity* was developed (Melton et al. 1987).

Broadly viewed, diminished capacity permits the accused to introduce medical and psychological evidence that relates directly to the *mens rea* for the crime charged, without having to assert a defense of insanity (Melton et al. 1987). For example, in the crime of assault with the intent to kill, psychiatric testimony would be permitted to address whether the offender acted with the purpose of committing homicide at the time of the assault. When a defendant's *mens rea* for the crime charged is nullified by psychiatric evidence, the defendant is acquitted only of that charge. In the preceding example, the prosecutor may still try to convict the defendant of another offense requiring a lesser *mens rea*, such as manslaughter (Melton et al. 1987). Patients suffering from psychiatric disorders who commit criminal acts may be eligible for a diminished capacity defense.

GUILTY BUT MENTALLY ILL

In a number of states, an alternative verdict of *guilty but mentally ill* (GBMI) has been established. Under GBMI statutes, if the defendant pleads not guilty by reason of insanity, this alternative verdict is available to the jury (Slovenko 1982). Under an insanity plea, the verdict may be

- Not guilty
- Not guilty by reason of insanity
- Guilty but mentally ill
- Guilty

The problem with GBMI is that it is an alternative verdict that is not different from finding the defendant plain guilty. The court must still impose a sentence on the convicted person. Although the convicted person will receive special treatment if necessary, this treatment provision is also available to any other prisoner. Moreover, the frequent unavailability of appropriate psychiatric treatment for prisoners adds an additional element of spuriousness to the GBMI verdict.

EXCULPATORY AND MITIGATING DISORDERS

Psychotic disorders of differing etiology form the most common basis for an insanity defense. In addition to the major psychiatric and organic brain disorders, however, a number of other conditions may provide a foundation for an insanity or diminished capacity defense.

Automatisms

For conviction of a crime, there must be not only a criminal state of mind (*mens rea*) but also the commission of a prohibited act (*actus reus*). The physical movement necessary to satisfy the *actus reus* requirement must be conscious and volitional. In addition to statutory and common law in many jurisdictions, Section 2.01(2) of the Model Penal Code (1962) specifically excludes from the *actus reus* the following:

> (a) a reflex or convulsion; (b) a bodily movement during unconsciousness or sleep; (c) conduct during hypnosis or resulting from hypnotic suggestion; [and] (d) a bodily movement that otherwise is not the product of the effort or determination of the actor . . .

A defense claiming that the commission of a crime was an involuntary act usually is referred to as an "automatism defense." The classic, though rare, example is the person who commits an offense while "sleepwalking." Courts have held that such an individual does not have conscious control of his or her physical actions and therefore acts involuntarily (*Fain v. Commonwealth* 1879; *H. M. Advocate v. Fraser* 1878). A conscious, reflexive action carried out under stressful circumstances may qualify for an automatism defense. For example, a driver who is being attacked in his car by a bee loses control in attempting to swat the insect. The car strikes a pedestrian, who is killed. An automatism defense exists to charges of vehicular homicide. Other situations relevant to psychiatry in which the defense might be used arise when a crime is committed during a state of altered consciousness caused by a concussion following a head injury, involuntary ingestion of drugs or alcohol, hypoxia, metabolic disorders such as hypoglycemia, or epileptic seizures (Low et al. 1982).

There are, however, limitations to the automatism defense. Most notably, some courts have held that if the person asserting the automatism defense was aware of the condition prior to the offense and failed to take reasonable steps to prevent the criminal occurrence, the defense is not available. For example, if a defendant with a known history of uncontrolled epileptic seizures loses control of a car during a seizure and kills someone, that defendant will not be permitted to assert the defense of automatism.

Intoxication

Ordinarily, intoxication is not a defense to a criminal charge. Because intoxication, unlike mental illness, mental retardation, and most neuropsychiatric conditions, is usually the product of a person's own actions, the law is naturally cautious about viewing it as a complete defense or mitigating factor. Most states view voluntary alcoholism as relevant to the issue of whether the defendant possessed the *mens rea* necessary to commit a specific intent crime or whether there was premeditation in a crime of murder. Generally, however, the mere fact that the defendant was voluntarily intoxicated will not justify a finding of automatism or insanity. A distinct difference arises when, because of chronic, heavy use of alcohol, the defendant suffers from an alcohol-induced psychotic disorder, withdrawal delirium, amnestic disorder, or dementia. If competent psychiatric evidence is presented that an alcohol-related neuropsychiatric disorder caused significant cognitive or volitional impairment, a defense of insanity or diminished capacity could be upheld.

Temporal Lobe Seizures

Another "mental state" defense occasionally raised by defendants regarding assault-related crimes is that the assaultive behavior was involuntarily precipitated by abnormal electrical patterns in the defendant's brain. This condition is frequently diagnosed as temporal lobe epilepsy (Devinsky and Bear 1984). Episodic dyscontrol syndrome (Elliott 1978, 1982) has also been advanced as a neuropsychiatric condition causing involuntary aggression. Studies have hypothesized that there are "centers of aggression" in the temporal lobe or limbic system—primarily the amygdala. This hypothesis has promoted the idea that sustained aggressive behavior by these persons may be primarily the product of an uncontrollable, randomly occurring, abnormal brain dysrhythmia. Hence, the legal argument is raised that these individuals should not be held accountable for their actions. Despite its simplicity and occasional success in the courts, few empirically significant data exist to support this theory at the present time (Blumer 1984).

Metabolic Disorders

Defenses based on metabolic disorders have also been tried. In 1979, the so-called Twinkie defense was used as part of a successful diminished capacity defense of Dan White in the murders of San Francisco Mayor George Moscone and Supervisor Harvey Milk. This defense was based on the theory that the ingestion of large amounts of sugar contributed to a state of temporary insanity (*People v. White* 1981). The forensic psychiatric report stated that the defendant had been "filling himself up with Twinkies and Coca-Cola" (Blinder 1981–1982, p. 16). A jury found

White guilty only of voluntary manslaughter. In 1981, California repealed the defense of diminished capacity (Slovenko 1995).

Hypoglycemic states also may be associated with significant psychiatric impairment (Droba and Whybrow 1989, pp. 1219–1220). When substantial glucose depletion occurs, a wide variety of responses may occur including episodic and repetitive dyscontrol, temporary amnesia, depression, and hostility with spontaneous recovery (i.e., quick recovery following the consumption of appropriate nutrients). The degree of mental abnormality associated with hypoglycemic states varies from mild to severe according to the blood glucose level. It is the degree of disturbance, not the mere presence of an etiological metabolic component, that is determinative in a mental state defense. This principle also applies to mental dysfunctions produced by disorders originating in the hepatic, renal, adrenal, and neuroendocrine systems (e.g., premenstrual syndrome; B. L. Parry and Berga 1991).

POSTTRAUMATIC STRESS DISORDER

In criminal cases, defendants have pleaded not guilty by reason of insanity secondary to posttraumatic stress disorder (PTSD; Sparr 1990). The diagnosis of PTSD has been alleged in criminal proceedings by prosecutors to bolster the credibility of the victim or by experts who attempt to argue backward from PTSD symptoms to establish the occurrence of a traumatic stressor (e.g., rape). Victims of criminal acts who develop PTSD or other psychiatric disorders may sue under criminal injuries compensation acts. PTSD has bolstered the supporters of "victim rights," whose advocacy poses a threat to the constitutional rights of defendants (Stone 1993). An insanity defense based on PTSD is more likely to succeed if it can be shown that the individual committed a crime while experiencing a dissociative behavioral reenactment of a prior traumatic event. Guidelines for the assessment of PTSD in litigation have been proposed (Simon 1995).

PERSONAL INJURY LITIGATION

ASSESSMENT OF SEXUAL HARASSMENT

Psychiatrists perform evaluations of litigants and provide testimony in court in a number of areas of civil litigation. As an example, civil suits alleging sexual harassment are burgeoning. Psychiatrists are being called on to testify in these cases, which present emerging, complex psychological and social issues.

The statutory basis for sexual harassment claims is found in Title VII of the Civil Rights Act of 1964. Section 703(a)(1) of Title VII, 42 U.S.C. § 2000e-2(a), reads as follows:

It shall be an unlawful employment practice for an employer . . . to fail or refuse to hire or to discharge any individual, or otherwise to discriminate against any individual with respect to his compensation, terms, conditions, or privileges of employment, because of such individual's race, color, religion, sex, or national origin.

In 1980, the Equal Employment Opportunity Commission (EEOC) issued guidelines that declared sexual harassment to be a violation of Section 703 of Title VII. The guidelines propounded criteria for determining unwelcome conduct of a sexual nature that constituted sexual harassment, defined the circumstances under which an employer may be held liable, and suggested affirmative steps that an employer should take to prevent sexual harassment (Guidelines on Discrimination Because of Sex, 29 C.F.R. § 1604.11).

In defining sexual harassment, Title VII does not proscribe all conduct of a sexual nature in the workplace. Only unwelcome sexual conduct that is a term or condition of employment constitutes a violation. The EEC's guidelines define two kinds of sexual harassment: "quid pro quo" and "hostile environment." Sexual conduct constitutes sexual harassment when "submission to such conduct is made either explicitly or implicitly a term or condition of an individual's employment" (29 C.F.R. § 1604.11[a][1]). Quid pro quo harassment takes place when "submission or rejection of such conduct by an individual is used as the basis for employment decisions affecting the individual" (29 C.F.R. § 1604.11[a][2]). The EEOC guidelines also recognize that unwelcome sexual conduct that "unreasonably interfere[s] with an individual's job performance" or creates an "intimidating, hostile, or offensive working environment" can constitute sex discrimination, even if it causes no tangible or economic job consequences (29 C.F.R. § 1604.11[a][3]).

The United States Supreme Court, in *Harris v. Forklift Systems, Inc.* (1993), ruled unanimously that a woman who claims she was sexually harassed on the job need not prove she was psychologically injured to win money damages. The Court defined unlawful harassment as creating a work environment that a reasonable person would find "hostile or abusive." The broadly written ruling will likely make it easier for employees to bring suits for sexual harassment.

Psychiatrists who become involved in sexual harassment litigation usually are asked to determine the veracity of harassment complaints, the psychological consequences of harassment, and the treatment needs and prognosis for women or men who have been sexually harassed. Binder (1992) presented examples of cases in which psychiatric testimony was provided to help decision making in assessing damages secondary to the psychological effects of sexual harassment. Guidelines have been proposed for conducting a credible forensic psychiatric evaluation in sexual harassment litigation (Simon 1996).

EXPERT TESTIMONY

Civil litigation in psychic injury and head trauma cases may require the evaluation and testimony of psychiatrists, often working in conjunction with neurologists, other physicians, psychologists, neuropsychologists, and allied mental health professionals. Psychiatrists become involved in litigation as witnesses in one of two ways: as treaters or as forensic experts.

The Treating Clinician

Psychiatrists who venture into the legal arena must be aware of the fundamentally different roles of the treating psychiatrist and the forensic psychiatric expert. Treatment and expert roles do not mix (Greenberg and Shuman 1997; Strasburger et al. 1997). For example, unlike the orthopedist, who possesses objective data such as the X ray of a broken limb to demonstrate physical damages in court, the treating psychiatrist must rely heavily on the subjective reporting of the patient. In the treatment context, psychiatrists are interested primarily in the patient's perception of his or her difficulties, not necessarily the objective reality. As a consequence, many treating psychiatrists do not speak to third parties or check pertinent records to gain additional information about a patient or to corroborate the patient's statements. The law, however, is interested only in testimony that is based on provable facts. Uncorroborated patient reportage is usually attacked in court as speculative, self-serving, and unreliable. The treating psychiatrist is vulnerable to these charges.

Credibility issues also abound. The treating psychiatrist is, and must be, an ally of the patient. This bias toward the patient is a proper treatment stance that fosters the therapeutic alliance. Furthermore, to be treated effectively, the patient should be reasonably "liked" by the psychiatrist. No practitioner can treat a patient who is disliked for long. Moreover, the psychiatrist looks for mental disorders to treat. This, again, is an appropriate bias for the treating psychiatrist.

In court, credibility is a critical commodity to possess when testifying. Opposing counsel will take every opportunity to portray the treating psychiatrist as a subjective mouthpiece for the patient-litigant, which may or may not be true. Also, court testimony by the treating psychiatrist may compel the disclosure of information that is not *legally* privileged but nonetheless is viewed as intimate and confidential by the patient. This disclosure by a trusted therapist is bound to cause psychological damage to the therapeutic relationship (Strasburger 1987). In addition, psychiatrists must be careful to inform patients about the consequences of releasing treatment information, particularly in legal matters. Section 4, Annotation 2 of the *Principles of Medical Ethics with Annotations Especially Applicable to Psychiatry* (American Psychiatric Association 1992a) states the following:

> The continuing duty of the psychiatrist to protect the patient includes fully apprising him/her of the connotations of waiving the privilege of privacy. This may become an issue when the patient is being investigated by a government agency, is applying for a position, or is involved in legal action. (p. 206)

Finally, when the treating psychiatrist testifies concerning the need for further treatment, a conflict of interest is readily apparent. In making such treatment prognostications, the psychiatrist stands to benefit economically from the recommendation of further treatment. Although this may not be the intention of the psychiatrist at all, opposing counsel is sure to point out that the psychiatrist has a financial interest in the case.

The American Academy of Psychiatry and the Law (1989, 1991), in its ethics statement, advises that "a treating psychiatrist should generally avoid agreeing to be an expert witness or to perform an evaluation of his patient for legal purposes because a forensic evaluation usually requires that other people be interviewed and testimony may adversely affect the therapeutic relationship" (p. xii).

The treating psychiatrist should attempt to remain solely in a treatment role. If it becomes necessary to testify on behalf of the patient, the treating psychiatrist should testify only as a fact witness rather than as an expert witness. As a fact witness, the psychiatrist will be asked to describe the number and length of visits, diagnosis, and treatment. Generally, no opinion evidence will be requested concerning the causation of the injury or the extent of damages. In some jurisdictions, however, the court may convert a fact witness into an expert at the time of the trial. Psychiatrists must remain ever mindful of the many double agent roles that can develop when mixing psychiatry and litigation (Simon 1987, 1992a).

The Forensic Expert

The forensic expert, on the other hand, is usually free from the preceding encumbrances. No doctor-patient relationship is created during forensic evaluation, with its treatment biases toward the patient. The forensic expert reviews a variety of records and likely speaks to a number of people who know the litigant. Furthermore, the forensic expert is not as easily distracted from considering exaggeration or malingering because of a clear appreciation of the litigation context and the absence of treatment bias. Finally, the forensic psychiatrist is not placed in a conflict-of-interest position of recommending treatment from which he or she would personally (i.e., financially) benefit. The forensic expert, however, is frequently viewed by opposing counsel as a "hired gun."

FORENSIC PSYCHIATRY

DEFINITION AND SCOPE

Forensic psychiatry is defined as "a subspecialty of psychiatry in which scientific and clinical expertise is applied to legal issues in legal contexts embracing civil, criminal, correctional or legislative matters" (American Academy of Psychiatry and the Law 1989, 1991). The subspecialty of forensic psychiatry is burgeoning. The past decade has witnessed enormous growth in interest in this specialty demonstrated by the proliferation of journals devoted exclusively to forensic psychiatry, the development of forensic psychiatry fellowships, and board certification. The American Board of Medical Specialties has recognized forensic psychiatry as a subspecialty of psychiatry. It authorized the American Board of Psychiatry and Neurology to conduct examinations for a certificate of added qualifications in forensic psychiatry beginning in 1994.

Just a few of the major areas in which forensic psychiatrists evaluate cases and provide testimony include malpractice litigation, will contests, personal injury litigation, competency determinations (both civil and criminal), criminal responsibility, and presentencing hearings. Many other areas of law and psychiatry, too numerous to list here, also require the professional services of the forensic psychiatrist. In the course of practice, the forensic psychiatrist often works on unusual, challenging cases that are not ordinarily found in the general outpatient or inpatient practice of psychiatry. A list of suggested readings in forensic psychiatry is provided following the references at the end of this chapter.

FORENSIC PSYCHIATRIC EVALUATION OF THE CLAIMANT

The forensic psychiatric evaluation of the injured *claimant* differs in a number of significant ways from the traditional psychiatric evaluation. In the litigation context, the distinction between the roles of treating psychiatrist and forensic evaluator must be firmly maintained. Problems invariably arise for the clinician when these roles are confused.

The psychiatrist who enters the legal arena must understand that equities usually exist on both sides of a legal case; otherwise the case would probably not have been brought to litigation. The fact that opposing experts disagree does not necessarily mean that one side or the other is wrong. The opinions of opposing experts should be carefully considered.

Team Approach

The comprehensive forensic psychiatric evaluation usually requires cooperation with a number of other practitioners and specialists. The forensic psychiatrist who is evaluating the claimant may require the input of a neurologist, psychologist, neuropsychologist, and internist or general practitioner. Depending on the complexities of the case, representatives of a number of other disciplines may need to be consulted. The forensic evaluator must also consider the findings of other examinations performed at the request of opposing counsel. The burgeoning number of ever-more-complicated brain studies currently available makes consultation with a qualified neurologist virtually a necessity in cases involving claims of brain injury.

Absence of Doctor-Patient Relationship

The psychiatrist should inform the claimant at the time of examination that no doctor-patient relationship will be formed. That is, the psychiatrist will not *treat* the claimant in any fashion. The psychiatrist should explain that he or she has been retained by [name the specific party] to perform an independent psychiatric examination. The sole purpose of the examination is to provide information to the party retaining the psychiatrist.

Absence of Confidentiality

The claimant must be informed that, unlike the usual doctor-patient relationship, confidentiality surrounding the forensic evaluation may not exist. Once the retaining attorney decides to disclose the findings of the evaluation in litigation, the information will be available to both sides and will likely become a public record.

Standard Diagnostic Schema

The diagnostic evaluation of claimants should be made according to the multiaxial classification system contained in DSM-IV. All five axes should be employed. Axis I permits the clinician to consider the major clinical psychiatric syndromes, either singly or multiply. It is not unusual for the claimant to have concurrent Axis I diagnoses. Concurrent Axis I disorders may have preexisted or been exacerbated.

Axis II forces the clinician to consider personality disorders that are often overlooked or ignored in the forensic evaluation of a claimant. The occurrence of significant head injuries is high in the violent criminal population, where there is a higher incidence of antisocial personality disorder (Lewis et al. 1986; Pétursson and Gudjónsson 1981).

On Axis III, the relationship of medical disorders and their treatments to the patient's clinical presentation on Axis I must be carefully evaluated. The claimant may have a number of injuries requiring extensive pharmacotherapy that may further complicate the clinical picture. Moreover, a host of medical disorders may present with or have associated symptoms of cerebral dysfunction. Prior head injuries or preexisting central nervous system (CNS) disorders must be considered. For example, young adults who have a history of learning disabilities or attention-deficit disorder are likely to develop serious incapacity when they sustain traumatic brain injury.

Axis IV permits the evaluation of a psychosocial stressor or multiple psychosocial stressors, usually occurring within the year preceding the current evaluation, that may have contributed to the development of a new mental disorder, recurrence of a prior mental disorder, or exacerbation of an already existing psychiatric disorder. Posttraumatic stress disorder can be an exception to the 1-year recommendation. The search for multiple psychosocial stressors must be carefully conducted. It is the rare claimant who has only one psychosocial stressor affecting his or her life. Injury often occurs in the context of other preexisting psychosocial stressors such as sustained interpersonal difficulties, financial problems, occupational distress, or other personal losses.

Finally, functional impairment should be assessed on Axis V according to the Global Assessment of Functioning Scale in combination with other standard methods of evaluation of psychiatric impairment discussed later.

DSM-IV contains a cautionary statement about its use in litigation. Lawyers and courts refer to DSM-IV extensively. Psychiatrists perform an important service by clinically informing the use of DSM-IV in the litigation context. Lawyers and courts have a tendency to cloak clinical guidelines and diagnostic manuals with a certainty more properly given to the reading of statutes and codes.

Collateral Sources of Information

In the treatment situation, the psychiatrist relies almost exclusively on the subjective reporting of the patient. The patient, who is suffering from a disorder, is presumed to be candid. No conscious, hidden agendas are usually present. In litigation, however, the claimant must naturally be expected to favor his or her own legal case. The possibility of malingering must always be kept in mind (Table 41–11). Malingering is not limited to the fabrication of symptoms. More often, malingering is manifested by the *exaggeration* or even *minimization* of symptoms. Thus, the psychiatrist must consider a broad array of information.

During the course of legal discovery by both parties to the suit, a great deal of information usually is developed. The forensic examiner should request that the retaining lawyer provide *all* relevant information. Proceeding to court with incomplete information will likely be exposed by opposing counsel, undercutting the psychiatrist's testimony and damaging the claimant's case irreparably. The forensic psychiatrist should review all data carefully before coming to a conclusion. The collateral sources of information listed in Table 41–12, although not exhaustive, indicate major areas for inquiry.

Traumatic Brain Injury

In evaluating the mental status of the traumatic brain injury (TBI) claimant, the psychiatrist must be able to con-

---

TABLE 41–11. Increased index of suspicion for malingering

Litigation context (financial compensation, evading criminal prosecution)

Marked discrepancy between clinical findings and subjective complaints

Lack of cooperation with evaluation and treatment

Antisocial personality traits or disorder

Overdramatization of complaints

History of recurrent accidents or injuries

Evidence of self-induced injuries

Vaguely defined symptoms

Poor work history

Unable to work but retains capacity for pleasurable activities

Source. Reprinted with permission from Simon RI: "Legal and Ethical Issues in Traumatic Brain Injury," in *Traumatic Brain Injury.* Edited by Silver JM. Washington, DC, American Psychiatric Press, 1994. Copyright 1994, American Psychiatric Press, Inc.

TABLE 41–12. Collateral sources of information

Other physicians and health care providers (reports, direct discussions)

Hospital records

Family

Other third parties

Military records

School records

Police records

Witness information

Work records

Work products (letters, work projects)

Legal discovery (depositions, legal documents)

Prior medical and psychiatric records

Prior psychological and neuropsychological evaluations

Source. Reprinted with permission from Simon RI: "Legal and Ethical Issues in Traumatic Brain Injury," in *Traumatic Brain Injury.* Edited by Silver JM. Washington, DC, American Psychiatric Press, 1994. Copyright 1994, American Psychiatric Press, Inc.

TABLE 41–13. Major factors influencing neuropsychological test findings

Original endowment

Environment (e.g., education, occupation, life experiences)

Motivation (effort)

Physical health

Psychological distress

Psychiatric disorders (e.g., depression, dissociative disorders)

Medications (e.g., anticonvulsants, psychotropics)

Qualifications and experience of neuropsychologist

Errors in scoring

Errors in interpretation

Source. Reprinted with permission from Simon RI: "Legal and Ethical Issues in Traumatic Brain Injury," in *Traumatic Brain Injury.* Edited by Silver JM. Washington, DC, American Psychiatric Press, 1994. Copyright 1994, American Psychiatric Press, Inc.

duct a thorough and reliable mental status examination. Moreover, the mental status assessment is an integral part of the psychiatric examination that cannot be delegated to others. Usually, it is better to conduct the examination in divided sessions over the course of 2 days because of possible fluctuations in the mental status of the TBI claimant. The practice of performing a perfunctory mental status examination or relying solely on the assessment of the neuropsychologist is unwarranted. Neuropsychological assessment can be a valuable adjunct to the neuropsychiatric assessment of the TBI claimant (Becker and Kay 1986). Nevertheless, the psychiatrist will have little basis for critically reviewing the neuropsychological findings unless he or she can perform a competent mental status examination. The mental status examination as described by Strub and Black (1985) provides a scored, comprehensive, reliable format for evaluation of mental status.

The role of neuropsychological testing must be critically evaluated in each case. Neuropsychological tests are not totally objective. The qualifications and experience of the neuropsychologist constitute a critical variable. Tests of behavior in neuropsychological testing are subject to the control of the person performing the task. Thus, the consideration of motivation is critical. Also, low test scores may be caused by factors other than brain damage (Table 41–13). Doctors, not tests, make diagnoses. A neuropsychological test score by itself cannot be used to point to a specific cause of the litigant's injury. Moreover, in litigation, causation is ultimately a matter for the finder of fact to determine.

Base rate neuropsychological deficits are typically demonstrated in the normal population. If impairments are noted without evaluation of the claimant's prior history and level of neuropsychological functioning, over-interpretation of the test data is likely. The critical review of school and work records to determine the prior level of intellectual functioning is important in establishing baseline performance. Neuropsychological impairments observed among a normal population increase with the age of the population. Lower IQ score and slower responses are also associated with normal aging.

Comorbidity and drug effects also must be considered when evaluating the results of neuropsychological test assessments. Questionable results will be obtained in the neuropsychological testing if the impact of concurrent psychiatric disorders and medications on the neuropsychological data is not considered.

Brain Injury Mimics

A number of psychiatric disorders may mimic traumatic brain injury. Some of the more common traumatic brain injury mimics include conversion, factitious, somatization, and depressive disorders presenting with symptoms of neurological and cerebral dysfunction. Conversion disorder symptoms classically mimic neurological disease. Dissociative symptoms may present with amnesia or atypical memory loss. Depressive pseudodementia is a commonly recognized clinical disorder in elderly patients. Posttraumatic stress disorder manifesting symptoms of difficulty in concentration and psychogenic amnesia may also mimic brain injury. Similarly, anxiety disorders may be associated with memory complaints secondary to the inability to concentrate. On the other hand, TBI may produce anxiety and depression.

To complicate matters, litigants may be receiving psychoactive substances. Neuroleptics, antidepressants, lithium, and particularly benzodiazepines can produce side effects that mimic neurological and brain disorders. Psychoactive substances may produce serious memory difficulties, either directly by acting on brain chemistry or indirectly through sedation. Unfortunately, the practice of polypharmacy by frustrated practitioners is common, particularly when the claimant appears refractory to treatment during the course of litigation. As a result, various combinations of medications may interact to produce a host of side effects that involve the CNS. Psychoactive drug abuse is also distressingly common in these cases, especially when the litigant complains of persistent pain. Narcotics and barbiturates, particularly when marketed in combination with nonnarcotic pain medications, are commonly abused.

Disability Determinations

In addition to the psychiatric diagnosis, an assessment of functional impairment and disability must be made. In litigation, it is the degree of functional impairment, not the psychiatric diagnosis per se, that determines the monetary damage award. The psychiatrist must also understand the difference between impairment and disability. An impaired individual may not necessarily be disabled. Psychiatric impairment is considered disabling only when a psychiatric disorder limits a person's capacity to meet the demands of living. The American Medical Association, in its *Guide to the Evaluation of Permanent Impairment* (1988, pp. 201–202), gives the example of the impact of the loss of the fifth finger on the left hand to illustrate this point. For a bank president, the occupational impact will likely be negligible; the concert pianist, however, will probably be totally disabled.

Similarly, a patient may have moderate impairment but only mild disability in social or occupational functioning owing to the development of compensatory coping mechanisms. On the other hand, practically every psychiatric clinician has seen patients who have little or no impairment but nevertheless are seriously disabled. This situation is particularly common in the litigation context. For claimants presenting such a picture, the psychiatrist should pay particular attention to the possible presence of concurrent Axis IV psychosocial stressors, comorbidity, polypharmacy, and the effect of litigation on the clinical presentation of the claimant.

Standard impairment assessment methods should be used in combination with the DSM-IV Axis V global assessment of functioning. The credible psychiatric assessment of functional impairment avoids strictly subjective, idiosyncratic, ex cathedra pronouncements about the examinee's impairment and the need for future treatment. Instead, whenever possible, the examinee's functional impairment and future treatment needs should be evaluated according to the American Medical Association's *Guide to the Evaluation of Permanent Impairment* (1993, pp. 291–302). The guide closely follows the Social Security Administration's guidelines to the assessment of disability. Assessment of permanent impairment should not be made until maximal medical improvement has been achieved.

Child Custody

Psychiatrists become involved in child custody cases throughout the separation and divorce process (Billick and Kerry 1994). Psychiatrists may be asked to give opinions in the following situations:

- Custody decisions (request by parents before litigation)
- Child custody litigation
- To assist a *guardian ad litem* (attorney appointed by court to represent a child)
- Child-care agency (usually court ordered following allegations of abuse)
- Divorce mediation procedures
- Visitation
- Psychiatric treatment of either parent or child

The guiding principle in child custody decisions is the recognition of children's rights through application of the "best interests of the child" standard. Psychiatrists who become involved in child custody decisions should have specialized training in child psychiatry. Adequately trained general psychiatrists may also be able to perform child custody evaluations. However, the general psychiatrist must recognize any limitations in training and experience in performing child psychiatric evaluations (Simon and Wettstein 1997). Consultation with a child psychiatrist may be necessary. The American Psychiatric Association (1982) provides guidelines for child custody evaluations.

When performing child custody evaluations, the psychiatrist should see both parties to the litigation. The eithical guidelines of the American Academy of Psychiatry and the Law (Section IV) state the following:

In custody cases, honesty and striving for objectivity require that all parties be interviewed, if possible, before an opinion is rendered. When this is not possible, or if for any reason not done, this fact should be clearly indicated in the forensic psychiatrist's report and testimony. Where one parent has not been seen, even after deliberate effort, it may be inappropriate to comment on that parent's fitness as a parent. Any comments on that parent's fitness should be qualified and the data for the opinion be clearly indicated.

Child custody disputes often result in hardball litigation. If one parent accuses the other of child sexual abuse, "nuclear warfare" breaks out. Many psychiatrists refuse to perform child custody evaluations because of their fears of being excoriated by aggressive attorneys. Forensically informed psychiatrists are usually able to function effectively in the litigation environment.

Child custody evaluation presents special challenges and rewards. Psychiatrists must be willing to commit the time necessary to do extensive interviewing as well as manage the emotional strain of child custody cases. Evaluators must be careful to identify and correct personal biases and not allow themselves to be influenced by importuning attorneys. Recommendations made by the psychiatrist will likely have a profound influence on the rest of the child's life. The psychiatrist must assiduously maintain a position of advocate for the child's needs. The professional and personal gratifications are great when the psychiatrist's evaluation provides the potential for healthy child development and a sound foundation for adult life.

After a divorce is final, one parent usually is granted custody of any minor children. The custodial parent holds the health care decision-making power. Psychiatrists may be asked to perform an examination or evaluation of a minor child at the request of a noncustodial parent. However, psychiatrists who perform such examinations expose themselves to legal action (Simon 1992a, p. 61). Although no court has found a psychiatrist liable for failure to obtain the custodial parent's consent prior to examination or evaluation, such decisions appear likely (Kuder 1986, pp. 8–9). Court decisions as well as statutory interpretations of the term *parent* have limited the use of that word to the parent awarded custody under a divorce decree's term (*Gary v. Gary*, 631 SW2d 781 [Tex Ct App 1982]; Texas Fam Code Ann § 14.08(C)(I)[Vernon 1990]). Before performing an evaluation or examination on a minor child, the psychiatrist should obtain the consent of the parent with legal custody.

CONCLUSIONS

The ethical and legal issues surrounding the treatment and management of psychiatric patients are challenging and complex. The legally informed psychiatrist is in a stronger position to provide good clinical care to the patient within the burgeoning regulation of psychiatry by the courts and through governmental legislation. Moreover, psychiatrists will be increasingly required to testify in court concerning psychiatric patients. Familiarity and comfort with the role of a fact or expert witness will facilitate competent psychiatric testimony.

REFERENCES

American Academy of Psychiatry and the Law: Ethical Guidelines for the Practice of Forensic Psychiatry. Adopted May 1987. Revised October 1989, 1991

American Medical Association: Guide to the Evaluation of Permanent Impairment, 3rd Edition. Chicago, IL, American Medical Association, 1988

American Medical Association: Guide to the Evaluation of Permanent Impairment, 4th Edition. Chicago, IL, American Medical Association, 1993

American Medical Association: Physician-Assisted Suicide. Code of Medical Ethics Reports, Vol. 5, No. 2. Chicago, IL, American Medical Association, July 1994, pp 269–275

American Medical Association: Report of the Council on Scientific Affairs. Evidence-Based Principles of Discharge and Discharge Criteria (CSA Report 4-A-96), Chicago, IL, American Medical Association, 1996

American Psychiatric Association: Child Custody Consultation. Washington, DC, American Psychiatric Association, 1982

American Psychiatric Association: The Psychiatric Uses of Seclusion and Restraint (APA Task Force Report No 22). Washington, DC, American Psychiatric Association, 1984

American Psychiatric Association: The Practice of Electroconvulsive Therapy: Recommendations for Treatment, Training, and Privileging: A Task Force Report of the American Psychiatric Association. Washington, DC, American Psychiatric Association, 1990

American Psychiatric Association: The Principles of Medical Ethics With Annotations Especially Applicable to Psychiatry. Washington, DC, American Psychiatric Association, 1992a

American Psychiatric Association: Tardive Dyskinesia: A Task Force Report of the American Psychiatric Association. Washington, DC, American Psychiatric Association, 1992b

American Psychiatric Association: Diagnostic and Statistical Manual of Mental Disorders, 4th Edition. Washington, DC, American Psychiatric Association, 1994

Appelbaum PS: Statutes regulating patient-therapist sex. Hosp Community Psychiatry 41:15–16, 1990

Appelbaum PS, Lidz CW, Meisel A: Informed Consent: Legal Theory and Clinical Practice. New York, Oxford University Press, 1987, pp 84–87

Appelbaum PS, Zonana H, Bonnie R, et al: Statutory approaches to limiting psychiatrists' liability for their patients' violent acts. Am J Psychiatry 146:821–828, 1989

Baxter P, Beck JC: The violent patient: minimize your risk, in Practicing Psychiatry Without Fear: Guidelines of Liability Prevention. Edited by Lifson LE, Simon RI. Cambridge, MA, Harvard University Press, 1998

Becker B, Kay GG: Neuropsychological consultation in psychiatric practice. Psychiatr Clin North Am 9:255–265, 1986

Benefacts. A Message from the APA-sponsored Professional Liability Insurance Program. Psychiatric News, April 19, 1996a, pp 1, 26

Billick SB, Kerry CD: Role of the psychiatric evaluator in child custody disputes, in Principles and Practice of Forensic Psychiatry. Edited by Rosner R. New York, Chapman & Hall, 1994, pp 271–281

Binder RL: Sexual harassment: issues for forensic psychiatrists. Bull Am Acad Psychiatry Law 20:109–118, 1992

Bisbing SB, Jorgenson LM, Sutherland PK: Sexual Abuse by Professionals: A Legal Guide. Charlottesville, VA, Michie, 1995

Black HC: Black's Law Dictionary, 6th Edition. St Paul, MN, West Publishing, 1990

Blackstone W: Commentaries, Vol 4, 1769, pp 24–25

Blinder M: My examination of Dan White. Am J Forensic Psychiatry 2:12–22, 1981–1982

Blumenthal SJ: An overview and synopsis of risk factors, assessment, and treatment of suicidal patients over the life cycle, in Suicide Over the Life Cycle. Edited by Blumenthal SJ, Kupfer DJ. Washington, DC, American Psychiatric Press, 1990, pp 685–733

Blumer D: Psychiatric Aspects of Epilepsy. Washington, DC, American Psychiatric Press, 1984

Brakel SJ, Parry J, Weiner BA: The Mentally Disabled and the Law, 3rd Edition. Chicago, IL, American Bar Foundation, 1985

Chiles JH, Strohsall K: The Suicidal Patient: Principles of Assessment, Treatment and Case Management. Washington, DC, American Psychiatric Press, 1995

Coke E: Third Institute 6, 6th Ed, 1680

Daniel DG, Zigun JR, Weinberger DR: Brain imaging in neuropsychiatry, in The American Psychiatric Press Textbook of Neuropsychiatry, 2nd Edition. Edited by Yudofsky SC, Hales RE. Washington, DC, American Psychiatric Press, 1992, pp 165–186

Devinsky O, Bear D: Varieties of aggressive behavior in temporal lobe epilepsy. Am J Psychiatry 141:651–656, 1984

Droba M, Whybrow PC: Endocrine and metabolic disorders, in Comprehensive Textbook of Psychiatry/V, Vol 2, 5th Edition. Edited by Kaplan HI, Sadock BJ. Baltimore, MD, Williams & Wilkins, 1989, pp 1209–1221

Elliott FA: Neurological aspects of antisocial behavior, in The Psychopath: A Comprehensive Study of Antisocial Disorders and Behaviors. Edited by Reid WH. New York, Brunner/Mazel, 1978, pp 146–189

Elliott FA: Neurological findings in adult minimal brain dysfunction and the dyscontrol syndrome. J Nerv Ment Dis 170:680–687, 1982

Emanuel EJ, Emanuel LL: Proxy decision making for incompetent patients—an ethical and empirical analysis. JAMA 267:2067–2071, 1992

Greenberg SA, Shuman DW: Irreconcilable conflict between therapeutic and forensic roles. Journal of Professional Psychology: Research and Practice 28:50–56, 1997

Grisso T: Evaluating Competencies: Forensic Assessments and Instruments. New York, Plenum, 1986

Grisso T, Appelbaum PS: Comparison of standards for assessing patients' capacities to make treatment decisions. Am J Psychiatry 152:1033–1037, 1995a

Grisso T, Appelbaum PS: The MacArthur treatment competence study, III: Abilities of patients to consent to psychiatric and medical treatments. Law and Human Behavior 19:149–174, 1995b

Gutheil TG, Appelbaum PS: Substituted judgement and the physician's ethical dilemma: with special reference to the problem of the psychiatric patient. J Clin Psychiatry 41:303–305, 1980

Gutheil TG, Simon RI: Risk management principles in recovered memory cases: the importance of the clinical foundation. Psychiatr Serv 48:1403–1407, 1997

Hassenfeld IN, Grumet B: A study of the right to refuse treatment. Bull Am Acad Psychiatry Law 12:65–74, 1984

Hoge SK, Jorgenson L, Goldstein N, et al: APA resource document: legal sanctions for mental health professional-patient sexual misconduct. Bull Am Acad Psychiatry Law 23:433–448, 1995

Johnson ID: Reports to the National Practitioner Data Bank. JAMA 265:407–411, 1991

Joint Commission on Accreditation of Healthcare Organizations: Comprehensive Accreditation Manual for Behavioral Health. Chicago, IL, Joint Commission on Accreditation of Healthcare Organizations, 1997

Kane JM, Weinhold P, Kinon B, et al: Prevalence of abnormal involuntary movements ("spontaneous dyskinesia") in the normal elderly. Psychopharmacology 77:105–108, 1982

Klawans HL, Barr A: Prevalence of spontaneous lingual-facial-buccal dyskinesia in the elderly. Neurology 32:558–559, 1982

Klein J, Onek J, Macbeth J: Seminar on Law in the Practice of Psychiatry. Washington, DC, Onek, Klein & Farr, 1983

Krouner LW: Shock therapy and psychiatric malpractice: the legal accommodation to a controversial treatment. J Forensic Sci 20:404–415, 1975

Kuder A: Legal alert: treatment and consent. Washington Psychiatric Society Newsletter, Summer 1986, pp 8–9

LaPuma J, Orentlicher D, Moss RJ: Advance directives on admission: clinical implications and analysis of the Patient Self-Determination Act of 1990. JAMA 266:402–405, 1991

Lazarus JA, Sharfstein SS: Changes in the economics and ethics of health and mental health care, in American Psychiatric Press Review of Psychiatry, Vol 13. Edited by Oldham JM, Riba MB. Washington, DC, American Psychiatric Press, 1994, pp 389–413

Leong GB, Eth S, Silva JA: The psychotherapist as witness for the prosecution: the criminalization of Tarasoff. Am J Psychiatry 149:1011–1015, 1992

Levinson W, Roter DL, Mullooly JP, et al: Physician-patient communication: the relationship with malpractice claims among primary care physicians and surgeons. JAMA 227:553–559, 1997

Lewis DO, Pincus JH, Feldman M, et al: Psychiatric, neurological, and psychoeducational characteristics of 15 death row inmates in the United States. Am J Psychiatry 143: 838–845, 1986

Link BG, Stueve A: Psychotic symptoms and the violent/illegal behavior of mental patients compared to community controls, in Violence and Mental Disorder: Developments in Risk Assessment. Edited by Monahan J, Steadman H. Chicago, IL, University of Chicago Press, 1994, pp 137–159

Lohr JB, Wisinewski A, Jeste DV: Neurological aspects of tardive dyskinesia, in Handbook of Schizophrenia, Vol 1: Neurology of Schizophrenia. Edited by Nasrallah H, Weinberger DR. Amsterdam, Elsevier, 1986, pp 97–119

Low P, Jeffries J, Bonnie R: Criminal Law: Cases and Materials. Mineola, NY, The Foundation Press, 1982, pp 152–154

The MacArthur Violence Risk Assessment Study. American Psychology Law Society News 16:3, 1996, pp 1–4

Marcus R: Court rules "right to die" depends on patient's intent. Washington Post, June 26, 1990, p A1, 8

Maris RW, Berman AL, Maltsberger JT, et al: Assessment and Prediction of Suicide. New York, Guilford, 1992

McGarry AL: Pathological gambling: a new insanity defense. Bull Am Acad Psychiatry Law 11:301–308, 1983

Melton GB, Petrila J, Poythress NG, et al: Psychological Evaluations for the Courts: A Handbook for Mental Health Professionals and Lawyers. New York, Guilford, 1987

Mishkin B: Decisions in Hospice. Arlington, VA, The National Hospice Organization, 1985

Mishkin B: Determining the capacity for making health care decisions, in Issues in Geriatric Psychiatry (Advances in Psychosomatic Medicine, Vol 19). Edited by Billig N, Rabins PV. Basel, Switzerland, S Karger, 1989, pp 151–166

Monahan J, Steadman H (eds): Violence and Mental Disorder: Developments in Risk Assessment. Chicago, IL, University of Chicago Press, 1994

O'Connell RA: A review of the use of electroconvulsive therapy. Hosp Community Psychiatry 33:469–473, 1982

Orentlicher D: The illusion of patient choice in end-of-life decisions. JAMA 267:2101–2104, 1992

Overman W Jr, Stoudemire A: Guidelines for legal and financial counseling of Alzheimer's disease patients and their families. Am J Psychiatry 145:1495–1500, 1988

Parry BL, Berga SL: Neuroendocrine correlates of behavior during the menstrual cycle (Chapter 58), in Psychiatry, Vol 3. Edited by Cavenar JO. Philadelphia, PA, JB Lippincott, 1991, pp 1–22

Parry HJ, Balter MB, Mellinger GD, et al: National patterns of psychotherapeutic drug use. Arch Gen Psychiatry 28:769–783, 1973

Perlin ML: Mental Disability Law: Civil and Criminal, Vol 3. Charlottesville, VA, Michie, 1989

Perr IN: Liability and electroshock therapy. J Forensic Sci 25:508–513, 1980

Perr IN: The clinical considerations of medication refusal. Legal Aspects of Psychiatric Practice 1:5–8, 1984

Pétursson H, Gudjónsson GH: Psychiatric aspects of homicide. Acta Psychiatr Scand 64:363–372, 1981

President's Commission for the Study of Ethical Problems in Medicine and Biomedical and Behavioral Research: Making Health Care Decisions, Vol 1: A Report on the Ethical and Legal Implications of Informed Consent in the Patient-Practitioner Relationship. Washington, DC, U.S. Government Printing Office, October 1982

Regan M: Protective services for the elderly: commitment, guardianship, and alternatives. William & Mary Law Review 13:569, 569–573, 1972

Reich J, Wells J: Psychiatric diagnosis and competency to stand trial. Compr Psychiatry 26:421–432, 1985

Robertson JD: The trial of a suicide case, in American Psychiatric Press Review of Clinical Psychiatry and the Law, Vol 202. Edited by Simon RI. Washington, DC, American Psychiatric Press, 1991, pp 423–441

Rosenthal RJ, Lorenz VC: The pathological gambler as criminal offender: comments on the evaluation and treatment. Psychiatr Clin North Am 15:647–660, 1992

Rutter P: Sex in the Forbidden Zone: When Therapists, Doctors, Clergy, Teachers and Other Men in Power Betray Women's Trust. Los Angeles, CA, JP Tarcher, 1989

Sale B, Powell DM, Van Duizend R: Disabled Persons and the Law: State Legislative Issues. 1982, p 461

Schoener GR, Milgrom JH, Gonsiorek JC, et al: Psychotherapists' Sexual Involvement With Clients. Minneapolis, MN, Walk-In Counseling Center, 1989

Schreiber J, Roesch R, Golding S: An evaluation of procedures for assessing competency to stand trial. Bulletin of the American Academy of Psychiatry and the Law 155: 187–203, 1987

Simon RI: The psychiatrist as a fiduciary: avoiding the double agent role. Psychiatric Annals 17:622–626, 1987

Simon RI: Sexual exploitation of patients: how it begins before it happens. Psychiatric Annals 19:104–112, 1989

Simon RI: Psychological injury caused by boundary violation precursors to therapist-patient sex. Psychiatric Annals 21: 614–619, 1991a

Simon RI: The suicide prevention pact: clinical and legal considerations, in American Psychiatric Press Review of Clinical Psychiatry and the Law, Vol 2. Edited by Simon RI. Washington, DC, American Psychiatric Press, 1991b, pp 441–451

Simon RI: Clinical Psychiatry and the Law, 2nd Edition. Washington, DC, American Psychiatric Press, 1992a

Simon RI: Clinical risk management of suicidal patients: assessing the unpredictable, in American Psychiatric Press Review of Clinical Psychiatry and the Law, Vol 3. Edited by Simon RI. Washington, DC, American Psychiatric Press, 1992b, pp 3–63

Simon RI: Concise Guide to Clinical Psychiatry and the Law. Washington, DC, American Psychiatric Press, 1992c

Simon RI: Treatment boundary violations: clinical, ethical, and legal considerations. Bull Am Acad Psychiatry Law 20:269–288, 1992d

Simon RI: Innovative Psychiatric Therapies and Legal Uncertainty: A Survival Guide for Clinicians. Psychiatric Annals, 23:473–379, 1993

Simon RI: Treatment boundaries in psychiatric practice, in Forensic Psychiatry: A Comprehensive Textbook. Edited by Rosner R. New York, Van Nostrand Reinhold, 1994

Simon RI (ed): Posttraumatic Stress Disorder in Litigation: Guidelines for Forensic Assessment. Washington, DC, American Psychiatric Press, 1995

Simon RI: The credible forensic psychiatric evaluation in sexual harassment litigation. Psychiatric Annals 26:139–148, 1996

Simon RI: Clinical Risk Management of the Rapid Cycling Bipolar Patient. Harvard Review of Psychiatry 4:245–254, 1997

Simon RI: Psychiatrists' duties in discharging sicker and potentially violent patients in the managed care era. Psychiatr Serv 49:62–67, 1998

Simon RI, Wettstein RM: Toward the development of guidelines for the conduct of forensic psychiatric examinations. Journal of American Psychiatry Law 25:17–30, 1997

Slovenko R: Commentaries on psychiatry and law: "guilty but mentally ill." Journal of Psychiatry and Law 10:541–555, 1982

Slovenko R: Assessing competency to stand trial. Psychiatric Annals 26:392–393, 397, 1995

Smith JT: Medical Malpractice: Psychiatric Care, Colorado Springs, CO, Shepard's/McGraw-Hill, 1986

Solnick PB: Proxy consent for incompetent nonterminally ill adult patients. J Leg Med 6:1–49, 1985

Strasburger LH: "Crudely, without any finesse": the defendant hears his psychiatric evaluation. Bull Am Acad Psychiatry Law 15:229–233, 1987

Strasburger LH, Jorgenson L, Randles R: Criminalization of psychotherapist-patient sex. Am J Psychiatry 148:859–863, 1991

Strasburger LH, Gutheil TG, Brodsky A: On wearing two hats: role conflict in serving as both psychotherapist and expert witness. Am J Psychiatry 154:448–456, 1997

Strub RL, Black FW: The Mental Status Examination in Neurology, 2nd Edition. Philadelphia, PA, FA Davis, 1985

Tardiff K: Concise Guide to Assessment and Management of Violent Patients, 2nd Edition. Washington, DC, American Psychiatric Press, 1989

Taylor MA, Sierles FS, Abrams R: The neuropsychiatric evaluation, in American Psychiatric Press Textbook of Neuropsychiatry. Edited by Hales RE, Yudofsky SC. Washington, DC, American Psychiatric Press, 1987, pp 3–16

Tischler GL: Utilization management of mental health services by private third parties. Am J Psychiatry 147:967–973, 1990

Tranel D: Functional neuroanatomy: neuropsychological correlates of cortical and subcortical damage, in The American Psychiatric Press Textbook of Neuropsychiatry, 2nd Edition. Edited by Yudofsky SC, Hales RE. Washington, DC, American Psychiatric Press, 1992, pp 70–75

U.S. Dept. of Health and Human Services: The Legal Status of Adolescents 1980. Washington, DC, U.S. Dept. of Health and Human Services, 1981

Walzer RS: Impaired physicians: an overview and update of legal issues. J Leg Med 11:131–198, 1990

Weiner RD: The psychiatric use of electrically induced seizures. Am J Psychiatry 136:1507–1517, 1979

Weir RF, Gostin L: Decisions to abate life-sustaining treatment for nonautonomous patients: ethical standards and legal liability for physicians after Cruzan. JAMA 264:1846–1853, 1990

Why Are Liability Premiums Rising? Psychiatric News, June 21, 1996, pp 1, 24–25

Wickizer TM, Lessler D, Travis KM: Controlling inpatient psychiatric utilization through managed care. Am J Psychiatry 153:339–345, 1996

Widiger TA, Trull TJ: Personality disorders and violence, in Violence and Mental Disorder: Developments in Risk Assessment. Edited by Monahan J, Steadman H. Chicago, IL, University of Chicago Press, 1994, pp 203–226

Woodward B, Duckworth K, Gutheil TG: The Pharmacotherapist-Psychotherapist Collaboration, in Annual Review of Psychiatry, Vol 12. Edited by Oldham J. Washington, DC, American Psychiatric Press, 1993

Yudofsky SC, Silver JM, Schneider SE: Pharmacologic treatment of aggression. Psychiatric Annals 17:397–407, 1987

Zeldow PB, Taub HA: Evaluating psychiatric discharge and aftercare in a VA medical center. Hosp Community Psychiatry 32:57–58, 1981

Zito JM, Lentz SL, Routt WW, et al: The treatment review panel: a solution to treatment refusal? Bull Am Acad Psychiatry Law 12:349–358, 1984

LEGAL CITATIONS

Aponte v United States, 582 FSupp 555, 566–69 (D PR 1984)

Bartling v Superior Court, 163 Cal App 3d 186, 209 Cal Rptr 220 (1984)

Bethea v United States, 365 A2d 64, (DC 1976), cert denied, 433 US 911 (1977)

Blanchard v Levine, No D 014550 Fulton Cty Super Ct (Ga 1985)

Bouvia v Superior Court, 179 Cal App 3d 1127, 225 Cal Rptr 297 (1986)

Callan v Norland, 114 Ill App 3d 196, 448 NE2d 651 (1983)

Canterbury v Spence, 464 F2d 772 (DC Cir), cert denied, Spence v Canterbury, 409 US 1064 (1972)

Chaires v St John's Episcopal Hospital, No 808/75 NY Cty Sup Ct (NY Feb 21, 1984)

Clifford v United States, No 82-5002 USDC (SD 1985)

Clites v State, 322 NW2d 917 (Iowa Ct App 1982)

Commonwealth v Robinson, 494 Pa 372, 431 A2d 901 (1981)

Cruzan v Director, Missouri Dept of Health, 497 U.S. 261 (1990)

Doerr v Hurley Medical Center, No 82-674-39 NM Mich Aug (1984)

Dovido v Vasquez, No 84-674 CA(L)(H) 15th Jud Dist Cir Ct, Palm Beach Cty (Fl Apr 4, 1986)

Dusky v United States, 362 U.S. 402 (1960)

Eighth Amendment and the execution of the presently incompetent. Stanford Law Review 32:765, 1980

Fain v Commonwealth, 78 Ky 183 (1879)

Ford v Wainwright, 477 US 399 (1986)

Frasier v Department of Health and Human Resources, 500 So 2d 858, 864 (La Ct App 1986)

Gary v Gary, 631 SW2d 781 (Tex Ct App 1982)

Gowan v United States, 601 FSupp 1297 (D Or 1985)

Gulf S I R Co. v Sullivan, 155 Miss 1, 119 So 501 (1928)

Harris v Forklift Systems, 510 U.S. 17 (1993)

Health Care Quality Improvement Act of 1986, 42 U.S.C. 11101 (Supp v 1987)

H M Advocate v Fraser, 4 Couper 70 (1878)

Holton v Pfingst, 534 SW2d 786, 789 (Ky 1976)

Howe v Citizens Memorial Hospital, 426 SW2d 882 (Tex Civ App 1968), rev'd, 436 SW2d 115 (Tex 1968)

Hyde v University of Michigan Board of Regents, 426 Mich 223, 393 NW2d 847 (1986), revised in accord with Ross v Consumer Power Company, 420 Mich 567, 363 NW2d 641 (1986)

Ill Ann Stat 1990

In re Boyer, 636 P2d 1085, 1089 (Utah 1981)

In re Conroy, 98 NJ 321, 486 A2d 1209, 1222-23 (1985)

In re Farrell, 108 NJ 335, 529 A2d 404 (1987)

In the Guardianship of John Roe, 411 MA 666 (1992)

In re Jobes, 108 NJ 365, 529 A2d 434 (1987)

In re Jobes, 108 NJ 394 (1987)

In re Peter, 108 NJ 365, 529 A2d 419 (1987)

In re Quinlin, 70 NJ 10, 355 A2d 647, cert denied, 429 US 922 (1976)

Jaffe v Redmond, U.S. Lexis 3879 (1996)

Jehovah's Witnesses v King County Hospital, 278 FSupp 488 (WD Wash 1967), affd, 390 US 598 (1968)

Karasik v Bird, 98 AD2d 359, 470 NYS2d 605 (1984)

Kilgore v County of Santa Clara, No 397-525 (Santa Clara Cty Super Ct Cal 1982)

Meek v City of Loveland, 85 Colo 346, 276 P 30 (1929)

Mental Aberration and Post Conviction Sanctions, 15 Suffolk UL Rev: 1219 (1981)

Minn Stat Ann 148 A.02 (West 1989)

M'Naughten's Case, 10 Cl F 200, 8 Eng Rep 718 (HL 1843)

Moran v Botsford General Hospital, No l 81-225-533, Wayne Cty Cir Ct (MI Oct 1, 1984)

Natanson v Kline, 186 Kan 393, 350 P2d 1093 (1960)

Neely v United States, 150 F2d 977 (DC Cir), cert denied, 326 US 768 (1945)

Nevada Revised Statutes

P.L. 98-473, 1984

Parham v JR, 442 US 584 (1979)

People v White, 117 Cal App 3d 270, 172 Cal Rptr 612 (1981)

Planned Parenthood v Danforth, 428 US 52, 74 (1976)

Radank v Heyl, No F4-2316 Wisc Comp Bd (1986)

Ramon v Farr, 770 P2d 131 (Utah 1989)

Rennie v Klein, 462 FSupp 1131 (D NJ 1978), remanded, 476 FSupp 1294 (D NJ 1979), affd in part, modified in part and remanded, 653 F2d 836 (3d Cir 1980), vacated and remanded, 458 U.S. 1119 (1982), 720 F2d 266 (3rd Cir 1983)

Restatement [second] of Torts 315(a) [1965]

Rivera v NYC Health and Hospitals, Reversed, 72 NY2d 1021; 531 N.E.2d 644 (1988)

Rogers v Commissioner of Dept of Mental Health, 390 Mass 489, 458 NE2d 308 (Mass 1983)

Scaria v St Paul Fire & Marine Ins Co, 68 Wis 2d 1, 227 NW2d 647 (1975)

Schloendorff v Society of New York Hospital, 211 NY 125, 105 NE 92 (1914), overruled, Bing v Thunig, 2 NY2d 656, 143 NE2d 3, 163 NYS2d 3 (1957)

Shaughnessy v Spray, Reversed and remanded, 55 ORE. App 42; 637 P2d 182 (1983)

Speer v United States, 512 FSupp 670 (ND Tex 1981), affd, Speer v United States, 675 F2d 100 (5th Cir 1982)

State v Hehman, 110 Ariz 459, 520 P2d 507 (1974)

Stone v Proctor, 259 NC 633, 131 SE2d 297 (1963)

Tarasoff v Regents of the University of California, 17 Cal 3d 425, 551 P2d 334, 131 Cal Rptr 14 (1976)

Texas Ct App 1982

Texas Fam Code Ann § 14.08 (C)(I)[Vernon 1990]

Truman v Thomas, 27 Cal 3d 285, 611 P2d 902, 165 Cal Rptr 308 (1980)

Tune v Walter Reed Army Medical Hospital, 602 FSupp 1452 (DDC 1985)

ULA 1974

Union Pacific Ry Co v Botsford, 141 US 250, 251 (1891)

United States v Brawner, 471 F2d 969 (DC Cir 1972), superseded by statute, see Shannon v United States, 512 U.S. 573 (1994)

United States v David, 511 F2d 355 (DC Cir 1975)

Wilson v Lehman, 379 SW2d 478,479 (Ky 1964)

Wilson v United States, 391 F2d 460, 463 (DC Cir 1968)

Witherell v Weimer, 148 Ill App 3d 32, 499 NE2d 46 (1986), rev'd on other grounds, 118 Ill 2d 515 NE2d 68 (1987)

Wright v State, No 83-5035 Orleans Parish Civ Dist Ct (LA April 1986)

Youngberg v Romeo (457 U.S. 307 (1982), on remand, Romeo v Youngberg, 687 F2d 33 (3rd Cir 1982)

SUGGESTED READINGS IN FORENSIC PSYCHIATRY

American Psychiatric Association: The Principles of Medical Ethics, With Annotations Especially Applicable to Psychiatry. Washington, DC, American Psychiatric Association, 1995

Appelbaum PS: Almost A Revolution: Mental Health Law and the Limits of Change. New York, Oxford University Press, 1994

Appelbaum PS, Gutheil TG: Clinical Handbook of Psychiatry and the Law, 2nd Edition. Baltimore, MD, Williams & Wilkins, 1991

Appelbaum PS, Lidz CW, Meisel A: Informed Consent: Legal Theory and Clinical Practice. New York, Oxford University Press, 1987

Appelbaum PS, Uyehara L, Elin M (eds): Trauma and Memory: Clinical and Legal Controversies. New York, Oxford University Press, 1997

Beck JC (ed): Confidentiality Versus the Duty to Protect: Foreseeable Harm in the Practice of Psychiatry. Washington, DC, American Psychiatric Press, 1990

Blumenthal SJ, Kupfer DJ (eds): Suicide Over the Life Cycle: Risk Factors, Assessment, and Treatment of Suicidal Patients. Washington, DC, American Psychiatric Press, 1990

Brakel SJ, Parry J, Weiner BA: The Mentally Disabled and the Law, 3rd Edition. Chicago, IL, American Bar Foundation, 1985

Chiles JH, Strohsall K: The Suicidal Patient: Principles of Assessment, Treatment and Case Management. Washington, DC, American Psychiatric Press, 1995

Dyer AR: Ethics and Psychiatry: Toward Professional Definition. Washington, DC, American Psychiatric Press, 1988

Felthous AR: The Psychotherapist's Duty to Warn or Protect. Springfield, IL, Charles C Thomas, 1989

Gabbard GO (ed): Sexual Exploitation in Professional Relationships. Washington, DC, American Psychiatric Press, 1989

Gutheil TG, Bursztajn HJ, Brodsky A, et al: Decision Making in Psychiatry and the Law. Baltimore, MD, Williams & Wilkins, 1991

Malcolm JG: Treatment Choices and Informed Consent: Current Controversies in Psychiatric Malpractice Litigation. Springfield, IL, Charles C Thomas, 1988

Maris RW, Berman AL, Maltsberger JT, et al: Assessment and Prediction of Suicide. New York, Guilford, 1992

Miller RD: Involuntary Civil Commitment of the Mentally Ill in the Post-Reform Era. Springfield, IL, Charles C Thomas, 1987

Monahan J, Steadman H (eds): Violence and Mental Disorder: Developments in Risk Assessment. Chicago, IL, University of Chicago Press, 1994

Perlin ML: Mental Disability Law: Civil and Criminal, Vols 1–3. Charlottesville, VA, Michie, 1989

Pope KS: Sexual Involvement With Therapist: Patient Assessment, Subsequent Therapy, Forensics. Washington, DC, American Psychological Association, 1994

Pope KS, Brown LS: Recovered Memories of Abuse: Assessment, Therapy, Forensics. Washington, DC, American Psychological Association, 1996

Reisner R, Slobogin C: Law and the Mental Health System, Second Edition. St Paul, MN, West Publishing, 1990

Schetky DH, Benedek EP: Clinical Handbook of Child Psychiatry and the Law. Baltimore, MD, Williams & Wilkins, 1992

Schoener GR, Milgrom JH, Gonsiorek JC, et al: Psychotherapists' Sexual Involvement With Clients. Minneapolis, MN, Walk-In Counseling Center, 1989

Shrier DK (ed): Sexual Harassment in the Workplace and Academia. Washington, DC, American Psychiatric Press, 1996

Simon RI (ed): American Psychiatric Press Review of Clinical Psychiatry and the Law, Vol 1. Washington, DC, American Psychiatric Press, 1990

Simon RI (ed): American Psychiatric Press Review of Clinical Psychiatry and the Law, Vol 2. Washington, DC, American Psychiatric Press, 1991

Simon RI (ed): American Psychiatric Press Review of Clinical Psychiatry and the Law, Vol 3. Washington, DC, American Psychiatric Press, 1992

Simon RI: Clinical Psychiatry and the Law, 2nd Edition. Washington, DC, American Psychiatric Press, 1992

Simon RI, Sadoff RL: Psychiatric Malpractice: Cases and Comments for Clinicians. Washington DC, American Psychiatric Press, 1992

Slovenko R: Psychiatry and Criminal Culpability. New York, Wiley, 1995

Tardiff K: Concise Guide to Assessment and Management of Violent Patients. Washington, DC, American Psychiatric Press, 1996

CHAPTER 42

PUBLIC PSYCHIATRY AND PREVENTION

H. RICHARD LAMB, M.D.

Public psychiatry today is far different from the much publicized and much criticized community psychiatry of the 1960s. This changing role has given rise to the need for a new term—hence the widespread and increasing use of the term *public psychiatry*. Community psychiatry of the 1960s generally neglected the chronically and severely mentally ill and instead focused on less sick patients (the healthy but unhappy, or the "worried well," as they have been characterized), primary prevention (with little evidence that such efforts were effective), and community activism in efforts to change the basic fabric of society. That focus gave rise to criticisms such as that community psychiatry "has branched out well beyond mental illness into problems that it is not especially qualified to handle—community, national, and international affairs; poverty, politics, and criminality. In each of these areas, we have responsibilities as citizens and human beings; we have yet to demonstrate any special competence as psychiatrists" (Kety 1974, p. 962). Moreover, issues such as those presented by the homeless mentally ill population have demonstrated major problems in the way that deinstitutionalization was implemented—problems for which the community psychiatry of past decades has to share the blame.

Modern-day public psychiatry generally recognizes that chronically and severely mentally ill persons should be given the highest priority in mental health efforts. Primary prevention has been brought into perspective; research is encouraged, but large-scale service programs with little evidence for their efficacy have been curtailed. Activism has mostly shifted to mental health issues within the expertise of psychiatrists, and efforts are under way to resolve the problems of deinstitutionalization. These are some of the larger issues that will be addressed in this chapter.

BRIEF HISTORICAL REVIEW

Public psychiatry and the community mental health movement have roots that go back to the 18th century, when the French psychiatrist Phillipe Pinel removed the chains from psychiatric patients, and to the 19th century, when the school of moral treatment in the United States stressed a humane and rehabilitative approach to mentally ill patients. Also playing a role were Dorothea Lynde Dix, who worked to better the lot of persons with mental illness in the mid-19th century, and Clifford Beers, founder of the National Committee for Mental Hygiene and author, in 1908, of *A Mind That Found Itself* (Beers 1908/1939), a description of his experiences as a mental hospital patient that has become a classic text. Although there is much more that could be said with regard to history, the historical focus here is on the contributions of military psychiatry to public psychiatry concepts and on the federal legislation that was crucial to the development of public psychiatry and deinstitutionalization.

THE CONTRIBUTION OF MILITARY PSYCHIATRY

Out of the experience of military psychiatrists in World Wars I and II (Cozza and Hales 1991; Hales and Gemelli 1987) came principles that were to have a major impact on public psychiatry for the civilian population (see Table 42–1). These included 1) proximity (i.e., treatment as close as possible to the combat zone); 2) immediacy (i.e., early identification and treatment of psychiatric disorder); 3) simplicity (i.e., providing rest, food, and social support); and 4) expectancy (i.e., the expectation of prompt return to duty). It was found that this approach was far more effective than evacuation of all psychiatric casualties to faraway hospitals from which few returned to duty.

The principle of treatment close to home became central to public psychiatry, as did the principles of early diagnosis and active treatment to effect prompt remission of acute psychiatric problems and avoid regression. The military experience also demonstrated that selected mental disorders are precipitated by stress and that identifying the precipitating stressors and finding ways of resolving them are extremely important. These principles proved useful in both the Korean and Vietnam conflicts and, more recently, in Operation Desert Storm (McDuff and Johnson 1992), further reinforcing the validity of these principles for both military and public psychiatry.

FEDERAL LEGISLATION

For more than half of the 20th century, the state hospitals fulfilled the function for society of keeping mentally ill persons out of sight and thus out of mind. Moreover, the controls and structure provided by the state hospitals, as well as the granting of almost total asylum, may have been necessary for many chronically and severely mentally ill patients before the advent of modern psychoactive medications. Unfortunately, the ways in which state hospitals

TABLE 42–1. Principles of combat psychiatry

Proximity

Immediacy

Simplicity

Expectancy

achieved this structure and asylum led to everyday abuses that left scars on the mental health professions as well as on the patients.

The stage was set for deinstitutionalization by periodic public outcries about the deplorable conditions in state hospitals, documented by journalists such as Albert Deutsch (1948). Mental health professionals and their organizational leaders also expressed growing concern. These concerns led ultimately to the passage of the Mental Study Act in 1955, which authorized the formation of the Joint Commission on Mental Illness and Health that same year. The commission's recommendations were published in 1961 as a widely read book, *Action for Mental Health* (Joint Commission on Mental Illness and Health 1961). These recommendations included the following:

1. That immediate care be made available in the community for acutely disturbed patients suffering major breakdowns
2. That major mental illness be recognized as the core problem and unfinished business of the mental health movement
3. That there be a fully staffed, full-time mental health clinic available to each 50,000 persons in the population
4. That smaller state hospitals, of 1,000 beds or less and suitably located for regional service, be made available for patients with major mental illness
5. That aftercare and rehabilitation services in the community be greatly expanded

It should also be noted that the National Institute of Mental Health was established in 1949; this marked the beginning of a significant federal role in mental health funding.

The process of deinstitutionalization was considerably accelerated by two significant federal developments in 1963. First, categorical Aid to the Disabled (ATD) became available to mentally ill persons, making such persons eligible for the first time for federal financial support in the community. Second, community mental health centers legislation was passed.

With ATD, psychiatric patients and mental health professionals acting on their behalf had access to federal grants-in-aid, in some states supplemented by state funds, which enabled patients to support themselves or to be supported either at home or in facilities such as board-and-care homes or old hotels at comparatively little cost to the state. Although the amount of money available to patients under ATD was not a princely sum, it was sufficient to allow a low standard of living in the community. Thus the states, even those that provided generous ATD supplements, found that it cost far less in terms of state funds to maintain patients in the community than in the hospital. (ATD is now called Supplemental Security Income, or SSI, and is administered by the Social Security Administration.)

The second significant federal development of 1963 was the passage of the Mental Retardation Facilities and Community Mental Health Centers Construction Act, amended in 1965 to provide grants for the initial costs of staffing the newly constructed centers. This legislation was a strong incentive to the development of community programs with the potential to treat people whose main resource previously had been the state hospital. The centers were required to provide five basic services: 1) inpatient treatment, 2) emergency services, 3) partial hospitalization, 4) outpatient services, and 5) consultation and education.

In 1975 Congress passed the Community Mental Health Centers Amendments, which established the principle of continuing federal responsibility for the treatment and prevention of mental disorder, with community mental health as the basic federal activity in this area. This law established the requirement for 12 services instead of the previous 5 services. The added services were 1) services for children, 2) services for the aged, 3) follow-up services for patients who were formerly in institutions, 4) screening before admission to state hospitals, 5) alcoholism services, 6) drug abuse services, and 7) transitional housing. The law further required that quality assurance programs and utilization review be built into each center. However, this legislation was not accompanied by any significant increase in funding.

In 1977 the President's Commission on Mental Health was formed. Its report, which was completed in 1978, led to the Mental Health Systems Act, which was passed in 1980 but never implemented. The act emphasized coordination of services, patients' rights and advocacy, and a number of grant programs for underserved populations.

PUBLIC PSYCHIATRY PRINCIPLES

A number of community (i.e., public) psychiatry principles were proposed in the 1960s (Caplan and Caplan 1967). These principles, listed in Table 42–2, have proven to be useful and valid, although only to varying degrees, and have undergone considerable rethinking and change in the succeeding decades. Moreover, new concepts and knowledge have been added over the past three decades as described throughout this chapter. Prevention and mental

health consultation, discussed in considerable detail later, are not addressed here. Linkages to health and human services are discussed in several places in the chapter, especially in the section on community treatment for patients who are chronically and severely mentally ill.

RESPONSIBILITY TO A POPULATION

The concept of a *catchment area*—that is, a geographic area in which a community mental health center takes responsibility for the total population—has great appeal. This approach was adopted by federal legislation, in which a catchment area was defined as a geographic area that includes 75,000–200,000 people. Theoretically, a community mental health center would identify all the mental health needs of its catchment area, formulate a plan to meet these needs, and provide services based on the needs of the population rather than on the staff's preferences for engaging in specific kinds of mental health activity. These needs would be determined by both citizens and staff and would take into account the cultural backgrounds of the population.

The catchment area concept has worked well when the catchment area includes a discrete area, both politically and geographically. There have been many problems, however, when this concept has been applied in large metropolitan or sparsely populated rural areas. In metropolitan areas, the boundaries are often artificial, and when boundaries are rigidly adhered to, persons moving from one part of a city to another find themselves transferred to a whole new treatment system. Continuity of care is interrupted, and patients and staff have to begin anew the process of getting to know each other. Many patients, especially those who are chronically and severely mentally ill, do not or cannot make this transition and become lost to treatment. A catchment area may not reflect political boundaries and natural

TABLE 42–2.   Community psychiatry principles as conceptualized in the 1960s

Responsibility to a total population (catchment areas)

Treatment close to the patient's home

Comprehensive services

Multidisciplinary team approach

Continuity of care

Consumer participation

Program evaluation and research

Prevention

Mental health consultation

Linkages to health and human services

communities, and as a result professionals may have difficulty serving its population.

In rural areas, a minimum population of 75,000 may result in a catchment area so large geographically that great distances make the rational provision of services unwieldy. (This problem is discussed in greater detail later, in the subsection on rural areas.) Clearly, flexibility is needed in determining the size of catchment areas, in increasing the ability of community mental health centers to share resources, in relaxing the requirement that patients transfer to another center when they move within a city, and in devising catchment areas that make sense politically, geographically, and culturally.

TREATMENT CLOSE TO THE PATIENT'S HOME

As has already been mentioned, the principle of having treatment available close to patients' homes grew, at least in part, out of the military experience. Clearly, proximity facilitates use of treatment by the patient and his or her family. Sending patients to a hospital far from home severs patients' connections with their community and their families and discourages the families' involvement in treatment.

COMPREHENSIVE SERVICES

It became apparent early on that the traditional inpatient and outpatient clinic services are insufficient to meet the needs of many patients. This was recognized in the original requirement for five basic services (i.e., inpatient, emergency, partial hospitalization, outpatient, and consultation/education) and in the seven services added later (services for children, services for the aged, alcoholism services, drug abuse services, aftercare, preadmission screening, and transitional housing). In recent years, additional services such as case management and a variety of housing services have been recognized. These are described later in this chapter.

MULTIDISCIPLINARY TEAM APPROACH

Each mental health discipline has something unique to add to the treatment of mentally ill patients. In the early days of community mental health, there was much emphasis on role blurring—that is, minimizing the differences between the disciplines and having professionals from the different disciplines tending to fulfill similar roles. This approach caused considerable confusion to both staff and patients, encouraged turf battles, and often resulted in inefficient use of skilled staff. Although some role blurring is inevita-

ble in a multidisciplinary team approach, in recent years there has been a greater recognition of the importance of taking full advantage of the unique skills of professionals in each discipline.

CONTINUITY OF CARE

It is obvious that a relationship between a patient and an individual psychiatrist or a treatment facility should, if possible, be a continuous one. Patients and staff come to know and to trust one another. Staff become familiar with the patients and their individual patterns of reacting to stress. Thus, crises can be dealt with early, and staff are familiar with what "works" with each patient. Having to change therapists or treatment centers can be traumatic for patients, especially for those who are chronically and severely mentally ill. An exacerbation of illness may be precipitated or the patient may be lost to treatment.

Whether the therapeutic relationship should be with an individual or a treatment agency has been a matter of some discussion. Chronically and severely mentally ill persons may have great difficulty in tolerating interpersonal closeness and may benefit from an institutional alliance (sometimes referred to as an *institutional transference*), in which the patient's relationship may be with the institution more than with an individual professional. The team treatment approach (Test 1979) can have the same result. The team approach has been described as having additional advantages. It can provide more continuous coverage because it does not depend on the availability of one individual, and it allows more points of view to be brought to bear on the solution of difficult problems. Also, especially in dealing with emotionally draining patients, it helps to prevent staff burnout.

Finally, a discussion of continuity of care would not be complete without mentioning the importance of monitoring the patient; obviously, continuous care cannot be given to a patient who tends not to keep appointments and whose whereabouts are unknown.

CONSUMER PARTICIPATION

Mental health services can be more effective and relevant to a population when there is input from community members, including both persons who have themselves experienced mental illness and family members of mentally ill persons, rather than when mental health needs and programs are defined only by professionals. However, the issue of participation is much more complex than it might appear at first. The involvement of the citizens of a small city or town with their mental health center may indeed be quite positive. The mental health staff become known and trusted in the community, the needs of the community are articulated to the professionals, and the services become more relevant. Mental health concepts are better understood and accepted, and citizens may provide important assistance to the center and to its patients.

Consumer participation has not been as successful in many large cities. Citizen advisory boards may seem to be representative of a city or a part of a city in terms of ethnicity, race, geographic area, and a host of other factors. However, these groups may not be as cohesive in the cities as is often assumed, and persons representing them may, in fact, be representing themselves primarily and not their group or the city as a whole. Or the mental health director may "pack" the citizen advisory board with persons known to be sympathetic to his or her policies, and such a group may represent the mental health director rather than the community. Thus, the appearance and the reality of consumer participation may be quite different. In recent years an important source of citizen input has been from families of patients with major mental illness (i.e., schizophrenia, schizoaffective disorder, bipolar disorder, and major depression). Families have organized, developed a new self-concept, and effectively devoted themselves to advocacy for the needs and rights of the chronically mentally ill population (Lefley and Johnson 1990). The formation of their organization, the National Alliance for the Mentally Ill, has been a major step in this process. This positive development has caused community treatment centers to give higher priority to chronically and severely mentally ill persons.

PROGRAM EVALUATION AND RESEARCH

Program evaluation—the use of scientific techniques to measure the value of an agency's work—is, or should be, a major concern in public psychiatry, and indeed in all of psychiatry.

Every program—national, regional, state, or local—needs to be objectively evaluated. Objectivity must be stressed, because without it, professionals become dependent on subjective impressions, and we are influenced by our biases. We remember what fits in with our preconceptions and forget what is in conflict with our beliefs. Most health and welfare workers feel that their work is important and has a positive influence on their patients. One of the purposes of scientific research methods is to minimize such subjective bias so that conclusions can be based on hard data. It is known that every mental health professional, whatever his or her theoretical orientation and therapeutic methods, has some patients who improve and some who do

not; no therapist is successful with every patient. Therapists employ various treatment methods, depending on the needs of patients as well as on their own preferences, orientations, and needs. Objective evaluation, however, can determine which methods are helpful for which therapists and with which patients, as well as whether the therapy itself has resulted in improvement. Moreover, there has been increased emphasis in recent years on mental health and substance abuse service systems routinely and continuously monitoring the outcomes of the treatment and rehabilitation they provide (Steinwachs et al. 1996).

Evaluative research that determines the effectiveness with which a program serves particular patients is not enough. Effort must be directed toward objectively examining the overall efficacy of the program. The research must examine not only how well patients are served but also how great a contribution the program makes to solving a particular mental health problem or to meeting a particular need. For example, one problem is the need for sheltered housing for patients returning from mental hospitals to the community. A halfway house may serve 2 such persons a month out of the 20 who return to the community. If, on the average, 1 of these patients per month moves into a more independent living situation, the agency shows a superficially impressive 50% success rate, but it is actually making only a 5% (1 in 20) contribution to meeting the housing needs of all the patients who return from mental hospitals to the community during this period.

Ideally, evaluation should be conducted within a controlled research framework. At a minimum, program goals must be explicit and formulated in a manner that permits objective evaluation of the program. We must be prepared to terminate programs that do not produce evidence of their worth.

PROBLEMS IN PUBLIC PSYCHIATRY

Problems in implementing the catchment area concept, citizen participation, and program evaluation have already been discussed. Here the focus is on some other major problems.

CHRONICALLY AND SEVERELY MENTALLY ILL PATIENTS

Interest in working with persons who are chronically and severely mentally ill revived in the 1980s (Talbott 1987); after decades of neglect, this was a welcome development. A leading factor in bringing about this revival of interest has been the homeless mentally ill population, whose plight constitutes one of the greatest problems of present-day society and one that cannot be ignored. The public and the media, as well as mental health professionals, are confronted daily by the sight of these severely ill individuals and the wretched circumstances of their lives. Another increasingly important factor has been the activities and changing attitudes of families of mentally ill persons. Families have organized and effectively devoted themselves to advocacy for the needs and rights of chronically and severely mentally ill individuals (often referred to as *seriously mentally ill*).

What precisely is meant by the term *chronically and severely mentally ill*? The term, as used here, refers to patients with major mental illnesses—schizophrenia, schizoaffective disorder, bipolar disorder, or major depression—and the resulting functional impairment, social and vocational. Another way to define this population (which includes some patients diagnosed as having severe personality disorders) is as persons who, before deinstitutionalization, would have lived out their lives in state hospitals.

Psychiatry has had the technology to treat and rehabilitate these patients for some years. We know about the importance of case management; of antipsychotic medications; of supervised housing; of adequate, comprehensive, and accessible psychiatric and rehabilitation services; of less restrictive laws governing involuntary treatment; of better coordination of community services; and of structured, ongoing 24-hour care for that small proportion of patients in need of it. What has been lacking has been the willingness of both society and the mental health professions to provide the resources necessary to employ this technology.

NEEDS FORMERLY MET BY STATE HOSPITALS

In the midst of valid concerns about the shortcomings and antitherapeutic aspects of state hospitals, it was not appreciated that these hospitals fulfilled some essential functions for patients who were chronically and severely mentally ill. The term *asylum* was in many ways an appropriate one, for these imperfect institutions did provide asylum and sanctuary from the pressures of the world, with which, in varying degrees, most of these patients were unable to cope (Lamb and Peele 1984). Furthermore, these institutions provided services such as medical care, patient monitoring, respite for the patient's family, and a social network for the patient, as well as food, shelter, and needed support and structure (Wing 1990).

In the state hospitals, the treatment and services that existed were in one place and under one administration. In the community, the situation is different. Services and treatment are under various administrative jurisdictions and in various locations. Even mentally healthy individuals have difficulty in dealing with a number of bureaucracies, both governmental and private, and in getting their needs met. Furthermore, patients can more easily get lost in the community than in a hospital, where they may have been neglected but at least their whereabouts were known. It is these problems that have led to the recognition of the importance of case management. Many homeless mentally ill persons would probably not be on the streets if they were on the caseload of a professional or a paraprofessional trained to deal with the problems of the chronically and severely mentally ill population, monitor them (with considerable persistence when necessary), and facilitate their receiving services. (See the subsection on community treatment for the chronically and severely mentally ill for a fuller discussion of case management.)

HOMELESS MENTALLY ILL PERSONS

Homeless mentally ill persons constitute one of the greatest challenges to public mental health and to society generally. Two American Psychiatric Association (APA) task forces on the homeless mentally ill (Lamb 1984; Lamb et al. 1992) concluded that this problem is the result not of deinstitutionalization per se but of the way it has been implemented. Homelessness among chronically and severely mentally ill persons is symptomatic of the grave problems facing these persons generally in this country. Thus, the problem of homelessness will not be resolved until the basic underlying problems of the chronically and severely mentally ill population are addressed and a comprehensive and integrated system of care for them is established. The solutions for the problem of homelessness among the mentally ill, therefore, are the same solutions enumerated later in the subsection on community treatment for persons who are chronically and severely mentally ill.

How do chronically and severely mentally ill individuals become homeless? Clearly, there are many pathways to the streets, and it is useful to look briefly at some of them. Chronically and severely mentally ill persons are not proficient at coping with the stresses of this world; therefore, they are vulnerable to eviction from their living arrangements, sometimes because of an inability to deal with difficult or even ordinary landlord-tenant situations, and sometimes because of circumstances in which they play a leading role. In the absence of an adequate case management system, these individuals are out on the streets and on their own. Many, especially the young, have a tendency to drift away from their families or from a board-and-care home;

they may be trying to escape the pull of dependency and may not be ready to come to terms with living in a sheltered, low-pressure environment. If they still have goals, they may find an inactive lifestyle extremely depressing. Or they may want more freedom to drink or use street drugs. Some chronically and severely mentally ill persons may regard leaving their comparatively static milieu as a necessary part of the process of realizing their goals, but this is a process that exacts its price in terms of homelessness, crises, decompensation, and hospitalizations.

Thus, once mentally ill persons are out on their own, they will more than likely stop taking their medications; after a while they will lose touch with the Social Security Administration and will no longer be able to receive their SSI checks. Their poor judgment and the state of disarray associated with their illness may cause them to fail to notify the Social Security Administration of a change of address or to fail to appear for a redetermination hearing. The lack of medical care on the streets and the effects of alcohol and other drug abuse are additional serious complications. These persons may become too disorganized to extricate themselves from living on the streets—except by exhibiting blatantly bizarre or disruptive behavior that leads to their being taken to a hospital or jail.

There is still another factor. Evidence is beginning to emerge that homeless mentally ill persons have a greater severity of illness than do mentally ill persons in general. At Bellevue Hospital in New York City, approximately 50% of inpatients who were homeless are transferred to state hospitals for long-term care, as opposed to 8% of other Bellevue psychiatric inpatients (Marcos et al. 1990).

CRIMINALIZATION

As a result of deinstitutionalization, there are now large numbers of mentally ill persons in the community. At the same time, community psychiatric resources, including hospital beds, are limited. Society has a limited tolerance of mentally disordered behavior, and the result is pressure to put persons who need 24-hour care into whatever institutions have room, including jail. Indeed, several studies describe a criminalization of mentally disordered behavior—a shunting of mentally ill persons in need of treatment into the criminal justice system instead of the mental health system (Lamb and Weinberger 1998; Teplin 1990; Torrey 1997). Rather than hospitalization and psychiatric treatment, mentally ill persons often are subject to inappropriate arrest and incarceration. Legal restrictions placed on involuntary hospitalization appear to result in the diversion of some patients to the criminal justice system.

Studies of 203 county jail inmates—102 men and 101 women—referred for psychiatric evaluation (Lamb and Grant 1982, 1983) shed some light on the issues of both criminalization and homelessness. This population had extensive experience with both the criminal justice and mental health systems, were characterized by severe acute and chronic mental illness, and generally functioned at a low level. Homelessness was common; at the time of arrest, 39% had been living on the streets, on the beach, in missions, or in cheap, transient skid-row hotels. Clearly, the problems of homelessness and criminalization were interrelated.

Almost half of the men and women charged only with misdemeanors had been living on the streets or the beach, in missions, or in cheap, transient hotels, compared with one-fourth of those charged with felonies. One can speculate as to possible explanations. Persons living in such places have a minimum of community supports; committing a minor offense may frequently be a way of asking for help. It is also possible that many of these minor criminal acts are manifestations of these persons' illness, their lack of treatment, and the lack of structure in their lives. Certainly, these were the clinical impressions of the investigators as they talked to these inmates and their families and read the police reports.

PROBLEMS IN TREATING CHRONICALLY AND SEVERELY MENTALLY ILL PATIENTS

It is useful to explore individual and systems problems that have made mental health professionals and society generally unenthusiastic and often unwilling to provide the care and treatment needed by the chronically and severely mentally ill population (see Table 42–3).

It is essential that mental health professionals have realistic expectations in their clinical work with chronically and severely mentally ill patients. If, instead, professionals proceed as if these patients can function at levels beyond

TABLE 42–3. Problems in treating patients who are chronically and severely mentally ill

Unrealistic expectations

Preconceived ideology

Amount of gratification from working with this population not recognized

Potential for independence overestimated

The overselling of treatment and rehabilitation programs with goals of high functioning

Neglect of the lower functioning segment of this population

their capabilities, the result will often be exacerbation of psychosis, dysphoria, and perhaps homelessness (Lamb 1986). Thus, psychiatrists may want their chronically and severely mentally ill patients to be independent, to be free, and to function at higher levels. If, instead, these patients need to be dependent and controlled, and are able to be only marginally functional, their increased symptoms reveal these limitations in no uncertain terms.

Ideology, then, must often give way to pragmatism. The experience with vocational rehabilitation can serve as an example. Everyone wants chronically and severely mentally ill patients to experience the heightened self-esteem and gratification that come from a life of employment, of feeling needed, and of being productive; in fact, many of these persons can achieve sheltered or competitive employment (Lehman 1995). However, the needs and ideology of mental health professionals must not obscure the clinical reality that the majority of severely and chronically mentally ill patients cannot handle the stress of competitive employment and that, for the minority who can, entry-level, low-stress jobs most often should be the goal, at least initially. Otherwise, the patient is simply given another experience of failure, which further lowers his or her self-esteem.

Mental health professionals, then, face a great temptation to try to transform these patients. The reality that the great majority of chronically and severely mentally ill patients have considerable limitations in their potential for higher functioning is difficult to accept, but psychiatrists must learn to accept these limitations. This problem tends to be greater in working with younger patients, for it has been shown that the course of schizophrenia in the middle and later years tends to be more benign and far less stormy (Bleuler 1974; Harding et al. 1987); both patients and mental health professionals often have come to terms with the illness by this time. Moreover, the gratification that can be derived from working with chronically and severely mentally ill patients at any age must not be overlooked. Without necessarily achieving high levels of functioning for their patients, psychiatrists can help to change chaotic, dysphoric lifestyles into lives characterized by stability and at least some contentment and satisfaction.

Another problematic issue is the matter of independence. All psychiatrists highly value independence. It is a quality permitting negotiation and free give-and-take with others. Yet nothing is more difficult for the chronically and severely mentally ill person to attain and sustain. For example, psychiatrists want to see their patients living in their own apartments and managing on their own, perhaps with some outpatient support. But psychiatrists have learned from hard experience that most chronically and severely

mentally ill persons living in unsupervised settings in the community find the ordinary stresses of managing on their own more than they can handle; these persons tend, after a while, to stop taking their medications, to neglect their nutrition, to let their lives unravel and become disorganized, and eventually to find their way back to the hospital (Lamb 1982). Patients also highly value independence, but they often underestimate their dependency needs. Professionals must be realistic about their patients' potential for independence, even if the patients are not.

Psychiatrists read and hear about exciting, innovative treatment and rehabilitation programs with impressive outcomes as measured by vocational and social functioning. They are told that these programs and these outcomes can easily be replicated in their own communities with their own patients. Yet the reality is that only the higher functioning chronically and severely mentally ill patients can handle the demands of such programs. Moreover, the numbers served are relatively small. These treatment and rehabilitation programs are too often oversold. The majority of chronically and severely mentally ill patients in the community disappoint professionals by "failing" in such programs or refusing to participate in them at all. They live with their families or in board-and-care homes or single-room-occupancy hotels. They need simpler, less ambitious programs calibrated to their needs, and many will not even participate in these types of programs. In any case, simpler programs that emphasize maintenance rather than entering the "mainstream" of society do not excite and sometimes do not even interest many professionals (Lamb 1986). The result is that the lower functioning segment of the chronically and severely mentally ill population is frequently underserved and neglected.

DEPENDENCY AND ASYLUM

Dependency brings up another host of problems. Professionals, as products of their culture and society, tend to disapprove morally of persons who have "given in" to their dependency needs, who have adopted a passive, inactive lifestyle, and who have accepted public support instead of working (Lamb 1982). Perhaps this moral disapproval helps to explain why programs that claim to accomplish rehabilitation to high levels of functioning (i.e., "mainstreaming") attract the most attention and the most funding. Vigorous attempts may be made to reverse low-functioning adaptations to the pressures of life without making a realistic appraisal of the capabilities of chronically and severely mentally ill persons; in the process, an acute exacerbation of psychosis may result. Probably no problems are more difficult for professionals in the treatment of chronically and severely mentally ill persons than to come to terms with their patients' dependency. But come to terms with it they must if the treatment of chronic and severe mental illness is not to fade again into oblivion.

The fact that chronically and severely mentally ill persons have been deinstitutionalized does not mean they no longer need social support and protection, as well as relief, either periodic or continuous, from the pressures of life. In short, they need asylum and sanctuary *in the community* (Lamb and Peele 1984). Unfortunately, because the old state hospitals were called "asylums," the word took on a pejorative, almost sinister connotation. Only in recent years has the word again become a respectable part of the language, by which one can denote the function of *providing asylum*, rather than *conceiving of asylum as a place*.

The concepts of asylum and sanctuary are important. Whereas some chronically and severely mentally ill patients eventually attain high levels of social and vocational functioning, many others cannot meet simple demands of living on their own, even with long-term rehabilitative help. Many consciously limit their exposure to external stimuli and pressure, not from laziness but from a well-founded fear of failure. Professionals must realize that whatever degree of rehabilitation is possible for each patient cannot take place unless support and protection—whether from family, treatment program, therapist, or board-and-care home—are provided at the same time. If this need for asylum and sanctuary in the community is not taken into account, living in the community may not be possible for many patients.

It has been shown that the treatment of chronically and severely mentally ill patients cannot be time limited; if it is not ongoing, most patients will regress (Fairweather 1980; Stein and Test 1985). Thus, it is important to guard against termination of treatment of chronically and severely mentally ill patients with the idea that they are cured; their need for a support system has not ended even though they may appear intact. When the treatment of a chronically and severely mentally ill person is undertaken, it should be understood that an ongoing, long-term commitment is being made to that patient.

FAMILIES OF THE CHRONICALLY AND SEVERELY MENTALLY ILL

Psychiatrists have learned that chronically and severely mentally ill persons and their families need advice. Many of the patients themselves lack the ability to cope with the routine stressors of life and need tutelage and specific guidance about what to do in many areas of their lives. For instance, a chronically and severely mentally ill patient may find him- or herself in a situation that will, if not resolved, precipitate an exacerbation of acute psychosis. Although it may be clear to a psychiatrist what the patient needs to do to extricate him- or herself, the patient may be overwhelmed and immobilized by what he or she perceives as the complexity of it all. It is crucial for psychiatrists to give advice and assistance.

Managing major mental illness in a relative at home is an immensely difficult task. Families can, and often do, learn by trial and error over a period of years how to help stabilize their mentally ill relative by encouraging the avoidance of excessive stress, having realistic expectations, setting appropriate limits, understanding the patient's problem in tolerating social stimulation, learning how to react to psychotic symptoms, and encouraging the taking of medications. But families learn this at great emotional cost, which can be avoided if they are assisted by knowledgeable professionals. Clearly, families deserve better. If psychiatrists themselves learn how to manage chronically and severely mentally ill persons at home, the families can be advised, and their lives, and the lives of their mentally ill relatives, can be made immeasurably better.

Psychiatrists can also use families' abilities in an important way in the treatment process. Psychiatrists have to learn to help families set limits and take charge of their households (Kanter 1985); psychiatrists have to feel comfortable in telling the family that schizophrenia and other major mental illnesses are biological illnesses and that the family has not caused them; psychiatrists have to be unambivalent about the use of psychoactive medications and in advising families to urge their relatives to take them; psychiatrists have to work with the families and the patients to determine what are realistic goals. Psychiatrists need to help relatives understand that social withdrawal may be a necessary defense for patients against too much stress or social stimulation but that excessive withdrawal may lead to a form of institutionalism in the home. A balance must be struck.

MODEL PROGRAMS: A SOLUTION?

Much attention has been paid to glamorous, innovative, and "successful" pilot treatment and rehabilitation programs with dedicated staff whose enthusiasm is infectious. The publicizing of these demonstration programs has led to one proposed remedy for the problems of the deinstitutionalized chronically and severely mentally ill patient: the mass cloning of these "model programs." This "solution" demands scrutiny, for it presents serious problems.

One problem in replicating these new programs for

the chronically and severely mentally ill population is that what works in one community may not work in another. Some programs are well suited to urban areas but not to rural areas, and vice versa; some programs that work well in small- or medium-sized cities are not feasible in inner-city settings. In addition, programs that are highly successful in one community may fail or be rejected in what appears to be an entirely comparable set of circumstances elsewhere. Cultural, political, and socioeconomic factors specific to each community must be taken into account.

It is instructive, however, for program planning to look at the eight elementary principles common to successful model programs as conceptualized by Bachrach (1980). These principles are listed in Table 42–4.

COMMUNITY TREATMENT FOR CHRONICALLY AND SEVERELY MENTALLY ILL PATIENTS

Clearly, a comprehensive and integrated system of care for chronically and severely mentally ill patients, with designated responsibility, accountability, and adequate fiscal resources, must be established. Following is a discussion of the components of such a system (see Table 42–5).

Adequate, comprehensive, and accessible psychiatric and rehabilitative services must be available and, when necessary, must be provided assertively through outreach services. First, there must be adequate direct psychiatric services that provide 1) outreach contact with the mentally ill persons in the community; 2) psychiatric assessment and evaluation; 3) crisis intervention, including hospitalization; 4) individualized treatment plans; 5) psychoactive medication and other somatic therapies; and 6) psychosocial treatment. Second, there must be adequate rehabilitative services that provide socialization experiences, training in the skills of everyday living, and social and vocational rehabilitation. Third, both treatment and rehabilitative services must be provided assertively—for instance, by going out to patients' living settings if they do not or cannot come to a centralized program location. Fourth, the difficulty of working with some of these patients must not be underestimated.

Crisis services must be available and accessible. Too often, chronically and severely mentally ill persons who are in

TABLE 42–4. Elementary principles common to successful model programs

Assign top priority to the care of the most severely impaired.

Provide realistic linkage with other resources in the community.

Provide out-of-hospital alternatives for the full range of functions performed in hospital settings.

Individually tailor treatment for each patient.

Provide cultural relevance and specificity—that is, tailoring programs to conform to the local realities of the community in which they are located.

Involve trained staff who are attuned to the unique survival problems of chronic mental patients living in noninstitutional settings.

Provide access to a complement of hospital beds, because there are some patients for whom periods of hospital care continue to be a necessity.

Incorporate an ongoing internal assessment mechanism that permits continuous self-monitoring.

TABLE 42–5. Components of a comprehensive system of care for chronically and severely mentally ill patients

Direct psychiatric services
Psychiatric assessment
Crisis intervention, including acute hospitalization
Acute and subacute day treatment
Psychoactive medications
Assertive outreach
Psychosocial treatment
Individual and group therapy
Social and vocational rehabilitation
Adequate number of trained professionals and paraprofessionals
Housing
Supervised housing (needed for most of this population)
Range of supervision and structure
Case management
One mental health professional or paraprofessional responsible for care of each patient
Families
Consider families as important allies in the patient's treatment
Give families adequate support
Legal and administrative procedures
Acute care: commitment laws need to be less restrictive
Long-term care: make increased use of conservatorship, guardianship, commitment to outpatient treatment, and treatment as a condition of probation
Increased coordination and integration of community agencies
General social services
Ongoing structured intermediate and long-term 24-hour care when indicated

crisis situations are put into inpatient hospital units, when rapid, specific interventions such as medication or crisis housing would have been more effective and less costly. Others in need of acute hospitalization are denied it because of shortages of hospital beds or restrictive commitment laws.

An adequate number of professionals and paraprofessionals must be trained for community care of chronically and severely mentally ill persons. An adequate number and ample range of graded, stepwise, supervised community housing settings must be established. Some small proportion of chronically and severely mentally ill persons can graduate to independent living. For the majority, however, mainstream low-cost housing is not appropriate. Housing settings that require people to manage entirely by themselves are generally beyond the capabilities of chronically and severely mentally ill persons. Instead, there must be settings that offer different levels of supervision, both more and less intensive, including quarterway and halfway houses, board-and-care homes, satellite housing, foster or family care, and crisis or temporary hostels.

A system of responsibility for chronically and severely mentally ill persons living in the community must be established, with the goal of ensuring that each patient ultimately has one mental health professional or paraprofessional (i.e., a case manager) who is responsible for his or her care. In such a case management system, each patient's case manager would ensure that the appropriate psychiatric and medical assessments are carried out; formulate, together with the patient, an individualized treatment and rehabilitation plan, including the proper pharmacotherapy; monitor the patient; and assist the patient in receiving services.

Clearly, the shift of psychiatric care from institutional to community settings does not in any way eliminate the need to continue the provision of comprehensive services to mentally ill persons. As a result, society must declare a public policy of responsibility for mentally ill persons who are unable to meet their own needs, governments must designate programs in each region or locale as core agencies responsible and accountable for the care of the chronically and severely mentally ill individuals living there, and the staff of these agencies must be assigned individual patients for whom they are responsible.

For the more than 50% of the chronically and severely mentally ill population living at home or who have positive ongoing relationships with their families, programs and respite care must be provided to enhance the family's ability to provide a support system. When the use of family systems is not feasible, the patient must be linked with a formal community support system. In any case, the entire burden of deinstitutionalization must not be allowed to fall on families.

Basic changes must be made in legal and administrative procedures to ensure continuing community care for chronically and severely mentally ill persons. In the 1960s and 1970s, more stringent commitment laws and patients' rights advocacy remedied some serious abuses in public hospital care. However, patients' rights to high-quality, comprehensive community care as well as the rights of their families and society were neglected. New laws and procedures must be developed to ensure provision of psychiatric care in the community—that is, to guarantee a right to treatment in the community.

For outpatients who are so gravely disabled or who have such impaired judgment that they cannot care for themselves in the community without legally sanctioned supervision, it must become easier to obtain mental health conservatorship status (Lamb and Weinberger 1992). Involuntary commitment laws must be made more humane to permit prompt return to active inpatient treatment for patients when acute exacerbation of their illnesses make their lives in the community chaotic and unbearable. Involuntary treatment laws should be revised to allow the option of outpatient civil commitment (Miller 1992), whereby the court, instead of committing the patient to a hospital, orders the patient to participate in outpatient treatment. In states that already have provisions for such a mechanism, it should be more widely used. Finally, advocacy efforts should be focused on making available competent care in the community, rather than simply focusing on "liberty" for patients at any cost.

A system of coordination among funding sources and implementation agencies must be established. Because the problems of chronically and severely mentally ill persons must be addressed by multiple public and private authorities, coordination, which was so lacking in the deinstitutionalization process, must become a primary goal. Territorial and turf issues have often been at the root of this problem, and different agencies serving the same patients have often worked at cross-purposes. The ultimate objectives must include a true system of care, rather than a loose network of services, and an ease of communication among different types of agencies (e.g., psychiatric, social, vocational, and housing).

Ongoing structured 24-hour care should be available for that small proportion of chronically and severely mentally ill persons who do not respond to current methods of treatment and rehabilitation. Some persons, even with high-quality treatment and rehabilitation efforts, remain dangerous or gravely disabled. For these persons, there is a pressing need for ongoing 24-hour care in long-term settings, whether in hospitals, including state mental hospitals (Bachrach 1996), or in intermediate facilities such as California's locked Institutes for Mental Disease (Lamb 1997).

UNDERSERVED POPULATIONS: RURAL AREAS

In addition to the chronically and severely mentally ill population, other groups whose needs have not been adequately addressed by public psychiatry include children, minority groups, the elderly, and those living in rural communities. I focus here on rural populations. It is generally held that the risks of psychiatric illness are at least as great in rural as in urban settings and that rural individuals tend to be exposed to a variety of stressors that can result in a need for psychiatric care (President's Commission on Mental Health 1978). Physical isolation, low levels of education, inadequate funding, and ignorance of psychiatric problems and of techniques for addressing them further inhibit optimal use of psychiatric services. Thus, rural populations in the United States are considered to have a substantial need for, but generally poor access to, psychiatric services (Bachrach 1983).

In terms of space, the sheer dimensions of rural service areas can be overwhelming. Most rural mental health catchment areas, for example, exceed 5,000 square miles. The largest mental health catchment area in the United States, located in Arizona, consists of 60,000 square miles. In conjunction with conditions of physical isolation, low population density, a limited tax base, and personnel shortages, space may create major barriers to providing care.

There generally is an urban bias in health and human services planning. Most social planners live in metropolitan areas, and their theoretical convictions derive from a literature and a perspective that is primarily drawn from the urban experience (Hollingsworth et al. 1993). The concept of designing mental health catchment areas consisting of 75,000– 200,000 people is strictly an urban notion. To include populations that large in a service area in most of the rural United States usually means ignoring natural and social boundaries and planning for jurisdictions of such large geographical proportions that realistic program planning is thwarted. Urban residents typically have at least potential access to a multiplicity of private and public psychiatric services, but rural residents may have only one psychiatric facility available within a reasonable distance. Even when such facilities exist in rural areas, the scope of available treatment modalities may be limited by a small staff and inadequate funding (Sullivan et al. 1996). Residential facilities for persons discharged from state hospitals may be particularly scarce.

Working in a rural area can present many problems for psychiatrists and other mental health professionals. They may have to provide a variety of services and thus be service generalists. They may be cultural outsiders, and that, together with the fact that they are mental health professionals, may make them suspect in the local community. They may experience professional isolation with the problems of lack of peer support and lack of opportunity to learn from fellow mental health professionals. Furthermore, rural service agencies tend to be understaffed, and as a result workloads may be excessive. All of these personnel issues can combine to cause job dissatisfaction and staff burnout.

There are also advantages in rural areas. The rural sense of community may provide a potential source of support for mental health efforts that is rarely found in urban areas. Tolerance of deviance may also be greater. There must, of course, be sensitivity to the local culture, but the rural social organization, when properly used, may well be an advantage in the delivery of psychiatric services (Bachrach 1983). There is evidence that rural mental health centers may be most helpful by providing brief therapy for immediate short-term interventions (Mooney and Johnson 1992). This approach also maximizes use of limited staff. Seriously ill psychiatric patients may have high visibility in a rural area, but this has the advantage of causing these patients to get help sooner than they might in a more anonymous urban culture. Moreover, rural psychiatrists may learn more about their patients in the normal course of conversation and everyday life in a rural community.

GOVERNANCE PROBLEMS

Some issues of governance have been discussed previously in the subsection on consumer participation, in which it was seen that consumer participation either can be an important asset or, especially in the larger cities, can be subverted.

Unfortunately, there is a tendency today for mental health directors to be other than psychiatrists; these directors may be psychologists, social workers, or psychiatric nurses. This has come about in part because of the reluctance of psychiatrists to assume purely administrative positions, in part because nonpsychiatrists command a considerably lower salary, and in part because of interdisciplinary rivalries and the active seeking out of administrative positions by nonpsychiatrists (see the subsection that follows concerning the decreasing number of psychiatrists working in public psychiatry).

There is, in addition, a growing tendency to appoint to high administrative mental health posts persons who are not mental health professionals at all, but instead are primarily trained as professional managers. This situation presents serious problems, because persons without training and experience in providing treatment cannot begin to appreciate the enormity, variety, and complexity of the task of caring for mentally ill patients.

In addition to the importance of sound management and of such issues as the efficient collection of data, both to determine cost effectiveness and to provide the kinds of data needed by clinicians (e.g., being able to track their patients through management information systems), there are other concerns. Elpers (1986) described the dilemma of public mental health professionals who, on the one hand, feel that they should advocate increased funding and services and point out to both public and political leaders the deficiencies in their systems and, on the other hand, feel concern about jeopardizing their own job security or effectiveness. Elpers has indicated that many political leaders and top budget officers seem to prefer administrators who have little or no professional or personal investment in the well-being of chronically and severely mentally ill patients, or of patients generally. These administrators fail to remind political leaders of the needs of mentally ill persons and instead cover up the inadequacies of the system.

UNSTABLE FUNDING

"The dollar does not follow the patient" has become a catchphrase in public psychiatry. Yet it describes a crucial problem in almost every state in the United States, where, in the process of deinstitutionalization, the numbers of patients in state hospitals have been dramatically reduced, but the funding of the state hospitals has not been transferred to community programs to provide treatment to the hundreds of thousands of patients who now live in the community (Talbott 1985). In many cases, state hospital budgets have not decreased because of the states' attempts to bring the hospitals up to the standards of the Joint Commission on Accreditation of Healthcare Organizations in order to achieve accreditation and because of union pressures to maintain hospital jobs. Another factor is the states' desire to save money. The result is insufficient funds and services to treat chronically and severely mentally ill patients in the community.

Adequate funding is clearly the first, but not the only, consideration. How efficient are community programs? Some states that spend considerably less per capita than the average have mental health systems that are far superior to those of states that spend much more per capita. An example is the high quality of community programs and the low per capita costs in Wisconsin (Stein and Test 1985).

How high are the administrative costs? In some jurisdictions, especially the largest cities, such costs reach 40% of the budget. Reasons for this include excessive bureaucracy and inefficiency, and in some cases it is a way to siphon mental health funds into non–mental health governmental activities.

What are the priorities of community programs? The answer to this question can have a major effect on services to subpopulations. For instance, if funding is adequate but chronically and severely mentally ill persons have a low priority, this population will not be well served.

FEWER PSYCHIATRISTS

The number of psychiatrists working in public psychiatry has decreased both in actual numbers and as a percentage of the total number of mental health professionals in public mental health. One factor is the reluctance to offer competitive salaries to psychiatrists. Often there is resentment from other professionals of the "high" salaries of psychiatrists. Conversely, these "high" salaries cannot compete with the remuneration that psychiatrists receive in the private sector. Many times representatives of community programs believe that they can save money by hiring nonpsychiatrists instead of psychiatrists. This shortsighted approach overlooks what is often a sacrifice in quality of both leadership and clinical work when psychiatrists are not actively recruited and adequately compensated.

Another major problem has been a tendency in many community programs to use psychiatrists primarily for functions for which they cannot be substituted, namely, to write prescriptions, instead of using their clinical skills for the full range of treatment and for consultation with other staff. It is not surprising that psychiatrists treated in this way feel underused and move on to more professionally rewarding settings. Still another problem has been that of role blurring (discussed earlier in the section on public psychiatry principles)—the notion that all mental health professionals have similar skills in the evaluation and management of mental disorder. This is demoralizing not only to psychiatrists but to all mental health professionals, for it denies the uniqueness of each discipline. Unfortunately, much of this problem can be laid at the doorstep of psychiatrists who in the 1960s stressed an "egalitarian" approach, which held that professionals from all mental health disciplines should have the same amount of power and similar duties. The result has been that psychiatrists have been pushed aside from positions of leadership, both administrative and clinical, much to the detriment of public mental health. Efforts are now under way to reverse this process;

most psychiatrists have learned from the mistakes of the 1960s.

THE IMPACT OF MANAGED CARE

As was seen in the discussion of deinstitutionalization, the fact that services are now out in the community and not systematically managed has created a number of problems in public-sector mental health systems. Hoge et al. (1994) observed that these problems include difficulties for patients in finding and accessing services, denial of services to patients who need them, lack of accountability and follow-up for individual patients, absence of coordination among providers, lack of continuity in treatment planning, little if any incentive for efficiency or cost saving, and inadequate systems for monitoring the necessity, appropriateness, and effectiveness of care. In recent years a number of methods, some of which are commonly used in managed care, have been employed to address these problems.

As already discussed, case management was introduced into public mental health, especially for chronically and severely mentally ill persons, to deal with many of the above problems. For instance, case management establishes single-point accountability for the care of individual patients, improves access to services, and promotes continuity of treatment planning and of care. Case management has also been widely used in the private sector of the health care system as part of managed care in an attempt to achieve the same goals and to facilitate cost containment.

Capitation is an arrangement whereby an agency is given a fixed amount of money to provide all aspects of needed mental health care for a particular patient (Mechanic and Aiken 1989). Capitation has also become a cornerstone of managed care in the area of physical health, in both the private and the public sectors. Usually the agency is given considerable flexibility as to how these funds are spent as long as the needs of the patient are met. In the field of mental health, capitation is most often used to encourage providers to serve the most seriously ill. This funding mechanism is another way to establish single-point accountability for care. Moreover, because capitation involves giving an agency a fixed amount of money per patient, it provides strong incentives for cost efficiency, including the incentive to provide early treatment and crisis intervention to avert costly psychiatric hospitalization. Capitation should also facilitate coordination because all services are delivered or purchased by one provider (Lehman 1987).

Assertive community treatment (Burns and Santos 1995) is another way of managing care in public mental health. Multidisciplinary teams are used to provide services directly to patients in the community. Staff work closely together in small teams, providing single-point accountability for the care of individual patients and improving coordination and continuity of care. The teams respond to crises around the clock, if need be, reducing the use of hospitalization. These teams go, on a regular basis, to see the patients wherever they are in the community and assist them in making adjustments to vocational, living, social, and recreational situations. Medication monitoring is another important function.

Another strategy for managing care in the public sector is to set up local mental health authorities in which administrative, fiscal, and clinical responsibility are combined in one local organizational entity. The purpose is to consolidate mental health funding so that scarce resources can be efficiently and flexibly used to meet the needs of a targeted population, most often the chronically and severely mentally ill, and to enable the mental health authorities to insist on coordination and collaboration among the various service units (Goldman et al. 1990). Care must be taken, however, to prevent political considerations from limiting the effectiveness of local mental health authorities (Elliott 1996).

Managed care often involves the shifting of responsibility for providing mental health care to a population (e.g., the chronically and severely mentally ill) from the public to the private sector. This shift is based on the belief, backed up by recent evidence, that the private sector, unencumbered by the bureaucratic inefficiencies of government, can provide mental health services at a lower cost (Shore 1996). Even if this is so, a system that was grossly underfunded when public may be equally underfunded when privatized. In addition, capitation, if not closely monitored, can result in undertreatment or lower-quality treatment, because the agency receives a fixed amount of money per patient regardless of what services or how few or how many services are provided to the patient. Moreover, a managed care approach may reduce or even eliminate patient choice with respect to type of treatment.

PREVENTION

Primary prevention (i.e., the avoidance of the occurrence of cases of mental illness) must be distinguished from the other forms of prevention with which it is often confused. Public health practitioners divided preventive activities into primary, secondary, and tertiary forms (Table 42–6);

TABLE 42–6. Prevention

Level	Definition
Primary prevention	Avoidance of the occurrence of cases of mental illness
Secondary prevention (i.e., treatment)	Enables people to regain their normal level of functioning and prevents further development of illness after its occurrence
Tertiary prevention (i.e., rehabilitation)	Prevents or reverses the sequelae of illness—that is, disability

these terms were later adopted by mental health practitioners (Caplan 1964). *Secondary prevention* (i.e., treatment) involves enabling people to regain their normal level of functioning and preventing further development of illness after its occurrence; early diagnosis and treatment is a sine qua non of secondary prevention. *Tertiary prevention* (i.e., rehabilitation) involves preventing or reversing the sequelae of illness—in other words, disability.

Secondary and tertiary prevention, despite their importance, do not have the glamour for some professionals that primary prevention has, especially with regard to treating the major mental illnesses such as schizophrenia, nor do these levels of prevention offer the same potential for alleviating these disorders. The situation is analogous to that of physical illnesses. In the case of smallpox, for example, secondary and tertiary prevention do not hold out the same promise of widespread relief of suffering for a relatively small amount of effort that is provided by vaccination, the primary preventive measure. It should also be noted that the terms *primary*, *secondary*, and *tertiary* prevention have proved confusing over the years. It might well have been better had these terms from public health not been adopted for the mental health field; instead, the three categories might have been referred to simply as *prevention*, *treatment*, and *rehabilitation*.

PRIMARY PREVENTION

Many past and present primary prevention efforts have been attempted through indirect services, as exemplified by consultation with teachers, welfare workers, or the police, who have personal contact with the patient or potential patient (Talbott 1988), as opposed to direct services, in which the professional treats the patient. Probably the best known classification of types of consultation was developed by Caplan (1964), who described four types. In *client-centered case consultation*, the consultant helps the consultee to understand the patient's problems and then to find the most effective treatment by discussion of case ma-

terial with the consultee and/or examination of the patient. In *consultee-centered case consultation*, the consultant identifies the consultee's difficulties in handling the case and remedies these difficulties, whether they stem from insufficient skill or knowledge, or from a lack of objectivity caused by countertransference problems. In *program-centered administrative consultation*, the consultant's primary goal is to suggest some actions the consultee might take to develop, expand, or modify a clinical or agency program. In *consultee-centered administrative consultation*, the consultant focuses on difficulties within the consultee that limit his or her effectiveness in instituting program change.

In the 1960s and early 1970s, it was often implied (and sometimes promised) by many in the field of community mental health that techniques of primary prevention, such as consultation and mental health education, would result in a significant reduction of mental illness and would eventually drastically reduce the numbers of patients requiring conventional treatment (Becker et al. 1971; Caplan 1964). Although some of these techniques, such as mental health consultation, have proved useful, there is, unfortunately, no evidence that the incidence of mental illness has decreased. Advocates remain just as enthusiastic about primary prevention, but they have become more careful in their wording. More important, there has been a tendency for the goals of primary prevention to become more realistic—that is, preventing exacerbation in persons who have already suffered mental illness (which is really secondary prevention), rather than preventing the underlying illness itself, and focusing on areas in which primary prevention has been shown to be effective (see the subsection "Prevention: Proven and Probable"). In any case, the disillusionment with primary prevention that occurred in the 1970s has given way to another upsurge of interest (Albee and Ryan-Finn 1993; Blair 1992).

The disenchantment of the 1970s seems to have resulted from a combination of factors: the absence of hard evidence to confirm the effectiveness of most primary preventive efforts, the recognition that primary prevention had been seriously oversold, and the shifting of interest to newer fads (Lamb and Zusman 1981). Nevertheless, a considerable number of workers believe that primary prevention will now come into its own, and many articles, reviews, and books describing or advocating various types of preventive programs are again appearing. Still, the uncomfortable question has not been answered: Is primary prevention of mental illness possible? This crucial question too often goes unanswered, or even unasked, during discussions of mental health program planning.

A FIELD IN DISARRAY

Much of the debate over primary prevention relates to the lack of clarity of the concepts and definitions underlying the issues (Lamb and Zusman 1981). Unless care is taken to distinguish prevention of mental illness from prevention of unhappiness, feelings of distress, or social incompetence, discussants will often be examining several different phenomena while thinking that they are focusing on one.

Much of the general interest in prevention undoubtedly stems from the expectation of reducing the number of seriously ill and disabled individuals, not simply from the belief that prevention may lead to a happier life for the average person. It is primarily on the basis of preventing mental illness and thereby reducing the need for treatment resources that the allocation of a large proportion of limited mental health funds and personnel for "preventive" efforts can be justified. If professionals are to keep their goals in focus and make intelligent decisions about priorities and the allocation of scarce funds, it is crucial that the distinction between preventing diagnosable mental illness and preventing general emotional distress remain clear.

Professionals concerned with primary prevention in the mental health field face a complex problem of definition: determining the boundaries of mental health. Public health practitioners almost always use the word *prevention* in regard to illness. Mental health practitioners, on the other hand, usually deal not only with individuals who have a diagnosable illness but also with those who have no recognized psychiatric illness but want help instead with interpersonal problems and concerns of everyday living that cause them distress and unhappiness. Meaningful and reasonable objective exploration of "prevention" and "mental illness" requires that the discussion be confined to diagnosable mental illness, including the neuroses and personality disorders.

Some mental health specialists seek to expand the definition of primary prevention further, believing that mental health services should be concerned with resolving basic social problems and improving the quality of life for everyone. Indeed, many advocates of community mental health in the 1960s and early 1970s felt its scope is and should remain without boundaries (Dinitz and Beran 1971). Even today some continue to take this position. However, the cause-and-effect relationship between social conditions and mental illness is extremely questionable (see the discussion following on genetic factors). It may well stretch the definitions of mental health and mental illness and the public health concept of prevention beyond their useful limits to relate these definitions and concepts to basic social problems. The concepts, techniques, and expertise necessary for effective resolution of social problems are in no way related to those used by clinicians. The resolution of social problems also requires a mandate to intervene, a mandate that mental health professionals have not been given.

Can investigators demonstrate that primary prevention is effective? There seems to be general agreement that research has only begun to reveal something about the causes of most mental illnesses. Without knowledge of cause, primary prevention programs can only be shots in the dark. Of course, shots in the dark may occasionally hit the mark, but with the pressing demands for scarce mental health funds, can spending hundreds of millions of dollars on such programs be justified?

Modern research has increasingly suggested the operation of genetic and biochemical factors in the causation of mental illness. The results of family studies, adoption studies, and twin studies (Kendler and Diehl 1994) have indicated that schizophrenia is, for the most part, genetically determined. The same is true for bipolar disorder and major depression (Gershon 1990; Tsuang and Faraone 1990). The effect of genetic traits can be reduced, of course, through measures such as genetic counseling, but that is not what most proponents of primary prevention have in mind. It also seems possible that the expression of genetic traits—the actual precipitation of the full-blown illness—may be related to environmental stress. It is not yet clear that measures to prevent the expression of a genetic trait should be labeled *primary prevention* and directed at entire populations rather than only at individuals known to be mentally ill, either overtly or in remission (which would be secondary prevention; see the discussion in the next subsection).

When one leaves the subject of major mental illness, one enters an area that is even less clear. Some researchers believe that minor mental illnesses, such as neuroses and character disorders, could be prevented by modifying environmental factors that produce stress, and they uncritically embrace this possibility as a commonsense idea (Cardoza et al. 1975). However, a growing body of research indicates that there are genetic factors in alcoholism, drug abuse, antisocial personality, generalized anxiety disorder, and minor psychiatric disturbances such as symptoms of anxiety and depression (Gordis 1996; Kendler et al. 1986, 1992; Lyons et al. 1995; Smith et al. 1992). Researchers have generally concluded that both environmental and genetic factors interact in these disorders.

CRISIS INTERVENTION AS PREVENTION

The lack of knowledge about specific causation as well as the mounting genetic evidence for etiology has probably laid the conceptual groundwork for more recent trends in prevention. Some leading proponents of primary prevention have come to believe that a patient's current reality may be a more important determinant of mental disorders than his or her past traumas (Bloom 1981). They question whether there should be a movement away from consideration of causative and predisposing factors in mental illness toward a focus on precipitating factors—that is, stressful life events thought to be associated with the precipitation of mental illness. Thus, crisis intervention has been considered a fertile area for efforts in primary prevention. Although focusing on precipitating stressors might avert acute exacerbation in persons already known to be mentally ill (overtly or in remission), it should be recognized that crisis intervention with this segment of the population constitutes secondary prevention: the provision of treatment services to persons whose ability to cope with stress is known to be impaired.

MENTAL HEALTH PROMOTION

Primary prevention has been subdivided into two categories: 1) activities that promote health generally and thereby increase resistance to disease and 2) activities that are aimed against the occurrence of specific illnesses. Promotion of general physical health is an easily understandable concept that seems valid in practice. Yet in the area of mental health, most, if not all, successful primary preventive activities have been aimed at specific diseases; in contrast to physical health, there is no evidence that "general mental health" can be promoted or strengthened and therefore that resistance to mental illness can be increased by preventive activities. Despite massive efforts to combat poverty, to increase social welfare and Social Security benefits, and to change the educational systems and methods of child rearing, there is no indication that the incidence of any of the functional (i.e., nonorganic) mental illnesses has decreased. Nor is there evidence that countries with stronger social welfare systems and different child-rearing practices have different rates of mental illness. Thus, the major functional mental illnesses (as well as the frequently occurring diagnosable minor illnesses) remain untouched by efforts to strengthen mental health. Nevertheless, "mental health promotion" has become one of the contemporary catchphrases.

Many programs that have been called "preventive" are geared toward the development of competence in individuals. However, although developing competence (e.g., interpersonally, vocationally, educationally) is a worthy goal in and of itself, there is no evidence that it prevents mental disorder. For instance, many emotionally disturbed persons are educationally incompetent, an observation that has led some researchers to believe that a cause-and-effect relationship exists (i.e., that educational incompetence causes emotional disturbance). Findings from the Head Start program are often cited to support this relationship: reports have shown that the program does in fact improve early school achievement, and presumably this would in turn enhance self-esteem. However, even if it can be shown that building competence prevents distress-inducing problems (e.g., school failure and low self-esteem), there is a need to distinguish such problems from mental illness.

SOCIAL PROBLEMS AND PREVENTION

Some researcher-clinicians have argued strongly that there is a causal relationship between the environment and mental illness, and studies have been conducted to provide data in support of this hypothesis. There can be no doubt that the prevalence of symptoms associated with mental illness as well as the rates of admission to state hospitals and of diagnosis of the major mental illnesses are higher among the poor. What remains to be unequivocally demonstrated, however, is that poverty is somehow causative. For example, persons who are ill or on the verge of illness may gravitate toward poverty-stricken neighborhoods (i.e., downward drift).

In addition to this fundamental lack of evidence for a causal relationship between societal factors and mental illness, there is another important problem associated with primary prevention. If one grants, for the sake of discussion, that a causal relationship exists, it remains to be demonstrated that the types of preventive efforts that could be undertaken by mental health professionals would be the most effective and appropriate ones. For example, one variable of concern for prevention is quality of education, including student-teacher relationships. Can a commonly prescribed preventive intervention—mental health consultation in the schools—have a significant effect on such variables? Could more powerful approaches be devised, such as augmenting or modifying teacher training programs, to attain the same results? Such activities may fall outside the jurisdiction of mental health professionals, but the results of such activities may well be more to the point and their effectiveness greater.

PREVENTION: PROVEN AND PROBABLE

Some primary prevention techniques in psychiatry have been shown to be extremely effective. Psychiatric complications of syphilis and vitamin deficiency are seldom seen today in developed nations. Decreased rates of birth injury and improved prenatal care have lowered the incidence of major psychiatric problems that result from congenital brain damage. Other common neuropsychiatric disorders such as stroke and head injury have been shown to be highly preventable. Elimination of lead from house paint has reduced the number of children suffering from organic brain syndromes, and control of industrial toxins has virtually eliminated "mad hatter's disease" and other such problems.

More recent preventive programs should also reduce the incidence of certain illnesses. For instance, counseling prospective mothers not to delay pregnancy until the later childbearing years is likely to reduce the incidence of Down's syndrome. Other programs show promise but await solid research findings demonstrating their effectiveness. Interventions directed toward abusing parents, such as Parents Anonymous, seem likely to prove effective in breaking the cycle of child abuse, which has been shown to be socially transmitted from generation to generation. Raising infants in impersonal institutions or without a consistent mother figure over a long period of time has been demonstrated to be harmful. Programs to replace institutions for homeless children with long-term, high-quality foster care or adoption should help to prevent personality disturbance. With the mounting evidence of genetic influence on the occurrence of schizophrenia and bipolar disorder, the appropriate use of birth control and genetic counseling should be effective in preventing the births of individuals who would be at high risk for development of these illnesses.

Sound, well-conceived research in prevention based on controlled studies is sorely needed. The prevention of mental illness is a vitally important goal, and generous funding of research is needed to reach it. Applied programs, however, except on a pilot basis, should await the outcome of further research. Finally, there is as yet no easy solution—such as primary prevention—to the problem of mental illness. Difficult patients will not magically go away. Professionals will have to struggle with discouraging and often overwhelming obstacles to overcoming mental illness and resist the temptation of uncritically embracing simple solutions that are proposed.

REFERENCES

Albee GW, Ryan-Finn KD: An overview of primary prevention. Journal of Counseling and Development 72:115–123, 1993

Bachrach LL: Overview: model programs for chronic mental patients. Am J Psychiatry 137:1023–1031, 1980

Bachrach LL: Psychiatric services in rural areas: a sociological overview. Hosp Community Psychiatry 34:215–226, 1983

Bachrach LL: The state of the state mental hospital in 1996. Psychiatr Serv 47:1071–1078, 1996

Becker A, Wylan L, McCourt W: Primary prevention—whose responsibility? Am J Psychiatry 128:412–417, 1971

Beers CW: A Mind That Found Itself (1908). New York, Doubleday, 1939

Blair A: The role of primary prevention in mental health services: a review and critique. Journal of Community and Applied Social Psychology 2:55–94, 1992

Bleuler M: The long-term course of the schizophrenic psychoses. Psychol Med 4:244–254, 1974

Bloom BL: The logic and urgency of primary prevention. Hosp Community Psychiatry 32:839–843, 1981

Burns BJ, Santos AB: Assertive community treatment: an update of randomized trials. Psychiatr Serv 46:669–675, 1995

Caplan G: Principles of Preventive Psychiatry. New York, Basic Books, 1964

Caplan G, Caplan RB: Development of community psychiatry concepts, in Comprehensive Textbook of Psychiatry. Edited by Freedman AM, Kaplan HI. Baltimore, MD, Williams & Wilkins, 1967, pp 1499–1516

Cardoza VG, Ackerly WC, Leighton AH: Improving mental health through community action. Community Ment Health J 11:215–227, 1975

Cozza KI, Hales RE: Psychiatry in the Army: a brief historical perspective and current developments. Hosp Community Psychiatry 42:413–418, 1991

Deutsch A: The Shame of the States. New York, Harcourt Brace, 1948

Dinitz S, Beran N: Community mental health as a boundaryless and boundary-busting system. J Health Soc Behav 12:99–108, 1971

Elliott RL: Mental health reform in Georgia, 1992 to 1996. Psychiatr Serv 47:1205–1211, 1996

Elpers JR: Dividing the mental health dollar: the ethics of managing scarce resources. Hosp Community Psychiatry 37:671–672, 1986

Fairweather GW (ed): The Fairweather Lodge: A Twenty-Five Year Retrospective (New Directions for Mental Health Services, No 7). San Francisco, CA, Jossey-Bass, 1980

Gershon ES: Genetics, in Manic-Depressive Illness. Edited by Goodwin FK, Jamison KR. New York, Oxford University Press, 1990, pp 373–401

Goldman HH, et al: Form and function of mental health authorities at RWJ Foundation program sites: preliminary observations. Hosp Community Psychiatry 41:1222–1230, 1990

Gordis E: Alcohol research: at the cutting edge. Arch Gen Psychiatry 53:199–201, 1996

Hales RE, Gemelli RR: Psychiatric education in the military. Psychiatric Annals 17:536–538, 1987

Harding CM, Brooks GW, Ashikaga T, et al: The Vermont Longitudinal Study of Persons With Severe Mental Illness, II: long-term outcome of subjects who retrospectively met DSM-III criteria for schizophrenia. Am J Psychiatry 144:727–735, 1987

Hoge MA, Davidson L, Griffith EEH, et al: Defining managed care in public-sector psychiatry. Hosp Community Psychiatry 45:1085–1089, 1994

Hollingsworth EJ, Pitts MK, McKee D: Staffing patterns in rural community support programs. Hosp Community Psychiatry 44:1076–1081, 1993

Joint Commission on Mental Illness and Health: Action for Mental Health: Final Report of the Commission. New York, Basic Books, 1961

Kanter JS (ed): Clinical Issues in Treating the Chronic Mentally Ill (New Directions for Mental Health Services, No 27). San Francisco, CA, Jossey-Bass, 1985

Kendler KS, Diehl SR: The genetics of schizophrenia: a current genetic-epidemiologic perspective. Schizophr Bull 19:261–285, 1994

Kendler KS, Heath A, Martin NG, et al: Symptoms of anxiety and depression in a volunteer twin population: the etiologic role of genetic and environmental factors. Arch Gen Psychiatry 43:213–221, 1986

Kendler KS, Neale MC, Kessler RC, et al: Major depression and generalized anxiety disorder: same genes, (partly) different environments? Arch Gen Psychiatry 49:716–722, 1992

Kety SS: From rationalization to reason. Am J Psychiatry 131:957–963, 1974

Lamb HR: Treating the Long-Term Mentally Ill. San Francisco, CA, Jossey-Bass, 1982

Lamb HR (ed): The Homeless Mentally Ill: A Task Force Report of the American Psychiatric Association. Washington, DC, American Psychiatric Association, 1984

Lamb HR: Some reflections on treating schizophrenics. Arch Gen Psychiatry 43:1007–1011, 1986

Lamb HR: The new state hospitals in the community. Psychiatr Serv 48:1307–1310, 1997

Lamb HR, Grant RW: The mentally ill in an urban county jail. Arch Gen Psychiatry 39:17–22, 1982

Lamb HR, Grant RW: Mentally ill women in a county jail. Arch Gen Psychiatry 40:363–368, 1983

Lamb HR, Peele R: The need for continuing asylum and sanctuary. Hosp Community Psychiatry 35:798–802, 1984

Lamb HR, Weinberger LE: Conservatorship for gravely disabled psychiatric patients: a four-year follow-up study. Am J Psychiatry 149:909–913, 1992

Lamb HR, Weinberger LE: Persons with severe mental illness in jails and prisons: a review. Psychiatr Serv 49:483–492, 1998

Lamb HR, Zusman J: A new look at primary prevention. Hosp Community Psychiatry 32:843–848, 1981

Lamb HR, Bachrach LL, Kass FI (eds): Treating the Homeless Mentally Ill: A Report of the Task Force on the Homeless Mentally Ill. Washington, DC, American Psychiatric Association, 1992

Lefley HP, Johnson DL (eds): Families as Allies in Treatment of the Mentally Ill: New Directions for Mental Health Professionals. Washington, DC, American Psychiatric Press, 1990

Lehman AF: Capitation payment and mental health care: a review of opportunities and risks. Hosp Community Psychiatry 38:31–38, 1987

Lehman AF: Vocational rehabilitation in schizophrenia. Schizophr Bull 21:645–656, 1995

Lyons MJ, True WR, Eisen SA, et al: Differential heritability of adult and juvenile antisocial traits. Arch Gen Psychiatry 52:906–915, 1995

Marcos LR, Cohen NL, Nardacci D, et al: Psychiatry takes to the streets: the New York City initiative for the homeless mentally ill. Am J Psychiatry 147:1557–1561, 1990

McDuff DR, Johnson JL: Classification and characteristics of Army stress casualties during Operation Desert Storm. Hosp Community Psychiatry 43:812–815, 1992

Mechanic D, Aiken LH (eds): Paying for Services: Promises and Pitfalls of Capitation (New Directions for Mental Health Services, No 43). San Francisco, CA, Jossey-Bass, 1989

Miller RD: An update on involuntary civil commitment to outpatient treatment. Hosp Community Psychiatry 43:79–81, 1992

Mooney DK, Johnson RD: Rural mental health appointment adherence: implications for therapy. Community Ment Health J 28:135–139, 1992

President's Commission on Mental Health: Report of the Task Panel on Rural Mental Health, Vol 3. Washington, DC, U.S. Government Printing Office, 1978

Shore MF (ed): Managed Care, the Private Sector, and Medicaid Mental Health and Substance Abuse Services (New Directions for Mental Health Services, No 72). San Francisco, CA, Jossey-Bass, 1996

Smith SS, O'Hara BF, Persico AM, et al: Genetic vulnerability to drug abuse: the D_2 dopamine receptor taq I B1 restriction fragment length polymorphism appears more frequently in polysubstance abusers. Arch Gen Psychiatry 49:723–727, 1992

Stein LI, Test MA (eds): The Training in Community Living Model: A Decade of Experience (New Directions for Mental Health Services, No 26). San Francisco, CA, Jossey-Bass, 1985

Steinwachs DM, Flynn LM, Norquist GS, et al. (eds.): Using Client Outcomes Information to Improve Mental Health and Substance Abuse Treatment. (New Directions for Mental Health Services, No 71). San Francisco, CA, Jossey-Bass, 1996

Sullivan G, Jackson CA, Spritzer KL: Characteristics and service use of seriously mentally ill persons living in rural areas. Psychiatr Serv 47:57–61, 1996

Talbott JA: The fate of the public psychiatric system. Hosp Community Psychiatry 36:46–50, 1985

Talbott JA: The chronically mentally ill: what do we now know, and why aren't we implementing what we know? in The Chronic Mental Patient, Vol 2.Edited by Menninger WW, Hannah GT. Washington, DC, American Psychiatric Press, 1987, pp 1–29

Talbott JA: The Perspective of John Talbott (New Directions for Mental Health Services, No 37). San Francisco, CA, Jossey-Bass, 1988

Teplin LA: The prevalence of severe mental disorder among male urban jail detainees: comparison with the Epidemiologic Catchment Area program. Am J Public Health 80:663–669, 1990

Test MA: Continuity of care in community treatment, in Community Support Systems for the Long-Term Patient. Edited by Stein LI (New Directions for Mental Health Services, No 2). San Francisco, CA, Jossey-Bass, 1979, pp 15–23

Torrey EF: Out of the Shadows. New York, Wiley, 1997

Tsuang MT, Faraone SV: The Genetics of Mood Disorder. Baltimore, MD, Johns Hopkins University Press, 1990

Wing JK: The functions of asylum. Br J Psychiatry 157: 822–827, 1990

APPENDIX: MULTIPLE CHOICE QUESTIONS FOR CME

1. Which one of the following is incorrect?
   Community psychiatry in the 1960s
   a. Emphasized primary prevention.
   b. Encouraged community activism to change the basic fabric of society.
   c. Involved itself in the community, national and international affairs, poverty, and politics.
   d. Gave high priority to chronically and severely mentally ill patients.
   e. Emphasized services to children.

2. Which of the following is correct?
   Principles learned from military psychiatry in World War II included
   a. Early identification of psychiatric disorder.
   b. Prompt treatment as close as possible to the combat zone.
   c. Active psychotherapeutic techniques.
   d. Social support.
   e. The expectation of prompt return to duty.

3. Which one of the following is incorrect?
   Deinstitutionalization was facilitated by
   a. Aid to the disabled being made available to the mentally ill.
   b. The abundance of community resources for the mentally ill.
   c. The community mental health centers legislation.
   d. The introduction of phenothiazines.
   e. The states' desire to shift costs of the mentally ill population to the federal government.

4. Which one of the following is incorrect?
   The original community psychiatry principles included
   a. Responsibility to a population.
   b. Treatment close to the patient's home.
   c. Comprehensive services.
   d. The primacy of psychiatry among the mental health disciplines.
   e. Continuity of care.

5. Which one of the following is incorrect?
   The initial community mental health centers legislation mandated five basic services:
   a. Inpatient treatment.
   b. Outpatient services.
   c. Drug and alcohol abuse services.
   d. Partial hospitalization.
   e. Consultation-education.

6. Which one of the following is incorrect?
   Problems in treating the chronically and severely mentally ill include
   a. Unrealistic expectations.
   b. Dealing with dependency.
   c. Providing asylum and sanctuary in the community.
   d. Reluctance to give practical advice to patients and families.
   e. Not making treatment time-limited.

7. Which of the following are incorrect?
   Case management should include
   a. Every chronically and severely mentally ill person is on the caseload of a mental health worker who has specific responsibility for that person.
   b. Monitoring the patient.
   c. A psychiatric and medical assessment.
   d. An individualized treatment and rehabilitation plan.
   e. Assisting the patient in receiving services.

8. Which one of the following is incorrect?
   Providing psychiatric services in rural areas is impeded by
   a. Increased tolerance of deviance.
   b. Large geographic areas.
   c. Limited psychiatric resources.
   d. Professional isolation.
   e. Excessive workloads.

9. Which one of the following is incorrect?
   Problems in public psychiatry include
   a. Dollar not following the patient.
   b. The catchment area concept frequently not working well.
   c. Lack of linkage among community services.
   d. Too many psychiatrists.
   e. Insufficient program evaluation.

10. Which one of the following is incorrect?
    Excluding genetic counseling, primary prevention is possible in
    a. Tertiary syphilis.
    b. Schizophrenia.
    c. Pellagra.
    d. Birth injury.
    e. Down's syndrome.

Answers: 1. d; 2. all 5; 3. b; 4. d; 5. c; 6. e; 7. all 5; 8. a; 9. d; 10. b.

CHAPTER 43

ADMINISTRATIVE PSYCHIATRY

STEPHEN RACHLIN, M.D.
STUART L. KEILL, M.D.

The psychiatrist in an administrative role, by choice or by assignment, usually finds the role, with its perquisites such as autonomy, power, and personal growth, challenging and even enjoyable. This feeling, which may be surprising to some, stems from a mastery of the knowledge and skills that constitute the art and science of administration. One wonders then why so many individuals, unfamiliar with these areas of psychiatry, consider administration to be mundane paper-shuffling and leave the direction of the organization to others while expressing dissatisfaction with their management.

There are numerous reasons. First, early-career psychiatrists, particularly those immersed in residency training programs, tend to be more committed to and interested in patient care. They seek to heal the ill, or they enjoy teaching others. Their role models are gifted clinical supervisors. The generally more distant executives are identified with the "impersonal" systems they direct.

After training, however, psychiatrists may find themselves running a ward, a clinic, or some other program that requires administrative expertise. Lacking relevant knowledge and experience, they may perceive management tasks as unrewarding and fraught with difficulties and they may react by fleeing from administrative positions. As a result, less qualified personnel often fill the vacuum created. This chapter provides a brief introduction to the essence of administration in psychiatry. We hope that the chapter, through focusing on what Levinson and Klerman (1972) referred to as the "Clinician Executive," encourages more psychiatrists to increase participation in leadership activities.

HISTORY

There is a long tradition of interest in the more effective management of systems to deal with psychiatric illness (S. L. Keill 1981). The Book of Jeremiah in the Old Testament includes a description of plans by Zephaniah (630 B.C.) to design procedures to take place in a prison setting for the treatment of "mad men and prophetizers." Later, Nebuchadnezzar (609 B.C.) benefited from the concept of asylum after his psychotic episode. Fourteenth-century England saw the Bethlehem Hospital (the source of the term *bedlam*) expand its mission from serving as a cloister for the religious to providing care for psychiatric patients. In the sixteenth century, the brilliant philosopher/executive Thomas More in his *Apologia* recommended "beating and correcting" patients at that hospital to enhance treatment effectiveness. In sixteenth-century Spain, Juan Ciudad instituted an organization to provide care for the mentally ill (with satellite facilities throughout western Europe) that assumed the responsibility for training what were then seen as mental health professionals. In 1783, Benjamin Rush, the only psychiatrist to sign the Declaration of Independence, founded the first general hospital psychiatry unit at the Pennsylvania Hospital. In the nineteenth century, Pinel in France, Tuke in England, and Amariah Brigham made major reforms in programs of psychiatric patient care. These individuals, with the public support of Dorothea Dix, one of the original consumer revolutionaries, humanized the organizational approach to patients with psychiatric disorders. In the twentieth century, Clifford Beers continued the education of state and federal officials as a mental health and patients' advocate.

The introduction of the professions of social work and occupational therapy by Adolf Meyer and an enhancement of the concept of therapeutic community by Harry Stack Sullivan contributed to the increasing complexity and multimodal organizational approach to the psychiatric patient.

Although these pioneers had an impact on the delivery of clinical psychiatric services, there was no formalized approach to management of these programs. Until recent years, little interest was shown by our leading academicians in learning and teaching the skills, strategies, and interventions needed for improving the systems in which delivery of psychiatric services takes place. Yet the opportunity to influence the direction of programs is one of the principal rewards of administrative psychiatry.

It is logical that psychiatrists be the ones to assume responsibility for providing structure, leadership, and direction to psychiatric programs. With our knowledge of basic and clinical science, we are probably in the best position to influence and lead systems for delivery of mental health care. However, training and experience in management are necessary to enhance our capacities to assume administrative roles.

EDUCATION AND TRAINING

Most psychiatrists in management positions do not obtain graduate degrees in business, public, or hospital administration, although some complete master of public health programs that have notable administrative components. Fellowships in public psychiatry, such as the one at Columbia University (Ranz et al. 1996), may include an emphasis

on developing leadership and managerial skills, and clinical rotations as well as didactic presentations with these foci may be offered.

To learn the basics of administration and management, the more serious student can enroll in individual courses at a nearby university. Mini courses in administrative psychiatry also are available periodically in several geographic locations. Most such courses are well advertised in professional newspapers and journals. Study on one's own should be viewed not as a substitute but as a supplement.

Organizations concerned with the education and training of clinicians in management are another source of seminars. The American College of Mental Health Administration, whose members are elected, is made up of the four predominant clinical professionals: psychiatrists, social workers, nurses, and psychologists. The American Association of Psychiatric Administrators, which, like the American Psychiatric Association (APA), is an outgrowth of a network of state hospital directors, features open membership to psychiatrists interested in the field and offers educational programs nationally as well as through its local chapters. That there is a body of knowledge in psychiatric administration is also attested to by the presentation of various symposia, workshops, and lectures at the two annual, national meetings sponsored by the APA.

For more than 40 years, the APA has had a structure in place for credentialing psychiatrists in administration. The process is overseen by the Committee on Psychiatric Administration and Management and begins with peer evaluation of the candidates' education, training, and experience. A written examination is administered first, and those who pass take an oral examination given immediately before the annual May meeting. Several hundred psychiatrists have obtained certification. In a survey of this group, Rodenhauser et al. (1995) found that the perceived best benefits of the process were self-satisfaction and an increase in skills, especially among the younger members. These psychiatrists relied mostly on self-study and continuing medical education courses to learn their craft, whereas older psychiatrists depended more on their mentors.

The APA examination covers four areas. The first area, *administrative theory and human resources*, encompasses personnel issues, management structures, and the like. Kraft (1983), who noted that there is no single coherent theory of organizational dynamics, wrote a summary of administrative theory and compiled a bibliography to guide the reader to the classics in the field. Additional historical readings have been gathered by Shafritz and Hyde (1987). We will not discuss this aspect further. *Psychiatric care management* includes such matters as managed care, utilization review, and quality assessment, all of which are addressed in this chapter. *Public psychiatric care and prevention of psychiatric illness* are covered in Chapter 42. The third area, *law and ethics*, likewise is addressed in other chapters (see Chapters 41 and 45). Finally, *fiscal management*—which includes but is not limited to such issues as budgeting, sources of revenue, and other related topics—will be examined later in this chapter.

With the increase in use of computers by administrative psychiatrists, systems of information management have become more and more important and are a vital tool for the future. Software can be developed in house, purchased from commercial sources, adapted from general medical systems, or shared among colleagues in the mental health professions. Indeed, professionals at different facilities learn from each other what types of data are best entered in the computer (Taintor et al. 1997).

THE ADMINISTRATOR AS LEADER

A variety of tasks confront the psychiatrist-administrator. Barton and Barton (1983) stated that the psychiatrist-administrator should be able to plan, organize, staff, direct, control, communicate, innovate, and represent. These authors go on to characterize the capacity for leadership as including the abilities to decide, prioritize, resolve conflicts, coordinate the work of others, expedite task completion, motivate staff, use power wisely, and delegate authority to others. Various additional skills could be added to this prototypical list, and we will expand on several of these items shortly.

Before proceeding further, we would like to distinguish, after Talbott (1987), the related concepts of management, administration, and leadership. *Management* is a hands-on process, and its goal is to keep the organization running smoothly. *Management* refers to the work done by those persons who occupy middle management positions and concern themselves with procedures. *Administration* is a broader concept, involving overseeing and taking executive charge. Administrators are concerned with policy and ensuring that tasks of the organization are performed well.

Leadership, in contrast, involves giving direction (as opposed to providing directions) and has something of a visionary component. Leaders promote and protect the values of the organization and involve, inspire, and nurture staff. There is an oft-repeated saying that the administrator does things right and the leader does the right things. The effective leader does not get bogged down in all the day-to-day crises but rather delegates to subordinates, whom he or she then helps develop toward assuming additional responsibility.

Menninger (1992) added that the leader must provide clear and consistent direction. It is essential for the leader to communicate and resolve conflict, because uncertainty and loss of control lead to poor morale. The person in charge must help the individuals within the organization to be aware of the overall goal of their work, to see that the goal is worthwhile and desirable, and to sense that their contributions are important. *Power* should not be considered a pejorative term when it is used constructively (Lipton and Loutsch 1985). Particularly if there is some instability in the organization, the leader is obligated to use power in a rational and planned manner.

Although a chairperson, chief of service, or department head may well be the "front office" to the staff on the clinical service, that same person is a middle manager to the chief executive officer, dean, commissioner, or other individual to whom he or she is accountable. Juggling these sometimes-competing roles and responsibilities takes skill. In all we do as health care providers, we are part of an open system that interacts with many other systems. Managing the many exchanges across these boundaries is yet another challenge for those persons in executive positions.

One final note before concluding this section: We strongly believe that an additional obligation of those in leadership positions is active involvement in professional associations. It is not only the networking with colleagues that is important, but also the sharing of experiences and expertise with others in the psychiatric field—the patient being the ultimate beneficiary of advances in mental health care delivery.

ADMINISTRATIVE STYLES AND SKILLS

The personality and style of the individual directing an organization will affect the organization's tone and output. Staff will adjust to a variety of personal styles and traits, although extremes are likely to create problems. Marcos and Silver (1988) demonstrated that most executives in our profession place high values both on the tasks at hand and on the interpersonal relationships necessary to accomplish them. In essence, participatory decision making facilitates selling the task to those charged with carrying it out.

With their tongues only slightly in cheek, Talbott and Keill (1980) created a typology of state hospital directors, one that could just as readily apply to psychiatrist-executives in any other organization. These authors delineated seven personae, with their mottoes, as seen in Table 43–1.

Perusal of Table 43–1 may lead the reader to identify

TABLE 43–1. Psychiatrist-executive personae

Label	Modus operandi
Saintly	*Try* to do as I do.
Renaissance	Judge me by my publications.
Lunatic Fringe	What crusade shall we promote this week?
Grandfather	You *know* I know best, now just do as I say.
Old Guard	The good old days were better and we'd better go slow now.
Uninvolved	It's not bad because it never happened.
Cynical	What have these *fools* in the state capital done now?

specific colleagues. When these personae were first presented, a large audience of psychiatrist-administrators bubbled over with a variety of named examples for each type.

Although every individual is of course different in personality and style, some common traits characterize effective leaders. As with all positive relationships, the staff and the supervisor's relationship is based on mutual respect and trust. The leader's behaviors consistently convey ethical integrity, a commitment to the goals of the organization, and a primary focus on the needs and the rights of patients, as well as a valuing of staff performance. Staff members work with more security when they believe in the reliability of the leader and his or her intentions to seek the resources that are needed to carry out the work. Commitments to action must be honored and breaches explained. Excellent performance is valued, poor performance rejected.

Administrators make decisions with a sense of timeliness. Many day-to-day decisions can be made quickly and easily, because occasional errors can be corrected. Major decisions require more data and deliberation, including input from those affected by the decisions. A fine balance needs to be maintained between the need for input and the need for timeliness of decision making. The old saying "No decision is after all a decision, but a bad one" is true.

The leader's actions and decisions have credibility when they are rooted in a broad body of knowledge about the clinical aspects of psychiatric treatment, rehabilitative systems, patient and family needs, gaps in the available resources, the community, the strengths and weaknesses of staff members' performance, and the effectiveness of the program.

The successful psychiatrist-administrator has insight into his or her own behavior and its motivations, dynamics, and impact on others, just as the clinical psychiatrist is aware of transference-countertransference phenomena. In professional work relationships as well, self-understanding is used to correct distortions in perception and in assessment of situations so that rational strategies for action can be formulated and struggles for control and no-win positions avoided.

The supervisor also teaches, directs, and provides a role model for the staff. He or she seeks input from staff about patients' needs and about ways to improve services to patients and families. The collegial administrator develops structures for ongoing feedback, input, and problem solving by frontline staff. This approach results not only in professional collegiality and interdependence but also in high morale and productivity. Staff members "own" the program with this administrative style. Such an administrative approach may at first seem time consuming, but the investment is amply returned in synergy.

Inculcating the concept of genuine collaboration among the staff fosters commitment to a common goal. Collaboration differs from *cooperation*, which is a willingness to help one another. *Collaboration* means sharing a responsible concern for outcome. Departmental structures for ongoing communication about planning, patient care, and other functions should foster the concept of shared ownership of programs and problems.

Optimism is another important quality for a leader. The administrator must believe that his or her leadership makes a difference. He or she also must maintain positive expectations for change, even in the face of setbacks. Staff members need to experience the optimism of their leader.

The competent leader has confidence in his or her abilities and is not threatened by, but indeed welcomes, the fact that some of his or her subordinates will be more competent in many activities. The leader cannot be expert in all areas but learns from and looks to the other experts in his or her program.

PLANNING

Planning is perhaps the most important function of organizational leadership. It ensures continuing vitality and growth, with the recognition that change is inevitable. If services are neither increased nor improved, they are in danger of losing their relevance. In planning, there is a high potential for frustration, because only a percentage of good ideas ultimately get translated into real programs. Even a cutback or reduction of a part of one's operation requires substantial effort to ensure that continuing treatment is provided for those patients who need additional care.

The accepted starting point in the planning process is the development of a mission statement. Actions by subdivisions must reflect these goals of the parent body. Basic to shaping the organization's future is a *strategic plan*. By definition, a strategic plan is long-range in nature, often 5 years, and provides the guideposts or overarching principles. Budgets, to be discussed in a succeeding section, should reflect the strategic plan and may be rejected if they do not. No plan is so static that it is immune from change, as long as direction remains intact.

Change may come from a variety of sources, both internal and external. Examples of the latter are alterations in state mental health laws, modifications in the requirements of accrediting bodies, community demands, and changes in availability of funding for special projects. Internal stimuli include, among others, the hiring of a new staff member with special interests (or the development of skills by existing personnel), a crisis in existing units or programs, and the appointment of a new leader. To be sure, there are barriers to effective planning—most prominently, lack of resources, either monetary or personnel, as well as regulatory constraints and unavailability of other supports. The kinds and numbers of staff also directly affect the process. Although all staff cannot be part of plan development, implementation will have an impact on each individual.

A PLANNING CYCLE

The acronym *DIME* is useful for conceptualizing and describing how one goes about planning—especially for the shorter term, with which most of us are more familiar and involved. The four-stage planning cycle includes *d*esign, *i*nitiation, *m*anagement, and *e*valuation. It can be used for a new program or for modification of one that is ongoing (Table 43–2).

The first stage, *design*, includes a study of the mission and a measurement of available resources. A draft plan is articulated that is based on an appropriate balance. In this phase there must be sensitivity toward changes in the needs of the patient population and the community. A basic first step is to determine who will be involved. Planning that is done by a single individual has great potential for failure because of lack of support. There should be group representation from professional and paraprofessional staff of the organization, the anticipated consumers of the services, advocacy organizations, and those to whom the program will be accountable. This ad hoc team is then charged with the responsibility of assessing both the needs and the existing or expected resources. If the plan that emanates from this process is consonant with the mission and strategic plan of the parent body, and funding (either existing or ad-

ditional) and staffing seem adequate, it is likely to be approved.

The next step is *initiation*, the creation of the actual structure. This is a particularly rewarding time, with high levels of staff excitement and enthusiasm. Managers select and train staff. Old procedures are modified, and support is developed in part by dissemination of information to interested collaborating services. Some resistance to change is inevitable, given the presence of a level of contentment with what is known and familiar. Such resistance should be anticipated and accepted as a natural dynamic, and sensitive strategies should be developed to deal with the phenomenon. Differences need to be talked about and resolved so that all groups can in some part "own" and sponsor the new effort. Investments in achieving consensus pay dividends in staff morale.

Management involves overseeing of the ongoing program, and the program's success depends on good management. Many clinical and administrative decisions will need to be made. Foreseen and unforeseen difficulties are dealt with; the wheels are greased to reduce friction and increase efficiency. Meeting common and important managerial challenges calls for a range of skills, chief among them the ability to develop forums for ongoing communication among staff, for airing differences and conflicts in a risk-free ambiance, for eliciting input from a number of perspectives, and for problem solving and building agreement.

The process of *evaluation*, in reality, needs to be introduced at the very beginning of the management phase. Records are kept and data collected; resources are balanced and reports made. Program evaluation is the measurement of effectiveness and efficiency of the defined program. Through analysis of this information, judgments can be made regarding continuing management and a course for

TABLE 43–2. DIME planning cycle

Phase	Actions
Design	Study mission, assess needs and resources, create and present plan
Initiation	Create structure, modify plant, and recruit staff, publicize program and elicit consensus
Management	Oversee operation, tune process, solve problems
Evaluation	Collect data including statistics and subjective responses by staff and consumers, measure effectiveness and efficiency, identify deficiencies

the future. If goals are being met and patients are being cared for, anticipated monies have been generated, and staff morale is good, the program should be maintained or expanded. If deficiencies are noted, depending on their nature, it may be worthwhile for the design group to consider relevant changes. Among the options for redesign are improving the performance of some staff, altering professional (or other staff)-to-patient ratios, extending or shortening length of stay, and improving communication with providers or consumers. The searching out of new techniques and the encouragement of creativity continue the cycle. Few provider organizations have all the resources necessary for the full spectrum of patient care services; thus, coordination, cooperation, and collaboration among entities are required. The different systems—all of which are under varying auspices, both public and private—have their own needs and priorities. Interorganizational agreements must be drawn up, and each party will need to adjust to a degree of change. Because decisions made by a single provider have a ripple effect on others, we are accountable to them. Open negotiations will define and resolve potential problems; trust at the executive level is at the core of this process. We believe that the future will bring even more interaction among service providers as we strive to create integrated systems for continuity of patient care.

ACCOUNTABILITY

All mental health agencies, and indeed human services in general, are accountable in a variety of ways to the three branches of government. The legislature enacts laws that govern the operations of hospitals, clinics, and the like and that provide for the licensing of professional staff. The executive branch, operating through state and/or local departments of mental health or hygiene, has the authority to issue regulations on many aspects of psychiatric treatment, and these regulations have the force of law. Finally, if we are unfortunate enough to be subjects of lawsuits, judicial decrees may have a substantial influence on how the job gets done. Even absent this degree of intervention, it is the courts that interpret the foregoing laws and regulations and, in so doing, directly affect what we do. In our day-to-day lives, most of us report to several different individuals or groups for various aspects of our systems.

TO THE GOVERNMENT

Depending on the institution's auspices, program directors may be accountable to municipal, state, or federal officials. One or another of these has statutory responsibility for approving and licensing of institutions or components

thereof, both initially and throughout their operation. Obtaining such certification from government, to which funding is tightly tied, involves a process of external evaluation of mission, staffing patterns, recruiting techniques, life safety factors, patients' rights, quality assurance, fiscal responsibility, and documentation in individual clinical records. There should never be any underestimation of the central role documentation plays in all types of certification and accreditation. Perhaps there will be other requirements, such as that a percentage of those treated come from certain geographic areas or that patients of lower income levels and appropriate ethnic groups be served. Generally, these site visits for evaluation occur at 2- or 3-year intervals, assuming that no serious deficiencies are uncovered. Different levels of government may be involved in this process if they contribute funds, to ensure appropriate utilization of public expenditures.

Site visits for evaluation can be helpful. Identification of service gaps and operating problem areas can result in a gaining of allies for their correction. Sometimes the visibility of such problem areas to regulatory bodies mobilizes additional administrative support and resources for correction. Naturally, when values and priorities of the evaluating team and the program staff differ, some tension can result. It is hard for the provider team to be "exposed"—to feel in a defensive, explanatory position. The psychiatrist-administrator should take the lead in easing this communication dynamic.

If the psychiatrist-executive, abashed by an apparent lack of understanding of clinical issues by a surveyor, takes a critical, adversarial stance, this almost invariably leads to disadvantages for the program and the staff. Antagonizing well-intentioned, powerful individuals can only lead to no-win conflicts, and the ultimate victim is the patient. It is often effective to attempt to understand and appreciate the site visitor's position and point of view. This individual may in turn appreciate the psychiatrist-administrator's concern about clinical issues, and benefits to the program may result.

TO THE COMMUNITY

For many years, both providers and consumers have perceived that the major systems for the delivery of health care in this country are *of* the community as well as *in* the community. It is therefore helpful for the program, educational for the staff, and important for the executive to work with informed and interested consumers and advocates. It is consistent with American philosophy for individuals to participate in decision making that affects them. There is a clear current trend toward open communication between the public, health delivery systems, and the government.

A comfortable way to begin such dialogue is with sophisticated groups such as the Alliance for the Mentally Ill or local and state mental health associations. These groups have a genuine dedication to enhancing mental health services and a real potential for increasing the staff's knowledge about myriad problems of patients and families. They are also helpful in sponsoring hearings to provide information to the community and to influence legislators to increase funding for clinical services. There will inevitably be areas of disagreement between community groups and professional staff about objectives, methods, and priorities, but the tensions created by different points of view can be invigorating and discussions of these differences can be of mutual benefit. The community's ability to articulate its needs and wishes, combined with the knowledge, skills, and dedication of the professional staff, can make for powerful and effective psychiatric programs. The community needs the skilled professional program, which in turn needs the community's resources. The value of this interdependence increases when it is acknowledged and nurtured.

Most large organizations, including hospitals and other health care institutions, are directed by a board of directors, trustees, managers, or governors. Prominent members of the community are appointed or elected to serve. In other than public programs, they may have substantial responsibility for raising funds. In government-sponsored facilities, although such boards may exist, the chief executive is additionally accountable to an appointed or elected official. Many board members are capable, knowledgeable, and administratively well versed. Mutual respect, plus continuing and open communications, can provide major benefits to patients.

TO THE MEDIA

Because the press, radio, and television influence the public, and therefore governmental figures, they can have a powerful effect on programs. The populace is interested in coverage of new techniques for dealing with psychiatric and other health care problems. Given the nature of many public psychiatric facilities, there is always a potential for various kinds of scandal. Those in the field of news reporting may find this useful as a way of enhancing the sale of newspapers or their own careers as "action reporters." It is essential, therefore, that the psychiatrist-administrator maintain a mutually respectful relationship with key figures in the media. Doing so not only protects the administrator and his or her organization but also allows the psychiatric establishment view of controversial public issues to be aired. It also provides an opportunity for a positive

and constructive influence on funding figures for the enhancement of programs. The executive must develop experience in dealing with those in the media whose priorities may be different but whose good intentions and ethical values may prove important in the mission of enhancement of programs for our patients.

STRATEGIES FOR INFLUENCE

Politics, like power, is not a dirty word. It is, most simply, a set of strategies for influencing others. This, in turn, is important to help improve systems of care for our patients, and should be honest, goal directed, rationally planned, and ideologically clear. Political skills are legitimate assets; they can and should be polished just as the other professional assets used in leading a program are. Among the groups and individuals we need to influence are governmental bodies, both executive and legislative; labor organizations; peer and professional groups; consumers; the media; accrediting bodies; immediate supervisors; and our organizations' comptrollers (S. L. Keill 1991). The psychiatrist in administration must of course maintain his or her own professional and ethical standards and not become so politically preoccupied that ideology and clinical skills are lost.

The term *politics* implies the use of power to accomplish goals. Politics also, by definition, involves adversarial situations. Other programs or individuals are inevitably and legitimately competing for the same resources, space, funds, or personnel. The psychiatrist committed to improving the care of patients will use skills, energies, talents, and resources to enhance the system of care and positively influence program development, even in the face of opposition. Public officials and legislators have a host of societal concerns, of which mental health is only one. The chief executive of a general hospital is responsible for many departments in addition to psychiatry. Politics involves influencing others to give one's needs priority. This may entail convincing hospital leaders to expend funds to enhance staffing on one inpatient unit instead of to build a new parking lot; it might mean convincing a local community group to support the development of a satellite clinic in a new neighborhood; or it might be a combined attempt with many allies to convince the state commissioner and the governor that several million additional dollars are needed for the state mental health budget.

Particularly important in these processes is the evaluation of the opposition. Knowledge of the opposition's strength, structure, style, resources, and vulnerability can make the difference between success and failure. The state official who might be able to provide additional funds for a psychiatric program has a basic and legitimate concern about costs and economy. An appropriate strategy with this individual may be to emphasize how the program actually saves money by eliminating duplication and expanding the tax base. In taking this tack, the psychiatrist-executive has not abdicated the humanistic perspective but rather is helping both the state official and himself or herself maintain priorities.

It is important to ration resources for influencing, to select a few targets of importance, and to eschew dissipation of energy by spreading oneself too thin. Strategic planning for influencing others increases one's power and image but also, most important, fosters the ability to help groups of patients and their families receive the care they need.

FISCAL PRACTICES

In health care organizations, personnel accounts for the lion's share of expenditures. The percentage varies by type of service provider but can be as much as 80% of annual outlays. Staff salaries, plus the cost of fringe benefits, make up this component. Other costs include rent, utilities, janitorial services, travel, postage, and telephone service. These monies must be monitored, and a budget is the mechanism for doing this, much as it may be in a family.

THE BUDGET

First and foremost, a budget is a financial plan. It flows from, and is consonant with, the overall mission statement and strategic plan discussed earlier. It thus supports the goals and objectives of the organization and takes into account that resources are finite. The overall plan drives the budget, not the reverse.

Warren (1992) discussed other functions of the budget as well. It is a policy document, balancing competing priorities and providing a framework for their implementation. It also obviously has a control function.

Performance can be studied and measured against allocations, and any type of variance can be noted. Doing so also allows feedback to be given to program directors so that corrections may be made midstream.

Accountability can be ensured, because it is the responsibility of the administrator to see to it that resources are used in a responsible and responsive fashion. The administrator need not be an accountant, but he or she must be able to deal with and understand the language of the financial division.

There are various types of operational budgets in use (Table 43–3) and all are oriented toward the future. Gov-

ernmental entities commonly operate with a *fixed ceiling, or lump sum, appropriation.* The executive has some flexibility in moving dollars from one project to another but cannot exceed the preset limit. By contrast, the *line item, or object, budget* includes a specific amount for each particular expenditure and perhaps also for every staff position in the agency. This type of budget is a rigid method that vests all spending authority in the funding body.

A *program budget* defines what is to be accomplished, by unit or division. This budget, also known as a PPBS (i.e., planning programming budget system), is complicated and produces a matrix-like structure containing objectives that allow for measurable units of performance. A *zero base budget* requires that all expenditures be examined each year. The entire request (including the salary of the psychiatrist-administrator) must be justified in detail, with priorities noted. Literally every dollar must be shown to be necessary. Finally, there is the *incremental budget.* This budget simply adjusts upward or downward from the previous year, depending on service demand and utilization, cost-of-living allowances, and the like. Little creativity is required in preparing, drafting, and putting together this type of budget.

Other concepts to keep in mind are the distinctions between various types of costs (Table 43–4). *Fixed costs,* salaries being an example, are those that remain the same regardless of volume of services produced. By contrast, *variable costs* are directly proportional to output numbers. In surgery, for example, the cost of supplies increases as more operations are performed. *Step-variable costs* are not as directly proportional to volume; they include the cost to maintain the facility.

Finally, all institutions have both direct and indirect costs. *Direct costs* are those that arise out of operation of the programs, such as salaries and supplies. On the other hand,

TABLE 43–3.   **Operational budgets**

Type	Characteristic
Lump sum	Appropriation of fixed amount for program
Line item	Specific amount for each expenditure
Program (PPBS)	Matrix of objectives and measurable performance units
Zero base	Each expenditure must be justified, beginning at base level
Incremental	Upward or downward adjustment from previous cycle based on demand and costs

Note.   PPBS = planning programming budget system.

TABLE 43–4. **Types of costs**

Type	Example	Definition
Fixed	Salaries	Static regardless of service volume
Variable	Supplies	Proportional to volume of service
Step-variable	Facility upkeep	Not directly related to volume
Direct	Supplies	Arise out of program operation
Indirect	Utilities	Necessary but not unique to program

indirect costs, such as housekeeping and utilities, are for necessities but are not unique to the program. They need to be allocated in a budget, the most common method being by unit or division. The directors of each service may disagree with each other about the correct proportions to be used, each wanting not to appear the big spender.

Usually, items such as construction of new facilities or extensive rehabilitation of old facilities and purchase of equipment are separately considered in a capital budget.

Once the budget is prepared, it must be submitted for approval to a higher authority, to a board of directors, to a governmental entity, or perhaps to all, depending on the type of facility. Our discussion thus far has focused on the expenditure side, but this represents only half the picture. The executive, or the financial officer with whom he or she is working, must be careful to avoid the trap of saving money by cutting staff if a program generates more in reimbursement than it costs to operate. It is to the income side that we next turn.

FINANCING OF SERVICES

By long tradition, state governments have financed mental health care through wholly owned and operated hospitals and clinics, as well as with grants to other agencies to care for psychiatric patients. No such well-developed system exists for the physically ill, although municipal and charity hospitals have been in existence for some years. Although many state systems are presently downsizing, partly in response to deinstitutionalization, they still provide an enormous amount of direct care and may be part of the types of cooperative and collaborative systems discussed earlier in the section on planning.

The federal government has also been a service provider for select populations. Medical-surgical care, as well as psychiatric care, has been provided at military facilities, at Department of Veterans Affairs medical centers, and through the Indian Health Service and the Public Health Service.

Through other means, Washington, DC (and Baltimore, MD, where the Social Security Administration is headquartered), now provides a substantial amount of the money used to fund programs for the elderly, the poor, and the disabled. Medicare and Medicaid were created by the 1965 amendments to the social security law. Medicare was originally enacted to provide medical care for the elderly (persons over age 65) who might be receiving retirement benefits. Part A, supported by taxes, pays for the cost of hospital treatment. Part B, optional and paid for in part by recipients, covers physician care and home health needs, among other items. Inpatient treatment may be reimbursed (unless it is provided in federal facilities), but there is a lifetime cap of 190 days for freestanding psychiatric hospitals. This limitation does not apply to care administered in general hospital settings. Outpatient psychotherapy is subjected to a 50% copayment, whereas other health services require only a 20% copayment. Disabled persons under age 65 with a work history are eligible to receive Supplemental Security Disability Income, and therefore Medicare, as are members of a few other narrowly defined groups.

Medicaid, on the other hand, is a federally sponsored program in association with the various states. Overall, the federal government pays half the costs and the states (and perhaps localities) pay the other half, but the exact proportions vary depending on the relative wealth of the states. Beneficiaries of public assistance are categorically eligible for Medicaid, and others whose incomes are above the cutoff level for welfare eligibility but insufficient for taking care of medical needs may also be eligible. The level of income required for participation, as well as the range of benefits provided, varies by state and is the product of discretionary decisions made by legislative and executive bodies. Medicaid also has special exclusions relative to psychiatry. It does not pay for psychiatric inpatient treatment for adults under age 65 unless the treatment is provided in a general hospital. Freestanding psychiatric hospitals, state facilities, and psychiatric skilled nursing homes may receive federally funded Medicaid only for those inpatients under age 22 or over age 65. Those persons who are chronically disabled and receiving Supplemental Security Income are eligible for Medicaid as well.

Psychiatric facilities have come to rely a great deal on

these sources of income, and virtually all health care entities are supported by multiple streams of revenue. In making this observation, Dorwart et al. (1992) noted how the mix of public entitlements and private funds must be managed to ensure financial viability. Commercial insurers, Blue Cross being the largest, cover many workers and their dependents through employer contributions, now increasingly supplemented by employee payroll deductions. The Federal Employees Health Benefits Program takes care of that group, whereas military families and retirees have their health needs covered by the Civilian Health and Medical Program for the Uniformed Services. And finally, some employers self-insure, a few patients are wealthy enough to do the same, and a huge number of Americans have no insurance whatsoever. For this last group, self-pay may be a euphemism for no pay, or a route to bankruptcy when large amounts of care are needed.

Each plan or program of insurance has different benefit levels, which makes for a bewildering array for any reimbursement manager or program administrator. An agency benefits when it is able to maximize its share of well-insured patients. If plans are being made to expand geriatric outpatient services at a hospital, for example, it is well to remember that Medicare pays little for ambulatory psychiatric services, although recent changes have substantially increased the annual cap and have made possible the full 80% reimbursement for physician-provided medical management services (typically psychopharmacological). Yet Medicare reimbursement for inpatient psychiatric care is presently adequate for most hospitals.

Further complicating the picture is that payment may be made retrospectively or prospectively. The traditional fee-for-service indemnity insurance pays after the services are rendered, basing payment on a bill submitted. However, various prospective plans impose limits, up front, on what will be paid for and at what level. For example, many health maintenance organizations limit inpatient care to 30 days annually and outpatient treatment to 20 visits per year. The service recipient is personally responsible for the balance. In regulating these types of operations, many states have enacted statutes mandating coverage of certain services at defined levels, which, unfortunately for our patients, may be inadequate. Self-insured groups are exempt, by federal preemption, from such requirements.

COST CONTROL

Society in general and elected officials in particular are expressing concern about the cost of health care and the percentage of the gross national product it is consuming. In response to this concern, several years ago the Health Care Financing Administration—that arm of government charged with the responsibility of operating and regulating federal entitlement programs— developed the payment system known as *diagnosis-related groups* (DRGs) for Medicare-funded hospital care. All illnesses are classified into one of several hundred diagnostic categories, and a fixed amount is paid for the hospital treatment of that illness. Allowances are made for complications and co-morbidity. If a hospital successfully treats a patient for less than the specified dollar amount, as by shortening the length of stay, it gets to keep the so-called change. But if this payment level is exceeded by costs, the facility itself is responsible for the difference. The patient cannot be billed.

This scheme proved extremely difficult to implement for psychiatric patients, because diagnosis alone serves to explain only a small amount of the variability in resources consumed or length of stay. Psychiatric hospitals (as well as rehabilitation facilities and children's hospitals) are categorically eligible for exemption from these prospective payment mechanisms. Psychiatric units in general hospitals can apply for an exemption, but an annual site visit is required to ensure compliance with the conditions of participation set forth by the Health Care Financing Administration. The process of this survey is typically contracted out to state agencies.

Physicians themselves have not been immune to the rate-setting zeal of government. A complicated set of rules—whereby such factors as the amount of professional work involved, the complexity of the procedure or medical decision to be made, local costs, and malpractice insurance rates—produces a set of values to be multiplied by a specific financial amount. This has resulted in what is known as the *Resource-Based Relative Value Scale*. Many of our colleagues are unhappy with the result, in part because the reimbursement codes do not accurately reflect all of the variables, particularly the range and diversity of services we generally provide to our patients.

Psychiatric services provided to patients are coded for reimbursement purposes according to the *Physicians' Current Procedural Terminology* (American Medical Association 1997). Governmental programs and commercial insurance companies have allowable fee schedules corresponding to each of several thousand categories, encompassing all interventions made by physicians and other health care professionals. A Relative Value Unit is assigned to every code and, when multiplied by a conversion factor, generates the amount of the practitioner's fee. These work values may be increased or decreased from time to time, and they may also be used by various payers with their own multipliers.

Billing categories distinguish between inpatient treatment (including partial hospitalization and treatment in residential care settings) and outpatient treatment and allow differential payment depending on whether medical evaluation and management services are an additional feature of the psychotherapy. Presumably, most psychotherapy performed by psychiatrists has an evaluation and management component as an integral feature, because it includes such things as ongoing diagnostic evaluation, pharmacotherapy, interpretation of laboratory and radiological studies, and overall treatment planning responsibility. Evolution and management is also associated with a higher reimbursement rate because of the additional work involved. For illustrative purposes, several selected procedural codes are listed in Table 43–5.

One positive step psychiatrist-administrators can take, although a bit foreign to our training and experience, is marketing of services. This is of ever-increasing importance. Consumer groups, insurers, and any other payers must be made aware of and encouraged in the appropriate use of those services, both general and special, that we provide, so that resource utilization is maximized and downtime is avoided.

UTILIZATION MANAGEMENT

Cost containment is not only a priority for government-sponsored methods of payment for health care, but also almost a national obsession. Private insurers and other payers are equally concerned, because the cost of health insurance continues to increase. Employers are limiting the amount they are willing to pay for employee medical care, and the period of charging what the traffic will bear is over. One common method of cutting insurance costs is to increase the annual deductible that the individual and family must pay before the company will reimburse expenses. In addition, and this is all too frequently applied to mental health care, there is the technique of increasing the copayment for which the insured is personally responsible. This is accomplished either by raising the percentage of copayment or by lowering the maximum amount that will be reimbursed per treatment visit.

Utilization review has been around for many years, in part as a cost control. Originally required for Medicare, it is now applied to all payers and patients and is necessary for hospital accreditation. Performance of this function may be prospective (i.e., in the form of preadmission certification), concurrent (i.e., while the patient is hospitalized), or retrospective (i.e., after discharge). Utilization review serves to ensure that the treatment is indicated and that the services are provided in an efficient manner. The consensus is that little real money has been saved by utilization review alone.

For the 1990s, and probably beyond, "the practice of psychiatry has been transformed by those who pay the bill" (Sharfstein 1992, p. vii). The use of resources is more carefully overseen by third-party payers such as insurance companies and now by so-called fourth parties (i.e., utilization management companies under contract to approve, deny, and monitor care rendered to beneficiaries). A system of case-by-case allocation, known as *utilization management*, is created.

When utilization management is combined with a select network of providers, both institutions and individuals, the result is a system of service delivery called *managed care* (American Psychiatric Association, Committee on Managed Care 1992). Traditional mental health and substance abuse services are commonly combined under the rubric of behavioral health care.

Pretreatment authorization provides an advance evaluation of proposed services in terms of both the site (hospital, office) and the level of intensity. Duration of treatment and the particular modalities to be used must be specified. Even then, approval may be given for no more than initial procedures for evaluation and creation of a treatment plan. Only those interventions that are consistent with the treatment plan will be approved, and finite (i.e., short) intervals for additional review will be delineated. More expensive items such as inpatient admission undergo greater scrutiny,

TABLE 43–5. **Examples of procedural codes**

CPT code	Description
90801	Psychiatric diagnostic interview examination . . .
90806	Individual psychotherapy . . . in an office or outpatient facility, approximately 45 to 50 minutes face-to-face with the patient
90807	. . . with medical evaluation and management services
90816	Individual psychotherapy . . . inpatient . . . 20 to 30 minutes face-to-face with the patient
90817	. . . with medical evaluation and management services
90862	Pharmacologic management . . . with no more than minimal medical psychotherapy
90865	Narcosynthesis for psychiatric diagnostic and therapeutic purposes
90870	Electroconvulsive therapy (includes necessary monitoring); single seizure

Source. Adapted from American Medical Association 1997.

but ambulatory services are subjected to authorization procedures as well.

While the patient is receiving care, the treatment is reviewed concurrently. In the case of inpatient care, this review could be performed as frequently as every few days but rarely exceeding a week; whereas treatment for psychiatric outpatients might be reviewed every 10 sessions. Scrutinized are treatment plan updates and other modifications, progress notes, and even special forms and summaries created by the third and fourth parties solely for this purpose. The provider will need to demonstrate that progress toward treatment goals is being made and that, regardless of modality, the inpatient is moving in the direction of fulfilling the criteria for discharge readiness. Some review organizations provide case managers to assist this process, but many of our colleagues view this as an unhelpful intrusion into the doctor-patient relationship.

To ensure approval of treatment, the provider must at a minimum demonstrate medical necessity. This is defined as that which is adequate and essential for evaluation and/or treatment of disease, is reasonably expected to improve the patient's condition or level of functioning, and is in keeping with accepted standards of psychiatric practice (American Psychiatric Association, Committee on Managed Care 1992). Some consider this to be cost effectiveness, whereas others look at it simply as "no frills" care.

By now the reader may be wondering why any facility or practitioner would become part of managed care. Why agree in advance to such utilization management, limited referral sources, and use of specified hospitals and consultants only? The answer is deceptively simple: to survive. As collaboration is replaced by competition and as more and more entities are moving in the direction of managed care, there are fewer and fewer patients not covered by one or another such plan. Hospitals make no money from empty beds, and therapists do not get paid for unfilled hours. Increasingly, also, practitioners' existing patients are being switched to managed care plans, as employers or insurers bite at the lure of cost containment.

IS IT WORKING?

Utilization management as a cost-cutting paradigm is controversial among health care professionals. Three recent studies suggest that the system may have gotten out of control before it was adequately tested and evaluated.

Warres et al. (1996) looked at initial and subsequent authorization by utilization reviewers for ongoing treatment. They found a low rate of outright denial but observed that fewer sessions than requested were usually authorized, and they concluded that much of the time and

money spent on intrusive review was squandered. Particularly troublesome were the detrimental effects on the treatment process, most prominently manifested as interference with the process of termination. In two-thirds of the cases in which authorization was denied, the providers judged that decision to be unreasonable or dangerous.

Wickizer et al. (1996) found that the modal outcome of the preadmission process was approval, but approval for fewer days than had been sought. The vast majority of admissions were approved for 1 week. The average total number of hospital days was 16.8, only 71% of the 23.5 days requested by the treating practitioners. Wickizer and colleagues also noted a lack of length-of-stay variability, even within diagnoses, and commented on the loss in physician and nurse productivity through time spent negotiating and documenting the need for additional time authorization.

Goldman et al. (1997) examined the validity of several widely used psychiatric utilization management criteria sets for inpatient admission and continued stay. Few differences were found in terms of admission judgments, but some of the criteria sets in wide use were found to be unsatisfactory for determining continued stay. The authors suggested modification and subsequent presentation of evidence for the validity of these utilization management schemata and questioned their continued use to assess appropriate levels of care.

One of us (Rachlin 1992) examined how the legal system has responded to situations in which patient harm resulted after third and fourth parties denied continued hospital stay. There have been only a few reported cases thus far, but it appears that a practitioner is not likely to be protected from liability for adverse outcomes resulting from economic constraints. We remain fully accountable for our clinical decisions, which must be made in the best interest of the patient.

Insurers will continue to be held to a legal standard of good faith and fair dealing, and they will be required to do their reviews responsibly and in accordance with accepted standards. The professions, however, are held to a higher level, that of ethics. This makes it the responsibility of the psychiatrist not to abandon her or his patient but to continue to provide necessary care, at least until an acceptable arrangement can be made, even in the absence of reimbursement.

Finally, there is the particularly invidious vulnerability of public sector services to cost-containment activities (Rachlin 1992; Tischler 1990). If, for example, continued hospitalization is deemed indicated by the staff of a private facility but the utilization management system disagrees and refuses to pay, the options are to continue to treat while incurring substantial financial loss or to attempt to arrange a transfer to a government-sponsored hospital. It may be presumed that the latter course will be pursued more often than not. As for outpatient care, what happens when additional psychotherapy is needed by patients and continuing reimbursement is denied? Can these patients simply be sent to public clinics, which surely will not relish taking responsibility for individuals whose coverage has run out? We are also aware of the limitations of the public sector, in which there is often inadequate financial support from governments strapped for cash.

The issues raised in this section affect not only administrative psychiatrists, but also clinical practitioners in all areas of the healing profession. Further, there is major overlap with issues raised by managed care, the focus of Chapter 47.

QUALITY ASSESSMENT AND IMPROVEMENT

Despite the fiscal constraints just delineated, patients and payers both want to know that the treatment they receive is of high or at least professionally acceptable quality. The ethics of medicine require no less of us as psychiatrists. The very finest care possible cannot truly be delivered for pennies, but we owe it to our patients to strike an equitable balance, however difficult that may be. The process of quality assurance is partially intended to approach this goal.

Quality assessment is today an established part of American culture. It is required not only by third and fourth parties but also by virtually every accrediting or regulatory agency with which we come into contact.

Quality assessment has not been a static entity, having had a series of modifications over the years, and it is destined to evolve further. As previously mentioned, perhaps the first phase of quality management was utilization review: looking at the necessity for, and efficiency and utilization of, health care resources. Federally mandated peer review organizations came on the scene not only to ensure quality in situations where taxes were funding treatment, but to attempt to contain costs as well.

Understanding quality assurance requires learning a new vocabulary. Fauman (1989) and Wilson and Phillips (1992) provided valuable dictionaries and other information on the process. Use of the phrase *quality care* implies that there is optimal outcome through the use of appropriate and available resources, that the provider meets explicit or implicit standards, and that the type of facility and kinds of services are relevant to the patient's diagnosis and clinical needs. *Standards* are established principles that are expected or required and against which measurement may be made. *Norms* are qualitative or quantitative measures of aspects of practice. Standards and norms combine to produce the criteria used to make quality-of-care judgments, because they define the appropriateness of care. These criteria need to be elucidated by professionals, from experience and the literature, and applied by peers once a review is triggered by internal or external request. Criteria can pertain to structure (Does the provider have appropriate resources and mechanisms?), process (How is care actually provided?), or outcome (What are the actual results for the patient?).

Quality assurance applies to medical staffs, hospital-wide functions, and individual clinical and support service activities. There are many things a department of psychiatry might choose to monitor, including psychopharmacological practices and discharges against medical advice. At a minimum one should study interventions that are problem prone, high risk, or used in high volume. If such monitoring fails to reveal problems, it would be wise to move on to something else for a while. One gets no credit for blind perseverance, nor does one improve patient care by not looking at problems. Such approaches would turn the whole process into meaningless movement of paper. So-called sentinel events, such as a suicide attempt or elopement from a locked unit, are of sufficient magnitude to warrant investigation of each occurrence. Review of appropriateness of seclusion and restraint usage is also expected.

EVOLUTIONARY CHANGES

There is a clear trend in quality assurance away from process toward outcome monitoring—that is, determining whether a high level of care is actually provided. Mirin and Namerow (1991) argued that despite difficulty in design and implementation, outcome study is crucial so that we modify our clinical practices in accordance with knowledge of which modalities are essential, which are useful, and which are ineffective. There are many treatment-related variables and a complicated system of mental health delivery, yet Mirin and Namerow wondered if the future might not tie reimbursement to outcome data. Incidentally, it is not just clinical status but patients' interpersonal relationships, their ability to function in society, and their quality of life that can and should be examined.

A postulated ideal system for evaluating outcome was offered by Sederer and colleagues (1997). It would be clinically relevant (useful and timely), sensitive to change, culturally sensitive, and of low burden and low cost; would involve the patient; would be built into standard operating procedures; and would meet the requirements of quality improvement, regulatory agencies, payers, and the community. The object is to relate interventions (e.g., inpatient days, partial hospitalization days, and outpatient visits) to clinical outcome (e.g., patient well-being, functioning, and/or symptoms), which can then be linked to cost (dollars per unit of service). One needs also to control for demographics and clinical variables such as diagnosis, legal status, and concomitant substance abuse. Patient satisfaction is a particularly pertinent outcome that we strive to achieve. Choosing tools for assessment involves determining whom, what, where, when, and how to measure. Recent publications attest to the fact that evaluation along the dimension of outcome has come of age in the field of mental health (Lyons et al. 1997; Sederer and Dickey 1996).

Kinzie et al. (1992) described how they applied traditional mortality-morbidity conferences to psychiatry. These sessions also served a risk management function. *Risk management* is the subdivision of quality improvement concerned with identification, analysis, and actions to deal with potential legal liability. Kinzie and colleagues reviewed deaths, major medical complications, seclusion and restraint, extended length of stay, early readmission, suicide attempts, and violence and presented the first 100 undesirable outcomes. A fair number of these events were judged at least potentially avoidable; the authors stressed that this process is just one component of their overall program.

A related aspect is the development of *clinical practice guidelines*, also known as *practice parameters*. Although practice guidelines may reduce variations in treatment and enhance quality, they may just as well not result in lowered utilization or costs. Variances should be assessed to assure that they have not resulted in the diminution of quality. Further details are to be found in Chapter 48, which is devoted to the subject of practice guidelines.

CONTINUOUS QUALITY IMPROVEMENT

The quality (performance) improvement process involves, in an ongoing manner, a broad view of the overall system rather than a focus on individual practitioner aberrances. There is less emphasis on the occasional, unusual event and more emphasis on common problems. Communication of results to all staff is an essential ingredient. In the best circumstances, the process is cross-disciplinary and interdepartmental.

Traditional quality assurance and the newer continuous quality improvement (CQI) are further differentiated by Paul (1996). As his table demonstrates (Table 43–6), there has been a notable change in focus in the last decade.

The prior emphasis (that is, in quality assurance) was somewhat punitive and regulatory, whereas there is a recognition in CQI that system issues are the principal cause of quality problems. CQI is concurrent and future oriented and distinguishes common from special causes of variation. Quality assurance may well identify events for which the quality improvement process should be applied.

CQI can be considered a method of improving the quality of care by strengthening organizational systems and processes, which then lead to improved outcome and better performances across all levels of staff. Stated a bit differently, organizational functions (activities) are composed of goal-directed and interrelated series of processes (actions to achieve a result), the performance of which leads to outcomes, those which we ultimately strive to improve.

Consider for example the function of assessment of patients, which includes 1) collecting data about each patient's physical and psychosocial status and health history, 2) analyzing the data to determine each patient's treatment needs and to identify any additional required information, and 3) making individualized care decisions based on the data. Further, it is necessary to distinguish between common (inherent) causes of variation and special (unpredictable, external) causes, because we can better reduce the former by modifying the program. Staff teams, regardless of

TABLE 43–6. Comparative characteristics of quality assessment tools

Quality assurance	Quality improvement
Identifies a problem	Cross-disciplinary team focus
Sets a performance standard	Considers all causes of variation
Screens to insure compliance with standard	Patient and customer focused
Identifies individual deficiencies	Applies statistical thinking
Takes corrective action to achieve performance standard	Data driven
Focuses on structure, process, and outcome	Benchmarks to "best practice"
Has a punitive component	Focuses on system improvement
Targets high-volume, high-risk services	De-emphasizes individual blame
Targets special causes of variation	
Limited use of statistical thinking	

Source. Reprinted with permission from Paul L: "Comparative characteristics of quality assessment tools." *The Physician Executive* 22:18, 1996. Copyright 1996, American College of Physician Executives.

discipline, department, or rank, study aspects of care with which they are involved on a day-to-day basis to identify that which can be improved and how such improvement may best be accomplished. A special cause of variation, although potentially an opportunity to reduce errors, should not be the impetus for a change in process, because it is not representative of the usual course of events.

Improvement opportunities must be prioritized, so that more attention is given to that which may have the greatest impact on performance and outcome. Various process improvement models, all cyclical, were compared by P. Keill and Johnson (1994), who added one of their own, labeled with the acronym *PRIDE*: choose a *p*rocess to improve, measure *r*elevant dimensions of performance, *i*nterpret and evaluate variance, *d*esign or redesign the process, and *e*xecute an improvement plan and validate by remeasuring.

The Joint Commission on Accreditation of Healthcare Organizations (1996) pays close attention to efforts at improving organization performance, which includes not only doing the right thing but doing the right thing well. We are expected to continuously design, quantify, assess, and improve both process and outcome measures. Further, these efforts are to be patient centered, performance focused, and organized around functions common to health care organizations.

To understand how this operates in real life, we turn to instructive examples provided by Coker et al. (1997). Their service began to admit increasing numbers of seriously and persistently mentally ill involuntary patients, individuals who had minimal family involvement but multiple social service needs and who presented threatening and disturbing behaviors. To better serve these patients, they undertook a process of management as a team effort, using data to guide their reasoning, thereby improving services and satisfying their patients.

In the first part of this effort, Coker's group responded to staff perceptions that the process of transferring patients from the crisis intervention site to the inpatient unit involved unnecessary delays. Time was lost between approval for admission and transfer to the ward, and there were even additional waits outside the door to the ward. Simply investigating the process produced enough improvement that no corrective measures were required; it was also determined that the problems were actually less serious than the staff had believed.

More concrete results were obtained by the authors' efforts to review and revise treatment planning. There were two separate documents, one produced by nursing and the other by the rest of the staff. The team developed a single list of patient care problems in 11 broad categories.

Corresponding goals and objectives, at least one per problem, were written. Although goals were general, objectives were discipline specific, as were treatment interventions. There emerged a comprehensive interdisciplinary plan, both general and specific, involving weekly updates and patient participation.

CONCLUSIONS

This chapter is intended to encourage readers to enhance their knowledge of psychiatric administration. We believe that this should increase the pool of psychiatrists who are able and willing to provide personal and professional leadership and who have executive skills, which in turn should improve the care our patients receive. The subjects addressed are those that need to be understood by all who are engaged in psychiatry as practiced in organized care settings. This chapter is not intended to provide complete knowledge or expertise in the field. Such understanding can only come from experience, further reading, and learning from colleagues. We urge the reader to study the previously mentioned relevant chapters of this textbook and the suggested readings listed at the end of this chapter.

Systems for the delivery of psychiatric services are becoming so complex that leadership of these programs is more important than ever. The executive role must be occupied by clinicians who possess a comprehensive understanding of the nature and management of mental illness, garnered through first-hand experience in actual treatment and through extensive education and training in its biopsychosocial phenomena. A fundamental skill of a successful leader—that of understanding interpersonal relationships—is already part of the psychiatrist's professional armamentarium.

There are monotonous aspects of the administrative psychiatrist's position, but these are outweighed by the excitement and challenges. It is our firm belief that leadership is at least as exciting and rewarding as any other opportunity available to the physician. Improving the delivery of treatment services is one of the ultimate responsibilities of the dedicated clinician and has clear potential for changing the lives of men and women with mental illness.

REFERENCES

American Medical Association: Physicians' Current Procedural Terminology/CPT '98 (Professional Edition); 4th Edition, 19th Revision. Chicago, IL, American Medical Association, 1997

American Psychiatric Association, Committee on Managed Care: Utilization Management: A Handbook for Psychiatrists. Washington, DC, American Psychiatric Association, 1992

Barton WE, Barton GM: The psychiatrist-administrator, in Psychiatric Administration: A Comprehensive Text for the Clinician-Executive. Edited by Talbott JA, Kaplan SR. New York, Grune & Stratton, 1983, pp 179–185

Coker M, Sharp J, Powell H, et al: Implementation of total quality management after reconfiguration of services on a general hospital unit. Psychiatr Serv 48:231–236, 1997

Dorwart RA, Chartock L, Epstein S: Financing of services, in Textbook of Administrative Psychiatry. Edited by Talbott JA, Hales RE, Keill SL. Washington, DC, American Psychiatric Press, 1992, pp 313–346

Fauman MA: Quality assurance monitoring in psychiatry. Am J Psychiatry 146:1121–1130, 1989

Goldman RL, Weir CR, Turner CW, et al: Validity of utilization management criteria for psychiatry. Am J Psychiatry 154:349–354, 1997

Joint Commission on Accreditation of Healthcare Organizations: Comprehensive Accreditation Manual for Hospitals: The Official Handbook. Oakbrook Terrace, IL, Joint Commission on Accreditation of Healthcare Organizations, 1996

Keill P, Johnson T: Optimizing performance through process improvement. J Nurs Care Qual 9 (1):1–9, 1994

Keill SL: Recurring issues in psychiatric administration: a 3,500-year perspective. Journal of the American Association of Psychiatric Administrators 4 (1):6–7, 1981

Keill SL: Strategies of influence: the psychiatrist-executive as a political being, in Administrative Issues in Public Mental Health (New Dir Ment Health Serv No 49). Edited by Keill SL. San Francisco, CA, Jossey-Bass, 1991, pp 79–89

Kinzie JD, Maricle RA, Bloom JD, et al: Improving quality assurance through psychiatric mortality and morbidity conferences in a university hospital. Hosp Community Psychiatry 43:470–474, 1992

Kraft AM: Behavioral and organizational theories, in Psychiatric Administration: A Comprehensive Text for the Clinician-Executive. Edited by Talbott JA, Kaplan SR. New York, Grune & Stratton, 1983, pp 123–133

Levinson D, Klerman G: The clinician-executive and the clinician-executive revisited. Administration in Mental Health 3:52–67, 1972

Lipton AA, Loutsch E: A reconsideration of power in psychiatric administration. Hosp Community Psychiatry 36:497–503, 1985

Lyons J, Howard K, O'Mahoney M, et al: The Measurement and Management of Clinical Outcomes in Mental Health. Washington, DC, American Psychiatric Press, 1997

Marcos LR, Silver MA: Psychiatrist-executive management styles: nature or nurture? Am J Psychiatry 145:103–106, 1988

Menninger WW: Hope and morale: critical elements in organizational function. Paper presented at the annual meeting of the American Psychiatric Association, Washington, DC, May 1992

Mirin SM, Namerow MJ: Why study treatment outcome? Hosp Community Psychiatry 42:1007–1013, 1991

Paul L: Quality assessment tools add value. Physician Executive 22 (10):16–19, 1996

Rachlin S: The psychiatrist-administrator in the economic crossfire, in American Psychiatric Press Review of Clinical Psychiatry and the Law, Vol 3. Edited by Simon RI. Washington, DC, American Psychiatric Press, 1992, pp 209–218

Ranz J, Rosenheck S, Deakins S: Columbia University's fellowship in public psychiatry. Psychiatr Serv 47:512–516, 1996

Rodenhauser P, Hatchette RK, Arce AA: A survey of psychiatrists with APA certification in administrative psychiatry. Psychiatr Serv 46:1278–1282, 1995

Sederer LI, Dickey B (eds): Outcomes Assessment in Clinical Practice. Baltimore, MD, Williams & Wilkins, 1996

Sederer LI, Dickey B, Eisen SV: Assessing outcomes in clinical practice. Psychiatr Q 68:316–325, 1997

Shafritz JM, Hyde AC (eds): Classics of Public Administration, 2nd Edition. Chicago, IL, Dorsey Press, 1987

Sharfstein SS: Foreword, in Utilization Management: A Handbook for Psychiatrists. Washington, DC, American Psychiatric Association, 1992, p vii

Taintor Z, Schwarz M, Miller M: Computers and patient care, in American Psychiatric Press Review of Psychiatry, Vol 16. Edited by Dickstein LJ, Riba MB, Oldham JM. Washington, DC, American Psychiatric Press, 1997, pp 15–60

Talbott JA: Management, administration, leadership: what's in a name? Psychiatr Q 58:229–242, 1987

Talbott JA, Keill SL: A typology of state hospital directors, in State Mental Hospitals: Problems and Potentials. Edited by Talbott JA. New York, Human Sciences Press, 1980, pp 88–105

Tischler GL: Utilization management of mental health services by private third parties. Am J Psychiatry 147:967–973, 1990

Warren SJ: Budget, in Textbook of Administrative Psychiatry. Edited by Talbott JA, Hales RE, Keill SL. Washington, DC, American Psychiatric Press, 1992, pp 287–312

Warres NE, Soderstrom P, Marcus LA, et al: The impact of managed care and utilization review: a cross sectional study in Maryland. Psychiatr Serv 47:1319–1322, 1996

Wickizer TM, Lessler D, Travis KM: Controlling inpatient psychiatric utilization through managed care. Am J Psychiatry 153:339–345, 1996

Wilson GF, Phillips KL: Concepts and definitions used in quality assurance and utilization review, in Manual of Psychiatric Quality Assurance: A Report of the American Psychiatric Association Committee on Quality Assurance. Edited by Mattson MR. Washington, DC, American Psychiatric Association, 1992, pp 23–30

SUGGESTED READINGS

Barton WE, Barton GM: Mental Health Administration: Principles and Practice. New York, Human Sciences Press, 1983

Greenblatt M (ed): Anatomy of Psychiatric Administration: The Organization in Health and Disease. New York, Plenum, 1992

Keill SL (ed): Administrative Issues in Public Mental Health (New Dir Ment Health Serv No 49). San Francisco, CA, Jossey-Bass, 1991

Talbott JA, Kaplan SR (eds): Psychiatric Administration: A Comprehensive Text for the Clinician-Executive. New York, Grune & Stratton, 1983

Talbott JA, Hales RE, Keill SL (eds): Textbook of Administrative Psychiatry. Washington, DC, American Psychiatric Press, 1992

CHAPTER 44

PSYCHIATRIC EDUCATION

JONATHAN F. BORUS, M.D.
WILLIAM H. SLEDGE, M.D.

Psychiatric education is a broad area involving many different teachers and learners. Teachers use didactic and experiential opportunities to help learners acquire 1) a knowledge base about normal and abnormal human behavior, 2) clinical skills to understand and therapeutically intervene to relieve suffering and restore function, and 3) appropriate attitudes and empathic sensitivity to interact successfully with patients to understand and treat their emotional disorders. Many forces affect psychiatric education, including the academic settings in which much of the education occurs, organizations accrediting individual learners and educational programs, professional and public interest groups concerned about both the education and its products, and economic and political influences on the profession that shape its educational possibilities.

This chapter will focus on the influence of these forces on undergraduate (medical student) education, graduate (resident) education and training, subspecialty (fellowship) training, continuing psychiatric education for psychiatric practitioners, and education of nonpsychiatric physicians as well as nonphysician mental health professionals during training and practice. Although important, education of the public, including policy makers and families of mentally ill persons, will not be addressed.

LEARNING PRINCIPLES IN MEDICAL AND PSYCHIATRIC EDUCATION

Education in medicine, as in other areas, is an interactive process between teachers and learners that is based on educational principles (Table 44–1). A first principle is that there are many different teaching and learning methods and styles, and thus the alliance and congruence between teacher and learner are important variables (for example, a teacher who insists on lecturing to a visual learner will not be successful). Too often in psychiatry, as in other medical disciplines, exposure to information is considered sufficient to produce learning. Most curricula require only that learners sit through a course of lectures, attend a defined seminar series, and/or see a specific number of patients. The fact that such exposure to information and practice issues is deemed adequate betrays a naive conception of how people learn.

A second educational principle is that learners not only must be exposed to new information but also must incorporate it (a process often aided by multimodal exposure and repetition), integrate the new material with existing ideas and skills, and master the newly integrated knowledge through putting it to use in their professional and personal activities (Borus 1993a).

TABLE 44–1.   Four principles of medical and psychiatric education

1. There are many different teaching and learning methods and styles; therefore, the alliance and congruence between teacher and learner are important variables.

2. For learning to occur, the learner must be *exposed* to new information, *incorporate* it, *integrate* it with existing knowledge or skills, and *gain mastery* by using the new knowledge.

3. The learner is given progressively increasing responsibility for patient care as he or she gains knowledge, skills, and experience.

4. The learner must appreciate the powerful emotions in the patient-doctor relationship and understand how to monitor, control, and utilize them to advance the treatment.

Medical education is also based on the principle of progressively increasing the learner's responsibility as he or she gains knowledge, skills, and experience (Accreditation Council for Graduate Medical Education 1996; Association of American Medical Colleges 1984; Ludmerer 1985). In medical education this progression begins with presentation of basic information to provide a knowledge base for the learner to understand a problem, and the progression continues with demonstration of the problem and its treatment by an experienced clinician, work by the learner under direct supervision, individual work by the learner with collateral (indirect) supervision, and, finally, work by the learner alone without ongoing supervision but with lifelong, self-initiated, continuing education. A specific problem in this paradigm for psychiatry is that to ensure confidentiality, the psychiatrist often works in a dyadic relationship with the patient without a supervisor's directly observing the patient-doctor interaction. Whether in psychotherapy, consultation on a medical ward, or in an emergency room setting, there is a danger that a neophyte psychiatric learner may be put into a situation in which he or she is overwhelmed by or harmful to the patient. Psychiatric educators must develop ways to monitor directly, as well as supervise collaterally, psychiatry trainees so that this pitfall is avoided.

In medicine, the terms *education* and *training* are often used interchangeably. However, these terms properly refer to different kinds of learning (Eaton 1980). *Education* is the development of the capacity for understanding, analysis, and problem solving in unique and novel circumstances. It may involve the study of topics and areas that seem to have little direct relevance to particular clinical problems. *Training*, also a type of learning, refers to the capacity to carry out specific behaviors and apply particular skills in a prescribed and standardized manner. Surgeons are trained to make precise incisions and educated about infection, anatomy, and physiological function. Psychiatrists are educated to understand depression and trained to prescribe antidepressants and carry out electroconvulsive therapy.

A fourth principle of medical education, having special implications for psychiatry, is the professionalization of intimacy (Parsons 1951). Physicians are sanctioned to explore intimate bodily areas and functions, and psychiatrists are expected to share in patients' most intimate thoughts and feelings as well. Therefore, psychiatric educators must help their learners understand the powerful emotional issues in the patient-doctor relationship and how to monitor, control, and use them to the advantage of the patient. Psychiatric professionals also must become intimately acquainted with themselves as evaluative and therapeutic "instruments," to understand, and intervene in, patients' disturbed behaviors and emotions. Facilitating the concurrent learning by trainees about themselves and their patients is a major task in psychiatric education.

THE CURRICULUM AND ITS EVALUATION

The curriculum is the heart of any educational endeavor. In medical and psychiatric education and training, the curriculum at the medical school and graduate levels is shaped by national regulatory agencies that accredit medical schools and residency programs. There are several aspects of a curriculum: educational philosophy; goals and objectives; teaching content and methods; learning resources including students, teachers, and materials; and evaluation.

Educational philosophy is the set of guiding principles and beliefs, such as those described in the previous section, that characterize the educational vision of those educators responsible for the development of the curriculum. Every curriculum has an educational philosophy, although that philosophy may not be explicit or sophisticated. Goals and objectives are more concrete accounts of what is intended to be achieved during and at the end of the learning experience. Terminal objectives are the final learning outcome and are often expressed in behavioral terms. Enabling objectives are the building blocks that compose the final outcome and are usually expressed as attitudes, knowledge, skills, and/or behaviors.

Methods for teaching psychiatry are many and diverse, but the methods used to teach a particular content area must be consistent with the learning goals in that area. For example, if a terminal objective is to teach trainees to conduct an initial psychiatric interview with a psychotic person, then the methods must include performing an interview. It would be inappropriate to rely solely on lectures to accomplish this objective; however, lectures may serve other important objectives by exposing the learner to basic information. Teaching methods in psychiatry include didactic lectures and demonstrations, supervision, small group discussions and seminars, rounds and small group clinical demonstrations, use of videotapes and audiotapes, and computer-aided instruction (Block 1996; Fauman 1989; Jachna et al. 1993; Powsner and Byck 1991).

Resources include students, teachers, time, settings, materials, and other valuable commodities such as money. A curriculum's goals and objectives must be consistent with the opportunities afforded by and limitations posed by the available resources.

Evaluation strategies must reflect and be consistent with the goals and methods of teaching. An evaluation may be of teachers, learners, programs, or all three at once. Evaluation measures include pretests and posttests to determine what was learned (usually in the form of cognitive knowledge but sometimes also in that of problem-solving capability), demonstration of certain clinical skills, and assessment of attitudes observed directly in the conduct of an intervention or indirectly through the reports of others (including patients) or with psychometric instruments. Other outcome measures used to assess psychiatric educational programs include accounts of what students do with their careers when they finish the program and what they liked or did not like about the training experience.

Students' assessments can be both an invaluable, easily obtained form of teacher evaluation and an integral aspect of program evaluation. Student reports of faculty effectiveness, collected blindly and prospectively, can be useful as a means of indicating the value of faculty members' teaching efforts. Graduating residents can be asked to name and describe the faculty who were particularly important to their growth and development as residents. When faculty members are proposed for reappointment or promotion review, former students and residents can be asked to reflect on the enduring value of the teaching of a particular faculty member. Ongoing evaluation by faculty and trainees of all aspects of the educational curriculum (philosophy, goals and objectives, teaching content and methods, resources, and the evaluation itself) is essential to the curriculum's continuing development (Borus and Yager 1986).

PSYCHIATRY IN THE ACADEMIC MEDICAL CENTER

The modern medical university has become the primary context in which psychiatric education and training are carried out in the United States. Although in the period before World War II psychiatric specialty training was largely based in state and private psychiatric hospitals, psychiatric education at the undergraduate level has always been carried out within medical school settings. Today, psychiatry residency training programs require a medical school affiliation for full accreditation (Accreditation Council for Graduate Medical Education 1996), and most continuing education also takes place within university medical centers and their closely affiliated institutions.

The location of psychiatric education and training in academic departments has had many effects. First, it has been one element in the remedicalization of our field that has seen an increased emphasis on psychiatry's biological underpinnings and a concomitant increase in biologically oriented research. In academic medical centers, research productivity that is understood and respected by colleagues from other medical disciplines is essential to faculty advancement and tenure. Not only have psychiatry faculty become more biological and descriptive in their intellectual orientation, but their advancement has come to depend increasingly on their research production, publication, and the ability to compete successfully for limited research funds (Carter 1992). In this milieu, education may become a secondary demand on the time and devotion of faculty (Borus 1993a).

Increasingly, academic psychiatrists must not only direct their efforts toward the establishment of a viable academic career as investigator/scholar and teacher, but also help fill the income needs of their departments. Since psychiatric reimbursement is primarily based on direct practitioner-patient contact rather than tests or procedures that can be administered by others, earning money for one's department is a demanding proposition, especially in these days of managed care and unprecedented cost-cutting efforts aimed at all aspects of psychiatry.

Within the modern university medical center, with its demanding tasks and complex social structures, it is important that psychiatry faculty have good relations not only with peer and mentoring colleagues within their own department but also with colleagues in other medical school departments. Such interdepartmental connections reduce isolation and increase access to opportunities for clinical program development, research, and teaching. Most nonpsychiatric academic clinicians welcome help in thinking about and dealing with the complex biopsychosocial forces that shape today's medical practice. Psychiatrists' grounding in psychological, social, and cultural disciplines provides them with the conceptual and clinical background to help other physicians deal more effectively with vexatious patient problems. Furthermore, with the expansion of neurobiological knowledge within psychiatry, professionals in other disciplines have found it increasingly beneficial to collaborate with psychiatrists. For example, the developing imaging techniques frequently make collaborators of psychiatry, nuclear medicine, and diagnostic radiology faculty. Similarly, opportunities in neural cell transplantation, basic neuroscience, and pharmacology have led psychiatrists, neuroscientists, and pharmacologists into effective collaborations.

REGULATION OF PSYCHIATRIC EDUCATION

Education in the field of psychiatry, as in all other medical specialties, is embedded in regulatory systems established to create public accountability and maintain professional standards through regular review and certification. Such regulation includes medical licensing, which is performed at the state level. In addition, regulation is aimed toward individuals through certification by the American Board of Psychiatry and Neurology (ABPN), and other psychiatry subspecialty boards; and toward programs through accreditation by the Liaison Committee on Medical Education (LCME) for undergraduate education, the Psychiatry Residency Review Committee (RRC) of the Accreditation Council for Graduate Medical Education (ACGME) for residency programs, and the Accreditation Council for Continuing Medical Education (ACCME) for continuing education programs.

Certification is the means by which individuals demonstrate that their skills and knowledge meet the standards of competency of the profession. Certification is voluntary, but it is increasingly linked to managed care credentialing and institutional compensation. The ABPN performs this certification function for the specialty fields of general psychiatry, child and adolescent psychiatry, and neurology and has begun certifying subspecialists in some psychiatric areas such as addictions, forensic, and geriatric psychiatry. The ABPN is an independent board whose members are nominated by its sponsoring organizations, the American Medical Association (AMA), the American Psychiatric Association (APA), the American Neurological Association, and the American Academy of Neurology (American Board of Psychiatry and Neurology 1996; Scheiber 1989). The ABPN is a member of the American Board of Medical Specialties (ABMS), which sets standards and serves as an advocacy organization for all medical specialty boards. The ABPN offers graduates of accredited residency programs in general psychiatry or child and adolescent psychiatry a written test of knowledge and a clinical test of skills, knowl-

edge, and attitudes for those who pass the written test. Applicants for subspecialty certification in addictions, forensic, and geriatric psychiatry must be ABPN certified in general psychiatry and are assessed with a written examination only. All ABPN certifications in psychiatry and its subspecialties attained after October 1, 1994, are time limited and recertification is required every 10 years. The ABPN also has provisions for double certification in neurology and psychiatry, and internal medicine and psychiatry, and a "triple board" project whereby highly selected applicants are eligible for board certification in pediatrics, psychiatry, and child and adolescent psychiatry with a 5-year training program at a limited number of approved training centers.

Independent groups carry out certifications in other subspecialty areas of psychiatry as well. For example, the APA conducts written and oral certifying examinations in administrative psychiatry. The oldest certification process is that of the American Psychoanalytic Association (APsA), in which graduates of APsA-accredited psychoanalytic institute training programs submit written accounts of their psychoanalytic work and are orally examined about these cases as part of the certification process.

Accreditation is the process whereby programs are reviewed and measured against programmatic standards and requirements set by independent accrediting agencies. The LCME sets standards for accreditation of schools granting medical degrees in the United States and Canada and monitors accredited medical schools with written reviews and site visits every 7 years (Liaison Committee on Medical Education 1997). The ACGME sets general standards for all institutions with medical specialty training programs and conducts periodic institutional reviews to see that these standards are met. It has specialty-specific RRCs that write and monitor residency and fellowship program requirements for the appropriate specialty (Accreditation Council for Graduate Medical Education 1996). Each RRC is composed of nominees from that specialty's professional societies, the ACGME parent organizations (the AMA, the Association of American Medical Colleges, the ABMS, and the American Hospital Association), the federal government, and the public. The RRCs set specialty-specific requirements and carry out accreditation reviews of residency and fellowship programs; however, the ACGME has the final authority for policy and accreditation actions. The Psychiatry RRC is composed of 10 members: four from the ABPN (three directors and the ABPN's executive vice president), three from the APA, and three from the AMA's Council on Medical Education. Each sponsoring organization selects two general psychiatrists and one child and adolescent psychiatrist. The programmatic requirements for residency accreditation in general psychiatry and in child and adolescent psychiatry—as well as the requirements for fellowship accreditation in addictions, forensic, and geriatric psychiatry—are listed in the annual *Directory of Graduate Education Programs* (Accreditation Council for Graduate Medical Education 1996). Finally, the ACCME is the agency that sets policy and reviews programs seeking to offer continuing medical education.

In addition to the accrediting and certifying bodies noted here, there are a variety of other organizations that have particular interests in and/or influence on the conduct of psychiatric education, as described in the appendix to this chapter.

UNDERGRADUATE MEDICAL EDUCATION IN PSYCHIATRY

The Flexner Report of 1910 introduced major changes in the ways undergraduate medical students were taught (Flexner 1910), and within a decade it led to a basic restructuring of the context in which that education was provided (Ludmerer 1985). Students became more active participants in their education as teaching moved beyond the lecture hall to laboratories and hospital clinics. The context for education became the academic medical center with its full-time faculty and its strong emphasis on the generation of new knowledge. The fundamental paradigm and goals of undergraduate medical education have changed little since the 1920s. In the 1950s, as academic psychiatry blossomed with federal funding, the call for more teaching of psychiatry and behavioral sciences to medical students was heeded by departments of psychiatry (Rosenfeld 1976; Werkman 1966).

The psychiatric curriculum in undergraduate education has three basic domains of knowledge to convey to medical students (Lidz and Edelson 1970; Werkman 1966): psychopathology, the psychological and social aspects of medicine in general, and the biological underpinnings of behavior. Psychiatry is unique within the medical school curriculum in that students must learn both *basic science material* (social and behavioral sciences such as psychology, sociology, and anthropology, as well as basic biological sciences such as molecular genetics and neurobiology of behavior) and *clinical material* (e.g., psychopathology, psychopharmacology, normative response to illness, doctor-patient relationship). Psychiatry has its own domain of pathological conditions (i.e., severe mental illness) that virtually no other medical discipline shares, as well as a range of conditions that also overlap with other

areas of medicine (e.g., dementias, normative responses to illness, the nature of the doctor-patient relationship, the roles of the character of the patient and the physician in the medical encounter). Psychiatry is often allied with other departments (e.g., pharmacology, pediatrics, internal medicine, neurology, neurosciences) and is an integrative and problem-solving discipline. Most skills, knowledge, and professional attitudes in psychiatry do not rely on technology (the imaging methods are an exception) and are frequently process oriented. Psychiatry's domain represents some of the most cherished ideals of modern medical education, namely, that the student learn to think for himself or herself and relate helpfully to distressed patients.

The LCME states that the undergraduate medical curriculum "must include the sciences basic to medicine, a variety of clinical disciplines, and ethical, behavioral, and socioeconomic subjects pertinent to medicine" (Liaison Committee on Medical Education 1997, p. 13). The National Board of Medical Examiners (NBME), in its role as developer of the national student evaluation and licensing examination (the United States Medical Licensing Examination [USMLE; Federation of State Medical Boards of the United States and the National Board of Medical Examiners]), exerts substantial informal influence on what is included in the average curriculum. The psychiatric topic areas covered by the NBME in the USMLE are listed in Table 44–2. With the emphasis on the need to teach and learn massive quantities of biomedical information, some medical faculties and students are intolerant of the process orientation of modern psychiatry. The 1984 General Professional Education of the Physician (GPEP) Report (Association of American Medical Colleges 1984) focused medical educators on the need to reexamine the educational process and stimulate active faculty and student participation in general medical education. Medical schools have begun exploring problem-based, small-group teaching that integrates basic science and clinical materials, and psychiatrists have played prominent roles in several of these new ventures (Block 1996; Schmidt 1984; Tiberius 1990; Tosteson 1990). Generally, however, the medical school curriculum is still divided into 1) preclinical material that provides the basic science underpinnings for medical practice, 2) introduction to clinical medicine courses, and 3) clinical rotations with both required and elective clerkships.

THE PSYCHIATRIC CURRICULUM

In the preclinical curriculum, departments of psychiatry are frequently tasked with providing an introduction to the behavioral sciences. Such courses typically address phe-

TABLE 44–2.   United States Medical Licensing Examination (USMLE) topics in psychiatry

Step 1 Examination

Psychosocial, cultural, and environmental influences on behavior, health, and disease processes

    Progression through life cycle (birth through senescence)

        Cognitive and language development

        Motor skills development

        Sexual development (e.g., puberty, menopause)

        Social and interpersonal development

    Psychological and social factors influencing patient behavior

        Personality

        Psychodynamic and behavioral factors, related past experience

        Family and cultural factors, including socioeconomic status

        Adaptive behavioral responses to stress and illness

        Maladaptive behavioral responses to stress and illness (in general for each organ system)

        Interactions between patient and physician or health care system (e.g., transference)

    Patient interviewing, consultation, and interactions with family

        Establishing and maintaining rapport

        Gathering of data

        Approaches to patient education

        Approaches to encourage patients to make life-style changes

        Communicating bad news

    Medical ethics, jurisprudence, and professional behavior

        Consent and informed consent to treatment

        Physician-patient relationships (e.g., ethical conduct, confidentiality)

        Death and dying

        Birth-related issues

        Issues related to patient participation in research

Organization and cost of health care delivery

Pharmacodynamic and pharmacokinetic processes

    Central and peripheral nervous systems

        Abnormal processes (listed here are those specific for psychiatry)

            Psychopathological disorders or processes and their evaluation

                Early-onset disorders (e.g., mental retardation, motor skills and learning disorders, communication disorders)

                Disorders (intoxication, abuse, dependence, withdrawal) related to substance use (e.g., ethanol, nicotine, cocaine, opioids)

                Schizophrenia and other psychotic disorders

                Mood disorders

                Anxiety disorders

                Somatoform disorders

                Personality disorders

                Physical and sexual abuse of children, adults, and elders

                Other disorders (e.g., dissociative, impulse control, factitious)

    Psychosocial, cultural, and environmental considerations (of each organ system pathology)

        Influence of emotional, behavioral factors on disease prevention, progression, and treatment (e.g., diet, depression, immune system)

        Influence of disease and treatment on person, family, and society (e.g., child leukemia)

Step 2 Examination

Mental disorders

    Health maintenance

    Mechanisms of disease

    Diagnosis

    Principles of management

Source.   Data from Federation of State Medical Boards of the United States and the National Board of Medical Examiners 1997.

nomenclature such as anxiety and depression, human development from the perspective of emerging psychological capacities and social roles, and the impact on behavior of culture, race, family, and social roles. A psychodynamic or psychoanalytic perspective may also be presented. Because of the growth of biological psychiatry, psychiatry faculty often also collaborate with pharmacology faculty in the presentation of material that addresses the effects of agents on the brain, and with neurology and basic neuroscience faculties in the presentation of materials that relate

neurobiology to particular affective states and motivated behavior. Changes in general medical education since the GPEP have also stimulated collaborations between psychiatrists and primary care internists in courses focused on the sick role, the patient-doctor relationship, and psychosocial development throughout the life cycle.

In the introduction to the clinical medicine portion of the medical school curriculum, psychiatrists have the responsibility for teaching psychopathology, the diagnostic skills necessary to recognize mental illness, and appropriate treatment approaches. During this portion of the curriculum, psychiatrists are frequently called on to provide basic instruction in patient interviewing techniques and assessment of the patient's mental status.

The LCME lists psychiatry as a required clinical clerkship. This experience is usually conceptualized as a means to convey to the future nonpsychiatric medical practitioner knowledge of the manifestations of defined mental illness and available treatment approaches, as well as the skills to recognize and diagnose mental disorders and refer mentally ill patients for specialty treatment (Reiser et al. 1988). The clerkship also offers opportunities to practice psychiatric interview techniques and initiate brief treatment efforts under close supervision. Students who are considering a career in psychiatry or who want to learn more psychiatric skills may opt for advanced elective clerkships that provide more clinical responsibility, independence, and opportunities to learn about the field.

The settings and methods of teaching psychiatry in the undergraduate curriculum are best determined by the educational goals of the curriculum. Lectures to large groups are primarily useful in organizing vast quantities of material, orienting students to what is more and less important, and introducing factual material as a guide to knowledge of an area. Lectures in psychiatry should be accompanied by well-organized notes, references, and the opportunity to put to use the material covered. In general, the process-oriented material of psychiatry should be presented in settings in which it can be demonstrated, discussed, and applied. A combination of lectures, small discussion groups, seminars, workshops, and supervised clinical experiences can be an effective and well-accepted means of conveying much of the material taught in psychiatry in the undergraduate curriculum.

RECRUITMENT INTO PSYCHIATRY

There has been a marked decrease over the last several years in the number of American medical school graduates going into psychiatry, and psychiatric educators are concerned with recruitment of medical students into the field. Many students enter medical school interested in psychiatry but find themselves drifting away in the face of large personal debt, the fiscal uncertainties of our field in the era of managed care, and the continued stigmatization of psychiatry by other specialties (Borus 1993b). It is imperative that all psychiatric educators strive to present the work of psychiatry in a positive manner so that students become acquainted with the many satisfactions of a psychiatric career (Kay 1991; Kay and Bienenfeld 1992; Taintor and Robinowitz 1980).

In very few medical schools do more than 5% of the graduating students become psychiatrists. This means that the bulk of undergraduate psychiatric education is oriented toward students who will not become psychiatrists but who, under many managed care systems, will control access to psychiatric specialist care. The psychiatric educator must therefore constantly consider the view of psychiatry through the eyes of the primary care practitioner and present psychiatry as an integral part of medicine (Kaltreider et al. 1994). Psychiatric concepts and terminology should be made accessible and not exotic, overly jargonistic, or pedantic; emphasis should be placed on issues of recognition, diagnosis, and treatment or referral for psychiatric specialist care of primary care patients with mental disorders; and time should be devoted to demonstrating the roles of personality, defenses, and coping styles in patients presenting with medical and surgical illness. Furthermore, the psychiatric educator should demonstrate the value of psychological knowledge and skills in caring for nonpsychiatric patients.

GRADUATE PSYCHIATRIC EDUCATION (RESIDENCY TRAINING)

Residency in general psychiatry is a 4-year program of learning and experiential education and training through supervised clinical practice that begins after graduation from medical school. The Psychiatry RRC of the ACGME prescribes the following:

> An approved residency program in psychiatry must provide an educational experience designed to assure that its graduates will possess sound clinical judgement, requisite skills, and a high order of knowledge about the diagnosis, treatment, and prevention of all psychiatric disorders and the common medical and neurological disorders that relate to the practice of psychiatry. While residents cannot be expected to achieve the highest possible degree of expertise in all of the diagnostic and treatment procedures used in psychiatry in 4 years of training, those individuals who satisfactorily complete residency programs in psychiatry must be competent to render effective professional care to patients. Furthermore, they must have a keen awareness of their own strengths and limitations and of the necessity for continuing their own professional development. (Accreditation Council for Graduate Medical Education 1996, p. 246)

In its "Special Essentials" for psychiatry training, the Psychiatry RRC provides both broad and specific guidelines for residency program design. A minimum of

4 months of training in a primary medical care specialty (internal medicine, family practice, and/or pediatrics) and 2 months of training in neurology are required during the 4-year residency, preferentially during the first postgraduate year (PGY-I). Psychiatry programs alternately may choose to devote the full PGY-I to medicine and neurology and begin formal training in psychiatry in PGY-II. Also specified by the Psychiatry RRC are a minimum of 9 months of inpatient psychiatry, 1 year of outpatient psychiatry, 2 months of child and adolescent psychiatry, 2 months of consultation-liaison psychiatry, and a variety of clinical experiences with different patient populations and settings, the lengths of which are not specified. The latter include experiences in community, emergency, geriatric, addictions, and forensic psychiatry; individual, group, couple, and family psychotherapy; psychopharmacology; psychiatric investigation; and elective opportunities. In many programs the curriculum is structured to provide most of the required clinical experiences in the first 3 years to achieve a broad foundation in psychiatry, while allowing time in PGY-IV for the senior resident to focus on particular areas of interest.

RESIDENT SELECTION IN PSYCHIATRY

Residents are selected almost exclusively through the National Residency Matching Plan (NRMP), which runs a computerized match for postgraduate medical training in the United States. Under a single entry agreement implemented in 1988 and monitored by the national Psychiatry Match Review Board, medical students applying for residency positions in psychiatry at either the PGY-I level (in 4-year programs) or the PGY-II level (after obtaining their own PGY-I internship or after completing another medical specialty training program) do so through the NRMP, which performs a two-stage match for psychiatry and announces the results in mid-March.

TYPES OF RESIDENCIES

Robert Michels (personal communication, 1982) has heuristically described three types of psychiatry residencies that aim at producing different kinds of psychiatrists. The first is the "scientific residency," which aims to produce research psychiatrists (Table 44–3). Bright, creative, and, at times, eccentric applicants are recruited for these programs, which are loosely structured with few requirements and ample elective time to facilitate research production during residency. Leaders of such programs realize that the residents may not become excellent psychiatric clinicians and may even drop out of training to pursue full-time

TABLE 44–3. **Three types of psychiatry residencies**

Scientific residency

Aim	To produce research psychiatrists
Recruits	Creative applicants with research track records
Curriculum	Minimal clinical requirements, maximal elective time for research
Strength	Provides time and resources to develop future research psychiatrists
Weakness	Does not provide superior clinical training

Apprenticeship residency

Aim	To produce "master craftsmen" in one particular type of psychiatric practice
Recruits	Applicants interested in that specific area of psychiatry
Curriculum	Focuses most of training on residents' learning, under close supervision from expert practitioners, that one area
Strength	Provides intensive clinical knowledge and experience in that area
Weakness	Does not provide a broad base of psychiatric knowledge or skill

Professional residency

Aim	To produce broad-based psychiatrists possessing a variety of theoretical orientations and clinical skills
Recruits	Applicants with broad interests and excellent clinical track records in medical school
Curriculum	Required core curriculum teaching the breadth of modern psychiatry
Strength	Provides education and training in all important aspects of psychiatry
Weakness	Allows less time to focus on a single area of psychiatry or to devote to research

Source. Adapted from R. Michels, personal communication, 1982.

research; however, these programs see their role as providing the intellectual "venture capital" for development of the scientific basis of psychiatry, and risks are taken willingly because of the potential for producing a few innovative scientific leaders.

A second program type is the "apprenticeship residency," which aims to produce "master craftsmen" in the program's particular type of psychiatry. Applicants recruited are interested in a specific area of psychiatry (be it psychoanalytic psychotherapy or biological psychiatry) that the department specializes in, and these programs provide the majority of their training in that one area. Such departments usually give only lip service to other areas of psychiatry, and training is an apprenticeship in which the resident, working with expert preceptors, learns to do one thing very well under expert supervision. Graduates of such programs have intensive clinical knowledge and skills in a specific area but do not have a broad base of expertise outside that area and often have shown little interest in exploring that area scientifically.

The third type of program, the "professional residency," aims at producing broadly versed psychiatrists who understand a variety of theoretical orientations and therapeutic interventions. Applicants recruited have excellent medical school track records in clinical medicine and psychiatry. The residents are provided with a structured training program featuring a required core curriculum of didactic and clinical learning experiences in which they are taught the breadth of the profession. The goal of such programs is that graduates will be capable of meeting at least minimum requirements of all aspects of the profession. These graduates have a broader foundation in psychiatry than do graduates of the other two types of programs, but they have not had as much time during residency either to devote to research productivity or to become experts in any single area of psychiatry. With the increasing breadth and specificity of the RRC's requirements, most programs in psychiatry are becoming "professional" in nature (Borus and Yager 1986; Yager et al. 1988).

RESIDENCY DESIGN

In most psychiatry residencies, PGY-I consists of between 4 and 10 months of internal medicine, 2 months of neurology, and any remaining months (if not in medicine) devoted to inpatient psychiatry or other activities at the interface of psychiatry and medicine (e.g., geriatric psychiatry, substance abuse, emergency psychiatry). PGY-II in most programs is an inpatient psychiatry year in which residents, often in more than one setting (mental hospital, general hospital psychiatric unit, public sector hospital, or community mental health center inpatient unit), learn to perform a comprehensive evaluation of inpatients, make descriptive and dynamic diagnoses and formulations of their problems, and design and implement inpatient treatment plans related to follow-up outpatient care. In many programs, a small number of outpatients are begun in treatment during PGY-II to allow a modest 3-year longitudinal outpatient psychiatry experience. Some programs also include training experiences in emergency psychiatry/crisis intervention and/or partial hospital settings in PGY-II.

Outpatient treatment is often the emphasis of PGY-III, with focus on a variety of long- and short-term, individual, group, couple, and family psychotherapies. In PGY-III, many programs also have major rotations in consultation-liaison and child and adolescent psychiatry. In the former rotation, residents under supervision provide psychiatric expertise and interventions for medical, surgical, and obstetric/gynecological inpatients. Child and adolescent psychiatry training is often outpatient based (but in some programs remains a "block" inpatient rotation) and usually focuses on diagnostic evaluation of children and their families rather than on longitudinal treatment. This provides future general psychiatrists with the skills necessary to evaluate and refer the children of their adult patients and to understand childhood issues in their adult patients' developmental histories.

PGY-IV in most programs combines continued longitudinal outpatient clinical experiences with elective or selective opportunities to focus more intensively on a particular area or areas of psychiatry. Many residents also use part of this year to take on senior or chief residency responsibilities that provide experiences in psychiatric clinical administration and teaching. Others undertake research during PGY-IV as a step toward becoming psychiatric investigators. With the trend toward subspecialization in psychiatry, PGY-IV provides an opportunity to solidify areas of interest in preparation for a formal subspecialty fellowship after residency. Especially in "professional programs," selecting an area of focus—in the final year of residency—from the broad psychiatric foundation gained in the first 3 years of residency is an important step toward choosing a practice area. Residents in the other two types of residencies, who have had a more singular focus (be it research—in a "scientific program"—or a particular mode of practice, in an "apprenticeship program"), often use PGY-IV to continue in-depth work in their area (Sledge et al. 1990b). Transition-to-practice seminars in PGY-IV are valuable opportunities in which residents are encouraged to explore a variety of practice possibilities within themselves and the external world before committing to a postresidency position (Borus 1978, 1982; Hales et al. 1982, 1985).

TEACHING AND SUPERVISION IN RESIDENCY

As the term *residency training* implies, all graduate medical education is a mixture of education and on-the-job skill training of resident physicians through the delivery of clinical care. To define an appropriate balance between these at times conflicting tasks is a challenge for both programs and residents. The excellent residency will offer a series of core didactic learning experiences to provide the resident with knowledge about modern psychiatry (including its neuroscience and psychological bases, evaluation and treatment methodologies, and psychiatry's sociopolitical roles) as well as the opportunity to become skilled in applying such knowledge through clinical practice under the close supervision of experienced faculty members. The resident in psychiatry, more so than in other fields of medicine, is a vital interpersonal "instrument" in diagnosing, understanding, and treating the patient, and thus close supervision of the resident's clinical practice is a crucial component of the resident's professional learning and development (Thorbeck 1992).

Supervision in psychiatry can be direct or collateral. Opportunities for a supervisor to observe directly the interactions of resident and patient most often occur in inpatient and emergency room settings as well as during consultations on medical and surgical inpatients, all situations in which it is not unusual for more than one psychiatrist to see a patient. In outpatient and intensive inpatient psychotherapeutic clinical experiences, which are usually based on the dyadic relationship between the (resident) therapist and patient, most supervision occurs on a collateral basis. After the clinical encounter, a verbal, audiotape, and/or videotape presentation is made to the supervisor, who provides feedback, increased understanding, and direction to the resident (Betcher and Zinberg 1988). Availability of direct, on-site supervision of clinical interactions and the regularity and expertise of collateral supervision are important aspects of any psychiatry residency. Residents should receive supervision from faculty with differing orientations and expertise who can help the residents integrate a multiplicity of perspectives and potential interventions into a specific treatment plan for each patient.

EVALUATION

Regular evaluation of residents, faculty, and the training program itself is crucial in the development of high-quality psychiatric practitioners (Borus 1997; Borus and Yager 1986). Evaluation of residents should be both formative and summative. Ongoing informal formative feedback to the resident from his or her clinical unit chiefs and supervisors about strengths and weaknesses should occur throughout the course of a clinical rotation or of supervised psychotherapy. Intermittent scheduled summative evaluation should occur through formal supervisory reports, end-of-service unit chief evaluations, and tests of cognitive and clinical skills. The Psychiatry RRC requires annual examinations of cognitive knowledge and an evalu-

ation of clinical skills at least twice during the 4 years of training (Accreditation Council for Graduate Medical Education 1996). Most programs use the Psychiatry Resident In-Training Examination (PRITE), a national examination of resident knowledge, to meet the cognitive examination requirement. Sponsored by the American College of Psychiatrists, the PRITE provides residents and their training directors with feedback on each resident's performance in nine content areas as well as a comparison of each resident's performance with others in his or her residency class, the total residency program, and other residents throughout the country who have had similar amounts of training (Smeltzer and Jones 1990; Strauss et al. 1982). To meet the second requirement, most programs conduct a "mock board" clinical examination in which the resident is directly observed by faculty examiners when he or she is evaluating a patient and the resident is asked to discuss his or her evaluation, diagnosis, formulation, and treatment plan for this patient and similar cases. It is vital that evaluation of residents' progress and problems be undertaken at least semiannually and the resulting determinations be shared with the residents directly by the training director or designated faculty members so that deficiencies can be identified early on for remediation and strengths can be recognized and built on.

Similarly, training programs should require regular resident feedback and evaluation of teachers, supervisors, clinical rotations, and overall structure and content of the residency program. Because psychiatric education depends on the collaboration between teachers and learners, it is important for faculty to understand their strengths and deficiencies in facilitating the learning and professional development of residents so that they may make strides to be more helpful. Such formal evaluations by their students can be used as one measure of teaching quality by faculty promotions committees (Borus 1993a). Residents' feedback about deficiencies in the training program should be viewed by faculty as important information that can improve the program (Sledge 1978). Although no program or resident is optimally strong in all areas of psychiatry, the goal of continuous improvement should be shared by both teachers and learners (Berwick 1989).

PSYCHIATRIC EDUCATION OF NONPSYCHIATRIC RESIDENTS

Educating nonpsychiatric residents about psychiatric issues is also an important role for psychiatric educators. Nonpsychiatric physicians are notoriously poor at recognizing and correctly diagnosing defined mental disorders in their patients (Borus et al. 1988; Jencks 1985). However, studies have shown that more patients with mental and addictive disorders in this country receive care from the general medical sector than from mental health and addictions specialist providers (Narrow et al. 1993; Shapiro et al. 1984). Also, in many managed care and capitated plans primary care physicians determine which patients are allowed to receive specialist evaluation and treatment. It is therefore vital that psychiatrists participate in the education of these physicians about psychiatric disorders and the psychosocial aspects of medical care.

Nonpsychiatric physicians need teaching to recognize when their patients have mental disorders, to diagnose the disorders correctly, and to learn when to treat the disorders within their practices and when to refer the patients for treatment to psychiatrists or other mental health specialists. Much of this teaching of primary care residents has been done by psychologists who have focused on improving residents' patient-interviewing skills (Burns et al. 1983) while paying inadequate attention to psychiatric diagnosis or psychopharmacological treatment, both of which should be part of the clinical armamentarium of the general physician (Borus 1985).

In a 1988 study, internists rated the emotional disorders of patients they had just seen in their offices, and these ratings were matched against psychiatrist and psychologist evaluations of the same patients with the Structured Clinical Interview for DSM-III-R (SCID) (Borus et al. 1988). In a sample of 100 patients, the general physicians missed six of the seven cases of current depression, the majority of cases of current anxiety disorders, and all four cases of current substance abuse disorders. When these diagnostic discrepancies were discussed, the internists acknowledged they did not understand psychiatric diagnosis, were unclear what criteria were necessary to define a disorder that required treatment, and thought that within the limited time available for their patient encounters it would be difficult to arrive at a definitive psychiatric diagnosis. In addition, they were concerned that making such a diagnosis might open a Pandora's box of problems and feelings that would require time and expertise to handle that they did not have.

Such studies suggest it is important that psychiatrists teach nonpsychiatric residents how, within the time limitations of general medical practice, to assess patients for psychiatric disorders and make definitive diagnoses. A method used by one of us (J.F.B.) was to teach busy internists the current major depression module of the SCID. If the answer to one of the two screening questions about persistent sadness or loss of interest is positive, the physician can fol-

low up with the additional questions about appetite and weight, guilt and feelings of worthlessness, energy, concentration, suicidality, sleep, and psychomotor agitation or retardation. The two screening questions add only a minute to the physician's review of systems, and the additional questions necessary to make a definitive diagnosis of major depression can be asked and answered in 5 minutes, a time allotment compatible with medical office practice that can result in ruling in or out an illness with high morbidity and mortality for which effective treatment is available (Wells et al. 1989). It is also important in working with nonpsychiatric residents to discuss the presentation of prevalent mental disorder in their patient population (often with somatic symptomatology as the "tickets of admission"), to stress the importance of these disorders to the patient's overall health (psychiatric disorders are not minor disorders and do require treatment), and to emphasize that there are successful treatments for many psychiatric disorders, some of which treatments can be provided as part of general medical care.

The psychiatric education of the nonpsychiatric resident should also include a basic course in psychopharmacology so that appropriate uses of antidepressant, antianxiety, neuroleptic, and sedative medications are understood. Although general physicians are the most frequent prescribers of benzodiazepines and selective serotonin reuptake inhibitors, they often overuse antianxiety medications and underdose antidepressive and neuroleptic medications. In recognition of the crucial roles of primary care physicians in recognizing mental and addictive disorders, directly providing mental health care, and longitudinally treating the physical problems of patients with mental disorders, some psychiatry residencies have initiated "primary care psychiatry" rotations to train psychiatrists to become effective consultants to and collaborators with primary care physicians (Greenberg and Paulsen 1996).

We do not mean to suggest, in the discussion of these priorities, that the teaching of psychologically informed patient-interviewing techniques is not important. Further, primary care residents should be taught to recognize difficulties in the doctor-patient relationship, specifically the roles played by patients' fear, shame, humiliation, demoralization, and character style, as well as the resident's own subjective response to caring for very ill patients (Sledge et al. 1987, 1990a).

FELLOWSHIPS AND SUBSPECIALIZATION

As the knowledge base in psychiatry expands and as reimbursement potential is increasingly linked to expertise in ever-narrowing areas, subspecialization has become a fact in our field. However, the degree to which this subspecialization should or will be formalized has been the subject of considerable debate. Some argue that subspecialization will lead to fragmentation of the field and undermine core graduate education (Weissman and Bashook 1989). Others believe that subspecialization is desirable because it will lead to enhancement of knowledge and skills related to patient care (Yager 1989) and will be driven by the needs of the marketplace and not by the preferences of the profession (Taintor 1989).

The decision by the AMA to place a moratorium on the creation of new medical subspecialty boards has slowed but not halted the development of subspecialty areas within psychiatry. The four current subspecialty areas with ABPN certification and ACGME accreditation are addictions psychiatry, child and adolescent psychiatry, forensic psychiatry, and geriatric psychiatry (Accreditation Council for Graduate Medical Education 1996; American Board of Psychiatry and Neurology 1996). Administrative psychiatry has an APA-sponsored certifying examination, and both consultation-liaison and community psychiatry have a strong cadre of psychiatrists but, to date, lack a formal certifying process.

Subspecialization is linked to the provision of formal fellowship programs leading to eligibility for certification within a particular subspecialty area. Child and adolescent psychiatry has the oldest subspecialty training accreditation and certification processes. The 2-year child and adolescent psychiatry training requirements are established by a subcommittee of the Psychiatry RRC. Residents may elect to enter child and adolescent psychiatry training as early as PGY-IV and, after successfully completing 2 additional years of training in this field, are eligible for board certification in child and adolescent psychiatry. Addictions, forensic, and geriatric psychiatry are other subspecialty areas with formal RRC fellowship program requirements for eligibility for ABPN certification. In addition, other less formal fellowship programs offer in-depth postresidency experience within a particular circumscribed clinical area of the field and/or opportunities for research over a 1- or 2-year period. Although a PGY-IV elective may resemble a PGY-V fellowship, the ABPN is clear that with the exception of child and adolescent psychiatry training PGY-IV subspecialty experiences cannot count toward eligibility for subspecialty certification. With the elimination of required military service, the knowledge expansion in psychiatry and its subspecialty areas, and the growing difficulty of establishing a practice without membership in managed care panels (many of which have board certification as the credentialing criterion), postresidency

fellowships are becoming increasingly popular among graduates who want to pursue a particular line of subspecialty work or become established in a new geographic area while obtaining their initial board certification.

Psychoanalytic training, the oldest subspecialty of psychiatry, is carried out as a part-time training activity under the auspices of independent educational institutes. Psychoanalytic institutes associated with the APsA are rigorously evaluated and accredited in much the same way as are medical schools and residencies. Psychoanalytic training accredited by the APsA has three components: a formal didactic curriculum addressing the basic theoretical, technical, historical, and clinical aspects of psychoanalysis; close supervision of selected cases; and a personal analysis. Many psychoanalytic institutes also sponsor continuing education activities that address assessment and treatment of patients from a psychoanalytic or psychodynamic perspective for psychiatrists and other mental health professionals who do not undergo full psychoanalytic training.

PSYCHIATRIC EDUCATION OF NONPHYSICIAN MENTAL HEALTH PROFESSIONALS

The practice of psychiatry is becoming increasingly multidisciplinary. With the development of community-based managed care and capitated systems, the delivery of mental health care is carried out in a wide range of settings in which providers from the disciplines of psychiatry, psychology, social work, and nursing must work together in a harmonious, collaborative manner. Much of this work is carried out in teams in which each discipline member performs functions specific to that discipline as well as functions and roles that overlap those of other disciplines.

Although there remains interprofessional conflict between psychiatry and psychology at the national organization level, academic psychologists and psychiatrists collaborate at the local institutional level along many dimensions of service delivery, research, and education. Psychologists and psychiatrists teach each other's trainees. Psychologists are frequently well represented on academic department of psychiatry faculties and tasked with the responsibilities of teaching behavioral sciences to medical students and the basics of psychological testing to psychiatric residents. Most psychologists involved in patient care hold a Ph.D., Psy.D., or Ed.D., and clinical psychology training programs are accredited by the American Psychological Association Office of Accreditation (American Psychological

Association Committee on Accreditation 1995). Licensing requirements vary from state to state, but most states require specified clinical experience following the award of the doctorate.

Psychiatric social work is a mental health discipline that is growing in prominence with the increasing acceptance of both managed care and community-based public sector services and in political strength as the number of its practitioners increase. Schools of social work offer bachelor's (B.S.W.), master's (M.S.W.), and doctoral (D.S.W.) degrees. The Council on Social Work sets national standards for social work accreditation, and state licensing and certification requirements vary (Council on Social Work, Division on Standards and Accreditation 1991).

As a profession, nursing combines a traditional background of medication administration with a commitment to holistic and continuous personal care delivered in a flexible, pragmatic fashion. In some states, nurses are licensed to prescribe medications under a physician's general guidance. The psychiatric nurse specialist is a master's-prepared nurse specializing in mental health. The American Nurses' Association (1994) sets standards for the psychiatric and mental health nurse specialist as well as standards of practice.

These allied disciplines are playing an increasing role in mental health service delivery. Psychiatrists can be of assistance in educating and training members of these disciplines through either formal or in-service, on-the-job training programs that teach general mental health skills as well as areas of particular psychiatric expertise, such as the use of psychoactive medications, the interface between medical and psychological processes, and some forensic and legal issues. Such education and training can increase the caregiving capacity of the other disciplines and fosters good working alliances with psychiatry for integrated care delivery. For these reasons, psychiatrists should seek ways to assist in the training of colleagues in the other mental health disciplines.

CONTINUING PSYCHIATRIC EDUCATION

CONTINUING MEDICAL EDUCATION FOR PSYCHIATRISTS

Psychiatric practitioners must stay up to date on meaningful developments in the field to avoid obsolescence. This has become increasingly important as managed care organizations and third-party insurers change the rules of psychiatric practice and shift the focus to short-term interventions rarely emphasized in residencies in the past. The rapidly growing neuroscience knowledge base in psychiatry; refinements in traditional psychotherapeutic, psychopharmacological, and psychosocial techniques; and exciting new imaging aids to diagnosis of serious mental disorders all require sophisticated education and, for some, additional training for the clinician to understand and appropriately integrate into his or her clinical repertoire. Many states require continuing medical education (CME) for license renewal. Another impetus to continuing psychiatric education was created by the ABPN's decision to provide only time-limited certifications; psychiatrists certified after October 1994 must demonstrate continuing competence for recertification every 10 years. Finally, the ultimate reason for continuing psychiatric education is the desire of practitioners to continue to learn and develop professionally to maintain an up-to-date understanding of the field and the best possible treatment armamentarium.

CME is divided into different categories. The most stringent is Category I, which requires that lectures, seminars, or self-instruction materials be sponsored by an institution accredited by the ACCME or a state medical society (Anderson 1991). The accredited sponsor is responsible for ensuring that the offering has clear objectives aimed at meeting CME needs of individual or groups of physicians, uses teaching/learning methods suitable to meet its goals, evaluates the quality and relevance of the educational effort, and documents physicians' participation. Category I continuing education in psychiatry is available in many forms (e.g., lectures, courses, tape series, World Wide Web offerings, newsletters with study guides). Academic departments of psychiatry, national psychiatric organizations, and some entrepreneurs offer courses that qualify for Category I credit. The most successful of such courses have paired excellent lectures with written study materials that contain an outline of the lecture and pertinent references to help the learner explore an area further. Adequate time for questioning and interaction with the teachers also seem to be key ingredients of well-received CME courses.

One advantage of a part-time affiliation with an academic department of psychiatry for many community-based practitioners is the opportunity to take part in the department's educational activities, such as grand rounds and case conferences. These educational opportunities help the practitioner avoid the isolation of private practice, maintain his or her knowledge and skill level, and often share his or her clinical experience and expertise through teaching or supervising medical students, psychiatric residents, or nonphysician mental health professionals. Some departments have focused specific CME opportunities for different segments of their part-time faculty as a reward for donated teaching time (Swiller and Davis 1992).

With the rapid development of our field, CME limited to such didactic information transfer may not enable the practicing psychiatrist to avoid clinical obsolescence. One might question whether periodic retraining, with both intensive acquisition of new knowledge and supervised practice of new diagnostic and treatment methods, should be a required part of the continuing education of psychiatrists. Providing such opportunities requires major additional teaching and supervisory efforts by faculty. The faculty costs of such efforts might be offset by the clinical care provided by retraining psychiatrists as they expand their expertise, or the opportunities might be funded by special institutional initiatives. Although there are many obstacles to such required, periodic (perhaps the equivalent of 6 months every decade) retraining, practitioners may not be able to provide their patients with the most effective treatment without it.

CONTINUING MEDICAL EDUCATION IN PSYCHIATRY FOR NONPSYCHIATRIC PHYSICIANS

Out of residency and no longer under the influence of the academic medical center, the increasingly time-stressed practicing physician gatekeeper is unlikely to recognize or focus on his or her patients' psychiatric disorders. Three developments—National Institute of Mental Health (NIMH)–sponsored initiatives on depression and anxiety, Agency for Health Care Practice and Research (AHCPR) guidelines, and the Diagnostic and Statistical Manual of Mental Disorders, Fourth Edition, Primary Care Version (DSM-IV-PC 1995)—may assist in the continuing psychiatric education of practicing physicians.

The Depression Awareness Recognition and Treatment (DART) initiative (Regier et al. 1988) and a subsequent similar NIMH initiative on anxiety disorders provide specific materials for educating nonpsychiatric physicians about the appropriate assessment, care, and referral of their depressed and anxious patients. In addition, AHCPR has developed and disseminated practice guidelines for primary care physicians on the detection, diagnosis, and treatment of depression in the medical setting (Depression Guideline Panel 1993a, 1993b).

Out of a desire to make DSM-IV (American Psychiatric Association 1994) more relevant and user-friendly for primary care physicians, the APA hosted an interspecialty consortium of major professional organizations of internists, family practitioners, pediatricians, and obstetricians/gynecologists to write a focused DSM-IV-PC emphasizing the mental disorders most prevalent in and relevant to primary medical and pediatric practice that

could be addressed in the residency training and continuing education of nonpsychiatric physicians (American Psychiatric Association 1995). The primary care organizations' recognition that psychiatric disorders are an important part of the knowledge base of their specialties should raise the priority of primary care physicians' recognition of psychiatric disorders, and DSM-IV-PC provides a schema for diagnosing such disorders within their practices. The publication of DSM-IV-PC does not lessen the responsibility of psychiatrists to educate nonpsychiatric physicians; on the contrary, the existence of this manual should bring about an increase in the demand for psychiatrists to teach nonpsychiatric physicians about their patients' psychiatric disorders.

CURRENT ISSUES RELEVANT TO THE FUTURE OF PSYCHIATRIC EDUCATION

The future of psychiatric education, of course, will be intimately linked to the future of the practice of psychiatry. Although forecasting the future is problematic, some general predictions about the profession are necessary to address the educational dimensions of what the future might hold.

Psychiatric practice is increasingly moving out of institutional settings and into community-based systems of care, heavily emphasizing management of limited resources, and utilizing more specific and time-limited treatments for some conditions and more rehabilitative treatments for others (Borus 1989). These systems of care are characterized by a multidisciplinary approach, with psychiatrists playing substantive clinical leadership roles by supervising treatment planning and providing consultation and advice. In the future, psychiatrists are likely to provide direct services primarily to patients requiring pharmacotherapy and to patient groups with special needs such as those relating to forensic issues, psychiatric and medical comorbidity, and refractory illness. An emphasis on the cost-effectiveness of psychiatric care is fostering this move of psychiatrists away from direct service provision to clinical leadership roles involving oversight, supervision, teaching, and the care of special patient populations. Psychiatrists increasingly will be collaborators with colleagues in general medicine and the nonmedical mental health disciplines.

As we look to the psychiatric education necessary to prepare our field for the future, several issues not previously addressed become apparent: the funding of psychiatric education; workforce issues in psychiatry, including the special needs of women and international medical graduates; educational research; and teacher development.

FUNDING OF PSYCHIATRIC EDUCATION

Although there was strong support by government funds for the quarter century following World War II, federal funding for psychiatric education and academic departments of psychiatry has dwindled substantially. The federal government continues to provide direct medical education payments and support through (declining) medical education adjustments to its Medicare payments (Fishman 1996; Magen and Banazak 1995), and state governments provide some funding for psychiatry faculty and trainees through their state medical schools and the public sector care facilities aligned with these schools.

With costs increasingly falling on medical schools and their fiscally strapped affiliated teaching hospitals, support for psychiatric education has become more difficult to sustain (Borus 1994; Meyer 1993). The emergence of managed care efforts to limit utilization of inpatient care—the one area for which many psychiatric patients had reasonable insurance, and therefore the endeavor from which psychiatry departments derived much of their reimbursement revenues to subsidize less reimbursable outpatient, emergency, and consultation-liaison training—has led to a crisis in the ability of medical centers to support trainee stipends and faculty salaries. Although in the past residents served as an inexpensive source of physician care for psychiatric disorders, Medicare and some other insurers now require faculty to bear direct clinical responsibility for patient care, at times making the resident redundant and jeopardizing the fiscal stability of residency training. Some managed care organizations explicitly exclude residents as providers of either inpatient or outpatient care, refusing to reimburse them for their services.

These financial forces are leading to changes in psychiatric education, both in funding current education and training and in preparing for the psychiatric practice of the future (Borus 1994). Faculty and residents are developing innovative methods to share patient care without disrupting the therapeutic alliance. Specific training is being devoted to teaching residents crisis intervention, short-term focused outpatient therapies, psychopharmacological interventions, group therapies, multidisciplinary care, and other resource-efficient treatment methods. Although there is a fear that these emphases will skew psychiatry (Brenneis 1994), such skills will be needed to practice in the future. As capitation becomes a major method of funding health care, academic psychiatry departments that take on financial risk are developing multilevel care networks to treat mental and substance abuse disorders. These academic departments must insist of insurers that well-supervised residents and other trainees be allowed to take clinical roles in such care networks congruent with both their training status and their developing skills. By providing defined prospective budgets and the freedom to use resources efficiently, capitation may help academic institutions make funding psychiatry trainees an integral part of an effective care network.

WORKFORCE ISSUES

In recent years the number of applicants for psychiatry residency has sharply decreased, and there is specific concern about the lower number of American medical school graduates entering the specialty (Weissman and Bashook 1991) (Table 44–4). After a decrease in the number of American graduates choosing psychiatry in the late 1970s, there was a gradual increase to a peak in 1988 of 5.5% (745) of American medical school seniors matching into psychiatry and filling 67.9% of the 1097 first-year psychiatry positions (Graettinger 1988). This number has decreased markedly since, and in 1996 only 3.3% (448) of American seniors chose psychiatry, filling only 48.9% of the 917 first-year psychiatry positions offered in the Match (Randlett and Creighton 1996). Speculated causes of this decrease in recruitment into psychiatry include concerns about the economic pressures on and monetary rewards of psychiatry compared with other specialties; the length of psychiatry residency training and the trend toward subspecialization; encroachment by both managed care systems and other mental health disciplines on the domain of psychiatry; and confusion about the image and roles of our specialty (Borus 1993b).

In times of decreased recruitment, leaders of training programs are concerned that unfilled positions will leave major holes in their clinical service programs. Residency directors are sometimes tempted to fill positions with less-than-optimal candidates to ensure service provision. The program that takes an unqualified applicant to fill a service need will regret this decision, because most such applicants will become residents who cannot perform adequately. In the case of an unqualified resident, enormous resources are consumed, over a long period, in monitoring and attempting to remediate inadequate performance, in determining whether training should be terminated or graduation should occur, and so forth. It is our experience as former training directors that a service vacancy is a temporary problem but an incompetent resident becomes an enduring albatross for the training program.

WOMEN IN PSYCHIATRY

The increased numbers of women in psychiatry during the 1980s—women chose psychiatry disproportionately to

TABLE 44–4. Entry of American graduates into psychiatry via the National Residency Matching Plan

	1979	1980	1981	1982	1983	1984	1985	1986	1987	1988	1989	1990	1991	1992	1993	1994	1995	1996
Percentage of all U.S. senior students choosing psychiatry via the NRMP	3.6	3.3	3.8	4.2	3.9	3.7	4.4	4.7	5.0	5.5	5.5	5.1	4.9	4.1	3.7	3.3	3.5	3.3
Number of PGY-I psychiatry positions filled by U.S. senior students via the NRMP	441	409	489	541	496	497	600	651	675	745	722	664	641	526	477	438	476	448
Percentage of offered PGY-I psychiatry positions filled by U.S. senior students via the NRMP				58.7	57.2	56.5	66.5	69.8	68.4	67.9	65.9	58.5	58.3	48.6	45.2	43.9	49.6	48.9

Note. NRMP = National Residency Matching Plan; PGY = postgraduate year.
Source. National Resident Matching Program.

other medical specialties—had a substantial impact on psychiatric education programs (DeTitta et al. 1992; Fenton et al. 1987). In 1995, 43.9% of all psychiatric residents were women (American Medical Association 1996). The increased total number of women in psychiatry has made them a substantial presence in psychiatric educational programs as trainees and faculty.

Although the influence of the larger number of women in psychiatry has been complex and difficult to quantify (Seiden 1980), several effects are clear. The presence of women trainees and faculty has increased sensitivity to, and understanding of, women's life experiences and thereby enriched the therapeutic capacities of all. The presence of women who want to and do have children during training has forced residency programs to develop innovative programs and more flexible training structures to accommodate dual training and parenting roles. Maternity leave, flexible rotations, part-time hours, and funding arrangements are available in many programs. Although at times accompanied by strain, such flexible arrangements, when negotiated with good faith and carried through with responsibility and competence, have had a consciousness-raising function (Braun and Susman 1992).

A salient issue for women trainees in psychiatry today is the limited availability of senior female faculty mentors and role models (Krener 1994; Liebenluft et al. 1993). Although it is clearly desirable for female medical students, residents, and junior faculty to have mentors who are women, the capacity of male faculty to act as mentors for women entering psychiatry until a sufficient number of women can assume these roles must be developed to facilitate the success of women in academic psychiatry (Reiser et al. 1993). Continued recruitment of women to psychiatry, vital to the future of our field, will in part depend on our success in fostering the retention and advancement of women in academic psychiatry.

INTERNATIONAL MEDICAL GRADUATES IN PSYCHIATRY

International medical graduates also have disproportionately chosen psychiatry over other medical specialties. In 1995, 41.4% of all psychiatric residents were international medical graduates (American Medical Association 1996). With notable exceptions, most international medical graduates have been recruited to fill less desirable training positions in public sector settings. In such settings they at times have been exploited by programs with large service demands, inadequate faculties, and meager educational programs that do not adequately prepare them to practice or to pass their board examinations. When not familiar with American culture or fluent in the language, they experience difficulties in responding empathically to the needs of their patients, who are frequently among the most complex and severely disturbed.

Regulatory policies have had an impact on the training of international residents in psychiatry. The Psychiatry RRC requires PGY-I training in an ACGME-accredited program, which ensures that the minimum of 4 months of primary medical care training and 2 months of neurology training will be undertaken in accordance with American standards of medical care and training. The RRC also requires specific instruction and special training for international medical graduates concerning American cultures, attitudes, values, and norms.

Psychiatry residency programs in the United States are likely to continue to want to train international medical graduates. Improved methods for selecting international medical graduates likely to succeed as residents and practicing psychiatrists, as well as further methods for facilitating their acculturation, must be developed (Rao et al. 1991, 1994). However, despite the current focus on decreased recruitment into psychiatry, we must continue to oppose inadequate training for any residents, whether graduates of medical schools in the United States or graduates of foreign medical schools, and eliminate residency programs that cannot provide an appropriate balance of education and service or an adequate amount of supervision and teaching. Given the changing medical marketplace, in which psychiatrists play more defined roles in multidisciplinary service systems, we should also question how many residents we presently need to train to meet the more limited psychiatric workforce needs of the future (Verhulst and Tucker 1995; Yager and Borus 1987).

EDUCATIONAL RESEARCH

Research into psychiatric education and training is a marginally developed and supported area within academic medicine and psychiatry. Despite a rich literature in the areas of general education, child development, and learning, there is little connection between this literature and professional education and training (Miller 1980). Some medical schools have developed units dedicated to the pursuit of new knowledge in medical education. When one considers the time and effort that go into medical education and the latter's high-stakes outcome, it is surprising that there is not more academic attention to the medical education process. Scholarly work in medical education has been concerned primarily with program efficacy, workforce and career choice activity, and the process of learning and teaching.

Program efficacy studies assess whether a particular educational effort or program has had the intended effects. Frequently such studies attempt to ascertain the critical ingredients and process that produce an effective outcome. These studies, analogous to treatment or psychotherapy outcome research efforts, are often limited in their generalizability from the specific site or circumstance of the educational program assessed.

What trainees do after being exposed to a particular educational sequence is a matter of substantial concern to policy makers. Studies that address these areas can help forecast career choice and formulate workforce policies (Sledge et al. 1990b). There also is considerable need to understand better the process of professional socialization in psychiatry as well as the best ways to teach and learn complex material that is not only technical and cognitive in nature but also subtle and psychological. For example, learning empathic responsiveness requires supervised interpersonal contact and cannot be achieved through classroom lectures or computer-aided instruction (Cooper 1989; Winer and Mostert 1988). Clearly, more research into the process of psychiatric education will be necessary to improve its effectiveness with limited teaching resources.

Further exploration of new educational technologies will be essential. Technologies now exist for complex evaluation and problem-solving strategies that can be learned at the student's own pace and convenience. Audiotapes and videotapes are excellent tools for studying and learning from clinical interactions (Goin et al. 1978). Computers not only can simulate clinical encounters, and thereby cause students to enter real clinical situations better prepared (Jachna et al. 1993), but also can carry out routine tasks related to education that would be otherwise prohibitively expensive in time or energy, such as literature searches, information storage and retrieval, and report preparation and review (Powsner and Byck 1991; Zak et al. 1993). Electronic mail, the World Wide Web, and telemedicine are having an impact on communication and information retrieval. "Distant" education, teaching, and consultation are feasible with real-time telecommunication and electronic mail. Through the World Wide Web, with its multimedia and interactive features, new forms of patient care–related information can be made available to learners (Powsner and Tufte 1994).

DEVELOPMENT OF TEACHERS

Despite the opportunities presented by the aforementioned technologies, the future of academic psychiatry and psychiatric education will largely depend on the quality of our teachers.

In many departments of psychiatry, teachers are an endangered species (Borus 1993a; Cooper 1989). Faced with decreasing support for psychiatric education, teachers of psychiatry have had to devote their primary efforts to earning their salary through a mix of clinical, administrative, and research tasks. Devoting time to teaching decreases one's academically rewarding research efforts or monetarily rewarding clinical work. In some medical schools, it is felt that teaching cannot be rigorously evaluated and therefore cannot be a major promotion criterion, and educational research has a lower valence than "more scientific" basic or clinical research efforts.

To stimulate medical students, recruit residents, and prepare for the increasingly complex practice world of the future, high priority must be accorded to teaching itself and the development of teachers of psychiatry. Residents, the primary teachers and role models for medical students in clerkships who are considering their career choice, can be helped to develop their teaching capabilities as part of the residency curriculum (Katzelnick et al. 1991). Faculty thrust unprepared into teaching and supervising positions can learn about the art of teaching from written sources (Whitman 1982) and from discussions with their more experienced faculty peers. Seasoned teachers can learn to apply new teaching methods (e.g., problem-based learning [Block 1996; Schmidt 1984]) to psychiatry as a way to continue their own professional development and more fully involve students and residents in the learning task.

The career development of psychiatric teachers can be fostered by greater valuation of carefully conducted educational research. Faculty who devote a sizable portion of their efforts to psychiatric education, such as residency training directors and directors of medical student education, should be given the resources to investigate their education programs rigorously (Borus and Woods 1991; Yager and Borus 1990). Teaching and educational innovations should be evaluated by defined criteria that can be used to assess whether the teacher's students have learned and how helpful the students believe the teacher was in facilitating their learning. Expert peer review should take place of the process and content of the teaching itself and of teaching innovations and materials developed by the teacher (Borus 1993a). Such evaluations must be given substantive weight in promotions decisions if we expect talented psychiatrists to devote their energies to the psychiatric education of the next generation of students and residents (Glaser 1989).

In the final analysis, it will be the teachers of psychiatry who impart the essential elements of our field to future generations through their example of commitment to learning, scientific investigation, high-quality clinical care, and devotion to the education of others. The investment we make now in psychiatric education and educators will be a major determinant of our profession's future.

REFERENCES

Accreditation Council for Graduate Medical Education: Directory of Graduate Medical Education Programs 1996–1997. Chicago, IL, American Medical Association, 1996

American Board of Psychiatry and Neurology: Information for Applicants. Deerfield, IL, American Board of Psychiatry and Neurology, 1996

American Medical Association: Appendix II: graduate medical education. JAMA 276:740, 1996

American Nurses' Association: Standards of Psychiatric and Mental Health Nursing Practice. Washington, DC, American Nurses' Association, 1994

American Psychiatric Association: Diagnostic and Statistical Manual of Mental Disorders, Fourth Edition. Washington, DC, American Psychiatric Association, 1994

American Psychiatric Association: Diagnostic and Statistical Manual of Mental Disorders, Fourth Edition, Primary Care Version. Washington, DC, American Psychiatric Association, 1995

American Psychological Association Committee on Accreditation: Accreditation Handbook. Washington, DC, American Psychological Association, 1995

Anderson AK: Massachusetts requirements for continuing medical education in risk management. Forum of the Risk Management Foundation of the Harvard Medical Institutions 12:10–11, 1991

Association of American Medical Colleges: Physicians for the Twenty-First Century: The GPEP Report: Report of the Panel on the General Professional Education of the Physician and College Preparation for Medicine. Washington, DC, Association of the American Medical Colleges, 1984

Berwick DM: Continuous improvement as an ideal in health care. N Engl J Med 320:53–56, 1989

Betcher RW, Zinberg NE: Supervision and privacy in psychotherapy training. Am J Psychiatry 145:796–803, 1988

Block SD: Using problem-based learning to enhance the psychosocial competence of medical students. Academic Psychiatry 20:65–75, 1996

Borus JF: The transition to practice seminar. Am J Psychiatry 135:1513–1516, 1978

Borus JF: The transition to practice. Journal of Medical Education 57:593–601, 1982

Borus JF: Psychiatry and the primary care physician, in Comprehensive Textbook of Psychiatry/IV, 4th Edition, Vol 2. Edited by Kaplan HI, Sadock BJ. Baltimore, MD, Williams & Wilkins, 1985, pp 1302–1308

Borus JF: How will new practice settings change psychiatry? in The Future of Psychiatry as a Medical Specialty. Edited by Yager J. Washington, DC, American Psychiatric Press, 1989, pp 17–22

Borus JF: Teaching and learning psychiatry. Academic Psychiatry 17:3–11, 1993a

Borus JF: Where have all the residents gone? Harvard Review of Psychiatry 1:66–67, 1993b

Borus JF: Economics and psychiatric education: the irresistible force meets the moveable object. Harvard Review of Psychiatry 2:15–21, 1994

Borus JF: Recognizing and managing residents' problems and problem residents. Academic Radiology 4:527–533, 1997

Borus JF, Woods SM: Career development of the residency training director, in Handbook of Psychiatry Residency Training. Edited by Kay J. Washington, DC, American Psychiatric Association, 1991, pp 205–218

Borus JF, Yager J: Ongoing evaluation in psychiatry: the first step towards quality. Am J Psychiatry 143:1415–1419, 1986

Borus JF, Howes MJ, Devins NP, et al: Primary health care providers' recognition and diagnosis of mental disorders in their patients. Gen Hosp Psychiatry 10:317–321, 1988

Braun D, Susman VL: Pregnancy during psychiatry residency: a study of attitudes. Academic Psychiatry 16:177–183, 1992

Brenneis CB: The skewing of psychiatry. Academic Psychiatry 18:71–80, 1994

Burns BJ, Scott JE, Burke JD, et al: Mental health training of primary care residents: a review of recent literature (1974–1981). Gen Hosp Psychiatry 5:157–169, 1983

Carter R: Criteria for the academic promotion of medical school based psychiatrists. Academic Psychiatry 16: 147–152, 1992

Cooper AM: The teacher: an endangered species? Academic Psychiatry 13:13–22, 1989

Council on Social Work, Division on Standards and Accreditation: Handbook of Accreditation Standards and Procedures. Washington, DC, Council on Social Work Education, 1991

Depression Guideline Panel: Depression in Primary Care, Vol 1: Detection and Diagnosis (Clinical Practice Guideline No 5; AHCPR Publ No 93-0550). Rockville, MD, U.S. Department of Health and Human Services, Public Health Service, Agency for Health Care Policy and Research, 1993a

Depression Guideline Panel: Depression in Primary Care, Vol 2: Treatment of Major Depression (Clinical Practice Guideline No 5; AHCPR Publ No 93-0551). Rockville, MD, U.S. Department of Health and Human Services, Public Health Service, Agency for Health Care Policy and Research, 1993b

DeTitta M, Robinowitz C, More W: The future of psychiatry: psychiatrists of the future. Am J Psychiatry 148:853–858, 1992

Eaton JS: The psychiatrist and psychiatric education, in Comprehensive Textbook of Psychiatry/III, 3rd Edition, Vol 3. Edited by Kaplan HI, Freedman AM, Sadock BJ. Baltimore, MD, Williams & Wilkins, 1980, pp 2926–2946

Fauman MA: The new information technologies. Academic Psychiatry 13:119–131, 1989

Federation of State Medical Boards of the United States and the National Board of Medical Examiners: USMLE, Steps 1 and 2: General Instructions, Content Description and Sample Items. Philadelphia, PA, Federation of State Medical Boards of the United States and National Board of Medical Examiners, 1997

Fenton WS, Robinowitz CM, Leaf P Jr: Male and female psychiatrists and their patients. Am J Psychiatry 144:358–361, 1987

Fishman LE: Medicare payments with an educational label: fundamentals and the future. Washington, DC, Association of American Medical Colleges, Division of Health Care Affairs, 1996

Flexner A: Medical education in the United States and Canada: a report to the Carnegie Foundation for the Advancement of Teaching (Bulletin No 4). New York, Carnegie Foundation for the Advancement of Teaching, 1910

Glaser RJ: The academic recognition of clinician teachers (editorial). Pharos 52:33, 1989

Goin MK, Kline F, Zimmerman W: The use of videotape in teaching supervision. Journal of Psychiatry Education 2:189–196, 1978

Graettinger JS: Results of the NRMP for 1988. Journal of Medical Education 63:491–494, 1988

Greenberg WE, Paulsen RH: Moving into the neighborhood: preparing residents to participate in a primary care environment. Harvard Review of Psychiatry 4:107–109, 1996

Hales RE, Baker FW, Borus JF, et al: Preparing Army physicians for practice, I: a survey of hospital commander and physician attitudes. Mil Med 147:554–557, 1982

Hales RE, Baker FW, Borus JF: Preparing Army physicians for practice, II: a transition to practice seminar. Mil Med 150:91–96, 1985

Jachna JS, Powsner SM, McIntyre PJ, et al: Teaching consultation psychiatry through computerized case simulation. Academic Psychiatry 17:36–42, 1993

Jencks SF: Recognition of mental distress and diagnosis of mental disorder in primary care. JAMA 253:1903–1907, 1985

Kaltreider NB, Lu FG, Thompson TL: Student education and recruitment into psychiatry: a synergistic proposal. Academic Psychiatry 18:154–161, 1994

Katzelnick DJ, Gonzales JJ, Conley MC, et al: Teaching psychiatric residents to teach. Academic Psychiatry 15:153–159, 1991

Kay J (ed): Handbook of Psychiatry Residency Training. Washington, DC, American Psychiatric Association, 1991

Kay J, Bienenfeld D: The role of the residency training director in psychiatric recruitment. Academic Psychiatry 16: 127–133, 1992

Krener P: Gender differences in career paths in psychiatry. Academic Psychiatry 18:1–21, 1994

Liaison Committee on Medical Education: Functions and Structure of a Medical School. Chicago, IL, Association of American Medical Colleges and the American Medical Association, 1997

Lidz T, Edelson M (eds): Training Tomorrow's Psychiatrist: The Crisis in Curriculum. New Haven, CT, Yale University Press, 1970

Liebenluft E, Haviland MG, Dial TH, et al: Sex differences in faculty retention and rank attainment in academic departments of psychiatry. Academic Psychiatry 17:73–76, 1993

Ludmerer K: Learning to Heal: The Development of American Medical Education. New York, Basic Books, 1985

Magen JG, Banazak DA: Graduate medical education financing in psychiatry. Academic Psychiatry 19:6–11, 1995

Meyer RE: The economics of survival for academic psychiatry. Academic Psychiatry 17:149–160, 1993

Miller GE: Educating Medical Teachers. Cambridge, MA, Harvard University Press, 1980

Narrow WE, Regier DA, Rae DS, et al: Use of services by persons with mental and addictive disorders: findings from the National Institute of Mental Health Epidemiologic Catchment Area Program. Arch Gen Psychiatry 50:95–107, 1993

Parsons T: Social structure and dynamic process: the case of modern medical practice, in Social System. Edited by Parsons T. New York, Free Press, 1951, pp 428–479

Powsner S, Byck R: Implementing a computer system for psychiatric training: the electric resident. Academic Psychiatry 15:100–105, 1991

Powsner SM, Tufte ER: A graphical summary of patient status. Lancet 344:386–389, 1994

Randlett RR, Creighton KP: Results of the National Resident Matching Program for 1996. Acad Med 71:697–699, 1996

Rao NR, Meinzer AE, Primavera LH, et al: Psychiatry residency selection criteria for American and foreign medical graduates: a comparative study. Academic Psychiatry 15:69–79, 1991

Rao NR, Meinzer AE, Berman SS: Perspectives on screening and interviewing international medical graduates for psychiatric residency training programs. Academic Psychiatry 18:178–188, 1994

Regier DA, Hirshfeld RM, Goodwin FK, et al: The NIMH depression awareness, recognition and treatment program: structure, aims, and scientific basis. Am J Psychiatry 145:1351–1357, 1988

Reiser L, Sledge W, Edelson M: Four year evaluation of a clerkship: 1982–1986. Am J Psychiatry 145:1122–1126, 1988

Reiser LW, Sledge WH, Fenton WH, et al: Beginning careers in academic psychiatry for women: Bermuda triangle? Am J Psychiatry 150:1392–1397, 1993

Rosenfeld AH (ed): Psychiatric Education: Prologue to the 1980s. Washington, DC, American Psychiatric Association, 1976

Scheiber SC: Graduate psychiatric education, in Comprehensive Textbook of Psychiatry/V, 5th Edition, Vol 2. Edited by Kaplan H, Sadock B. Baltimore, MD, Williams & Wilkins, 1989, pp 2099–2106

Schmidt HG: Problem-based learning: rationale and description. Med Educ 17:11–16, 1984

Seiden AE: The roles of women in psychiatry, in Comprehensive Textbook of Psychiatry/III, 3rd Edition, Vol 3. Edited by Kaplan HI, Freedman AM, Sadock BJ. Baltimore, MD, Williams & Wilkins, 1980, pp 2950–2960

Shapiro S, Skinner EA, VonKorff M, et al: Utilization of health and mental health services: three epidemiologic catchment area sites. Arch Gen Psychiatry 41:971–982, 1984

Sledge WH: Resource identification: a use of resident evaluations of faculty. Journal of Medical Education 53:149–151, 1978

Sledge WH, Lieberman PB, Reiser L: Teaching about the doctor-patient relationship in the first postgraduate year. Journal of Medical Education 62:187–190, 1987

Sledge WH, Lieberman PB, Wolf HL, et al: Distress among interns. Acad Med 65:608, 1990a

Sledge WH, Leaf P, Fenton W, et al: The effect of training on career: the experience of the Yale advanced track program. Arch Gen Psychiatry 47:82–88, 1990b

Smeltzer DJ, Jones BA: Reliability and validity of the Psychiatry Resident In-Training Examination. Academic Psychiatry 14:115–121, 1990

Strauss GD, Yager J, Strauss GE: Assessing assessment: the content and quality of the psychiatry in-training examination. Am J Psychiatry 139:85–88, 1982

Swiller HI, Davis KL: Continuing education in psychotherapy as a method to attract and involve voluntary faculty in an academic department of psychiatry. Academic Psychiatry 16:187–192, 1992

Taintor Z: Reflections on the future, in The Future of Psychiatry as a Medical Specialty. Edited by Yager J. Washington, DC, American Psychiatric Press, 1989, pp 121–133

Taintor Z, Robinowitz C: The career choice of psychiatry: a national conference on recruitment into psychiatry. Journal of Psychiatric Education 4:323–326, 1980

Thorbeck J: The development of the psychodynamic psychotherapist in supervision. Academic Psychiatry 16:72–82, 1992

Tiberius RG: Small Group Teaching. Toronto, Ontario Institute for Studies in Education Press, 1990

Tosteson DC: New pathways in general medical evaluation. N Engl J Med 332:234–238, 1990

Verhulst J, Tucker G: How many psychiatrists do we need? Academic Psychiatry 19:219–223, 1995

Weissman S, Bashook P: The future psychiatrist as a generalist: arguments against credentials for subspecialists, in The Future of Psychiatry as a Medical Specialty. Edited by Yager J. Washington, DC, American Psychiatric Press, 1989, pp 23–33

Weissman SH, Bashook PG: Forty year trends in selecting a psychiatric career. Psychiatr Q 62:81–93, 1991

Wells KB, Stewart A, Hays RD, et al: The functioning and well-being of depressed patients: results from the medical outcomes study. JAMA 262:914–919, 1989

Werkman S: The Role of Psychiatry in Medical Education. Cambridge, MA, Harvard University Press, 1966

Whitman NA: There Is No Gene for Good Teaching: A Handbook on Lecturing for Medical Teachers. Salt Lake City, UT, University of Utah School of Medicine, 1982

Winer JA, Mostert M: Evaluation of residents' dynamic psychotherapy skills. Journal of Psychiatric Education 12: 329–337, 1988

Yager J: Subspecialization in psychiatry, in The Future of Psychiatry as a Medical Specialty. Edited by Yager J. Washington, DC, American Psychiatric Press, 1989, pp 33–47

Yager J, Borus JF: Are we training too many psychiatrists? Am J Psychiatry 144:1042–1048, 1987

Yager J, Borus JF: A survival guide for psychiatric residency training directors. Academic Psychiatry 14:180–187, 1990

Yager J, Borus JF, Robinowitz CB, et al: Developing minimal national standards for clinical experience in psychiatric training. Am J Psychiatry 145:1409–1413, 1988

Zak J, Sheehan H, Roth D, et al: Palmtop computer residency log. Academic Psychiatry 17:143–148, 1993

APPENDIX: NATIONAL ORGANIZATIONS INVOLVED IN MEDICAL AND PSYCHIATRIC EDUCATION

American Association of Chairmen of Departments of Psychiatry (AACDP). The psychiatry chairmen's group is vitally interested in all aspects of psychiatric education, as well as in other academic, research, and clinical service issues.

American Association of Directors of Psychiatric Residency Training (AADPRT). This organization of training directors formulates and sponsors policies and procedures that influence residency training and serves an educational function for training directors and other academicians. With the AAP it runs and cosponsors the journal *Academic Psychiatry*.

American College of Psychiatrists (ACP). The ACP sponsors a variety of continuing education efforts, as well as the Psychiatry Resident In-Training Examination (PRITE), the annual written examination of psychiatric knowledge, administered to almost every psychiatric resident in the country, which provides evaluative feedback to individual residents and training programs.

American Medical Association (AMA). This national professional organization addresses undergraduate, graduate, and continuing medical education through its Council on Medical Education. In the *Journal of the American Medical Association*, the Council publishes an annual report of the status of medical education. The AMA is a sponsor or participant in almost all medical education accrediting and certifying agencies, including the Liaison Committee on Medical Education, the Accreditation Council for Graduate Medical Education, the Accreditation Council for Continuing Medical Education, and the American Board of Medical Specialties.

American Psychiatric Association (APA). As the major specialty society for psychiatry, the APA focuses on all aspects of psychiatric education through components of its Council on Medical Education and Career Development.

Association for Academic Psychiatry (AAP). This organization of teachers of psychiatry supports the development and dissemination of innovative teaching methods and programs in undergraduate, graduate, and continuing education in psychiatry. With the AADPRT, it cosponsors the journal *Academic Psychiatry*.

Association of American Medical Colleges (AAMC). This large, complex organization has five membership components, all of which have different types of constituents and consequently different agendas: the Council of Deans (COD), the Council of Teaching Hospitals (COTH), the Council of Academic Societies (CAS), the Organization of Student Representatives, and the Organization of Resident Representatives. The COD is broadly interested in all of medical education but is particularly concerned with undergraduate medical education. The COTH is oriented toward issues related to teaching hospitals and focuses on the financing of medical education, house staff roles, fellowship programs, and welfare issues of graduate education. The CAS, comprising specialty and subspecialty societies, is concerned with graduate and postgraduate education. The AAMC also sponsors research into medical education; the National Residency Matching Program, which oversees placement of graduating medical students into residency positions; the Medical College Admissions Test; the American Medical College Application Service; a loan assistance program (MEDLOANS); and other policy, educational, and informational services related to medical education.

Association of Directors of Medical Student Education in Psychiatry (ADMSEP). This society of medical student teachers focuses on issues in undergraduate psychiatric education.

National Board of Medical Examiners (NBME). The NBME develops and administers the comprehensive national medical student evaluation and licensing examination and the United States Medical Licensing Examination (USMLE).

CHAPTER 45

ETHICS AND PSYCHIATRY

ALLEN R. DYER, M.D., PH.D.

Ethics is born in conflict. People turn to ethics in the hope of resolving conflict when values clash. Ethics is often used as a tool to justify one's own position. Sometimes an appeal is made to ethics to resolve a dilemma when a decision maker is torn between alternatives. Some have suggested that one of the roles of ethicists in medical centers is to justify the high technology used to control people's lives. Others—perhaps those made most uncomfortable by the feelings associated with conflict—hope that rational analysis will solve problems that might otherwise lead to heated emotions. At its best, ethics—like psychotherapy—offers insight into conflict, a clarification of competing motives, drives, and values. At its best, ethics offers insight into the mind and the culture.

Ethics is at the center of human experience. Because it is concerned with what is right and what is wrong, the term *ethics* is often used synonymously with the term *morality*. Sometimes, however, a distinction is made between *ethics*, the systematic approach to understanding right and wrong, and *morality*, the forces that govern right conduct. Ethics is a fundamental aspect of human identity and of one person's relationships with others. It touches on the political, the social, the psychological, the spiritual, and even the biological aspects of human existence. In a time of cultural change, the appeal to ethics becomes an important aspect of both civic life and self-understanding. For the professions, psychiatry among them, ethical codes and ethical traditions are important in defining the norms of professional conduct and even in defining what it means for a profession to be a profession. Insofar as ethics deals with intellectual attempts to understand right and wrong (reason),as well as the affective impact of struggling with moral issues (emotion), psychiatric thinking offers an important perspective on ethics. This chapter deals with both ethics in psychiatry and psychiatry's contributions to ethics.

A BRIEF HISTORY OF MEDICAL ETHICS

The ethical traditions of the medical profession go back some 2,400 years to the fourth century B.C.E. and the writings of a Pythagorean cult, which have come to be known as the *Hippocratic corpus*. This is notable because it includes the oath of Hippocrates, sworn by a band of healer-craftsmen, which has come to symbolize the ethical ideals of the medical profession. The Hippocratic oath was not in widespread use until the 19th century, when first the British Medical Association and subsequently the American Medical Association (AMA) and professional organizations in other countries began to adopt formal codes of ethics. These codes of ethics were modeled on the principles first articulated in the oath of Hippocrates, most notably the principle of patient benefit. Throughout most of the history of medicine, this paternalistic emphasis on patient benefit has been the central tenet of medical ethics, as indicated in Table 45–1.

By the mid-1960s a number of factors in medicine and society had converged in a way that began to change the values underlying the doctor-patient relationship. Most notable was the emergence of new technologies, which began to change the way people thought about medicine and even what it meant to be human: genetic engineering, organ transplantation, advanced life support, safe abortion and birth control, medical and surgical treatments based on clinical research. No longer was medical care primarily palliative. No longer could it be assumed that the patient necessarily wanted what the doctor might offer (Dyer 1997b).

Also in this era, several social movements began to change the way society thought about assumed relationships. The civil rights movement, which was about much more than race (landmark: Civil Rights Act of 1964), the women's movement, and the consumer movement all began to place more emphasis on the right of the autonomous person to self-determination. Informed consent came to be the key to medical ethics and medical decision making. Autonomy came to be the ethical principle that guided thinking about medical decision making. *Medical ethics* became *bioethics* in this era as it came to be realized that the decisions in medicine were not just decisions faced by doctors but decisions in which society had a stake.

By the 1970s, economics increasingly became a part of thinking about ethics. Benefits were often seen in economic terms, and ethical issues were often translated into economic terms. Allocation of resources became a concern, and the question was often asked, "Can health costs be contained without rationing care?" No longer were the decisions of doctors and patients the only thing to be considered. Society's interests (especially economic interests) became a greater concern. The principle of justice eventually superseded beneficence and autonomy in ethical discourse, and justice was discussed as fair distribution of medical resources (Table 45–2).

In 1975 the Supreme Court rendered a decision, *Goldfarb v. Virginia State Bar Association*, that changed the way professions were to be considered and regulated. *Goldfarb* ended the "learned professions exemption" under the Sherman Antitrust Act. Before 1975 it was held that the Sherman Act applied only to businesses or trades and the learned professions were exempt. Mr. Goldfarb, an attorney himself, sued the Virginia Bar because he found that all attorneys in Fairfax County, where he wanted to buy a house, were charging the same fees to conduct a title search. He contended that this was restraint of trade, and the Supreme Court agreed with him.

Not long after the *Goldfarb* decision was announced, the Federal Trade Commission (FTC) sued the AMA, holding that the AMA was in restraint of trade because its code of ethics prohibited advertising. This case was decided by the Supreme Court in 1982 in favor of the FTC, thereby ending any ban on professional advertising and furthermore requiring the AMA to get approval from the FTC for any subsequent additions to its code of ethics (Greenhouse 1982). Medicine in effect ceased to be a profession—at least in the traditional sense of an autonomous association self-regulated by a code of ethics—and became a trade (Table 45–3).

THE ETHICS OF ADVERTISING

Professional organizations such as the AMA can no longer formally constrain physicians from advertising. Most physicians are not inclined to seek patients though advertising. Health care organizations, however, which employ physicians, may make their appeal through advertising, especially in a market-driven health care economy. The 1957 version of the AMA *Principles* in effect at the time of the Federal Trade Commission suit prohibited "solicitation" of patients, by which was meant "obtaining patients by deception," or making false claims (American Medical Association 1957). The interest of the FTC was primarily in promoting competition and thereby lowering health costs. The FTC was also interested in regulating advertising by requiring that claims be measurable. For example, to claim that a mouthwash "killed germs on contact by millions," it would be necessary to demonstrate a method for measuring millions of killed germs. To claim a success rate,

TABLE 45–1.   **Brief history of medical ethics**

4th century B.C.E.—1965	Age of medical paternalism
1965—1982	Age of patient autonomy
1982— ?	Age of bureaucratic regulation
21st century— ?	Age of partnership and community

TABLE 45–2.   **Evolution of ethical priorities**

1950s–1960s	1970s–1980s	1990s
Beneficence	Autonomy	Justice
Autonomy	Beneficence	Autonomy
(Justice)	(Justice)	Beneficence

TABLE 45–3. Time line for professional ethics

4th century B.C.E.	Oath of Hippocrates
1804	Percival's *Medical Ethics* (a basis for British Medical Association and American Medical Association codes)
1847	American Medical Association founded
1895	Sherman Antitrust Act
1975	*Goldfarb* decision ends learned professions exemption
1975	*Federal Trade Commission v. American Medical Association*
1982	Supreme Court decides in favor of Federal Trade Commission

one would need to have both a measurable numerator and a measurable denominator.

Advertising has two basic goals: dissemination of information and product differentiation. For physicians, providing information about services offered and fees charged is consistent with patient benefit, but attempts to differentiate the product are suspect. Licensing, accrediting, and credentialing organizations assume the role of maintaining standards. Beyond the activities of individual practitioners, the larger ethical question for advertising concerns truthfulness. The barrage of advertising in the media says little about the products being sold; instead, products are identified with desirable images, appealing to and manipulating unconscious fantasies of sex, power, status, and pleasure. Much advertising is antithetical to professional goals of patient benefit. Notable is the advertising of unhealthy products, especially alcohol and tobacco, often providing no information but associating the products with strong men, liberated women, and cool teenagers. One of the problems open markets always have to contend with is dangerous drugs. To the extent that dangerous drugs are not regulated and tightly controlled, one is likely to find either commercial promotions or gangsterism—as was the case in the distribution of alcohol during Prohibition and of most other dangerous drugs currently (see Dyer 1985a, 1995, 1997a).

THE PLACE OF ETHICS IN THE DEFINITION OF A PROFESSION

What makes a profession a profession instead of a trade? What makes medicine a profession? Are medicine (and psychiatry) better considered professions or technologies?

Clearly medicine has aspects of business, but medicine should be more than a business. If so, what are the essential characteristics of a profession? The emphasis on the commerce of technology in medicine in recent years may obscure the centrality of an ethical attitude toward the patient that has traditionally been considered the defining feature of a professional life (Table 45–4).

A profession may be defined by its knowledge, technology, and expertise, on the one hand, or by its ethics and values. The habits of modern thought might lead one to believe that this is an either/or choice. Clearly for psychiatry, as for most of medicine, technology has become important and perhaps even central in some people's minds. Medicine is usually understood to mean *allopathic* treatment. Drugs and procedures are technologies of choice. The recent primary care thrust has reopened consideration of medicine as a more holistic approach to healing. Talking again has become an important part of healing. It is important to recognize that ethics is more fundamental to professional definition than is technology. Technology is useful as long as it serves ethical ends but not as an end in itself. It might be better to recognize that knowledge, technology, and expertise are not merely commodities to be bartered in the marketplace but skills that may be used to ethical ends. Medical technology falls under the purview of professional values.

Ethics is central to professional life. All aspects of professional development involve ethics. Entry into the profession—usually through admission to professional school—involves ethics, at least implicitly. in that candidates are chosen who have demonstrated a work ethic in achieving good grades. Perhaps ethics is involved explicitly as well in attempts to select candidates of character, who

TABLE 45–4. A professional checklist

1. The professional is engaged in social service that is essential and unique.
2. The professional has developed a high degree of knowledge.
3. The professional has developed the ability to apply the special body of knowledge.
4. The professional is part of a group that is autonomous and claims the right to be self-regulating.
5. The professional recognizes and affirms a code of ethics.
6. The professional exhibits strong self-discipline and accepts personal responsibility for actions and decisions.
7. The professional's primary concern and commitment is to communal interest rather than merely to the self.
8. The professional is more concerned with services rendered than with financial rewards.

Source. Modified from Campbell 1982.

reflect the values of the profession. Ethics may be a formal part of the curriculum, but its role is more implicit in the socialization to the norms of the profession. Finally, ethics is involved in professional discipline, which may result in exit (expulsion) from the profession for members who violate the codes of ethics.

THE HIPPOCRATIC OATH AND THE HIPPOCRATIC TRADITION

If one accepts the view that medicine is a profession defined by its ethics, one must make some attempt to articulate those ethics. Although much of a profession's ethics is implicit—the rules of a culture learned by living in it—professional organizations all have formal codes of ethics. Most professional codes of ethics are derived in some way from the Hippocratic oath, which serves as a paradigm code for the organization of a profession. For the medical profession, the Hippocratic oath also serves as a symbol of the profession's ongoing identification with an ethical outlook toward the patient (Figure 45–1).

The Hippocratic oath is a remarkable document, not so much because it answers the ethical questions posed by modern medicine, but because it frames those questions. It is often said that the oath is anachronistic and offers little useful guidance to the modern physician. People who hold this view might be expecting the oath to function as an administrative list of rules. The oath does indeed offer little to those with such expectations. The oath is much more useful in defining the ends or goals of medicine. It articulates principles, most notably the principle of patient benefit, which is often helpful to physicians in sorting out where their allegiances lie. Taken together with its corollary, the principle of nonmaleficence (*primum non nocere*—first, do no harm), the principle of beneficence puts the patient at the center of ethical decision making. At a time when many other considerations (especially economic ones) lay claim to the physician's attention, the greatest liability of the Hippocratic oath ironically may be its greatest asset, namely its antiquity. The Hippocratic oath provides an ethical perspective that calls into question many of the assumptions of modern culture. It provides a vantage point for an ethical perspective that transcends the pressures of political expediency.

The first paragraph of the oath introduces the idea of sacredness in its invocation of all the gods and goddesses. The oath is not just a list of rules, but a set of ideals that define the character of the healer. It is not just a promise, although it is that, but also a covenant with whatever is held sacred.

OATH OF HIPPOCRATES

1. I SWEAR BY Apollo Physician and Asclepius and Hygieia and Panaceia and all the gods and goddesses, making them my witnesses, that I will fulfill according to my ability and judgment this oath and this covenant:

2. To hold him who has taught me this art as equal to my parents and to live my life in partnership with him, and if he is in need of money to give him a share of mine, and to regard his offspring as equal to my brothers in male lineage and to teach them this art—if they desire to learn it—without fee and covenant; to give a share of precepts and oral instruction and all the other learning to my sons and to the sons of him who has instructed me and to pupils who have signed the covenant and have taken an oath according to the medical law, but to no one else.

3. I will apply dietetic measure for the benefit of the sick according to my ability and judgment; I will keep them from harm and injustice.

4. I will neither give a deadly drug to anybody if asked for it, nor will I make a suggestion to this effect. Similarly I will not give to a woman an abortive remedy. In purity and holiness I will guard my life and my art.

5. I will not use the knife, not even on sufferers from the stone, but will withdraw in favor of such men as are engaged in this work.

6. Whatever houses I may visit, I will come for the benefit of the sick, remaining free of all intentional injustice, of all mischief and in particular of sexual relations with both female and male persons, be they free or slaves.

7. What I may see or hear in the course of the treatment or even outside of the treatment in regard to the life of men, which on no account one must spread abroad, I will keep to myself holding such things shameful to be spoken about.

8. If I fulfill this oath and do not violate it, may it be granted to me to enjoy life and art, being honored with fame among all men for all time to come; if I transgress it and swear falsely, may the opposite of all this be my lot.

FIGURE 45–1. Oath of Hippocrates.
Source. Edelstein 1943.

In the second paragraph are the origins of what has come to be understood as the professional organization of physician-healers. The profession is organized around its teachers, and the relationship between teacher and student is like family, including the bonds of dependency. The oath is sometimes criticized as exclusionary (by those who view medicine as a commodity) for not making instruction available to everyone. Again, this may be more of a virtue than a shortcoming, for it makes "signing the covenant and taking an oath according to medical law" a requirement of receiving instruction. Entry into the profession requires a commitment to shared values.

The third paragraph provides the context for medical care. Medical care is viewed as primarily dietetic; the main thing ancient physicians had to offer was their recommendations about proper diet. Pharmacy (giving drugs) is also mentioned as an acceptable activity of physicians. Cutting is considered an activity that should be left to those trained to do it (i.e., barbers), not an acceptable activity for the physician in Hippocratic times. Talking therapy is not mentioned explicitly in the oath, but therapy of the word (*logos*) was an implicit part of ancient medicine and healing (Laín Entralgo 1970). Doctor and patient related primarily through the medium of language. The patient-benefit principle is stressed here. The physician is to strive "according to his ability and judgment" to keep his patients from harm and injustice. The tone is paternalistic; the physician is expected to behave as a benevolent father toward his patients as well as his students.

The fourth paragraph is controversial to modern ears; it requires the physician to forswear euthanasia and abortion. What is striking in this paragraph, seen in historical context, is the emergence of a unique kind of healer. Medicine, emerging from a shamanistic tradition, in which the medicine man might make someone better or worse for moral or social reasons, focuses solely on making people better. More precisely, the physician now focuses on helping the body heal itself through natural means. Anthropologist Margaret Mead (Levine 1972) noted that this was the first time in the history of the world that the power to heal was vested in a practitioner who was not also a shaman with the power to harm. According to Mead, the Hippocratic oath marked one of the turning points in human history: "For the first time in our tradition there was a complete separation between killing and curing. Throughout the primitive world the doctor and the sorcerer tended to be the same person. He with power to kill had power to cure, including and especially the undoing of his own killing activities. He who had power to cure would necessarily also be able to kill." (Levine 1972, pp. 324–325)

"With the Greeks," according to Mead, "the distinction was made clear. One profession, the followers of Aesculapius, were to be dedicated completely to life under all circumstances, regardless of rank, age, or intellect—the life of a slave, the life of the Emperor, the life of a foreign man, the life of a defective child." Mead observed that "[this] is a priceless possession which we cannot afford to tarnish." However, society is always attempting to make the physician into a killer—to kill the defective child at birth, to leave sleeping pills beside the bed of the cancer patient (currently discussed as "physician-assisted suicide")—and Mead was convinced that "it is the duty of society to protect the physician from such requests." (Levine 1972, p. 324)

The fifth paragraph might also sound antiquated if read as a rule rather than as a principle. Should we understand that the Hippocratic oath does not apply to surgeons or that surgeons should not be considered part of the medical family? The principle underlying the admonition not to cut on the stone is that one should practice within the limits of one's competence, doing what one is trained to do. That principle endures quite well.

The sixth paragraph speaks to the conduct of physicians, introducing character, or virtue, in a way that was unique for the times. The physician was expected to follow forbearance, or restraint, in a way that was not expected of most citizens. The physician entered houses not just for a brief "house call" but for extended periods of time. He was an itinerant who lived in the household while he tended to the sick. He also advised on preventive measures. In ancient Greece it was not uncommon for the master of the house to offer slaves or free men or women or even his own children as a gesture of hospitality. The oath defines a different relationship between the healer and those served, and the Hippocratic physician forswears such "mischief" and does so equally for males and females.

The seventh paragraph is the confidentiality paragraph. In the context of the oath, secrecy was part of a special relationship between the healer and those with whom he dealt. Spreading secrets is not only prohibited, it is "shameful." The constraint on the physician is not just externally imposed; it is part of how he sees himself and feels about himself.

The eighth paragraph links with the first to provide the frame for the promises made in the other paragraphs. The reward for following a life of forbearance and restraint is honor and fame, a reputation that defines who one is or how one is perceived. The result of following the code is a reputation for character or predictability, which reflects on the individual and the larger family (the profession as a whole).

THE CONTEMPORARY RELEVANCE OF THE HIPPOCRATIC OATH

A reading of the Hippocratic oath reveals many phrases that responsible physicians might not want to follow literally. Even in ancient Greece, the oath called the physician to standards of behavior that were not required of ordinary citizens and that might put the physician at odds with the larger society. Medicine was delineated as a higher calling, a covenant with the gods. The oath provided a relationship with a like-minded family of individuals who shared certain values and self-understanding. It defined the physician's life in a beneficial relationship to those served. Its paternalism was questioned when society emphasized individualistic autonomy, but the oath's emphasis on justice foreshadowed a larger concern for community interests.

A physician is a citizen, subject to cultural norms and political forces. The Hippocratic tradition has at various times and places served as an ethical reference, external to immediate expediency, by which physicians may gauge their behavior and to which they can appeal (or by which they may be judged by their colleagues). An extreme example of the lapse of ethical behavior is provided by the activities of Nazi physicians, but there are several other notable examples as well. The World Psychiatric Association has censured the practices of psychiatrists in the former Soviet Union and other Eastern European countries for the detention of political dissidents. Such mislabeling with psychiatric diagnoses, when the profession is used for ends other than patient benefit, is referred to as the "political abuse of psychiatry" (Bloch 1991; Bloch and Reddaway 1977). Many physicians have been used by military governments in Latin America and elsewhere to assist in torture. Medical societies organized as governmental agencies rather than independent professional associations have had difficulty enforcing sanctions against state-supported physician involvement in interrogations. The existence of such extreme abuses makes a case, which is not always appreciated, for autonomous professional organizations self-regulated by a code of ethics rather than serving the interests of society. Society's interests, as represented by governments, are of necessity conflicted and caught up in political striving for power or influence.

Less dramatic examples make a more subtle point. Physicians could be involved in capital punishment; they have the skills to perform lethal injections, for example, and states would be willing to pay them, but such activities are outside the healing role. The forensic psychiatrist in giving court testimony does not have the same allegiance to a patient as a treating psychiatrist does. Analogous is the expectation that physicians will be agents of cost containment or rationing of health care. Physicians control much of health expenditures, and their interest is primarily in patient benefit. The Hippocratic oath is an ever-present reminder that acting in the interest of someone other than the patient creates a conflict, which is often experienced internally by the physician.

HONOR IN MEDICINE[1]

The Hippocratic oath speaks of honor, holiness, and purity. All these higher virtues allude to the character, ethics, and integrity of the physician. The good name and respect of both the practitioner and the profession are to be earned through consistent application of the ethical principles, and the code provides guidance. Good conduct becomes "characteristic" of the professional, and a code of conduct is a way of organizing one's thinking about good conduct both symbolically and in practical matters. In this sense medicine is like the military, the profession of arms. The warrior, like the physician, lives by a code that is internalized as a way of life. For example, this code was so deeply internalized that the ancient Japanese samurai warrior understood that violation of the code required death at one's own hand. Physicians often live by a warrior's ideal, and medicine is often spoken of in military analogy. Disease is the enemy. Hard work defends a noble cause. Practice is experienced and described as being "in the trenches."

The role of the military officer is not just to win battles but also to provide moral leadership. Thus, honor codes identify the higher principles by which more routine decisions can be made. What can be said about such ineffable ideals? How can moral aspirations be articulated? "An officer will not lie, cheat, or steal," say the military honor codes, to which is sometimes added the phrase "or tolerate anyone who does" (thereby indicating a responsibility in honor for the reputation of the group). "Thou shalt not kill" is a high commandment that is not often articulated in either military or medical circles. "Primum non nocere" (Hippocrates). "Do unto others as you would have them do unto you" (Jesus). "Act only according to that maxim that you would at the same time will to be a universal principle" (Kant).

---

[1] I owe an enormous debt to two military friends, who in conversations over the years have helped me appreciate the importance of a sense of honor in the professions as much as anything that has been written about medicine. Lieutenant General Sir Sam Cowan, Commander of the British Empire, Commander of Knights Bath, has recently been awarded a knighthood for his role in educating British and NATO officers in the importance of moral responsibility in the military in a democracy. Sensei Dale Scott Kirby, Sr., Vietnam veteran, sixth-degree black belt, U.S. National Weapons and Karate Champion, and master teacher, has helped a generation of warrior-athletes find the spiritual path in athletic training, competition, and cooperation. I believe it is such life-defining commitments to a set of ideals that Sir William Osler intended when, in 1913, he spoke of medicine as "a way of life" (Osler 1913/1969).

Part of the motivation for acting ethically is the honor of associating with a body that brings high regard and defining purpose for right action. However, the military metaphor is rapidly being replaced by the market metaphor. The market has its own ideals, which create tensions for those with a sense of honor: "caveat emptor"—let the [autonomous] consumer beware.

THE FIDUCIARY PRINCIPLE

The doctor-patient relationship is spoken of sacredly as a fiduciary relationship, a relationship based on trust. This conception derives from a sense of honor and the sense that the physician must be worthy of the trust, faith, and belief invested in the healer by the patient. That trust must be earned, first by the hard work required to acquire the skills necessary to apply the art. It must also be continuously earned by the consistent application of attentive response to the patient's needs, what is called "responsibility." There is an important distinction between the fiduciary relationship in medicine and that in law or business, where the trustee may act *for* the client. In medicine the physician must act *with* the patient and with the patient's consent. That action may be paternalistic in the best sense, that of the concern for the child or dependent; if that concern verges on control, however, the modern patient may well lose trust and confidence. In medicine the fiduciary principle is best understood as implying a partnership between doctor and patient.

A HIPPOCRATIC OATH FOR PSYCHIATRISTS

Maurice Levine (1972) articulated a Hippocratic oath for psychiatrists with some uniquely important insights about the values of this profession. In focusing on high ideals he suggested a standard transcending the minimalist requirements of administrative documents that should be very much part of the self-set moral ideals of any psychiatrist. Levine's oath demands competence but recognizes that human beings are not perfect. His code stresses an important principle about the value of self-knowledge, self-awareness, and constant self-scrutiny. This would be understood in Levine's era and now as recognizing the need for personal therapy or psychoanalysis for those doing such work. Levine stressed the need for psychiatrists to recognize in ourselves the feelings that such work can stir up, particularly working with seductive patients, and the importance of getting consultation or supervision, not just in training but whenever it might be necessary. This is a useful reminder at a time when many treatments are briefer and more biologically oriented. Many of the complaints of unethical conduct received by the American Psychiatric Association (APA) come from patients whose doctors did not sufficiently deal with their own feelings and acted out in treatment situations. It might be easier to justify self-disclosure in therapy, giving advice, accepting a gift, or socializing outside of therapy if the therapy were understood as merely a physiological intervention. At the same time, it becomes hard for a psychiatrist to defend against accusations of boundary violations if the feelings involved for both doctor and patient are not carefully considered in the therapy. Self-reflection is an important ethical tradition, not only in psychiatric and psychoanalytic circles, but throughout Western culture, dating back to the Socratic admonition to "know thyself." Physician Otto Guttentag (1963) articulated it nicely: "We exist as epistemological peers with our patients; we know no more about our patients than we know about ourselves." (p. 200)

CONTEMPORARY CODES OF ETHICS (AMA AND APA)

The second paragraph of the oath of Hippocrates presents the form of a profession organized around its code of ethics. When the AMA was founded in 1847, it adopted a code based largely on the Hippocratic principles of beneficence and honor. This code, *The Principles of Medical Ethics* (Figure 45–2), has been revised every few decades (most recently in 1957 and 1980). When the American Psychiatric Association adopted its first code in 1973, it decided to use the AMA *Principles* (because psychiatrists are physicians) with annotations especially applicable to psychiatry. The preamble of the AMA principles explicitly states that the principles "are not laws but standards of conduct, which define the essentials of honorable behavior for the physician" (Figure 45–2). The principles should be read teleologically as principles, not deontologically as rules. The requirement of honorable behavior of the physician applies to the physician's character and virtue and cannot be reduced to a list of rules. The physician must understand the principles in terms of a higher calling and act in accord with the dictates of conscience. Nonetheless, physicians look to the codes, principles, or annotations for guidance in specific situations. Because there may be sanctions for misconduct, physicians read the perspective of the AMA (American Medical Association 1997) and the APA (American Psychiatric Association 1995a) perspective to see what may be permitted or prohibited.

Principles of honor transcend the written word, which at best is a distillation of accumulated wisdom, stories, and

PRINCIPLES OF MEDICAL ETHICS OF THE AMERICAN MEDICAL ASSOCIATION

PREAMBLE The medical profession has long subscribed to a body of ethical statements developed primarily for the benefit of the patient. As a member of this profession, a physician must recognize responsibility not only to patients but also to society, to other health professionals, and to self. The following Principles, adopted by the American Medical Association, are not laws but standards of conduct, which define the essentials of honorable behavior for the physician.

SECTION 1 A physician shall be dedicated to providing competent medical service with compassion and respect for human dignity.

SECTION 2 A physician shall deal honestly with patients and colleagues, and strive to expose those physicians deficient in character or competence, or who engage in fraud or deception.

SECTION 3 A physician shall respect the law and also recognize a responsibility to seek changes in those requirements which are contrary to the best interests of the patient.

SECTION 4 A physician shall respect the rights of patients, of colleagues, and of other health professionals, and shall safeguard patient confidences within the constraints of the law.

SECTION 5 A physician shall continue to study, apply, and advance scientific knowledge, make relevant information available to patients, colleagues, and the public, obtain consultation, and use the talents of other health professionals when indicated.

SECTION 6 A physician shall, in the provision of appropriate patient care, except in emergencies, be free to choose whom to serve, with whom to associate, and the environment in which to provide medical services.

SECTION 7 A physician shall recognize a responsibility to participate in activities contributing to an improved community.

FIGURE 45-2. Principles of Medical Ethics, American Medical Association.
Source. Reprinted by permission of American Medical Association: *Code of Medical Ethics* (150th Anniversary Edition). In *Current Opinions with Annotations of the Council on Ethical and Judicial Affairs.* Chicago, IL, American Medical Association. Copyright 1997, American Medical Association.

feelings. To appreciate honor fully, the professional must internalize the norms of a culture by living them and understanding what a teacher or a parent would approve or disapprove of and why. In this sense a code is minimalist but essential. One of the motivating factors for the APA in articulating its annotations in 1973 was to respond to complaints of misconduct against its members. Physicians

should know the difference between right and wrong, but if sanctions were to be applied, it would be necessary to spell out the grounds for applying them. Treating the profession as a corps, the code serves as a tool for professional discipline. The entrepreneurial physician may see the medical license licentiously, as sanctioning whatever he or she might choose to do, but ethics provides a fundamental basis for accountability.

The APA (American Psychiatric Association 1995b) may impose four possible sanctions for misconduct:

1. Admonishment—an informal warning
2. Reprimand—a formal censure
3. Suspension (for a period not to exceed 5 years)
4. Expulsion

The Ethics Committee of the APA has given much thought to the procedures needed to ensure due process, particularly the procedures for holding a hearing, and the articulation of the various annotations. In the minimalist or legalistic perspective, a psychiatrist should know what is specified in the code because he or she might be subject to sanctions. Membership in the professional organization entails a promise to abide by the code just as it did for the Hippocratic physician. The modern physician should also understand the principles that underlie the code to be able to act in situations that have not been explicitly spelled out. The following discussions illustrate the constant tension between rule and principle and the importance of the physician's acting in the upward perspective to strive for virtuous action.

SEXUAL MISCONDUCT AND BOUNDARY VIOLATIONS

Sexual contact with a patient is unethical. This is one of the least ambiguous sections of the ethical code. It is a tradition that goes back to the oath of Hippocrates, which speaks of such conduct as "mischief." It is important for psychiatrists because the intimacy of the treatment activates strong feelings and fantasies in the doctor-patient relationship, the discussion of which may be essential to healing. In psychiatry, especially, feelings the patient has for the doctor (understood as *transferences*, i.e., derived from significant relationships in the past and activated in the treatment) and feelings the doctor has for the patient (understood as *countertransferences*) receive close scrutiny. Scrutiny of these feelings is no less important for other physicians, other therapists, or other professionals.

It is sometimes argued that sexual contact is proscribed because of the power differential, an argument that applies equally to employers and employees, supervisors and supervisees, teachers and students. Fundamentally, the importance of trust in the therapeutic relationship requires the treater to maintain forbearance, particularly when the mode of therapy is talking to understand rather than acting to alter feelings. Some professionals prefer to think of their relationships with patients (or clients) as contractual (rather than covenantal). This outlook implies more autonomy on the part of the client and gives the client more control and choice in what goes on. In the case of sexual behavior with a professional, however, even the choices of a consenting adult do not justify crossing sexual boundaries. Those more legalistically inclined might wonder whether erotic feelings may be acted on if the professional relationship were terminated. Because transferences endure over time, the interests of the patient/client can never be served by crossing this boundary. The APA *Principles of Medical Ethics With Annotations Especially Applicable to Psychiatry* (American Psychiatric Association1995b) spells this out: "Sexual activity with a current or former patient is unethical." How could a psychiatrist who became sexually involved with a patient or former patient ever defend him- or herself against a subsequent claim that the feelings acted on were feelings activated in therapy, which should have been addressed as therapeutic issues? The possible exception to this, which rarely gets consideration (and rarely happens), is when the two parties enter a covenantal relationship of marriage. Other examples of boundary violations, which rest on similar considerations, are conducting business with a patient, using the professional relationship to make other contacts, and profiting from information gained from the therapeutic relationship.

Table 45–5 compares the numbers of ethical complaints received by the APA in three periods.

THE BOUNDARY BETWEEN ETHICS AND LAW

Ethics and the law share a similar concern for right and wrong, but the ethical requirements of professionals are

TABLE 45–5. Numbers of ethical complaints received by the American Psychiatric Association in three time periods

	1950–1973	1972–1983	1991–1995
Charges made	82	382	211
Number (%) found unethical	12 (15%)	86 (23%)	82 (38%)
Number of expulsions	6	27	8

Source. Adapted from data of Moore 1985 and Lazarus, personal communication, 1997.

not identical to the requirements of all citizens. The oath of Hippocrates held physicians to a standard that was not required of all citizens. The AMA *Principles* and APA *Annotations* recognize this tension and expect physicians to "respect the law" (Figure 45–2) and "seek changes in those requirements which are contrary to the best interests of the patient" (American Psychiatric Association 1995b, p. xiv). Criminal behavior is usually unethical as well, but there may be situations in which it is not. Civil disobedience against unjust laws is a respected ethical tradition. A physician is a citizen whose professional role requires adherence to principles such as patient benefit. The *Principles* and *Annotations* both recognize an affirmative obligation to take part in activities contributing to the improvement of the community.

CONFIDENTIALITY

Confidentiality, understood as secrecy, in the doctor-patient relationship is one of the most fundamental principles of professional ethics. In the Hippocratic oath it is spoken of as "shameful to noise abroad what I may hear or see in the course of treatment." Confidentiality has its roots in the confidence or trust that is placed in the physician and on which the treatment depends. Confidentiality is one of the most fragile tenets in the contemporary era. As more and more people and agencies are involved in medical treatment and health care, it becomes increasingly difficult to safeguard confidentiality. Insurance companies, managed care organizations, other providers, courts, and sometimes families claim a right to know what is going on in patients' treatments. Mandatory reporting of suspected child abuse is an example in which the interest of the state in protecting children legally supersedes the physician's duty to maintain secrecy. Similarly, the *Tarasoff* decision (now precedent) obligates a psychotherapist who has knowledge that a patient or client may intend harm to a third party to notify that third party of the potential risk. These are examples of principles in conflict, and they speak to the insufficiency of relying absolutely on a principle as a rule. However, in a larger context the erosion of confidentiality threatens to undermine the possibility of a kind of therapy that requires developing openness to another person in which the patient may be confident that what is disclosed is only for his or her benefit.

THE DOUBLE AGENT PROBLEM

Double agents work both sides. The whole weight of tradition in professional ethics focuses the physician's responsibility on the patient. The physician works for the patient and is guided by the patient's needs and interests. This is especially the case in fee-for-service financial arrangements, even those buffered by insurance reimbursement. There are situations, however, in which the physician works for someone other than the patient, and there may be a conflict between the patient and the physician's employer, resulting in a divided allegiance. The classic case is the physician who works for the military. In such situations confidentiality may be compromised. Psychiatrists dealing with combat neuroses trying to get soldiers back into combat have faced the ethical dilemma of helping someone get into a situation in which he may get killed. This is ethically analogous to treating the psychotic prisoner who is incompetent to face execution. The student health psychiatrist doing an evaluation for the dean and the psychiatrist doing a prearraignment examination have loyalties that go beyond the patient's best interest and require at the least disclosure of the purpose of the examination and how the information will be used. Increasingly, physicians working for corporations, health maintenance organizations, and managed care organizations have interests that radically transform the nature of the relationship between doctor and patient.

FEES, BILLING, AND REIMBURSEMENT

The financial arrangements for medical service strike at the heart of the ethical issues concerning how medicine is valued. Not all values are economic, but ethics is often turned into economics. Inevitably there must be some sort of exchange for the services rendered, and inescapably there are some sort of feelings about the monetary transaction. In the dyadic doctor-patient relationship, there is a direct transaction, although it may be buffered by insurance companies, billing clerks, credit cards, or electronic transactions. In Hippocratic times, the physician was likely to be an itinerant who was housed and fed by the families of those he cared for. In horse-and-buggy days, farm produce or manual labor may have substituted for the fee. European academic robes had pockets in the hoods for tuition coins to be placed out of sight, so shameful was the monetary transaction. Not everyone could afford to pay equally, so often the paying patients subsidized the care of the poor. Patient benefit and fee-for-service have traditionally gone hand in hand, and the fee (alongside honor and duty, of course) has helped focus the physician's attention on the recipient of his treatment. One of the general criticisms often leveled against traditional Hippocratic medical ethics is that it does not deal with the physician's larger obligations to society and particularly to the distribution of medical services.

One financial arrangement that sometimes is questioned is the practice of charging for missed sessions. The APA *Annotations* has specifically addressed this issue: "It is ethical for the psychiatrist to make a charge for a missed appointment when this falls within the terms of the specific contractual agreement with the patient" (Section 2, paragraph 6). The idea of patients having responsibility for the treatment and ultimately for their health and wellness is not something usually considered in medical ethics, but it goes beyond the idea of medicine as technology that the doctor delivers and stresses the patient's investment and commitment to the healing process.

Another financial arrangement that is addressed throughout the AMA *Opinions* and APA *Annotations* is fee-splitting. Physicians should receive remuneration for the work they do, and they should obtain patients by referral based on the quality of their work and the reputation they earn in the eyes of satisfied patients and other physicians. Any incentive such as splitting the fee with a referring physician is considered unethical. It offers a temptation to place monetary gain above the best interest of the patient. Fee-splitting arrangements have largely been considered in the context of fee-for-service arrangements, but new financial arrangements in physician reimbursement often provide incentives for physicians to be paid for limiting care or otherwise acting in the interest of someone other than their patient.

THE TASKS AND METHODS OF ETHICS

Throughout the discussion of the codes of professional ethics and their application to particular situations, there is a tension between an understanding of the codes as precise rules and an understanding of their statements as more general principles. In a homogeneous culture, tribe, or community, morality is tacitly understood with little need for formal reflection or articulation. One learns the rules of culture by living in that culture and not by being taught abstract and explicitly formulated rules. In a heterogeneous group, what is called a "pluralistic society," there may be little adhesion to shared principles. In a stable culture, moral norms are internalized, and ethics are thought of as matters of conscience. In a changing culture, the internalized morality of a particular subgroup or individual may be in conflict with other mores, and people may not trust that the dictates of individual conscience are an adequate safeguard of right conduct. Increasingly, in this society we are moving away from informal standards of both personal and professional ethics, from broad and tacitly indwelling general principles developed over centuries, toward a civilly enforced body of laws and administrative regulations. This change has been interpreted as resulting from a deep mistrust of all "assumed relationships," that is, the breakdown of *gemeinschaft* (a community of feeling that results from likeness and shared life experience) into *gesellschaft* (a more rational, more mechanistic way of life, with greater structure and more written and explicit rules and regulations; Toennies 1940). Broad ethical principles no longer serve as shared values, and there is an attempt to make moral principles explicit as behavioral guidelines.

DEONTOLOGICAL ETHICAL THEORIES

Ethical theory identifies the tension between rules and principles by the terms *deontological* (rule-based) and *teleological* (from the Greek *telos*, meaning end or goal; Frankena 1963). Deontological ethical theories maintain that there are rules of action that have moral validity independent of the consequences and that one must act in accordance with these rules. Deontological theories assert that there are considerations other than goodness or badness on which to base decisions—such as keeping a promise, maintaining justice, or adhering to a commandment of God or the state—which are important regardless of the consequences of the action. One finds deontological theories in well-defined communities, such as religious communities, where one of the ethical considerations is preservation of the social order. Duty, obligation, obedience, and loyalty are the values that define deontological functioning. Professional standards of ethics have such deontological features, where the rule may be applied to exclude or coerce the deviant member to maintain the reputation of the group. Because of possible ambiguity in interpretation of the laws, there is often a complex corpus of interpretation and devoted study such as in Talmudic scholarship or in American constitutional law or in the opinions concerning professional codes (see the discussion that follows). The problem of interpreting ambiguity can be avoided if an overarching rule that is basic to all situations can be identified. The most successful example of such a pure deontological rule is Kant's famous categorical imperative: " Act only according to that maxim that you would at the same time will to be a universal principle." This formula assumes a highly motivated moral agent who will decide on a course of action by rational reflection.

TELEOLOGICAL ETHICAL THEORIES

Teleological theories are based on more general principles. *The Principles of Medical Ethics* of the American Medical Association (American Medical Association 1997), on which the American Psychiatric Association's standards are based, states explicitly that these principles "are not laws but standards of conduct, which define the essentials of honorable behavior for the physician" (Figure 45–2). Teleological ethical theories hold that the ultimate standard by which an act is judged morally right, wrong, obligatory, or correct is the general happiness of all people concerned or the greatest net balance of good over evil. This is often identified as the principle of utility or beneficence, which implies that good and bad are capable of being measured and balanced in some quantitative or mathematical way ("the greatest good for the greatest number"). Thus teleological theories often go by the name of *utilitarianism*. They are represented by such philosophers as Jeremy Bentham, John Stuart Mill, and G. E. Moore, and more recently by Joseph Fletcher (1966), whose *situation ethics* employs as its central principle "agape, the love for humanity, or general goodwill." Situation ethics is an example of another form of ethical reasoning, called the *consequentialist* approach, in which an action is judged to be morally right or wrong through an assessment of the consequences of the action. Much of clinical medicine is consequentialist in that the goodness of actions is judged by their outcomes. It should be noted, of course, that not all teleologists are utilitarians. Plato, Augustine, and even Aristotle all strove to articulate principles of conduct, but they would be horrified by the mathematical connotations of utilitarianism. Decision trees in Figures 45–3 and 45–4 outline the deontological and consequentialist forms of teleological ethical thinking (modified from Brody 1981).

Deontological and teleological theories are not just options to choose from on an ethical smorgasbord; their use depends greatly on what one is trying to accomplish. In Table 45–6, I draw a distinction between the upward perspective and the downward perspective in the tasks of ethics (Dyer 1988). The upward perspective is that of the individual moral agent in relation to the larger culture. The downward perspective is the view of the individual from the perspective of the norms of the culture or group. The upward perspective refers to the highest standards of ethical conduct to which anyone might aspire—ethical ideals, ideals of moral perfection. The task of ethics in the downward perspective is the regulation of abuse. In terms of a profession, the downward perspective concerns the profession's policing of itself. The upward perspective is that of the individual (practitioner) seeking to ensure that his or her own conduct is the highest possible. The upward perspective presupposes the mutual trust of the physician and patient in their collaboration. There is no maximum limit on mutual responsibility of the patient and physician in their partner-

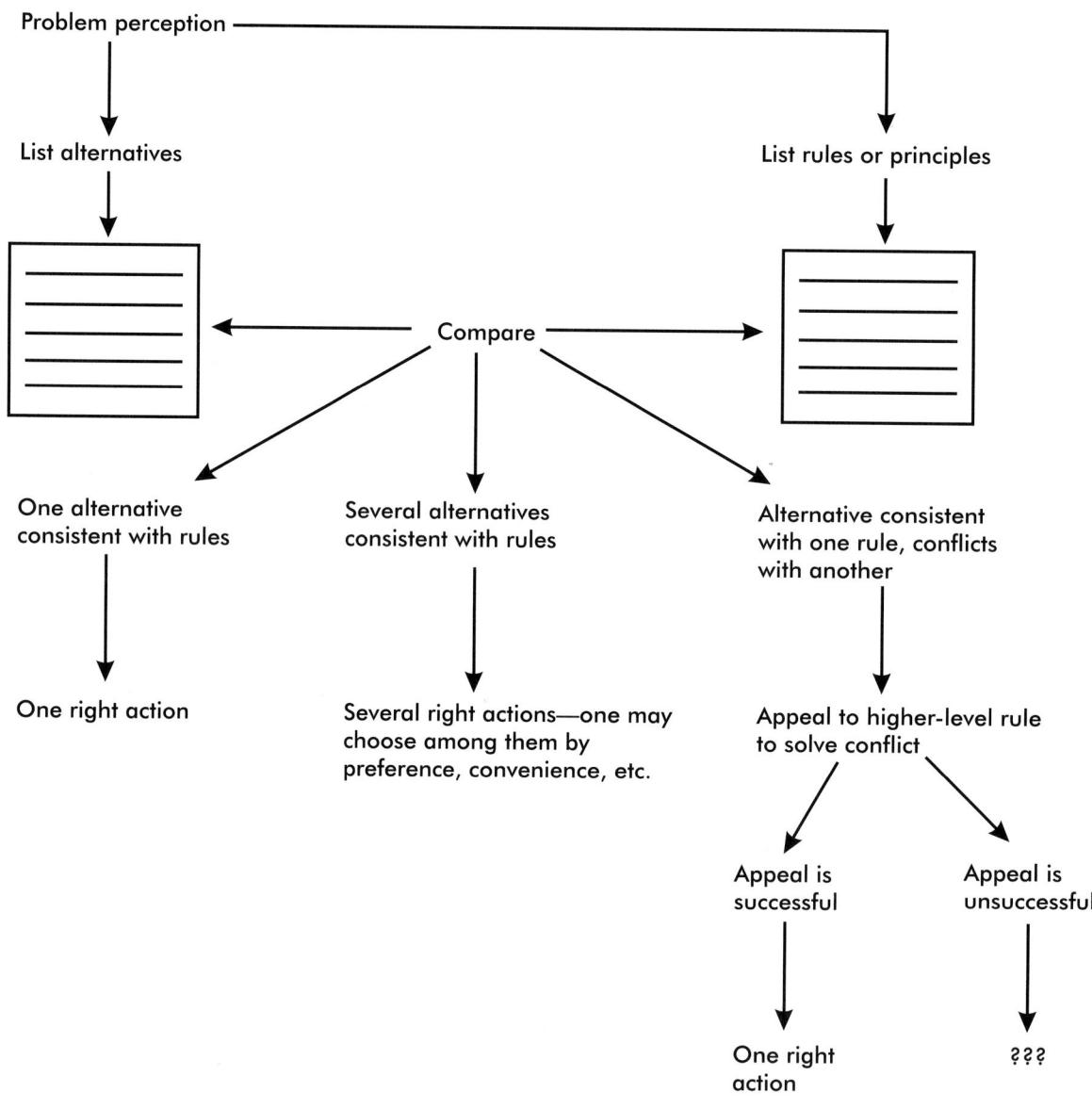

FIGURE 45–3.   Deontological ethical method.
Source.   Modified from Brody 1981.

ship, but there are minimum limits. The downward perspective is that of the regulatory agency or professional society seeking to ensure that the behavior of a particular individual does not fall below certain minimum standards, which are articulated as well as possible.

ETHICS OF VIRTUE AND CHARACTER

Both teleological and deontological approaches to ethics have one serious shortcoming. They depend on the activities of the rational mind of a motivated moral agent to apprehend right and wrong. Moral philosophers and psychiatrists alike appreciate that not everyone is motivated to be

moral, that even good people sometimes do bad things, and that people are capable of rationalizing self-interest (see Dyer 1985b; Hauerwas 1977, 1981; Pincoffs 1971, 1980). Whatever place Freudian thought assumes in contemporary psychiatry and in modern culture, Freud's explication of moral psychology is inescapable in understanding moral process. Human beings have impulses that they don't necessarily act on even though they may be tempted to. The urges of the *id* are constrained by the restrictions of society internalized as the *superego* and mediated by the more or less rational *ego*.

A delineation of obligations, however essential, is not the whole picture of ethics. Virtue, character, and integrity

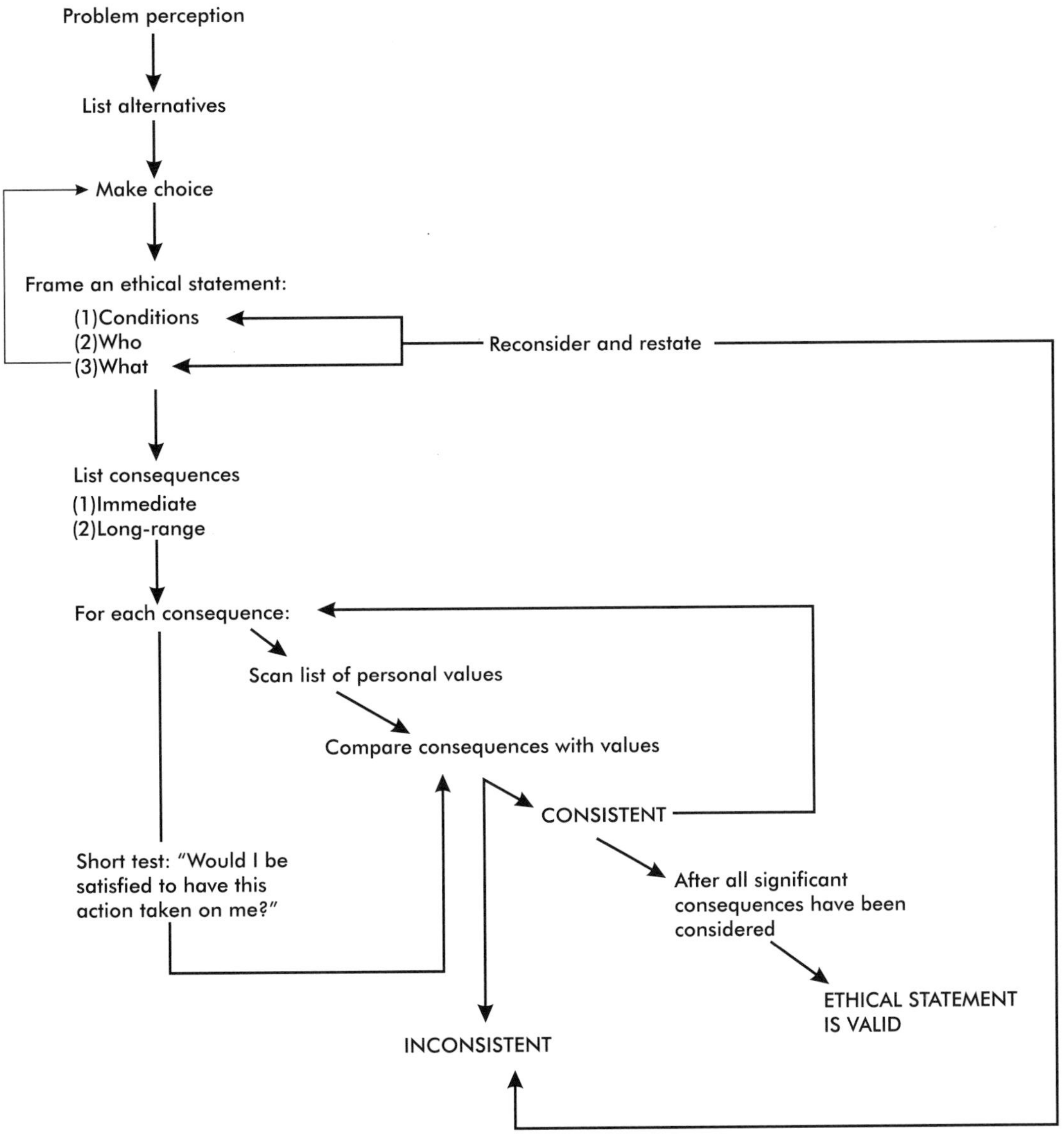

Problem perception

↓

List alternatives

↓

→ Make choice

↓

Frame an ethical statement:
    (1)Conditions ←
    (2)Who
    (3)What ←   — Reconsider and restate —

↓

List consequences
(1)Immediate
(2)Long-range

↓

For each consequence: ←

    ↘ Scan list of personal values

        ↘ Compare consequences with values

Short test: "Would I be
satisfied to have this
action taken on me?"

CONSISTENT —

After all significant
consequences have been
considered

INCONSISTENT

ETHICAL STATEMENT
IS VALID

FIGURE 45–4.   Teleological ethical method.
Source. Modified from Brody 1981.

are every bit as important in understanding right conduct. For the professions especially, integrity in concrete situations is the hallmark of virtuous life.

THE ETHICS OF MANAGED CARE

The current revolution in health care financing is calling into question not only many of the traditional assumptions of medical ethics, but assumptions about the doctor-patient relationship, the nature of health, and even the role of persons in a society. It is not just about economic values; it is about human values. The most fundamental

change to be noted is the departure from a dyadic person-to-person doctor-patient relationship:

doctor←→patient

Doctors in the new environment are being transformed into "providers"; patients are transformed into "consumers"; and any number of third parties may claim an interest in what goes on in that relationship:

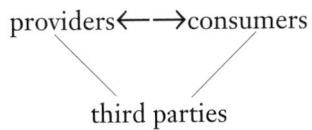

providers←→consumers

third parties

TABLE 45–6.   **The tasks of ethics**

Upward perspective	Downward perspective
Moral inspiration	Regulation of abuse
Affective	Cognitive
Self-reflective	Critical
Teleological (end-based, goal-based)	Deontological (rule-based)
Fiduciary relationship (based on trust)	Adversary relationship (based on control)
Tacit	Explicit

The metaphor of health care as an industry radically transforms the healing process. In the economic model of marketplace transactions, much more is at stake than how the payment is to be allotted. Health care is reduced to physiological interventions that take place in a delimited period of time. Physicians become not merely providers but technicians, and patients become not merely consumers but recipients of technology. Providers and consumers are likely to be strangers to one another. Medicine is transformed from a human service into a commodity.

In the interest of efficiency or economy (i.e., cost savings), these transformations might seem warranted, but the practices currently witnessed in the name of managed care must themselves be subjected to ethical scrutiny. Certainly much of what is going on is not ethically justifiable, nor are the intended ends served.

The transformation of medicine from a profession to a trade by the Federal Trade Commission was justified as a cost-saving measure on the grounds that increasing consumer choice (through advertising) would lower costs. The value placed on autonomy set the stage for a transformation that reduces the amount of choice consumers have in the health care they receive. Health care has become an investment opportunity in which vast amounts of money have been siphoned away from service delivery into the pockets of executives and shareholders of megacorporations. The market solution has been a nonsolution up until now in that it has succeeded only in lowering costs without adequately addressing quality of service or the distribution and allocation of services. The current anarchy in health care of the free market or unregulated (or underregulated) market resembles the lawlessness of the post-Civil War American frontier or of the early stages of industrialization, when efficiencies and wealth were achieved by the robber barons at the cost of environmental pollution and human suffering.

The ethical physician is inevitably in tension with a system designed to limit the care given to his or her patients or deny care altogether. Recognizing that resources are finite, the ethical physician must struggle to do the best possible for individual patients without compromising integrity. Many of the practices of managed care are fraudulently unethical, such as gag rules prohibiting physicians from discussing treatment options with their patients. Such policies do not enhance consumer choice (even the choice of paying for treatment out of pocket) but diminish patient autonomy. They are directly counter to the goal of informed consent, which has been such a key feature of the ethics of autonomy. Such gag rules place the physician in the position of a double agent without the possibility of disclosure. It is difficult for the physician to say, "Trust me," and difficult also for him or her to say, "Consumer, beware." Many of the practices of managed care are more subtly unethical, such as use of misleading advertising or incomplete disclosure, and some, such as limiting who may serve on panels, may be in restraint of trade. They are certainly not pro-competitive. Managed care is an ethically unstable response to the health care financing dilemma and must be subjected to thoroughgoing ethical evaluation. A just society must demand accountability for its citizens.

PREPARING FOR A POSTMODERN FUTURE IN MEDICINE AND PSYCHIATRY

It is not an exaggeration to suggest that a revolution in health care is taking place. It is probably also true that the revolution in health care is part of a larger revolution in social thinking. Many are suggesting that what is taking place is a paradigm shift of the sort Thomas Kuhn described in *The Structure of Scientific Revolutions* (1970). It is also being suggested that the current cultural change is a transition from modern culture to postmodern culture (see Eberle 1994; Gergen 1991; Jameson 1991; Kolb 1992). There is little consensus, however, as to what postmodern culture might entail. It is too soon to tell. For the medical profession to make an appropriate response to these new challenges, it should begin to reconceptualize the issues it faces. Physicians should do as the great hockey player Wayne Gretzky does: skate to where the puck is going to be. We shall be required to understand historical change as it occurs. We shall be required to understand our own cultural assumptions.

Although there can be no consensus on what the postmodern future will hold, one can recognize certain features of modernity as well as the fact that the assumptions of the old modern age are no longer valid. Table 45–7 summarizes features that have come to be associated with modernity: secular society, free market, constitutional democ-

TABLE 45-7.   The old modern age

Secular society
Free market
Constitutional democracy
Civil rights
Nationalism
Bureaucratic administration
Industrialization and efficiency
Capitalism
Science and technology
Rational thought
Progress

racy, civil rights, nationalism, bureaucratic administration, industrialization/efficiency, capitalism, science and technology, rational thought, and progress. Many of the tensions experienced in professional ethics and bioethics stem from tensions concerning how to think about and experience the process of valuing in the modern paradigm. Whereas many of the features of the old modern age are familiar and comfortable and perhaps worth defending, they cannot be taken for granted.

There are at least two distinct strains of postmodernism. The intellectual movement most often identified with postmodernism is called *deconstructionism*. Deconstructionism seeks to undermine the unities and certainties found in modern thought on the grounds that they are artificial constructions of a false and impersonal scientism in which human experience is made the object of detached analysis. Often using linguistic innovations, such as talking about "psychiatries" rather than "psychiatry" to emphasize the plurality of opinion within a discipline, deconstructionism seeks to attack traditional values and break traditional restrictions. Deconstructionism's postmodernism is postindividual, postcolonial, postpatriarchal, and posthumanist. Deconstructionism is either unnerving or exciting, depending on one's vantage point.

An alternative form of postmodernism may be called "postcritical" after the philosophy of Michael Polanyi (1958). Polanyi recognized that modern science, as it was usually understood, purported to be objective with a detached, value-neutral observer. In fact, real science never proceeded in this manner, but depended on the judgments of a committed knower. Science was neither objective nor subjective, but rather personal. Hence Polanyi called his major work *Personal Knowledge: Toward a Post-Critical Philosophy*. In Polanyi's philosophy, tradition (i.e., scientific tradition) plays an important role in the understanding of

the scientific community, and it lays the ground for respecting a variety of cultural traditions.

These epistemological theories have an important bearing on how ethics is to be understood. Ethics explicitly articulated (the deontological ambition) is always in tension with more tacitly understood principles (the teleological tradition). Ethics understood as conflict may be appreciated in the context of the larger cultural tensions of which such conflicts are in fact manifestations.

The goal of autonomy is very much a feature of the modern outlook. The yearning for explicitness is very much a feature of the modern outlook. But these approaches—as useful as they are, as far as they go—do not go far enough. Ethics must also deal with the nuances of human experience. Table 45–8 highlights this postmodern outlook. To the list in this figure should be added a key feature of postmodernism, namely, the toleration of ambiguity.

One may anticipate the postmodern by identifying the distinguishing features of modernity. However, one may better appreciate the paradigm shift now being experienced by looking at what preceded modernity. Table 45–9 suggests a perspective on this development. Notable in premodern thinking is the focus on human experience and the human dimension. In the more deconstructive approaches to postmodernism, this dimension drops out; however, in approaches that stress the role of tradition (such as Polanyi's postcritical philosophy), the recovery of the human dimension lost in modernity becomes an important part of the postmodern enterprise. It is notable that in postmodern approaches to art and architecture, one sees the reintroduction of the human form and human scale.

Premodern art was representational. Pictures told stories. Modern art abandoned these representations in favor of more abstract and expressionistic ideas in painting. Postmodern art reintroduces the human form. Classical (premodern) architecture was built around the human

TABLE 45-8.   The functions of ethics

Modern account	Postmodern (postcritical) account
Universal	Contextual
Impersonal	Personal
Atemporal	Historical
Acultural	Cultural
Based on obligation	Based on integrity
Enforced by control, suasion, or sanction	Enforced by willing assent, trust in a convivial order, or community

TABLE 45–9.   A perspective on modernity

Premodern thinking	Prescientific, ecclesiastical authority, magical thinking, focus on human experience
Modern thinking	Emphasizes the individual and the search for a systematic, scientific *certitude*
Postmodern thinking	*Deconstructive:* undermines the unities and closures found in modern thought
	Postcritical: makes use of modern achievement; offers new freedoms

form. Modern architecture, grand and impersonal, forced humans to adapt to monolithic skyscrapers, huge black boxes in which humans were but cogs in the machine. Postmodern architecture reintroduces the human element in building. It does this by whimsical elements such as oversized arches, pediments, columns, and windows, which even in large buildings serve as reminders that the buildings are human meeting places. Postmodern buildings often exist in relationship to their surroundings and community, respecting the traditions of their neighbors by borrowing (mirroring) elements such as classical (Greek) columns, Gothic arches, or Victorian ornamentation.

It is such humanistic, communitarian, historical elements in continuity with tradition that offer hopeful and exciting possibilities for the future of medicine (Table 45–10). Medicine in the modern paradigm has been a technological marvel, but focusing on the body as a machine has left an impersonal coldness that has created the host of ethical dilemmas that have come to be associated with the domain of bioethics; it also has created an economic nightmare. The possibility of recovering the human dimension in medicine suggests a useful direction for postmodernism in medicine. It must be acknowledged, however, that this is not necessarily the way things are

TABLE 45–10.   Modern and postmodern medical practice

Old paradigm (modern)	New paradigm (postmodern)
Acute illness (hospital based)	Chronic illness (community based)
Curative	Preventive
Physician centered	Doctor-patient partnership
Individual patient	Health of population
Prototype: young, white male	Cultural diversity

headed if present trends are extrapolated into the future. The value of individual life is already threatened by capitated economic systems that focus on the well-being of the population.

Looking back at the contributions of the premodern classical age allows an appreciation for the place of the Hippocratic oath and the Hippocratic tradition in contemporary medicine. Although these ideas are sometimes criticized for being anachronistic, their value becomes apparent. The Hippocratic tradition in medicine provides a perspective of enduring values by which the shortcomings of modern expediency may be judged.

REFERENCES

American Medical Association: Opinions and Reports of the Judicial Council. Chicago, IL, American Medical Association, 1957

American Medical Association: Code of Medical Ethics (150th Anniversary Edition): Current Opinions with Annotations of the Council on Ethical and Judicial Affairs. Chicago, IL, American Medical Association, 1997

American Psychiatric Association: Opinions of the Ethics Committee on the Principles of Medical Ethics With Annotations Especially Applicable to Psychiatry. Washington, DC, American Psychiatric Press, 1995a

American Psychiatric Association: The Principles of Medical Ethics With Annotations Especially Applicable to Psychiatry. Washington, DC, American Psychiatric Press, 1995b

Bloch S: The political misuse of psychiatry in the Soviet Union, in Psychiatric Ethics, 2nd Edition. Edited by Bloch S, Chodoff P. New York, Oxford University Press, 1991

Bloch S, Reddaway P: Psychiatric Terror: How Soviet Psychiatry is Used to Suppress Dissent. New York, Basic Books, 1977

Brody H: Ethical Decisions in Medicine, 2nd Edition. Boston, MA, Little, Brown, 1981

Dyer AR: Ethics, advertising, and the definition of a profession J Med Ethics 11:72–78, 1985a

Dyer AR: Virtue and medicine: a physician's analysis, in Virtue and Medicine. Edited by Shelp E. Dordrecht, The Netherlands, D. Reidel, 1985b, pp 223–235

Dyer AR: Ethics and Psychiatry: Toward Professional Definition. Washington, DC, American Psychiatric Press, 1988

Dyer AR: Advertising, in Encyclopedia of Bioethics, 2nd Edition. Edited by Reich W. New York, Macmillan, 1995

Dyer AR: Ethics, advertising, and assisted reproduction: the goals and methods of advertising. Women's Health, May/June 1997a

Dyer AR: Ethics of human genetic intervention: a postmodern perspective. Exp Neurol 144:168–172, 1997b

Eberle G: The Geography of Nowhere: Finding One's Self in the Postmodern World, Kansas City, MO, Sheed & Ward, 1994

Edelstein L: The Hippocratic oath: Text, translation, and interpretation. Bull Hist Med (suppl 1), 1943

Fletcher J: Situation Ethics. Philadelphia, PA, Westminster Press, 1966

Frankena W: Ethics. Englewood Cliffs, NJ, Prentice-Hall, 1963

Gergen KJ: The Saturated Self: Dilemmas of Identity in Contemporary Life. New York: Basic Books, 1991

Greenhouse J: Justices uphold right of doctors to solicit trade. The New York Times, March 24, 1982, p 10

Guttentag OE: On defining medicine. The Christian Scholar 46:200–211, 1963

Hauerwas S: Community and Character. Notre Dame, IN, University of Notre Dame Press, 1981

Hauerwas S: Truthfulness and Tragedy: Further Investigations Into Christian Ethics. Notre Dame, IN, University of Notre Dame Press, 1977

Jameson F: Postmodernism, or, the Cultural Logic of Late Capitalism, Durham, NC, Duke University Press, 1991

Kant I: Fundamental Principles of the Metaphysics of Morals (1797) (The Library of Liberal Arts). Indianapolis, IN, Bobbs-Merrill, 1949

Kolb D: Postmodern Sophistications: Philosophy, Architecture, and Tradition, Chicago, IL, University of Chicago Press, 1992

Kuhn TS: The Structure of Scientific Revolutions, 2nd Edition. enlarged with postscript. Chicago, IL, Chicago University Press, 1970. [2nd Edition includes postscript.]

Laín Entralgo P: The Therapy of the Word in Classical Antiquity. New Haven. CT, Yale University Press, 1970

Levine M: Psychiatry and Ethics. New York, Holt, Rinehart & Winston, 1972

Osler W: A Way of Life: An Address to Yale Students, Sunday Evening, April 29, 1913. Springfield, IL, Charles C Thomas, 1969

Pincoffs E: Quandary Ethics. Mind 75:552–571, 1971

Pincoffs E: Virtue, the quality of life and punishment. The Monist 63(2):23–27, 1980

Polanyi M: Personal Knowledge: Towards a Post-Critical Philosophy. London, Routledge & Kegan Paul, 1958

Toennies F: Fundamental Concepts of Sociology. Translated by Loomis C. New York: American Book Company, 1940

CHAPTER 46

PSYCHIATRY AND PRIMARY CARE

DONALD M. HILTY, M.D.
MARK E. SERVIS, M.D.

Substantial changes in the organization and delivery of health care are taking place. A major transition in health care has been the shift from inpatient to outpatient services. Health care costs and technological advances have facilitated this process, and the result has been decreased hospital utilization rates and lengths of stay. The goal for both medical and psychiatric hospitalization is now stabilization of the patient in an acute state. Patients become outpatients while on complex treatment regimens and while their conditions are still acute. Psychiatrists with consultation-liaison skills will continue to play a vital role in hospital settings and will be increasingly important in the primary care setting because of the need for follow-up care and for managing behaviors that affect compliance and medical stability.

The primary care provider is becoming increasingly important in the delivery of mental health care in the primary care setting. Primary care practices serve as the de facto mental health network, providing the sole contact for more than 50% of patients with mental illness (Regier et al. 1978, 1993). This percentage is likely to grow, given the increased emphasis on outpatient care and the administrative arrangements that encourage initial management of psychiatric disorders by primary care physicians. These pro-viders need standardized treatment protocols, access to psychiatric consultation, and an administrative infrastructure to manage patients with mental health care needs.

Psychiatric care in the primary care setting is being carefully evaluated because of concerns about rising health care costs. In this era of managed care, payers have attempted to reduce costs by prospective payment, increased utilization review, and case management. A new service is not developed unless a clear benefit can be shown in reducing costs. Cost-offset analyses, which have been used in the past to justify funding for psychiatric care in medical settings, measure whether overall medical costs are reduced by psychiatric consultation. However, currently any new treatment is generally more expensive in its direct and indirect costs than its predecessors. A conceptual shift is called for in light of reimbursement changes, particularly given that capitated payment systems require the provider to share financial risk for patient care. Cost-benefit analysis, which assesses the gain from each treatment in comparison with each dollar spent, has already begun to show the benefits of psychiatric care in primary care settings for patients with depression (Katon et al. 1997). If risk is shared among providers in different specialties and the health system, all involved may be more willing to consider how a patient's psychosocial issues affect health and illness.

There is a marked need for research in the primary care setting. Leaders in the field have proposed guidelines for randomized, controlled trials that are necessary to determine how best to evaluate and treat patients with mental disorders in the primary care setting (Katon et al. 1994a; Schulberg et al. 1993). These patients' illnesses are less homogeneous than those seen in psychiatric settings and are frequently comorbid with medical illnesses. Because treatments in primary care are less intensive than those in mental health care, questions arise regarding their efficacy, how to maintain compliance, and how best to organize treatment resources. Primary care patients may also be more ambivalent about obtaining care, and therefore the study of expectations and satisfaction should be undertaken.

In this chapter, we begin with a comprehensive review of the epidemiology of common psychiatric disorders in the primary care setting. Next is a discussion of the undertreatment of these disorders because of inadequate recognition and treatment, along with a report of the results of randomized clinical trials in which attempts were made to improve treatment. A summary of conceptual models for psychiatric consultation is followed by a section on detecting psychiatric illness in the primary care setting, and the chapter concludes with a discussion of the basic principles for the management of common psychiatric disorders in this setting.

EPIDEMIOLOGY OF PSYCHIATRIC DISORDERS IN THE PRIMARY CARE SETTING

A review of investigations from several decades reveals that mental disorders are present in approximately 25% of patients in the primary care setting (Schulberg and Burns 1988). Overall, approximately 60%–70% of patients with anxiety, mood, somatoform, and chemical dependency disorders are seen within the primary care setting and only about one-fifth of these patients are referred to mental health specialists (Shapiro et al. 1984). Primary care physicians estimate that they spend between 20% and 50% of their time treating psychiatric problems (Fauman 1983; Stoudemire et al. 1982–1983). Primary care physicians write the majority of prescriptions for antidepressants (Simon and Von Korff 1993) and anxiolytic medications (Mellinger et al. 1984).

DEPRESSIVE AND ANXIETY DISORDERS

Epidemiologic studies in primary care typically show that 10%–15% of patients have anxiety or depressive disorders (Eisenberg 1992). Depression has been best studied in the primary care setting. When structured interview schedules were used to detect major depression, 5%–10% of ambulatory medical patients met criteria for a current mood disorder (Katon and Schulberg 1992). The prevalence of generalized anxiety disorder in the primary care setting is estimated to be 1.6%–11.9% (Barrett et al. 1988; Hoeper et al. 1979; Shear et al. 1994; Zinbarg et al. 1994) and that of panic disorder is estimated to be 1.6%–11% (Angst et al. 1990; Katon et al. 1986; Shear et al. 1994; Zinbarg et al. 1994). Of patients meeting criteria for a major depression, 75% had a lifetime history of comorbid anxiety disorder (Schulberg et al. 1995b). Of patients meeting criteria for panic disorder or generalized anxiety disorder, 80% reported a history of major depression (Shear et al. 1994). In the primary care sites of the DSM-IV (American Psychiatric Association 1994) field trial for mixed anxiety-depression, the prevalence of other anxiety disorders was 1.2% for obsessive-compulsive disorder, 4.5% for posttraumatic stress disorder, 10.4% for simple phobia, and 13.0% for social phobia (Zinbarg et al. 1994). A mixed anxiety-depression disorder was proposed for DSM-IV (but was not accepted) for patients who do not meet criteria for major depression or generalized anxiety disorder but who have a substantial number of clinically relevant symptoms (Katon and Roy-Byrne 1991). The prevalence of the disorder is 5.1%–6.6% (Fifer et al. 1994; Roy-Byrne et al. 1994; Zinbarg et al. 1994).

FUNCTIONAL SOMATIC DISORDERS

Other disorders commonly found in the primary care setting include the somatoform disorders. The lifetime risk for somatization disorder is estimated to be approximately 2%–3% in women (Cloninger et al. 1984). The Epidemiologic Catchment Area (ECA) study prevalence of 0.2%–0.3% of women is likely an underestimate, because of the use of different diagnostic criteria and the reliance on interviews by nonphysicians (Escobar et al. 1987). A somatization syndrome has been proposed—to be diagnosed using the Somatic Symptom Index—defined as the presence of four somatic symptoms for males and six somatic symptoms for females. Prevalence of this syndrome would have been 12% in the ECA population (Escobar et al. 1989) and is 26% in another primary care setting (Kirmayer and Robbins 1991). The prevalence of hypochondriasis is estimated to be between 0.5% and 6.3% in the primary care setting (Barsky et al. 1990; Escobar 1996). The prevalence of hypochondriasis was not assessed by the ECA study. With more narrow definitions of hypochondriasis, figures range from 3% to 13% in different cultures (Kenyon 1965).

SUBSTANCE USE DISORDERS

The prevalence of substance use disorders has been studied less extensively. Alcohol is the most common drug of abuse in most primary care settings. Epidemiologic studies have found that 5%–15% of patients abuse alcohol, with higher prevalence rates in urban clinics serving patients of lower socioeconomic status (Hoeper et al. 1979; Johnson et al. 1993; Schulberg et al. 1985; Simon and Von Korff 1991; Von Korff et al. 1987). The frequency of other substance use disorders ranges from 5.0% to 7.1% (Hoeper et al. 1979; Schulberg et al. 1985; Von Korff et al. 1987). Current and lifetime substance use disorders are more prevalent in patients with major depression and other depressive disorders (Coyne et al. 1994).

DISABILITY AND COST OF DISORDERS

Psychiatric disorders cause marked disability in patients in the primary care setting. Depression profoundly limits social and vocational functioning (Broadhead et al. 1990; Mintz et al. 1992; Von Korff et al. 1992). Depression is associated with more functional disability than are most chronic illnesses (Wells et al. 1989b), and the number of reports of medically unexplained symptoms associated with depression is increasing (Katon 1982). Depression can increase the morbidity and mortality associated with a variety of medical disorders (Rodin and Voshart 1987; Rovner et al. 1991). Studies show that anxiety disorders and mixed anxiety-depression cause at least mild impairment in social and occupational roles (Roy-Byrne 1996). Patients with unrecognized anxiety report notably worse functioning on both physical and emotional measures, levels of functioning in ranges reported for patients with chronic physical illnesses (Fifer et al. 1994). The economic impact of depression in all settings is estimated to exceed $43 billion per year (Greenberg et al. 1993) and the impact of anxiety disorders is estimated to be more than $46 billion annually (DuPont et al. 1995).

Epidemiologic studies highlight the value of diagnosis and treatment of mental disorders in the primary care setting. Appropriate care for depression improves functional outcomes and is associated with increased cost (Katon et al. 1997; Sturm and Wells 1995). Inadequate treatment of mental health disorders by the primary care physician worsens outcomes and is linked with reduced cost (Sturm and Wells 1995). Compared with nondepressed control subjects, patients with a diagnosis of depression have higher annual health care costs and higher costs for every aspect of care (e.g., primary care, medical specialty care, medical inpatient care, pharmaceuticals, laboratory work), even when adjustments are made for differences in the number and severity of medical illnesses (Simon et al. 1995b). In addition, the costs associated with the greater utilization of medical services by depressed patients exceed the treatment costs for depression. In another similar study, overall health care costs for patients with depressive and anxiety disorders were also higher than for controls (Simon et al. 1995a).

INADEQUATE TREATMENT OF PSYCHIATRIC DISORDERS

There is a substantial literature about the inadequate treatment of psychiatric disorders, particularly depression. The National Depressive and Manic-Depressive Association prepared a consensus statement on the undertreatment of depression, which describes a gap between our knowledge of depression and implementation of treatment (Hirschfeld et al. 1997). This gap has been attributed to patient, provider, and administrative factors. Methods of improving the treatment of mental disorders in patients in the primary care setting must take all of these factors into account, rather than simply focusing on improving knowledge and skills of primary care physicians (Cole and Raju 1996). Psychiatrists detect most cases of depression (Wells et al. 1989a) and in the Medical Outcomes Study were likely to prescribe antidepressant medications, particularly in more severe cases (Wells et al. 1994).

Patient Factors

Patients do not recognize they have symptoms of depression and instead focus on somatic etiologies. Patients and their family members underestimate the severity of depression and therefore do not pursue treatment (Endicott and Blumenthal 1995). They may view depression as an expected response to a life situation. Results of a poll regarding what Americans do for minor health problems indicated a great reluctance to take a medication for relief of depression (Roper Poll 1986). Patients who recognize the importance of their problem may face limited access to treatment, especially in areas that are underserved by physicians and by providers of mental health care. Finally, there are also substantial problems with adherence to a medical regimen.

Provider Factors

The undertreatment of depression is linked in many ways to the provider of mental health care. Interestingly, 84% of primary care physicians feel strongly that they should care for the emotional problems of their patients (Harr et al.

1972), but they may not be adequately prepared. Medical school training in psychiatry and residency training do not allow ample time for trainees to learn a full range of treatments. After residency training, only 10% of primary care physicians receive any form of continuing medical education in psychiatry (Fink 1980). Other provider factors that contribute to the undertreatment of psychiatric illnesses include the physician's limited amount of time with a patient, barriers to prescribing newer medication, lack of reimbursement for services rendered for the treatment of mental disorders, and the belief that others should manage a patient's mental health problem or that mental disorders are not legitimate medical problems.

Administrative Factors

A number of health care system factors also contribute to the undertreatment of depression and other psychiatric disorders. In a busy practice, primary care physicians are unable to offer structured psychotherapy, and hence efficacious approaches are ignored (Jarrett and Rush 1994). Health plans do not facilitate detection of illness, can discourage proper monitoring of medication, and may not offer reimbursement to primary care physicians for the treatment of depression (Hirschfeld et al. 1997).

Studies of the Adequacy of Treatment

A number of studies in the literature delineate the inadequate treatment of mental disorders in the primary care setting, revealing both a failure of recognition and inadequate trials of antidepressant medication. In a study of nearly 2,000 consecutive patients entering a primary care clinic, only two-thirds of depressed patients were considered by their primary care physicians to be distressed and only 56% of those patients filled prescriptions for antidepressant medications within 3 months (Simon and Von Korff 1995). In a study of nearly 1,500 depressed patients, 35% of patients dropped out of treatment within the first 60 days and only 35% of patients studied continued taking acute-phase medication for 6 months or more (Katon and Schulberg 1992). In a study of high utilizers of primary care services, 55% of depressed patients had not received antidepressants in the year before evaluation and only 10% received an adequate dose of antidepressants for an adequate duration (Katon et al. 1992b).

According to a recent report, an estimated 5% of patients with depression receive an antidepressant for a 6-month maintenance phase after appropriate acute treatment (Katzelnick 1997). The following assumptions were made in determining this figure: depression is appropriately diagnosed in 50% of patients; one-fourth of those

with the diagnosis receive adequate treatment (12.5% of the overall sample); two-thirds respond to the medication trial (8.5% of the overall sample); and less than two-thirds of those who respond to the trial continue taking the medication for 6 months (5% of the overall sample).

Data from the Medical Outcomes Study are also revealing (Wells et al. 1994). Minor tranquilizers were used more commonly for depressed patients than were antidepressants—30% and 23%, respectively. Overall, 39% of patients treated with antidepressants received subtherapeutic doses, as judged by criteria used by Katon et al. (1992a) and by applying the clinical practice guidelines of the Agency for Health Care Policy and Research (AHCPR) (Depression Guideline Panel 1993b). Of the patients treated by psychiatrists, sicker patients were more likely to be prescribed medication; that did not hold true for similar patients treated by nonphysicians (i.e., the sicker patients were neither recognized nor referred for medication treatment).

The literature reveals conflicting findings regarding the outcome for those patients who undergo inadequate trials of medication. In a study of only 47 depressed patients, 63% received an antidepressant (Rost et al. 1995). Only 11% received an antidepressant in accordance with AHCPR guidelines, and those treated adequately showed more improvement at 5-month follow-up. For patients with severe depression, outcome is definitely worse with inadequate treatment (Katon et al. 1994b; Schulberg et al. 1987b). The outcome for inadequately treated patients may not differ from that for patients whose illnesses go unrecognized, because the latter group often have a milder and more self-limited form (Simon and Von Korff 1995; Simon et al. 1995c). This finding is consistent with the results of another study, which revealed that the outcome of unrecognized cases was similar to the outcome of cases that were recognized (Simon and Von Korff 1993). In a secondary analysis of the data, it was discovered that persons with unrecognized illness had milder symptoms of depression and were less disabled. In addition, severity of illness does not always correspond with use of services. Finally, two other studies found that compared with control subjects, patients in whom the disorder was not recognized were noted to have substantially more social impairment and disability at follow-up but used health care services less often (Ormel et al. 1991).

RECOGNITION OF PSYCHIATRIC DISORDERS IN THE PRIMARY CARE SETTING

The research literature suggests there are major shortcomings in the recognition of psychiatric disorders in the primary care setting. In one review of studies using structured criteria from DSM-III (American Psychiatric Association 1980) or DSM-III-R (American Psychiatric Association 1987), it was reported that between 33% and 79% of mental disorders in the primary care setting are not recognized, depending on the criteria used for recognition (Higgins 1994). According to studies assessing the underrecognition of specific disorders, 40%–50% of depression is not recognized by treating primary care physicians (Ormel et al. 1990; Schulberg et al. 1985; Simon and Von Korff 1993; Von Korff et al. 1987). Anxiety disorders are not recognized 41%–60% of the time and somatic disorders are not recognized 51% of the time (Anderson and Harthorn 1989).

PATIENT PRESENTATION OF ILLNESS

Recognition of psychiatric disorders is difficult in the primary care setting for many reasons. Depression is thought by physicians to be of lesser severity among medical patients than among psychiatric patients (Sireling et al. 1985). The interaction of medical and psychiatric illness is often more complex among medical patients than among mental health sector patients (Schulberg et al. 1987a). Another hypothesis about underrecognition is that primary care physicians encounter more diverse affective and anxiety illnesses (Shepherd and Wilkinson 1988). Ambulatory medical patients often present more somatic symptoms than affective symptoms (Katon 1982). The recognition of depression is related to the degree of somatization in the patient's presentation (Figure 46–1) (Kirmayer et al. 1993).

The diagnosis of anxiety disorders can be particularly difficult because patients may have comorbid depression or may not present with anxiety symptoms. One study found that 83% of patients with anxiety or depression presented with somatic complaints, whereas only 17% of patients with anxiety or depression presented with psychological symptoms (Bridges and Goldberg 1985). Another study found that family physicians correctly diagnosed anxiety or depressive disorders in 77% of patients who presented with psychological complaints but in only 22% of patients with somatic complaints (Kirmayer et al. 1993). The number of physical complaints is correlated with the prevalence of anxiety disorders (Kroenke et al. 1994). Prevalence rates of anxiety disorders were 1% for patients with one or no symptoms, 7% for those with two to three symptoms, 13% for those with four to five symptoms, 30% for those with six to eight symptoms, and 48% for those with nine or more symptoms.

GUIDELINES FOR DIAGNOSING DEPRESSION IN MEDICALLY ILL PATIENTS

The literature offers some guidelines to aid the clinician in distinguishing whether depressive symptoms are due to major depressive illness or are manifestations of physical illness. Generally, the presence of affective and cognitive symptoms is a better determinant of depressive illness in medically ill patients (Cavanaugh 1984). Symptoms of irritability, sadness, dissatisfaction, discouragement about the future, and difficulty with decisions are often manifestations of the psychological reaction to illness and hospitalization, unless they are persistent or severe (Cavanaugh 1983). Some psychiatrists suggest taking a *substitutive approach*, whereby depressive symptoms frequently seen in the medically ill population are replaced with other symptoms (Endicott 1984). For example, social withdrawal could replace sleep disturbance in a patient with pain and insomnia, or self-pity or pessimism could replace fatigue in a patient with viral hepatitis. Others advocate an *inclusive approach* to diagnosing depression, in which depression is diagnosed based on the presence of standardized criteria (Cohen-Cole et al. 1993). The argument is that if a symptom could be due to physical illness or major depression, it should nevertheless be counted toward the diagnosis of depression. The approach would likely result in false-positive diagnoses, but studies show the risk of overdiagnosis of depression in the medical setting to be only 1.5%–8% (Fedoroff et al. 1991; Kathol et al. 1990).

PATIENT POPULATIONS AT INCREASED RISK FOR MENTAL DISORDERS

Physicians in the primary care setting and emergency rooms must contend with complex presentations of illness and high utilizers of services. In a study of distressed frequent attenders to primary care settings, it was discovered that 23.5% had major depression, 16.8% dysthymia, 21.8% generalized anxiety disorder, and 20.2% somatization disorder (Katon et al. 1990). Among patients identified as "frustrating" by their physicians, there is a higher incidence of somatization, generalized anxiety, and depressive disorders (Lin et al. 1991). Among patients presenting to the emergency room, 31% had panic disorder, 23% had generalized anxiety disorder, and 23% had major depression (Wulsin et al. 1991).

The prevalence of anxiety and depressive disorders is much higher in specific medical populations than in community populations. Therefore, the presence of a medical condition should increase suspicion of the presence of a mental disorder. The epidemiology of and the diagnostic

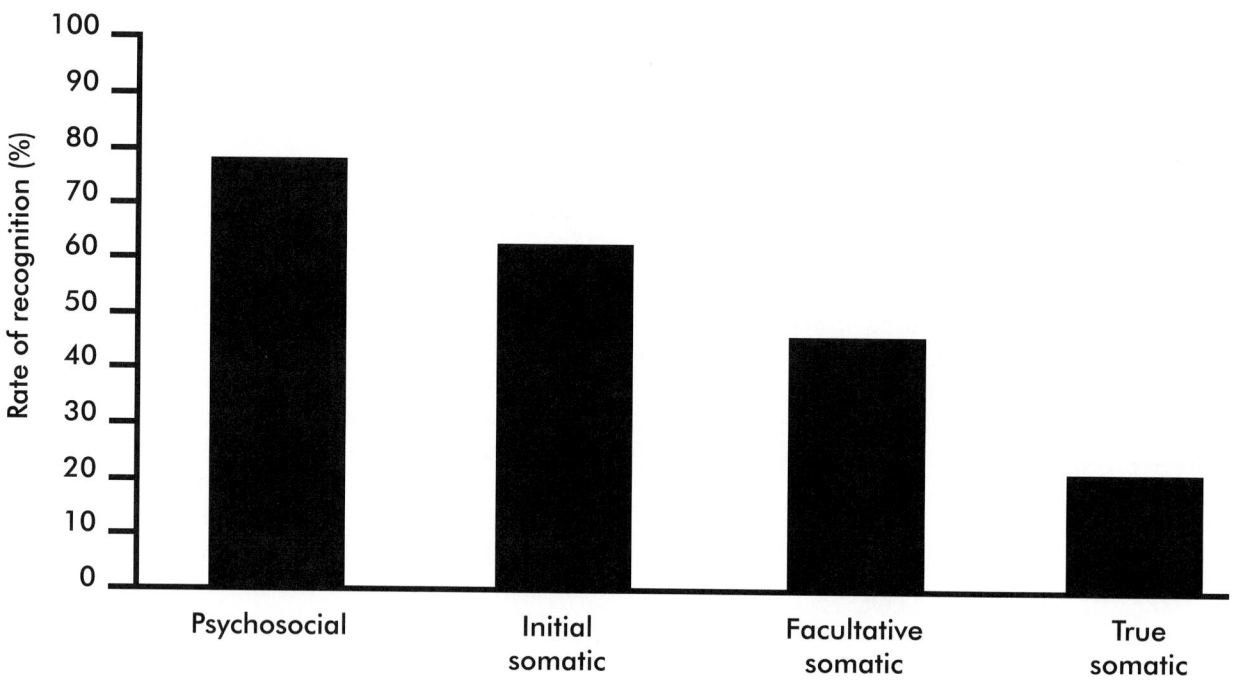

FIGURE 46-1.   Effect of type of patient presentation on recognition of depression in primary care setting. Reprinted with permission from Docherty J: "Barriers to the diagnosis of depression in primary care." *J Clin Psychiatry* 58 (suppl 1):5–10, 1997. Copyright 1997, Physician Postgraduate Press, Inc.

considerations and treatment approaches for medically ill patients have been succinctly reviewed (Wise and Rieck 1993; Wise and Taylor 1990). Depressive symptoms and disorders occur at rates of 18%–39% in patients with cancer, 10%–37% in patients with Parkinson's disease, 20%–50% in patients who have had strokes, 15%–19% in patients who have had myocardial infarctions, 5%–11% in patients with diabetes mellitus, and 13% in patients with rheumatoid arthritis (Cohen-Cole et al. 1993). Anxiety symptoms and disorders occur at increased rates in patients with chronic obstructive pulmonary disease, hyperthyroidism, Parkinson's disease, diabetes mellitus, irritable bowel syndrome, myocardial infarction, and other chronic medical illnesses (R. J. Goldberg 1995; Wise and Rieck 1993).

USE OF INTERVENTIONS TO IMPROVE RECOGNITION

Attempts have been made in a number of controlled studies to improve the recognition and treatment of mental illness by primary care physicians (Table 46–1). In 8 studies, each physician in the intervention group was given the results of a screen completed by the patient before the visit, an action referred to as *notification*. In 4 studies the physicians were educated through either instruction or psychi-

atric consultation. Of the 10 studies that assessed physician recognition, 8 found improved physician recognition of mental illness in the treatment group. Of the 8 studies that assessed physician treatment, 6 found increased mental health treatment in the intervention group. The treatments and actions assessed included psychotherapy, filling of prescriptions, and mental health referrals. When the data from all 12 studies were pooled, it was determined that 8 of 12 notification interventions and 4 of 4 education interventions were successful.

EFFECT OF INTERVENTIONS ON PATIENT OUTCOME

The impact of interventions on the clinical outcome for patients has been measured in several studies (Table 46–2). These studies, in which outcome is measured in a controlled manner, take into account recognition of disorders, treatment, and patient compliance with treatment. The data collected reveal whether recognition affects outcome. Outcome is generally divided into outcome with regard to patient symptoms, to health care use, and to cost. Generally, interventions had a positive impact on symptom outcome, but no impact was found in terms of the use of health services.

Two other reports complement the studies summa-

TABLE 46–1. Controlled studies in primary care with a goal of improving recognition and treatment of mental illness by primary care physicians

| Source, y | Setting | Intervention | Participants, No. | | Effect on Recognition | Effect on Treatment |
			Physicians	Patients		
Johnstone and Goldberg 1976	Solo general practice in Birkenshaw, England	Notification: results of GHQ for patients with unrecognized psychiatric disorders were randomly assigned to the physician	1	179	—	Increased treatment and psychiatric consultation
Moore et al. 1978	Duke Family Medicine Center, Durham, NC	Notification: results of Zung Scale were randomly assigned to the physicians	Not reported	212	Increased recognition of depression noted on chart	—
Goldberg et al. 1980	Medical University of South Carolina Family Medicine Center, Charleston	Education: family medicine residents were instructed in psychiatric assessment during four sessions with videotape review	24	1440 patient encounters	Improved correlation with GHQ-28 results	—
Linn and Yager 1984	University of California–Los Angeles Ambulatory Care Center	Notification: results of Zung Scale were randomly assigned to physicians	Not reported	150	Increased recognition of depression noted on chart	No difference
Zung et al. 1983	Duke Family Medicine Center	Notification: results of Zung Scale and *DSM-III* checklist for major depression were randomly assigned to physicians	Not reported	72	Increased recognition of depression noted on chart	—
Hoeper et al. 1984	Marshfield (Wis) Medical Clinic	Notification: results of GHQ were randomly assigned to physicians	14	1452	No difference in recognition	—
Shapiro et al. 1987	The Johns Hopkins Internal Medicine Associates Clinic, Baltimore, MD	Notification: results of GHQ were randomly assigned to physicians	45	1242	No difference in recognition	No difference

(continued)

TABLE 46-1. Controlled studies in primary care with a goal of improving recognition and treatment of mental illness by primary care physicians *(continued)*

Source, y	Setting	Intervention	Participants, No. Physicians	Participants, No. Patients	Effect on Recognition	Effect on Treatment
Rand et al. 1988	Family medicine residency center, University of Alabama, Tuscaloosa	Education: family medicine residents at one site were trained in interpretation of GHQ, which was then given to all patients at that site	32	1040 patient encounters	Increased recognition at study site	Increased antidepressant prescriptions
Magruder-Habib et al. 1990	Durham Veterans Affairs General Medical Clinic	Notification: results of Zung Scale and *DSM-III* depression screen were randomly assigned to physicians	9 (and 3 physician assistants)	112	Increased recognition of depression noted on chart	Increased treatment of depression
Katon et al. 1992	Group Health Cooperative of Puget Sound (Wash)	Education: study was limited to distressed, high utilizers; intervention group received psychiatric consultation	18	232	—	Increased filling of prescriptions for antidepressants
Mathias et al. 1994	Health maintenance organization in central Colorado	Notification: intervention physicians received summarized information about patients' anxiety levels and functional status	75	573	Increased recognition of anxiety noted on chart	Increased psychotropic prescriptions and mental health referrals
Roter and Hall 1991	The Johns Hopkins School of Hygiene and Public Health	Education: physicians were randomly assigned to an interviewing skills seminar or a control group	69	652	Increased correlation between physicians' rating of emotional distress and patients' GHQ results in intervention physicians	Increased use of the specific interviewing skills in which intervention physicians had been trained

Note. Empty cells indicate that the parameter was not evaluated (or researched).
Source. Reprinted from Higgins ES: "A Review of Unrecognized Mental Illness in Primary Care: Prevalence, Natural History, and Efforts to Change the Course." *Archives of Family Medicine* 3:908–917, 1994. Copyright 1994, American Medical Association. Used with permission.

TABLE 46–2. Controlled studies examining interventions that improved recognition of mental illness by primary care physicians and effect on patient symptoms and use of general medical health care

Source, y	Setting	Method	Participants, No. Physicians	Participants, No. Patients	Effect on Symptoms	Effect on Health Care Use
Johnstone and Goldberg 1976	Solo general practice in Birkenshaw, England	Results of GHQ for patients' with unrecognized psychiatric disorders were randomly assigned to the physician	1	179	Increased percentage judged well at 3, 6, and 9 months but not at 12 months; decreased duration of episode in identified group	No difference in rate of health care appointments over 12 months after initial visit
Zung et al. 1983	Duke Family Medicine Center, Durham, NC	Results of Zung Scale and DSM-III checklist for major depression were randomly assigned to physicians	Not reported	72	Increased percentage of patients in identified group "improved" after 4 weeks	—
Magruder-Habib et al. 1989	Durham Veterans Affairs General Medical Clinic	Results of Zung Scale and DSM-III depression screen were randomly assigned to the physicians	9 (and 3 physician assistants)	112	No difference in depressive symptoms at 3, 6, 9, and 12 months	—
Katon et al. 1992	Group Health Cooperative of Puget Sound (Wash)	Study was limited to distressed, high utilizers; intervention group received psychiatric consultation	18	232	No difference in anxiety or depression at 6 and 12 months	No difference in use of health care services at 6 and 12 months
Mathias et al. 1994	Health maintenance organization in central Colorado	Intervention physicians received summarized information about patients' anxiety levels and functional status	75	573	No difference in anxiety at 5 months	No difference in office visits at 5 months
Roter and Hall 1991	The Johns Hopkins School of Hygiene and Public Health, Baltimore, MD	Physicians were randomly assigned to an interviewing skills seminar or a control group	69	652	Significantly greater improvement in GHQ results of patients with intervention physicians at 6 months	No difference in use of health care services at 3 and 6 months

Note. Empty cells indicate that the parameter was not evaluated (or researched).
Source. Reprinted from Higgins ES: "A Review of Unrecognized Mental Illness in Primary Care: Prevalence, Natural History, and Efforts to Change the Course." *Archives of Family Medicine* 3:908–917, 1994. Copyright 1994, American Medical Association. Used with permission.

rized in Table 46–2. In one study, physicians rated initial psychopathology in an attempt to affect outcome. The results indicated that recognition of depression and anxiety disorders did not lead to a better outcome (Tiemens et al. 1996). This finding was attributed to the fact that in addition to the capability of recognition, primary care physicians must have the skills and resources to perform adequate interventions. These results paralleled those of other studies that failed to find an association between recognition and better outcome (Schulberg et al. 1987a; Simon et al. 1995c). A study of a health maintenance organization showed that notification provided to primary care physicians increased the number of chart notations of mental illness, referrals to mental health specialists, and outpatient visits with the primary care physician (Mazonson et al. 1996). Notification did not lead to an increase in the use of psychotropic medications or in the rate of hospitalization.

PSYCHIATRIC CONSULTATION IN THE PRIMARY CARE SETTING

CONCEPTUAL MODELS

The principal clinical interface for psychiatry with primary care is psychiatric consultation, usually in an ambulatory clinic setting. Several models of psychiatric consultation have been described (Katon et al. 1995; Pincus 1987; Strathdee 1987). These models include the following:

- The traditional referral or replacement model, in which the psychiatrist is the principal provider of mental health services and there is limited communication between primary care physician and psychiatrist.
- The consultation care model, in which the primary care physician is the principal provider of mental health services and is in close communication with the psychiatrist.
- The collaborative care model or liaison-attachment model, in which mental health services are provided jointly by the primary care physician and the psychiatrist and there are joint sessions with the patient and frequent communication between providers.

These three models are on a continuum in which the critical variable is the amount of direct contact that the consultant has with the patient.

Psychiatrists in Great Britain have looked at the utilization of these three models of psychiatric consultation in the primary care setting. All three models are employed in Great Britain, with the slight majority of psychiatrists functioning in the traditional referral model, fewer psychiatrists using the collaborative care model, and the fewest using the consultation model (Strathdee 1987). Strathdee (1987) and Bailey et al. (1994) surveyed general practitioners and psychiatrists on the practice patterns of psychiatric consultation in ambulatory clinic settings in Great Britain. Younger psychiatrists were more likely than older psychiatrists to be involved in some form of consultation with primary care physicians. Psychiatrists were more likely than primary care physicians to have been the initiators of consultation or the prime movers in setting up consultation arrangements (Bailey et al. 1994). Approximately one-third of the psychiatrists doing primary care consultation were involved in some formal educational activity at their primary care site. The majority of primary care physicians favored the collaborative care model, although traditional referral with crisis intervention services or short-term treatment was also favored. Administrative problems such as record keeping and lack of office space were frequently cited by psychiatrists and primary care physicians as obstacles to effective consultation. There was nearly unanimous support from both primary care physicians and psychiatrists of the concept that the consultation process is improved by physically locating the psychiatrist in the primary care clinic setting. In a study on collaborative treatment of depression in primary care settings, Katon (1997) found that 100% of primary care physicians preferred on-site treatment of depression to referral of depressed patients to a specialty clinic.

Few studies have compared the clinical efficacy, quality, or cost of psychiatric consultation. The results of one Scandinavian study on psychiatric consultation supported the concept of a collaborative care model's long-term effectiveness with regard to identifying and treating depression and lowering the risk of suicide in patients (Rutz et al. 1992). Katon et al. (1995) and Wells et al. (1989a) independently looked at models of psychiatric consultation in the primary care setting in the United States. Katon and colleagues (1995) studied the collaborative care model using a multifactorial treatment approach to depression in a primary care clinic setting. They found a measurable effect on the clinical outcome of major depression and a more modest effect on the treatment of minor depression as compared with usual care. Wells and co-workers (1989a) examined psychiatric consultation in primary care settings from the perspective of administrative motives in managed care systems. They described a "for profit" system and a "for quality" system approach to psychiatric consultation and mental health services. The "for quality" system consultation model builds stable copractice systems that are closest to those created in the collaborative care model and is associated with clinical outcomes superior to those associated with the "for profit" system. The "for profit" consultation model is closest to the consultation care model, in which patient access to psychiatrists is severely limited. Not surprisingly, the "for profit" system provides impressive short-term cost savings, but less effective clinical interventions may have undesirable long-term cost effects because of poor patient outcomes.

ADMINISTRATIVE CONSIDERATIONS

A number of administrative factors affect the nature and effectiveness of psychiatric consultation in a primary care clinic. Key administrative factors include location of the consulting psychiatrist, the predominant primary care practice in the clinic, the presence or absence of trainees in the clinic, the continuity of the consulting psychiatrist, organizational elements, and fiscal or reimbursement mechanisms.

Location

The location of the consulting psychiatrist has a notable impact on the psychiatric consultation process for patients as well as for referring primary care physicians. The most advantageous location is the primary care clinic itself. Many patients are more comfortable seeing a psychiatrist in the familiar surroundings of their primary care clinic, as opposed to seeing him or her in a freestanding psychiatric clinic. Some patients who are resistant to psychological explanations for their problems or symptoms may be less likely to resist a referral to their medical clinic. Referring physicians also benefit from the proximity of a consulting psychiatrist. Opportunities for communication and follow-up are greatly enhanced, more effective face-to-face communication is possible, and joint sessions with patients can be arranged. "Curbside consultation" and informal discussions about patients not requiring formal referrals can occur. The collaborative care model is the prototypical model of consultation in which the physical presence of a consulting psychiatrist in the primary care clinic is required in order for effective joint clinical management of patients to be established. Consulting psychiatrists benefit as well by witnessing firsthand the workings of the clinic and the practice styles of the referring physicians. A better understanding of the patient's experience in the clinic enhances the consulting psychiatrist's effectiveness.

Psychiatrists providing consultation in freestanding psychiatric clinics or separate offices must establish effective lines of communication with primary care physicians

to offset the absence of face-to-face communication. Advantages of separate locations for psychiatric consultation include a greater sense of confidentiality for the patient, less travel for the consulting psychiatrist, less time spent learning new administrative systems, and, usually, office space that is more appropriate for psychiatric interviews.

Telemedicine—the use of telecommunications technology to link health care professionals with isolated areas for diagnosis, treatment, consultation, transfer of medical data, and education—allows patients to be seen in the office of the primary care physician and facilitates consultation and ongoing care by specialists. Telemedicine was first used for medical purposes for telepsychiatry consultation (Wittson et al. 1961). A spectrum of technologies are available, including facsimile, medical data transmission, audio-only format (telephone and radio), transmission of still images, and full-motion video (Perednia and Allen 1995). The format most applicable to psychiatry is live, two-way audio, two-way video transmission (known as interactive television [IATV]). Telemedicine has already been considered a partial solution to the problems of delivering medical care to remote areas or to areas underserved by physicians (Preston et al. 1992), including the inner city (Straker et al. 1976). Telemedicine can help the academic department of psychiatry meet the needs of patients, primary care physicians, and the health system by complementing other psychiatric services (Hilty et al. 1997).

There has been a proliferation of telemedicine services used to provide mental health care nationwide, in nearly every state. In 1995, according to results of a recent survey on services provided in that year, 50 IATV programs were in use, 6,267 physician-patient consultations took place, the average duration of consultations was 33.4 minutes, and telepsychiatry was the most common consultation performed (Allen and Scarbrough 1996). The expansion of telemedicine for the provision of psychiatric care has been accompanied by discussion of its effect on patient satisfaction (Dongier et al. 1986; McCloskey Armstrong 1997), reliability and validity (telemedicine versus live interviews) (Baer et al. 1995), legal ramifications (Klein and Manning 1995; Savkar and Waters 1996), and economic issues (Bashshur 1995).

Consultee

The consultee's primary care specialty or the nature of the consultee's practice in the clinic often affects the choice of consultation model used by the consulting psychiatrist. Family practice physicians and general practitioners are frequently more comfortable with collaborative care or consultation care models in which the primary care physician plays a substantial role in the provision of mental health services. Physicians in internal medicine and pediatrics are often more comfortable with a traditional referral model of care. Mixtures of primary care physicians, common in many clinic settings, may require flexibility on the part of the consulting psychiatrist in the provision of services to individual clinicians.

Trainees

Trainees exert a largely positive effect on the psychiatric consultant's role in the primary care clinic. In a designated teaching setting, it is easier for the consultant to develop and expand educational activities for primary care physicians. Trainees also invigorate the physicians and staff with their interest in the psychiatric issues of patient care, with the result that the referring clinician's receptivity to the work of a consulting psychiatrist is increased. The presence of trainees in these settings adds complexity to the role of the consulting psychiatrist, who must both attend to the needs of the referring physicians and trainees and ensure excellent patient care. To be successful, the consultant must not overlook any of these tasks.

Continuity

The continuity of the consulting psychiatrist also has a powerful effect on psychiatric consultation provided to primary care physicians. Rapid turnover of consulting psychiatrists disrupts the process of collaborative care of patients. Liaison work involves the building of relationships with and confidence and trust in primary care clinicians over time. Consulting psychiatrists need time to learn about the clinic culture and how best to meet the needs of the referring primary care physicians.

Organizational Elements

Organizational elements that influence the consultation process include the mechanism of patient referral; the means of communication, charting, and other transfers of clinical information used in the clinic; arrangements for follow-up of patients and the use of inpatient psychiatric services and other ancillary mental health services; and staff support and space available to the consulting psychiatrist. These critical elements of effective consultation are best addressed proactively and in an ongoing manner as the consulting psychiatrist's understanding of the primary care clinic grows and the consultation role evolves. Administrative problems around organizational elements are frequently cited by primary care physicians and by consulting psychiatrists as the primary obstacle to effective

psychiatric consultation (Bailey et al. 1994; Strathdee 1987).

Financial Factors

Finally, fiscal issues have powerful effects on psychiatric consultation in primary care clinics. The absence of effective reimbursement mechanisms for psychiatric consultation will eventually defeat even the otherwise best-organized and best-planned consultation effort. Managed care systems are often reluctant to reimburse liaison and educational elements of consultation, which usually predominate in effective collaborative clinical care. Cost-offset effects of psychiatric consultation as well as improved treatment outcome and patient satisfaction can be cited to support a collaborative consultation approach (Katon 1997; G. R. Smith et al. 1986a; Sturm and Wells 1995). Fiscal accountability also drives the consulting psychiatrist to develop more cost-effective use of available psychiatric time and to refine skills and time-limited treatments that are favored by referring physicians.

DETECTION OF PSYCHIATRIC DISORDERS IN THE PRIMARY CARE SETTING

Detection of psychiatric disorders may be facilitated by the use of patient self-report questionnaires and/or clinician-administered rating scales. Detection of mental health disorders in the primary care setting is often referred to as *screening* but is better defined as *case finding* or *case identification* (Sackett and Holland 1975). Self-report questionnaires can be valuable as case identification tools. They are easily administered, are low-cost, and are usually sensitive with regard to detecting illness. Patient responses to these instruments cannot be used directly to formulate a diagnosis of an disorder. If a patient does not score positive on a screening questionnaire, no further evaluation need be done unless obvious clinical clues are present. However, a high score warrants a clinical interview based on standardized criteria. Many questionnaires and rating scales have been developed for the primary care setting, and those developed for the mental health setting are being researched for applicability to the primary care setting. Still to be established, through further research and randomized clinical trials, are thresholds for a positive score for each questionnaire that are specific to primary care populations.

SELF-REPORT QUESTIONNAIRES

Self-report questionnaires are summarized in Table 46–3. There are a number of self-report questionnaires that screen for many psychiatric disorders, including the General Health Questionnaire (D. P. Goldberg and Blackwell 1970), the Mental Health Inventory (Ware and Johnston 1979), and the Hopkins Symptom Checklist—90 (HSCL; Derogatis et al. 1974) (Table 46–3).

Depression

The Agency for Health Care Policy and Research (AHCPR) developed clinical practice guidelines for detection and diagnosis of depression in the primary care setting (Depression Guideline Panel 1993a). The guidelines serve as a review of symptoms, risk factors, screening instruments, and the differential diagnosis of depression. The AHCPR Task Force advocates screening for depression in high-risk populations.

The majority of information in the literature about case identification instruments regards the detection of depression, and Coulehan et al. (1989) and Feightner and Worrall (1990) reviewed the information in a succinct fashion. Patient questionnaires specifically designed to detect depression include the Beck Depression Inventory (BDI; Beck 1961; Beck et al. 1988), the Center for Epidemiological Studies Depression Scale (Radloff 1977), and the Zung Self-Rating Depression Scale (Zung 1965) (Table 46–3).

The BDI is the best-studied questionnaire for depression. It was designed to identify depression as well as measure its severity. The BDI measures cognitive, affective, motivational, and physiological types, takes less than 10 minutes to complete, and is well received by ambulatory patients (Rucker et al. 1986). In this 21-item scale, each question's response is graded from 0 to 3 on a scale of severity. A score of 13 is considered to indicate positivity. In a primary care population, a BDI score of 13 showed a sensitivity of 0.79 and a specificity of 0.77 compared with a psychiatrist's interview (Nielsen 1980). An abbreviated version consists of 13 items and is well correlated with the 21-item version (Beck and Beck 1972). The Beck Depression Inventory–Primary Care (BDI-PC; Beck 1996) is a newly developed guide for assessing the severity of symptoms.

Anxiety Disorders

Two patient questionnaires can be used to detect anxiety disorders in the primary care setting (Table 46–3). The

TABLE 46–3. Patient self-report questionnaires for detection of mental illness

Instrument	Use	Description
General Health Questionnaire (GHQ)	Depression, anxiety, social impairment, hypochondriasis	60-item original version; 28- and 12-item versions useful
Mental Health Inventory (MHI)	Multiple symptoms and disorders'	38-item original version used in medical outcome study; 18- and 5-item versions useful
Hopkins Symptom Checklist (HSCL)	Multiple symptoms and disorders, including somatization	90-item original version; 25-item version used for assessment of depression and anxiety only
Beck Depression Inventory (BDI)	Depression	21 items scored 0–3, positive score of 13 for primary care; 13-item and primary care versions
Center for Epidemiological Studies Depression Scale	Depression	20 items scored 0–3, positive score of 16 for primary care
Zung Self-Rating Depression Scale	Depression	20 items scored 0–4, positive score of 50–60 for primary care
Zung Self-Rating Anxiety Scale (ZSAS)	Anxiety	20 items scored 0–4, positive score of 45 for primary care
Beck Anxiety Inventory (BAI)	Anxiety	21 items scored 0–4, positive score for primary care being researched
Michigan Alcoholism Screening Test (MAST)	Alcoholism	24 items that are answered yes/no; 13-item version, positive score of 2
Alcohol Use Disorders Identification Test (AUDIT)	Alcohol consumption, drinking behavior	10 items scored 0–4, positive score of 8
Illness Behavior Questionnaire (IBQ)	Hypochondriasis	Assesses attitudes associated with illness behavior
Whitely Index	Hypochondriasis	13 items on attitudes, beliefs, and fear of disease

Zung Self-Rating Anxiety Scale (ZSAS; Zung 1971) is a 20-item questionnaire. A score of 45 is considered indicative of notably severe anxiety. The Beck Anxiety Inventory (BAI; Beck and Steer 1990) is a 21-item questionnaire that assesses severity of anxiety symptoms. Both scales are being studied for use in the primary care setting.

Functional Somatic Disorders

Several scales have been specifically developed for the assessment of somatic symptoms and patient attitudes about illness (Table 46–3). The Hopkins Symptom Checklist—90 somatization subscale is commonly used. For identifying hypochondriasis, the Illness Behavior Questionnaire (Pilowsky and Spence 1981) and the Whitely Index (Pilowsky et al. 1979) are useful. The latter has been shown to identify patients with hypochondriasis as defined by DSM-III (Barsky et al. 1986a), and elevated scores are associated with increased use of medical services (Barsky et al. 1986b). For measuring change by self-report, it has also been modified into a 6-point scale called the Heightened Illness Concern Questionnaire (Fallon et al. 1993).

Substance Use Disorders

There is a paucity of information about the use of questionnaires for detection of substance abuse and/or dependence in the primary care setting. Most physicians prefer informal clinical screening to questionnaires (Townes and Harkley 1994), and up to 90% of cases of substance use disorders in inpatients and outpatients go undetected (Maly 1993). Many physicians ask a single question regarding a patient's use of alcohol, but more questions must be asked if detection is to increase (Crum and Ford 1994).

The CAGE questionnaire was specifically designed for use in primary care (Ewing 1984; Mayfield et al. 1974). (The acronym *CAGE* is derived from the following questions: 1) Have you ever felt that you should *C*ut down your drinking? 2) Have you ever been *A*nnoyed by criticism of your drinking? 3) Have you ever felt *G*uilty about your drinking? 4) Do you ever drink in the morning—an *E*ye opener?) Compared with DSM-III-R in a primary care setting, the CAGE questionnaire had a sensitivity and a specificity of 0.94 and 0.97, respectively, for detection of a problem in the past year and a sensitivity and a specificity of 0.91 and 0.84, respectively, for detection of a problem over a lifetime (Wenrich et al. 1995). It appears that alcohol use disorders are not mistakenly classified as other psychiatric disorders (Crum et al. 1994).

Two other screening questionnaires are commonly used (Table 46–3). The Michigan Alcoholism Screening Test (MAST) is a 24-item, yes-or-no questionnaire (Selzer 1971). The Short Michigan Alcoholism Screening Test (SMAST) is a 13-item, yes-or-no questionnaire (Selzer et al. 1975). In a study in a primary care setting, a SMAST positivity criterion of 2 optimized the sensitivity (0.72) and specificity (0.64), compared with the usual criterion of 5 for hospital settings (sensitivity 0.56, specificity 0.83) (Fleming and Barry 1991). The Alcohol Use Disorders Identification Test (AUDIT) is a 10-item questionnaire that was developed from a six-country World Health Organization collaborative project (Saunders and Aasland 1987). Responses to questions are scored from 0 to 4, and a total score of 8 indicates a high likelihood of hazardous or harmful consumption. In the collaborative study involving 1,888 patients, sensitivity was 0.92 and specificity was 0.94 (Saunders et al. 1993).

RATING SCALES AND STRUCTURED CLINICAL INTERVIEWS

Clinician-administered rating scales are summarized in Table 46–4.

Recently, the Diagnostic and Statistical Manual of Mental Disorders, Fourth Edition, Primary Care Version (DSM-IV-PC; American Psychiatric Association 1995) was published. The traditional DSM is organized according to major subclasses of disorders, many of which are rarely seen in primary care, and it assumes the user knows which section to refer to. Therefore, DSM-IV-PC with its symptom-based clinical algorithm, as established by both psychiatrists and primary care physicians, is of more utility than are DSM-III and DSM-III-R (Pincus et al. 1995).

Another method for diagnosing mental disorders in primary care is the Primary Care Evaluation of Mental Disorders (PRIME-MD; Williams and Spitzer 1992). One part of the PRIME-MD is a 1-page patient questionnaire that is completed before the patient sees the physician. The other part is a 12-page clinician evaluation guide, which is a structured interview form that the physician uses to follow up on positive responses on the patient questionnaire. A study of the utility of the PRIME-MD found that the average time required of the primary care physician to complete the PRIME-MD evaluation was 8.4 minutes and a new treatment referral was initiated for 62% of the 125 patients whose condition was diagnosed using the PRIME-MD and who were not already being treated (Spitzer et al. 1994).

The Symptom Driven Diagnostic System for Primary Care (SDDS-PC; Olfson et al. 1995) is a new computerized clinical procedure that assists primary care physicians in diagnosing mental disorders during the course of routine practice. It has three components: a 5-minute, 16-item

TABLE 46–4. Clinician-administered rating scales for detection of mental illness

Instrument	Use	Description
DSM-IV–Primary Care Version (DSM-IV-PC)	Common mental disorders in primary care	Symptoms lead to 9 algorithms with steps to rule out/rule in diagnoses
Primary Care Evaluation of Mental Disorders (PRIME-MD)	Mood, anxiety, alcohol use, somatoform, and eating disorders	26-item patient questionnaire scored yes/no; 12-page clinician guide to evaluate yes answers
Symptom Driven Diagnostic System for Primary Care (SDDS-PC)	Depression; panic, alcohol use, obsessive-compulsive, and anxiety disorders; suicidal ideation	5-minute, 16-item patient questionnaire scored yes/no; six 5-minute clinician modules to evaluate yes answers
Hamilton Rating Scale for Depression	Depression and somatic symptoms	17-item version scored 0–4, positive score of 13
Hamilton Anxiety Scale	Anxiety and somatic symptoms	17-item version scored 0–4, not yet standardized for primary care
Anxiety Disorders Interview Scale for DSM-IV (ADIS-IV)	Anxiety, depression, psychosis, substance use disorders	Structured interview administered by trained staff (not primary care physician)
Structured Clinical Interview for DSM-III-R (SCID)	Alcohol and substance use disorders	30- to 60-minute structured interview administered by trained staff (not primary care physician)
Addiction Severity Index (ASI)	Substance use disorders	40- to 60-minute semistructured interview to determine stresses and suitability for treatment programs; not standardized for primary care
Recovery Attitude and Treatment Evaluator (RAATE)	Substance use disorders	30-minute initial evaluation of patient resistance to treatment; 15-minute follow-up evaluation not standardized for primary care

screening questionnaire completed by the patient, six 5-minute physician-administered diagnostic interview modules based on DSM-III-R criteria, and a longitudinal tracking form. The sensitivity, specificity, and positive predictive value of the SDDC-PC have been evaluated (Broadhead et al. 1995). Surveys of providers revealed important considerations. The diagnostic interviews were found useful by all 16 participating physicians, with 87% reporting that they had diagnosed a new mental problem (Weissman et al. 1995). However, 26% thought the procedure was too time consuming, and 80% believed reimbursement would be necessary for routine use.

Depressive and Anxiety Disorders

A number of rating scales can be used by the clinician to detect depressive and anxiety disorders (Table 46–4). The Hamilton Rating Scale for Depression (Hamilton 1967) is commonly used. Two rating scales have been specifically designed to measure anxiety disorders. The Hamilton Anxiety Scale (Hamilton 1959) has been used in original form. Further assessment is needed regarding its applica-

tion to the primary care setting. In the DSM-IV field trial for mixed anxiety-depression, a revised form was used to detect physical symptoms and symptoms consonant with DSM-III-R criteria and to determine duration of symptoms (Zinbarg et al. 1994). Recently, the Anxiety Disorders Interview Schedule for DSM-IV (ADIS-IV) was developed (T. A. Brown et al. 1994). This structured interview is used for identifying current episodes of anxiety disorders and also has sections to briefly identify mood, somatoform, and substance use disorders. The ADIS-IV is typically administered by psychiatric staff or by others who have had training in using the scale.

Functional Somatic Disorders

Many scales are used to detect functional disorders in the primary care setting. The somatic factor of the Hamilton Anxiety Scale is a valid, sensitive, and extensively used rating scale (Uhlenhuth et al. 1982). The Illness Attitude Scale was designed to measure attitudes responsible for hypochondriacal behavior and to distinguish hypochondriacal patients from other psychiatric patients

(Kellner 1986). The Brief Rating Scale of Hypo-chondriasis is a scale of disease conviction with high interrater reliability (Kellner 1982). The hypochondriasis subscale of the Minnesota Multiphasic Personality Inventory (MMPI; McKinley and Hathaway 1940) has been distilled to a scale referring only to somatic symptoms (Welsh 1952). A structured clinical interview for hypochondriasis (SCIH) based on DSM-III-R has also been developed (Barsky et al. 1992).

Substance Use Disorders

Three scales that identify substance use disorders may be used for the primary care setting (Table 46–4). The Structured Clinical Interview for DSM-III-R (SCID; Spitzer et al. 1992) has a substance disorder module that can be completed in 30–60 minutes. The Addiction Severity Index (ASI; McClellan et al. 1980), a semistructured interview, gathers information about areas of a patient's life that contribute to substance use. It takes 40–60 minutes to administer and can be used for ongoing evaluation. Finally, the Recovery Attitude and Treatment Evaluator (RAATE; Mee-Lee 1988) is designed to quantitatively assess patient resistance and impediments to treatment. It takes 30 minutes to complete initially and 15 minutes to complete in follow-up evaluations. None of these scales has been extensively evaluated in primary care populations.

PRINCIPLES FOR TREATMENT OF PSYCHIATRIC DISORDERS IN THE PRIMARY CARE SETTING

ISSUES FOR PHYSICIANS

The most common providers of psychiatric treatment are primary care physicians, who vary in terms of knowledge, skill, and comfort with such treatment. Often, no provider of mental health care is available for consultation or to provide nonpharmacologic care. Psychiatric patients in the primary care setting have more medical comorbidity than do psychiatric patients elsewhere, which can affect the choice of, compliance with, and efficacy of treatments. Primary care physicians can apply basic principles for choosing and administering treatment in the primary care setting (Table 46–5). Primary care physicians must also know when to seek consultation or a second opinion on complex cases (Table 46–6).

TABLE 46–5. **Principles for and questions to ask when choosing and administering psychiatric treatment in the primary care setting**

A patient's full treatment plan must be based on his or her history of illness.

What treatments, if any, have been successfully or unsuccessfully used in the past?

What symptom (e.g., suicidal ideation), comorbid psychiatric disorder, or comorbid medical disorder must be taken into account?

Which treatments can be administered by the available staff in a particular setting?

Which treatments are both comfortably and skillfully administered by providers?

Which treatments have the greatest likelihood of efficacy for a specific disorder?

Given that relapse or recurrence will follow symptom remission if a treatment is not continued, which treatment can the patient tolerate and comply with during all phases of the illness? The physician and patient should collaborate on the decision as much as possible.

What time frame is to be used to judge success or failure for a given treatment?

How often should visits occur to monitor the illness and treatment?

TABLE 46–6. **Situations that might warrant a second opinion from mental health professionals**

1. Diagnostic consultation
2. Recommended medication management
3. Need for psychotherapy
4. Need for crisis intervention, involuntary commitment, or hospitalization
5. Need for maintenance medication
6. Severe, recurrent, or psychotic illness
7. Presence of complex general medical problems
8. Poor adherence
9. Partial response to initial treatment(s)
10. Patient request
11. Symptom breakthrough after a positive acute phase response

Source. Adapted from Kathol et al. 1994.

PATIENT AND FAMILY ISSUES

Psychiatric patients and their families should receive a description of the cause, symptoms, and natural history of the illness, followed by an explanation of treatment options, in which indications, mechanisms of action, costs, risks, and benefits are addressed. A discussion should occur regarding the anticipated outcomes in terms of symptom relief, functional ability, and quality of life. Potential difficulties with regard to compliance should be identified, along with strategies for management. The early warning signs of relapse or recurrence should be reviewed. Specific counseling on compliance may be indicated for patients with histories of poor compliance, substance use or personality disorders, unfounded negative attitudes toward the selected treatment, or marked lack of understanding about the illness. A review of treatment compliance also indicated that intensive contact with patients during the acute phase of treatment, ongoing patient and family education, and development of an alliance with the family facilitated compliance by the patient (Frank 1997). At least seven studies found that patient education helps ensure treatment compliance in depressed outpatients (Depression Guideline Panel 1993b).

PRINCIPLES FOR TREATMENT OF DEPRESSION

Depression is one of the few disorders for which clinical practice guidelines have been developed (Depression Guideline Panel 1993b). Guidelines by the AHCPR have been summarized recently (Kathol et al. 1994; Katon 1996). Effective management depends on accurate diagnosis and adequate treatment with medication. Depressive syndromes due to medical illnesses or medication use must be ruled out, and if they are discovered, they must be treated rapidly. The course of depression and the three distinct phases of treatment have been described (Figure 46–2).

Acute Phase

Acute-phase treatment of depression includes treatment with medications and/or psychotherapy. Antidepressant therapy is recommended as the initial treatment for patients with more severe and more chronic depression, those with psychotic, melancholic, or recurrent depression, and those with a strong family history of depression. Newer medications such as serotonin reuptake inhibitors are associated with less risk of fatal overdose, have more tolerable side effects, require less dosage adjustment, and cost more than tricyclic antidepressants. The guidelines suggest that patients be seen every 2 weeks for reevaluation of symptoms, checking for side effects, and adjustment of dosage if necessary during the acute phase of treatment. Assessment of outcome should occur at 6 weeks. If a patient has a partial response, treatment should be continued for a total of 12 weeks. If there is a lack of response at 6 weeks or a partial response at 12 weeks, a switch to another agent is recommended. Alternatively, if a partial response occurs at a maximal dose of a medication, augmentation with other medications can be considered. A review of seven studies involving depressed medical outpatients revealed a median response rate to tricyclic antidepressants of 65% (range 38%–73%) (Schulberg et al. 1993).

Psychotherapy may play a valuable role in the treatment of depression. In the Medical Outcomes Study, only a third of the patients in general medical practices received even 3 minutes of counseling for depression (Wells et al. 1989b). Psychotherapy, when available, is recommended for patients with less severe, less chronic, nonpsychotic, and nonmelancholic depression. It may be added to the treatment in those with a partial response to medication, particularly if residual symptoms are largely psychological (e.g., low self-esteem). Interpersonal, cognitive, behavioral, brief dynamic, and marital psychotherapies have been shown to benefit patients in research trials.

A review of controlled trials revealed that approximately 50% of psychiatric outpatients improved over the course of 12 weeks when undergoing these therapies (Depression Guideline Panel 1993b). Findings of a review of psychosocial treatments generally support the efficacy of these treatments for patients in primary care settings (C. Brown and Schulberg 1995). The authors of this review noted deficiencies in the randomized controlled trials of psychosocial treatments, including nonstructured assessment of patients' diagnoses, potentially differing attrition patterns that affect analysis of clinical efficacy, and lack of standardized criteria for assessing treatment response. Of 10 other studies using nonstructured assessment, only studies using manualized treatments found that psychotherapy produces significantly greater reduction in psychological symptoms than does "usual care," no treatment, or pharmacotherapy. Of six studies using structured assessment and manualized treatments, five found psychotherapy more efficacious than placebo, no treatment, or usual care. Few studies have been performed on the benefit of psychotherapy continuing beyond 20 sessions.

Continuation Phase

The AHCPR guidelines also specify that treatment of depression with medication should be continued in the continuation phase. In double-blind trials, patients had a

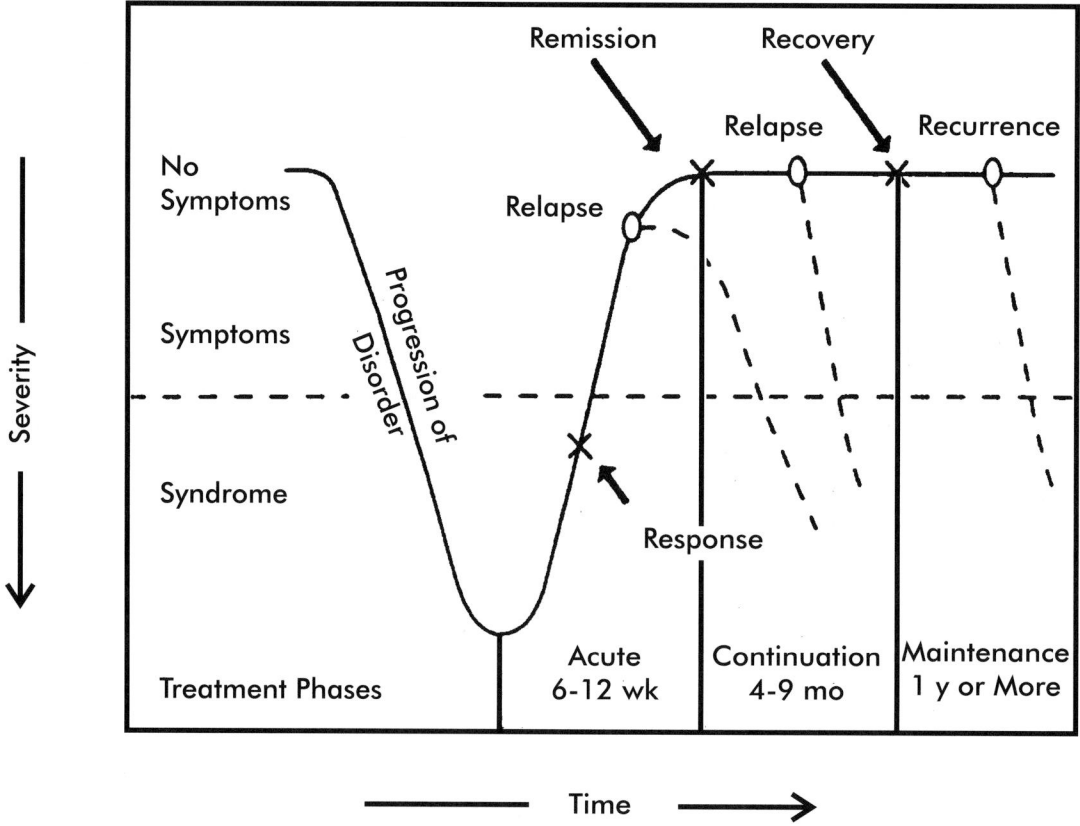

FIGURE 46–2.   Phases of treatment for major depression. Reprinted with permission from Katon W: "Practical Guidelines for the Treatment of Depression in a Managed Care Environment." Paper presented at the 148th annual meeting of the American Psychiatric Association, Miami Beach, FL, May 1995. Copyright 1995, American Psychiatric Association.

higher rate of relapse when taking placebo than when taking antidepressants for 3-, 6-, and 9-month periods (NIMH/NIH Consensus Development Conference Statement 1985). It is recommended that patients have a 6- to 9-month course of antidepressant treatment once they are in remission. The decision to implement continuation-phase psychotherapy depends on the patient's residual symptoms, psychosocial problems, and history of psychological functioning between episodes and the patient's and the practitioner's judgment.

Maintenance Phase

Maintenance-phase treatment of depression usually continues for 1 year or more. Patients with three or more episodes of depressive disorder should be strongly considered for maintenance antidepressant management, because the rate of relapse is fourfold for such patients taking placebo (Frank et al. 1987). Other patients who should be strongly considered for maintenance medication treatment include those with two or more episodes and a positive family history, a history of recurrence within a year after medication

therapy was discontinued, early onset (before age 20) of the first episode, double depression (dysthymia and major depression), or at least two depressive episodes in the past 3 years that were severe, sudden, or life-threatening. The decision to implement maintenance-phase psychotherapy depends on the patient's residual symptoms, psychosocial problems, and history of psychological functioning between episodes and the patient's and the practitioner's judgment. In addition, psychotherapy may be indicated for women who wish to become pregnant and bear a child in a drug-free condition.

Studies of Patient Care With Regard to AHCPR Guidelines

Many patients do not receive the treatment they need. It is estimated that only 30%–40% of primary care patients with major depression undergo antidepressant treatment according to AHCPR guidelines (Katon et al. 1997). Treatment within the guidelines is feasible but complex, and primary care physician adherence to protocols is moderate (Schulberg et al. 1995a). Treatment provided to patients with major depression according to the guidelines is effective, but only 33% of patients in one study completed the entire medication treatment and 42% completed the psychotherapy treatment (Schulberg et al. 1996). In a rural primary care setting, only 11% of patients with major depression received pharmacotherapy according to guidelines (Rost et al. 1995).

A collaborative care model, in which depression treatment guidelines are followed, was studied in a randomized controlled trial (Katon et al. 1995). Over a 12-month period, 217 patients were recognized as depressed by their primary care physicians. Patients in the intervention group had four visits over a 4- to 6-week period (visits 1 and 3 by a primary care physician and visits 2 and 4 by a psychiatrist). Patient education was supplemented by videotaped and written materials. The control group had "usual care." The groups were assessed for compliance with short-term (30-day) and long-term (90-day) therapy with antidepressants at guideline doses, satisfaction with care and medication, and reduction in depressive symptoms. Compared with patients in the control group, patients in the intervention group exhibited greater compliance with medication therapy, rated the quality of care more highly, and were more likely to rate medications as helpful. In the case of patients with major depression—but not in the case of patients with minor depression—outcome was better for those in the intervention group. Cost-effective analysis revealed that the cost per successful outcome was $1,783 for the intervention group and $1,940 for the control group (Katon et al. 1997).

PRINCIPLES FOR TREATMENT OF ANXIETY

No formal clinical practice guidelines have been developed for the treatment of anxiety disorders in the primary care setting, but a number of treatment algorithms, strategies, and suggestions have been published. Effective treatment rests on accurate diagnosis. Anxiety syndromes due to medical illnesses or medication use must be ruled out, and if they are found, they must be treated quickly. The efficacy and feasibility of treatments used in the mental health settings have not been studied in the primary care setting. Treatment options include treatment with medication, psychotherapy, and other somatic therapies.

In diagnostic and treatment algorithms, anxiety disorders have been divided into acute and persistent anxiety, because many primary care physicians rarely use DSM-IV (Hales et al. 1997). Figure 46–3 shows the diagnostic algorithm, which focuses on generalized anxiety disorder, adjustment disorder with anxiety, and panic disorder. Figure 46–4 shows the treatment algorithm, in which first-line

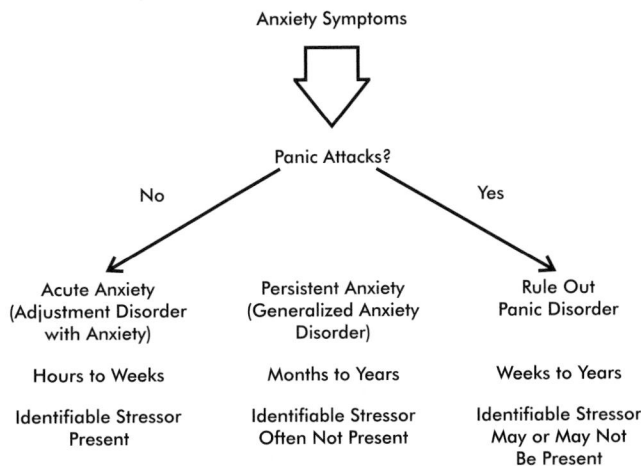

FIGURE 46–3. Diagnostic algorithm for categorizing anxiety in primary care practice. Reprinted with permission from Hales RE, Hilty DM, Wise MG: "A Treatment Algorithm for the Management of Anxiety in Primary Care Practice." *Journal of Clinical Psychiatry* 58 (suppl 3):76–80, 1997. Copyright 1997, Physicians Postgraduate Press, Inc.

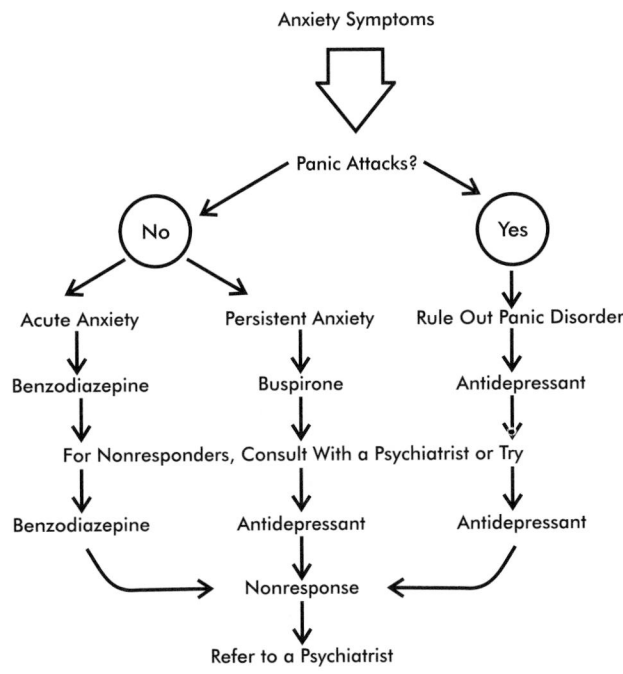

FIGURE 46–4. Treatment algorithm for the management of anxiety in primary care practice. Reprinted with permission from Hales RE, Hilty DM, Wise MG: "A Treatment Algorithm for the Management of Anxiety in Primary Care Practice." *Journal of Clinical Psychiatry* 58 (suppl 3):76–80, 1997. Copyright 1997, Physicians Postgraduate Press, Inc.

treatments and reasons for consultation or referral are specified. Recommended are acute, continuation, and maintenance phases of treatment, which parallel the treatment phases of depression. Patients with treatment refractive anxiety should be evaluated for adequacy of medication treatment and for comorbid medical, substance use, or psychiatric disorders (Hollander and Cohen 1994).

Treatment of anxiety in primary care settings is derived to a notable degree from the treatment of anxiety in mental health settings. The efficacy of specific treatments in the primary care setting has been evaluated in a small number of uncontrolled trials. A three-session cognitive-behavioral intervention has been used (Barkham 1989). Brief problem-solving therapy has been as effective as benzodiazepine therapy for treating generalized anxiety disorder in some patients (Mynors-Wallis and Gath 1992). A review of outcome studies since 1980 suggests that patients in primary care settings have better outcomes than patients in mental health settings (Durham and Allan 1993). Interestingly, studies reveal a trend toward clinical outcome's not being related to the intensity of mental health treatment. Patients with minor illnesses may improve regardless of treatment, and severely ill patients may need intensive services available only in mental health settings (Ormel et al. 1990).

PRINCIPLES FOR TREATMENT OF FUNCTIONAL SOMATIC SYMPTOMS

The presence of medically unexplained symptoms is a frequent reason for psychiatric consultation in the primary care setting. Patients may meet criteria for somatization disorder or have a subsyndromal presentation, both of which are associated with substantial morbidity, disability, and use of health services (Katon et al. 1990; G. R. Smith et al. 1986a). Many patients have a comorbid personality disorder (Rost et al. 1992). In addition, a number of patients have strictly somatic presentations of depression and anxiety disorders (Kirmayer and Robbins 1991) or comorbid somatization with a depressive or anxiety disorder (Katon et al 1990; Kellner 1985).

The management of functional somatic symptoms in the primary care setting is similar to that in the outpatient psychiatric setting, the exception being that the psychiatrist collaborates with primary care physicians. Many physicians continue to work up patients with somatic complaints despite the existence of an atypical history and may not feel comfortable diagnosing somatization if not completely sure of the diagnosis (Quill 1985). Often this leads to the patient's going to another physician because his or her needs have not been met or to the physician's deciding

the patient is unworthy of further effort because evaluations never uncover a medical cause. Efforts have been made to educate these physicians (Lipsitt 1992) in the essentials of psychosocial assessment, interviewing, and psychiatric diagnosis. Approaches have been developed for dealing with somatizing patients, and attempts have been made to improve the referral skills of primary care physicians. An overall approach to these patients involves the development of a good physician-patient relationship, performance of a physical examination at each visit, techniques of behavior modification, engagement of the patient at the somatic level but including life stresses among the issues to be addressed, treatment of comorbid conditions, and regularly scheduled brief visits irrespective of symptoms (R. C. Smith 1985). Primary care physicians may need to be reminded that clinical outcome goals are decreased morbidity, use of medical services, and cost expenditures.

Specific interventions for patients with somatization disorder have been evaluated in a number of randomized controlled trials. Two studies showed that a psychiatric consultation and an instructive letter to the physician about diagnostic and therapeutic measures resulted in sharp reduction in health care charges with no change in patient satisfaction (Rost et al. 1994; G. R. Smith et al. 1986b). In a follow-up study, those findings were replicated and sustained improvement at 1-year follow-up was reported (G. R. Smith et al. 1995). Short-term group psychotherapy (eight sessions) reduced health care costs and patients reported substantially better physical and mental health at 1-year follow-up (Kashner et al. 1995).

The treatment of hypochondriasis in the primary care setting is comparable to that in the hospital and in mental health outpatient settings. The key to treatment of hypochondriasis, like somatization disorder, is recognition of the illness.

PRINCIPLES FOR TREATMENT OF SUBSTANCE USE DISORDERS

Substance use disorders are usually not treated in the primary care setting. After the primary care physician diagnoses the disorder, he or she encourages the patient to obtain treatment. The patient is referred to community self-help programs, to a psychiatrist or another mental health professional for ongoing individual or group psychotherapy, and/or to a residential treatment program.

CONCLUSIONS

The primary care setting is a site of vital importance in the provision of medical and mental health care. The prevalence, difficulties of recognition, and inadequacy of treatment of psychiatric disorders call for systematic improvements in clinical, educational, administrative, and research methods. Changes in the organization and delivery of health care add a compelling economic consideration for all who work in the primary care setting. Collaboration between psychiatrists and primary care physicians is vital to determining the most efficient methods of organizing care. Consultation-liaison psychiatrists are uniquely qualified for playing a key role in improving patient care by facilitating the integration of care and fostering collaboration.

The gap must be narrowed between knowledge and treatment of mental disorders in the primary care setting. Although treatment guidelines by the AHCPR, the American Psychiatric Association, and other organizations are an important first step, protocols for standard treatments must be devised to direct primary care and mental health clinicians, and treatment must also fit patients' needs. Randomized controlled trials are necessary to evaluate psychopharmacological and psychotherapeutic treatments that have been developed and that have proved to be effective in specialty care (Katon et al. 1994a; Schulberg et al. 1993); however, without the use of standard treatments in these trials, findings may not be generalizable for primary care settings because of epidemiologic differences in patients, differences in skills of providers, and differences in the structure of care. Standard treatments will also facilitate health plans' monitoring of provision of care in the future. Comprehensive evaluations of care will include clinical, health service, pharmaceutical, and other administrative data. Increased collaboration between primary care physicians and mental health clinicians is necessary, particularly in light of the shift of specialty care to the primary care physician. Finally, mental health professionals must continue to develop a continuum of outpatient services and help primary care physicians refer patients to these services. There is a need to implement and study innovations such as telemedicine, which broaden the possibilities for patient care and education.

REFERENCES

Allen A, Scarbrough ML: 3rd annual program review. Telemedicine Today July/August:10–17, 1996

American Psychiatric Association: Diagnostic and Statistical Manual of Mental Disorders, 3rd Edition. Washington, DC, American Psychiatric Association, 1980

American Psychiatric Association: Diagnostic and Statistical Manual of Mental Disorders, 3rd Edition, Revised. Washington, DC, American Psychiatric Association, 1987

American Psychiatric Association: Diagnostic and Statistical Manual of Mental Disorders, 4th Edition. Washington, DC, American Psychiatric Association, 1994

American Psychiatric Association: Diagnostic and Statistical Manual of Mental Disorders, Fourth Edition, Primary Care Version. Washington, DC, American Psychiatric Association, 1995

Anderson SM, Harthorn BH: The recognition, diagnosis, and treatment of mental disorders by primary care physicians. Med Care 27:869–886, 1989

Angst J, Vollrath M, Merikangas KR, et al: Co-morbidity of anxiety and depression in the Zurich Cohort Study of Young Adults, in Comorbidity of Mood and Anxiety Disorders. Edited by Maser JD, Cloninger CR. Washington, DC, American Psychiatric Press, 1990, pp 123–138

Baer L, Cukor P, Jenike MA, et al: Pilot studies of telemedicine for patients with obsessive-compulsive disorder. Am J Psychiatry 152:1383–1385, 1995

Bailey J, Black M, Wilkin D: Specialist outreach clinics in general practice. BMJ 308:1083–1086, 1994

Barkham M: Brief prescriptive therapy in two-plus-one sessions: initial cases from the clinic. Behavioral Psychotherapy 17:161–175, 1989

Barrett JE, Barrett JA, Oxman TE, et al: The prevalence of psychiatric disorders in a primary care practice. Arch Gen Psychiatry 45:1100–1106, 1988

Barsky AJ, Wyshak G, Klerman GL: Hypochondriasis: an evaluation of the DSM-III criteria in medical outpatients. Arch Gen Psychiatry 43:493–500, 1986a

Barsky AJ, Wyshak G, Klerman GL: Medical and psychiatric determinants of outpatient medical utilization. Med Care 24:548–560, 1986b

Barsky AJ, Wyshak G, Klerman G, et al: The prevalence of hypochondriasis in medical outpatients. Soc Psychiatry Psychiatr Epidemiol 25:89–94, 1990

Barsky AJ, Cleary PD, Wyshak G, et al: A structured diagnostic interview for hypochondriasis: a proposed criterion standard. J Nerv Ment Dis 180:20–27, 1992

Bashshur RL: Telemedicine effects: cost, quality, and access. J Med Syst 19:81–91, 1995

Beck AT: The Beck Depression Inventory for Primary Care. San Antonio, TX, Psychological Corporation, 1996

Beck AT, Beck RW: Screening for depressed patients in family practice: a rapid technique. Postgrad Med 52:81–85, 1972

Beck AT, Steer RA: The Beck Anxiety Inventory. San Antonio, TX, Psychological Corporation, 1990

Beck AT, Ward CH, Mendelson M: An inventory for measuring depression. Arch Gen Psychiatry 18:561–567, 1961

Beck AT, Steer RA, Garbin MG: Psychometric properties of the Beck Depression Inventory: twenty-five years of evaluation. Clinical Psychology Review 8:77–100, 1988

Bridges KW, Goldberg DP: Somatic presentation of DSM-III psychiatric disorders in primary care. J Psychosom Res 29:563–569, 1985

Broadhead WE, Blazer DG, George LK, et al: Depression, disability days, and days lost from work in a prospective epidemiologic survey. JAMA 264:2524–2528, 1990

Broadhead WE, Leon AC, Weissman MM, et al: Development and validation of the SDDS-PC screen for multiple disorders in primary care. Arch Fam Med 4:211–219, 1995

Brown C, Schulberg HC: The efficacy of psychosocial treatments in primary care. Gen Hosp Psychiatry 17:414–424, 1995

Brown TA, Di Nardo PA, Barlow DH: Anxiety Disorders Interview Schedule for DSM-IV (ADIS-IV). Albany, NY, Graywind Publications, 1994

Cavanaugh SVA: The prevalence of emotional and cognitive dysfunction in a general medical population: using MMSE, GHQ, and BDI. Gen Hosp Psychiatry 5:15–24, 1983

Cavanaugh SVA: Diagnosing depression in the hospitalized patient with chronic medical illness. J Clin Psychiatry 45:13–16, 1984

Cloninger CR, Sigvardsson S, von Knorring AL, et al: An adoption study of somatoform disorders, II: identification of two discrete somatoform disorders. Arch Gen Psychiatry 41:863–871, 1984

Cohen-Cole SA, Brown FW, McDaniel JS: Assessment of depression and grief reactions in the medically ill, in Psychiatric Care of the Medical Patient. Edited by Stoudemire A, Fogel BS. New York, Oxford University Press, 1993, pp 53–69

Cole SA, Raju M: Overcoming barriers to integration of primary care and behavioral health care: focus on knowledge and skills. Behavioral Healthcare Tomorrow 5:30–37, 1996

Coulehan JL, Schulberg HC, Block MR: The efficiency of depression questionnaires for case finding in primary medical care. J Gen Intern Med 4:541–547, 1989

Coyne JC, Fechner-Bates S, Schwenk TL: Prevalence, nature, and comorbidity of depressive disorders in primary care. Gen Hosp Psychiatry 16:267–276, 1994

Crum RM, Ford DE: The effect of psychiatric symptoms on the recognition of alcohol disorders in primary care patients. Int J Psychiatry Med 24:63–82, 1994

Depression Guideline Panel: Depression in Primary Care, Vol 1: Detection and Diagnosis (Clinical Practice Guideline No 5; AHCPR Publ No 93-0550). Rockville, MD, U.S. Department of Health and Human Services, Public Health Service, Agency for Health Care Policy and Research, 1993a

Depression Guideline Panel: Depression in Primary Care, Vol 2: Treatment of Major Depression (Clinical Practice Guideline No 5; AHCPR Publ No 93-0551). Rockville, MD, U.S. Department of Health and Human Services, Public Health Service, Agency for Health Care Policy and Research, 1993b

Derogatis LR, Lipman RS, Rickels K, et al: The Hopkins Symptom Checklist (HSCL): a self-report symptom inventory. Behav Sci 19:1–15, 1974

Docherty J: Barriers to the diagnosis of depression in primary care. J Clin Psychiatry 58 (suppl 1):5–10, 1997

Dongier M, Tempier R, Lalinec-Michaud M, et al: Telepsychiatry: psychiatric consultation through two-way television: a controlled study. Can J Psychiatry 31:32–34, 1986

DuPont RL, Rice DP, Shiraki S, et al: Economic costs of obsessive-compulsive disorder. Medical Interface 8:102–109, 1995

Durham RC, Allan T: Psychological treatment of generalized anxiety disorder: a review of the clinical significance of results in outcome studies since 1980. Br J Psychiatry 163:19–26, 1993

Eisenberg L: Treating depression and anxiety in primary care: closing the gap between knowledge and practice. N Engl J Med 326:1080–1084, 1992

Endicott J: Measurement of depression in patients with cancer. Cancer 53:2243–2248, 1984

Endicott J, Blumenthal R: Barriers to seeking treatment for major depression. Paper presented at the Annual Scientific Meeting of the New York State Office of Mental Health, Albany, NY, December 1995

Escobar JI: Overview of somatization: diagnosis, epidemiology, and management. Psychopharmacol Bull 30:589–596, 1996

Escobar JI, Burnam M, Karno M, et al: Somatization in the community. Arch Gen Psychiatry 44:713–718, 1987

Escobar JI, Rubio-Stipec M, Canino G, et al: Somatic Symptom Index (SSI): a new and abridged somatization construct. J Nerv Ment Dis 177:140–146, 1989

Ewing JA: Detecting alcoholism: the CAGE questionnaire. JAMA 252:1905–1907, 1984

Fallon BA, Liebowitz MR, Salman E, et al: Fluoxetine for hypochondriacal patients without major depression. J Clin Psychopharmacol 13:438–441, 1993

Fauman MA: Psychiatric components of medical and surgical practice, II: referral and treatment of psychiatric disorders. Am J Psychiatry 140:760–763, 1983

Fedoroff JP, Starkstein SE, Parikh RM, et al: Are depressive symptoms nonspecific in patients with acute stroke? Am J Psychiatry 148:1172–1176, 1991

Feightner JW, Worrall G: Early detection of depression by primary care physicians. Can Med Assoc J 142:1215–1220, 1990

Fifer SK, Mathias SD, Patrick DL, et al: Untreated anxiety among adult primary care patients in a health maintenance organization. Arch Gen Psychiatry 51:740–750, 1994

Fink PJ: Psychiatry and the primary care physician, in Comprehensive Textbook of Psychiatry, 3rd Edition. Edited by Kaplan HI, Freedman AM, Sadock BJ. Baltimore, MD, Williams & Wilkins, 1980

Fleming MF, Barry KL: The effectiveness of alcoholism screening in an ambulatory care setting. J Stud Alcohol 52:33–36, 1991

Frank E: Enhancing patient outcomes: treatment adherence. J Clin Psychiatry 58 (suppl 1):11–14, 1997

Frank E, Kupfer DJ, Jacob M, et al: Personality measure and response to treatment in recurrent depression. Journal of Personality Disorders 1:14–26, 1987

Goldberg RJ: Diagnostic dilemmas presented by patients with anxiety and depression. Am J Med 98:278–284, 1995

Goldberg DP, Blackwell B: Psychiatric illness in general practice: a detailed study using a new method of case identification. BMJ 1:439–443, 1970

Goldberg DP, Steele JJ, Smith C, et al: Training family doctors to recognize psychiatric illness with increased accuracy. Lancet 2:521–523, 1980

Greenberg PS, Stiglin LE, Finkelstein SN, et al: The economic burden of depression in 1990. J Clin Psychiatry 54: 405–418, 1993

Hales RE, Hilty DM, Wise MG: A treatment algorithm for the management of anxiety in primary care practice. J Clin Psychiatry 58 (suppl 3):76–80, 1997

Hamilton M: The assessment of anxiety states by rating. Br J Med Psychol 32:50–55, 1959

Hamilton M: Development of a rating scale for primary depressive illness. Br J Soc Clin Psychol 6:278–296, 1967

Harr E, Green M, Hyam L, et al: Varied needs of primary physicians for psychiatric resources, II: subjective factors. Psychosomatics 13:255–264, 1972

Higgins ES: A review of unrecognized mental illness in primary care: prevalence, natural history, and efforts to change the course. Arch Fam Med 3:908–917, 1994

Hilty DM, Hales RE, Nesbitt T, et al: A comparative study of telemedicine psychiatric care versus usual care for the diagnosis and treatment of depression in primary care. Paper presented at the annual meeting of the Psychiatric Research Society, Park City, UT, February 1997

Hirschfeld RMA, Keller MB, Panico S, et al: The National Depressive and Manic-Depressive Association Consensus Statement on the Undertreatment of Depression. JAMA 277:333–340, 1997

Hoeper E[W], Nycz GR, Cleary P, et al: Estimated prevalence of RDC mental disorder in primary medical care. International Journal of Mental Health 8:6–15, 1979

Hoeper EW, Nycz GR, Kessler LG, et al: The usefulness of screening for mental illness. Lancet 1:33–35, 1984

Hollander E, Cohen LJ: The assessment and treatment of refractory anxiety. J Clin Psychiatry 55 (suppl 1):27–31, 1994

Jarrett RB, Rush AJ: Short-term psychotherapy of depressive disorders: current status and future directions. Psychiatry 57:115–132, 1994

Johnson J, Spitzer RL, Williams JB, et al: Alcohol abuse/dependence diagnosed by primary care physicians: recognition rate, psychiatric comorbidity, and functional impairment. Paper presented at the 7th annual National Institute of Mental Health International Research Conference on Mental Health Problems in the General Health Sector, McLean, VA, September 1993

Johnstone A, Goldberg D: Psychiatric screening in general practice: a controlled trial. Lancet 1:605–608, 1976

Kashner TM, Rost K, Cohen B, et al: Enhancing the health of somatization disorder patients: effectiveness of short-term group therapy. Psychosomatics 36:462–470, 1995

Kathol RG, Mutgi A, Williams J, et al: Major depression diagnosed by DSM-II, DSM-III-R, RDC, and Endicott criteria in patients with cancer. Am J Psychiatry 147:1021–1024, 1990

Kathol R, Katon W, Smith GR, et al: Guidelines for the diagnosis and treatment of depression for primary care physicians. Psychosomatics 35:1–12, 1994.

Katon W: Depression: somatic symptoms and medical disorders in primary care. Compr Psychiatry 23:274–287, 1982

Katon W: Cost-effectiveness of collaborative intervention to improve the primary care treatment of depression (abstract). American Psychiatric Association 1997 Annual Meeting New Research Program and Abstracts. Washington, DC, American Psychiatric Association, 1997, p 106

Katon W, Roy-Byrne PP: Mixed anxiety and depression. J Abnorm Psychol 100:337–345, 1991

Katon W, Schulberg HC: Epidemiology of depression in primary care. Gen Hosp Psychiatry 14:237–247, 1992

Katon W, Vitaliano PP, Russo J, et al: Panic disorder: epidemiology in primary care. J Fam Pract 23:233–239, 1986

Katon W, Von Korff M, Lin E, et al: Distressed high utilizers of medical care: DSM-III-R diagnoses and treatment needs. Gen Hosp Psychiatry 12:355–362, 1990

Katon W, Von Korff M, Lin E, et al: Adequacy and duration of antidepressant treatment in primary care. Med Care 30:67–76, 1992a

Katon W, Von Korff M, Lin E, et al: A randomized trial of psychiatric consultation with distressed high utilizers. Gen Hosp Psychiatry 14:86–98, 1992b

Katon W, Von Korff M, Lin E, et al: Methodological issues in randomized trials of liaison psychiatry in primary care. Psychosom Med 56:97–103, 1994a

Katon W, Lin E, Von Korff M, et al: The predictors of persistence of depression in primary care. J Affect Disord 31:81–90, 1994b

Katon W, Von Korff M, Lin E, et al: Collaborative management to achieve treatment guidelines. JAMA 273:1026–1031, 1995

Katon W, Von Korff M, Lin E, et al: Collaborative management to achieve depression treatment guidelines. J Clin Psychiatry 58 (suppl 1):20–24, 1997

Katzelnick D: Research perspectives, in Psychiatry and Primary Care: Managed Care Models Course. Paper presented at the annual meeting of the American Psychiatric Association, San Diego, CA, May 1997

Kellner R: Scoring Instruction for the Brief Rating Scale of Hypochondriasis. Albuquerque, NM, University of New Mexico, 1982

Kellner R: Functional somatic symptoms and hypochondriasis: a survey of empirical studies. Arch Gen Psychiatry 42:821–833, 1985

Kellner R: Somatization and Hypochondriasis. New York, Praeger, 1986

Kenyon FE: Hypochondriasis: a survey of some historical, clinical, and social aspects. BMJ 38:117–133, 1965

Kirmayer LJ, Robbins JM: Three forms of somatization in primary care: prevalence, co-occurrence, and sociodemographic characteristics. J Nerv Ment Dis 179:647–655, 1991

Kirmayer LJ, Robbins JM, Dworkind M, et al: Somatization and the recognition of depression and anxiety in primary care. Am J Psychiatry 150:734–741, 1993

Klein SR, Manning WL: Telemedicine and the law. Journal of Healthcare Information Management 9:35–40, 1995

Kroenke K, Spitzer RL, Williams JBW, et al: Physical symptoms in primary care: predictors of psychiatric disorders and functional impairment. Arch Fam Med 3:774–779, 1994

Lin EH, Katon W, Von Korff M, et al: Frustrating patients: physician and patient perspectives among distressed high users of medical services. J Gen Intern Med 6:241–246, 1991

Linn LS, Yager J: Recognition of depression and anxiety by primary physicians. Psychosomatics 25:593–600, 1984

Lipsitt DR: Challenges of somatization: diagnostic, therapeutic and economic. Psychiatric Medicine 10:1–12, 1992

Magruder-Habib HK, Zung WW, Feussner JR, et al: Management of general medical patients with symptoms of depression. Gen Hosp Psychiatry 11:201–207, 1989

Magruder-Habib K, Zung WW, Feussner JR: Improving physicians' recognition and treatment of depression in general medical care. Med Care 28:239–250, 1990

Maly RC: Early recognition of chemical dependence. Prim Care 20:33–50, 1993

Mathias SD, Fifer SK, Mazonson PD, et al: Necessary but not sufficient: the effect of screening and feedback on outcomes of primary care patients with untreated anxiety. J Gen Intern Med 9:606–615, 1994

Mayfield DG, McLoed G, Hall P: The CAGE questionnaire: validation of a new alcoholism screening instrument. Am J Psychiatry 131:1121–1123, 1974

Mazonson PD, Mathias SD, Fifer SK, et al: The mental health patient profile: does it change primary care physicians' practice patterns? J Am Board Fam Pract 9:336–345, 1996

McClellan AT, Luborsky L, Woody GE: An improved diagnostic evaluation instrument for substance abuse patients: the Addiction Severity Index. J Nerv Ment Dis 168:26–33, 1980

McCloskey Armstrong T: Rural psychiatric collaborative care via telemedicine. American Psychiatric Association 1995 Annual Meeting New Research Program and Abstracts. Washington, DC, American Psychiatric Association, p 106, 1997

McKinley JC, Hathaway SR: A multiphasic personality schedule (Minnesota), II: a differential study of hypochondriasis. J Psychol 10:255–268, 1940

Mee-Lee D: An instrument for treatment progress and matching: the Recovery Attitude and Treatment Evaluator (RAATE). J Subst Abuse Treat 5:183–186, 1988

Mellinger G, Balter M, Uhlenhuth E: Prevalence and correlates of the long-term use of anxiolytics. JAMA 251:375–379, 1984

Mintz J, Mintz L, Arruda M, et al: Treatments of depression and the functional capacity to work. Arch Gen Psychiatry 49:761–768, 1992

Moore JT, Silimperi DR, Bobula JA: Recognition of depression by family medicine residents: the impact of screening. J Fam Pract 7:509–513, 1978

Mynors-Wallis LM, Gath DH: Brief psychological treatments. International Review of Psychiatry 4:301–305, 1992

Nielsen AC III, Williams TA: Prevalence by self-report questionnaire and recognition by nonpsychiatric physicians. Arch Gen Psychiatry 37:999–1004, 1980

NIMH/NIH Consensus Development Conference statement: mood disorders: pharmacologic prevention of recurrences. Am J Psychiatry 142:469–476, 1985

Olfson M, Leon AC, Broadhead WE, et al: The SDDS-PC: a diagnostic aid for multiple mental disorders in primary care. Psychopharmacol Bull 31:415–420, 1995

Ormel J, van den Brink W, Koeter MW, et al: Recognition, management, and outcome of psychological disorders in primary care: a naturalistic follow-up study. Psychol Med 20:909–923, 1990

Ormel J, Koeter MW, van den Brink W, et al: Recognition, management, and course of anxiety and depression in general practice. Arch Gen Psychiatry 48:700–706, 1991

Perednia DA, Allen A: Telemedicine technology and clinical applications. JAMA 273:483–488, 1995

Pilowsky I, Spence ND: Manual for the Illness Behavior Questionnaire (IBQ). Adelaide, South Australia, University of Adelaide, 1981

Pilowsky I, Murrell PGC, Gordon A: The development of a screening method for abnormal illness behavior. J Psychosom Res 23:203–207, 1979

Pincus HA: Patient-oriented models for linking primary care and mental health care. Gen Hosp Psychiatry 9:95–101, 1987

Pincus HA, Vettorello NE, McQueen LE, et al: Bridging the gap between psychiatry and primary care: the DSM-IV-PC. Psychosomatics 36:328–335, 1995

Preston J, Brown FW, Hartley B: Using telemedicine to improve health care in distant areas. Hosp Community Psychiatry 43:25–32, 1992

Quill TE: Somatization disorder: one of medicine's blind spots. JAMA 254:3075–3079, 1985

Radloff LS: The CES-D Scale: a self-report depression scale for research in the general population. Applied Psychological Measure 1:385–401, 1977

Rand EH, Badger LW, Coggins DR: Toward a resolution of contradictions: utility of feedback from the GHQ. Gen Hosp Psychiatry 10:189–196, 1988

Regier DA, Goldberg ID, Taube CA: The de facto US mental health services system: a public health perspective. Arch Gen Psychiatry 35:685–693, 1978

Regier DA, Narrow WE, Rae DS, et al: The de facto US mental and addictive disorders service system: Epidemiologic Catchment Area prospective 1-year prevalence rates of disorders and services. Arch Gen Psychiatry 50:85–94, 1993

Rodin G, Voshart K: Depressive symptoms and functional impairment in the medically ill. Gen Hosp Psychiatry 9:251–258, 1987

Roper Poll: To Medicate: What People Do for Minor Health Problems. (Roper Reports 86–8.) New York, NY, Roper Organization, 1986

Rost K, Akins RN, Brown FW, et al: The comorbidity of DSM-III-R personality disorders in somatization disorder. Gen Hosp Psychiatry 14:322–326, 1992

Rost K, Kashner TM, Smith GR Jr: Effectiveness of psychiatric intervention with somatization disorder patients: improved outcomes at reduced costs. Gen Hosp Psychiatry 16:381–387, 1994

Rost K, Williams C, Wherry J, et al: The process and outcomes of care for major depression in rural family practice settings. Journal of Rural Health 11:114–121, 1995

Roter D, Hall J: Recruitment and training of primary care physicians in interviewing skills to identify and address psychosocial distress, in Primary Care Research Program: The Fifth Annual NIMH International Research Conference on Mental Health Problems in the General Health Sector. Bethesda, MD, National Institute of Mental Health, 1991

Rovner BW, German PS, Brant LJ, et al: Depression and mortality in nursing homes. JAMA 265:993–996, 1991

Roy-Byrne PP: Generalized anxiety disorder and mixed anxiety-depression: association with disability and health care utilization. J Clin Psychiatry 57 (suppl 7):86–91, 1996

Roy-Byrne PP, Katon W, Broadhead WE, et al: Subsyndromal ("mixed") anxiety-depression in primary care. J Gen Intern Med 9:507–512, 1994

Rucker L, Frye EB, Cygan RW: Feasibility and usefulness of depression screening in medical outpatients. Arch Intern Med 146:729–731, 1986

Rutz W, von Knorring L, Walinder J: Long term effects of an educational program for general practitioners given by the Swedish Committee for the Prevention and Treatment of Depression. Acta Psychiatr Scand 85:83–88, 1992

Sackett DL, Holland WW: Controversy in the detection of disease. Lancet 2:357–359, 1975

Saunders JB, Aasland OG: WHO Collaborative Project on Identification and Treatment of Persons With Harmful Alcohol Consumption, Phase I: Development of a Screening Instrument (MHN/DAT/86.3). Geneva, World Health Organization, 1987

Saunders JB, Aasland OG, Babor TF, et al: Development of the Alcohol Use Disorders Identification Test (AUDIT): WHO Collaborative Project on Identification and Treatment of Persons With Harmful Alcohol Consumption, Phase II. Addiction 88:791–804, 1993

Savkar S, Waters RJ: Telemedicine—implications for patient confidentiality and privacy, in The Telemedicine Sourcebook 1996–1997. Edited by Allen A. New York, Faulkner & Gray, 1996, pp 351–354

Schulberg HC, Burns BJ: Mental disorders in primary care: epidemiological, diagnostic, and treatment research directions. Gen Hosp Psychiatry 10:79–87, 1988

Schulberg HC, Saul M, McClelland M, et al: Assessing depression in primary medical and psychiatric practices. Arch Gen Psychiatry 42:1164–1170, 1985

Schulberg H[C], McClelland M, Burns M, et al: Depression and physical illness: the prevalence, causation, and diagnosis of comorbidity. Clinical Psychology Review 7:145–167, 1987a

Schulberg HC, McClelland M, Gooding W: Six-month outcomes for medical patients with major depressive disorders. J Gen Intern Med 2:312–317, 1987b

Schulberg HC, Coulehan JL, Block MR, et al: Clinical trials of primary care treatments for major depression: issues in design, recruitment, and treatment. Int J Psychiatry Med 23:29–42, 1993

Schulberg HC, Block MR, Madonia MJ, et al: Feasibility of clinical pharmacotherapy guidelines for major depression in primary care settings. Arch Fam Med 4:106–112, 1995a

Schulberg HC, Madonia MJ, Block MR, et al: Major depression in primary care practice: clinical characteristics and treatment implications. Psychosomatics 36:129–137, 1995b

Schulberg HC, Block MR, Madonia MJ, et al: Treating major depression in primary care practice: eight-month clinical outcomes. Arch Gen Psychiatry 53:913–919, 1996

Selzer ML: Michigan Alcoholism Screening Test: the quest for a new diagnostic instrument. Am J Psychiatry 127:1653–1658, 1971

Selzer ML, Vinokur A, van Rooijen L: A self-administered Short Michigan Alcoholism Screening Test (SMAST). J Stud Alcohol 36:117–126, 1975

Shapiro S, Skinner EA, Kessler LG, et al: Utilization of health and mental health services: three Epidemiologic Catchment Area sites. Arch Gen Psychiatry 41:971–978, 1984

Shapiro S, German PS, Skinner EA, et al: An experiment to change detection and management of mental morbidity in primary care. Med Care 25:327–339, 1987

Shear MK, Schulberg HC, Madonia M: Panic and generalized anxiety disorder in primary care. Paper presented at a meeting of the Association for Primary Care, Washington, DC, September 1994

Shepherd M, Wilkinson G: Primary care as the middle group for psychiatric epidemiology. Psychol Med 18:263–267, 1988

Simon GE, Von Korff M: Somatization and psychiatric disorders in the NIMH Epidemiologic Catchment Area Study. Am J Psychiatry 148:1494–1500, 1991

Simon GE, Von Korff M: Management and outcome of depression in primary care, in Primary Care Research Program: The Seventh Annual NIMH International Research Conference on Mental Health Problems in the General Health Sector. Bethesda, MD, National Institute of Mental Health, 1993, p 65

Simon GE, Von Korff M: Recognition, management, and outcomes of depression in primary care. Arch Fam Med 4:99–105, 1995

Simon GE, Ormel J, Von Korff M, et al: Health care costs associated with depressive and anxiety disorders in primary care. Am J Psychiatry 152:352–357, 1995a

Simon GE, Von Korff M, Barlow W: Health care costs of primary care patients with recognized depression. Arch Gen Psychiatry 52:850–856, 1995b

Simon GE, Lin EH, Katon W, et al: Outcomes of "inadequate" antidepressant treatment. J Gen Intern Med 10:663–670, 1995c

Sireling L, Freeling P, Paykel E, et al: Depression in general practice: clinical features and comparison with outpatients. Br J Psychiatry 147:119–126, 1985

Smith GR Jr, Monson RA, Ray DC: Patients with multiple unexplained symptoms: their characteristics, functional health, and health care utilization. Arch Intern Med 146:69–72, 1986a

Smith GR Jr, Monson RA, Ray DC: Psychiatric consultation in somatization disorder: a randomized controlled study. N Engl J Med 314:1407–1413, 1986b

Smith GR Jr, Rost K, Kashner TM: A trial of standardized psychiatric consultation on health outcomes and costs in somatizing patients. Arch Gen Psychiatry 52:238–243, 1995

Smith RC: A clinical approach to the somatizing patient. J Fam Pract 21:294–301, 1985

Spitzer RL, Williams JBW, Gibbon M, et al: The Structured Clinical Interview for DSM-IIIR (SCID), I: history, rationale, and description. Arch Gen Psychiatry 49:624–629, 1992

Spitzer RL, Williams JB, Kroenke K, et al: Utility of a new procedure for diagnosing mental disorders in primary care: the PRIME-MD 1000 study. JAMA 272:1749–1756, 1994

Stoudemire A, Thompson TL II, Mitchell WD, et al: Family physicians' perceptions of psychosocial disorders: pilot survey report and educational implications. Int J Psychiatry Med 12:281–287, 1982–1983

Straker N, Mostyn P, Marshall C: The use of two-way TV in bringing mental health services to the inner city. Am J Psychiatry 133:1202–1205, 1976

Strathdee G: Primary care–psychiatry interaction: a British perspective. Gen Hosp Psychiatry 9:102–110, 1987

Sturm R, Wells KB: How can care for depression become more cost-effective? JAMA 273:51–58, 1995

Tiemens BG, Ormel J, Simon GE: Occurrence, recognition, and outcome for psychological disorders in primary care. Am J Psychiatry 153:636–644, 1996

Townes PN, Harkley AL: Alcohol screening practices of primary care physicians in eastern Carolina. Alcohol 11:489–492, 1994

Uhlenhuth EH, Glass RM, Haberman SJ, et al: Relative sensitivity of clinical measures in trials of anxiety agents, in Quantitative Techniques for the Evaluation of the Behavior of Psychiatric Patients. Edited by Burdock EI, Gershon S. New York, Marcel Dekker, 1982, pp 393–410

Von Korff M, Shapiro S, Burke JD, et al: Anxiety and depression in a primary care clinic: comparison of Diagnostic Interview Schedule, General Health Questionnaire, and practitioner assessments. Arch Gen Psychiatry 44:152–156, 1987

Von Korff M, Ormel J, Katon W, et al: Disability and depression among high utilizers of health care: a longitudinal analysis. Arch Gen Psychiatry 49:91–100, 1992

Ware JE, Johnston SA: Conceptualization and Measurement of Health for Adults, Vol 3: Mental Health. (Health Insurance Study, Publ No R-1987/3-HEW). Santa Monica, CA, Rand, 1979

Weissman MM, Olfson M, Leon AC, et al: Brief diagnostic interviews (SDDS-PC) for multiple mental disorders in primary care: a pilot study. Arch Fam Med 4:220–227, 1995

Wells KB, Hays R, Burman MA, et al: Detection of depressive disorder for patients receiving prepaid or fee-for-service care: results from the Medical Outcomes Study. JAMA 262:3298–3302, 1989a

Wells KB, Stewart A, Hays R, et al: The functioning and well-being of depressed patients: results from the Medical Outcomes Study. JAMA 262:914–919, 1989b

Wells KB, Katon W, Rogers B, et al: Use of minor tranquilizers and antidepressant medication by depressed outpatients: results from the Medical Outcomes Study. Am J Psychiatry 151:694–700, 1994

Welsh GS: A factor study of the MMPI using scales with item overlap eliminated. Am Psychol 7:341–347, 1952

Wenrich MD, Paauw DS, Carline JD, et al: Do primary care physicians screen patients about alcohol intake using the CAGE questions? J Gen Intern Med 10:631–634, 1995

Williams JB, Spitzer RL: PRIME-MD: a new system for the evaluation of mental disorders in primary care, in Primary Care Research Program: The Sixth Annual NIMH International Research Conference on Primary Care Mental Health Research. Bethesda, MD, National Institute of Mental Health, 1992

Wise MG, Rieck SO: Diagnostic considerations and treatment approaches to underlying anxiety in the medically ill. J Clin Psychiatry 54 (suppl 5):22–26, 1993

Wise MG, Taylor SE: Anxiety and mood disorders in medically ill patients. J Clin Psychiatry 51 (suppl 1):27–32, 1990

Wittson CL, Affleck DC, Johnson V: Two-way television group therapy. Mental Hospitals 12:22–23, 1961

Wulsin LR, Arnold LM, Hillard JR: Axis I disorders in ER patients with atypical chest pain. Int J Psychiatry Med 21:37–46, 1991

Zinbarg RE, Barlow DH, Liebowitz M, et al: The DSM-IV field trial for mixed anxiety-depression. Am J Psychiatry 151:1153–1162, 1994

Zung WWK: A self-rating depression scale. Arch Gen Psychiatry 12:63–70, 1965

Zung WWK: A rating instrument for anxiety disorders. Psychosomatics 12:371–379, 1971

CHAPTER 47

MANAGED CARE AND PSYCHIATRY

DOUGLAS F. ZATZICK, M.D.

This chapter is an overview of managed care and its relationship to psychiatry. It begins with the definition of managed care and the tracing of the historical development of managed care delivery systems within psychiatry. The reader is then updated on changes in mental health care delivery brought about by managed care. The chapter also includes a review of psychiatric research into managed care; the findings of some of the key studies are briefly discussed and the challenges to empirical research in the area of managed mental health care are clarified. The chapter concludes with an assessment of models and perspectives that are important for the understanding of psychiatry's future survival in managed care environments. Throughout the chapter are definitions of new terms and concepts in the psychiatric lexicon that derive from managed care's impact on psychiatry.

WHAT IS MANAGED CARE?

The essence of managed care is cost containment in conjunction with the monitoring of the quality and outcomes of care (M. F. Shore and Beigel 1996; Wells et al. 1995). The central technique of managed care involves containment of costs through enrollment of patients in prepaid service plans. Before the advent of managed care, psychiatrists and other mental health professionals were reimbursed through the traditional *fee-for-service* mechanism. Under fee-for-service, practitioners were reimbursed directly by third-party payers, such as private insurance or the government, for services provided to individual patients.

In managed care, fee-for-service reimbursement is replaced by *capitation*. Through capitation, practitioners are paid a specific sum of money for the ongoing care of a person or a group of people for a particular period (Berwick 1996). Capitation forces mental health practitioners to focus on the treatment needs of an entire enrolled population, not just the immediate concerns of those patients seeking services. Managed care therefore causes a shift in the practice of medicine from a patient-based focus to a population-based focus (Brook et al. 1996a; M. F. Shore and Beigel 1996). From the clinician's perspective, managed care can be defined as clinical practice that takes into account the costs of care (M. F. Shore and Beigel 1996).

In managed mental health care, capitated services are provided to populations through a variety of institutional structures. Health maintenance organizations (HMOs) are institutions that combine insurers and providers; in an HMO, those administering the coverage and those providing the care are within the same organization. The group or staff model HMO combines insurers, providers, and hospitals in one organization (e.g., the Kaiser-Permanente Medical Care Program or Group Health HMO). In this model, inpatient and outpatient benefits are provided by one organization. Independent practice associations are networks of practitioners and hospitals that operate outside one institution (Bodenheimer and Grumbach 1994). An independent practice association might contract with an insurer to provide outpatient services for a designated population at a set fee.

The institutional structure of managed care delivery is currently in flux and is evolving new forms. This rapid change makes clear definition of managed care's many organizational structures difficult at times (Bachrack 1995; Mechanic 1996).

HISTORICAL DEVELOPMENT OF MANAGED CARE

Managed care has its origins in attempts to contain costs and represents the growth of economic forces in medicine (Drake 1997). Managed care was initially a response to pressure from private and public purchasers of medical care to slow medical expenditures; large corporations buying medical benefits for their employees and the United States government purchasing medical care through programs such as Medicare and Medicaid were concerned about rapidly increasing health care costs. Between 1960 and 1990, spending for health care increased almost 6% each year, more than double the growth rate of the rest of the economy. If health care spending had continued at this rate for another three decades, it would have accounted for nearly 30% of America's economic output (Fuchs 1997).

The origins of prepaid group practice in America can be traced back to the 1920s; the Kaiser Permanente and Group Health staff model HMOs developed in the 1930s and 1940s (Shapiro 1996; Smillie 1991). The earliest, most notable progenitor of managed mental health care may have been the community mental health movement (M. F. Shore 1996). Community mental health centers, which became established in the 1960s, had fixed budgets to provide treatment for previously delineated populations and thus resembled the capitated systems of today's managed mental health care. Many of the techniques for cost control that are essential to the practice of managed behavioral health care—including case management, decreased utilization of inpatient services, and the development of partial hospitalization and prevention programs—derive from the community mental health movement (M. F. Shore 1996).

The rise of managed behavioral health care appears to have been a response, at least in part, to the expansion of inpatient and outpatient mental health expenditures in the 1980s. For example, spending by employers for services related to substance abuse increased by an average of 50% from 1986 to 1990 (Iglehart 1996; M. F. Shore 1996). Managed behavioral health care may have been a reaction to entrepreneurial efforts by owners of private hospitals in the late 1980s who exploited the expanding benefits of fee-for-service insurance reimbursement (Iglehart 1996).

Thus, managed behavioral health care arose out of a need to contain costs. The expectation that managed behavioral health care techniques could limit costs derived from observations that practice patterns for psychiatric disorders varied widely, a great deal of unnecessary and prolonged psychiatric hospitalization occurred, and a small proportion of patients accounted for a high proportion of visits. A key condition enabling purchasers of care to force cost controls on providers has been an excess in the numbers and types of providers in many health care markets (Fuchs 1997), including mental health.

IMPACT OF MANAGED CARE

ETHICAL DILEMMAS FOR THE PRACTITIONER

The shift from fee-for-service reimbursement to capitation brings into conflict two ethical principles that underlie the practice of medicine: beneficence and distributive justice (Bodenheimer and Grumbach 1995; Halpern 1994; Sabin 1996). *Beneficence*, as it relates to medicine, is the obligation of health professionals to do all they can for an individual patient. In the fee-for-service system of care, individual practitioners could focus without conflict on doing all they could for the patient. However, with the advent of managed care, practitioners must now also consider the principle of *distributive justice*, that is, the fair and equitable distribution of limited medical resources to the entire population of patients under care. In this system of care, the resources are not unlimited and the provider must consider that care delivered to one patient may limit the amount of resources available for others. This shift in provider responsibility from the care of the individual patient to the care of the entire population has a number of far-reaching implications for the delivery of mental health care.

QUALITY OF CARE

The tensions between population-based practice and the delivery of care to individual patients have brought concerns about the quality of care to the forefront of medical practice and research (Berwick 1996; Blumenthal 1996a, 1996b; Blumenthal and Epstein 1996; Brook et al. 1996a, 1996b; Chassin 1996). Managed care has been effective in controlling costs, but its impact on the quality of care remains unclear (Fuchs 1997).

Although what constitutes high-quality care is currently being debated, there is some consensus that high-quality care should contribute to the improvement or maintenance of a particular patient's *quality of life* (American Medical Association 1986). Quality of life can be viewed as encompassing three domains of an individual's experience: functional status, access to resources and opportunities, and well-being (Lehman 1995).

High-quality care can also be viewed as it relates to the attributes and results of care (Blumenthal 1996a). In this context, quality is defined by the nature of the interaction between the patient and the physician. Thus, high-quality care requires adequate doctor-patient trust and communication, as well as an ability on the part of the physician to make adequate technical decisions and to intervene appropriately on the patient's behalf (Blumenthal 1996a).

Another important aspect to consider in the assessment of quality of care is the satisfaction of health care consumers' expectations of and desires for care; thus, *patient satisfaction* is another component of high-quality care (Lewis 1994). Quality of care may also be viewed from the perspective of health care plans and organizations; because population-based measures of accessibility and cost containment (i.e., accessibility of health care services to consumers and affordability of services for purchasers) can lead to improvements in quality of care, high-quality care involves such measures (Blumenthal 1996a).

The shift from fee-for-service to capitated systems of care may have negative impacts on the quality of care (Berwick 1996; Spencer et al. 1996). In the fee-for-service system, there was no incentive for providers to limit the amount of care delivered to a particular patient (McFarland 1993). However, when a provider is delivering care to a capitated population, there are financial incentives to treat healthier patients and provide less care. These incentives may translate into a series of practices that could threaten the quality of care in managed behavioral health plans; these practices include selecting patients who require less care, transferring costly patients to the public sector, and designing systems of care that limit access. In theory, the quality of managed mental health care might be ensured through the ability of consumers to shift plans if not satisfied with the services provided. However, in reality, the delivery of mental health care and the very nature of mental illness make this ideal less attainable (Spencer et al. 1996).

This is not to say that capitated systems of care do not have the potential to improve the quality of care. Managed care that is appropriately monitored and accountable may positively affect quality by encouraging innovations in the design and delivery of care (M. F. Shore 1997).

ACCOUNTABILITY

M. F. Shore (1997) suggested that although the greatest impact of managed care to date has been cost containment, the lasting consequences of the managed behavioral health care revolution will be the impact on professional accountability. The essence of *accountability* is attention to how medical resources are distributed, as well as attention to the outcomes of these resource allocation decisions. Before the arrival of managed care, the clinical work of psychiatrists and other mental health professionals was for the most part a private matter without external accountability (M. F. Shore 1997). Quality was defined in idiosyncratic terms, and consumer satisfaction with the patient-provider relationship often sufficed as a measure of clinical outcomes. M. F. Shore (1997) argued that managed care brings an expansion of accountability, to include responsibilities at the organizational level. "The evolution to external accountability was likely inevitable, for it was irresistibly driven by the increasing technical sophistication required of responsible practitioners, by the abundance of research findings available to improve care, by the demonstrated problems of practice variability and medical error, and by the lure of information technology, which promised to assist physicians and other health professionals to improve the personal care of their patients" (M. F. Shore 1997, p. 310).

PRACTICE OF PSYCHIATRY

Managed care has had a tremendous impact on the day-to-day practice of clinical psychiatry, so much so that some authors have asked, "Are psychiatrists replaceable?" (Fink 1996) and "Is the private practice of psychiatry compatible with managed care?" (Pomerantz et al. 1996) These authors are referring to the trend of hiring less expensive clinicians (e.g., social workers with master's degrees, clinicians with Ph.D.'s) to function in clinical roles that do not absolutely demand a physician. Most managed care companies will not reimburse psychotherapy at psychiatric rates; thus, psychotherapy involving relatively high functioning patients—a form of therapy that was once a mainstay of psychiatric practice—is increasingly becoming the territory of nonmedical clinicians. Long-term, intensive psychodynamic psychotherapy is becoming obsolete for all but the wealthiest patients.

In containing costs, managed care organizations have redefined the principal aim of treatment, which is now the reestablishment of a reasonable level of functioning and the prevention of recurrence (M. F. Shore and Beigel 1996). *Functioning* or *functional status* has been defined as an individual's ability to perform physical activities, such as activities of daily living (physical functioning); to perform in particular social roles (social functioning); or to perform in particular roles at work, at home, or at school (occupational functioning) (Stewart and Ware 1992). It is now well established that impaired functioning is associated with a broad spectrum of psychiatric disorders; large-scale, population-based reports have established that functional morbidity is associated with depressive, anxiety, substance abuse, and posttraumatic stress disorders (Ormel et al. 1994; Sherbourne et al. 1996; Spitzer et al. 1995; Wells et al. 1989; Zatzick et al. 1997).

Functional outcomes assessment represents a major shift away from traditional psychiatric treatment models that targeted assessments and amelioration of clinical symptoms (Hales and Zatzick 1997; M. F. Shore and Beigel 1996). Comprehensive assessments of managed mental health care will need to include methodologically rigorous assessments of the individual, institutional, and societal outcomes associated with changes in the delivery of mental health care.

A further challenge to psychiatric practitioners who operate within a managed care environment is that the treatment of patients with mental disorders is shifting to the primary care sector (Pardes 1996). The majority of patients with mental illness initially present to and are treated in the primary care setting (Kessler et al. 1985; Regier et al. 1978). However, in contrast to the fee-for-service era, psychiatrists are now actively pursuing methods of addressing the treatment needs of patients with mental disorders in the primary care setting. Katon and colleagues (1995, 1996) developed *collaborative models of care* in which mental health professionals work side by side with general medical providers in primary care clinics. Schulberg and co-workers (1996b) demonstrated that standard psychotherapeutic and psychopharmacological treatments developed in the sector of specialty mental health care are equally efficacious applied to depressed patients in the primary care setting.

ACADEMIC CENTERS AND PSYCHIATRIC TRAINING

These changes in the practice of psychiatry raise a number of serious questions for academic departments of psychiatry and psychiatry residency programs. Academic centers

have traditionally been hospital-based institutions committed to a number of activities that are poorly reimbursed, including teaching, research, treatment of severely ill patients, and care of the indigent (Riba and Carli 1996). These centers are now having to revise their service delivery in order to survive financially in the new and competitive behavioral mental health care marketplace. In addition, academic centers must redesign psychiatry training programs to educate residents about the changes occurring in psychiatric practice. The breadth of these changes and the rapidity at which these changes are being made have led some authors to ask whether academic psychiatry will survive managed care (Riba and Carli 1996).

HEALTH SERVICES AND TREATMENT OUTCOMES RESEARCH

Managed care has brought about a resurgence of interest in health services and treatment outcomes research. *Mental health services research* is the branch of psychiatric inquiry that focuses on the interrelationships between the structure, process, and outcomes of service delivery (Starfield 1973; Wells et al. 1995). Health services research is by nature interdisciplinary, incorporating economic, historical, anthropological, and clinical investigative methodologies and perspectives. Mental health services research encompasses a broad spectrum of investigation and includes research related to the costs of mental disturbance, research into access to care in underserved mentally ill populations, identification and treatment of psychiatric disorders in primary care, and, perhaps most important, studies of the quality and outcomes of care for psychiatric patients treated through managed care.

Outcomes assessment refers to a broad area of health services research in which attempts are made to assess the impact of a particular treatment or system of care on a variety of individual, institutional, and societal outcomes. Examples of *individual outcomes* include clinical symptom levels (e.g., depression, anxiety, somatization); physical, role, or social functioning; and individual patient satisfaction. Perhaps the best examples of *institutional outcomes* are the use of clinical services and the costs of providing care. Assessment of *societal outcomes* may involve measures of return to work after psychiatric illness and rates of interpersonal violence or incarceration.

When assessing editorial and research reports in the area of health services research on managed care, it is extremely important to understand the perspective from which the reports derive (Pincus et al. 1996). Investigations funded by large foundations or the federal government tend to represent a societal perspective, because they are free from proprietary interests; these studies are often most useful in informing public policy. It has been argued that researchers should strive for this impartiality in their evaluations of managed care (Wells et al. 1995). Corporate or institutional investigations tend to focus on cost reduction or ways of increasing market share. These investigations are most useful in aiding individual corporations in making decisions regarding allocation of internal resources. Reports from the perspective of providers tend to focus on the interests of health care workers within the shifting economic arena of managed care, whereas reports from the patient's perspective focus on the needs and concerns of consumers of health care. Investigations conducted from these different perspectives may have varying aims and draw contrasting conclusions.

HEALTH SERVICES RESEARCH INTO MANAGED CARE

Recently, a number of senior health services researchers commented on the challenges inherent in designing methodologically rigorous investigations into managed mental health care (Mechanic 1996; Pincus et al. 1996; Wells et al. 1995). A primary and formidable obstacle to designing high-quality, generalizable investigations is the rapidly changing, dynamic nature of the managed care marketplace. Investigators must question what the health care delivery systems for which they are designing studies will be like in 5–10 years. A related difficulty is that the diversity of managed care arrangements limits the generalizability of any one study undertaken in a particular system of care.

In addition, access to data is often limited because of the proprietary nature of many managed care databases. Plan administrators may be cautious about releasing information, fearing that study results—if published or disseminated—could disrupt or decrease plan enrollments. Therefore, concerns regarding confidentiality extend beyond the usual issues of patient and firm privacy to issues of how outcomes data may detract from or benefit the proprietary interests of the organization. Furthermore, data sets are often incomplete and may not contain, for example, information on out-of-plan utilization. Finally, businesses are often not interested in experimental designs, because of the potential disruption of organizational routines.

There are conceptual challenges for health services and treatment outcomes in the managed care environment as well. Many of the current measures of quality require further research and development. For example, patient satisfaction is now being used as a measure of overall quality of care. A number of authors have critiqued available measures of satisfaction as overly general, simplistic, and unable to provide a deeper understanding of the experiences and meanings patients derive from their clinical encounters (Williams 1994; Williams and Wilkinson 1995). (Similar concerns have been raised regarding other outcomes, such as self-reported quality of life [Gill and Feinstein 1994].) Furthermore, patient satisfaction, although correlated with mood state (Eyers et al. 1994), is not strongly associated with improved functioning over time and thus may not be an adequate independent measure of quality of care in the case of psychiatric disorders (Wells et al. 1996).

The differences between efficacy and effectiveness trials are also important to consider in a discussion of health services research. Traditionally, clinical *efficacy trials* in psychiatry have maximized the *internal validity* of the investigation; such trials strengthen the design of the study so that a causal link can be made between an isolated treatment intervention and outcomes. Techniques often used in efficacy trials to enhance causal attribution include strict inclusion and exclusion criteria, randomized design, blinding, and treatment protocols followed by expert clinicians (Begg et al. 1996).

Health services researchers have noted that although efficacy trials maximize internal validity, they leave much to be desired with regard to external validity. *External validity* concerns the extent to which the results of a trial can be generalized to real-world treatment settings. The very factors that strengthen the causal link between predictor and outcome in a particular study, such as adherence to a strict protocol by expert clinicians, may limit generalizability of the findings to the managed mental health care or primary care sectors. Therefore, researchers have begun to design and implement investigations in which the actual effectiveness of treatments in real-world settings is evaluated (Schulberg et al. 1996a). *Effectiveness trials* incorporate a number of methodological innovations, including randomization to usual care, and multimodal interventions, rather than isolated treatments, that target not only patients but also providers and systems of care. Studies of treatment effectiveness also employ nonrandomized designs (Wells et al. 1996).

EMPIRICAL INVESTIGATIONS INTO MANAGED CARE

Empirical investigations into managed mental health care have focused on a number of areas, including costs, outcomes, and service delivery. This section is an overview of some of the major research findings, within both the sector of specialty mental health care and the primary care sector.

In a series of investigations into managed care, in which differences in clinical outcomes, functional status, service utilization, and health care costs were assessed, patients were randomized to either prepaid capitated services or fee-for-service care. The RAND Health Insurance Experiment, an experimental trial conducted between 1974 and 1982, included a total 6,970 patients (Manning et al. 1984, 1987; Newhouse 1974; Wells et al. 1990). In one part of the study, more than 2,000 general medical patients in the Group Health Cooperative were randomized to fee-for-service or prepaid HMO care (Manning et al. 1984). The study results demonstrated that the rate of hospital admissions for HMO patients was 40% less than that for fee-for-service patients. Rates of expenditures were 25% less for HMO patients than for fee-for service patients.

Other components of the RAND Health Insurance Experiment addressed the use of mental health services. Wells et al. (1990) reported that no clinically meaningful differences in outcomes were detected between the group of 1,080 patients enrolled in Group Health and the group of 1,026 patients randomized to fee-for-service care. These results have been called into question, however, because the outcome measures were extremely general and the randomized trial did not include a substantial proportion of patients with chronic mental illness (Mechanic 1996). A further observation was that HMO patients were equally likely as comparable fee-for-service patients, or more likely than such patients, to take advantage of the mental health benefits supplied by their employers (Manning et al. 1987).

Beginning in 1986, the Health Care Financing Administration sponsored a series of model systems in which Medicaid recipients in Minnesota were enrolled in prepaid plans (Christianson et al. 1992; Lurie et al. 1992). Random samples of individuals with severe mental illness were assigned to fee-for-service or prepaid plans. Individuals in each of the plans were compared across a broad profile of outcomes, including psychiatric symptoms status, physical functioning, social functioning, and patterns of service utilization. No major differences were observed between the prepaid-plan group and the fee-for-service group with regard to psychiatric symptoms, general health status, or patterns of participation in community mental health programs. Members of the prepaid-plan group were less frequently victims of crime than were fee-for-service enrollees. However, Global Assessment Scale scores were significantly lower in the prepaid-plan group than in the fee-for-service group. A number of concerns have been raised regarding the generalizability of this study; one such concern is that the majority of study subjects were followed for less than a year, with no longer-term outcome assessments (Mechanic 1996).

The Medical Outcomes Study (Stewart and Ware 1992; Wells et al. 1996), a nonrandomized effectiveness investigation, examined differences in a broad profile of outcomes between patients with depression who were enrolled in fee-for-service plans and depressed patients enrolled in prepaid plans. The study included more than 11,000 patients treated in group or solo practices in Boston, Chicago, or Los Angeles. The patients had a number of chronic conditions, and approximately 2,500 patients in the study screened positive for depressive symptoms. A subsample of these patients was followed longitudinally and a comparison was made between treatment in fee-for-service and treatment in prepaid practice settings. Depressed patients in both practice settings had significantly greater functional impairment than did patients with chronic medical illness (Wells et al. 1989). In 617 depressed patients followed for 2 years, functional outcomes were poorer in some prepaid practice settings. Also, compared with psychiatrists, general medical providers were found to provide lower-quality care for depression at reduced costs (Sturm and Wells 1995).

Norquist and Wells (1991), using data from the National Institute of Mental Health's Epidemiologic Catchment Area study, reported that seriously mentally ill subjects in an HMO population were more likely to receive their mental health care from general practitioners and that overall the rates of outpatient visits were approximately 40% lower in the HMO population than in the fee-for-service population, despite the fact that prevalences of psychiatric disorders were similar in the two groups. Norquist and Wells (1991) attributed these differences to a "less intensive style of care" among HMOs for seriously mentally ill patients.

In summary, there is evidence that patients enrolled in prepaid plans are treated at lower costs than are patients in fee-for-service plans. What remains unclear and requires further intensive investigation is whether the quality of care for patients with mental illness suffers in prepaid plans.

A number of empirical investigations have shown the effectiveness of innovative treatment strategies that successfully adapt to the changes in the delivery of mental health care brought about by managed care. Collaborative models of care are one such innovation.

Katon and colleagues (1995, 1996) developed *collaborative treatment models* for the treatment of depression in HMO primary care clinics. Patients with major depression and patients with minor depression (i.e., two to four symptoms of depression nearly every day for 2 weeks) visiting Group Health primary care clinics were recruited into the study. The intervention consisted of distribution of video and written materials describing depressive symptoms and antidepressant medications; didactic education and as-needed consultation for primary care physicians providing the interventions; four to six sessions of cognitive-behavioral psychotherapy treatment for depression; antidepressant therapy; individual case supervision by a psychiatrist, with the option of a single session patient-psychiatrist consultation regarding medications; regular psychiatric feedback to primary care providers; and a relapse prevention plan at the last patient-provider encounter combined with telephone follow-up 24 weeks after the last visit.

Patients in the intervention group demonstrated increased compliance with antidepressant therapy and improved satisfaction with treatment compared with patients receiving usual care. Intervention patients with major depression showed significantly greater improvement of depressive symptoms than did control subjects; there were no significant differences in depressive outcomes in the group of patients with minor depression. Also, there were no substantial differences in use of primary care services between the intervention and control groups. This investigation demonstrated that a multifaceted intervention improves the overall quality of care among depressed patients in an HMO primary care clinic. However, there was no evidence that this improvement in the quality of care was offset by a reduction in the number of primary care visits or was accompanied by an overall offset of cost.

Smith and colleagues (1985, 1995) reported that in the case of patients with somatization disorder or high levels of somatic symptoms, a single psychiatric consultation significantly reduces use of health care services. In this group's most recent randomized trial (Smith et al. 1995), primary care physicians treating patients with somatization disorder received a single letter describing the chronic relapsing course of the disorder. Additionally, the letter recommended regularly scheduled appointments with the patients and avoidance of costly workups and hospitalizations. Subjects receiving the intervention demonstrated statistically significant improvements in physical functioning. Also, a 33% decrease in costs was observed for intervention patients; this reduction in costs remained stable for the 2 years after intervention and was likely due to a reduction in hospitalizations.

MANAGED CARE AND PSYCHIATRY: FUTURE PERSPECTIVES

The advent of managed care has brought about radical and what appear to be lasting changes in psychiatry. In re-

sponse to these dramatic shifts in the structure of psychiatric practice, training, and research, a number of models have been proposed with the hope of sustaining psychiatry as an autonomous clinical and investigative specialty. Bloom (1996) suggested three potential directions for psychiatry: the community mental health model, the primary care model, and the clinical neuroscience model.

The community mental health model applies principles of treatment derived from the community mental health movement—such as psychiatric consultation to nonmedical mental health providers, primary prevention, and delivery of services to capitated severely mentally ill populations—to HMOs. In the primary care model, psychiatrists are seen as delivering both primary care and psychiatric treatments. Proponents of this model envision the development of combined psychiatry/primary care residencies (J. H. Shore 1996).

Advocates of the clinical neuroscience model suggest that psychiatry needs to be reinvented as a biological specialty with close ties to neurology (Detre and McDonald 1997). According to these authors, psychiatrists must understand that their specialty is and always will be a consulting specialty: psychiatrists will not be able to define themselves as primary care practitioners and should therefore prepare for clinical roles as consultants. In this capacity, psychiatrists can anticipate treating the most difficult and refractory patients. Psychiatric research and practice will therefore need to incorporate increasing knowledge of the biological sciences and neurosciences. Simultaneously, psychiatrists would shed their nonmedical knowledge and activities. In this model, the nonmedical care of mentally ill persons is administered by practitioners such as social workers and psychologists.

Perhaps the most important point to be distilled from these three perspectives is that psychiatrists of the future are likely to be practicing in multiple capitated environments and interacting with a diverse array of care providers. Therefore, rather than focusing on practice in a particular environment or developing a narrow set of skills, psychiatric educators, clinicians, and investigators may do well to ask what the guiding principles are for psychiatrists in an era of managed care.

The essence of the changes brought about by managed care are first and foremost socioeconomic; no amount of additional focused biological or clinical training will elucidate for psychiatrists how to resolve conflicts inherent in moving from a fee-for-service to a population-based practice. Wherever they practice, psychiatrists will need to make informed decisions about medical resource allocation and be able to think clearly about outcomes assessments for the interventions they provide. Furthermore, these decisions are likely to be made in the context of an increasingly diverse and pluralistic American society.

In this rethinking of psychiatry (Kleinman 1988), what may be most important is the incorporation of multidisciplinary models that include economic, ethical, and historical perspectives as well as perspectives that address culturally competent care (Sue 1988). These diverse perspectives are potentially embodied by a *health services research and practice model* of psychiatry. As a branch of psychiatric inquiry, psychiatric services research is by nature interdisciplinary, incorporating social scientific perspectives and employing both quantitative and qualitative research methodologies (Inui 1996). Incorporation of a health services model would allow psychiatric practitioners a flexible integrated approach to patient care and problem solving that could inform any number of interactions, including the collaborative management of patients with primary care practitioners, the supervision of treatments provided by nonmedical mental health practitioners, and clinical and investigative relationships with other medical specialists. Thus, this evolving health services model may help guide future psychiatrists as they face the multifaceted challenges of managed mental health care.

REFERENCES

Aday LA, Andersen R: A framework for the study of access to medical care. Health Serv Res 1:208–220, 1974

American Medical Association, Committee of Medical Service: Quality of care. JAMA 256:1032–1034, 1986

Bachrack LL: Managed care, I: delimiting the concept. Psychiatr Serv 46:1229–1230, 1995

Begg C, Cho M, Eastwood S, et al: Improving the quality of reporting of randomized controlled trials: the CONSORT statement. JAMA 276:637–639, 1996

Berwick DM: Quality of health care, part 5: payment by capitation and the quality of care. N Engl J Med 335:1227–1231, 1996

Bloom JD: Psychiatry: three models in search of a future. Psychiatr Serv 47:874–875, 1996

Blumenthal D: Quality of health care, part 1: quality of care—what is it? N Engl J Med 335:891–894, 1996a

Blumenthal D: Quality of health care, part 4: the origins of the quality-of care-debate. N Engl J Med 335:1146–1149, 1996b

Blumenthal D, Epstein AM: Quality of health care, part 6: the role of physicians in the future of quality management. N Engl J Med 335:1328–1331, 1996

Bodenheimer TS, Grumbach K: Reimbursing physicians and hospitals. JAMA 272:971–977, 1994

Bodenheimer TS, Grumbach K: Medical ethics and the rationing of health care, in Understanding Health Policy: A Clinical Approach. Norwalk, CT, Appleton & Lange, 1995, pp 173–194

Brook RH, Kamberg CJ, McGlynn EA: Health system reform and quality. JAMA 276:476–480, 1996a

Brook RH, McGlynn EA, Cleary PD: Quality of health care, II: measuring quality of care. N Engl J Med 335:966–970, 1996b

Chassin MR: Quality of health care, part 3: improving the quality of care. N Engl J Med 335:1060–1063, 1996

Christianson JB, Lurie N, Finch M, et al: Use of community-based mental health programs by HMOs: evidence from a Medicaid demonstration. Am J Public Health 82:790–796, 1992

Detre T, McDonald MC: Managed care and the future of psychiatry. Arch Gen Psychiatry 54:201–213, 1997

Drake DF: Managed care: a product of market dynamics. JAMA 277:560–563, 1997

Eyers K, Brodaty H, Roy K, et al: Patient satisfaction with a mood disorder unit: elements and components. Aust N Z J Psychiatry 28:279–287, 1994

Fink PJ: Are psychiatrists replaceable? in Controversies in Managed Mental Health Care. Edited by Lazarus A. Washington, DC, American Psychiatric Press, 1996, pp 3–16

Fuchs VR: Managed care and merger mania. JAMA 277: 920–921, 1997

Gill TM, Feinstein AR: A critical appraisal of the quality of quality-of-life measurements. JAMA 272:619–626, 1994

Hales RE, Zatzick DF: What is PTSD? Am J Psychiatry 154:143–145, 1997

Halpern J: What ethical frameworks shape the development of practice guidelines? Paper presented at the Robert Wood Johnson Clinical Scholars 22nd Annual Meeting, Fort Lauderdale, FL, November 9–12, 1994

Iglehart JK: Health policy report: managed care and mental health. N Engl J Med 334:131–135, 1996

Inui TS: What are the sciences of relationship-centered primary care? J Fam Pract 42:171–177, 1996

Katon W, Von Korff M, Lin E, et al: Collaborative management to achieve treatment guidelines: impact on depression in primary care. JAMA 273:1026–1031, 1995

Katon W, Robinson P, Von Korff MV, et al: A multifaceted intervention to improve treatment of depression in primary care. Arch Gen Psychiatry 53:924–932, 1996

Kessler LG, Cleary PD, Burke JD: Psychiatric disorders in primary care: results of a follow-up study. Arch Gen Psychiatry 42:583–587, 1985

Kleinman AK: Rethinking Psychiatry: From Cultural Category to Personal Experience. New York, Free Press, 1988

Lehman A: Measuring quality of life in a reformed health system. Health Aff (Millwood) 14:90–101, 1995

Lewis JR: Patient views on quality care in general practice: literature review. Soc Sci Med 39:655–670, 1994

Lurie N, Moscovice IS, Finch M, et al: Does capitation affect the health of the chronically mentally ill? results from a randomized trial. JAMA 267:3300–3304, 1992

Manning WG, Leibowitz A, Goldberg GA, et al: A controlled trial of the effect of a prepaid group practice on use of services. N Engl J Med 310:1505–1510, 1984

Manning WG, Wells KB, Benjamin BS: Use of outpatient mental health services over time in a health maintenance organization and fee-for-service plans. Am J Psychiatry 144:283–287, 1987

McFarland B: Capitation and mental health. Focus on Mental Health Research 6:1–8, 1993

Mechanic D: Can research on managed care inform practice and policy decisions? in Controversies in Managed Behavioral Health Care. Edited by Lazarus A. Washington, DC, American Psychiatric Press, 1996, pp 197–211

Newhouse JP: A design for a health insurance experiment. Inquiry 1:5–27, 1974

Norquist G, Wells KB: How do HMOs reduce outpatient mental health care costs? Am J Psychiatry 148:96–101, 1991

Ormel J, Von Korff M, Ustun TB, et al: Common mental disorders and disability across cultures: results from the WHO Collaborative Study on Psychological Problems in General Health Care. JAMA 272:1741–1748, 1994

Pardes H: A changing psychiatry for the future. Am J Psychiatry 153:1383–1386, 1996

Pincus HA, Zarin DA, West JC: Peering into the 'black box': measuring outcomes of managed care. Arch Gen Psychiatry 53:870–877, 1996

Pomerantz JM, Liptzin B, Carter A, et al: Is private practice compatible with managed care? in Controversies in Managed Mental Health Care. Edited by Lazarus A. Washington, DC, American Psychiatric Press, 1996, pp 17–28

Regier DA, Goldberg ID, Taube CA: The de facto US mental health services system: a public health perspective. Arch Gen Psychiatry 35:685–689, 1978

Riba MB, Carli TC: Will academic psychiatry survive managed care, in Controversies in Managed Mental Health Care. Edited by Lazarus A. Washington, DC, American Psychiatric Press, 1996, pp 81–98

Sabin JE: Is managed care ethical care? in Controversies in Managed Behavioral Health Care. Edited by Lazarus A. Washington, DC, American Psychiatric Press, 1996, pp 115–126

Schulberg HC, Magruder KM, deGruy F: Major depression in primary medical care practice: research trends and future priorities. Gen Hosp Psychiatry 18:395–406, 1996a

Schulberg HC, Block MR, Madonia MJ, et al: Treating major depression in primary care practice: eight month clinical outcomes. Arch Gen Psychiatry 53:913–919, 1996b

Shapiro S: An historical perspective on the roots of managed care. Curr Opin Pediatr 8:159–163, 1996

Sherbourne CD, Wells KB, Judd LL: Functioning and well-being of patients with panic disorder. Am J Psychiatry 153:213–218, 1996

Shore JH: Psychiatry at a crossroad: our role in primary care. Am J Psychiatry 153:1398–1405, 1996

Shore MF: An overview of managed behavioral health care. New Dir Ment Health Serv 72:3–12, 1996

Shore MF: A lesson in history, circa 2047. Am J Psychiatry 154:307–311, 1997

Shore MF, Beigel A: The challenges posed by managed behavioral health care. N Engl J Med 334:116–118, 1996

Smillie JG: Can Physicians Manage the Quality and Costs of Health Care? The Story of the Permanente Group. New York, McGraw-Hill, 1991

Smith GR, Monson RA, Ray DC: Psychiatric consultation in somatization disorder: a randomized controlled study. N Engl J Med 314:1407–1413, 1985

Smith GR, Rost K, Kashner TM: A trial of the effect of a standard psychiatric consultation on health outcomes and costs in somatizing patients. Arch Gen Psychiatry 52:238–243, 1995

Spencer CS, Frank RG, McGuire TG: How should the profit motive be used in managed care? in Controversies in Managed Mental Health Care. Edited by Lazarus A. Washington, DC, American Psychiatric Press, 1996, pp 279–290

Spitzer R, Kroenke K, Linzer M, et al: Health-related quality of life in primary care patients with mental disorders: results from the PRIME-MD study. JAMA 274:1511–1517, 1995

Starfield B: Health services research: a working model. N Engl J Med 289:132–135, 1973

Stewart A, Ware J: Measuring Functioning and Well-Being: The Medical Outcomes Study Approach. Durham, NC, Duke University Press, 1992

Sturm R, Wells KB: How can care for depression become more cost-effective? JAMA 273:51–58, 1995

Sue S: Psychotherapeutic services for ethnic minorities. Am Psychol 43:301–308, 1988

Wells KB, Stewart A, Hays RD, et al: The functioning and well-being of depressed patients: results from the Medical Outcomes Study. JAMA 262:914–919, 1989

Wells KB, Manning WG, Valdez BR: The effects of a prepaid group practice on mental health outcomes. Health Serv Res 25:615–625, 1990

Wells KB, Astrachan BM, Tischler GL, et al: Issues and approaches in evaluating managed mental health care. Milbank Q 73:57–75, 1995

Wells KB, Sturm R, Sherbourne CD, et al: Caring for Depression. Cambridge, MA, Harvard University Press, 1996

Williams B: Patient satisfaction: a valid concept? Soc Sci Med 38:509–516, 1994

Williams B, Wilkinson G: Patient satisfaction in mental health care: evaluating an evaluative method. Br J Psychiatry 166:559–562, 1995

Zatzick DF, Marmar CR, Weiss DS, et al: Posttraumatic stress disorder, and functioning and quality of life outcomes in a nationally representative sample of male Vietnam veterans. Am J Psychiatry 154:1690–1695, 1997

PRACTICE GUIDELINES IN PSYCHIATRY AND A PSYCHIATRIC PRACTICE RESEARCH NETWORK

DEBORAH A. ZARIN, M.D.
JOHN S. MCINTYRE, M.D.
HAROLD ALAN PINCUS, M.D.
LESLIE SEIGLE, B.A.

Over the past two decades, the field of psychiatry has moved systematically toward the goal of evidence-based clinical practice. Central to its progress has been the American Psychiatric Association's (APA's) development, on the platform of a criteria-based nomenclature (American Psychiatric Association 1980, 1994a), of evidence-based practice guidelines. An additional effort that will strengthen further the evidence-based foundations of clinical psychiatry is a psychiatric practice research network, which was begun in the mid-1990s (Zarin et al. 1997). This chapter addresses both of these initiatives; we describe in detail the APA's practice guideline project and offer a brief review of the development of the APA's practice research network.

PRACTICE GUIDELINES IN MEDICINE

Practice guidelines are systematically developed strategies of patient care that are developed to assist clinicians (and patients) in clinical decision-making (McIntyre and Talbott 1990). Eddy (1990) considered the meaning of the term *parameters* to encompass standards, guidelines, and options. In Eddy's schema, *standards* are instructions that should be followed in essentially all cases; exceptions to standards should be infrequent and strongly justified. *Guidelines* are recommendations that should be followed in the majority of cases. Exceptions to guidelines are more common and require only minimal justification. *Options* present strategies for use in clinical contexts in which there is no clearly preferred course of action. Using these definitions, the APA chose the term *guidelines* to describe its recommendations in this arena, and that is the term used throughout his chapter.

Practice guidelines have proliferated over the past decade throughout medicine and health care, and they continue to be developed by professional associations, insurance companies, health maintenance organizations, provider groups, state governments, and the federal government. Guidelines will play an increasing role in accreditation processes (American Medical Association 1997) and are beginning to influence psychiatric curricula. Most important, for clinicians and patients, well-constructed guidelines permit a critical review and synthesis of a rapidly expanding treatment literature; provide a framework for clinical decision-making and, within it, recommendations for treating a "typical" patient with a given diagnosis; and allow consideration, in light of research data, of the implications of specific clinical features for treatment recommendations.

As suggested above, explicit reasons exist for the heightened interests in the development of practice guidelines:

- The scientific foundation of medicine has grown exponentially in recent decades. Specialist physicians experience increasing difficulty in staying abreast of the latest research findings, and for the generalist the problem is greatly magnified. Even when one is knowledgeable about current studies, it is not always easy to translate new data into an optimal clinical strategy for an individual patient. Research findings must be evaluated, synthesized, and incorporated into a patient care strategy.

- Because the knowledge explosion has contributed to the introduction of expensive new technologies, health care costs have risen dramatically, and cost containment has become a pervasive concern. Identifying effective and cost-effective treatments is an economic imperative.

- Numerous studies have demonstrated substantial regional variation in treatment approaches for the same illness (Chassin et al. 1986; Lewis 1969). National guidelines are one way to address this issue.

- Increasingly, patients, potential patients, and payers are involved in decisions concerning choice of treatment. Their participation necessitates a clear description of treatment options and the evidence supporting the various choices.

Although these disparate factors recently have converged, triggering a surge in guideline development, pa-

rameters of care are not new. In 1851–1852, the young APA exercised its influence over psychiatric care with 40 "propositions" regarding the construction and organization of hospitals for the insane (Standing Committee 1851, 1853). Although these early practice parameters were agreed to by nationally recognized experts, no attempt was made to provide data that supported the recommendations. More recently, APA Task Force reports on the use of laboratory tests in psychiatry (Task Force on the Use of Laboratory Tests 1985) and clinical use of benzodiazepines (American Psychiatric Association 1990) cited research evidence as the basis for recommendations, but there was lacking the formal, systematic process for collecting and rating evidence that is used in developing contemporary APA practice guidelines. Psychiatry's experience historically parallels that of medicine generally. More than 50 years ago, for example, the American Academy of Pediatrics issued statements on immunization that resemble guidelines.

By the mid-1980s, the propensity of various medical groups to keep modifying and refining the processes used for guideline development prompted calls for some standardization of guideline development—guidelines for guidelines! The American Medical Association (AMA) and the Institute of Medicine (IOM) each have developed a series of principles to be followed in the development of practice guidelines. The AMA described six attributes of effective guidelines (Office of Quality Assurance 1996) (Table 48–1). In a separate issuance, the IOM (1992) identified eight attributes of "good" guidelines, listed in Table 48–2. Today, the practice guideline attributes suggested by the AMA and the IOM essentially constitute national standards for guideline efforts.

The broad involvement of physician organizations today in guideline development and dissemination belies the depth of resistance early on—resistance that continues, at a lower level—that was based principally on a concern that guidelines promote cookbook medicine: sterile, oversim-

TABLE 48–1. American Medical Association attributes of effective guidelines

Be developed by or in conjunction with physician organizations

Use reliable methodologies that integrate relevant research findings and clinical expertise

Be as comprehensive and specific as possible

Be based on current information

Be widely disseminated

Include outcomes research, goals, and measures

Source. Adapted from Office of Quality Assurance 1996.

TABLE 48–2. Institute of Medicine attributes of "good" guidelines

Validity
Reproducibility
Clinical applicability
Clinical flexibility
Clarity
Multidisciplinary process
Scheduled review

Source.   Adapted from Institute of Medicine 1992.

plified, and rigid treatment that does not take into account individual symptoms in patient illnesses and ignores subtleties in clinical work ("Legislated Clinical Medicine" 1990). Others have warned that guidelines will limit opportunities and incentives to innovate in practice and, at the same time, will increase professional liability exposure. Concerns that overly strict adherence to guidelines might diminish clinical innovation, retarding the development of novel approaches to patient care, may have a measure of validity, but well-developed guidelines minimize this possibility by not permitting overstatement of evidence from research or clinical consensus and by allowing clear identification of areas of relative uncertainty. As discussed later in this chapter, the APA's guideline development process is evidence based and open and involves a large number of clinicians; among psychiatrists who have made their thoughts known, most have experienced the completed guidelines as flexible and appropriately attending to the many variables in the expression of illness and the strategies for care.

At this writing, the impact of guidelines on professional liability exposure remains unclear. Recently, Hyams et al. (1995) reported that plaintiffs' attorneys, more frequently than defense attorneys, cite practice guidelines in malpractice litigation. A favorable impact may be seen, however, in a significant (25%) reduction in anesthesiologists' professional liability insurance premiums and similar reductions in obstetricians' and gynecologists' premiums when the respective national associations for these specialties accepted guidelines (Holzer 1990; "OB-GYN Premiums Decrease Drastically" 1993). Moreover, pilot programs underway in some jurisdictions (e.g., Maine) mandate that compliance with guidelines be used only as an affirmative malpractice defense. The prediction that guidelines will result in decreased professional liability exposure seems to be increasingly favored. Further protection for the clinician results from a clear qualifying description of the intent and limitations of guidelines. The first

paragraph of this statement of intent, which appears prominently at the front of each APA published guideline is as follows:

> This practice guideline is not intended to be construed or to serve as a standard of medical care. Standards of medical care are determined on the basis of all clinical data available for an individual case and are subject to change as scientific knowledge and technology advances and patterns evolve. These parameters of practice should be considered guidelines only. Adherence to them will not ensure a successful outcome in every case nor should they be construed as including all proper methods of care or excluding other acceptable methods of care aimed at the same results. The ultimate judgement regarding a particular clinical procedure or treatment plan must be made by the psychiatrist in light of the clinical data presented by the patient and the diagnostic and treatment options available.

In an effort to minimize misinterpretation or misuse of the guideline, the second paragraph of the statement of intent characterizes those involved in the development of the guideline and describes the process for dealing with potential and perceived conflicts of interest.

AMERICAN PSYCHIATRIC ASSOCIATION PRACTICE GUIDELINE PROJECT

The process for developing a guideline consists of eight stages: topic selection, work group appointment, scope determination and outline development, evidence definition, draft development, draft review, dissemination and implementation, evaluation, and revision (Table 48–3). Each step is discussed here.

TOPIC SELECTION

The APA Steering Committee on Practice Guidelines selects topics for practice guidelines according to the following criteria: 1) public health importance, as defined by prevalence and seriousness of the condition; 2) relevance to psychiatric practice; 3) availability of information and relevant data; and 4) availability of results of work already done that would be useful in the development of a practice guideline.

WORK GROUP APPOINTMENT

Following topic selection, a four- to six-member work group is appointed. Work group members must be in active clinical practice and are chosen because of their exper-

TABLE 48–3. American Psychiatric Association practice guidelines development process

Topic selection
Work group appointment
Scope determination and outline development
Evidence definition
Draft development
Draft review
Dissemination and implementation
Evaluation
Revision

Source. Adapted from Zarin et al. 1993.

tise in the area that is the focus of the guideline. Some members are primarily involved in academic and/or research efforts, but all must be involved in the care of patients. All members are asked to declare that there are no conflicts of interest that would affect their ability to maintain objectivity toward the guideline recommendations.

SCOPE DETERMINATION AND OUTLINE DEVELOPMENT

After a topic has been selected, the standard outline is customized as warranted. The first step in this process is determining the scope of the guideline. The bipolar disorder guideline, for example, was limited to recommendations for the care of individuals with bipolar I disorder. However, within this framework were discussed all treatments that might be useful for these patients, including psychosocial treatments that were considered adjunctive to pharmacological mood stabilizer therapies. Careful definition of the scope of the guideline facilitates the transition from evidence tables to initial draft.

EVIDENCE DEFINITION

The delineation of evidence supporting treatment strategies is key to the development of a high-quality guideline. Evidence is derived from two sources—research studies and clinical consensus. Because of the importance of the supporting evidence, the details of the literature review—basic search strategy, sources used, criteria for selecting publications, review methods, and means of cataloging reported outcomes—are described explicitly for each guideline. Although evidence tables are created to aid the work group in writing the guideline, these tables generally are not included in the published guidelines. The APA process uses a coding system to describe the type of

evidence being cited (Table 48–4).

Advances in psychiatry's research database notwithstanding, many questions crucial for clinical decision-making must be answered by consensus of expert clinicians. Organizing this input and shaping its focus are major challenges in guideline development. A new tool, the practice research network (described in a later section), will eventually be able to provide some of the necessary answers in a generalizable and systematic manner.

DRAFT DEVELOPMENT

With evidence thus laid out, the work group, assisted by APA Office of Research staff, begins the arduous task of writing the guideline, integrating the data into clinical strategies. A *process document*, which contains many of the items discussed in this chapter, offers a starting point for understanding guideline development and serves as a resource document throughout the ensuing process (American Psychiatric Association 1996b).

DRAFT REVIEW

Guideline development is an iterative process in which multiple successive drafts are reviewed by a larger circle of

TABLE 48–4. American Psychiatric Association coding system for references

A. Randomized clinical trial: A study of an intervention in which subjects are followed prospectively over time, there are treatment and control groups, subjects are randomly assigned to the two groups, and both the subjects and the investigators are blind to the assignments

B. Clinical trial: A prospective study in which an intervention is made and the results of that intervention are tracked longitudinally; the study does not meet standards for a randomized clinical trial

C. Cohort or longitudinal study: A study in which subjects are followed prospectively over time without any specific intervention

D. Case-control study: A study in which a group of patients is identified in the present and information about them is pursued retrospectively or backward in time

E. Review with secondary data analysis: A structured analytic review of existing data (e.g., a meta-analysis or a decision analysis)

F. Review: A qualitative review and discussion of previously published literature without a quantitative synthesis of the data

G. Other: Textbooks, expert opinion, case reports, and other reports not included above

experts and clinicians. Whereas the first draft is reviewed by the approximately 20 members of the APA Steering Committee on Practice Guidelines, the third draft is reviewed by several hundred APA members, other experts, and representatives of other organizations. Reviewers include experts from other mental health disciplines, patient and patient advocate organizations, nonpsychiatric physicians, and other health care professionals. The completed guideline is approved by the APA Assembly, a representative body of approximately 200 individuals, and the APA Board of Trustees.

DISSEMINATION AND IMPLEMENTATION

The impact of a guideline clearly is influenced by the effectiveness with which the guideline is disseminated. Each APA guideline is published initially as a supplement to the *American Journal of Psychiatry* and subsequently by the American Psychiatric Press. Several studies (Asaph et al. 1991; Greco and Eisenberg 1993) concluded, however, that simply publishing guidelines does not change physician behaviors. In Ontario, Canada, Lomas and colleagues (1991) examined the impact of an obstetrical guideline on vaginal deliveries after cesarean delivery. A major objective of the guideline, which was endorsed strongly and disseminated widely by the Society of Obstetricians and Gynecologists of Canada, was to increase the frequency of a trial of vaginal delivery in women who had had a prior cesarean delivery. In selected "intervention hospitals," opinion leaders—recognized excellent clinicians highly regarded by their peers—organized special sessions to review and discuss the guideline and its implications. When the impact of the guideline was evaluated after 24 months, the researchers found no significant change in rates of trial of labor and vaginal births in the hospitals in which the physicians received feedback after the intervention—that is, the obstetricians' behavior was not influenced by the availability of the guideline. In the intervention hospitals, however, substantial change in the direction encouraged by the guideline was detected.

Another dissemination strategy of demonstrated effectiveness is to incorporate the guideline into teaching programs at all levels: medical student, resident, and continuing education. Questions concerning the APA guidelines are now included in the Psychiatric Residents in Training Examination (PRITE) examination, and the guidelines are the primary source material in the recertification process in geriatric psychiatry, conducted by the American Board of Psychiatry and Neurology. Furthermore, through the involvement of several hundred members in development of a guideline, the APA process

itself aids in dissemination. Of course, formal approval by the APA carries weight and increases the guideline's acceptance by APA members. In a survey of internists, Tunis et al. (1994) found that respondents similarly were more likely to accept guidelines developed by their professional associations than those developed by others, especially insurance companies.

Devising effective dissemination strategies will be an increasingly urgent and important task over the next several years. In 1996, the New York State Psychiatric Association, in collaboration with the APA, the RAND Corporation, the National Alliance for the Mentally Ill, and the National Depressive and Manic-Depressive Association (NDMDA), launched a study of the effectiveness of a "high-intensity" dissemination strategy of the APA major depressive disorder guideline. The approach involves the use of opinion leaders like those used in the study by Lomas et al. (1991). If this dissemination strategy is shown to be effective in New York State, similar approaches will be considered in other parts of the country and for other guidelines. Interactive computer programs and other dissemination strategies influenced by knowledge of how practicing psychiatrists learn will be studied as well.

Guidelines also are being incorporated into residency training programs as part of the basic readings in core psychopathology treatment seminars and as part of the clinical supervision process.

Although guidelines are developed primarily to assist clinicians, the utility of guidelines and the advantages of effective dissemination ought to be viewed with two other audiences in mind: policy makers and patients. Guidelines are a promising tool for educating policy makers that there exist specific treatments for specific psychiatric disorders and that substantial evidence documents the efficacy and effectiveness of these treatments. By addressing these poorly understood facts, guidelines may demythologize all too common perceptions and directly influence policy level discussions, including those regarding reimbursement. In addition, the process of developing guidelines makes information gaps apparent and thus lays out an agenda for research. In fact, a section of guidelines concerned with future research directions is specifically intended to suggest policy directions for research funding and development.

Guidelines also support the priority of providing patients and their families with information about treatment options. The ready availability of comprehensible information about the strategies and objectives of psychiatric treatment improves treatment compliance and strengthens the doctor-patient relationship. In collaboration with patient and patient advocacy organizations, the APA guideline project has begun to develop patient brochures that present the guidelines in considerable detail.

EVALUATION

An essential aspect of guideline development from a quality-improvement perspective, evaluation should contribute to improvements in the content of the guideline as well as the development process. Guidelines should be measured along four major parameters: reliability/validity, utilization, psychiatrist behaviors, and patient outcomes. Clearly, guidelines should accurately reflect the research literature and the existing clinical consensus. The process should be reliable, meaning that another group focusing on the same data and using a similar process should arrive at similar recommendations. Further, the recommendations must speak to the issues that clinicians need addressed. The material must be presented in a format that is useful to clinicians, and there must be included indications of the ease with which the guidelines may be incorporated into clinical practice. Evaluation must ascertain whether clinicians actually use the guidelines and, if the guidelines are not followed, what modifications might increase their use. When guidelines receive a high rate of use, clinicians' behaviors in the targeted areas of the recommendations are more likely to be influenced. Studies such as the New York State project described previously will help assess whether this objective is being met.

Because the ultimate purpose of guidelines is to improve patient care, evaluation of guidelines must eventually include measurement of patient outcomes. To that end, the AMA recently added the sixth attribute for effective guidelines (Table 48–1)—namely, that guideline development should include outcomes research, goals, and measures.

REVISION

The rapid expansion of psychiatry's knowledge base and the need to incorporate refinements indicated by the evaluation processes dictate the need for regular revisions of practice guidelines. The APA plans to revise guidelines at intervals no longer than 5 years. If there are insufficient data to warrant a revision of the entire guideline, a more focused revision will be done within 5 years and a complete revision within 10 years.

STRUCTURE AND CONTENT OF AMERICAN PSYCHIATRIC ASSOCIATION GUIDELINES

In the standardized format that the APA developed for its guidelines, the statement of intent that prefaces each guideline is followed by the eight sections listed in Table 48–5. Each section is discussed here.

I. Executive summary: This section provides an overview of the guideline, with major recommendations succinctly presented. The executive summary is not intended to stand by itself, and in the summary the reader is explicitly encouraged to consult the relevant portions of the guideline for more information concerning the recommendations. In this section and throughout the guideline, each recommendation is weighted by the following levels of endorsement:

1. Recommended with substantial clinical confidence: These recommendations are usually based on several well-controlled clinical trials that reported similar findings or featured key principles of clinical psychiatric care with broad expert consensus.
2. Recommended with moderate clinical confidence: These recommendations are usually based on a few studies with positive findings or on less consistent data from many sources.
3. Recommended with lower clinical confidence or recommended on a base of individual circumstances: These recommendations usually have not been adequately tested or are associated with conflicting reports concerning efficacy but are consistent with expert opinion and with accepted principles of treatment.

II. Disease definition, epidemiology, and natural history: This section begins with a brief discussion of diagnoses, using the current DSM criteria; differential diagnoses; and appropriate diagnostic procedures. Also included in this section is a limited review of epidemiologic data and aspects of the natural history of the disorder, with an emphasis on those issues having important treatment implications.

TABLE 48–5. American Psychiatric Association standard guideline sections

I. Executive summary
II. Disease definition, epidemiology, and natural history
III. Treatment principles and alternatives
IV. Formulation and implementation of a treatment plan
V. Clinical features influencing treatment
VI. Research directions
VII. Individuals and organizations that submitted comments
VIII. References

III. Treatment principles and alternatives: Specific treatment approaches are described within three broad categories: 1) psychiatric management, 2) psychosocial interventions, and 3) somatic interventions. The section synthesizes available data on the indications, safety, and efficacy of each approach. During the writing of the first six guidelines, the meaning of the term *psychiatric management* has evolved. The psychiatric management section addresses all clinical considerations that a well-trained psychiatrist would entertain for essentially every patient with a particular disorder, whatever the phase of illness. It includes, for example, approaches and techniques that may be included in the concept of "supportive psychotherapy." It includes aspects of the doctor-patient relationship and issues important in developing a therapeutic alliance. Recommendations for psychiatric management encompass three levels of specificity: 1) principles and techniques that are important for all physicians, 2) principles and techniques that are important for psychiatrists, and 3) principles and techniques that are important for psychiatrists treating all patients with the particular disorder.

With the practice guideline for bipolar disorder used as an example, the components of psychiatric management include 1) establishing and maintaining a therapeutic alliance, 2) monitoring the patient's psychiatric status, 3) providing education regarding bipolar disorder, 4) enhancing treatment compliance, 5) promoting regular patterns of activity and wakefulness, 6) promoting understanding of and adaptation to the psychosocial effects of bipolar disorder, 7) identifying new episodes early, and 8) reducing the morbidity and sequelae of bipolar disorder.

IV. Formulation and implementation of a treatment plan: This section assists the psychiatrist in making decisions concerning the individual "typical" patient. Whereas section III is organized around treatment strategy, the organizing principle in this section is the patient—and when pertinent information exists, the patient in a particular phase of the illness. In the bipolar disorder guideline, for example, section III describes numerous effective treatments and section IV delineates how to select from the broad array of effective treatments to meet the needs of a particular patient in each phase of illness (i.e., manic, depressive, maintenance). Figure 48–1 illustrates the interplay of patient characteristics and treatment factors that underlie identification of an appropriate treatment strategy and regimen for a given patient. For most treatments, only a few of the cells in this figure will contain useful data. Clinical judgment is required in many instances to fill in the other cells, in order to make appropriate clinical decisions.

V. Clinical features influencing treatment: This section addresses psychiatric, general medical, and demographic and other psychosocial variables (e.g., ethnicity, cross-cultural issues, gender, age, socioeconomic issues) that modify the treatment recommendations discussed in section IV and thus may be relevant to formulation of a treatment plan. Comorbidities are considered in this section. A large percentage of patients have more than one illness (Kessler et al. 1994). This reality presents a major challenge in writing guidelines that are relevant and specific for patients with multiple disorders. In the APA guidelines, the only aspects of the comorbid disorder that are considered are those having specific treatment implications for the patient with the disorder being addressed by the guideline. For further details about the treatment of the comorbid psychiatric disorder, the reader is referred to the appropriate guideline for that disorder.

VI. Research directions: An important benefit of developing practice guidelines is the identification of gaps in the database that impede the formulation of clear and specific treatment recommendations. In terms of the APA process, a goal is to be able to describe more level 1 (i.e., "substantial clinical confidence") recommendations. In this section of the guideline, the research that is necessary to achieve this goal is identified. An intent is that this information will influence policy decisions concerning research funding and priorities.

VII. Individuals and organization that submitted comments: This section lists the typically large number of individuals and organizations who reviewed, commented on, and provided specific recommendations on drafts of a guideline.

VIII. References: A particular value of the extensive reference section of each guideline is annotation of each citation by the coding designation described earlier.

Adhering to the principles and format discussed here, the APA has approved and published (through 1998) nine guidelines (American Psychiatric Association 1993a, 1993b, 1994b, 1995a, 1995b, 1996a, 1997a, 1997b, 1998). Four guidelines are now under development (Table 48–6).

Patient Factors	TREATMENT FACTORS				
	Type	Dose	Frequency	Duration	Combinations
Age					
Gender					
Setting					
Ethnicity					
Comorbidities					
Severity					

FIGURE 48–1.   Factors in clinical decision making.

NATIONAL AND INTERNATIONAL COLLABORATION

In addition to the work with the AMA that focuses especially on process issues in guideline development, the APA also collaborates with others on content issues. The American Academy of Child and Adolescent Psychiatry (AACAP) has published a number of guidelines since 1991. The leaders of the APA and the AACAP projects work closely together to avoid duplication and to support each other's efforts. The Royal College of Psychiatrists in Australia and New Zealand published its first practice guidelines in psychiatry in 1981, and many other countries are developing evidence-based guidelines. The APA has established dialogue with several of these countries to promote collaborative efforts on guideline development. For example, the Royal College of Psychiatrists in the United Kingdom, after extensive consultation, has initiated a practice guidelines program in large part modeled on that of the APA.

PRACTICE RESEARCH NETWORK

The evolution and elaboration of the practice guideline project have underscored the existence of a number of limitations in psychiatry's existing database.

■ Major gaps persist in the research data regarding many key clinical issues facing psychiatrists. For example, in the case of a patient with major depressive disorder for whom an antidepressant appears warranted but who does not respond to the first antidepressant prescribed, no systematic data are available to help the clinician select a second antidepressant.

■ Questions about the generalizability of the research data that do exist are common. Of particular interest is the similarity or dissimilarity of those patients who are seen in most psychiatrists' daily practices and patients who are subjects in traditional research protocols. Most randomized clinical trials are conducted in tertiary care centers with rarefied patient referral

TABLE 48–6. American Psychiatric Association practice guidelines completed or in development: topics

Eating disorders

Major depressive disorder

Bipolar disorder

Substance use disorders

Psychiatric evaluation

Nicotine dependence

Schizophrenia

Alzheimer's disease

Panic disorder

Delirium

Geriatric care

Borderline personality

HIV/AIDS

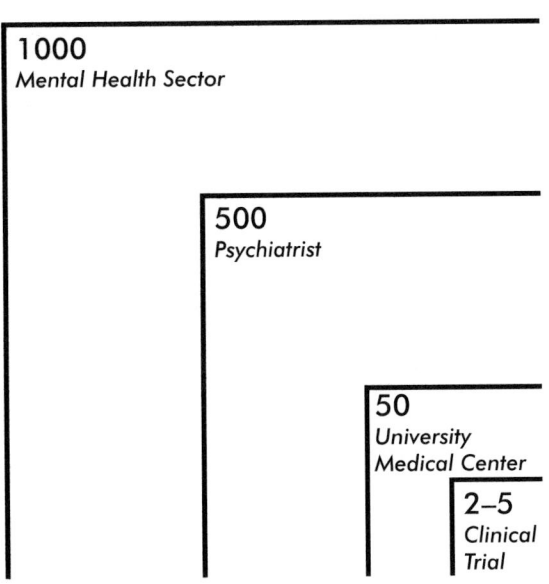

FIGURE 48–2. Ecology of mental health care.
Source. Adapted from White et al. 1961.

patterns. Figure 48–2 illustrates part of the problem. For every 1,000 patients seen in the mental health sector, it is estimated that fewer than 50 would be seen in a university medical center and only a small percentage of this group would be eligible to participate in a clinical trial. A single exclusion criterion of absence of comorbid psychiatric disorders (which is very common in most randomized clinical trials) by itself eliminates a large number of patients.

■ There is no mechanism to assess clinical experience systematically. Although the practice guidelines process incorporates broad clinical input throughout the development of drafts, there is no assurance that this input accurately and objectively represents the full range of clinical experience.

When evidence-based guidelines first were being developed, the recognition of these and other gaps in the knowledge base prompted an exploration of how the needed information could be captured. At the same time, there was also a growing recognition of the potential usefulness of a national research and monitoring system that would help inform major policy debates about health care services, including issues of access and reimbursement.

A practice research network (PRN) offers a means of meeting both objectives. A PRN is a group of practicing clinicians who cooperate to collect data and to conduct research studies on a variety of clinical and service delivery issues. In the United States, more than two dozen networks were formed by the early 1990s to study the patterns and outcomes of primary care in the community and to assess these findings in light of those derived from academic, ter-

tiary care research settings (Niebauer and Nutting 1994). Among the largest and most active practice-based networks in the United States are the Pediatric Research in Office Settings (PROS) network, developed in 1986 by the American Academy of Pediatrics (Wasserman et al. 1992), and the Ambulatory Sentinel Practice Network (ASPN), developed in 1981 by the American Academy of Family Physicians and the University of Colorado (Green et al. 1984) At this writing in 1998, ASPN had 838 national members, and approximately 1,500 pediatricians in 500 practices make up the PROS network.

In 1993, the APA established a national practice-based research network of psychiatrists, who collaborate to collect data and conduct clinical and health services research. This PRN serves as a "national psychiatric research laboratory." Its aim is to strengthen and expand the clinical services and health services research base in psychiatry in a manner that has direct bearing on the improvement of psychiatric treatments and outcomes of care for persons with mental disorders (Zarin et al. 1997).

One of the primary goals of this initiative is to bridge the gap between current clinical research and the practical needs of clinicians and patients (Zarin et al. 1993). Because of the network's "observational" or "naturalistic" research design, the effectiveness of psychiatric treatments provided in routine practice are assessed, rather than the efficacy of treatments under optimal circumstances. The network is designed to collect ongoing data regarding clinical status, treatments provided, and outcomes (Davies et al. 1994).

By the end of 1998, the APA's PRN will include 750 APA members representative of American psychiatry and the range of public and private psychiatric treatment settings. Members must spend at least 15 hours per week providing direct face-to-face care; this requirement that ensures that PRN members are substantially engaged in treating patients. Once fully established, the network will involve 1,000 members and will provide a nationally representative sample of psychiatrists, settings, patients, and treatments to yield statistically significant subsamples for many areas of interest.

CONCLUSIONS

The practice guideline project promotes the development of and enhances the dissemination and practice of evidence-based psychiatry. By contributing to the scientific information database for the revision of DSM-IV (American Psychiatric Association 1994a) and for new and revised practice guidelines, the PRN is helping bridge gaps in the current clinical and health services research base in psychiatry. Both the APA's PRN and practice guidelines projects provide clinically useful and generalizable information that physicians will need to practice medicine in the twenty-first century.

REFERENCES

American Medical Association: Board of Trustees Report 39—A97: American Medical Accreditation Program. Chicago, IL, American Medical Association, 1997

American Psychiatric Association: Diagnostic and Statistical Manual of Mental Disorders, 3rd Edition. Washington, DC, American Psychiatric Association, 1980

American Psychiatric Association: Benzodiazepine: Dependence, Toxicity, and Abuse: A Task Force Report of the American Psychiatric Association. Washington, DC, American Psychiatric Association, 1990

American Psychiatric Association: Practice guideline for eating disorders. Am J Psychiatry 150(2):212–228, 1993a

American Psychiatric Association: Practice guideline for major depressive disorder in adults. Am J Psychiatry 150(4):1–26, 1993b

American Psychiatric Association: Diagnostic and Statistical Manual of Mental Disorders, 4th Edition. Washington, DC, American Psychiatric Association, 1994a

American Psychiatric Association: Practice guideline for the treatment of patients with bipolar disorder. Am J Psychiatry 151(12, suppl):1–36, 1994b

American Psychiatric Association: Practice guideline for the psychiatric evaluation of adults. Am J Psychiatry 152(11, suppl):67–80, 1995a

American Psychiatric Association: Practice guideline for the treatment of patients with substance use disorder, alcohol, cocaine, opioids. Am J Psychiatry 152(11, suppl):1–55, 1995b

American Psychiatric Association: Practice guideline for the treatment of patients with nicotine dependence. Am J Psychiatry 153(10, suppl):1–31, 1996a

American Psychiatric Association: Practice Guidelines. Washington, DC, American Psychiatric Association, 1996b

American Psychiatric Association: Practice guideline for the treatment of patients with Alzheimer's disease and other dementias of late life. Am J Psychiatry 154(5, suppl):1–39, 1997a

American Psychiatric Association: Practice guideline for the treatment of patients with schizophrenia. Am J Psychiatry 154(4, suppl):1–63, 1997b

American Psychiatric Association: Practice guideline for the treatment of patients with panic disorder. Am J Psychiatry 155(5, suppl): 1–34, 1998

Asaph JW, Janoff K, Wayson K, et al: Carotid endarterectomy in a community hospital: a change in physicians' practice patterns. Am J Surg 161:616–618, 1991

Chassin M, Brook R, Park R, et al: Variations in the use of medical and surgical services by the Medicare population. N Engl J Med 314:285–290, 1986

Davies AE, Doyle MA, Lansky D, et al: Outcomes assessment in clinical settings: a consensus statement on principles and best practices in project management. Journal of Quality Improvement 20:6–16, 1994

Eddy DM: Clinical decision making: from theory to practice. Practice policies—what are they? JAMA 263:877–878, 1990

Greco PJ, Eisenberg JM: Changing physician practices. N Engl J Med 329:1271–1273, 1993

Green LA, Wood M, Becker LA, et al: The Ambulatory Sentinel Practice Network: purpose, methods, and policies. J Fam Pract 18:275–280, 1984

Holzer JF: The advent of clinical standards for professional liability. Quality Review Bulletin 16:71–79, 1990

Hyams AL, Brandenberg BA, Lipsitz SR, et al: Practice guidelines and malpractice litigation: a two-way street. Ann Intern Med 122:450–455, 1995

Institute of Medicine: Guidelines for Clinical Practice From Development to Use. Edited by Field MJ, Lohr KN. Washington, DC, National Academy Press, 1992

Kessler RC, McGonagle KA, Zhao S, et al: Lifetime and 12-month prevalence of DSM-III-R psychiatric disorders in the United States. Results from the National Comorbidity Survey. Arch Gen Psychiatry 51:8–19, 1994

Legislated clinical medicine (editorial). Lancet 335:1004–1006, 1990

Lewis CE: Variations in the incidence of surgery. N Engl J Med 1969:281:880–885

Lomas J, Enkin M, Anderson GM, et al: Opinion leaders vs audit and feedback to implement practice guidelines. Delivery after previous cesarean section. JAMA 265:2202–2207, 1991

McIntyre J, Talbott J: Developing practice parameters. Hosp Community Psychiatry 41:1103–1105, 1990

Niebauer LJ, Nutting PA: Primary care practice-based research networks active in North America. J Fam Pract 38:425–426, 1994

OB-GYN premiums decrease drastically. American Medical Association News, February 2, 1993, p 31

Office of Quality Assurance: Attributes to Grade the Development of Practice Parameters. Chicago, IL, American Medical Association, 1996

Standing Committee (APA): Report on the Construction of Hospitals for the Insane. American Journal of Insanity 8:79–81, 1851

Standing Committee (APA): Report on the Organization of Hospitals for the Insane. American Journal of Insanity 10:67–69, 1853

Task Force on the Use of Laboratory Tests in Psychiatry: Tricyclic antidepressants—blood level measurements and clinical outcome: an APA Task Force report. Am J Psychiatry 142:155–162, 1985

Tunis SR, Hayward RS, Wilson MC, et al: Internists' attitudes about clinical practice guidelines. Ann Intern Med 120:956–963, 1994

Wasserman RC, Croft CA, Brotherton SE: Preschool vision screening in pediatric practice: a study from the Pediatric Research in Office Settings (PROS) Network. Pediatrics 89:834–838, 1992

White KL, Williams TF, Greenberg BG: The ecology of medical care. N Engl J Med 265:885–892, 1961

Zarin DA, Pincus HA, McIntyre JS: Practice guidelines (editorial). Am J Psychiatry 150:175–177, 1993

Zarin DA, Pincus HA, West JC, et al: Practice-based research in psychiatry. Am J Psychiatry 154:1199–1208, 1997

CHAPTER 49

CLINICAL NEUROPSYCHIATRY

JEFFREY L. CUMMINGS, M.D.

MICHAEL R. TRIMBLE, M.D., F.R.C.P., F.R.C.PSYCH.

ROBERT E. HALES, M.D., M.B.A.

Neuropsychiatry and behavioral neurology are clinical disciplines devoted to understanding and treating behavioral disturbances associated with brain dysfunction. Detection and characterization of brain disorders require a careful clinical assessment as well as application of selected neurodiagnostic procedures. In this chapter, clinical examination as well as neuropsychological testing, laboratory tests, electrophysiological techniques, and brain imaging are discussed. Four main categories of neuropsychiatric disorders are presented: epilepsy and limbic system disorders, movement disorders, stroke and brain tumors, and head injury. The reader is referred to more comprehensive textbooks of neuropsychiatry listed at the end of the chapter and to the recently published *Concise Guide to Neuropsychiatry* (Cummings and Trimble 1996), on which the material in this chapter is based.

NEUROPSYCHIATRIC ASSESSMENT

DEFINITIONS

Symptoms are the complaints of the patient that are reported spontaneously or determined through the taking of the clinical history. *Signs* are observed by the physician, the patient, or the patient's friends or relatives and indicate the presence of abnormal functioning of one or more body systems. A *syndrome* is a constellation of signs and symptoms that coalesce to form a recognizable entity with defining characteristics. Syndromes may be classified, and they are the clinical manifestations of illness. *Illness* is what brings the patient clinical attention and is typically the expression of disease. However, the presentation of an illness depends on many factors, including environmental and personality variables.

CLINICAL EXAMINATION

Initial Observations

In a clinical examination, the physician should observe first and then listen and examine. The patient's dress may reveal the eccentricity caused by frontal lobe dysfunction or the flamboyance brought on by mania or may hint at the dishevelment associated with schizophrenia or dementia. Eye contact might not be maintained. The posture may be the flexed position of the depressed or parkinsonian patient or the stilted stance of a person with schizophrenia.

Disturbances of motor activity may aid diagnosis. In catatonia, muscle tone is high, leading to resistance, and in flexibilitas cerea ("waxy flexibility"), limbs and postures can be maintained for hours at a time. *Gegenhalten* is the passive resistance to movement of a limb that increases in direct relation to the force applied by the examiner.

The gait may suggest an extrapyramidal disorder. For example, smaller steps and poverty of accessory movements are observed in parkinsonism. Akinesia, with poverty of movement, is seen in patients treated with conventional antipsychotic medications. The patient with akathisia may not be able to sit for longer than a few minutes, whereas the patient with agitation paces, rummages, and has outbursts. Mannerisms (exaggerated components of the usual behavioral repertoire), stereotypies (repeated complex sequences of purposeless movement), and choreoathetoid writhing may be noted. Mannerisms and stereotypies are common in schizophrenia; choreoathetoid writhing occurs in several extrapyramidal conditions. Tics (frequent stereotyped repetitive movements) may suggest Tourette's syndrome. Vocal tics and excessive sniffing or clearing of the throat are also characteristic of this disorder. The mouth may writhe, as in tardive dyskinesia, or assume more sustained abnormal forms, as in a dystonia. The lips may exhibit the lesions of vitamin deficiency, the scars of self-mutilation, or the dryness of anxiety.

The hands may tremble in cases of anxiety or extrapyramidal disease. The physician should look for evidence of muscle wasting (loss of muscle bulk generally or in specific areas). The patient's fingers may show evidence of nicotine addiction, and bitten nails may suggest an anxiety disorder. On shaking the patient's hand, the clinician may detect the clammy sweat of anxiety or the tremor of an underlying extrapyramidal tremor. Handshaking also provides the opportunity to test for a grasp reflex. Lefthandedness should be noted; it may suggest atypical cerebral organization.

The patient's speech should be studied for form and content. The slowing of speech in cases of depression contrasts with the pressured overactivity of mania. Dysarthria, due to impairment of the neuromuscular mechanisms of speech, may hint at intoxication or pyramidal or cerebellar damage. A stammer may occur in congenital syndromes or be due to anxiety; paraphasias and neologisms may indicate aphasia or schizophrenia. Attention and concentration, the ability to maintain a stream of thought, and the ability to converse coherently should be noted. Prosody, the melodic intonation of speech, may be lost in cases of schizophrenia or after development of right-hemisphere and subcortical lesions.

Formal thought disorder—disorganization and concretization of thought processes—is suggestive of either schizophrenia or a neurological disease with schizophrenia-like manifestations. Slowing of the train of thought is seen with the psychomotor slowing of depression and with the bradyphrenia of many neurological disorders, such as head injury, Parkinson's disease, epilepsy, and multiple sclerosis. Viscosity is exhibited by some patients with epilepsy; such patients engage in sticky interpersonal interactions. *Circumstantiality* refers to a persistent tendency to wander slowly over the irrelevant details of a subject before reaching a final conclusion.

Delusions are unshakable beliefs that are manifestly incorrect, even when the patient's cultural surrounding is taken into account. Autochthonous delusions arise suddenly, fully formed and spontaneously. They are bizarre and nearly always signify schizophrenia. *Hallucinations* are percepts without objects, and *illusions* are abnormal distortions of sensory stimuli.

Hyperesthesia, especially acoustic hyperesthesia, is not uncommon in anxious patients; hypoesthesia is frequent in depression. Anesthesia, along with anesthetic patches or hemianesthesia, may be seen in patients with hysteria (conversion disorder), peripheral neuropathy, or syphilis.

Conditions in which the perceived size of objects is altered, such as micropsia and macropsia, may suggest ophthalmological disease, epilepsy, or migraine. *Derealization* and *depersonalization*, in which the world and the patients themselves, respectively, feel different, unreal, empty, or two-dimensional, are noted in a variety of conditions but particularly in anxiety disorders (depersonalization disorder and panic disorder), in migraine, and as an aura in temporal lobe epilepsy. In *déjà vu* experiences, patients feel that everything they are experiencing has happened before. *Jamais vu* is the opposite, an abnormal feeling of unfamiliarity. These memory distortions occur in temporal lobe epilepsy.

Careful attention should be paid to the patient's mood and to whether delusions are congruent or incongruent to the mood state. Mood-incongruent delusions are more frequently associated with schizophrenia. Apathy is common after cerebral damage, and it is seen in a wide range of neuropsychiatric disorders. *Emotional lability* is noted when the patient is unable to control his or her emotional expressions, laughing at the hint of a joke or crying at the hint of sadness. *Pseudobulbar palsy* is a common form of affective lability. This condition is contrasted with the empty euphoria of patients with multiple sclerosis and the meaningless, playful *witzelsucht* of frontal lobe dysfunction. Inappropriate affect is more characteristic of schizophrenia.

Whenever possible, another person who knows the patient should be interviewed to confirm the accuracy of the patient's account of his or her illness. Family history should always be sought, and any potential genetic diseases should be noted. A review of early upbringing may reveal earlier behavior problems relevant to the clinical presentation. These problems include sleepwalking, enuresis, stammering, tics, phobias, and hyperactivity. Inquiries should be made concerning developmental delay, especially with regard to motor development, speaking, and language. Attention-deficit/hyperactivity disorder, conduct disorder, oppositional defiant disorder, and autistic behavior should be noted.

Insight into the patient's illness should be noted. The clinician should observe whether the patient displays awareness of his or her abnormalities or depends on family members to report details.

Mental Status Testing

Although formal testing is done in the laboratory, clinical mental status testing can be valuable, and in many patients it is an essential part of the initial screening. This clinical testing is outlined in Table 49–1. These tests should be done routinely, but any suspicion of cognitive dysfunction may be better defined by more formal neuropsychological testing. It is necessary to specify the kind of deficit anticipated; for example, the clinician might ask that frontal lobe function be carefully assessed. Selected laboratory, imaging, and electrophysiological tests (described later in this chapter) may be required to establish a specific diagnosis.

Patients with confusional states cannot be reliably tested, but the degree, content, and variability of their mental state must be noted. Patients with typical *delirium* seem confused and are disoriented for time and possibly also for place. Simple mental arithmetic is poorly performed, and memory is unreliable. Hallucinations are predominantly visual, complex, and silent. Delusions are often paranoid. Typically, the severity of the symptoms fluctuates with time.

Attention can be tested by repetition of digits or by the serial 7s (or serial 3s) subtraction test. Attention for longer periods *(vigilance)* is tested by reading to the patient a series of letters and asking him or her to tap every time a certain letter is heard.

Memory is tested clinically by assessing recall of three or four items given by the examiner or recall of items from a short story (standardized stories are available). Nonverbal learning can be tested by asking the patient to reproduce simple figures drawn earlier in the examination as part of testing of constructions. Items of general knowledge

TABLE 49–1. Bedside mental status testing

Assess level of consciousness

Observe and assess orientation for time, place, and person

Assess attention and vigilance

   Digit repetition

   Serial 7 subtraction

   Digit reversal

   Days or months in reverse order

Test verbal output

   Rate, rhythm, syntax, and semantics

   Speech errors

Ask patient to point to objects in the environment named by the examiner

Ask patient to perform simple commands

Ask patient to name objects, body parts, and colors

Ask patient to

   Read a passage of simple text (e.g., from a newspaper); test comprehension

   Write his or her name and a short paragraph on a subject of interest to him or her

Test memory ability

   Ask patient to repeat the Babcock sentence ("The one thing a nation needs in order to be rich and great is a large secure supply of wood" or "The clouds hung low in the valley and the wind howled among the trees as the men went on through the rain")

   Ask patient to repeat a story

   Ask patient to remember four words

   Test general knowledge for recent events

   Test knowledge for remote events

Test for constructional ability

   Ask patient to copy circle, cross, and cube and to draw a clock

Test for ideomotor and ideational apraxia

   Ask patient to perform tasks on command: to complete complex sequence of actions

Test executive function

   Verbal fluency: number of animals named in 1 minute or number of words that begin with a certain letter in 1 minute

   Perseveration: fist-palm-side test

Test for right-left disorientation

Test calculation

Test proverb interpretation

Test understanding of similarities

Retest memory: ask patient to recall items of earlier memory tests

Test cognitive estimates

should be tested, relevant to the patient's cultural and intellectual background. The ability accurately to recall events from the more distant past *(remote memory)* should also be tested. Questions about general knowledge of news items and famous people or events should be asked.

Anosognosia, denial of hemiparesis, most commonly accompanies right-hemisphere disease. *Finger agnosia* is the inability to recognize different fingers, either the patient's own or those of the examiner. *Autotopagnosia* is similar to finger agnosia except that it involves any body part. Finger agnosia, right-left disorientation, acalculia, and agraphia (Gerstmann's syndrome) indicate a left-hemisphere lesion.

Tests of constructional ability require the patient to draw a familiar object, such as a clock or a house. Poor performance, especially in the form of small or disorganized reproductions, suggest cerebral disease. *Neglect* of one-half of the drawing is seen with contralateral-hemisphere lesions. Neglect is more common and more severe with right-hemisphere lesions.

Neurological Examination

All patients should undergo a neurological examination. A screening examination for neurological disease is described in Table 49–2. This brief examination takes 10 minutes; if abnormalities are revealed, more detailed testing is needed.

Formal Tests of Neuropsychological Function

Formal tests of neuropsychological function are listed in Table 49–3.

LABORATORY EXAMINATION

Metabolic and Biochemical Investigations

The following measurements, counts, and tests are commonly performed when patients present with neurological signs or symptoms whose etiology is unclear:

- Hemoglobin, red blood cell count, and related indices (hematocrit, mean corpuscular volume [MCV], and mean corpuscular hemoglobin concentration [MCHC])
- White cell and platelet counts
- Sedimentation rate
- Serum electrolytes
- Tests of liver function (alanine aminotransferase [ALT], alkaline phosphatase, aspartate aminotransferase [AST])
- Tests of renal function (blood urea nitrogen [BUN], creatinine)

TABLE 49–2. Brief neurological screening examination

Stance and gait
    Observe walking and turning
    Ask patient to balance with feet together and eyes closed (Romberg's test)

Cranial nerves[a]
    Check ability to smell (especially in head trauma) (I)
    Check visual fields by quadrant (II)
    Examine fundus (II)
    Visual pursuit (III, IV, VI) (patient follows the examiner's finger in horizontal and vertical directions)
    Bulk of temporalis and masseter muscles (V) (patient opens jaw against force; muscle bulk on tight bite)
    Observe grimace of patient showing teeth (VII)
    Rub finger and thumb an inch from the patient's ears and check for deafness (VIII)
    Observe palate; ask patient to say "ah" (IX, X)
    Ask patient to push chin against the examiner's hand and test bulk of sternocleidomastoids (XI)
    Observe tongue for abnormal movements or deviation on protrusion (XII)

Motor system
    Test tone, power, and reflexes, and note muscle bulk (test in all four limbs)
        Tone: patient holds arms out, palms down; observe any wrist drop; rotate leg at knee and note foot movements
        Power: patient holds arms out, palms down, and is asked to "play the piano"; with patient's palms up, watch for any flexion, pronation, or drift; ask patient to elevate legs from couch and then see whether they can be maintained in the air against examiner's pressure; patient taps floor rapidly with soles of the feet
        Reflexes: muscle stretch (biceps, triceps, supinator, knee, ankle); pathological (plantar [Babinski sign])
    Coordination
        Finger-nose test
        Rapid movements (patient taps quickly the back of one hand with the palm of the other)
    Sensory testing
        Stroke skin on representative parts of the body, especially distal extremities
    Other reflexes
        Palmomental (draw a stick across the palm from the thenar eminence and watch for a reflex contraction of the ipsilateral mentalis muscle; the skin puckers)
        Grasp (stroke the patient's palm, firmly moving outward)
        Jaw jerk
        Snout and pout reflexes (tap lips)

[a]Numeral in parentheses refers to the cranial nerve tested.

TABLE 49-3. **Some formal neuropsychological tests**

Wechsler Adult Intelligence Scale (WAIS)—11 subtests, widely used to assess IQ

Halstead-Reitan Neuropsychological Test Battery— developed to detect structural lesions

Nelson Adult Reading Test (NART)—used to determine premorbid IQ

Wechsler Memory Scale—tests various components of memory

Progressive Matrices—a test of nonverbal intelligence, useful for those with language problems

Trail Making Test—patient connects ascending numbers (1, 2, etc.) and letters (a, b, etc.), then numbers alternating with letters (1-a, 2-b, etc.)

Wisconsin Card Sorting Test—tests patient's ability to infer rules and shift sets

- Thyroid-stimulating hormone (TSH)
- Blood glucose (if abnormal, glucose tolerance test is performed)

The following measurements and tests are done in selected cases:

- Vitamin B_{12}
- Iron and total iron–binding capacity
- Creatinine clearance test
- Calcium and phosphorus estimations
- Drug screen (for illicit drugs)
- Syphilis serology (Venereal Disease Research Laboratory [VDRL] or fluorescent treponemal antibody absorption [FTA-ABS])
- Human immunodeficiency virus (HIV) serology and T_4 cell counts or T_4-to-T_8 ratio
- Prolactin (increased by neuroleptics; increased transiently by seizures)
- Cholesterol and fatty acids
- Heavy metal screen

The following measurements and tests are performed in association with specific diagnoses:

- Alcoholism: red cell transketolase, serum γ-glutamyltransferase (SGGT), serum alcohol
- Systemic lupus erythematosus: lupus erythematosus cells and serum antinuclear or anti-DNA antibodies, antiphospholipid antibodies
- Fatigue: Paul-Bunnell test (test for infectious mononucleosis), brucellosis and borreliosis antibody titers
- Polydipsia: plasma and urine osmolality

- Porphyria: urinary or fecal porphyrins
- Movement disorders: serum copper and ceruloplasmin
- Muscle weakness: serum creatine kinase

Lumbar puncture is performed to diagnose central nervous system infections such as cerebral syphilis, to facilitate differential diagnosis in some cases of dementia, and to diagnose multiple sclerosis (cerebrospinal fluid is examined for the presence of oligoclonal bands).

Electroencephalography

The first electroencephalogram (EEG) recorded in humans was performed by the psychiatrist Hans Berger in 1929. The electroencephalographic signal is created by the average of electrical currents from the surface dendrites of neurons.

The international 10–20 system of electrode placement allows coverage of only 20% of the cortical surface. Additional electrodes, in the following placements, may improve the detection of abnormalities and may be useful in selected clinical circumstances:

- Sphenoidal (in the region of the foramen ovale)
- Nasopharyngeal (in the nasopharynx at the base of the skull)
- Intracranial (subdural or intracerebral)

Activation procedures facilitate detection of abnormal rhythms. These procedures include hyperventilation, photic stimulation, sleep induction or deprivation, and, occasionally, administration of drugs (e.g., pentylenetetrazol).

Waveforms. There are four main types of waveforms:

- Beta: faster than 13 cycles per second (cps); increased by many psychotropic drugs, especially sedatives and hypnotics
- Alpha: 8–13 cps, maximal occipitally, blocked by eye opening
- Theta: 4–7 cps
- Delta: slower than 4 cps, in the alert state often a sign of pathology

These waveforms are influenced by genetics, age, sleep, drugs, and disease. Theta and delta waves are more common in the very young. Orthodox (non–rapid eye movement [REM]) or slow-wave sleep is dominated by slow rhythms. Paradoxical (REM) sleep is characterized by fast desynchronized activity—similar to that shown in the waking recording, but the patient is asleep—and muscle activity is diminished.

During the night, there are usually six periods of REM sleep, lasting up to 30 minutes each and spaced about 40–60 minutes apart; these periods account for approximately 20%–25% of total sleep time. The first REM period has its onset after about 40 minutes (the REM latency). This period may be altered in disease states; for example, depressed patients have a short REM latency. Dreaming typically occurs during REM sleep.

The EEG plays an important role in the workup of patients with epilepsy and those who present with paroxysmal behavioral disorders. Recordings during the period of the ictus are of most value. The EEG is helpful in diagnosing tumors, some types of dementia (particularly Creutzfeldt-Jakob disease), and delirium.

Evoked potentials. The technique of evoked potentials allows the very small potentials generated by a stimulus to be exaggerated and studied. The responses generated by many similar stimuli are averaged, and the signal-to-noise ratio is thus enhanced. The waveform is derived from computer analysis of the data; a series of positive and negative waves is detected. The latency (interval between stimulus and response) of these waves is one index used to indicate pathology. Usually, visual, auditory, or somatosensory evoked potentials are recorded.

Potentials also can be evoked by endogenous events, including the contingent negative variation (CNV or expectancy wave), the P300 wave, and premotor potentials such as the Bereitschaftspotential. The CNV arises out of anticipation of an expected response. It is a slow negative shift in the vertex and frontal regions. The P300 wave is thought to relate to a process of cognitive appraisal of a stimulus.

Other electroencephalographic techniques. *Ambulatory monitoring* involves placing electrodes on the head (or heart), signals from which are continuously recorded onto a small cassette recorder that the patient carries. The patient can walk around wearing this recorder, and recordings can be made over several days, for example, while the patient is at home. In *videotelemetry*, a picture of the patient's behavior is recorded simultaneously with the EEG, and both are replayed simultaneously on a television screen. The behavior and the EEG can be directly compared.

Computerized electroencephalographic mapping produces topographical images of the brain's electrical activity by means of computerized analysis of the electroencephalographic waveforms or evoked potentials.

Magnetoencephalography

Magnetoencephalography involves the detection of magnetic source fields in the brain. Because magnetic signals are not interfered with by the skull, magnetoencephalography provides better spatial resolution and detection of fields beneath the surface than does electroencephalography.

Brain Imaging

Skull X rays. Skull X rays are of little value when other imaging techniques are available. They may reveal skull fractures following trauma.

Computed tomography. Computed tomography (CT) provides a computerized image of brain structure. It is essential that a structural image of the brain be obtained in any case of suspected focal cerebral lesion. CT also aids in the evaluation of many conditions (e.g., dementia) in which more diffuse pathology is expected.

In CT, X rays are projected through the brain in many directions around the patient's head. Those X rays interacting with intrinsic brain electrons are captured or scattered and do not reach the detectors; the number detected depends on the tissue density. The result is a matrix display of brain density, represented as squares that reflect the average density of the tissue lying within the imaged area. The square is the *pixel*; the volume of tissue represented is the *voxel*.

The partial volume effect is an important source of error. If a voxel contains an admixture of tissue and air or tissue and bone, the average result may suggest pathology where none is present.

Contrast media are administered that are efficient at electron capture, delete X rays, and enhance the image of pathological tissue.

CT remains the examination tool of first choice in many centers, especially where magnetic resonance imaging (MRI) is unavailable. A CT scan should always be requested if there is any suspicion of intracranial pathology.

Magnetic resonance imaging. The principle of MRI is examination of the physicochemical environment of the brain's protons.

An object (a proton) with a charge and velocity provokes a magnetic field adjacent to it. Because a proton spins around its axis at random, the sum total of magnetization in an area of the brain is zero. On application of an external magnetic field, the particles and their charges align, like the compass needle of a small compass in the earth's magnetic field.

The aligned protons can now be excited by the momentary application of a radio signal at their specific frequency, a process that can be likened to a tuning fork's provoking resonation in a guitar string tuned to it. When the signal is turned off, a signal is returned (in the analogy, the guitar string continues to resonate) and can be detected and analyzed. Thus, after the application of the radiofrequency pulse, the magnetization returns exponentially to its preexcitement level: the relaxation. This process is defined by two time constants known as T_1 and T_2. A T_1-weighted image is referred to as the *inversion recovery image*. The T_2-weighted image is referred to as the *spin-spin relaxation time image*. A variant image is the *spin echo image*.

Each tissue has specific T_1 and T_2 values. In the brain, the measured proton behavior relates to the hydrogen nucleus, most commonly water. Heightened contrast between these tissues is achieved by exploiting relaxation times of different tissues. The derived image has a high spatial resolution (in some machines, 1.5 mm). Most pathological tissues increase the length of T_1 and T_2. On T_1-weighted images, this lengthening is darker; on T_2-weighted images, the lengthening is lighter.

The advantages and disadvantages of MRI are shown in Table 49–4.

Magnetic resonance spectroscopy (MRS) involves quantitation of the physicochemical spectra that are derived through MRI. The main techniques are phosphorus-31 MRS, which yields information about membrane phospholipid and high-energy phosphate metabolism, and hydrogen-1 (proton) MRS, with a broader spectrum encompassing choline and some amino acids, including neurotransmitters such as glutamate and γ-aminobutyric

acid (GABA). Different disease states produce different chemical changes in the brain that may be detected by MRS.

More modern techniques allow good quantitation of neuronal structures—for example, accurate assessment of hippocampal volumes. It is also possible to capture functional images, using functional or echoplanar MRI. This technique relies on the principle that active neurons convert more hemoglobin to oxyhemoglobin, increasing the relaxation time (T_2); determination of this ratio over two closely related periods provides an assessment of blood flow.

Single photon emission computed tomography and positron-emission tomography. In contrast to the imaging methods previously discussed, which (apart from newer MRI techniques) assess brain structure, single photon emission computed tomography (SPECT) and positron-emission tomography (PET) assess brain function.

Cerebral blood flow (CBF) and metabolism are normally closely linked; therefore, assessment of CBF may provide an indirect measure of neuronal activity. In SPECT, a patient is given a dose of a radioactive tracer that specifically interacts with brain tissue. Commonly used is technetium Tc 99m hexamethyl propylenamine oxime (HMPAO), which is taken up by tissue and then trapped. Radiation is detected by rotating gamma cameras, and, by a process of back-projection and tomographic reconstruction, an image of blood flow is obtained.

PET is primarily a research tool. Radioactive isotopes are created by a cyclotron. Each of these isotopes essentially is a compound that gains a proton, which becomes unstable. In tissue, the proton unites with an electron, and the two particles convert their mass into radiation energy. The particles annihilate, releasing two coincident gamma rays at 180° to each other. These rays are detected by a scanner, and, through computerized reconstruction of the data, an image is created.

Several different positron emitters are available, but the most used are carbon 11, fluorine 18, and oxygen 15. The resulting images are of CBF or metabolism.

With both PET and SPECT, it is possible to label ligands for a variety of drugs and neuroreceptors—for example, the serotonin and dopamine receptors.

TABLE 49–4. Advantages and disadvantages of magnetic resonance imaging

Advantages	Disadvantages
No radiation	Noise discomfort
Minimal risk[a]	Claustrophobia
Good gray/white contrast	Limited discrimination between pathologies
Less degradation of image with movement	Length of scan time
No bone artifacts	Artifacts from ferromagnetic material (e.g., tooth fillings)
Clear structural images	Expensive
Ability to visualize several planes	Limited availability
Very sensitive to some types of pathology	

[a]Patients with cardiac pacemakers or intracranial magnetic clips or in the first trimester of pregnancy should not be scanned.

EPILEPSY AND LIMBIC SYSTEM DISORDERS

A number of conditions may affect the limbic areas of the brain and lead to behavior disorders. Among these conditions is one form of epilepsy, *temporal lobe epilepsy* (TLE), in which the seizure focus is in the medial limbic portions of that lobe. The following discussion of epilepsy includes special reference to TLE.

EPILEPSY

Epilepsy is a cerebral disorder in which the patient has recurrent seizures. Not all seizures indicate the presence of epilepsy; 1 person in 20 has a seizure in his or her lifetime, and the prevalence of epilepsy is about 0.5%.

The currently used classification of seizures is shown in Table 49–5. *Partial seizures* are those in which clinical and electroencephalographic changes suggest a focal onset. Further classification depends on whether consciousness is impaired during the attack. *Generalized seizures* are seizures in which the first clinical and electroencephalographic changes suggest bilateral abnormalities with widespread disturbance in both hemispheres. *Absence seizures* are usually associated with regular 3-Hz-per-second spike and slow-wave activity on electroencephalography. *Tonic-clonic seizures* are classic grand mal episodes; *myoclonic seizures* are sudden, brief, jerklike contractions that may be focal or generalized. Running takes place during *cursive seizures*, and *gelastic seizures* involve laughing. *Automatisms* are automatic motor acts carried out in a state of altered consciousness during or after seizures, for which there is usually amnesia. Automatisms generally last less than 15 minutes. Persistent focal seizures are referred to as *epilepsia partialis continua*. *Rasmussen's syndrome* is a viral encephalitis that presents as persistent focal seizures and is associated with slow neurological deterioration and brain atrophy, usually unilateral.

Status epilepticus is defined by recurrent seizures without return of consciousness between attacks. In nonconvulsive status epilepticus, patients present with prolonged episodes of abnormal behavior due to continuous seizures of either the complex-partial or absence type. Schizophrenia-like states, associated with variable degrees

of confusion (sometimes only slight), may be seen.

The classification of the epilepsies is essentially one of syndromes, not diseases. *West's syndrome* consists of infantile spasms in association with hypsarrhythmia, a specific electroencephalographic pattern. Hypsarrhythmia is characterized by high-amplitude slow waves at frequencies of 17 Hz, mixed with sharp waves and spikes of varying amplitude, morphology, and duration and arising from varying sites. The time of onset is the first year of life. The *Lennox-Gastaut syndrome* occurs in children up to about age 8 years and presents with multiple seizure types, a markedly disturbed EEG, and mental handicap. In the *reflex epilepsies*, seizures are provoked by cognitive, emotional, sensory, or motor events.

Psychiatric Disorders of Epilepsy

A classification of psychiatric disorders encountered in patients with epilepsy is shown in Table 49–6. The distinction between *ictal* and *interictal* syndromes is useful but not always clear. In some patients, prolonged postictal psychotic states occur, merging into interictal psychoses in the setting of clear consciousness.

There are few epidemiologic studies of the incidence and prevalence of interictal psychopathology. It is estimated that approximately 20%–30% of epileptic patients demonstrate psychopathology at some time, mainly anxiety and depression. The lifetime prevalence for an episode of psychosis is approximately 4%–10%; this prevalence increases to 10%–20% in patients with TLE.

The *interictal personality syndrome* is characterized by the features given in Table 49–7. Aggression is not a specific component. High-risk factors for the latter include

---

TABLE 49-5.   Classification of seizures

1. Partial (focal, local) seizures

    Simple-partial (retention of consciousness)

    Complex-partial (may begin with simple-partial)

    Partial seizures evolving to secondarily generalized seizures

2. Generalized seizures

3. Unclassified seizures

Source.   Adapted from International League Against Epilepsy 1981.

TABLE 49-6.   Classification of psychiatric disorders of epilepsy

Seizure related

Peri-ictal (including auras and prodromes)

Parictal (associated with increased seizures and clusters)

Forced normalization (associated with sudden cessation of seizures)

Postictal (associated with a disorganized electroencephalogram and clouding of consciousness following a seizure)

Interictal

Schizophrenia-like psychoses

Paranoid states

Affective disorders

Anxiety states

Personality disorders

TABLE 49–7. **Features of the interictal personality syndrome**

Hyperreligiosity, philosophical and mystical preoccupation

Disordered sexual function

Hypergraphia (tendency for excessive and compulsive writing)

Irritability

Viscosity (stickiness of thought—bradyphrenia)

mental retardation, low socioeconomic class, and a dysfunctional family.

In *episodic dyscontrol syndrome* there are sudden episodes of spontaneously occurring violence, often with minimal provocation, that are brief and terminate abruptly. These episodes may be precipitated by small amounts of alcohol, and patients later show remorse. Evidence of subtle cerebral damage may be present, including an abnormal EEG with slow rhythms (theta waves) over the temporal lobes and neuroimaging evidence of medial temporal lobe pathology. The condition may be associated with epilepsy but is clearly distinct from it. The term *epileptic equivalent* is not useful; a patient either has epilepsy or does not.

Depression is the most common interictal syndrome. However, many patients present with a chronic dysphoria accompanied by high anxiety levels and irritability rather than with a typical major affective disorder. Suicide is higher in epileptic populations, particularly patients with TLE, than in nonepileptic populations. The following have been associated with depression in epilepsy: barbiturates and drugs acting at the GABA-benzodiazepine receptor complex, low serum and red cell folate levels, late-onset epilepsy, and a decrease in the frequency of seizures.

The psychoses typically have a paranoid or schizophrenia-like presentation. The latter often include schneiderian first-rank symptoms in the absence of personality deterioration, affective warmth being maintained. This presentation is most often seen with TLE, especially with left-sided or bilateral seizure foci. Risk factors for the development of psychoses in patients with epilepsy are given in Table 49–8.

Many patients with TLE can be shown to have a specific pathology, that is, *mesial temporal sclerosis*. This condition is often unilateral, and there is loss of neurons, with gliosis in the hippocampus and related structures. The CA$_1$ region is especially vulnerable. Mesial temporal sclerosis is associated with prolonged febrile convulsions of childhood. Hamartomas and tumors also occur in temporal lobe regions and may cause TLE. Hamartomas arise from disordered cell differentiation and migration during development and resemble tumors but are not neoplastic. Schizophrenia is associated with cellular architectural abnormalities at the same sites. It is therefore of substantial interest that the development of a schizophrenia-like psychosis is associated with TLE. A difference between the pathology associated with idiopathic schizophrenia and that associated with schizophrenia-like states of epilepsy is that the pathology of schizophrenia does not include gliosis. The similarities are 1) the disorganization of neuronal ensembles; 2) the involvement primarily of the hippocampus; 3) the fact that in both syndromes the pathology is established in very early life, whereas the main manifestations appear years later, particularly in late adolescence and early adulthood; and 4) the fact that both syndromes present with a wide range of psychological and behavioral symptoms and signs.

The term *forced normalization* refers to the observation that certain patients develop psychiatric symptoms when their seizures come under control. Originally, forced normalization was thought to involve only psychoses, but other behaviors are now recognized in this setting, including depression, anxiety, agitation, and conversion disorders. In children, attention-deficit/hyperactivity disorder or conduct disturbance can result. The EEG normalizes during the behavior disturbances, and as behavior improves, the EEG becomes abnormal again.

The phenomenon is usually of acute onset, but in some patients, an interictal psychosis gradually emerges over time as seizure frequency decreases. This psychosis is usually precipitated by anticonvulsant drugs, especially benzodiazepines, barbiturates, ethosuximide, lamotrigine, and vigabatrin.

TABLE 49–8. **Risk factors for the development of psychoses in epilepsy**

Age at onset: around puberty

Interval: period between onset of seizures and onset of psychosis is around 14 years

Sex: bias to females

Seizure type: complex-partial; automatisms

Seizure frequency: may be diminished; forced normalization in a subgroup

Epilepsy syndrome: localization related, symptomatic

Seizure focus: temporal, especially left-sided or bilateral

Neurology: left-handed; abnormal neurological examination

Pathology: gangliogliomas and hamartomas

Electroencephalogram: mediobasal focus

NONEPILEPTIC SEIZURES

The term *pseudoseizures* is problematic. The seizures of patients who do not have epilepsy are better described as *nonepileptic seizures* or *pseudoepileptic seizures*, and the condition might be called *nonepileptic attack disorder*.

In some cases, the clinical pattern so resembles epilepsy that videotelemetry is essential before a diagnosis can be made. After generalized tonic-clonic seizures, prolactin levels reliably increase dramatically (to more than 1,000 IU/L) from a normal baseline, but levels fail to do so after a pseudoseizure. This test is less reliable for complex-partial seizures and is not reliable for simple-partial seizures and status epilepticus. Blood must be sampled within 20 minutes of an attack for an increase in prolactin levels to be detected.

Patients with *frontal lobe epilepsies* may present with sudden-onset, short-duration seizures that look bizarre, with much motor movement that is often wild and with little or no postictal mental confusion. The EEG may be remarkably normal. Conditions to consider in the nonpsychiatric differential diagnosis of pseudoseizures are listed in Table 49–9.

OTHER TEMPORAL LOBE DISORDERS

Although TLE is the most common temporal lobe syndrome seen in neuropsychiatry, other pathologies also may damage the limbic system. Three viruses that often affect this region of the brain are those causing *rabies*, those causing *herpes encephalitis*, and those causing *encephalitis lethargica*. Herpes encephalitis is caused by herpes simplex virus type 1 and has a high mortality rate; survivors often display psychopathology. Part or all of the *Klüver-Bucy syndrome* (see Table 49–10) may be present. In addition, there is often severe amnesia, irritability, distractibility, and dysphoria with apathy.

Cerebral tumors and tumorlike masses include gliomas and hamartomas. The latter occur anywhere in the brain but seem to be more associated with psychopathology, especially psychosis, when they occur in the temporolimbic areas.

Limbic encephalitis has been associated with systemic carcinoma.

Some patients have temporal lobectomies for relief of intractable TLE. A number of patients develop postoperative psychiatric syndromes, including transient or more severe mood disorders, anxiety states, and psychoses. Suicide is one cause of postoperative death.

MOVEMENT DISORDERS

Movement disorders are produced by dysfunction of the basal ganglia, and these deep gray-matter structures are increasingly recognized as being critically important in cognition and emotion as well as in motor function. There are three important corollaries with respect to the role of the basal ganglia in mental function: 1) basal ganglia disorders are frequently accompanied by abnormalities of intellectual function, mood, motivation, and personality; 2) many psychotropic agents affect the basal ganglia and produce movement disorders as side effects; and 3) many idiopathic psychiatric disorders have motor manifestations.

In this section are described the neuropsychiatric disturbances that accompany common movement disorders. Parkinson's disease (PD) and parkinsonian syndromes are discussed first, followed by the hyperkinetic movement disorders and tremors.

TABLE 49–9. **Conditions to consider in the nonpsychiatric differential diagnosis of nonepileptic seizures**

Hypoglycemia

Syncope and vasovagal attacks

Migraine, especially basilar migraine

Vertebrobasilar ischemia

Transient ischemic attacks

Transient global amnesia

Sleep disorders

  Parasomnias

    REM related

      REM behavior disorder

      Nightmares

    Non–REM related

      Night terrors

      Somnambulism

  Hypersomnias

    Narcolepsy

    Cataplexy

Note. REM = rapid eye moment.

TABLE 49–10. **Main components of the Klüver-Bucy syndrome**

Hypermetamorphosis (overattention to external stimuli)

Tendency to explore objects orally

Agnosia

Inappropriate sexual activity

Tameness, loss of fear

PARKINSON'S DISEASE

Demography

PD is an idiopathic degenerative disease that affects selected nuclei of the brain stem (substantia nigra, ventral tegmental area, locus coeruleus) and produces depletion of neurotransmitters (dopamine, norepinephrine) from neurochemical systems originating in these nuclei. The prevalence of PD in the general population is 100–200 in 100,000. The mean age at onset of PD is between 58 and 62 years, and the duration of illness averages 13–14 years. Men are slightly more likely than women to have PD; little genetic risk for the disorder exists.

Clinical Features

The cardinal motor features of PD are bradykinesia, rigidity, and rest tremor. *Bradykinesia* is manifested by hesitation before initiating movements, slowness in executing movements, and a paucity of spontaneous movement and gesture. Reduced arm swing when walking and a tendency to take several small steps when turning are additional manifestations of bradykinesia. Hypophonia, an expressionless (masked) face, and micrographia are also manifestations of bradykinesia. Two types of *rigidity* occur in PD. Most patients exhibit a plastic type of rigidity with increased resistance to passive flexion and extension of the limbs. In addition, if tremor is present, a cogwheel type of ratchet resistance can be detected while tone is being assessed. The typical *rest tremor* of PD is a large-amplitude, 4- to 6-cycles-per-second (cps), alternating flexion-extension movement that usually involves the fingers and wrist but may involve other body parts (lips, tongue, legs). Rest tremor is most apparent when the patient is in a state of alert repose; the tremor disappears with action of the involved limb and is absent in sleep. Tremor is exaggerated by stress. An *action tremor* (small amplitude, 10–12 cps) that appears with motion and disappears with rest occurs in some patients with PD.

In PD, findings of structural neuroimaging such as CT and MRI are normal or indicate mild to moderate cerebral atrophy. Glucose metabolism demonstrated by PET and cerebral perfusion imaged by SPECT are usually normal. Fluorodopa-PET scans reveal diminished transmitter uptake into the basal ganglia.

Pathology

The substantia nigra, ventral tegmental area, and locus coeruleus are routinely affected in PD. There is depigmentation and Lewy body formation in the substantia nigra and locus coeruleus and loss of neurons from the involved structures. The nucleus basalis of Meynert, a basal forebrain nucleus, is involved in some but not all patients, and some patients have Alzheimer-type pathology of the cerebral cortex. Lewy bodies are common in a restricted distribution in the cerebral cortex of patients with PD, and a few patients have widespread cortical Lewy bodies.

Several types of neurochemical changes are present in PD. Dopamine is synthesized in the substantia nigra and transported to the putamen, caudate, and medial temporal and medial frontal lobe regions. In PD, dopamine depletion is most marked in the putamen. Norepinephrine is synthesized in the locus coeruleus, and the pathological changes in this region in PD are associated with variable cortical noradrenergic deficits. Serotonin is reduced in the striatum, substantia nigra, and hippocampus in PD. Acetylcholine is synthesized by choline acetyltransferase, which is manufactured by neurons in the nucleus basalis. Cholinergic function is reduced in patients with PD who have atrophy of nucleus basalis.

Treatment

PD responds to treatment with dopaminergic agents, and failure of a patient to improve with therapy challenges the accuracy of the diagnosis. Two treatment approaches are currently pursued: treatment that slows the progress of the disease and delays or prevents cell death and treatment that provides relief of symptoms but has no effect on the underlying disease process. *Selegiline* is a monoamine oxidase B (MAO-B) inhibitor that inhibits the formation of hydroxy radicals generated in the course of the catabolism of dopamine and exogenous toxins suspected to play a role in the pathogenesis of PD. These hydroxyl molecules damage cell members and lead to cell death; thus, MAO-B inhibition reduces oxidative damage, preserves cell membranes, and enhances cell survival. Unanimity on whether this is selegiline's principal mode of action has not been achieved.

Symptomatic relief in PD can be provided by anticholinergic agents, dopamine precursors (levodopa, usually administered in a fixed combination with carbidopa [Sinemet] to prevent peripheral metabolism of the levodopa), amantadine (which facilitates dopamine release and inhibits reuptake), and dopamine receptor agonists (bromocriptine, pergolide, pramipexole, ropinirole). Table 49–11 lists drugs used in the treatment of PD, their dosages, and their principal side effects.

TABLE 49–11.   Agents used in the treatment of Parkinson's disease

Class and agent	Usual dosage	Side effects of the class
Monoamine oxidase B inhibitor		
Selegiline	5 mg po in A.M.; 5 mg at noon	Insomnia, hallucinations, delusions
Anticholinergics		
Benztropine	2–6 mg/day	Urinary retention, constipation, blurred vision, confusion
Trihexyphenidyl	4–8 mg/day	
Dopamine release facilitation		
Amantadine	200–300 mg/day	Hallucinations, delusions
Dopamine precursor		
Levodopa	300–2,000 mg/day	Hallucinations, delusions, euphoria, mania, hypersexuality, confusion
Sinemet[a]	10/100 tid to 25/250 qid	
Dopamine receptor agonist		
Bromocriptine	6–30 mg/day	Hallucinations, delusions, euphoria, mania, hypersexuality, confusion
Pergolide	1–5 mg/day	

Note.   [a]Sinemet is a fixed combination of levodopa and carbidopa; the latter is a dopamine β-hydroxylase inhibitor that prevents the peripheral metabolism of levodopa.

Dementia and Cognitive Alterations

Intellectual impairment is common in PD. Approximately 40% of patients with PD meet routine mental status examination criteria for overt dementia, and an additional 30% have more subtle cognitive impairments. Many of the patients with mild cognitive decline exhibit the characteristics of subcortical dementia. The causes of intellectual deterioration in PD are multiple. Severe dopamine deficiency can produce the syndrome of subcortical dementia. Patients with pathological changes in the nucleus basalis and the brain-stem dopaminergic nuclei have combined cholinergic and dopaminergic deficits and are reported to have more severe dementia than patients with changes limited to the dopaminergic nuclei. Patients with widespread cortical Lewy bodies also show evidence of dementia, and patients with Alzheimer-type cortical pathology have the clinical features of both PD and Alzheimer's disease.

Depression

Dysphoric mood is frequent in PD, occurring in nearly half of patients. Sadness and feelings of hopelessness and helplessness are common, but guilt and self-deprecation are rare. Anxiety is common in conjunction with depression; suicide and psychotic depression are infrequent. Depressed patients tend to have lower levels of 5-hydroxyindoleacetic acid (5-HIAA), the principal me-

tabolite of serotonin, in their cerebrospinal fluid. PET studies have shown that glucose metabolism of the frontal lobes is decreased in depressed compared with nondepressed patients with PD. The depression does not correlate with the severity of the motor deficit and must be treated separately with antidepressant agents or electroconvulsive therapy (ECT).

Other Neuropsychiatric Disorders

Anxiety is common in both depressed and nondepressed patients with PD. Apathy is the most frequent personality alteration of PD and has been identified in both depressed and nondepressed patients. Psychosis is uncommon in PD except after treatment with dopaminergic or anticholinergic agents; psychosis occurs primarily in patients with dementia.

Drug-induced neuropsychiatric disorders.   Dopamine is one of the most powerful psychoactive agents in clinical use. The drug functions in a variety of nervous system circuits that mediate motor, cognitive, and emotional activities. Dopamine has the ability to produce a resurrection of motor abilities in patients with PD but can also produce a panoply of motoric and behavioral side effects. Chorea, tics, and myoclonus are motor expressions of dopamine excess in PD. Hallucinations occur in 30% of PD patients treated with dopaminergic agents, and delusions occur in 10%; anxiety occurs in 10%, euphoria in 10%, and hypersexuality in 1%. These complications usually occur in the absence of delirium, although high doses of dopaminergic agents can produce an acute confusional state. Hallucinations and delusions are associated with dementia. Most of these manifestations are best managed by reducing the dose of the dopaminergic drug. Dopaminergic psychosis can be managed by administering low doses of a neuroleptic agent such as thioridazine or by using atypical antipsychotic agents such as clozapine, olanzapine, risperidone, or quetiapine. PD patients are unusually sensitive to the sedating effects of clozapine, and doses in the range of 25–100 mg may be adequate to control the psychosis and will not produce intolerable side effects. Risperidone also is sedating, and doses of 0.5–3 mg are usually sufficient to control drug-related psychosis. Extrapyramidal symptoms may be exaggerated by risperidone. When behavioral changes are induced by anticholinergic agents, the patient is usually in a delirium, with marked attentional deficits, fluctuating arousal, and reduced coherence of thought.

PARKINSONIAN SYNDROMES

Parkinsonian syndromes resemble PD but lack the cardinal features or deviate from PD in some other important way. Patients with parkinsonian syndromes typically demonstrate bradykinesia and rigidity but often lack tremor. Patients also tend to respond poorly to dopaminergic therapy. The most common parkinsonian syndromes are described briefly in this section, and conditions to consider in the differential diagnosis are given in Table 49–12.

Progressive Supranuclear Palsy

Progressive supranuclear palsy (PSP) is manifested by *supranuclear gaze palsy*, *axial rigidity*, *pseudobulbar palsy*, and *dementia*. Supranuclear gaze palsy is characterized by the loss of vertical gaze (downward gaze is compromised before upward gaze, and volitional saccadic eye movements are impaired before pursuit movements). In axial rigidity, increased tone in truncal and neck muscles causes the patient to have an extended posture. Marked dysarthria is a symptom of pseudobulbar palsy in PSP. The dementia of PSP has subcortical features. Depression and obsessive-compulsive disorder (OCD) have been described in PSP patients. Treatment is with antiparkinsonian agents (described previously), but the response is modest at best. At autopsy, patients are found to have cell loss, neurofibrillary tangles, and granulovacuolar degeneration involving the neurons of the midbrain, globus pallidus,

TABLE 49–12. **Conditions to consider in the differential diagnosis of parkinsonism**

Parkinsonian syndrome	Key clinical features
Parkinson's disease	Bradykinesia, rigidity, rest tremor, treatment responsive
Postencephalitic parkinsonism	Followed encephalitis lethargica epidemic (1918–1926); occasional current cases, oculogyric crises, asymmetric motor changes, prominent neuropsychiatric alterations
Progressive supranuclear palsy	Axial rigidity, vertical gaze paralysis, pseudobulbar palsy
Rigid Huntington's disease	Early onset, family history, minor choreiform movements
Shy-Drager syndrome	Prominent impotence, postural hypotension, incontinence
Striatonigral degeneration	Similar to Parkinson's disease but unresponsive to treatment
Olivopontocerebellar atrophy	Cerebellar and pyramidal system abnormalities
Cortical-basal degeneration	Asymmetric onset, marked apraxia, and visuospatial deficits
Cortical Lewy body disease	Dementia similar to Alzheimer's disease with visual hallucinations and fluctuations in disability
Rett syndrome	Autism, ataxia, stereotyped hand movements in girls
Wilson's disease	Kayser-Fleischer corneal rings, low serum ceruloplasmin
Idiopathic basal ganglia calcification	Calcified basal ganglia on CT, normal serum calcium
Hallervorden-Spatz disease	Globus pallidus mineralization on CT and MRI
Vascular parkinsonism	Spastic rigidity, asymmetric reflexes, Babinski signs
Dementia pugilistica	Extensive history of boxing
Hydrocephalus	Markedly enlarged ventricles on CT or MRI
Creutzfeldt-Jakob disease	Rapid progression, pyramidal signs, periodic electroencephalographic pattern
Syphilis	Positive serum FTA-ABS and CSF VDRL
Drug-induced parkinsonian syndromes	Neuroleptic treatment, tremor absent or minimal

(continued)

TABLE 49–12. Conditions to consider in the differential diagnosis of parkinsonism *(continued)*

Parkinsonian syndrome	Key clinical features
Carbon monoxide poisoning	Carbon monoxide exposure, globus pallidus lesions on CT
Hypoparathyroidism	Calcified basal ganglia on CT, reduced serum calcium level

Note. CSF = cerebrospinal fluid; CT = computed tomography; FTA-ABS = fluorescent treponemal antibody absorption; MRI = magnetic resonance imaging; VDRL = Venereal Disease Research Laboratory.

and thalamus. Neuroimaging (CT or MRI) may reveal brain-stem atrophy, and SPECT or PET usually demonstrates diminished perfusion or metabolism of the frontal lobes.

Vascular Parkinsonism

Vascular parkinsonism occurs in patients with multiple small vessel occlusions that produce infarctions in the basal ganglia and the deep hemispheric white matter. The most common causes of the small vessel disease are sustained hypertension (leading to lipohyalinosis of arterioles) and diabetes. Patients typically exhibit subcortical dementia, parkinsonism with gait changes and bradykinesia but little tremor, and pyramidal tract signs (spasticity, exaggerated muscle stretch reflexes, pseudobulbar palsy, and Babinski signs). Occasional patients may improve with antiparkinsonian agents. Depression, psychosis, apathy, and irritability are the most common neuropsychiatric features of vascular parkinsonism. The terms *lacunar state* and *Binswanger's disease* are used in cases when infarctions or ischemic injury predominate in the basal ganglia and white matter, respectively.

Drug-Induced Parkinsonian Syndromes

Parkinsonian syndromes may be induced by dopamine-blocking agents including neuroleptics (phenothiazines, butyrophenones) and agents used to control gastrointestinal disorders (prochlorperazine maleate [Compazine], metoclopramide). Patients typically manifest bradykinesia and rigidity and are less likely to exhibit tremor. Older patients are more susceptible to this side effect than are younger patients. Amelioration of the syndromes is usually accomplished by reducing the dosage of the inciting agent and temporarily treating the patient with anticholinergic agents or amantadine. Levodopa and dopamine-receptor agonists are used in the treatment of drug-induced parkinsonian syndromes only if motor symptoms are extreme. These agents may exacerbate a psychotic disorder.

HUNTINGTON'S DISEASE

Clinical Features

Huntington's disease (HD) is an autosomal-dominant neurodegenerative disease associated with a triplicate repeat mutation on chromosome 4. The disease commonly begins between ages 35 and 40 years and duration is 12–16 years. Late-onset (after age 50 years) and juvenile-onset (before age 20 years) cases occur. The disease is equally common in men and women; inheritance from the father is more likely among early-onset cases.

HD is a hyperkinetic disorder with choreic movements affecting the proximal and distal limbs, trunk, face, and speech musculature. Gait abnormalities and dysarthria are prominent. A supranuclear gaze palsy occurs in a majority of patients. A rigid variant with parkinsonian syndrome is much less common and is most frequent in the juvenile form of the disease. Structural imaging (CT, MRI) typically reveals atrophy of the caudate nuclei in HD, and PET demonstrates reduced metabolism in these nuclei.

Neuroleptic medications suppress the chorea. No treatment is available that retards the course of the disease or improves the accompanying dementia.

Pathology

Autopsy reveals marked cell loss in the caudate nuclei and the putamina, moderate loss of cells from thalamic nuclei, and variable neuronal dropout in the cerebral cortex. Medium-sized spiny neurons are disproportionately affected in the striatum. GABA is depleted in the affected regions in HD. Concentrations of substance P, cholecystokinin, and met-enkephalin are also severely reduced.

Neuropsychiatric Manifestations

A variety of neuropsychiatric disorders occur in HD. All patients with HD manifest subcortical dementia, and the cognitive alterations are the earliest manifestations in some cases. Personality changes are ubiquitous throughout the illness and include irritability, disinhibition, and conduct disorders. Patients may have personality alterations closely resembling intermittent explosive disorder or antisocial personality disorder. Depression occurs in 40%–50% of patients, and mania is present in approximately 2%. Suicide is a major complication of the depressive disorder. Psychosis is present in 5%–15% of patients. OCD has been observed in some cases. Behavioral alterations precede the onset of the chorea in approximately one-third of cases. Treatment of the behavioral disorders of HD involves the use of conventional psychotropic agents. Carbamazepine is usually superior to lithium for the management of mania in HD.

NON–HUNTINGTON'S DISEASE CHOREAS

Chorea occurs in a wide array of neurological and systemic disorders. Three common causes of chorea are described here.

Tardive Dyskinesia

Tardive dyskinesia (TD) is a choreiform disorder that occurs after chronic administration of dopamine-blocking agents. For a diagnosis of TD to be made, the patient must have had a cumulative exposure of at least 3 months to a neuroleptic or other dopamine-blocking agent and other causes of chorea must be excluded. The movements of TD are typically small-amplitude choreic jerks involving the tongue, lips, and fingers. Truncal dyskinesia and foot and toe movements also are common. The chorea is present at rest and increased by distraction; the chorea is reduced by action of the affected limb, direction of attention to the movements, and the patient's volitional suppression of the movements. There is little subjective awareness of TD. Once TD occurs, the disorder remains stable in a majority of patients, although in a small number TD progresses to severe chorea and disability. Resolution may occur if the patient is able to discontinue taking dopamine-blocking agents for 1–2 years. The disorder may be permanent, and failure to resolve is particularly common in elderly patients. TD is suppressed by reintroducing or increasing the dose of dopamine-blocking drugs. Patients may improve with reserpine, propranolol, or clonazepam therapy. A syndrome identical to TD may occur in elderly patients with no history of exposure to dopamine-blocking agents.

Chorea With Systemic Lupus Erythematosus

Chorea may occur in systemic lupus erythematosus (SLE). Chorea is most common in women whose disease begins early (around age 18 years). The disease is most frequent in SLE patients who have antiphospholipid antibodies and may also occur in patients with antiphospholipid antibodies who lack other evidence of SLE. Recurrent bouts of hemichorea and asymmetric chorea are common. SLE may be complicated by a variety of neuropsychiatric disor-

ders, including psychosis, depression, and seizures. The diagnosis of SLE is supported by positive antinuclear antibody (ANA) test results and, more specifically, by positive anti–double-stranded DNA test results. Antiphospholipid antibodies include lupus anticoagulant and anticardiolipin A and B.

Sydenham's Chorea and Chorea Gravidarum

Sydenham's chorea follows group A streptococcal infections, although the original episode may not be recognized clinically. The chorea typically begins 1–6 months after the original infection. Sydenham's chorea is a small-amplitude chorea affecting primarily the distal muscles (hands and fingers). Sedimentation rate and anti-streptolysin-O titer may be normal; a serological test for anti-DNase B usually yields positive results. The chorea typically resolves in 4–6 months but may occasionally persist. Sydenham's chorea is accompanied by irritability, and both the acute and the postchoreic states may be associated with obsessional and compulsive symptoms and mood disorders.

Most patients who exhibit chorea during pregnancy (chorea gravidarum) or when taking oral contraceptives have a previous history of Sydenham's chorea, and these disorders represent reactivation of a latent movement disorder.

DYSTONIC DISORDERS

Dystonia refers to sustained muscle contraction that results in slow contortions or a continuously sustained abnormal posture. In the early stages of a dystonic disorder, the dystonia may occur only when the involved limb is used, and intermittent muscle contraction may result in an action tremor. Dystonia may involve any muscles and may affect a single body part (focal dystonia), adjacent body parts (segmental dystonia), or essentially all muscle groups (generalized dystonia). Hereditary dystonia often begins in childhood. This form of dystonia begins in the legs and progresses gradually, eventually affecting all body regions. Spontaneous remissions may occur. Adult-onset idiopathic dystonia is usually focal or segmental, involving the neck (torticollis), jaw and eyelids (Meige's syndrome), or hand during writing (writer's cramp). Dystonia accompanies many choreic and parkinsonian syndromes (e.g., HD, PD), and tardive dystonia frequently occurs with TD.

No neuropsychiatric disorders are commonly associated with idiopathic dystonia, although when the illness begins, patients are often incorrectly considered to have conversion disorders.

TIC SYNDROMES AND DISORDERS

Tourette's syndrome (TS) is one of several tic syndromes (see Table 49–13). TS is characterized by onset of body and vocal tics before age 18 years. The tics wax and wane over time and persist throughout life. The components of the tic syndrome also vary over time, changing from one location to another and varying in complexity. The vocal tics may be unformed (e.g., throat clearing, sniffing) or formed (words); coprolalia (cursing) occurs in less than 50% of patients. There are no imaging or laboratory abnormalities in TS. Neuropathological studies suggest that there is an increased number of dopamine receptors in the caudate nucleus and putamen. The tics can usually be suppressed by neuroleptic agents (e.g., haloperidol, pimozide), and some patients improve with clonidine or clonazepam therapy.

Two principal neuropsychiatric disorders accompany TS: attention-deficit/hyperactivity disorder (ADHD) in childhood and OCD. ADHD occurs in approximately half of all TS patients in childhood, and TS sometimes first becomes evident when the child with ADHD is treated with stimulants and tics are precipitated. OCD occurs in about half of all TS patients; these patients typically respond to treatment with conventional anti-OCD agents such as clomipramine and fluvoxamine. Self-mutilation and exhibitionism are occasional manifestations of OCD. In some families, OCD and TS are inherited in an autosomal-dominant manner, with some members having OCD, others manifesting TS, and some developing both OCD and TS.

More limited idiopathic tic syndromes and disorders may occur in childhood or adulthood. Clinically, these syndromes and disorders are manifested by single or multiple tics without vocalizations. The tics are stable and unchanging over time. Tics may also be induced by a variety of drugs and can occur with other movement disorders.

TREMOR

Tremors have no specific neuropsychiatric associations but may be induced by drugs that are commonly used in neuropsychiatry. Table 49–14 lists the features of two major types of tremor and their etiologies and treatments.

CATATONIA

Catatonia is a complex motor disorder that occurs in psychiatric, neurological, medical, and drug-induced conditions (Table 49–15). *Catatonia* refers to a variety of disordered movements, including stereotypy (repetitive non–goal-directed movements), mannerisms (repetitive goal-oriented but bizarre or exaggerated movements), sustained postures, waxy flexibility, catatonic unresponsiveness, automatic obedience, echolalia, and echopraxia. Treatment with benzodiazepines may be helpful and sometimes produces dramatic relief. ECT is usually beneficial as well.

NEUROLEPTIC-INDUCED MOVEMENT DISORDERS

Several of the disorders discussed in this section can be induced by dopamine-blocking drugs. The widespread use of neuroleptic-type dopamine-blocking agents to treat psychotic and agitated patients results in a plethora of drug-induced movement abnormalities, of which the clinician must be aware.

STROKE AND BRAIN TUMORS

Cerebrovascular disease is one of the most common causes of neuropsychiatric syndromes in adults. With the marked expansion of the cerebral cortex that occurred in human evolution, the cerebral vasculature was stretched and contorted, creating border zones and end arterial zones with little collateral circulation and a consequent vulnerability to ischemic injury. Moreover, the lateralization of cogni-

---

TABLE 49–13. **Classification of tic syndromes and disorders**

Idiopathic tic disorders

Tourette's syndrome

Chronic multiple motor tic or phonic tic disorder

Chronic single tic disorder

Transient tic disorder

Nonspecific tic disorder

Symptomatic tic disorders

Postrheumatic tics (after rheumatic fever)

Tics due to carbon monoxide exposure

Neurodegenerative syndromes

Neuroacanthocytosis

Lesch-Nyhan syndrome

Drug-induced tics

Tardive tic disorders

Tics induced by stimulants (amphetamines, methylphenidate)

Tics induced by levodopa

Tics induced by anticonvulsants (phenytoin, carbamazepine, phenobarbital)

TABLE 49–14.   Characteristics of tremors (cerebellar intention-type tremors not included)

Characteristic	Rest tremor	Action tremor
Amplitude	Large	Small
Frequency	4–6 cps	10–12 cps
Present at rest	Yes	No
Increased by action	No	Yes
Reduced by alcohol	No	Yes
Increased by stress	Yes	Yes
Associated disorders	Parkinson's disease and parkinsonian syndromes	Benign essential tremor, tremor associated with dystonia, exaggerated physiological tremor
Drugs that induce the tremor	Neuroleptics	Lithium, tricyclic antidepressants, stimulants, ephedrine, caffeine, valproate
Treatment	Reduce dosage of neuroleptic, administer anticholinergic or dopaminergic agents	Propranolol, primidone, clonazepam

Note.   cps = cycles per second.

tive functions in humans reduced redundancy and further increased the chance of intellectual dysfunction from focal lesions. These two themes in human evolution converge to make the brain vulnerable to ischemic injury and create a high likelihood of disability after stroke.

Tumors are a less common but important cause of neurological disability and behavioral change in both adults and children. This section includes a description of common stroke syndromes and their behavioral correlates and a discussion of brain tumors and their associated neuropsychiatric morbidity.

CEREBROVASCULAR DISEASE AND STROKE

Types of Cerebrovascular Disease

In the United States, there are approximately 400,000 new cases of stroke annually, and the total number of Americans who have had stroke is 1.7 million. Stroke is age related, becoming increasingly common among older individuals. The annual incidence of stroke rises from approximately 100/100,000 among 45- to 54-year-olds to approximately 2,000/100,000 in those older than 75 years. Men are at greater risk for stroke than women (1.33:1 ratio). Seventy percent of stroke survivors have a permanent occupational disability, and approximately 25% have vascular dementia.

There are several major types of stroke syndromes (Table 49–16). Atherothrombotic occlusions result from atherosclerotic (large vessels) or arteriosclerotic (arterioles) in situ obstruction of cerebral vessels. Cerebral emboli arise from the heart and are carried distally in the arterial circulation to the brain. Emboli occasionally arise from plaques in the carotid, vertebral, and basilar arteries. Intracerebral hemorrhage is typically associated with hypertension and rupture of small arteriole aneurysms in the deep gray nuclei of the brain. Subarachnoid hemorrhage results from rupture of congenital aneurysms of the circle of Willis at the base of the brain. Transient ischemic attacks (TIAs) are produced by temporary interruption of the blood supply to the brain, usually caused by disease of the carotid arteries. TIAs occasionally happen with occlusion of small vessels and mark the occurrence of a lacunar infarction in deep-brain structures.

The type of stroke syndrome observed clinically depends on the size of the cerebral vessel involved. Occlusion of the carotid arteries usually leads to a border-zone infarction at the junction of the middle cerebral artery territory and the territories of the anterior and posterior cerebral arteries or an infarction in the combined territories of the middle and anterior cerebral arteries. Occlusion of a stem or surface branch of the anterior, middle, or posterior cerebral artery produces a regional syndrome (aphasia, aprosodia, homonymous hemianopia). Occlusion of the proximal branches of the intracerebral vessels that supply the basal ganglia, thalamus, and deep white matter produces lacunar infarctions and white-matter ischemic injury. Vertebral or basilar compromise produces brain-stem and posterior cerebral artery signs (e.g., nystagmus, dysarthria, diplopia). Figures 49–1 and 49–2 illustrate where ischemic and hemorrhagic strokes, respectively, typically occur.

TABLE 49–15. Etiologies of catatonia

Psychiatric disorders

Depression

Mania

Schizophrenia

Neurological disorders

Encephalitis (especially herpes encephalitis)

Subacute sclerosing panencephalitis

General paresis

Parkinson's disease

Globus pallidus lesions

Thalamic infarction

Medial frontal infarctions or hemorrhage

Epilepsy

Systemic disorders

Diabetic ketoacidosis

Hypercalcemia

Hepatic encephalopathy

Uremia

Thrombocytopenic purpura

Systemic lupus erythematosus

Mononucleosis

Drug-induced catatonia

Amphetamines

Phencyclidine (PCP)

Neuroleptics

Neuroleptic malignant syndrome

TABLE 49–16. Relative frequency of types of stroke syndromes

Syndrome	Frequency (%)
Atherothrombotic vascular occlusion	60
Cerebral embolus	15
Intracerebral hemorrhage	5
Subarachnoid hemorrhage	10
Transient ischemic attacks	7
Other	3

sidered in younger individuals who have a stroke syndrome.

Assessment of the Stroke Patient

Evaluation of the stroke patient should include a complete blood count; determination of prothrombin time, partial thromboplastin time, and erythrocyte sedimentation rate; measurement of electrolytes and blood sugar, blood urea nitrogen (BUN), and serum cholesterol concentrations; electrocardiography; and CT or MRI. Diffusion-weighted MRI demonstrates areas of recent stroke dramatically. Patients who sustain strokes but have no identifiable risk factors or who have a history of spontaneous abortions or migraine should be studied for the antiphospholipid antibody syndrome through obtaining anticardiolipin antibodies. Patients with TIAs may be candidates for carotid endarterectomy and should undergo Doppler studies of the carotid arteries, magnetic resonance angiography, or angiography. Echocardiography may be necessary to identify a source of emboli within the heart. SPECT and PET usually reveal areas of diminished cerebral perfusion or metabolism that are larger than the areas of structural change demonstrated by CT or MRI.

Treatment of Cerebrovascular Disease

Treatment in the acute phase consists of maintaining blood pressure in the high normal range and providing anticoagulation therapy if the stroke is evolving or if the stroke is small and is thought to have resulted from a cardiac embolus. Long-term anticoagulation therapy should be provided for patients with cardiac disorders such as atrial fibrillation. Other patients with atherothrombotic strokes should be treated with aspirin. Patients who are intolerant of aspirin or who have additional strokes despite aspirin should be considered for treatment with ticlopidine. Physical therapy, speech therapy, and occupational therapy will optimize outcome.

Risk Factors for Cerebrovascular Disease

The most potent risk factor for stroke is hypertension. Congestive heart failure, coronary artery disease, and electrocardiographic abnormalities are also highly correlated with stroke occurrence. Elevated blood lipid concentrations, cigarette smoking, diabetes, obesity, and elevated hematocrit also contribute to stroke risk. Cerebral emboli arise from the heart as a consequence of valvular disease, myocardial infarction with mural thrombus, cardiac arrhythmia (particularly atrial fibrillation), and cardiac surgery.

Among younger patients, a history of migraine and use of oral contraceptives are risk factors for stroke. Nonatherosclerotic vascular disorders such as collagen vascular diseases are also more common in younger stroke patients. Table 49–17 provides a list of disorders to be con-

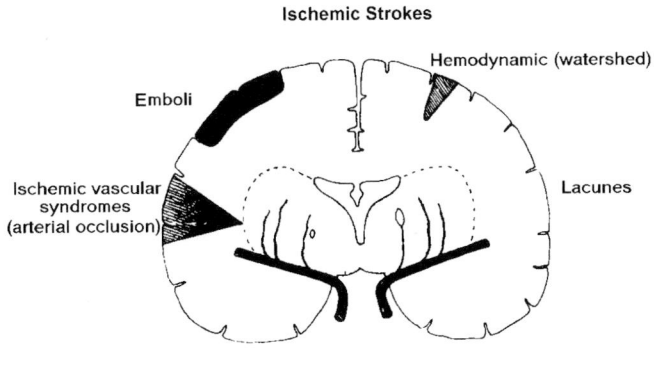

FIGURE 49-1. Locations of ischemic strokes.
Source. Reprinted with permission from Hachinski V, Norris JW: *The Acute Stroke.* Philadelphia, PA, FA Davis, 1985, p. 98.

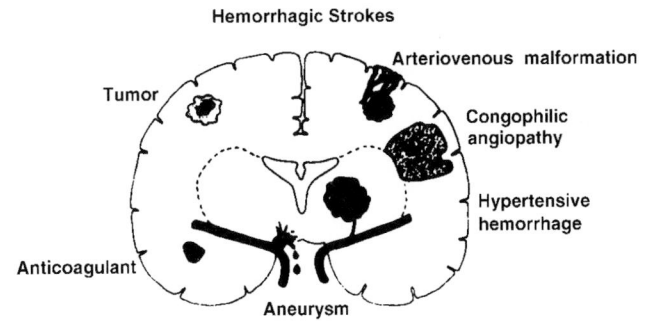

FIGURE 49-2. Locations of hemorrhagic strokes.
Source. Reprinted with permission from Hachinski V, Norris JW: The Acute Stroke. Philadelphia, PA, FA Davis, 1985, p. 98.

Neuropsychiatric Consequences of Stroke

The neuropsychiatric consequences of stroke depend on the location and extent of the brain injury, whether other ischemic damage exists, and the premorbid intellectual and emotional functioning of the individual. Stroke-related frontal lobe syndromes, aphasia, visuospatial disorders, memory disorders, and vascular dementia are frequent complications. In this section, abnormalities of mood and emotional function after a stroke are emphasized. Neuropsychiatric disorders may be accompanied by motor and sensory abnormalities or may be the only manifestations of ischemic brain injury. Emotional and cognitive disorders may coexist or may occur independently.

Depression is the most common neuropsychiatric consequence of stroke and occurs in 30%–50% of stroke patients within 2 years of the initial event. About half of the patients meet criteria for major depressive episode, and half have minor depression similar to dysthymic disorder. Major depression is not correlated with the degree of disability, whereas minor depression is more closely related to the patient's deficit syndrome. Depression is most common with lesions that affect the frontal lobes (dorsolateral prefrontal cortex and head of the caudate nucleus), and the frequency and severity of depression increase with increasing proximity of the lesion to the frontal pole. Lesions producing depression are more commonly found in the left frontal lobe than in the right frontal lobe; PET reveals bilateral frontal hypometabolism in patients who manifest a mood disorder. Anxiety accompanies cortical, but not subcortical, lesions that produce depression. Poststroke depression and anxiety respond to conventional psychotropic agents. Several recent studies using MRI found an increased prevalence of periventricular white-matter lesions in patients with late-onset idiopathic depression. The changes may be vascular in origin, which suggests that the associated depression is a manifestation of subtle ischemic brain injury.

Mania is much less common than depression after stroke and occurs almost exclusively with lesions of the right hemisphere. The lesions may affect the inferior medial frontal cortex, caudate nucleus, thalamus, or basal temporal region. Many of these patients have a family history of affective disorder. Cortical lesions produce single manic events; subcortical lesions may initiate a series of relapsing depressive and manic episodes similar to those of idiopathic bipolar disorder.

Psychosis is a rare complication of single strokes and may occur with lesions of the left temporal region that produce Wernicke's aphasia, lesions of the right temporoparietal region, and subcortical lesions affecting the caudate nuclei. Right-sided lesions are often accompanied by visual hallucinations and delusions. Seizures are common in patients who manifest poststroke psychosis. Psychosis is more common with bilateral cerebrovascular lesions. Poststroke delusions are treated with antipsychotic agents used to treat idiopathic psychotic disorders.

Visual hallucinations occur with retinal ischemia in amaurosis fugax, optic nerve lesions in ischemic optic neuritis, midbrain lesions in the syndrome of peduncular hallucinosis, and lesions of the geniculocalcarine radiations that produce homonymous visual-field defects (release hallucinations). Stroke-related seizures of the temporal, parietal, or occipital cortex may produce visual hallucinations. *Auditory hallucinations* may occur with pontine or temporal lobe ischemic injuries and may accompany poststroke delusions.

TABLE 49–17. Etiologies of stroke in young individuals

Systemic disorders

Hypertension
Diabetes

Cardiac disorders

Rheumatic heart disease
Prosthetic mitral valve
Atrial myxoma
Mitral valve prolapse
Marantic endocarditis
Atrial fibrillation
Cardiomyopathy
Patent foramen ovale

Trauma

Carotid artery dissection

Vasculitis

Systemic lupus erythematosus
Antiphospholipid antibody syndrome
Polyarteritis nodosa
Behçet's disease
Sarcoidosis
Disseminated intravascular coagulation
Thrombotic thrombocytopenic purpura
Sneddon's syndrome (seronegative vasculitis with livido reticularis)
Takayasu's disease
Granulomatous angiitis
Microangiopathy of retina and brain

Medication and drug induced

Oral contraceptives
Ergot derivatives
Cocaine (oral or intravenous)
Heroin (intravenous)
Pentazocine lactate (intravenous)
Methylphenidate (intravenous)

Hematologic disorders

Sickle-cell disease
Polycythemia vera
Leukemia with leukocytosis
Hypercoagulation (idiopathic or with systemic cancer)
Waldenström's macroglobulinemia
Dysproteinemias

Infectious arteritis

Syphilis
Chronic basal meningitis

Inherited metabolic defects

Homocystinuria
Fabry's disease
Mitochondrial encephalopathy

Cerebral venous thrombosis

(may occur during pregnancy)

Migraine

Arteriovenous malformation

Fibromuscular dysplasia

Moyamoya disease

Ehlers-Danlos syndrome

Pseudoxanthoma elasticum

Neoplastic angioendotheliosis

BRAIN TUMORS

Intracranial neoplasms can present with neuropsychiatric disturbances, or behavioral alterations may evolve as the tumor enlarges. Detection of an underlying tumor is important because increased intracranial pressure can be life threatening and immediate treatment may be required. Some tumors are benign and can be removed completely, whereas others are malignant and only palliative treatment is possible.

Types of Brain Tumors

The major types of brain tumors and the relative frequency of their occurrence are presented in Table 49–18. Gliomas arise from the nonneural central nervous system cells, including astrocytes (gliomas, astrocytomas), arachnoid cells (meningiomas), ependymal cells (ependymomas), oligodendrocytes (oligodendrogliomas), and embryonic cerebellar cells (medulloblastomas). Gliomas and menin-giomas usually occur around age 50 years; medulloblastomas occur before age 20 years. Gliomas are the most malignant and the most common intracranial tumors. Survival after diagnosis rarely exceeds 2 years, even with aggressive surgical management, radiation, and chemotherapy. Astrocytomas are much less malignant, and some patients survive for several decades. Meningiomas are benign tumors but may recur after surgical resection if removal is incomplete or if tumor fragments are left in place because of their proximity to critical structures. Medulloblastomas usually occur in the first decade of life and are highly radiosensitive. Metastases arise from carcinomatous tumors occurring in the lung, breast, skin (melanomas), gastrointestinal tract, and kidney (in decreasing order of frequency). Breast and prostate tumors and multiple myeloma often metastasize to the skull and dura. The discovery that the patient has more than one intracranial tumor favors the diagnosis of metastatic disease.

TABLE 49-18.   Relative frequency of types of brain tumors

Tumor type	Frequency (%)
Glioblastoma multiforme	20
Meningioma	15
Astrocytoma	10
Pituitary adenoma	7
Neurinoma	7
Metastatic tumors	6
Ependymoma	6
Oligodendroglioma	5
Medulloblastoma	4
Craniopharyngioma and related tumors	4
Other	16

Clinical Features

Headaches are prominent in one-third of patients with tumors. The headache is typically nonpulsatile and intermittent. Seizures are very common in conjunction with intracranial tumors, occurring in 30%–40% of patients with gliomas, 60%–70% of patients with astrocytomas, and up to half of patients with meningiomas. Increased intracranial pressure produces papilledema characterized by obscuring of the optic disk margins, disk hyperemia, retinal hemorrhages, cotton-wool spots, and venous engorgement. Vision is not affected by papilledema, although the physiological blind spot may be enlarged. Unilateral weakness, sensory loss, ataxia, or homonymous visual-field defects may be present, depending on the location of the tumor.

Neuropsychiatric Consequences of Brain Tumors

Tumors produce behavioral disturbances similar to those that occur with stroke, but the disturbances are usually less discrete because neoplasms and their associated edema and increased intracranial pressure tend to produce more extensive dysfunction. Mental status changes characteristic of mild delirium (slowness of thought, reduced attention, and impaired comprehension) are typical of patients with intracranial tumors. Irritability is also common. These symptoms may be combined with more focal symptoms such as aphasia. Meningiomas sometimes develop from the floor of the anterior cranial fossa, producing orbitofrontal compression and a progressive frontal lobe syndrome. Frontal lobe tumors are particularly likely to cause depression; temporal lobe tumors produce psychosis or atypical mood disturbances with euphoria, hypomania, and lability. Diencephalic tumors may cause hypomania.

Treatment

Steroids are used to reduce edema associated with intracranial tumors. The role of surgery, radiation therapy, and chemotherapy is dictated by the tumor type. Seizures are treated with carbamazepine, phenytoin, gabapentin, lamotrigine, or valproate. Behavioral disturbances are treated with conventional psychotropic agents. Increased intracranial pressure is a contraindication to the use of ECT.

HEAD INJURY AND ITS SEQUELAE

The incidence of head injury in the United States is estimated to be between 175 and 367/100,000. Of these injuries, 7% may be considered severe. The most common causes are falls, traffic accidents, and assaults. However, head injuries are not randomly distributed in the population. In the United States, 20% are due to the use of firearms, and semiskilled and unskilled workers are overrepresented, as are individuals who engage in substance abuse. Head injury accounts for 1% of all deaths but also leads to considerable morbidity. The morbidity depends on a number of factors, including the site and the severity of the injury, the premorbid status of the patient, and whether complications such as epilepsy exist.

There are several ways to assess the severity of a head injury. One commonly used method involves determining the duration of posttraumatic amnesia (PTA) (Table 49–19). Another method involves determining the depth of any coma, sometimes easier than gauging the duration of PTA. A coma that lasts more than 6 hours is indicative of a severe injury. Several validated rating scales are used to assess head injury. The Glasgow Coma Scale assesses eye opening, verbal responses, and motor responses; higher scores correspond to less severe injury (Table 49–19).

The pathogenesis of the trauma is either direct or indirect. In cases of direct trauma, an object or torn meninges or fractured skull impinge on brain tissue. Effects include contusions and brain lacerations. Shearing forces injure the long white-matter fibers, leading to diffuse axonal injury. The higher the velocity at which the head injury occurs, the more likely it is that shearing of white-matter tracts will take place. The anterior poles of the frontal and temporal cortices are tightly held by the rigid anterior fossae of the skull, and damage is more apt to occur at these sites. These poles are the areas most

TABLE 49–19.   Methods used to assess head injury

Duration of posttraumatic amnesia

<5 min = very mild

≥5 min to <1 h = mild

≥1 h to <24 h = moderate

≥24 h to <1 wk = severe

≥1 wk = very severe

Glasgow Coma Scale[a]

Eye opening	Motor response	Verbal response
1. Nil	1. Nil	1. Nil
2. To pain	2. Extensor	2. Groans
3. To speech	3. Flexor	3. Inappropriate
4. Spontaneously	4. Withdrawal	4. Confused
	5. Localizing	5. Oriented
	6. Voluntary	

Note.   [a]1–4 = very severe; 5–8 = severe; 9–12 = moderate; ≥13 = mild.

likely to show effects of contrecoup injuries.

Indirect injury arises from shearing forces that lead to parenchymatous damage. This damage occurs in part because of rotational movements of the brain, which lag behind movements of the skull, setting up destructive intracranial forces. Where the glide of the brain inside the skull is greatest, small dural tears and bleeding of the surface blood vessels occur usually in the parieto-occipital regions.

Other causes of indirect injury are cerebral bleeding and thrombosis, hypoxia, raised intracranial pressure, and herniation of brain tissue. The hippocampus is particularly affected by *transtentorial herniation.*

There is debate over the long-term consequences of boxing. The term *punchdrunk* suggests that patients have dysarthria, ataxia, and cognitive changes. *Dementia pugilistica* is an alternative diagnosis. This state, which occurs after repeated sublethal blows to the brain, is associated with pathological changes to the subcortical midline structures and cerebellum. Damage to the substantia nigra results in parkinsonism. At autopsy, patients with dementia pugilistica are found to have abundant intracellular neurofibrillary tangles without Alzheimer-type neuritic plaques.

The most common neurological complications of head injury are intracranial hematoma, infection, and epilepsy. The epilepsy is usually focal but may present as a secondarily generalized seizure. The chances of developing epilepsy correlate with three factors: the length of the PTA, the presence or absence of an early seizure, and the presence or absence of a depressed skull fracture.

Imaging studies are relevant for the assessment of head injury. MRI may show intracranial lesions that are not revealed by CT, and perfusion deficits may be demonstrated by SPECT. There is an association between persistent neuropsychological deficits and both ventricular dilation and deep white-matter lesions on MRI.

PERSONALITY CHANGES DUE TO NEUROLOGICAL INJURY

After head injury, three independent mechanisms operate to shape the resulting personality. These are the premorbid personality, a generalized cerebral disturbance, and the results of any focal deficits, especially frontal lobe damage.

The premorbid personality may become exaggerated. An excessively tidy person may develop overt obsessional tendencies; a person with a sociopathic personality may manifest explosive violence.

The generalized deficits plus frontal lobe injury lead to a regular pattern of symptoms that are often subtle and at first may not be attributed to the underlying brain damage (Table 49–20). In general, there is poor tolerance of environmental change, stimulus boundedness (the patient becomes more dependent on external stimuli for action), concretization and loss of mental flexibility, and affective change with irritability, lability, and explosiveness. When damage is more severe, extremes of this profile are seen, with social disorganization, loss of interest in the self, explosive irritability, and a shallow, labile, blunted affect.

TABLE 49–20.   Generalized disturbance of cerebral function that may be seen after head trauma

Activity influenced more by external stimuli

Impaired ability to use abstract concepts

Concretization

Disturbed attention and concentration

Disturbed spontaneity

Poverty of ideas

Posttraumatic orderliness

Posttraumatic slovenliness

Disturbed and labile affect

Psychomotor slowing

Fatigability

Memory complaints

Diminished social awareness

Indecision

Loss of intellectual flexibility

These personality changes may be intertwined with the effects of focal damage and posttraumatic stress disorder (PTSD).

OTHER NEUROPSYCHIATRIC CONSEQUENCES OF TRAUMA

Cognitive changes after trauma are also both generalized and focal. There is blunting of overall performance on standardized IQ tests, with a decline from estimated premorbid levels. The patient's premorbid IQ is often assessed by using the educational history of the patient combined with a test of word reading ability such as the National Adult Reading Test. Focal deficits reflect those areas of the cortex that are directly damaged. Memory disturbance is common, with impaired learning of new material and slowing of retrieval. Psychomotor slowing (bradyphrenia) is common with more severe injury. These neurocognitive deficits may be compounded in patients who engage in substance abuse and continue to use alcohol.

Psychoses are not common. When they occur, they are often schizophrenia-like, with paranoid features. These psychoses are more common with left-sided injuries, especially if the temporal lobes are involved. As in many organic psychotic states, affect may be preserved in the presence of a florid delusional disorder.

Mania is not frequent. It is more frequent after right-hemisphere (especially limbic) lesions. Depression is common (20%–50% prevalence). There is evidence that left dorsolateral frontal cortical lesions and left basal ganglia lesions are associated with major depression more often than are lesions in other brain areas. Among causes of death, suicide is overrepresented; 14% of all deaths are suicide.

POSTCONCUSSIONAL SYNDROME

The nosologic status of this condition remains in doubt. However, many patients who have had head injury complain of headache, dizziness, diplopia, fatigue, sensitivity to noise, and poor concentration. Most of the patients become asymptomatic within a few weeks of the injury. A small percentage remain symptomatic. In some patients, there may be signs of central nervous system damage: for example, auditory evoked-potential changes, abnormal caloric test results, and acute vertigo and nystagmus on suddenly lying down. These symptoms may become persistent and blend in with those of anxiety, depression, and often PTSD.

There are several etiological factors underlying the chronic nonpsychotic disorders of cerebral trauma. The emotional impact of a head injury is variable. However, the head does play a special role in body image; consequently, head injury poses a threat that does not apply to other body parts. Furthermore, the circumstances of the accident may not be straightforward and may have personal consequences for patients, leading to unresolved conflict or guilt (e.g., when a friend or relative is killed).

The development of PTSD after head injury is common. It is partially true that the more severe the head injury is, the less likely it is that PTSD will develop. This is because patients with marked brain damage are more likely to have an amnesia for the psychological trauma of the accident. However, many patients with severe head injuries have PTSD, but the disorder is often overlooked in the setting of more obvious cognitive and physical changes.

Other posttraumatic syndromes include *posttraumatic anxiety*, with or without phobias and panic attacks; *posttraumatic conversion disorder* (including pseudoseizures); and *posttraumatic obsessional states.*

In a setting where financial compensation is involved, the possibility of malingering must be considered. There are no diagnostic tests useful to unequivocally identify malingering.

The management of the behavioral complications of head injury is complicated and requires a multidisciplinary approach. Substance abuse must be treated, and psychotropic drugs should be used with care. Seizures are an ever-present risk, and psychotropic drugs may precipitate convulsions. Behavioral techniques, cognitive retraining, and psychotherapy all form part of remedial therapy. In the case of more severely disabled patients, the relatives and caregivers usually need help and support to cope with the changed personality and behavior of the injured person.

CONCLUSIONS

This chapter provides an overview of the neuropsychiatric assessment of patients, including laboratory tests and neuroimaging techniques that may assist the clinician in arriving at diagnoses of and treatment plans for common neuropsychiatric disorders. Because the field of neuropsychiatry is so vast and overlaps considerably with psychiatry, only the neuropsychiatric disorders most frequently encountered in clinical practice were summarized: epilepsy and limbic system disorders, movement disorders, stroke and brain tumors, and head injury.

SUGGESTED READINGS

NEUROPSYCHIATRIC ASSESSMENT

Andreasen NC (section ed): Brain imaging, in American Psychiatric Press Review of Psychiatry, Vol 12. Edited by Oldham JM, Riba MB, Tasman A. Washington, DC, American Psychiatric Press, 1993, pp 315–510

George MS, Ring HA, Costa DC, et al: Neuroactivation and Neuroimaging With SPECT. New York, Springer-Verlag, 1991

Grant I, Adams KM: Neuropsychological Assessment of Neuropsychiatric Disorders, 2nd Edition. New York, Oxford University Press, 1994

Roberts JKA: Differential Diagnosis in Neuropsychiatry. Chichester, UK, Wiley, 1984

Rosse RB, Giese AA, Deutch SI, et al: Concise Guide to Laboratory and Diagnostic Testing in Psychiatry. Washington, DC, American Psychiatric Press, 1989

Strub RL, Black FW: The Mental Status Examination in Neurology, 3rd Edition. Philadelphia, PA, FA Davis, 1993

Trimble MR: Biological Psychiatry, 2nd Edition. Chichester, UK, Wiley, 1994

EPILEPSY AND LIMBIC SYSTEM DISORDERS

Bear D: Behavioural changes in TLE: conflict, confusion, challenge, in Aspects of Epilepsy and Psychiatry. Edited by Trimble MR, Bolwig T. Chichester, UK, Wiley, 1986, pp 19–30

Corsellis JAN, Goldberg GJ, Norton AR: Limbic encephalitis, and its association with carcinoma. Brain 91:481–496, 1968

Davison K, Bagley CR: Schizophrenia-like psychoses associated with organic disorders of the CNS, in Current Problems in Neuropsychiatry. Edited by Herrington RN. Kent, UK, Headley Brothers, 1969, pp 113–184

Fenwick P: Precipitation and inhibition of seizures, in Epilepsy and Psychiatry. Edited by Reynolds EH, Trimble MR. Edinburgh, Churchill Livingstone, 1981, pp 242–263

Fenwick P: Aggression and epilepsy, in Aspects of Epilepsy and Psychiatry. Edited by Trimble MR, Bolwig T. Chichester, UK, Wiley, 1986, pp 31–60

Glaser G, Pincus JH: Limbic encephalitis. J Nerv Ment Dis 149:59–68, 1969

Heath RG: Common characteristics of epilepsy and schizophrenia. Am J Psychiatry 118:1013–1026, 1962

International League Against Epilepsy: Proposal for a revised clinical and electroencephalographic classification of epileptic seizures. Epilepsia 22:489–501, 1981

International League Against Epilepsy: Proposal for a classification of the epilepsies and epileptic syndromes. Epilepsia 26:268–278, 1985

Monroe R: Episodic Behavior Disorders. Boston, MA, Harvard University Press, 1970

Perez MM, Trimble MR: Epileptic psychosis diagnostic comparison with process schizophrenia. Br J Psychiatry 137:245–249, 1984

Robertson MM, Trimble MR: Depressive illness in patients with epilepsy: a review. Epilepsia 24 (suppl 2):S109–S116, 1983

Scheibel A: Are complex partial seizures a sequela of temporal lobe dysgenesis? in Neurobehavioral Problems in Epilepsy. Edited by Smith DB, Treiman DM, Trimble MR. New York, Raven, 1991, pp 59–78

Slater E, Beard AW: The schizophrenia-like psychoses of epilepsy. Br J Psychiatry 109:95–150, 1963

Taylor DC: Factors influencing the occurrence of schizophrenia-like psychoses in patients with epilepsy. Psychol Med 5:249–254, 1975

Trimble MR: The Psychoses of Epilepsy. New York, Raven, 1991

Waxman SG, Geschwind N: The interictal behavior syndrome of TLE. Arch Gen Psychiatry 32:1580–1586, 1975

Wolf P, Trimble MR: Biological antagonism and epileptic psychosis. Br J Psychiatry 146:272–276, 1985

MOVEMENT DISORDERS

Cummings JL: Clinical Neuropsychiatry. New York, Grune & Stratton, 1985

Cummings JL: Intellectual impairment in Parkinson's disease: clinical, pathologic, and biochemical correlates. J Geriatr Psychiatry Neurol 1:24–36, 1988

Cummings JL: Behavioral complications of drug treatment in Parkinson's disease. J Am Geriatr Soc 39:708–716, 1991

Cummings JL: Depression in Parkinson's disease. Am J Psychiatry 149:443–454, 1992

de Bruin VMS, Lees AJ: The clinical features of 67 patients with clinically definite Steele-Richardson-Olszewski syndrome. Behavioural Neurology 5:229–232, 1992

Folstein SE: Huntington's Disease: A Disorder of Families. Baltimore, MD, Johns Hopkins University Press, 1989

Frankel M, Cummings JL, Robertson MM, et al: Obsessions and compulsions in Gilles de la Tourette's syndrome. Neurology 36:378–382, 1986

Grafton ST, Mazziotta JC, Pahl JJ, et al: A comparison of neurological, metabolic, structural, and genetic evaluations in persons at risk for Huntington's disease. Ann Neurol 28:614–621, 1990

Joseph AB, Young RR (eds): Movement Disorders in Neurology and Psychiatry. Boston, MA, Blackwell Scientific, 1992

Koller WC (ed): Handbook of Parkinson's Disease, 2nd Edition. New York, Marcel Dekker, 1992

Lees AJ: Tics and Related Disorders. New York, Churchill Livingstone, 1985

Mayeux R, Denaro J, Hemenegildo N, et al: A population-based investigation of Parkinson's disease with and without dementia. Arch Neurol 49:492–497, 1992

Menza M, Harris D: Benzodiazepines and catatonia: an overview. Biol Psychiatry 26:842–846, 1989

Rogers D: Motor Disorder in Psychiatry. New York, Wiley, 1992

Taylor MA: Catatonia: a review of a behavioral neurologic syndrome. Neuropsychiatry Neuropsychol Behav Neurol 3:48–72, 1990

The Tourette Syndrome Classification Study Group: Definitions and classification of tic disorders. Arch Neurol 50:1013–1016, 1993

Trimble M: Psychopathology and movement disorders: a new perspective on the Gilles de la Tourette syndrome. J Neurol Neurosurg Psychiatry Suppl 1989, pp 90–95

Weiner WJ, Lang AE: Movement Disorders: A Comprehensive Survey. Mount Kisco, NY, Futura Publishing, 1989

Weiner WJ, Lang AE (eds): Drug-Induced Movement Disorders. Mount Kisco, NY, Futura Publishing, 1992

Wirshing WC, Cummings JL: Tardive movements disorders. Neuropsychiatry Neuropsychol Behav Neurol 3:23–35, 1990

STROKE AND BRAIN TUMORS

Adams RD, Victor M: Principles of Neurology, 5th Edition. New York, McGraw-Hill, 1993

Beckson M, Cummings JL: Neuropsychiatric aspects of stroke. Int J Psychiatry Med 21:1–15, 1991

Bornstein RA, Brown G (eds): Neurobehavioral Aspects of Cerebrovascular Disease. New York, Oxford University Press, 1991

Caplan LR, Stein RW: Stroke: A Clinical Approach. Boston, MA, Butterworths, 1986

Cascino GD, Adams RD: Brainstem auditory hallucinations. Neurology 36:1042–1047, 1986

Cummings JL, Miller BL: Visual hallucinations: clinical occurrence and use in differential diagnosis. West J Med 146:46–51, 1987

Gorman DG, Cummings JL: Neurobehavioral presentations of the antiphospholipid antibody syndrome. J Neuropsychiatry Clin Neurosci 5:37–42, 1993

Hachinski V, Norris JW: The Acute Stroke. Philadelphia, PA, FA Davis, 1985

Kolmel HW: Complex visual hallucinations in the hemianopic field. J Neurol Neurosurg Psychiatry 48:29–38, 1985

Lepore FE: Spontaneous visual phenomena with visual loss: 104 patients with lesions of retinal and neural afferent pathways. Neurology 40:444–447, 1990

McKee AC, Levine DN, Kowall NW, et al: Peduncular hallucinosis associated with isolated infarction of the substantia nigra pars reticulata. Ann Neurol 27:500–504, 1990

Robinson RG, Starkstein SE: Current research in affective disorders following stroke. J Neuropsychiatry Clin Neurosci 2:1–14, 1990

Starkstein SE, Robinson RG: Depression in cerebrovascular disease, in Depression in Neurologic Disease. Edited by Starkstein SE, Robinson RG. Baltimore, MD, Johns Hopkins University Press, 1993, pp 28–49

Starkstein SE, Robinson RG: Neuropsychiatric aspects of stroke, in Textbook of Geriatric Neuropsychiatry. Edited by Coffey EC, Cummings JL. Washington, DC, American Psychiatric Press, 1994, pp 457–477

Starkstein SE, Pearlson GD, Boston J, et al: Mania after head injury. Arch Neurol 44:1069–1073, 1987

HEAD INJURY AND ITS SEQUELAE

American Psychiatric Association: Diagnostic and Statistical Manual of Mental Disorders, 4th Edition. Washington, DC, American Psychiatric Association, 1994

Corsellis JAN: Boxing and the brain. Br Med J 298:105–109, 1989

Federoff JP, Starkstein SE, Forrester AW, et al: Depression in patients with head injury. Am J Psychiatry 149:918–923, 1992

Goldstein K: After Effects of Brain Injuries in War. New York, Grune & Stratton, 1942

Jennett B, Teasdale G: Assessment of head injuries, in Management of Head Injuries. Philadelphia, PA, FA Davis, 1981, pp 301–316

Jorge RE, Robinson RG, Starkstein SE, et al: Depression and anxiety following traumatic brain injury. J Neuropsychiatry Clin Neurosci 5:369–374, 1993

Kraus JF: Epidemiology of head injury, in Head Injury, 2nd Edition. Edited by Cooper P. Baltimore, MD, Williams & Wilkins, 1987, pp 1–19

Levin HS, Benton AL, Grossman RG: Neurobehavioral Consequences of Head Injury. New York, Oxford University Press, 1982

Lishman WA: Organic Psychiatry, 2nd Edition. Oxford, UK, Blackwell Scientific, 1987, pp 137–186

Starkstein SE, Pearlson GD, Boston J, et al: Mania after brain injury. Arch Neurol 44:1069–1073, 1987

NEUROPSYCHIATRY TEXTBOOKS

Cummings JL, Trimble MR: Concise Guide to Neuropsychiatry and Behavioral Neurology. Washington, DC, American Psychiatric Press, 1995

Lishman WA: Organic Psychiatry, 2nd Edition. Oxford, UK, Blackwell Scientific, 1987

Trimble MR: Biological Psychiatry, 2nd Edition. Chichester, UK, Wiley, 1996

Yudofsky SC, Hales RE (eds): American Psychiatric Press Textbook of Neuropsychiatry, 3rd Edition. Washington, DC, American Psychiatric Press, 1997

CHAPTER 50

THE FUTURE OF PSYCHIATRY

MELVIN SABSHIN, M.D.

The last quarter century has been characterized by enormous changes in almost every aspect of psychiatry in the United States. From my perspective, many of these changes have resulted from the interaction of new research and new economics. Although this interaction between science and economics has been most dramatic in North America and western Europe, similar changes have begun to occur throughout the world. Certainly, economic pressures have had a great impact on psychiatry throughout the twentieth century. At times, the field has grown in influence and power with surges of fiscal support. In the United States, such a spurt occurred after World War II. Both public and private support grew rapidly; many people sought treatment, and plans for reformation of our mental health care system began to take shape. During that time, however, the field of psychiatry in the United States was subdivided among several divergent treatment ideologies. Each point of view was advocated by separate leadership, and these leaders rarely consulted with each other. The charisma of much of this leadership sometimes obscured the fact that the therapeutic approaches were often not founded on good evidence, and ultimately confidence in the field began to weaken (Sabshin 1990).

During the past quarter century, the domination of American psychiatry by ideological groupings began to change. Evidence-based psychiatry became more powerful, and empirically based treatment became the rule rather than the exception. These changes occurred in the context of radical changes in the economic principles affecting our entire medical system. Health care in the United States has changed from being offered through an almost free market to being heavily regulated. Today, for treatment to be reimbursed, approval of the treatment must be obtained in advance from the managed care company. Length of hospitalization is severely limited and alternative care systems are preferred. In the mental health field, an effort is often made by these intermediaries to have treatment conducted by psychologists or social workers, who, it is assumed, will charge less than psychiatrists.

The pressure to limit length of hospital stay and the pressure to produce more rapid results in outpatients have reinforced the use of psychopharmacological agents in clinical practice. Recent developments in psychopharmacology have supported psychiatry's efforts to cope with the external economic pressures. On the other hand, psychosocial treatments have been made more difficult to support in the world of managed care. The future of psychotherapeutic work by psychiatrists is under attack from several fronts, and strong efforts will need to be made to prevent atrophy of psychiatrists' psychotherapeutic skills. Several other danger signals to American psychiatry have appeared; indeed, this chapter on the future of psychiatry is being written at a time when much of American psychiatry faces irrational external regulation and constraint.

When I first came to the American Psychiatric Association in 1974, I had a vision concerning how the field might be united and how we as psychiatrists might deal with the many challenges of that time (Sabshin 1976, 1977). Similarly, in this chapter I have emphasized steps that psychiatry might take to facilitate coping with the new challenges. Some of the predictions are based on developments already in progress. Others represent aspirations of new directions that will require much work if they are to be achieved. The list is not intended to be a complete formulation; rather, I have chosen several areas in which I have a special interest.

DEVELOPMENTS IN DIAGNOSIS AND RELATED MEASURES

American psychiatrists' interest in nosology has undergone dramatic change during the last quarter of the twentieth century. The status of nosology in the United States was somewhat de-emphasized following World War II, but interest in diagnosis has now become a central feature of American psychiatry (Frances et al. 1989). Indeed, DSM-III (American Psychiatric Association 1980), DSM-III-R (American Psychiatric Association 1987), and DSM-IV (American Psychiatric Association 1994) have had enormous worldwide impact and, along with ICD-10 (World Health Organization 1992), have contributed to a scientific resurgence in the entire nosological arena. No issue dramatizes change in American psychiatry more than the relative importance of diagnostic methodology in the past half century. Psychiatrists' capacity or incapacity to make reliable diagnoses had become a matter of public policy concern. The great scientific progress during the last 25 years has increased the credibility of psychiatry for the general public and for decision makers.

Much work remains to be done in refining the diagnostic categories. It is to be hoped that by the second half of the twenty-first century there will have been more progress in developing an etiologically and pathogenetically based nosology. Such a nosology has been a fundamental goal of psychiatry for a long time, and its systematic evolution will help to define an evidence-based psychiatry.

An important step in achieving greater scientific precision will involve increased use of all of the multiaxial categories in diagnosis. I believe that psychobiological understanding of adaptation will be enhanced in the first quarter of the twenty-first century and will help researchers and clinicians to explain why some people are more or less vulnerable to disorder. Those individuals who have greater psychobiological predilection to cope will be less vulnerable. More attention to data about the best level of adaptation experienced by patients should also be helpful in understanding the clinical implications of adaptation.

One of the most important current needs involves an understanding of the level of disability found in patients with each psychiatric disorder (Massel et al. 1990). The development of disability indices should indeed be a high priority for American psychiatry; such assessment has notable social and economic implications, as well as clinical importance.

DEVELOPMENT OF PRACTICE GUIDELINES AND NETWORKS

During the last decade, much progress in American psychiatry has occurred with the publication of practice guidelines. These efforts will continue in the twenty-first century, and it is anticipated that such guidelines will be formulated for almost all nosological entities. The interaction between nosological advances and guidelines is vital, and evidence-based treatment has depended on systematic evolution of a modern diagnostic system. After their original formulation, these guidelines will continue to be amended as new methods are introduced and new results are determined for each treatment.

In addition to the development of practice guidelines, the organization of a practice research network in the United States has great potential (Zarin et al. 1997). Such a network will complement the traditional methods of evaluating new treatments under controlled conditions. This control may make it necessary to concentrate on conditions in which patients have one clear diagnosis and are treated by one specific approach. Given the prevalence of comorbidity in the case of psychiatric conditions and given the need to test treatments in a variety of contexts, a treatment network may provide much additional information. I look forward to the organization of such networks in many specialties and many countries. Each of them will be composed of practitioners representing multiple areas of interest. Embedded within this concept is the concern that current systems of assessing treatment may, in some cases, be somewhat constrained and insufficiently reflective of actual practice. Clearly, both controlled and network-generated data have special purposes and should complement one another.

The emergence of networks across the world will be a

major step toward a more sophisticated transnational comparative analysis of psychiatry. Similarities and differences of findings by different networks will be very important. The maturation of an evidence-based international psychiatry will be one of the most exciting aspects of our field throughout the twenty-first century.

I predict a continued evolution of nosology, which, in turn, should facilitate a rational evolution of treatment guidelines. The emergence of treatment research networks will reflect and facilitate the new guidelines and the new treatments. Ultimately, new treatments will evolve in a more sophisticated manner.

COMBINED USE OF PSYCHOTHERAPY AND PHARMACOTHERAPY BY PSYCHIATRISTS

Many patients with psychiatric disorders are now treated with a combination of medication and psychotherapy (Beitman and Klerman 1991). Often, however, these treatments are provided by different therapists and there is relatively little communication about the therapeutic interactions. When a single therapist employs both psychopharmacotherapy and psychotherapy today, most often these treatments are used additively rather than integratively. The future practice of psychiatry will be influenced meaningfully by efforts at genuine integration of these treatments.

Traditionally, pharmacotherapy and psychotherapy have developed under separate auspices. Indeed, in the era of ideological domination, there often were conflicts between proponents of pharmacotherapy and those who advocated psychotherapy (Klerman 1991). More recently, many psychiatrists have recognized that patients may require medication before they can respond adequately to psychotherapy. Conversely, many psychopharmacologists have recognized that psychotherapy may enhance and prolong the effects of medication. In my judgment, this recognition is an early step in understanding that many types of interaction between the treatments are possible. The effects of psychotherapy and pharmacotherapy, when better understood, should be complementary and reinforcing. Various types of medications will have different kinds of effects when used with different types of psychotherapy, and various types of psychotherapy will have different effects when used with different kinds of medication.

The current separation of psychotherapy and pharmacotherapy reflects their divergent historical roots. Integration will require educational programs in which the teaching of both is combined. Ultimately, individual educators should be able to teach about the combined treatment and individual psychiatrists should be able to provide integrated rather than separate or additive treatment.

Most current discussion of psychiatrists' role in providing psychotherapy fails to include consideration of the implications for combined use of psychotherapy and pharmacotherapy.

The psychiatrist who is untrained in psychotherapy will not, of course, be able to provide the combined treatment. It should be obvious that a psychiatrist without experience in psychotherapy will not be able to supervise treatment by this method. Nevertheless, it has been advocated that such supervision could be provided by psychiatrists even if they do not conduct psychotherapy themselves.

The combined treatment will have many economic implications. One psychiatrist providing such combined treatment will increase his or her efficiency and, I believe, will also have better long-term results. I predict that this kind of integrated treatment will become the type of service provided by the psychiatrist by the middle of the twenty-first century. I also predict that the combined treatment will differentiate the psychiatrist from colleagues in primary care medicine and colleagues in other mental health fields. To accomplish this goal in a successful fashion, a large number of educational and service delivery changes will be required. It is hoped that some of these changes will begin now with efforts designed to preserve and improve psychiatrists' skills in various kinds of psychotherapy. These skills will be the bedrock for the combined treatments.

BIOLOGICAL AND PSYCHOLOGICAL MARKERS

In medical specialties other than psychiatry, predilection or vulnerability to various illnesses may be ascertained by specific tests long before signs or symptoms of the disorder make their appearance. In psychiatry, such accurate predictions of vulnerability are rare (Bunney et al. 1986). In part, the paucity of specific markers relates to our lack of information about the pathophysiology of most psychiatric disorders. At times, however, we have come close to proposing hypotheses about blood tests, radiographic signs, or identification of genetic findings that might predict the later emergence of specific disorders or parts thereof. Unfortunately, we have not yet found reliable predictors.

I have already mentioned that a nosological system based on pathogenesis or etiology should be present by the latter part of the twenty-first century. Such a system should facilitate the discovery of laboratory findings that precede and hence predict the onset of disorder. Of course, relevant prediction should lead to preventive steps that might be taken to block the pathological tendencies.

These biological markers will include indicators of genetic predilection to disorder as well as vulnerabilities that develop later. Molecular genetics will become an even more important basic science for psychiatric progress.

One variant of these markers will involve measurement of factors that may reduce the chance for a specific disorder or disorders to develop. For example, those processes that enhance coping and/or adaptation may also be measurable and this measurement may become one of the most important aspects for the future of psychiatry. Markers indicating lowered vulnerability to disorders may be as important as those predicting the development of disorders.

In psychiatry, psychological markers should also emerge in conjunction with biological and physical markers. The subject of psychological markers has been very much affected by theories and hypotheses throughout the twentieth century that have formulated a relationship between childhood trauma and adult illnesses. Psychiatric researchers have often questioned the scientific basis of many of these earlier hypotheses and prefer to emphasize the need for hypotheses that can be tested and validated or invalidated. Psychobiological markers that predict vulnerability to disorder or predict capacity to deal effectively with impending disorder will become a major part of psychiatry by the middle of the twenty-first century. The psychological component of those markers will include personality traits, subsyndromal symptomatology, and developmental deficits. These psychological markers should also include a new language of coping and adaptational criteria.

The biopsychosocial psychiatry (some prefer the term *psychobiological*) of the latter part of the twenty-first century will also lend itself to a different kind of nosological system for psychiatry that takes etiology and pathogeneses into consideration. The markers used in predicting vulnerability and immunity will be important in the new etiologically based diagnostic system. Studies of markers that may indicate a capacity to reduce vulnerability to illness have important theoretical as well as practical implications. The psychosomatic medicine of the twenty-first century may be affected substantially by study of these mechanisms. The knowledge that some people are highly unlikely to develop peptic ulcers or hypertension, for example, may be as important as good predictors of specific vulnerability.

STUDIES OF THE LIFE CYCLE

During the twentieth century, it has been logical to separate child/adolescent psychiatry as a subspecialty of psychiatry. Subsequently, it also was logical that geriatric psychiatry became a subspecialty. It was not logical, however, to think of general psychiatry simply as psychiatry geared toward the time between adolescence and old age. General psychiatry always included chronological components, but time did not necessarily serve as the central feature of general psychiatry, even when the term *adult psychiatry* was employed. Adulthood does not have the same relatively clearly delineated chronological characteristics as do childhood and older age. I predict, however, that there will be a better formulation of adult development in the twenty-first century.

I believe that the total life cycle will be reexamined in the twenty-first century, with the development of new hypotheses related to vulnerabilities and also the capacity to deal with these vulnerabilities. Throughout the twentieth century there have been important debates about the continuity or discontinuity of psychopathology (Chess and Alexander 1990). Continuity or discontinuity of adaptive methods and styles has undergone less study but should become a much more important topic. Adaptation will be studied directly, not simply through studying people who demonstrate low scores on a scale of maladaptation. Understanding why and how some people adapt over a full life cycle should have many implications for new types of treatment and prevention of illness. New types of treatment that facilitate adaptation rather than combat illness, as in the approach taken in oncology, could become a central part of psychiatry. Also, the understanding of chronic illness should be facilitated by data about the continuity or discontinuity of symptomatology during various phases of the life cycle.

TECHNOLOGICAL ADVANCES

There are several contexts in which new technology will have a notable impact on the field of psychiatry.

The technology of psychopharmacology has had a remarkable developmental history in the last four decades. There is good reason to expect that developments in neuroscience and psychopharmacology will continue. As the underlying psychobiological basis of disorders unfolds, new forms of psychopharmacological treatment will be developed. The psychopharmacological treatments facilitating adaptation will also become a new form of therapy.

I predict an emerging psychopharmacological industry with a new model, one emphasizing reinforcement of adaptive capacity rather than the combating of disorder.

A variety of new approaches and hypotheses will also refine the current techniques employed in psychotherapy. Combined use of pharmacotherapy and psychotherapy will facilitate the focusing of attention on new possibilities in psychotherapy. In the past, psychotherapeutic techniques have been used to support "defenses" (e.g., rationalization); the implicit concept of this approach is a method to shore up less than optimal techniques. The concept of adaptation is different from the concept of defense mechanism, and this concept should affect psychotherapeutic techniques substantially. A new technology of psychotherapy should emerge.

New technology can also have other special implications for psychotherapy and psychiatric rehabilitation. Telepsychiatry and cyberspace techniques will probably revolutionize interpersonal treatment during the next quarter century. The therapist's office has been the site of much outpatient treatment. Twenty-five years from now, therapist and patient will have many other options. It will be possible to treat a patient by therapeutic techniques in settings almost fully approximating current sensory reality—even when the patient is thousands of miles away from the therapist. It may also be possible to administer medication and perform other medical treatments through cyberspace. The implications for follow-up treatment after patient or therapist changes residence are enormous, as is the problem of licensing and credentialing. All of these new techniques may seem somewhat strange for those raised earlier in the twentieth century but will be easier for those raised in an environment in which such use of the Internet and telemedicine is much more common.

Telepsychiatry is already useful for reminding people to take their medications and for reinforcing treatment. The use of such methods for elderly and incapacitated patients has begun but has many implications that will be expanded as new techniques are implemented. There are many practical implications of these new technological advances, including increase in efficiency and cost-effectiveness.

PREVENTION OF MENTAL ILLNESS

Throughout the twentieth century there have been many programs designed to prevent the onset of mental illness (primary prevention) or intended to provide effective therapeutic early intervention (secondary prevention). Some of these programs have been very effective. For example, the psychoses associated with vitamin deficiency have been prevented by better nutrition, and pellagra has become less common as well. In the middle of the twentieth century, syphilis had a major impact and affected psychiatry throughout the world. Tertiary syphilis was associated with psychotic syndromes that were common and diverse. The effectiveness of penicillin in treating central nervous system syphilis, and, even more important, in preventing tertiary symptoms, has been one of the great preventive achievements of the century. Indeed, the decrease in prevalence of many infectious diseases has had important ramifications for psychiatry. However, new infectious diseases have now emerged that have a powerful impact on the central nervous system. HIV infection has had a major effect on the psychiatry of the turn of the century (Checkley et al. 1996; Rosenbaum 1994).

General principles of better child care, adequate education, better treatment for many medical illnesses, careful attention to a variety of toxic reactions (including the effects of many medications), and better public health have had a positive impact on mental illnesses with generic types of primary prevention. In some countries, after social upheaval or revolution, it was hoped that improvement in the implementation of these measures would eradicate mental illness. Unfortunately, even after effective general preventive actions, severe mental illnesses continue to occur, as do some less severe illnesses, and many of these illnesses continue to create major health problems throughout the world.

Primary prevention of most severe mental illnesses is limited without better understanding of their causes and also awaits improvement of methods for early diagnosis and early intervention. Schizophrenia has been studied intensively, but achieving a full understanding of its pathogenesis will require much work in the new century; in many cases, however, reduction of residual symptomatology in schizophrenic patients is now possible. Further, once a diagnosis of depression has been made, secondary preventive treatment results in patients with this disorder are very good ("Health Care Reform for Americans With Severe Mental Illnesses" 1993). Primary prevention for most severe mental illnesses, however, is a goal that will not be attained until late in the twenty-first century. I anticipate that a resurgence of preventive psychiatry will occur by the first quarter of the century and that preventive psychiatry will gain a more solid footing as the century goes on.

INTEGRATION OF THEORY AND PRACTICE

During the third quarter of the twentieth century, there was an efflorescence of theoretical concepts, many of which were attached to specific ideologies within psychiatry. In the last 25 years, however, there has been a marked tendency toward a pragmatism almost devoid of theory. In my judgment, American psychiatry has attempted to compensate for its earlier immersion in theory by emphasizing an evidence-based approach in developing new hypotheses. I believe that the current lack of theory will begin to have a negative impact when new efforts are made to integrate biological, psychological, and social data. Throughout this chapter, I have discussed the need for a scientific rationale of treatment. New theoretical formulation of levels and sequences of integration between biological and psychological data will be very important as long as they lead to hypotheses that can be tested. It is my opinion that there will be a gradual increase in willingness and ability to formulate new psychosomatic theories and new theories designed to help the understanding of the interaction between vulnerability and adaptation.

There is already some increased interest in psychiatric theory. The new journal *Philosophy, Psychiatry, & Psychology* has gained many subscribers in both the United Kingdom and America. I believe that the journal's popularity will increase and will help lead us out of the current atheoretical period.

GRADUAL DECLINE OF STIGMA

In the United States, there has been a substantial decline in stigma against psychiatric patients and psychiatrists in the last 25 years. Various surveys have indicated that the majority of the public now believes that mental illness is diagnosable and treatable (Clements 1993). In the middle of the twentieth century, by contrast, there was much skepticism about diagnosis and treatment. Even earlier in the century, much more stigma existed, represented by gross distortions of psychiatric illness. There was also gross distortion about what psychiatrists actually did with patients.

During the 1990s, extensive debate took place in the United States Congress regarding legislation designed to provide parity of care for patients with psychiatric illness (Mental Health Parity Act of 1996, 1996). The arguments against this legislation involved concern about increased costs of such efforts. Connected with this concern, however, was old-fashioned stigma. It was asserted repeatedly that mental illness could not be diagnosed accurately, and it was also stated that treatments had little success and tended to be employed interminably. These allegations illustrate that progress against stigma may be reversed under the stress of seeking parity of care for the mentally ill. Further-

more, the Domenici-Wellstone amendment did not provide for parity for those who engage in substance abuse. A very special kind a stigma still exists in the arena of care for substance abusers.

Stigma against psychiatrists has also been reduced in the last decade. The fact that a substantial number of psychiatrists have become deans of American medical schools demonstrates that there is widespread respect for certain psychiatrists. Nevertheless, among the medical colleagues of psychiatrists, substantial stigma still exists against most psychiatrists. When a medical student tells classmates or professors that he or she plans to seek a residency in psychiatry, the reaction is often negative.

As widespread awareness of psychiatric research spreads in many sectors of public understanding, however, stigma against psychiatric patients and psychiatrists diminishes. I believe that this trend will continue into the twenty-first century and that there will be a continuing gradual decline of stigma. There still will be some stigma, however, even at the end of an enlightened new century. Dealing with irrational and occasionally unpredictable behavior will always stir up questions and misunderstanding.

Psychiatrists' alliances with patients and family groups will become stronger, and such alliances will play a beneficial role in many areas and will also play a role in reducing stigma. The continuing reduction of stigma will occupy much attention of the mental health/mental disorder/brain disease alliances of the twenty-first century.

CHANGES IN DELIVERY OF PSYCHIATRIC SERVICES

There is enormous variation in the way in which psychiatric services are delivered in different countries today. In some nations, primitive systems continue and reform will take many years to accomplish. In the United States, during the past decade, there has been tremendous change in the regulation of all medical care, including psychiatric treatment. A determined effort has been mounted through managed care to control health costs; included in this effort is an attempt to limit reimbursement to those clinical approaches that are perceived to be efficient and/or cost-effective (Bartlett 1994). There is currently a backlash against managed care. Some practitioners stay outside the system by limiting their practice to patients who pay for care entirely out of their own pockets. I predict that there will also be increased attempts at local levels to regulate and control egregious practices of managed care. Suits initiated by practitioners to combat bad managed care will be another effort to combat bad practice.

One of the most important political and economic developments related to care of psychiatric patients in the United States has been the parity movement. The middle 1990s saw the emergence of a determined effort to raise the level of reimbursement for psychiatric treatment so that the reimbursement was equivalent to that for treatment of other medical illnesses. The Domenici-Wellstone amendment was a major step toward achieving partial parity (Sabshin 1997). Although the amendment's provisions were limited and involved annual and lifetime caps for psychiatric care to become equivalent, under certain conditions, to other medical caps, the passage of the amendment was notable. In the debate before the president signed the legislation, those opposing the Domenici-Wellstone amendment used old-fashioned, stigma-related approaches, including questioning the reliability of psychiatric diagnoses and the effectiveness of psychiatric treatment. Those arguments failed.

I believe that parity legislation at the national level will continue to be passed and will bring about equality for psychiatric treatment compared with the rest of medical treatment by the second decade of the twenty-first century (Sabshin 1997). The implication of this prediction is that a majority of decision makers will join together to support parity despite residual opposition by a strong group who will nevertheless find themselves in a minority. For the first time in history, a series of political decisions will be made supporting parity of care for the mentally ill in the face of vigorous public discussion, including opposition.

In the United States, the debate regarding parity will also occur in each state. Support for the mentally ill will spread throughout the United States by the end of the first decade of the new century. In accomplishing this purpose, families of the mentally ill will join with citizens' groups and professional groups. The increasing effectiveness of this coalition will have much impact on the parity movement. In addition, I predict that this coalition will ultimately make a difference in the debate about equity in reimbursement for treatment of mental illness.

One of the most important current questions involves how mental illness is defined for purposes of reimbursement. Some groups advocate the limitation of reimbursement to those with severe and persistent mental illness. I believe that this approach will dominate the national and state parity efforts for the next decade. I also predict that by the second decade of the twenty-first century, there will be a resurgence of interest in those people with less severe mental illnesses that nevertheless have a substantial impact in the workplace and in family life. Also, those disorders that affect children will receive increased attention. The fact that many individuals who engage in substance abuse also have a comorbid mental illness will receive much more attention as better treatments are more widely appreciated early in the new century.

PSYCHIATRIC WORKFORCE

Projections regarding the number of psychiatrists needed in particular countries depend on a variety of assumptions and definitions (Scully 1995). When a limited definition of mental illness is employed and when it is assumed that most of the less severely ill patients will continue to be treated by nonpsychiatrists, the projected number of psychiatrists needed is low.

Projections based on just the opposite assumptions are also made today. These assumptions include a very broad definition of mental illness that encompasses substance abuse and the treatment of notable comorbidity. Under these conditions the need for psychiatrists is greater. There is also the question of the extent of needs in the subspecialty areas of psychiatry; the demand for practitioners increases with the increase in needs across many subspecialties. Very much related to these projections is how the definition of mental illness is handled in particular reimbursement schemes. As demand for treatment for those individuals with psychiatric problems affecting work and family life increases, the need for psychiatrists to be part of these treatment efforts will rise. Of course, other mental health workers will be involved in such programs as well, but psychiatrists will provide very special combinations of psychotherapy and pharmacotherapy. Earlier in this chapter I discussed this increased use of conjoint psychotherapy and pharmacotherapy by one practitioner—namely, the psychiatrist. If this prediction is correct, the need for psychiatrists will be greater.

The potential workforce in mental health is diverse and large. I believe that physicians other than psychiatrists will become increasingly involved in providing pharmacotherapeutic care for many psychiatric patients. I believe also that mental health workers other then psychiatrists will provide psychotherapeutic care for a larger sample of the population. Psychotherapy and pharmacotherapy will, however, become even more integrated, and psychiatrists will be especially qualified for providing such combined treatment.

Workforce projections will also be affected by new technological possibilities—namely, those of treating people who reside in other parts of the world. Licensing and credentialing will be important issues in telepsychiatry.

Nevertheless, workforce demands in the United States will be affected by worldwide psychiatric needs in the twenty-first century.

In the United States, there is one area in which there is an enormous need for psychiatrists, and this need is likely to grow in the next two decades. Forensic psychiatry has expanded far beyond previous projections in almost all of its divisions. Policy decisions will determine what kind of support will be provided for prisoners with overt and serious mental problems. Provision of psychiatric treatment to prisoners is a major societal issue, one that will demand discussion and could affect educational programs and workforce projections.

RIGHTS OF PSYCHIATRIC PATIENTS

Human rights issues have very special meaning for psychiatric patients and for the individuals who treat them. When psychiatric patients are treated under authoritarian conditions, numerous problems affect the process and the outcome. The authoritarianism may result from political, religious, economic, or other social circumstances. All of these variables affect the confidentiality of treatment, the conditions under which treatment is administered, the relationship between the patient and the persons and institutions providing treatment, and the basis for hospitalization and discharge. Democracy and human rights have particular impacts on the mental health field, more perhaps than on any other area of medicine (Sabshin 1995). It is to be hoped that in the twenty-first century a broader understanding of this relationship will exist and efforts will be made around the world to guarantee the rights of patients with mental illness.

At the same time, there needs to be an awareness that antipsychiatry groups have entered this arena of patients' rights. These groups argue for human rights from a libertarian or scientology perspective. Scientologists are very much against psychiatry and have tended to portray psychiatrists as despicable villains. The problems with psychiatry, from this group's perspective, are the providers and the treatment itself, and scientologists are a strong force in the struggle against all mental health care. Libertarians also argue against treatment (especially involuntary treatment) and question whether commitment to mental institutions is still necessary. Despite antipsychiatry, democratic principles have been promulgated widely to support better psychiatric treatment in many countries. Psychiatric abuses still occur, however, and efforts to expose these abuses and improve care will continue to make a large difference.

Rights for psychiatric patients are fundamental to good practice and development of these rights will be part of psychiatric advances in the twenty-first century.

CONCLUSIONS

This chapter has included discussion and future projections of some of the major issues facing psychiatry. Some predictions have been made as well. I have focused on an increasingly evidence-based psychiatry that will recognize its dependence on a good mixture of science, humanistic clinical practice, and democratic conditions. New technology could help psychiatric patients and psychiatrists in a number of ways—for example, through provision of treatment to patients living far from their therapists. The psychiatrist in the twenty-first century might concentrate on providing combined psychotherapy and pharmacotherapy, an exciting area of psychiatry that awaits additional refinement. Many economic constraints have recently been placed on the psychiatrist and psychiatric patients. It is to be hoped that these constraints will diminish with the advent of more enlightened policies of parity and equity regarding psychiatric treatment.

REFERENCES

American Psychiatric Association: Diagnostic and Statistical Manual of Mental Disorders, 3rd Edition. Washington, DC, American Psychiatric Association, 1980

American Psychiatric Association: Diagnostic and Statistical Manual of Mental Disorders, 3rd Edition, Revised. Washington, DC, American Psychiatric Association, 1987

American Psychiatric Association: Diagnostic and Statistical Manual of Mental Disorders, 4th Edition. Washington, DC, American Psychiatric Association, 1994

Bartlett J: The emergence of managed care and its impact on psychiatry. New Dir Ment Health Serv 63:25–34, 1994

Beitman BD, Klerman GL (eds): Integrating Pharmacotherapy and Psychotherapy. American Psychiatric Press, Washington, DC, 1991

Bunney WE, Garland-Bunney B, Patel SB: Biological markers in depression. Psychopathology 19 (suppl 2):72–78, 1986

Checkley GE, Thompson SC, Crofts N, et al: HIV in the mentally ill (review). Aust N Z J Psychiatry 30:184–194, 1996

Chess S, Alexander T: Continuities and discontinuities in temperament, in Straight and Devious Pathways From Childhood to Adulthood. Edited by Robins LN, Rutter M. Cambridge, England, Cambridge Press, 1990, pp 205–220

Clements M: What we say about mental illness. Parade, October 31, 1993, pp 4–6

Frances AJ, Widiger TA, Pincus HA: The development of DSM-IV. Arch Gen Psychiatry 46:373–375, 1989

Health care reform for Americans with severe mental illnesses: report of the National Advisory Mental Health Council. Am J Psychiatry 150:447–465, 1993

Klerman GL: Ideological conflicts in integrating pharmacotherapy and psychotherapy, in Integrating Pharmacotherapy and Psychotherapy. Edited by Beitman BD, Klerman GL. American Psychiatric Press, Washington, DC, 1991, pp 3–19

Massel HK, Liberman RP, Mintz J, et al: Evaluating the capacity to work of the mentally ill. Psychiatry 53:31–43, 1990

Mental Health Parity Act of 1996. U.S. Public Law 104-204, 1996

Rosenbaum M: Similarities of psychiatric disorders of AIDS and syphilis: history repeats itself. Bull Menninger Clin 58:375–382, 1994

Sabshin M: Medical Director's Report. Am J Psychiatry 133: 1236–1240, 1976

Sabshin M: Medical Director's Report. Am J Psychiatry 134: 1194–1199, 1977

Sabshin M: Turning points in twentieth-century American psychiatry. Am J Psychiatry 147:1267–1274, 1990

Sabshin M: Authoritarianism and the practice of psychiatry. Paper presented at the Institute on Psychiatric Services, October 1995

Sabshin M: Parity for mental illness: the half-full glass. Molecular Psychiatry 2:177, 1997

Scully JH: Determining workforce needs. Paper presented at the 148th annual meeting of the American Psychiatric Association, Miami, FL, May 20–25, 1995

World Health Organization: International Classification of Diseases, 10th Revision. Geneva, World Health Organization, 1992

Zarin DA, Pincus HA, McIntyre JS: Practice based research in psychiatry. Am J Psychiatry 154:1199–1208, 1997

INDEX

Page numbers printed in **boldface** type refer to tables or figures.